THE COLOR ATLAS OF PEDIATRICS

NOTICE

THE COLOR ATLAS OF PEDIATRICS

EDITORS

Richard P. Usatine, MD
Professor of Family and Community Medicine
Professor of Dermatology and Cutaneous Surgery
Assistant Director, Medical Humanities Education
University of Texas Health Science Center at San Antonio
Medical Director, Skin Clinic, University Health System
San Antonio, Texas

Camille Sabella, MD
Associate Professor of Pediatrics
Vice Chair for Education, Pediatric Institute
Center for Pediatric Infectious Diseases
Cleveland Clinic Children's
Cleveland, Ohio

Mindy Ann Smith, MD
Clinical Professor
Department of Family Medicine
Michigan State University
East Lansing, Michigan

E.J. Mayeaux, Jr., MD
Professor and Chairman, Department of Family and Preventive Medicine
Professor of Obstetrics and Gynecology
University of South Carolina School of Medicine
Columbia, South Carolina

Heidi S. Chumley, MD
Executive Dean and Chief Academic Officer
American University of the Caribbean

Elumalai Appachi, MD, MRCP (UK)
Department of Pediatric Critical Care
Cleveland Clinic Children's
Cleveland, Ohio

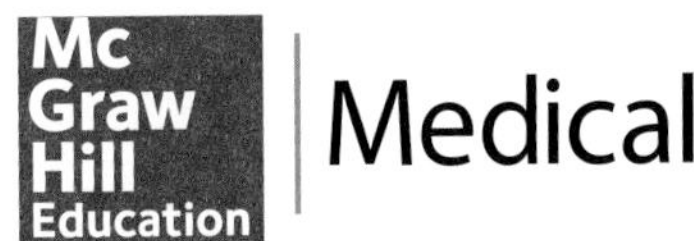

New York Chicago San Francisco Athens London Madrid Mexico City
Milan New Delhi Singapore Sydney Toronto

The Color Atlas of Pediatrics

1 2 3 4 5 6 7 8 9 0 CTP/CTP 18 17 16 15 14

ISBN: 978-0-07-176701-9
MHID: 0-07-176701-0

This book was set in Perpetua by Aptara®, Inc.
The editors were Alyssa Fried and Karen G. Edmonson.
The production supervisor was Rick Ruzycka.
Project management was provided by Aptara®, Inc.
The cover designer was Thomas Di Pierro.
China Translation & Printing Services, Ltd. was printer and binder.

This book is printed on acid-free paper.

Library of Congress Cataloging-in-Publication Data

The color atlas of pediatrics / editors, Richard P. Usatine, Camille Sabella, Mindy Ann Smith, E.J. Mayeaux, Jr., Heidi S. Chumley, Elumalai Appachi. – Second edition.
p. ; cm.
Includes index.
ISBN 978-0-07-176701-9 (hardcover : alk. paper) – ISBN 0-07-176701-0 (hardcover : alk. paper)
I. Usatine, Richard, editor.
[DNLM: 1. Pediatrics–Atlases. WS 17]
RJ48.5
618.9200022′2–dc23

2014007213

DEDICATION

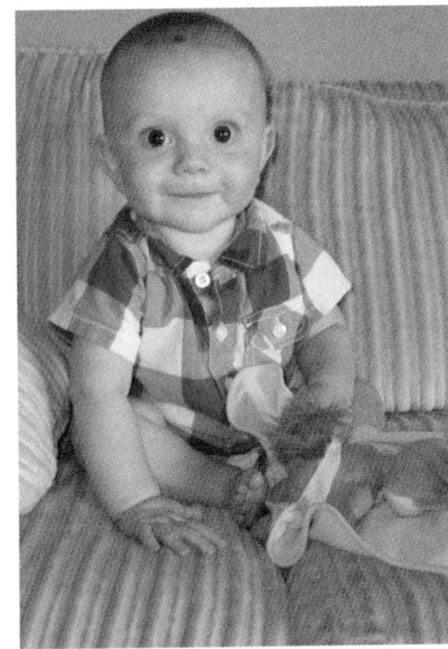
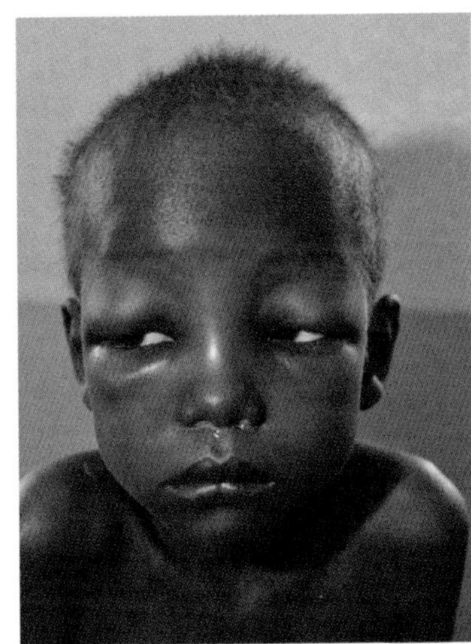
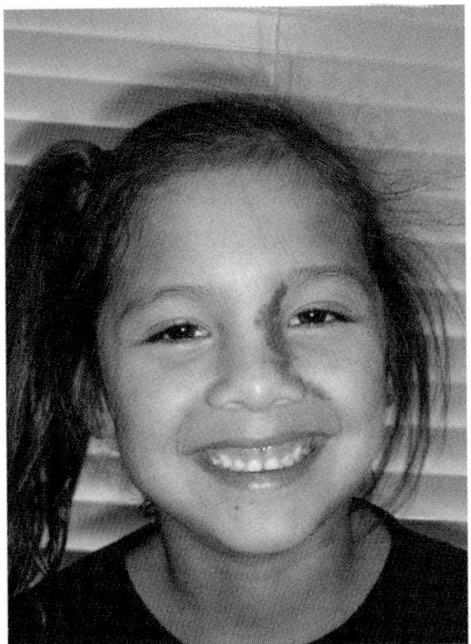
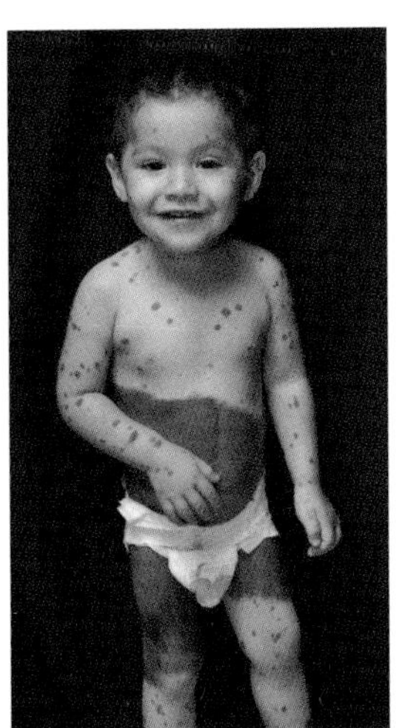
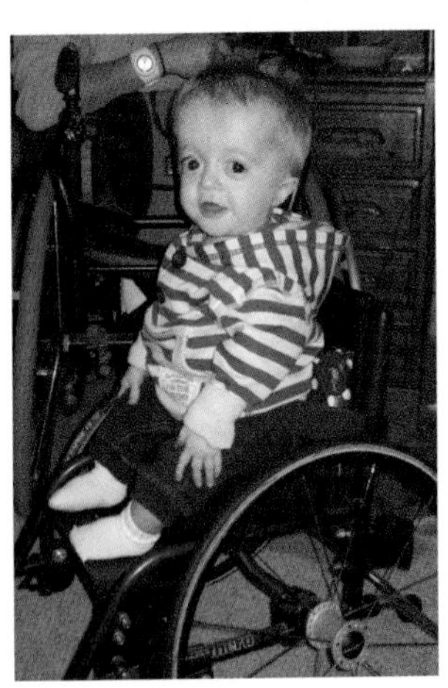
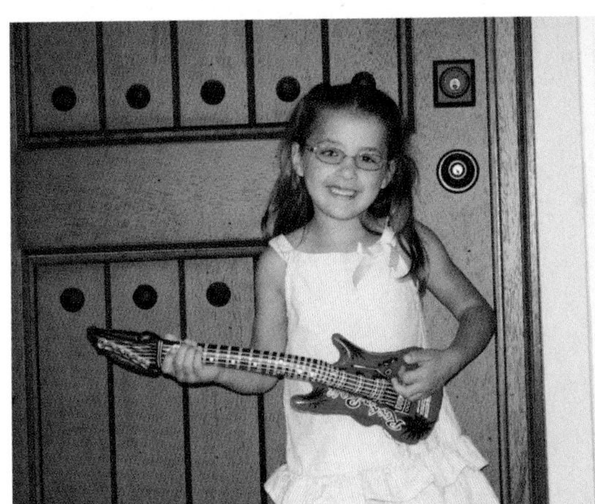
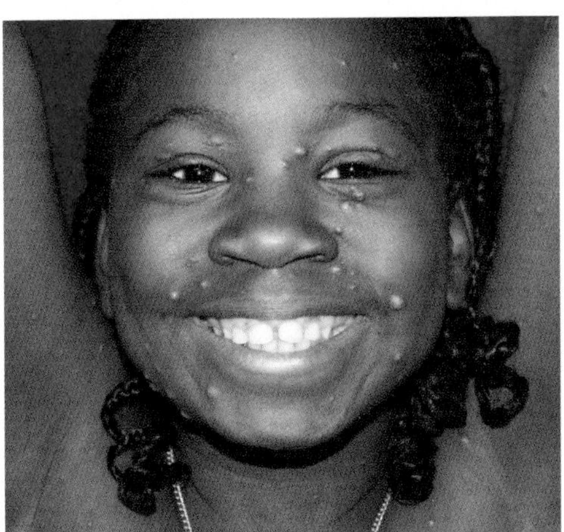

To our patients who unselfishly agreed to let us display their diseases and afflictions to the world to enhance the study and practice of medicine. We are honored by this trust. We have learned much from our patients as they continue to help us teach the next generation of health care providers.

Sincerely,

Richard P. Usatine, MD
Camille Sabella, MD
Mindy Ann Smith, MD
E.J. Mayeaux, Jr., MD
Heidi S. Chumley, MD
Elumalai Appachi, MD, MRCP (UK)

CONTENTS

CONTENTS

PART 18

NEUROLOGY

PART 19

HEMATOLOGY-ONCOLOGY

PART 20

ALLERGY AND IMMUNOLOGY

PART 21

GENETIC DISORDERS

PART 22

SUBSTANCE ABUSE

APPENDIX

Nazha Abughali, MD
Department of Pediatrics
Metrohealth Medical Center
Case Western Reserve University
Cleveland, Ohio

Shoghik Akoghlanian, MD
Fellow, Pediatric Rheumatology
University Hospitals Case Medical Center
Rainbow Babies & Children's Hospital
Cleveland, Ohio

Sophia Ali, MD
Department of Pediatric Gastroenterology and Hepatology
Cleveland Clinic Children's
Cleveland, Ohio

Naim Alkhouri, MD
Department of Pediatric Gastroenterology and Hepatology
Cleveland Clinic Children's
Cleveland, Ohio

Anna Allred, MD
Resident Physician
Department of Neurological Surgery
University of Texas South Western Medical Center
Dallas, Texas

Homa Amini, DDS, MPH, MS
Postdoctoral Program Director and Associate Professor of Pediatric Dentistry
Division of Pediatric Dentistry and Community Oral Health
The Ohio State University and Nationwide Children's Hospital
Columbus, Ohio

James Anderst, MD, MS
Division of Child Abuse and Neglect
Associate Professor
Children's Mercy Hospital
UMKC School of Medicine
Kansas City, Missouri

Samantha Anne, MD, MS
Assistant Professor of Surgery
Pediatric Otolaryngology
Head & Neck Institute, Cleveland Clinic
Cleveland, Ohio

Elumalai Appachi, MD, MRCP
Department of Pediatric Critical Care
Cleveland Clinic Children's
Cleveland, Ohio

Swathi Appachi, BS
Medical Student
Cleveland Clinic Lerner College of Medicine
Case Western Reserve University
Cleveland, Ohio

Marjan Attaran, MD
The Cleveland Clinic
Womens' Health Institute
Head Pediatric and Adolescent Gynecology
Cleveland, Ohio

Hend Azhary, MD
Assistant Professor
Department of Family Medicine
Michigan State University College of Human Medicine
East Lansing, Michigan

Peter Aziz, MD
Pediatric Electrophysiology
Department of Pediatric Cardiology
Cleveland Clinic Children's
Cleveland, Ohio

Michael Babcock, MD
Colorado Springs Dermatology Clinic
Colorado Springs, Colorado

Keith Bachmann, MD
Orthopedic Surgery Resident
Department of Orthopedic Surgery
Cleveland Clinic
Cleveland, Ohio

Yoon-Soo Cindy Bae-Harboe, MD
Boston University Hospital
Medical Center Department of Dermatology
Boston, Massachusetts

R. Tracy Ballock, MD
Department of Orthopedic Surgery
Cleveland Clinic
Cleveland, Ohio

Luke Baudoin, MD
Associate Professor of Family Medicine
LSUHSC Shreveport
Shreveport, Louisiana

Ruth E. Berggren, MD
Professor of Medicine
Division of Infectious Diseases
University of Texas Health Science Center
San Antonio, Texas

Steven N. Bienvenu, MD, FAAP
Associate Clinical Professor of Pediatrics
Chief, Section of Ambulatory Care
Director, LSU Children's Clinic
Department of Pediatrics
Louisiana State University Health Sciences Center
Shreveport, Louisiana

James R. Boynton, DDS, MS
Clinical Associate Professor and Director
Pediatric Dentistry
Department of Orthodontics and Pediatric Dentistry
University of Michigan School of Dentistry
Ann Arbor, Michigan

Allison W. Brindle, MD
Staff Pediatrician
Department of General Pediatrics
Cleveland Clinic Children's
Cleveland, Ohio

Margaret L. Burks, MD
Student Affiliate School of Medicine
University of Texas Health Science Center at San Antonio
San Antonio, Texas

Timothy Campbell, MD
Allergy and Immunology Fellow
Cleveland Clinic
Cleveland, Ohio

Kevin Carlisle, MD
Resident
Department of Family Medicine
Louisiana State University
Shreveport, Louisiana

Nancy Carst, MSW
Nancy Carst, MSW
Bereavement Specialist
Haslinger Family Center for Pediatric Palliative Care
Akron Children's Hospital
Akron, Ohio

Julie Cernanec, MD, FAAP
Julie Cernanec, MD FAAP
Department of Pediatric Hospital Medicine
Cleveland Clinic Children's
Cleveland, Ohio

Melissa M. Chan, MD
Family Practicioner
Sutter East Bay Medical Foundation
Albany, California

Pierre Chanoine, MD
Drexel University School of Medicine
Philadelphia, Pennsylvania
St. Christopher's Hospital for Children
Philadelphia, Pennsylvania

Alia Chauhan, MD, FAAP
Assistant Professor
Department of Pediatrics
Hofstra North Shore-LIJ School of Medicine
New Hyde Park, New York

Debby Chuang, MD
Urology Institute
University Hospitals of Cleveland
Case Western Reserve University
Cleveland, Ohio

Heidi S. Chumley, MD
Executive Dean and Chief Academic Officer
American University of the Caribbean

Joshua Rai Clark, MD
Family Medicine House Officer 2
Louisiana State University Health Sciences Center
Shreveport, Louisiana

Sigrid M Collier, MD
Med Derm Resident
University of Minnesota
Minneapolis, Minnesota

Thomas J. Corson, DO
Emergency Medicine Resident
University of Connecticut School of Medicine
Hartford Hospital
Hartford, Connecticut

Lara Danziger-Isakov, MD, MPH
Associate Professor of Pediatrics
Division of Infectious Disease
Cincinnati Children's Hospital Medical Center
Cincinnati, Ohio

Kshama Daphtary, MBBS, MD, FAAP
Department of Pediatric Critical Care
Cleveland Clinic Children's
Cleveland, Ohio

John DiFiore, MD
Department of Pediatric Surgery
Cleveland Clinic Children's
Cleveland, Ohio

Gregor Dückers, MD
Helios Clinic Krefeld Children's Hospital
Department for Pediatric Immunology
Krefeld, Germany

David S. Ebenezer, MD
Department of Orthopaedic Surgery
Cleveland Clinic
Cleveland, Ohio

Brian Elkins, MD
Associate Professor of Clinical Family Medicine
LSU Health Sciences Center
Department of Family Medicine and Comprehensive Care
Shreveport, Louisiana

Katharine Eng, MD
Department of Pediatric Gastroenterology and Hepatology
Cleveland Clinic Children's
Cleveland, Ohio

Gavin A. Falk, MD
Resident Surgeon
Department of General Surgery
Cleveland Clinic Foundation
Cleveland, Ohio

Angela M. Fals, MD, FAAP
Diplomate, American Board of Obesity Medicine
Medical Director
Florida Hospital for Children
Center for Child and Family Wellness
Orlando, Florida

Cristina Fernandez, MD
Associate Professor of Pediatrics
Creighton University Children's Physicians Medical Director
HEROES Program, Associate Program Director
UNMC/ Creighton Univeristy/Children's Hospital and Medical Center, Omaha, Nebraska

Lindsey B. Finklea, MD
Dermatologist
San Antonio, Texas

Aron Flagg, MD
Department of Pediatric Hematology and Oncology
Cleveland Clinic Children's
Cleveland, Ohio

Anthony Todd Flowers, MD
Family Physician
Louisiana State University Health Sciences Center
Shreveport, Louisiana

Charles B. Foster, MD
Associate Professor of Pediatrics
Center for Pediatric Infectious Diseases
Cleveland Clinic Children's
Cleveland, Ohio

Kelli Hejl Foulkrod, MS
Psychotherapist/Yoga Teacher
Psychology Center of Austin
Austin, Texas

Jeremy A. Franklin, MD
Director, Medical Sciences
MedImmune LLC.
Lubbock, Texas

Sarah Friebert, MD
Director
Haslinger Family Center for Pediatric Palliative Care
Akron Children's Hospital
Akron, Ohio

Neil Friedman, MBChB
Pediatric Neurologist
Staff Physician, Center for Pediatric Neurology
Neurological Institute
Cleveland Clinic
Cleveland, Ohio

Kimberly Giuliano, MD
Assistant Professor of Pediatrics
Department of General Pediatrics
Cleveland Clinic Children's
Cleveland, Ohio

Wanda C. Gonsalves, MD
Professor and Vice Chair
Department of Family and Community Medicine
University of Kentucky College of Medicine, Lexington, Kentucky

Blanca E. Gonzalez, MD
Assistant Professor of Pediatrics
Center for Pediatric Infectious Diseases
Cleveland Clinic Children's
Cleveland, Ohio

Ryan C. Goodwin, MD
Center Director, Pediatric Orthopaedics and Scoliosis Surgery
Fellowship Director, Pediatric Orthopaedics and Scoliosis Surgery
Associate Residency Program Director
Department of Orthopedic Surgery
Cleveland Clinic
Cleveland, Ohio

Elizabeth Sutton Gosnell, DMD, MS
Assistant Professor of Clinical Dentistry
Director, Pre-Doctoral Pediatric Dentistry
The Ohio State University College of Dentistry
Nationwide Children's Hospital
Columbus, Ohio

Kelly Green, MD
Ophthalmology, Private Practice
Marble Falls Texas
Clinical Assistant Professor
Department of Ophthalmology
University of Texas Health Science Center
San Antonio, Texas

Justin Greiwe, MD
Allergy and Immunology Fellow
Cleveland Clinic
Cleveland, Ohio

Heather M. Guillot, MD
Assistant Professor of Clinical Family Medicine
LSU Health Sciences Center
Department of Family Medicine and Comprehensive Care
Shreveport, Louisiana

David Gurd, MD
Director of Pediatric Spinal Deformity
Staff Physician, Department of Orthopedic Surgery
Cleveland Clinic
Cleveland, Ohio

Meredith Hancock, MD
Preliminary Resident Internal Medicine
Loyola University Medical Center
Maywood, Illinois

Jimmy H. Hara, MD, FAAFP
Professor of Clinical Family Medicine
David Geffen School of Medicine at UCLA
Los Angeles, California

Tara Harwood, MS, RD, CSP, LD
Pediatric Dietitian
Cleveland Clinic Children's
Cleveland, Ohio

Karen Hawley, MD
Otolaryngology, Resident Physician
Head and Neck Institute
Cleveland Clinic
Cleveland, Ohio

John H. Haynes, Jr., MD
Family Physician
Rural Family Practice Program Director
Chief of Staff, North Caddo Medical Center
Vivian, Louisianna

David Henderson, MD
Associate Dean, Medical Student Affairs
Associate Professor
Department of Family Medicine
University of Connecticut School of Medicine
Farmington, Connecticut

Nathan Hitzeman, MD
Faculty, Sutter Health Family Medicine Residency Program
Sacramento, California

Janalee Holmes, MD
Resident Physician
Head and Neck Institute
Cleveland Clinic
Cleveland, Ohio

Ashley D. Hopkins, MD
Fellow
Child Abuse Pediatrics
The Children's Mercy Hospital
Kansas City, Missouri

Anne Hseu, MD
Head and Neck Institute
Cleveland Clinic
Cleveland, Ohio

Karen A. Hughes, MD
Associate Director
North Mississippi Center Family Medicine Residency Program
Tupelo Mississippi

Khalilah Hunter-Anderson, MD
Assistant Professor
Department of Traumatology & Emergency Medicine
University of Connecticut Health Center
Farmington, Connecticut

Sabine Iben, MD
Assistant Professor
Department of Neonatology
Pediatric Institute
Cleveland Clinic Children's
Cleveland, Ohio

Edward A. Jackson, MD
Covenant Medical Group
Saginaw Medicine
Clinical Professor of Family Medicine
Michigan State University College of Human Medicine
Hemlock, Michigan

Meghan Drayton Jackson, DO
Chief Pediatric Resident
Cleveland Clinic Children's
Cleveland, Ohio

Halima S. Janjua, MD
Center for Pediatric Nephrology
Cleveland Clinic Children's
Cleveland, Ohio

Adeliza Jimenez, MD
Staff Physician
Southern California Permanente Medical Group
Downey, California

Brooke Johnston, MD
Fellow
Haslinger Family Center for Pediatric Palliative Care
Akron Children's Hospital
Akron, Ohio

Skyler Kalady, MD
Assistant Professor of Pediatrics
Department of General Pediatrics
Cleveland Clinic Lerner College of Medicine of Case Western Reserve University,
Cleveland Clinic Children's
Cleveland, Ohio

Jonathan B. Karnes, MD
Assistant Clinical Professor
Dartmouth School of Medicine
Main Dartmouth Family Medicine Residency
Augusta, Maine

Jennifer A. Keehbauch, MD, FAAFP
Director of Research, Graduate Medical Education
Florida Hospital
Assistant Director, Family Medicine, Residency, Florida Hospital
Director, Women's Medicine Fellowship, Florida Hospital
Orlando, Florida

Nancy D. Kellogg, MD
Professor of Pediatrics
Chief, Division of Child Abuse
University of Texas Health Science Center at San Antonio
San Antonio, Texas

Amor Khachemoune, MD
Attending Physician, Dermatologist
Mohs Surgeon and Dermatopathologist
Veterans Affairs Medical Center
Brooklyn, New York

Joel Kolmodin, MD
Resident, Department of Orthopedic Surgery
The Cleveland Clinic
Cleveland, Ohio

Catherine Kowalewski, DO
Assistant Chief of Dermatology STVHCS
Assistant Professor Dermatology
University of Texas San Antonio
San Antonio, Texas

Robert Kraft, MD
Clinical Assistant Professor
Department of Family and Community Medicine
University of Kansas School of Medicine
Wichita, Wichita, Kansas

Paul Krakovitz, MD
Vice Chairman Surgical Operations
Section Head of Pediatric Otolaryngology
Head and Neck Institute
Cleveland Clinic
Cleveland, Ohio

Jennifer Krejci-Mannwaring, MD
Assistant Professor
Division of Dermatology
University of Texas Health Science Center at San Antonio
San Antonio, Texas

Ashok Kumar, DDS, MS
Associate Professor of Pediatric Dentistry
Division of Pediatric Dentistry and Community Oral Health
The Ohio State University and Nationwide Children's Hospital
Columbus, Ohio

Charles Y. Kwon, MD
Center for Pediatric Nephrology
Cleveland Clinic Children's
Cleveland, Ohio

Katherine B. Lee, MD
Assistant Professor of Surgery
Cleveland Clinic Lerner College of Medicine of
Case Western Reserve University
Cleveland Clinic Breast Center
Cleveland Clinic
Cleveland, Ohio

Jose Lozada, MD
Resident – General Surgery
Cleveland Clinic
Cleveland, Ohio

Megha Madhukar, MD
Resident
Department of Radiology
Penn State Hershey Radiology
Hershey, Pennslyvania

Lori A. Mahajan, MD
Fellowship Director
Department of Pediatric Gastroenterology
Cleveland Clinic Children's
Cleveland, Ohio

Amara Majeed, MBBS
The Aga Khan University Medical College,
Karachi, Pakistan

Prashant Malhotra, MD, FAAP
Prashant Malhotra, MD, FAAP
Department of Otolaryngology Head and Neck Surgery
Nationwide Children's Hospital
Assistant Professor, Ohio State University
Columbus, Ohio

Bridget Malit, MD
Pediatric Resident
Department of Pediatrics
Weil Cornell Medical College
New York, New York

David Mandell, MD
Clinical Associate Professor
NOVA Southestern University College of Osteopathic Medicine
Division of Otolaryngology
Davie, Florida

Andreas Marcotty, MD
Assistant Clinical Professor
Cleveland Clinic Lerner School of Medicine
Cole Eye Institute, Cleveland Clinic
Section, Pediatric Ophthalmology
Cleveland, Ohio

Michaela R. Marek, MD
Dermatology Resident
University of Texas Health Sciences Center
San Antonio, Texas

Michelle Marks, DO, FAAP, FHM
Chair, Department of Pediatric Hospital Medicine
Cleveland Clinic Children's
Cleveland, Ohio

Nathan Scott Martin, MD
Chief Resident in Emergency Medicine/Family Medicine Combined Program
LSU Health Sciences Center
Shreveport, Louisiana

Raed Bou Matar, MD
Center for Pediatric Nephrology
Cleveland Clinic Children's Hospital
Cleveland, Ohio

Jessie Maxwell, MD
Department of Pediatrics
Metrohealth Medical Center,
Case Western Reserve University
Cleveland, Ohio

Rachna May, MD FAAP
Department of Pediatric Hospital Medicine
Cleveland Clinic Children's
Cleveland, Ohio

E.J. Mayeaux, Jr., MD, DABFP, FAAFP
Professor and Chairman
Department of Family and Preventive Medicine
Professor of Obstetrics and Gynecology
University of South Carolina School of Medicine
Columbia, South Carolina

Maria D. McColgan, MD
Assistant Professor
Departments of Pediatrics and Emergency Medicine
Director, Child Protection Program
Drexel University College of Medicine
Philadelphia, Pennslyvania

Stacy McConkey, MD, FAAP
Pediatric Residency Program Director
Florida Hospital for Children
Orlando, Florida

Carolyn Milana, MD
Assistant Professor of Pediatrics
Stony Brook Long Island Children's Hospital
Stony Brook, New York

William A. Miller, MD, MPH, MSc
Resident Physician
Department of Neurological Surgery
University of Texas Southwestern Medical Center
Dallas, Texas

Shashi Mittal, MD
Family Physician
MedFirst Northeast Primary Care Clinic
San Antonio, Texas

Arunkumar Modi, MD MPH
Department of Pediatric Hematology and Oncology
Cleveland Clinic Children's
Cleveland, Ohio

Jonathan Moses, MD
Department of Pediatric Gastroenterology
Cleveland Clinic Children's
Cleveland, Ohio

Melissa Muszynski, MD
Resident, Department of Dermatology
Georgetown University Hospital
Washington Hospital Center, Washington DC

Todd D. Nebesio, MD
Associate Professor of Clinical Pediatrics
Department of Pediatrics
Section of Pediatric Endocrinology/Diabetology
Indiana University School of Medicine
Riley Hospital for Children
Indianapolis, Indiana

Lisanne Newton, MD
Department of Allergy and Immunology
Cleveland Clinic Children's
Cleveland, Ohio

Tim Niehues, MD
Professor of Pediatrics
Helios Clinic Krefeld Children's Hospital
Department for Pediatric Immunology
Krefeld, Germany

Vera Okwu, MD
Department of Pediatric Gastroenterology
Cleveland Clinic Children's
Cleveland, Ohio

Kyra Osborne, MD
Otolaryngology, Resident Physician
Head and Neck Institute
Cleveland Clinic
Cleveland, Ohio

Asif Padiyath, MD
Pediatric Resident
Cleveland Clinic Children's
Cleveland, Ohio

Rita Pappas, MD, FAAP, FHM
Staff, Department of Pediatric Hospital Medicine
Cleveland Clinic Children's
Cleveland, Ohio

Ellen Park, MD
Department of Pediatric Radiology
Cleveland Clinic Children's
Cleveland, Ohio

Nisha Patel, MD
Department of Pediatric Gastroenterology and Hepatology
Cleveland Clinic Children's
Cleveland, Ohio

Denise Powers-Fabian, MSSA, LISW-S
Social Worker
Haslinger Family Center for Pediatric Palliative Care
Akron Children's Hospital
Akron, Ohio

Matthew Prine, MD
Chief Resident
Rural Family Practice Program
Louisiana State University Health Sciences Center
Shreveport, Louisania

Athar M. Qureshi, MD
Associate Director
CE Mullins Catheterization Laboratories
Texas Children's Hospital,
Associate Professor of Pediatrics
Baylor College of Medicine
Houston, Texas

Karthik Rajasekaran, MD
Head and Neck Institute
Cleveland Clinic
Cleveland, Ohio

Vidya Raman, MD
Assistant Professor
Section of Pediatric Rheumatology
Nationwide Children's Hospital
Columbus, Ohio

Rachel M. Randall
Center for Pediatric Orthopaedics
Orthopaedic and Rheumatology Institute
Cleveland Clinic
Cleveland, Ohio

Brian Z. Rayala, MD
Assistant Professor
Department of Family Medicine
University of North Carolina School of Medicine
Chapel Hill, North Carolina

Samiya Razvi, DCH, MD
Pediatric Pulmonologist
Department of Pediatrics
Apollo Hospitals, Jubilee Hills
Hyderabad, India

Katie Reppa, MD
Resident
University of Pittsburgh
Pittsburgh, Pennsylvania

Olvia Revelo, MD
Family Physician
Houston, Texas

Peter Revenaugh, MD
Head and Neck Institute
Cleveland Clinic
Cleveland, Ohio

Karl T. Rew, MD
Assistant Professor of Family Medicine and Urology
University of Michigan Medical School
Ann Arbor, Michigan

Paul J. Rychwalski, MD
Associate Professor of Ophthalmology and Pediatrics
Cleveland Clinic Lerner College of Medicine
Case Western Reserve University
Staff Ophthalmologist
Cole Eye Institute, Cleveland Clinic
Cleveland, Ohio

Camille Sabella, MD
Associate Professor of Pediatrics
Vice Chair for Education, Pediatric Institute
Center for Pediatric Infectious Diseases
Cleveland Clinic Children's
Cleveland, Ohio

Paula Sabella, MD, FAAP
Assistant Professor of Pediatrics
Department of Emergency Medicine
Akron Children's Hospital
Akron, Ohio

Paul M. Saluan, MD
Director, Pediatric and Adolescent Sports Medicine
Department of Orthopaedic Surgery
Cleveland Clinic
Cleveland, Ohio

M. Jason Sanders, MD
Assistant Professor
Division of Community and General Pediatrics
Department of Pediatrics
UT Health Medical School at Houston
Houston, Texas

Khashayar Sarabi, MD
Internal & Integrative Medicine
Irvine, California

Rebecca Schein, MD
Pediatric Infectious Diseases
Department of Pediatrics
MetroHealth Medical Center
Cleveland, Ohio

Melissa A. Scholes, MD
Assistant Professor Pediatric Otolaryngology
Department of Otolaryngology
University of Colorado
Aurora, Colorado

Brian Schroer, MD
Associate Professor of Pediatrics
Lerner College of Medicine Cleveland Clinic
Staff Pediatrics and Respiratory Institutes, Cleveland Clinic
Cleveland, Ohio

Emily Gale Scott, MD
Pediatric Emergency Medicine Attending Physician
Medical Director, Suture Program
Akron Children's Hospital
Akron, Ohio

Adriana Segura DDS, MS
Professor
Department of Comprehensive Dentistry
Associate Dean for Student Affairs
University of Texas Health Science Center at San Antonio
Dental School
San Antonio, Texas

Federico G. Seifarth, MD
Department of Pediatric Surgery
Cleveland Clinic Children's
Cleveland, Ohio

Andrew Shedd, MD
Emergency Medicine Resident
Department of Emergency Medicine
Advocate Christ Medical Center
Oak Lawn, Illimois

Arun Singh, MD
Director, Ophthalmic Oncology
Cole Eye Institute
Cleveland Clinic
Cleveland, Ohio

Abdul-Karim Sleiman
Faculty of Medicine and Medical Center
American University of Beirut
Beirut, Lebanon

Mindy A. Smith, MD, MS
Clinical Professor, Department of Family Medicine
Michigan State University
East Lansing, Michigan
Deputy Editor, Essential Evidence Plus
Associate Medical Editor, FP Essentials

Linda M. Speer, MD
Professor and Chair Department of Family Medicine
University of Toledo, College of Medicine and Life Sciences
Toledo, Ohio

Anthony Stallion, MD
Chief of Pediatric Surgery
Pediatric Surgeon-in-Chief
Levine Children's Hospital
Jeff Gordon Children's Hospital
Carolinas Healthcare System
Concord, North Carolina

Ahila Subramanian, MD, MPH
Allergy and Immunology Fellow
Cleveland Clinic
Cleveland, Ohio

Di Sun, BS, MPH
Cleveland Clinic Lerner College of Medicine
Case Western Reserve University
Cleveland, Ohio

Joan Tamburro, DO
Pediatric Dermatology Staff
The Dermatology and Plastic Surgery Institute
Cleveland Clinic
Cleveland, Ohio

Dimitris N. Tatakis, DDS, PhD
Diplomate, American Board of Periodontology
Professor and Director, Advanced Education Program in Periodontics
Division of Periodontology, College of Dentistry, The Ohio State University
Columbus, Ohio

Julie Scott Taylor, MD, MSc
Associate Professor of Family Medicine
Director of Clinical Curriculum
Alpert Medical School of Brown University
Providence, Rhode Island

Stephen Taylor, MD
Associate Professor of Family Medicine
Louisiana State University Health Sciences Center
Family Medicine Rural Track
Shreveport, Louisiana

Danyal Thaver, MBBS
Otolaryngology, Resident Physician
Head and Neck Institute
Cleveland Clinic
Cleveland, Ohio

Sarat Thikkurissy, DDS, MS
Professor & Director, Residency Program
Department of Pediatric Dentistry and Orthodontics
Cincinnati Children's Hospital
Cincinnati, Ohio

Stefanie Thomas, MD
Department of Pediatric Hematology and Oncology
Cleveland Clinic Children's
Cleveland, Ohio

Margaret C. Thompson, MD, PhD
Department of Pediatric Hematology and Oncology
Cleveland Clinic Children's
Cleveland, Ohio

Carla Torres-Zegarra, MD
Chief Pediatric Resident
The Pediatric Institute
Cleveland Clinic Children's
Cleveland, Ohio

Elias I. Traboulsi, MD
Head, Department of Pediatric Ophthalmology and Strabismus
Director, The Center for Genetic Eye Diseases
Cole Eye Institute
Cleveland Clinic
Cleveland, Ohio

Victor E. Uko, MD
Department of Pediatric Gastroenterology
Cleveland Clinic Children's
Cleveland, Ohio

Richard P. Usatine, MD
Professor of Family and Community Medicine
Professor of Dermatology and Cutaneous Surgery
Assistant Director, Medical Humanities Education
University of Texas Health Science Center at San Antonio
Medical Director, Skin Clinic, University Health System
San Antonio, Texas

Neil Vachhani, MD
Chair, Section of Pediatric Radiology
Cleveland Clinic Children's
Cleveland, Ohio

Ernest Valdez, DDS
Assistant Professor
Department of Oral and Maxillofacial Surgery
The University of Texas Health Science Center at San Antonio
San Antonio, Texas

Frits van der Kuyp, MD
Department of Medicine
Metrohealth Medical Center,
Case Western Reserve University
Cleveland, Ohio

Allison Vidimos, MD
Dermatology Department Chair and Dermatology staff
The Dermatology and Plastic Surgery Institute
Cleveland Clinic
Cleveland, Ohio

Holly H. Volz, MD
Resident Physician
The University of Texas Health Science Center at San Antonio
San Antonio, Texas

Eugene K. Vortia, MD
Department of Pediatric Gastroenterology
Cleveland Clinic Children's
Cleveland, Ohio

Yu Wah, MD
Assistant Professor
Department of Family and Community Medicine
University of Texas Health Science Center at Houston
Houston, Texas

Brian Williams, MD
Brian J. Williams Dermatology, Private Practice
Midvale, Utah

Lynn L. Woo, MD
Assistant Professor of Pediatric Urology
Case Western ReserveUniversity
Rainbow Babies & Children's Hospital
University Hospitals of Cleveland
Cleveland, Ohio

Matthew Wyneski, MD
Department of Pediatric Gastroenterology and Hepatology
Cleveland Clinic Children's
Cleveland, Ohio

Congjun Yao, MD
Adjunct Assistant Professor
Department of Family and Community Medicine
University of Texas Health Science Center
San Antonio, Texas

Dawood Yusef, MD
Center for Pediatric Infectious Diseases
Cleveland Clinic Children's
Cleveland, Ohio

Abbas H. Zaidi, MB, BS
Senior Clinical Fellow Cardiology
Department of Cardiology
Boston Children's Hospital
Boston, MA

Andrew Zeft, MD, MPH
Center for Pediatric Rheumatology
Cleveland Clinic Children's
Cleveland, Ohio

Pediatricians see a wide variety of genetic and congenital disorders, infections, skin conditions, and many other problems that span the pediatric spectrum. It is clear that a comprehensive atlas that aids in diagnosis using visible signs and internal imaging will be of tremendous value. We have assembled more than 1,900 outstanding clinical images for this very purpose and are proud to present the first edition of a modern comprehensive atlas of pediatrics. Some photographs will amaze you and all will inform you about the various conditions that befall our patients.

It took a number of people many years to create the first edition of *The Color Atlas of Pediatrics*. For us, it has been a life long inspired by many great mentors, who taught us the importance of physical examination findings in caring for our patients. We have been fortunate to compile many photographs of our patients over the years, which we have used to teach medical students and residents. We now have the honor of sharing these images with the readers of this atlas. We are grateful to the many outstanding contributors to this textbook who have unselfishly shared with us their patient stories and images, and their vast knowledge of the disease processes, which has allowed us to compile this truly comprehensive pediatric atlas.

The Color Atlas of Pediatrics is written for pediatricians and all healthcare providers involved in providing care to children and adolescents. It can be invaluable to medical students, residents, nurse practitioners, physician assistants, family physicians and dermatologists.

The Color Atlas of Pediatrics is also for anyone who loves to look at clinical photographs for learning, teaching, and practicing medicine. The first chapter begins with an introduction to learning with images and digital photography. The core of the book focuses on medical conditions organized by anatomic and physiologic systems. This book covers healthcare from birth to adulthood. There are special sections devoted to the essence of pediatrics, physical/sexual abuse, newborn and adolescent health, dermatology, and genetic disorders.

The collection of clinical images is supported by evidence-based information that will help the healthcare provider diagnose and manage a wide spectrum of common and not so common pediatric problems. The text is concisely presented with many easy to access bullets as a quick point-of-care reference. Each chapter begins with a patient story that ties the photographs to the real life stories of our patients. The photographic legends are also designed to connect the images to the people and their human conditions. Strength of recommendation ratings are cited throughout so that the science of medicine can be blended with the art of medicine for optimal patient care.

The first edition of *The Color Atlas of Pediatrics* is available electronically on iPad, iPhone, iPod touch, all Android devices, Kindle, and on the web through Access Pediatrics. These electronic versions will allow healthcare providers to access the images and the content rapidly and at the point-of-care.

Because knowledge continues to advance after any book is written, we recommend that you use the online resources presented in many of the chapters to keep up with the most current changes in medicine. Care deeply about your patients and enjoy your practice, as it is a privilege to be a healthcare provider and healer.

The Editors

Strength of Recommendation (SOR)	Definition
A	Recommendation based on consistent and good-quality patient-oriented evidence.*
B	Recommendation based on inconsistent or limited-quality patient-oriented evidence.*
C	Recommendation based on consensus, usual practice, opinion, disease-oriented evidence, or case series for studies of diagnosis, treatment, prevention, or screening.*

*See Appendix A on pages 1320–1322 for further information.

ACKNOWLEDGMENTS

This book could not have been completed without the contributions of many talented physicians, healthcare professionals, and photographers. We received photographs from people who live and work across the globe. Each photograph is labeled and acknowledges the photographer and contributor. There are some people who contributed so many photographs it is appropriate to acknowledge them upfront in the book. The dermatology division at University Of Texas Health Sciences Center San Antonio contributed much of their expertise in photography, writing, and reviewing the extensive dermatology section. During the last few years, I was fortunate to work closely with the dermatology faculty and residents and they contributed generously to our book. Dr. Eric Kraus, the program director, gave us many wonderful photographs, especially for the section on bullous diseases. He also gave us open access to the 35-mm slides collected by the Division of Dermatology. Drs. Jeff Meffert and John Browning also contributed photographs to many chapters. Dr. Jack Resneck, Sr., from Louisiana, scanned his slides from more than 40 years of practice and gave them to Dr. E.J. Mayeaux, Jr., for use. Dr. Resneck's vast dermatologic experiences add to our atlas.

The UTHSCSA Head and Neck Department contributed many photographs for this book. We especially thank Dr. Frank Miller and Dr. Blake Simpson for their contributions. UTHSCSA pediatrics faculty contributed to our chapters on child abuse and otitis media. We are fortunate to have Dr. Nancy Kellogg contribute her photographs and expertise in caring for abused children to the book. Dr. Dan Stulberg, a family physician from New Mexico, with a passion for photography and dermatology, contributed many photographs throughout our book.

We thank our learners, many of whom coauthored chapters with us. UTHSCSA medical students and residents and fellows from Michigan State University's Primary Care Faculty Development Fellowship program coauthored chapters and contributed photographs with great enthusiasm to the creation of this work. It was a pleasure to mentor these young writers and experience with them the rewards of authorship. Dr. Usatine is thankful for the contributions of his "Underserved Dermatology Fellows". Working closely with such brilliant and caring doctors in our Skin Clinic and free outreach clinics allowed me to learn from them while doing my best to advance their academic and humanistic careers.

Of course, we would have no book without the talented writing and editing of my coeditors, Drs. Camille Sabella, Elumalai Appachi, Mindy A. Smith, E.J. Mayeaux, and Heidi Chumley. They each bring years of clinical and educational experience to the writing of the *Atlas*. Drs. Sabella, Appachi and Mayeaux contributed many of their own photographs. We also thank the chapter and photograph contributions of the many physicians at the Cleveland Clinic Children's Hospital. It has been a real pleasure to work with this dedicated group of individuals. We thank them for their expertise, perseverance, and devotion to teaching. We also want to thank the late Dr. Robert Mercer, one of the founding fathers of pediatrics at the Cleveland Clinic, who was responsible for the Cleveland Clinic Children's Hospital Photo Files, and whose photos are featured throughout this book. Dr. Mercer was a devoted clinician and educator, and we are indebted to him for his contributions to the field of pediatrics. We would like to also recognize Dr. Daniel Shapiro, who was responsible for collecting, safeguarding, and stressing the use of the photo files for educational purposes.

Most of all we need to thank our patients who generously gave their permission for their photographs to be taken and published in this book. While some photos are not recognizable, we have many photos of the full face that are very recognizable and were generously given to us by our patients with full written permission to be published as is. For photographs that were taken decades ago in which written consents were no longer available, we have used bars across the eyes to make the photos less recognizable—verbal consent was always obtained for these images.

I (Dr. Richard Usatine) thank my family for giving me the support to see this book through. It has taken much time from my family life and my family has supported me through the long nights and weekends it takes to write a book while continuing to practice and teach medicine. I am fortunate to have a loving wife, wonderful daughter, successful son, great son-in-law and one very cute grandson who add meaning to my life and allowed me to work hard on the creation of this *Color Atlas*. I personally want to thank Dr. Camille Sabella for his strong work ethic, warmth and good humor during the whole process. It is rare to find such superb collaborators in life. In every step of this journey, we worked together with mutual respect, kindness and consideration.

Dr. Camille Sabella would like to thank his wife Paula, and his three children, Carmen, Julia, and Annmarie, for their unwavering support, love, and encouragement. The sense of humor they provided also was instrumental in helping maintain a good balance throughout the process. He would like to personally thank Dr. Richard Usatine for sharing his knowledge, wisdom and experience, and for the selflessness he has shown in creating this *Color Atlas*. He would also like to thank his colleagues at the Cleveland Clinic Children's Hospital for their dedication to their patients and to the scholarly mission.

Dr. Mindy Smith adds, "I thank my husband, Gary, and daughter, Jenny, for their support and willingness to listen when I struggle with phrasing and wording in my writing and editing. I also thank several colleagues who have helped me to establish myself as an editor and supported my continued growth in this field—Drs. Barry Weiss, Mark Ebell, Richard Usatine, Suzanne Sorkin, and Leslie Shimp."

Dr. E.J. Mayeaux would like to thank his wife and family for understanding the many hours of work and computer time it takes to produce this work. He would like to dedicate this work to Mr. Bob (Papa Bob) Mitchell who can always find the funny angle to any situation and who gave him his partner and love of his life. I would also like to thank my new work family at the Department of Family and Preventive Medicine at the University of South Carolina School of Medicine in Columbia. We are going to do great things!

Dr. Heidi Chumley adds, "I want to thank my husband, John Delzell, who has brought love and peace to my often chaotic life, and my children, Cullen, Sierra, David, Selene, and Jack, who give me joy and provide the incentive to stay on task. Each one, in turn, has cheerfully pitched in to help a grumpy and tired mom who stayed up most of the night working on one of many chapters. I have been very blessed."

Dr Elumalai Appachi states that "I would like to thank all my teachers and patients who taught me the art of clinical pediatrics and how to show compassion for sick children. I want to take this opportunity to recognize my parents who always wanted me to be a physician and serve sick children. Finally I want to thank my family who has supported me to be sane and focused. Finally, I want to thank Camille Sabella who has given me opportunity to share what I learnt."

Finally, we all thank James Shanahan, Alyssa Fried and Karen Edmonson from McGraw-Hill for believing in this project and never giving up as our book grew larger and more comprehensive over time.

PART 1

LEARNING WITH IMAGES AND DIGITAL PHOTOGRAPHY

Strength of Recommendation (SOR)	Definition
A	Recommendation based on consistent and good-quality patient-oriented evidence.*
B	Recommendation based on inconsistent or limited-quality patient-oriented evidence.*
C	Recommendation based on consensus, usual practice, opinion, disease-oriented evidence, or case series for studies of diagnosis, treatment, prevention, or screening.*

*See Appendix A on pages 1320–1322 for further information.

1 AN ATLAS TO ENHANCE PATIENT CARE, LEARNING, AND TEACHING

Richard P. Usatine, MD

People only see what they are prepared to see.

—Ralph Waldo Emerson

Whether you are viewing **Figure 1-1** in a book, in an aquarium, or in the sea, you immediately recognize the image as a fish. Those of you who are more schooled in the classification of fish might recognize that this is an angelfish with the tail resembling the head of the angel and the posterior fins representing the wings. If you are truly prepared to see this fish in all its splendor, you would see the blue circle above its eye as the crown of the queen angelfish.

Making a diagnosis in medicine often involves the kind of pattern recognition needed to identify a queen angelfish. This is much the same as recognizing a beautiful bird or the painting of a favorite artist. If you are prepared to look for the clues that lead to the identification (diagnosis), you will see what needs to be seen. How can we be best prepared to see these clues? There is nothing more valuable than seeing an image or a patient who has the condition in question at least once before you encounter it on your own. The memory of a powerful visual image can become hardwired into your brain for ready recall.

In medicine, it also helps to know where and how to look to find the clues you may need when the diagnosis cannot be made at a single glance. For example, a 3-year-old girl presents with bad seborrheic dermatitis of the scalp and hand dermatitis that is not responding to typical treatments with selenium based shampoos and topical steroids (**Figures 1-2** and **1-3**). The prepared clinician knows that not all scaly erythematous rashes on the scalp and hands are dermatitis and looks for clues of psoriasis such as nail changes (**Figure 1-4**) or scaling erythematous plaques around the elbows and knees (**Figure 1-5**). Knowing where to look and what to look for is how an experienced clinician makes the diagnosis of psoriasis.

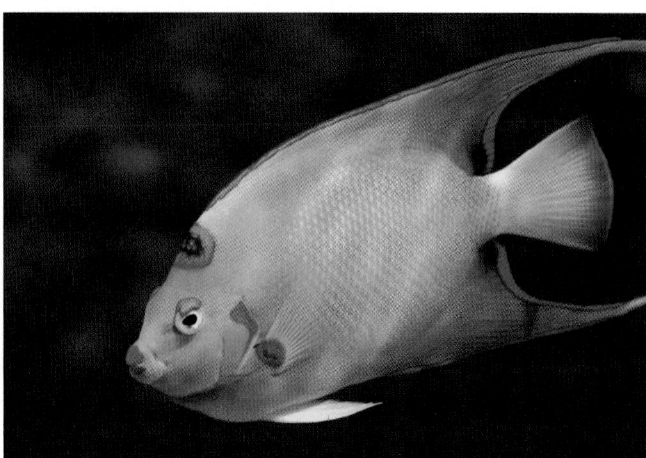

FIGURE 1-1 Queen angelfish (*Holacanthus ciliaris*). (*Used with permission from Sam Thekkethil. http://www.flickr.com/photos/natureloving.*)

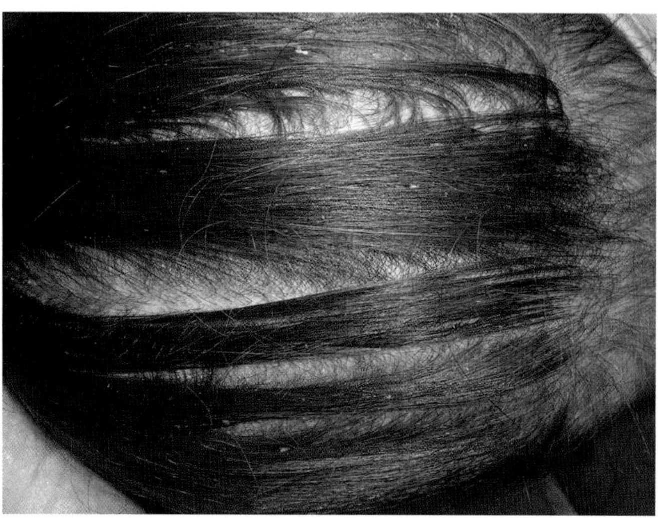

FIGURE 1-2 Scaling on the scalp of this 3-year-old girl was thought to be seborrheic dermatitis for one year. When the cradle cap did not go away with appropriate treatment another clinician looked for other clues of disease to determine that this was psoriasis. (*Used with permission from Richard P. Usatine, MD.*)

USING OUR SENSES

As physicians we collect clinical data through sight, sound, touch, and smell. Although physicians in the past used taste to collect data, such as tasting the sweet urine of a patient with diabetes, this sense is rarely, if ever, used in modern medicine. We listen to heart sounds, lung sounds, bruits, and percussion notes to collect information for diagnoses. We touch our patients to feel lumps, bumps, thrills, and masses. We occasionally use smell for diagnosis. Unfortunately, the smells of disease are rarely pleasant. Even the fruity odors of *Pseudomonas* are not like the sweet fruits of a farmers' market. Of course, we also use the patient's history, laboratory data, and more advanced imaging techniques to diagnose and manage patients' illnesses.

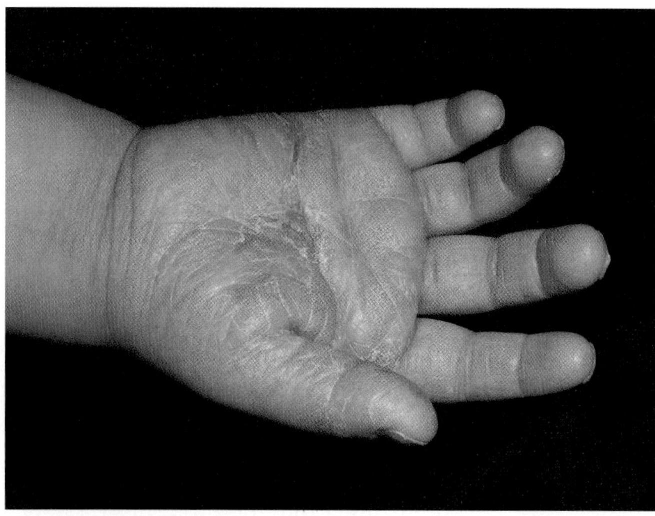

FIGURE 1-3 The same 3-year-old girl with scaling and cracking of the hands thought to be atopic dermatitis. It was not until another clinician looked carefully at the nails and knees that the correct diagnosis of psoriasis was made. Knowing where to look for the clues is critical to making the correct diagnosis. (*Used with permission from Richard P. Usatine, MD.*)

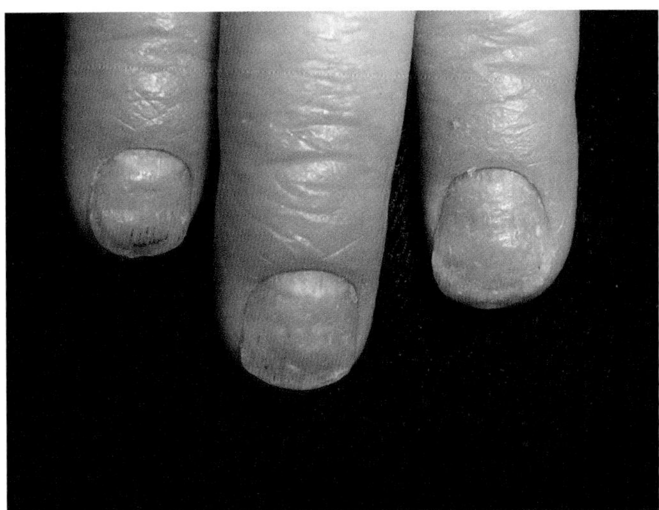

FIGURE 1-4 When the diagnosis of psoriasis is being considered, look at the nails for pitting or other nail changes such as splinter hemorrhages, onycholysis, or oil spots. This is a good example of nail pitting and splinter hemorrhages in a 3-year-old girl with psoriasis. (*Used with permission from Richard P. Usatine, MD.*)

It was our belief in the value of visual imagery that led to the development of this first *Color Atlas of Pediatrics*. We are pleased to provide more than 2,000 images to you and doctors around the world as a large color textbook and also as an interactive electronic application for easy use on the iPhone, iPod touch, iPad, and all Android devices.

EXPANDING OUR INTERNAL IMAGE BANKS

The larger our saved image bank in our brain, the better clinicians and diagnosticians we can become. The expert clinician has a large image bank stored in memory to call on for rapid pattern recognition. Our image banks begin to develop in medical school when we view pictures in lectures, textbooks, and electronic media. We then begin to develop our own clinical image bank by our clinical experiences. Our references are printed color atlases and those color atlases are available on the Internet and electronically.

Studying and learning the patterns from any atlas can enhance your expertise by enlarging the image bank stored in your memory. An atlas takes the clinical experiences of clinicians over decades and gives it to you as a single reference. We offer you a modern comprehensive pediatric color atlas, which includes all areas of pediatrics from head to toe with special areas of focus on newborn and adolescent health, dermatology, and genetic disorders.

USING IMAGES TO MAKE A DIAGNOSIS

We all see visible clinical findings on patients that we do not recognize. When this happens, open this book and look for a close match. Use the Topic Index, Table of Contents, or Subject Index to direct you to the section with the highest yield photos. If you find a direct match, you may have found the diagnosis. Read the text and see if the history and physical examination match your patient. Perform or order tests to confirm the diagnosis, if needed.

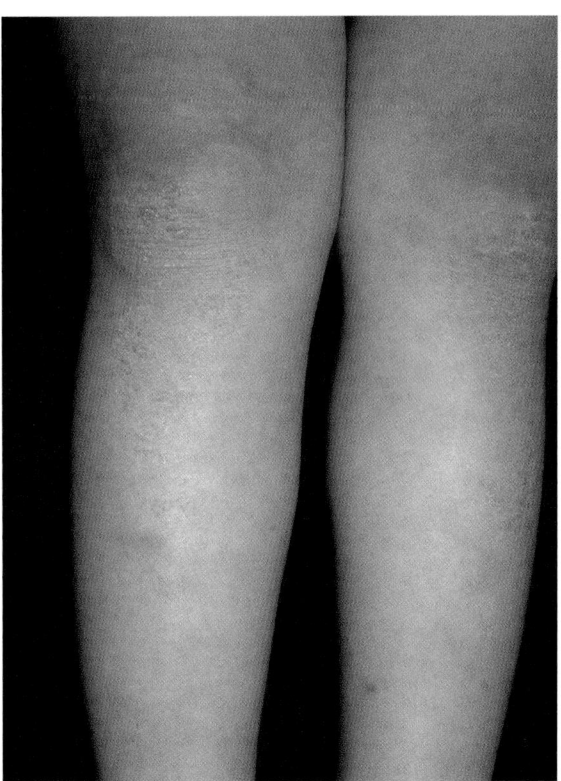

FIGURE 1-5 Subtle plaques over the knees and extensor surfaces of the lower legs in a 3-year-old girl with psoriasis. (*Used with permission from Richard P. Usatine, MD.*)

If you cannot find the image in our book try the Internet and Google's search engine. Try a Google image search and follow the leads. Of course, this is easiest to do if you have a good differential diagnosis and want to confirm your impression. If you do not have a diagnosis in mind, you may try putting in descriptive words and look for an image that matches what you are seeing. If the Google image search does not work, try a Web search and look at the links for other clues.

Finally, there are dedicated atlases on the Internet for organ systems that can help you find the needed image. Most of these atlases have their own search engines, which can help direct you to the right diagnosis.

Table 1-1 lists some of the best resources currently available online.

USING IMAGES TO BUILD TRUST IN THE PATIENT–PHYSICIAN RELATIONSHIP

If you are seeing a patient with a mysterious illness that remains undiagnosed and you figure out the diagnosis, you can often bridge the issues of mistrust and anxiety by showing the patient and their family the picture of another person with the diagnosis. Use our atlas for that purpose and supplement it with the Internet. This is especially important for a patient who has gone undiagnosed or misdiagnosed for some time. "Seeing is believing" for many patients. Ask the patient or parents first if they would want to see some pictures of other persons with a similar condition; most will be very interested. The parents and the patient can see the similarities between their condition and the other images, and feel reassured that your diagnosis is correct. Write down the name of the diagnosis and use your patient education skills.

TABLE 1-1 Excellent Clinical Image Collections on the Internet

Derm Atlas	www.dermatlas.org	Johns Hopkins University
DermIS	www.dermis.net	Derm Information Systems from Germany
Dermnet	www.dermnet.com	Skin Disease Image Atlas
Interactive Derm Atlas	www.dermatlas.net	From Richard P. Usatine, MD
ENT	www.entusa.com	From an ENT physician
Eye	www.eyerounds.org	University of Iowa
Figure Search	www.figuresearch.askhermes.org	University of Wisconsin
Images of all types	www.commons.wikimedia.org	Wikimedia Commons
	www.consultant360.com	Consultant Image Database
Infectious Diseases	www.phil.cdc.gov	CDC Public Health Image Library
Radiology	http://rad.usuhs.edu/medpix/	MedPix
Skinsight	www.skinsight.com/html	Logical Images

Do be careful when searching for images on the Web in front of patients. Sometimes what pops up is not "pretty" (or, for that matter, G or PG rated). I turn the screen away from the patient and their family before initiating the search and then censor what I will show them. I also explain that the images in a book or on the Internet may be the worst cases so that they may appear more severe than what your patient has. This can help blunt the anxiety of whether the child will go on to develop a worse case.

If you teach, model this behavior in front of your students. Show them how reference books and the Internet at the point of care can help with the care of patients.

TAKING YOUR OWN PHOTOGRAPHS

Images taken by you with your own camera of your own patients complete with their own stories are more likely to be retained and retrievable in your memory because they have a context and a story to go with them. We encourage our readers to use a digital camera (within a smartphone or a stand-alone camera) and consider taking your own photos. Of course, always ask permission before taking any photograph of a patient. Explain how the photographs can be used to teach other doctors and to create a record of the patient's condition at this point in time. If the photograph will be identifiable, ask for written consent; for patients younger than age 18 years, always ask the parent to sign. Store the photos in a manner that avoids any Health Insurance Portability and Accountability Act (HIPAA) privacy violations, such as on a secure server or on your own computer with password protection and data encryption. These photographs can directly benefit the patient when, for example, following various chronic diseases or skin conditions for changes.

Digital photography is a wonderful method for practicing, teaching, and learning medicine. You can show patients pictures of conditions on parts of their bodies that they could not see without multiple mirrors and some unusual body contortions. You can also use the zoom view feature on the camera or smartphone to view or show a segment of the image in greater detail. Children generally love to have their photos taken and will be delighted to see themselves on the screen of your camera/phone. If the child is old enough to be self-conscious about the condition that is "not normal," consider asking to take a picture of a healthy aspect of the child first. Most children will smile for a photograph of their face when they are feeling well and then be less puzzled or disturbed by a photograph of their foot or other involved area.

The advent of digital photography makes the recording of photographic images less expensive, easier to do, and easier to maintain. Digital photography also gives you immediate feedback and a sense of immediate gratification. No longer do you have to wait for a roll of film to be completed then processed before finding out the results of your photography. Not only does this give you instant gratification to see your image displayed instantaneously in the camera, but also alerts you to poor-quality photographs that can be retaken while the patient is still in the office. This speeds up the learning curve of the beginning photographer in a way that could not happen with film photography.

OUR GOALS

Many of the images in this atlas are from my collected works over the past 30 years of my practice in medicine. My patients have generously allowed me to photograph them so that their photographs would help the physicians and patients of the future. To these photos, we have added images that represent decades of experiences by other physicians and specialists. The Cleveland Clinic Children's Hospital photo files have been a real treasure for the rare conditions not seen regularly by the practicing pediatrician. For those photos, I thank my co-author and co-editor Dr. Camille Sabella for all the work that went into cataloguing and providing these treasured images for this atlas.

It is the goal of this atlas to provide you with a wide range of images of common and uncommon conditions, and provide you with the knowledge you need to make the diagnosis and initiate treatment. We want to help you be the best diagnostician you can be. We may aspire to be a clinician like Sir William Osler and have the detective acumen of Sherlock Holmes. The images collected for this atlas can help move you in that direction by making you prepared to see what you need to see.

PART 2

THE ESSENCE OF PEDIATRICS

Strength of Recommendation (SOR)	Definition
A	Recommendation based on consistent and good-quality patient-oriented evidence.*
B	Recommendation based on inconsistent or limited-quality patient-oriented evidence.*
C	Recommendation based on consensus, usual practice, opinion, disease-oriented evidence, or case series for studies of diagnosis, treatment, prevention, or screening.*

*See Appendix A on pages 1320–1322 for further information.

2 DOCTOR—PATIENT RELATIONSHIP

Camille Sabella, MD

PATIENT STORY

Patient and family stories, particularly if we listen attentively and nonjudgmentally, provide us with a window into their lives and experiences. These stories help us to know our patients and families in powerful ways, and that knowledge about the patient, as someone special, provides the context, meaning, and clues about their symptoms and illnesses that can lead to healing. At our best, we serve as witness to their struggles and triumphs, supporter of their efforts to change and grow, and guide through the medical maze of diagnostic and therapeutic options. Sometimes, their stories become our own stories—those patients who we will never forget because their stories have changed our lives and the way we practice medicine (**Figures 2-1** and **2-2**).

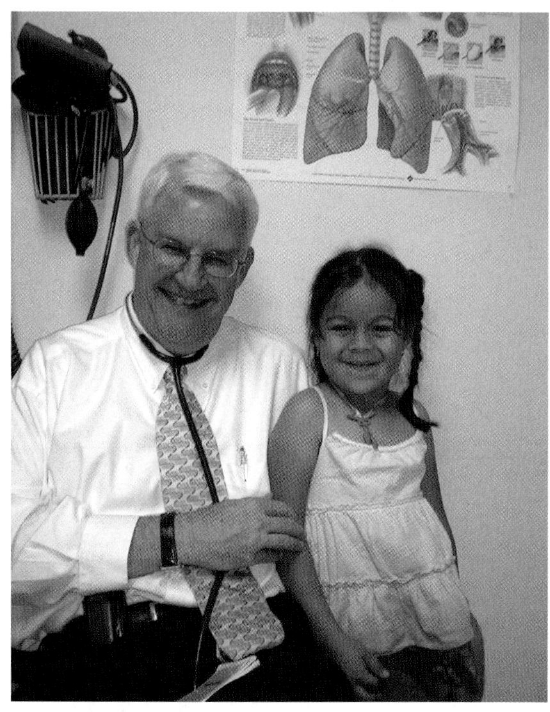

FIGURE 2-1 Dr. Jim Legler caring for a young girl in a free clinic within a transitional housing village for homeless families. He is a pediatrician who volunteers every week to care for the families working their way out of homelessness. He had been caring for Kimberly and her family for many months at the time this photograph was taken. Dr. Legler serves as a role model for students interested in primary care of the underserved. He is known for his kindness and compassion to all his patients.

WHAT FAMILIES WANT FROM THEIR PEDIATRIC PROVIDERS

- In a study of families of pediatric patients under 13 years of age in a large outpatient clinic, three elements were shown to be essential for effective physician-parent-child communication from a parent perspective.[1] These included:
  - Informativeness—Parents place considerable importance on the quality and quantity of information provided by the physician regarding their child's health.
  - Interpersonal sensitivity—Parents highly value physicians who were supportive and sensitive to the child's and parent's feelings and concerns.
  - Partnership building—The extent to which the physician involves the parent and child in the care of the child.
- Yet, traditionally, there has been little emphasis placed on building interpersonal skills in pediatric practice and training. This led to an American Academy of Pediatrics (AAP) report in 2001, which stated that "there is a need to better learn how to elicit information, including a narrative interview approach, allowing the child, adolescent, and parents to tell their stories" and that "there is a need to communicate empathy."[2]

BENEFITS OF EFFECTIVE COMMUNICATION

- The pediatric encounter is complex and unique because it:
  - Involves the physician-parent-child and other family members.
  - Is influenced by the developmental and cognitive stage of the child.
  - Needs to cover medical issues, emotional concerns, behavioral issues, anticipatory guidance, immunizations, and parent and child education.
- Dealing with these unique aspects in an effective manner requires that the physician be flexible in adjusting the history and physical exam to gain the most information and provide the most education efficiently.
- Communicating with patients and families is essential for quality care; effective physician-parent communication has been shown to be essential in securing:
  - An accurate diagnosis.

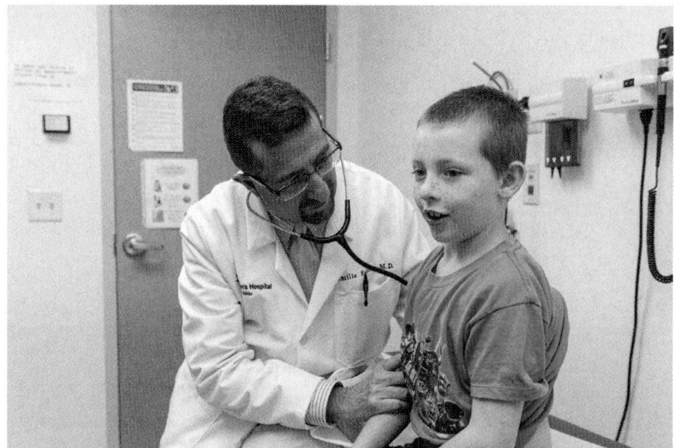

FIGURE 2-2 Dr. Camille Sabella examines a child recovering from osteomyelitis of the femur. This child required 6 weeks of antimicrobial therapy, which was accomplished successfully. Because this is a common and "routine" infection for a pediatric infectious diseases physician, it is easy to forget the considerable psychosocial effect that this infection had on this boy and his mother. Close follow-up, careful listening, education regarding the expectations and prognosis, and engaging the child in his own care all are important for a successful outcome.

  - Parental satisfaction with care.
  - Implementation and adherence to treatment recommendations.
  - Improved patient knowledge.
  - Enhanced discussion of psychosocial issues leading to improved psychological and behavioral outcomes.
- Effective communication is essential for patient-centered and family-centered care, which is endorsed by the AAP as a cornerstone for care.

COMMUNICATION WITH THE CHILD PATIENT

- A unique aspect of pediatric care is the approach to the child patient.
- Communication with the child patient is important if we expect the child to be an active participant in their care because it shows respect for the child's abilities and capacities, enhances their skill in making future health decisions, and enables their input in situations where there is more than one method of diagnosis or treatment. This is especially relevant for older children and adolescents.
- Treating the child as a partner results in improved adherence to the treatment plan and resultant outcome.[3,4]
- Despite the importance of direct communication with children, this appears to be limited in outpatient medical visits. In an older study from the Netherlands, children's contributions were limited to 4 percent of the encounters, although pediatricians directed 1/4 of their statements to the child.[5] In addition, only a small portion of medical information (13%) was directed at children.
- To help physician-child communication, pediatricians and primary care providers caring for children need to develop strategies for engaging children in the outpatient setting.
- To encourage participation of children in the medical encounter, physicians can ask children social questions early in the visit, phrase questions as requiring a yes-no response, and direct their gaze at the child when asking questions.[5]
- Other suggested strategies may include:[6]
  - Speak with the child—Not at or to him/her.
  - Setting should be private—Especially with the adolescent patient where confidentiality is critical.
  - Begin with a nonthreatening topic.
  - Listen actively.
  - Pay attention to body language and tone of voice.
  - Use drawings, games, or other creative communication techniques.
  - Elicit fears and concerns by reference to self or a third party.

FAMILY-ORIENTED CARE

- Ten years ago, the American Academy of Pediatric appointed a Task Force on the Family, in part to assist pediatricians in promoting well-functioning families.[7] This type of care was referred to as "family-oriented care" or "family pediatrics" and was strongly endorsed as a way to provide pediatric care in a context that promotes successful families and good outcomes for children.
- Family-oriented care is also important in addressing psychosocial issues, which accounts for 65 percent of primary care visits and requires a holistic approach by the clinician. It has been shown that a majority of parents welcome or do not mind being asked about emotional and psychosocial stressors.[8] It is clear that disclosure of psychosocial issues are likely to occur when the pediatrician:
  - Shows interest and attention while listening.
  - Directly asks questions.
  - Shows interest in managing parenting and behavioral concerns.[9]
- Caring is also an essential feature of family oriented care. Caring, as connectedness with a patient, evolves from the relationship. Within the context of this relationship, the clinician makes the patient and family feel known, pays attention to the meaning that a symptom or illness has in the family's life, expresses real feeling (separate from reflecting back the patient's feelings), and practices devotion (e.g., a willingness at times to do something extra for the patient and family).[10] To provide caring to patients, clinicians must take care of themselves.

CONCLUSION

The physician-parent-child interaction is complex and unique, and requires the provider to address multiple aspects of care, including medical diagnosis, treatment plan, anticipatory guidance, family education, and attention to psychosocial aspects. Genuine caring, empathy, support, and respect for the patient and family provide the foundation for an effective and long lasting physician-family relationship.

REFERENCES

1. Street, RL. Communication. Physician's communication and parents' evaluations of pediatric consultations. *Medical care* 1991;29:1146-1152.
2. American Academy of Pediatrics, Committee on psychosocial aspects of child and family health. The new morbidity revisited: a renewed commitment to the psychosocial aspects of pediatric care. *Pediatrics* 2001;108:1227-1230.
3. Rushforth H. Practitioner review: communicating with hospitalized children: review and application of research pertaining to children's understanding of health and illness. *J child Pediatr Psychol Psychiatry* 1999;40:683-69.
4. Tates K, Meeuwesen L. Doctor-parent-child communication. A review of the literature. *Soc Sci Med* 2001;52:839-851.
5. Van Dulmen AM. Children's contributions to pediatric outpatient encounters. *Pediatrics* 1998;102:563-568.
6. Lask B. Talking with children. *Br J Hosp Med* 1992;47:688-690.
7. American Academy of Pediatrics. Family Pediatrics. *Report of the Task Force on the Family Pediatrics* 2003;111(S2):1541-1571.
8. Kahn RS, Wise PH, Finkelstein JA, et al. The scope of unmet maternal health needs in pediatric settings. *Pediatrics*. 1999;103: 576-581.
9. Wissow LS. Pediatrician interview style and mothers' disclosure of psychosocial issues. *Pediatrics*. 1994;93:289-295.
10. Rider EA. Communication and relationships with children and parents. In: Novack DH, Clark W, Saizow R, Daetwyler C, eds. *doc.com: an interactive learning resource for healthcare comm. unication. 2006. Available at: http://webcampus.drexelmed.edu/doccom/user/.* Accessed February 9, 2008.

3 PATIENT- AND FAMILY-CENTERED CARE

Michelle Marks, DO, FAAP, FHM
Rita Pappas, MD, FAAP, FHM

PATIENT STORY

A 15-month-old boy is admitted with fever, rash, and conjunctivitis. Kawasaki disease is suspected and he is transferred to the inner city academic hospital from the community hospital. The mother of the boy is very concerned about the child and the diagnosis. Family Centered Rounds occur in the morning (**Figures 3-1** to **3-4**). During rounds, the health care team is introduced and a plan of care is initiated with input from the mother.

SYNONYMS

Family centered care; Family centered rounds.

DEFINITION

An innovative approach to the planning, delivery, and evaluation of health care that is grounded in a mutually beneficial partnership among patients, families, and providers, all of whom recognizes the importance of the family in the patient's life.[1,2]

It is an approach to health care that shapes policies, programs, facility design, and staff day-to-day interactions. It leads to better health outcomes, wiser allocation of resources, and greater patient and family satisfaction.

It should be noted that the term "Patient- and Family-Centered Care" has replaced "Family-Centered Care" to more explicitly capture the importance of engaging the family and the patient in a developmentally supportive manner, as essential members of the health care team.

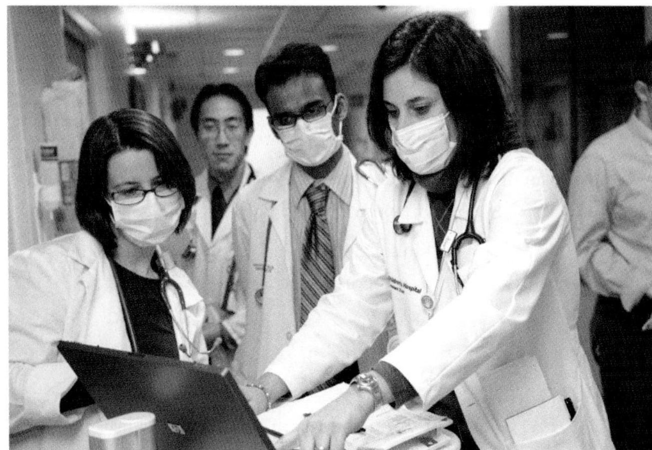

FIGURE 3-1 Patient-and Family-Centered Care. The pediatric team is preparing to enter the room by pre-rounding prior to entering the room.

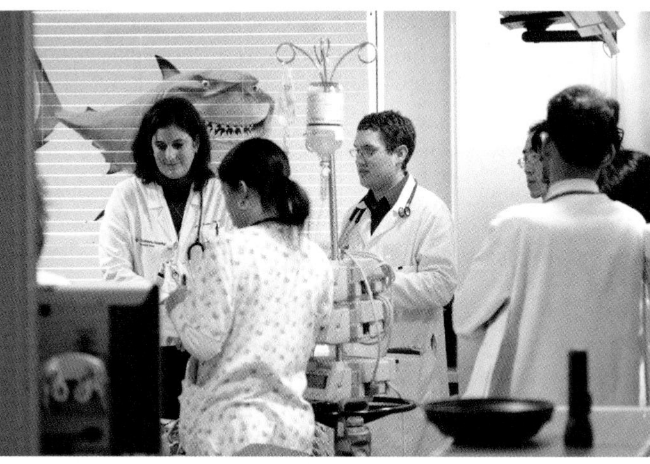

FIGURE 3-2 The pediatric team includes nursing, residents, medical students, and attending staff. It is vital to patients and families to include all involved in the care of the child and family.

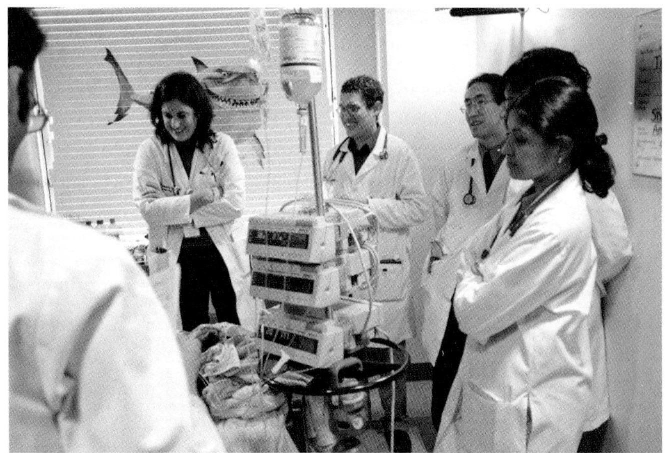

FIGURE 3-3 In the patient room, all participants need to be engaged and participate in the discussion.

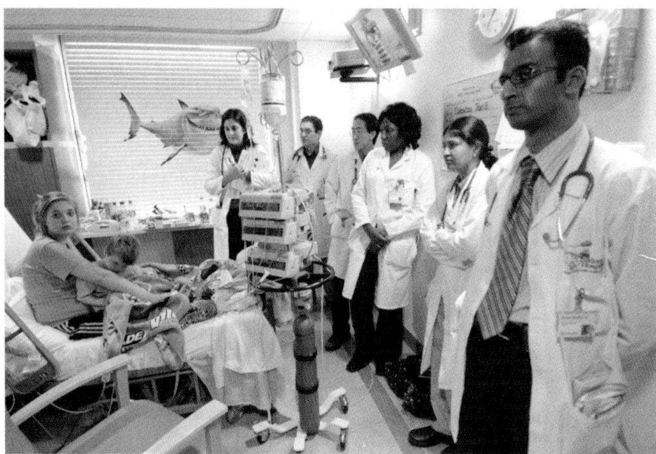

FIGURE 3-4 The pediatric team conducting rounds in the patient's room. The parents should be offered the choice to round inside of the patient room or outside of the patient room.

CORE PRINCIPLES OF PATIENT AND FAMILY-CENTERED CARE[1,2]

1. Listening to and respecting each child and his or her family, and honoring various types of backgrounds and family experiences. Patient and family knowledge, values, beliefs, and cultural backgrounds are incorporated into the planning and delivery of care.
2. Ensuring flexibility in the practice of the team so that services can be tailored to the needs, beliefs, and cultural values of each child and family, thus facilitating choice for the child and family about approaches to care.
3. Sharing complete, honest, and unbiased information with patients and their families on an ongoing basis, and in ways they find useful and affirming. Patients and families should receive timely, complete, and accurate information in order to effectively participate in care and decision-making. Health information for children and families should be available in the appropriate health literacy. In hospitals, conducting physician rounds in the patients' rooms with nursing staff and family present will enhance the exchange of information and encourage the involvement of the family in decision-making.
4. Providing and/or ensuring formal and informal support (e.g., peer-to-peer support) for the child and family during each phase of the child's life. Patients and families are encouraged and supported in participating in care and decision-making at the level they choose.
5. Collaborating with patients and families at all levels of health care: in the delivery of care to the individual child; in professional education, policy making, program development, implementation, and evaluation; and in health care facility design. In the area of medical research, patients and families should have voices at all levels in all facets of research.

HISTORY/INTRODUCTION

- Patient- and family-centered care emerged as an important concept in health care during the second half of the 20th century. Much of the early work focused on hospitals; for example, as research emerged about the effects of separating hospitalized children from their families, many institutions adopted policies that welcomed family members to be with their child around the clock and also encouraged their presence during medical procedures.
- The Maternal and Child Health Bureau of the Health Resources and Service Administration played an active role in furthering the involvement of families and the support of family issues and service needs.
- Federal legislation of the late 1980s and 1990s, much of it targeted at children with special needs, provided additional validation of the importance of family-centered principles.
- Family-centered care has long been a characteristic of an effective medical home. Founded in 1992, Family Voices comprises advocates for family-centered, community-based services for children with special health care needs.
- Building on work started in the previous decade, the Institute for Family- Centered Care (now the Institute for Patient- and Family-Centered Care) was also founded in 1992 to foster the development of partnerships among patients, families, and health care professionals, and to provide leadership for advancing the practice of family centered care in all settings.
- Patient- and family-centered care is supported by a growing body of research and by prestigious organizations, such as the Institute of Medicine (IOM), which in its 2001 report, "Crossing the Quality Chasm: A New Health System for the 21st Century," emphasized the need to ensure the involvement of patients in their own health care decisions, to better inform patients of treatment options, and to improve patients' and families' access to information.[3]
- In 2006, the Institute for Family-Centered Care and the Institute for Health care Improvement (IHI) brought together leadership organizations and patient and family advisors to advance the practice of patient- and family-centered care and ensure that there are sustained, effective partnerships with patients and families in all aspects of the health care system.[2,4,5]
- The American Academy of Pediatrics (AAP) has incorporated many of the principles of patient- and family centered care into several policy statements and manuals.[1,6] In 2006, the AAP Board of Directors approved a Parent Advisory Group pilot program under the section on Home Care. Members of the Parent Advisory Group all share a special interest in patient- and family-centered care, have personal experience with children with special health care needs, and serve as advisors and leaders for patient- and family-centered pediatric care within their own communities and at the national level.
- Founded in 1991, the IHI is an independent organization to improve health care throughout the world. Among its core values is patient and family centeredness. The National Institute for Children's Health care Quality (NICHQ) was launched as an IHI program in 1999. The NICHQ is dedicated to improving the quality of health care provided to children. One component of its 4-part improvement agenda is promoting evidence-based patient and family-centered care for children with chronic conditions.[7]
- There now have been several studies published in the literature, which demonstrate the benefits of patient and family-centered care.
- In the hospital environment, patient and family-centered care is associated with a decreased length of stay, reduced medical errors, and improved staff satisfaction.[8,9]
- There is also a significant link between patient and family satisfaction as well as hospital safety and communication, which is a fundamental part of this type of care.[8–10]
- Overall, this model of care can improve patient and family outcomes, improve the patient's and family's experience, increase patient and family satisfaction, build on child and family strengths, increase professional satisfaction, decrease health care costs, and lead to more effective use of health care resources.

RECOMMENDATIONS FOR IMPLEMENTATION[1]

1. As leaders of the child's medical home, pediatric providers should ensure that true collaborative relationships with patients and families as defined in the core concepts of patient- and

family-centered care are incorporated into all aspects of their professional practice. The patient and family are integral members of the health care team. They should participate in the development of the health care plan and have ownership of it.

2. Pediatric providers should unequivocally convey respect for families' unique insights into the understanding of their child's behavior and needs, should actively seek out their observations, and should appropriately incorporate family preferences into the care plan.
3. In hospitals, conducting attending physician rounds (i.e., patient presentations and discussions) in the patients' rooms with nursing staff and the family present should be standard practice.
4. Parents or guardians should be offered the option to be present with their child during medical procedures and offered support before, during, and after the procedure.
5. Families should be strongly encouraged to be present during hospitalization of their child, and pediatric providers should advocate for improved employer recognition of the importance of family presence during a child's illness.
6. Pediatric providers should share information with and promote the active participation of all children, including children with disabilities, if capable, in the management and direction of their own health care. The adolescent's and young adult's capacity for independent decision-making and right to privacy should be respected.
7. In collaboration with patients, families, and other health care professionals, pediatric providers should modify systems of care, processes of care, and patient flow as needed to improve the patient's and family's experience of care.
8. Pediatric providers should share medical information with children and families in ways that are useful and affirming. This information should be complete, honest, and unbiased.
9. Pediatric providers should encourage and facilitate peer-to-peer support and networking, particularly with children and families of similar cultural and linguistic backgrounds or with the same type of medical condition.
10. Pediatric providers should collaborate with patients and families and other health care providers to ensure a transition to good-quality, developmentally appropriate, patient- and family-centered adult health care services.
11. In developing job descriptions, hiring staff, and designing performance appraisal processes, pediatric providers should make explicit the expectation of collaboration with patients and families and other patient- and family-centered behaviors.
12. Pediatric providers should create a variety of ways for children and families to serve as advisors for and leaders of office, clinic, hospital, institutional, and community organizations involved with pediatric health care.
13. The design of health care facilities should promote the philosophy of patient- and family-centered care, such as including single room care, family sleeping areas, and availability of kitchen and laundry areas and other areas supportive of families. Providers should advocate for children and families to participate in design planning of health care facilities.
14. Education and training in patient and family-centered care should be provided to all trainees, students, and residents as well as staff members.
15. Patients and families should have a voice in shaping the research agenda, and they should be invited to collaborate in pediatric research programs. This should include determining how children and families participate in research and deciding how research findings will be shared with children and families.
16. Providers should advocate for and participate in research on outcomes and implementation of patient- and family-centered care in all venues of care.
17. Incorporating the patient- and family-centered care concepts into patient encounters requires additional face-to-face and coordination time by pediatricians. This time has value and is an investment in improved care, leading to better outcomes and prevention of unnecessary costs in the future. Payment for time spent with the family should be appropriate and paid without undue administrative complexities.

PROVIDER RESOURCES

- Johnson BH: Family-centered care: four decades of progress. *Fam Syst Health*. 2000;18(2):133-156.
- Johnson B, Abraham M, Conway J, et al. *Partnering With Patients and Families to Design a Patient- and Family-Centered Health Care System: Recommendations and Promising Practices*. Bethesda, MD: Institute for Family-Centered Care; 2008.
- Institute for Healthcare Improvement. Available at: http://www.ihi.org/ihi, accessed September 13, 2013.
- American Hospital Association. *Strategies for Leadership: Patient- and Family-Centered Care. Chicago, IL: American Hospital Association*; 2004. Available at: http://www.aha.org/aha/issues/Communicating-With-Patients/pt-family-centered-care.html, accessed May 12, 2013.
- Institute of Medicine, Committee on Quality Health Care in America. *To Err is Human: Building a Safer Health System*. Washington, DC: National Academies Press; 1999.
- Tearing down the walls. *Healthc Exec*. 2005;1(5):2-6.
- Sodomka P, Scott HH, Lambert AM, Meeks BD: *Patient and family centered care in an academic medical center: informatics, partnerships and future vision*. In: Weaver CA, Delaney CW, Weber P, Carr R, eds. Nursing and Informatics for the 21st Century: An International Look at Practice, Trends and the Future. Chicago, IL: Healthcare Information and Management Systems Society; 2006:501-506.
- Dowling J, Vender J, Guilianelli S, Wang B: A model of family-centered care and satisfaction predictors: the Critical Care Family Assistance Program. Chest. 2005;128(3):81S-92S.

REFERENCES

1. Patient- and Family-Centered Care and the Pediatrician's Role. *Pediatrics* February 1, 2012;129(2): 394-404.
2. Institute For Patient-And Family-Centered Care. Available at: http//www.ipfcc.org, accessed May 22, 2013.

3. Institute of Medicine. *Committee on Quality Health Care in America. Crossing the Quality Chasm: A New Health System for the 21st Century*. Washington, DC: National Academies Press; 2001.

4. Conway J, Johnson BH, Edgman-Levitan S, et al. *Partnering with patients and families to design a patient- and family-centered health care system: a roadmap for the future—a work in progress*. Bethesda, MD: Institute for Family-Centered Care and Institute for Healthcare Improvement; 2006.

5. Muething SE, Kotagal UR, Schoettker PJ, Gonzalez del Rey J, DeWitt TG. *Family-centered bedside rounds: a new approach to patient care and teaching. Pediatrics*. 2007;119(4):829-832.

6. American Academy of Pediatrics. Family pediatrics. Report of the Task Force on the Family. *Pediatrics*. 2003;111(s2):1539-1587.

7. National Initiative for Children's Healthcare Quality. Available at: http://www.nichq.org/nichq, accessed May 12, 2013.

8. Britto MT, Anderson JM, Kent WM, et al. Cincinnati Children's Hospital Medical Center: transforming care for children and families. *Jt Comm J Qual Patient Saf*. 2006;32(10): 541-548.

9. Cooley WC, McAllister JW. Building medical homes: improvement strategies in primary care for children with special health care needs. *Pediatrics*. 2004;113(5):1499-1506.

10. MacKean GL, Thurston WE, Scott CM. Bridging the divide between families and health professionals' perspectives on family-centered care. *Health Expect*. 2005;8(1):74-85.

4 THE BIRTH OF A CHILD

Sabine Iben, MD

PATIENT STORY

Mary and Joe are expecting their first baby. The pregnancy has been without complications; routine prenatal screens and ultrasounds have been negative including the screen for Mary's Group B Streptococcal (GBS) status, the Quad screen for fetal anomalies and cystic fibrosis carrier status. Mary is happy to report strong fetal movements. One week before her due date Mary experiences strong contractions. She is admitted in active labor, membranes rupture spontaneously within 2 hours after arrival in the hospital. Labor progresses uneventfully, pain relief is provided by epidural anesthesia. Ten hours later a vigorous baby girl is born. The only intervention provided for resuscitation is drying followed by skin-to-skin placement on mother's chest for bonding. Initial physiologic cyanosis is resolved by 5 minutes of life (**Figure 4-1**). APGAR scores of 8 at 1 min and 9 at 5 min are assigned. Her weight shows that she is appropriate for gestational age. Erythromycin eye ointment is applied to both eyes for prophylaxis of ophthalmia neonatorum, an injection of Vitamin K intramuscularly is given for prophylaxis of hemorrhagic disease of the newborn. Mary chooses to breastfeed that is initiated shortly after delivery with the aid of a lactation consultant. Over the next couple of days, the newborn is breastfeeding about 10 times a day, voiding several times a day and has passed her first meconium stool by 14 hours of life. On day of life # 2 she has lost 6 percent of her birthweight and appears mildly jaundiced. A bilirubin level shows a value within the physiologic range. She is discharged at about 50 hours of life with her mother and a follow-up visit with her pediatrician is arranged for 2 days after discharge.

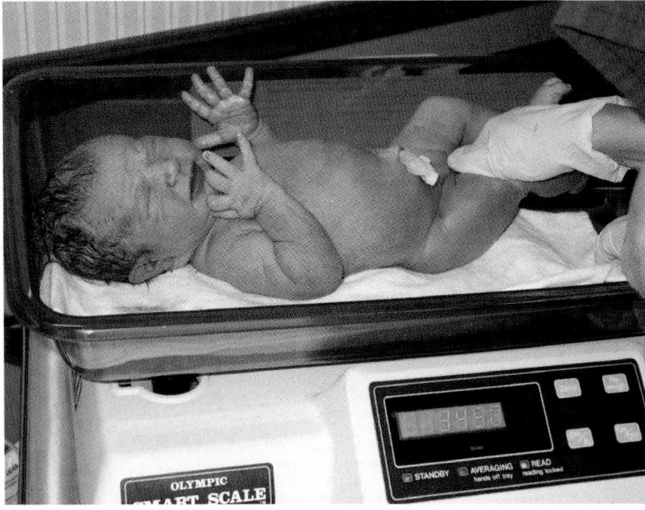

FIGURE 4-1 Acrocyanosis of hands and feet in a newborn is physiologic and not a sign of hypoxia. (*Used with permission from Dr. Sabine Iben.*)

EPIDEMIOLOGY

- According to the Center for Disease Control,[1] in the US in 2011 there were:
  - a total of 3,953,593 births recorded.
  - 32.8 percent of infants delivered by Cesarean Section.
  - 11.72 percent of infants preterm.
  - 8.1 percent of low birthweight (<2500g).
- The neonatal mortality rate in 2011 was 4.04 neonatal deaths/1,000 live births/year, resulting in ca. 24,000 deaths per year.[2]
- The leading causes of neonatal deaths are preterm related (ca. 35%) and due to congenital malformations, most commonly heart defects.[3]
- Overall, 3 percent of all infants in the US are born with a major structural or genetic birth defect.[4]
- Ten percent of newborns require some degree of assistance in the delivery room; less than 1 percent require extensive resuscitation measures.[5]

ETIOLOGY AND PATHOPHYSIOLOGY

- A baby's due date (Estimated date of Confinement [EDC]) is calculated at 40 weeks after the Last Menstrual Period (LMP).
- A baby born at <37 weeks gestational age (GA) is considered preterm; borderline of viability is considered 22 to 23 weeks GA.
- Irrespectively of gestational age, a baby weighing less than 2500 g is considered low birthweight; less than 1500 g very low birthweight; and less than 750 g extremely low birthweight.
- Transition from intrauterine to extrauterine life.
  - Intrauterine fetal circulation (**Figure 4-2**):
    - Gas exchange occurs through the placenta, which represents the path of lowest resistance in fetal circulation.
    - Non-ventilated high-resistance lungs are bypassed by the foramen ovale and the patent ductus arteriosus and receive only minimal perfusion.
  - Uncomplicated transition is characterized by:
    - Increase in systemic pressure promoted by clamping of the cord and removal of the low resistance placenta.
    - Surfactant secretion which decreases the surface tension in the alveoli.
    - Loss of fetal lung fluid.
    - Establishment of a Functional Residual capacity (FRC) facilitated by the first breaths.
    - Functional closure of physiologic shunts (Foramen ovale and Ductus arteriosus).
    - These changes result in a decrease in pulmonary vascular resistance and increase in pulmonary artery blood flow.
  - Failure of appropriate transitioning into the newborn circulation may result in Persistent Pulmonary Hypertension of the Newborn (PPHN) characterized by hypoxemia due to persistently high pulmonary vascular resistance and decreased pulmonary blood flow.

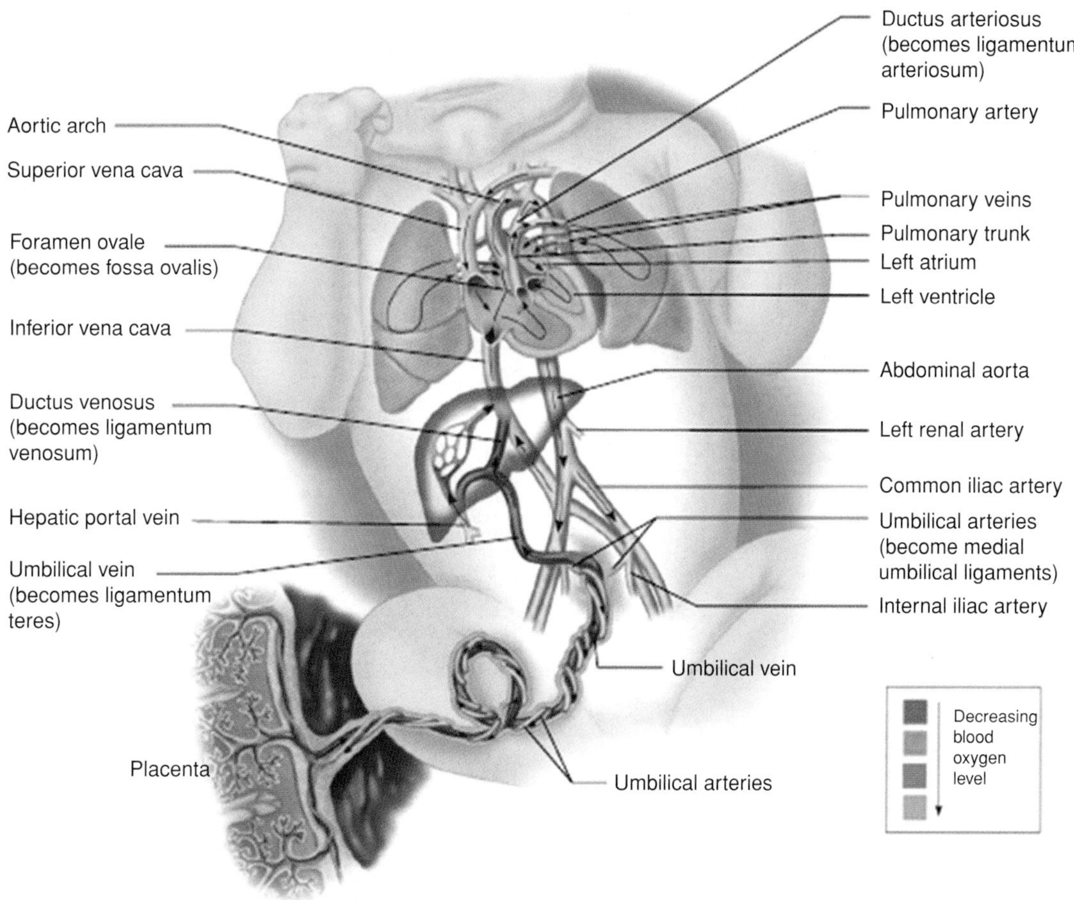

FIGURE 4-2 Illustration of the fetal circulation. Blood is oxygenated in the placenta, bypassing the lungs through physiologic shunts (Ductus arteriosus, Foramen ovale). (*Used with permission from Hole's* Human Anatomy and Physiology, *12e, McGraw-Hill.*)

RISK FACTORS

Common prenatal factors that may result in a need for neonatal intervention at delivery or further intensive care include:

- Fetal malformations/chromosomal anomalies.
- A variety of hereditary familial disorders.
- Multiple gestation (**Figure 4-3**).
- Placental insufficiency due to maternal hypertension/preeclampsia, abnormal cord insertion, placental infarcts, chronic abruption (**Figure 4-4**).
- Exposure to certain maternal medications or illicit drugs.
- Poor maternal nutrition.
- Maternal obesity/diabetes.
- Poor prenatal care.
- Inappropriate fetal growth (intrauterine growth retardation or macrosomia).
- Known blood group incompatibility.
- Untreated maternal sexually transmitted diseases.
- Abnormal fetal monitoring (fetal decelerations, poor reactivity, tachycardia).

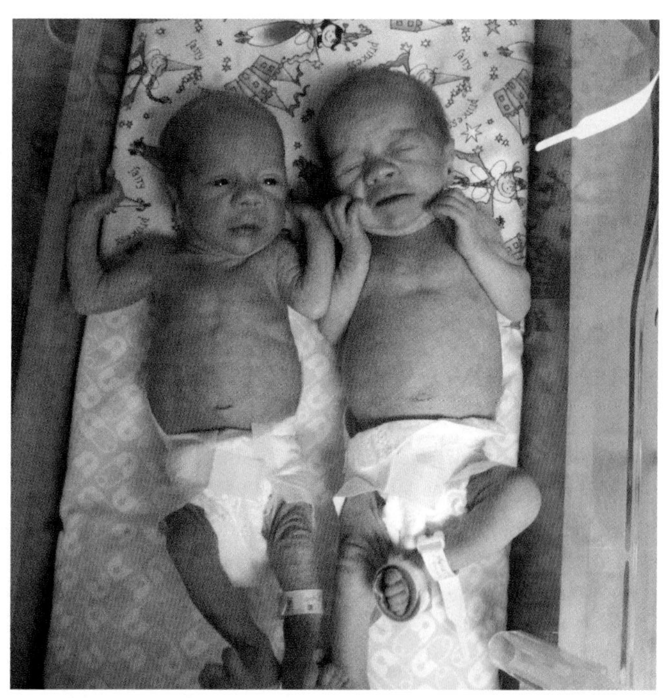

FIGURE 4-3 Monoamniotic, dichorionic twin girls with a 10 percent growth discrepancy, born premature at 31 weeks. (*Used with permission from Dr. Sabine Iben.*)

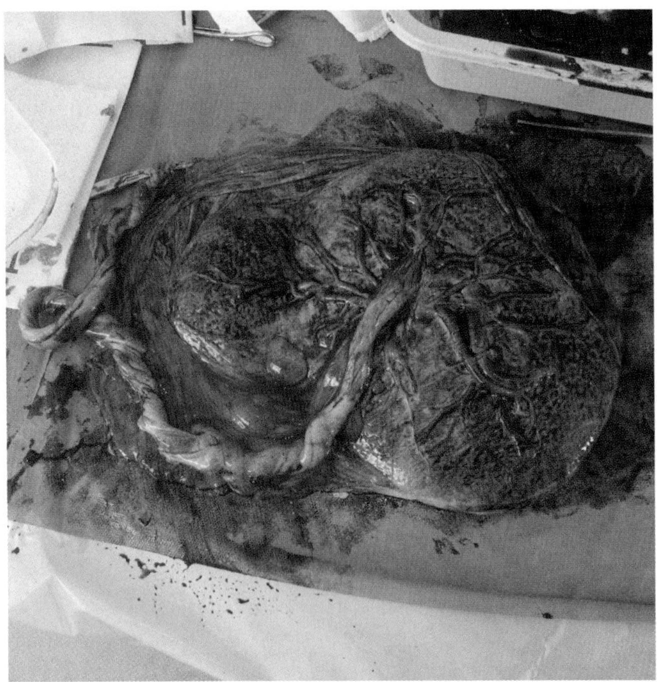

FIGURE 4-4 Bilobate placenta, rarely of clinical significance. Placental anomalies or abnormal cord insertions can be associated with poor fetal outcome. (*Used with permission from Dr. Sabine Iben.*)

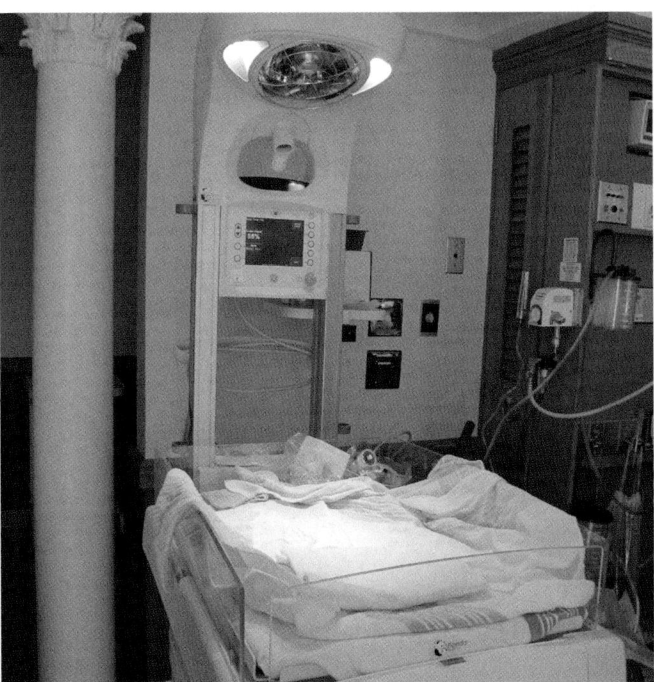

FIGURE 4-5 Resuscitation table set up for newborn resuscitation: heat source is turned on, several blankets prepared for drying the newborn, suction devices (bulb and wall suction), bag/mask, oxygen source and intubation equipment all available and checked. (*Used with permission from Dr. Sabine Iben.*)

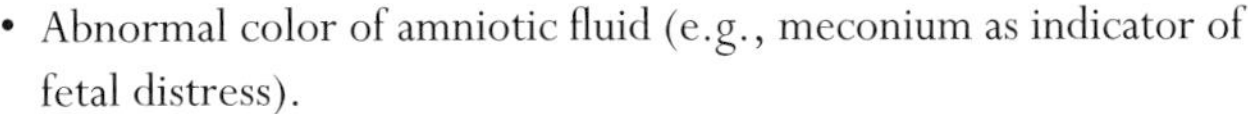

- Abnormal color of amniotic fluid (e.g., meconium as indicator of fetal distress).
- Maternal fever.
- Maternal colonization with pathogens—GBS, *Escherichia coli.*
- Prolonged rupture of membranes.
- Preterm labor.
- Abnormal fetal lie.
- Cesarean delivery.

DIAGNOSIS

Assessment of the newborn in the delivery room (**Figures 4-5** to **4-8**) include:

- Detailed maternal history.
- Determination of the gestational age by history.
- Identification of risk factors for conditions that require additional monitoring or intervention.
- Assignment of APGAR scores by the team attending the delivery:
  - At 1 minute reflecting the assessment at birth.
  - At 5 minutes reflecting the response to resuscitation.
  - At 10 minutes if score at 5 minutes is less than 7.[6]
- A cursory physical examination. Findings of a normal transition may include peripheral cyanosis and mild tachypnea.

Initial assessment in the newborn nursery include:

- Length, head circumference, and weight measurements.
- Vital signs including temperature, heart rate (HR), and respiratory rate.
- Categorization into SGA (small for gestational age, weight <10th percentile), AGA (appropriate for gestational age, weight 10–90th percentile), and LGA (large for gestational age, weight >90th percentile).

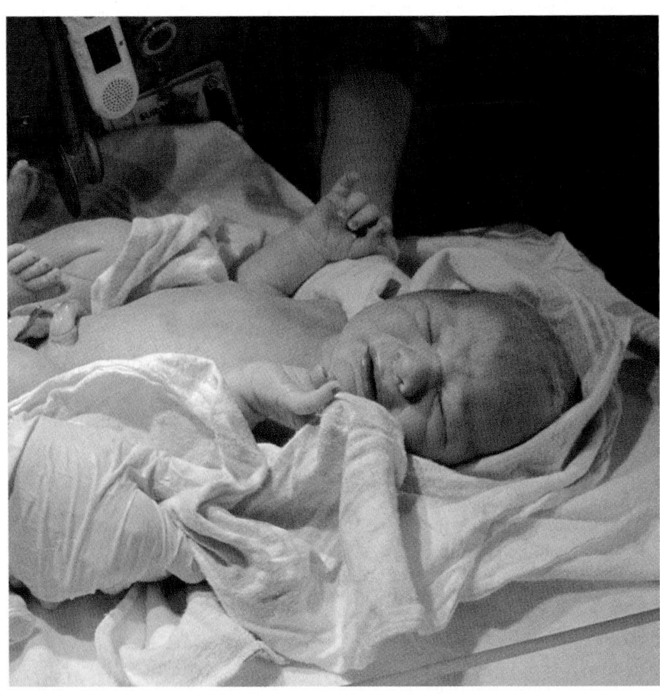

FIGURE 4-6 Vigorous newborn at 1 minute of age, no resuscitation needed other than drying. (*Used with permission from Dr. Sabine Iben.*)

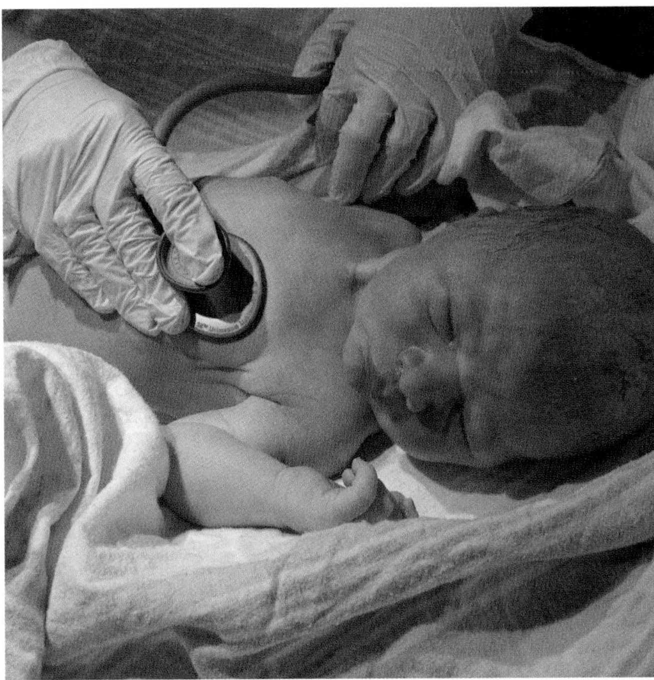

FIGURE 4-7 An initial physical examination is part of the newborn assessment. (*Used with permission from Dr. Sabine Iben.*)

- Complete physical examination.
- Review of maternal medical history, prenatal screens, and prenatal imaging.
- Screen for hypoglycemia as indicated:
  - Infants with risk factors only, asymptomatic: 30 minutes after the first feed. Risk factors include LGA or SGA, infant of diabetic mother (IDM), and prematurity. Symptomatic infants need to be screened earlier.

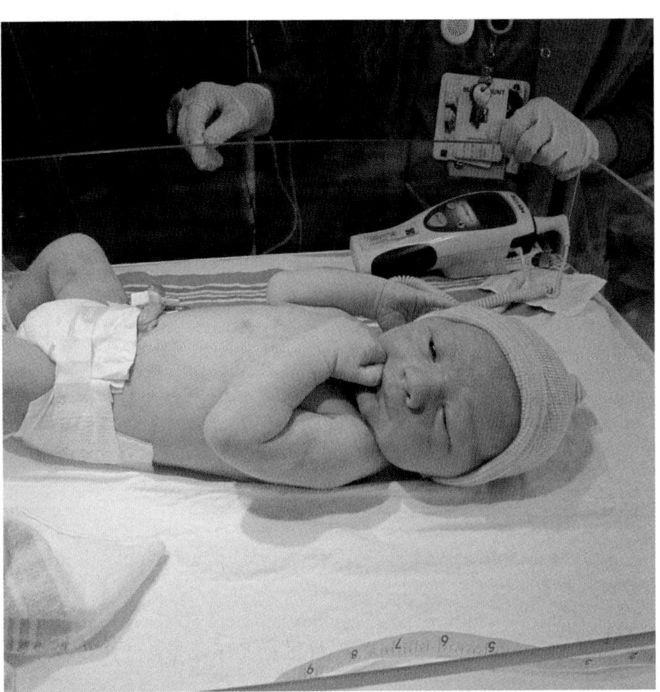

FIGURE 4-8 A hat helps to minimize heat loss. The baby is in no distress and ready to spend time with mom. (*Used with permission from Dr. Sabine Iben.*)

  - Target glucose concentration is ≥45 mg/dl; babies should be followed before feedings for 12 (IDM) to 24 hours of life (preterm, SGA)[7]. SOR Ⓒ
- Ballard exam[8] if gestational age is unknown or uncertain. Of note, gestational age is most accurately determined by early ultrasound or LMP. The estimated gestational age by Ballard exam may be inaccurate by as much as 2 weeks.
- Screening complete blood count with differential, blood culture as recommended by the CDC algorithm for prevention of early GBS sepsis[9] or if risk factors for sepsis are present.[10]
- Assess for risk factors for jaundice, which includes the verification of maternal blood type. Most facilities routinely obtain the infants blood type on cord blood, either universally or selectively if maternal blood type is O, Rh negative, or direct antibody positive.

MANAGEMENT

In the delivery room:

- Newborn resuscitation according to NRP guidelines.[11] SOR Ⓒ
- Vitamin K 0.5 to 1mg intramuscularly for prophylaxis of hemorrhagic disease of the newborn.[12] SOR Ⓐ
  - Incidence is 0.25 to 1.7 percent without prophylaxis.
  - Oral Vitamin K may not prevent late-onset hemorrhagic disease of the newborn.
- Eye prophylaxis with erythromycin 0.5 percent ointment for prevention of gonococcal ophthalmia neonatorum.[13] SOR Ⓐ
- Identification band on baby, mother, and second adult (father or other support person designated by mother).
- Application of security device/sensor if available.
- Determination of appropriate further care (newborn nursery, transitional care, neonatal intensive care unit).

In the newborn nursery:

- Recording of birth parameters on growth charts.
- Bath/sponge bath with mild, non-medicated soap after temperature is stable.
- Encourage breastfeeding and educate mothers about benefits.
- Assess for contraindications for breastfeeding (active herpes simplex virus lesions on the breast, maternal human immunodeficiency virus [HIV] infection, treatment with antimetabolites, chemotherapeutic or radioactive agents, some metabolic disorders in the infant). If in doubt, consult with lactation consultant or neonatologist:
  - Estimation of intake and output by recording duration of breastfeeding, amount of formula, number of wet diapers, and meconium.
  - Eecording of vital signs.
  - Maintain temperature.
  - Daily weight.
  - Appropriate positioning (supine on flat surface).
  - Regular assessment for signs and symptoms of withdrawal using a narcotic abstinence scoring system if exposed to opiates prenatally.[14]

- Exam by physician at least by 24 hours of age, within 24 hours before discharge.
- Circumcision care
  - Cleaning of surgical site and application of petroleum jelly with each diaper change for 4 to 7 days after circumcision.[15]
  - Foreskin should not be forcibly retracted in uncircumcised penis. Adhesions are physiologic.
- Cord care
  - Cord should be kept clean and dry.
  - Antiseptic agents (alcohol, triple dye, chlorhexidine) not indicated in developed countries. SOR Ⓐ
- Assess maternal hepatitis B surface antigen (HepBsAg) status and follow recommendations per CDC[16]; early immunization is effective in preventing acquisition of Hepatitis B. SOR Ⓐ
  - If maternal screen is positive the infant will require Hepatitis B vaccine AND Hepatitis B immunoglobulin (HBIG) within first 12 hours of life.
  - If Hep B status cannot be determined within first 12 hours of life the baby will need Hepatitis B vaccine within that timeframe as well as immunoglobulin within 7 days of life if the maternal screen returns positive or remains unknown.
  - If Hepatitis B status is unknown and the baby's birthweight is less than 2000g, both the vaccine and immunoglobulin should be given within first 12 hours of life.

Some problems can be managed in the newborn nursery while many require monitoring and treatment in the neonatal intensive care unit.

- Dehydration as indicated by excessive weight loss and/or poor urine output:
  - If bottle-feeding, observe feeding technique. Consider change in nipple or feed more frequently.
  - Lactation consultation for breastfeeding moms.
  - Consider transient supplements with formula.
  - Bottle versus tube extension to the breast, finger feeding, or cup feeding.
- Jaundice
  - Assess need for phototherapy (**Figure 4-9**) using American Academy of Pediatrics recommended phototherapy levels and guidelines.[17,18]
    - May be provided in the newborn nursery as long as there is no excessive rise and/or impending need for exchange transfusion.
    - Assure optimal skin exposure while closely monitored for hypothermia.
    - Devices include phototherapy banks and biliblankets that may provide continuous phototherapy while breastfeeding and enable maximal skin surface exposure.
    - Efficacy of phototherapy lights can be measured with a commercially available radiometer.
    - Depending on the rate of rise Serum Bilirubin should be checked every 6 to 24 hours.
    - Transcutaneous measurements cannot be used during and up to 48 hours after receiving phototherapy.
    - Eyes have to be covered with eye patches. SOR Ⓒ
    - Infant can be removed for a limited time for feeding and bonding after decrease in bilirubin is documented.
    - Dehydration should be avoided, supplementation of breastfeeding infants can be considered.

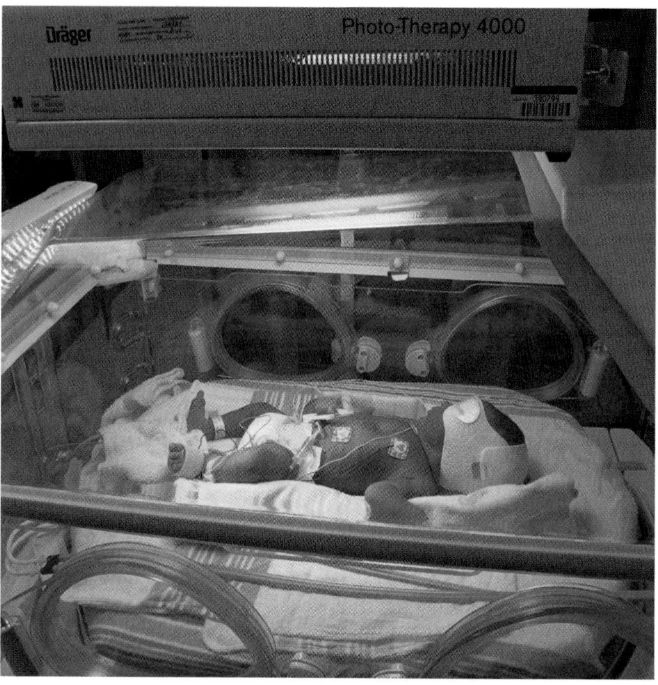

FIGURE 4-9 Maximized phototherapy in a newborn with ABO-incompatibility and hemolytic jaundice. Several banks of phototherapy may be used including a biliblanket. The baby is in an Isolette to prevent heat loss while clothing is removed to maximize exposed body surface area. (*Used with permission from Dr. Sabine Iben.*)

- Hypothermia
  - Investigate causes.
  - Add additional blankets.
  - Optimize environmental temperature.
- Hypoglycemia
  - Encourage oral (po) feeds, feed every 2 to 3 hours
  - Consider supplements.
  - Consider IV fluids.
  - Regular monitoring BEFORE feeds.
  - Work-up for causes of persistent hypoglycemia with endocrinology input.
- Failure to pass meconium by 48 hours.
  - Avoid rectal stimulation/suppositories.
  - Obtain plain abdominal radiograph.
  - Detailed exam to make sure anus is patent.
  - Specialty consultation (neonatology, pediatric surgery) for suspected bowel obstruction.
- Emesis
  - Assess volume/frequency.
  - Physical exam.
  - Consider radiographic studies (abdominal x-ray).
  - Bilious vs. non-bilious.
  - Bilious emesis ALWAYS requires work-up including abdominal x-ray, Upper GI, subspecialty consultation; this finding could be the only symptom of a volvulus and may present a surgical emergency because of the risk of bowel necrosis.
- Neonatal withdrawal
  - Elevated narcotic abstinence scores on an assessment scale.[14]
  - Encourage breastfeeding.

- Initiate comfort measures (swaddling, holding, minimal stimulation, or dark room).
- May require pharmacologic treatment.

Discharge criteria:

- Most states and US Congress enacted legislation that ensures hospital stay for up to 48 hours for a vaginal delivery and up to 96 hours after Cesarean delivery.
- The following criteria should be met:[19]
  - Physiologic stability.
  - Family competence to provide newborn care at home.
  - Assessment of family, environmental and social risk factors with actions taken if needed.
  - Completed teaching about care of the newborn.
  - Access to the health care system and resources, follow-up appointments have been made.
  - No excessive weight loss.
  - No significant jaundice.
  - Feeding appropriately.

PREVENTION AND SCREENING

- Hearing screen.
  - The incidence of hearing loss is approximately 1 to 3/1000 newborns (20 to 40/1000 in the NICU population).
  - Benefits of early detection and intervention include higher receptive and expressive language skills.
  - Hearing screens at discharge by otoacustic emissions (OAE) or automated auditory brainstem response (ABR) are mandatory in most states[20] following the recommendations of the Joint Committee of Infant Hearing by the American Academy of Audiology.[21]
- Screening for critical congenital heart disease by pulse oximetry.
  - Recommended by Health and Human Services since September 2011 and endorsed by the AAP.[22]
  - Goal is to identify infants with critical congenital heart disease before infant becomes symptomatic, cardiac work-up is pursued after positive screen.[23]
- Newborn metabolic state screen.
  - Obtained between 24 to 48 hours of life by heelstick.
  - Included disorders vary by state.[24,25]
- Car safety seat testing for premature infants at less than 37 weeks gestational age.
  - Preterm infants are more prone to hypoxic events in a semi-upright position.
  - Car safety seat monitoring involves infant being placed in infant car seat and monitored by pulse oximetry for a set amount of time, a minimum of 90 to 120 minutes or longer if expected to spend longer periods in a car.[26]
- Initiation of Hepatitis B vaccination per CDC childhood immunization schedule.[27]
- Vitamin D supplements for breastfeeding babies (400 IU/day) to start in the first few days of life.[28]
- Male circumcision before discharge if parental preference.
  - Circumcision rates in the US vary widely by region; overall, 55 percent of newborn males are currently being circumcised.[29]
  - The American Academy of Pediatrics currently justifies a medical indication for circumcision based on preventive health benefits including a decreased incidence of urinary tract infection in first year of life, heterosexual acquisition of HIV and other sexually transmitted diseases, and for penile cancer in circumcised males, outweighing the risks of the procedure.[30]
- Screening for developmental dysplasia of the hip by physical exam.[31] Risk factors include female gender, breech birth, or positive family history.

PROGNOSIS

- Readmission rates have been shown to be higher with earlier discharges.[32]
- Readmissions most frequently related to jaundice, dehydration, and feeding difficulties.[33]

FOLLOW-UP

Follow-up with the primary care provider within 2 to 3 days or earlier if there are specific concerns. The follow-up visit should include:

- Tracking the infant's weight.
  - Weight loss beyond 3 days of age, >7 percent of birthweight or failure to regain birthweight by 10 days of age warrants evaluation of feeding technique/breastfeeding adequacy.
- Assessment of jaundice.
- Answering parental questions and concerns.

PATIENT EDUCATION

Routine discharge teaching should include education about:

- Appropriate urination and stooling pattern.
- Transition from meconium to yellow around 3 to 4 days of age.
- Umbilical cord, skin, and genital care.
- Temperature assessment and measurement with a thermometer.
- Signs of illness and common newborn problems.
- Infant safety and SIDS education:[34]
  - Use of an appropriate car safety seat.
  - Supine positioning ("Back to sleep") for sleeping with supervised tummy time while awake.
  - Firm sleeping surface.
  - "Bare crib," no loose blankets, or soft objects.
  - No positioning devices in cribs.
  - Avoid smoke exposure, alcohol and illicit drug use before and after birth.
  - Breastfeeding.
  - Avoid overheating.
  - Room sharing, but no bed sharing.

  - Pacifier use during sleep.
  - Safe handling—never shaking.
- Hand hygiene as a way to reduce infection.
- Instructions to follow in the event of a complication or emergency.

PROVIDER RESOURCES

- American Academy of Pediatrics and the American College of Obstetricians and Gynecologists: *Guidelines for Perinatal Care*, edited by Riley LE, Stark AR. Elk Grove Village, WA; 2012.
- American Heart Association and American Academy of Pediatrics. *Neonatal Resuscitation Textbook*, edited by Kattwinkel JK. American Academy of Pediatrics and the American Heart Association: 2011.

PARENT RESOURCES

- Shelov, SP, Altman TR: *Caring for Your Baby and Young Child Birth to Age 5*. American Academy of Pediatrics. Elk Grove Village, WA: 2009.
- Meek JY: New Mother's Guide to Breastfeeding, American Academy of Pediatrics, Elk Grove Village, WA: 2011. http://www.marchofdimes.com/baby/bringinghome_indepth.html.

REFERENCES

1. US Department of Health and Human Services, Centers for Disease Control and Prevention: Births: Preliminary data for 2011. *National Vital Statistics Reports*. 2012;61(5):1-13.
2. US Department of Health and Human Services, Centers for Disease control and Prevention. Deaths: Preliminary Data for 2011. *National Vital Statistics Reports*. 2012;61(6):1-11.
3. US Department of Health and Human Services, Centers for Disease control and Prevention: Infant Mortality Statistics From the 2008 Period Linked Birth/Infant Death Data Set. *National Vital Statistics Reports*. 2012;60(5):1-13.
4. US Department of Health and Human Services, Centers for Disease control and Prevention: Update on Overall Prevalence of Major Birth Defects-Atlanta, Georgia, 1978-2005. *MMWR*. 2008;57(01):1-5.
5. American Heart Association: *American Academy of Pediatrics: Neonatal Resuscitation Textbook*, edited by Kattwinkel JK. American Heart Association and the American Academy of Pediatrics: 2011.
6. American Academy of Pediatrics, The American College of Obstetricians and Gynecologists: Care of the Newborn, in American Academy of Pediatrics. *The American College of Obstetricians and Gynecologists: Guidelines for Perinatal Care*, edited by Riley LE, Stark AR. Elk Grove Village, WA; 2012:274.
7. Adamkin DH. Committee on Fetus and Newborn: Postnatal Glucose Homeostasis in Late- Preterm and Term Infants. *Pediatrics* 2011;127(3):575-579.
8. Ballard, JL, Khoury, JC, Wedig, K et al. New Ballard Score, expanded to include extremely premature infants. *J. Pediatr.* 1991;119(3):417-423.
9. Committee on Infectious Diseases and Committee on Fetus and Newborn: Policy statement- Recommendations for the Prevention of Perinatal Group B Streptococcal (GBS) Disease. Pediatrics 2011;128:611-616.
10. Polin, RA. Committee on Fetus and Newborn: Management of Neonates with Suspected or Proven Early- Onset Bacterial Sepsis. *Pediatrics* 2012;129:1006-1015.
11. American Heart Association: *American Academy of Pediatrics: Textbook of neonatal resuscitation 6th edition*, edited by Kattwinkel JK. Elk Grove Village,IL: 2011.
12. American Academy of Pediatrics Committee on Fetus and Newborn: Controversies Concerning Vitamin K and the Newborn. Pediatrics. 2003;112(1):191-192.
13. Hammerschlag MR, Cummings C, Roblin PM, et al. Efficacy of Neonatal Ocular Prophylaxis for the Prevention of Chlamydial and Gonococcal Conjunctivitis. *N Engl J Med.* 1989;320(12):769-772.
14. Finnegan LP, Connaughton JF Jr, Kron RE, et al. Neonatal abstinence syndrome: assessment and management. *Addict. Dis.* 1975;2(1-2):141-58.
15. American Academy of Pediatrics: The American College of Obstetricians and Gynecologists: Care of the Newborn, in American Academy of Pediatrics, The American College of Obstetricians and Gynecologists: Guidelines for Perinatal Care, edited by Riley LE, Stark AR. Elk Grove Village, WA: 2012:286-287.
16. American Academy of Pediatrics: Red Book: 2012 Report of the Committee on Infectious Diseases. Edited by Pickering LK. American Academy of Pediatrics, Elk Grove Village, IL: 2012:369-390.
17. Bhutani VK. Committee on Fetus and Newborn American Academy of Pediatrics: Phototherapy to prevent severe neonatal hyperbilirubinemia in the newborn infant 35 or more weeks of gestation. *Pediatrics.* 2011;128(4):e1046-52.
18. American Academy of Pediatrics Subcommittee on Hyperbilirubinemia: Management of Hyperbilirubinemia in the Newborn Infant 35 or More Weeks of Gestation. *Pediatrics.* 2004;114(1):297-316.
19. Committee on Fetus and Newborn: Policy statement: Hospital Stay for Healthy Term Newborns. *Pediatrics.* 2010;125(2):405-409.
20. National Conference of State legislatures: Newborn hearing screening laws, http://www.ncsl.org/issues-research/health/newborn-hearing-screening-state-laws.aspx, Washington, DC: 2011.
21. Joint Committee on Infant Hearing: Principles and guidelines for early hearing detection and intervention programs. *Pediatrics.* 2007;120(4):898-921.
22. American Academy of Pediatrics Section on Cardiology and Cardiac Surgery Executive committee: Policy Statement- Endorsement of health and human services recommendation for pulse oximetry screening for critical congenital heart disease. *Pediatrics.* 2012;129(1):190-192.
23. Kemper AR, Mahle WT, Martin GR, et al. Strategies for Implementing Screening for Critical Congenital Heart Disease. *Pediatrics.* 2011;128(5):e1259-e1267.

24. Kaye CI. American Academy of Pediatrics Committee on Genetics: Newborn screening fact sheets. *Pediatrics.* 2006;118 (3):e934-63.

25. American Academy of Pediatrics Newborn Screening Authoring Committee: Newborn screening expands: recommendations for pediatricians and medical home- implications for the system. *Pediatrics.* 2008;121(10):192-217.

26. Bull MJ, Engle WA, the Committee on Injury, Violence and Poison Prevention, et al. Safe transportation of preterm and low birth weight infants at hospital discharge. *Pediatrics.* 2009;123(5):1424-1429.

27. AAP Committee on Infectious Diseases: Policy statement. Recommended Childhood and Adolescent Immunization Schedules-United States. *Pediatrics.* 2012;129(2):385-386.

28. Wagner CL, Greer FR, American Academy of Pediatrics Section on Breastfeeding, et al. Prevention of rickets and vitamin D deficiency in infants, children, and adolescents. *Pediatrics.* 2008;122(5):1142-52.

29. Maeda JL, Chari R, Elixhauser A. *Healthcare Cost and Utilization Project (HCUP): Circumcisions Performed in U.S. Community Hospitals, 2009: Statistical Brief #126.* http://www.hcup-us.ahrq.gov/reports/statbriefs/sb126.jsp. Rockville, MD: 2012.

30. American Academy of Pediatrics Task Force on Circumcision: Male circumcision. *Pediatrics.* 2012;130(3):e756-85.

31. Committee on Quality Improvement, Subcommittee on Developmental Dysplasia of the Hip: American Academy of Pediatrics: Clinical practice guideline: early detection of developmental dysplasia of the hip. *Pediatrics.* 2000;105(4 Pt 1): 896-905.

32. Datar A, Sood N. Impact of postpartum hospital-stay legislation on newborn length of stay, readmission, and mortality in California. *Pediatrics.* 2006;118(1):63-72.

33. Escobar GJ, Greene JD, Hulac P., et al. Rehospitalization after birth hospitalization: patterns among infants of all gestations. *Arch. Dis. Child.* 2005;90(2):125-131.

34. Task force on Sudden Infant Death Syndrome: Policy Statement: SIDS and Other Sleep- Related Deaths: Expansion of Recommendations for a Safe Infant Sleeping Environment. *Pediatrics.* 2011; 128(5):1030-1039.

5 PEDIATRIC PALLIATIVE CARE

Brooke Johnston, MD
Denise Powers-Fabian, MSSA, LISW-S
Nancy Carst, MSW
Sarah Friebert, MD

PATIENT STORY

At 7 months of age, Blake (**Figure 5-1**) was diagnosed with a rare, progressive malignancy. His initial admission was prompted by swelling of his left lower extremity, and imaging studies revealed an extra-renal rhabdoid tumor. His family experienced a rapid indoctrination into the world of childhood cancer. Blake had a central line placed and chemotherapy begun; his parents faced the accompanying challenges of work absence, needs of their other child, the responsibilities of communicating complicated information to supportive communities, and the fear of losing their infant son. Six weeks later, Blake was admitted for emesis and the detection of brain metastases lent new gravity to his prognosis. A ventriculoperitoneal shunt was placed and bone marrow studies performed. The Palliative Care service met Blake, his parents, and 4 year-old sister shortly thereafter. Blake's family sought support in managing anticipatory grief, supporting and preparing his sister, decision-making discussions, end-of-life planning, as well as in planning for life after his death. The Palliative Care service also provided symptom control consultation for Blake's disease-related pain and agitation. Music and art therapies were helpful for diversion and expression of difficult emotions, particularly for Blake's sister. Blake received palliative chemotherapy which was temporarily quite efficacious and resulted in marked clinical improvement. He would play, smile, engage those around him, and grant his family an unexpected gift of treasured time. Between admissions for chemotherapy, his family was supported by local hospice, as well as the on-call oncology and palliative care staff. Upon admission for a fourth round of high-dose chemotherapy it became evident that the hydration therapy necessary for chemotherapy administration would worsen Blake's already tenuous respiratory status. His parents, who had clearly expressed that they desired only therapies that would be beneficial for Blake, wished to discontinue chemotherapy. Supportive measures, including opioid treatment for pain and dyspnea, and benzodiazepine infusion for anxiety and dyspnea, were titrated to address clinical symptoms. Team members supported the family through this decision-making process, and offered discussions regarding common occurrences at the end of life. His parents elected to have Blake's end of life in the hospital setting as they felt most comfortable with the resources there. He died peacefully in the company of his family. The Palliative Care team continues to provide bereavement support.

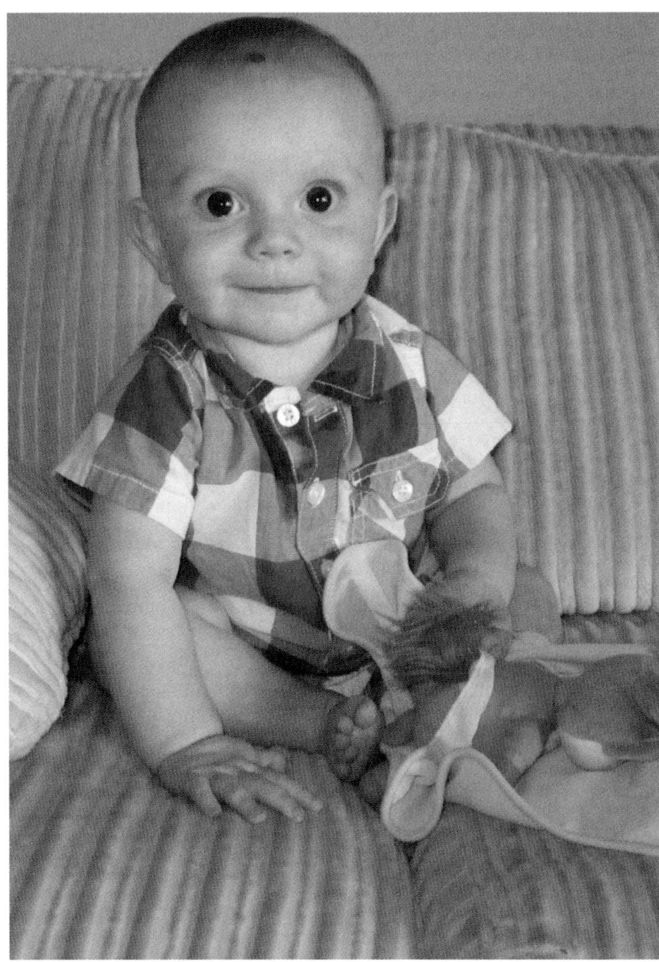

FIGURE 5-1 Blake was diagnosed with an extra-renal rhabdoid tumor. Blake appears healthy in his home at an early stage of his disease. His parents elected to have Blake's end of life in the hospital setting as they felt most comfortable with the resources there. He died peacefully in the company of his family. The Palliative Care team remains involved. *(Used with permission from Blake's family.)*

INTRODUCTION

Pediatric palliative care (PPC) is comprehensive, interdisciplinary, compassionate, inclusive, adaptive and effective. Ideally, it begins at the time a child or adolescent is diagnosed with a life-threatening illness (including prenatally) whether or not the etiology is completely understood. It comprises a community of professionals trained in medical, spiritual and psychosocial arenas. PPC provides support during the unpredictable course of an illness, attends to needs at the time of death, and supports grieving persons for the years leading up to and following the death of a child.

EPIDEMIOLOGY

- According to National Summary of Vital Statistics data, there were 2,437,163 deaths in the US during the year 2009.[1] Of these deaths, 48,033 were among persons under the age of 19 years.
- It is difficult to compare statistics involving pediatric deaths, as the ages of inclusion often vary. Some studies include children and adolescents up to 19 years of age, while others include participants up to 24 years of age.[2]
- Overall, deaths among children are decreasing in number in the US and worldwide.[3,4]
- Over half of all pediatric deaths occur in the first year of life.[3]

- Antepartum losses (not included in the above statistics) occur at a rate of more than one million per year. In 2008, the most recent year for which data is available, 1,118,000 pregnancies ended in pregnancy loss. Over one million pregnancies in the same year were electively terminated.[5]
- The US infant mortality rate (IMR), or total number of deaths of all children under the age of one year divided by the number of live births, was 6.39 in 2009.[1] Preliminary 2010 data predict a decrease of IMR to 6.14.[6]
  - IMR, while decreasing in the US, continues to be markedly higher among black and Hispanic populations. IMR among whites was 5.30 for the same year, while non-whites had a rate of 10.02. The highest IMR was among black families, at a rate of 12.64.[6]
  - The US has higher IMRs than Hong Kong (1.7), Ireland (3.3), Netherlands (3.8), the United Kingdom (4.7), or Croatia (5.3).[3]
- Causes of death in the US pediatric population vary with age group.
  - Congenital malformations and chromosomal abnormalities are the most frequent cause of death among infants.
  - Among children greater than one year of age, the most common cause of death is unintentional injury.
  - Malignant neoplasm is a common cause of pediatric death, particularly for children under 14 years of age, and represents the most common cause of disease-related death.
  - Homicide and suicide are the second and third leading causes of death in adolescents aged 15 to 19 years, respectively.
- Internationally, the WHO reports that:
  - Twelve million children under the age of 5 years died in 1990. In 2011, deaths in this age group declined to fewer than 7 million, a decrease of 41 percent.[7]
  - Half of these deaths occurred in India, Nigeria, Pakistan, China, and the Democratic Republic of the Congo.
  - Rates of death of children under 5 years of age have steadily decreased since 1990, by about 2.5 percent per year. The decline is associated with increasing disparity, as American and Western Pacific countries have much greater decline than African and Southeast Asian countries.
  - Worldwide, leading causes of death decreasing order are under-nutrition, pneumonia, preterm birth complications, diarrhea, and malaria.[7]
  - Most recent WHO information regarding adolescent mortality is from 2004. In that year, 2.6 million persons aged 10 to 24 died worldwide, with common causes including maternal conditions (15%), traffic accidents (14% in males and 5% in females), violence (12% males), and suicide (6%).[4]
  - A 2012 report on international adolescent health observed maternal mortality as a significant contributor to adolescent mortality. Remarkable variation in mortality rates from causes such as suicide, traffic injury and violence—even among high-income nations—was also noted.[8]
- Location of death has been shown to be important to parents of children dying with cancer Parents who have the opportunity to choose are more prepared for and comfortable with their child's end of life.[9]
- Of children who die in the US, most die in the hospital. While the precise number of children who die at home in the US is not known, studies of children with complex chronic diseases (CCCs) have shown the number of home deaths to be increasing in that population.[10] A Canadian study of children receiving PPC, in an area offering pediatric hospice facility services, showed an even distribution of number of deaths among hospital, pediatric hospice facility and home.[11]
- In a study of Florida children who died between 2003 and 2006, 65 percent died at home. Among hospice enrollees included in the study, 55 percent died at home; 15 percent of children not enrolled in hospice died at home.[12]
- The same study showed minority populations enrolling in hospice at reduced rates when compared to whites. Authors proposed distrust, cultural insensitivity, or lack of staff diversity as causes.[12] In addition, home deaths among black and Hispanic children with chronic illness were found to be significantly fewer than those among white children.[10]
- Persons under the age of 24 accounted for 0.4 percent of the 963,000 hospice admissions in 2009.[2] A Michigan survey of pediatric providers with experience in end-of-life care cited medical and non-medical support, preparation for death, care coordination and dignified death as benefits of hospice care. Detractors were a sense of intrusion, loss of hope, and distrust.[13]
- A 2007 survey of a small number of hospice agencies showed that 78 percent of hospice agencies care for children. Over 30 percent have pediatric programs and more than 20 percent have specialized staff members who care exclusively for children.[2] An upcoming survey conducted by the Center to Advance Palliative Care (CAPC) will detail more specifically PPC services that are available in hospitals.
- It is estimated that 100,000 parents suffer the death of a child each year. Such grief has been shown to be more intense and of longer duration than that experienced when mourning the loss of a parent or spouse. Approximately 19 percent of people in the US have been affected by the loss of a child in their nuclear or extended family.[14]

ETIOLOGY AND PATHOPHYSIOLOGY

- As mentioned previously, etiologies of pediatric death vary with age group.
- Prematurity and low birth weight (LBW).
  - Following a 16-year trend of increasing frequency, the rate of preterm birth (<37 weeks gestation) in the US declined from 2007 to 2009.[1]
  - LBW incidence has not declined, likely as a result of an increase in multiple compared to singleton births, early obstetric intervention, advanced maternal age and increased utilization of treatments for infertility.[1]
- Chromosomal abnormalities and congenital malformations.
  - According to the March of Dimes, the most common serious birth defects are congenital heart defects, neural tube defects such as anencephaly and encephalocele, and hemoglobin disorders such as sickle cell disease and thalassemia. The US experienced a 46 percent decline in birth defect-related mortality between the years of 1980 and 2001. Such declines have been

observed in other nations with similar income levels; 95 percent of the 3.3 million annual deaths due to birth defects occur in middle or low-income nations.[15]
  - Most deaths due to congenital heart disease occur in the first year of life or after the age of 18 years.[16] Congenital heart malformations resulted in a death rate among infants of 38.8 annually.[1] Between the years 1999 and 2006 there was a decrease in infant mortality due to congenital heart disease attributed to improved surgical and catheter-based interventions.[16]
  - Mortality due to sickle cell disease has decreased a result of identification with newborn screening and the routine administration of pneumococcal vaccine and penicillin prophylaxis.[17]
  - Neural tube defects resulted in a death rate of 5.9/100,000 live births in 2009. The rate decreased after 1998, when guidelines mandating fortification of foods with folic acid were instituted.[18]
- Unintentional injury.
  - Among persons between the ages of 1 and 19 years, the death rate due to unintentional injury declined 29 percent between the years 2000 and 2009.[19]
  - Infant deaths from unintentional injury increased, primarily as a result of the increase in incidence of deaths due to suffocation. In 2009, 907 infants died as a result of suffocation.[19]
  - SIDS, or Sudden Infant Death Syndrome, is the most common cause of sudden unexpected infant death (SUID). SIDS occurs in a child under one year of age and investigation including autopsy does not reveal an etiology.[20] Over 2000 children died from SIDS in 2009, a decrease of more than 50 percent since 1990.[20] It is believed that safe sleeping recommendations such as supine positioning have resulted in this decrease, as well as identification of tobacco smoke exposure, bed sharing, overheating, prematurity and LBW, soft sleeping surfaces, and loose bedding as risk factors.[21] In addition, accurate diagnosis of other causes such as suffocation, have caused a decline in the incidence of SIDS.[22]
  - Poisonings among 15- to 19-year-olds nearly doubled between 2000 and 2009, associated with an increase in prescription drug misuse and deaths associated with prescription drugs.[19]
  - Increased seat belt and child safety seat usage, decreases in alcohol impaired driving, improved vehicle and road design and licensing requirements are credited with a 41 percent decline in traffic-related deaths since 2000. Despite this, traffic-related deaths remain the most frequent cause of death due to unintentional injury for persons aged 5 to 19 years.[19]
  - Males and American Indian/Alaskan Natives are more likely to die from unintentional injuries and great variation in death rates exists between states.[19]
  - Deaths due to unintentional injuries occur more often in the US than in countries of similar economic status.[19]
- Assault
  - In 2010, the Department of Health and Human Services reported 1,537 childhood deaths as a result of maltreatment such as neglect, physical, or sexual abuse. The majority of children who died as a result of maltreatment suffered multiple types of abuse. Almost 80 percent of deaths occurred in children under the age of 4 years, with 40 percent of these in children under one year of age. Over 12 percent of families had been previously referred to Child Protective Services. Parents are most commonly the perpetrators.[23]
  - Deaths from homicide in 10 to 24 year-olds occurred at a rate of 14.1 per 100,000 in 1990. In 2009 the rate for 15-24 year-olds was 11.3 per 100,000. Males are more likely than females to commit or become a victim of homicide. Over 80 percent of homicides involve a firearm and deaths due to homicide are most common among non-Hispanic black adolescents.[24]
- Suicide
  - Suicide occurred at a rate of 10.1 per 100,000 15 to 24 year-olds in 2009.[1] More suicides are attempted by women than men, and 7 percent of high school students had attempted suicide in 2007. On the other hand, more suicide completions occur in men (24). Approximately 4,600 adolescents and young adults die of self-inflicted harm each year.[25]
  - Risk factors for suicide include a history of substance abuse, suicide of a family member, child maltreatment, physical or mental illness, isolation, and access to means of committing an act of self-harm.
  - Protective factors include support from family and care providers, problem-solving skills, and cultural or religious beliefs that preclude suicide.[26]
- Malignant neoplasms
  - Surveillance, Epidemiology, and End Results (SEER) data from 1975 to 2006 show the incidence of childhood cancer to be increasing, most prominently in acute lymphoblastic leukemia (ALL). Brain tumor incidence has stabilized since increasing in the 1980s.[27]
  - Prognosis is more favorable with malignancies such as ALL, NHL, Wilm's tumor, non-CNS germ cell tumors, and Hodgkin's lymphoma than for solid tumors such as Ewing sarcoma, rhabdomyosarcoma, or osteosarcoma.[27]
  - Overall, the survival rates for childhood cancers have been increasing for the last forty years. Of children diagnosed with a pediatric malignancy, 80 percent will survive for at least five years from the time of diagnosis.[28] This represents a 50 percent decline in death rates from childhood malignancy between 1975 and 2006.[27] These advances are attributed to the increased use of combination and multimodal therapies, enhanced knowledge regarding molecular underpinnings of malignancy, and the customization of treatment regimens including advances in imaging and neurosurgical techniques.[29]
  - With increased survival comes the reality of a new population of persons living with long-term effects of cancer treatment. Cancer survivors have an increased risk of death from cancer-related illness for as long as 30 years after diagnosis and an increased risk of death from illnesses not related to their primary oncologic diagnosis.[28]
  - Infants typically have poorer outcomes due to inadequate therapy response, increased treatment-related morbidity, and therapy limitations due to known adverse effects.[29]
  - Despite advances, most cancer deaths are due to leukemias, followed by malignancies of the central nervous system. Total deaths from childhood cancers in 2006 numbered 2,035.[27]
  - Decreased survival rates can result from unfavorable genetic features and cancer subtypes, delayed detection and decreased likelihood of receiving therapy in accordance with a pediatric treatment regimen.[29]

- Multiple studies have described ethnic disparity in cancer survival. Proposed explanations include differences in access, genetic predisposition to unfavorable subtypes, tendency toward poor therapy response, co-morbidities, and inadequate monitoring.[29,30]

- Complex Chronic Conditions (CCCs)
  - Some studies have distinguished characteristics of deaths among children with chronic illness from those of children without health issues. The death rate among children with CCCs, such as cancer, metabolic disorders and neuromuscular disorders, is double that of age-matched peers without disease. At the same time, the number of children with CCCs appears to be increasing, largely as a result of improved technology and supportive care.[10]

DIAGNOSIS

- Factors predictive of pediatric death have not yet been determined. Scoring tools such as PRISM, Pediatric Risk of Mortality Score, have accurately predicted death in some populations.[31] The tool accounts for factors such as mechanical ventilation, parenteral nutrition, vasoactive medication dependence, presence of hospital-acquired infection, and duration of hospitalization.
- A recent study of new admissions to six US palliative care programs included children with genetic/congenital (40.8%), neuromuscular (39.2%), oncologic (19.8%), respiratory 12.8%), and gastrointestinal (10.7) diagnoses[32] (**Figure 5-2**).
- Criteria developed in the United Kingdom by the Association for Children with Life-threatening or Terminal Conditions and their Families characterize children with life-limiting conditions into four groups by prognosis and treatment availability. See **Table 5-1** for descriptions of the categories created and clinical examples of each. Such categorization illustrates that patients and families will likely utilize palliative care services in different ways over the trajectory of their diseases and grieving processes and that each family has needs unique to the experience.[33]
- CAPC has developed assessment tools to identify adult or pediatric patients and families who would benefit from palliative care services.[34,35]
- As illness trajectory is uncertain, particularly in pediatrics, it is essential that families are introduced to PPC at the time of diagnosis. Furthermore, early establishment of a relationship gives parents and patients access to resources for symptom management, financial and practical concerns, bereavement, decision-making and spiritual support. These services should be offered alongside curative efforts.
- Unfortunately, many children do not receive PPC until curative efforts are ceased, or until they are very near death.[36] Barriers such as uncertain prognosis, language barriers and time constraints, as well as inability of a family to accept illness as incurable have been identified. Limited staff resources, insufficient knowledge of palliative care and absence of staff members trained in palliative care have also been identified as barriers.[37] However, it has been proposed that situations of diagnostic and prognostic uncertainty benefit greatly from early palliative care support, precisely because the disease trajectory is unknown. In addition, many illnesses are of unknown etiology and additional knowledge does not change treatment course.[38]

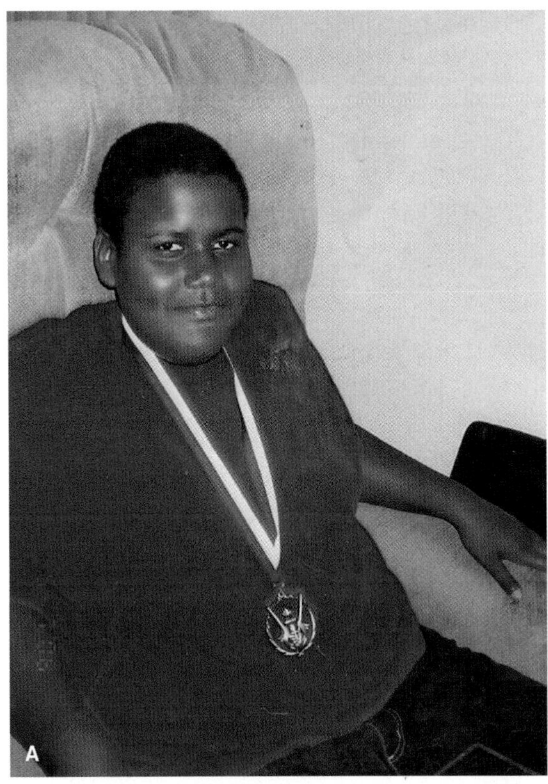

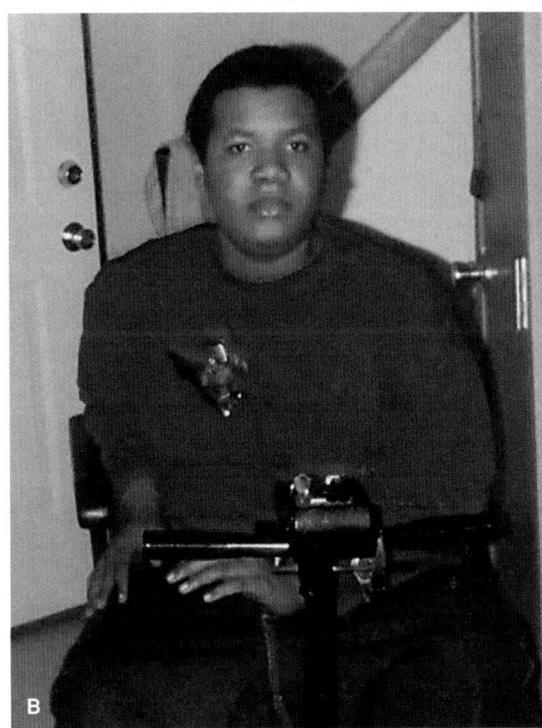

FIGURE 5-2 Brothers who died from complications of Becker's Muscular Dystrophy. The older brother Bobby **(A)** died first. The younger brother Rayshawn **(B)** having observed the decline and death of Bobby needed special support measures. (*Used with permission from Bobby and Rayshawn's family.*)

TABLE 5-1 Categorization of life-limiting Illnesses in Children

Group	Inclusion Criteria	Examples
1	Life-threatening: Curative treatment exists but prognosis uncertain	Cancer, irreversible organ failure, complex congenital heart disease, trauma, sudden severe illness, extreme prematurity
2	Life-limiting: Intensive life-prolonging treatment permits typical lifestyle; early death characteristic of disease	Cystic fibrosis, hypoplastic left heart disease with surgical palliation, muscular dystrophy, HIV/AIDS, severe short-gut (TPN-dependent)
3	Long-term progressive disease without cure: treatment is exclusively palliative and may extend over many years	Spinal muscular atrophy type 2, adrenoleukodystrophy, severe mitochondrial disease, trisomies 13 and 18, other lethal genetic syndromes
4	Neurological disability with increased susceptibility to disease and unpredictable course	Traumatic brain injury, severe multiple disabilities following brain or spinal cord malformations (hydranencephaly, holoprosencephaly, severe hypoxic ischemic encephalopathy)

Adapted from Royal College of Pediatrics and Child Health and Association for Children with Life-Threatening or Terminal Conditions and Their Families' A Guide to the Development of Pediatric Palliative Care Services, 1997.

CLINICAL FEATURES

- Certain symptoms are common in PPC and at end of life. Estimates of prevalence vary among studies, but most frequently reported are pain, fatigue, dyspnea, anorexia and depression, nausea and vomiting, diarrhea, and constipation.[39,40] Many children also suffer from anxiety, agitation, sleep disturbances, pruritus, cough, seizures, and decubitus ulcers.[41]
- Needs of caregivers for children near the end of life are numerous. They are faced with social isolation, financial burdens, responsibilities for complicated medical care, obligations to other children and communities, as well as physical and psychological challenges that accompany their predicament.[42]

MANAGEMENT

- The following distinguish palliative care services for children from those of adults:
  - Wide range of ages and varied diagnoses, including patients with prenatal diagnoses as well as adults suffering from childhood illnesses.[2]
  - Unpredictable trajectory of illness—Due to the small numbers of children with terminal illnesses, relative to adults, it is difficult to establish standardized expectations.[2] Most children survive for more than a year after being referred to pediatric palliative medicine services.[32] In contrast, hospice studies have observed decreasing lengths of service, with almost 50 percent of patients dying or being discharged within 2 weeks of service initiation.[43]
  - Challenging symptom management—Many medications are not tested in pediatric populations, and their use in children is off-label. In addition, symptom assessment can be challenging because of limits in communication ability, either age-appropriate or due to disease or treatment.
  - Ethical concerns—In contrast to competent adults, a child relies upon parents or a community to make decisions in his or her best interest.[2] Children and adolescents have varying abilities to participate in decision-making regarding their care though many children desire to be active in such discussions.[44]
  - Personnel and resource needs—Children require size-appropriate equipment and personnel trained in their care. In addition, children are dependent upon others for medical as well as non-medical needs.[2] Interdisciplinary support of the child and family requires a diverse staff capable of providing spiritual, psychosocial, bereavement, medical, and decision-making support.
  - Other distinctions include a relative paucity of literature to guide assessment and management, increased use of in-home care and decreased use of long-term care facilities, loss of anticipated life of normalcy, increased use of life-sustaining technology that requires discontinuation prior to death, and varied models of care delivery.[45]
- Communication Facilitation and Decision-Making Support
  - At the time of diagnosis, establishment of a supportive therapeutic relationship involving honest, open, and respectful communication commences. Initial meetings may involve:
  - Introduction of palliative care services and staff members as well as patient and family members.
  - Opportunities for patient and/or family to share the story of their illness experience and other information about the persons involved, if desired by patient and family.
  - Information exchange. After assessing information needs, provide:
    - Name of the child's illness and its etiology, if known.
    - Prognosis and illness trajectory.
    - Benefits and burdens associated with treatment options.
    - Symptoms and complications along with available interventions.
    - Sources of support for predicted changes in family life (38).
  - It is preferable to discuss these matters in a series of conversations, the first of which could include diagnosis and general prognosis information, as well as other information as desired by patient and family.[38]

- Periods of silence may serve as opportunities for processing of information as well as invitations for patients and family members to express emotion, information need or other concerns.
- It is helpful for meetings to conclude with a discussion of next steps and a plan for future communication. Thorough documentation ensures that all providers understand the plan of care and associated family priorities.
- Clarification and reevaluation of goals of care (i.e., longevity of life, freedom from mechanical ventilation, school participation, opportunity to take a trip or experience a specific life event) may enhance the decision-making process.
- For some parents, hope for cure is a means of coping.[46] Understanding this motivation may allow providers to identify with parents who comprehend the unlikelihood of cure but who are unwilling to discontinue curative therapies.
- Updated advance directives reflect preferences in regard to medical treatment. Decisions may include the allowance of natural death, the discontinuation of medically-provided nutrition and hydration, continuation of antibiotic therapy to treat infection, or the refusal of chest compressions and medications for cardiac resuscitation. Preferences should be documented and shared with other medical providers, schools, and local emergency medical services.
- Parent-child relationships continue within the context of a child's illness. A child's preferences may be affected by a desire to please her parents.[47] In contrast, a desire to establish control and independence may predispose an adolescent to make choices that do not mimic those of his parents.

- Psychosocial
  - Families with an ill child continue to deal with demands of daily life, though now with increased financial and emotional stressors and decreased time and resources.[46] The extent to which a serious illness strains the constructs of a family system cannot be overestimated. Families encounter previously unimagined challenges to marital, sibling and parent-child relationships as well as to those with extended family and other communities. Medical expenses and missed work can result in significant financial hardship. The demands of caring for an ill child can result in decreased attention to other family members by the primary caregiver, as well as insufficient opportunity to care for him or herself.
  - Support may include assistance with living expenses and transportation needs; child care, school absence and processing needs of siblings and parents as well as anticipatory grief work; work absence/Family Medical Leave Act processing; and assistance navigating the extensive web of available resources.
    - Child life specialists utilize play to facilitate communication of medical information to a patient, as well as to address anxiety of patients and siblings.[41]
    - Expressive Therapies involve writing, artwork, music, dance, spoken word, film and any medium that is meaningful to patients and families. They permit processing of difficult circumstances by individuals of differing abilities and interests. As an example, **Figure 5-3** shows prayer flags made by Brandon, a teenage patient with Spinal Muscular Atrophy. Such modalities are particularly helpful for children and patients who have communication limitations, as well caregivers facing limited time to process the coming loss.[48]

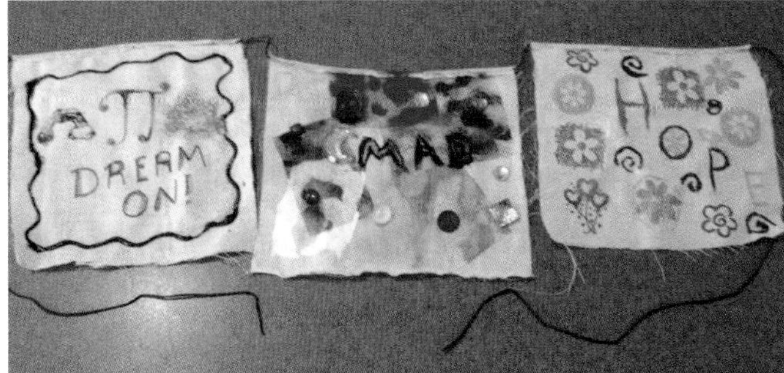

FIGURE 5-3 Prayer flags as expressive therapy for a child coping with the threat of death from an incurable disease.

- Bereavement
  - Grief work begins at the time of diagnosis, as families mourn the loss of the life they had envisioned for themselves and their children. Bereavement specialists may establish relationships with families and begin the lifelong process of grieving. These staff members may also assist with funeral planning, sibling support, memory-making, and preparing families for what is to come. Anticipatory grief work is particularly important in families where serious illness and death has been encountered previously; for Rayshawn (**Figure 5-2B**), who knew what his future held from watching his older brother Bobby (**Figure 5-2A**) die of muscular dystrophy, nonpharmacologic outlets for his anxiety, depression and grief/loss were particularly important interventions from the palliative care team.
  - Memory-making may include tangible reminders such as plaster molds or ink prints of hands or feet, photographs of special events or family members with the child, songs, poems or writings, or videos, voice recordings and letters that allow patients to preserve special messages. See the photograph of Camden (**Figure 5-4**), who died shortly after birth, due to prenatally-diagnosed renal agenesis.
  - Complicated grief may involve inability to engage in life activities, depression, isolation, compromised self-esteem, or even suicidal ideation.[48]

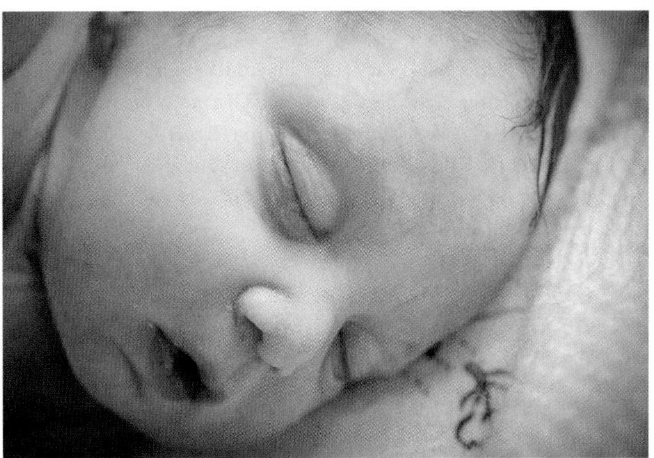

FIGURE 5-4 Camden died shortly after birth, due to prenatally-diagnosed renal agenesis. The family had this special photograph taken to provide a lasting memory of their child. (*Photo by Brent Watkins, Sylvart Studios.*)

- Spiritual care
  - Staff members trained to listen and respond to spiritual concerns of patients and families may provide needed support, learn about culture-specific needs at the time of death, and provide space for discussion of difficult questions raised by such challenging circumstances.[49] In addition, some families desire baptisms, blessings or other rituals at or in preparation for the end of life or simply the presence of a spiritual care provider.
- Medical care during the dying phase involves preparation, support, and effective symptom management, and documentation of events.
  - Adequate personnel, medications and supplies will ensure timely care and enhance symptom management. For a list of common symptoms at the end of life as well as options for management, see **Table 5-2**.
  - Over 1/2 of hospice patients discharged in 2007 utilized complementary and alternative therapies while receiving hospice care. Some hospices offer massage, pet, guided imagery, aromatherapy, expressive arts, and therapeutic touch therapies.[50]
  - Families differ in their methods of supporting and grieving a dying child. Efforts should be made to accept and accommodate varied means of expression.
  - In some cases, allowance of a natural death involves discontinuation of life-sustaining therapies that are no longer beneficial. Benefits and burdens of mechanical ventilation, medically-provided hydration and nutrition, chemotherapy regimens, dialysis, and other interventions should be discussed with patients and families.
  - Also considered is the desired location for death. Planned discontinuation of no-longer beneficial life-sustaining therapy may occur in a private area of a hospital, allowing families time during and after death to be with their loved one. With the help of an area hospice or other service provider, the process can occur in the home as well. Whatever the setting, it is essential to anticipate symptoms likely to accompany the change in support and ensure access to appropriate treatments.
- Pronouncement of death entails confirmation of patient identity and a physical exam to confirm lack of response to respectful tactile stimulation, absent pulse, respiratory effort, or pupillary response.
- Documentation requirements vary by state. In general, a death certificate must be completed by a physician and include cause of death and time of death recorded. A note recording end-of-life events is also crucial.
- Autopsy regulations also vary according to location. However, in situations of unexpected death, suspected harm, or unknown cause of death, an autopsy will likely be required. Regardless of regulations, families should be offered an autopsy; autopsies can answer families' questions regarding cause of death and indicate if testing of family members is indicated.[51]

PATIENT AND FAMILY EDUCATION AND SUPPORT

- Communicating with children about death—be they a patient, sibling, or friend of a dying child—involves assessing what they already understand and what they wish to know.[51] Expressive arts, role-playing and play-based therapies can be helpful. It is of note that withholding information may produce more anxiety in children, who are apt to create their own explanations for what they observe.
- Persons caring for children at the end of life are susceptible to guilt and exhaustion. The stressful circumstance can exacerbate existing struggles such as marital or financial strain. Caregivers may be responsible for other children or family members. Respite services provided by facilities or community members may relieve some of this strain. Caregivers may also be helped by supportive providers who identify home health, transportation, financial, and spiritual resources that meet existing and future needs.[52]
- Numerous challenges face siblings of an ill child, including divided parental attention, travel for hospitalization(s), guilt, fear of "catching" the illness, embarrassment, social isolation and lifestyle change, and observing sibling suffering.[52] Helpful interventions can be designed to fit a sibling's developmental level and needs. Conversations to discuss information at the sibling's level of understanding are helpful, some with parents and some with trusted team members such as bereavement coordinators, child life specialists, or medical care providers, including the child's primary care physician. Maintenance of these relationships after the death is helpful as siblings re-experience their grief through stages of development. Siblings may also benefit from support groups, appropriate engagement in research and decision-making, memory-making, or simply the option to participate in activities that were important prior to life changes due to illness.[52]
- The network of available resources for families with dying children is extensive and complicated. Financial difficulties can result from medical expenses and the need to cease working to care for an ill child. Families dealing with illness also need services related to respite care, home nursing, housing that can accommodate medical equipment, child care for siblings, and transportation. Some things that a child wishes to accomplish before his or her death are facilitated by wish organizations or local charities.[52] In short, families who have had adequate resources for their life before illness often find these same resources insufficient for their "new normal." Contact information for organizations and information sources are listed in the resources sections later in this chapter.
- Advance directives discussion tools such as "My Wishes" booklets facilitate communication about a child's preferences regarding treatment plans, comfort measures, how a child would like to be treated by those around him or her and what the child would like to communicate to caregivers and loved ones.[53]
- Families may benefit from descriptions of what the child will look like, what symptoms he/she may experience (color change, noisy breathing, gasping) and how family members may support him/her during the dying phase. Soliciting specific concerns will allow them to be addressed adequately.
- Organ donation is an option that may benefit families of eligible donors. Deaths of patients desiring to donate heart valves and cornea tissue may occur at home; if donation of solid organs is desired the death must occur in the hospital.[54]
- Primary medical doctors (PMDs) can be a resource for families of children with serious illness. Small studies suggest that PMDs play a diminished role, likely due to assumption of care by hospital-based physicians and lack of training in end-of-life care for primary medical doctors. However, funeral attendance and attention to grieving siblings were noted as significant by some parents.

TABLE 5-2 Common Symptoms in Pediatric End of Life

Symptom	Causes	Management
Agitation	Medications, infection, pain, environment	Review medications, decrease stimulation; benzodiazepines, haloperidol, phenobarbital
Anorexia	Malignancy, loss of muscle mass	Appetite stimulants (megestrol acetate, medroxyprogesterone acetate, cannabinoids)
Anxiety	Apprehension, grief, pain	Hypnotherapy, CBT, expressive therapies, benzodiazepines, SSRIs
Constipation	Dehydration, lack of dietary fiber, opioids	Stool softener, laxative, osmotic agent, enema. Opioid antagonist
Cough	GERD, pericardial or pleural irritation, aspiration, malignant compression, airway irritants, bronchospasm	Opioids, positioning, assisted cough, bronchodilators, nebulized saline, mucolytic medications
Depression	Isolation, fatigue, circumstance	Selective serotonin reuptake inhibitors, tricyclic antidepressants, psychological counseling
Diarrhea	Medications, infection, fiber supplementation	Anticholinergics, opioids, octreotide for secretory diarrhea
Dyspnea	Air hunger	Environmental therapies such as repositioning or increasing ambient air flow; supplemental oxygen +/– positive pressure, bronchodilator, mucolytic, opioid, benzodiazepine
Fatigue	Anemia, increased work of breathing, medications, poor nutrition, insomnia	Treat underlying cause, stimulants (methylphenidate)
Nausea/ Vomiting	Chemotherapy, constipation, heart failure, anxiety, organ failure, dysmotility	Antiemetics, treatment of underlying causes, integrative therapies such as biofeedback, acupuncture or aromatherapy
Pain	Metastases, muscle spasm, tissue injury, vaso-occlusive event, immobility, compression, infection	General: opioids, integrative therapies such as music, massage, imagery Appropriate adjuvants Neuropathic pain: anticonvulsants, NMDA antagonists, antidepressants Muscle spasm: baclofen, dantrolene, benzodiazepines Bone pain: NSAIDs, radiation, bisphosphonates
Pressure ulcers	Moisture, decreased sensation, friction, decreased mobility, poor nutritional status	Specialized mattress and bedding, regular repositioning, barrier creams, optimized nutrition status
Pruritis	Medications, malignancy, cholestasis	Antihistamine, topical emollient, cholestyramine/ rifampicin for cholestasis, steroids in malignancy
Seizures	CNS malignancy, fever, electrolyte abnormality, medication, metabolic disease	AED appropriate for seizure type, benzodiazepines, surgery for refractory seizures
Sleep Difficulty	Brain injury, daytime sedating medications, environment	Give sedating medications at night, sleep hygiene, melatonin, diphenhydramine, benzodiazepine (for short-term use only)

AED – antiepileptic drug; CBT – cognitive behavioral therapy; CNS – central nervous system; GERD – gastroesophageal reflux disease; NSAID – non-steroidal anti-inflammatory drug; NMDA – N-methyl-D-aspartate; SSRIs – selective serotonin reuptake inhibitors.

TABLE 5-3 Components of Psychosocial Assessment for Families of a Child with Life-Threatening Illness

Components of Psychosocial Assessment
Living arrangements
Family composition
Persons living in home
Marital status of patient and caregivers
Guardianship/custody issues
Safety/accessibility
Family characteristics
Decision-making practices
Cultural considerations
Health status of family members
Strengths
Sources of income
Medical technology utilization (feeding, lines, respiratory equipment)
Accessed supports
Hospice
Waiver/insurance
Social service agencies
Education plans/schools
Therapies/rehabilitation needs
Leisure/respite practices
Social networks
Sources of strength
Spiritual practices, beliefs, associations
Understanding of illness
Coping mechanisms
Life changes and losses associated with illness
Predominant concerns and challenges
Practical considerations
Activities of daily living assistance needed
Transportation
Proximity to resources (therapies, faith community, supportive persons)
Caregiver employment
Legal matters

- Hospice services offer extensive support and assistance with medical and psychosocial needs. With the passage and upholding of the Patient Protection and Affordable Care Act, children receiving Medicaid are eligible for the hospice benefit even if receiving curative therapies. This is substantially different from the restrictions upon adults receiving hospice care, who exclusively receive supportive care.
- A list of considerations for psychosocial assessment for a family of a child with life-threatening illness is found in **Table 5-3**.

FOLLOW-UP

- Ensure private space for caregivers to spend final moments with their child, as this is a valuable part of the grieving process. They may appreciate the opportunity to bathe, dress, or simply hold their child.[48,55]
- After the death of a child, families experience a drastic change in relationship to providers who were involved.[48] It may be appropriate for a member of the staff to contact the family a few days after the death. Some sources recommend phone calls or visits at predicted intervals such as 3 months, 6 months, 1 year, and beyond as families desire.[42] Continued support may take the form of funeral attendance, phone calls, letters commemorating a birthday or day of death, or hosting an annual memorial service for grieving families.
- Subsequent meetings may include autopsy review, discussions regarding the death of a child and the care received, opportunities to share a child's story with new staff members or learners, or conversations with subspecialty providers involved in a child's care.

CONCLUSION

Children with life-threatening conditions and their families are likely to encounter physical, psychosocial, spiritual, emotional, and practical challenges. Interdisciplinary PPC services offer support for families facing such challenges and are integral whether illness ends in cure or death and bereavement. PPC involvement beginning at the time of diagnosis provides an extra layer of support for children and families throughout their difficult journeys.

PATIENT AND FAMILY RESOURCES

- **www.wish.org**
- **www.starlight.org**
- **www.togetherforshortlives.org**
- **www.familyvoices.org**
- Children's Hospice and Palliative Care Coalition—**www.chpcc.org**

PROVIDER RESOURCES

- Center to Advance Palliative Care (CAPC)—**www.capc.org**.
- American Academy of Hospice and Palliative Medicine (AAHPM)—**www.aahpm.org**.
- American Academy of Pediatrics Section on Hospice and Palliative Medicine—**www.aap.org-section**.
- National Hospice and Palliative Care Organization (NHPCO)—**www.nhpco.org/pediatrics**.
- *When Children Die: Improving Palliative and End-of-Life Care for Children and Their Families*, a report published by The National Academies; 2003.
- *Palliative Care for Infants, Children and Adolescents*, a textbook edited by B Carter, M Levetown, and S Friebert. The National Academies Press is the publisher: 2011.
- American Academy of Pediatrics statement on Pediatric Palliative Care—**http://pediatrics.aappublications.org/content/106/2/351.full**.

REFERENCES

1. Kochanek KD, Xu J, Murphy SL, Minino AM, Hsiang-Ching K. Deaths: Final data for 2009. *National Vital Statistics Reports*. 2011; 60:1-117.
2. Friebert S. *NHPCO facts and figures: Pediatric palliative and hospice care in America*. 2009 National Hospice and Palliative Care

Organization; 2009. http://www.nhpco.org/sites/default/files/public/quality/Pediatric_Facts-Figures.pdf, accessed December 1, 2013.

3. Kochanek KD, Kirmeyer SE, Martin JA, Strobino DM, Guyer B. Annual summary of vital statistics. *Pediatrics*. 2012;129:338-348.
4. World Health Organization: Global Health Observatory: Under-five mortality. http://www.who.int/gho/child_health/mortality/mortality_under_five_text/en/index.html, Geneva, Switzerland 2012.
5. Ventura SJ, Curtin SC, Abma J, Henshaw SK. Estimated pregnancy rates and rates of pregnancy outcomes for the United States, 1990-2008. *National Vital Statistics Reports*. 2012;60:1-22.
6. Minino AM, Murphy SL. Death in the United States, 2010. *NCHS Data Brief*. 2012;99:1-8.
7. World Health Organization. Levels and trends in child mortality report 2011. http://childinfo.org/files/Child.Mortality_Report_2011.pdf, accessed December 1, 2013.
8. Patton GC, Coffey C, Cappa C, et. al. Health of the world's adolescents: a synthesis of internationally comparable data. *Lancet*. 2012;379:1665-1775.
9. Dussel V, Kreicbergs U, Hilden JM, et al. Looking beyond where children die: determinants and effects of planning a child's location of death. *Journal of Pain and Symptom Management*. 2009;37:33-43.
10. Feudtner C, Feinstein JA, Satchell M, Zhao H, Kang TI. Shifting place of death among children with complex chronic conditions in the United States, 1989-2003. *JAMA*. 2007;297:2725-2732.
11. Siden H, Miller M, Straatman L, Omesi L, Tucker T, Collins JJ. A report on location of death in paediatric palliative care between home, hospice and hospital. *Palliative Medicine*. 2008;22:831-834.
12. Knapp CA, Shenkman EA, Marcu Mi, Madden VL, Terza JV. Pediatric palliative care: describing hospice users and identifying factors that affect hospice expenditures. *Journal of Palliative Medicine*. 2009;12:223-229.
13. Dickens DS. Comparing pediatric deaths with and without hospice support. *Pediatr Blood Cancer*. 2010;54:746-750.
14. Hendrickson KC. Morbidity, Mortality and parental grief: A Review of the literature on the relationship between the death of a child and the subsequent health of parents. *Palliative and Supportive Care*. 2008;7:109-119.
15. Christianson A, Howson CP, Modell B. *Executive summary of March of Dimes global report on birth defects: the hidden toll of dying and disabled children*. March of Dimes Birth Defects Foundation White Plains, New York, NY; 2006.
16. Gilboa SM, Salemi JL, Nembhard WN, Fixler DE, Correa A. Mortality resulting from congenital heart disease among children and adults in the United States, 1999 to 2006. *Circulation*. 2010; 122:2254-2263.
17. Yanni E, Grosse SD, Yang O, et al. Trends in pediatric sickle cell disease-related mortality in the United States 1983-2002. *Journal of Pediatrics*. 2008;154:541-545.
18. Centers for Disease Control and Prevention: Spina bifida and anencephaly before and after the folic acid mandate-United States 1995-1996 and 1999-2000. *MMWR*. 2004;53:362-365.
19. Centers for Disease Control and Prevention. Vital signs: Unintentional injury deaths among persons aged 0-19 years-United States, 2000-2009. *MMWR*. 2012;61:1-7.
20. Centers for Disease Control and Prevention. Sudden unexpected infant death. http://www.cdc.gov/sids./Atlanta, GA; 2012.
21. Centers for Disease Control and Prevention. Eliminate disparities in infant mortality. http://www.cdc.gov/omhd/amh/factsheets/infant.htm. Atlanta, GA; 2007.
22. Christian CW, Sege RD. Child fatality review. *Pediatrics*. 2010; 126:592-596.
23. Department of Health and Human Services. Child Maltreatment 2010. Available at http://archive.acf.hhs.gov/programs/cb/pubs/cm10/cm10.pdf, accessed November 12, 2012.
24. Mulye TP, Park MJ, Nelson CD, Adams SH, Irwin CE, Brindis CD. Trends in adolescent and young adult health in the United States. *Journal of Adolescent Health*. 2009;45:8-24.
25. Centers for Disease Control and Prevention: Suicide Prevention. http://www.cdc.gov/ViolencePrevention/pub/youth_suicide.html. Atlanta, GA; 2012.
26. Centers for Disease Control and Prevention. Suicide: risk and protective factors. http://www.cdc.gov/ViolencePrevention/suicide/riskprotectivefactors.html. Atlanta, GA; 2012.
27. Smith M, Seibel NL et al. Outcomes for children and adolescents with cancer: challenges for the twenty-first century. *Journal of Clinical Oncology*. 2010;28:2625-2634.
28. Armstrong Gt, Liu Q, Yutaka Y, Neglia JP, Leisenring W, Robison LL. Mertens AC. Late mortality among 5-year survivors of childhood cancer: A summary from the childhood cancer survival study. *Journal of Clinical Oncology*. 2009;27:2328-2338.
29. Linabery AM, Ross JA. Childhood and adolescent cancer survival in the US by race and ethnicity for the diagnostic period 1975-1999. *Cancer*. 2008;113:2575-2596.
30. Bhatia S. Disparities in Cancer Outcomes: Lessons learned from children with cancer. *Pediatr Blood Cancer*. 2011;56:994-1002.
31. Costa GA, Delgado AF, Ferraro A, Okay TS. Application of the Pediatric Risk of Mortality Score (PRISM) score and determination of mortality risk: factors in a tertiary pediatric intensive care unit. *Clinics*. 2010;65:1087-1092.
32. Feudtner C, Kang T, Hexem KR et al. Pediatric palliative care patients: A prospective multicenter cohort study. *Pediatrics*. 2011;127:1094-1101.
33. Association for Children with Life-threatening or Terminal Conditions and their Families and the Royal College of Paediatrics and Child Health: *A guide to the development of children's palliative care services: report of the joint working party*. Bristol, UK; 1997.
34. Weissman MD. Identifying patients in need of a palliative care assessment in a hospital setting: a consensus report from the Center to Advance Palliative Care. *Journal of Palliative Medicine*. 2011;14:1-8.
35. Center to Advance Palliative Care: Consult triggers. http://www.capc.org/signup?tool=/clinical-tools/consult-triggers. New York, NY; 2012.

36. Thompson LA, Knapp, Madden V, Shenkeman E. Pediatricians' Perceptions of and Preferred Timing for Pediatric Palliative Care. *Pediatrics*. 2009;123;e777.

37. Davies B, Sehring SA, Partridge JC, et al. Barriers to palliative care for children: Perceptions of pediatric health care providers. *Pediatrics*. 2008;121:282-288.

38. Graham RJ, Levetown M, Comeau M. *Decision Making, in Palliative Care for Infants, Children and Adolescents*, edited by B Carter, M Levetown, S Friebert. Baltimore: Johns Hopkins University Press; 2011:139-168.

39. Wolfe J, Holcombe EG, Klar N et al. Symptoms and suffering at the end of life in children with cancer. *The New England Journal of Medicine*. 2000;342:326-333.

40. Wolfe J, Hammel JF, Edwards KE et al. Easing of suffering in children with cancer at the end of life; is care changing? *Journal of Clinical Oncology*. 2008;26:1717-1723.

41. Graham RJ, Zeltzer L, Hellsten M. Holistic Management of Symptoms, in Palliative Care for Infants, Children and Adolescents, edited by B Carter, M Levetown, S Friebert. Baltimore: Johns Hopkins University Press; 2011:244-274.

42. Hudson P, Remedios C, Zordan R, et al. Guidelines for the Psychosocial and Bereavement support of family caregivers of palliative care patients. *Journal of Palliative Medicine*. 2012;15:696-702.

43. National Hospice and Palliative Care Organization: NHPCO Facts and Figures: Hospice Care in America; 2009 edition.

44. Taylor S, Haase-Casanovas S, Weaver T, Kiddy J. Garralda EM. Child involvement in the pediatric consultation: a qualitative study of children and carers' views. *Child Care Health Dev*. 2010;36:678-85.

45. Friebert S, Bower KA, Lookabaugh B. *Caring for Pediatric Patients, in UNIPAC: A resource for Hospice and Palliative Medicine Physicians*, edited by CP Storey. Glenview, IL; 2012:5-7.

46. Zelcer S, Cataudella D, Calmey E, Bannister SL. Palliative care of children with brain tumors: a parental perspective. *Arch Pediatric Adolesc Med*. 2010;164:225-230.

47. Knapp C, Komatz K. Preferences for end-of-life care for children with cancer. *CMAJ*. 2011;183:e1250-1251.

48. Orloff SF, Toce SS, Sumner L, Grimes LA. Bereavement, in Palliative Care for Infants, Children and Adolescents, edited by B Carter, M Levetown, S Friebert. Baltimore: Johns Hopkins University Press; 2011:275-308.

49. Dexter L, Morrison W, Koch KD, Feudtner C. Spiritual Dimensions, in Palliative Care for Infants, Children and Adolescents, edited by B Carter, M Levetown, S Friebert. Baltimore: Johns Hopkins University Press; 2011:227-243.

50. Bercovitz A, Sengupta M, Jones A, Jones A, Harris-Kojetin LD. Complementary and Alternative Therapies in Hospice: The National Home and Hospice Care Survey: United States, 2007. *National Health Statistics Reports*. 2011:33.

51. Levetown M, Meyer EC, Gray D. Communication skills and relational abilities, in Palliative Care for Infants, Children and Adolescents, edited by B Carter, M Levetown, S Friebert. Baltimore: Johns Hopkins University Press; 2011:169-201.

52. Orloff SF, Jones B, Ford K. Psychosocial needs of the child and family, in Palliative Care for Infants, Children and Adolescents, edited by B Carter, M Levetown, S Friebert. Baltimore: Johns Hopkins University Press; 2011:202-226.

53. *Aging With Dignity. Five Wishes Resources: Pediatric My Wishes.* http://agingwithdignity.org/catalog/product_info.php?products_id=85. Tallahassee, FL; 2012.

54. Dominica SF. After the child's death: family care, in Oxford Textbook of Palliative Care for Children, edited by A Goldman, R Hain, S Liben. Oxford: Oxford University Press; 2006: 183.

55. Committee on Palliative and End-of-Life Care for Children and Their Families: Care and caring from diagnosis through death and bereavement. When Children Die: Improving Palliative and End-of-Life Care for Children and Their Families. Washington, DC: The National Academies Press; 2003:151.

6 SOCIAL JUSTICE

Mindy A. Smith, MD, MS
Richard P. Usatine, MD

Of all the forms of inequality, injustice in health care is the most shocking and inhumane.

—Martin Luther King, Jr.

The first question which the priest and the Levite asked was: "If I stop to help this man, what will happen to me?" But . . . the Good Samaritan reversed the question: "If I do not stop to help this man, what will happen to him?"

—Martin Luther King, Jr.

PATIENT STORIES

At only 5.5 pounds (10 pounds less than the fifth percentile for weight on the World Health Organization's growth chart), an 8-month-old boy suffered from severe malnutrition. In the summer of 2003, amidst the height of Liberia's civil war, his aunt brought him to the Médecins Sans Frontières/Doctors Without Borders hospital for treatment. Because of the war, his family had been forced to flee from their home, leaving behind their usual methods of getting food. Dr. Andrew Schechtman was there to help the day the child was brought to the clinic in Liberia (**Figure 6-1**). Despite the best available treatment for the malnutrition and concurrent pneumonia, the boy died on his third hospital day.

OUR STORIES AS CARING CLINICIANS

Those of us who become pediatricians or other health care providers do so for many reasons. One reason is because of a desire to help someone else.

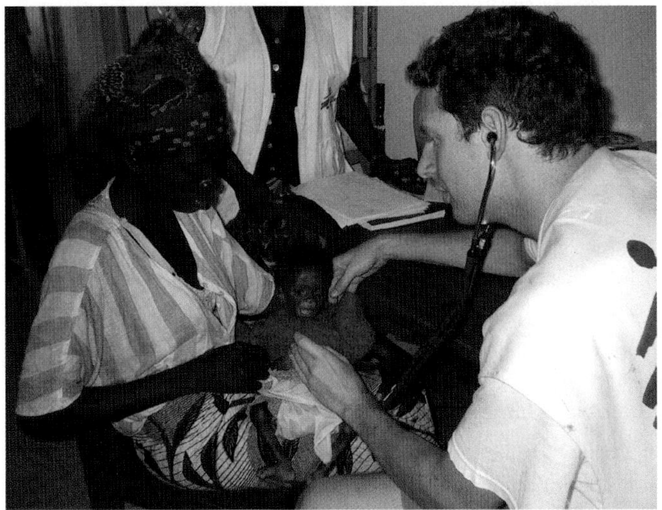

FIGURE 6-1 Dr. Andrew Schechtman was there to help the day a severely malnourished child was brought to the clinic in war-torn Liberia. Despite the best available treatment that could be provided in the Doctors Without Borders hospital, the child died of complications of malnutrition and pneumonia—a casualty of war and poverty. (*Used with permission from Andrew Schechtman, MD.*)

Along the way, we sometimes lose ourselves in the day-to-day struggles, disappointments, obligations, fatigue, and the profound helplessness that descends upon us after a particularly bad day. But we are still here, and if we listen with our hearts we are still capable of great and small things.

We are privileged in so many ways and we must recognize our power over ourselves and over the communities that we serve. It is easy to become overwhelmed by the problems that we face as clinicians and as fellow human beings. Our health care system is in shambles, our natural world is being poisoned, our nations are continually at war, and yet, as this chapter highlights, there is so much that we can do—we can listen, we can observe, we can witness, we can bring aid, we can touch, we can love, and we can lead.

The text that follows highlights just a few examples of the ways in which our colleagues are challenging themselves to find creative solutions to the many problems faced by those who are underserved, displaced, or suffering.

DOCTORS WITHOUT BORDERS (ANDREW SCHECHTMAN, MD)

EPIDEMIOLOGY

The United Nations (UN) High Commissioner for Refugees reported that in 2011 there were 10.9 million refugees (those displaced across an international border) and 27.5 million internally displaced persons (IDPs, those displaced within their own country).[1] At the end of 2010, the UN refugee agency was caring for an estimated 14.7 million of these IDPs. During times of a complex humanitarian emergency (defined as a humanitarian crisis in a country, region, or society where there is a breakdown of authority resulting from internal or external conflict and which requires an international response that goes beyond the mandate or capacity of any single agency and/or the ongoing UN country program), the following usually occur:[2]

- Civilian casualties.
- Populations besieged or displaced.
- Serious political or conflict-related impediments to delivery of assistance.
- Inability of people to pursue normal social, political, or economic activities.
- High security risks for relief workers.

ETIOLOGY

People can be displaced from their homes by manmade (war or persecution) or natural disasters (tsunami, earthquake, or hurricane). War is responsible for most of the displacement. Some of the source countries accounting for the most refugees are Afghanistan, Sudan, Somalia, the Palestinian territories, and Iraq.

- Communicable diseases usually cause the most illness and deaths in humanitarian emergencies in less-developed countries. Children younger than 5 years of age are the most vulnerable.[2] Other priority areas include provision of adequate safe water, food, shelter, and protection from violence.

- In addition to the usual causes of illness and death in emergency-affected populations in less-developed countries (measles, malaria, pneumonia, and diarrhea), crowded settlements may be prone to outbreaks of cholera, meningitis, and other diseases, which can be rapidly spread. Such outbreaks may be explosive and cause many deaths in a relatively short period of time.

PROBLEM IDENTIFIED

In times of stability, writes Dr. Andrew Schechtman, many of the poorest people in the world succeed in their struggle to meet basic needs for shelter, food, and water. When displaced from their homes by man-made or natural disaster, communities and extended families are disrupted, access to food and water are lost, and marginal circumstances become desperate. Displaced people are often dependent on the support of the international aid community to meet their basic needs.

BEING PART OF THE SOLUTION

When infrastructure collapses as a result of manmade or natural disasters, access to health care can be limited or nonexistent. Serving as a volunteer physician with Médecins Sans Frontières (Doctors Without Borders) allowed Dr. Schechtman to provide medical care to people in desperate circumstances who had nowhere else to turn for assistance. Bearing witness to tragedies such as the case described in **Figure 6-1** gave him another means to help, that is, the authority to speak out on behalf of victims like this child, focus public attention on the situation, and encourage political pressure to bring the fighting to an end.

GLOBAL HEALTH: PERU HEALTH OUTREACH PROJECT (SANGEETA KRISHNA, MD)

EPIDEMIOLOGY

Global health can be defined as the health of populations, which transcends national and international borders. As such, global health involves the perspectives of economics, epidemiology, medicine, public health, and many of the social sciences for measuring, understanding, and providing care to improve health and achieve equity in health for all people. The health issues faced on a global scale are staggering. Worldwide, one billion people lack access to health care systems.[3] Non-communicable diseases such as cardiovascular disease, cancer, chronic lung disease, and diabetes cause about 36 million deaths per year, and communicable diseases including AIDS/HIV, tuberculosis, malaria, and measles cause about 6.7 million deaths annually. Over 7.5 million children under the age of 5 years die from malnutrition and mostly preventable diseases each year.[3]

Global health experiences can complement and enhance physician training in many ways. For the student, these experiences can bring new interpersonal and technical skills, teach cultural competency, and enhance their knowledge base about health issues faced by their host country and management of many of these health problems. Students express great interest in these experiences. In a survey of medical students at Sanford School of Medicine, University of South Dakota, almost 95 percent of students indicated they were either very interested or somewhat interested in serving internationally during medical school or later during their career.[4] Following these experiences, students report having greater clinical skills, being more culturally competent, and are more likely to choose a primary care specialty and/or a public service career.[5,6]

ETIOLOGY

Peru, as the host country, is a nation of 29,988,000 people. The gross national income per capita is $9,440, making it one of the poorest nations in the region. Peru's total per capita expenditure on health also falls far below its neighbors, by nearly tenfold, and the health workforce of 9.2 physicians per 10,000 population and 12.7 nurses and midwives per 10,000 population is inadequate to meet the nation's health care needs. Based on the World Health Organization database, more people die of communicable disease in Peru than the regional average (37% versus 20%, 2008 data) and the probability of dying under age 5 years, although greatly improved since 1990 is 18/1000 live births, similar to the regional average. Communicable diseases such as infectious diarrhea, tuberculosis, hepatitis, dengue fever, and typhoid fever are widely seen, and malaria, bartonellosis, leishmaniasis, and yellow fever are endemic in specific areas of the country. All are potentially preventable through vaccinations and preventive health measures.

As global citizens, we can't ignore these health issues, particularly those of us in wealthier nations living in relative affluence. The brave among us actively work for change. While many schools offer global health experiences, the challenge to educators in the academic institution, medical care providers in the host country, and policy makers is to create regulatory frameworks and curricula that are current and relevant.[8] This requires a level of understanding of globalization on medical education, and the underlying ethical, cultural, and health issues to prepare students for the planned experience and to practice competently in a globalized world. The following should be considered in creating global health electives for medical students or residents:

- Balancing the provision of a fulfilling educational experience with honoring the integrity of medically underserved populations.[9]
- Offering training that is appropriate for the educational level of the learner, and different types of training for the types of physicians preparing to work in the global health community—the "globalized doctor," "humanitarian doctor," and the "policy doctor."[10]
- Taking the time to observe and study the structure and function of the health care delivery system in the host country.
- Considering the safety of the health team, travel and lodging, and adequately preparing them prior to going to the host country on the nature of the host country culture, health care system, and assignment site.[11]
- Securing financial support.

- Preparing participating faculty members, who may have limited experience, to enable them to support and guide students during their global experience.

PROBLEM IDENTIFIED

Dr. Krishna's involvement in "global health" began when, as a medical student in India, she witnessed a cholera epidemic in the neighboring country of Bangladesh. Overnight there was an influx of sick, dehydrated refugees at the doorsteps of the hospital where she was training. Intravenous lines were inserted before histories were taken. As the epidemic spread into the local communities, the vaccine fell into short supply and populations at risk received only one dose instead of the 2 recommended doses of Cholera vaccine. This left her with many unanswered questions regarding the efficacy of a single vaccine dose, the ethics of "good enough," and how to dive into such issues when the opportunity arose. Now on staff at the Cleveland Clinic, Dr. Krishna had the opportunity to participate in and subsequently direct the Peru Health Outreach Project (PHOP), a formal elective for medical students at her institution.

BEING PART OF THE SOLUTION

The PHOP was started in 2007 by four medical students at the Lerner College of Medicine (Cleveland Clinic) and Case Western Reserve University School of Medicine. The mission of this student-led staff-mentored project is to collaborate with health care professionals in Peru to provide ethical and sustainable medical care to the underserved in the Sacred Valley of Peru. Since inception, it has continued to grow exponentially due to student interest and participation. Students participate in clinics; vision screening; well child checks (**Figures 6-2** and **6-3**); diabetes screening; counseling regarding hygiene including dental, lifestyle modifications, healthy diet; prophylaxis for Vitamin A deficiency (**Figure 6-4**); and research. In collaboration with physicians in Peru, the students also organize and hold a 2-day educational symposium for local health care workers. Speakers have included staff members and students with topics ranging from CPR to recognition of high-risk pregnancies and common respiratory illnesses in children.

Students continue to provide very positive feedback from this elective. As one student wrote, "I learned a great deal about cross-cultural communication and humility. In terms of global health, I've learned that there's a lot that needs fixing out in the world, particularly in the Sacred Valley of Peru, and that we need to search for a sustainable mechanism to help that involves and empowers the local residents to take charge of their own health and that of their neighbors. In terms of leadership, I've learned a lot about working with a team of people from all different backgrounds toward a common goal. I've learned that it can be extremely challenging at times but that the best way to come to a compromise is to encourage and use effective communication. Overall, I would say the Peru Trip has been one of the greatest learning experiences for me during my first two years of medical school, teaching me lessons I will take with me through the rest of my career and life.

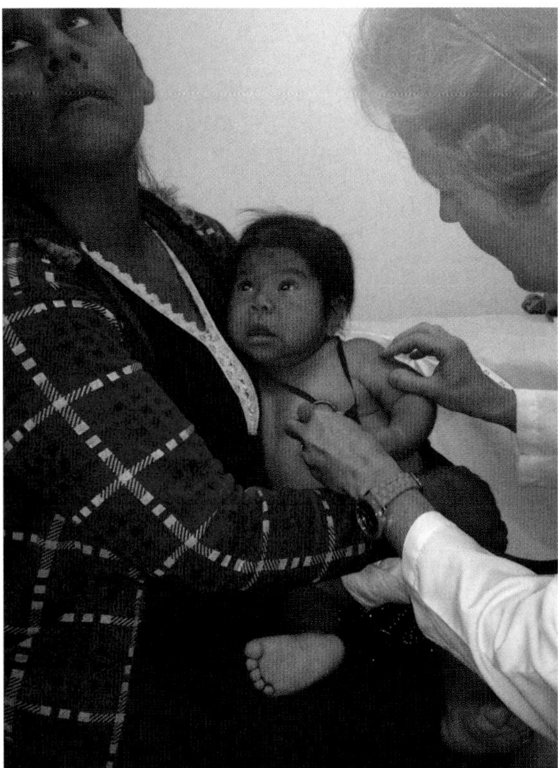

FIGURE 6-2 A 3-year-old girl with no prior medical care arrived at the free clinic in Chincha, Peru. She was unable to sit up without support, or say a few words. Her exam was significant for global developmental delay, hypotonia and an umbilical hernia. An elevated TSH, which was obtained at a subsidized price by the clinic, confirmed our suspicion of congenital hypothyroidism. She was referred to an endocrinologist in a tertiary care hospital in the capital city of Lima and started on thyroid hormone supplement. (*Used with permission from Sangeeta Krishna, MD.*)

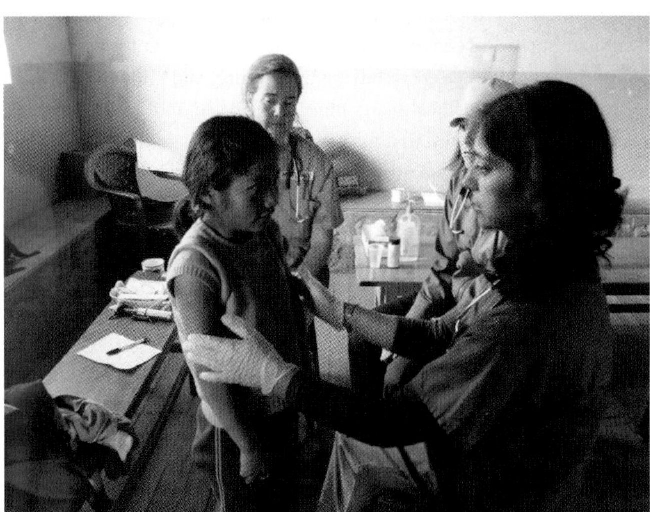

FIGURE 6-3 Dr. Sangeeta Krishna is examining an 11-year-old girl from a remote community of 200 people in Andean Peru where a health care worker was available only once a year. She had been involved in an accident that left her left arm partially paralyzed. She lacked access to medical care for years. She was taught strengthening exercises with the help of a physical therapist. (*Used with permission from Sangeeta Krishna, MD.*)

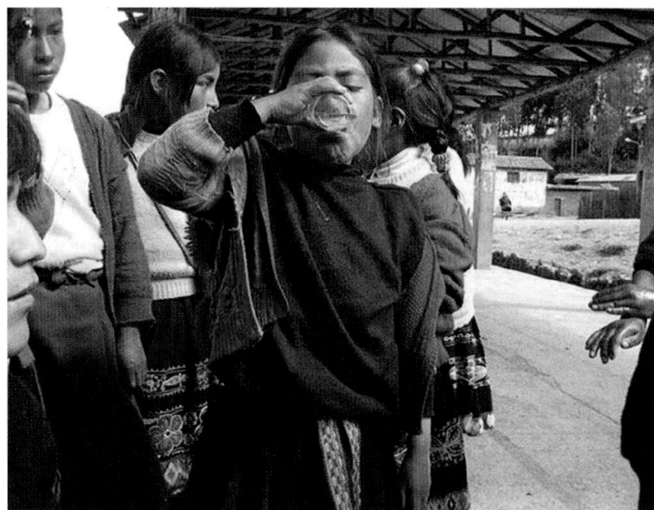

FIGURE 6-4 Vitamin A prophylaxis being provided for the schoolchildren of this remote Peruvian village. Vitamin A deficiency is common in developing countries and can result in blindness along with an increased risk of infection and death. (*Used with permission from Sangeeta Krishna, MD.*)

It has been truly life-changing."—Andrea Grosz, Case Western Reserve University School of Medicine, class of 2014.

The Project leadership has also established a seminar series at the Cleveland Clinic for the benefit of current and future participants addressing topics such as ethics in clinical practice and research, cultural sensitivity, and exploring the standards of care in international rural outreach clinics. Speakers include experienced residents, Fellows, invited faculty from the local institutions, and Case Western Reserve University.

Dr. Krishna warns that these experiences just might change your life! Involvement in this work can be humbling, meaningful, and fulfilling. There are unexpected ethical dilemmas along the way, with no right or wrong answers necessarily. We strive not to set standards and expectations that cannot be sustained by us or the host community when we leave. Understanding the local health system, making appropriate contacts in the community and getting the support of local health authorities are vital to success. Staying aware of ethnocentricity, of the "mzungu" effect, studying the culture, and understanding local factors affecting health and illness are not an option, they are a necessity (mzungu is an African word for a white person). Empowering the community is the ultimate goal. Research if undertaken, should be such that it is acceptable to the community, respectful, and the results should be fed back to "close the loop" and hopefully drive local health care policy decision. Intervention based on the research builds community trust. Above all, we should strive to do no harm.

INTERNATIONAL HUMANITARIAN EFFORTS: ETHIOPIA (RICK HODES, MD)

EPIDEMIOLOGY

Chronic food deficits affect about 792 million people in the world, including 20 percent of the population in developing countries. Malnutrition greatly increases the risk of disease and early death, particularly in young children where protein-energy malnutrition plays a major role in half of all deaths of children under age 5 years annually in developing countries.[12] Worldwide, malnutrition affects one in three people and is especially common among the poor and those with inadequate access to health education, clean water, and good sanitation. About 26 percent of children with protein-energy malnutrition live in Africa. Severe forms of malnutrition include marasmus, iodine deficiency, which can result in cretinism and irreversible brain damage, and vitamin A deficiency, which can result in blindness and increased risk of infection and death.[12]

Worldwide, 2.4 billion people will remain without improved sanitation in 2015 and in 2011, 768 million people relied on unimproved drinking-water sources. In most of Africa, sanitation coverage is less than 50 percent.[13] Ethiopia and its neighbor Somalia are among the few remaining countries in Africa with <50 percent of the population using improved sources of drinking water.[13] Piped drinking water supplies, associated with the best health outcomes, are present for only 1 to 10 percent of Ethiopia's population.

ETIOLOGY

Ethiopia has a population of over 91 million people. The gross national income per capita is $1100, making it one of the poorest nations in the world. The probability of dying under age 5 years is 68/1000 live births, in part due to the low percentage of women attending antenatal care and only 10 percent of births being attended by skilled health personnel. 14 The health workforce is nearly nonexistent with 0.3 physicians per 10,000 population and 2.5 nurses and midwives per 10,000 population. Health problems in Ethiopia include maternal mortality, malaria, tuberculosis and HIV/AIDS compounded by malnutrition and lack of access to clean water and sanitation.

PROBLEM IDENTIFIED

Rick Hodes is a physician who has lived and worked in Ethiopia for over 20 years. As an Orthodox Jew, he always aspired to serve others and even as a child, his favorite books were about doctors who went to remote places to help people. He first went to Ethiopia in 1984 to do famine relief work. His experience of working at a mission in Ethiopia run by Mother Theresa changed his life. He returned to Ethiopia on a Fulbright Fellowship and in 1990 was hired by the American Jewish Joint Distribution Committee as the medical adviser for the country. His original position was to care for 25,000 potential immigrants to Israel but he is continually drawn back to Ethiopia to provide care to patients. When asked once if he would prefer to work in the US rather than Africa with its poverty and lack of resources, Hodes said, "It would be less frustrating—but it would also be less inspiring."

BEING PART OF THE SOLUTION

As senior consultant at a Catholic mission, Dr. Hodes helps patients with heart disease (rheumatic and congenital) (**Figure 6-5**), spinal disease (TB and scoliosis) (**Figures 6-6** and **6-7**), infectious disease (**Figure 6-8**) and cancer. He has worked with refugees in Rwanda, Zaire, Tanzania, Somalia, and Albania in addition to Ethiopia. Dr. Hodes is part of a team at the

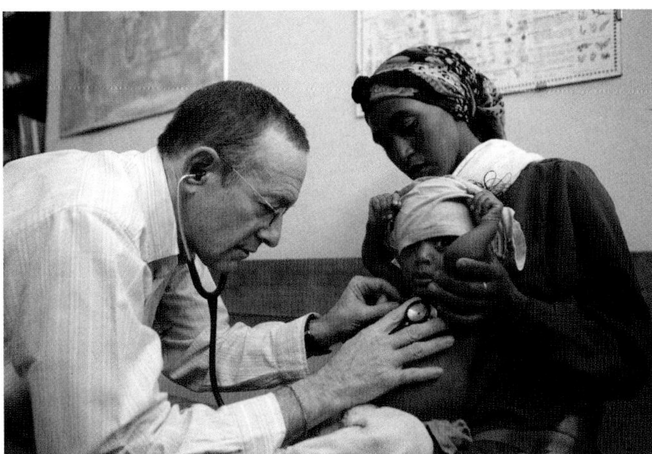

FIGURE 6-5 Dr. Hodes examining a young Ethiopian girl with heart disease secondary to rheumatic fever. (*Used with permission from Mark Tuschman.*)

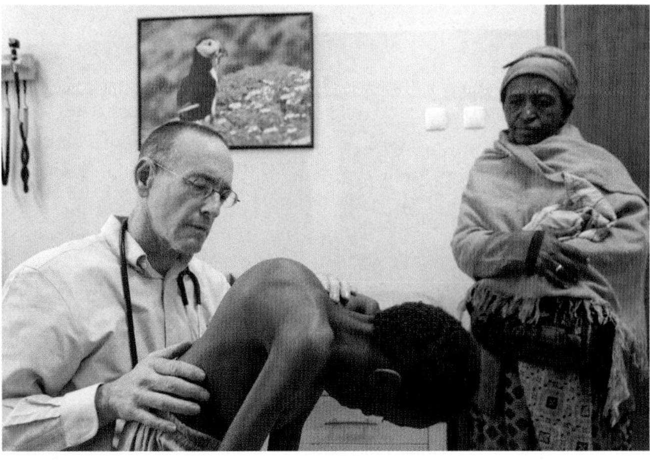

FIGURE 6-6 Dr. Hodes examining an Ethiopian boy with severe kyphoscoliosis secondary to TB of the spine. (*Used with permission from Richard Lord.*)

American Jewish Joint Distribution Committee (JDC), a Jewish humanitarian assistance organization founded in 1914 that provides needed services in more than 70 countries. Among his JDC duties has been providing medical care for thousands of Ethiopian Jews preparing to immigrate to Israel. In addition to its assistance to the Ethiopian Jewish community, the JDC has served tens of thousands of Ethiopians, Jews and non-Jews, through clinics, immunization, nutrition programs, family planning, and community health (**Figure 6-9**).

Dr. Hodes has worked primarily in Ethiopia for the JDC since 1990. In addition to providing direct patient care, he has arranged for

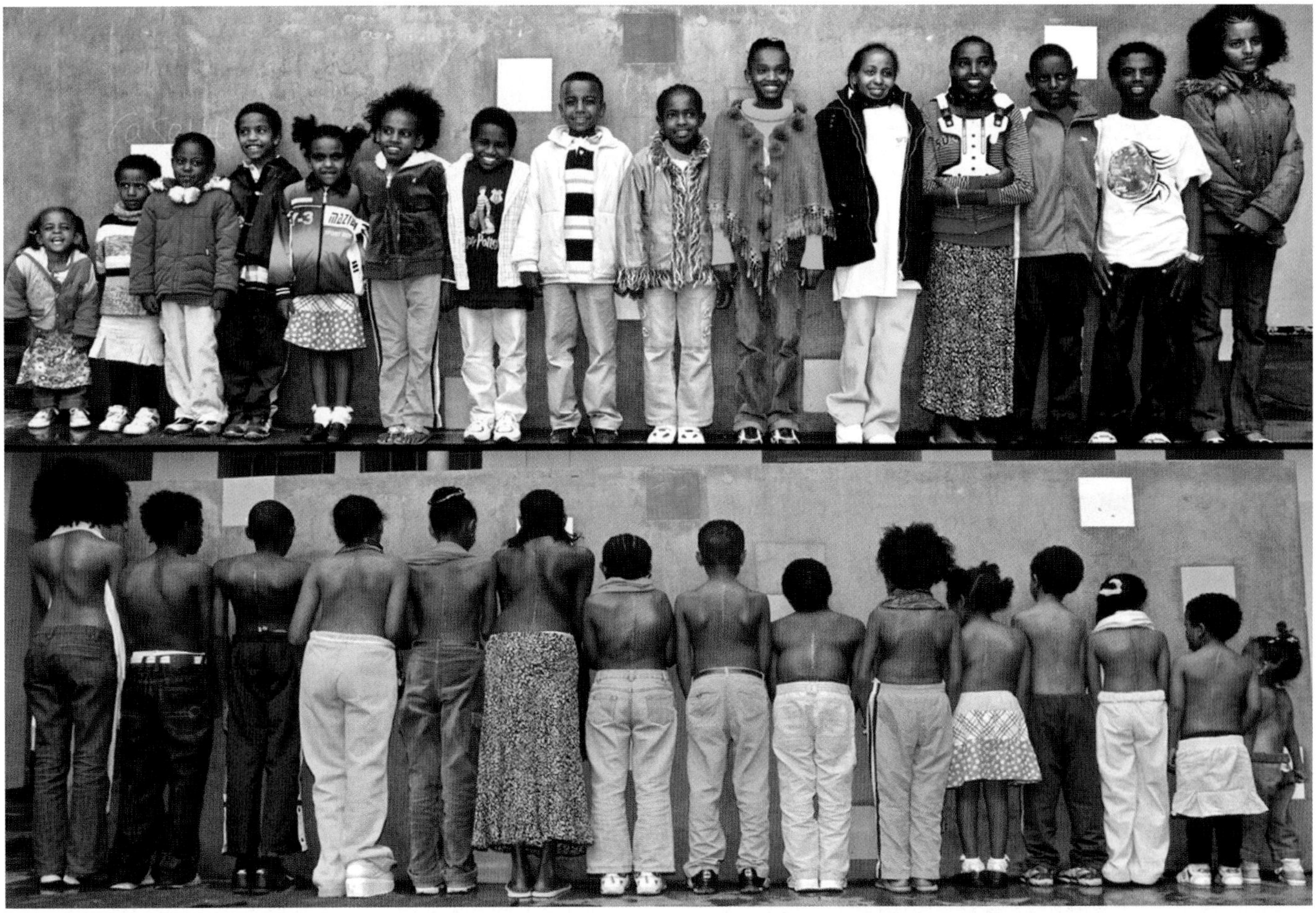

FIGURE 6-7 Ethiopian children with a variety of spine diseases after returning from spine surgery in Ghana Africa. Medical evaluation and funding was arranged by Dr. Rick Hodes and the American Jewish Joint Distribution Committee. They can look forward to improved lives with straighter spines. (*Used with permission from Rick Hodes, MD.*)

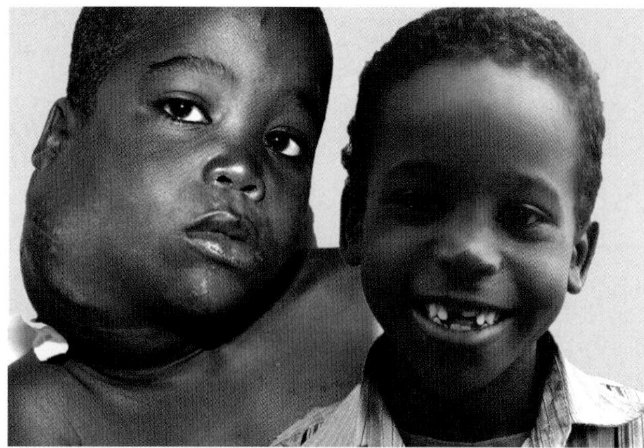

FIGURE 6-8 The same Ethiopian child before and after chemotherapy for Hodgkin's lymphoma. Dr. Hodes diagnosed and treated this young boy. (*Used with permission from Rick Hodes, MD.*)

specialized care for hundreds of children in need with neurosurgeons and orthopedic surgeons in the US and Ghana. He has fostered numerous orphaned children and adopted four children, providing needed medical care with his own insurance. Some of these children are now attending schools and colleges around the US. He has also led teams of doctors, who come to work with him as volunteers (**Figure 6-10**). In one interview, Dr. Hodes said, "Getting free medical care in a Catholic hospital by a Jewish doctor is like the whole world coming together. It's the way the world should work."

CARING FOR THOSE WITH DISABILITIES (LAURIE WOODARD, MD)

EPIDEMIOLOGY

Approximately 54 million Americans currently live with at least 1 disability and the vast majority (52 million) live in their communities (**Figure 6-11**).[15]

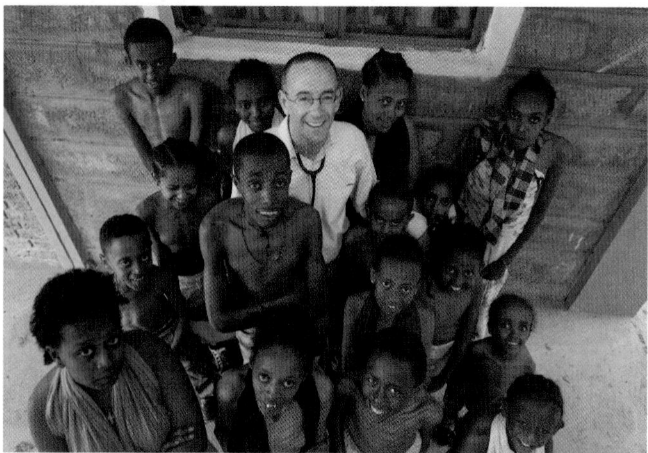

FIGURE 6-9 Dr. Hodes with some of his Ethiopian patients that have spine disease. (*Used with permission from Richard Lord.*)

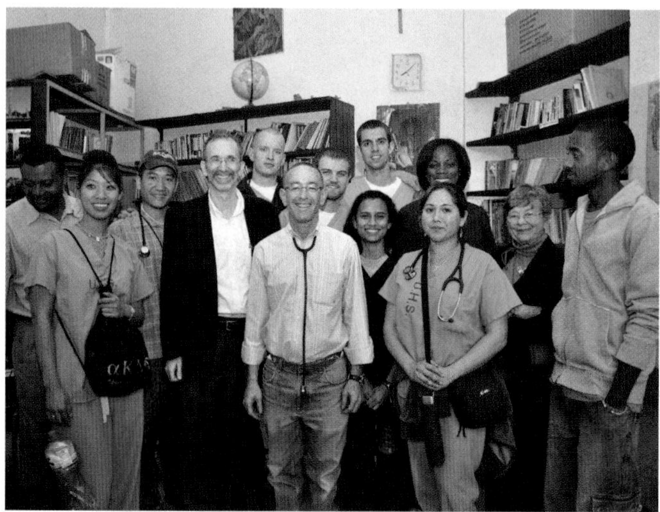

FIGURE 6-10 Dr. Hodes hosting a group of US medical students and doctors in his clinic at the Mother Teresa mission in Ethiopia. (*Used with permission from Richard P. Usatine, MD.*)

- According to data from 1999, the prevalence rate of disability was 24 percent among women and 20 percent among men.[16] Approximately 32 million adults had difficulty with 1 or more functional activities, and approximately 16.7 million adults had a limitation in

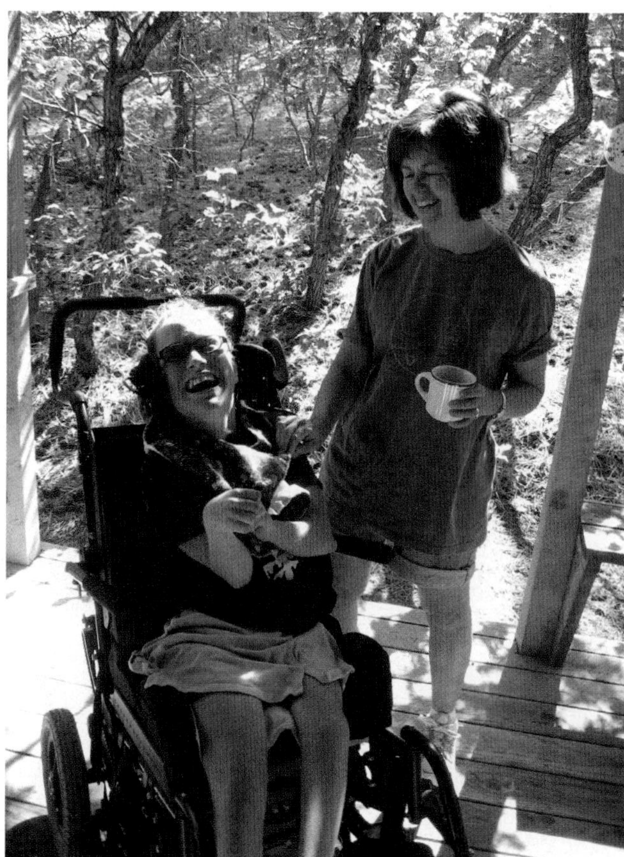

FIGURE 6-11 Dr. Laurie Woodard and her daughter Anika share a good laugh following breakfast while on vacation in New Mexico. Although Anika is dependent for all her activities of daily living and is nonverbal because of spastic quadriparetic cerebral palsy, she loves to travel and has a wonderful sense of humor.

the ability to work around the house. Two million adults used a wheelchair and 7 million used a cane, crutches, or a walker.

- Of children ages 3 to 17 years, 4.9 million were told that they have some type of learning disability and 12.8 percent (9.4 million) have special health care needs.[15]
- Racial and ethnic minorities have higher rates of disabilities than whites or Asian Americans; 7.3 million individuals (ages 15 to 65 years) with disabilities are of racial or ethnic minorities.
- In 2005, the surgeon general issued a Call to Action to improve the health and wellness of persons with disabilities underscoring the need in this population.[15]

ETIOLOGY

Challenges to a person's health can happen at any age and at any time. Disabilities are not illnesses, rather they are limitations related to a medical condition that have an influence on essential life functions such as walking, seeing, or working.[15] Furthermore, disabilities do not affect all people in the same way.

- Of all the adults with disabilities, 41.2 million (93.4%) reported that their disability was associated with a health condition including arthritis and rheumatism (17.5%), back or spine problems (16.5%), heart trouble/hardening of the arteries (7.8%), lung or respiratory problems (4.7%), deafness or hearing problems (4.2%), mental or emotional problems (3.7%), blindness or visual problems (3.4%), and intellectual disability (2%).[16]
- Rates of disability are increasing in part because of the aging population, better survival of catastrophic illnesses and trauma, and advances in preventing infant and child mortality.

PROBLEM IDENTIFIED

As a mother of a child with profound disabilities, Dr. Laurie Woodard found that her medical training did little to prepare her for caring for her child or finding help (**Figure 6-11**). She became acutely aware that people with disabilities had great difficulty finding physicians and those who provided care often seemed afraid of them. She said, "I couldn't imagine someone not wanting to care for her because she had a disability." Physicians tend to focus on the medical condition and not the whole person and their families; when confronted with the patient's health care needs and functional issues, the feeling of acting more like a social worker than a physician caused them to fall back into medical model framework. In addition, societal support for those with disabilities, particularly disabilities acquired as an adult, are fragmented and the primary care physician needs to become the link.

BEING PART OF THE SOLUTION

Dr. Woodard began to care for increasing numbers of patients with disabilities, training herself through reading, experience, and asking patients what worked. As she worked with individual students she planned for a time when she could break into the medical student curriculum to provide this training. Eight years ago, when the curriculum for third-year students underwent major reform, she saw her opportunity. Within the primary care 12-week experience, a curriculum on special populations was planned and Laurie made sure that it included teaching about persons with disabilities. Her curriculum, implemented in 2005 with goals ranging from sensitivity training to understanding both the capabilities and needs of individuals with disabilities, contains the following components:

- Clinic-like experience with 8 to 10 patients with physical disabilities (e.g., cerebral palsy, communication issues, wheelchair users) where pairs of students complete brief interview and physical examination under video monitoring. The session ends with a debriefing circle wrap up with students and patients.
- Panel discussion with patients with varying abilities who usually represent an advocacy agency or organization. Special emphasis is placed on community services and opportunities including the arts and sports.
- Home visits where student pairs (2 medical students or a medical student and physical therapy student) receive a preparation sheet and checklist, and learn how disability affects individuals and their family. Following the visit, students prepare reflection plus research reports that are posted on blackboard; part of the assignment is to read and comment on all the papers.
- Service learning project where students give presentations on health topics (e.g., first aid, influenza) selected by staff at an adult daycare facility for individuals with intellectual disabilities or the high school group noted above, or assist in the recreational activities for individuals with disabilities (e.g., free physicals for riders in therapeutic horseback riding program).
- An objective structured clinical examination (OSCE) case involving a manual wheelchair user with shoulder pain; the standardized patients are individuals who are wheelchair users.
- Sensitivity training session, run by Parks and Recreation where students are randomly assigned a disability (e.g., using a wheelchair or other assistive device or blindfold) and complete tasks followed by watching the movie *Murderball* (an informative and proactive documentary about the Paralympics sport, quadriplegic rugby, and its players). A speech pathologist also provides a hands-on assistive/augment communication device tutorial.

"The students learn to see the patient first," she says, "that caring for these individuals requires recognizing the patient's expertise about their disability and problem solving together. For most students, even the most jaded, this is simply an eye opening experience as the patients are usually quite physically impaired but lead full and active lives" (**Figure 6-12**).

Dr. Woodard has expanded this program and is co-teaching with faculty from the School of Physical Therapy (PT) so that medical and PT students interview and examine patients together. In addition, she will begin providing training within the courses Doctoring 1 and Doctoring 2 to first- and second-year medical students (the home visit and panel discussion will be moved to the first year) allowing more complex and challenging issues to be addressed during the clerkship. Finally, she is also involved with Alliance for Disability in Health Education, a group mainly out of the Northeast whose mission is to get the American Association of Medical Colleges (AAMC) to require the topic of disability in the curriculum.

Since the initial publication of this chapter, Dr. Woodard's daughter graduated from high school in June 2011. The family is working on

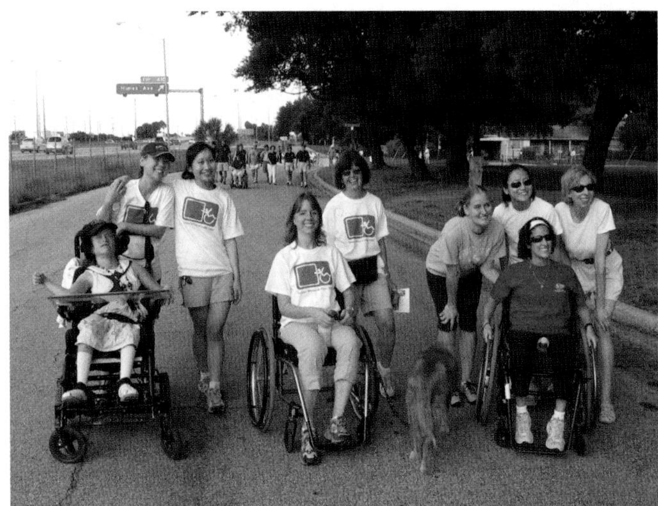

FIGURE 6-12 Dr. Woodard, daughter Anika, and dog Nikki are part of a team of University of South Florida (USF) medical students, faculty, and family who participated in a "wheel-a-thon" to raise money for Tampa's first fully accessible playground. Teaching medicals students the therapeutic value of sports and recreation for people with disabilities is an important aspect of the USF curriculum.

helping her structure her day and move beyond the interminable wait list for services to which she is entitled. She is happy and healthy, and the family members consider themselves lucky to have good, affordable caregivers and companions to assist her.

CARING FOR THE HOMELESS (RANDAL CHARLES CHRISTENSEN, MD, MPH)

EPIDEMIOLOGY

At least 643,000 persons were homeless on any given night in 2009 and 1 in every 200 Americans (approximately 1.56 million people) spent at least 1 night in a shelter during that year.[17] Of those who were homeless in one study, 3 percent reported having HIV/AIDS and 26 percent reported other acute health problems, including tuberculosis and other sexually transmitted infections.[18]

Causes of death were investigated in one study of 40 homeless people for more than a 1-year period (1985 to 1986) conducted by the Fulton County Medical Examiner in Georgia. It was thought at that time that between 4,000 and 7,000 individuals were homeless, so the crude death rate for that year was estimated at 5.7 to 10 per 1,000.[19]

- Black males accounted for 19 (48%) of the 40 deaths, white males for 18 (45%), and black females for 3 (8%). The median age for 36 individuals whose age was known was 44 years (range = 21 to 70 years).
- Twenty-two individuals (55%) died or were found dead outdoors. Of the 18 persons who died indoors, 7 were found in vacant buildings and 5 died at shelters.
- Cause of death, based on the medical history, investigation scene information, circumstances of death, and autopsy and toxicologic studies (when performed) was classified as natural (16), accidental (19), or homicide (4) or suicide (1). Natural deaths included alcohol related (9 including 3 with seizures likely from alcohol withdrawal), heart disease (4), and lung disease (3). Accidental deaths were primarily a result of acute alcohol toxicity (7), fire (6), hypothermia (2), and pedestrian–motor vehicle incidents (2). No deaths were attributed to drugs other than alcohol.

ETIOLOGY

Homeless persons are often extremely poor and socially isolated, the latter is considered a significant contributor to being homeless. Many medical conditions are caused by or exacerbated by the adverse living conditions and lack of health care experienced by the homeless. These include:

- Psychiatric illnesses (affecting as many as 40% of homeless persons).
- Physical health problems, including injuries from trauma, respiratory disease (e.g., tuberculosis), scabies and pediculosis infestations, and chronic illnesses such as diabetes.

PROBLEM IDENTIFIED

Dr. Randal Christensen earned both a medical degree and MPH from Tufts University School of Medicine followed by a four-year combined Pediatrics and Internal Medicine program in Phoenix, Arizona. Medical education became a priority for him and he wanted to find a way to combine the provision of medical care to underserved populations while teaching and inspiring students to get involved with their communities. Throughout his career, Dr. Christensen has maintained a strong desire to care for children who have no voice.

BEING PART OF THE SOLUTION

Dr. Christensen began working for Phoenix Children's Hospital as the Medical Director of the Crews'n Healthmobile, a mobile medical van that delivers medical care to homeless youth and teens (**Figures 6-13** and **6-14**). As a Clinical Assistant Professorship at the University of Arizona College of Medicine and the Arizona State University School of Nursing, he was in an ideal position to expand this program serving homeless children in Phoenix and the surrounding communities. This mobile medical center provides comprehensive medical and social services; it is essentially a doctor's office on wheels. Dr. Christensen and his team reach out to thousands of children and adolescents living in poverty on the streets of Arizona (**Figures 6-15** to **6-17**). Systems and procedures set up by his team are still in place today and in multiple other mobile medical centers around the country.

Dr. Christensen has also exercised his leadership abilities on behalf of many community organizations. As the Medical Director for Camp AZDA, one of the largest camps in the US for children with diabetes, he has taken a team approach to expanding numbers of children and staff at camp while providing a safe and perhaps life changing experience for these children. Other memberships include the Executive Board for VisionQuest 20/20 (an organization with a mission to insure all children have proper vision screening through enhanced technology), and the Advisory Board for Health care for the

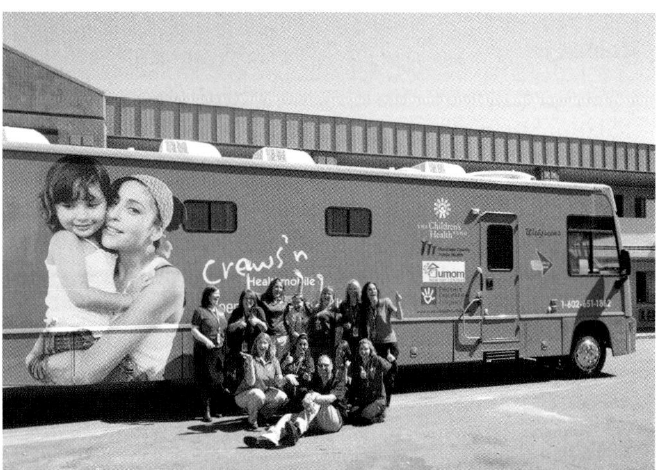

FIGURE 6-13 Dr. Randy Christensen with his team and Healthmobile getting ready to go out on the streets of Phoenix to deliver free health care to homeless and at-risk children and teens. This mobile medical van, nicknamed "Big Blue," is outfitted with three exam rooms and the latest technology. (*Photography used with permission by Phoenix Children's Hospital.*)

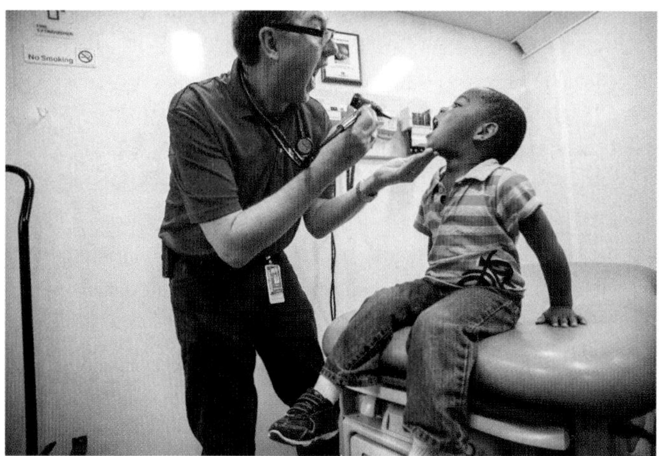

FIGURE 6-14 "Say ahhh!" Dr. Christensen visits with Jacob for a routine health check-up inside the Crews'n Healthmobile. In the 12 years Dr. Christensen has been operating the van, he has completed more than 32,000 medical encounters. (*Photography used with permission by Phoenix Children's Hospital. Photography by Desert Ridge Photography/ Charles Siritho.*)

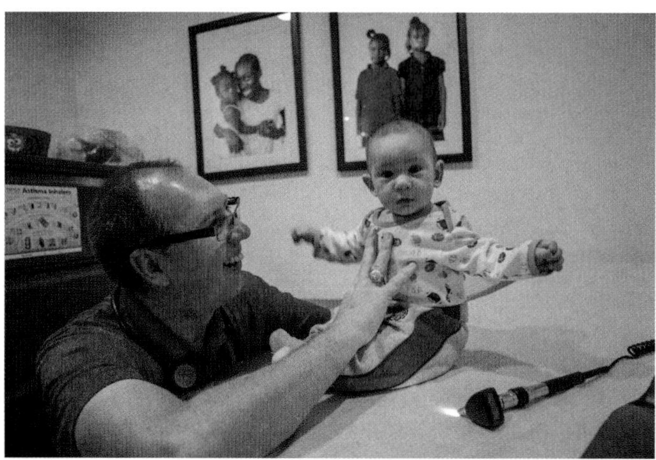

FIGURE 6-15 Dr. Christensen examines this cute baby at a local homeless shelter. (*Photography used with permission by Phoenix Children's Hospital. Photography by Desert Ridge Photography/Charles Siritho.*)

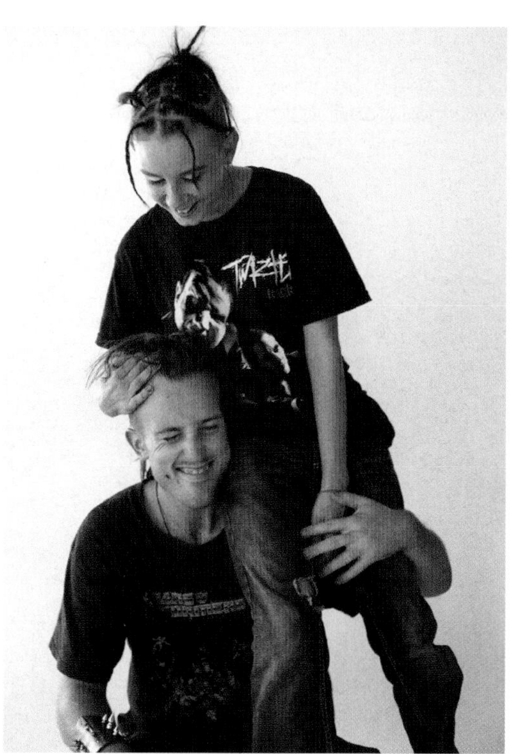

FIGURE 6-16 The Crews'n Healthmobile visits multiple sites around the Phoenix area where homeless teens gather. This teenage couple was happy to pose for photos that are displayed on the site: http://www.askmewhyihurt.com/big-blue/faces-of-crews/.

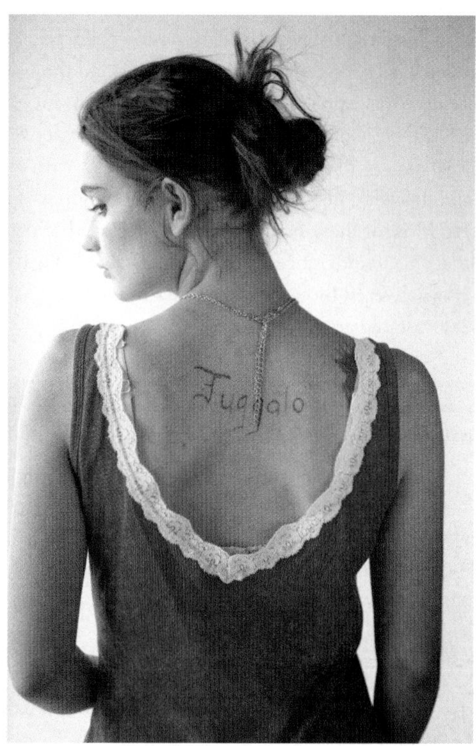

FIGURE 6-17 This teen is showing us her tattoo. Many teens come to the healthmobile after getting a tattoo or piercing to have their skin checked to make sure they "don't get an infection". During those times Dr. Christensen and his team try very hard to establish a rapport and encourage follow up. As trust builds then so does the chance for the teens' success to graduate and get meaningful work (http://www.askmewhyihurt.com/big-blue/faces-of-crews/).

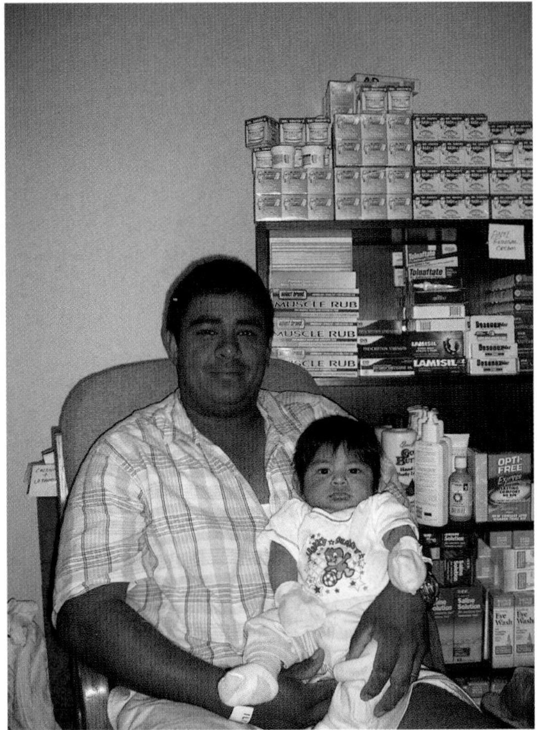

FIGURE 6-18 Father and daughter receiving medical care after being evacuated from New Orleans post Hurricane Katrina. (*Used with permission from Richard P. Usatine, MD.*)

Homeless. His efforts to help underserved populations include yearly trips to Washington, DC, to advocate for children.

Dr. Christensen's contributions extend far beyond the walls of Phoenix Children's Hospital. When Hurricane Katrina hit New Orleans in 2006, Dr. Christensen organized a team to deliver medical care within 10 days of the storm. His team was meet with officials in Louisiana and provided needed health care during more than 330 clinical visits. Most of these families were in dire need of primary care and had not seen a doctor since the hurricane started (**Figure 6-18**). The team also delivered thousands of dollars of medications and supplies to the devastated area.

PROVIDER RESOURCES

International Humanitarian Efforts

- Doctors Without Borders—**www.doctorswithoutborders.org.**
- International Health Volunteers (IHVO)—**www.internationalhealthvolunteers.org**.
- Rick Hodes website—**www.rickhodes.org**.

Disabled Persons

- US Department of Justice—**www.usdoj.gov/crt/ada/cguide.htm**.
- Social Security Administration—**www.ssa.gov/disability** (information on benefits).
- Information on sports events for the disabled—**www.dsusa.org**.
- **www.disabilityinfo.gov**.

Homeless

- National Coalition for the Homeless—**http://www.nationalhomeless.org**.
- National Alliance to End Homelessness—**http://www.naeh.org**.
- US Department of Housing and Urban Development—**www.hud.gov/homeless/index.cfm**.
- Veterans Affairs—**www1.va.gov/homeless/**.
- **www.askmewhyihurt.com**.

REFERENCES

1. United Nations High Commissioner for Refugees (UNHCR). http://www.unhcr.org/pages/49c3646c11.html, accessed April 26, 2012.
2. Center for Disease Control (CDC). http://www.cdc.gov/globalhealth/gdder/ierh/FAQ.htm#What health issues are most important early in an emergency?, accessed April 26, 2012.
3. Global Health Overview. http://www.globalissues.org/article/588/global-health-overview, accessed October 2013.
4. Liebe S, Elliott A, Bien M. Student interest and knowledge concerning global health electives: a USD Sanford School of Medicine study. *S D Med*. 2013;66(6):231-233.
5. Thompson MJ, Huntington MK, Hunt DD, et al. Educational effects of international health electives on U.S. and Canadian medical students and residents: a literature review. *Acad Med*. 2003;78(3):342-347.
6. Jeffrey J, Dumont RA, Kim GY, Kuo T. Effects of international health electives on medical student learning and career choice: results of a systematic literature review. *Fam Med*. 2011;43(1):21-28.
7. World Health Organization. *Peru*. http://www.who.int/countries/per/en/, accessed October 2013.
8. Martimianakis MA, Hafferty FW. The world as the new local clinic: a critical analysis of three discourses of global medical competency. *Soc Sci Med*. 2013;87:31-38.
9. Rassiwala J, Vaduganathan M, Kupershtok M, et al. Global Health Educational Engagement-A Tale of Two Models. *Acad Med*. 2013;25.
10. Rowson M, Smith A, Hughes R, et al. The evolution of global health teaching in undergraduate medical curricula. Global Health. 2012;13:8:35.
11. Imperato PJ. A third world international health elective for U.S. medical students: the 25-year experience of the State University of New York, Downstate Medical Center. *BMC*. 2004;29(5):337-373.
12. World Health Organization. Water-Related Diseases. *Malnutrition*. http://www.who.int/water_sanitation_health/diseases/malnutrition/en/, accessed October 2013.
13. World Health Organization. *Progress on Sanitation and Drinking Water: 2013 Update*. http://apps.who.int/iris/bitstream/10665/81245/1/9789241505390_eng.pdf, accessed October 2013.

14. World Health Organization African Region. *Ethiopia*. http://www.who.int/countries/eth/en/, accessed November 2013.

15. Department of Health and Human Services. *The Surgeon General's Call to Action to Improve the Health and Wellness of Persons with Disabilities.*, http://www.ncbi.nlm.nih.gov/books/NBK44667/pdf/TOC.pdf, accessed April 25, 2007.

16. Prevalence of disabilities and associated health conditions among adults—United States, 1999. *MMWR Morb Mortal Wkly Rep*. 2001;50(07):120-125.

17. Centers for Disease Control and Prevention. *National Prevention Information Network*, http://www.cdcnpin.org/scripts/population/homeless.asp, accessed May 1, 2012.

18. National Resource Center on Homelessness and Mental Illness. *Who Is Homeless?* http://homeless.samhsa.gov/Resource/View.aspx?id=32511.

19. Centers for Disease Control and Prevention: Enumerating deaths among homeless persons: comparison of medical examiner data and shelter-based reports—Fulton County, Georgia, 1991. *MMWR Morb Mortal Wkly Rep*. 1993;42(37):719, 725-726.

7 GLOBAL HEALTH

Ruth E. Berggren, MD
Richard P. Usatine, MD

COMMUNITY STORY

Common River is a US-based nongovernmental organization (NGO) implementing a community development program in Aleta Wondo, Ethiopia. This NGO is founded on the principle of positive deviance, in which local best practices are identified and replicated to maximize agricultural production (organically grown coffee is produced in this region), as well as to improve the nutritional status, health, and education of orphaned and vulnerable children. Since 2009, a group from the University of Texas School of Medicine has travelled annually to Aleta Wondo to provide school health screening and free health care, including treatment of endemic helminth infections, trachoma, and skin diseases, while collaborating with and supporting the local government-sponsored health clinic (**Figures 7-1A** and **B**). In **Figure 7-1C**, the schoolchildren of Common River are looking at the new group of American medical students that have just arrived in Africa. In the coming week, these children will receive oral albendazole to treat intestinal parasites and have complete physical exams to detect and treat other common conditions, such as head lice, tinea capitis, trachoma, and foot infections. Note that many of the children are barefoot. In **Figure 7-1D**, a group of women have just completed their woman's literacy class for the day. Improving women's literacy can improve the health of the entire community.

WHAT IS GLOBAL HEALTH?

For years, the term *international health* has described health work in resource-limited settings with an emphasis on tropical diseases,

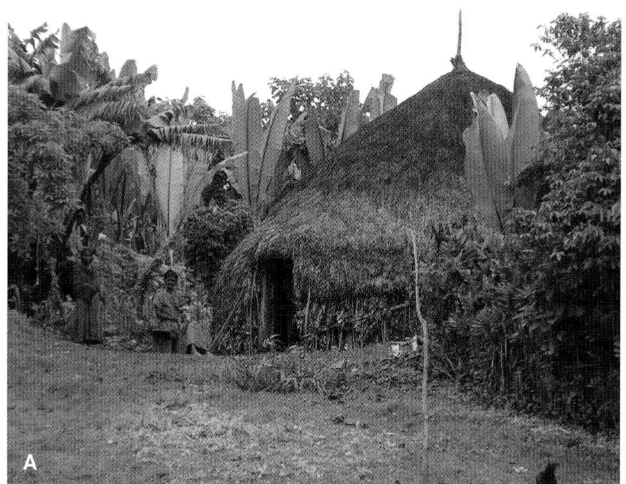

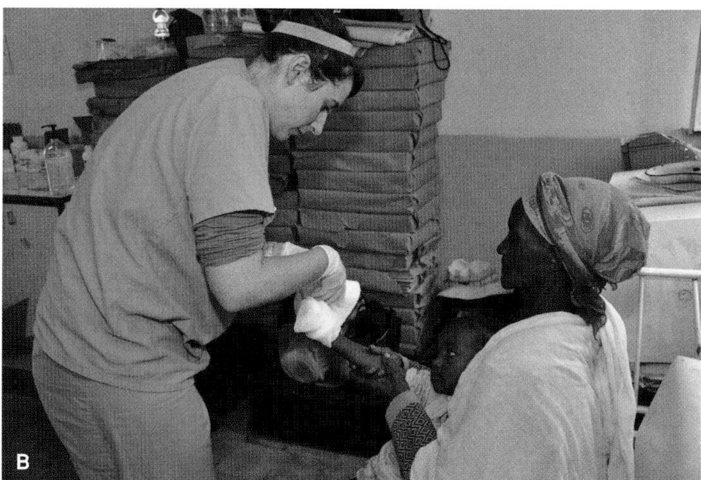

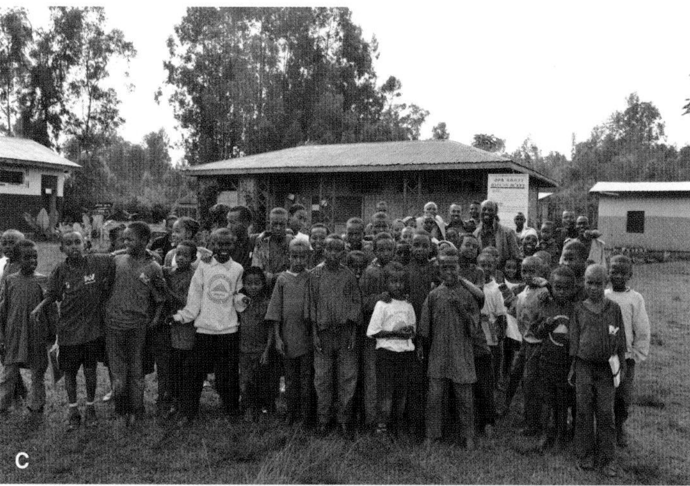

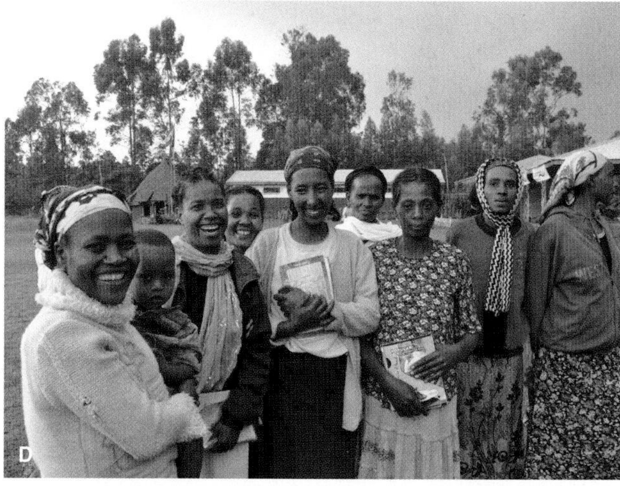

FIGURE 7-1 **A.** Many people still live in extreme poverty with no running water and electricity. This is a typical hut in Ethiopia. This one is inhabited by a grandmother, her grandchild, and a cow. The photograph was taken after a home visit to provide IM ceftriaxone to the child after her release from the local hospital where she was treated for a neck abscess and cellulitis. The medical team was staying at Common River and originated from the University of Texas. **B.** A University of Texas medical student is bandaging the hand of a 2-year-old girl in Aleta Wondo. The medical team had just drained an abscess of her hand. **C.** The schoolchildren of Common River in rural Ethiopia greet the new group of American medical students that have just arrived in Africa. **D.** Smiling women that have just completed their woman's literacy class for the day. Improving woman's literacy is a great way to raise the health status of the community. (*Used with permission from Richard P. Usatine, MD.*)

communicable diseases, and illness caused by poor nutrition and inadequate access to water, sanitation, and maternal care.[1] More recently, *global health* is commonly used to emphasize mutual sharing of experience and knowledge, in a bilateral exchange between industrialized nations and resource-limited countries, and the emphasis is expanding to include noncommunicable diseases and chronic illness.[2] One definition of global health, proposed by the Consortium of Universities for Global Health Executive Board, is "an area for study, research, and practice that places a priority on improving health and achieving equity in health for all people worldwide."[1] This chapter focuses on a few conditions commonly encountered in developing nations, emphasizing communicable diseases and malnutrition.

Ethical dilemmas abound when professionals from resource-rich settings leave their familiar environment and apply their practices in a severely resource-limited setting. Consider, for example, breastfeeding guidelines in the setting of maternal-to-child HIV prevention. National protocols differ depending on resource availability. In some settings, telling an HIV-positive mother not to breastfeed (because breast-milk can transmit HIV) may sentence her infant to near-certain death from diarrhea. If a program overturns local teaching about exclusive breastfeeding, it must ensure a safe and sustainable alternative form of infant feeding. Imposing the standards of industrialized nations in a community that cannot afford to continue to provide these standards can undo years of program development. Care must be taken not to undermine the trust a community has placed in local health providers, as this can ultimately increase morbidity rather than relieve suffering. Working with local health providers is essential so that a short trip can result in extended benefits to the community (**Figure 7-2**).

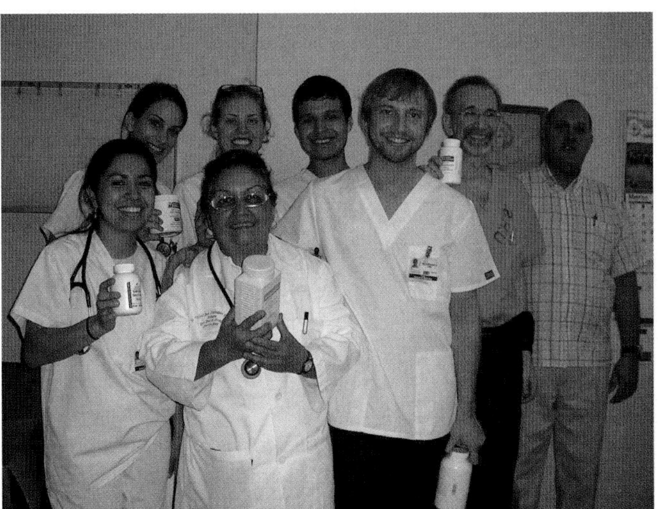

FIGURE 7-2 The physician in the front of this picture is pleased to receive medications that are unavailable to her hospital in rural Panama. Before shipping or bringing medications abroad, it is essential to learn what practicing physicians need. Bringing redundant or nearly expired meds or short-term supplies of expensive brand medications causes more harm than good. Donated medications should be locally relevant generics that are not expired. The WHO list of essential medications may be helpful in planning (http://www.who.int/medicines/publications/essentialmedicines/en/index.html). (*Used with permission from Richard P. Usatine, MD.*)

This chapter briefly introduces some of the relevant subject areas with which global health providers should familiarize themselves when preparing for international work. Statistics that aid in understanding the state of a nation's health relative to other countries are the mortality rate of children younger than age of 5 years old and adult life expectancy. Least-developed countries report that as many as 112 of 1,000 children die before age 5 years, compared to 8 per 1,000 in developed countries,[3] and adult life expectancy ranges from 48 or 49 years at birth (Chad, Swaziland) to 88 or 89 years (Japan, Monaco).[3] Another important parameter by which to compare the health status of countries is that of maternal mortality, defined as the number of maternal deaths per 100,000 livebirths. These figures, together with basic epidemiology of disease provide important insights into public health priorities for populations.

What statistics do not provide, however, is the level of importance ascribed to a particular health issue by a community. It is necessary to acknowledge and address the needs expressed by communities themselves, in order of their own priorities, so as to achieve sustained improvements in health outcomes. All health improvements ultimately rely on long-term behavioral changes, whether dietary, pill taking, physical activity, or hygiene related. Group behavioral change requires buy-in from the population with approbation and influence of local leadership.

A useful method of creating a positive impact is to make use of ongoing peer-to-peer adult education techniques through the introduction of community health clubs. This can be effective for empowering resource-limited communities to develop their priorities, and to advocate for their community health and development needs.[4] It is best to learn about and collaborate with the local and governmental community health activities before launching any intervention, be it clinical, infrastructural, or preventive.

WATER AND SANITATION

Many diseases in resource-poor settings are traceable to deficits in clean water supply and storage, lack of soap for bathing, and lack of functioning infrastructure to manage human waste (e.g., garbage collection and latrines) (**Figure 7-3**). Some of the most important ones include typhoid fever, cholera, and intestinal parasites.

Lack of governmental and public health infrastructure in the developing world leads to large populations living without clean running water. World Health Organization (WHO) and UNICEF estimate that 780 million persons are without access to improved water sources and 2.5 billion (37% of the world's population) people are without access to improved sanitation sources.[6]

Water and sanitation deficiencies are responsible for most of the global burden of diarrheal disease. The most common diarrheal disease of returning travelers is caused by enterotoxigenic *Escherichia coli*. All over the world, young and malnourished children die of preventable diarrhea caused by rotavirus, *E. coli*, *Salmonella*, *Shigella*, and *Campylobacter*.

Diseases that are particularly deadly as a result of lack of access to clean water include typhoid fever and cholera. Intestinal parasites, while usually not deadly, do lead to chronic problems with malnutrition and anemia, which themselves contribute to cyclical poverty and disease because they lead to impaired learning, reduced productivity, and vulnerability to other infectious diseases.

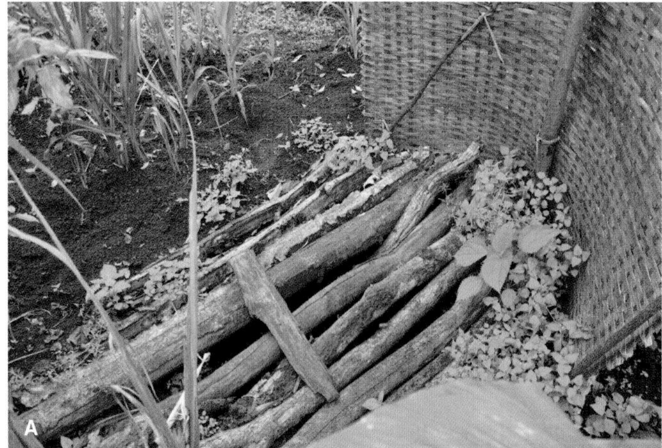

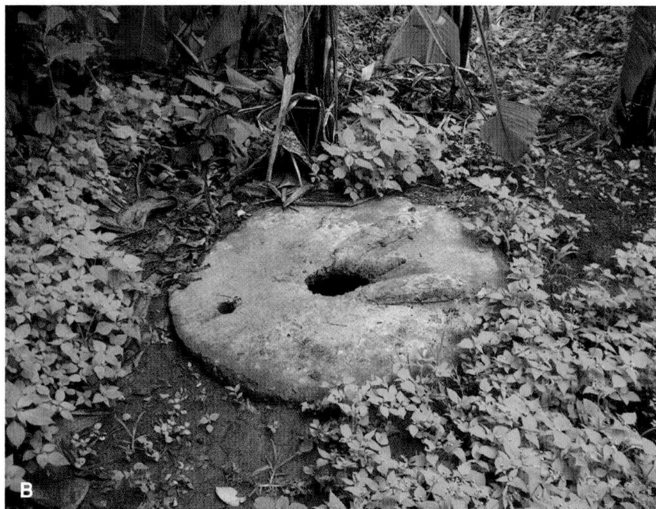

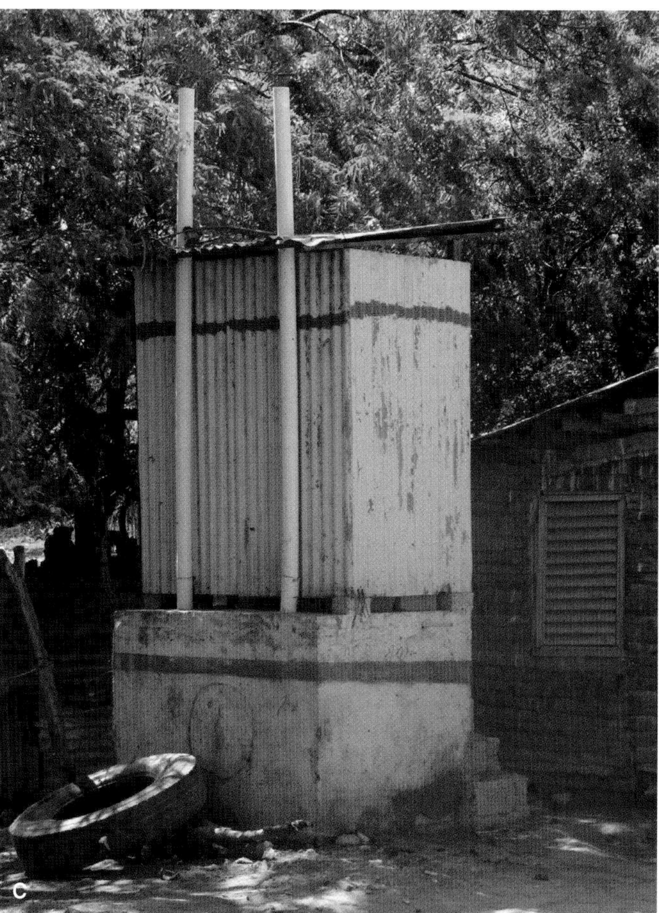

FIGURE 7-3 A. A covered pit latrine serving the needs of an Ethiopian family. The latrine is located on the edge of the garden near their home and presents a fall hazard for young children. (*Used with permission from Richard P. Usatine, MD.*) **B.** An Ethiopian pit latrine, which offers no mitigation for flies and is situated in proximity to the water table below. Heavy rains will lead to contamination of the water supply with fecal pathogens. (*Used with permission from Richard P. Usatine, MD.*) **C.** An elevated, ventilated improved pit latrine can protect the water table and reduce flies. Air circulates down the squat hole, into the pit and up through the pipe. To ensure unhindered flow of air, the top of the vent pipe must be 0.5 meters above the top of the shelter. The latrine interior is kept dark so the main light source in the pit comes from the vent pipe. Flies are attracted to the light, but the pipe has a fly-proof screen at the top, so they cannot escape and eventually die.[5] Many countries consider the ventilated improved pit latrine to be the minimum standard for improved sanitation. (*Used with permission from Jason Rosenfeld, MPH.*)

TYPHOID FEVER

Typhoid fever, also known as enteric fever, is an acute systemic illness caused by the invasive bacterial pathogen, *Salmonella typhi*. *Salmonella* is ingested in contaminated water or food, invades the mucosal surface of the small intestine, and causes bacteremia, with seeding of the liver, spleen, and lymph nodes.

EPIDEMIOLOGY

Typhoid fever is mainly found in countries with poor sanitary conditions. Because most such countries do not routinely confirm the diagnosis with blood cultures, the disease is highly underreported. Outbreaks of typhoid are often seen in the rainy season, and in areas where human fecal material washes into sources of drinking water. Shallow water tables and improperly placed latrines are environmental risk factors for typhoid. Globally there are 16 to 33 million cases annually, with up to a half a million deaths every year.[7]

CLINICAL PRESENTATION

Patients develop an acute systemic illness with prolonged fever, malaise, and abdominal pain after ingesting contaminated food or water. This truly nonspecific syndrome may include headache, mild cough, and constipation, with nausea and vomiting. Diarrhea may be present but it is not the rule. After a 10- to 20-day incubation period, there is a stepwise progression of fever over a period of 3 weeks, and the patient may display a transient rash described as rose spots (2- to 4-mm pink macules on the torso, which fade on pressure). Temperature pulse dissociation with relative bradycardia despite high fever may be noted in fewer than 25 percent of patients. In the second week, the patient becomes more toxic and may develop hepatosplenomegaly. Untreated, typhoid can progress to include delirium, neurologic complications and intestinal perforation caused by a proliferation of *Salmonella* in the Peyer patches (lymphoid tissue) of the intestinal mucosa. Although the mortality rate for untreated typhoid is 20 percent, early antibiotic therapy can decrease mortality. Approximately 1 percent to 4 percent of those who recover from acute typhoid fever become carriers of the disease who continue to shed *Salmonella* in their stool despite not being ill.[7]

DIAGNOSIS

Culture of blood, stool, rectal swab, or bone marrow.[8]

DIFFERENTIAL DIAGNOSIS[9]

- Malaria (often clinically indistinguishable from typhoid; empiric therapy for both malaria and typhoid may be warranted if diagnostic testing is unavailable).
- Enteroinvasive *E. coli*.
- *Campylobacter*.
- Paratyphoid fever (*Salmonella para typhi*, other less virulent *Salmonellae*).
- Dengue fever (mosquito borne arbovirus infection spread by *Aedes aegypti*).
- Rickettsial diseases (typhus, spotted fever, Q fever).
- Brucellosis.
- Leptospirosis.
- Heat stroke.

MANAGEMENT

Prompt diagnosis and initiation of antibiotic therapy is essential and life-saving. Oral rehydration therapy should be initiated first, followed by IV fluids if vomiting cannot be controlled and for patients with altered mental status or hypovolemic shock. Antibiotic resistance patterns differ with geographic location.

For Africa and resource-limited settings in the Americas, the first choice is chloramphenicol or ciprofloxacin. Historically, trimethoprim-sulfamethoxazole has been used,[8] but there has been increasing drug resistance to sulfa in these areas. In Asia, where multidrug resistant *S. typhi* strains are well described, ciprofloxacin, ceftriaxone, or azithromycin may be used for 7 to 14 days.[8–10] Azithromycin should only be used in mild disease. Some guidelines advocate the use of dexamethasone, 3 mg/kg IV followed by 1 mg/kg every 6 hours for 2 days in the setting of shock or altered mental status.[8] See vaccine information at the end of this chapter.

CHOLERA

Cholera is an acute, diarrheal disease caused by *Vibrio cholerae*. It is usually transmitted by contaminated water or food, and is associated with pandemics in countries that lack public health infrastructure and resources for sanitation. Although the infection is often mild or asymptomatic, in 5 to 10 percent of patients it can be severe and life-threatening.[14]

EPIDEMIOLOGY

V. cholerae reservoirs occur in brackish and salt water as well as estuaries. Although the organism occurs in association with copepods and zooplankton, its largest reservoir is in humans. Cholera pandemics have been reported in south Asia, Africa, and Latin America. Characteristically, cholera outbreaks occur in countries that have suffered destruction of public health infrastructure (collapse of water supplies, sanitation, and garbage collection systems). The 2010 outbreak in postearthquake Haiti has been traced to UN peace-keeping soldiers, whose waste contaminated a major Haitian river used for bathing, irrigation, and drinking water. In just 10 months, 300,000 cases were reported, of whom 4500 died, and the outbreak has continued to wax and wane with the rainy seasons for years.[11] A large infective dose is necessary for infection, and although only approximately 10 percent of those infected fall ill, the infection can be fatal for young children, elderly, and malnourished individuals.

PATHOPHYSIOLOGY

V. cholerae is a motile, gram-negative rod. After ingestion via contaminated water or food, it must survive the acid environment of the stomach before colonizing the mucosal surface of the small intestine. The organism is noninvasive and not associated with bloody diarrhea. Rather, it makes a potent toxin causing massive secretion of electrolyte-rich fluid into the gut lumen. Human to human contact spread virtually never occurs. Transmission through contaminated food or water is the rule.[12]

Clinical presentation ranges from mild watery diarrhea to acute, fulminant watery diarrhea which looks like rice water. After an incubation period of 18 to 40 hours, patients may lose up to 30 L of fluid daily, with resulting metabolic acidosis and electrolyte disturbances. Severe dehydration can lead to death in a matter of hours. Vomiting, when present, starts after the onset of diarrhea. Profoundly dehydrated patients present with decreased skin turgor, sunken eyes, and lethargy. Children, but not adults, may have mild fever. Cramping caused by loss of calcium and potassium is common.[12]

DIFFERENTIAL DIAGNOSIS AND LABORATORY TESTS

Early presentation may resemble enterotoxigenic *E. coli*; however, the syndrome is quickly distinguishable because of the extreme volume of "rice water" secretory diarrhea that is the result of cholera toxin. *V. cholerae* may be confirmed by stool culture, polymerase chain reaction (PCR) for toxin genes, or dark-field microscopy with specific antisera, which immobilizes the *V. cholerae*.[13] The Centers for Disease Control and Prevention (CDC) recommends confirmation of cholera by stool specimen culture or rectal swab. For transport, Cary Blair media is used, and for identification, thiosulfate-citrate-bile-salts (TCBS) agar is recommended.[14]

MANAGEMENT

Water, sanitation, and hygiene education is essential, as is education about recognizing the symptoms and immediately seeking medical attention while initiating oral rehydration. Optimally, rehydration should commence with reconstitution of WHO-distributed oral rehydration salts (ORS), which is available in all but the most remote areas of the world. Hydration is the mainstay of therapy, and replacement of fluids should be calibrated to match losses. ORS should be prepared with previously boiled water and consumed within 24 hours of reconstitution. IV or intraosseous hydration with Ringer lactate solution should be initiated if the patient is vomiting or in danger of hypovolemic shock. The volume needed to rehydrate a cholera patient is often underestimated; for this reason, collection and

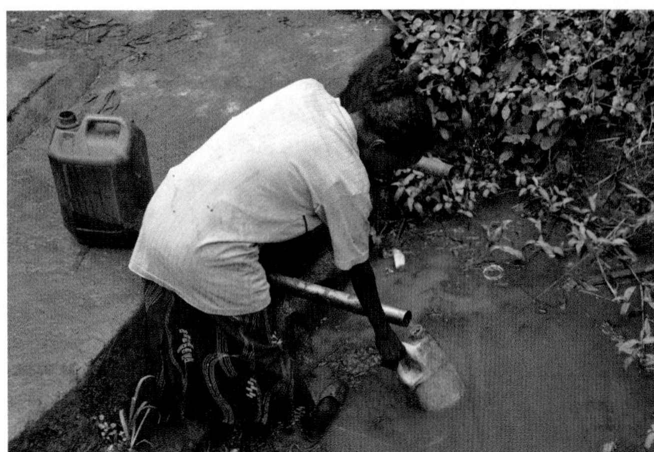

FIGURE 7-4 In this Ethiopian community without running water, water is collected in Jerry cans. Thousands of women carry these heavy, filled cans for miles after filling them up from this single pipe. The local town has provided one single pipe as the water source for the community. Although there is muddy water below, the water coming from the pipe appears clear, although it is likely to harbor bacteria and parasites. *(Used with permission from Richard P. Usatine, MD.)*

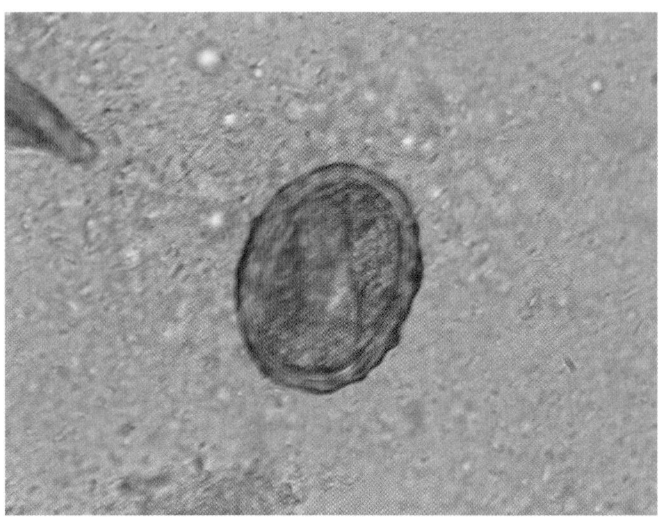

FIGURE 7-5 *Ascaris* egg found in the stool of a child with intestinal parasites. In most developing countries *Ascaris* is treated empirically with albendazole; stool studies are not always available or may not be cost effective. *(Used with permission from Richard P. Usatine, MD.)*

measurement of the watery stool in a bucket placed under the cholera cot is recommended.

Antibiotics are recommended for severe cases of cholera; options include doxycycline, azithromycin, ciprofloxacin, and furazolidone.[15]

PREVENTION OF DISEASES SECONDARY TO CONTAMINATED WATER

Drinking purified or treated water, good handwashing practices, and avoidance of contaminated food are essential. Travellers should be reminded not to brush their teeth with tap water and to avoid having potentially contaminated ice added to their beverages. Carbonated beverages are safe as the carbonation process is bactericidal. Community education about handwashing and treatment of water is essential. In communities lacking running water (**Figure 7-4**), home storage of drinking water should be in containers with protective lids. Local guidelines regarding addition of chlorine to home stored water containers should be followed.

INTESTINAL PARASITES

EPIDEMIOLOGY AND GEOGRAPHIC DISTRIBUTION

1/3 of the world's population is infected with intestinal parasites, and although many parasitic infections are asymptomatic, some have serious health consequences. Especially affected are pregnant women and children, for whom hookworm-associated anemia results in maternal mortality, low-birth-weight babies, growth stunting, and impaired learning. The CDC recommends predeparture albendazole treatment as a single 600-mg dose for all refugees from sub-Saharan Africa and South Asia. While this treatment will eradicate most of the nematodes, it is insufficient for *Strongyloides stercoralis* and schistosomiasis.[16]

CLINICAL PRESENTATION

Abdominal pain, cramps, bloating, anorexia, anemia, fatigue, growth stunting of children, and hepatomegaly (schistosomiasis).

DIAGNOSIS

Stool for ova and parasite studies (**Figure 7-5**). Note that these will not reliably detect *Strongyloides* or schistosomiasis; serologic testing is available for the latter. Eosinophilia is an important diagnostic clue for the presence of parasites; the finding of persistent eosinophilia warrants a careful diagnostic evaluation for parasitic infection.

TREATMENT

▶ Older Children and Adults

Albendazole 400 mg orally as single dose will eradicate hookworm, and *Ascaris*, but not *Trichuris* in most people.[17] Eradication of *Trichuris trichiura* requires 3 daily doses of albendazole or adding ivermectin to mebendazole.[18]

▶ Children 12 months to 2 years

Albendazole 200 mg orally as a single dose is recommended by the WHO.[19] *S. stercoralis* requires 7 days of albendazole at 400 mg twice daily. For schistosomiasis, praziquantel is effective against all species of schistosomes. Give 2 doses of 20 mg/kg PO 4 to 6 hours apart (3 doses 4 hours apart for *Schistosoma japonicum*).[20]

PREVENTION

Preventative measures include proper management of human waste, handwashing after defecation and before cooking, and wearing shoes (prevents hookworm and *Strongyloides*). WHO guidelines recommend mass treatment of school children in endemic areas with single-dose albendazole therapy once every 6 months.

MALNUTRITION

Types of malnutrition include:

- Kwashiorkor
- Marasmus
- Micronutrient deficiencies

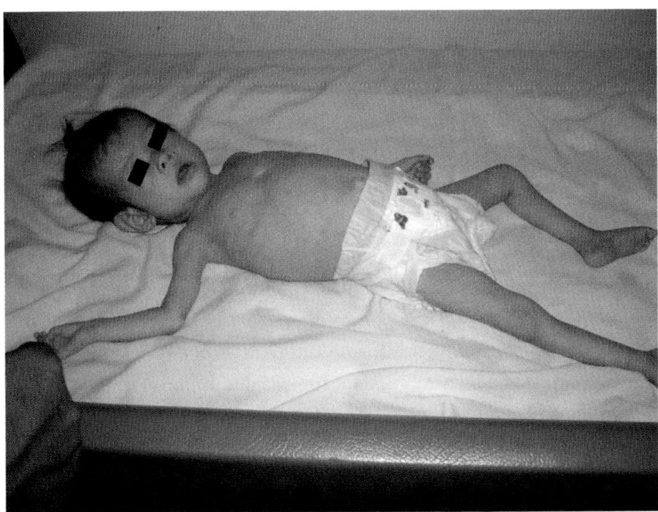

FIGURE 7-6 This 12 month-old Bolivian child with marasmus presented to medical attention with pneumonia. She has severe growth stunting, atrophied limbs, and looks miserable. Her presentation highlights the association between malnutrition and infection. (*Used with permission from Carolina Clark.*)

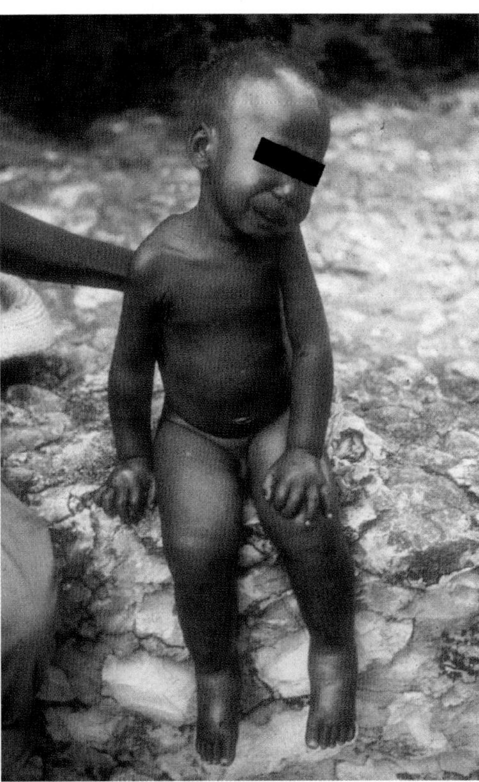

FIGURE 7-7 This 2-year-old child presented with classic signs and symptoms of kwashiorkor, a severe form of protein-energy malnutrition. The word *kwashiorkor*, from a Ghanaian language, refers to the sickness a child develops when it is weaned from breastfeeding. In countries with limited protein sources, newly weaned children are especially vulnerable to this disease. They present with depigmentation, red discoloration of the hair, distended abdomens, and peripheral edema. (*Used with permission from Ruth Berggren, MD.*)

A global shift is underway, from diseases of undernutrition to overnutrition in tandem with industrialization and advances in transportation and technology. In spite of this global shift, about a quarter of the world's preschool children demonstrate growth stunting caused by nutritional deficiencies. In resource-poor countries, adult obesity and childhood undernutrition may coexist within the same families. The causes of this seeming paradox include many factors associated with poverty: the vulnerability of preschool children to infection when sanitation is inadequate, lack of nutrition education, decreased physical activity with increasing availability of technology and transportation, and mass marketing of inexpensive, calorie-rich foods.

Two classic presentations of malnutrition in children are important to recognize because they signal a patient who is immunocompromised and vulnerable not only to infection but also to preventable developmental delay. The accompanying photographs show an emaciated child with marasmus (severe, nonedematous malnutrition caused by calorie deprivation; **Figure 7-6**), and a puffy child with kwashiorkor (severe, edematous protein energy malnutrition; **Figure 7-7**). Marasmic kwashiorkor is another descriptor, illustrating the high level of overlap in the etiology and presentation of these extreme forms of malnutrition.[21] Whenever possible, one should avoid hospitalizing these children for nutritional rehabilitation as hospitalization will expose them to many infectious pathogens that could be lethal during their vulnerable period of "nutritional AIDS."[22]

DIAGNOSIS

Growth chart monitoring is important for earliest detection of weight loss, growth stunting, or failure to gain height and weight over time. In most resource-poor countries, growth monitoring is implemented by trained community health workers, who refer mothers for nutrition and education programs upon detecting faltering growth in children younger than the age of 5 years. Children often fail to gain weight normally after an episode of infectious diarrhea or malaria; this should be followed by a period of rapid catchup growth. If a child becomes reinfected before catchup growth is complete, the child will fall further behind on the growth curve.

Depending on the relative protein content of the diet, patients develop marasmus (calorie deprivation), characterized by emaciation and listlessness (**Figure 7-6**), or kwashiorkor, "the disease of weaning"—protein-energy malnutrition. Kwashiorkor is characterized by red discoloration of the hair (**Figure 7-8**), which is also brittle, puffy eyes, bloated bellies, and pitting edema of the extremities (**Figure 7-7**). These children feel miserable and are lethargic and uninterested in food. The differential diagnosis of kwashiorkor includes nephrotic syndrome, renal failure, or right-side congestive heart failure.

PATHOPHYSIOLOGY

Childhood malnutrition, and especially kwashiorkor, may begin when a breastfeeding mother weans her child from the breast. Deprived of protective maternal antibodies and protein source, weaning infants begin sampling their contaminated environments and ingesting pathogens. Production of cytokines such as tumor necrosis factor (TNF)-α during infectious episodes suppresses appetite and impedes nutritional recovery.[22]

Micronutrient deficiencies coexist,[21] and deficiencies of vitamin A and zinc, in particular, predispose children to increased morbidity from subsequent infections. When parents are unable to replace

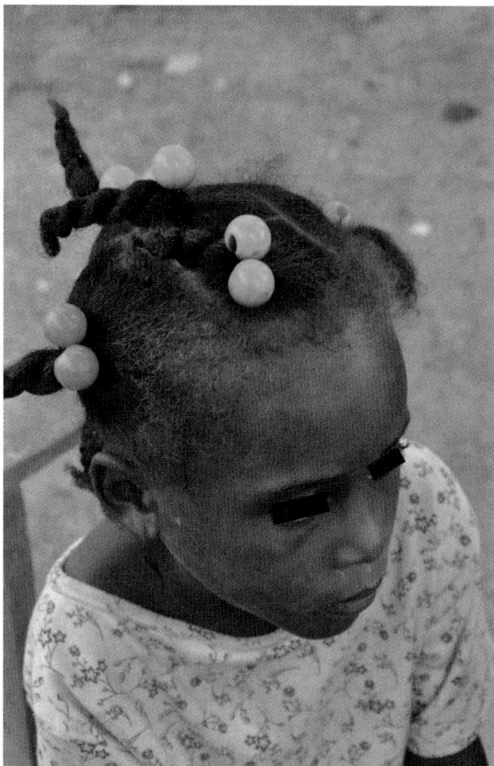

FIGURE 7-8 Child with kwashiorkor, protein-calorie malnutrition and red hair. The red hair is a result of the kwashiorkor. (*Used with permission from Richard P. Usatine, MD.*)

protein requirements of weaning infants, children eat whatever locally available calorie sources (grains, cereals, bread, fruit) they can find. The poor in many developing countries lack protein sources and toddlers are frequently not prioritized when meat, milk, or eggs become available.

As a result of severe protein deficiency, hypoalbuminemia and decreased intravascular oncotic pressure lead to edema, and the classic puffy appearance of the child with kwashiorkor. For years, it was believed that children with kwashiorkor are disproportionately deprived of protein, whereas children with marasmus are deprived of both protein and carbohydrate calories proportionally; it now appears there is a great deal of overlap between these two presentations of severe malnutrition.[21]

MANAGEMENT

The endless cycle of infection leading to poor appetite and weight loss leading to malnutrition and further risk of infection[22] can be difficult to break unless mothers of malnourished children are taught to introduce calorie-dense weaning food supplements and snacks. Many countries have locally produced ready-to-use therapeutic foods (RUTF),[21] offering products like Plumpy'nut, or Haiti's Nourimanba, made from peanut butter, milk powder, vegetable oil, sugar, and a vitamin mix.[23]

These therapeutic foods are a useful adjunct to breaking the cycle of infection, anorexia, weight loss and malnutrition, but they are not a substitute for educating mothers about how to rehabilitate their malnourished child using locally available and affordable foods. Nonmeat protein substitutes, such as red beans, and locally available green leafy vegetables are easier for mothers to obtain than meat, cow's milk, or expensive imported food supplements.

MICRONUTRIENT DEFICIENCIES

VITAMIN A DEFICIENCY

In contrast to marasmus and kwashiorkor, growth stunting is a more subtle syndrome affecting 200 million children who are younger than the age of 5 years. A variety of micronutrient deficiencies are believed to contribute to stunting syndrome and to accompany developmental delays, reduced cognitive function, impaired immunity, and future risk of obesity and hypertension.[24] There are 4 micronutrient deficiencies of global importance, each with associated clinical syndromes that should be recognized. All can be associated with growth stunting in children, who may present with abnormally short stature but relatively normal weight for height.

Vitamin A is a critical regulator of immune function, which is required for maintaining the integrity of mucosal surfaces. Vitamin A supplementation in countries with malnutrition reduces blindness (from xerophthalmia) as well as the morbidity of infectious diseases (especially measles, diarrhea, and respiratory infections). **Figure 7-9** shows a photograph of blindness caused by vitamin A deficiency. In 2009, the WHO estimated that clinical vitamin A deficiency (night blindness) and biochemical vitamin A deficiency (serum retinol concentration <0.70 μmol/L) affected 5.2 and 190 million preschool-age children, respectively.[26] About 250,000 children develop blindness caused by vitamin A deficiency every year, and half of these die within 12 months of losing sight.[27]

▶ Clinical presentation

The earliest presentation of vitamin A deficiency is poor night vision, which may progress to night blindness, xerophthalmia, ulceration, and scarring of the cornea, with ultimate blindness. Vitamin A deficiency is also associated with anemia, and is particularly dangerous in patients with measles, for whom mortality rates are high.

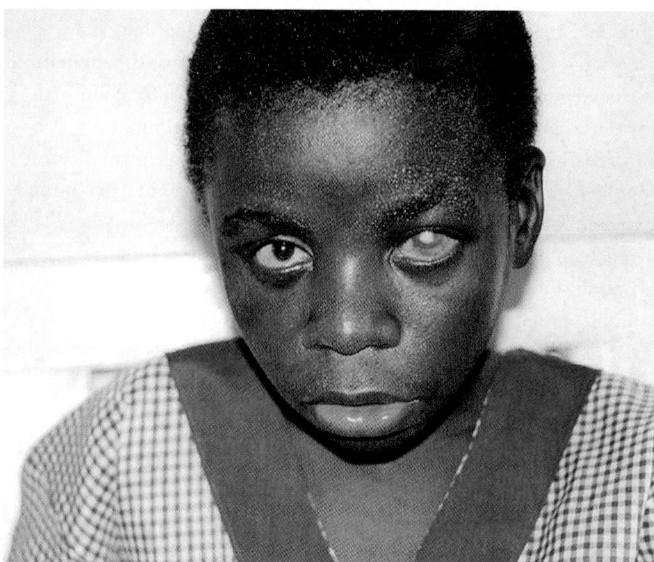

FIGURE 7-9 Child with severe xerophthalmia of the left eye secondary to vitamin A deficiency.[25] (*Used with permission from SIGHT AND LIFE www.sightandlife.org.*)

▶ Management

A metaanalysis of 43 trials involving 216,000 children younger than the age of 5 years who were given vitamin A supplements revealed striking reductions in mortality and morbidity. Seventeen of these trials reported a 24 percent reduction in mortality, and 7 trials reported a 28 percent reduction in mortality associated with diarrhea. Vitamin A reduced diarrhea and measles incidence. Vitamin A significantly reduces morbidity, mortality, and eye disease. Vitamin A supplements are recommended to all children who are at risk in low- and middle-income countries.[28] Most countries implement WHO guidelines for vitamin A supplementation synchronized with childhood vaccine schedules.

ZINC DEFICIENCY

Zinc plays a central role in cellular growth, differentiation, and metabolism. It is necessary for physical growth, GI, and immune function. Many zinc studies show improved growth of children and decreased infections when supplements are given to vulnerable populations. Studies suggest that the global prevalence of zinc deficiency approaches 31 percent, especially in Africa, the eastern Mediterranean, and South Asia.[29]

▶ Clinical presentation

The most common presentation of zinc deficiency is nonspecific and may include growth stunting, delayed sexual maturation, dermatitis, and defective immunity. Zinc deficiency is associated with decreased macrophage chemotaxis, decreased neutrophil activity, and decreased T-cell responses.[22] It is widely acknowledged that zinc deficiency contributes significantly to child mortality from pneumonia, diarrhea, and malaria. A rare but characteristic presentation of profound zinc deficiency is acrodermatitis enteropathica (**Figure 7-10**).

▶ Diagnosis

Because there is no good biomarker for zinc deficiency, diagnosis must rest on clinical suspicion and documentation of therapeutic response to supplementation.

▶ Management

WHO guidelines for diarrhea recommend use of low concentration ORS together with routine zinc supplementation for 10 to 14 days. Children older than age 6 months should get 20 mg daily; infants younger than age 6 months should get 10 mg daily.[30] Zinc supplementation decreases the duration and volume of diarrheal stools by 25 percent and 30 percent, respectively. More importantly, 14 days of zinc supplementation for a diarrheal episode reduces the incidence of diarrhea and pneumonia in the subsequent 2 to 3 months, reduces hospital admissions for diarrhea, and brings approximately a 50 percent reduction in noninjury deaths in the year following the treatment.[31] Unfortunately, zinc supplementation benefits are still not widely known by health care workers in developing countries.[32]

IRON

Iron deficiency is the most common micronutrient deficiency in the world, and 2 billion people (nearly 1/3 of the global population) are anemic. In resource-limited countries, iron-deficiency anemia is

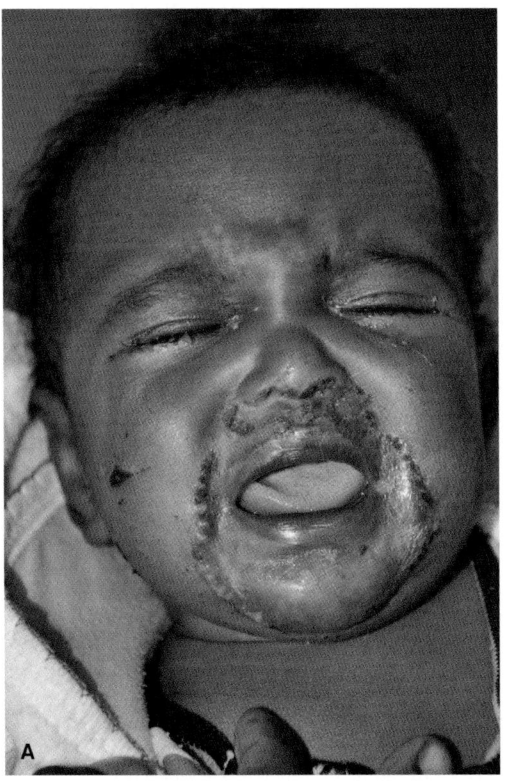

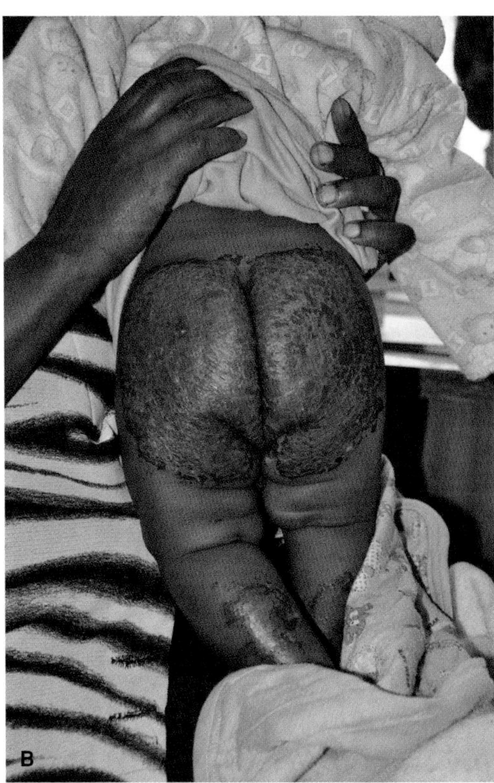

FIGURE 7-10 Acrodermatitis enteropathica caused by a zinc deficiency. Zinc supplementation is a standard recommendation from WHO in treatment of childhood diarrhea. Even children who do not have skin findings of zinc deficiency benefit with reduced duration of diarrhea and reduced mortality from all infectious causes in the ensuing months after receiving supplementation. Note the typical lesions around the **(A)** mouth and **(B)** buttocks. (*Used with permission from Richard P. Usatine, MD.*)

either caused or aggravated by malaria, intestinal parasites such as hookworm, and other chronic infections such as HIV, tuberculosis, or schistosomiasis. Iron deficiency causes enormous morbidity and contributes to 20 percent of global maternal mortality. Because the consequences include impaired cognition and physical development, increased risk of illness in children and reduced work productivity, iron deficiency is a real barrier to economic development in resource-poor countries.[33] As with zinc and vitamin A, iron deficiency can be detrimental to host immunity, causing decreased neutrophil chemotaxis.[22]

▶ Interventions

The WHO has developed a three-pronged strategy for addressing global iron deficiency: increasing iron uptake through dietary diversification and supplementation, improvement of nutritional status, and controlling infections, especially worms. In countries with significant iron-deficiency anemia, malaria, and helminth infections, these interventions can restore individual health as well as raise national productivity levels, thereby interrupting the cycle of poverty and disease.[33]

IODINE

Insufficient dietary iodine can significantly lower the IQ of whole populations and is the leading preventable cause of brain damage. Although iodine deficiency is easily solved through food fortification costing 2 cents per person annually, prevalences of 60 percent to 90 percent iodine deficiency among school-age children are observed in multiple African, Asian, and eastern Mediterranean countries. There is tremendous variance of iodine deficiency within individual countries and deficiency is not linked to poor or disadvantaged districts.[34] Iodine deficiency occurs where the soil has low iodine content because of past glaciation or repeated leaching effects of precipitation. Food crops grown in iodine-deficient soil provide inadequate dietary iodine.[35]

▶ Clinical presentation

Because iodine is required for thyroid hormone synthesis, iodine deficiency results in hypothyroidism and goiter (**Figure 7-11**). Congenital iodine deficiency results in a form of profound cognitive impairment known as *cretinism*. Other consequences include stillbirths, deaf mutism, subclinical hyper- or hypothyroidism, impaired mental function, and retarded physical development.[35]

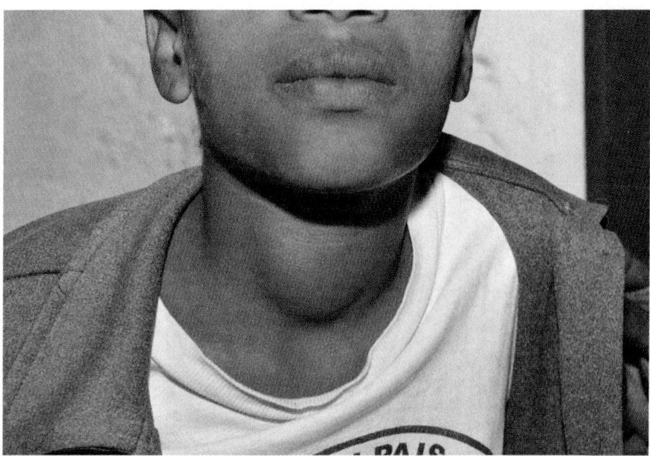

FIGURE 7-11 A goiter caused by iodine deficiency in this teen from a country in Africa where iodine is not routinely supplemented in the diet and goiter is endemic. (*Used with permission from Richard P. Usatine, MD.*)

▶ Interventions

Iodine may be supplied in tablets or liquid form and taken daily; in adults, 150 μg/day is sufficient for thyroid function and an adult multivitamin typically contains 150 μg of iodine per tablet, but this is impractical. Population-based interventions should include iodization of salt, and in some developing countries, eradication of iodine deficiency has been accomplished by adding iodine drops to well water.

VECTOR BORNE DISEASES

MALARIA

Malaria is a protozoan infection spread by the *Anopheles* mosquito vector in endemic areas. Of the four species of malaria (*Plasmodium falciparum*, *Plasmodium ovale*, *Plasmodium malariae*, and *Plasmodium vivax*), *P. falciparum* is the most important to address, because if unrecognized and untreated, it can be rapidly fatal. Only *P. falciparum* exhibits high levels of parasitemia in blood, and it is the only type of malaria that causes sequestration of parasitized erythrocytes in microvasculature. This unique feature of *P. falciparum* is responsible for the severe end-organ damage, including renal failure, acute respiratory distress syndrome, and coma that is seen with untreated disease.[36]

▶ Epidemiology and geographic distribution

There are more than 200 million cases of malaria in the world every year. According to the WHO, up to 1 million people worldwide die annually from malaria, with 89 percent of these deaths occurring in Africa. Most of the deaths caused by malaria occur in children younger than age 5 years. *P. falciparum*, *P. vivax*, *P. malariae*, and *P. ovale* are globally distributed in the tropics. *P. vivax* is more common in Asia, South America, Oceania, and India. *P. ovale* is found mainly in West Africa, and *P. malariae* is much less common than *P. vivax* or *P. falciparum*.

The risk for malaria varies greatly within a given country, and depends on altitude (higher altitudes have lower risk), season (greatest risk in rainy season), and urbanization (rural areas have greater risk than urban areas). Thus, travelers should be aware of these differences and plan for prophylaxis accordingly.

The CDC publication, *Health Information for International Travel*, is available online at http://www.cdc.gov/travel/ and should be consulted for updates about regional patterns of malaria risk, as well as drug resistance and guidelines, which are subject to frequent changes.[37]

▶ Clinical presentation

After a 1- to 3-week incubation period following the bite of an infected female mosquito, patients develop a nonspecific syndrome of high fever, headache, myalgia, and shaking chills. This syndrome is frequently accompanied by nausea, vomiting, and back pain, and occasional diarrhea. Splenomegaly and anemia (related to hemolysis) are common in all four types of malaria.

As untreated *P. falciparum* progresses, there is a risk of cerebral malaria, which is caused by parasitized erythrocytes sequestered in the capillaries of the brain, with secondary metabolic consequences. Cerebral malaria is characterized by severe headache and altered

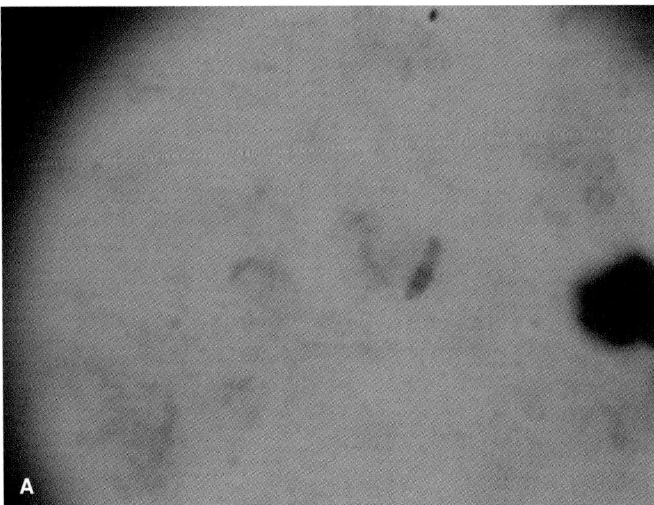

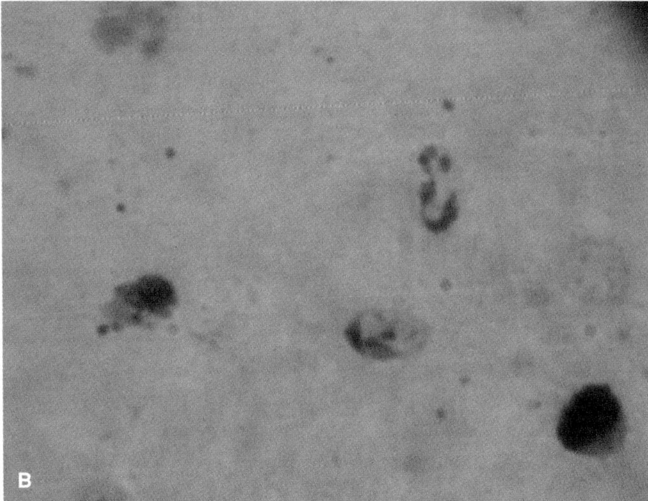

FIGURE 7-12 **A.** *Plasmodium falciparum* with a banana-shaped gametocyte. Of all the species of malaria, *P. falciparum* is the most likely to cause severe morbidity and mortality. **B.** *Plasmodium falciparum* with chromatin in rings. (*Used with permission from Richard P. Usatine, MD.*)

consciousness. These patients may also develop acute respiratory distress syndrome (ARDS), hypoglycemia, acidosis, and shock in the setting of hyperparasitemia. Untreated patients with cerebral malaria ultimately progress to coma, respiratory failure, and death.[38]

▶ Differential diagnosis

The initial presentation of malaria is so nonspecific that it mimics influenza (without the respiratory symptoms), enteric fever (see section on typhoid), dengue fever, rickettsial infections, brucellosis, and leishmaniasis. If hemolysis has been extensive, the patient may present with jaundice, and viral hepatitis or leptospirosis may also be on the differential diagnosis.[36]

▶ Laboratory diagnosis

Malaria is usually diagnosed by light microscopy of peripheral blood smears prepared with a Giemsa, Field, or modified Wright stain (**Figures 7-12** and **7-13**). A thick-and-thin smear should be obtained whenever possible in every febrile patient in whom malaria is suspected, especially from febrile travelers returning from malaria endemic areas. Thin smears allow relative quantification and speciation of parasites when the parasitemia is high; thick smears are useful to rule in malaria, especially when parasitemia is low. Because a single negative smear does not rule out malaria, the test must be repeated on at least three occasions at 12- to 24-hour intervals.[39] Patients with high levels of parasitemia (>5%) have a worse prognosis and should be considered for inpatient care.

Other diagnostic modalities include the fluorochrome acridine orange stain for fluorescence microscopy and PCR (not yet widely available but helpful for very low levels of parasitemia). Rapid antigen assays using fingerstick blood samples on cards impregnated with specific antibodies are alternative methods for laboratory diagnosis of malaria. In the US, the US Food and Drug Administration has approved the BinaxNOW Malaria test, which, although costly, is convenient for rapid field use. Unfortunately, this and other immunochromatographic strip assays are not able to determine parasite load.[37]

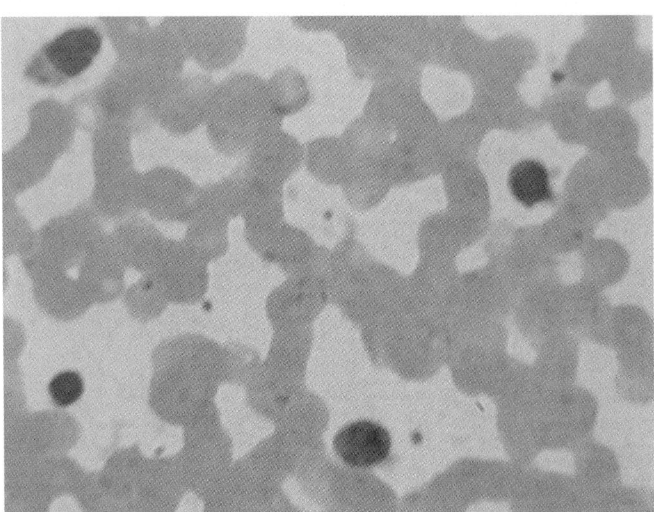

FIGURE 7-13 Blood smear for malaria diagnosis showing *Plasmodium vivax*. Rapid field tests are now available but still more expensive than microscopy. (*Used with permission from Richard P. Usatine, MD.*)

▶ Treatment

Many cases of malaria can be treated effectively with oral medication and parenteral therapy is reserved for severe disease or for patients who are vomiting. Before prescribing therapy, determine which species is most likely involved based on microscopy or rapid diagnostic test; consider the geographic area and local drug resistance patterns.

After the patient has been given the first dose of medication, the patient should be observed for an hour. Vomiting can be managed with metoclopramide, 10 mg orally, and if the vomiting occurs within 30 minutes, the full initial dose can be repeated. The WHO recommends artemisinin-based combination treatments as first-line for uncomplicated *P. falciparum*: artemether-lumefantrine 1 dose at hours 1, 8, 24, 36, 48, and 60 based on body weight: 5 to 14 kg: 1 tablet per dose; 15 to 24 kg: 2 tablets per dose; 25 to 34 kg: 3 tablets per dose; >34 kg: 4 tablets per dose.

Other artemisinin combinations can be used as follows: artesunate plus amodiaquine, artesunate plus mefloquine, and artesunate plus sulfadoxine-pyrimethamine. The combination of choice depends on the level of resistance of the partner medication in a given region. Artemisinin and derivatives should not be given as monotherapy.

For US-returning travelers, the choice of malaria chemotherapy is based on the infecting species, possible drug resistance, and severity of disease. Options for therapy include atovaquone-proguanil, quinine in combination with tetracycline, artemether-lumefantrine, mefloquine, or artesunate.

Treatment of severe *P. falciparum*

All cases of severe malaria should be managed as medical emergencies. Give IV or IM artesunate, artemether, or quinine dihydrochloride (not available in the US).

In the US, give quinidine gluconate, 10 mg base/kg (up to 600 mg) in 0.9 percent saline by rate-controlled IV infusion over 1 to 2 hours, followed by a maintenance dose of 0.02 mg base/kg per minute with electrocardiogram (ECG) monitoring until patient can take oral drugs. Quinine and quinidine must never be given by IV bolus because of the potential for fatal hypotension. For patients with severe malaria in the US who do not tolerate or cannot easily access quinidine, intravenous artesunate has become available through a CDC investigational new drug protocol. Clinicians may contact the physician on call through the CDC malaria hotline (770-488-7788, Monday–Friday, 9:00 AM–5:00 PM Eastern Time; or 777-488-7100 at all other times) for additional information and release of the drug.

Patients with cerebral malaria should undergo lumbar puncture to rule out bacterial meningitis (**Figure 7-14**) and their blood glucose should be checked every 4 hours because of the significant risk of hypoglycemia in severe malaria. Careful hemodynamic monitoring and management of seizures (with intravenous benzodiazepines) are essential.

▶ Prevention

Prevention measures are a public health priority and should include mosquito control, elimination of standing water in households and gardens, insect repellant containing at least 10 percent to 50 percent diethyltoluamide (DEET; 30 percent DEET provides 6 to 8 hours of protection), and permethrin-impregnated bed nets. Since 2000, prevention and control measures have reduced malaria mortality by more than 25 percent globally and by 33 percent in Africa.[40]

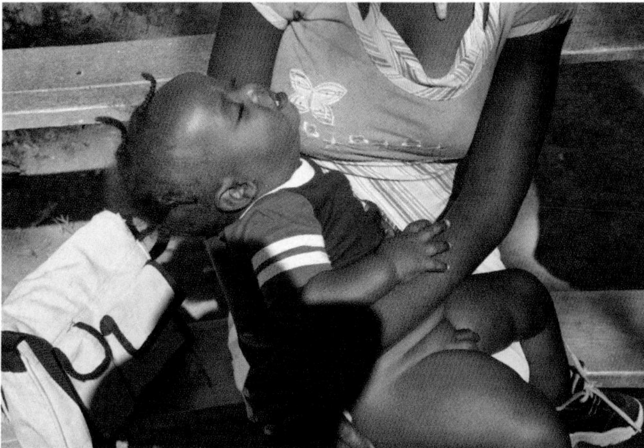

FIGURE 7-14 Meningitis in a child with a very rigid neck. Cerebral malaria should be in the differential diagnosis for this child. Most bacterial meningitis in children can now be prevented by vaccines frequently still not available in developing countries. (*Used with permission from Richard P. Usatine, MD.*)

Prevention for travelers

Choice of chemoprophylaxis depends on drug resistance patterns for *P. falciparum* in the country being visited. Generally, prophylaxis should start 1 week before arrival and should continue through 4 weeks after leaving the endemic area. In the case of atovaquone-proguanil, prophylaxis may start the day before arrival and end 7 days after departure. Drugs commonly used in prophylaxis include atovaquone-proguanil (Malarone, which is expensive in the US), mefloquine (may cause central nervous system side effects), and doxycycline (causes photosensitivity). Chloroquine can be used only in a few areas; chloroquine-susceptible malaria is restricted to the Caribbean, Central America, and parts of the Middle East.

LEISHMANIASIS

Leishmaniasis is a vector-borne disease transmitted by the sandfly. It can be divided into two major forms, a cutaneous form, which is the most common, and the visceral form. There is also a more rare mucocutaneous form that can cause significant facial disfigurement around the nose and mouth.

▶ Synonyms

Kala-azar is another name for visceral leishmaniasis.

▶ Epidemiology

- New World leishmaniasis is found in Mexico, Central America, and South America. Old World leishmaniasis is found in India, Africa, the Middle East, southern Europe, and parts of Asia.
- Most leishmaniasis diagnosed in the US occurs in travelers returning from endemic areas including military personnel who served in Iraq or Afghanistan.
- Some cutaneous leishmaniasis cases acquired in the US have been reported in Texas and Oklahoma.[41]
- Ninety percent of cutaneous leishmaniasis occurs in Afghanistan, Algeria, Iran, Saudi Arabia, Syria, Brazil, Colombia, Peru, and Bolivia.[41]
- Ninety percent of visceral leishmaniasis cases occur in parts of India, Bangladesh, Nepal, Sudan, Ethiopia, and Brazil.[41]

▶ Etiology and pathophysiology

- Leishmaniasis is caused by more than 20 species of the protozoan genus *Leishmania*.
- Leishmaniasis is transmitted to people through the bite of the sandfly.
- The intracellular amastigotes of *Leishmania* replicate within macrophages.
- The disease can also be transmitted like any bloodborne infection, but human-to-human transmission is rare.

▶ Risk factors

- Living in and traveling to endemic countries.
- Rural areas have a higher prevalence of disease in the endemic countries.
- Not protecting the skin from sandfly bites during the time from dusk to dawn.
- Blood transfusions, needle sharing in injection-drug users, needle-stick injuries, and congenital transmission also are all reported risk factors for visceral leishmaniasis.[42]

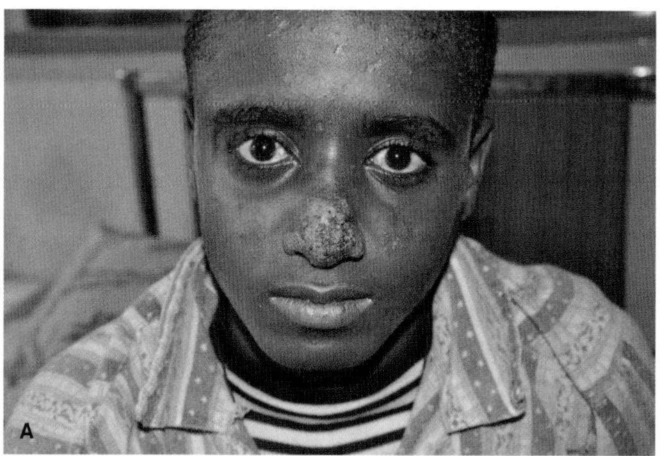
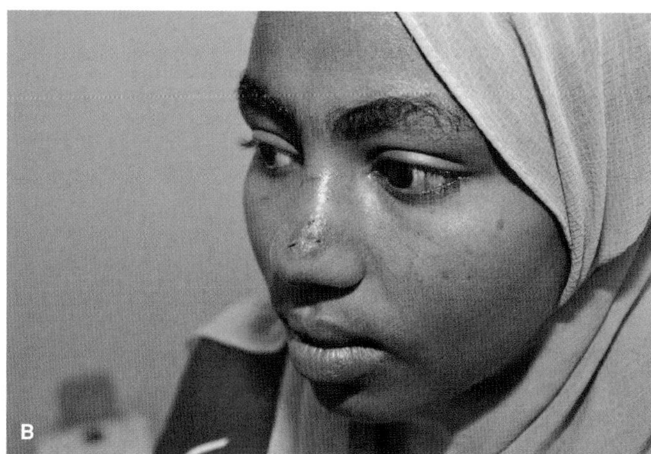

FIGURE 7-15 Examples of leishmaniasis on the face. Lesions emerge in the site of the sandfly bite; the nose is commonly affected as seen in the children in figures **A** and **B** from Africa. (*Used with permission from Richard P. Usatine, MD.*)

Diagnosis

Clinical features

- Six weeks after a sandfly bite, the cutaneous form may be localized to a single ulcer or nodule (**Figure 7-15**) or may be disseminated widely (**Figure 7-16**).
- After a 2- to 6-month incubation period, the visceral form can involve the liver, spleen, and bone marrow and causes systemic illness. The patient may present with fever, anemia, night sweats, weight loss, and an enlarged abdomen because of hepatosplenomegaly.[43]
- Mucocutaneous leishmaniasis affects the nose and mouth and may affect the nasal septum and palate (**Figure 7-17**). This form may occur months to years after what appears to be healing of cutaneous leishmaniasis.

Distribution

- A cutaneous form of leishmaniasis has a predilection for the nose and face (**Figure 7-15**).
- Cutaneous leishmaniasis is also commonly seen on the extremities. Note that the sandfly would generally have more access to bite the face and extremities where clothing is less likely to be a protective barrier.
- Disseminated cutaneous leishmaniasis can be seen from the head to the toes (**Figure 7-16**).

Laboratory testing

- Cutaneous leishmaniasis may be diagnosed by clinical appearance and a biopsy or a scraping of the ulcer. A Giemsa stain will demonstrate parasites in the skin smears taken from the edge of an active ulcer.[43] In some centers, PCR is available and is considered the method of choice.[44]
- Visceral leishmaniasis is diagnosed from a blood sample or a bone marrow biopsy. Several serologic agglutination tests (direct agglutination test [DAT] or fluorescent allergosorbent test [FAST]) are highly sensitive for detection of leishmania antibodies. Culture of a bone marrow aspirate or PCR improve diagnostic yield.[43]

Differential diagnosis

- The differential diagnosis of cutaneous leishmaniasis includes leprosy, sarcoidosis, pyoderma gangrenosum, primary syphilis, and venous stasis ulcers.
- The differential diagnosis of visceral leishmaniasis includes malaria, typhoid fever, and lymphoma.

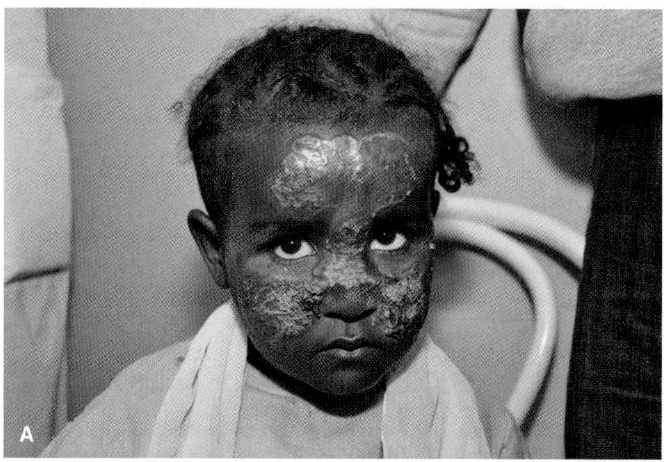
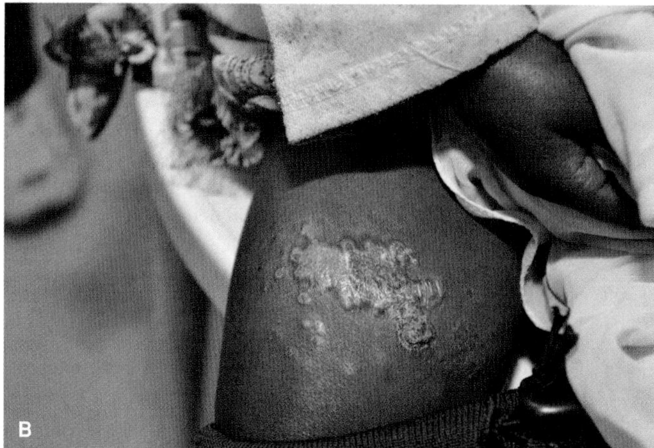

FIGURE 7-16 Widespread leishmaniasis in a young African girl with involvement from the face and trunk. The multiple nodules on the face could be lepromatous leprosy or lupus but by skin snip testing, the diagnosis of leishmaniasis was confirmed. Figures **A** shows a type of leishmaniasis that is called lupoid leishmania. (*Used with permission from Richard P. Usatine, MD.*)

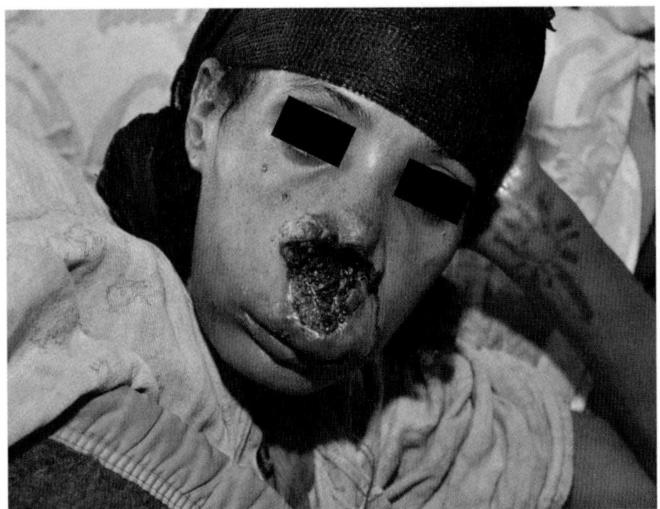

FIGURE 7-17 Severe mucocutaneous leishmaniasis causing destruction of the nose. (*Used with permission from Richard P. Usatine, MD.*)

▶ Management

Nonpharmacologic

- Wound care for ulcers.

Medications

- The main drugs used to treat leishmaniasis include sodium stibogluconate (available from the CDC) and meglumine antimonate.[45,46] Other medications used include miltefosine (the only oral drug for leishmaniasis) fluconazole and liposomal amphotericin b (this is the only drug with FDA approval for visceral leishmaniasis in the US).[45,46] Amphotericin b is the standard of care in India because of antimonial resistance.[44]

Surgery

- Plastic surgery may be used to treat the disfigurement of mucocutaneous or cutaneous leishmaniasis.

PREVENTION OF VECTOR-BORNE DISEASES

Prevention is a public health priority that must include vector (mosquito and sandfly) control, elimination of standing water in households and gardens, insect repellant containing 20 percent to 30 percent DEET, and permethrin-coated bednets. Sandflies and *Anopheles* mosquitoes bite from dusk to dawn, but the *Aedes aegypti* vector of dengue fever bites any time during the day, making daytime use of mosquito repellant especially important in dengue-endemic areas.

PROGNOSIS

- Cutaneous leishmaniasis does resolve spontaneously in some cases and in other cases it may persist and resist treatments. The prognosis is related to the severity of the case and the community of the host. Even in those cases that resolve scarring is frequent.
- Visceral leishmaniasis is fatal if not diagnosed and treated.

EYES—TRACHOMA

EPIDEMIOLOGY AND GEOGRAPHIC DISTRIBUTION

Chlamydia trachomatis is the leading infectious cause of blindness, accounting for 3 percent of the world's blindness. Globally, 21.4 million people have trachoma, and of these, 1.2 million are blind.[47] Trachoma is associated with poor sanitation, inadequate water supply, and lack of personal hygiene. It is transmitted from person to person via unwashed fingers, flies, and close family contact (sharing of face towels and bedclothes). Trachoma is endemic in Africa (especially in the driest regions) India, South Asia, Australia, and parts of South America.

CLINICAL PRESENTATION

Patients experience inflammation of the eye with watery discharge, itching, burning, and blurry vision. Examination of the tarsal conjunctiva reveals follicles (round swellings that are paler than the surrounding conjunctiva, at least 0.5 mm in diameter). With progression, intense trachomatous inflammation develops, producing inflammatory thickening of the tarsal conjunctiva, which appears red and thickened with numerous follicles (**Figure 7-18**).

Eventually, trachoma causes scarring, with white lines or bands in the tarsal conjunctiva as well as trichiasis, in which eyelashes turn inward and begin to rub against the cornea, and entropion, or inward turning of the eyelid itself. With time, this chronic rubbing causes corneal opacity and blindness (**Figure 7-19**).

DIAGNOSIS

Although laboratory diagnostic testing is available for staining *C. trachomatis* in scrapings from the tarsal plate, most settings where trachoma is endemic do not offer this resource, and visual inspection of the everted upper eyelid must suffice. Each eye should be examined for trichiasis and corneal opacities. The upper eyelid is everted by asking the patient to look down, holding eyelashes between thumb and finger, and everting the lid using a cotton-tipped applicator. The everted lid is then checked for follicles, inflammation, and scarring.

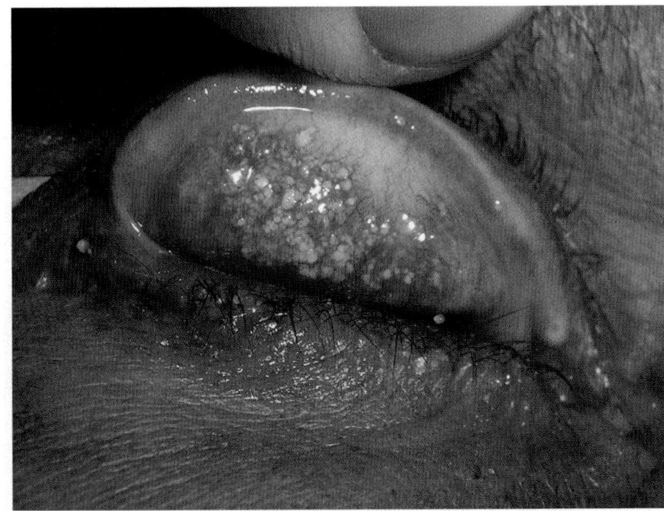

FIGURE 7-18 Trachoma causing prominent follicles on the upper eyelid in a person infected with *C. trachomatis*. Note how flipping the eyelid is needed to see the follicles under the upper eyelid. (*Used with permission from Richard P. Usatine, MD.*)

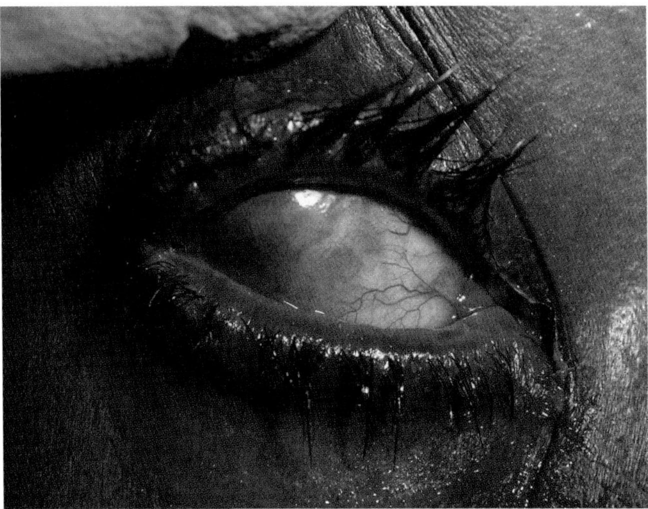

FIGURE 7-19 Blindness caused by untreated trachoma. Although this is one of the most common causes of blindness worldwide, trachoma is easily treatable with a single dose of oral azithromycin. Prevention is achieved through better access to water and soap, together with education about the three "Fs": flies, fingers, facial hygiene. (*Used with permission from Richard P. Usatine, MD.*)

The differential diagnosis of trachoma includes allergic conjunctivitis (which can also produce follicles of the tarsal plate), and bacterial or viral conjunctivitis.

MANAGEMENT

- Azithromycin, 1 g single oral dose for adults and 20 mg/kg for children in a single dose.
- In pregnancy: erythromycin 500 mg twice daily for 7 days.
- Less effective: topical erythromycin and tetracycline.[10]
- In some settings, surgery is available to correct entropion and trichiasis.

PREVENTION

Preventive measures include community hygiene education, use of soap and water for washing hands and faces, and control of flies through use of ventilated improved pit (VIP) latrines. The WHO has developed the acronym "SAFE" for the global elimination of trachoma:

S Surgery for entropion and trichiasis

A Antibiotics for infectious trachoma

F Facial cleanliness to reduce transmission

E Environmental improvements such as control of disease-spreading flies and access to clean water[48]

SKIN

INFECTIOUS SKIN DISEASES

Many of the skin diseases encountered in resource-limited countries are secondary to crowded living conditions and lack of clean water and soap. Scabies mites and human lice are endemic in many populations that are unable to wash frequently. If clean water is scarce, it is more likely to be used for drinking and cooking than bathing. In developed countries, we take clean running water (hot and cold), soap, and shampoo for granted. In developing countries, even if water is available, it may not be accessible as warm running water for showers or baths.

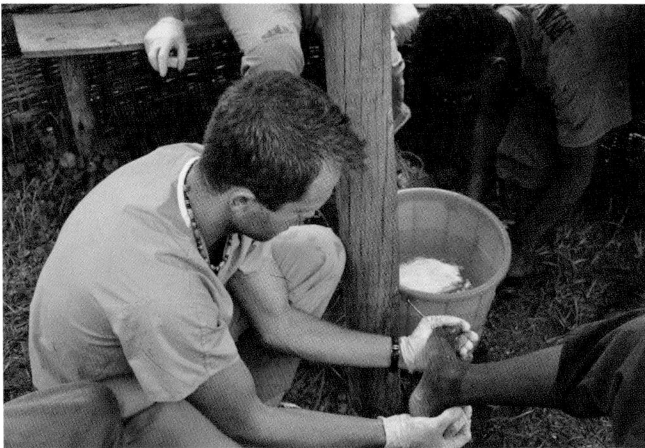

FIGURE 7-20 An American medical student is washing the feet of Ethiopian schoolchildren to treat skin infections and to educate them on preventive hygiene measures. (*Used with permission from Richard P. Usatine, MD.*)

When an intervention as simple as mass distribution of free soap for personal hygiene draws enormous crowds to a mobile clinic, the vastness of inequality in access to basic health measures around the world becomes painfully obvious. Although people recognize the importance of access to soap and clean water, the absence of this luxury results in skin infections and infestations that are highly prevalent and spread from person-to-person (**Figure 7-20**).

We can divide the skin diseases into infestations, bacterial, viral, and fungal infections. All of these skin infections are covered in the dermatology section of this book. Here we highlight some cases seen in developing countries.

Scabies (see Chapter 128, Scabies) is caused by a human mite that burrows under the skin causing itching and leading to scratching. The itching and scratching may keep the person awake at night and may lead to bacterial superinfections (**Figure 7-21**). Scabies is spread by

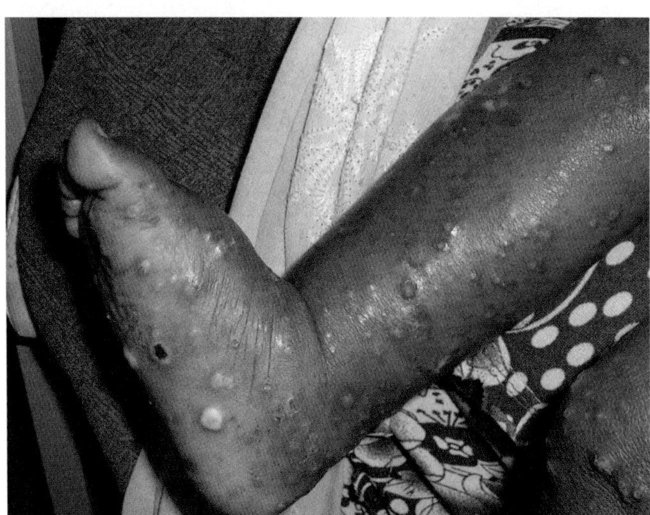

FIGURE 7-21 Badly superinfected scabies with pustules and crusting sores on this young child's leg. (*Used with permission from Richard P. Usatine, MD.*)

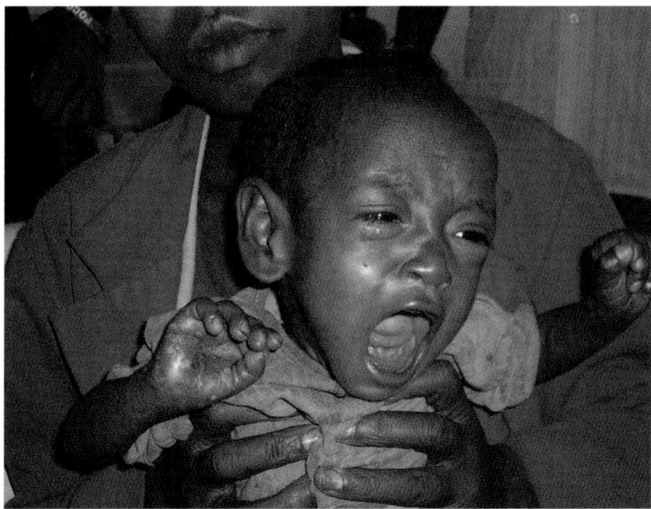

FIGURE 7-22 A malnourished baby with marasmus is infested with scabies seen on the hands and arms. Lack of adequate nutrition also is a risk factor for many infections and diseases. The scabies infestation is a marker for scarcity of clean water; the consequences of both may be contributing to the child's irritability and poor feeding. (*Used with permission from Richard P. Usatine, MD.*)

direct skin contact (**Figures 7-22** and **7-23**), shared bedding and clothing, and occasionally by fomites.

Human lice (see Chapter 127, Lice) exist as 3 separate species that are known as head lice, body lice, and pubic lice. Schoolchildren are particularly at risk for head lice, and in areas with limited head washing, the majority of kids may be infested. Body lice live on clothing and feed on the blood of their host. Body lice are more prevalent on adults that bathe rarely and wear the same unwashed clothing day after day. Pubic lice are transmitted through sexual contact and are not known to be more prevalent in developing countries. Water and hygiene issues do predispose to increased head and body lice in developing countries.

Bacterial infections of the skin (see Chapter 99, Impetigo) are ubiquitous throughout the world. Impetigo is a superficial bacterial

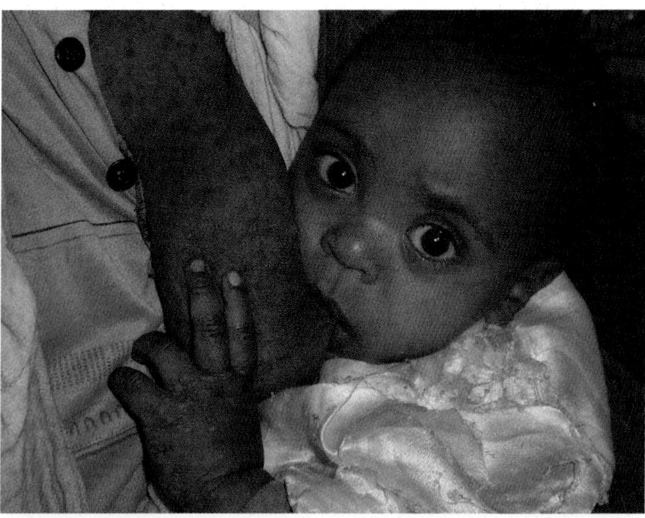

FIGURE 7-23 Scabies infestation covering the mother's breast and her baby's hand. With poor access to health care, this infestation would likely remain untreated, and could lead to bacterial superinfection and impetigo on the baby's skin. (*Used with permission from Richard P. Usatine, MD.*)

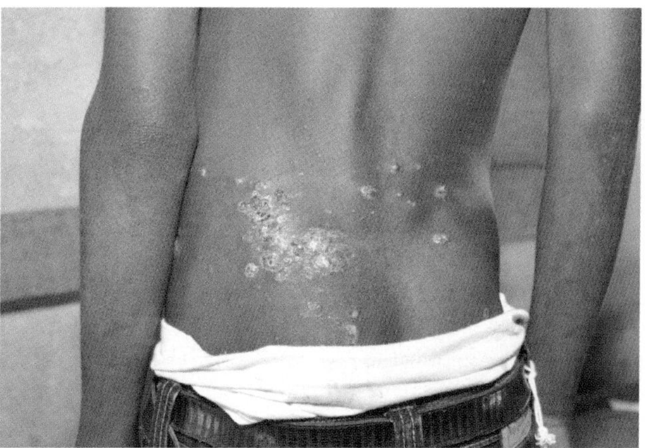

FIGURE 7-24 Impetigo caused by a bacterial infection on the buttocks of this child in Haiti. Impetigo is more prevalent when there is inadequate hygiene and lack of access to health care. (*Used with permission from Richard P. Usatine, MD.*)

infection that presents with honey crusts (**Figure 7-24**) or bullae. Good hygiene can prevent impetigo and therefore is not surprising that many cases of impetigo will be seen in countries that lack access to soap and clean water. Impetigo is often secondary to other skin diseases such as scabies or fungal infections that create breaks in the skin barrier function. Cases of secondarily infected scabies and tinea are seen commonly in developing countries.

Viral infections of the skin (see Chapters 108, Varicella; 109, Zoster; 110, Zoster Ophthalmicus; 111, Measles; 112, Fifth Disease; 113, Hand Foot and Mouth Disease; 114, Herpes Simplex; 115, Molluscum Contagiosum; 116, Common Warts; 117, Flat Warts; 118, Genital Warts; and 119, Plantar Warts) include herpes simplex, varicella zoster, molluscum contagiosum, and human papilloma virus infections. These infections are seen commonly in HIV-infected persons who are not receiving optimal antiretroviral therapy. In countries with a high prevalence of HIV-infected persons, a severe case of molluscum, warts, or shingles in a young person should prompt a clinician to consider HIV testing, if possible. Molluscum infections and warts are so ubiquitous throughout the world that it is important to realize that healthy people with healthy immune systems can get these infections too. Viral exanthems caused by such diseases as varicella and measles may be more prevalent in countries where vaccinations are less available.

Fungal infections of the skin (see Chapters 120, Fungal Overview; 121, Candidiasis; 122, Tinea Capitis; 123, Tinea Corporis; 124, Tinea Cruris; 125, Tinea Pedis; and 126, Tinea Versicolor) can occur from the head down to the toes. Heat, humidity, and lack of bathing are predisposing factors to fungal skin infections. Therefore, tropical developing countries provide good environments for tinea capitis (**Figure 7-25**), tinea corporis, and tinea pedis.

MYCOBACTERIUM (LEPROSY AND TUBERCULOSIS-HIV COINFECTION)

LEPROSY

▶ Patient story

A young boy presents with significant changes to his face (**Figure 7-26**). The boy and his father are from rural Africa, and it is obvious to the

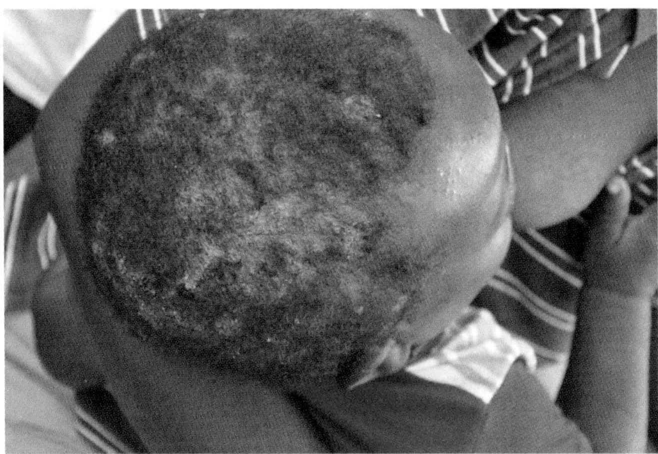

FIGURE 7-25 Tinea capitis in this young boy living in a developing country. Many children live with untreated tinea capitis in developing countries because of limited hygiene resources and poor access to health care. (*Used with permission from Richard P. Usatine, MD.*)

physician that the boy has lepromatous leprosy. The father is also examined and he has more subtle signs of leprosy present (several patches of hypopigmented anesthetic skin). A slit skin exam is performed on the ear lobe of the boy and many acid-fast bacilli, characteristic of *Mycobacterium leprae*, are found. The boy is started on the WHO-standard multidrug therapy using rifampin, clofazimine, and dapsone. The father is also examined and treated.

Introduction

Leprosy (Hansen disease) is caused by *M. leprae* and is still endemic in many parts of the developing world where there is poverty and poor access to clean water. At one time, persons with leprosy were called "lepers" and isolated to leper colonies because the disease was disfiguring and the communities were afraid that it was highly contagious. Current science and epidemiology tell us that leprosy is transmitted via droplets from the nose and mouth during close and frequent contact over a period of years, and not by casual contact. Thus doctors working with patients who have leprosy are at no real risk of becoming infected. Issues related to stigma and discrimination still do exist.

Epidemiology

- There were 219,075 new cases reported in the world by 105 countries in 2011.[49]
- The US reported 173 new cases reported in 2011.[49]
- Since 1990, more than 14 million leprosy patients have been cured, about 4 million from 2000 to 2010.[50]

Etiology and pathophysiology

- The clinical manifestations of leprosy depend upon the immunologic reaction to the infection. The 2 opposite ends of the spectrum consist of:
  - Lepromatous leprosy in which there is a strong antibody response and a poor cell-mediated community resulting in larger amounts of *M. leprae* in the tissues (**Figure 7-26**).

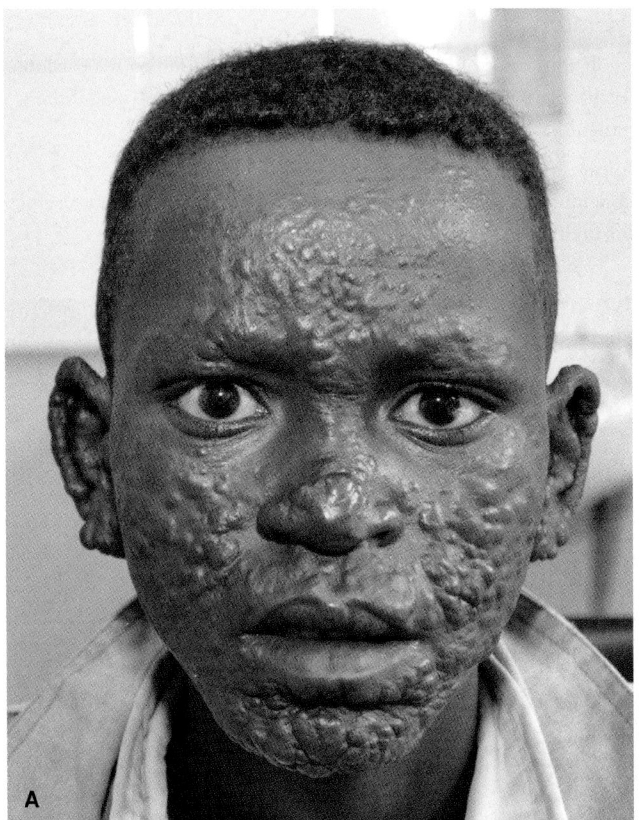

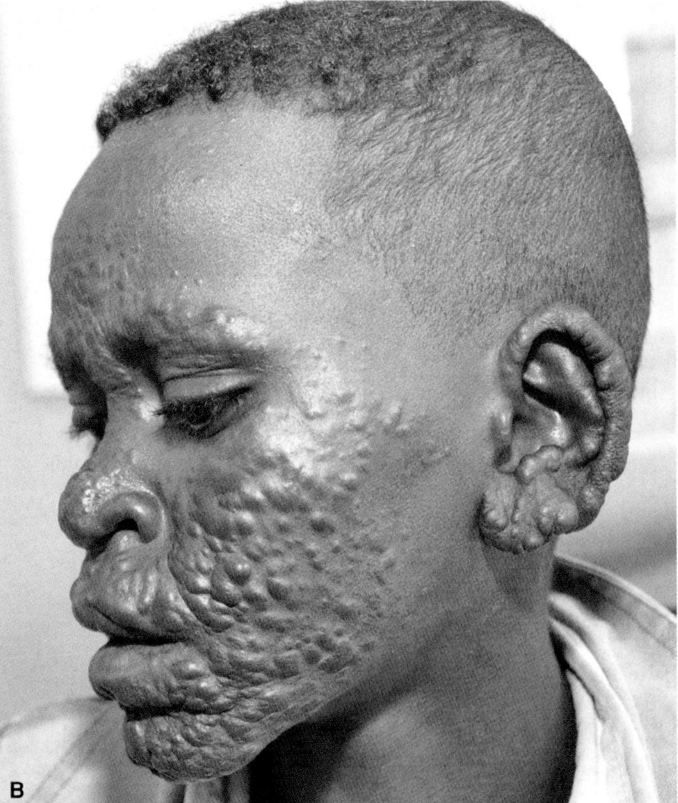

FIGURE 7-26 Lepromatous leprosy with leonine facies in a young boy. **A.** Note the loss of eyebrows called madarosis. **B.** Also note the prominent ear involvement. (*Used with permission from Richard P. Usatine, MD.*)

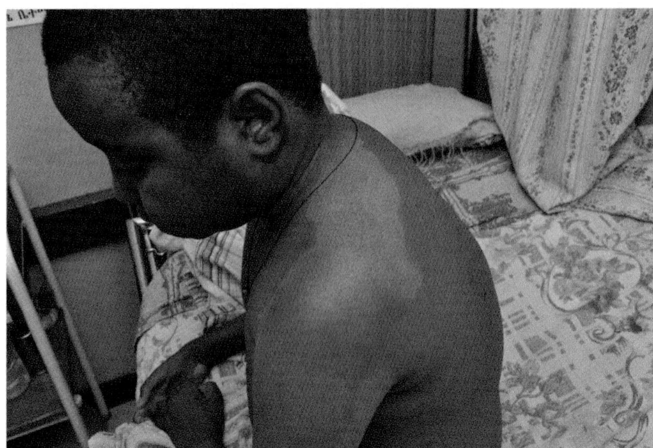

FIGURE 7-27 Leprosy with hypopigmented patches on the back of this young boy. These patches are numb due to cutaneous nerve damage from mycobacterial infection. He also has a Bell's palsy. (*Used with permission from Richard P. Usatine, MD.*)

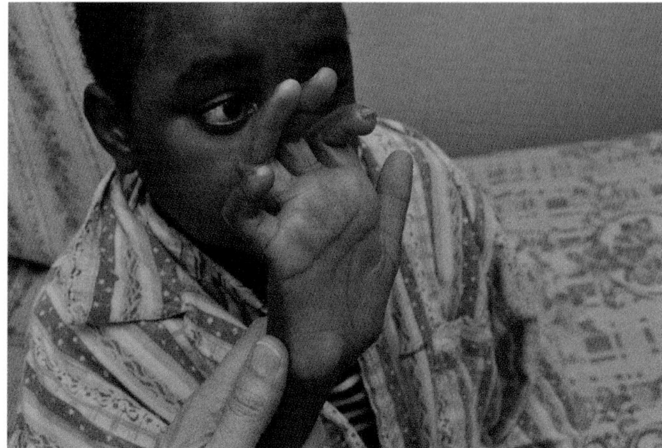

FIGURE 7-28 Clawhand caused by the neurological damage of leprosy in the same boy as in the previous photo. This condition may be amenable to surgical intervention involving tendon transfer. (*Used with permission from Richard P. Usatine, MD.*)

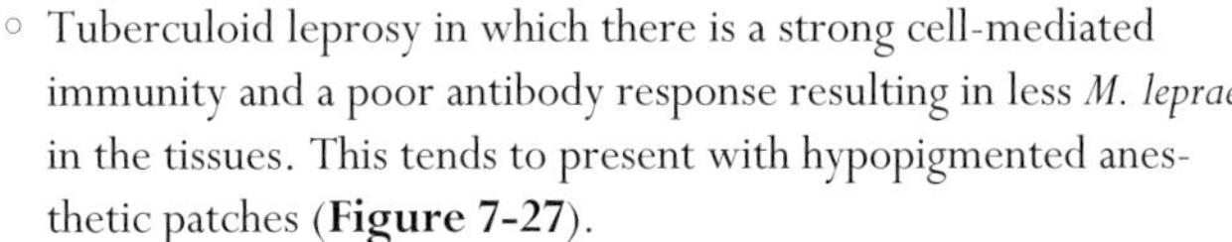

- Tuberculoid leprosy in which there is a strong cell-mediated immunity and a poor antibody response resulting in less *M. leprae* in the tissues. This tends to present with hypopigmented anesthetic patches (**Figure 7-27**).

- There is also borderline leprosy in which there is a mixed cell-mediated immunity and antibody response showing features of both lepromatous leprosy and tuberculoid leprosy.
- Treatment regimens differ depending on whether the patient has paucibacillary (fewer organisms) or multibacillary leprosy. Lepromatous leprosy and borderline lepromatous leprosy are most likely to be multibacillary.

Risk factors

- Poverty and living in an endemic area.
- Inadequate access to clean water and poor hygiene.
- Living in the household of an infected person.
- Eating or handling armadillos as these animals are natural hosts for *M. leprae*.

Diagnosis

Clinical features

- Facial features include leonine facies, madarosis (loss of eyebrows as seen in **Figure 7-26**), elongated and dysmorphic earlobes, and saddle-nose deformities from destruction of the nasal cartilage and bone.
- Visible skin changes include nodules in lepromatous leprosy, hypopigmented patches in tuberculoid (**Figure 7-27**) and borderline leprosy, and annular saucer-like lesions in borderline leprosy.
- Nerve involvement can cause a clawhand (flexion contractures of the fingers as seen in **Figure 7-28**), wristdrop, footdrop, Bell's palsy, hammertoes, and sensory neuropathy leading to neurotropic ulcers and traumatic blisters.
- Eye involvement can cause corneal anesthesia, keratitis, episcleritis, lagophthalmos (the inability to close the eyelid completely), and blindness.
- Advanced untreated leprosy can lead to shortening and/or loss of fingers as a result of bone resorption in hands that have become anesthetic and not protected from repeated trauma (**Figure 7-29**).

Distribution

The nodules of lepromatous leprosy are mostly seen on the face and ears but can be seen in other areas. Hypopigmented patches can be seen anywhere on the body including the face.

Laboratory testing

- In obvious cases of leprosy, the slit skin exam done on the ear lobe for bacillary index is the most important test to determine if the patient has multibacillary or paucibacillary leprosy.
- In cases that are suspicious for leprosy (especially outside of endemic areas), a skin punch biopsy of a suspicious lesion is useful for finding *M. leprae* in the tissues.

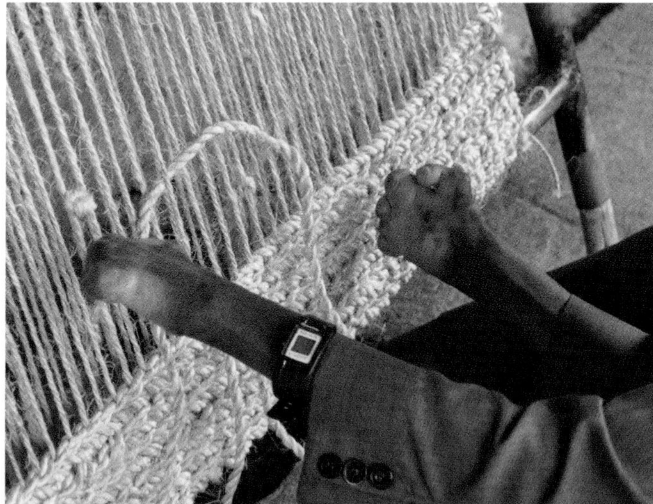

FIGURE 7-29 Leprosy has caused this older man to lose his fingers but he continues to lead a productive life weaving rugs for sale at a leprosy hospital. (*Used with permission from Richard P. Usatine, MD.*)

▶ Differential diagnosis

Superficial mycoses, vitiligo, and cutaneous filariasis all cause changes in pigmentation similar to leprosy. Infiltrated lesions that resemble leprosy include those of leishmaniasis, psoriasis, and sarcoidosis.[52]

▶ Management

Early diagnosis and multidrug therapy are essential to reducing the disease burden of leprosy worldwide. The WHO has supplied multidrug therapy free of cost to leprosy patients in all endemic countries.[51]

- Leprosy is curable and treatment in an early stage can prevent disability.
- Multidrug therapy is a combination of rifampin, dapsone, and clofazimine for multibacillary leprosy patients, and rifampin and dapsone for paucibacillary patients.
- Duration of multidrug therapy is 12 to 24 months for multibacillary and 6 months for paucibacillary patients.[52]
- Treatment with a single antileprosy drug will always result in development of drug resistance to that drug and is therefore an unethical practice.
- Strategies to increase early access to care and provide easy-to-obtain free multidrug treatment are essential to eliminating leprosy in the world. Research on a preventive vaccine continues in tandem with *Mycobacterium tuberculosis* vaccine research.[53]
- Comprehensive treatment of advanced cases with neuropathy should include foot and hand care to prevent further damage to these insensitive limbs.[52]
- Surgical management for some leprosy-associated problems, such as tendon transfer to correct the clawhand, may be available in some centers.[54]

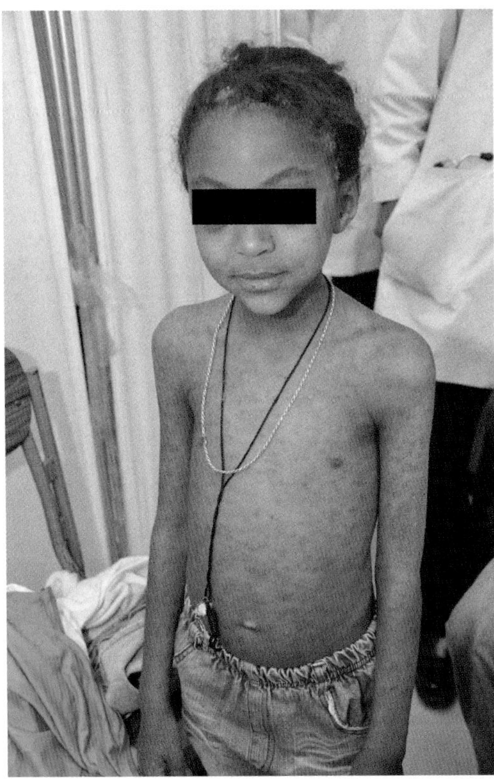

FIGURE 7-30 Young girl who acquired HIV at birth and now has papular pruritic eruption. One in three children born to HIV-infected mothers may be infected; mother-to-child transmission is preventable with simple and affordable antiviral regimens. Fortunately this girl had no signs or symptoms of tuberculosis. (*Used with permission from Richard P. Usatine, MD.*)

TUBERCULOSIS AND HIV

▶ Epidemiology

Tuberculosis (TB) is a very common HIV-associated infection, and causes at least 13 percent of HIV-associated deaths worldwide.[55] In 2010 alone, the WHO estimated there were 1.1 million HIV-associated new cases of TB, the majority of who live in sub-Saharan Africa (**Figure 7-30**). Globally, about 1/3 of HIV-infected people are co-infected with TB (at least 11 million people) (**Figure 7-31**).[56]

▶ Pathogenesis

TB is transmitted by aerosolized respiratory droplet nuclei (see Chapter 186, Pediatric Tuberculosis). Weakened cell-mediated immunity in HIV-infected individuals allows more rapid disease progression and causes higher mortality rates from TB. At the same time, untreated TB infection accelerates immunologic decline in HIV infection. Because these two diseases preferentially afflict populations with reduced access to medications and supportive care, the emergence of multidrug resistant TB has become an increasing threat.

▶ Clinical presentation

The clinical presentation of TB in an HIV-infected person with a relatively preserved immune system (CD4+ T-cell count greater than 350 cells/μL) is identical to that seen in HIV-negative patients. With increasing immunodeficiency, however, TB often presents atypically. Chest radiographs may not demonstrate classic findings of upper lobe fibronodular or cavitary disease, and extrapulmonary presentations (lymphadenitis, pleuritis, pericarditis, or meningitis) are seen. Tuberculous lymphadenitis and cutaneous TB (designated scrofula when it affects the neck) are illustrated in **Figures 7-31** and **7-32**. Tuberculous lymphadenitis and

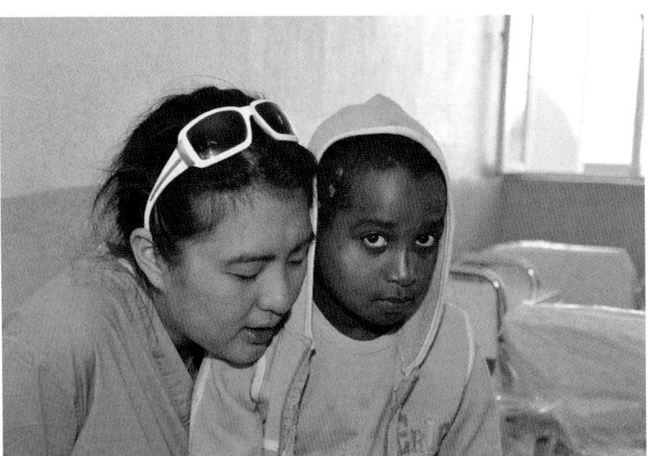

FIGURE 7-31 Young Ethiopian girl with HIV since birth who has neck swelling secondary to tuberculosis. She also has tinea capitis. HIV is a highly stigmatizing disease in most cultures, and clinicians can play an important role in mitigating community stigma by modeling compassionate care. (*Used with permission from Richard P. Usatine, MD.*)

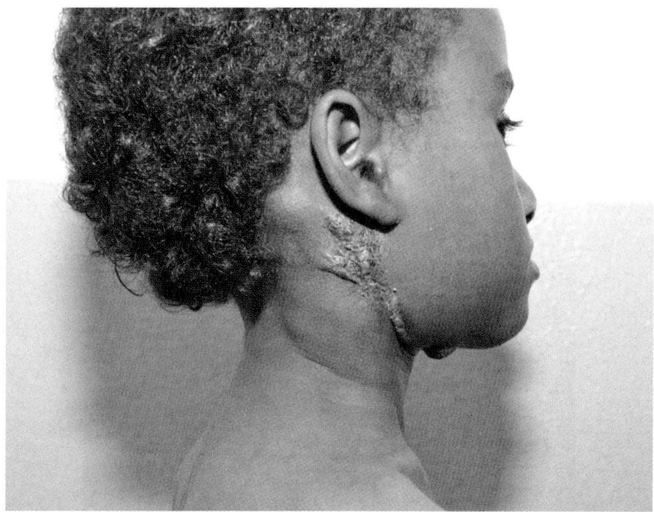

FIGURE 7-32 Scrofula of the neck caused by *M. tuberculosis* in a child. Chronic drainage and fistulous tract formation are commonly associated with this entity, and therapy is the same as for pulmonary tuberculosis. (*Used with permission from Richard P. Usatine, MD.*)

cutaneous TB can also affect the inguinal lymph nodes and groin (**Figures 7-33** and **7-34**).

▶ Diagnosis

HIV screening should be performed in all patients diagnosed with TB, and HIV-infected patients should be screened annually for *M. tuberculosis* with purified protein derivative (PPD) skin testing, chest x-ray, and/or blood test for interferon-γ release assay (IGRA) depending on availability. Patients with low CD4 cell counts and percentages, as defined by age, commonly have poorly reactive skin tests for TB, and thus need a careful history of exposures, review of symptoms, physical examinations, and monitoring of the chest x-ray for evidence of active disease, with repeat TB screening when the CD4 cell count rises above reference levels for age.

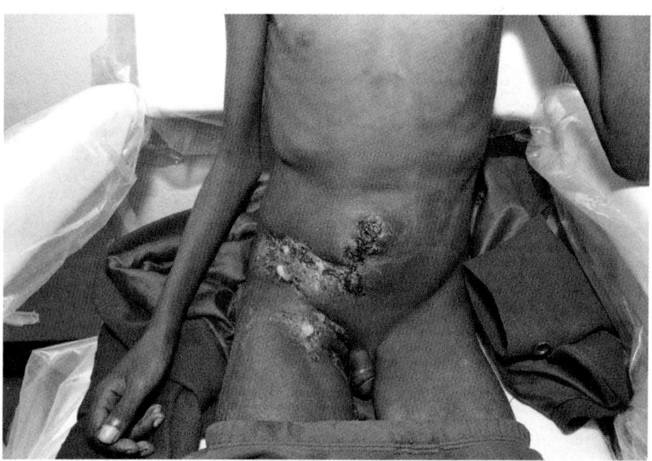

FIGURE 7-33 Scrofula in the inguinal area caused by *M. tuberculosis*. The patient appears systemically ill with weight loss. (*Used with permission from Richard P. Usatine, MD.*)

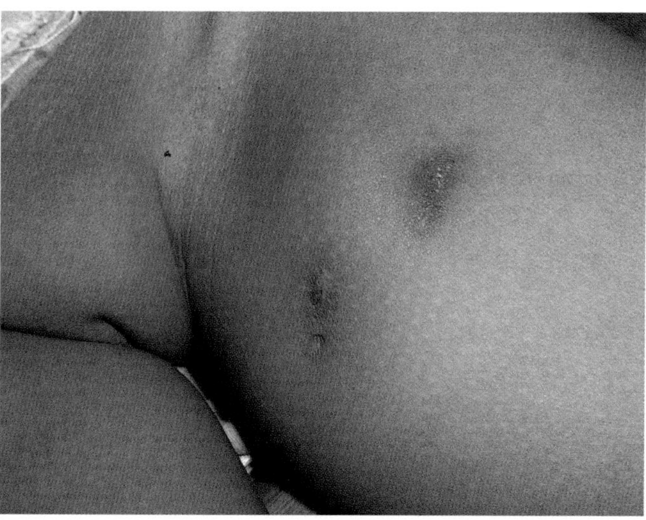

FIGURE 7-34 Scrofula of the groin caused by *M. tuberculosis* in 4-year-old girl. This is an early case and rapid recognition should lead to early treatment. (*Used with permission from Richard P. Usatine, MD.*)

▶ Management

Management of TB in HIV-positive adolescents is generally similar to adults and is discussed in the following section. Optimal treatment regimens for younger children however have not been established.

Latent TB infection

HIV-positive patients with latent tuberculosis infection (LTBI) should have a chest x-ray and three sputum smears or gastric aspirates for acid-fast bacilli to rule out active disease. Once active TB is ruled out, isoniazid prophylaxis should be initiated regardless of age for any HIV-positive person with the following characteristics: (a) a positive diagnostic test for LTBI, (b) a negative LTBI test but with evidence of old or poorly healed fibrotic lesions on chest x-ray, or (c) negative LTBI diagnostic test in a close contact of a person with infectious pulmonary TB.

Duration of LTBI prophylaxis: Isoniazid 300 mg daily or twice weekly for 9 months given with vitamin B6 (pyridoxine 25 mg daily). An alternative regimen of 12 doses of once weekly isoniazid-rifapentine has recently been validated. Pyridoxine prevents isoniazid-associated peripheral neuropathy.[57]

Active M. tuberculosis disease

Any HIV-positive patient with cough and pulmonary infiltrates should be placed in respiratory isolation until TB is ruled out by 3 separately obtained sputum smears (Ziehl-Neelsen) with cultures sent for acid-fast bacilli. This rule applies even when the chest radiograph does not demonstrate cavitary or upper lobe infiltrates. Smear-negative, culture-positive *M. tuberculosis* is not uncommon.

Treatment regimens for HIV-TB coinfected patients are largely identical to those of TB mono-infected patients. It is important not to start antiretroviral therapy (ART) and TB therapy simultaneously, to avoid confusion about drug allergies and side effects. In addition, there is a risk of immune reconstitution syndrome (IRIS [immune reconstitution inflammatory reaction]: inflammatory response that worsens manifestations of any opportunistic infection) when ART is started too soon after initiating TB medication.

Guidelines for ART in TB coinfection are specific. If the CD4 cell count is less than 50, ART should start within 2 weeks of TB therapy. If the CD4 count is greater than 50, ART should start within 8 to 12 weeks of TB therapy. If IRIS does occur, both ART and TB treatment should be continued while managing the IRIS.[58]

Directly observed therapy (DOT) for TB is strongly recommended for HIV-TB coinfected patients.

PROVIDER AND PATIENT RESOURCES

- Traveler's Health from the Centers for Disease Control and Prevention is a comprehensive site that includes information on more than 200 international destinations, travel vaccinations, diseases related to travel, illness and injury abroad, finding travel health specialists, insect protection, safe food and water, and a survival guide—**http://wwwnc.cdc.gov/travel/**.
- The Yellow Book 2012 is available online as a reference for those who advised international travelers about health risks—**http://wwwnc.cdc.gov/travel/page/yellowbook-2012-home.htm**.
- Detailed vaccine information for travel can be obtained at the CDC website on vaccinations. This includes information on yellow fever vaccine, typhoid vaccine, and routine vaccines—**http://wwwnc.cdc.gov/travel/page/vaccinations.htm**.
- Vaccine information can be looked up by specific destination on the traveler's health website—**http://wwwnc.cdc.gov/travel/**.
- U. S. Department of State International Travel Site, including country specific information, travel alert, and travel warnings—**http://travel.state.gov/travel/travel_1744.html**.
- Centers for Disease Control and Prevention. *Malaria*—**http://www.cdc.gov/malaria**.
- World Health Organization. **http://www.who.int/malaria/en/**.
- PubMed Health. *Leishmaniasis*—**http://www.ncbi.nlm.nih.gov/pubmedhealth/PMH0002362/**.
- Centers for Disease Control and Prevention. *Parasites–Leishmaniasis*—**http://www.cdc.gov/parasites/leishmaniasis/**.

CONCLUSION

Medical students and health professionals are increasingly drawn to global health for reasons ranging from the desire for enhanced cultural understanding, to the mission to work for global health equity, to alleviate suffering, or to broaden medical experience beyond geographic boundaries. Whatever one's personal motivation, such experiences should never be undertaken without disciplined preparation. Medical professionals should learn in advance of their travels about the culture, language, and expressed needs and priorities of the local government and health providers and their service populations. In addition, they need to learn about the diagnoses and locally appropriate management of prevalent diseases in the population they plan to serve. Equally important, they should take appropriate preventive measures (vaccines and malaria prophylaxis) to protect their own health. Lack of personal and professional preparation can easily turn the tide from net benefit to major burdens for host country organizations. Ultimately, well-prepared medical educators and clinicians, wherever they may come from, are uniquely positioned to share knowledge that saves lives and leads to a more equitable world.

REFERENCES

1. Kaplan JP, Bond TC, Merson MH, et al. Towards a common definition of global health. *Lancet*. 2009;373:1993-1995.
2. Brown TM, Cueto M, Fee E. The World Health Organization and the transition from "international" to global" public health. *Am J Public Health*. 2006;96:62-72.
3. Central Intelligence Agency. *The World Factbook*. www.cia.gov/library/publications/the-world-factbood/geos/cy.html, accessed September 20, 2012.
4. Waterkeyn J, Carincross S. Creating demand for sanitation and hygiene through community health clubs: a cost-effective intervention in two districts in Zimbabwe. *Soc Sci Med*. 2005;61(9):1958-1970.
5. World Health Organization. *VIP and ROEC latrines*. www.who.int/water_sanitation_health/hygiene/emergencies/fs3_5.pdf, accessed September 21, 2012.
6. UNICEF and WHO. *Progress on Drinking Water and Sanitation 2012 Update*. www.wssinfo.org/fileadmin/user_upload/resources/JMP-report-2012-en.pdf, accessed September 21, 2012.
7. Epstein J, Hoffman S. Typhoid fever. In: Guerrant, RL, Walker DH, Weller PF, eds. *Tropical Infectious Diseases; Principles, Pathogens & Practice*. 2nd ed. Philadelphia, PA: Elsevier; 2006:220-240.
8. Araujo-Jorge T, Callan M, Chappuis F, et al. Multisystem diseases and infections. In: Eddleston M, Davidson R, Brent A, Wilkinson R, eds. *Oxford Handbook of Tropical Medicine*. 3rd ed. New York, NY: Oxford University Press; 2008:665-739.
9. Boggild AK, Van Voorhis WC, Liles WC. Travel-acquired illnesses associated with fever. In: Jong E, Sanford E, eds. *Travel and Tropical Medicine Manual*. 4th ed. Philadelphia, PA: Saunders Elsevier; 2008.
10. Gilbert D, Moellering R, Eliopoulos G, Chambers H, Saag M. *The Sanford Guide to Antimicrobial Therapy*. 41st Ed. Sperryville, VA: Antimicrobial Therapy; 2011.
11. Cravioto A, Lanata CF, Lantagne DS, Nair GB. *Final Report of the Independent Panel of Experts on the Cholera Outbreak in Haiti 2011*. http://www.un.org/News/dh/infocus/haiti/UN-cholera-report-final.pdf, accessed September 21, 2012.
12. Levine MM, Gotuzzo E, and Sow SO. Cholera Infections. In: Guerrant RL, Walker DH, Weller, PF. eds. Tropical Infectious Diseases; Principles, Pathogens & Practice, 2nd Ed Philadelphia, PA: Elsevier; 2006:273-282.
13. Penny ME. Diarrhoeal Diseases. In: Eddleston M, Davidson R, Brent A, Wilkinson R. eds. Oxford Handbook of Tropical Medicine 3rd Ed. New York, NY: Oxford University Press; 2008:213-267.
14. Centers for Disease Control and Prevention. *Cholera Diagnosis and Testing*. http://www.cdc.gov/cholera/diagnosis.html, accessed September 21, 2012.

15. Centers for Disease Control and Prevention. *Recommendations for the Use of Antibiotics for the Treatment of Cholera*. http://www.cdc.gov/cholera/treatment/antibiotic-treatment.html, accessed September 21, 2012.
16. Centers for Disease Control and Prevention. *Domestic Intestinal Parasite Guidelines*. http://www.cdc.gov/immigrantrefugeehealth/guidelines/domestic/intestinal-parasites-domestic.html, accessed September 21, 2012.
17. Keiser J, Utzinger J. Efficacy of current drugs against soil-transmitted helminth infections: systematic review and meta-analysis. *JAMA*. 2008;299(16):1937-1948.
18. Knopp S, Mohammed K, Speich B, et al. Mebendazole administered alone or in combination with ivermectin against *Trichuris trichiura*: a randomized controlled trial. *Clin. Infect. Dis.* 2010;51(12):1420-1428.
19. World Health Organization. *Model Formulary for Children, 2010*. http://www.who.int/selection_medicines/list/WMFc_2010.pdf, accessed September 21, 2012.
20. Mendelson M. Gastroenterology. In: Eddleston M, Davidson R, Brent A, Wilkinson R, eds. *Oxford Handbook of Tropical Medicine*. 3rd ed. New York, NY: Oxford University Press; 2008:269-327.
21. Alderman H, Shekar M. Nutrition, food security and health. In: Kliegman RM, Behrman RE, Jenson HB, Bonita, Stanton, eds. *Nelson Textbook of Pediatrics*. 19th ed. St. Louis, MO: Saunders; 2011.
22. Kosek M, Black R, Keusch G. Nutrition and micronutrients in tropical infectious diseases. In: Guerrant, RL, Walker DH, Weller PF, eds. *Tropical Infectious Diseases; Principles, Pathogens & Practice*. 2nd ed. Philadelphia, PA: Elsevier; 2006:36-52.
23. Diop el HI, Dossou NI, Ndour MM, Briend A, Wade S. Comparison of the efficacy of a solid ready-to-use food and a liquid, milk-based diet for the rehabilitation of severely malnourished children: a randomized trial. *Am J Clin Nutr*. 2003;78:302-307.
24. Branca F, Ferrari M. Impact of micronutrient deficiencies on growth: the stunting syndrome. *Ann Nutr Metab*. 2002;46 Suppl 1:8-17.
25. Burgess A. Mother and child undernutrition—vitamin A deficiency. *So. Sudan. Med. J.* 2008;1:13. http://www.southsudanmedicaljournal.com/assets/images/Articles/feb08/image2.jpg, accessed September 21, 2012.
26. World Health Organization. *Global Prevalence of Vitamin A Deficiency in Populations at Risk 1995-2005*. In: WHO Global Database on Vitamin A Deficiency. http://whqlibdoc.who.int/publications/2009/9789241598019_eng.pdf, accessed Sept 21, 2012.
27. World Health Organization. *Micronutrient Deficiencies: Vitamin A Deficiency*. http://www.who.int/nutrition/topics/vad/en/index.html, accessed Sept 21, 2012.
28. Mayo-Wilson E, Imdad A, Herzer K, Yakoob MY, Bhutta ZA. Vitamin A supplements for preventing mortality, illness, and blindness in children aged under 5: systematic review and meta-analysis. *BMJ*. 2011;343:d5094.
29. Brown K, Wuehler S, Peerson J. The importance of zinc in human nutrition and estimation of the global prevalence of zinc deficiency. *Food Nutr Bull*. 2001;22:113-169.
30. World Health Organization. *Implementing the New Recommendations of the Clinical Management of Diarrhea. Guidelines for Policy Makers and Programme Managers*. Geneva, Switzerland: World Health Organization; 2006. http://whqlibdoc.who.int/publications/2006/9241594217_eng.pdf, accessed September 21, 2012.
31. Baqui AH, Black RE, Shams EA, et al. Effect of zinc supplementation started during diarrhoea on morbidity and mortality in Bangladeshi children: community randomised trial. *BMJ*. 2002;325:1059.
32. Brown K, Wuehler S, Peerson J. The importance of zinc in human nutrition and estimation of the global prevalence of zinc deficiency. *Food Nutr Bull*. 2001. http://archive.unu.edu/unupress/food/fnb22-2.pdf, accessed September 21, 2012.
33. World Health Organization. *Micronutrient Deficiencies. Iron Deficiency Anaemia*. http://www.who.int/nutrition/topics/ida/en/index.html, accessed September 21, 2012.
34. Horton S, Miloff, A. Iodine status and availability of iodized salt: an across-country analysis. *Food Nutr. Bull.* 2010;31: 214-220.
35. World Health Organization. *Iodine Status Worldwide*. http://whqlibdoc.who.int.publications/2004/9241592001.pdf, accessed September 21, 2012.
36. Day N. Malaria. In: Eddleston M, Davidson R, Brent A, Wilkinson R, eds. *Oxford Handbook of Tropical Medicine*. 3rd ed. New York, NY: Oxford University Press; 2008:31-65.
37. Ashley E, White N. Malaria diagnosis and treatment. In: Jong E, Sanford E, eds *Travel and Tropical Medicine Manual*. 4th ed. Philadelphia, PA: Saunders Elsevier; 2008:303-321.
38. Hoffman S, Campbell C, White N. Malaria. In: Guerrant, RL, Walker DH, Weller PF, eds. *Tropical Infectious Diseases; Principles, Pathogens & Practice*. 2nd ed. Philadelphia, PA: Elsevier; 2006:1024-1062.
39. Centers for Disease Control. *Treatment of Malaria (Guidelines for Clinicians)*. April 2011. http://www.cdc.gov/malaria/resources/pdf/clinicalguidance.pdf, accessed September 21, 2012.
40. World Health Organization. *10 Facts on Malaria*. http://www.who.int/features/factfiles/malaria/en/index.html, accessed September 21, 2012.
41. Centers for Disease Control and Prevention. *Parasites—Leishmaniasis*. http://www.cdc.gov/parasites/leishmaniasis/, accessed September 15, 2012.
42. Singh S. New developments in diagnosis of leishmaniasis. *Indian J Med Res* 2006;123:311-330.
43. Ryan T. Dermatology. In: Eddleston M, Davidson R, Brent A, Wilkinson R, eds. *Oxford Handbook of Tropical Medicine*. 3rd ed. New York, NY: Oxford University Press; 2008:566.
44. Schwartz E. Leishmaniasis: In: Jong E, Sanford E, eds. *Travel and Tropical Medicine Manual*. 4th ed. Philadelphia, PA: Saunders Elsevier; 2008:532-542.
45. Pub Med Health. *Leishmaniasis*. http://www.ncbi.nlm.nih.gov/pubmedhealth/PMH0002362/, accessed September 15, 2012.
46. Pearson R, Weller P, Guerrant R. Chemotherapy of parasitic diseases. In: Guerrant, RL, Walker DH, Weller PF, eds. *Tropical Infectious Diseases; Principles, Pathogens & Practice*. 2nd ed. Philadelphia, PA: Elsevier; 2006:142-168.
47. World Health Organization. *Prevention of Blindness and Visual Impairment, Priority Eye Diseases: Trachoma*. http://www.who.int/blindness/causes/priority/en/index2.html, accessed September 21, 2012.

48. Yorston D. Ophthalmology. In: Eddleston M, Davidson R, Brent A, Wilkinson R, eds. *Oxford Handbook of Tropical Medicine.* 3rd ed. New York, NY: Oxford University Press; 2008:523.

49. Global Leprosy Situation, 2012. *Wkly Epidemiol Rec.* 2012;87(34): 317-328.

50. World Health Organization. *Leprosy; Fact Sheet No.101.* http://www.who.int/mediacentre/factsheets/fs101/en/index.html, accessed August 26, 2012.

51. World Health Organization. *Leprosy Elimination. WHO Multidrug Therapy.* http://www.who.int/lep/mdt/en/index.html, accessed August 26, 2012.

52. Meyers W. Leprosy. In: Guerrant, RL, Walker DH, Weller PF, eds. *Tropical Infectious Diseases; Principles, Pathogens & Practice.* 2nd ed. Philadelphia, PA: Elsevier; 2006:436.

53. Gormus BJ, Meyers WM. Under-explored experimental topics related to integral mycobacterial vaccines for leprosy. *Expert Rev Vaccines.* 2003;2(6):791-804.

54. Sapienza A, Green S. Correction of the claw hand. *Hand Clin* 2012;28(1):53-66.

55. National Institutes of Health Clinical Guidelines Portal. *Federally Approved HIV/AIDS Medical Practice Guidelines.* http://www.aidsinfo.nih.gov/contentfiles/lvguidelines/adult_oi_041009.pdf, accessed September 21, 2012.

56. World Health Organization. *TB/HIV FACTS 2011-2012.* http://www.who.int/tb/publications/TBHIV_Facts_for_2011.pdf, accessed September 21, 2012.

57. Johnson J, Ellner J. Tuberculosis and atypical mycobacterial infections. In: Guerrant, RL, Walker DH, Weller PF, eds. *Tropical Infectious Diseases; Principles, Pathogens & Practice.* 2nd ed. Philadelphia, PA: Elsevier; 2006:411.

58. National Institutes of Health Clinical Guidelines Portal. *Considerations for Antiretroviral Use in Patients with Coinfections; Mycobacterium Tuberculosis Disease with HIV Coinfection.* http://www.aidsinfo.nih.gov/guidelines/html/1/adult-and-adolescent-treatment-guidelines/27/, accessed September 21, 2012.

PART 3

PHYSICAL AND SEXUAL ABUSE

Strength of Recommendation (SOR)	Definition
A	Recommendation based on consistent and good-quality patient-oriented evidence.*
B	Recommendation based on inconsistent or limited-quality patient-oriented evidence.*
C	Recommendation based on consensus, usual practice, opinion, disease-oriented evidence, or case series for studies of diagnosis, treatment, prevention, or screening.*

*See Appendix A on pages 1320–1322 for further information.

8 CHILD PHYSICAL ABUSE

James Anderst, MD, MS
Ashley D. Hopkins, MD

PATIENT STORIES

CASE 1

A 1-month-old child was seen in the emergency department for bruising. Physical examination revealed bruises to the buttocks, chest, and eye. The parents reported that the child received the buttock bruise (**Figure 8-1**) after being dropped by the father, that the chest bruise was from the child's seat belt, and the eye bruise from accidentally hitting the child with an elbow while co-sleeping. The social worker was consulted and found no concerning "red flags" in the family. The emergency department physician felt the findings were because of inexperienced parents. The child was sent home with the parents and the emergency department later reported the case to Child Protective Services (CPS) in hopes of providing the family with support services. A child abuse pediatrician (CAP) was consulted by CPS to review the case the next day. The CAP requested that the child be brought back to the hospital emergently for further evaluation. At that time, a skeletal survey, including oblique views of the ribs, showed a healing fracture of the eighth posterior rib (**Figure 8-2**). A head CT and liver function tests were performed to screen for occult trauma and laboratory tests were done to evaluate for a bleeding diathesis. All were negative. Law enforcement was contacted and coinvestigated with CPS. The child was placed in the home of a relative. Two weeks later, a repeat skeletal survey showed new bone formation over the right femur, indicating a healing fracture.

CASE 2

A 15-month-old child is brought to the emergency department by the police after a relative called 911. The child and his mother attended a family gathering where concerned relatives viewed the mother's story that the child "falls a lot" with suspicion. On examination there were many signs of physical abuse (**Figures 8-3** to **8-5**). His face was covered with bruises, especially around the right eye and cheek (**Figure 8-3**). His axilla showed signs of being gouged with fingernails (**Figure 8-4**). Although an initial skeletal survey did not show any fractures, a repeat skeletal survey and oblique views of the ribs were done 2 weeks later. The second skeletal series showed eight healing rib fractures. Repeat skeletal surveys are recommended in children younger than 4 years of age, who are confirmed or suspected victims of abuse (**Figure 8-5**). The child was admitted to the

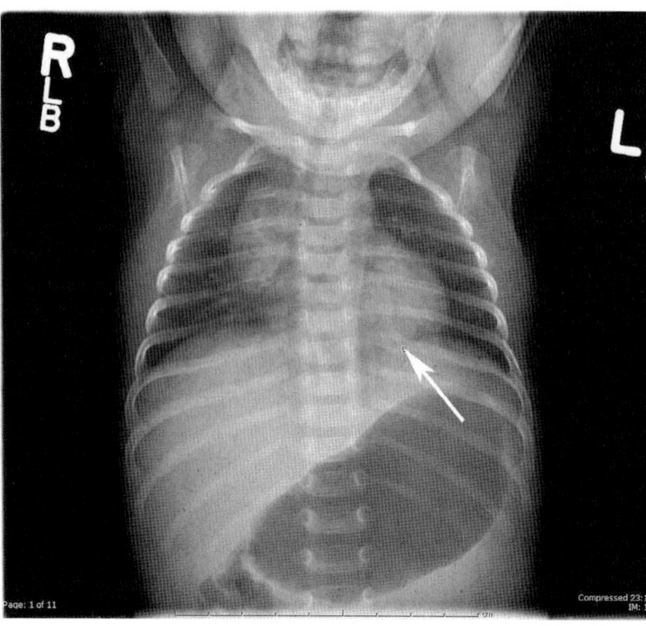

FIGURE 8-2 Healing eighth posterior rib fracture in the same child from Figure 8-1. A skeletal survey is indicated in any child younger than 2 years of age where suspicions of physical abuse exist. (*Used with permission from James Anderst, MD, MS.*)

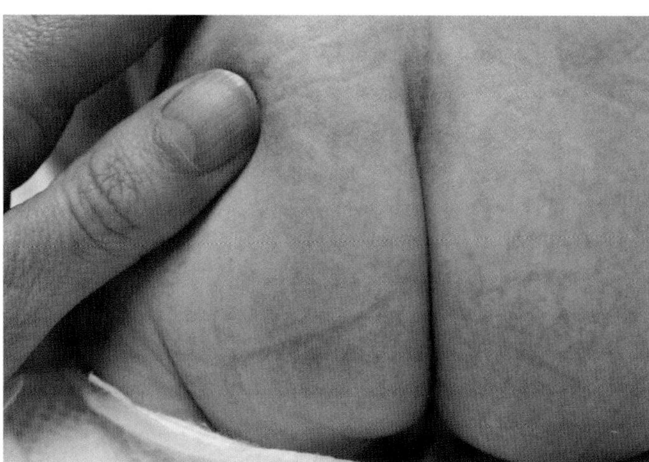

FIGURE 8-1 Bruising to the left buttock noted in a 1-month-old child. Any bruising on an immobile child is highly concerning for child physical abuse. Bleeding disorders must be considered in the differential diagnosis. (*Used with permission from James Anderst, MD, MS.*)

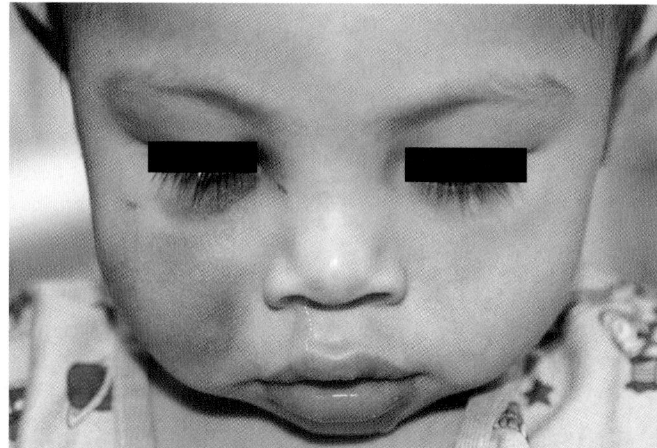

FIGURE 8-3 A 15-month-old boy who has been physically abused by his mother's boyfriend for several weeks. There is bruising under both eyes, with the greatest degree of bruising seen under the right eye and on the right cheek. The boy is in the emergency department after concerned relatives called the police. (*Used with permission from James Anderst, MD, MS.*)

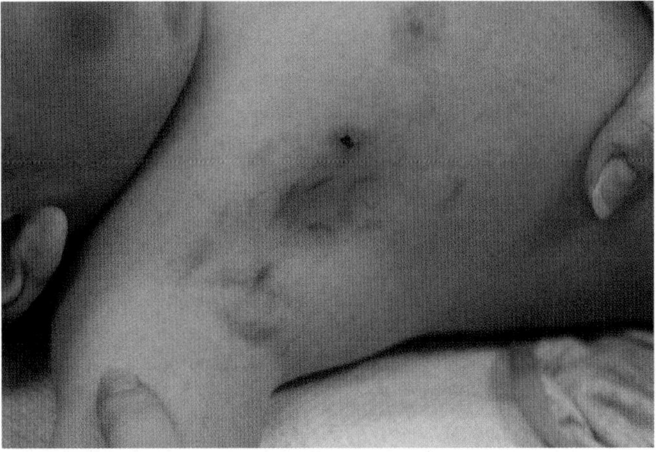

FIGURE 8-4 Same 15-month-old boy from Figure 8-3 with multiple fingernail gouges in his right axilla. Some are fresh and one appears to be older and somewhat crusted. Injuries in different stages of healing may indicate chronicity of abuse. (*Used with permission from James Anderst, MD, MS.*)

hospital and the police, hospital social workers, and CPS were notified. In the emergency department, the child was evaluated by a forensic nurse examiner trained in child-abuse photo documentation. The child was then referred to a CAP who assessed mechanisms of injuries, reexamined the child, and interpreted the initial and follow-up skeletal surveys.

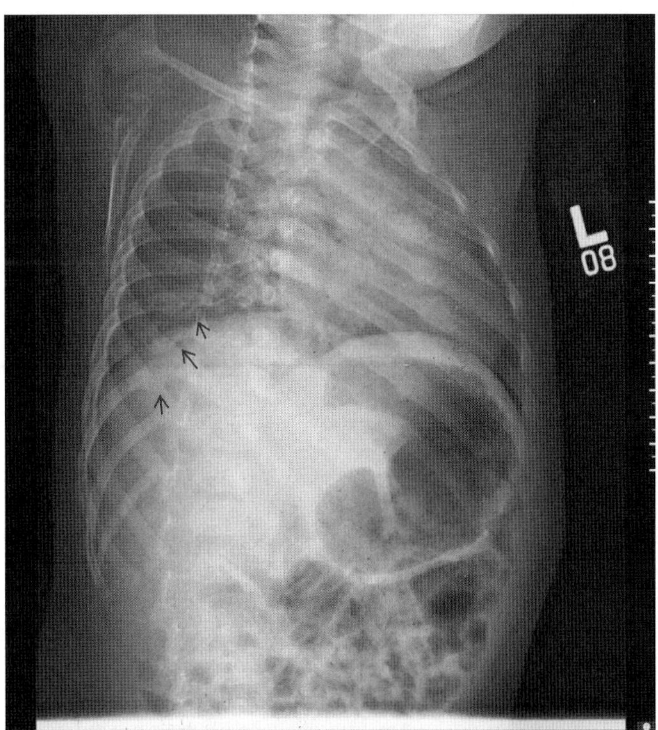

FIGURE 8-5 Same boy from Figure 8-3 with oblique x-ray showing healing rib fractures with callus in eight different locations as marked by the *arrows*. The degree of callus formation shows that these rib fractures are not new. Oblique radiographs should be requested in addition to a "skeletal survey" because lateral rib fractures are best seen with this view. (*Used with permission from James Anderst, MD, MS.*)

INTRODUCTION

The appropriate identification of child physical abuse is critical. Misdiagnoses in either direction (missed abuse or inappropriate diagnosis of abuse) are extremely harmful to the child and family. A careful evaluation of each case, coupled with an application of the existing scientific data on child physical abuse, may result in improved outcomes for the child and family.

EPIDEMIOLOGY

- Occurs in 9.2 per 1000 children, with highest rate of victimization in the birth to 1 year age group (20.6 per 1000).
- The Department of Health and Human Services compilation of State CPS Child Maltreatment 2010 had 3.3 million CPS reports filed in 2010, with 695,000 confirmed child victims.[1] Of these:
  - Seventy-eight percent were neglected.
  - Eighteen percent were physically abused.
  - Nine percent were sexually abused.
  - Eight percent were psychologically abused.
- Nearly 81 percent of victims were abused by a parent acting alone or with another person.
- Medical personnel made only 8.2 percent of the referrals to CPS.

RISK FACTORS

Caregiver factors associated with child abuse include the following:[2–4]

- Inappropriate parental expectations of the child.
- Lack of empathy toward the child's needs.
- The parent's belief in physical punishment.
- Parental role reversal.
- Caregiver's personal history:
  - Was abused during childhood.
  - Parents' rearing practices modeled.
  - Mental illness or substance abuse.

Factors specific to the child that are associated with abuse:[2]

- Prematurity.
- Disabilities.
- Difficult temperament.

Environmental factors associated with abuse:

- Domestic violence.
- Financial, family, or work stressors.
- Housing issues.

DIAGNOSIS

CONCERNING HISTORY[5]

- History inconsistent with child's developmental stage.
- Injuries inconsistent with history given.

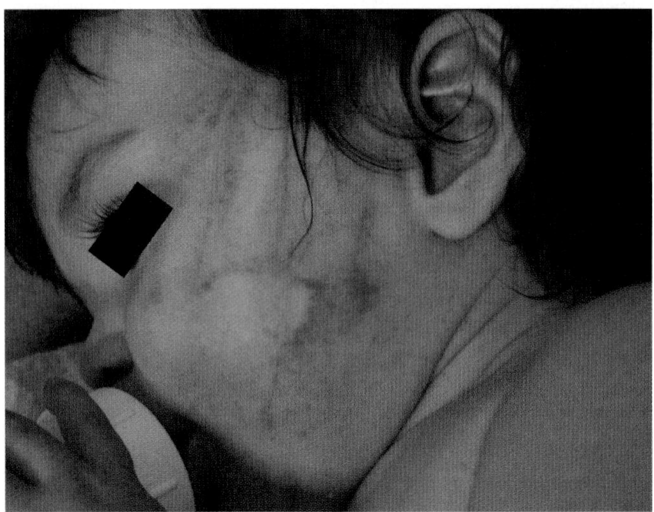

FIGURE 8-6 Linear ecchymosis on the cheek of a baby who was slapped in the face by an abusive parent. (*Used with permission from James Anderst, MD, MS.*)

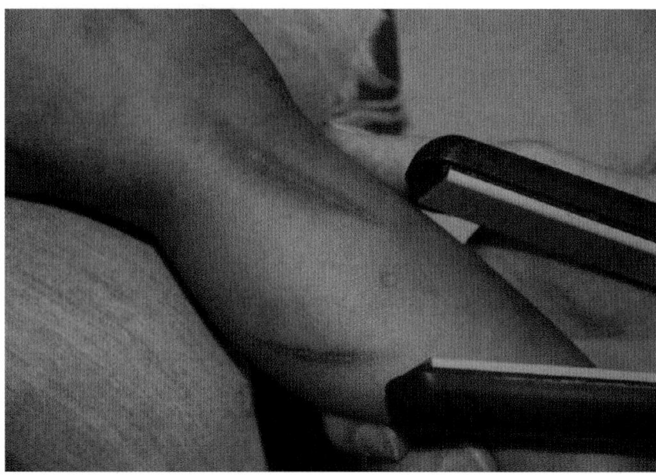

FIGURE 8-7 Toddler being seen for a burn caused by hair straightener. The family claimed the iron fell onto the leg but further investigation seemed to indicate that the iron was applied to the child by an angry parent to control a crying child. Although the iron falling could explain the injury on the calf, it does not explain the additional injury higher up on the leg. (*Used with permission from James Anderst, MD, MS.*)

- History changes over time.
- History differs among witnesses.
- Delay in seeking medical care (must consider family's access to care and availability of transportation).
- Sibling blamed.
- Magical injury—No one knows how it happened.

CLINICAL FEATURES

- Bruising:[6]
  - In children who are not independently mobile.
  - Seen away from boney prominences.
  - To the face, hands, ears, buttocks, back, abdomen, and arms.
  - In the shape of an imprint of an object or hand, or a ligature (**Figure 8-6**).
  - Multiple bruises in clusters.
- Burns:[7]
  - Inconsistent with history (**Figure 8-7**).
  - Stocking/glove distribution.
  - Well-demarcated edges.
  - Symmetrical burns.
  - No splash marks.
- Fractures:[8]
  - Rib fractures.
  - Fractures in immobile children that are not attributable to birth injury.
  - Multiple fractures and/or multiple fractures of different ages.
  - Fractures in the absence of a history of trauma.
  - Any fracture that is inconsistent with the reported mechanism.
- Intracranial injury:
  - Highly variable clinical presentation; however, presence of apnea, retinal hemorrhages, and/or rib fractures is more strongly associated with inflicted (versus noninflicted) intracranial injury.[9,10]
  - Mild abusive head injury may present with isolated vomiting or fussiness.[11]
- Oral lesions—Torn frenula, palatal petechiae, contusions, or lacerations (typically from a bottle, finger, or other object forced into the child's mouth).[12]
- Failure to thrive and signs of malnutrition as a result of intentional withholding of food and/or liquids.

LABORATORY STUDIES AND IMAGING

- Concerning bruising that is not obviously abusive—Prothrombin time/partial thromboplastin time (PT/PTT), complete blood count (CBC), von Willebrand testing, factor 8 and factor 9 levels. Testing best done in collaboration with a CAP or pediatric hematologist.[13]
- Detection of occult abdominal trauma—Liver function tests (LFTs), amylase, lipase, urinalysis; CT of abdomen recommended if laboratory results are elevated or urinalysis positive for blood.[14]
- Detection of occult fractures—Skeletal survey (including oblique views of the ribs) in children younger than 2 years of age or nonverbal children; consider radionuclide bone scan to look for acute fractures, or a follow-up skeletal survey 2 weeks after initial presentation.[15]
- Detection of occult intracranial injury—CT/MR of head in all young children, even if there are no clinical signs of intracranial injury; ophthalmology examination for retinal hemorrhages.[16]

DIFFERENTIAL DIAGNOSIS

- Bruises and other skin findings:
  - Accidental bruises—Any bruising in an infant or precruiser is very concerning for abuse. Accidental bruising is much more common in cruising or walking children.[17] Any inflicted bruising or skin markings (including those from spanking or other punishment) lasting more than 24 hours constitutes abuse.[18] Ear bruising is very specific for abuse (**Figure 8-8**).[19] It is not

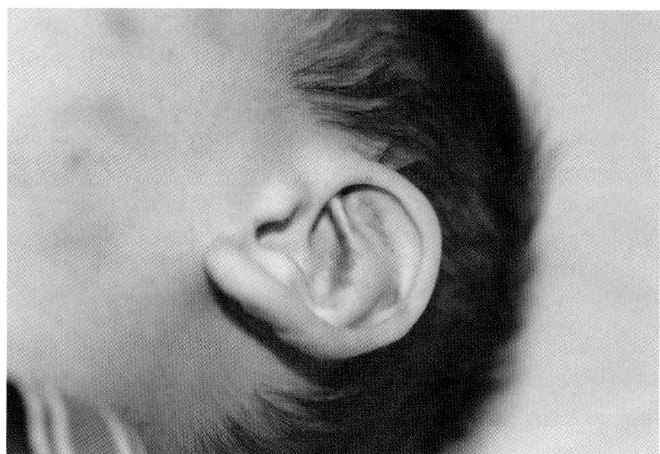

FIGURE 8-8 Bruising of the ear in a young boy who was physically abused by a parent. Ear bruising is rarely accidental. The additional bruising on the cheek suggests this child was hit with a hand or another object to produce the bruising seen in this photo. (*Used with permission from James Anderst, MD, MS.*)

possible to accurately date bruises.[20] Accidental bruising is typically located on the shins, lower arms, under chin, forehead, hips, elbows, ankles, and bony prominences. Loop-like bruising is suspicious for blows with a cord or a looped belt (**Figure 8-9**).

- ◦ Bruising with tracking of blood (subgaleal hematoma) can be seen with severe injuries to the head from violent hair pulling (**Figure 8-10**).
- ◦ Bleeding disorders—Familial history, abnormal coagulation laboratory test results, vitamin K deficiency.
- ◦ Other rare diseases associated with bruising—Ehlers-Danlos, Henoch-Schönlein purpura, phytophotodermatitis (skin reaction to psoralens, most commonly found in limes), osteogenesis imperfecta (brittle bones).

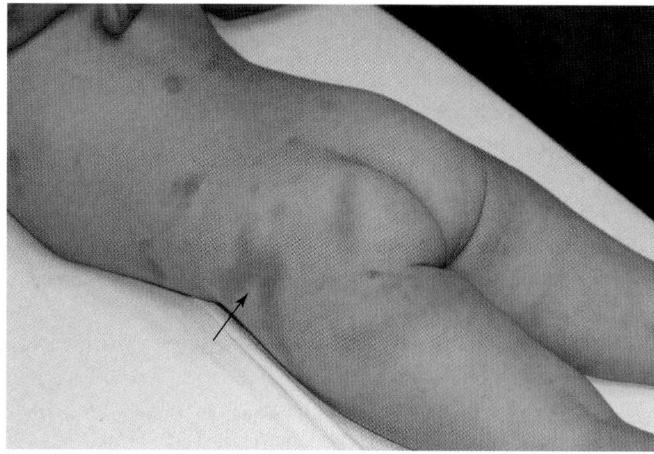

FIGURE 8-9 Young girl with linear bruising on the back, buttocks, and thigh from being hit with a belt. One bruise appears to have a loop-like form (*arrow*) and was likely caused by blows with a cord or a looped belt. Blows with flexible objects produce patterns that tend to conform to the curved surfaces of the body, whereas inflexible objects may produce a discontinuous pattern over curved surfaces. (*Used with permission from Nancy Kellogg, MD.*)

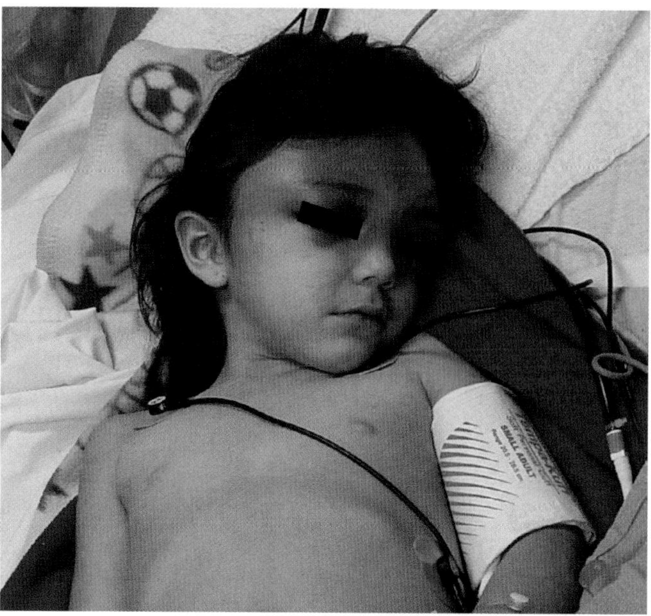

FIGURE 8-10 Young girl with severe subgaleal hematoma with extensive blood tracking into the upper face after being lifted off the ground by her hair. Blood tracking after significant injury is most commonly seen on the face, although some injuries to the genitals may also track into the perineum. (*Used with permission from James Anderst, MD, MS.*)

- ◦ Skin discoloration—Common examples are allergic shiners (dark, puffy lower eyelids) and Mongolian spots (macular blue-gray pigmentation usually on the sacral area of normal infants, usually present at birth or appear within the first weeks of life; see Chapter 92, Normal Skin Changes).

- Burns:
  - ◦ Accidental burns (splash marks usually seen).
  - ◦ Bullous impetigo, cellulitis, scalded skin syndrome, diaper rash.
  - ◦ Chemical burn caused by senna containing laxatives.
  - ◦ Drug reaction.
- Fractures from other diseases occurring in infants and young children:
  - ◦ Osteogenesis imperfecta—A congenital disorder with bone fragility; patients may have repeated fractures after mild trauma that heal readily. Other features seen in some cases include blue sclera, easy bruising, and deafness (see Chapter 225, Osteogenesis Imperfecta).
  - ◦ Rickets—Usually from vitamin D deficiency, consider in exclusively breastfed infants, dark-skinned children, children with little sun exposure. The metaphyses show widening and cupping with irregular calcification as a result of poor calcification of osteoid (see Chapter 198, Rickets).
- Failure to thrive from other causes including improper mixing of formula, breastfeeding difficulty, organic diseases such as cystic fibrosis, HIV, metabolic disorders, celiac disease, and renal disease[21] (see Chapter 53, Failure to Thrive).

Intracranial bleeding—Other causes include accidental injury, infection, coagulation disorders, birth injury, and rare metabolic conditions (glutaric aciduria).

Cultural practices—Coining (**Figure 8-11**), cupping, moxibustion (cultural practice of burning herbs on skin).

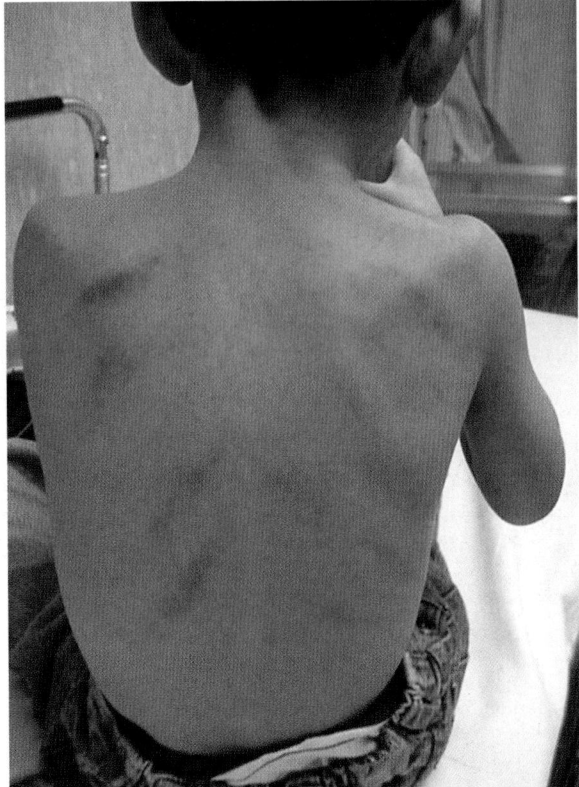

FIGURE 8-11 Young boy with the marks of coining on his back. A coin was rubbed across his back leaving ecchymoses over bony prominences with the intent to help the child heal from an acute illness. This cultural practice is more common among Asian immigrants to this country and mimics child abuse. (*Used with permission from Maria McColgan, MD.*)

MANAGEMENT

- Emergent care first; treat injuries, burns, failure to thrive accordingly.
- Careful examination of the skin and oral cavity, palpation for bony tenderness or callus formation, signs of abdominal trauma or neurologic abnormalities, ophthalmologic evaluation for retinal hemorrhages.
- Document the history provided by caregivers and physical findings accurately, including pictures.
- Consider consultation with a CAP or a family physician with additional training or expertise. Child abuse pediatrics is a new subspecialty of pediatrics requiring an additional 3 years of fellowship training.
- In cases where the injury was truly caused by an accidental mechanism, the role of neglect must be considered.
- Mandated reporting:
  - All 50 states require that all professionals who work with children report suspected child abuse and neglect.
  - Reporter of abuse is granted legal immunity.
  - Once the case is reported, further collaboration with CPS or law enforcement is usually necessary to ensure appropriate outcomes.[22]

PATIENT EDUCATION

- Prevention programs:
  - Home visitation programs have been shown to reduce child abuse and child mortality.[23]
  - Nursery-based prevention of abusive head trauma.[24]
  - Specific models of primary care may reduce abuse.[25]
  - Population-based prevention.[26]
  - Parent–child interactive therapy (PCIT) reduces repeat abuse.[27]

FOLLOW-UP

- If there is suspicion of fractures, obtain repeat skeletal x-ray in 2 weeks to look for evidence of healing fractures.
- Siblings of abused children should be interviewed and examined for findings concerning abuse.
- Counseling for child and family as appropriate.
- Frequent follow-up with primary care provider to evaluate for signs of abuse and neglect.
- Report to CPS.

PATIENT RESOURCES

- Child Help—**http://childhelp.org/**.
- Prevent Child Abuse America—**http://www.preventchildabuse.org/index.shtml**.

PROVIDER RESOURCES

- Mechanisms of Injury in Childhood phone app/computer program—**http://www.childrensmercy.org/mic/**.
- The American Academy of Pediatrics Evaluation of Suspected Child Physical Abuse—**http://pediatrics.aappublications.org/cgi/content/full/119/6/1232**.
- The American Professional Society on the Abuse of Children—**www.apsac.fmhi.usf.edu/index.asp**.
- Child Abuse Evaluation & Treatment for Medical Providers—**http://www.childabusemd.com/index.shtml**.

REFERENCES

1. U.S. Department of Health and Human Services, Administration for Children and Families, Administration on Children, Youth and Families, Children's Bureau. 2010. *Child Maltreatment 2009.* http://www.acf.hhs.gov/programs/cb/stats_research/index.htm#can, accessed March 2012.
2. Giardino AP, Alexander R. *Child Maltreatment: A Clinical Guide and Reference*. St. Louis, MO: G.W. Medical; 2005.
3. Bavolek S. *The Nurturing Parent Programs*. Washington, DC: Office of Juvenile Justice and Delinquency Prevention, U.S. Department of Justice; 2000.
4. Helfer RM. The etiology of child abuse. *Pediatrics.* 1973;51 (4):777-779.

5. Kellogg ND. American Academy of Pediatrics, Committee on Child Abuse and Neglect. Evaluation of suspected child physical abuse. *Pediatrics.* 2007;119(6):1232-1241.
6. Maguire S, Mann MK, Sibert J, Kemp A. Are there patterns of bruising in childhood which are diagnostic or suggestive of abuse? A systematic review. *Arch Dis Child.* 2005;90:182-186.
7. Maguire S, Moynihan S, Mann M, et al. A systematic review of the features that indicate intentional scalds in children. *Burns.* 2008;34(8):1072-1081.
8. Maguire S. Which injuries may indicate child abuse? *Arch Dis Child Educ Pract Ed.* 2010;95:170-177.
9. Maguire S, Pickerd N, Farewell D, et al. Which clinical features distinguish inflicted from non-inflicted brain injury? A systematic review. *Arch Dis Child.* 2009;94:860-867.
10. Maguire S, Kemp AM, Lumb R, Farewell D. Estimating the probability of abusive head trauma: A pooled analysis. *Pediatrics.* 2011; 128(3):e550-e564.
11. Jenny C, Hymel KP, Ritzen A, et al. Analysis of missed cases of abusive head trauma. *JAMA.* 1999;282(7):621-626.
12. Kellogg ND. American Academy of Pediatrics, Committee on Child Abuse and Neglect. Oral and dental aspects of child abuse and neglect. *Pediatrics.* 2005;116(6):1565-1568.
13. Jackson J, Carpenter S, Anderst J. Challenges in the evaluation for possible abuse: presentations of congenital bleeding disorders in childhood. *Child Abuse Negl.* 2012;36:127-134.
14. Lindberg D, Makoroff K, Harper N, et al. Utility of hepatic transaminases to recognize abuse in children. *Pediatrics.* 2009;124(2): 509-516.
15. American Academy of Pediatrics Section on Radiology. Diagnostic imaging of child abuse. *Pediatrics.* 2009;123(5):1430-1435.
16. Rubin DM, Christian CW, Bilaniuk L, et al. Occult head injury in high risk abused children. *Pediatrics.* 2003;111(6):1382-1386.
17. Sugar NF, Taylor JA, Feldman KW. Bruises in infants and toddlers: those who cruise rarely bruise. *Arch Pediatr Adolesc Med.* 1999;153: 399-403.
18. American Academy of Pediatrics, Committee on Child Abuse and Neglect: When inflicted skin injuries constitute child abuse. *Pediatrics.* 2002;110(3):644-645.
19. Dunstan FD, Guildea ZE, Kontos K, et al. A scoring system for bruise patterns: a tool for identifying abuse. *Arch Dis Child.* 2002; 86:330-333.
20. Maguire S, Mann MK, Sibert J, Kemp A. Can you age bruises accurately in children? A systematic review. *Arch Dis Child.* 2005;90:187-189.
21. Block RW, Krebs NF. Failure to thrive as a manifestation of child neglect. *Pediatrics.* 2005;116(5):1234-1237.
22. Anderst J, Kellogg N, Jung I. Is the diagnosis of physical abuse changed when Child Protective Services consults a Child Abuse Pediatrics subspecialty group as a second opinion? *Child Abuse Negl.* 2009;33(8):481-489.
23. American Academy of Pediatrics, Council on Child and Adolescent Health. The role of home-visitation programs in improving health outcomes for children and families. *Pediatrics.* 1998;101(3):486-489.
24. Barr RG, Barr M, Fujiwara T, et al. Do educational materials change knowledge and behavior about crying and shaken baby syndrome? A randomized controlled trial. *CMAJ.* 2009; 180(7):727-733.
25. Dubowitz H, Feigelman S, Lane W, Kim J. Pediatric primary care to help prevent child maltreatment: the safe environment for every kid (SEEK) model. *Pediatrics.* 2009;123(3):858-864.
26. Prinz RJ, Sanders MR, Shapiro CJ, et al. Population-based prevention of child maltreatment: the U.S. triple p system population trial. *Prev Sci.* 2009;10(1):1-12.
27. Timmer SG, Urquiza AJ, Zebell NM, McGrath JM. Parent-child interaction therapy: application to maltreating parent-child dyads. *Child Abuse Negl.* 2005;29(7):825-842.

9 CHILD SEXUAL ABUSE

Nancy D. Kellogg, MD
Maria D. McColgan, MD

PATIENT STORY

A 12-year-old girl is being seen for chronic abdominal pain by her family physician. The physician asks the mother to step out of the room and does a complete history including the HEADSS (home life, education level, activities, drug use, sexual activity, suicide ideation/attempts) questions. The girl tearfully reports that her stepfather has been touching her in her private areas when her mother is not home. On examination with a female nurse chaperone in the room, the physician finds that the girl's hymen initially appears normal (**Figure 9-1**). However, when the girl is more carefully examined with a cotton-tip applicator, a healed posterior hymenal transection is seen (**Figure 9-2**). When the girl is asked whether any other types of sexual abuse occurred with her stepfather, she admits to repeated penile penetration. Although rare, sometimes the examination reveals more than what the child is willing to disclose about the abuse. Partial disclosures of abuse are common in children. In addition, the findings of sexual abuse tend to be subtle and are easily missed if a careful examination and special techniques are not used. Attempts are made to reassure the girl that this should never happen and that this is not her fault. Her mother is brought back into the room and after a sensitive discussion, the police are called and Child Protective Services (CPS) notified.

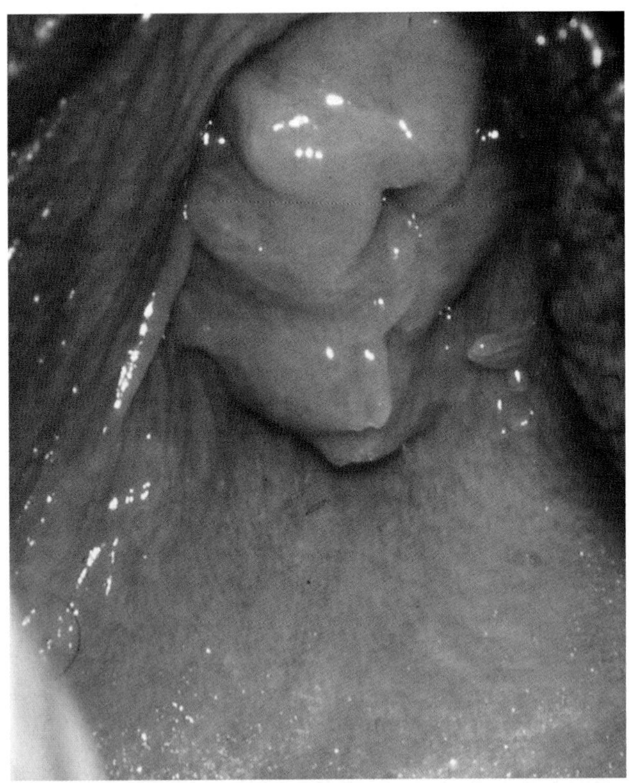

FIGURE 9-1 Typical appearance of the hymen and perihymenal tissues in a 12-year-old girl. Once females have entered puberty, the hymen becomes redundant with overlapping folds and is more difficult to examine for subtle signs of acute or healed injury. (*Used with permission from Nancy D. Kellogg, MD.*)

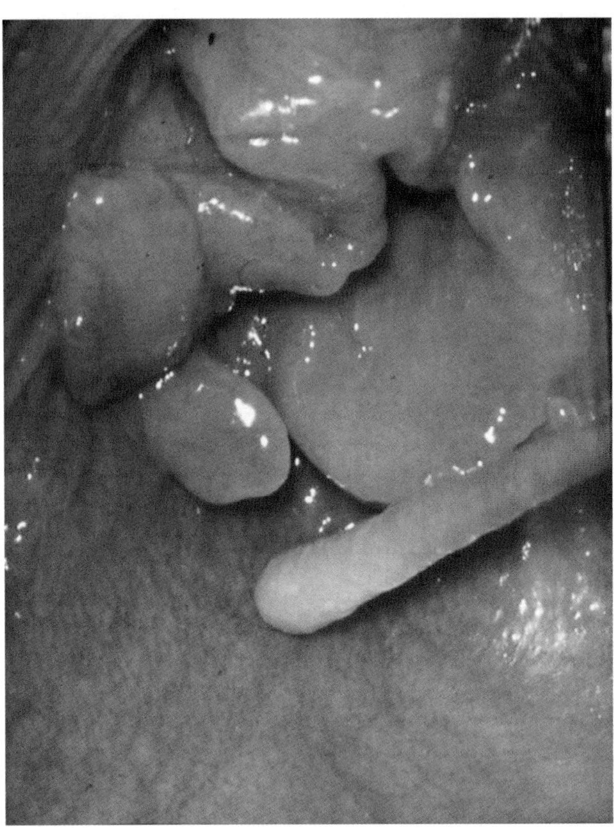

FIGURE 9-2 Hymenal cleft visible when the girl in **Figure 9-1** is more carefully examined using a saline moistened cotton-tip applicator to gently separate and demonstrate the edges of the hymen. This injury was caused by sexual abuse and may have been missed without the more careful examination. (*Used with permission from Nancy D. Kellogg, MD.*)

HEADSS is an acronym that provides a framework for interviewing adolescents and children about health risks. The questions start from easiest and least sensitive to more sensitive questions that need to be asked:

H—home

E—education

A—activities

D—depression and drugs

S—sex and sexual abuse

S—suicide

EPIDEMIOLOGY

- The US Department of Health and Human Services compilation of CPS data from 48 states in 2008 indicates there were 772,000 children confirmed as victims of abuse.[1] Of these, 9 percent were victims of sexual abuse. Not included in these numbers are several thousand additional victims who are sexually assaulted by nonfamily members; these cases are reported to law enforcement but not CPS.

- Sexual abuse of girls occurs at much higher rate than boys: 2.3 per 1000 females versus 0.6 per 1000 males.[2]
- Up to 50 percent of abusive sexual acts involve penetration of the vagina, anus, or oral cavity, or oral–genital contact.[3] In general, penetrative types of abuse are associated with poorer medical and mental health outcomes.

ETIOLOGY AND PATHOPHYSIOLOGY

Child sexual abuse occurs when a child is involved in sexual activities that he or she cannot comprehend, for which the child is developmentally unprepared and cannot or does not give consent, and/or that violate laws. All states have laws that require physicians to report a suspicion of abuse to child protection or law enforcement agencies.

Most sexual abuse involves an adult perpetrator the child knows and is expected to trust who uses deception and position of authority to gain the child's acquiescence and accommodation to the abuse;[4] it is not unusual for the abuse to progress from less to more severe and intrusive sexual acts, and for the child to wait months or years to disclose the abuse.

DIAGNOSIS

CLINICAL FEATURES

- Child victims of sexual abuse may have behavior changes, depression, increased sexual behaviors, somatic complaints (e.g., headaches or abdominal pain, constipation, enuresis/encopresis, genital/anal pain), or may be asymptomatic.
- Child may present to a medical provider for the following reasons:
  - Child has disclosed abuse (most common); it is rare for the abuse to be witnessed. Referrals to specialized programs with clinicians trained in the assessment of child sexual abuse is recommended, and are generally accessible in most areas of the US.
  - Caregiver suspects abuse and presents to the clinician because of behavioral or physical symptoms.
  - Child is brought for routine care and sexual abuse is suspected based on clinical findings (e.g., acute or healed genital injuries, vaginal discharge in a prepubertal child, lesions suggestive of human papillomavirus [HPV] or herpes simplex virus [HSV]).
- Recent studies show that less than 5 percent of child sexual abuse victims have physical examination findings indicative of penetrative trauma because the type of sexual act either does not result in tissue damage or because when tissue damage occurs, most injuries heal quickly and completely.[5–7] In a study of 36 pregnant adolescents, only two had evidence of penetrative trauma.[8] The medical diagnosis relies predominantly on the child's history and clinicians should remember that "normal" does not mean "nothing happened."
- Tips for doing the physical examination:
  - The anogenital inspection should utilize optimal direct light source, magnification, and appropriate examination positions and techniques.
  - Recommended examination positions include supine frogleg or lithotomy and prone knee-chest; the latter position is particularly important to confirm any posterior (between the 4 and 8 o'clock positions of the hymen in supine) defects of the hymen that are seen in supine position.
  - Various examination techniques include labial separation and traction (gently pulling the labia outward and inferiorly), gluteal lifting in prone knee-chest, and using cotton-tipped applicator for separating tissues.
  - In some cases, it may help to have an assistant gently squirt a small amount of nonbacteriostatic saline onto the hymen as the examiner uses gentle labial traction; this procedure is used to free folded hymenal edges.
  - A speculum examination and use of a cotton-tipped applicator to separate hymenal edges are traumatic procedures for prepubertal females and should not be used.
  - Most findings of anal trauma can be visualized by gently spreading the anal folds.
- Physical findings concerning for abuse include:[9]
  - Abrasions or bruising of the hymen, perihymenal structures, or anus (**Figures 9-3** and **9-4**).
  - Acute or healed tear in the posterior aspect of the hymen extending to, or nearly to, the base of the hymen or further to the posterior vestibule (**Figure 9-2**).
  - Anal bruising or lacerations (**Figure 9-5**).
  - Petechiae or bruising on the soft palate following a history of forced oral penetration.

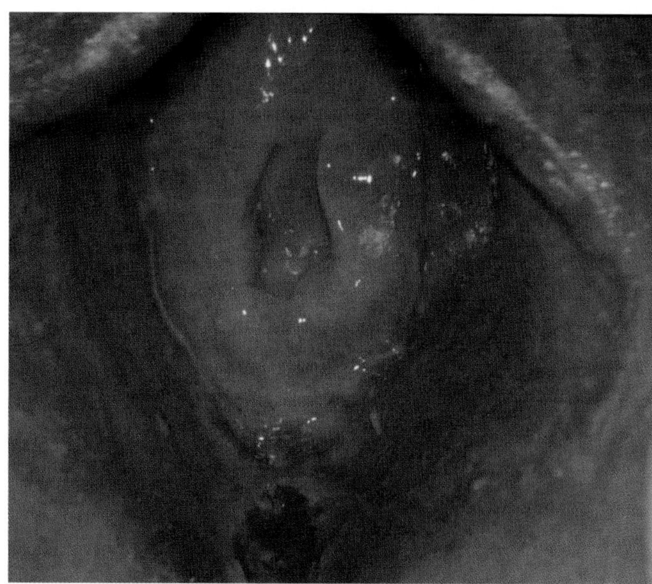

FIGURE 9-3 A 10-year-old girl with an acute tear of the posterior vestibule after recent sexual assault by a stranger. The posterior vestibule is the most common location for acute penetrative trauma in females. *(Used with permission from Nancy D. Kellogg, MD.)*

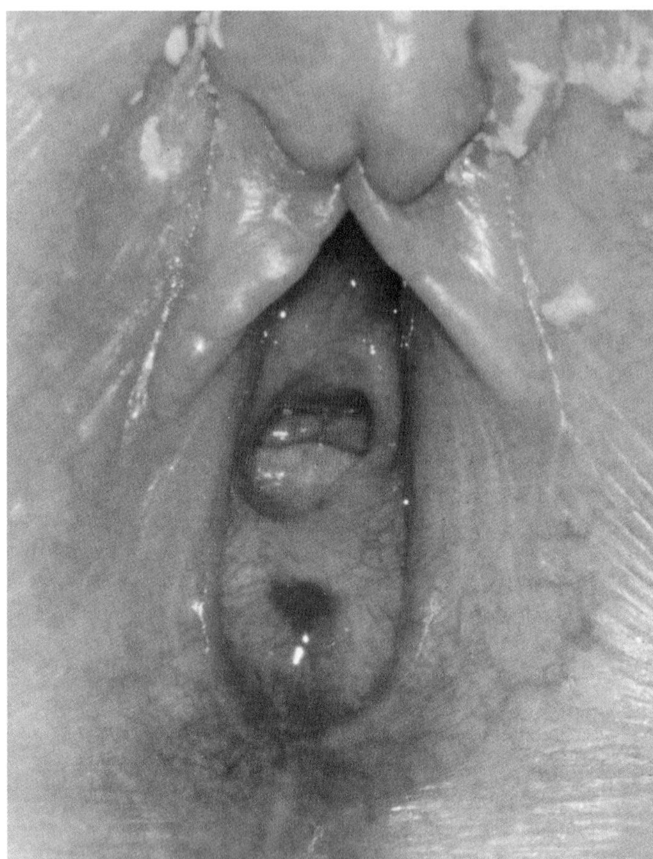

FIGURE 9-4 Acute hymenal hematoma in a prepubertal girl from penile penetration/contact. One reason why the considerable majority of examinations are normal may be that contact is more common than complete penetration and injuries resulting from penile contact are uncommon or are minor injuries that heal quickly and completely within days. (*Used with permission from Nancy D. Kellogg, MD.*)

LABORATORY TESTS AND IMAGING

- Forensic evidence collection if sexual assault occurred less than 72 to 96 hours (protocols vary from region to region) prior to clinical presentation (consider referring to an emergency department or rape crisis center skilled in performing forensic evidence collection on children).
- Approximately 5 percent of sexually abused children and adolescents acquire a sexually transmitted infection (STI) from the abuse[9] (**Figure 9-6**).
- Consider STI testing in all postpubescent patients and in prepubescent children with a history of genital contact with any orifice.
- HIV, hepatitis B (if unimmunized), rapid plasma reagin (RPR) (for syphilis), cultures or nucleic acid amplification tests (with confirmation) for chlamydia, and gonorrhea and culture or polymerase chain reaction (PCR) for trichomonas.
- Culture or PCR for HSV1 and HSV2 if ulcers or vesicles are present (**Figure 9-6**).
- Condylomata acuminata is a clinical diagnosis and biopsy is required only if lesions are atypical or resistant to treatment (molluscum contagiosum is a mimic and not sexually transmitted in children).

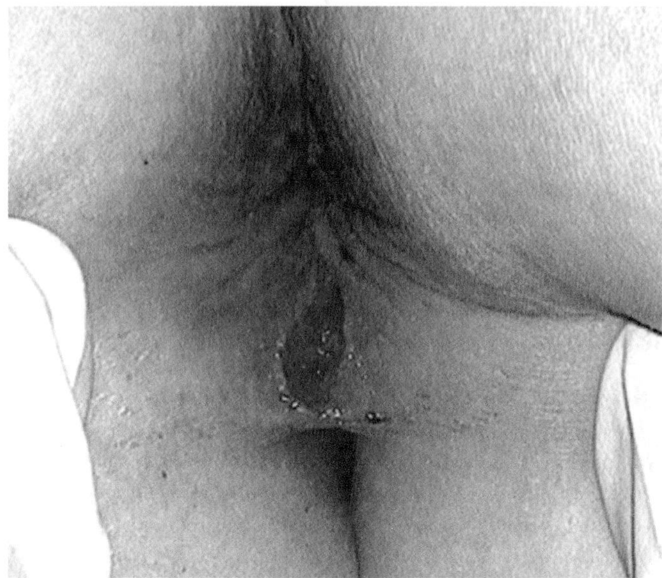

FIGURE 9-5 Acute rectal laceration in a young boy who was sexually abused by a relative. More than 95 percent of anal examinations in children with a history of anal penetration are normal or nonspecific. (*Used with permission from Nancy D. Kellogg, MD.*)

- Pregnancy testing in postpubescent children; consider prophylaxis (e.g., plan B) if the event occurred less than 96 hours prior to evaluation.
- Follow-up examinations 2 to 3 weeks after an acute assault to complete testing for STIs with prolonged incubation periods (especially HPV), assess resolution of injuries, and ensure emotional recovery.

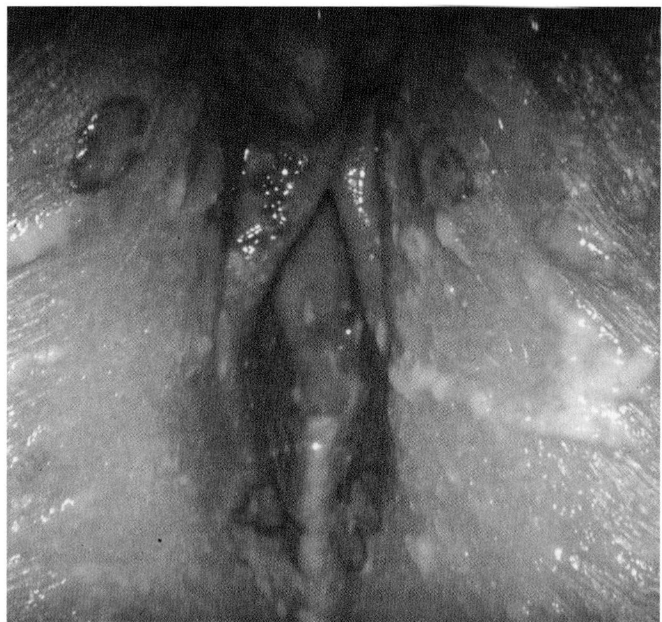

FIGURE 9-6 Herpes simplex virus (HSV) type 1 infection on the vulva of the prepubertal girl caused by sexual abuse. HSV type 1 of the genitals from sexual contact is increasing in prevalence relative to HSV type 2 infections of the genitals. (*Used with permission from Nancy D. Kellogg, MD.*)

DIFFERENTIAL DIAGNOSIS

In females, the following may be confused with abuse:

- Straddle injury (or other accidental trauma)—This occurs when a child falls onto an object. Bruising or lacerations to the labia majora, labia minora, or posterior fourchette may be seen. Although rare, accidental penetrating injury involving perihymenal tissues occurs, but rarely.
- Anatomic variants of normal, including shallow hymenal notches, anterior hymenal clefts, midline vestibule white lines, perineal defects, and narrow hymenal rims.
- Vulvar dermatitis—This may be caused by atopy, contact irritation, or seborrhea.
- Vulvovaginitis (e.g., nonspecific vaginal flora, shigella, streptococcus, poor hygiene, candidiasis)—Complaints include vaginal irritation or itching and vaginal discharge; wet prep and/or culture may be helpful.
- Lichen sclerosus et atrophicus is a cutaneous disease not caused by sexual abuse. It may present with bleeding, bruising, and/or vulvar itching, and the examination shows subepidermal hemorrhages and/or atrophic changes with areas of hypopigmentation over the vulva, perineum, and/or anus, an "hourglass" configuration (**Figure 9-7**).
- Anogenital irritation or bleeding—Causes may be infectious (pinworms, candidiasis, group B streptococcal infection), irritative (overgrowth of normal flora, sensitivity to laundry detergent or fabric softeners, sequelae of pubic hair shaving) or anatomic (urethral prolapse, dehiscence of a labial adhesion) (**Figure 9-8**).

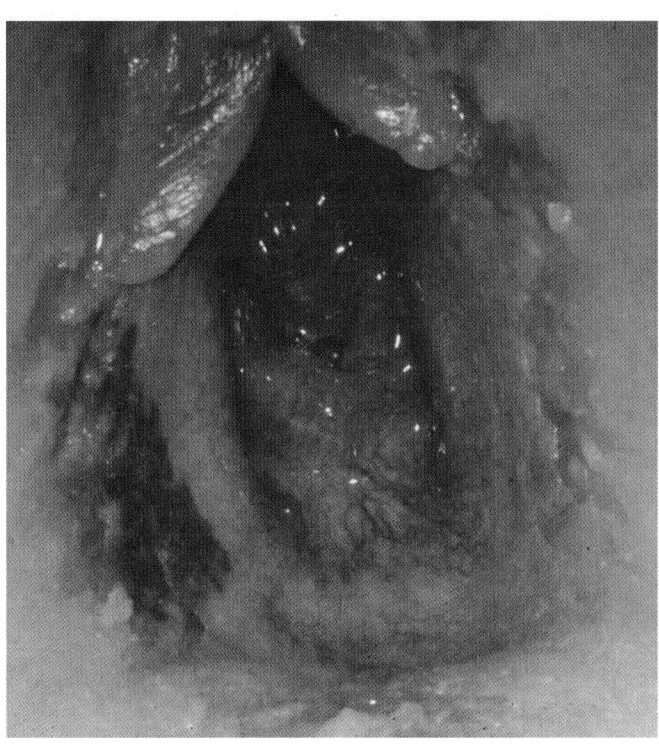

FIGURE 9-7 Lichen sclerosus et atrophicus in a young girl. This is a cutaneous disease, but commonly confused with sexual abuse because of the subepidermal hemorrhages. (*Used with permission from Nancy D. Kellogg, MD.*)

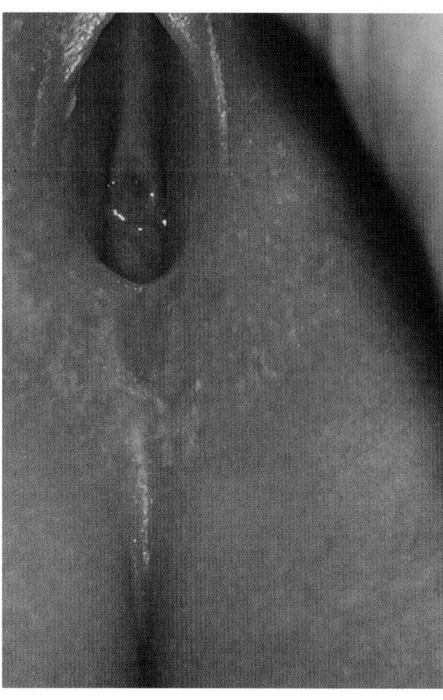

FIGURE 9-8 Labial adhesion can be confused with scarring secondary to child sexual abuse. This acquired condition is common in prepubertal girls and thought to be related to hygiene, irritation, and possibly trauma. The young girl is in supine frog-leg position. (*Used with permission from Nancy D. Kellogg, MD.*)

- Normal physiologic leukorrhea—Scant, whitish tenacious discharge in pubertal females. Wet mount is normal.

In males, the following may be confused with abuse:

- Accidental trauma (e.g., penis caught in zipper)—History should support pattern of injury. Most intentionally inflicted injuries of male genitals are physical, not sexual, abuse.
- Phimosis—Unretractable foreskin. Irritation and redness occurs as a result of trapped debris.
- Additional findings that may be confused with abuse:
- Anal fissure(s), which is a superficial excoriation or tear that extends from the anal verge into the anal canal, may or may not cause pain or bleeding during bowel movements. Sometimes, but not always, associated with diarrhea or constipation.
- Perianal venous pooling is sometimes mistaken for bruising.

MANAGEMENT

- Children may present with nonspecific behavioral and physical symptoms (but no disclosure of abuse) that include chronic stomachaches or headaches, school difficulties, mood changes, and sleeping difficulties. These children should be questioned in a careful and nonleading manner about the possibility of sexual abuse. For example, the clinician may state: "I treat other children who have problems like you do with school and headaches. Some of these children have told me about things that have happened to their body or feelings that made them sad, scared, or confused. Has anything like that ever happened to you?"

- Take a history from the child if necessary to make a medical diagnosis and to determine appropriate testing, treatment, and the need to report suspected abuse to child protection or law enforcement. The clinician may opt not to take a history if the child was or will be interviewed elsewhere; in this case, information necessary to determine what type of medical assessment and testing should be obtained from other sources.
  - Ensure that the parent is not in the room for the history. Parents may be present for the physical examination.
  - Use open-ended questions, such as "What happened?" or "Tell me more . . ." as opposed to suggestive questions such as "Did Daddy touch your private parts?"
  - Take careful notes and document with quotations whenever possible.
- Conduct a full physical examination including genitalia. Elicit cooperation from the child by explaining all procedures and earning his or her trust.
- Consider STI and pregnancy prophylaxis for postpubertal patients.
- Withhold STI treatment in asymptomatic prepubescent children until STI tests are confirmed positive, as the incidence of STI in asymptomatic prepubertal children is relatively low.
- Consult with an infectious disease specialist regarding HIV prophylaxis. If HIV prevalence is high in local regions, assailant risk factors are unknown or high for HIV, and if the child is evaluated within 72 hours of a high-risk exposure, then HIV prophylaxis may be appropriate.
- Examine closely for signs of physical and emotional abuse and neglect.

FOLLOW-UP

- Laws vary by state; however, all states have mandated reporting laws (see Child Welfare Information Gateway—http://www.childwelfare.gov/).
- All victims of sexual abuse and their families should be referred to local counseling agencies and to a Children's Advocacy Center, or other child abuse agency if available in the community.

PATIENT EDUCATION

At well-child visits, provider should discuss touches that make children sad, scared, or confused, or that give them an "uh-oh" feeling inside, and encourage parents to reinforce these themes at home.

PATIENT RESOURCES

- Child Help—**http://childhelp.org/**.
- National Child Abuse Hotline—**1-800-422-4453**.
- Prevent Child Abuse America—**http://www.preventchildabuse.org/index.shtml**.
- National Center for Missing and Exploited Children—**http://www.missingkids.com/**.

PROVIDER RESOURCES

- The American Academy of Pediatrics Guidelines for the Evaluation of Sexual Abuse of Children—**http://pediatrics.aappublications.org/content/103/1/186.full**.
- National Guideline Clearing House—When to suspect child maltreatment. **http://www.guideline.gov/content.aspx?id=15523**.
- Child Welfare Information Gateway provides state statutes on child abuse and neglect—**http://www.childwelfare.gov/systemwide/laws_policies/state/can/**.

REFERENCES

1. U.S. Department of Health and Human Services: Administration of Children, Youth and Families. *Child Maltreatment: 2008*. Washington, DC: Government Printing Office; 2010.
2. U.S. Department of Health and Human Services, Youth and Families: *Child Maltreatment 1998*. Washington, DC: Government Printing Office; 1999.
3. Finkelhor D. Current information on the scope and nature of child sexual abuse. *Future Child.* 1994;4(2):31-53.
4. Summit R. Child sexual abuse accommodation syndrome. *Child Abuse Negl.* 1983;7(2):177-193.
5. Berenson AB, Chacko MR, Weimann CM, et al. A case-control study of anatomic changes resulting from sexual abuse. *Am J Obstet Gynecol.* 2000;182(4):820-831.
6. Heger A, Ticson L, Velasquez O, et al. Children referred for possible sexual abuse: Medical findings in 2384 children. *Child Abuse Negl.* 2002;26(6–7):645-659.
7. Adams JA, Harper K, Knudson S, Revilla J. Examination findings in legally confirmed child sexual abuse: It's normal to be normal. *Pediatrics.* 1994;94(3):310-317.
8. Kellogg ND, Menard SW, Santos A. Genital anatomy in pregnant adolescents: "normal" does not mean "nothing happened." *Pediatrics.* 2004;113(1):e67-e69.
9. Kellogg ND. The evaluation of sexual abuse in children. *Pediatrics.* 2005;116(2):506-512.

PART 4

OPHTHALMOLOGY

Strength of Recommendation (SOR)	Definition
A	Recommendation based on consistent and good-quality patient-oriented evidence.*
B	Recommendation based on inconsistent or limited-quality patient-oriented evidence.*
C	Recommendation based on consensus, usual practice, opinion, disease-oriented evidence, or case series for studies of diagnosis, treatment, prevention, or screening.*

*See Appendix A on pages 1320–1322 for further information.

10 HORDEOLUM AND CHALAZION

Heidi Chumley, MD

PATIENT STORY

A 5-year-old girl presented with a tender nodule on the lower eyelid for 3 days (**Figure 10-1**). The clinician diagnosed an external hordeolum (stye) and recommended that the mother apply warm moist compresses to the affected eyelid 4 times a day. Her hordeolum resolved within 7 days.

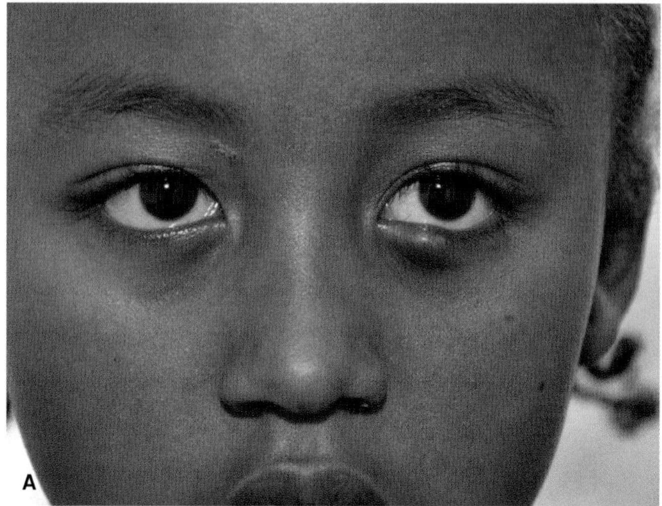

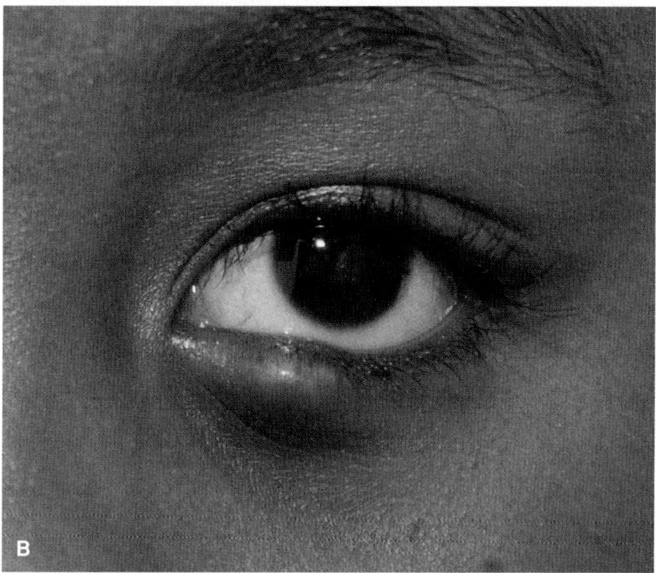

FIGURE 10-1 **A.** External hordeolum on the lower eyelid of a 5-year-old girl. **B.** Close-up showing eyelid swelling. (*Used with permission from Richard P. Usatine, MD.*)

INTRODUCTION

A hordeolum is an acute painful infection of the glands of the eyelid, usually caused by bacteria. Hordeola can be located on the internal or external eyelid. Internal hordeola that do not completely resolve become cysts called chalazia. External hordeola are commonly known as styes.

SYNONYMS

Stye (external hordeolum).

EPIDEMIOLOGY

- Unclear incidence or prevalence in the US, but often stated to be more common in school-age children.
- In one study of school-age children in Brazil, the prevalence of chalazion was found to be 0.2 percent and that of hordeolum was 0.3 percent.[1]

ETIOLOGY AND PATHOPHYSIOLOGY

HORDEOLUM (ACUTELY TENDER NODULE IN THE EYE)

- Infection in the meibomian gland (internal hordeolum), often resolves into a chalazion (**Figure 10-1**).
- Infection in the Zeiss or Moll gland (external hordeolum) (**Figures 10-2** and **10-3**).
- *Staphylococcus aureus* is the causative agent in most cases.

CHALAZION

- Meibomian gland becomes blocked, often in a patient with blepharitis.
- Blocked meibomian gland's duct releases gland contents into the soft tissue of eyelid.
- Gland contents cause a lipogranulomatous reaction (**Figure 10-4**).

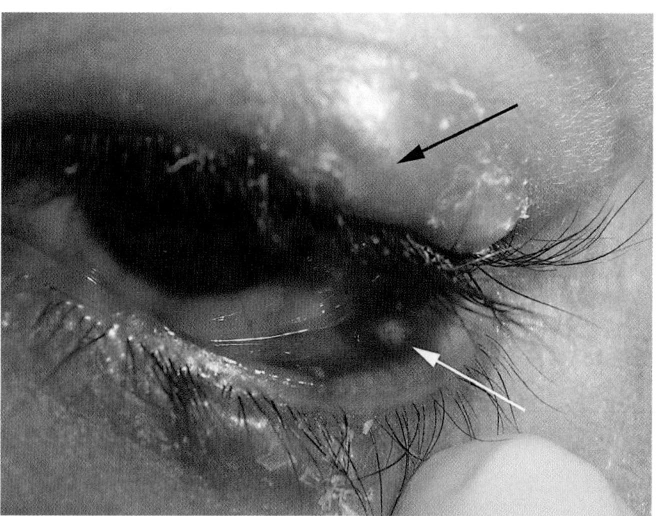

FIGURE 10-2 External hordeolum (*black arrow*) and an internal hordeolum (*white arrow*). (*Used with permission from Richard P. Usatine, MD.*)

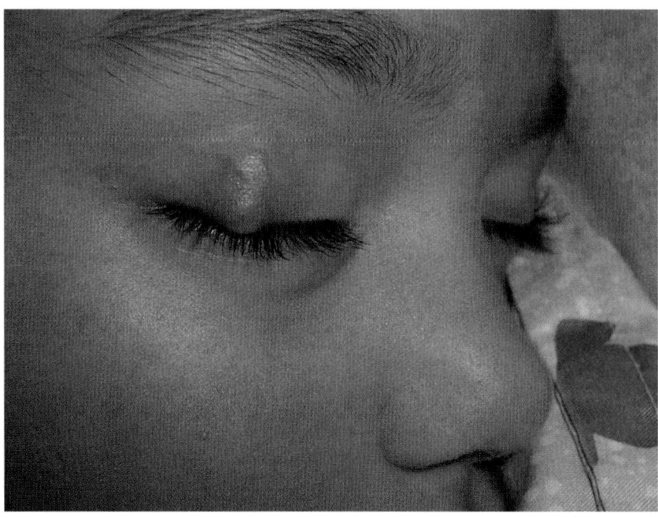

FIGURE 10-3 External hordeolum with disruption of the normal contour of the eyelid. (*Used with permission from Richard P. Usatine, MD.*)

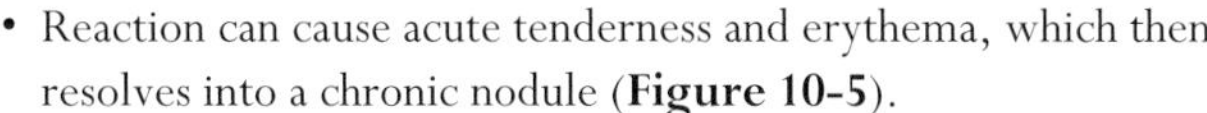

- Reaction can cause acute tenderness and erythema, which then resolves into a chronic nodule (**Figure 10-5**).

RISK FACTORS

- Hordeolum: *S. aureus* blepharitis, previous hordeolum.
- Chalazion: Seborrheic blepharitis and rosacea.

DIAGNOSIS

- Chalazion and hordeolum are clinical diagnoses.
- Chalazion is a nontender nodule on the eyelid.
- Hordeolum.

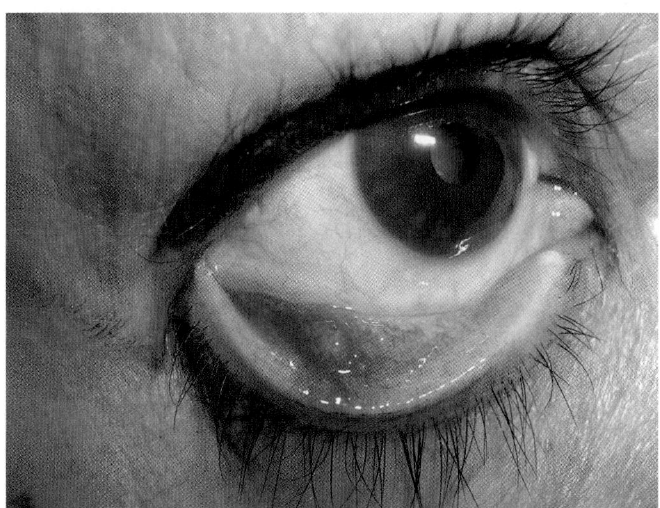

FIGURE 10-4 Chalazion viewed from internal eyelid showing the yellow lipogranulomatous material. (*Used with permission from Richard P. Usatine, MD.*)

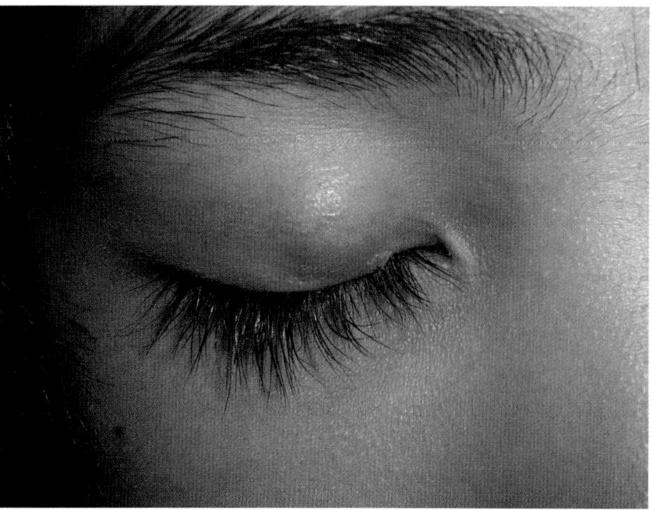

FIGURE 10-5 Chalazion present for 4 months on the upper eyelid of a young girl with minimal symptoms but cosmetically unappealing. (*Used with permission from Richard P. Usatine, MD.*)

  - Tenderness and erythema localized to a point on the eyelid (**Figures 10-1** to **10-3**).
  - Conjunctival injection may be present.
  - Fever, preauricular nodes, and vision changes should be absent.
  - Laboratory tests are generally not indicated.

DIFFERENTIAL DIAGNOSIS

- Xanthelasma—Yellowish plaques, generally near medial canthus (see Chapter 193, Hyperlipidemia).
- Molluscum contagiosum—Waxy nodules with central umbilication; generally multiple (see Chapter 115, Molluscum Contagiosum).

MANAGEMENT

- Hordeolum (internal):
  - No studies of nonsurgical interventions (compresses, lid scrubs, antibiotics, or steroids) met criteria for inclusion in a Cochrane study. No evidence for or against nonsurgical interventions for acute internal hordeolum.[1] SOR Ⓐ
  - Treat as described in the following section for external hordeolum.
- Hordeolum (external):
  - Warm soaks, 3 to 4 times a day for 15 minutes, will elicit drainage in most cases. SOR Ⓒ
  - Topical antibiotics (e.g., bacitracin ophthalmic ointment) may be beneficial for recurrent or spontaneously draining hordeolum. SOR Ⓒ
  - Cases that do not respond to warm soaks or that are extremely painful and swollen may be incised and drained with a small incision using a #11 blade. Make the incision on either the internal or external eyelid depending on where the hordeolum is pointing. A chalazion clamp can be used to protect the globe from damage. SOR Ⓑ

 - Antibiotics do not provide benefit after incision and drainage.[3] SOR B
 - Systemic antibiotics are usually not needed unless patient has preseptal cellulitis. SOR C
- Chalazion
 - Can be treated conservatively with lid hygiene and warm compresses. Warm compresses can be applied 2 to 3 times daily but may take weeks to months to work. SOR C
 - One study demonstrated a 58 percent response rate of 1 percent topical chloramphenicol with warm compresses.[3] SOR B
 - Higher percentages of resolution can be achieved with either incision and curettage or injection with steroid (e.g., 0.3 mL triamcinolone acetonide) (80% to 92%).[4–6] SOR B The chalazion is usually drained from the internal eyelid using a chalazion clamp to protect the globe. After anesthetizing the area, a #11 blade is carefully used to open the chalazion. A chalazion curette helps to scoop out the lipogranulomatous material. No suturing is needed.
 - A study of 106 patients compared triamcinolone injection, incision and curettage, and warm compresses, and found resolution rates of 84 percent, 87 percent, and 46 percent, respectively.[6] SOR B
 - One study demonstrated a better response to incision and curettage in the following situations: patients 35.1 years of age or older, with lesion duration equal to or greater than 8.5 months and size equal to or greater than 11.4 mm.[5] SOR B

REFERRAL

Refer to an ophthalmologist if the hordeolum or chalazion is interfering with vision and not responding to therapy. If a surgical intervention is needed and you lack experience doing such a procedure, refer to ophthalmology. Recurrent chalazia due to underlying blepharitis raises a concern for ocular rosacea and should prompt a referral to ophthalmology (see Chapter 97, Rosacea).

PREVENTION

Eyelid hygiene (keeping the area around the eyelid clean) may prevent hordeola.

PROGNOSIS

Chalazia can persist for years if untreated (**Figure 10-6**). Some patients are prone to recurrence of hordeola and chalazia.

FOLLOW-UP

A hordeolum with significant purulence and swelling should be reevaluated in 2 to 3 days or referred to an ophthalmologist. Warm compresses are slow to work for a chalazion, so follow-up should be no sooner than 1 month if nonsurgical treatment is prescribed.

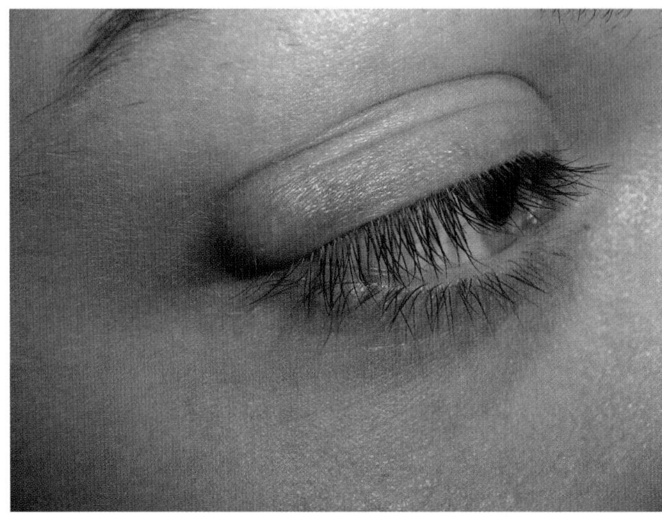

FIGURE 10-6 Chalazion in a 14-year-old girl. This eyelid swelling had been there for one year at the time of presentation. She had no pain but was unhappy with the appearance. (*Used with permission from Richard P. Usatine, MD.*)

PATIENT EDUCATION

Hordeolum commonly responds to warm soaks and topical antibiotics. It often recurs and can develop into a chronic chalazion, which may need to be treated with surgical removal or a steroid injection.

PATIENT RESOURCES

- The American Academy of Ophthalmology—**http://www.geteyesmart.org/eyesmart/diseases/chalazion-stye/index.cfm**.
- The American Academy of Family Physicians has a patient handout in English or Spanish on stye—**www.familydoctor.org/familydoctor/en/diseases-conditions/sty.html.**

PROVIDER RESOURCES

- *Hordeolum and Stye in Emergency Medicine*—**www.emedicine.medscape.com/article/798940**.
- *Chalazion*—**http://emedicine.medscape.com/article/1212709**.
- *Chalazion Injection Demonstration*—**www.youtube.com/watch?v=yYCCkDZwKgg**.
- *Chalazion Incision and Curettage*—**www.youtube.com/watch?v=tdKw_zjYCf8**.

REFERENCES

1. Garcia CA, Pinheiro FI, Montenegro DA, et al. Prevalence of biomicroscopic findings in the anterior segment and ocular adnexa among schoolchildren in Natal, Brazil. *Arq Bras Oftalmol.* 2005;68(2):167-170.

2. Lindsley K, Nichols JJ, Dickersin K. Interventions for acute internal hordeolum. *Cochrane Database Syst Rev.* 2010;(9):CD00742.
3. Hirunwiwatkul P, Wachirasereechai K. Effectiveness of combined antibiotic ophthalmic solution in the treatment of hordeolum after incision and curettage: a randomized, placebo-controlled trial: a pilot study. *J Med Assoc Thai.* 2005;88(5):647-650.
4. Chung CF, Lai JS, Li PS. Subcutaneous extralesional triamcinolone acetonide injection versus conservative management in the treatment of chalazion. *Hong Kong Med J.* 2006;12(4):278-281.
5. Ahmad S, Baig MA, Khan MA, et al. Intralesional corticosteroid injection vs surgical treatment of chalazia in pigmented patients. *J Coll Physicians Surg Pak.* 2006;16(1):42-44.
6. Goawalla A, Lee V. A prospective randomized treatment study comparing three treatment options for chalazia: triamcinolone acetonide injections, incision and curettage and treatment with hot compresses. *Clin Experiment Ophthalmol.* 2007;35(8):706-712.
7. Dhaliwal U, Bhatia A. A rationale for therapeutic decision-making in chalazia. *Orbit.* 2005;24(4):227-230.

11 CORNEAL FOREIGN BODY AND CORNEAL ABRASION

Heidi Chumley, MD
Kelly Green, MD

PATIENT STORY

An 8-year-old boy was poked in the eye with a small branch while hiking with his cub scout pack. He presented with pain, tearing, photophobia, and a foreign body sensation. Fluorescein application demonstrated a green area under cobalt-blue filtered light (**Figure 11-1**). Careful inspection with magnification, including eversion of the upper eyelid, revealed no foreign body. He was treated with antibiotic eye drops. He showed improvement the next day and over time had complete resolution.

INTRODUCTION

Corneal abrasions are often the result of eye trauma and can cause an inflammatory response and significant pain. Corneal abrasions are detected using fluorescein and a UV light. A corneal foreign body can be seen during a careful physical examination with a good light source or slit lamp. Nonpenetrating foreign bodies can be removed by an experienced physician in the office using topical anesthesia. Refer all penetrating foreign bodies to an ophthalmologist.

SYNONYMS

Corneal abrasion is sometimes referred to as a corneal epithelial defect.

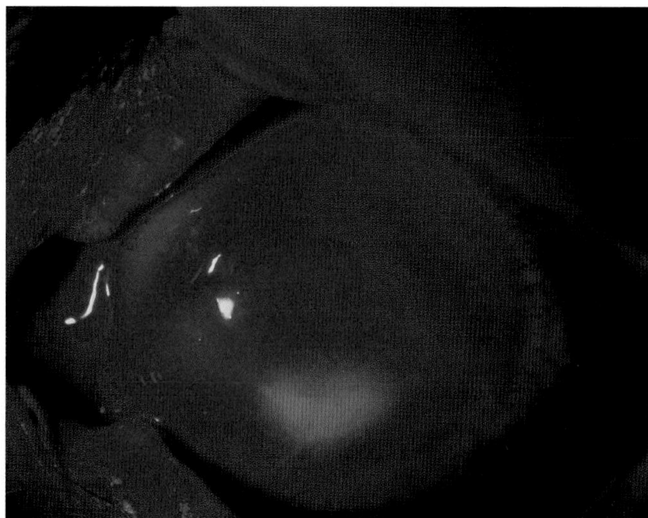

FIGURE 11-1 Fluorescein stains green, indicating corneal abrasion. *(Used with permission from Paul D. Comeau.)*

EPIDEMIOLOGY

- Corneal abrasion with or without foreign body is common; however, the prevalence or incidence of corneal abrasion in the general pediatric population is unknown.
- Corneal abrasion is the most common eye injury for children presenting to an emergency room.[1]

ETIOLOGY AND PATHOPHYSIOLOGY

- The cornea overlies the anterior chamber and iris and provides barrier protection, filters UV light, and refracts light onto the retina.
- Abrasions in the cornea are typically caused by direct injury from a foreign body, resulting in an inflammatory reaction.
- The inflammatory reaction causes the symptoms and can persist for several days after the foreign object is out. Typically in children, the corneal abrasion heals more rapidly than in adults.

RISK FACTORS

- Participation in sports such as hockey, lacrosse, or racquetball raises the risk of corneal abrasions from ocular trauma.[2]
- Ventilated neonates (as a result of mask pressure on the orbit) or sedated patients (as a result of disruption of the blink reflex, and subsequent corneal exposure) are at increased risk for corneal abrasions.[2]

Contact lenses, especially soft extended wear, increase the risk of developing an infected abrasion that ulcerates.[2] Any contact lens wearer with a corneal abrasion should see an ophthalmologist, due to the high risk of permanent vision loss due to infection.

DIAGNOSIS

CLINICAL FEATURES

▶ History and physical

- History of ocular trauma or eye rubbing (although corneal abrasions can occur with no trauma history and young children may not accurately report trauma).
- Symptoms of pain, eye redness, photophobia, and a foreign-body sensation.
- Foreign body seen with direct visualization or a slit lamp (**Figures 11-2** and **11-3**).
- Fluorescein application demonstrates green area (which represents the disruption in the corneal epithelium) under cobalt-blue filtered light (**Figure 11-1**).
- History of contact lens wear.
- History of ocular or perioral herpes virus infection.

LABORATORY TESTING

- Culture by an ophthalmologist if an abrasion with infection (corneal ulcer) is suspected.

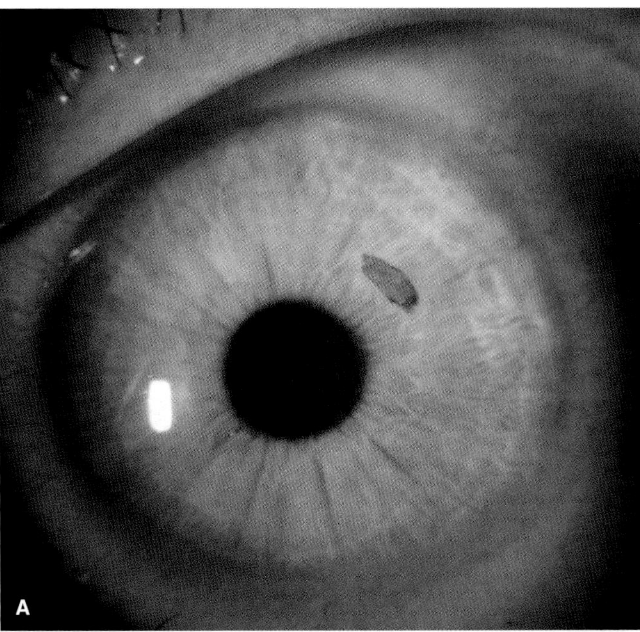

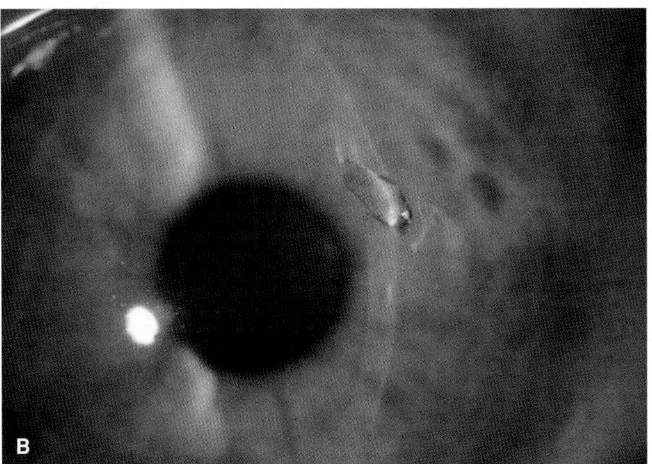

FIGURE 11-2 **A.** Wood chip is visible in the cornea on close inspection of the eye. **B.** Slit-lamp examination reveals this wood chip has penetrated the cornea. (*Used with permission from Paul D. Comeau.*)

IMAGING

- If physical examination is equivocal, imaging may be useful to determine if a foreign body has perforated the cornea. An object that has fully perforated the cornea has passed through the cornea and will be located in the anterior segment or posterior segment of the eye, making it difficult to see without imaging technology. The most important question to answer is the following: what is the mechanism of injury? If there is a chance of an intraocular foreign body, proceed with imaging. On exam, it is important to note apparent disruption of other ocular structures, such as the iris. If there is gross blood in the anterior chamber with history of mechanism of injury which could lead to intraocular foreign body, consider imaging.
- CT or spiral CT can detect nonmetallic and metallic foreign bodies.
  - A metallic foreign body can be seen on an orbital radiograph. Avoid MRI if the history suggests the foreign body may be metallic. Ultrasound and ultrasound biomicroscopy can also aid in visualization of intraocular foreign bodies and may be useful in some cases.

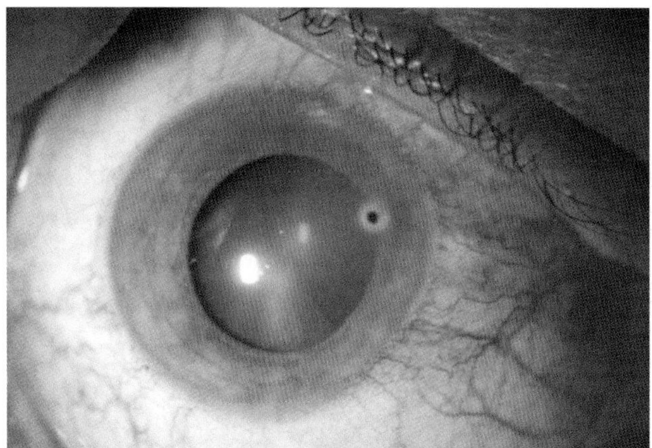

FIGURE 11-3 Metallic foreign body with rust ring within the corneal stroma and conjunctival injection. (*Used with permission from Paul D. Comeau.*)

DIFFERENTIAL DIAGNOSIS

- Uveitis or iritis—Usually no history of trauma, with unilateral 360-degree perilimbal injection, eye pain, photophobia, and vision loss (see Chapter 13, Uveitis and Iritis).
- Keratitis or corneal ulcerations—Diffuse erythema with ciliary injection often with miosis; eye discharge; pain, photophobia, and vision loss depending on the location of ulceration (**Figures 11-4** and **11-5**). There is often a history of trauma, herpes simplex virus (HSV), or contact lens wear. Patients should see an ophthalmologist urgently.
- Conjunctivitis—Conjunctival injection; eye discharge; gritty or uncomfortable feeling; no vision loss, history of respiratory infection, or contacts with others who have red eyes (see Chapter 12, Conjunctivitis).

MANAGEMENT

NONPHARMACOLOGIC

- Confirm diagnosis with fluorescein and a UV light (for abrasion) if no foreign body is readily visible (see **Figure 11-4**).

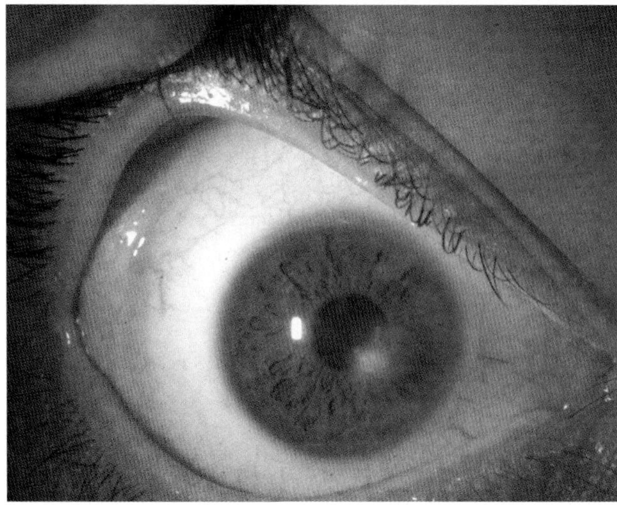

FIGURE 11-4 Small corneal ulcer in the visual axis. (*Used with permission from Paul D. Comeau.*)

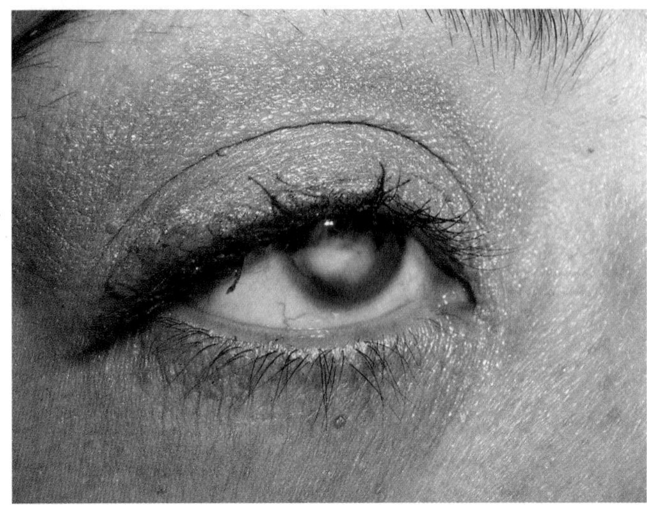

FIGURE 11-5 Large corneal scar from previous ulcerations secondary to contact lens use. The scar obscures the visual axis and this young patient is awaiting a corneal transplant. (*Used with permission from Richard P. Usatine, MD.*)

- Carefully inspect for a foreign body. Evert the upper eyelid for full visualization. Slit-lamp visualization may be needed to determine if the cornea has been penetrated (see **Figure 11-2**). Note that foreign bodies can frequently lodge in the superior tarsal conjunctiva and must be removed, lest they continue to abrade the cornea.
- Remove (or refer for removal) nonpenetrating foreign bodies. Apply a topical anesthetic, such as proparacaine or tetracaine. Remove with irrigation, a wet cotton-tipped applicator, or a fine-gauge needle at the slit lamp.
- Remove contact lenses until cornea is healed.[3] SOR Ⓒ
- Avoid patching in corneal abrasions smaller than 10 mm; it does not help.[4] SOR Ⓐ

MEDICATIONS

- Consider topical ophthalmic NSAIDs for pain if needed.[5,6] SOR Ⓐ While the evidence for this intervention of pain relief is relatively good, there are some risks to their use and these medications can be costly. They do not speed healing and oral analgesics can be used for pain.
- Consider topical antibiotics. SOR Ⓒ Chloramphenicol ointment reduced the risk of recurrent ulcer in a prospective, non-placebo, controlled trial.[7] Although chloramphenicol is rarely used in the US, other ophthalmic antibiotics, such as erythromycin ointment, are used for corneal abrasions. SOR Ⓒ While there is an epithelial defect, there is risk for infection/ulceration. The choice of whether or not to use antibiotics can be based upon the mechanism of injury. Small abrasions can be treated with lubrication with artificial tears and over-the-counter ophthalmic ointments until the abrasion heals.

REFERRAL

- Refer penetrating foreign bodies to an experienced eye surgeon.

PREVENTION

Eye protection should be worn for high-risk occupational and recreational activities.

PROGNOSIS

Prognosis is generally good. Development of infection or a rust ring worsens prognosis.

FOLLOW-UP

See all patients in 24 hours for reassessment. If there is no improvement, look for an initially overlooked foreign body or a full-thickness injury. Do not hesitate to refer to ophthalmology if the patient is not improving.

PATIENT EDUCATION

- Advise children (and their parents) who play sports, such as racquetball or hockey, to wear eye protection for primary prevention.
- Advise patients with corneal abrasions that healing usually occurs within 2 to 3 days, and they should report persistent pain, redness, and photophobia.
- Patients should be advised not to sleep in contact lenses, even if labeled "extended wear."

PATIENT RESOURCES

- FamilyDoctor.org. Patient handout on *Corneal Abrasions*—**http://familydoctor.org/familydoctor/en/prevention-wellness/staying-healthy/first-aid/corneal-abrasions.html**.

PROVIDER RESOURCES

- Cao C. *Corneal Foreign Body Removal*—**http://emedicine.medscape.com/article/82717**.

REFERENCES

1. Michael JG, Hug D, Dowd MD. Management of corneal abrasion in children: a randomized clinical trial. *Ann Emerg Med*. 2002;40:67-72
2. Wilson SA, Last A. Management of corneal abrasions. *Am Fam Physician*. 2004;1(70):123-128.
3. Weissman BA. *Care of the Contact Lens Patient: Reference Guide for Clinicians*. St Louis, MO: American Optometric Association; 2000.
4. Turner A, Rabiu M. Patching for corneal abrasion. *Cochrane Database Syst Rev*. 2006 Apr 19;(2):CD004764.
5. Smith CH, Goldman RD. Topical nonsteroidal anti-inflammatory drugs for corneal abrasions in children. *Can Fam Physician*. 2012;58(7):748-9.
6. Calder LA, Balasubramanian S, Fergusson D. Topical nonsteroidal anti-inflammatory drugs for corneal abrasions: meta-analysis of randomized trials. *Acad Emerg Med*. 2005 May;12(5):467-73.
7. Upadhyaya MP, Karmacharyaa PC, Kairalaa S, et al. The Bhaktapur eye study: ocular trauma and antibiotic prophylaxis for the prevention of corneal ulceration in Nepal. *Br J Ophthalmol*. 2001;85: 388-392.

12 CONJUNCTIVITIS

Heidi Chumley, MD
Richard P. Usatine, MD
Kelly Green, MD

PATIENT STORY

A 4-year-old boy woke up with one eye matted shut. The child's parents cleared the matted material with a warm washcloth and brought the child into the doctor's office. The child indicates discomfort but not pain. The child and the parents believe the child's vision is fine. On examination, the child is afebrile with conjunctival injection, lid swelling and purulent discharge in the left eye (**Figure 12-1**). Vision testing is normal. Based on the age of the child and the purulence of the discharge, bacterial conjunctivitis was diagnosed and antibiotic drops were prescribed.

INTRODUCTION

Conjunctivitis, inflammation of the membrane lining the eyelids and globe, presents with injected pink or red eye(s), eye discharge ranging from mild to purulent, eye discomfort or gritty sensation, and no vision loss. Conjunctivitis is most commonly infectious (viral or bacterial) or allergic, but can be caused by irritants. Diagnosis is clinical, based on differences in symptoms and signs.

SYNONYMS

Pink eye.

EPIDEMIOLOGY

- Infectious conjunctivitis is common and often occurs in outbreaks, making the prevalence difficult to estimate.
- In the US, the estimated annual incidence rate for bacterial conjunctivitis is 135 per 10,000 people, with 23 percent, 28 percent and 13 percent of cases occurring in children ages 0 to 2, 3 to 9, and 10 to 19, respectively.[1]
- Viral conjunctivitis is far more common than bacterial conjunctivitis.
- Allergic conjunctivitis in children and adults had a point prevalence of 6.4 percent and a lifetime prevalence of 40 percent in a large population study in the US from 1988 to 1994.[2]

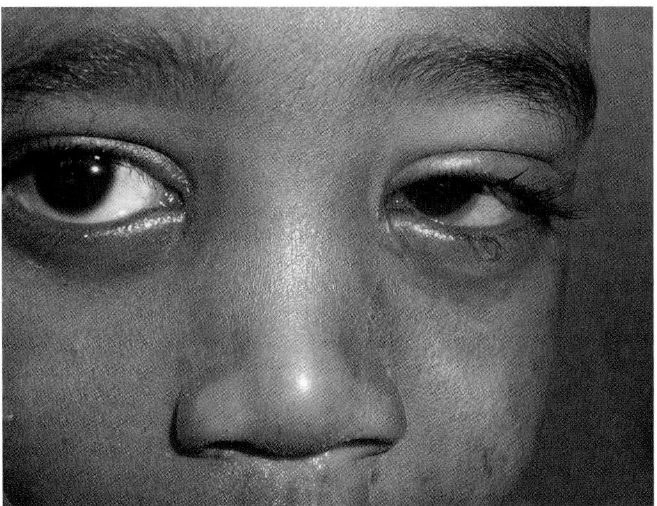

FIGURE 12-1 Unilateral conjunctivitis in a 4-year-old child. The child's age and purulent discharge are consistent with a bacterial etiology. *(Used with permission from Richard P. Usatine, MD.)*

ETIOLOGY AND PATHOPHYSIOLOGY

Conjunctivitis is predominately infectious (bacterial or viral) or allergic, and the most common etiologies vary by age.

- Neonatal conjunctivitis is often caused by *Chlamydia trachomatis* and *Neisseria gonorrhoeae*.[3]
- Children younger than 6 years are more likely to have a bacterial than viral conjunctivitis. In the US, the most common bacterial causes are *Haemophilus* species and *Streptococcus pneumoniae* accounting for almost 90 percent of cases in children.[4,5]
- Children age 6 years or older are more likely to have viral or allergic causes for conjunctivitis.[4] Adenovirus is the most common viral cause.

DIAGNOSIS

- To distinguish conjunctivitis from other causes of a red eye, ask about pain and check for vision loss. Patients with a red eye and intense pain or vision loss that does not clear with blinking are unlikely to have conjunctivitis and should undergo further evaluation.
- Always ask about contact lens use as this can be a risk factor for all types of conjunctivitis, including bacterial conjunctivitis. Any patient who uses contact lenses should remove the lenses from both eyes in the event of any sort of red eye complaint. The patient should see an ophthalmologist.
- Typical clinical features of any type of conjunctivitis may include eye discharge, gritty or uncomfortable feeling, one or both pink eyes, and no vision loss. The infection usually starts in one eye, and progresses to involve the other eye days later.
- Viral conjunctivitis often presents with two pink eyes and minimal discharge (**Figure 12-2**).
- Bacterial conjunctivitis (**Figures 12-1**, **12-3**, and **12-4**) has a more purulent discharge than viral or allergic conjunctivitis.
- In one study, 96 percent of children, presenting to an emergency room, with a history of gluey or sticky eyelids and a purulent discharge noted on physical examination had bacterial conjunctivitis.[5]
- Allergic conjunctivitis is typically bilateral and accompanied by eye itching. Giant papillary conjunctivitis is a type of allergic reaction, most commonly seen in patients who wear soft contact lenses (**Figure 12-5**).

LABORATORY TESTING

- An in-office rapid test for adenoviral conjunctivitis (RPS Adeno Detector) has a sensitivity of 88 percent and a specificity of 91 percent compared to viral cell culture with confirmatory immunofluorescence staining.[6] Since adenoviral conjunctivitis is self-limited, and is usually diagnosed based on history and physical examination, the test is rarely performed.

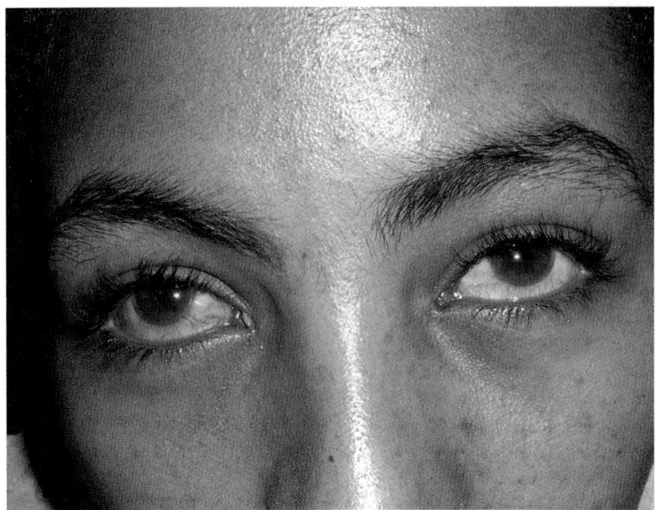

FIGURE 12-2 Viral conjunctivitis demonstrating bilateral conjunctival injection with little discharge. (*Used with permission from Richard P. Usatine, MD.*)

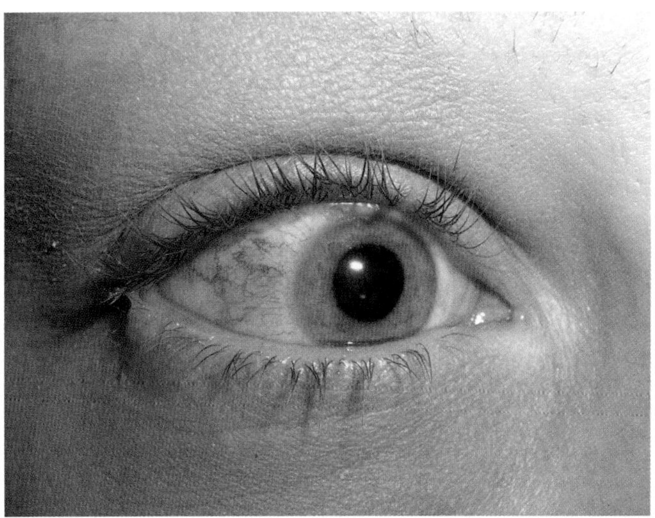

FIGURE 12-3 Bacterial conjunctivitis with visible discharge on the lateral eyelids. The conjunctivitis was bilateral. (*Used with permission from Richard P. Usatine, MD.*)

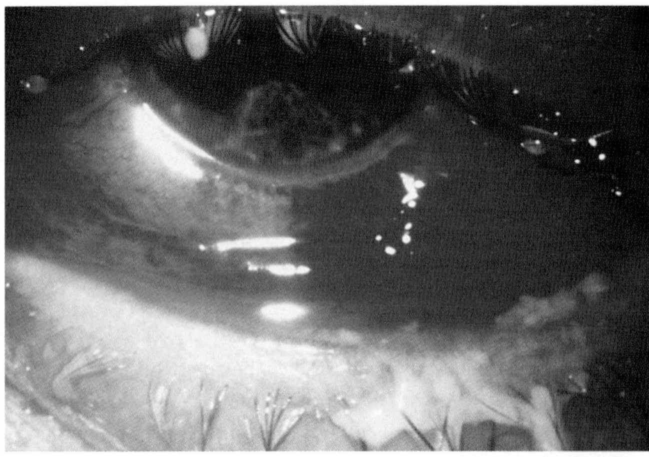

FIGURE 12-4 Gonococcus conjunctivitis has a copious discharge. This severe case resulted in partial blindness. (*Used with permission from Disease Control and Prevention [CDC].*)

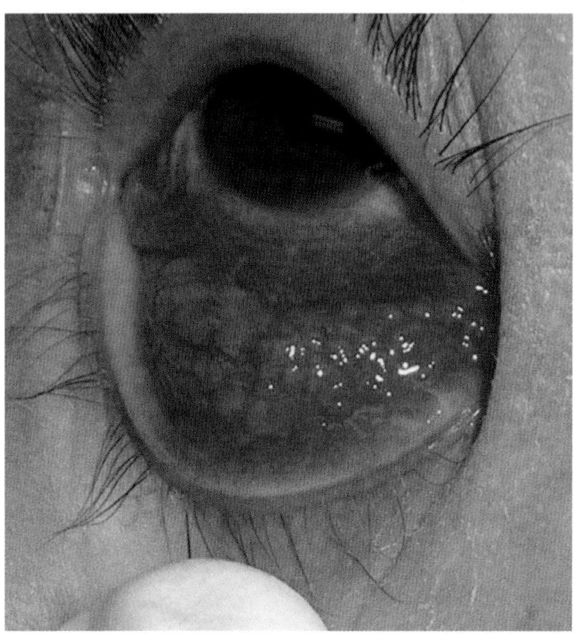

FIGURE 12-5 Giant papillary conjunctivitis in a contact lens wearer. (*Used with permission from Mike Johnson, MD.*)

DIFFERENTIAL DIAGNOSIS

- Nasolacrimal duct obstruction in newborns typically presents with excess tearing. Erythema and inflammation may be present at the nasal and inferior lid. The obstruction may occasionally lead to the development of infectious conjunctivitis (see also Chapter 14, Nasolactrimal Duct Obstruction).
- Keratitis or corneal ulcerations—Diffuse conjunctival injection, often with miosis (constriction of pupil), eye discharge, pain, photophobia, and vision loss depending on the location of ulceration. Herpes keratitis is a diagnosis that should not be missed (**Figures 12-6** and **12-7**). The use of fluorescein and a UV light can help identify dendritic ulcers or other corneal damage and prompt an emergent referral to an ophthalmologist (**Figure 12-7**). Contact lens wearers should urgently see an ophthalmologist for keratitis.
- A foreign body in the eye can cause conjunctival injection and lead to a bacterial superinfection. If the foreign body is not easily dislodged with conservative measures, or appears to be superinfected

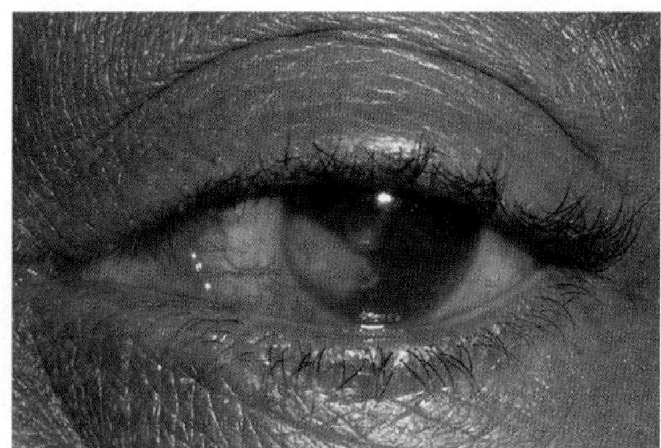

FIGURE 12-6 Herpetic keratitis in a woman staying in a shelter after Hurricane Katrina. (*Used with permission from Richard P. Usatine, MD.*)

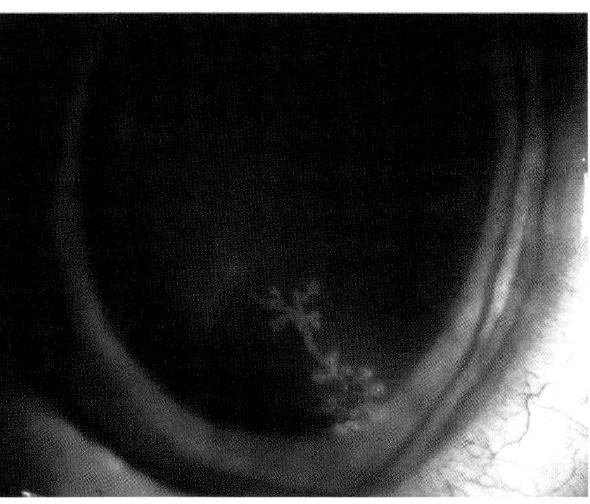

FIGURE 12-7 Slit-lamp view of a dendritic ulcer with fluorescein uptake from herpetic keratitis. (*Used with permission from Paul D. Comeau.*)

with ulceration or leukocyte infiltrate, prompt referral to an ophthalmologist is required (**Figure 12-8**).

- Uveitis or iritis—360-degree perilimbal injection, eye pain, photophobia, and vision loss. Frequently treated initially as conjunctivitis without resolution (see also Chapter 13, Uveitis and Iritis).
- Trachoma is an eye infection caused by *C. trachomatis* that is rare in the US but common in the rural areas of some developing countries. It is a leading cause of blindness in the developing world. Poverty and poor hygiene are major risk factors. Once the eye is infected, follicles can be seen on the upper tarsal conjunctiva upon eyelid eversion (**Figure 12-9**). Superior tarsal conjunctival scarring leads to entropion, which causes corneal scarring and ultimately blindness.
- Vernal conjunctivitis is a severe recurrent form of allergic conjunctivitis that is more common in the summer (not the spring). The term *vernal* refers to the spring time, and therefore it is now referred to as "warm weather conjunctivitis" rather than "spring catarrh." Giant papillae that look like a cobblestone pattern may be seen in this condition. It occurs primarily in young boys, and typically ceases to recur seasonally with age.

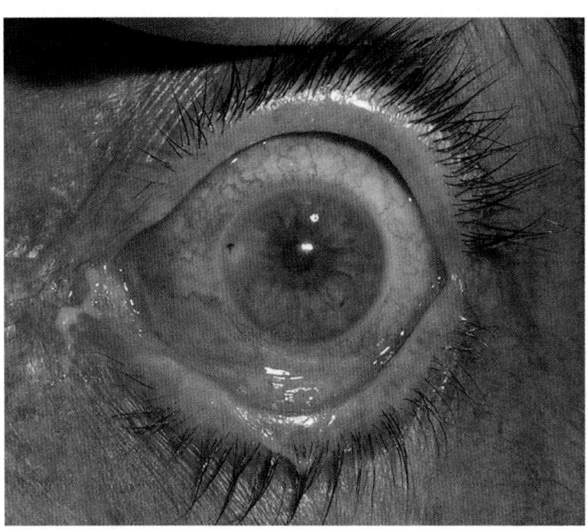

FIGURE 12-8 Conjunctivitis caused by a foreign body in the eye. The ground metal speck is seen on the cornea, and the corneal infiltrate, along with a purulent discharge, indicate a bacterial superinfection. (*Used with permission from Richard P. Usatine, MD.*)

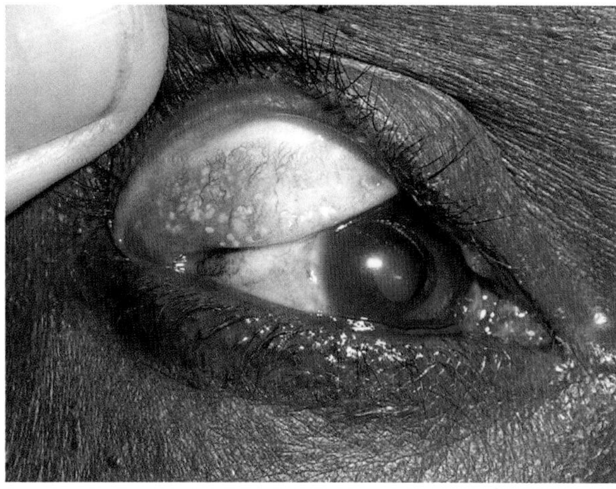

FIGURE 12-9 Trachoma showing many white follicles on the underside of the upper eyelid. (*Used with permission from Richard P. Usatine, MD.*)

MANAGEMENT

- Hand hygiene can control the spread of infectious conjunctivitis.
- Children younger than age 6 years.[4]
  - Azithromycin 1.5 percent ophthalmic solution twice daily for 3 days resulted in a clinical and microbiologic cure in more than 80 percent of children.[7,8] SOR A This dosing regimen provides equivalent efficacy to 4 times a day dosing of tobramycin.[7,8] SOR B
  - A combination of polymixin B and trimethoprim (Polytrim) is effective and widely used for the treatment of bacterial conjunctivitis.
  - Erythromycin can also be used for bacterial conjunctivitis although its utility may be limited by resistance of *Haemophilus* and *Moraxella* species.
- Any patient with significant purulent ocular discharge should be treated for bacterial conjunctivitis.
- Many agents can be used to treat bacterial conjunctivitis. Studies show that more than 80 percent of patients show improvements with 0.3 percent ciprofloxacin, tobramycin, norfloxacin, or gentamicin, and 0.6 percent besifloxacin.[9–12]
- Moxifloxacin (Vigamox 0.5% solution) is a new generation fluoroquinolone that has been shown to be effective for the treatment of bacterial conjunctivitis.[13–15] It has a near neutral pH (6.8), so is well tolerated by children.[15] It is FDA approved for use in children over age 1 year. The dosing is 1 drop in the affected eye(s) three times daily for one week. SOR B
- Aminoglycosides, such as tobramycin and gentamicin, are very effective against gram negative infections but not generally effective against streptococci.
- Allergic conjunctivitis can be treated with antihistamines, mast-cell stabilizers, nonsteroidal antiinflammatory agents, corticosteroids (only if under the care of an ophthalmologist), and immunomodulatory agents.[16]

REFERRAL

- Refer patients who have vision loss, copious purulent discharge (this could represent gonococcal disease, which must be cultured, and which can cause vision loss), severe pain, lack of response to therapy, or a history of herpes simplex or zoster eye disease to an ophthalmologist. In the case of any child who has copious purulent

discharge, one should consider the possibility of sexual abuse. Obtain cultures immediately.
- Any patient who may need ocular steroid should be seen by an ophthalmologist. There is a severe risk for complications (elevated eye pressure, cataract, and corneal perforation) with the use of ocular steroids.

PREVENTION

Good hygiene practices with washing of the hands and face with soap and water.

FOLLOW-UP/RETURN TO SCHOOL

- Routine follow-up is generally not needed if symptoms resolve in 3 to 5 days.
- State health departments have no consensus on when children with conjunctivitis can return to school. A literature-based review suggests the best strategy is excluding children from school until they are asymptomatic.[17]

PATIENT EDUCATION

- Most children older than age 6 years have a nonbacterial cause of conjunctivitis, except those with a history of gluey eyes and a purulent discharge seen on physical examination.
- Remove contact lenses until conjunctivitis has resolved.
- Avoid touching the face or rubbing the eyes and wash hands immediately afterwards.
- Do not share face towels, eye makeup, or contact lens cases.
- Inform your physician immediately if your child experiences eye pain or vision loss.

PATIENT RESOURCES

- PubMed Health. *Conjunctivitis*—**www.ncbi.nlm.nih.gov/pubmedhealth/PMH0002005/**.
- American Academy of Ophthalmology has patient information under For Patients and the Public—**www.aao.org**.
- American Academy of Ophthalmology. *Conjunctivitis: What Is Pink Eye?*—**www.geteyesmart.org/eyesmart/diseases/conjunctivitis.cfm**.
- Centers for Disease Control and Prevention has patient information in English and Spanish—**www.cdc.gov**.
- Centers for Disease Control and Prevention. *Conjunctivitis (Pink Eye)*—**www.cdc.gov/conjunctivitis/index.html**.
- The Livestrong foundation has auditory patient information on YouTube. *Conjunctivitis Health Byte*—**www.youtube.com/watch?v=O8LkDfbLCaY**; and *A Healthy Byte: Pink Eye*—**www.youtube.com/watch?v=Hp28hS7XYCo& feature=relmfu**.

PROVIDER RESOURCES

- Agency for Healthcare Research and Quality. *Conjunctivitis guidelines*—**www.guidelines.gov/content.aspx?id=13501**.

REFERENCES

1. Smith AF, Waycaster C. Estimate of the direct and indirect annual cost of bacterial conjunctivitis in the United States. *BMC Ophthalmol.* 2009;9:13.
2. Singh K, Axelrod S, Bielory L. The epidemiology of ocular and nasal allergy in the United States, 1988-1994. *J Allergy Clin Immunol.* 2010;126(4):778-783.
3. Gigliotti F, Williams WT, Hayden FG, et al. Etiology of acute conjunctivitis in children. *J Pediatr.* 1981;98(4):531-536.
4. Meltzer JA, Kunkov D, Crain EF. Identifying children at low risk for bacterial conjunctivitis. *Arch Pediatr Adolesc Med.* 2010;124:263-267.
5. Patel PB, Diaz MC, Bennett JE, Attia MW. Clinical features of bacterial conjunctivitis in children. *Acad Emerg Med.* 2007;14(1):1-5.
6. Sambursky R, Tauber S, Schirra F, et al. The RPS adeno detector for diagnosing adenoviral conjunctivitis. *Ophthalmology.* 2006; 113(10):1758-1764.
7. Bremond-Gignac D, Mariani-Kurkdjian P, Beresniak A, et al. Efficacy and safety of azithromycin 1.5% eye drops for purulent bacterial conjunctivitis in pediatric patients. *Pediatr Infect Dis J.* 2010;29(3):222-226.
8. Cochereau I, Meddeb-Ouertani A, Khairallah M, et al. 3-day treatment with azithromycin 1.5% eye drops versus 7-day treatment with tobramycin 0.3% for purulent bacterial conjunctivitis: multicentre, randomized and controlled trial in adults and children. *Br J Ophthalmol.* 2007;91(4):465-469.
9. Gross RD, Hoffman RO, Lindsay RN. A comparison of ciprofloxacin and tobramycin in bacterial conjunctivitis in children. *Clin Pediatr (Phila).* 1997;36(8):435-444.
10. Miller IM, Vogel R, Cook TJ, Wittreich J. Topically administered norfloxacin compared with topically administered gentamicin for the treatment of external ocular bacterial infections. The Worldwide Norfloxacin Ophthalmic Study Group. *Am J Ophthalmol.* 1992;113(6):638-644.
11. DeLeon J, Silverstein BE, Allaire C, et al. Besifloxacin ophthalmic suspension 0.6% administered twice daily for 3 days in the treatment of bacterial conjunctivitis in adults and children. *Clin Drug Investig.* 2012;32(5):303-317.
12. Szaflik J, Szaflik JP, Kaminska A. Clinical and microbiological efficacy of levofloxacin administered three times a day for the treatment of bacterial conjunctivitis. *Eur J Ophthalmol.* 2009;19(1):1-9.
13. Williams L, Malhotra Y, Murante B, et al. A single-blinded randomized clinical trial comparing polymyxin B-trimethoprim and moxifloxacin for treatment of acute conjunctivitis in children. *J Pediatr.* 2013 Apr;162(4):857-861.
14. Keating GM. Moxifloxacin 0.5% ophthalmic solution: in bacterial conjunctivitis. *Drugs.* 2011;71(1):89-99.
15. Benitez-Del-Castillo J, Verboven Y, Stroman D, Kodjikian L. The role of topical moxifloxacin, a new antibacterial in Europe, in the treatment of bacterial conjunctivitis. *Clin Drug Investig.* 2011;31(8):543-557.
16. Mishra GP, Tamboli V, Jwala J, Mitra AK. Recent patents and emerging therapeutics in the treatment of allergic conjunctivitis. *Recent Pat Inflamm Allergy Drug Discov.* 2011;5(1):26-36.
17. Ohnsman CM. Exclusion of students with conjunctivitis from school: policies of state departments of health. *J Pediatr Ophthalmol Strabismus.* 2007;44(2):101-105.

13 UVEITIS AND IRITIS

Heidi Chumley, MD

PATIENT STORY

A 16-year-old boy presents with sudden onset of a red right eye, severe eye pain, tearing, photophobia, and decreased vision. He denies eye trauma. His review of systems is positive for knee and ankle pain over the previous 6 months. On examination, he has a ciliary flush (**Figure 13-1**) and decreased vision. He is referred to an ophthalmologist who confirms the diagnosis of acute anterior uveitis. He is also referred to a pediatric rheumatologist who makes the diagnosis of juvenile onset spondyloarthritis. His uveitis is treated with topical steroids.

INTRODUCTION

Uveitis is inflammation of any component of the uveal tract: iris (anterior), ciliary body (intermediate), or choroid (posterior). Most uveitis is anterior and is also called iritis. Uveitis is caused by trauma, inflammation, or infection and the most common etiologies vary by location in the uveal tract. Patients present with vision changes and, if uveitis is anterior, eye pain, redness, tearing, and photophobia. All patients with uveitis should be referred to an ophthalmologist.

SYNONYMS

Anterior uveitis includes iritis and iridocyclitis. *Iritis* is when the inflammation is limited to the iris. If the ciliary body is involved too, then it is called *iridocyclitis*. Posterior uveitis includes choroiditis and chorioretinitis.

EPIDEMIOLOGY

- Annual incidence of uveitis is 17 to 52 per 100,000 population and prevalence is 38 to 714 per 100,000 population.[1]
- Occurs at any age, but most commonly between 20 and 59 years.[1]
- Anterior uveitis (iritis) accounts for approximately 90 percent of uveitis as seen in primary care settings.[1]
- Eighty percent of uveitis cases seen in children are caused by juvenile idiopathic arthritis.[2]
- In the US, noninfectious uveitis accounts for 10 percent of legal blindness.[3]

ETIOLOGY AND PATHOPHYSIOLOGY

- Uveitis in children is predominantly associated with juvenile idiopathic arthritis, but can also be caused by trauma, infections, inflammation, or, rarely, neoplasms. Most likely causes differ by location.[4]
- Iritis—Autoimmune disorders, especially juvenile idiopathic arthritis, and trauma are more common (**Figure 13-2**). Infection, malignancy and idiopathic causes are less common. Infections include herpes, syphilis, and tuberculosis.[4]
- Intermediate—Most are idiopathic[4] (**Figure 13-3**).
- Posterior—In infants, congenital infections (toxoplasmosis, rubella, cytomegalovirus, herpes simplex virus, and syphilis) are common causes. In toddlers, Toxocara canis or Toxocara cati acquired from ingestion of contaminated soil can cause a unilateral posterior uveitis. Cytomegalovirus is the most common in immunocompromised children. It may also be autoimmune, trauma, malignancy or idiopathic.
- Panuveitis (affecting all layers)—Idiopathic (22% to 45%) and sarcoidosis (14% to 28%).[4] Unilateral panuveitis is often endophthalmitis (endogenous or related to trauma or surgery). Bilateral panuveitis can be caused by sarcoidosis or syphilis.

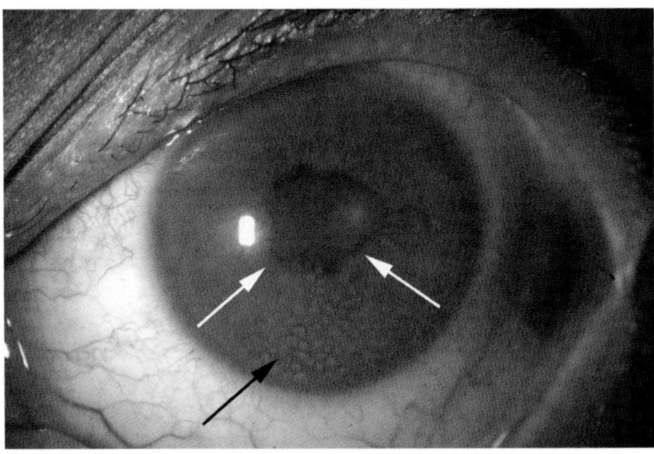

FIGURE 13-1 Acute anterior uveitis with corneal endothelial white cell aggregates (*black arrow*) and posterior synechiae formation (iris adhesions to the lens, *white arrows*). (*Used with permission from Paul D. Comeau.*)

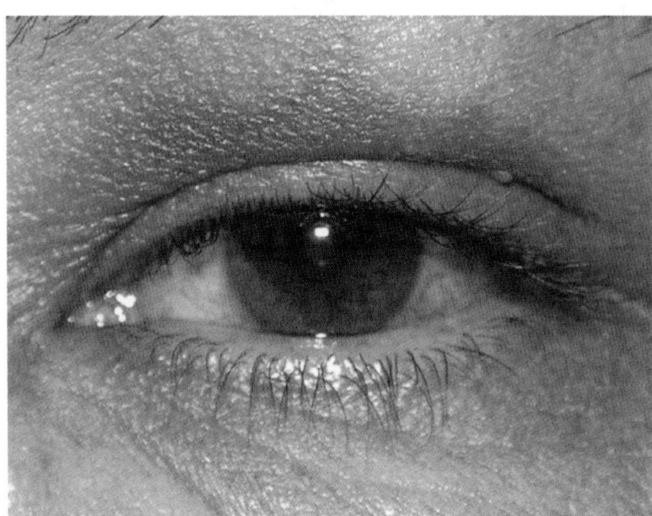

FIGURE 13-2 Traumatic iritis (anterior uveitis) after being hit in the eye with a baseball. He has photophobia and eye pain. (*Used with permission from Richard P. Usatine, MD.*)

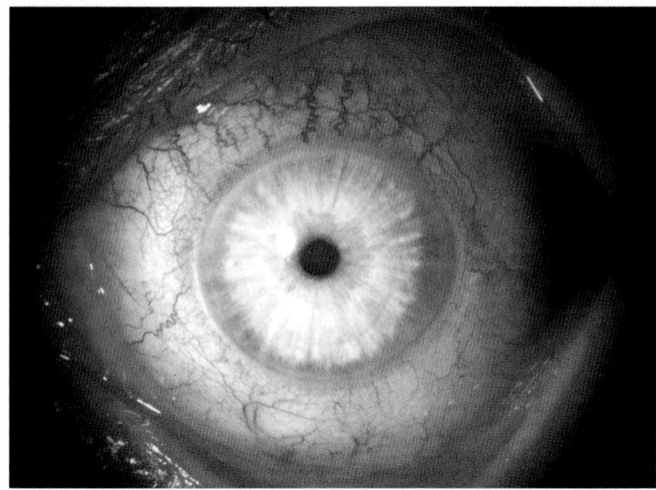

FIGURE 13-3 Idiopathic intermediate uveitis. The ciliary flush is perilimbal injection from dilation of blood vessels adjacent to the cornea, extending 3 mm into the sclera. Perilimbal injection may appear as a violet hue around the limbus with blurring of individual vessels. (*Used with permission from Paul D. Comeau.*)

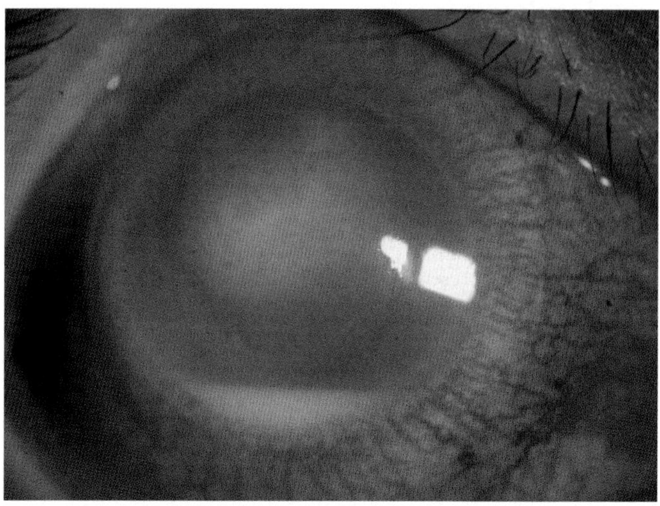

FIGURE 13-4 Hypopyon with severe anterior uveitis, showing layering of leukocytes and fibrinous debris in the anterior chamber. May be sterile or infectious. An intense ciliary flush is seen. Most commonly seen in HLA-B27-positive patients with uveitis. Hypopyon may also be a presenting sign of malignancy (retinoblastoma and lymphoma). (*Used with permission from Paul D. Comeau.*)

RISK FACTORS

Patients with Behçet disease and ankylosing spondylitis have uveitis more commonly than the general population (relative risk of 4 to 20) because of human leukocyte antigen (HLA) associations.[5] Congenital infections and immunodeficiency raise the risk of infectious uveitis.

DIAGNOSIS

CLINICAL FEATURES

Anterior acute uveitis presents with:

- Usually unilateral eye pain, redness, tearing, photophobia, and decreased vision.
- 360-Degree perilimbal injection, which is most intense at the limbus (**Figures 13-1**, **13-2**, and **13-4**).
- History of eye trauma, an associated systemic disease, or risk factors for infection.
- Severe anterior uveitis may cause a hypopyon from layering of leukocytes and fibrous debris in the anterior chamber (**Figure 13-4**). Behçet syndrome and HLA-B27 disease are the only two common noninfectious causes of hypopyon.

Intermediate and posterior uveitis:

- Presents with altered vision or floaters.
- Often, there is no pain, redness, tearing, or photophobia.

Sarcoid uveitis presents with:

- Panuveitis (anterior, intermediate, and posterior).
- Gradual and usually a bilateral onset.
- Few vision complaints unless cataracts or glaucoma develops.
- Characteristic findings on slit-lamp examination (i.e., mutton-fat keratic precipitates, posterior iris synechiae).[6]

Typical distribution

- Anterior uveitis is typically unilateral and sarcoid uveitis is typically bilateral.

DIFFERENTIAL DIAGNOSIS

Causes of red eye, other than uveitis:

- Scleritis—Segmental or diffuse inflammation of sclera (dark red, purple, or blue color); severe, boring eye pain often radiating to head and neck; and photophobia and vision loss.
- Episcleritis—Segmental or diffuse inflammation of episclera (pink color), mild or no discomfort but can be tender to palpation, and no vision disturbance.
- Keratitis or corneal ulcerations—Diffuse erythema with ciliary injection often with constricted pupil; eye discharge; and pain, photophobia, and vision loss depending on the location of ulceration. Frequently associated with trauma, a history of herpes simplex virus (HSV) infection, or contact lens wear. Needs urgent evaluation by an ophthalmologist. There will be staining of the cornea with fluorescein.
- Conjunctivitis—Conjunctival injection, eye discharge, gritty or uncomfortable feeling, and no vision loss (see Chapter 12, Conjunctivitis). Recent history of red eye contacts or URI symptoms.

MANAGEMENT

Refer patients for any red eye along with loss of vision to an ophthalmologist. Patients with uveitis warrant additional examinations by the ophthalmologist.

- Traumatic uveitis—Dilated funduscopy for other ocular trauma, measurement of intraocular pressure, gonioscopy to evaluate for

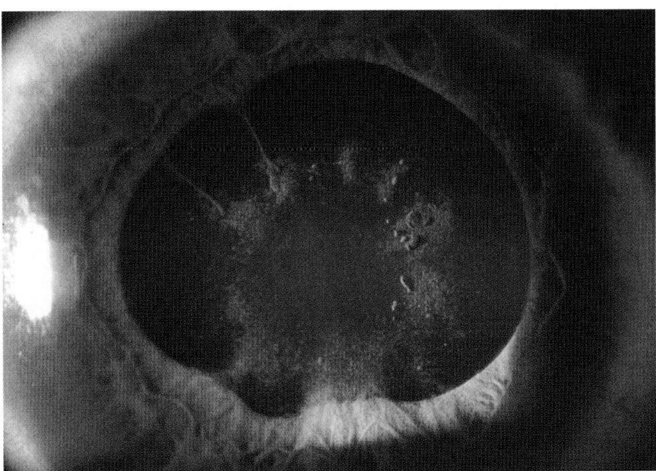

FIGURE 13-5 This patient with uveitis had posterior synechiae that are attachments of the iris to the anterior capsule of the lens. Therapeutic dilation broke the synechiae, but left residual pigment on the anterior capsule. (*Used with permission from Paul D. Comeau.*)

angle recession and risk for future glaucoma, and treatment may include steroid and/or cycloplegics for comfort.

- Nontraumatic uveitis—Slit-lamp examination and laboratory tests to assist with diagnosis of underlying cause; treatment is based on underlying cause but is usually topical steroid drops with or without cycloplegia.
- Therapeutic dilation is used to break the posterior synechiae that can occur (**Figure 13-5**).

PROGNOSIS

Uveitis causes vision loss, cataract, and often glaucoma if treatment is delayed or not provided. HLA-B27 disease is the most common etiology for anterior uveitis, and is associated with recurrent, bilateral anterior uveitis.

FOLLOW-UP

Appropriate follow-up is based on the underlying cause.

PATIENT EDUCATION

- See a physician immediately for a red eye with loss of vision.
- A series of tests may be performed to determine the cause of the uveitis; however, the underlying cause is often elusive.

PATIENT RESOURCES

- **http://www.ncbi.nlm.nih.gov/pubmedhealth/PMH0002000/**.

PROVIDER RESOURCES

- **http://emedicine.medscape.com/article/798323**.

REFERENCES

1. Wakefield D, Chang JH. Epidemiology of uveitis. *Int Ophthalmol Clin.* 2005;45(2):1-13.
2. Foster CS. Diagnosis and treatment of juvenile idiopathic arthritis-associated uveitis. *Curr Opin Ophthalmol.* 2003;14(6):395-398.
3. Gritz DC, Wong IG. Incidence and prevalence of uveitis in northern California; the Northern California Epidemiology of Uveitis Study. *Ophthalmology.* 2004;111(3):491-500.
4. Brazis PW, Stewart M, Lee AG. The uveo-meningeal syndromes. *Neurologist.* 2004;10(4):171-134.
5. Capsi RR. A look at autoimmunity and inflammation in the eye. *J Clin Invest.* 2010;120(9):3073-3083.
6. Uyama M. Uveitis in sarcoidosis. *Int Ophthalmol Clin.* 2002;42(1):143-150.

14 NEONATAL NASOLACRIMAL DUCT OBSTRUCTION

Andreas Marcotty, MD

PATIENT STORY

A 6-month-old child is brought to the pediatrician with a history of tearing, drainage, crusting of the eyelashes and lids, perhaps of both eyes and most notably upon awakening. The tearing occurs without distress and is worse with outside air exposure, especially if it is cold and windy. There is no associated fever or discomfort. Despite the increase in tearing, there is no light sensitivity.[1] Most notable is the chronically increased tear film meniscus (**Figure 14-1**). The baby has a chronic problem since shortly after birth with constant tearing, mucoid debris and a couple of episodes of increased debris, suggestive of conjunctivitis.

Examination demonstrates no photophobia by penlight or indication of pain. There is mild erythema to the lower lids. Notable is the increased tear lake bilaterally, dried mucous on the skin and mucoid debris in the tear film. The eyes show no conjunctival injection or inflammation. There is a normal and symmetrical red reflex by ophthalmoscopy. Fluorescein dye disappearance test demonstrates prolonged retention of the dye in the tear film of each eye longer than 5 minutes.[2,3] Massage of the tear sac can result in expression of copious amount of mucopurulent material but did not in this case. The child was diagnosed with neonatal nasolacrimal duct obstruction (NLDO).

INTRODUCTION

Neonatal nasolacrimal duct obstruction (NLDO) presents with the parents stating that the eye is always crying. The eye remains wet leading to debris and crusting. NLDO may look like infectious conjunctivitis and occasionally leads to the development of true conjunctivitis.

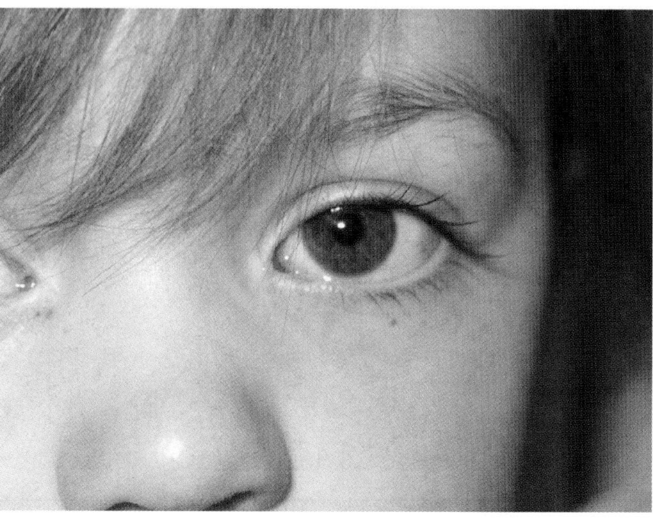

FIGURE 14-1 Nasolacrimal Duct Obstruction with an increased tear film and no evidence of infection (conjunctival injection, purulent debris). (*Used with permission from Andreas Marcotty, MD.*)

SYNONYMS

Dacrocystitis is when the NLDO is infected. Epiphora is the overflow of tears.

EPIDEMIOLOGY

- In a large cohort by Peterson and Robb published in 1978, 50 percent had resolution by the age of 4 months and 89 percent resolved without surgical therapy.[4]
- There is no sex predilection and no genetic predisposition. The blockage can be unilateral or bilateral.
- Range of spontaneous resolution (including the use of massage) is from 65 percent to 95 percent by the age of 10 months.[5–7]
- The natural history of resolution helps to determine the optimal age of surgical intervention (**Table 14-1**).

TABLE 14-1 Natural Progression of Nasolacrimal Duct Obstruction

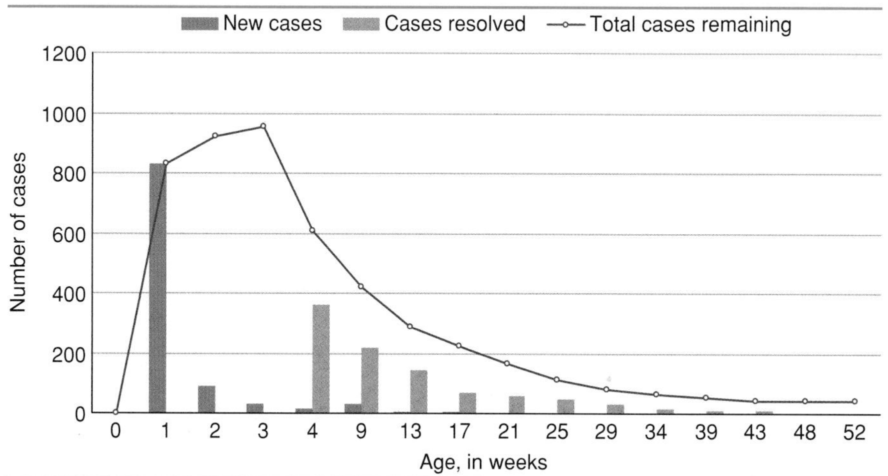

Data adapted from: MacEwen CJ and Young DH: Epiphora During the First Year of Life. *Eye.* 1991;5:596-600.

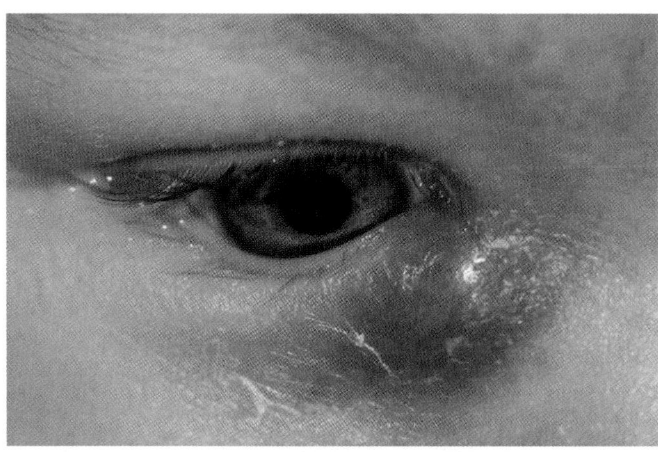

FIGURE 14-2 Dacryocystitis with probable dacryocystocele. There is erythema of skin, fullness to lower lid and an increased tear film. (*Used with permission from Andreas Marcotty, MD.*)

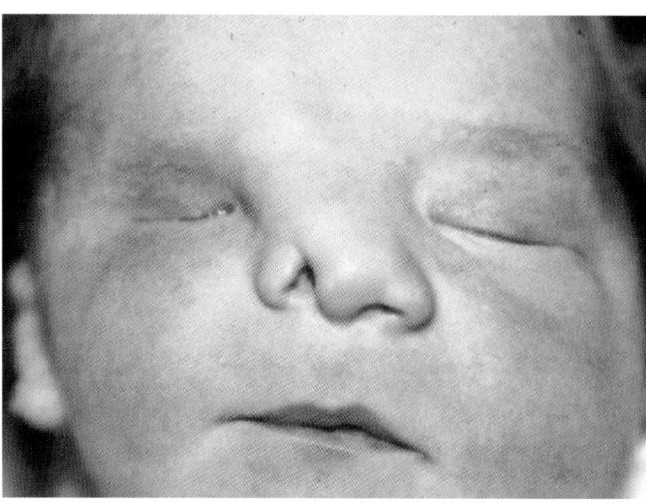

FIGURE 14-3 Midline craniofacial abnormality with secondary tear duct abnormalities. There is an abnormal medial canthus of the right eye and a cleft involving the nasal bone to the right nares. (*Used with permission from Andreas Marcotty, MD.*)

ETIOLOGY

- NLDO can result from Congenital Impatency of Nasolacrimal System. Canalization of the nasolacrimal duct (NLD) is usually complete by 8 months of gestation.[8]
- Most frequent location for impatency is the distal end of NLD at the valve of Hasner beneath the inferior turbinate of the nose.
- Both upper and lower system obstructions can occur.
- May present as an amniocele or dacryocystocele and be associated with the infection Dacryocystitis (**Figure 14-2**).
- May have fluid filled cyst within the nasal cavity.
- NLDO can be acquired as a consequence of conjunctivitis.
- Less common presentations include:
  - Generalized ductal stenosis.
  - Imperforate nasolacrimal puncta.
  - Canalicular abnormalities.

RISK FACTORS

NLDO is associated with craniofacial abnormalities and syndromes such as:

- Trisomy 21, Crouzon, Treacher-Collins, ectodermal dysplasia, Hay-Wells syndrome, Saethre-Chotzen syndrome, Kallmann syndrome, Nager syndrome, frontonasal dysplasia, branchio-oculofacial syndrome, CHARGE syndrome, and velocardiofacial syndrome (**Figure 14-3**).[9–11]

DIAGNOSIS

HISTORY

- Parents state that the eye is "always crying."
- The eye remains wet leading to debris and crusting.

PHYSICAL EXAMINATION

Presentation can range from simple tearing to an acute dacryocystitis. Key findings include:

- Erythema of surrounding skin with the primary location of inflammation at the nasal and inferior lid.
- An increased tear film meniscus with tears frequently resting on the skin temporally (**Figure 14-4**).
- Occasionally a fluctuant or a cystic mass at the inner lower lid (**Figure 14-5**).
  - May also have a cystic lesion present upon nasal endoscopy (**Figure 14-6**).
- Tenderness of the localized mass.
- Expression of mucopurulent debris with compression of the sac.

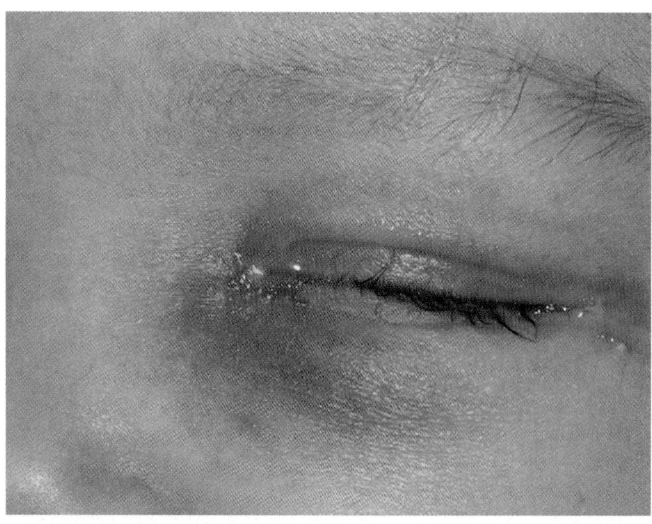

FIGURE 14-4 Acute dacryocystitis. Note the erythema of the skin that is not localized, tearing and mucopurulent debris. (*Used with permission from Andreas Marcotty, MD.*)

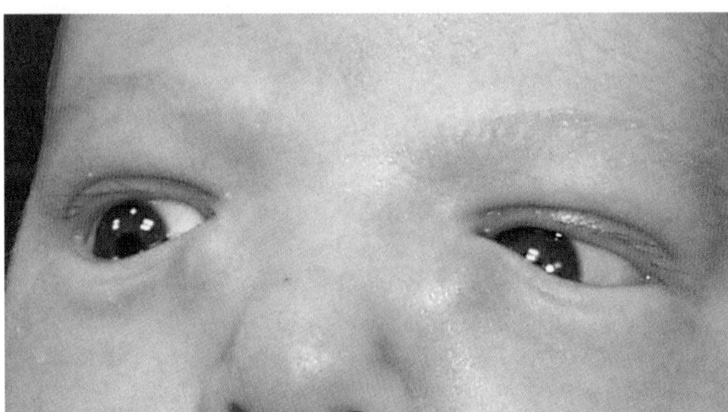

FIGURE 14-5 Bilateral dacryocystoceles demonstrating blueish discoloration of the skin at the medial canthus, as well as cystic swelling of the nasal aspect to both lower lids. (*Used with permission from Elias Traboulsi, MD.*)

TESTING

- Compression of the sac with regurgitation of tears and debris.
- Fluorescein dye retention test.[3,4] Using a fluorescein strip, stain the tears (in the cul-de-sac of the eyelid) with a small amount of fluorescein, dab the excess, and wait 5 minutes. Using a Woods lamp or ultraviolet light, illuminate the eyes and lids, looking for the green fluorescence.
  - A negative test will reveal little to no residual dye fluorescence.
  - A positive test will show an increased tear lake with green fluorescence.

IMAGING

- While imaging is usually not needed, a CT or MRI scan could show an enlarged tear sac/duct on the orbital views and additional structural changes involving the nasal bone.

DIFFERENTIAL DIAGNOSIS

- Epiblepharon is a developmental anomaly caused by an abnormal insertion of muscle fibers of the lower or upper lid resulting in a fold of skin which presses against the lashes, rolling them inward, causing them to rub on the cornea and conjunctiva. This creates a foreign body sensation and secondary tearing (**Figure 14-7**).
- Congenital Glaucoma is a structural abnormality involving Schlemm's canal and the trabecular meshwork resulting in decreased outflow from the anterior chamber and the secondary increase of the intraocular pressure. It occurs in approximately 1/10000 births (**Figure 14-8**). The presentation of congenital glaucoma includes: epiphora, photophobia (**Figure 14-9**), corneal opacification/haze, and buphthalmos also known as enlarged eye.
  - Primary occurs when there are no other abnormalities causing the outflow to be obstructed. Associated with autosomal recessive genetic abnormalities, approximately 10 percent are inherited.
  - Secondary is when there are other anterior segment abnormalities such as aniridia (absence of the iris) or systemic disorders leading to the congenital glaucoma.
- One anterior segment dysgenesis syndrome is Axenfeld-Rieger Syndrome/Peter's anomaly (**Figure 14-10**).

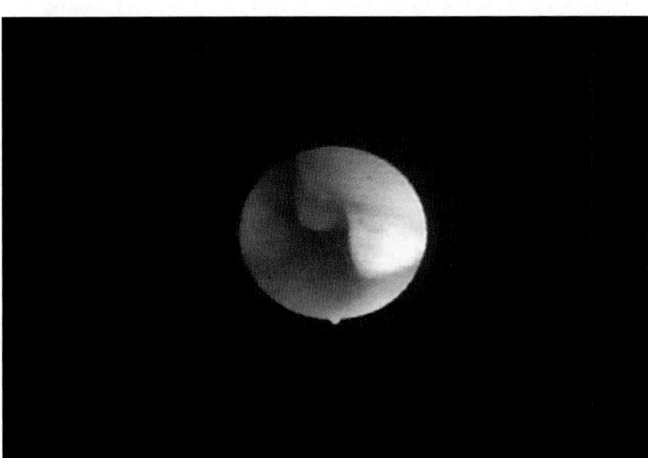

FIGURE 14-6 Intranasal cyst found with a dacryocystocele using endoscopy. (*Used with permission from Paul Krakovitz, MD.*)

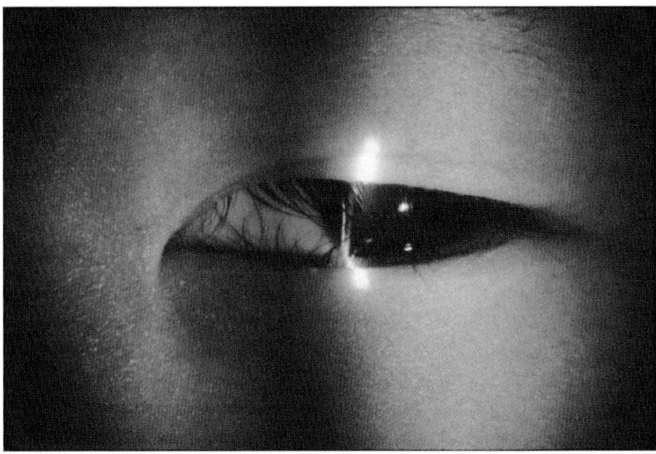

FIGURE 14-7 Congenital epiblepharon typified by in-turned upper and lower lid lashes, with corneal and conjunctival touch. Photograph taken during slit-lamp exam. (*Used with permission from Andreas Marcotty, MD.*)

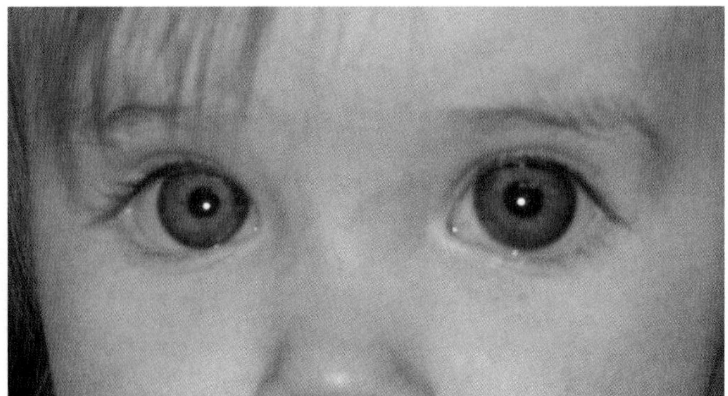

FIGURE 14-8 Congenital glaucoma with epiphora. Note the asymmetrically enlarged corneas, epiphora, and absence of corneal edema. (*Used with permission from Andreas Marcotty, MD.*)

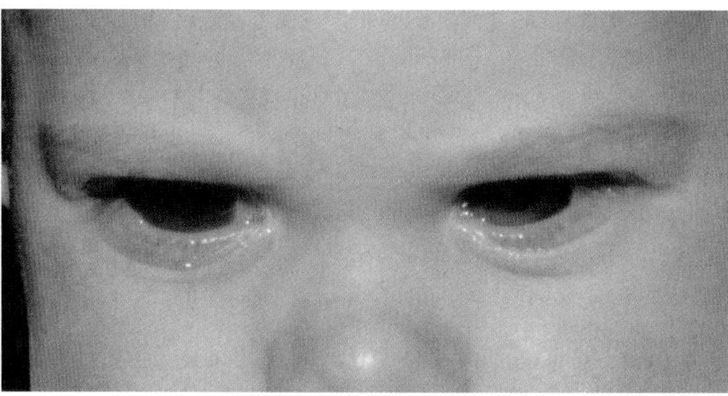

FIGURE 14-9 Congenital Glaucoma with epiphora and photophobia. Note the head down posture, epiphora and enlarged corneas with fluorescein staining of tears. (*Used with permission from Andreas Marcotty, MD.*)

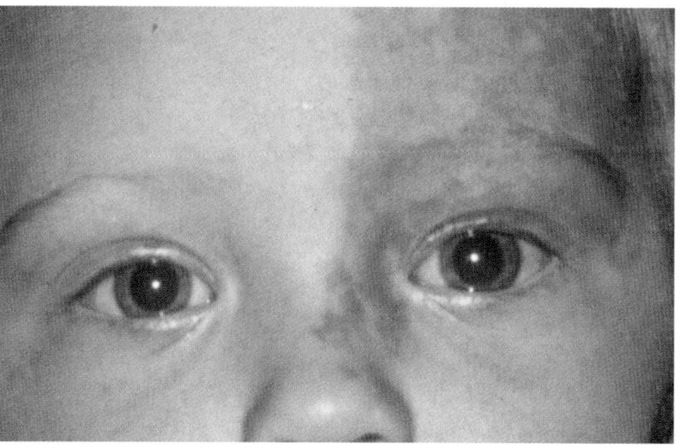

FIGURE 14-11 Encephalotrigeminal hemangiomatosis is also called Sturge-Weber disease when there are neurological abnormalities accompanying the vascular malformation. Note the "Port Wine stain" on the face with lid involvement and scleral injection, but no glaucomatous changes. Glaucoma can occur at birth with this disease. (*Used with permission from Andreas Marcotty, MD.*)

- Congenital infections (TORCH) and neurocutaneous disorders can cause congenital glaucoma. One neurocutaneous disorder is known as Sturge-Weber disease (**Figure 14-11**).
- External infections include: Conjunctivitis (viral or bacterial; see Chapter 12, Conjunctivitis).
- Internal infections include: Congenital Viral Infection, Toxocara, Congenital Syphilis, or TORCH infections.
- Corneal ulcer, which could be secondary to an infection or trauma (**Figure 14-12**).
- Corneal abrasion (**Figure 14-13**; see Chapter 11, Corneal Foreign Body and Corneal Abrasion).

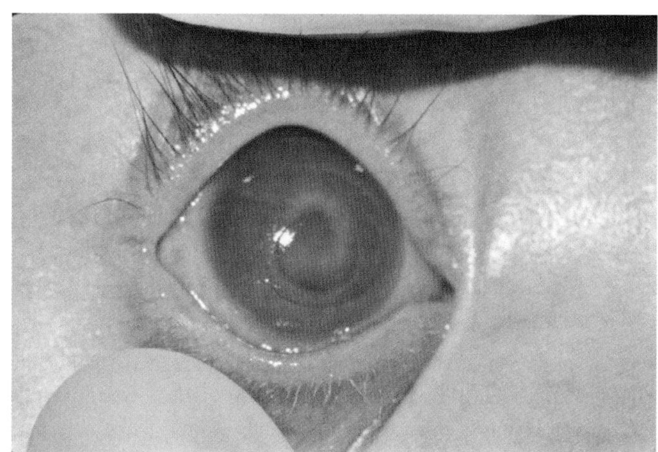

FIGURE 14-12 Sterile corneal ulcer in Familial Dysautonomia with a central epithelial defect and raised edges. (*Used with permission from Andreas Marcotty, MD.*)

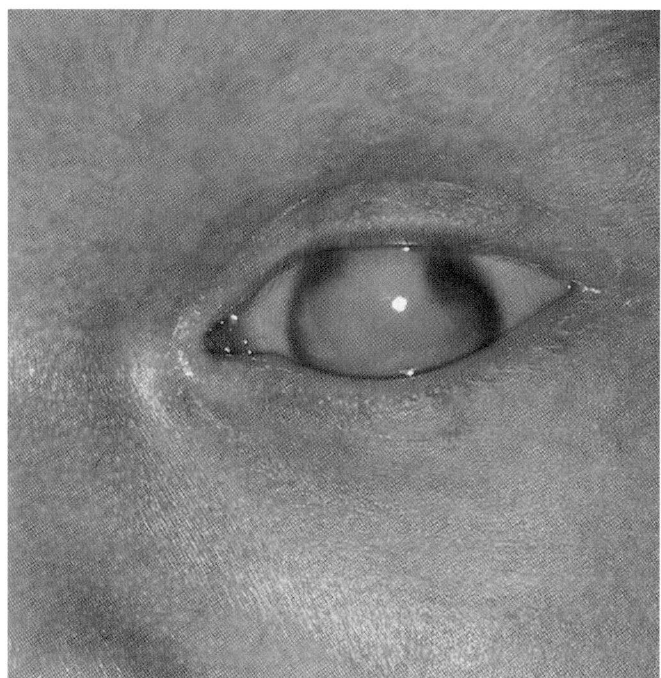

FIGURE 14-10 Peter's Anomaly showing opacification of the cornea. This may be associated with glaucoma. (*Used with permission from Andreas Marcotty, MD.*)

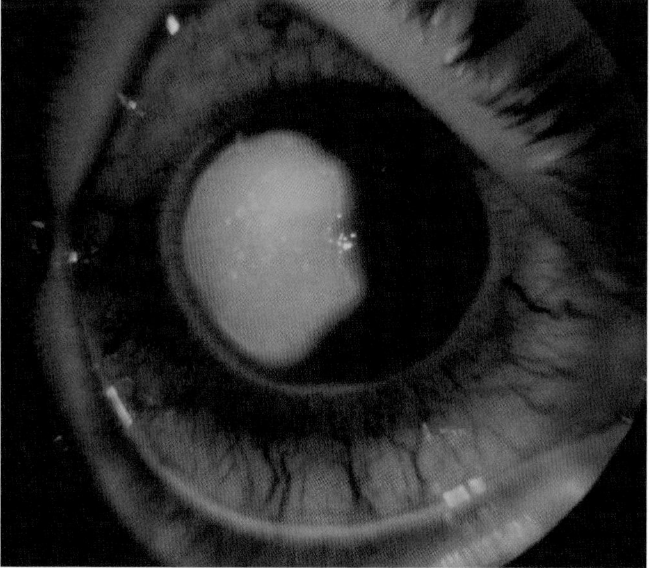

FIGURE 14-13 Corneal abrasion stained with fluorescein and illuminated with a Wood's lamp (ultraviolet light). (*Used with permission from Andreas Marcotty, MD.*)

MANAGEMENT

ANTIBIOTICS ONLY WHEN NEEDED

- Initially, the distinction between tearing as a consequence of an obstruction of the outflow system versus an insult to the eye with secondary tearing must be made. This differentiation is critical in the successful management of tearing and to the health of the visual system and child. Occasionally, there may an infectious component in NLDO.
- If cultures are taken when there is a NLDO, there was a 25 percent chance of infection with *Haemophilus influenzae*, *Staphylococcus aureus*, or *Moraxella catarrhalis*. If there is an associated dacryocystitis, the organisms isolated have been reported to be coagulase-negative Staphylococcus and non-pneumococcal α-Streptococcus.[12]
- Conjunctival culture is not indicated unless there are signs of significant infection.
- If there is an infection, an antibiotic ophthalmic preparation should be prescribed. Antibiotics that have the appropriate therapeutic antibacterial spectrum include: Erythromycin, Polymyxin-trimethoprim sulfate, Azithromycin, Quinolones (Gatifloxacin, Ciprofloxacin, Ofloxacin, Levofloxacin), and Gentamicin.

MASSAGE

- Traditionally, the management of tear duct obstruction without complication is primarily one of observation, with massage.
- The massage technique is described in an article by Crigler[13] and restated by Kushner.[14]
- Anatomically, the nasolacrimal sac and duct sit very nasal and begin in the superior nasal corner of the orbit. The lacrimal sac and duct then travel straight downward alongside the posterior and nasal edge of the caruncle of the medial canthus and into the lacrimal bone, where it can no longer be massaged.

MASSAGE TECHNIQUE

Compression begins at the superior, nasal site with a steady pressure, squeezing the lacrimal sac between the fingertip and the nasal bone. The finger is then rolled downward and posteriorly against the frontal and lacrimal bones, finishing the massage, when the lower edge of the orbit is felt.

SURGERY

- In infants without spontaneous resolution, surgical treatment with Probe and Irrigation (P&I) can result in a cure rate of 78 percent to 96 percent with the variability reflecting the age of probing and the selection bias of the surgeon or the complexity of the case.[7,14–16] SOR Ⓐ
- The younger the age of the infant in the series, the more successful the procedure. Some studies show a dramatic decrease in surgical success after 13 months of age and others only after 36 months of age.[15,16] SOR Ⓑ
- Given the success that early treatment can achieve, some advocate in-office P&I under local anesthesia, with general anesthesia necessary for older children (older than 6 months).
- If primary treatment with P&I fails, the secondary procedure may be repeat probing, placing a stent, or performing a balloon catheter dilation. Early stenting was performed using a silicone tube looped through both the upper and lower canalicular systems with the ends knotted and secured in the nasal cavity.
- Stenting is currently done through one canaliculus using a Monoka™ stent, decreasing the risk of trauma to both punta and canaliculi if the tube becomes dislodged.
- Balloon catheter dilation is another procedure, which combines dilation and a stent. An inflatable stent is passed into the nasolacrimal duct and filled with a saline solution, enlarging the canal with rupture of the obstruction as well as dilation of the canal. Balloon catheter dilation has also been performed as a primary treatment with an 82 percent success rate in children under four years age.[18] SOR Ⓑ Notably, it has a higher cost due to the material and equipment as well as a requirement of general anesthesia. As a secondary procedure, following a primary treatment of P&I, balloon catheter dilation is as successful as the placement of any type of temporary indwelling tube, into the lacrimal system to create permanent patency.[19]
- Finally, the last procedure to consider would be lacrimal duct bypass surgery, also called a dacryocystorhinostomy (DCR), which is destructive to the natural anatomy of the system and therefore the final option.

PROGNOSIS

The natural history of resolution and the success of surgery by age vary according to the series. Spontaneous resolution with massage occurs in 54 percent to 89 percent of infants.[5,7,15,17] SOR Ⓐ

FOLLOW-UP

Simple NLDO without a dacrycystitis or dacryocystocele can be followed less closely as it is common and has a minor risk of complication. Dacryocystitis is a more serious problem and close management with appropriate antibiotics oral or intravenous therapy is needed. Dacryocystocele is important to recognize early, as it may require very early surgery with P&I and possible ENT endoscopic assistance to look for and manage an intranasal cyst.

PATIENT EDUCATION

The most important educational information to provide to parents is that of appropriate massage technique and the need to persist in this treatment, as time generally will allow for resolution. If the family is concerned, early therapy with in-office surgery can be undertaken, although not to the exclusion of tear duct massage.

PATIENT RESOURCES

- *American Association for Pediatric Ophthalmology and Strabismus*—**http://www.aapos.org/terms/conditions/72.**
- **Children's Hospital Colorado—http://www.childrenscolorado.org/wellness/info/parents/21306.aspx.**

PROVIDER RESOURCES

- *EyeWiki*—**http://eyewiki.aao.org/Congenital_Nasolacrimal_Duct_Obstruction**.

  Contains videos of the surgical procedures along with referenced text on NLDO.

REFERENCES

1. Lee, KA. Congenital Nasolacrimal Duct Obstruction. Available at: http://eyewiki.aao.org/Congenital_Nasolacrimal_Duct_Obstruction, accessed January 22, 2013.
2. Zappia RJ, Milder B. Lacrimal Drainage Function 2. The Flourescein Dye Disappearance Test. *Am J Ophthalmol.* 1972;74(1):160-2.
3. MacEwen, CJ, Young, JDH. The fluorescein disappearance test (FDT): an evaluation of its use in infants. *J Pediatr Ophthalmol and Strabismus.* 1991;28:302-305.
4. Peterson, RA, Robb, RM. The Natural Course of Congenital Obstruction of the Nasolacrimal Duct. *J Pediatr Ophthalmol and Strabismus.* 1978;15:246-250.
5. MacEwen, CJ, Young, JDH. Epiphora During the First Year of Life. *Eye.* 1991;5:596-600.
6. Paul, TO, Shepard, R. Congenital Nasolacrimal Duct Obstruction: Natural History and the Timing of Optimal Intervention. *J Pediatr Ophthalmol Strabismus.* 1994;31:362-367.
7. Guerry D, Kendig EL. Congenital Impatency of the Nasolacrimal Duct. *Arch Ophthalmol.* 1948;39:193-204.
8. Cassady JV. Developmental Anatomy of Nasolacrimal Duct. *Arch Ophthalmol.* 1952;47:141-158.
9. Coats D, Brady McCreery KM, Plager et al: Outflow Drainage Anomalies in Down's Syndrome. *Ophthalmol.* 2003;110:1437-1441.
10. Ahn Yuen SJ, Oley C, Sullivan TJ. Lacrimal Outflow Dysgenesis. *Ophthalmol.* 2004;111:1782-1790.
11. Prabhakaran VC, Davis G, Wormald PJ, Selva D. Congenital Absence of the Nasolacrimal Duct in Velocardiofacial Syndrome. *J AAPOS.* 2008;12:85-86.
12. Baskin DE, Reddy AV, Chu YI, Coats DK. The timing of antibiotic administration in the management of infant dacryocystitis. *J AAPOS.* 2008;12:456-459.
13. Crigler L. The treatment of congenital dacryocystitis. *JAMA.* 1923;81:21-4.
14. Kushner BJ. Congenital nasolacrimal system obstruction. *Arch Ophthalmol.* 1982;100:597-600.
15. Katowtiz JA, Welsh, MG. Timing of Initial Probing and Irrigation in Congenital Nasolacrimal Duct Obstruction. *Ophthalmol.* 1987; 94:698-705.
16. Pediatric Eye Disease Investigator Group. Primary Treatment of Nasolacrimal Duct Obstruction with Probing in Children Younger than 4 Years. *Ophthalmol.* 2008;115:577-584.
17. Pediatric Eye Disease Investigator Group. Resolution of Congenital Nasolacrimal. Duct Obstruction With Nonsurgical Management. *Arch Ophthalmol.* 2012;130:730-734.
18. Pediatric Eye Disease Investigator Group. Primary treatment of Nasolacrimal Duct Obstruction With Balloon Catheter Dilation in Children Less than Four Years Old. *JAAPOS.* 2008: 12:451-455.
19. Pediatric Eye Disease Investigator Group. Balloon Catheter Dilation and Nasolacrimal Intubation for Treatment of Nasolacrimal Duct Obstruction Following a Failed Probing. *Arch Ophthalmol.* 2009;127: 633-639.

15 STRABISMUS AND PSEUDOSTRABISMUS

Paul J. Rychwalski, MD

PATIENT STORY

A 5-month-old infant is brought to your office by her mother. The mother reports that the child has a "lazy eye." On further inquiry, the mother describes a 1-month history of the child's eyes turning inward toward the nose. This occurs intermittently and is not noticed by the child's father. The mother shows several photographs that are inconclusive. The infant's maternal uncle had strabismus surgery as a child. On examination, the infant protests when either eye is covered, and seems to have an inward deviation of the right eye, more pronounced when looking to the left (**Figures 15-1A,B,C**). The patient is able to move the eyes easily in all directions.

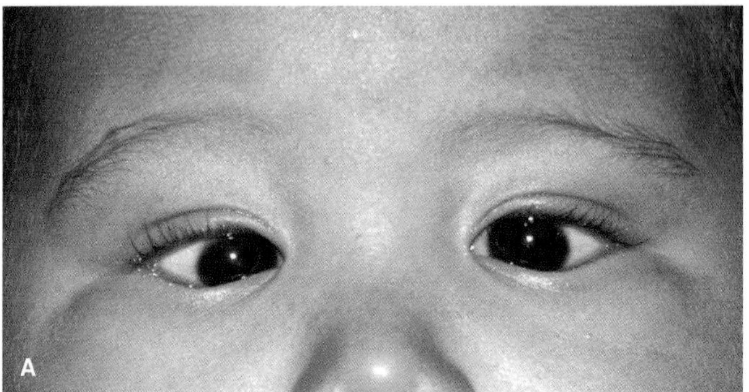

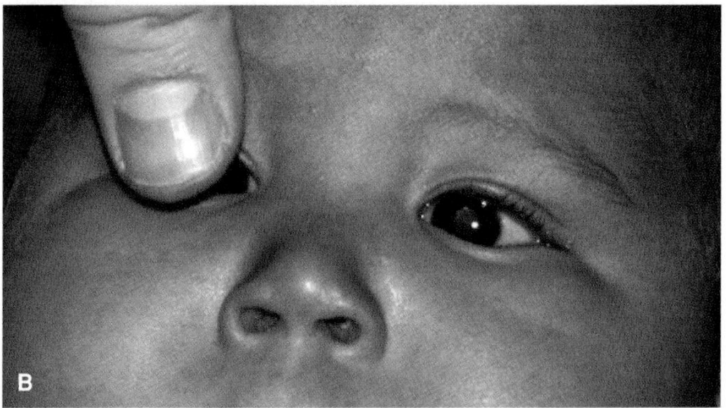

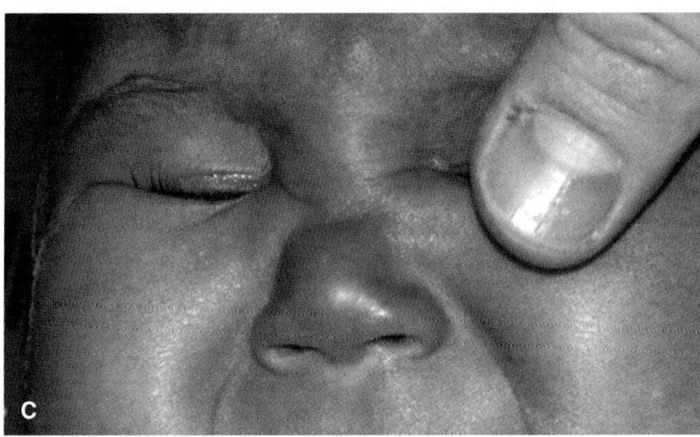

FIGURE 15-1 **A.** Congenital or infantile esotropia. Demonstrates cross-fixation with left eye preference. **B.** Infant tolerates right eye blockage. **C.** Infant upset to have left eye covered. (*Used with permission from Paul J. Rychwalski, MD.*)

INTRODUCTION

Strabismus refers to any misalignment of the eyes. It can be further categorized based on the direction of the deviating eye(s): 1) esotropia—the eye turns inward; 2) exotropia—the eye turns outward; 3) hyper- and hypotropia—the eye turns upward or downward respectively; and 4) cyclotropia or torsional—the eye is rotated clockwise or counterclockwise. Further, the terms used to describe strabismus also depend upon the conditions under which it is present (constant or intermittent) and whether it changes with the position of gaze (comitant or incomitant).

SYNONYMS

Squint, lazy-eye, cross-eye, walleye, or crooked eye.

EPIDEMIOLOGY

- There is geographical variation in the prevalence of strabismus.
- Esotropia is more common in Western populations whereas exotropia is more common in Eastern populations.
- US population-based studies have found an annual incidence per 100,000 population of 64 in exotropia (corresponding to a prevalence of 1 percent of children aged <11 years), 111 in esotropia (corresponding to a prevalence of 2 percent of children aged <6 years), and 12.9 in hypertropia (corresponding to a prevalence of 0.26 percent of children aged <19 years).
- In the US, the incidence of esotropia is highest in children younger than 7 years, whereas the incidence of exotropia is highest in children aged 6 to 9 years, and is also high in adolescents and adults with sensory strabismus.
- The prevalence of strabismus is higher in those with intellectual disabilities (44.1%) compared with the general population. The prevalence in white people is 2 percent to 4 percent, but may be lower in Asian populations.[1–3] Among Hispanic and Latino children, prevalence is:
    - 2 percent at ages six to 11 months.
    - 2.6 percent at ages 36 to 47 months.
    - 2.8 percent at ages 60 to 72 months.
- Among African-American children, prevalence:
    - 1.1 percent at ages six to 11 months.
    - 1.9 percent at ages 36 to 47 months.
    - 3.9 percent at ages 60 to 72 months.[4]

ETIOLOGY AND PATHOPHYSIOLOGY

Proper alignment of the eyes is guaranteed by a normally functioning sensory and motor fusion mechanism. If either of these two systems is perturbed, strabismus may result.

- Sensory:
  - All the nervous impulses that reach the eyes. These factors include the movements of extraocular muscles, psycho-optical reflexes (poorly understood fusional impulses), external influences on muscle tone (endolymph, vestibular system, possible reflexes from neck muscles), and influences of the several nuclear and supranuclear areas that govern ocular motility.
- Motor:
  - Second, there are *anatomical factors,* which consist of orientation and shape of the orbits; size and shape of the globes; volume of the retrobulbar tissue; functioning of the eye muscles as determined by their insertion, length, elasticity, and structure; and anatomical arrangement of connective tissue, ligaments, and pulleys of the orbit.[5]

RISK FACTORS

- Positive family history.
- Prematurity.
- Developmental delay.
- Neurologic disease.
- Genetic abnormalities.
- Vision loss.

DIAGNOSIS

The diagnosis is made with a careful history and physical examination as outlined in the following sections.

- History
  - Age of onset, especially during perinatal period.
  - Birth history.
  - Family history.
  - Associated illness or trauma, especially neurologic.
  - Associated signs including nystagmus, headache, ptosis, anisocoria.
  - Constant vs. intermittent.
  - Change of deviation based on direction or distance of fixation.
- Physical examination.
  - General health and neurologic status.
  - Head position—ocular torticollis may be induced by ocular misalignment.
  - Vision, eyelid position, or pupils.
  - Corneal light reflex or Hirschburg test.
    - The projected light reflex will be centered on each eye if they are aligned. In esotropia, the light on the inwardly deviated eye will be displaced temporally and in exotropia it will be displaced nasally.
  - Cover and cover/uncover test.
    - Cover the apparently straight/fixating eye and observe the fellow eye for a refixation movement.
    - An esotropic eye will have a refixation movement from nasal to temporal in order to pick up fixation and vice versa.
  - Ductions and versions.
    - Check eyes separately and together for ability to move completely.
  - Penlight exam.
    - Look for ocular abnormalities of the cornea, iris or lens.
  - Red reflex test.
  - Complete ophthalmologic examination including cycloplegic refraction and dilated fundus examination.

CLINICAL FEATURES

It is important to distinguish between congenital or infantile and acquired strabismus, as some forms of acquired strabismus can be caused by a life-threatening or vision-threatening condition.

- Causes of primary strabismus include idiopathic infantile or congenital esotropia (**Figure 15-1**) and intermittent exotropia (**Figure 15-2**). These are usually comitant.
- Secondary strabismus can be caused by retinoblastoma (sensory strabismus), head trauma with cranial nerve palsies or orbital fracture, myasthenia gravis, and Graves' disease.
- Acute onset of acquired strabismus may occur with increased intracranial pressure due to intracranial hemorrhage, abscess, encephalitis, shunt failure, and tumors (intracranial, intraocular, or intraorbital).

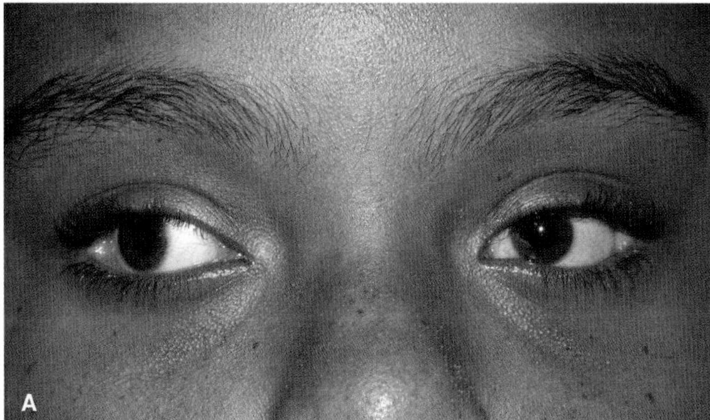

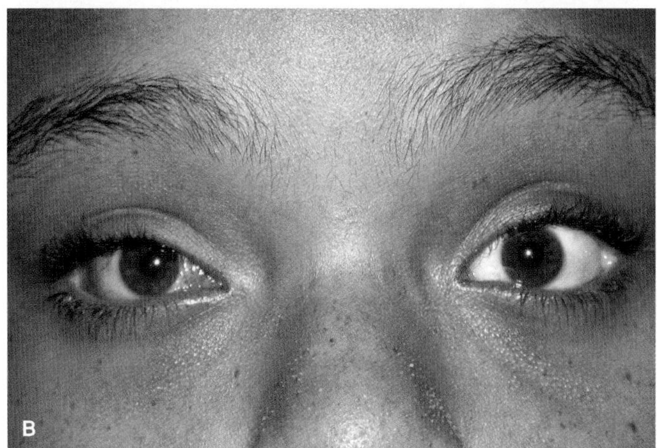

FIGURE 15-2 **A.** Constant exotropia of right eye. **B.** Exotropia surgically corrected with bilateral lateral rectus recession. (*Used with permission from Paul J. Rychwalski, MD.*)

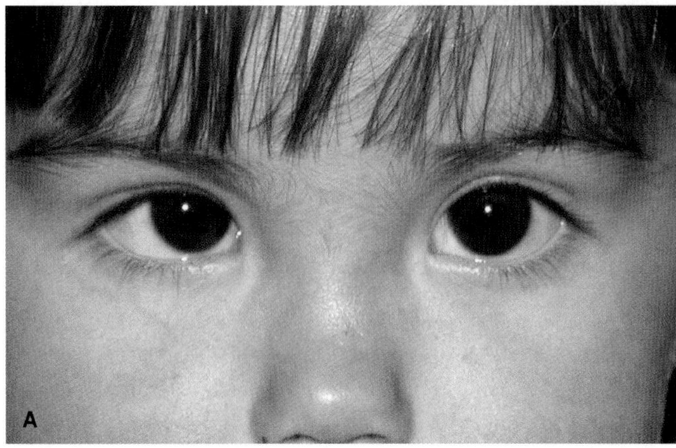

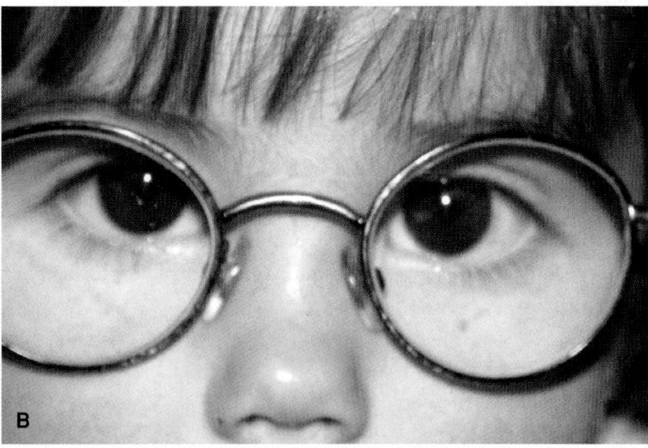

FIGURE 15-3 **A.** Accommodative esotropia. **B.** Corrected with glasses. *(Used with permission from Paul J. Rychwalski, MD.)*

- Forms of esodeviations include accommodative and refractive esotropia (**Figure 15-3**) due to high hyperopia or a high accommodative convergence to accommodation (AC/A) ratio, idiopathic infantile esotropia, esotropic Duane (**Figure 15-4**), or dysinnervation syndrome Moebius syndrome, sensory esotropia, and abducens nerve palsy.
- Forms of exodeviations include intermittent exotropia, oculomotor nerve palsy (usually seen with ptosis and mydriasis on the ipsilateral side), and exotropic Duane syndrome.
- Causes of vertical deviations include trochlear nerve palsy, oculomotor nerve paresis, orbital fracture, thyroid-related ophthalmopathy, and Brown or superior oblique tendon syndrome (**Figure 15-5**).

IMAGING

- Neurologic imaging: In general, a fat-suppression MRI of the brain and orbits with and without contrast is indicated if the results of the history and physical examination point to a possible neurologic cause. Several features warrant investigation with imaging:
  - Abrupt onset.
  - History of trauma.
  - Associated neurologic signs such as anisocoria, ptosis, nystagmus, seizures, or headache.
  - Incomitance.
  - Craniofacial abnormalities.

DIFFERENTIAL DIAGNOSIS

- Pseudostrabismus (**Figure 15-6**).
  - Prominent epicanthal folds.
  - Flat nasal bridge.
  - More apparent on lateral gaze.
  - Normal pupillary light reflex and cover tests.
  - Normal eye exam including refraction, anterior segment and retina.
- Infantile ocular instability.
  - Normal, variable deviation of the eyes seen in the first several weeks of life; usual exotropic.

MANAGEMENT

- Pseudostrabismus.
  - Complete visual and ocular examination.
  - Reassurance.
  - Repeat examination in 4 to 6 months looking for true strabismus. underlying the pseudostrabismus.
- Strabismus.
  - The treatment depends upon the etiology. The goal is to restore normal ocular alignment, preserve vision and binocular vision and stereopsis.

NONPHARMACOLOGIC

- Optical correction and amblyopia therapy (patching or other forms of occlusion) if indicated.[6–8] SOR Ⓐ
- Prism glasses. SOR Ⓒ

MEDICATIONS

- Miotic drops may induce accommodation (Phospholine iodide). SOR Ⓒ
- Cycloplegics may be used in order to blur the stronger eye in amblyopia treatment (Atropine 1%).[6–9] SOR Ⓐ

COMPLIMENTARY/ALTERNATIVE THERAPY

- Orthoptic exercises may be beneficial, especially in some smaller exodeviations. SOR Ⓒ

SURGERY

- In sensory strabismus, surgery is indicated to correct conditions that cause obstruction of the visual axis (ptosis repair, cataract removal, or capillary hemangioma treatment).[10–13] SOR Ⓐ
- Strabismus surgery.
  - Recession: move the "over-working" muscle posteriorly in order to weaken it (**Figure 15-7**).
  - Resection: remove a segment and reattach a relatively underacting muscle in order to strengthen it.

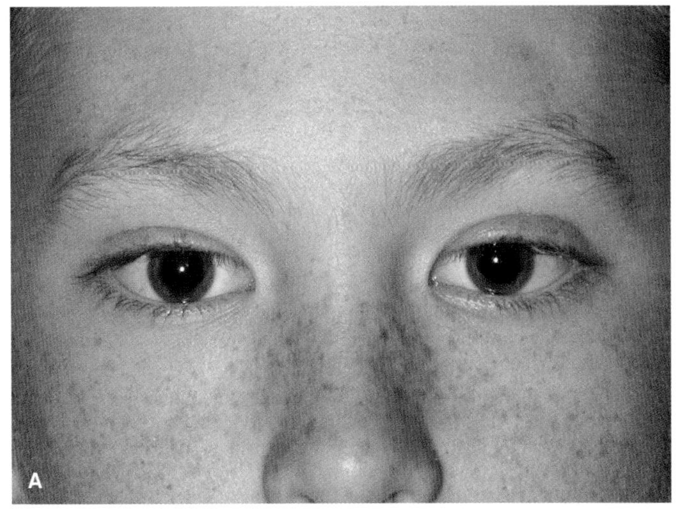

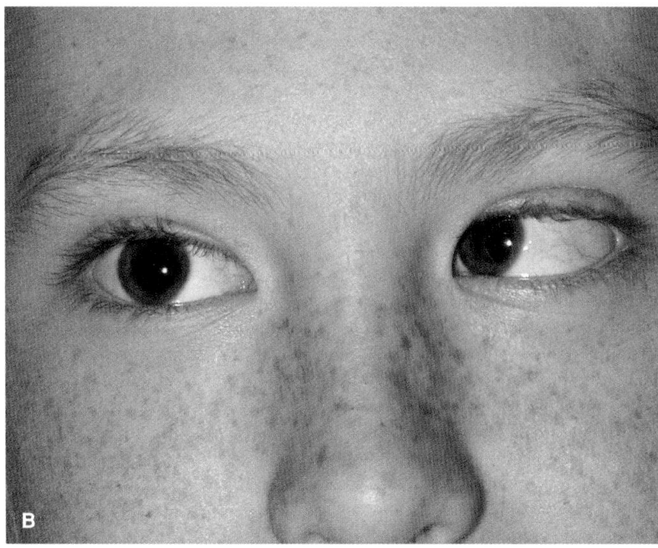

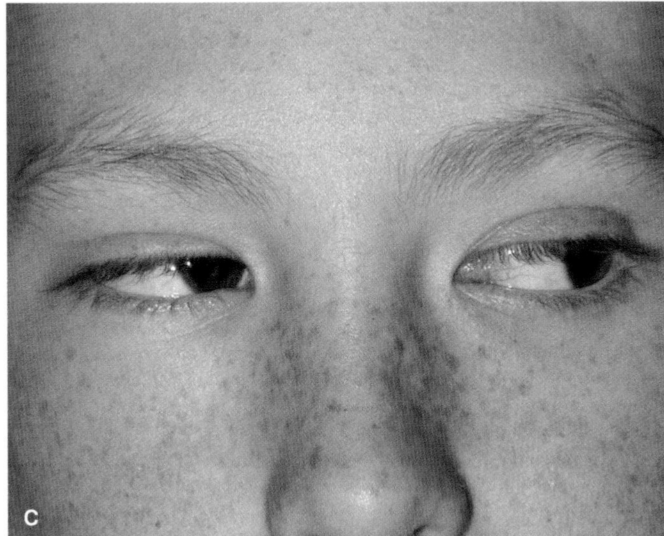

FIGURE 15-4 Duane syndrome. **A.** Eyes are straight in primary position. **B.** Reduced abduction of the right eye with a left esotropia. **C.** Normal adduction of the right eye but globe retraction and palpebral fissure narrowing of the right eye in adduction. (*Used with permission from Paul J. Rychwalski, MD.*)

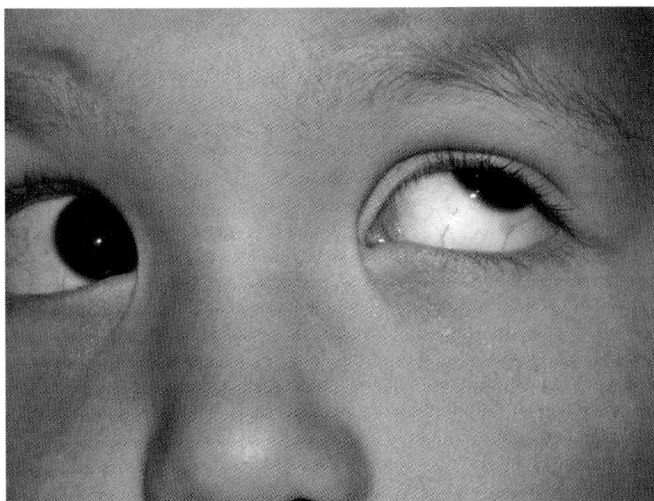

FIGURE 15-5 Right Brown syndrome (superior oblique tendon syndrome). Note restricted upgaze of right eye in adduction and apparent over-elevation of the left eye in abduction. (*Used with permission from Paul J. Rychwalski, MD.*)

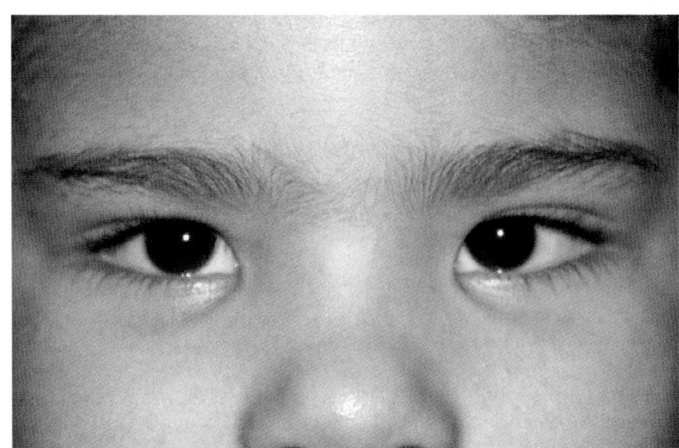

FIGURE 15-6 Pseudostrabismus. Note centered light reflexes, wide nasal bridge and prominent epicanthal folds. (*Used with permission from Paul J. Rychwalski, MD.*)

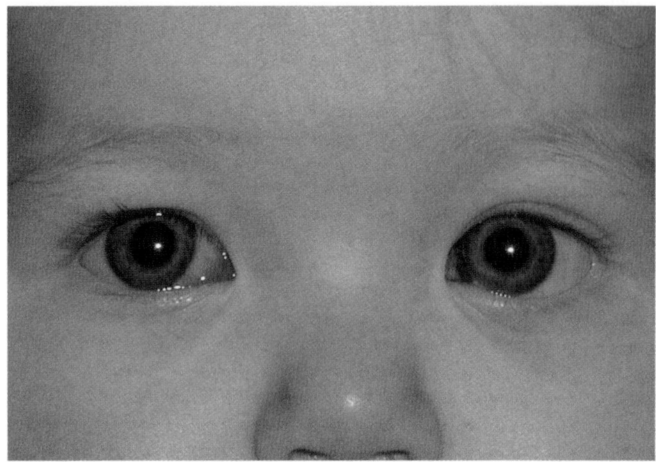

FIGURE 15-7 Eyes now in alignment one week after bilateral medial rectus recession for congenital esotropia. Note the remaining subconjunctival hemorrhages. (*Used with permission from Paul J. Rychwalski, MD.*)

REFERRAL

Indications for referral to a pediatric ophthalmologist include:

- Constant esotropia at any age.
- The corneal light reflection test or cover test demonstrates deviation.
- Incomitant deviations (deviations that change depending upon the position of gaze). This could be a cranial nerve palsy, trauma or extraocular muscle syndrome.
- Torticollis that may be ocular.
- Parental concern exists about ocular alignment despite reassurance.
- Strong family history of strabismus or amblyopia.

PREVENTION AND SCREENING

- Vision screening is a very important way to identify vision problems.
- Children with a family history of childhood vision problems are more likely to have eye problems.
- The American Academy of Ophthalmology and the American Academy of Pediatrics recommend that children have their eyes checked by a pediatrician at the following ages:[14,15]
- Newborn.
    - All babies should have their eyes checked for infections, defects, cataracts, or glaucoma before leaving the hospital. This is especially true for premature babies, babies who were given oxygen for an extended period, and babies with multiple medical problems.
- By 6 months of age.
    - As part of each well-child visit, eye health, vision development, and alignment of the eyes should be checked.
- At 3 to 4 years of age.
    - Eyes and vision should be checked for any abnormalities that may cause problems with later development.
- At 5 years of age and older.
    - Vision in each eye should be checked separately every year. If a problem is found during routine eye exams, referral to a pediatric ophthalmologist may be required.
- Learning disabilities.
    - Learning disabilities are quite common in childhood years and have many causes. The eyes are often suspected but are almost never the cause of learning problems. Vision therapy will not improve a learning disability. A referral for a thorough evaluation by an educational specialist may be indicated.[8]

PROGNOSIS

- Early identification is crucial for a good visual outcome. Adherence to amblyopia therapy remains a significant barrier to success even in cases of strabismus caught and treated early.

FOLLOW-UP

Follow-up is typically conducted every 2 to 3 months if the child is patching. In younger children, close follow-up is recommended, as the risk of amblyopia is higher during the critical period of visual development. Children otherwise at risk are seen at 6 and 12 month intervals.

PATIENT EDUCATION

- Early screening for problems and possible referral to a pediatric ophthalmologist is important.
- Adherence to the recommended therapies are critical to successful correction of any problem.

PATIENT AND PROVIDER RESOURCES

- American Association for Pediatric Ophthalmology and Strabismus—**www.aapos.org**.
- Children's Eye Foundation—**www.childrenseyefoundation.org**.
- American Academy of Pediatrics—Ophthalmology sub-section—**www.aap.org**.
- American Academy of Ophthalmology—**www.aao.org**.

REFERENCES

1. Abrahamsson M, Magnusson G, Sjöstrand J. Inheritance of strabismus and the gain of using heredity to determine populations at risk of developing strabismus. *Acta Ophthalmol Scand.* 1999; 77:653.
2. Greenberg AE, Mohney BG, Diehl NN, Burke JP. Incidence and types of childhood esotropia: a population-based study. *Ophthalmology.* 2007;114:170.

3. Williams C, Northstone K, Howard M, et al. Prevalence and risk factors for common vision problems in children: data from the ALSPAC study. *Br J Ophthalmol*. 2008;92:959.
4. Varma R, et al. Prevalence of Amblyopia and Strabismus in African-American and Hispanic Children Aged 6 Months to 72 Months: The Multi-Ethnic Pediatric Eye Disease Study. *Ophthalmology*. 2008;115(7):1229-1236.
5. Von Noorden, GK, Campos, EC. Binoculer: Vision and Ocular Motility, Sixth edition, St. Louis: Mosby; 2002:134.
6. Gunton, KB. Advances in amblyopia: what have we learned from PEDIG trials? *Pediatrics*. 2013;131(3):540-547.
7. Repka, MX, Wallace, DK, Beck, RW, Kraker, RT, Birch, EE, Cotter, SA, Donahue, S., et al. Two-year follow-up of a 6-month randomized trial of atropine vs patching for treatment of moderate amblyopia in children. *Archives of ophthalmology*. 2005b; 123(2):149-157.
8. Scheiman, MM, Hertle, RW, Beck, RW, Edwards, AR, Birch, E, Cotter, S A, Crouch, ERJ, et al. Randomized trial of treatment of amblyopia in children aged 7 to 17 years. *Archives of ophthalmology*. 2005;123(4), 437-447.
9. Repka, MX, Holmes, JM, Melia, BM, Beck, RW, Gearinger, MD, Tamkins, SM, & Wheeler, DT. The effect of amblyopia therapy on ocular alignment. *Journal of AAPOS*. 2005a;9(6):542-545.
10. Gusek-Schneider, G, & Boss, A. Results following eye muscle surgery for secondary sensory strabismus. *Strabismus*. 2010;18(1), 24-31.
11. Hopker, LM, & Weakley, DR. Surgical results after one-muscle recession for correction of horizontal sensory strabismus in children. *Journal of AAPOS*. 2013;17(2):174-176.
12. Lennerstrand, G. Strabismus and eye muscle function. *Acta ophthalmologica Scandinavica*. 2007;85(7):711-723.
13. Repka, MX, Holmes, JM, Melia, BM, Beck, RW, Gearinger, MD, Tamkins, SM, & Wheeler, DT. The effect of amblyopia therapy on ocular alignment. *Journal of AAPOS*. 2005;9(6): 542-545.
14. American Academy of Pediatrics. Eye examination in infants, children, and young adults by pediatricians. *Pediatrics*. 2003;Apr;111(4,1): 902-907.
15. American Academy of Pediatrics. Instrument-based pediatric vision screening policy statement. *Pediatrics*. 2012;130(5):983-6.

16 RETINOBLASTOMA AND THE DIFFERENTIAL DIAGNOSIS OF LEUKOCORIA

Abdul-Karim Sleiman
Arun Singh, MD
Elias I. Traboulsi, MD

PATIENT STORY

A 14-month-old boy was referred by his pediatrician because a whitish reflex from his left pupil (**Figure 16-1**) was noticed by his parents in certain directions of gaze. It was also noted on a few recent photographs. His pediatrician had checked the pupillary light reflex and indeed noted a dimmer and tan-colored reflex from the left pupil as opposed to a brighter and more reddish reflex in the left eye. She referred the child for further evaluation and management. Dilated fundus examination revealed a single large tumor in the left eye, occupying more than 50 percent of the globe. Ultrasonography showed a pattern consistent with calcifications within the tumor, and suggestive of retinoblastoma. A magnetic resonance imaging (MRI) scan showed no evidence of optic nerve or intracranial involvement. There were no other tumors in either eye. There was no family history of retinoblastoma. A decision was made to enucleate the eye because of the size of the tumor.

INTRODUCTION

Leukocoria means a white (*leuko*) reflex from the pupil (*coria*). Leukocoria is a sign observed by the naked eye or with a scope, often detected incidentally on routine eye examination, or in photographs; it is not a diagnosis. The most feared cause of a white reflex in the pupil is retinoblastoma, the most common intraocular tumor of childhood. Other conditions can manifest themselves initially with leukocoria. Precise diagnosis ensures appropriate and early treatment to prevent irreversible blindness from primary pathology, secondary amblyopia, or life-threatening malignancies.

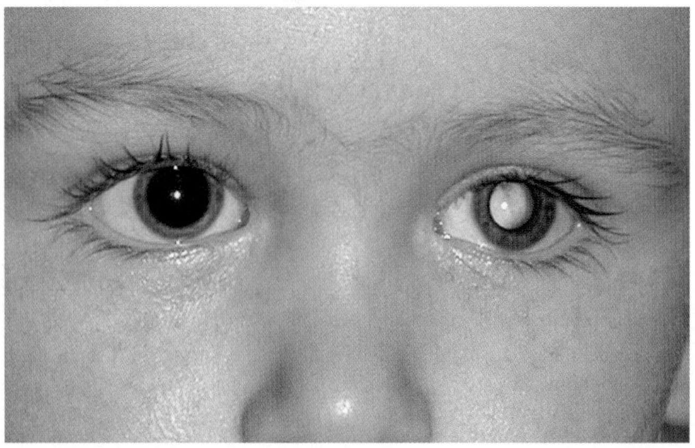

FIGURE 16-1 Leukocoria in the left eye of this infant with retinoblastoma. The tumor can actually be visualized behind the clear lens. (*Used with permission from Elias Traboulsi, MD.*)

SYNONYMS

White pupillary reflex. White pupil.

EPIDEMIOLOGY

- Retinoblastoma is diagnosed in 47 percent of children who are referred with leukocoria to tertiary centers.[1]
- The majority (32 to 73%) of children with retinoblastoma present with leukocoria.[2,3]
- Retinoblastoma occurs as rarely as in 1:13,000 to 1:20,000 live births, with an annual incidence of 11.8 per million children between zero and four years of age in the US and similar statistics in Europe.[4]
- Other causes of leukocoria are slightly more common but exact estimates of their incidence are not available.

ETIOLOGY AND PATHOPHYSIOLOGY

- The direct cause underlying leukocoria that is common to the different conditions that cause it is an interference with the normal red reflex from opacities or abnormalities that occur strictly anywhere from the crystalline lens and posteriorly, hence excluding corneal opacities.
- Leukocoria from retinoblastoma is caused by the whitish well-circumscribed retinal mass.
- The tumor develops when a negative regulator of the cell cycle (pRB) is inactive or absent secondary to mutations in both alleles of the tumor suppressor gene *RB1* in a retinal progenitor cell.[5]
- The "two-hit" theory (first germline, second somatic; or both somatic) explains both heritable and non-heritable forms of retinoblastoma.
- Other conditions are listed in the differential diagnosis (see **Table 16-1**).

RISK FACTORS

- The presence of a germinal mutation in the retinoblastoma gene confers up to 90 percent risk of developing retinoblastoma.
- A family history of retinoblastoma is a strong risk factor for offspring and siblings.
- Radiation exposure predisposes to second malignant neoplasms in hereditary retinoblastoma.
- The 13q deletion predisposes to bilateral disease with multiple other malformations including facial dysmorphism.
- The Children's Oncology Group (COG) trials for retinoblastoma are currently evaluating histopathologic risk factors, familial and

TABLE 16-1 Differential Diagnosis and Features of Entities that Can Simulate Retinoblastoma or Cause a Whitish Reflex from the Pupil

Entity	Definition & Epidemiology	Leukocoria	Causes and Risk Factors	Clinical Features	Management	Prognosis	Prevention, Screening, & Education
Cataract	Progressive opacification of the lens. Congenital: ~2 per 10,000. Infantile: 1 to 15 per 10,000.	Opacity in the lens. Noticed by primary carephysician or parents, by naked eye, on red reflex evaluation or in photos.	Genetically determined in 50 percent of cases; mostly autosomal dominant. Could be a sign of systemic or infectious process, or the result of an injury.	Decreased visual acuity. Nystagmus. Strabismus. Photophobia. Family history of hereditary cataract. Features of genetic disorders associated with cataract (galactosemia, Down's, etc). Labs for infections or metabolic causes. Genetic testing and/or karyotype.	If extra-axial or small & good vision, conservative: close follow up during age of visual development (until 8 to 9 years). Otherwise, prompt surgical extraction with optical rehabilitation (intraocular lens or postoperative contact lens) + near vision glasses + frequent adjustment of prescription with growth. Occlusion therapy (patching) if amblyopia ensues.	Untreated, amblyogenic and causing partial or total blindness. With early diagnosis and treatment, visual acuities of 20/40 to 20/20 can be achieved in many cases. Poor prognostic factors: nystagmus, strabismus, and unilateral infantile or congenital cataract.	Red reflex screening for all children in every exam. Regardless of leukocoria, all high risk children (positive family history, personal history of ionizing radiation exposure, long-term use of systemic steroids, or a systemic disorder associated with cataracts) require referral and yearly ophthamologic follow-up.
Persistent fetal vasculature (PFV) or Persistent hyperplastic vitreous (PHPV).	Congenital malformation resulting from failure of regression of the primary vitreous and hyaloid vascular system. Rare in the population. PFV is in up to 63 percent of children presenting with leukocoria.	Rudimentary vascular stalk in vitreous associated to plaque-like opacity retrolental fibrovascular tissue. Usually unilateral (**Figure 16-4**).	Arrest of normal involution of the embryonic vascular connective tissue that normally occurs after 4 months gestation. Non hereditary.	Microphthalmia. Strabismus. Cataract. Vascularized white retrolental tissue. Prominent iridial vessels. Elongated ciliary processes Glaucoma. Other malformations (intralenticular hemorrhage, uveal coloboma, etc) Posterior features (retinal fold, hypoplastic macula &/or optic nerve, traction retinal detachment + stalk to optic disc)	Ocular ultrasound: persistent hyaloid remnants with hyaloid artery or canal from disc into vitreous towards lens + confirmation of other clinical findings. CT or MRI: same as ultrasound. With contrast: hypervascular vitreous. Treatment: Lens extraction and anterior vitrectomy; can be complex. Enucleation in severe cases with no vision and malformed small globe.	High risk of: glaucoma, cataract, intraocular hemorrhage, and retinal detachment. Visual prognosis limited by associated optic nerve or macular disease. Long term: enucleation for terminal glaucoma, intraocular hemorrhage, retinal detachment, phthisis bulbi.	Red reflex screening for all children in every exam. No preventive measures available due to sporadic nature of the abnormality. Has been diagnosed on fetal ultrasound.

(continued)

TABLE 16-1 Differential Diagnosis and Features of Entities that Can Simulate Retincblastoma or Cause a Whitish Reflex from the Pupil (*Continued*)

Entity	Definition & Epidemiology	Leukocoria	Causes and Risk Factors	Clinical Features	Management	Prognosis	Prevention, Screening, & Education
Extensive myelination of the nerve fiber layer	Abnormal myelination of nerve fibers of the retina. Almost in 1 percent of the population.	Lesion follows distribution of nerve fibers, typically striated white or gray myelinated nerve fibers patches with feathery borders (**Figure 16-5**).	Most cases are sporadic. Can occur in the context of some syndromes such as Gorlin syndrome (basal cell nevus syndrome).	Mostly asymptomatic. Usually normal vision (scotomas or enlarged blind spots may occur). In extensive cases has been associated with a higher incidence of amblyopia, myopia, and strabismus. Optic nerve may also be hypoplastic.	Visual field test. Asymptomatic cases: no treatment required. Symptomatic cases: prompt treatment of coexisting conditions that are associated with negative prognosi such as high myopia and amblyopia.	Generally stable. Poor vision from amblyopia in some cases.	Typically stable and benign disease. No preventive measures available.
Retinopathy of prematurity (ROP).	Developmental vascular disorder with uncontrolled vasoproliferation of incompletely vascularized retinas of premature infants. Affects around 21 percent to 36 percent of preterm infants.	Opaque mass behind lens (retrolental fibroplasia) in advanced and untreated cases of ROP and retinal detachment.	Prematurity <32 weeks Decreasing gestational age and birth weight. Assisted ventilation (>1 week). Surfactant therapy. Blood transfusions. Severity of illness. Hyperglycemia and insulin therapy. Sepsis. Elevated arterial oxygen tension. Fluctuations in blood gas measurements. Intraventricular hemorrhage. Bronchopulmonary dysplasia.	Detected on screening by an experienced ophthalmologist: location and retinal changes noted. The AAP/AAO/AAPOS 2006 recommendations for screening: 1- all infants with a birth weight <1500 g or gestational age ≤32 weeks 2- selected infants weighing: 1500 to 2000 g or gestational age >32 weeks with an unstable clinical course 3- infants at high risk according to their attending pediatrician or neonatologist.	Prethreshold ROP: elective treatment for prevention of progression. Threshold ROP: ablation of peripheral abnormal retina with laser photocoagulation (better than cryotherapy). Severe ROP without retinal detachment + ocular opacities (photocoagulation not possible): Bevacizumab (anti-VEGF) off-label (optimal timing and dose unknown). Retinal detachment: urgent surgical treatment. Post-treatment follow-up exam: weekly or biweekly for 1 to 2 months then less frequently depending on clinical course.	Irregular progression. Spontaneous regression in vast majority in 4 months. Poor visual acuity or fundus structural abnormalities in 5.1 percent. Blindness in children <1000 g birth weight. Poor visual prognosis in untreated severe ROP. High risk for: vitreous hemorrhages, preretinal membrane, tractional retinal detachment, strabismus, anisometropia, future myopia.	First screening examination: sufficient if both retinas fully vascularized. Screening examinations should continue until ROP regresses and the vessels mature, or until treatment is needed. Prevention targeted at oxidant injury (vitamins, penicillamine, and limiting light exposure): tested but not supported by evidence. Recommendations: avoiding episodes of physiologic instability.

Toxocariasis	Ocular infection caused by a zoonotic parasite: the dog or cat ascarid *Toxocara* (*canis* or *catis*). Most common in children aged 1 to 5 years. Leukocoria is the presenting sign in 15 percent of the cases. 98 percent of the cases have a history negative for visceral larva migrans syndrome.	Subretinal granuloma: whitish, 1 to 2 disc diameters, located anywhere in the retina. Nematode endophthalmitis: large inflammatory mass (with prominent vitreous inflammation). Both lesions may have calcification & be confused with retinoblastoma.	Ocular lesion: caused by inflammatory response to the second-stage larva. Human infection: due to accidental ingestion of infective eggs and tissue invasion of second stage larvae. Transmission: by con- taminated food or geophagia. Factors influencing onset of ocular disease are unknown, but the inflammatory reaction is mainly associated with larval death.	The only manifestation of the disease may be ocular. Unilateral. Subretinal granuloma (alone, in a quiet eye). Retinal damage: folds, elevation, detachment. Strabismus. Decreased vision. Chronic endophthalmitis. Uveitis (posterior). Macular and optic nerve disversion. Positive serum IgG (ELISA): confirmatory. Negative serum IgG: does not rule Toxocariasis out. Aqueous humor antibodies demonstrate intraocular production.	Peripheral granuloma (silent, minimal inflammation) does not require treatment. Anthelmintics (tiabendazole or diethylcarbamazepine) are controversial: larvae death may increase inflammation. Steroid umbrella (systemic or periocular) with anhelmintics to reduce inflammation, or alone to control vitreoretinal tractional membranes. Vitreoretinal surgery: for vitreous opacities, epiretinal membranes, and retinal detachment. Laser photocoagulation: to kill mobile visible larva, under "steroid umbrella." Other ophthalmologic procedures to improve vision.	56 percent suffer permanent vision loss. Poor visual prognostic factors are: Severe vitreitis. Cystoid macular edema. Tractional retinal detachment.	No screening (no need for treatment if silent). Prevention by reducing oral transmission to humans: periodic deworming treatment of pets (especially lactating females), timely disposal of pet feces, and good hygiene practices. Education to patients at risk: to prevent infection in pets, and to avoid exposure to potentially contaminated soil.
Optic disc and uveal coloboma.	Cleft of the optic disc secondary to failure of the fetal fissure to close inferiorly. Rare.	White sharp decentered excavation in the optic disk. May extend inferiorly to retina and choroid (rarely affects the entire disc; **Figure 16-6**).	Sporadic or inherited. Isolated or part of a syndrome: Renal coloboma syndrome (autosomal dominant, PAX2 gene on 10q). CHARGE syndrome. Other syndromes (Walker-Warburg, Aicardi, Goldenhar, linear sebaceous nevus, Noonan, focal dermal hypoplasia).	Unilateral or bilateral. Thin neuroretinal rim. Iris & ciliary coloboma. Orbital cyst. Iris heterochromia. Retinal venous malformations. Renal coloboma findings (VU reflux, renal hypoplasia, renal failure, chronic nephritis). CHARGE syndrome (+PHPV, microphthalmos, facial palsy, facial dysmorphism, TE fistula, renal, cardiovascular and CNS abnormalities.)	Renal ultrasound to rule out significant renal disease. Rule out CHARGE syndrome (Colobomas, Heart defects, Choanal Atresia, Retarded growth, Genital abnormalities, Ear abnormalities) with echocardiography, nasal catheter (or CT sinuses) and hearing test.	Visual acuity ranges form normal to complete visual loss (not predictable by appearance of the lesion). Best visual prognostic factor: sparing of the fovea by associated chorioretinal coloboma.	Red reflex screening for all children in every exam. No preventive measures available due to nature of the abnormality.

(*continued*)

TABLE 16-1 Differential Diagnosis and Features of Entities that Can Simulate Retinoblastoma or Cause a Whitish Reflex from the Pupil (*Continued*)

Entity	Definition & Epidemiology	Leukocoria	Causes and Risk Factors	Clinical Features	Management	Prognosis	Prevention, Screening, & Education
Coats disease	Primary retinal telangiectasias, a rare exudative retinopathy usually affecting young males (80% are 5 to 10 years old).	Luminous leukocoria from massive yellow exudates on/in edematous retina (pseudotumor; **Figure 16-7**).	Idiopathic, congenital, and nonhereditary. Somatic mutation in NDP gene, causing deficiency of norrin (protein product) in the developing retina. No known associated systemic problems.	90 percent unilateral. Decreased visual acuity. Strabismus. Retinal telangiectasia: usually peripheral strings of fusiform aneurysmal dilatations of the retinal vessels (tiny light bulbs). Pseudo-tumoral exudates, predilection for macula. Exudative (partial or total) retinal detachment. Iridis rubeosis. Neovascular glaucoma. Cataract. Uveitis. Phthisis bulbi.	Treatment goal: arresting vascular progression. Cryotherapy or laser photocoagulation: limited success. Avoided if lesions around optic nerve. Enucleation is an option for further complicated cases.	Variable evolution. Spontaneous stabilization or regression is occasional and may be temporary or permanent, but usually with loss of central vision (macular deposits). Retinal exudation can cause retinal detachment. Progressive retinal damage and eventual definitive blindness.	As precise origin is unknown, disease cannot be prevented.
Morning Glory syndrome	Congenital anomaly: funnel shaped excavation of the fundus and the optic nerve head with a ring of chorioretinal pigment around the disk. Uncommon, but more common in females.	Central white glialtuft of tissue at center of optic cup, surrounded by vessels radiating out like spikes from an enlarged optic nerve head.	Unknown. Sporadic occurrence in great majority of cases. Some underlying genetic defect must be present (see associated malformations).	Unilateral. Usually isolated. Retinal detachment up to 1/3 of cases. Association to midline cranial defects with symptoms of mouth-breathing, snoring, and rhinorrhea. Baasal cephaloceles Reported associations with capillary hemangiomas, carotid circulation abnormalities such as Moyamoya disease, and renal disease.	MRI: transsphenoidal encephalocele may be seen affecting the nasopharynx. MRAs are essential to rule out associated Moyamoya disease that could be treatable.	Serous retinal detachment retinal folds, and subretinal neovascularization may contribute to a poor visual prognosis. Usually severely reduced visual acuity (20/200 to finger counting). But occasionally better.	No preventive measures available for malformation itself.

Congenital Toxoplasmosis	Ocular infection with the protozoa *Toxoplasma* causing uveitis, vitritis, and focal necrotizing retinochoroiditis. Congenital cases show chorioretinal scars (Figure 16-8), may also have optic atrophy, cataract, and microphthalmos.	Fluffy whitish lesion + retinal edema: necrosis, usually involving inner layers of the retina where the primary site of multiplying parasites is. Possible sites of contiguous inflammation: choroid and sclera.	Transplacental transmission from infected mother to fetus, highest in 3rd semester. Maternal infection from ingestion of undercooked or contaminated dairy products and meat, or (directly or indirectly) cat feces. Immune deficient state primes for infection or reactivation of toxoplasmosis (HIV or medical immune suppression).	No clinical signs in 90 percent of congenital infections. Symptomatic infection: Chorioretinitis (in 80 percent of congenital cases, and usually bilateral), intracranial Calcification, convulsions, as well as cerebral palsy, mental retardation, microcephaly or hydrocephaly. Accounts for up to 50 percent of cases of posterior uveitis cases. Panuveitis, optic atrophy, microphthalmos, cataract. Retinal destruction & thickening from retinal vasculitis. Elevated IgM in neonate (ELISA).	Fluorescein angiography: hypofluorescence, followed by progressive leakage. Indocyanine angiography: dark small spots around the lesions implying retinal involvement is greater than initially seen. Useful for follow up after treatment. Pharmacologic therapies: Triple: pyrimethamine, sulfadiazine, & prednisone. Quadruple: add clindamycin. + folinic acid to avoid hematologic complications of pyrimethamine. Duration of therapy depends on clinical response: usually 4 to 6 weeks. Goals: to eradicate parasite and suppress inflammation.	Poor prognostic factor: earlier infection in pregnancy. Indications to treat: Lesions involvement of the optic disc, papillomacular bundle, or macula. Active large lesions. Immunocompromised patient.	Cooking food to safe temperatures and other habits that reduce risk from food, as well as keeping pregnant women away form litter boxes and other behaviors that reduce risk from the environment are recommended by the CDC and the USDA.

environmental factors, multimodality treatments (including chemotherapies, stem cell therapy and viral oncolysis) for extraocular retinoblastoma and associated tumors, and late complications in survivors.[6–8]

DIAGNOSIS

Securing a firm diagnosis frequently necessitates examination under anesthesia with ocular, orbital and brain imaging as well as ocular photography.

CLINICAL FEATURES

- Common presenting signs of retinoblastoma include leukocoria, strabismus, poor vision, family history alone, and ocular inflammation.[2,3]
- The tumor may grow subretinally (exophytic) with later exudative retinal detachment, and/or towards the vitreous (endophytic) with possible intravitreal seeding.
- Patients with hereditary retinoblastoma are at risk of second malignant neoplasms.

DISTRIBUTION

- Unilateral unifocal retinoblastoma is usually non-hereditary.
- Hereditary retinoblastomas are in general either bilateral or unilateral and multifocal and occur early in infancy. They carry a high risk of second extraocular tumors.
- Extraocular disease consists of trilateral retinoblastoma (bilateral disease with pinealoblastoma), second malignancies (sarcomas), or metastasis.
- Based on its size, position in the globe, and dissemination, retinoblastoma is classified according to the International Intraocular Retinoblastoma Classification (ICRB), with the aim of accurate prognostication of globe salvage.[9]

LABORATORY TESTING

- Molecular genetic testing requires prior genetic counseling (see the following section).
- Histopathology of retinoblastoma (if enucleation is performed) is indispensable for detecting microscopic infiltration of the optic nerve or choroid, classification of the tumor, and subsequent decision regarding adjuvant chemotherapy.[10]
- Additional tests are individualized upon the planned mode of treatment; baseline blood chemistries and complete blood count before chemotherapy.

IMAGING

- Digital fundus photography is needed for documentation and classification (**Figure 16-2**).
- Ocular ultrasonography demonstrates the solid intraocular mass, usually with calcifications, and evaluates the surrounding orbital tissues (**Figure 16-3**).
- Computed tomography (CT) scanning also exhibits the characteristic intratumoral calcified foci, but it is avoided for the associated increased long-term risk for cancer. CT is reserved for diagnostically challenging cases.
- MRI differentiates retinoblastoma from Coats disease, in the presence of exudative retinal detachment.
- During workup and follow-up, MRI precisely ascertains tumor size, optic nerve and choroid involvement, and any associated brain tumors.

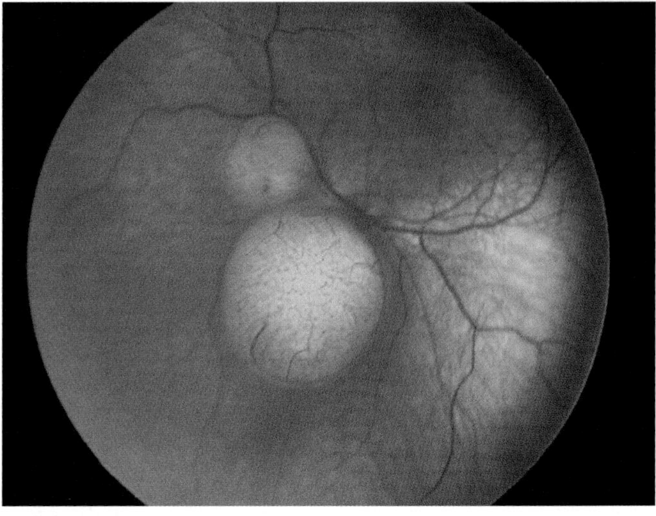

FIGURE 16-2 Wide-angle fundus photograph reveals two retinoblastoma tumors nasal to the optic nerve head. (*Used with permission from Elias Traboulsi, MD.*)

DIFFERENTIAL DIAGNOSIS

- The differential diagnosis of leukocoria in a child is the differential diagnosis of retinoblastoma (see **Table 16-1**).

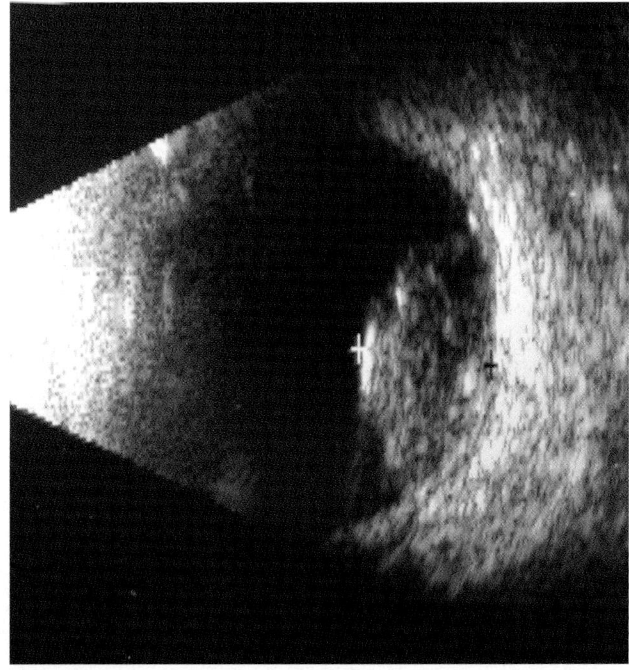

FIGURE 16-3 Ocular B-scan ultrasonogram of a single medium sized intraocular tumor. The areas of increased echodensity (white areas) within the mass correspond to foci of calcification. (*Used with permission from Elias Traboulsi, MD.*)

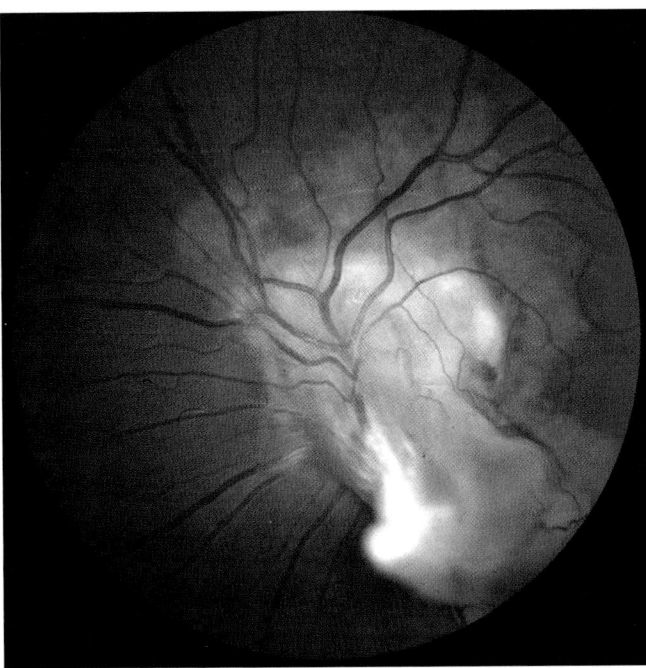

FIGURE 16-4 Persistent hyperplastic primary vitreous. The posterior portion of the retained and proliferated fetal vitreous is attached to the optic nerve head. Anteriorly these patients have a whitish mass occupying the posterior aspect of the lens and dragging the ciliary processes towards the lens. (*Used with permission from Elias Traboulsi, MD.*)

MANAGEMENT

- The management includes (1) ruling out extraocular extension or other tumors, (2) treatment of the intraocular tumor, (3) long-term follow-up, and (4) genetic counseling.

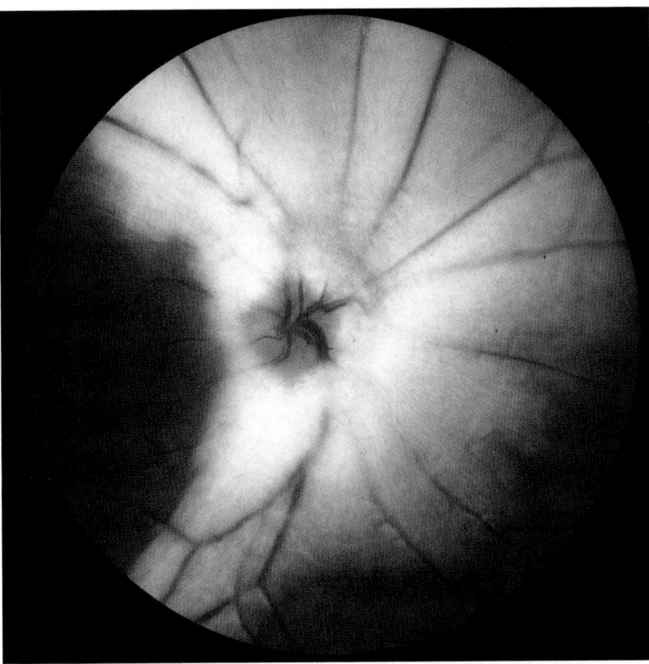

FIGURE 16-5 Extensive myelination of the optic nerve fibers in this right eye. Note fluffy edges and partial obstruction of the view of the optic nerve head by the white opaque myelinated axons. (*Used with permission from Elias Traboulsi, MD.*)

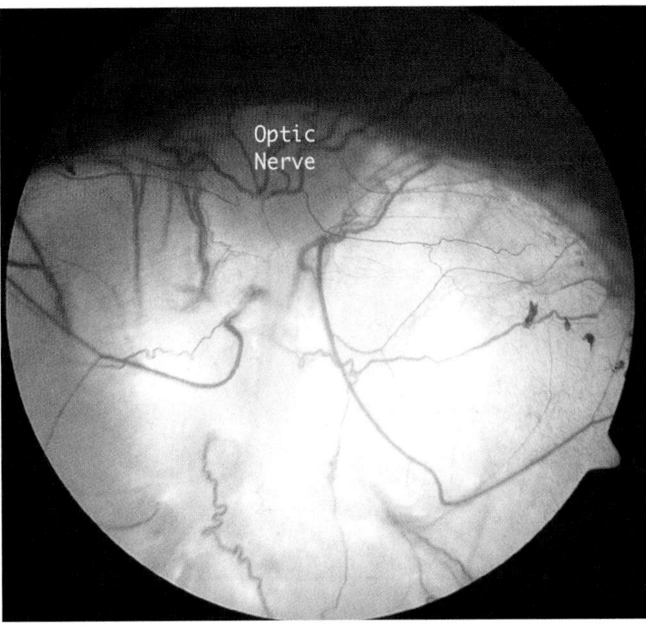

FIGURE 16-6 Large chorioretinal coloboma involving the optic nerve head and the inferior part of the fundus. This will cause a white pupillary reflex. (*Used with permission from Elias Traboulsi, MD.*)

- With modern treatment techniques, the ICRB proved to be the best predictor of treatment outcomes, especially first-line chemotherapy and adjuvant focal therapy.[9]
- The treatment plan is tailored to age, laterality, potential for vision, intraocular tumor burden, and tumor extent beyond the eye.
- Treatment aims at (1) saving the child's life by eradicating the tumor, (2) maximizing preserved vision, and (3) decreasing the adverse effects of therapy.[6]

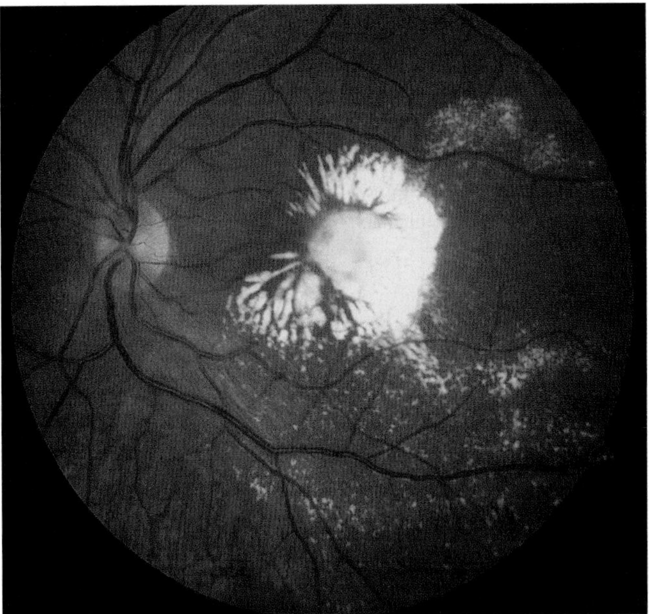

FIGURE 16-7 Yellowish macular elevated lesion made of cholesterol exudates from an abnormal leaky vascular aneurysm (not evident on this photo). The aneurysm can be in the peripheral part of the retina and the leakage will pool in the posterior pole. (*Used with permission from Elias Traboulsi, MD.*)

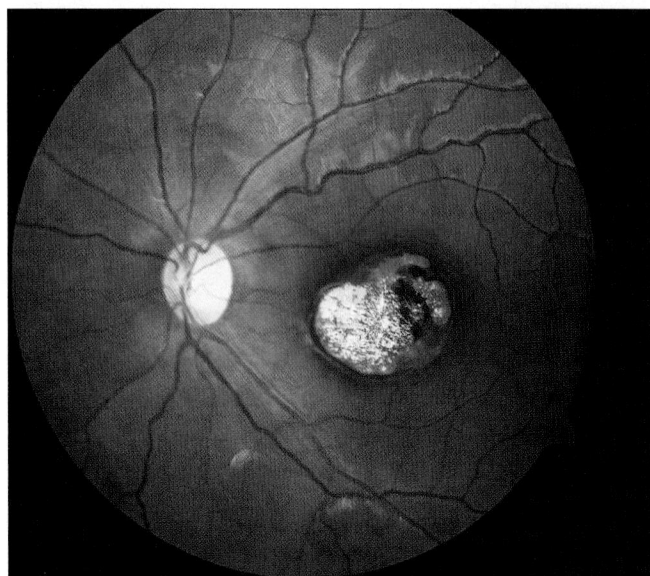

FIGURE 16-8 Macular chorioretinal scar from congenital toxoplasmosis. The white is sclera and the black is proliferated retinal pigment epithelium during the healing phase of the infections and inflammatory process. This is a typical location for congenital toxoplasmosis. (*Used with permission from Elias Traboulsi, MD.*)

NONPHARMACOLOGIC

- Ablation of small tumors with local consolidative measures (cryotherapy, laser photocoagulation or transpupillary thermotherapy) can salvage the eye.
- In larger tumors, ablation may be used in conjunction with chemotherapy.[6] SOR Ⓐ
- Cryotherapy (through the sclera) is used for anteriorly located small tumors.
- Laser photocoagulation targets feeding vessels of small posterior tumors.
- Transpupillary thermotherapy directs infrared waves at the tumor mass, heats it up, and destroys it.
- Failures of the preceding therapies or recurrences are treated with episcleral radioactive plaques, external beam radiotherapy, or enucleation.

MEDICATIONS

- Chemotherapy is a safer alternative to radiation in retinoblastoma.
- Carboplatin alone can cause the tumor to shrink, however, most standard multi-agent regimens also include vincristine ± etoposide for 6 cycles.[6,11] SOR Ⓑ
- Success rates depend on regimen, tumor thickness, extent, and seeding.[12]
- Chemoreduction reduces tumor size to make it amenable to focal therapy.
- Local chemotherapy modalities, such as sub-Tenon (subconjunctival) carboplatin injection, are evolving as treatments for larger tumors. SOR Ⓒ

COMPLEMENTARY/ALTERNATIVE THERAPY

- External-beam radiation therapy (EBRT) aims at globe sparing, but it is avoided for major risk of inducing second neoplasms in hereditary disease.
- Brachytherapy (plaque radiotherapy) has excellent outcomes with minimal complications, especially for localized tumors.[13] SOR Ⓐ
- In extensive disease, combining chemoreduction with radiotherapy makes globe salvage more likely than when applying either modality alone.[13] SOR Ⓐ

SURGERY

- Enucleation is indicated for advanced unilateral intraocular tumors when the affected eye is unsalvageable, that is, hope of useful vision in it is very low to null, or when previous "globe-conserving" treatments have failed.[14] SOR Ⓐ
- Adjuvant chemotherapy should be considered after enucleation, if the pathology indicates high-risk features. SOR Ⓑ
- Approximately 6 weeks postoperatively, an ocular prosthesis can be placed.

REFERRAL

- All patients with suspected leukocoria need urgent referral to an ophthalmologist.
- Often, different specialists need to be involved in the work-up of leukocoria.
- Ophthalmologists and ocular oncologists evaluate the metastatic risk from the clinical features, the imaging, and the histopathology.
- Once the diagnosis of retinoblastoma is established, a pediatric oncologist needs to be involved in the management.
- The National Cancer Institute recommends referral of all pediatric and adolescent patients with malignancy to a medical center where the treatment plan can be developed under the care of a multidisciplinary team.[6]

PREVENTION AND SCREENING

- Newborns with a family history need prompt ophthalmologic evaluation with close follow up screening until age of 6 or until negative genetic test for *RB1*.[14]
- Risk prediction for patients and relatives is improved if genetic testing is used to distinguish asymptomatic children at risk from relatives without the mutation.[5,15]
- Relatives (parent, siblings, and offsprings) of individuals with documented germline mutations should undergo close surveillance.

PROGNOSIS

- Obvious external findings often predict enucleation and evidently poor visual prognosis.[16]
- Intraocular staging according to the ICRB predicts the ocular salvage rate (success of chemoreduction, no enucleation, no EBRT).[16–18]

- Relapse in the orbit is associated with systemic disease.[19]
- Metastatic risk is assessed from clinical features, imaging, and histopathology.
- Patients with extraocular involvement carry worse survival prognosis.
- The overall 5-year survival of retinoblastoma is around 94 percent in the US.[20]
- Survivors of the hereditary form have up to 35 percent risk for second malignancies in adulthood.[21]

FOLLOW-UP

- After diagnosis, periodic exams are performed to rule out asynchronous bilaterality.[6]
- Ophthalmologic follow-up consists of periodic careful examinations with or without MRI.
- After enucleation, a 2-year follow-up is needed to rule out orbital relapse.[19]
- In survivors, lumps or bone pain may indicate soft tissue or bone sarcomas.[5]

PATIENT EDUCATION

- Genetic testing requires counseling since it implies disclosure of critical information.
- A geneticist or genetic counselor provides information on the nature, inheritance, and consequences of a genetic disorder to individuals and families for better decision-making.
- Tumor laterality, family history, and molecular genetic diagnosis determines the risk to offsprings.
- Potential genetic risks, reproductive options, and prenatal testing are discussed with young adults who are affected or at risk, optimally prior to pregnancy.
- Survivors must avoid carcinogenic behaviors (smoking and DNA-damaging exposures).

PATIENT RESOURCES

- Retinoblastoma Treatment (PDQ®), Patient Version, from the National Cancer Institute at the National Institutes of Health—**http://cancer.gov/cancertopics/pdq/treatment/retinoblastoma/patient**.
- Understanding Cancer Series, Gene Testing, from the National Cancer Institute at the National Institutes of Health—**http://cancer.gov/cancertopics/understandingcancer/genetesting**.
- Retinoblastoma, from the American Cancer Society—**http://www.cancer.org/cancer/retinoblastoma/index**.

PROVIDER RESOURCES

- Approach to the child with leukocoria, UpToDate—**www.uptodate.com/contents/approach-to-the-child-with-leukocoria**.
- Overview of retinoblastoma, UpToDate—**www.uptodate.com/contents/overview-of-retinoblastoma**.
- Retinoblastoma Treatment (PDQ®), Health Professional Version, from the National Cancer Institute at the National Institutes of Health—**http://cancer.gov/cancertopics/pdq/treatment/retinoblastoma/HealthProfessional**.

REFERENCES

1. Traboulsi EI, ed: *Genetic Diseases of the Eye*, second ed. New York: Oxford UP; 2012.
2. Singh A. *Clinical Ophthalmic Oncology*, first ed., Saunders: Philadelphia, PA; 2007.
3. Boubacar T, Fatou S, Fousseyni T, et al. A 30-month prospective study on the treatment of retinoblastoma in the Gabriel Toure Teaching Hospital, Bamako, Mali. *Br J Ophthalmol*. 2010;94:467-469.
4. Broaddus E, Topham A, Singh AD. Incidence of retinoblastoma in the USA: 1975–2004. *Br J Ophthalmol*. 2009;93:21-23.
5. Lohmann DR, Gallie BL. Retinoblastoma. In: *GeneReviews at GeneTests: Medical Genetics Information Resource* (database online). Pagon RA, Bird TD, Dolan CR, et al., eds. University of Washington, Seattle. 1997-2012. www.ncbi.nlm.nih.gov/books/NBK1452, accessed on December 24, 2012.
6. *Retinoblastoma Treatment (PDQ®) Health Professional Version—Intraocular Retinoblastoma Treatment*. Retinoblastoma Treatment (PDQ®)—National Cancer Institute. http://cancer.gov/cancertopics/pdq/treatment/retinoblastoma/HealthProfessional/page5, accessed December 1, 2013.
7. National Institutes of Health. National Cancer Institute. *Clinical Trials Search Results*. Search: Retinoblastoma, COG. http://www.cancer.gov/clinicaltrials/search/results?protocolsearchid=11288725, acessed December 1, 2013.
8. Esmaeli B, ed. Ophthalmologic Oncology. In: *MD Anderson Solid Tumor Oncology Series*, Pollock, RE, ed., New York: Springer Science+Business Media, LLC; 2011.
9. Linn MA. Intraocular retinoblastoma: the case for a new group classification. *Ophthalmol Clin North Am*. 2005;18(1):41-53.
10. Chawla B, Sharma S, Sen S, et al. Correlation between clinical features, magnetic resonance imaging, and histopathologic findings in retinoblastoma: a prospective study. *Ophthalmology*. 2012;119:850-856.
11. Abramson DH, Lawrence SD, Beaverson KL, et al. Systemic carboplatin for retinoblastoma: change in tumour size over time. *Br J Ophthalmol*. 2005;89:1616-1619.
12. Shields CL, Mashayekhi A, Cater J, et al. Chemoreduction for retinoblastoma. Analysis of tumor control and risks for recurrence in 457 tumors. *Am J Ophthalmol*. 2004;138:329-337.
13. Shields CL, Ramasubramanian A, Thangappan A, et al. Chemoreduction for group E retinoblastoma: comparison of chemoreduction alone versus chemoreduction plus low-dose external radiotherapy in 76 eyes. *Ophthalmology*. 2009;116:544-551.

14. Hurwitz RL, Shields CL, Shields JA, et al. Retinoblastoma. In: *Principles and Practice of Pediatric Oncology*, 6th ed, Pizzo PA, Poplack DG, eds. Lippincott Williams & Wilkins, Philadelphia, PA; 2011:809.

15. Howard GM, and Ellsworth RM. Differential diagnosis of retinoblastoma. A statistical survey of 500 children. I. Relative frequency of the lesions which simulate retinoblastoma. *Am J Ophthalmol*. 1965;60:610-618.

16. Shields CL, Gorry T, and Shields JA. Outcome of eyes with unilateral sporadic retinoblastoma based on the initial external findings by the family and the pediatrician. *J Pediatr Ophthalmol Strabismus*. 2004;41:143-149.

17. Shields CL, Mashayekhi A, Au AK, et al. The International Classification of Retinoblastoma predicts chemoreduction success. *Ophthalmology*. 2006;113:2276-2280.

18. Shields CL, Mashayekhi A, Demirci H, et al. Practical Approach to Management of Retinoblastoma. *Arch Ophthalmol*. 2004;122:729-735.

19. Kim JW, Kathpalia V, Dunkel IJ, et al. Orbital recurrence of retinoblastoma following enucleation. *Br J Ophthalmol*. 2009;93:463-467.

20. Broaddus E, Topham A, and Singh AD. Survival with retinoblastoma in the USA: 1975-2004. *Br J Ophthalmol*. 2009;93:24-27.

21. Kleinerman RA, Schonfeld SJ, and Tucker MA. Sarcomas in hereditary retinoblastoma. *Clin Sarcoma Res*. 2012;4;2:15.

17 PRESEPTAL (PERIORBITAL) CELLULITIS

Dawood Yusef, MD
Camille Sabella, MD

PATIENT STORY

A 1-year-old unimmunized boy is brought to the emergency department by his mother because of fever, eyelid swelling, and erythema for the past 24 hours. On examination, the child is febrile to 39°C and irritable. The right upper and lower eyelids are swollen and erythematous, with no proptosis (**Figure 17-1**). His extraocular movements are intact. A blood culture and complete blood count are drawn and the patient is admitted to the hospital for preseptal cellulitis and treated with intravenous antibiotics. Twenty-four hours later, the blood culture grows *Haemophilus influenzae* type b. He was treated with intravenous antibiotics and recovered completely.

INTRODUCTION

Preseptal (or periorbital) cellulitis is a bacterial infection of the eyelid anterior to the orbital septum that can result from bacteremia or from direct extension from the surrounding skin. It should always be distinguished from orbital cellulitis, which involves the tissue posterior to the septum (**Figure 17-2**).

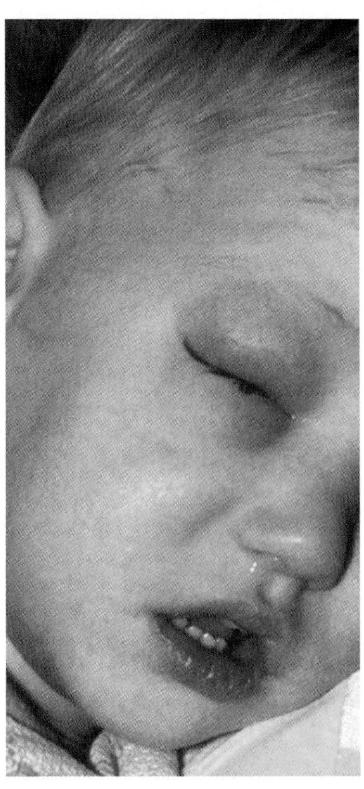

FIGURE 17-1 A 1-year-old boy with bacteremic periorbital cellulitis. *(Used with permission from Sabella C, Cunningham RJ III.* Intensive Review of Pediatrics, *4th edition. Lippincott Williams Wilkins, p 417, Figure 50.1.)*

SYNONYMS

Periorbital cellulitis or preseptal cellulitis.

EPIDEMIOLOGY

- Preseptal cellulitis is most common in young children, occurring at a mean age of 21 months.[1,2]
- Because there are multiple modes of infection, periorbital cellulitis is more common than orbital cellulitis.[3,4]

ETIOLOGY AND PATHOPHYSIOLOGY

- The source of infection and mode of transmission can predict the bacteriology of the infection.
- The most common route of infection is from a breech in the skin overlying the eyelid or face, such as external trauma to the eye, an insect bite, or dacryocystitis (**Figure 17-3**).
- *Staphylococcus aureus* (including community-associated methicillin-resistant *S aureus* [MRSA]) and *Streptococcus pyogenes* (Group A) are the most common pathogens when the route of infection is secondary to direct spread from the skin.[3]
- Community acquired-MRSA has become an emerging pathogen causing preseptal cellulitis.[5]
- Sinusitis can be associated with preseptal cellulitis, although orbital cellulitis is the more common complication of sinusitis. When sinusitis is the source of infection, the usually causative organisms are *Streptococcus pneumoniae*, *H influenzae*, and anaerobes.[2,4]
- Hematogenous spread (bacteremia) is another route of infection and mainly occurs in infants less than 2 years of age. In these cases,

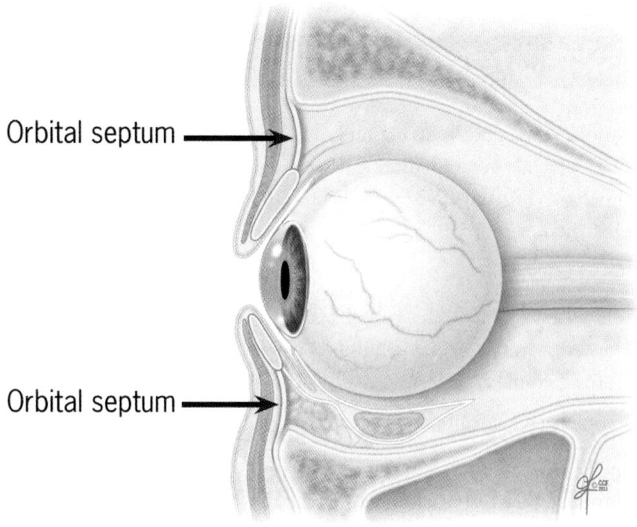

FIGURE 17-2 Illustration of a sagittal section of the orbit. Orbital septum is the anatomical landmark used to differentiate orbital (or postseptal) from preseptal cellulitis. *(Reprinted with permission, Cleveland Clinic Center for Medical Art & Photography © 2013. All Rights Reserved.)*

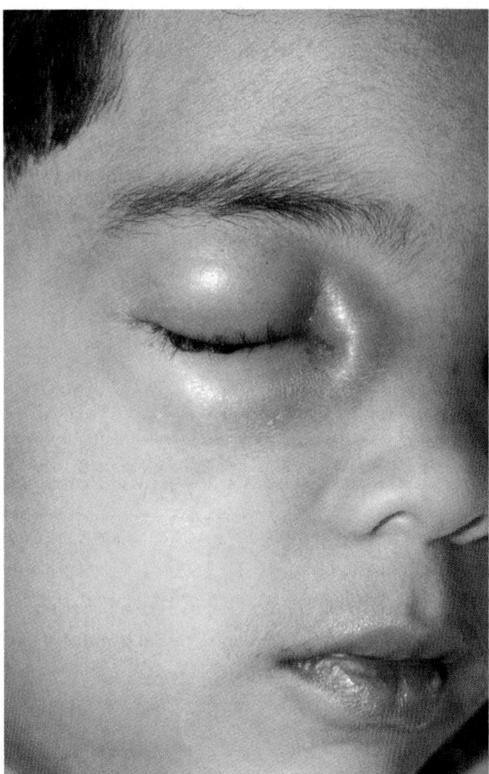

FIGURE 17-3 Dacryocystitis as a cause of periorbital cellulitis. (*Used with permission from Johanna Goldfarb, MD.*)

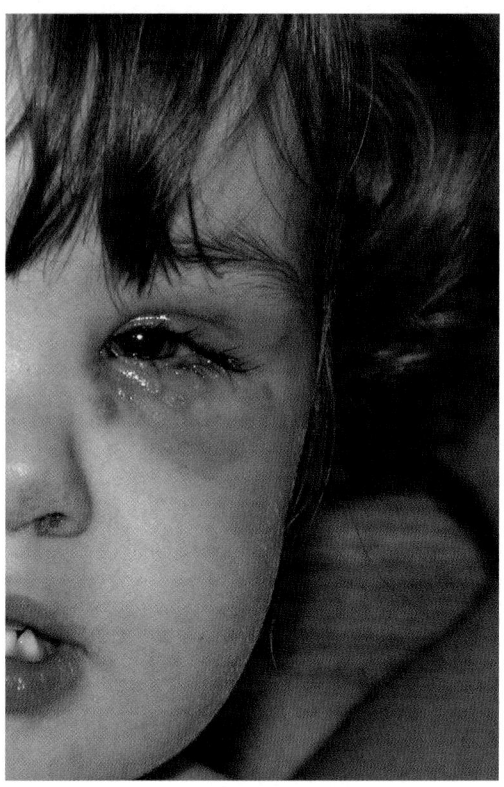

FIGURE 17-4 Periorbital cellulitis complicating herpes simplex virus infection of the face. (*Used with permission from Paul Rychwalski, MD.*)

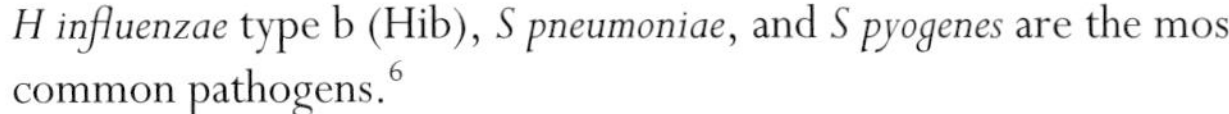

H influenzae type b (Hib), *S pneumoniae*, and *S pyogenes* are the most common pathogens.[6]

- The incidence of bacteremic preseptal cellulitis has decreased significantly because of widespread immunization with HIB vaccine. However, HIB infection should always be considered in unimmunized children (**Figure 17-1**).[4]

RISK FACTORS

- Nasolacrimal duct obstruction is a risk factor for acute dacryocystitis, which is inflammation and secondary infection of the nasolacrimal sac (**Figure 17-3**; see Chapter 14, Nasolacrimal Duct Obstruction).[7]
- Insect bite.
- Impetigo (see Chapter 99, Impetigo).
- Herpetic viral preseptal cellulitis (**Figure 17-4**; see Chapter 114, Herpes Simplex).
- Varicella (see Chapter 108, Varicella).
- Trauma.
- Upper respiratory tract infection including sinusitis (see Chapter 26, Sinusitis).
- Recent eyelid surgery.
- Chalazion—Inflammation of the eyelid due to obstructed meibomian gland (see Chapter 10, Hordeolum and Chalazion).

DIAGNOSIS

CLINICAL FEATURES

- The diagnosis can usually be made clinically.
- Unilateral eyelid swelling, pain, and erythema are the main features of preseptal cellulitis. Fever may or may not be present.
- In contrast to orbital cellulitis, visual impairment, ophthalmoplegia, and proptosis are usually absent in preseptal cellulitis.
- History and physical exam may reveal any of the risk factors previously mentioned and is helpful in making the diagnosis.
- Buccal cellulitis, like periorbital cellulitis, is a potential complication of bacteremia secondary to *H influenzae* type b or *S pneumoniae* (**Figure 17-5**).

DISTRIBUTION

- Unilateral involvement is typical.

LABORATORY TESTING

- Laboratory testing is not usually required when the clinical presentation is mild and the route of spread is clear and benign.
- If the condition is difficult to differentiate from orbital cellulitis, a complete blood count with differential and a blood culture may be helpful.
- A blood culture should be obtained whenever systemic signs or symptoms are present, or if there is concern about hematogenous route of spread.[1,2]

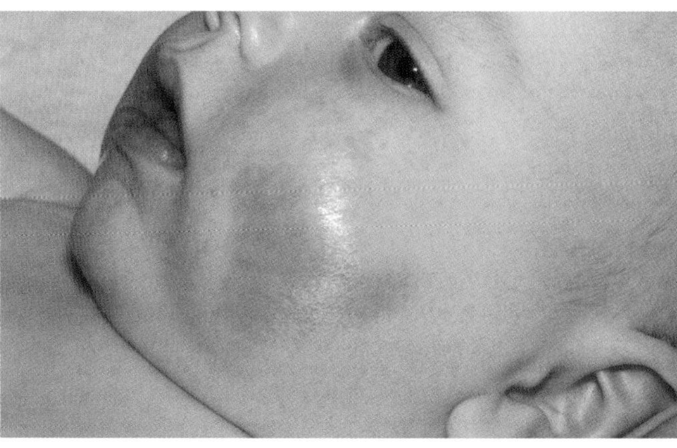

FIGURE 17-5 Buccal cellulitis in a 6-month-old infant with pneumococcal bacteremia. (*Used with permission from Sabella C, Cunningham RJ III. Intensive Review of Pediatrics, 4th edition. Lippincott Williams Wilkins, p 417, Figure 50.2.*)

- Gram stain and culture from fluid or purulent material from the periorbital area should be obtained whenever possible.
- Examination of the cerebrospinal fluid should be considered when bacteremic disease is confirmed or suspected. Infants with bacteremic preseptal cellulitis secondary to HIB have a high incidence of meningitis.[8]

IMAGING

- Imaging of the orbit may be required to distinguish preseptal from postseptal cellulitis (see Chapter 18, Orbital Cellulitis). In most cases, this distinction is made clinically so that imaging is not.
- Imaging should be considered when systemic signs and symptoms are present, when there is ophthalmoplegia or impaired vision, or in cases where clinical improvement is not achieved within 24 to 48 hours after initiation of appropriate antimicrobial therapy.
- Computed tomography is the most appropriate imaging study to differentiate preseptal from postseptal cellulitis.

DIFFERENTIAL DIAGNOSIS

- Orbital cellulitis can at times be difficult to differentiate from preseptal cellulitis (see Chapter 18, Orbital Cellulitis).
- Eye trauma with subsequent erythema and swelling in the periorbital area can usually be distinguished by the history (see Chapter 19, Eye Trauma—Hyphema).
- Allergic reaction may be difficult to distinguish from preseptal cellulitis. The presence of pruritis, bilateral involvement, and response to H2-blockers are suggestive of allergic reaction.
- Insect bite with local reaction—diagnosis can be made clinically and with a good history.
- Eyelid edema due to hypoproteinemia or end organ failure is usually bilateral.
- Hordeolum (stye) is a localized infection of the hair follicles of eye lashes or the eyelid glands—can be distinguished by the lack of significant eyelid erythema and edema, but may be complicated by cellulitis (see Chapter 10, Hordeolum and Chelazion).
- Chalazion is inflammation of the eyelid due to obstructed meibomian gland (see Chapter 10, Hordeolum and Chalazion).

MANAGEMENT

MEDICATIONS

- Because an organism is rarely isolated, treatment is usually empiric and targeted against the most common causative organisms, predicted by the suspected route and source of infection.
- The route of therapy should be based on the severity of infection and the likelihood of bacteremic infection.
- When the source of infection is from local trauma or from an adjacent infection like dacryocystitis, a first-generation cephalosporin an anti-staphylococcal penicillin, or clindamycin may be used as initial empiric therapy. SOR Ⓒ
- The need for empiric coverage for MRSA depends on local prevalence and epidemiology.
- Intravenous therapy with ceftriaxone can be used when a bacteremic route of spread is suspected or proven, such as that seen with *H influenzae* type b infections.[9] SOR Ⓐ
- For uncomplicated preseptal cellulitis, the usual duration of therapy is 7 to 10 days, depending on clinical response. SOR Ⓒ
- If significant clinical improvement is not observed within 24 to 48 hours of initiating appropriate antimicrobial therapy, a CT scan of the orbit to rule out orbital cellulitis and initiation of IV antibiotics should be considered. SOR Ⓒ

REFERRAL

- If the diagnosis is in doubt, or if there is poor response to initial therapy, consultation with ophthalmology, infectious diseases, and/or otolaryngology should be considered.

PROGNOSIS

- Most patients how have preseptal cellulitis do well with appropriate therapy. Complications such as local abscess formation, retro-orbital, and intra-cranial extension are extremely rare.

FOLLOW-UP

- Adequate follow up is essential, especially in the first 24 to 48 hours after initiation of therapy.

PATIENT EDUCATION

- Redness and/or swelling around the eye should be considered a potential serious problem and warrants medical attention.
- Close follow-up is needed with the provider to assure that the infection is resolving in an expected manner.

PATIENT RESOURCES

- **Periorbital Cellulitis—www.ncbi.nlm.nih.gov/pubmedhealth/PMH0001971/.**

PROVIDER RESOURCES

- **Periorbital and Orbital Cellulitis—http://pedsinreview.aappublications.org/content/31/6/242.full.**
- **Preseptal Cellulitis—http://emedicine.medscape.com/article/1218009.**
- **Periorbital Infections—http://emedicine.medscape.com/article/798397.**

REFERENCES

1. Isreale V, Nelson JD. Periorbital and orbital cellulitis. *Pediatr Infect Dis J.* 1987;6(4):404-410.
2. Hauser A, Fogarasi S. Periorbital and Orbital Cellulitis. *Pediatrics in Review.* 2010;31:242.
3. Botting AM, McIntosh D, Mahadevan M. Pediatric pre- and post-septal peri-orbital infections are different diseases. A retrospective review of 262 cases. *Int J Pediatr Otorhinolaryngol.* 2008;72:377.
4. Ambati BK, Ambati J, Azar N, et al. Periorbital and orbital cellulitis before and after the advent of Haemophilus influenzae type B vaccination. *Ophthalmology.* 2000;107:1450-1453.
5. Blomquist PH. Methicillin-resistant Staphylococcus aureus infections of the eye and orbit. *Trans Am Ophtha lmol Soc.* 2006;104:322-345.
6. Smith TF, O'Day D, Wright PF. Clinical implications of preseptal (periorbital) cellulitis in childhood. *Pediatrics.* 1978;62:1006.
7. Chaudhry IA, Shamsi FA, Elzaridi E, et al. Inpatient preseptal cellulitis: experience from a tertiary eye care centre. *Br J Ophthalmol.* 2008;92:1337.
8. Baker RC, Bausher JC. Meningitis complicating acute bacteremic facial cellulitis. *Pediatr Infect Dis.* 1986;5(4):421-423.
9. American Academy of Pediatrics: Haemophilus influenzae infections. In: Pickering LK, Baker CJ, Kimberlin DW, Long SS, eds. Red Book: 2012 Report of the Committee on Infectious Diseases. Elk Grove Village, IL: American Academy of Pediatrics. 2012:345-352.

18 ORBITAL CELLULITIS

Dawood Yusef, MD
Camille Sabella, MD

PATIENT STORY

A 12-year-old boy is brought to the emergency room with progressive eye lid swelling and redness associated with blurring of vision for the past 24 hours. Physical examination is significant for left eye lid swelling, erythema, ptosis, and painful eye movements. A computed tomography (CT) scan of the orbit shows opacification of the paranasal sinuses with retro-orbital extension and abscess formation (**Figure 18-1**). He is diagnosed with orbital cellulitis and orbital abscess and he is admitted to the hospital for intravenous antibiotics, and otolaryngology and ophthalmologic evaluation. His orbital abscess is surgically drained and he completes a 3-week course of antibiotic therapy and recovers completely.

INTRODUCTION

Orbital cellulitis is a serious infection of the orbit that involves the tissue located posterior to the orbital septum (postseptal cellulitis). Orbital cellulitis most commonly results as a complication of sinusitis, and should be distinguished from preseptal (periorbital) cellulitis, which involves the anterior portion of the septum (**Figure 18-2**).[1,2]

SYNONYMS

- Post-septal cellulitis; orbital subperiosteal abscess.

EPIDEMIOLOGY

- Orbital cellulitis is mostly a disease of children, although it can be seen at any age.
- Most commonly occurs during the winter months because of the close association between upper respiratory viral infections, rhinosinusitis, and orbital cellulitis.

ETIOLOGY AND PATHOPHYSIOLOGY

- Orbital cellulitis in children is usually a complication of rhinosinusitis, especially ethmoidal sinusitis, which results in direct extension of the inflammation to the orbit.[1,3,4]
- The ethmoid sinuses are separated from the orbit by a thin and fenestrated bony structure called lamina papyracea. Loss of integrity of the lamina papyracea from inflammation results in orbital extension (**Figure 18-1**).
- Less common pathogenic causes of orbital cellulitis include penetrating trauma to the orbit, infection of the orbit following eye surgery, and bacteremic disease.

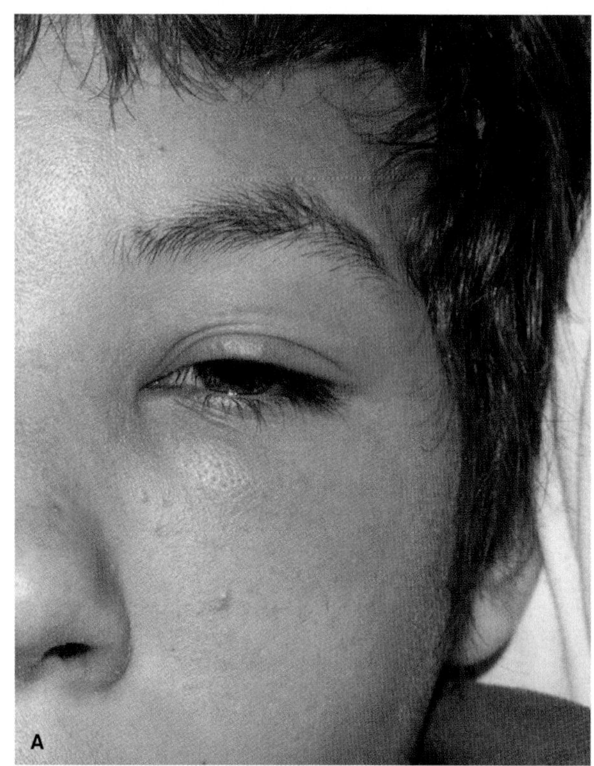

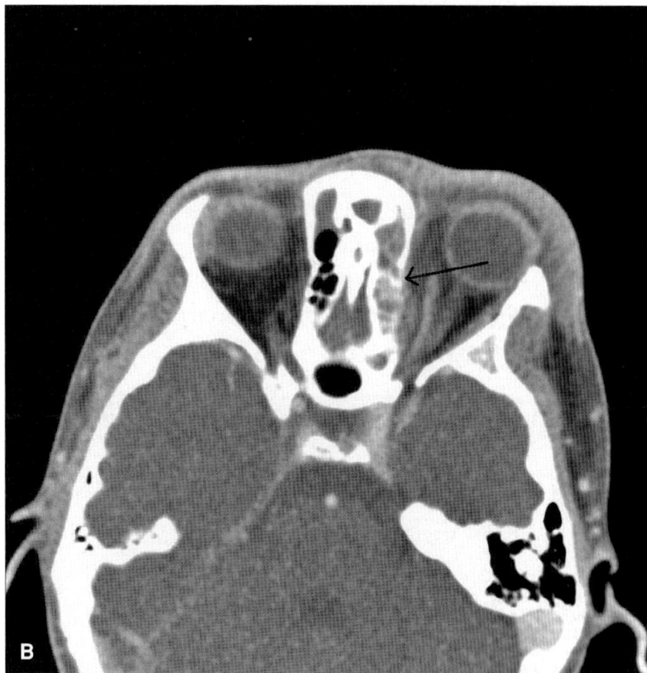

FIGURE 18-1 **A.** Left eyelid swelling and edema in a 12-year-old boy. **B.** Computed tomography (CT) scan of the orbit revealed left ethmoidal sinusitis with extensive adjacent post septal cellulitis and destruction of the lamina papyracea (arrow), the thin bony structure separating the ethmoid sinus from the orbit. (*Used with permission from Camille Sabella, MD.*)

- The etiologic agent implicated depends on the mechanism of infection. *Streptococcus pneumoniae* is the most likely pathogen complicating acute sinusitis. *Staphylococcus aureus, Streptococcus anginosus,* and anaerobic bacteria warrant consideration when orbital cellulitis complicates chronic sinusitis. These pathogens as

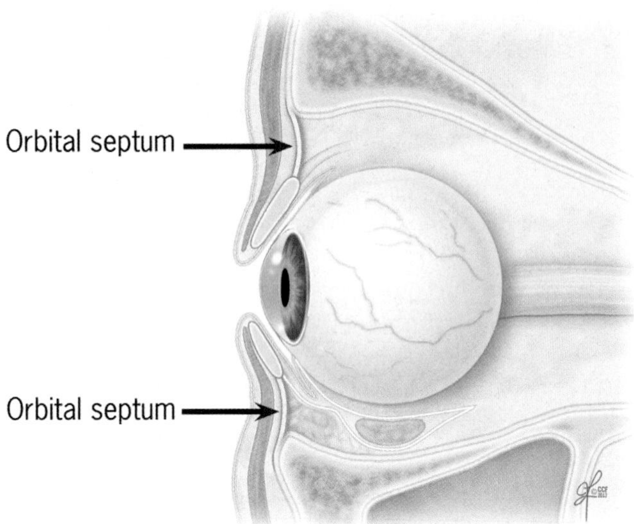

FIGURE 18-2 Illustration of a sagittal section of the orbit. The orbital septum is the anatomical landmark used to differentiate orbital (post-septal) from periorbital (preseptal) cellulitis. (*Reprinted with permission, Cleveland Clinic Center for Medical Art & Photography © 2013. All Rights Reserved.*)

well as gram-negative aerobes need to be considered when the process is secondary to penetrating trauma.[1,3]

- At one time a very common pathogen, *Haemophilus influenzae* type b (Hib) has become a very rare cause of orbital cellulitis since the introduction of the Hib vaccine. However, this organism should always be considered as a potential cause of orbital cellulitis in unimmunized children.[5]
- Community-acquired methicillin-resistant *S aureus* (CA-MRSA) is an emerging pathogen causing orbital cellulitis.[6,7]
- Fungal infection (i.e., Aspergillus or mucormycosis) is a rare but life threatening cause of orbital cellulitis, occurring exclusively in immunocompromised hosts.

RISK FACTORS

- Ethmoidal sinusitis or pansinusitis.
- Upper respiratory tract infections.
- Incomplete or unimmunization.
- Eye surgery or trauma to the orbit.

DIAGNOSIS

- The diagnosis is usually made clinically and confirmed by the appropriate imaging study.

CLINICAL FEATURES

- Fever, unilateral eye pain, and eye lid swelling and erythema are the main features of orbital cellulitis (**Figures 18-1, 18-3, 18-4**).[1,4,7]
- Visual impairment, ophthalmoplegia, chemosis, and proptosis are distinctive clinical features that help distinguish orbital from preseptal cellulitis.[1,4]

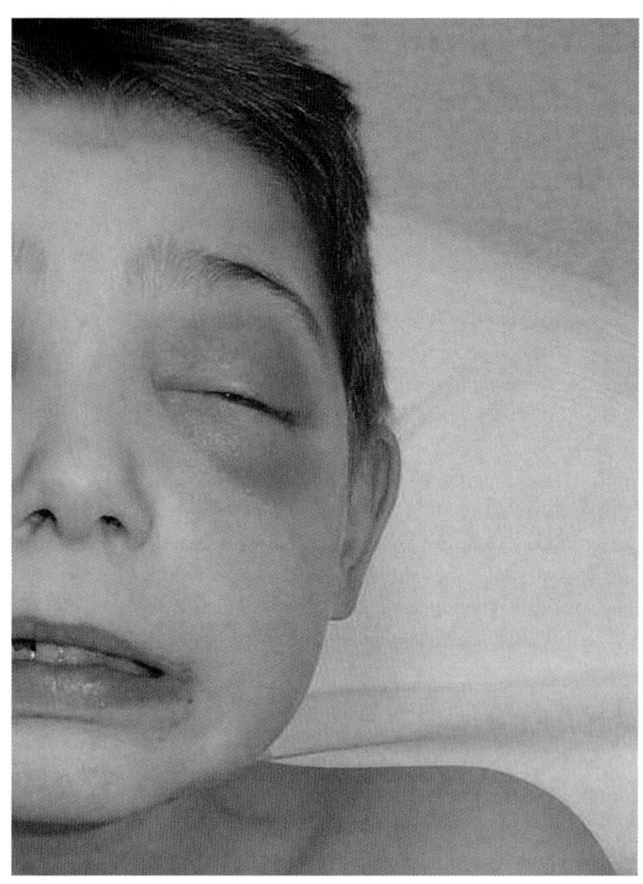

FIGURE 18-3 Orbital cellulitis in a 7-year-old boy. (*Used with permission from Camille Sabella, MD.*)

- A history of sinus or upper respiratory tract infection, previous eye surgery, or trauma may help identifying the source of the infection.
- Headache, lethargy, altered mental status, or other signs of central nervous system involvement may indicate meningitis or intracranial extension.

DISTRIBUTION

- Almost always unilateral.

LABORATORY TESTING

- Peripheral leukocytosis is more common in orbital than in periorbital cellulitis.[1,2,6] However, this is neither a sensitive or specific marker for orbital cellulitis.
- Bacteremia is rare and is more common in children less than 2 years of age. These infants may have more systemic symptoms and/or peripheral leukocytosis.
- Eye drainage (clear or purulent) is not always present, and when present, culture of the material often is not predictive of the etiologic agent.
- No organism is isolated in the majority of cases, especially if surgical drainage is not performed.

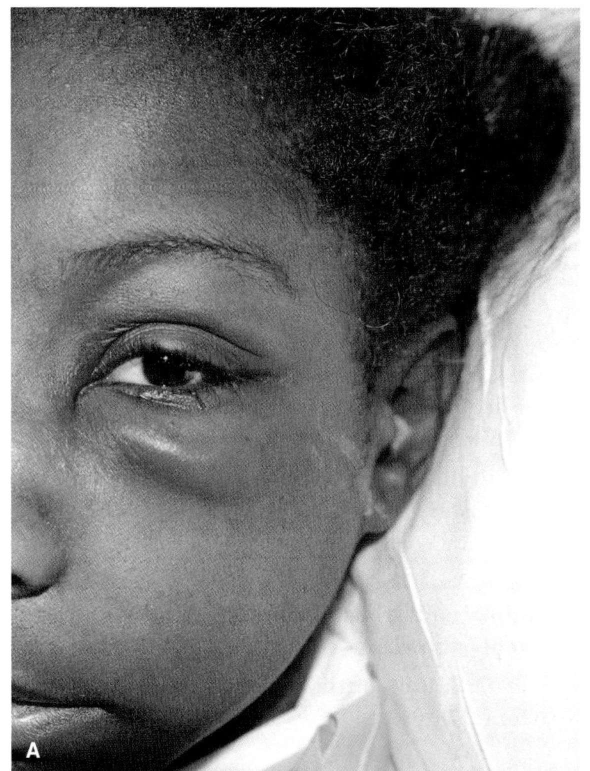

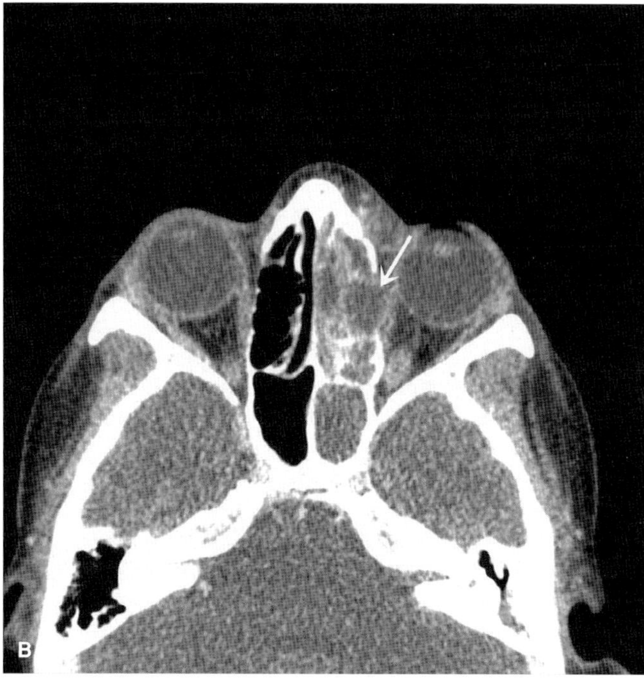

FIGURE 18-4 **A.** Left lower eyelid swelling and edema in a 9-year-old girl. **B.** CT scan revealed orbital cellulitis with a subperiosteal abscess (arrow) and extensive left-sided ethmoidal sinusitis. (*Used with permission from Camille Sabella, MD.*)

IMAGING

- CT scan or magnetic resonance imaging of the orbit is used to confirm the diagnosis of orbital cellulitis.
- The presence of extensive inflammation of the retro-orbital space, especially adjacent to the ethmoid sinuses, confirms the diagnosis of orbital cellulitis (**Figures 18-1** and **18-4**).
- Orbital cellulitis may progress into a subperiosteal or an orbital abscess (**Figure 18-4**).
- Sinus involvement (sinus mucosal thickening or sinus opacification), especially of the ethmoidal sinuses, is usually present; a break in the integrity of the lamina papyracea is often appreciated (**Figures 18-1** and **18-4**).

DIFFERENTIAL DIAGNOSIS

- Preseptal cellulitis is an infection of the tissue anterior to the orbital septum, and can usually be distinguished from orbital cellulitis by the absence of proptosis and ophthalmoplegia (see Chapter 17, Preseptal (Periorbital) Cellulitis).
- Eye trauma, which may result in orbital cellulitis, is usually evident from the history.
- An allergic reaction usually results in bilateral swelling and pruritus, and the absence of fever and systemic signs of infection.
- An insect bite may result in preseptal cellulitis and can be distinguished clinically and by history.
- Eyelid edema due to hypoproteinemia or end organ failure usually is bilateral; history of chronic disease helpful in differentiating this entity.
- Hordeolum (stye)—Localized infection of the hair follicles of eye lashes or the eyelid glands, usually does not lead to significant swelling (see Chapter 10, Hordeolum and Chalazion).

MANAGEMENT

MEDICATIONS

- Children with orbital cellulitis should be hospitalized and empirically treated with broad spectrum parenteral antibiotics aimed at the most likely pathogens, based on the most likely mechanism of infection.
- A third generation cephalosporin such as ceftriaxone or cefotaxime is often combined with an antistaphylococcal agent such as clindamycin when the process is secondary to sinusitis.[1,3,7] SOR C
- The need for empiric coverage against CA-MRSA depends on local prevalence and epidemiology.[6,8] SOR C
- When the process is secondary to penetrating trauma or after a surgical procedure, more broad coverage may be required. In these situations, vancomycin is often combined with an antipseudomonal agent such as ceftazidime and/or gentamicin. SOR C
- The spectrum of antimicrobial therapy can be narrowed if culture results and susceptibilities are available.

- Intravenous therapy should be continued until the patient is nearly normal clinically. In uncomplicated orbital cellulitis, completing therapy with oral antibiotics may be appropriate. The usual duration is 2 to 3 weeks, depending on the clinical response.[1,3,6,7] SOR Ⓒ

SURGERY

- Surgical drainage may be required in cases of orbital or subperiosteal abscess, or in cases where there is a poor initial response to intravenous broad- spectrum antibiotics.[1,3,7] SOR Ⓒ
- Surgical drainage of the sinuses may also be needed in some cases.[6] SOR Ⓒ
- The drainage from purulent material obtained at the time of surgery should be sent for gram stain and culture to help guide antimicrobial therapy.

REFERRAL

- Ophthalmology, infectious diseases, and otorhinolaryngology often collaborate in cases of orbital cellulitis to determine optimal management.

PROGNOSIS

- Most patients with orbital cellulitis recover completely with antibiotic therapy and appropriate surgical intervention, when needed.
- Patients who develop severe complications, such as intracranial extension, cavernous sinus thrombosis, or vision loss, have a more guarded prognosis.[1,7]

FOLLOW-UP

- Close monitoring of the infection for complications and to assess for the possible need for surgical intervention are important.
- Although clinical assessment is most important, repeat imaging studies may be required, especially if the response to therapy is slow.
- Long-term management of sinusitis may be required in some patients after recovery of the orbital process.

PATIENT EDUCATION

- Children who have redness or swelling around the eye, especially when associated with fever, impaired vision, or bulging of the eye, need immediate medical attention.
- Children who have signs and symptoms of sinusitis, such as severe and/or prolonged nasal congestion and cough, should be evaluated by their primary care physician.

PATIENT RESOURCES

- **Orbital Cellulitis—www.uptodate.com/contents/orbital-cellulitis-the-basics?source=search_result&search=orbital+cellulitis&selectedTitle=3~24.**
- **Orbital Cellulitis—www.ncbi.nlm.nih.gov/pubmedhealth/PMH0002007.**

PROVIDER RESOURCES

- **Periorbital and Orbital Cellulitis—http://pedsinreview.aappublications.org/content/31/6/242.extract.**
- **Orbital Cellulitis—http://emedicine.medscape.com/article/1217858.**

REFERENCES

1. Hauser A and Fogarasi S. Periorbital and Orbital Cellulitis. *Pediatrics in Review*. 2010;31;242.
2. Botting AM, McIntosh D, Mahadevan M. Pediatric pre- and post-septal peri-orbital infections are different diseases. A retrospective review of 262 cases. *Int J Pediatr Otorhinolaryngol*. 2008;72:377.
3. Seltz LB, Smith J, Durairaj VD, Enzenauer R, Todd J. Microbiology and Antibiotic Management of Orbital Cellulitis. *Pediatrics*. 2011;127;e566.
4. Swift AC, Charlton G. Sinusitis and the acute orbit in children. *J Laryngol Otol*. 1990;104:213.
5. Ambati BK, Ambati J, Azar N, et al. Periorbital and orbital cellulitis before and after the advent of Haemophilus influenzae type B vaccination. *Ophthalmology*. 2000;107:1450-1453.
6. Bilyk JR. Periocular infection. *Current Opinion in Ophthalmology*. 2007;18:414-423.
7. Nageswaran S, Woods CR, Benjamin DK Jr, et al. Orbital cellulitis in children. *Pediatr Infect Dis J*. 2006;25:695.
8. McKinley SH, Yen MT, Miller AM, Yen KG. Microbiology of pediatric orbital cellulitis. *Am J Ophthalmol*. 2007;144:497.

19 EYE TRAUMA—HYPHEMA

Heidi Chumley, MD

PATIENT STORY

A 14-year-old boy was hit in the eye with a baseball and presented to the emergency department with eye pain, redness, and decreased visual acuity. There was a collection of blood in his anterior chamber (**Figure 19-1**) and he was diagnosed with a hyphema. He was given an eye shield for protection, advised to take acetaminophen for pain, and counseled not to engage in sporting activities until his hyphema resolved. He was referred urgently to ophthalmology and the eye was otherwise healthy. His hyphema resolved in 5 days.

INTRODUCTION

Hyphema, blood in the anterior chamber, can be seen following eye trauma or as a result of clotting disturbances, vascular abnormalities, or mass effects from neoplasms. Traumatic hyphema occurs more often in boys and men, often related to work or sports. Hyphema typically resolves in 5 to 7 days, but some cases are complicated by rebleeding.

EPIDEMIOLOGY

- Hyphema occurs in 17 to 20 per 100,000 persons per year in the US.[1]
- Sixty percent of hyphemas result from sports injuries.[2] Sports with higher risk for eye injuries include paintball, baseball/softball, basketball, soccer, fishing, ice hockey, racquet sports, fencing, lacrosse, and boxing.

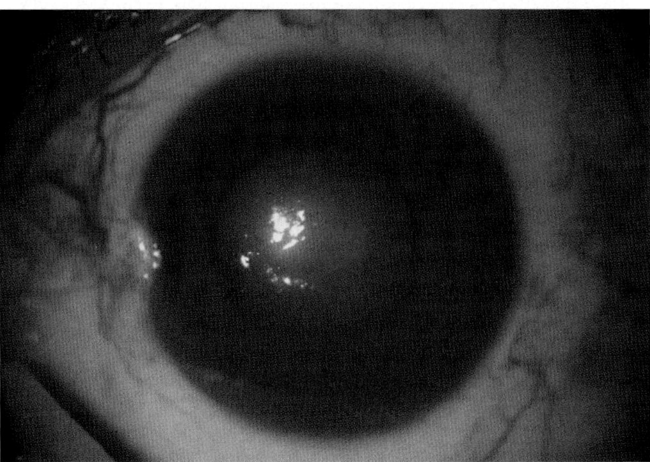

FIGURE 19-1 Layering of red blood cells in the anterior chamber following blunt trauma. This grade 1 hyphema has blood filling in less than 1/3 of the anterior chamber. (*Used with permission from Paul D. Comeau.*)

ETIOLOGY AND PATHOPHYSIOLOGY

- A hyphema is a collection of blood, mostly erythrocytes, that layer within the anterior chamber.
- Trauma is the most common cause, often resulting from a direct blow from a projectile object such as a ball, air pellet or BB, rock, or fist.
- Direct force to the eye (blunt trauma) forces the globe inward, distorting the normal architecture.
- Intraocular pressure rises instantaneously causing the lens/iris/ciliary body to move posteriorly, thus disrupting the vascularization with resultant bleeding.
- Intraocular pressure continues to rise and bleeding stops when this pressure is high enough to compress the bleeding vessels.
- A fibrin-platelet clot forms and stabilizes in 4 to 7 days; this is eventually broken down by the fibrinolytic system and cleared through the trabecular meshwork.

DIAGNOSIS

The diagnosis of hyphema is clinical, depending on the classic appearance of blood layering in the anterior chamber.

CLINICAL FEATURES

History and physical:

- Layered blood in the anterior chamber.
- History of eye trauma or risk factor for nontraumatic hyphema.
- Increased intraocular pressure (32%).
- Decreased vision.
- Hyphemas are classified according to the amount of blood in the anterior chamber:[1]
    - Grade 1: Less than 1/3 of the anterior chamber (see **Figure 19-1**); 58 percent of all hyphemas.
    - Grade 2: 1/3 to 1/2 of the anterior chamber; 20 percent of all hyphemas.
    - Grade 3: 1/2 to almost completely filled anterior chamber; 14 percent of all hyphemas.
    - Grade 4: Completely filled anterior chamber; 8 percent of all hyphemas.
- Eye trauma without hyphema (**Figures 19-2** and **19-3**) can lead to subconjunctival hemorrhage, anterior uveitis, and/or distortion of the normal architecture, including globe rupture.

LABORATORY TESTING (INCLUDE ANCILLARY TESTING, TOO)

- Consider laboratory tests to evaluate for bleeding disorders: Bleeding time, electrophoresis for sickle cell trait, platelet count, prothrombin and partial thromboplastin time, and liver tests.

IMAGING

- Consider CT imaging if a mechanism of injury suggests an associated orbital fracture or concern for orbital or intraocular foreign body.

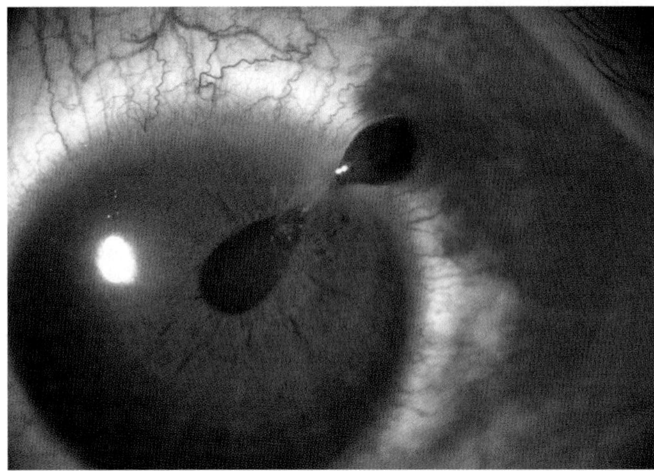

FIGURE 19-2 This young patient was hit in the eye with the corner of a laminated name card. The sharp edge perforated the cornea and pulled a portion of the iris out of the wound. Note the abnormal configuration of the pupil (dyscoria). No hyphema noted. This patient required emergent surgical repair. (*Reprinted with permission from Lo MW, Chalfin S. Retrobulbar anesthesia for repair of ruptured globes. Am J Ophthalmol. 1997;123(6):833–835. Photo by Paul D. Comeau.*)

DIFFERENTIAL DIAGNOSIS

Hyphema is an unmistakable physical examination finding that can be caused by any of the following:

- Trauma—History of trauma, including nonaccidental trauma (i.e., child abuse).
- Blood clotting disturbances—Personal or family history of bleeding disorder, little or no trauma, and black race (increased incidence of sickle trait and disease).
- Medication-induced anticoagulation—Chronic use of aspirin or warfarin and little or no trauma.
- Neovascularization—Diabetes with diabetic retinopathy, history of other ocular disease (central retinal vein occlusion), or history of prior eye surgery (cataract); without trauma, often painless, sudden, blurry vision.
- Melanoma or retinoblastoma—Variety of presentations depending on the size and location; hyphema occurs when mass effect sheers the lens/iris/ciliary body causing bleeding.
- Abnormal vasculature, that is, juvenile xanthogranuloma—Red to yellow papules and nodules in the eyes, skin, and viscera, most often present by 1 year of age.

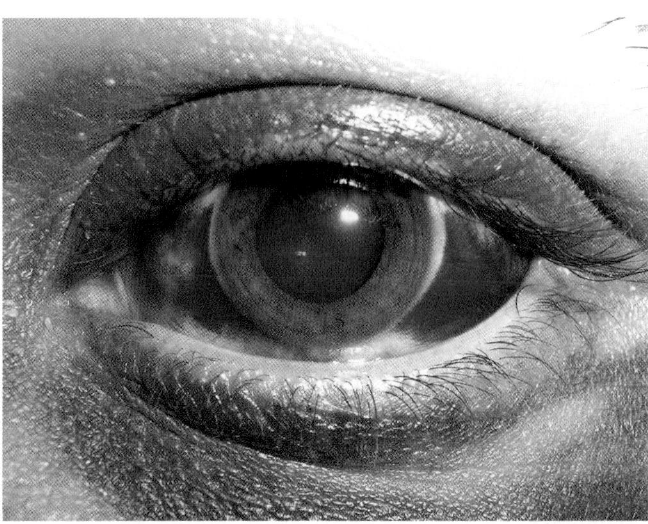

FIGURE 19-3 Subconjunctival hemorrhage and eyelid ecchymosis following accidental trauma. There was no hyphema present. (*Used with permission from Richard P. Usatine, MD.*)

MANAGEMENT

- Most hyphemas resolve in 5 to 7 days; management strategies protect the eye and decrease complications, including rebleeding.
- Evaluate or refer for evaluation for elevated intraocular pressure and other associated injuries. Urgent referral if concern for globe rupture.

A recent Cochrane review evaluated these interventions: antifibrino-lytic agents, corticosteroids, cycloplegics, miotics, aspirin, conjugated estrogens, eye patching, head elevation, and bed rest.

- No interventions had a significant effect on visual acuity.
- Aminocaproic acid (antifibrinolytic) use resulted in a slower resolution of the primary hyphema.
- Antifibrinolytics: aminocaproic acid, tranexamic acid, and aminomethylbenzoic acid reduced the rate of secondary hemorrhage.[3]

NONPHARMACOLOGIC

- Eye patching, head elevation, and bed rest do not independently affect visual acuity. However, experts recommend to patch and shield the injured eye and allow the patient to remain ambulatory as part of a comprehensive treatment plan.[1] SOR C

MEDICATIONS

- Although controversy remains about the best treatment, each of the following has been demonstrated to lower the risk of rebleeding in randomized-controlled trials:
  - Oral antifibrinolytic agents (aminocaproic acid 50 mg/kg every 4 hours for 5 days, not to exceed 30 g/day, or tranexamic acid 75 mg/kg per day divided into 3 doses).[4] SOR C
  - Topical aminocaproic acid (30% in a gel vehicle 4 times a day) is as effective as oral.[4] SOR C
  - Avoid aspirin and NSAIDs, which have been associated with higher rates of rebleeding.
  - Use acetaminophen, if needed, for pain.

REFERRAL OR HOSPITALIZATION

- Signs of a violated globe, such as a perforation of the cornea, conjunctiva or sclera, distorted ocular architecture, or exposed and/or distorted uveal tissue such as the iris (causing a peaked pupil), require immediate surgical evaluation and repair (see **Figure 19-2**).
- Surgical intervention has been recommended for patients with persistent total hyphema or prolonged elevated intraocular pressure.

- Outpatient management is acceptable for children if patient and parents are likely to be able to follow treatment plan.[4,5] SOR Ⓑ

PREVENTION

Ninety percent of sports-related eye injuries can be prevented with appropriate eyewear.[6]

PROGNOSIS

The percentage of patients who regain 20/40 vision varies by severity of the hyphema: grade I, 80 percent; grade III, 60 percent; grade IV, 35 percent.[1]

FOLLOW-UP

Patients should be monitored daily for the first 5 or more days by a provider familiar with caring for hyphemas. Patient with a hyphema should be followed subsequently for signs of angle recession and high intraocular pressure, which predisposes the patient to traumatic glaucoma, an insidious cause of blindness in patients with a history of trauma.

PATIENT EDUCATION

- Complications include rebleeding, decreased visual acuity, posterior or peripheral anterior synechiae, corneal bloodstaining, glaucoma, and optic atrophy. Patients may need surgical or medical management for glaucoma.
- Patients who are more likely to rebleed include black patients (irrespective of sickle cell/trait status),[7,8] patients with a grade 3 or 4 hyphema, and patients with high initial intraocular pressure.
- Warn patients that they may have angle recession from traumatic causes of the hyphema. This will predispose the patient to a lifetime risk of traumatic glaucoma, which can cause blindness without any symptoms. These patients need to be monitored regularly by an ophthalmologist for increased pressure and glaucomatous nerve changes.

PATIENT RESOURCES

- The National Eye Institute has information for children, parents, teachers, and coaches—**www.nei.nih.gov/sports**.
- Play Hard Play Safe Web site has recommended eye protection by sport—**www.lexeye.com**.

PROVIDER RESOURCES

- Coalition to prevent eye injuries has a variety of handouts suitable for displaying or giving to patients—**www.sportseyeinjuries.com**.

REFERENCES

1. Sheppard J. Hyphema. *Medscape Reference.* http://emedicine.medscape.com/article/119016, accessed June 15, 2012.
2. Schein OD, Hibberd PL, Shingleton BJ, et al. The spectrum and burden of ocular injury. *Ophthalmology*. 1988;95(3):300-305.
3. Gharaibeh A, Savage HI, Scherer RW, et al. Medical interventions for traumatic hyphema. *Cochrane Database Syst Rev*. 2011;19(1):CD005431.
4. Walton W, Von HS, Grigorian R, Zarbin M: Management of traumatic hyphema. *Surv Ophthalmol*. 2002;47(4):297-334.
5. Rocha KM, Martins EN, Melo LA Jr, Moraes NS: Outpatient management of traumatic hyphema in children: Prospective evaluation. *J AAPOS*. 2004;8(4):357-361.
6. Harrison A, Telander DG: Eye injuries in the youth athlete: a case-based approach. *Sports Med*. 2002;131(1):33-40.
7. Lai JC, Fekrat S, Barron Y, Goldberg MF: Traumatic hyphema in children: risk factors for complications. *Arch Ophthalmol*. 2001;119(1):64-70.
8. Spoor TC, Kwitko GM, O'Grady JM, Ramocki JM: Traumatic hyphema in an urban population. *Am J Ophthalmol*. 1990;109(1):23-27.

PART 5

EAR, NOSE, AND THROAT

Strength of Recommendation (SOR)	Definition
A	Recommendation based on consistent and good-quality patient-oriented evidence.*
B	Recommendation based on inconsistent or limited-quality patient-oriented evidence.*
C	Recommendation based on consensus, usual practice, opinion, disease-oriented evidence, or case series for studies of diagnosis, treatment, prevention, or screening.*

*See Appendix A on pages 1320–1322 for further information.

SECTION 1 EAR

20 PREAURICULAR TAGS

Linda French, MD

PATIENT STORY

A 7-year-old boy comes into the office with his mother with complaint of a fleshy growth in front of his left ear (**Figure 20-1**). It has been present since birth. He passed his newborn hearing screen and the parents were told that it was nothing to worry about. Recently, other children have teased him about it and mom inquires about having it removed. He has no other congenital abnormalities evident to date and no chronic medical problems.

INTRODUCTION

Preauricular tags are benign congenital abnormalities consisting of epithelial mounds or pedunculated skin located near the front of the ear that can be associated with other conditions.

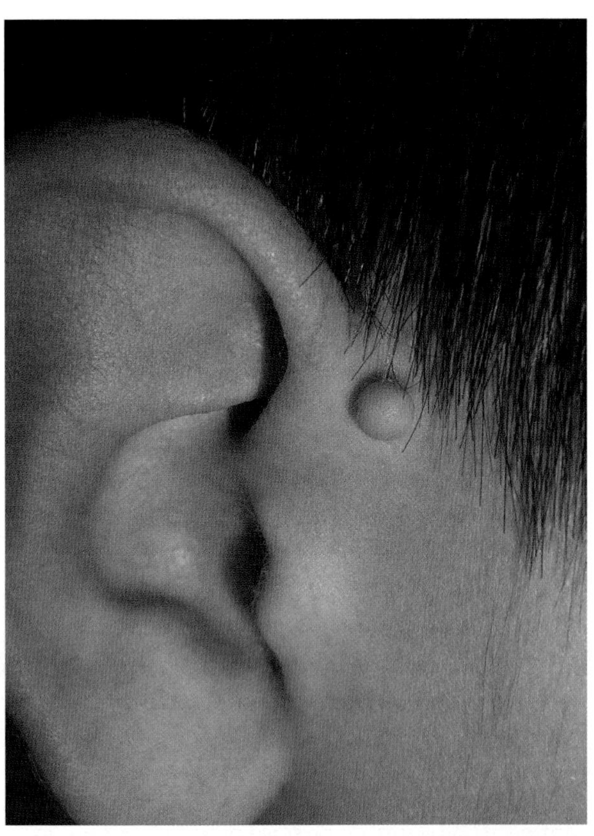

FIGURE 20-1 A preauricular skin tag in a 7-year-old boy. *(Used with permission from Richard P. Usatine, MD.)*

EPIDEMIOLOGY

- Occur in approximately 1 of 10,000 to 12,500 births without predilection for gender or race.
- Ear malformations may occur in isolation or as part of a constellation of abnormalities, often involving the renal system. Children have a five-fold risk of hearing impairment (8 of 10,000 vs. 1.5 of 10,000).[1]
- Postnatal hearing loss has not been associated with preauricular tags.[2]
- Several chromosomal abnormalities include preauricular tags as one of the phenotypic expressions.
- The Goldenhar syndrome includes preauricular skin tags, bilateral limbal dermoids of the eye and eyelid colobomas (see Chapter 34, Congenital Anomalies of the Head and Neck).

ETIOLOGY AND PATHOPHYSIOLOGY

- Arise from remnants of supernumerary brachial hillocks.[3]
- Early stage embryology involves the formation of several slit-like structures on the side of the head, the branchial clefts. The three hillocks between the first four clefts eventually form the structure of the outer ear. Preauricular tags are generally minor malformations arising from remnants of supernumerary branchial hillocks.[4]

DIAGNOSIS

- Based on physical examination.

CLINICAL FEATURES OF PREAURICULAR TAGS

- Fleshy knob in front of the ear (**Figures 20-1** to **20-5**).
- May be 2 tags on one side of similar or different sizes (**Figures 20-2**, **20-4**, and **20-5**).
- Present from the time of birth.
- Generally asymptomatic.

TYPICAL DISTRIBUTION

- Preauricular tags may be unilateral or bilateral, more often present on the left.

BIOPSY

- Not indicated for preauricular tag.

DIFFERENTIAL DIAGNOSIS

- The key issue in the diagnosis of preauricular tags is whether the ear tags are an isolated anomaly or part of a syndrome involving vital organs, especially the kidneys. There is no consensus about whether children with ear tags who otherwise appear to be healthy should be evaluated with renal ultrasound.[4,5]

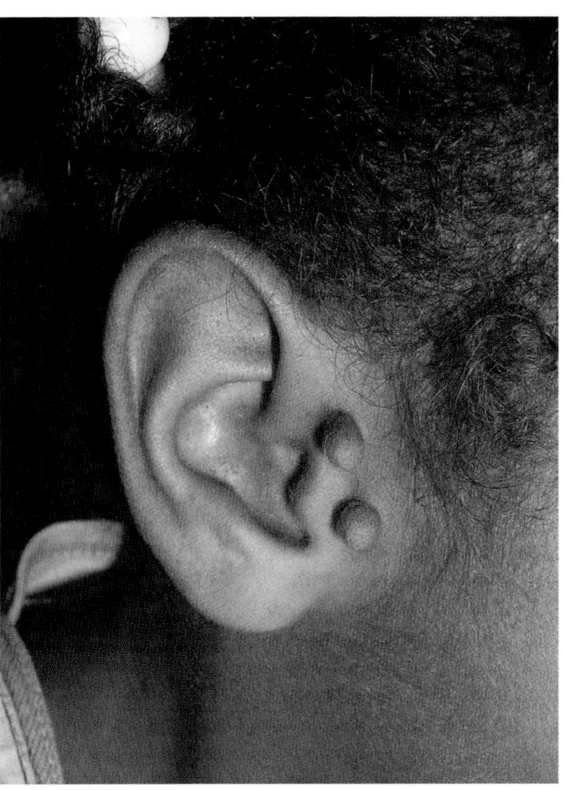

FIGURE 20-2 Two preauricular tags in a young black girl. (*Used with permission from Richard P. Usatine, MD.*)

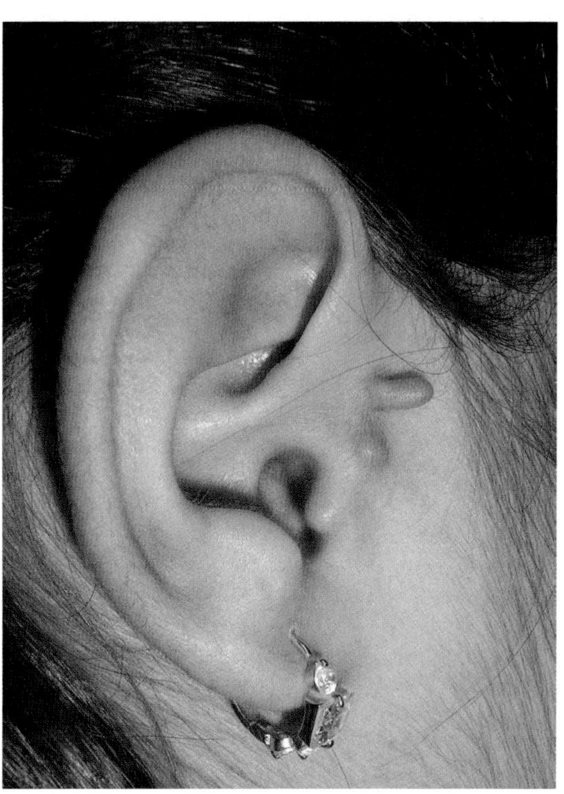

FIGURE 20-4 Two preauricular tags in a 4-year-old girl. (*Used with permission from Richard P. Usatine, MD.*)

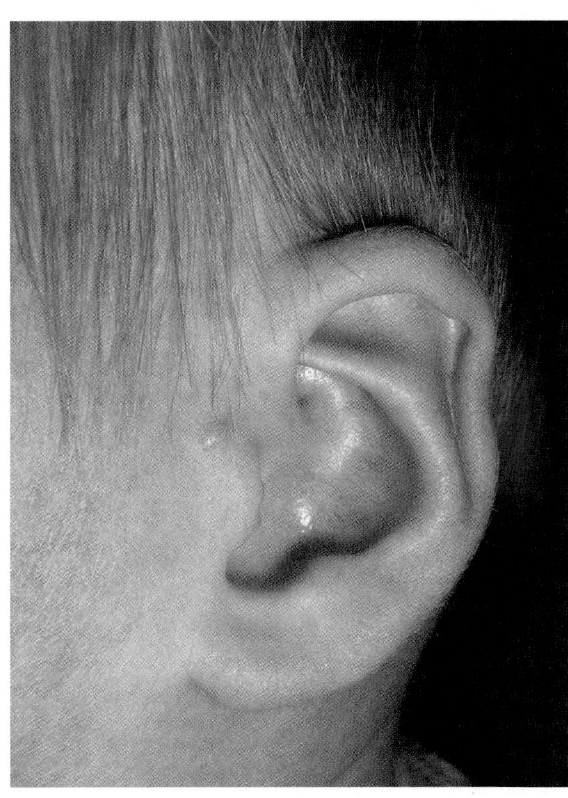

FIGURE 20-3 Preauricular tag in a 1-year-old boy. (*Used with permission from Richard P. Usatine, MD.*)

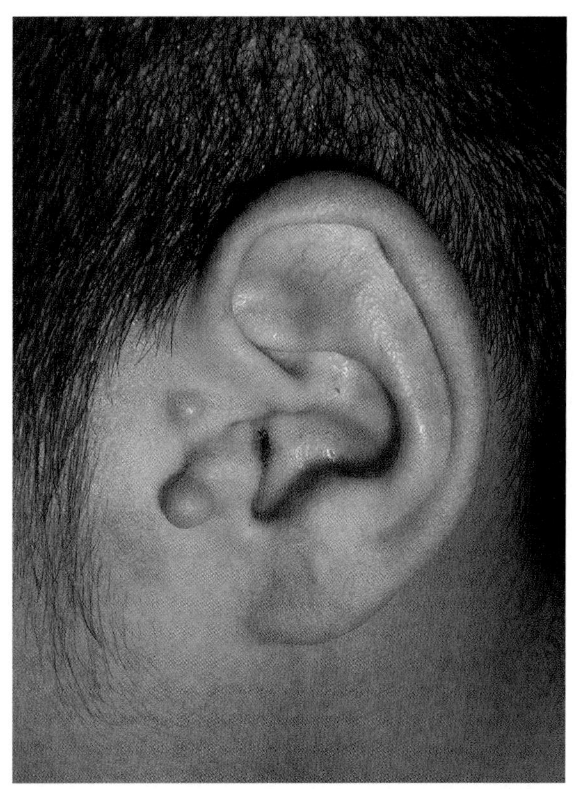

FIGURE 20-5 Two preauricular tags in a young boy. The lower preauricular tag may be considered an accessory tragus. (*Used with permission from Richard P. Usatine, MD.*)

- Accessory tragus is a preauricular tag that is adjacent to the normal tragus and may contain cartilage. The lower preauricular tag in **Figure 20-5** may be considered an accessory tragus.

MANAGEMENT

- Elective removal can be performed for cosmesis.

PATIENT RESOURCES

- Preauricular tags—**http://nlm.nih.gov/medlineplus/ency/article/003304.htm**.

PROVIDER RESOURCES

- Preauricular tags—**http://emedicine.medscape.com/article/845288.**

REFERENCES

1. Roth DA, Hildesheimer M, Bardenstein S, et al. Preauricular skin tags and ear pits are associated with permanent hearing impairment in newborns. *Pediatrics.* 2008;122(4):e844-e890.
2. Beswick R, Discoll C, Kei J. Monitoring for postnatal hearing loss using risk factors: a systematic literature review. *Ear Hear.* 2012; 33(6):745-56.
3. Ostrower ST. Preauricular cysts, pits, and fissures. http://emedicine.medscape.com/article/845288-overview#a05, accessed July 20, 2011.
4. Deshpande SA, Watson H. Renal ultrasound not required in babies with isolated minor ear abnormalities. *Arch Dis Child Fetal Neonatal Ed.* 2006;91:F29-F30.
5. Kohelet D, Arbel E. A prospective search for urinary tract abnormalities in infants with isolated preauricular tags. *Pediatrics.* 2000; 105:E61.

21 OTITIS EXTERNA

Brian Z. Rayala, MD
Camille Sabella, MD

PATIENT STORY

An 11-year-old girl with a history of psoriasis presented to her pediatrician with a 2-day history of ear pain and drainage from her right ear canal. On physical examination, she is well appearing and afebrile. She has exquisite pain on movement of her right pinna and dried drainage visible at the opening of her external auditory canal (EAC). Her EAC is erythematous and mildly edematous, but the tympanic membrane is visualized and appears normal. She also has psoriatic lesions around her ear and scalp as currently her psoriasis is not under control (**Figure 21-1**). The pediatrician makes the diagnosis of otitis externa and prescribes once daily ofloxacin drops for 7 days. The girl has a prompt response and recovers completely.

INTRODUCTION

Otitis externa (OE) is common in all parts of the world. OE is defined as inflammation, often with infection, of the EAC.[1]

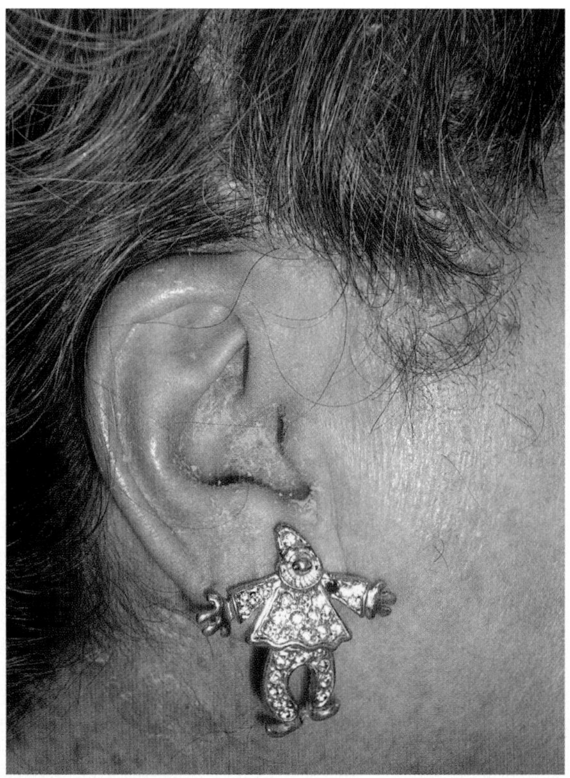

FIGURE 21-1 Dried drainage at the opening of the external ear canal in a girl with otitis externa. Note the psoriatic lesions, which predisposed this girl to otitis externa. (*Used with permission from Richard P. Usatine, MD.*)

SYNONYMS

Swimmer's ear.

EPIDEMIOLOGY

- Incidence of OE is not known precisely; its lifetime incidence was estimated at 10 percent in one study.[2]
- In temperate climates, it is more common in the summer.
- Associated with head immersion in water.

ETIOLOGY AND PATHOPHYSIOLOGY

- Common pathogens, which are part of normal EAC flora, include aerobic organisms predominantly (*P. aeruginosa and Staphylococcus aureus*) and, to a lesser extent, anaerobes (*Bacteroides* and *Peptostreptococcus*). Up to 1/3 of infections are polymicrobial. A small proportion (2% to 10%) of OE is caused by fungal overgrowth (e.g., *Aspergillus niger* usually occurs with prolonged antibiotic use).[1]
- Pathogenesis of OE includes the following:
  - Trauma, the usual inciting event, leads to breach in the integrity of EAC skin.
  - Skin inflammation and edema ensue, which, in turn, leads to pruritus and obstruction of adnexal structures (e.g., cerumen glands, sebaceous glands, and hair follicles).
  - Pruritus leads to scratching, which results in further skin injury.
  - Consequently, the milieu of the EAC is altered (i.e., change in quality and quantity of cerumen, increase in pH of EAC, and dysfunctional epithelial migration).
  - Finally, the EAC becomes a warm, alkaline, and moist environment—ideal for growth of different pathogens.

RISK FACTORS[3]

- Environmental factors:
  - Moisture—Macerates skin of EAC, increases pH, and washes away protective cerumen layer (e.g., swimming, sweating, humid environments).
  - Trauma—Leads to injury of EAC skin (e.g., cotton buds, fingernails, hearing aids, ear plugs, paper clips, match sticks, mechanical removal of cerumen).
  - Warm environments.
- Host factors:
  - Anatomical—Buildup of wax and debris that lead to retained moisture (e.g., a narrow ear canal, hairy ear canal).
  - Cerumen—Paucity of or excessive production of cerumen (results in disappearance of the protective layer and retained moisture, respectively).
  - Chronic skin disorder—for example seborrheic dermatitis, psoriasis, atopic dermatitis (**Figures 21-1** and **21-2**).
  - Immunocompromise—for example HIV/AIDS, chemotherapy, diabetes, neutropenia.

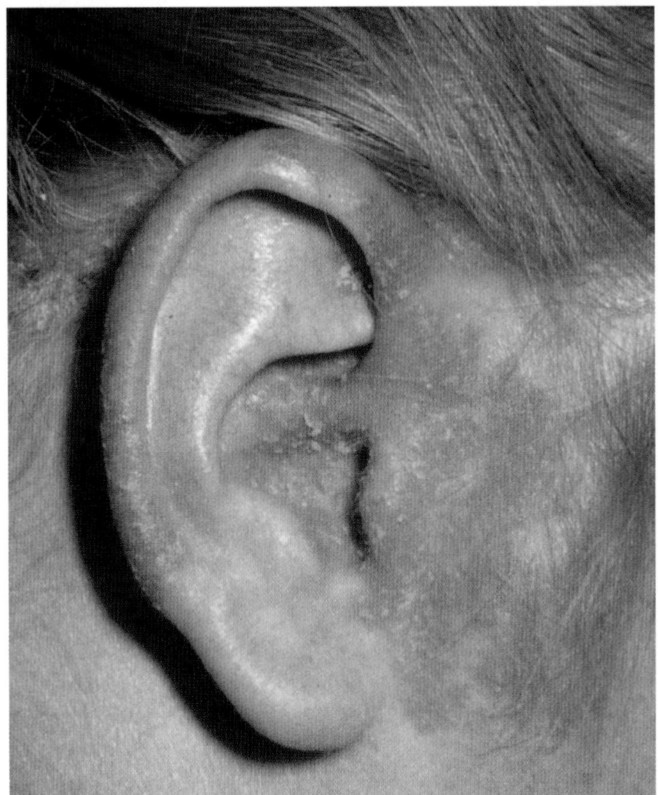

FIGURE 21-2 Seborrheic dermatitis causing erythema and greasy scale of the external ear and ear canal. The seborrheic dermatitis itself causes breaks in the skin and the coexisting pruritus may lead the patient to damage their own ear canal. All this can become secondarily infected. (*Used with permission from Eric Kraus, MD.*)

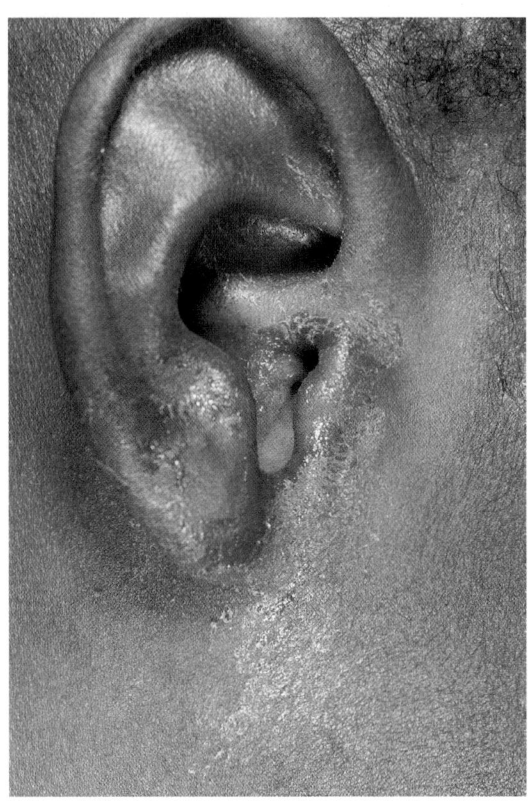

FIGURE 21-3 Purulent otorrhea in a child with otitis externa. (*Used with permission from Strange GR, Ahrens WR, Schafermeyer RW, Wiebe RA. Pediatric Emergency Medicine, 3rd edition: http://www.accessemergencymedicine.com.*)

DIAGNOSIS

CLINICAL FEATURES

- OE can either be localized, like a furuncle, or generalized (**Figures 21-1** to **21-3**). The latter is known as "diffuse OE," or simply OE. Seborrheic dermatitis of the external ear and EAC can be diffuse or generalized (**Figures 21-1** and **21-2**).
- Forms of (diffuse) OE:[1]
  - Acute (<6 weeks; **Figures 21-3** and **21-4**).
  - Chronic (>3 months)—May cause hearing loss and stenosis of the EAC (**Figure 21-5**).
  - Necrotizing or malignant form—Defined by destruction of the temporal bone, usually in diabetics or immunocompromised people; often life-threatening (**Figure 21-6**).
- Key historical features include:
  - Otalgia, including pruritus.
  - Otorrhea (**Figures 21-3** to **21-5**).
  - Mild hearing loss.
- Key physical findings include:
  - Pain with tragal pressure or pain when the auricle is pulled superiorly; this may be absent in very mild cases.
  - Signs of EAC inflammation (edema, erythema, aural discharge) (**Figures 21-3** to **21-5**).

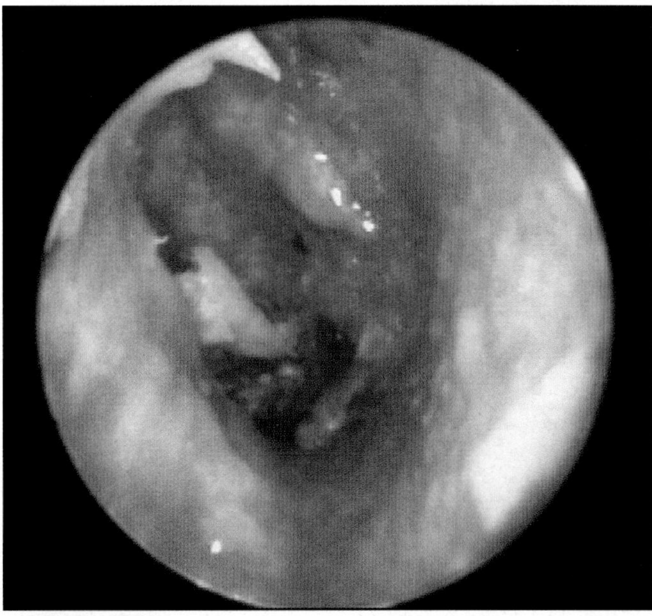

FIGURE 21-4 Acute otitis externa showing purulent discharge and narrowing of the ear canal. (*Used with permission from Roy F. Sullivan, PhD. Audiology Forum: Video Otoscopy, www.rcsullivan.com.*)

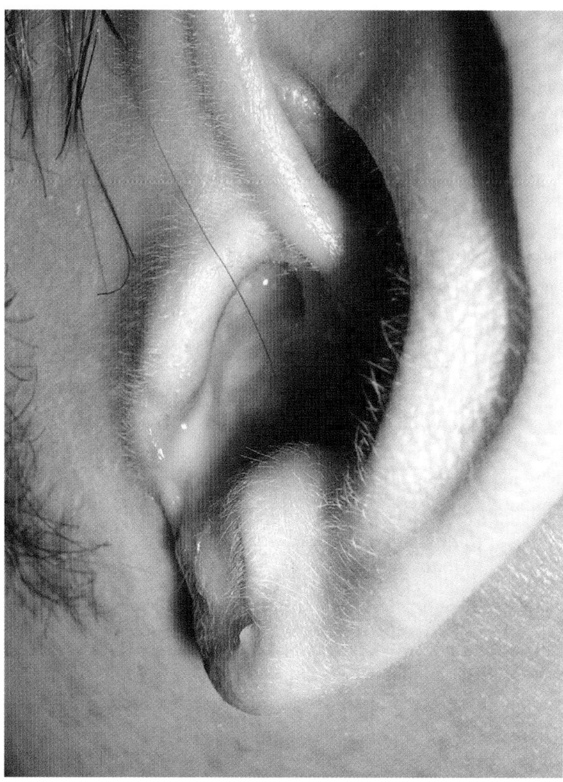

FIGURE 21-5 Chronic suppurative otitis media with purulent discharge chronically draining from the ear of this young man. This image could be seen in acute otitis media with perforation of the tympanic membrane or in a purulent otitis externa. (*Used with permission from Richard P. Usatine, MD.*)

  - Fever, periauricular erythema, and lymphadenopathy point to severe disease.
  - Complete obstruction of EAC occurs in advanced OE.
- Establishing the integrity of the tympanic membrane (TM) (through direct visualization) and the absence of middle-ear effusion (through pneumatic otoscopy) is crucial in differentiating OE from other diagnoses (e.g., suppurative otitis media, cholesteatoma).

LABORATORY AND IMAGING

- Because OE is essentially a clinical diagnosis, diagnostic testing has a limited role. When a patient fails to respond to empiric treatment, obtaining a culture of aural discharge may help guide choice of treatment (antibacterial versus antifungal agents).
- If necrotizing or malignant OE is suspected, CT or MRI of the ear/skull base is warranted.

DIFFERENTIAL DIAGNOSIS

- Chronic suppurative otitis media—Otoscopy shows TM perforation; history reveals a chronically draining ear and recurrent middle-ear infections with or without hearing loss (**Figure 21-5**). At times, it is difficult to differentiate this from otitis externa because of edema and drainage in the EAC. In these cases, close follow-up in necessary in ensuring the integrity of the tympanic membrane.
- Seborrheic dermatitis involving the external ear and EAC can lead to inflammation and breaks in the skin (**Figures 21-1** and **21-2**).

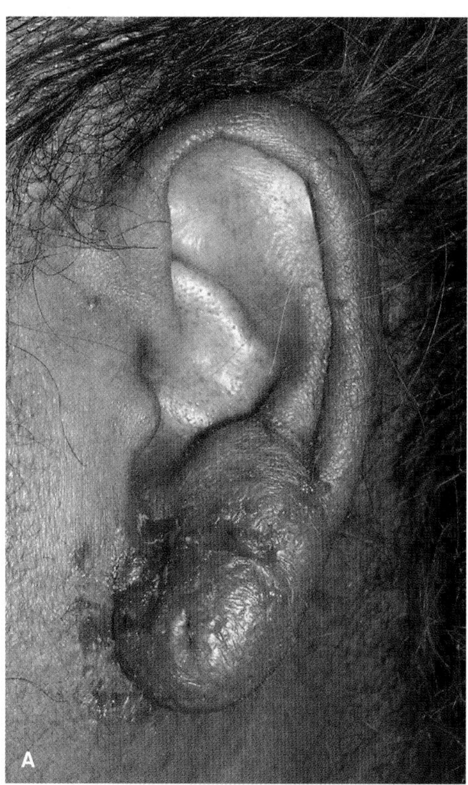

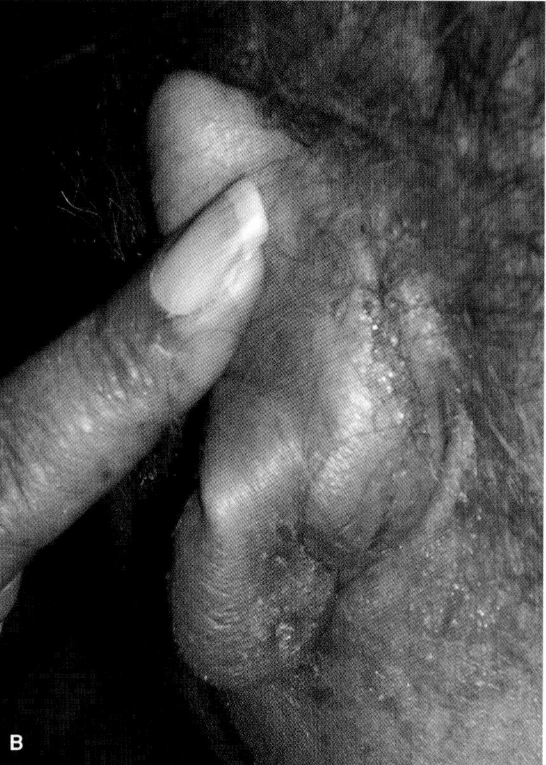

FIGURE 21-6 **A.** Malignant/necrotizing otitis externa in a young woman with diabetes. Note the swelling and honey-crusts of the pinna. The external auditory canal and temporal bone were involved. **B.** Posterior view of the swollen and infected ear. (*Used with permission from E.J. Mayeaux, MD.*)

The coexisting pruritus can lead the patient to damage their own ear canal. This can all become secondarily infected.

- Acute otitis media with perforated TM—Presents with purulent drainage from the canal in the setting of ear pain and clinical signs or symptoms of acute illness such as fever. If the TM is visible, it will be red with a perforation.
- Foreign body in the EAC—Otoscopy, with or without aural toilet, confirms presence of foreign body (that incites an inflammatory response, leading to otalgia and otorrhea; see Chapter 24, Ear—Foreign Body).
- Otomycosis—Pruritus is generally more prominent and EAC inflammation (otalgia and otorrhea) is less pronounced; fungal organisms have a characteristic appearance in the EAC.
- Contact dermatitis—Usually caused by ototopical agents (e.g., neomycin, benzocaine, propylene glycol) or jewelry; prominent clinical features include pruritus, erythema of conchal bowl, crusting, and excoriations.

MANAGEMENT

NONPHARMACOLOGIC

- The effectiveness of ear cleaning is unknown.[3] SOR Ⓑ
- The effectiveness of specialist aural toilet (use of operating microscope to mechanically remove material from external canal) for treating OE is unknown.[1] SOR Ⓑ

MEDICATIONS

- The management of acute OE should include an assessment of pain. The clinician should recommend analgesic treatment based on the pain severity.[4] SOR Ⓑ
- Topical treatments alone are effective for uncomplicated acute OE. Additional oral antibiotics are not required.[3] SOR Ⓑ
- There is very limited evidence supporting the use of steroid-only drops for acute OE.[3] SOR Ⓑ
- Since most topical medications for OE are equally efficacious, choosing the appropriate treatment is influenced by other factors including cost, availability, dosing frequency, risk of ototoxicity, risk of contact sensitivity, and risk of developing resistance.[3] SOR Ⓑ
  - Evidence from one trial of low quality found no difference in clinical efficacy between quinolone and nonquinolone drops. Quinolones are more expensive than nonquinolones.[3] SOR Ⓑ
  - Topical mixtures of antibiotics and steroids may reduce swelling, redness, drainage, and use of pain medications compared to preparations without steroids. High-potency steroids may be more effective in treating pain, inflammation and swelling than low-potency steroids.[3] SOR Ⓑ
  - Acetic acid appears to be as effective as an antibiotic-steroid topical mixture after a week of therapy. In patients requiring extended therapy (>1 week). However, acetic acid was less effective and required a longer duration of treatment (i.e., 2 extra days).[3] SOR Ⓑ
  - Topical aluminum acetate may be comparable to topical antibiotic-steroid medications in terms of cure rates for acute OE.[1] SOR Ⓑ
- Patients can remain symptomatic for the first 6 days of therapy with topical antibiotic-steroid medications. The typical duration of therapy is 7 to 10 days. Since this standard approach may overtreat some patients and undertreat others, a good rule-of-thumb is to instruct patients to use antibiotic-steroid drops for a minimum of 1 week and to extend therapy, up to a maximum of 1 extra week, until resolution of symptoms.[3] SOR Ⓑ
- The use of topical antifungal agents in OE, alone or with steroids, is not supported by evidence.[1] SOR Ⓑ
- Necrotizing or malignant otitis externa: Management generally involves surgical debridement to remove necrotic tissue and intravenous antibiotics directed toward coverage of *P aeruginosa* and *S aureus* initially. An antipseudomonal agent such as piperacillin-tazobactam, ceftazidime, or cefipime, is often combined with gentamicin to treat *P aeruginosa*, and vancomcyin is used initially to cover *S aureus*. SOR Ⓒ Results of cultures and histology obtained at the time of surgical debridement can guide subsequent therapy.

PREVENTION

- Prophylactic treatments to prevent OE (topical acetic acid, topical corticosteroids, or water exclusion) have not been evaluated in clinical trials.[1] SOR Ⓑ

PROGNOSIS

- Acute OE often resolves within 6 weeks but can recur.

FOLLOW-UP

- If the patient fails to respond to empiric therapy within 48 to 72 hours, the clinician should reassess the patient to confirm the diagnosis of OE and to exclude other causes of illness.[4] SOR Ⓑ
- Patients with symptoms that last more than 2 weeks have likely failed their initial therapy and should be considered for alternative therapy.[3] SOR Ⓑ

PATIENT EDUCATION

- To avoid recurrent infections:[5]
  - Recommend that patients not use cotton swabs inserted into the ear canal.
  - Avoid frequent washing of the ears with soap as this leaves an alkali residue that neutralizes the normal acidic pH of the ear canal.
  - Avoid swimming in polluted water.
  - Ensure that the canals are emptied of water after swimming or bathing—This can be done by turning the head or holding a facial tissue on the outside of the ear to act as a wick.
- Consider ear drops for swimmers who get frequent OE. A combination of a 2:1 ratio of 70 percent isopropyl alcohol and acetic acid can be used after each episode of swimming to assist in drying and acidifying the ear canal.[5] SOR Ⓒ

- Do not use earplugs while swimming because they may cause trauma to the ear canal leading to OE.[5]

PATIENT RESOURCES

- **www.familydoctor.org/online/famdocen/home/common/ear/657.html.**
- **www.healthychildren.org/English/health-issues/conditions/ear-nose-throat/Pages/Swimmers-Ear-in-Children.aspx.**

PROVIDER RESOURCES

- **www.emedicine.medscape.com/article/84923**
- **www.emedicine.medscape.com/article/763918**

REFERENCES

1. Hajioff D, MacKeith S. Otitis externa. *Clin Evid (Online).* 2010;pii:0510.
2. Raza SA, Denholm SW, Wong JC. An audit of the management of otitis externa in an ENT casualty clinic. *J Laryngol Otol.* 1995;109:130-133.
3. Kaushik V, Malik T, Saeed SR. Interventions for acute otitis externa. *Cochrane Database Syst Rev.* 2010;(1):CD004740.
4. Rosenfeld RM, Brown L, Cannon CR, et al. American Academy of Otolaryngology—Head and Neck Surgery Foundation. Clinical practice guideline: acute otitis externa. *Otolaryngol Head Neck Surg.* 2006;134(4):S4-S23.
5. Garry JP, Bhalla SK. Otitis Externa. Updated November 12, 2012. http://emedicine.medscape.com/article/84923-overview, accessed on February 28, 2013.

22 OTITIS MEDIA—ACUTE OTITIS AND OTITIS MEDIA WITH EFFUSION

Brian Z. Rayala, MD

PATIENT STORY

A 15-month-old boy is brought by both parents to his pediatrician with a 2-day history of fever, irritability, and frequent tugging of his left ear. This was preceded by a 1-week history of nasal congestion, cough, and rhinorrhea. On otoscopy, his left tympanic membrane (TM) appears erythematous, cloudy, bulging, and exudative (**Figure 22-1**). His left TM fails to move on pneumatic otoscopy. The physician diagnoses acute otitis media and decides with the parents to prescribe a 10-day course of amoxicillin; the child recovers uneventfully.

In follow-up 2 months later, the child appears healthy and is meeting all his developmental milestones. On otoscopic examination, air–fluid levels are seen in the right ear (**Figure 22-2**). The physician explains the diagnosis of otitis media with effusion to the parents and arranges follow-up. Three months later the effusion is completely resolved.

INTRODUCTION

Acute otitis media (AOM) is the most common diagnosis for acute office visits for children.[1] AOM is characterized by middle-ear effusion in a patient with signs and symptoms of acute illness (e.g., fever, irritability, otalgia). Otitis media with effusion (OME) is a disorder characterized by fluid in the middle ear in a patient without signs and symptoms of acute ear infection; it is also very common in childhood.

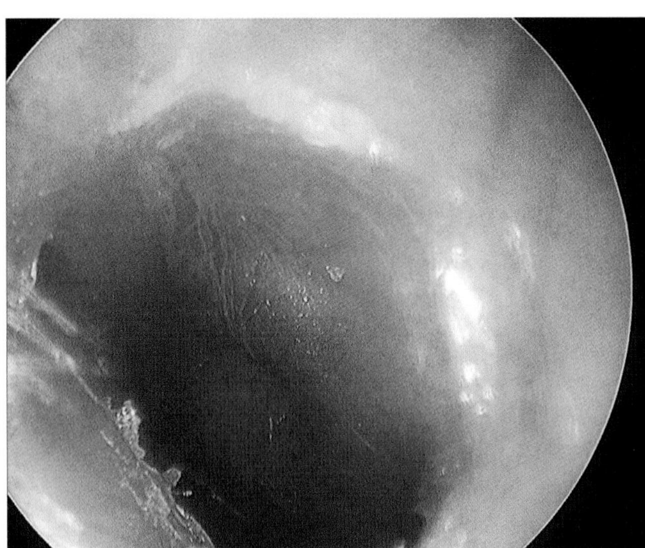

FIGURE 22-1 Acute otitis media in the left ear of a 15-month-old patient with marked erythema and bulging of the tympanic membrane. The malleus and light reflex are not visible. (*Used with permission from William Clark, MD.*)

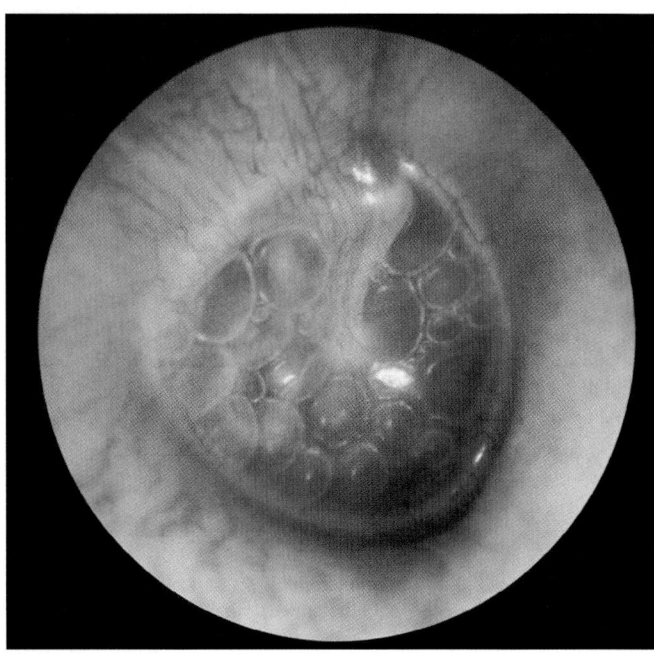

FIGURE 22-2 Otitis media with effusion (OME) in the right ear. Note multiple air–fluid levels in this slightly retracted, translucent, nonerythematous tympanic membrane. (*Used with permission from Frank Miller, MD.*)

EPIDEMIOLOGY

- AOM accounted for $5 billion of the total national health expenditure in 2000; more than 40 percent was incurred for children between 1 and 3 years of age.[1]
- It is estimated that 60 percent to 80 percent of children in the US develop AOM by 1 year of age and that 80 percent to 90 percent develop AOM by 2 to 3 years of age.[2,3]
- The highest incidence occurs between 6 and 24 months of age.[2,3]
- AOM is the most common reason for outpatient antibiotic treatment in the US.[4] A national survey in 1992 revealed that 30 percent of all antibiotics prescribed for children younger than age 18 years was for treatment of AOM.[5]
- OME is diagnosed in 2.2 million children yearly in the US.[6]
- Approximately 90 percent of children (80% of individual ears) have OME at some time before school age, most often between ages 6 months and 4 years.[6]
- The combined direct and indirect health care costs of OME amount to $4 billion annually.[6]

ETIOLOGY AND PATHOPHYSIOLOGY

AOM is often preceded by upper respiratory symptoms such as cough and rhinorrhea.

- Pathogenesis of AOM includes:[7]
  - Eustachian tube dysfunction (usually a result of an upper respiratory infection) and subsequent tube obstruction.
  - Increased negative pressure in the middle ear.
  - Accumulation of middle-ear fluid.

- Microbial growth.
- Suppuration (that leads to clinical signs of AOM).

- Most common pathogens in the US and United Kingdom are:[8,9]
  - Strains of *Streptococcus pneumoniae* not in the heptavalent pneumococcal vaccine (PCV7) (after introduction of PCV7 vaccine in 2000).
  - Nonencapsulated (nontypeable) *Haemophilus influenzae* (NTHi).
  - *Moraxella catarrhalis.*
  - *Staphylococcus aureus.*
- Viruses account for 16 percent of cases. Respiratory syncytial viruses, rhinoviruses, influenza viruses, and adenoviruses have been the most common isolated viruses.[10]

OME most commonly follows AOM; it may also occur spontaneously.

- Fluid limits sound conduction through the ossicles and results in decreased hearing.
- Reasons for the persistence of fluid in otitis media remain unclear, although potential etiologies include allergies, biofilm, and physiologic features.
- "Glue ear" refers to extremely viscous mucoid material within the middle ear and is a distinct subtype of OME.

RISK FACTORS

- The most important risk factors for AOM include young age and attendance at a child care center.
- Other risk factors include:[11]
  - White race.
  - Male gender.
  - History of enlarged adenoids, tonsillitis, or asthma.
  - Multiple previous episodes.
  - Bottle feeding.
  - History of ear infections in parents or siblings.
  - Use of a soother or pacifier.
- Second-hand smoke is a risk factor when parents smoke at home.
- Risk factors for OME include age 6 years or younger, large number of siblings, low socioeconomic group, frequent upper respiratory tract infection, tobacco exposure, daycare attendance, and bottle feeding.[12]

DIAGNOSIS

CLINICAL FEATURES OF AOM

- To diagnose AOM, the clinician should confirm a bulging TM using otoscopy, verify the acuteness of symptoms, *and* identify objective signs of middle-ear effusion (MEE) using pneumatic otoscopy and/or tympanometry.[6,13] SOR Ⓒ
- Elements of the definition of AOM are:[6,13]
  - Signs or symptoms of middle-ear inflammation as indicated by:
    - Moderate to severe bulging of the TM *or* new otorrhea not attributable to acute otitis externa.
    - Mild bulging of the TM *and* recent onset (≤48 hours) of ear pain *or* intense erythema of the TM (**Figure 22-1**) in contrast to the normal TM (**Figure 22-5**).
  - The presence of MEE. Although MEE is often presumed by bulging of the TM (**Figure 22-1**) or air–fluid level behind the TM (**Figure 22-2**), guidelines stress the use of objective measures of confirming MEE such as:
  - Limited or absent mobility of the TM established by pneumatic otoscopy—The TM does not move during air insufflation; often initially seen as retraction of the TM (**Figures 22-3** and **22-4**).
  - Tympanometry demonstrating reduced or flat waveforms.

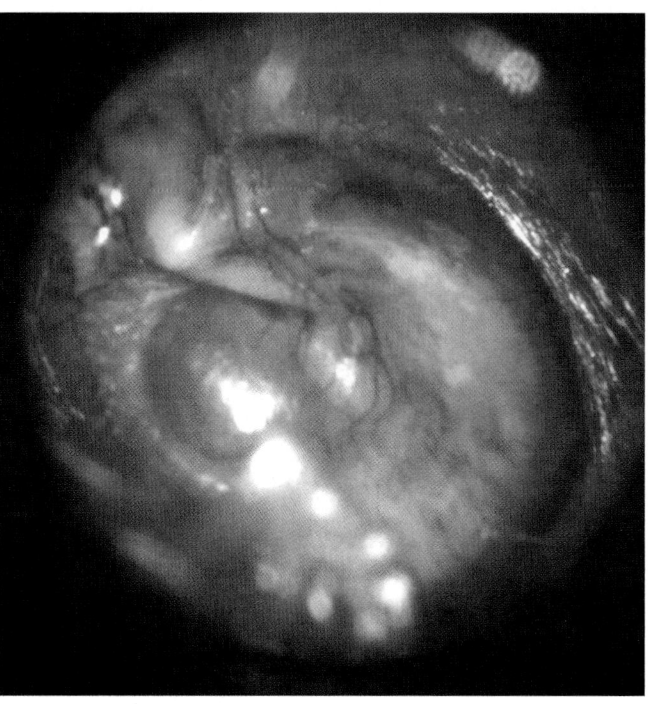

FIGURE 22-3 Otitis media with effusion in the left ear showing retraction of the tympanic membrane (TM) and straightening of the handle of the malleus as the retraction pulls the bone upward. (*Used with permission from Glen Medellin, MD.*)

CLINICAL FEATURES OF OME

- The most common symptom, present in more than half of patients, is mild hearing loss. This is usually identified when parents express concern regarding their child's behavior, performance at school, or language development.[12]
- Absence of signs and symptoms of acute illness assists in differentiating OME from AOM.
- Common otoscopic findings include:
  - Air–fluid level or bubble (**Figure 22-2**).
  - Cloudy TM (**Figures 22-4** and **22-6**) in contrast to the normal TM (**Figure 22-5**).
  - Redness of the TM is present in approximately 5 percent of ears with OME.
- Clinicians should use pneumatic otoscopy as the primary diagnostic method for OME.[14] SOR Ⓐ
  - Impaired mobility of the TM is the hallmark of MEE.

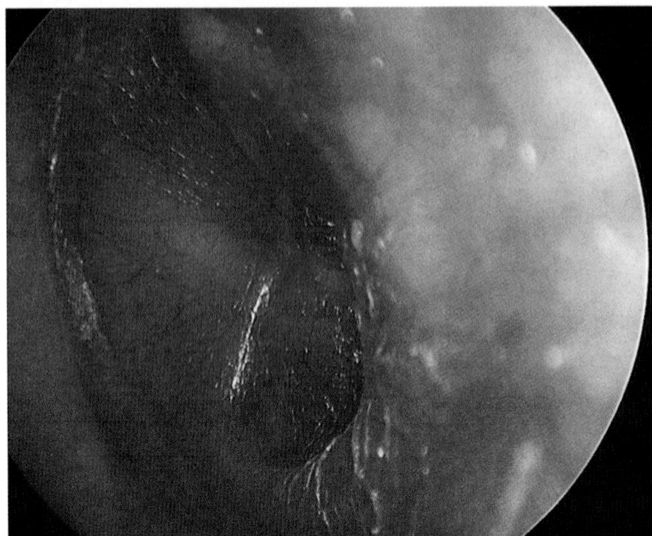

FIGURE 22-4 Early acute otitis media at the stage of eustachian tube obstruction. Note the slight retraction of the tympanic membrane (TM), the more horizontal position of the malleus, and the prominence of the lateral process. (*Used with permission from William Clark, MD.*)

- According to a metaanalysis, impaired mobility on pneumatic otoscopy has a pooled sensitivity of 94 percent and specificity of 80 percent, and positive likelihood ratio of 4.7 and negative likelihood ratio of 0.075.[14]

LABORATORY TESTS AND IMAGING

- Because AOM and OME are clinical diagnoses, diagnostic testing has a limited role. When clinical presentation and physical examination (including otoscopy) do not establish the diagnosis, the following can be used as adjunctive techniques:

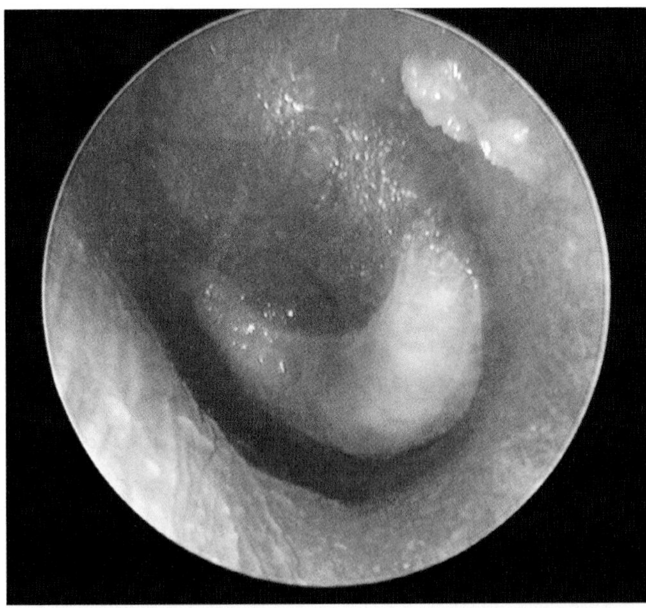

FIGURE 22-5 Acute otitis media, stage of suppuration. Note presence of purulent exudate behind the tympanic membrane (TM), the outward bulging of the TM, prominence of the posterosuperior portion of the drum, and generalized TM edema. The *white area* is tympanosclerosis from a previous infection. (*Used with permission from William Clark, MD.*)

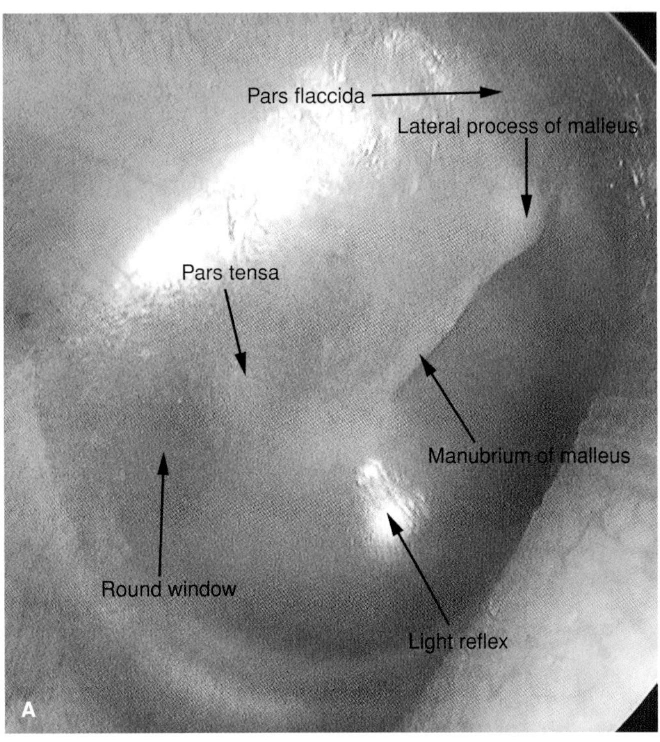

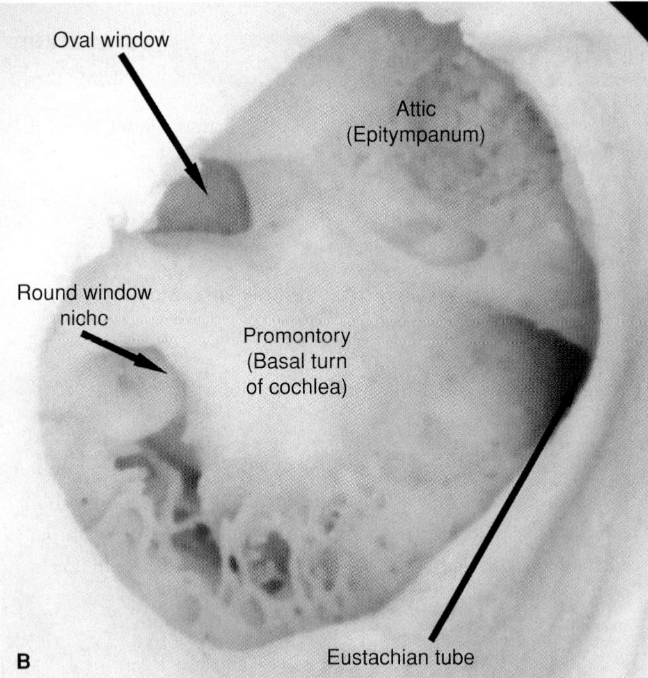

FIGURE 22-6 **A.** Normal right tympanic membrane with comparison using. **B.** Normal bony landmarks of the inner ear. The ossicles were removed in this dissection. (*Used with permission from William Clark, MD.*)

- Tympanometry—This procedure records compliance of the TM by measuring reflected sound. AOM and OME will plot as a reduced or flat waveform. This technique requires patient cooperation but provides more objective data.
- Acoustic reflectometry—This procedure, very similar to tympanometry, measures sound reflectivity from the middle ear. With this test, the clinician is able to distinguish air- or fluid-filled space without requiring an airtight seal of the ear canal.

- Middle ear aspiration—For patients with AOM, aspiration may be warranted if patient is toxic, immunocompromised, or has failed prior courses of antibiotics.

DIFFERENTIAL DIAGNOSIS

The key differentiating feature between AOM and OME is the absence of signs and symptoms of acute illness in OME (e.g., fever, irritability, otalgia). Otoscopic findings may be similar. Other clinical entities that can be confused with AOM and OME include:

- Otitis externa—Otitis externa presents with otalgia, otorrhea and mild hearing loss, all of which can be present in AOM. Tragal pain on physical exam and signs of external canal inflammation on otoscopic exam differentiate it from AOM. Careful ear irrigation if tolerated may be helpful to visualize the TM to differentiate otitis externa from AOM (see Chapter 21, Otitis Externa).
- Otitic barotrauma—This often presents with severe otalgia. Key historical features include recent air travel, scuba diving, or ear trauma, preceded by an upper respiratory infection.
- Cholesteatoma—Unlike AOM, this is a clinically silent disease in its initial stages. Presence of white keratin debris in the middle ear cavity (on otoscopy) is diagnostic (**Figures 22-7** and **22-8**).
- Foreign body—A foreign body may present with otalgia. Otoscopy reveals presence of foreign body (see Chapter 24, Ear—Foreign Body).
- Bullous myringitis—Bullous myringitis is often associated with viral or mycoplasma infection as well as usual AOM pathogens; in approximately 1/3 of patients, there is a component of sensorineural hearing loss. Otoscopy shows serous-filled bulla on the surface of the TM (**Figure 22-9**). Patients present with severe otalgia.
- Chronic suppurative otitis media (CSOM)—Otoscopy shows TM perforation and otorrhea; history reveals a chronically draining ear and recurrent middle-ear infections with or without hearing loss.

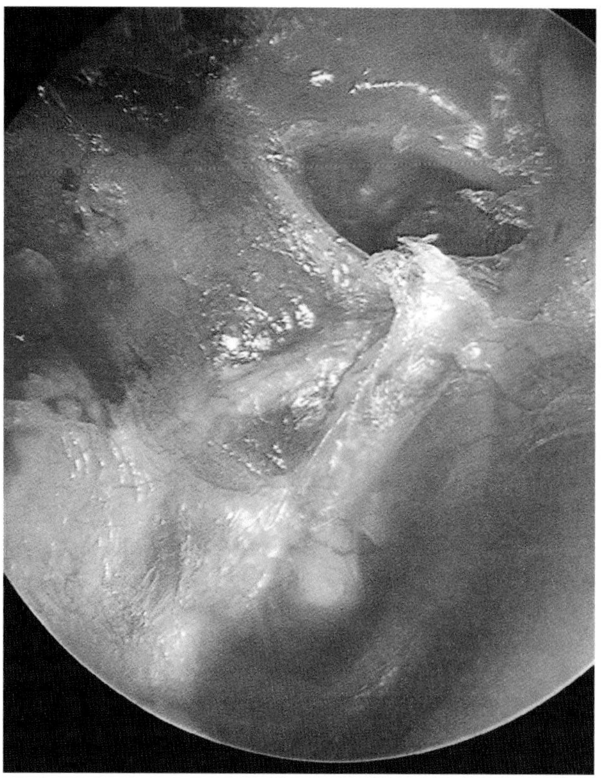

FIGURE 22-8 Primary acquired cholesteatoma with debris removed from the attic retraction pocket. (*Used with permission from William Clark, MD.*)

- Referred otalgia—This is rare in children and in cases of bilateral otalgia. Should be considered in cases of otalgia that do not fit clinical features of AOM. Referred pain is usually from other head and neck structures (e.g., teeth, jaw, cervical spine, lymph and salivary glands, nose and sinuses, tonsils, tongue, pharynx, meninges).

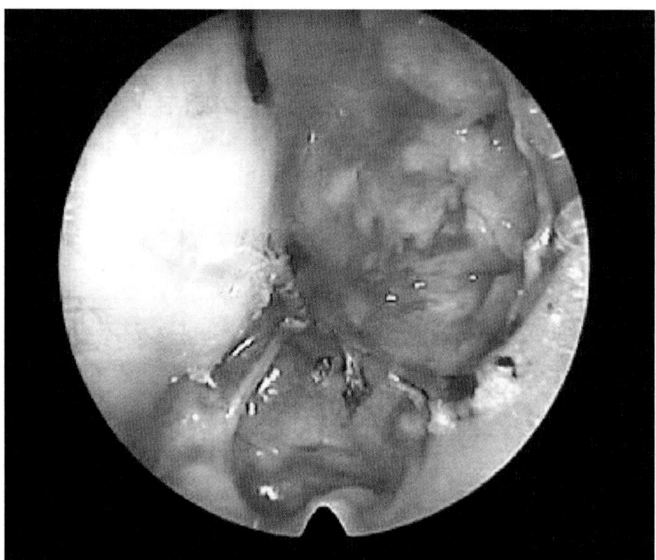

FIGURE 22-7 Cholesteatoma. (*Used with permission from Vladimir Zlinsky, MD, in Roy F. Sullivan, PhD. Audiology Forum: Video Otoscopy, www.rcsullivan.com.*)

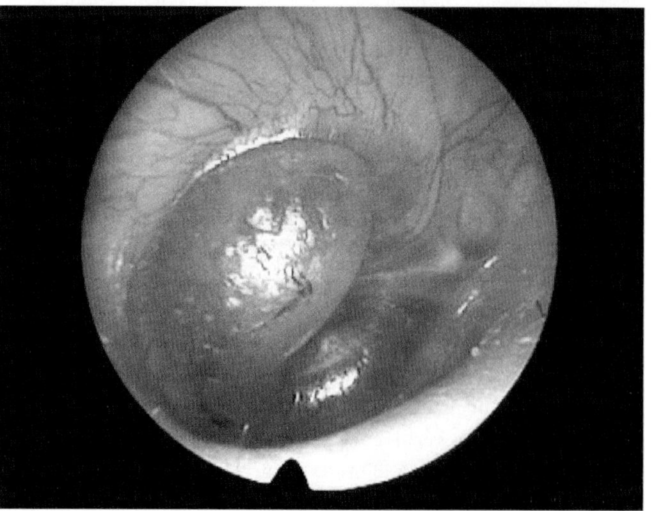

FIGURE 22-9 Bullous myringitis can be differentiated from otitis media with effusion by identifying serous-filled bulla on the surface of the tympanic membrane (TM). (*Used with permission from Vladimir Zlinsky, MD, in Roy F. Sullivan, PhD. Audiology Forum: Video Otoscopy, www.rcsullivan.com.*)

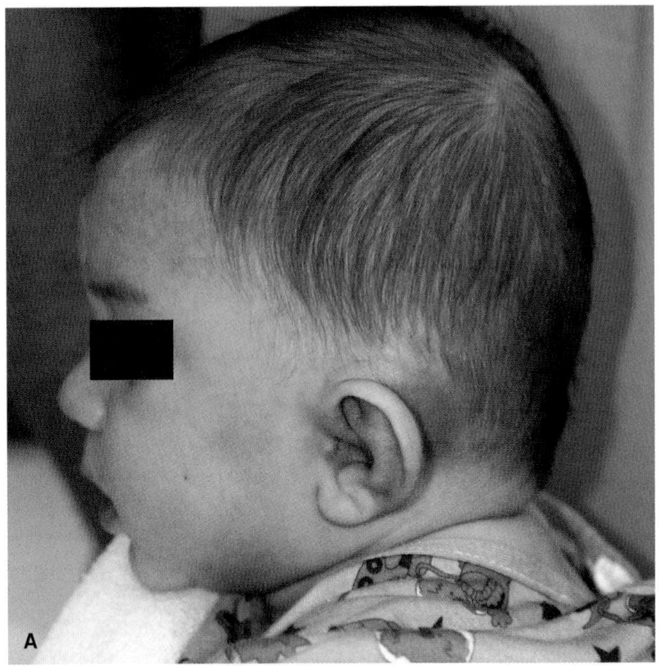

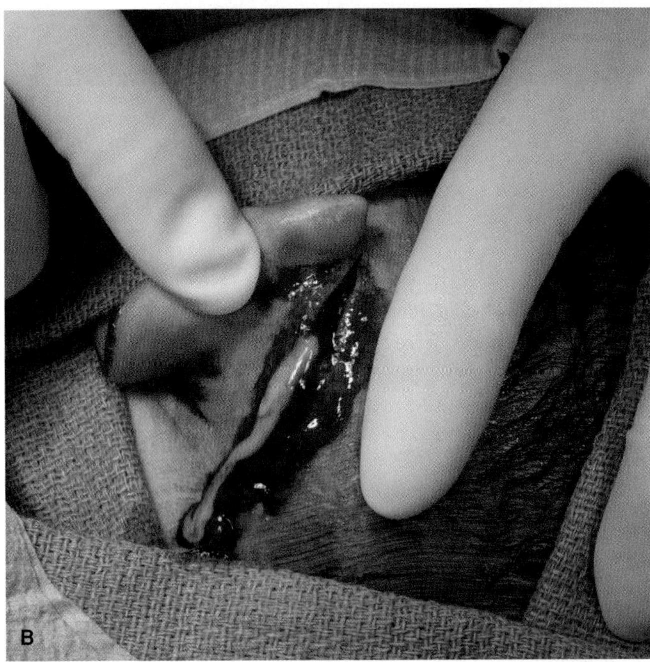

FIGURE 22-10 **A.** Mastoiditis in a young boy with recurrent otitis media. Note the erythema and swelling behind the ear. The ear is sticking out more than the other side. **B.** Surgical drainage was performed. *(Used with permission from William Clark, MD.)*

- Mastoiditis—Mastoiditis can be differentiated from simple AOM by the presence of increasing pain, erythema, and tenderness over mastoid bone in a patient with AOM who has not been treated with antibiotics or recurrence of mastoid pain and tenderness in patients treated with antibiotics. Recurrence or persistence of fever as well as progressive otorrhea are other historical clues. The mastoid swelling can cause the pinna to protrude further than normal (**Figure 22-10**).
- Traumatic perforation of the TM (**Figure 22-11**)—A hole in the TM is seen without purulent drainage.

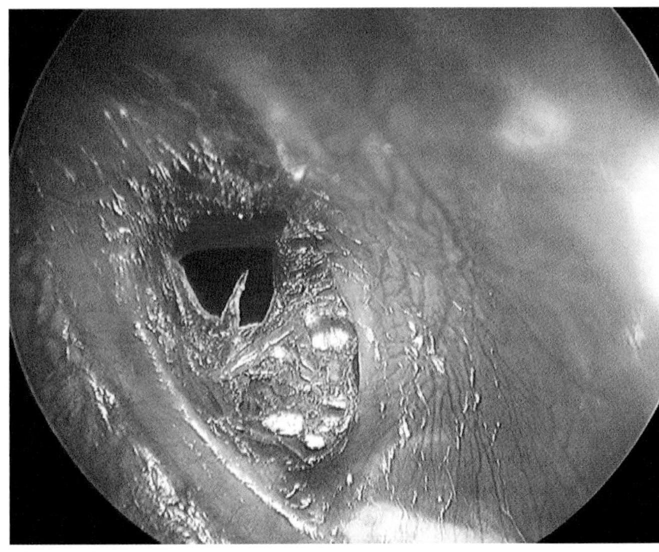

FIGURE 22-11 Traumatic perforation of the left tympanic membrane. *(Used with permission from William Clark, MD.)*

MANAGEMENT

NONPHARMACOLOGIC

Management of OME primarily consists of watchful waiting. Most cases resolve spontaneously within 3 months; only 5 percent to 10 percent last 1 year or longer. Treatment depends on duration and associated conditions. The following options should be considered:

- Document the laterality, duration of effusion, and presence and severity of associated symptoms at each assessment of the child with OME.[6] SOR Ⓒ
- Distinguish the child with OME who is at risk for speech, language, or learning problems from other children with OME and more promptly evaluate hearing, speech, language, and need for intervention in children at risk.[6] SOR Ⓒ Risk factors for developmental difficulties include:
    - Permanent hearing loss independent of OME.
    - Suspected or diagnosed speech and language delay or disorder.
    - Autism-spectrum disorder and other pervasive developmental disorders.
    - Syndromes (e.g., Down syndrome) or craniofacial disorders that include cognitive, speech, and language delays.
    - Blindness or uncorrectable visual impairment.
    - Cleft palate with or without associated syndrome.
    - Developmental delay.
- Manage the child with OME who is not at risk with watchful waiting for 3 months from the date of effusion onset (if known) or diagnosis (if onset is unknown).[6] SOR Ⓑ
- Hearing testing is recommended when OME persists for 3 months or longer or at any time if language delay, learning problems, or significant hearing loss is suspected in a child with OME.[6] SOR Ⓑ
- Autoinflation methods that attempt reopening the eustachian tube by increasing intranasal pressure may have some short-term benefits for

restoring hearing in patients with OME. These methods include forced exhalation through closed nose and mouth (which may be impractical for young children), inflatable intranasal balloon, or an anesthetic mask. Acute side effects are rare and the cost is not prohibitive; however, long-term adverse effects are unknown.[12] SOR Ⓑ

MEDICATIONS

- Oral acetaminophen (paracetamol) and ibuprofen can reduce earache when given with antibiotics.[16] Anesthetic ear drops (e.g., amethocaine, benzocaine, or lidocaine) can be effective in reducing pain among children ages 3 to 18 years with AOM when used with oral analgesics.[17] SOR Ⓑ
- Antibiotics seem to be most beneficial in children ages 6 to 23 months with bilateral AOM, otorrhea, or severe signs and symptoms (e.g., moderate to severe otalgia, persistent otalgia greater than 48 hours, temperature 39 °C [102.2 °F] or higher). For most other children with mild, unilateral disease, an observational policy based on shared decision-making seems justified.[13,15,18] SOR Ⓑ
- Antibiotics can lead to more rapid reduction in symptoms of AOM, but increase the risk of adverse effects, including diarrhea, vomiting, and rash.[16] SOR Ⓑ
  - Antibiotics seem to reduce pain at 2 to 7 days, and may prevent development of contralateral AOM, but increase the risks of adverse effects compared with placebo.[14]
  - There is insufficient effectiveness data regarding which antibiotic regimen is better than another.[14,16]
  - Antibiotics found to be effective in AOM include amoxicillin, amoxicillin-clavulanic acid, and cephalosporins. Amoxicillin is a good first-line treatment because it is inexpensive and children tolerate the bubblegum taste well.[13]
  - For children who have been treated with amoxicillin within the past 30 days, or with superimposed conjunctivitis suggestive of *H. influenzae*, or who previously failed amoxicillin in the setting of recurrent AOM, adding beta-lactamase coverage is recommended (e.g., amoxicillin-clavulanate). Alternative treatment for non-anaphylactic penicillin-allergic patients include 2nd-generation (e.g., cefuroxime) and 3rd generation cephalosporins (e.g., cefdinir, cefpodoxime, or ceftriaxone).[13]
  - Longer (8- to 10-day) courses of antibiotics reduce short-term treatment failure but have no long-term benefits compared with shorter regimens (5-day courses).[16,19]
  - An observational approach substantially reduces unnecessary use of antibiotics in children with AOM and may be an alternative to routine use of antimicrobials for treatment of such children.[20]
- Immediate antibiotic treatment (i.e., given at initial consultation) may reduce the duration of symptoms of AOM, but increases the risk of vomiting, diarrhea, and rash compared with delayed treatment (i.e., given after 72 hours).[16] SOR Ⓑ
- Treatment of AOM with decongestants and antihistamines is not recommended.[21] SOR Ⓑ
- Antihistamines and decongestants are not effective for OME.[6] Furthermore, they may cause harm in children younger than 5 years.[22] SOR Ⓐ
- Antimicrobials, oral corticosteroids, and intranasal steroids are not recommended for OME.[6,23] SOR Ⓐ

COMPLEMENTARY AND ALTERNATIVE THERAPY

- Current evidence is unclear on the effectiveness of zinc supplementation to prevent otitis media in young, healthy children in developing countries.[24] SOR Ⓑ

REFERRAL

- Refer to a specialist (otolaryngologist, audiologist, or speech-language pathologist) if there is:[6] SOR Ⓒ
  - Persistent fluid for 4 or more months with persistent hearing loss.
  - Associated speech delay.
  - Structural damage to TM or middle-ear.
- Tympanostomy tubes (or grommets) for children with recurrent AOM (3 or more episodes of AOM in 6 months, or 4 or more AOM in 1 year) diminish AOM recurrences for up to six months. Because long-term effectiveness is uncertain, clinicians should weigh this immediate benefit alongside potential adverse outcomes from the surgery.[25] SOR Ⓑ
- Insertion of tympanostomy tubes in young children with persistent middle-ear infection does not improve cognitive development, language acquisition, or speech development compared with waiting 6 to 9 months for the effusion to resolve before placing the tubes.[26] Moreover, delayed insertion of tubes helps children avoid getting tubes altogether and does not result in worse developmental outcomes.[27] SOR Ⓐ
- When a child becomes a surgical candidate, tympanostomy tube insertion is the preferred initial procedure; adenoidectomy should not be performed unless a distinct indication exists (e.g., nasal obstruction or chronic adenoiditis).[6] SOR Ⓑ
- Repeat surgery consists of adenoidectomy plus myringotomy, with or without tube insertion. Tonsillectomy alone or myringotomy alone should not be used to treat OME.[6] SOR Ⓑ

PREVENTION

- At best, the previously licensed PCV7 was only marginally effective in preventing AOM as an infant vaccine. However, this 6 percent to 7 percent reduction in incidence of AOM was justifiable from a public health perspective considering the significant disease burden. The PCV7 vaccine was not effective in preventing AOM in older children with prior history of AOM.[28] SOR Ⓐ
- There are insufficient data to determine the effectiveness of the currently licensed 13-valent pneumococcal vaccine (PCV13) given its recent licensure and use.
- Influenza vaccination may decrease the incidence of AOM but rigorous systematic reviews are needed to evaluate the magnitude of this effect.[13] SOR Ⓑ
- For at-risk children, long-term oral antibiotics administered for at least 6 weeks reduces the incidence of AOM while on therapy from 3 to 1.5 episodes per year. This benefit needs to be balanced against the potential side effects and the risks of antibiotic resistance.[16,29] SOR Ⓐ This practice is no longer considered routine.
- Xylitol chewing gum, lozenge or syrup prophylactically given 3 to 5 times daily among healthy children at daycare centers can prevent AOM recurrence by 25 percent. However, the safety of giving a

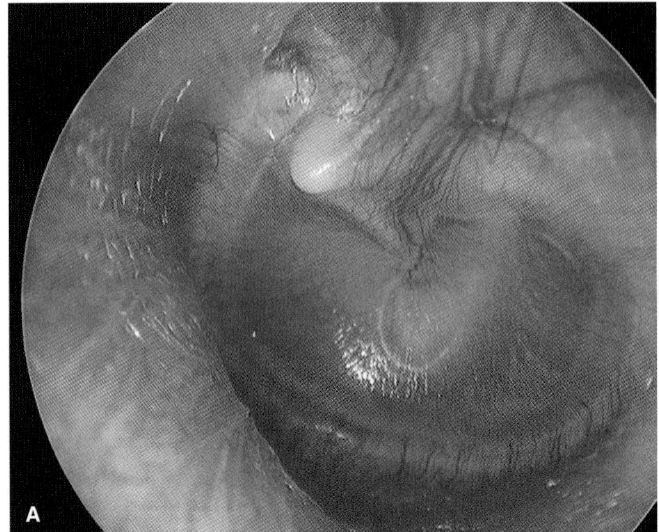

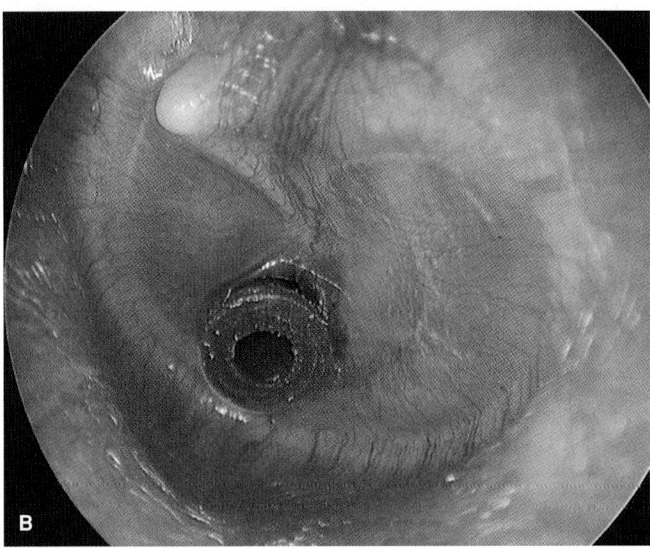

FIGURE 22-12 **A.** Left tympanic membrane (TM) of a 9-year-old girl with recurrent acute otitis media and chronic TM retractions prior to polyethylene (PE) tube placement. The circular area near the center of the TM is caused by the TM being retracted against the promontory of the medial wall of the middle ear. **B.** A fluoroplastic polyethylene (PE) tube is placed in the anterior-inferior quadrant of the TM of a 9-year-old girl with recurrent acute otitis media. It is black because it is impregnated with silver oxide to retard the growth of bacterial microfilms. (*Used with permission from William Clark, MD.*)

gum or lozenge to a young child, coupled with the compliance issues raised by its frequent administration, renders it an unrealistic preventive option.[30] SOR Ⓑ

- Exclusive breastfeeding for at least 6 months appears to diminish occurrence of AOM, hence should be encouraged.[13] SOR Ⓑ
- Tympanostomy tubes lead to short-term reduction in the number of episodes of AOM but increase the risk of complications (i.e., tympanosclerosis; **Figures 22-12** and **22-13**).[16] SOR Ⓑ

PROGNOSIS

- Without antibiotics, AOM resolves within 24 hours in approximately 60 percent of children and within 3 days in approximately 80 percent of children. Rate of suppurative complications if antibiotics are withheld is 0.13 percent.[31]
- Most cases of OME resolve spontaneously within 3 months; only 5 percent to 10 percent last 1 year or longer. However, effusion will recur in 30 percent to 40 percent of patients.[6]

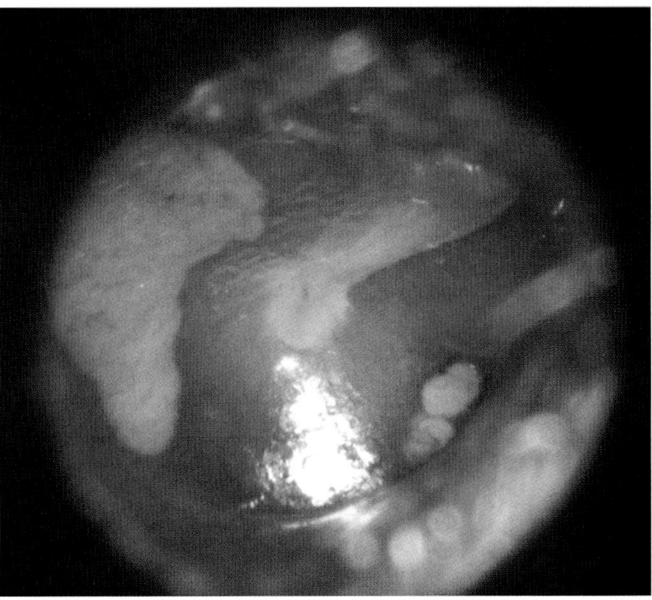

FIGURE 22-13 Tympanosclerosis as the result of previous recurrent episodes of otitis media and polyethylene (PE) tube placement. (*Used with permission from Glen Medellin, MD.*)

FOLLOW-UP

- If a patient with AOM fails to respond to the initial management option within 48 to 72 hours, the clinician should reassess the patient to confirm AOM and exclude other causes of illness. If AOM is confirmed in a patient initially managed with observation, the clinician should begin antibiotics. If the patient was initially managed with antibiotics, the clinician should change antibiotics.[6] SOR Ⓑ
- Potentially serious complications of AOM, such as mastoiditis or facial nerve involvement, require urgent referral.
- There is no consensus in the medical community regarding timing of posttreatment follow-up of AOM or who should receive follow-up. There is some evidence that parents can be reliable predictors in the resolution or persistence of AOM following antibiotic treatment.[32]
- Children with persistent OME who are not thought to be at significant risk should be reexamined at 3- to 6-month intervals until the effusion is gone, significant hearing loss is identified, or structural abnormalities of the eardrum or middle ear are suspected.[6] SOR Ⓑ

PATIENT EDUCATION

- Patient education should focus on identification, prevention, and control of risk factors.
- Parents should be made aware of the high rates of spontaneous resolution of AOM and potential adverse effects of antibiotics. Providing a prescription for an antibiotic at the initial visit but

advising delay of initiation of medication (i.e., observational approach for up to 48 hours) is an alternative to immediate treatment and is associated with lower antibiotic use.[20]

- Patients should be informed that the natural history of OME is spontaneous resolution.
  - Periodic follow-up to monitor resolution of MEE is extremely important.
  - If MEE is persistent and signs and symptoms of hearing loss, language difficulties, and learning problems arise, additional treatment may be considered.

PATIENT RESOURCES

AOM

- **www.nlm.nih.gov/medlineplus/ency/article/000638.htm.**
- **www.nidcd.nih.gov/health/hearing/earinfections.**
- **www.familydoctor.org/online/famdocen/home/common/ear/055.html.**
- **www.kidshealth.org/PageManager.jsp?dn=familydoctor&lic=44&article_set=22743.**
- **www.nhs.uk/conditions/Otitis-media/Pages/Introduction.aspx.**

OME

- **http://familydoctor.org/online/famdocen/home/common/ear/330.html.**
- **http://www.nlm.nih.gov/medlineplus/ency/article/007010.htm.**

PROVIDER RESOURCES

AOM

- Clinical Practice Guideline: The diagnosis and management of acute otitis media from the American Academy of Pediatrics. *Pediatrics*. 2013;131;e964-e99.
- Guideline: diagnosis and management of acute otitis media. Clinical Practice Guideline by the American Academy of Family Physicians, American Academy of Otolaryngology-Head and Neck Surgery, and American Academy of Pediatrics Subcommittee on Management of Acute Otitis Media. *Pediatrics*. 2004;113:1451-1465.
- British Columbia Guidelines for AOM—**http://www.bcguidelines.ca/pdf/otitaom.pdf.**

OME

- Guideline: otitis media with effusion. Clinical Practice Guideline by the American Academy of Family Physicians, American Academy of Otolaryngology-Head and Neck Surgery, and American Academy of Pediatrics Subcommittee on Otitis Media With Effusion. *Pediatrics*. 2004;113:1412-1429.
- British Columbia Guidelines for OME—**http://www.bcguidelines.ca/pdf/otitome.pdf.**

REFERENCES

1. Bondy J, Berman S, Glazner J, Lezotte D. Direct expenditures related to otitis media diagnoses: extrapolations from a pediatric medicaid cohort. *Pediatrics*. 2000;105(6):E72.
2. Teele DW, Klein JO, Rosner BA. Epidemiology of otitis media during the first seven years of life in children in greater Boston: a prospective, cohort study. *J Infect Dis*. 1989;160(1):83-94.
3. Paradise JL, Rockette HE, Colborn DK, et al. Otitis media in 2253 Pittsburgh-area infants: prevalence and risk factors during the first two years of life. *Pediatrics*. 1997;99(3):318-333.
4. Del Mar C, Glasziou P, Hayem M. Are antibiotics indicated as initial treatment for children with acute otitis media? A meta-analysis. *BMJ*. 1997;314:1526-1529.
5. Nyquist AC, Gonzales R, Steiner JF, Sande MA. Antibiotic prescribing for children with colds, upper respiratory tract infections, and bronchitis. *JAMA*. 1998;279:875.
6. Guideline: otitis media with effusion. Clinical practice guideline by the American Academy of Family Physicians, American Academy of Otolaryngology-Head and Neck Surgery, and American Academy of Pediatrics Subcommittee on Otitis Media With Effusion. *Pediatrics*. 2004;113:1412-1429.
7. Rovers MM, Schilder AG, Zielhuis GA, Rosenfeld RM. Otitis media. *Lancet*. 2004;363:465.
8. Casey JR, Adlowitz DG, Pichichero ME. New patterns in the otopathogens causing acute otitis media six to eight years after introduction of pneumococcal conjugate vaccine. *Pediatr Infect Dis J*. 2010;29(4):304-309.
9. McEllistrem MC. Acute otitis media due to penicillin-nonsusceptible *Streptococcus pneumoniae* before and after the introduction of the pneumococcal conjugate vaccine. *Clin Infect Dis*. 2005;40(12):1738-1744.
10. Ruuskanen O, Arola M, Heikkinen T, Ziegler T. Viruses in acute otitis media: increasing evidence for clinical significance. *Pediatr Infect Dis J*. 1991;10:425.9.
11. Froom J, Culpepper L, Jacobs M, et al. Antimicrobials for acute otitis media? A review from the International Primary Care Network. *BMJ*. 1997;315:98-102.
12. Perera R, Haynes J, Glasziou PP, Heneghan CJ. Autoinflation for hearing loss associated with otitis media with effusion. Cochrane Database Syst Rev. 2006;(4):CD006285.
13. Lieberthal AS, Carroll AE, Chonmaitree T, et al. The diagnosis and management of acute otitis media. *Pediatrics*. 2013;131;e964-e99.
14. Takata GS, Chan LS, Morphew T, et al. Evidence assessment of the accuracy of methods of diagnosing middle ear effusion in children with otitis media with effusion. *Pediatrics*. 2003;112:1379-1387.
15. Gamboa S, Park MK, Wanserski G, Lo V. Clinical inquiries. Should you use antibiotics to treat acute otitis media in children? *J Fam Pract*. 2009;58(11):602-604.
16. Damoiseaux RA, Rovers MM. AOM in children. *Clin Evid (Online)*. 2011 May 10;2011. pii: 0301.
17. Foxlee R, Johansson AC, Wejfalk J, et al. Topical analgesia for acute otitis media. *Cochrane Database Syst Rev*. 2006;3:CD005657.

18. Rovers MM, Glasziou P, Appelman CL, et al. Antibiotics for acute otitis media: a meta-analysis with individual patient data. *Lancet.* 2006;368:1429-1435.

19. Kozyrskyj AL, Klassen TP, Moffatt M, Harvey K. Short-course antibiotics for acute otitis media. *Cochrane Database Syst Rev.* 2010;(9):CD001095.

20. Spiro DM, Tay KY, Arnold DH, et al. Wait-and-see prescription for the treatment of acute otitis media: a randomized controlled trial. *JAMA.* 2006;296:1235-1241.

21. Coleman C, Moore M. Decongestants and antihistamines for acute otitis media in children. *Cochrane Database Syst Rev.* 2008;3:CD001727.

22. Griffin G, Flynn CA. Antihistamines and/or decongestants for otitis media with effusion (OME) in children. *Cochrane Database Syst Rev.* 2011;(9):CD003423.

23. Simpson SA, Lewis R, van der Voort J, Butler CC. Oral or topical nasal steroids for hearing loss associated with otitis media with effusion in children. *Cochrane Database Syst Rev.* 2011;(5):CD001935.

24. Gulani A, Sachdev HS. Zinc supplements for preventing otitis media. *Cochrane Database Syst Rev.* 2012; (4):CD006639.

25. McDonald S, Langton Hewer CD, Nunez DA. Grommets (ventilation tubes) for recurrent acute otitis media in children. *Cochrane Database Syst Rev.* 2008;(4):CD004741.

26. Paradise JL, Dollaghan CA, Campbell TF, et al. otitis media and tympanostomy tube insertion during the first three years of life: developmental outcomes at the age of four years. *Pediatrics.* 2003;112:265-277.

27. Paradise JL, Feldman HM, Campbell TF, et al. Tympanostomy tubes and developmental outcomes at 9 to 11 years of age. *N Engl J Med.* 2007;356:300-302.

28. Jansen AGSC, Hak E, Veenhoven RH, Damoiseaux RAMJ, Schilder AGM, Sanders EAM. Pneumococcal conjugate vaccines for preventing otitis media. *Cochrane Database Syst Rev.* 2009;(2):CD001480.

29. Leach AJ, Morris PS. Antibiotics for the prevention of acute and chronic suppurative otitis media in children. *Cochrane Database Syst Rev.* 2006;(4):CD004401.

30. Azarpazhooh A, Limeback H, Lawrence HP, Shah PS. Xylitol for preventing acute otitis media in children up to 12 years of age. *Cochrane Database Syst Rev.* 2011;(11):CD007095.

31. Rosenfeld RM. Natural history of untreated otitis media. *Laryngoscope.* 2003;113:1645-1657.

32. Raimer PL. *Parents Can Be Reliable Predictors in the Resolution or Persistence of Acute Otitis Media Following Antibiotic Treatment.* University of Michigan Department of Pediatrics Evidence-based Pediatrics Web site. 2005. http://www.med.umich.edu/pediatrics/ebm/cats/omparent.htm, accessed February 2012.

23 MASTOIDITIS

Samantha Anne, MD, MS

PATIENT STORY

A 12-month-old girl presents to your office with 1-day history of fever and increasing swelling and redness behind her left ear. On examination, the left auricle is protruding and there is marked erythema, swelling, tenderness, and fluctuance overlying the left mastoid bone (**Figure 23-1**). Otoscopy reveals a purulent middle ear effusion. A computed tomography (CT) scan of the temporal bones reveals opacification of the mastoid air cells. A diagnosis of acute mastoiditis is made and the girl undergoes urgent myringotomy and tympanostomy tube placement and mastoidectomy. Postoperatively, she is treated with intravenous antibiotics and recovers completely.

INTRODUCTION

Mastoiditis is a complication of otitis media, characterized by a suppurative infection of the mastoid air cells.[1] Acute mastoiditis refers to the finding of acute otitis media on otoscopy in conjunction with local inflammatory findings in the mastoid including erythema, edema, and auricular protrusion, with duration of symptoms less than one month. Coalescent mastoiditis occurs when there is an acute otitis media which progresses into an acute infection of mastoid with osteolytic changes in the bone and destruction of the mastoid air cells. Chronic mastoiditis is defined by the presence of long-standing infection in the presence of tympanic membrane perforation or tympanostomy tube or as a complication of cholesteatoma. Chronic mastoiditis follows an indolent course of infection.

SYNONYMS

Mastoid inflammation or Mastoid infection.

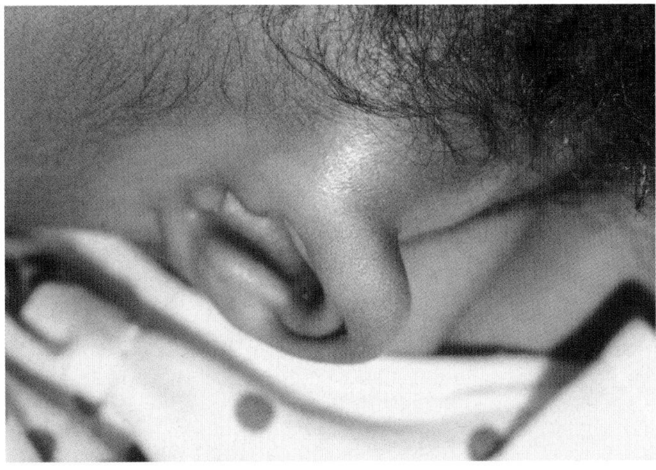

FIGURE 23-1 12-month-old girl with protrusion of the auricle and erythema and swelling in the left mastoid area. (*Used with permission from Johanna Goldfarb, MD.*)

EPIDEMIOLOGY

- The epidemiology of acute mastoiditis is similar to that of otitis media. Thus, acute and coalescent mastoiditis occurs most frequently in children less than 4 years of age.[2]
- Although recurrent otitis media is a risk factor for mastoiditis, a significant percentage of cases of mastoiditis occur in young children who do not have a prior history of OM.[2]
- Few studies on the incidence of mastoiditis are population based; thus it is difficult to estimate the true incidence and whether the incidence is increasing.
- Chronic mastoiditis tends to occur in children with chronic otitis media, chronic otorrhea thru tympanic membrane perforation, and/or cholesteatoma.[1]

ETIOLOGY AND PATHOPHYSIOLOGY

- Acute and coalescent mastoiditis may occur in children with well pneumatized mastoids with little or minimal prior history of otitis media.
- These acute infections also occur in younger children with more immature immune systems.[2]
- The infectious process usually begins with an acute otitis media that causes edema of the mucoperiosteal lining of the mastoid air cells and middle ear. This blocks the aditus of the mastoid and the Eustachian tube thereby disrupting the normal aeration.[1,3] This leads to worsening purulence and inflammation and eventually development of localized acidosis and bony septa decalcification. In addition, osteoclastic activity cases further destruction of bony septa in the mastoid causing eventual coalescence.
- Eventually as the pressure continues to increase in the mastoid, the infection progresses to either intracranial extension or thru lateral cortical bone destruction into the neck and soft tissue postauricularly.
- The microbiologic agents responsible for acute and coalescent mastoiditis include *Streptococcus pneumoniae*, *Streptococcus pyogenes*, *Staphylococcus aureus* [including methicillin-resistant strains (MRSA)] and rarely, *Pseudomonas aeruginosa*.
- S pneumoniae serotype 19A, which can be a multidrug resistant organism, has emerged as an important pathogen causing acute mastoiditis.[4]
- The microbiology of chronic mastoiditis includes *P. aeruginosa*, *S. aureus* (including MRSA), Proteus sp., and anaerobes including Peptostreptococcus, and Bacteroides.

RISK FACTORS

- Otitis media, young age, and altered immunity are risk factors for mastoiditis.
- A history of recurrent otitis media is a risk factor for acute mastoiditis.[5]
- Cholesteatoma is a risk factor for chronic mastoiditis.

DIAGNOSIS

- The diagnosis of acute mastoiditis is a clinical diagnosis based on the characteristic clinical findings.[6]
- The diagnosis of coalescent mastoiditis can be made in the appropriate clinical setting when osteolytic changes in the bone and destruction of the mastoid air cells are present.
- The diagnosis of chronic mastoiditis relies on the presence of a chronic suppurative process and evidence of inflammatory changes in the mastoid.

CLINICAL FEATURES

- Postauricular tenderness, erythema, swelling, and fluctuance are the hallmarks of acute mastoiditis.[7]
- Protrusion of the auricle is common (**Figure 23-2**); the displacement is usually downward and outward in young children and upward and outward in older children.
- Fever, ear pain, or irritability in younger children may be present.
- Otoscopic examination commonly reveals signs of acute otitis media (bulging or erythematous tympanic membrane; **Figure 23-3**).[6]

LABORATORY TESTING

- A complete blood count with differential may reveal a leukocytosis with a left shift.[8]
- Inflammatory markers are usually elevated with acute mastoiditis, although they may be normal early in the course and in cases of chronic mastoiditis.[9,10]
- A blood culture has low yield for ascertaining the etiologic organism, but when positive is very helpful in the specific bacteriologic diagnosis.

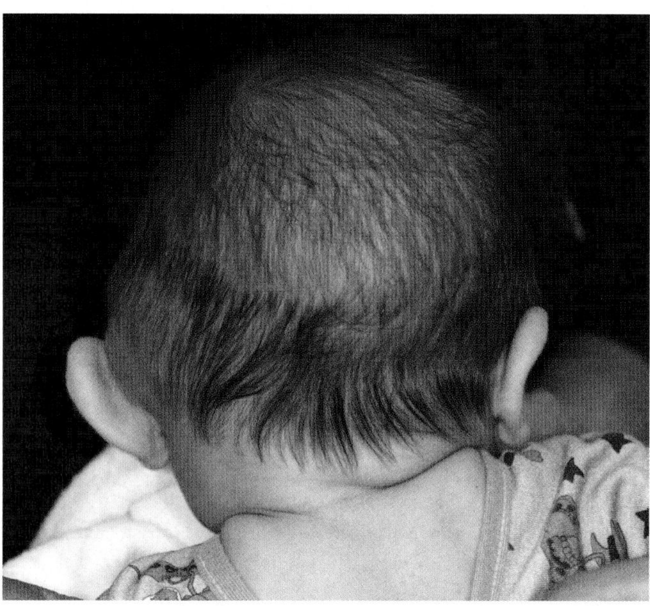

FIGURE 23-2 Mastoiditis in a young boy with recurrent otitis media. Note the erythema and protrusion of the left ear. (*Used with permission from William Clark, MD.*)

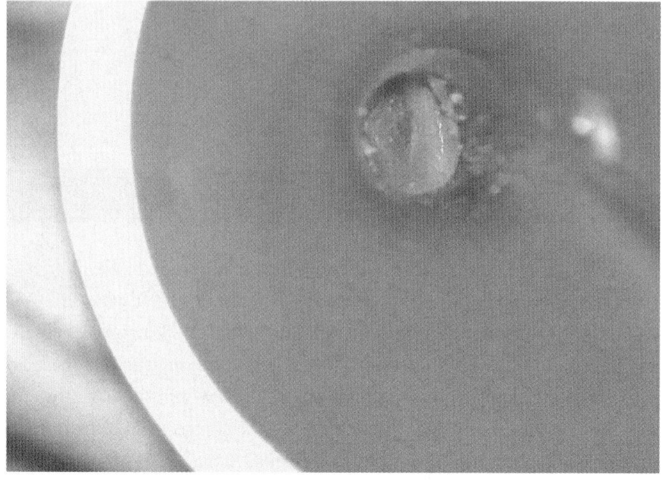

FIGURE 23-3 Picture of tympanic membrane with purulent effusion in a child about to undergo myringotomy with tube placement with coalescent mastoiditis. (*Used with permission from Prashant Malhotra, MD.*)

- Middle ear and mastoid cultures attained surgically are very helpful in directing the initial antimicrobial therapy and subsequent follow-up.

IMAGING

- Imaging is not required to make the diagnosis of acute mastoiditis in children who have classic clinical manifestations. However, imaging is helpful in cases that are not classic, and in assessing for coalescent mastoiditis and other complication of acute mastoiditis.[11]
- Imaging is also helpful in planning a management course for a patient with acute mastoiditis.
- A contrast enhanced CT of the temporal bones is the best imaging modality for acute mastoiditis. Findings include opacification of mastoid air cells, cortical bone erosion, coalescence of air cells, and post auricular fluid collections (**Figures 23-4** and **23-5**).
- If there is concern for intracranial complication, cranial magnetic resonance imaging with gadolinium is more sensitive than CT and recommended.[12]

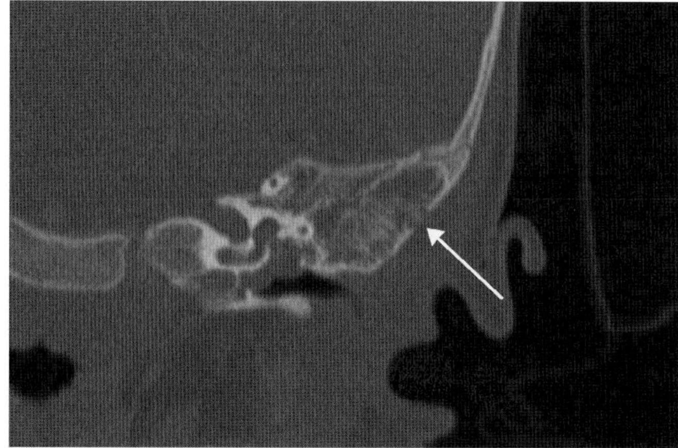

FIGURE 23-4 Computed tomography (CT) scan of the temporal bone showing localized bony destruction along the lateral margin (arrow) of the left mastoid air cells.

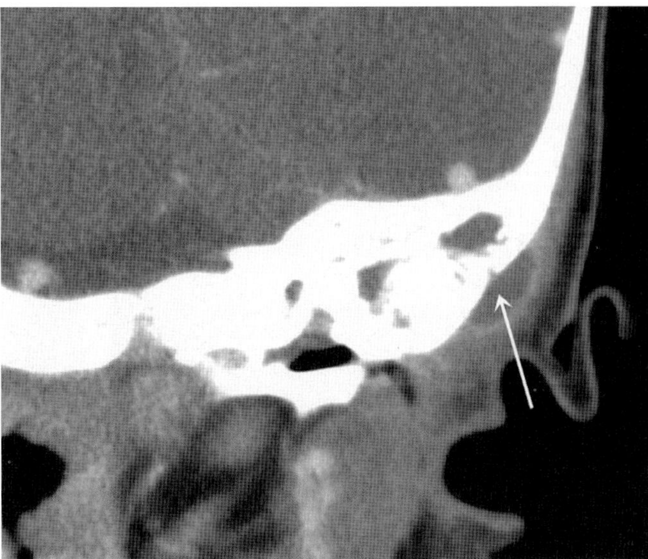

FIGURE 23-5 Computed tomography (CT) scan of the temporal bone showing prominent soft tissue thickening (arrow) overlying the posterior left temporal region with central abscess formation.

- Imaging findings with chronic mastoiditis include cholesteatoma and erosion of the cortical mastoid bone (**Figure 23-6**).

DIFFERENTIAL DIAGNOSIS

- Otitis externa can also cause cellulitic changes in the post auricular region which can mimic acute mastoiditis. The appearance of the external canal and the degree of tenderness of the auricle itself, rather than the postauricular area can be helpful in differentiating these entities. CT of the temporal bones also can help differentiate otitis externa from mastoiditis in that there usually will not be opacification of mastoid air cells and will reveal mostly soft tissue changes in the ear canal.
- Trauma can also cause skin discoloration, edema, and changes in postauricular area. However, the normal tympanic membrane, the lack of constitutional symptoms, lack of leukocytosis along with clinical history and imaging should easily differentiate trauma from acute mastoiditis.
- Postauricular lymphadenopathy from a viral infection or from a scalp infection may cause postauricular swelling and erythema. However, the normal auricle, tympanic membrane, and often palpable lymph node help distinguish this from mastoiditis.

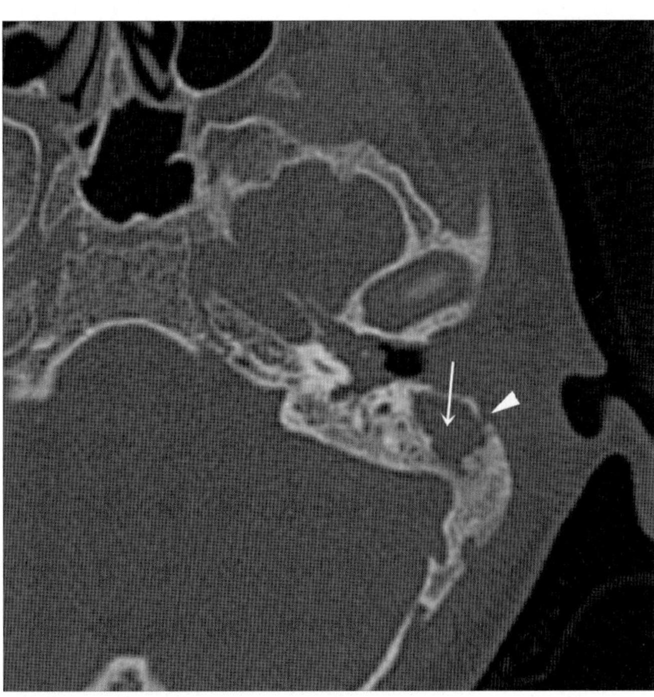

FIGURE 23-6 Chronic mastoiditis and cholesteatoma in 16 year-old. Note the soft tissue seen filling middle ear and mastoid (arrow) with erosion of lateral mastoid cortical bone (arrowhead) and posterior external auditory canal.

MANAGEMENT

- In general, acute mastoiditis and coalescent mastoiditis can be treated with parenteral antibiotics and myringotomy with or without placement of a tympanostomy tube. SOR Ⓒ
- This conservative approach is not always successful, as evidenced by one study, which showed that nearly 1/4 to 1/3 of these patients eventually required further surgical intervention.[13]
- Acute mastoiditis with intracranial complications and other suppurative complications is treated with intravenous antibiotics, myringotomy with or without placement of tympanotomy tubes, and mastoidectomy. SOR Ⓒ
- Chronic mastoiditis, in general, fails to resolve with medical therapy alone and often requires mastoidectomy.

NONPHARMACOLOGIC

- If there is a tympanic membrane perforation, dry ear precautions may be necessary to prevent further infection.

MEDICATIONS

- Empiric antibiotics directed against the most likely agents must be administered. More specific therapy can be administered once the etiologic agent has been isolated.[14]
- For acute mastoiditis, a third generation cephalosporin such as Ceftriaxone is a good empiric option. Vancomycin is often added to the regimen, especially if there is high index of suspicion for a Staphylococcal infection. SOR Ⓒ
- Alternative agents that have been used include penicillin with a beta-lactamase inhibitor (e.g., ampicillin-sulbactam), cefepime, and piperacillin-tazobactam.
- For chronic mastoiditis, vancomycin often is used with an anti-pseudomonal agent such as ceftazidime, cefepime or an aminoglycoside. SOR Ⓒ
- Parenteral therapy should be given initially for cases of acute mastoiditis. The duration of parenteral and total antimicrobial therapy depends on clinical improvement, resolution of the findings, and the microbiology; a 3- to 4-week total course of antibiotics is commonly prescribed. SOR Ⓒ

- In addition, ototopical agents such as ofloxacin or ciprofloxacin with dexamethasone can be used as an adjunct. SOR C

SURGERY

- Myringotomy with or without tympanotomy tube placement is important to perform in order to drain purulence, attain culture material, and to relieve pain.
- Mastoidectomy is important to remove diseased bone postauricularly especially in setting of acute and/or coalescent mastoiditis.
- Mastoidectomy is generally required for chronic mastoidectomy.

REFERRAL

Early consultation to otolaryngology is important to determine need for surgical intervention and to aid in attaining cultures. If intracranial involvement is present, neurosurgery consultation is important. An infectious diseases specialist is often involved in the care of these patients to direct antimicrobial therapy.

PREVENTION AND SCREENING

- Close follow-up for otitis media, surveillance for cholesteatoma, and aggressive management of worsening symptoms and signs is important in preventing progression to mastoiditis.

PROGNOSIS

- Complications of mastoiditis are related to the spread of infection to contiguous structures, and occur in approximately 10 percent to 30 percent of patients with acute mastoiditis.[6,15]
- Mastoiditis can extend posteriorly to cause sigmoid sinus thrombosis, laterally to produce subperiosteal abscess, superiorly to cause intracranial infections, or inferiorly to form a Bezold abscess, which is a neck abscess located beneath the sternocleidomastoid and digastric muscles.[16]
- Other complications of mastoiditis include facial nerve paralysis, hearing loss, labyrinthitis, and osteomyelitis of the bones of the skull.
- Intracranial complications of mastoiditis include meningitis, brain abscess, epidural or subdural abscess, and venous sinus thrombosis.
- Intracranial complications of mastoiditis, such as a brain abscess, may be the presenting complaint (**Figure 23-7**).

FOLLOW-UP

- Children who are diagnosed with mastoiditis require very close follow-up to assure they respond appropriately and to limit complications.
- The timing and need for follow-up studies are determined by the type of treatment used, whether surgical and medical, and the response to treatment.

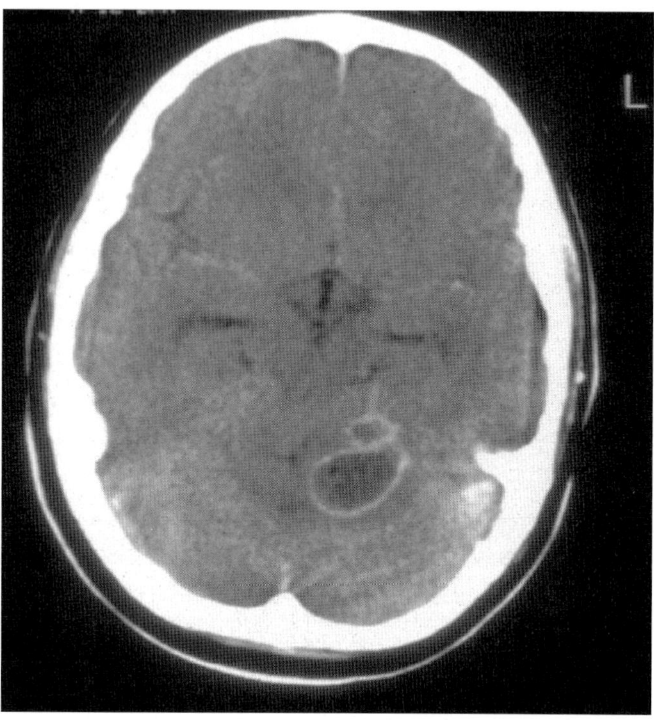

FIGURE 23-7 This adolescent presented with headache and fever and was found to have a brain abscess, which was the result of chronic otitis media and mastoiditis. (*Used with permission from Camille Sabella, MD.*)

PATIENT EDUCATION

- Worsening otalgia, protrusion of the auricle, and/or erythema and tenderness behind the ear warrants immediate medical attention.

PATIENT RESOURCES

- **www.webmd.com/cold-and-flu/ear-infection/mastoiditis-symptoms-causes-treatments.**

PROVIDER RESOURCES

- *Pocket guide to antimicrobial therapy in otolaryngology and head and neck surgery*, 13th edition, 2007—**www.entnet.org/EducationAndResearch/upload/AAO-PGS-9-4-2.pdf.**

REFERENCES

1. Lewis K, Shapiro NL, Cherry JD. Mastoiditis. In: Feigin RD, Cherry JD, Demmler- Harrison GJ, Kaplan SL, eds. *Textbook of Pediatric Infectious Diseases, 6th ed.*, Philadelphia, PA: Saunders; 2009: 238.
2. Ghaffar FA, Wördemann M, McCracken GH Jr: Acute mastoiditis in children: a seventeen-year experience in Dallas, Texas. *Pediatr Infect Dis J.* 2001; 20:376.
3. Anderson KJ. Mastoiditis. *Pediatr Rev.* 2009;30:233.
4. Ongkasuwan J, Valdez TA, Hulten KG, et al. Pneumococcal mastoiditis in children and the emergence of multidrug-resistant serotype 19A isolates. *Pediatrics.* 2008;122:34.

5. Luntz M, Brodsky A, Nusem S, et al. Acute mastoiditis—the antibiotic era: a multicenter study. *Int J Pediatr Otorhinolaryngol.* 2001;57:1.

6. van den Aardweg MT, Rovers MM, de Ru JA, et al. A systematic review of diagnostic criteria for acute mastoiditis in children. *Otol Neurotol.* 2008;29:751.

7. Wald ER, Conway JH. Mastoiditis. In: Long SS, Pickering LK, Prober CG, eds. *Principles and Practice of Pediatric Infectious Diseases, 4th ed*, Edinburgh: Elsevier Saunders; 2012:222.

8. Katz A, Leibovitz E, Greenberg D, et al. Acute mastoiditis in Southern Israel: a twelve year retrospective study (1990 through 2001). *Pediatr Infect Dis J.* 2003;22:878.

9. Bilavsky E, Yarden-Bilavsky H, Samra Z, et al. Clinical, laboratory, and microbiological differences between children with simple or complicated mastoiditis. *Int J Pediatr Otorhinolaryngol.* 2009;73: 1270.15.

10. Oestreicher-Kedem Y, Raveh E, Kornreich L, et al. Complications of mastoiditis in children at the onset of a new millennium. *Ann Otol Rhinol Laryngol.* 2005;114:147.

11. Tamir S, Schwartz Y, Peleg U, et al. Acute mastoiditis in children: is computed tomography always necessary? *Ann Otol Rhinol Laryngol.* 2009;118:565.

12. Bluestone CD. Clinical course, complications, and sequelae of acute otitis media. *Pediatr Inf Dis J.* 2000;19:S37.

13. Ionnis M, Psarommatis A, Charalampos V, et al. Algorithmic management of pediatric acute mastoiditis. *Int J Pediatr Otorhinolaryngol.* 2012;(76):791-796.

14. Moore JA, Wei JL, Smith HJ, et al. Treatment of pediatric suppurative mastoiditis: Is peripherally inserted central catheter (PICC) antibiotic therapy necessary? *Otolaryngol Head Neck Surg.* 2006; 135;(1):106-110.

15. El-Kashlan HK, Harker LA, Shelton C, et al. Complications of temporal bone infections. In: Flint, PW, Haughey, BH, Lund, VJ, Niparko, JK, Richardson, MA, Robbins, KT, and Thomas, JR. *Otolaryngology-Head & Neck Surgery*, Elselvier: Maryland Heights, MO; 2010:1979-1998.

16. Leskinen K. Complications of acute otitis media in children. *Curr Allergy Asthma Rep.* 2005;5:308.

24 EAR—FOREIGN BODY

Brian Z. Rayala, MD

PATIENT STORY

A 3-year-old girl is brought by her parents to an urgent care facility after a day of crying, irritability, scant otorrhea, and frequent pulling of her right ear. Otoscopy reveals an erythematous, swollen external auditory canal (EAC) where a bead is wedged (**Figure 24-1**). The patient is referred to an otolaryngologist and the bead is removed using an operating microscope for visualization.

INTRODUCTION

- Children with ear foreign bodies (FBs) usually present with otalgia, otorrhea, or decreased hearing. At times, symptoms may be non-specific, like irritability and crying. Other times, presentation may be asymptomatic.

EPIDEMIOLOGY

- Ear FBs are commonly seen in children aged 1 to 6 years.[1–3]
- Equal male-to-female ratio in the pediatric population.[4]

ETIOLOGY AND PATHOPHYSIOLOGY

- Most common FBs in children include:[5]
  - Inanimate objects such as beads (**Figure 24-1**), cotton tips, paper, toy parts, crayons (**Figure 24-2**), eraser tips, food, or organic matter, including sand (**Figure 24-3**), sticks, and stones.
  - Insects (**Figure 24-4**).

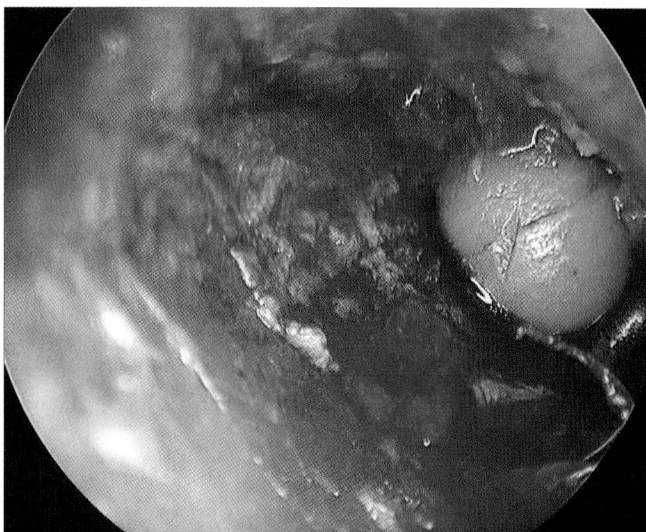

FIGURE 24-1 Foreign body (bead) in the ear canal of a 3-year-old girl with reactive tissue around it. (*Used with permission from William Clark, MD.*)

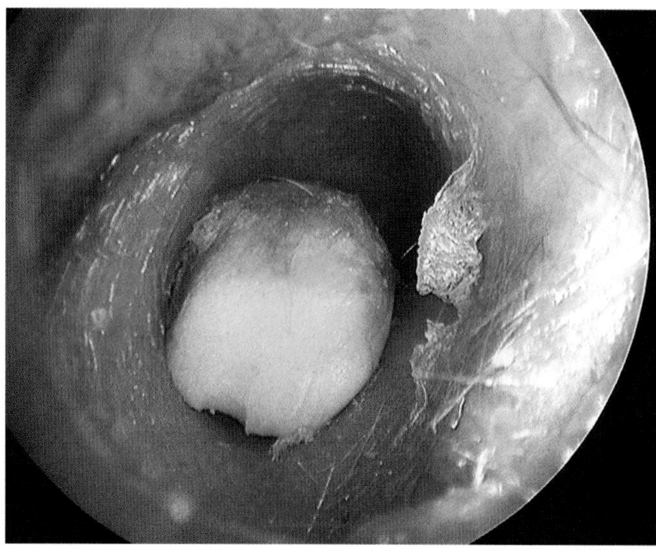

FIGURE 24-2 Piece of a crayon in the ear canal of a 4-year-old boy. (*Used with permission from William Clark, MD.*)

- Pathogenesis includes some of the key elements of otitis externa (see Chapter 21, Otitis Externa):
  - Initial breakdown of the skin-cerumen barrier (caused by presence of FB).
  - Skin inflammation and edema leading to subsequent obstruction of adnexal structures (e.g., cerumen glands, sebaceous glands, and hair follicles).
  - FB reaction leading to further skin injury.
  - In the case of alkaline battery electrochemical reaction, severe alkaline burns may occur.

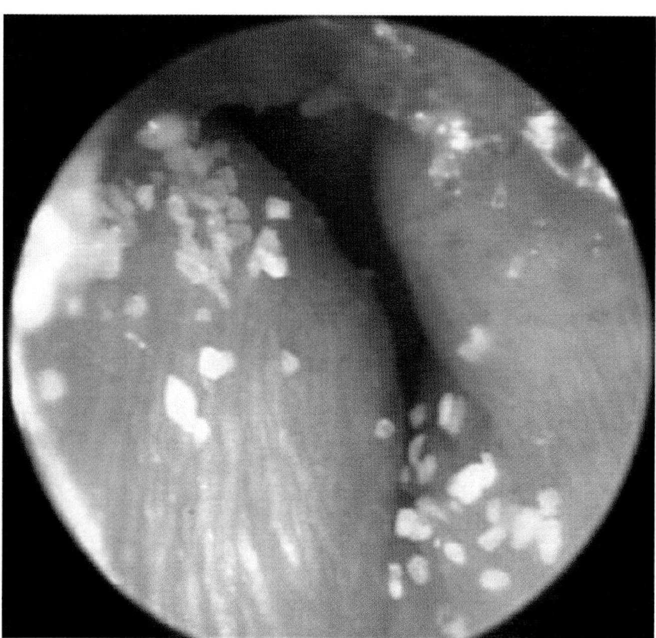

FIGURE 24-3 Beach sand granules with exostosis in the ear of a cold water surfer. The exostoses are common in cold water swimmers and surfers. (*Used with permission from Roy F. Sullivan, PhD. Audiology Forum: Video Otoscopy, www.rcsullivan.com.*)

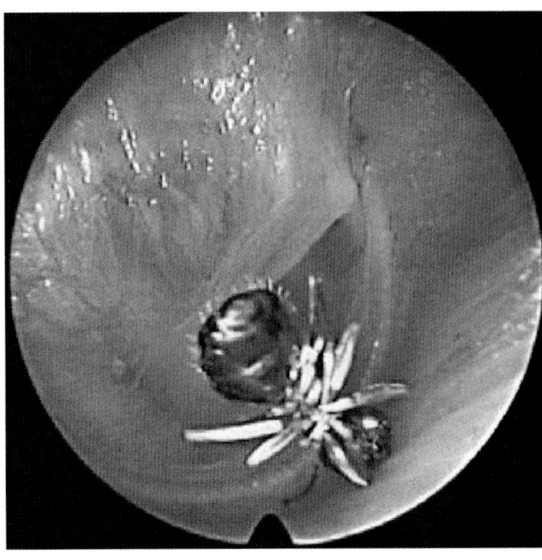

FIGURE 24-4 Ant in the ear canal. (*Used with permission from Vladimir Zlinsky, MD in Roy F. Sullivan, PhD. Audiology Forum: Video Otoscopy, www.rcsullivan.com.*)

RISK FACTORS

- Children with attention deficit hyperactivity disorder (ADHD) may be more likely to self-insert FBs and ADHD should be considered in children with ear FBs who are older than age 5 years.[6]

DIAGNOSIS

CLINICAL FEATURES

- Key historical features include:
  - Otalgia.
  - Otorrhea or otorrhagia.
  - Mild hearing loss.
  - Irritability or crying.
  - History suspicious for FB insertion or witnessed FB insertion.
- Some children are asymptomatic.
- Hallmark of diagnosis includes visualization of FB on otoscopy (**Figures 24-1** through **24-4**).
- Otoscopy can reveal signs of EAC inflammation (e.g., edema, erythema, or aural discharge) (**Figure 24-1**).

LABORATORY AND IMAGING

- Aural FB is a clinical diagnosis. Laboratory and imaging studies have very limited use.

DIFFERENTIAL DIAGNOSIS

- Otitis externa—Presents with otalgia, otorrhea, and mild hearing loss, all of which can be present in ear FB. Absence of FB (on otoscopic exam) is the key differentiating factor (see Chapter 21, Otitis Externa).
- Acute otitis media (with or without perforated tympanic membrane [TM])—Otoscopy shows absence of FB and presence of middle-ear inflammation and effusion (i.e., bulging, erythematous, cloudy, or immobile TM). Patients present with clinical signs or symptoms of acute illness like fever (see Chapter 22, Otitis Media—Acute Otitis and Otitis Media with Effusion).
- Chronic Suppurative Otitis Media—Otoscopy shows absence of FB and presence of TM perforation; history reveals a chronically draining ear and recurrent middle-ear infections with or without hearing loss.

MANAGEMENT

PROCEDURES

- Adequate immobilization of the child (sedation if necessary) and proper instrumentation allow the uncomplicated removal of many ear FBs in the pediatric population.[7] SOR C
  - The use of general anesthesia is preferred in very young children and in children of any age with ear FBs whose contour, composition, or location predispose to traumatic removal in the ambulatory setting.[7] SOR C
- Ear FBs can be removed by irrigation, suction, or instrumentation. The type of procedure depends on the type of FB being removed.
  - Small inorganic objects can be removed from the EAC by irrigation. Contraindication to irrigation includes:
    - Perforated TM.
    - Vegetable matter—Irrigation causes swelling of the vegetable matter, which leads to further obstruction.
    - Alkaline (button) battery—Irrigation enhances leakage and potential for liquefaction necrosis and severe alkaline burns.
  - Objects with protruding surfaces or irregular edges can be removed with alligator forceps under direct visualization.
  - Objects that are round or breakable can be removed using a wire loop, a curette, or a right-angle hook that is slowly advanced beyond the object and carefully withdrawn.
  - Cyanoacrylate adhesive (e.g., "superglue") has been used to remove tightly wedged, smooth, or round FBs.
  - Live insects should be killed before removing them (by irrigation or forceps). Instilling alcohol or mineral oil into the auditory canal can kill them.

REFERRAL

Referral to otolaryngology should be considered if:

- More than one attempt has been carried out without success.[8]
- More than one instrument is needed for removal.[7]
- Patients who have firm, rounded FBs (**Figure 24-1**).[9]
- Patients who have FBs with smooth, non-graspable surfaces (**Figure 24-1**).[10]

PREVENTION

- Efforts should focus on preventing small children from access to tiny objects (e.g., beads, small toys, etc.).

PROGNOSIS

- Several retrospective studies from urban emergency departments showed that emergency physicians successfully removed most FBs (53% to 80%) with minimal complications and no need for operative removal.[7,8–10]

FOLLOW-UP

- Follow-up is very important, especially in cases where EAC inflammation or infection is likely (e.g., numerous attempts, use of numerous instruments, protracted exposure to the FB).

PATIENT EDUCATION

- Parents should be informed that successful removal depends a great deal on the length of time that the FB has remained in the EAC.

PATIENT RESOURCES

- **www.emedicinehealth.com/foreign_body_ear/article_em.htm.**
- **www.webmd.com/a-to-z-guides/foreign-body-in-the-ear.**

PROVIDER RESOURCES

- **www.entusa.com/external_ear_canal.htm.**
- **www.nlm.nih.gov/medlineplus/ency/article/000052.htm.**
- **http://emedicine.medscape.com/article/763712-overview.**

REFERENCES

1. Balbani AP, Sanchez TG, Butugan O, et al. Ear and nose foreign body removal in children. *Int J Pediatr Otorhinolaryngol.* 1998;46:37-42.
2. Mishra A, Shukla GK, Bhatia N. Aural foreign bodies. *Indian J Pediatr.* 2000;67:267-269.
3. Ansley JF, Cunningham MJ. Treatment of aural foreign bodies in children. *Pediatrics.* 1998;101:638-641.
4. Baker MD. Foreign bodies of the ears and nose in childhood. *Pediatr Emerg Care.* 1987;3:67-70.
5. Ryan C, Ghosh A, Wilson-Boyd B, et al. Presentation and management of aural foreign bodies in two Australian emergency departments. *Emerg Med Australas.* 2006;18:372-378.
6. Perera H, Fernando SM, Yasawardena AD, et al. Prevalence of attention deficit hyperactivity disorder (ADHD) in children presenting with self-inserted nasal and aural foreign bodies. *Int J Pediatr Otorhinolaryngol.* 2009;73(10):1362-1364.
7. Ansley JF, Cunningham MJ. Response to O'Donovan. Glue ear and foreign body. *Pediatrics.* 1999;103(4):857.
8. Marin JR, Trainor JL. Foreign body removal from the external auditory canal in a pediatric emergency department. *Pediatr Emerg Care.* 2006;22:630-634.
9. Thompson SK, Wein RO, Dutcher PO. External auditory canal foreign body removal: management practices and outcomes. *Laryngoscope.* 2003;113:1912-1915.
10. DiMuzio J Jr, Deschler DG. Emergency department management of foreign bodies of the external ear canal in children. *Otol Neurotol.* 2002;23:473-475.

SECTION 2 NOSE AND SINUS

25 NASAL POLYPS

Linda French, MD

PATIENT STORY

A 14-year-old boy complains of unilateral nasal obstruction for the past several months of gradual onset. On examination of the nose, a nasal polyp is found (**Figure 25-1**).

INTRODUCTION

Nasal polyps are benign lesions arising from the mucosa of the nasal passages including the paranasal sinuses. They are most commonly semitransparent and pale in appearance.

EPIDEMIOLOGY[1]

- Prevalence of 0.1 percent of children of all races and classes.
- Nasal polyps are rare in children younger than 10 years old; peak age of onset is age 20 to 40 years.
- Associated with the following conditions:
  - Nonallergic and allergic rhinitis and rhinosinusitis.
  - Asthma—In 20 percent to 50 percent of patients with polyps.
  - Cystic fibrosis.
  - Aspirin intolerance—In 8 percent to 26 percent of patients with polyps.

ETIOLOGY AND PATHOPHYSIOLOGY

- Nasal polyposis is an inflammatory process. The precise cause is unknown, but genetic associations have been identified.[2]
- Infectious agents causing desquamation of the mucous membrane can play a triggering role. Presence of *Helicobacter pylori* was identified in nasal flora in all 25 patients in one case series.[3]
- Activated epithelial cells appear to be the major source of mediators that induce an influx of inflammatory cells, including eosinophils prominently; these in turn lead to proliferation and activation of fibroblasts.[4] Cytokines and growth factors play a role in maintaining the mucosal inflammation associated with polyps.
- Food allergies including milk allergy are strongly associated with nasal polyps.

DIAGNOSIS

CLINICAL FEATURES

- The appearance is usually smooth and rounded (**Figure 25-1**).
- Moist and translucent (**Figure 25-2**).
- Variable size.
- Color ranging from nearly none to deep erythema.

TYPICAL DISTRIBUTION

- Nasal polyps arise most commonly from the ethmoid sinus and middle meatus.

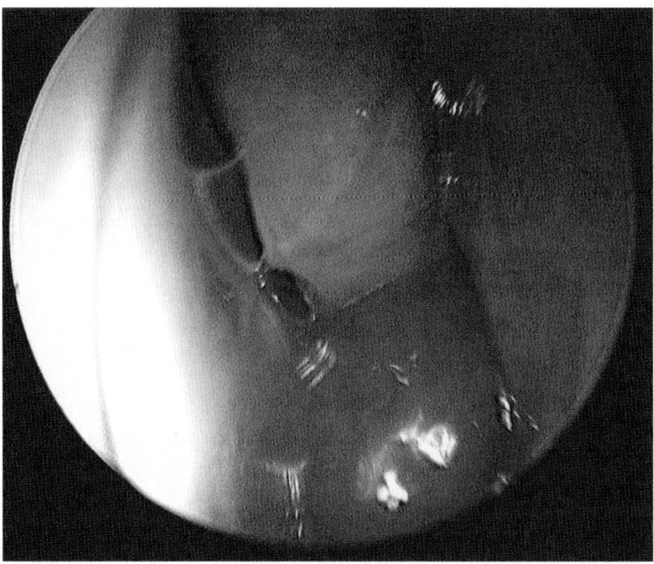

FIGURE 25-1 Nasal polyp in left middle meatus with normal surrounding mucosa. *(Used with permission from William Clark, MD.)*

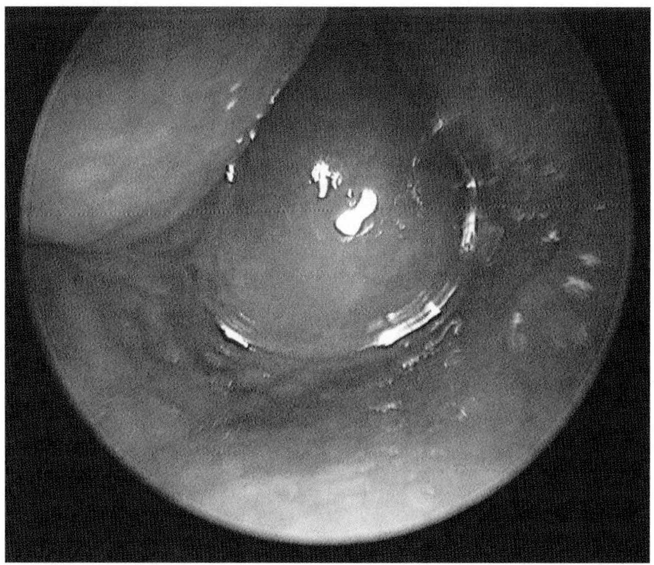

FIGURE 25-2 Nasal polyp in right nasal cavity in a patient with inflamed mucosa from allergic rhinitis. *(Used with permission from William Clark, MD.)*

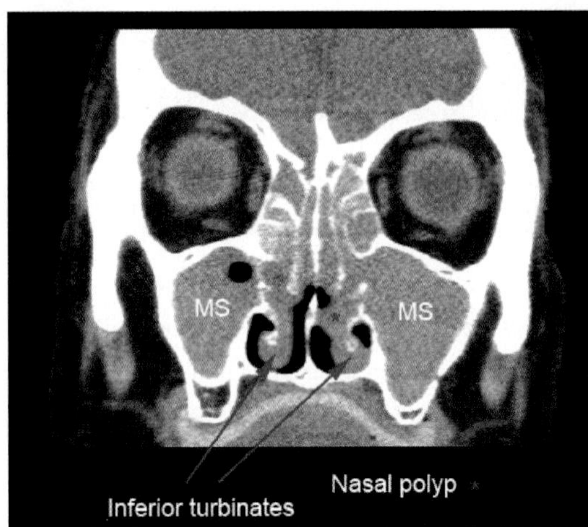

FIGURE 25-3 Computed tomography (CT) scan showing polyps (*asterisk*) and bilateral opacified maxillary sinuses (*MS*). Note the nasal polyp appears to be coming from the left maxillary sinus and is above the inferior turbinate. (*Used with permission from Richard P. Usatine, MD.*)

LABORATORY AND IMAGING

- Consider allergy testing.
- In children with multiple polyps, order sweat test to rule out cystic fibrosis.
- A competed tomography (CT) of the nose and paranasal sinuses may be indicated to evaluate extent of lesion(s) (**Figure 25-3**).

BIOPSY

- Not usually indicated. Histology typically shows pseudostratified ciliary epithelium, edematous stroma, epithelial basement membrane, and proinflammatory cells with eosinophils present in 80 percent to 90 percent of cases.

DIFFERENTIAL DIAGNOSIS

Many relatively rare conditions can cause an intranasal mass including:

- Rhabdomyosarcoma—Malignant tumor of childhood originating from striated muscle.
- Dermoid tumor—Inclusion cysts of ectodermal epithelial elements, usually manifest before 20 years of age; they can grow slowly.
- Hemangioma—Congenital, abnormal proliferation of blood vessels that can occur in any vascularized tissue (see Chapter 93, Childhood Hemangiomas and Vascular Malformations).
- Neuroblastoma—Unusual presentation of relatively common malignancy of childhood.
- Meningoencephalocele—Grayish gelatinous appearance.
- Angiofibroma—Locally-invasive neoplasm that appears as a firm grayish mass. Bleeds easily. Occurs in adolescent males, ages 14 to 18 years old. Undetermined etiology.[5]
- Pyogenic granuloma (see Chapter 142, Pyogenic Granuloma).[6]

MANAGEMENT

MEDICATIONS

- Medical treatment consists of intranasal corticosteroids.[7,8] SOR Ⓐ
- An initial short course (2 to 4 weeks) of oral steroids may be considered in severe cases.[9,10] SOR Ⓐ
- Steroid treatment reduces polyp size, but does not generally resolve them. Corticosteroid treatment is also useful preoperatively to reduce polyp size.
- Oral doxycycline can be considered for adolescents; 100 mg daily for 20 days was shown to decrease polyp size, providing benefit for 12 weeks in one randomized controlled trial.[11] SOR Ⓑ
- Topical nasal decongestants can provide some symptom relief, but do not reduce polyp size.[12] SOR Ⓑ
- Montelukast reduces symptoms when used as an adjunct to oral and inhaled steroid therapy in patients with bilateral nasal polyposis.[13] SOR Ⓑ

PROCEDURES

- Surgical excision is indicated when medical treatment fails. Postoperative topical nasal steroid and/or oral montelukast treatment helps prevent recurrence.[14]
- Consider immunotherapy for patients with allergies.

PROGNOSIS

Lesions are benign but tend to recur.

FOLLOW-UP

- Periodic reevaluation is recommended because recurrence rates are high.[15]

PATIENT EDUCATION

- Patients should be informed about the benign nature of nasal polyps and their tendency to recur.

PATIENT RESOURCES

- **www.mayoclinic.com/health/nasal-polyps/DS00498.**
- **Nasal Polyps—www.nlm.nih.gov/medlineplus/ency/article/001641.htm.**

PROVIDER RESOURCES

- **Nasal Polyps—www.emedicine.medscape.com/article/994274.**
- **Nonsurgical Treatment of Nasal Polyps—www.emedicine.medscape.com/article/861353.**

REFERENCES

1. McClay JE. *Nasal Polyps*. Available at http://emedicine.medscape.com/article/994274, accessed July 20, 2011.
2. Bae JS, Pasaje CF, Park BL, et al. Genetic associations of CIITA variations with nasal polyp pathogenesis in asthmatic patients. *Mol Med Report*. 2012 [epub ahead of print].
3. Burduk OK, Kaczmarek A, Budzynska A, et al. Detection of Helicobacter pylori and cagA gene in nasal polyps and benign laryngeal diseases. *Arch Med Res*. 2011;42:686-689.
4. Pawliczak R, Lewandowska-Polak A, Kowalski ML. Pathogenesis of nasal polyps: an update. *Curr Allergy Asthma Rep*. 2005;5:463-471.
5. Tewfik TL. *Angiofibroma*. Available at http://emedicine.medscape.com/article/872580, accessed July 20, 2011.
6. Hoving EW. Nasal encephaloceles. *Childs Nerv Syst*. 2000;16:702-706.
7. Rudmik L, Schlosser RJ, Smith TL, Soler ZM. Impact of tropical nasal steroid therapy on symptoms of nasal polyposis: a meta-analysis. *Laryngoscope*. 2012;122:1431-1437.
8. Joe SA, Thambi R, Huang J. A systematic review of the use of intranasal steroids in the treatment of chronic rhinosinusitis. *Otolaryngol Head Neck Surg*. 2008;139(3):340-347.
9. Martinez-Devesa P, Patiar S. Oral steroids for nasal polyps. *Cochrane Database Syst Rev*. 2011;6(7):CD005232.
10. Vaidyanathan S, Barnes M, Williamson P, et al. Treatment of chronic rhinosinusitis with nasal polyposis with oral steroids followed by topical steroids: a randomized trial. *Ann Intern Med*. 2011;154(5):293-252.
11. Van Zele T, Gevaert P, Holtappels G, et al. Oral steroids and doxycycline: two different approaches to treat nasal polyps. *J Allergy Clin Immunol*. 2010;125(5):1069-1076.e4.
12. Johansson L, Oberg D, Melem I, Bende M. Do topical nasal decongestants affect polyps? *Acta Otolaryngol*. 2006:126:288-290.
13. Stewart RA, Ram B, Hamilton G, et al. Montelukast as an adjunct to oral and inhaled steroid therapy in chronic nasal polyposis. *Otolaryngol Head Neck Surg*. 2008;139(5):682-687.
14. Vento SI, Blomgren K, Hytonen M, et al. Prevention of relapses of nasal polyposis with intranasal triamcinolone acetonide after polyp surgery: a prospective, double-blind, placebo-controlled, randomized study with a 9-month follow-up. *Clin Otolaryngol*. 2012:37:117-123.
15. Vento SI, Ertama LO, Hytonen ML, et al. Nasal polyposis: clinical course during 20 years. *Ann Allergy Asthma Immunol*. 2000;85:209-214.

26 SINUSITIS

Mindy Smith, MD, MS
Camille Sabella, MD

PATIENT STORY

A 6-year-old is brought in by his mother for persistent rhinorrhea. He had what appeared to be a cold about 2 weeks prior but continues to have a stuffy nose and a constant cough, which is worse at night. He has no fever but his mother says that he appears more tired than usual and has a decreased appetite. On examination, the child has a purulent nasal discharge, nasal mucosal erythema, and allergic shiners (**Figure 26-1**); he otherwise appears healthy. You diagnose acute bacterial sinusitis (ABS) and prescribe oral amoxicillin-clavulanate. You discuss the lack of benefit of antihistamines and decongestants but offer a prescription for nasal corticosteroids, which the parent declines.

INTRODUCTION

Sinusitis is symptomatic inflammation of the sinuses, nasal cavity, and their epithelial lining. Mucosal edema blocks mucous drainage creating a culture medium for viruses and bacteria. Sinusitis is classified by duration as acute (<4 weeks), subacute (4-12 weeks), or chronic (>12 weeks).

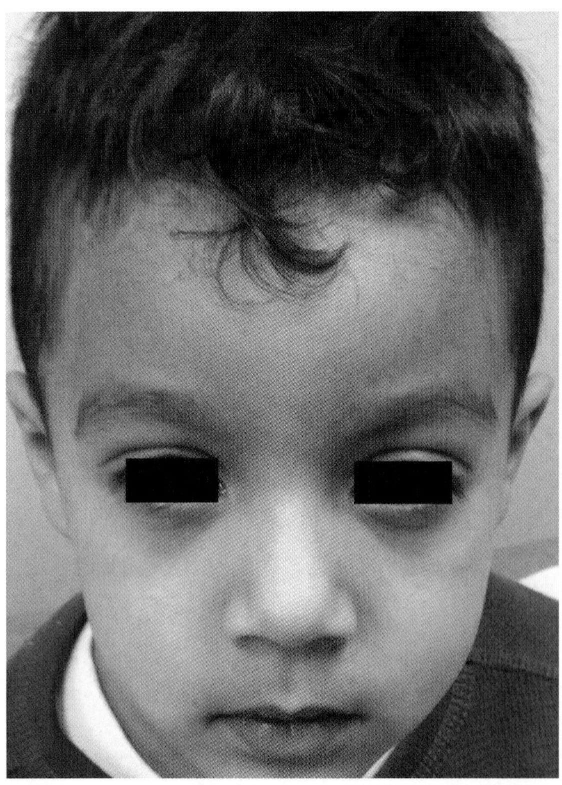

FIGURE 26-1 Allergic shiners in a child with acute bacterial sinusitis. Allergy is a risk factor for the development of acute bacterial sinusitis. (*Used with permission from Camille Sabella, MD.*)

EPIDEMIOLOGY

- Approximately 1 percent of children per year develop sinusitis, accounting for 20 million antibiotic prescriptions; 6 percent to 7 percent of children seeking care for respiratory symptoms have acute bacterial sinusitis.[1]
- Children average six to eight colds per year. Of those, 0.5 percent to 8 percent will develop a sinus infection.[2,3]
- Risk factors include viral upper respiratory tract infection (URI) (about 80% of cases are preceded by a viral URI),[2] allergy,[4] and day care attendance.[5]
- Only 1/3 to 1/2 of primary care patients with symptoms of sinusitis actually have bacterial infection.[6]

ETIOLOGY/PATHOPHYSIOLOGY

- Sinus cavities are lined with mucus-secreting respiratory epithelium. The mucus is transported by ciliary action through the sinus ostia (openings) to the nasal cavity. Under normal conditions, the paranasal sinuses are sterile cavities and there is no mucus retention.
- The maxillary and ethmoid sinuses are present at birth and the frontal sinuses develop from the ethmoid sinuses by age 5 to 6 years.
- ABS occurs when ostia become obstructed or ciliary action is impaired, causing mucus accumulation and secondary bacterial overgrowth.
- The causes of sinusitis include:
  - Infection—Most commonly viral (e.g., rhinovirus, parainfluenza, and influenza) followed by bacteria infection (e.g., *Streptococcus (S) pneumoniae*, *Haemophilus influenzae*, *Moraxella catarrhalis*). In the past 10 years, *S. pneumoniae* has become less common and *Haemophilus influenzae* more common as the etiologic agent of acute bacterial sinusitis in children.[2] In immunocompromised patients, fulminant fungal sinusitis can occur.
  - Noninfectious obstruction—Allergic, polyposis, barotrauma (e.g., airplane travel), chemical irritants, tumors, and conditions that alter mucus composition (e.g., cystic fibrosis).

DIAGNOSIS

- The diagnosis of ABS is clinical. Symptoms arising from a viral URI generally peak by day 5 or before and resolve by day 10.[1,2] ABS is diagnosed when:
  - Symptoms are present for 10 days or longer without improvement but less than 30 days.
  - Symptoms worsen after initial stability or improvement ("double worsening" or "double sickening").
  - There are unusually severe signs and symptoms (high fever [>39°C], purulent rhinorrhea) present for at least 3 consecutive days.
- Sinusitis can be presumed when there are extra-sinus manifestations of infection (periorbital inflammation, orbital cellulitis, orbital or brain abscess), although these complications of sinusitis are infrequent (**Figures 26-2** and **26-3**).[2]

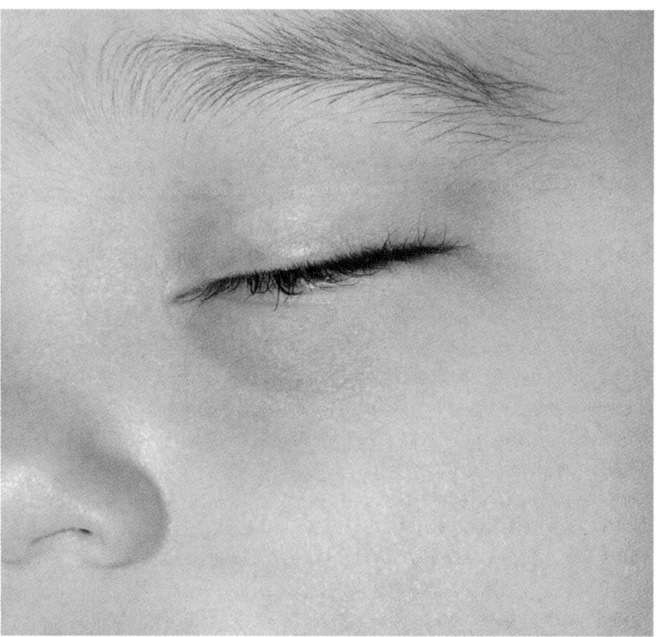

FIGURE 26-2 Periorbital erythema and swelling in a 1-year-old child with pansinusitis and left orbital abscess. (*Used with permission from Camille Sabella, MD.*)

CLINICAL FEATURES

- Most cases occur as a complication of a viral URI or allergic inflammation.[2]
- Symptoms of URI and ABS overlap to a great extent; thus, it is the persistence of symptoms without improvement that suggests the diagnosis of ABS.
- These symptoms include nasal discharge (can be watery, mucoid, purulent or discolored) and daytime cough, which may be worse at night.
- Nonspecific symptoms include halitosis, fever, fatigue, headache, and decreased appetite.
- Physical examination findings are not particularly helpful in making the diagnosis of ABS. Erythema and swelling of the nasal mucosa are nonspecific findings.

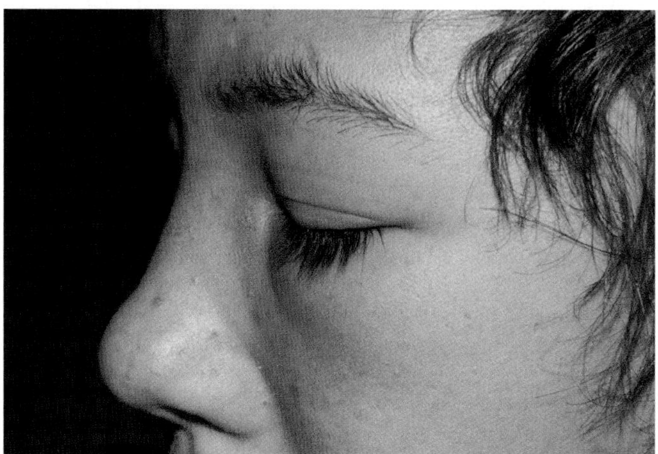

FIGURE 26-3 Periorbital swelling in a 12-year-old boy with left orbital cellulitis as a complication of acute bacterial sinusitis. (*Used with permission from Camille Sabella, MD.*)

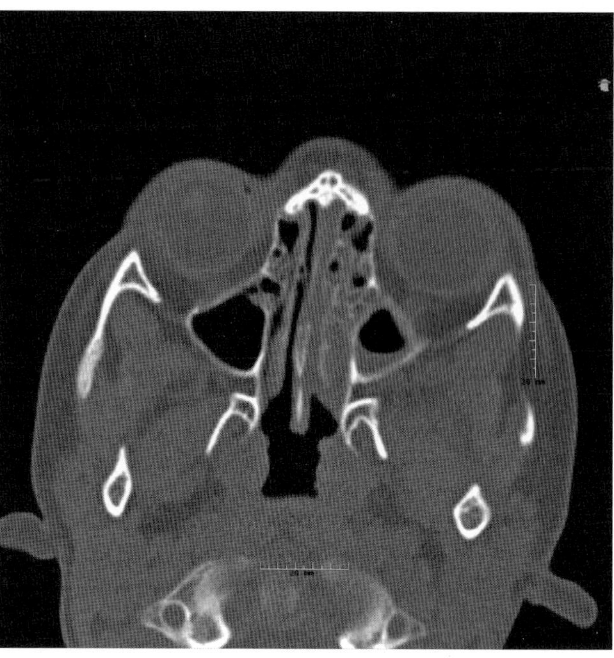

FIGURE 26-4 Opacification of the left ethmoidal and maxillary sinuses in a 5-year-old boy with acute bacterial sinusitis. Note the air-fluid level in the left maxillary sinus. (*Used with permission from Camille Sabella, MD.*)

- Complications of sinusitis are suspected in children with severe headache, seizures, focal neurologic deficits, periorbital edema, or erythema (**Figures 26-2** and **26-3**), proptosis, or abnormal intra-ocular muscle function.[2]

TYPICAL DISTRIBUTION

- Most sinus infections involve the maxillary sinus followed in frequency by the ethmoid (anterior), frontal, and sphenoid sinuses; however, most cases involve more than one sinus (**Figures 26-4** to **26-6**).[4]

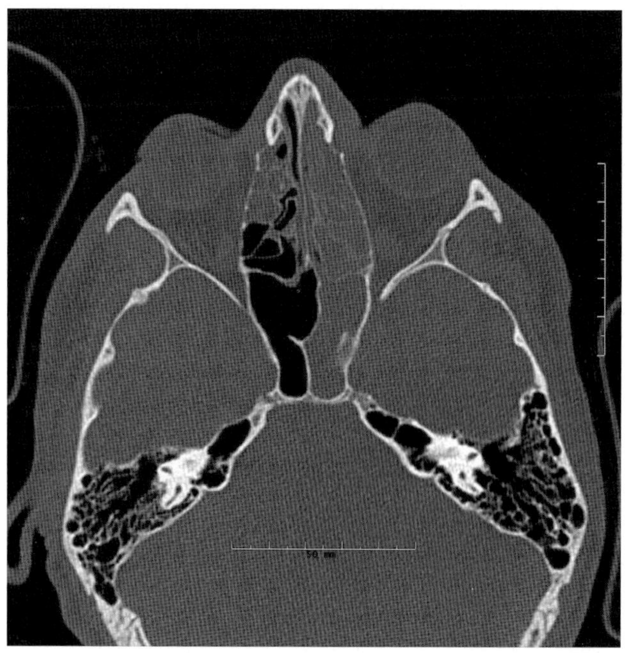

FIGURE 26-5 Opacification of the ethmoidal and sphenoid sinuses in a 16-year-old boy with acute bacterial sinusitis. (*Used with permission from Camille Sabella, MD.*)

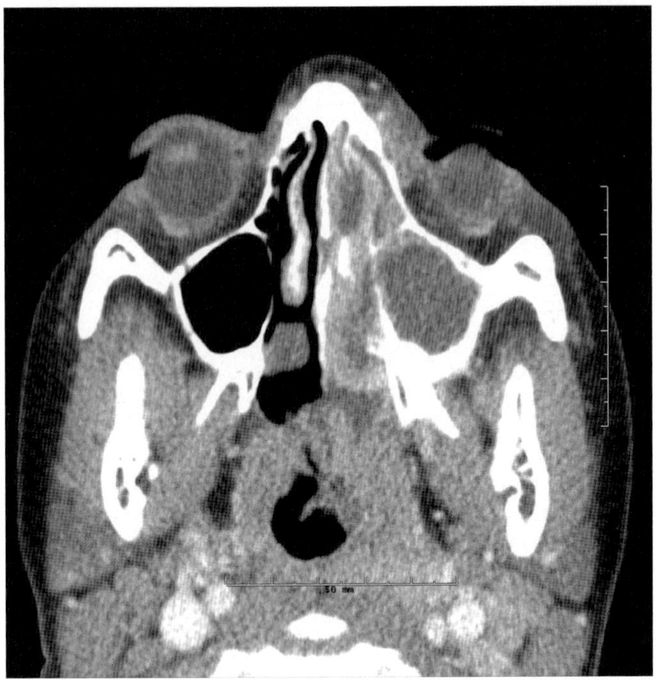

FIGURE 26-6 Opacification of the left ethmoidal and maxillary sinuses in a young girl who developed orbital cellulitis as a complication of acute bacterial sinusitis. (*Used with permission from Camille Sabella, MD.*)

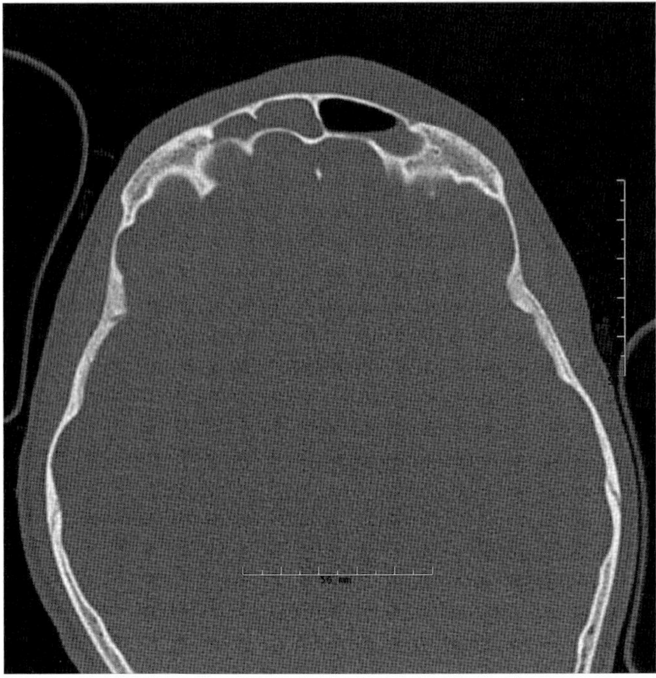

FIGURE 26-7 Air fluid level in left frontal sinus and proptosis of the frontal bone in an adolescent who developed Pott's puffy tumor and a subdural empyema from acute bacterial sinusitis. (*Used with permission from Camille Sabella, MD.*)

- Children are more likely to have inflammation in the posterior ethmoid and sphenoid sinuses.[7]

LABORATORY AND IMAGING

- Culture of nasal or nasopharyngeal secretions is not recommended as these do not differentiate between URI and ABS.[1]
- If culture is needed due to suspected bacterial resistance or persistent infection, a meta-analysis in adult patients found endoscopically-directed middle meatal cultures to be reasonably sensitive (80.9%), specific (90.5%), and accurate (87.0%; 95% confidence interval, 81.3% to 92.8%) compared with maxillary sinus taps.[8]
- There are no trials comparing meatal cultures to maxillary sinus aspirates in children with ABS. Given that the middle meatus in children is commonly colonized with the pathogens that cause sinusitis, it is difficult to ascertain the accuracy of meatal cultures in children without comparative trials.
- The Infectious Disease Society of America (IDSA) recommends direct sinus aspiration for specimens for culture rather than nasopharyngeal swabs.[9]
- Radiography should not be obtained routinely for patients meeting diagnostic criteria for ABS, unless a complication (**Figures 26-2, 26-3, 26-6, 26-7**) or alternate diagnosis is suspected. In these cases, CT or MRI is warranted.[1]
    - In children with persistent ABS despite treatment, recurrent, or chronic sinusitis, the American College of Radiology recommends CT of the paranasal sinuses without contrast.[10]
    - In children with orbital or intracranial complications of ABS, the American Academy of Pediatrics recommend a contrast enhanced CT or MRI with contrast of the head and/or orbits and paranasal sinuses.
- Nasal endoscopy can be considered in patients with chronic rhinosinusitis. In one case series of adult patients with suspected chronic rhinosinusitis, the addition of endoscopy to symptom criteria had similar sensitivity (88.7% versus 84.1%) but significantly improved specificity (66% vs. 12.3%) using CT as the gold standard.[11]

REFER OR HOSPITALIZE

- Patients who are seriously ill, immunocompromised, continue to deteriorate clinically despite extended courses of antimicrobial therapy, or have recurrent bouts of ABS should be referred to a specialist.[10]
- Hospitalize patients with potentially life threatening complications including subperiosteal orbital abscess (**Figure 26-2** and **26-3**), meningitis, epidural or cerebral abscess, and cavernous sinus thrombosis. An estimated 2 percent to 30 percent of patients hospitalized with ABS have complications; most complications occur in males.[12]
    - The risks of frontal sinusitis include eroding through the frontal bone forward causing a Pott's puffy tumor (**Figure 26-7**), or inward and spreading into the brain and cavernous sinuses. In a small case series (N = 25, mostly adolescents), epidural abscess (N = 13) was the most common intracranial complication of ABS followed by subdural empyema (N = 9), meningitis (N = 6), encephalitis (N = 2), brain abscess (N = 2), and dural sinus thrombophlebitis (N = 2).[13]
    - Infection in the ethmoid sinuses is responsible for the majority of orbital complications.[13] Periorbital cellulitis is the most common complication of ABS in children, accounting for 80 percent to 90 percent of all extracranial complications.[13] Orbital complications should be suspected in children with ophthalmoplegia and/or proptosis.[13] Orbital abscess is highly dangerous and can also be the result of spread from the frontal sinuses.

- In immunocompromised patients, fulminant fungal sinusitis may cause orbital swelling, cellulitis, proptosis, ptosis, impairment of extra-ocular motion, nasopharyngeal ulceration, and epistaxis. Bony erosion can occur. Nasal mucosa might appear black, blanched white, or erythematous.

DIFFERENTIAL DIAGNOSIS

- Upper respiratory tract infections—These are common infections, primarily viral (most commonly rhinovirus), that cause six to eight infections per year in children. Infections are self-limited (lasting approximately 7 to 10 days) and typical symptoms include rhinorrhea, nasal congestion, sore throat, and cough. URI often precedes acute sinusitis.
- Post-nasal drip—Lack of fever, clear discharge, cough occurring only at night.
- Reactive airway disease—History of asthma or atopy, wheezing, cough occurs at night.
- Allergic rhinitis—Sneezing, itching, watery rhinorrhea.
- Tumor—Rare; unilateral epistaxis or discharge and obstruction, recurrent sinusitis, sinus pain.

MANAGEMENT

Duration of illness assists in decision making, as most patients improve without specific treatment; a period of watchful waiting for up to 10 days is consistent with guidelines.[10] Treatment of symptoms, including pain, is important.

NON-PHARMACOLOGIC

- There is no evidence supporting the use of nasal saline irrigation for ABS in children.[14] In adults with chronic sinusitis, nasal saline irrigation provides symptom relief, both alone and as an adjunct to nasal steroids, and is well tolerated.[15] SOR B

MEDICATIONS

- Analgesics (acetaminophen or non-steroidal anti-inflammatory drugs) should be used for pain.
- No benefit in symptom relief and significant toxicity from ABS has been demonstrated with the use of antihistamines and decongestants in children.[2,10] SOR A
- Antihistamines should not be used for ABS, although they may be helpful in reducing allergic symptoms in children with atopy who develop ABS. SOR C
- Intranasal corticosteroids appear to be of benefit in improvement and resolution of symptoms of ABS in adolescents and adults.[16] SOR B The benefit of intranasal corticosteroids in young children with ABS has not been proven.[1]
- There have been no clinical trials of mucolytics reported in non-atopic children or adults with ABS. However, they may be useful in preventing crust formation and liquefying secretions. SOR C
- Patients who fail to improve with symptomatic treatment, have severe symptoms or worsening of symptoms should be offered oral antibiotics. SOR B Of five randomized controlled trials in children with acute sinusitis, three showed benefit; however, in the remaining two trials the antimicrobial treatment dose was suboptimal and in one, the presence of asthma and allergic conditions may have compromised accurate diagnosis or determination of treatment response.[2]
    - In the most recent trial, provision of antibiotics (90 mg of amoxicillin and 6.4 mg of clavulanate per kilogram of body weight per day, administered in two doses) was associated with reduced treatment failure (14% versus 68% on placebo) with a number needed to treat of three.[17] The clinical success rate for the drug and clinical failure rate for placebo in this trial, however, are high. In the older Wald et al. trial, cure rate was 67 percent for amoxicillin, 64 percent for amoxicillin-clavulanate potassium, and 43 percent for placebo.[18]
- Choice of antibiotics and dosing should be made considering local resistance patterns to *S. pneumoniae* (commonly 10% to 15%) and other risk factors for bacterial resistance.
    - Amoxicillin–clavulanate (45–90 mg per kilogram per day of amoxicillin administered in two doses) rather than amoxicillin alone is recommended as empiric antimicrobial therapy for ABS in children by the IDSA.[10]
    - The American Academy of Pediatric recommends amoxicillin as the first line treatment of uncomplicated ABS when antimicrobial resistance is not suspected.[1]
    - Amoxicillin and amoxicillin-clavulanate have been best studied but there are no studies demonstrating comparative effectiveness of one antibiotic over another.[2] Macrolides and trimethoprim-sulfamethoxazole should not be used.[10]
    - High dose amoxicillin-clavulanate or amoxicillin (2 g orally twice daily or 90 mg/kg/day twice daily of amoxicillin component) is recommended as first-line therapy for children in areas where bacterial resistance rates are 10 percent or higher and for those in day care, those <2 years of age, those with comorbidities or immune compromise, and those who have been hospitalized in the past 5 days or treated with antibiotics in the past month.[10] SOR C
    - A single-dose of intramuscular or intravenous ceftriaxone can be used for children who are unable to tolerate oral medication or unlikely to be adherent to oral therapy.[1]
    - Second-line therapy for children recommended by IDSA and AAP includes **a** third-generation oral cephalosporin (cefixime or cefpodoxime) with or without clindamycin in cases with non–type I penicillin allergy or in regions with high endemic rates of bacterial resistance.[1,10] SOR C
    - Levofloxacin may be considered for children with a history of type I hypersensitivity to penicillin, although allergy referral for penicillin and cephalosporin skin testing is encouraged in this situation.[1,10] SOR C
    - Recommended treatment duration is 10 to 14 days or 7 days after a child is symptom-free (per AAP).[1,10] SOR C
- In a Cochrane review of fifty-nine trials evaluating antibiotic treatment for acute maxillary sinusitis, antibiotics decreased clinical failure by about 10 percent.[19] Comparisons between classes of antibiotics showed no significant differences; therefore narrow-spectrum antibiotics were recommended.[20]
- The modest benefit of antibiotics for improving rates of clinical cure or symptom improvement should be weighed against the risks of harm (primarily gastrointestinal but also skin rash, headache, dizziness, and fatigue). In the most recent Wald et al. trial, adverse effects (primarily diarrhea) occurred in 44 percent (versus 14%

with placebo) and three children (11%) discontinued treatment due to medication side effects.[18]

- Intravenous antibiotics are used for complications of sinusitis with therapy dictated by culture and local resistance patterns. Combination therapy with vancomycin, ceftriaxone, and metronidazole provides coverage for most intracranial pathogens complicating ABS.[13]

PROCEDURES

- In ABS, surgery is primarily used to obtain cultures or drain fluid collections.[13]
- Immunocompromised patients with fungal sinusitis are treated with aggressive debridement and adjunctive antifungal agents.[20]
- Authors of a Cochrane review of adenoidectomy to treat chronic nasal symptoms in children found only two studies (one of recurrent otitis media); both did not show benefit.[21]
    - The presence of biofilm in adenoid samples from children with chronic rhinosinusitis compared with children who had adenoidectomy for sleep apnea (95% versus 2%) provides some rationale for removing adenoids in children prior to proceeding to endoscopic sinus surgery.[22]
- For patients with chronic sinusitis, authors of a Cochrane review found endoscopic sinus surgery was not superior to medical treatment; in one study there was a lower relapse rate (2.4% versus 5.6% without surgery).[23] SOR Ⓑ In an older meta-analysis of eight published papers (not randomized trials) and unpublished data, functional endoscopic surgery in children was highly successful (88.7% positive outcomes) with a 0.6 percent complication rate.[24] SOR Ⓒ
- Smoking and exposure to smoke increase the risk of sinusitis. Thus, avoidance will help to lower the risk of sinusitis, especially in children with a history of allergies, who are already at higher risk for developing ABS.

PROGNOSIS

- Based on a Cochrane review, cure or improvement rate for acute sinusitis within two weeks was high in both the placebo group (80%) and the antibiotic group (90%).[19] In the trials conducted with children, cure rates were 64 percent to 86 percent on antibiotics and cure rates on placebo were an absolute rate of 20 percent lower.[2]
- An unknown number of children develop chronic rhinosinusitis.[25]

FOLLOW-UP

- For children who fail first-line antibiotic treatment after 3 to 5 days, a nonbacterial cause or resistant organism should be considered and antibiotic coverage should be broadened or a different antibiotic class should be chosen (e.g., amoxicillin-clavulanate, respiratory fluoroquinolone).[1,10] SOR Ⓒ
- If the child still fails to improve, refer to a specialist and consider imaging (CT or MRI to investigate non-infectious causes or complications) and direct sinus aspirate or meatal cultures.[10]
- The role of bacteria and inflammatory mediators in chronic rhinosinusitis is unclear; none-the-less, antibiotics (e.g., amoxicillin-clavulanate) for 3 to 4 weeks and intranasal steroids are often used.[26] Assessing children for allergy and systemic predisposing factors (e.g., cystic fibrosis, primary ciliary dyskinesia) can help direct treatment.

PATIENT EDUCATION

- Persistent nasal congestion and rhinitis (more than 10 days after a cold) or worsening or severe symptoms (fever, facial pain) following a cold may indicate a sinus infection and patients should see their primary provider. Symptoms due to a cold usually abate within one week.
- Methods to improve sinus drainage (oral and nasal decongestants and nasal saline irrigation) have not been shown to work in children but intranasal steroids may prove useful.

PATIENT RESOURCES

- **http://www.niaid.nih.gov/topics/sinusitis/Pages/Index.aspx**.
- **http://kidshealth.org/parent/infections/bacterial_viral/sinusitis.html#**.

PROVIDER RESOURCES

- Clinical Practice Guideline for the Diagnosis and Management of Acute Bacterial Sinusitis in Children Aged 1 to 18 Years—**www.pediatrics.aappublications.org/content/early/2013/06/19/peds.2013-1071**.
- Chow AW, Benninger MS, Brook I, et al. IDSA clinical practice guideline for acute bacterial rhinosinusitis in children and adults. *Clin Infect Dis*. 2012;54(8):e72-e112. http://cid.oxfordjournals.org/content/54/8/1041.long.

REFERENCES

1. DeMuri GP, Wald ER. Acute bacterial sinusitis in children. *N Engl J Med*. 2012;367:1128-34.
2. Ramadan HH. Pediatric sinusitis: update. *J Otolaryngol*. 2005;34(1):S14-7.
3. Revai K, Dobbs LA, Nair S, et al. Incidence of acute otitis media and sinusitis complicating upper respiratory tract infection: the effect of age. *Pediatrics*. 2007;119(6):e1408-1412.
4. Chen CF, Wu KG, Hsu MC, Tang RB. Prevalence and relationship between allergic diseases and infectious diseases. *J Microbiol Immunol Infect*. 2001;34:57-62.
5. Wald ER, Guerra N, Byers C. Upper respiratory tract infections in young children: duration of and frequency of complications. *Pediatrics*. 1991;87:129-133.
6. Holleman DR Jr, Williams JW Jr, Simel DL. Usual care and outcomes in patients with sinus complaints and normal results of sinus roentgenography. *Arch Fam Med*. 1995;4:246-251.
7. Gordts F, Clement PA, Destryker A, et al. Prevalence of sinusitis signs on MRI in a non-ENT pediatric population. *Rhinology*. 1997;35:154-157.
8. Benninger MS, Payne SC, Ferguson BJ, et al. Endoscopically directed middle meatal cultures versus maxillary sinus taps in

acute bacterial maxillary rhinosinusitis: a meta-analysis. *Otolaryngol Head Neck Surg*. 2006;134(1):3-9.

9. Chow AW, Benninger MS, Brook I, et al. IDSA clinical practice guideline for acute bacterial rhinosinusitis in children and adults. *Clin Infect Dis*. 2012;54(8):e72-e112.
10. Karmazyn BK, Gunderman R, Coley BD, et al. *ACR Appropriateness Criteria® sinusitis – child*. Available at http://www.guideline.gov/content.aspx?id=15752&search=rhinosinusitis, accessed October 2012.
11. Bhattacharyya N, Lee LN. Evaluating the diagnosis of chronic rhinosinusitis based on clinical guidelines and endoscopy. *Otolaryngol Head Neck Surg*. 2010;143(1):147-151.
12. DeMuri GP, Wald ER. Complications of acute bacterial sinusitis in children. *Pediatr Infect Dis J*. 2011;30:701-702.
13. Germiller JA, Monin DL, Sparano AM, et al. Intracranial complications of sinusitis in children and adolescents. *Arch Otolaryngol Head Neck Surg*. 2006;132:969–976.
14. Shaikh N, Wald ER, Pi M. Decongestants, antihistamines and nasal irrigation for acute sinusitis in children. *Cochrane Database Syst Rev*. 2012;(9):CD007909.
15. Harvey R, Hannan SA, Badia L, Scadding G. Nasal saline irrigations for the symptoms of chronic rhinosinusitis. *Cochrane Database Syst Rev*. 2007;(3):CD006394.
16. Zalmanovici Trestioreanu A, Yaphe J. Intranasal steroids for acute sinusitis. *Cochrane Database Syst Rev*. 2009, Issue 4. Art. No.: CD005149.
17. Wald ER, Nash D, Eickhoff J. Effectiveness of amoxicillin-clavulanate potassium in the treatment of acute bacterial sinusitis in children. Pediatrics. 2009;124:9-15.
18. Wald ER, Chiponis D, Ledesma-Medina J. Comparative effectiveness of amoxicillin and amoxicillin-clavulanate potassium in acute paranasal sinus infections in children: a double-blind, placebo-controlled trial. *Pediatrics*. 1986;77:795-800.
19. Ahovuo-Saloranta A, Rautakorpi U-M, Borisenko OV, et al. Antibiotics for acute maxillary sinusitis. Cochrane Database Syst Rev. 2008;(2):CD000243.
20. Thorp BD, McKinney KA, Rose AS, Ebert CS Jr: Allergic fungal sinusitis in children. *Otolaryngol Clin North Am*. 2012;45(3):631-642.
21. van den Aardweg MTA, Schilder AGM, Herkert E, et al. Adenoidectomy for recurrent or chronic nasal symptoms in children. *Cochrane Database Syst Rev*. 2010;(1):CD008282.
22. Zuliani G, Carron M, Gurrola J, et al. Identification of adenoid biofilms in chronic rhinosinusitis. *Int J Pediatr Otorhinolaryngol*. 2006;70(9):1613–1617.
23. Khalil HS, Nunez DA. Functional endoscopic sinus surgery for chronic rhinosinusitis. Cochrane Database Syst Rev. 2006;3: CD004458.
24. Bebert RL 2nd, Brent JP 3rd. Meta-analysis of outcomes of pediatric functional endoscopic sinus surgery. *Laryngoscope*. 1998;108(6):796-9.
25. Ramadan HH. Chronic rhinosinusitis in children. *Int J Pediatr*. 2012;2012:573942. Epub 2011 Oct 5.

27 COMPLICATIONS OF SINUSITIS

Janalee Holmes, MD
Prashant Malhotra, MD, FAAP

PATIENT STORY

A 10-year-old girl has a 2-week history of daily headaches and rhinorrhea. She is admitted from the emergency department to the pediatric intensive care unit for a 2-day history of worsening left frontal headache, mental status changes including lethargy and slurred speech, nausea, and mild periorbital edema. Computed tomography (CT) demonstrates opacification of bilateral frontal, maxillary, and anterior ethmoid sinuses as well as pneumocephalus (**Figure 27-1A**). Magnetic resonance imaging demonstrated extensive left sided subdural empyema (worse frontal and temporal) and diffuse bilateral dural enhancement (**Figure 27-1B**). She is urgently treated via a combined surgical approach with pediatric otolaryngology for bilateral endoscopic sinus surgery and pediatric neurosurgery for left craniotomy. She subsequently had 10 weeks of intravenous antimicrobial therapy. Her immediate postoperative course was complicated by seizures; she has now made a full recovery and is doing well.

INTRODUCTION

Complications of acute sinusitis are typically extensions of infection beyond the paranasal sinuses into adjacent structures and can have devastating consequences, including blindness, neurologic morbidity, and even death.

SYNONYMS

Periorbital cellulitis, subperiosteal abscess, orbital cellulitis, orbital abscess, cavernous sinus thrombosis, meningitis, subdural abscess, subdural empyema, pyocele, mucopyocele, intracranial abscess, or invasive fungal sinusitis.

EPIDEMIOLOGY

- Orbital complications account for 90 percent of acute complications from sinusitis and approximately 3 percent of all acute rhinosinusitis.[1]
- Children younger than age 7 years of age develop isolated orbital complications associated with acute ethmoiditis.[2]
- Children older than 7 years, mostly teenage males, are more likely to develop intracranial complications.[2,3] This is likely related to the age related development of the frontal and sphenoid sinuses.

ETIOLOGY AND PATHOPHYSIOLOGY

- Children have a high rate of upper respiratory infections (URI) and viral rhinosinusitis.
- Congenital or traumatic dehiscences in the lamina papyracea and skull base provide potential routes for direct spread.

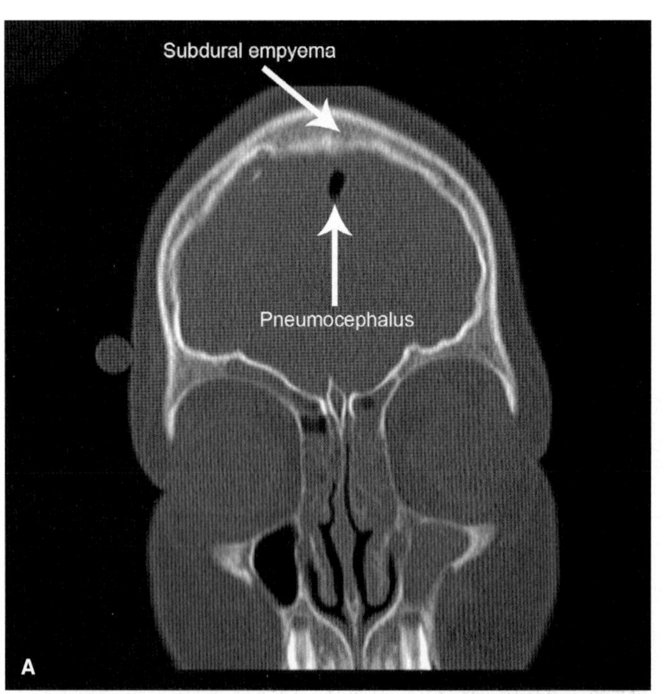

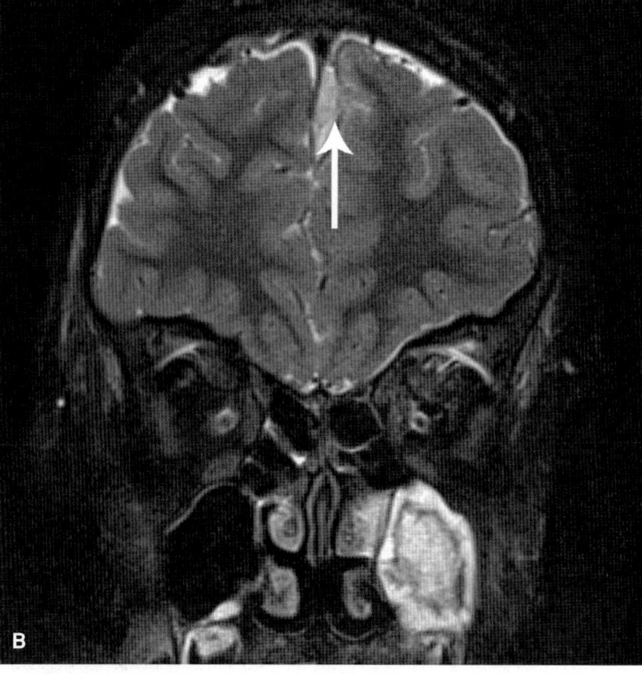

FIGURE 27-1 **A.** Coronal CT scan demonstrating bilateral ethmoid and left maxillary sinus opacification along pneumocephalus, in a 10-year-old with intracranial extension from frontal sinusitis leading to subdural empyema. **B.** Same patient, coronal T2 MRI demonstrating a hyperintense extra-axial collection (arrow) along the falx to the left of midline and uniform dural enhancement overlying both cerebral hemispheres. *(Used with permission from Prashant Malhotra, MD.)*

TABLE 27-1 Chandler Classification of Orbital Complications[4]

I	Preseptal cellulitis
II	Subperiosteal abscess
III	Orbital cellulitis
IV	Orbital abscess
V	Cavernous sinus thrombosis

- The diploic veins of the skull and ethmoid bone as well as the ophthalmic veins are valveless and allow for communication between the nose, sinuses, face, orbit, cavernous sinus, and intracranial system.
- The combination of phlebitis and direct entry of bacteria into perivascular structures results in a continuum of inflammatory and infectious changes.
- The valveless intracranial venous system allows for further spread of thrombophlebitis and septic emboli.
- Complications can be orbital (**Table 27-1**),[4] intracranial, or involving adjacent bone.
- Intracranial complications can include meningitis, epidural or subdural abscess or empyema, and intracerebral abscess or venous sinus thrombophlebitis.
- Culprit bacteria in children include the usual acute rhinosinusitis bacteria (*Streptococcus pneumoniae, Haemophilus influenzae,* and *Moraxella catarrhalis*); however, suppurative complications are also associated with other Streptococcus species, *Staphylococcus aureus*, anaerobes (such as *Bacteroides* and *Fusobacterium* species), and polymicrobial infections.[9]
- Local bony complications include mucocele, pyocele, or mucopyocele, as well as osteomyelitis.

RISK FACTORS

- Children with immune deficiencies, cystic fibrosis, and ciliary dyskinesias are more likely to develop acute bacterial rhinosinusitis.[5,6]
- Orbital complications are associated with ethmoiditis in 86 percent of cases.[1]
- Intracranial complications are more likely in children with frontal sinusitis, adolescent age, and male gender.[3,7]

DIAGNOSIS

CLINICAL FEATURES

- Every patient with a possible complication of sinusitis should have an examination with anterior rhinoscopy or nasal endoscopy to evaluate for polyps or purulent drainage in the middle meatus.
- Endoscopy can also assist in identifying local complications and anatomic abnormalities such as mucopyocele.
- The eye must be assessed for visual acuity, extraocular movements, and proptosis. Upper and lower lid edema and erythema are common, and conjunctiva should be assessed for chemosis. Fluctuance of lids consistent with abscess is rare (**Figure 27-2A,B**).

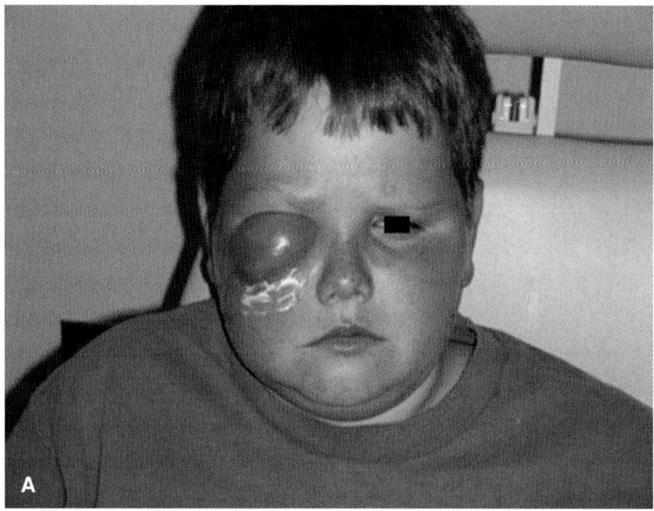

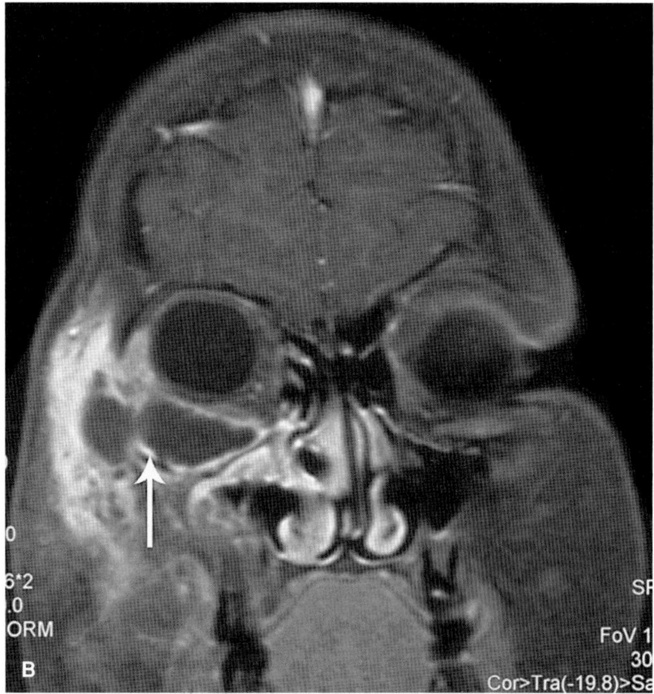

FIGURE 27-2 **A.** Eleven-year-old male with right ethmoid sinusitis, subperiosteal abscess who developed lower eyelid abscess. **B.** Same patient, coronal CT scan demonstrating lower eyelid abscess (arrow). (*Used with permission from Paul Krakovitz, MD.*)

- The orbital septum is a fascial continuation of the periosteum extending into the upper and lower eyelids, and is a physiologic barrier to the orbit. When post-septal involvement is suspected an ophthalmologic consultation should be obtained immediately to help with surgical planning.
- Generalized symptoms indicative of increased intracranial pressure include frontal or retro-orbital headache, nausea and vomiting, altered mental status, nuchal rigidity, abducent nerve palsy, and papilledema.
- Late intracranial findings include seizures, hemiparesis, and focal neurologic findings.[8]

TABLE 27-2 Complications of Sinusitis and Their Corresponding Clinical Findings

Complication	Clinical Findings
Preseptal cellulitis	Eyelid edema, erythema, and tenderness (**Figure 27-3**). No deficits in extraocular movement or visual acuity.
Subperiosteal abscess	Eyelid edema, erythema, and tenderness, and possibly proptosis and impaired extraocular muscle movement. Can have downward and laterally displaced globe (**Figures 27-4** and **Figure 27-5**).
Orbital cellulitis	Eyelid edema and erythema, proptosis, chemosis, limited or no impairment of extraocular movements or vision. Normal visual acuity.
Orbital abscess	Significant exophthalmos, chemosis, ophthalmoplegia, and visual impairment (**Figures 27-6**).
Cavernous sinus thrombosis	Bilateral orbital pain, chemosis, proptosis, ophthalmoplegia, cranial neuropathies (IV, V1, V2, and VI), picket-fence fevers, meningismus, lethargy.
Meningitis	Headache, neck stiffness, and high fever, vomiting.
Epidural abscess	Headache, fever, and local pain and tenderness. Unenhanced CT reveals a hypodense or isodense crescent-shaped area adjacent to the inner table of the skull.
Subdural abscess	Headache, fever, meningismus, focal neurologic deficits, and lethargy with rapid deterioration. MRI demonstrates a low signal on T1 images and high signal on T2 images with peripheral contrast enhancement (**Figures 27-1**).
Intracerebral abscess	Fever, headache, vomiting, lethargy, seizures and focal neurologic deficits. Frontal deficits can include changes in mood and behavior. Lumbar puncture can be life threatening. MRI demonstrates a cystic lesion with a distinct hypointense strongly enhancing capsule on T2 images.
Venous sinus thrombosis	Extremely ill with meningeal signs or other serious neurologic symptoms. Picket fence fevers. MRI may reveal focal defects of enhancement. MR angiogram and venogram can further delineate.
Pott's puffy tumor or frontal bone osteomyelitis	"Puffy" fluctuant forehead swelling, frontal pain, fever (**Figures 27-7**).
Mucocele, pyocele, mucopyocele	Proptosis and impaired extraocular muscle movement (**Figure 27-8**).

- Specific complications of sinusitis and their common clinical findings are summarized in **Table 27-2**.

LABORATORY TESTING

- A white blood cell count is helpful in evaluating for leukocytosis.
- Lumbar puncture should be considered when there is concern for intracranial infection.

IMAGING

- Contrast-enhanced CT is indicated whenever there is suspicion of post-septal involvement or an intracranial complication.
- CT should also be considered when preseptal inflammation progresses in 24 to 48 hours despite treatment, symptoms are severe (ill appearing, high fevers), or in patients who are immunocompromised.
- Contrast-enhanced magnetic resonance imaging (MRI) is performed when intracranial complications is suspected and should include axial and coronal T1 and T2 images.

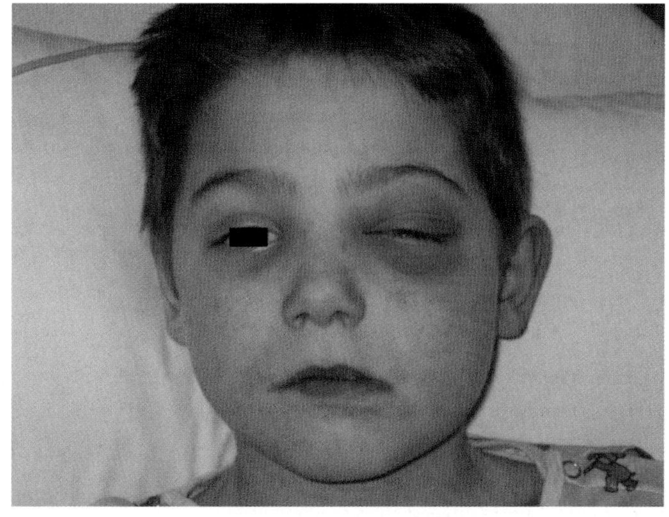

FIGURE 27-3 Preseptal cellulitis in the setting of acute ethmoid sinusitis. This resolved with antibiotic therapy alone. (*Used with permission from Paul Krakovitz, MD.*)

DIFFERENTIAL DIAGNOSIS

- Trauma—History and lack of sinusitis on examination and imaging will help to differentiate from sinusitis complication.
- Foreign body—Same as for trauma.
- Eyelid infection—Physical examination findings and lack of sinusitis on examination and imaging will help to differentiate.
- Invasive fungal sinusitis—see the following.
- Orbital hematoma—Diagnosis based on characteristic appearance on examination and imaging.
- Otitis media—Often present concurrently with sinusitis (see Chapter 22, Otitis Media—Acute and OME).
- Nasal polyposis—Usually evident on examination and nasal endoscopy.

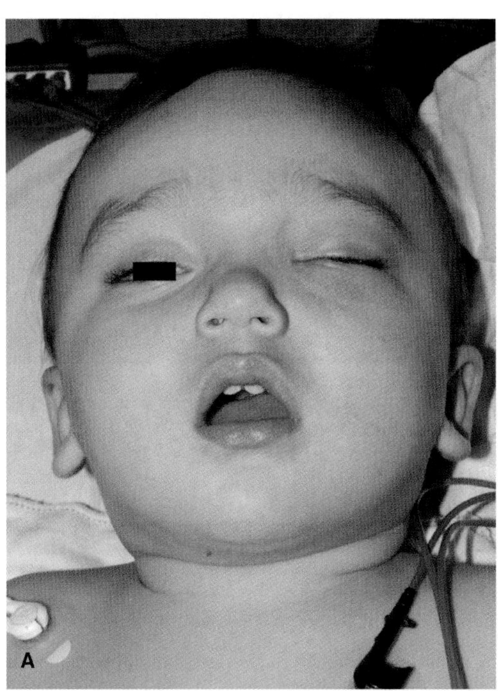

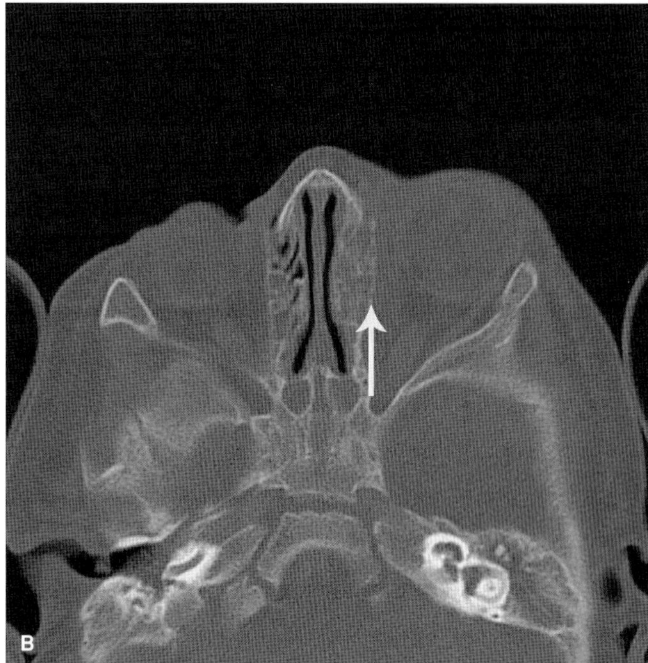

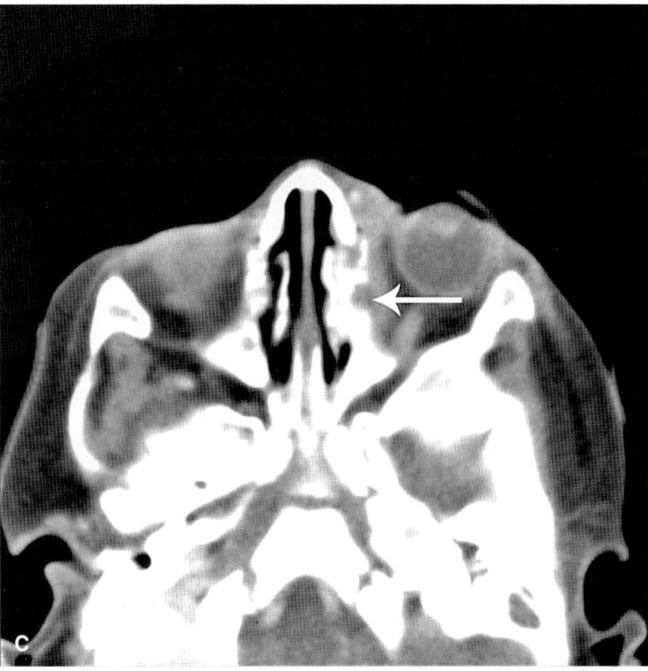

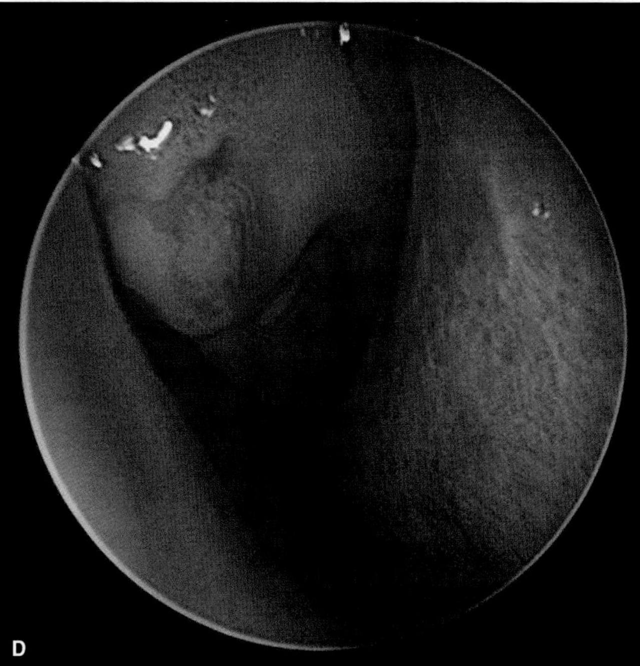

FIGURE 27-4 **A.** Ten-month-old with pansinusitis and left subperiosteal abscess. Has periorbital edema, erythema with intact extraocular mobility. **B.** Same patient, axial CT scan (bone windows) demonstrating dehiscence in lamina papyracea (arrow). **C.** Same patient, axial CT scan (soft tissue windows) demonstrating subperiosteal abscess (arrow). **D.** Same patient, intraoperative nasal endoscopy demonstrating middle turbinate edema. *(continued)*

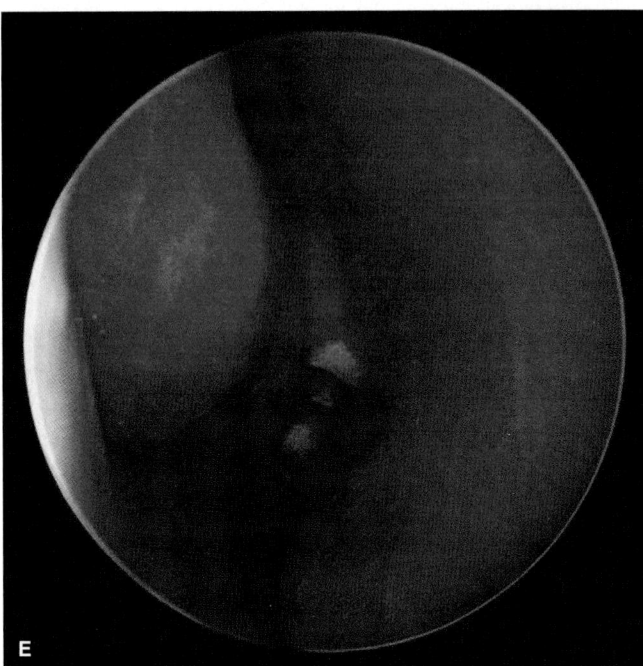

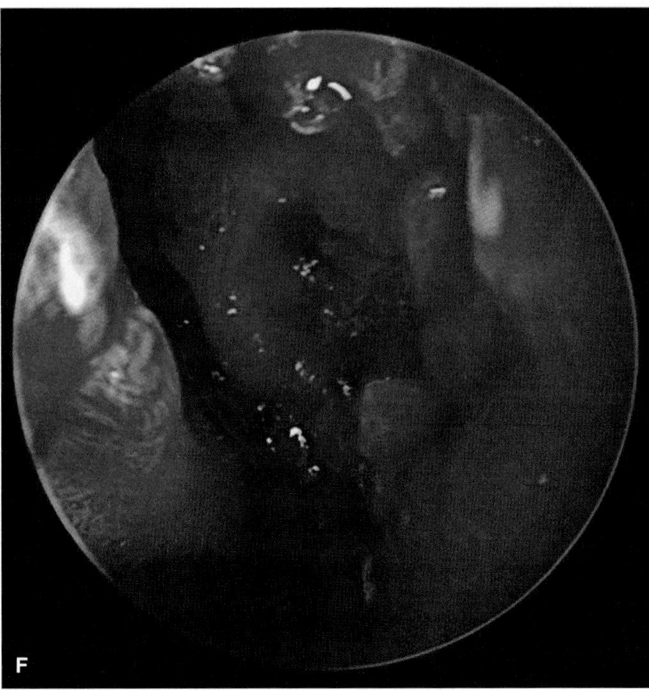

FIGURE 27-4 (*Continued*) **E.** Same patient, intraoperative nasal endoscopy demonstrating purulent drainage in middle meatus after removal of uncinate process. **F.** Same patient, intraoperative nasal endoscopy demonstrating abscess cavity, dehiscent bone, and exposed periorbita. (*Used with permission from Prashant Malhotra, MD.*)

- Sinonasal mass—Usually evident on examination, imaging, and nasal endoscopy.
- Orbital mass—Imaging and intraoperative findings will help to differentiate.

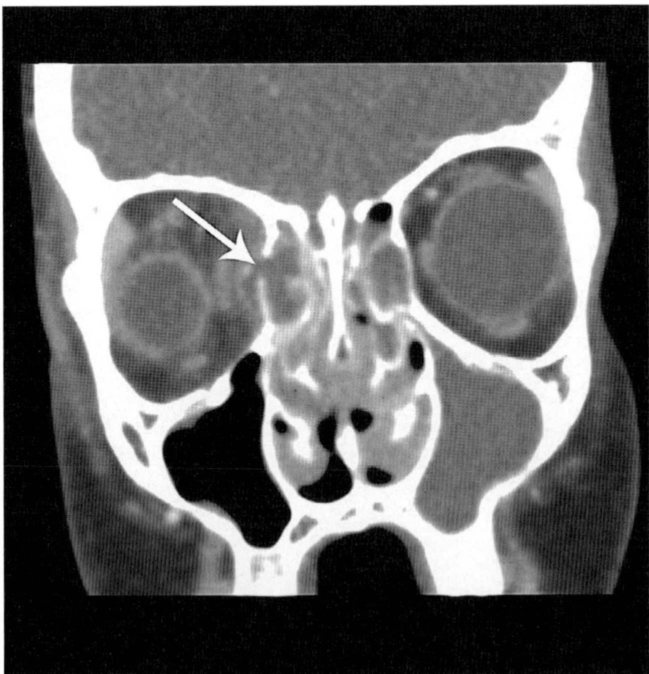

FIGURE 27-5 Coronal CT scan demonstrating a right medial subperiosteal abscess with dehiscence of the lamina (arrow). (*Used with permission from Paul Krakovitz, MD.*)

MANAGEMENT

MEDICATIONS

- Prompt identification and initiation of treatment is critical.
- Preseptal cellulitis often can be treated with oral antibiotics as an outpatient and with close follow-up (see Chapter 17, Preseptal (Periorbital) Cellulitis).
- The other complications require initial medical treatment with broad-spectrum intravenous antibiotics (often followed by oral therapy). SOR Ⓒ
- Topical nasal decongestant and saline irrigations are frequently used, but utility is debated. SOR Ⓒ
- Antibiotics that cross the blood–brain barrier should be used when there is intracranial involvement.
- Corticosteroids and anticonvulsants can be administered to treat any secondary cerebral edema. SOR Ⓒ
- The use of anticoagulants in venous thrombosis is controversial.

SURGERY

- Surgical intervention is recommended in cases where there is loss in visual acuity on initial evaluation, severe orbital complications, intracranial abscess, progression of orbital signs, symptoms despite medical treatment, or lack of improvement within 48 hours despite aggressive medical treatment. SOR Ⓒ
- Functional endoscopic sinus surgery or conventional open sinus surgery to drain the involved sinuses is performed on a case-by-case basis. SOR Ⓒ

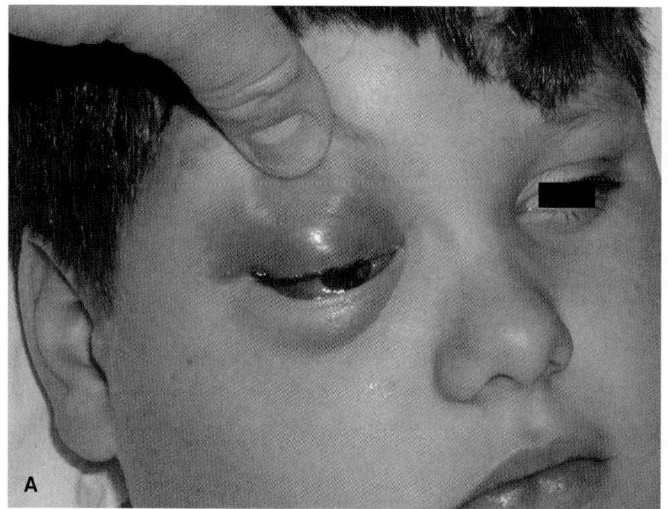

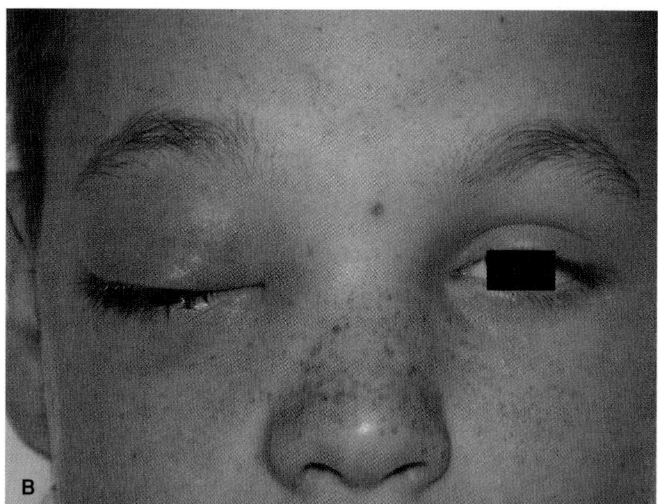

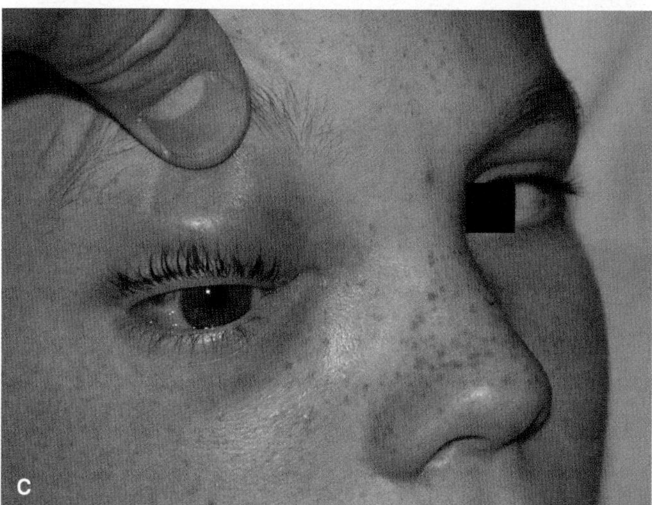

FIGURE 27-6 **A.** Young boy with periorbital edema, erythema, chemosis, proptosis, and restricted extraocular mobility from superior orbital abscess. **B.** Same patient, frontal view demonstrating hypoglobus. **C.** Same patient, frontal view demonstrating chemosis, purulent drainage, and gaze restriction. (*Used with permission from Paul Rychwalski, MD.*)

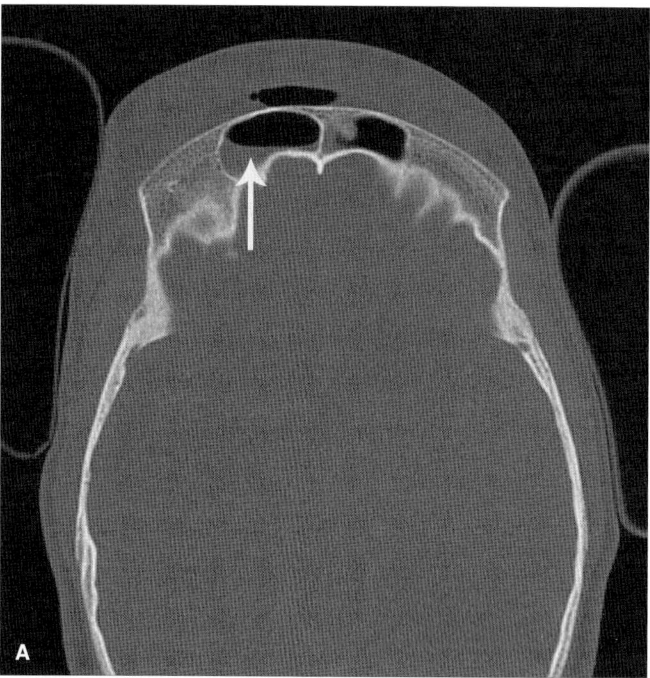

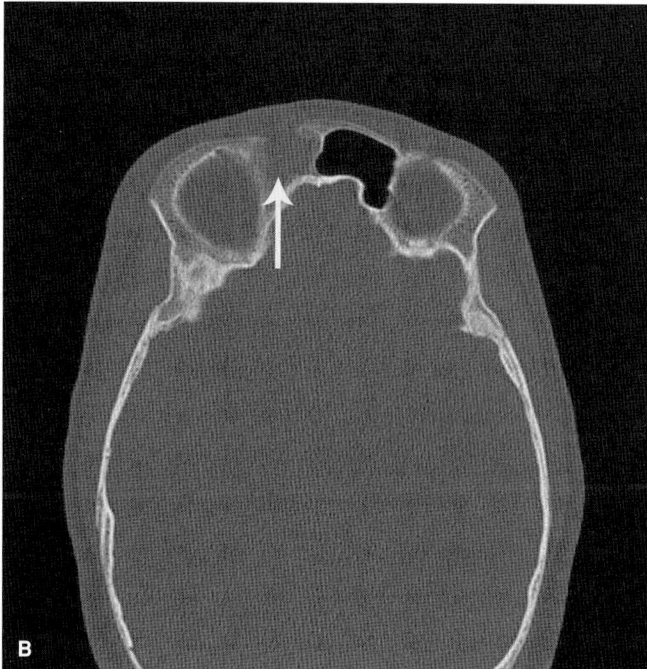

FIGURE 27-7 **A.** Axial CT scan demonstrating an air-fluid level in the right frontal sinus with associated subgaleal abscess (arrow). **B.** Axial CT scan 8 weeks after subgaleal abscess treatment, now with erosion of the frontal table and complete opacification of the sinus (arrow). (*Used with permission from Paul Krakovitz, MD.*)

- Drainage of subperiosteal abscesses should be done in the same setting either by endoscopic techniques, medial canthal, or via a transconjunctival incision depending on the location of the abscess.[10] SOR C
- The CT dimensions of a subperiosteal abscess that can be treated medically have been debated; when the abscess is wider than 10 mm, decision to proceed immediately for drainage can be considered.[11]

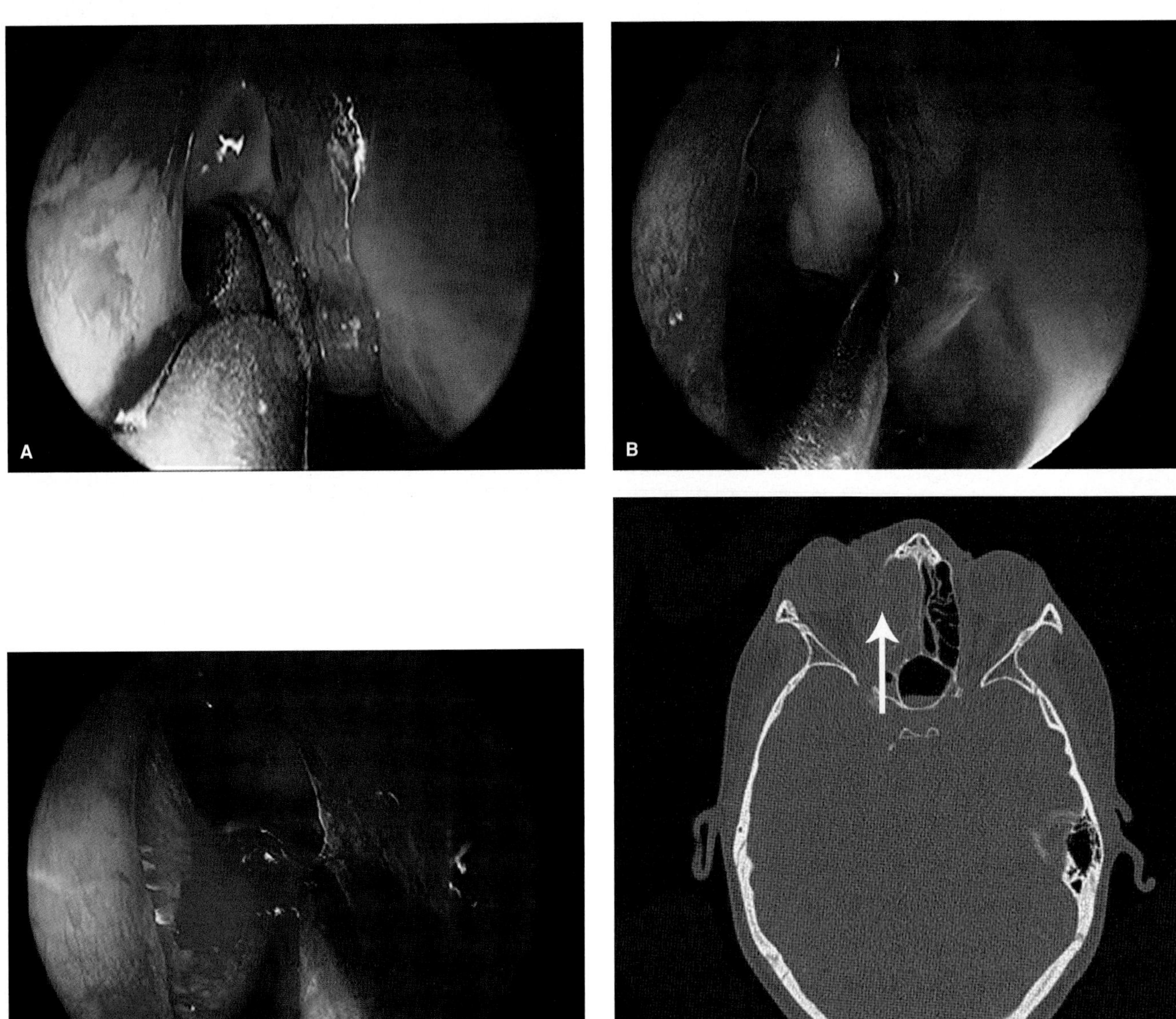

FIGURE 27-8 **A.** Mucopyocele of right ethmoid sinus, endoscopic view before rupture. **B.** Same patient, endoscopic view after rupture. **C.** Same patient, endoscopic view after rupture with empty cavity seen. **D.** Same patient, CT scan. Note expansion and erosion of right ethmoid cells as well as dehiscence of lamina papyreacea (medial orbital wall) (arrow). (*Used with permission from Prashant Malhotra, MD.*)

- Treatment of Pott's puffy tumor includes drainage of the abscess with removal of infected bone followed by at least 6 weeks of antibiotics. SOR Ⓒ
- Neurosurgical management of intracranial infection can be done concurrently with sinus surgery.

REFERRAL

- Ophthalmologic evaluation should be performed if orbital cellulitis, orbital abscess, or subperiosteal abscess is present, or if there is any change in vision or ocular mobility. Visual acuity, intraocular pressures, and complete ophthalmologic exam should be documented prior to surgical intervention.
- Neurosurgical evaluation should be performed if there are any concerns for intracranial extension.
- Pediatric otolaryngology evaluation should be considered if any complications of sinusitis are encountered, for medical and possible surgical intervention of source infection, as well as possibility of endoscopic transnasal approaches to abscesses.
- Infectious disease consultation, to guide antimicrobial choice and length of therapy, is suggested if suppurative complications are present.

PREVENTION AND SCREENING

- Appropriate management of acute bacterial rhinosinusitis is the most effective means of prevention.
- This can be made according to guidelines such as those from the 2012 Infectious Diseases Society of America.[12]

PROGNOSIS

- Children with intracranial extension are typically hospitalized and treated for longer durations than those with intraorbital extension; however, the risk of persistent sequelae is not higher.[13]
- Persistent sequelae include diplopia, vision loss, hemi-paresis, aphasia, and other neurologic deficits; this is reported to occur in about 3 to 23 percent of cases.[11–14]

FOLLOW-UP

- The timing of follow-up is determined by the severity of the disease process.
- Patients with complications other than preseptal cellulitis will be managed in the inpatient setting.
- Close follow-up is required in all patients to prevent progression and visual impairment.
- Patients are typically seen at 1 week following endoscopic sinus surgery for debridement.

INVASIVE FUNGAL SINUSITIS

- Invasive fungal sinusitis is a unique and important complication where prompt recognition can be lifesaving and deserves special mention. This devastating infection can occur in children in immunocompromised states such as hematologic or lymphoid malignancies, post-transplant, immunodeficiency disorders, or poorly controlled type 1 diabetes mellitus.
- Invasive fungal sinusitis may be heralded by fever, facial pain, numbness in trigeminal distribution, sinus symptoms (congestion, rhinorrhea), palatal fistula, overlying skin changes, or signs of orbital or intracranial extension.[15,16]
- Nasal endoscopy and biopsy should be promptly performed as soon as there is concern for invasive fungal sinusitis. Fungal hyphal elements with submucosal infiltration, angio-invasion, and necrosis are diagnostic.[15–17]
- Contrast enhanced CT scan and MRI is performed when invasive fungal sinusitis are suspected and includes axial and coronal T1 and T2 images (**Figures 27-9A,B**).
- Treatment usually requires multi-agent parenteral antifungal therapy along with radical surgical debridement.[15,17] Surgical treatment is aggressive, often disfiguring.
- Mortality rates are high and range from 50 to 90 percent.[17–19]

PATIENT EDUCATION

- Severe or prolonged congestion, nasal drainage, facial pain, and/or fever requires medical attention.
- Blurry or double vision, eye pain, neck stiffness, severe headaches, or changes in mental status should be evaluated urgently.
- Nonresponse to therapy for sinus infections also warrants medical attention.

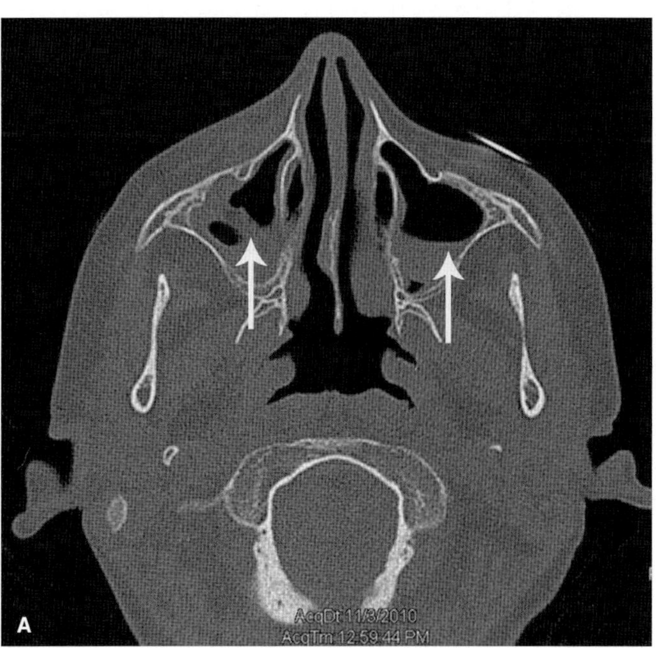

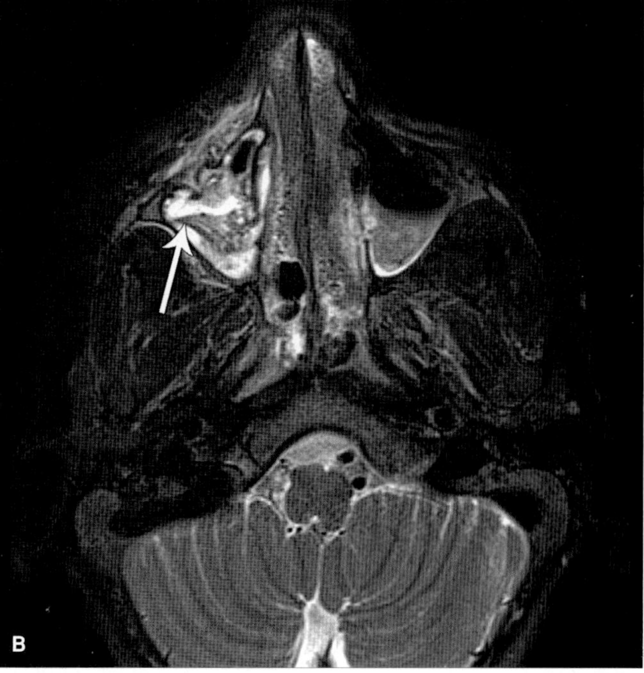

FIGURE 27-9 **A.** Mild maxillary air-fluid levels bilaterally (arrows) on axial CT scan in a 9-year-old boy with combined variable immunodeficiency, and aplastic anemia, who presented with nasal congestion and malar pain and numbness on the right. Nasal endoscopy and biopsy demonstrated invasive *Aspergillus* infection. **B.** Same patient, T2-weighted MRI scan demonstrating extension of invasive fungal sinusitis along infraorbital nerve into soft tissues of cheek (arrow). This patient and his family elected medical and palliative therapy instead of radical, disfiguring surgery and died 3 months later. (*Used with permission from Prashant Malhotra, MD.*)

PATIENT RESOURCES

- University of Maryland Medical Center—**www.umm.edu/patiented/articles/what_symptoms_of_sinusitis_000062_4.htm.**
- —**www.boogordoctor.com/2010/04/8-complications-of-sinusitis-3-that-can-kill/.**

PROVIDER RESOURCES

- Clinical practice guideline: management of sinusitis. *Pediatrics*. 2001;108(3):798-808. Available at **www.pediatrics.aappublications.org/content/108/3/798.full,** *accessed October 2012.*
- Chow AW, Benninger MS, Brook I, et al. IDSA clinical practice guideline for acute bacterial rhinosinusitis in children and adults. *Clin Infect Dis*. 2012;54(8):e72-e112.

REFERENCES

1. Botting AM, McIntosh D, Mahadevan M, et al. Paediatric pre- and post-septal peri-orbital infections are different diseases: a retrospective review of 262 cases. *Int J Pediatr Otorhinolaryngol*. 2008;72:377-383.
2. Herrmann BW, Forsen JW Jr: Simultaneous intracranial and orbital complications of acute rhinosinusitis in children. *Int J Pediatr Otorhinolaryngol*. 2004;68:619-625.
3. Rosenfeld EA, Rowley AH. Infectious intracranial complications of sinusitis, other than meningitis, in children: 12-year review. *Clin Infect Dis*. 1994;18:750-754.
4. Chandler JR, Langenbrunner DJ, Stevens ER. The pathogenesis of orbital complications in acute sinusitis. *Laryngoscope*. 1970;80: 1414-1428.
5. Duse M, Caminiti S, Zicari AM. Rhinosinusitis: prevention strategies. *Pediatr Allergy Immunol*. 2007;18(18):71-74.
6. Principi N, Esposito S. New insights into pediatric rhinosinusitis. *Pediatr Allergy Immunol*. 2007;18(18):7-9.
7. El Hakim et al. *Int J Pediatr Otorhinolaryngol*. 2006;70: 1383-1387.
8. Pelton RW, Smith ME, Patel BC, et al. Cosmetic considerations in surgery for orbital subperiosteal abscess in children: Experience with a combined transcaruncular and transnasal endoscopic approach. *Arch Otolaryngol Head Neck Surg*. 2003;129:652-655.
9. Edmundson, N, Parikh S. Complications of Acute Bacterial Sinusitis in Children. *Pediatr Ann*. 2008;37(10):680-685.
10. Hicks CW, Weber JG, Reid JR, and Moodley M. Identifying and Managing Intracranial Complications of Sinusitis in Children. *Pediatr Infect Dis J* 2011;30:3.
11. Ryan JT, Preciado DA, Bauman N, et al. Management of pediatric orbital cellulitis in patients with radiographic findings of subperiosteal abscess. *Otolaryngol Head Neck Surg*. 2009;140:907-911.
12. Chow AW, Benninger MS, Brook I, et al. IDSA clinical practice guideline for acute bacterial rhinosinusitis in children and adults. *Clin Infect Dis*. 2012;54(8):e72-e112.
13. Goytia VK, Giannoni CM, and Edwards MS. Intraorbital and Intracranial Extension of Sinusitis: Comparative Morbidity. *J Pediatr* 2011;158:3:486-491.
14. Fokkens W, Lund V, Mullol J. EP3OS. European position on rhinosinusitis and nasal polyps 2007. *Rhinology*. 2007;20:1-139.
15. Park AH, Muntz HR, Smith ME, Afify Z, Pysher T, Pavia A. Pediatric invasive fungal rhinosinusitis in immunocompromised children with cancer. *Otolaryngol Head Neck Surg*. 2005;133(3):411-416.
16. Idris N, Lim LH. Nasal eschar: a warning sign of potentially fatal invasive fungal sinusitis in immunocompromised children. *J Pediatr Hematol Oncol*. 2012;34(4):e134-136.
17. Kasapoglu F, Coskun H, Ozmen OA, Akalin H, Ener B. Acute invasive fungal rhinosinusitis: evaluation of 26 patients treated with endonasal or open surgical procedures. *Otolaryngol Head Neck Surg*. 2010;143(5):614-620.
18. Blitzer A, Lawson W, Meyers BR, et al. Patient survival factors in paranasal sinus mucormycosis. *Laryngoscope* 1980;90:635-648.
19. Johnson PJ, Lydiatt WM, Huerter JV, et al. Invasive fungal sinusitis following liver or bone marrow transplantation. *Am J Rhinol*. 1994;8:77-83.

SECTION 3 MOUTH AND THROAT

28 SCARLET FEVER AND STRAWBERRY TONGUE

M. Jason Sanders, MD
Linda French, MD

PATIENT STORY

A 7-year-old boy is brought to the pediatrician's office with a rough red rash on his trunk (**Figures 28-1** and **28-2**) along with fever and a sore throat. The sandpaper rash and signs that are consistent with strep pharyngitis lead the physician to diagnose scarlet fever. The physician explains the diagnosis to the mother and oral penicillin V is prescribed. The boy feels markedly better by the next day and the mother continues to give the penicillin for the full 10 days, as directed, to prevent rheumatic fever.

INTRODUCTION

Scarlet fever is an illness caused by toxin-producing group A β-hemolytic *streptococcus* (strep) infection. Most commonly, scarlet fever evolves from an exudative pharyngitis.

Strawberry tongue may be observed in patients with scarlet fever and usually develops within the first 2 to 3 days of illness. A white or yellowish coating usually precedes the classic red tongue with white papillae (**Figure 28-3**).

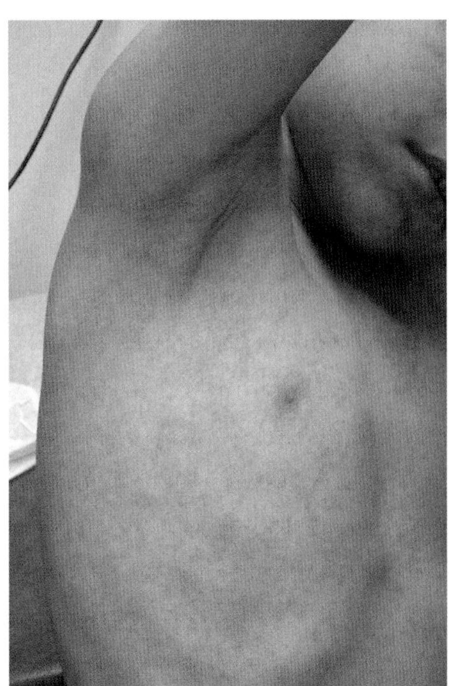

FIGURE 28-1 Sandpaper rash on the trunk and in the axilla of a 7-year-old boy with scarlet fever. (*Used with permission from of Richard P. Usatine, MD.*)

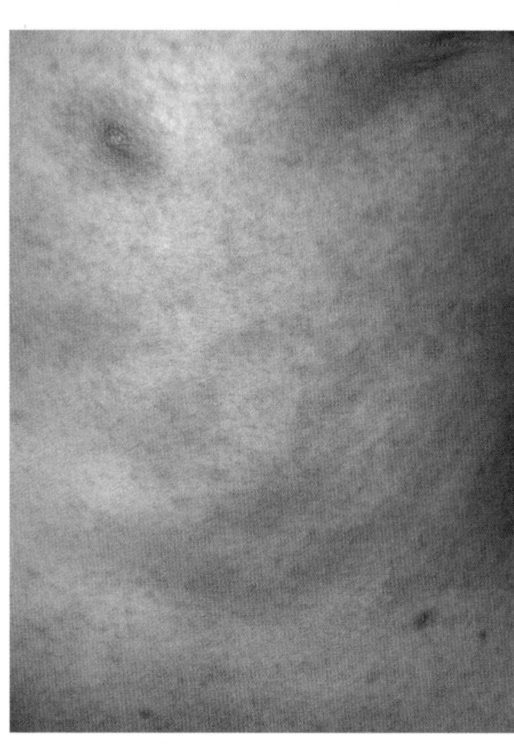

FIGURE 28-2 Scarlatiniform rash comprising small papules and erythema on the trunk of a febrile child with strep pharyngitis. (*Used with permission from Richard P. Usatine, MD.*)

EPIDEMIOLOGY

- Scarlet fever is predominately seen in school-age children with no gender predilection.
- Majority related to strep pharyngitis, with 1 in 10 developing scarlet fever (**Figures 28-1**, **28-2**, and **28-4**).
- Prevalent in late fall to early spring.
- Strawberry tongue (**Figure 28-4**) is most commonly seen in children in association with scarlet fever or Kawasaki disease.
- Can be present with other group A strep infection.
- In cases of strep, a white membrane through which the papillae are seen can initially cover the tongue followed by desquamation of the membrane (with the appearance as in **Figure 28-4**).

ETIOLOGY AND PATHOPHYSIOLOGY

- Transmission of *Streptococcus pyogenes* (Group A) (GAS) occurs via respiratory secretions.
- Virulent GAS incubates over 2 to 7 days. M protein serotypes of GAS are typically more invasive, with greater potential for progression to rheumatic fever or acute glomerulonephritis if untreated.[1]

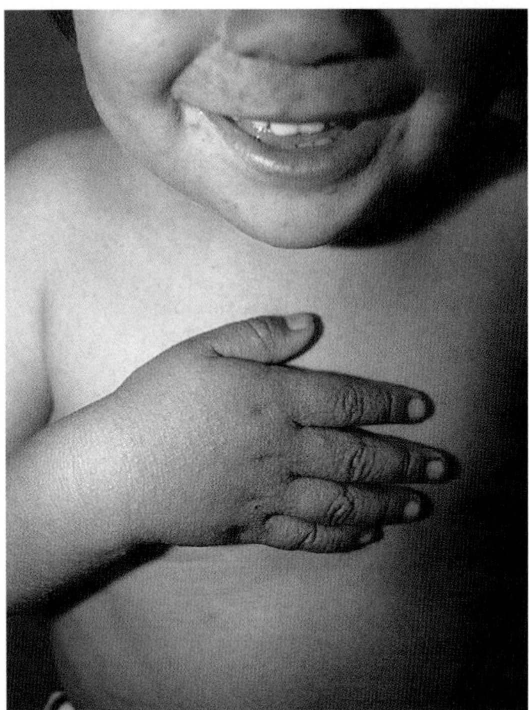

FIGURE 28-3 Sandpaper rash (scarlatiniform) seen prominently on the hand of a child recovering from strep pharyngitis. (*Used with permission from Richard P. Usatine, MD.*)

- Fever and rash are related to pyrogenic A–C and erythrogenic exotoxins produced by GAS.[2]
- Infection can originate from other sites like skin (e.g., cellulitis) and seed blood (bacteremia) or organ systems (e.g., pneumonia).
- Strawberry tongue results from a general inflammatory response during the early course of the disease.

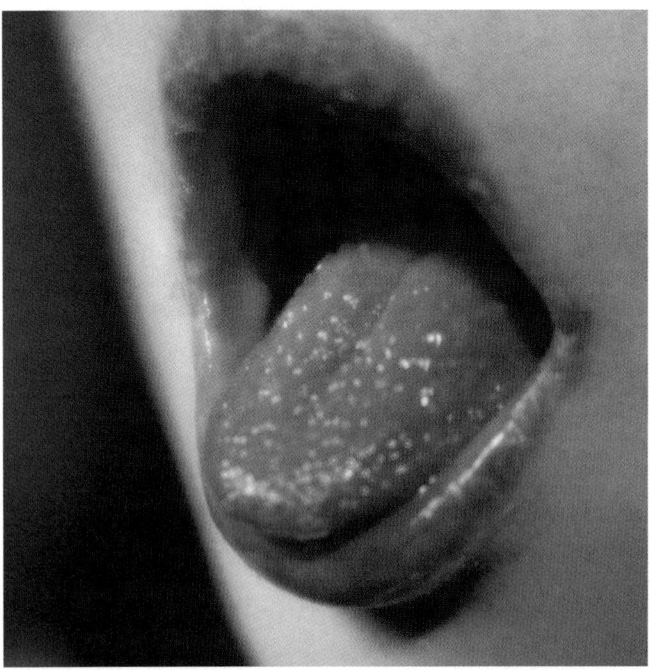

FIGURE 28-4 Strawberry tongue in a child with scarlet fever caused by strep pharyngitis; note marked erythema and prominent papillae. (*Used with permission from of Richard P. Usatine, MD.*)

DIAGNOSIS

CLINICAL FEATURES

- Headache, sore throat, cervical lymphadenopathy, abdominal pain, nausea and vomiting, decreased oral intake, malaise, and fever can precede rash. Cough and rhinorrhea are usually not present.
- Oropharyngeal findings include:
  - Strawberry tongue—Erythematous and sometimes edematous tongue with prominent papillae (**Figure 28-4**).
- Tongue is sometimes covered by a white membrane/coating through which the papillae can be seen.
- Not typically painful.
- Forchheimer spots—Palatal and uvular petechiae and erythematous macules.
- Initial sandpaper rash, associated with blanching erythema and occasional pruritus, erupts in 1 to 2 days (**Figures 28-1** to **28-3**).[2]
- Pastia's lines are pink or red lines seen in the body folds (especially elbows and axilla) during scarlet fever. Linear hyperpigmentation can persist after the rash fades (**Figure 28-1**).
- Desquamation of the skin (especially of the hands and feet) ensues in 3 to 4 days as rash fades and can persist for 2 to 4 weeks.[1]

TYPICAL DISTRIBUTION

- Progresses centrally (torso) to peripherally (extremities) and can be prominent on the face, chest, palms, fingers, and toes.[1]

LABORATORY TESTS AND IMAGING

- Throat swab for rapid strep testing (screening) and/or culture (confirmation) is usually performed.
- Complete blood count (CBC), if indicated, to look for:
  - Elevation of white blood cell count with left shift.
  - Elevated platelet count—Seen with Kawasaki disease (after 1 week).
- Antistreptolysin-*O* titer is obtained to confirm prior infection or support suspected poststreptococcal complication, such as rheumatic fever.[3]
- Acute phase reactants (C-reactive protein [CRP] and erythrocyte sedimentation rate [ESR]) can be elevated, and is useful in monitoring nonsuppurative complications such as rheumatic fever.[4]
- If Kawasaki disease is suspected, two-dimensional echocardiography or angiography is obtained to detect coronary artery abnormalities. The initial echocardiogram should be performed as soon as the diagnosis is suspected to establish a baseline for longitudinal follow-up of coronary artery morphology, left ventricular and left valvular function, and the evolution and resolution of pericardial effusion when present.[4] SOR Ⓒ

DIFFERENTIAL DIAGNOSIS

The rash of scarlet fever can be confused with the following:

- Allergic/contact dermatitis—Often localized to areas of contact; prominent pruritus and skin vesicles often in linear streaks (see Chapter 130, Atopic Dermatitis and Chapter 131, Contact Dermatitis).

- Viral exanthem—Many viral exanthems have prodromal phases with fever followed by skin rashes that can be macular or maculopapular including measles (see Chapter 111, Measles), rubella (tender retroauricular, cervical, and occipital lymphadenopathy; rash starts on face and spreads and fades quickly), and roseola (rash occurs at the end of a period of 3 to 5 days of high fever). Lack of sandpaper feel and oral findings help distinguish.
- Staphylococcal scalded skin syndrome (see Chapter 105, Staphylococcal Scalded Skin Syndrome)—Rash can also follow a prodrome of malaise and fever but is macular, brightly erythematous, and initially involves the face, neck axilla, and groin. Skin is markedly tender and large areas of the epidermis peel away.
- Erythema toxicum—Rash of newborns; often blotchy, evanescent, macular erythema that can include pale yellow or white wheals or papules on an erythematous base (see Chapter 92, Normal Skin Changes).

The differential diagnosis for strawberry tongue includes:

- Kawasaki disease (**Figure 28-5**)—Fever persists at least 5 days and there must be the presence of at least four principal features including the following (see Chapter 177, Kawasaki Disease):[4]
    - Changes in extremities—Acute: Erythema of palms and soles; edema of hands and feet. Subacute: Periungual peeling of fingers and toes in weeks 2 and 3.
    - Polymorphous exanthem.
    - Bilateral bulbar conjunctival injection without exudate.
    - Changes in lips and oral cavity—Erythema, lips cracking, strawberry tongue, diffuse injection of oral, and pharyngeal mucosae.
    - Cervical lymphadenopathy (>1.5 cm diameter), usually unilateral.
- Viral stomatitis with eruptive lingual papillitis—Lack of other features for scarlet fever or Kawasaki's will assist in differentiating.
- Red-colored food dyes—History is helpful; edema and prominent papillae will be absent.

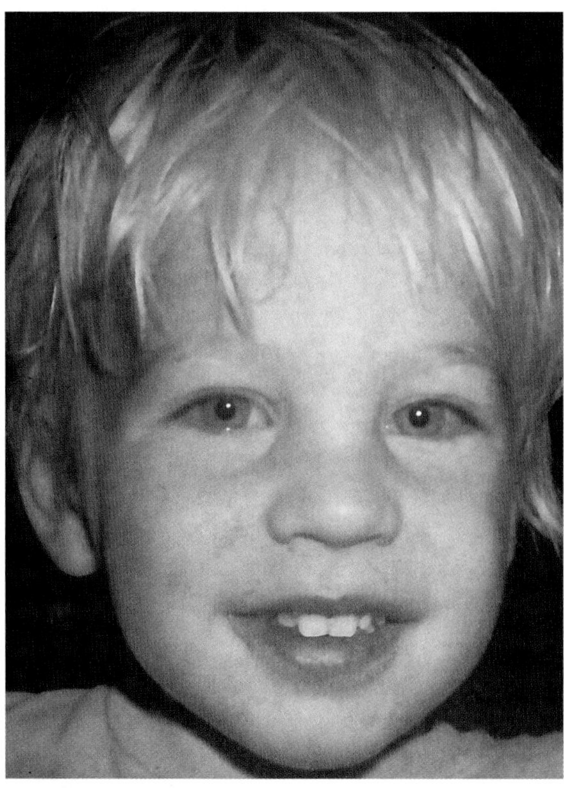

FIGURE 28-5 Child recovering from Kawasaki disease. Note the conjunctival injection that still remains. (*Used with permission from Greg Thompson, MD.*)

MANAGEMENT

NONPHARMACOLOGICAL

- Supportive care with oral fluids and age-appropriate symptomatic measures, such as salt-water gargles, and an antipyretic as needed are recommended.

MEDICATIONS

- For scarlet fever and strawberry tongue caused by group A *Streptococcus*:
    - Oral penicillin (penicillin V 25 to 50 mg/kg per day for 10 days [maximum 1500 mg per day] or amoxicillin 50 mg/kg per day [maximum 1200mg per day]).
    - Macrolide (azithromycin 12 mg/kg per day once daily on day 1 [maximum 500 mg per day], followed by 6 mg/kg per day once daily on days 2 to 5 [maximum 250 mg per day]) or clindamycin 20 mg/kg per day for 10 days (maximum 1800 mg per day) in penicillin-allergic patients.[5] SOR Ⓐ
    - Cephalosporins are an efficacious alternative if no history of immediate penicillin hypersensitivity (cefuroxime axetil 20 mg/kg per day for 10 days [maximum 500mg per day]); cephalosporins were more effective than penicillin in a metaanalysis.[6] SOR Ⓐ
    - Symptoms typically resolve in 4 to 7 days.
- For strawberry tongue caused by Kawasaki disease (also see Chapter 177, Kawasaki Disease):
    - Intravenous gammaglobulin (IVIG), 2 g/kg in a single infusion, within 7 to 10 days of onset for Kawasaki disease to reduce subsequent coronary artery abnormalities.[4] Additional IVIG infusion may be considered if defervescence is not achieved in the first 1 to 2 days.[7] SOR Ⓐ
    - In the acute phase, aspirin is also administered at 80 to 100 mg/kg per day in 4 doses with IVIG followed by low-dose aspirin (3 to 5 mg/kg per day) until the patient shows no evidence of coronary changes by 6 to 8 weeks after the onset of illness.[4] SOR Ⓒ

REFERRAL OR HOSPITALIZE

- Hospitalization should be considered if a patient is dehydrated or exhibits cardiorespiratory instability. It should also be considered for cases of complicated scarlet fever, streptococcal toxic shock, staphylococcal scalded skin syndrome, rheumatic fever, acute glomerulonephritis, or Kawasaki disease (when suspected).
- Cardiology, infectious disease, or nephrology consultation should be considered in severe cases.

PROGNOSIS

Scarlet fever usually follows a benign course. Rarely, it is complicated by septic shock and multi-organ failure, suppurative complications such as peritonsillar abscess, or nonsuppurative complications such as rheumatic fever or poststreptococcal glomerulonephritis.

FOLLOW-UP

- Routine follow-up is not required unless the illness is protracted or a complication is suspected.
- For patients with uncomplicated Kawasaki disease, echocardiographic evaluation should be performed at the time of diagnosis, at 2 weeks, and at 6 to 8 weeks after onset of the disease.[4] Recent studies show that repeat echocardiography performed 1 year after the onset of the illness is unlikely to reveal coronary artery enlargement in patients whose echocardiographic findings were normal at 4 to 8 weeks.[4] SOR Ⓒ

PATIENT EDUCATION

- Contact your physician for fever recurrence, atypical or persistent rash, and new symptoms or potential complications (meningitis, sinusitis, otitis media, oropharyngeal abscess, pneumonia, acute glomerulonephritis, or rheumatic fever).
- Completion of a prescribed antibiotic course is encouraged to decrease the incidence of recurrence and potential complications.[3]

REFERENCES

1. Cunningham MW. Pathogenesis of group A streptococcal infections. *Clin Microbiol Rev.* 2000;13(3):470-511.
2. Cherry JD. Contemporary infectious exanthems. *Clin Infect Dis.* 1993;16(2):199-205.
3. Hahn RG, Knox LM, Forman TA. Evaluation of poststreptococcal illness. *Am Fam Physician.* 2005;71(10):1949-1954.
4. Newburger JW, Takahashi M, Gerber MA, et al. Diagnosis, treatment, and long-term management of Kawasaki disease: a statement for health professionals from the committee on rheumatic fever, endocarditis and Kawasaki disease, council on cardiovascular disease in the young, American Heart Association. *Circulation.* 2004;110(17):2747-2771.
5. Pickering LK, Baker CJ, Kimberlin DW, Long SS, et al. In: *Red Book: 2012 Report of the Committee on Infectious Diseases.* 29th ed. American Academy of Pediatrics; Elk Grove, IL; 2012.
6. Casey JR, Pichichero ME. Meta-analysis of cephalosporin versus penicillin treatment of group A streptococcal tonsillopharyngitis in children. *Pediatrics.* 2004;113(4):866-882.
7. Freeman AF, Shulman ST. Kawasaki disease: summary of the American Heart Association guidelines. *Am Fam Physician.* 2006;74(7):1141-1148.

29 UPPER RESPIRATORY INFECTIONS INCLUDING PHARYNGITIS

Brian Williams, MD
Melissa A. Scholes, MD
Richard P. Usatine, MD
Mindy A. Smith, MD
Camille Sabella, MD

PATIENT STORY

A mother brings her nine year-old daughter to the pediatrician's office with complaints of sore throat, fever, and malaise for 2 days. The girl has not had cough or runny nose. The mother is concerned about strep throat because a classmate of the daughter's was just diagnosed with this. On exam, the girl has erythematous tonsillar pillars, palatal petechiae, and impressive cervical lymphadenopathy (**Figure 29-1**). A throat swab for rapid streptococcal antigen is positive and the girl is treated with penicillin VK for 10 days and recovers completely.

INTRODUCTION

Upper respiratory tract infection (URI), also known as the common cold, and pharyngitis, inflammation and pain of the pharyngeal tissues, including the pharynx, tonsils and adenoids are among the most common illnesses of childhood. URIs are characterized by rhinorrhea, nasal congestion, and sore or scratchy throat. They are caused by viruses. Symptoms and signs of pharyngitis include throat soreness or scratchiness, fever, headache, malaise, rash, joint and muscle pains, and cervical lymphadenopathy. Viruses are responsible for the majority of cases of pharyngitis in infants and children, although Group A β-hemolytic streptococci (GABHS) are important causes of pharyngitis because of their ability to cause suppurative (peritonsillar and parapharyngeal abscesses) and non-suppurative (acute rheumatic fever and glomerulonephritis) complications.

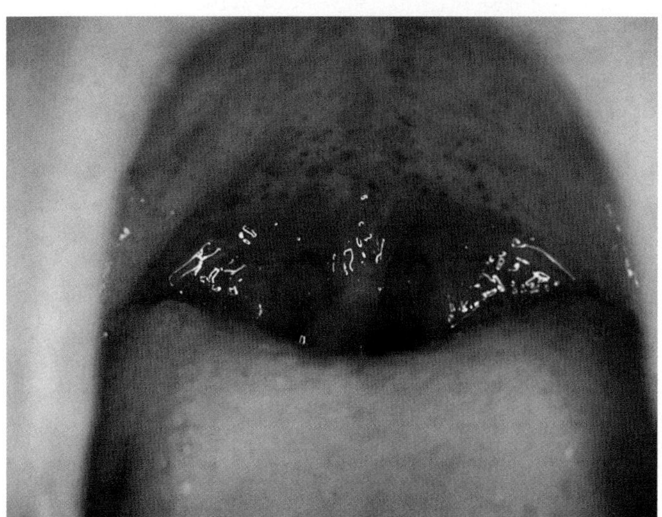

FIGURE 29-1 Erythema and edema of the pharynx, and palatal petechiae in a child with Group A Streptococcal pharyngitis. *(Used with permission from CDC/Public Health Image Library/Heinz F. Eichenwald, MD.)*

EPIDEMIOLOGY

- Acute URI and pharyngitis account for 3.4 percent and 1 percent of primary care visits, respectively.[1]
- Viral infections account for the vast majority of cases of URI and 60 to 90 percent of cases of pharyngitis in children. GABHS is responsible for the majority of bacterial pharyngitis.
- In temperate climates, the highest prevalence of URI and pharyngitis occurs from autumn until spring. This corresponds directly with circulating viruses over this period of time.
- Frequency of URIs varies with age: highest frequency is in children 1 to 5 years of age, who experience 7 to 8 colds per year; infants less than one year of age average 6.5 colds a year; adolescents average 4.5 colds per year.[2]
- Highest incidence of GABHS pharyngitis is in school-aged children and adolescents.
- Acute rheumatic fever is rare in the US (see Chapter 45, Acute Rheumatic Fever).
- Viruses causing URIs and pharyngitis can be spread via small particle aerosol (Influenza and Coronaviruses), large particle droplet (Rhinoviruses), or direct hand-to-hand transmission (Rhinoviruses and RSV).
- Up to 14 percent of deep neck infections result from pharyngitis.[3]

ANATOMY

- The lingual tonsils on the base of tongue, the lateral palatine tonsils ("tonsils") and the superior pharyngeal tonsils ("adenoids") together make up Waldeyer's ring. This ring of lymphoid tissue is favorably located for airborne and food-related antigen exposure.
- Adenoids and tonsils are predominantly B-cell organs and immunologically most active between the ages of 4 and 10 years.[4,5] Overall, data show that adenotonsillectomy does not significantly affect the immune system adversely.

ETIOLOGY AND PATHOPHYSIOLOGY

- Rhinoviruses are the most common cause of URIs and pharyngitis in children; other viruses implicated include coronaviruses, respiratory syncytial virus (RSV), human metapneumovirus, influenza virus, parainfluenza viruses, adenovirus, enteroviruses (i.e., herpangina), and human bocavirus.[6]
- Herpes simplex virus, human immunodeficiency virus, syphilis, and *Neisseria gonorrhoeae* are causes of pharyngitis in sexually active adolescents.
- Viruses that infect nasal epithelial cells release cytokines and other inflammatory mediators, producing an inflammatory response of polymorphonuclear cells such as albumin and bradykinins that are responsible for the clinical symptoms of URI.
- The paranasal sinuses and middle ear are commonly involved during uncomplicated URIs. Thus, it is common to have abnormal CT and MRI scans of the sinuses and middle ear fluid during URIs.[7,8]

- Some viruses, such as adenovirus, cause inflammation of the pharyngeal mucosa by direct invasion of the mucosa or secondary to suprapharyngeal secretions.[9] Other viruses, such as rhinovirus, cause pain through stimulation of pain nerve endings by mediators, such as bradykinin.
- GABHS accounts for 15 to 30 percent of pharyngitis cases in children and up to 38 percent of cases of tonsillitis.
- GABHS releases exotoxins and proteases. Erythrogenic exotoxins are responsible for the development of the scarlatiniform exanthem (**Figure 29-2**).[10]
- Secondary cross-reacting antibody formation during GABHS pharyngitis can result in rheumatic fever and valvular heart disease.[11] Antigen–antibody complexes can lead to acute poststreptococcal glomerulonephritis. These are the nonsuppurative complications of GABHS infection.
- GABHS pharyngitis can result in suppurative complications including bacteremia, otitis media, meningitis, mastoiditis, cervical lymphadenitis, endocarditis, pneumonia, or deep neck abscess formation (**Figure 29-3**).

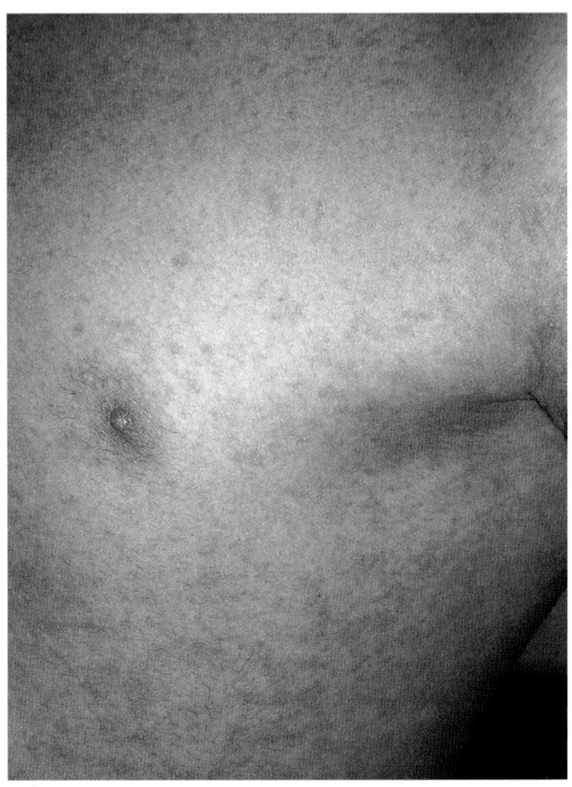

FIGURE 29-2 Scarlatiniform rash in scarlet fever. This 7-year-old boy has a typical sandpaper rash with his strep throat and fever. The erythema is particularly concentrated in the axillary area. (*Used with permission from Richard P. Usatine, MD.*)

RISK FACTORS

- Immune deficiency.

DIAGNOSIS

CLINICAL FEATURES

- Infants and young children with URI commonly manifest fever, nasal congestion, irritability, and rhinorrhea, which may be clear or

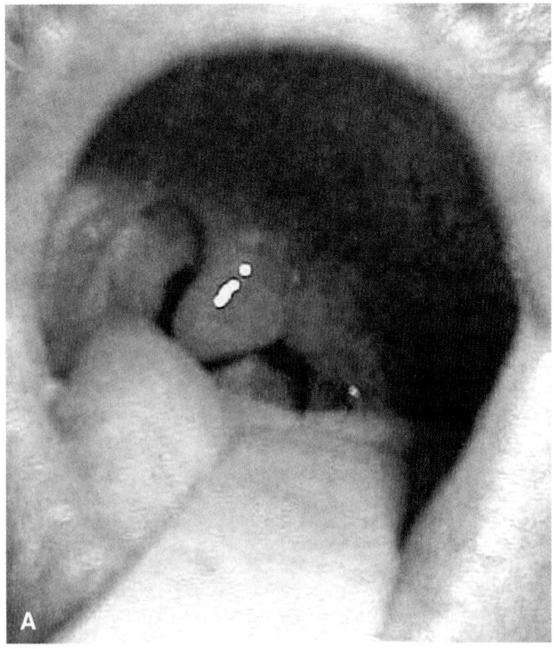

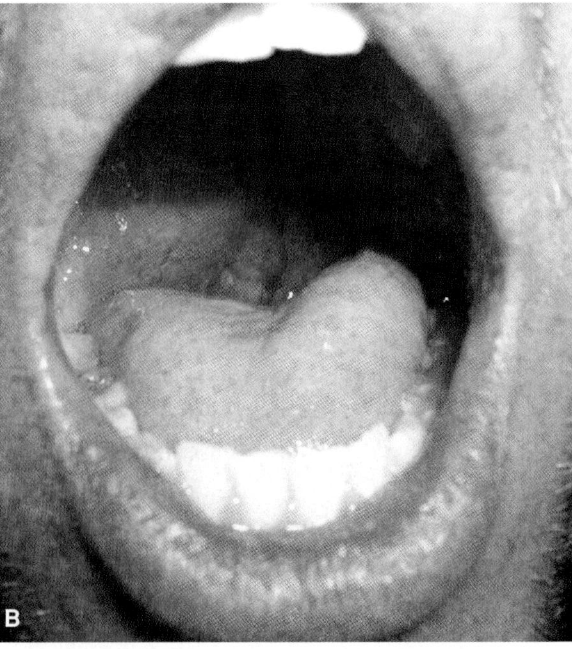

FIGURE 29-3 **A.** Peritonsillar abscess on the left showing uvular deviation away from the side with the abscess. **B.** Peritonsillar abscess with swelling and anatomic distortion of the right tonsillar region. (*Used with permission from Charlie Goldberg, MD, and The Regents of the University of California.*)

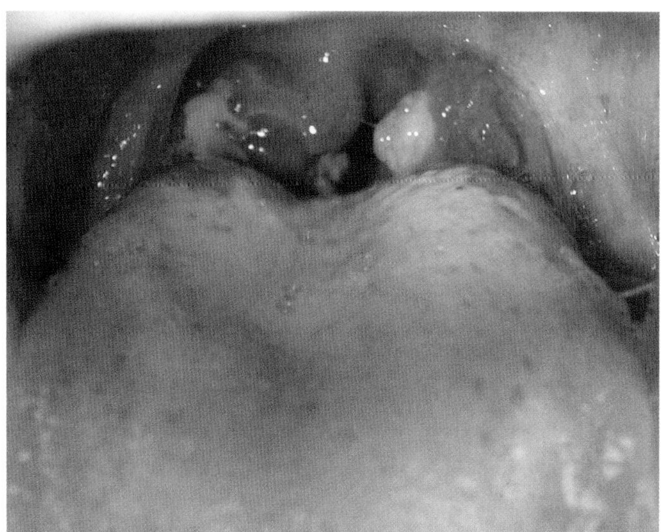

FIGURE 29-4 Mononucleosis with considerable tonsillar exudate. (*Used with permission from Tracey Cawthorn, MD.*)

purulent. Mild to moderate enlargement of the anterior cervical lymph nodes may be present.

- Older children and adolescents commonly manifest rhinorrhea, sore or scratchy throat, sneezing, sinus fullness, malaise, and hoarseness. Physical exam findings are minimal and may include mild erythema of the pharyngeal or nasal mucosa.
- Rapid onset of odynophagia, tonsillar exudates, anterior cervical lymphadenopathy, and fever are consistent with streptococcal pharyngitis. Headache and abdominal pain are common in children who have streptococcal pharyngitis.
- Not all tonsillar exudates are caused by streptococcal pharyngitis. Mononucleosis and other viral causes of pharyngitis commonly produce tonsillar exudates in children (**Figures 29-4** and **29-5**). The positive predictive value for tonsillar exudate in strep throat is only 31 percent; that is, 69 percent of patients with tonsillar exudate will have a nonstreptococcal cause.

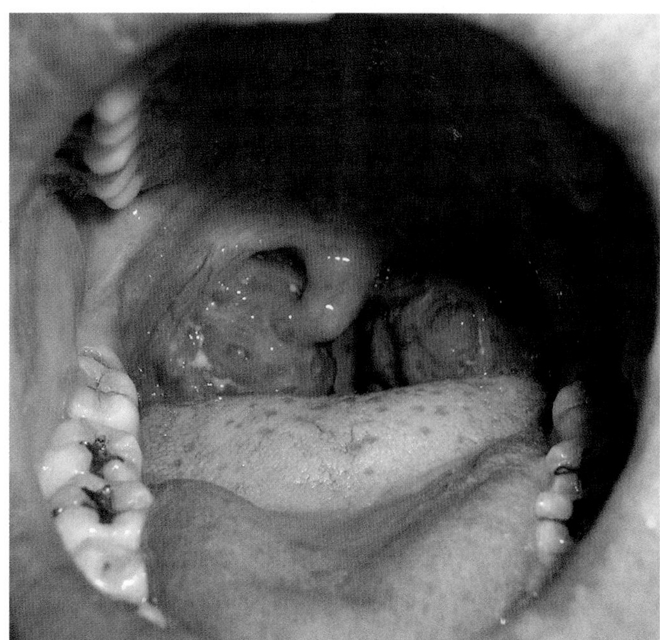

FIGURE 29-5 Viral pharyngitis showing enlarged cryptic tonsils with some erythema and exudate. (*Used with permission from Richard P. Usatine, MD.*)

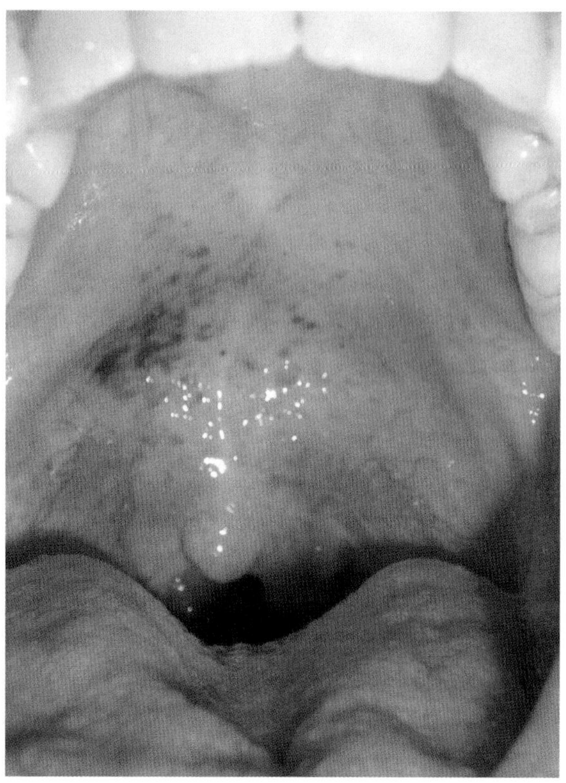

FIGURE 29-6 Viral pharyngitis with visible palatal petechiae. Palatal petechiae can be seen in all types of pharyngitis. (*Used with permission from Richard P. Usatine, MD.*)

- Para- and supratonsillar edema with medial and/or anterior displacement of the involved tonsil and uvular displacement to the contralateral side suggest peritonsillar abscess (**Figure 29-2**). Trismus and anterior cervical lymphadenopathy with severe tenderness to palpation are additional findings.
- Palatal petechiae can be seen in all types of pharyngitis (**Figures 29-1** and **29-6**).
- A sandpaper rash is suggestive of scarlet fever (**Figure 29-2**, and Chapter 28, Scarlet Fever and Strawberry Tongue). Strawberry tongue frequently accompanies scarlet fever (**Figure 28-4**).
- Lymphoid hyperplasia from viral infections, gastroesophageal reflux disease (GERD), or allergies can cause a cobblestone pattern on the posterior pharynx or palate (**Figure 29-7**). Although it usually is more suggestive of a viral infection or allergic rhinitis, lymphoid hyperplasia can be seen in strep pharyngitis (**Figure 29-8**).
- The presence of rhinorrhea and nasal congestion indicate a viral URI infection and are not consistent with GABHS infection.

LABORATORY TESTS AND IMAGING

- The diagnosis of viral URI is made clinically; testing for specific viral etiologies is not indicated for most cases.
- Children who are at high risk for complications from viral URI (i.e., immunodeficient patients), or who require hospitalization,

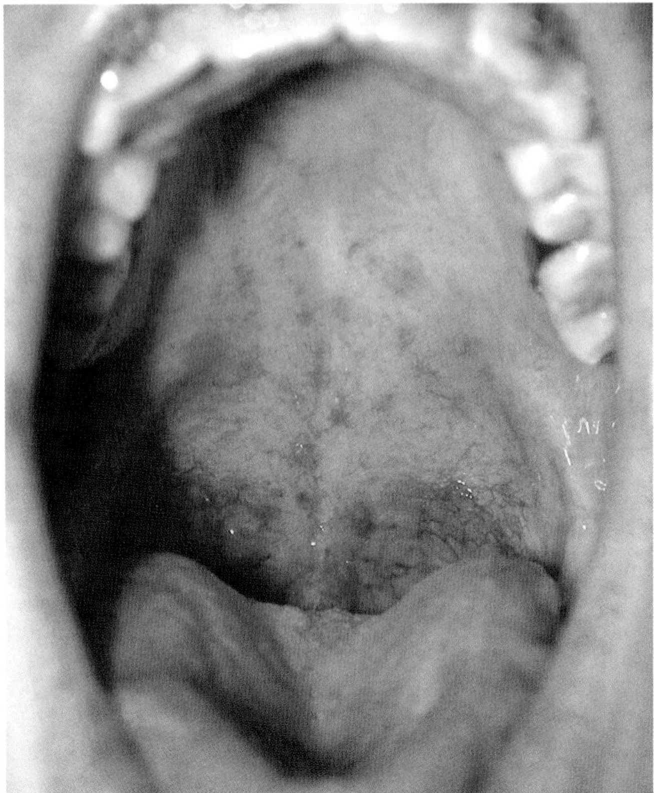

FIGURE 29-7 Viral pharyngitis with prominent vascular injection of the soft palate and lymphoid hyperplasia. (*Used with permission from Richard P. Usatine, MD.*)

may benefit from having a specific viral etiology identified. In these cases, a nasopharyngeal swab or washing for respiratory viruses can be obtained. Direct fluorescent antibody tests, real-time polymerase chain reaction testing, or viral cultures are the most commonly used modes of viral detection in these settings.

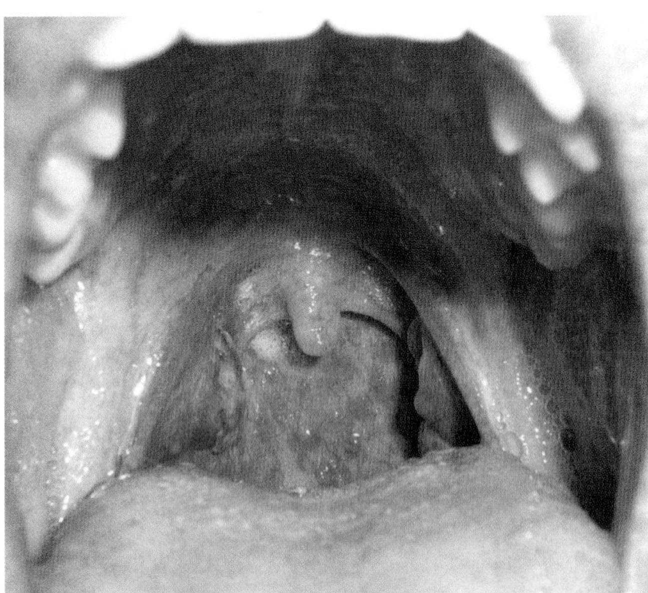

FIGURE 29-8 Strep pharyngitis with dark necrotic area on right tonsil and prominent lymphoid hyperplasia in a cobblestone pattern on the posterior pharynx. (*Used with permission from Richard P. Usatine, MD.*)

- Swabbing the throat and testing for GABHS pharyngitis by rapid antigen detection test (RADT) and/or culture should be performed because the clinical features alone do not reliably discriminate between GABHS and viral pharyngitis. In children and adolescents, negative RADT should be backed up by a culture. A positive RADT does not require a backup culture.[12]
- Diagnostic studies for GABHS are not indicated in children <3 years of age because these infections are uncommon in this age group.[12]
- Diagnostic studies for GABHS are not indicated in children who have symptoms that are consistent with a viral URI, such as rhinorrhea, nasal congestion, and hoarseness.
- Test options for RADT include enzyme immunoassays, latex agglutination, liposomal method, and immunochromatography assays; the latter has the highest reported sensitivity (0.97), specificity (0.97), and positive (32.3) and negative (0.03) likelihood ratios.[12]
- False-positive tests for streptococcal infection can occur when the patient is colonized with GABHS but the bacteria are not the cause of the acute disease (carrier state). GABHS is part of the normal oropharyngeal flora in many school-aged children and the diagnosis of acute streptococcal pharyngitis must include both the clinical signs of acute infection and a positive throat culture. Distinguishing GABHS infection versus colonization can be challenging; the history and physical findings of pharyngitis should be used to determine whether a throat culture should be performed.
- False-negative tests for streptococcal infection can occur when poor sampling technique with the throat swab fails to recover the streptococcal organism despite being the cause of the acute infection.
- Laboratory testing helps confirm the diagnosis of infection with EBV with a differential blood count characteristically showing 50 percent lymphocytosis and 10 percent atypical lymphocytes. Serologic studies include a monospot and serum heterophil antibody titer. Testing may initially be negative and should be repeated in two weeks if clinical suspicion is high.[13]
- Viral cultures from vesicles can be obtained in Coxsackievirus and herpes infections, but the diagnosis is usually based on clinical suspicion and findings.
- Head-neck CT scan or ultrasonography can assist in the diagnosis and localization of peritonsillar abscess and should be obtained if further extension into the deeper neck is suspected such as a parapharyngeal or retropharyngeal abscess.[14]

DIFFERENTIAL DIAGNOSIS

- Allergic rhinitis—Can have similar clinical symptoms as URI but without constitutional symptoms; usually seasonal in nature and family history of allergies is common. Physical exam findings of allergic "shiners" and "nasal salute" can help in the diagnosis (see Chapter 215, Allergic Rhinitis).
- Acute bacterial sinusitis—May complicate URI and manifests as prolonged duration of URI symptoms (greater than 10 to 14 days) or severe symptoms of fever, purulent nasal congestion present for at least 3 to 4 consecutive days in a child who appears ill.
- Infectious mononucleosis—Nausea, anorexia without vomiting, uvular edema, generalized symmetric lymphadenopathy,

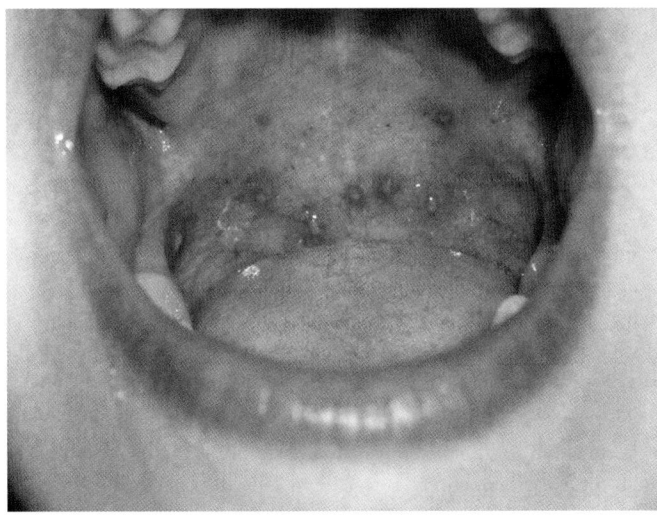

FIGURE 29-9 Herpangina caused by Coxsackievirus virus. (*Used with permission from Emily Scott, MD.*)

and lethargy particularly in teenagers and young adults, is more suggestive of acute mononucleosis (Epstein-Barr virus [EBV]) although the pharyngeal examination has a similar appearance to GABHS (**Figure 29-4**). Tonsils often appear dirty-gray. Hepatosplenomegaly is indicative of EBV in this group. Management is symptomatic and recovery can take weeks. Upper airway obstruction can occur because of enlarged tonsils and adenoids and can be managed with a nasal trumpet and high-dose steroids. Children and adolescents should avoid any physical activity for 4 to 5 weeks because of the risk of splenic rupture[15] (see Chapter 184, Infectious Mononucleosis).

- Herpangina/Coxsackievirus infection—Oropharyngeal vesicles and ulcers indicate herpangina, which is caused by Coxsackievirus A16 in the majority of cases (**Figure 29-9**).
- Oral *Candida*—Whitish plaques of the oropharyngeal mucosa indicate oral *Candida*/thrush, which is mainly found in infants (see Chapter 121, Candidiasis). Risk factors include antibiotic use, immunodeficiency, and use of steroid inhalers.
- Sexually transmitted infections must be considered in the adolescent population—Primary human immunodeficiency virus, gonococcal and syphilitic pharyngitis can all present with the symptom of sore throat. *Neisseria gonorrhoeae* has been detected in 6 percent of adolescents with acute pharyngitis and can manifest with acute exudative tonsillitis.[16] Although uncommon, these diagnoses should be considered in high-risk populations.
- Primary herpes gingivostomatitis causes oral ulcers and pain in the mouth. The wide distribution of ulcers with the first case of herpes simplex virus (HSV)-1 distinguishes this infection from other types of pharyngitis (see Chapter 39, Herpes Simplex Virus Gingivostomatitis and 114, Herpes Simplex).
- *Cytomegalovirus* (CMV)—Primary CMV infection in the immunocompetent host is usually asymptomatic. In the immunocompromised host, CMV can present with a mononucleosis-like syndrome clinically indistinguishable from EBV infection.
- Epiglottitis—Rapid-onset fever, malaise, sore throat, and drooling in the absence of coughing characterize acute epiglottitis, especially when presenting in children. Progression of the disease can lead to life-threatening airway obstruction. Fortunately, this is a rare condition because of the preventive effect of the *Haemophilus influenzae* type b (HIB) vaccine.
- Supraglottitis—Similar symptoms to epiglottitis, although typically seen in adults this can occur in children and adolescents. Sore throat and painful swallowing are the most common presenting symptoms, seen in more than 90 percent of cases. Muffled voice and drooling, dyspnea, stridor, and cough reported in less than 50 percent of cases. No definite organism is identified in the majority of cases. Unlike epiglottitis in children, HIB is responsible for less than 20 percent of supraglottitis cases but still accounts for the majority of positive cultures. Supraglottitis is currently more common than epiglottitis, because of HIB vaccine. Mortality rates have been reported up to 20 percent.
- Diphtheria—A rare condition in the US today, as most patients have been immunized. However, it needs to be considered, especially in unvaccinated and immigrant populations. Pharyngeal diphtheria presents with sore throat, low-grade fever, and malaise. The pharynx is erythematous with a grayish pseudomembrane that cannot be scraped off. Complications include myocarditis resulting in acute and severe congestive heart failure (CHF), endocarditis, and neuropathies.
- Other bacterial causes—Non–group A *Streptococcus*, *Fusobacterium necrophorum*, *Mycoplasma pneumoniae*, *Chlamydophila pneumoniae*, and *Arcanobacterium haemolyticum* have all been isolated as bacterial causes of pharyngitis.
- PFAPA syndrome—The association of periodic fever, aphthous stomatitis, pharyngitis, and cervical adenitis was first described by Marshall et al. in 1987.[17] The hallmark of this condition is the periodicity of its occurrence and abrupt onset high fevers lasting 3 to 7 days and recurring every 3 to 6 weeks. The fever cycle is associated with one or more of the following: aphthous stomatitis, pharyngitis, and cervical adenitis. PFAPA syndrome can also be associated with rashes, headaches, abdominal pain, and arthralgias. Between episodes the child is asymptomatic. On physical exam, the child usually exhibits an erythematous pharynx or tonsils and culture is usually GABHS negative. Treatment with steroids has been used which does shorten the febrile cycle. However, the asymptomatic periods between fevers also shortens. Treatment is usually tonsillectomy; a recent case series showed resolution of symptoms in 99 of 102 patients undergoing this surgery.[18]

MANAGEMENT

NONPHARMACOLOGIC

- Hydration with plenty of liquids.
- Saltwater gargles.

MEDICATIONS

- Age-appropriate dosing of acetaminophen and ibuprofen can be used for symptomatic relief of discomfort, fever, and pain. Doses can be alternated as needed. Aspirin should be avoided in children.

- Antihistamines, decongestants, antitussives, and expectorants are not helpful for the treatment of URI in children and are not recommended.[2]
- Over-the-counter cold and cough medications should not be given to infants because of the risk of life-threatening adverse effects.
- Zinc gluconate has not been shown to be effective for the treatment of URI.[19]
- Steroids (e.g., dexamethasone single 10-mg injection) are recommended for children with infectious mononucleosis who have severe tonsillitis causing airway obstruction. SOR Ⓒ However, there is no strong evidence to recommend steroids for patients with infectious mononucleosis who do not have airway obstruction.[20]
- For suspected or proven GABHS, penicillin V, 250 mg two or three times daily in children weighing less than 27 kg and 500 mg two or three times daily for children and adolescents weighing greater than 27 kg is first-line therapy. Treatment in penicillin allergic individuals should consist of a 10-day course of a first generation cephalosporin if no history of anaphylaxis is noted, or 10 days of clindamycin or clarithromycin or 5 days of azithromycin.[12] In some cases, amoxicillin 50 mg/kg per day in divided doses every 12 hours is preferred over penicillin V because of palatability.
- Various regimens for peritonsillar abscess may be used including Penicillin G in combination with metronidazole, ampicillin-sulbactam, amoxicillin-clavulanate, and clindamycin. Route and duration of therapy varies according to severity, need for surgical drainage, and response to therapy.[21]

COMPLICATIONS

- Bacterial sinusitis and otitis media may complicate URI. New-onset fever and earache may be signs of bacterial otitis media, while persistent nasal symptoms or development of severe purulent nasal drainage for 3 to 4 consecutive days may indicate bacterial sinusitis.
- Viral URI can be an important trigger for an asthma exacerbation in a child with underlying reactive airway disease.
- Peritonsillar abscess—More commonly occurs in patients with recurrent or chronic tonsillitis that is inadequately treated. Infection from the tonsil spreads from the superior pole to the potential space between the tonsil and tonsillar capsule. These usually occur unilaterally and have a characteristic appearance of swelling superiolaterally to the tonsil and deviation of the uvula to the opposite side. Pain is usually severe and involves the ipsilateral ear. Dysphagia, odynophagia, trismus, and drooling are common. Treatment is drainage, usually via needle aspirate or open incision and drainage. If a patient has two or more occurrences, a tonsillectomy is recommended.[22]
- Deep neck infections—A cervical mass, poor range of motion of the neck, high fevers, and any displacement if the pharyngeal walls should raise suspicion. Associated shortness of breath may be a warning sign of impending airway obstruction. Other complications include aspiration, thrombosis, mediastinitis, and septic shock.[14]
- Scarlet fever is secondary to acute streptococcal tonsillitis or pharyngitis with production of endotoxins by the bacteria.[23] An erythematous rash, sore throat, cervical lymphadenopathy, vomiting, headache, fever, erythematous tonsils, and pharynx sometimes associated with a yellow exudate and tachycardia are common manifestations. An enlarged, erythematous tongue with a rash and enlarged papillae is also a common sign (strawberry tongue; see Chapter 28, Scarlet Fever and Strawberry Tongue). Treatment is similar to the treatment of streptococcal pharyngitis.
- Post-streptococcal glomerulonephritis can be seen after pharyngeal or skin infections. The incidence is 24 percent after exposure to nephrogenic strains, but these strains account for less than 1 percent of pharyngeal strains.[23] The condition is due to the presence of a common antigen of the glomerulus with the streptococcus and occurs 2 weeks after the initial infection.
- Pediatric Autoimmune Neuropsychiatric Disorders associated with Streptococcal Infections (PANDAS)—This disorder is characterized by a tic disorder or obsessive-compulsive disorder postulated to be associated with GABHS infection during childhood. Children can also exhibit abnormal movements and other neurologic symptoms. It is postulated that this entity occurs from cross-reaction of antibodies to the basal ganglia, similar what is seen in rheumatic fever movement disorders. It is more common in boys and younger children. The association with GABHS has not been proven however, and antibiotics do not seem to be beneficial. Immunoglobulin, plasma exchange, and tonsillectomy have been proposed for treatment, but there is little evidence for their benefit.[24,25]

REFERRAL

- If signs of airway impairment are present, the patient should be immediately transported to an emergency department. Intubation can be extremely difficult and risky.
- Refer patients with peritonsillar abscess or deep neck abscess to ear, nose, and throat (ENT). Incision and drainage is the treatment of choice in addition to using systemic antibiotics.
- Consider ENT referral for tonsillectomy in proven recurrent or chronic GABHS cases, or under certain other conditions (e.g., antibiotic allergies/intolerances) with recurrence.[26] However, there is no evidence to support tonsillectomy for isolated cases of GABHS.[27]

PREVENTION AND SCREENING

- Influenza vaccine is routinely recommended for all children 6 months and older.

PROGNOSIS

- URI and pharyngitis, regardless of the cause, is typically self-limiting. Typical symptoms last for 10 to 14 days in infants and children.
- Antibiotics shorten the duration of illness in GABHS infection by approximately one day and help to prevent transmission. Most importantly, antibiotic treatment for GABHS pharyngitis greatly reduces the risk of rheumatic fever.[21]

FOLLOW-UP

- Follow-up for new onset of symptoms following a URI may indicate a bacterial superinfection.
- There is no role for test of cure in asymptomatic children following treatment for streptococcal pharyngitis. This practice is likely to lead to identification of streptococcal carriage (which is benign and not associated with sequelae or transmission) rather than true infection.[28]
- Follow-up if clinically deteriorating, especially if swallowing or breathing becomes more difficult or severe headache develops.

PATIENT EDUCATION

- The treatment for most cases of URI and non-GABHS pharyngitis is education. Explain to patients or parents the difference between a viral and a bacterial infection to help them understand why antibiotics were prescribed or not prescribed. Antibiotic treatment for a patient with an obvious viral infection is inappropriate, despite patient or parental requests. Studies demonstrate that spending time to explain the disease process is associated with greater patient satisfaction than prescribing an antibiotic.[29,30]
- Rest, liquids, and analgesics should be encouraged.
- Patients receiving antibiotics should be reminded to complete the entire course, even if symptoms improve. Common antibiotic side effects, like rash, nausea, and diarrhea should be reviewed.
- Patients with mononucleosis and splenomegaly should be warned to avoid contact sports because of the risk of splenic rupture.

PATIENT RESOURCES

- **www.familydoctor.org/familydoctor/en/diseases-conditions/sore-throat.html**.
- **www.nlm.nih.gov/medlineplus/ency/article/000639.htm**.
- Mononucleosis information for patients—**www.nlm.nih.gov/medlineplus/infectiousmononucleosis.html**.

PROVIDER RESOURCES

- Shulman ST, Bisno AL, Clegg HW, et al. Clinical practice guideline for the diagnosis and management of group A streptococcal pharyngitis: 2012 update by the Infectious Diseases Society of America. *Clin Infect Dis*. 2012;55(10):1279-1282.
- **www.aapredbook.aappublications.org/content/**.
- Modified Centor Score for Strep Pharyngitis. Estimates probability that pharyngitis is streptococcal in nature, and suggests management course—**www.mdcalc.com/modified-centor-score-for-strep-pharyngitis**.
- The Modified Centor criteria are:
  - History of fever or temperature of 38°C (100.4°F) (1 point).
  - Absence of cough (1 point).
  - Tender anterior cervical lymph nodes (1 point).
  - Tonsillar swelling or exudates (1 point).
  - Age:
    - <15 years (1 point).
    - 15 to 45 years (0 points).
    - >45 years (–1 point).

The probability of GABHS is approximately 1 percent with –1 to 0 points and approximately 51 percent with 4 to 5 points.[31] Although this scoring system does not adequately predict the presence of GABHS pharyngitis, it does predict the low likelihood of GABHS when the score is low. This may help determine the need for a throat culture or RADT test.

REFERENCES

1. Vital Health and Statistics. US Department of Health and Human Services, Series 13, Number 169 April 2011; Ambulatory Medical Care Utilization Estimates for 2007.
2. Pappas DE, Hendley JO. The Common Cold. In: Long SS, Pickering LK, Prober CG, eds. Principles and Practice of Pediatric Infectious Diseases. 4th edition. Philadelphia, PA: Elsevier/Saunders; 2012.
3. Bottin R, Marioni G, Rinaldi R, et al. Deep neck infection: A present-day complication. A retrospective review of 83 cases (1998-2001). *Eur Arch Otorhinolaryngol*. 2003;260(10):576-579.
4. Richtsmeier WJ, Shikhari AM. The physiology and immunology of the pharyngeal lymphoid tissue. *Otolaryngol Clin North Am*. 1987;20:219-228.
5. Richtsmeier WJ. Human interferon production in tonsil and adenoid tissue cultures. *Am J Otolaryngol*. 1983;4(5):325-333.
6. Ruohala A, Waris M, Allander T, et al. Viral etiology of common cold in children, Finland. *Emerg Infect Dis*. 2009;15:344-345.
7. Gwaltney JM Jr, Phillips CD, Miller RD, et al. Computed tomographic study of the common cold. *N Engl J Med*. 1994;330:25-30.
8. Kristo A, Uhari M, Luotonen J, et al. Paranasal sinus findings in children during respiratory infection evaluated with magnetic resonance imaging. *Pediatrics*. 2003;111:e586-e589.
9. Aung K, Ojha A, Lo C. *Viral Pharyngitis*. http://emedicine.medscape.com/article/225362-overview, accessed March 2013.
10. Halsey ES. *Bacterial Pharyngitis*. Available at http://emedicine.medscape.com/article/225243-overview, accessed March 2013.
11. Guilherme L, Kalil J, Cunningham M. Molecular mimicry in the autoimmune pathogenesis of rheumatic heart disease. *Autoimmunity*. 2006;39(1):31-39.
12. Shulman ST, Bisno AL, Clegg HW, et al. Clinical practice guideline for the diagnosis and management of group A streptococcal pharyngitis: 2012 update by the Infectious Diseases Society of America. *Clin Infect Dis*. 2012 Nov 15;55(10):1279-1282.
13. Ebell MH. Sore throat. In: Sloane PD, Slatt LM, Ebell MH, Jacques LB, eds. *Essentials of Family Medicine*. Baltimore, MD. Lippincott Williams & Wilkins; 2002:727-738.
14. Wang LF, Kuo WR, Tsai SM, Huang KJ. Characterizations of life-threatening deep cervical space infections: a review of one hundred ninety-six cases. *Am J Otolaryngol*. 2003;24(2):111-117.
15. Papesch M, Watkins R. Epstein-Barr virus infectious mononucleosis. *Clin Otolaryngol Allied Sci*. 2001;26(1):3-8.

16. Wiesner PJ. Gonococcal pharyngeal tonsillar infections. *Clin Obstet Gynecol.* 1981;18:121-128.

17. Marshall GS, Edwards KM, Butler J, Lawton AR. Syndrome of periodic fever, pharyngitis, and aphthous stomatitis. *J Pediatr.* 1987;110(1):43-46.

18. Licameli G, Lawton M, Kenna M, Dedeoglu F. Long-term surgical outcomes of adenotonsillectomy for PFAPA syndrome. *Arch Otolaryngol Head Neck Surg.* 2012;138(10):902-906.

19. Caruso TJ, Prober CG, Gwaltney JM Jr: Treatment of naturally acquired common colds with zinc: A structured review. *Clin Infect Did.* 2007;45:569-574.

20. Candy B, Hotopf M. Steroids for symptom control in infectious mononucleosis. *Cochrane Database Syst Rev.* 2006;3:CD004402.

21. Spinks A, Glasziou PP, Del Mar CB. Antibiotics for sore throat. *Cochrane Database Syst Rev.* 2006;(4):CD000023.

22. Sugita R, Kawamura S, Icikawa G, et al. Microorganisms isolated from peritonsillar abscess and indicated chemotherapy. *Arch Otolaryngol Head Neck Surg.* 1982;108:655-658.

23. Palumbo FM. Pediatric considerations of infections and inflammations of Waldeyer's ring. *Otolaryngol Clin North Am.* 1987;20(2):311-316.

24. Perlmutter SJ, Leitman SF, Garvey MA, et al. Therapeutic plasma exchange and intravenous immunoglobulin for obsessive-compulsive disorder and tic disorders in childhood. *Lancet.* 1999;354(9185):1153-1158.

25. Orvidas LJ, Slattery MJ. Pediatric autoimmune neuropsychiatric disorders and streptococcal infections: role of otolaryngologist. *Laryngoscope.* 2001;111(9):1515-1519.

26. Baugh RF, Archer SM, Mitchell RB, et al. Clinical practice guideline: tonsillectomy in children. *Otolaryngol Head Neck Surg.* 2011; 144(1):S1-S30.

27. Neill RA, Scoville C. Clinical inquiries. What are the indications for tonsillectomy in children? *J Fam Pract.* 2002;51(4):314.

28. American Academy of Pediatrics. Group A Streptococcal infections. In: Pickering LK, Baker CJ, Kimberlin DW, Long SS, eds. Red Book: 2012 Report of the Committee on Infectious Diseases. 29th ed. Elk Grove Village, IL: American Academy of Pediatrics; 2012:668-680.

29. Hamm RM, Hicks RJ, Bemben DA. Antibiotics and respiratory infections: Are patients more satisfied when expectations are met. *J Fam Pract.* 1996;43(1):56-62.

30. Ong S, Nakase J, Moran GJ, et al. Antibiotic use for emergency department patients with upper respiratory infections: prescribing practices, patient expectations, and patient satisfaction. *Ann Emerg Med.* 2007;50(3):213-220.

31. McIsaac WJ, Goel V, To T, Low DE. The validity of a sore throat score in family practice. *CMAJ* 2000;163:811-815.

30 ACUTE UPPER AIRWAY OBSTRUCTION

Kshama Daphtary, MBBS, MD, FAAP

PATIENT STORY

A 9-month-old infant is brought to the emergency department because of a 1-hour history of a barky cough and difficulty breathing, which followed a 2-day history of rhinorrhea and low-grade fever. He does not appear toxic, but is tachypneic, and has inspiratory stridor and suprasternal retractions. He is not drooling and has no change in voice. A dose of nebulized epinephrine is administered while awaiting the results of his neck x-ray. The frontal view of an x-ray of the soft tissues of the neck shows narrowing of the subglottic space (Steeple sign) (**Figure 30-1**). A diagnosis of croup is made and the infant is given a dose of dexamethasone orally. Thirty minutes later, his stridor and retractions have resolved.

INTRODUCTION

Upper airway obstruction refers to blockage of any portion of the airway above the thoracic inlet or the extrathoracic airway. It is one of the most daunting emergencies faced by a physician and, if not promptly diagnosed and managed, can progress to hypoxia and can lead to cardio-respiratory arrest and irreversible brain damage. Stridor, suprasternal retractions, and change of voice are the sentinel signs of upper airway obstruction.

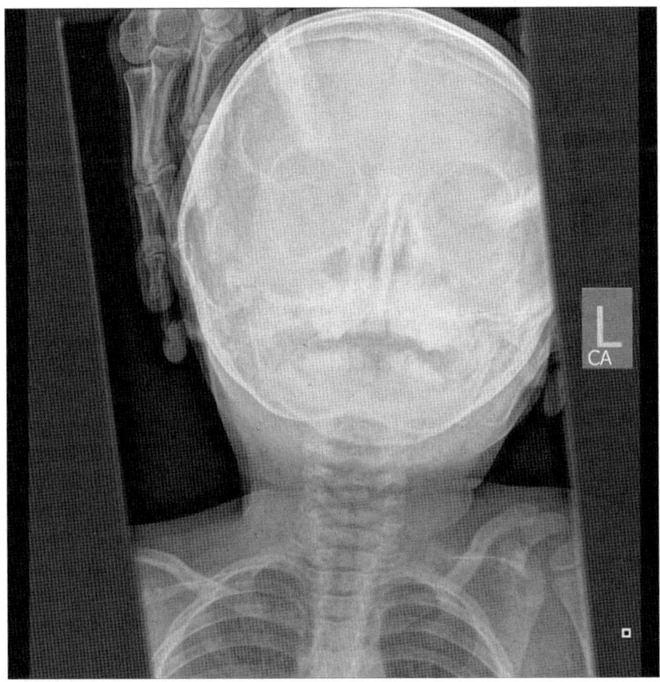

FIGURE 30-1 Subglottic narrowing ("steeple sign") of croup on frontal x-ray of the neck. *(Used with permission from Kshama Daphtary, MBBS, MD.)*

SYNONYMS

- Upper airway obstruction is often referred to as extra-thoracic airway obstruction.
- Croup is also known as laryngotracheobronchitis.
- Epiglottitis is used synonymously with supraglottitis.
- Bacterial tracheitis is also known as bacterial laryngotracheobronchitis or pseudomembranous croup.

EPIDEMIOLOGY

- Upper airway obstruction is one of the most common life-threatening emergencies in children, accounting for up to 15 percent of visits to the emergency department.[1]
- Croup is the most common infection that causes acute upper airway obstruction and has an annual incidence of 18 per 1,000 children in the US; children between the ages of 6 months and 4 years are primarily affected, with a peak incidence of 60 per 1,000 among children 1 to 2 years of age. Although sporadic cases occur throughout the year, croup is epidemic in early fall and winter.[2]
- The incidence of epiglottitis has decreased dramatically, since the introduction of the conjugated *Haemophilus influenzae* type b vaccine, from 41 cases per 100,000 children in 1987 to 1.3 per 100,000 in 1997.[2,3]
- Bacterial tracheitis has an estimated incidence of approximately 0.1 cases per 100,000 children per year and has a peak incidence in fall and winter. Although it affects all age groups, it occurs more frequently in children between the ages of 6 months and 8 years. Retropharyngeal abscess is more common in young children, with the vast majority of cases occurring in patients younger than 6 years of age.[2]
- Peritonsillar abscess is usually a disease of older children and adolescents.
- Foreign body aspiration is a common pediatric problem that has the potential to cause partial or complete airway obstruction. The majority of cases involve the toddler age group. Common foods aspirated are peanuts, popcorn, hotdog, candy, and grapes.

ETIOLOGY AND PATHOPHYSIOLOGY

- Although upper airway obstruction can occur at different levels of the airway, obstruction at the level of the larynx and subglottis assumes the greatest importance because the subglottis is the narrowest portion; therefore, even small lesions can become symptomatic.
- The subglottic region is completely encircled by the cricoid cartilage and cannot expand in diameter. Should inflammation and edema develop, the subglottic airway caliber is substantially reduced as it contains loosely attached connective tissue.
- Narrowing of the airway has an exponential effect on airflow. Poiseulle's law for laminar airflow states that $\Delta P = (Q)\ (8\ \eta l/\ \pi r4)$ where ΔP is the pressure gradient between 2 ends of a tube

TABLE 30-1 Common Causes of Acute Upper Airway Obstruction

Congenital
- Choanal atresia
- Pierre-Robin sequence
- Cystic hygroma
- Laryngeal web
- Vascular ring (**Figure 30-2**)
- Subglottic stenosis (**Figure 30-3**)

Infections
- Croup—Parainfluenza virus type 1 most common, although parainfluenza types 2 and 3, influenza A and B, respiratory syncytial virus, adenovirus, *Mycoplasma pneumoniae*, herpes simplex type 1, and other organisms have also been implicated.
- Bacterial tracheitis—*Staphylococcus aureus* is the most common cause, but *Streptococcus pyogenes*, *Streptococcus pneumoniae*, other alpha hemolytic streptococcal species, *Moraxella catarrhalis*, and anerobes are all possible causes.
- Epiglottitis—*Haemophilus influenzae* type b is the most common causative organism of epiglottitis, although many other agents have been reported, including *S pyogenes*, *S. pneumoniae*, *S. aureus*, *Klebsiella* sp, *Pseudomonas aeruginosa*, and *Candida* sp (**Figure 30-4**).
- Retropharyngeal abscess—Polymicrobial flora including *Staphylococcus aureus*, various streptococcal species, and anaerobes (**Figure 30-5**).
- Peritonsillar abscess—Most often caused by *S pyogenes* (**Figure 30-6**).
- Acute tonsillopharyngitis—Most commonly caused by *S pyogenes*. Polymicrobial infections and viral pathogens are also important sources of infection.
- Infectious mononucleosis—Epstein-Barr virus commonly. The differential diagnosis also includes cytomegalovirus.
- Ludwig's angina—*S aureus*, alpha-haemolytic streptococci, and anaerobes such as bacteroides, peptococci, and peptostreptococci.
- Laryngeal papillomatosis—Human papilloma virus (HPV), usually types 6 and 11 (**Figure 30-7**).

Foreign bodies
- Airway
- Esophageal (**Figure 30-8**).

Vocal cord paralysis
- Secondary to neurological disorders such as Chiari malformation.
- Following surgeries especially cardio-thoracic procedures such as ligation of patent ductus arteriosus and trachea-esophageal fistulas and thyroid surgeries.

Trauma

Burns, inhalational injury

Allergic
- Anaphylaxis
- Angioedema—Allergic, pseudoallergic (secondary to drugs), nonallergic (such as hereditary angioedema with C1 inhibitor deficiency), and idiopathic.

Neoplasms
- Hemangiomas
- Cysts (**Figures 30-9** and **30-10**).

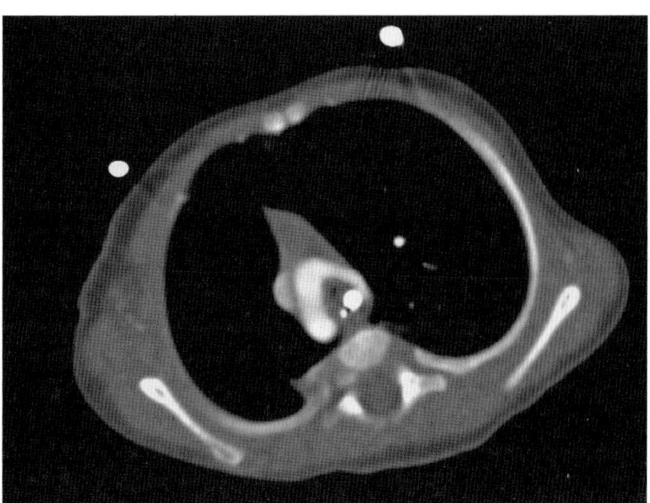

FIGURE 30-2 Vascular ring (double aortic arch) on CT of the chest. This is a cause of congenital upper airway obstruction. (*Used with permission from Kshama Daphtary, MBBS, MD.*)

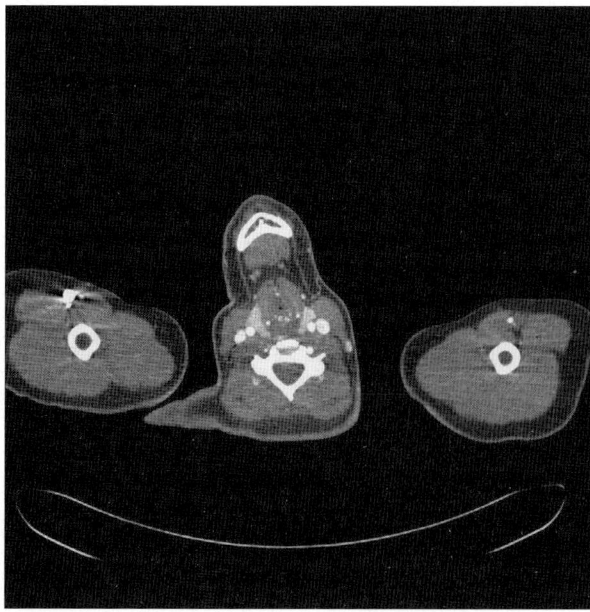

FIGURE 30-3 Subglottic stenosis, another congenital cause of upper airway obstruction, seen on CT scan. (*Used with permission from Kshama Daphtary, MBBS, MD.*)

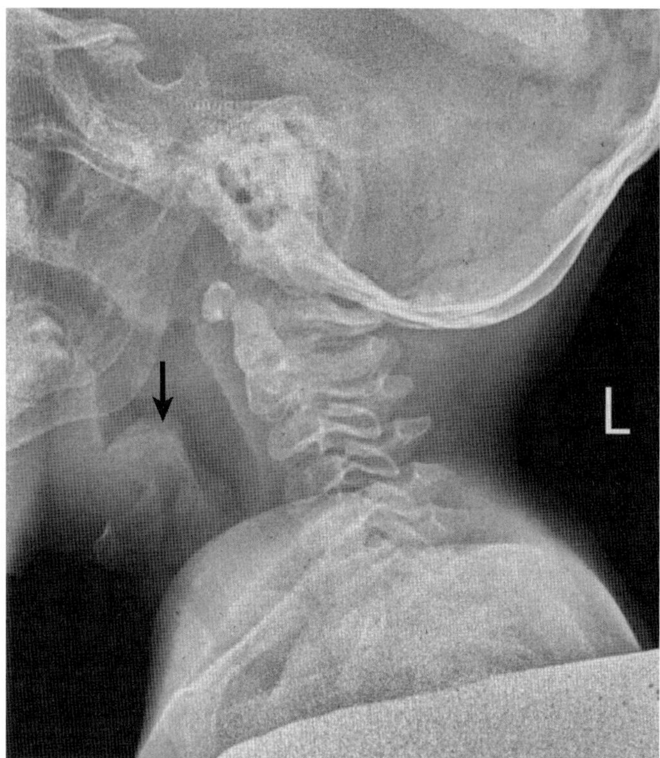

FIGURE 30-4 Epiglottitis characterized by a round, thick epiglottis ("thumb sign") (arrow), loss of the vallecular air space and thickening of the aryepiglottic folds on lateral neck film. (*Used with permission from Kshama Daphtary, MBBS, MD.*)

(airway); Q is the volume of air passing through the tube per unit time (or velocity of flow); r is the radius; η is the viscosity of the medium; and l is the length. Rearranging this equation gives us the determinants of the resistance to laminar airflow, which is $\Delta P/Q = (8\ \eta l/\pi r4)$. However, when airway diameter is reduced, airflow becomes turbulent and the resistance to turbulent flow is inversely proportional to the fifth power of the radius of the lumen of the airway. Thus, a small decrease in the radius of the airway results in a marked increase in resistance to airflow and work of breathing.

- **Table 30-1** shows the common causes of acute upper airway obstruction. The etiology of upper airway obstruction differs by age group with congenital abnormalities predominating in neonates, and infectious agents accounting for the majority of cases in infancy and early childhood.

RISK FACTORS

Acute symptomatic upper airway obstruction can affect a normal airway or one that has chronic but asymptomatic narrowing. Children with the following conditions are at higher risk for developing symptomatic upper airway obstruction:

- Craniofacial anomalies (maxillary hypoplasia, nasal septal deviation, micrognathia, retrognathia (**Figures 30-11** and **30-12**), platybasia, or macroglossia).
- Previous tracheal intubation.
- Neuromuscular diseases.

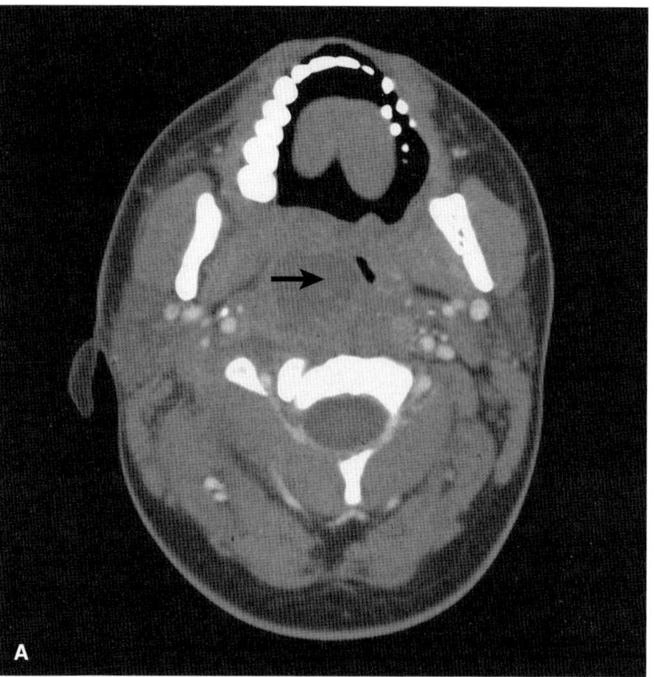

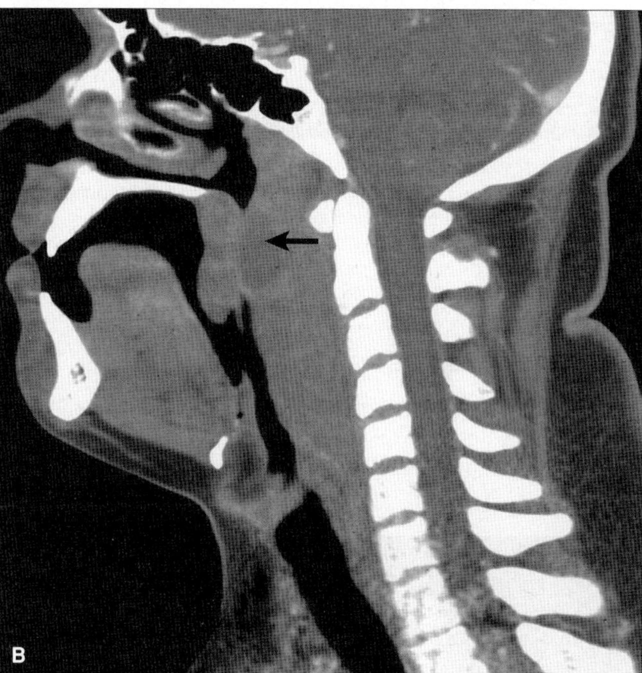

FIGURE 30-5 Retropharyngeal abscess (arrow) on axial cut (**A**) and sagittal cut (**B**) CT scan. (*Used with permission from Kshama Daphtary, MBBS, MD.*)

DIAGNOSIS

CLINICAL FEATURES

Clinical presentation varies depending on the cause, but some features are common to all types of upper airway obstruction. A quick evaluation should be performed to determine the site and cause of obstruction, the severity of obstruction, and the need to establish an airway urgently.

- Patients with upper airway obstruction usually present with stridor, tachypnea, and increased work of breathing.

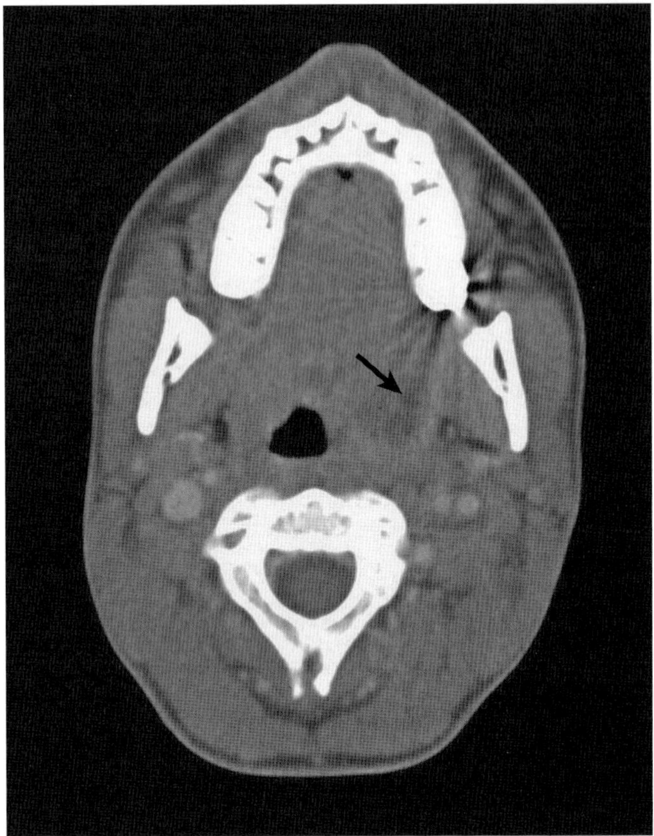

FIGURE 30-6 Peritonsillar abscess (arrow) on CT scan in a child who developed this as a complication of group A streptococcal pharyngitis. (*Used with permission from Kshama Daphtary, MBBS, MD.*)

- A history of choking should be obtained to exclude foreign body aspiration.
- The physician should also enquire about a history of trauma.
- The pattern, severity and duration of fever, change in voice, inability to swallow, presence of drooling, exposure to allergens, and immunization history may offer clues about the etiology.

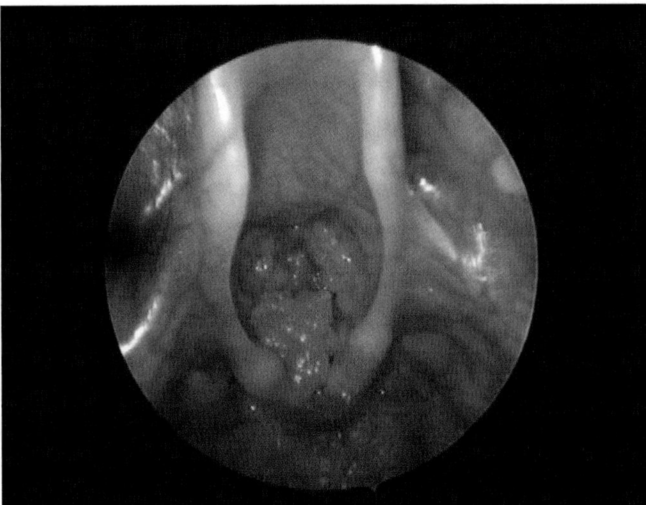

FIGURE 30-7 Laryngeal papilloma (papillomatosis) in an infant exposed to human papilloma virus at birth. (*Used with permission from Paul Krakovitz, MD.*)

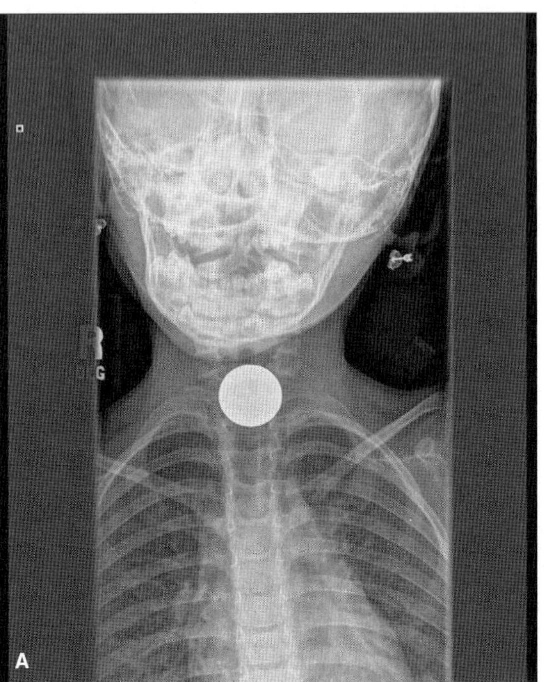

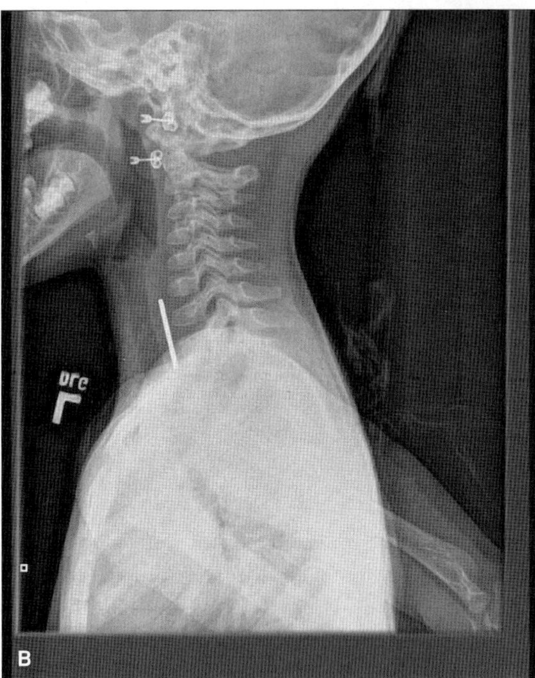

FIGURE 30-8 Esophageal foreign body on Frontal (**A**) and lateral (**B**) views of a chest x-ray in a child who swallowed a coin. (*Used with permission from Kshama Daphtary, MBBS, MD.*)

- Physical examination should be performed preferably with the child sitting on the parent's lap with the chest and neck exposed to minimize disturbing the patient.
- Key physical findings that help in determining the site and cause of obstruction include the physical appearance of the child, the position of comfort that the child assumes, the character of the noisy breathing, characteristics of the voice, the inability to handle secretions, presence of swelling over the face or neck, the use of accessory muscles of respiration, and craniofacial anomalies.

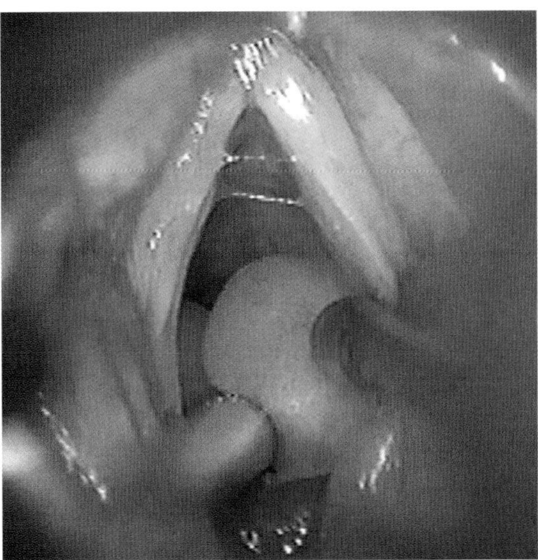

FIGURE 30-9 Subglottic cyst causing upper airway obstruction in a child. (*Used with permission from Paul Krakovitz, MD.*)

- Agitation, confusion, panic, altered state of consciousness, paradoxical breathing, sternal retractions, gasping respiration, and decrease in oxygen saturation are signs of impending respiratory arrest.
- Sudden total obstruction is not infrequent in patients with epiglottitis and foreign body aspiration, and may be precipitated by examination of the pharynx, the supine position or stressful procedures (e.g., intravenous canula insertion). If these conditions are deemed to be unlikely, examination of the pharynx may be carried out.
- Direct visualization of the airway may be necessary and should only be performed by a skilled and experienced practitioner. Flexible fiberoptic nasopharyngolaryngoscopy can be done at the bedside. Alternatively, flexible or rigid laryngoscopy and bronchoscopy may be performed in the operating room and may also prove therapeutic (e.g., removal of a foreign body).
- In an unconscious patient, the first sign of airway obstruction is the inability to ventilate with a bag-valve mask or a jaw-thrust that does not open the airway.

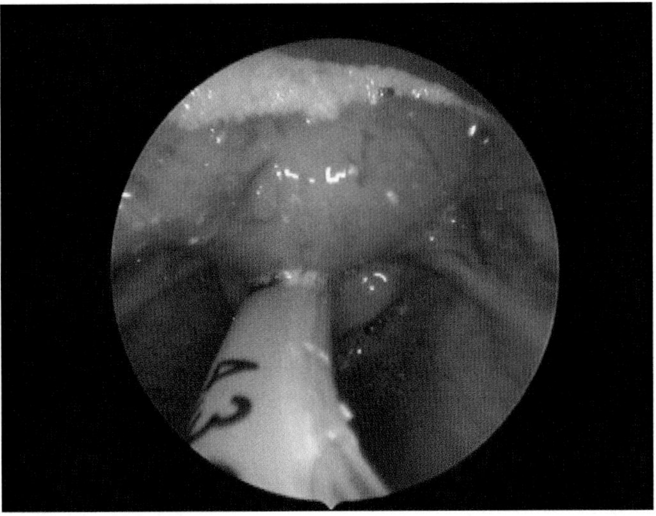

FIGURE 30-10 Vallecular cyst causing upper airway obstruction in an infant. (*Used with permission from Paul Krakovitz, MD.*)

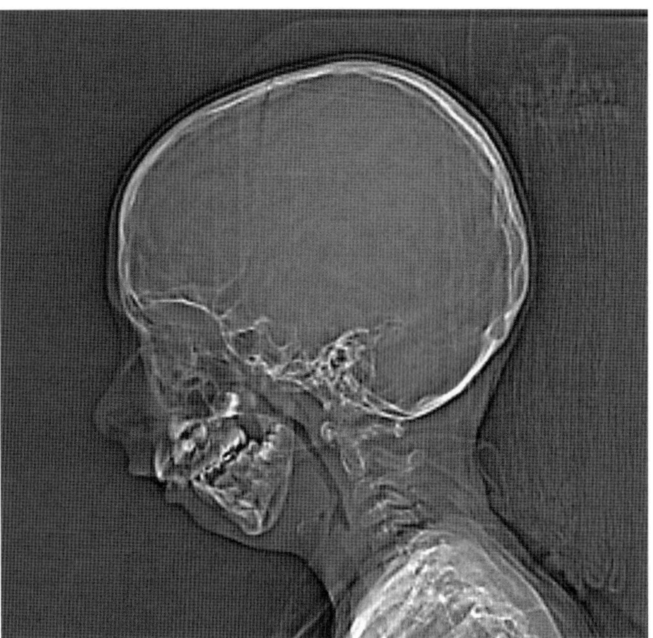

FIGURE 30-11 Retrognathia on scout CT scan. (*Used with permission from Kshama Daphtary, MBBS, MD.*)

LABORATORY TESTING

- No investigation is warranted until the airway is stabilized.
- Blood cultures are generally negative in patients with retropharyngeal abscesses, epiglottitis and bacterial tracheitis.
- Cultures of the affected area usually yield the causative organism.
- The white blood cell count, C-reactive protein and erythrocyte sedimentation rate may be elevated in patients with these infections.
- Blood gas analysis is rarely useful.
- Routine laboratory studies are not indicated in the evaluation of most patients with acute urticaria or angioedema. However, patients with recurrent angioedema without concomitant hives, including patients with angioedema associated with angiotensin-converting enzyme inhibitor should have assays of C4, C1 inhibitor antigen, and C1 inhibitor function. Serum C4 levels are reduced in patients with C1 inhibitor deficiency (hereditary angioedema).[4]

IMAGING

- Imaging should be postponed until the airway is secured in patients who are unstable.
- A physician who is competent in providing airway support should accompany stable patients to the radiology department.
- Plain films of the neck and chest may be useful to identify radio-opaque foreign bodies and to screen for infections that cause upper airway obstruction.
- Computed tomography is useful to diagnose abscesses, magnetic resonance imaging for vascular anomalies; these two tests and echocardiography have replaced barium swallow to diagnose vascular rings.
- The steeple sign or narrowing of the subglottic area on the frontal view of an x-ray of the neck or chest is the classic radiographic finding in croup (**Figure 30-1**).

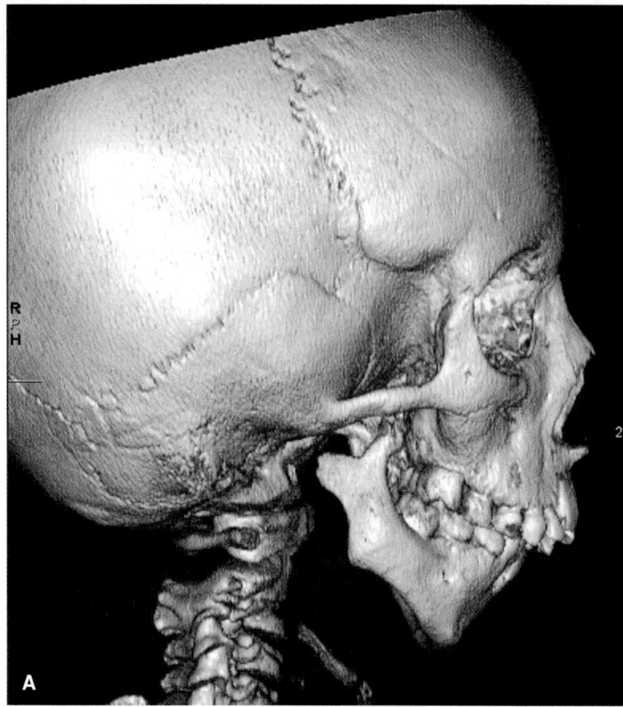

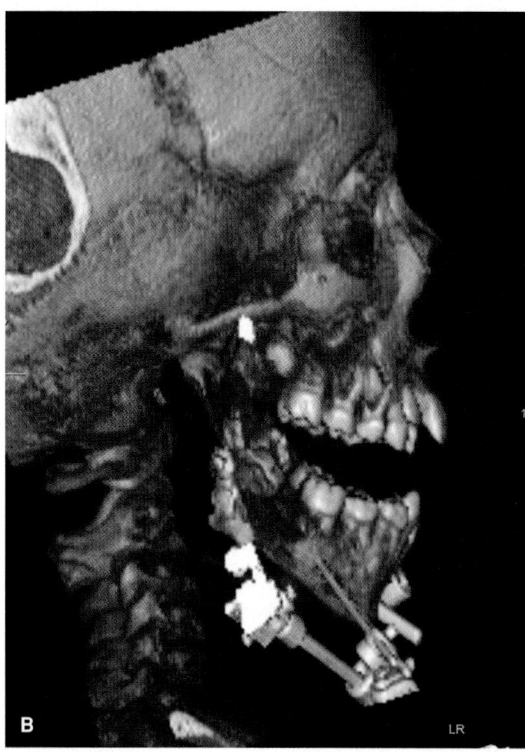

FIGURE 30-12 CT 3D reconstruction of retrognathia before (**A**) and after (**B**) mandibular distraction. (*Used with permission from Kshama Daphtary, MBBS, MD.*)

- A round and thickened epiglottitis (thumb sign), loss of the vallecular air space, and thickening of the aryepiglottic folds are the classic findings on a lateral neck x-ray taken during inspiration with hyperextension of the neck (**Figure 30-4**).
- Bacterial tracheitis may be indistinguishable from croup on x-ray, but in some cases, the tracheal column appears hazy with multiple irregularities within the lumen.
- Increased thickness of the pre-vertebral soft tissue, with or without presence of gas or air-fluid levels and loss of normal cervical lordosis, in a lateral x-ray taken during inspiration with extension of the neck suggests a retropharyngeal abscess.
- Radio-opaque foreign bodies can be readily diagnosed on plain x-rays. Foreign bodies that are flat that are lodged in the esophagus usually assume a coronal orientation (**Figure 30-8**). Esophageal foreign bodies generally obstruct immediately distal to the pyriform sinus, at the level of the aortic arch or at the cardia.

DIFFERENTIAL DIAGNOSIS

Common causes of acute upper airway obstruction can be differentiated on the basis of age of the patient, onset of illness, prodrome, symptoms and signs (**Table 30-2**).

MANAGEMENT

- A child with a respiratory compromise should never be left unattended.
- Efforts should be taken to minimize disturbing the patient unless airway obstruction is life-threatening. Initial evaluation should be directed to making triage decisions about management and further evaluation.
- The unstable child must be evaluated and treated rapidly, with emergency stabilization of the airway receiving the highest priority.
- Patients with airway obstruction leading to respiratory arrest should promptly be ventilated with a combination of bag-valve-mask technique and proper head positioning (slight neck extension, chin lift and jaw thrust maneuvers). Oral and nasopharyngeal airways should be available for use in case of difficulty in bag-valve-mask ventilation.
- A patent airway should then be established under optimal conditions by the physician most experienced in handling difficult airways.
- The stable child with signs and symptoms of airway compromise should be carefully monitored and offered supplemental oxygen in a nonthreatening manner, keeping the patient as calm as possible while definitive treatment is instituted.
- Patients with epiglottitis, Ludwig's angina, facial burns, and smoke inhalation should be intubated early in a controlled atmosphere by an experienced practitioner with a specialist capable of performing a tracheostomy present.

NONPHARMACOLOGICAL

▶ Cool humidified oxygen or air

Cold humidified oxygen or air has been advocated for patients with croup. However, there is evidence showing that there is no benefit.[5–7] SOR Ⓐ

▶ Heliox

- Heliox or helium-oxygen mixture reduces the work of breathing by decreasing airway resistance to turbulent flow across the obstructed airway.

TABLE 30-2 Differential Diagnosis of Common Causes of Acute Upper Airway Obstruction

	Croup	Bacterial Tracheitis	Epiglottitis	Retropharyngeal Abscess	Foreign Body
Age	6 m – 4 y	6 m–8 y	6 m – 4 y	<6 y	Toddlers
Onset	Gradual	Intermediate	Rapid	Intermediate	Sudden
Fever	Usually low	Usually high	High	High	None
Prodrome	Upper respiratory	Upper respiratory	Usually none	Upper respiratory	Choking
Cough	Barking, brassy	Brassy	None	Unusual	Croupy
Appearance	Sick but nontoxic	Toxic	Toxic, assumes 'tripod' position	Sick, muffled voice, neck stiffness, trismus	Nontoxic
Drooling	No	No	Usually	Usually	Variable
Course	Usually benign	May acutely decompensate	Fulminant	Insidious	Occasionally life-threatening
Sore throat	None	Usually absent	Usually severe	Usually	None
Radiographic appearance	Narrowing of the subglottic space (steeple sign) on frontal view	Narrowing of subglottic space, tracheal air column may be hazy, intraluminal irregularities may be present	Round and thick epiglottis (thumb sign), loss of vallecular space, thickening of aryepiglottic folds on lateral view	Increase prevertebral soft tissue space	Flat objects assume coronal orientation when lodged in the esophagus

- It has been used to provide temporary support and management in several conditions that cause airway obstruction including croup and post-extubation subglottic edema.[8] To be effective, the helium: oxygen ratio should be at least 60:40. SOR B

MEDICATIONS

▶ Racemic epinephrine

- Nebulized epinephrine is effective in reducing airway edema due to its vasoconstrictive effect on the vasculature of the airway musculature.
- It leads to a rapid (within 30 minutes) but transient improvement in symptoms for croup.[9] SOR A

▶ Corticosteroids

- Glucocorticoids have been used in the treatment of airway obstruction secondary to edema as a result of infection, allergy, and trauma.[10]
- Glucocorticoids are effective in relieving symptoms of croup within 6 hours.[11]
- The effect lasts about 12 hours and has been found to reduce the need for other drugs and decrease the length of hospital stay or return visits.[11] SOR A
- Glucocorticoids are commonly used to prevent or treat post-extubation stridor.[12] SOR B

▶ Antibiotics

- Third-generation cephalosporins are the preferred agents for epiglottitis. SOR C
- A combination of a penicillin-beta-lactamase inhibitor, such as ampicillin-sulbactam, is the preferred agent for peritonsillar and retropharyngeal abscess. Clindamycin or metronidazole, combined with a third-generation cephalosporin, are alternative therapies for such conditions. SOR C
- Additional coverage against *S aureus* is often required for bacterial tracheitis. In these situations, clindamycin or a penicillinase-resistant penicillin (such as oxacillin or nafcillin) is often combined with a third generation cephalosporin. Vancomycin may be used in patients that appear toxic, have multiorgan involvement, or if methicillin-resistant *S. aureus* is prevalent in the community. In most cases, clinical improvement should be seen within 24 to 48 hours. SOR C

▶ Other

- Patients with angioedema should be treated with histamine blockers (H1 and H2), corticosteroids, and epinephrine if symptoms are severe.
- Drugs that may be responsible for angioedema, such as non-steroidal anti-inflammatory drugs and angiotensin-converting enzyme inhibitors, should be discontinued. Hereditary angioedema may be refractory to this treatment.
- For patients with hereditary angioedema, plasma-derived C1 esterase inhibitors should be administered.[13–15] Recombinant C1 esterase inhibitors, ecallantide and icatibant are recommended in adults but are not currently approved for use in children.[16] If no other treatment that has been proved to be effective is available, fresh frozen plasma should be used.[17] SOR C

- Recurrent laryngeal papillomata are treated with laser or surgical resection. Adjuvant pharmacotherapy with interferon-alfa and antivirals given systemically or intralesional cidofovir may be considered.[18,19] Quadrivalent human papilloma virus vaccine has been used successfully in one patient.[20] SOR B

SURGERY

- Cricothyroidotomy and tracheostomy may rarely be required to establish a secure airway.
- Patients with bacterial tracheitis often require a bronchoscopy for diagnostic and therapeutic purposes.
- Retropharyngeal and peritonsillar abscesses will require surgical drainage.
- Airway and esophageal bodies require removal in the operating room.
- Cysts, webs, hemangiomas, and papillomas will also require surgical intervention.

REFERRAL

- If epiglottitis or Ludwig's angina are suspected, arrangements should be made for immediate evaluation by an anesthesiologist and otolaryngologist to secure the airway in the operating room.
- An otolaryngologist should also be consulted whenever retropharyngeal or peritonsillar abscesses, foreign bodies, subglottic stenosis, vocal cord palsy, or other causes of airway obstruction are suspected that need further evaluation and surgical intervention.
- An allergy and immunology specialist should be consulted whenever hereditary angioedema is suspected.
- A pediatric intensivist should be consulted for all patients with moderate to severe airway obstruction as they need to be monitored in the intensive care unit because of the potential for decompensation.

PREVENTION AND SCREENING

- Most infections can be prevented by maintain good hand hygiene such as frequent hand washing.
- Epiglottitis can be prevented by immunization with the *H. influenzae* type b vaccine.[3] SOR A
- Patients with hereditary angioedema should be counseled and educated about their disease with attention to the identification and avoidance or elimination of precipitating factors that may trigger acute attacks such as trauma, mental stress, infections, angiotensin converting enzyme inhibitors, and estrogen contraceptives.[14,16]
- Patients with hereditary angioedema may require short-term prophylaxis with a plasma-derived C1 inhibitor prior to undergoing a procedure likely to precipitate an attack.[14,16] SOR C
- Regular therapy with plasma-derived C1 inhibitor is the preferred treatment for long-term prophylaxis in hereditary angioedema. Attenuated androgens may be used in children over 16 years of age. The antifibrinolytic drugs, ε-aminocaproic and tranexamic acid, although less effective, may offer some benefit.[16,21]
- Since recurrent respiratory papillomatosis is caused by human papilloma virus, most commonly types 6 and 11, and is transmitted from the mother to the child either in utero or at the time of birth, quadrivalent human papilloma virus vaccine holds promise for preventing recurrent respiratory papillomatosis.[22]

PROGNOSIS

- All patients with upper airway obstruction are at risk of developing pulmonary edema once the obstruction is relieved and should be carefully monitored.[23]
- Once the patient is past the acute phase, complete recovery is expected in most cases of upper airway obstruction.
- Most patients with croup have resolution of symptoms within 48 hours.
- One to eight percent of children with croup are hospitalized and less than 3 percent of the hospitalized patients are intubated.[1] Mortality is low.
- The mortality rate for bacterial tracheitis has been reported as high as 18 to 40 percent. Associated morbidity includes pneumonia, ARDS, septic shock, and multiple organ dysfunction syndrome.[24,25]
- Lemierre's syndrome is an uncommon complication of pharyngotonsillar infections caused most commonly by *Fusobacterium necrophorum* and characterized by ipsilateral internal jugular vein thrombosis and septic emboli most commonly affecting the lung and causing pulmonary abscesses.
- Patients with recurrent respiratory papillomatosis require repeated surgeries, often 20 procedures during their lifetimes.[19] The risk of malignant transformation is less than 1 percent.[26]

PATIENT RESOURCES

- Acute Upper Airway Obstruction—**www.nlm.nih.gov/medlineplus/ency/article/000067.htm**.
- Bacterial Tracheitis—**www.ncbi.nlm.nih.gov/pubmedhealth/PMH0001983**.
- Hereditary Angioedema—**www.nlm.nih.gov/medlineplus/ency/article/001456.htm**.

REFERENCES

1. Zoorob R, Sidani M, Murray J. Croup: an overview. *Am Fam Physician.* 2011;83(9):1067-1073.
2. Rotta AT, Wiryawan B. Respiratory emergencies in children. *Respir Care.* 2003;48(3):248-260.
3. Progress toward eliminating Haemophilus influenzae type b disease among infants and children—United States, 1987–1997. *MMWR Morb Mortal Wkly Rep.* 1998;47(46):993-998.
4. Lang DM, Aberer W, Bernstein JA, Chng HH, Grumach AS, Hide M, et al. International consensus on hereditary and acquired angioedema. *Ann Allergy Asthma Immunol.* 2012;109(6):395-402.
5. Scolnik D, Coates AL, Stephens D, Da Silva Z, Lavine E, Schuh S. Controlled delivery of high vs low humidity vs mist therapy for croup in emergency departments. *JAMA.* 2006;295(11):1274-1280.
6. Moore M, Little P. Humidified air inhalation for treating croup. *Cochrane Database Syst Rev.* 2010;(9):CD002870.

7. Moore M, Little P. Humidified air inhalation for treating croup. *Fam Pract.* 2007;24(4):295-301.

8. Frazier MD, Cheifitz IM. The Role of Heliox in Paediatric Respiratory Disease. *Paediatr Respir Rev.* 2010 Mar;11(1):46-53.

9. Bjornson C, Russell KF, Vandermeer B, Durec T, Klassen TP, Johnson DW. Nebulized epinephrine for croup in children. *Cochrane Database of Systematic Reviews* 2011, Issue 2.

10. de Benedictis FM, Bush A. Corticosteroids in respiratory diseases in children. *Am J Respir Crit Care Med.* 2012;185(1):12-23.

11. Russell KF, Liang Y, O'Gorman K, Johnson DW, Klassen TP. Glucocorticoids for croup. Cochrane Database of Systematic Reviews 2011, Issue 1.

12. Khemani RG, Randolph A, Markovitz B. Corticosteroids for the prevention and treatment of post-extubation stridor in neonates, children and adults. *Cochrane Database of Systematic Reviews* 2009, Issue 3.

13. Cicardi, M., Bork, K., Caballero, T., Craig, T., Li, H. H., Longhurst, H., Reshef, A., Zuraw, B. and on behalf of HAWK (Hereditary Angioedema International Working Group): Evidence-based recommendations for the therapeutic management of angioedema owing to hereditary C1 inhibitor deficiency: consensus report of an International Working Group. *Allergy* 2012;67:147-157.

14. Hsu D, Shaker M. An update on hereditary angioedema. *Curr Opin Pediatr.* 2012;24(5):638-646.

15. Schneider L, Hurewitz D, Wasserman R, Obtulowicz K, Machnig T, Moldovan D, Reshef A, Craig TJ. C1-INH concentrate for treatment of acute hereditary angioedema: a pediatric cohort from the I.M.P.A.C.T. studies. *Pediatr Allergy Immunol.* 2013;24:54-60.

16. Longhurst HJ, Farkas H, Craig T, Aygören-Pürsün E, Bethune C, Bjorkander J et al. HAE international home therapy consensus document. *Allergy, Asthma & Clinical Immunology* 2010;6:22.

17. Lang DM, Werner A, Bernstein JA, Chng HH, Grumach AS, Hide M, et al. International consensus on hereditary and acquired angioedema. *Ann Allergy Asthma Immunol.* 2012;109:395-402.

18. Chadha NK, James A. Adjuvant antiviral therapy for recurrent respiratory papillomatosis. Cochrane Database of Systematic Reviews 2012, Issue 12.

19. Venkatesan NN, Pine HS, Underbrink MP. Recurrent Respiratory Papillomatosis. *Otolaryngol Clin North Am.* 2012;45(3):671-ix.

20. Mudry P, Vavrina M, Mazanek P, Machalova M, Litzman J, Sterba J. Recurrent laryngeal papillomatosis: successful treatment with human papillomavirus vaccination. *Arch Dis Child.* 2011;96: 476-477.

21. Larson DA, Derkay CS. Epidemiology of recurrent respiratory papillomatosis. APMIS 2012;118:450-454.

22. Oudjhane K, Bowen A, Oh KS, Young LW. Pulmonary edema complicating upper airway obstruction in infants and children. *Can Assoc Radiol J.* 1992;43(4):278-282.

23. Lang SA, Duncan PG, Shephard DA, Ha HC. Pulmonary oedema associated with airway obstruction. *Can J Anaesth.* 1990;37(2): 210-8.

24. Seigler RS. Bacterial tracheitis: recognition and treatment. *J S C Med Assoc.* 1993;89:83–87.

25. Shargorodsky J, Whittemore KR, Lee GS. Bacterial tracheitis: a therapeutic approach. *Laryngoscope* 2010;120:2498-2501.

26. Cook JR, Hill DA, Humphrey PA. Squamous cell carcinoma arising in recurrent respiratory papillomatosis with pulmonary involvement: emerging common pattern of clinical features and human papillomavirus serotype association. *Mod Pathol.* 2000;13:914-918.

31 CHRONIC UPPER AIRWAY OBSTRUCTION—LARYNGOMALACIA

Anne Hseu, MD
Paul Krakovitz, MD

PATIENT STORY

A 4-month-old infant presents to your office with noisy breathing. His mother notes it began at a few weeks of life and has gradually worsened. The noise is described as a high-pitched wheeze with inspiration. It worsens when the baby is feeding, crying, or supine. Laryngoscopy confirms the diagnosis of laryngomalacia (**Figure 31-1**). The infant is treated with acid suppression therapy. The infant's symptoms resolve by 18 months of age.

INTRODUCTION

Laryngomalacia is a congenital abnormality of the larynx. It results in dynamic collapse of supraglottic structures leading to airway obstruction.

SYNONYMS

Laryngomalacias, Larynx chondromalacia.

EPIDEMIOLOGY

- Most common cause of stridor in newborns, affecting 45 to 75 percent of all infants with congenital stridor.[1]

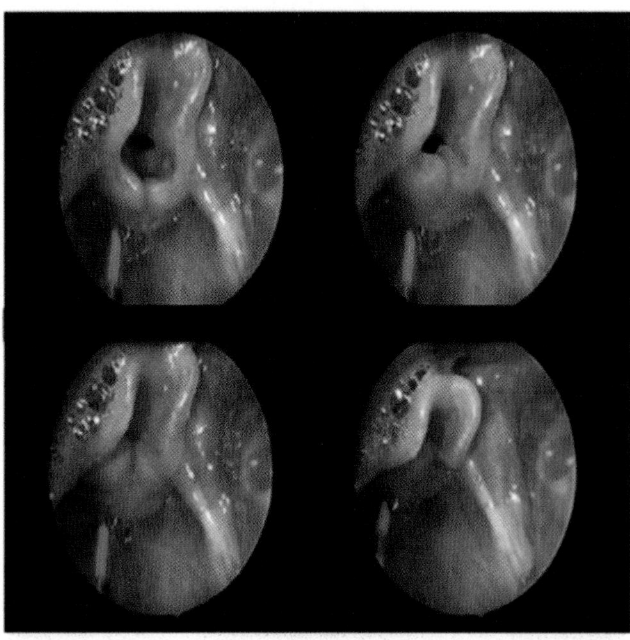

FIGURE 31-1 Multiple views of laryngomalacia in one infant. Note the omega-shaped epiglottis and prolapse of redundant supraglottic tissue into the airway. *(Used with permission from Paul Krakovitz, MD.)*

ETIOLOGY AND PATHOPHYSIOLOGY

- Exact etiology of laryngomalacia is unknown.
- Theories include anatomic displacement of flaccid tissue, immaturity of cartilage, neurologic underdevelopment affecting laryngeal function, and tone.[1]

RISK FACTORS

- Gastroesophageal and laryngopharyngeal reflux.
- Neurologic disease.
- Secondary airway lesions.
- Congenital heart disease.
- Congenital abnormalities/genetic disorders.

DIAGNOSIS

CLINICAL FEATURES

- Presents with inspiratory stridor that typically worsens with feeding, crying, supine, or positioning.
- Symptoms begin within first few weeks of life, peak at 6 to 8 months, and usually resolve by 12 to 24 months.
- Common associated symptoms include regurgitation, coughing, choking, and slow feeding.
- Less common symptoms include respiratory distress, cyanosis, pectus excavatum, and failure to thrive.

PROCEDURES

- Diagnosis suspected by clinical history and confirmed by awake dynamic flexible laryngoscopy.
- Typical features include supraglottic tissue prolapse during inspiration, omega-shaped epiglottis, retroflexed epiglottis, foreshortened aryepiglottic folds, and redundant arytenoid tissue (**Figure 31-1**).
- Based on history, patients may need to be screened for secondary, synchronous airway lesions.

LABORATORY TESTING AND IMAGING

- Usually not indicated. If there is concern for a synchronous airway lesion, may consider bronchoscopy or imaging.

DIFFERENTIAL DIAGNOSIS

- Subglottic stenosis—Congenital or acquired narrowing of the subglottic airway (**Figure 31-2**).
- Tracheomalacia—Flaccidity of tracheal cartilage leading to tracheal collapse especially with increased airflow (**Figure 31-3**).
- Vocal cord paresis or paralysis—Weakness or immobility of one or both vocal cords (**Figure 31-4**).

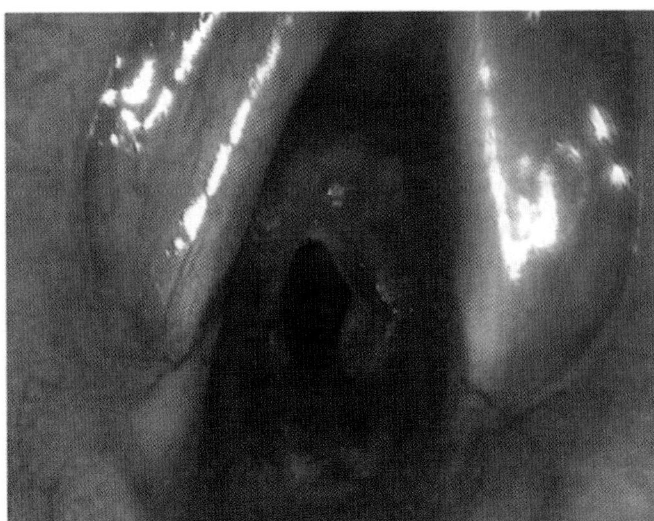

FIGURE 31-2 Subglottic stenosis. Note the true vocal cords laterally and the area of airway narrowing seen just distally in the subglottis. (*Used with permission from Paul Krakovitz, MD.*)

MANAGEMENT

Management depends on categorization of mild, moderate, or severe disease. This is based on associated feeding and obstructive symptoms, not severity of stridor. Factors that are associated with disease severity and progression include APGAR scores, number of medical co-morbidities, presence of secondary airway lesions, and baseline resting oxygen saturation average. Gestational age at birth, birth weight, gender, and race have not been found to influence disease severity.[2]

NONPHARMACOLOGIC

- At the time of disease presentation, approximately 40 percent of infants will have mild disease.[1]
- Seventy percent of these patients will have self-limiting disease and can be managed expectantly.

MEDICATIONS

- Infants with moderate disease are often described as fussy and difficult to feed. Treatment with acid suppression therapy may improve symptoms and shorten the duration of laryngomalacia's natural course.[3] SOR Ⓒ
- Acid suppressive therapy options include H2 blockers such as ranitidine or proton pump inhibitors such as omeprazole.

SURGERY

- Approximately 5 to 20 percent of infants with laryngomalacia present with severe disease and require surgical intervention.[4,5]
- Indications for surgery include recurrent cyanosis, obstructive apneas, aspiration or feeding difficulties, failure to thrive, and cor pulmonale.[4] SOR Ⓐ
- Surgical treatment includes supraglottoplasty where obstructive tissue is removed endoscopically (**Figure 31-5**). Surgery should also include a thorough airway assessment to rule out secondary airway pathology.
- Tracheotomy is usually reserved for supraglottoplasty failures and patients with multiple medical comorbidities. SOR Ⓒ

REFERRAL

- Pediatric otolaryngology consultation for patients who are thought to have moderate to severe disease.

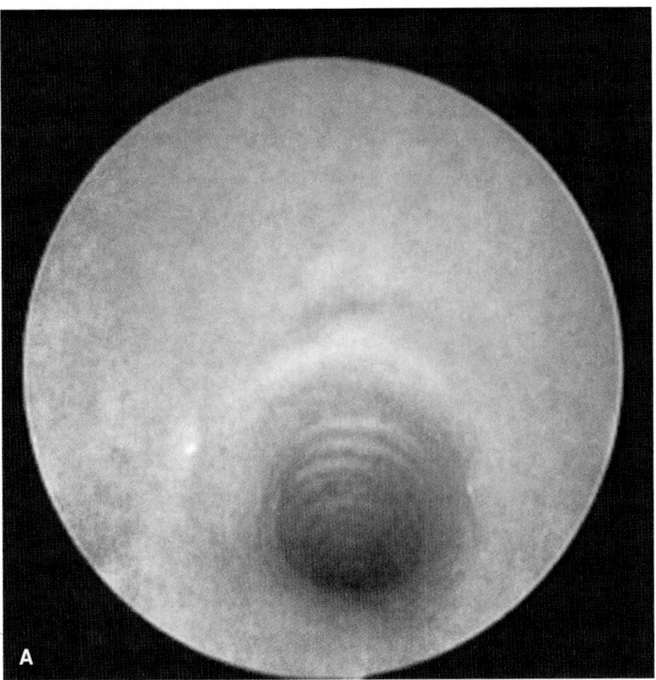

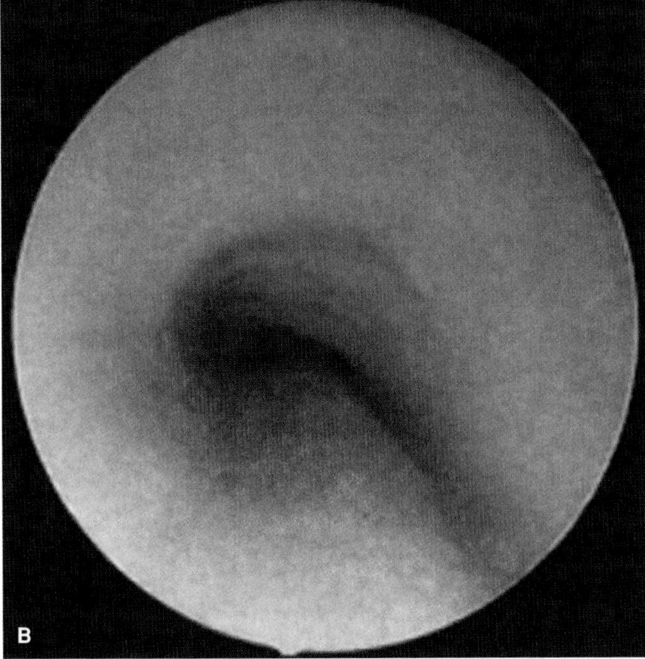

FIGURE 31-3 **A.** Endoscopic view of a normal trachea. **B.** Endoscopic view of tracheomalacia. Note the anterior-posterior collapse of the trachea seen just above the carina. (*Used with permission from Paul Krakovitz, MD.*)

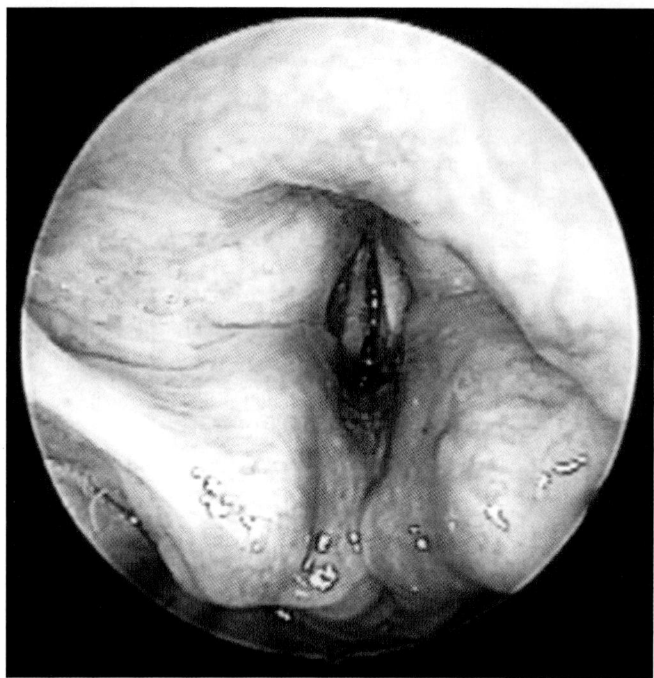

FIGURE 31-4 Bilateral vocal cord paralysis with right and left true vocal cords sitting in a paramedian position. (*Used with permission from Paul Krakovitz, MD.*)

PREVENTION AND SCREENING

- Identify patient factors and symptoms associated with moderate and severe disease that may warrant otolaryngology consultation.

FOLLOW-UP

- Patients with risk factors for severe symptoms and progression warrant close follow-up with otolaryngology.

PATIENT EDUCATION

- Infants with noisy breathing should have a medical evaluation.

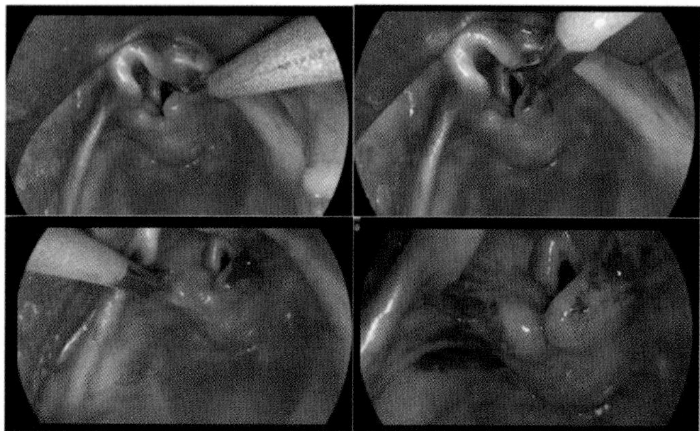

FIGURE 31-5 Supraglottoplasty. Foreshortened aryepiglottic folds are divided bilaterally. (*Used with permission from Soham Roy, MD.*)

PATIENT RESOURCES

- **www.emedicine.medscape.com/article/1002527-overview**.

PROVIDER RESOURCES

- **www.ncbi.nlm.nih.gov/pmc/articles/PMC3299329**.

REFERENCES

1. Landry AM, Thompson DM. Laryngomalacia: disease presentation, spectrum, and management. *Int J Pediatr*. 2012;2012: 753526. Epub 2012 Feb 27.
2. Thompson DM. Abnormal sensorimotor integrative function of the larynx in congenital laryngomalacia: a new theory of etiology. *Laryngoscope*. 2007;117(6):1-33.
3. Thompson DM. Laryngomalacia: factors that influence disease severity and outcomes of management. *Curr Opin Otolaryngol Head Neck Surg*. 2010;18(6):564-570.
4. Richter GT, Thompson DM. The surgical management of laryngomalacia. *Otolaryngol Clin North Am*. 2008;41(5):837-864, vii.
5. Wright CT, Goudy SL. Congenital laryngomalacia: symptom duration and need for surgical intervention. *Ann Otol Rhinol Laryngol*. 2012;121(1):57-60.

SECTION 4 NECK

32 THYROGLOSSAL DUCT CYST AND OTHER HEAD AND NECK MASSES

Karthik Rajasekaran, MD
Peter Revenaugh, MD
Paul Krakovitz, MD

PATIENT STORY

A 6-year-old boy is brought to his pediatrician with a 2-day history of fevers and cough. During the exam, the pediatrician notes a mass in the neck. His father first noticed it this morning. The mass is approximately 2 × 2 cm in size and located at the level of the hyoid in the midline of his neck (**Figure 32-1**). It is well circumscribed, with erythematous, and tender overlying skin. The mass moves when the boy swallows. The pediatrician suspects a thyroglossal duct cyst and refers to pediatric otolaryngology. The surgeon recommends complete excision to the father. After the upper respiratory infection has resolved, the thyroglossal duct cyst is removed completely under general anesthesia with no complications. The boy recovers completely.

INTRODUCTION

Thyroglossal duct cyst is a congenital neck mass that occurs during development, as the thyroid descends from the base of the tongue to its paratracheal location.

SYNONYMS

Ectopic cervical thyroid.

EPIDEMIOLOGY

- It is reported that 7 percent of the population have thyroglossal duct cysts.[1]
- The most common congenital anomaly of the neck in children, representing more than 75 percent of congenital midline neck masses.[2]

ETIOLOGY AND PATHOPHYSIOLOGY

- Between the 3rd and 4th week of gestation, the thyroid gland descends from the base of tongue to its paratracheal location and remains connected by the thyroglossal duct, which involutes between the 7th and 10th week. Failure to involute results in persistence of a portion of this duct, which is known as a thyroglossal duct cyst.
- Thyroglossal duct anomalies commonly present when they become acutely infected as a tender mass in the midline neck near the level of the hyoid. It is postulated that lymphoid tissue of the neck close to the thyroglossal structures reacts to repeated upper respiratory infections and this infectious irritation may stimulate epithelial remnants to undergo cystic change.[3]

RISK FACTORS

- There are no risk factors identified that predispose a child to acquiring this mass.

DIAGNOSIS

A good history of the present illness is paramount in the diagnosis and management of a neck mass. Important details include age that the mass was first noted, clinical signs, rate of growth and constitutional symptoms, recent travel outside of the US, and cat exposure.

CLINICAL FEATURES

- Typically presents after an upper respiratory infection as a painful, erythematous, and tender midline neck mass (**Figures 32-1** and **32-2**).
- It can also appear as a mobile, painless mass in the midline of the neck.
- Associated symptoms that may develop include fever, dysphagia, dysphonia, and/or a discharging sinus.
- Average size is 2 to 4 cm in diameter.
- Movement of the cyst with swallowing is often cited as a reliable diagnostic sign because of the thyroglossal duct's close association with the hyoid bone and foramen cecum.[4]

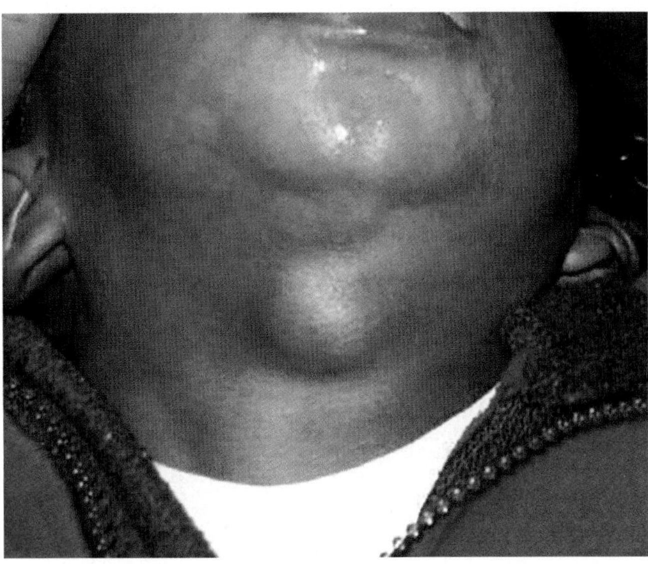

FIGURE 32-1 Thyroglossal duct cyst in a 6-year-old boy. The mass is in central portion of the neck. (*Used with permission from Paul Krakovitz, MD.*)

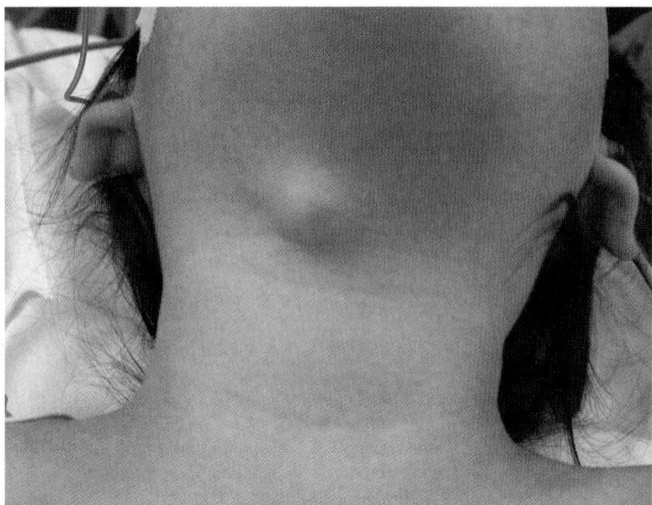

FIGURE 32-2 A thyroglossal duct cyst in a young girl. Note how it is close to the midline. These will move up with swallowing. (*Used with permission from Frank Miller, MD, and Usatine R. Dermatologic and Cosmetic Procedures in Office Practice. Elsevier, 2012.*)

LABORATORY TESTING

- A complete blood count may be useful in identifying an infectious etiology.
- Other laboratory tests that are not particularly required for the evaluation of a midline neck mass but may be helpful in the work-up of other pediatric neck masses are:
  - *Bartonella* titers—To rule out cat scratch disease.
  - *Toxoplasma* titers.
  - Cytomegalovirus (CMV) titers.
  - Epstein-Barr virus (EBV) titers.
  - Monospot.

IMAGING

- Ultrasonography is the investigation of choice for a clinically suspected thyroglossal duct cyst (**Figure 32-3**). It is helpful prior to removal of the cyst to ensure that there is normal thyroid tissue and that the cyst does not represent an ectopic thyroid.
- CT and MRI play a supplementary role to more accurately delineate the anatomy of large cysts, and MRI may be utilized to define a residual sinus tract in cases of recurrent disease.

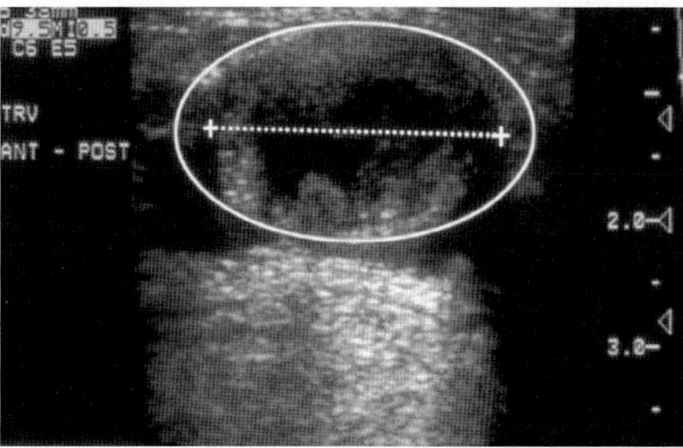

FIGURE 32-3 Thyroglossal duct cyst on ultrasound of the neck. (*Used with permission from Camille Sabella, MD.*)

DIFFERENTIAL DIAGNOSIS

- Mass location may help determine the diagnosis:
  - Midline neck mass.
    - Dermoid—Epithelium entrapped in tissue during embryogenesis. Dermoids are usually attached to the skin.
  - Lateral neck mass.
    - Branchial cyst—Second most common congenital neck mass, which arise from incomplete obliteration of the pharyngeal pouches and clefts during embryogenesis (**Figure 32-4**).
    - Represents 20 percent of congenital pediatric head and neck masses.[5]
    - Similar clinical presentation as thyroglossal duct cyst—Usually presents after an upper respiratory infection as a painful, erythematous neck mass.
    - Imaging and diagnostic work up similar to thyroglossal duct cyst.
    - Treatment is complete surgical excision (**Figure 32-5**).
  - Cystic lymphangioma:
    - Most common lymphatic malformation, usually soft, and fluctuant (**Figure 32-6**).
    - Represents a congenital hamartomatous malformation of the lymphatic system that typically presents during infancy, and has a tendency to grow unless it is completely excised.
    - About 75 percent of all cases are localized in the neck region.[6]
    - Imaging and diagnostic work up similar to thyroglossal duct cyst.
    - Treatment of choice is complete surgical excision.

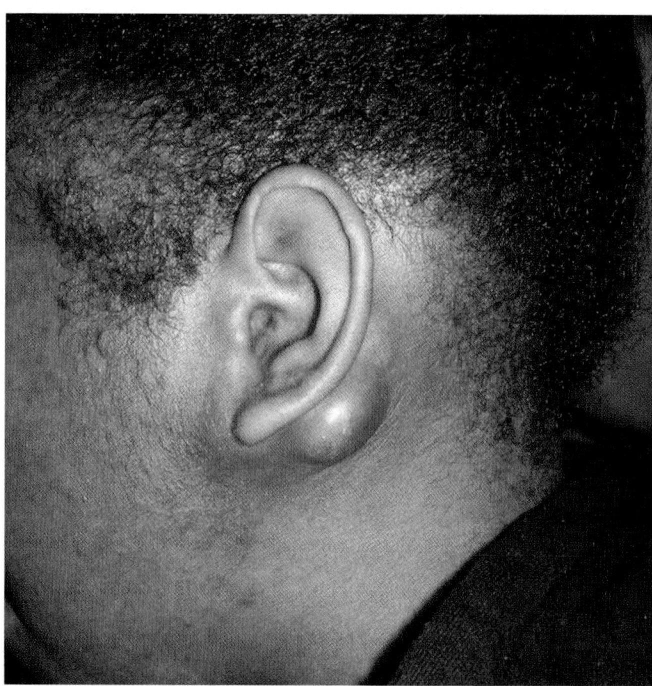

FIGURE 32-4 Type I branchial cleft cyst in the post-auricular area of this child. Typically, these occur in a peri-auricular pattern, more commonly anterior and inferior and down to the jaw line. Differential diagnosis for this location includes lymphovascular anomalies, mastoiditis, dermoid, or epidermal inclusion cysts. The recurrent nature of the abscesses and imaging on this child pointed to the diagnosis of a branchial cleft cyst. (*Used with permission from Paul Krakovitz, MD.*)

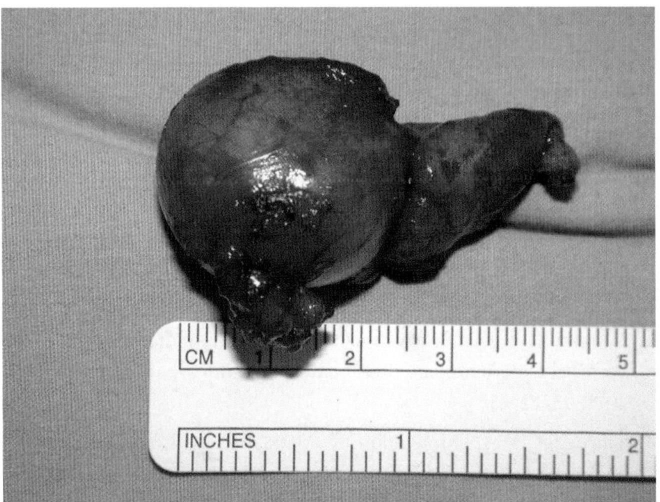

FIGURE 32-5 A branchial cleft cyst after removal. (*Used with permission from Frank Miller, MD and Usatine R. Dermatologic and Cosmetic Procedures in Office Practice. Elsevier, 2012.*)

- Entire neck.
  - Hemangioma—Represents the majority of vascular tumors and present as red or bluish soft multi-locular masses (**Figure 32-7**).
  - Venous Malformation—Lesion that is made up of dilated veins in a disorganized fashion, which readily expand in a dependent position and with raised venous pressure (**Figure 32-8**).
  - Inflammatory adenopathy: most common cause of pediatric cervical adenopathy that comprises a wide variety of clinical conditions (see Chapter 33, Lymphadenopathy).

MANAGEMENT

NONPHARMACOLOGIC

- At the time of presentation, treatment of any acute infection, basic lab work, and possibly imaging would be appropriate first steps.
- Once the infection has resolved, imaging, if not already obtained, can be acquired.

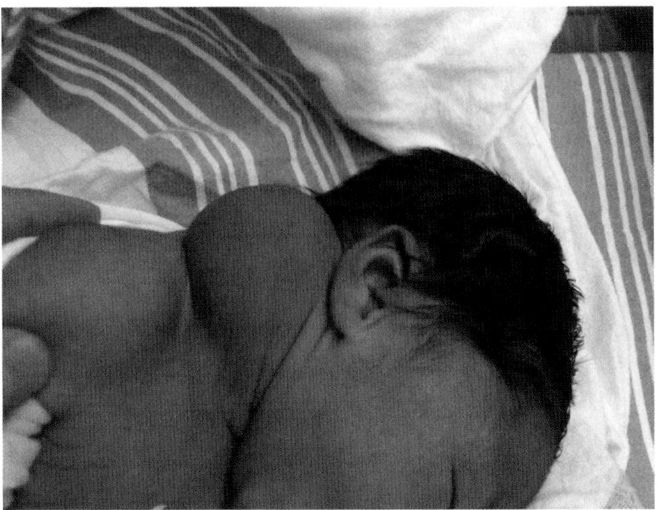

FIGURE 32-6 Cystic lymphangioma in an infant. Note the soft and fluctuant appearance. (*Used with permission from Federico Seifarth, MD.*)

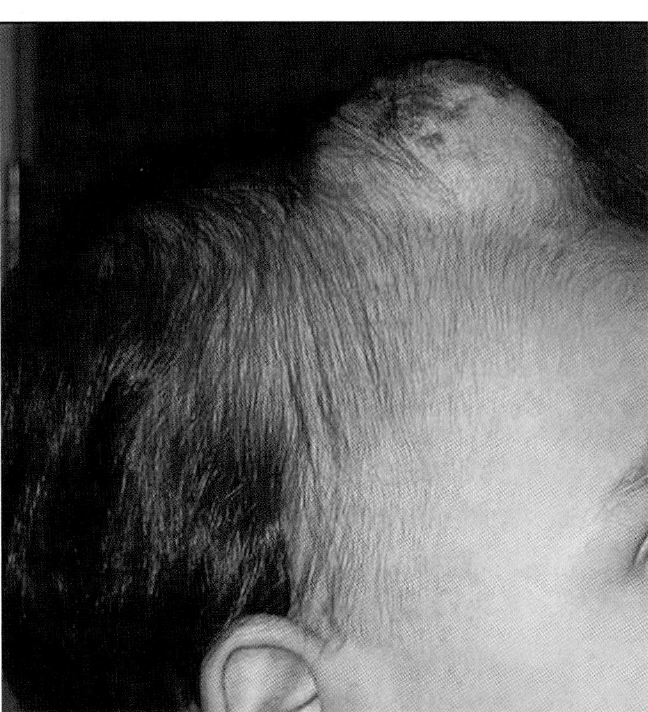

FIGURE 32-7 Classic hemangioma with erythematous cutaneous plaques on a soft tissue mass. (*Used with permission from Paul Krakovitz, MD.*)

MEDICATIONS

- There are no medications that can treat a thyroglossal duct cyst. However, medical treatment of an infection prior to surgical resection is reported to help decrease the rates of post-surgical recurrence.[7] SOR B

SURGERY

- Complete excision is the treatment of choice. Removal of the entire cyst including the central portion of the hyoid bone and focused tongue base excision of the foramen cecum (commonly known as the Sistrunk procedure) is necessary.[4] SOR B

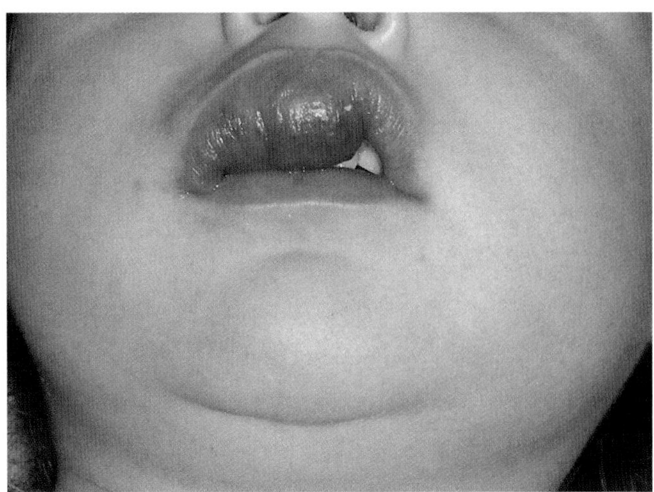

FIGURE 32-8 Venous malformation. Appearance can be similar to hemangioma. However, they have different characteristics on imaging and do not "regress" like a hemangioma. (*Used with permission from Paul Krakovitz, MD.*)

REFERRAL

- Referral to Pediatric otolaryngology is advised when the diagnosis is made or suspected.
- Neck masses that have not resolved with antibiotics may warrant otolaryngology consultation.

PROGNOSIS

- Following complete excision of the thyroglossal duct cyst with the Sistrunk procedure, patients frequently do very well.
- Recurrences after Sistrunk operation are reported to occur in 0 to 12.2 percent of patients, in the most recent literature.[8,9]
- Failure to surgically excise the thyroglossal duct cyst can lead to repeated infections, dysphagia, dysphonia, and/or draining sinus.

FOLLOW-UP

- Only routine follow-up is needed following surgery, provided there is no further evidence of infection or clinical evidence of recurrence.

PATIENT RESOURCES

- **www.thyroidcancer.com/thyroglossal-duct-cyst.html**.

PROVIDER RESOURCES

- Agarwal AK, Kanekar: Imaging of Head and Neck Spaces for Diagnosis and Treatment Submandibular and Sublingual Spaces. *Otolaryngol Clinics of North Am*. 2012;45(6):1311-1323.

REFERENCES

1. Ellis PD, van Nostrand AW. The applied anatomy of thyroglossal tract remnants. *The Laryngoscope*. 1977;87:765-770.
2. Tunkel DE, Domenech EE. Radioisotope scanning of the thyroid gland prior to thyroglossal duct cyst excision. *Archives of otolaryngology—head & neck surgery*. 1998;124:597-599; discussion 600-591.
3. Allard RH. The thyroglossal cyst. *Head & neck surgery*. 1982;5: 134-146.
4. Mondin V, Ferlito A, Muzzi Eet al. Thyroglossal duct cyst: personal experience and literature review. *Auris, nasus, larynx*. 2008;35:11-25.
5. Schroeder JW Jr, Mohyuddin N, Maddalozzo J. Branchial anomalies in the pediatric population. *Otolaryngol Head Neck Surg*. 2007; 37:289-295.
6. Gilbey LK, Girod CE. Blue Rubber bleb nevus syndrome: endobronquial involvement presenting as chronic cough. *Chest*. 2003;124:760-763.
7. Marianowski R, Ait Amer JL, Morisseau-Durand MP, Manach Y, Rassi S. Risk factors for thyroglossal duct remnants after Sistrunk procedure in a pediatric population. *International journal of pediatric otorhinolaryngology*. 2003;67:19-23.
8. Turkyilmaz Z, Sonmez K, Karabulut Ret al. Management of thyroglossal duct cysts in children. *Pediatrics international: official journal of the Japan Pediatric Society*. 2004;46:77-80.
9. Brousseau VJ, Solares CA, Xu M, Krakovitz P, Koltai PJ. Thyroglossal duct cysts: presentation and management in children versus adults. *International journal of pediatric otorhinolaryngology*. 2003;67:1285-1290.

33 LYMPHADENOPATHY

Samantha Anne, MD, MS
David Mandell, MD

PATIENT STORY

A 2-year-old girl presented to her pediatrician with a one month history of swollen glands in her neck and under her arms. Physical examination revealed non-tender firm lymphadenopathy in the anterior and posterior lymph node chains bilaterally (**Figure 33-1**). Work-up revealed anemia, neutropenia and thrombocytopenia. Biopsy of the lymph nodes and bone marrow biopsy showed acute lymphoblastic leukemia. She underwent induction chemotherapy and has responded well.

INTRODUCTION

Lymphadenopathy refers to nodes that are abnormal in either size, consistency, or number. In children, causes of lymphadenopathy can be divided into two large groups-inflammatory versus malignant. Cervical adenopathy due to inflammatory causes is by far the most common. Malignancy is less common but must be considered in the differential diagnosis based on certain concerning features in the history and physical exam.

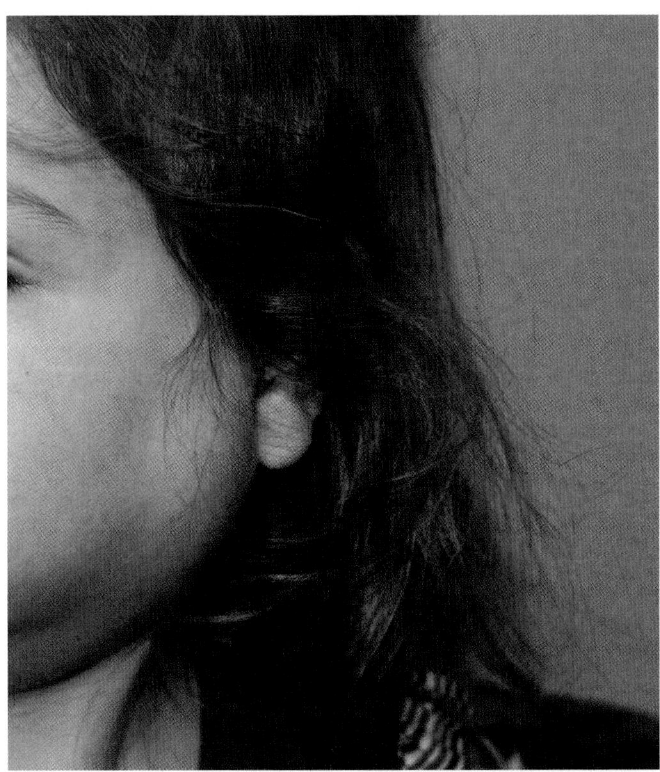

FIGURE 33-1 Firm, nontender pre-auricular and posterior cervical lymphadenopathy in a 2-year-old girl. This, along with pancytopenia, were the presenting features of acute leukemia. (*Used with permission from Camille Sabella, MD.*)

SYNONYMS

Lymphadenitis, lymph node enlargement.

EPIDEMIOLOGY

- Almost all children develop lymphadenopathy at some point during childhood with nearly 2/3 of them developing enlarged nodes within infancy.[2]

ETIOLOGY AND PATHOPHYSIOLOGY

- Lymph nodes are organized centers of immune cells that filter antigenic material such as infectious agents from lymphatics draining from areas of inflammation.
- When activated due to infection or antigenic stimulation, the nodes enlarge in size largely due to proliferation of cells intrinsic to the node such as plasma cells, macrophages, and others.
- Enlargement of nodes can also occur due to infiltration of malignant cells.[2]

RISK FACTORS

- Risk factors for inflammatory causes of lymphadenopathy are most commonly associated with exposure to pathogens.
- Viral illnesses that lead to lymphadenopathy are common in childcare centers.
- Parasitic and atypical infections can occur from a variety of exposures, including *Bartonella henselae* infection from a cat scratch and toxoplasmosis from exposure to cat feces.
- Lymphadenopathy associated with human immunodeficiency virus (HIV) infection can result from perinatal exposure, exposure to intravenous drug use, or unprotected sexual behavior.
- Certain infectious etiologies of lymphadenopathy can be regional in nature, such as exposure to coccidiomycosis in the southwest US and histoplasmosis exposure in the southeastern or central US.
- Medications, such as phenytoin or penicillin, can be associated with the development of lymphadenopathy.
- Odontogenic infections may cause a lymphadenopathy adjacent to the site of the infection.
- Risk factors for malignant causes of lymphadenopathy include exposures to Epstein-Barr virus (EBV) in cases of lymphoma or nasopharyngeal carcinoma.

DIAGNOSIS

CLINICAL FEATURES

- Localized lymphadenopathy occurs in 75 percent of the cases and generalized lymphadenopathy in the rest of the cases.

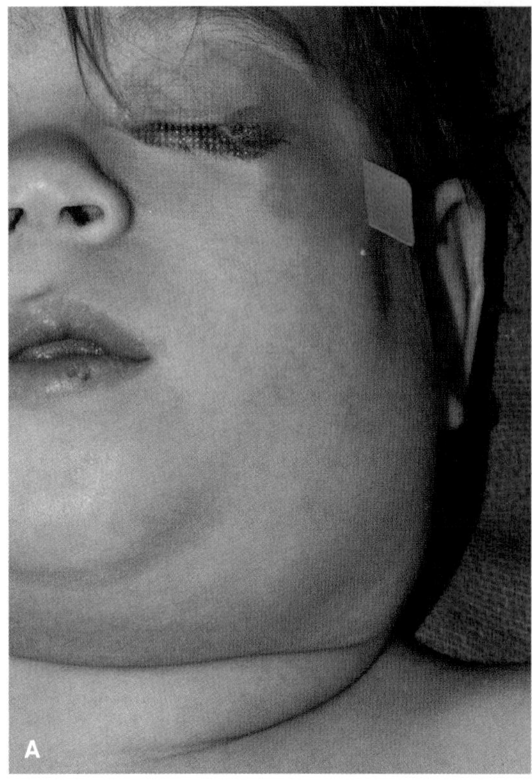

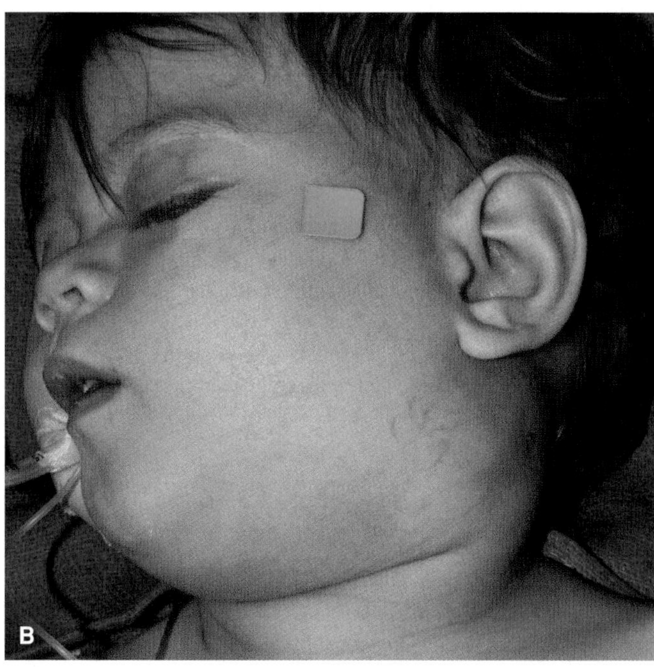

FIGURE 33-2 Unilateral left-sided fullness with confirmed abscess formation in a child about to undergo drainage procedure (**A**). Note the skin blanching due to underlying abscess formation (**B**). (*Used with permission from Prashant Malhotra MD.*)

- Of all the locations that localized lymphadenopathy can occur, head and neck manifestation occurs in 55 percent of the cases.[1]
- Acute unilateral adenopathy is most likely due to streptococcal, staphylococcal, or viral infections (**Figures 33-2** and **33-3**).
- Acute bilateral adenopathy tends to be due to systemic infections, such as infectious mononucleosis or viral upper respiratory infections (**Figure 33-4**).

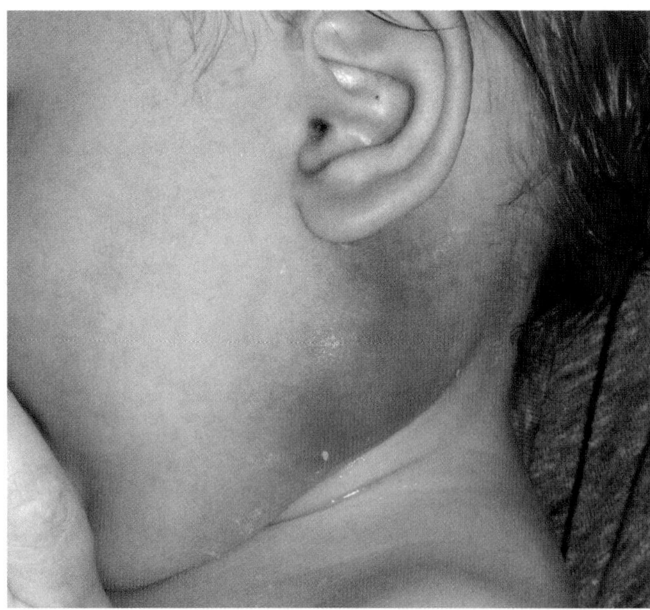

FIGURE 33-3 Acute lymphadenitis and abscess in a 9-month-old infant. (*Used with permission from Emily Scott, MD.*)

- Subacute or chronic lymphadenopathy usually occurs due to slow-growing bacterial or viral infections such as cat-scratch disease or nontuberculous mycobacterial infection (**Figures 33-5** and **33-6**).
- Inflammatory masses are generally tender and mobile. Exceptions include some of the causes of subacute or chronic lymphadenopathy, such as nontuberculous mycobacterial infection, which is usually a nontender lymphadenopathy with fixation of the node to the skin (see **Figure 33-5** and **33-6**).
- Features that may raise concern for the possible presence of malignancy include persistent nontender adenopathy with a size greater than 2 cm, constitutional symptoms such as fevers, night sweats, or

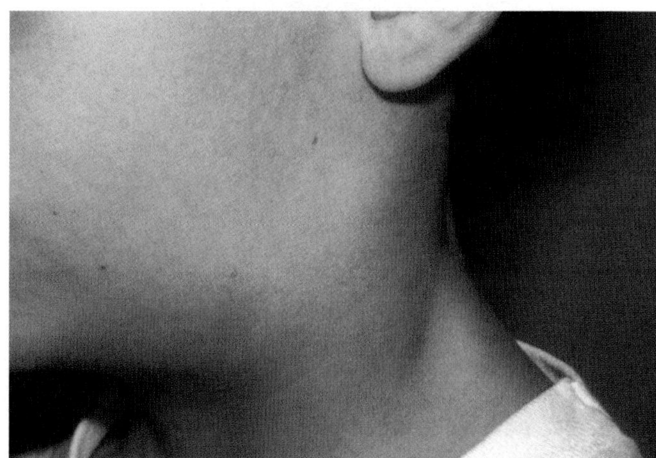

FIGURE 33-4 Anterior and posterior cervical lymphadenopathy in a school-aged child. This is most commonly of viral etiology. (*Used with permission from Johanna Goldfarb, MD.*)

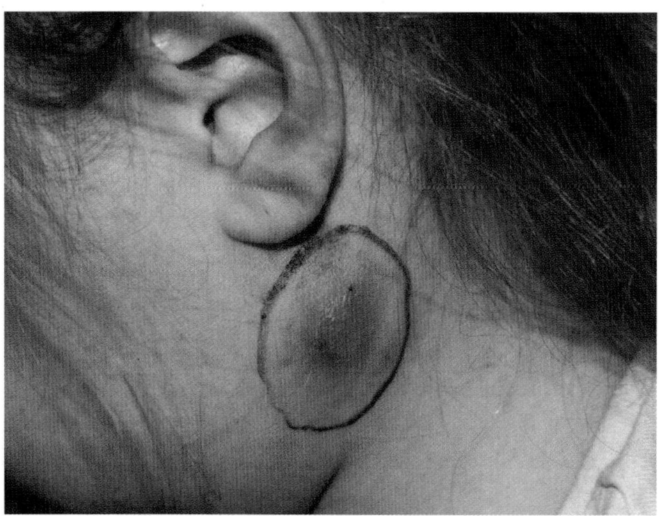

FIGURE 33-5 Subacute, cervical lymphadenopathy in a 3-year-old girl. Note the discoloration and proximity of the lymph node to the skin. This can be caused by cat scratch disease or nontuberculous mycobacteria. (*Used with permission from Camille Sabella, MD.*)

weight loss, and adenopathy in certain unusual locations such as the supraclavicular region and in some cases, the posterior neck.[3]

- In addition, firm, rapidly enlarging, fixed nodes should alert concern for malignancy (**Figure 33-7**).

DISTRIBUTION

- Lymphadenopathy can be divided into level I including submental and submandibular nodes; level II, III, and IV, which include superior, middle, and inferior internal jugular nodes, respectively; level V, which is the posterior triangle, level VI which are the jutavisceral nodes; and, finally, level VII, which are nodes in the tracheoesophageal groove.
- Supraclavicular nodes have traditionally been felt to have a higher incidence of malignancy than other more common cervical locations and further evaluation should be considered even if the size is less than 2 centimeters.

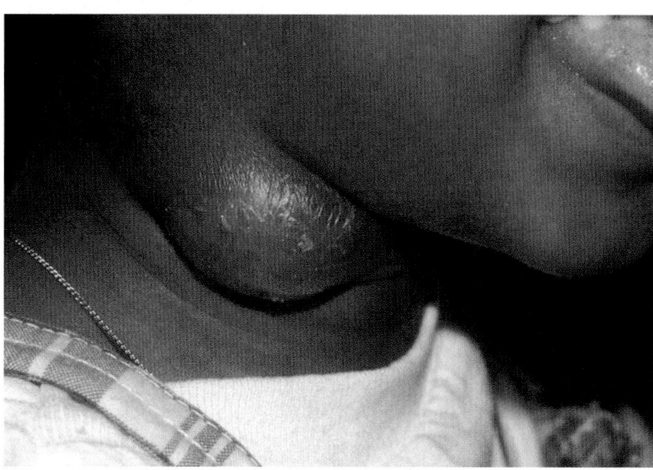

FIGURE 33-6 Nontuberculous mycobacterial adenitis in a young girl. Note the discoloration and the close proximity of the node to the skin. (*Used with permission from Johanna Goldfarb, MD.*)

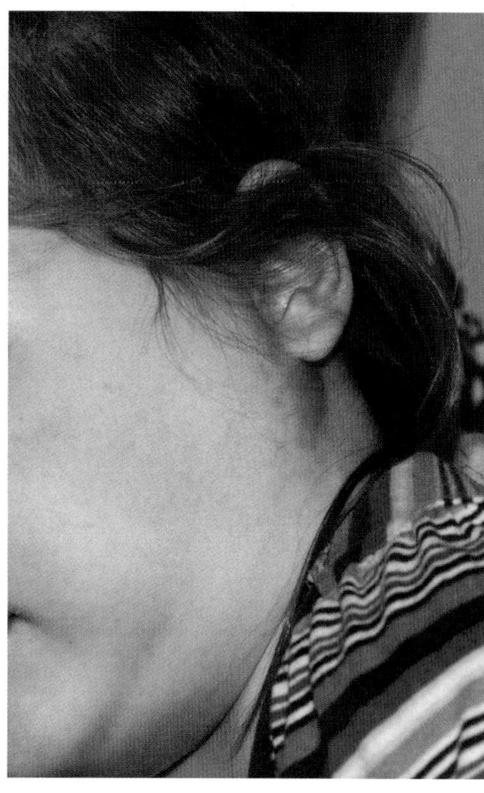

FIGURE 33-7 Rapidly enlarging lymph nodes in the same girl as in **Figure 33-1**. Note the discoloration, likely due to stasis from large matted lymphadenopathy. (*Used with permission from Camille Sabella, MD.*)

LABORATORY TESTING

- Complete Blood Count with differential, serologic testing for EBV, CMV, cat-scratch disease, toxoplasmosis, HIV, and syphilis can be attained based on clinical suspicion.
- Cultures of infected tissue would be helpful in choosing appropriate medications.
- In addition, serum Lactate Dehydrogenase (LDH) can be attained in evaluation for lymphoma and urine VMA when there is concern for neuroblastoma.
- Pathology of the incised lymph node is helpful in ascertaining a definitive diagnosis, especially when malignancy needs to be excluded.

IMAGING

- Chest x-ray is helpful in the evaluation of malignancies, tuberculosis, HIV, and sarcoidosis.
- Computed tomography (CT) of the neck can be attained for infections to differentiate lymphadenitis and cellulitis from suppuration and abscess formation.
- Ultrasound can also make this differentiation and can be a less expensive alternative to CT. The attainment and interpretation of ultrasound results can be significantly operator-dependent (**Figure 33-8**).

DIFFERENTIAL DIAGNOSIS

- Differential diagnosis of lymphadenopathy is extensive but can be differentiated into inflammatory versus malignant causes.

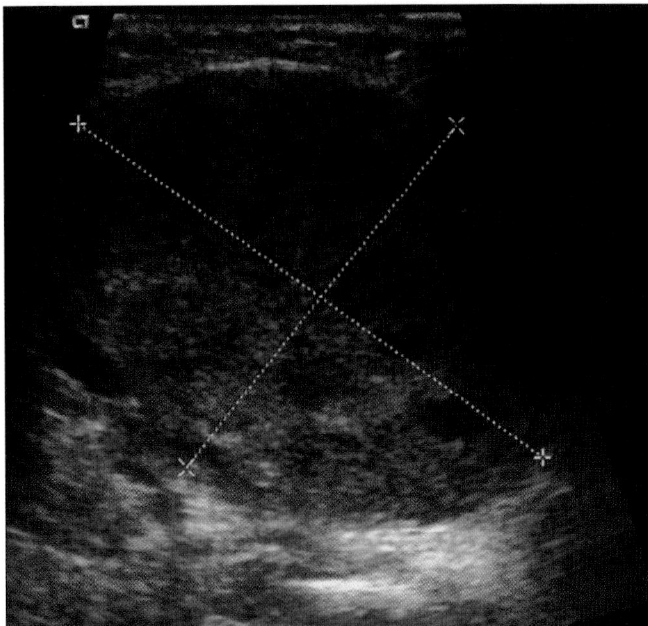

FIGURE 33-8 Heterogeneous enlarged lymph node between the left parotid and submandibular glands on ultrasound in a child with non-tuberculous mycobacterial infection. (*Used with permission from Camille Sabella, MD.*)

- The most common inflammatory causes are due to viral infections, which commonly cause nonspecific, reactive lymphadenopathy and infections with cytomegalovirus (CMV) or EBV or Varicella-zoster virus (VZV).
- The most common bacterial causes of adenopathy are streptococcal or staphylococcal upper respiratory infections, mycobacterial or atypical mycobacterial, cat scratch disease, and bacterial adenitis.
- Fungal infections, especially tinea capitis, can cause lymphadenopathy (**Figure 33-9**).
- Non-infectious inflammatory causes include Kawasaki disease (see Chapter 177, Kawasaki Disease), Kimura disease, histiocytosis, and PFAPA syndrome (see Chapter 176, Periodic Fever Syndromes).[2]
- The most common malignant causes include lymphoma, leukemia, rhabdomyosarcoma, neuroblastoma, and nasopharyngeal carcinoma.

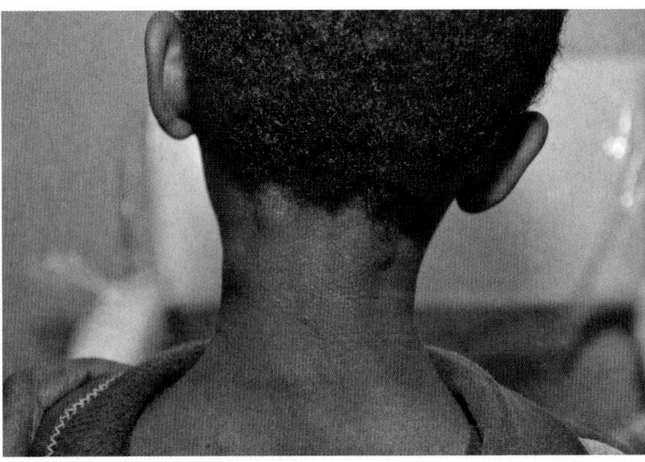

FIGURE 33-9 Occipital lymphadenopathy secondary to tinea capitis. (*Used with permission from Richard Usatine, MD.*)

MANAGEMENT

- Treatment in general is directed toward underlying etiology.
- Early biopsy should be considered when there is involvement of supraclavicular nodes, systemic symptoms, fixation or hard masses, abnormal chest x-ray findings, or rapid enlargement or increase in adenopathy in the absence of obvious infection.[2] SOR C

NONPHARMACOLOGICAL

- Observation and conservative management including rest, hydration, and pain control is reasonable in acute adenopathy from viral causes and with no concerning features in the history and physical exam.
- Reassurance is important to family members since the majority of cases of acute lymphadenopathy, especially in children, are due to transient, self-limited diseases, such as viral upper respiratory infections, that resolve within 4 to 6 weeks without sequelae.

MEDICATIONS

- Treatment of viral lymphadenitis ranges from observation to antiviral medication, depending on the type of virus, the severity of the symptoms, and the immune status of the host.
- Treatment of bacterial lymphadenitis often requires antibiotics, and sometimes surgical drainage.
- Subacute infections, including atypical mycobacterial infection, cat-scratch disease, protozoan and fungal infections, as well as sexually transmitted diseases, may be treated medically and occasionally surgically, depending on the infecting organism, the severity of the symptoms, and the immune status of the patient.
- Autoimmune disorders and malignancies are managed according to current treatment protocols specific for each disease.

SURGERY

- Options include needle aspiration, incision and drainage, incision and curettage, and excision/excisional biopsy (**Figure 33-10**).
- Small unilocular abscesses can resolve with needle aspiration itself followed by antimicrobial/antifungal therapy based on culture results.
- Larger abscesses or abscesses associated with airway compromise, impending complications, or severe systemic illnesses should undergo incision and drainage.[2] SOR B
- Excision of nodes or excisional biopsies should be considered in cases of nontuberculous mycobacterial adenopathy due to incidence of sinus tracts and development of chronic drainage whenever there is concern for malignancy.[2,4] SOR B

REFERRAL

- For head and neck lymphadenopathy, early consult to otolaryngology is important to determine need for surgical intervention and to aid in attaining cultures.
- If concern for malignancy is present, hematology/oncology consultation is important.

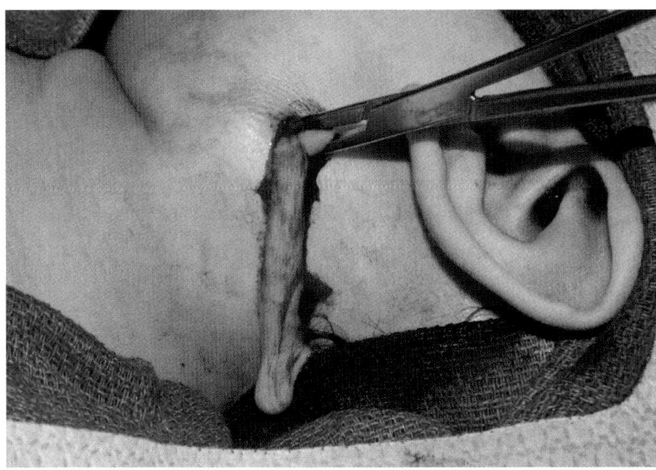

FIGURE 33-10 Abscess of the child in **Figures 33-2**, surgically incised with resultant copious purulent drainage elicited. (*Used with permission from Prashant Malhotra MD.*)

PREVENTION AND SCREENING

- Avoiding sick contacts (including in childcare centers) may reduce the incidence of benign reactive lymphadenitis in children.
- Appropriately timed vaccinations can prevent childhood illnesses associated with lymphadenopathy such as rubella, rubeola, and varicella.

PROGNOSIS

- Complications of poorly managed infectious causes of lymphadenopathy can result in progression of illness resulting in systemic toxicity, suppuration, vascular complications such as venous thrombosis, and/or airway compromise.
- Delay in diagnosis of malignancy can result in progression in stage and worsened prognosis.

FOLLOW-UP

- The type of treatment used, whether surgical or medical, and response to treatment will determine the timing of follow-up and need for further testing.

PATIENT EDUCATION

- Patients (and parents) should be advised to notify their physician with increasing size and number of lymph nodes, development of constitutional symptoms in addition to lymphadenopathy, and with persistence of enlarged lymph nodes.

PATIENT RESOURCES

- **www.webmd.com/a-to-z-guides/swollen-lymph-nodes-topic-overview**.

PROVIDER RESOURCES

- Pocket Guide to Antimicrobial Therapy in Otolaryngology. Head and Neck Surgery. 13th edition, 2007, The American Academy of Otolaryngology.
- Head and Neck Surgery Foundation—**www.entnet.org/EducationAndResearch/upload/AAO-PGS-9-4-2.pdf**.

REFERENCES

1. Ferrer R. Lymphadenopathy: Differential diagnosis and Evaluation. *Am Fam Physician*. 1998;58(6):1313-1320.
2. Rosenfeld RM. Cervical Adenopathy. In: *Pediatric Otolaryngology*. Charles D. Bluestone, Sylvan E. Stool, Cuneyt M. Alper, Ellis M. Arjmand, Margaretha L. Casselbrant, Joseph E. Dohar, and Robert F. Yellon, eds. Philadelphia, PA: Elselvier; 2003:1665-1680.
3. Wetmore RF and Potsic WP. Differential Diagnosis of Neck Masses. In: *Otolaryngology-head & neck surgery*. Paul W. Flint, Bruce H. Haughey, Valerie J. Lund, John K. Niparko, Mark A. Richardson, K. Thomas Robbins, and J. Regan Thomas, eds. Maryland Heights, MO. Elselvier; 2010:1979-1998.
4. Lindeboom JA, Kuijper EJ, Bruijnesteijn van Coppenraet ES, Lindeboom R, Prins JM. Surgical excision versus antibiotic treatment for nontuberculous mycobacterial cervicofacial lymphadenitis in children: a multicenter, randomized, controlled trial. *Clin Inf Dis*. 2007;44:1057-1064.

34 CONGENITAL ANOMALIES OF THE HEAD AND NECK

Karen Hawley, MD
Kyra Osborne, MD
Prashant Malhotra, MD, FAAP

PATIENT STORY

A newborn male, day of life 0, presented with respiratory distress requiring intubation. He was noted to have low set ears, micrognathia, and a cleft palate. Upon closer examination, he was also noted to have a right-sided complete aural atresia and the left canal is stenotic. His midface appeared hypoplastic and he was noted to have a cleft palate. A genetics consult was obtained and the patient was diagnosed with Treacher Collins syndrome (**Figure 34-1**). Surgical repair of palate was performed at 10 months of age, and a softband bone conduction device was provided in infancy for hearing habilitation. The family was counseled regarding ultimate options for reconstruction of microtia and aural atresia.

INTRODUCTION

Congenital anomalies in the head and neck are numerous and varied. In this chapter, we provide a general approach to the diagnosis and management of children with these anomalies and then outline an anatomic approach to considering these abnormalities using some illustrative photographs of those commonly encountered or unique entities.

Consensus terminology is critical for discussion. An anomaly is a structural or functional defect, which is present at the time of birth. A malformation is a major defect that is the result of incorrect morphogenesis. A sequence is a series of defects that occur in a nonrandom fashion. A single event then leads to a series of malformations. Pierre-Robin sequence is an example of a sequence. An association is encountered when there is a tendency of some malformations to occur together more commonly than would be expected by chance, but are not considered to be a part of an established malformation syndrome. An example is the CHARGE association, which includes coloboma, heart anomaly, choanal atresia, retarded growth, genital, or ear anomalies.[1]

DIAGNOSIS

CLINICAL FEATURES

- Congenital anomalies in the head and neck are common and a thorough head and neck examination is recommended.
- An initial airway evaluation for signs of distress or obstruction is essential. This includes observation of retractions and desaturations, listening for stridor, stertor, as well as evaluation of the voice. Stridor is generally a higher pitched sound and can occur during inspiration, expiration, or both. Stertor sounds more like snoring and occurs on inspiration, and is more indicative of obstruction in the nasal cavity, nasopharynx, or oropharynx.

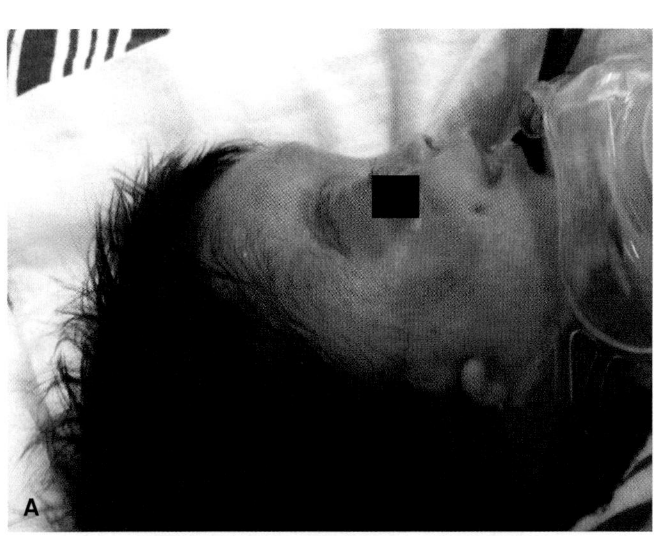

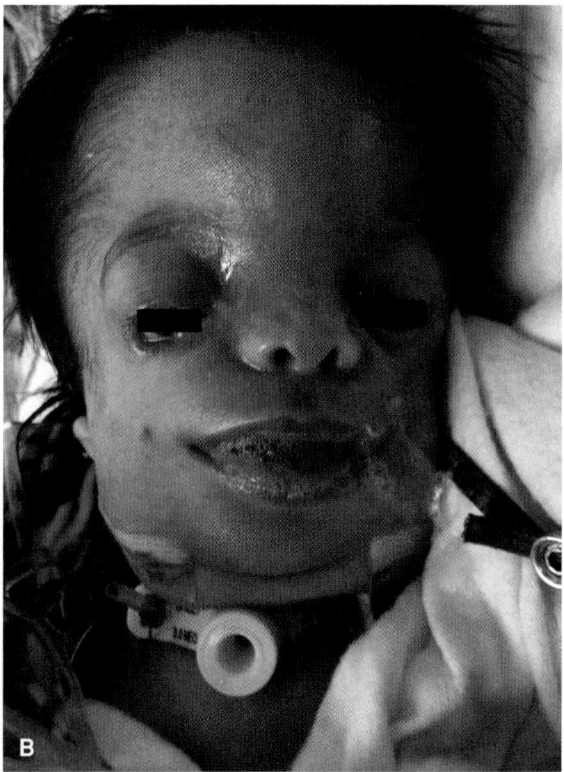

FIGURE 34-1 Treacher Collins syndrome in an infant with severe manifestations, as seen on lateral (**A**) and frontal (**B**) views. Note the microtia (underdeveloped pinna) and aural atresia. Severe maxillary and zygomatic hypoplasia leads to downsloping lateral canthi. This infant also has a facial pit and cleft palate. (*Used with permission from Prashant Malhotra, MD.*)

A hoarse, quiet, or raspy cry may indicate vocal cord pathology such as cord immobility or mass.

- Noting abnormalities in the general appearance of the infant such as facial asymmetry, low set ears, or down-slanting palpebrae may help to identify syndromic pathology. Skin changes such as skin tags, sinuses, and vascular malformations should be noted.
- The ear exam should include not only evaluation of the pinnae, but also assessment of canal patency for atresia. Routine examination of the tympanic membrane and middle ear is also critical. A newborn hearing screen with consideration of both auditory brainstem responses and otoacoustic emissions testing should be discussed with an audiologist or neonatologist if appropriate.
- External nasal examination should include evaluation for pits or central hair, which could be indicative of a nasal dermoid. Anterior nasal rhinoscopy can be performed using an otoscope to assess for nasal mass or lesion. If there is suspicion for nasal obstruction, a 5 or 6 French catheter should be passed. If resistance is met, this may indicate intranasal obstruction. The need for nasal endoscopy can be determined by referral to a pediatric otolaryngologist.
- An oral exam should include visual inspection of the whole oral cavity and posterior oropharynx as well as bimanual palpation of the floor of mouth and assessment of the infant's lip and palate.
- The neck should be evaluated for masses, pits, or draining sinuses.
- As several craniofacial syndromes are associated with ocular abnormalities, routine exam of the eyes should be performed and ophthalmology consultation obtained if needed.
- Any infant with suspected upper airway anomaly should be examined by a pediatric otolaryngologist. In the patient who is awake, a bedside flexible nasolaryngoscopy allows for a dynamic airway exam. If warranted, a complete airway evaluation in the operating room includes a direct laryngoscopy with rigid and/or flexible bronchoscopy. The need for such an exam depends on the clinical scenario and is a decision to be made by the consulting otolaryngologist.

LABORATORY DATA

- Various laboratory data and genetic testing may be obtained depending upon the identified anomaly. This is tailored to the patient and made in conjunction with neonatology, genetics, and other specialty team members.

MANAGEMENT

- The management of congenital abnormalities is specific to each pathologic process.
- A genetics consultation should be initiated if multiple anomalies are identified or if a syndrome is otherwise suspected.
- The appropriate consultations to an otolaryngologist, ophthalmologist, plastic surgeon, or other pediatric specialists will guide nonsurgical and surgical management.
- While cosmetic concerns may be most immediately apparent, functional anomalies related to airway, feeding, vision, and hearing should be prioritized.

HEAD AND NECK ANOMALIES BY ANATOMIC SITE

The more common head and neck anomalies will be discussed by anatomic site. A tabular summary will include basic epidemiology, evaluation, and management.

Congenital Nasal Anomalies (**Table 34-1; Figures 34-2** to **34-4**)

- **Embryology**—At approximately 3 weeks of gestation, the nasal placodes develop as invaginations of neural crest cells from the frontal prominence into nasal pits. These deepen to eventually create medial and lateral nasal prominences. Posteriorly, the nasobuccal membrane forms to separate the nasal and oral cavity. Failure of this membrane to degenerate causes choanal atresia.[2–4]
- The medial nasal prominence will fuse in the midline forming the columella, philtrum, and primary palate. The maxillary prominences fuse in the midline posteriorly creating the secondary palate (posterior to the incisive foramen) and to the medial nasal prominences anteriorly forming the upper lateral lip. Failure of all three fusions to occur (medial nasal prominence to maxillary prominences, left and right, and maxillary prominences in the midline) will create a bilateral complete cleft lip and palate.[2–4]
- Between the superior aspect of the nasal bone and the inferior aspect of the frontal bone there is a transient fontanelle. A pyramidal shaped extension of dura extends inferiorly toward the osseocartilaginous junction of the nasal bridge. This is temporarily congruent with the epidermal elements of the nasal dorsum and protrudes through the skull base at the foramen cecum. Failure of these layers to separate can cause a variety of midline nasal masses such as dermoids and neurogenic nasal deformities.[3,5]

Congenital Ear Anomalies (**Table 34-2; Figures 34-5** and **34-6**)

- **Embryology**—The otic placode is present at the third week of gestation. The auricle is derived from the six hillocks of His, from the first and second branchial arches, that are present by the sixth week of gestation. These form the tragus, antitragus, antihelix, helix, lobule, and the helical crus. The hillocks have fused by week 12. Cartilage formation begins in the 7th week of gestation.[6]

Congenital Oral/Oropharyngeal Anomalies (**Table 34-3; Figures 34-7** through **34-13**)

- **Embryology**—The mandible is derived from Meckel's cartilage, which is the lower portion of the first branchial arch. Development takes place from the 4th to 10th week of gestation. The tongue is actually derived from branchial arches 1 to 4 as well as occipital stomites (masses of mesoderm along sides of neural tube). The tongue originally forms in the nasal cavity and as the palatine shelves join in the midline, the tongue is pushed inferiorly into the oral cavity. See the preceding nasal/oral embryology for more detail. In the setting of Pierre Robin Sequence, it is hypothesized that relative macroglossia prevents the palatine shelves of the maxillary prominences from fusing, creating a midline cleft palate.[12]

Congenital Cervical Anomalies (**Table 34-4; Figures 34-14** through **34-18**)

- **Embryology**—The thyroid gland forms from a diverticulum arising between the anterior 2/3 and posterior 1/3 muscle tongue. This

TABLE 34-1 Congenital Nasal Anomalies[2]

Anomaly	Epidemiology	Presentation	Evaluation	Treatment
Pyriform Aperture Stenosis Narrowing of anterior bony openings to nasal passages from overgrowth of nasal processes of maxilla (**Figure 34-2**)	• Rare; case reports and series	• Respiratory distress • Cyclical cyanosis • Apnea • Poor feeding • Narrow anterior nasal openings • Central solitary central maxillary incisor (SCMI)	• CT scan • Look for solitary central maxillary incisor (SCMI) • If SCMI present, MRI to r/o holoprosencephaly or other midline defects • Pediatric ENT consult • Consider genetics consult	• Conservative (oral airway, decongestants) vs. surgical opening of pyriform aperture
Choanal Atresia Failure of bucconasal membrane to degenerate, with failure to develop choanal openings in posterior nasal cavity (**Figure 34-3**)	• 1:8000 births • 50 percent have associated congenital anomalies • 2/3 are unilateral	• Respiratory distress • Cyclical cyanosis • Apnea • Poor feeding • May be normal in unilateral atresia • Failure to pass 5 or 6 Fr catheter	• Endoscopic evaluation • CT scan to see bony/membranous • Pediatric ENT consult • Genetics consult to evaluate for CHARGE or other associated syndrome	• Unilateral may be able to be managed conservatively • Bilateral usually requires intubation and early surgical opening of choanae vs. tracheostomy
Nasolacrimal Duct Cyst Cyst formation from distal nasolacrimal duct obstruction – commonly from an imperforate nasolacrimal duct opening	• 8:10,000 • F > M	• Respiratory distress • Cyclical cyanosis • Canthal swelling • Bluish mass • Epiphora	• Endoscopic evaluation • CT scan • Pediatric ENT consult	• Can managed conservative, usually surgical especially when bilateral
Nasal Dermoid Cyst formation from failure of involution of dural diverticulum, with trapping of epithelial remnants (including glands and hair) (**Figure 34-4**)	• 1:20,000–1:40,000 newborns	• Nasal obstruction • Visible mass – can be from glabella to columella • Midline pit +/– hair • Not pulsatile, does not transilluminate	• CT scan • MRI to r/o intracranial extension and differentiate glioma/encephalocele • Pediatric ENT consult • Possible neurosurgery consultation	• Surgical excision

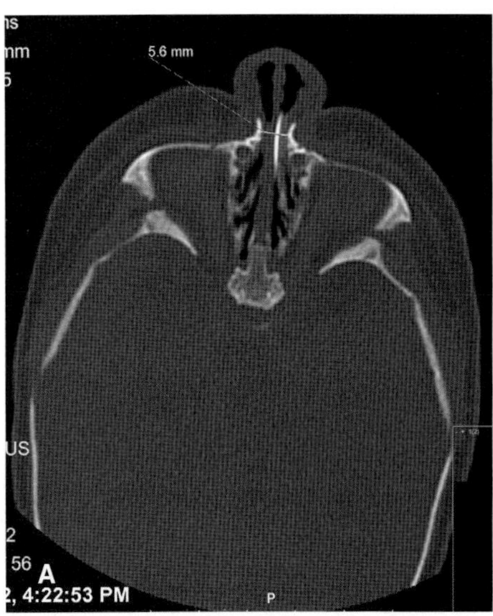

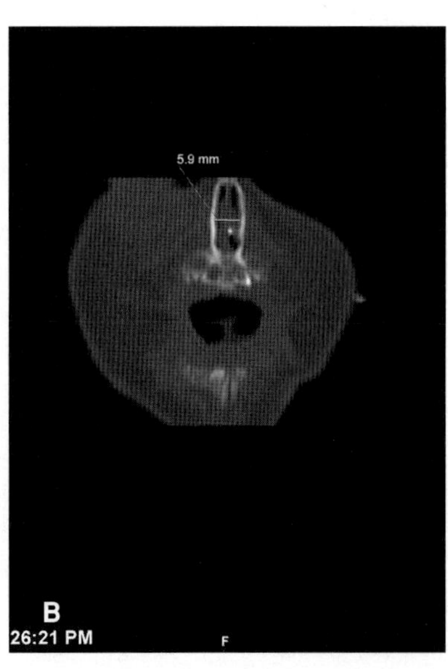

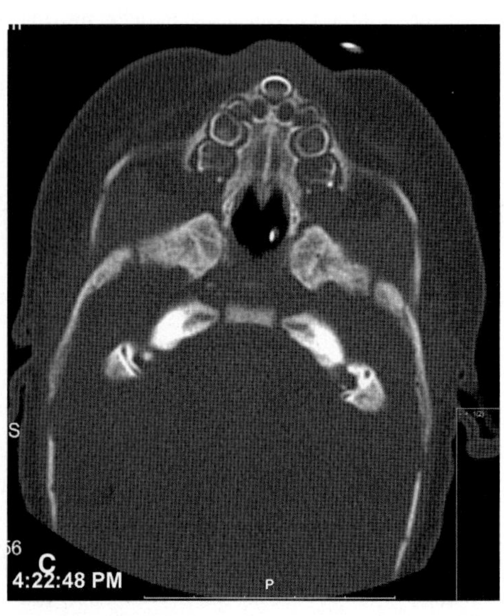

FIGURE 34-2 Pyriform Aperture Stenosis seen on axial (**A**), and coronal (**B**) CT scan in a 2-week-old infant who presented with neonatal respiratory distress and feeding difficulty. A solitary central maxillary incisor seen on axial CT (**C**). (*Used with permission from Prashant Malhotra, MD.*)

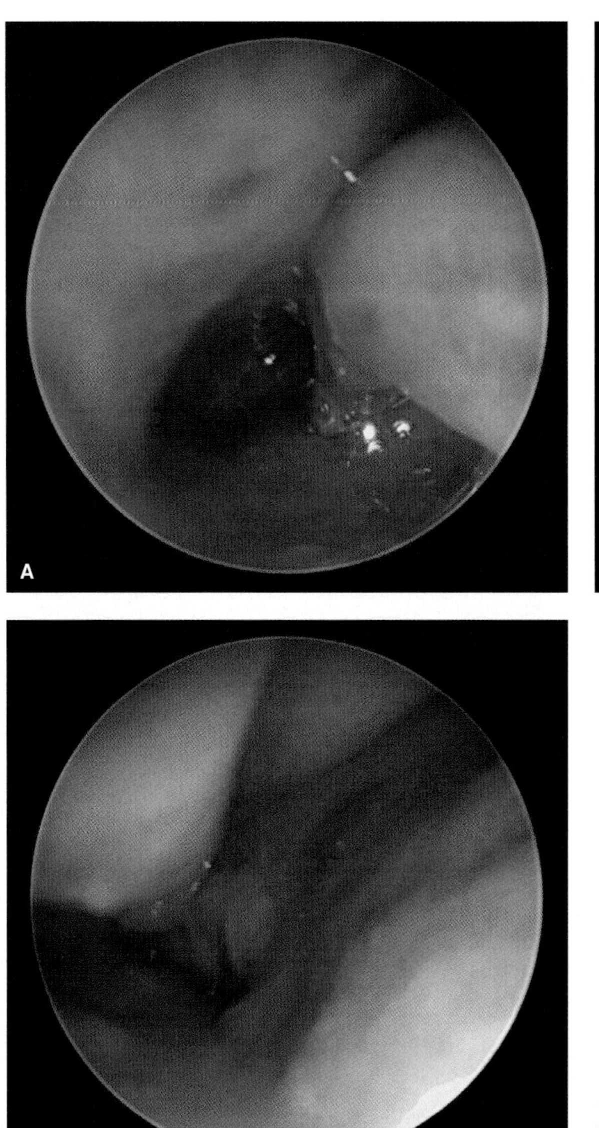

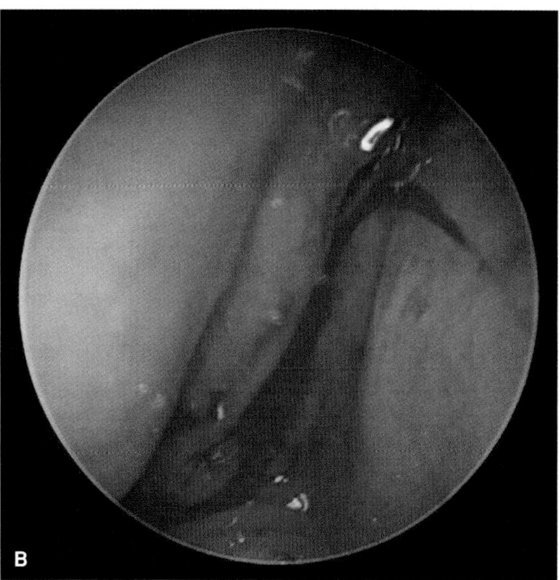

FIGURE 34-3 Left unilateral choanal atresia seen on endoscopy (**A**, **B**). Note inferior turbinate laterally (**A**). The right side is unaffected (**C**) with a patent choanal opening seen behind the turbinate. (*Used with permission from Prashant Malhotra, MD.*)

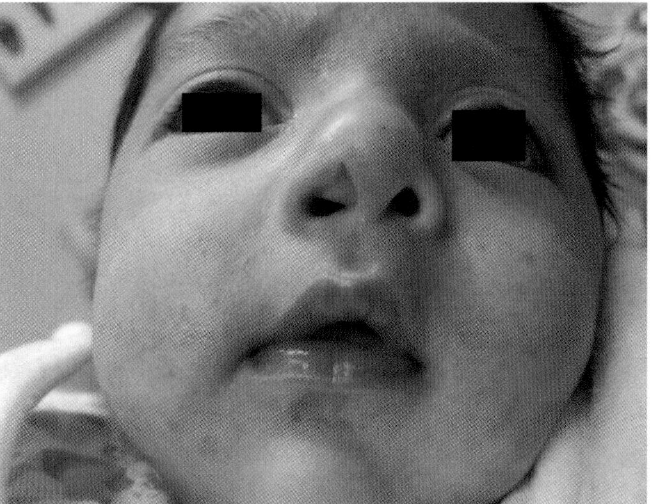

FIGURE 34-4 Predominantly nasal dermoid in an infant causing unilateral nasal obstruction. No intracranial extension was noted. Note the small dimple on nasal tip. (*Used with permission from Prashant Malhotra, MD.*)

TABLE 34-2 Congenital Ear Anomalies[6]

Anomaly	Epidemiology	Presentation	Evaluation	Treatment
Microtia Abnormal development of auricle of ear, from altered development of auricular hillocks (1st and 2nd branchial arches) (**Figures 34-1, 34-5,** and **34-24**)	• 1:10-20,000 births • Unilateral > Bilateral • M > F • ↑ in Japanese, Hispanic, Native American	• Malformed auricle	• Can occur with aural atresia • Associated with other anomalies 50 percent of time • Comprehensive audiologic evaluation • Pediatric ENT/Plastic consult • Genetics consult	• Elective surgical repair usually age 6–7y if desired (for cosmesis) vs. prosthesis
Aural Atresia Failure of external auditory canal to develop, from failure of canalization of epidermal plug in first branchial groove (**Figures 34-1** and **34-24**)	• 1:10–20,000 births • Unilateral > Bilateral • M > F	• Absent or blind external meatus • Conductive hearing loss	• Comprehensive audiologic evaluation • Pediatric ENT consult • CT scan by age 4 yrs (anatomic eval and r/o cholesteatoma)	• Early: Consideration of bone anchored conduction device (for conductive hearing loss) • Critical for bilateral atresia • Age 5–7: Consideration of surgical repair of atresia or implanted bone anchored hearing aid
Prominent Ears Abnormal development of the hillocks of His (**Figure 34-6**)	• 5 percent of caucasians	• Lack of antihelical fold • Overdevelopment of conchal cartilage	• Complete otologic examination	• Otoplasty: age 6–7y

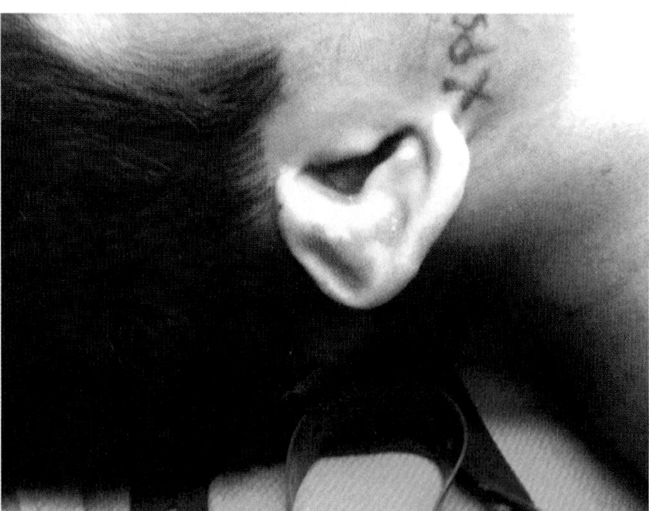

FIGURE 34-5 Microtia (underdeveloped pinna) in a child. (*Used with permission from Prashant Malhotra, MD.*)

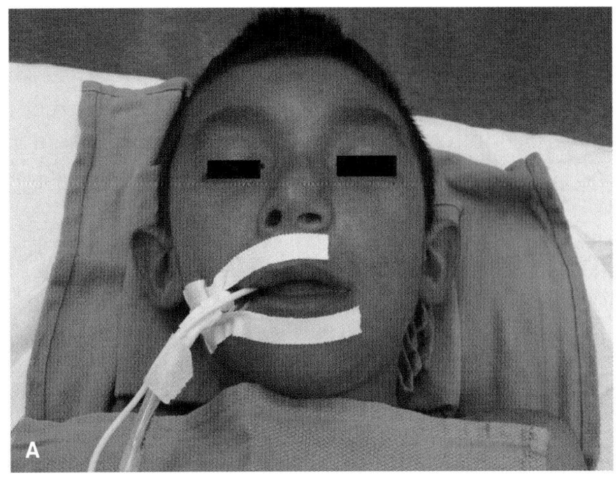

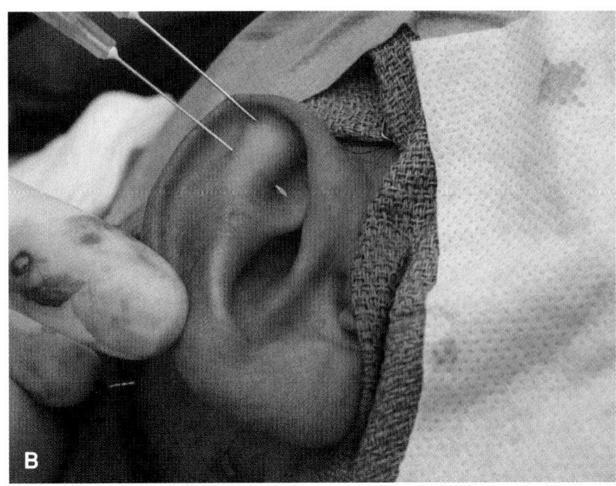

FIGURE 34-6 Prominent, protruding ears (**A**) in a child presenting for elective bilateral otoplasty (**B**). Protrusion typically results from absence of antihelical fold and excessive conchal bowl cartilage. Otoplasty involves intraoperative creation of an antihelical fold, to be secured with sutures. (*Used with permission from Prashant Malhotra, MD.*)

TABLE 34-3 Congenital Oral/Oropharyngeal Anomalies[7]

Anomaly	Epidemiology	Presentation	Evaluation	Treatment
Micrognathia Small mandible (**Figures 34-7** and **34-8**)	• Can occur in isolation or as part of syndrome • Pierre Robin Sequence (PRS) occurs in about 1/8,500 births	• Most are asymptomatic, but can present with significant airway obstruction if associated with Pierre-Robin sequence	• Monitor airway • Monitor weight gain • Pediatric ENT and craniofacial surgery consults	• Conservative—prone positioning or nasal airways • Surgical treatment: tongue-lip adhesion, tracheostomy or mandibular distraction osteogenesis
Ankyloglossia Short, fibrous lingual frenulum or a highly attached genioglossus muscle (**Figure 34-9**)	• Incidence 0.04–0.1 percent • Equal female to male ratio	• "Tongue-tie" • Feeding difficulties • Speech articulation difficulties • Tongue cannot contact the hard palate • Cannot protrude more than 1–2 mm past the teeth	• Consider speech therapy evaluation	• Speech therapy • Surgical treatment includes division of the frenulum (timing debated)
Macroglossia Enlargement of the tongue	Associated with: • vascular malformations, • congenital hypothyroidism • Beckwith-Wiedemann syndrome, • Down syndrome	• Difficulty feeding, stridor, airway obstruction • Diffuse enlargement of the tongue	• Consider ultrasound (evaluate floor of mouth for mass)	• Depends on severity • Surgical reduction may be indicated in severe cases.
Lingual thyroid Failure of the thyroid to descend from the foramen cecum[8]	• 1:4–10,000 • Female:Male = 4:1	• Presents in early childhood, adolescence or menopause • Airway obstruction • Pink, firm mass at base of tongue • Dysphagia, dysphonia or dyspnea	• U/S to assess for other areas of ectopic thyroid (In 75% of patients, this is the only functioning gland) • CT, MRI and technetium Tc-99m can also be used • Thyroid function tests; 50 percent of patients will be hypothyroid	• Debated - some authors argue for excision due to malignant potential. • If asymptomatic, may choose to follow clinically • Treat hormone dysfunction medically, as needed

(*continued*)

TABLE 34-3 Congenital Oral/Oropharyngeal Anomalies[7] (*Continued*)

Anomaly	Epidemiology	Presentation	Evaluation	Treatment
Natal Teeth Infant is born with a tooth or teeth[9]	• 1:3000 births	• Neonate will have normal appearing tooth • Function and structure of the tooth may not be normal • Can be either early eruption or supernumerary	• Referral to dentist • Monitor for any oral mucosa or tongue ulceration from the tooth	• Possible extraction if supernumerary or if concern for aspiration from highly mobile tooth
Congenital Epulis Granular cell tumor of the gingiva; benign mesenchymal tumor[9,10] (**Figure 34-10**)	• Female:Male = 8:1 • 5–16 percent exist in multiple sites	• Firm, mucosal covered lesion, more commonly along the maxillary gingival • Airway obstruction • Maxillary to mandibular ratio is 3:1	• CT demonstrates regular, prominent margins without associated bony tissue • Consult to pediatric ENT or oral surgeon	• Surgical excision
Dermoid Cystic lesion of the floor of mouth comprised of skin appendages with a squamous epithelial lining[11] (**Figure 34-11**)	• 7 percent of dermoids occur in the head and neck • 11.5 percent of dermoids in the head and neck are in the floor of mouth	• Midline slow growing mass • Cystic lesion of the floor of the mouth, rarely in the tongue • Can occur superior or inferior to the mylohyoid muscle	• CT scan or ultrasound • Consult pediatric ENT	• Medical management +/– incision and drainage in the setting of an acute infection • 5 percent risk of malignant transformation • Surgical excision

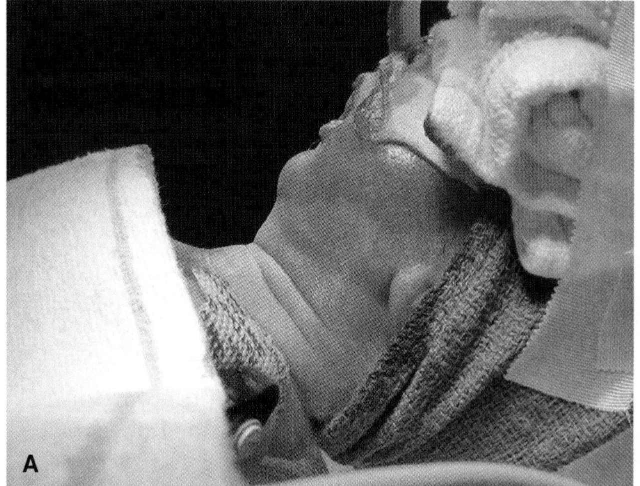

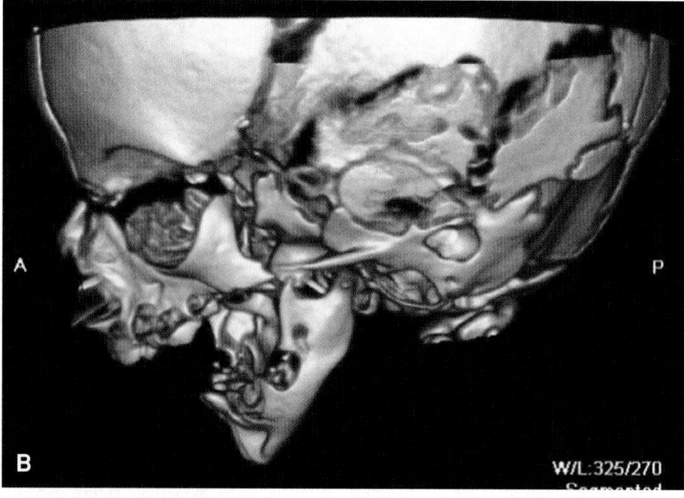

FIGURE 34-7 3 week old infant with severe micrognathia and upper airway obstruction, prior to mandibular distraction, on preoperative, profile view (**A**) and on CT scan with 3D reconstruction (**B**). (*Used with permission from Jonathan Grischkan, MD*)

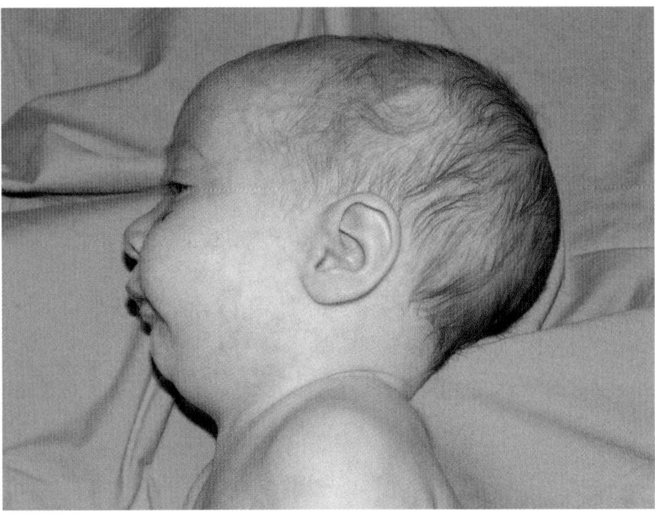

FIGURE 34-8 Micrognathia in an infant, which ultimately required mandibular distraction for persistent respiratory distress and poor growth. (*Used with permission from Prashant Malhotra, MD.*)

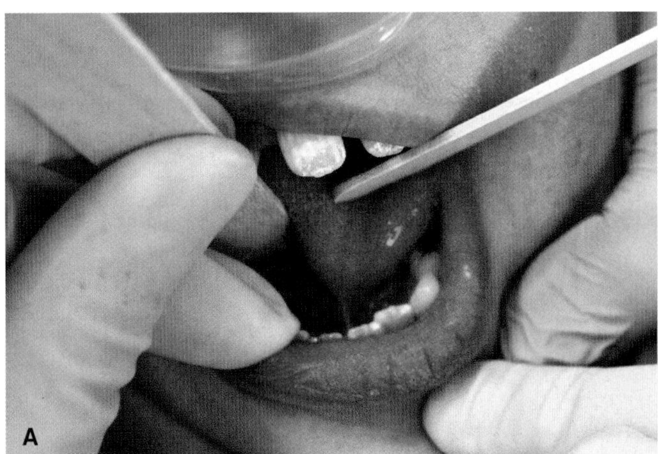

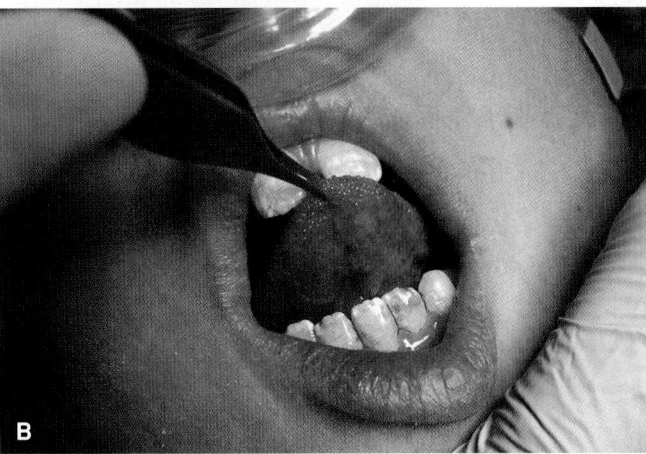

FIGURE 34-9 Ankyloglossia in an 8-year-old boy with speech articulation disorder and membranous ankyloglossia, preoperatively (**A**). Patient was unable to pass tongue tip beyond mandibular teeth. Note the extent of the release after frenuloplasty (**B**). Patient is also able to now protrude tongue tip well past mandibular teeth. (*Used with permission from Prashant Malhotra, MD.*)

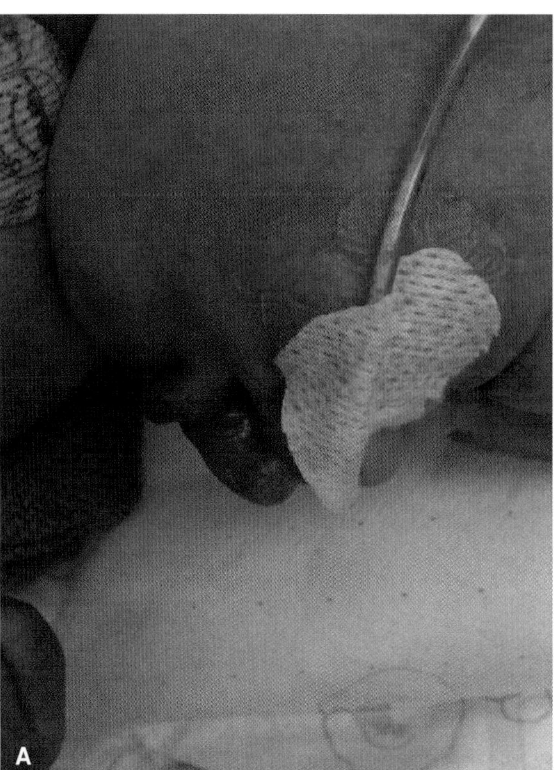

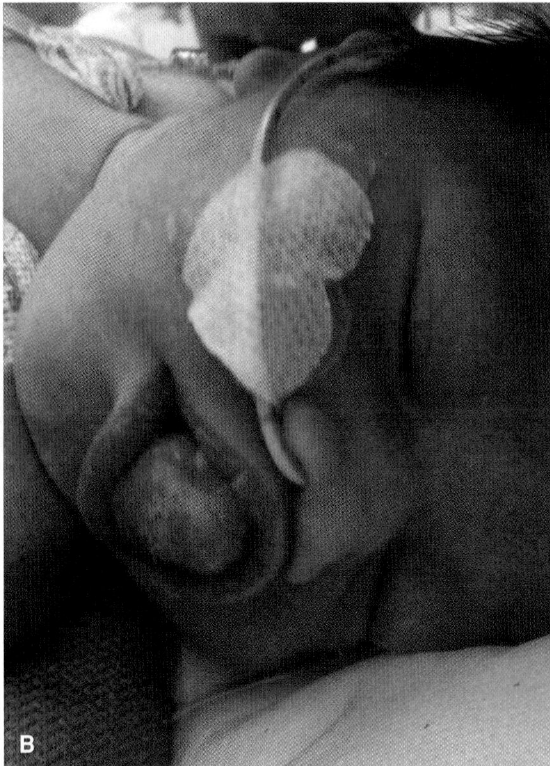

FIGURE 34-10 Congenital epulis (benign tumor on the gingival or alveolar mucosa) arising from maxillary alveolar ridge in a newborn, on lateral (**A**) and primarily frontal (**B**) views. (*Used with permission from Prashant Malhotra, MD.*)

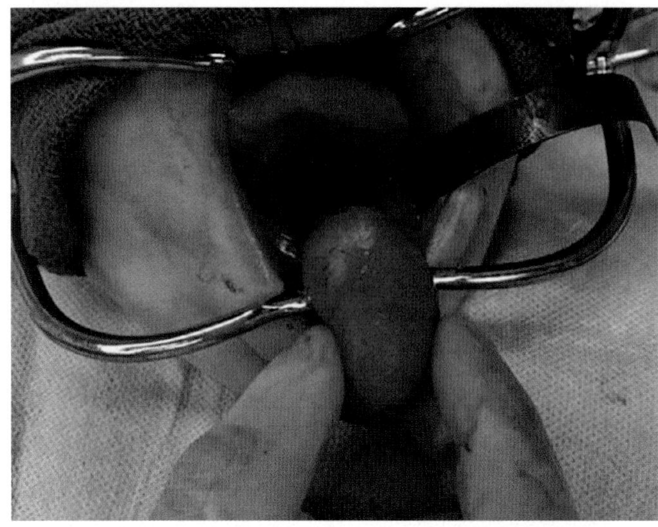

FIGURE 34-11 Oral dermoid cyst in a 2-year-old child being surgically excised from the floor of the mouth. (*Used with permission from Prashant Malhotra, MD.*)

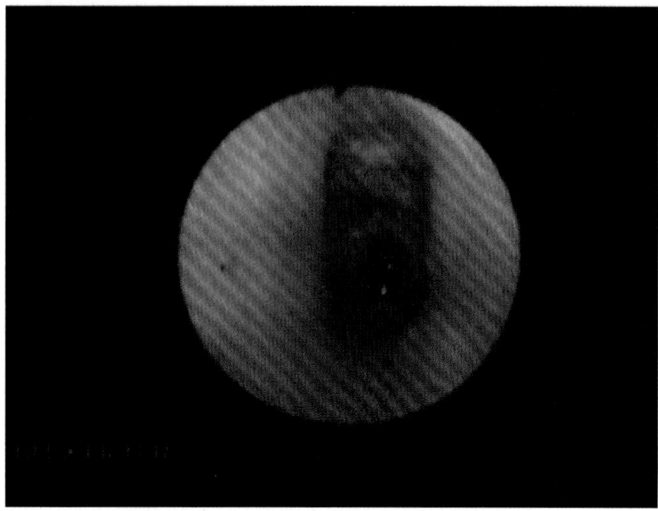

FIGURE 34-12 Naso-oropharyngeal soft tissue stenosis in a young child with Mobius syndrome. Endoscopic view with flexible scope shows narrowed caliber, normal larynx in the distance. (*Used with permission from Prashant Malhotra, MD.*)

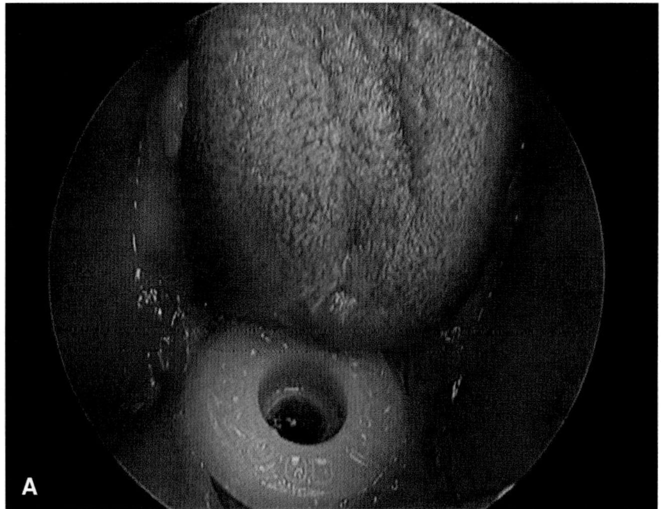

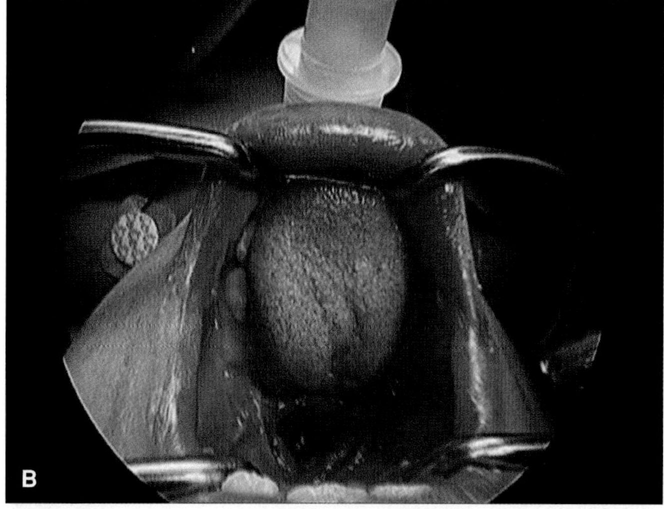

FIGURE 34-13 Pharyngeal aplasia with (**A**) and without (**B**) a stent in place. There was no oropharyngeal opening until created surgically. Oropharyngeal stent in place through surgically created opening. Soft tissue was serially resected/ablated with ultimate restoration of patency. (*Used with permission from Prashant Malhotra, MD.*)

TABLE 34-4 Congenital Cervical Anomalies[13]

Anomaly	Epidemiology	Presentation	Evaluation	Treatment
Thyroglossal Duct Cyst (TGDC) Failure of obliteration of caudally descended median thyroid anlage, or thyroglossal duct (**Figures 34-14** and **34-15**; see Chapter 32, Thyroglossal Duct Cyst and Other Head and Neck Masses)	• 7 percent in lifetime • Half are identified <10 years age	• Anterior midline neck mass, usually painless • Usually moves with swallow or tongue protrusion • Possible infected mass or draining sinus	• Ultrasound to evaluate thyroid gland (r/p TGDC as only ectopic thyroid tissue)	• Elective surgical resection via Sistrunk procedure (middle 1/3 of hyoid removed along with entire tract)
Branchial Anomaly (cysts, sinuses or fistulae) First Cleft Anomaly (1%) • Type 1 (ectoderm only) • Type 2 (ecto + mesoderm) Second Cleft Anomaly (95%) Third Cleft Anomaly (rare) Fourth Cleft Anomaly (rare) (**Figures 34-16** to **34-18**; see Chapter 32, Thyroglossal Duct Cyst and Other Head and Neck Masses)	• 30 percent of congenital neck masses	• Neck mass • External auditory canal fistula • Draining sinus around ear • Draining sinus in neck	• CT scan • Upper airway endoscopy to r/o pharyngeal fistula	• Surgical excision of entire cyst, sinus, or fistula
Dermoid Entrapped epithelial (ectodermal and endodermal) elements	• 20 percent of head and neck dermoids occur in neck	• Painless, superficial/subcutan-eous mass in anterior neck • Gradual increase in size	• Ultrasound neck	• Surgical excision (plan Sistrunk as if TGDC if adjacent to hyoid)

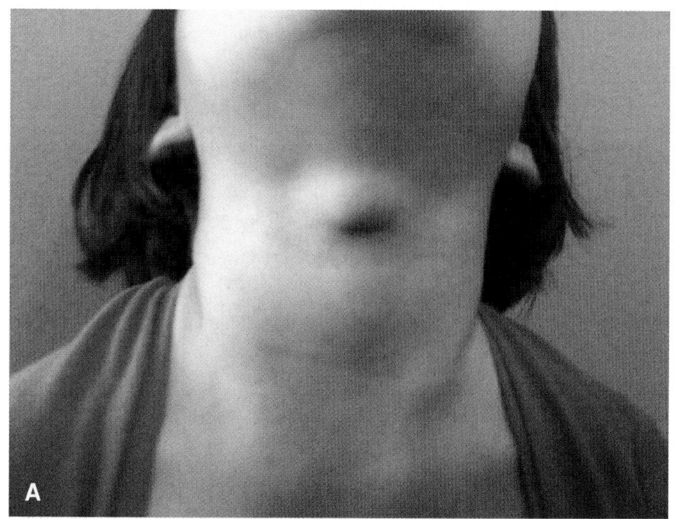

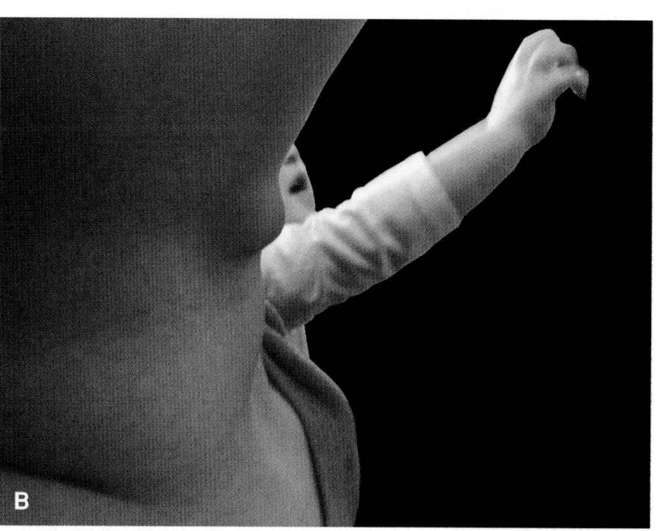

FIGURE 34-14 Thyroglossal duct cyst in a 2-year-old girl, as seen on frontal (**A**) and lateral (**B**) views. (*Used with permission from Prashant Malhotra, MD.*)

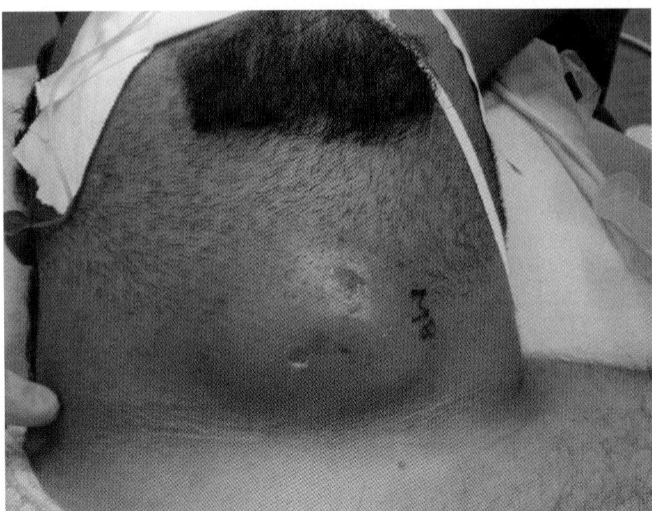

FIGURE 34-15 Acutely infected thyroglossal duct cyst in a teenager. This required incision and drainage prior to definitive Sistrunk procedure (excision of cyst with tract and middle third of hyoid bone). (*Used with permission from Prashant Malhotra, MD.*)

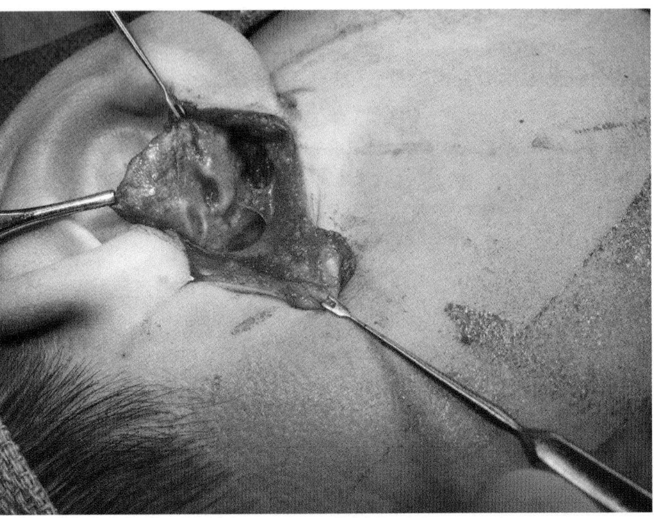

FIGURE 34-17 First Branchial Anomaly. Intraoperative view of Type 1 first branchial anomaly with duplicated cartilage and sinus. This was excised along with small cyst and external canal reconstructed. (*Used with permission from Prashant Malhotra, MD.*)

descends caudally, anterior to the hyoid, and fuses with fourth and fifth branchial pouches to form the thyroid.[13] The branchial arches are responsible for much of the musculoskeletal and neural development of the head and neck. Branchial anomalies result from incomplete obliteration of the clefts and pouches, and are classified by the cleft or pouch of origin. The origin affects the location of associated fistulae and relationship to nerves, arteries, and muscles. This has clear relevance for surgical resection. Branchio-oto-renal syndrome is a classic example of a genetic cause for congenital branchial arch abnormalities.

- Branchial anomalies can present as cysts, sinuses, or fistulae. Cysts have no external opening, sinuses open to the skin, and fistulae have a skin opening and an opening into the pharynx.

Other Anomalies and Syndromes

- **Cleft lip/palate**—Orofacial clefting occurs in approximately 1/700 live births with a higher prevalence in Native Americans and Asians, and a lower prevalence in African Americans. It is the second most common birth deformity (second to club foot) and 2/3 of these children have other associated abnormalities.[14] Cleft lip is associated with cleft palate in 68 to 86 percent of cases and a unilateral cleft is more common than bilateral.[4] Management is best orchestrated in the context of a multidisciplinary Cleft-Craniofacial team (**Figures 34-19** and **34-20**).
- **Vascular anomalies**—These include vascular tumors such as hemangiomas as well as malformations such as capillary and venous malformations, arteriovenous malformations (AVM), and lymphatic malformations. Other than focal hemangiomas, they are best managed by a multidisciplinary vascular anomalies team, consisting of dermatology, plastic surgery, otolaryngology, radiology, and other specialists. A brief discussion follows for selected lesions.

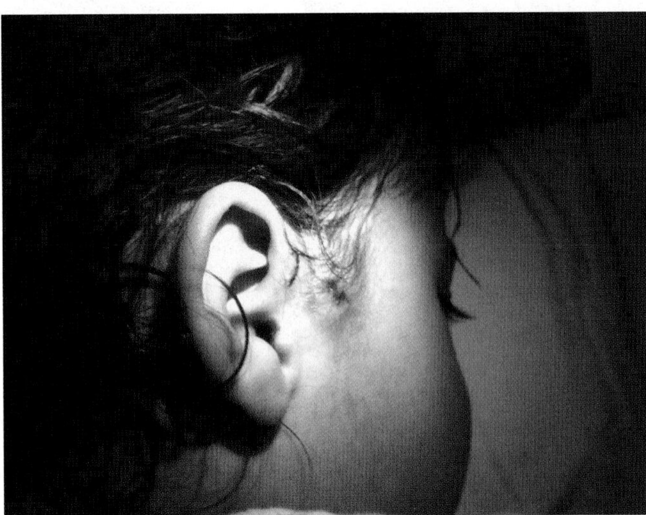

FIGURE 34-16 Infected right preauricular sinus with abscess in a young girl. (*Used with permission from Prashant Malhotra, MD.*)

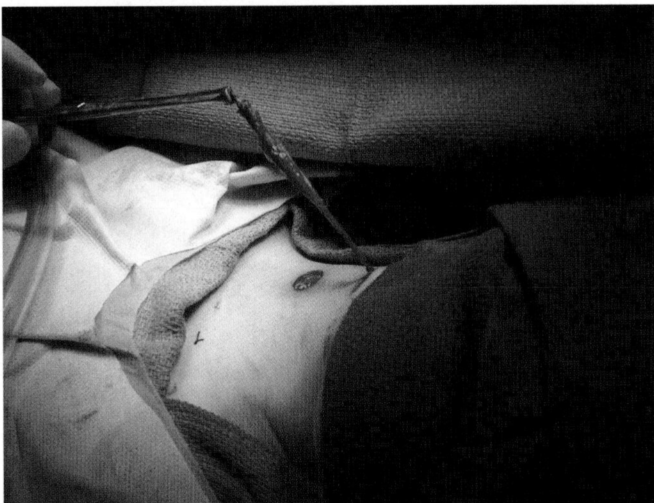

FIGURE 34-18 Stairstepping horizontal incisions demonstrate characteristic tract of 2nd branchial anomaly as it traverses between the carotid bifurcation, superficial to CN IX and toward the tonsillar fossa. (*Used with permission from Prashant Malhotra, MD.*)

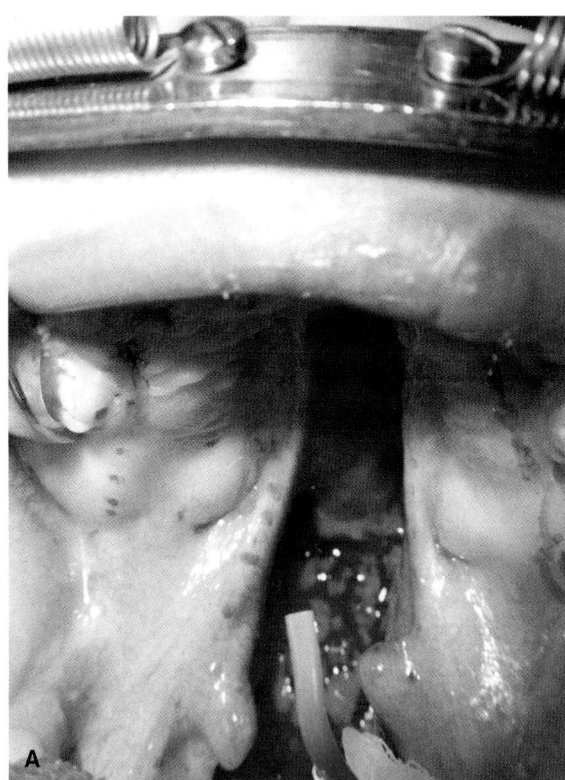
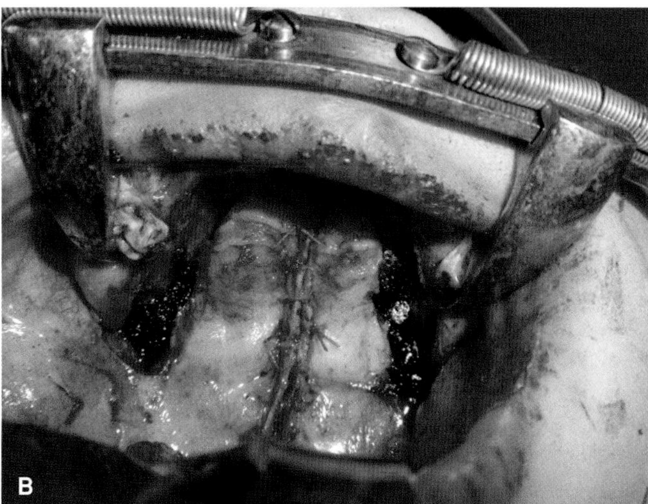

FIGURE 34-19 Cleft palate as seen intraoperatively prior to repair (**A**) and immediately after repair (**B**). (*Used with permission from Prashant Malhotra, MD.*)

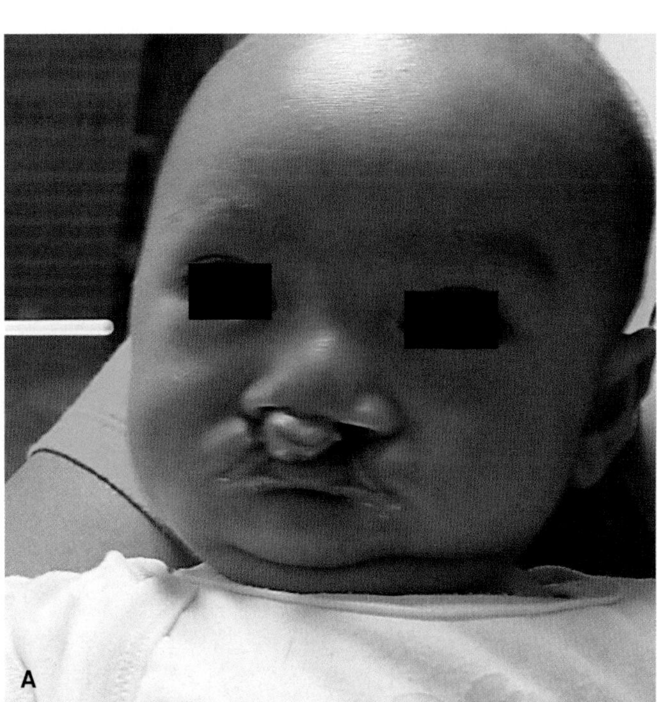
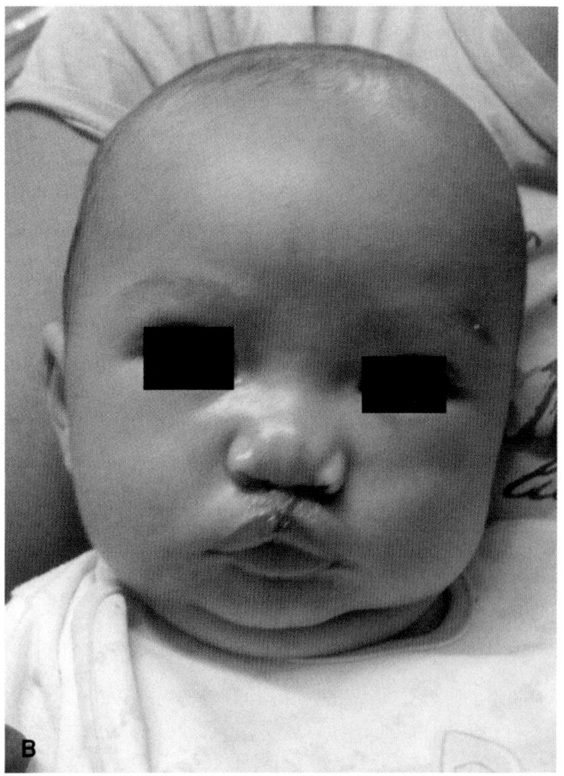

FIGURE 34-20 Bilateral cleft lip with prominent premaxilla, prior to repair (**A**) and 1 week after repair (**B**). (*Used with permission from Prashant Malhotra, MD.*)

- Hemangiomas: These common benign neoplasms are composed of proliferating endothelial type cells, and affect the head and neck in 60 percent of cases. They typically develop after birth and have a characteristic proliferate phase, plateau phase, and subsequent involutional phase. They have varied presentations and treatment is individually tailored. If they have no complications (ulceration or bleeding) or a threat to function (vision, airway, cosmesis, etc.), they may be observed. First line medical therapy previously consisted of systemic corticosteroids, but the use of propranolol has supplanted this. Surgery has a role for aggressive proliferative or function threatening lesions, or after incomplete involution.[15]
- Venous Malformations (VMs)—VMs are benign malformations made up of ectatic veins. They differ from hemangiomas, as they are present at birth, grow proportionally with the child, and are not proliferative lesions. MRI can help confirm diagnosis and determine extent of lesion. They are low-flow lesions that are isointense to muscle on T1-weighted images and enhance brightly on T2. Conservative management, injection sclerotherapy, and laser therapy are usually first line options, with surgery reserved for persistent symptomatic disease (**Figure 34-21**).[16]
- Lymphatic Malformations (LMs, previously known as cystic hygroma or lymphangioma)—These are rare vascular anomalies, common in the head and neck, from aberrant formation of peripheral lymphatic vessels or fusion with venous structures, occurring in 1 to 4/10,000 births. They are categorized as macrocystic, microcystic, or combined lesions depending on the size of the fluid filled compartments. They present as asymptomatic masses or with functional difficulties such as dysphagia or airway difficulties. MRI is imaging modality of choice, typically with low signal intensity on T1-weighted images, high signal intensity with well demarcated margins on T2-weighted images. LMs may be identified on antenatal ultrasound and appropriate airway planning should be anticipated. LMs are difficult to treat. Medical therapy with antibiotics and anti-inflammatory may be used if they acutely worsen. Definitive treatment varies based on de Serres staging, affected site and type of lesion, and is individualized. Observation, surgery, and injection sclerotherapy are options for macrocystic lesions. These same options exist for microcystic lesions, which are more difficult to treat (**Figures 34-22** and **34-23**).[17]

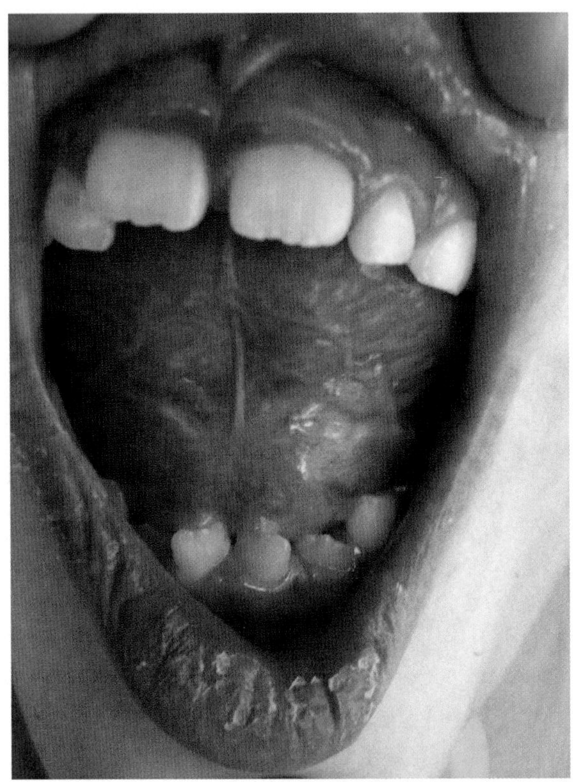

FIGURE 34-21 Venolymphatic Malformation in a 10-year-old with bilateral, symmetric, floor of mouth fullness. Imaging and pathology after excision demonstrated combined venous and lymphatic (venolymphatic) malformation. (*Used with permission from Prashant Malhotra, MD.*)

- **Syndromic associated anomalies**—Congenital anomalies of the head and neck can be associated with numerous genetic abnormalities and syndromes (**Figures 34-1** and **34-24**). **Table 34-5** lists some of those, which are more commonly encountered. Head and neck, other findings, and the causes are listed.

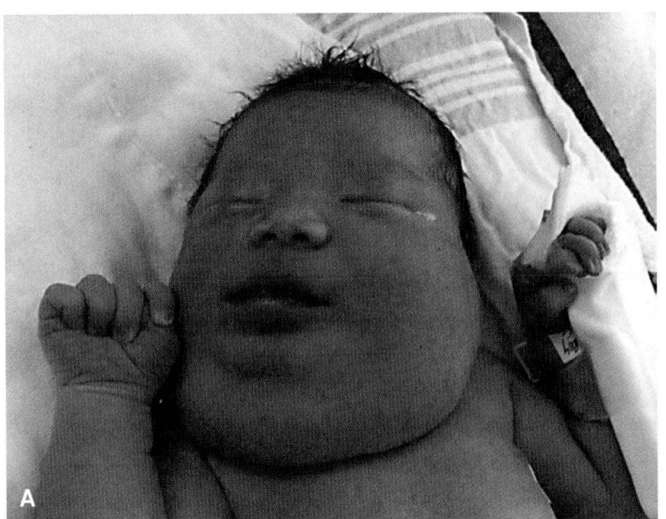

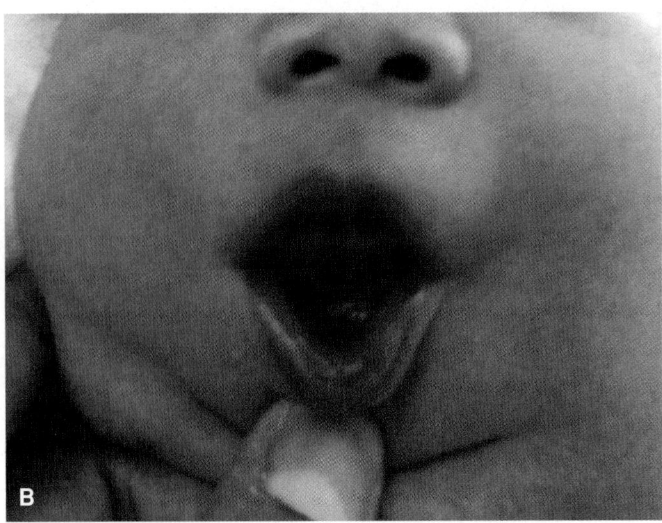

FIGURE 34-22 Massive Lymphatic Malformation (LM) in a 1-day-old newborn involving suprahyoid and infrahyoid spaces, floor of mouth, tongue, pharynx, supraglottic larynx, and into mediastinum (**A**). LM was combined microcystic and macrocystic. Note the tense floor of mouth and tongue involvement (**B**), with mouth pushed upwards to palate. (*Used with permission from Prashant Malhotra, MD.*)

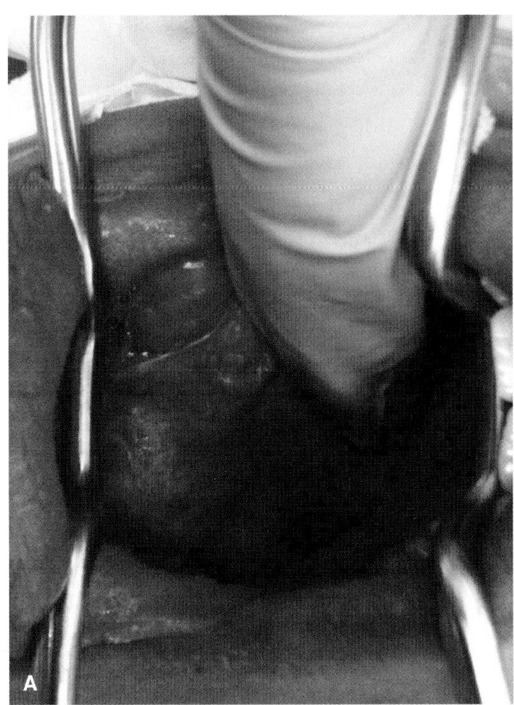

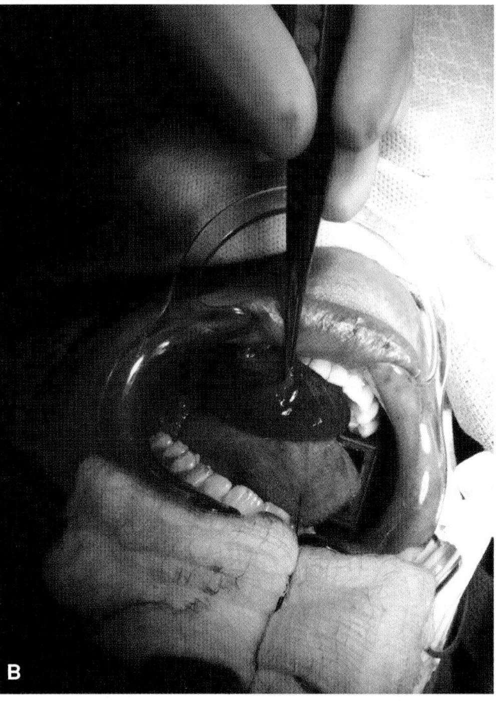

FIGURE 34-23 Lymphatic malformation on the right floor of mouth in a 10-year-old child (**A**). Tongue is pushed to the right to expose left lateral tongue and floor of mouth. Note bluish discoloration. Intraoperative view (**B**) of well circumscribed macrocystic LM. (*Used with permission from Prashant Malhotra, MD.*)

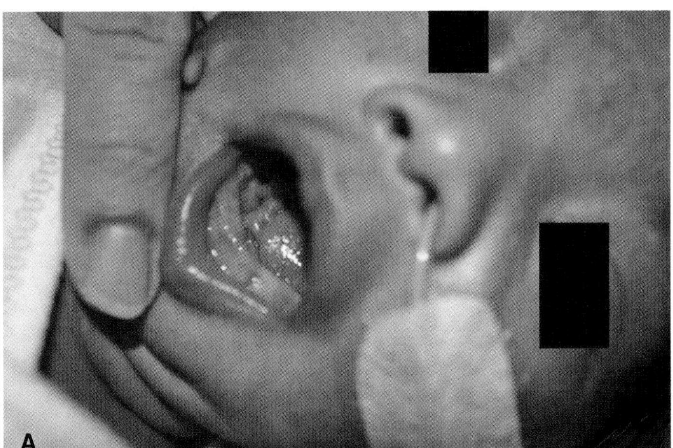

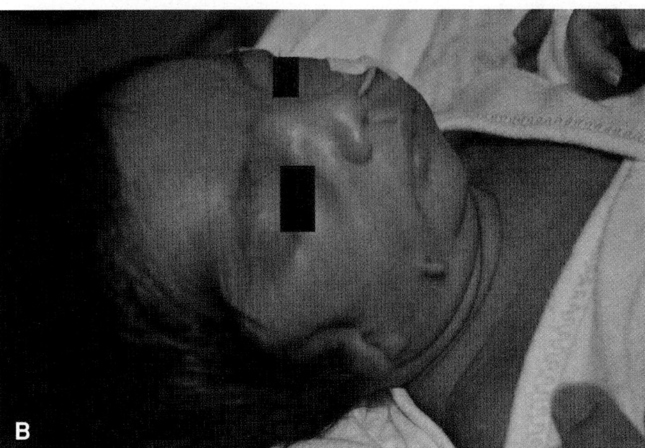

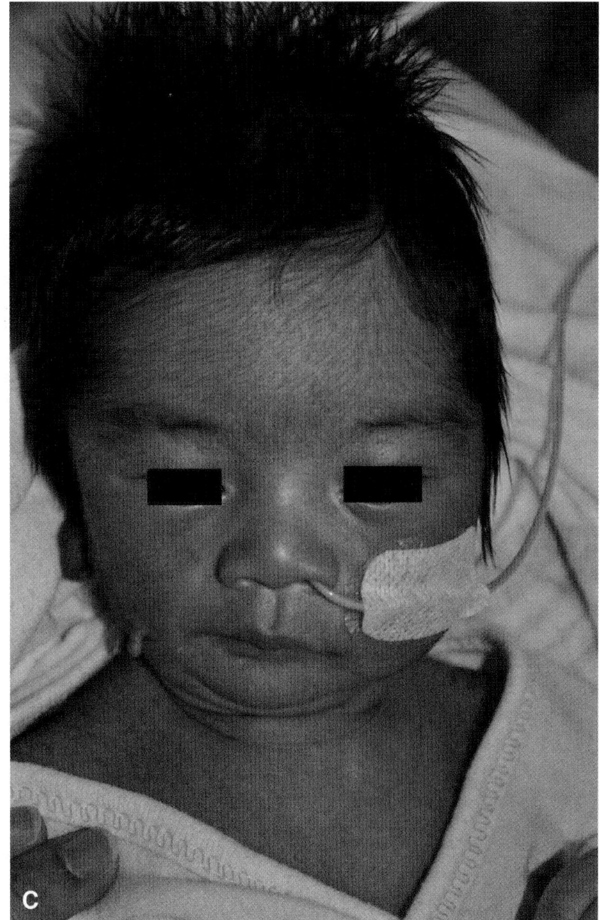

FIGURE 34-24 Hypoplastic right hemi-tongue in an infant with oculoauricularvertebral spectrum (OAVS or Goldenhar syndrome) on superior (**A**), lateral/oblique (**B**) and frontal (**C**) views. Note microtia (underdeveloped pinna), aural atresia, accessory skin tag, along with mastoid tip, malar, maxillary and mandibular hypoplasia (hemifacial microsomia) in views B and C. (*Used with permission from Prashant Malhotra, MD.*)

TABLE 34-5 Syndromes Associated with Head and Neck Findings

Syndrome	Head & Neck Findings	Other Findings	Cause
Treacher Collins[18] (**Figure 34-1**)	Down slanting palpebral fissures, lower eyelid colobomas, maxillary hypoplasia, microtia, atresia of external auditory canal	None	AD; TCOF1 on chromosome 5
Oculo-Auriculo-Vertebral Spectrum (Goldenhar Syndrome included; **Figure 34-24**)[18]	Hemifacial microsomia, epibulbar dermoids, upper eyelid colobomas, macrostomia, facial clefts, ear malformations	Vertebral, cardiac, renal defects	Can be non-genetic (diabetes, teratogens) or genetic (chromosomes 5, 18, 22, X)
Stickler's[2]	Ophthalmic abnormalities, flattened midface, depressed nasal bridge, SNHL, mandibular hypoplasia, cleft palate	Skeletal abnormalities	AD; COL2A1 gene on chromosome 12 – type II collagen
Crouzon's[2,19]	Craniosynostosis (usually coronal suture), midface hypoplasia, atresia of the nasopharynx, proptosis, hypertelorism	Cerebellar herniation, hydrocephalus, jugular foramen stenosis	AD; FSFR2 gene mutation on chromosome 10q26
Velocardiofacial[20] (see Chapter 216, DiGeorge Syndrome)	Thyroid dysfunction/malformation, aplasia/hypoplasia parathyroids, abnormal thymus, cleft palate, velopalatal insufficiency, laryngotracheal abnormalities, dysphagia/esophageal dysmotility	Heart and renal defects, impaired immunity, growth retardation, skeletal abnormalities, mental illness	Deletion 22q11 (band 11.2 on chromosome 22)
Branchio-Oto-Renal[21]	Branchial arch abnormalities, hearing loss, preauricular pits, external/middle/inner ear abnormalities, facial asymmetry, cleft palate	Renal abnormalities	AD; EYA1 long arm of chromosome 8, SIX1 or SIX5 gene
Fetal Alcohol Syndrome[22]	Short palpebral fissures, smooth philtrum, thin upper vermillion border, maxillary hypoplasia, microcephaly	Growth retardation, CNS dysfunction	Maternal alcohol consumption

PATIENT RESOURCES

- Cleft Palate Foundation—**www.cleftline.org**.
- Vascular Birthmarks Foundation—**www.birthmark.org**.

PROVIDER RESOURCES

- American Cleft Palate-Craniofacial Association (ACPCA)—**www.acpa-cpf.org**.
- Cleft Palate Foundation—**www.cleftline.org**.

REFERENCES

1. Isaacson G. An Approach to Congenital Malformations of the Head and Neck. *Otolaryngol Clin N Am*. 2007;40:1-8.
2. Szeremeta W, Parikh TD, Widelitz JS. Congenital nasal malformations. *Otolaryngol Clinic North Amer*. 2007;40:97-112.
3. Lee WT, Koltai PJ. Nasal deformity in neonates and young children. *Ped Clinic North Amer*. 2003;50:459-467.
4. Arosarena OA. Cleft lip and palate. *Otolaryngol Clin N Am*. 2007; 40:27-60.
5. Sreetharan V, Kangesu L, Sommerlad BC. Atypical congenital dermoid of the face: a 25-year experience. *Journal of Plast, Reconst Aesth Surg*. 2007;60:1025-1029.
6. Kelley P. Microtia and Congenital Aural Atresia. *Otolaryngol Clin N Am*. 2007;40:61-80.
7. Mueller et al. Congenital malformations of the oral cavity. *Otolaryngol Clin N Am*. 2007;40:141-160.
8. Toso A, Colombani F, Averono G, Aluffi P, Pia F. Lingual thyroid causing dysphagia and dyspnoea. Case reports and review of the literature. *Acta Otorhinolaryng Italica*. 2009;29:213-217.
9. Nield LS, Stenger JP, Kamat D. Common pediatric dental dilemmas. *Clinical Pediatrics*. 2008;47(2):99-105.
10. Hasanov A, Musayev J, Onal B et al. Gingival granular cell tumor of the newborn: a case report and review of the literature. *Turkish J of Pathology* 2011;27(2):161-163.
11. Koeller KK, Alamo L, Adair CF et al. Congenital cystic masses of the neck: radiologic-pathologic correlation. *Radiographics* 1999;19:121-146.
12. Cummings CW et al. Cummings: Otolaryngology: Head and Neck Surgery. 4th Ed. Ch 171 Developmental Anatomy. Elsevier Inc. 2005 US MD Consult
13. Acierno SP et al. Congenital cervical cysts, sinuses, and fistulae. *Otolaryngol Clin N Am*. 2007;40:161-176.
14. Eppley BL, Van Aalst JA, Robey A, Havlik RJ, Sadove MA. The spectrum of orofacial clefting. *Plast Reconstr Surg*. 2005;115:101e-114e.

15. Hartzell et al. *Otolaryngol Clin North Am.* 2012;45(3):545-56, vii.

16. Buckmiller L. Update on hemangiomas and vascular malformations. *Curr Opin Otololaryngol Head Neck Surg.* 2004;12:476-487.

17. Adams et al. Head and neck malformation treatment. *Otolaryngol Head Neck Surg.* 2012;147(4):627-639.

18. Passos-Bueno MR, Ornelas CC, Fanganiello RD. Syndromes of the first and second branchial arches: a review. *Am J of Med Genet Part A.* 2009;149A:1853-1859.

19. Katzen JT, McCarthy JG. Syndromes involving craniosynostosis and midface hypoplasia. *Otolaryngol Clin N Am.* 2000;33(6):1257-1284.

20. Marom T, Roth Y, Goldfarb A, et al. Head and neck manifestations of 22q11.2 deletion syndromes. *Eur Arch Otorhinolaryngol.* 2012;269:381-387.

21. Senel E, Kocak H, Akbiyik F et al. From branchial fistula to a branchiootorenal syndrome: a case report and review of the literature. *J of Pediatric Surgery.* 2009;44:623-625.

22. Riley EP, Infante MA, Warren KR. Fetal alcohol spectrum disorders: an overview. *Neuropsychol Rev.* 2011;21:73-80.

23. Isaacson G. An Approach to Congenital Malformations of the Head and Neck. *Otolaryngol Clin N Am.* 2007;40:1-8.

PART 6

ORAL HEALTH

Strength of Recommendation (SOR)	Definition
A	Recommendation based on consistent and good-quality patient-oriented evidence.*
B	Recommendation based on inconsistent or limited-quality patient-oriented evidence.*
C	Recommendation based on consensus, usual practice, opinion, disease-oriented evidence, or case series for studies of diagnosis, treatment, prevention, or screening.*

*See Appendix A on pages 1320–1322 for further information.

35 GEOGRAPHIC TONGUE

Ernest Valdez, DDS
Richard P. Usatine, MD
Wanda C. Gonsalves, MD

PATIENT STORY

A 4-year-old girl is brought to the pediatrician's office because the mother is concerned about her child's tongue having a "strange appearance." She denies pain or discomfort and is unsure how long the lesions have been present. The lesions seem to change areas of distribution on the tongue. The examination reveals large, well-delineated, shiny and smooth, erythematous spots on the surface of the tongue (**Figure 35-1**). The diagnosis is geographic tongue (benign migratory glossitis). The physician explains that it is benign and that no treatment is needed unless symptoms develop.

INTRODUCTION

Geographic tongue is a recurrent, benign, usually asymptomatic, inflammatory disorder of the mucosa of the dorsum and lateral borders of the tongue. Geographic tongue is characterized by circinate, irregularly shaped erythematous patches bordered by a white keratotic band. The central erythematous patch represents loss of filiform papillae of tongue epithelium. Geographic tongue can, although rarely, present as symptomatic.

SYNONYMS

Benign migratory glossitis or geographic stomatitis.

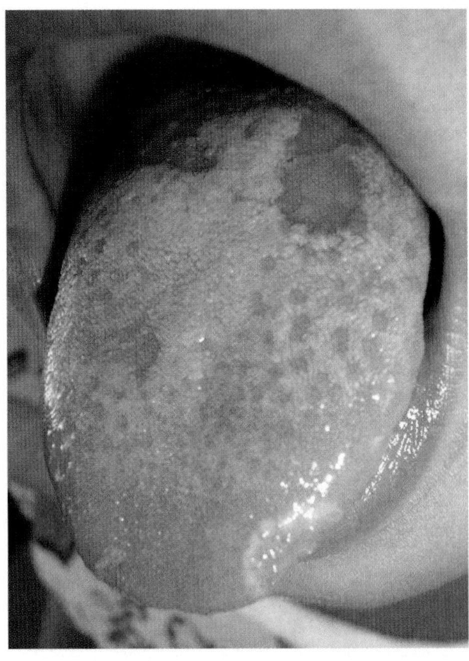

FIGURE 35-1 Geographic tongue (benign migratory glossitis) in a 4-year-old girl. Note the pink continent among the white ocean. (*Used with permission from Richard P. Usatine, MD.*)

EPIDEMIOLOGY

- Geographic tongue has an estimated prevalence of 1 to 3 percent of the population.[1]
- It may occur in either children or adults and exhibits a female predilection.
- Geographic tongue in the US has a greater prevalence among white and black persons than among Mexican Americans.[2]

ETIOLOGY AND PATHOPHYSIOLOGY

- Geographic tongue is a common oral inflammatory condition of unknown etiology.
- Some studies have shown an increased frequency in patients with allergies, pustular psoriasis, stress, type 1 diabetes, fissured tongue, and hormonal disturbances.[3]
- Histopathologic appearance resembles psoriasis.[4]

DIAGNOSIS

CLINICAL FEATURES

- The diagnosis is made by visual inspection and history of the lesion. The lesions are suggestive of a geographic map (hence geographic tongue) with pink continents surrounded by whiter oceans (**Figure 35-1**).
- Geographic tongue consists of large, well-delineated, shiny, and smooth, erythematous patches surrounded by a white halo (**Figure 35-2**).

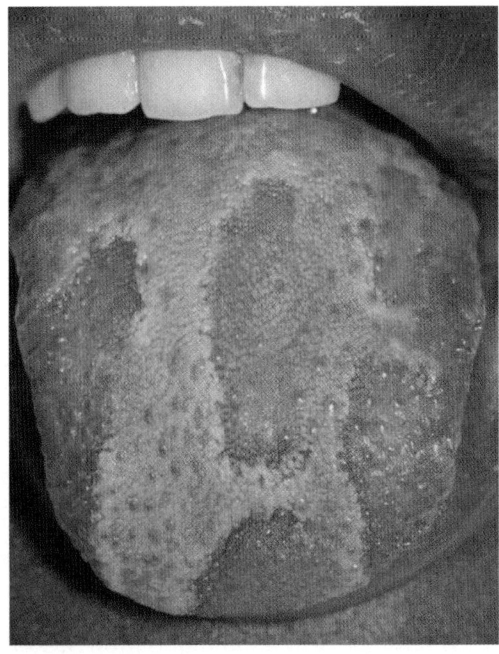

FIGURE 35-2 Geographic tongue (benign migratory glossitis). Note the pink continents among the white oceans. (*Reprinted with permission from Gonsalves WC, Chi AC, Neville BW. Common oral lesions: part II. Am Fam Phys 2007;75(4):501-508. Copyright © 2007 American Academy of Family Physicians. All rights reserved.*)

- Tongue lesions exhibit central erythema because of atrophy of the filiform papillae and are usually surrounded by slightly elevated, curving, white-to-yellow elevated borders (**Figures 35-1** and **35-2**).
- The condition typically waxes and wanes over time so the lesions appear to be migrating (hence migratory glossitis).
- Lesions may last days, months, or years. The lesions do not scar.
- Most patients are asymptomatic, but some patients may complain of pain or burning, especially when eating spicy foods.
- Suspect systemic intraoral manifestations of psoriasis or reactive arthritis if the patient has psoriatic skin lesions or has conjunctivitis, urethritis, arthritis, and skin involvement suggestive of reactive arthritis.

TYPICAL DISTRIBUTION

- The lesions are typically found on the anterior 2/3 of the dorsal tongue mucosa.
- Geographic tongue usually affects the tongue, although other oral sites may be involved such as the buccal mucosa, the labial mucosa, and, less frequently, the soft palate.[3]

DIFFERENTIAL DIAGNOSIS

- Lichen planus—Reticular forms are characterized by interlacing white lines commonly found on the buccal mucosa, or erosive forms, characterized by atrophic erythematous areas with central ulceration and surrounding radiating striae (see Chapter 138, Lichen Planus).
- Psoriasis—Intraoral lesions have been described as red or white plaques associated with the activity of cutaneous lesions (see Chapter 136, Psoriasis).
- Reactive arthritis—A condition characterized by the triad of "urethritis, arthritis, and conjunctivitis," may have rare intraoral lesions described as painless ulcerative papules on the buccal mucosa and palate.
- Fissured tongue—An inherited condition in which the tongue has fissures that are asymptomatic. Although it has been called a *scrotal tongue* in the past, the term *fissured tongue* is preferred by patients (**Figure 35-3**).

MANAGEMENT

Most individuals are asymptomatic and do not require treatment (**Figure 35-4**).

- For symptomatic cases, several treatments have been proposed for adults but not proven effective with good clinical trials:[6,7]
  - Topical steroids such as triamcinolone dental paste (Oralone or Kenalog in Orabase). SOR C
  - Supplements such as zinc, vitamin B_{12}, niacin, and riboflavin. SOR C
  - Antihistamine mouth rinses (e.g., diphenhydramine elixir 12.5 mg per 5 mL diluted in a 1:4 ratio with water). SOR C
  - Topical anesthetic rinses.[6,7] SOR C
- Because of safety concerns, these therapies are not recommended for young children.

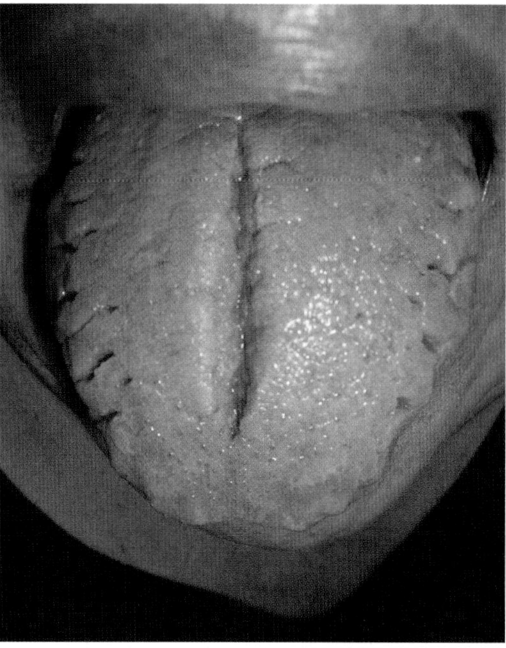

FIGURE 35-3 Fissured tongue present since birth. Although this has also been called a *scrotal tongue*, the preferred terminology is now *fissured tongue*, for obvious reasons. (*Used with permission from Richard P. Usatine, MD.*)

Geographic tongue can rarely present as persistent and painful (**Figure 35-5**). In one case report, 0.1 percent tacrolimus ointment was applied twice daily for 2 weeks with significant improvement of symptoms.[8] SOR C

No treatment has been proven to be uniformly effective.[9]

FOLLOW-UP

Instruct the parent to contact you if the symptoms continue past 10 days and to go to the emergency department immediately if:

- The tongue swells significantly.

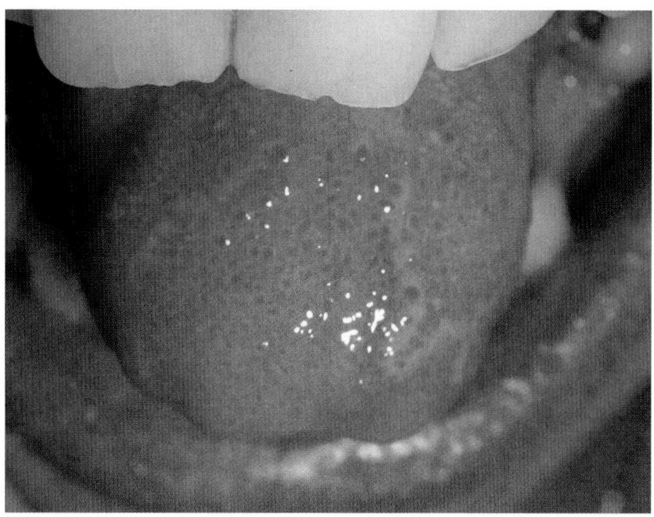

FIGURE 35-4 A mild asymptomatic case of geographic tongue. Note the atrophic filiform papillae and the subtle white halo. (*Used with permission from Richard P. Usatine, MD.*)

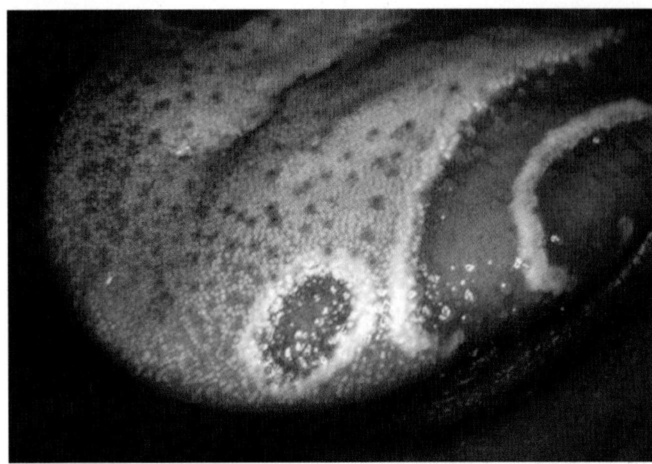

FIGURE 35-5 Geographic tongue with more severe symptomatology, including pain and a burning sensation when eating spicy foods. The contrast between the normal tongue tissue and the pink atrophic papillae is striking. (*Used with permission from Ellen Eisenberg, DMD.*)

- The patient has trouble breathing.
- The patient has trouble talking or chewing/swallowing.

PATIENT EDUCATION

Patients and parents should be reassured of the condition's benign nature. Tell patients with geographic tongue to avoid irritating spicy foods and liquids.

PATIENT RESOURCES

- Children's Physician Network. *Geographic Tongue*—**www.cpnonline.org/CRS/CRS/pa_gtongue_hhg.htm**.
- Medline Plus. *Geographic Tongue*—**www.nlm.nih.gov/medlineplus/ency/article/001049.htm**.

PROVIDER RESOURCES

- Medscape. *Geographic Tongue*—**www.emedicine.medscape.com/article/1078465**.
- Mayo Clinic. *Geographic Tongue*—**www.mayoclinic.com/health/geographic-tongue/DS00819**.

REFERENCES

1. Redman RS. Prevalence of geographic tongue, fissured tongue, median rhomboid glossitis, and hairy tongue among 3,611 Minnesota schoolchildren. *Oral Surg Oral Med Oral Pathol.* 1970;30:390-395.
2. Shulman JD, Carpenter WM. Prevalence and risk factors associated with geographic tongue among US adults. *Oral Dis.* 2006;12:351-356.
3. Assimakopoulos D, Patrikakos G, Fotika C, Elisaf M. Benign migratory glossitis or geographic tongue: an enigmatic oral lesion. *Am J Med.* 2002;113:751-755.
4. Espelid M, Bang G, Johannessen AC, et al. Geographic stomatitis: report of 6 cases. *J Oral Pathol Med.* 1991;20:425-428.
5. Darwazeh AM, Almelaih AA. Tongue lesions in a Jordanian population. Prevalence, symptoms, subject's knowledge and treatment provided. *Med Oral Patol Oral Cir Bucal.* 2011;16:e745-e749.
6. Abe M, Sogabe Y, Syuto T, et al. Successful treatment with cyclosporin administration for persistent benign migratory glossitis. *J Dermatol.* 2007;34:340-343.
7. Reamy BV, Derby R, Bunt CW. Common tongue conditions in primary care. *Am Fam Physician.* 2010; 81:627-634.
8. Ishibashi M, Tojo G, Watanabe M, et al. Geographic tongue treated with topical tacrolimus. *J Dermatol Case Rep.* 2010;4:57-59.
9. Gonsalves W, Chi A, Neville B. Common oral lesions: part 1. Superficial mucosal lesions. *Am Fam Physician.* 2007;75:501-507.

36 EARLY CHILDHOOD CARIES

Adriana Segura DDS, MS
Wanda C. Gonsalves, MD

PATIENT STORY

A mother brings her 18-month-old son to the physician's clinic for his well-child examination. He is almost weaned from his bottle, but still drinks from a bottle to go to sleep. During the day, he uses a sippy cup to drink everything—from milk to soda. His mother has started giving him apple juice in the bottle instead of milk because he tends to get constipated. On performing an oral examination, the physician notices that several of his teeth have "white spots" (**Figure 36-1**). The physician discusses dental hygiene and treats him with topical fluoride gel.

INTRODUCTION

Dental caries continues to be the most prevalent chronic disease problem facing infants and children. The American Academy of Pediatric Dentistry, American Academy of Pediatrics, and American Dental Association recommend that a child's first visit to a dentist should occur 6 months after the eruption of the first tooth or at 1 year of age. Providing a dental home by age 1 year allows the health provider to complete a risk assessment, provide an introduction to dentistry, and provide anticipatory guidance. It is important to be able to recognize disease and to provide prevention strategies early on to the parents/caregivers.

SYNONYMS

Nursing bottle caries or baby bottles caries.

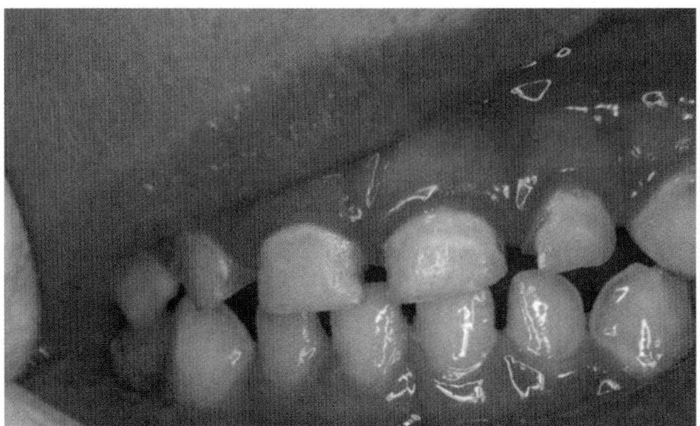

FIGURE 36-1 Demineralization at gingiva margins characterized by whitish discolorations. (*Used with permission from Gerald Ferretti, DMD.*)

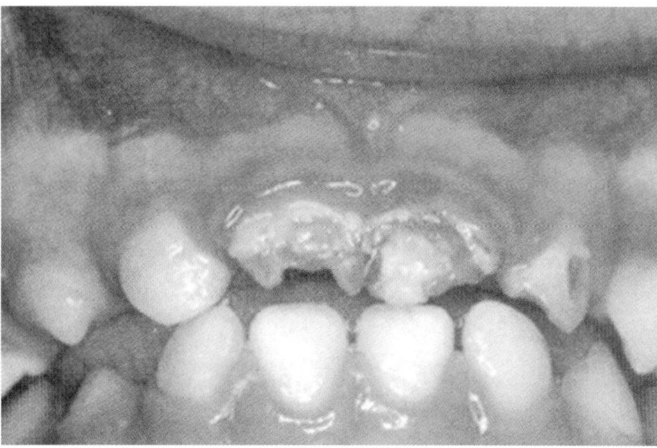

FIGURE 36-2 Central maxillary incisors with severe tooth decay, and bilateral maxillary lateral incisors with demineralized area near gingival line (yellow-brownish discolorations). The upper incisors are often the first teeth involved in nursing bottle caries. (*Used with permission from Gerald Ferretti, DMD.*)

EPIDEMIOLOGY

- Early childhood caries (ECC; tooth decay) is the single most common chronic childhood disease. It is 5 times more common than asthma and 7 times more common than hay fever among children 5 to 7 years of age.[1]
- Tooth decay affects more than 25 percent of US children between 2 and 5 years of age and about half of those 12 to 15 years of age.
- Disparities in oral health exist—In 2002, 32 percent of Mexican American and 27 percent of non-Hispanic black children 2 to 11 years of age had untreated decay in their primary teeth, compared to 18 percent of non-Hispanic white children.[2,3]
- ECC is defined as "the presence of one or more decayed (noncavitated or cavitated lesions), missing (as a consequence of caries), or filled tooth surfaces in any primary tooth in a child 71 months of age or younger (**Figures 36-2** to **36-4**)."[4]

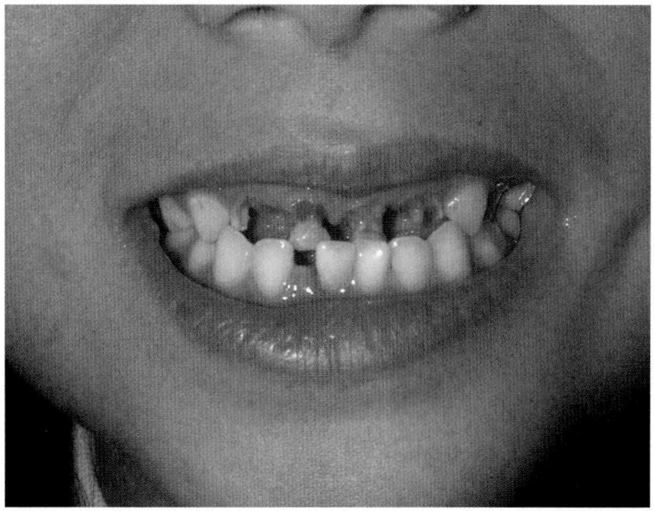

FIGURE 36-3 Severe ECC in a 4-year-old with severe decay of all four maxillary incisors. (*Used with permission from Richard P. Usatine, MD.*)

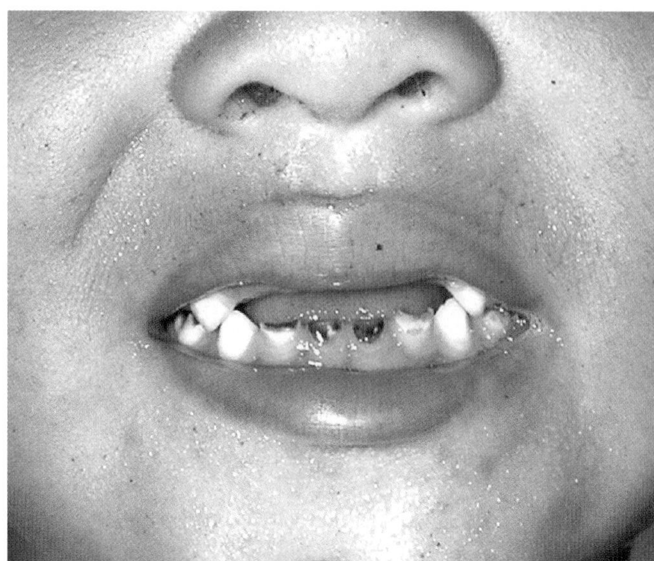

FIGURE 36-4 Severe ECC in a 3-year-old with multiple areas of cavitary lesions involving the mandibular incisors and missing maxillary incisors secondary to decay. *(Used with permission from Richard P. Usatine, MD.)*

- Consequences of ECC include poor self-esteem, diminished physical development, decreased ability to learn, higher risk of new caries, and added cost.[4]

ETIOLOGY AND PATHOPHYSIOLOGY

- Dental caries is a multifactorial, infectious, communicable disease caused by the demineralization of tooth enamel (**Figure 36-1**) in the presence of a sugar substrate and acid-forming cariogenic bacteria, *Streptococcus mutans* (also known as *mutans streptococci*), which is considered to be the primary strain causing decay that are found in the soft gelatinous biofilm.
- Caries can develop at any time after tooth eruption. Early teeth are principally susceptible to caries caused by the transmission of *S. mutans* from the mouth of the caregiver or sibling(s) to the mouth of the infant or toddler. This type of tooth decay is called baby bottle tooth decay, nursing bottle caries, or ECC.

RISK FACTORS

Risk factors for caries development include:

- Frequent consumption of liquids.
- Repetitive use of a "sippy cup" containing sugars (juice, milk, formula, or soda).
- Consumption of sticky foods.
- Human breast milk is uniquely superior in providing the best possible nutrition to infants and, by itself, has been shown to be noncariogenic.[3]
- Nighttime bottle feeding and caregiver with caries.
- Drinking unfluoridated community water or bottled water, which usually lacks fluoride.
- Low socioeconomic status.
- Taking medications that contain sugar or cause dryness.

Lack of good oral hygiene practices.

Subnormal saliva and function.

DIAGNOSIS

CLINICAL FEATURES

- Demineralized areas develop on the tooth surfaces, between teeth, and on pits and fissures. These areas are painless and appear clinically as opaque or brown spots (**Figure 36-1**). White-spot lesions are the first indication the demineralization has started.
- Infection that is allowed to progress forms a cavity that can spread to and through the dentin (the component of the tooth located below the enamel) and to the pulp (composed of nerves and blood vessels; an infection of the pulp is called pulpitis) causing pain, necrosis, and, perhaps, an abscess.

TYPICAL DISTRIBUTION

Demineralized (white or brown spots) and carious lesions generally occur at the margins of the gingiva upper incisors, and later first and second molars in pits and grooves of occlusal surfaces. Lower incisors are rarely affected.

LABORATORY AND IMAGING

Demineralized lesions may not be seen on radiographs, but advanced carious lesions between and on the occlusal surfaces are detected by x-ray.

MANAGEMENT

- Counsel patients about the importance of good oral hygiene practices and perform a caries risk assessment during well-child examination visits.[5,6] SOR B
- Refer to the dental health professional for the application of pit and fissure sealants.[5,6] SOR B
- Before prescribing supplemental fluoride, the primary care provider must determine the fluoride concentration in the child's primary source of drinking water. If fluoridated water is not available in the community, natural sources of fluoride are well water exposed to fluorite minerals and certain fruits and vegetables grown in soil irrigated with fluoridated water.[7] SOR B
- Fluoride supplementation is not recommended for use by persons who live in communities whose water is optimally fluoridated (0.7 to 1.2 parts per million [ppm] or >0.6 mg/L). See **Table 36-1** for fluoride supplementation.[7] SOR A
- Advise the caregiver to take the child to a dentist by age 1 year.[6] SOR C
- Application of fluoride varnishes twice per year in moderate to high-risk children have been shown to prevent caries in demineralized enamel.[8] SOR A

TABLE 36-1 Supplemental Fluoride Dosage Schedule

	Concentration of Fluoride in Water		
Age	<0.3 ppm F	0.3 to 0.6 ppm F	>0.6 ppm F
Birth to 6 months	0	0	0
6 months to 3 years	0.25 mg	0	0
3 to 6 years	0.50 mg	0.25 mg	0
6 to at least 16 years	1.00 mg	0.50 mg	0

Source: Guideline on Fluoride Therapy. Pediatric Dentistry, Volume 35 (6):2013-2014. American Academy of Pediatric Dentistry. http://www.aapd.org/media/Policies_Guidelines/G_fluoridetherapy.pdf

FOLLOW-UP

Ensure that any child whose teeth have "white spots" or visible caries is taken to a dentist for evaluation and treatment so the teeth can be saved from decay or repaired.

PATIENT EDUCATION[6]

- Give the child's caregiver anticipatory guidance that is appropriate to the child's age and dental development. Before the teeth erupt, the caregiver should use a washcloth or cotton gauze to clean a baby's mouth and to transition the child to tooth brushing. SOR C
- A "smear" of fluoridated toothpaste (approximately 0.1 mf fluoride) should be considered for children younger than 2 years of age who are at moderate risk or high risk for caries (**Figure 36-5**).[6] SOR B
- A "pea size" amount of toothpaste (approximately 0.2 mg fluoride) is appropriate for children 2 through 5 years of age.[6] SOR B
- The caregiver should brush the child's teeth until the child is capable of doing an adequate job (usually around age 7 years).
- Educate caregivers about the benefits of fluoride and fluorosis, and the possible side effects of using too much fluoride (see **Table 36-1**).
- Advise caregivers to teach the child to drink from a "sippy cup" as soon as possible and to avoid giving the child milk, juice, or soda in either a bottle or sippy cup when putting the child to bed.

Breastfeeding by itself is noncariogenic but when supplemented with other carbohydrates can place the child at risk for caries.[9,10]

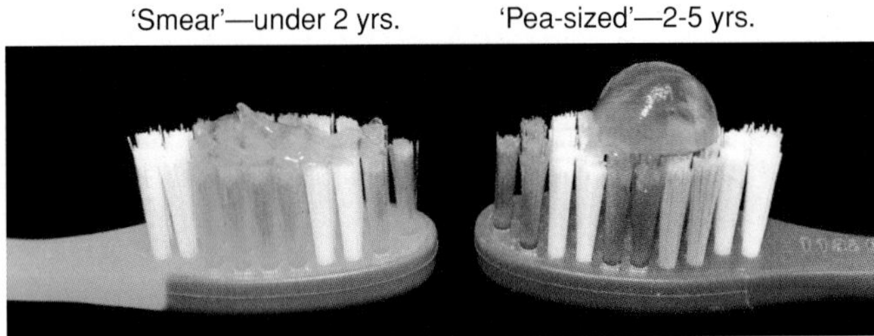

FIGURE 36-5 Comparison of a "smear" (*left*) with a "pea-sized" (*right*) amount of toothpaste. (*Used with permission from Richard P. Usatine, MD.*)

The American Academy of Pediatric Dentistry (AAPD) promotes breastfeeding for infants but recommends cessation of ad libitum breastfeeding as the first primary tooth begins to erupt and other dietary carbohydrates are introduced.[9] SOR C

PATIENT RESOURCES

- Centers for Disease Control and Prevention. *Brush Up on Healthy Teeth*—**www.cdc.gov/OralHealth/pdfs/BrushUpPoster.pdf**.
- Douglass JM, Douglass AB, Silk HJ: Your baby's teeth. *Am Fam Physician*. 2004;70:2121. **www.aafp.org/afp/20041201/2121ph.html**.
- **www.mychildrensteeth.org/education/**.
- **www.mouthhealthy.org/en/babies-and-kids/**.

PROVIDER RESOURCES

- American Academy of Pediatric Dentistry—**www.aapd.org/**.
- Smiles for Life: A National Oral Health Curriculum—**www.smilesforlifeoralhealth.org/**.
- Centers for Disease Control and Prevention. *Preventing Cavities, Gum Disease, Tooth Loss, and Oral Cancers at a Glance 2011*—**www.cdc.gov/chronicdisease/resources/publications/AAG/doh.htm**.

REFERENCES

1. U.S. Department of Health and Human Services. *Oral Health in America: A Report of the Surgeon General-Executive Summary*. Rockville, MD: US Department of Health and Human Services, National Institute of Dental and Craniofacial Research, National Institutes of Health, 2000. http://www.nidr.nih.gov/sgr/execsumm.htm, accessed April 20, 2012.
2. Centers for Disease Control and Prevention. *Oral Health: Preventing Cavities, Gum Disease, and Tooth Loss, and Oral Cancers*. http://www.cdc.gov/chronicdisease/resources/publications/AAG/doh.htm, accessed April 20, 2012.
3. Centers for Disease Control and Prevention. *Oral Health Resources: New Report Finds Improvements in Oral Health of Americans*. http://www.cdc.gov/oralhealth/publications/library/pressreleases/improvements.htm, accessed April 20, 2012.

4. American Academy of Pediatric Dentistry. Council on Clinical Affairs. *Policy on Early Child Caries (ECC: Classifications, Consequences, and Prevention Strategies) (Revised 2011)*. http://www.aapd.org/media/policies_guidelines/p_eccclassifications.pdf, accessed April 20, 2012.

5. National Institutes of Health. Consensus Development Conference Statement, March 26-28, 2001. *Diagnosis and Management of Dental Caries Throughout Life*. http://consensus.nih.gov/2001/2001DentalCaries115html.htm, accessed April 20, 2012.

6. American Academy of Pediatric Dentistry. Clinical Affairs Committee—Infant Oral Health Subcommittee. *Guideline on Infant Oral Health Care (Revised 2011)*. http://www.aapd.org/media/policies_guidelines/g_infantoralhealthcare.pdf, accessed April 20, 2012.

7. American Academy of Pediatric Dentistry. Liaison with Other Groups Committee, Council on Clinical Affairs. *Guideline on Fluoride Therapy*, p. 90. http://www.aapd.org/media/Policies_Guidelines/G_FluorideTherapy.pdf, accessed April 20, 2012.

8. Adair SM. Evidence base use of fluoride in contemporary pediatric dental medicine. *Pediatr Dent*. 2006;28(2):133-142, discussion 192-198.

9. American Academy of Pediatric Dentistry, Council on Clinical Affairs. *Policy on Dietary Recommendation for Infants, Children and Adolescents (Revised 2008)*. http://www.aapd.org/media/policies_guidelines/p_dietaryrec.pdf, accessed April 20, 2012.

10. Iada H, Auinger P, Billings RJ, Weitzman M. Association between infant breast feeding and early childhood caries in the United States. *Pediatrics*. 2007;120(4):936-952.

37 DENTAL COMPLICATIONS: HARD TISSUE (TEETH)

Homa Amini, DDS, MPH, MS
Ashok Kumar, DDS, MS
James R. Boynton, DDS, MS

PATIENT STORY

A 9-year-old boy presents to his pediatrician after suffering trauma to his face 45 minutes ago while jumping on a trampoline (**Figure 37-1**). The mother presents with a tooth folded in a wet napkin. There are no signs or symptoms of trauma to other craniofacial structures nor signs of neurological trauma. Upon examination, a fully rooted permanent tooth is noted to have been lost from its socket and the adjacent tooth is fractured. He is diagnosed with avulsion of the maxillary right central incisor. After a call to the child's dentist, the pediatrician reimplanted the tooth as directed (**Figure 37-2**). The boy was then sent directly to the dentist for evaluation and stabilization.

INTRODUCTION

Dental trauma may involve a tooth fracture or the traumatic displacement of a whole tooth. Intraoral and extraoral soft tissue (involving the gingiva, oral mucosa, and the tongue) may be injured as well.

EPIDEMIOLOGY

- Dental trauma is most common among children with a slight male predilection; the most commonly traumatized teeth are the maxillary central incisors.[1]

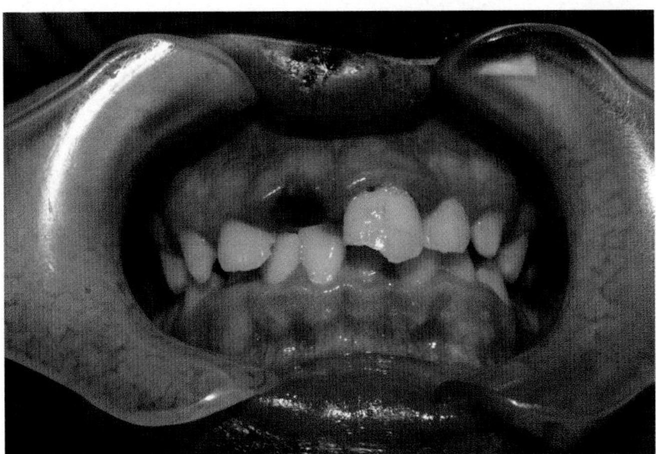

FIGURE 37-1 Maxillary right central incisor is completely avulsed out of its socket and maxillary left central incisor is fractured involving enamel and dentin. (*Used with permission from the Division of Pediatric Dentistry and Community Oral Health, The Ohio State University.*)

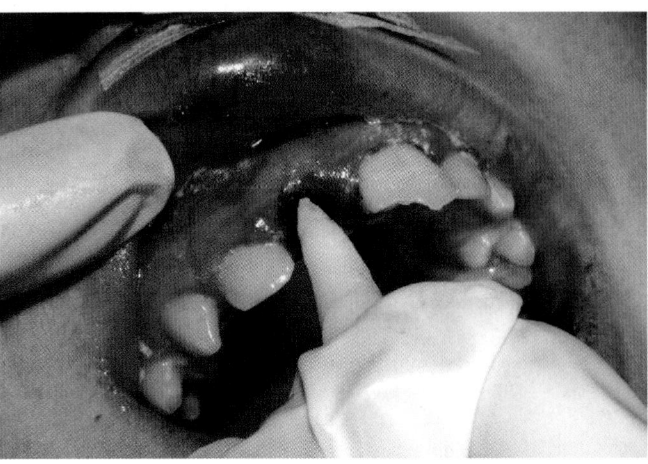

FIGURE 37-2 Avulsed permanent teeth should be reimplanted as soon as possible. Handle the tooth by the crown and avoid touching the root. (*Used with permission from the Division of Pediatric Dentistry and Community Oral Health, The Ohio State University.*)

ETIOLOGY AND PATHOPHYSIOLOGY

- Most incidents of trauma are caused by accidents in or around the home or at school.
- The impact of the injury may cause damage to the hard tissue of the tooth, the pulpal tissue within the tooth, the periodontal ligament which holds the tooth in the arch, the alveolar bone, intraoral soft tissue, the maxilla/mandible, or other craniofacial structures.
- Dental trauma, or delayed treatment of a traumatized tooth, may cause necrosis of the pulp tissue within the tooth necessitating root canal therapy or inflammation of the periodontal ligament, which can result in resorption of the root.
- After ruling out neurological and damage to other craniofacial structures, referral to a dentist is necessary for a thorough clinical and radiographic intraoral examination.

RISK FACTORS

- Malocclusion of maxillary/mandibular teeth.
- Lower socioeconomic status.
- Risk-taking children.
- Children being bullied or under emotionally stressful conditions.
- Children with obesity or ADHD.[2]

DIAGNOSIS

CLINICAL FEATURES

- Tooth fractures:
  - Enamel fracture—Fracture confined to the outer enamel surface without exposing the underlying dentin. Normally asymptomatic, although fracture site may be rough to the touch.

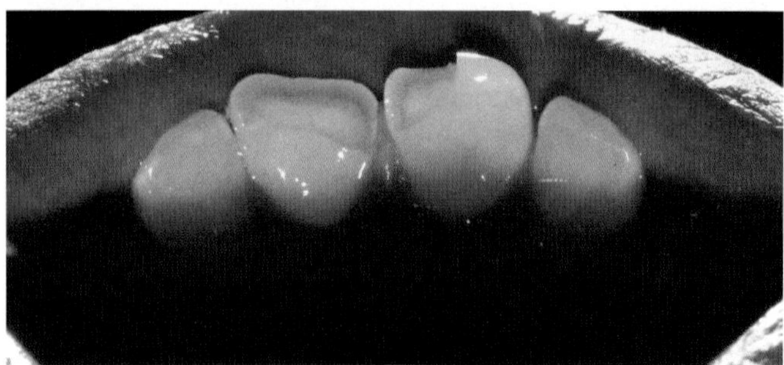

FIGURE 37-3 Tooth fracture involving the outer enamel and inner, more yellow-colored dentin. (*Used with permission from the Division of Pediatric Dentistry and Community Oral Health, The Ohio State University.*)

   - Enamel/dentin fracture—Fracture involving the outer enamel and inner, more yellow-colored dentin. Normally moderate to severely sensitive to heat or cold (**Figure 37-3**).
   - Enamel/dentin/pulp fracture—Fracture involving the enamel and dentin, which exposes the underlying vascular pulp tissue. Symptoms may range from no symptoms to sensitivity to heat and cold (**Figure 37-4**).
- Tooth displacement injuries:
   - Concussion/subluxation—Injuries to a tooth resulting in tooth mobility and/or sensitivity without displacement from the socket. Teeth may be sensitive to touch or abnormally loose, but the tooth remains in its prior position.
   - Luxation—Displacement of a tooth from its position in its socket. Teeth may be luxated laterally from the socket, intruded into the socket, or extruded partially out of the socket. These injuries are often associated with damage to the supporting alveolar bone (**Figures 37-5** and **37-6**).
   - Avulsion—Complete loss of tooth from socket. Tooth will be lost and a blood clot will form in the socket (**Figure 37-1**).
- Intraoral soft tissue trauma:
   - Laceration, abrasion, contusion of gingival, labial or lingual tissue, visible upon clinical examination (**Figure 37-7**).

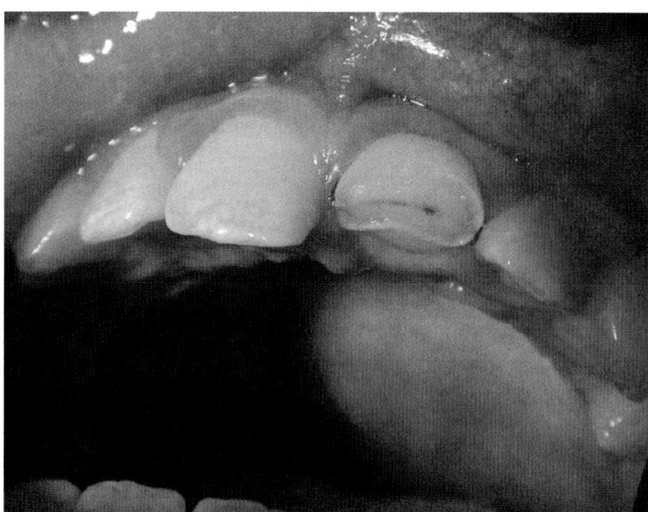

FIGURE 37-4 Tooth fracture resulting in pulpal exposure. (*Used with permission from the Division of Pediatric Dentistry and Community Oral Health, The Ohio State University.*)

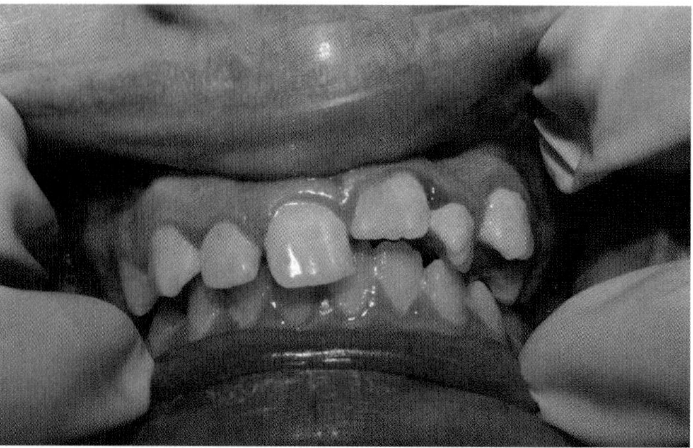

FIGURE 37-5 Traumatic dental injury resulting in intrusion of the tooth into the socket. (*Used with permission from the Division of Pediatric Dentistry and Community Oral Health, The Ohio State University.*)

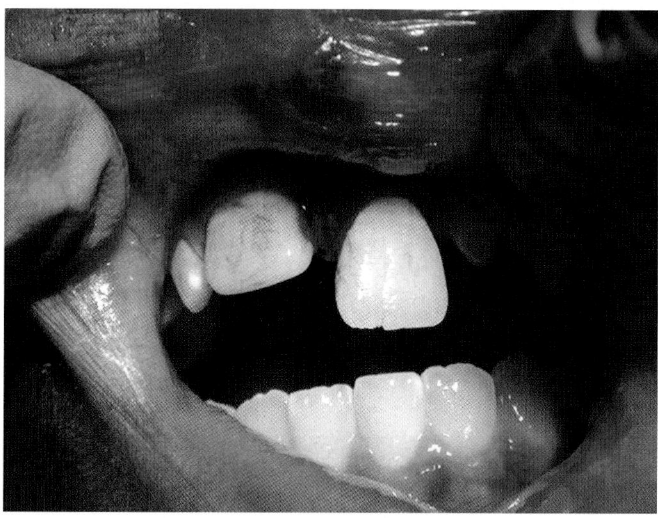

FIGURE 37-6 Traumatic dental injury resulting in partial extrusion of the tooth out of its socket. (*Used with permission from the Division of Pediatric Dentistry and Community Oral Health, The Ohio State University.*)

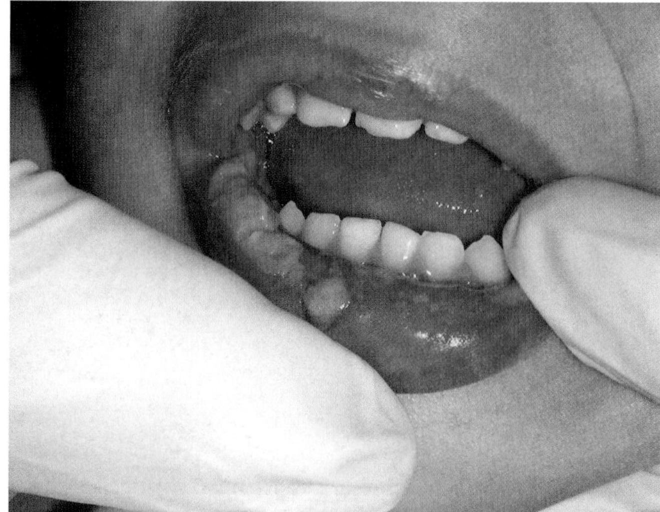

FIGURE 37-7 Soft tissue trauma of the lower lip associated with lip chewing following the use of local anesthesia in a 4-year-old child. (*Used with permission from the Division of Pediatric Dentistry and Community Oral Health, The Ohio State University.*)

IMAGING

To evaluate the extent of dental trauma, intraoral dental radiographs are exposed and evaluated by a dentist. A panoramic radiograph may be useful to evaluate suspected fracture of the mandible. Other head and neck radiographs, CT scans, and other imaging tests are not routinely ordered unless specifically indicated.

DIFFERENTIAL DIAGNOSIS

- Rule out child abuse, as approximately half of child abuse cases involve injuries to the head and neck.[3]
- Dental trauma may occur in conjunction with trauma to other head and neck structures; a thorough evaluation is critical to determine neurological trauma or trauma to other areas of the craniofacial complex.

MANAGEMENT

- Tooth fractures should be urgently referred to a dentist for clinical and radiographic evaluation and treatment. Treatment options for primary and permanent teeth are the same and may involve restoration of the fractured tooth surface and pulp therapy (**Figure 37-8**). Some fractured teeth are unable to be restored and must be extracted.
- Tooth displacement injuries should be urgently/immediately referred to a dentist for clinical and radiographic evaluation and treatment. Treatment for primary teeth may range from observation to extraction of the traumatized tooth. Treatment for permanent teeth may involve observation, repositioning, or extraction of the traumatized tooth.
- Avulsion injuries:
  - Primary tooth—Do not attempt to replace in socket. Refer to dentist for further evaluation.
  - Permanent tooth—Handle the tooth by the crown. Avoid touching the root. If the root has debris on it, rinse gently for a few seconds and then reimplant the tooth in its socket as quickly as possible. Have the patient bite on a washcloth to hold the tooth in place and refer to a dentist for urgent evaluation and stabilization of the tooth (**Figures 37-2** and **37-9**).

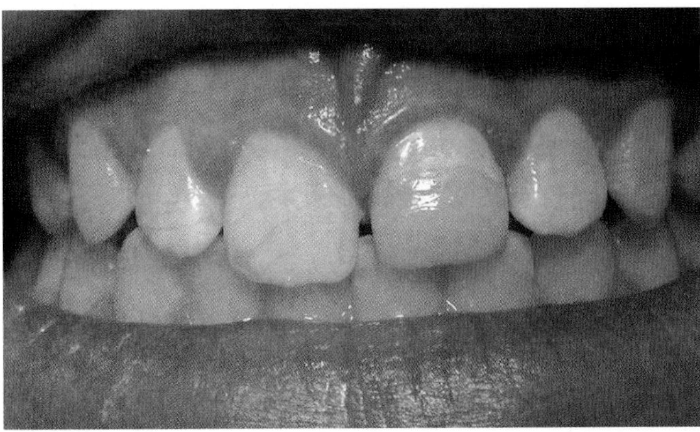

FIGURE 37-8 The left maxillary central incisor is restored with dental materials to its original form after a crown fracture. (*Used with permission from the Division of Pediatric Dentistry and Community Oral Health, The Ohio State University.*)

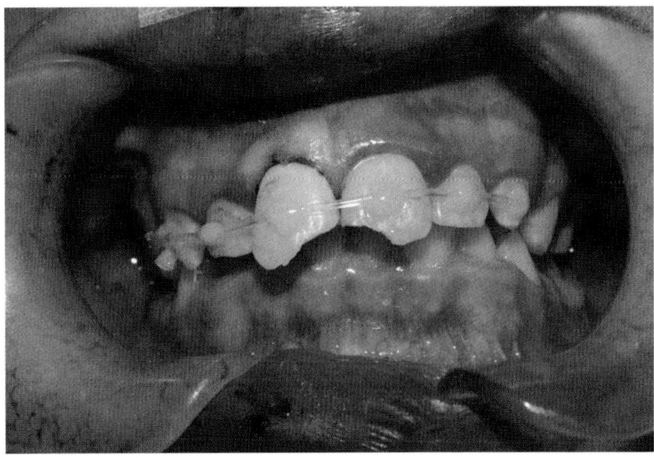

FIGURE 37-9 The avulsed teeth are stabilized by a splint after reimplantation. (*Used with permission from the Division of Pediatric Dentistry and Community Oral Health, The Ohio State University.*)

  - If not able to reimplant, tooth should be placed in a storage medium such as milk, Hank's Balanced Salt Solution, or normal saline for transport, and the child should be immediately seen by a dentist for urgent evaluation and reimplantation.[4]
- Soft tissue injuries—Clean the wound with saline irrigation. Sutures may be indicated. Intraoral radiographs may be indicated to rule out foreign body impaction. Refer to dentist for evaluation and treatment.

MEDICATIONS

- Ibuprofen or acetaminophen as needed for pain.
- Chlorhexidine Gluconate Oral Rinse, 0.12 percent, rinse twice daily for 1 week.

PREVENTION AND SCREENING

- Wear a mouthguard when playing sports.
- Childproof the home (cover table corners and install safety gates near stairs).

PROGNOSIS

- Prognosis is dependent on the nature of the injury. Minor tooth fractures have a good prognosis after restoration of the fracture whereas extensive fractures do not. Minor displacement injuries have a good prognosis, whereas intrusion and avulsion of a tooth have the most guarded prognosis of dental injuries. Intraoral soft-tissue injuries typically have a good prognosis.

FOLLOW-UP

The patient's dentist will follow-up with the patient on a routine schedule with clinical and radiographic examinations to evaluate the response of the pulp and periodontal ligament following the traumatic event.

PATIENT EDUCATION

Provide anticipatory guidance for prevention of traumatic dental injuries. Promote use of mouth guards for sport activities and advise parents to childproof their home.

PATIENT RESOURCES

- American Dental Association—**www.mouthhealthy.org/en/az-topics/d/dental-emergencies.aspx**.
- *Dental Injuries: A Field Side Guide for Parents, Athletic Trainers, and Dentists*—**www.sickkids.ca/pdfs/Dentistry/12902-DentalInjuries.pdf**.

PROVIDER RESOURCES

- International Association of Dental Traumatology guidelines—**www.iadt-dentaltrauma.org/GUIDELINES_Book.pdf**.
- American Academy of Pediatric Dentistry Guideline on Management of Acute Dental Trauma—**www.aapd.org/media/Policies_Guidelines/G_Trauma.pdf**.

REFERENCES

1. Bastone EB, Freer TJ, McNamara JR. Epidemiology of Dental Trauma: A Review of the Literature. *Aust Dent J*. 2000;(45)1:2-9.
2. Glendor U. Aetiology and risk factors related to traumatic dental injuries—a review of the literature. *Dent Traumatol*. 2009;25:19-31.
3. Needleman HL. Orofacial trauma in child abuse: types, prevalence, management, and the dental profession's involvement. *Pediatr Dent*. 1986;8:71-80.
4. The Dental Trauma Guide. http://dentaltraumaguide.org/ Copenhagen, Denmark, 2010.

38 DENTAL COMPLICATIONS—SOFT TISSUE (GINGIVA AND MUCOSA)

Sarat Thikkurissy, DDS, MS
Elizabeth Sutton Gosnell, DMD, MS
Dimitris N. Tatakis, DDS, PhD

ANKYLOGLOSSIA

PATIENT STORY

A 2-year-old male child presents with a chief complaint per mother of "not being able to stick out his tongue." (**Figure 38-1**). On examination, the child could not protrude the tip of the tongue over the mandibular anterior teeth and could not effectively lick his upper lip. Neither gingival recession nor speech pathology was noted. A diagnosis of ankyloglossia was made. Frenectomy was suggested and delayed until child's age made feasible necessary behavioral management in the dental chair.

INTRODUCTION

Ankyloglossia refers to a congenital abnormality, where a short and/or thick lingual frenum may restrict tongue movement (**Figure 38-2**).[1] Severity may vary significantly.

SYNONYM

Tongue-Tie.

EPIDEMIOLOGY

- Reported prevalence varies from 0.1 to 10.7 percent, dependent on age population surveyed.[1]

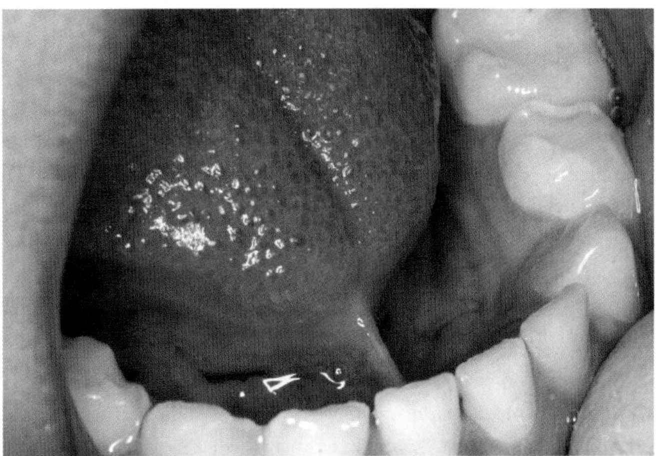

FIGURE 38-1 Ankyloglossia characterized by a short and thick frenum. (*Used with permission from Dimitris N. Tatakis DDS, PhD.*)

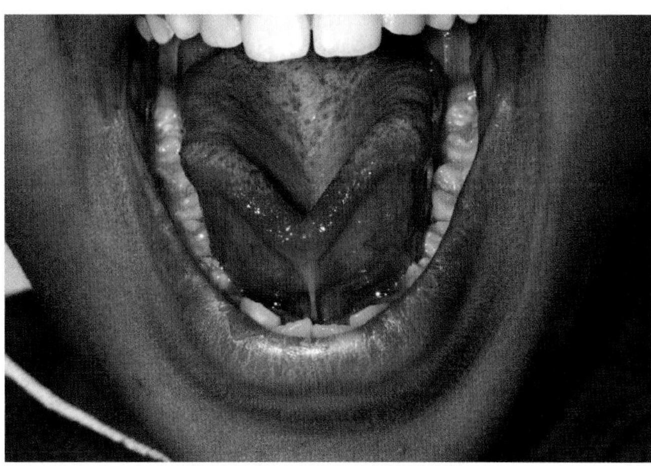

FIGURE 38-2 Ankyloglossia in a child restricting movement of the tongue. (*Used with permission from Dimitris N. Tatakis DDS, PhD.*)

- It has been reported as being more prevalent in males, although this is a controversial and inconclusive finding.[2]

ETIOLOGY AND PATHOPHYSIOLOGY

- This is a developmental, congenital condition.
- There have been reports associating ankyloglossia with specific syndromes such as X-linked cleft palate.[3]
- However, most incidences of ankyloglossia occur in individuals without any other congenital disease.
- A positive family history of ankyloglossia was noted in a wide range (10% to 53%) of families surveyed in a 2002 study,[4] while it has been strongly associated with maternal cocaine use.[5]

RISK FACTORS

- Family history.
- Maternal cocaine use (3.2 times the increased risk).[5]

DIAGNOSIS

CLINICAL FEATURES

- Variably short and thick lingual frenum with concomitant limitation of tongue mobility (range of motion) and/or functionality.
- Clinical diagnosis is typically made during early feeding disturbances in children, in which severe ankyloglossia prevents/impedes completion of a sufficient oral seal during nursing.
- Initial diagnosis in neonates and young infants might be made by lactation consultants.
- A randomized controlled trial demonstrated in 2005 that 95 percent of infants receiving surgical correction had improved feeding, compared to <10 percent in the control group.[6]

DIFFERENTIAL DIAGNOSIS

- Feeding and speech difficulties may be associated with other intrinsic behaviors and causative factors.
- Therefore, a comprehensive review is required to determine the possible contribution of ankyloglossia and the need for management.

MANAGEMENT

- Management approaches, which are surgical, are often based on the severity of the ankyloglossia and its impact (i.e., effects on feeding, speech, peer acceptance, social life and self image). SOR B
- A comprehensive evaluation of the severity of the problem and the impact of the problem on the child's pathology is important prior to any surgical correction.
- It should be noted that the literature reflects possible recurrence of ankyloglossia due to excessive scar tissue formation.[7]
- Surgical Options
  - Frenotomy—Surgical release of frenal constriction.
  - Frenectomy—Complete excision of entire frenum.
  - Frenuloplasty—Surgical rearrangement of frenal attachments and extension.

PATIENT EDUCATION

Parents should be advised to seek consultations from a pediatric dentist (or dentist familiar with ankyloglossia in young children), lactation consultant (if nursing is a specific issue), and speech pathologist (if speech is affected) to have a comprehensive evaluation of the child's limitations, to ensure that ankyloglossia is a contributing factor to child's pathology, prior to referring the child for surgical correction.

PATIENT RESOURCES

- **www.nlm.nih.gov/medlineplus/ency/article/001640.htm**.
- **www.ncbi.nlm.nih.gov/pubmedhealth/PMH0002606/**.
- **pediatrics.aappublications.org/content/110/5/e63.full**.

GINGIVITIS

PATIENT STORY

A 13-year-old female presents to your office because of persistent "bleeding" from her gums. The bleeding occurs most often during brushing of her teeth. She has no other history of bleeding or other contributory medical history. Her gingiva appear edematous and friable (**Figure 38-3**).

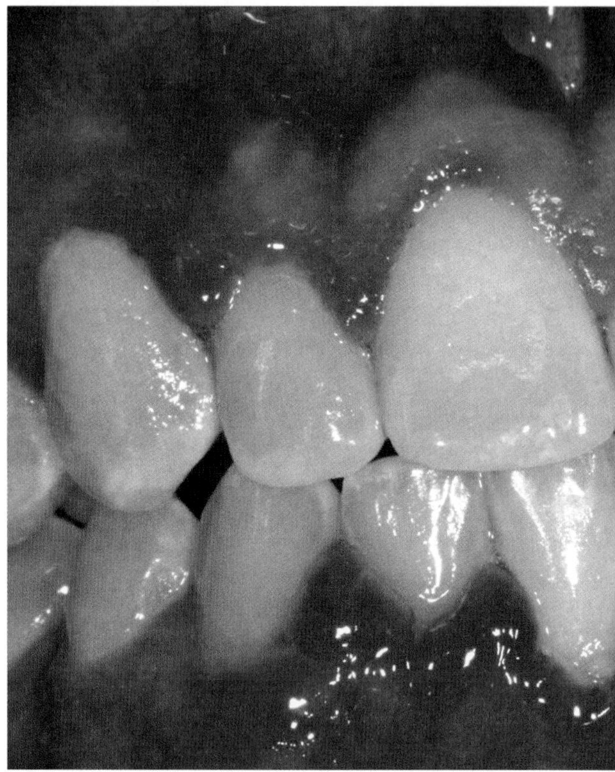

FIGURE 38-3 Gingivitis in an adolescent characterized by erythematous and edematous gingiva. (*Used with permission from Dimitris N. Tatakis DDS, PhD.*)

INTRODUCTION

Gingivitis refers to a reversible and (classically) bacterial-plaque mediated gingival inflammation. There are other sub-genres of gingivitis that may have additional etiologic factors (such as pregnancy gingivitis). Gingivitis does not include the broad spectrum of periodontal diseases in children (those associated with loss of soft and hard (alveolar bone) tissue support around the teeth).

SYNONYM

Gum disease or gingival disease.

EPIDEMIOLOGY

- Epidemiologic studies suggest a nearly universal prevalence of gingivitis in children and adolescents, beginning in the primary dentition and peaking during puberty.[8,9]
- The lingual surfaces of primary and permanent molars are most often affected by gingivitis.[8]
- The American Academy of Periodontology International Workshop on Classification of Periodontal diseases and conditions lists dental plaque-induced gingival disease as a distinct category of disease that affect "young individuals." There are specific conditions (namely puberty and diabetes) that can modify the gingival response to bacterial plaque.[11]

ETIOLOGY AND PATHOPHYSIOLOGY

- Gingivitis is a plaque-induced, bacterial mediated condition. Commonly isolated pathogens associated with gingivitis include *Actinomyces* sp. and *Capnocytophaga* sp.[10]
- However, irrespective of specific bacterial colonization, the progression of gingivitis is typically associated with poor oral hygiene and plaque-accumulation.
- Fluctuations in gonadotrophic hormone levels associated with puberty may modify the gingival inflammatory response, increasing susceptibility to gingivitis.
- Unfavorable insulin levels in diabetic patients may also have this effect.[12,13]
- The presence of local factors that favor plaque accumulation (e.g., tooth crowding or orthodontic appliances) or prevent proper oral hygiene (e.g., erupting teeth) may predispose areas to gingivitis development.

RISK FACTORS

- Bacterial plaque accumulation.
- Poor oral hygiene.
- Poor control of diabetes.
- Circumpubertal hormone changes.
- Mouthbreathing.

DIAGNOSIS

CLINICAL FEATURES

- Typically painless, erythematous and edematous marginal (and papillary) gingiva with shiny surface appearance.
- Increased severity of inflammation is associated with greater prevalence of bleeding upon provocation (e.g., during toothbrushing).

DIFFERENTIAL DIAGNOSIS

- Pyogenic granuloma—Typically localized gingival enlargement that may be painful; often associated with pregnancy.
- Gingival abscess—Painful, localized gingival swelling; typically sudden onset and classically associated with a foreign body of some type.
- Acute necrotizing ulcerative gingivitis—Gingivitis characterized by pain, bleeding, and necrotic (punched out) interdental (papillary) and/or marginal gingiva; typically sudden onset; associated with smoking and stress-inducing conditions.
- Vitamin C deficiency associated gingivitis—Typically accompanied by systemic manifestations (petechiae, ecchymoses, or impaired wound healing); rare in populations with adequate food supply.
- Leukemia—Inflamed gingiva (shiny, red, and edematous) with bleeding a common feature; systemic symptoms may include fever, malaise, easy bruising or bleeding, and bone or joint pain.

MANAGEMENT

- Daily, attentive and effective oral hygiene habits are paramount.
- Younger children (those 10 and younger) will often require some form of direct parental involvement in performing oral hygiene procedures.
- Use of oral hygiene adjuncts, such as mouthrinses, may help.[14] SOR Ⓐ

PREVENTION & PATIENT EDUCATION

- The American Academy of Pediatric Dentistry/American Academy of Pediatrics' position is that all children should visit a dentist by the age of one or eruption of first tooth.
- During this visit, anticipatory guidance will help caregivers understand how to assess whether oral hygiene is adequate.

PATIENT RESOURCES

- **www.perio.org/consumer/children.htm**.
- **www2.aap.org/ORALHEALTH/pact/ch13_sect2.cfm**.
- **www.aapd.org/media/Policies_Guidelines/E_PeriodontalDisease.pdf**.
- **www.emedicine.medscape.com/article/763801-overview**.

MUCOCELE

PATIENT STORY

An 11-year-old boy presents with a chief complaint of a "bump" on his lip that has been there for about 1 month. The lesion has fluctuated in size, and is painless, unless he bites on it, which sometimes happens when he is playing. A mucocele was the working clinical diagnosis (**Figure 38-4**). The lesion was excised and the child healed uneventfully.

INTRODUCTION

Traumatic injury or pathologic alteration of minor salivary glands in the lip may result in mucous accumulation (pseudocyst). This may result in a swelling on the lip that alters in size due to mucous accumulation and extravasation.

SYNONYM

Mucous retention cyst/phenomena; Ranula (when on floor of mouth); Mucocele of Glands of Blandin-Nuhn (ventral tongue surface).

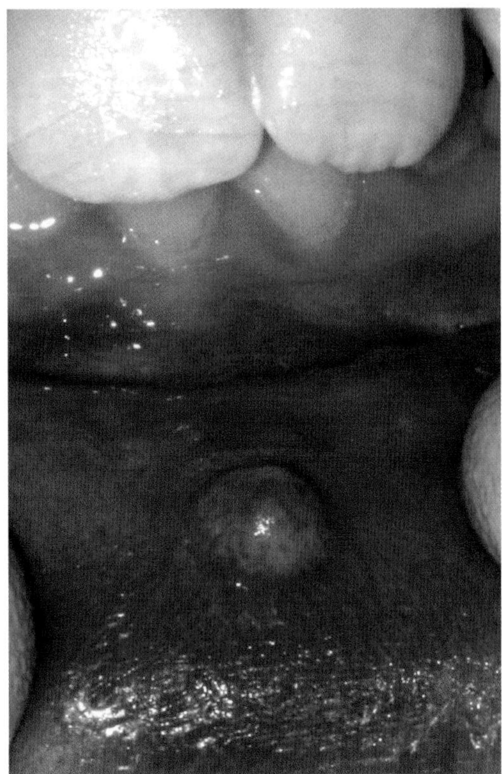

FIGURE 38-4 Mucocele apparent on the lower lip of this boy. (*Used with permission from Dimitris N. Tatakis DDS, PhD.*)

EPIDEMIOLOGY

- Most often occurs in the second decade of life,[15] with no gender predilection.
- Studies have reported average progression time to be about 6 months.
- A large retrospective analysis determined the overall prevalence to be 16 percent of lesions found in over 4,000 children during a 30-year period.[18]

ETIOLOGY AND PATHOPHYSIOLOGY

- Traumatic injury of minor salivary gland ducts in the lip, leading to mucous extravasation into adjacent tissues.[16]
- Size fluctuations are directly related to mucin accumulation within the lesion. Lip lesions are often related to the bite (occlusion) (**Figure 38-5**).

RISK FACTORS

- Self-injurious behaviors, such as lip biting.
- Previous history of mucocele.
- Lichen Planus (associated with multiple mucoceles).
- Graft versus host disease.

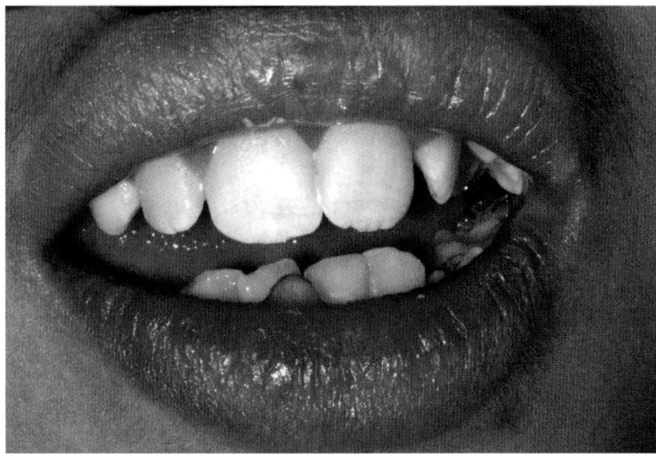

FIGURE 38-5 Mucocele on the lower lip of this child. (*Used with permission from Dimitris N. Tatakis DDS, PhD.*)

DIAGNOSIS

CLINICAL FEATURES

- Typically painless, soft/fluctuant papule, translucent, or pink to bluish color, smooth surface; may acquire nodular appearance if persisting for longer periods.
- While it is common to have a working clinical diagnosis, final diagnosis can only be made following histological examination, which reveals mucin and minor salivary gland components.

DIFFERENTIAL DIAGNOSIS

- Lymphangioma.
- Hemangioma.
- Traumatic hematoma.
- Irritation (traumatic) fibroma.
- Verucca Vulgaris wart—Often present on other sites of body as well.

MANAGEMENT

- Typically, surgical excision.
- Aspiration is not an effective treatment.
- Incomplete lesion removal or further trauma to the minor salivary glands may result in recurrence.
- Recent literature has suggested that conventional surgical excision is a definitive treatment of mucoceles.[17] SOR B
- Reported recurrence rates vary between 4 to 8 percent.[17,18]

PREVENTION

- As these lesions are often traumatically induced, prevention is challenging.
- Children with large overjet (protruding maxillary teeth) may be more prone to lip biting as well as those patients with self-injurious biting behaviors.

PATIENT EDUCATION

Encourage patients to avoid any self-injurious behaviors.

PATIENT RESOURCES

- **www.ncbi.nlm.nih.gov/pubmedhealth/PMH0002605**.

GINGIVAL FIBROMA

PATIENT STORY

A 7-year-old female presents with a parental chief complaint of "pink bump on her gums" (**Figure 38-6**). The child has adequate oral hygiene, a regular dentist and no clinical evidence of dental caries. An excisional biopsy was performed and a diagnosis of gingival fibroma was made.

INTRODUCTION

Gingival fibroma may be classified as a localized reactive gingival lesion, characterized by connective tissue hyperplasia, resulting of chronic irritation. It is a benign lesion, but due to potential severity of differential diagnoses, histopathological examination is warranted.[19]

SYNONYM

Traumatic fibroma or irritation fibroma.

EPIDEMIOLOGY

- In a population-based study of over 25,000 biopsies, approximately 7 percent were localized reactive gingival lesions.[20]
- Fibromas, potentially occurring on any mucosal surface, are among the most common oral lesions.

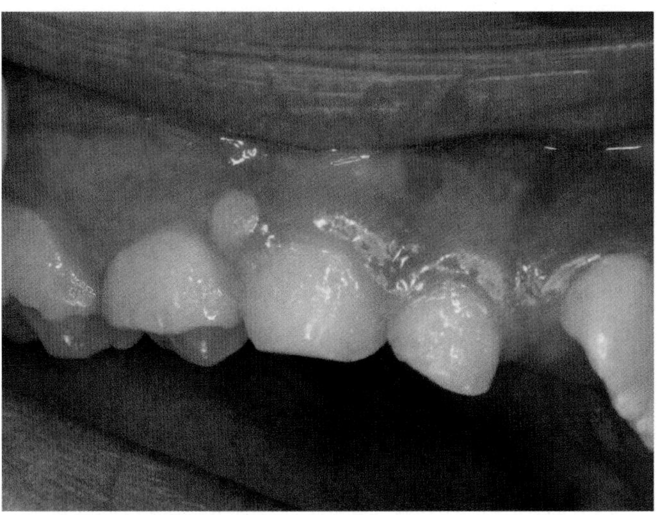

FIGURE 38-6 Fibroma seen on the upper gingiva of a child. (*Used with permission from Dimitris N. Tatakis DDS, PhD.*)

ETIOLOGY AND PATHOPHYSIOLOGY

- The etiology of gingival fibroma is considered to be chronic irritation or persistent trauma.
- In children, there is the possibility that improper oral hygiene or oral habits may contribute to chronic irritation.

RISK FACTORS

- Chronic irritation/trauma.
- Tuberous Scelerosis—Demosplastic fibroma variant.

DIAGNOSIS

CLINICAL FEATURES

- Typically normal or pale pink color, smooth surface, firm to rubbery consistency, and sessile base.
- Definitive diagnosis is made based on histologic examination and history.

DIFFERENTIAL DIAGNOSIS

- Pyogenic Granuloma (may be associated with pregnancy).
- Peripheral Giant Cell Granuloma.
- Peripheral Ossifying Fibroma (may present with characteristic radiographic appearance of mixed radiopaque and radiolucent lesion).

MANAGEMENT

- Excisional biopsy, along with removal of source of irritation, is a conservative and highly effective method of management. SOR Ⓑ
- Failure to eliminate/control local irritant may lead to recurrence.

PREVENTION

- Elimination/correction of identified local irritants or sources of chronic trauma.

PATIENT EDUCATION

- Cessation of any self-injurious behaviors or habits.

PATIENT RESOURCES

- **www.emedicine.medscape.com/article/1080948-overview**.

REFERENCES

1. VGA Suter, MM Bornstein: Ankyloglossia: Facts and Myths in Diagnosis and Treatment. *J Periodontol.* 2009;80:1204-1219.
2. Jorgenson RJ, Shaprio SD, Salinas CF, Levin LS. Intraoral Findings and anomalies in neonates. *Pediatrics.* 1982;69:577-582.
3. Bjornsson A, Arnason A, Tippet P. X-linked Cleft palate and ankyloglossia in an Icelandic Family. *Cleft Palate J.* 1989;26:3-8.
4. Ballard JL, Auer CE, Khoury JC. Ankyloglossia: Assessment, incidence and effect of frenuloplasty on the breastfeeding dyad. *Pediatrics.* 2002;110:e63.
5. Harris EF, Friend GW, Tolley EA. Enhanced prevalence of ankyloglossia with maternal cocaine use. *Cleft Palate Craniofac J.* 1992;9:72-76.
6. Hogan M, Westcott C, Griffiths M. Randomized controlled trial of division of tongue-tie in infants with feeding problems. *J Paediatr Child Health.* 2005;41:246-250.
7. Wright JE. Tongue-tie. *J Paediatr Child Health.* 1995;31:276-278.
8. Jenkins WMM, Papapanou PN. Epidemiology of Periodontal Disease in Children and Adolescents. *Periodontology.* 2000;26:16-32.
9. Kelly JE, Sanchez MJ. Periodontal disease and oral hygiene among children. United States. *Vital Health Stat 1.* 1972;11(117):1-28.
10. Moore W, Holdeman L, Smibert R, et al. Bacteriology of experimental gingivitis in children. *Infect Immun.* 1984;46:1-6.
11. Nakagawa S, Fujii H, Machida Y, Okuda K. A longitudinal study from prepuberty to puberty of gingivitis. Correlation between the occurrence of *Prevotella intermedia* and sex hormones. *J Clin Periodontol.* 1994;21:658.
12. De Pommereau V, Dargent-Par C, Robert JJ, Brion M. Periodontal status in insulin-dependent diabetic adolescents. *J Clin Periodontol.* 1992;19:628-632.
13. KN Varlinkova, R Kabaktchieva: Oral health Status Assessment Indicators in a Child Dental Patient. *Journal of IMAB.* 2008;14(2): 1-101.
14. American Academy of Pediatric Dentistry. http://www.aapd.org/media/Policies_Guidelines/E_PeriodontalDisease.pdf, accessed March 27, 2013.
15. MM Nico, SV Lourenco, JH Park: Mucocele in Pediatric Patients: Analysis of 36 Children. *Pediatric Dermatology.* 2008;25(3); 308-311.
16. LA Alves, R DiNicolo, L Shintome, CS Barbosa: Retention mucocele on the lower lip associated with inadequate use of pacifier. *Dermatol Online J.* 2010;16(7):9.
17. RN Bahadure, P Fulzele, N Badole, S Baliga: Conventional surgical Treatment of Oral Mucocele: A series of 23 cases. *Eur J Paediatric Dent.* 2012;13(2):143-146.
18. IM Martinez, C Bonet-Coloma, J Ata-Ali-Mahmud, et al. Clinical Characteristics, Treatment and Evolution of 89 Mucoceles in Children. *J Oral Maxillfac Surg.* 2010:68(10);2468-2471.
19. A Buchner, A Shnaiderman, M Vared: Pediatric localized reactive gingival lesions: A retrospective study from Israel. *Pediatric Dentistry.* 2010;32:486-492.
20. A Buchner, A Shnairderman-Shapiro, M Vered: Relative Frequency of Localized Reactive Hyperplastic Lesions of the Gingiva; A Retrospective study of 1675 cases from Israel. *J Oral Pathol Med.* 2010;39:631-638.

39 HERPES SIMPLEX VIRUS GINGIVOSTOMATITIS

Camille Sabella, MD

PATIENT STORY

A 12-month-old previously healthy boy is seen in the office with a 3-day history of fever and ulcerative lesions on his lips and mouth. Over the past day the lesions had spread to his face and around his eye (**Figure 39-1**). His mother has noted that the lesions have evolved from flat to raised lesions to fluid-filled ulcers. The boy has been irritable, and over the past day, has refused to eat and drink. He appears dehydrated and is admitted to the hospital for intravenous fluid hydration.

INTRODUCTION

Primary herpes simplex virus (HSV) infection occurs commonly in infants and children. While most infections are asymptomatic, the most common clinical manifestation of primary HSV infection is gingivostomatitis. This infection in otherwise healthy infants and children is self-limited, but can occasionally lead to dehydration and hospitalization. Immunocompromised individuals who are infected with HSV may have more severe and systemic manifestations.

SYNONYMS

Oro-labial HSV infection; cold sores; fever blisters; herpetic stomatitis.

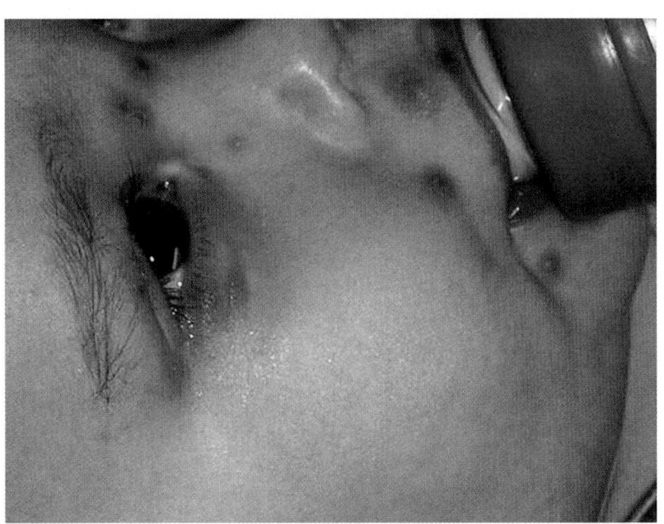

FIGURE 39-1 Vesicular lesions of primary HSV infection in a 12-month-old infant. (*Used with permission from Johanna Goldfarb, MD.*)

EPIDEMIOLOGY

- Most perioral HSV infections are asymptomatic; thus, manifestations of HSV infections are apparent in a small proportion of patients who become infected.[1]
- Primary infection with HSV-1 usually occurs in infants and children.[2]
- Acquisition occurs after mucocutaneous contact between a susceptible host and a contact who is shedding the virus.
- Transmission occurs commonly from an asymptomatic individual who is shedding the virus after primary infection or after reactivation of the virus.
- Incubation period is 3 to 4 days.

ETIOLOGY AND PATHOPHYSIOLOGY

- Most infections are caused by HSV-1.
- Primary infection occurs when the virus penetrates through abraded skin or mucosal surfaces.
- HSV enters cutaneous neurons and then migrates to the sensory ganglia, where the virus replicates and then returns to the inoculation site via peripheral sensory ganglia.[3]
- Skin and mucous membrane changes are more severe following primary infection than following reactivation of the virus.
- Establishment of lifelong latency is a hallmark feature of all herpes viruses; latency is established in the trigeminal ganglia.
- Periodic reactivation of the virus occurs, resulting in spread of the virus down the neuroaxis, causing shedding of the virus and possible recurrent skin lesions.

RISK FACTORS

- Possible triggers of reactivation of HSV include stress, exposure to ultraviolet light, intercurrent infections, manipulation of nerve roots, dental manipulation, hormonal changes, and immunosuppression.

DIAGNOSIS

CLINICAL FEATURES

Primary infections

- Fever, irritability, and tender submandibular lymphadenopathy are common in symptomatic patients.
- Vesiculo-ulcerative lesions can occur on the palate, gingiva, tongue, lip, and face (**Figures 39-2** and **39-3**).[4]
- Lesions are associated with pain and intraoral edema (**Figure 39-4**).
- Involvement of the peri-orbital area can occur via autoinoculation or as a manifestation of the primary infection (**Figure 39-5**).
- Lesions evolve from vesicles to shallow ulcers on an erythematous base.

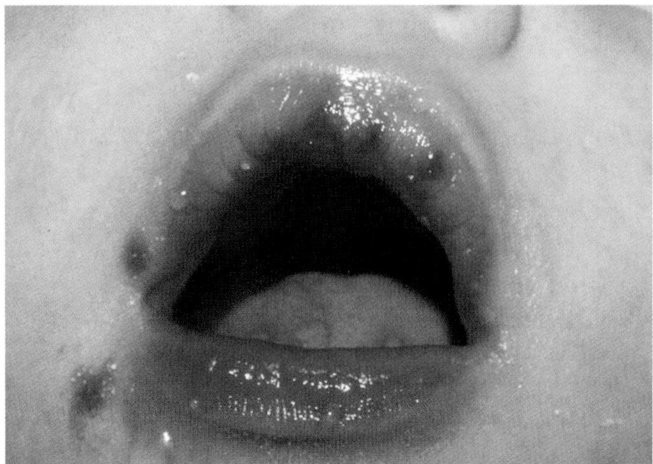

FIGURE 39-2 HSV stomatitis in an infant. Note the cluster of vesicles on the upper lip. (*Used with permission from Johanna Goldfarb, MD.*)

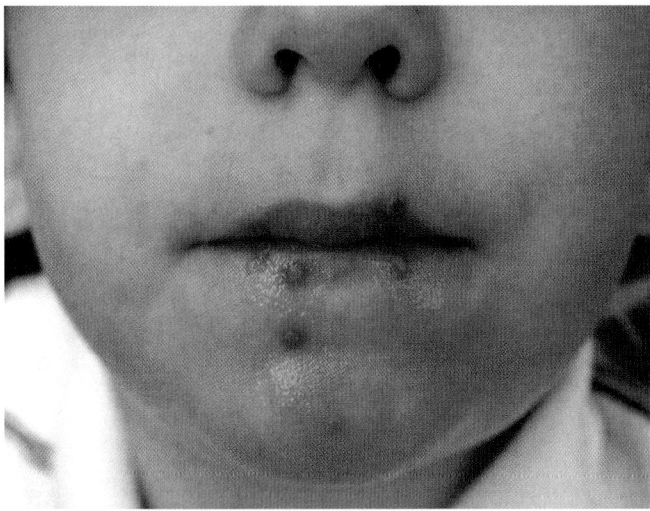

FIGURE 39-3 HSV stomatitis in a school-aged child. (*Used with permission from Camille Sabella, MD.*)

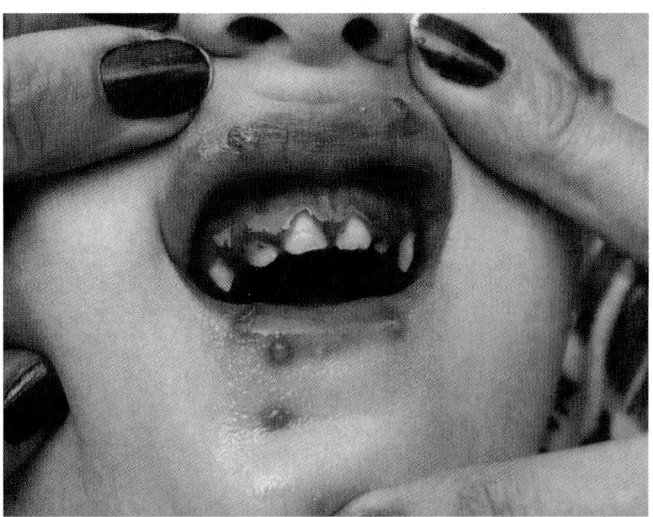

FIGURE 39-4 HSV stomatitis in the same child. Note the marked gingival edema, characteristic of a primary HSV infection. (*Used with permission from Camille Sabella, MD.*)

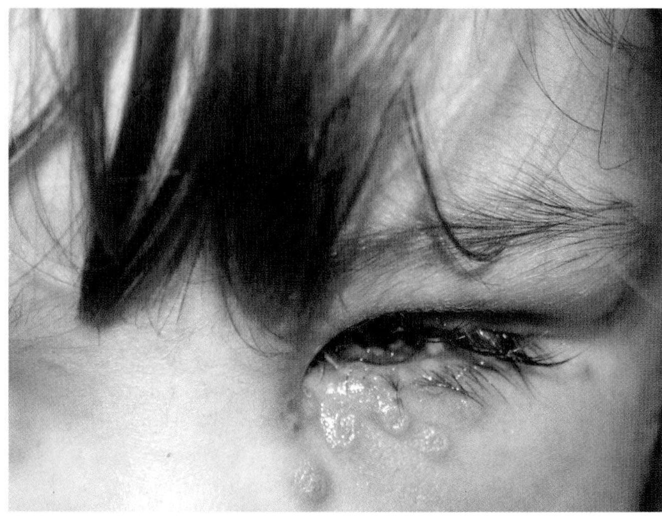

FIGURE 39-5 Periorbital vesiculo-bullous HSV lesions in a toddler. (*Used with permission from Paul Rychwalski, MD.*)

- Lesions may last 2 to 3 weeks.
- Inability to take oral liquids and solids is common.
- Most common cause of hospitalization is dehydration.
- Immunocompromised patients may have more severe involvement of the mouth and face, and may evolve into disseminated disease (**Figure 39-6**).

Reactivation

- Most reactivation of HSV from the trigeminal ganglia results in asymptomatic infection/shedding.
- Signs and symptoms in those who are symptomatic are mild: prodromal burning, pain, tingling may precede the eruption by 1 to 2 days.[5]
- On average, three to five lesions are present.
- Lesions begin as vesicles, evolve into pustules or ulcers in 1 to 2 days, and heal completely within 7 to 10 days.

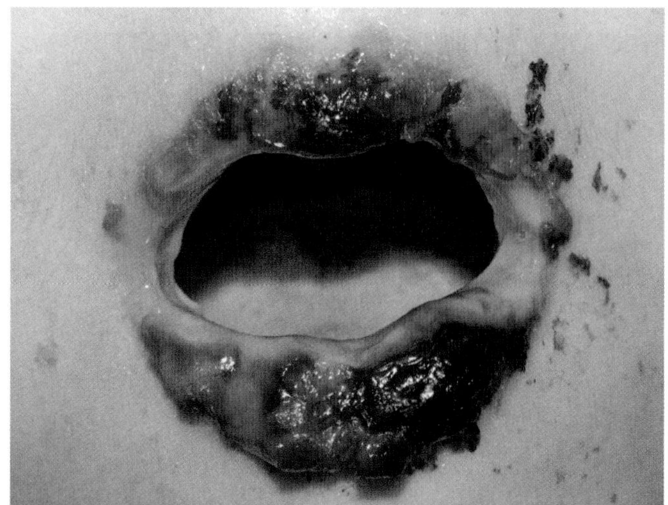

FIGURE 39-6 HSV stomatitis in a child who has acute leukemia. Note the widespread involvement of the infection. (*Used with permission from Camille Sabella, MD.*)

DISTRIBUTION

- In primary infections, lesions may occur on the palate, gingival, tongue, lips, and facial areas.
- Outer edge of the vermillion border is the most common site of reactivation.

LABORATORY TESTING

- Often a clinical diagnosis based on classic signs and symptoms.
- When a virologic diagnosis is required, samples of the skin should be obtained by aspirating contents of intact skin lesions or by swabbing the base of the denuded skin lesions.
- Culture of HSV from skin lesions is the most sensitive and specific method of diagnosing an active HSV infection.[6]
- Yield of recovery of HSV by culture very high when taken from a vesicular lesions and much lower from a crusted lesion.[6]
- The average time to positive culture for HSV utilizing cytopathic effect is 2 to 5 days. However, immunofluorescent staining of tissue cell cultures can rapidly confirm the presence of HSV and distinguish between HSV-1 and HSV-2.
- Direct immunofluorescent staining of infected cells (obtained by unroofing a lesion and removing cells from the base of the lesion) is 80 to 90 percent sensitive and very specific. This can provide a rapid diagnosis.[7,8]
- A Tzank test less sensitive and specific than culture and direct immunofluorescent staining.

DIFFERENTIAL DIAGNOSIS

- Aphthous stomatitis is frequently confused with HSV; this most commonly occurs inside the mouth rather than on the lips and external to the mouth.
- Erythema multiforme/Stevens Johnson syndrome usually manifests with more systemic manifestations, such as rash and eye involvement, as well as more severe oral involvement with necrosis and sloughing of the mucosa (**Figure 39-7**). HSV is a recognized cause of erythema multiforme/Stevens Johnson syndrome.

MANAGEMENT

MEDICATIONS

- For primary infections, oral acyclovir shortens duration of oral lesions, and results in earlier disappearance of fever, extraoral lesions, and drinking and eating difficulties.[9] SOR Ⓐ
- Some experts treat hospitalized children who have primary HSV infection with intravenous acyclovir. SOR Ⓒ
- For HSV reactivation, topical acyclovir is not effective; oral acyclovir is marginally effective in immunocompetent hosts.[10,11] SOR Ⓑ
- Prophylactic administration of oral acyclovir reduces the number of recurrences in adults with frequent recurrent orolabial HSV infection.[12–14] Pediatric studies are lacking.

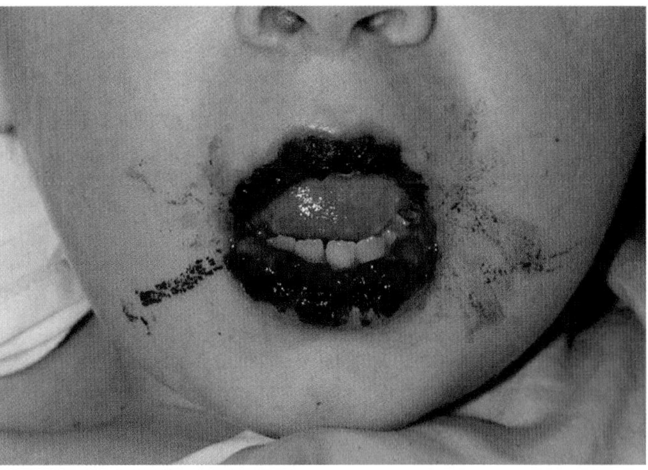

FIGURE 39-7 Stevens-Johnson syndrome, characterized by necrosis and sloughing of the mucosa. (*Used with permission from Camille Sabella, MD.*)

REFERRAL

Healthy children who have frequent recurrences of HSV gingivostomatitis may be referred to a pediatric infectious diseases specialist to discuss possible suppressive therapy.

PROGNOSIS

- The infection is self-limited in immunocompetent hosts.
- Immunocompromised hosts have higher risk of disseminated disease.

PATIENT EDUCATION

Parents should be counseled that oral HSV infections in otherwise healthy children are benign and self-limited, are often asymptomatic, and require symptomatic care.

PATIENT RESOURCES

- **www.healthychildren.org/English/health-issues/conditions/skin/Pages/Herpes-Simplex-Virus-Cold-Sores.aspx**.
- **http://www.nlm.nih.gov/medlineplus/coldsores.html**.

PROVIDER RESOURCES

- American Academy of Pediatrics. Herpes simplex virus infections. In: Pickering LK, Baker CJ, Kimberlin DW, Long SS, eds. *Red Book: 2012 Report of the Committee on Infectious Diseases.* Elk Grove Village, IL: American Academy of Pediatrics; 2012:398-408.

REFERENCES

1. Prober CG. Herpes simplex virus. In: Long S, Pickering L, Prober, C, eds. *Principles and practice of pediatric infectious diseases*. Livingstone Elsevier. Philadelphia; 2008:1012-1021.
2. Whitley RJ, Roizman B. Herpes simplex virus infections. *Lancet* 2001;357:1513.

3. Stanberry LR, Kern ER, Richards JT, et al. Genital herpes in guinea pigs: Pathogenesis of the primary infection and description of recurrent disease. *J Infect Dis.* 1983;146:397.
4. Kuzushima K, Kimura H, Kino Y, et al. Clinical manifestations of primary herpes simplex virus type 1 infection in a closed community. *Pediatrics.* 1991;87:152.
5. Spruance SL, Overall JC, Kern ER, et al. The natural history of recurrent herpes simplex labialis: Implications for antiviral therapy. *N Engl J Med.* 1977;297:69.
6. Moseley RC, Corey L, Benjamin D, et al. Comparison of viral isolation, direct immunofluorescence, and indirect immunoperoxidase techniques for detection of genital herpes simplex virus infection. *J Clin Microbiol.* 1981;13:913.
7. Goldstein LC, Corey L, McDougall JK, et al. Monoclonal antibodies to herpes simplex viruses: Use in antigenic typing and rapid diagnosis. *J Infect Dis.* 1983;147:829.
8. Pouletty P, Chomel JJ, Thouvenot D, et al. Detection of herpes simplex virus in direct specimens by immunofluorescence assay using a monoclonal antibody. *J Clin Microbiol.* 1987;25:958.
9. Amir J, Harel L, Smetana Z, et al. Treatment of herpes simplex gingivostomatitis with acyclovir in children: A randomised double blind placebo controlled study. *BMJ.* 1997;314:1800.
10. Spruance SL, Stewart JCB, Rowe NH, et al. Treatment of recurrent herpes simplex labialis with oral acyclovir. *J Infect Dis.* 1990;161:185.
11. Spruance SL, Schnipper LE, Overall JC Jr, et al. Treatment of herpes simplex labialis with topical acyclovir in polyethylene glycol. *J Infect Dis.* 1982;146:85.
12. Rooney JF, Straus SE, Mannix ML, et al. Oral acyclovir to suppress frequently recurrent herpes labialis: A double-blind, placebo-controlled trial. *Ann Intern Med.* 1993;118:268.
13. Spruance SL, Freeman DJ, Steward JC, et al. The natural history of ultraviolet radiation-induced herpes simplex labialis and response to therapy with peroral and topical formulation of acyclovir. *J Infect Dis.* 1991;163:728.
14. Spruance SL, Hamill ML, Hoge WS. Acyclovir prevents reactivation of herpes simplex labialis in skiers. *JAMA.* 1988;260:1597.

40 APHTHOUS ULCER

Richard P. Usatine, MD

PATIENT STORY

A 5-year-old girl is in her pediatrician's office for her school physical and immunizations when her mother asks about her child's complaint of mouth pain. The girl is otherwise healthy and on physical examination a small round ulcer is seen on the nonkeratinized mucosa above the upper teeth (**Figure 40-1**). The necrotic center with slightly raised borders and surrounding erythema were easily recognized features of an aphthous ulcer. The pediatrician reassured the mother that this will go away spontaneously without medication or treatment. She suggested to avoid giving the child acidic or spicy foods in the coming days and to be careful to not traumatize the ulcer further with vigorous toothbrushing.

INTRODUCTION

Aphthous ulcers are painful ulcerations in the mouth, which can be single, multiple, occasional, or recurrent. These ulcers can be small or large but are uniformly painful and may interfere with eating, speaking, and swallowing. Oral trauma, stress, and systemic diseases can contribute to the occurrence of these ulcers but no precise etiology is apparent. Recurrent aphthous stomatitis (RAS) is a frustrating condition that merits aggressive treatment aimed at pain relief and prevention.

SYNONYMS

Canker sores, aphthous stomatitis, aphthae, recurrent aphthous ulcer (RAU), or recurrent aphthous stomatitis (RAS).

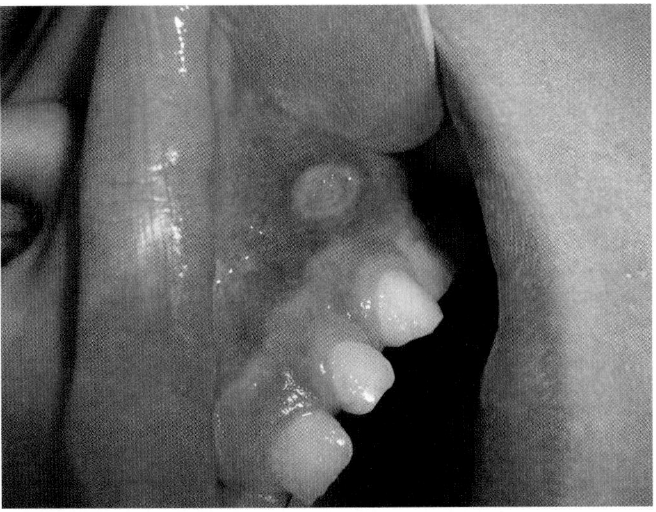

FIGURE 40-1 Aphthous ulcer located on unkeratinized (movable) mucosa in a 5-year-old girl. It is slightly raised, round, with a white-yellow necrotic center and surrounding erythema. (*Used with permission from Richard P. Usatine, MD.*)

EPIDEMIOLOGY

- Twenty percent of the general population are reported to have aphthous ulcers.[1]
- One and 1/2 percent of children and adolescents have been reported to have RAUs.[2]
- RAS is more common in females, in people younger than age 40 years, in whites, in nonsmokers, and in people of high socioeconomic status.[2]

ETIOLOGY AND PATHOPHYSIOLOGY

- The precise etiology and pathogenesis of this condition remains unknown, although a variety of host and environmental factors have been implicated.
- A positive family history is seen in about 1/3 of RAS patients. A genetic predisposition is suggested by an increased frequency of HLA types A2, A11, B12, and DR2.[2]
- In one study, Th1 (T-helper subtype 1) activation was more intense in the patients with RAUs. Many conditions that increase the incidence of RAUs, such as psychologic stress, NSAIDs, Crohn disease, and celiac disease, also shift the immune response toward the Th1 subtype. Conditions and medications that inhibit the Th1 immune response pathway, such as pregnancy, thalidomide, glucocorticoids, and tetracycline, decrease the incidence of RAUs.[3]
- Another study found a significantly higher-than-normal serum level of tumor necrosis factor (TNF)-α in 20 to 39 percent of patients in the ulcerative stage of RAUs.[3] Medications that have anti–TNF-α effects, such as pentoxifylline, levamisole, and thalidomide, have also been found to be useful in the treatment of RAUs.[2–4]
- Although studies show that there are active immune mechanisms associated with RAUs, there is still much to learn regarding their etiology and pathogenesis.

RISK FACTORS

- Oral trauma.
- Stress and anxiety.
- Systemic diseases (celiac disease, Crohn disease, Behçet syndrome, HIV, or reactive arthritis).
- Medications (NSAIDs, β-blockers, or angiotensin-converting enzyme inhibitors [ACEIs]).
- Vitamin deficiencies (zinc, iron, B_{12}, or folate).
- Food and chemical sensitivities.

DIAGNOSIS

CLINICAL FEATURES

History:

- Symptoms may begin with a burning sensation and the pain is exacerbated by moving the area affected by the ulcer.

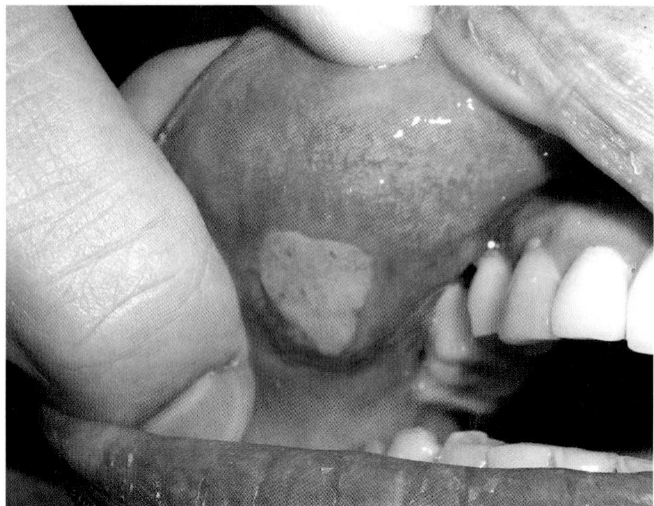

FIGURE 40-2 Major aphthous ulcer on the buccal mucosa of a man who has been suffering with recurrent aphthous stomatitis for the past year. (*Used with permission from Richard P. Usatine, MD.*)

- Eating often hurts, especially foods and drinks with a high acidic content.
- Ask about recurrences and onset in relation to the use of medications.
- Ask about GI symptoms, genital ulcers, HIV risk factors, and joint pain.

Physical:

- Three clinical variations are described based on the size of the ulcers:
  1. Minor (3 to 10 mm) (**Figure 40-1**)—most common.
  2. Major (>10 mm) (**Figure 40-2**).
  3. Herpetiform (<3 mm and multiple ulcers) —least common.
- The most common minor form appears as rounded, well-demarcated, single, or multiple ulcers less than 1 cm in diameter that usually heal in 10 to 14 days without scarring.

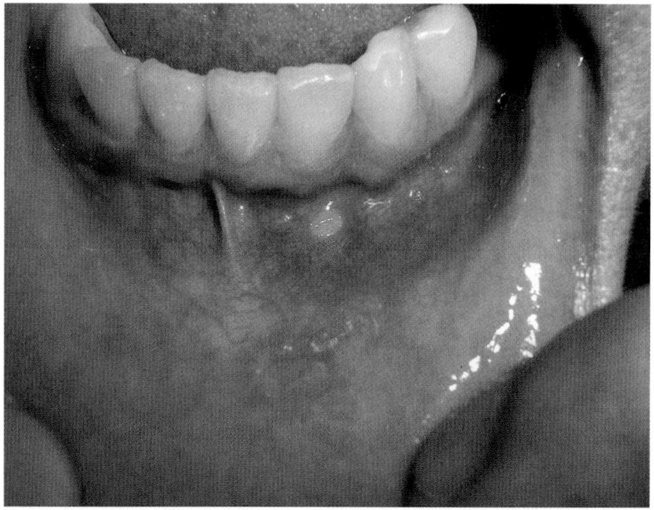

FIGURE 40-3 One small aphthous ulcer on the lower labial movable mucosa of a child. (*Used with permission from Richard P. Usatine, MD.*)

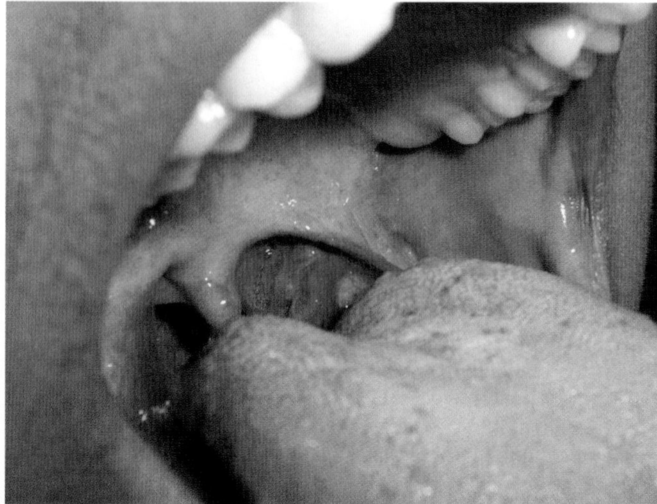

FIGURE 40-4 Aphthous ulcer near the tonsillar mucosa in a young boy with a sore throat. (*Used with permission from Richard P. Usatine, MD.*)

- Herpetiform aphthae usually do not present until the second or third decade of life.[1]
- The ulcers are solitary or multiple covered by a gray or tan pseudomembrane and surrounded by an erythematous halo (**Figure 40-1**).

TYPICAL DISTRIBUTION

Aphthous ulcers usually involves nonkeratinizing mucosa (e.g., labial mucosa, buccal mucosa, or ventral tongue) (**Figure 40-3**). Aphthous ulcers spare the attached gingiva and the hard palate (nonmovable mucosa). Aphthous ulcers can even appear adjacent to the tonsillar mucosa (**Figure 40-4**).

CLASSIFICATION

Simple aphthosis—Aphthae are few at a time, not associated with systemic diseases, and occurs only 2 to 4 times per year.

Complex aphthosis—Aphthae are associated with systemic diseases, there are many lesions at one time, which can include genital aphthous ulcers, or there is a continuous disease activity with new ulcers developing as older lesions heal or the ulcers recur more often than 4 times per year. Behçet disease is one example of a complex aphthosis.

LABORATORY TESTS

The diagnosis of a single episode of aphthous ulcers is usually based on history and physical examination. If there is RAS, consider complete blood count (CBC), ferritin, B_{12}, folate, erythrocyte sedimentation rate (ESR), viral culture, biopsy, and/or HIV testing, if indicated. If there is evidence of malabsorption, consider testing for celiac disease (see Chapter 60, Celiac Disease).

DIFFERENTIAL DIAGNOSIS

- Primary oral herpes simplex virus (primary gingivostomatitis)—Begins as vesicular lesions, which quickly ulcerate on all mucosal lesions in the mouth. It is accompanied by systemic manifestations such as fever, malaise, anorexia, and sore throat. The ulcers are located on movable and nonmovable oral mucosa (includes attached gingiva and hard palate). Lesions may also appear on keratinized surfaces such as the lip (see Chapter 39, HSV Gingivostomatitis and Chapter 114, Herpes Simplex).

- Hand, foot, and mouth disease presents as mucocutaneous lesions involving the hand, foot, and mouth caused by enterovirus. Any area of oral mucosa may be involved. Lesions resolve within 1 week (see Chapter 113, Hand Foot, and Mouth Disease).
- Herpangina causes multiple ulcers in the mouth, especially on the soft palate and the anterior fauces (**Figure 29-9**). It is caused by coxsackievirus A16 in most cases. The distribution of the ulcers is different than in aphthous ulcers.
- Thrush—White plaque, when removed, appears red. Scrape the white plaque with a tongue depressor and add KOH to the slide and the preparation will be positive for pseudohyphae and/or budding yeast (see Chapter 121, Candidiasis).
- Erythema multiforme (EM)—Mucocutaneous lesion preceeded by infection of herpes simplex virus (HSV), *Mycoplasma pneumoniae*, or exposure to certain drugs or medications. Oral lesions begin as patches and evolve into large shallow erosions and ulcerations with irregular borders. Common sites include the lip, tongue, buccal mucosa, floor of the mouth, and soft palate. The presence of targetoid skin lesions should help differentiate EM from RAS (see Chapter 151, Erythema Multiforme, Stevens-Johnson Syndrome, and Toxic Epidermal Necrolysis).
- Behçet disease was originally characterized by three conditions: 1) recurrent oral aphthous ulcers (**Figure 40-5**), 2) genital ulcers, and 3) uveitis. The aphthous ulcers appear no different from those found in people without Behçet disease. The recurrent genital ulcers are painful and heal with scarring. Diagnosis is now based on agreed clinical criteria that require recurrent oral ulcers and two of the following: recurrent genital ulcers, ocular inflammation, defined skin lesions, and pathergy.[5] Behçet disease is a type of complex aphthosis. If Behçet disease is suspected, refer the patient to an ophthalmologist to look for signs of uveitis or retinal vasculitis. Behçet disease is a multi-system vasculitis and referral to a rheumatologist may also be helpful (see Chapter 75, Mucosal Ulcerative Disorders).

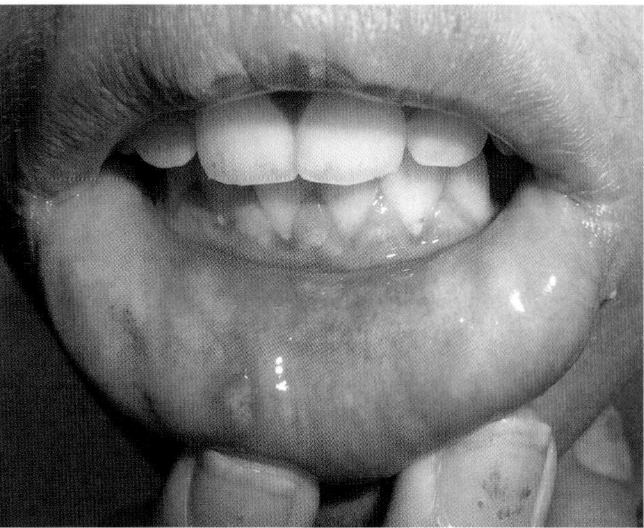

FIGURE 40-5 Behçet disease characterized by recurrent oral and genital ulcers in a 17-year-old girl. (*Used with permission from Richard P. Usatine, MD.*)

- PFAPA syndrome (periodic fever, aphthae, pharyngitis, and adenitis) is also a complex aphthosis condition with systemic symptoms and multiple areas of involvement (see Chapter 176, Periodic Fever Syndromes).

MANAGEMENT

Identify and treat any vitamin deficiency, systemic disease, or recurrent oral trauma. Stress management is reasonable for all persons. See **Table 40-1** for an evidence-based summary of treatments.

TABLE 40-1 Evidence-based Summary of Treatments

Treatment	Route/Comparison	Total Patients Studied	Outcomes	Benefit
Amlexanox 5 percent paste[6]	Topical qid/placebo	1335	Pain-free by Day 3 Ulcer resolution at prodromal stage Ulcer healed by Day 3	NNT = 5 (42% vs 22%; *P* < .05) NNT = 1.6 (97% vs 35%; *P* < .01) NNT = 7 (47% vs 21%; *P* < .05)
Corticosteroids (various)[7]	Topical qid	116	Pain reduction	3 of 4 clinical trials show benefit
Silver nitrate[9]	1-time topical application/placebo	97	Pain reduction by Day 1	NNT = 1.7 (70% vs 10%; *P* < .001)
Debacterol[10]	1-time topical application/placebo	60	Complete ulcer resolution by Day 6	NNT = 1.4 (100% vs 30%; *P* < .01)
Chlorhexidine[13]	Mouthwash qid	77	Reduction in total days with ulcers	2 of 3 trials show benefit
Vitamin B_{12}[14]	Oral daily for prophylaxis	58	No new ulcers by 6 months	NNT = 2.3 (74% vs 32%; *P* < .01)

Adapted from: Bailey J, McCarthy C, Smith RF. Clinical inquiry. What is the most effective way to treat recurrent canker sores? *J Fam Pract.* 2011;60:621-632. With permission from Frontline Medical Communications.

NONPHARMACOLOGIC

Most isolated aphthae require no treatment or only periodic topical therapy.

MEDICATIONS

- Amlexanox 5 percent paste (Aphthasol) reduces ulcer size, pain duration, and healing time.[6] It is nonprescription and the paste is applied directly to ulcers four times a day until ulcers heal.[6] SOR Ⓑ
- Topical corticosteroids, such as clobetasol gel or fluocinonide gel, can promote healing and lessen the severity of RAS.[7] Patients should be instructed to dab the area of ulcer dry, apply the gel, paste, or cream after rinsing, and avoid eating or drinking for at least 30 minutes. SOR Ⓑ
- Lidocaine 1 percent cream applied to aphthous ulcers was found to reduce pain intensity compared to the placebo cream.[8] SOR Ⓑ
- Silver nitrate cautery can lessen the pain of an aphthous ulcer with a single application. The application is painful and probably would only be acceptable to a teen wanting immediate relief of the pain. This must be performed by the physician in the office. The time to healing does not change.[9]
- Debacterol is another topical agent that reduces pain in one day and requires a prescription. It is also painful on application so its use is limited.[10]

COMPLEMENTARY AND ALTERNATIVE THERAPY

Vitamin C was shown to reduce the frequency of minor RAS and the severity of pain by 50 percent in a small group of teens. They were given 2000 mg/m^2 per day of ascorbate.[11]

REFERRAL

Consider referring children with periodic fever with aphthous stomatitis, pharyngitis, and adenitis (PFAPA) syndrome for tonsillectomy or adenotonsillectomy. A meta-analysis found little evidence to support surgery, but the authors concluded that surgery is an option when symptoms markedly interfere with the child's quality of life and medical treatment has failed.[12] SOR Ⓒ

PREVENTION

- Chlorhexidine mouth rinse was shown to reduce the total days with recurrent aphthous ulcers in two of three studies.[13] SOR Ⓑ
- Oral vitamin B_{12} was studied in a RCT of adults. A sublingual dose of 1000 mcg of vitamin B_{12} was used by patients in the intervention group for 6 months. During the last month of treatment more participants in the intervention group reached a status of "no aphthous ulcers" (74.1% vs. 32.0%; $P < 0.01$). The treatment worked regardless of the serum vitamin B_{12} level.[14] SOR Ⓑ This could be used as a treatment in older and/or adult-size teens.

PATIENT EDUCATION

Foods that are spicy or acidic worsen pain and should be avoided during outbreaks. Recommend the use of a soft bristled toothbrush as trauma from a firm toothbrush could precipitate an aphthous ulcer.

PATIENT RESOURCES

- MedicineNet.com. *Canker Sores (Aphthous Ulcers)*—**www. medicinenet.com/canker_sores/article.htm**.

PROVIDER RESOURCES

- Dermnet NZ. *Aphthous Ulcers*—**www.dermnetnz.org/site-age-specific/aphthae.html**.
- eMedicine. *Aphthous Ulcers*—**www.emedicine.medscape.com/article/867080**.
- eMedicine. *Aphthous Stomatitis*—**www.emedicine.medscape.com/article/1075570**.
- Keogan MT. Clinical Immunology Review Series: an approach to the patient with recurrent orogenital ulceration, including Behçet's syndrome. *Clin Exp Immunol.* 2009. **http://www.ncbi.nlm.nih.gov/pmc/articles/PMC2674035/**.

REFERENCES

1. Femiano F, Lanza A, Buonaiuto C, Gombos F, Nunziata M, Piccolo S, and Cirillo N. Guidelines for diagnosis and management of aphthous stomatitis. *Pediatr Infect Dis J.* 2007;26(8): 728-732.
2. Messadi DV, Younai F. Aphthous ulcers. *Dermatol Ther.* 2010;23: 281-290.
3. Borra RC, Andrade PM, Silva ID, et al. The Th1/Th2 immune-type response of the recurrent aphthous ulceration analyzed by cDNA microarray. *J Oral Pathol Med.* 2004;33:140-146.
4. Sun A, Wang JT, Chia JS, Chiang CP. Levamisole can modulate the serum tumor necrosis factor-alpha level in patients with recurrent aphthous ulcerations. *J Oral Pathol Med.* 2006;35: 111-116.
5. Keogan MT. Clinical Immunology Review Series: an approach to the patient with recurrent orogenital ulceration, including Behçet's syndrome. *Clin Exp Immunol.* 2009;156(1):1-11.
6. Bell J. Amlexanox for the treatment of recurrent aphthous ulcers. *Clin Drug Investig.* 2005;25:555-566.
7. Rodriguez M, Rubio JA, Sanchez R. Effectiveness of two oral pastes for the treatment of recurrent aphthous stomatitis. *Oral Dis.* 2007;13:490-494.
8. Descroix V, Coudert AE, Vige A, et al. Efficacy of topical 1% lidocaine in the symptomatic treatment of pain associated with oral mucosal trauma or minor oral aphthous ulcer: a randomized, double-blind, placebo-controlled, parallel-group, single-dose study. *J Orofac Pain.* 2011;25:327-332.
9. Alidaee MR, Taheri A, Mansoori P, et al. Silver nitrate cautery in aphthous stomatitis: a randomized controlled trial. *Br J Dermatol.* 2005;153:521-525.
10. Rhodus NL, Bereuter J. An evaluation of a chemical cautery agent and an anti-inflammatory ointment for the treatment of recurrent aphthous stomatitis: a pilot study. *Quintessence Int.* 1998;29:769-773.

11. Yasui K, Kurata T, Yashiro M, et al. The effect of ascorbate on minor recurrent aphthous stomatitis. *Acta Paediatr*. 2010;99: 442-445.
12. Garavello W, Pignataro L, Gaini L, et al. Tonsillectomy in children with periodic fever with aphthous stomatitis, pharyngitis, and adenitis syndrome. *J Pediatr*. 2011;159:138-142.
13. Meiller TF, Kutcher MJ, Overholser CD, et al. Effect of an antimicrobial mouthrinse on recurrent aphthous ulcerations. *Oral Surg Oral Med Oral Pathol*. 1991;72:425-429.
14. Volkov I, Rudoy I, Freud T, et al. Effectiveness of vitamin B12 in treating recurrent aphthous stomatitis: a randomized, double-blind, placebo-controlled trial. *J Am Board Fam Med*. 2009;22:9-16.

PART 7

THE HEART AND CIRCULATION

Strength of Recommendation (SOR)	Definition
A	Recommendation based on consistent and good-quality patient-oriented evidence.*
B	Recommendation based on inconsistent or limited-quality patient-oriented evidence.*
C	Recommendation based on consensus, usual practice, opinion, disease-oriented evidence, or case series for studies of diagnosis, treatment, prevention, or screening.*

*See Appendix A on pages 1320–1322 for further information.

41 CLUBBING AND CYANOSIS

Danyal Thaver, MBBS
Athar M. Qureshi, MD

PATIENT STORY

A 9-year-old boy from rural Asia was brought to the clinic by his parents for complaints of being tired and "blue." Further history reveals that he has had frequent episodes of squatting after exertion which relieves some of the symptoms temporarily. On exam, he has clubbing of the fingers and toes with cyanosis of the lips and oral mucous membranes (**Figure 41-1**). A harsh systolic ejection murmur is best heard at the left mid and upper sternal border. An echocardiogram confirms the diagnosis of tetralogy of Fallot.

INTRODUCTION

Clubbing is the enlargement of the distal fingers or toes along with the formation of convex shaped fingernails or toenails.

Cyanosis is the bluish discoloration of the skin or mucous membranes due to increased quantity of deoxyhemoglobin in the blood. Unless otherwise specified, cyanosis in this chapter refers to central cyanosis.

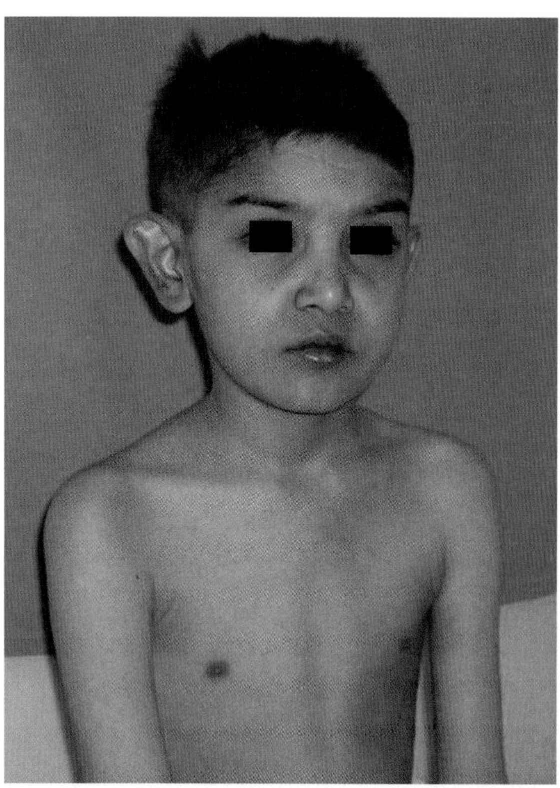

FIGURE 41-1 Central cyanosis of the lips in this 9-year-old boy with unrepaired Tetralogy of Fallot. (*Used with permission from Athar M. Qureshi, MD.*)

SYNONYMS

Clubbing: Hypertrophic osteoarthropathy.

Cyanosis: Central cyanosis or hypoxemia.

EPIDEMIOLOGY

- Clubbing and cyanosis are disease manifestations seen worldwide and their incidence is difficult to discern.
- Chronic cyanosis as a result of unrepaired congenital heart disease is seen mainly in developing nations.

ETIOLOGY AND PATHOPHYSIOLOGY

- The exact etiology of clubbing is unknown. However, it has been hypothesized that it may result from megakaryocytes that have bypassed the pulmonary vascular bed and entered the systemic circulation or from platelet clumps that form and/or enter the systemic circulation. They then release platelet-derived growth factor causing clubbing.[1,2]
- A right to left cardiac shunt or significant lung disease easily allows platelets to bypass the lungs and hence cause clubbing. Conditions that result in platelet excess, that is, inflammatory bowel disease, may also result in clubbing.
- Cyanosis occurs due to reduced capillary blood oxygen saturation and becomes apparent when deoxyhemoglobin in the blood exceeds a value of 3 to 5 g/dL (corresponding arterial saturations of 70 to 85 percent).[3]

RISK FACTORS

▶ Clubbing

- Lung disease including chronic infections or malignancies.
- Cyanotic congenital heart disease (most common cause in children), endocarditis.
- Chronic gastrointestinal disorders, i.e., inflammatory bowel disease, liver cirrhosis.
- Hereditary.

▶ Cyanosis

- Cyanotic heart disease.
- Lung disorders.

DIAGNOSIS

CLINICAL FEATURES

▶ Clubbing

- Fluctuation and softening of the nail bed can be appreciated early. Enlargement of the distal segments of affected extremities that is usually painless develops (**Figures 41-2** and **Figure 41-3**).

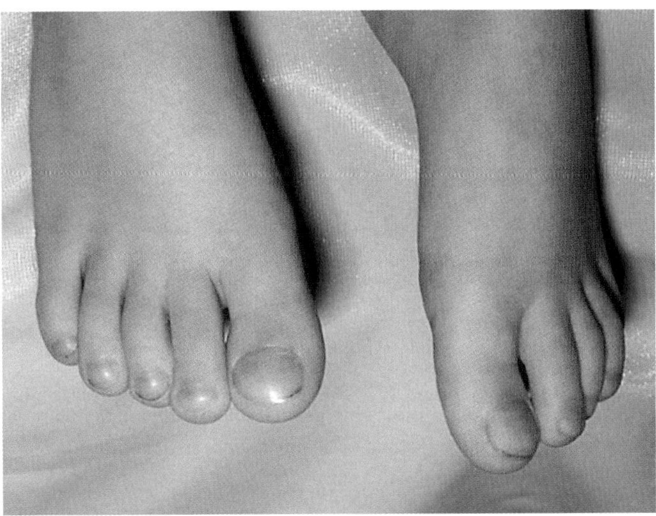

FIGURE 41-2 Clubbing of the toes in this 3.5 year old with severe immune deficiency and chronic lung disease—note the convex shaped toenails. (*Used with permission from Johanna Goldfarb, MD.*)

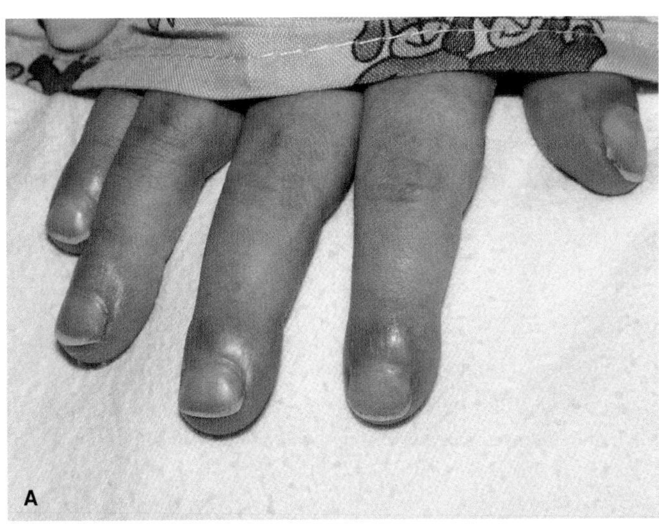

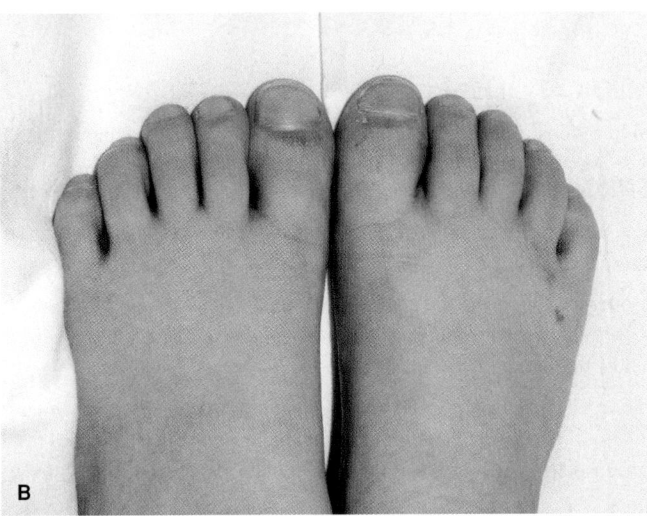

FIGURE 41-3 Clubbing of the fingers (**A**) and toenails (**B**) in a 4-year-old with cyanotic heart disease consisting of tricuspid atresia and a Glenn circulation. As opposed to the child in **Figure 41-2**, note the cyanotic nail beds. (*Used with permission from Athar M. Qureshi, MD.*)

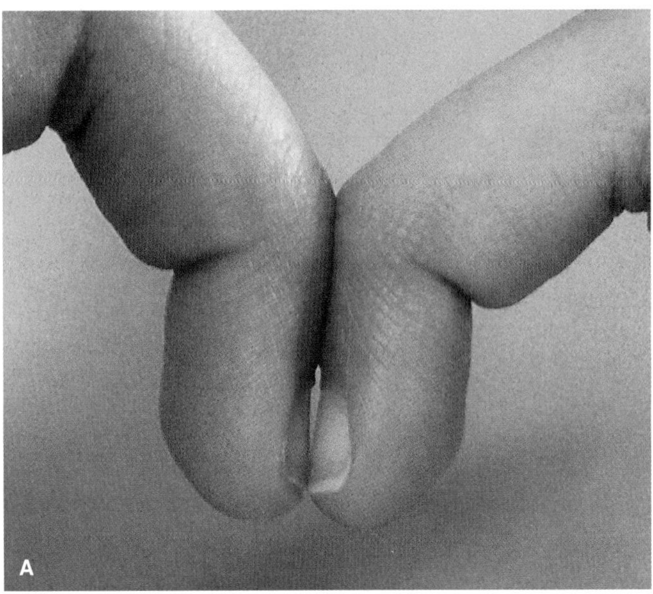

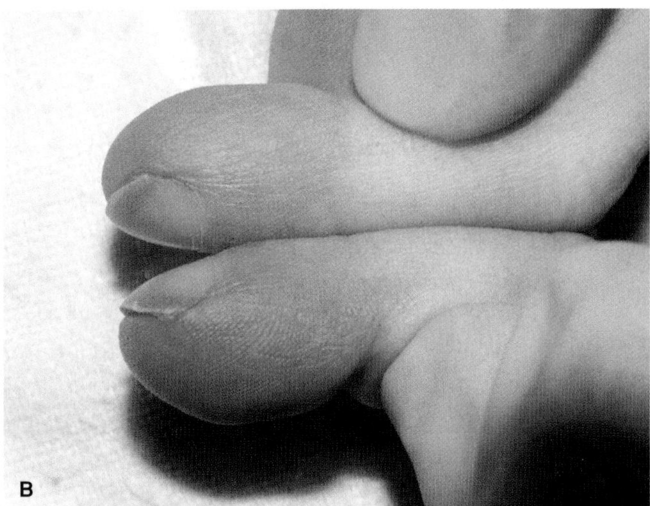

FIGURE 41-4 Schamroth sign. Normal diamond shaped space when corresponding right and left digits are opposed as seen in this healthy 6-year-old girl (**A**). This space is obliterated in patients with significant clubbing (**B**) as seen in this 4-year-old boy with tricuspid atresia and a Glenn circulation. (*Used with permission from Athar M. Qureshi, MD.*)

- Reduction in the angle between the nail plate and the finger. When the nail beds of corresponding right and left digits are opposed, the diamond-shaped space is obliterated ("Schamroth sign") (**Figure 41-4**).
- In later stages, distal segments of the digits may develop a typical "drumstick" appearance (**Figure 41-5**).

▶ Cyanosis

- Patients have symptoms such as dyspnea or fatigue.
- Oxygen saturations are low.
- A thorough examination should be performed seeking an etiology based on common risk factors (see the previous section).

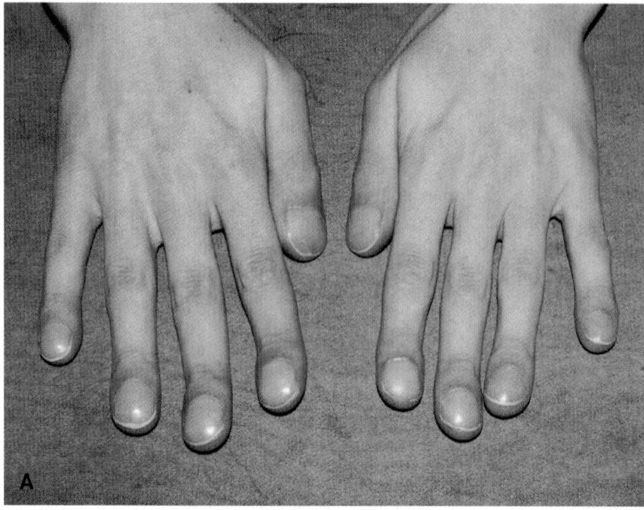

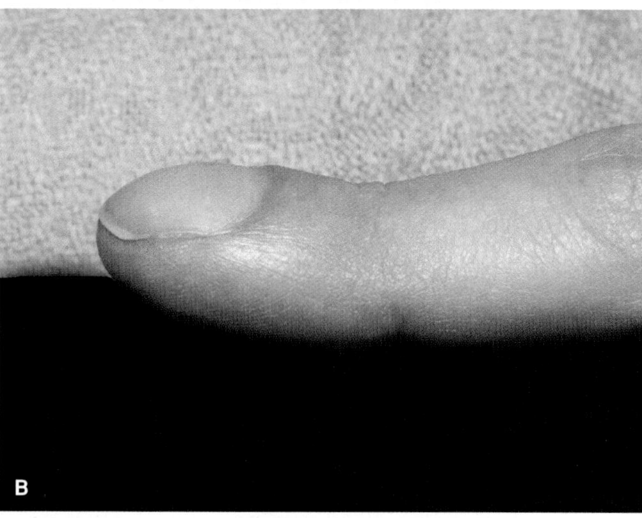

FIGURE 41-5 Prominent clubbing with cyanosis of the nailbeds of the hands is seen in this 25-year-old with uncorrected cyanotic congenital heart disease (**A**). Drumstick like appearance of an index finger can be seen in a side profile view (**B**). (*Used with permission from Athar M. Qureshi, MD.*)

DISTRIBUTION

- Clubbing is present in distal segments of fingers and toes.
- In patients with central cyanosis, bluish discoloration is most evident in the nail beds, lips (**Figure 41-1**), and mucous membranes of the oral cavity or conjunctivae.

LABORATORY TESTING

- Systemic oxygen saturation should be measured. A congenital heart disease is strongly suggested if the oxygen saturation (and pO2) does not significantly increase.
- Methemoglobin levels should be obtained if methemoglobinemia is suspected.

IMAGING

- The need for imaging depends on suspected etiology.
- A chest x-ray should be performed to detect any cardiac or lung disease. A chest CT or MRI may then be ordered if necessary.
- Echocardiography helps the diagnosis of unrepaired congenital cardiac defects.
- Abdominal imaging including ultrasound and endoscopy may be needed for gastrointestinal causes.

DIFFERENTIAL DIAGNOSIS

▶ Clubbing

- See risk factors.

▶ Cyanosis

- Hemoglobin abnormalities, for example, methemoglobinemia. In this condition, (congenital or acquired) cyanosis and low saturations are present with a normal pO2.
- Peripheral cyanosis or "acrocyanosis" (sparing of mucous membranes) is due to sluggish blood flow and may occur with normal arterial blood saturation. This occurs in the extremities of babies due to vasospasm when they are cold and is usually transient. (see Chapter 4, Birth of a Child, Figure 4-1).
- Circumoral cyanosis occurs around the lips due to prominent veins. Prominent veins can also be seen on the forehead giving the impression of cyanosis. This is a benign finding.

MANAGEMENT

Definitive treatment of both clubbing and cyanosis is to treat the underlying cause.

NONPHARMACOLOGIC

- Supplemental oxygen if hypoxemia is the cause of cyanosis.
- Patients who develop Eisenmenger's syndrome (as a result of irreversible pulmonary hypertension from an unrepaired congenital cardiac defect causing a right to left shunt) or who have chronic cyanosis from other reasons are at increased risk of polycythemia.[4]
- Phlebotomies may be needed to treat hyperviscosity, although this may result in iron deficiency.

MEDICATIONS

Medications, as appropriate, are used to treat the underlying cause.

SURGERY

- A variety of surgical procedures may be indicated depending on the cause.
- Surgery (or cardiac interventional catheterization procedures) may be indicated to repair congenital heart defects (as long as irreversible pulmonary hypertension is not present).
- Surgery may be indicated for lung pathology (i.e., resection of lung tumors) and for treatment of inflammatory bowel disease. Liver transplant may be needed for end stage liver cirrhosis.

REFERRAL

Referrals to a cardiologist, pulmonologist, gastroenterologist and other specialists may be required depending on the etiology.

PREVENTION AND SCREENING

- Early diagnosis of cardiac, pulmonary, gastrointestinal, or other chronic diseases.
- Fetal ultrasounds may detect cardiac lesions in utero.

PROGNOSIS

Prognosis depends on the underlying condition and symptoms may be reversed by treating the cause early in the disease course.

FOLLOW-UP

These patients need frequent follow-up visits due to the chronic nature of their underlying illnesses.

PATIENT EDUCATION

Patients should be educated about the implications of chronic cyanosis and polycythemia, that is, potential cerebrovascular accidents or brain abscess formation in cardiac lesions with right to left shunts.

PATIENT RESOURCES

- **www.news-medical.net/health/Symptoms-of-cyanosis.aspx**.

PROVIDER RESOURCES

- **www.emedicine.medscape.com/article/1105946**.

REFERENCES

1. Dickinson CJ, Martin JF. Megakaryocytes and platelet clumps as the cause of finger clubbing. *Lancet*. 1987;330(8573):1434-1435.
2. Dickinson CJ. The aetiology of clubbing and hypertrophic osteoarthropathy. *Eur J Clin Invest*. 1993;23(6):330-338.
3. Nadas AS and Fyler DC. Hypoxemia. In: Keane JF, Lock JE and Fyler DC, eds. *Nadas' Pediatric Cardiology, 2nd ed*. Elsevier, 2006;97-101.
4. Brickner ME, Hillis LD, Lange RA. Congenital heart disease in adults. Second of two parts. *N Engl J Med*. 2000;342(5):334-342.

42 ACYANOTIC CONGENITAL HEART DISEASE

Asif Padiyath, MD
Peter Aziz, MD

The three most important and common types of acyanotic congenital heart disease are:

- Atrial septal defect.
- Ventricular septal defect.
- Patent ductus arteriosus.

All three conditions are covered sequentially in this chapter.

ATRIAL SEPTAL DEFECT

PATIENT STORY

A 4-year-old recent immigrant from Nicaragua presents to her pediatrician for a well-child examination. She does not have any significant past medical history. On examination, she was found to have a normodynamic precordium, widely split and fixed S2 and a grade 2/6 systolic ejection murmur in the pulmonary auscultation area. She is diagnosed with an atrial septal defect (ASD) (**Figure 42-1**).

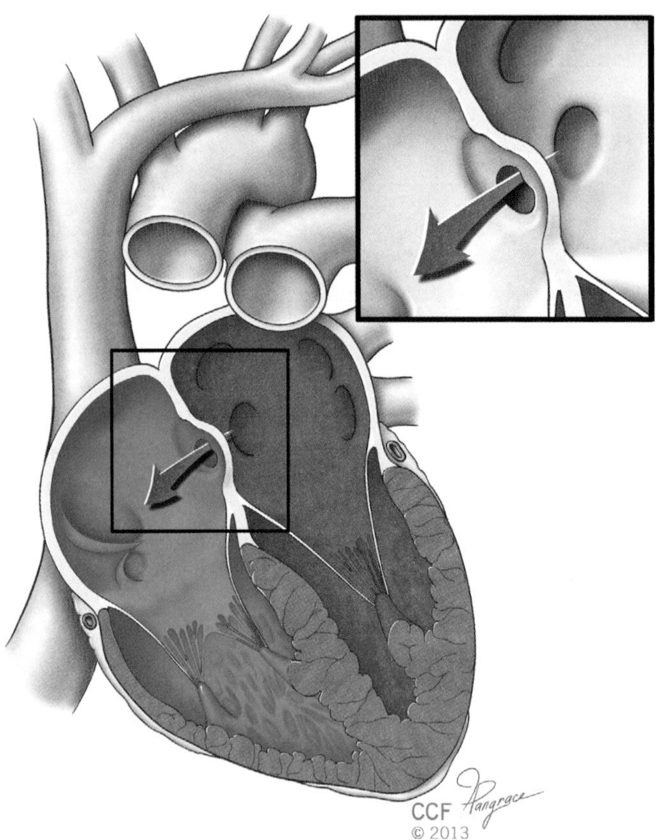

FIGURE 42-1 Atrial septal defect with flow from the left atrium to the right atrium as depicted by the red arrow. *(Reprinted with permission, Cleveland Clinic Center for Medical Art & Photography © 2012. All Rights Reserved.)*

INTRODUCTION

Any opening in the atrial septum is described as an ASD. Although many of these defects close spontaneously, early diagnosis and follow-up is essential in preventing sequelae from undiagnosed ASD's.

EPIDEMIOLOGY

- Atrial septal defects (ASD) account for 10 percent of all congenital heart disease and as much as 20 to 40 percent of congenital heart disease presenting in adulthood.[1,2]

ETIOLOGY AND PATHOPHYSIOLOGY

- There are three major types of atrial septal defects.
  - Ostium secundum defect is the most common type of ASD. It results from incomplete adhesion between the flap valve associated with the foramen ovale and the septum secundum after birth. It also includes patent foramen ovale, which results from abnormal resorption of the septum primum during the formation of the foramen secundum.
  - Ostium primum defects are the second most common type of ASD. This is a form of atrioventricular septal defect and is commonly associated with mitral valve abnormalities. These defects are caused by incomplete fusion of septum primum with the endocardial cushion.
  - Sinus venosus defect is the least common of the three. The defect is located along the superior (SVC type) or inferior (IVC type) aspect of the atrial septum. Anomalous connection of the right-sided pulmonary veins is common and should be expected in the SVC type. Abnormal fusion between the embryologic sinus venosus and the atrium causes these defects.
    - A clinically significant moderate to large defect, if undiagnosed and untreated, can cause enlargement of right atrium and right ventricle.
    - Dilation of the right atrium can also lead to the development of atrial arrhythmias.
    - Older patients may develop pulmonary vascular disease leading to Eisenmenger syndrome, which is the most significant long-term complication of an ASD.

RISK FACTORS

- ASDs may occur on a familial basis.
- Holt-Oram syndrome and Ellis van Creveld syndrome are associated with ASDs.

DIAGNOSIS

CLINICAL PRESENTATION

- ASD can go undiagnosed for decades due to subtle physical examination findings and lack of symptoms.
- Defects which are even moderate-to-large typically do not cause symptoms in childhood as in the previous vignette described.
- Some patients however may manifest symptoms of easy fatigability, recurrent respiratory infections, or exertional dyspnea.

PHYSICAL EXAMINATION

- Patients can have a hyperdynamic right ventricular impulse due to increased diastolic filling and large stroke volume.
- A dilated pulmonary artery can cause a palpable pulsation and an ejection click.
- S_2 is often widely split and fixed because of persistence of left to right shunting during inspiration as well as expiration causing delayed closure of the pulmonary valve.
- A systolic ejection murmur heard in the pulmonary area is a result of increased right ventricular stroke volume across the pulmonary outflow tract.
- The blood flow across the ASD does not cause a murmur at the site of the shunt because no substantial pressure gradient exists between the atria.

ECG FINDINGS

- Patients with untreated clinically significant ASDs can have right axis deviation, RSR' pattern suggestive of right bundle branch block of various degrees and right atrial enlargement (tall 'p' waves in the limb leads >2.5 mm).
- The "crochetage" pattern is described as the presence of a notch in the apex of R waves in the inferior leads which is characteristic of an ASD (**Figure 42-2**).

IMAGING

- Definitive diagnosis is made with a transthoracic echocardiogram.
- Doppler and contrast echocardiography can provide additional confirmation by visualizing atrial shunting.

DIFFERENTIAL DIAGNOSIS

- Physical exam findings of systolic murmur over the pulmonary area with a widely split (but not fixed) S2 can be found in patients with pulmonary stenosis.

MANAGEMENT

- For practical purposes, any defect 8 mm or larger with evidence of left to right shunt should be closed when identified, even at a very young age, because such defects will likely never close spontaneously.[3–5] SOR Ⓐ
- Smaller defects (<3 mm) in asymptomatic patients can be followed clinically as a majority of them spontaneously close.[6] SOR Ⓐ
- Closure can be achieved surgically or with device closure via catheterization.
- The size of the lesion is the major determining factor regarding the type of closure, which can be used.

REFERRAL

- Children diagnosed with an ASD require referral to a pediatric cardiologist.

PROGNOSIS

- The prognosis for patients who are diagnosed with ASD and do not develop pulmonary vascular disease is generally good.

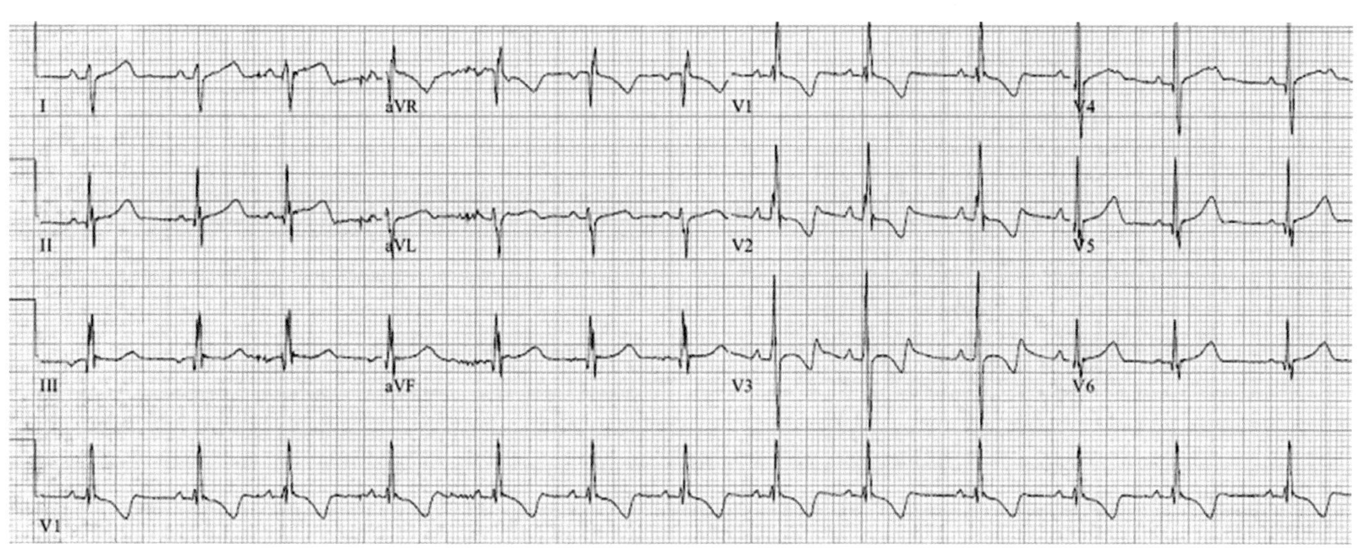

FIGURE 42-2 ECG in a patient with an ASD. Note the RSR' pattern in V1 (incomplete RBBB) and the "crochetage pattern" in the inferior leads (II, III, aVF). (*Used with permission from Peter Aziz, MD.*)

FOLLOW-UP

- Close follow-up of patients diagnosed with an ASD is essential in determining the need for an intervention or continued observation.

PATIENT RESOURCES

- **www.my.clevelandclinic.org/disorders/atrial_septal_defect/hic_atrial_septal_defect_asd.aspx.**

PROVIDER RESOURCES

- **www.ncbi.nlm.nih.gov/pubmedhealth/PMH0001210.**
- **www.cdc.gov/ncbddd/heartdefects/index.html.**

VENTRICULAR SEPTAL DEFECT

PATIENT STORY

A full-term, 2-month-old male infant with an unremarkable perinatal history presents for a well-child examination. He is gaining weight appropriately. On physical exam, he is found to have a grade IV/VI holosystolic murmur in the left lower parasternal area. He did not have a documented murmur during the examination performed in the newborn nursery. A ventricular septal defect (**Figure 42-3**) is suspected and he is referred to a pediatric cardiologist, who confirms the diagnosis by echocardiography.

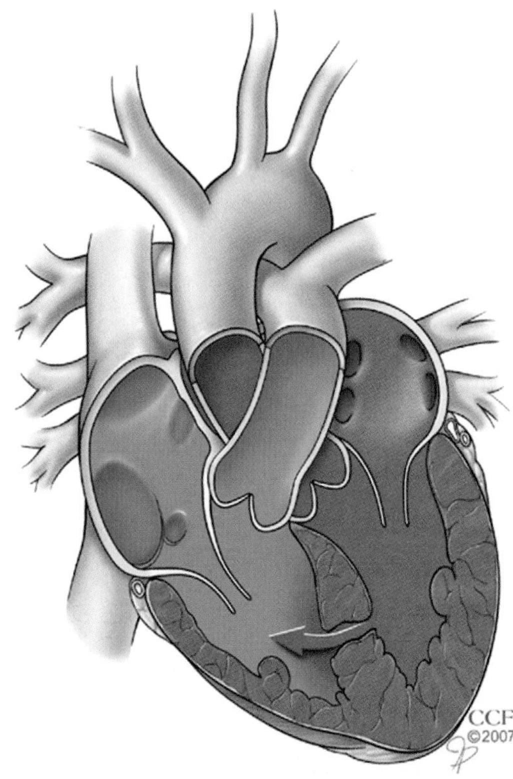

FIGURE 42-3 Ventricular septal defect with flow from the left ventricle to the right ventricle as depicted by the red arrow. *(Reprinted with permission, Cleveland Clinic Center for Medical Art & Photography © 2012. All Rights Reserved.)*

INTRODUCTION

The term ventricular septal defect (VSD) describes an opening in the ventricular septum.

EPIDEMIOLOGY

- A VSD is the most common lesion seen in congenital heart disease overall.
- In the recent years, a prevalence rate of 2.5 per 1000 live births has been determined.[7]

ETIOLOGY AND PATHOPHYSIOLOGY

- Ventricular septal defects result from a delay in closure of the interventricular septum beyond the first 7 weeks of intrauterine life.
- The ventricular septum has four parts: inlet septum, trabecular septum, infundibular septum/outlet septum, and membranous septum.
- Overall, VSDs can be classified into four broad categories.
  - Conoventricular defects—A defect in the small translucent structure located immediately superior to the division of the septal band and adjacent to the commissure between the anterior and septal leaflet of the tricuspid valve.
  - Muscular defect—This type may be located anywhere in the muscular part of the septum.
  - Conoseptal hypoplasia defect—This type of defect is located just under the pulmonary valve. The adjacent right coronary aortic valve cusp often prolapses into the VSD with or without aortic regurgitation.
  - Inlet defect—This type of defect often involves AV valves and has a strong association with Down syndrome.
- The size of the defect and the pulmonary vascular resistance usually determines the hemodynamics in these patients.
- As the drop occurs in the high fetal pulmonary arteriolar resistance in the immediate postnatal life, left to right shunting begins.
- With larger defects, pulmonary artery pressure remains high resulting in right ventricular failure.

RISK FACTORS

- VSD can be associated with a genetic syndrome or as a part of a constellation of heart defects.

DIAGNOSIS

CLINICAL PRESENTATION

- Most infants with small defects remain asymptomatic and the murmur will not be evident until the pulmonary artery pressures significantly decrease.

- Smaller defects can produce the classic murmur of VSD, which is a loud, holosystolic murmur in the left, lower parasternal area.
- Larger defects can manifest as congestive failure resulting in poor feeding, diaphoresis with feeds, tachypnea, and poor growth.
- Physical exam can show signs of cardiac failure, tachypnea, hyperdynamic precordium, and hepatomegaly.
- In larger defects since there no pressure gradient between the ventricles, the classic holosystolic murmur may not be present.

IMAGING AND OTHER INVESTIGATIONS

- Electrocardiography—Most of the children with small VSDs have normal ECGs. Those with larger defects can show biventricular hypertrophy. In endocardial cushion defects, superior axis deviation can be seen.
- Echocardiography—Two-dimensional imaging with color flow Doppler can accurately identify the defects and degree of shunting.

DIFFERENTIAL DIAGNOSIS

- Tricuspid regurgitation and mitral regurgitation can be distinguished by definitive echocardiographic studies.

MANAGEMENT

- Medical management.
    - Maximizing growth and feeding is critical
    - Diuretics, digoxin, and angiotensin-converting enzyme inhibitors may be used to treat congestive heart failure symptoms. SOR Ⓒ
- Surgical management.
    - Surgical management is largely guided by the size and location/type of the defect and should be individualized. In general, if surgery is needed, it is performed between 3 and 6 months of age to prevent long-standing pulmonary hypertension.
- Small defects in clinically asymptomatic patients older than1 year of age should be followed up every 1 to 2 years. SOR Ⓒ
- Larger defects with unrestrictive flow should undergo surgical closure during early infancy. SOR Ⓒ
- Larger defects with restrictive flow can be followed medically given that many defects will decrease in size. SOR Ⓒ

REFERRAL

- All patients with VSDs need to be evaluated by a pediatric cardiologist.

PROGNOSIS

- Asymptomatic, small muscular VSDs have excellent prognosis and spontaneous closure is common.
- If no pulmonary vascular disease is present, large-sized defects also carry an excellent prognosis post-repair.

FOLLOW-UP

- Patients with VSDs, especially the ones with moderate to large-sized VSDs need close follow-up to monitor for adequate weight gain in order to nutritionally prepare them for a possible surgical intervention if deemed necessary.
- Older patients with unrepaired VSDs should be followed for any progression to cardiac failure

PATIENT EDUCATION

- Parents should be educated on the options for potential surgical vs medical management and watchful waiting of VSD's.

PATIENT RESOURCES

- **www.my.clevelandclinic.org/heart/disorders/congenital/septal.aspx**.

PROVIDER RESOURCES

- **www.emedicine.medscape.com/article/892980-overview**.

PATENT DUCTUS ARTERIOSUS

PATIENT STORY

A 16-day-old boy, born prematurely at 24 weeks gestational age is in the neonatal intensive care unit and has just been started on primer feeds. He develops abdominal distention. An abdominal radiograph shows pneumatosis intestinalis suggestive of necrotizing enterocolitis. On physical examination, he has a blood pressure of 66/18 mm Hg, bounding pulses in the femoral arteries and a grade II/VI continuous murmur in the left 2nd intercostal space. Echocardiography confirms the diagnosis of a patent ductus arteriosus (PDA) (**Figure 42-4**).

INTRODUCTION

Patent ductus arteriosus (PDA) represents a persistent communication between the aorta and the pulmonary artery that results from failure of normal physiologic closure of the fetal ductus arteriosus (**Figure 42-4**).

EPIDEMIOLOGY

- Reported prevalence of PDA in infants ranges from 0.138 to 0.8 per 1000 live births.[7,8]
- PDA persists longer among premature infants and prematurity also accounts for some of the PDAs seen long after infancy.

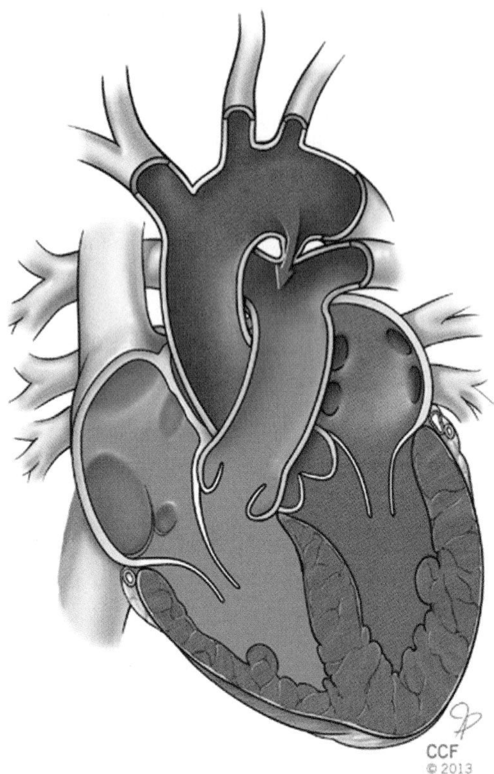

FIGURE 42-4 Patent ductus arteriosus with flow from the aorta to the pulmonary artery as depicted by the red arrow. (*Reprinted with permission, Cleveland Clinic Center for Medical Art & Photography © 2012. All Rights Reserved.*)

ETIOLOGY AND PATHOPHYSIOLOGY

- With the first respiratory gasps after birth, the ductus arteriosus closes through muscular constriction; later with thickening of the endothelium and occlusion via thrombosis.
- When the closure does not take place, there is a persistent runoff from the aorta to the pulmonary artery, with excessive blood flow to the lungs, left atrium, left ventricle, and to the ascending aorta.

RISK FACTORS

- Prematurity is the major risk factor.
- Antenatal rubella infection around the time of conception can cause PDA in the infant.
- Also children born at high altitude have a higher prevalence of PDAs compared those born at sea level.

DIAGNOSIS

CLINICAL FEATURES

- Symptoms and signs are proportionate to the amount of blood passing into the pulmonary circulation.
- With a small shunt in a full-term newborn, a crescendo systolic murmur in the second left intercostal space might be the only feature.
- In a newborn with a larger shunt, during the diastolic flow there could be runoff to the pulmonary circulation causing wide pulse pressures as illustrated in the vignette.
- Bounding peripheral pulses might be palpable for the same reason. The murmur can be softer due to less turbulent flow through the PDA.
- Older children typically have the "classic" cardiac exam of PDA consisting of a crescendo systolic murmur peaking in intensity at aortic closure and continuing into diastole as a high-frequency, decrescendo diastolic murmur in the second left intercostal space.

IMAGING

- Echocardiography—PDA are easily visualized with 2 D echocardiography.

DIFFERENTIAL DIAGNOSIS

- Continuous murmur of a PDA needs to be differentiated from:
  - Venous hum—More prominent with patient sitting rather that lying down with evanescent quality.
  - Coronary artery fistula to one of the cardiac chambers—Usually not the loudest at the second left intercostal space.
  - Ruptured sinus of Valsalva—New murmur, location might be similar to that of PDA.

MANAGEMENT

- PDA can be managed medically, surgically or by cardiac intervention.
- Medical management.
  - In premature patients (those weighing less 1000 g) indomethacin is recommended even in the absence of a clinically significant left to right shunt.[9] SOR Ⓐ
  - For those weighing greater than 1000 g, when signs relating to a significant shunt appear, indomethacin is recommended.[10] SOR Ⓐ
- Surgical Management
  - Surgically repair is performed by open thoracotomy or via Video Assisted Thoracic Surgery (VATS).
- Cardiac Intervention
  - Closure with cardiac catheterization employing coils (or special devices for larger defects) have comparable results with that of VATS treated patients.[11] SOR Ⓐ

REFERRAL

- In the neonatal age group, this patient group is usually managed by a neonatologist or a cardiac surgeon.
- Older children with a persistent ductus arteriosus, require referral to a pediatric cardiologist for management.

PREVENTION

- Prevention of maternal rubella by widespread immunization is one way of preventing PDA in the neonate.
- Use of prophylactic indomethacin in the absence of a ductus in those weighing less than 1000 g is controversial and is generally not recommended.[9,12] SOR Ⓑ

PROGNOSIS

Patients with isolated PDA have excellent prognosis. Spontaneous closure occurs in >34 percent in extremely low-birth-weight neonates.[13]

FOLLOW-UP

Patients who have had permanent closure do not require a follow-up by Pediatric Cardiologist.

PATIENT RESOURCES

- **www.my.clevelandclinic.org/childrens-hospital/health-info/diseases-conditions/heart/hic-Patent-Ductus-Arteriosus.aspx**.

PROVIDER RESOURCES

- Moss and Adams' Heart Disease in Infants, Children, and Adolescents: Including the Fetus and Young Adult, Section VI, Chapter 31.[14]

REFERENCES

1. Wang ZJ, Reddy GP, Gotway MB, Yeh BM, Higgins CB. Cardiovascular shunts: Mr imaging evaluation1. *Radiographics*. 2003;23(1):S181-S194.
2. Feldt RH, Avasthey P, Yoshimasu F, Kurland LT, Titus JL. Incidence of congenital heart disease in children born to residents of olmsted county, minnesota, 1950-1969. *CORD Conference Proceedings*. 1971;46(12):794-799.
3. Radzik D, Davignon A, van Doesburg N, Fournier A, Marchand T, Ducharme G. Predictive factors for spontaneous closure of atrial septal defects diagnosed in the first 3 months of life. *Journal of the American College of Cardiology*. 1993;22(3):851-853.
4. Helgason H, Jonsdottir G. Spontaneous closure of atrial septal defects. *Pediatr Cardiol*. 1999;20(3):195-199.
5. McMahon CJ, Feltes TF, Fraley JK, Bricker JT, Grifka RG, Tortoriello TA, Blake R, Bezold LI. Natural history of growth of secundum atrial septal defects and implications for transcatheter closure. *Heart*. 2002;87(3):256-259.
6. Senocak F, Karademir S, Cabuk F, Onat N, Koc S, Duman A. Spontaneous closure of interatrial septal openings in infants: An echocardiographic study. *Int J Cardiol*. 1996;53(3):221-226.
7. Botto LD, Correa A, Erickson JD. Racial and temporal variations in the prevalence of heart defects. *Pediatrics*. 2001;107(3):E32.
8. Report of the new england regional infant cardiac program. *Pediatrics*. 1980;65(2):375-461.
9. Mahony L, Carnero V, Brett C, Heymann MA, Clyman RI. Prophylactic indomethacin therapy for patent ductus arteriosus in very-low-birth-weight infants. *N Engl J Med*. 1982;306(9):506-510.
10. Ellison RC, Peckham GJ, Lang P, Talner NS, Lerer TJ, Lin L, Dooley KJ, Nadas AS. Evaluation of the preterm infant for patent ductus arteriosus. *Pediatrics*. 1983;71(3):364-372.
11. Jacobs JP, Giroud JM, Quintessenza JA, Morell VO, Botero LM, van Gelder HM, Badhwar V, Burke RP. The modern approach to patent ductus arteriosus treatment: Complementary roles of video-assisted thoracoscopic surgery and interventional cardiology coil occlusion. *The Annals of thoracic surgery*. 2003;76(5):1421-1427; discussion 1427-1428.
12. Schmidt B, Davis P, Moddemann D, Ohlsson A, Roberts RS, Saigal S, Solimano A, Vincer M, Wright LL. Long-term effects of indomethacin prophylaxis in extremely-low-birth-weight infants. *N Engl J Med*. 2001;344(26):1966-1972.
13. Koch J, Hensley G, Roy L, Brown S, Ramaciotti C, Rosenfeld CR. Prevalence of spontaneous closure of the ductus arteriosus in neonates at a birth weight of 1000 grams or less. *Pediatrics*. 2006;117(4):1113-1121.
14. Allen HD. *Moss and adams heart disease in infants, children, and adolescents: Including the fetus and young adult*. Philadelphia, PA: Wolters Kluwer Health/Lippincott Williams & Wilkins; 2013.

43 CYANOTIC CONGENITAL HEART DISEASE

Amara Majeed, MBBS
Athar M. Qureshi, MD

PATIENT STORY

A 20-day-old baby boy is brought into the emergency department by his parents who noticed that he was "blue." On examination, he is alert and is cyanotic with an oxygen saturation of 83 percent. His cardiac exam reveals a mild right precordial heave with a harsh, long-grade 3/6 systolic ejection murmur at left upper sternal border. In the ED, he becomes more cyanotic (oxygen saturation of 60%), irritable and his murmur becomes softer. An echocardiogram was performed which identified cyanotic congenital heart disease (Tetralogy of Fallot) (**Figure 43-1**). He was treated medically and then underwent palliative surgery with a Blalock Taussig shunt. He was discharged in stable condition to be followed up on an outpatient basis until he could have further corrective surgery at a later date.

INTRODUCTION

Cyanotic congenital heart disease is an anatomic malformation of the heart or great vessels which occurs during intrauterine development (resulting in a right to left shunt) and manifests as cyanosis in the neonatal period.

EPIDEMIOLOGY

- Congenital heart defects are the most common type of birth defect in the US, affecting nearly 1 percent of newborns, although this number is variable depending on methodology.[1]
- A significant portion of patients with potentially fatal forms of congenital heart disease have cyanotic defects.
- The most common forms of cyanotic congenital heart disease are:[2]
  - Tetralogy of Fallot (**Figure 43-1**), transposition of the great arteries (**Figure 43-2**), truncus arteriosus, tricuspid atresia, total anomalous pulmonary venous return, or pulmonary valve stenosis (severe or critical pulmonary valve stenosis).
  - Other examples: Ebstein's anomaly, double outlet right ventricle, pulmonary atresia, or multiple single ventricle variants.

ETIOLOGY AND PATHOPHYSIOLOGY

- Most cases are due to an unknown etiology and are multifactorial.
- Systemic venous blood bypasses the pulmonary circulation, resulting in a right to left shunt, systemic arterial desaturation and clinical cyanosis.

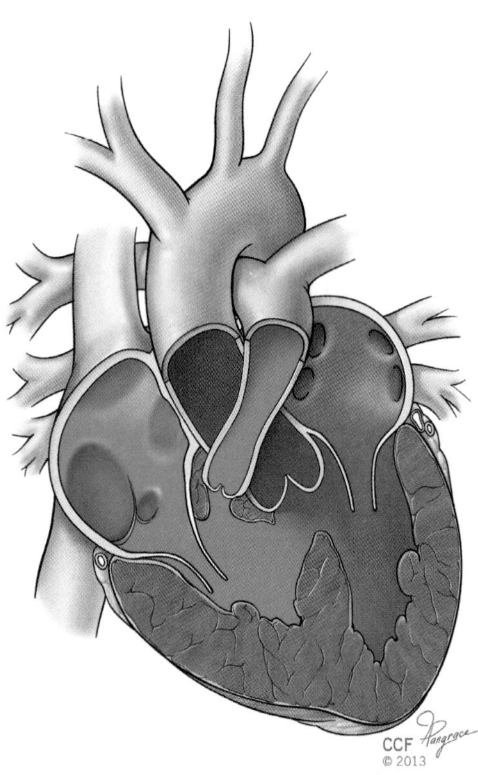

FIGURE 43-1 Tetralogy of Fallot. Note the four components, "anterior-malaligned" VSD, pulmonary stenosis, over-riding aorta and right ventricular hypertrophy. *(Reprinted with permission, Cleveland Clinic Center for Medical Art & Photography © 2012. All Rights Reserved.)*

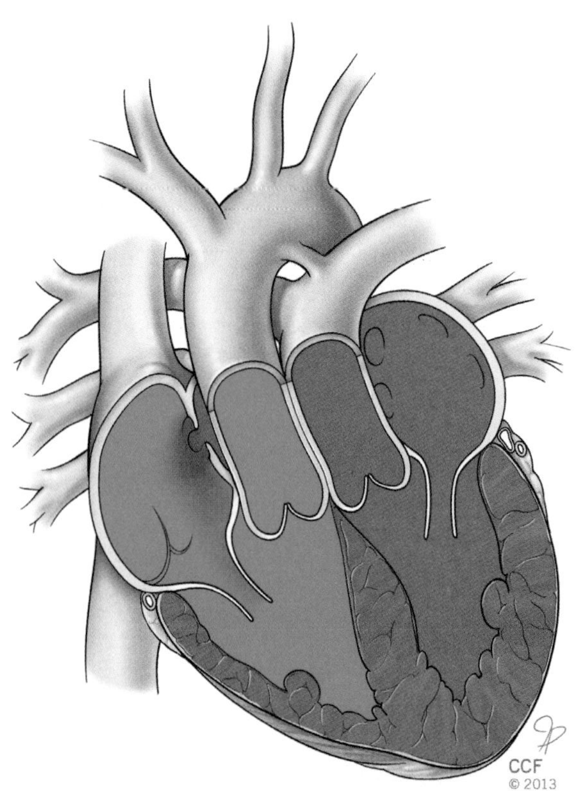

FIGURE 43-2 Transposition of the great arteries with the aorta arising from the right ventricle and the pulmonary artery arising from the left ventricle. Mixing (via an atrial septal defect, ventricular septal defect or patent ductus arteriosus) is essential for survival before corrective surgery. *(Reprinted with permission, Cleveland Clinic Center for Medical Art & Photography © 2012. All Rights Reserved.)*

- Depending on the predominant physiology, cyanosis may be variable and not the primary underlying problem.

RISK FACTORS

Hereditary or genetic risk factors

- Relatives with congenital heart disease.
- Genetic syndromes, which include congenital heart disease as a feature (i.e., DiGeorge syndrome).[1,3]

Maternal risk factors

- In vitro fertilization.
- Cardiac teratogen exposure (e.g., alcohol, lithium, isotretinoin, anticonvulsants, thalidomide, organic solvents).[4]
- Maternal illness (e.g., diabetes, phenylketonuria, rubella).[4]

Fetal risk factors

- Includes extra cardiac anomalies in the fetus, aneuploidy, hydrops, abnormal fetal situs, chromosomal abnormality, and monochorionic twins.

DIAGNOSIS

CLINICAL FEATURES

- Clinical features are highly variable depending on the particular lesion.
- Central cyanosis is present.
- Respiratory distress, hypercyanotic spells, poor feeding, or failure to thrive may be present depending on the specific lesion.
- Vital signs may show tachycardia, tachypnea, decreased oxygen saturation, and hypotension.
- A difference between preductal and postductal oxygen saturations may be present.
- Blood pressures in all four extremities may detect a coexistent coarctation of aorta.
- Cardiac exam may reveal abnormal heart sounds and a pathological murmur depending on the type of lesion.
- Signs of congestive heart failure may be present, that is, tachypnea, subcostal retractions, and hepatomegaly.

LABORATORY TESTING

- Hyperoxia test is done to distinguish cardiac from respiratory cause of cyanosis. The oxygen saturation and Po_2 does not significantly increase with cyanotic congenital heart disease.
- Complete blood count, arterial blood gas, and a blood culture to rule out sepsis are generally indicated.

IMAGING

- Chest x-ray (**Figure 43-3**).
- Electrocardiogram.
- Echocardiogram.

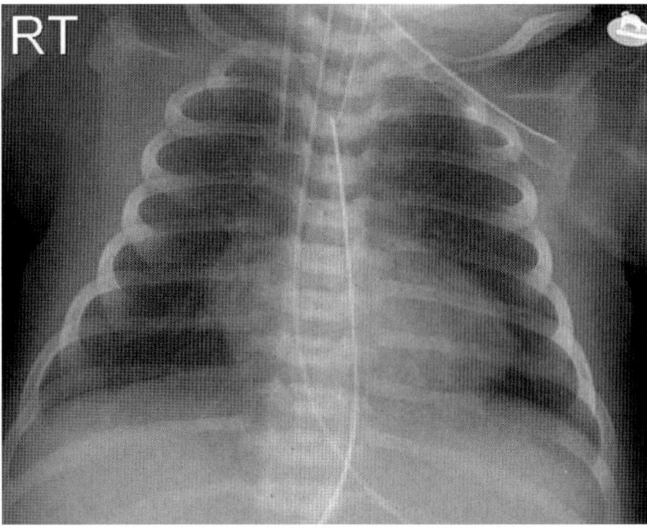

FIGURE 43-3 CXR (AP view) of an infant with tetralogy of Fallot. Note the upturned cardiac apex and concave pulmonary shadow representing a "boot-shaped heart." Relatively dark lung fields from decreased pulmonary blood flow are also seen. (*Used with permission from Athar M. Qureshi, MD.*)

DIFFERENTIAL DIAGNOSIS

- Pulmonary disorders including pulmonary hypertension can be excluded with the previous history and imaging studies.
- Poor peripheral perfusion due to sepsis, hypoglycemia, dehydration, and hypoadrenalism.
- Abnormal hemoglobin, for example, methemoglobinemia.

MANAGEMENT

NONPHARMACOLOGICAL

- Supportive care with cardiorespiratory support and vigilant monitoring to ensure adequate perfusion and oxygenation.
- Maintain neutral thermal environment.
- Provide supplemental oxygen or mechanical ventilation as required.
- Increased caloric intake.

MEDICATIONS

- Prostaglandin E1 infusion is indicated where there is a suspicion of having ductal dependent physiology.
- Correction of metabolic derangements and acid-base balance.
- Diuretics, digoxin, and angiotensin converting enzyme inhibitors may be used depending on the physiology present.
- Vasopressors to correct hypotension.

SURGERY

- Cardiac catheterization, which can be diagnostic or therapeutic.
- Balloon atrial septostomy can be done to create a connection between the left and right atria in patients with transposition

of the great arteries or left sided obstructive lesions (**Figure 43-4**).

- Balloon valvuloplasty can be done in valvular pulmonary stenosis to increase blood flow across the valve (**Figure 43-5**).
- The final treatment for most common causes of cyanotic congenital heart disease is cardiac surgery. The timing of the surgical procedures is variable depending on the type of lesion. For each of the common lesions the surgical procedure most commonly performed are the following:
  - Tetralogy of Fallot—Ventricular septal defect (VSD) closure and relief of obstruction to pulmonary flow (**Figure 43-6**).
  - Transposition of the great arteries—arterial switch operation (**Figure 43-7**).
  - Tricuspid atresia—Blalock Taussig shunt placement, Glenn operation, and then Fontan operation.
  - Total anomalous pulmonary venous return—Redirection of common pulmonary venous confluence to the left atrium.
  - Truncus arteriosus—VSD closure with right ventricle to pulmonary artery conduit placement.

REFERRAL

- Pediatric cardiologist, cardiothoracic surgeon, maternal-fetal medicine specialist, obstetrician, neonatologist, or geneticist.

PREVENTION AND SCREENING

PREVENTION

- Preventive measures include genetic counseling, control of maternal disease, and avoiding teratogen exposure during pregnancy.

SCREENING

- Basic obstetrical ultrasound examination should be performed at 18 to 22 weeks of gestation.
- A full fetal echocardiogram is indicated in pregnancies with risk factors (see preceding section) for congenital heart anomalies.
- The identification of a fetal cardiac defect should prompt a search for any associated abnormalities.

PROGNOSIS

- Most cyanotic congenital heart diseases have a poor prognosis if left untreated. With prompt diagnosis and treatment, however, the prognosis is favorable for most lesions.
- Untreated and chronic cyanotic congenital heart diseases have been associated with stroke, organ damage, impaired muscle performance, thrombosis, and vascular damage amongst other devastating consequences.[5]

FOLLOW-UP

Regular and periodic follow-up after surgical or interventional correction is necessary to address continued medical management and long term complications associated with corrected circulations.

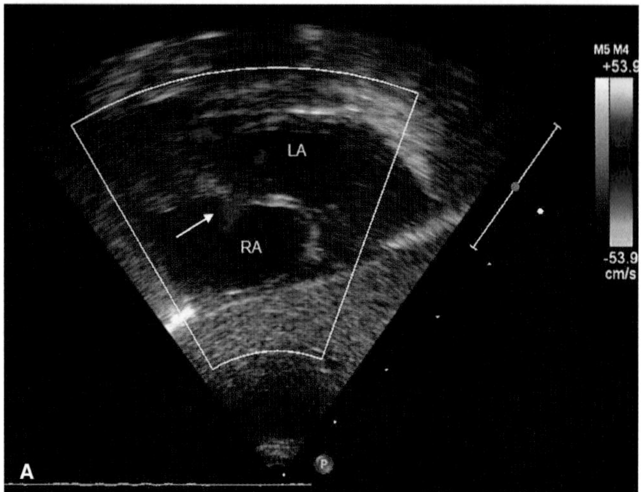

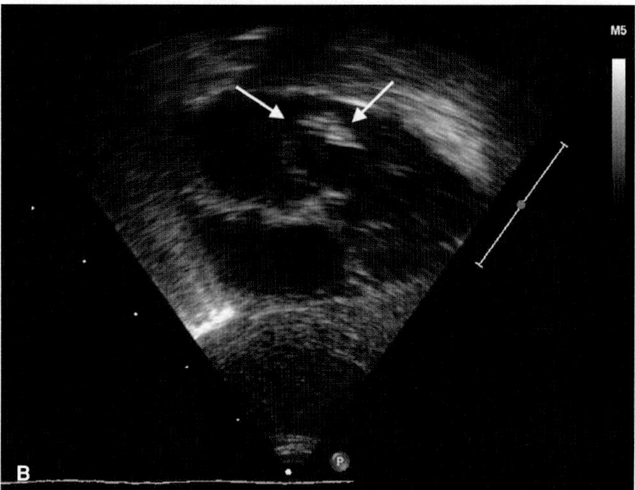

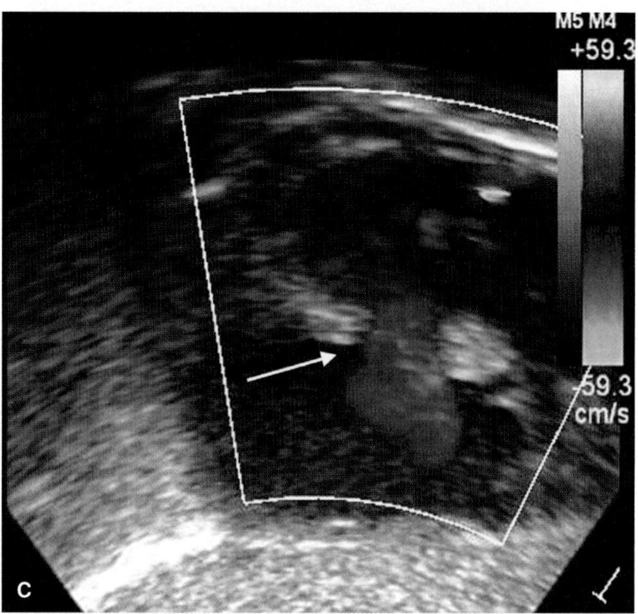

FIGURE 43-4 Transthoracic echocardiogram of an infant with severe cyanosis from transposition of the great arteries (TGA). **A.** There is minimal flow across the ASD (arrow) initially (4-a). **B.** Following a catheter-based balloon (arrows) atrial septostomy (4-b). **C.** There is much improved flow and a larger ASD (arrow) (4-c). This procedure is critical for many patients with TGA and allows survival until corrective surgery can be performed. (RA = right atrium, LA = left atrium). (*Used with permission from Athar M. Qureshi, MD.*)

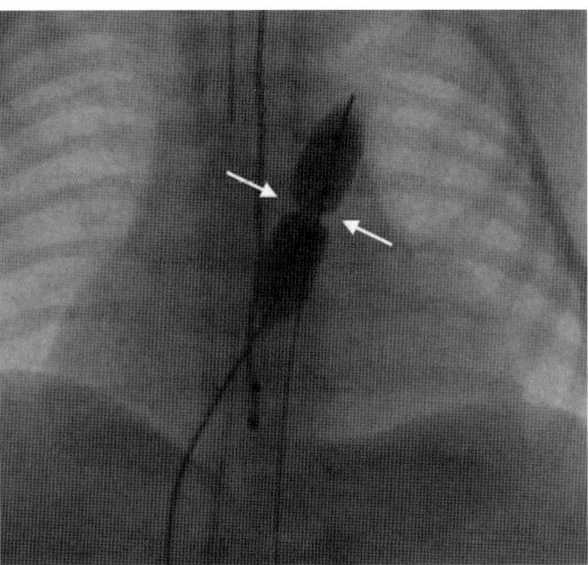

FIGURE 43-5 Balloon valvuloplasty in the cardiac catheterization laboratory in a newborn with critical pulmonary valve stenosis and cyanosis. Note the "waist" in the balloon (arrows) that corresponds to the narrow valve orifice. This will be eliminated with full balloon inflation. (*Used with permission from Athar M. Qureshi, MD.*)

PATIENT EDUCATION

Patients with congenital heart disease need complex and multifaceted care in order to ensure their continued survival and improve their quality of life. Teams of specialists are needed to care for families and patients prior to conception, in childhood and in adulthood.

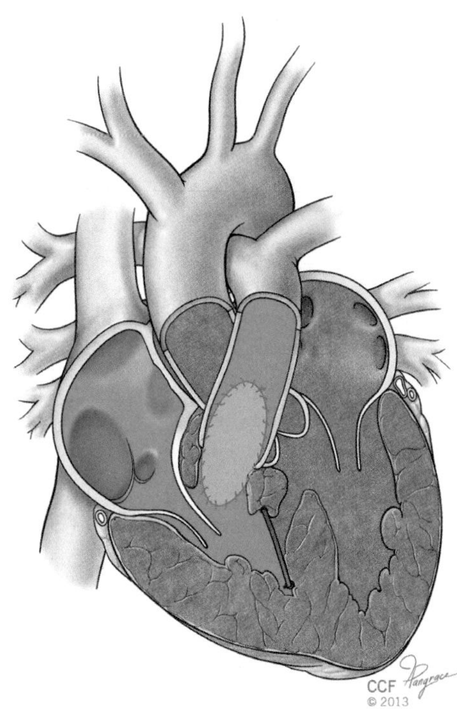

FIGURE 43-6 Complete repair for tetralogy of Fallot, involving VSD closure, and relief of the pulmonary stenosis (in this case with a "transannular patch" across the pulmonary valve annulus). (*Reprinted with permission, Cleveland Clinic Center for Medical Art & Photography © 2012. All Rights Reserved.*)

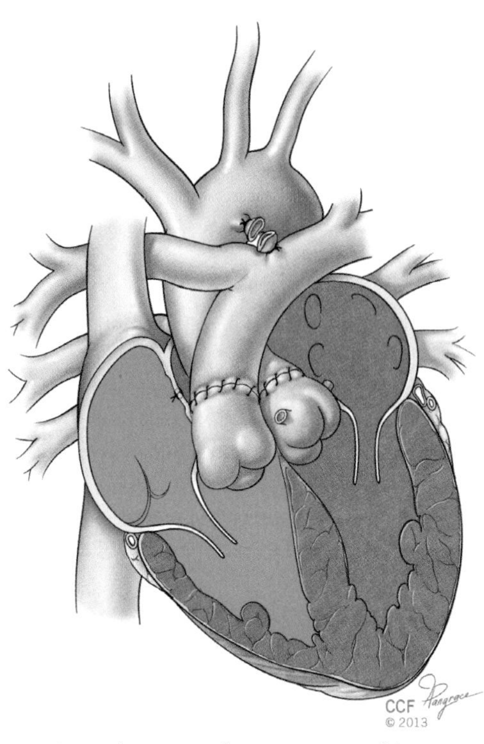

FIGURE 43-7 Surgical correction for transposition of the great arteries (TGA)—the arterial switch operation, which establishes a physiologic and anatomic correction of the defect. The great vessels are "switched" and coronary artery buttons are created and moved over to the "neo" aorta. (*Reprinted with permission, Cleveland Clinic Center for Medical Art & Photography © 2012. All Rights Reserved.*)

PATIENT RESOURCES

- Congenital Heart Disease. John Hopkins University—**www.pted.org**.
- **www.my.clevelandclinic.org/childrens-hospital/health-info/diseases-conditions/heart/hic-pediatric-congenital-heart-defects.aspx**.

PROVIDER RESOURCES

- **www.emedicine.medscape.com/article/900574**.

REFERENCES

1. Hoffman JL, Kaplan S. The incidence of congenital heart disease. *J Am Coll Cardiol*. 2002;39(12):1890-1900.
2. Silberbach M, Hannon D. Presentation of congenital heart disease in the neonate and young infant. *Pediatr Rev*. 2007;28(4): 123-131.
3. Lacro RV. Dysmorphology and Genetics. In: Keane JF, Lock JE and Fyler DC, eds. *Nadas' Pediatric Cardiology, 2nd ed*. Elsevier, 2006;49-72.
4. Jenkins KJ, Correa A, Feinstein JA, et al. Noninherited risk factors and congenital cardiovascular defects: current knowledge: a scientific statement from the American Heart Association Council on Cardiovascular Disease in the Young: endorsed by the American Academy of Pediatrics. *Circulation*. 2007;115:2995-3014.
5. Rachael L. Cordina and David S. Celermajer: Chronic cyanosis and vascular function: implications for patients with cyanotic congenital heart disease. *Cardiology in the Young* 2010;242-253.

44 BACTERIAL ENDOCARDITIS

Heidi Chumley, MD
Camille Sabella, MD

PATIENT STORY

A 14-year-old girl with a history of mitral regurgitation that complicated rheumatic heart disease was brought in by her parents after two weeks of intermittent low-grade fevers, fatigue, weakness, arthralgias, and myalgias. On examination, she appeared ill, was febrile, and had a heart murmur. Her funduscopic examination revealed Roth spots (**Figures 44-1** and **44-2**). Her blood cultures grew *Streptococcus mitis*. An echocardiogram demonstrated a vegetation on the mitral valve. She was hospitalized and treated for bacterial endocarditis.

INTRODUCTION

Bacterial endocarditis is a serious infection that in the pediatric population is seen most commonly in patients with congenital heart disease, prosthetic valves, injection drug users, and patients with indwelling central venous catheters. The diagnosis is made based on the Duke Criteria. The rate of cure with appropriate antibiotics and surgical management, when indicated, is high, and facilitated by prompt diagnosis and vigilance in recognizing complications.

EPIDEMIOLOGY

- 0.34 to 0.64 cases per 100,000 patient-years.[1]
- 1 case per 1000 pediatric hospital admissions.

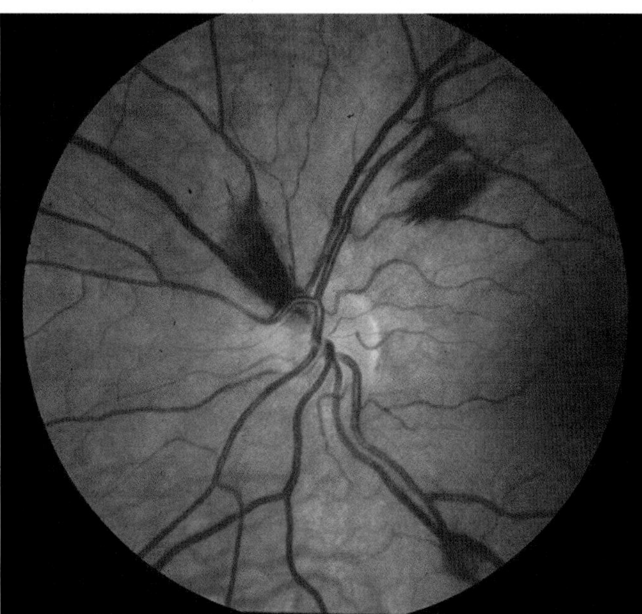

FIGURE 44-1 Roth spots that are retinal hemorrhages with white centers seen in bacterial endocarditis. These can also be seen in leukemia and diabetes. (*Used with permission from Paul D. Comeau.*)

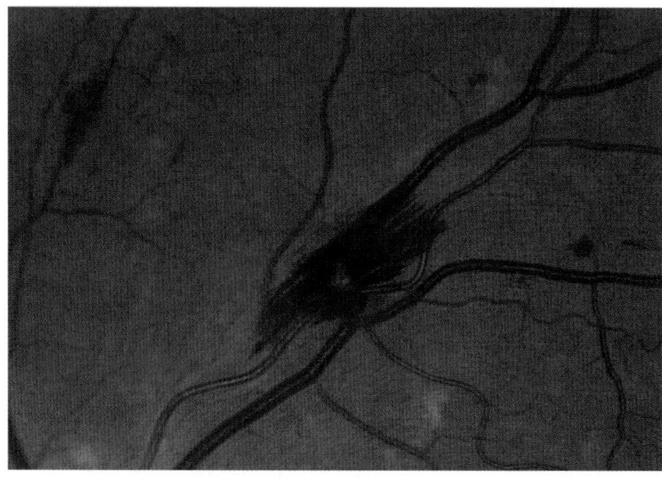

FIGURE 44-2 Close-up of a Roth spot, which is actually a cotton-wool spot surrounded by hemorrhage. The cotton-wool comes from ischemic bursting of axons and the hemorrhage comes from ischemic bursting of an arteriole. (*Used with permission from Paul D. Comeau.*)

- 46 percent of cases in ages 0 to 1, followed by 23 percent, 20 percent, and 12 percent in ages 12 to 18, 5 to 12, and 1 to 5 years, respectively.[2]
- 58 percent of cases in male patients.[2]
- 68 percent of patients hospitalized with infective endocarditis (IE) had some type of congenital heart disease.[2]
- 2007 AHA guidelines for IE prophylaxis have not changed IE admissions.[2]

ETIOLOGY AND PATHOPHYSIOLOGY

- Flow through an abnormal valve or abnormal communication between systemic and pulmonary circulation (as in various congenital heart diseases) damages endothelium.
- Platelets and fibrin adhere to damaged endothelium initiating a sterile thrombus.
- Microbes adhere to compromised endothelium during transient bacteremia.
- Common organisms include viridans Streptococci (such as *Streptococcus mitis* and *Streptococcus oralis*) *Staphylococcus aureus*, coagulase-negative *Staphylococci*, *Enterococci*, *Candida spp*, and rarely *Streptococcus pneumoniae*.
- Viridans streptococci are more commonly associated with rheumatic fever, unrepaired congenital heart disease, and late postoperative endocarditis.
- Staphylococcal species, including methicillin-resistant *S aureus* (MRSA) and coagulase-negative Staphylococci, are commonly associated with endocarditis after cardiac surgery and with prosthetic valves; *S aureus* is also common as a cause of endocarditis in individuals who have normal hearts and in intravenous drug users.
- Fungal causes of endocarditis, such as *Candida* spp., are especially common in those who have hospital-acquired endocarditis, those with central venous catheters, those with prosthetic valves, and in neonates.
- Fastidious agents, known as the HACEK group, are rare causes of endocarditis in the pediatric population and include *Haemophilus*,

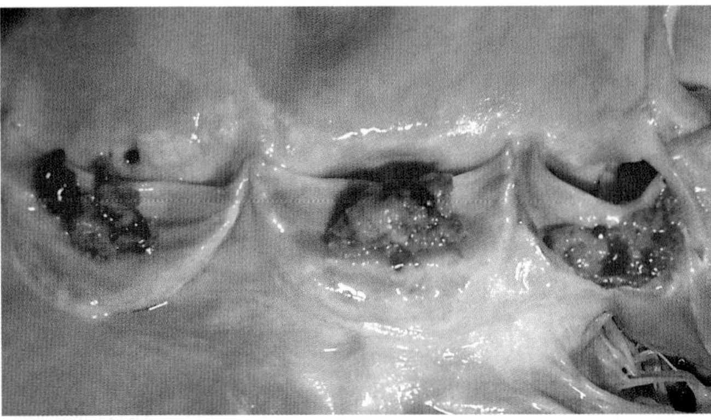

FIGURE 44-3 Pathology specimen of a patient who died of bacterial endocarditis. Bacterial growth can be seen on the three cusps of this heart valve. *(Used with permission from Larry Fowler, MD.)*

Actinobacillus, Cardiobacterium, Eikenella, and *Kingella (neonates* and *immunocompromised).*

- Blood contacts subendothelial factors, which promotes coagulation.
- Pathogens bind and activate monocyte, cytokine, and tissue factor production, enlarging the vegetations on the heart valves.
- The vegetations enlarge and damage the heart valves (**Figure 44-3**). This process can lead to death if not treated adequately in time.
- Septic emboli can occur, most commonly in the brain, spleen, or kidney.[3]

RISK FACTORS[4]

- Congenital heart disease.
- Prosthetic valve.
- Injection drug use.
- Rheumatic fever.
- Prior episode of bacterial endocarditis.
- Central venous catheters (neonates).
- Prior heart surgery with resultant valvulopathy or systemic to pulmonary shunt.

DIAGNOSIS

- The Duke criteria use a combination of history, physical examination, laboratory, and echocardiogram findings, and across several studies, have a sensitivity of approximately 80 percent.[5]
- The diagnosis is considered definite when patients have two major, one major and three minor, or five minor criteria.[5]
- The diagnosis is considered possible when one major and one minor or three minor criteria are present.[5]
- Major criteria include:[5]
    - Two separate blood cultures positive with:
        - viridans *Streptococci*, S aureus, HACEK group, or enterococci.
        - Persistently positive blood cultures.
        - Single positive culture or high IgG titer for *Coxiella burnetti* (Q fever).

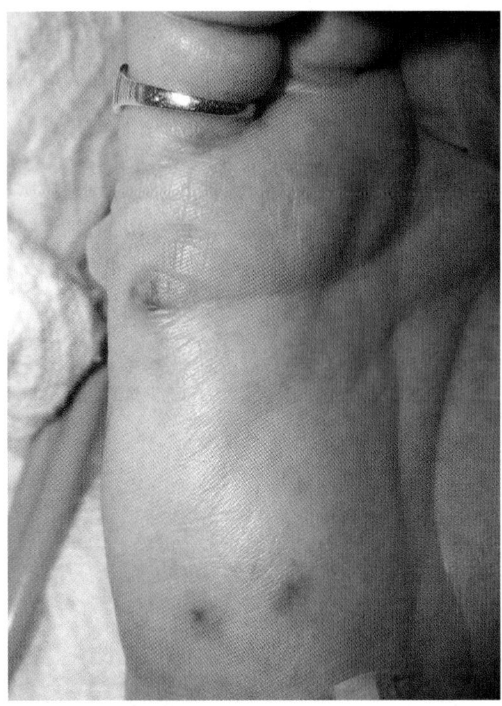

FIGURE 44-4 Janeway lesions on the palm of a woman hospitalized with acute bacterial endocarditis. These were not painful. *(Used with permission from David A. Kasper DO, MBA.)*

    - Echocardiogram evidence of vegetation, abscess, or new partial dehiscence of a prosthetic valve.
        - New valvular regurgitation.
- Minor criteria include:[5]
    - Predisposition (e.g., heart condition such as a congenital or acquired valvular defect, injection drug use, prior history of endocarditis).
    - Temperature >38°C (100.4°F).
    - Clinical signs: arterial emboli, septic pulmonary infarcts, mycotic aneurysms, intracranial hemorrhages, splinter hemorrhages, Osler nodes, Roth spots, or Janeway lesions (**Figures 44-1, 44-2**, and **44-4** to **44-7**).
    - Glomerulonephritis.
    - Positive rheumatoid factor.
    - Positive blood culture not meeting major criteria.
    - Echocardiographic findings consistent with infective endocarditis that do not meet major criteria.

CLINICAL FEATURES

- Fever—Seen in 75 to 99 percent of patients, and is typically low-grade.
- New or changing heart murmur—Seen in 20 to 80 percent of patients.
- Splenomegaly may be in 50 to 75 percent of patients.
- Petechiae seen in up to 50 percent of patients (**Figure 44-5**).
- Septic emboli—Seen in up to 50 percent, largely dependent on the size (>10 mm) and mobility of the vegetation.
- Intracranial hemorrhages—Seen in 30 to 40 percent of patients, bleeding from septic emboli or cerebral mycotic aneurysms.

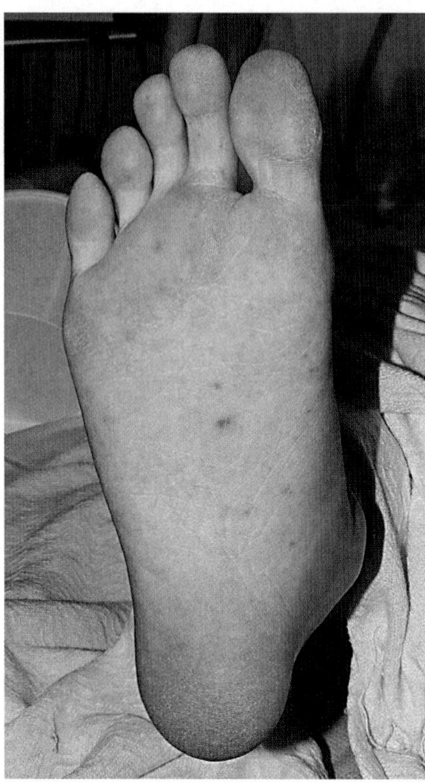

FIGURE 44-5 Janeway lesions and petechial lesions on the sole of a 17-year-old boy who was hospitalized with *S aureus* bacteremia and endocarditis. (*Used with permission from Blanca Gonzalez, MD.*)

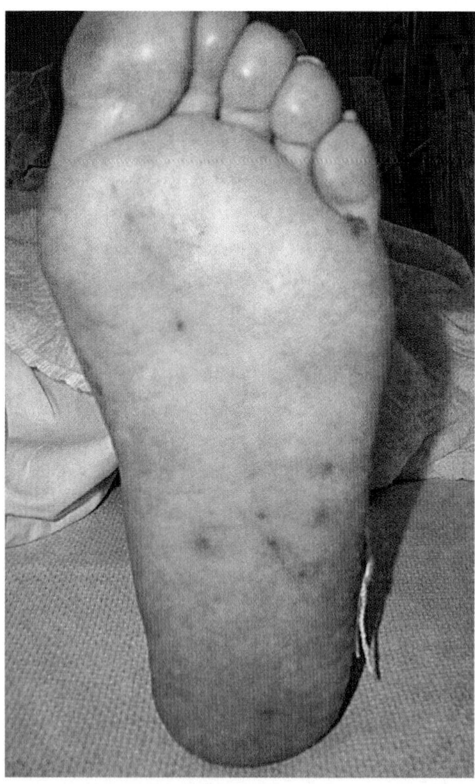

FIGURE 44-6 Osler node causing pain within pulp of the big toe in the same woman hospitalized with acute bacterial endocarditis. (Osler nodes are painful—remember "O" for Ouch and Osler.) Note the multiple painless flat Janeway lesions over the sole of the foot. (*Used with permission from David A. Kasper DO, MBA.*)

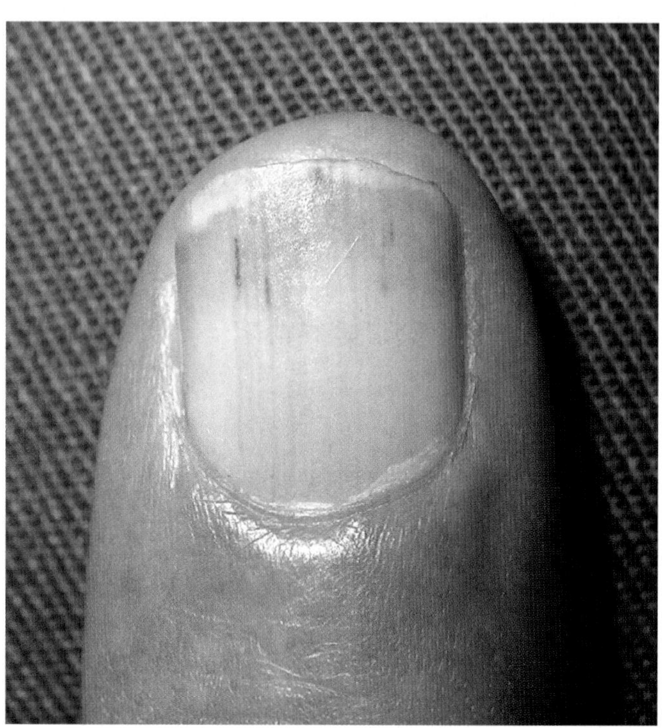

FIGURE 44-7 Splinter hemorrhages appearing as red linear streaks under the nail plate and within the nail bed. Although endocarditis can cause this, splinter hemorrhages are more commonly seen in psoriasis and trauma. (*Used with permission from Richard P. Usatine, MD.*)

- Mycotic aneurysms—Aneurysms resulting from infectious process in the arterial wall, most commonly in the thoracic aorta, also found in the cerebral arteries.
- Splinter hemorrhages—Red, linear streaks in the nail beds of the fingers or toes (**Figure 44-7**).
- Janeway lesions—Very rare, flat, painless, red to bluish-red spots on the palms, and soles (**Figures 44-4** and **44-5**).
- Glomerulonephritis—Immune mediated that can result in hematuria and renal insufficiency, occurs in approximately 15 percent of patients with endocarditis.
- Osler nodes—Tender, subcutaneous nodules in the pulp of the digits (**Figure 44-6**).
- Roth spots—Retinal hemorrhages from microemboli, seen in approximately 5 percent of cases of endocarditis (**Figures 44-1** and **44-2**).

TYPICAL DISTRIBUTION

- Native endocarditis—Mitral valve (prior rheumatic fever or mitral valve prolapse), followed by aortic (prior rheumatic fever, calcific aortic stenosis of bicuspid valve).
- Prosthetic valve endocarditis—Site of any prosthetic valve.
- In IV drug users—Tricuspid valve, followed by aortic.

LABORATORY AND ANCILLARY TESTING

- Positive blood cultures (75% to 100% of patients), anemia (75% to 90%) and an elevated erythrocyte sedimentation rate (ESR) (seen in 75% to 100%) are the most common laboratory findings.

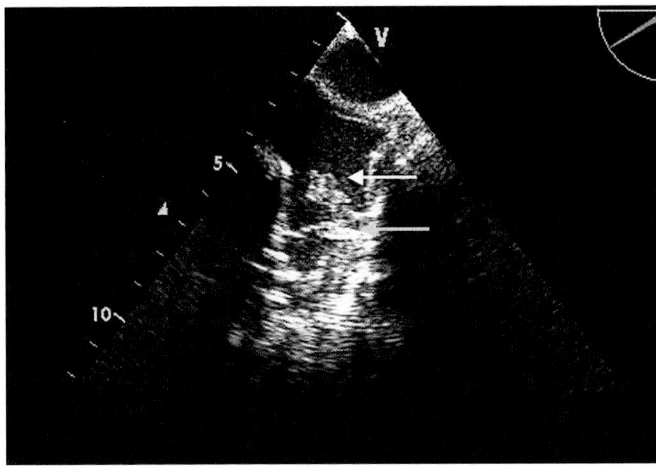

FIGURE 44-8 Transesophageal echocardiogram in a teenage boy with endocarditis of a prosthetic right ventricle to pulmonary artery conduit. Note the vegetation (white arrow) attached to the pulmonary valve leaflets (yellow arrow). *(Used with permission from Athar Qureshi, MD.)*

- A positive rheumatoid factor is found in 25 to 50 percent of patients with endocarditis.
- Hematuria is found in 25 to 50 percent of patients with endocarditis.
- Positive blood culture—First two sets of cultures are positive in 90 percent.[3]

IMAGING

- Abnormal transthoracic echocardiogram.
- Transthoracic echocardiogram has a sensitivity of 80 percent in children under 60 kg; Transesophageal echocardiogram is rarely indicated in the pediatric population but is occasionally required for adolescent and young adults[6] (**Figure 44-8**).

DIFFERENTIAL DIAGNOSIS

Fever without a clear cause may be seen with:

- Connective tissue disorders—Typically with other signs depending on the disorder, negative blood cultures, normal echocardiogram.
- Fever of unknown origin—Negative blood cultures or positive cultures with atypical organisms, normal echocardiogram in non-cardiac causes.
- Intraabdominal infections—Fever and positive blood cultures, normal echocardiogram.
- Acute leukemias—Fever and systemic symptoms, abnormal CBC

Echocardiogram findings similar to bacterial endocarditis may be seen with:

- Noninfective vegetations—No fever and negative blood cultures.
- Cardiac tumors—Embolic complications, right or left heart failure, often located off valves in cardiac chambers, negative blood cultures.
- Cusp prolapse—No fever and negative blood cultures.
- Myxomatous changes—Extra connective tissue in the valve leaflets.
- Lamb excrescences—Stranding from wear and tear on the valve, most commonly aortic, no fever, and negative blood cultures.

MANAGEMENT

- Two or three sets of blood cultures should be obtained when the diagnosis is suspected. Patients with suspected endocarditis should be admitted to the hospital.
- The decision to give antibiotics empirically depends on the clinical findings and suspicion for endocarditis. It is critical that appropriate blood cultures are obtained prior to the start of intravenous antibiotics. SOR Ⓒ

MEDICATIONS

- Empiric coverage for endocarditis must take into account the most likely organism based on the age, risk factor, preexisting heart disease, recent surgery, clinical presentation, and most likely mode of acquisition.
- Coverage for viridans Streptococci in native valve endocarditis usually includes penicillin G with or without gentamicin. The treatment duration is 2 to 4 weeks.
- Coverage for *Staphylococcus* in IV drug abusers includes nafcillin with or without gentamicin; Vancomycin should be given instead of nafcillin when there is concern about methicillin-resistant *Staphylococcus aureus* (MRSA) or when a prosthetic valve in involved (with gentamicin). The typical treatment duration is 4 to 6 weeks.
- Definitive antimicrobial therapy should be based on culture and susceptibility results.
- Treatment of Gram-positive infections should include a β-lactam when the organism is susceptible; current evidence does not support adding an aminoglycaside.[7] SOR Ⓐ
- Surgical consultation should be obtained when:
  - Congestive heart failure is severe with mitral or aortic regurgitation.
  - Fever and/or bacteremia persist for 7 to 10 days despite adequate antibiotic therapy, abscesses or perivalvular involvement occurs, or fungal organisms are identified.
  - Embolic events recur on adequate antibiotic therapy or the risk of embolic events is high because of vegetations larger than 10 mm. SOR Ⓒ
- Anticoagulation and aspirin are not indicated for infective endocarditis and are contraindicated with cerebral complications or aneurysms.

PREVENTION

- Bacterial endocarditis is a serious life-threatening disease requiring long-term antibiotics and close follow-up.
- Patients who are at high risk for endocarditis should be educated regarding the importance of prophylactic antibiotics before certain procedures. The following are the 2007 American Heart Association recommendations:[8]

- Prophylactic antibiotics should be prescribed only to patients at the highest risk: SOR B
  - Patients with prosthetic cardiac valves.
  - Patients with previous bacterial endocarditis.
  - Cardiac transplant recipients with cardiac valvuloplasty.
  - Patients with these congenital heart defects (CHDs): unrepaired cyanotic CHD; CHD repaired with prosthetic material within the last 6 months; repaired CHD with a residual defect at or adjacent to the site of a prosthetic device.
- Prophylactic antibiotics are *no longer recommended* for patients with mitral valve prolapse.
- Prophylactic antibiotics should be prescribed only to patients undergoing one of the following:
  - Any dental procedure that involves manipulation of gingival tissue or the periapical region of teeth or perforation of the oral mucosa. SOR C
  - Respiratory procedures involving incision or biopsy of the respiratory mucosa such as a tonsillectomy or adenoidectomy. SOR C
  - Procedures on infected skin or musculoskeletal tissue.
- Endocarditis prophylaxis is *no longer recommended* for patients undergoing gastrointestinal or genitourinary procedures. SOR B
- A one-dose regimen to be taken 30 minutes to 1 hour before the procedure should be prescribed:[8]
  - Amoxicillin 50 mg/kg up to 2.0 g orally.
  - If unable to take oral medications: ampicillin 50 mg/kg up to 2.0 g IM or IV 30 minutes before the procedure; *or* cefazolin or ceftriaxone 50 mg/kg up to 1 g IM or IV.
  - Penicillin allergic: clindamycin 20 mg/kg up to 600 mg po, IM, or IV; *or* azithromycin or clarithromycin 15 mg/kg up to 500 mg po. If allergy to penicillin is *not* anaphylaxis, angioedema, or urticaria, may also use cephalexin 50 mg/kg up to 2.0 g po; *or* cefazolin or ceftriaxone 50 mg/kg up to 1 g IM or IV.

PROGNOSIS

Bacterial endocarditis requires early detection and aggressive antibiotic therapy to decrease mortality. Overall mortality varies according to the pathogen and underlying condition but may be as high as 16 to 25 percent.

FOLLOW-UP

- Most patients with bacterial endocarditis will require 4 to 6 weeks of IV antibiotics.
- Depending on the antibiotics, some patients will need to have medication levels monitored.
- Repeat blood cultures are important to ensure response to therapy.
- An echocardiogram at the end of treatment provides baseline imaging, as patients with endocarditis are at risk for another episode.[9] SOR C

PATIENT EDUCATION

- Bacterial endocarditis is a serious disease with a significant mortality rate.
- Finish all antibiotics and keep follow-up appointments to ensure adequate treatment.
- Mortality remains elevated even 6 months after an episode.
- Recurrence is common, especially if risk factors remain (i.e., continued immunosuppression or IV drug use).

PATIENT RESOURCES

- The American Heart Association has information about who is at risk for bacterial endocarditis and a printable wallet card for at-risk patient, available in English or Spanish—**www.heart.org/HEARTORG/Conditions/CongenitalHeartDefects/TheImpactofCongenitalHeartDefects/Infective-Endocarditis_UCM_307108_Article.jsp**.

PROVIDER RESOURCES

- The American Heart Association guidelines on endocarditis prophylaxis—**www.circ.ahajournals.org/content/116/15/1736.full.pdf**.
- Guidelines on Infective Endocarditis: Diagnosis, Antimicrobial Thherapy, and Management of Complications—**www.circ.ahajournals.org/content/111/23/e394.full**.
- MedCalc has an interactive Web site with Duke criteria for Infective Endocarditis—**www.medcalc.com/endocarditis.html**.

REFERENCES

1. Knirsch W, Nadal D. Infective endocarditis in congenital heart disease. *Eur J Pediatr.* 2011;170(9):1111-1127.
2. Pasquali SK, Xia H, Zeinab M, et al. Trends in endocarditis hospitalizations at US children's hospitals: Impact of the 2007 American Heart Association Antiobiotic Prophylaxis Guidelines. *Amer Heart J.* 2012;163(5):894-899.
3. Prendergast BD. The changing face of infective endocarditis. *Heart.* 2006;92(7):879-885.
4. Gewitz MH. *Pediatric Bacterial Endocarditis.* http://emedicine.medscape.com/article/896540, accessed May 17, 2011.
5. Habib G. Management of infective endocarditis. *Heart.* 2006; 92(1):124-130.
6. Penk JS, Webb CL, Shulman ST, Anderson EJ. Echocardiography in pediatric infective endocarditis. *Pediatr Infect Dis J.* 2011;3(12): 1109-1111.
7. Falagas ME, Matthaiou DK, Bliziotis IA. The role of aminoglycosides in combination with a beta-lactam for the treatment of bacterial endocarditis: a meta-analysis of comparative trials. *J Antimicrob Chemother.* 2006;57(4):639-647.
8. Wilson W, Taubert KA, Gewitz M, et al. Prevention of infective endocarditis: a guideline from the American Heart Association. *Circulation.* 2007;116:1736-1754.
9. Baddour LM, Wilson WR, Bayer AS, et al. American Heart Association Scientific Statement on Infective Endocarditis. *Circulation.* 2005; 111:e394-e434.

45 ACUTE RHEUMATIC FEVER

Abbas H. Zaidi, MB, BS
Athar M. Qureshi, MD

PATIENT STORY

An 11-year-old girl was referred for evaluation of a heart murmur. She has right knee pain and swelling that was preceded by right ankle pain and swelling. Three weeks prior to the presentation, she had a fever and sore throat. On exam, she has swelling and tenderness of her right knee, a hyperdynamic precordium with a pansystolic murmur heard best at the apex. She has an elevated Anti-streptolysin O (ASO) titer. Her echocardiogram confirms severe mitral regurgitation (**Figure 45-1**). She was diagnosed with acute rheumatic fever and admitted to the hospital. She was treated with penicillin, aspirin, and bed rest with significant clinical improvement. She was discharged from the hospital within a week and over the course of the next few months, her mitral regurgitation improved.

INTRODUCTION

Acute rheumatic fever (ARF) is an inflammatory disease that affects susceptible children and adolescents, (most commonly aged 3 to 19 years). It is mediated by humoral and cellular autoimmune responses that occur as delayed sequelae of *Streptococcus pyogenes* (group A) (GAS) pharyngitis. The manifestations of ARF usually manifest 2 to 4 weeks after the initial infection.

SYNONYMS

- Sydenham's chorea is also called St. Vitus' dance. It is only one manifestation of ARF and is addressed in the following section.

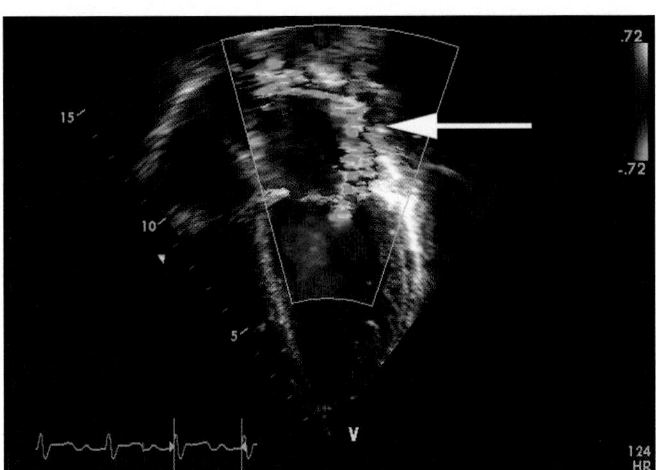

FIGURE 45-1 Transthoracic echocardiogram (apical four-chamber view) in an 11-year-old with acute rheumatic fever and severe mitral regurgitation (arrow). (*Used with permission from Athar M. Qureshi, MD.*)

EPIDEMIOLOGY

- Rheumatic heart disease has a prevalence of at least 15.6 million cases, with 282,000 new cases and 233,000 deaths each year.[1]
- The disease today mostly occurs in developing countries.
- There has been a dramatic decline in the incidence of ARF in the US over the past few decades. Although the reasons for this decline are not entirely clear, a shift in the prevalence from circulating rheumatologic to nonrheumatologic strains of GAS likely has played an important role.[2]
- Nevertheless, outbreaks of acute ARF have continued to occur in the US over the past three decades.[3,4]

ETIOLOGY AND PATHOPHYSIOLOGY

- Mimicry between group A streptococci and host antigens has been proposed as a mechanism for the development of the manifestations observed in ARF.
- GAS possess antigens and superantigens, which stimulate B and T cells to respond to self.

RISK FACTORS

Risk factors for RF can be categorized as being:

- Socioeconomic factors such as poverty, crowding, lack of education, and poor access to health care.
- Biological factors such as failure to diagnose the infection and genetic susceptibility.
- Lifestyle factors, such as poor nutrition.

DIAGNOSIS

CLINICAL FEATURES

According to revised Jones criteria,[5,6] the diagnosis can be made when two major criteria, or one major and two minor criteria are present, along with evidence of streptococcal infection, that is, elevated or rising ASO titer or DNAase.

Major criteria

- Polyarthritis—A migrating and temporary inflammation of joints, which usually starts in the legs and involves large joints.
- Carditis—Inflammation of the heart, which may present as valvular heart disease (**Figure 45-1**), pericarditis, or congestive heart failure due to myocarditis.
- Subcutaneous nodules (**Figure 45-2**).
- Erythema marginatum (**Figure 45-3**).
- Sydenham's chorea (St. Vitus' dance)—A characteristic rapid movement of the extremities, which is involuntary and may be associated with facial grimacing. This can occur late in the disease up to a few months from the onset of the infection.

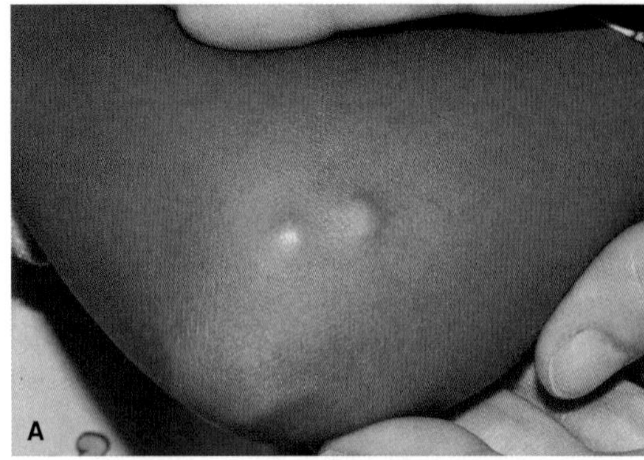

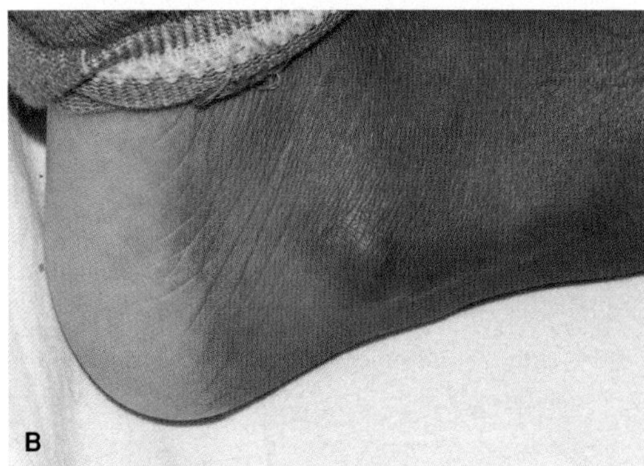

FIGURE 45-2 Painless subcutaneous nodules of acute rheumatic fever over the dorsal forearm/elbow (A) and lateral foot (B) in a 3-year-old girl who presented with fever, migratory arthritis, new-onset mitral regurgitation, elevated erythrocyte sedimentation rate and very elevated antistreptolysin O titer. (Used with permission from Blanca Gonzalez, MD)

Minor criteria

- High fever ranging from 38.2 to 38.9 °C (101 to 102°F).
- Arthralgia—Joint pain without any significant signs of swelling or redness. (A diagnosis of polyarthritis eliminates arthralgia from the criteria.)
- Elevated erythrocyte sedimentation rate or C-reactive protein.
- Leukocytosis.

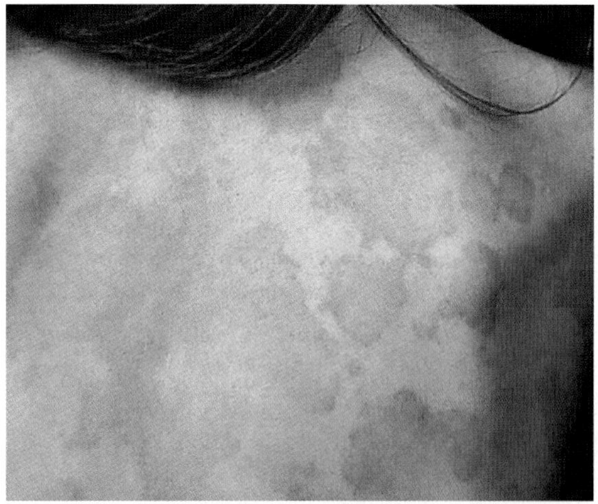

FIGURE 45-3 Erythema marginatum. This photosensitive rash begins on the central areas of the body as macules, and spreads more distally. The macules clear out from the center to form rings, which can sometimes coalesce to form a serpentine pattern on the body. (*Used with permission from Cleveland Clinic Hospital Photo File.*)

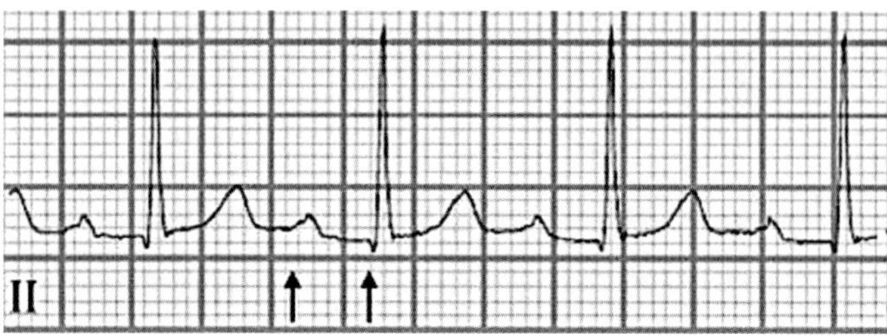

FIGURE 45-4 First-degree heart block with prolonged PR interval (interval between arrows), which may be present as a minor criterion for acute rheumatic fever. (*Used with permission from Athar M. Qureshi, MD.*)

- Electrocardiogram (ECG) with features of heart block, that is, a prolonged PR interval (**Figure 45-4**). (Cannot be included if carditis is a major finding.)
- Prior episode of rheumatic fever or inactive heart disease.

LABORATORY TESTING

- Throat culture for GAS.
- ASO titer or DNAse titer.
- Erythrocyte sedimentation rate and C-reactive protein.

IMAGING

- CXR is recommended to evaluate heart size.
- ECG is recommended to assess for PR prolongation.
- Echocardiography is recommended to confirm and characterize cardiac involvement.

DIFFERENTIAL DIAGNOSIS

- Poststreptococcal reactive arthritis—Typically occurs after a shorter latent period (7 to 10 days) and is usually not migratory in nature.
- Infectious arthritis—Monarticular arthiritis with a positive joint aspirate fluid analysis and culture for organisms (not present in ARF).
- Rheumatoid arthritis—Longer lasting and commonly also involves small joints (see Chapter 172, Juvenile Rheumatoid Arthritis).

MANAGEMENT

NONPHARMACOLOGIC

- Avoidance of vigorous activity during the acute phase is recommended. SOR Ⓒ
- If the patient presents with congestive heart failure, management involves salt and water restriction, and upright posture.
- Injury protection during episodes of chorea.

MEDICATIONS

- Patients with ARF should be treated with antibiotics to eradicate GAS carriage regardless of culture status.[7] SOR Ⓐ

- Patients should receive either 10 days of oral penicillin or a single intramuscular injection of benzathine penicillin.[7] SOR Ⓐ
- Household contacts should have throat cultures performed and those with a positive throat culture should be treated with antibiotics. SOR Ⓒ
- Salicylates (i.e., aspirin) are the major anti-inflammatory agents for relief of arthritis symptoms due to acute rheumatic fever.[8] This results in the prompt relief of arthritis symptoms. SOR Ⓐ
- Patients with significant heart failure from carditis should be treated with conventional therapy for heart failure.
- Anti-inflammatory agents such as aspirin are used in the acute management of rheumatic carditis. The role of corticosteroids and other anti-inflammatory agents in rheumatic carditis is uncertain.[9] SOR Ⓒ
- The rash associated with ARF is temporary and does not require specific treatment, although antihistamines may help to alleviate pruritus.
- Although chorea is a self-limited disease, the emotional distress can be alleviated with valproic acid, phenobarbital, or valium. SOR Ⓒ

SURGERY/INTERVENTIONAL CARDIOLOGY TREATMENT

Cardiac surgery or percutaneous treatment via cardiac catheterization is usually not needed in the acute phase, but may be needed for chronic valvular heart disease.[10,11]

REFERRAL

- Pediatric Cardiology, Infectious Disease and Rheumatology referral is warranted for most cases of ARF.

PREVENTION AND SCREENING

PRIMARY PREVENTION

- Prompt diagnosis and treatment of streptococcal pharyngitis is the key to primary prevention.
- Any child presenting with manifestations of GAS pharyngitis should have a throat culture performed, and if GAS is isolated, should be treated with antibiotics.

SECONDARY PREVENTION

- Patients who have a history of ARF and develop subsequent GAS pharyngitis are at high risk for rheumatic heart disease or exacerbation of existing rheumatic heart disease.[7]
- Thus, patients with a history of ARF should receive prophylactic antibiotics to prevent streptococcal pharyngitis.[7]
- Duration of antibiotic prophylaxis for those with a history of ARF depends on whether or not cardiac involvement was present initially and whether there is active cardiac disease.

PROGNOSIS

- The cardiac manifestations of ARF are associated with significant morbidity and mortality.
- Noncardiac manifestations of ARF ultimately resolve without sequelae.

FOLLOW-UP AND PATIENT EDUCATION

Patients should be educated about ARF and on the consequences of not treating acute streptococcal pharyngitis. After the diagnosis of ARF is made, patients should be counseled about the need for prevention of acute streptococcal pharyngitis and the need for long term follow-up for rheumatic carditis.

PATIENT RESOURCES

- **www.www.ncbi.nlm.nih.gov/pubmedhealth/PMH0004388/.**

PROVIDER RESOURCES

- **www.my.americanheart.org/professional/General/Rheumatic-Fever-and-Strep-Throat_UCM_423927_Article.jsp.**
- **www.who.int/cardiovascular_diseases/resources/trs923/en.**

REFERENCES

1. Carapetis, J.R., et al. The global burden of group A streptococcal diseases. *Lancet Infect Dis*. 2005;(11):685-694.
2. Markowitz M, Kaplan EL. Reappearance of rheumatic fever. In: Barness LA, ed. *Advances in Pediatrics*. Chicago, Year Book Medical Publishers;1989:39-66.
3. Veasy LG, Wiedmeier SE, Orsmond GS, et al. Resurgence of acute rheumatic feve in the intermountain area of the US. *N Engl J Med*. 1987;316:421-427.
4. Wald ER, Dashefsky B, Feidt C, et al. Acute rheumatic fever in Western Pennsylvania and the tri-state area. *Pediatrics*. 1987;80:371-374.
5. Dajani AS, Ayoub E, Bierman FZ, et al. Guidelines for the diagnosis of rheumatic fever: Jones criteria, updated 1992. *Circulation*. 1993;87:302-307.
6 Ferrieri, P. Proceedings of the Jones Criteria workshop. *Circulation*. 2002;106(19):2521-2523.
7. Gerber, M.A., et al. Prevention of rheumatic fever and diagnosis and treatment of acute Streptococcal pharyngitis: a scientific statement from the American Heart Association Rheumatic Fever, Endocarditis, and Kawasaki Disease Committee of the Council on Cardiovascular Disease in the Young, the Interdisciplinary Council on Functional Genomics and Translational Biology, and the Interdisciplinary Council on Quality of Care and Outcomes Research: endorsed by the American Academy of Pediatrics. *Circulation*. 2009;119(11):1541-1551.
8. United Kingdom and United States Joint Report: The treatment of acute rheumatic fever in children. *Circulation*. 1955;11:343.
9. Cilliers A, Manyemba J, Adler AJ, Saloojee H. Anti-inflammatory treatment for carditis in acute rheumatic fever. *Cochrane Database of Systematic Reviews* 2012;6.
10. Cilliers, AM. Rheumatic fever and its management. *BMJ*. 2006;333:1153.
11. Skoularigis J, Sinovich V, Joubert G, Sareli P. Evaluation of the long-term results of mitral valve repair in 254 young patients with rheumatic mitral regurgitation. *Circulation*. 1994;90:II167.

46 COMMON DYSRHYTHMIAS

Asif Padiyath, MD
Peter Aziz, MD

Three important dysrhythmias in the pediatric population include:

- Wolff-Parkinson-White syndrome.
- Long QT syndrome.
- Complete Heart Block.

All three conditions will be covered sequentially in this chapter.

WOLFF-PARKINSON-WHITE SYNDROME

PATIENT STORY

A previously healthy 14-year-old female presents with a 1-month history of rapid onset, rapid offset palpitations without any identifiable precipitating factors. The physical examination is unremarkable. The electrocardiogram (ECG) showed a delta wave, wide QRS, and short PR interval (**Figure 46-1**).

INTRODUCTION

Wolff-Parkinson-White (WPW) syndrome is a congenital abnormality involving the presence of abnormal conduction tissue, or accessory pathway, between the atria and the ventricles in association with supraventricular tachycardia (SVT).[1]

SYNONYM

Pre-excitation or WPW syndrome.

EPIDEMIOLOGY

- In large-scale general population studies involving children and adults, the prevalence of WPW is estimated to be 1 to 3 in 1000.[2]

ETIOLOGY AND PATHOPHYSIOLOGY

- Ventricular pre excitation occurs due to electrical conduction down an accessory pathway (AP).
- AP conduction circumvents the usual conduction delay between the atria and ventricles, which occurs at the AV node (AVN), and predisposes the patient to develop reentrant tachycardia.
- The most common type of supraventricular tachycardia seen in patients with WPW is orthodromic reentrant tachycardia (ORT; **Figure 46-2**).
- Most commonly precipitated by a premature atrial contraction (PAC), the cardiac impulse travels down the AV node to the ventricles and then back to the atria via the accessory pathway.Rarely, antidromic reciprocating tachycardia (ART) occurs due to antegrade conduction down the accessory pathway and retrograde conduction up the AVN.

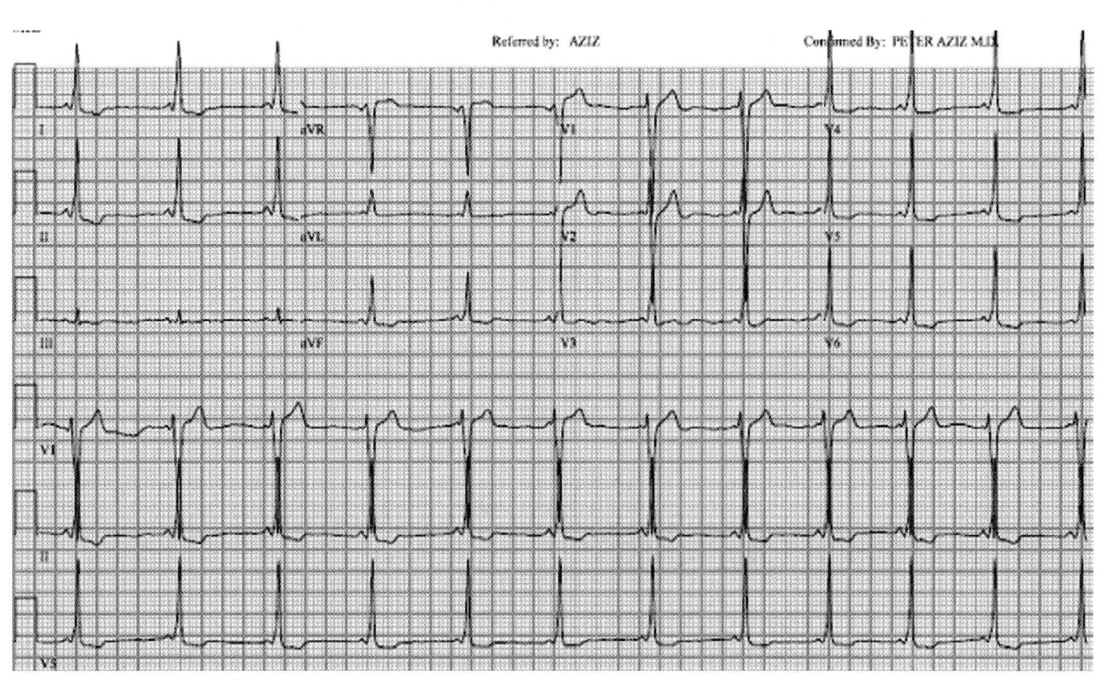

FIGURE 46-1 ECG showing delta wave, wide QRS, and shortened PR interval (Wolff-Parkinson-White). (*Used with permission from Peter Aziz, MD.*)

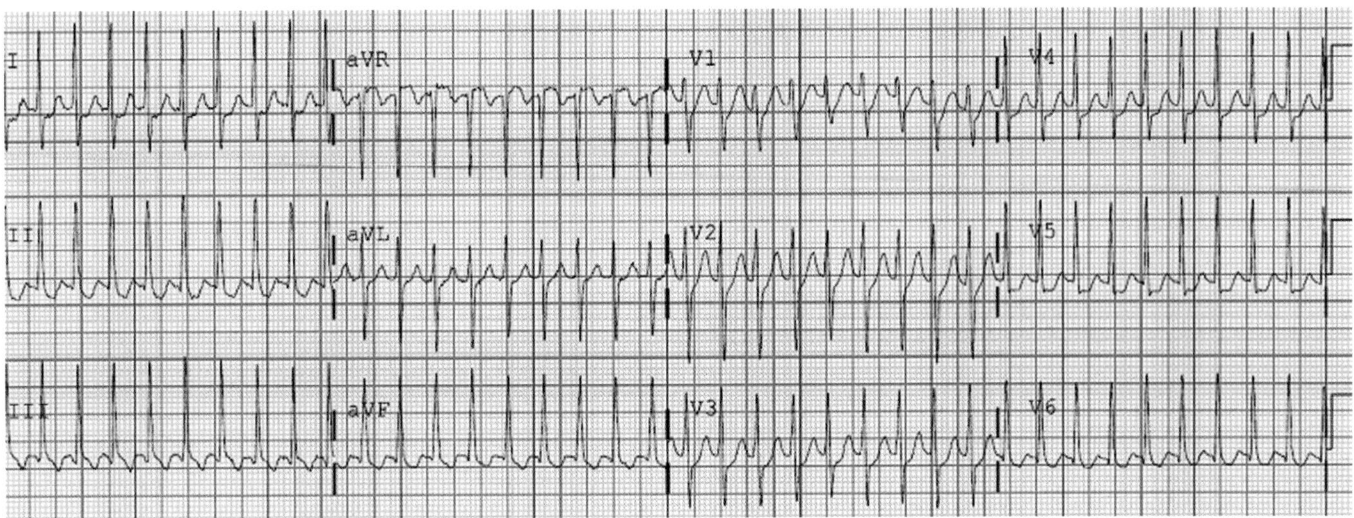

FIGURE 46-2 Orthodromic reciprocating tachycardia (ORT) via a left lateral pathway. Note the narrow complex QRS seen in patients during supraventricular tachycardia. (*Used with permission from Peter Aziz, MD.*)

RISK FACTORS

- Mutations in the PRKAG2 gene can cause familial WPW syndrome.
- Congenital anomalies such as Ebsteins and hypertrophic cardiomyopathy are associated with WPW.

DIAGNOSIS

CLINICAL FEATURES

- Patients with WPW can be asymptomatic.
- The most common clinical manifestation is palpitations.
- Syncope or sudden death is rare and associated with rapid ventricular conduction of atrial fibrillation.
- Physical exam is usually unremarkable. During periods of SVT, tachycardia can be noted with a decrease in blood pressure. If the episode has been untreated for several hours, patients can manifest poor perfusion, hepatomegaly, and cardiac failure.
- Stigmata of associated congenital anomalies such as Ebstein anomaly should be excluded.

IMAGING

- The ECG will show classic findings of WPW: (1) short PR interval, (2) delta wave, and (3) wide QRS complex.
- In patients with atrial fibrillation and rapid accessory pathway conduction, an ECG will show an irregularly, irregular, wide complex tachycardia (**Figure 46-3**). This is the cause of sudden death in patients with WPW.

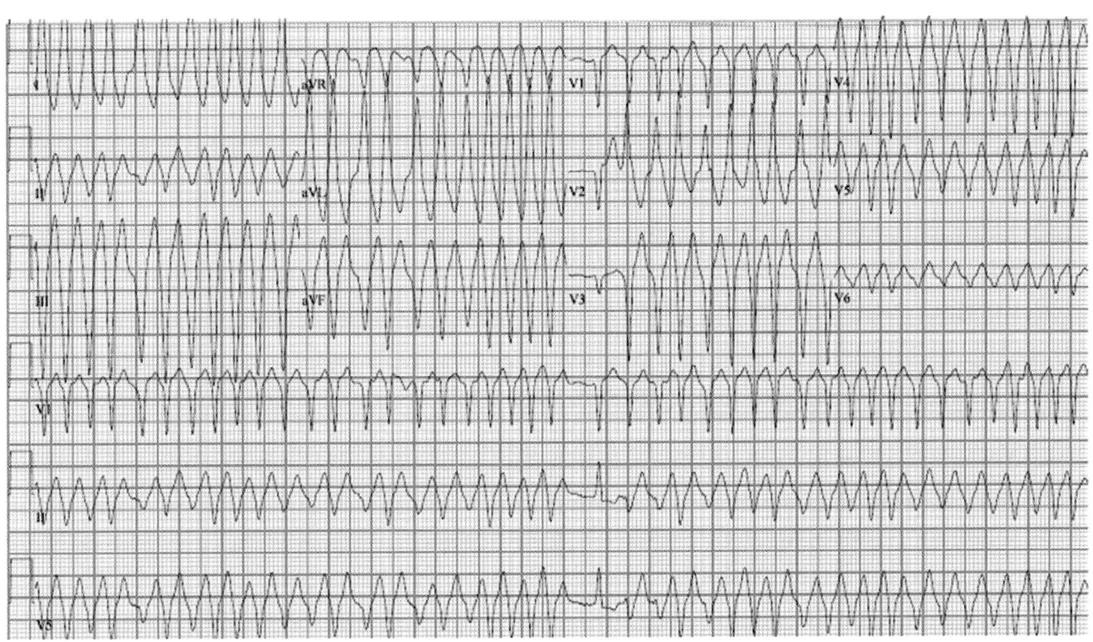

FIGURE 46-3 Atrial fibrillation with rapid ventricular response in a patient with WPW. ECG shows an irregularly irregular wide complex tachycardia. This phenomenon is the cause of sudden cardiac death in WPW patients. (*Used with permission from Peter Aziz, MD.*)

DIFFERENTIAL DIAGNOSIS

- Other types of arrhythmias (AVNRT, atrial tachycardia, or ventricular tachycardia) are typically excluded by an ECG during the tachycardia.
- Other rare pre-excitation subtypes (Mahain fibers, permanent junctional reciprocating tachycardia) can also be distinguished by ECG findings.

MANAGEMENT

- Treatment must be individualized for each patient and should include individual risk assessment.
- Reentrant SVT will terminate with vagal maneuvers (Valsalva or carotid message) or adenosine.
- Two main treatment approaches to WPW syndrome are pharmacotherapy and electrophysiology study (EPS) with catheter ablation.
  - EPS with catheter ablation is the first-line treatment for symptomatic WPW syndrome.[3] SOR Ⓐ
  - AVN blocking agents (digoxin, calcium channel blockers) are contraindicated in patients with WPW.[3,4] SOR Ⓑ

REFERRAL

- Patients with WPW require an evaluation by a pediatric electrophysiologist.

PREVENTION AND SCREENING

- No preventive modalities currently exist since mostly WPW is congenital in origin.
- No established screening is being currently used in the US.

PROGNOSIS

- Once identified and appropriately treated, WPW syndrome has an excellent prognosis.
- Mortality is rare and is related to Sudden Cardiac Death (SCD). Incidence of mortality in SCD in WPW syndrome is found to be 1 in 100 symptomatic patients when followed up to 15 years.[5]

FOLLOW-UP

- Regular follow-up is needed to assess for recurrence of arrhythmia, adverse reaction to medicines, and to assess the effectiveness of therapy.

PATIENT EDUCATION

- Close follow-up with patients diagnosed with WPW syndrome is essential to assess the need and timing of interventions.

PATIENT RESOURCES

- **http://my.clevelandclinic.org/heart/disorders/electric/wpw.aspx.**

PROVIDER RESOURCES

- **http://www.hrsonline.org/News/Press-Releases/2012/05/Management-Of-Asymptomatic-Patients-With-Wolff-Parkinson-White#axzz2VWWD0EKU.**

LONG QT SYNDROME

PATIENT STORY

A 12-year-old female presents with recent syncope. She was swimming during a family vacation on a beach. She lost consciousness and was unresponsive for 30 seconds. She does not recall a prodrome prior to the syncopal event. She had started a decongestant medication for Upper respiratory tract infection symptoms the day prior. Her mother and grandmother have also had syncopal events in the past associated with exercise. Her ECG shows QTc prolongation (**Figure 46-4**).

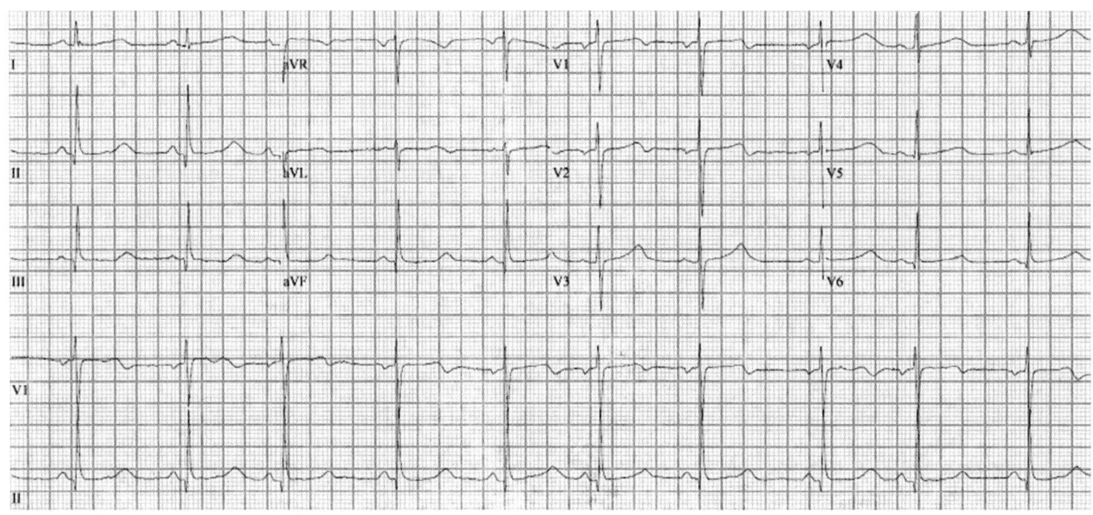

FIGURE 46-4 ECG showing QTc prolongation (QTc=570ms). This patient had the classic long QT syndrome presentation of syncope during swimming consistent with long QT type 1. (*Used with permission from Peter Aziz, MD.*)

INTRODUCTION

Long QT syndrome (LQTS) is an ion channelopathy characterized by a prolonged QTc interval, syncope, ventricular arrhythmias and sudden death.[6,7]

SYNONYMS

Jervell and Lange-Nielson syndrome and Romano Ward Syndrome refer to specific types of LQTS.

EPIDEMIOLOGY

- The estimated prevalence of LQTS is about 1:5000.[8]
- There are presumably many patients with LQTS that are asymptomatic or have not yet been diagnosed.

ETIOLOGY AND PATHOPHYSIOLOGY

- LQTS is caused by ion channel mutations that result in delayed ventricular repolarization.
- This delay in ventricular repolarization subjects myocardial cells to arrhythmias as after depolarizations are propagated between cells.
- Catecholamines play an important role in precipitating these after depolarizations and patients with LQTS are particularly at risk during periods of exercise or excitement.
- The hallmark arrhythmia for LQTS is torsade de pointes (**Figure 46-5**).

RISK FACTORS

- The majority of LQTS cases are inherited in an autosomal dominant fashion. As such, children of parents with LQTS have a 50 percent chance of having the same gene defect.
- Patients with syncope, particularly during exertion, should under an ECG to assess for LQTS.
- Though uncommon, an autosomal recessive form of LQTS (Jervell and Lange-Nielson syndrome) is associated with congenital deafness therefore patients with hearing loss should also undergo ECG evaluation.

DIAGNOSIS

- The ECG is the hallmark of the diagnosis in LQTS and should be performed in any patient with a family history of LQTS or with symptoms of LQTS. The ECG has important limitations, however.
- Some patients with LQTS (depending on the specific genotype) will have abnormal repolarization responses to exercise. Therefore, the exercise stress test has been employed as a diagnostic tool.[9]
- The Schwartz criteria provide a point system based on various risk factors known to be associated with LQTS.[7]
- Genetic testing has become commercially available for LQTS and most insurance companies provide coverage for testing. There are currently 13 identified LQT genes.

DIFFERENTIAL DIAGNOSIS

- All causes of syncope and sudden cardiac death should be considered including hypertrophic cardiomyopathy, anomalous coronary origin, Wolff-Parkinson-White syndrome, catecholaminergic polymorphic ventricular tachycardia (CPVT), Brugada syndrome, and arrhythmogenic right ventricular cardiomyopathy (ARVC).
- These diagnoses can typically be excluded during the evaluation by a cardiologist or electrophysiologist.

MANAGEMENT

- The management of LQTS is predicated on beta-blocker therapy, specifically nonselective types such as nadolol or propranolol.[10] SOR Ⓐ
- Patients who continue to have symptoms (syncope or aborted cardiac arrest) while on therapy should undergo implantation of an implantable cardioverter-defibrillator (ICD).[11] SOR Ⓐ
- Other therapies such as ganglionectomy have also been used in high-risk patients.[12] SOR Ⓑ

REFERRAL

- Patients with long QT syndrome need a referral to a pediatric electrophysiologist.

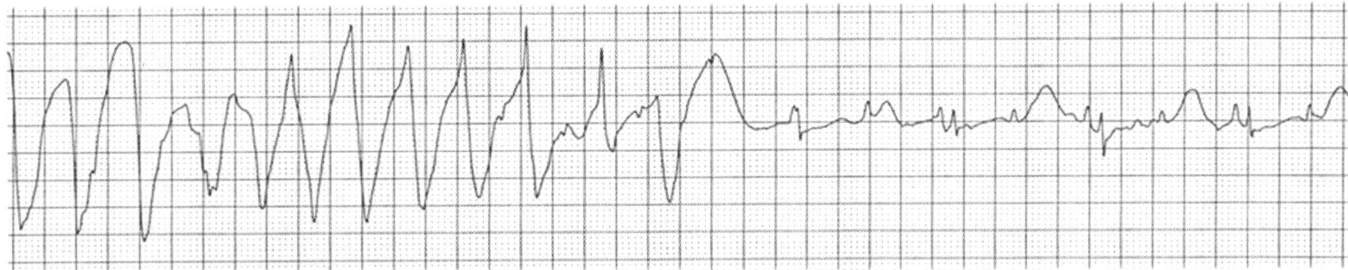

FIGURE 46-5 Rhythm strip showing torsade de pointes in an infant with long QT syndrome. The rhythm disturbance spontaneously terminated in this patient. (*Used with permission from Peter Aziz, MD.*)

PREVENTION AND SCREENING

- All drugs known to cause a prolongation in the QT interval should be avoided. A current list of these drugs can be found on www.qtdrugs.org.
- If congenital long QT syndrome is suspected, all first degree relatives should undergo genetic screening.[13,14] SOR A

PROGNOSIS

- Generally, the prognosis for LQTS patients who are compliant with medication is excellent. Few patients considered high-risk will continue to have symptoms despite therapy.

FOLLOW-UP

- Patients with Long QT syndrome need to be followed up closely by a pediatric electrophysiologist.

PATIENT EDUCATION

- Patients with long QT syndrome should be educated appropriately to avoid QTc prolonging drugs.
- They should also be encouraged to have their immediate family members screened for Long QT syndrome.

PATIENT RESOURCES

- **http://my.clevelandclinic.org/heart/disorders/electric/longqtsyndrome.aspx.**

PROVIDER RESOURCES

- 2013 HRS/EHRA/APHRS Expert Consensus Statement on the Diagnosis and Management of Patients with Inherited Prima-ryArrhythmia Syndromes. Developed in partnership with the Heart Rhythm Society (HRS), the European Heart Rhythm, Association (EHRA), a registered branch of the European Society of Cardiology, and the Asia Pacific Heart Rhythm Society (APHRS); and in collaboration with the American College of Cardiology Foundation (ACCF), the American Heart Association (AHA), the Pediatric and Congenital Electrophysiology Society (PACES) and the Association for European Pediatric and Congenital Cardiology (AEPC).

COMPLETE HEART BLOCK

PATIENT STORY

A 15-month-old boy is seen by his pediatrician for failure to thrive. The patient has had poor growth since a viral infection consisting of rhinorrhea and cough about 4 months ago. His activity level has decreased. His physical examination is remarkable for hepatomegaly and bradycardia (heart rate 50 beats per minute). An ECG is performed showing AV dissociation (**Figure 46-6**).

INTRODUCTION

Complete heart block (CHB) occurs when the atrioventricular node (AVN) is unable to conduct an electrical impulse from the atrium to the ventricle. Congenital complete heart block is the most common indication for pacemaker implantation in the pediatric population in the absence of congenital heart disease. Approximately 20 to 30 percent of pacemakers in the pediatric population are implanted for this

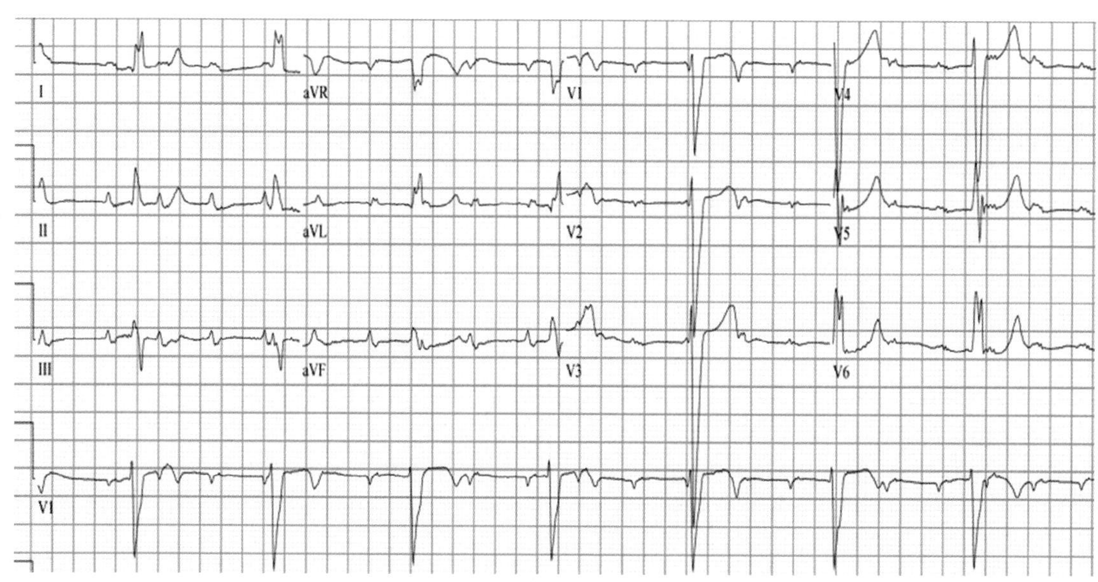

FIGURE 46-6 ECG showing complete heart block. The ECG is notable for bradycardia, AV dissociation, and a wide complex ventricular escape rhythm. (*Used with permission from Peter Aziz, MD.*)

indication. Although maternal lupus antibody exposure is the most common cause of CHB, most cases are idiopathic. Isolated CHB in the absence of congenital heart disease carries an excellent prognosis.[15,16]

SYNONYM

Atrioventricular dissociation or atrioventricular block.

EPIDEMIIOLOGY

The prevalence of CHB is between 0.04 and 0.02 percent.[17]

ETIOLOGY AND PATHOPHYSIOLOGY

- Fibrosis or scarring of the AVN can occur for a variety of reasons.
- In the absence of structural heart disease, lupus antibodies SS-A (Ro) and SS-B (La) cause damage to the AVN resulting in complete heart block.
- Mothers can transmit these antibodies through the placenta causing fetal AVN damage.
- Acquired CHB can occur spontaneously in patients with specific types of congenital heart disease (see the following section) or as the result of surgical correction of congenital heart disease.
- Occasionally acquired CHB is the sequelae of viral infections as in the patient described in this scenario.
- CHB is also a known, though transient, consequence of Lyme disease.

RISK FACTORS

- Infants at risk for CHB include those exposed to maternal lupus antibodies.
- Children undergoing surgical correction of heart disease, particularly those with ventricular septal defects, are at risk for developing acquired CHB.
- Patients with L-transposition of the great arteries (L-TGA), heterotaxy syndrome and atrioventricular canal defects can develop CHB spontaneously, in the absence of surgical manipulation of the AVN.

DIAGNOSIS

- The ECG is diagnostic of complete heart block.
- Ambulatory monitoring (Holters) can offer insight into the severity of disease.
- Echocardiograms should be performed in any patient with CHB to assess for congenital heart disease and cardiomyopathy.

DIFFERENTIAL DIAGNOSIS

- The differential for bradycardia in the absence of complete heart block includes hypervagatonia, which is common in young athletes.

MANAGEMENT

- Complete heart block requires a thorough investigation by a pediatric electrophysiologist.
- The acute management of CHB depends on symptoms. In a symptomatic patient, administration of isoproterenol or atropine can increase the ventricular escape rate and relieve symptoms.[18] SOR Ⓐ Transcutaneous pacing is rarely indicated.
- Typically an asymptomatic patient does not require acute treatment. SOR Ⓒ
- Pacemaker implantation depends on disease severity and the presence of congenital heart disease. Most patients that are asymptomatic with normal cardiac function can be followed closely.
- Patients with low average heart rates or a wide escape rhythm should undergo pacemaker implantation (**Figures 46-7** and **46-8**).[19] SOR Ⓑ
- Patients with post-surgical heart block can be monitored for 7 to 10 days as spontaneous resolution can occur.[20] SOR Ⓐ

REFERRAL

- Patients diagnosed with CHB irrespective of the etiology, need immediate referral, evaluation, and management by a pediatric electrophysiologist.

PREVENTION AND SCREENING

- Patients with known risk factors such as maternal history of lupus should be screened with a post natal ECG.
- Use of steroids prenatally in SLE in the setting on maternal SLE has been evaluated but has not been found to be effective.[21]

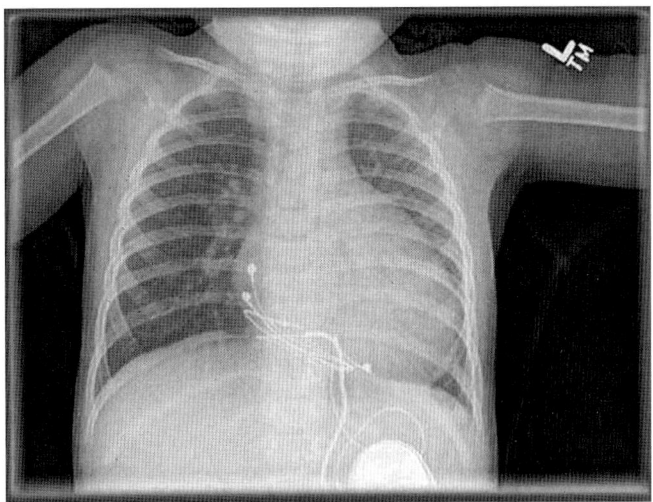

FIGURE 46-7 Chest radiograph post-implantation of an epicardial, dual-chamber pacemaker. The chest radiograph is significant for cardiomegaly. The pacemaker is implanted surgically in the abdomen and the pacemaker leads are sutured on the surface of the atrial and ventricular myocardium. (*Used with permission from Peter Aziz, MD.*)

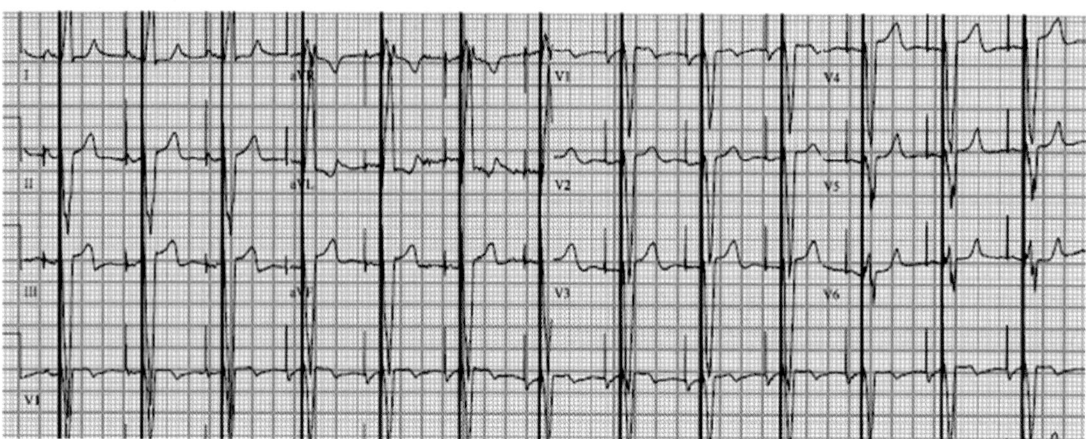

FIGURE 46-8 ECG after pacing of patient in Figure 46-7 showing sequential atrioventricular pacing denoted by the large pacing spikes prior to the P wave and the QRS. This patient has sinus node dysfunction in addition to complete heart block. (*Used with permission from Peter Aziz, MD.*)

PROGNOSIS

- Short-term prognosis is generally good in newborns with CHB born to mothers with Lupus antibodies unless the clinical picture is complicated by prematurity, development of hydrops or abnormal cardiac anatomy.[22] But in the long term, 32 percent of the unpaced eventually develop symptoms, including 5 percent who experience sudden cardiac death.[23]
- Prognosis of CHB secondary to an open heart surgery, is mostly transient but can be permanent depending on the degree of the damage to the AV node during surgery.

FOLLOW-UP

- Close follow-up is needed once the diagnosis is made. Patients with CHB need routine assessment including cardiac examinations, echocardiograms and ECGs.

PATIENT EDUCATION

- Appropriate anticipatory counseling should be offered to a pregnant mother with a fetus diagnosed with CHB.

PATIENT RESOURCES

- **http://www.chop.edu/service/cardiac-center/heart-conditions/heart-block.html.**

PROVIDER RESOURCES

- **http://emedicine.medscape.com/article/894596-overview.**

REFERENCES

1. Calkins H, Sousa J, el-Atassi R, Rosenheck S, de Buitleir M, Kou WH, Kadish AH, Langberg JJ, Morady F. Diagnosis and cure of the wolff-parkinson-white syndrome or paroxysmal supraventricular tachycardias during a single electrophysiologic test. *N Engl J Med*. 1991;324(23):1612-1618.
2. Hiss RG, Lamb LE. Electrocardiographic findings in 122,043 individuals. *Circulation*. 1962;25:947-961.
3. Cohen MI, Triedman JK, Cannon BC, Davis AM, Drago F, Janousek J, Klein GJ, Law IH, Morady FJ, Paul T, Perry JC, Sanatani S, Tanel RE. Paces/hrs expert consensus statement on the management of the asymptomatic young patient with a wolff-parkinson-white (wpw, ventricular preexcitation) electrocardiographic pattern: Developed in partnership between the pediatric and congenital electrophysiology society (paces) and the heart rhythm society (hrs). Endorsed by the governing bodies of paces, hrs, the american college of cardiology foundation (accf), the american heart association (aha), the american academy of pediatrics (aap), and the canadian heart rhythm society (chrs). *Heart Rhythm*. 2012;9(6):1006-1024.
4. Bromberg BI, Lindsay BD, Cain ME, Cox JL. Impact of clinical history and electrophysiologic characterization of accessory pathways on management strategies to reduce sudden death among children with wolff-parkinson-white syndrome. *Journal of the American College of Cardiology*. 1996;27(3):690-695.
5. Sarubbi B, Scognamiglio G, Limongelli G, Mercurio B, Pacileo G, Pisacane C, Russo MG, Calabrò R. Asymptomatic ventricular preexcitation in children and adolescents: A 15 year follow up study. *Heart*. 2003;89(2):215-217.
6. Ackerman MJ, Clapham DE. Ion channels—basic science and clinical disease. *New England Journal of Medicine*. 1997;336(22): 1575-1586.
7. Schwartz PJ, Moss AJ, Vincent GM, Crampton RS. Diagnostic criteria for the long qt syndrome. An update. *Circulation*. 1993;88(2):782-784.
8. Goldenberg I, Moss AJ. Long qt syndrome. *Journal of the American College of Cardiology*. 2008;51(24):2291-2300.
9. Aziz PF, Wieand TS, Ganley J, Henderson J, Patel AR, Iyer VR, Vogel RL, McBride M, Vetter VL, Shah MJ. Genotype- and mutation site–specific qt adaptation during exercise, recovery, and postural changes in children with long-qt syndrome. *Circulation: Arrhythmia and Electrophysiology*. 2011;4(6):867-873.

10. Roden DM. Long-qt syndrome. *New England Journal of Medicine*. 2008;358(2):169-176.

11. Epstein AE, DiMarco JP, Ellenbogen KA, Estes NAM, Freedman RA, Gettes LS, Gillinov AM, Gregoratos G, Hammill SC, Hayes DL, Hlatky MA, Newby LK, Page RL, Schoenfeld MH, Silka MJ, Stevenson LW, Sweeney MO. 2012 accf/aha/hrs focused update incorporated into the accf/aha/hrs 2008 guidelines for device-based therapy of cardiac rhythm abnormalities: A report of the american college of cardiology foundation/american heart association task force on practice guidelines and the heart rhythm society. *Circulation*. 2013;127(3):e283-e352

12. Schwartz PJ, Priori SG, Cerrone M, Spazzolini C, Odero A, Napolitano C, Bloise R, De Ferrari GM, Klersy C, Moss AJ, Zareba W, Robinson JL, Hall WJ, Brink PA, Toivonen L, Epstein AE, Li C, Hu D. Left cardiac sympathetic denervation in the management of high-risk patients affected by the long-qt syndrome. *Circulation*. 2004;109(15):1826-1833.

13. Behr E, Wood DA, Wright M, Syrris P, Sheppard MN, Casey A, Davies MJ, McKenna W. Cardiological assessment of first-degree relatives in sudden arrhythmic death syndrome. *The Lancet*. 2003;362(9394):1457-1459.

14. Ackerman MJ, Priori SG, Willems S, Berul C, Brugada R, Calkins H, Camm AJ, Ellinor PT, Gollob M, Hamilton R, Hershberger RE, Judge DP, Le Marec H, McKenna WJ, Schulze-Bahr E, Semsarian C, Towbin JA, Watkins H, Wilde A, Wolpert C, Zipes DP. Hrs/ehra expert consensus statement on the state of genetic testing for the channelopathies and cardiomyopathies: This document was developed as a partnership between the heart rhythm society (hrs) and the european heart rhythm association (ehra). *Europace*. 2011;13(8):1077-1109.

15. Silvetti MS, Drago F, Grutter G, De Santis A, Di Ciommo V, Ravà L. Twenty years of paediatric cardiac pacing: 515 pacemakers and 480 leads implanted in 292 patients. *Europace*. 2006;8(7):530-536.

16. Sachweh JS, Vazquez-Jimenez JF, Schöndube FA, Daebritz SH, Dörge H, Mühler EG, Messmer BJ. Twenty years experience with pediatric pacing: Epicardial and transvenous stimulation. *European Journal of Cardio-Thoracic Surgery*. 2000;17(4):455-461.

17. Kojic EM, Hardarson T, Sigfusson N, Sigvaldason H. The prevalence and prognosis of third-degree atrioventricular conduction block: The reykjavik study. *J Intern Med*. 1999;246(1):81-86.

18. Gilchrist AR. The action of atropine in complete heart-block. *QJM*. 1933;2(4):483-498.

19. Friedman RA. Congenital av block: Pace me now or pace me later? *Circulation*. 1995;92(3):283-285.

20. Aziz P, Serwer G, Bradley D, LaPage M, Hirsch J, Bove E, Ohye R, Dick M, II. Pattern of recovery for transient complete heart block after open heart surgery for congenital heart disease: Duration alone predicts risk of late complete heart block. *Pediatr Cardiol*. 2013;34(4):999-1005.

21. Brucato A. Prevention of congenital heart block in children of ssa-positive mothers. *Rheumatology*. 2008;47(suppl 3):iii35-iii37.

22. Esscher E. Congenital complete heart block. *Acta Pædiatrica*. 1981;70(1):131-136.

23. Sholler GF, Walsh EP. Congenital complete heart block in patients without anatomic cardiac defects. *American Heart Journal*. 1989;118(6):1193-1198.

47 SYNDROMES ASSOCIATED WITH HEART DISEASE

Asif Padiyath, MD
Peter Aziz, MD

Infants and children with genetic syndromes frequently have associated cardiovascular abnormalities. It is important to recognize the cardiovascular anomalies associated with these genetic syndromes, as they account for significant morbidity and mortality. In this chapter, important genetic syndromes that are associated with cardiovascular manifestations are presented successively and include:

- Down syndrome.
- Turner syndrome.
- DiGeorge syndrome.
- Williams syndrome.
- Marfan syndrome.

The focus of this chapter is on the cardiovascular abnormalities. For further clinical information on these genetic syndromes, please refer to Chapters 216, DiGeorge Syndrome; 221, Down Syndrome; 222 Turner Syndrome; and 223, Marfan Syndrome.

DOWN SYNDROME

PATIENT STORY

A 35-week premature infant of a 42-year-old mother is delivered due to premature labor. A prior fetal echocardiogram showed an atrioventricular (AV) canal defect. The patient's mother had denied amniocentesis and chromosomal testing during pregnancy. Post-natal examination of the infant reveals simian creases, macroglossia and sandal gap toe. The diagnosis of Down syndrome is made clinically and the diagnosis of AV canal defect is confirmed on echocardiogram (**Figure 47-1**). Surgery to repair the AV canal defect was scheduled at 3 to 6 months of age.

INTRODUCTION

Down syndrome (Trisomy 21) is associated with a significant risk of congenital heart disease. Every infant with Down syndrome must be evaluated for the presence of congenital heart disease.

SYNONYMS

Trisomy 21

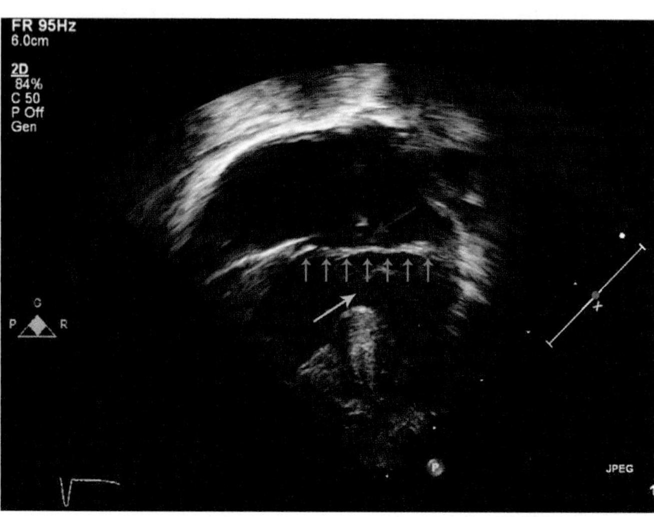

FIGURE 47-1 Apical four chamber view of a complete atrio-ventricular canal defect in an infant on echocardiogram. Note the atrial and ventricular septal defects (red and blue arrows respectively). The common atrioventricular valve (green arrows) sits in a horizontal plane along the atrioventricular groove which is characteristic of this defect. (*Used with permission from Peter Aziz, MD.*)

EPIDEMIOLOGY

- Cardiovascular malformations are found in 40 to 50 percent of individuals with Down syndrome.[1]

ETIOLOGY AND PATHOPHYSIOLOGY

- A spectrum of endocardial cushion defects is common in Down syndrome and its prevalence is higher in patients with Down syndrome compared to that of general population.
- The most common cardiac anomalies associated with Down syndrome include common AV canal, ventricular septal defect (VSD), tetralogy of Fallot and patent ductus arteriosus.

RISK FACTORS

- Advanced maternal age.

DIAGNOSIS

- The diagnosis of Down syndrome is frequently made antenatally with first trimester screening lab tests and ultrasound appearance of increased nuchal cord thickness.
- Diagnosis is often confirmed by chromosomal analysis from amniocentesis.
- Antenatal diagnosis of cardiac defects in Down syndrome fetuses is accomplished by fetal echocardiography in the second trimester.
- Newborn infants with AV canal defects are typically asymptomatic. They typically manifest symptoms at 3 to 6 months of age when the pulmonary vascular resistance decreases.

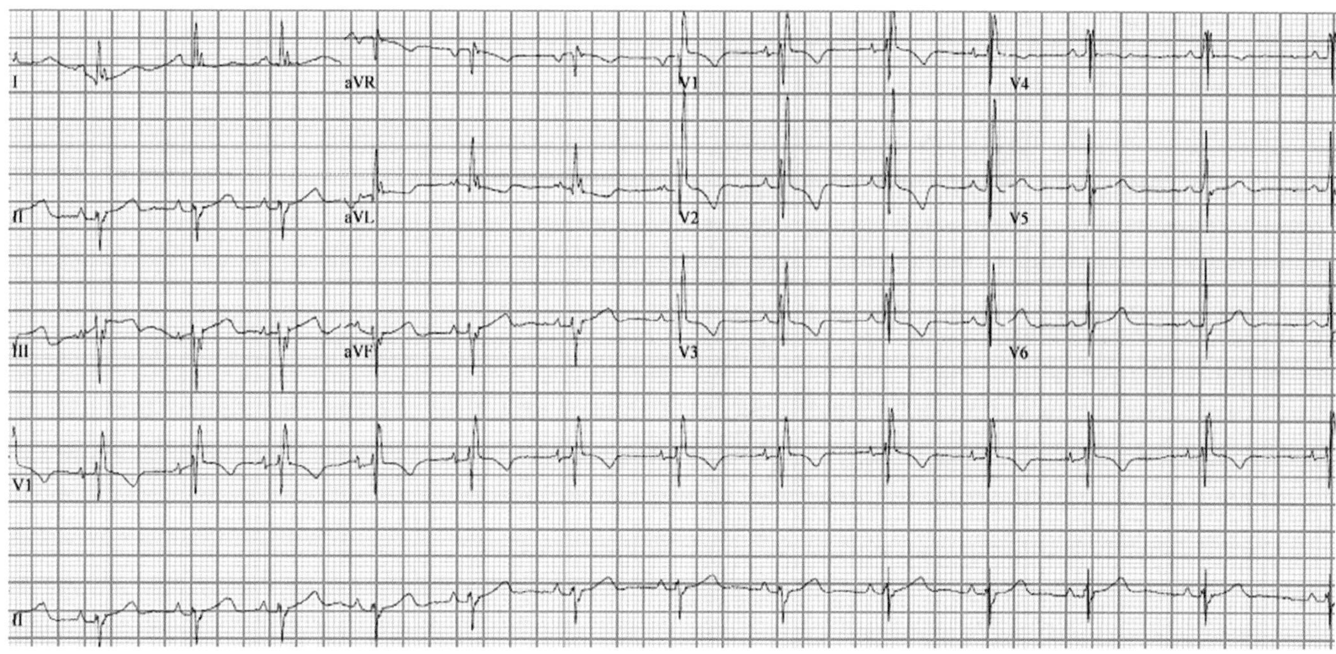

FIGURE 47-2 Superior axis (negative QRS in aVF), characteristic of common atrioventricular canal defect on electrocardiogram. The patient also has a right bundle branch block (RSR′ in V1 and wide QRS) as the result of surgical closure of the canal type ventricular septal defect. (*Used with permission from Peter Aziz, MD.*)

IMAGING

- Electrocardiogram should be obtained and will reveal abnormalities associated with the specific cardiac defects (**Figure 47-2**).
- Echocardiography.

MANAGEMENT

- Management of each cardiac lesion in Down syndrome is addressed in Chapter 42, Acyanotic Congenital Heart Disease, and Chapter 43, Cyanotic Congenital Heart Disease.

REFERRAL

- Many of the cardiac defects are detected by antenatal screening ultrasounds and appropriate referral to a fetal cardiologist for further evaluation with a fetal echocardiogram is commonplace.

PREVENTION AND SCREENING

- Screening for a cardiac anomaly is usually performed by prenatal ultrasounds in the second trimester.

PROGNOSIS

- The prognosis depends on the specific cardiac anomaly detected.

FOLLOW-UP

- Once a cardiac anomaly is detected prenatally or postnatally, careful follow-up by a pediatric cardiologist is required.

PATIENT RESOURCES

- **www.ndss.org/Resources/Health-Care/Associated-Conditions/The-Heart–Down-Syndrome/.**

PROVIDER RESOURCES

- **http://www.ndss.org/Resources/Health-Care/Associated-Conditions/The-Heart--Down-Syndrome/.**

TURNER SYNDROME

PATIENT STORY

A 16-year-old female is seen by her primary care physician for primary amenorrhea. On examination she is noted to have short stature, a webbed neck, and widely spaced nipples. Her upper limb blood pressures are above the 95th percentile for her height and four-extremity blood pressures show a systolic gradient of 50 mm Hg between the upper and lower limbs. She has brachiofemoral delay. On chest auscultation she has a grade II/VI systolic ejection murmur in the base of the heart and in the left interscapular region. She also has a continuous murmur audible almost all over the rib cage. A diagnosis of coarctation of the aorta is made via echocardiography and CT angiography (**Figure 47-3**). Chromosomal testing confirms the diagnosis of Turner syndrome. She undergoes surgical repair of the coarctation without complications.

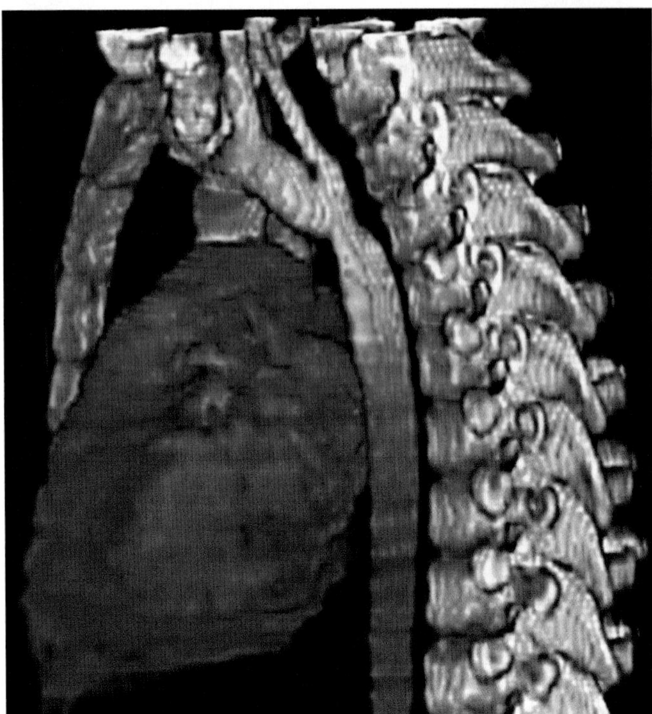

FIGURE 47-3 Discrete coarctation of the aorta just distal to the left subclavian artery on CT angiogram in a patient with Turner syndrome. (*Used with permission from Kenneth Zahka, MD.*)

INTRODUCTION

Turner syndrome is caused by an absence of one sex chromosome yielding the 45,X genotype. Turner syndrome is associated with coarctation of the aorta.

SYNONYMS

45X syndrome, Bonnevie-Ullrich syndrome, Monosomy X, Ullrich-Turner syndrome.

EPIDEMIOLOGY

- The incidence of Turner syndrome is approximately 1 in 2000 liveborn female infants[2]
- Twenty to 40 percent of girls born with Turner syndrome have cardiovascular anomalies.

ETIOLOGY AND PATHOPHYSIOLOGY

- The most common cardiovascular malformation is coarctation of the aorta, although bicuspid aortic valve and aortic stenosis are also common.
- Patients with Turner syndrome can have a spectrum of left heart obstructive lesions ranging from bicuspid aortic valve to hypoplastic left heart syndrome, although the latter is quite rare.

DIAGNOSIS

- Unlike Down syndrome, Turner syndrome is usually diagnosed postnatally. Once the diagnosis of Turner syndrome is made, a clinical and echocardiographic evaluation for cardiac defects should be performed.
- Complete or near complete obstruction occurring from coarctation of the aorta can result in left sided heart failure.
- Milder forms of coarctation may go unnoticed for many years and become apparent during evaluation of "primary" hypertension.
- As described in the case, uncomplicated coarctation of the aorta will have clinical signs of hypertension, lower blood pressures in the lower limbs, brachiofemoral delay and a systolic ejection murmur in the left interscapular region.
- A long-standing coarctation can cause collateral flow through the intercostal arteries resulting in continuous murmurs.
- Patients with a bicuspid aortic valve can have a systolic click and/or a systolic ejection murmur in the aortic area radiating to the carotid arteries.

IMAGING

- A chest radiograph can show rib notching due to collateral artery formation in aortic coarctation. This finding is uncommon in young children.
- An echocardiogram offers definitive diagnosis of the cardiac manifestations, although MRI and CT angiography may be utilized to help demonstrate the level of the obstruction, especially in older patients.

DIFFERENTIAL DIAGNOSIS

- Associated left-sided cardiac anomalies should be excluded when a coarctation is diagnosed in a patient with Turner syndrome.

MANAGEMENT

- The mainstay of management is surgical repair of aortic coarctation.[3] SOR Ⓐ
- Balloon angioplasty or stent placement can also be used in select patient groups.[4] SOR Ⓑ

REFERRAL

- All patients with Turner syndrome should have evaluation performed by a pediatric cardiologist.

PROGNOSIS

- The prognosis is excellent following successful complete surgical repair.
- Sports participation is generally permitted with the exception of high static (isometric) activities.[6] SOR Ⓑ

- Systolic blood pressures should be monitored closely after coarctation repair, as hypertension may develop.

FOLLOW-UP

- Depending on the diagnosis and timing of repair, close follow-up with a pediatric cardiologist is required to look for a recurrence or for development of complications such as hypertension.

PATIENT EDUCATION

- A collaborative approach of management in this patient group involving a geneticist, pediatric endocrinologist and general pediatrician should be planned and patients should be provided with anticipatory information regarding prognosis and follow-up.

PATIENT RESOURCES

- **http://my.clevelandclinic.org/childrens-hospital/health-info/diseases-conditions/endocrinology/hic-turner-syndrome.aspx**.

PROVIDER RESOURCES

- **http://pediatrics.aappublications.org/content/123/5/1423.full**.

DIGEORGE SYNDROME

PATIENT STORY

A 38-week gestation infant girl who was diagnosed antenatally with Truncus arteriosus (**Figure 47-4**) is transferred to the neonatal intensive care unit for stabilization soon after delivery. At 3 hours of life, the girl has a generalized seizure and is found to have serum calcium level of 4.5 mg/dL. The diagnosis of DiGeorge syndrome is suspected based on the cardiac lesion and the hypocalcemia, and confirmed by chromosomal testing. She undergoes surgical repair of her heart lesion at 8 days of life and recovers after a long hospitalization.

INTRODUCTION

DiGeorge syndrome (DGS) is caused by deletion or mutation of the long arm of chromosome 22 (22q11.2).

SYNONYMS

Velo-cardio-facial syndrome, Shprintzen syndrome, conotruncal anomaly face syndrome, Strong syndrome, congenital thymic aplasia/hypoplasia.

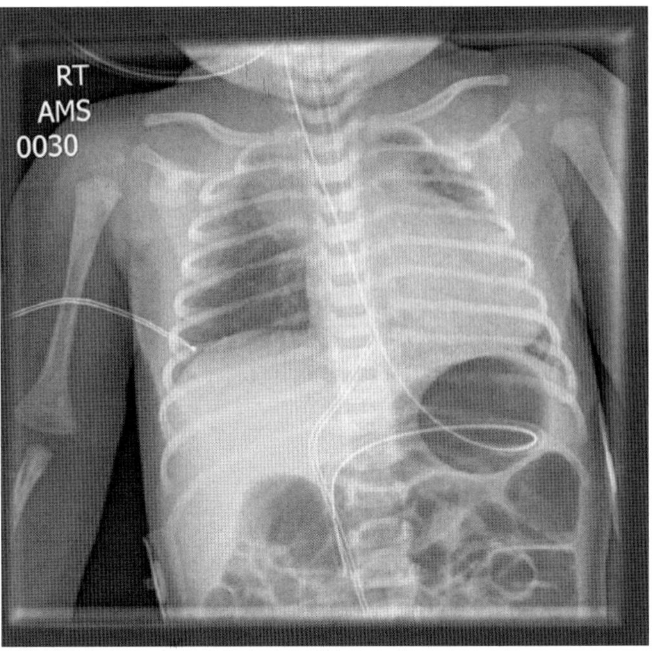

FIGURE 47-4 Profound cardiomegaly and right sided aortic arch in a newborn infant with Truncus arteriosus and DiGeorge syndrome. (*Used with permission from Camille Sabella, MD.*)

EPIDEMIOLOGY

- The incidence of DGS in the general population is 1 in 2000 to 4000 persons.
- Congenital heart defects are observed in 74 to 80 percent of affected patients.[7]

ETIOLOGY AND PATHOPHYSIOLOGY

- DiGeorge syndrome results from deletion of the 22q11.2 segment.
- Most of the manifestations of this syndrome are a result of defective migration of neural crest cells.
- Since neural crest cells contribute to the formation and septation of the outflow tract of the heart, lack of migration results in a spectrum of conotruncal malformations.

RISK FACTORS

- Gestational diabetes is thought to be associated with DiGeorge syndrome.[8]

DIAGNOSIS

- The most common cardiac anomalies associated with DGS include truncus arteriosus, tetralogy of Fallot, and interrupted aortic arch.
- These cardiac anomalies, especially when they are associated with craniofacial features should make one suspect DGS.

- Rarer cardiac anomalies associated with DiGeorge syndrome include vascular ring anomaly, transposition of great arteries with VSD, coarctation of the aorta, atrial septal defect (ASD), pulmonary stenosis, hypoplastic left heart syndrome, and patent ductus arteriosus.
- Neonatal hypocalcemia and absence of a thymic shadow on chest x-ray also warrants genetic evaluation for DiGeorge syndrome.

DIFFERENTIAL DIAGNOSIS

- Cayler syndromes—Caused by paresis of the depressor anguli oris muscle and can also be associated with cardiac anomalies.

MANAGEMENT

- The management of the cardiac manifestations of DGS depends on the specific heart lesion.

REFERRAL

- All patients clinically suspected of having DGS should have an evaluation by a pediatric cardiologist.

PREVENTION AND SCREENING

- An echocardiogram to screen for cardiac anomalies is required for all patients with DGS.

PROGNOSIS

The prognosis of patient with a cardiac anomaly in the setting of DGS varies widely and depends on the severity of the defect.

FOLLOW-UP

- Close outpatient follow-up is needed by a pediatric cardiologist; the frequency determined based on the severity of the lesion.

PATIENT EDUCATION

Ongoing genetic counseling should be offered to educate parents about possible recurrence with future pregnancies.

PATIENT RESOURCES

- **http://ghr.nlm.nih.gov/condition/22q112-deletion-syndrome**.

PROVIDER RESOURCES

- Practical Guidelines for Managing Patients with 22q11.2 Deletion Syndrome—**www.sciencedirect.com/science/article/pii/S0022347611002447**.

WILLIAMS SYNDROME

PATIENT STORY

A 10-year-old girl with failure to thrive is referred to a pediatric cardiologist because of asystolic murmur heard during a routine physical examination. She was small for gestational age (SGA) at birth and was born at 38 weeks gestation. She has history of multiple ear infections in the past. On exam she has facial features consisting of a short upturned nose, flat nasal bridge, long philtrum, and wide mouth (**Figure 47-5**). On cardiovascular exam, she has an ejection systolic murmur in the right 2nd intercostal space, which radiates to the carotids. An echocardiogram revealed supravalvular aortic stenosis. Based on the cardiac findings, a diagnosis of Williams syndrome was suspected and confirmed with chromosomal testing. She is scheduled for very close follow-up with the pediatric cardiologist.

INTRODUCTION

Williams syndrome is characterized by a distinct facial appearance, supravalvular aortic stenosis, idiopathic hypercalcemia, and a characteristic neurodevelopmental and behavioral profile.

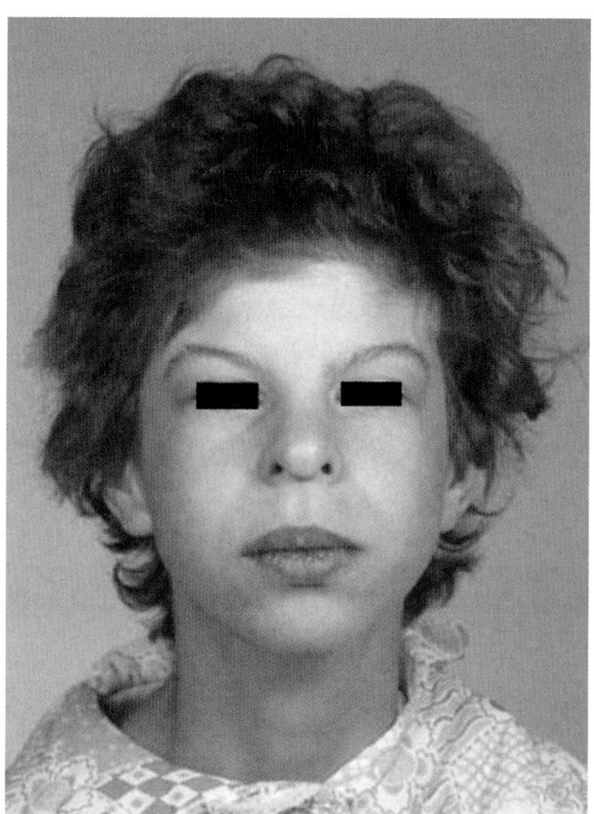

FIGURE 47-5 Typical facies of a patient with Williams syndrome. Note the presence of a short upturned nose, flat nasal bridge, long philtrum, and wide mouth. (*Used with permission from Cleveland Clinic Children's Hospital photo file.*)

SYNONYMS

Williams–Beuren syndrome (WBS), Elfin facies syndrome.

EPIDEMIOLOGY

- The reported prevalence of Williams syndrome is 1 per 7,500 to 20,000 births.[10]

ETIOLOGY AND PATHOPHYSIOLOGY

- Haploinsufficiency (loss of 1 of 2 copies) due to a deletion at chromosome band 7q11.23 that involves the elastin gene (ELN) is implicated in the etiology of Williams syndrome.[11]
- Cardiac defects account for most of the morbidity and mortality in this syndrome.

DIAGNOSIS

- Chromosomal testing showing a 7q11.23 deletion provides a confirmatory diagnosis.
- Clinical features include prenatal and postnatal growth delay, short stature, mild to moderate mental retardation, facial features as described in the case, hypercalcemia, developmental delay, learning disabilities, excessive social personality, and interest and enthusiasm for music.
- Cardiac manifestations include diffuse stenosis of medium sized or large sized arteries, most commonly involving the ascending aorta (supravalvular aortic stenosis), or pulmonary arteries.
- Coronary artery involvement leading to myocardial ischemia and brachiocephalic and cerebral artery involvement leading to stroke in young patients can occur.[12,13]
- Hypertension occurs in 50 percent of patients, which may be secondary to renal artery involvement.[14]
- QTc prolongation is also reported in patients with Williams syndrome.[15]

DIFFERENTIAL DIAGNOSIS

- Isolated aortic valve stenosis—May be seen without Williams syndrome. The distinguishing features of Williams syndrome are absent.
- Attention deficit hyperactivity disorder—These children do not have the clinical, genetic, cardiovascular, and metabolic manifestations of Williams syndrome.

MANAGEMENT

- Management of the cardiac manifestations of Williams syndrome depends on the extent of supravalvular aortic stenosis and other cardiac manifestations.
- Treatment of hypertension will depend on the cause and the presence of co-morbid cardiovascular problems.

REFERRAL

- Patients diagnosed with Williams syndrome require evaluation and follow-up with a pediatric cardiologist.
- Patients with hypercalcemia and renal artery stenosis often require referral and follow-up with a pediatric nephrologist and/or pediatric endocrinologist.

PREVENTION AND SCREENING

- Close monitoring of blood pressures should be performed during office visits as patients with Williams syndrome can have hypertension from renal artery involvement.
- Screening and surveillance with serial echocardiograms should be performed.

PROGNOSIS

- Patients with supravalvular aortic stenosis have good long-term prognosis if gradients during infancy are low. Those with gradients above 20 mm Hg tend to have an increase in gradient as they grow and 60 percent of them require surgical relief.[16] SOR Ⓐ
- Sudden cardiac death is also a well-known risk in patients with William Syndrome.

FOLLOW-UP

- Annual or more frequent follow-up is needed with a pediatric cardiologist.
- Follow-up with a pediatric nephrologist or pediatric endocrinologist will depend on the presence and extent of renal and metabolic problems.

PATIENT EDUCATION

- Parents need to be given anticipatory counseling about the possibility of having renal artery involvement in future.
- Education regarding the risk of sudden cardiac death should also be discussed with the family.

PATIENT RESOURCES

- **www.williams-syndrome.org/what-is-williamssyndrome**
- **http://www.williams-syndrome.org/what-is-williams-syndrome**.

PROVIDER RESOURCES

- **www.orpha.net/consor/cgi-bin/OC_Exp.php?Lng=GB&Expert=904.0.**

MARFAN SYNDROME

PATIENT STORY

A 16-year-old previously healthy boy presenting for a sports physical to his pediatrician is found to have a mid to late systolic murmur in the apex with a mid-systolic click, which becomes more prominent with standing. The family history is significant for sudden death in a paternal uncle. His height is at the 99th percentile for his age, he is slender, has long fingers, hypermobile joints, and pectus excavatum (**Figures 47-6** and **47-7**). The diagnosis of Marfan syndrome was suspected and he was referred to a geneticist and cardiologist. He was found to have a mutation in the fibrillin-1 gene and dilatation of the aorta.

INTRODUCTION

Marfan syndrome is the most common and best characterized form of connective tissue disorder and is associated with serious cardiovascular manifestations.

EPIDEMIOLOGY

- The estimated incidence of Marfan syndrome is 1 in 5,000 to 2 to 3 in 10,000 persons.[17]

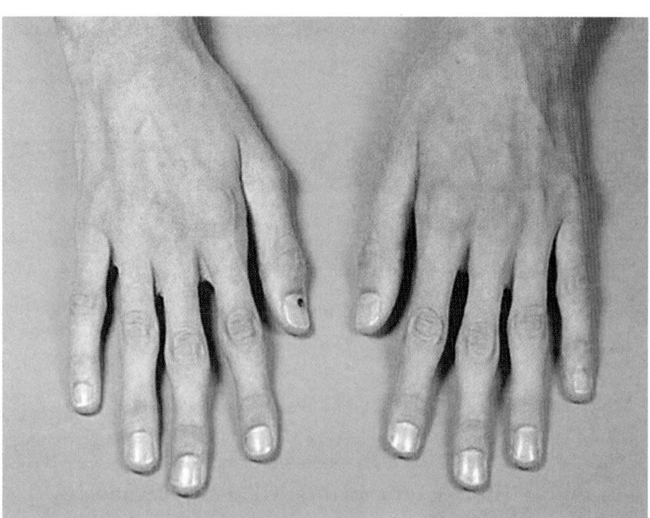

FIGURE 47-6 Arachnodactyly (long, slender fingers) in a patient with Marfan syndrome. (*Used with permission from Cleveland Clinic Children's Hospital photo file.*)

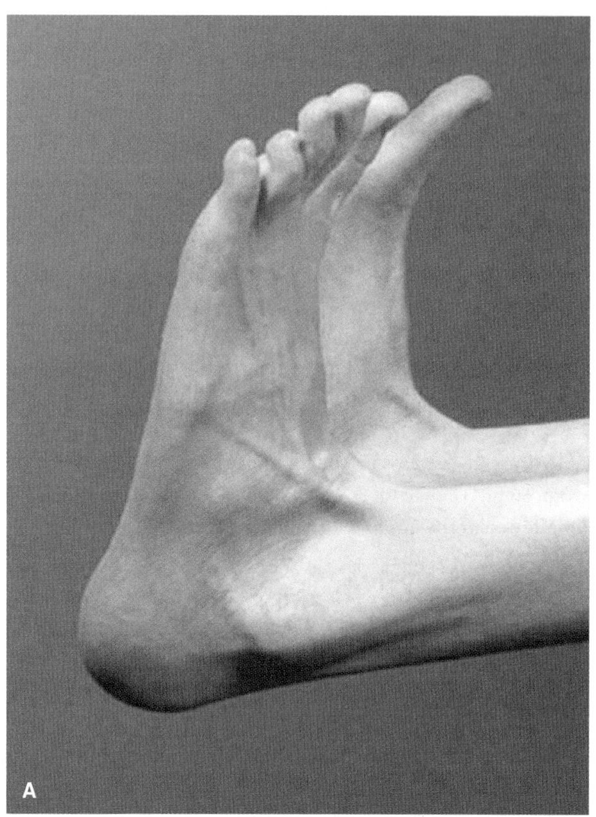

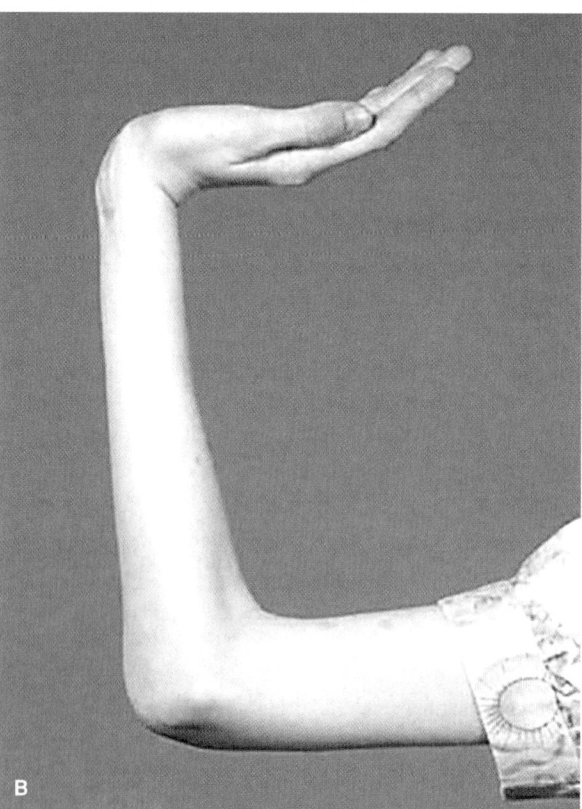

FIGURE 47-7 Hypermobility of the ankle (**A**) and wrist (**B**) joints in a patient with Marfan syndrome. (*Used with permission from Cleveland Clinic Children's Hospital photo file.*)

ETIOLOGY AND PATHOPHYSIOLOGY

- Autosomal dominant inherited, multisystem disorder with serious cardiovascular manifestations.[18]
- Mutations involving the FBN1 gene for the connective tissue protein fibrillin-1 have been identified as the genetic defect causing Marfan syndrome.

RISK FACTORS

- Family history of Marfan syndrome.
- Autosomal dominant inheritance.

DIAGNOSIS

- The clinical diagnosis of Marfan syndrome is usually made using the revised Berlin criteria, or Ghent criteria, both of which take into consideration skeletal, cardiovascular, ocular, skin and integumental, pulmonary system and family history.[19,20]
- Confirmatory diagnosis is usually made with gene testing for a mutation in the FBN1 gene.
- Cardiovascular manifestations include:
    - Dilation of the ascending aorta (**Figure 47-8**) with or without regurgitation.
    - Dissection of the ascending/thoracic/abdominal aorta.
    - Mitral valve prolapse with or without regurgitation.
    - Dilatation of main pulmonary artery in the absence of valvular or peripheral pulmonary stenosis or any other obvious causes and calcification of mitral valve annulus.

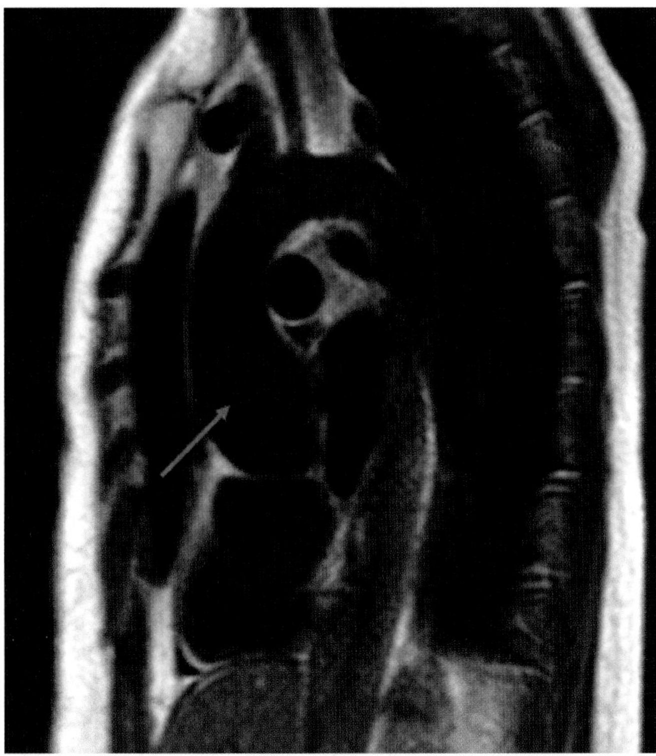

FIGURE 47-8 Sagittal plane MRI image of the aorta (arrow) in a patient with Marfan syndrome. The aorta is dilated at the level of the sinuses of valsalva while the remainder of the aorta is normal in size. *(Used with permission from Peter Aziz, MD.)*

DIFFERENTIAL DIAGNOSIS

- Loeys-Dietz syndrome can present with aortic root dilation similar to Marfan syndrome and is caused by mutation of transforming growth factor beta receptor 1 (TFFBR1) or 2 (TFFBR2).[21]
- Ehlers Danlos syndrome can also manifest with aortic root dilation and mitral regurgitation[22] (see Chapter 224, Ehlers Danlos Syndrome).

MANAGEMENT

- B-blockers, which reduce hemodynamic stress on the aortic wall, are often prescribed for patients with Marfan syndrome. SOR Ⓒ
- Afterload reduction agents can be used to decrease the stress on the aortic and mitral valves and aortic roots.[23] SOR Ⓑ
- Animal studies and a small clinical study have shown that Losartan can improve the contractile function of the aorta.[24,25] SOR Ⓑ
- Clinically significant mitral valve prolapse would necessitate replacement of the valve.[26] SOR Ⓐ
- Similarly, dilated ascending aorta/root >5.5 cm in those without family history of dissection and >5 cm in those with family history of dissection (applies to adults only) may require surgical repair as well.[27] SOR Ⓑ

REFERRAL

- Patients suspected of having Marfan syndrome patients should be managed using a multidisciplinary approach involving a pediatrician, pediatric cardiologist, pediatric ophthalmologist, geneticists, and pediatric surgeon.
- Referral to a pediatric cardiologist should be made if diagnosis is suspected.

PREVENTION AND SCREENING

- Genetic counseling should be provided to families who have a child with Marfan syndrome.

PROGNOSIS

- Patients with Marfan syndrome have a life expectancy similar to that of persons without Marfan because of advancement in pharmacotherapy and improvement in surgical outcome. However, cardiovascular compromise is the most common cause of patient death from sudden death in a previously undiagnosed patient.

FOLLOW-UP

- Close follow-up with a pediatric/adult cardiologist is needed to closely follow-up the status of aortic root to determine need for a surgical repair.

PATIENT EDUCATION

- Patients need to be educated about having other family members screened for Marfan and to have them undergo an evaluation by a cardiologist.

PATIENT RESOURCES

- **http://my.clevelandclinic.org/heart/disorders/aorta_marfan/default.aspx**.

PROVIDER RESOURCES

- **http://circ.ahajournals.org/content/121/13/e266.full**.
- 2013 Updated guidelines on Health Supervision for Children with Marfan Syndrome from the Committee on Genetics of the American Academy of Pediatrics—**http://pediatrics.aappublications.org/content/132/4/e1059.abstract**.

REFERENCES

1. Irving CA, Chaudhari MP. Cardiovascular abnormalities in down's syndrome: Spectrum, management and survival over 22 years. *Archives of disease in childhood*. 2012;97(4):326-330.
2. Donaldson MD, Gault EJ, Tan KW, Dunger DB. Optimising management in turner syndrome: From infancy to adult transfer. *Archives of disease in childhood*. 2006;91(6):513-520.
3. Zehr KJ, Gillinov AM, Redmond JM, Greene PS, Kan JS, Gardner TJ, Reitz BA, Cameron DE. Repair of coarctation of the aorta in neonates and infants: A thirty-year experience. *The Annals of thoracic surgery*. 1995;59(1):33-41.
4. Hellenbrand WE, Allen HD, Golinko RJ, Hagler DJ, Lutin W, Kan J. Balloon angioplasty for aortic recoarctation: Results of valvuloplasty and angioplasty of congenital anomalies registry. *The American journal of cardiology*. 1990;65(11):793-797.
5. Bondy CA. Care of girls and women with turner syndrome: A guideline of the turner syndrome study group. *The Journal of clinical endocrinology and metabolism*. 2007;92(1):10-25.
6. Graham TP, Jr., Driscoll DJ, Gersony WM, Newburger JW, Rocchini A, Towbin JA. Task force 2: Congenital heart disease. *Journal of the American College of Cardiology*. 2005;45(8):1326-1333.
7. Shprintzen RJ. Velo-cardio-facial syndrome: 30 years of study. *Dev Disabil Res Rev*. 2008;14(1):3-10.
8. Wilson TA, Blethen SL, Vallone A, Alenick DS, Nolan P, Katz A, Amorillo TP, Goldmuntz E, Emanuel BS, Driscoll DA. Digeorge anomaly with renal agenesis in infants of mothers with diabetes. *Am J Med Genet*. 1993;47(7):1078-1082.
9. Bassett AS, McDonald-McGinn DM, Devriendt K, Digilio MC, Goldenberg P, Habel A, Marino B, Oskarsdottir S, Philip N, Sullivan K, Swillen A, Vorstman J. Practical guidelines for managing patients with 22q11.2 deletion syndrome. *The Journal of pediatrics*. 2011;159(2):332-339.e331.
10. Stromme P, Bjornstad PG, Ramstad K. Prevalence estimation of williams syndrome. *J Child Neurol*. 2002;17(4):269-271.
11. Nickerson E, Greenberg F, Keating MT, McCaskill C, Shaffer LG. Deletions of the elastin gene at 7q11.23 occur in approximately 90% of patients with williams syndrome. *Am J Hum Genet*. 1995; 56(5):1156-1161.
12. Soper R, Chaloupka JC, Fayad PB, Greally JM, Shaywitz BA, Awad IA, Pober BR. Ischemic stroke and intracranial multifocal cerebral arteriopathy in williams syndrome. *J Pediatr*. 1995;126(6): 945-948.
13. Wessel A, Gravenhorst V, Buchhorn R, Gosch A, Partsch CJ, Pankau R. Risk of sudden death in the williams-beuren syndrome. *Am J Med Genet A*. 2004;127A(3):234-237.
14. Broder K, Reinhardt E, Ahern J, Lifton R, Tamborlane W, Pober B. Elevated ambulatory blood pressure in 20 subjects with williams syndrome. *Am J Med Genet*. 1999;83(5):356-360.
15. Collins RT, 2nd, Aziz PF, Gleason MM, Kaplan PB, Shah MJ. Abnormalities of cardiac repolarization in williams syndrome. *The American journal of cardiology*. 2010;106(7):1029-1033.
16. Wessel A, Pankau R, Kececioglu D, Ruschewski W, Bürsch JH. Three decades of follow-up of aortic and pulmonary vascular lesions in the williams-beuren syndrome. *American Journal of Medical Genetics*. 1994;52(3):297-301.
17. Ammash NM, Sundt TM, Connolly HM. Marfan syndrome-diagnosis and management. *Curr Probl Cardiol*. 2008;33(1): 7-39.
18. McKusick VA. The defect in marfan syndrome. *Nature*. 1991; 352(6333):279-281.
19. De Paepe A, Devereux RB, Dietz HC, Hennekam RC, Pyeritz RE. Revised diagnostic criteria for the marfan syndrome. *Am J Med Genet*. 1996;62(4):417-426.
20. Loeys BL, Dietz HC, Braverman AC, Callewaert BL, De Backer J, Devereux RB, Hilhorst-Hofstee Y, Jondeau G, Faivre L, Milewicz DM, Pyeritz RE, Sponseller PD, Wordsworth P, De Paepe AM. The revised ghent nosology for the marfan syndrome. *J Med Genet*. 2010;47(7):476-485.
21. Loeys BL, Schwarze U, Holm T, Callewaert BL, Thomas GH, Pannu H, De Backer JF, Oswald GL, Symoens S, Manouvrier S, Roberts AE, Faravelli F, Greco MA, Pyeritz RE, Milewicz DM, Coucke PJ, Cameron DE, Braverman AC, Byers PH, De Paepe AM, Dietz HC. Aneurysm syndromes caused by mutations in the tgf-beta receptor. *N Engl J Med*. 2006;355(8):788-798.
22. Wenstrup RJ, Meyer RA, Lyle JS, Hoechstetter L, Rose PS, Levy HP, Francomano CA. Prevalence of aortic root dilation in the ehlers-danlos syndrome. *Genet Med*. 2002;4(3):112-117.
23. Ahimastos AA, Aggarwal A, D'Orsa KM, Formosa MF, White AJ, Savarirayan R, Dart AM, Kingwell BA. Effect of perindopril on large artery stiffness and aortic root diameter in patients with

marfan syndrome: A randomized controlled trial. *JAMA : the journal of the American Medical Association*. 2007;298(13):1539-1547.

24. Yang HH, Kim JM, Chum E, van Breemen C, Chung AW. Long-term effects of losartan on structure and function of the thoracic aorta in a mouse model of marfan syndrome. *British journal of pharmacology*. 2009;158(6):1503-1512.
25. Brooke BS, Habashi JP, Judge DP, Patel N, Loeys B, Dietz HC III. Angiotensin II blockade and aortic-root dilation in Marfan's syndrome. *N Engl J Med.* 2008; 358: 2787-2795.
26. Bhudia SK, Troughton R, Lam BK, Rajeswaran J, Mills WR, Gillinov AM, Griffin BP, Blackstone EH, Lytle BW, Svensson LG. Mitral valve surgery in the adult marfan syndrome patient. *The Annals of thoracic surgery*. 2006;81(3):843-848.
27. Vardulaki KA, Prevost TC, Walker NM, Day NE, Wilmink ABM, Quick CRG, Ashton HA, Scott RAP. Growth rates and risk of rupture of abdominal aortic aneurysms. *British Journal of Surgery*. 1998;85(12):1674-1680.

PART 8

THE LUNGS

Strength of Recommendation (SOR)	Definition
A	Recommendation based on consistent and good-quality patient-oriented evidence.*
B	Recommendation based on inconsistent or limited-quality patient-oriented evidence.*
C	Recommendation based on consensus, usual practice, opinion, disease-oriented evidence, or case series for studies of diagnosis, treatment, prevention, or screening.*

*See Appendix A on pages 1320–1322 for further information.

48 BRONCHIOLITIS

Rachna May, MD, FAAP
Julie Cernanec, MD, FAAP

PATIENT STORY

A 5-month-old full-term female infant presents to your office with 3 days of fever and cough. On examination, you note a frequent wet cough and appreciate bilateral wheezes. Pulse oximetry reveals a normal oxygen saturation. You reassure the mom that her daughter has bronchiolitis and needs supportive care only (**Figure 48-1**). She agrees to follow up with you in 1 to 2 days.

INTRODUCTION

Bronchiolitis is inflammation of the bronchioles typically caused by a viral illness that frequently affects young children.[1]

SYNONYMS

Respiratory Syncytial Virus (RSV) or lower respiratory tract infection (LRTI).

EPIDEMIOLOGY

- Most common lower respiratory tract infection in children less than 1 year of age.[1]
- Annual hospitalizations for bronchiolitis account for greater than half a billion dollars in health care expenditures.[2]

ETIOLOGY AND PATHOPHYSIOLOGY

- Viral etiology, most frequently RSV.
- Other viruses implicated include influenza, parainfluenza, adenovirus, and human metapneumovirus.

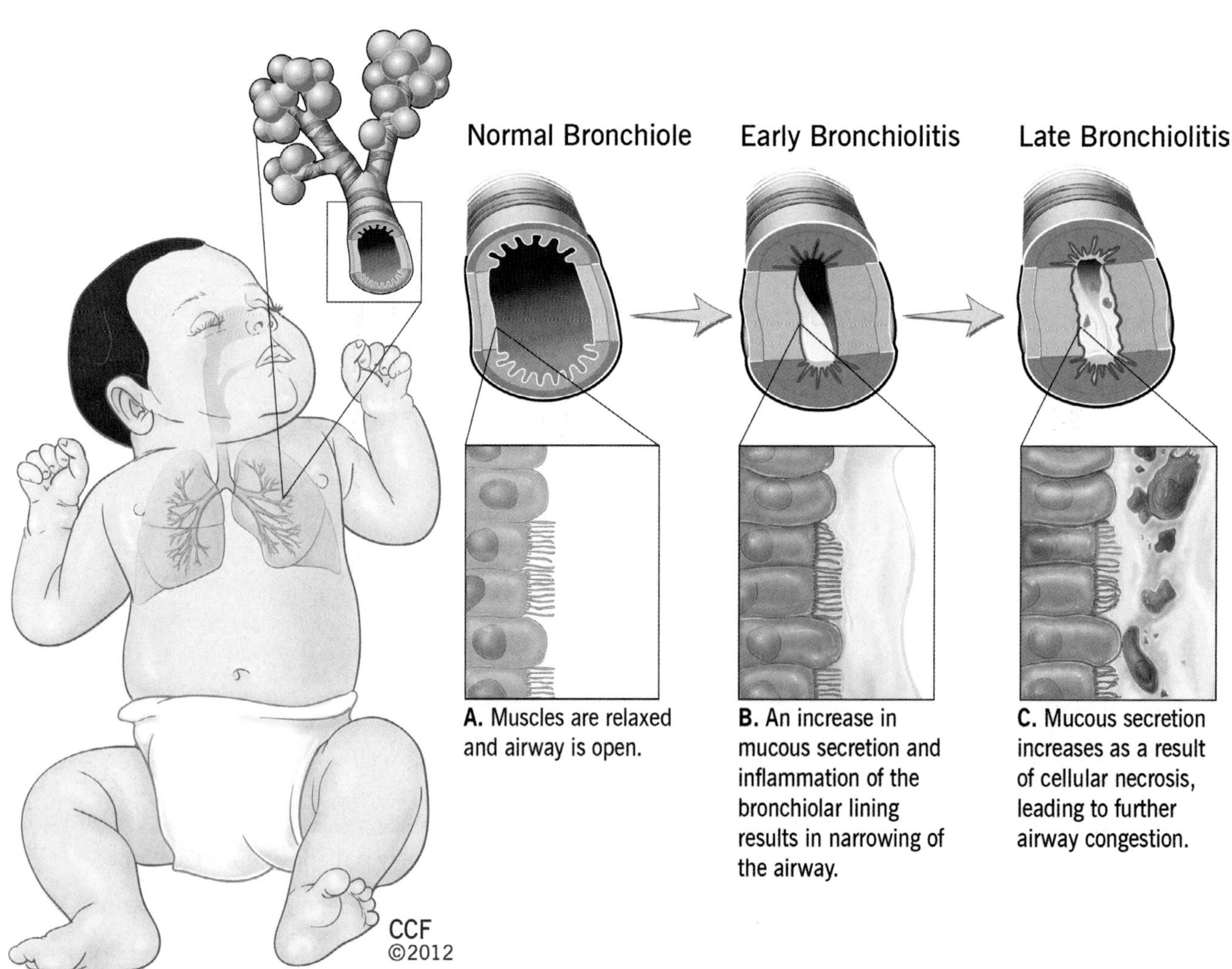

FIGURE 48-1 Bronchiolitis illustration with captions embedded. (*Reprinted with permission, Cleveland Clinic Center for Medical Art & Photography © 2012. All Rights Reserved.*)

* Inflammation, edema, and necrosis of epithelial cells lining bronchioles (**Figure 48-1**).
* Leads to increased mucus production and bronchospasm.

RISK FACTORS

* Up to 90 percent of infants will have had an RSV infection by the age of 2 years.[1]
* Infants with exposure to child care center populations, school-aged siblings, and smoke are at higher risk for developing bronchiolitis.[3]
* Risk factors for severe disease include:
    * Prematurity of less than 35 weeks gestation.
    * Chronic lung disease or congenital airway malformations.
    * Cyanotic congenital heart disease.
    * Severe neuromuscular disease.
    * Immunocompromised state.[4]

DIAGNOSIS

CLINICAL FEATURES

* Bronchiolitis is a clinical diagnosis.
* Signs and symptoms include rhinorrhea, cough, tachypnea, bilateral wheezing, and signs of increased work of breathing such as use of accessory muscles and/or nasal flaring.

LABORATORY TESTING

* Laboratory testing is not routinely indicated.
* Respiratory viral testing can be obtained if necessary for epidemiologic surveillance and research but the results do not change the management of the disease.

IMAGING

* As most chest x-rays obtained in patients with bronchiolitis are found to be normal, routine chest radiography is *not* recommended for patients with bronchiolitis (**Figure 48-2**).
* Nonspecific findings such as hyperinflation, perihilar markings, or central bronchial thickening can be seen in some patients (**Figure 48-3** to **48-5**).
* Chest radiography may be necessary if the patient experiences a severe course or does not improve as expected based on the natural history of disease.

DIFFERENTIAL DIAGNOSIS

* Reactive Airway Disease—Asthma-like condition in toddlers, presenting with wheezing and airway hyperreactivity, and may be exacerbated by viral illness (see Chapter 49, Asthma).
* Pneumonia—Infection of the lung most commonly caused by viral or bacterial infection (see Chapter 50, Community-Acquired Pneumonia).

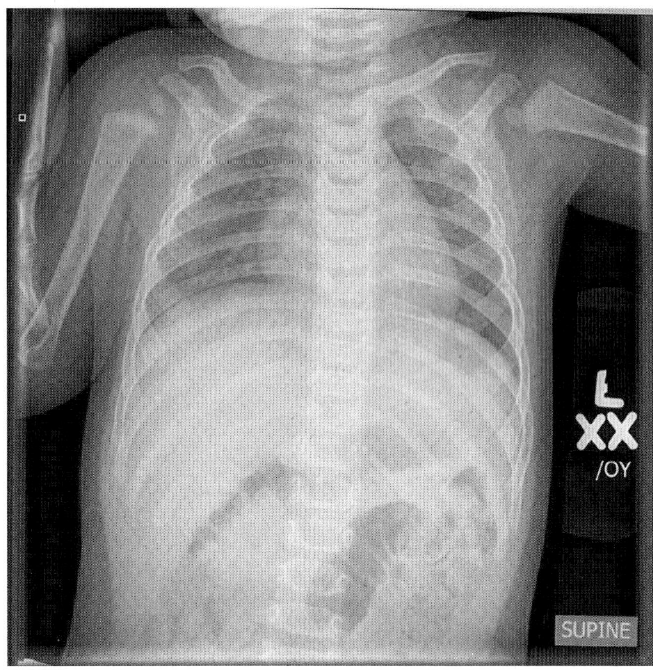

FIGURE 48-2 Normal chest x-ray of an 8-month old infant. (*Used with permission from Rachna May, MD.*)

MANAGEMENT

NONPHARMACOLOGIC

* Supportive care with supplemental oxygen, suction, and fluid resuscitation as indicated by the patient's clinical status is the mainstay of treatment.

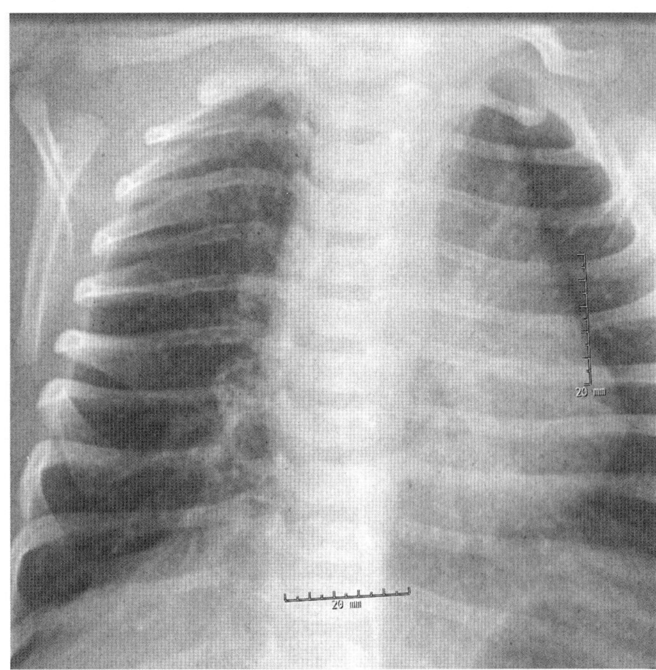

FIGURE 48-3 Hyperinflation secondary to air trapping and mild atelectasis seen in some patients with bronchiolitis. (*Used with permission from Rachna May, MD.*)

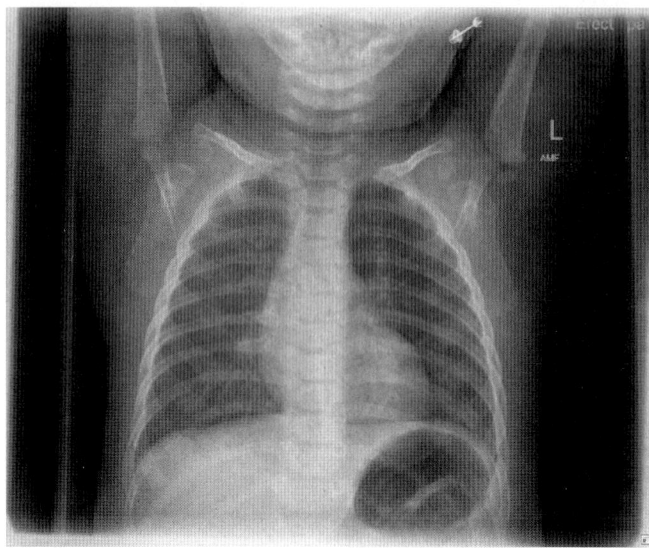

FIGURE 48-4 Increased perihilar markings, a non-specific sign often seen with viral infections. (*Used with permission from Rachna May, MD.*)

- IV fluid therapy is usually indicated when feeding is compromised in the setting of severe tachypnea.

MEDICATIONS

- Bronchodilators are not routinely recommended for wheezing in bronchiolitis. However, it is reasonable to attempt a single dose to assess the patient's response, after which the decision can be made to continue the therapy. Studies suggest that up to 25 percent of patients may benefit from bronchodilator treatment.[1] SOR Ⓑ
- Systemic or high-dose inhaled steroids are also not recommended for treatment of bronchiolitis.[1] SOR Ⓑ
- The use of hypertonic saline is controversial and requires further study.[2]

REFERRAL

- Inpatients that require supplemental oxygen beyond the typical length of stay of approximately 3 days may benefit from a pulmonology consultation for further evaluation of underlying reactive airway disease or structural abnormality.

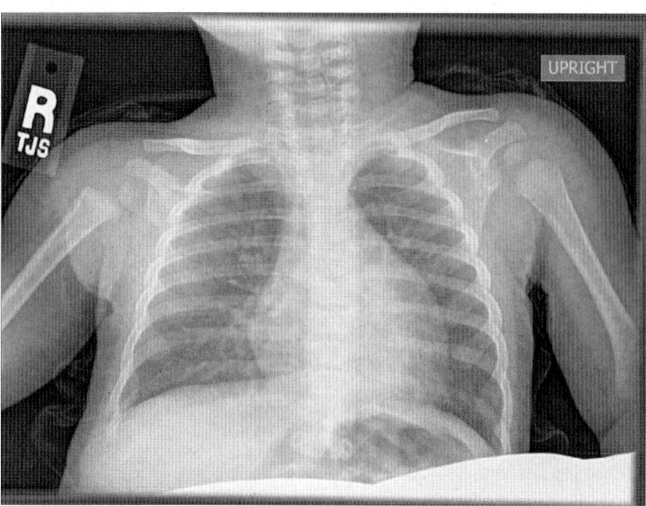

FIGURE 48-5 Central bronchial thickening, a nonspecific sign often seen with viral infections. (*Used with permission from Rachna May, MD.*)

PREVENTION AND SCREENING

- Effective handwashing is the best prevention for viral respiratory infections that cause bronchiolitis.[1]
- Palivizumab, a monoclonal antibody against RSV, may be given to infants who qualify based on risk factors for severe RSV infection, including but not limited to prematurity, chronic lung disease, and cyanotic congenital heart disease.[1] Palivizumab has been shown to reduce the risk of hospitalization in infants who are at risk for severe RSV infection.[5–7] SOR Ⓐ

PROGNOSIS

Most infants and children recover without long-term adverse effects.

FOLLOW-UP

- Most children who are otherwise healthy may continue routine follow-up with their primary care pediatrician.
- Children with underlying medical conditions such as chronic lung disease or reactive airway disease will benefit from follow-up with the appropriate subspecialist.

PATIENT EDUCATION

- If the diagnosis of bronchiolitis is made in the outpatient setting, parents should be counseled on reasons to seek further emergency medical care, including tachypnea, retractions, cyanosis, and dehydration.

REFERENCES

1. American Academy of Pediatrics Subcommittee on Diagnosis and Management of Bronchiolitis: Diagnosis and management of bronchiolitis. *Pediatrics*. 2006;118(4):1774-1793.
2. Alverson, B and Ralston, SL. Management of Bronchiolitis: Focus on Hypertonic Saline. *Contemporary Pediatrics*. 2011;30-36.
3. McConnochie KM, Roghmann KJ. Parental smoking, presence of older siblings, and family history of asthma increase risk of bronchiolitis. *Am J Dis Child*. 1986;140(8):806-812.
4. Meissner, CH. Selected populations at increased risk from respiratory syncytial virus infection. *The Pediatric Infectious Disease Journal*. 2003;22(2):S40-S45.
5. The IMpact-RSV study group: Palivizumab, a humanized respiratory syncytial virus monoclonal antibody, reduces hospitalization from respiratory syncytial virus infection in highrisk infants. *Pediatrics*. 1998;102:531-537.
6. Feltes TF, Cabalka AK, Meissner HC, et al. Palivizumab prophylaxis reduces hospitalization due to respiratory syncytial virus in young children with hemodynamically significant congenital heart disease. *J Pediatr*. 2003;143:532-540.
7. Romero JR. Palivizumab prophylaxis of respiratory syncytial virus disease from 1998 to 2002: results from four years of palivizumab usage. *Pediatr Infect Dis J*. 2003;22(2 suppl):S46-S54.

49 ASTHMA AND PULMONARY FUNCTION TESTING

Mindy A. Smith, MD, MS

PATIENT STORY

A 7-year-old boy with a history of atopic dermatitis as an infant, presents with an episode of continued cough and wheezing 2 weeks following a recent cold. The cough is keeping the family up at night. This is his third episode this winter and has gone on longer than the others. He has otherwise been quite healthy. He appears comfortable but is coughing intermittently. His examination is significant for mild inspiratory and expiratory wheezing but no crackles. His mother mentions that she had asthma as a child and is worried that this might be asthma. The pediatrician prescribes an inhaled bronchodilator and refers the child for spirometry before and after an inhaled bronchodilator.

The spirometry results in **Table 49-1** show a mild to moderate baseline defect with marked improvement post bronchodilator. The flow volume loops provide graphical demonstration of the same data (**Figure 49-1**). This confirms the diagnosis of asthma and an asthma treatment plan is developed.

Interpretation: mild to moderate baseline defect with marked improvement post bronchodilator.

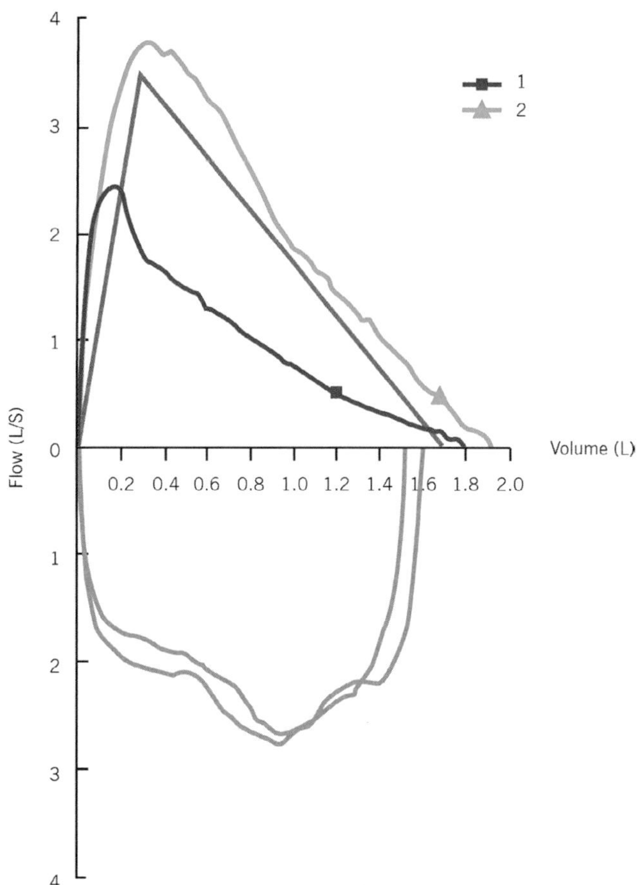

FIGURE 49-1 Pulmonary Function Tests (PFTs) showing flow volume loop in a 7-year-old boy with newly diagnosed asthma. He has a mild to moderate baseline defect with marked improvement post bronchodilator. See **Table 49-1** for specific numbers. Blue—pre-bronchodilator. Green—post-bronchodilator. Red—predicted.

INTRODUCTION

Asthma is a chronic inflammatory airway disorder with variable airflow obstruction and bronchial hyperresponsiveness that is at least partially reversible, spontaneously or with treatment (e.g., beta-2 agonist treatment). Patients with asthma have recurrent episodes of wheezing, breathlessness, chest tightness, and cough (particularly at night or in the early morning).

EPIDEMIOLOGY

- About one in 12 people (25 million or 8% of the population) had asthma in 2009, including about one in 10 children.[1] Rates of asthma are increasing; the greatest rise in rates is among black children, an almost 50 percent increase between 2001 and 2009.[1]
- The number of deaths linked to asthma in 2007 was 3,447.[1] Using the 2006 to 2008 Nationwide Emergency Department (ED) Sample database, the estimated overall annual number of in-hospital asthma-related deaths was 1,144 (0.06%).[2] Most patients died as inpatients (N = 1043) but 101 died in the ED. There were 37 asthma-related deaths per year among children.
- Asthma was the first-listed diagnosis for 479,000 hospital discharges in 2009 with an average length of stay of 4.3 days.[1]
- Asthma-associated medical expenses increased from $48.6 billion in 2002 to $50.1 billion in 2007.[1] Many uninsured people with asthma (about 40%) and about 1 in 9 insured people could not afford their prescription drugs.[1] In one retrospective study based

TABLE 49-1 Pulmonary Function Tests: 7-year-old boy. Weight 30.7 Kg; Height 131 cm (see Table 49-2 for key to abbreviations)

	Predicted	Pre-bronchodilator	% Predicted	Post-bronchodilator	% Predicted
FVC (L)	1.70	1.80	105.6	1.92	112.9
FEV1 (L)	1.45	1.17	81.0	1.67	115.5
FEV % FVC (%)	88.00	65.36	74.5	87.11	99.2
PEF (L/s)	3.49	2.43	69.6	3.76	107.9
FEF 25/75 (L/s)	1.67	0.76	45.5	1.88	112.1

Pulmonary Function Tests: 9-year-old boy. Weight 46 Kg; Height 141 cm (see Table 49-2 for key to abbreviations)

	Predicted	Pre-bronchodilator	% Predicted	Post-bronchodilator	% Predicted
FVC (L)	2.32	1.58	67.9	2.02	87.0
FEV1 (L)	2.01	0.97	48.3	1.44	71.5
FEV % FVC (%)	87.41	61.53	70.4	71.11	81.4
PEF (L/s)	5.07	2.62	51.8	4.23	83.4
FEF 25/75 (L/s)	2.33	0.52	22.5	0.93	39.8

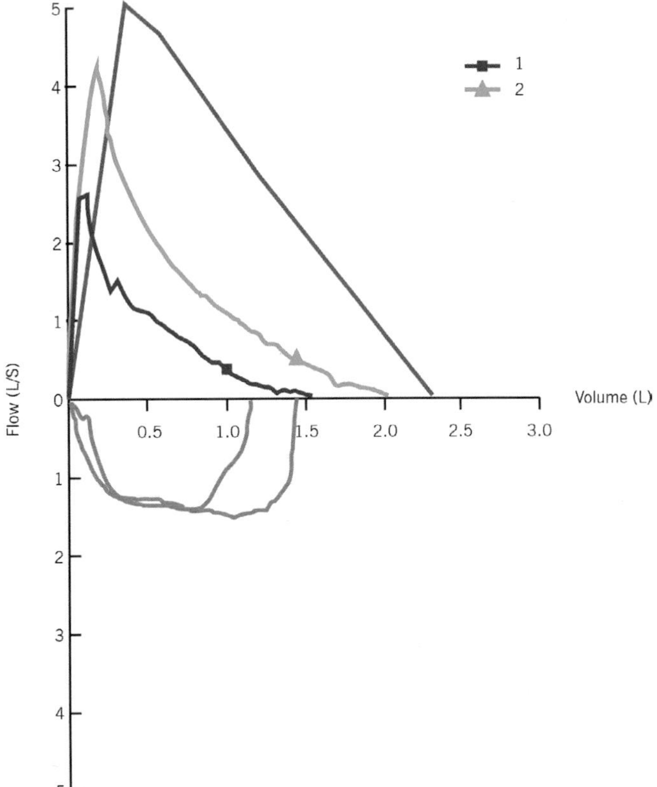

FIGURE 49-2 Pulmonary Function Tests (PFTs) showing flow volume loop in a 9-year-old boy with ongoing asthma. He has a moderate baseline obstruction defect with marked improvement in the FEV1 and FEF 25/75 post-bronchodilator but not to predicted levels. Blue—pre-bronchodilator. Green—post-bronchodilator. Red—predicted.

on insurance claims for children with asthma who initiated asthma control therapy between 1997 and 2007 (N = 8834), the mean annual out-of-pocket asthma medication cost was \$154 (95% CI, \$152-\$156) among children aged 5 to 18 years and slightly lower (mean \$151) among younger children.[3] In this study, asthma-related hospitalization was higher for children aged 5 to 18 years who were in the top quartile of out-of-pocket costs (2.4 [95% CI, 1.9 to 2.8] hospitalizations per 100 children versus 1.7 [95% CI, 1.3 to 2.1] per 100 in the bottom quartile).

- More than half (59%) of children and 1/3 (33%) of adults who had an asthma attack missed school or work because of asthma in 2008; on average, children missed 4 days of school.[1]

ETIOLOGY AND PATHOPHYSIOLOGY

- Although the precise cause is unknown, early exposure to airborne allergens (e.g., house dust-mite, cockroach antigens) and childhood respiratory infections (e.g., respiratory syncytial virus, parainfluenza) are associated with asthma development. In one prospective cohort study, 50 percent of children who experienced severe RSV bronchiolitis at age 12 months or less had a subsequent asthma diagnosis.[4]
- In addition to environmental factors, asthma has an inherited component, although the genetics involved remain complex.[5] The gene ADAM 33 (A Disintegrin And Metalloproteinase) may increase risk of asthma as metalloproteinases appear to effect airway remodeling.[6] A recent nested case-control study found that genetic variation in the ATPAF1 gene predisposed children of different racial backgrounds to asthma.[7]
- In the Copenhagen Prospective Studies on Asthma in Childhood (N = 411 at-risk children followed prospectively from birth using spirometry), children with asthma by age 7 years (14%) had a significant airflow deficit as neonates.[8] It was estimated that approximately 40 percent of the airflow deficit associated with asthma was present at birth and the remainder developed with clinical disease.

TABLE 49-2 Pulmonary Function Tests (Key to Abbreviations)

FVC (L)	Forced vital capacity
FEV1(L)	Forced vital capacity at one second
FEV1/FVC %	FEV1 divided by FVC
FEF 25–75% (L/sec)	Forced expiratory flow between 25% and 75% of capacity—same as maximal mid expiratory flow (MMFR)
FEF max (L/sec)	Forced expiratory flow maximum
FEF 25% (L/sec)	Forced expiratory flow rate when 25% of the FVC has been exhaled (slope of FVC curve at 25% exhaled)
FEF 50% (L/sec)	Forced expiratory flow rate when 50% of the FVC has been exhaled
FEF 75% (L/sec)	Forced expiratory flow rate was 75% of the FVC has been exhaled
FITC (L)	Forced inspiratory vital capacity
FIF 50% (L/sec)	Forced inspiratory flow at 50% capacity
SVC (L)	Slow vital capacity
TLC (L)	Total lung capacity
RV (L)	Residual volume
RV/TLC	Residual volume divided by total lung capacity
TGV (L)	Thoracic gas volume
Raw	Airway resistance
ERV (L)	Expiratory reserve volume
IC (L)	Inspiratory capacity
DLCO	Diffusing capacity of lung (using carbon monoxide measuring)
VA (L)	Alveolar volume
DL/VA	Diffusing capacity divided by alveolar volume

- The pulmonary obstruction characterizing asthma results from combinations of mucosal swelling, mucous production, constriction of bronchiolar smooth muscles and neutrophils (the latter, particularly important in smokers or those with occupational asthma).[4] The smaller airways of children make them particularly susceptible.
- Over time, airway smooth muscle hypertrophy and hyperplasia, remodeling (thickening of the sub-basement membrane, subepithelial fibrosis and vascular proliferation and dilation), along with mucous plugging complicate the disease.[4]
- Allergen-induced acute bronchospasm involves immunoglobulin-E (IgE)-dependent release of mast cell mediators.[4]

RISK FACTORS

Based on a cohort study, early life (first 5 years) risk factors for diagnosed asthma at age 10 years includes:[9]

- Family history of asthma (maternal [odds ratio (OR) 2.26; 95% confidence interval (CI) 1.24 to 3.73); paternal [OR 2.30; 95% CI 1.17 to 4.52]; sibling [OR 2.00; 95% CI 1.16 to 3.43]).
- Recurrent chest infections at 1 year of age (OR 2.67; 95% CI 1.12 to 6.40) and 2 years of age (OR 4.11; 95% CI 2.06 to 8.18).
- Atopy at 4 years of age (OR 7.22; 95% CI 4.13 to 12.62).
- Parental smoking at 1 year of age (OR 1.99; 95% CI 1.15 to 3.45).
- Male gender (OR 1.72; 95% CI 1.01 to 2.95).
- Recent use of acetaminophen has also been associated with asthma symptoms in adolescents (OR 1.43; 95% CI 1.33 to 1.53 and OR 2.51; 95% CI 2.33 to 2.70 for at least once a year and at least once a month use versus no use, respectively).[10] One possible mechanism is through acetaminophen reducing the immune response and prolonging rhinovirus infection.[11]
- Environmental mold is also a risk factor; in one study the OR was 1.8 (95% CI 1.5 to 2.2) for asthma diagnosed at age 7 years for a 10-unit increase in the Environmental Relative Moldiness Index value in the child's home in infancy.[12]
- In one study, consumption of salty snacks (OR 4.8; 95% CI 1.50 to 15.8) was strongly associated with the presence of asthma symptoms, especially in children with television/video-game viewing of >2 hours/day.[13]
- In a prospective study of children following an episode of severe bronchiolitis, risk factors for physician-diagnosed asthma by age 7 years included maternal asthma (OR 5.2; 95% CI 1.7 to 15.9), exposure to high levels of dog allergen (OR 3.2; 95% CI 1.3 to 7.7), aeroallergen sensitivity at age 3 years (OR 10.7; 95% CI 2.1 to 49.0), recurrent wheezing during the first 3 years of life (OR 7.3; 95% CI 1.2 to 43.3), and CCL5 mRNA expression in nasal epithelia during acute RSV infection (OR 3.8; 95% CI 1.2 to 2.4).[4]
- Obesity has also been associated with risk of wheezing in children (OR 1.62, 95% CI 1.13 to 2.32).[14]
- Not surprisingly, in patients with severe or difficult-to-treat asthma, recent exacerbation history was the strongest predictor of future asthma exacerbations.[15] High concentrations of pollen also increase the risk of asthma- and wheeze-related ED visits by up to 15 percent.[16]

DIAGNOSIS

The diagnosis of asthma is made on clinical suspicion (presence of symptoms of recurrent and partially reversible airflow obstruction and airway hyperresponsiveness) and confirmed with spirometry.[5] Alternative diagnoses should be excluded.

CLINICAL FEATURES

Asthma's most common symptoms are recurrent wheezing, difficulty breathing, chest tightness, and cough. An absence of wheezing or normal physical exam does not exclude asthma.[3] In fact, up to

25 percent of patients with asthma have normal physical examinations even though abnormalities are seen on pulmonary function testing.[4] As part of the diagnosis of asthma, ask about the following:[3]

- Pattern of symptoms and precipitating factors. Symptoms often occur or worsen at night and during exercise, viral infection, exposure to inhalant allergens or irritants (e.g., tobacco smoke, wood smoke, or airborne chemicals), changes in weather, strong emotional expression (laughing hard or crying), menstrual cycle, and stress.[3]
- Family history of asthma, allergy or atopy in close relatives.
- Social history (e.g., daycare, workplace, or social support).
- History of exacerbations (e.g., frequency, duration, or treatment), and impact on patient and family. The preschool-aged asthmatic population tends to be characterized as exacerbation prone with relatively limited impairment while older children and adolescents have more impairment-dominant disease.[13]

Findings on physical exam may include:[3]

- Upper respiratory tract—Increased nasal secretion, mucosal swelling, and/or nasal polyp.
- Lungs—Decreased intensity of breath sounds is the most common (33% to 65% of patients).[4] Additional findings may include wheezing, prolonged phase of forced exhalation, use of accessory respiratory muscles, appearance of hunched shoulders, and chest deformity. During a severe exacerbation of asthma, minimal airflow may result in no audible wheezing.
- Skin—Atopic dermatitis and/or eczema (see Chapters 130, 132, and 133). There is a strong association between asthma, allergic rhinitis and atopic dermatitis (**Figure 49-3**). The "atopic triad" with the coexistence of all three conditions at one time (Figure **49-3**) is less common. Children with asthma are also more likely to develop pityriasis alba, a chronic skin disorder characterized by patches of lighter skin mainly on the face (**Figure 49-4**). In a US study of children with physician-confirmed atopic dermatitis (N = 2270), 38.0 percent reported symptoms of asthma and allergic rhinitis on a survey;[17] similarly in a population study in Taiwan using the National Insurance register, of the 66,446 individuals diagnosed with atopic dermatitis, about half had a concomitant diagnosis of allergic rhinitis and/or asthma.[18] Data support a sequence of atopic manifestations beginning typically with atopic dermatitis in infancy followed by allergic rhinitis and/or asthma in later stages.[19]

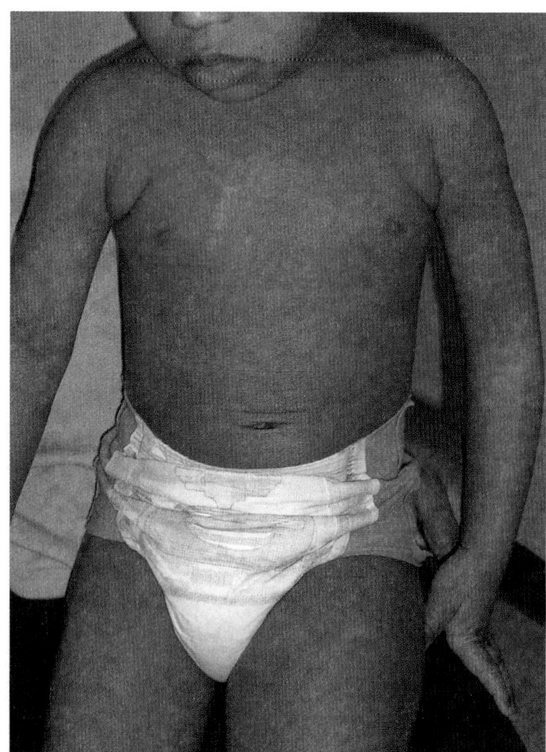

FIGURE 49-3 Two-year-old boy with the "atopic triad" showing skin manifestations of atopic dermatitis. (*Used with permission from Richard P. Usatine, MD.*)

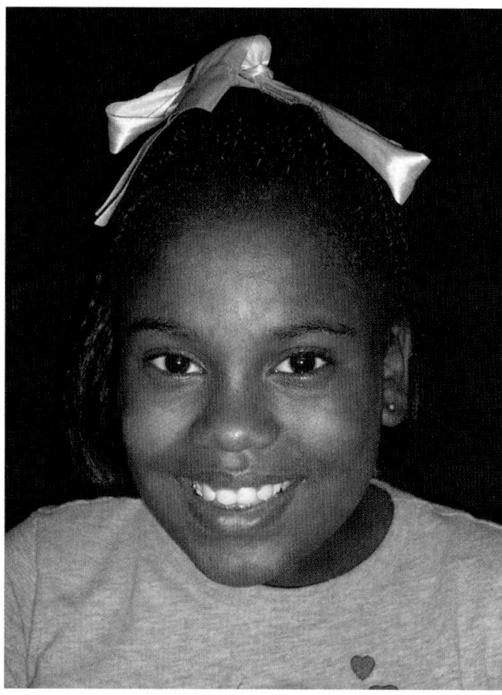

FIGURE 49-4 Ten-year-old girl with pityriasis alba, atopic dermatitis, and asthma under control. (*Used with permission from Richard P. Usatine, MD.*)

Findings in patients with status asthmaticus (prolonged/severe asthma attack that is not responsive to standard treatment) may include:[4]

- Tachycardia (heart rate >120 beats/minute) and tachypnea (respiratory rate >30 breaths/minute).
- Use of accessory respiratory muscles.
- Pulsus paradoxus (inspiratory decrease in systolic blood pressure >10 mm Hg).
- Mental status changes (due to hypoxia and hypercapnia).
- Paradoxical abdominal and diaphragmatic movement on inspiration.

LABORATORY TESTING

Spirometry is recommended by NAEP for all patients over 4 years of age to determine airway obstruction that is at least partially reversible (**Figures 49-1, 49-2, 49-5,** and **49-6**).[3] SOR B The British Thoracic Society also recommends an assessment of the reversibility of airway obstruction in response to an inhaled bronchodilator.

- In preschool-aged children diagnosis is most often based on symptom patterns, presence of risk factors, and therapeutic responses.[13]

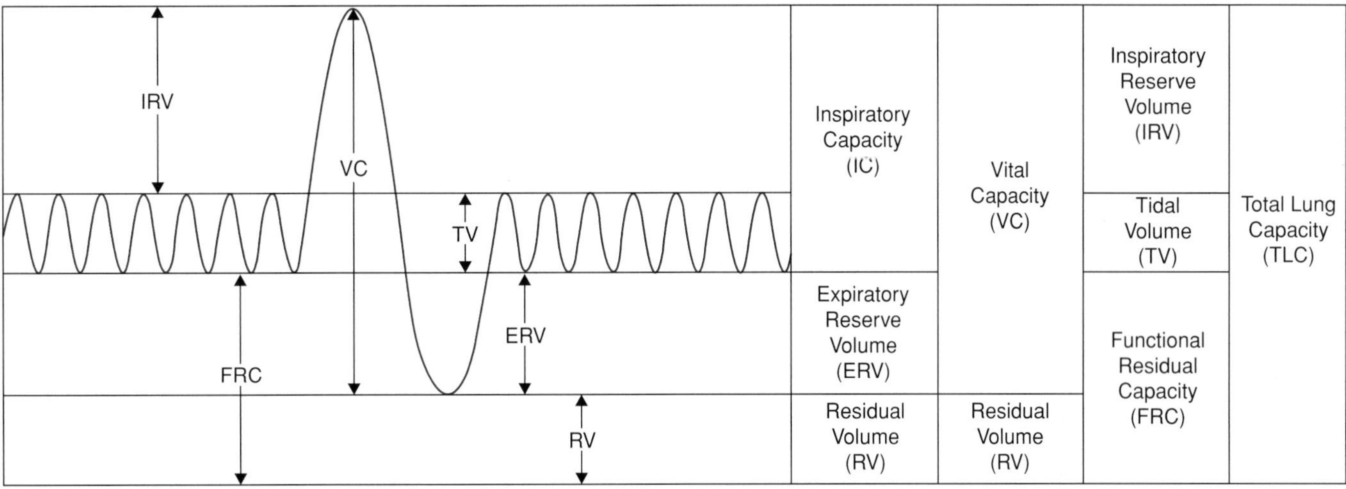

FIGURE 49-5 Graph of lung volumes showing the relationship of tidal volume to vital capacity and other important lung volumes.

Assess severity:

- Severity is defined as the intrinsic intensity of the disease process.[3] The NAEP divides severity into four groups for youths age 12 and up and adults: intermittent, persistent-mild, persistent-moderate, and persistent-severe.
- For younger children, the Composite Asthma Severity Index (CASI) has been proposed for assessment of control, including both impairment and risk.[20] CASI was developed by members of the National Institutes of Health-supported Inner City Asthma Consortium through a modified Delphi consensus process and subjected to factor analysis and validation using the Inner City Anti-IgE Therapy for Asthma trial. CASI includes five domains that are scored and summed for a final score of up to 20 points for most severe; scores might be useful for determining treatment and monitoring response to therapy:
    - Day symptoms and albuterol use in the past 2 weeks (scored 0 [0 to 3 symptoms and albuterol use] to 3 [daily symptoms and use]).
    - Night symptoms in the past 2 weeks and albuterol use (scored 0 [0 to 1 night] to 3 [5 to 14 nights]).
    - Lung function (scored 0 [FEV1% >85] to 3 [FEV1% <70]).
    - Controller treatment (scored 0 [none] to 5 [high dose ICS]).
    - Exacerbations (scored 2 for prednisone burst and 4 for prednisone burst plus hospitalization).
- Initially, severity can be assessed in the office, urgent or emergency care setting with predicted forced expiratory volume in 1 second (FEV1) or PEF; a value of <40 percent indicates a severe exacerbation. A value of >=70 percent predicted FEV1 or PEF is a goal for discharge from the emergency care setting.
- Once asthma control is achieved, severity can also be assessed by the step of care required for control (i.e., amount of medication; see the following list).

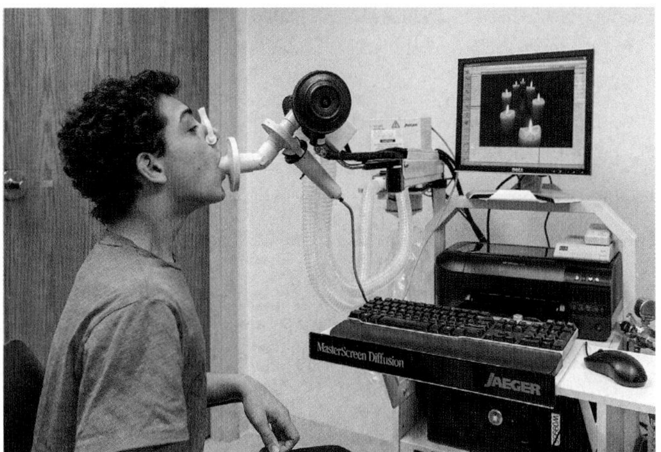

FIGURE 49-6 Boy having PFTs measured. Note the good seal around the mouth and the screen with candles to be blown out for motivational purposes. (*Used with permission from John Carl, MD.*)

Additional tests that may be useful include:[3]

- Pulmonary function testing if a diagnosis of restrictive lung disease or vocal cord dysfunction is considered.
- Bronchoprovocation (using methacholine, histamine, cold air or exercise challenge) if spirometry is normal or near-normal and asthma is still suspected; a negative test is helpful in ruling out asthma.
- Pulse oximetry or arterial blood gas if hypoxia is suspected (e.g., cyanosis, rapid or respiratory rate).
- In preschool-aged children, consider allergen sensitization, increased IgE levels, or presence of blood eosinophilia to help in establishing a diagnosis of asthma.[21] In the PARIS birth cohort study, the risk of severe wheeze was increased in infants having eosinophilia (OR 1.76, 95% CI 1.21 to 2.49) or being sensitized to ≥2 allergens (OR 1.88; 95% CI 1.13 to 3.14).[14]
- The fraction of exhaled nitric oxide (FENO), a biomarker for eosinophilic airway inflammation, has also been used to detect future uncontrolled asthma in patients on corticosteroids.[22] In addition, in a post-hoc analysis, daily FENO (performed at home) was shown to increase before moderate (but not severe) exacerbations in children with asthma.[23]

IMAGING

A CXR is not useful for diagnosis but is helpful for excluding other diseases (e.g., pneumonia) or identifying comorbidity (e.g., heart failure).

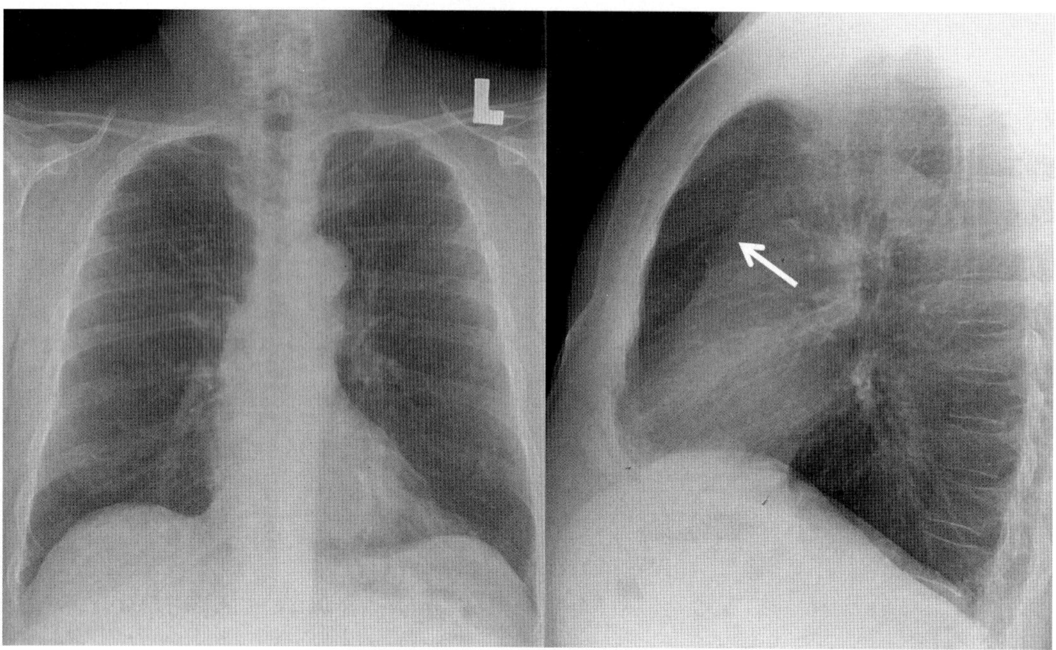

FIGURE 49-7 Acute asthma exacerbation with increased lung volumes on chest x-ray. The lateral projection reveals enlargement of the retrosternal clear space (*arrow*). (*Used with permission from Carlos Santiago Restrepo, MD.*)

The main finding on CXR is hyperinflation (occurring in about 45% of patients with asthma).[4] Hyperinflation is manifested by the following:

- Lung hyperexpansion and abnormal lucency (**Figure 49-7**).
- Increased AP diameter.
- Increased retrosternal air space (**Figure 49-8**).
- Infracardiac air.
- Low-set flattened diaphragms (best assessed in lateral chest) (**Figure 49-7**).
- Vertical heart (**Figure 49-7**).

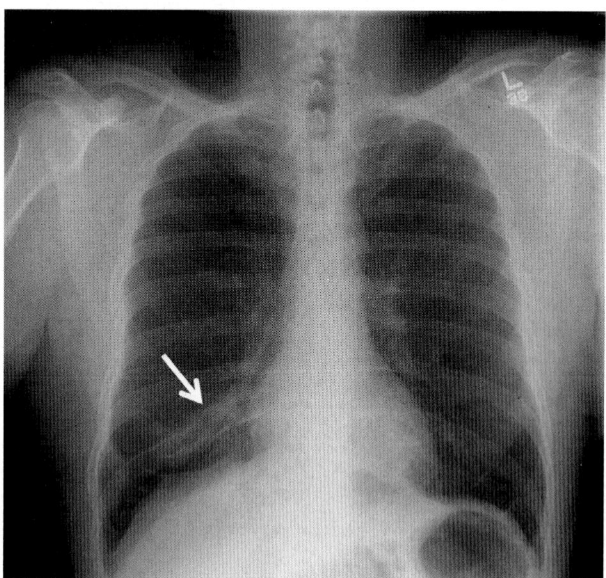

FIGURE 49-8 Acute asthma exacerbation in a young man. Frontal chest radiograph demonstrates increased lung volumes and ill-defined opacity in the right infrahilar region consistent with middle lobe segmental atelectasis (*arrow*). (*Used with permission from Carlos Santiago Restrepo, MD.*)

- Atelectasis is another finding seen during acute severe episodes (**Figure 49-8**).

DIFFERENTIAL DIAGNOSIS

The differential diagnosis of an infant or child with wheezing includes:[3]

- Upper airway disease (e.g., allergic rhinitis, sinusitis)—Exam or imaging helps differentiate.
- Airway obstruction (foreign body, vascular rings, vocal cord dysfunction, tracheal stenosis, enlarged lymph node or tumor, infection, cystic fibrosis, or heart disease)—Imaging helps differentiate.
- Other causes such as recurrent cough or reflux. Cough-variant asthma (only cough) occurs especially in young children.
- Rarely, cardiac causes such as shunts, outflow obstruction, coronary artery disease, and cardiomyopathy can cause exertional dyspnea; electrocardiography and echocardiography can help distinguish these causes.[24]
- Asthma may occur in conjunction with these conditions.

MANAGEMENT

NAEP outlines four components of care: assessment and monitoring, provision of education, control of environmental factors and comorbid conditions, and use of medications.[3] The goals of asthma therapy are twofold:[3]

- Reduce impairment—Prevent chronic symptoms, require infrequent (<= twice weekly) use of rescue inhaler, maintain near normal pulmonary function, maintain normal activity levels, meet patient and family expectations, and satisfaction with care.

- Reduce risk—Prevent recurrent exacerbations and minimize need for emergency or hospital care, prevent loss of lung function (for children, prevent reduced lung growth), and provide optimal pharmacotherapy while minimizing side effects and adverse effects.

In the future, it may be possible to better tailor therapy to asthma phenotype, based on a child's clinical signs and use of health care resources. Three phenotypes have been recently described—mild, nonatopic severe, and severe atopic.[25] In this study conducted during the 18-month examination (N = 1831), most children (69.4%) had a low prevalence respiratory symptoms or allergy followed by a group of 306 (16.7%) with a mild phenotype, 195 (11%) with nonatopic severe phenotype, including 88 percent of the children with recurrent wheezing, and atopic severe (N = 59 [3.2%]), including 78 percent with atopic dermatitis and 61 percent with allergic sensitization; in the latter group, 49 children also had wheezing.

NONPHARMACOLOGIC

- Exercise should be encouraged. In a randomized clinical trial (RCT) of aerobic exercise in patients with persistent asthma, the group randomized to exercise showed significant improvements in physical limitations, frequency of symptoms, health-related quality of life, number of asthma-symptom-free days, and anxiety and depression levels over the control group (education and breathing exercises only).[26]
- For patients exposed to secondhand smoke in the home, use of high-efficiency, particulate-arresting (HEPA) air cleaners was shown in one RCT to decrease unscheduled asthma visits for children ages 6 to 12 years; there was no difference between groups in parent-reported symptoms.[27]
- Dietary changes may also be useful. In a cross-sectional study of children, greater adherence to a Mediterranean-type diet was associated with a lower prevalence of asthma symptoms.[28]
- Provide patient education. SOR Ⓐ Pediatric asthma education was shown in a meta-analysis to reduce mean number of hospitalizations and emergency department (ED) visits and the odds of an emergency department visit for asthma;[29] there was no influence of education on the odds of hospitalization or mean number of urgent physician visits. Reduction in hospital and ED visits and missed work/school has also been shown for self-management education with written asthma action plans and physician review.[4]
    - In several RCTs of adolescents, peer-led asthma education was associated with more positive attitudes at 6 months,[30] greater improvements in quality of life,[30,31] and greater self-efficacy to resist smoking and knowledge of asthma self-management.[31]
    - In another study, a school-based program for primarily minority race high school students resulted in greater confidence in managing asthma, more preventive steps taken, greater use of controller medication and written treatment plans, and improved control (e.g., fewer night awakenings, days with activity limitation, school absences); in addition, there were fewer asthma acute care visits, ED visits, and hospitalizations.[32] Authors of a meta-analysis of school-based asthma education programs, however, found consistent results demonstrating improved asthma knowledge, self-efficacy, and self-management behaviors but fewer studies showing reduced symptoms days (5 of 11 studies), reduced nights with symptoms (2 of 4 studies), and school absences (5 of 17 studies).[33]

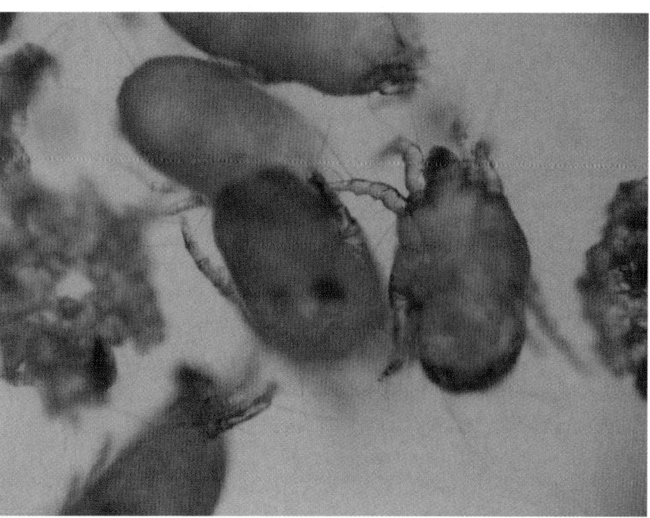

FIGURE 49-9 Dust mites under the microscope. Dust mites are a common allergen for patients who suffer from asthma and allergic rhinitis. Environmental control to minimize dust mite exposure can help control asthma for some individuals. (*Used with permission from Richard P. Usatine, MD.*)

- Consider interventions to control home environmental triggers; comprehensive individual programs may reduce symptom days.[4] SOR Ⓑ
    - Many people who have asthma are allergic to dust mites (**Figure 49-9**). Two relatively easy interventions to decrease dust mite exposure are: encase pillows and mattresses in special dust-mite proof covers and wash the sheets and blankets on the bed each week in hot water.[3]
    - Other suggestions for reducing environmental triggers can be found in the NAEP reference.[5]

MEDICATIONS

To determine appropriate medication management, assess severity based on symptoms, medication usage, exacerbations, and lung function (as discussed in Laboratory Testing). For children, severity is usually assessed through symptoms, night-time awakenings, interference with normal activity, and lung function; the latter if over age 4 years. Children are also categorized as controlled, not-well controlled, or very poorly controlled with steps of care associated with each category. Several charts for children are available in the NAEP reference to facilitate these assessments and include treatment protocols by age group divided into 6 steps of care as described in the following:[5]

- **Step 1:** For all aged patients with intermittent asthma, an inhaled short-acting beta-2 agonist (SABA) is recommended. SOR Ⓐ Metered dose inhalers with spacers are at least as effective (with fewer side effects) as nebulized treatment for most patients.
- **Step 2:** Low-dose inhaled corticosteroids (ICS) are the preferred long-term control therapy for all ages with persistent asthma. SOR Ⓐ Alternatives for young children (ages 0 to 4 years) include cromolyn inhaler and montelukast and for older children (ages 5 to 11 years) cromolyn, leukotriene receptor antagonist (LTRA), nedocromil, or theophylline
    - LTRAs are less effective than ICS but better than placebo.[5] SOR Ⓐ
    - In a RCT of preschool-aged children with recurrent wheezing (N = 278), intermittent budesonide inhalation suspension (1 mg twice daily for 7 days, starting early during a predefined

respiratory tract illness) was as effective as a daily low-dose regimen (0.5 mg nightly) in preventing acute exacerbations (about 1 fewer per patient-year) while reducing mean exposure to budesonide.[34]

- **Step 3:** For children ages 0 to 4 years not well controlled on low dose ICS, medium dose ICS is recommended. For children over age 4 years, combination low-dose ICS and long-acting beta-2 agonist (LABA) or medium-dose ICS are equally preferred options.[5] SOR Ⓐ Alternatives include low-dose ICS plus LTRA (less effective than ICS and LABA), theophylline, or zileuton. Theophylline requires monitoring serum concentration levels. Zileuton is less desirable due to limited supporting data and need to monitor liver function. Authors of a Cochrane review found the combination ICS/LABA modestly more effective in reducing the risk of exacerbations requiring oral corticosteroids than higher dose ICS for adolescents and adults, but a trend toward increased risks of exacerbation and hospitalization among children.[35]
    - For patients ages 4 years and younger, low-dose ICS and LABA can be used followed by increasing ICS dose if persistent low lung function and >2 days per week of impairment;[5] ICS/LABA combination may not reduce exacerbations but appears to improve PEF and growth.[36] Although serious asthma-related events (asthma-related deaths, intubations, and hospitalizations) attributable to LABAs appear to be greatest among children, in a meta-analysis there was no statistically significant difference in serious events by age group for the subgroup on both ICS and LABA.[37]
    - One trial of step-up therapy for children with not-well controlled persistent asthma on ICS found that although combination ICS/LABA was most likely to result in a best response, some children had a best response to doubling ICS or combination ICS/ LTRA.[38] In a systematic review of medium (300-400 μg/d) vs. low dose (200 μg/d or less) steroids in children with mild-moderate persistent asthma, although medium dose steroids provided a small but significant improvement in FEV1 (mean difference 0.11 [95% CI, 0.01 to 0.21), there were no differences in any other outcome (e.g., symptom scores).[39]
- **Step 4:** For children with poorly controlled asthma, combination medium-dose ICS and LABA are recommended along with consultation with an asthma specialist. Alternatives are combination medium-dose ICS plus LTRA (or theophylline or zileuton in older children).
- **Step 5:** Combination high-dose ICS and LABA.
- **Step 6:** Combination high-dose ICS and LABA plus oral corticosteroid. For children presenting to the ED with moderate or severe asthma, investigators of an observational study (N = 406) found early administration of systemic corticosteroids reduced the odds of admission by 0.4 (95% confidence interval 0.2 to 0.7) and the length of active treatment by 0.7 hours (95% confidence interval −1.3 to −0.8 hours), with no significant effect on relapse.[40]

Other drug options:

- Omalizumab can be considered for patients over 11 years of age who have allergies.[3] In a RCT with inner-city children, adolescents, and young adults (N = 419) with persistent asthma, omalizumab reduced symptom days and the proportion of subjects who had one or more exacerbations (30.3% versus 48.8% on placebo).[41]
- To assist with smoking cessation, consider nicotine replacement therapy (bupropion [150 mg, twice daily], varenicline [1 mg twice daily], nortriptyline [75–100 mg daily], or nicotine replacement [gum, inhaler, spray, patch]), and supportive counseling and follow-up; using these interventions improves rates of smoking cessation by up to twofold.[42–44] SOR Ⓐ
- In patients with persistent asthma attributed to allergies, consider allergy immunotherapy.[5] SOR Ⓑ One meta-analysis concluded that specific immunotherapy for patients with positive skin tests resulted in a reduction in need for increased medications (number needed to treat = 5) and another study in patients with high IgE found immunotherapy reduced exacervations.[4]
- The use of proton-pump inhibitor therapy is not likely to add significant benefit.[45] Among children with uncontrolled asthma on ICS but without gastrointestinal reflux symptoms, the addition of a lansoprazole (versus placebo) resulted in no improvement in symptoms or lung function but increased adverse events.[46]

For patients with an *exacerbation* of asthma, SABAs and sometimes oral corticosteroids are used for home management of patients with a mild exacerbation (dyspnea with activity, PEF >=70 percent predicted or personal best) following their action plan. NAEP does not recommend doubling the dose of ICS for home management versus oral steroids for exacerbations.[3] A Cochrane review concluded that a short course of oral steroids was effective in reducing the number of relapses to additional care, hospitalizations, and use of SABA without an apparent increase in side effects.[47]

- Moderate exacerbation (dyspnea interferes with usually activity, PEF 40% to 69% predicted or personal best)—Usually requires office or ED visit; SABA and oral corticosteroids (typically 40–60 mg prednisone for adults and 1-2 mg/kg/day of prednisolone liquid in two divided doses) are recommended for 3 to 10 days. SOR Ⓐ SABA can be administered every 20 minutes as needed and the addition of inhaled ipratropium bromide may reduce the need for hospitalization (0.68–0.75).[4] SOR Ⓐ Symptoms usually abate in 1 to 2 days.
- Severe exacerbation (dyspnea at rest, PEF <40% predicted or personal best)—Usually requires ED visit and hospitalization likely; combination SABA/anticholinergic nebulized treatment hourly or continuously as needed, oral corticosteroids, adjunctive treatment as needed (see the following bullet). Symptoms last for >3 days after treatment begins.
- Life-threatening exacerbation (too dyspneic to speak, diaphoresis, PEF <25% predicted or personal best)—ED/hospitalization, consider intensive care unit; SABA/anticholinergic, intravenous corticosteroids, and adjunctive therapies.
- Oxygen therapy—Use to correct hypoxia in patients with moderate to life-threatening exacerbations; maintain O_2 saturation above 90 percent.[3,4] SOR Ⓒ
- Consider intravenous magnesium sulfate or heliox-driven albuterol nebulization if severe exacerbation and unresponsive to treatment after initial assessments.
- Monitor response to treatment with serial assessments of FEV1 or PEF. Pulse oximetry may be useful in children for assessing initial severity—A result <92–94 percent after 1 hour is an indication for hospitalization.[3]

- Patients with severe or life-threatening exacerbation unresponsive to initial treatments may require intubation and mechanical ventilation. Drowsiness may be a symptom of impending respiratory failure.
- The following should not be used as they have no supporting evidence and may delay effective treatment: drinking large volumes of liquids; breathing warm, moist air; using nonprescription products, such as antihistamines or cold remedies, and pursed-lip and other forms of breathing.[3] In addition, NAEP does not recommend use of methylxanthines, antibiotics (except as needed for comorbid conditions), aggressive hydration, chest physical therapy, mucolytics, or sedation in the ED or hospital setting.[3]

REFERRAL

- Consider referral to an asthma specialist if signs and symptoms are atypical, there are problems in assessing other diagnoses, or if additional specialized testing is needed.
- Referral or consultation should aalso be considered if there are difficulties achieving or maintaining control of asthma, if the patient required >2 bursts of oral systemic corticosteroids in 1 year or has an exacerbation requiring hospitalization, or if immunotherapy or omalizumab is considered.[3]
- Consultation with an asthma specialist should be conducted for patients with persistent asthma requiring step 4 care or higher and considered if a patient requires step 3 care.[3]

PREVENTION AND SCREENING

- Smoking cessation and avoidance of second-hand smoking, limiting occupational exposures, and exposure to indoor air pollution may be preventive.
- In the Danish National Birth Cohort, maternal intake of peanuts and tree nuts during pregnancy was inversely associated with asthma in children at 18 months (OR 0.79 95% CI, 0.65 to 0.97 OR 0.75; 95 percent CI, 0.67 to 0.84, respectively).[48]
- Breastfeeding protects against asthma, especially among children with atopy; in one study, in children with atopy, exclusive breastfeeding for 3 or more months reduced current asthma at ages 4 to 6 years by more than 50 percent.[49]
- Influenza and pneumococcal vaccination are recommended.[3] SOR B
- Despite limited data, vitamins A, D, and E; zinc; fruits and vegetables; and a Mediterranean diet may be useful for the prevention of asthma.[50] In addition, raw cow's milk consumption appears protective (adjusted OR, 0.59; 95% CI, 0.46 to 0.74).[51]

PROGNOSIS

- More than half of children with asthma will no longer have symptoms by age 6 years.[4]
- In a meta-analysis, maternal asthma was associated with an increased risk of low birthweight (RR, 1.46; 95% CI 1.22 to 1.75), small for gestational age (RR, 1.22; 95% CI 1.14 to 1.31), preterm delivery (RR, 1.41; 95% CI 1.22 to 1.61) and pre-eclampsia (RR, 1.54; 95% CI 1.32 to 1.81).[52] The RR of preterm delivery and preterm labor became nonsignificant by active asthma management. Pregnancy does not appear to increase asthma severity, provided women continue to use their prescribed medications.[53]
- Among children, factors predictive of an asthma exacerbation include bronchiolitis or pneumonia during infancy, maternal eczema, paternal history of hay fever, asthma symptoms ≥3 months/year, more than four scheduled physician visits for asthma in the previous year, and use of certain medications (SABAs, antiinflammatory medications, and one or more courses of oral steroids) in the prior year.[36] A 17-item checklist assessing asthma symptoms, use of medications and health care services, and history has been demonstrated to be helpful for identifying children at high or low-risk for asthma exacerbations.[54]
- For patients with an asthma exacerbation, the following factors place a patient at higher risk of asthma-related death; these patients should be advised to seek medical care early during an exacerbation:[3]
    - Previous severe exacerbation (e.g., intubation or ICU admission for asthma).
    - Two or more hospitalizations or >3 ED visits in the past year.
    - Use of >2 canisters of SABA per month.
    - Difficulty perceiving airway obstruction or the severity of worsening asthma.
    - Low socioeconomic status or inner-city resident.

FOLLOW-UP

- Many patients have asthma that is not well controlled. In a cross-sectional study of 29 pediatric practices (N = 2429), 46 percent reported uncontrolled asthma (defined as a Childhood Asthma Control Test (C-ACT) or the Asthma Control Test (ACT)<or = 19).[55] One of the new aspects of the NAEP 2007 guideline is the focus on monitoring asthma severity and control, the latter defined as the degree to which manifestations of asthma are minimized by therapeutic interventions and the therapy goals are met.
- At each visit, ask about frequency and intensity of symptoms and functional limitations currently or recently experienced (impairment). A self-assessment sheet for follow-up visits is available in the NAEP document and a simple symptom checklist can be downloaded from **http://www.qvar.com/asthma/asthma-symptoms-checklist.aspx**. SOR C
- In addition, at each visit, assess the likelihood of either asthma exacerbations, progressive decline in lung function (or lung growth for children) or risk of medication adverse effects. A patient self-assessment sheet rating asthma control (e.g., symptoms or PEF) and medication use is available in the NAEP reference.[3] Provision of a visually standardized, interpreted peak flow graph to assist in understanding when to add medication or contact a health provider may reduce need for oral steroids and urgent care visits.[56]
- For patients on medications, monitor treatment effectiveness ("have you noticed a difference, for example less breathlessness") and side effects. Observe inhaler technique at least once to ensure optimal delivery.
- For smokers, encourage cessation.

- Document exacerbations/hospitalizations—This may indicate a need for additional treatment.
- Monitor for comorbidities (e.g., heart disease, chronic lung disease) and maximize control of those conditions.
- Measurement of fractional nitric oxide (NO) concentration in exhaled breath (Fe(NO)) is a quantitative, noninvasive method of measuring airway inflammation.[57] It is under investigation as a complementary tool to other ways of assessing airways disease, including asthma.
- Post-hospital discharge management was investigated in a recent before and after study of implementing the Joint Commission's three Children's Asthma Care (CAC) measures in a tertiary care children's hospital.[58] The measures were (1) percentage of patients who received beta agonists, (2) percentage of patients who received systemic steroids during their hospital stay, and (3) percentage of patient's discharged with a home management care plan including quick reliever and controller drugs, follow-up appointment, environmental or other trigger control, and a written action plan. Compliance with the first two measures was extremely high before and after (99% versus 100%, CAC-1; 100% versus. 100%, CAC-2) but compliance with the third measure increased from 0 to 87 percent. There was an associated small but significant decrease in readmissions from an average of 17 to 12 percent post implementation.

For patients who appear well controlled, step-down therapy can be considered. Authors of one study found that although daily ICS was associated with the lowest rates of exacerbations (28%) and treatment failure (2.8%), no daily medication with rescue albuterol and ICS was a reasonable alternative (exacerbations 35%, treatment failure 8.5%) and did not affect linear growth (versus 1.1 cm less).[59] Combined rescue performed better than albuterol rescue alone.

PATIENT EDUCATION

- Smoking cessation should be strongly and repeatedly encouraged; passive smoking can trigger asthma exacerbations.[60] Exercise should also be encouraged along with weight loss, if obese, or maintenance of a healthy weight.
- The NAEP suggests that key educational messages include basic facts about asthma, the role of medications (i.e., rescue/short-term vs. control/long-term), and patient skills (e.g., correct inhaler technique, self-monitoring).
- Creation of an asthma action plan can be helpful in promoting self-management and greater understanding of warning signs of worsening asthma. An example of an action plan can be found in the NAEP document.[3] Asthma action plans usually use three zones, similar to traffic lights, with green zone representing good control (e.g., few symptoms, PEF 80% to 100%), yellow zone representing worsening or not well-controlled asthma (e.g., mild to moderate symptoms, PEF 50% to 80%), and red zone representing an alert or warning (severe symptoms, PEF $<50\%$) with advice to seek emergency care if not better after 15 minutes of rescue medication use and unable to reach their care provider. Each zone contains instructions for management, which the primary care provider can modify.

PATIENT RESOURCES

For general information, these sites are helpful:

- American Lung Association—**www.lung.org/lung-disease/asthma/**.
- National Library of Medicine—**www.nlm.nih.gov/medlineplus/asthma.html**.

PROVIDER RESOURCES

- National Asthma Education and Prevention Program—**www.nhlbi.nih.gov/guidelines/asthma/asthsumm.pdf**.
- Centers for Disease Control and Prevention—**www.cdc.gov/nchs/fastats/asthma.htm**.

REFERENCES

1. Centers for Disease Control and Prevention. Asthma in the US. Available at http://www.cdc.gov/VitalSigns/Asthma/index.html, accessed December 2012.
2. Tsai CL, Lee WY, Hanania NA, Camargo CA Jr: Age-related differences in clinical outcomes for acute asthma in the United States, 2006-2008. *J Allergy Clin Immunol*. 2012;129(5):1252-1258.
3. Karaca-Mandic P, Jena AB, Joyce GF, Goldman DP. Out-of-pocket medication costs and use of medications and health care services among children with asthma. *JAMA*. 2012;307(12):1284-1291.
4. Bacharier LB, Cohen R, Schweiger T, et al. Determinants of asthma after severe respiratory syncytial virus bronchiolitis. *J Allergy Clin Immunol*. 2012;130(1):91-100.
5. National Asthma Education and Prevention Program Expert Panel Report 3 (2007). Available at http://www.nhlbi.nih.gov/guidelines/asthma/asthsumm.pdf, accessed February 2012.
6. Roett MA, Gillespie C. Asthma. In: Sloane PD, Slatt LM, Ebell MH, Smith MA, Power D, Viera AJ, eds. *Essential of Family Medicine*. Philadelphia, PA: Lippincott Williams & Wilkins; 2011: 607-623.
7. Schauberger EM, Ewart SL, Arshad SH, et al. Identification of ATPAF1 as a novel candidate gene for asthma in children. *J Allergy Clin Immunol*. 2011;128(4):753-760.
8. Bisgaard H, Jensen SM, Bønnelykke K. Interaction between asthma and lung function growth in early life. *Am J Respir Crit Care Med*. 2012;185(11):1183-1190.
9. Arshad SH, Kurukulaaratchy RJ, Fenn M, Matthews S. Early life risk factors for current wheeze, asthma, and bronchial hyperresponsiveness at 10 years of age. *Chest*. 2005;127(2):502-508.
10. Beasley RW, Clayton TO, Crane J, et al. Acetaminophen use and risk of asthma, rhinoconjunctivitis, and eczema in adolescents: International Study of Asthma and Allergies in Childhood Phase Three. *Am J Respir Crit Care Med*. 2011;183(2):171-178.
11. Holgate ST. The acetaminophen enigma in asthma. *Am J Respir Crit Care Med*. 2011;183(2):147-151.
12. Reponen T, Lockey J, Bernstein DI, et al. Infant origins of childhood asthma associated with specific molds. *J Allergy Clin Immunol*. 2012;130(3):639-644.

13. Arvaniti F, Priftis KN, Papadimitriou A, et al. Salty-snack eating, television or video-game viewing, and asthma symptoms among 10- to 12-year-old children: the PANACEA study. *J Am Diet Assoc.* 2011;111(2):251-257.

14. Herr M, Just J, Nikasinovic L, et al. Influence of host and environmental factors on wheezing severity in infants: findings from the PARIS birth cohort. *Clin Exp Allergy*. 2012;42(2):275-283.

15. Chipps BE, Zeiger RS, Borish L, et al. Key findings and clinical implications from The Epidemiology and Natural History of Asthma: Outcomes and Treatment Regimens (TENOR) study. *J Allergy Clin Immunol*. 2012;130(2):332-342.

16. Darrow LA, Hess J, Rogers CA, et al. Ambient pollen concentration and emergency department visits for asthma and wheeze. *J Allergy Clin Immunol*. 2012;130(3):630-638.

17. Kapoor R, Menon C, Hoffstad O, et al. The prevalence of atopic triad in children with physician-confirmed atopic dermatitis. *J Am Acad Dermatol*. 2008;58(1):66-73.

18. Hwang CY, Chen YJ, Lin MW, et al. Prevalence of atopic dermatitis, allergic rhinitis and asthma in Taiwan: a national study 2000-2007. *Acta Derm Venereol*. 2010;90(6):589-594.

19. Spergel JM. From atopic dermatitis to asthma. *Ann Allergy Asthma Immunol*. 2010;105(2):99-106.

20. Wildfire JJ, Gergen PJ, Sorkness CA, et al. Development and validation of the Composite Asthma Severity Index-an outcome measure for use in children and adolescents. *J Allergy Clin Immunol*. 2012;129(3):694-701.

21. Bacharier LB, Guilbert TW. Diagnosis and management of early asthma in preschool-aged children. *J Allergy Clin Immunol*. 2012; 130(2):287-296.

22. Zeiger RS, Schatz M, Zhang F, et al. Elevated exhaled nitric oxide is a clinical indicator of future uncontrolled asthma in asthmatic patients on inhaled corticosteroids. *J Allergy Clin Immunol*. 2011;128(2):412-414.

23. van der Valk R, Baraldi E, Stern G, et al. Daily exhaled nitric oxide measurements and asthma exacerbations in children. *Allergy*. 2012;67(2):265-271.

24. Jenkins C, Seccombe L, Tomlins R. Investigating asthma symptoms in primary care. *BMJ*. 2012;344:e2734.

25. Herr M, Just J, Nikasinovic L, et al. Risk factors and characteristics of respiratory and allergic phenotypes in early childhood. *J Allergy Clin Immunol*. 2012;130(2):389-396.

26. Mendes FA, Goncalves RC, Nunes MP, et al. Effects of aerobic training on psychosocial morbidity and symptoms in patients with asthma: a randomized clinical trial. *Chest*. 2010;138(2): 331-337.

27. Lanphear BP, Hornung RW, Khoury J, et al. Effects of HEPA air cleaners on unscheduled asthma visits and asthma symptoms for children exposed to secondhand tobacco smoke. *Pediatrics*. 2011; 127(1):93-101.

28. Arvaniti F, Priftis KN, Papadimitriou A, et al. Adherence to the Mediterranean type of diet is associated with lower prevalence of asthma symptoms, among 10–12 years old children: the PANACEA study. *Pediatr Allergy Immunol*. 2011;22(3):283-289.

29. Coffman JM, Cabana MD, Halpin HA, Yelin EH. Effects of asthma education on children's use of acute care services: a meta-analysis. Pediatrics. 2008;121(3):575-586.

30. Rhee H, Belyea MJ, Hunt JF, Brasch J. Effects of a peer-led asthma self-management program for adolescents. *Arch Pediatr Asolesc Med*. 2011;165(6):513-519.

31. Al-sheyab N, Gallagher R, Crisp J, Shah S. Peer-led education for adolescents with asthma in Jordan: a cluster-randomized controlled trial. *Pediatrics*. 2012;129(1):e106-112.

32. Bruzzese JM, Sheares BJ, Vincent EJ, et al. Effects of a school-based intervention for urban adolescents with asthma: a controlled trial. *Am J Respir Crit Care Med*. 2011;183(8):998-1006.

33. Coffman JM, Cabana MD, Yelin EH. Do school-based asthma education programs improve self-management and health outcomes? *Pediatrics*. 2009;124(2):729-742.

34. Zeiger RS, Mauger D, Bacharier LB, et al. Daily or intermittent budesonide in preschool children with recurrent wheezing. *N Engl J Med*. 2011;365(21):1990-2001.

35. Ducharme FM, Ni Chroinin M, Greenstone I, Lasserson TJ. Addition of long-acting beta2-agonists to inhaled steroids versus higher dose inhaled steroids in adults and children with persistent asthma. *Cochrane Database Syst Rev*. 2010;(4):CD004933.

36. Ni Chroinin M, Lasserson TJ, Greenstone I, Ducharme FM. Addition of long-acting beta-agonists to inhaled corticosteroids for chronic asthma in children. *Cochrane Database Syst Rev*. 2009;(3):CD007949.

37. McMahon AW, Levenson MS, McEvoy BW, et al. Age and risks of FDA-approved long-acting β_2-adrenergic receptor agonists. *Pediatrics*. 2011;128(5):e1147-1154.

38. Lemanske RF Jr, Mauger DT, Sorkness CA, et al. Step-up therapy for children with uncontrolled asthma receiving inhaled corticosteroids. *N Engl J Med*. 2010;362(11):975-985.

39. Zhang L, Axelsson I, Chung M, Lau J. Dose response of inhaled corticosteroids in children with persistent asthma: a systematic review. *Pediatrics*. 2011;127(1):129-138.

40. Bhogal SK, McGillivray D, Bourbeau J, et al. Early administration of systemic corticosteroids reduces hospital admission rates for children with moderate and severe asthma exacerbation. *Ann Emerg Med*. 2012;60(1):84-91.

41. Busse WW, Morgan WJ, Gergen PJ, et al. Randomized trial of omalizumab (anti-IgE) for asthma in inner-city children. *N Engl J Med*. 2011;364(11):1005-1015.

42. Hughes JR, Stead LF, Lancaster T. Antidepressants for smoking cessation. *Cochrane Database Syst Rev*. 2007;(1):CD000031.

43. Stead LF, Perera R, Bullen C, Mant D, Lancaster T. Nicotine replacement therapy for smoking cessation. *Cochrane Database Syst Rev*. 2008;(1):CD000146.

44. Stead LF, Bergson G, Lancaster T. Physician advice for smoking cessation. *Cochrane Database Syst Rev*. 2008;(2):CD000165.

45. Chan WW, Chiou E, Obstein KL, et al. The efficacy of proton pump inhibitors for the treatment of asthma in adults: a meta-analysis. *Ann Intern Med*. 2011;171(7):620-629.

46. Writing Committee for the American Lung Association Asthma Clinical Research Centers, Holbrook JT, Wise RA, Gold BD,

et al. Lansoprazole for children with poorly controlled asthma: a randomized controlled trial. *JAMA*. 2012;307(4):373-381.

47. Rowe BH, Spooner CH, Ducharme FM, et al. Corticosteroids for preventing relapse following acute exacerbations of asthma. *Cochrane Database Syst Rev*. 2007;(3):CD000195.

48. Maslova E, Granström C, Hansen S, et al. Peanut and tree nut consumption during pregnancy and allergic disease in children-should mothers decrease their intake? Longitudinal evidence from the Danish National Birth Cohort. *J Allergy Clin Immunol*. 2012;130(3):724-732.

49. Silvers KM, Frampton CM, Wickens K, et al. Breastfeeding protects against current asthma up to 6 years of age. *J Pediatr*. 2012;160(6):991-996.

50. Nurmatov U, Devereux G, Sheikh A. Nutrients and foods for the primary prevention of asthma and allergy: systematic review and meta-analysis. *J Allergy Clin Immunol*. 2011;127(3):724-733.e1-30.

51. Loss G, Apprich S, Waser M, et al. The protective effect of farm milk consumption on childhood asthma and atopy: the GABRIELA study. *J Allergy Clin Immunol*. 2011;128(4):766-773.e4.

52. Murphy VE, Namazy JA, Powell H, et al. A meta-analysis of adverse perinatal outcomes in women with asthma. *BJOG*. 2011; 118(11):1314-1323.

53. Belanger K, Hellenbrand ME, Holford TR, Bracken M. Effect of pregnancy on maternal asthma symptoms and medication use. *Obstet Gynecol*. 2010;115(3):499-567.

54. Forno E, Fuhlbrigge A, Soto-Quiros ME, et al. Risk factors and predictive clinical scores for asthma exacerbations in childhood. *Chest*. 2010;138(5):1156-1165.

55. Liu AH, Gilsenan AW, Stanford RH, et al. Status of asthma control in pediatric primary care: results from the pediatric Asthma Control Characteristics and Prevalence Survey Study (ACCESS). *J Pediatr*. 2010;157(2):276-281.

56. Janson SL, McGrath KW, Covington JK, et al. Objective airway monitoring improves asthma control in the cold and flu season: a cluster randomized trial. *Chest*. 2010;138(5):1148-1149.

57. Dweik RA, Boggs PB, Erzurum SC, et al. An official ATS clinical practice guideline: interpretation of exhaled nitric oxide levels (FENO) for clinical applications. *Am J Respir Crit Care Med*. 2011;184(5):602-615.

58. Fassl BA, Nkoy FL, Stone BL, et al. The Joint Commission Children's Asthma Care quality measures and asthma readmissions. *Pediatrics*. 130(3):482-491.

59. Martinez FD, Chinchilli VM, Morgan WJ, et al. Use of beclomethasone dipropionate as rescue treatment for children with mild persistent asthma (TREXA): a randomized, double-blind, placebo-controlled trial. *Lancet*. 2011;377(9766): 650-657.

60. Britton J. Passive smoking and asthma exacerbation. *Thorax*. 2005;60:794-795.

50 COMMUNITY-ACQUIRED PNEUMONIA

Mindy A. Smith, MD, MS

PATIENT STORY

Max is a 4-year-old boy who presents with a 2-day history of cough, fever, and chills. He tells you that his tummy hurts. On examination, he appears moderately ill and his breathing is rapid (about 55 breaths per minute); his oxygen saturation on room air is 94 percent. You hear decreased breath sounds and crackles on the left side of his chest and possibly on the right. You obtain a chest x-ray which is concerning for bacterial pneumonia. (**Figures 50-1** and **50-2**). You admit him to the hospital with a diagnosis of probable bacterial pneumonia and prescribe intravenous antibiotics. He improves considerably over 48 hours and is discharged home on oral antibiotics.

INTRODUCTION

Pneumonia refers to an infection in the lower respiratory tract (distal airways, alveoli, and interstitium of the lung). Community-acquired pneumonia (CAP) has traditionally referred to pneumonia occurring outside of the hospital setting. A subgroup of CAP that is associated with health care risk factors (e.g., prior hospitalization, dialysis, immunocompromised state) has been classified as health care-associated pneumonia.

CAP can be caused by a wide variety of viral, bacterial, and "atypical" pathogens. The age and immune status of the host are important in considering the potential causes and management of pneumonia in the pediatric population.

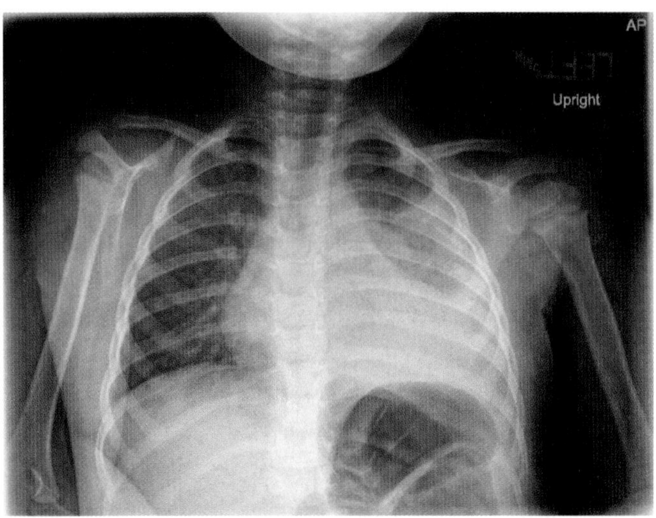

FIGURE 50-1 Left lower and partial left upper lobe consolidation and pleural effusion on PA chest x-ray in a 4-year-old child, concerning for bacterial pneumonia. (*Used with permission from Camille Sabella, MD*).

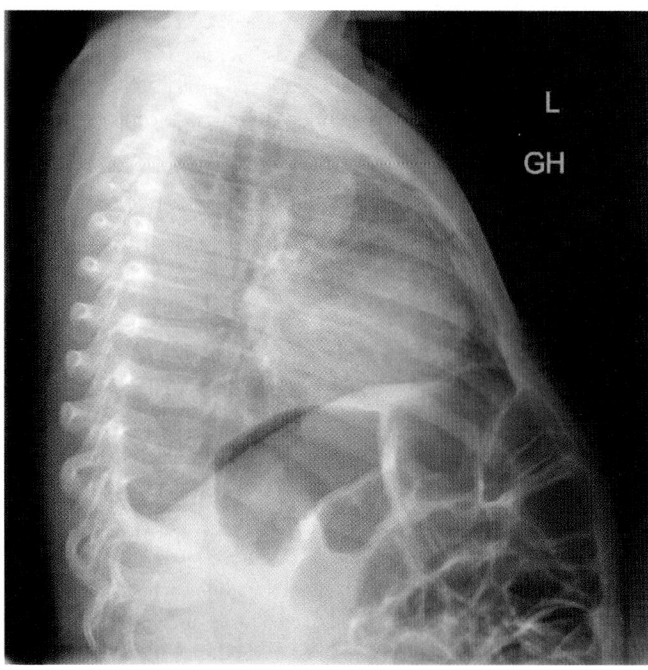

FIGURE 50-2 Lateral chest x-ray in the same child. (*Used with permission from Camille Sabella, MD.*)

EPIDEMIOLOGY

- The incidence rate of CAP among children in the first 5 years of life is 10 to 40 cases/1000,[1] with an incidence rate of 6 to 12 cases/1000 in children older than 9 years in North America.[2]
- In the National Hospital Discharge Survey (2006) of 1,232 first-listed pneumonia discharges from short-stay hospitals, 172 (14%) were children aged <15 years.[3]
- The distribution of the pneumococcal vaccine in 2000 has resulted in an approximately 35 percent decrease in all-cause pneumonia hospitalizations in US children since 1997–1999, with incident rates in 2005 and 2006 for children aged <2 years of 9.1/1,000 and 8.1/1,000, respectively.[4] For pneumococcal pneumonia, rates of hospitalizations between 1997–1999 and 2004 in an employer-based population study of children <age 2 years declined from 0.6 to 0.3 per 1000 children (57.6% decline) and rates of ambulatory visits declined from 1.7 to 0.9 per 1000 children (46.9% decline).
- CAP is the most frequent cause of death due to infectious disease in the US and the eighth leading cause of death overall (2007).[5,6]
- Deaths in 2009 from influenza and pneumonia occurred in 5.9/50,000 children <age 1 year, 0.9/50,000 for children aged 1 to 4 years, 0.6/50,000 for children aged 5 to 14 years and 1.0/50,000 for those aged 15 to 24 years.[7]

ETIOLOGY AND PATHOPHYSIOLOGY

- *Streptococcus (S) pneumoniae* is the most important pathogen at all ages.[8] Age, however, is an important consideration: in the first 20 days of life, most cases of pneumonia are secondary to Group B *Streptococci* or gram negative enteric bacteria while among young children with CAP, respiratory syncytial virus (RSV), influenza, and rhinovirus are common.[9] *Mycoplasma pneumoniae* and *Chlamydophila pneumoniae* are common in school-aged children and adolescents.[89] *Mycoplasma pneumoniae* is the single most common cause of CAP is school-aged children. Newly identified microbes in childhood pneumonia include human metapneumovirus, human bocavirus, and Simkania negevensis (an intracellular bacterium).[8]

- For children who are immunocompromised, other pathogens such as *Pneumocystis jiroveci* and *Mycobacterium tuberculosis* should be considered.[9]
- In a study of children hospitalized with CAP (N = 254), the cause of the disease (identified in 85% of cases) was most often viral (62%, with 30% having evidence of both viral and bacterial pathogens).[10] The most common identified pathogens were *S. pneumoniae* (37%), RSV (29%), and rhinovirus (24%). Dual bacterial infections were found in 19 patients; only one patient of 125 tested had a positive blood culture.
- In a retrospective study of children with unresponsive or recurrent CAP undergoing flexible bronchoscopy with bronchoalveolar lavage, an infectious agent was detected in the majority (76%) of cases with aerobic bacteria identified in about half including non-typeable *Haemophilus influenzae* (75%), *Moraxella catarrhalis* (28.9%), and *S. pneumoniae* (13.3%).[11]
- The most common route of infection is microaspiration of oropharyngeal secretions colonized by pathogens.[12] In this setting, *S. pneumoniae* and *Haemophilus influenza* are the most common pathogens.
- Pneumonia can also occur secondary to gross aspiration (postoperatively or in those with central nervous system disorders) where anaerobes and gram-negative bacilli are common pathogens.[12]
- Hematogenous spread, most often from the urinary tract, can result in *Escherichia coli* pneumonia and hematogenous spread from intravenous catheters or in the setting of endocarditis may cause *Staphylococcus aureus* pneumonia.[12]
- *Mycobacterium tuberculosis* (TB), fungi, *legionella,* and many respiratory viruses are spread by aerosolization.
- Etiology is unknown in up to 70 percent of cases of CAP.

RISK FACTORS[13,14]

Among children <5 years of age, risk factors include:

- History of recurrent respiratory infections during the past year (odds ratio [OR] 5.5) or previous chest infections (2.31; 95% confidence intervals [CI], 1.55–3.43).
- History of wheezing episodes (OR 5.3).
- History of otitis media and tympanocentesis before the age of 2 years (OR 3.6).
- Lower weight for height (OR 1.28; 95% CI, 1.10–1.51).
- Spending less time outside (1.96; 95% CI, 1.11–3.47).
- Mold in the child's bedroom (1.93, 95% CI, 1.24–3.02).

Among older children, risk factors include:

- History of recurrent respiratory infections during the previous year (OR 3.0).
- History of wheezing periods at any age (OR 2.1).

DIAGNOSIS

CLINICAL FEATURES

- Constellation of symptoms includes fever (88% to 96%), cough (76% to 88%), dyspnea (37% to 40%), chills, pleuritic chest pain, and sputum production.[8] Children may also complain of fatigue, myalgia, and headache.[9]
- Patients with viral or atypical pathogens (e.g., mycoplasma or chlamydia) often present with low-grade fever, nonproductive cough, and constitutional symptoms developing over several days.[9]
- About half of children report nonspecific signs like vomiting and abdominal pain.[8]
- Wheezing is most frequently associated with viral or atypical pathogens and bacterial infection is less likely when true wheezing is present.[9]
- Signs of pneumonia include increased respiratory rate, dullness to percussion, bronchial breathing, egophony, crackles, wheezes, and pleural-friction rub. Nonspecific crackles were reported in two recent Italian studies in 1/3 to half of children with CAP.[15,16] Lung findings in atypical pneumonia may be more diffuse. Pleural effusion is common and appears to increase the risk of a bacterial etiology.[9]
- In one emergency department case series of children >12 months of age with suspected pneumonia, respiratory rates >50 breaths per minute and oxygen saturation below 96 percent had a high specificity (97%) for predicting radiographic evidence of pneumonia.[17] In another study, tachypnea was present in 50 percent to 80 percent of pediatric radiologically-confirmed CAP cases.[18]
- Signs of respiratory distress in children include tachypnea (defined as age 0 to 2 months: >60 breaths per minute, age 2 to 12 months: >50 breaths per minute, age 1–5 years: >40 breaths per minute, and age >5 years: >20 breaths per minute), apnea, altered mental status, dyspnea, grunting, nasal flaring, pulse oximetry <90 percent on room air or retractions.[19]

LABORATORY STUDIES[12]

- Routine complete blood count (CBC) and acute phase reactants (e.g., erythrocyte sedimentation rate, C-reactive protein, procalcitonin) are not necessary for children with suspected CAP managed as outpatients but should be considered for children with more serious disease, if deemed useful.[19] SOR Ⓒ
- In one RCT of hospitalized children with CAP, use of procalcitonin (admission level <0.25 ng/mL) reduced antibiotic prescriptions (85.8% versus 100%).[20]
- Acute phase reactants should not be used as the sole determinant for distinguishing between viral and bacterial CAP.[19] SOR Ⓐ
- CBC should be obtained in children hospitalized for severe pneumonia (interpreted in the context of other tests).[19] SOR Ⓒ
- Sputum culture and gram stain should be obtained in hospitalized children who can produce sputum.[19] SOR Ⓒ Tracheal aspirates for gram stain, culture, and viral pathogens (as appropriate) should be obtained at the time of initial endotracheal tube placement in children requiring mechanical ventilation.[19] SOR Ⓒ

- Blood cultures are not recommended routinely for nontoxic, fully immunized children with CAP managed in the outpatient setting.[19] SOR Ⓑ In developing the microbial testing strategy for the Pneumonia Etiology Research for Child Health (PERCH) study, investigators found that only 1 percent to 5 percent of children with CAP have documented bloodstream infections; prevalence is higher among children with severe infection.[21]
- Blood cultures should be obtained in children who fail to demonstrate clinical improvement and in those who have progressive symptoms or clinical deterioration after initiation of antibiotics.[19] SOR Ⓑ
- Blood cultures are recommended for children requiring hospitalization for presumed bacterial CAP that is moderate to severe, particularly those with complicated pneumonia.[19] SOR Ⓒ
- Sensitive and specific tests for the rapid diagnosis of influenza virus and other respiratory viruses should be used in the evaluation of children with CAP.[19] A positive influenza test may decrease both the need for additional diagnostic studies and antibiotic use, while guiding appropriate use of antiviral agents in both outpatient and inpatient settings.[19] SOR Ⓐ Serology (fourfold rise in IgM titer) may also be useful in diagnosing *Mycoplasma pneumoniae*, *Chlamydophilaia pneumoniae*, legionnaires, and other viral pneumonia.[19] SOR Ⓒ
- Urinary antigen detection tests are not recommended for the diagnosis of pneumococcal pneumonia in children, as false-positive tests are common.[19] SOR Ⓐ
- Pulse oximetry should be performed in patients with pneumonia and suspected hypoxemia. The presence of hypoxemia should guide decisions regarding site of care and further diagnostic testing.[19] SOR Ⓑ

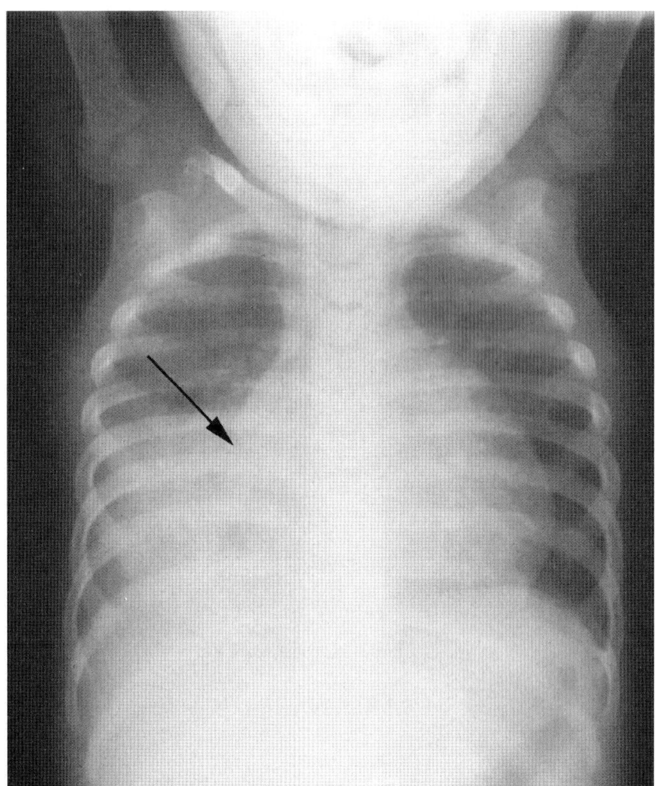

FIGURE 50-3 Right middle lobe infiltrate in an infant with bacterial pneumonia. Note the obliteration of the right heart border (arrow) characteristic of a right middle lobe process. (*Used with permission from Camille Sabella, MD.*)

IMAGING

- Routine chest x-ray (CXR) is not necessary for the confirmation of suspected CAP in children treated in the outpatient setting.[19] SOR Ⓐ
- CXR, posteroanterior and lateral, should be obtained in patients with suspected or documented hypoxemia, significant respiratory distress, those who failed initial antibiotic therapy, and hospitalized patients.[19] SOR Ⓑ
- In one RCT in Pakistan of treatment of CAP in young children (2 to 59 months), CXRs were normal in most children (82%) with a clinical diagnosis of pneumonia.[22]
- There are four general patterns of pneumonia seen on CXR;[12] however, they do not differentiate causative agents in CAP[19]:
    - Lobar—Consolidation involves the entire lobe (**Figures 50-1** to **50-5**). Early, especially with pneumococcal pneumonia in children, infiltrates can appear as round and can be mistaken for a pulmonary or mediastinal mass (**Figures 50-6** and **50-7**).[23] In young children, the thymic shadow can be mistaken as a pneumonic infiltrate (**Figure 50-8**).
    - Bronchopneumonia—Patchy involvement of one or several lobes that may be extensive, usually in the dependent lower and posterior lungs. Although bilateral patchy infiltrate with hilar lymphadenopathy are commonly associated with atypical pneumonia, lobar consolidation is not uncommon (**Figures 50-9** to **50-11**).
    - Interstitial pneumonia—Inflammatory process involves the interstitium and is usually patchy and diffuse (**Figure 50-12**). Viral pneumonia in children often appears radiographically as parihilar

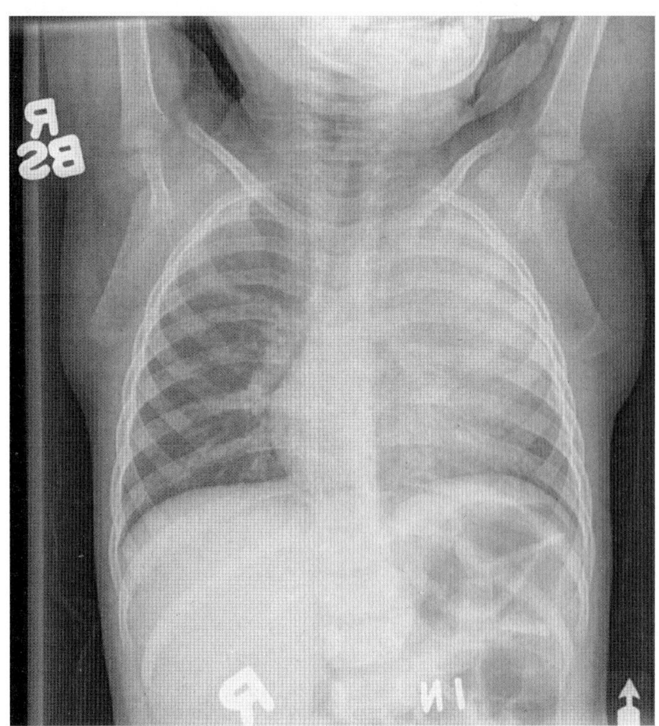

FIGURE 50-4 Left upper lobe consolidation on PA chest x-ray in a 1-year-old infant. (*Used with permission from Camille Sabella, MD.*)

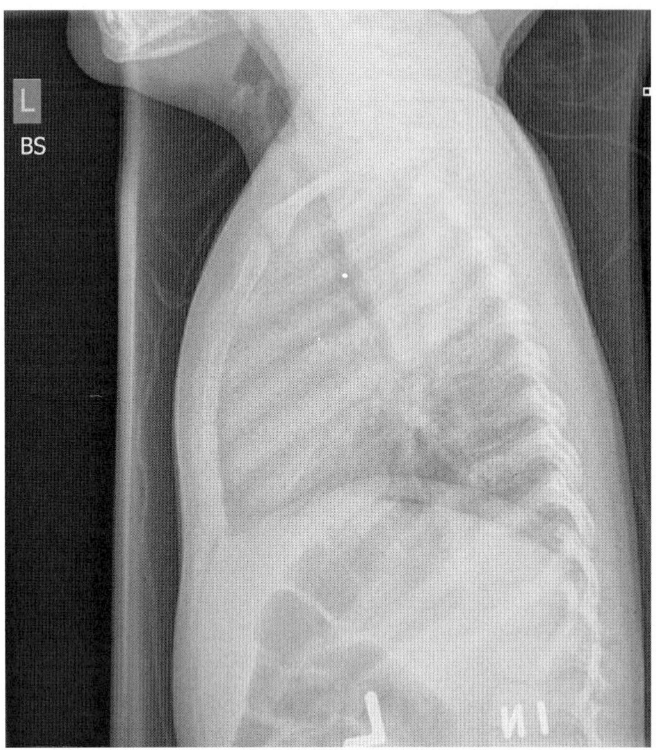

FIGURE 50-5 Left upper lobe consolidation on lateral chest x-ray in the same infant as previous figure 50-4. (*Used with permission from Camille Sabella, MD.*)

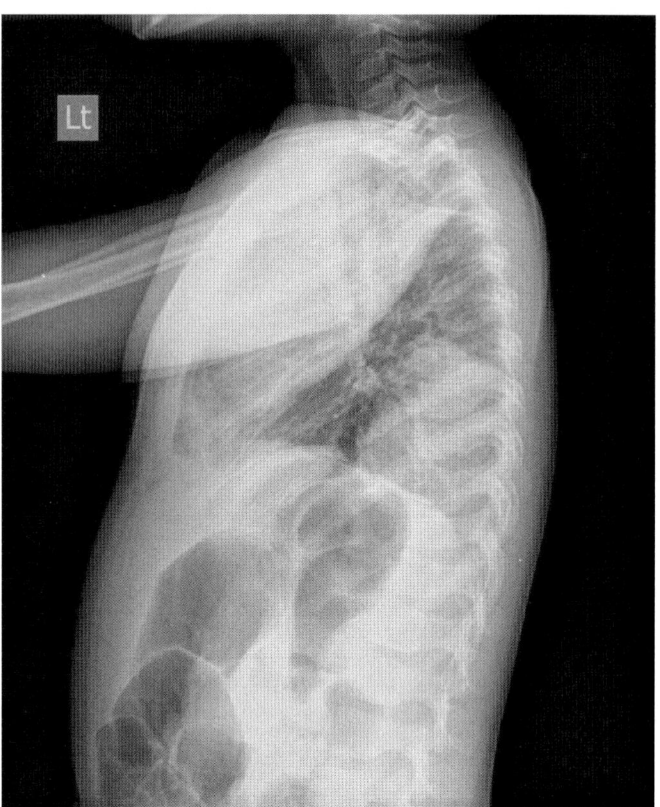

FIGURE 50-7 Pneumonia involving the right upper lobe on lateral chest x-ray in the same girl as previous figure 50-6. (*Used with permission from Camille Sabella, MD.*)

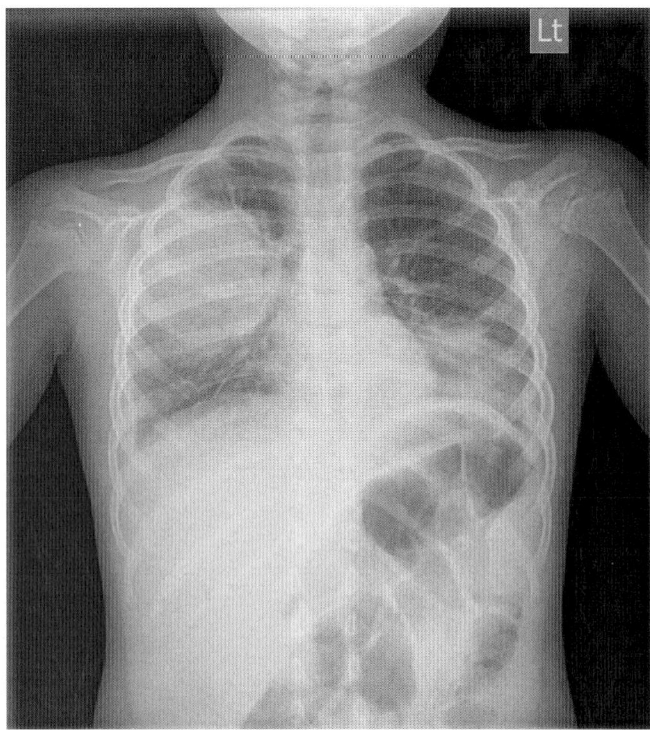

FIGURE 50-6 Round pneumonia involving the right upper lobe on a PA chest x-ray in a 4-year-old girl. This infection was presumed to be due to *S pneumoniae* and she responded well to appropriate antibiotics. (*Used with permission from Camille Sabella, MD.*)

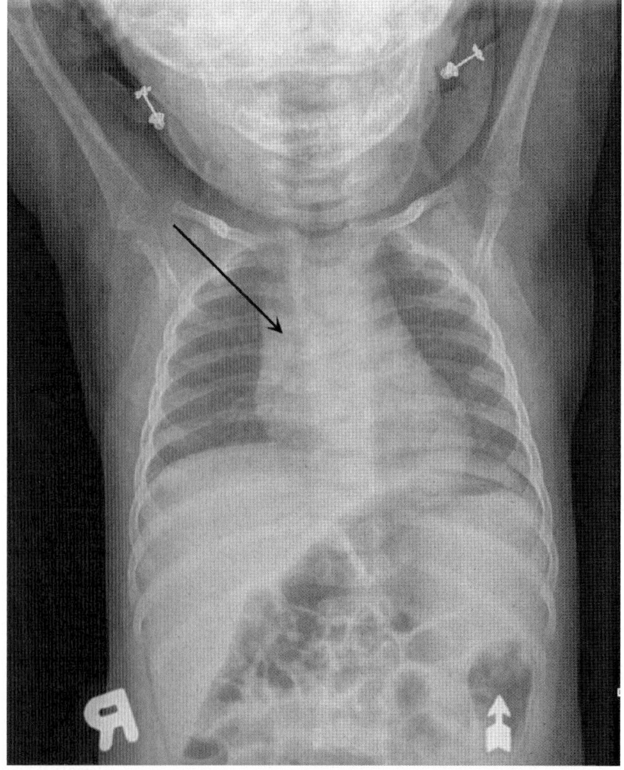

FIGURE 50-8 Thymic shadow (arrow) on a chest x-ray of a young infant, which can be mistaken for pneumonia. (*Used with permission from Camille Sabella, MD.*)

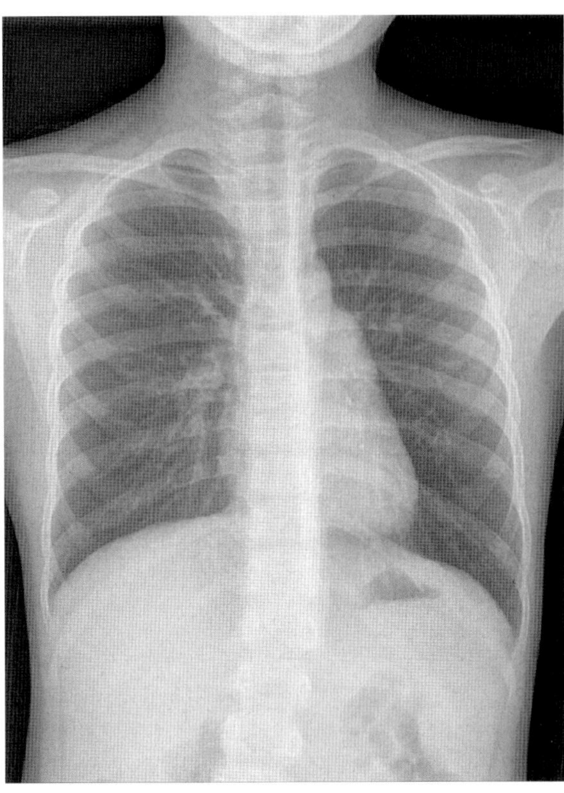

FIGURE 50-9 Bilateral diffuse infiltrates in a 9-year-old child with *Mycoplasma* pneumonia. (*Used with permission from Camille Sabella, MD.*)

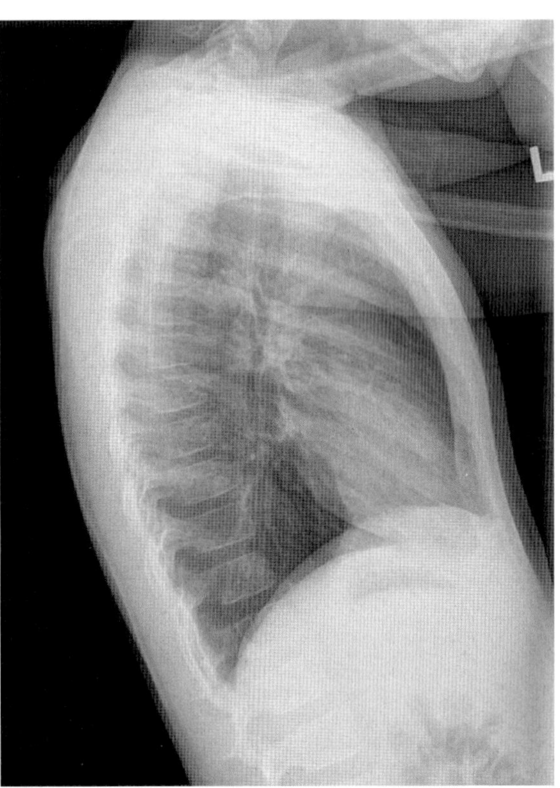

FIGURE 50-10 Bilateral diffuse infiltrates on lateral CXR in a 9-year-old with *Mycoplasma* pneumonia. Same child as in Figure 50-9. (*Used with permission from Camille Sabella, MD.*)

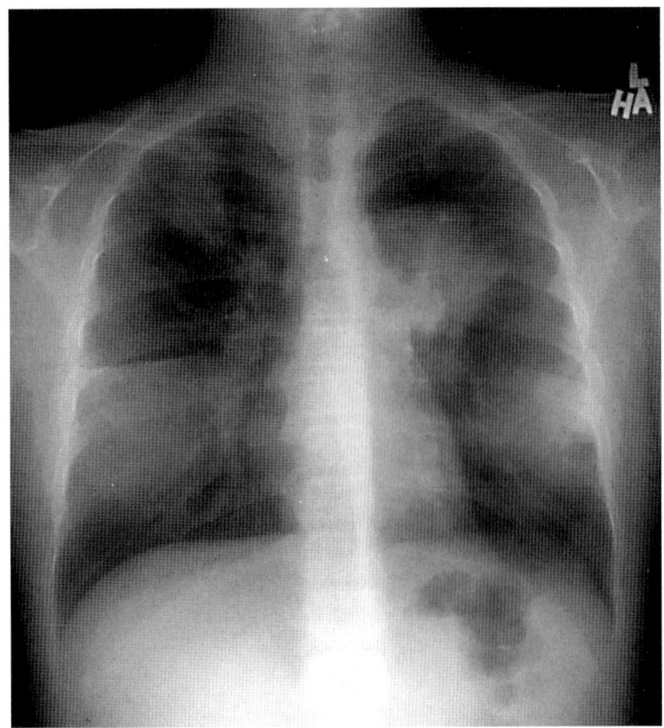

FIGURE 50-11 Multilobar infiltrate in a school-aged child with *Mycoplasma* pneumonia. Although the classic radiographic finding of *Mycoplasma* is a bibasilar diffuse infiltrate, a lobar and multilobar pattern can be seen. (*Used with permission from Camille Sabella, MD.*)

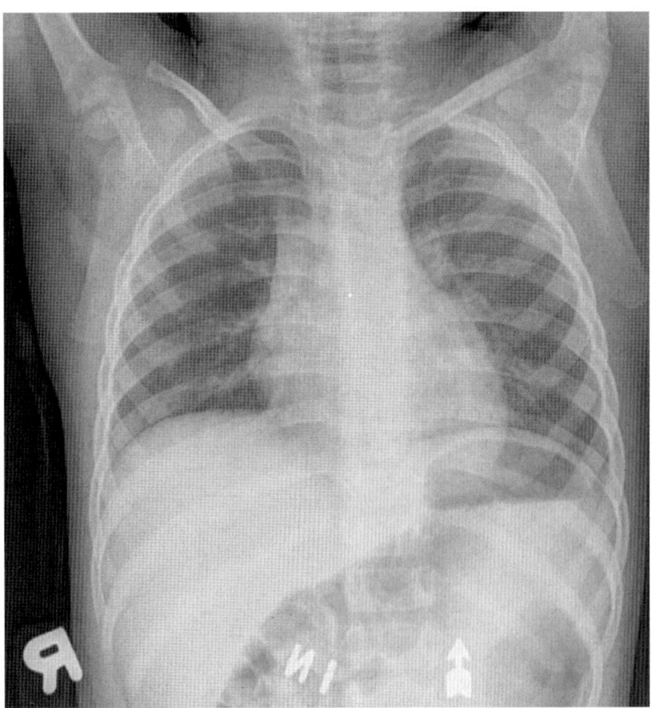

FIGURE 50-12 Central peribronchial thickening and pathy infiltrates in an infant with viral pneumonia. (*Used with permission from Camille Sabella, MD.*)

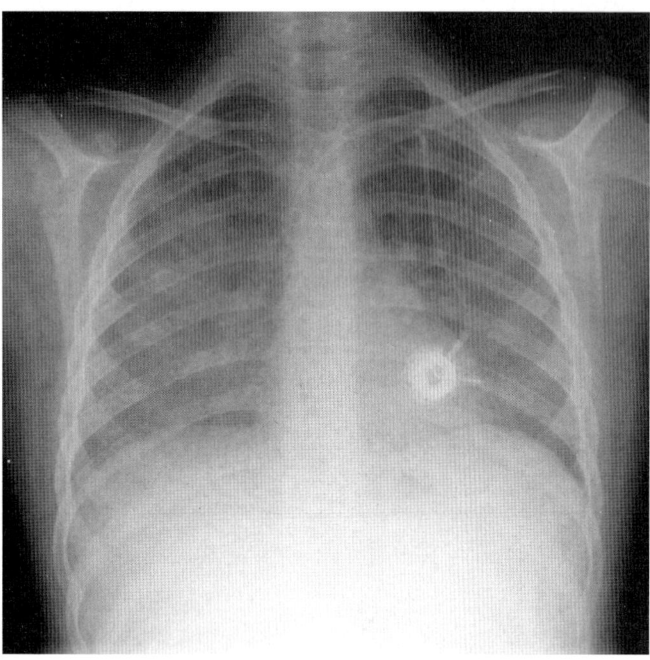

FIGURE 50-13 Diffuse interstitial pattern in child with *Pnemocystis jiroveci* pneumonia. This child's predisposition for this infection is acute leukemia. Note the presence of a central venous catheter to treat his underlying leukemia. (*Used with permission from Camille Sabella, MD.*)

peribronchial infiltration in a diffuse reticular pattern; the heart's borders may appear shaggy due to adjacent peribronchial inflammation.[23] *Pneumocystis* pneumonia can be represented by any type of radiographic pattern, but a diffuse interstitial pattern has classically been described (**Figure 50-13**).

  - Miliary pneumonia—Numerous discrete lesions from hematogenous spread (see Chapter 186, Tuberculosis).

- Parapneumonic effusions and empyema, as well as necrotizing pneumonia, can often be appreciated on CXR (**Figure 50-14**).

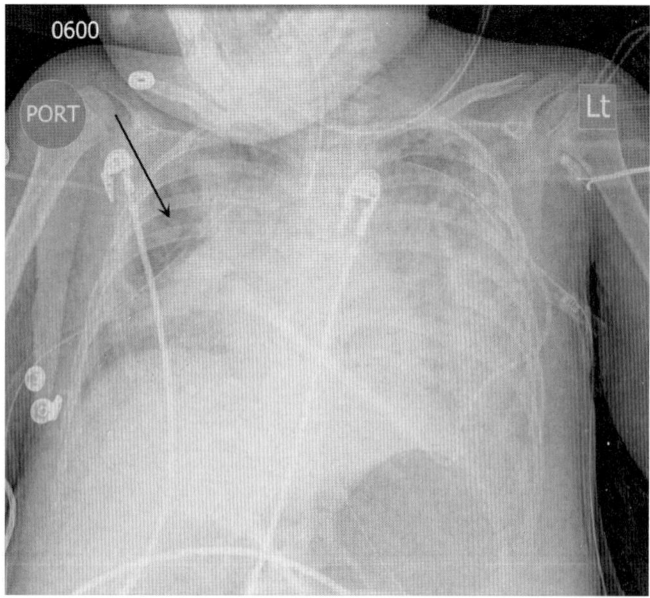

FIGURE 50-14 Necrotizing pneumonia (arrow) in the right upper lobe and large pleural effusion on the left side caused by *S pneumoniae* in a 4-year-old girl. (*Used with permission from Camille Sabella, MD.*)

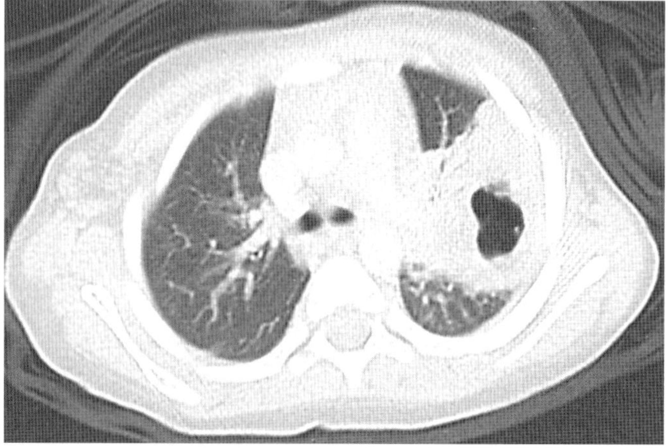

FIGURE 50-15 CT scan of the chest showing left lobar consolidation and cavitation from necrotizing pneumonia in a previously healthy 15-month-old child. (*Used with permission from Camille Sabella, MD.*)

- Ultrasound may be useful for evaluation of pleural effusion.[24]
- Computed tomography (CT) may be useful in the evaluation of complications of pneumonia, such as parapneumonic effusions, empyema, and necrotizing pneumonia (**Figures 50-15** and **50-16**).

DIFFERENTIAL DIAGNOSIS

- Upper respiratory illnesses, including bronchitis, can cause cough, fever, chills, and sputum production with a negative CXR.
- Asthma can cause cough, wheezing, dyspnea, and hypoxia; CXR is negative unless mucous plugging causes collapse of airways (see Chapter 49, Asthma and Pulmonary Function Testing).

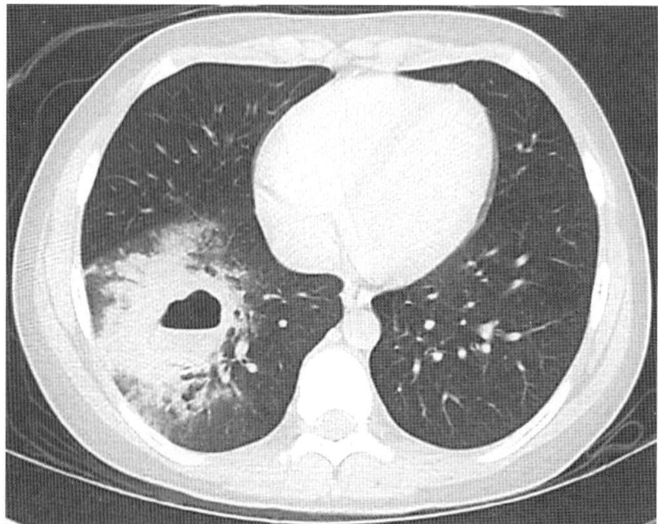

FIGURE 50-16 CT scan of the chest showing right lobar consolidation and cavitation from necrotizing pneumonia caused by *S pneumoniae* in a previously healthy 9-year-old child. (*Used with permission from Camille Sabella, MD.*)

MANAGEMENT

Initial determination of hypoxia and clinical severity of illness is used to identify children with CAP who may be candidates for inpatient treatment (see the following section "Hospitalize"). Children should be admitted to an Intensive Care Unit (ICU) if they require invasive ventilation SOR A or have a pulse oximetry measurement of <92 percent on inspired oxygen of ≥0.50. Children should be admitted to either an ICU or a unit with continuous cardiorespiratory monitoring capabilities for any of the following:[19]

- Requirement for noninvasive positive pressure ventilation. SOR A
- Impending respiratory failure. SOR B
- Sustained tachycardia, inadequate blood pressure, or need for pharmacologic support of blood pressure or perfusion. SOR B
- Altered mental status. SOR C

There is no existing pediatric severity of illness score for CAP in children but items in the adult CAP severity score can be considered, including need for assisted ventilation (invasive or non-invasive positive pressure), shock, respiratory distress, multilobar infiltrates or effusion, comorbid conditions, and unexplained metabolic acidosis. In the PERCH study focused on hospitalized children aged 1 to 59 months with pneumonia, children defined with severe pneumonia had lower chest wall indrawing and those with very severe pneumonia had symptoms and signs including central cyanosis, difficulty breastfeeding/drinking, vomiting everything, convulsions, lethargy, unconsciousness, or head nodding.[25] The Pediatric Infectious Diseases Society (PIDS) and the Infectious Diseases Society of America (IDSA) guideline, however, recommends that a severity score alone should not be used as the sole criteria for ICU admission but should be used in the context of other clinical, laboratory, and radiologic findings.[19]

NONPHARMACOLOGIC

- Based on three clinical trials, chest physiotherapy (PT) did not improve outcomes for children with CAP.[26] In one RCT (N = 72 children aged 1 to 12 years), there were no differences in respiratory rate, decrease in severity score or days of hospitalization for children randomized to standardized chest PT versus the group randomized to non-mandatory request to breathe deeply, expectorate sputum, and maintain a lateral body position once a day.[27]
- Drainage procedures for children with pneumonia complicated by parapneumonic effusion include chest tube without fibrinolysis, chest tube with fibrinolysis, video-assisted thoracoscopic surgery (VATS), and thoracotomy. In one multihospital case series (N = 3500), there was no difference in length of stay (median 10 days) by type of procedure and outcomes were similar in patients undergoing initial chest tube placement with or without fibrinolysis.[28] Children undergoing VATS in this study received fewer additional drainage procedures.

MEDICATIONS

Antimicrobial therapy is not routinely required for preschool-aged children with CAP because of the high proportion with viral disease.[19] SOR A When antibiotics are prescribed, treatment courses of 10 days are recommended.[19] Recommended and alternate treatments for CAP based on a known bacterial pathogen are summarized in **Table 50-1**.

- Amoxicillin should be used as first-line therapy for previously healthy, appropriately immunized infants and preschool children with mild to moderate CAP suspected to be of bacterial origin.[19] SOR B A Cochrane review supported use of amoxicillin (or co-trimoxazole) as first-line therapy with amoxicillin clavulanate and cefpodoxime considered as alternative second-line drugs; limited data were available on other antibiotics.[29]
- Amoxicillin is also recommended for previously healthy, appropriately immunized school-aged children and adolescents with mild to moderate CAP with consideration of atypical pathogens.[19] SOR B If atypical pathogens are suspected clinically, macrolide antibiotics should be prescribed and diagnostic testing performed (**Table 50-1**). Authors of a Cochrane review were unable to determine whether macrolides were superior to other agents for pneumonia due to Mycoplasma as most trials found no differences in clinical response with the exception of a single trial where macrolides were associated with higher clinical resolution (100% vs. 77% for those not treated with azithromycin).[30]
- Influenza antiviral therapy should be administered as soon as possible (within 48 hours) to children with moderate to severe CAP consistent with influenza virus infection during widespread local circulation of influenza viruses.[19] SOR B
- For children with CAP who are inpatients, ampicillin or penicillin G should be administered to the fully immunized infant or school-aged child when local epidemiologic data document lack of substantial high-level penicillin resistance for invasive *S. pneumoniae*.[19] Empiric therapy with a third-generation parenteral cephalosporin (ceftriaxone or cefotaxime) should be prescribed for hospitalized infants and children who are not fully immunized, in regions where local epidemiology of invasive pneumococcal strains documents high-level penicillin resistance, or for infants and children with life threatening infection.[19] SOR B
- For children who are inpatients, empiric combination therapy with a macrolide (oral or parenteral) in addition to a β-lactam antibiotic should be prescribed when *M. pneumoniae* and *C. pneumoniae* are significant considerations; diagnostic testing should be performed.[19] SOR B
- Vancomycin or clindamycin (based on local susceptibility data) should be provided in addition to β-lactam therapy for hospitalized children if clinical, laboratory, or imaging characteristics are consistent with infection caused by *S. aureus*.[19] SOR C
- Among children hospitalized with CAP, adjunctive steroids appear to reduce hospital stay but only in children on concomitant β-agonist therapy (i.e., likely only children with acute wheezing benefit).[31] SOR B For others, steroid use increased length of stay and readmission.
- It is not known whether cough medications (mucolytics or cough suppressants) provide relief in reducing cough severity for patients with pneumonia.[32] SOR C

COMPLEMETARY AND ALTERNATIVE THERAPY

- Zinc adjuvant therapy might be useful for children with severe pneumonia. In one large RCT (N = 610 children in Nepal), zinc (10 mg in 2- to 11-month-olds and 20 mg in older children) was not

TABLE 50-1 Antimicrobial Therapy for Pediatric Community-Acquired Pneumonia

Pathogen	First-line Agent (oral)	Alternate Agent	If Hospitalized (parenteral)
S. Pneumoniae	Amoxicillin (90 mg/kg/day in 2 doses)	Second- or third-generationcephalosporin (e.g., cefuroxime) OR levofloxacin[b], if susceptible	Ampicillin (150–200 mg/kg/day every 6 h) OR penicillin (200,000–250,000 U/kg/day every 4–6 h)
S. Pneumoniae penicillin resistant[a]	Levofloxacin[b], if susceptible OR linezolid[c]	Clindamycin (30–40 mg/kg/day in 3 doses)	Ceftriaxone (100 mg/kg/day every 12–24 h)
Group A *streptococcus*	Amoxicillin (50–75 mg/kg/day in 2 doses), OR penicillin V (50–75 mg/kg/day in 3 or 4 doses)	Clindamycin (40 mg/kg/day in 3 doses)	Penicillin (100,000–250,000 U/kg/day every 4–6 h) OR ampicillin (200 mg/kg/day every 6 h)
Staphylococcus aureus, methicillin sensitive	Cephalexin (75–100 mg/kg/day in 3 or 4 doses)	Clindamycin (30–40 mg/kg/day in 3 or 4 doses)	Cefazolin (150 mg/kg/day every 8 h) OR semisynthetic penicillin (e.g., oxacillin) (150–200 mg/kg/day every 6–8 h)
Staphylococcus aureus, methicillin resistant	Clindamycin (30–40 mg/kg/day in 3 or 4 doses) or oral linezolid[c], if clindamycin resistant	Linezolid[c]	Vancomycin (40–60 mg/kg/day every 6–8 h or dosing to achieve an AUC/MIC ratio of >400) OR clindamycin (40 mg/kg/day every 6–8 h)
Haemophilus influenzae	Amoxicillin (75–100 mg/kg/day in 3 doses) if β-lactamase negative OR amoxicillin clavulanate (amoxicillin component, 90 mg/kg/day in 2 doses) if β-lactamase producing	Cefdinir, cefixime, cefpodoxime, OR ceftibuten	Ampicillin (150–200 mg/kg/day every 6 h) if β-lactamase negative, ceftriaxone (50–100 mg/kg/day every 12–24 h) if β-lactamase producing, OR cefotaxime (150 mg/kg/day every 8 h)
Mycoplasma pneumoniae, Chlamydia trachomatis OR *Chlamydophila pneumoniae*	Azithromycin (10 mg/kg followed by 5 mg/kg/day once daily on days 2–5)	Clarithromycin (15 mg/kg/day in 2 doses) OR erythromycin; for adolescents with skeletal maturity, levofloxacin (500 mg once daily) OR moxifloxacin	Azithromycin (10 mg/kg on days 1 and 2 of therapy; transition to oral therapy if possible)

[a]MIC (minimum inhibitory concentration) ≥4.0 μg/mL.
[b]16–20 mg/kg/day in 2 doses for children 6 months to 5 years and 8–10 mg/kg/day once daily for children 5–16 years, maximum daily dose, 750 mg.
[c]30 mg/kg/day in 3 doses for children <12 years; 20 mg/kg/day in 2 doses for children >12 years.
Abbreviations: h = hours.
Information in this table is adapted from reference 19.

significantly better than placebo in reducing recovery time or response to treatment[33] while in another RCT (N = 352 children in Uganda), zinc at similar dosing reduced the case fatality rate (4% versus 11.9%), especially among children with human immunodeficiency virus.[34]

HOSPITALIZATION[19]

- Children and infants who have moderate to severe CAP, as defined by several factors including respiratory distress and hypoxemia (sustained saturation of peripheral oxygen [SpO2] <90% at sea level), should be hospitalized for management (skilled pediatric nursing care). SOR A
- Infants less than 3 to 6 months of age with suspected bacterial CAP. SOR C
- Children and infants with suspected or documented CAP caused by a high virulence pathogen (e.g., community-acquired MRSA). SOR C
- Children and infants for whom there is concern about careful observation at home or who are unable to comply with therapy or follow-up. SOR C

PREVENTION

- Vaccination—Children should be immunized with vaccines for bacterial pathogens including *S. pneumoniae*, *Haemophilus influenzae* type b, and pertussis to prevent CAP.[19] SOR A The use of pneumococcal conjugate vaccine is associated with an overall decreased incidence of invasive disease among children <age 5 years (from approximately 99 cases per 100,000 population (1998–1999) to 21 cases per 100,000 population (2008).[35]
- All infants ≥6 months of age, children, adolescents, persons ≥50 years of age, others at risk for influenza complications, and health care workers should be immunized annually with vaccines for influenza virus to prevent CAP.[12,19] SOR A Vaccination status should be assessed at the time of hospital admission for all patients and appropriate vaccines offered at discharge.[12] SOR C
- Smoking cessation assistance should be offered to adolescents and children who smoke. Parents who smoke around their children should be counseled about the adverse health consequences that this poses for their children.
- To prevent spread of respiratory pathogens, respiratory hygiene measures should be practiced.[12] These include the coughing into the elbow and use of hand hygiene and masks or tissues for patients with cough, particularly in outpatient settings and EDs.

PROGNOSIS

- Patients on adequate therapy for CAP should demonstrate clinical (and laboratory) signs of improvement within 48 to 72 hours.[19]
- Complications of CAP include pulmonary (e.g., pleural effusion, empyema or abscess, pneumothorax, bronchopleural fistula), metastatic (e.g., meningitis or brain abscess, peri- or endocarditis, osteomyelitis, septic arthritis), and systemic (e.g., sepsis, hemolytic uremic syndrome).[12]
- Most US children with CAP recover. In a case series from Sweden (N = 277), 4 percent of children hospitalized with CAP died; the most important factor independently associated with death was an initial low serum albumin concentration.[36] Elevated interleukin-6 was also associated with mortality.
- In a systematic review of 13 papers on long term sequelae from childhood pneumonia, the risk of at least one major sequelae (restrictive lung disease, obstructive lung disease, bronchiectasis) was 5.5 percent (95% CI, 2.8–8.3%) in non-hospitalized children and 13.6 percent (95% CI, 6.2–21.1%) in hospitalized children.[37] Adenovirus pneumonia was associated with the highest risk of sequelae.

FOLLOW-UP

- Assess need and provide pneumococcal and influenza vaccination at hospital discharge and/or follow-up.
- Monitor improvement and treat comorbid illness (which may worsen).
- Repeat blood cultures to document resolution of bacteremia in children with bacteremia caused by S. aureus, regardless of clinical status.[19] SOR C Otherwise, repeat blood cultures in children with clear clinical improvement are not needed.[19] SOR C
- Acute phase reactants can be useful in conjunction with clinical findings to assess response to treatment for children who are hospitalized with CAP of have pneumonia-associated complications.[19] SOR C
- Repeat CXRs (inpatient or outpatient) are not routinely required if recovery from an episode of CAP is uneventful.[19] SOR B Follow-up chest radiographs should be obtained in patients with complicated pneumonia with worsening respiratory distress or clinical instability, or in those with persistent fever that is not responding to therapy over 48 to 72 hours or with clinical deterioration.[19] SOR C
- Repeated CXR at 4 to 6 weeks after the diagnosis of CAP should be obtained in patients with recurrent pneumonia involving the same lobe and in patients with lobar collapse at initial CXR with suspicion of an anatomic anomaly, chest mass, or foreign body aspiration.[19] SOR B

PATIENT EDUCATION

- Improvement is expected in healthy outpatients in 48 to 72 hours with return to school in approximately 4 to 5 days and complete improvement within 2 weeks.

PATIENT RESOURCES

- **www.healthychildren.org/English/health-issues/conditions/chest-lungs/Pages/Pneumonia.aspx**.
- **www.nhlbi.nih.gov/health/health-topics/topics/pnu/**.
- **www.nlm.nih.gov/medlineplus/pneumonia.html**.

PROVIDER RESOURCES

- **http://pediatrics.aappublications.org/content/128/6/e1677.full**.

REFERENCES

1. Esposito S, Cohen R, Domingo JD, et al. Antibiotic therapy for pediatric community-acquired pneumonia: do we know when, what and for how long to treat? *Pediatr Infect Dis J*. 2012;31(6):e78-85.
2. Mullholland K. Magnitude of the problem of childhood pneumonia. *Lancet*. 1999;354:590-592.
3. Buie VC, Owings MF, DeFrances CJ, Golosinskiy A. National Hospital Discharge Survey: 2006 summary. National Center for Health Statistics. *Vital Health Stat*. 13(168). 2010. Available at http://www.cdc.gov/nchs/data/series/sr_13/sr13_168.pdf, accessed October 2012.
4. Centers for Disease Control and Prevention. Pneumonia hospitalizations among young children before and after introduction of pneumococcal conjugate vaccine–United States, 1997-2006. *MMWR*. 2009;58(1):1-4.
5. File TM. Case studies of lower respiratory tract infections: community-acquired pneumonia. *Am J Med*. 2010;123:4 Suppl):S4-15.
6. Xu J, Kochanek MA, Murphy SL, Tejada-Vera B. Deaths: final data for 2007. *Natl Vital Stat Rep*. 2010;58(19):1-136.
7. Kochanek KD, Xu JQ, Murphy SL, Miniño AM, Kung H. Deaths: Final Data for 2009. National Vital Statistics Reports; vol 60 no 3. Hyattsville, MD: National Center for Health Statistics. 2011. Available at http://www.cdc.gov/nchs/data/nvsr/nvsr60/nvsr60_03.pdf, accessed October 2012.
8. Don M, Canciani M, Korppi M. Community-acquired pneumonia in children: what's old? What's new? *Acta Paediatr*. 2010;99(11):1602-1608.
9. Stein RT, Marostica PJC. Community-acquired pneumonia: a review and recent advances. *Pediatr Pulmonol*. 2007;42:1095-1103.
10. Juvén T, Mertsola J, Waris M, et al. Etiology of community-acquired pneumonia in 254 hospitalized children. *Pediatr Infect Dis J*. 2000;19(4):293-298.
11. De Schutter I, De Wachter E, Crokaert F, et al. Microbiology of bronchoalveolar lavage fluid in children with acute nonresponding or recurrent community-acquired pneumonia: identification of nontypeable Haemophilus influenzae as a major pathogen. *Clin Infect Dis*. 2011;52(12):1437-1444.
12. Marrie TJ, Campbell GD, Walker DH, Low DE. Pneumonia. In: Kasper DL, Braunwald E, Fauci AS, Hauser SL, Longo DL, Jameson JL eds. *Harrison's Principles of Internal Medicine,* 16th ed. New York: McGraw-Hill, 2005:1528–1541.
13. Heiskanen-Kosma T, Korppi M, Jokinen C, Heinonen K. Risk factors for community-acquired pneumonia in children: a population-based case control study. *Scand J Infect Dis*. 1997;29(3):281-285.
14. Grant CC, Emery D, Milne T, et al. Risk factors for community-acquired pneumonia in pre-school-aged children. *J Paediatr Child Health*. 2012;48(5):402-412.
15. Juven T, Ruuskanen O, Mertsola J. Symptoms and signs of community-acquired pneumonia in children. *Scand J Prim Health Care*. 2003; 21: 52-56.
16. Korppi M, Don M, Valent F, Canciani M. The value of clinical features in differentiating between viral, pneumococcal and atypical bacterial pneumonia in children. *Acta Paediatr*. 2008;97: 943-947.
17. Mahabee-Gittens EM, Grupp-Phelan J, Brody AS, et al. Identifying children with pneumonia in the emergency department. *Clin Pediatr (Phila)*. 2005;44:427-435.
18. Palafox M, Guiscafré H, Reyes H, et al. Diagnostic value of tachypnoea in pneumonia defined radiologically. *Arch Dis Child*. 2000;82: 41-45.
19. Bradley JS, Byington CL, Shah SS, et al. The management of community-acquired pneumonia in infants and children older than 3 months of age: clinical practice guidelines by the Pediatric Infectious Diseases Society and the Infectious Diseases Society of America. *Clin Infect Dis*. 2011;53(7):e25-76.
20. Esposito S, Tagliabue C, Picciolli I, et al. Procalcitonin measurements for guiding antibiotic treatment in pediatric pneumonia. *Respir Med*. 2011;105(12):1939-1945.
21. Murdoch DR, O'Brien KL, Driscoll AJ, et al. Laboratory methods for determining pneumonia etiology in children. *Clin Infect Dis*. 2012;54(S2):S146-152.
22. Hazir T, Nisar YB, Qazi SA, et al. Chest radiography in children aged 2–59 months diagnosed with non-severe pneumonia as defined by World Health Organization: Descriptive multicentre study in Pakistan. *BMJ*. 2006;333:629.
23. Butler K, Pusic M. Pediatric Considerations. *In*: Schwartz DT, Reisdorff EJ eds. *Emergency Radiology*. New York: McGraw-Hill, 2000:610-615.
24. Reynolds JH, McDonald G, Alton H, Gordon SB. Pneumonia in the immunocompetent patient. *Br J Radiol*. 2010;83(996):998-1009.
25. Scott JAG, Wonodi C, Moisi JC, et al. The definition of pneumonia, the assessment of severity and clinical standardization in the Pneumonia Etiology Research For Child Health Study. *Clin Infect Dis*. 2012;54(S2):S109-116.
26. Gilchrist FJ. Is the use of chest physiotherapy beneficial in children with community-acquired pneumonia? *Arch Dis Child*. 2008;93(2):176-178.
27. Lukrafka JL, Fuchs SC, Fischer GB, et al. Chest physiotherapy in paediatric patients hospitalized with community-acquired pneumonia: a randomised clinical trial. *Arch Dis Child*. 2012; 97(11):967-971.
28. Shah SS, Hall M, Newland JG, et al. Comparative effectiveness of pleural drainage procedures for the treatment of complicated pneumonia in childhood. *J Hosp Med*. 2011;6(5):256-263.
29. Kabra SK, Lodha R, Pandey RM. Antibiotics for community-acquired pneumonia in children. *Cochrane Database of Syst Rev*. 2010;(3):.CD004874.
30. Mulholland S, Gavranich JB, Gillies MB, Chang AB. Antibiotics for community-acquired lower respiratory tract infections secondary to Mycoplasma pneumoniae in children. *Cochrane Database Syst Rev*. 2012;(9):CD004875.
31. Weiss AK, Hall M, Lee GE, et al. Adjunct corticosteroids in children hospitalized with community-acquired pneumonia. *Pediatrics*. 2011;127(2):e255-263.
32. Chang CC, Cheng AC, Chang AB. Over-the-counter (OTC) medications to reduce cough as an adjunct to antibiotics for acute

pneumonia in children and adults. *Cochrane Database Syst Rev*. 2012;(2):CD006088.

33. Basnet S, Shrestha PS, Sharma A, et al. A randomized controlled trial of zinc as adjuvant therapy for severe pneumonia in young children. *Pediatrics*. 2012;129(4):701-708.
34. Srinivasan MG, Ndeezi G, Mboijana CK, et al. Zinc adjunct therapy reduces case fatality in severe childhood pneumonia: a randomized double blind placebo-controlled trial. *BMC Med*. 2012 Feb 8;10:14.
35. Centers for Disease Control and Prevention. Pneumococcal disease. Available at http://www.cdc.gov/vaccines/pubs/pinkbook/pneumo.html, accessed February 2012.
36. Hedlund J. Community-acquired pneumonia requiring hospitalisation. Factors of importance for the short-and long term prognosis. *Scand J Infect Dis Suppl*. 1995;95:1-60.
37. Edmond K, Scott S, Korczak V, et al. Long term sequelae from childhood pneumonia; systematic review and meta-analysis. *PLoS One*. 2012;7(2):e31239.

51 CYSTIC FIBROSIS

Di Sun, BS, MPH
Elumalai Appachi, MD, MRCP

PATIENT STORY

A 9-month-old girl presents to her pediatrician for persistent cough, failure to gain weight and a bulging mass from her rectum. Her mother reports that the girl has had two episodes of "pneumonia" requiring hospitalization at the age of 3 and 5 months. Since that time, she has not gained much weight and is noted to be at the 10th percentile for weight and length. On examination, the patient has course breath sounds and wheezes throughout the lung fields, and has rectal prolapse (**Figure 51-1**). The pediatrician suspects cystic fibrosis and orders a sweat chloride test, which is 120 mEq/L. This confirms the suspected diagnosis, as a result greater than 60 mEq/L is diagnostic for cystic fibrosis. The family is referred to a comprehensive cystic fibrosis center.

INTRODUCTION

- Cystic fibrosis (CF) is an autosomal recessive disorder caused by a mutation in the CF transmembrane conductance regular gene that alters the composition of mucus secreted in the lungs, pancreas, sweat glands, digestive tract, and vas deferens. This leads to obstructive lung disease and pancreatic insufficiency leading to malabsorption and malnutrition in affected children.

SYNONYMS

CF, fibrocystic disease of pancreas, mucoviscidosis.

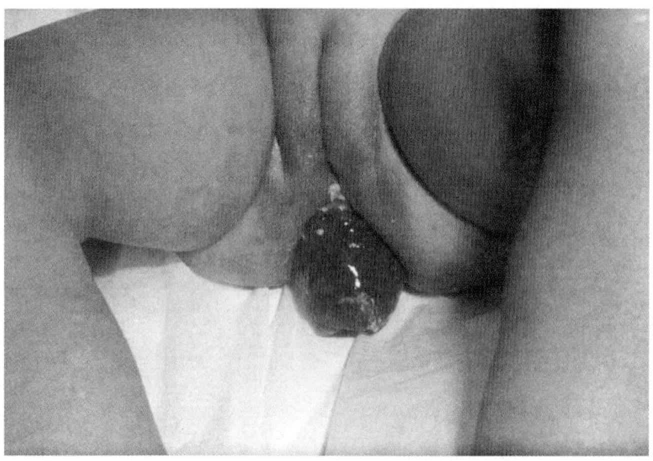

FIGURE 51-1 Rectal prolapse in an infant with cystic fibrosis. (*Used with permission from Elumalai Appachi, MD.*)

EPIDEMIOLOGY

- Incidence of CF is 1 in 3200 newborns in the US.[1]
- CF is the most common fatal inherited disorder among Caucasians.
- Current median life expectancy of patients diagnosed with CF in the US is between 30 to 40 years.[2]
- CF is most common among Caucasians; 4 to 5 percent of Caucasians in North America are heterozygous for CF.[1,3]
- CF incidence among Hispanics ranges from 1:9200 to 1:13500 individuals.[4]
- CF has an incidence of 1:15,000 in African Americans and 1:31,000 in Asian Americans.[3]

ETIOLOGY AND PATHOPHYSIOLOGY

- CF is caused by a mutation in the cystic fibrosis transmembrane conductance regulator (*CFTR*) gene on chromosome 7.
- The *CFTR* gene is a 250 kb, 27 exon gene encoding an ATP binding cassette transporter found on the apical surface of mucosal epithelial cells. This protein is responsible for regulating chloride entrance into mucosal cells.[5]
- Mutations in CFTR are divided into several classes:[3,5]
  - Class 1 mutations—Premature transcription termination signal leading to a defective protein.
  - Class 2 mutations—Protein misfolding leading to premature degradation of CFTR and absence of CFTR expression at the apical surface of mucosal epithelial cells.
  - Class 3 mutations—Defective regulation of CFTR at the apical surface despite intact ability to traffic CFTR to the cell surface.
  - Class 4 mutations—Defective CFTR channel conductance of chloride.
  - Class 5 mutations—Decreased synthesis of functional CFTR due to splicing abnormalities.
  - Class 6 mutations—Increased turnover of CFTR at the apical surface.
- Class 1, 2, and 3 mutations are associated with more severe disease, while class 4 and 5 mutations tend to demonstrate pancreatic insufficiency and milder pulmonary disease.[3]
- The most common mutation in CF is ΔF508, a class 2 mutation that is present in 70 percent of CF patients.[1]
- The pathophysiology of CF lies in the importance of CFTR in regulating the chloride conductance across the apical membrane of mucosal cells, which impacts sodium and water transport. The end result is a thick, viscous mucus that leads to inflammation, obstruction, and finally fibrosis of organs expressing CFTR in its mucosal cells.[6]
- Pulmonary manifestations of CF are due to increased viscosity of the airway surface liquid, which leads to impaired ciliary beating and thus decreased mucociliary clearance.[5]
- In addition to alteration of the airway surface liquid, pulmonary disease in CF is also characterized by an impaired immune response to pathogens because of decreased opsonization, decreased pH, and inactivation of antimicrobial peptides.[5,7]

- CFTR protein is also hypothesized to serve as a binding site for *Pseudomonas aeruginosa* which leads to phagocytosis and clearance via desquamation.[5]
- Another important manifestation of CF is pancreatic insufficiency, which results from thickened secretions from epithelial mucosal cells in the pancreas and leads to destruction of pancreatic β cells. Although insulin secretion is decreased, there is still some endogenous production, preventing the development of ketosis. In addition, the inflammation in the pancreas also reduces α cell mass, which leads to decreased glucagon. Insulin resistance is present in some patients with more severe disease, possibly due to increased inflammation. As patients develop diabetes, slight peripheral insulin resistance also develops.[6]

RISK FACTORS

- Family history of CF or carrier state.
- Caucasian.

DIAGNOSIS

CLINICAL FEATURES

- Pulmonary symptoms are the most common presenting manifestations of CF. Thick airway mucus and impaired clearance of pathogens leads to colonization of the airways and inflammation. This culminates in obstructive lung disease, specifically bronchiectasis, and leads to clinical findings such as diminished breath sounds, tachypnea, and increased chest diameter.[1]
- Common pathogens colonizing the airways early in life include *Staphylococcus aureus* and *Haemophilus influenzae.*
- Eventually, almost all patients acquire and become permanently colonized with *P aeruginosa*.
- Patients with more severe disease may also be colonized with *Burkholderia cepacia*, which is associated with a poor prognosis.
- Pulmonary complications, although uncommon, can become life threatening and include massive hemoptysis, spontaneous pneumothorax, and pulmonary hypertension.
- Digital clubbing is apparent even with only mildly reduced lung function (**Figure 51-2**).

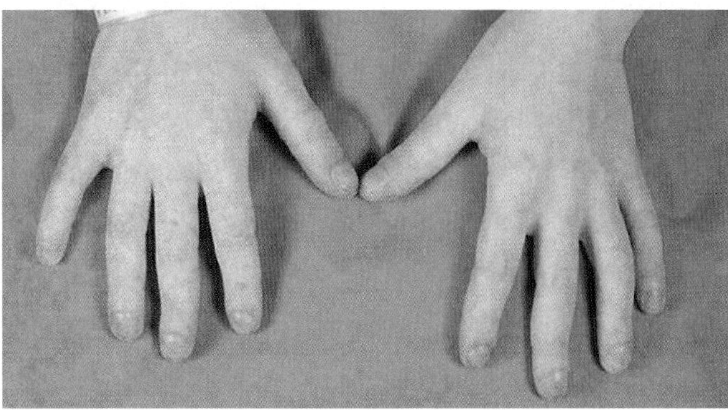

FIGURE 51-2 Digital clubbing in a boy with cystic fibrosis. (*Used with permission from Cleveland Clinic Children's Hospital Photo Files.*)

- Pancreatic disease in children with CF is characterized by obstruction of pancreatic ducts, which can lead to pancreatitis and eventual loss of pancreatic exocrine function. Consequently, children are unable to digest fat and protein, leading to greasy, foul-smelling stool, abdominal distention, and cramping. This can also lead to malnutrition and failure to thrive. Loss of pancreatic endocrine function can also lead to diminished insulin secretion and thus diabetes.[6]
- Twenty to thirty percent of newborns with CF present with meconium ileus due to obstruction from thick intestinal secretions. Older infants and children can develop distal intestinal obstruction syndrome (DIOS) when stool becomes firm and accumulates at the ileocecal valve.
- Rectal prolapse occurs in about 20 percent of infants and children and usually occurs early in life (**Figure 51-1**). This is caused by bowel obstruction, malnutrition, and loss of anal sling musculature.
- Hepatobiliary disease occurs from thickened biliary secretions which can lead to acalculous cholecystitis. Liver disease occurs in about a third of children who have CF and a small percentage of them will develop cirrhosis and eventual liver failure.
- Pansinusitis is present in almost all children, while nasal polyposis occurs in about 25 percent children with CF. Children less than 12 years of age who have nasal polyposis should be screened for CF.
- Infertility is common in males due to absence of the vas deferens. Women with CF may also have decreased fertility due to thickened mucus obstructing the cervix.

LABORATORY TESTING

- Newborn screening is increasingly used in the US to identify newborns with CF. Newborns are identified by testing for immunoreactive trypsinogen (IRT), an inactive pancreatic enzyme that is elevated in the serum of infants with CF. Infants who are positive on this initial screen will then undergo either a DNA mutation analysis (IRT/DNA) or a second IRT (IRT/IRT), depending on state policy.[8]
- Infants who have a positive newborn screen (2 positive IRT screens or a positive IRT screen and DNA mutation analysis) should be referred to a CF center and undergo sweat chloride testing or definitive genetic testing to confirm the diagnosis.
- Sweat chloride testing remains the gold standard for diagnosis and involves using quantitative pilocarpine iontoelectrophoresis. Pilocarpine is applied to stimulate sweat glands. Sweat is collected and analyzed for chloride content.
  - A chloride concentration greater than 60 mEq/L is diagnostic for CF, whereas a concentrations less than 40 mEq/L is normal. A concentration between 40–60 mEq/L (30–60 mEq/L in infants less than 2 months) is considered indeterminate.
  - Infants and children with indeterminate tests should undergo genotype analysis.
- DNA testing for known CF mutations can also be used to diagnose CF. This requires identifying two known CF-causing mutations in the *CFTR* gene. Current DNA tests identify >90 percent *CFTR* mutations. Thus, a diagnosis of CF cannot be totally excluded using genetic testing. Uncharacterized *CFTR* mutations are more

common in non-Caucasian CF patients. Thus, DNA testing may be more likely to miss a mutation in these patients.[1]

- In general, genetic testing for CF should be reserved for patients in whom sweat testing is logistically difficult or has yielded indeterminate results.
- The function of the CFTR protein in respiratory epithelium can also be assessed directly in vivo by measuring the bioelectric voltage difference across nasal epithelium (the "nasal potential difference"), which is available in a few specialized CF centers.[9] This test can be used for children who have clinical symptoms of CF but who have normal sweat chloride and genetic testing.

IMAGING

- Chest x-ray may be normal early in the course of the disease.
- Persistent obstruction and inflammation leads to bronchiectasis that is visible on routine chest x-ray as the disease process progresses (**Figures 51-3** to **51-5**).
- Chest-x-ray is important in identifying complications such as pneumothorax and pulmonary hemorrhage (**Figure 51-6**).
- CT scan can further define the extent of bronchiectasis and other complications of CF (**Figures 51-7** to **51-9**).
- Testicular ultrasonography can be used to determine the presence of the vas deferens.
- Abdominal x-rays and contrast studies can be used to identify bowel obstruction.
- Right upper quadrant ultrasound is useful in diagnosing biliary disease.

DIFFERENTIAL DIAGNOSIS

- CF is easily recognized in any infant or child who has the classic triad of chronic pulmonary disease, steatorrhea, and growth failure.
- Recurrent pneumonia due to other causes, such as aspiration pneumonia due to dysphagia or gastroesophageal reflux, anatomic abnormalities such as bronchogenic cysts, congenital airway malformations, immunodeficiencies, sickle cell disease, asthma, right middle lobe syndrome, and foreign body aspiration should always be considered.[10]
- The lack of other features of CF, such as growth failure and gastrointestinal manifestations, help to differentiate these entities from CF. However, a sweat chloride test should be part of the

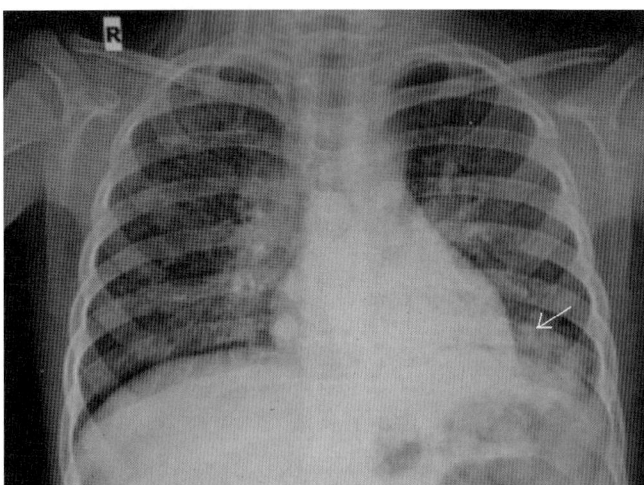

FIGURE 51-3 Marked peribronchial thickening, chronic left lower lobe collapse/consolidation (arrow), bronchiectatic changes, and mucus plugging of bronchioles on chest x-ray in a 6-year-old girl with a homozygous delta F508 mutation of cystic fibrosis. (*Used with permission from Samiya Razvi, MD.*)

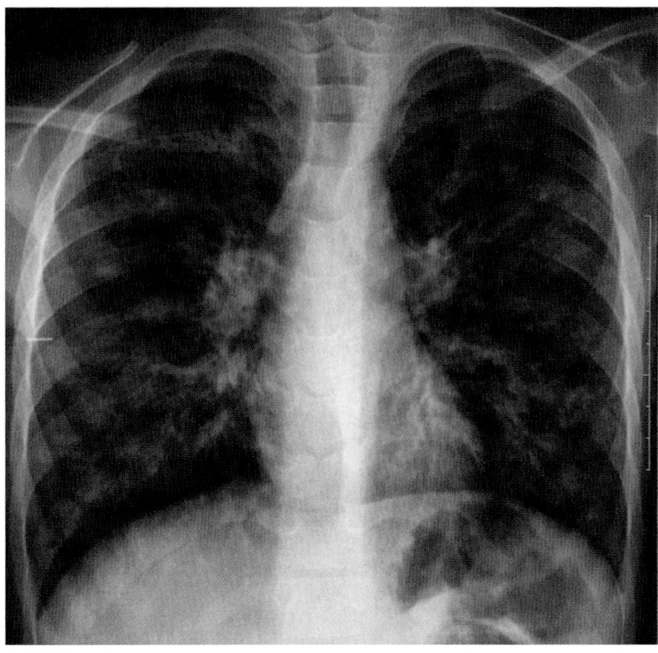

FIGURE 51-4 Bilateral patchy opacities, marked peribronchial thickening extending into the lung peripheries, and hyperinflation indicating airway obstruction and air trapping on chest x-ray in a 10-year-old boy with cystic fibrosis, homozygous delta F508. (*Used with permission from Samiya Razvi, MD.*)

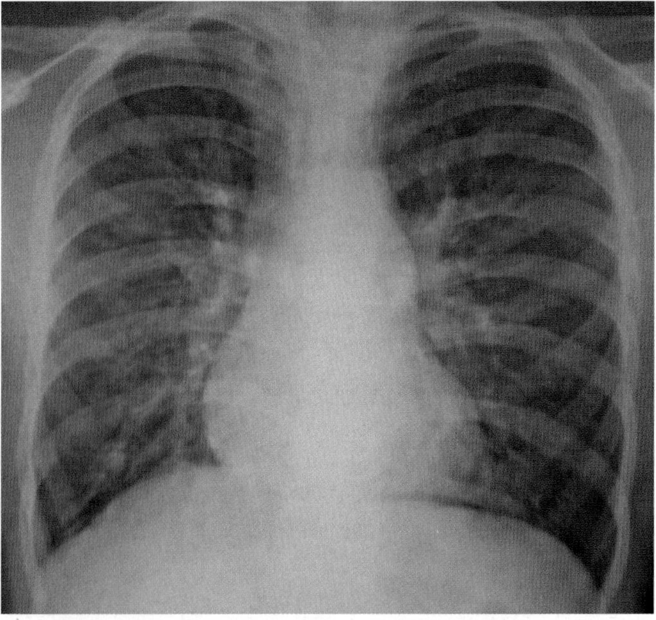

FIGURE 51-5 Increased bronchovascular markings, peribronchial thickening and cystic changes of bronchiectasis on chest x-ray in a 13-year-old boy with cystic fibrosis. (*Used with permission from Samiya Razvi, MD.*)

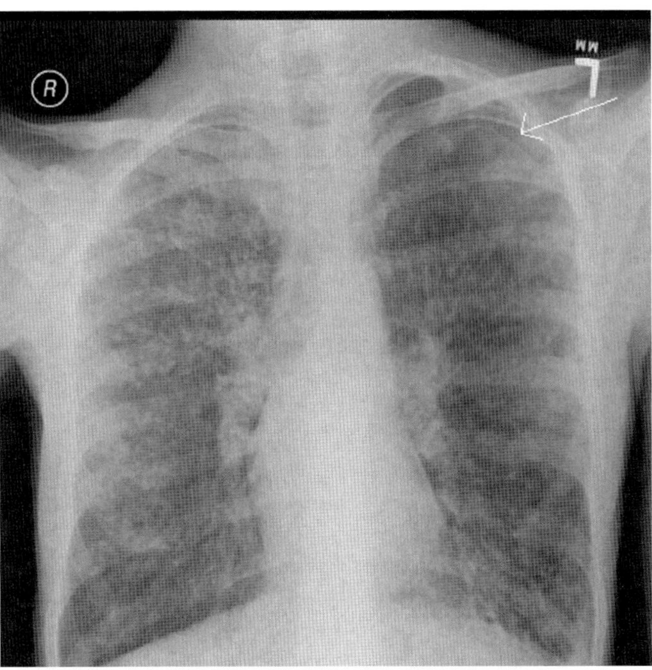

FIGURE 51-6 Increased interstitial markings, peribronchial thickening, bronchiectasis in the left lower lobe and an acute small left apical pneumothorax with visible left lung margin (arrow) on chest x-ray in a 20-year old patient with cystic fibrosis. (*Used with permission from Samiya Razvi, MD.*)

work up of a child with recurrent pneumonia to definitively exclude CF.

MANAGEMENT

- Management of CF should focus on slowing the course of the disease. This requires educating family members, particularly families of infants identified through the newborn screen. Infants identified at birth may often not have clinical manifestations, but it is imperative to educate families that early intervention can result in better outcomes.
- After diagnosis, all patients should be referred to an accredited CF care center with coordination of care between all health care providers, especially the primary care physician.
- The goal of care is to maintain normal growth and delay the development of pulmonary disease.
- Delaying onset of pulmonary disease:
  - Ensure that the patient is in a smoke-free environment.
  - Airway clearance.
    - These regimens take considerable time with adults reporting spending a mean of 108 min/day on all CF therapies.[11] This makes adherence an issue for many CF patients.

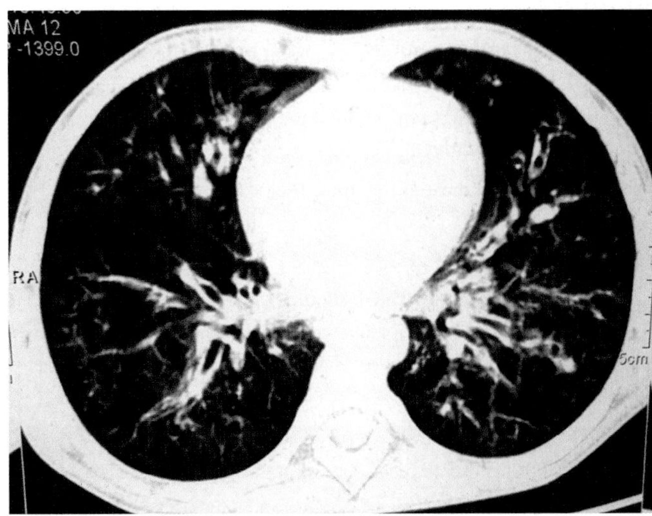

FIGURE 51-7 Peribronchial thickening, increased interstitial markings, and cylindrical bronchiectasis on axial CT scan of the same boy as in **Figure 51-4**. (*Used with permission from Samiya Razvi, MD.*)

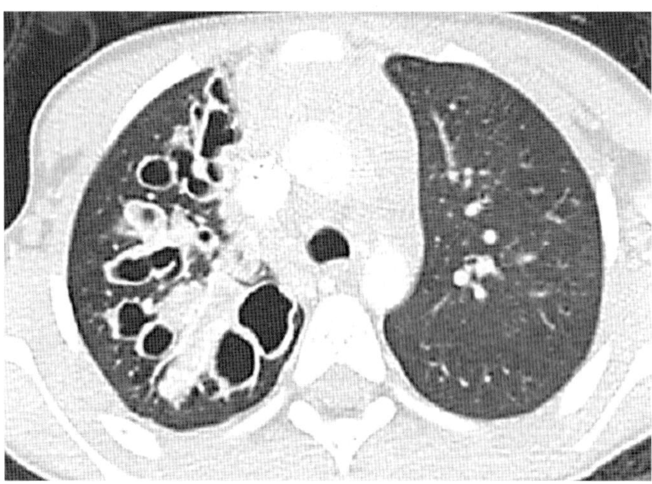

FIGURE 51-8 Saccular bronchiectasis of the right upper lobe with cavitary changes and peribronchial thickening on axial chest CT scan in a 7-year-old boy with cystic fibrosis. This boy had a history of chronic productive cough, hemoptysis during pulmonary exacerbations, and sputum cultures positive for multidrug resistant *Pseudomonas aeruginosa*. (*Used with permission from Samiya Razvi, MD.*)

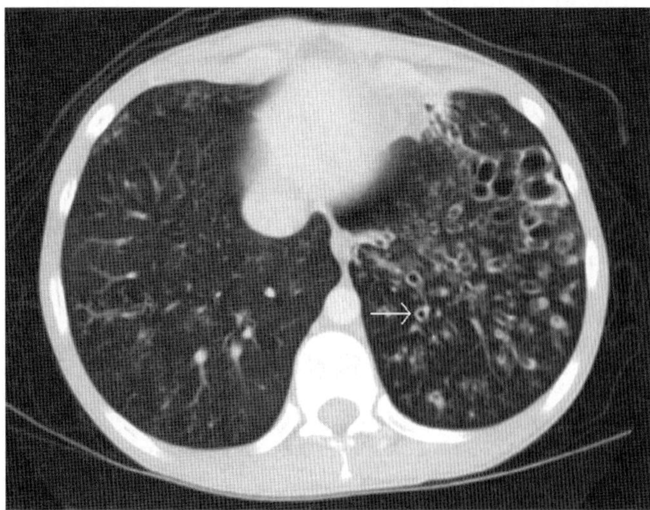

FIGURE 51-9 Saccular bronchiectasis of the left lower lobe, peribronchial thickening and signet ring sign (arrow) demonstrating dilatation and enlarged diameter of bronchiole compared to the accompanying pulmonary blood vessel on axial chest CT scan in a 17-year-old girl with cystic fibrosis. (*Used with permission from Samiya Razvi, MD.*)

- For infants <2 years of age, the recommended method of mucociliary clearance is percussion followed by postural drainage.
- In older children, there are many mechanical devices for airway clearance including: positive expiratory pressure masks, Flutter, Acapella, and high-frequency chest wall oscillation (Vest). No trials have demonstrated the superiority of one device over another; treatment should be individualized to the patient.
- Children >6 years of age should also receive inhaled daily Dornase Alfa (recombinant Human DNase) and twice daily 7 percent hypertonic saline after bronchodilator pretreatment.[12,13] SOR Ⓐ
- Azithromycin given three times a week is recommended for children >6 years of age colonized with *P aeruginosa*, based on trials showing increased pulmonary function and increased length of time between infectious exacerbations.[14,15] SOR Ⓐ The precise mechanism of action of azithromycin in this setting in not known, although an anti-inflammatory effect is postulated. The long-term benefit of such treatment is not clear.
  - Pulmonary function tests (PFTs) should be performed to monitor progression of lung disease.
  - Aerobic exercise should also be encouraged.

- Prevention of infection.
  - Patients should receive:
    - Influenza vaccine annually if >6 months of age.
    - Palivizumab for infants <2 years of age to prevent severe respiratory syncytial virus infections.
  - Upon diagnosis in infants <2 years of age, all patients should undergo oropharyngeal cultures every 3 months.
  - A variety of antimicrobial prophylactic antimicrobial agents are used in different CF centers. Treatment is individualized taking into consideration potential benefits and risks.
  - Infants <2 years of age who are colonized with *P aeruginosa* should receive primary treatment aimed at eradicating the pathogen.[11,16] SOR Ⓒ
  - Patients chronically infected with *P aeruginosa* should receive inhaled antibiotic treatment. Although prior recommendations were to receive inhaled tobramycin every other month, recently centers have switched to continuous inhaled tobramycin treatment or alternating inhaled tobramycin with colistin.[12] SOR Ⓒ
  - In clinic and in the hospital, CF patients should not come into contact with each other to prevent spread of colonizing agents among patients.
- Maintaining normal growth.
  - CF children should be maintained at the 50th percentile in weight-for-length by 2 years of age. This is associated with improved pulmonary function in later life. Although breast milk is recommended, infants who are formula-fed have similar weights to breast milk-fed babies. Standard infant formula can be used as there are no benefits from hydrolyzed formula.[17]
  - Infants and children failing to gain adequate weight can be supplemented with fortified human milk, formulas with higher calories, or complementary foods. Enteral supplements may be necessary to improve weight gain.[17]
  - CF patients often have more behavioral issues regarding food. Early intervention with parents consistently praising children for trying new foods or eating independently, ignoring behavior when children refuse to eat, and limiting meal times to 15 minutes while increasing the frequency of snacks can help with this issue.[17]
  - Pancreatic insufficiency (PI) is present in 60 percent of patients with CF at birth even if patients are asymptomatic. The fecal elastase assay, which is low in patients with PI, can be used in infants >2 weeks of age to check for PI. Patients with symptoms of PI or who have diagnosed PI should be started on nongeneric pancreatic enzyme replacement therapy (PERT).[17]
    - If patients have 2 CFTR mutations associated with PI, nongeneric PERT should also be started even if they are asymptomatic.
    - Asymptomatic patients with at least one copy of a pancreatic sufficient genotype should not be started on PERT.
  - All patients should be started on age-appropriate doses of fat soluble vitamins (A, D, E, K). Vitamin levels should be measured every two months the first year and annually afterward.
  - In infants <2 years of age who fail to grow despite adequate intake and PERT, a trial of zinc supplementation can be initiated.[17]
  - Other supplementations for infants under age 2 years include salt (1/8 tsp daily and increased to 1/4 tsp daily at 6 months of age) and fluoride 0.25 mg/dl if the water supply contains <0.3 ppm fluoride.[17]
  - Patients who develop CF-related diabetes should be managed by an endocrinologist.[12]

- Acute exacerbation of pulmonary disease:
  - Frequent comprehensive clinical evaluation of patients, including microbiological examination of respiratory tract flora by a laboratory that is experienced in detecting pathogens of cystic fibrosis, is critical for the management of patients with CF.
  - Clinical symptoms of acute pulmonary exacerbation include increased cough, increased sputum production, dyspnea, chest pain, hemoptysis, loss of appetite, weight loss, and decline in PFTs.
  - In general, patients who are having a pulmonary exacerbation should be admitted to the hospital for intravenous and inhaled antibiotic administration.
  - Antimicrobial agents are chosen based on the colonizing strains and their susceptibilities.
  - During this acute exacerbation, airway clearance regimens may be intensified. Patients may also require additional support including supplemental oxygen and bronchodilators.

SURGERY

- Lung transplantation has been successful for a limited number of patients with cystic fibrosis and end-stage pulmonary disease. A recent study, however, questioned the benefit of lung transplantation for children with CF.[18]
- Surgery may be indicated for sinus disease and polyposis.

REFERRAL

- All patients diagnosed with CF should be referred to a certified CF center. Care should be coordinated between the CF center, the patient's PCP, and any other specialties (e.g., endocrine).

PREVENTION AND SCREENING

- Newborn CF screening is increasingly utilized in the US.
- Children with any clinical manifestations of CF such as recurrent pulmonary infections, nasal polyposis, failure to thrive, or

pancreatic dysfunction should be tested for CF using the sweat chloride test.

PROGNOSIS

- Currently, the life expectancy for CF is 30 to 40 years, a dramatic improvement from a life expectancy of 25 years in 1985.[1,2]
- Most children with CF can participate in normal childhood activities with 90 percent of CF patients completing high school.[1]

FOLLOW-UP

- A comprehensive clinical evaluation including PFT testing and microbiologic cultures of respiratory flora should be carried out on a regular basis at a CF center.
- Patients should continue to follow-up with their primary care physicians. All routine vaccinations should be given at age appropriate times.

PATIENT EDUCATION

- CF requires a coordinated effort from the family to manage the time-consuming airway clearance therapies. Families should be provided with education on the importance of adhering to these regimens.
- As children transition to adolescents and adults, they must also learn to take charge of their own therapies. This often requires additional training and support from the provider.

PATIENT RESOURCES

- CF foundation—**www.cff.org**.
- NIH CF website—**www.nhlbi.nih.gov/health/health-topics/topics/cf**.
- CF community support resources—**www.cfri.org/cfsupport.shtml**.
- CF gene mutations—**www.cftr2.org**.

PROVIDER RESOURCES

- **http://pedsinreview.aappublications.org/content/30/8/302.full?sid=a05fb5ed-0219-4bc0-a89c-dc92cbe6a5dc**.
- CF gene database—**www.cftr2.org/browse.php**.
- European CF guidelines—**www.ecfs.eu/ecfs_guidelines**.

REFERENCES

1. Montgomery GS, Howenstine M: Cystic fibrosis. *Pediatr Rev Am Acad Pediatr*. 2009;30(8):302-309; quiz 310.
2. *Cystic Fibrosis Foundation—Patient Registry Report*. Bethesda, MD; 2011. Available at: http://www.cff.org/livingwithcf/qualityimprovement/patientregistryreport/, accessed September 3, 2013.
3. Strausbaugh SD, Davis PB: Cystic fibrosis: a review of epidemiology and pathobiology. *Clin Chest Med*. 2007;28(2):279-288.
4. Rohlfs EM, Zhou Z, Heim RA, et al. Cystic Fibrosis Carrier Testing in an Ethnically Diverse US Population. *Clin Chem*. 2011; 57(6):841-848.
5. Gibson RL, Burns JL, Ramsey BW: Pathophysiology and management of pulmonary infections in cystic fibrosis. *Am J Respir Crit Care Med*. 2003;168(8):918-951.
6. Moran A, Becker D, Casella SJ, et al. Epidemiology, pathophysiology, and prognostic implications of cystic fibrosis-related diabetes: a technical review. *Diabetes Care*. 2010;33(12):2677-2683.
7. Goss CH, Ratjen F: Update in cystic fibrosis 2012. *Am J Respir Crit Care Med*. 2013;187(9):915-919.
8. Wagener JS, Zemanick ET, Sontag MK: Newborn screening for cystic fibrosis. *Curr Opin Pediatr*. 2012;24(3):329-335.
9. Knowles M, Gatzy J, Boucher R: Increased bioelectric potential difference across respiratory epithelia in cystic fibrosis. *N Engl J Med*. 1981;305:1498-1495.
10. Panitch HB: Evaluation of recurrent pneumonia. *Pediatr Infect Dis J*. 2005;24(3):265-266.
11. Sawicki GS, Tiddens H: Managing treatment complexity in cystic fibrosis: challenges and opportunities. *Pediatr Pulmonol*. 2012;47(6):523-533.
12. Cohen-Cymberknoh M, Shoseyov D, Kerem E: Managing Cystic Fibrosis: Strategies That Increase Life Expectancy and Improve Quality of Life. *Am J Respir Crit Care Med*. 2011;183(11):1463-1471.
13. Harms HK, Matouk E, Tournier G, et al., on behalf of DNase International Study Group. Multicenter, open-label study of recombinant human DNase in cystic fibrosis patients with moderate lung disease. *Pediatr Pulmonol*. 1998;26:155-161.
14. Saiman L, Marshall BC, Mayer-Hamblett N, Burns JL, Quittner AL, Cibene DA, Coquillette S, Fieberg AY, Accurso FJ, Campbell PW 3rd, et al. Azithromycin in patients with cystic fibrosis chronically infected with Pseudomonas aeruginosa: a randomized controlled trial. *JAMA*. 2003; 290(13):1749-1756.
15. Southern KW, Barker PM, Solis-Moya A, Patel L: Macrolide antibiotics for cystic fibrosis. *Cochrane Database Syst Rev*. 2011;(12):CD002203. Epub 2011 Dec 7.
16. Fredericksen B, Koch C, Hoiby N: Antibiotic treatment of initial colonization with *Pseudomonas aeruginosa* postpones chronic infection and prevents deterioration of pulmonary function in cystic fibrosis. *Pediatr Pulmonol*. 1997;23:330-335.
17. Cystic Fibrosis Foundation, Borowitz D, Robinson KA, et al. Cystic Fibrosis Foundation evidence-based guidelines for management of infants with cystic fibrosis. *J Pediatr*. 2009;155(6):S73-93.
18. Liou TG, Adler FR, Cox DR, Cahill BC: Lung transplantation and survival in children with cystic fibrosis. *N Engl J Med*. 2007;357:2143-2152.

52 CONGENITAL PULMONARY MALFORMATIONS

Samiya Razvi, DCH, MD
Ellen Park, MD

Congenital pulmonary malformations are relatively rare entities that can cause a wide variety of pulmonary findings in infants and children. In this chapter, we review the clinical and radiographic features of the most important malformations, including:

1. Congenital absence of the pulmonary vein
2. Tracheal bronchus
3. Bronchial cyst
4. Congenital lobar emphysema
5. Congenital cystic adenomatoid malformation
6. Pulmonary sequestration
7. Pulmonary agenesis

CONGENITAL ABSENCE OF THE PULMONARY VEIN

PATIENT STORY

A 5 year-old-girl is hospitalized for respiratory distress and hypoxemia. This is her third episode of right-sided pneumonia. She is thinly built; both height and weight are at the 25th percentile for age. Chest auscultation reveals fine alveolar crackles over the entire right lung without wheeze; the left lung is clear. Heart sounds are normal without a murmur. Her chest x-ray shows haziness of the entire right lung, with patchy opacity in the right lower zone; the left lung is normal. She is treated with parenteral antibiotics and improves. Blood and sputum cultures are negative. She is evaluated further for recurrent pneumonia. Serum immunoglobulin profile is normal. Sweat chloride is within normal limits. Chest CT scan with contrast shows Swiss cheese appearance of the entire right lung with cystic lucencies and septal thickening; the left lung is normal (**Figure 52-1**). Further cardiac evaluation with Echocardiography shows no intra-cardiac defect. Cardiac catheterization and pulmonary angiography reveal normal pulmonary artery anatomy, with isolated absence of the right main pulmonary vein. She is followed closely and her subsequent respiratory illnesses are treated early with antibiotics and bronchodilators. She remains asymptomatic with exercise tolerance and growth appropriate for age.

INTRODUCTION

Unilateral absence of the pulmonary vein is a rare congenital abnormality thought to be due to atresia of the pulmonary vein during development in the prenatal period. This results in abnormal venous drainage of the affected lung and significant ventilation perfusion mismatch.

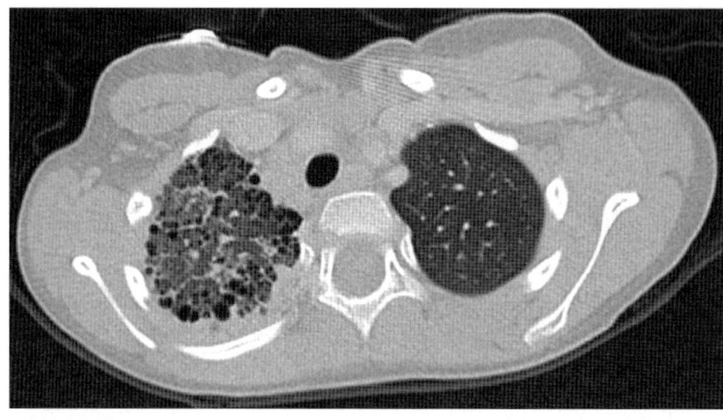

FIGURE 52-1 Congenital absence of the right pulmonary vein: Axial cut of chest CT scan with contrast showing classical findings of ground glass changes, interlobular and interstitial septal thickening of the right lung as compared to the normal left lung. (*Used with permission from Samiya Razvi, DCH, MD and Ellen Park, MD.*)

SYNONYM

Congenital unilateral pulmonary vein agenesis.

EPIDEMIOLOGY

- Congenital absence of the pulmonary vein is a rare congenital anomaly, found in about 0.5 percent of autopsies performed in children.
- May occur as an isolated lesion or associated with other congenital cardiac defects in about 30 to 50 percent of cases.
- Mortality rate approaches 50 percent if untreated.

ETIOLOGY AND PATHOPHYSIOLOGY

- Rare developmental abnormality, in which there is absence of the right or left pulmonary vein or both.
- Thought to result from failure of incorporation of the pulmonary vein into the left atrium.
- There is a spectrum of disease: lesser degrees of venous atresia result in pulmonary vein stenosis with narrowing, venous obstruction and anatomic variations in the pulmonary vessels that drain the affected lung to complete absence of the affected pulmonary vein.
- Pulmonary venous obstruction from the intra-uterine period affects normal development and architecture of the lung, leading to engorgement of bronchial veins, chronic pulmonary edema, lymphatic dilatation, inter-alveolar septal thickening, patchy interstitial fibrosis, cystic changes, and development of collateral vessels.
- Inadequate gas exchange occurs at the alveolar level of the entire affected lung, resulting in large dead space ineffective ventilation and significant ventilation perfusion mismatch.

DIAGNOSIS

The diagnosis is often elusive and difficult to make; it requires a high index of suspicion when a patient presents with the clinical history of recurrent pneumonia together with asymmetry of lung aeration with reticular interstitial infiltrates on imaging. This should prompt further investigation with CT scan and pulmonary angiography.

CLINICAL FEATURES

- Presentation is often in infancy or early childhood (usually less than 5 years age).
- Typical symptoms include recurrent unilateral respiratory infections/ pneumonia and exercise intolerance with dyspnea on exertion.[1]
- Occasionally, hemoptysis may be a presenting symptom.
- As the pulmonary circulation is suboptimal, infections can spread rapidly within the lung parenchyma with suppuration; repeated infections lead to bronchiectasis and chronic lung disease.
- Rarely, mildly symptomatic cases without associated cardiac defects or pulmonary hypertension can remain undetected and present later in adulthood.[2]
- Mortality approaches 50 percent if untreated.
- Complete atresia of the common pulmonary vein has been reported in the neonatal period presenting with severe respiratory distress, refractory hypoxemia, acidosis, pulmonary hypertension, and death, with diagnosis made at autopsy.

IMAGING

Chest x-ray—Shows haziness of the entire affected lung with reticular opacities and septal prominence. The affected lung is reduced in volume with ipsilateral mediastinal shift at baseline. Opacification of the affected lung or lobar involvement with consolidation or suppuration may occur when symptomatic with lower respiratory infection.

Chest CT scan

- Shows asymmetry with small hemithorax due to reduced lung volume, and ground-glass haziness with interlobular septal thickening throughout the affected lung (**Figure 52-1**).
- Interstitial fibrosis can occur secondary to pulmonary venous infarction and chronic pulmonary edema.
- There may be an ipsilateral small pulmonary artery with aberrant systemic arterial supply to the affected lung.
- The bronchial anatomy and patency are normal.[3]
- Of note, multidetector CT noninvasively demonstrates the anatomy and may obviate the need for invasive angiography.[4]

Magnetic resonance imaging—Confirms hypoplasia of affected lung, with diffuse interstitial thickening, pulmonary edema, and engorgement of pulmonary lymphatics.

Ventilation perfusion scan—Shows marked reduction in ventilation and perfusion to the affected side without air trapping.

Bronchoscopy—Shows normal tracheal and bronchial anatomy.

Cardiac catheterization—Pulmonary angiography is used for definitive diagnosis with characteristic findings: markedly increased pulmonary capillary wedge pressures, small ipsilateral pulmonary artery, and absence of the pulmonary vein on venous phase imaging.[5]

HISTOPATHOLOGY

The pulmonary parenchyma shows patchy interstitial fibrosis, pulmonary arteries show medical muscular hypertrophy. The pulmonary veins show medial muscular hypertrophy with intimal fibrosis and luminal narrowing without inflammatory change.

DIFFERENTIAL DIAGNOSIS

- Pulmonary lymphangiectasia—Usually distinguished by the radiographic appearance of the lymphatic malformation.

MANAGEMENT

NONPHARMACOLOGIC

- Attention to nutritional intake for optimal somatic and lung growth and development and recovery from infection.
- Chest physiotherapy for airway clearance with respiratory illnesses.
- Inhaled bronchodilators if there is associated bronchospasm or wheeze.
- Immunization—In addition to routine childhood immunizations, annual influenza vaccine after age 6 months, 23-valent pneumococcal vaccine for children aged >2 years every 5 years.

MEDICATIONS

- Early appropriate antibiotic therapy for lower respiratory infections; antibiotics tailored to known bacterial pathogens according to age.
- Aggressive approach in treating respiratory infections is essential to avoid suppurative complications; parenteral antibiotics when dictated by clinical presentation and radiological findings on chest x-ray.

SURGERY

- Anastomosis of the atretic pulmonary vein to the left atrium is a theoretical consideration but may not be possible due to complex and abnormal vascular anatomy.
- Pneumonectomy is recommended if there are recurrent or chronic suppurative complications or if the affected lung becomes a nidus of infection.[6] Pneumonectomy effectively eliminates the dead space and left to right shunt that may have developed.

REFERRAL

- Pediatric Cardiology—For (1) echocardiography to screen for associated congenital heart defects and (2) Cardiac catheterization and pulmonary angiography, measurement of pulmonary capillary wedge pressures for definitive diagnosis.
- Pediatric Pulmonology—To effectively manage recurrent respiratory infections, chest physiotherapy for airway clearance and to monitor pulmonary function longitudinally.

PREVENTION AND SCREENING

Maintain high index of suspicion and screen children with history of recurrent unilateral pneumonia with or without hemoptysis in early infancy or childhood with chest CT with contrast.

PROGNOSIS

- Prognosis following pneumonectomy is excellent with good functionality.
- Post-pneumonectomy, there is potential for scoliosis to develop in the growing child. Plombage (in which the empty hemithorax is filled with an inert material, e.g., sterile Lucite balls) is an option to maintain thoracic volume and prevent/minimize scoliosis.
- Mortality approaches 50 percent if left untreated.

FOLLOW-UP

- Optimize nutrition for lung growth and development.
- Annual cardiac screening with ECHO to monitor for pulmonary hypertension and right heart strain secondary to repeated lung infections.

PROVIDER RESOURCES

- Vyas HV, Greenberg SB, Krishnamurthy R: MR Imaging and CT Evaluation of Congenital Pulmonary Vein Abnormalities in Neonates and Infants. *RadioGraphics*. 2012;32:87-98.

TRACHEAL BRONCHUS

PATIENT STORY

A 17-year-old boy with Type 1 neurofibromatosis, seizure disorder, developmental delay, and dysphagia presents in winter with high-grade fever, cough, and respiratory distress. On examination he appears toxic and is tachycardic and tachypneic with intercostal and subcostal retractions. He requires oxygen via facemask at 5 liters/minute to maintain pulse oximetry saturations above 92 percent. Chest auscultation reveals scattered crackles and expiratory rhonchi over both lung fields. Rapid viral screen for influenza (H1N1) virus is positive. Chest x-ray shows right upper lobe consolidation and bibasilar patchy infiltrates. Laboratory investigations show an elevated white count and blood culture is negative. He is treated with broad spectrum parenteral antibiotics, oral oseltamivir, inhaled bronchodilators, and aggressive chest physiotherapy for airway clearance. He improves with weaning in his oxygen requirement to room air. Serial chest x-rays show right upper lobe collapse, which persists despite clinical improvement, even a month after discharge home. Further imaging with chest CT with contrast is done, which shows a tracheal bronchus supplying the right upper lobe, with a mucus plug obstructing the aberrant tracheal bronchus lumen (**Figure 52-2**). As he is asymptomatic and clinically stable, he is continued on chest physiotherapy with manual clapping and inhaled bronchodilators. A follow-up chest x-ray 2 months later shows resolution of the right upper lobe atelectasis with well aerated lung fields bilaterally.

INTRODUCTION

Tracheal bronchus describes a variety of bronchial anomalies, which arise from the main trachea proximal to the carina. An aberrant tracheal bronchus to the right upper lobe of the lung arises directly from the trachea itself proximal to the carina, unlike its typical origin after tracheal bifurcation, from the right main bronchus.

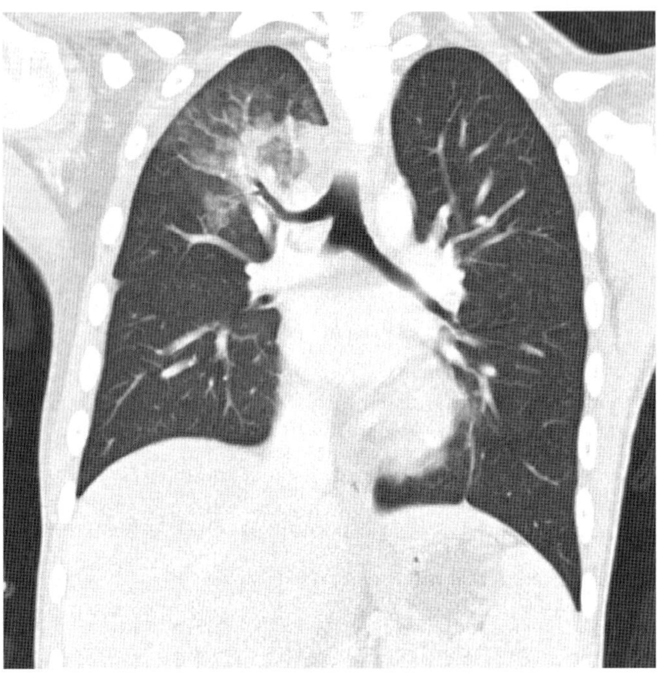

FIGURE 52-2 Aberrant right tracheal bronchus arising from the trachea proximal to its bifurcation, and supplying the right upper lobe, on coronal view chest CT scan. The carina, both right and left mainstem bronchi and their bronchial divisions are normal. (*Used with permission from S. Pinar Karakas, MD.*)

SYNONYMS

Bronchus suis, Pig bronchus.

EPIDEMIOLOGY

- An aberrant tracheal bronchus is often detected incidentally on CT imaging of the chest or bronchoscopy, and occurs in about 2 percent of the population.
- The right tracheal bronchus may be displaced in its origin to arise from the mainstem of the trachea proximal to the carina (a "pig bronchus" with all three segmental branches from it with no connection of the right upper lobe to the right main bronchus) or it may consist of only the right upper lobe apical bronchus with anterior and posterior segmental upper lobe branches arising from the right main bronchus.
- A prevalence of 0.1 to 2 percent for right tracheal bronchus and 0.3 to 1 percent for left tracheal bronchus have been reported in bronchoscopic and imaging studies.[7]
- Very rarely, bilateral tracheal bronchi may occur directed to both upper lobes of the lung.
- Tracheal bronchus has been found in association with other congenital anomalies including trachea-esophageal fistula, tracheal stenosis,

VATER syndrome (vertebral anomalies, anal atresia, trachea-esophageal fistula, esophageal atresia, renal defects), and Trisomy 21.

ETIOLOGY AND PATHOPHYSIOLOGY

- Embryogenic hypotheses for this congenital bronchial abnormality are the reduction, selection and theories of bronchial bud development (that the final anatomy is the result of shrinkage, suppression of portions of the original distribution and movement/migration from the initial location to arise from new origins) resulting in local disturbances in morphogenesis.[7]
- Altered drainage of the affected right upper lobe can result in localized pulmonary problems: partly due to the more horizontal direction of the tracheal bronchus, which impairs airway clearance as compared to the more vertical and gravitationally assisted normal configuration of the right upper lobe bronchus.
- This may result in localized or persistent atelectasis of the right upper lobe and recurrent infections with potential for suppurative changes and development of bronchiectasis.
- Both the pulmonary and bronchial vascular supply to the affected lobe of the lung are normal.

DIAGNOSIS

Tracheal bronchus is now diagnosed with increased frequency as a result of advances in and availability of chest CT imaging. Bronchoscopic examination of the airways is definitive, clearly demonstrating the tracheal origin of the aberrant bronchus.

CLINICAL FEATURES

- Often asymptomatic; may be detected incidentally on imaging or bronchoscopic examination.
- May cause recurrent infection, atelectasis, or consolidation of the right upper lobe due to mucus plugging and/or retained airway secretions.[8]
- Persistent cough may be a symptom. Occasionally hemoptysis may occur.
- Bronchiectatic changes may occur with repeated infections.
- If unrecognized, it may be the cause of persistent right upper lobe atelectasis/collapse in intubated patients due to occlusion of the orifice of the aberrant tracheal bronchus by the endotracheal tube.[9] Occasionally, inadvertent intubation of the aberrant bronchus may occur resulting in impaired ventilation.

IMAGING

- Chest x-ray—Right upper lobe atelectasis/collapse with lobar opacification that may be recurrent or persistent in nature.
- Chest CT scan—Shows the origin of the aberrant tracheal bronchus proximal to the carina; the rest of the bronchial anatomy is normal with normal lung parenchyma.[10] CT virtual bronchoscopy is a non-invasive alternative for diagnosis.
- Bronchoscopy—Definitive diagnosis rests on bronchoscopic examination of the airway, and visualization of the origin of the aberrant bronchus from the tracheal lumen proximal to the carina.[11]

DIFFERENTIAL DIAGNOSIS

- Supernumerary tracheal bronchus—This occurs in addition to the normally originating right upper lobe bronchus arising from the right main bronchus.
- Accessory bronchus—Will be seen on radiographic imaging.

MANAGEMENT

- Although asymptomatic and often incidentally detected, if present it can impact the care of children undergoing anesthesia and intubation and post-operative recovery. This airway anomaly must be kept in mind when chronic right upper lobe atelectasis/collapse is noted.[9]
- Management is based on the severity and frequency of associated symptoms.
- Surgical resection of the anomalous bronchus and lobe is indicated if recurrent suppurative infections occur.
- In asymptomatic or infrequently symptomatic patients, conservative and expectant management with antibiotics, chest physiotherapy and airway clearance are preferred.

NONPHARMACOLOGIC

- Care must be taken when intubation is being performed especially in children with conditions known to be associated with tracheal bronchus, including Down syndrome, foregut malformations, and tracheal stenosis.
- Chest physiotherapy regimen for airway clearance.

MEDICATIONS

- Inhaled bronchodilators may be used to aid mucociliary clearance and augment chest physiotherapy maneuvers.

SURGERY

- Right upper lobectomy is indicated if there is recurrent suppurative lung disease secondary to bronchial obstruction and impaired drainage of secretion.

REFERRAL

Physiotherapist—To teach parent/caregiver chest physiotherapy for airway clearance, instruct patient in use of airway clearance devices using positive end-expiratory pressure, that is, Acapella or Flutter device.

PREVENTION AND SCREENING

Tracheal bronchus should be screened for in children presenting with recurrent right upper lobe pneumonia or collapse, particularly if there are other associated congenital malformations of the heart, vertebrae, and gastrointestinal tract.

PROGNOSIS

Risk of recurrent respiratory infections due to obstruction of tracheal bronchus. Prognosis is good following surgical intervention with lobectomy.

PROVIDER RESOURCES

- Congenital malformations of the Trachea—**www.emedicine.medscape.com/article/837827**.

BRONCHOGENIC CYST

PATIENT STORY

A healthy, athletic 16-year-old-girl presented with acute right lower abdominal pain and vomiting for one day. She was evaluated with an abdominal CT scan with contrast which ruled out acute appendicitis. Incidentally, the lower thoracic cuts of the CT scan showed a low density mass inferior to the left mainstem bronchus (**Figure 52-3**). There were no lung parenchymal abnormalities, no adenopathy or effusion noted. She reported no symptoms, her lungs were clear on auscultation and spirometry revealed normal lung function and capacities. A chest MRI was done which showed a 40 × 30 × 37 mm mass with increased signal intensity located between the left inferior pulmonary vein and the descending thoracic aorta without contrast enhancement following administration of gadolinium (**Figure 52-4**). This cystic infrahilar mass appeared most compatible with a bronchogenic cyst. Elective surgical resection of the cyst was done successfully via thoracotomy; histopathology showed ciliated respiratory epithelium with goblet cells without metaplasia. She recovered uneventfully, was asymptomatic and returned to sport with normal exercise tolerance.

INTRODUCTION

- Bronchogenic cysts result from abnormal branching or budding of the ventral diverticulum of the foregut during embryologic development of the tracheobronchial tree.[12]

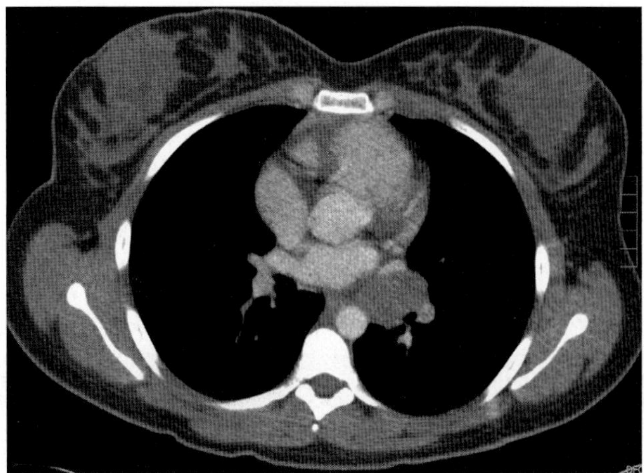

FIGURE 52-3 Cystic homogenous infratracheal lesion on chest CT without contrast, axial cut. (*Used with permission from Samiya Razvi, DCH, MD and Ellen Park, MD.*)

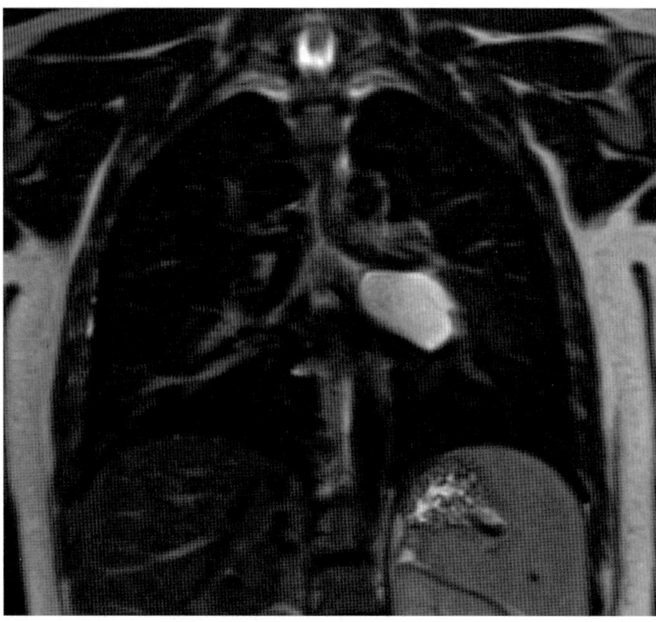

FIGURE 52-4 MRI chest with gadolinium demonstrating uniform fluid density cystic lesion inferior to left mainstem bronchus. (*Used with permission from Samiya Razvi, DCH, MD and Ellen Park, MD.*)

- Most often unilocular and lined with pseudo-stratified columnar respiratory epithelium, with a fibrovascular connective tissue wall of hyaline cartilage, smooth muscle and mucus glands.
- Do not usually communicate with the bronchial tree and therefore not typically air filled. They contain fluid (water), with variable amounts of proteinaceous material.

SYNONYMS

- Foregut duplication cyst.

EPIDEMIOLOGY

- Bronchogenic cysts comprise approximately 6 percent to 15 percent of primary mediastinal masses. Most often detected incidentally upon routine chest radiography.
- Tend to be detected more commonly in the right chest and more often in males.[1]

ETIOLOGY AND PATHOPHYSIOLOGY

- Bronchogenic cysts are characteristically oval or round in shape and occur in various locations depending on the stage of embryogenesis in which their formation occurs.
- Most commonly located in the mediastinum (paratracheal, pericarinal), intrapulmonary, and extrathoracic (para-esophageal and even subdiaphragmatic).
- Often asymptomatic, but have the potential to enlarge and compress adjacent structures in the mediastinum.
- Infection and rupture of the cyst can result in mediastinitis.

DIAGNOSIS

Usually suspected from its appearance on chest radiograph as a well marginated opacity of fluid attenuation. Definitive diagnosis can only be made by surgical excision and histopathological confirmation of the cyst lining as pseudo-stratified ciliated epithelium and wall containing cartilage, smooth muscle, or mucus glands.

CLINICAL FEATURES

- Usually benign congenital masses, which are asymptomatic; most commonly mediastinal in location.
- Clinical presentation varies from asymptomatic with incidental detection on imaging, to symptomatic large masses causing compression of adjacent structures.[13]
- Complete bronchial obstruction due to compression can lead to atelectasis of the lung; or air trapping if partial bronchial obstruction.
- Potential for infection of the cyst, resulting in fever, cough, dyspnea, and chest pain. Occasionally life-threatening hemoptysis or mediastinitis may occur.[13] Repeated cyst infection and inflammation can result in pericystic adhesions, ulceration of the cyst wall, and fistulous connection with the bronchial tree.
- Rarely, metaplasia may occur in the cyst lining, with malignant degeneration, and potential for development of bronchioalveolar carcinoma.

DISTRIBUTION

- Bronchogenic cysts can be broadly classified as mediastinal and intrapulmonary.
- Most common location is middle mediastinum (2/3)—Typically these cysts do not communicate with the tracheobronchial tree, and can be hilar, paratracheal, or subcarinal in location.
- Intrapulmonary or parenchymal (1/3)—Typically perihilar with a predilection for the lower lobes of the lung, and cyst lumen may communicate with the tracheobronchial tree.

IMAGING

- Prenatal diagnosis—With ultrasound imaging confirmed by fetal MRI at birth and then by Chest CT scan at age 1 month.
- Chest x-ray—Plain films reveal homogenous mass lesions, occasionally an air fluid level or peripheral calcification in the wall are noted.
- Chest CT scan with contrast—Selected thin slices delineate the cyst in relation to adjacent structures which aids preoperative planning. On CT imaging, the cyst is usually round or oval in shape with well circumscribed smooth or lobulated margins. The cyst typically has homogenous fluid density/consistency and hypoattenuation without contrast enhancement.[14]
- Magnetic resonance imaging with gadolinium—Differentiates these cysts from solid mediastinal masses. Simple bronchogenic cysts are fluid filled and characterized by very low intensity signals on T1 weighted images, in combination with markedly high signal intensity on T2 weighted images depending on the proteinaceous content.[14] There is usually no enhancement with contrast.

DIFFERENTIAL DIAGNOSIS[15]

- Esophageal duplication cyst, pericardial cyst.
- Thymic mass or cyst.
- Neurenteric cyst.
- Cystic teratoma.
- Cystic hygroma, lymphangioma.
- Infected bulla of lung, lung abscess, or fungal ball.
- Enlarged lymph node.
- These can be differentiated by the radiographic appearance, but ultimately definite diagnosis is made by histopathologic confirmation.

MANAGEMENT

Although the clinical course is uncertain, surgical excision is recommended even in asymptomatic patients to prevent complications including compression, infection, hemorrhage and malignant degeneration. The optimal timing for surgical resection is debated, as cysts tend to grow with age (likely due to mucus secretion), increasing the need for open thoracotomy as compared minimally invasive procedures (video assisted thoracoscopic surgery).[16]

With prenatal detection on ultrasonography, early thoracoscopic resection between the ages of 6 to 12 months is reported to better conserve lung parenchyma with lower risk of inflammatory/infectious complications.

SURGERY

- Complete surgical excision is recommended for mediastinal bronchogenic cysts and if required, lobectomy for intrapulmonary bronchogenic cysts.
- If excision is incomplete due to adhesion to surrounding tissues, partial excision with de-epithelization must be done in order to prevent recurrence at a later date.
- Surgical approach varies from open thoracotomy to video assisted thoracic surgery (VATS) with favorable outcomes for both with regard to duration of surgery and overall complications.[17]

REFERRAL

Pediatric cardiothoracic surgery.

PROGNOSIS

- If left untreated, the risk of morbidity (infections, inflammation, rupture, compression of adjacent structures) is estimated to be about 20 percent, and untreated cysts would need to be followed with periodic CT imaging, resulting in cumulative radiation dose exposure.
- Surgical excision is well tolerated; extended surgical dissection is required in complicated cysts, which have been infected resulting in adhesions to surrounding tissues.

PROVIDER RESOURCES

- Pediatric Bronchogenic Cyst—**www.emedicine.medscape.com/article/1005440**.
- Bronchogenic Cyst Imaging—**www.emedicine.medscape.com/article/354447**.

CONGENITAL LOBAR EMPHYSEMA

PATIENT STORY

A 10 month-old-male infant presents with history of recurrent wheezing episodes with intercurrent viral infections. Each episode begins with upper respiratory symptoms, cough, low grade fever, and rapidly escalates to severe respiratory distress and hypoxemia necessitating hospitalization. Review of his serial chest x-rays show persistent localized hyperlucency of the right upper lobe of the lung (**Figure 52-5**). Chest CT scan is done and reveals isolated hyperinflation of the right upper lobe with emphysematous appearance, reduced vascularity, and herniation across the mediastinum with contralateral mediastinal shift (**Figure 52-6**). There is ipsilateral compression and atelectasis of the right lower lobe of the lung. The tracheobronchial anatomy is normal. Surgical consultation is obtained and an elective right upper lobectomy is performed. Histopathological examination of the resected lobe of the lung shows overinflation of alveoli with emphysematous changes, and destruction and paucity of interalveolar septae (**Figure 52-7**). He recovers well postoperatively without complication. Over the next several months, he continues to have mild residual airway hyperreactivity and wheezing with respiratory illnesses; however this responds satisfactorily to inhaled bronchodilator treatments and does not progress to severe respiratory distress and decompensation as before. He continues to do well at follow-up with good growth and development with well aerated lung fields on follow-up chest x-ray.

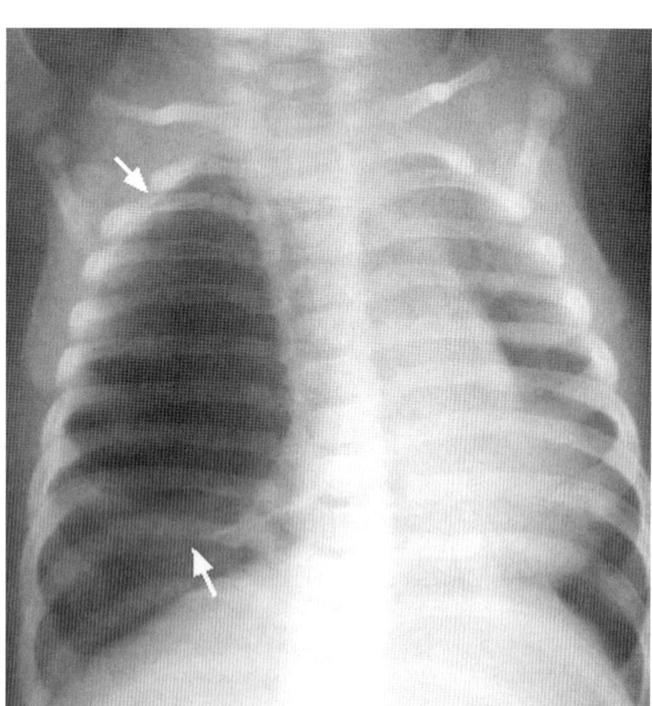

FIGURE 52-5 Plain chest x-ray demonstrating asymmetry in lung aeration (arrows), emphysematous right upper lobe, with herniation across the midline and compression of right lower lobe. (*Used with permission from Nitin Mehta, MD.*)

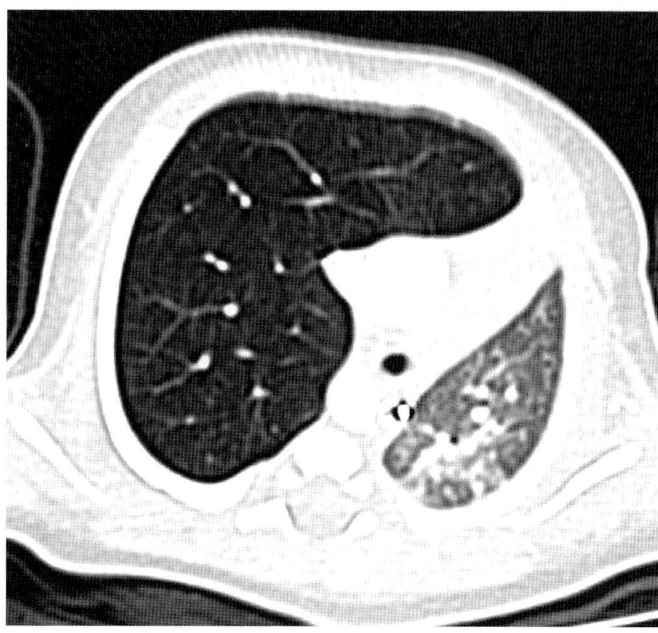

FIGURE 52-6 Chest CT scan showing emphysematous, hyperlucent right upper lobe with herniation across the midline. The bronchial anatomy and vascular supply to the lung is normal. (*Used with permission from Nitin Mehta, MD.*)

INTRODUCTION

Congenital lobar emphysema is a rare congenital abnormality caused by localized hyperinflation of a histologically normal single lobe of the lung with herniation of the emphysematous lobe and mediastinal shift

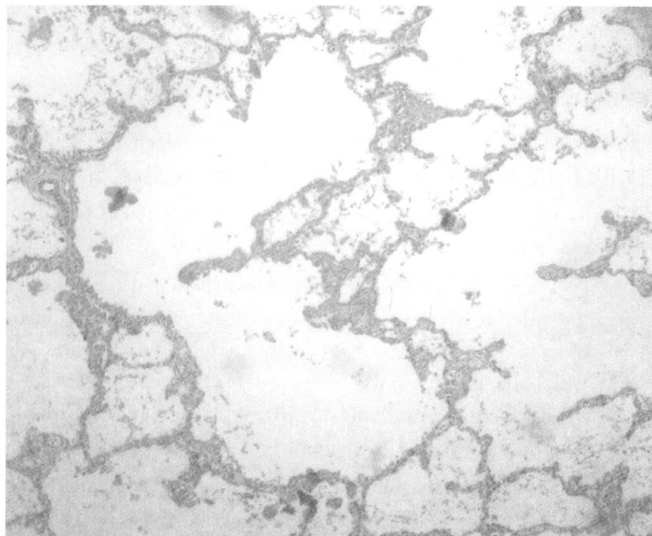

FIGURE 52-7 Histopathologic section with diagnostic findings of emphysematous change, overinflation of alveoli with destruction and paucity of interalveolar septae. (*Used with permission from the Department of Pathology, Christian Medical College Hospital, Vellore, India.*)

to the contralateral side and compressive atelectasis of the ipsilateral adjacent lung lobes.[18] There may be varying degrees of respiratory distress, and occasionally this condition may be mistaken for pneumothorax. This entity was first reported in 1932.

SYNONYMS

Infantile lobar emphysema.

EPIDEMIOLOGY

- Typically, symptoms occur in infancy, with tachypnea, retractions, wheeze, and respiratory distress with in infants less than 6 months age.
- Approximately twice as common in males as compared to females.[18]
- Fourteen to forty percent of cases are noted to be associated with congenital anomalies, most often congenital heart disease.
- Rarely, this may be discovered as an incidental finding in an asymptomatic older child or adult.

ETIOLOGY AND PATHOPHYSIOLOGY

- Pathogenetic factors implicated as causes for congenital lobar emphysema include developmental anomalies of the bronchus supplying the affected lobe.
- Cartilaginous dysplasia, bronchomalacia, or deficiency of the bronchial cartilaginous rings cause the bronchus to collapse during expiration resulting in ball valve effect and air trapping causing emphysematous changes of the affected lobe.[19]
- In some cases, there is intraluminal bronchial obstruction due to bronchial mucosal proliferation or extrinsic bronchial compression from aberrant vessels.

DIAGNOSIS

Congenital lobar emphysema is diagnosed based on clinical and radiologic findings with histological confirmation in patients who have undergone surgical removal of the affected lung lobe.

CLINICAL FEATURES

- Typically presentation occurs in the newborn period or infancy.
- Neonatal presentation can occur with respiratory distress, which may be severe; about half the cases are reported to be symptomatic in the first few weeks of life.
- Intercurrent respiratory illnesses precipitate onset of respiratory failure/distress in infancy.
- On auscultation, breath sounds are decreased over the affected lobe.
- Respiratory symptoms range from asymptomatic tachypnea, recurrent episodes of wheezing to severe respiratory decompensation and respiratory failure.
- Emphysematous changes in the affected lobe result in tachypnea at baseline due to increase in dead space ventilation, progressive distension and hyperinflation of the affected lobe with respiratory distress.
- Rarely, may remain asymptomatic until detected in adulthood.[20]

DISTRIBUTION

- The left upper lobe is more often affected than the right upper lobe; next in frequency is the right middle lobe and involvement of the lower lobes is rare.

LABORATORY TESTING

- Arterial blood gas analysis shows hypoxemia when symptomatic and hypercarbia due to increased dead space ventilation.

IMAGING

- Improved resolution in prenatal ultrasound techniques can detect unilateral hypoechoic lesion in the lung.[21]
- Chest x-ray—Hyperlucency of the affected lobe with herniation across the midline to opposite side, mediastinal shift, and compressive atelectasis of adjacent ipsilateral lung lobes. There may be a widening of the rib spaces as well as flattening of the hemidiaphragm on the affected side.
- Chest CT scan—Provides definitive diagnosis, by delineating normal bronchial anatomy with stretched attenuated vessels in the affected emphysematous lobe and herniation across the mediastinum to the opposite side.[22]
- Bronchoscopy—Can rule out bronchial luminal obstruction, bronchial structural anomalies, bronchial stenosis, or an obstructing mucus plug.
- Ventilation perfusion scan with technetium 99m—Shows reduced ventilation and perfusion in the affected lobe. This technique also establishes whether the lobe affected by CLE is nonfunctional, and whether the compressed lung is functioning normally.

HISTOPATHOLOGY

Shows emphysematous change, overinflation of alveoli with destruction, and paucity of interalveolar septae (**Figure 52-7**).

DIFFERENTIAL DIAGNOSIS

- Tension pneumothorax in grossly distended lobe; differentiated by presence of lung markings in CLE.

MANAGEMENT

Treatment is based on the acuity of presentation and severity of respiratory distress. Traditionally, surgical resection of the affected lobe is recommended, either electively in the mildly symptomatic infant or urgently when there is life-threatening respiratory decompensation and failure.[23]

Some patients with mild symptoms have been treated conservatively without surgical intervention and are reported to have done well. However the long-term impact of conservative treatment is yet undetermined and needs further evaluation.

SURGERY

- Lobectomy is recommended early in order to prevent potentially life-threatening respiratory distress.
- During anesthesia these patients may tolerate positive pressure ventilation poorly with risk for air trapping, further distension of the affected lobe with cardiorespiratory compromise for which they must be carefully monitored.[23]
- Rapid thoracotomy may be necessary and the surgeon present at anesthetic induction; the abnormal lobe herniates through the thoracotomy while the remaining lung is atelectatic.
- Following lobectomy, the remaining lobe of the ipsilateral lung expands to fill the hemithorax.

REFERRAL

Pediatric cardiothoracic surgery. Pediatric pulmonology to follow lung function and development longitudinally.

PROGNOSIS

- Lobectomy is safe and effective therapy, and tolerated well.[24]
- Growth and expansion of the remaining lung tissue occurs in children up to the age of 6 to 8 years, resulting in near normal lung volume and function.

FOLLOW-UP

- Postoperative chest x-rays are near normal with good potential for lung growth and development in young children.[24]
- Serial pulmonary function testing to assess lung capacities and to screen for small airway obstruction/airway hyperreactivity can be done in older children.

PATIENT RESOURCES

- **www.emedicinehealth.com/emphysema_congenital_lobar-health/article_em.htm**.

PROVIDER RESOURCES

- Imaging in Congenital Lobar Emphysema—**www.emedicine.medscape.com/article/407635**.

CONGENITAL CYSTIC ADENOMATOID MALFORMATION (CCAM)

PATIENT STORY

A 35-year-old-woman, with history of 4 previous spontaneous abortions (all occurring in the first trimester of pregnancy) is followed closely at the obstetric high risk clinic. Prenatal ultrasound screening of the fetus, detects a cystic lesion of the right lung at 20 weeks gestation, which occupies about 40 percent of the right hemithorax. There are no associated congenital abnormalities and fetal growth and developmental parameters are normal. On serial ultrasound imaging, the cystic lesion of the right lung is noted to be progressively smaller with fetal growth, and is reduced in size to about 10 percent of the right lung towards term. The infant is born normally at 40 weeks gestation, a male with birth weight 3.5kg, and Apgar scores 9 and 10, and 1 and 5 minutes respectively. There are no respiratory symptoms or distress. The neonate is asymptomatic, feeding and sucking well, with comfortable respirations and normal oxygenation on pulse oximetry. Physical examination is normal and his lungs are clear on auscultation. Chest x-ray taken on the first day of life shows normal well aerated lung fields bilaterally without any masses or opacity noted.

The infant is followed closely and remains well without any respiratory symptoms. He has mild gastroesophageal reflux in the first 3 months but normal weight gain. Chest x-rays are repeated at regular intervals at age 1, 3, and 6 months and are normal. A chest CT scan with contrast is planned and done electively at age 12 months, given the history of the prenatally detected cystic right lung lesion. The chest CT scan shows a cystic lesion of the right lower lobe, with hyperlucent loculation, normal bronchial anatomy and normal blood supply (**Figure 52-8**).

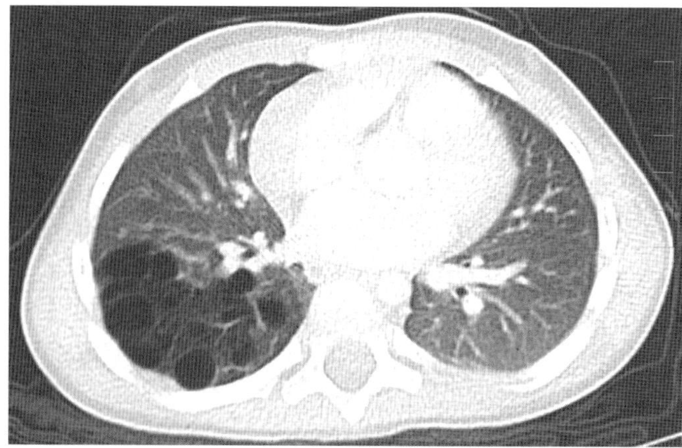

FIGURE 52-8 CT axial view showing cystic lucencies in the right lower lobe of the lung diagnostic of congenital cystic adenomatoid malformation (CCAM). *(Used with permission from Samiya Razvi, DCH, MD and Ellen Park, MD.)*

Diagnosis of a congenital cystic adenomatoid malformation (CCAM) is made, and elective right lower lobectomy is performed via thoracotomy. He tolerates the surgery well, without complications. On long-term follow-up, he has normal growth and development, is active with good exercise tolerance, and no respiratory symptoms.

INTRODUCTION

CCAM is a rare developmental abnormality of lung, first described by Chin and Tang in 1949. This malformation is considered to be a benign hamartomatous or dysplastic lung tumor. CCAM occurs as a result of cessation of bronchial maturation, and characteristic overgrowth of mesenchymal elements, which produce the adenomatoid appearance with reduction in the number of alveoli.[25]

SYNONYMS

Congenital pulmonary airway malformation (CPAM).

EPIDEMIOLOGY

- Incidence is reportedly between 1:11,000 and 1:35,000 live births.
- Slightly more predominant in males than females.

ETIOLOGY AND PATHOPHYSIOLOGY

- Overgrowth, hyperplasia, and hamartoma formation have been proposed as etiology. Failure in the interaction between mesenchyma and epithelial elements during lung development and maturation may result in the discordance in vascularity and proliferation of lung tissue.
- Traditionally, one classification based on the size of the cysts and histopathology by Stocker et al. [26] is as follows:
    - Type I—Macrocystic adenomatoid malformation usually affecting a single lobe, with cysts usually greater than 2 cm in diameter. Cyst walls have a lining of respiratory epithelium and communicate with the proximal airways and distal lung parenchyma.
    - Type II—Microcystic adenomatoid malformation resulting from obstruction of the airways during development resulting in multiple small cysts less than 1 cm in diameter.
    - Type III—Solid airless mass consisting of mostly bronchiolar elements with respiratory epithelial lining, and some alveolar elements.

DIAGNOSIS

A significant proportion are detected on antenatal ultrasound screening as cystic or solid fetal lung lesions. If detected postnatally on chest x-ray, chest CT scan imaging is definitive. CCAMs should be suspected in cases of unilateral recurrent pneumonia, or when there is persistent localized opacification noted on serial chest x-rays.

CLINICAL FEATURES

- Prenatal ultrasound detects hypoechoic lung lesions in the fetus, which are then confirmed postnatally by chest CT scan in those who are liveborn.[27]
- Majority (80%) present in the neonatal period with respiratory distress, especially if large cystic lesions. Significant cardiorespiratory compromise can occur due to associated pulmonary hypoplasia, which can be severe, as a result of mass effect of the lesion during intrauterine development. [27]
- Smaller cystic or solid CCAMS may be asymptomatic and go undetected in early infancy, and may present later in childhood or even adulthood as unilateral recurrent pneumonia, lung abscess, persistent localized chest opacity on chest x-ray or rarely with malignant transformation.[27]

DISTRIBUTION

- Usually unilateral involving only one lobe of the lung; rarely bilateral lesions have been reported.

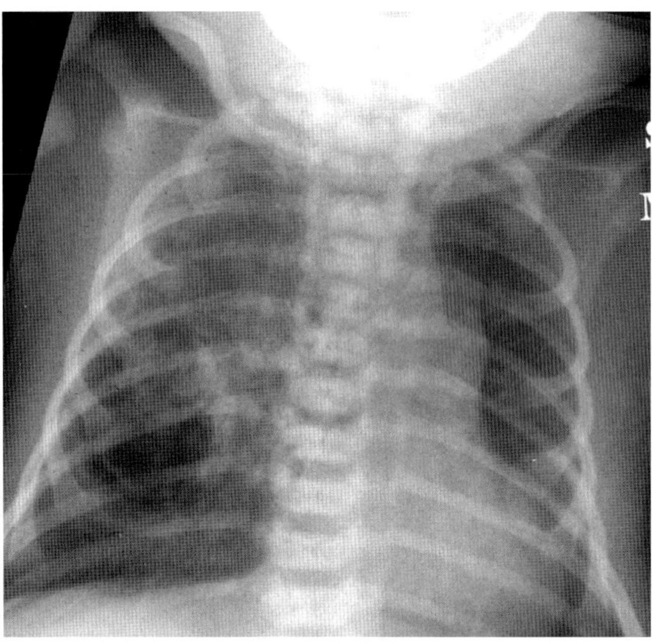

FIGURE 52-9 Chest radiograph in a newborn with congenital cystic adenomatoid malformation (CCAM) shows large cystic areas in the right lower lobe with some mass effect and depression of the hemidiaphragm. *(Used with permission from S. Murthy Chennapragada, MD.)*

- Left sided lesions are more common than right.
- Coexistence of a pulmonary sequestration occurs in up to half the patients in some reports.

IMAGING[28]

- High resolution ultrasound can detect CCAMs on prenatal screening, as hypoechoic or cystic fetal lung lesions, depending on the relative amounts of cystic and solid tissue. Fetal MRI provides additional detail on structure of the lesion and reliably distinguishes CCAM from congenital diaphragmatic hernia. Color Doppler ultrasound is used to identify the absence of a systemic feeding vessel, which differentiates this from pulmonary sequestration.
- Chest x-ray findings vary and may show no abnormality, a large air filled cystic lesion, cystic lesions interspersed with parenchymal opacity or a solid appearing lung mass (**Figures 52-9** and **52-10**).
- Chest CT scan with contrast is the imaging modality of choice in the postnatal evaluation of infants suspected to have a congenital lung lesion (**Figures 52-11** and **52-12**).

DIFFERENTIAL DIAGNOSIS

- These entities can usually be distinguished by the classic appearance of CCAM on Chest CT:
    - Pulmonary sequestration.
    - Congenital diaphragmatic hernia.
    - Teratoma.
    - Bronchogenic or enteric duplication cyst.
    - Congenital lobar emphysema.

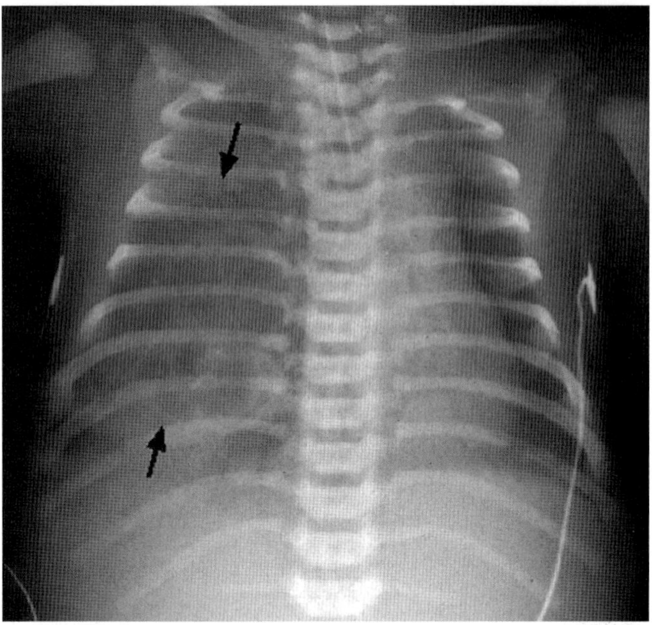

FIGURE 52-10 Plain CXR of a newborn showing cystic lesions with soap bubble appearance in right lung (arrows), with poorly defined margins. This is another example of congenital cystic adenomatoid malformation. (*Used with permission from Nitin Mehta, MD.*)

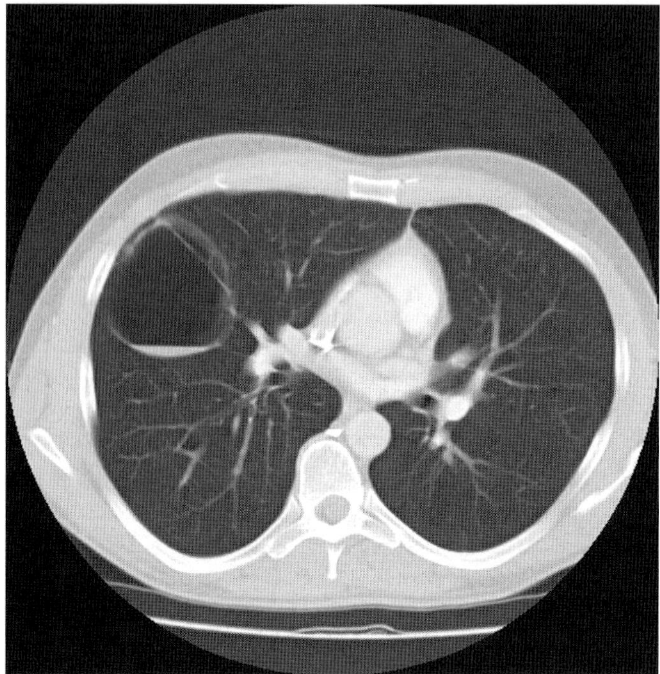

FIGURE 52-12 Axial cut chest CT showing single large cystic lesion with well-defined wall in right lung consistent with congenital cystic adenomatoid malformation. (*Used with permission from Nitin Mehta, MD.*)

MANAGEMENT

- Congenitally diagnosed lung masses have been reported to decrease in size toward term on serial ultrasonography and "disappear"; controversy exists whether postnatal imaging should be done for such infants. Several authors have shown that significant abnormalities do remain in such cases, and CT imaging is essential to delineate the presence, location, and size of the lung lesion.[29]
- Surgical resection is now the standard of care, even if asymptomatic, given the risk of complications which include sudden respiratory compromise, pneumothorax, infection, compression of adjacent structures, rupture, and malignant degeneration.

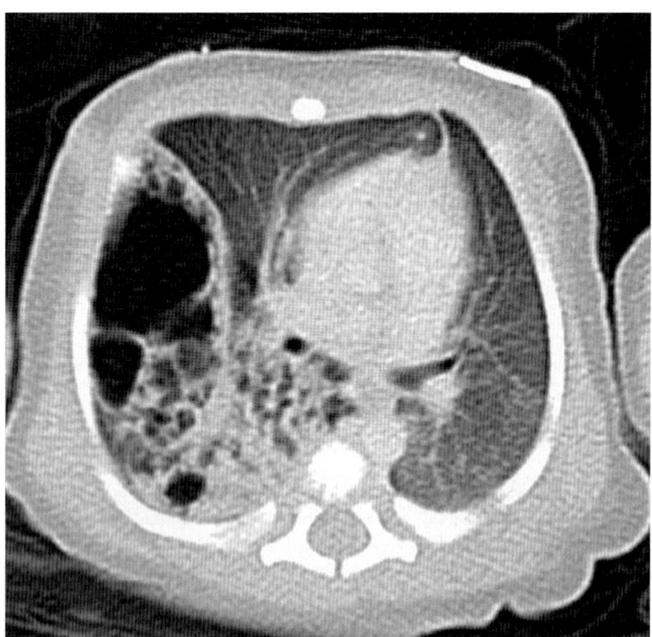

FIGURE 52-11 Congenital pulmonary airway malformation Type 1. Chest CT showing multiple cysts of varying sizes replacing the right lower lobe. The dominant ones measure >2 cm and are surrounded by multiple smaller cysts. (*Used with permission from S. Murthy Chennapragada, MD.*)

SURGERY

- Lobectomy is the procedure of choice and well tolerated; occasionally emergency resection may be needed. Video-assisted thoracoscopic surgery is minimally invasive, safe, and effective. The optimal timing for elective surgery is not well delineated, and is often recommended in the latter half of infancy to reduce anesthetic and surgical risks.[29]
- Debate exists whether segmental resection of the lung can be done as a parenchymal sparing technique to conserve normal pulmonary remnants for subsequent growth and development. However, it has been described that the preoperative CT is not predictive of extension of the malformation to the rest of the lobe. Segmental resection (subtotal lobectomy or segmentectomy) would therefore risk leaving remnants of the CCAM and may also be associated with greater incidence of postoperative complications such as air leak and infections requiring repeat surgery and lobectomy.[30]

REFERRAL

Pediatric Cardiology to evaluate for associated cardiac anomalies or intracardiac defects.

PREVENTION AND SCREENING

Prenatal high resolution ultrasound screening and serial evaluation; fetal MRI when indicated.

PROGNOSIS

- Perinatal mortality varies greatly depending on the size of the lesion from 9 to 49 percent, with complications resulting from severe respiratory distress in symptomatic neonates.
- Lobectomy overall provides good symptom relief and excellent long-term outcomes. Infants and children tolerate lobectomy well with continued lung growth resulting in near normal lung volumes and gas exchange capacity.
- Type I CCAMs have the best prognosis, whereas Type III lesions have worse outcomes.
- Poor prognosis is associated with bilateral lesions, presence of associated pulmonary hypoplasia and cardiac anomalies.

FOLLOW-UP

- Residual mild respiratory symptoms including airway hyperreactivity and wheeze may be present on long-term follow-up in some patients.
- Serial pulmonary function testing may be done in older patients to monitor lung function.

PROVIDER RESOURCES

- Cystic Adenomatoid Malformation Treatment and Management—**www.emedicine.medscape.com/article/1001488-overview**.
- Imaging in Congenital Cystic Adenomatoid Malformation—**www.emedicine.medscape.com/article/407407-overview**.

PULMONARY SEQUESTRATION

PATIENT STORY

A 13-year-old-African American girl presents with history of intermittent colicky, abdominal pain for several weeks with acid reflux symptoms. She also has exercise induced asthma, which is well controlled with inhalers. She has a history of pneumonia once at the age of 5 years; her previous Cx-rays are unavailable. Cx-ray shows cystic lesion in the right lower lobe with well-defined wall, central lucency, and an air fluid level (**Figure 52-13**). She is evaluated with an upper GI series for the abdominal pain, which detects intestinal malrotation without acute obstruction. CT scan of the abdomen is done and shows polysplenia. Chest CT shows a dense contrast enhancing opacity of the right lower lobe, with mixed solid and cystic characteristics supplied by an aberrant artery from the descending thoracic aorta

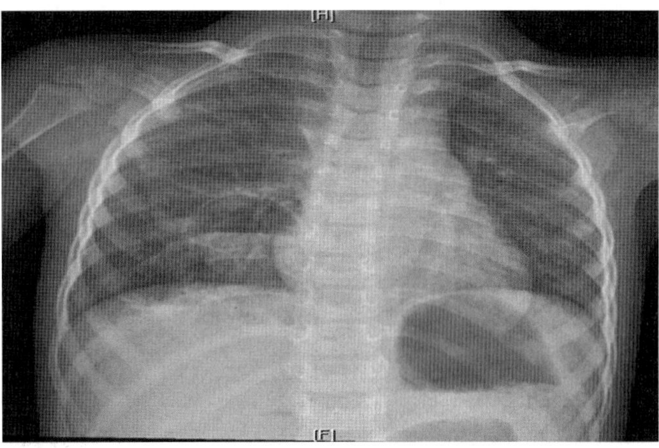

FIGURE 52-13 Plain CXR showing cystic lesion in the right lower lobe, with well circumscribed wall and central lucency with air fluid level. (*Used with permission from Sneha Varki, MD.*)

(**Figure 52-14**). There are no other anomalous vessels. She first undergoes surgical correction of the intestinal malrotation with relief of her abdominal symptoms. Elective surgical resection of the right lower lobe lesion with interruption and ligation of the anomalous supplying artery is done successfully at a later date, with an uneventful postoperative course. Histopathological examination of the resected lung lobe shows features characteristic of intrapulmonary sequestration (**Figure 52-15**). On follow-up, she is asymptomatic with normal chest x-ray and normal lung function as assessed by spirometry.

INTRODUCTION

Pulmonary sequestration occurs as a localized abnormality of the lung parenchyma that is nonfunctioning, lacks communication with the tracheobronchial tree, and has aberrant arterial blood supply directly from the aorta. Sequestration can be either intralobar sequestration (ILS) or extralobar sequestration (ELS) depending on whether the affected lung tissue is within the normal lung lobe or outside.[31]

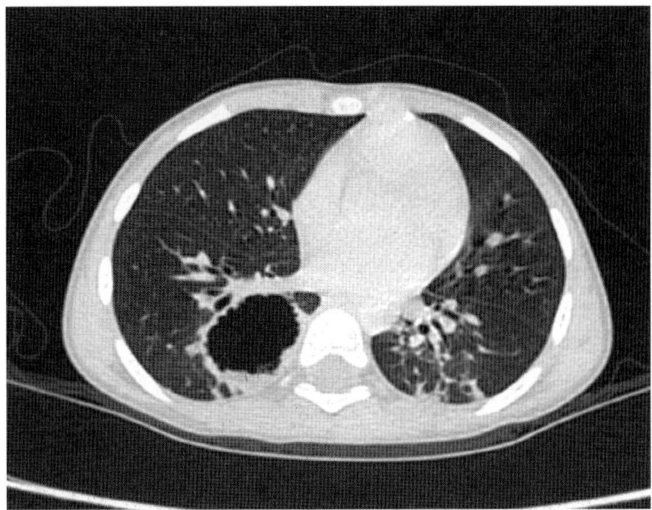
FIGURE 52-14 CT scan axial cut of the same lesion in Figure 52-13 showing cystic nature of intralobar sequestration contained within the right lower lobe of the lung. (*Used with permission from Sneha Varki, MD.*)

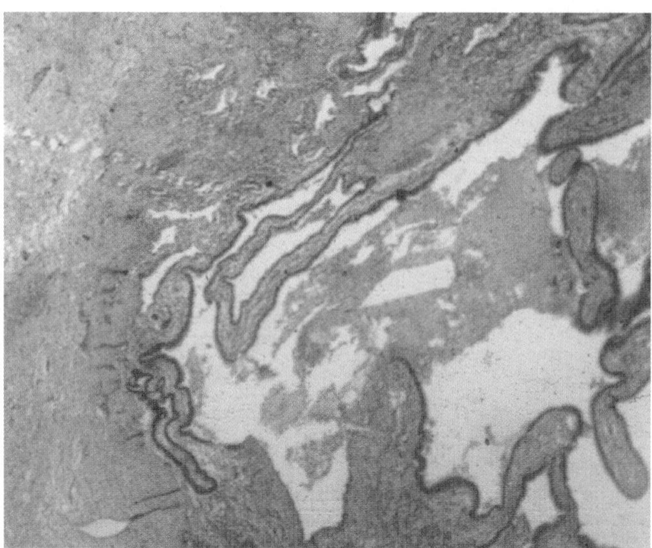

FIGURE 52-15 Histopathological section of intrapulmonary sequestered lobe- demonstrating well circumscribed lesion, dilated bronchi with moderate mononuclear cell infiltrate in the bronchial wall, dilated alveoli, a few of which contain foamy histiocytes as well as hemosiderophages within the lumen. The blood vessels have thick muscular walls and there is moderate interstitial fibrosis. (*Used with permission from the Department of Pathology, Christian Medical College Hospital, Vellore, India.*)

SYNONYMS

Bronchopulmonary sequestration.

EPIDEMIOLOGY[31]

- Second most common congenital pulmonary malformation, with the frequency of intralobar (ILS) to extralobar sequestration (ELS) being about 3:1.
- Anomalies of the chest wall, spine, diaphragm, intestinal tract, and heart associated more often with ELS (65%) and fewer with ILS (11%). Most common anomalies associated with ELS include congenital diaphragmatic hernia and CCAM.

ETIOLOGY AND PATHOPHYSIOLOGY

- Pulmonary sequestration occurs due to abnormalities in development during branching and proliferation of the bronchial structures, with separation of the affected lobe and loss of communication with the tracheobronchial tree.[32]
- Intralobar sequestration (ILS) is contained with the lung and the affected lobe does not have its own pleura.
- Extralobar sequestration (ELS) has its own covering with visceral pleura and thus is anatomically separate from adjacent lung tissue.
- Both ILS and ELS have systemic arterial blood supply arising from the aorta. The venous drainage of ELS is usually into the systemic veins, whereas the ILS drains into the pulmonary veins.
- Large sequestration lesions may compress residual lung tissue during development, increasing the risk of pulmonary hypoplasia.
- Connections to the gastrointestinal tract (stomach, esophagus) may be present and increase the risk of infection.

DIAGNOSIS

CLINICAL FEATURES

- ILS usually are symptomatic early in infancy, whereas ELS usually have a silent clinical course and may be asymptomatic (10%) until incidentally detected in the older child or adult.[33]
- May present as recurrent pneumonia localized to the affected lobe and persistent opacity on chest x-ray prompting further imaging with CT.
- High output cardiac failure may occur due to left to right shunting in the affected lobe with increased pulmonary blood flow via the aberrant systemic arterial blood supply.
- Congenital anomalies such as diaphragmatic hernia, CCAM, foregut duplication cysts, pectus excavatum, and congenital heart defects are reported in about 60 percent of ELS cases.[34]
- Serious complications include infection with formation of lung abscess, massive hemoptysis due to erosion of the systemic artery supplying the sequestered lobe, and malignant degeneration.

DISTRIBUTION

- ILS occurs equally in both genders, whereas ELS has a slight male predominance (3:1).
- Occurs more commonly in the left lung (55% of ILS and 65% of ELS).
- Most common location for ILS is the posterior basal segment of the left lower lobe and for EPS is below the left lower lobe.

IMAGING

- Demonstration of a systemic arterial blood supply is essential for diagnosis of pulmonary sequestration, either by Doppler ultrasound, CT, or MRI angiography.[35]
- Chest x-ray—Nonspecific and may show a homogenous opacity in the lower lobes of the lung; areas of cavitation may occur with infection and communication with the tracheobronchial tree.
- Ultrasound—Both ILS and ELS appear as solid, well-circumscribed, and echogenic masses on ultrasound. Color Doppler can demonstrate the aberrant systemic feeding artery to the sequestered lobe.
- Angiography—Traditionally considered the gold standard for diagnosis by depiction of the arterial and venous anatomy. However, it is invasive, with radiation exposure and need for sedation in young children and has been replaced by noninvasive multidetector CT or MR angiography.
- **Chest CT scan with contrast**—Now the diagnostic modality of choice. CT noninvasively confirms the diagnosis, delineates the anatomical location of the sequestered lobe, its lack of communication with the bronchial system, and clear demonstration of the aberrant systemic arterial supply to the affected lobe (**Figure 52-16**).

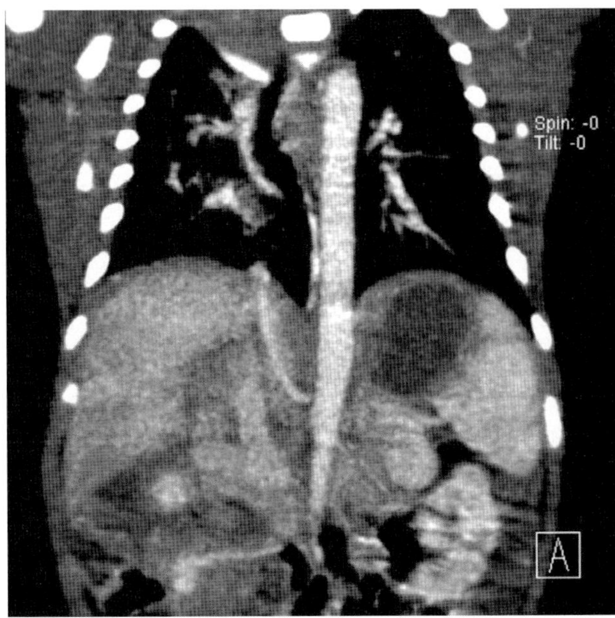

FIGURE 52-16 Coronal Chest CT scan post contrast images in the arterial phase demonstrate an aberrant artery arising from the abdominal aorta and supplying the sequestered lung in the right lower lobe; the venous drainage is into the pulmonary veins: intralobar sequestration. (*Used with permission from S. Murthy Chennapragada, MD.*)

HISTOPATHOLOGY

Microscopy shows dilated bronchioles, alveoli, and air spaces lined with respiratory epithelium. There may be changes of chronic infection or inflammation and fibrosis.

DIFFERENTIAL DIAGNOSIS

- CCAM—See previous section.
- Teratoma—Usually detected by radiographic manifestations.

MANAGEMENT

SURGERY

- Definitive treatment for both ILS and ELS is surgical resection of the mass, even if asymptomatic, to prevent complications.
- Preoperatively, it is imperative to delineate the anomalous blood vessels to the sequestered lobe to minimize the risk of hemorrhage during surgery.
- Lobectomy is indicated since the anomalous vasculature may be difficult to delineate intra-operatively, making resection challenging for the surgeon and the risk for significant and massive bleeding given the systemic arterial supply.
- As recurrent infection results in inflammatory changes and adhesions, which may obliterate intersegmental planes, early elective resection is recommended.
- Arterial embolization of the sequestered lobe with subsequent reduction in size on CT imaging has been reported, but does not exclude the presence of residual dysplastic tissue with risk for malignant degeneration.
- Traditionally, thoracotomy is used as it provides adequate exposure for lobectomy. Minimally invasive techniques are an alternative approach in minimizing surgical trauma, morbidity, and postoperative pain.[36]

PREVENTION AND SCREENING

Serial prenatal ultrasound imaging for monitoring fetal lung lesions is recommended at 1- to 3-week intervals until stability of the lesion has been established, and then typically monthly thereafter. Fetal MRI imaging is useful to delineate vascular anatomy and other associated congenital anomalies.

PROGNOSIS

Overall, the outcome is good with resolution of symptoms and complications including heart failure due to left to right shunting. As the lung tissue in the sequestered lobe is nonfunctional, the functional consequences are insignificant after postoperative recovery. With the increasing use of minithoracotomies and minimally invasive techniques, the long-term sequelae on thoracic wall growth and development are reduced.

PROVIDER RESOURCES

- Pulmonary sequestration Imaging—**www.emedicine.medscape.com/article/412554-overview**.

PULMONARY AGENESIS

PATIENT STORY

A term male infant is born by elective Caesarean section, to a third gravida mother with gestational diabetes mellitus and history of two previous Caesarean sections. The infant is pink, vigorous at birth with good cry and tone; Apgar scores are 8 and 9 at 1 and 5 minutes, respectively. His birth weight is 3000 grams. At 24 hours age, he is noted to have mild respiratory distress with a respiratory rate of 50/min and subcostal retractions. His pulse oximetry saturations are 96 percent on room air. He is afebrile, sucking and feeding well. On auscultation of the chest, breath sounds appear diminished over the right chest. Heart sounds are normal and there is no murmur. A chest x-ray is ordered and shows opacification of the right hemithorax, with shift of the mediastinum to the right. The left lung is hyperinflated and extends across the midline to the right upper chest. The cardiac silhouette is normal. An echocardiogram is done and shows no intracardiac defect, the great vessels are normal. A chest CT scan is done and shows absence of the right lung and right main bronchus (**Figures 52-17** and **52-18**). The left lung bronchial anatomy and lung parenchyma are normal. Virtual bronchoscopy using reconstructive images confirms the findings of normal trachea, and absent right main bronchus, normal left bronchial anatomy. He is diagnosed to have complete agenesis of the right lung. There are no other congenital abnormalities; renal ultrasound is normal. He is followed closely after discharge from hospital. He continues to have mild tachypnea with retractions at rest, but is otherwise well and gaining weight.

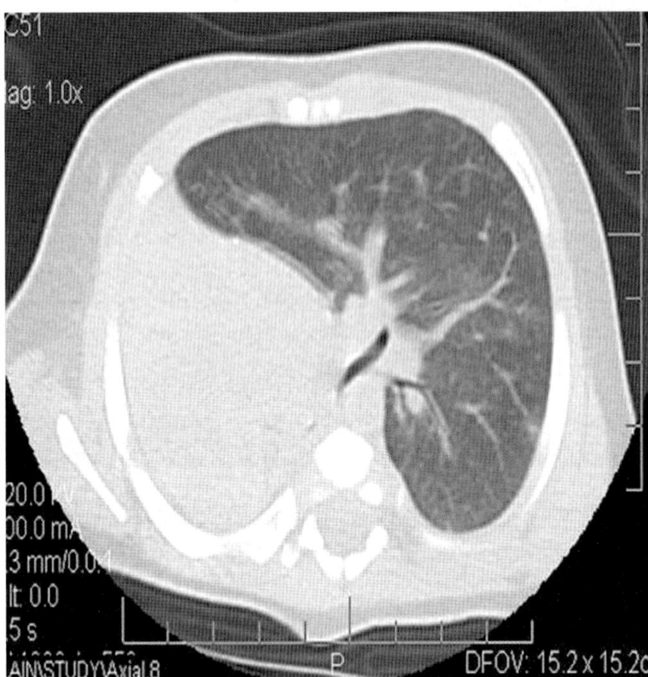

FIGURE 52-17 Axial cut of chest CT of right pulmonary agenesis with classical findings of no definable lung tissue, pulmonary artery or main bronchus on the affected side. There is ipsilateral shift of the heart and mediastinum. (*Used with permission from Nadeem Ahmed, MD, DNB.*)

INTRODUCTION

Pulmonary agenesis (PA) is a rare developmental defect in which there is unilateral or bilateral complete absence of the lung, its bronchus and vascular supply. Schneider and Schwalbe classified the

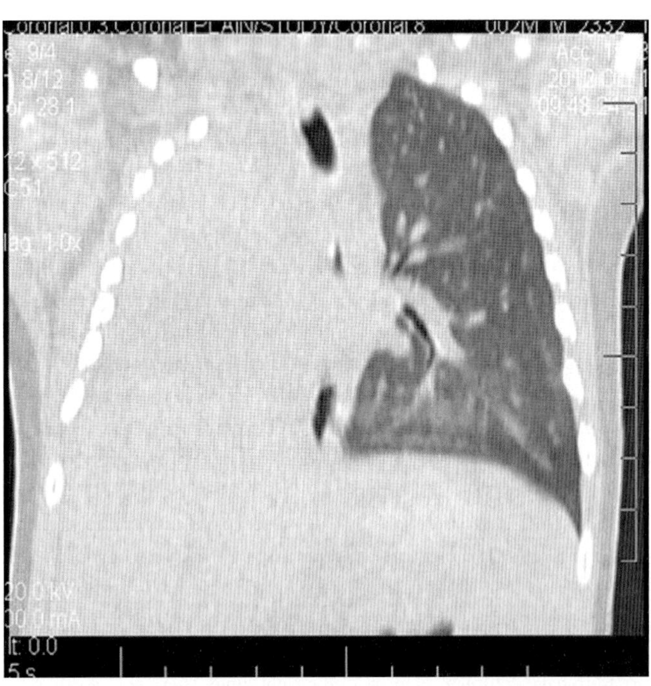

FIGURE 52-18 Chest CT scan coronal view showing complete absence of right lung, including right main bronchus and right pulmonary artery with opacification of the affected hemithorax. (*Used with permission from Nadeem Ahmed, MD.*)

anomaly into 3 categories: (1) agenesis: complete absence of a lung, bronchus and pulmonary vasculature (2) aplasia: there is a blind-ending rudimentary bronchus coming off the trachea without lung tissue or pulmonary vasculature (3) hypoplasia: there is a rudimentary bronchus and hypoplastic lung, airways, alveoli and pulmonary vessels are decreased in size and number.[37]

EPIDEMIOLOGY

- Rare congenital anomaly estimated to occur in approximately 1 per 15,000 pregnancies and frequently associated with other abnormalities. The true incidence may be higher as 50 percent of cases are stillborn and more than 20 percent die at birth or during their first few months.[37]

ETIOLOGY AND PATHOPHYSIOLOGY

- Occurs as a result of complete failure of development of one of the lung buds. It has been hypothesized that abnormal blood flow in the dorsal aortic arch during the 4th week of gestation (embryonic phase) causes pulmonary agenesis.
- There is mediastinal shift with compensatory hyperexpansion of the contralateral normal lung.
- Tracheal compression can be caused by the displaced aorta; there may also be intrinsic tracheobronchial anomalies including tracheal stenosis and tracheomalacia.
- Cardiac failure or pulmonary hypertension can occur in survivors; due to associated congenital heart disease and/or pulmonary vascular anomalies.
- Esophageal anomalies such as tracheoesophageal fistula and gastroesophageal reflux can occur; pulmonary agenesis can be a part of VACTERL sequence.[38]

DIAGNOSIS

CLINICAL FEATURES

- Variable clinical presentation; may be asymptomatic and incidentally detected.[39]
- Symptoms range from mild dyspnea on exertion, recurrent respiratory infections to severe distress with respiratory failure requiring mechanical ventilatory support in the neonatal period.
- Associated anomalies involving cardiovascular, GI, skeletal, and urogenital systems are present in about half the cases.
- Agenesis of the right lung is associated with a higher frequency of anomalies than agenesis of the left lung.
- Tracheal compression can be caused by a deviated aorta, dilated pulmonary artery, or cardiac chamber or vascular ring. Tracheal stenosis and tracheomalacia can occur.

DISTRIBUTION

- Slight preponderance in females.
- Right and left lungs are absent with equal frequency.

IMAGING

- Ultrasound—Prenatal diagnosis is characterized by unilateral hyperechogenicity of the affected lung.[40]
- Chest x-ray—Shows complete opacification or white-out of the affected hemithorax suggestive of collapse consolidation. There is asymmetry in the lung volumes and configuration with overexpansion of the contralateral normal lung often causing mediastinal shift. The definitive diagnosis is made via pulmonary angiography, which shows the pulmonary artery to the affected side to be absent.
- Chest CT scan with contrast—Provides precise anatomical delineation with no definable lung tissue, pulmonary artery, or main bronchus on the affected side with ipsilateral shift of the heart and mediastinum. Vascular compression of the major airways can also be detected.
- MRI—Accurately defines the airway and vascular anatomic abnormalities and has replaced conventional angiocardiography in patient management and surgical planning.
- Bronchoscopy—Reveals a blind-ending main bronchus on the affected side.

MANAGEMENT

Asymptomatic patients do not require surgical intervention especially in the absence of associated anomalies. Respiratory infections should be treated early and aggressively as there is low respiratory reserve. Pulmonary hypertension can occur due to reduction in the pulmonary vascular bed, and if associated with left to right intracardiac shunts can progress to irreversible vascular disease.

SURGERY

- Surgery may also be indicated to relieve significant bronchial obstruction (aortopexy, division of vascular rings, and resection of stenotic and malacic bronchus) or for stabilization of the mediastinum (relocation of diaphragm and insertion of prosthesis).
- Associated cardiac and esophageal anomalies will require surgical correction.[37]

REFERRAL

Pediatric Cardiology to rule out associated congenital heart disease.

PROGNOSIS

- Survival has improved with advancements in neonatal and surgical management; survival into adulthood is reported.
- Right-sided agenesis has poor outcome attributed to greater shift of heart and mediastinum with consequent distortion of the vascular structures and airway, and a higher incidence of associated cardiac and vascular anomalies.[37]

FOLLOW-UP

- Patients should be closely monitored for growth retardation and scoliosis; major airway compression may lead to symptoms of stridor.
- Serial pulmonary function tests can help assess and monitor lung capacities, lung volumes and airway flow rates in older children and adults.

PROVIDER RESOURCES

- Congenital lung malformations—**www.emedicine.medscape.com/article/905596-overview**.

REFERENCES

1. Beerman, LB, Oh KS, Park SC, Freed MD, Sondheimer HM, Fricker FJ, Mathews RA, Fischer DR. Unilateral Pulmonary Vein Atresia: Clinical and Radiographic Spectrum. *Pediatric Cardiology*. 1983;4(2):105-112.
2. Kim Y, Yoo IR, Ahn MI, Han DH. Asymptomatic adults with isolated unilateral right pulmonary vein atresia: multidetector CT findings. *British Journal of Radiology*. 2011;84(1002):e109-e113.
3. Heyneman LE, Nolan RL, Harrison JK, McAdams HP. Congenital Unilateral Pulmonary vein atresia radiologic findings in 3 adult patients. *Am J Roentgenol.* 2001;177(3):681-685.
4. Mataciunas M, Gumbiene L, Cibiras S, Tarutis V, Tamosiunas AE. CT angiography of mildly symptomatic, isolated, unilateral right pulmonary vein atresia. *Pediatr Radiol.* 2009;39(10):1087-1090.
5. Cullen S, Deasy PF, Tempany E, Duff, DF. Isolated pulmonary vein atresia. *British Heart Journal* 1990;63:350-354.
6. Pourmoghadam KK, Moore JW, Khan M, Geary EM, Madan N, Wolfson BJ, et al. Congenital unilateral pulmonary venous atresia: definitive diagnosis and treatment. *Pediatr Cardiol.* 2003; 24:73-79.
7. Ghaye B, Szapiro D, Fanchamps JM, Dondelinger RF. Congenital bronchial anomalies revisited. *RadioGraphics*. 2001;21:105-119.
8. McLaughlin FJ, Strieder DJ, Harris GB, Vawter GP, Eraklis AJ. Tracheal bronchus: association with respiratory morbidity in childhood. *J Pediatr.* 1985;106(5):751-755.
9. O'Sullivan BP, Frassica JJ, Rayder SM. Tracheal bronchus: a cause of prolonged atelectasis in intubated children. *Chest.* 1998; 113(2):537-540.
10. Gower WA, Mc-Grath-Morrow SA, MacDonald KD, Fishman EK. Tracheal bronchus in a 6-month-old infant identified by CT with three-dimensional airway reconstruction. *BMJ Case Rep*. 2009; bcr2006071100.
11. Doolittle AM, Mair EA. Tracheal bronchus: Classification, endoscopic analysis and airway management. *Otolaryngol Head Neck Surg*. 2002;126(3):240.
12. Petroze R, McGahren ED. *Pediatric chest II: Benign tumors and cysts. Surg Clin North Am*. 2012;92(3):645-658.
13. Limaïem F, Ayadi-Kaddour A, Djilani H, Kilani T, El Mezni F. Pulmonary and mediastinal bronchogenic cysts: a clinicopathologic study of 33 cases. *Lung*. 2008;186(1):55-61.
14. McAdams HP, Kirejcyzk WM, Rosado-de-Christenson ML, Matsumoto S. Bronchogenic cyst: imaging features with clinical and histopathological correlation. *Radiology*. 2000;217:441–446.

15. Jeung MY, Gasser B, Gangi A et al. Imaging of cystic masses of the mediastinum. *Radiographics.* 2002;22:S79-93.
16. Fievet L, D'Journo XB, Guys JM, Thomas PA, De Lagausie P. Bronchogenic cyst: best time for surgery? *Ann Thorac Surg.* 2012;94(5):1695-1699.
17. Nasr A, Bass J. Thoracoscopic versus open resection of congenital lung lesions: a meta-analysis. *J Pediatr Surg.* 2012;47(5): 857-861.
18. Mendeloff EN. Sequestrations, Congenital Cystic Adenomatoid Malformations and Congenital Lobar Emphysema. *Semin Thorac Cardiovasc. Surg.* 2004;16:209-214.
19. R Ulku, Onat S, Ozcelik C. Congenital lobar emphysema: Differential diagnosis and therapeutic approach. *Pediatrics International.* 2008;50:658-661.
20. Sadaqat M, Malik JA, Karim R. Congenital lobar emphysema in an adult. *Lung India.* 2011;28:67-69.
21. Epelman M, Kreiger PA, Servaes S, Victoria T, Hellinger JC. Current imaging of prenatally diagnosed congenital lung lesions. *Semin Ultrasound CT MR.* 2010;31(2):141-157.
22. Lee EY, Boiselle PM, Cleveland RH. Multidetector CT evaluation of congenital lung anomalies. *Radiology.* 2008; 247(3):632-648.
23. Olutoye OO, Coleman BG, Hubbard AM, Adzick NS. Prenatal diagnosis and management of congenital lobar emphysema. *J Pediatr Surg.* 2000; 35(5):792-795.
24. Ozçelik U, Göçmen A, Kiper N, Doğru D, Dilber E, Yalçin EG. Congenital lobar emphysema: evaluation and long-term follow-up of thirty cases at a single center. *Pediatr Pulmonol.* 2003;35(5): 384-391.
25. Azizkhan RG, Crombleholme TM. Congenital cystic lung disease: contemporary antenatal and postnatal management. *Pediatr Surg Int.* 2008;24:643-657.
26. Stocker JT, Madewell JE, Drake RM. Congenital cystic adenomatoid malformation of the lung. *Hum Pathol.* 1977;8:155-171.
27. Aslan AT, Yalcin E, Soyer T, Dogru D, Talim B, Ciftci AO, Ozcelik U, Kiper N. Prenatal period to adolescence: The variable presentations of congenital cystic adenomatoid malformation. *Pediatr Int.* 2006;48(6):626-630.
28. Winters WD, Effmann EL. Congenital masses of the lung: prenatal and postnatal imaging evaluation. *J Thorac Imaging.* 2001;16(4): 196-206.
29. Eber E. Antenatal diagnosis of congenital thoracic malformations: early surgery, late surgery, or no surgery? *Semin Respir Crit Care Med.* 2007;28(3):355-366.
30. Muller CO, Berrebi D, Kheniche A, Bonnard A. Is radical lobectomy required in congenital cystic adenomatoid malformation? *J Pediatr Surg.* 2012;47(4):642-645.
31. Corbett HJ, Humphrey GME. Pulmonary sequestration. *Paediatric Respiratory Reviews.* 2004;5:59-68.
32. Guidry C, McGahren ED. Pediatric chest I: Developmental and physiologic conditions for the surgeon. *Surg Clin North Am.* 2012;92(3):615-643.
33. Bratu I, Flageole H, Chen MF, Di Lorenzo M, Yazbeck S, Laberge JM. The multiple facets of pulmonary sequestration. *J Pediatr Surg.* 2001;36(5):784-790.
34. Mendeloff EN. Sequestrations, congenital cystic adenomatoid malformations, and congenital lobar emphysema. *Semin Thorac Cardiovasc Surg.* 2004;16(3):209-214.
35. Abbey P, Das CJ, Pangtey GS, Seith A, Dutta R, Kumar A. Imaging in bronchopulmonary sequestration. *Journal of Medical Imaging and Radiation Oncology* 2009; 53:22-31.
36. Kestenholz PB, Schneiter D, Hillinger S, Lardinois D, Weder W. Thoracoscopic treatment of pulmonary sequestration. *Eur J Cardiothorac Surg.* 2006;29(5):815-818.
37. Nazir Z, Qazi SH, Ahmed N, Atiq M, Billoo AG. Pulmonary agenesis—vascular airway compression and gastroesophageal reflux influence outcome. *J Pediatr Surg.* 2006;41(6):1165-1169.
38. Cunningham ML, Mann N. Pulmonary agenesis: a predictor of ipsilateral malformations. *Am J Med Genet.* 1997;70(4):391-398.
39. Thomas RJ, Lathif HC, Sen S, Zachariah N, Chacko J. Varied presentations of unilateral lung hypoplasia and agenesis: a report of four cases. *Pediatr Surg Int.* 1998;14(1-2):94-95.
40. Meller CH, Morris RK, Desai T, Kilby MD. Prenatal diagnosis of isolated right pulmonary agenesis using sonography alone: case study and systematic literature review. *J Ultrasound Med.* 2012; 31(12):2017-2023.

PART 9

THE GASTROINTESTINAL TRACT AND NUTRITIONAL DISORDERS

Strength of Recommendation (SOR)	Definition
A	Recommendation based on consistent and good-quality patient-oriented evidence.*
B	Recommendation based on inconsistent or limited-quality patient-oriented evidence.*
C	Recommendation based on consensus, usual practice, opinion, disease-oriented evidence, or case series for studies of diagnosis, treatment, prevention, or screening.*

*See Appendix A on pages 1320–1322 for further information.

53 FAILURE TO THRIVE

Vera Okwu, MD
Lori A. Mahajan, MD

PATIENT STORY

A 12-year-old African American boy with cerebral palsy-quadriplegia was brought to clinic as mother was having progressive difficulty feeding him (**Figure 53-1**). He had not been seen in the office since age 9 years when he plotted at the 20th percentile for both weight and length on the cerebral palsy-quadriplegia growth chart. Mother stated that she was having difficulty obtaining his supplemental 1.5cal/cc supplement that had been prescribed and her son was becoming progressively more selective regarding intake of solids. School officials also reported feeding difficulty. On examination, he appeared emaciated. Length, weight, and BMI were far below the 5th percentile. Labs including a celiac antibody panel, comprehensive metabolic panel, CBC with differential, sedimentation rate, and thyroid function studies were normal with the exception of mild lymphopenia and a low pre-albumin. Swallow evaluation showed oropharyngeal dysphagia characterized by residuals and delay in swallow onset. A trial of nasogastric (NG) feeds resulted in rapid weight gain with good tolerance.

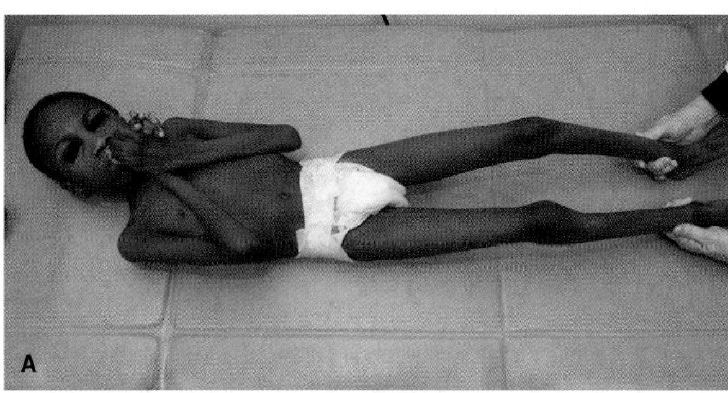

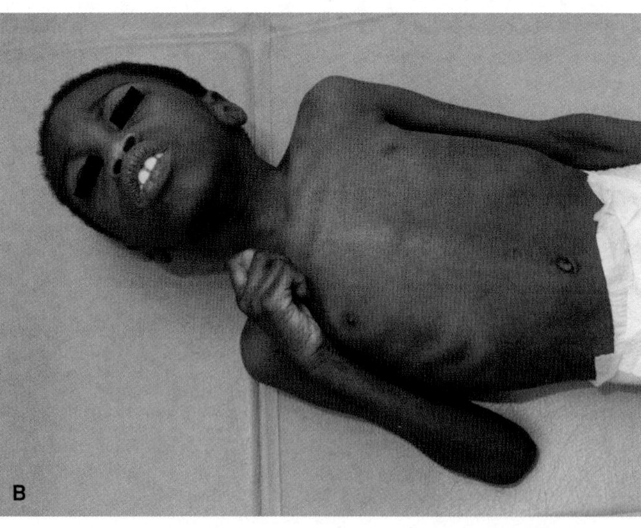

FIGURE 53-1 Cerebral palsy, quadriplegia and severe protein-calorie malnutrition in a 12-year-old boy. **A.** Note the extremely thin extremities. **B.** Close-up of the spasticity and extreme emaciation seen in his chest. *(Used with permission from Lori Mahajan, MD.)*

A gastrostomy was subsequently placed for supplemental feeds. Close follow-up was scheduled with the nutritional support team, his physician, and social services.

INTRODUCTION

Failure to thrive (FTT) is a clinical sign, rather than a diagnosis. A wide variety of medical conditions and psychosocial factors contribute to FTT. Potential long-term complications of FTT include permanent cognitive impairment with decreased IQ, short stature, and serious infections due to immune deficiency.

SYNONYMS

Malnutrition, nutritional insufficiency, growth failure.

EPIDEMIOLOGY

- Occurs more commonly in children living in poverty.
- Affects 5 to 10 percent of children in the primary care setting.[1]
- Up to 50 percent of children with FTT are not identified by health care providers.

ETIOLOGY AND PATHOPHYSIOLOGY

- More than 90 percent of cases are purely nutritional, with no identifiable underlying medical condition.
- Causes of FTT are currently classified into the following categories: inadequate caloric intake, inadequate absorption or increased losses, increased metabolic needs, or ineffective utilization.[1,2]

INADEQUATE CALORIC INTAKE

- Behavioral problems interfering with meals/inappropriate feeding habits.
- Dysfunctional parent-child relationship.
- Neglect (**Figure 53-2**).
- Poverty.
- Inadequate lactation.
- Improper formula preparation.
- Suck/swallow dysfunction (esophageal motility dysfunction, CNS, neuromuscular, anatomic-cleft lip, or palate) (**Figure 53-3**).
- Feeding fatigue (anemia, genetic syndrome, cerebral palsy, neuromuscular disease, CNS structural abnormality).
- Feeding refusal (reflux or eosinophilic esophagitis, aspiration).
- Recurrent emesis.

INADEQUATE CALORIC ABSORPTION

- Necrotizing enterocolitis.
- Protein malabsorption (cow milk protein allergy, enterokinase deficiency).

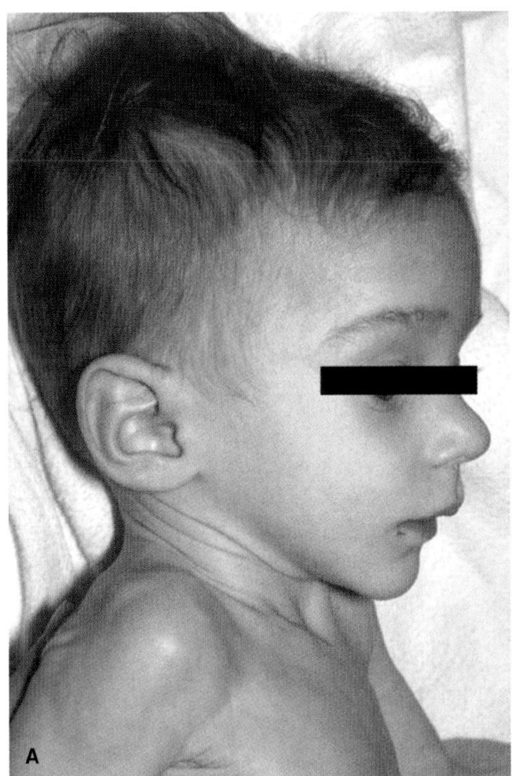

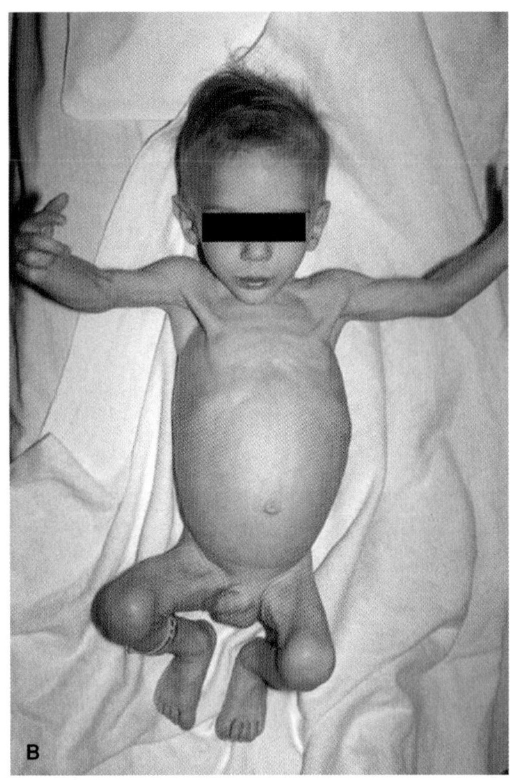

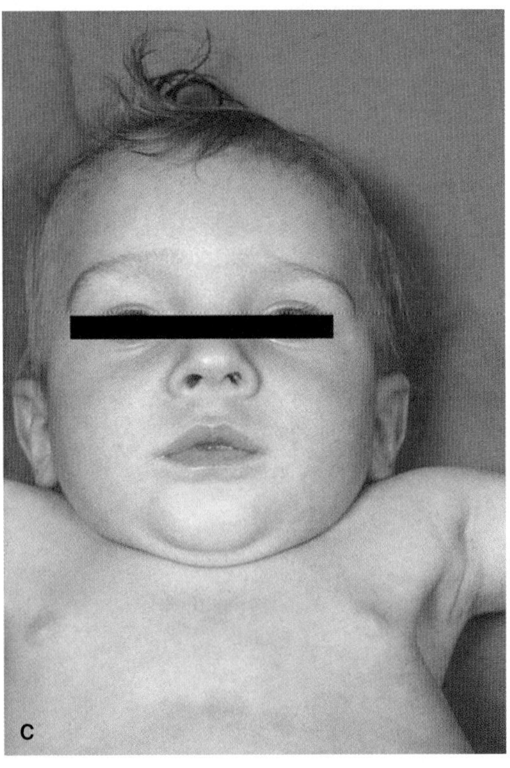

FIGURE 53-2 **A** and **B.** Thin, cachectic infant who is failing to thrive due to psychosocial neglect. **C.** Same infant after one month of adequate calorie intake. *(Used with permission from Cleveland Clinic Children's Photo Files.)*

- Pancreatic insufficiency (cystic fibrosis, chronic pancreatitis, Shwachman-Diamond syndrome).
- Liver disease.
- Celiac disease—See Chapter 60, Celiac Disease.
- GI tract infections.
- Carbohydrate malabsorption.
- Short bowel syndrome.
- Inflammatory bowel disease—See Chapter 59, Inflammatory Bowel Disease.

INCREASED CALORIC NEEDS

- Congenital heart disease—See Chapters 42 and 43, Acyanotic Congenital Heart Disease and Cyanotic Congenital Heart Disease.

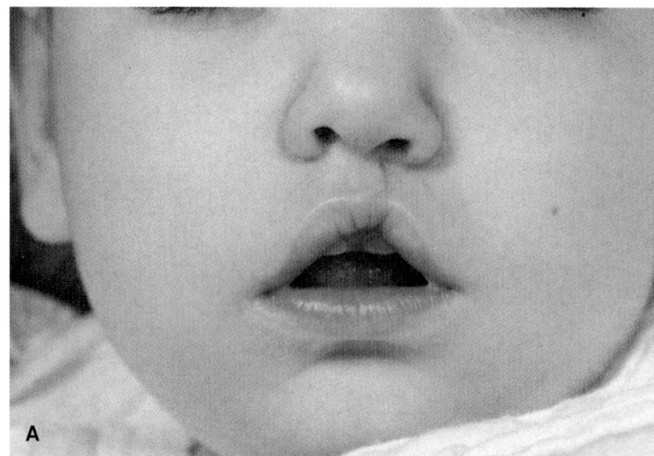

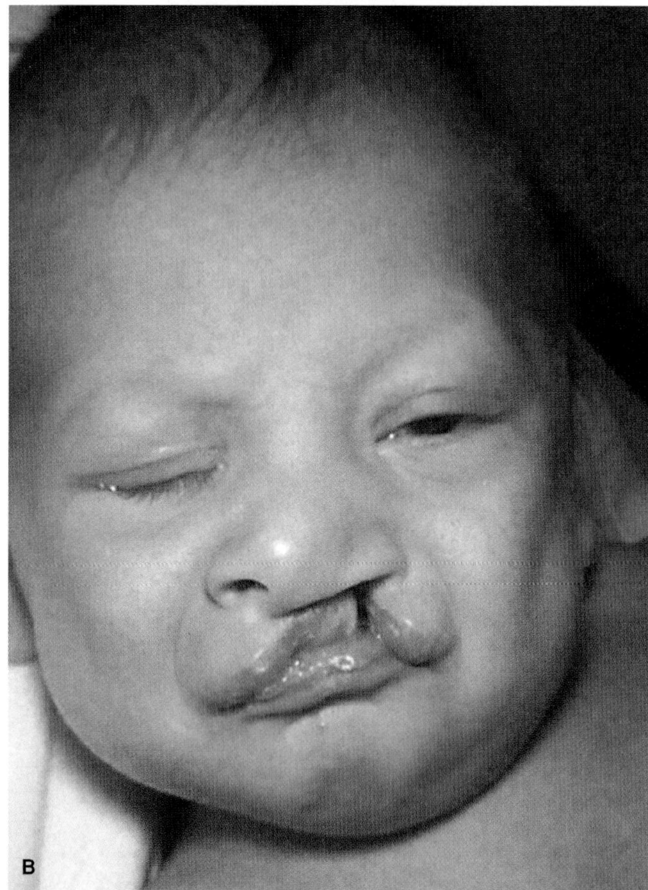

FIGURE 53-3 Incomplete (**A**) and complete (**B**) cleft lip and palate in two infants with failure to thrive due to suck and swallowing dysfunction. (*Used with permission from Cleveland Clinic Children's Photo Files.*)

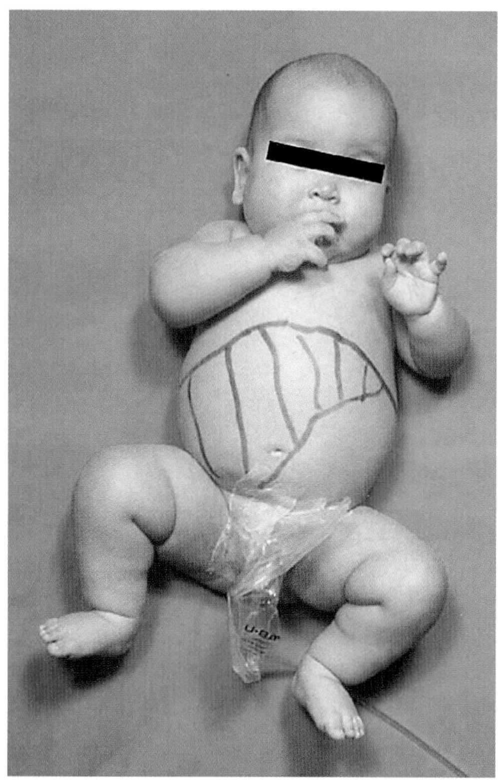

FIGURE 53-4 Hepatomegaly and growth failure in an infant who was found to have a glycogen storage disease. The presence of physical findings such as hepatomegaly should raise concern for an organic etiology for failure to thrive. (*Used with permission from Cleveland Clinic Children's Photo Files.*)

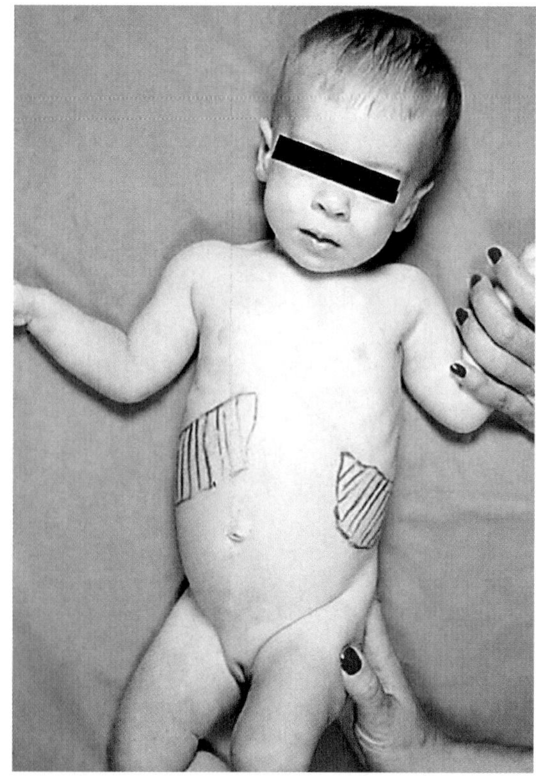

FIGURE 53-5 Hepatosplenomegaly and abdominal distension in a young infant who has severe developmental delay. This infant was diagnosed with Niemann-Pick syndrome, a lysosomal storage disorder. (*Used with permission from Cleveland Clinic Children's Photo Files.*)

- Chronic lung disease.
- Chronic systemic infection (congenital infections, HIV)—See Chapter 187, Congenital Infections.
- Chronic metabolic disorder (adrenal insufficiency, diabetes mellitus, hyperthyroidism, inborn errors of metabolism) (**Figures 53-4** and **53-5**).
- Kidney disease (renal tubular acidosis).
- Chronic systemic disease (systemic lupus erythematosus, juvenile idiopathic arthritis)—See Chapters 172 and 173,

Juvenile Idiopathic Arthritis and Lupus—Systemic and Cutaneous.

- Malignancy.
- Inflammatory bowel disease—See Chapter 59, Inflammatory Bowel Disease.
- Genetic Syndromes (Trisomy 21, Turner, Russell-Silver syndromes)—See Chapters 221 to 228.

RISK FACTORS

- Hostile intrauterine environment (exposure to alcohol, illicit drugs, infection, anticonvulsants).
- Prematurity.
- Concomitant syndrome or congenital abnormality (cleft lip, cleft palate, congenital heart disease, etc.).
- Developmental delay.
- Any condition that interferes with adequate intake, interferes with intestinal absorption, or increases the underlying metabolic rate.
- Psychosocial factors including poverty, first born status of infant, poor parenting skills or feeding techniques, parental substance or physical abuse, or erroneous nutrition practices (administration of dilute formula, prolonged exclusive breastfeeding, and intentional caloric restriction due to fear of obesity).

DIAGNOSIS

CLINICAL FEATURES

- Precise measurement of weight and length/height are essential.
- Common anthropometric criteria for FTT include:
  - Weight < 2nd percentile for gestation-corrected age and gender on > one occasion.
  - Weight < 80th percentile of ideal weight-for-age on a standard growth chart.
  - Weight to length ratio < 10th percentile.
  - Body mass index for age < 5th percentile.
- The World Health Organization growth charts should be used to assess the growth of children in the US under the age of 24 months.[3]
- Growth charts for prematurity should be used until 24 months.
- Genetic syndrome-specific (Achondroplasia, Cornelia de Lange Syndrome, Marfan Syndrome, Prader-Willi Syndrome, Rubinstein Taybi Syndrome, Trisomy 21, Turner Syndrome, Williams Syndrome) growth charts and special needs (Cerebral Palsy-Quadriplegic) growth charts exist and should be used.
- Growth standards for children < age 2 years are based on recumbent length; a stadiometer with fixed headboard and sliding footboard should be used.
- An accurate wall mounted stadiometer should be used for children ≥2 years of age.
- Degree of malnutrition is categorized by different systems as mild, moderate, severe (**Table 53-1**).[4]

TABLE 53-1 Grading of Malnutrition by Waterlow Classification[4]

Grade	Acute Malnutrition* (% weight for height)	Chronic Malnutrition** (% height for age)
Mild	<90	<95
Moderate	<80	<90
Severe	<70	<85

*To **calculate % weight for height**, divide child's measured weight by the 50th percentile value of weight for child's actual height age and multiply by 100. Height age equals the age for which child's measured height plots on the 50th percentile of the growth curve.
To **calculate % height for age, divide child's measured height by the 50th percentile value of height for child's age and multiply by 100.

- Decline in weight gain or height velocity due to underlying nutritional or endocrine etiologies need to be differentiated from constitutional causes (**Figure 53-6**).
- A careful and detailed history, including dietary history, feeding history, medical/surgical history, family history, and social history should be obtained.

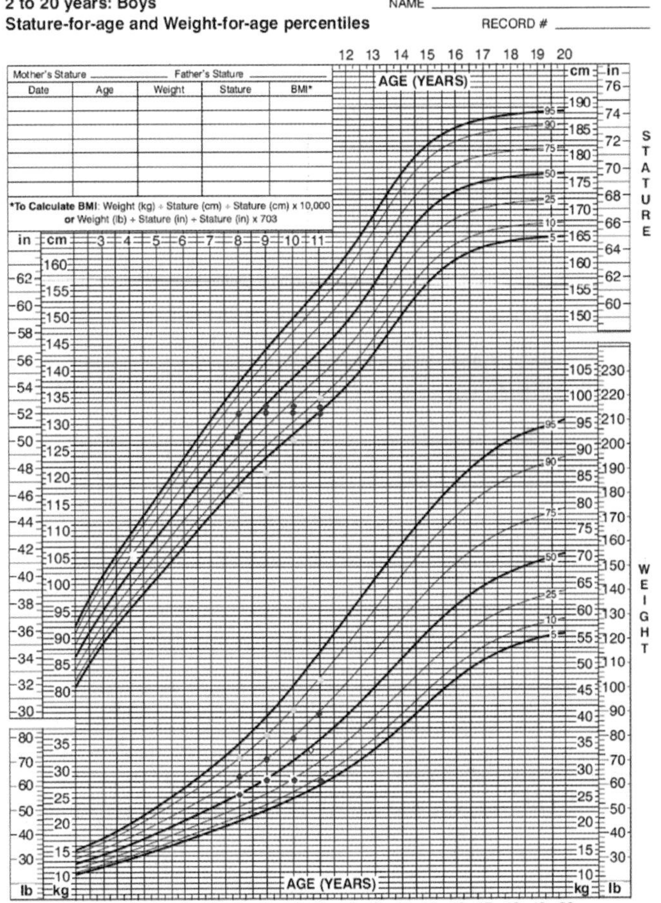

FIGURE 53-6 Typical growth curves seen in malnutrition (blue), growth hormone deficiency (red) and constitutional growth delay (yellow). (*Used with permission from Lori Mahajan, MD.*)

- The interaction between the parent and the child as well as attempted feeding should be observed.
- Careful physical examination may uncover findings that support an underlying condition (**Table 53-2**).[5]

LABORATORY TESTING

- Should be guided by the findings from the history and physical examination.
- No standard laboratory studies recommended as the majority of studies in FTT are normal.

TABLE 53-2 Physical Examination Red Flags in Evaluation of Failure to Thrive

	Red Flag	Diagnostic Consideration
Vital Signs	Tachycardia	Anemia/increased metabolic demand
	Tachypnea	Pulmonary disease/infection
	Hypotension	Thyroid or adrenal insufficiency
	Hypertension	Renal or cardiac disease
General Appearance	Poor Hygiene	Neglect; limited resources
	Dysmorphic	Underlying genetic syndrome
Head	Microcephalic	Congenital infection, neurologic disorder, genetic syndrome
	Widened anterior fontanelle or delayed closure	Hypothyroidism, Hydrocephalus Vitamin D deficiency
	Alopecia	Thyroid disorder, fungal infection, systemic lupus erythematosus, diabetes mellitus, iron-deficiency anemia, vitamin A toxicity, trichotillomania
	Cataracts	Congenital infection, galactosemia
	Aphthous stomatitis	Crohn's disease
	Milk bottle carries	Neglect
	Horizontal brown lines on permanent teeth	Celiac disease
	Structural abnormalities: high arched or cleft palate, enlarged tongue, enlarged tonsils	Mechanical feeding impairment
	Drooling	Oromotor dysphagia
Neck	Thyroid enlargeçment	Thyroid disease
Lungs	Crackles, wheezes	Reactive airway disease, cystic fibrosis, chronic infection
Cardiovascular	Murmur	Congenital heart disease
	Digital clubbing	Cardiac disease, pulmonary disease or inflammatory bowel disease
Abdomen	Increased bowel sounds, distension	Malabsorption
	Hepatosplenomegaly	Primary liver or biliary disease, malignancy, glycogen storage disease
	Enlarged kidney(s)	Urinary obstruction, neuroblastoma
Rectal	Anal tags or fistula	Crohn's
	Empty vault with stool explosively expelled upon withdrawal of digit	Hirschsprung disease
Genitourinary	Ambiguous genitalia	Endocrinopathy
Neurologic	Accentuated deep tendon reflexes	Cerebral palsy, central lesion, hyperthyroidism
	Hypotonia	May cause ineffective latch
Skin/Nails	Bruising	Abuse
	Candidiasis	Immunodeficiency
	Orificial rash	Acrodermatitis enteropathica
	Nail spooning	Iron deficiency

- If FTT persists despite nutritional intervention, a complete blood count, comprehensive metabolic panel, thyroid function tests, celiac panel, lead level, and a urinalysis may be obtained. Sweat chloride testing to rule out cystic fibrosis and pancreatic function tests may be indicated. Specific labs for macro- and micronutrient deficiencies should be based on physical findings.

IMAGING

- Recommended only if indicated by clinical history or examination.
- Studies that may be helpful include:
  - Pyloric ultrasound—To rule out pyloric stenosis in young infant with recurrent emesis.
  - Upper GI series—To rule out intestinal malrotation.
  - Modified barium swallow with speech pathologist present, gastric emptying scan.

DIFFERENTIAL DIAGNOSIS

- Most cases are due to psychosocial factors.
- Other considerations are listed under etiology and pathophysiology.

MANAGEMENT

NONPHARMACOLOGIC

- Treatment is customized according to identified physical, psychiatric, and socioeconomic contributing factors.
- A three day food diary may be required for assessment of baseline caloric intake.
- Age-appropriate nutritional therapy with close follow-up is advised if patient has inadequate intake for catch-up growth.
- Aggressiveness of repletion is dictated by the severity of malnutri tion and can be managed in the outpatient setting in most cases.
- Inpatient observed feeding may be necessary when psychosocial contributing factors are suspected.
- For breastfed infants, frequent breastfeeding should be encouraged to stimulate milk production as well as consultation and close follow-up with a lactation consultant. Formula supplementation may be needed until catch-up growth has occurred.
- For formula-fed infants, information on how to concentrate the formula, and adding cereal or oils (vegetable, canola, or coconut) to increase caloric intake should be provided.
- For older children, adding butter, cream, oils, cheese, or peanut butter as dietary additives to increase the caloric density of foods and fluids should be attempted.
- Regularly scheduled outpatient and/or home visits should be arranged.
- Feeding techniques may need modified. If aspiration is a risk, feeds may need to be thickened and speech and occupational therapists consulted to work on swallowing techniques. Noises and distractions such as television may need removal during mealtime. Eating schedules need to be established with limits placed on snacks and length of times set for meals.

MEDICATIONS

- Medications should be prescribed for identified underlying medical conditions.
- Cyproheptadine is currently clinically used as an appetite stimulant for children with failure to thrive without underlying organic disease; however, no randomized control trials in this patient population have been completed to date. In a small trial, cyproheptadine was shown to be an effective appetite stimulant with minimal side effects in children and adults with cystic fibrosis.[6] SOR Ⓑ

SURGERY

- Some underlying anatomic/physiological etiologies for failure to thrive may be corrected surgically (e.g., pyloric stenosis, intestinal malrotation, Hirschsprung's, etc.).
- If adequate calories cannot be safely or effectively consumed orally in the long term, consideration should be given to placement of a gastrostomy following a trial of nasogastric feeding. SOR Ⓒ
- Central line placement may also be considered for parenteral nutrition if enteral feeds cannot be tolerated. SOR Ⓒ

REFERRAL

- Multi-disciplinary approach is encouraged in the management of failure to thrive.
- Referral to Pediatric Gastroenterology, Pediatric Nutrition, and Social Work for persistent failure to thrive is important.
- Referral to other specialists is dependent on the etiology of failure to thrive.

PREVENTION AND SCREENING

- Appropriate anticipatory guidance, nutritional counseling, and close monitoring of the trend of the child's growth chart at each well child visit may prevent some cases.
- Early consultation with pediatric dietician, social work, and home visiting nurse for ongoing evaluation and support for children/families of children at increased risk of failure to thrive.

PROGNOSIS

- Children with a history of failure to thrive are at increased risk for a recurrence.
- Nutritional deprivation in the infant and toddler age group can have permanent effects on growth and brain development.[7]

FOLLOW-UP

- Very close follow-up advised until catch-up growth has occurred. After catch-up growth achieved, follow-up should still occur 3 to 4 times per year for several years given the increased risk of recurrence.

PATIENT EDUCATION

- Parents should be educated early and often regarding appropriate nutrition for their children.
- Parents should also be educated on the importance of keeping well child visits.

PATIENT RESOURCES

- **www.gikids.org/content/33/en/Digestive-Topics**.
- **http://kidshealth.org** › Parents › Growth & Development
- **http://www.livestrong.com** › ... › Malnutrition

PROVIDER RESOURCES

- **www.emedicine.medscape.com/article/985140-overview**.
- **www.clinicalkey.com/topics/pediatrics/failure-to-thrive.html**.
- **www.dhs.wisconsin.gov/wic/WICPRO/CYSHCN/08-charts.pdf**.

REFERENCES

1. Daniel M, Kleis L, Pinar Cemeroglu A. Etiology of Failure to Thrive in Infants and Toddlers Referred to a Pediatric Endocrinology Outpatient Clinic. *Clin Pediatr.* 2008;47(8):762-765.
2. Levy Y, Levy A, Zangen T, et al. Diagnostic clues for identification of nonorganic vs organic causes of food refusal and poor feeding. *J Pediatr Gastoenterol Nutr.* 2009;48(3):355-362.
3. de Onis M, Garza C, Onyango AW, et al. Comparison of the WHO child growth standards and the CDC 2000 growth charts. *J Nutr.* 2007;137(1):144-148.
4. Waterlow JC. Classification and Definition of Protein Calorie Malnutrition. *Br Med J.* 1972;3:566-569.
5. Cole S, Lanham J. Failure to Thrive: An Update. *Am Fam Physician.* 2011;83(7):829-834.
6. Homnick DN, Homnick BD, Reeves AJ, et al. Cyproheptadine is an effective appetite stimulant in cystic fibrosis. *Pediatr Pulmonol.* 2004;38(2):129-34.
7. Rudolf MC, Logan S. What is the long term outcome for children who fail to thrive? A systematic review. *Arch Dis Child.* 2005; 90(9):925-931.

54 ESOPHAGEAL DISORDERS: GASTROESOPHAGEAL REFLUX DISEASE AND EOSINOPHILIC ESOPHAGITIS

Sophia Ali, MD
Matthew Wyneski, MD

PATIENT STORIES

A 6-month-old boy presents with a history of gagging and emesis shortly after formula feedings. During these episodes, the child arches his back and becomes fussy according to his worried parents. His mother relates that the emesis is mostly partially-digested formula, and is non-bloody and non-bilious. These episodes occur 2 to 3 times per day, and the parents are very concerned because their child looks very uncomfortable during these episodes. His vital signs are stable. On physical exam, the pediatrician notes a well-nourished baby who is growing appropriately along the 50th percentile for all parameters, is happy and playful. The pediatrician diagnoses gastroesophageal reflux (**Figure 54-1**) and prescribes acid-suppression with an H2-blocker at a weight-appropriate dosing. His episodes of emesis, arching, and discomfort improve significantly.

A 12-year-old boy presents with a chief complaint of "food sticking in his throat." He feels that it happens with several foods, and his mother states that his diet mostly consists of peanut butter sandwiches and steak. His past history is only significant for seasonal allergies. He feels that he has heartburn constantly. Trials of H2-blockers and proton pump inhibitors in the past resulted in little improvement of his symptoms. An endoscopy is performed and demonstrates white patches and concentric rings in the esophagus, with pathology results confirming a diagnosis of eosinophilic esophagitis (**Figures 54-2** and **54-3**).

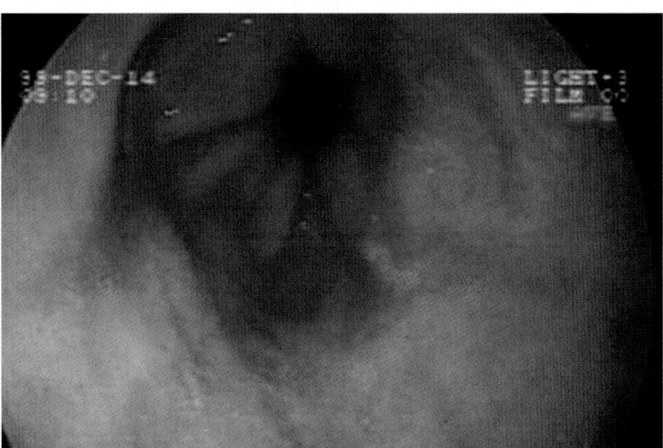

FIGURE 54-1 Reflux esophagitis seen on endoscopy. (*Provided by The NASPGHAN Foundation for Children's Digestive Health and Nutrition and the North American Society for Pediatric Gastroenterology, Hepatology and Nutrition. www.naspghanfoundation.org and www.naspghan.org.*)

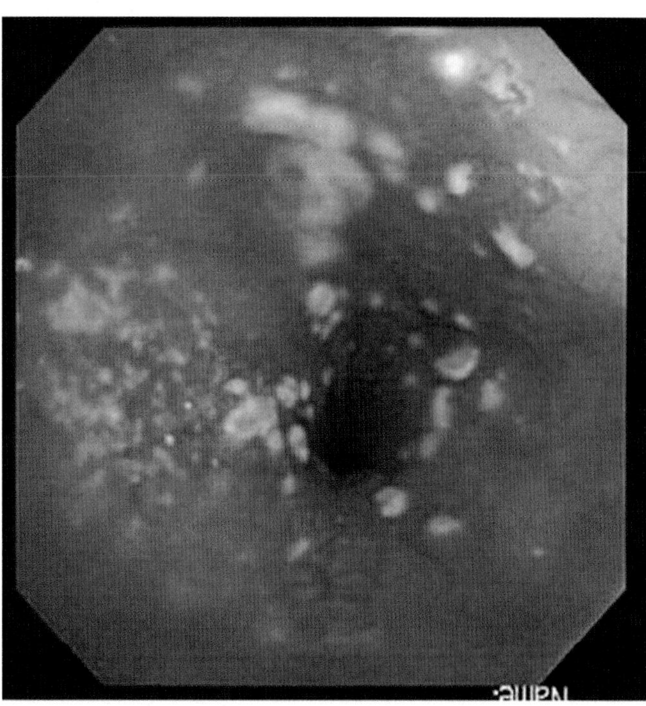

FIGURE 54-2 Classic eosinophilic microabscesses seen in the esophagus of a patient with eosinophilic esophagitis. (*Used with permission from Matthew Wyneski, MD.*)

INTRODUCTION

Gastroesophageal reflux disease (GERD) is a common pediatric problem in general practice. The manifestations and mechanisms of reflux vary between infants, children, and adolescents, and is brought to attention due to the discomfort it causes in all three age ranges. GERD is defined as the passage of gastric contents into the esophagus due to relaxation of the lower esophageal sphincter.

Eosinophilic esophagitis (EoE) is a Th-2 cell mediated immune disease which causes epithelial eosinophilia in the esophagus, leading to

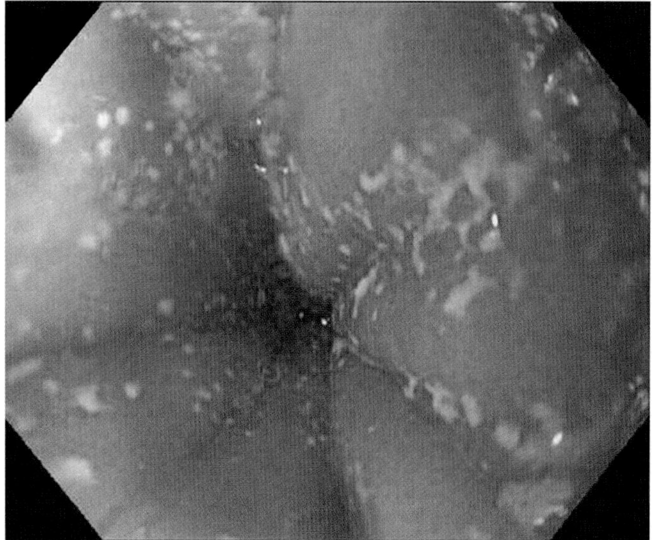

FIGURE 54-3 Microabscesses and trachealization (concentric esophageal rings) in a patient with eosinophillic esophagitis. (*Used with permission from Jonathan Moses, MD.*)

symptoms of dysphagia and reflux symptoms refractory to acid suppression.

SYNONYMS

Reflux, gastroesophageal reflux, acid reflux, heartburn.

Eosinophilic gastroenteritis.

EPIDEMIOLOGY

- Approximately 50 to 67 percent of infants aged 3 to 4 months have reflux as reported by parents.[1]
- Prevalence decreases to 5 percent at 12 months.[1]
- Approximately 7 to 8 percent of older children and adolescents experience reflux symptoms.[2]
- GERD is more common in children with neurologic impairment and has been reported in up to 77 percent in this population.[3]
- The estimated prevalence of EoE is reported in children to be around 1 in 10,000.[4]

ETIOLOGY AND PATHOPHYSIOLOGY

- Reflux results from inappropriate relaxation of the lower esophageal sphincter, allowing gastric juices and contents to reflux back into the esophagus.
- EoE is a chronic immune/antigen mediated disease which causes the build-up of eosinophils in the esophageal mucosa, leading to dysphagia, foreign body impaction, and refractory reflux symptoms.

RISK FACTORS

- Reflux risk factors include age, genetic predisposition, spicy foods, caffeine consumption, cigarette smoking, neurologic conditions such as cerebral palsy or seizure disorders, and Down Syndrome.
- EoE risk factors include other atopic diseases (asthma, eczema, or allergic rhinitis) as well as allergies to food antigens. Genetics also play a role in EoE; in 6.8 percent of cases, there is a family member with similar symptoms.[5]

DIAGNOSIS

CLINICAL FEATURES

- Reflux in infants—Regurgitation, hematemesis, feeding difficulties, wheezing or stridor, cough, apnea, irritability, and hoarseness.
- Reflux in children—Heartburn, emesis, dysphagia, chest pain, abdominal pain, persistent cough or wheezing, stridor, dental erosions, and hoarseness.
- EoE—Dysphagia, nausea, vomiting, retrosternal chest pain, regurgitation, food refusal, choking/gagging, throat pain, food impactions, or persistent reflux symptoms unresponsive to therapy.

DISTRIBUTION

- Both EoE and GERD are distributed in the esophageal regions, and reflux can manifest in the stomach as well.

LABORATORY TESTING

- For GERD, no specific laboratory workup is required.
- For EoE, eosinophilia on CBC or IgE testing is neither sensitive nor specific for the disease.
- May consider *Helicobacter pylori* stool antigen tests or breath testing when the diagnosis is not clear.

IMAGING/PATHOLOGIC TESTING

- Upper GI series may be performed to rule out other causes of emesis, including achalasia, hiatal hernia, malrotation, or gastric outlet obstruction, but should NOT be used to diagnose GERD.
- For reflux, esophageal pH impedance probe is the gold standard and can detect acid and nonacid reflux.
- Abdominal ultrasound can rule out pyloric stenosis, pancreatitis, and gallstones.
- Gastric emptying study can detect esophageal reflux, aspiration, gastroparesis, or gastric outlet obstruction; however, specificity ranges are not as high as pH impedance probe.[6]
- Endoscopy can reveal reflux esophagitis (**Figure 54-1**) but is usually performed to rule out other causes that can mimic reflux, such as stricture, peptic ulcer disease, and infectious esophagitis.
- In EoE, endoscopic biopsies demonstrating >15 eosinophils per high-powered field are diagnostic (**Figure 54-4**).

DIFFERENTIAL DIAGNOSIS

- Malrotation—Usually presents acutely with bilious vomiting and ill appearance.
- *H. pylori* infection—Can mimic symptoms of reflux but contributes to peptic ulcer disease (see Chapter 55, Peptic Ulcer Disease).

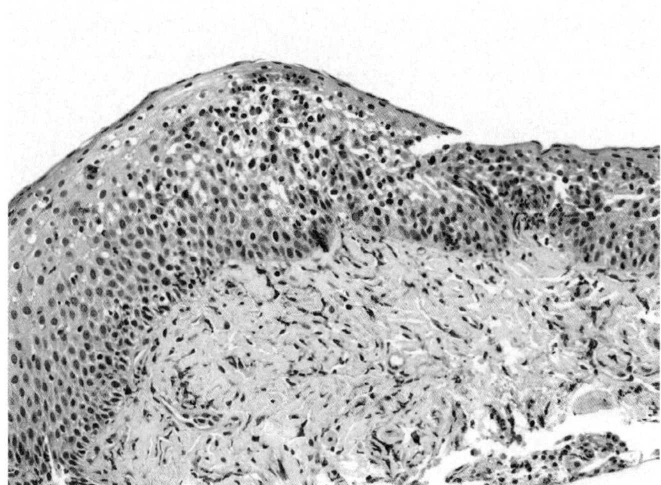

FIGURE 54-4 Eosinophilic infiltration characteristic of eosinophilic esophagitis. (*Used with permission from Thomas Plesec, MD.*)

- Foreign body impaction—May mimic EoE, but history and acuity are helpful in differentiating from EoE.
- Pyloric stenosis—Presents very early in life with projectile vomiting (see Chapter 57, Pyloric Stenosis).
- Pancreatitis—Usually associated with more severe abdominal pain.
- Celiac Disease—Often presents with growth abnormalities along with the gastrointestinal symptoms (see Chapter 60, Celiac disease).
- Inflammatory Bowel Disease—Usually can be differentiated on the severity of symptoms and growth disturbances (see Chapter 59, Inflammatory Bowel Disease).
- Spinal muscular atrophy syndrome—Presents early in life with generalized weakness.

MANAGEMENT

NONPHARMACOLOGIC

- For reflux, recommendations include lifestyle modifications include avoiding spicy foods, caffeinated beverages, chocolate, high-fat foods, overuse of non-steroidal anti-inflammatory drugs, acidic foods, juices, and carbonated beverages.[1,2] SOR A
- For infants with reflux, propping up for 30 minutes after feeds and starting rice cereal or oatmeal at 4 months do not decrease esophageal acid exposure but do decrease the frequency of regurgitation.[7]
  - For eosinophilic esophagitis, avoiding foods that are allergen inducing, including peanuts, soy, eggs, and milk.[8] SOR B
  - Eosinophilic esophagitis has also been shown to respond well to an elemental diet with nasogastric feedings of amino acid based formula.[8] SOR B

MEDICATIONS

Reflux

- Reflux medications are indicated when dietary modification and nonpharmacologic therapy are not sufficiently controlling symptoms.
- Options for medical therapy include:
  - Proton pump inhibitors, including omeprazole, lansoprazole, and esomeprazole.
    - Work to block H2-Na-K ATPase and stop acid production by parietal cells.
    - Side effects include headache, nausea, and diarrhea.
  - Histamine H-2 blockers, including famotidine and ranitidine.
    - Bind to H-2 receptors in the parietal cell in the stomach and block acid production.
    - Generally less effective than proton pump inhibitors.
    - Side effects include headaches and irritability.
  - Prokinetic agents including erythromycin and metoclopramide (Reglan):
    - Cause stomach to empty more rapidly.
    - Erythromycin is associated with hypertrophic pyloric stenosis in infants, and with prolonged QT syndrome in older children.
    - Metoclopramide may cause extrapyramidal side effects including tardive dyskinesia.
  - Sucralfate is a topical agent that contains sucrose, sulfate, and aluminum.
    - Binds to eroded regions of the stomach and is used more often for gastric ulcers than GERD or EoE.
    - Side effects include aluminum toxicity and bezoar formation.
  - Antacids (liquid or chewable forms) to decrease acid production may be used in older children. These may contain calcium, magnesium, or aluminum as the active ingredient.
    - Aluminum-containing antacids should be used with caution, as they have been associated with osteopenia, rickets, microcytic anemia, and neurotoxicity.

Eosinophilic esophagitis

- Budesonide or fluticasone.[9] SOR B
  - Liquid preparation mixed with honey or sugar taken orally to coat the esophagus.
  - Inhaled preparation is administered into the mouth and swallowed.
- Elemental diet has been shown to decrease EoE; however, this is very restrictive and difficult to implement.[8] SOR B
- Elimination of food allergens has also proven effective.[8] SOR B

SURGERY

- Fundoplication is only considered for the most refractory cases of GERD as it is major surgery with significant risks. SOR C
  - Fundoplication can now be performed with laparoscopy. This procedure increases the lower esophageal sphincter pressure and elongates the esophagus.
  - Risk of complications is as high as 10 percent postoperatively.[6]
  - Prospective trials needed to explore success of fundoplication surgery.

PREVENTION AND SCREENING

- Prevention in infants and children can be achieved with proper and frequent burping, sitting child up for 30 minutes following feeds, and propping infant up at an angle when lying.
- In older children and adolescents, dietary changes are most effective in preventing reflux.
  - Avoiding caffeinated beverages, chocolate, acidic foods, spicy foods, and juices can be effective.
- For EoE, prevention of symptoms can be achieved by avoiding allergenic foods and transitioning to an elemental diet if needed.

PROGNOSIS

- Cases of Barrett's esophagus have been reported in patients with EoE.[4]
- Reflux generally resolves by 9 to 12 months of age in infants.[6]
- Severe GERD can lead to complications including Barrett's esophagus, esophagitis, adenocarcinoma, and esophageal strictures.[6]
- Treatment with proton-pump inhibitors and topical corticosteroid therapy can improve long-term outcome of EoE.

PATIENT EDUCATION

- Advise and encourage patients and their parents to follow recommended dietary and positional changes to improve symptoms, and correct other predisposing factors.

PATIENT RESOURCES

- **www.ncbi.nlm.nih.gov/pubmedhealth/PMH0001311/.**
- **http://digestive.niddk.nih.gov/ddiseases/pubs/gerinchildren/.**
- **www.gikids.org/content/8/en/Reflux-GERD.**
- **www.gikids.org/content/5/en/eosinophilicesophagitis.**
- **http://digestive.niddk.nih.gov/ddiseases/pubs/gerdinfant/index.aspx.**

PROVIDER RESOURCES

- **www.naspghan.org/user-assets/Documents/pdf/PositionPapers/FINAL%20-%20JPGN%20GERD%20guideline.pdf.**
- **www.naspghan.org/user-assets/Documents/pdf/CDHNF%20Old%20Site/Eosinophilic%20Esophagitis%20Medical%20Professional%20Resources/EoEinChildrenandAdults_SystematicReview_DiagnosisandTreatment.pdf.**
- **http://emedicine.medscape.com/article/930029.**

REFERENCES

1. Nelson SP, Chen EH, Syniar GM, Christoffel KK. Pediatric Practice Research Group. Prevalence of symptoms of gastroesophageal reflux during infancy. A pediatric practice-based survey. *Arch Pediatr Adolesc Med.* 1997;151(6):569-572.
2. Nelson SP, Chen EH, Syniar GM, Christoffel KK. Pediatric Practice Research Group. Prevalence of symptoms of gastroesophageal reflux during childhood: a pediatric practice-based survey. *Arch Pediatr Adolesc Med.* 2000 Feb;154(2):150-154.
3. Gössler A, Schalamon J, Huber-Zeyringer A, Höllwarth ME. Gastroesophageal reflux and behavior in neurologically impaired children. *J Pediatr Surg.* 2007;42(9):1486-1490.
4. Heine RG, Nethercote M, Rosenbaum J, Allen KJ. Emerging management concepts for eosinophilic esophagitis in children. *J Gastroent Hepat.* 2011;26(7):1106-1113.
5. Straumann A, Aceves SS, Blanchard C, Collins MH, Furuta GT, Hirano I, Schoepfer AM, Simon D, Simon H-U. Pediatric and adult eosinophilic esophagitis: similarities and differences. *Allergy.* 2012;67:477-490.
6. Sullivan, J and Sundaram, Shikha S. Gastroesophageal Reflux. *Pediatrics in Review.* 2012;33;243.
7. Vandplas, Y. Thickened infant formula does what it has to do: decrease regurgitation. *Pediatrics.* 2009;123(3).
8. Markowitz JE, Spergel JM, Ruchelli E,Liacouras CA. Elemental diet is an effective treatment for eosinophilic esophagitis in children and adolescents. *Am J Gastroenterol.* 2003;98:777-782.
9. Dohil R, Newbury R, Fox L, Bastian J,Aceves SS. Oral viscous budesonide is effective in children with eosinophilicesophagitis in a randomized, placebo-controlled)trial. *Gastroenterology.* 2010; 139(2):418-429.

55 PEPTIC ULCER DISEASE

Mindy A. Smith, MD, MS
Hend Azhary, MD

PATIENT STORY

A 10-year-old boy is brought in by his mother because of several episodes of vomiting. The most recent episode was small volume and had some brown-colored material in it. The boy tells you that he has had stomach pain off and on in the past few months and feels nauseated. He has not been having difficulty in school but his mother tells you that they will likely need to move soon as his father lost his job recently and has been unable to find work. The patient is the oldest of the 3 boys and shares a room with his brothers. He worries about his dad and hopes that he will be able to stay at his school. You discuss your concerns and recommend that the patient undergo esophagogastroduodenoscopy (EGD). His mother states that the children have health insurance through a state program and agrees to the testing. You start the patient on generic ranitidine. His EGD reveals a small pyloric ulcer and the biopsy specimens test positive for *Helicobacter pylori* (**Figure 55-1**). You prescribe 10 days of triple therapy with bismuth salts, amoxicillin, and metronidazole as the child's insurance does not cover the more expensive alternative medications.

INTRODUCTION

Peptic ulcer disease (PUD) is a disease of the gastrointestinal (GI) tract characterized by a break in the mucosal lining of the stomach or duodenum secondary to pepsin and gastric acid secretion; this damage is greater than 5 mm in size and with a depth reaching the submucosal layer.[1] PUD can be either primary or secondary; the latter most often due to severe systemic illness (e.g., sepsis) or from ulcerogenic drug ingestion (e.g., nonsteroidal antiinflammatory drugs (NSAIDs) or steroids).

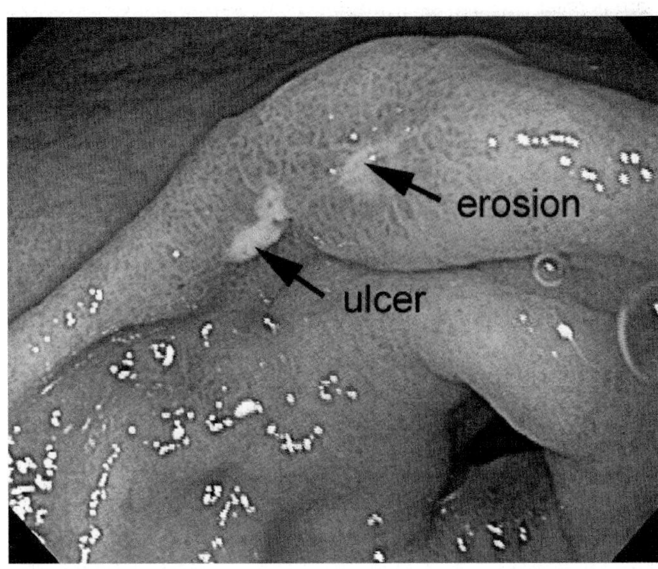

FIGURE 55-1 Endoscopic view of a pyloric ulcer and an erosion of the mucosa. (*Used with permission from Marvin Derezin, MD.*)

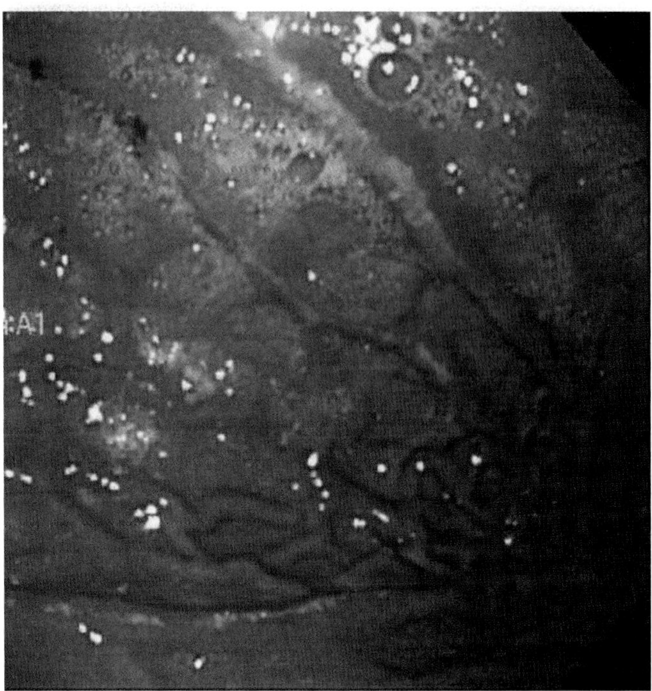

FIGURE 55-2 Gastric ulcers, characterized by whitish linear gastric ulcerations along the rugae, in a young child. (*Used with permission from Matthew Wyneski, MD.*)

EPIDEMIOLOGY

- PUD is a common disorder affecting approximately 4.5 million people annually in the US. It encompasses both gastric and duodenal ulcers (**Figures 55-1** to **55-4**).[2]

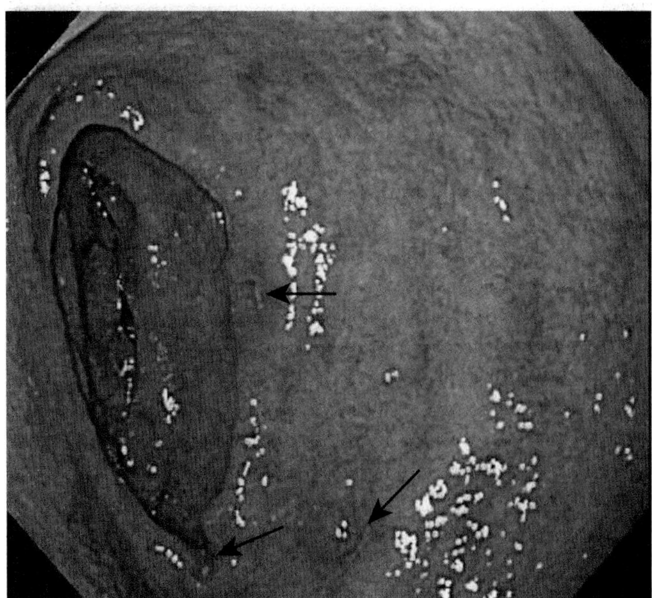

FIGURE 55-3 Several focal, deep ulcers (arrows) noted in the second portion of the duodenum in a patient with Crohn disease. (*Used with permission from Jonathan Moses, MD.*)

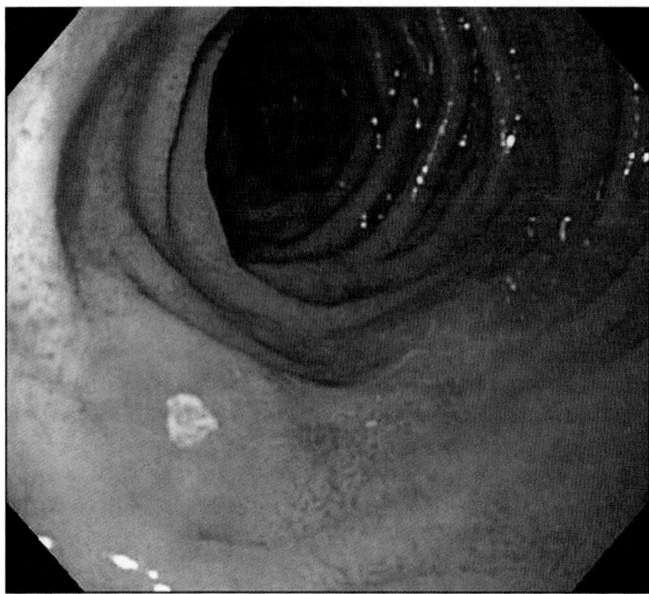

FIGURE 55-4 Solitary, large ulceration noted in the second portion of the duodenum in a patient with Crohn disease. (*Used with permission from Jonathan Moses, MD.*)

- One-year point prevalence is 1.8 percent, and the lifetime prevalence is 10 percent in the US.[2]
- Prevalence is similar in both sexes, with increased incidence with age.[1]
- PUD is less common in children. In an Israeli study of 751 symptomatic children referred for endoscopy, peptic ulcers were found in 51 patients (6.8%).[3] *H. pylori* was positive in 112 (66.3%) patients and *H. pylori*-associated ulcers were more common in children older than age 10 years. A similar rate was demonstrated in a Chinese case series where 43 of 619 children (6.9%) undergoing upper endoscopy for investigation of upper gastrointestinal symptoms had primary PUD.[4] Authors of an Italian study (N = 2234 endoscopies in children) reported a lower rate of 3.4 percent positive endoscopies for PUD, rates similar to those reported in older endoscopy studies performed on symptomatic children (1.8% to 3.6%).[5] This is in somewhat less than the 8 percent prevalence of PUD in adults with dyspepsia who undergo endoscopy.[6]
- Rates of non-*H. pylori*-associated ulcers and erosions appear to be increasing among children.[7]
- Utilizing a US inpatient pediatric database (2008), the estimated incidence of peptic ulcer bleeding ranged from 0.5 to 4.4/100,000 individuals, with a total number of cases between 378 and 3250.[8]

ETIOLOGY AND PATHOPHYSIOLOGY

- Causes of PUD include:
  - Nonsteroidal antiinflammatory drugs (NSAIDs), chronic *H. pylori* infection, and acid hypersecretory states such as Zollinger-Ellison syndrome.[2]
  - Uncommon causes include *Cytomegalovirus* (especially in transplant recipients), systemic mastocytosis, Crohn disease (**Figures 55-3** and **55-4**), lymphoma, and medications other than NSAIDs (e.g., alendronate).[2]
  - Children with chronic renal failure (CRF) have been shown to have high basal levels of gastrin; in one study of children with CRF on continuous ambulatory peritoneal dialysis (N = 19), almost three quarters had abnormal upper gastrointestinal endoscopic findings including hemorrhagic gastritis or gastroduodenitis, gastric nodular gastritis, and polyps.[9]
- In a 5-year Canadian retrospective study of children admitted to a tertiary care center with PUD (N = 36, aged 3 months to 17 years), about half the cases were secondary; most of these resulting from severe underlying illness (11/17).[10] All children under age 10 years had secondary PUD.
- Infection with *H. pylori*, a short, spiral-shaped, microaerophilic Gram-negative bacillus, occurs in about half of the world's population and is the leading cause of PUD in adults. *H. pylori* infection is associated with up to 70 to 80 percent of duodenal ulcers in adults.[2] In patients who do not use NSAIDS, infection rates are lower at about 60 percent of those with ulcers.[11]
- *H. Pylori* infection is also associated with iron-deficiency anemia, gastric ulcer, gastric mucosa-associated lymphoid tissue (MALT) lymphoma, and distal gastric cancer.[12] In one study of school-aged Andean children, chronic *H. Pylori* infection was associated with slowed growth (0.022 cm/month [95% confidence interval 0.008 to 0.035] slower than H. pylori-negative children).[13]
- The role of *H. Pylori* infection in childhood PUD is unclear as infection less frequently causes clinical disease in this population. It is estimated that, at adolescence, approximately 65 percent of children in developing countries (range 7% to 87%) are infected with *H. pylori*.[12] Vertical transmission appears to occur, although maternal *H. pylori* IgG transfer may be protective.[14]
- In an older retrospective study of 40 children endoscopically diagnosed with gastritis, gastric ulcer, or duodenal ulcer, *H. pylori* was found in about half (48%) and was more commonly detected among those with primary gastritis (88%) than either primary (22%) or secondary (50%) duodenal ulcers.[15] This is similar to the rate of 53.5 percent *H. pylori*-positive PUD found in the Chinese study[4] but lower than rates reported in older studies where 73 to 80 percent of childhood peptic ulcers were associated with either NSAIDs or *H pylori*.[16,17]
- In a more recent European study of 518 children aged 1 to 14 years with *H. pylori* infection, 454 children (87.6%) had endoscopically proven gastritis and only 64 had an ulcer (12.3%).[5] Ulcer disease, however, was more common among Russian children in this sample than the remainder of European children (35% versus 6.7%, respectively).
- *H. pylori* colonize the deep layers of the gel that coats the mucosa and disrupt its protective properties causing release of certain enzymes and toxins. These make the underlying tissues more vulnerable to damage by digestive juices and thus cause injury to the stomach (**Figures 55-1** and **55-2**) and duodenum cells (**Figures 55-3** and **55-4**).[1] One theory is that children's developing immune system mounts a lesser inflammatory response reducing the risk of disruption to the gastric mucosa.[12] In the Chinese case series, all children with *H. pylori* disease had evidence of chronic active gastritis on the biopsy specimens.[4]
- NSAIDs are the second most common cause of PUD in adults and account for many *H. pylori*-negative cases. NSAIDs and aspirin

inhibit mucosal cyclooxygenase activity reducing the level of mucosal prostaglandin causing defects in the protective mucous layer.

- There is a 10 to 20 percent prevalence of gastric ulcers and a 2 to 5 percent prevalence of duodenal ulcers in long-term NSAID users.[2] The annual risk of a life-threatening ulcer-related complication is 1 percent to 4 percent in long-term NSAID users, with older patients having the highest risk.[18]
- Polymorphisms of IL-1 gene cluster are associated with histological changes and IL-1β expression in the gastric mucosa in adults and children. In one study of Chinese children with peptic symptoms (N = 128), 60.7 percent of children with moderate or severe gastritis or gastric ulcer had the IL-1B-511TT/-31CC genotype.[19]

RISK FACTORS

- Severe physiologic stress—Burns, central nervous system trauma, surgery, and severe medical illness increase the risk for secondary (stress) ulceration.[11]
- Childhood physical abuse—In a Canadian population study, childhood physical abuse, reported by 1020 individuals (7.3%), was associated with diagnosed peptic ulcers (6.6% of those reporting abuse versus 2.7% of those not reporting abuse [OR 1.68; 95% CI 1.22-2.32]).[20]
- Smoking—Evidence that tobacco use is a risk factor for duodenal ulcers in not conclusive, with several studies producing contradictory findings. However, smoking in the setting of *H. pylori* infection may increase the risk of relapse of PUD.[21] A recent US population study reported an odds ratio (OR) of 1.99 for current and 1.55 for former tobacco use.[22]
- Alcohol use—Ethanol is known to cause gastric mucosal irritation and nonspecific gastritis. Evidence that consumption of alcohol is a risk factor for duodenal ulcer is inconclusive.[21] The preceding population study reported an OR of 1.29 for former alcohol use.[22]
- Medications—Corticosteroids alone do not increase the risk for PUD; however, they can potentiate ulcer risk in patients who use NSAIDs concurrently.[11]
- Other risk factors for gastrointestinal ulcers include, African-American race (OR 1.20), obesity (OR 1.18), chronic renal insufficiency (OR 2.29), and three or more doctor visits in a year (OR 1.49).[22] There appears to be an association between duodenal ulceration and celiac disease.[23]
- Risk factors for *H. pylori* infection include socioeconomic factors such as lower family income, household crowding, number of children sharing the same room, parents' education, and sharing a bed with children.[12]

DIAGNOSIS

CLINICAL FEATURES

- Symptoms of *H. pylori*-related PUD in children are nonspecific and include epigastric pain, nausea and/or vomiting, anorexia, iron deficiency anaemia, and hematemesis.[12]
- In the Chinese case series, thirty children (70%) presented with acute gastrointestinal bleeding and only 19 had a history of epigastric pain.[4] This was not true in either the study of Italian children where only 21 percent with *H. pylori*-positive PUD had acute bleeding (eight required emergency surgery)[5] or the Canadian study where only one child with primary PUD required emergency surgery.[10] These figures are similar to a 10-year US study of 61 children with PUD of whom 31 had primary PUD, most commonly presenting as abdominal pain or bleeding; in this study, one third required surgery for intractable pain, perforation, or massive recurrent hemorrhage.[24]
- Reported differences between *H. pylori*-positive and *H. pylori*-negative PUD in children include male predominance, older age at presentation, and lower recurrence rates in the former.[5]

TYPICAL DISTRIBUTION

- Most duodenal ulcers occur in the first portion of the duodenum.[1] In the Chinese case series, most children had duodenal ulcers (N = 37/43) with 30 (81%) occurring in the first portion of the duodenum.[4] In the Canadian study, duodenal ulcers were nearly three times more common than gastric ulcers.[10]
- Of the six gastric ulcers found in the Chinese study, four were central and two were pyloric.[4]

LABORATORY STUDIES

- Routine laboratory tests are not helpful in most patients with uncomplicated PUD.[11]
- Noninvasive tests include serum *H. pylori* antibody detection, fecal antigen tests, and ^{13}C-urea breath tests (C-UBT); the latter two, if positive, indicate active disease.[25] Although a large number of high quality pediatric studies have demonstrated high accuracy, sensitivity and specificity of C-UBT and stool antigen testing, a positive test does not confirm or exclude the presence of an ulcer, gastritis or other pathology and endoscopy continues to be standard care in children with suspected PUD.[12]
- Evidence-based guidelines from the European and North American Societies of Pediatric Gastroenterology, Hepatology and Nutrition (ESPGHAN and NASPGHAN) do not recommend testing for *H. pylori* infection in children with functional abdominal pain, as infection has not been shown to be associated with recurrent abdominal pain[12] and the primary goal of clinical investigation is to determine the underlying cause of the gastrointestinal symptoms and not solely the presence of *H. pylori* infection.[26]
  - Testing for *H. pylori* infection should be considered in children with first-degree relatives with gastric cancer and those with refractory iron-deficiency anemia.[26] SOR C
  - For children undergoing esophagogastroduodenoscopy (EGD), gastric biopsies (antrum and corpus) for histopathology should be obtained for the diagnosis of *H. pylori* infection.[26] However, initial diagnosis of *H. pylori* infection can be based on either positive histopathology + positive rapid urease test or a positive culture. SOR B
  - The ^{13}C-urea breath test (SOR A) or stool antigen test (SOR B) can be used to determine whether *H. pylori* has been eradicated.[26]
- In a prospective cohort study of 50 symptomatic children aged 2 to 18 years, invasive rapid urease test (via endoscopy with gastric biopsy) combined with non-invasive serology was the optimum

approach to the diagnosis of *H. pylori* infection in symptomatic children.[27]

- Serum enzyme-linked immunosorbent assay (ELISA) is the least accurate test and is useful only for diagnosing the initial infection.
- Serum gastrin testing may be useful in patients with recurrent, refractory, or complicated PUD and in patients with a family history of PUD to screen for Zollinger-Ellison syndrome.[1]

IMAGING

- Upper endoscopy is the procedure of choice for the diagnosis of duodenal and gastric ulcers (**Figures 55-1** to **55-4**).[2]
- Endoscopy provides better diagnostic accuracy than barium radiography and affords the ability to biopsy for the presence of malignancy and *H. pylori* infection. Endoscopy is usually reserved for the following situations:[18]
- Patients with red flag signs (e.g., bleeding, dysphagia, severe pain, abdominal mass, recurrent vomiting, weight loss).
  - Patients who fail initial therapy.
  - Patients whose symptoms recur after appropriate therapy.
- Barium upper gastrointestinal (UGI) series is an acceptable alternative to endoscopy but is not as sensitive for the diagnosis of small ulcers (<0.5 cm) and does not allow for biopsy with gastric ulcer.[25]

DIFFERENTIAL DIAGNOSIS

Disease processes that may present with "ulcer-like" symptoms include:

- Nonulcer or functional dyspepsia (FD)—The most common diagnosis among patients seen for upper abdominal discomfort; it is a diagnosis of exclusion. Dyspepsia has been reported to occur in up to 30 percent of the US population.
- Recurrent abdominal pain of childhood (RAP)—Also a diagnosis of exclusion, defined as three episodes of abdominal pain occurring in the space of three months, severe enough to affect daily activities. Associated with stressful life events, proposed etiologies include gastrointestinal motility disorders, food sensitivities/allergy, and abdominal migraine.[28]
- Gastroesophageal reflux—Classic symptoms are heartburn (i.e., substernal pain that may be associated with acid regurgitation or a sour taste) aggravated by bending forward or lying down, especially after a large meal. Endoscopy is considered if symptoms fail to respond to treatment (e.g., histamine-2-receptor agonist, proton pump inhibitor [PPI]) or red flag signs and symptoms occur; see Chapter 54, Esophageal Disorders).
- Gastroduodenal Crohn disease—Symptoms include epigastric pain, nausea, and vomiting. On endoscopy, patients often have *H. pylori*-negative gastritis or duodenal ulcers (**Figures 55-3** and **55-4**), and may develop gastric outlet obstruction. Extraintestinal manifestations include erythema nodosum, peripheral arthritis, conjunctivitis, uveitis, and episcleritis. Endoscopy shows an inflammatory process with skip lesions, fistulas, aphthous ulcerations, and rectal sparing. Small bowel involvement is seen on imaging with longitudinal and transverse ulceration (cobblestoning) in addition to segmental colitis and frequent stricture (see Chapter 59, Inflammatory Bowel Disease).

MANAGEMENT

- The approach to children with PUD includes use of H_2-receptor antagonists (e.g., cimetidine, ranitidine) and antibiotic treatment for *H. pylori* eradication when present.
- An early case series from Hong Kong using surveillance endoscopy demonstrated the effectiveness of 6-week therapy with H_2-receptor antagonists with complete ulcer healing in 22/29 children with duodenal ulcers and all 3 children with gastric ulcer.[29] Recurrence rates for duodenal ulcer (35%) were much lower for children on nightly maintenance therapy (1/9 versus 8/17). Ranitidine should be used with caution in low birthweight infants as use is associated with increased risk of infection, necrotizing enterocolitis, and mortality.[30]
- For all patients with PUD, counsel to avoid smoking, alcohol, and NSAIDs.
- The goals of treatment of active *H. pylori*-associated ulcers are to relieve dyspeptic symptoms, promote ulcer healing, and to eradicate *H. pylori* infection. Eradication of *H. pylori* is better than ulcer-healing drug therapy for duodenal ulcer healing[8] and greatly reduces the incidence of ulcer recurrence.
- First-line eradication regimens are: 12,26 SOR Ⓑ
  - Triple therapy with a proton pump inhibitor [PPI] (1–2 mg/kg/day) + amoxicillin (50 mg/kg/day, maximum 2 g/day) + metronidazole (20 mg/kg/day, maximum 1 g/day) given twice daily for 10 to 14 days.
  - PPI + amoxicillin + clarithromycin (20 mg/kg/day) given twice daily for 10 to 14 days.
  - Bismuth salts (8 mg/kg/day) + amoxicillin + metronidazole.
  - Sequential therapy: PPI + amoxicillin for 5 days followed by PPI + amoxicillin + metronidazole for 5 days.
- The worldwide empiric use of traditional triple therapy with PPI, clarithromycin, and amoxicillin in adults no longer provides an acceptable cure rate (cure rate below 80%) because of the increasing prevalence of clarithromycin resistance.[9] For children, the ESPGHAN and NASPGHAN recommend antibiotic susceptibility testing for clarithromycin before initial clarithromycin-based triple therapy in areas/populations with a known high resistance rate (>20%) of *H. pylori* to clarithromycin.[26]
- If initial treatment for *H. pylori* fails, ESPGHAN and NASPGHAN recommend one of the following:[26]
  - EGD, with culture and susceptibility testing to guide therapy if not performed before initial treatment.
  - Fluorescence in situ hybridization (FISH) on previous paraffin-embedded biopsies if clarithromycin susceptibility testing has not been performed before initial treatment.
  - Modify therapy by adding an antibiotic (quadruple therapy), using different antibiotics (e.g. PPI, amoxicillin, levofloxacin [10 mg/kg/day, maximum 500 mg/day]),[12] adding bismuth, and/or increasing dose (e.g., PPI at 2 mg/kg/day), and/or duration (14 days) of therapy.

- Fluoroquinolone resistance is an emerging problem in the adult population; levofloxacin should be cautiously used in children who were previously exposed to this drug.[12]
- Treat NSAID-induced ulcers with cessation of NSAIDs, if possible, and an appropriate course of standard ulcer therapy with a H_2-receptor antagonist or a PPI. If NSAIDs are continued, prescribe a PPI. SOR Ⓐ

PREVENTION

- Authors of a metaanalysis found the use of prophylactic H_2 blockers to prevent stress ulcers in adults was not necessary in patients receiving enteral nutrition and that such therapy was associated with pneumonia and higher risk of hospital mortality.[31] In another meta-analysis of adult patients, PPIs were similar to H_2-receptor antagonists in terms of stress-related UGI bleeding prophylaxis, pneumonia, and mortality among patients admitted to intensive care units.[32]
- Because *H. pylori* infection is often acquired during childhood, a vaccine would be optimal for preventing many cases of gastritis and PUD. Thus far, however, human vaccine trials have shown only moderate effectiveness and adjuvant-related adverse effects.[12]

PROGNOSIS

- In the Canadian retrospective study, most children (67%) with primary duodenal ulcer disease had recurrent symptoms and 40 percent of them required surgery for intractable disease.[10] None of the children with secondary PUD had chronic or recurrent disease.
- In other studies, the recurrence rate of endoscopically-proven peptic ulcers in children was 43 percent within one year[33] and 47 percent among children monitored until adulthood.[34] In the more recent Chinese study, the annual ulcer recurrence rates were much lower at 5.2 percent (95% CI 4.2–6.3) for children with *H. pylori*-positive and 11.4 percent (95% CI 9.1–13.6) for children with *H. Pylori*-negative ulcers.[4] In this study, multivariate logistic regression suggested *H pylori*–negative status and ulcer size >1 cm were independent risk factors for recurrence.[4] As with adults, eradication of *H. pylori* infection dramatically reduces recurrence.[12]
- The incidence of perforation is approximately 0.3 percent per patient year and the incidence of obstruction is approximately 0.1 percent per patient year.[11]

FOLLOW-UP

- Although not recommended in adult patients with uncomplicated ulcers due to infection, confirmation of *H. pylori* eradication is recommended in children, preferably with C-UBT.[12,26] Stool sampling can be used for confirmation in small children in whom collecting breath samples is difficult. Based on adult studies, discontinue antibiotics for at least 4 weeks and acid-suppressive drugs, particularly PPIs, for at least 2 weeks prior to testing.[12]
- Persistent *H. pylori* infection requires additional treatment.
- Children with non-*H. pylori* PUD with continued symptoms should be considered for maintenance antisecretory therapy.

PATIENT EDUCATION

- Patients with PUD should be encouraged to eat balanced meals at regular intervals, avoid alcohol use, smoking, and NSAIDs; stress reduction counseling might be helpful in individual cases.
- Parents should be advised to contact their health provider if their child experiences sudden sharp, persistent pain, bloody/tarry stools, or bloody or coffee ground emesis.

PATIENT RESOURCES

- Kidshealth—**http://kidshealth.org/parent/medical/digestive/peptic_ulcers.html**.
- National Digestive Diseases Information Clearing House—**http://digestive.niddk.nih.gov/ddiseases/pubs/pepticulcers_ez/index.htm**.

PROVIDER RESOURCES

- **http://emedicine.medscape.com/article/181753-overview**.

REFERENCES

1. Del Valle J. Peptic ulcer disease and related disorders. In: Kasper DL, Braunwald E, Fauci AS, Hauser SL, Longo DL, Jameson JL, eds. *Harrison's Principles of Internal Medicine*, 16th ed. New York, NY: McGraw-Hill; 2005:1746-1762.
2. McPhee SJ, Papadakis MA, Tierney LW Jr: *Current Medical Diagnosis and Treatment*. New York, NY: McGraw-Hill; 2007.
3. Shaoul R, Levine A. Letter to the Editor. Non-helicobacter, non-NSAIDs peptic disease in children. *J Pediatr Gastroenterol Nutr*. 2010;51(5):685.
4. Tam YH, Lee KH, To KF, et al. *Helicobacter pylori*–positive versus *Helicobacter pylori*-negative idiopathic peptic ulcers in children with their long term outcomes. *J Pediatr Gsatroenterol Nutr*. 2009; 48:299-305.
5. Oderda G, Mura S, Valori A, Brustia R. Idiopathic peptic ulcers in children. *J Pediatr Gsatroenterol Nutr*. 2009;48:268-270.
6. Ford AC, Marwaha A, Lim A, Moayyedi P. What is the prevalence of clinically significant endoscopic findings in subjects with dyspepsia? Systematic review and meta-analysis. *Clin Gastroenterol Hepatol*. 2010;8(10):830-837.
7. Sýkora J, Rowland M. Helicobacter pylori in pediatrics. *Helicobacter*. 2011;16(1):59-64.
8. Brown K, Lundborg P, Levinson J, Yang H. Incidence of peptic ulcer bleeding in the US pediatric population. *J Pediatr Gsatroenterol Nutr*. 2011;33(5-6):221-226.
9. Urganci N, Ozcelik G, Kalyoncu D, et al. Serum gastrin levels and gastroduodenal lesions in children with chronic renal failure on continuous ambulatory peritoneal dialysis: a single-center experience. *Eur J Gastroenterol Hepatol*. 2012;24(8):924-928.
10. Drumm B, Rhoads JM, Stringer DA, et al. Peptic ulcer disease in children: etiology, clinical findings, and clinical course. *Pediatrics*. 1988;82(3 Pt 2):410-414.

11. Anand BS, Bank S, Qureshi WA, et al. *Peptic Ulcer* Disease. http://emedicine.medscape.com/article/181753-overview, accessed January 2013.

12. Ertem D. Clinical Practice: *Helicobacter pylori* infection in childhood. *Eur J Pediatr*. 2012; DOI 10.1007/s00431-012-1823-4.

13. Goodman KJ, Correa P, Mera R, et al. Effect of Helicobacter pylori infection on growth velocity of school-age Andean children. *Epidemiology*. 2011;22(1):118-126.

14. Khanna B, Banatvala N, Israel NR, Gold BD. Helicobacter pylori acquisition in infancy following decline of maternal passive immunity: an IgG and IgM response. *J Pediatr Gastroenterol Nutr*. 1995;21(3):342.

15. Chong SKF, Eizember L, Lou O, et al. Peptic Ulcer disease in children is infrequently associated with helicobacter pylori infection. *J Pediatr Gsatroenterol Nutr*. 1995;21:342.

16. Hassal E, Dimmick JE. Unique features of Helicobacter pylori disease in children. *Dig Dis Sci*. 1991;36:417-423.

17. Elitsur Y, Lawrence Z. Non-Helicobacter pylori related duodenal ulcer disease in children. *Helicobacter*. 2001;6:239-243.

18. Ramakrishnan K, Salinas RC. Peptic ulcer disease. *Am Fam Physician*. 2007;76(7):1005-1012.

19. Li J, Wang F, Zhou Q, et al. IL-1 polymorphisms in children with peptic symptoms in South China. *Helicobacter*. 2011;16(3):246-251.

20. Fuller-Thomson E, Bottoms J, Brennenstuhl S, Hurd M. Is childhood physical abuse associated with peptic ulcer disease? Findings from a population-based study. *J Interpers Violence*. 2011;26(16):3225-3247.

21. Aldoori WH, Giovannucci EL, Stampfer MJ, et al. A prospective study of alcohol, smoking, caffeine, and the risk of duodenal ulcer in men. *Epidemiology*. 1997;8(4):420-424.

22. Garrow D, Delegge MH. Risk factors or gastrointestinal ulcer disease in the US population. *Dig Dis Sci*. 2010;55(1):66-72.

23. Veres G, Korponay-Szabó I, Maka E, et al. Duodenal ulceration in a patient with celiac disease and plasminogen I deficiency: coincidence or cofactors? *Pediatrics*. 2011;128(5):e1302-1306.

24. Tolia V, Dubois RS. Peptic ulcer disease in children and adolescents: a ten year experience. *Clin Pediatr (Phila)*. 1983;22(10):665-669.

25. Chey WD, Wong BCY. Practice Parameters Committee of the American College of Gastroenterology. American College of Gastroenterology guideline on the management of *Helicobacter pylori* infection. *Am J Gastroenterol*. 2007;102:1808-1825.

26. Koletzko S, Jones NL, Goodman KJ, et al. H pylori Working Groups of ESPGHAN and NASPGHAN. Evidence-based guidelines from ESPGHAN and NASPGHAN for Helicobacter pylori infection in children. *J Pediatr Gastroenterol Nutr*. 2011;53(2):230-243.

27. Abdulqawi K, El-Mahalaway AM, Abdelhameed A, Abdelwahab AA. Correlation of serum antibody titres with invasive methods for rapid detection of Helicobacter pylori infections in symptomatic children. *Int J Exp Pathol*. 2012;93(4):295-304.

28. Plunkett A, Beattie RM. Recurrent abdominal pain in childhood. *J R Soc Med*. 2005;98(3):101-106.

29. Tam PKH, Saing H. The use of H_2-receptor antagonist in the treatment of peptic ulcer disease in children. *J Pediatr Gastroenterol Nutr*. 1989;8:41-46.

30. Terrin G, Passariello A, De Curtis M, et al. Ranitidine is associated with infections, necrotizing enterocolitis and fatal outcome in newborns. *Pediatrics*. 2012;129(1):e40-45.

56 FOREIGN BODY INGESTION

Eugene K. Vortia, MD
Lori A. Mahajan, MD

PATIENT STORY

A 2-year-old boy presented to his primary care physician's office with decreased oral intake and cough of 4 days duration. He had been very irritable with a markedly decrease in intake of solids. He was seen in an urgent care 2 days prior and was discharged home with a prescription for an antibiotic but his symptoms did not improve. On examination, he had a low-grade fever with increased oral secretions and transmitted upper airway sounds but no localized wheezing. A chest radiograph performed to assess for pneumonia revealed a coin in the proximal esophagus (**Figure 56-1**). Due to increased oral secretions and the duration of symptoms, he was referred for immediate endoscopy. The coin was removed with ulceration of the underlying esophageal mucosa at the site of impaction noted. Oral intake soon returned to normal. He was prescribed a 1-week course of sucralfate with no long-term complications noted.

INTRODUCTION

- Foreign body ingestion is a frequent cause of emergency room visits in children and is accidental in most cases. Fortunately, 90 percent of ingested foreign bodies pass spontaneously without complication. Most children with an impacted foreign body have no underlying gastrointestinal anomalies. Food is classified as a foreign body when it leads to impaction, particularly in the esophagus. Steak, hotdogs, and chicken are the primary cause of esophageal foreign body impaction in teenagers and adults.

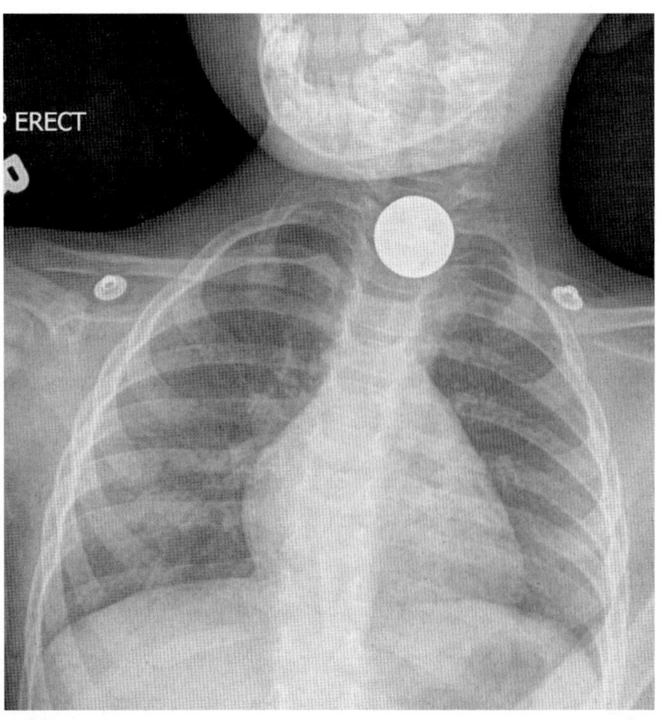

FIGURE 56-1 Coin in the proximal esophagus of a 2-year-old boy (AP view). It was causing a cough over the previous 4 days. It was impacted at the upper esophageal sphincter. (*Used with permission from Eugene Vortia, MD.*)

SYNONYMS

- Gastrointestinal foreign bodies.
- Swallowed foreign bodies.
- Esophageal food impaction.

EPIDEMIOLOGY

- More than 100,000 instances of foreign body ingestion were reported in 2010, with most of these cases reported in children and adolescents.[1]
- 75 percent of all foreign body ingestions occur in children, with a peak incidence between the ages of 6 months and 6 years.[2]
- 90 percent of all ingested foreign bodies in children are coins.
- Most ingested foreign bodies result in an uneventful outcome, with a complication rate of less than 1 percent.
- Only 10 percent of ingested foreign bodies require intervention to remove them.
- There were more than 3,300 reported cases of button battery ingestion in the US between 2008 to 2010 with 50 major complications and 7 deaths, all in children less than 6 years of age.[3]
- An estimated 1,700 ingestions of magnets from magnet sets were treated in US emergency departments between January 1, 2009 and December 31, 2011, with 70 percent of the victims less than 12 years of age and 20 patients requiring surgery.[4]

ETIOLOGY AND PATHOPHYSIOLOGY

- Ingestion of button batteries (**Figure 56-2**) is of particular concern given the high risk of severe complications and possible death.
- Small powerful "rare earth" magnets (**Figure 56-3**) marketed as adult desk toys, stress relievers, and science kits present the potential for serious complications when two or more are swallowed within a short period of time.
- Impaction and obstruction often occurs at areas of anatomical narrowing (strictures, surgical anastomoses, duodenal C-loop) or physiologic sphincters (upper and lower esophageal sphincters, pylorus, ileocecal valve).

ESOPHAGUS

- There are three areas of anatomical narrowing in the esophagus where foreign bodies are most likely to become impacted in children:

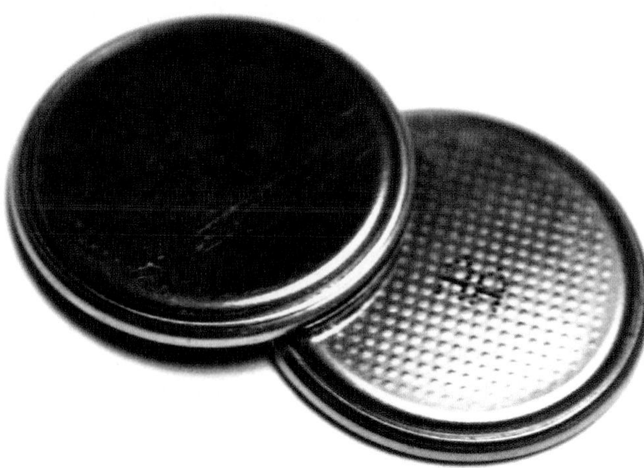

FIGURE 56-2 Button batteries are commonly swallowed by children and present a high risk of severe complications and possible death. *(Used with permission from Eugene Vortia, MD.)*

- Upper esophageal sphincter (70% of cases; **Figure 56-4**).
- Mid-esophagus (at the aortic indentation; **Figure 56-5**).
- Lower esophageal sphincter (LES) (**Figure 56-6**).

STOMACH AND LOWER GASTROINTESTINAL TRACT

- Swallowed objects that reach the stomach pass spontaneously and uneventfully through the gastrointestinal tract in 90 percent of cases.
- As a general rule, objects >2 cm in diameter or >6 cm in length are not likely to make it past the pylorus or the duodenum and will require endoscopic removal.[5]

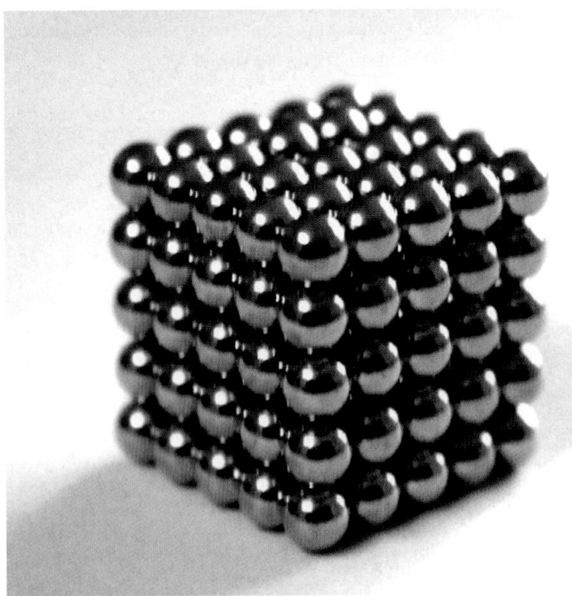

FIGURE 56-3 Rare earth magnets or Neodymium magnets are particularly dangerous when swallowed, especially if more than one is swallowed within a short period of time. *(Used with permission from Vera Okwu, MD.)*

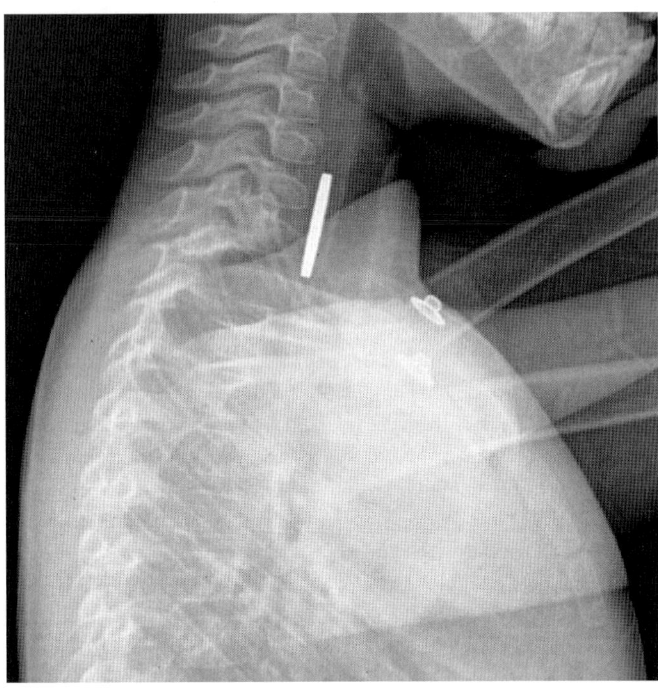

FIGURE 56-4 Lateral view of coin in proximal esophagus. *(Used with permission from Eugene Vortia, MD.)*

- With the possible exception of multiple magnet ingestion and some sharp objects, the vast majority of objects that successfully reach the small or large intestine will pass without complications.

RISK FACTORS

- Poor parental supervision or neglect.
- Psychological disorders.

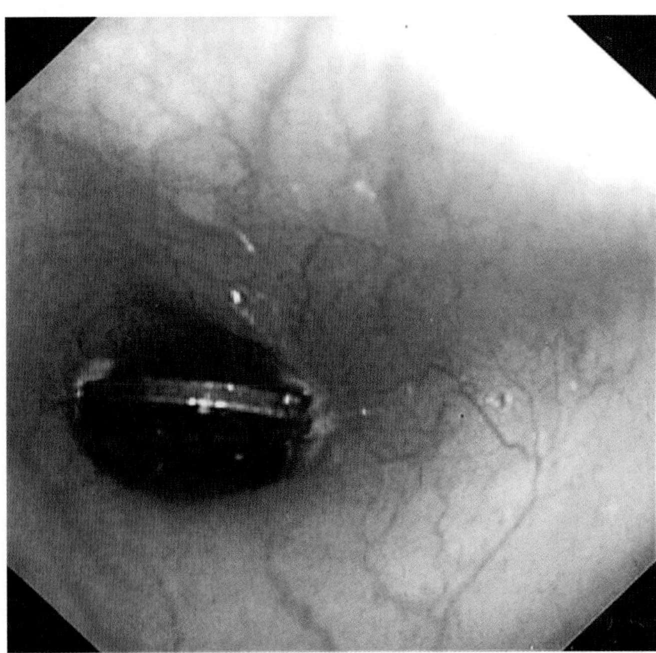

FIGURE 56-5 Endoscopic view of coin impacted in mid-esophagus. *(Used with permission from Katharine Eng, MD.)*

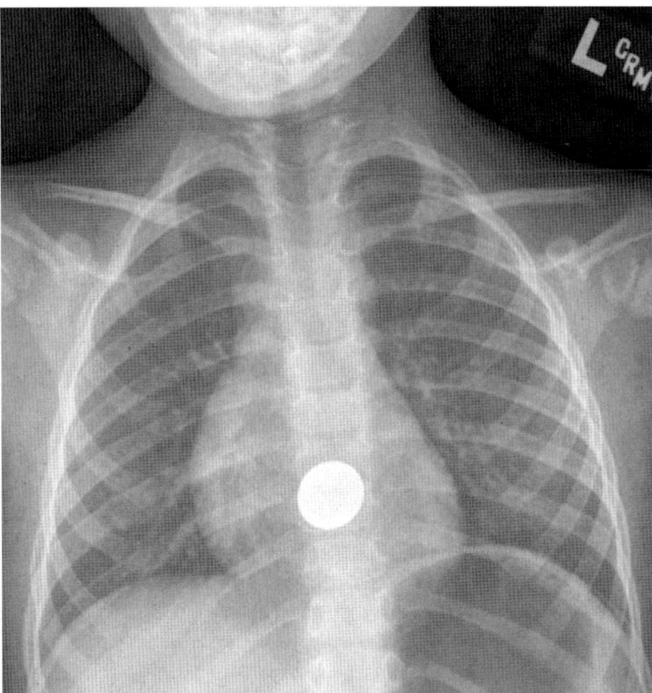

FIGURE 56-6 Coin in lower esophagus (PA view). It was impacted at the lower esophageal sphincter. (*Used with permission from Katharine Eng, MD.*)

- Attention seeking behavior (in older children).
- Certain factors increase the likelihood of impaction in the gastrointestinal tract after foreign body ingestion:
  - Age less than 3 years.
  - Large foreign bodies (>2 cm in diameter or >6 cm in length).
  - Functional and structural abnormalities of the esophagus:[6–8]
    - Eosinophilic esophagitis.
    - Esophageal strictures from previous esophageal surgery or reflux disease.
    - Achalasia.
    - Esophageal webs/rings.

DIAGNOSIS

CLINICAL FEATURES

- Presentation is usually straightforward but may be subtle, causing delayed diagnosis.
- The site of impaction is often not accurately localized and does not correlate with the area of discomfort in younger children.
- The nature of the presenting symptom is most often based on the type of foreign body ingested, the size and location of the foreign body, and the duration of the impaction.
- Younger children often present with drooling, poor feeding, vomiting, choking, coughing, and respiratory distress.
- Persistent mild respiratory symptoms and "recurrent" aspiration pneumonias in young children may in some cases precede identification of an esophageal foreign body during routine radiography.
- Older children often present with dysphagia, odynophagia, choking, and chest pain.
- Massive, life-threatening gastrointestinal hemorrhage due to erosion of a long-standing retained esophageal foreign body into adjacent vascular structures has been reported.
- Serious complications (perforation or strictures) are more commonly associated with ingestion of button batteries, large sharp objects, or multiple magnets.
- Proximal esophageal perforation may lead to pneumomediastinum with neck erythema, swelling, crepitus, or tenderness.
- Peritonitis or symptoms related to small-bowel obstruction may be present in rare cases.

LABORATORY TESTING

- Laboratory testing is not usually required except in the case of ingestion of foreign bodies composed of or coated with toxic substances such as lead.

IMAGING

- Initial evaluation of children with known or suspected foreign body ingestion should include biplane radiographs (posteroanterior and lateral) of the chest and abdomen to locate, enumerate and confirm the type and size of the ingested object(s).
- Esophageal coins (**Figures 56-1**, **56-4**, and **56-6**) most often appear in a coronal alignment on a posteroanterior radiograph view, whereas coins lodged in the trachea usually appear "enface" on the lateral view.
- A "double-contour" configuration or a "halo" on plain radiograph may distinguish a disk battery from a coin (**Figure 56-7**).
- In cases of magnet ingestion, the radiograph should be examined carefully to assess for the presence of multiple magnets in close proximity which may mimic a single magnet (**Figure 56-8**).

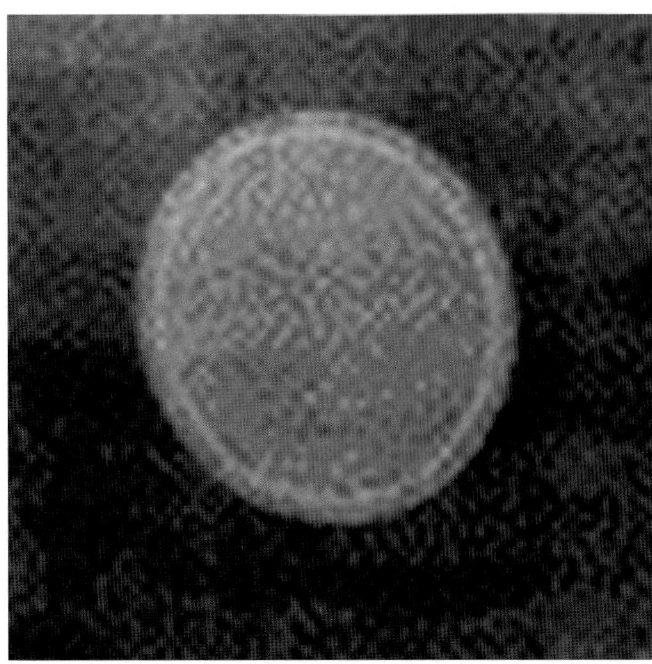

FIGURE 56-7 Radiograph of a button battery showing the "double contour" or "halo." (*Used with permission from Nisha Patel, MD.*)

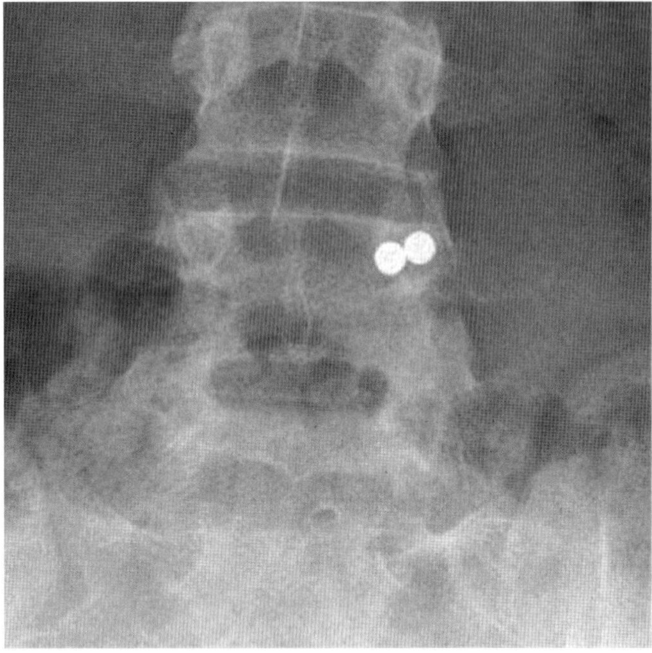

FIGURE 56-8 Radiograph showing two magnets in close proximity in the small bowel. It may not be possible to tell if they are attached across the bowel wall or within the bowel lumen. (*Used with permission from Vera Okwu, MD.*)

- A contrast examination should not be performed because of increased aspiration risk and the potential of complicating planned endoscopic procedures.

DIFFERENTIAL DIAGNOSIS

There are numerous differential diagnoses that must be considered in the case of reported foreign body ingestion. In addition, other predisposing disorders may be brought to light after an ingested foreign body has been retained in the gastrointestinal tract. These include:

- Tracheal Foreign Bodies—Can usually be differentiated from esophageal foreign bodies on radiographs as previously discussed.
- Acute bronchiolitis (see Chapter 48, Bronchiolitis)—Usually URI symptoms and fever are present.
- Reactive Airway Disease (see Chapter 49, Asthma)—History of previous wheezing episode can be elicited.
- Aspiration Pneumonia—History of choking and an infiltrate on CXR is present.
- Eosinophilic esophagitis (see Chapter 54, Esophageal Disorders).
- Munchausen Syndrome—Should be suspected with unusual ingestions or when the history does not align with the findings.
- Pica.
- Parental neglect.

MANAGEMENT

- Support airway with suctioning of secretions and supplemental oxygen if indicated.
- Ensure that patients with esophageal impaction remain fasting until foreign body removal can be performed to decrease the risk of aspiration.
- Under the following circumstances, emergent specialty consultation is indicated:
  - Signs or symptoms of airway compromise.
  - Evidence of esophageal obstruction such as the inability to swallow secretions.
  - Signs or symptoms of intestinal obstruction such as abdominal pain or vomiting.
  - Esophageal foreign body presentation 24 or more hours after presumed time of ingestion, or an unknown time of ingestion.
  - Multiple magnet ingestions within a short time.
  - Retained disk battery in the esophagus (within 2 hours).
  - Sharp objects (nonstraight pins, needles, razors, or multiple straight pins).
  - Long objects (>6 cm).
- With the exception of cases involving multiple magnets, disk batteries in the esophagus and sharp objects, asymptomatic patients able to handle oral secretions may have the procedure delayed for up to 24 hours.
- In asymptomatic patients with an esophageal foreign body, repeat radiograph immediately prior to endoscopic intervention if significant delay after initial assessment has occurred to establish that the object has not passed to the stomach.
- In most cases, with the exception of cases involving multiple magnets, large objects (>2 cm in diameter or >6 cm in length) and sharps, objects confirmed to pass into or beyond the stomach can be managed with an expectant approach since they are likely to successfully pass through the intestines and out the body without complication.
- Referral for endoscopic removal is required if symptoms such as persistent abdominal pain or vomiting develop as these may indicate pyloric obstruction.
- If there is no evidence of gastric/intestinal foreign body passage in the stool by 4 weeks post-ingestion, repeat abdominal x-ray is recommended. Referral for further evaluation is indicated if the foreign body is still present.

SPECIAL SITUATIONS

▶ Battery ingestions

Button batteries (**Figures 56-2** and **56-7**) result in high rates of serious complications due to discharge of current and leakage of caustic material. They must be immediately removed as esophageal perforation may occur within 4 hours or less of ingestion.

- For batteries confirmed to be in the stomach, follow-up radiographs should be performed after 48 hours. Referral for endoscopic removal is indicated if the battery is still in the stomach.

▶ Sharp foreign bodies

- Presence of a sharp foreign body (**Figure 56-9**) requires immediate referral for consideration of surgical or endoscopic retrieval.

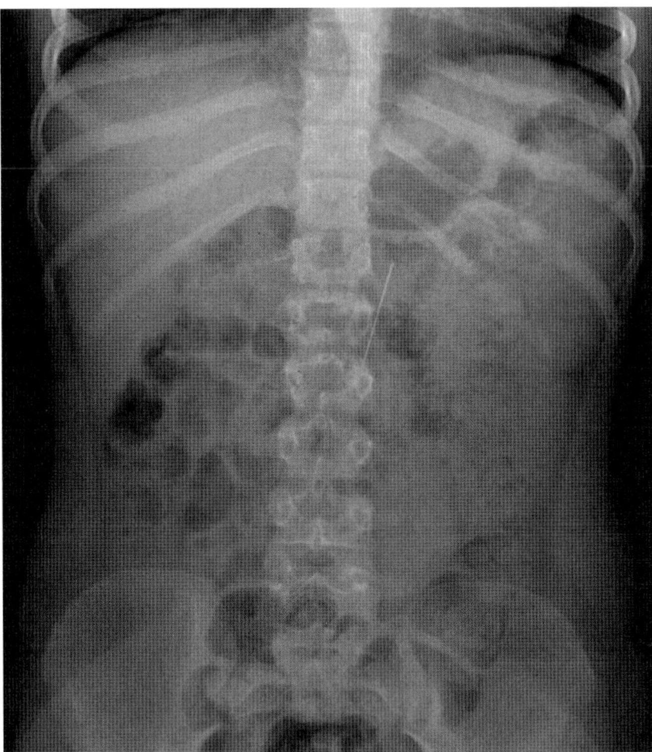

FIGURE 56-9 Straight pin on abdominal radiograph (PA view). (*Used with permission from Nisha Patel, MD.*)

- Single straight pins with a bulbous head will most often successfully navigate the gastrointestinal tract by peristaltic action without injury, with the blunt end leading and the sharp end trailing. Expectant management with close follow-up is recommended.

▶ Magnets

- Confirmed single magnet ingestions result in few gastrointestinal complications and may be clinically followed. Care should be taken to not mistake multiple magnets in close proximity as a single magnet (**Figure 56-8**).
- Ingestion of multiple magnets may result in the magnets attracting each other through the bowel wall and causing pressure necrosis with perforation or entero-enteric fistula formation. Early referral for possible endoscopic or surgical intervention is, therefore, indicated.

▶ Food impaction

- Meat impacted in the esophagus should be removed within 12 hours to minimize mucosal damage. Referral for consultation recommended even if esophageal food impaction resolves spontaneously due to the high rate of underlying pathology.

▶ Non-radio-opaque foreign bodies

- Management of non-radio-opaque foreign bodies (**Figure 56-10**) most often depends on adequate history regarding the length, size and sharpness of the object as well as the presence of symptoms.
- Having an identical copy of the ingested foreign body can be helpful to guide management.

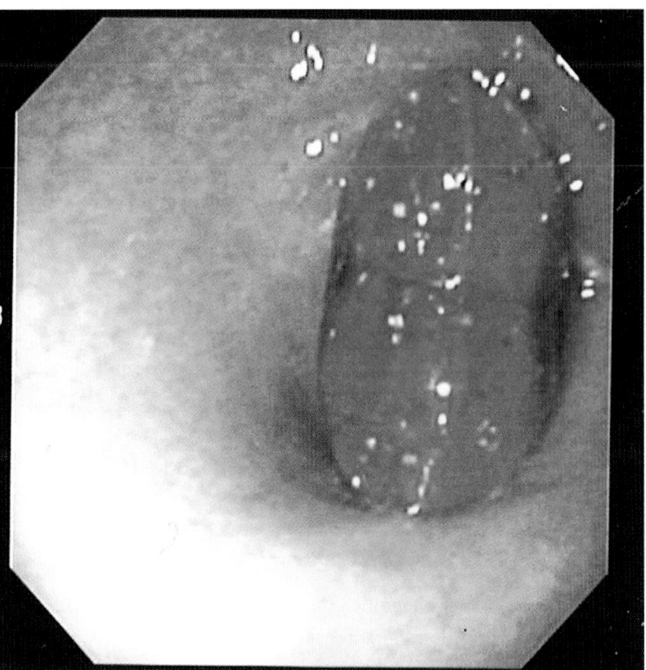

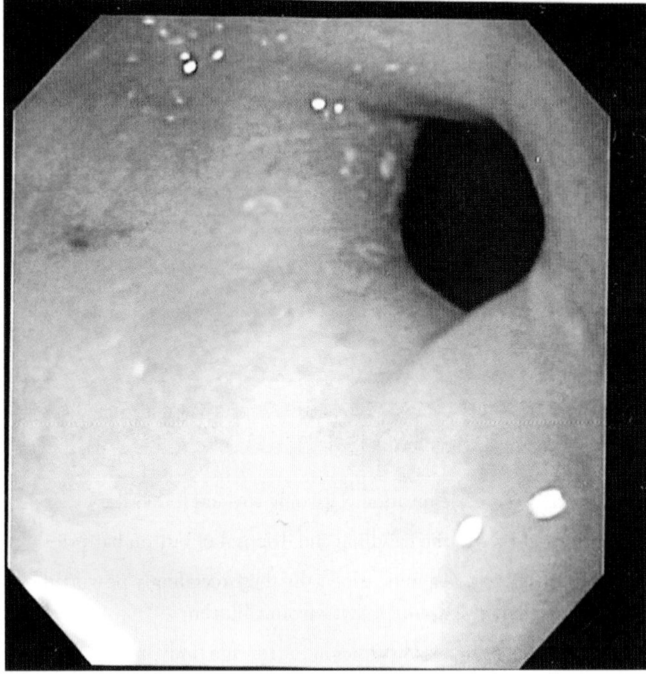

FIGURE 56-10 Large radiolucent foreign body obstructed at the pylorus. The first view shows a heart shaped plastic toy obstructed at the pylorus. The second view represents the view after endoscopic extraction of the plastic toy. (*Used with permission from Eugene Vortia, MD.*)

- Abdominal CT scan or ultrasound may be considered to provide more information.

MEDICATIONS

- Smooth muscle relaxants such as glucagon have been used with success in adults with foreign bodies impacted at lower esophageal sphincter but this approach has not been uniformly successful in children. SOR Ⓒ

- The use of laxatives to hasten transit of ingested foreign bodies through intestinal tract does not lead to an improved clinical outcome and is not recommended. SOR Ⓒ
- Meat tenderizers for esophageal meat impaction are **contraindicated** due to the risk of hypernatremia and esophageal injury.
- Administration of a pro-emetic such as ipecac is **contraindicated**.

SURGERY

- Surgical intervention may be needed if endoscopic retrieval is not possible:
  - Multiple magnets attracting each other through the bowel wall are not able to traverse the gastrointestinal tract.
  - After ingestion of multiple sharp straight pins or other sharp objects.
  - Any object obstructing the gastrointestinal tract that cannot be endoscopically removed.
- Patients with life-threatening complications from foreign body ingestion (perforation/hemorrhage).

REFERRAL

- Refer all cases of foreign body impaction to an appropriate specialist or referral center for retrieval.
- For button batteries in the esophagus, patients should be transported to a referral center within 2 hours regardless of symptoms in order to decrease the risk of serious complication.
- Any child with suspected multiple-magnet ingestion, ingestion of a multiple straight pins, or double-ended sharp objects should be emergently referred for consideration of endoscopic or surgical retrieval.

PREVENTION AND SCREENING

- Improve caregiver education regarding toy and food safety.
- Use special care in the handling and disposal of button batteries.
- Ensure that small magnets, especially the exceedingly powerful rare earth magnets are kept away from children.
- Maintain a high index of suspicion for foreign body ingestion, especially if the eating pattern of a child abruptly changes.
- Inform families to promptly report all foreign body ingestions, particularly magnets, button batteries, and sharp objects to their physician or proceed to the emergency room for further evaluation.

PROGNOSIS

- The prognosis is excellent in most cases of foreign body ingestion.
- Patients with ingestion of multiple magnets, multiple straight pins, large sharp objects, and button batteries generally do well after treatment but have a more guarded prognosis because of an increased incidence of late complications.

FOLLOW-UP

- Patients with ingestion of multiple magnets, multiple straight pins, large sharp objects, and button batteries require follow-up because of the risk of late complications.
- After removal of an esophageal foreign body most asymptomatic patients do not need further follow-up unless significant underlying esophageal mucosal disease was identified at endoscopy.
- All patients who develop new gastrointestinal symptoms after conservative therapy should be referred for specialist evaluation.
- With the exception of large, sharp or long objects and magnets, asymptomatic patients with gastric foreign bodies should monitor their stool for the object and if confirmed to pass, require no further follow-up.
- Abdominal radiographs may be used to localize objects that have not passed in 4 weeks.

PATIENT RESOURCES

- NASPGHAN patient hand-out on rare earth magnets—**www.naspghan.org/user-assets/Documents/Magnet%20patient%20education%20handout%20with%20picture%20July%202012(3)%20%20(2).pdf**.
- United States Consumer Products Safety Commission patient information on magnets—**www.cpsc.gov/info/magnets/index.html**.
- SAFEKIDS.ORG—**www.safekids.org/our-work/blog/magnet-poisoning.html**.
- National Capital Poison Center patient information on button batteries—**www.poison.org/battery**.

PROVIDER RESOURCES

- National Capital Poison Center provider guideline on management of button batteries—**www.poison.org/battery/guideline.asp**.
- NASPGHAN Issue Brief—Preventing Magnet Ingestions by Children, June 2012—**www.naspghan.org/user-assets/Documents/pdf/Advocacy/July%202012/Magnet%20Ingestion%20One%20Pager.pdf**.
- Management of ingested foreign bodies and food impactions. ASGE Standards of Practice Committee. *Gastrointest Endosc*. 2011;73(6):1085-1091.

REFERENCES

1. Bronstein AC, Spyker DA, Cantilena LR Jr, Green JL, Rumack BH, Dart RC. 2010 Annual Report of the American Association of Poison Control Centers' National Poison Data System (NPDS): 28th Annual Report. *Clin Toxicol (Phila)*. 2011;49(10):910-941.
2. Cheng W, Tam PK. Foreign-body ingestion in children: experience with 1265 cases. *J Pediatr Surg*. 1999;34:1472-1476.
3. Litovitz T, Whitaker N, Clark L, White NC, Marsolek M. Emerging battery ingestion hazard: Clinical implications. *Pediatrics*. 2010; 125(6):1168-1177.

4. Garland, S. Memorandum, subject: NEISS estimates and analysis of reported incidents related to ingestion of small, strong magnets that are part of a set of magnets of various sizes. Bethesda, MD: Division of Hazard Analysis, Directorate for Epidemiology, U.S. Consumer Product Safety Commission; 2012.
5. Kay M, Wyllie R. Pediatric foreign bodies and their management. *Curr Gastroenterol Rep*. 2005;7(3):212-218.
6. Chandra S, Hiremath G, Kim S, Enav B. Magnet ingestion in children and teenagers: an emerging health concern for pediatricians and pediatric subspecialists. *J Pediatr Gastroenterol Nutr*. 2012; 54(6):828.
7. Lao J, Bostwick HE, et al. Esophageal food impaction in children. *Pediatr Emerg Care*. 2003:19:402-407.
8. ASGE Standards of Practice Committee, Ikenberry SO, Jue TL, Anderson MA, Appalaneni V: Management of ingested foreign bodies and food impactions. *Gastrointest Endosc*. 2011;73(6): 1085-1091.

57 PYLORIC STENOSIS

Skyler Kalady, MD
Neil Vachhani, MD

PATIENT STORY

A 4-week-old male presents to outpatient clinic with vomiting, which began two weeks ago and has become progressively worse. He is now vomiting after every feed. The vomit is projectile, non-bilious, and non-bloody. He seems hungry but over the past day, he has become fussy and urine output has decreased. He has no fever, respiratory symptoms, diarrhea, or rashes.

On examination, the infant appears alert but mildly dehydrated. His exam reveals fullness in the epigastric region. A quiet, a peristaltic wave is noted (**Figure 57-1**).

Ultrasound of the abdomen confirms the diagnosis of pyloric stenosis. Laboratory studies reveal hypochloremic, hypokalemic, and metabolic alkalosis. He is admitted for intravenous hydration and undergoes laparoscopic pyloromyotomy the following day. He is discharged home a day later, tolerating breast milk with resolution of his vomiting.

INTRODUCTION

Pyloric stenosis is defined as the progressive thickening and elongation of the pyloric channel ultimately resulting in partial or complete gastric outlet obstruction.

SYNONYMS

Infantile hypertrophic pyloric stenosis (IHPS).

EPIDEMIOLOGY

- IHPS occurs in 0.5–4/1000 live births. Estimates vary by region and surveillance method.[1]

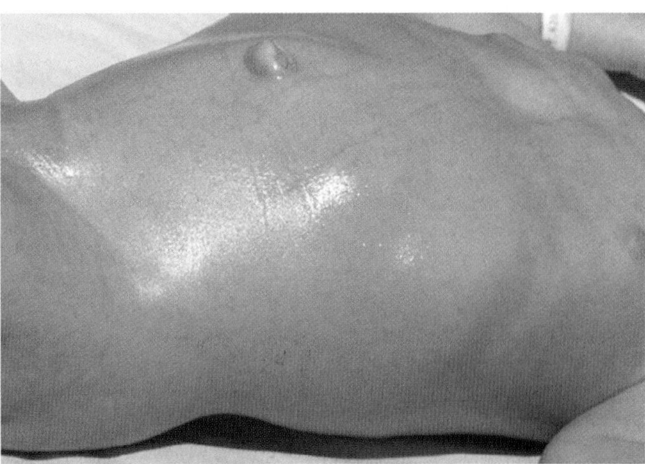

FIGURE 57-1 A peristaltic wave was visualized in this infant with pyloric stenosis. (*Used with permission from Cleveland Clinic Children's Hospital Photo File*)

- There is a clear gender bias with males affected more than females 4 to 5: 1.[1-4]
- A genetic component is theorized with increased rates in twins and other relatives.[1,2]
- First-born children are affected more often.[1]
- Maternal race and/or ethnicity alter prevalence. IHPS is more common in white and Hispanic families than African or Asian descent.[1]
- IHPS is the most common condition requiring surgery in early infancy.[2]

ETIOLOGY AND PATHOPHYSIOLOGY

- The underlying etiology of IHPS remains unknown.
- Causes are likely multifactorial with genetic and environmental contributions.
- Pyloric sphincter function is abnormal. The muscle fails to relax due to decreased nitric oxide synthase production and abnormal smooth muscle receptors.[1]
- Over time and with activation of local growth factors, the pylorus gradually thickens producing outlet obstruction. In compensation, the stomach dilates, thickens, and peristalses leading to emesis with every feed.

RISK FACTORS

- Genetic factors clearly play a role. There is a 200-fold increase in monozygotic twins and a 20-fold increase in dizygotic twins and siblings, as compared to individuals without affected relatives.[2]
- Erythromycin treatment used for pertussis prophylaxis increases risk for IHPS up to 10-fold perhaps due to its action as a motilin agonist.[1,4]
- Additional relative risk factors including maternal smoking during pregnancy, preterm delivery, small weight for gestational age, cesarean section, congenital malformations, and bottle feeding have been recently implicated.[3,5]
- Smith-Lemli-Opitz and Cornelia de Lange syndromes confer a great risk of IHPS.[4]

DIAGNOSIS

CLINICAL FEATURES

- Symptoms classically occur between 3 to 6 weeks of age, rarely starting after 12 weeks.
- The patient develops projectile, nonbilious, nonbloody emesis immediately following feeds.
- The patient remains vigorous and hungry until hydration is compromised.
- When the abdomen is relaxed following emesis, a pyloric "olive" or mass may be palpable by the skilled examiner.
- With dehydration and weight loss, a gastric peristaltic wave may be visualized moving from left to right in the upper abdomen prior to emesis (**Figure 57-1**).
- Jaundice is seen in 5 to 14 percent of cases.[4,6]

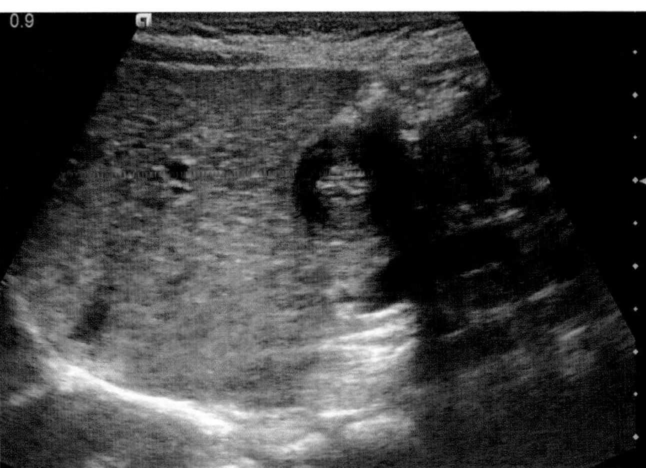

FIGURE 57-2 Transverse ultrasound through the pylorus showing thickening of the muscular wall (red marks). (*Used with permission from Neil Vachhani, MD.*)

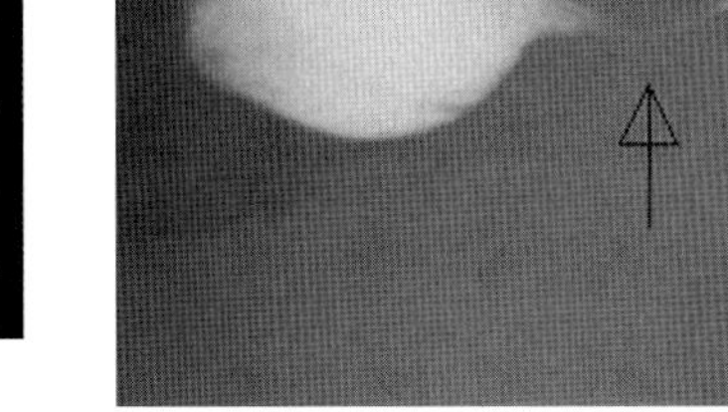

FIGURE 57-4 Lateral view from an Upper GI examination shows a small amount of barium passing through the pyloric channel (arrow) known as the "string sign." (*Used with permission from Neil Vachhani, MD.*)

LABORATORY TESTING

- Laboratory testing is adjunctive but not diagnostic.
- An electrolyte panel typically reveals hypochloremic, hypokalemic, or metabolic alkalosis. However, with increased clinician awareness and advances in imaging, many patients are now diagnosed prior to developing electrolyte abnormalities.
- Unconjugated hyperbilirubinemia is relatively common likely due to transiently decreased levels of hepatic glucuronoyl transferase from poor feeding.

IMAGING

- Ultrasound is currently the imaging modality of choice when performed by an experienced operator.[4,7] It is highly sensitive and specific and does not utilize radiation. Findings include thickening of the pyloric muscle and elongation of the pyloric channel (**Figures 57-2** and **57-3**).

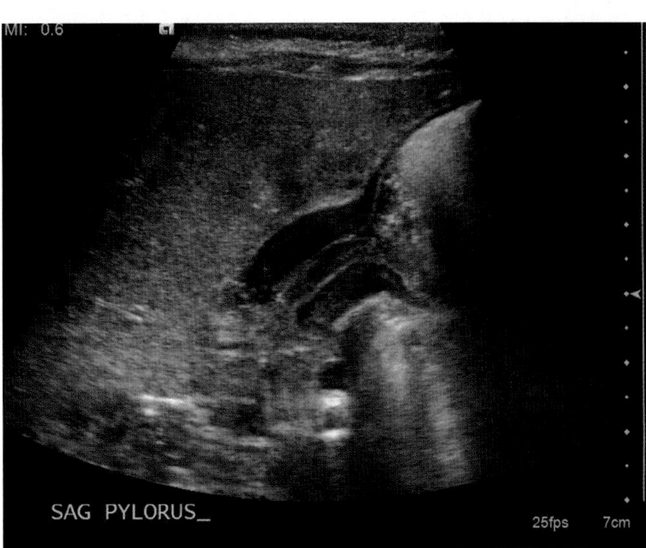

FIGURE 57-3 Longitudinal ultrasound through the pylorus showing elongation of the pyloric channel (red dots) and thickening of the muscular wall. (*Used with permission from Neil Vachhani, MD.*)

- Upper GI examination is less operator-dependent and can be used when there is limited ultrasound experience.[7] It also has high sensitivity and specificity but utilizes ionizing radiation. It demonstrates delayed passage of contrast as well as a small amount of contrast traversing the pyloric channel (string sign; **Figure 57-4**).
- Abdominal radiograph is not sensitive for diagnosing pyloric stenosis and is not routinely indicated. If obtained, it often shows a distended stomach with a paucity of distal bowel gas.[7] Undulation of the stomach contour can be seen due to hyperperistalsis (caterpillar sign; **Figure 57-5**).

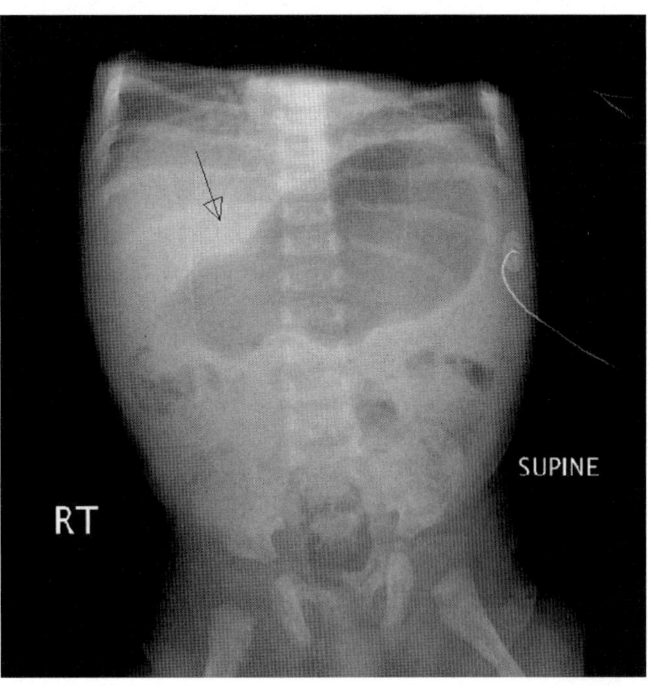

FIGURE 57-5 Supine anteroposterior abdominal radiograph shows a gas filled distended stomach. Undulation of the gastric contour, known as the "caterpillar sign" (arrow) is due to gastric hyperperistalsis. (*Used with permission from Neil Vachhani, MD.*)

DIFFERENTIAL DIAGNOSIS

Common entities:

- Gastroesophageal reflux (GER)—Similar to IHPS, patients have non-bilious emesis following feeds. However, patients with GER should not have projectile vomiting or develop dehydration (see Chapter 54, Esophageal Disorders).
- Milk protein allergy—Emesis may be related to feeds but ultimately signs of colitis predominate with hematochezia rather than projectile vomiting and dehydration.
- Gastroenteritis—Viral infection can typically be differentiated from IHPS with presence of a sick contact, diarrhea and self resolution over a few days.

Less common entities with important differences in the history:

- Doudenal atresia/stenosis—Signs of obstruction should be present from birth.
- Hirschsprung's Disease—Delayed passage of meconium followed by emesis should differentiate this entity (see Chapter 62, Anal and Rectal Disorders).
- Adrenal crisis—Patients should present with lethargy, poor feeding, and vomiting and become progressively ill. Labs reveal hyperkalemic, metabolic acidosis. Many states have newborn screening programs to aid in diagnosing this condition.
- Infection—Presence of fever or temperature instability in an ill patient with vomiting could suggest UTI, bacteremia, or meningitis.
- Malrotation with volvulus should be considered immediately with any bilious emesis.

MANAGEMENT

SURGERY

- Pyloromyotomy is the definitive treatment for IHPS.[4] SOR Ⓐ
- Infants with dehydration or electrolyte derangement require volume resuscitation and correction of electrolyte abnormalities via intravenous fluids prior to surgery.[4] SOR Ⓐ
- Both laparoscopic and open pyloromyotomy are well studied and effective. However, recent meta-analyses suggest the laparoscopic approach is preferable with less wound infection, decreased length of stay and shorter time to feeding.[8,9] SOR Ⓐ
- Patients are generally discharged home after 24 to 48 hours once they are tolerating feeds without emesis.[4]

NONPHARMACOLOGIC

Prolonged nasoduodenal feeds were studied in the remote past, but good surgical outcomes render this prior approach outdated and impractical.[10]

MEDICATIONS

- In rare instances when a patient cannot undergo surgery, successful treatment with intravenous followed by oral atropine sulfate has been described.[11]

REFERRAL

Referral to a medical center staffed by pediatric anesthesiologists and surgeons is the current standard of care.

PREVENTION AND SCREENING

- Research into genetic and environmental factors will lead to further insight in this arena.
- Currently, avoidance of erythromycin therapy in young infants is recommended.

PROGNOSIS

- Prognosis for patients with pyloric stenosis is excellent following surgical correction.
- One study reported an increased chance of developing chronic abdominal pain in patients with IHPS as compared to controls (25% versus 5.8%).[12]

FOLLOW-UP

Routine follow-up with a primary care physician is recommended.

PATIENT EDUCATION

Projectile vomiting in a newborn requires urgent medical attention.

PATIENT RESOURCES

- Healthychildren.Org from the American Academy of Pediatrics—**www.healthychildren.org/English/health-issues/conditions/abdominal/Pages/Infant-Vomiting.aspx**.
- **www.nlm.nih.gov/medlineplus/ency/article/000970.htm**.

PROVIDER RESOURCES

- Aspelund G, Langer JC: Current management of hypertrophic pyloric stenosis. *Semin Pediatr Surg*. 2007;16(1):27-33.

REFERENCES

1. Ranells S, Carver J, Kirby, R. Infantile Hypertrophic Pyloric Stenosis: Epidemiology, Genetics and Clinical Update. *Advances in Pediatrics*. 2011;(58):195-206.
2. Krogh C, Fischer TK, Skotte L, et al. Familial aggregation and heritability of pyloric stenosis. *JAMA*. 2010;303:2393-2399.
3. Krogh C, Gortz S, Wohlfahrt J, Biggar R, Melbye M, Fischer TK. Pre-and Perinatal Risk Factors for Pyloric Stenosis and Their Influence on the Male Predominance. *Am J Epidemiol*. 2012; 176(1):24-31.

4. Pandya S & Heiss K. Pyloric Stenosis in Pediatric Surgery: An Evidence- Based Review. *Surg Clin N Am*. 2012;92:527-539.
5. Krogh C, Biggar R, Fischer T et al. Bottle-feeding and the Risk of Pyloric Stenosis. *Pediatrics*. 2012;130(4): 1-7.
6. Hua L, Shi D, Bishop PR, et al. The role of UGT1A1*28 mutation in jaundiced infants with hypertrophic pyloric stenosis. *Pediatr Res*. 2005;58(5):881-884.
7. Hernanz-Schulman M, Berch BR, Neblett III W. Imaging of Infantile Hypertrophic Pyloric Stenosis (IIHPS). In: Medina LS, Blackmore CC editors. *Evidence-Based Imaging: Optimizing Imaging in Patient Care.* New York: Springer; 2010:447-457.
8. Sola JE, Neville HL. Laparoscopic vs open pyloromyotomy: a systematic review and meta-analysis. *J Pediatr Surg*. 2009;44(8): 1631-1637.
9. Oomen, MW, Hoekstra LT et al. Open Versus Laparoscopic Pyloromyotomy for Hypertrophic Pyloric Stenosis: A Systematic Review and Meta-Analysis Focusing on Major Complications. *Surg Endosc*. 2012;26: 2104-2110.
10. Yamashiro Y, Mayama H, Yamamoto K, et al. Conservative Management of infantile pyloric stenosis by nasoduodenal feeding. *Eur J Pediatr*. 1981;136:187.
11. Kawahar H, Takama Y et al. Medical Treatment of Infantile Hypertrophic Pyloric Stenosis: Should We Always Slice the Olive? *J Pediatr Surg*. 2005;40(12):1848-1851.
12. Saps M, Bonilla S. Early life events: infants with pyloric stenosis have a higher risk of developing chronic abdominal pain in childhood. *J Pediatr* 2011;159(4):551-4 e1.

58 INTUSSUSCEPTION

Allison W. Brindle, MD
Ellen Park, MD
John DiFiore, MD

PATIENT STORY

An 11-month-old previously healthy male infant is brought to the Emergency Department (ED) for a 1-day history of fussiness and vomiting. His parents report that throughout the day he has had periods of crying and has been inconsolable, drawing his knees in towards his chest. Crying episodes last for about 20 minutes. Between episodes, he had been content. He then developed vomiting immediately after an episode of crying. He passed a bowel movement that appeared to have blood and mucus in the stool. He became more lethargic between crying episodes and his parents have become quite concerned. In the ED, he appeared moderately dehydrated, appeared sleepy, and was noted to have tenderness on palpation of the abdomen. After stabilization with intravenous fluids the physician ordered an abdominal ultrasound, which was concerning for intussusception (**Figure 58-1A–C**). The pediatric radiologist was able to reduce the intussusception with an air enema under fluoroscopic guidance. The patient tolerated the procedure well and recovered completely.

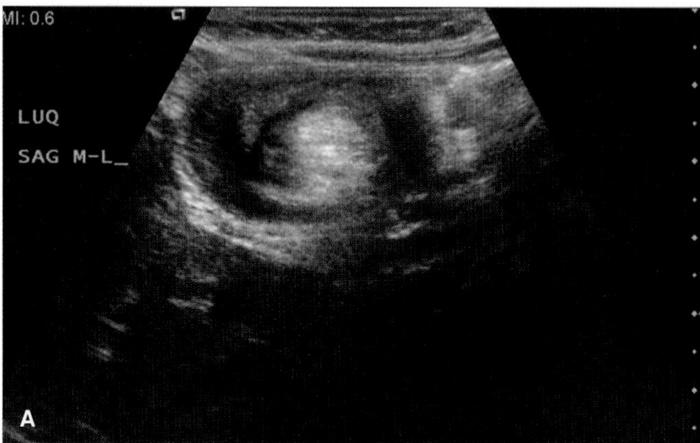

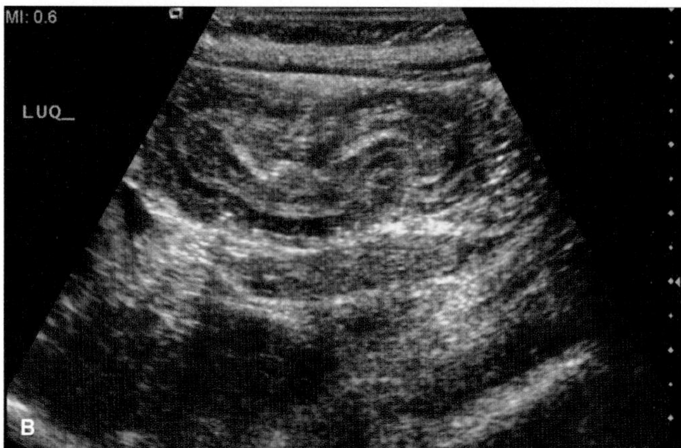

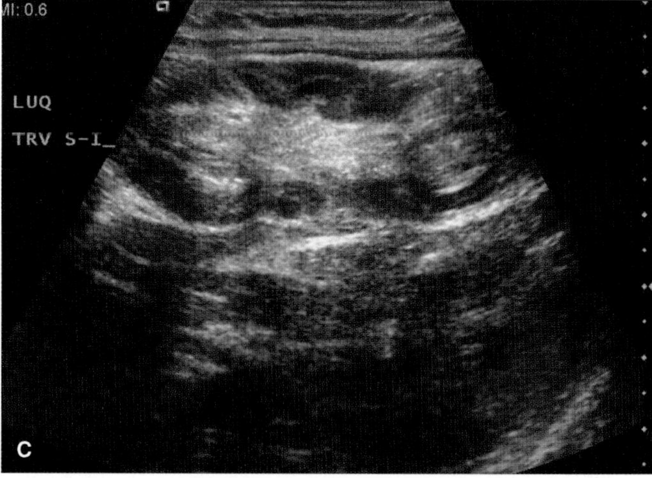

FIGURE 58-1 **A.** Intussusception in an 11-month-old infant. Transverse plane ultrasound images demonstrates a typical "target sign" with alternating concentric hypoechoic and hyperechoic bands of intussuscepted bowel walls. **B.** Sagittal plane ultrasound image of intussusception in the same patient demonstrating alternating layers of hypoechoic bowel wall and hyperechoic mesentery. **C.** Oblique sagittal plane ultrasound image of intussusception in the same patient demonstrates a typical "pseudokidney sign" with hypoechoic bowel wall mimicking the appearance of renal cortex and hyperechoic mesentery the renal sinus fat. (*Used with permission from Ellen Park, MD.*)

INTRODUCTION

Intussusception refers to the "telescoping" or invagination of one portion of the intestine (the intussusceptum) into a more distal portion, the intussuscipiens. It leads to an intestinal obstruction.

EPIDEMIOLOGY

- Most commonly diagnosed in children between the ages of 3 months and 36 months.
- It is the most common form of intestinal obstruction in children less than 2 years of age.[1–3]
- Male predominance.
- Between 1998 and 1999, there was an increased incidence of intussusception in infants who had received the tetravalent rhesus—based rotavirus vaccination (RotaShield, Wyeth Laboratories, Inc., Marietta, PA).[4] This vaccine was then taken off the market.
- Post marketing surveillance of RotaTeq™, a currently available pentavalent rotavirus vaccine, did not show an increased incidence of intussusception, and rotavirus immunization continues to be a recommended immunization in the primary immunization series.[5,6]

ETIOLOGY AND PATHOPHYSIOLOGY

- Most cases of intussusception are idiopathic.
- It is thought that lymphoid hyperplasia of the Peyer's Patches can act as a lead point in idiopathic cases.

- Seasonal variation of the incidence of intussusception suggests a correlation with common gastrointestinal viruses, such as adenovirus.
- The most common type of intussusception is ileocolic when the ileum enters the cecum. Ileoileocolic, colocolic, or small bowel-small bowel intussusceptions have also been described, but are less frequent.
- When the intussusceptum invaginates into the intussuscipiens, the surrounding mesentery is pulled with it. This leads to intestinal edema.
- Complications of intussusception include intestinal ischemia, perforation, peritonitis, and death.
- Lead points for the intussusception are more common in children older than 2 years of age. Lead points may include: Meckel's diverticulum, polyp, cyst, hematoma, or lymphoma.

RISK FACTORS

- Henoch-Schonlein purpura can cause a small bowel hematoma, which acts as a lead point for intussusception.
- Cystic fibrosis: thick inspissated stool is the lead point.
- Post-operative intussusception: within several days of intra-abdominal surgery (**Figure 58-2**).
- Prior intussusception: Intussusception can recur in 5 to 10 percent of idiopathic cases.

DIAGNOSIS

CLINICAL FEATURES

- Key Historical Features
  - Common historical features of intussusception are:
    - Lethargy[7]
    - Abdominal Pain—The pain typically occurs in colicky paroxysms and can be quite severe.[8]
    - Emesis—Usually emesis begins as nonbilious. However, as the disease progresses, bilious emesis can occur.

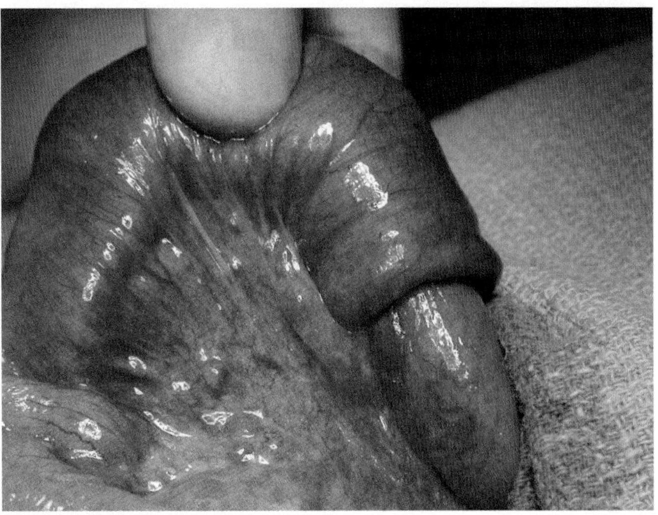

FIGURE 58-2 Small bowel-small bowel post-operative intussusception (intussusception within the small bowel after previous abdominal surgery). This was successfully reduced in the operating room without bowel resection. (*Used with permission from John DiFiore, MD.*)

    - "Currant Jelly" Stools (containing gross blood and mucus) can be seen in up to 50 to 60 percent of patients.
    - Fever may be present, but typically is a later finding.

PHYSICAL EXAMINATION FINDINGS

- Usually the patients are ill-appearing and very irritable, although the child may have alternating episodes of appearing well.
- Abdominal Mass—"Sausage" shaped mass in the right lower quadrant may be palpated.
- Guaiac positive stool on rectal examination.

IMAGING

- Plain film radiographs are not diagnostic of intussusception. However, they can be used to guide the need for further imaging studies. A study of the use of three view radiographs (supine, prone, and left lateral decubitus views) showed that the presence of air in the ascending colon on all 3 views of the series can decrease the likelihood of intussusception in a patient with an otherwise low clinical index of suspicion.[9] Free intraperitoneal air on abdominal x-ray is a contraindication for performing therapeutic enema.
- Ultrasound is the imaging modality of choice to diagnose intussusception with greater than 98 percent sensitivity (**Figure 58-1A–C**). Using ultrasound as a diagnostic tool will reduce radiation exposure in children who do not have intussusception and increase the likelihood of successful reduction in those who do.
- CT scan—Intussusception can be visualized on CT scan and has a higher sensitivity for detection of lead points. However, because CT is not also a therapeutic modality (as is ultrasound) and because it has a higher radiation exposure for the child, it is not the imaging study of choice.
- Fluoroscopy combined with hydrostatic or pneumatic enema can be both diagnostic and therapeutic.

DIFFERENTIAL DIAGNOSIS

- Gastroenteritis or enterocolitis—Children with gastroenteritis can have abdominal pain and diarrhea. However, the colicky character of pain associated with intussusception as well as the development of bloody stools is less typical of viral gastroenteritis. Patients with bacterial enterocolitis look persistently ill between episodes of cramps and diarrhea.
- Meckel's diverticulum—Although this may cause bloody stool, it is typically painless.
- Small bowel obstruction—Other etiologies of small bowel obstruction should also be considered. However, since most of these are fixed, they lack the intermittent, colicky nature of intussusception.

MANAGEMENT

- Initial treatment of intussusception in clinically stable and fluid-resuscitated patients is nasogastric decompression and emergent reduction. Spontaneous reduction may occur in approximately 5 percent of patients.

- Non-operative reduction of ileocolic intussusception can be completed with either hydrostatic or pneumatic enema using fluoroscopic guidance achieving an 80 to 95 percent success rate (**Figure 58-3A–E**).[10] SOR Ⓐ Ultrasound may be used to guide the procedure as well.
- Contraindications for therapeutic enema reduction are peritonitis, sepsis/shock, and free intraperitoneal air on radiographs.
- The primary risk of nonoperative reduction is perforation of the bowel (overall rate of perforation is less than 1%), and in

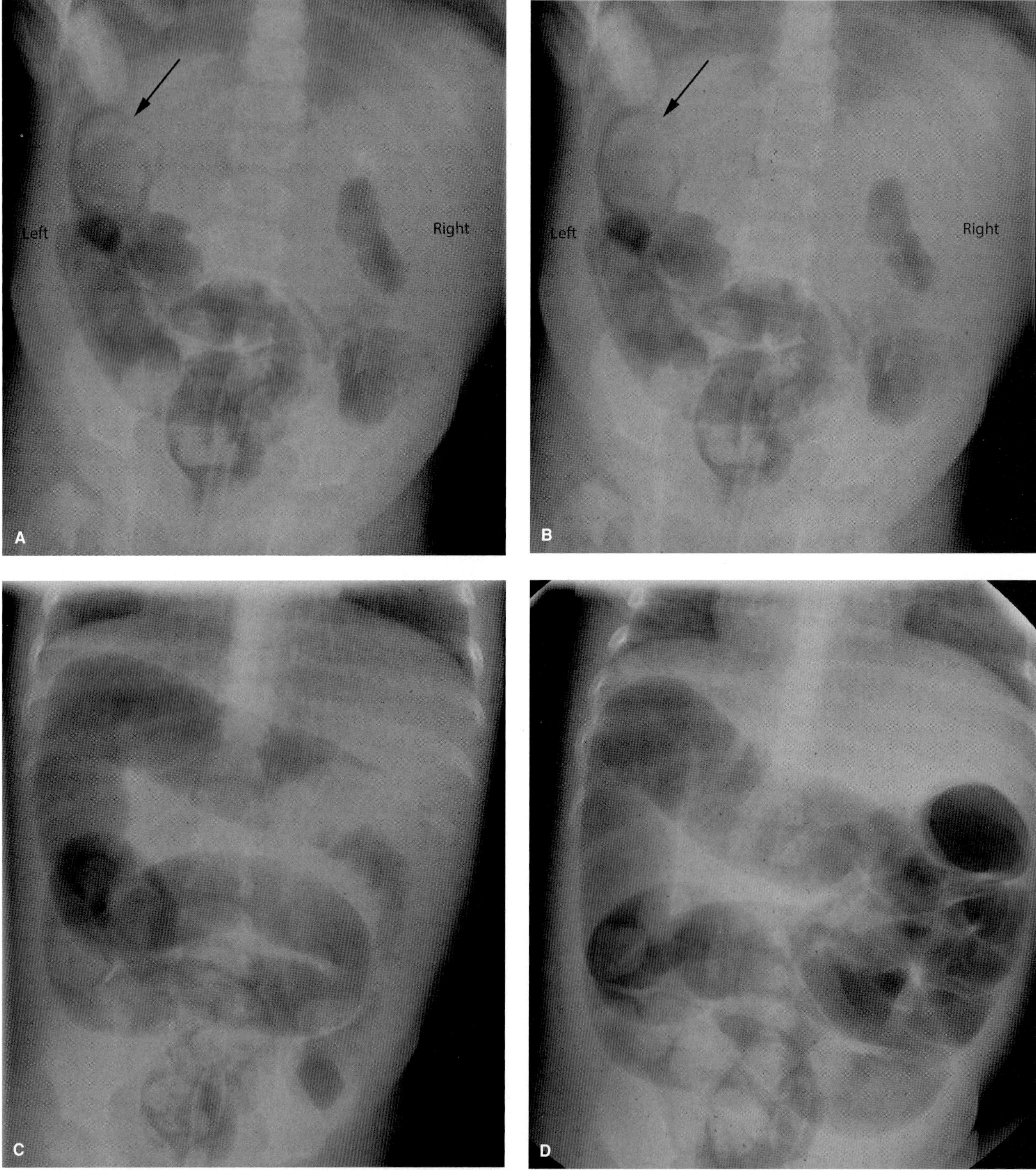

FIGURE 58-3 **A–E.** Air contrast enema reduction of an ileocolic intussusception in an 11-month-old boy obtained in prone position. Intussusception is initially demonstrated as a soft tissue mass (arrow) at the level of the splenic flexure (**A**). With continued air insufflation, intussusception is seen to move toward the cecum, and air eventually freely refluxes into the distal ileum as the ileocolic intussusception is reduced (**B–E**). (*Used with permission from Ellen Park, MD*). (*continued*)

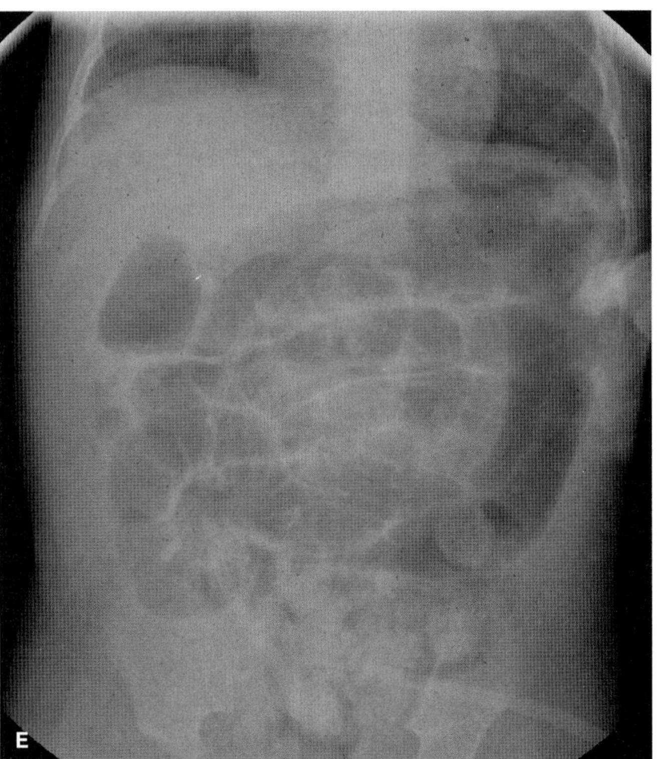

FIGURE 58-3 (Continued)

pneumatic reduction there is increased risk for tension pneumoperitoneum.

SURGERY

- A pediatric surgical team should be available for all attempts of non-operative therapeutic enema reduction in the event of perforation (approximately 1% of attempted reductions).
- Surgery may be indicated if an enema procedure fails to reduce the intussusception.
- Surgical reduction and possible resection is necessary for ileo-ileo intussusception (**Figure 58-2**).
- Surgery is also necessary in patients who are acutely ill and patients with perforation.
- Manual reduction may be attempted during the surgical procedure, but more likely will be a resection with anastomoses.
- Surgery may be necessary to resect an identified lead point.

REFERRAL

- Suspected or diagnosed intussusception should be managed at a medical center staffed with pediatric radiology and pediatric surgery services.

PROGNOSIS

- The usual course of untreated intussusception is bowel obstruction, perforation, peritonitis, sepsis, and shock.
- Nonsurgical reduction in spontaneous ileocolic intussusception is successful in 80 to 95 percent of patients, especially if treated within the first 24 to 48 hours.
- Morbidity and mortality rates increase if the intussusception has been present for more than 48 hours.
- Recurrence rate of intussusception is 10 percent; more than 50 percent of these will occur during the first 48 hours after successful reduction. Each recurrence can be managed as if it were the initial instance. However, multiple recurrences may be associated with a pathologic lead point.

FOLLOW-UP

- Patients should be observed in the hospital for approximately 24 hours post reduction.
- Gastric decompression with nasogastric suction is often continued until bowel function has returned and the patient has had a bowel movement.
- Upon the return of bowel function, feeding can be advanced.

PATIENT EDUCATION

- Parents should be aware that abdominal pain and irritability in a young child warrants medical attention.
- Most cases of intussusception on infants and children are idiopathic and not associated with a lead point.
- Recurrences occur in 10 percent of patients after successful nonsurgical reduction.

PATIENT RESOURCES

- **www.nlm.nih.gov/medlineplus/ency/article/000958.htm**.

PROVIDER RESOURCES

- **www.nlm.nih.gov/medlineplus/ency/article/000958.htm**.
- Kennedy M and Liacouras CA: Intussusception. Nelson Textbook of Pediatrics, 19th ed, edited by Kliegman RM, Stanton BM, St. Geme JW, Schor NF, Behrman RE. Philadelphia, Elsevier Inc.; 2011, p. 1287-1289.
- **www.accesspediatrics.com/videoplayer.aspx?aid=8146025**.

REFERENCES

1. Stringer MD, Pablot SM, Brereton RJ. Paediatric intussusception. *Br J Surg*. 1992;79:867-876.
2. Bines J, Ivanoff B. *Acute Intussusception in Infants and Children*. Geneva, Switzerland: World Health Organization; 2002. Report 02.19
3. Hutchison IF, Olayiwola B, Young DG. Intussusceptionin infancy and childhood. *Br J Surg*. 1980;67:209-212.
4. Intussusception Among Recipients of Rotavirus Vaccine—United States, 1998–1999. Centers for Disease Control and Prevention. *MMWR Morb Mortal Wkly Rep*. 1999;48(27):577-581.

5. Centers for Disease Control and Prevention. Postmarketing Monitoring of Intussusception After RotaTeq™ Vaccination–United States, February 1, 2006–February 15, 2007. *MMWR Morb Mortal Wkly Rep*. 2007;56(10);218-222.

6. Shui IM, Baggs, J, Patel M, Parashar UD, Rett M, Belongia EA, Hambidge SJ, Glanz JM, Klein NP, Weintraub E. Risk of intussusception following administration of a pentavalent rotavirus vaccine in US infants. *JAMA*. 2012;307(6)598-604.

7. Weihmiller SN, Buonomo C, and Bachur R. Risk Stratification of Children Being evaluated for Intussusception. *Pediatrics*. 2011:127(2):e296-e303.

8. Mandeville K, Chien M, Willyerd FA, Mandell G, Hostetler MA, Bulloch B. Intussusception: clinical presentations and imaging characteristics. *Pediatr Emerg Care*. 2012;28(9): 842-844.

9. Roskind CG, Kamdar G, Ruzal-Shapiro CB, Bennett JE, Dayan PS. Accuracy of plain radiographs to exclude the diagnosis of intussusception. *Pediatr Emerg Care*. 2012;28(9):855-858.

10. van den Ende ED, Allema JH, Hazebroek FW, Breslau PJ. Success with hydrostatic reduction of intussusception in relation to duration of symptoms. *Arch Dis Child*. 2005;90(10): 1071-1072.

59 INFLAMMATORY BOWEL DISEASE

Nisha Patel, MD
Naim Alkhouri, MD

PATIENT STORY

A 12-year-old female presents with cramping abdominal pain, a ten pound weight loss, diarrhea, and bloody stools. Physical examination is remarkable for oral aphthous ulcers, mild right lower quadrant tenderness, and perianal skin tag at six o'clock position. Further laboratory work up reveals anemia (hemoglobin 7.2 g/dL) and elevated erythrocyte sedimentation rate (41 mm/hr). She was referred to pediatric gastroenterology and underwent an esophagogastroduodenoscopy and colonoscopy, which was visually and histologically remarkable for gastritis, duodenitis, pan-colitis, and terminal ileitis (**Figure 59-1** and **59-2**). She was diagnosed with Crohn disease.

INTRODUCTION

Inflammatory bowel disease (IBD) refers to two chronic conditions of the gastrointestinal tract: Crohn disease (CD) and ulcerative colitis (UC), that frequently have their presentations in the late childhood and adolescence. IBD is one of the most common chronic diseases of childhood and adolescents.

SYNONYMS

Crohn's Disease, Ulcerative Colitis (UC), Indeterminate Colitis.

EPIDEMIOLOGY

- Pediatric-onset inflammatory bowel disease (IBD) has been significantly increasing in prevalence and incidence worldwide over the past few decades.[1]
- It is currently estimated that as many as 1.4 million persons in the US and 2.2 million persons in Europe suffer from these diseases.[2] More than 20 percent of patients present during childhood and diagnosed before the age of 10 years and fewer than 5 percent diagnosed before age 5 years.[3]
- The mean age at diagnosis of pediatric IBD in the US is 12.5 years.[3]

ETIOLOGY AND PATHOPHYSIOLOGY

- IBD is characterized by chronic inflammation of the gastrointestinal tract and encompasses two entities: CD and UC.
- The pathogenesis of IBD remains elusive, but involves an interaction between a genetic predisposition, defects of host immunoregulation, environmental factors, and an imbalance in the intestinal microbiota (dysbiosis). Dysbiosis (also called dysbacteriosis) is considered crucial for the development of chronic intestinal inflammation.

RISK FACTORS

- Up to 25 percent of children who develop IBD have a positive family history of IBD. Children who have a first-degree relative affected by either UC or CD have a 10 to 13 times higher risk for developing IBD.[4]
- Monozygotic twin concordance is approximately 50 percent for CD and nearly 20 percent for UC.[5]

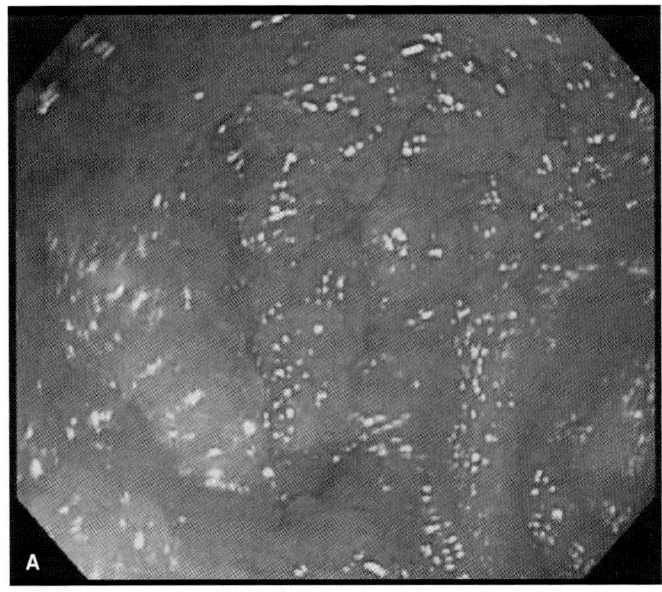

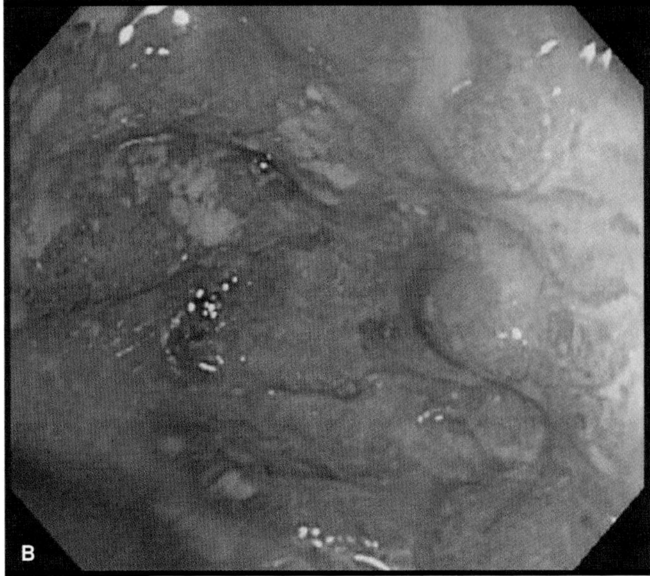

FIGURE 59-1 **A.** Normal terminal ileum. Note the Peyer's patches and nodularity. **B.** Crohn ileitis. Note the edematous mucosa with aphthous ulcerations and mucopurulent exudate. *(Used with permission from Nisha Patel, MD.)*

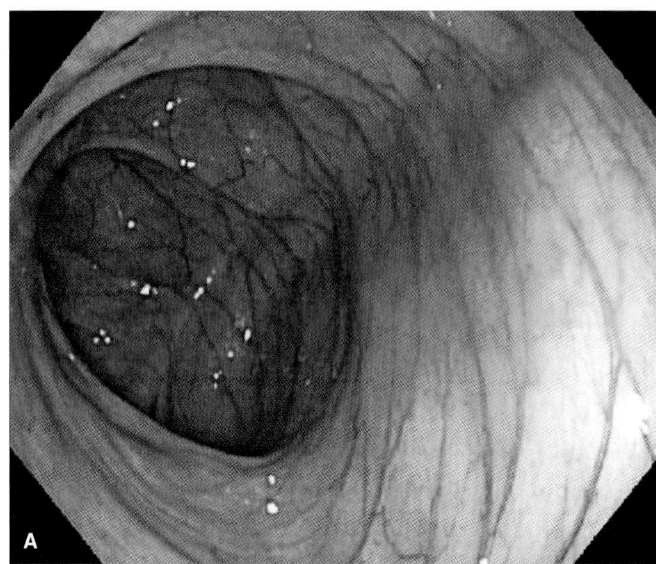

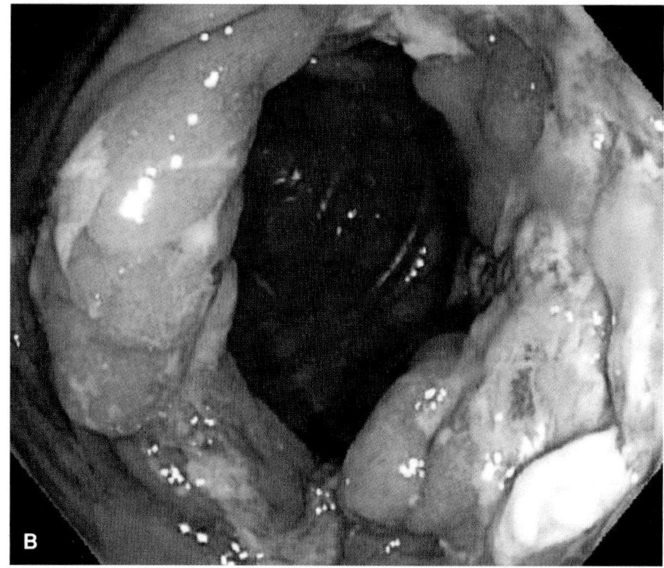

FIGURE 59-2 **A.** Normal colonic mucosa is shiny, with normal folds and normal vascular pattern. **B.** Severe Crohn disease with deep ulcerations, erythema, friability, and patchy cobblestoning pattern with exudates. (*Used with permission from Nisha Patel, MD.*)

- Genetic linkage analyses and genome-wide association studies have identified numerous IBD candidate genes. *NOD2/CARD15* gene, located on chromosome 16q has been associated with CD.
- Anti-Saccharomyces cerevisiae antibody (ASCA) is found in 50 to 60 percent of patients who have CD.
- Perinuclear antineutrophil antibody (pANCA) is detected in approximately 70 percent of patients with UC.

DIAGNOSIS

CLINICAL FEATURES

- Both CD and UC have overlapping features, but the cardinal symptoms of CD are:
  - Cramping abdominal pain, which can be diffuse or localized to the right lower quadrant.
  - Diarrhea (urgency, tenesmus, and nighttime awakening for bowel movements).
  - Weight loss.
  - Recurrent aphthous-stomatitis.
  - Growth failure.
  - Perianal disease (tags, fissures, fistulae, and abscesses).
- The classic presentation of UC is diarrhea, hematochezia, and abdominal cramping associated with fecal urgency.
- One third of patients with IBD can present with extraintestinal manifestations prior to manifesting intestinal symptoms (**Table 59-1**).

DISTRIBUTION

- CD can involve any portion of the gastrointestinal tract from the mouth to anus. It predominately affects the distal ileum and colon and can present in a patchy or discontinuous pattern. The inflammation is typically transmural and can be associated with intestinal granulomas (pathognomonic), strictures, fistulas, and abscesses (**Figures 59-1** and **59-2**).

TABLE 59-1 Extraintestinal Manifestations of IBD

Liver	Nonspecific elevation of aminotransferases, autoimmune hepatitis, primary sclerosing cholangitis (UC > CD) (**Figure 59-5**), cholelithiasis, fatty liver disease
Joints	Arthralgias, arthritis (**Figure 59-6**), ankylosing spondylitis, sacroiliitis
Skin	Erythema nodosum (Chapter 152), pyoderma gangrenosum (**Figure 59-7**), aphthous ulcers (Chapter 40)
Eye	Uveitis (Chapter 13), episcleritis, keratitis
Bone	Digital clubbing (hypertrophic osteoarthropathy), osteopenia, osteoporosis, aseptic necrosis
Pancreas	Acute pancreatitis
Renal	Nephrolithiasis (oxalate stones)
Hematologic	Anemia (iron deficiency, folate deficiency, vitamin B12 deficiency, or autoimmune hemolytic anemia), thrombocytosis, thrombocytopenic purpura
Vascular	Hypercoagulability (thrombosis, thrombophlebitis, thromboembolism)
Endocrine	Growth failure, pubertal delay
Malignancy	Dysplasia, increased risk of colon cancer
Other	Recurrent fevers, malaise, anorexia

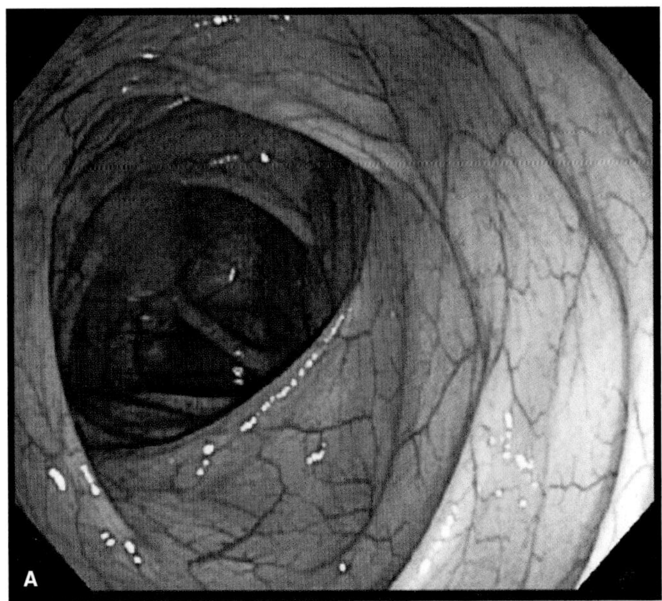

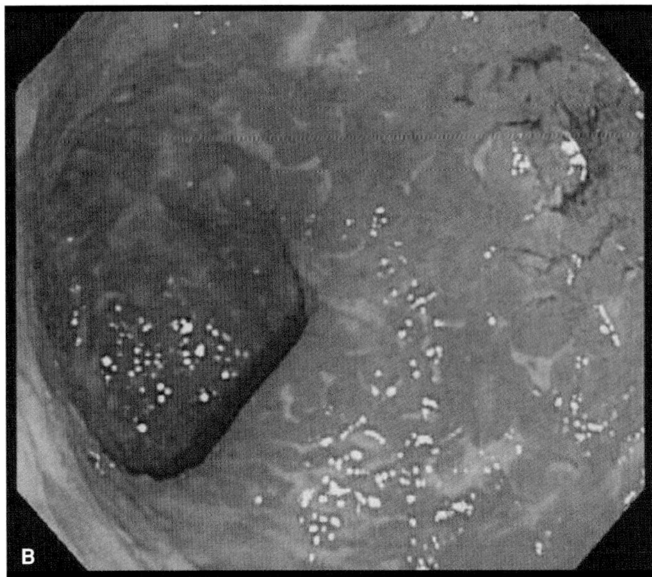

FIGURE 59-3 **A.** Normal colon. **B.** Severe ulcerative colitis. Note the continuous pattern of erythema, loss of vascularity, superficial ulcerations and exudate with friability in areas of endoscope contact. (*Used with permission from Nisha Patel, MD.*)

- UC involves the rectum and colon in a continuous pattern and the inflammation is typically confined to the superficial mucosa. Crypt abscesses are common in UC (**Figure 59-3**).

LABORATORY STUDIES

- Complete blood count (CBC) with differential, complete metabolic profile, erythrocyte sedimentation rate, C-reactive protein, and albumin.
- Stool studies (culture, *Clostridium difficile*, ova, & parasite) to exclude infectious etiologies, fecal calprotectin, and lactoferrin.
- Ancillary tests—IBD serologic panels: pANCA, ASCA, Anti Omp C (outer membrane protein of *Escherichia coli*).
    - IBD serologic panels are not recommended for screening or as an isolated diagnostic tool. False-positive results can create unwarranted anxiety and lead to excessive invasive testing. It should be noted that nearly 1/3 of patients who have a positive serologic panel do not have IBD. Serologic panels are most useful in children who have indeterminate colitis to differentiate CD from UC.[1]

IMAGING

- Upper gastrointestinal series—Can assess areas or stenosis and abnormal separation of bowel loops
- Computed Tomography Enterography scan (**Figure 59-4**)—Can assess for intestinal wall thickening and acute complications of IBD, such as abscess formation and fistulizing or stricturing disease.
- Magnetic resonance imaging (MRI) or MR enterography (MRE)—No radiation exposure and has greater than 90 percent sensitivity and specificity for detecting small bowel disease.

Wireless video capsule endoscopy (VCE)—Can assess small bowel which is not accessible routine endoscopy.

ENDOSCOPY

- Endoscopy including esophagogastroduodenoscopy and colonoscopy with biopsy is gold standard for diagnosing IBD.
- Noncaseating granulomas on pathology are pathognomonic for CD (**Figure 59-8**).

DIFFERENTIAL DIAGNOSIS

- Infectious enterocolitis—Enteric pathogens such as *Salmonella, Shigella, Campylobacter, Escherichia coli* 0157:H7, *Yersinia,* and

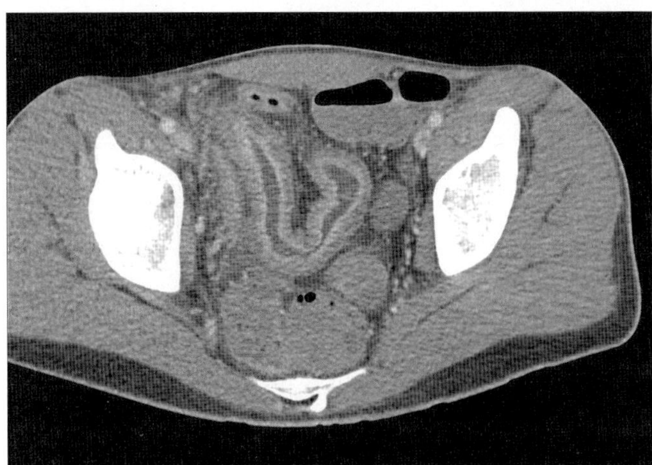

FIGURE 59-4 CT scan showing transmural thickening of the terminal ileum in a patient with Crohn disease. (*Used with permission from Nisha Patel, MD.*)

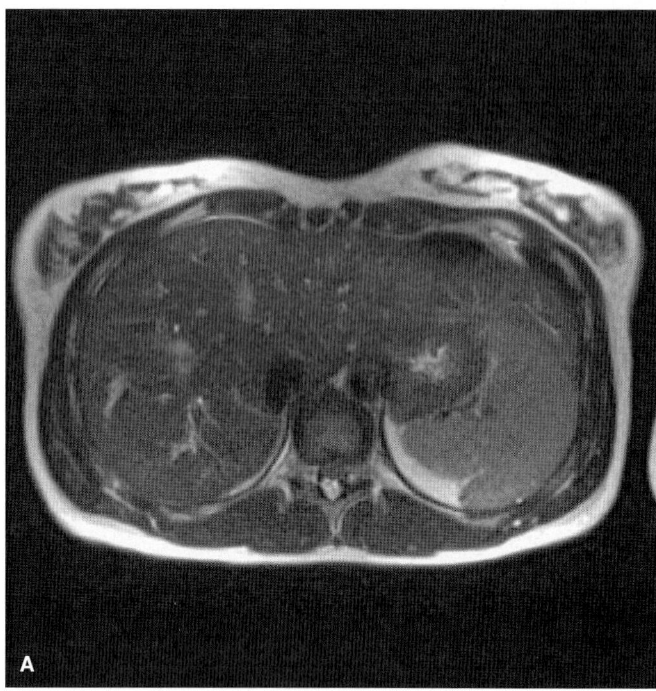

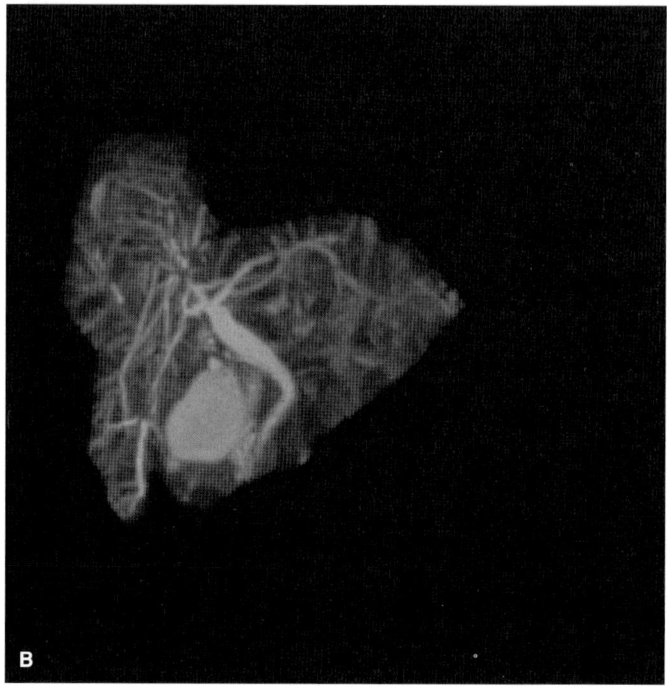

FIGURE 59-5 Magnetic resonance cholangiopancreatography (MRCP): Primary Sclerosing Cholangitis (PSC). Typical symptoms include chronic fatigue, anorexia, pruritus, and jaundice. Elevated gammaglutamyltranspeptidase and alkaline phosphatase values along with results of cholangiography and liver biopsy help confirm the diagnosis. Note the areas of intrahepatic bile duct strictures alternating with normal-caliber ducts (**A**) forming a "beaded appearance" (**B**). Close-up of the biliary tree showing same "beaded" appearance. (*Used with permission from Nisha Patel, MD.*)

Aeromonas—These usually cause more acute symptoms than IBD and are not associated with growth failure.

- Pseudomembranous colitis *(Clostridium difficile)*—Usually associated with antibiotic use and produces more acute symptoms.
- Lymphocytic colitis—Can be seen as a complication of opportunistic infection in immunocompromised hosts and can be differentiated from IBD based on epidemiology and pathology.

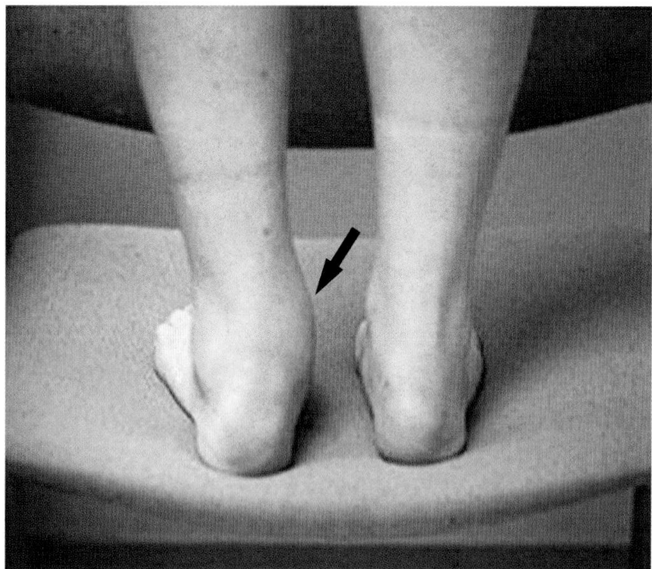

FIGURE 59-6 Seronegative spondyloarthropathy in the ankle of a patient with Crohn disease. Note the swelling (arrow) of the left ankle that is a due to joint effusion and enthesopathy. (*Used with permission from Andrew Zeft, MD.*)

- Eosinophilic enterocolitis—Most commonly affects the stomach and small intestine but can extend to the colon. Peripheral eosinophilia and biopsy of the bowel can differentiate this from IBD.
- Henoch-Schonlein purpura—Can usually be differentiated because of the presence of palpable purpura and arthritis (see Chapter 179, Henoch Schonlein Purpura).
- Hemolytic-uremic syndrome—Differentiated by the presence of hemolytic anemia, thrombocytopenia and acute renal failure (see Chapter 69, Hemolytic Uremic Syndrome).
- Periodic fevers syndromes, such as TRAPS (TNF receptor-associated periodic syndrome) and PFAPA (periodic fever, aphthous stomatitis, pharyngitis, and cervical adenitis)—Usually associated with significant diarrhea, but abdominal pain and fever can be common (see Chapter 176, Periodic Fever Syndromes).
- Rheumatologic disorders—Many characteristics overall with pediatric IBD, such as weight loss, malaise, recurrent fevers, and joint involvement.
- Intestinal tuberculosis and CD have similar clinical, radiographic, and endoscopic features and can be remarkably difficult to differentiate. Intestinal tuberculosis typically involves the ileocolonic region, and the ulcerative form is most common. A patient who has risk factors for tuberculosis should have a tuberculin skin test placed.

MANAGEMENT

The main goals of therapy are:

- Induction and maintenance of remission.

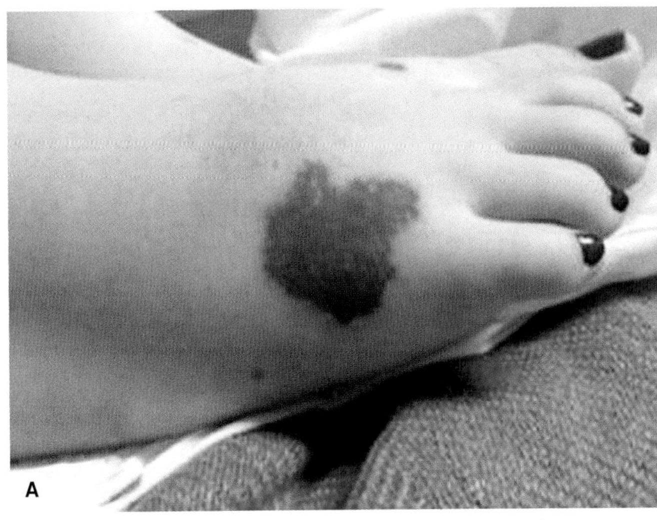

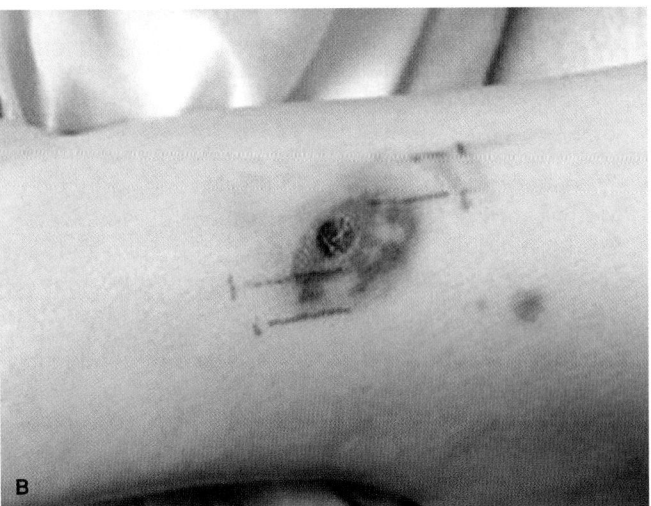

FIGURE 59-7 Pyoderma gangrenosum (PG) is a rare noninfectious neutrophilic dermatosis which starts as a sterile pustule that rapidly progress and turns into painful ulcers of variable depth and size with violaceous borders. Lower extremities are most commonly affected. **A.** A small ulcer is barely visible within the violaceous area on the foot in this early case of PG. **B.** Visible ulcer on the lower leg in PG. (*Used with permission from Michael J. Nowicki, MD.*)

- Prevention of disease complications (fistula, stricture, abscess, and cancer).
- Maintenance of normal growth and development.

NONPHARMACOLOGIC

- Nutritional therapy is more effective in CD than UC, may consist of polymeric or elemental diets, and may result in remission of disease.[6]
- Nutritional fatigue and/or inability to sustain diet are common, often limiting the response of diet therapy alone.

MEDICATIONS

- Medications are chosen based on the disease severity and location.
- Classes of IBD medications include corticosteroids, 5-aminosalicylates (5-ASA), immunomodulators, biologic agents, antibiotics, and probiotics (**see Table 59-2**).

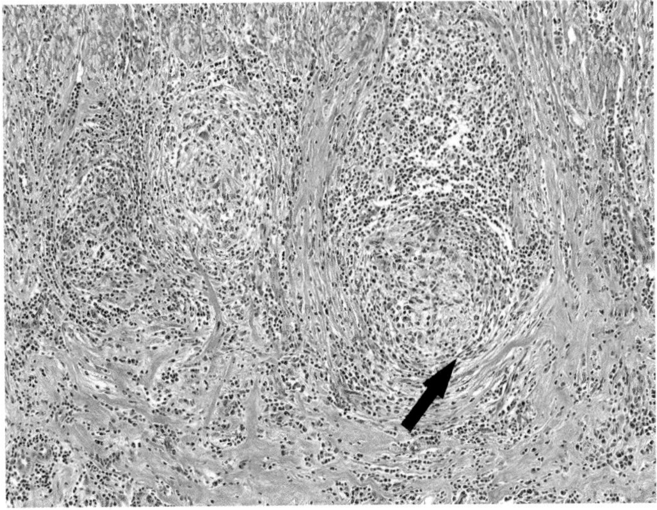

FIGURE 59-8 Noncaseating granulomas on histopathology is diagnostic of Crohn disease. (*Used with permission from Thomas Plesec, MD.*)

- In general, therapy for mild disease involves the use of 5-aminosalicylic acid (5-ASA) agents. SOR Ⓒ
- For patients with more severe disease or who do not respond to 5-ASA therapy, corticosteroids are typically added. These are usually effective in establishing remission but are not effective in maintaining remission.[7,8] SOR Ⓐ
- Methotrexate may be useful in management especially if there are concurrent joint symptoms. SOR Ⓒ
- Immunomodulators, such as azathioprine, 6-mercaptopurine, and methotrexate are utilized for the treatment of steroid refractory disease and as maintenance therapy. SOR Ⓒ
- Antibiotics such as ciprofloxacin and metronidazole are often used in the management. Their precise mechanism of action and role in the management is not clear. SOR Ⓒ
- Monoclonal antibodies to tumor necrosis factor alpha, such as infliximab (given as intravenous infusions), have been shown to be highly effective in achieving clinical improvement and remission and are especially helpful in healing perianal and other fistulas.[9] SOR Ⓐ

SURGERY

- Indications for surgery for patients with IBD include the inability to control the inflammatory conditions despite optimal medical management, intestinal perforation, abscess, bowel obstruction, enterocutaneous fistula, or hemorrhage.[10]
- Surgery is not a cure for CD, but is aimed at providing relief from symptoms and treating disease complications.
- Unlike surgery for CD, surgery for UC may be curative and is used when optimal medical management fails or when there are complications of disease, such as bleeding, perforation, or toxic megacolon.

PREVENTION AND SCREENING

- Baseline bone density scan because of the risk of osteoporosis (especially with long term systemic steroids).

TABLE 59-2 Management of Inflammatory Bowel Disease

Medication Class	Indications	Adverse Effects
Aminosalicylates (Mesalamine, Sulfasalazine)	Mild CD and mild to moderate UC	Headache, arthralgias, fever, rash, photosensitivity, bloody diarrhea
Corticosteroids (Prednisone, Methylprednisolone, Budesonide)	Prednisone: induction of remission for moderate to severe CD or UC Budesonide: mild to moderately active CD involving the ileum and ascending colon Enemas or suppositories: distal UC	Cushingoid facies, weight gain, acne, stretch marks, growth suppression, osteopenia, hypertension, hyperglycemia, cataracts
Immunomodulators (Azathioprine, 6-mercaptopurine, Methotrexate)	AZA or 6-MP: induction of remission and maintenance therapy for moderate to severe CD or UC, steroid dependent/refractory MTX: induction of remission and maintenance therapy for CD	Leukopenia, elevated aminotransferases, pancreatitis, increased risk of infections
Antibiotics (Metronidazole, Ciprofloxacin)	Fistulizing disease with perianal abscesses, pouchitis	Peripheral neuropathy, nausea
Probiotics (Lactobacillus GG, Saccharomyces boulardii)	Adjuvant therapy	None
Biologic therapy (Infliximab, Adalimumab, Certolizumab)	Induction of remission and maintenance therapy for moderate to severe CD or UC who are steroid dependent/refractory or have failed immunomodulator therapies or with severe fistula	Acute or delayed hypersensitivity reactions, serious infections, reactivation of TB or histoplasmosis or varicella, malignancy (including fatal lymphoma), autoimmune diseases
Anti-integrin (Natalizumab)	Induction of remission and maintenance therapy for moderate to severe CD	Progressive multifocal leukomalacia
Surgery	Refractory to medical therapy, small bowel obstruction, gastrointestinal hemorrhage, perforation or dysplasia	

- Annual ophthalmology examination.
- IBD patients who are not on immunosuppressive therapy (steroids, immunomodulators, biologics) should follow routine vaccination schedule.
- Live vaccines (measles-mumps-rubella, varicella, oral polio vaccine, intra-nasal influenza) are contraindicated in immunocompromised patients. Killed vaccines can be given according to recommended schedules.

PROGNOSIS

- 1/3 of patients may experience an IBD flare at 1 year and more than half at 2 years after initiation of therapy.
- Patients with IBD are at increased risk for colorectal cancer and the risk depends on the extent and duration of the disease.

FOLLOW-UP

- Routine surveillance colonoscopy to screen for dysplasia beginning 8 years after initial diagnosis and 1 to 2 years thereafter.

PATIENT EDUCATION

- Patients with manifestations of IBD require a careful and thorough evaluation by a gastroenterologist.
- Adherence to dietary and medical management is of paramount importance in achieving a sustained response.

PATIENT RESOURCES

- Crohn's & Colitis Foundation of America (CCFA)—**www.ccfa.org**.
- **www.webmd.com/ibd-crohns-disease/crohns-disease/inflammatory-bowel-syndrome**.
- Inflammatory Bowel Disease—**www.gastro.org/patient-center/digestive-conditions/inflammatory-bowel-disease#Inflammatory Bowel Disease**.

PROVIDER RESOURCES

- Glick S., Carvalho R: Inflammatory Bowel Disease. *Pediatrics in Review* 2011;32:14.
- **www.cdc.gov/ibd**.

REFERENCES

1. Glick S., Carvalho R. Inflammatory Bowel Disease. *Pediatrics in Review.* 2011;32;14.
2. Loftus EV, Jr: Clinical epidemiology of inflammatory bowel disease: Incidence, prevalence, and environmental influences. *Gastroenterology*. 2004;126:1504-1517.
3. Kugathasan S, Judd RH, Hoffmann RG, et al. Epidemiologic and clinical characteristics of children with newly diagnosed inflammatory bowel disease in Wisconsin: a statewide population-based study. *J Pediatr.* 2003;143:525-531.
4. Weinstein TA, Levine M, Pettei MJ, Gold DM, Kessler BH, Levine JJ. Age and family history at presentation of pediatric inflammatory bowel disease. *J Pediatr Gastroenterol Nutr.* 2003;37:609-613.
5. Halfvarson J, Bodin L, Tysk C, Lindberg E, Jarnerot G. Inflammatory bowel disease in a Swedish twin cohort: a long-term follow-up of concordance and clinical characteristics. *Gastroenterology*. 2003;124:1767-17736.
6. Kleinman RE, Baldassano RN, Caplan A, et al. Nutrition support for pediatric patients with inflammatory bowel disease: a clinical report of the North American Society for Pediatric Gastroenterology, Hepatology and Nutrition. *J Pediatr Gastroenterol Nutr.* 2004;39:15-27.
7. Benchimol EI, Seow CH, Steinhart AH, et al. Traditional corticosteroids for induction of remission in Crohn's disease. *Cochrane Database Syst Rev.* 2008;16:CD006792.
8. Seow CH, Benchimol EI, Griffiths AM, et al. Budesonide for induction of remission in Crohn's disease. *Cochrane Database Syst Rev.* 2008;16:CD000296.
9. Behm BW, Bickston SJ. Tumor necrosis factoralpha antibody for maintenance of remission in Crohn's disease. *Cochrane Database Syst Rev.* 2008:CD006893.
10. Telander RL, Schmeling DJ. Current surgical management of Crohn's disease in childhood. *Semin Pediatr Surg.* 1994;3: 19-27.

60 CELIAC DISEASE

Jonathan Moses, MD
Tara Harwood, MS, RD, CSP, LD

PATIENT STORY

A 2-year-old male presents with weight loss. The mother states his pediatrician first noticed impaired growth around 12 months of age. The mother also noticed his abdomen looked more distended over the last few months and he is more irritable than usual. She describes a vague history of looser stools without overt hematochezia. Pediatric gastroenterology was consulted and sent blood work which was remarkable for mild anemia and positive anti-tissue transglutaminase immunoglobulin A antibodies (TTG IgA). The patient underwent an upper endoscopy with biopsies, which was visually remarkable for erythematous duodenal mucosa with scalloping of the intestinal folds (**Figures 60-1** and **60-2**).

Histology demonstrated increased intra-epithelial lymphocytes (IEL) with villous blunting, confirming the diagnosis of celiac disease (**Figure 60-3**). The patient was placed on a gluten free diet and has had improved growth and normalization of laboratory values.

INTRODUCTION

Celiac disease is an autoimmune disorder related to the ingestion of gluten containing foods in genetically susceptible individuals. If unrecognized and untreated celiac disease can result in gastrointestinal symptoms, growth disturbances, and potential long-term complications.

SYNONYMS

Celiac Sprue; Gluten Enteropathy; Gluten-sensitive Enteropathy; Nontropical Sprue.

EPIDEMIOLOGY

- Worldwide distribution has been demonstrated despite the incorrect historical view that celiac disease was limited to the Caucasian population.[1]
- Incidence of various countries:[2]
  - US—1:100 to 1:200.
  - Europe—1:88 to 1:262.
  - Middle East—1:87 to 1:166.
  - South America—1:67 to 1:681.
  - India—1:100 to 1:310.
- True incidence likely unknown given wide variation in presentation, as illustrated by the "celiac iceberg" (**Figure 60-4**).

ETIOLOGY AND PATHOPHYSIOLOGY

- Celiac disease is an autoimmune disorder related to the ingestion of gluten containing foods (wheat, barley, and rye) in genetically susceptible individuals.[3,4]
- Genetic predisposition linked to human leukocyte antigen (HLA)-DQ2 and DQ8.[3,4]
  - More than 95 percent of patients with celiac disease have the HLA-DQ2 heterodimer, with the remainder positive for the HLA-DQ8.

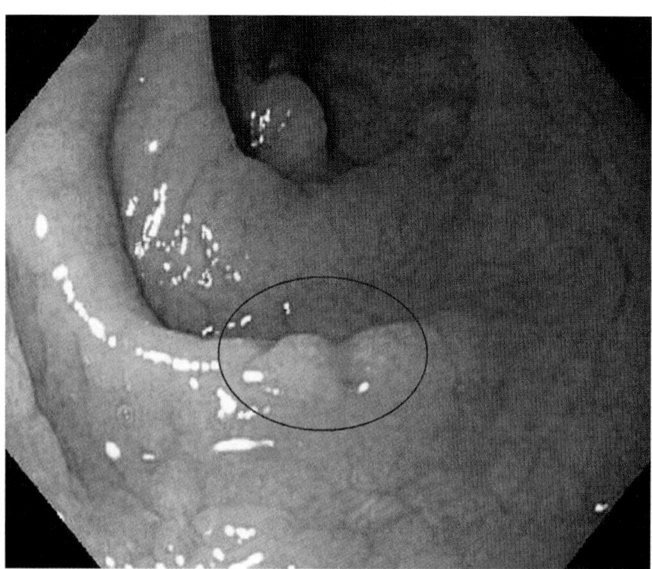

FIGURE 60-1 Endoscopic findings of scalloping in celiac disease. Note the notching of the mucosal folds (red circle). The mucosal surface also demonstrates a mosaic pattern found in celiac disease. (*Used with permission from Jonathan Moses, MD.*)

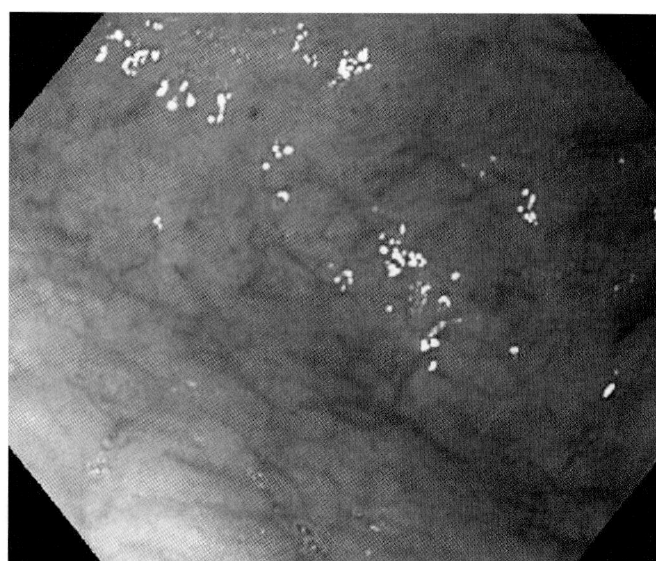

FIGURE 60-2 Endoscopic findings of nodularity in celiac disease. The duodenal mucosa shows a diffuse, nodular pattern which is an abnormality found in celiac disease. There is also significant erythema of the duodenal mucosa due to the inflammation. (*Used with permission from Jonathan Moses, MD.*)

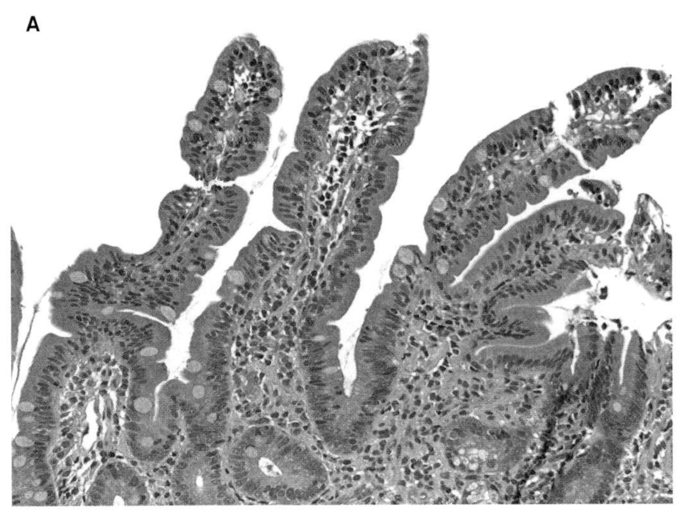

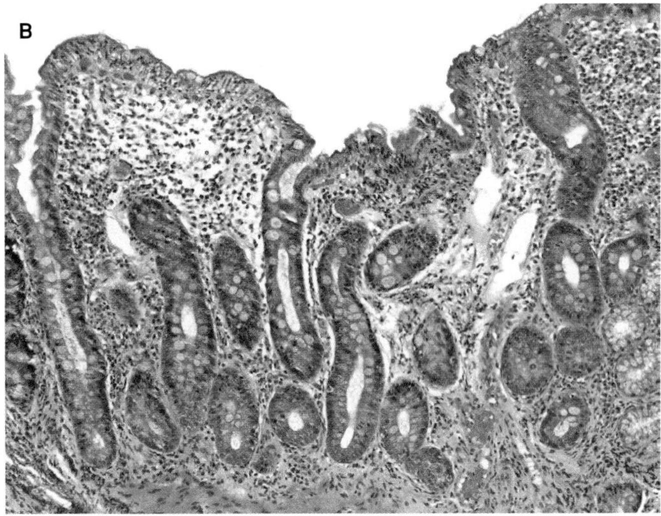

FIGURE 60-3 Histological findings in celiac disease. **A.** Marsh grade I changes with increased intraepithelial lymphocytes and intact villi. **B.** Marsh III changes with increased intraepithelial lymphocytes, crypt hyperplasia, and villous atrophy. (*Used with permission from Thomas Plesec, MD.*)

 - Presence of the HLA-DQ2 molecules does not necessarily confer disease as 30 to 40 percent of the Caucasian population possesses this genetic background, without developing celiac disease.
- Upon ingestion of gluten containing foods, activation of the immune system occurs as follows:[5,6]
  - Deamidation of the gluten proteins by tissue transglutamine 2 (TG2) and formation of an antigen complex, which includes DQ2 and DQ8.
  - This antigen complex is presented to T cells, which become activated T cells and release antibodies to TG2 and gliadin peptides, along with pro-inflammatory cytokines.

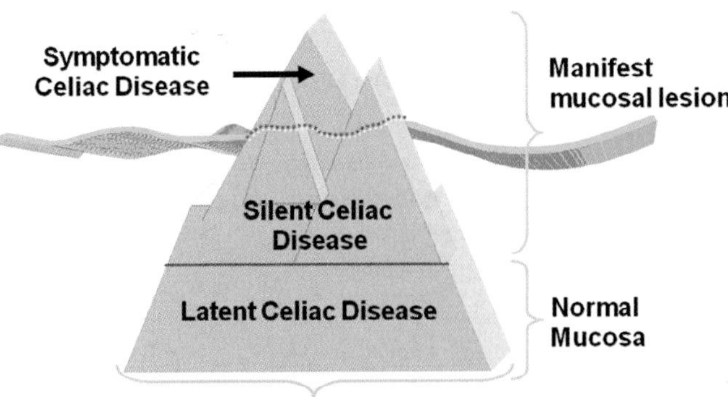

FIGURE 60-4 The "celiac iceberg" as an illustration of the various manifestations of celiac disease. The top level represents symptomatic patients with typical mucosal lesions. The middle level represents asymptomatic patients with typical mucosal lesions. The bottom level represents asymptomatic patients with normal mucosa who will likely develop celiac disease at some point in their lifetime. The common denominator is the genetic predisposition of HLA-DQ2 and DQ8. (*Provided by The NASPGHAN Foundation for Children's Digestive Health and Nutrition and the North American Society for Pediatric Gastroenterology, Hepatology and Nutrition. www.naspghanfoundation.org and www.naspghan.org.*)

RISK FACTORS

- The presence of other disorders places patients at-risk of developing of celiac disease.[3,7] These disorders with associated prevalence rates are:
  - Type I diabetes (8%).
  - Autoimmune thyroiditis (2%).
  - Down's Syndrome (5 to 12%).
  - Turner Syndrome (4.1 to 8.1%).
  - Williams Syndrome (8.2%).
  - Selective IgA deficiency (1.7 to 7.7%).
- In a study by Fasano et al., the prevalence of celiac disease in a not at-risk population was 1:133 and increased to 1:22 in first degree relatives of patients with established celiac disease.[8]

DIAGNOSIS

CLINICAL FEATURES

- Classic presentation is a child between the ages of 6 to 24 months with growth issues, irritability, and diarrhea.[3] The clinical presentation of celiac disease has evolved over time as the diagnosis has become better recognized and testing more ubiquitous, with it being diagnosed across all ages.
- Gastrointestinal symptoms at presentation can include:[3]
  - Diarrhea.
  - Failure to thrive.
  - Abdominal pain.
  - Vomiting.
  - Constipation.
  - Anorexia.
  - Abdominal distention.
  - Malnutrition.

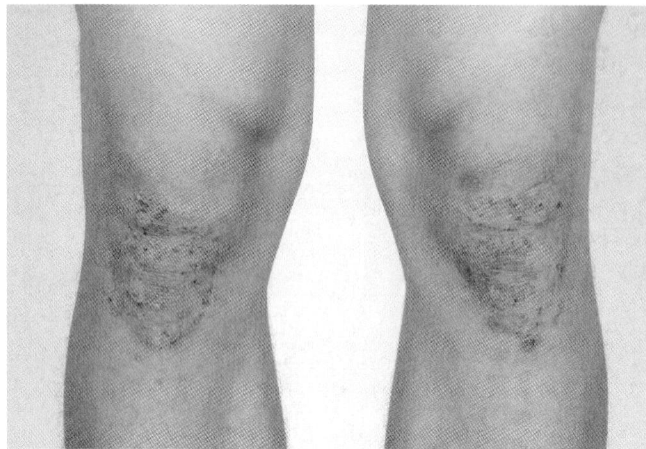

FIGURE 60-5 Dermatitis herpetiformis, an extraintestinal manifestation of celiac disease. This is characterized by a vesicular to pustular rash on an erythematous base. This lesion is symmetric and rarely asymptomatic, as patients present with severe pruritus. Correlates well with villous atrophy on endoscopy, but overt gastrointestinal symptoms may not be present. (*Used with permission from Janine Sot, Cleveland Clinic.*)

- Non-gastrointestinal symptoms at presentation can include:[3]
  - Dermatitis herpetiformis (**Figure 60-5**).
  - Dental enamel hypoplasia of permanent teeth (**Figure 60-6**).
  - Osteopenia/osteoporosis.
  - Short stature.
  - Delayed puberty.
  - Iron deficiency anemia unresponsive to oral supplementation.
  - Hepatitis.
  - Arthritis.
  - Epilepsy with occipital calcifications.
- Asymptomatic patients are increasingly being recognized and generally fall into the at-risk population, along with first-degree relatives of patients with celiac disease.

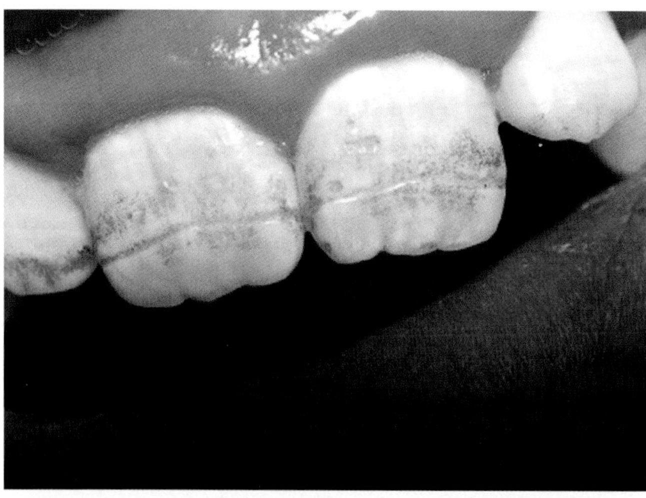

FIGURE 60-6 Dental enamel defects, another extraintestinal manifestation of celiac disease. This generally involves the secondary dentition and may be the only presenting sign of celiac disease. (*Provided by The NASPGHAN Foundation for Children's Digestive Health and Nutrition and the North American Society for Pediatric Gastroenterology, Hepatology and Nutrition. www.naspghanfoundation.org and www.naspghan.org.*)

- Celiac crisis is the rare presentation of severe diarrhea, metabolic and electrolyte abnormalities, and hypoproteinemia. It is considered a life-threatening syndrome.[1]

LABORATORY STUDIES

- Laboratory abnormalities can include iron deficiency anemia on complete blood count (CBC) and hypoalbuminemia on metabolic panel.
- First line testing should include a TTG IgA with a total IgA level. TTG IgA provides a high level and sensitivity (98%) and specificity (98%), which is ideal for screening purposes.[9]
- Additional celiac antibodies available include:
  - Anti-endomysium IgA and IgG antibodies (EMA IgA and IgG).
  - Anti-deamidated gliadin IgA and IgG antibodies (DGA IgA and IgG).
  - Anti-gliadin IgA and IgG antibodies (AGA IgA and AGA IgG).
- EMA IgA provides excellent specificity and have a role as confirmatory testing when the TTG IgA results are unclear.[1]
- In patients with IgA deficiency, IgG testing is indicated with DGA IgG performing the best.[1,9]
- AGA IgA and IgG do not provide adequate accuracy and are not recommended for screening purposes.[3]
- Genetic testing for HLA DQ2 and DQ8 status may play a role in cases of uncertain diagnosis. There may also be a role in at-risk populations to eliminate frequent screening, if both HLA DQ2 and DQ8 are negative.[3,4]

ENDOSCOPY

- The gold standard for diagnosis of celiac disease remains upper endoscopy with small bowel biopsies, specifically from the duodenum.
- Characteristic macroscopic findings include:
  - Scalloping (**Figure 60-1**).
  - Mosaicism (**Figure 60-1**).
  - Nodularity (**Figure 60-2**).
  - Erythematous mucosa (**Figure 60-2**).
  - Flattening of intestinal villi.
- Characteristic microscopic findings on biopsy include:
  - Presence of intraepithelial lymphocytes (**Figure 60-3**).
  - Villous atrophy (**Figure 60-3**).
  - Crypt hyperplasia (**Figure 60-3**).
- These histological findings are the basis of the Marsh criteria used to confirm the diagnosis of celiac disease.[10]

DIFFERENTIAL DIAGNOSIS

- Infectious diarrhea, commonly *Giardia lamblia*—may manifest with similar symptoms but can be ruled out with appropriate testing of stool and by microscopic examination of the small intestine (see Chapter 179, Gastrointestinal Infections (including diarrhea)).
- Nonspecific diarrhea of childhood (toddler's diarrhea)—Usually related to ingestion of large amounts of fluids and not associated with growth disturbances.

- Inflammatory bowel disease—Usually presents later in life and associated with more severe symptoms and possible extraintestinal manifestations (see Chapter 59, Inflammatory Bowel Disease).
- Autoimmune enteritis—Can be differentiated on histopathology of the small intestine.
- HIV enteropathy—Usually manifests with other signs of HIV such as lymphadenopathy and recurrent infections early in life.
- Non-steroidal anti-inflammatory drug-induced enteropathy—Can be differentiated by history, laboratory, and histopathology of celiac disease.
- Eosinophilic gastroenteritis—Usually manifests with peripheral eosinophilia and eosinophilia on histopathology of the small intestine (see Chapter 54, Esophageal Disorders).
- Food protein induced enterocolitis syndromes—Can be distinguished by appropriate laboratory and histopathologic work-up for celiac disease.
- Immunodeficiency—Usually associated with other findings such as recurrent infections.

MANAGEMENT

NONPHARMACOLOGIC

- Initiation of a gluten free diet remains the cornerstone for treatment of celiac disease.[3,11] SOR Ⓐ
- Elimination of wheat, barley, and rye is advised. Elimination of oats is less clear due to concerns of gluten contamination during processing.[3]
- Acceptable dietary alternatives include rice and corn (maize), with a complete list in **Table 60-1**.[11]
- Secondary lactose intolerance is not common. When suspected a 2- to 4-week lactose elimination course could be instituted. SOR Ⓒ
- Commonly overlooked sources of gluten:[11]
  - Prescription and over-the-counter medications.
  - Lipstick.
  - Candy.
  - Communion wafers.
  - Beer and lagers.
  - Playdoh (proper hand washing advised, does not pass through skin).
  - Soy sauce.
  - Luncheon meats.
  - Gloss and balms.

REFERRAL

- Patients with typical gastrointestinal symptoms, non-gastrointestinal symptoms, in the at-risk groups, or with first degree relatives who have established celiac disease should be screened with a TTG IgA and total IgA level. If positive for TTG IgA with normal total IgA levels, clinical suspicion persists despite negative TTG IgA, or if IgA deficient, referral to a pediatric gastroenterologist is warranted.

TABLE 60-1 List of Grains Allowed and Not Allowed As Part of a Gluten Free Diet

Allowed	Not Allowed
• Amaranth	• Barley (malt, malt flavoring, and malt vinegar are usually made from barley)
• Arrowroot	• Bulgur
• Buckwheat	• Couscous
• Corn (maize)	• Durum
• Flax	• Einkorn
• Flours made from nuts, beans, and seeds	• Emmer
• Millet	• Fraina
• Montina	• Faro
• Potato Starch	• Graham flour
• Potato Flour	• Kamut
• Quinoa	• Matzo flour/meal
• Rice	• Orzo
• Rice Bran	• Panko
• Sago	• Rye
• Sorghum	• Seitan
• Soy	• Semolina
• Tapioca	• Spelt
• Teff	• Triticale (a cross between wheat and rye)
	• Udon
	• Wheat (including bran, germ, and starch)

SCREENING

- Patients in the at-risk group should be actively screened (**see Risk Factors**), along with first-degree relatives of patients with established celiac disease.

PROGNOSIS

- Patients who maintain a lifelong gluten free diet are expected to have a normal life expectancy.
- Untreated Celiac disease can lead to long term complications:
  - Osteoporosis.[1]
  - Increased risk of gastrointestinal malignancies.[12]

FOLLOW-UP

- Repeat TTG IgA at 6 months after institution of a gluten free diet.[3]
- Repeat TTG IgA for patients with continued symptoms and to monitor compliance with the gluten free diet.

- Once stable and developed good understanding of a gluten free diet without symptoms, follow-up is every 1 year with the pediatric gastroenterologist, which includes:
  - Assessment of growth.
  - Recheck TTG IgA.
  - Monitoring for associated conditions, such as osteoporosis or autoimmune thyroid disease.[1]

PATIENT EDUCATION

- Instructions should be given to the patient and family to continue their current diet and not implement a gluten free diet before consultation with the pediatric gastroenterologist. Initiation of a gluten free diet prior to diagnostic endoscopy can lead to false negative results on biopsy specimens.
- Newly diagnosed celiac patients should meet with a registered dietitian to review institution of a gluten free diet.

PATIENT RESOURCES

- Green, P, Jones R. *Celiac Disease: A Hidden Epidemic. New York, NY: Harper Collins; 2010.*
- Gluten-Free Diet—**www.glutenfreediet.ca**.
- Korn, D. *Kids with Celiac Disease: A Family Guide to Raising Happy, Healthy, Gluten-free Children. Bethesda: Woodbine House; 2001.*
- Korn, D. *Living Gluten-Free for Dummies. 2nd edition. Hoboken; Wiley Publishing; 2010.*

PROVIDER RESOURCES

- GIKids—**www.gikids.org/content/3/en/Celiac-Disease**.
- National Institutes of Health Celiac Disease Awareness Campaign—**www.celiac.org**.
- **www.naspghanfoundation.org**.
- **www.naspghan.org**.

REFERENCES

1. Fasano A, Catassi C. Celiac disease. *N Engl J Med.* 2012;367:2419.
2. Gujral N, Freeman HJ, and Thomson ABR. Celiac disease: Prevalence, diagnosis, pathogenesis and treatment. *World J. Gastroenterol.* 2011;18:1636.
3. Hill ID, Dirks MH, Liptak GS, et al. Guideline for the diagnosis and treatment of celiac disease in children: Recommendations of the North American Society of Pediatric Gastroenterology, Hepatology, and Nutrition. *J. Pediatr. Gastroenterol. Nutr.* 2005;40:1.
4. Husby S, Koletzko S, Korpany-Szabo IR, et al. European Society of Pediatric Gastroenterology, Hepatology, and Nutrition guidelines for the diagnosis of celiac disease. *J. Pediatr. Gastroenterol. Nutr.* 2012;54:136.
5. A-Kader HH, Alexander F, Alonso EM, et al. Pediatric Gastrointestinal and Liver Disease, edited by R Wyllie and JS Hyams. Philadelphia, Saunders Elsevier Inc.; 2006, 520.
6. Plenge RM. Unlocking the pathogenesis of celiac disease. *Nat. Genet.* 2010;42:281.
7. Fasano A. Systemic autoimmune disorders in celiac disease. *Curr Opin Gastroenterol.* 2006;22:674.
8. Fasano A, Berti I, Gerarduzzi T, et al. Prevalence of celiac disease in at-risk and not at-risk groups in the United States. *Arch. Intern. Med.* 2003;163:286.
9. Leffler DA, Schuppan D. Update on Serologic Testing in Celiac Disease. *Am. J. Gastroenterol.* 2010;105:2520.
10. Oberhuber G, Granditsch G, and Vogelsang H. The histopathology of coeliac disease: time for a standardized report scheme for pathologists. *Eur. J. Gastroenterol. Hepatol.* 1999;11:1189.
11. North American Society for Pediatric Gastroenterology, Hepatology and Nutrition. GIKids. http://www.gikids.org/content/3/en/Celiac-Disease, accessed on December 1, 2013.
12. Askling J, Linet M, Gridley G, et al. Cancer Incidence in a Population-Based Cohort of Individuals Hospitalized With Celiac Disease or Dermatitis Herpetiformis. *Gastroenterology.* 2002;123:1428.

61 NEONATAL CHOLESTASIS

Katharine Eng, MD
Naim Alkhouri, MD

PATIENT STORY

A 4-week-old full-term female is seen for routine follow-up with her pediatrician. Her mother reports that she has been taking breast milk well with good weight gain. She has no specific concerns; however does report she noticed lighter colored stools recently. On physical exam, jaundice and scleral icterus are noted, along with dark urine in her diaper. The pediatrician orders labs drawn urgently and calls the pediatric gastroenterologist for immediate assistance. The work-up is expedited and she is found to have biliary atresia (**Figures 61-1** and **61-2**). The Kasai portoenterostomy procedure is performed to treat the cholestatic jaundice. This surgery involves exposing the porta hepatis and attaching part of the small intestine to the exposed liver surface to allow bile to drain out of the liver into the intestines.

INTRODUCTION

- Neonatal jaundice can be a common finding in the first 2 weeks of life.
- Majority of cases are caused by *physiologic jaundice* and *breast milk jaundice*, characterized by *unconjugated hyperbilirubinemia*, which can spontaneously resolve.
- However, neonatal jaundice persisting after the 2nd week of life is concerning and requires urgent investigation to differentiate *unconjugated hyperbilirubinemia* from the less frequent, but pathological and more serious condition of *cholestatic jaundice*.
- *Cholestatic jaundice* is characterized by the *elevation of conjugated bilirubin*, indicating impaired hepatobiliary function.
- Conjugated hyperbilirubinemia has been defined as (1) direct bilirubin >1 mg/dL if total bilirubin is <5 mg/dL or (2) direct bilirubin >20 percent of the total bilirubin if the total bilirubin >5 mg/dL.[1]
- Neonatal cholestatic jaundice can be serious and requires early detection by the primary care physician with prompt referral to a pediatric gastroenterologist to ensure timely diagnosis and appropriate treatment for a favorable prognosis.

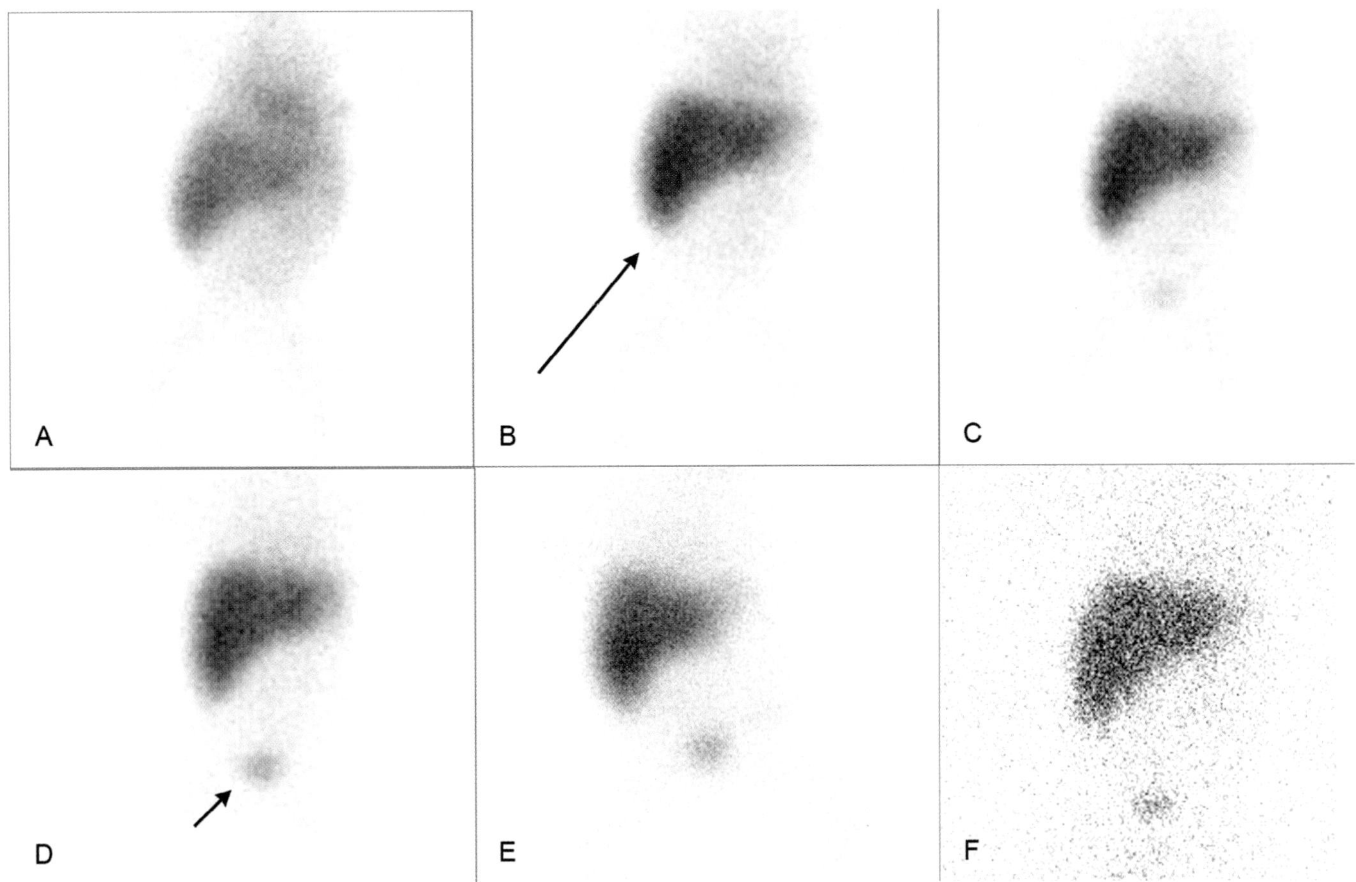

FIGURE 61-1 Biliary atresia on a hepatobiliary nuclear scintigram. Selected static images of the abdomen and pelvis seen here show good uptake of Tc-99m mebrofenin radiotracer in the liver (*large arrow*); however, there is no evidence of excretion into the biliary tree, gallbladder, or intestines. Images are taken at 1 min (**A**), 15 min (**B**), 30 min (**C**), 60 min (**D**), 4 hrs (**E**), and 24 hrs (**F**) after tracer injection. There is excretion into the bladder (*small arrow*) via the kidneys from backup of tracer in the blood pool. Lack of bowel visualization on 24-hour images is suggestive of biliary atresia. *(Used with permission from Shyam Srinivas, MD.)*

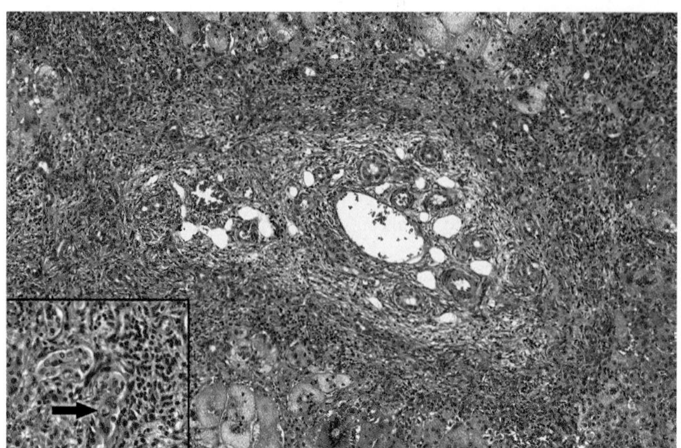

FIGURE 61-2 Biliary atresia on a liver biopsy. The typical changes seen on liver biopsy (hematoxylin and eosin stain) in a patient with biliary atresia. Note the characteristic portal edema, marked bile ductular proliferation, and chronic cholestatic changes to the periportal hepatocytes. In the inset, ductular cholestasis can be appreciated with bile duct plugging (*arrow*). (*Used with permission from Thomas Plesec, MD.*)

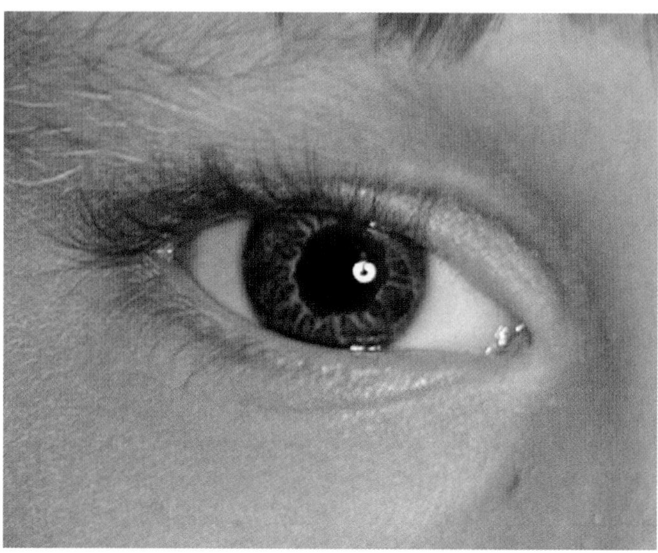

FIGURE 61-3 Scleral icterus, or yellowing of the conjunctiva of the eye, in a pediatric patient with hyperbilirubinemia. (*Used with permission from Naim Alkhouri, MD.*)

- Early intervention for underlying infectious or metabolic causes for cholestasis can be crucial, and in particular, timely surgical management of extra-hepatic biliary obstruction is of paramount importance.

SYNONYM

Neonatal cholestasis, neonatal conjugated hyperbilirubinemia.

EPIDEMIOLOGY

- Neonatal cholestasis is estimated to affect about 1 in every 2,500 infants.[2]
- There are many causes for neonatal cholestasis, with the most common cause being biliary atresia.
- The incidence of biliary atresia is estimated to be between 1 in 8,000 to 1 in 21,000 live births.[3]
- Neonatal cholestasis is caused by:
  - Biliary atresia in about 1/3 of cases.
  - Idiopathic neonatal hepatitis is estimated to comprise about 10 to 15 percent.
  - Alpha-1-antitrypsin deficiency about 10 percent.
  - Inborn errors of metabolism about 20 percent.
  - Various inherited forms of cholestasis 10 to 20 percent.
  - Congenital infections about 5 percent of cases.[3,4]

ETIOLOGY

- Cholestasis is a result of either reduced bile formation by hepatocytes or obstruction of bile flow through the intra- or extrahepatic biliary tree. This can lead to accumulation of biliary substances in the liver, extrahepatic tissue, and blood.

DIAGNOSIS

CLINICAL FEATURES

- Cholestasis may be recognized by findings of jaundice, scleral icterus (**Figure 61-3**), pale (or acholic) stools, and/or dark urine. Hepatomegaly can also be found on exam.
- Infants may sometimes initially present with gastrointestinal blood loss, intracranial hemorrhage, bleeding from umbilical stump, or bruising as a result of a coagulopathy from poor hepatic synthetic function and vitamin K deficiency.
- Ascites (**Figure 61-4**) and edema can also be seen in the setting of impaired hepatic function with advanced disease such as cirrhosis. Splenomegaly may be found in the setting of advanced disease, but can also be found in the presence of infection.
- The clinical presentation of neonatal cholestasis may vary depending on the underlying etiology.
- Infants with biliary atresia may present with jaundice, acholic stools, and/or dark urine, and they can often be healthy appearing and asymptomatic until later in their disease progression
- Poor feeding, irritability, lethargy, and vomiting may be seen in metabolic disorders such as galactosemia and tyrosinemia, but also may be a sign of generalized infections causing cholestasis.
- Infants with cholestasis secondary to congenital infections may present with low birth weight, microcephaly, chorioretinitis, and purpura.
- Dysmorphic facial features (**Figure 61-5**), heart murmur, and anomalies of vertebrae, eyes, and kidneys may be found in Alagille syndrome.[5]

LABORATORY STUDIES[3]

▶ Initial laboratory studies

- Initial laboratory tests should always include a fractionated bilirubin to establish the presence of cholestasis, along with a total bilirubin.

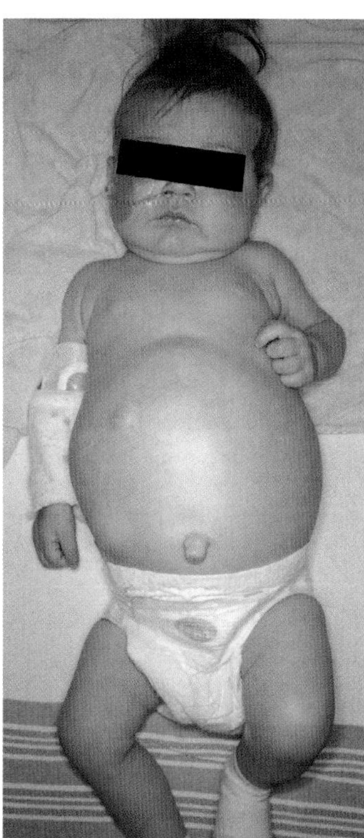

FIGURE 61-4 Ascites with abdominal distention is visible here in a 7-month-old female with history of biliary atresia, with a now failing Kasai portoenterostomy. A small incisional scar and incisional hernia are noted in the right upper quadrant region of her abdomen from her prior procedure. (*Used with permission from Naim Alkhouri, MD.*)

- Tests of hepatic synthetic function: ammonia, albumin, serum glucose levels, or coagulation studies (partial thromboplastin time, prothrombin time and INR, coagulation factor levels).
- Serum hepatic chemistry: ALT, AST, alkaline phosphatase, or gamma glutamyl transferase.

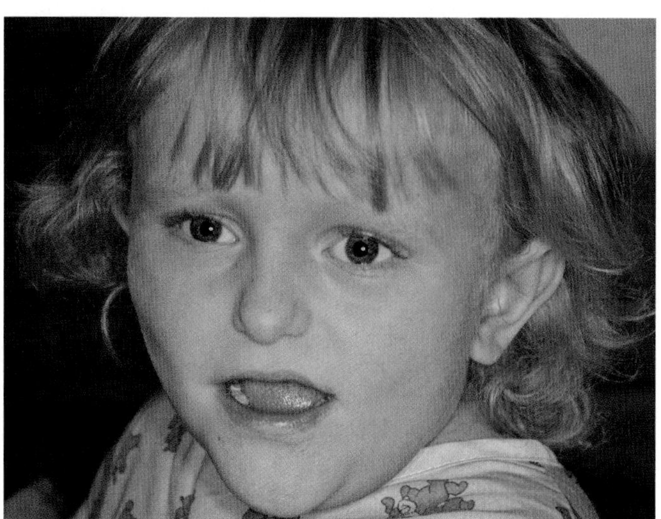

FIGURE 61-5 Alagille syndrome in a 3-year-old girl with the classic dysmorphic facial features. Note the prominent forehead, straight nose with flattened tip, deep-set eyes, and pointed chin. (*Used with permission from Naim Alkhouri, MD.*)

- Complete blood count.
- Blood and urine culture if indicated.

More specific laboratory studies to be considered based on the differential diagnosis:

- Serum alpha-1-antitrypsin level and phenotype.
- Sweat chloride analysis.
- Serology and culture for infection (TORCH, viral hepatitis, parvovirus, or HIV).
- Urine and serum bile acid analysis.
- Metabolic screen (urine reducing substances, urine and serum amino acids and organic acids, galactose-1-phosphate uridylyltransferase activity).
- Endocrinologic studies (TSH, free T4, or consider work-up for hypopituitarism).
- Genetic testing (Alagille syndrome, cystic fibrosis, or progressive familial intrahepatic cholestasis).

IMAGING

- Ultrasound—Can be useful to identify structural causes of cholestasis, such as the presence of gallstones, sludge in biliary tree or gallbladder, or choledochal cyst. A small or absent gallbladder would be suggestive (but not diagnostic) of biliary atresia, however, the presence of the gallbladder does not exclude biliary atresia.
- Hepatobiliary scintigraphy—Can be useful to differentiate biliary atresia from nonobstructive causes of cholestasis. While hepatobiliary scintigraphy has a high sensitivity for biliary atresia, it is important to note that the specificity is low, thus diagnosis should not be made solely on this test (**Figure 61-1**).[6]

INVASIVE TESTS

- Percutaneous liver biopsy—Thought to be the most reliable diagnostic procedure in the evaluation of neonatal cholestasis (**Figures 61-2** and **61-6**).[6]
- If biliary atresia cannot be excluded from initial studies, an exploratory laparotomy and intra-operative cholangiography should be performed.

DIFFERENTIAL DIAGNOSIS

OBSTRUCTIVE CHOLESTASIS

- Biliary atresia—Most common cause of neonatal cholestasis and critical to identify as early as possible.
- Choledochal cyst—A rare congenital bile duct anomaly that may manifest with cholestasis and diagnosed with imaging.
- Alagille syndrome—An autosomal dominant genetic disorder with variable expression is associated with abnormalities in liver, heart, skeleton, eye, kidneys, and with distinct facial features (**Figure 61-5**).
- Cholelithiasis or biliary sludge—Rarely presents early in life.
- Cystic fibrosis—Cholestasis may be a result of abnormally viscous bile resulting in obstruction of bile ducts (see Chapter 51, Cystic Fibrosis).

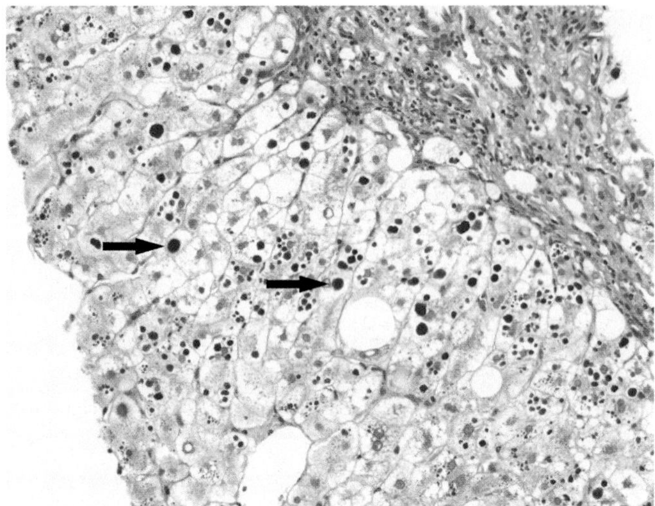

FIGURE 61-6 Alpha-1-antitrypsin on a liver biopsy. A PAS with diastase stain has been performed on this liver biopsy specimen in a patient with alpha-1-antitrypsin deficiency. Note the presence of PAS-positive diastase-resistant pink periportal intracytoplasmic globules (*arrows*), which is characteristic of this disease. (*Used with permission from Thomas Plesec, MD.*)

- Congenital hepatic fibrosis—May be associated with other congenital defects; more frequently associated with polycystic kidney disease (see Chapter 66, Polycystic Kidneys).

HEPATOCELLULAR CHOLESTASIS

- Idiopathic neonatal hepatitis—Features of hepatocellular cholestasis but without a specific etiology found.
- Genetic/metabolic disorders.
  - Alpha-1-antitrypsin deficiency—Most common hereditary cause of liver disease in children.
  - Disorders of bile acid secretion and metabolism—Related to deficiency in enzymes necessary for bile acid synthesis/metabolism or defects in biliary epithelial transporters.
  - Cystic fibrosis—See the preceding discussion.
  - Galactosemia—A rare metabolic disorder that affects the ability to metabolize the sugar galactose appropriately; cholestasis may be the initial manifestation.
  - Tyrosinemia—An inherited metabolic disorder in which the body lacks the enzyme to metabolize tyrosine, an amino acid found in most proteins.
  - Hereditary fructosemi—A metabolic disorder that affects the ability to metabolize the sugar fructose appropriately; key identifying feature is the appearance of symptoms following the introduction of fructose into the diet.
  - Other inborn errors of metabolism.
- Endocrine disorders—Cholestasis may be the initial manifestation of hypothyroidism or hypopituitarism.
- Infectious—Cholestasis and hepatitis is a common manifestation of any infection in the neonate and always warrant consideration because the manifestations of these infections are nonspecific:
  - Viral infection (cytomegalovirus, HIV, herpesvirus, coxsackie virus, echovirus, rubella, or parvovirus).
  - Bacterial infection (urinary tract infection, sepsis, or syphilis).
  - Toxoplasmosis.
- Vascular disorders.
  - Budd-Chiari—Occlusion of the hepatic veins or outflow of blood from the liver.
  - Cardiac insufficiency—May compromise blood flow to the liver and biliary tract.
  - Shock, hypoperfusion—May compromise blood flow to the liver and biliary tract.
- Toxic/secondary.
  - Parenteral nutrition-associated cholestasis—In neonates who are in the neonatal intensive care unit receiving parenteral nutrition for various reasons.
  - Drugs (maternal or used in intensive care)—Hepatotoxic drugs or medications used by the mother or the infant.

MANAGEMENT

- Recognition of neonatal cholestasis by the primary care physician is critical, and prompt referral to a pediatric gastroenterologist for further work-up is necessary.
- It is important to address medical and surgical emergencies immediately when evaluating a neonate with cholestasis.
- Specific management of neonatal cholestasis is often dependent on the underlying diagnosis, and it is important to identify those diseases that are amenable to early surgical intervention (e.g., biliary atresia, choledochal cyst) or specific medical therapy (e.g., hypothyroidism, galactosemia, infections).
- Early diagnosis of biliary atresia is crucial to a good outcome. Observational evidence and expert recommendations suggest that infants referred for Kasai portoenterostomy before 45 to 60 days of age have the greatest likelihood of re-establishing bile flow and longer term survival of their native liver.[1,7–10] SOR Ⓐ Some studies do suggest that there is no contraindication to performing a Kasai portoenterostomy for biliary atresia in children over 75 days of age and up to 100 days.[11,12] One study by Wong et al. showed performing the Kasai portoenterostomy between the age of 60 and 100 days was not associated with a worse outcome.[12]
- In addition to treating specific disorders, general management for neonatal cholestasis is mainly supportive, working towards optimal nutrition and growth, correcting fat soluble vitamin deficiencies if present, and treating complications such as hypercholesterolemia, pruritus, portal hypertension, cirrhosis, and liver failure.[4]

REFERRAL

- Cholestasis in the pediatric population requires evaluation by a pediatric gastroenterologist.
- Further referral may be required depending on the specific etiology of the cholestasis.

PROGNOSIS

- The specific prognosis depends on the etiology for the cholestasis.
- The preponderance of the evidence shows that infants with biliary atresia who undergo portoenterostomy prior to 60 days of age have a better prognosis than those diagnosed after this time period.[7–10]

FOLLOW-UP

- The need for and specific timing for follow-up depends on the specific diagnosis and should be directed by the appropriate subspecialists.

PATIENT EDUCATION

- Parents should be educated regarding the possible etiologies and work-up for cholestasis.
- Once the specific etiology is found, support for the family can be provided, as many of the causes of cholestasis are chronic in nature.

PATIENT RESOURCES

- **www.naspghan.org/user-assets/documents/pdf/positionpapers/cholestaticjaundiceininfants.pdf**.
- **http://emedicine.medscape.com/article/927029-overview**.

PROVIDER RESOURCES

- **http://accesspediatrics.com/abstract/55944887**.
- **http://accesspediatrics.com/content/55943109**.
- Chardot C, Carton M, Spire-Bendelac N, Le Pommelet C, Golmard JL, Auvert B: Prognosis of biliary atresia in the era of liver transplantation: French national study from 1986 to 1996. *Hepatology*. 1999;30:606-611.
- Shneider BL, Brown MB, Haber B, et al. A multicenter study of the outcome of biliary atresia in the US, 1997 to 2000. *J Pediatr*. 2006;148:467-474.

REFERENCES

1. Moyer V, Freese DK, Whitington PF, Olson AD, Brewer F, Colletti RB, et al. Guideline for the evaluation of cholestatic jaundice in infants: Recommendations of the North American Society for Pediatric Gastroenterology, Hepatology and Nutrition. *J Pediatr Gastroenterol Nutr*. 2004;39(2):115-128.
2. Dick MC, Mowat AP. Hepatitis syndrome in infancy—an epidemiological survey with 10 year follow up. *Arch Dis Child*. 1985;60(6):512-516.
3. Suchy FJ. Neonatal cholestasis. *Pediatr Rev*. 2004;25(11):388-396.
4. De Bruyne R, Van Biervliet S, Vande Velde S, Van Winckel M. Clinical practice: Neonatal cholestasis. *Eur J Pediatr*. 2011;170(3): 279-84.
5. Vajro P, Ferrante L, Paolella G. Alagille syndrome: An overview. *Clin Res Hepatol Gastroenterol*. 2012;36(3):275-277.
6. Miethke A, MD, Balistreri W. Approach to neonatal cholestasis. *In*: Walker's Pediatric Gastrointestinal Disease, Fifth edition, edited by Kleinman R, Goulet O, Mieli-Vergani G, et al. Shelton, CT. People's Medical Publishing House, 2008; 789-799.
7. Chardot C, Carton M, Spire-Benelac N, et al. Is the Kasai operation still indicated in children older than 3 months diagnosed with biliary atresia? *J Pediatr*. 2001;138:224-228.
8. Mieli-Vergani G, Howard ER, Portman B, et al. Late referral for biliary atresia–missed opportunities for effective surgery. *Lancet*. 1989;1:421-423.
9. Altman RP, Lilly JR, Greenfeld J, et al. A multivariable risk factor analysis of the portoenterostomy (Kasai) procedure for biliary atresia. *Ann Surg*. 1997;226:348-353.
10. Mowat AP, Davidson LL, Dick MC. Earlier identification of biliary atresia and hepatobiliary disease: selective screening in the third week of life. *Arch Dis Child*. 1995;72:90-92.
11. Schoen BT, Lee H, Sullivan K, Ricketts RR. The Kasai portoenterostomy: when is it too late? *J Pediatr Surg*. 2001;36(1):97-99.
12. Wong KK, Chung PH, Chan IH, Lan LC, Tam PK. Performing Kasai portoenterostomy beyond 60 days of life is not necessarily associated with a worse outcome. *J Pediatr Gastroenterol Nutr*. 2010;51(5):631-634.

62 ANAL AND RECTAL DISORDERS

Federico G. Seifarth, MD
Gavin A. Falk, MD

It is important to recognize the various anal and rectal disorders in infants and children. In this chapter, the following disorders are discussed in succession:

1. Hirschprung disease
2. Imperforate anus
3. Rectal prolapse
4. Anal fissure
5. Anal abscess and Fistula in ano

HIRSCHSPRUNG DISEASE

PATIENT STORY

An 8-week-old girl is brought to your office with abdominal distention and constipation. On digital examination of her anus she has an episode of explosive diarrhea and flatus. A plain radiograph shows stool impaction and a contrast enema reveals a transition zone in the sigmoid colon (**Figure 62-1**). A suction biopsy confirms the diagnosis of Hirschsprung disease. An enema regimen was started and 3 weeks later she underwent a primary pull through operation.

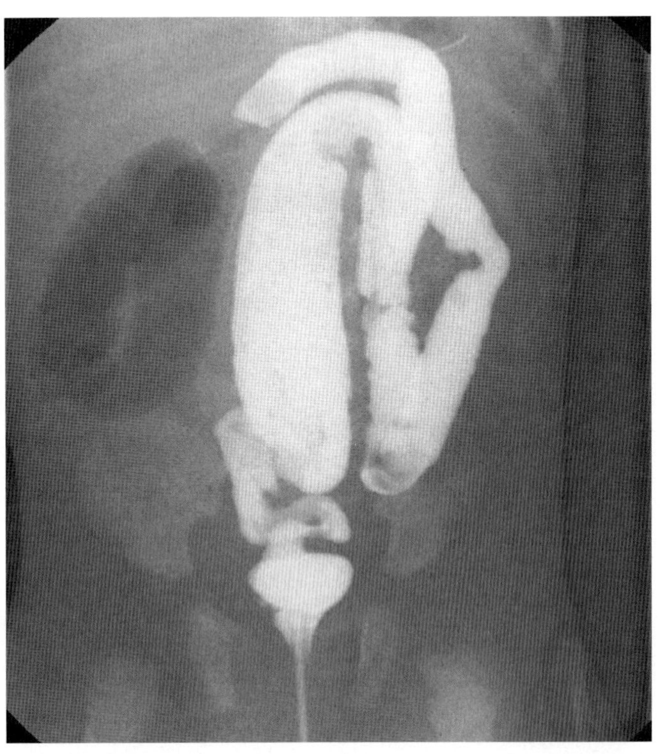

FIGURE 62-1 Hirschprung disease on a water-soluble contrast enema demonstrating a transition zone at the splenic flexure. (*Used with permission from Oliver S. Soldes, MD.*)

INTRODUCTION

Hirschsprung disease is a developmental disorder of the enteric nervous system characterized by absence of ganglion nerve cells in the myenteric and submucosal plexuses of the distal intestine.

SYNONYMS

Hirschsprung disease; partial or total aganglionosis; congenital megacolon.

EPIDEMIOLOGY

- US: 1 case per 5400 to 7200 newborns.
- Worldwide: 1 case per 1500 to 7000 newborns.[1]
- Most cases are diagnosed by 2 years of age.

ETIOLOGY AND PATHOPHYSIOLOGY

- Congenital aganglionosis of the distal bowel leads to impaired bowel peristalsis with constipation. The aganglionosis usually begins in the anus and continues proximally for a variable distance.
- There are two theories for the aganglionosis: The incomplete migration of ganglion cells from the neural crest to the distal bowel or the dysfunctional maturation or apoptosis of primitive nerve cells. There is increasing evidence that mutations in a variety of genes, including the RET proto-oncogene, may play a key role in the etiology.[2,3]

RISK FACTORS

- Race: No racial predilection.
- Sex: Male to Female ratio 4:1.
- About 10 percent of patients have a positive family history.
- Trisomy 21.

DIAGNOSIS

HISTORY

- Neonatal period.
    - Consider the diagnosis in any newborn with delayed passage of first meconium. beyond the first 24 hours, abdominal distention, and repeated vomiting.
    - Signs of intestinal obstruction with bilious vomiting, poor feeding, and failure to thrive.
- Children.
    - Chronic constipation, abdominal distension since birth.
    - Soiling and overflow incontinence.
- Enterocolitis.
    - Ten percent of all patients present with fever, abdominal distension, and diarrhea caused by enterocolitis, which can progress to colonic perforation and life-threatening sepsis.

CLINICAL FEATURES

- Physical examination may reveal a distended abdomen and/or a hypertonic anus with empty rectum.
- Digital rectal examination may result in explosive expulsion of stool.

RECTAL BIOPSY

- Definitive diagnosis is made by histologic evaluation of a rectal biopsy.
- A *suction* rectal biopsy that samples rectal mucosa and submucosa is routinely used in neonates and small children and can be performed at the bedside.
- Alternatively, full-thickness rectal biopsies are taken under general anesthesia in the OR.

LABORATORY TESTING

- White blood cell count and C-reactive protein may be elevated in children with enterocolitis.
- Chemistry panel: Electrolytes are usually normal. Children with diarrhea may have findings consistent with dehydration.

IMAGING

- Plain abdominal radiographs may show distended bowel without air in the rectum.
- Contrast enema—A narrowed distal colon representing the pathologic segment with proximal dilation of the normal bowel is the classic finding (**Figure 62-1**).

ANORECTAL MANOMETRY

- Demonstrates decreased relaxation of the diseased segment.
- May not be available in all facilities and is not routinely used for neonates.
- Most useful in the evaluation of an older child with chronic constipation to rule out Hirschsprung disease.

DIFFERENTIAL DIAGNOSIS

- Functional constipation—Usually not associated with systemic symptoms, failure to thrive and bilious vomiting.
- Cystic fibrosis—Can present with meconium ileus early in life (see Chapter 51, Cystic Fibrosis).
- Hypothyroidism—Constipation is often a manifestation along with other systemic findings.
- Intestinal obstruction—May present with similar symptoms and may need to rely to imaging studies to determine the location of the obstruction.
- Ileus—Usually more acute and does not present with systemic manifestations such as failure to thrive.
- Neonatal sepsis—Always need to be considered in the newborn, but signs other than constipation usually evident (see Chapter 187, Congenital and Perinatal Infections).
- Intestinal Motility Disorders—May present with symptoms similar to Hirschsprung but without the systemic manifestations.
- Low imperforate anus with large perineal fistula opening—Usually can be seen on physical examination.

MANAGEMENT

- Definitive treatment is surgical—To remove the aganglionic portion of bowel, which can be performed semielectively.[4,5] SOR Ⓐ
- Preoperative considerations include treatment of complications of unrecognized or untreated disease until reconstructive surgery can be performed:
  - Constipation—Rectal stimulation, enemas, laxatives.
  - Dehydration—Resuscitation with intravenous fluids.
  - Bowel obstruction—Naso-/orogastric tube decompression.
  - Enterocolitis—Colonic irrigations, broad-spectrum antibiotics.

MEDICATIONS

- Antimicrobial therapy—Perioperatively and in cases of enterocolitis. SOR Ⓒ
- Laxatives. SOR Ⓒ

SURGERY

- Surgical treatment options:
  - Primary pull-through procedure without diverting colostomy.
  - Diverting colostomy with secondary definitive repair.
- Contraindications to a one-stage procedure include very distended proximal bowel, enterocolitis, bowel perforation, and malnutrition.

REFERRAL

- Pediatric surgeon.
- Pediatric gastroenterologist.
- Geneticist if associated with a syndrome.

PREVENTION AND SCREENING

- Hirschsprung disease can be associated with different syndromes, including trisomy 21.[6]

PROGNOSIS

- Left untreated, Hirschsprung disease results in a high rate of mortality.
- Common postoperative problems include obstructive symptoms, fecal soiling, and enterocolitis.[7]
- Constipation can be caused by mechanical obstruction, residual aganglionosis, motility disorder, or habitual stool-holding behavior.
- The long-term outcome after definitive pull-through procedure is good.[4,5] SOR Ⓑ
- Most adolescents and adults with Hirschsprung disease report normal sexual function.

FOLLOW-UP

- Despite proper corrective surgery patients remain at high risk of developing constipation, soiling, and enterocolitis.[7]

PATIENT RESOURCES

- **www.digestive.niddk.nih.gov/ddiseases/pubs/hirschsprungs_ez.**
- **www.cincinnatichildrens.org/health/h/hirschsprung.**

PROVIDER RESOURCES

- **www.aafp.org/afp/2006/1015/p1319.html.**

ANORECTAL MALFORMATIONS—IMPERFORATE ANUS

PATIENT STORY

A newborn boy is found to have noticeably flat buttocks and no anal opening on his first physical examination (**Figure 62-2**). The pediatric surgeon is consulted and the child is given nothing by mouth (NPO). The following day fecal particles are noted in his urine. A cross-table radiograph shows a rectal stump above the coccyx (**Figure 62-3**). A high rectourethral fistula is suspected and the surgeon takes the neonate to the operating room for colostomy formation. Three months later the child undergoes definitive imperforate anus repair and later colostomy takedown.

INTRODUCTION

Imperforate anus is a congenital anomaly in which the natural anal opening is absent. The presentation is highly variable with inconsistent findings of fistulas to skin or the urogenital tract. The term "anorectal malformations" integrates various forms of imperforate anus.

EPIDEMIOLOGY

- Approximately 1 newborn per 5000 live births.[8]
- Slight male preponderance.

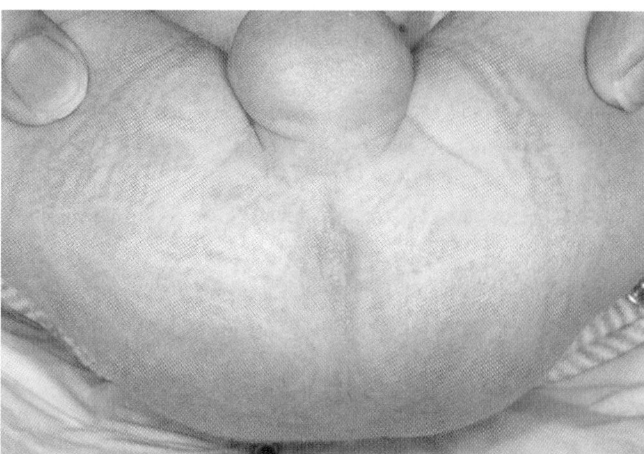

FIGURE 62-2 Newborn boy with imperforate anus and rectourethral fistula. (*Used with permission from Federico Seifarth, MD.*)

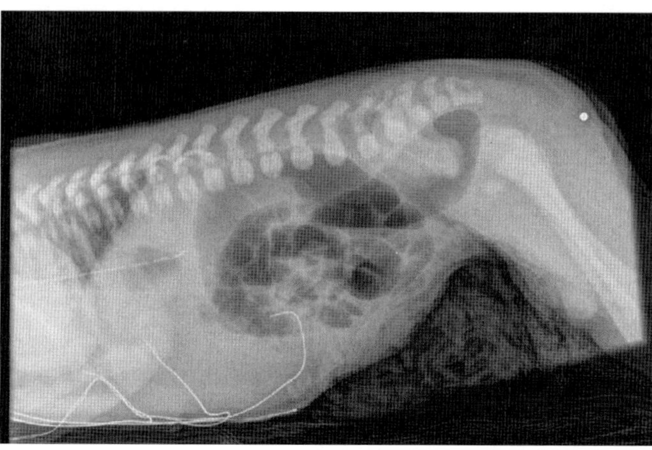

FIGURE 62-3 Cross-table lateral radiograph showing a high rectal stump. The radiopaque pellet marks the imperforate anal skin. (*Used with permission from Federico Seifarth, MD.*)

ETIOLOGY AND PATHOPHYSIOLOGY

- Defects in the early urogenital and anorectal development, normally completed by 9 weeks gestation, account for the described abnormalities of imperforate anus.[9]

RISK FACTORS

- There are no known risk factors.
- Most cases are sporadic, but geographic clustering and families with cases in succeeding generations have been described.

DIAGNOSIS

- Usually identified at first physical examination in newborn age. More subtle cases of imperforate anus with large perineal fistulas may be missed and manifest later with chronic constipation.

CLINICAL FEATURES

- Usually discovered within 24 hours—At first physical exam or when the neonate develops abdominal distention and fails to pass meconium.
- May present with flat buttocks, malformed sacrum, perineal fistula opening, or no visible signs of meconium filled fistula tract.[10]
- Lesions are classified as *low* or *high* based on the termination of the rectum in relation to the levator muscles or more recently according to clinical relevance and fistula anatomy.

LABORATORY TESTING

- Urinalysis.

IMAGING

- Directed to identify associated anomalies: cardiac, gastrointestinal, spinal/sacral/vertebral, or urogenital.[11]
  - Babygram—Vertebral anomalies.
  - Sacral radiography—Sacral defects.

- Abdominal ultrasonography—Genitourinary tract anomalies.
- Spinal ultrasonography—Spinal malformations.
- Echocardiogram—Cardiac defects.
- Cross-table lateral radiograph—Elevated, prone lateral radiograph to determine level of sacral pouch if no fistula is evident on second day of life (**Figure 62-3**).

MANAGEMENT

- Assessment of type of malformation, level of rectal pouch, and identification of rectal fistula, which is present in the majority of cases.
- Naso-/orogastric tube decompression and NPO.
- Workup for associated malformations.
- Planning of surgical management according to the level of the rectal pouch: *high* versus *low*.

MEDICATIONS

- Newborns with imperforate anus should not be fed and need intravenous hydration. SOR Ⓑ

SURGERY

- Primary repair versus colostomy and definitive repair in a staged fashion.[12] SOR Ⓑ
  - High lesions (high position of rectal pouch and urogenital fistulas) may require initial colostomy (**Figure 62-4**).
  - Low lesions with visible fistulas at skin level may be primarily repaired.
- The preferred surgical approach for anal reconstruction is the posterior sagittal anorectoplasty (PSARP; **Figure 62-5**).[12] SOR Ⓑ

REFERRAL

- Immediate consultation of Pediatric surgeon.
- Neurosurgeon, if a tethered spinal cord is present (25% of all cases).

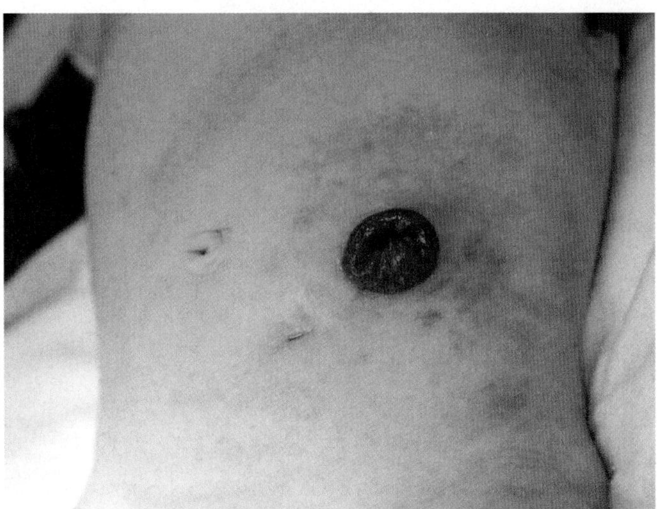

FIGURE 62-4 Descending sigmoid colostomy with distal mucous fistula in a patient with an imperforate anus/recto-bladder neck fistula. (*Used with permission from Federico Seifarth, MD.*)

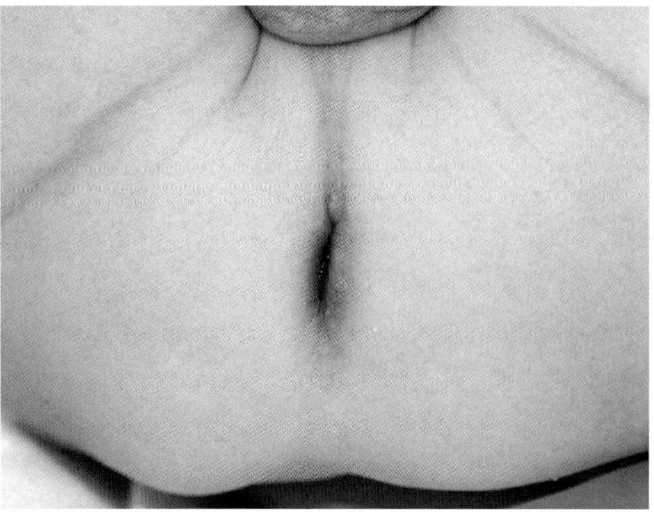

FIGURE 62-5 New functional anus after operative reconstruction of an imperforate anus/recto-bladder neck fistula. (*Used with permission from Federico Seifarth, MD.*)

PROGNOSIS

- Patients with anorectal malformations may suffer from long-term sequelae like constipation and fecal soiling.

FOLLOW-UP

- Long-term close follow-up is required to early identify and treat complications such as soiling and constipation. Some patients need lifelong bowel management and dietary modifications.[13]

PATIENT RESOURCES

- **www.pullthrough.org**.
- **www.pediatricsurgerymd.org/AM/Template.cfm?Section=Resources_for_Parents&TEMPLATE=/CM/ContentDisplay.cfm&CONTENTID=1535**.
- **www.cincinnatichildrens.org/health/a/anorectal-malformations**.

PROVIDER RESOURCES

- **www.ncbi.nlm.nih.gov/pmc/articles/PMC1971061**.

RECTAL PROLAPSE

PATIENT STORY

A 3-year-old boy is brought to your office. He was recently potty trained and has been complaining of anal pain after defecation for the last two days. His mother noted a mass protruding from his anus after bowel movements (**Figure 62-6**). On further discussion, the mother

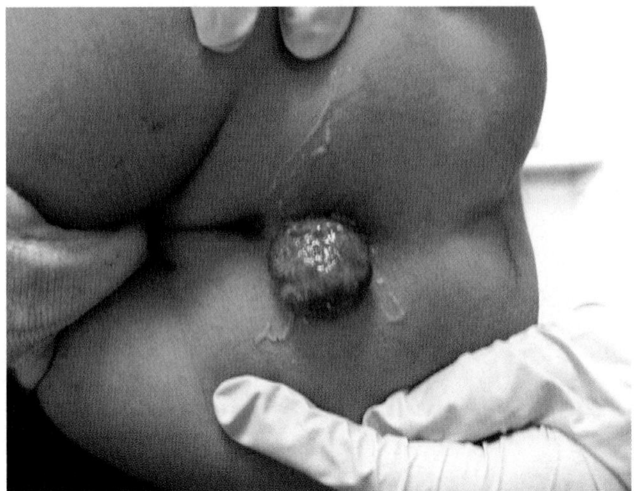

FIGURE 62-6 Mucosal rectal prolapse in a child. (*Used with permission from Thomas J Abramo, MD, From* ***Figure 72-7*** *Pediatric Emergency Medicine, 3rd edition. www.accessemergency medicine.com.*)

reports that her son has an aversion to using the potty. Potty training was delayed, and the mother was educated on importance of a high fiber/fluid diet to promote regular, soft bowel movements. On follow up, the prolapse had resolved.

INTRODUCTION

Rectal prolapse in a child is relatively common and the vast majority of patients do not have any predisposing factors. It may involve only a small ring of mucosa or all layers of the rectum (full thickness prolapse).

EPIDEMIOLOGY

- Relatively common with peak incidence between 1 to 3 years of age.

ETIOLOGY AND PATHOPHYSIOLOGY

- Idiopathic.
- Postoperative—Mucosal rectal prolapse is common after imperforate anus repair (PSARP).
- Predisposing conditions:
  - Constipation—Controversial. Only 3 percent of patients with chronic constipation have rectal prolapse.[14]
  - Cystic fibrosis (CF)—More than 20 percent of CF patients suffer from rectal prolapse.
  - Myelomeningocele—Dysfunctional levator ani complex.
  - Connective tissue disorders—Ehler-Danlos.
  - Behavioral disorders—Withholding stool with subsequent increased intraabdominal pressure.
  - Rectal polyps may act as leading point.

RISK FACTORS

- See Etiology.

DIAGNOSIS

- Usually noticed by parents shortly after or during defecation.

CLINICAL FEATURES

- A rosette of rectal mucosa is seen after defecation and usually reduces spontaneously.
- Radial folds of mucosa are suggestive of mucosal prolapse.
- Concentric circles of mucosa are seen with full-thickness prolapse (**Figure 62-7**).
- Easy manual reduction.

DIFFERENTIAL DIAGNOSIS

- Prolapsing rectal polyp—Can usually be differentiated by appearance of the tissue.
- Hemorrhoids—Unusual in the pediatric population. Can usually be differentiated by the characteristic appearance.
- Intussusception—Usually associated with abdominal pain and bloody/mucus stools (see Chapter 58, Intussusception).
- Proctitis—Usually associated with systemic manifestations.

MANAGEMENT

- Nonoperative management—Prompt manual reduction.

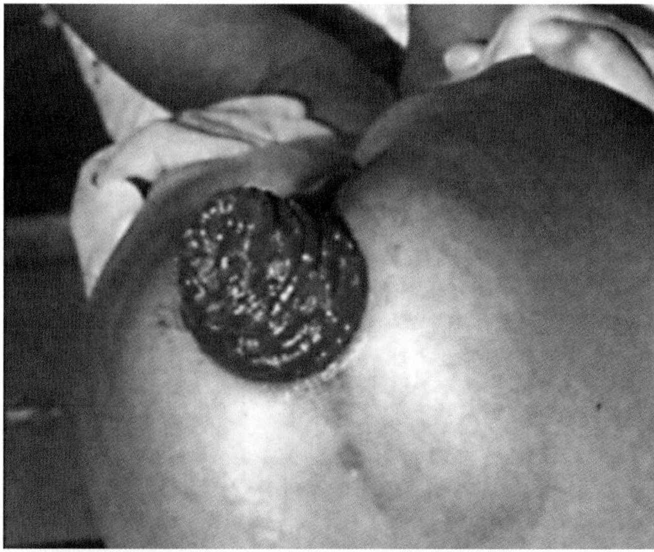

FIGURE 62-7 Full thickness rectal prolapse with concentric rings. The concentric rings in the prolapsed mucosa are a sign of a full thickness rectal prolapse. (*Used with permission from Rudolph Textbook of Pediatrics, 22nd edition.* ***Figure 416-1****. www.accesspediatrics.com.*)

NONPHARMACOLOGIC

- Biofeedback in patients with chronic straining or paradoxical contractions of the anal sphincters. SOR Ⓒ
- Behavioral modification.

MEDICATIONS

- Treat diarrhea or constipation if present.

SURGERY

- Reserved for chronic prolapse in children older than 4 years of age or for complicated cases with recurrent, painful, ulcerated, or bleeding prolapse. SOR Ⓒ
- Surgical options include transanal treatments such as sclerotherapy, thermocauterization, or excision of redundant mucosa. SOR Ⓑ
- Laparoscopic suspension of the rectum to anterior sacrum or resection of the sigmoid colon may be rarely necessary.[15] SOR Ⓑ

REFERRAL

- Pediatric surgeon—Gastroenterologist.

PREVENTION AND SCREENING

- Screen for Cystic fibrosis.[16]
- Proctosigmoidoscopy to rule out rectal polyps or other lesions.

PROGNOSIS

- High rate of spontaneous resolution.[17] SOR Ⓑ
- Patients older than 4 years of age require surgery much more frequently than younger children.[18] SOR Ⓑ
- Low recurrence rate for patients who require surgery.[19] SOR Ⓑ

FOLLOW-UP

- Routine well child visits by primary care physician.

PATIENT EDUCATION

- Parents need to be educated regarding the role of constipation in the etiology of rectal prolapse.

PATIENT RESOURCES

- **www.livestrong.com/article/220449-rectal-prolapse-in-children**.

PROVIDER RESOURCES

- **www.patient.co.uk/doctor/Rectal-Prolapse.htm**.

ANAL FISSURE

PATIENT STORY

An 11-month-old baby boy presents with blood in his diaper. Examination of his anal region reveals longitudinal skin lesions (**Figure 62-8**). The differential is discussed with the parents and sitz baths were recommended. Dietary changes are advised in order to promote regular, soft bowel movements. Three weeks later at follow-up, the child's anal fissure has healed.

INTRODUCTION

An anal fissure is a longitudinal tear in the distal anal canal epithelium that extends from the dentate line to the anal verge. It is the most common cause of rectal bleeding in childhood and a frequent cause of anal pain.

EPIDEMIOLOGY

- Anal fissures may occur at any age but most commonly occur in children aged 12 to 24 months.

ETIOLOGY AND PATHOPHYSIOLOGY

- The pathogenesis of anal fissures is not completely understood.
- A mechanical tear caused by hard stools is the suspected etiology in children.
- Avoidance of painful defecation can worsen the fissure and prevent healing.
- May become infected and develop into a chronic ulcer.

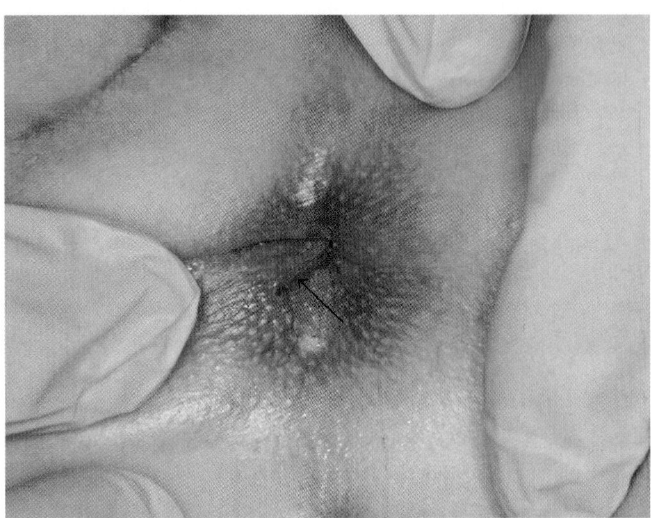

FIGURE 62-8 Anal fissure in an 11-month-old boy who presented with diarrhea and streaks of blood in his stool. (*Used with permission from Federico Seifarth, MD.*)

RISK FACTORS

- Constipation.
- Habitual stool withholding.

DIAGNOSIS

HISTORY

- Painful bowel movements, with bright red blood on stool, diaper or toilet paper.
- Diagnosis is made by inspection.

CLINICAL FEATURES

- Gentle retraction of the perianal skin reveals a longitudinal tear usually in the posterior midline.
- Digital examination should be avoided as it will cause pain and sphincter spasm.
- Usually posterior midline (90%) but may be seen in the anterior midline or lateral.
- A classic sentinel skin tag in the posterior midline can develop from a healed fissure. This is due to epithelialized granulation tissue from chronic inflammation.

IMAGING

- Abdominal flat radiograph to evaluate grade of constipation may be obtained.

DIFFERENTIAL DIAGNOSIS

- Pruritus ani—Usually differentiated based on history of pruritis and evidence of more widespread irritation.
- Inflammatory bowel disease—Usually more chronic or recurrent and associated with systemic manifestations (see Chapter 59, Inflammatory Bowel Disease).
- Immunologic disorders—Usually involved other mucosal surfaces and other manifestations usually present, such as failure to thrive and recurrent infections (see Chapter 221, Combined B and T cell Immunodeficiencies).
- Sexual abuse—Should be suspected based on the history and extent of the involvement (see Chapter 9, Child Sexual Abuse).

MANAGEMENT

NONPHARMACOLOGIC

- Nonsurgical management includes dietary modification, stool softeners, sitz baths, and increasing fluid consumption and fiber intake. SOR C

MEDICATIONS

- Botulinum toxin injections into the anal sphincter muscles to reduce pressure for chronic fissures.[20] SOR A

SURGERY

- Surgical therapies are rarely necessary.
- Reported surgical options for chronic anal fissure in children include fissurectomy, anal dilatation, and lateral internal sphincterotomy.[21] SOR A

PREVENTION AND SCREENING

- Adequate hydration, high fiber diet, and avoid constipation and straining. SOR B

PROGNOSIS

- Symptoms usually resolve in 10 to 14 days with medical management.[22]
- In 50 percent of cases, idiopathic fissures heal in 6 to 8 weeks with conservative management, and 25 percent of these will have a recurrence in 5 years.[23] SOR B

FOLLOW-UP

- Dietary modifications, stool softeners, and sitz baths should be continued for several weeks after operative treatment.
- A follow-up visit is scheduled for 2 to 3 weeks after the procedure.

PATIENT EDUCATION

- Parents should be educated regarding the importance of adequate hydration and avoidance of constipation.
- Reassurance should be provided to the parents that anal fissures are usually benign and resolve with adequate attention to prevent dehydration and constipation.

PATIENT RESOURCES

- **www.patient.co.uk/health/Anal-Fissure.htm**.

PROVIDER RESOURCES

- **www.cpnonline.org/CRS/CRS/pa_analfis_hhg.htm**.

PERIANAL ABSCESS AND FISTULA IN ANO

PATIENT STORY

A 5-month-old boy presents with an area of cellulitis and obvious fluctuance in his perianal region (**Figure 62-9**). He undergoes and incision and drainage under general anesthesia (**Figures 62-10** and **62-11**). Two months later, he still suffers from recurrent drainage from the

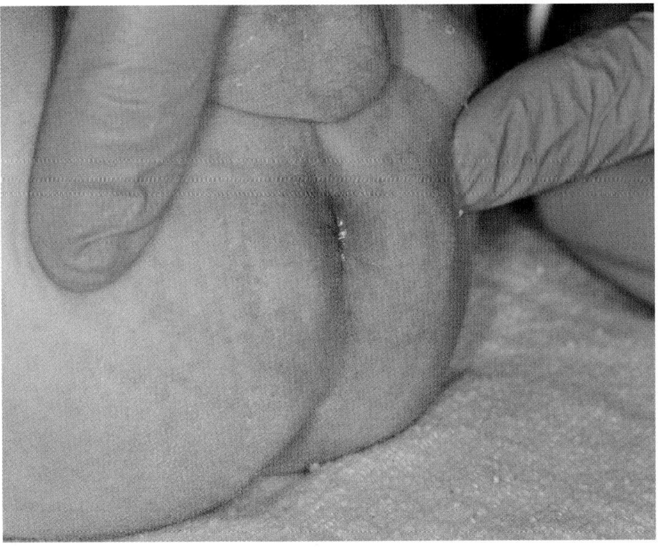

FIGURE 62-9 Perianal abscess at 9 o'clock position in lithotomy position. Note the induration at the site. (*Used with permission from Federico Seifarth, MD.*)

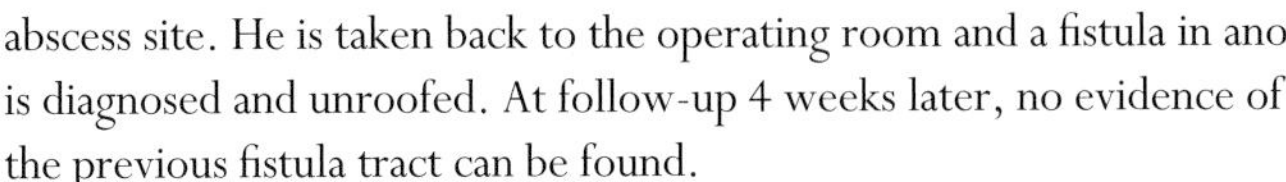

abscess site. He is taken back to the operating room and a fistula in ano is diagnosed and unroofed. At follow-up 4 weeks later, no evidence of the previous fistula tract can be found.

INTRODUCTION

Perianal abscesses are common and typically present between 6 and 12 months of age. After spontaneous rupture or incision and drainage, the condition may progress to a fistula in ano in 10 to 20 percent of patients.[24]

EPIDEMIOLOGY

- More common in males.

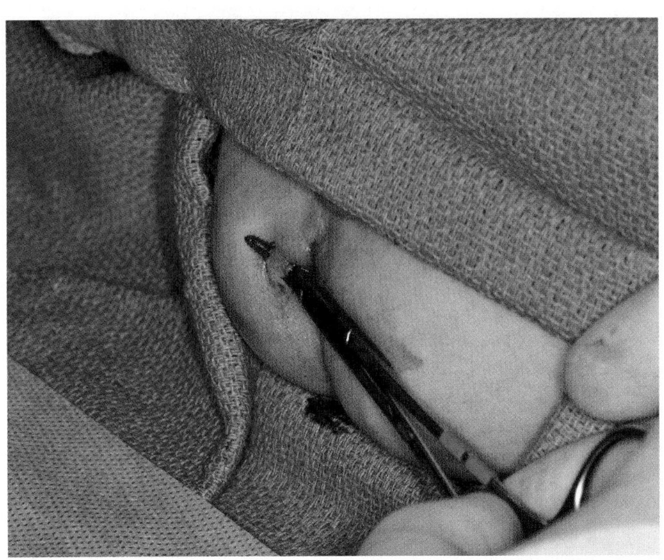

FIGURE 62-10 Incision and counterincision of perianal abscess. (*Used with permission from Federico Seifarth, MD.*)

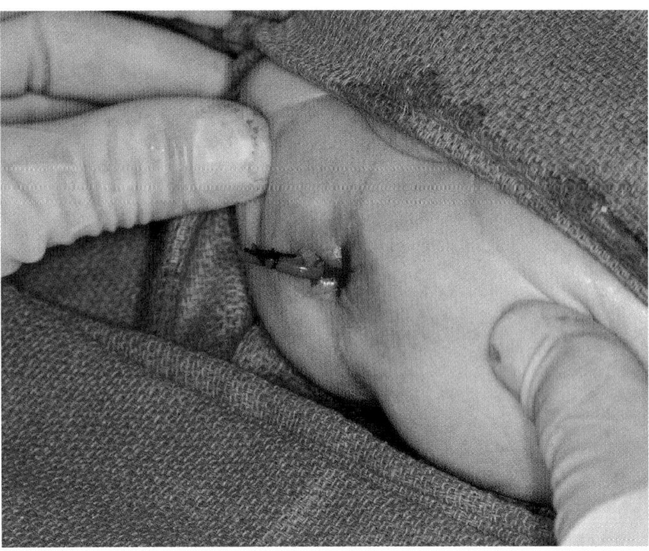

FIGURE 62-11 Perianal abscess with red vessel loop drain in place. (*Used with permission from Federico Seifarth, MD.*)

ETIOLOGY AND PATHOPHYSIOLOGY

- Perianal abscesses are caused by infected anal crypts.
- Epithelization of draining abscesses can lead to development of anal fistulas. They traverse from the affected crypt through the subcutaneous external sphincter to the perianal skin.
- A congenital etiology has been suggested for infant anal fistulas.[25]
- A proposed relationship to androgens resulting in congenital deep, epithelialized crypts may explain the predominant occurrence in male infants.[26]

RISK FACTORS

- Male gender.

DIAGNOSIS

A careful physical examination of the perianal region is the key to the diagnosis.

CLINICAL FEATURES

- Abscess—Tender erythematous perianal swelling with or without spontaneous drainage.
- Anal fistula—Draining fistulous tract opening or perianal pustule (**Figure 62-12**). The tract is typically subcutaneous, extrasphincteric, and straight.

DISTRIBUTION

- The fistulas are usually distributed evenly around the anal circumference.
- Multiple lesions occur in 15 to 20 percent of cases.[27]

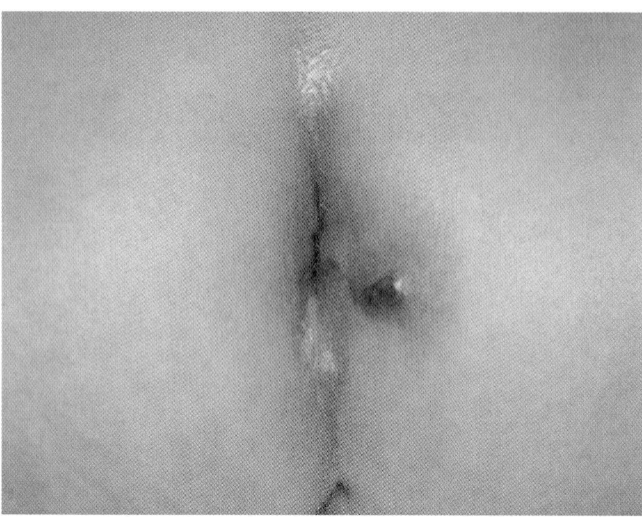

FIGURE 62-12 Fistula in ano following a perianal abscess. This infant presented with a recurrent pustule at the site of the previously drained abscess. (*Used with permission from Federico Seifarth, MD.*)

DIFFERENTIAL DIAGNOSIS

- Anal fissure—see previous discussion.
- Diaper rash and dermatitis, fungal infection—Usually more widespread involvement (see Chapter 121, Candidiasis).
- Sexual abuse—Should be suspected based on the history and other findings (see Chapter 9, Child Sexual Abuse).
- Inflammatory bowel disease in older children (**Figure 62-13**) (see Chapter 59, Inflammatory Bowel Disease).

MANAGEMENT

- Initially nonsurgical therapy: SOR C
  - Sitz baths.
  - Warm packs.

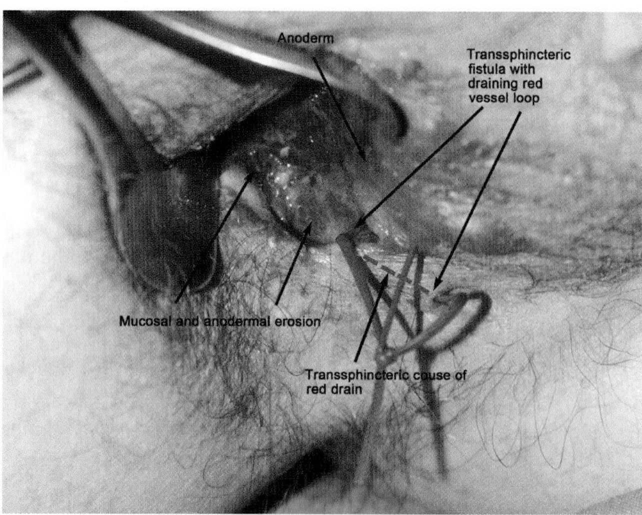

FIGURE 62-13 Transsphincteric anal fistula in a patient with Crohn disease. (*Used with permission from David K. Magnuson, MD.*)

  - Frequent diaper changes and hygienic measures.
  - Expression of pus collections.

MEDICATIONS

- Antibiotic therapy Definitive choice of agent can be guided by culture and susceptibility information obtained at the time of surgical drainage.

SURGERY

- Perianal abscess—Incision and drainage (**Figures 62-10** and **62-11**) vs. antibiotic therapy alone.[24]
- Anal fistula—Deroofing of the fistula tract and fistulotomy (**Figure 62-14**).
- Recent reports have advocated expectant treatment for asymptomatic anal fistulas.[28]
- Treatment of adolescent anal fistulae is similar to adults. The fistulous tract is incised and left open to granulate or excised with primary closure.

PREVENTION AND SCREENING

- Crohn's disease should be ruled out in all children who present outside the typical age groups.

PROGNOSIS

- Most fistulas heal within 12 to 24 months without further sequelae.
- Surgery—Recurrent fistulas are seen in 10 to 20 percent of cases.

FOLLOW-UP

- By primary care physician and pediatric surgeon.

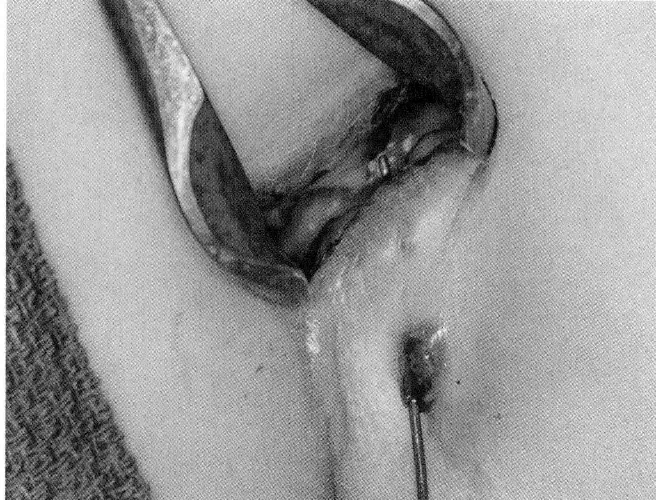

FIGURE 62-14 Fistula in ano in the same infant as in Figure 62-12, as seen with metal probing at the time of surgical excision. Note the fistulous tract extending from the perianal skin to inner opening at the anal crypt. (*Used with permission from Federico Seifarth, MD.*)

PATIENT EDUCATION

- The expected course and management options should be reviewed with the parents.

PATIENT RESOURCES

- **www.pedsurg.ucsf.edu/conditions–procedures/perirectal-abscessfistula.aspx**.

PROVIDER RESOURCES

- **www.patient.co.uk/doctor/Ano-rectal-Abscess.htm**.

REFERENCES

1. Russell MB, Russell CA, Niebuhr E. An epidemiological study of Hirschsprung's disease and additional anomalies. *Acta Paediatr.* 1994;83(1):68-71.
2. Amiel J, Lyonnet S. Hirschsprung disease, associated syndromes, and genetics: a review. *J Med Genet.* 2001;38(11):729-739.
3. Bordeaux MC, Forcet C, Granger L, Corset V, Bidaud C, Billaud M, et al. The RET proto-oncogene induces apoptosis: a novel mechanism for Hirschsprung disease. *EMBO J.* 2000;19(15):4056-4063.
4. Dasgupta R, Langer JC. Transanal pull-through for Hirschsprung disease. *Semin Pediatr Surg.* 2005;14(1):64-71.
5. Tannuri U, Romao RL. Transanal endorectal pull-through in children with Hirshsprung disease-technical refinements and comparison of results with the Duhamel procedure. *J Pediatr Surg.* 2009;44(4):767-772.
6. Moore SW. The contribution of associated congenital anomalies in understanding Hirschsprung's disease. *Ped Surgery Int.* 2006; 22(4):305-315.
7. Dasgupta R, Langer JC. Evaluation and management of persistent problems after surgery for Hirschsprung disease in a child. *J Pediatr Gastroenterol Nutr.* 2008;46(1):13-19.
8. Spouge D, Baird PA. Imperforate anus in 700,000 consecutive liveborn infants. *Am J Med Genet Suppl.* 1986;2:151-161.
9. Stephens FD. Embryology of the cloaca and embryogenesis of anorectal malformations. *Birth Defects Orig Artic Ser.* 1988;24(4): 177-209.
10. Levitt MA, Peña A. Pediatric Surgery. In: Coran AG, Caldamone A, Adzick NS, Krummel TM, Laberge J-M, Shamberger R, eds. *Expert Consult—Online and Print.* Mosby;2012:848.
11. Smith ED, Saeki M. Associated anomalies. *Birth Defects Orig Artic Ser.* 1988;24(4):501-549.
12. deVries PA, Peña A. Posterior sagittal anorectoplasty. *Journal of Pediatric Surgery.* 1982;17(5):638-643.
13. Levitt MA, Kant A, Peña A. The morbidity of constipation in patients with anorectal malformations. *J Pediatr Surg.* 2010;45(6): 1228-1233.
14. Abrahamian FP, Lloyd-Still JD. Chronic constipation in childhood: a longitudinal study of 186 patients. *J Pediatr Gastroenterol Nutr.* 1984;3(3):460-467.
15. Koivusalo A, Pakarinen M, Rintala R. Laparoscopic suture rectopexy in the treatment of persisting rectal prolapse in children: a preliminary report. *Surg Endosc.* 2006;20(6):960-963.
16. Kopel FB. Gastrointestinal manifestations of cystic fibrosis. *Gastroenterology.* 1972;62(3):483-491.
17. Rintala R, Lindahl H, Louhimo I. Anorectal malformations—results of treatment and long-term follow-up in 208 patients. *Ped Surgery Int.* 1991.
18. Antao B, Bradley V, Roberts JP, Shawis R. Management of rectal prolapse in children. *Dis Colon Rectum.* 2005;48(8):1620-1625.
19. Ashcraft KW, Garred JL, Holder TM, Amoury RA, Sharp RJ, Murphy JP. Rectal prolapse: 17-year experience with the posterior repair and suspension. *Journal of Pediatric Surgery.* 1990; 25(9):992-995.
20. Husberg B, Malmborg P, Strigård K. Treatment with botulinum toxin in children with chronic anal fissure. *Eur J Pediatr Surg.* 2009; 19(5):290-292.
21. Cohen A, Dehn TC. Lateral subcutaneous sphincterotomy for treatment of anal fissure in children. *Br J Surg.* 1995;82(10): 1341-1342.
22. Nelson R. Non surgical therapy for anal fissure. *Cochrane Database Syst Rev.* 2006;(4):CD003431.
23. Kenny SE, Irvine T, Driver CP, Nunn AT, Losty PD, Jones MO, et al. Double blind randomised controlled trial of topical glyceryl trinitrate in anal fissure. *Arch Dis Child.* 2001;85(5):404-407.
24. Macdonald A, Wilson-Storey D, Munro F. Treatment of perianal abscess and fistula-in-ano in children. *Br J Surg.* 2003;90(2):220-221.
25. Fitzgerald RJ, Harding B, Ryan W. Fistula-in-ano in childhood: a congenital etiology. *Journal of Pediatric Surgery.* 1985;20(1):80-81.
26. Shafer AD, McGlone TP, Flanagan RA. Abnormal crypts of Morgagni: the cause of perianal abscess and fistula-in-ano. *Journal of Pediatric Surgery.* 1987;22(3):203-204.
27. Watanabe Y, Todani T, Yamamoto S. Conservative management of fistula in ano in infants. *Ped Surgery Int.* 1998;13(4):274-276.
28. Rosen NG, Gibbs DL, Soffer SZ, Hong A, Sher M, Peña A. The nonoperative management of fistula-in-ano. *Journal of Pediatric Surgery.* 2000;35(6):938-939.

63 NUTRITIONAL DISORDERS IN CHILDREN

Victor E. Uko, MD
Lori A. Mahajan, MD

PATIENT STORY

An 18-month-old female was brought in for evaluation of a pale appearance. She was described as an active toddler with no recent fatigue, melena, or hematochezia. She was described as a picky eater and has averaged 30 to 40 ounces of milk intake per day for the past 6 months. Family history and past medical histories were noncontributory. On exam, height and weight were at the 50th percentile. Examination was normal except for a pale appearance, spooning of her nails (**Figure 63-1**), mild tachycardia, and a grade II/VI systolic ejection murmur heard best over the left lower sternal border. Labs were significant for the following: Hgb 7.0 g/dl, Hct 21.0 percent, MCV 52 fL, RDW 18 percent, reticulocyte count 1.9 percent, total iron 10 ug/dL (30 to 140 ug/dL), transferrin saturation 9 percent (11 to 46%), and ferritin 16 ng/mL (18–300 ng/mL). Peripheral smear showed microcytosis, hypochromia, mild anisocytosis, and polychromasia.

She was diagnosed with iron deficiency anemia and started on oral iron with concomitant reductions in her daily consumption of milk to no more than 18 to 20 ounces a day. At follow-up appointment one month later, she looked well and her appetite had improved with consumption of a wider variety of foods. Repeat Hgb was 9.5 g/dL and her MCV 69 fL. Three months later, her hemoglobin had completely normalized.

INTRODUCTION

Nutritional disorders in children include both deficiency and excess states. Protein energy malnutrition remains one of the leading causes of death in children in underdeveloped countries. Obesity has emerged as one of the most common nutritional disorders in children worldwide. Children who have a body mass index (BMI) in the 85th to 94th sex- and age-specific percentile are considered overweight. Those with a BMI at or above the 95th percentile are considered obese.

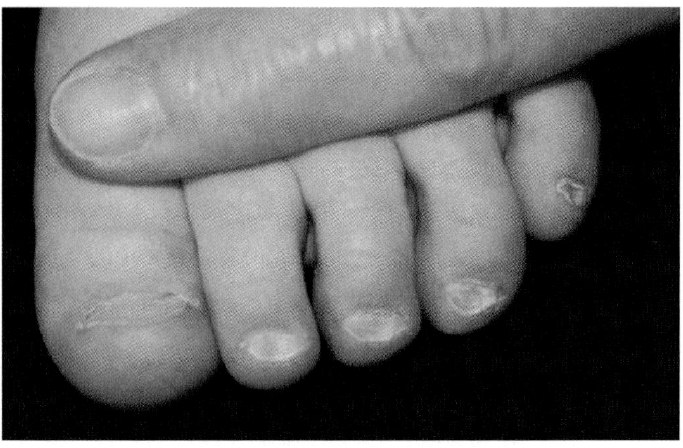

FIGURE 63-1 Koilonychia due to iron deficiency. (*Used with permission from Rudolph CD, Rudolph AM, Lister GE, First LR, Gershon AA: Rudolph's Pediatrics, 22nd edition: www.accesspediatrics.com.*)

EPIDEMIOLOGY

- Severe protein-energy malnutrition is uncommon in the US and other developed countries.
- Childhood obesity rates have risen steadily, with current global estimates at approximately 17 percent, disproportionately affecting minority youth. Overweight and obesity are now on the rise in low- and middle-income countries, particularly in urban settings. Almost 35 million overweight children live in developing countries and 8 million in developed countries.
- Overweight and obesity are linked to more deaths worldwide than malnutrition.

ETIOLOGY AND PATHOPHYSIOLOGY

- Nutritional deficiency states may occur as a result of poor dietary intake, increased nutrient loss, or increased nutrient and energy requirements as seen in patients with chronic illness.
- The small intestine is the predominant site of absorption of nutrients from the gastrointestinal tract. Any disease that interrupts bile flow, digestive enzyme excretion, or small bowel mucosal integrity, may result in a variety of nutritional deficiencies (**Table 63-1**).
- Deficiencies in fat soluble vitamins (A, D, E, and K) can be seen in patients with poor oral intake and diseases that cause malabsorption

TABLE 63-1 Possible Nutritional Deficiencies in Gastrointestinal Disease

Disease	Vitamin(s)	Mineral	Trace Element
Cystic fibrosis/Pancreatic Insufficiency	A, D, E, K, B_{12}	Magnesium	Iron, Selenium, Zinc
Cholestasis	A, D, E, K, B_{12}	Calcium	
Celiac disease	A, D, E, K, B_{12}, Folate	Calcium	Iron, Copper
Crohn's disease	A, D, E, K, B_{12}, Folate	Magnesium	Iron, Copper, Selenium, Zinc
Ulcerative colitis	D, Folate	Magnesium	Iron, Zinc

including pancreatic disorders and cholestatic liver disease. Vitamin D deficiency can also result from lack of sun exposure.[1]

- Iron deficiency is the most common nutritional deficiency in childhood. It can be seen secondary to poor oral intake, poor absorption, and in cases of chronic blood loss.
- Vitamin B_1 (thiamin) is found in milk, meats, eggs, legumes, and fruits. Deficiency results from inadequate intake or poor absorption due to intestinal or liver disease.
- Vitamin B_2 (riboflavin) deficiency is seen in patients on long term barbiturates, disorders of intestinal malabsorption, and in patients who avoid dairy products which are a good source of this vitamin.
- Vitamin B_3 (niacin) deficiency is seen in patients with carcinoid syndrome and Hartnup disease (autosomal recessive disorder of tryptophan metabolism). It is also seen with prolonged use of certain medications such as isoniazid, azathioprine, and phenobarbital.[2]
- Vitamin B_6 (pyridoxine) deficiency is uncommon. Low levels of pyridoxal phosphate can be seen in patients with chronic illnesses such as diabetes, asthma, and sickle cell anemia.
- Vitamin B_9 (folic acid) is essential to numerous bodily functions including DNA synthesis and repair as well as to act as a cofactor in certain biological reactions. It is especially important in aiding rapid cell division and growth, and is required to produce healthy red blood cells and prevent anemia. Lack of adequate intake leads to folate deficiency, which is now uncommon.
- Vitamin B_{12} is bound to intrinsic factor in the stomach and is absorbed primarily in the terminal ileum. Deficiency typically results from inadequate intake (vegan mothers and in their breast fed infants), surgery involving the stomach or terminal ileum, or lack of excretion of intrinsic factor in the stomach (pernicious anemia).
- Vitamin C (ascorbic acid) deficiency occurs in severely malnourished patients and in those who consume a diet devoid of fruits and vegetables. Deficiency leads to impaired collagen and chondroitin sulfate formation. The tendency to hemorrhage, presence of defective tooth dentin, and loosening of teeth caused by deficient collagen is known as scurvy.
- Copper deficiency can be seen in patients after gastric bypass surgery and also in those with malabsorption such as patients with untreated celiac disease. Premature infants receiving milk without adequate copper supplementation and those on long-term total parenteral nutrition (TPN) can also develop copper deficiency.
- Zinc deficiency can occur in patients with pancreatic insufficiency (pancreatic enzymes are needed for the release of dietary zinc), chronic inflammatory diseases and those on long term total parenteral nutrition (TPN). Acrodermatitis enteropathica results in zinc deficiency due to malabsorption.[3]
- Selenium deficiency is rare, but can occur in patients receiving long-term parenteral nutrition without supplementation.[4]
- Nutrient toxicity states are more commonly seen with fat soluble vitamins as well as minerals and are due to excess ingestion or administration.
- The causes of obesity can be attributed to both genetic and environmental factors.[5] The most common cause is overconsumption of calories as compared to amount of calories used.

RISK FACTORS FOR NUTRITIONAL DEFICIENCY STATES

- Poor nutritional intake.
- Low socioeconomic status.
- Patients on long-term TPN.
- Malabsorption syndromes and chronic disorders (**Table 63-1**).

RISK FACTORS FOR NUTRITIONAL TOXICITY STATES AND OBESITY

- Excessive intake.
- Sedentary lifestyle.

DIAGNOSIS

CLINICAL FEATURES

- The clinical manifestations of malnutrition and overweight/obesity can be assessed using anthropometric measurements (standardized growth charts), specific physical examination findings, and confirmatory laboratory measurements.
- Common clinical features of nutrient deficiency and excess states are listed in **Tables 63-2** and **63-3**.
- Iron deficiency leading to anemia is the most prevalent mineral deficiency in children. Chronic deficiency may lead to spooning and pallor of the nail beds (**Figure 63-1**).
- Vitamin A deficiency presents with night blindness (earliest symptom), xerosis (dry eyes), and the development of Bitot's spot—triangular areas of abnormal squamous cell proliferation and keratinization of the conjunctiva (**Figure 63-2**).[6]
- Vitamin B_1 (Thiamin) is classically associated with symptoms of cardiac dysfunction (cardiomyopathy) along with neurological symptoms, which may include polyneuropathy and seizures. Wernicke-Korsakoff syndrome (characterized by a triad of nystagmus, ophthalmoplegia, and ataxia) is only rarely seen in the pediatric age group.
- Vitamin B_2 (Riboflavin) deficiency is characterized by angular stomatitis, glossitis and seborrheic dermatitis (**Figure 63-3**).
- Zinc deficiency is characterized by perioral and perianal dermatitis (**Figure 63-4**). Other clinical manifestations include an increased susceptibility to infections, diarrhea, and growth failure.
- Obese children should be carefully evaluated for hypertension. Other commonly associated signs include hepatomegaly from fatty liver disease and acanthosis nigricans (associated with insulin resistance). Signs of possible reversible causes of obesity should also be sought including deep purple striae and the "buffalo hump" of Cushing's syndrome (a rare secondary cause of obesity).

LABORATORY TESTING

- Should be tailored based on clinical history and physical exam findings.

TABLE 63-2 Clinical Features of Vitamin Deficiency and Excess States

Vitamin	Deficiency State	Excess State
Vitamin A	Nyctalopia (night blindness) Xerophthalmia Bitot Spots	Nausea and vomiting Bone and muscle pain Hepatomegaly/hepatic fibrosis Pseudotumor cerebri
Vitamin D	Rickets/osteomalacia Dental caries	Pseudotumor cerebri Bone pain/cortical hyperostosis Hypertension Ectopic calcification
Vitamin E	Neurologic changes: decreased DTRs, wide-based gait, ocular palsy, spinocerebellar degeneration Anemia/hemolysis	Prolonged PT/vitamin K antagonism
Vitamin K	Coagulopathy Hemorrhagic disease of newborn	Shock, anaphylaxis with IV Hemolysis
Vitamin B_1 (Thiamin)	Beriberi Cardiac failure/ neuropathy Korsakoff's syndrome/ Wernicke's encephalopathy	Nausea/anorexia/lethargy or anaphylaxis from parenteral form
Vitamin B_2 (Riboflavin)	Seborrheic dermatitis Cheilitis Glossitis	
Vitamin B_3 (Niacin)	Pellagra: dermatitis, diarrhea, dementia	Flushing Burning, stinging hands
Vitamin B_6	Decreased tryptophan to niacin conversion Personality changes	Seizures Peripheral neuropathy
Vitamin B_9 (Folate)	Macrocytic anemia/leukopenia	
Vitamin B_{12}	Cheilitis Glossitis Peripheral neuropathy Macrocytic anemia/hypersegmented neutrophils	
Vitamin C	Scurvy Poor wound healing	Gastritis Diarrhea

- Fat-soluble vitamins (A and E) are measured directly in the serum.
- Vitamin D—Evaluated by measuring 25-dihydroxyl vitamin D (25 OH Vit D) levels in serum.
- Vitamin K—Evaluated by measuring prothrombin time and international normalized ratio (INR) in the serum.
- B group of vitamins—Laboratory tests are specific for each vitamin in this group.
- Most trace elements can be measured directly in the serum. Twenty-four hour urine collection for copper is preferred to copper analysis test in Wilson's disease. Low alkaline phosphatase levels are seen in patients with zinc deficiency.
- Laboratory testing recommended for children with a body mass index between the 85th and 94th percentiles but who have no obesity-related illnesses (hypertension, known dyslipidemia, increased blood pressure) include a fasting lipid profile should be done. Children with a BMI between the 85th and 94th percentiles and risk factors should have a fasting lipid profile, and measurement of alanine transaminase and aspartate transaminase levels (to detect fatty liver disease) and fasting blood glucose (to detect type 2 diabetes).[7] Children whose BMI is above the 95th percentile should have the same tests plus measurement of blood urea nitrogen and creatinine to detect impaired renal function (which may develop from long-standing hypertension or diabetes).
- Karyotype (with fluorescence in situ hybridization [FISH] for Prader-Willi [15q-]), only when indicated by clinical history and physical examination (**Figure 63-5**).

TABLE 63-3 Clinical Features of Mineral/Trace Element Deficiency and Excess States

Mineral/Trace Element	Deficiency State	Excess State
Calcium	Bone demineralization Tetany/seizures Cardiac arrhythmia	Nephrocalcinosis (milk-alkali syndrome)
Copper	Hypochromic anemia, neutropenia skin depigmentation CNS dysfunction	Hepatic necrosis Hemolysis Renal failure Coma/death
Fluoride	Increased dental carries Osteoporosis	Mottled enamel (chronic)
Iron	Hypochromic microcytic anemia Pica	Coagulopathy GI bleeding
Iodine	Goiter Cretinism	Thyrotoxicosis
Magnesium	Cardiac arrhythmia Seizures	Laxative effect Heart block Flaccid quadriplegia Respiratory paralysis
Manganese	Decreased nail and hair growth Depressed clotting factors Dermatitis	
Selenium	Cardiomyopathy Fatigue/hypothyroidism	Alopecia Garlic odor to breath
Zinc	Rash (perianal/perioral), poor wound healing, Immune dysfunction	Nausea/dyspepsia/vomiting Hypercholesterolemia

DIFFERENTIAL DIAGNOSIS

- Potential causes of nutritional deficiencies are many with the most common cause being poor oral intake. Other important considerations are listed in **Tables 63-1** to **63-3**.

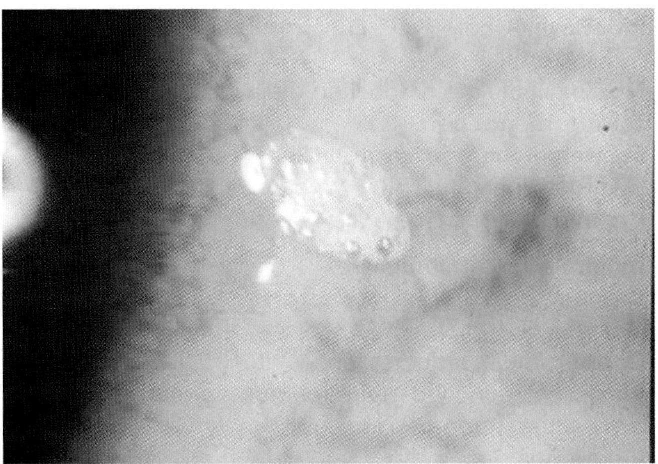

FIGURE 63-2 Bitot's spot on the conjunctiva due to vitamin A deficiency. It is associated with conjunctival xerosis. (*Used with permission from Lueder GT: Pediatric Practice Ophthalmology www.accesspediatrics.com.*)

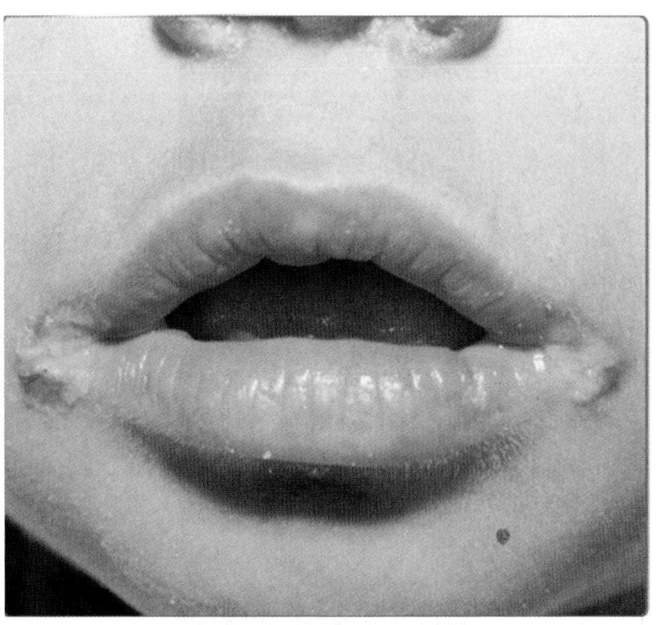

FIGURE 63-3 Angular Stomatitis due to vitamin B2 (riboflavin) deficiency. (*Used with permission from Goldsmith LA, Katz SI, Gilchrest BA, Paller AS, Leffell DJ, Wolff K: Fitzpatrick's Dermatology in General Medicine, 8th edition: www.accessmedicine.com.*)

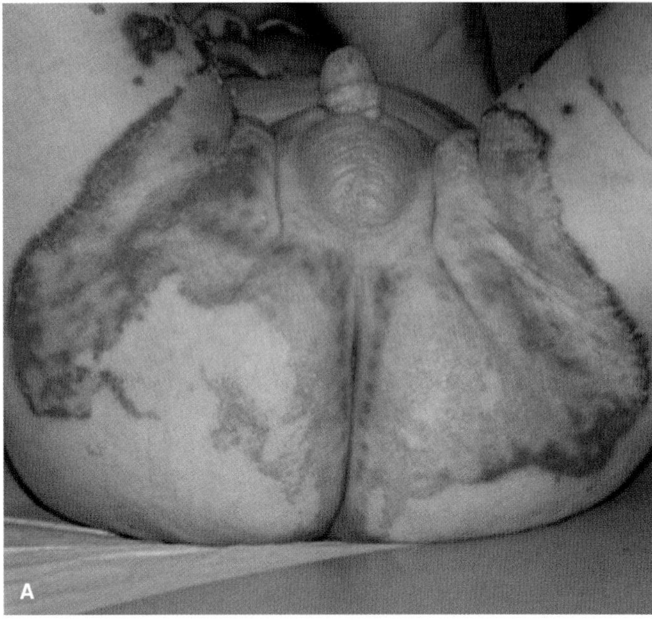

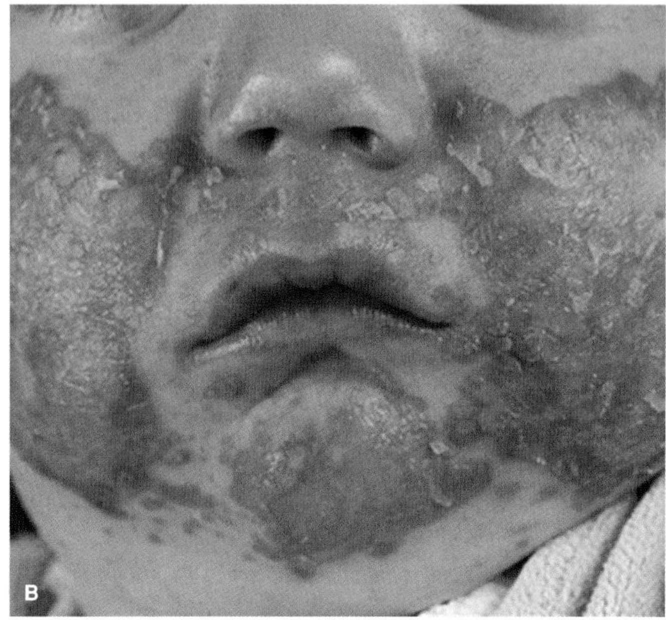

FIGURE 63-4 Perianal (**A**) and perioral (**B**) dermatitis due to zinc deficiency. Known as acrodermatitis enteropathica. (*Used with permission from Goldsmith LA, Katz SI, Gilchrest BA, Paller AS, Leffell DJ, Wolff K: Fitzpatrick's Dermatology in General Medicine, 8th edition: www.accessmedicine.com.*)

MANAGEMENT

NONPHARMACOLOGIC

- Appropriate dietary counseling (recommend intake or avoidance depending on deficiency or excess state; see **Table 63-4**).

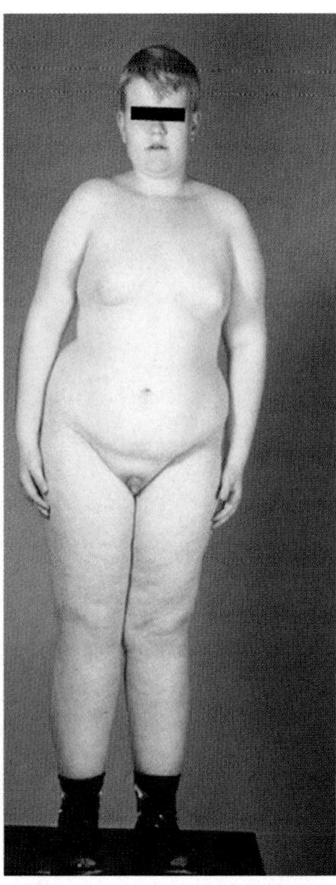

FIGURE 63-5 Prader Willi Syndrome in an 11-year-old boy. (*Used with permission from Cleveland Clinic Children's Hospital Photo File.*)

TABLE 63-4 Dietary Sources Rich in Nutrients

Fat Soluble Vitamins
Vitamin A: egg, liver, fortified milk, dark green and yellow fruits & vegetables
Vitamin D: fortified milk, egg yolk, fish, sunlight
Vitamin E: nuts, soybeans, green leafy vegetables, corn or canola oil, olives
Vitamin K: green leafy vegetables, herbs, prunes
Water-Soluble Vitamins
Thiamin: whole grain/enriched grain products, meat, milk, legumes
Riboflavin: whole grain/enriched grain products, meat, milk, eggs
Niacin: whole grain/enriched grain products, meat, fish, green vegetables
Folate: fortified grains, green leafy vegetables, bean sprouts, peanuts
Vitamin B_{12}: meat (particularly seafood), milk, eggs
Minerals/Trace Elements
Calcium: dairy, tofu, almonds, green leafy vegetables, herring
Copper: meat, legumes, chocolate
Iron: meat, enriched grains, pumpkin/squash seeds, sun-dried tomatoes/apricots
Iodine: seafood, iodized salt
Magnesium: seafood, nuts, green vegetables
Zinc: meat, dark chocolate, peanuts

- The issue of weight should be addressed with all children at least once a year.
- A four-stage approach to treatment of childhood obesity as set forth by the American Medical Association is summarized as follows:[8]

Stage 1 (Prevention-plus protocol)

- Eat ≥5 servings of fruits and vegetables daily.
- Use television and computer ≤2 hours per day.
- No television in child's bedroom.
- ≥60 minutes of moderate to vigorous physical activity per day.
- No sugar-sweetened beverages.
- Eat breakfast daily.
- Limit meals outside the home.
- Family meals ≥ five times per week.
- Allow child to self-regulate food intake and avoid food restriction (e.g., a child should be permitted to eat portions of food until satiated, no more, or less).

Stage 2 (Structured weight-management protocol)

- A more structured plan that includes structured meals, supervised physical activity of at least 60 minutes daily, one hour or less screen time per day, and increased self-monitoring of these behaviors through log completion. If no improvement in BMI takes place after three to six months, Stage 3 is appropriate.

Stage 3 Comprehensive, Multidisciplinary Intervention

Stage 4 Tertiary-Care Intervention

MEDICATIONS

- Replacement of the deficient micronutrient or mineral should be instituted.
- Treatment should be instituted for any underlying disorder that has led to the nutritional deficient state.

SURGERY

- Patients with nutritional deficiencies and/or underlying disease may require surgical procedures for placement of feeding tubes or central venous lines for parenteral nutrition. SOR Ⓒ
- Weight loss surgery (gastric banding, bypass procedures) should be considered for adolescents with extreme obesity (BMI ≥40) and other comorbidities associated with long-term risks who are unresponsive to dietary and lifestyle modification. SOR Ⓒ

REFERRAL

- Consultation with a pediatric dietitian to provide appropriate dietary counseling.
- Consultation with a pediatric gastroenterologist to address any underlying gastrointestinal causes for nutritional deficiencies.
- The overweight or obese patient should have a multidisciplinary team assembled as indicated (dietitian, gastroenterologist, endocrinologist, counselor, trainer, etc.).

PREVENTION AND SCREENING

- Supplementation of fat soluble vitamins (A,D,E,K) is required for patients with cholestatic disease or fat malabsorption. They should also be periodically screened for insufficient levels of these vitamins even though supplemented.
- To prevent vitamin D deficiency, adequate sun exposure (30 minutes per week for infants clothed in diapers or 2 hours per week when fully clothed) is recommended. Dark-skinned infants require at least threefold longer periods of sunlight exposure.
- Daily vitamin D intake of 400 units/day for exclusively breast fed infants and those consuming less than 1 liter of infant formula each day is recommended.[9]
- Vitamin K administration to infants at or around the time of birth is recommended to prevent hemorrhagic disease of the newborn.
- Vitamin B_{12} supplementation is required for pregnant women who are strict vegans especially those who intend to exclusively breast feed their babies.
- Breast fed babies should start iron supplementation at 4 months of age. Infants (6 months and older) should have at least 2 iron fortified cereal feeds each day along with at least one feeding per day of vitamin C rich foods such as citrus fruits, dark green vegetables, tomatoes.
- Children aged 1 to 5 years should not consume more than 600 mL (20 ounces) of milk per day.
- Universal screening for iron deficiency is recommended for all children at 9 to 12 months of age.
- Additional iron screening at 15 to 18 months and also at 5 to 8 years of age for high-risk patients (premature infants, children with chronic inflammatory disease, children with recurrent/chronic infections and those on restricted diets).
- Children should be screened for overweight/obesity states at least annually. Parents should be counseled at initial well child checks regarding healthy foods, healthy habits, setting a good example themselves, and living an active lifestyle.

PROGNOSIS

- This is dependent on the underlying cause for the nutritional deficiency state.
- Nutritional deficiencies due to poor intake have an excellent prognosis with successful replacement of the deficient nutrient.
- Treatment of obesity at any age is a challenge. Obese children are at high risk of becoming obese adults. Approximately 80 percent of children who are obese at 10 to 15 years of age remain obese as adults.

FOLLOW-UP

- Close follow-up is required after pharmacological or dietary interventions are instituted in patients with nutritional deficiencies or excesses.

PATIENT RESOURCES

- American Academy of Pediatrics (AAP). Right from the start: ABCs of Good Nutrition for Young Children—**www.patiented.aap.org/content.aspx?aid=5705**.
- **www2.aap.org/obesity**.

PROVIDER RESOURCES

- **www.health.gov/dietaryguidelines/dga2005/toolkit/default.htm**.
- **www.apps.nccd.cdc.gov/dnpabmi/**.
- Centers for Disease Control and Prevention. Trends in the Prevalence of Extreme Obesity Among US Preschool-Aged Children Living in Low-Income Families. 1998–2010. *JAMA*. 2012;308(24):2563-2565.

REFERENCES

1. Gordon CM, DePeter KC, Feldman HA, Grace E, Emans SJ. Prevalence of vitamin D deficiency among healthy adolescents. *Arch Pediatr Adolesc Med*. 2004;158(6):531-537.
2. Wan P, Moat S, Anstey A. Pellagra: a review with emphasis on photosensitivity. *Br J Dermatol* 2011;164(6):1188-1200.
3. Wang K, Pugh EW, Griffen S, Doheny KF, Mostafa WZ, al-Aboosi MM, et al. Homozygosity mapping places the acrodermatitis enteropathica gene on chromosomal region 8q24.3. *Am J Hum Genet*. 2001;68(4):1055-1060.
4. Ishida T, Himeno K, Torigoe Y, Inoue M, Wakisaka O, Tabuki T, et al. Selenium deficiency in a patient with Crohn's disease receiving long-term total parenteral nutrition. *Intern Med*. 2003;42(2):154-157.
5. Maffeis C. Aetiology of overweight and obesity in children and adolescents. *Eur J Pediatr*. 2000;159(1):S35-44.
6. Tanumihardjo SA. Assessing vitamin A status: past, present and future. *J Nutr*. 2004;134(1):290S-293S.
7. Krebs NF, Himes JH, Jacobson D, Nicklas TA, Guilday P, Styne D. Assessment of child and adolescent overweight and obesity. *Pediatrics*. 2007;120(4):S193-228.
8. Barlow SE, for the Expert Committee: Expert committee recommendations regarding the prevention, assessment, and treatment of child and adolescent overweight and obesity: summary report. *Pediatrics*. 2007;120(4):S164-S192.
9. Misra M, Pacaud D, Petryk A, Collett-Solberg PF, Kappy M, Drug and Therapeutics Committee of the Lawson Wilkins Pediatric Endocrine Society: Vitamin D deficiency in children and its management: review of current knowledge and recommendations. *Pediatrics*. 2008;122(2):398-417.

PART 10

THE GENITORURINARY SYSTEM AND KIDNEYS

Strength of Recommendation (SOR)	Definition
A	Recommendation based on consistent and good-quality patient-oriented evidence.*
B	Recommendation based on inconsistent or limited-quality patient-oriented evidence.*
C	Recommendation based on consensus, usual practice, opinion, disease-oriented evidence, or case series for studies of diagnosis, treatment, prevention, or screening.*

*See Appendix A on pages 1320–1322 for further information.

64 URINARY SEDIMENT/ URINARY TRACT INFECTIONS

Mindy A. Smith, MD, MS
Richard P. Usatine, MD

PATIENT STORY

A 10-year-old boy presented to the office with a 2-day history of "tea-colored" urine. Two weeks prior to this presentation, he had an upper respiratory infection that resolved without treatment. Two years ago, he had a similar episode of gross hematuria that developed after a viral infection, and at that time the diagnosis of IgA nephropathy was entertained. His urine now reveals hematuria (**Figure 64-1**) but no proteinuria.

INTRODUCTION

Examination of the urinary sediment is a test frequently done for evaluation of patients with suspected genetic/intrinsic (e.g., systemic lupus nephritis, sickle cell disease, glomerulonephritis, interstitial nephritis), anatomic (e.g., arteriovenous malformation), obstructive (e.g., posterior urethral valves, kidney stones), infectious, metabolic (e.g., coagulopathy), traumatic, or neoplastic disease of the urinary tract. Potential findings of red or white blood cells, casts, bacteria, or neoplastic cells help in directing further evaluation of a patient's problem.

EPIDEMIOLOGY

- Although there is no consensus on the definition of microscopic hematuria in children, 5 to 10 RBCs/HPF are considered significant.[1]

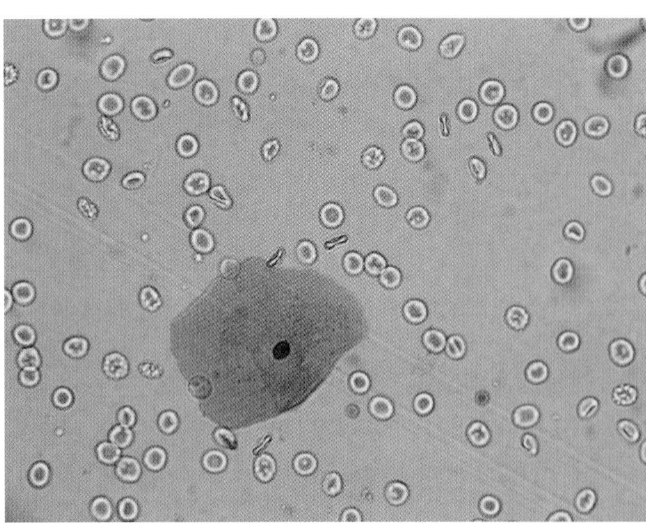

FIGURE 64-1 Red blood cells (RBCs) seen in the urine. Some of the RBCs are crenated and there is one epithelial cell visible. (*Used with permission from Richard P. Usatine, MD.*)

- Based on an older study (N = 8,954 unselected children ages 8 to 15 years), the incidence of microscopic hematuria found in one or more of four urine specimens was 4.1 percent; the incidence was 1.1 percent for hematuria present in two or more specimens.[2]
- Macroscopic (visible) or gross hematuria among children has an estimated incidence of 1.3/1000.[3]
- Isolated pyuria (>2 to 10 white blood cells per high-power field [WBCs/HPF]) is not uncommon in sick neonates and febrile children.
    - In a study of 110 consecutive infants admitted to a neonatal intensive care unit in Karachi, 35 had pyuria, of who 71.4 percent had no growth in urine cultures.[4]
    - In a case series of children with Kawasaki disease (KD; N = 210), 29.5 percent (N = 62) had pyuria including 34 with sterile pyuria and eight with bacterial pyuria.[5]
    - In another case series of children with acute KD compared to children with other febrile illnesses, 79.8 percent of KD and 54.0 percent of febrile children without KD had pyuria.[6] The median number of white blood cells in the urine was higher for children with KD (42 WBC/microL vs. 12 WBC/microL in febrile children).
- Urinary tract infections (UTIs) are common in children (8% of girls and 2% of boys by age 7 years) and WBCs on microscopy have 73 percent sensitivity and 81 percent specificity for the diagnosis.[7]
    - About 60 percent of children who have a febrile UTI are found to have defects on renal cortical scintigraphy (RCS) indicating acute pyelonephritis; of these, 10 to 40 percent will have permanent renal scarring.[8]
- In a laboratory study of greater than 11,000 urinalyses from 88 institutions, 62.5 percent of the tests received a manual microscopic evaluation of the urinary sediment, usually triggered by an abnormal urinalysis.9 New information was obtained 65 percent of the time as a result of the manual examination.

ETIOLOGY AND PATHOPHYSIOLOGY

- Hematuria (**Figure 64-1**) has many causes including:[1]
    - Idiopathic.
    - Glomerular disease (e.g., immunoglobulin [Ig]A nephropathy, post-streptococcal glomerulonephritis, membranoproliferative glomerulonephritis [MPGN]).
    - Interstitial and tubular disease (e.g., acute pyelonephritis, tuberculosis, hematologic disorders such as sickle cell, or thrombocytopenia).
    - Structural or congenital abnormalities (e.g., polycystic kidney disease).
    - Urinary tract (collecting system, ureters, bladder, or urethra) disease (e.g., bladder infection [*Escherichia coli* in about 85%],[7] stone, trauma [including recent catheterization], tumors, or exercise).
    - Metabolic abnormalities including hypercalcemia and hyperuricemia.
    - Medications (e.g., aminoglycosides, anticonvulsants, or aspirin).
    - Toxins (e.g., lead, turpentine).
    - Contamination (menstruation or bloody diarrhea).
    - The most common causes of hematuria in children are idiopathic, benign familial, idiopathic hypercalciuria, IgA nephropathy, and

sickle cell trait or anemia.[1] In the Vehaskari et al. study, of 28 children with hematuria (6 or more RBC/0.9 mm^3 or more than 100,000 RBC/hour) on two occasions who underwent renal biopsy, 12 children had normal biopsies, two children were diagnosed with IgA-IgG nephropathy, one with focal segmental sclerosis, one with extracapillary glomerulonephritis, and one with possible hereditary nephritis.[2]
  - The source of bleeding in children is most commonly glomerular (vs. urinary tract); RBCs cross the glomerular endothelial-epithelial barrier entering the capillary lumen through discontinuities in the capillary wall.[1]
  - A family history of hematuria, hypertension, renal disease (e.g., kidney stones, cystic disease), sickle cell, hemophilia, and dialysis or transplant can be helpful.[1] In one study of 500 children with beta-thalassemia major requiring transfusion, 10.6 percent had hematuria.[10]
- Hematuria with dysmorphic RBCs or RBC casts (**Figure 64-2**) and excess protein excretion (>500 mg/dL) suggests glomerulonephritis.
- Gross hematuria suggests a postrenal source in the collecting system, although recurrent episodes of gross hematuria occur in 10 to 20 percent of patients with MPGN.[11]
  - Bright red urine and/or visible clots with normal appearing RBCs on microscopy suggest bleeding from the urinary tract.[1]
  - Brownish-colored urine (described as tea or cola-colored) with RBC casts and dysmorphic RBCs suggest glomerular bleeding.[1]
- Pyuria (**Figure 64-3**) is often the result of urinary tract infection.
  - The presence of bacteria (>10^2 organisms per mL or >10^5 using a midstream urine specimen in older children and adults) suggests infection. A urinalysis with 10 bacteria per HPF is highly suggestive (specificity 99%) of infection (positive likelihood ratio [LR+] 85).[12]

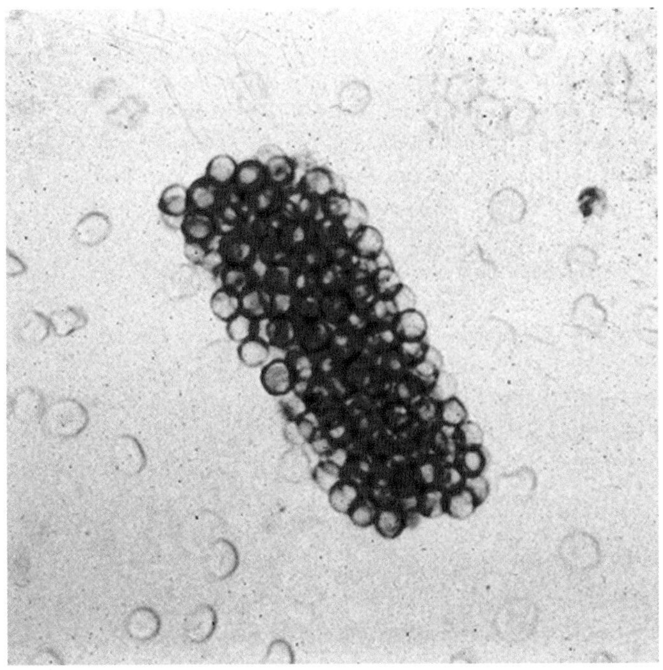

FIGURE 64-2 A RBC cast caused by bleeding into the tubule from the glomerulus. These casts are seen in glomerulonephritis, IgA nephropathy, lupus nephritis, Goodpasture syndrome, and Wegener granulomatosis. RBC casts are always pathologic.

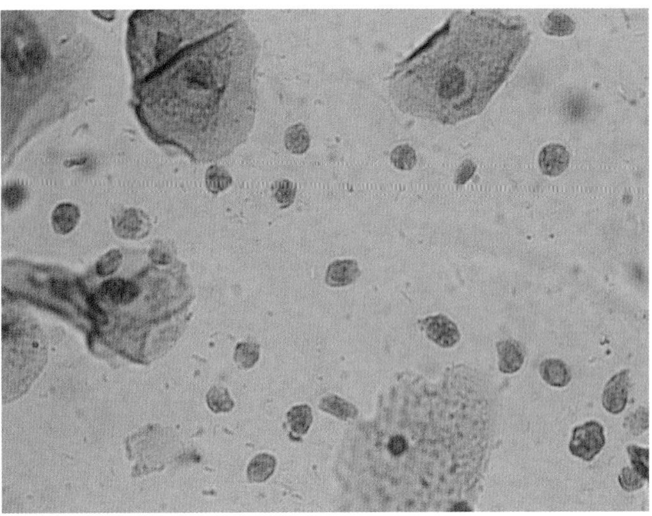

FIGURE 64-3 Pyuria and bacteriuria in a patient with a urinary tract infection. A simple stain was added to the wet mount of spun urine. Although there are epithelial cells present, the culture demonstrated a true urinary tract infection (UTI) and not merely contaminated urine. *(Used with permission from Richard P. Usatine, MD.)*

  - Asymptomatic bacteruria is found in 4 to 15 percent of pregnant women, usually *Escherichia coli*.
  - The presence of WBC casts (**Figure 64-4**) with bacteria indicates pyelonephritis.
- As previously noted, isolated (sterile) pyuria can also been seen in children with KD or tuberculosis.[5,6,13]
- WBCs and/or WBC casts can be seen in tubulointerstitial processes like interstitial nephritis, systemic lupus erythematosus, or transplant rejection.
- Urinary casts are formed only in the distal convoluted tubule (DCT) or in the collecting duct (distal nephron).
- Hyaline casts are formed from mucoprotein secreted by the tubular epithelial cells within the nephrons. These translucent casts are the most common type of cast and can be seen in normal persons after vigorous exercise or with dehydration. Low urine flow and

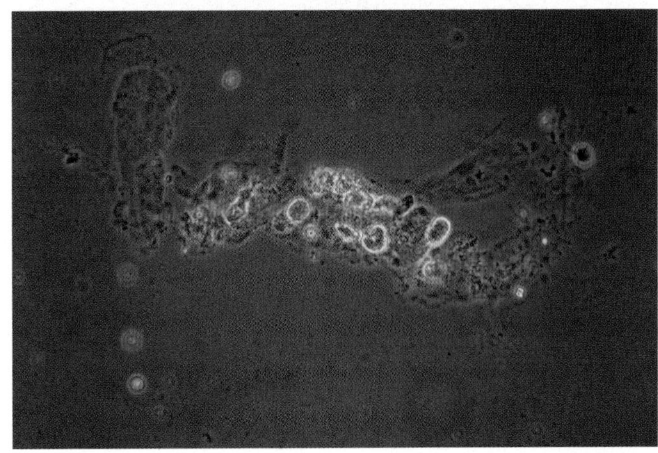

FIGURE 64-4 WBC casts seen in pyelonephritis. These can be differentiated from a clump of WBCs by their cylindrical shape and the presence of a hyaline matrix.

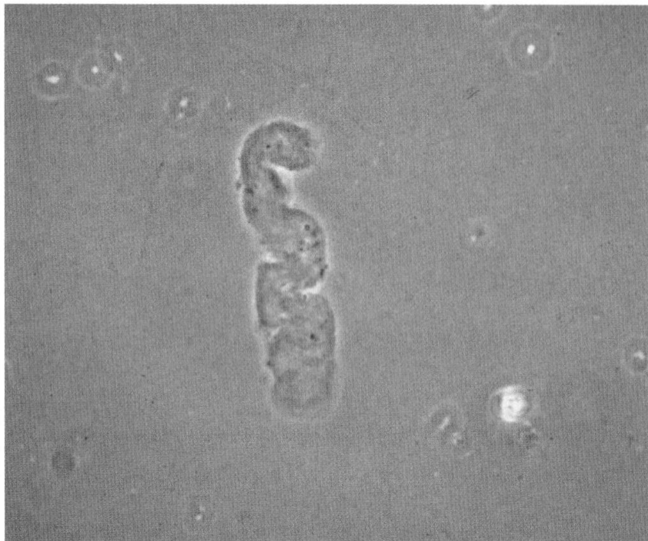

FIGURE 64-5 Hyaline casts are translucent and proteinaceous. These are the most common casts found in the urine and can be seen in normal individuals. Concentrated urine with low flow, usually caused by dehydration, exercise, and/or diuretics, can lead to hyaline cast formation.

concentrated urine from dehydration can contribute to the formation of hyaline casts (**Figure 64-5**).

- Granular casts are the second most common type of cast seen (**Figure 64-6**). These casts can result from the breakdown of cellular casts or the inclusion of aggregates of albumin or immunoglobulin light chains. They can be classified as fine or coarse based on the size of the inclusions. There is no diagnostic significance to the classification of fine or coarse.

RISK FACTORS

- Constipation (for UTI in children).
- Clinical factors associated with urinary tract infection in febrile children in one study were:[14]
  - Uncircumcised male (OR 10.4; 95% CI 4.7 to 31.4).
  - Temperature of > or = 39 degrees C (OR 2.4 per degree C; 95% CI 1.5 to 3.6).

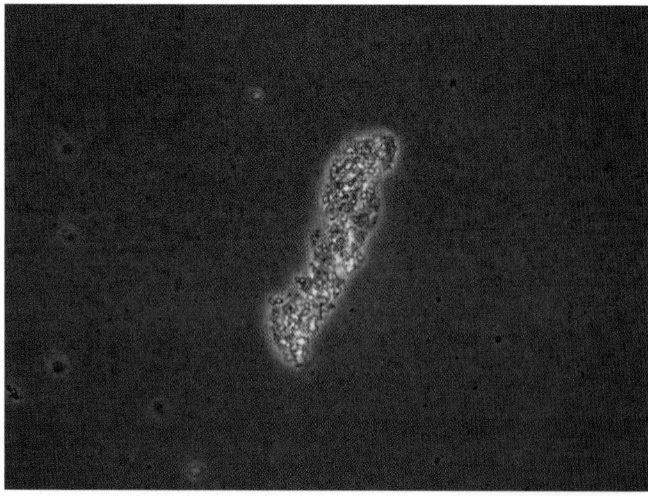

FIGURE 64-6 Coarse granular cast. All granular casts indicate underlying renal disease. These are nonspecific and may be seen in diverse renal conditions.

DIAGNOSIS

CLINICAL FEATURES

- Hematuria is often asymptomatic in patients with glomerular disease or metabolic abnormalities.
  - Important aspects of the history include prior or current infection (urinary tract, diarrhea, or strep throat), strenuous exercise, menstruation, tropical exposures, trauma, pain (bladder, flank, or joint), rash, or symptoms of UTI (frequency or dysuria).[1,18] Inquire about changes in urine volume. Also examine for foreign body insertion and occult trauma, including sexual abuse (e.g., genital bleeding).
  - Family history of sickle cell disease or hemophilia, stone disease, hearing loss, and familial renal disease, hematuria, and hypertension can be helpful.[18]
  - Signs and symptoms of glomerular disease include various degrees of renal failure, edema, oliguria, hypertension, and anemia out of proportion to the degree of renal failure. Ask about sore throat or skin infection within the last 4 weeks, suggesting post-infectious disease. Patients with MPGN present with one of the following patterns: nephrotic syndrome (40 to 70%); acute nephritic syndrome (20 to 30%); asymptomatic proteinuria and hematuria detected on routine urinalysis (20 to 30%); or recurrent episodes of gross hematuria (10 to 20%).[15] Hypertension is detected in 1/3 of patients with MPGN.[15]
  - In a case series of children with Henoch-Schönlein purpura (N = 223), nephritis occurred in 46 percent, most within 1 month of diagnosis.[16] Nephritis presented as isolated hematuria in 14 percent, isolated proteinuria in 9 percent, both hematuria and proteinuria in 56 percent, nephrotic-range proteinuria in 20 percent, and nephrotic-nephritic syndrome in 1 percent.
  - Renal stones can cause pain in the ipsilateral flank and/or abdomen with radiation to the ipsilateral groin, testicle, or vulva or irritative symptoms of frequency, urgency, and dysuria, if located in the bladder.
  - An abdominal mass may be caused by a tumor, hydronephrosis, multicystic dysplastic kidney, or polycystic kidney disease.[1]
  - Rash and/or arthritis can occur in patients with Henoch-Schönlein purpura or systemic lupus erythematosus.
- UTI in children is more likely in the presence of pain (abdominal pain [LR+ 6.3; 95% CI, 2.5 to 16.0] or back pain [LR+ 3.6; 95% CI, 2.1 to 6.1]) in addition to dysuria, frequency, or both (LR+ 2.2 to 2.8); new-onset urinary incontinence (LR+ 4.6; 95% CI, 2.8 to 7.6) also increases the likelihood of a UTI.[17]
  - In infants, findings of previous UTI (LR+ 2.3 to 2.9), fever higher than 40°C (104°F) (LR+ 3.2 to 3.3), and suprapubic tenderness (LR+ 4.4) were the findings most useful for identifying UTI.
- Symptoms of pyelonephritis include chills and rigor, fever, nausea and vomiting, and flank pain; positive likelihood ratios, however, are low (1.5 to 2.5).

LABORATORY TESTING AND IMAGING

- The work-up for microscopic hematuria in a child includes urinary sediment looking for dysmorphic cells or RBC casts (**Figure 64-2**) and a test for proteinuria (>2+ by dipstick).
  - If positive, suspect glomerular disease and consider a basic metabolic panel, complete blood count and platelet count, complement, albumin, streptozyme, and antibody testing (antistreptolysin O, antiglomerular basement membrane antibody, antineutrophil cytoplasmic antibody); a renal biopsy may be indicated.[1] Work-up for patients with suspected MPGN is covered elsewhere.[11]
  - If negative and the sediment contains WBCs (**Figure 64-3**) or WBC casts (**Figure 64-4**), suspect infection and obtain a urine culture and susceptibility test if pyelonephritis is suspected; *E. coli* is the most common organism.
  - If negative and no WBCs or symptoms, obtain a urinalysis (UA) from family members looking for hematuria (if positive, the diagnosis of benign familial hematuria is likely) or signs of glomerular disease, and a urine for calcium/creatinine ratio; if the diagnosis remains unclear, consider a 24-hour urine collection for protein, creatinine and calcium.[1] If these tests are also negative and hematuria persists, consider a hearing test, renal ultrasound, and hemoglobin electrophoresis.[1]
  - For a child with isolated hematuria, the American College of Radiology (ACR) recommends an ultrasound of the kidneys and bladder.[18] If the child has painful, nontraumatic hematuria, ACR recommends a computed tomography (CT) scan without contrast to evaluate for stones and an ultrasound of the kidneys and bladder. An x-ray of the abdomen and pelvis can also be considered.
- For a child with macroscopic hematuria, look for signs of glomerulonephritis (e.g., edema, hypertension, proteinuria, or RBC casts) and if present, consider tests previously noted for microscopic hematuria suspicious for glomerulonephritis.
  - If there is no trauma involved, obtain a urine culture and renal and bladder ultrasound.[1]
  - If the hematuria was caused by trauma, ACR recommends obtaining a CT of the abdomen and pelvis with contrast.[18] x-ray retrograde urography is considered in cases where blood is present at the urethral meatus or if there are pelvic fractures.[18]
  - For painful hematuria that is not infectious, a CT of the abdomen and pelvis without contrast and/or an ultrasound of the kidneys and bladder is most appropriate looking for stones or urologic conditions (e.g., tumor).[18]
  - Cystoscopic evaluation is helpful if bladder pathology is suspected or to localize bleeding during an episode of active bleeding.
  - If the preceding evaluation is negative, consider periodic follow-up.
- If RBC casts (**Figure 64-2**) are seen on UA in addition to proteinuria, also consider nephrotic syndrome caused by diabetes or amyloidosis (see Chapter 67, Nephrotic Syndrome).
- Note that RBC casts are fragile and are best seen in a fresh urine specimen (**Figure 64-2**).
- Based on older data, for a child with a suspected UTI, microscopy positive for pyuria and bacteruria (pooled LR+ 37.0; 95% CI 11.0 to 125.9) or a dipstick positive for both leukocyte esterase (LE) and nitrite (pooled LR+ 28.2; 95% CI: 17.3 to 46.0) are best for ruling in UTI.[19] Microscopy negative for both (pooled LR− 0.11; 95% CI: 0.05 to 0.23) or a dipstick negative for both LE and nitrite (pooled LR− 0.20, 95% CI, 0.16 to 0.26) can be used to rule out UTI.[11]
  - If the child is 3 years of age or younger, a urine sample for microscopy and culture is recommended; pyuria and positive bacteruria (at least 50,000 colonies per mL of a single uropathogenic organism in an appropriately collected specimen of urine) defines UTI.[20] Positive likelihood ratios are lower for dipstick testing in infants (LR+ 7.62; 95% CI 0.95 to 51.85).[21] For febrile infants, the urine specimen should be obtained before an antimicrobial agent is administered and through catheterization or suprapubic aspiration.[20]
  - For older children with a positive LE and nitrite, treatment can be initiated empirically and a urine culture obtained for confirmation and susceptibility testing. If only one of the dipstick tests is positive, a urine sample for microscopy and culture is indicated with treatment based on clinical and lab findings.[7]
- Following a UTI, imaging is recommended by ACR in the following cases:[22]
  - Age <2 months, febrile urinary tract infection—Ultrasound of kidneys and bladder with consideration of x-ray voiding cystourethrogram in boys and in the presence of an ultrasound abnormality.
  - Age >2 months and ≤3 years, febrile urinary tract infection with good response to treatment—Ultrasound of kidneys and bladder. The yield of this test decreases with increasing age and clinical judgement is needed for older children.
  - Atypical (poor response to antibiotics within 48 hours, sepsis, urinary retention, poor urine stream, raised creatinine, non-*E. coli* UTI), or recurrent febrile UTI—ultrasound of kidneys and bladder, x-ray voiding cystourethrogram (VCUG), and consideration of radionuclide cystography in girls.
- VCUG is also indicated for children if renal and bladder ultrasonography reveals hydronephrosis, scarring, or other findings that would suggest either high-grade VUR or obstructive uropathy.[20]

MANAGEMENT

Treatment will depend on the underlying etiology:

- If the child has glomerulonephritis, hyperkalemia or azotemia, stone disease, or a family history of renal failure, referral to a nephrologist is indicated.[1] Management of MPGN is covered elsewhere.[11]
- If the child with hematuria has sustained trauma or has obstructing stone disease, tumor, or structural abnormalities referral to an urologist is indicated. Such referral can also provide reassurance in cases where no cause of hematuria has been found.
- Cystitis is treated with appropriate antibiotics based on knowledge of the sensitivities of *E. coli* in the individual practice location (there is increasing resistance to amoxicillin).
  - First line choices are trimethoprim-sulfamethoxazole, amoxicillin/clavulanate, or cephalosporins such as cefixime.[7] Symptoms usually improve within 24 to 36 hours.
- Uncomplicated pyelonephritis can be treated with appropriate antibiotics as an outpatient (e.g., amoxicillin/clavulanate, cefixime, ceftibuten) for 10 to 14 days or with short-courses (two to four days) of intravenous therapy followed by oral therapy.[7,23] The urine

should always be cultured in pyelonephritis to help guide therapy. Pregnant women or children with complicated pyelonephritis may need hospitalization.

- See Chapter 68, Nephritic Syndromes and Chapter 70, Kidney Stones for management of patients with these conditions.

PREVENTION AND SCREENING

- According to the Institute for Clinical Systems Improvement, urinalysis for screening in children and adolescents is among tests considered of low predictive value and/or uncertain beneficial action for true positives and is not recommended.[24]
- A yearly screening urinalysis is recommended for certain populations such as survivors of childhood cancers exposed to radiation or some chemotherapeutic agents.[25]
- A national urine screening program of school children in Korea (1999–2008) resulted in over 5,000 children being referred to pediatric nephrologists.[26] Renal biopsies were performed on 1,478 children [28.79 % of total subjects; 26.77 % for isolated hematuria (IH), 9.09 % for isolated proteinuria (IP), and 51.19 % for both] with chronic glomerulonephritis identified in 25% (40% with IgA) nephropathy, 24% with mesangial proliferative and 13% with GN with thin basement membrane nephropathy).
- For healthy children following a first UTI, prophylactic antibiotics do not appear to reduce subsequent UTI, even in children with mild to moderate vesicoureteral reflux.[27,28]

PROVIDER RESOURCES

- *Urinalysis*—**www.library.med.utah.edu/WebPath/TUTORIAL/URINE/URINE.html**.

REFERENCES

1. Meyers KEC. Evaluation of hematuria in children. *Urol Clin North Am*. 2004;31:559-573.
2. Vehaskari VM, Rapola J, Koskimies O, et al. Microscopic hematuria in school children: epidemiology and clinicopathologic evaluation. *J Pediatr*. 1979;95(1):676-684.
3. Ingelfinger JR, Davis AE, Grupe WE. Frequency and etiology of gross hematuria in a general pediatric setting. *Pediatrics*. 1977;59: 557-561.
4. Rahmam AJ, Naz F, Ashraf S. Significance of pyuria in the diagnosis of urinary tract infections in neonates. *J Pak Med Assoc*. 2011; 61(1):70-73.
5. Jan SL, Wu MC, Lin MC, et al. Pyuria is not always sterile in children with Kawasaki disease. *Pediatr Int*. 2010;52(1):113-117.
6. Shike H, Kanegave JT, Best BM, et al. Pyuria associated with acute Kawasaki disease and fever from other causes. *Pediatr Infect Dis J*. 2009;28(5):440-443.
7. White B. Diagnosis and treatment of urinary tract infections in children. *Am Fam Physician*. 2011;83(4):409-415.
8. Montini G, Tullus K, Hewitt I. Febrile urinary tract infections in children. *N Engl J Med*. 2011;365:239-250.
9. Tworek JA, Wilkinson DS, Walsh MK. The rate of manual microscopic examination of urine sediment: a College of American Pathologists Q-Probes study of 11,243 urinalysis tests from 88 institutions. *Arch Pathol Lab Med*. 2008;132(12):1868-1873.
10. Fallahzadeh MH, Fallahzadeh MK, Shahriari M, et al. Hematuria in patients with Beta-thalassemia major. *Iran J Kidney Dis*. 2010; 4(2):133-136.
11. Alchi B, Jayne D. Membranoproliferative glomerulonephritis. *Pediatr Nephrol*. 2010;25:1409-1418.
12. Jones R, Charlton J, Latinovic R, Gulliford MC. Alarm symptoms and identification of non-cancer diagnoses in primary care: cohort study. *BMJ*. 2009;339:b3094. doi: 10.1136/bmj.b3094.
13. Chiang LW, Jacobsen AS, Ong CL, Huang WS. Persistent sterile pyuria in children? Don't forget tuberculosis! *Singapore Med J*. 2010;51(3):e48-50.
14. Zorc JJ, Levine DA, Platt SL. Clinical and demographic factors associated with urinary tract infection in young febrile infants. *Pediatrics*. 2005;116(3):644-648.
15. Alchi B, Jayne D. Membranoproliferative glomerulonephritis. *Pediatr Nephrol*. 2010;25:1409-1418.
16. Jauhola O, Ronkainen J, Koskimies O, et al. Renal manifestations of Henoch-Schonlein purpura in a 6-month prospective study of 223 children. *Arch Dis Child*. 2010;95(11)877-882.
17. Shaikh N, Morone NE, Lopez J, et al. Does this child have a urinary tract infection? *JAMA*. 2007;298(24):2895-2904.
18. Coley BD, Gunderman R, Bulas D, et al. *Expert Panel on Pediatric Imaging*. ACR Appropriateness Criteria® hematuria - child [online publication]. Reston, VA: American College of Radiology (ACR); 2009. Available at http://www.guideline.gov/content.aspx?id=15750&search=hematuria+children, accessed January 2013.
19. Whiting P, Westwood M, Watt I, et al. Rapid tests and urine sampling techniques for the diagnosis of urinary tract infection (UTI) in children under five years: a systematic review. *BMC Pediatr*. 2005;5(1):4.
20. Subcommittee on Urinary Tract Infection, Steering Committee on Quality Improvement and Management, Roberts KB, Downs SM, Finnell SM, et al. Urinary tract infection: clinical practice guideline for the diagnosis and management of the initial UTI in febrile infants and children 2 to 24 months. *Pediatrics*. 2011; 128(3):595-610.
21. Mori R, Yonemoto N, Fitzgerald A, et al. Diagnostic performance of urine dipstick testing in children with suspected UTI: a systematic review of relationship with age and comparison with microscopy. *Acta Paediatr*. 2010;99(4):581-584.
22. Karmazyn B, Coley BD, Binkovitz LA, et al. *Expert Panel on Pediatric Imaging*. ACR Appropriateness Criteria® urinary tract infection—child [online publication]. Reston, VA: American College of Radiology (ACR); 2012. Available at http://www.guideline.gov/content.aspx?id=37938&search=pyelonephritis+children, accessed January 2013.
23. Hodson EM, Willis NS, Craig JC. Antibiotics for acute pyelonephritis in children. *Cochrane Database Syst Rev*. 2007;(4): CD003772.

24. Institute for Clinical Systems Improvement (ICSI). *Preventive services for children and adolescents*. Bloomington, MN: Institute for Clinical Systems Improvement (ICSI); 2011. Available at http://www.guideline.gov/content.aspx?id=35090&search=urinalysis+and+screening, accessed January 2013.

25. Children's Oncology Group. *Long-term follow-up guidelines for survivors of childhood, adolescent, and young adult cancers*. Sections 38-91: radiation. Bethesda, MD: Children's Oncology Group; 2008 Oct. 117 p. [357 references]. Available at http://www.guideline.gov/content.aspx?id=15470&search=urinalysis+and+screening, accessed January 2013.

26. Cho BS, Hahn WH, Cheong HI, et al. A nationwide study of mass urine screening tests on Korean school children and implications for chronic kidney disease management. *Clin Exp Nephrol*. 2013;17:205-210.

27. Conway PH, Cnaan A, Zaoutis T, et al. Recurrent urinary tract infections in children: risk factors and association with prophylactic antimicrobials. *JAMA*. 2007;298(2):179-186.

28. Montini G, Rigon L, Zucchetta P, et al. IRIS Group. Prophylaxis after first febrile urinary tract infection in children? A multicenter, randomized, controlled, noninferiority trial. *Pediatrics*. 2008;122(5):1064-1071.

65 HYDRONEPHROSIS AND URETEROPELVIC JUNCTION OBSTRUCTION

Debby Chuang, MD
Lynn L. Woo, MD

PATIENT STORY

An otherwise healthy 7-year-old boy presents with a one day history of crampy left-sided abdominal and flank pain associated with nausea and non-bilious vomiting. He is afebrile and denies recent trauma. He is voiding and stooling normally. Exam is unremarkable except for some tenderness to palpation over the left costovertebral angle. Urinalysis is negative for blood or infection. Serum creatinine is within normal limits. Radiographic imaging reveals moderate left-sided hydronephrosis without ureteral dilation and an absence of stones or masses (**Figure 65-1**). The contralateral kidney and bladder are normal. Renal function testing is consistent with obstruction in the left kidney. The boy undergoes surgical repair for ureteropelvic junction obstruction (UPJO). On follow-up, he has resolution of hydronephrosis and his symptoms.

INTRODUCTION

Prenatal detection of congenital abnormalities has significantly increased in the past two decades with advancements in ultrasound technology and improvements in prenatal care. Common genitourinary abnormalities, such as hydronephrosis and UPJO, are not only being identified more frequently in the perinatal period but are also being managed effectively in children at younger ages. Earlier treatment of such conditions is believed to improve the growth and development of the genitourinary system in these children as they mature into adulthood.

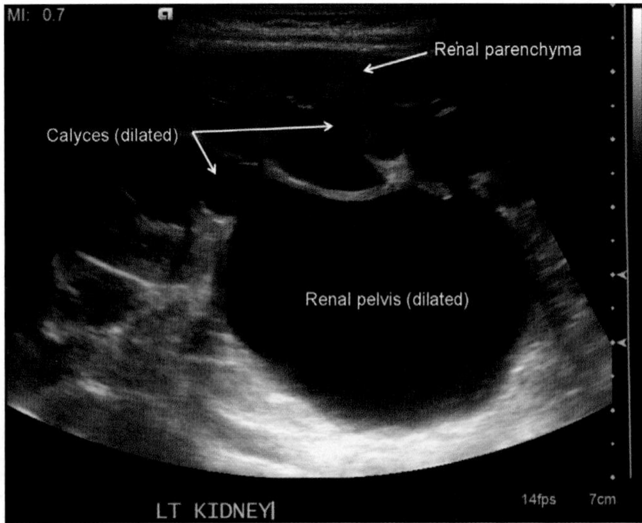

FIGURE 65-1 Ultrasound image of the left kidney. The findings of hydronephrosis with no dilation of the ureter are suggestive of ureteropelvic junction obstruction (UPJO). *(Used with permission from Lynn L. Woo, MD)*

SYNONYMS

- Pelviureteric junction obstruction.
- Proximal ureteral narrowing or stricture.
- Renal pelvic dilation.
- Pelviectasis.

EPIDEMIOLOGY

- Of all congenital abnormalities detected during pregnancy, approximately 20 to 30 percent involve the genitourinary system, with the majority being hydronephrosis.[1–4]
  - Hydronephrosis is defined as abnormal dilation of the renal pelvis, with the anteroposterior diameter of the renal pelvis measured to be ≥5 mm in the perinatal period.[5–7]
  - Hydroureteronephrosis is defined as abnormal dilation of the renal pelvis *and* ipsilateral ureter.
- UPJO is the most common cause of perinatal hydronephrosis, accounting for approximately 40 percent of cases.[8]
- Large population studies have demonstrated a predominance of UPJO in males, with the male-to-female ratio being greater than 2:1, as well as a predilection for occurrence on the left side, particularly among neonates.[9–12]
- Bilateral UPJO has been reported to range from 10 to 40 percent cases.[10,11,13]

RISK FACTORS

- While there have been case reports of UPJO occurring in families,[14–16] there is currently no established genetic predisposition for congenital UPJO.
  - However, recent studies have postulated that abnormalities in various factors involved in nephrogenesis, including bone morphogenetic proteins (BMP's), Wilm's Tumor (WT1) gene, and human leukocyte antigen (HLA) genes, may contribute to familial cases of UPJO.[15,17–19]
- UPJO may often present in association with other congenital renal and non-renal abnormalities.[20]
  - UPJO is found in ≥15 percent cases of horseshoe kidneys, and is reported to also occur with malrotated kidneys.[12,21–25]
  - More than 1/3 of cases of hydronephrosis in ectopic kidneys, particularly pelvic kidneys, are due to UPJO.[25,26]
  - Approximately 20 percent of children with VATER syndrome have UPJO.[27]

ETIOLOGY AND PATHOPHYSIOLOGY

- UPJO may be primary (congenital) or secondary.
- Primary UPJO (**Figure 65-2**).
  - Involves a congenital defect in which there is a narrowing of the ureteral lumen at the ureteropelvic junction that is associated with impairment of urinary transport and renal function.

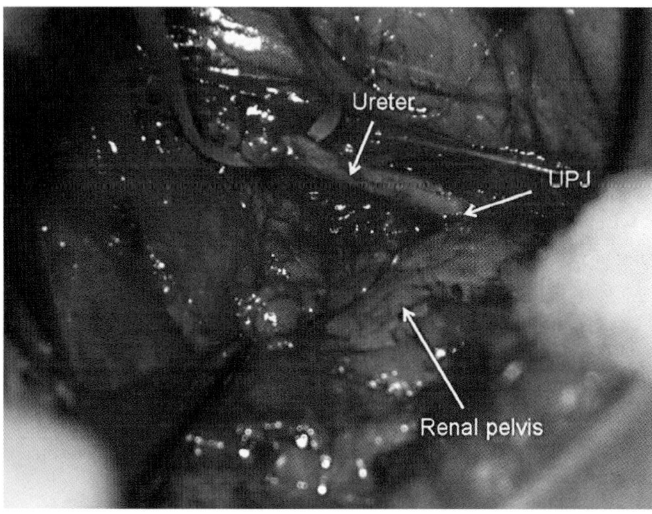

FIGURE 65-2 Intraoperative image of primary congenital UPJO. The ureter is found to be narrowed and kinked at the ureteropelvic junction. The renal pelvis is dilated and filled with urine. (*Used with permission from Lynn L. Woo, MD*)

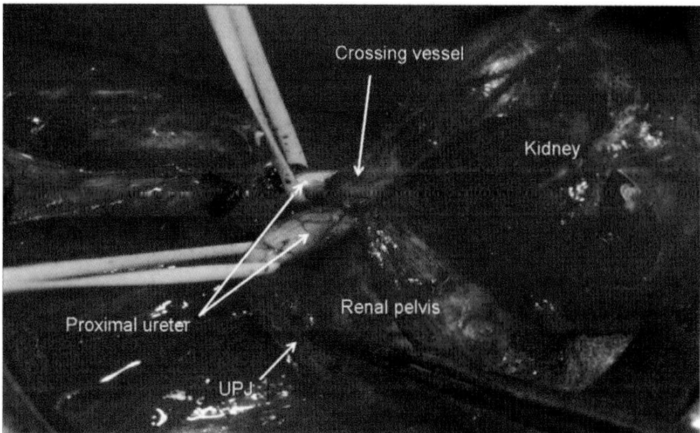

FIGURE 65-4 Intra-operative view of UPJO with crossing vessel. The ureter is identified by the yellow vessel loops, while the crossing vessel is denoted by the red vessel loop. Crossing vessels typically arise from the lower pole of the kidney and cross *anterior* to UPJ or proximal ureter, resulting in "kinking" of the ureter. Whether the aberrant vessel is the primary cause or a co-variable that is associated with intrinsic narrowing is unclear. (*Used with permission from Lynn L. Woo, MD*)

- True underlying etiology is still unknown but is believed to be likely multifactorial.[20,28]
  - Intrinsic factors (**Figure 65-3**).
    - Incomplete recanalization of the ureter during embryologic development.[29,30]
    - Abnormal ureteral muscle and fibrous tissue development that affects ureteral peristalsis.[31,32]
  - Extrinsic factors (**Figure 65-4**).
    - Mechanical obstruction from lower-pole crossing vessel, which can be seen in up to 63 percent cases of UPJO.[33,34]
- Secondary UPJO.
  - Obstruction develops as a result of kinking at the UPJ from a severely dilated and tortuous ureter. The ureteral dilation is most often secondary to severe vesicoureteral reflux or congenital megaureter.

DIAGNOSIS

CLINICAL FEATURES

- As many cases of hydronephrosis and UPJO are detected by prenatal ultrasound imaging, or incidentally during imaging for pediatric trauma, many infants and children will be asymptomatic.
  - Hydronephrosis identified in the prenatal period may spontaneously resolve in the immediate postnatal period.[35]
  - Hydronephrosis identified in the perinatal period may remain stable or spontaneously resolve as a child gets older, obviating the

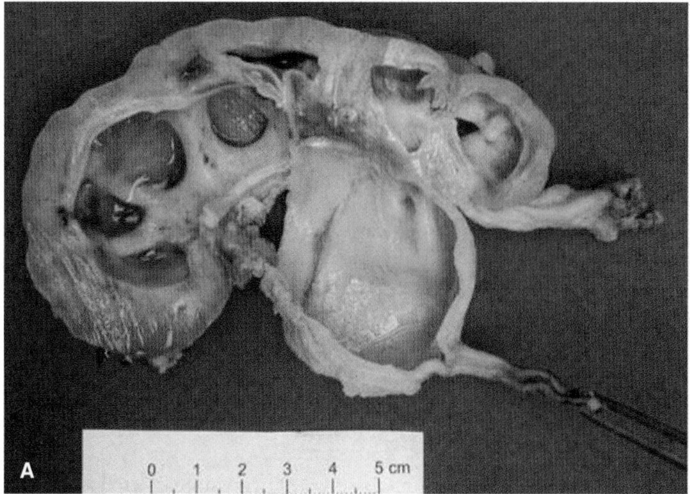

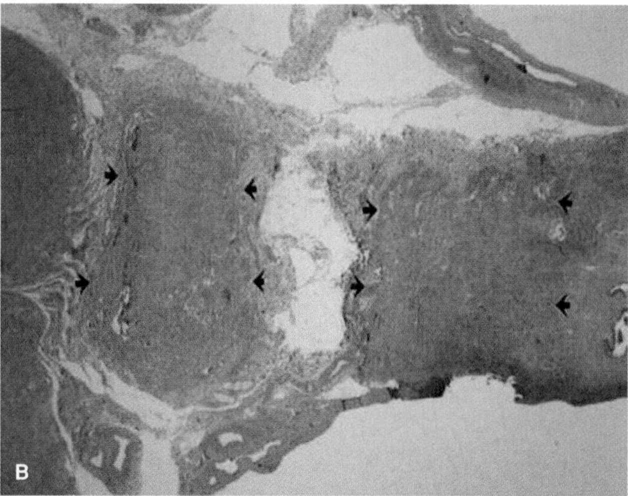

FIGURE 65-3 Pathology of congenital ureteropelvic junction obstruction (UPJO). **A.** Gross specimen of kidney with congenital UPJO. The renal pelvis and all calyces are dilated, and there is marked loss of renal parenchyma. The ureter distal to the UPJ is of normal caliber. **B.** Histologic view of congenital UPJO at lower power. Renal pelvic muscle is at far left. Muscle at the UPJ appears discontinuous, surrounded by two collars of muscle, as indicated by opposing sets of arrows, with disorganized muscle bundle orientation, separated by paucicellular collagenous areas. (*Used with permission from Lynn L. Woo, MD*)

need for any intervention, especially in the absence of symptoms.[36,37]
 - Hydronephrosis is not necessarily indicative of obstruction.
- Symptoms/Presentation.
 - Flank/abdominal pain.
 - Nausea/vomiting (non-bilious).
 - Hematuria.
 - Urinary tract infection.
 - Failure to thrive.
- *Dietl's crisis* describes a combination of episodic upper abdominal pain or flank pain with nausea/vomiting, particularly during diuresis, which is associated with UPJO.
- As children with UPJO may present with abdominal pain, nausea, and vomiting, they may often undergo prior evaluation for gastrointestinal or psychological etiologies before the genitourinary etiology is identified and a referral to a pediatric urologist is made.[38,39]
- Untreated UPJO may be associated with increased risk for failure of the affected renal unit, kidney atrophy, pain, recurrent infections, stone development, and/or hypertension in adulthood.

LABORATORY STUDIES

- Urinalysis may demonstrate gross or microscopic hematuria, thought to be due to rupture of mucosal vessels in the dilated renal pelvis.
- Basic metabolic panel may reveal renal insufficiency, although in the setting of a normal contralateral kidney, this would be unlikely.
 - In evaluating newborns, one must bear in mind that postnatal serum creatinine will reflect maternal serum creatinine until at least 48 hours after birth.

DIAGNOSTIC STUDIES

- Retrograde Pyelogram (**Figure 65-5**).
 - Anatomic study, typically performed at time of surgical repair.
 - Allows confirmation of anatomical abnormality and helps exclude the possibility that the hydronephrosis is actually from a more distal obstructive lesion.

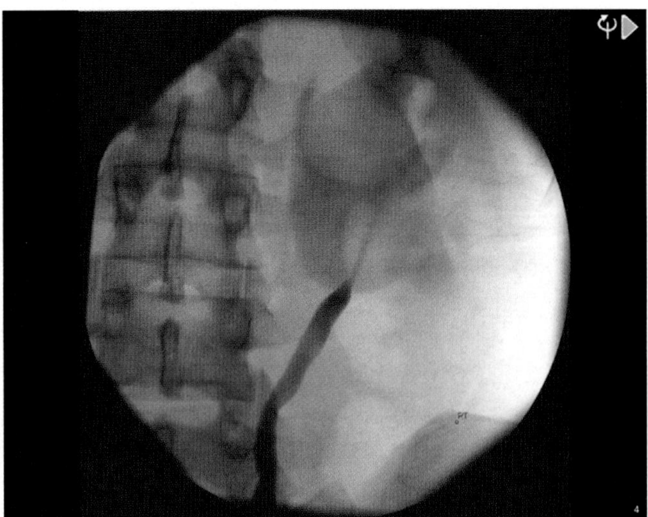

FIGURE 65-5 Retrograde pyelogram of left kidney. The pelvis appears massively dilated with blunted calyces. There is also an area of narrowing at the proximal ureter, consistent with ureteropelvic junction obstruction (UPJO). (*Used with permission from Lynn L. Woo, MD*)

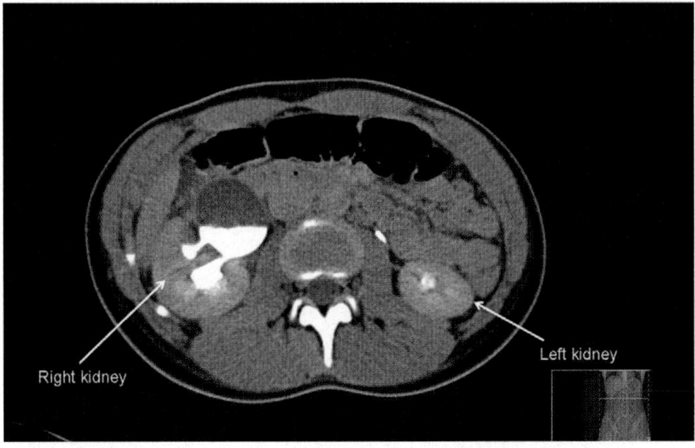

FIGURE 65-6 Computed Tomography of abdomen with intravenous contrast demonstrating right UPJO. The right renal pelvis and calyces are dilated, and contrast can be seen pooling dependently in the collecting system, while the normal left kidney shows normal excretion of contrast into the ureter. (*Used with permission from Lynn L. Woo, MD*)

  - Findings—Dilated renal pelvis with characteristic narrowing or kinking at the UPJ and a distal ureter of normal caliber.
- Ultrasound Imaging (US) (**Figure 65-1**).
 - Anatomic study.
 - Findings suggestive of UPJO:
  - Hydronephrosis or dilated renal pelvis; AP diameter ≥5 mm in children.
  - Non-visualization of the ureter is the rule (as a normal ureter is not dilated, it is usually not visible on US).
  - Thinned parenchyma.
  - Abnormal renal growth.
- Computed Tomography (CT) or Magnetic Resonance Imaging (with or without contrast) (**Figure 65-6**).
 - Anatomic and functional studies, more often used in older children.
 - CT involves considerable radiation exposure and should therefore be minimized in children.
 - Findings suggestive of obstruction:
  - Dilated renal pelvis +/− dilated calyces.
  - Narrowing of ureter at UPJ.
  - Crossing vessel.
  - Delayed uptake or excretion of contrast agent from the affected kidney.
- Diuretic Renography/Renal Flow Scan (**Figure 65-7**).
 - Functional nuclear medicine study.
 - Measures differential renal function as well as renal excretion and drainage.
  - Most commonly used radiotracer agent is technetium-99m. mercaptoacetyltriglycine (*MAG-3*).
  - Furosemide is administered during the study to promote diuresis of agent.
 - Findings suggestive of obstruction:
  - Differential renal function of <40 percent in affected kidney.
  - Impaired or lack of uptake and/or clearance of radiotracer agent.
- Time to clearance of 50 percent tracer agent ($T_{1/2}$).
 - Normal: <10 minutes.

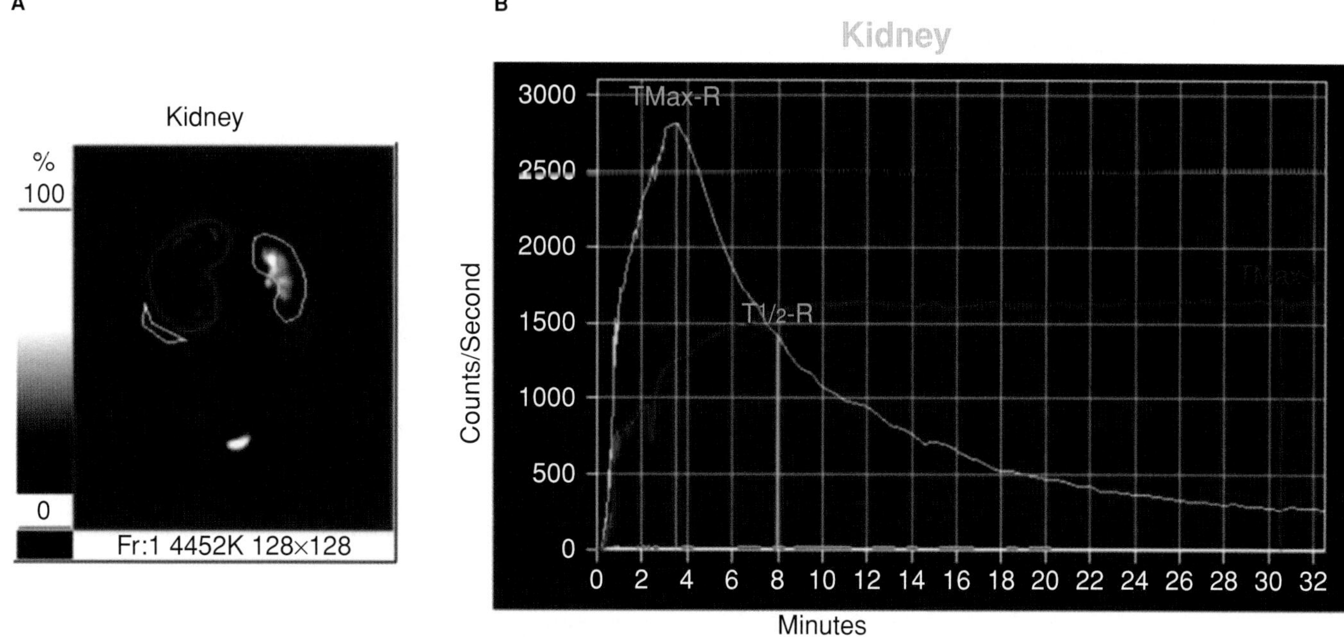

C

Table of Results (Summary)

Parameters	Left	Right	Total
Split Function (%)	28.0	72.0	
Kidney Counts (cpm)	58037	149203	207240
Time of Max (min)	30.5	3.502	
Time of 1/2 Max (min)		7.980	

FIGURE 65-7 MAG-3 Lasix Renal Scan (interpreted from a posterior view). **A.** Differential renal function. The radiotracer uptake is severely diminished in the left kidney (red outline), with the left kidney contributing only 28 percent to overall renal function, and the right kidney (yellow outline) contributing 72 percent to overall renal function. **B.** Renal uptake and excretion. The graph depicts the tracer uptake and excretion pattern for each kidney. The right kidney (yellow) quickly takes up and excretes the tracer. The time it takes to excrete ½ of the maximum tracer agent that was taken up is 7.98 minutes, which is consistent with normal renal function. The left kidney (red) takes up the agent, but does not excrete the agent in the documented time period (30 minutes), as demonstrated by the plateau, which is consistent with obstruction. **C.** Summary of renal differential function and T1/2. (*Used with permission from Lynn L. Woo, MD*)

- Indeterminate: 10 to 20 minutes.
- Obstructed: >20 minutes.

DIFFERENTIAL DIAGNOSIS (OF PEDIATRIC HYDRONEPHROSIS) (FIGURE 65-8)

- Transient/physiologic hydronephrosis.
- Vesicoureteral reflux (backflow of urine into upper collecting system).
- Posterior urethral valves (congenital obstruction of urethra or other bladder outlet obstruction).
- Congenital megaureter.
- Ureterovesical junction obstruction.
- Duplicated collecting system.
- Ectopic ureter (abnormal insertion of ureteral orifice).
- Ureterocele (cystic dilation of distal ureter).
- Obstructing urinary calculus, ureteral polyp or neoplasm.
- Multicystic dysplastic kidney.

MANAGEMENT

- As prenatal hydronephrosis may result from different etiologies and may be obstructive or nonobstructive, referral to a pediatric urologist and close follow-up are necessary for optimal management.
- With improvements in pediatric imaging technology, as well as the expansion in the field of pediatric urology, there has been a growing trend towards more conservative management for hydronephrosis and UPJO.[40,41] SOR C
  - More than 40 percent children with UPJO may not require surgical intervention.[42]
  - Current proposed indications for intervention.[43]
    - Persistent symptoms (pain, nausea, failure to thrive).
    - Significant obstruction on diuretic renal scan.
    - Impairment of overall renal function or abnormal renal growth.
    - Hypertension.
    - Worsening ipsilateral renal function.
    - Recurrent urinary tract infections.

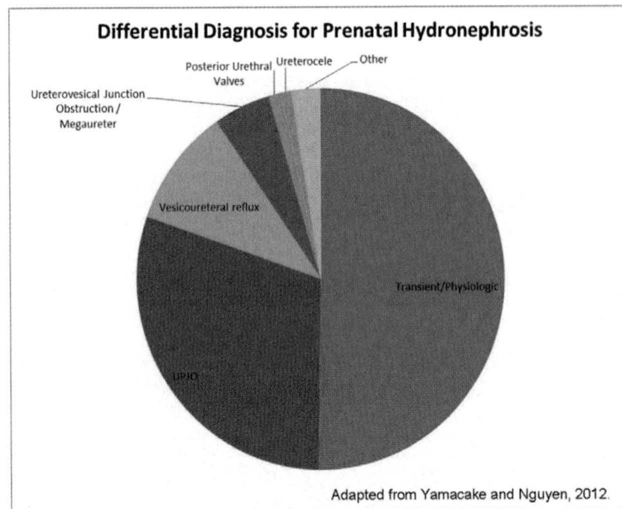

FIGURE 65-8 Differential diagnosis for prenatal hydronephrosis.[65] As most cases of prenatal hydronephrosis will resolve in immediate postnatal period, UPJO is the most common cause of persistent hydronephrosis in the perinatal period. (*Adapted from Yamacake KG, Nguyen HT: Current management of antenatal hydronephrosis. Pediatr Nephrol 2012;28(2):237-243. With kind permission from Springer Science and Business Media.*)

- Development of stone disease.
- Renal failure.

INTERVENTION

- Since its introduction in 1949, the Anderson-Hynes open dismembered pyeloplasty (**Figure 65-9**) has been considered the gold standard for treatment of pediatric UPJO, with success rates reported to be ≥98 percent.[44,45] SOR Ⓐ
    - Even about 90 percent of children with UPJO in poorly functioning kidneys (relative renal function <30%) will demonstrate persistent improvement in post-operative renal function more than three years after pyeloplasty.[46]
- The recent decade has seen a surge in advancement of laparoscopic and robotic pyeloplasty techniques, as well as in endoscopic procedures, all of which are becoming more accepted alternatives to the open dismembered pyeloplasty (**Figure 65-10**).
    - Recent studies have demonstrated that robotic and laparoscopic techniques are feasible and safe, and may have success rates of ≥97 percent.[47,48] SOR Ⓐ
    - Endopyelotomy has been reported to have a 65 percent success rate.[49]
- A ureteral stent is often placed during the pyeloplasty to assist with healing of the anastomosis.
    - Children with ureteral stents placed during the pyeloplasty will need to undergo a subsequent outpatient procedure for stent removal approximately 2 to 6 weeks after the pyeloplasty.

PREVENTION AND SCREENING

- As the etiology of UPJO is still unclear and may be multifactorial, there is currently no known prevention for the development of UPJO.
    - In children with severe VUR or megaureter concurrently with secondary UPJO, early surgical repair may help to prevent the development of symptoms and/or further renal deterioration.
- Most cases of hydronephrosis and UPJO are detected by routine prenatal ultrasound imaging, and patients may be referred to a

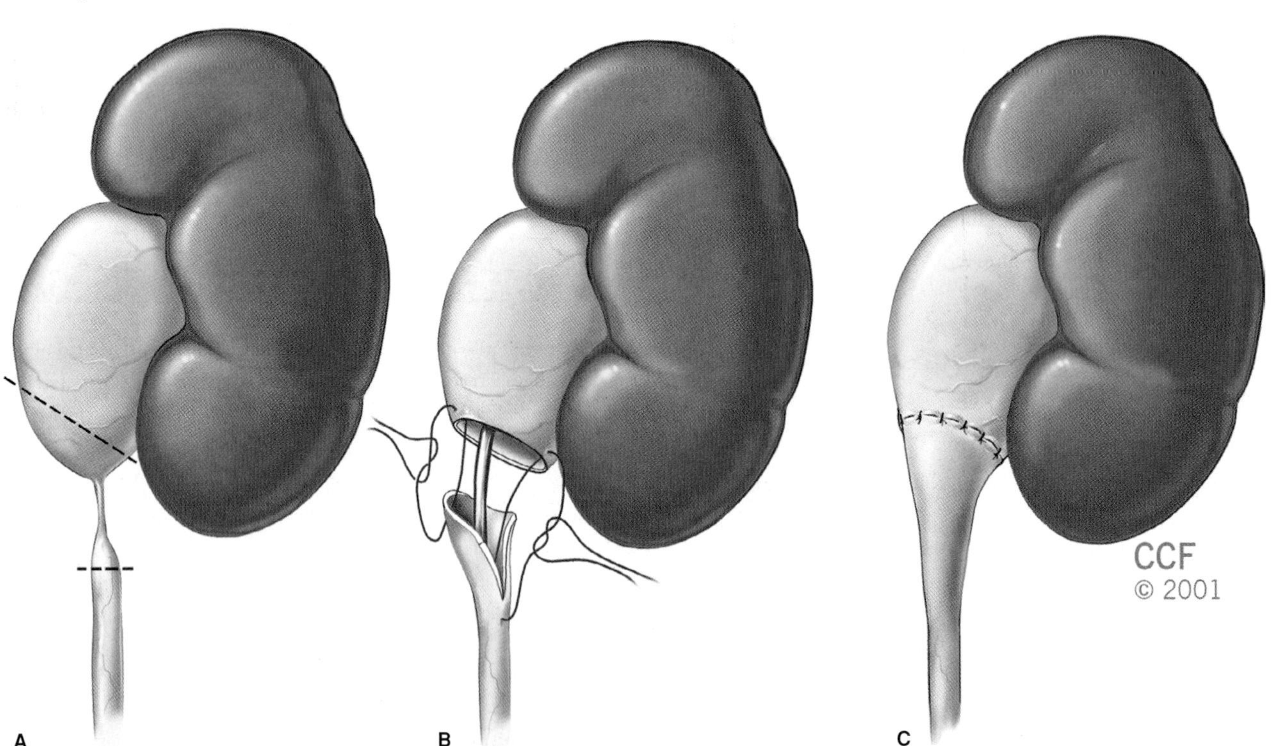

FIGURE 65-9 Illustration of dismembered pyeloplasty. **A.** The area of abnormal ureter is excised. **B.** The ureter is spatulated laterally. **C.** The renal pelvis is then re-anastomosed to the proximal ureter, re-establishing continuity of the UPJ. (Reprinted with permission, Cleveland Clinic Center for Medical Art & Photography © 2001-2013. All Rights Reserved.)

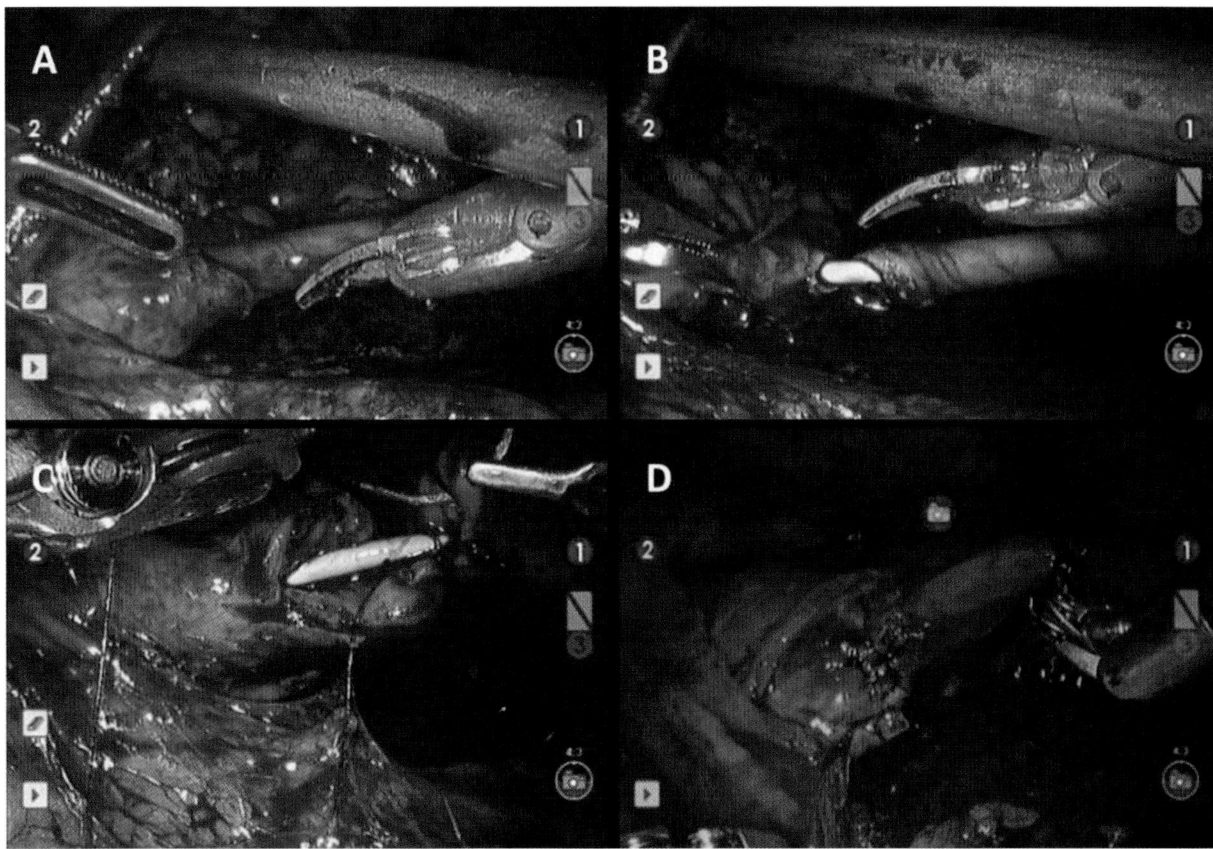

FIGURE 65-10 Robotic-assisted laparoscopic pyeloplasty. The principles of repair are identical to open dismembered pyeloplasty. In this case, a ureteral stent was placed initially. **A.** The UPJ is identified. **B.** The UPJ is transected, revealing narrowing at the renal pelvis. **C.** The pelvis and spatulated ureter are then re-anastomosed over the stent. **D.** The completed repair. (*Used with permission from Lynn L. Woo, MD*)

pediatric urologist for prenatal counseling or shortly after birth, as further imaging studies may be required. Cases of bilateral hydronephrosis should be followed closely in the prenatal period for potential oligohydramnios. There are no additional *screening* studies recommended for hydronephrosis or UPJO.

- Children with recurrent urinary tract infections, fevers, and/or flank or lateralizing abdominal pain should undergo evaluation for infection, as well as renal and bladder ultrasound imaging for detection of possible underlying abnormalities.
- Cases of newly diagnosed hydronephrosis from imaging studies should be referred to a pediatric urologist for further work-up and management.

PROGNOSIS

- The overall risk of obstruction recurrence after surgical repair with pyeloplasty is reported to be as low as 1.3 percent after 5 years.[50]
    - Complete resolution of obstruction is typically seen in up to 94 percent children within the first 3 to 6 months after pyeloplasty.[44,46,51]
    - Preservation of renal function has been reported to persist at least 6 to 19 years after surgery, even into adulthood.[52–54]
    - Risk factors for recurrence are cited to be younger age of initial surgery, prolonged urinary leakage, missed anatomical findings, lack of intra-operative retrograde pyelogram, and dorsal lumbotomy approach.[55,56]

FOLLOW-UP

- While the literature suggests that resolution of obstruction and renal function appears to be stabilized in the long term, there is still a lack of consensus on the optimal amount time needed for follow-up time after pyeloplasty.
    - Most pediatric urologists will follow children with serial ultrasound imaging and/or post-repair diuretic renography to ensure resolution of obstruction.[45,57]
    - With improved and stable renal function, children may be referred back to their pediatrician as early as 2 years after UPJO repair.[20]
- With recurrence of obstruction, a percentage of children may be referred back to a pediatric urologist for management.
    - Recurrent UPJO may result from development of scar tissue or stricture, redundant renal pelvis, and/or persistent or missed crossing vessel.
    - Children may be symptomatic or asymptomatic with recurrent obstruction.
        - Symptomatic children may present in a similar manner as their initial presentation for UPJO (pain, nausea/vomiting, renal insufficiency, or worsening hypertension).

- Imaging may demonstrate hydronephrosis and UPJ narrowing.
- Diuretic renography may reveal obstruction and/or decreased differential renal function.
- Indications for intervention are similar to those for initial UPJO repair.
- Management options.
  - Ureteral stent placement.
    - May provide symptomatic relief from obstruction as well as preserve renal function in the short-term, but not typically considered to be a long-term solution for children.
    - Retrograde pyelogram performed at the time of stent placement may help to delineate the extent of obstruction and length of ureter involved.
- Endopyelotomy.
  - The area of ureteral obstruction can be directly visualized with ureteroscopy and scar or stricture tissue may be excised with cold-knife incision, electrocautery, and/or laser ablation.[58]
  - Success rates have been reported to be as high as 70 percent.[59]
- Endoscopic balloon dilation.
  - Endoscopic dilation of scarred tissue at the ureteropelvic junction.
  - Success rates are variable when compared to endopyelotomy.[58,60]
- Repair of obstruction with re-do pyeloplasty or ureterocalicostomy.
  - Open, laparoscopic, and robotic techniques have been demonstrated to be safe, feasible, and effective, with success rates reported to be >83 percent.[60–63]
- Nephrectomy.
  - Indications for nephrectomy include severe obstruction with significant fibrosis that may prevent surgical repair, poor differential renal function (usually <20%), decreased renal growth/development, recurrent urinary tract infections, and/or persistent and severe symptoms.[64]
  - Considered to be the definitive management for recurrent and persistent UPJO in the setting of poor renal function.

PATIENT RESOURCES

- Your child has hydronephrosis. In: *National Kidney Foundation A to Z Health Guide-Children*. New York, NY: National Kidney Foundation, Inc.; 2012. **http://www.kidney.org/atoz/content/hydronephrosis.cfm**.
- *UPJ Obstruction*. The New York Times Health Guide. The New York Times Company, 2012. **http://health.nytimes.com/health/guides/disease/upj-obstruction/overview.html**.

PROVIDER RESOURCES

- Baskin LS: Congenital ureteropelvic junction obstruction. In: Rose BD (Ed), UpToDate, Watham, MA, 2012.
- Shulam PG: Ureteropelvic junction obstruction. In: Litwin MS, Saigal CS, eds. *Urologic Diseases in America*. US Department of Health and Human Services, Public Health Service, National Institutes of Health, National Institute of Diabetes and Digestive and Kidney Diseases. Washington, DC: US Government Printing Office, 2007: 323-332. **http://kidney.niddk.nih.gov/statistics/uda/Ureteropelvic_Junction_Obstruction-Chapter09.pdf**.

REFERENCES

1. Grisoni ER, Gauderer MW, Wolfson RN, Izant RJ, Jr: Antenatal ultrasonography: the experience in a high risk perinatal center. *J Pediatr Surg*. 1986;21(4):358-361.
2. Elder JS. Antenatal hydronephrosis. Fetal and neonatal management. *Pediatr Clin North Am*. 1997;44(5):1299-1321.
3. Damen-Elias HA, De Jong TP, Stigter RH, Visser GH, Stoutenbeek PH. Congenital renal tract anomalies: outcome and follow-up of 402 cases detected antenatally between 1986 and 2001. *Ultrasound Obstet Gynecol*. 2005;25(2):134-143.
4. Sairam S, Al-Habib A, Sasson S, Thilaganathan B. Natural history of fetal hydronephrosis diagnosed on mid-trimester ultrasound. *Ultrasound Obstet Gynecol*. 2001;17(3):191-196.
5. Coelho GM, Bouzada MC, Pereira AK, Figueiredo BF, Leite MR, Oliveira DS, et al. Outcome of isolated antenatal hydronephrosis: a prospective cohort study. *Pediatr Nephrol*. 2007;22(10):1727-1734.
6. Feldman DM, DeCambre M, Kong E, Borgida A, Jamil M, McKenna P, et al. Evaluation and follow-up of fetal hydronephrosis. *J Ultrasound Med*. 2001;20(10):1065-1069.
7. Scott JE, Renwick M. Antenatal renal pelvic measurements: what do they mean? *BJU Int*. 2001;87(4):376-380.
8. Brown T, Mandell J, Lebowitz RL. Neonatal hydronephrosis in the era of sonography. *AJR Am J Roentgenol*. 1987;148(5):959-963.
9. Johnston JH, Evans JP, Glassberg KI, Shapiro SR. Pelvic hydronephrosis in children: a review of 219 personal cases. *J Urol*. 1977;117(1):97-101.
10. Karnak I, Woo LL, Shah SN, Sirajuddin A, Ross JH. Results of a practical protocol for management of prenatally detected hydronephrosis due to ureteropelvic junction obstruction. *Pediatr Surg Int*. 2009;25(1):61-67.
11. Robson WJ, Rudy SM, Johnston JH. Pelviureteric obstruction in infancy. *J Pediatr Surg*. 1976;11(1):57-61.
12. Snyder HM ,3rd, Lebowitz RL, Colodny AH, Bauer SB, Retik AB. Ureteropelvic junction obstruction in children. *Urol Clin North Am*. 1980;7(2):273-290.
13. Kim YS, Do SH, Hong CH, Kim MJ, Choi SK, Han SW. Does every patient with ureteropelvic junction obstruction need voiding cystourethrography? *J Urol*. 2001;165(6):2305-2307.
14. Dwoskin JY. Ureteropelvic junction obstruction and sibling uropathology. *Urology*. 1979;13(2):153-154.
15. Karami H, Kazemi B, Jabbari M, Rahjoo T, Golshan A. Mutations in intron 8 and intron 9 of Wilms' tumor genes in members of family with ureteropelvic junction obstruction. *Urology*. 2009;74(1):116-118.
16. Cohen B, Goldman SM, Kopilnick M, Khurana AV, Salik JO. Ureteropelvic junction obstruction: its occurrence in 3 members of a single family. *J Urol*. 1978;120(3):361-364.
17. He JL, Liu JH, Liu F, Tan P, Lin T, Li XL. Mutation screening of BMP4 and Id2 genes in Chinese patients with congenital ureteropelvic junction obstruction. *Eur J Pediatr*. 2012;171(3):451-456.
18. Wang GJ, Brenner-Anantharam A, Vaughan ED, Herzlinger D. Antagonism of BMP4 signaling disrupts smooth muscle investment

of the ureter and ureteropelvic junction. *J Urol*. 2009;181(1): 401-407.

19. Klemme L, Fish AJ, Rich S, Greenberg B, Senske B, Segall M. Familial ureteral abnormalities syndrome: genomic mapping, clinical findings. *Pediatr Nephrol*. 1998;12(5):349-356.

20. Carr M, Casale P. Anomalies and surgery of the ureter in children. In: Wein A, Kavoussi L, Novick A, Partin A, Peters C, eds. *Campbell-Walsh Urology*, 10th ed.; 2011:3212-3235.

21. Pitts WR, Jr, Muecke EC. Horseshoe kidneys: a 40-year experience. *J Urol*. 1975;113(6):743-746.

22. Das S, Amar AD. Ureteropelvic junction obstruction with associated renal anomalies. *J Urol*. 1984;131(5):872-874.

23. Kolln CP, Boatman DL, Schmidt JD, Flocks RH. Horseshoe kidney: a review of 105 patients. *J Urol*. 1972;107(2):203-204.

24. Bove P, Ong AM, Rha KH, Pinto P, Jarrett TW, Kavoussi LR. Laparoscopic management of ureteropelvic junction obstruction in patients with upper urinary tract anomalies. *J Urol*. 2004; 171(1):77-79.

25. Jabbour ME, Goldfischer ER, Klima WJ, Stravodimos KG, Smith AD. Endopyelotomy after failed pyeloplasty: the long-term results. *J Urol*. 1998;160(3):690-693.

26. Gleason PE, Kelalis PP, Husmann DA, Kramer SA. Hydronephrosis in renal ectopia: incidence, etiology and significance. *J Urol*. 1994; 151(6):1660-1661.

27. Uehling DT, Gilbert E, Chesney R. Urologic implications of the VATER association. *J Urol*. 1983;129(2):352-354.

28. Yiee JH, Johnson-Welch S, Baker LA, Wilcox DT. Histologic differences between extrinsic and intrinsic ureteropelvic junction obstruction. *Urology* 2010;76(1):181-184.

29. Alcaraz A, Vinaixa F, Tejedo-Mateu A, Fores MM, Gotzens V, Mestres CA, et al. Obstruction and recanalization of the ureter during embryonic development. *J Urol*. 1991;145(2):410-416.

30. Ruano-Gil D, Coca-Payeras A, Tejedo-Mateu A. Obstruction and normal recanalization of the ureter in the human embryo. Its relation to congenital ureteric obstruction. *Eur Urol*. 1975; 1(6):287-293.

31. Hanna MK, Jeffs RD, Sturgess JM, Barkin M. Ureteral structure and ultrastructure. Part II. Congenital ureteropelvic junction obstruction and primary obstructive megaureter. *J Urol*. 1976; 116(6):725-730.

32. Gosling JA, Dixon JS. Functional obstruction of the ureter and renal pelvis. A histological and electron microscopic study. *Br J Urol*. 1978;50(3):145-152.

33. Richstone L, Seideman CA, Reggio E, Bluebond-Langner R, Pinto PA, Trock B, et al. Pathologic findings in patients with ureteropelvic junction obstruction and crossing vessels. *Urology*. 2009;73(4):716-719.

34. Zeltser IS, Liu JB, Bagley DH. The incidence of crossing vessels in patients with normal ureteropelvic junction examined with endoluminal ultrasound. *J Urol*. 2004;172(6):2304-2307.

35. Scott JE, Renwick M. Urological anomalies in the Northern Region Fetal Abnormality Survey. *Arch Dis Child*. 1993;68(1): 22-26.

36. Ulman I, Jayanthi VR, Koff SA. The long-term followup of newborns with severe unilateral hydronephrosis initially treated nonoperatively. *J Urol*. 2000;164(3):1101-1105.

37. Koff SA. Postnatal management of antenatal hydronephrosis using an observational approach. *Urology*. 2000;55(5):609-611.

38. Alagiri M, Polepalle SK. Dietl's crisis: an under-recognized clinical entity in the pediatric population. *Int Braz J Urol*. 2006; 32(4):451-453.

39. Flotte TR. Dietl syndrome: intermittent ureteropelvic junction obstruction as a cause of episodic abdominal pain. *Pediatrics*. 1988;82(5):792-794.

40. Heinlen JE, Manatt CS, Bright BC, Kropp BP, Campbell JB, Frimberger D. Operative versus nonoperative management of ureteropelvic junction obstruction in children. *Urology*. 2009; 73(3):521-525.

41. Ross SS, Kardos S, Krill A, Bourland J, Sprague B, Majd M, et al. Observation of infants with SFU grades 3-4 hydronephrosis: worsening drainage with serial diuresis renography indicates surgical intervention and helps prevent loss of renal function. *J Pediatr Urol*. 2011;7(3):266-271.

42. Chertin B, Pollack A, Koulikov D, Rabinowitz R, Hain D, Hadas-Halpren I, et al. Conservative treatment of ureteropelvic junction obstruction in children with antenatal diagnosis of hydronephrosis: lessons learned after 16 years of follow-up. *Eur Urol*. 2006;49(4): 734-738.

43. Nakada S, Hsu T. Management of upper urinary tract obstruction. In: Wein A, Kavoussi L, Novick A, Partin A, Peters C, eds. *Campbell-Walsh Urology, 10th ed*; 2011:1122-1168.

44. Salem YH, Majd M, Rushton HG, Belman AB. Outcome analysis of pediatric pyeloplasty as a function of patient age, presentation and differential renal function. *J Urol*. 1995;154(5):1889-1893.

45. Pohl HG, Rushton HG, Park JS, Belman AB, Majd M. Early diuresis renogram findings predict success following pyeloplasty. *J Urol*. 2001;165(6):2311-2315.

46. Bansal R, Ansari MS, Srivastava A, Kapoor R. Long-term results of pyeloplasty in poorly functioning kidneys in the pediatric age group. *J Pediatr Urol*. 2012;8(1):25-28.

47. Blanc T, Muller C, Abdoul H, Peev S, Paye-Jaouen A, Peycelon M, et al. Retroperitoneal Laparoscopic Pyeloplasty in Children: Long-Term Outcome and Critical Analysis of 10-Year Experience in a Teaching Center. *Eur Urol*. 2012;11.

48. Singh P, Dogra PN, Kumar R, Gupta NP, Nayak B, Seth A. Outcomes of robot-assisted laparoscopic pyeloplasty in children: a single center experience. *J Endourol*. 2012;26(3):249-253.

49. Kim EH, Tanagho YS, Traxel EJ, Austin PF, Figenshau RS, Coplen DE. Endopyelotomy for Pediatric Ureteropelvic Junction Obstruction: A Review of our 25-Year Experience. *J Urol*. 2012;188(4):1628-1633.

50. Psooy K, Pike JG, Leonard MP. Long-term followup of pediatric dismembered pyeloplasty: how long is long enough? *J Urol*. 2003 May;169(5):1809-1812; author reply 1812.

51. Almodhen F, Jednak R, Capolicchio JP, Eassa W, Brzezinski A, El-Sherbiny M. Is routine renography required after pyeloplasty? *J Urol*. 2010;184(3):1128-1133.

52. O'Reilly PH, Brooman PJ, Mak S, Jones M, Pickup C, Atkinson C, et al. The long-term results of Anderson-Hynes pyeloplasty. *BJU Int*. 2001;87(4):287-289.

53. Boubaker A, Prior JO, Meyrat B, Bischof Delaloye A, McAleer IM, Frey P. Unilateral ureteropelvic junction obstruction in children: long-term followup after unilateral pyeloplasty. *J Urol.* 2003;170(1):575-579.

54. Chertin B, Pollack A, Koulikov D, Rabinowitz R, Shen O, Hain D, et al. Does renal function remain stable after puberty in children with prenatal hydronephrosis and improved renal function after pyeloplasty? *J Urol*. 2009;182(4):1845-1848.

55. Braga LH, Lorenzo AJ, Bagli DJ, Keays M, Farhat WA, Khoury AE, et al. Risk factors for recurrent ureteropelvic junction obstruction after open pyeloplasty in a large pediatric cohort. *J Urol*. 2008;180(4):1684-1688.

56. Lim DJ, Walker RD, 3rd. Management of the failed pyeloplasty. *J Urol.* 1996;156(2):738-740.

57. Nirmal TJ, Singh JC. Follow-up after pyeloplasty: How long? *Indian J Urol*. 2008;24(3):429-430.

58. Park J, Kim WS, Hong B, Park T, Park HK. Long-term outcome of secondary endopyelotomy after failed primary intervention for ureteropelvic junction obstruction. *Int J Urol*. 2008;15(6):490-494.

59. Veenboer PW, Chrzan R, Dik P, Klijn AJ, de Jong TP. Secondary endoscopic pyelotomy in children with failed pyeloplasty. *Urology*. 2011;77(6):1450-1454.

60. Thomas JC, DeMarco RT, Donohoe JM, Adams MC, Pope JC, 4th, Brock JW, 3rd edition: Management of the failed pyeloplasty: a contemporary review. *J Urol.* 2005;174(6):2363-2366.

61. Shapiro EY, Cho JS, Srinivasan A, Seideman CA, Huckabay CP, Andonian S, et al. Long-term follow-up for salvage laparoscopic pyeloplasty after failed open pyeloplasty. *Urology* 2009;73(1): 115-118.

62. Sundaram CP, Grubb RL, 3rd, Rehman J, Yan Y, Chen C, Landman J, et al. Laparoscopic pyeloplasty for secondary ureteropelvic junction obstruction. *J Urol.* 2003;169(6):2037-2040.

63. Niver BE, Agalliu I, Bareket R, Mufarrij P, Shah O, Stifelman MD. Analysis of robotic-assisted laparoscopic pyleloplasty for primary versus secondary repair in 119 consecutive cases. *Urology*. 2012; 79(3):689-694.

64. Helmy TE, Sarhan OM, Hafez AT, Elsherbiny MT, Dawaba ME, Ghali AM. Surgical management of failed pyeloplasty in children: single-center experience. *J Pediatr Urol*. 2009;5(2):87-89.

65. Yamacake KG, Nguyen HT. Current management of antenatal hydronephrosis. *Pediatr Nephrol*. 2012.

66 POLYCYSTIC KIDNEYS

Mindy A. Smith, MD, MS

PATIENT STORY

A 17-year-old boy is seen in the office with mild abdominal pain and blood in his urine noticed after playing football with his friends. Exam is significant only for left flank tenderness and his vital signs, including blood pressure, are normal. His urine tests positive for blood (3+) and 1+ protein; microscopic urinalysis reveals numerous red blood cells but no white blood cells or casts. On further questioning, his mother reports that the boy's father and paternal aunt have some type of "kidney problem" but she and his father have been divorced for many years and he rarely sees his father. An ultrasound reveals bilateral enlarged kidneys with multiple cysts and a calculus in the left kidney. A CT scan confirms the diagnoses (**Figure 66-1**).

INTRODUCTION

Polycystic kidney disease (PKD) is a manifestation of a group of inherited disorders resulting in renal cyst development. In the most common form, autosomal-dominant polycystic kidney disease (ADPKD), extensive epithelial-lined cysts develop in the kidney; in some cases, abnormalities also occur in the liver, pancreas, brain, arterial blood vessels, or a combination of these sites. In autosomal recessive polycystic disease (ARPKD), the disease primarily causes enlarged cystic kidneys and hepatic fibrosis and usually presents in infancy. The cysts in ARPKD form only in the collecting tubule and are smaller and typically not visible on gross examination.

EPIDEMIOLOGY

- Most common tubular disorder of the kidney, affecting 1 in 300 individuals.
- Autosomal dominant in 90 percent of cases.[1] The majority of cases of ADPKD are diagnosed in adults but can be diagnosed at any age.[2] In a German population study, the overall prevalence of ADPKD was 32.7/100,000 reaching a maximum of 57.3/100,000 in the 6th decade of life.[3]
- Sporadic mutation in approximately 1:1000 individuals.
- ADPKD accounts for approximately 5 to 10 percent of cases of end-stage renal disease (ESRD) in the US.
- ADPKD is most frequently seen in the third and fourth decades of life, but can be diagnosed at any age.
- ARPKD is estimated to occur in 1:10,000 to 1:40,000 live births, although this may be an underestimate as severely affected neonates do not survive beyond the first few days of life and may not be correctly diagnosed.[2]
- Both diseases are seen in all races and ethnicities and affect males and females equally.

ETIOLOGY AND PATHOPHYSIOLOGY

- ADPKD results from mutations in either of 2 genes that encode plasma membrane–spanning polycystin 1 (PKD1) and polycystin 2 (PKD2).[4] Polycystins regulate tubular and vascular development in the kidneys and other organs (liver, brain, heart, and pancreas). PKD1 and PKD2 are colocalized in primary cilia and appear to mediate Ca^{2+} signaling as a mechanosensor, essential for maintaining the differentiated state of epithelia lining tubules in the kidney and biliary tract.[5]
- In ADPKD, few (1% to 5%) nephrons actually develop cysts. The remaining renal parenchyma shows varying degrees of tubular atrophy, interstitial fibrosis, and nephrosclerosis.
- ADPKD can also be a component of tuberous sclerosis.[2]
- In ADPKD, cysts are also found in other organs such as liver (**Figure 66-2**), spleen, pancreas, and ovaries; liver cysts are found

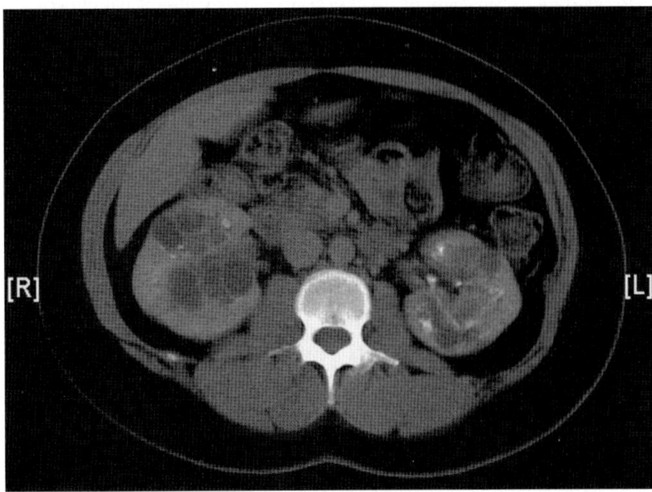

FIGURE 66-1 Polycystic kidneys in a patient with hematuria. (*Used with permission from Michael Freckleton, MD.*)

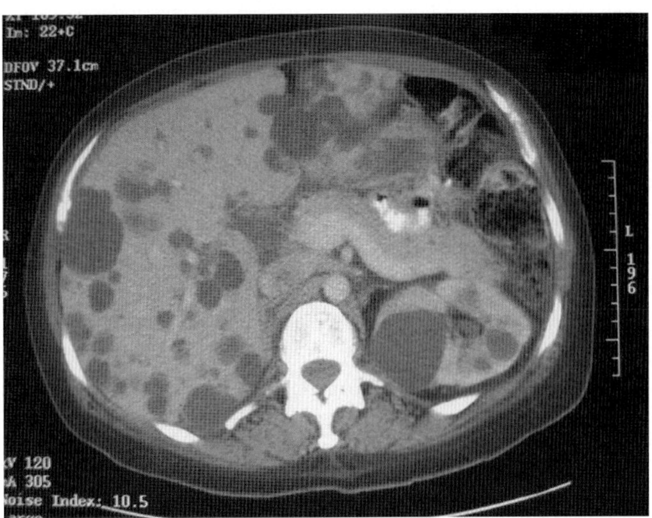

FIGURE 66-2 CT scan showing multiple liver cysts and multiple cysts in both kidneys in a patient with polycystic kidney disease. (*Used with permission from Vesselin Dimov, MD, Cleveland Clinic, ClinicalCases.org.*)

in up to 80 percent of patients with ADPKD.[3] There is also an increased incidence of intracranial aneurysms (5% to 12%).

- ARPKD, previously thought to be the neonatal form of PKD, is caused by genetic mutations in PKHD1 (polycystic kidney hepatic disease 1). This gene encodes the protein, fibrocystin/polyductin, that is localized to cilia/basal body and complexes with PKD2. This large, receptor-like protein is thought to be involved in the tubulogenesis and/or maintenance of duct-lumen architecture of epithelium.
- ARPKD can be associated with pulmonary hypoplasia, generally as a result of the oligohydramnios (Potter's) sequence.[2]
- In one study of young patients (mean age 16 years) with ADPKD, serum log(10) vascular endothelial growth factor was negatively correlated with creatinine clearance indicating a possible role for angiogenesis in the early progression of renal disease in these patients.[6]
- Rare syndromic forms of PKD include defects of the eye, central nervous system, digits, and/or neural tube.[5]
- A variant of PKD is glomerulocystic kidney (GCK), which refers to a kidney with greater than 5 percent cystic glomeruli.[7] This condition is usually diagnosed in young patients. Although PKD-associated gene mutations have been excluded in many cases, there is a familial form of GCK presenting with cystic kidneys, hyperuricemia, and isosthenuria (concentration similar to plasma).[7]

DIAGNOSIS

Family history is a useful tool for diagnosing early ADPKD.

CLINICAL FEATURES

- ADPKD is usually asymptomatic in children, diagnosed incidentally on imaging studies done for other reasons.[2]
- Chronic flank pain as a result of the mass effect of enlarged kidneys.
- Acute pain with infection, obstruction, or hemorrhage into a cyst.
- Enlarged liver.
- Hypertension is common in adults (75%) and is present in 10 to 30 percent of children. Left ventricular hypertrophy can be seen in adolescents/young adults even before overt hypertension is present.[2]
- Mitral valve prolapse (MVP) occurs in up to 15 percent of children and adults with ADPKD.[2]
- Gross hematuria or urinary tract infection; the former can effect up to 40 percent of patients.[2] Because renal cysts can be disconnected from the urinary tract, infection can result in abscess; persistent fever and flank pain should raise suspicion even if the urine culture is negative.[2]
- Kidney stones (calcium oxalate and uric acid) develop in 15 to 20 percent of affected individuals because of urinary stasis from distortion of the collecting system, low urine pH, and low urinary citrate. Kidney stones are uncommon in children, but have been reported in children as young as age 11 years.[8]
- Nocturia can also be present from impaired renal concentrating ability.
- In a Danish study, low birth weight was a risk factor for earlier onset of ESRD in patients with ADPKD as was male gender and increased mean arterial pressure.[9]
- Up to half the cases of ARPKD are diagnosed prenatally, usually with evidence of its sequelae (e.g., oligohydramnios, pulmonary hypoplasia).[2] Neonates and infants can present with palpable flank masses, hepatomegaly, hypertension, or respiratory distress due to pulmonary hypoplasia.[2]
- The diagnosis of children with ARPKD is clinical, based on the presence of enlarged, echogenic kidneys and one or more of the following: absence of renal cysts in both parents; history of a previously affected sibling; parental consanguinity; or clinical, laboratory, or pathologic features of hepatic fibrosis.[2]
- A small subset of patients with ARPKD present as older children or young adults with hepatic (portal hypertension, hepatomegaly) and/or renal disease.[2]
- In a case series of Brazilian patients with ARPKD ($N = 25$), median age at diagnosis was 61 months, half had arterial hypertension, 40 percent had urinary tract infections, almost 1/3 had portal hypertension, and about 1/4 had chronic kidney disease stage ≥2.[10]

LABORATORY TESTING

- Gross or microscopic hematuria (60% with ADPKD).[4] Obtain a urinalysis to document hematuria and a complete blood count or hemoglobin to identify anemia.
- Genetic testing is available for both disorders but is unnecessary in patients with a family history and typical appearance of bilateral renal cysts. Screening asymptomatic children with a family history of ADPKD is not recommended due to financial and psychosocial concerns and lack of disease-specific treatment; annual monitoring of blood pressure and urine (hematuria, proteinuria) should be considered, with additional evaluation as needed.[2] In one retrospective study, renal outcomes were similar between children with ADPKD diagnosed by screening or presenting with symptoms.[11]

IMAGING

- Diagnosis is often made with ultrasound. More than 80 percent of patients with ADPKD have cysts present by age 20 years and 100 percent by age 30 years. In one study, the sensitivity of ultrasound in at-risk individuals younger than age 30 years was 70 to 95 percent, depending on the type of PKD present.[12] For younger patients or those with small cysts, CT scan (**Figures 66-1** and **66-2**) or MRI can be helpful. Authors of one case series found MRI satisfactory for following total kidney and cyst volume in children with ADPKD.[13]
- In the neonatal period, ultrasound of patients with ARPKD shows markedly enlarged echogenic kidneys, indicating the presence of numerous microscopic cysts not discernible by ultrasound (**Figure 66-3**).[2] Larger cysts, more typical of ADPKD, are usually absent in neonates.
- Over time, the appearance of the kidneys in patients with ARPKD looks similar to ADPKD.[2]
- Children with ADPKD can have asymmetric involvement or even isolated unilateral cysts.[2] Because simple cysts are rare in children, the finding of a single cyst in a patient at-risk for ADPKD is considered diagnostic by some authors.
- If an infected cyst is suspected, positron emission tomography has been reported to be the optimal test.[14]

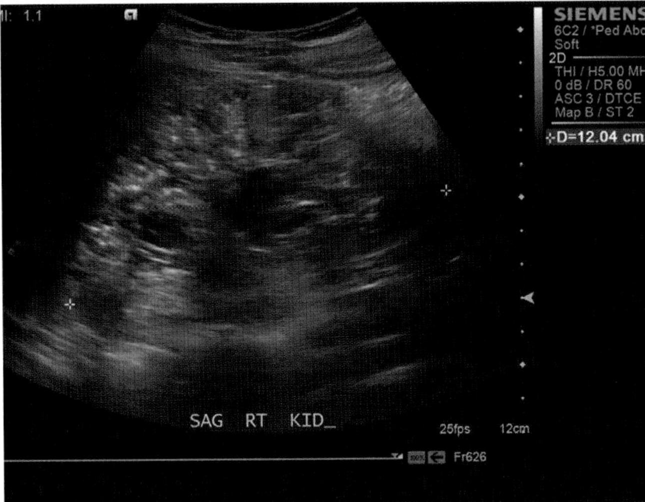

FIGURE 66-3 Autosomal-dominant polycystic kidney disease in an eight-year-old boy. Note the multiple bright echoes through both kidneys due to many interfaces of the numerous small cysts. *(Used with permission from Karl Rew, MD.)*

- In patients with ADPKD, cysts are commonly found in the liver (50% to 80%) (**Figure 66-2**), spleen, pancreas, and ovaries.
- Age-dependent ultrasound criteria have been established for both diagnosis and disease exclusion in subjects at risk of PKD1 (the more severe disorder),[15] but criteria for at-risk children have not been established.[2]
- Transient elastography can be useful in detecting liver fibrosis in cystic kidney diseases.[16]

DIFFERENTIAL DIAGNOSIS[2]

- Simple cyst—Diagnosed at any age; few cysts seen; benign features.
- Acquired cystic disease—Diagnosed in adulthood; few to many cysts; cyst development preceded by renal failure.
- Tuberous sclerosis—Diagnosed at any age; few to many renal angiomyolipomas; inherited nonmalignant tumors grow in the skin, brain/nervous system, kidneys, and heart.

MANAGEMENT

The current role of therapy in PKD is to slow the rate of progression of renal disease and minimize symptoms. However, specific treatments are on the horizon.

NONPHARMACOLOGIC

- Neither protein restriction nor tight blood pressure control decreased the decline in glomerular filtration rate (GFR) in clinical trials.[17,18] However, in a UK population study, increasing coverage (from 7% to 46% of the population prescribed an antihypertensive agent) showed a trend towards decreasing mortality, and increased intensity of antihypertensive therapy was associated with decreasing mortality in people with ADPKD.[19]
- Nutritional interventions in animal PKD studies shown to be beneficial are avoidance of caffeine, consumption of soy-based protein or flaxseed, and increased water consumption; none have been tested in human studies.[2]
- For episodes of gross hematuria, one author recommends bed rest, analgesics, and hydration sufficient to increase the urinary flow rate to 2 to 3 L/day; hematuria generally declines to microscopic levels in a few days.[4] SOR Ⓒ

MEDICATIONS

- Control blood pressure to reduce the risk of associated cardiovascular disease. SOR Ⓐ
- In one randomized controlled trial (RCT) (N = 46 patients with ADPKD and hypertension), no differences in renal function, urinary albumin excretion, or left ventricular mass index were detected between those treated with ramipril versus metoprolol, during 3 years of follow-up.[20] Renal function declined significantly in both groups. Angiotensin-converting enzyme (ACE) inhibitors and angiotensin receptor blockers are the traditionally used agents for children with chronic kidney disease, including ADPKD and ARPKD, and hypertension but have not been tested in this population. SOR Ⓒ Patients with ARPKD can require several medications to control hypertension.[2]
- There is an ongoing RCT of children and young adults with ADPKD already on an ACE inhibitor to assess the effect of pravastatin treatment on renal and cardiovascular disease progression.[21]
- Treat infection as early as possible. If pyocyst is suspected, agents that penetrate cysts such as trimethoprim-sulfamethoxazole and ciprofloxacin are used. SOR Ⓒ
- Future therapies focus on exploiting signaling mechanisms underlying disease pathogenesis. Experimental and observational studies suggest that the mammalian target of rapamycin (mTOR) pathway plays a critical role in cyst growth.
- A 2-year RCT of the mTOR inhibitor everolimus for patients with ADPKD (N = 46) demonstrated a slowing of the increase in total kidney volume over placebo but not the progression of renal impairment.[22] An open-label trial (N = 100 patients with ADPKD and early chronic kidney disease) of the mTOR inhibitor sirolimus did not show slowing of kidney growth or improved function over standard care.[23]
- In a RCT of octreotide (a long-acting somatostatin analog) versus placebo for patients with polycystic liver disease (some of whom had ADPKD), patients with ADPKD randomized to octreotide had a stabilization of kidney volume (versus an increase in the control group) and all patients randomized to treatment showed a reduced liver volume; there was no difference between groups in GFR.[24]

SURGERY AND OTHER PROCEDURES

- Cyst puncture and a sclerosing agent (i.e., ethanol) can be used for painful cysts. SOR Ⓒ Alternatives include decortication (unroofing of the cyst) or denervation.[2]
- For painful liver enlargement, partial hepatectomy can be performed, with good outcomes reported at experienced centers;[25] this is rarely a problem in children. SOR Ⓒ

- For patients with ESRD as a result of PKD, transplantation and dialysis are options.
- In a nationwide study of 15-year outcomes following renal transplantation (N = 534 patients with ADPKD and 4779 patients without ADPKD), patients with ADPKD had better graft survival and no difference in infections, but more thromboembolic complications, more metabolic complications, and increased incidence of hypertension.[26]
- Combined liver-kidney transplantation are also considered for patients with PKD and significant liver involvement.[2]

REFERRAL

- Patients with PKD with progressive renal failure and/or ESRD should be managed by a team of providers as they often require dialysis or kidney transplantation and can develop multiple complications; other considerations include anemia management, aneurysm screening pre-transplantation, and nephrectomy of the native ADPKD kidneys.[27] SOR Ⓒ
- Consider hospitalization for patients with PKD who develop acute pyelonephritis and symptomatic cyst infection.[4]

PROGNOSIS

- Approximately 50 percent of patients with ADPKD progress slowly to ESRD; kidney failure requiring renal-replacement therapy typically develops in the fourth to sixth decade of life.[26] Patients with ADPKD and ESRD seem to have more favorable outcomes compared to those with other causes of kidney failure.[28]
- The following are the characteristics that predict a faster rate of decline in GFR in persons with ADPKD:[29]
  - Greater serum creatinine (independent of GFR).
  - Greater urinary protein excretion.
  - Higher mean arterial pressure (MAP).
  - Young age.
  - Increased kidney volume (>1500 mL).[2]
  - Disease caused by PKD1 mutation.[2,30]
  - The presence of tubulointerstitial fibrosis.[31]
  - Urinary stones.[32]
- The vast majority of pediatric patients with ADPKD, however, have normal renal function throughout childhood.[2]
- ARPKD phenotype is highly variable ranging from causing neonatal death to causing minimal kidney disease presenting later in life.[5] Estimated mortality in the neonatal period is 30 percent; 10-year survival of children who survive the neonatal period is about 80 percent.[33] About one third progress to ESRD in the first decade of life and an additional 20 to 30 percent will progress during adolescence.[2] The renal survival rate is only 42 percent by adulthood.[2]
- In a small retrospective study of 14 patients aged 3 to 24 years with ARPKD who underwent renal transplantation with or without liver transplantation, first renal graft survival was 92 percent at 1 year but only 14 percent by 10 years post-transplantation. Mortality rate was 21 percent (3/14) and was directly related to infectious complications (recurrent angiocholitis) or severe dilatation of hepatic bile ducts.[34] Outcomes were better in another study of 15 combined liver kidney transplants performed in 14 pediatric patients (median age 8 years, of whom 7 had ARPKD).[35] Six patients had postoperative bleeding complications and three required operative revision for intra-abdominal bleeding. Half needed dialysis but 1- and 5-year patient survival was 100 percent and 1- and 5-year graft survival was 80 percent for the liver and 93 percent for the kidney allograft.
- Patients with ADPKD are more prone to kidney stones (Chapter 68, Kidney Stones)[36] and cerebral aneurysms (present in 10% to 12% of adults).[2]
- Neonates can develop respiratory distress, oliguria, fluid and electrolyte abnormalities and hypertension.[2] In the case series noted above of 25 children with ARPKD, after an average follow-up time of 152 months, arterial hypertension was detected in 76 percent of the cases (up from half), portal hypertension in 68 percent (up from 32%), CKD ≥2 in 44 percent (up from 24%), and UTI in 52 percent.[10]

FOLLOW-UP

- Monitor patient's renal function and watch for hypertension and posttransplantation diabetes mellitus; imaging to assess the rate of increased kidney and total cyst volume can be useful in prognosis.[37]
- For all patients with PKD with renal dysfunction, review medications to adjust for level of kidney function and avoid nephrotoxic drugs if possible. SOR Ⓒ
- Management of metabolic derangements (e.g., hyperkalemia, metabolic acidosis, anemia, metabolic bone disease) is also needed, particularly in children with ARPKD.[2]
- Attention to feeding is important, particularly for neonates with ARPKD where feeding can be hampered by massively enlarged kidneys impinging on the stomach and creating early satiety and gastroesophageal reflux. Enteral feedings are often needed to ensure adequate calories and nephrectomy is sometimes considered.[2]
- UTIs are common in patients with ADPKD (30% to 50%) and ARPKD, although cyst infection and abscess is uncommon in those with ARPKD (for whom standard antimicrobials are usually adequate).[2] In one retrospective study of 256 patients with ADPKD, the annual incidence of asymptomatic pyuria was 0.492 episodes/patient/year and those with persistent asymptomatic pyuria experienced an upper UTI more frequently (hazard ratio = 4.612; 95% confidence interval, 1.735 to 12.258 adjusted for gender and hypertension).[38]
- Children with ARPKD who survive the neonatal period but have congenital hepatic fibrosis (also called Caroli's disease) should be monitored yearly by a hepatologist for complications associated with portal hypertension, including periodic endoscopy for esophageal varices and monitoring for cholangitis.[2] These children are also prone to splenomegaly causing anemia, thrombocytopenia, and leukopenia and are at increased risk of cholangiocarcinoma.[2]
- Posttransplantation, patients with ADPKD may be more prone to the development of diabetes mellitus (odds ratio 2.3; 95% confidence interval, 1.008 to 5.14).[28]
- In the absence of a family history of aneurysm, screening is not routinely recommended for asymptomatic patients; diagnostic

testing should be considered in patients with ADPKD and new-onset or severe headache or other central nervous system symptoms or signs.[2]

PATIENT EDUCATION

- Explain the genetics (among patients with ADPKD disease will develop in half of their offspring) and prognosis to patients. Referral to a genetic counselor may be useful for patients considering childbearing. Preimplantation genetic screening for ARPKD is possible.[39]
- Hypertension is common and should be treated.
- Kidney dysfunction is also common and should be monitored.
- Avoid high-impact sports in which abdominal trauma may occur (e.g., boxing).[2]
- In otherwise healthy women with ADPKD, pregnancy is usually uncomplicated but the risks of severe hypertension and pre-eclampsia are higher than those in the general population when elevated blood pressure or renal insufficiency is present before conception.[40]

PATIENT RESOURCES

- National Kidney Foundation (800-622-9010)—**www.kidney.org**.
- National Kidney Disease Education Program—**www.nkdep.nih.gov**.
- National Institutes of Health, PubMed Health. *Polycystic Kidney Disease*—**www.ncbi.nlm.nih.gov/pubmedhealth/PMH0001531/**.

PROVIDER RESOURCES

- Roser T. *Polycystic Kidney Disease* **www.emedicine.medscape.com/article/244907-overview**.

REFERENCES

1. Asplin JR, Coe FL. Tubular disorders. In: Kasper DL, Braunwald E, Fauci AS, Hauser SL, Longo DL, Jameson JL, eds. *Harrison's Principles of Internal Medicine*, 16th ed. New York, NY: McGraw-Hill; 2005:1694-1696.
2. Dell KM. The spectrum of polycystic kidney disease in Children. *Adv Chronic Kidney Dis*. 2011;18(5):339-347.
3. NeumannHP, Jilg C, Bacher J, et al. Epidemiology of autosomal-dominant polycystic kidney disease: an in-depth clinical study for south-western Germany. *Nephrol Dial Transplant*. 2013 Jan 8. [Epub ahead of print].
4. Grantham JJ. Autosomal dominant polycystic kidney disease. *Ann Transplant*. 2009;14(4):86-90.
5. Harris PC, Torres V.. Polycystic kidney disease. *Annu Rev Med*. 2009;60:321-337.
6. Reed BY, Masoumi A, Elhassan E, et al. Angiogenic growth factors correlate with disease severity in young patients with autosomal dominant polycystic kidney disease. *Kidney Int*. 2011; 79(1):128-134.
7. Lennerz JK, Spence DC, Iskandar SS, et al. Glomerulocystic kidney: one hundred-year perspective. *Arch Pathol Lab Med*. 2010; 134(4):583-605.
8. Firinci F, Soylu A, Demir BK, et al. An 11-year-old child with Autosomal Dominant Polycystic Kidney Disease who presented with nephrolithiasis. *Case Rep Med*. 2012;2012:428749.
9. Orskov B, Christensen KB, Feldt-Rasmussen B, Strandgaard S. Low birth weight is associated with earlier onset of end-stage renal disease in Danish patients with autosomal dominant polycystic kidney disease. *Kidney Int*. 2012;81(9):919-924.
10. Dias NF, Lanzarini V, Onuchic LF, Koch VH. Clinical aspects of autosomal recessive polycystic kidney disease. *J Bras Nefrol*. 2010; 32(3):263-267.
11. Mekahli D, Woolf AS, Bockenhauer D. Similar renal outcomes in children with ADPKD diagnosed by screening or presenting with symptoms. *Pediatr Nephrol*. 2010;25(11):2275-2282.
12. Nicolau C, Torra R, Bandenas C, et al. Autosomal dominant polycystic kidney disease types 1 and 2: assessment of US sensitivity for diagnosis. *Radiology*. 1999;213(1):273-276.
13. Cadnapaphornchai MA, Masoumi A, Strain JD, et al. Magnetic resonance imaging of kidney and cyst volume in children with ADPKD. *Clin J Am Soc Nephrol*. 2011;6(2):369-376.
14. Sallee M, Rafat C, Zahar JR, et al. Cyst infections in patients with autosomal dominant polycystic kidney disease. *Clin J Am Soc Nephrol*. 2009;4(7):1183-1189.
15. Barua M, Pei Y. Diagnosis of autosomal-dominant polycystic kidney disease: an integrated approach. *Semin Nephrol*. 2010;30(4): 356-365.
16. Kummer S, Sagir A, Pandey S, et al. Liver fibrosis in recessive multicystic kidney diseases: transient elastography for early detection. *Pediatr Nephrol*. 2011;26(5):725-731.
17. Klahr S, Breyer JA, Beck GJ, et al. Dietary protein restriction, blood pressure control, and the progression of polycystic kidney disease. Modification of Diet in Renal Disease Study Group. *J Am Soc Nephrol*. 1995;6(4):1318.
18. Schrier R, McFann K, Johnson A, et al. Cardiac and renal effects of standard versus rigorous blood pressure control in autosomal-dominant polycystic kidney disease: results of a seven-year prospective randomized study. *J Am Soc Nephrol*. 2002;13(7): 1733-1739.
19. Patch C, Charlton J, Roderick PJ, Gulliford MC. Use of antihypertensive medications and mortality of patients with autosomal dominant polycystic kidney disease: a population-based study. *Am J Kidney Dis*. 2011;57(6):856-862.
20. Zeltner R, Poliak R, Stiasny B, et al. Renal and cardiac effects of antihypertensive treatment with ramipril vs metoprolol in autosomal dominant polycystic kidney disease. *Nephrol Dial Transplant*. 2008;23(2):573-579.
21. Cadnapaphornchai MA, George DM, Masoumi A, et al. Effect of statin therapy on disease progression in pediatric ADPKD: design and baseline characteristics of participants. *Contemp Clin Trials*. 2011;32(3):437-445.

22. Walz G, Budde K, Mannaa M, et al. Everolimus in patients with autosomal dominant polycystic kidney disease. *N Engl J Med.* 2010;363(9):830-840.
23. Serra AL, Poster D, Kistler AD, et al. Sirolimus and kidney growth in autosomal dominant polycystic kidney disease. *N Engl J Med.* 2010;363(9):820-829.
24. Hogan MC, Masyuk TV, Page LJ, et al. Randomized clinical trial of long-acting somatostatin for autosomal dominant polycystic kidney and liver disease. *J Am Soc Nephrol.* 2010;21(6): 1052-1061.
25. Park EY, Woo YM, Park JH. Polycystic kidney disease and therapeutic approaches. *BMB Rep.* 2011;44(6):359-368.
26. Jacquet A, Pallet N, Kessler M, et al. Outcomes of renal transplantation in patients with autosomal dominant polycystic kidney disease: a nationwide longitudinal study. *Transpl Int.* 2011;24(6): 582-587.
27. Alam A, Perrone RD. Management of ESRD in patients with autosomal dominant polycystic kidney disease. *Adv Chronic Kidney Dis.* 2010;17(2):164-172.
28. Jacquet A, Pallet N, Kessler M, et al. Outcomes of renal transplantation in patients with autosomal dominant polycystic kidney disease: a nationwide longitudinal study. *Transpl Int.* 2011;24(6): 582-587.
29. Klahr S, Breyer JA, Beck GJ, et al. Dietary protein restriction, blood pressure control, and the progression of polycystic kidney disease. Modification of Diet in Renal Disease Study Group. *J Am Soc Nephrol.* 1995;6(4):1318.
30. Pei Y. Practical genetics for autosomal dominant polycystic kidney disease. *Nephron Clin Pract.* 2011;118(1):c19-c30.
31. Norman J. Fibrosis and progression of autosomal dominant polycystic kidney disease (ADPKD). *Biochim Biophys Acta.* 2011;1812(10):1327-1336.
32. Ozkok A, Akpinar TS, Tufan F, et al. Clinical characteristics and predictors of progression of chronic kidney disease in autosomal dominant polycystic kidney disease: a single center experience. *Clin Exp Nephrol.* 2012 Oct 20. (Epub ahead of print)
33. Roy S, Dillon MJ, Trompeter RS, Barratt TM. Autosomal recessive polycystic kidney disease: long-term outcome of neonatal survivors. *Pediatr Nephrol.* 1997;11(3):302-306
34. Chapal M, Debout A, Dufay A, et al. Kidney and liver transplantation in patients with autosomal recessive polycystic kidney disease: a multicentric study. *Nephrol Dial Transplant.* 2012;27(5):2083-2088.
35. Herden U, Kemper M, Ganschow R, et al. Surgical aspects and outcome of combined liver and kidney transplantation in children. *Transpl Int.* 2011;24(8):805-811.
36. Nishiura JL, Neves RF, Eloi DR, et al. Evaluation of nephrolithiasis in autosomal dominant polycystic kidney disease patients. *Clin J Am Soc Nephrol.* 2009;4(4):838-844.
37. Bae KT, Grantham JJ. Imaging for the prognosis of autosomal dominant polycystic kidney disease. *Nat Rev Nephrol.* 2010;6(2): 96-106.
38. Hwang JH, Park HC, Jeong JC, et al. Chronic asymptomatic pyuria precedes overt urinary tract infection and deterioration of renal function in autosomal dominant polycystic kidney disease. BMC Nephrol. 2013; Jan 7;14:1. doi: 10.1186/ 1471-2369-14-1.
39. Lau EC, Janson MM, Roesler MR, et al. Birth of a healthy infant following preimplantation PKHD1 haplotyping for autosomal recessive polycystic kidney disease using multiple displacement amplification. *J Assist Reprod Genet.* 2010;27(7):397-407.
40. Vora N, Perrone R, Bianchi DW. Reproductive issues for adults with autosomal dominant polycystic kidney disease. *Am J Kidney Dis.* 2008;51(2):307-318.

67 NEPHROTIC SYNDROME

Charles Y. Kwon, MD
Raed Bou Matar, MD
Halima S. Janjua, MD

PATIENT STORY

A 3-year-old boy has had intermittent facial swelling for the past 3 weeks. Symptoms were self-limited and attributed to seasonal allergies. He awoke with significant periorbital and facial edema (**Figure 67-1**), and pitting edema to his mid-tibia bilaterally. He denies any abdominal pain, headache, rash, or gross hematuria. His evaluation reveals a normal blood pressure, normal renal function, and 4+ protein on a urine dipstick. He was presumptively diagnosed with minimal change disease and started on a course of prednisone. His edema gradually subsided (**Figure 67-2**) and his proteinuria resolved within the first two weeks of therapy.

INTRODUCTION

Nephrotic syndrome is a tetrad of signs and symptoms: proteinuria (>50 mg/kg/day), hypoalbuminemia (serum albumin <3 gm/dL), edema, and hyperlipidemia. Prognosis is largely dependent on the glomerular etiology of the proteinuria. Minimal change disease is by far the most common etiology of nephrotic syndrome in childhood and carries an excellent long-term renal prognosis.

SYNONYM

- Nephrosis.

EPIDEMIOLOGY

- Estimated incidence of minimal change disease is 5 per 100,000 children under the age of 16 with a median age of 2.5 years.
- Boys are more commonly affected.[1]
- Rare familial cases have been reported.

ETIOLOGY AND PATHOPHYSIOLOGY

- Nephrotic syndrome begins with a glomerular lesion, causing significant proteinuria. Protein losses result in hypoalbuminemia. This produces edema, typically facial, lower extremity, and genital. The etiology of the associated hyperlipidemia is not fully elucidated.
- Although minimal change disease is the most common cause of nephrotic syndrome, little is known about the disease etiology. The most common hypothesis involves an unidentified circulating factor.[2]

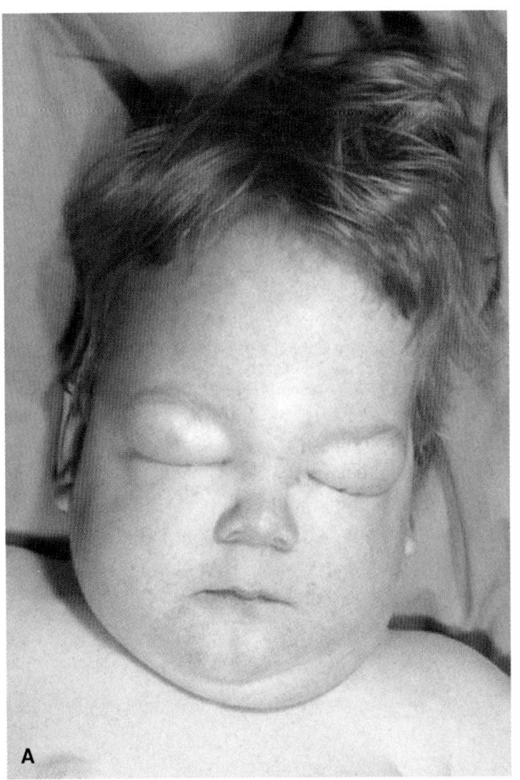

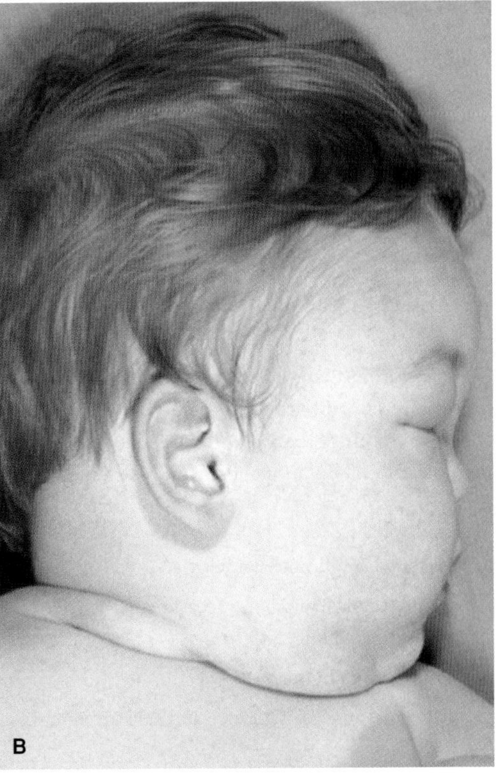

FIGURE 67-1 Significant facial edema on frontal (**A**) and lateral (**B**) views in a 3-year-old boy secondary to minimal change disease. (*Used with permission from Cleveland Clinic Children's Hospital Photo Files.*)

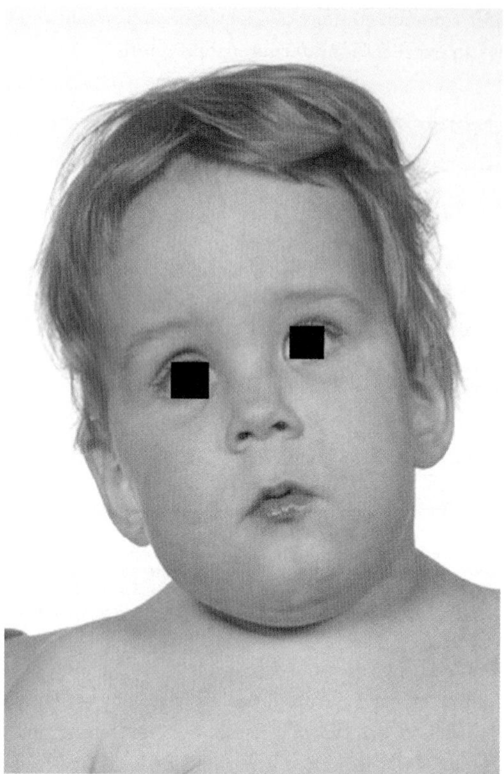

FIGURE 67-2 Resolution of facial edema in the same child from figure 67-1 following a course of prednisone. (*Used with permission from* Cleveland Clinic Children's Hospital Photo Files)

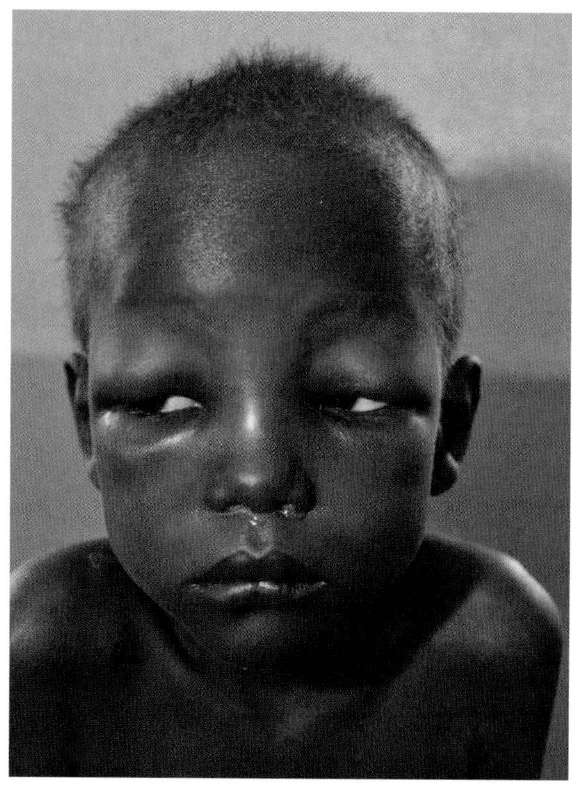

FIGURE 67-3 Young boy with nephrotic syndrome and malnutrition in Africa. Note the prominent periorbital edema from the low albumin due to the combination of renal protein loss and malnutrition. The red hair is a sign of kwashiorkor. (*Used with permission from Richard P. Usatine, MD.*)

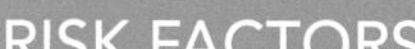

RISK FACTORS

- Most cases of minimal change disease are preceded by an acute illness, often an upper respiratory infection.

DIAGNOSIS

CLINICAL FEATURES

- Children typically present initially with edema (**Figures 67-1** and **67-3**).
- Urinary symptoms are rare. Microscopic hematuria can be seen in up to 10 percent of children with nephrotic syndrome. Gross hematuria has also been rarely described with minimal change disease and is more indicative of glomerulonephritis.[5]

LABORATORY TESTING

- A urine dipstick will show significant proteinuria.
- Urine microscopy is often unremarkable. Occasionally, it will show fatty casts (acellular casts containing fat droplets).
- Serum tests show low serum albumin.
- Renal function (BUN/creatinine) is typically normal in minimal change disease.
- Abnormal kidney function can be attributed to pre-renal injury secondary to significant third-spacing and decreased intravascular volume. It may also indicate a different etiology, such as focal segmental glomerulosclerosis (FSGS) or glomerulonephritis.[2,3]
- Lipid studies are abnormal. LDL, total cholesterol, and triglycerides are elevated. HDL can be normal or low.[3]

IMAGING

- Renal ultrasonography is most often normal and not pursued in nephrotic syndrome unless a biopsy is planned.
- Chest x-ray may show pulmonary edema (**Figure 67-4**).

DIFFERENTIAL DIAGNOSIS

- Primary/Idiopathic.
  - Minimal change disease.[1]
    - Up to 90 percent of nephrotic patients between 1 to 10 years.
    - Can be seen in all ages but likelihood decreases with age.
  - Focal segmental glomerulosclerosis—To be considered when renal function is not normal. Steroid resistant. Diagnosis made histologically (**Figure 67-5**).
- Secondary.
  - Most glomerulonephritic disorders can have associated nephrotic syndrome.
    - IgA nephropathy.
    - Post-streptococcal glomerulonephritis.
    - Systemic lupus erythematosus.

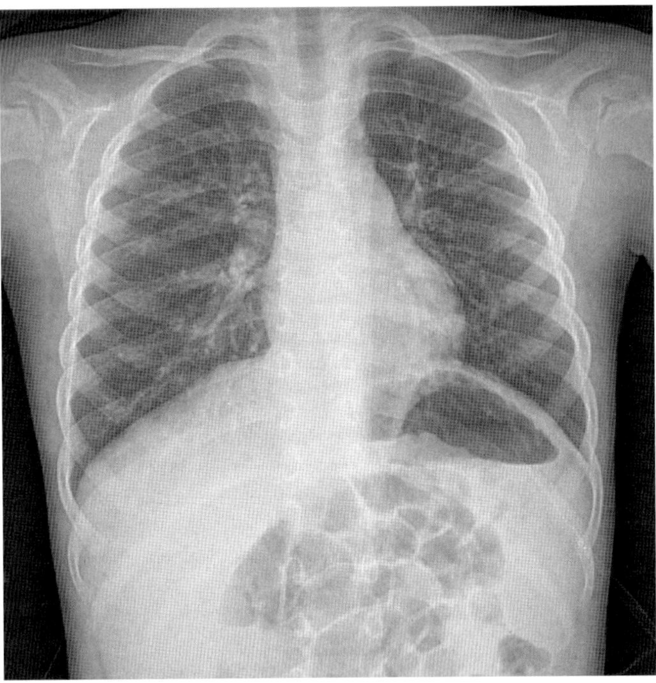

FIGURE 67-4 Mild pulmonary edema on chest x-ray of a 5-year-old girl with nephrotic syndrome. (*Used with permission from Camille Sabella, MD.*)

- Infection can have associated nephrosis.
  - Hepatitis B and C.
  - HIV.
  - Syphilis.
- Malignancy—Very rare cause of nephrotic syndrome.

- Congenital nephrotic syndrome.[6]
  - Should be considered in all patients under 1 year of age.
  - Etiology most often is a genetic defect leading to absence of a structural protein important in podocyte function.

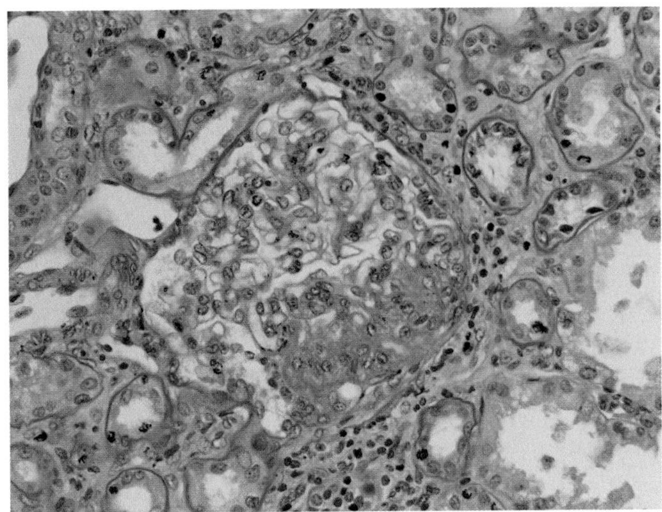

FIGURE 67-5 Focal segmental glomerulosclerosis seen on light microscopy. Note the collapsed and sclerotic tuft seen in the visualized glomerulus. (*Used with permission from Kemp, Burns, Brown, Pathology: The Big Picture. Figure 16-2. www.accessmedicine.com. McGraw-Hill*).

MANAGEMENT

SUPPORTIVE

- Sodium restriction is critical to limit edema. Fluid restriction plays a comparatively minor role and is typically not aggressively pursued except in patients who are hyponatremic.
- Diuretics should be used with caution in children due to a high risk of intravascular volume depletion.
- Diuretics with albumin can effectively remove fluid but the effect is transient.[4]
- Close monitoring for complications, such as spontaneous peritonitis and thrombotic disease, is important.

MEDICATIONS

- Prednisone is the first line therapy for children with presumed minimal change disease.
- Response to prednisone closely correlates with long-term outcome.[3,7] SOR Ⓐ
  - Steroid-responsive—Patients who respond and are successfully weaned off steroids. High likelihood of long-term remission.
  - Steroid-dependent—Patients who respond but cannot be fully weaned off steroids. Typically require alternative immunosuppression to maintain long-term remission.
  - Steroid-resistant—No response to steroids. Remission is difficult to achieve and risk of eventual chronic kidney disease is high.
- Patients with congenital nephrotic syndrome do not respond to immunosuppression.

SURGERY

- Renal biopsy (most often percutaneous) is considered in patients who are steroid-resistant or who present with evidence of glomerular injury (abnormal kidney function, hypertension, or cellular casts). SOR Ⓒ

REFERRAL

- Patients with nephrotic syndrome should be referred to a specialist with expertise in management of pediatric renal disorders.

SCREENING

- There is no indication for routine urinalysis screening in children. Diagnosis of nephrotic syndrome before the onset of edema does not alter patient outcomes.

FOLLOW-UP

- Patients who are steroid-responsive have >50 percent risk of relapse during their first year post-diagnosis. Relapses are typically triggered by acute illnesses. While these relapses typically do require additional steroids, the occurrence of a relapse does not alter the patients' favorable long-term prognosis.[7]

- Follow-up for potential complications of nephrotic syndrome, such as primary peritonitis and thrombotic disease, is important.

PATIENT RESOURCES

- Nephrotic Syndrome—**http://kidneyweb.net/handouts.htm**.
- **www.uptodate.com/contents/the-nephrotic-syndrome-beyond-the-basics**.

PROVIDER RESOURCES

- **http://emedicine.medscape.com/article/982920-overview**.

REFERENCES

1. Nephrotic syndrome in children: prediction of histopathology from clinical and laboratory characteristics at time of diagnosis. A report of the International Study of Kidney Disease in Children. *Kidney Int*. 1978;13(2):159-165.
2. Primary nephrotic syndrome in children: clinical significance of histopathologic variants of minimal change and of diffuse mesangial hypercellularity. A Report of the International Study of Kidney Disease in Children. *Kidney Int*. 1981;20(6):765-771.
3. Hogg RJ, Portman RJ, Milliner D, Lemley KV, Eddy A, Ingelfinger J. Evaluation and management of proteinuria and nephrotic syndrome in children: recommendations from a pediatric nephrology panel established at the National Kidney Foundation conference on proteinuria, albuminuria, risk, assessment, detection, and elimination (PARADE). *Pediatrics*. 2000;105(6):1242-1249.
4. Haws RM, Baum M. Efficacy of albumin and diuretic therapy in children with nephrotic syndrome. *Pediatrics*. 1993;91(6):1142-1146.
5. Butani L. Gross hematuria in minimal-change disease nephrotic syndrome. *Pediatr Nephrol*. 2006;21(11):1783.
6. Hinkes BG, Mucha B, Vlangos CN, Gbadegesin R, Liu J, Hasselbacher K, Hangan D, Ozaltin F, Zenker M, Hildebrandt F. Nephrotic syndrome in the first year of life: two thirds of cases are caused by mutations in 4 genes (NPHS1, NPHS2, WT1, and LAMB2). *Arbeitsgemeinschaft für Paediatrische Nephrologie Study Group. Pediatrics*. 2007;119(4):e907-919. Epub 2007.
7. Tarshish P, Tobin JN, Bernstein J, Edelmann CM Jr: Prognostic significance of the early course of minimal change nephrotic syndrome: report of the International Study of Kidney Disease in Children. *J Am Soc Nephrol*. 1997;8(5):769-776.

68 NEPHRITIC SYNDROMES

Raed Bou Matar, MD
Charles Y. Kwon, MD
Halima S. Janjua, MD

PATIENT STORY

An 8-year-old girl presents to the emergency room with severe headache and tea-colored urine of 2 days duration (**Figure 68-1**). She has just completed a 10-day course of amoxicillin for streptococcal pharyngitis. Her blood pressure upon arrival is 132/88. She is diagnosed with probable post-streptococcal glomerulonephritis and treated with salt restriction and a diuretic, and recovers.

INTRODUCTION

Nephritic syndrome is characterized by gross hematuria, acute kidney injury and retention of salt and water (manifested as hypertension with/without edema).

SYNONYMS

Acute glomerulonephritis, acute nephritis.

EPIDEMIOLOGY

- Peak incidence is between the age of 5 and 12 years.
- Post-streptococcal glomerulonephritis is uncommon in children less than 3 years of age.
- Incidence ranges from 9.5 to 28.5 per 100,000.[1]
- Post-streptococcal glomerulonephritis is far more common in the developing countries.[1]

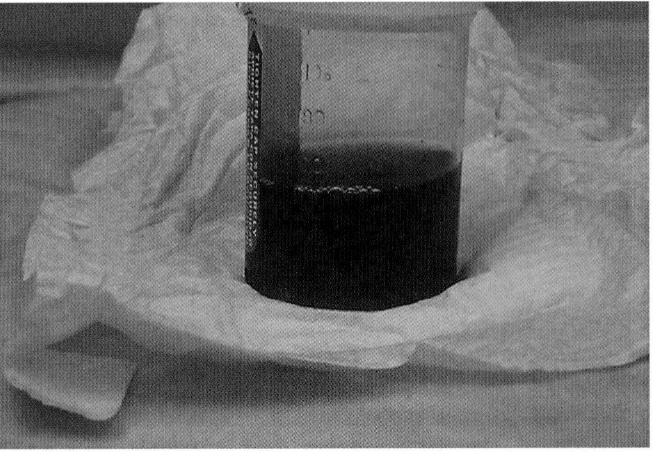

FIGURE 68-1 Tea-colored urine suggestive of glomerular gross hematuria. (*Used with permission from Rudolph's Pediatrics, 22nd edition, eFigure 467.1, McGraw-Hill.*)

ETIOLOGY AND PATHOPHYSIOLOGY

- Post-streptococcal glomerulonephritis is the most common cause of nephritic syndrome in children. It follows a pharyngeal or skin infection involving a nephritogenic strain of group A beta-hemolytic streptococci.
- Streptococcal antigens form immune complexes that activate a complement mediated cascade of inflammatory glomerular injury.[2]
- Less common etiologies for nephritic syndrome include: membranoproliferative glomerulonephritis, lupus nephritis, IgA nephropathy, Henoch-Schonlein purpura, infectious glomerulonephritis (commonly associated with endocarditis), and post-infectious glomerulonephritis due to other bacterial, viral, or parasitic etiologies.
- Rapidly progressive glomerulonephritis is a syndrome characterized by rapid loss of renal function (over a period of days to weeks) and the presence of glomerular crescents on renal biopsy (**Figure 68-2**). It represents the most severe presentation of any form of acute nephritis.[3]

DIAGNOSIS

CLINICAL FEATURES

- Nephritic syndrome classically presents with an abrupt onset of gross hematuria (tea-colored urine; **Figure 68-1**), oliguria, elevated blood pressure, and/or generalized edema.
- Onset of gross hematuria is 1 to 2 weeks following streptococcal pharyngitis and 3 to 6 weeks following streptococcal skin infection. In contrast, gross hematuria associated with IgA nephropathy commonly occurs concurrently with an upper respiratory infection.
- Mild (subclinical) cases of nephritis may be reflected by microscopic hematuria detected on urinalysis.[4]

LABORATORY TESTING

- Acute kidney injury is often present, manifested by variable elevation in serum creatinine.
- Urinalysis shows microscopic hematuria. Red blood cell casts confirm the glomerular origin of hematuria (**Figure 68-3**).

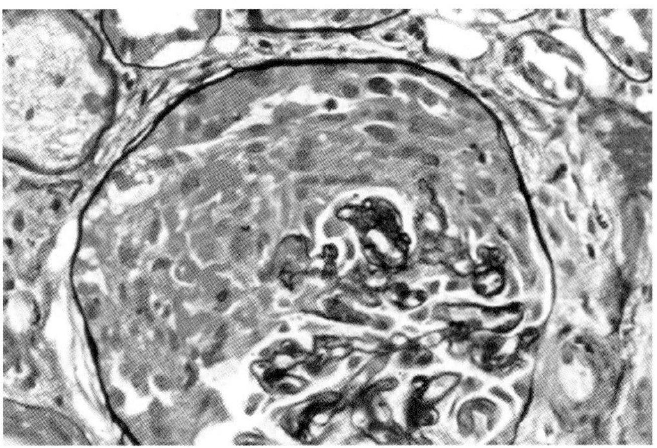

FIGURE 68-2 Cellular crescents. (*Used with permission from Harrison's Principles of Internal Medicine, 18th edition, Fig e14-14A, McGraw-Hill*).

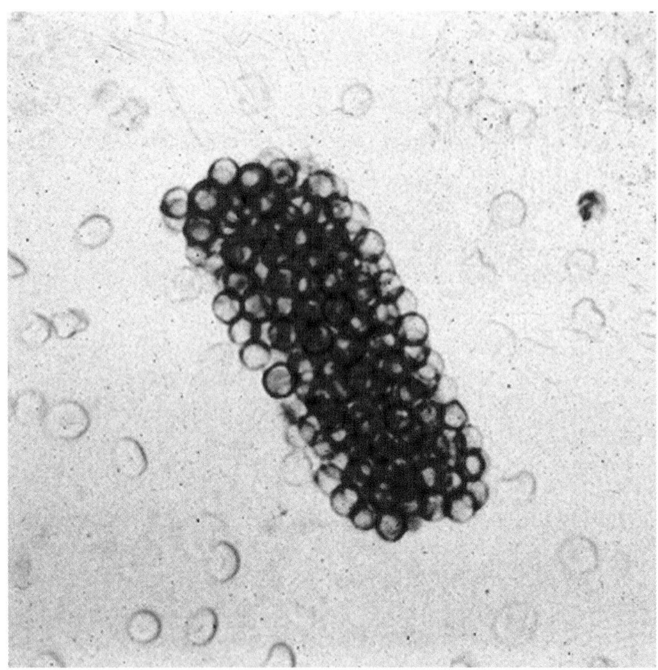

FIGURE 68-3 Red blood cell cast. (*Used with permission from Agnes B. Fogo, MD.*)

- Proteinuria may be present, but is usually low grade.
- Complement levels vary by etiology:
  - Transiently low C3 (for up to 8 weeks) with normal C4: post-streptococcal glomerulonephritis.
  - Chronically low C3—Membranoproliferative glomerulonephritis.
  - Low C3 and C4—Lupus nephritis.
  - Normal C3 and C4—IgA nephropathy or Henoch Schonlein purpura.
- Serology.
  - Streptozyme test measures five different streptococcal antibodies. It is highly sensitive for detecting evidence for a recent group A streptococcal infection.[5]
  - Positive ANA, anti-double stranded DNA, and/or anti-Smith antibodies suggest lupus nephritis.

RENAL BIOPSY

The diagnosis of post-streptococcal glomerulonephritis is typically based on clinical and laboratory findings. A renal biopsy is only indicated in atypical presentations or when an alternative etiology is suspected.

Characteristic histologic findings in post-streptococcal glomerulonephritis include diffuse (involving all glomeruli) cellular proliferation on light microscopy (**Figure 68-4**), coarse granular pattern of IgG & C3 deposits on immunofluorescence (**Figure 68-5**), and sub-epithelial hump-like immune deposits on electron microscopy (**Figure 68-6**). Presence of glomerular crescents (**Figure 68-2**) indicates rapidly progressive glomerulonephritis.

DIFFERENTIAL DIAGNOSIS

- Membranoproliferative glomerulonephritis (**Figure 68-7**): may be undistinguishable from post-streptococcal glomerulonephritis at disease onset. However, complement C3 levels remain persistently low beyond 8 weeks following the disease onset, indicating chronic immune complex deposition.
- Lupus nephritis—Distinguished by the systemic manifestations and the persistently low complement C3 and C4. Positive anti double stranded DNA antibodies and/or anti Smith antibodies confirms the diagnosis. Renal biopsy reveals glomerular deposition of immunoglobulins, C3 and C1q (Full house immunofluorescence).
- IgA nephropathy—Gross hematuria tends to occur concurrently with upper respiratory infections (In contrast, post-streptococcal glomerulonephritis presents following a 1- to 2-week latency period.) Complement levels are normal. Renal biopsy shows prominent mesangial deposition of IgA on immunofluorescence.
- Henoch-Schönlein purpura: characterized by a palpable purpuric rash commonly involving the lower extremities and buttocks. Complement levels are normal.

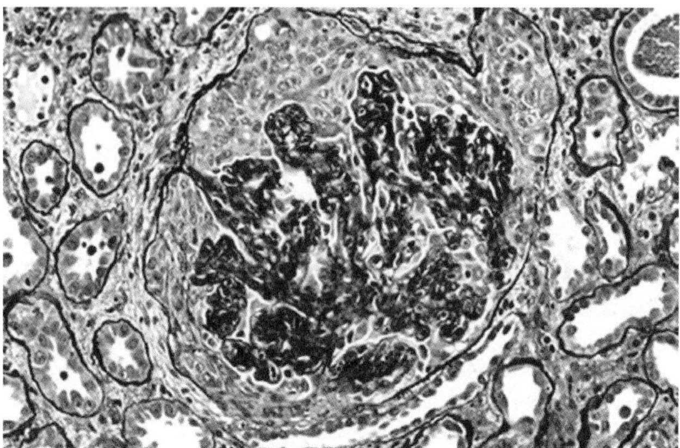

FIGURE 68-4 Post-streptococcal glomerulonephritis. Glomeruli show proliferative changes with an inflammatory infiltrate on light microscopy. (*Used with permission from Harrison's Principles of Internal Medicine, 18th edition, Fig e14-6A, McGraw-Hill.*)

MANAGEMENT

Post-streptococcal glomerulonephritis is generally self-limited. There is no known specific treatment and the management is generally supportive.

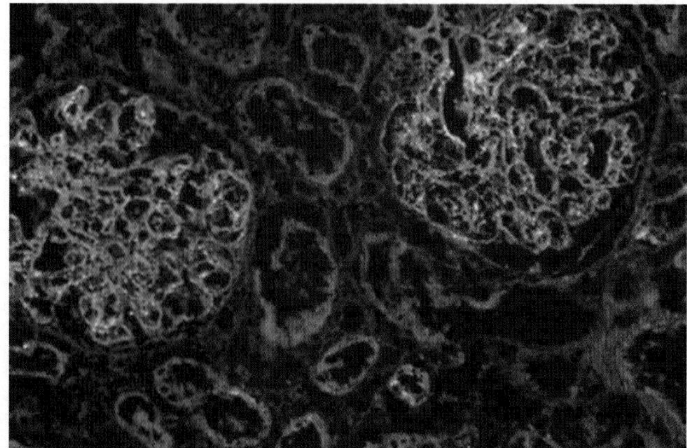

FIGURE 68-5 Post-streptococcal glomerulonephritis. Immunofluorescence shows C3 and IgG deposits localized to the mesangium and along the capillary walls. (*Used with permission from Harrison's Principles of Internal Medicine, 18th edition, Fig e14-6B, McGraw-Hill.*)

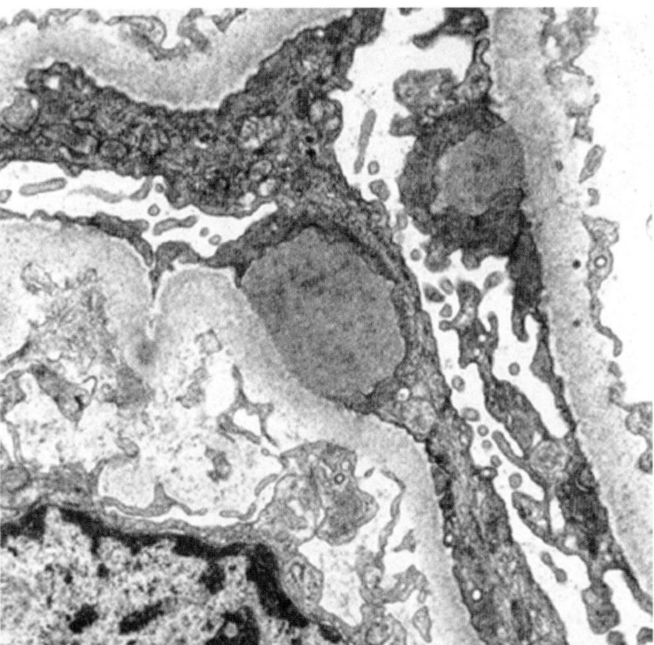

FIGURE 68-6 Post-streptococcal glomerulonephritis. Electron microscopy reveals the typical sub-epithelial hump-like immune deposits. (*Used with permission from Harrison's Principles of Internal Medicine, 18th edition, Fig e14-6C, McGraw-Hill.*)

NONPHARMACOLOGIC

- Dietary salt restriction may attenuate hypertension and generalized swelling. SOR Ⓒ

MEDICATIONS

- Diuretics effectively offset hypertension and salt retention during the acute illness. SOR Ⓒ
- Calcium channel blockers or vasodilators may be used for severe hypertension. SOR Ⓒ

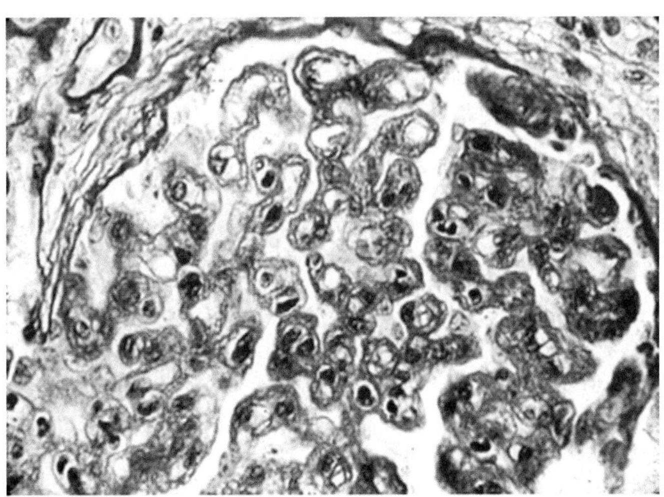

FIGURE 68-7 Membranoproliferative glomerulonephritis. Light microscopy shows mesangial expansion and endocapillary proliferation resulting in the typical "tram-track" duplication of glomerular basement membrane. (*Used with permission from Harrison's Principles of Internal Medicine, 18th edition, Fig e14-9, McGraw-Hill.*)

- Dialysis may be needed for electrolyte disturbances (like hyperkalemia), volume overload, or uremia. SOR Ⓒ
- High dose steroids may improve outcome in rapidly progressive glomerulonephritis.[6] SOR Ⓒ

REFERRAL

Patients with acute nephritis and significant hypertension or renal dysfunction should be referred to a specialist with expertise in management of renal disorders.

PREVENTION AND SCREENING

Antibiotic therapy has not been shown to decrease the risk of post-streptococcal glomerulonephritis, but may prevent the spread of nephritogenic group A streptococcal strains to other individuals.

PROGNOSIS

- Most children with post-streptococcal glomerulonephritis have an excellent prognosis with complete or near complete recovery from their disease.
- Children with rapidly progressive glomerulonephritis frequently progress to end-stage renal disease.[3]
- The prognosis of other forms of nephritis varies according to the nature and severity of the underlying etiology.

PATIENT RESOURCES

- **www.nlm.nih.gov/medlineplus/ency/article/000503.htm**.

PROVIDER RESOURCES

- **www.emedicine.medscape.com/article/240337-overview**.

REFERENCES

1. Rodriguez-Iturbe B, Musser JM. The current state of poststreptococcal glomerulonephritis. *J Am Soc Nephrol*. 2008;19(10):1855-1864.
2. Rodriguez-Iturbe B, Batsford S. Pathogenesis of poststreptococcal glomerulonephritis a century after clemens von pirquet. *Kidney Int*. 2007;71(11):1094-1104.
3. Jennette JC. Rapidly progressive crescentic glomerulonephritis. *Kidney Int*. 2003;63(3):1164-1177.
4. Rodríguez-Iturbe B, Rubio L, García R. Attack rate of poststreptococcal nephritis in families: a prospective study. *The Lancet*. 1981;317(8217):401-403.
5. Eison TM, Ault B, Jones D, Chesney R, Wyatt R. Post-streptococcal acute glomerulonephritis in children: clinical features and pathogenesis. *Pediatric Nephrology*. 2011;26(2):165-180.
6. Couser WG. Rapidly progressive glomerulonephritis: classification, pathogenetic mechanisms, and therapy. *Am J Kidney Dis*. 1988;11(6):449-464.

69 HEMOLYTIC UREMIC SYNDROME

Kshama Daphtary, MBBS, MD, FAAP

PATIENT STORY

A 4-year-old boy presents to his pediatrician because of swelling over the face, malaise, fatigue, and decreased appetite. On further questioning, his parents state that he appears pale and has reduced urine output. He recently finished a course of antibiotics for bloody diarrhea. On exam, he is found to be hypertensive and pale and has anasarca. Initial laboratory studies show a hemoglobin of 7 g/dL, platelet count of 44,000/mm^3, blood urea nitrogen of 39 mg/dL and creatinine of 2.9 mg/dL. Peripheral smear shows the presence of schistocytes and a paucity of platelets (**Figures 69-1** and **69-2**). He is admitted to the pediatric intensive care unit for hemolytic uremic syndrome. He is treated conservatively with close attention to fluid intake and output, restriction of sodium and fluid intake, and antihypertensive medications as needed. A stool culture obtained at the onset of his bloody diarrhea grows Escherichia coli and is identified as serotype O157:H7. Hemoglobin declines to 5.2 g/dL for which he is transfused packed red blood cells. Platelet count decreases over the next few days and then improves. He has no evidence of bleeding. Azotemia and oliguria improve over a week, appetite improves and anasarca resolves. He is discharged home with an excellent prognosis for full recovery.

INTRODUCTION

The hemolytic uremic syndrome (HUS) was first described in 1955 by Gasser et al.[1] HUS is a thrombotic microangiopathy characterized by a triad of hemolytic anemia, thrombocytopenia and acute kidney injury.

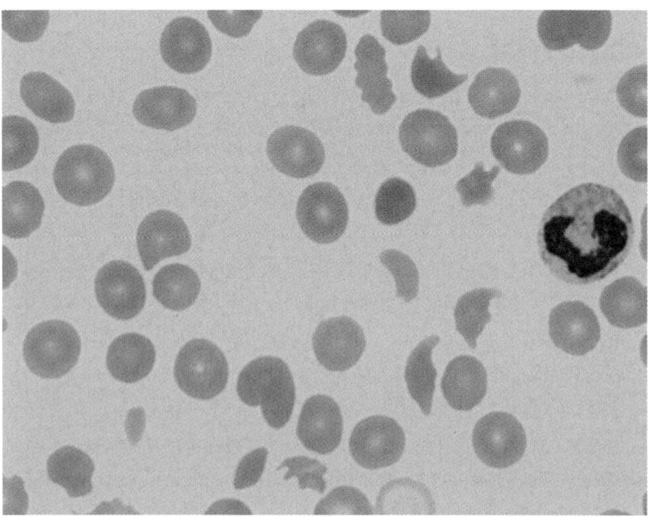

FIGURE 69-1 Schistocytes (fragmented "helmet" cells) and paucity of platelets, characteristic features of hemolytic uremic syndrome on blood peripheral smear, high magnification. (*Used with permission from Megan Nakashima, MD.*)

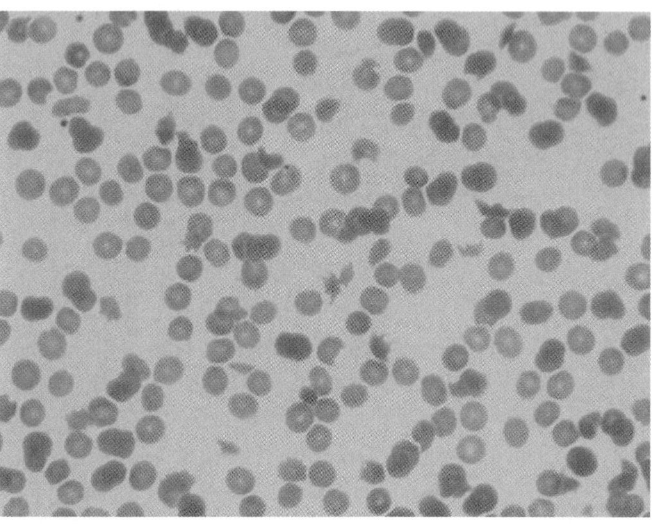

FIGURE 69-2 Schistocytes (fragmented "helmet" cells) and paucity of platelets, characteristic features of hemolytic uremic syndrome on blood peripheral smear, low magnification. (*Used with permission from Megan Nakashima, MD.*)

SYNONYMS

- Typical HUS is also known as D(+) HUS, Shiga toxin-producing *Escherichia* coli (STEC) HUS, verocytotoxin producing *Escherichia* coli (VTEC) HUS, or Shiga-like toxin associated (Stx) HUS.
- Atypical HUS is also referred to as D(−) HUS and non-Shiga-like toxin associated (non-Stx) HUS.

EPIDEMIOLOGY

- It is the most common cause of renal failure in childhood.[2]
- Worldwide, the incidence is 0.2 to 4 cases per 100,000 per year.[3]
- It is more common in children under 5 years with an incidence of approximately 6 cases per 100,000 per year.[4]
- There is also a geographical variation, with the highest incidence reported in Argentina.[5]

ETIOLOGY AND PATHOPHYSIOLOGY

- In 2006, the European Study Group for HUS proposed a classification for HUS, thrombotic thrombocytopenic purpura (TTP) and related disorders, which is summarized in **Table 69-1**.[6]
- The underlying histological lesion in HUS is thrombotic microangiopathy, characterized by thickening of arteriole and capillary walls, with prominent endothelial damage (swelling and detachment), subendothelial accumulation of proteins and cell debris, and fibrin and platelet-rich thrombi obstructing vessel lumina.
- In practice, HUS can be distinguished in a "typical" variety or diarrheal-associated form, termed as D(+) HUS, primarily triggered

TABLE 69-1 Classification of HUS, TTP and Related Disorders

Etiology Advanced

1. Infection-induced
   a. Shiga and Shiga-like toxin-producing bacteria (EHEC, S. dysenteriae type 1)
   b. *S. pneumoniae*
2. Disorders of complement regulation
   a. Genetic
   b. Acquired
3. ADAMTS13 deficiency
   a. Genetic
   b. Acquired
4. Defective cobalamin metabolism
5. Quinine-induced

Etiology Unknown

1. HIV infection
2. Malignancy, cancer chemotherapy, ionizing radiation
3. Calcineurin inhibitors and transplantation
4. Pregnancy HELPP syndrome, contraceptive pill
5. Systemic lupus erythematosus, anti-phospholipid antibody syndrome
6. Glomerulopathy
7. Familial not included in Box 1
8. Unclassified

Adapted with permission from Ariceta G, Besbas N, Johnson S, Karpman D, Landau D, Licht C, et al. Guideline for the investigation and initial therapy of diarrhea negative hemolytic uremic syndrome. Pediatr Nephrol. 2009;24(4):687-696.

by preceding diarrheal illness with Shiga toxin-producing *Ecoli*, mostly serotype O157:H7. This form accounts for 90 percent of all cases of HUS.[7]

- Ten percent of cases of HUS fall into the "atypical" category known as atypical HUS or D(−) HUS. It occurs in a familial as well as in a sporadic form.
- Atypical HUS (aHUS) is a heterogeneous group of disorders caused by defective complement regulation in the majority of cases.[7,8] Mutations have been identified in genes encoding the regulatory proteins of the complement alternative pathway, complement factor H (CFH), membrane cofactor protein (MCP or CD46), complement factor I (CFI) and complement factor H-related proteins (CFHR) as well as complement activators, complement factor B (CFB) and C3 as well as thrombomodulin (THBD). Inhibitory autoantibodies to CFH account for an additional 5 to 10 percent of cases and can occur in isolation or in association with these mutations.[7]
- Atypical HUS has an equal incidence in boys and girls.[9] Seventy percent of children have the first episode before the age of 2 years and approximately 25 percent before the age of 6 months.[9]
- In contrast, less than 5 percent of D(+) HUS occurs in children below the age of 6 months.[9]

RISK FACTORS

- Only 10 to 15 percent of children who are infected with *E coli* O157:H7 develop HUS.[10,11]
- Higher initial leukocyte counts, vomiting, and use of antibiotics are associated with subsequent development of HUS.[11]
- About 80 percent of cases of aHUS are also triggered by infections, either upper respiratory tract infections or gastroenteritis.[9] Other triggers reported are varicella, H1N1 influenza and, interestingly, Shigatoxin associated diarrheal illness.[9]

DIAGNOSIS

CLINICAL FEATURES

- Patients with D(+) HUS develop diarrhea about 2 to 5 days after contracting a Shiga toxin-producing bacterial infection.[4] The diarrhea is often profuse and bloody. Depending on the virulence of the strain, 10 to 15 percent (25% in the German outbreak of 2011 with *E coli* O104:H4) of cases present with features of HUS 3 to 8 days later.[12]
- Onset is generally sudden and symptoms consist of pallor (**Figure 69-3**), poor feeding, vomiting, fatigue, drowsiness, and sometimes generalized edema. Often, there is oliguria or anuria, hypertension, and signs of fluid overload and anemia.
- Three to forty-one percent of cases of aHUS develop signs of central nervous system involvement including irritability, altered level of consciousness, and seizures, which usually develop after the onset of HUS.[12]
- Atypical HUS is usually recognized after the diagnosis of HUS is made. Atypical HUS should be considered if the presentation is before 6 months of age, onset is insidious, and there is a history of previous episode of HUS, previous unexplained anemia, asynchronous family history of HUS or HUS following transplantation of any organ.[8]

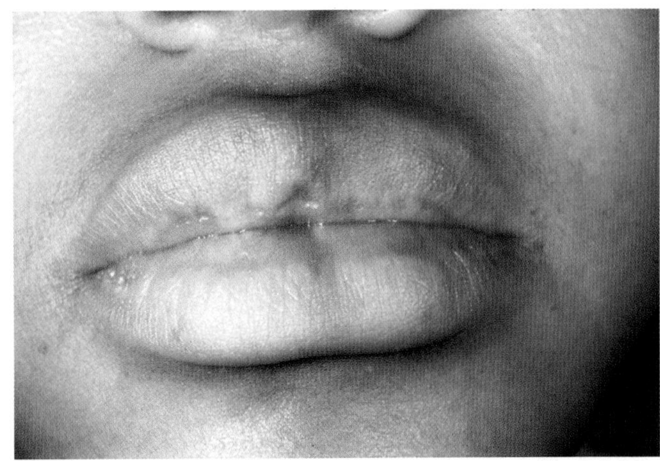

FIGURE 69-3 Lip pallor evident in this adolescent with hemolytic uremic syndrome and a hemoglobin of 5 g/dL. (*Used with permission from Binita R. Shah, MD, www.accessemergencymedicine.com.*)

LABORATORY TESTING

HUS is defined by the simultaneous appearance of:

- Hemolytic anemia (hemoglobin <10 g/dL). The presence of fragmented erythrocytes (schistocytes) (see **Figures 69-1** and **69-2**), undetectable haptoglobin levels and elevated lactate dehydrogenase (LDH) confirm the presence of intra-vascular hemolysis.
- Thrombocytopenia (platelets $<150{,}000/\text{mm}^3$).
- Renal impairment (serum creatinine > upper limit of normal for age).
- Hyperkalemia, metabolic acidosis and hyponatremia may also be seen.
- In children, a renal biopsy is not needed for the diagnosis.

Table 69-2 shows the investigative work up recommended for patients with HUS and is also a flowchart that aids in the recognition of aHUS.[8]

- Children older than 6 months who have a history of diarrhea or bloody diarrhea should be investigated for enterohemorrhagic *E coli* (EHEC) or *Shigella dysenteriae*. Even if there is no recent diarrheal illness or if there is recent diarrhea and the presence of atypical features, investigate for EHEC infection as unusual presentations have been known to occur. These patients also require a full investigation for alternative causes of HUS (see **Table 69-3**).[8]
- In infants (<6 months) presenting with HUS, CFH, CFI and C3 should be screened first, regardless of whether C3 plasma concentration is decreased or not. If onset is after infancy and C3 level is normal, MCP mutation should be investigated. Anti-CFH antibodies-HUS is common after the age of approximately 7 years and in pre-adolescents and adolescents. Patients in these age groups should be screened for anti-CFH antibodies especially if C3 concentration is decreased. At any age, if no mutation is found in CFH, CFI, MCP and C3, screening for CFB and THBD mutation should be undertaken.
- ADAMTS13 activity determination is required in all patients with aHUS as manifestations of aHUS and TTP may overlap. Blood must be collected before transfusion of fresh frozen plasma (FFP) or plasma exchange (PE). ADAMTS13 activity below 10 percent of normal is suggestive of TTP.
- Screening for defects of cobalamine metabolism (homocystinuria with methylmalonic aciduria) is mandatory.
- Patients with HELPP syndrome, post-partum HUS, and post-transplant HUS require an investigation of the complement system.

TABLE 69-2 Work Up for HUS and Recognition of Atypical HUS

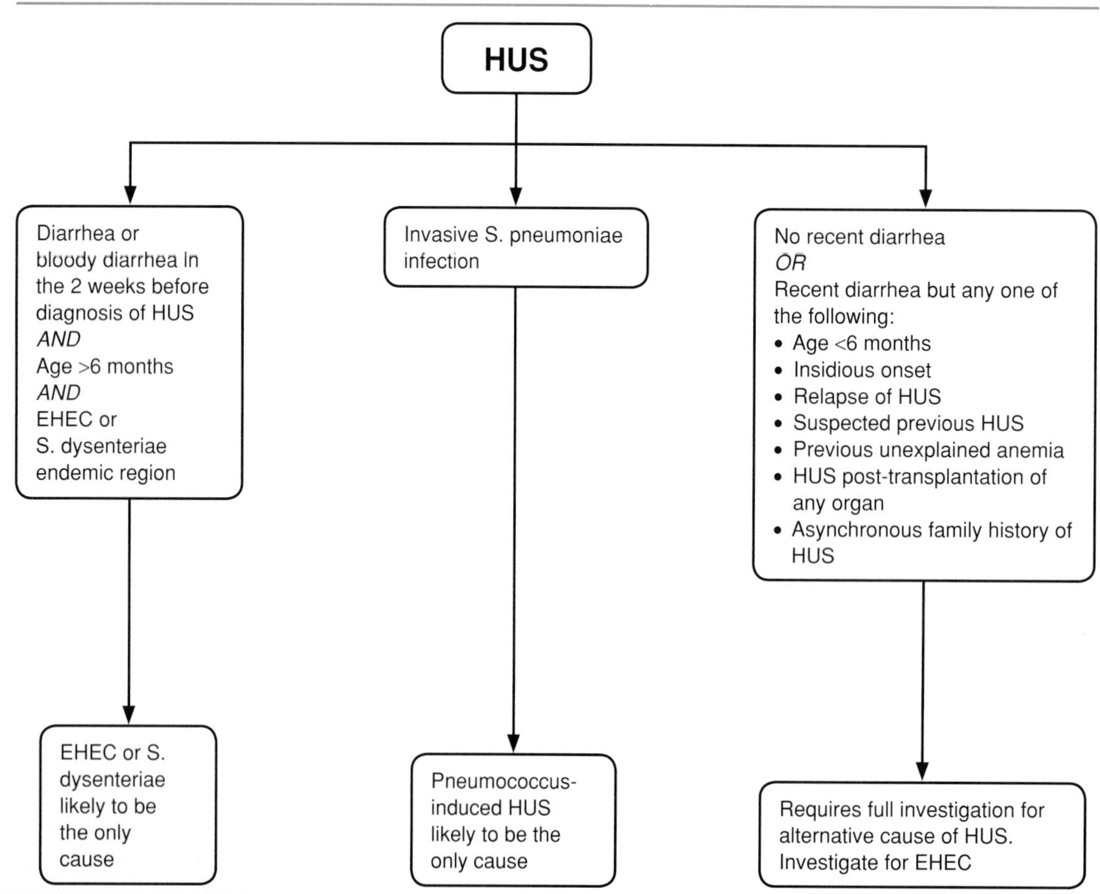

EHEC- enterohemorrhagic Escherichia coli.

Adapted with persmission from Ariceta G, Besbas N, Johnson S, Karpman D, Landau D, Licht C, et al. Guideline for the investigation and initial therapy of diarrhea negative hemolytic uremic syndrome. *Pediatr Nephrol.* 2009; 24(4):687-696.

TABLE 69-3 Investigations for Patients with Suspected Atypical HUS

Classification	Investigation
Disorders of complement regulation	C3 (plasma/serum) Factor H and Factor I (plasma/serum) Factor H autoantibody MCP (CD46) Gene mutation analysis in factor H, factor I, MCP, factor B and C3
ADAMTS13 (vWFcp) deficiency Inherited or acquired	Plasma vWF protease (ADAMTS13) activity ± inhibitor (plasma)
Cobalamin metabolism	Homocysteine, methylmalonic acd (plasma and urine) ± mutation analysis in MMACHC gene
HIV	Serology
Pregnancy HELPP syndrome	Pregnancy test, liver enzymes
Miscellaneous	Antinuclear antibody, lupus anticoagulant, anti-phospholipid antibodies

MCP- membrane cofactor protein.

Adapted with permission from Ariceta G, Besbas N, Johnson S, Karpman D, Landau D, Licht C, et al. Guideline for the investigation and initial therapy of diarrhea negative hemolytic uremic syndrome. *Pediatr Nephrol* 2009; 24(4):687-696.

DIFFERENTIAL DIAGNOSIS

- TTP may have similar symptoms. Traditionally, TTP and HUS were distinguished clinically, considering TTP to have predominant neurological involvement and HUS to primarily have renal dysfunction. Both share a common pathology of thrombotic microangiopathy and symptoms can overlap with neurological manifestations seen in HUS and renal problems seen in TTP. Therefore, TTP and HUS are often considered together.[6,13]

MANAGEMENT

NONPHARMACOLOGIC

- Most patients can be managed with close attention to fluid and electrolyte balance, management of hypertension, and nutritional support.
- Patient with more severe renal impairment and anuria are likely to require renal replacement therapy with either peritoneal dialysis or hemodialysis.
- Red blood cell transfusions may be given for anemia.
- Platelet transfusions should be limited to cases of severe thrombocytopenia or to cases of hemorrhage or in anticipation of an invasive procedure.
- Recently, the European Working Group on HUS published consensus guidelines with the aim of establishing a standardized approach to the initial management of aHUS.[8] SOR C Due to a lack of randomized controlled trials, these guidelines are based on combined personal experiences and published case reports.
    - Plasma exchange (PE) should be initiated within 24 hours of the initial presentation along with supportive treatment. Initially, 1.5 times (60 to 75 ml/kg) the expected plasma volume should be exchanged (replaced with FFP). Daily PE is recommended for the initial 5 days followed by five sessions a week for the next 2 weeks and then three sessions a week for the subsequent 2 weeks.
    - Blood counts, electrolytes, and serum creatinine should be monitored daily to determine the impact on degree of hemolysis and renal dysfunction.
    - In patients with low initial C3 levels, daily C3 levels should be measured.
    - PE can be discontinued if an alternative diagnosis is made that is not expected to respond to PE (such as cobalamin-C disorder), congenital ADAMTS13 deficiency, complications arise, or if remission is achieved.
    - Remission is achieved if platelet count is sustained above 150×10^9/l for 2 weeks and there is no evidence of hemolysis. A relapse is said to occur if there is recurrence of thrombocytopenia and hemolysis after 2 weeks of recovery. Reinstitution of PE is recommended if it had been successful initially.
    - If PE cannot be performed and the patient is not volume-overloaded or hypertensive and in cardiac failure, 10 to 20 mL/kg of body weight of FFP should be transfused (to replace a deficient factor).

MEDICATIONS

- Eculizumab, a humanized monoclonal antibody against C5, has recently been shown to be an effective treatment in aHUS.[7] There have been reported benefits of eculizumab in individual cases of aHUS and its efficacy has recently being evaluated in controlled clinical trials.[14] The Food and Drug Administration has approved the use of eculizumab in the treatment of pediatric and adult patients with aHUS.[15] SOR Ⓐ

- The initial success of eculizumab and the practical difficulties involved in PE demonstrate the potential for eculizumab to be used early in children in the near future. It is administered as an intravenous infusion. The most frequently reported adverse effects are hypertension, upper respiratory infection, diarrhea, headache, anemia, vomiting, urinary tract infection, and leukopenia.
- Although it has been used in patients with severe Shiga toxin-associated HUS, the safety and efficacy of eculizumab have not been established for, and it is not recommended for use in D(+) HUS.[15]
- Treatment with eculizumab has been associated with meningococcal infections.[15] Providers are required by the FDA to enroll in a registration program, certify that they will counsel and provide educational materials to patients about the risks of eculizumab, and agree to promptly report cases of meningococcal infection.[15] Patients should be immunized with a polyvalent meningococcal vaccine.
- Patients treated with eculizumab may be an increased risk of serious infections due to *S. pneumoniae* and *H. influenza* type b, and if not immunized, patients should receive vaccinations for the prevention of these infections. Patients may require antibiotic prophylaxis as well.

SURGERY

- Patients with HUS who reach end stage renal failure (ESRF) may be candidates for renal transplantation. There is a 30 to 100 percent risk of recurrence of aHUS after renal transplantation.[7]

REFERRAL

- Pediatric Nephrology for management and follow up.
- Pediatric Surgery for vascular access for hemodialysis or PE, or for placement of a catheter for peritoneal dialysis.

PREVENTION AND SCREENING

- There are no specific measures to prevent HUS. However, it is advisable to take precautions against EHEC and other foodborne illnesses by washing hands, utensils and food surfaces often, keeping raw food separate from read-to-eat food, thoroughly cooking meat, washing fruits and vegetables, avoiding unpasteurized milk, juice and cider, and avoiding swimming in water potentially contaminated with feces.

PROGNOSIS

- Typical HUS carries a mortality rate of up to 5 percent.[6,12] Patients with a milder course gradually improve with resolution of renal impairment over a few weeks. Approximately 25 percent have residual defects which range from persistent proteinuria and hypertension to end-stage renal disease.[12] Oligoanuria persisting for longer than 4 weeks increases the risk of a poorer prognosis.[16]
- Atypical HUS has a poorer prognosis than D(+) HUS with a 25 percent mortality rate.[7] It is characterized by frequent relapses and progression to end-stage renal failure in approximately 50 percent of cases.[16,17] Disease recurrence following isolated renal transplantation is high and has been reported to occur in up to 30 to 100 percent of aHUS patients depending on the underlying complement defect.[7]

PATIENT RESOURCES

- **www.kidney.niddk.nih.gov/kudiseases/pubs/childkidneydiseases/hemolytic_uremic_syndrome**.
- aHUS—**www.ghr.nlm.nih.gov/condition/atypical-hemolytic-uremic-syndrome**.

PROVIDER RESOURCES

- **http://emedicine.medscape.com/article/982025**.

REFERENCES

1. Gasser C, Gautier E, Steck A, Siebenmann RE, Oechslin R. Hemolytic-uremic syndrome: bilateral necrosis of the renal cortex in acute acquired hemolytic anemia (Article in German). *Schweiz Med Wochenschr*. 1955;85(38-39):905-909.
2. Gould LH, Demma L, Jones TF, et al. Hemolytic uremic syndrome and death in persons with Escherichia coli O157:H7 infection, Foodborne Diseases Active Surveillance Network sites, 2000–2006. *Clin Infect Dis*. 2009;49:1480-1485.
3. Verweyen HM, Karch H, Brandis M, Zimmerhackl LB. Enterohemorrhagic Escherichia coli infections: following transmission routes. *Pediatr Nephrol*. 2000; 14:73-83.
4. Scheiring J, Andreoli SP, Zimmerhackl LB. Treatment and outcome of Shiga-toxin -associated hemolytic uremic syndrome (HUS). *Pediatr Nephrol*. 2008;23:1749-1760.
5. Taylor CM. Enterohaemorrhagic Escherichia coli and Shigella dysenteriae type 1-induced haemolytic uraemic syndrome. *Pediatr Nephrol*. 2008;23:1425-1431.
6. Besbas N, Karpman D, Landau D, Loirat C, Proesmans W, Remuzzi G, et al. A classification of hemolytic uremic syndrome and thrombotic thrombocytopenic purpura and related disorders. *Kidney Int*. 2006;70:423-431.
7. Waters AM, Licht C. aHUS caused by complement dysregulation: new therapies on the horizon. *Pediatr Nephrol*. 2011;26(1):41-57. Erratum in: *Pediatr Nephrol*. 2013;28(1):165.
8. Ariceta G, Besbas N, Johnson S, Karpman D, Landau D, Licht C, et al. Guideline for the investigation and initial therapy of diarrhea negative hemolytic uremic syndrome. *Pediatr Nephrol*. 2009; 24(4):687-696.
9. Loirat C, Fremeaux-Bacchi V. Atypical hemolytic uremic syndrome. *Orphanet J Rare Dis*. 2011;6:60.
10. Tarr PI, Gordon CA, Chandler WL. Shiga-toxin-producing Escherichia coli and haemolytic uraemic syndrome. *Lancet*. 2005; 365:1073-1086.

11. Wong CS, Jelacic S, Habeeb RL, Watkins SL, Tarr PI. The risk of the hemolytic-uremic syndrome after antibiotic treatment of Escherichia coli O157:H7 infections. *N Engl J Med*. 2000;342: 1930–1936.

12. Keir LS, Marks SD, Kim JJ. Shigatoxin-associated hemolytic uremic syndrome: current molecular mechanisms and future therapies. *Drug Des Devel Ther*. 2012; 6:195-208.

13. Keir L, Coward RJM. Advances in our understanding of the pathogenesis of glomerular thrombotic microangiopathy. *Pediatr Nephrol*. 2011;26:523-533.

14. Legendre CM, Licht C, Muus P, Greenbaum LA, Babu S, Bedrosian C,et al. Terminal complement inhibitor eculizumab in atypical hemolytic-uremic syndrome. *N Engl J Med*. 2013; 368(23): 2169-2181.

15. US Food and Drug Administration, US Department of Health and Human Services. http://www.fda.gov/AboutFDA/CentersOffices/OfficeofMedicalProductsandTobacco/CDER/ucm273089.htm, accessed on 2013

16. Westra D, Wetzels JF, Volokhina EB, van den Heuvel LP, van de Kar NC. A new era in the diagnosis and treatment of atypical haemolytic uraemic syndrome. *Neth J Med*. 2012; 70(3): 121-129.

17. Noris M, Remuzzi G. Hemolytic uremic syndrome. *J Am Soc Nephrol*. 2005; 16:1035-1050.

70 PEDIATRIC KIDNEY STONES

Karl T. Rew, MD

PATIENT STORY

A 13-year-old girl presents with pain in the right flank and mid-abdomen. Several family members have had kidney stones. Her urinalysis shows blood but no signs of infection. A pregnancy test is negative. Abdominal x-ray reveals bilateral stones (**Figure 70-1**). A CT shows a right ureteral stone and a non-obstructing stone in the left kidney (**Figures 70-2** and **70-3**). She successfully passes and catches the symptomatic stone. Stone analysis shows calcium oxalate. A metabolic workup shows idiopathic hypercalciuria as the cause of her stones.

INTRODUCTION

A kidney stone is a solid mass that forms when minerals crystallize and collect in the urinary tract. Kidney stones can cause pain and hematuria, and may lead to complications such as urinary tract obstruction and infection.

SYNONYMS

Kidney stone, nephrolithiasis, renal calculus, renal stone, urinary tract stone, ureterolithiasis, urolithiasis.

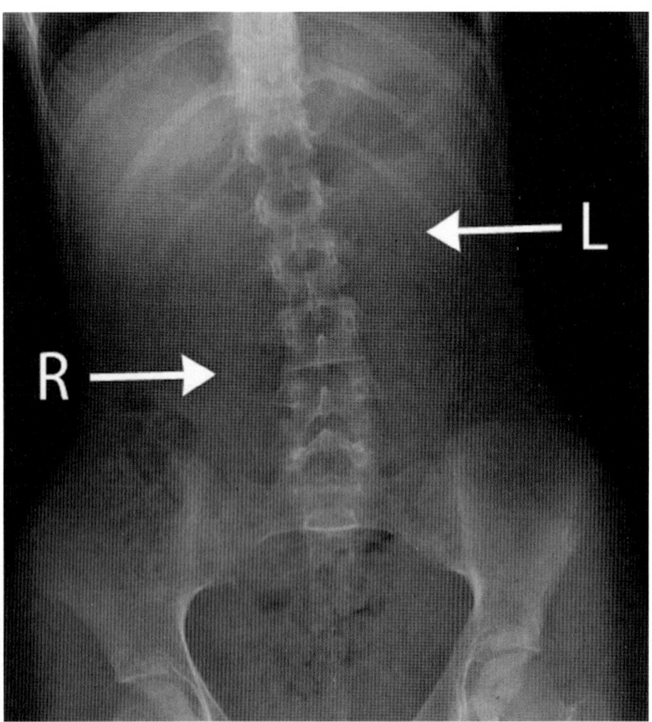

FIGURE 70-1 Plain abdominal x-ray showing with two subtle stones (arrows), one in the right ureter and one in the left kidney of a 13-year-old girl. (*Used with permission from Julian Wan, MD.*)

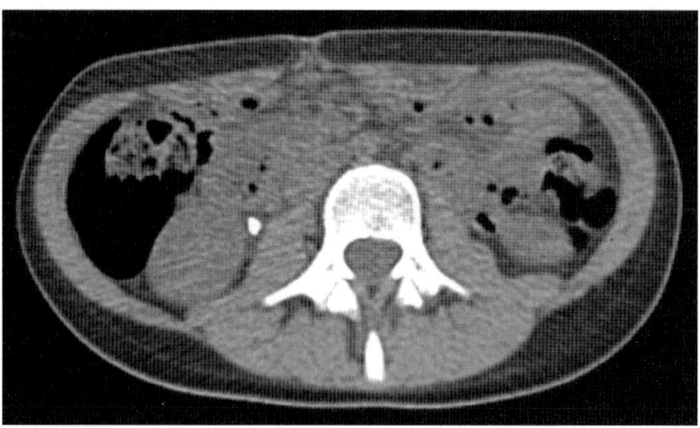

FIGURE 70-2 CT of the abdomen and pelvis of the same girl in **Figure 70-1**, showing a right ureteral stone. (*Used with permission from Julian Wan, MD.*)

EPIDEMIOLOGY

- The prevalence of kidney stones among children and adults in the US is increasing.[1] Part of this increase may be due to improvements in imaging techniques.[2,3] Although pediatric data are incomplete, children appear to be about 1/10 as likely to develop stones as adults.
- Kidney stones affect children of all ages but are most prevalent among adolescents, who are also more likely than younger children to present with symptomatic ureteral stones.[3,4]
- Boys and girls overall have similar rates of stone formation, although prevalence varies by age, type of stone, and geographic region.[5,6]
- African-American children have a lower rate of kidney stones than white children.[4,7]
- Genetic, metabolic, and anatomic disorders are the main causes of stones in children. Children are at higher risk of recurrent stones and subsequent renal dysfunction than adults for whom environmental and dietary causes are more common.[4] Obesity and weight gain increase the risk of stone formation in adults;[8] the effects of pediatric obesity are being studied.

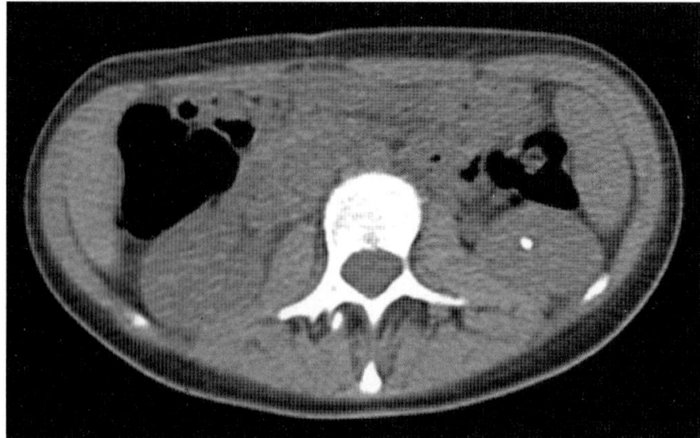

FIGURE 70-3 CT of the abdomen and pelvis of the same girl in **Figure 70-1**, showing a left kidney stone. (*Used with permission from Julian Wan, MD.*)

- Calcium oxalate and calcium phosphate stones are the most common in children, occurring in about 90 percent of cases. Struvite (magnesium ammonium phosphate) stones occur in about 5 percent of cases and are becoming less common. About 2 percent of pediatric stones are cystine stones. Uric acid stones are less common in children than adults, occurring in less than 1 percent of cases. Medication stones and other types of stones are rare.[6]

ETIOLOGY AND PATHOPHYSIOLOGY

- Kidney stones form when there is supersaturation of otherwise soluble materials, usually from increased excretion of these compounds or from dehydration. Idiopathic hypercalciuria is the most common abnormality found in adolescents. Low urinary citrate can increase the risk of calcium stone formation because citrate in the urine binds calcium and impedes stone formation in several other ways. Urine pH can affect stone formation: calcium phosphate and cystine stones form in more alkaline urine (pH >7), while uric acid stones form in acidic urine (pH <5.5).
- Struvite stones are caused by infection with urea-splitting bacteria, mainly *Proteus*.
- Cystine stones occur in patients with an inherited defect of dibasic amino acid transport. These stones can be pure cystine or cystine mixed with calcium oxalate.
- Uric acid stones form in patients with hyperuricemia from gout, myeloproliferative disorders, chemotherapy, or Lesch-Nyhan syndrome. Acidic urine due to a ketogenic diet or chronic diarrhea can increase the risk of uric acid stones.
- Struvite, cystine, and uric acid stones can grow large, filling the renal pelvis and extending into the calyces to form staghorn calculi (**Figure 70-4**).

RISK FACTORS

- Many kidney stones occur in patients with no known risk factors. However, a 24-hour urine collection often shows a low urine volume from inadequate fluid intake.

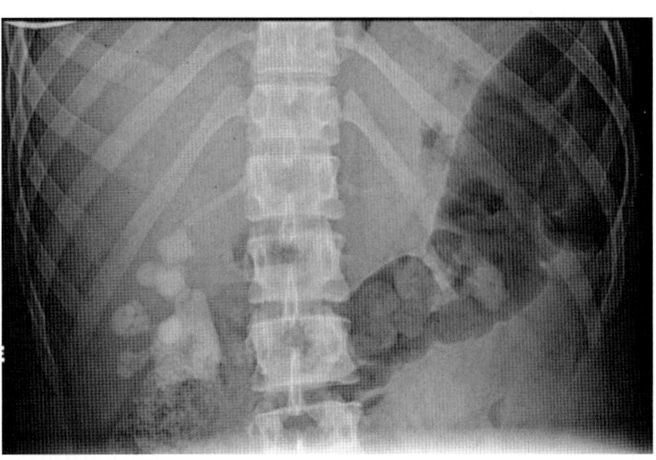

FIGURE 70-4 Plain abdominal x-ray of a 15-year-old girl with cystinuria and a large staghorn calculus in the right kidney. (*Used with permission from Julian Wan, MD.*)

- The risk of forming calcium stones has been shown in adults to be increased by obesity,[8] diabetes mellitus, metabolic syndrome, and by diets high in animal protein, salt, and oxalate-containing foods; these factors are being studied in children.
- Contrary to popular belief, calcium in the diet does not lead to calcium stones; in fact, dietary calcium can help prevent calcium oxalate stones by trapping oxalate in the GI tract.
- Patients with neurogenic bladder, anatomic anomalies causing poor urinary drainage, or long-term catheters are at risk for *Proteus* urinary tract infections and struvite stones.
- Cystine stones are found in families with an autosomal recessive defect in a protein that transports dibasic amino acids in the kidneys, increasing the concentration of insoluble cystine in the urine. All homozygotes and some heterozygotes are at risk for cystinuria and stones.
- Uric acid stones are most likely in patients who have hyperuricemia along with acidic urine from chronic diarrhea, diabetes mellitus, or a ketogenic diet.

DIAGNOSIS

CLINICAL FEATURES

- Stones in the kidneys can be asymptomatic. Such stones, found incidentally on imaging done for other reasons, sometimes remain in the kidneys for years without causing symptoms.
- Stone passage into the ureter usually causes pain and hematuria. The pain of renal colic in adolescents typically begins suddenly in the ipsilateral flank or abdomen and progresses in waves, gradually increasing in intensity over the next 20 to 60 minutes. As the stone moves downward, pain may be felt in the ipsilateral groin, testis, or vulva. Diagnosing urinary tract stones is often more difficult in younger children who may present with hematuria, nonspecific abdominal pain, or urinary tract infection.
- Obstructing stones cause hydronephrosis, often with an associated constant dull flank pain. Stones in the bladder can cause frequency, urgency, dysuria, or recurrent urinary tract infections.

LABORATORY

- Urinalysis usually reveals microscopic hematuria and limited pyuria. Gross hematuria is less common. Cystine crystals are pathognomonic for cystinuria.
- Urine culture should be done to assess for infection.
- Because treatment and prevention depend on stone type, stone capture and analysis is recommended. SOR Ⓒ Stones can be collected with a strainer in older children, and by examining diapers in younger children.
- Metabolic work-up is recommended for all children with a urinary tract stone.[9] This includes testing of urine (ideally with a 24-hour collection) for pH, volume, calcium, oxalate, and citrate, with simultaneous serum tests for calcium, uric acid, electrolytes, and creatinine. When a 24-hour urine cannot be collected, a random urine should be tested. In patients with elevated serum calcium, parathyroid hormone (PTH) should be measured.

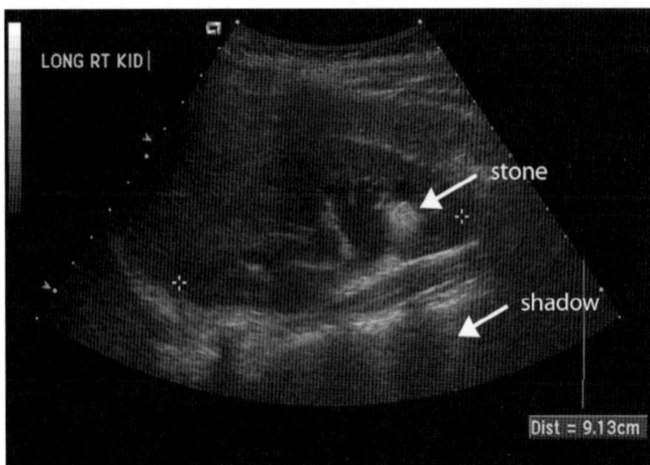

FIGURE 70-5 Ultrasound of right sided kidney stone (arrow) in an 8-year-old girl. Note the shadowing that occurs below the stone. *(Used with permission from Julian Wan, MD.)*

IMAGING

- Plain abdominal x-ray will demonstrate most calcium, struvite, and cystine stones. It is recommended for patients with a prior radiopaque stone (**Figures 70-1** and **70-4**).
- Ultrasound can be used to monitor uric acid stones (typically radiolucent), to assess hydronephrosis, or to limit exposure to x-rays (**Figure 70-5**). Ultrasound also may provide clues to diagnoses outside the urinary system.
- Noncontrast helical CT (**Figures 70-2** and **70-3**) is the preferred imaging approach for adults with stones and has largely replaced intravenous urography. However, in children, an adequate assessment can often be made using plain x-ray and ultrasound, reducing their radiation exposure. CT is effective for diagnosing stones in children and it may provide clues to diagnoses outside the urinary system, but the radiation exposure is 2 to 10 times that of a single plain abdominal x-ray.[10]

DIFFERENTIAL DIAGNOSIS

Other causes of flank and lower pelvic/groin pain:

- Gynecologic conditions in girls (e.g., ovarian torsion, cyst, or ectopic pregnancy) can often be distinguished on ultrasound. Pelvic inflammatory disease can also present with pain and is diagnosed based on clinical examination and culture.
- In boys, orchitis, epididymitis, or testicular torsion can cause pain that can be confused with kidney stones. Testicular tumors rarely cause pain. Physical examination can help differentiate these conditions.
- Urologic disorders that can cause pain include ureteropelvic junction obstruction, renal subcapsular hematoma, and renal cysts (see Chapter 65, Hydronephrosis and UPJ Obstruction and Chapter 66, Polycystic Kidneys). Imaging assists in differentiating these from kidney stones.

Abdominal pain from renal stones may be similar to pain caused by other diagnoses:

- Colitis or appendicitis—Systemic symptoms may include fever, diarrhea, rectal bleeding, tenesmus (i.e., urgency with a feeling of incomplete evacuation), passage of mucus, and cramping abdominal pain (see Chapter 59, Inflammatory Bowel Disease). GI symptoms with kidney stones are usually limited to nausea and vomiting from stimulation of the celiac plexus.
- Peptic ulcer disease is characterized by epigastric pain along with dyspeptic symptoms (see Chapter 55, Peptic Ulcer Disease). Upper endoscopy is the preferred procedure for diagnosing ulcers. Stool antigen test can confirm *Helicobacter pylori* infection.
- Urinary tract infection (UTI) can mimic stones within the bladder. Helpful indictors of UTI are a urine dipstick positive for nitrates (positive likelihood ratio [LR+] 26.5) and urinary sediment showing 10 or more bacteria/ high-power field (LR+ 85).

Hematuria can be seen in patients with:

- Infection including UTI, sexually transmitted infection or schistosomiasis.
- Renal disease such as glomerulonephritis, immunoglobulin [Ig] A nephropathy, lupus nephritis or hemolytic uremic syndrome (see Chapters 67, Nephrotic Syndrome; Chapter 68, Nephritic Syndromes; and Chapter 69, Hemolytic Uremic Syndrome).
- Trauma.

MANAGEMENT

NONPHARMACOLOGIC

- Adequate fluid intake is essential—2 to 3 L of water per day for most adolescent and adult patients.[11] SOR B
- Small stones are likely to pass spontaneously. About 3/4 of distal ureteral stones and about half of proximal ureteral stones will pass spontaneously.

MEDICATIONS

- Medical expulsive therapy, with α-adrenergic blockers (such as tamsulosin) or calcium-channel blockers, increases the chance of stone passage in adults and has been used successfully in children, although it is not currently FDA approved.[12] SOR B
- Effective pain control should be provided using NSAIDs and narcotics if needed. NSAIDs may need to be avoided if planning lithotripsy because of increased risk of perinephric bleeding.

COMPLEMENTARY AND ALTERNATIVE THERAPY

- For prevention of struvite stones, urine can be acidified with cranberry juice.[11] Drinking lemon juice daily can raise citrate levels in urine and help prevent calcium stones. Other supplements have been suggested as potentially protective against renal stones, but study results are conflicting.

PROCEDURES

- Stones that do not pass spontaneously or with medical expulsive therapy can be treated with extracorporeal shockwave lithotripsy or removed via ureteroscopy. Endoscopic retrograde lithotripsy and laser procedures have been increasingly successful, even in smaller children. Large stones may require percutaneous nephrolithotomy or open surgery.

REFERRAL

- Urgent urologic consultation is recommended for patients with stones and urosepsis, anuria, or renal failure. Urologic consultation is recommended for patients with refractory pain and nausea, extremes of age, major comorbidities, and stones >5 mm. SOR Ⓒ
- Nephrologic consultation is helpful to guide treatment for patients with acute kidney injury or chronic kidney disease.
- Both parents and patients can benefit from consultation with a dietician to help them adhere to a stone-prevention diet while maintaining adequate nutrition.
- Genetic consultation is recommended for those with cystinuria or other inherited risk factors.

PREVENTION

- High fluid intake and low sodium intake will help prevent most types of stones.
- Low-calcium diets should not be used in patients with calcium stones. A low-calcium diet can increase stone formation and decrease bone mineral density.
- Foods high in oxalate should be avoided by those who form calcium oxalate stones; food sources include rhubarb, spinach, Swiss chard, beets, apricots, figs, kiwi, many soy products, chocolate, and many nuts and seeds.
- Cystine stone formers should avoid methionine, found in higher-protein foods such as fish, meat, eggs, dairy products, and soybeans.
- Uric acid stones are prevented with a low-purine diet. High-purine foods to avoid include fish, shellfish, meats (especially game meats and organ meats), and protein supplements such as brewer's yeast. Daily allopurinol can help prevent uric acid stones.

Additional treatments may be warranted based on the type of stone:

- Patients with recurrent calcium-containing stones caused by idiopathic hypercalciuria can be treated with a thiazide diuretic, which may reduce recurrence by 50 percent over 3 years. Hypokalemia should be avoided because low potassium can reduce urinary citrate and increase stone formation.
- Idiopathic stone disease can be treated with fluids and potassium citrate. Potassium citrate is not FDA approved for use in children but European studies suggest an initial pediatric dose of 1 mEq/kg/d divided into 2 to 3 daily doses.[13]
- For cystine stones, increasing fluid intake, alkalinizing the urine to a pH ≥7.5, and a low-sodium diet are recommended. D-Penicillamine binds with cystine, helping to dissolve and prevent cystine stones, but it is not always well tolerated.

PROGNOSIS

- Half of patients with a first calcium-containing stone have a recurrence within 10 years. Twenty-five percent of struvite stones recur if there was incomplete removal of the stone. Cystine stones recur one or more times per year in most patients.
- Long-term complications can include hypertension and chronic kidney disease. The proportion of nephrolithiasis-related end-stage renal disease (ESRD) in patients of all ages is small (3.2%).

FOLLOW-UP

- A follow-up consultation to discuss kidney stone prevention is important for all patients with an initial stone. Patients started on medical therapy should be reevaluated with a 24-hour urine in 3 months. Those with a history of recurrent stones should be seen at least annually.

PATIENT EDUCATION

Increasing water intake to keep urine specific gravity around 1.005 (or about 2 to 3 L/day in adolescents) is recommended for most patients. In adults this has been shown to reduce stone recurrences by half. Dietary information is available (see the following section, "Patient Resources").

PATIENT RESOURCES

- National Kidney and Urologic Diseases Information Clearinghouse. *Kidney Stones in Children*—**http://kidney.niddk.nih.gov/KUDiseases/pubs/stoneschildren/**.
- National Kidney and Urologic Diseases Information Clearinghouse. *Diet for Kidney Stone Prevention*—**http://kidney.niddk.nih.gov/kudiseases/pubs/kidneystonediet/**.
- *The Oxalate Content of Food*—**www.ohf.org/docs/Oxalate2008.pdf**.

PROVIDER RESOURCES

- American Urologic Association. *2007 Guideline for the Management of Ureteral Calculi*—**www.auanet.org/content/clinical-practice-guidelines/clinical-guidelines.cfm?sub=uc**.
- European Association of Urology. *Guidelines on Urolithiasis*, update March 2011—**www.uroweb.org/gls/pdf/18_Urolithiasis.pdf**.

REFERENCES

1. VanDervoort K, Wiesen J, Frank R, et al. Urolithiasis in pediatric patients: a single center study of incidence, clinical presentation and outcome. *J Urology*. 2007;177:2300-2305.
2. Tanaka ST, Pope JC IV. Pediatric stone disease. *Curr Uro Rep*. 2009;10:138-143.
3. Dwyer ME, Krambeck AE, Bergstralh EJ, et al. Temporal trends in incidence of kidney stones among children: a 25-year population based study. *J Urology*. 2012;188:247-252.
4. Habbig S, Beck BB, Hoppe B. Nephrocalcinosis and urolithiasis in children. *Kidney Int*. 2011;80:1278-1291.

5. Gnessin E, Chertin L, Chertin B. Current management of paediatric urolithiasis. *Pediatr Surg Int*. 2012;28:659-665.

6. Gabrielsen JS, Laciak RJ, Frank EL, et al. Pediatric urinary stone composition in the United States. *J Urology*. 2012:187;2182-2187.

7. Sas DJ, Hulsey TC, Shatat IF, Orak JK. Increasing incidence of kidney stones in children evaluated in the emergency department. *J Pediatr*. 2010;157(1):132-136.

8. Taylor EN, Stampfer MJ, Curhan GC. Obesity, weight gain, and the risk of kidney stones. *JAMA*. 2005;293(4):455-462.

9. Worcester EM, Coe FL. Calcium kidney stones. *N Engl J Med*. 2010:363:954-963.

10. Johnson EK, Faerber GJ, Roberts WW, et al. Are stone protocol computed tomography scans mandatory for children with suspected urinary calculi? *Urology*. 2011;78:662-667.

11. Frasetto L, Kohlstadt I. Treatment and prevention of kidney stones: an update. *Am Fam Physician*. 2011;84(11):1234-1242.

12. Hollingsworth JM, Rogers MA, Kaufman SR, et al. Medical therapy to facilitate urinary stone passage: a metaanalysis. *Lancet*. 2006;368:1171-1179.

13. Tekin A, Tekgul S, Atsu N, et al. Oral potassium citrate treatment for idiopathic hypocitruria in children with calcium urolithiasis. *J Urology*. 2002;168(6):2572–2574.

71 RENOVASCULAR HYPERTENSION

Halima S. Janjua, MD
Raed Bou Matar, MD
Charles Y. Kwon, MD

PATIENT STORY

A 14-year-old girl presents to your office for a routine physical examination. She has history of chronic headaches and complains about abdominal pain after eating. Her vital signs reveal a blood pressure of 163/100 mm Hg. Repeat manual blood pressure is 152/98 mm Hg. You obtain laboratory studies, which reveal a normal serum creatinine, mild hypokalemia, and elevated plasma renin activity and aldosterone level. Her renal ultrasound with Doppler is suspicious for right renal artery stenosis. You start hypertension management with a calcium-channel blocker and refer her to a pediatric nephrologist, who obtains a computed tomography angiography (**Figure 71-1**) that reveals severe narrowing of right renal artery. Her blood pressure remains sub-optimally controlled with calcium-channel blockers. An angiotensin II receptor blocker is added to her hypertension management.

INTRODUCTION

Renovascular hypertension is hypertension that results from lesions that impair blood flow to one or both kidneys. It is an important cause of reversible hypertension in children.

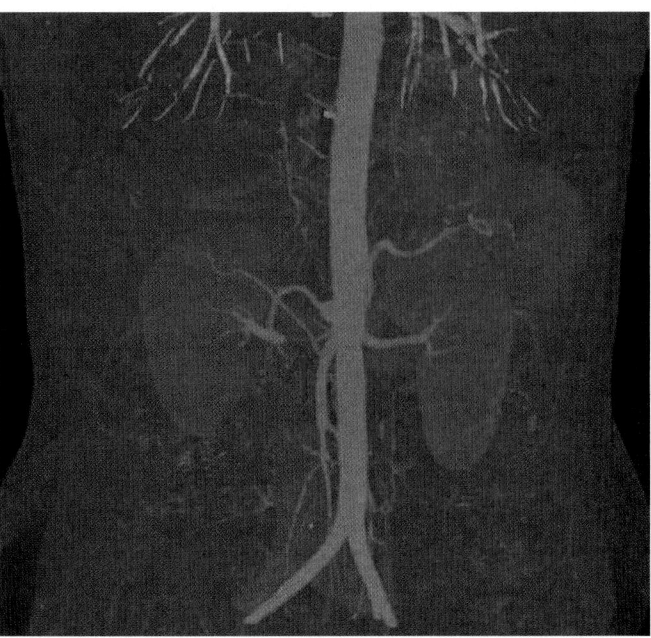

FIGURE 71-1 Stenosis of the right renal artery (arrow) on computed tomography angiography. (*Used with permission from Halima Janjua, MD.*)

SYNONYMS

Renal artery stenosis; renovascular disease.

EPIDEMIOLOGY

- Renovascular hypertension accounts for about 5 to 10 percent of hypertension in children.[1,2]

ETIOLOGY AND PATHOPHYSIOLOGY

- Renovascular hypertension is caused by the interplay of renin-mediated mechanisms, sodium-related volume expansion, and increased sympathetic nervous system activity.
- Specific causes of renovascular hypertension include:
  - Fibromuscular dysplasia.
  - Vasculitis (e.g., Takayasu's disease, Polyarteritis nodosa, or Kawasaki disease).
  - Syndromes (e.g., Neurofibromatosis type 1, Tuberous sclerosis, Williams syndrome, or Marfan syndrome).
  - Umbilical artery catheterization.
  - Mid-aortic syndrome.
  - Renal artery hypoplasia.
  - Extrinsic compression (e.g., Neuroblastoma, Wilms tumor).

DIAGNOSIS

CLINICAL FEATURES

- The clinical presentation of renovascular hypertension can be very variable.
- Children can be asymptomatic and incidentally found to have severe hypertension or they can present with symptoms secondary to end-organ damage from severe hypertension.
- An abdominal or flank bruit, signaling turbulent blood flow, may be heard on physical exam.

LABORATORY TESTING

- Increased plasma renin activity (PRA)—PRA may be elevated in children with renovascular hypertension.
- Hyperaldosteronism—Aldosterone may be elevated due to activation of rennin-angiotensin-aldosterone system.
- Hypokalemia—May be seen due to effect of aldosterone.
- Metabolic alkalosis—May be seen due to effect of aldosterone.

IMAGING

- Doppler Ultrasonography—Renal arteries and its branches can be viewed by color and pulsed-wave Doppler. Ultrasonography allows for measurement of peak systolic velocities in the intrarenal branches, although this study may not be sensitive enough to detect distal sites of stenosis.[3]
- Computed Tomography Angiography (CTA)—It provides three-dimensional images. It has better spatial resolution compared to

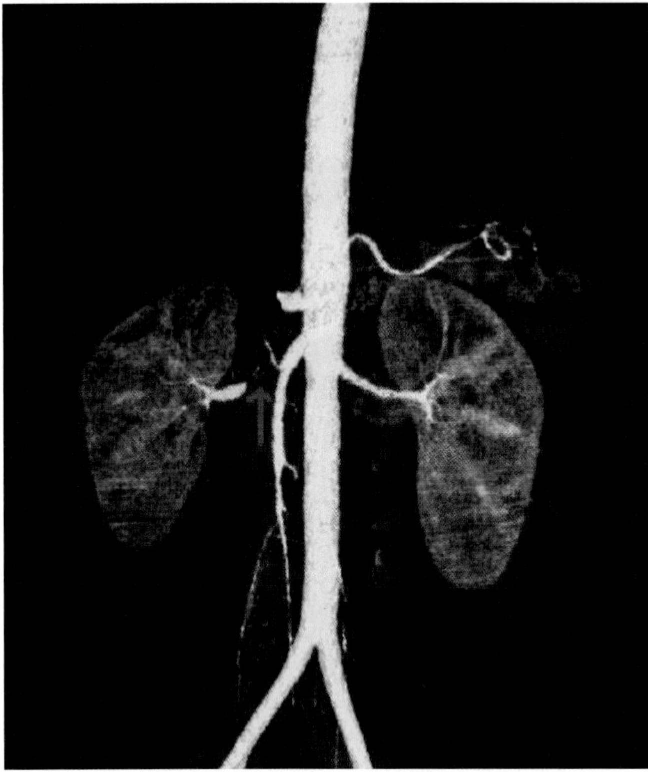

FIGURE 71-2 Right renal artery stenosis (arrow) on color-enhanced computed tomography angiography in the same patient as in **Figure 71-1**. (*Used with permission from Halima Janjua, MD.*)

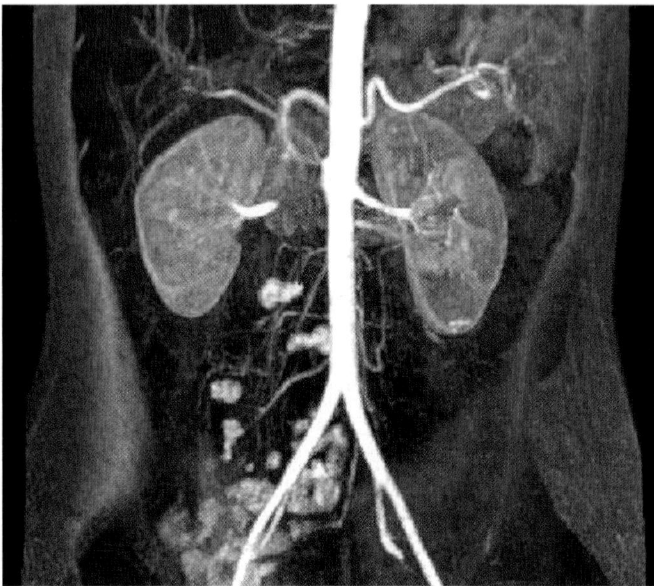

FIGURE 71-3 Magnetic Resonance Angiography of the patient in Figure 71-1 showing diffuse, long (2.4 cm) unilateral narrowing of the proximal/mid segments of the right renal artery (arrow) and mild-moderate narrowing of superior mesenteric artery above it. (*Used with permission from Halima Janjua, MD.*)

magnetic resonance angiography (MRA). This study can be conducted quickly and without general anesthesia though there is exposure to ionizing radiation (**Figures 71-1** and **71-2**).[4]

- Magnetic Resonance Angiography (MRA)—There is no exposure to ionizing radiation though gadolinium-based contrast is used that can lead to nephrogenic systemic fibrosis in children with glomerular filtration rates (GFR) of less than 30 mL/min/1.73 m^2. MRA also requires sedation or general anesthesia (**Figure 71-3**).
- Digital Subtraction Angiography (DSA)—It is considered the "gold standard" for diagnosing renovascular abnormalities. DSA can provide excellent images of the branches of renal arteries as well as show the "string of beads" sign of fibromuscular dysplasia. Presence of unilateral stenosis can be confirmed by sampling blood for renin from both renal veins. Another advantage of DSA is the endovascular treatment that can be performed by the interventional radiologist at the time of DSA. DSA requires higher radiation dose than CTA, general anesthesia, and a pediatric vascular surgical backup.

DIFFERENTIAL DIAGNOSIS

Other than renovascular hypertension, differential diagnosis for children with severe hypertension includes:

- Renal scarring—Usually a history of chronic urinary tract infections is apparent.
- Chronic glomerulonephritis—History of prior renal disease and signs of nephritis usually apparent (see Chapter 68, Nephritic Syndromes).
- Polycystic kidney diseases—Usually detected on imaging studies (see Chapter 66, Polycystic Kidneys).
- Hemolytic uremic syndrome—Suspected on basis on renal dysfunction, hemolytic anemia and thrombocytopenia (see Chapter 69, Hemolytic Uremic Syndrome).
- Chronic renal failure—Signs and symptoms will be apparent.
- Tumors—Detected on imaging studies.
- Vasculitis—Usually accompanied by other systemic manifestations.
- Coarctation of aorta—Apparent on a careful physical examination of all peripheral pulses.
- Pheochromocytoma—Manifests with severe hypertension, tachycardia, and systemic symptoms.
- Neuroblastoma—May be the presenting feature. Usually seen on imaging studies.
- Iatrogenic—Uncommon in infants and children.

MANAGEMENT

Children with renovascular hypertension usually have chronic high blood pressure, which must be lowered gradually.

MEDICATIONS

- Angiotensin-converting enzyme inhibitors (ACEi) and angiotensin II receptor blockers (ARBs) should be used with caution since they can reduce an already diminished glomerular filtration pressure. The resulting drop in glomerular filtration pressure may cause severe acute kidney injury in some patients with bilateral severe stenosis, high-grade stenosis in one kidney or advanced chronic kidney disease.[6] SOR Ⓒ

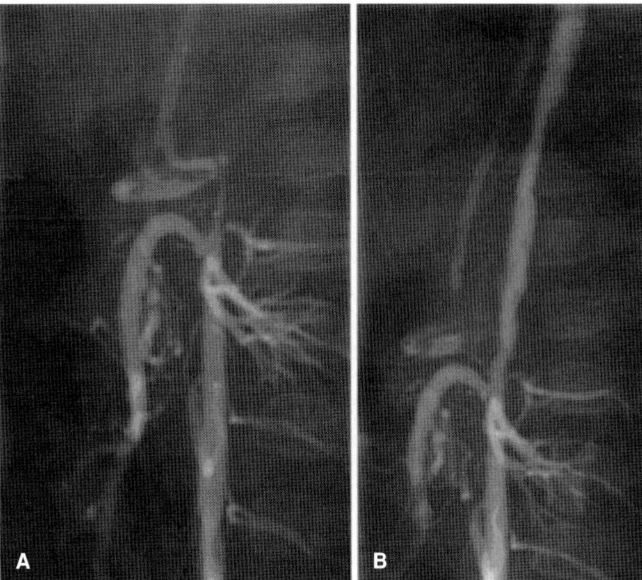

FIGURE 71-4 Severe midaortic syndrome. Note the narrowing of the abdominal aorta before angioplasty (**A**) that improved after angioplasty (**B**). (*Used with permission from Springer Science+Business Media, with kind permission: Clinical Hypertension and Vascular Diseases: Pediatric Hypertension, edited by: J. T. Flynn et al. DOI 10.1007/978-1-60327-824-9_20. Springer Science+Business Media, LLC 2011. Chapter 20. Fig. 2.*)

- Calcium-channel blockers and beta-blockers are relatively safe initial antihypertensive options. However, it not unusual for these children to require multiple antihypertensive medications to control their blood pressure leading to cautious use of ACEi or ARBs. SOR C

ENDOVASCULAR INTERVENTIONS

- Revascularization and restoration of renal blood flow is required in patients who either cannot tolerate antihypertensive medications or have refractory hypertension.
- Revascularization can be achieved via percutaneous angioplasty, segmental transarterial ethanol ablation, or surgery. In general, the choice of treatment depends on the age and size of the child, technical feasibility, extent of the disease process, and underlying cause.
- Percutaneous angioplasty, with or without stenting, is the most commonly used first line intervention. It has shown clinically significant improvement in about 50 percent of the cases and is associated with a high rate of restenosis (**Figures 71-4** and **Figure 71-5**). SOR C
- In cases of segmental branch stenosis, for which angioplasty is difficult to perform, segmental ethanol ablation may be a reasonable alternative.[9,10] SOR C

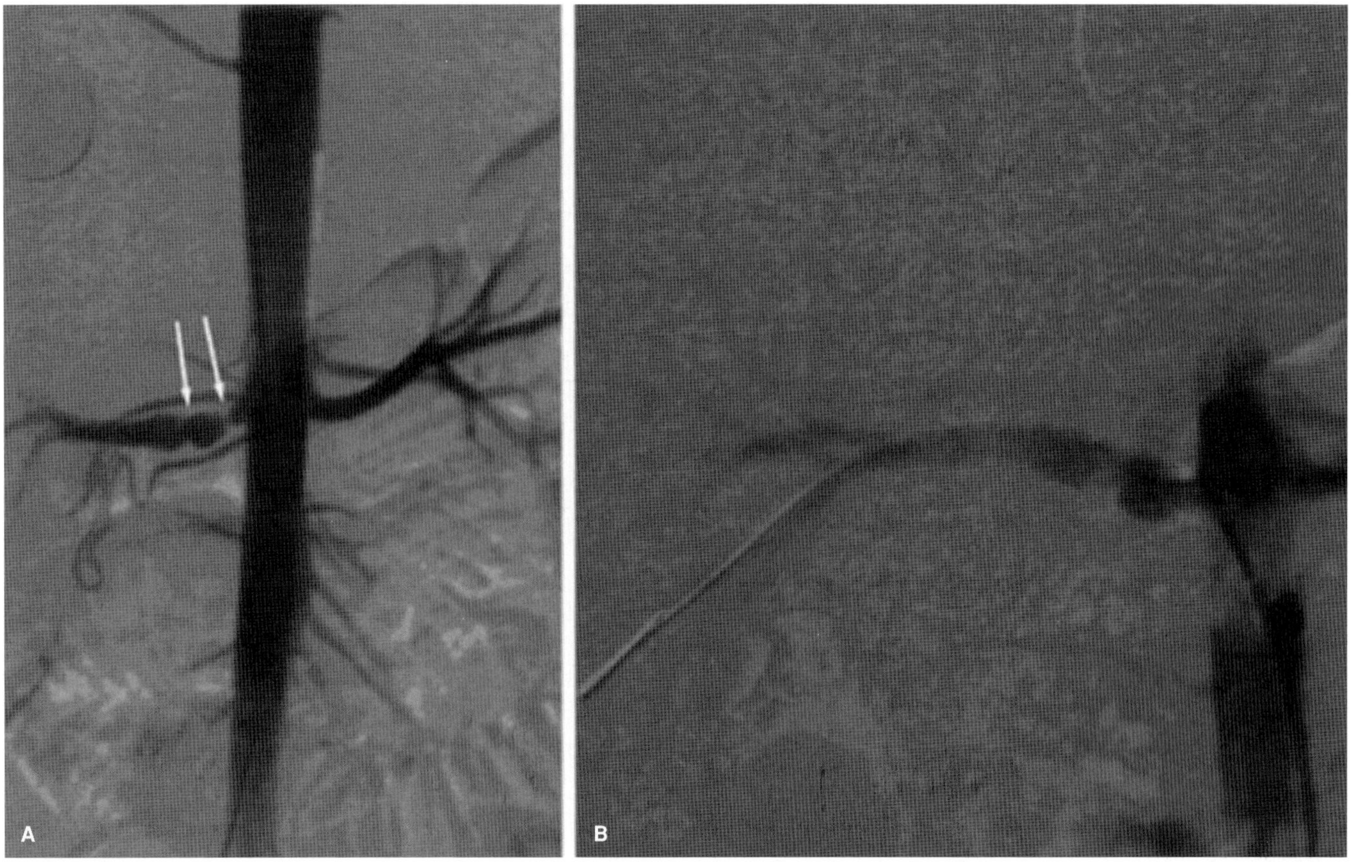

FIGURE 71-5 (**A**) Typical beaded appearance of a renal artery with severe stenosis. The arrows point to areas of stenosis between the beads. (**B**) After treatment with angioplasty. (*Used with permission from Springer Science+Business Media, Clinical Hypertension and Vascular Diseases: Pediatric Hypertension, edited by J. T. Flynn et al. DOI 10.1007/978-1-60327-824-9_20. Springer Science+Business Media, LLC 2011. Chapter 20. Fig. 3.*)

SURGERY

- Partial or complete unilateral nephrectomy or revascularization surgery with autologous or synthetic grafts is reserved for complicated cases or those with failed angioplasty or ethanol ablation. These surgical procedures have shown to be of clinical benefit in about 97 percent of the cases.[11] SOR C

REFERRAL

- Renovascular hypertension is best managed by a multidisciplinary team approach that may include pediatric nephrologist, interventional radiologist, and vascular surgeon.

SCREENING

- Blood pressure screening should begin at age 3 years and continue with each health care visit, as recommended by American Academy of Pediatrics.[12]
- Children with severe or stage 2 hypertension defined as blood pressure >5 mmHg above the 99th percentile should be evaluated for secondary causes of hypertension.

PROGNOSIS

- Long-term outcome of renovascular hypertension is not clear.

FOLLOW-UP

- Periodic blood pressure measurements are recommended in patients with history of renovascular hypertension due to a significant risk of restenosis or formation of new vascular lesions.

PATIENT RESOURCES

- **www.healthychildren.org/English/health-issues/conditions/heart/Pages/High-Blood-Pressure-in-Children.aspx.**
- **www.heart.org/HEARTORG/Conditions/HighBloodPressure/UnderstandYourRiskforHighBloodPressure/High-Blood-Pressure-in-Children_UCM_301868_Article.jsp.**
- **www.vasculardisease.org/renovascular-hypertension-ras.**

PROVIDER RESOURCES

- *Clinical Hypertension and Vascular Diseases*. Pediatric Hypertension, edited by J. T. Flynn et al. DOI 10.1007/978-1-60327-824-9_20.
- **www.emedicine.medscape.com/article/245140.**

REFERENCES

1. Gill DG, Mendes de Costa B, Cameron JS, et al. Analysis of 100 children with severe and persistent hypertension. *Arch Dis Child*. 1976;51:951-956.
2. Wyszynska T, Cichocka E, Wieteska-Klimczak A, et al. A single pediatric center experience with 1025 children with hypertension. *Acta Paediatrica*. 1992;81:244-246.
3. Marks SD, Tullus K. Update on imaging for suspected renovascular hypertension in children and adolescents. *Curr Hypertens Rep*. 2012;14:591-595.
4. Frush DP. Pediatric abdominal CT angiography. *Pediatr Radiol*. 2008;38(2):S259-66.
5. Tan KT, van Beek EJ, Brown PW, et al. Magnetic resonance angiography for the diagnosis of renal artery stenosis: A meta-analysis. *Clin Radiol*. 2002;57:617-624.
6. Wong H, Hadi M, Khoury T, et al. Management of severe hypertension in a child with tuberous sclerosis-related major vascular abnormalities. *J Hypertens*. 2006;24:597-598.
7. Shroff R, Roebuck DJ, Gordon I, et al. Angioplasty for renovascular hypertension in children: 20-year experience. *Pediatrics*. 2006;118:268-725.
8. Bayrak HA, Numan F, Cantasdemir M, et al. Percutaneous balloon angioplasty of renovascular hypertension in pediatric cases. *Acta Chir Belg*. 2008;6:708-714.
9. Klimberg IW, Locke DR, Hawkins IF, Jr., et al. Absolute ethanol renal angioinfarction for control of hypertension. *Urology*. 1989;33:153-158.
10. McLaren CA, Roebuck DJ. Interventional radiology for renovascular hypertension in children. *Techniques in Vascular & Interventional Radiology*. 2003;6:150-157.
11. Stanley JC, Criado E, Upchurch GR, Jr., et al. Pediatric renovascular hypertension: 132 primary and 30 secondary operations in 97 children. *Journal of Vascular Surgery*. 2006;44:1219-1229.
12. *American Academy of Pediatrics*, Bright Futures, 2013.

PART 11

NEWBORN

Strength of Recommendation (SOR)	Definition
A	Recommendation based on consistent and good-quality patient-oriented evidence.*
B	Recommendation based on inconsistent or limited-quality patient-oriented evidence.*
C	Recommendation based on consensus, usual practice, opinion, disease-oriented evidence, or case series for studies of diagnosis, treatment, prevention, or screening.*

*See Appendix A on pages 1320–1322 for further information.

72 NEONATAL CONJUNCTIVITIS

Dawood Yusef, MD
Camille Sabella, MD

PATIENT STORY

A 6-day-old girl is admitted to the hospital because of profuse yellowish drainage from both eyes. The infant was born at home after a 36-week gestation age to an 18-year-old mother. Maternal screens were not obtained during pregnancy due to poor prenatal care. On exam, the infant had profuse purulent drainage from both eyes with significant eyelid edema (**Figure 72-1**). Gram stain of the purulent drainage revealed gram-negative diplococci, consistent with *Neisseria gonorrhoeae* infection (**Figure 72-2**). Blood and cerebrospinal fluid cultures were negative. The infant was treated with one dose of intravenous ceftriaxone and frequent eye irrigations and recovered completely.

INTRODUCTION

- Neonatal conjunctivitis (Ophthalmia neonatorum) occurs in the first month of life, and may be infectious or noninfectious (chemical) in origin. Knowledge of the differential diagnosis is essential in early diagnosis and management.

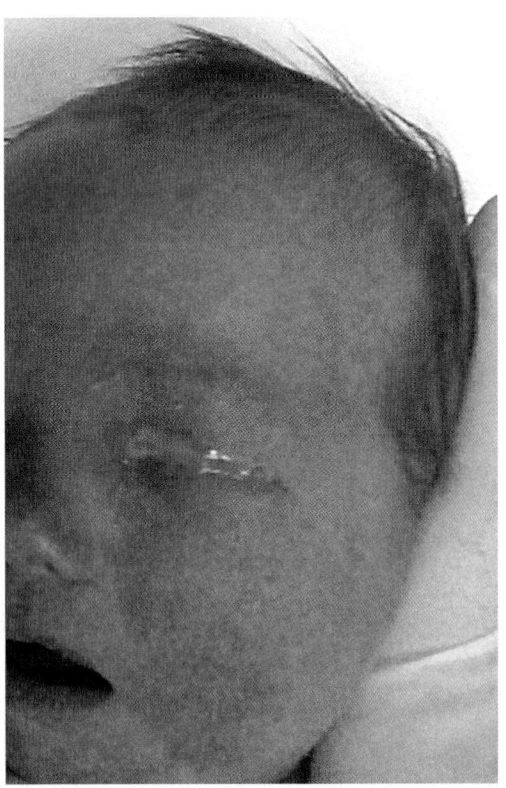

FIGURE 72-1 A 6-day-old infant with gonococcal conjunctivitis. *(Used with permission from Camille Sabella, MD.)*

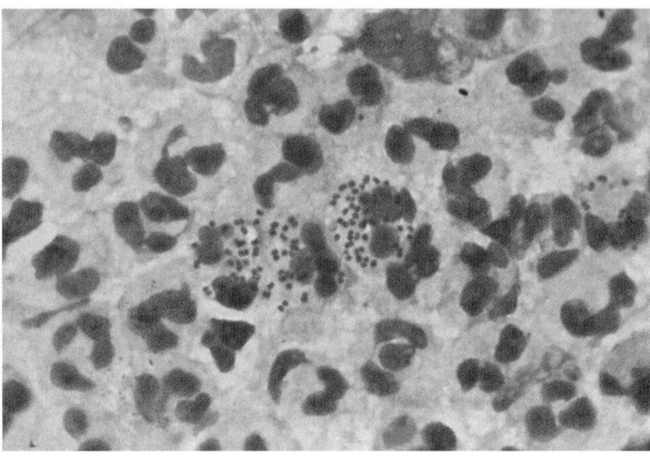

FIGURE 72-2 A Gram stain showing intracellular gram-negative diplococci of *Neisseria gonorrhoea*. *(Used with permissions from CDC/Bill Schwartz.)*

SYNONYMS

Ophthalmia neonatorum, inclusion (chlamydial) conjunctivitis.

EPIDEMIOLOGY

- Most infectious causes are acquired by the neonate during vaginal delivery.
- The risk of a newborn acquiring *Chlamydia trachomatis* from the infected mother is estimated to be 50 percent; up to half of these may develop conjunctivitis.[1]
- The incidence of gonococcal conjunctivitis has decreased dramatically since the introduction of newborn antimicrobial ocular prophylaxis.[2]
- Skin, eye, and mouth disease represents up to 45 percent of cases of neonatal herpes simplex infection,[3] which may present as neonatal conjunctivitis.

ETIOLOGY AND PATHOPHYSIOLOGY

- The most common cause of neonatal conjunctivitis is *Chlamydia trachomatis;* Other causative agents include *N gonorrhoeae* and Herpes simplex virus (HSV).[4]
- The role of bacterial agents other than *C trachomatis, N gonorrhoeae,* and HSV in the etiology of neonatal conjunctivitis is controversial; organisms such as *Staphylococcus aureus*, Group B Streptococci, and *Haemophilus influenzae,* which are occasionally isolated from newborns with conjunctivitis have been isolated from the conjunctivae of asymptomatic newborns.[1]
- Although rare, nosocomial neonatal conjunctivitis due to *Pseudomonas aeruginosa* can occur, and is related to prolonged stay in the neonatal intensive care unit.[5]
- Chemical conjunctivitis is a noninfectious cause of neonatal conjunctivitis, which most commonly occurs secondary to silver nitrate infant prophylaxis.

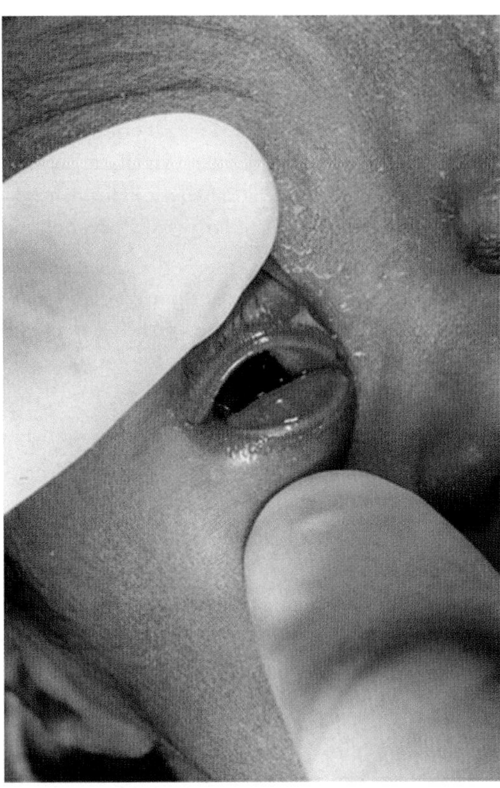

FIGURE 72-3 Chlamydia conjunctivitis in a neonate. (*Used with permission from Shah SS: Pediatric Practice: Infectious Diseases, www.accesspediatrics.com, and Shah BR, Lucchesi M. Atlas of Pediatric Emergency Medicine, McGraw-Hill.*)

RISK FACTORS

- Maternal infection with *C trachomatis, N gonorrhoeae* or HSV, especially during vaginal delivery, is the most important risk factor.[4]

DIAGNOSIS

CLINICAL FEATURES

- Signs and symptoms vary from mild erythema and watery eye discharge to severe eyelid swelling and purulent eye drainage, sometimes with chemosis (conjunctival edema) and formation of pseudomembranes (**Figures 72-1** to **72-4**).[4,6,7]
- Systemic signs or symptoms may indicate disseminated gonococcal infection, disseminated HSV infection, or sepsis.[3,6]
- *N gonorrhoeae* causes very severe infection and may lead to ulceration and scarring of the eye if untreated.
- Gonococcal conjunctivitis presents early in life (2 to 7 days of life), while conjunctivitis secondary to *C trachomatis* and other pathogens usually presents in the second week of life.[7]
- Chemical conjunctivitis usually occurs in the first 24 hours of life, and has been associated with eye prophylaxis with silver nitrate, which is no longer available for use in the US.[7]
- Neonatal HSV conjunctivitis may be the presenting feature of neonatal HSV infection involving the skin, eyes, and mucous membranes.[3]

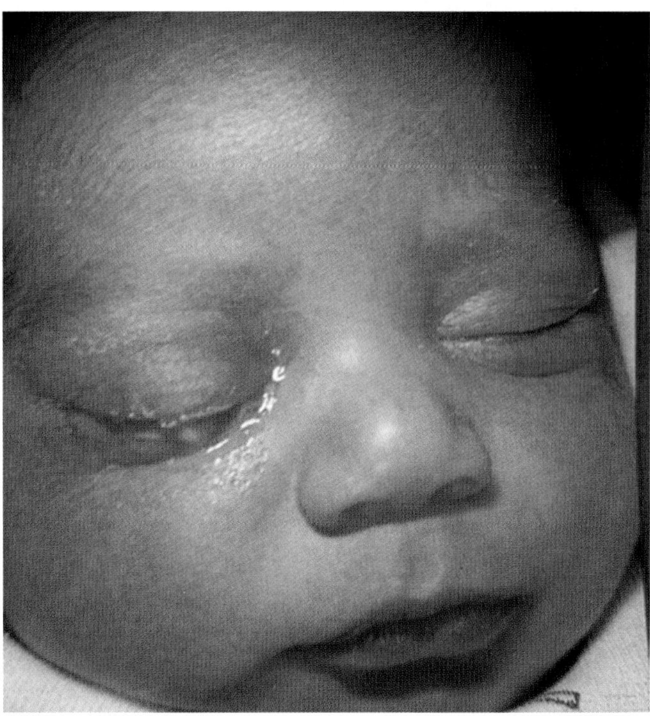

FIGURE 72-4 Neonate with gonococcal conjunctivitis. Note the purulent drainage and eyelid edema. (*Used with permission from Shah SS: Pediatric Practice: Infectious Diseases, www.accesspediatrics.com, and Shah BR, Lucchesi A. Atlas of Pediatric Emergency Medicine, McGraw-Hill.*)

DISTRIBUTION

- The conjunctivitis is usually bilateral, but can be unilateral.[4,6]
- Concurrent involvement of the skin and mucus membranes is common with HSV infection.

LABORATORY TESTING

- Gram stain of eye discharge that reveals intracellular gram-negative diplococci is highly suggestive of gonococcal conjunctivitis (**Figure 72-2**); culture of the organism confirms the diagnosis.
- Antigen detection tests for *C trachomatis*, such as Direct Fluorescent Antibody (DFA) and Enzyme Immunoassay have high specificity and sensitivity. These tests are approved by the US Food and Drug Administration (FDA) for the diagnosis of Chlamydial conjunctivitis.[9]
- Nucleic Acid Amplification Tests (NAAT) have not been approved by FDA for diagnosis of Chlamydial or gonococcal neonatal conjunctivitis.[7]
- Blood and cerebrospinal fluid cultures should be obtained when gonococcal infection is suspected or confirmed, to rule out disseminated disease.[4,7]
- Specimens from the conjunctivae and skin/mucus membranes lesions should be sent for HSV viral culture when HSV infection is suspected in a newborn. A DFA, which can provide a rapid diagnosis, can also be performed from suspicious lesions. DFA is highly specific but less sensitive than viral culture for detecting HSV.[3]

DIFFERENTIAL DIAGNOSIS

- Chemical conjunctivitis—Usually occurs in the first 24 hours of life, has a less severe course, and often resolves within 48 hours without specific treatment; a history of use of ocular silver nitrate prophylaxis is usually elicited.[7]

- Nasolacrimal duct obstruction—See Chapter 14, Nasolacrimal Duct Obstruction.
- Foreign body—Rarely can cause conjunctival erythema and drainage. History and unilateral presentation helpful in distinguishing from other causes.

MANAGEMENT

NONPHARMACOLOGICAL

- Frequent eye irrigation to prevent damage and scarring to the eye is essential in the management of gonococcal conjunctivitis.[4,6,7] SOR Ⓐ
- Chemical conjunctivitis is managed expectantly, and usually resolves spontaneously within 24 to 48 hours.

MEDICATIONS

- Oral erythromycin for 14 days is recommended by the American Academy of Pediatrics (AAP) for the treatment of *Chlamydial* conjunctivitis.[7] SOR Ⓐ
- Although an association between the use of erythromycin in neonates and infantile hypertrophic pyloric stenosis (IHPS) has been described,[10] there is a lack of adequate data with the use of other antimicrobial agents; thus, erythromycin continues to be the treatment of choice.
- Intravenous ceftriaxone is the treatment of choice for gonococcal conjunctivitis, given in a single dose for isolated ophthalmia neonatorum and for 7 to 14 days for disseminated gonococcal infection.[4,7] SOR Ⓐ
- The treatment of conjunctivitis caused by other pathogens depends on the likelihood of true infection and the pathogen involved.
- Neonatal HSV infection confined to the eyes, skin, and mucus membranes should be treated with intravenous acyclovir for a minimum of 14 days. A longer duration is required for disseminated or central nervous system involvement.[3,7] SOR Ⓐ

REFERRAL

- Ophthalmologists should be involved in the management of infants who have ophthalmia neonatorum.

PREVENTION AND SCREENING

- Maternal screening and treatment of maternal chlamydial and gonococcal infections during pregnancy decrease the rate of transmission to the newborn, and therefore, decrease the risk of neonatal conjunctivitis caused by these two pathogens.[8]
- Ocular prophylaxis for the neonate soon after birth is effective in preventing gonococcal conjunctivitis, but not chlamydial conjunctivitis. Topical agents used for this purpose include 0.5 percent erythromycin ointment, 1 percent tetracycline ointment, and 1 percent silver nitrate solution; however, only topical erythromycin ointment is currently available in the US.[2,8]
- Asymptomatic neonates born to mothers with untreated gonococcal infection should receive one dose of intravenous or intramuscular ceftriaxone or cefotaxime.[7,8] SOR Ⓐ
- Antibiotics are not indicated for newborns born to women with untreated *C trachomatis* because of unknown efficacy of such therapy and the risk of hypertrophic pyloric stenosis in neonates. Instead, the newborn should be monitored for signs of infection and careful follow-up ensured.[7] SOR Ⓒ
- Topical antibiotics are neither adequate nor necessary for treatment of gonococcal or chlamydia conjunctivitis when systemic antibiotics are used.[4,7] SOR Ⓐ

PROGNOSIS

- Generally, neonatal conjunctivitis has a good prognosis if treated promptly and appropriately.[4,6]
- Without adequate treatment, neonatal conjunctivitis may result in corneal scarring and vision impairment. This is especially true of conjunctivitis caused by *N gonorrhoeae* or HSV infection.[3,4,6,7]

FOLLOW-UP

- Newborns born to mothers who have *Chlamydia* infection should be followed closely for signs of conjunctivitis and treated accordingly if they develop such manifestations.
- *C trachomatis* may also cause pneumonia in the neonatal period, with or without history of conjunctivitis. Chlamydial pneumonitis, characterized by cough and tachypnea, usually becomes apparent at 4 to 12 weeks of life.[1,7]

PATIENT EDUCATION

- Parents are encouraged to seek medical advice immediately if a newborn baby develops signs or symptoms of conjunctivitis.
- The diagnosis of chlamydial or gonococcal conjunctivitis in a newborn warrants screening and appropriate treatment of sexually transmitted infections in the mother and her sexual partner.[8]

PATIENT RESOURCES

- **www.cdc.gov/conjunctivitis/newborns.html**.
- **www.uptodate.com/contents/newborn-conjunctivitis-the-basics?source=see_link**.

PROVIDER RESOURCES

- Committee on Infectious Diseases American Academy of Pediatrics. *Red Book: 2012 Report of the Committee on Infectious Diseases*, 29th, Pickering, LK, eds., American Academy of Pediatrics. Elk Grove Village, IL; 2012.

REFERENCES

1. Rours IG, Hammerschlag MR, Ott A, et al. Chlamydia trachomatis as a cause of neonatal conjunctivitis in Dutch infants. *Pediatrics*. 2008;121:e321.
2. Hammerschlag MR, Cummings C, Roblin PM, et al. Efficacy of neonatal ocular prophylaxis for the prevention of chlamydial and gonococcal conjunctivitis. *N Engl J Med*. 1989;320:769.
3. Kimberlin DW. Herpes simplex virus infections of the newborn. *Semin Perinatol*. 2007;31:19.
4. Hammerschlag MR. Neonatal conjunctivitis. *Pediatr Ann*. 1993;22 (6):346-351.
5. Shah SS, Gallagher PG. Complications of conjunctivitis caused by *Pseudomonas aeruginosa* in a newborn intensive care unit. *Pediatr Infect Dis J*. 1998;17(2):97-102.
6. Teoh DL, Reynolds S. Diagnosis and management of pediatric conjunctivitis. *Pediatr Emerg Care*. 2003 Feb;19(1):48-55.
7. Committee on Infectious Diseases American Academy of Pediatrics. Red Book: 2012 Report of the Committee on Infectious Diseases, 29th, Pickering, LK, eds., *American Academy of Pediatrics*. Elk Grove Village, IL; 2012.
8. Koumans EH, Rosen J, van Dyke MK, et al. Prevention of mother-to-child transmission of infections during pregnancy: implementation of recommended interventions, US, 2003-2004. *Am J Obstet Gynecol*. 2012;206:158.e1.
9. Black CM. Current methods of laboratory diagnosis of Chlamydia trachomatis infections. *Clin Microbiol Rev*. 1997;10:160.
10. Centers for Disease Control and Prevention (CDC). Hypertrophic pyloric stenosis in infants following pertussis prophylaxis with erythromycin–Knoxville, Tennessee, 1999. *MMWR Morb Mortal Wkly Rep*. 1999;48:1117.

73 ABDOMINAL WALL DEFECTS

Jose Lozada, MD
Anthony Stallion, MD

The normal abdominal wall is formed by infolding of the cranial, caudal, and two lateral embryonic folds. These folds form in the 4th week of development as a combination of the parietal layer of lateral plate mesoderm and overlying ectoderm. As they move ventrally to meet in the midline, rates of cell proliferation and fusion in the folds differ. This fusion process between the folds is complex, involving cell-to-cell adhesion, cell migration, and cell reorganization. Simultaneously, as the abdominal wall is forming, the rapid growth of the intestinal tract leads to its herniation through the umbilical ring into the yolk sac from the 6th to the 10th week of gestation. By the 10th to 12th week of gestation, the intestine returns to the abdominal cavity in a well-coordinated pattern. This results in normal intestinal rotation and fixation, followed by complete formation of the abdominal wall.[1]

Abnormal formation of the abdominal wall can result in omphalocele and possibly gastroschisis, which are discussed in succession.

GASTROSCHISIS

PATIENT STORY

A term newborn infant is found to have protrusion of the abdominal wall, involving the viscera (**Figure 73-1**). A prenatal diagnosis of gastroschisis had been made by ultrasound and the mother was referred to a high-risk obstetrical service for management. The infant was born via vaginal delivery and upon delivery was taken to the neonatal intensive care unit for immediate resuscitation and management. The family had met with the pediatric surgeon and neonatal intensive care team prior to the delivery. The infant underwent successful surgical repair for the defect. After a 5-week hospital course, the infant was discharged home with good bowel function.

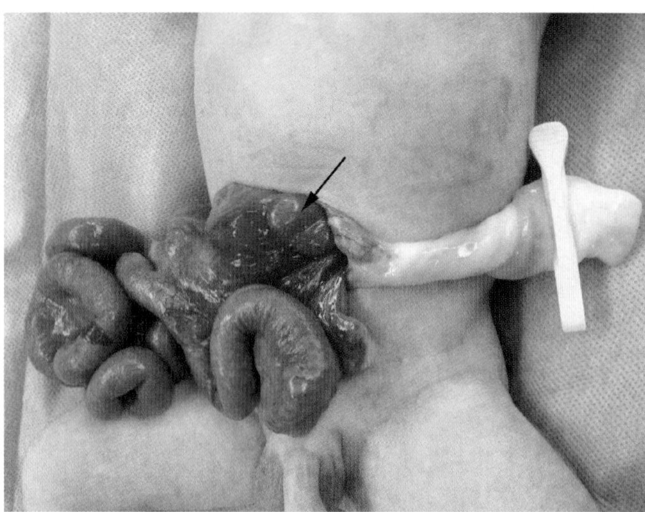

FIGURE 73-1 Newborn infant with gastroschisis. Note the evisceration occurring to the right of the umbilical cord. In addition to small intestine, his left testis (*arrow*) can also be appreciated as part of the exstrophy. (*Used with permission from Anthony Stallion, MD.*)

INTRODUCTION

Gastroschisis is a full-thickness defect in the abdominal wall, typically to the right of umbilical cord (**Figure 73-1**), where a variable amount of intestine and/or other organs may be herniated through the abdominal wall without a membrane or covering.[2,3]

EPIDEMIOLOGY

- The incidence of gastroschisis seems to be increasing worldwide and is approaching 3 to 4 per 10,000 births in endemic areas.[4]
- Recent epidemiologic studies have found a strong association between the occurrence of gastroschisis and young maternal age. However, a clear cause of gastroschisis has yet to be determined.[4,5]

ETIOLOGY AND PATHOPHYSIOLOGY

- The cause of a gastroschisis is unknown.
- Several theories have been proposed to explain the unique abdominal wall defect through which abdominal organs may eviscerate early in gestation.[6] These theories include:
  - Localized failure of mesoderm formation.
  - Rupture of the amnion at the umbilical ring.
  - Abnormal involution of the right umbilical vein.
  - Disruption of the right vitelline artery with subsequent localized body wall ischemia.
  - Abnormal body wall folding.
- Gastroschisis does not appear to be strongly associated with other congenital abnormalities. It is unclear if this represents evidence that gastroschisis is not a primary developmental defect.

RISK FACTORS

- Young maternal age.

DIAGNOSIS

PRENATAL DIAGNOSIS

- Abdominal wall defects are often diagnosed before birth by ultrasound. The specificity is greater than 95 percent, with sensitivity being more variable due to operator variability.[7]
- A study performed on pregnant women whose fetuses had known ventral wall defects found that there was an increase in serum alpha-fetoprotein levels.[8]

CLINICAL FEATURES

- About 10 percent of babies with gastroschisis will have intestinal stenosis or atresia likely stemming from vascular insufficiency to the bowel; this insufficiency could occur early at the time of gastroschisis development or later from volvulus or compression of the mesenteric vascular pedicle against a narrowing abdominal wall ring.
- Other associated anomalies, such as chromosomal abnormalities, are uncommon.[9,10]

DIFFERENTIAL DIAGNOSIS

- Omphalocele—see the following section.

MANAGEMENT

PRENATAL MANAGEMENT

- The most common associated risks for a fetus with gastroschisis include intrauterine growth retardation (IUGR), oligohydramnios, premature delivery, and fetal death.
- Because of these associated risks, the family should undergo high-risk obstetrics care connected to a specialized pediatric center to optimize the post-partum outcome.
- If prenatally diagnosed, the family should be introduced to the pediatric surgeon.
- While there are no current intrauterine interventions, this introduction allows the family to be counseled about the condition, its treatment and prognosis.

POST-PARTUM MANAGEMENT

- Initial airway, breathing, and circulation evaluation and intervention if necessary.
- Once this initial assessment and care has occurred, the next step involves placing the exposed viscera and entire lower half of the dried baby in a transparent plastic bag, commonly called a bowel bag. This allows the preservation of body heat and keeps the bowel moist. Care must be taken to support the bowel with moist gauze so that it does not fall to either side of the body and cause venous congestion and subsequent edema. This can hinder the ability to attain primary closure.
- A small hole can be made if necessary for a lower extremity to allow for intravenous access.
- Ensure appropriate gastric decompression.
- Given the risk of volume loss, aggressive hydration should be part of the initial management.

SURGERY

- If a primary closure is not possible, or if there are signs of bowel ischemia, a "silo" may be placed in the operating room (**Figure 73-2**). A "silo" is a tubular or inverted funnel-like structure with synthetic material to give temporary cover to the abdominal viscera and allow for serial reduction of the organs into the abdominal cavity. The "silo" protects the intestine and other viscera outside the abdomen while they are slowly reduced into the abdominal cavity with daily gentle pressure.

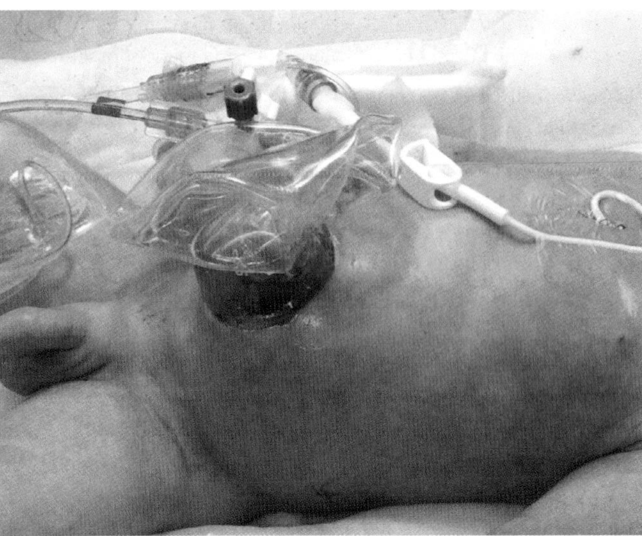

FIGURE 73-2 Intraoperative placed silo on same patient as **Figure 73-1**. *(Used with permission from Anthony Stallion, MD.)*

- This serial reduction of bowel has the goal of completely reducing the exposed viscera by the seventh to tenth day of life.
- Another approach that is being used more recently is the "pre-fashioned" or "pre-manufactured silo." A pre-fashioned silo is a tubularized synthetic material that comes formed from the manufacturer and does not require any suturing and can be placed at the bedside.
- This is followed by operative closure of the abdominal wall primarily or with a synthetic patch to avoid excessive intra-abdominal pressure.

REFERRAL

Referral to high-risk obstetrics care connected to a specialized pediatric center and pediatric surgery is imperative.

PREVENTION AND SCREENING

- Abdominal wall defects are often diagnosed before birth by ultrasound.

PROGNOSIS

- The outcome of patients with gastroschisis depends in great part to the condition of the bowel, size of the defect, and ability to reduce the viscera in a timely fashion.
- Survival has been reported to be between 90 and 95 percent, with the main cause of death being bowel loss and intestinal necrosis.[11]
- The risk for necrotizing enterocolitis is high, manifested by pneumatosis intestinalis (gas in the bowel wall) on radiographic imaging. This may occur in the postoperative period when feedings are being advanced.[12]
- The hospitalization period is usually long. This is mainly due to delayed return of bowel function and advancing to full enteral feedings, which is usually a combination of oral and tube feedings.

Many patients have some degree of difficulty nippling since they do not feed at birth and have a prolonged period without oral intake.

- Approximately 40 percent of patients are discharged within one month of surgical intervention, 36 percent between one to two months, and 25 percent greater than two months.[13]
- Overall, long-term gastrointestinal function is good. There are occasional patients with long-term intolerance of feedings, mainly due to dysmotility.[14] There is also a reported 5 to 10 percent long-term risk of adhesive obstructions.[15]

PATIENT RESOURCES

- **www.cdc.gov/ncbddd/birthdefects/Gastroschisis.html**.
- **www.nlm.nih.gov/medlineplus/ency/article/000992.htm**.

PROVIDER RESOURCES

- **www.ncbi.nlm.nih.gov/pubmed/19635303**.

OMPHALOCELE

PATIENT STORY

A diagnosis of omphalocele was made on fetal ultrasound in an infant who was delivered by Cesarean section at 37 weeks of gestation due to onset of labor. The newborn infant was noted to have a large midline abdominal wall defect with herniated intestines covered by a membrane. The umbilical vessels inserted directly into the membrane (**Figure 73-3**). The infant received immediate resuscitation including nasogastric compression and respiratory support. The infant's work-up included a chest x-ray, cardiac echocardiogram, and renal ultrasound to rule out associated congenital anomalies. The results of all these studies were normal. The patient was taken electively 24 hours after birth for surgical repair. The repair required placement of a biosynthetic patch to prevent excessive intra-abdominal pressure with closure. The skin was able to be closed primarily. The patient's postoperative course was uneventful except for a prolonged ileus. He was begun on enteral feeds on postoperative day #20. The patient reached full feeds on postoperative day #34 and was discharged home on all oral feedings on postoperative day #40.

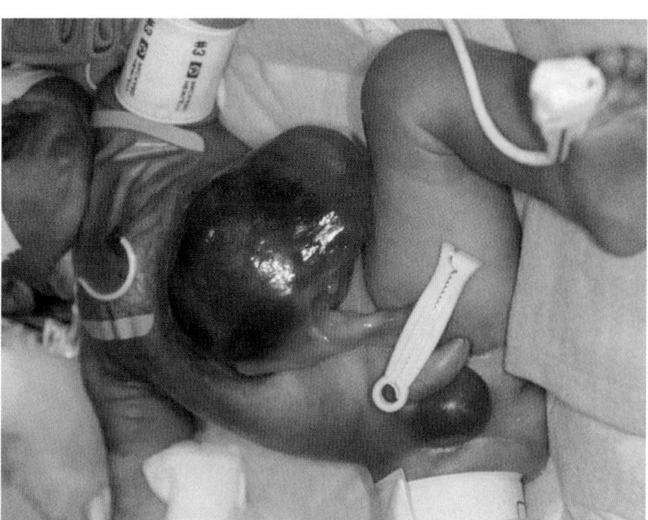

FIGURE 73-3 Newborn infant with an omphalocele. Note that the umbilical vessels insert directly into the membrane. (*Used with permission from Anthony Stallion, MD.*)

INTRODUCTION

An omphalocele is a midline abdominal wall defect of variable size in which the herniated viscera is covered by a membrane consisting of peritoneum on the inner surface, amnion on the outer surface, and Wharton's jelly between the layers. The umbilical vessels insert directly into the membrane and not on the abdominal wall. This is a true midline developmental defect. There is failure of complete closure of the two cranio-caudal and two lateral folds not fully meeting in the midline. The defect may be centered in the upper, middle, or lower abdomen. The herniated viscera within the omphalocele may include any abdominal organ and is largely dependent on the defect size and location.

SYNONYMS

Exomphalos.

EPIDEMIOLOGY

- The incidence of omphalocele ranges between 1.5 and 3 per 10,000 births.
- Most cases are sporadic but there are rare familial cases of omphalocele.[16]

ETIOLOGY AND PATHOPHYSIOLOGY

- In omphalocele, the intestine that is physiologically herniated into the umbilical cord in the 6th to 10th weeks does not return to the abdominal cavity.
- The cause of this failure of intestinal return to the abdomen is unknown but is thought to be associated with defects in body wall folding.
- As this is a true developmental defect, there is a high association of associated congenital anomalies.
- When there is a predominately cranial fold deficit, the result is an epigastric omphalocele. This abnormality may be associated with additional cranial fold abnormalities, particularly midline developmental defects, including anterior diaphragmatic hernias, sternal clefts, pericardial defects, and cardiac defects (Pentalogy of Cantrell).
- When there is a predominately caudal fold deficit, the omphalocele may be associated with bladder or cloacal exstrophy (**Figure 73-4**) or other anorectal malformations.

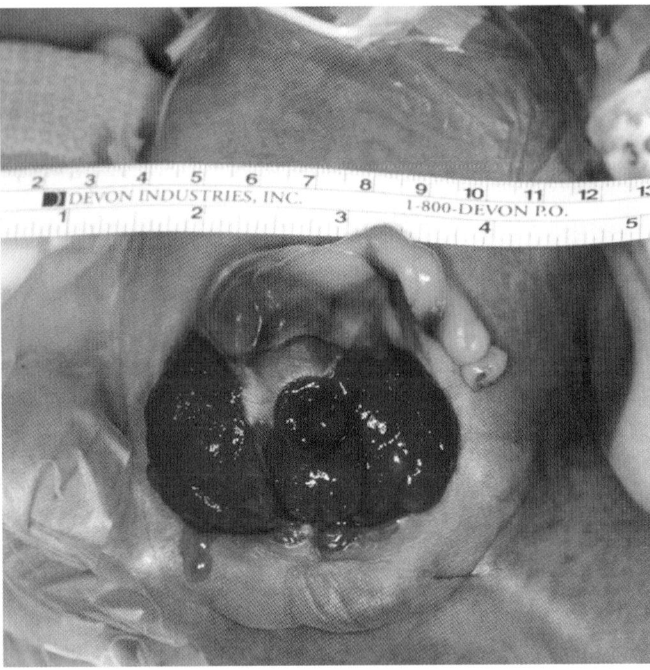

FIGURE 73-4 Omphalocele with predominately caudal fold deficit and an associated cloacal exstrophy. (*Used with permission from Anthony Stallion, MD.*)

DIAGNOSIS

PRENATAL DIAGNOSIS

- Similar to gastroschisis, prenatal ultrasound after the first trimester is the gold-standard for prenatal diagnosis with similar specificity and sensitivity.
- Elevated maternal serum AFP may alert the clinician performing the prenatal care that a referral for high level ultrasound is needed.

CLINICAL FEATURES

- Fifty to seventy percent of cases of omphalocele have an associated anomaly:[17]
  - Thirty percent of cases have associated chromosomal anomalies.
    - Trisomy 13, Patau syndrome.
    - Trisomy 14.
    - Trisomy 15.
    - Trisomy 18, Edwards syndrome.
    - Trisomy 21, Down syndrome.
  - Thirty to fifty percent have associated cardiac anomalies.
  - Syndromic anomalies may occur.
  - Beckwith-Wiedemann syndrome (10% of infants with omphalocele have this syndrome). This syndrome is an overgrowth syndrome that may present with macrosomia, macroglossia, visceromegaly, and renal abnormalities along with the omphalocele.
  - Pentalogy of Cantrell (omphalocele, anterior diaphragmatic hernias, sternal clefts, pericardial defects, and cardiac defects).
- Associated complications during pregnancy:
  - Intrauterine growth restriction (5 to 35%).
  - Premature delivery (5 to 60%).
  - Loss of pregnancy.

LABORATORY TESTING

- Chromosomal studies are warranted in all cases because of associated congenital anomalies.

IMAGING

- Ultrasound evaluation and fetal echocardiography for other structural defects is recommended.
- After delivery obtain an abdominal ultrasound and cardiac echocardiogram to confirm prenatal findings and rule out missed anomalies.

DIFFERENTIAL DIAGNOSIS

- Gastroschisis—see the previous section.

MANAGEMENT

PRENATAL MANAGEMENT

- Once discovered by fetal ultrasound, further diagnostic evaluation should include:
  - Fetal ultrasound evaluation for other structural defects.
  - Fetal echocardiography.
  - Chromosome determination.
- There is no indication for early delivery, although caesarian section is recommended for infants with a large omphalocele to prevent sac rupture or dystocia during labor.

NEWBORN RESUSCITATION

- Initial ABC resuscitation.
- Placement of nasogastric tube for gastric decompression.

SURGERY

- If the covering sac is intact, there is no urgency to perform operative closure.
- If intact, a complete evaluation for associated defects should be done before any operative intervention. The sac should be supported or suspended to prevent venous congestion of the viscera, edema, or ischemia. This will aid in later attempts at reduction.
- With small defects, the membrane can be excised, and the defect closed primarily. Any membrane adherent to the liver may be left in place.
- Larger defects can be treated similarly to gastroschisis, with excision of the external membrane, followed by the placement of a "silo" with serial reduction of the abdominal viscera over 7 to 10 days.
- For very large defects relative to the size of the infant, there may be resulting loss of abdominal domain and reduction may not be possible. In this instance, the membrane may be treated with a topical agent such as silver sulfadiazine to promote desiccation, contraction and epithelialization of the membrane. The visceral contents may be slowly reduced with loose elastic bandages over time with delayed closure up to 2 years after initial treatment.[18]

- Also, long-term consideration can be given to placement of tissue expanders and eventual component separation to assist in eventual closure of the giant defects.

REFERRAL

Referral to high-risk obstetrics care connected to a specialized pediatric center with pediatric surgery is imperative.

PREVENTION AND SCREENING

- Prenatal ultrasound after the first trimester is the gold-standard for prenatal diagnosis.
- Elevated maternal serum AFP may also be useful.

PROGNOSIS

- Overall, outcomes of children after omphalocele repair will depend largely on the presence of other congenital anomalies, especially cardiac anomalies, and other comorbidities.

PATIENT RESOURCES

- **www.cdc.gov/ncbddd/birthdefects/omphalocele.html**.
- **www.ncbi.nlm.nih.gov/pubmedhealth/PMH0001989/**.

PROVIDER RESOURCES

- **http://emedicine.medscape.com/article/975583**.
- **http://omphalocele.net/wordpress/wp-content/uploads/2010/03/sdarticle.pdf**.

REFERENCES

1. Sadler TW. The embryologic origin of ventral body wall defects. *Semin Pediatr Surg*. 2010;19(3):209-214.
2. Suver D, Lee SL, Shekherdimian S, et al. Left-sided gastroschisis: higher incidence of extraintestinal congenital anomalies. *Am J Surg*. 2008;195(5):663-666.
3. Owen A, Marven S, Johnson P, et al. Gastroschisis: a national cohort study to describe contemporary surgical strategies and outcomes. *J Pediatr Surg*. 2010;45(9):1808-1816.
4. Castilla EE, Mastroiacovo P, Orioli IM. Gastroschisis: international epidemiology and public health perspectives. *Am J Med Genet C Semin Med Genet*. 2008;148C(3):162-179.
5. Fillingham A, Rankin J. Prevalence, prenatal diagnosis and survival of gastroschisis. *Prenat Diagn*. 2008;28(13):1232-1237.
6. Feldkamp ML, Carey JC, Sadler TW. Development of gastroschisis: review of hypotheses, a novel hypothesis, and implications for research. *Am J Med Genet A*. 2007;143(7):639-652.
7. Fillingham A, Rankin J. Prevalence, prenatal diagnosis and survival of gastroschisis. *Prenat Diagn*. 2008;28(13):1232-1237.
8. Saller DN Jr, Canick JA, Palomaki GE, et al. Second-trimester maternal serum alpha-fetoprotein, unconjugated estriol, and hCG levels in pregnancies with ventral wall defects. *Obstet Gynecol*. 1994;84(5):852-855.
9. Ledbetter, DJ. Congenital abdominal wall defects and reconstruction in pediatric surgery. Gastroschisis and Omphalocele. *Surg Clin N Am*. 2012;92:713-727.
10. Ruano R, Picone O, Bernardes L, et al. The association of gastroschisis with other congenital anomalies: how important is it? *Prenat Diagn*. 2011;31(4):347-350.
11. Molik KA, Gingalewski CA, West KW, et al. Gastroschisis: a plea for risk categorization. *J Pediatr Surg*. 2001;36(1):51-55.
12. Oldham KT, Coran AG, Drongowski RA, et al. The development of necrotizing enterocolitis following repair of gastroschisis: a surprisingly high incidence. *J Pediatr Surg*. 1988;23(10):945-949.
13. Lao OB, Larison C, Garrison MM, et al. Outcomes in neonates with gastroschisis in U.S. children's hospitals. *Am J Perinatol*. 2010;27(1):97-101.
14. Davies BW, Stringer MD. The survivors of gastroschisis. *Arch Dis Child*. 1997;77(2):158-160.
15. van Eijck FC, Wijnen RM, van Goor H. The incidence and morbidity of adhesions after treatment of neonates with gastroschisis and omphalocele: a 30-year review. *J Pediatr Surg*. 2008;43(3):479-483.
16. Frolov P, Alali J, Klein MD. Clinical risk factors for gastroschisis and omphalocele in humans: a review of the literature. *Pediatr Surg Int*. 2010;26(12):1135-1148.
17. Stoll C, Alembik Y, Dott B, et al. Omphalocele and gastroschisis and associated malformations. *Am J Med Genet A*. 2008;146A(10):1280-1285.
18. Lee SL, Beyer TD, Kim SS, et al. Initial nonoperative management and delayed closure for treatment of giant omphaloceles. *J Pediatr Surg*. 2006;41(11):1846-1849.

PART 12

ADOLESCENT PROBLEMS

Strength of Recommendation (SOR)	Definition
A	Recommendation based on consistent and good-quality patient-oriented evidence.*
B	Recommendation based on inconsistent or limited-quality patient-oriented evidence.*
C	Recommendation based on consensus, usual practice, opinion, disease-oriented evidence, or case series for studies of diagnosis, treatment, prevention, or screening.*

*See Appendix A on pages 1320–1322 for further information.

74 OVERVIEW OF VAGINITIS

E.J. Mayeaux, Jr., MD

PATIENT STORY

An 18-year-old female presented to her physician with vulvar and vaginal itching associated with a vaginal discharge. On examination, the patient is noted to have redness and excoriations on her vulva (**Figure 74-1**). She also had a thick white discharge was seen covering cervix and vaginal sidewallson speculum exam. The pH of the discharge was 4.2, and <10 percent of the epithelial cells on her wet prep were clue cells (**Figure 74-2**), but yeast and hyphae were noted. She was diagnosed with candida vulvovaginitis and was treated with oral fluconazole.

INTRODUCTION

Vaginal discharge is a frequent presenting complaint in primary care. The three most common causes in adolescents and adults are bacterial vaginosis, candidiasis, and trichomoniasis. Providers must refrain from "diagnosing" a vaginitis based solely on the color and consistency of the discharge, as this may lead to misdiagnosis and may miss concomitant infections.[1]

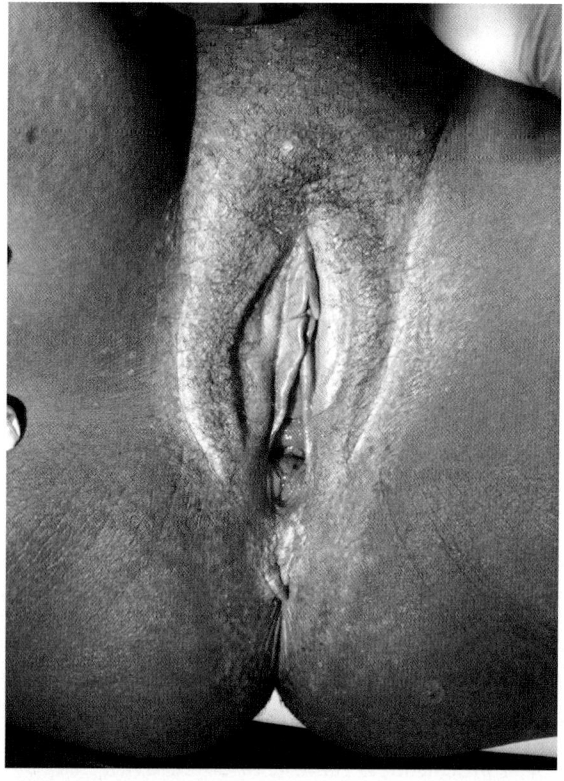

FIGURE 74-1 Candida vulvovaginitis in an 18-year-old female who complained of severe vaginal and vulvar itching. Her vulva demonstrated redness with excoriations. Note the satellite lesions near the borders of the inflamed areas. She was diagnosed with candida vulvovaginitis. (*Used with permission from E.J. Mayeaux, Jr., MD.*)

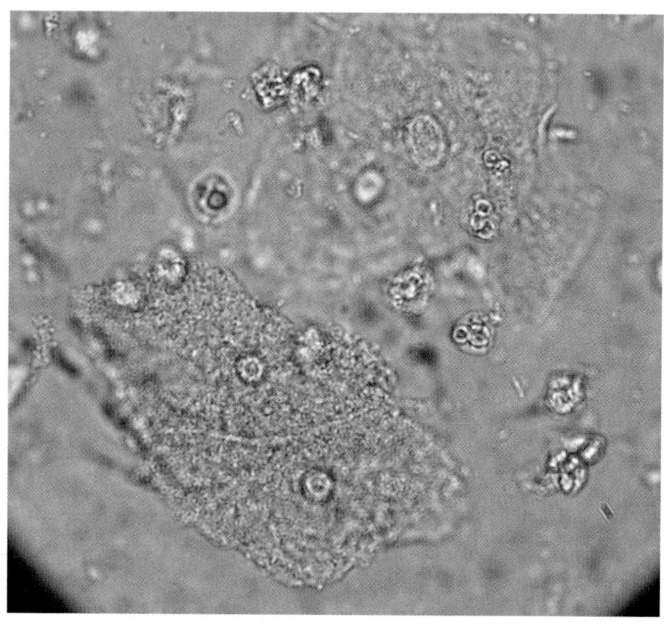

FIGURE 74-2 Clue cells on a wet mount of vaginal discharge in saline under high-power light microscopy. Note the presence of vaginal epithelial cells, smaller white blood cells (polymorphonucleocytes), and bacteria. The bacteria are the coccobacilli of *Gardnerella vaginalis* covering the cell membranes of the two vaginal epithelial cells near the lower end of the field. These are clue cells seen in patients with bacterial vaginosis. (*Used with permission from Richard P. Usatine, MD.*)

Vulvovaginal complaints in prepubertal children may be result from infection, congenital abnormalities, trauma, or dermatologic conditions. Vaginitis is the most commont gynecologic problem in prepubertal girls, often presenting with symptoms including vaginal discharge, erythema, soreness, pruritus, dysuria, or bleeding.[2]

Adolescence is a developmental period with rapid changes in physical characteristics, sexual development, emotional development, and sexual activity. These changes may result in potential increased risk for acquiring sexually transmitted diseases.

EPIDEMIOLOGY

The reported rates of chlamydia and gonorrhea are highest among females ages 15 to 19 years. Adolescents are at greater risk for sexually transmitted diseases (STDs) because they frequently have unprotected intercourse, are biologically more susceptible to infection, are often engaged in partnerships of limited duration, and face multiple obstacles to utilization of health care.[1]

Cross-sectional data from the 2003 to 2004 US National Health and Nutrition Examination Survey (NHANES) shows 24 percent of female adolescents (aged 14 to 19 years) had laboratory evidence of infection with human papillomavirus (HPV, 18%), Chlamydia trachomatis (4%), Trichomonas vaginalis (3%), herpes simplex virus type 2 (HSV-2, 2%), or Neisseria gonorrhoeae. Among girls who reported ever having had sex, 40 percent had laboratory evidence of one of the four STDs, most commonly HPV (30%) and chlamydia (7%).[3]

ETIOLOGY AND PATHOPHYSIOLOGY

- The quantity and quality of normal vaginal discharge in healthy adolescents vary. Physiologic leukorrhea refers to generally nonmalodorous, mucousy, white or yellowish vaginal discharge in the absence of a pathologic cause. It is not accompanied by signs and symptoms, such as pain, pruritus, burning, erythema, or tissue friability. However, slight malodor and irritative symptoms can be normal for some women at certain times.[4] Physiologic leukorrhea is usually a result of estrogen-induced changes in cervicovaginal secretions.
- Nonspecific vulvovaginitis accounts for 25 to 75 percent of vulvovaginitis in prepubertal girls.[5] Potential factors that increase their risk of vulvovaginitis in children include poor hygiene, lack of labial development, unestrogenized thin mucosa, more alkaline vaginal pH, bubble baths, deodorant soaps, obesity, and tight-fitting clothes.
- Foreign bodies in children can cause acute and chronic recurrent vulvovaginitis. Toilet paper is the most common foreign body found in the vaginas of children but small toys, hair bands, beads, and paper clips are also common.[6]
- Sexual abuse may also result in nonspecific vulvovaginitis. Not finding STDs does not rule out abuse.[7]
- Noninfectious causes of vaginitis include irritants (e.g., scented panty liners, spermicides, povidone-iodine, soaps and perfumes, and some topical drugs) and allergens (e.g., latex condoms, topical antifungal agents, and chemical preservatives) that produce hypersensitivity reactions.
- Before starting an examination, determine whether the patient douched recently, because this can lower the yield of diagnostic tests and increase the risk of pelvic inflammatory disease.[8] Patients who have been told not to douche will sometimes start wiping the vagina with soapy washcloths, which also irritates the vagina and cervix and may cause a discharge. Douching is associated with increases in bacterial vaginosis and acquisition of sexually transmitted infections when exposed. However, recent studies indicate that douching with plain water once a week or less did not disturb normal flora.[9,10]
- There are many causes of vaginitis. Infectious causes include bacterial vaginosis (40% to 50% of cases) (**Figure 74-2**), vulvovaginal candidiasis (20% to 25%) (**Figure 74-1**), and trichomonas (15% to 20%) (**Figure 74-3**).[11] Less common causes include atrophic vaginitis, cytolytic or desquamative inflammatory vaginitis, streptococcal vaginitis, ulcerative vaginitis, and idiopathic vulvovaginal ulceration associated with HIV infection.
- *Streptococcus pyogenes* is the most commonly identified pathogen in prepubertal girls occuring in about 20 percent of girls with vulvovaginitis.[7]
- Pinworms infestation can cause vulvar symptoms, especially itching (see Chapter 179, Intestinal Worms and Parasites). Children with recurrent episodes of vulvar and/or perianal itching, especially when most symptomatic at night, should be examined for pinworms and possibly treated empirically.[7]
- In addition to classic STDs, *Mycoplasma genitalium* infections are increasingly recognized as causes of sexually transmitted discharge in adolescents and young adults.[12]

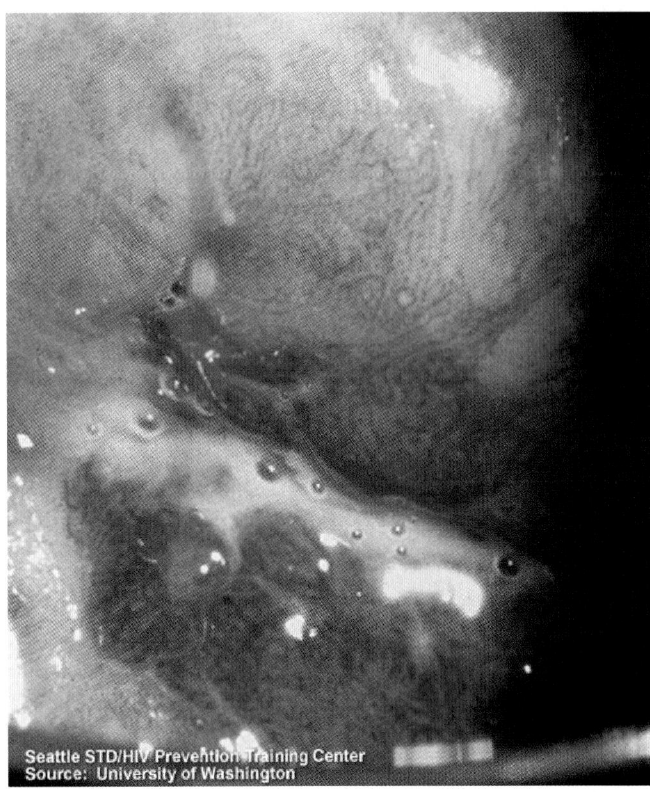

FIGURE 74-3 Colposcopic view of the cervix in a patient infected with trichomonas vaginalis. Note the frothy discharge with visible bubbles and the cervical erythema. (*Used with permission from Seattle STD/HIV Prevention Training Center, University of Washington.*)

- More rare noninfectious causes include chemicals, allergies, hypersensitivity, contact dermatitis, trauma, postpuerperal atrophic vaginitis, erosive lichen planus, collagen vascular disease, Behçet syndrome, and pemphigus syndromes.

DIAGNOSIS

CLINICAL FEATURES

- Examine the external genitalia for irritation or discharge (**Figure 74-1**). Speculum examination is done to determine the amount and character of the discharge (**Figure 74-3**). A chlamydia and gonorrhea test should always be done in sexually active females with a vaginal discharge. Look closely at the cervix for discharge and signs of infection, dysplasia, or cancer (**Figures 74-3** and **74-4**). Bimanual examination may show evidence of cervical, uterine, or adnexal tenderness. **Table 74-1** shows diagnostic values for examination of vaginitis.
- Vaginal pH testing can be helpful in the diagnosis of vaginitis. The pH can be checked by applying pH paper to the vaginal sidewall. Do not place the pH paper in contact with the cervical mucus. A pH above 4.5 is seen with menopausal patients, trichomonas infection, or bacterial vaginosis.
- Wet preps are obtained by applying a cotton-tipped applicator to the vaginal sidewall and placing the sample into normal saline. A drop of the suspension is then placed on a slide and examined for

TABLE 74-1 Diagnostic Values for Vaginal Infections

Diagnostic Criteria	Normal	Bacterial Vaginosis	Trichomonas Vaginitis	Candida Vulvovaginitis
Vaginal pH	3.8 to 4.2	>4.5	4.5	<4.5 (usually)
Discharge	White, thin, flocculent	Thin, white, gray	Yellow, green, or gray, frothy	White, curdy, "cottage cheese"
Amine odor "whiff" test	Absent	Fishy	Fishy	Absent
Microscopic	Lactobacilli, epithelial cells	Clue cells, adherent cocci, no white blood cells	Trichomonads, white blood cells >10/hpf	Budding yeast, hyphae, Pseudohyphae

Used with permission from E.J. Mayeaux, Jr., MD.

the presence and number of white blood cells (WBCs), trichomonads, candidal hyphae, or clue cells (**Figure 74-2**).

- A KOH prep is made by adding a drop of KOH solution to a drop of saline suspension of the discharge. The KOH lyses epithelial cells in 5 to 15 minutes (faster if the slide is warmed briefly) and allows easier visualization of candidal hyphae. The use of KOH with DMSO allows for quicker lyses of the epithelial cells and immediate examination of the smear.
- Another diagnostic procedure is the "whiff" test, which is performed by placing a drop of KOH on a slide of the wet prep and smelling for a foul, fishy odor. The odor is indicative of anaerobic overgrowth or infection. The "whiff" test is positive if the fishy amine odor is detected during the exam and it is then not necessary to add KOH and "whiff" again.

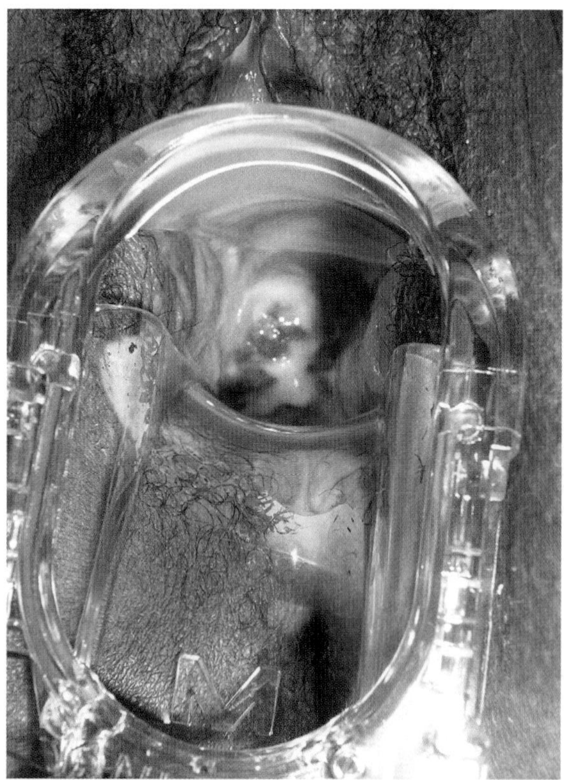

FIGURE 74-4 Speculum exam showing mucopurulent discharge with a friable appearing cervix in a patient with chlamydia cervicitis. (*Used with permission from Richard P. Usatine, MD.*)

LABORATORY TESTING

- Nucleic acid amplification tests are highly sensitive tests for *Neisseria gonorrhoeae*, *Chlamydia*, and *Chlamydia trachomatis* that can be performed on genital specimens or urine. Urine screening for gonorrhea, chlamydia, or both using nucleic acid amplification test can be used successfully in difficult-to-reach adolescents.[13]
- Newer tests are available using nucleic acid detection for multiple pathogens that cause vaginal discharge. These have the advantages of much higher sensitivity and are not affected by delays in microscopic assessment. They also do not require providers maintain microscopic proficiency testing. They take longer to perform than classic microscopic tests.[1]

MANAGEMENT

- Management is based on the identification of the causative agent.
- Management of vaginal irritants and allergens involves identifying and eliminating the offending agents. However, irritants and allergens can often be difficult to identify.
- Health food store lactobacilli are the wrong strain and do not adhere well to the vaginal epithelium. Ingestion of live-culture, nonpasteurized yogurt does not significantly change the incidence of candidal vulvovaginitis or bacterial vaginosis.[14]
- Treatment for physiologic leukorrhea is unnecessary.
- There are multiple recommendations for nonspecific vaginitis in children once a specific etiology has been excluded:
    - Avoid leotards and sleeper pajamas. Nightgowns allow air to circulate.
    - Use cotton underpants.
    - Double-rinse underwear after washing to avoid residual irritants. Do not use fabric softeners for underwear and swimsuits.
    - Avoid tights, leotards, and leggings for daytime use. Skirts and loose-fitting pants allow air to circulate.

- Daily warm bathing for 10 to 15 minutes. Use soap to wash regions other than the genitals just before exiting tub. Rinse the genital area well and gently pat dry.
- Do not use bubble baths or perfumed soaps.
- If the vulvar area is irritated, cool compresses may relieve the discomfort.
- Wet wipes can be used instead of toilet paper for wiping. Emollients may help protect skin.
- Review hygiene with the child. Emphasize wiping front-to-back after bowel movements.
- Avoid letting children sit in wet swimsuits for long periods of time after swimming.

- If symptoms persist beyond two to three weeks or recur, the possibility of a foreign body or specific infection should be examined.

MEDICATIONS

- Antibiotic therapy (amoxicillin PO; topical metronidazole; or topical clindamycin) may hasten the resolution of a purulent vaginal discharge that does not respond to hygiene measures and for which other diagnoses have been excluded.
- Occasionally, a short course of estrogen cream can thicken the vaginal mucosa and make it more resistant to recurrent nonspecific infections.
- A foreign body can often be removed with irrigation with warmed fluid. The introitus may be treated with a topical anesthetic agent such as Xylocaine jelly if necessary. Examination under sedation and/or anesthesia may be necessary for extraction of larger foreign bodies and those that cannot be removed with simple irrigation.[6]

PATIENT RESOURCES

- Centers for Disease Control and Prevention. *Sexually Transmitted Diseases* page—**www.cdc.gov/std/**.
- Planned Parenthood—**www.plannedparenthood.org/cameron-willacy/images/South-Texas/What_Every_Woman_Needs_to_Know_English.pdf**.
- Illinois Department of Public Health. *Vaginitis*—**www.idph.state.il.us/public/hb/hbvaginitis.htm**.

PROVIDER RESOURCES

- Centers for Disease Control and Prevention. *2010 Guidelines for Treatment of Sexually Transmitted Diseases*—**www.cdc.gov/std/treatment/2010/STD-Treatment-2010-RR5912.pdf**.
- Centers for Disease Control and Prevention. *Self-Study STD Module–Vaginitis*—**http://www2a.cdc.gov/stdtraining/self-study/vaginitis/default.htm**
- Centers for Disease Control and Prevention. Vaginitis slides—**http://www2a.cdc.gov/stdtraining/ready-to-use/vaginitis.htm**
- eMedicine—**www.emedicine.medscape.com/article/257141-overview**.
- American Family Physician—**www.aafp.org/afp/20000901/1095.html**.

REFERENCES

1. Centers for Disease Control and Prevention. *Guidelines for Treatment of Sexually Transmitted Diseases*. http://www.cdc.gov/std/treatment/2010/STD-Treatment-2010-RR5912.pdf, accessed December 24, 2011.
2. Joishy M, Ashtekar CS, Jain A, Gonsalves R. Do we need to treat vulvovaginitis in prepubertal girls? *BMJ*. 2005;330:186.
3. Forhan SE, Gottlieb SL, Sternberg MR, et al. Prevalence of sexually transmitted infections among female adolescents aged 14 to 19 in the United States. Pediatrics 2009;124:1505.
4. Anderson M, Karasz A, Friedland S. Are vaginal symptoms ever normal? A review of the literature. *MedGenMed*. 2004;6:49.
5. Garden AS. Vulvovaginitis and other common childhood gynaecological conditions. *Arch Dis Child. Educ Pract Ed*. 2011;96:73.
6. Stricker T, Navratil F, Sennhauser FH. Vaginal foreign bodies. *J Paediatr Child Health*. 2004;40(4):205-207.
7. Stricker T, Navratil F, Sennhauser FH. Vulvovaginitis in prepubertal girls. *Arch Dis Child*. 2003;88:324.
8. Zhang J, Thomas AG, Leybovich E. Vaginal douching and adverse health effects: A meta-analysis. *Am J Public Health*. 1997;87:1207-1211.
9. Hassan S, Chatwani A, Brovender H, et al. Douching for perceived vaginal odor with no infectious cause of vaginitis: a randomized controlled trial. *J Low Genit Tract Dis*. 2011;15(2):128-133.
10. Zhang J, Hatch M, Zhang D, et al. Frequency of douching and risk of bacterial vaginosis in African-American women. *Obstet Gynecol*. 2004;104(4):756-760.
11. Sobel JD. Vaginitis. *N Engl J Med*. 1997;337:1896-1903.
12. Tosh AK, Van Der Pol B, Fortenberry JD, et al. Mycoplasma genitalium among adolescent women and their partners. *J Adolesc Health*. 2007;40:412.
13. Monroe KW, Weiss HL, Jones M, Hook EW, 3rd: Acceptability of urine screening for *Neisseria gonorrheae* and *Chlamydia trachomatis* in adolescents at an urban emergency department. *Sex Transm Dis*. 2003;30:850-853.
14. Pirotta M, Gunn J, Chondros P, et al. Effect of lactobacillus in preventing post-antibiotic vulvovaginal candidiasis: A randomised controlled trial. *BMJ*. 2004;329:548.

75 MUCOSAL ULCERATIVE DISORDERS IN FEMALE ADOLESCENTS

Marjan Attaran, MD

Mucosal ulcerative disorders in adolescent females can be caused by sexually transmitted as well as nonsexually transmitted diseases. In this chapter, common mucosal ulcerative disorders are discussed sequentially and include:

1. Vulvar herpes simplex virus (HSV) infection
2. Syphilis in teenage females
3. Chancroid
4. Behcet Disease

VULVAR HERPES SIMPLEX

See Chapter 114, Herpes Simplex, for information on all types of herpes simplex infections.

PATIENT STORY

A 16-year-old girl presents with vulvar swelling, pain, and difficulty urinating. She admits to being sexually active. On examination, ulcerative lesions are noted on the inner aspects of the labia minora (**Figure 75-1**). She is treated with analgesics and oral acyclovir for presumed Herpes simplex virus type 2 (HSV-2). She is also tested for other STDs including blood tests for syphilis, HIV, and urine tests for gonorrhea and chlamydia. Her culture of the lesions is positive for HSV-2 as expected. Her other tests are all negative. Her lesions resolve after 2 weeks.

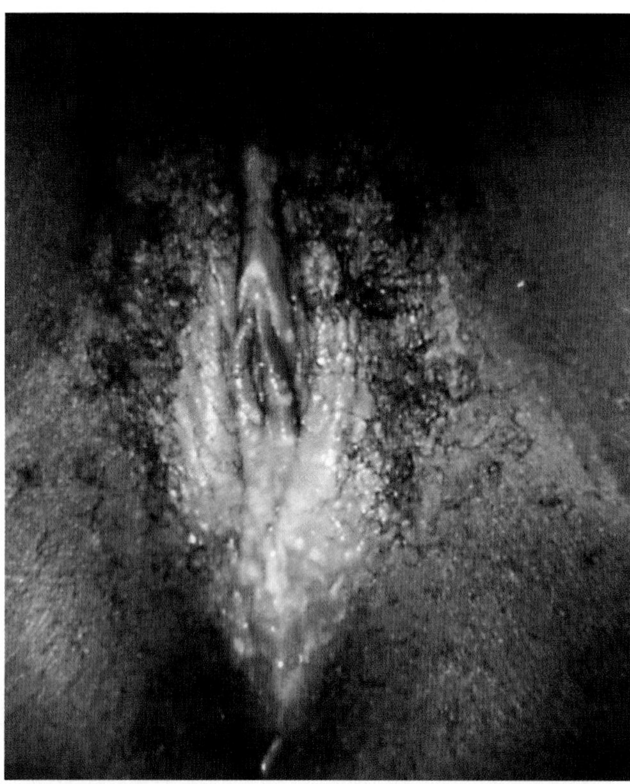

FIGURE 75-1 Tender ulcerative lesions on the vulva which are positive for herpes simplex virus infection. (*Used with permission from Centers for Disease Control/Susan Lindsley, MD.*)

INTRODUCTION

HSV-2 is a sexually transmitted infection that usually causes vesicles and ulcers in the genito-anal region. HSV-1 usually involves infections found extra-genitally. HSV-2 infections present with painful genital ulcerative lesions. HSV-1 can occur in the genito-anal region and HSV-2 can occur on the oral mucosa. There are many people with positive serologies for both types of herpes simplex that are not aware of having a "herpes infection" with symptoms.

EPIDEMIOLOGY

- The prevalence of HSV increases with age.[1–4]
- By age 15 years of age, 40 percent will be infected with HSV-1.[2]
- The prevalence of HSV-1 is greater than HSV-2 in most areas of the world and since HSV-2 is primarily sexually transmitted, it is not as common in children.
- Data from the Centers for Disease Control and Prevention (CDC) monitored through the National Health and Nutrition Examination Survey (NAHNES) found the overall prevalence of HSV-2 from 2005 to 2008 to be 16.2 percent; of those testing positive for HSV-2 infection, 81.1 percent said they had never been told by a doctor or health care professional that they had genital herpes.[2]
- In this study, seroprevalence increased with age, ranging from 1.4 percent among those aged 14 to 19 years to 26.1 percent among those aged 40 to 49 years.[2]
- HSV-2 seroprevalence is greater among women (20.9%) than men (11.5%).[2]

ETIOLOGY AND PATHOPHYSIOLOGY

- Genital herpes is usually caused by HSV-2 but may also be caused by HSV-1.
- Transmission occurs more commonly from an infected male to a female partner.
- Infection occurs as a result of exposure to mucosal tissue that has active lesions or as a result of exposure to the secretion of an individual who has active HSV infection.
- Incubation period is about 4 days but can range from 2 to 12 days.
- It may be divided into two categories: first episode versus recurrences. Patients experiencing their first outbreak may not have any antibodies to type 1 or 2 HSV or they may have an antibody to usually type 1.

- The virus usually remains in the sensory ganglia of the autonomic nervous system. Once triggered the virus can travel down the sensory nerve and reactivate the same region as the initial infection.

RISK FACTORS

- Found more commonly in females and African Americans.[2]
- Found more commonly in individuals with lower socioeconomic status.[1]

DIAGNOSIS

CLINICAL FEATURES

- Vesicles are noted on the labia minora and vestibule (**Figure 75-1**). Lesions may also be noted in the vagina and on the cervix.
- The vesicles are small, on an erythematous base, and rupture into painful shallow ulcerations.
- Skin lesions are usually preceded by prodromal symptoms that include: fever, malaise, burning, and paresthesia at the site, loss of appetite, and headaches. Lymphadenopathy may also be noted.
- Recurrences occur as a result of triggers such as stress, fatigue, and menstruation.

LABORATORY TESTING

- Viral culture may be obtained from an active lesion. In these cases, the base of the unroofed lesion must be swabbed vigorously. The cells are then evaluated for HSV infection.
- Direct fluorescent antibody (DFA)—This technique identifies the presence of viral antigens. It is rapid, sensitive, and relatively inexpensive. Tzanck smear-cells obtained from the base of a vesicle are stained and then assessed for multinucleated giant cells. This is not as specific as culture and DFA and only valuable if done by persons well trained in this testing.
- Polymerase chain reaction (PCR)—May be used to detect the presence of herpes virus DNA in the CSF when herpes encephalitis is suspected. It is used less often for genital herpes infections.
- Serologic assays—Used primarily for diagnosing recurrent infection. This is generally not helpful in acute diagnosis and management.

DIFFERENTIAL DIAGNOSIS

- Other sexually transmitted infections must be considered and include syphilis and chancroid.
- Other diagnoses to consider are candida infection, Behcet disease (as discussed in this chapter), lichen planus, lichen sclerosis, herpes zoster, and trauma. These entities can usually be distinguished based on their characteristic appearance and usual involvement in areas other than the genital tract.
- Prepubertal children who develop genital herpes must be evaluated for sexual abuse (see Chapter 9, Child Sexual Abuse).

MANAGEMENT

PREVENTION

- Patients must be educated about the mode of transmission and understand the concept of asymptomatic shedding.

MEDICATIONS

- Systemic antiviral drugs can modestly improve the signs and s ymptoms of herpes episodes when used to treat first clinical and recurrent episodes, or when used as daily suppressive therapy.[5]
- Antiviral drugs do not eradicate latent virus.
- Acyclovir, valacyclovir and famciclovir have been shown to provide clinical benefit for genital herpes.[5] SOR Ⓑ
- Oral acyclovir has been approved for use in children with primary genital HSV infection. The medication should be started within 6 days of onset of disease. Oral acyclovir may also be used in recurrent HSV within 2 days of onset.
- Recommended maximum dose is 80 mg/kg/day (1200 mg/day) for 7 to 10 days for a primary infection and 5 days for a recurrent infection.
- Supportive therapy may be necessary for control of pain associated with the lesions.
- At times chronic suppressive therapy may be necessary and may be more effective than episodic therapy for recurrent infection. The maximum dose is 1000 mg/day of acyclovir.

PROGNOSIS

- The treatment of genital herpes does not lead to cure.

PATIENT EDUCATION

- Patients have to be educated about the modes of transmission of herpes virus.
- Patients with active lesions need to avoid direct contact of their lesions with other individuals.
- Condoms should be used at all other times.
- They should be educated about the factors that may precipitate a recurrence.

PATIENT RESOURCES

- **www.cdc.gov/std/Herpes/STDFact-Herpes.htm.**
- **www.cdc.gov/std/herpes/STDFact-herpes-detailed .htm.**

PROVIDER RESOURCES

- **www.cdc.gov/std/treatment/2010/STD-Treatment-2010-RR5912.pdf.**
- **www.cdc.gov/std/treatment/2010/genital-ulcers .htm#hsv.**

SYPHILIS ON THE MUCOSAL SURFACES OF ADOLESCENT FEMALES

See Chapter 181, Syphilis, for information on all types of syphilis infections.

PATIENT STORY

A 16-year-old female noted several nonpainful bumps while shaving her vulvar area (**Figure 75-2**). She noted in the ensuing couple days that the surface of the some of the bumps eroded into ulcers. While this was not painful she was scared and presented to her physician for evaluation. She admitted to having had intercourse (unprotected) for the first time 6 weeks ago. The physician noted flat-topped raised plaques that could be condyloma lata or HPV. Her serum RPR test and confirmatory treponemal test were positive. She was treated with one dose of 2.4 million units of benzathine penicillin given intramuscularly. An HIV screen and an HIV DNA PCR were performed and fortunately, were negative.

INTRODUCTION

Syphilis is an infection caused by the spirochete *Treponema pallidum*. It causes ulcerative lesions on the external genitalia.

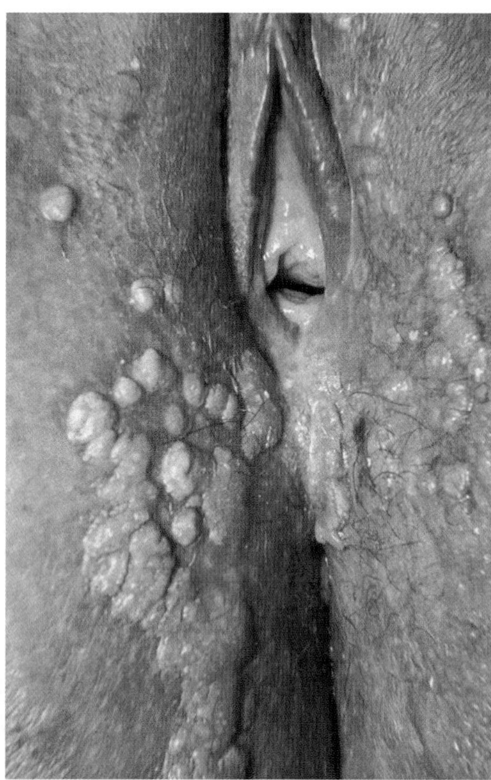

FIGURE 75-2 Condyloma lata lesions of secondary syphilis in a young female. (*Used with permission from Centers for Disease Control/Joyce Ayers, MD.*)

EPIDEMIOLOGY

- The rate of syphilis in the US in 2011 was 1.0 case per 100,000 adult population.[6]
- The rate of primary and secondary syphilis in 15 to 19 year olds in the US in 2011 was 2.4 per 100,000 population.[6]

ETIOLOGY AND PATHOPHYSIOLOGY

- Acquired syphilis is transmitted by direct contact with syphilis lesions. The spirochete enters through areas of micro trauma in the mucous membranes.
- Syphilis is categorized as early (primary, secondary and early latent <2 years of infection) versus late (>2 years of infection).

RISK FACTORS

- Persons in correctional facilities.
- Males having sex with males.
- Persons having multiple sexual partners.
- Persons using drugs and alcohol and participating in commercial or coerced sex.

DIAGNOSIS

CLINICAL FEATURES

- The chancre is typically single, painless and appears round and firm and lasts for 3 to 6 weeks. There is associated lymphadenopathy.
- The appearance of the chancre marks the first stage of syphilis. It appears about 3 weeks after transmission. It heals with or without treatment.
- Multisystem involvement is noted in the second stage of syphilis. The patient experiences skin rashes and mucous membrane lesions. Sometimes condyloma lata (large raised, gray, or white lesions) may develop in areas such as the mouth, under arms and groin area (**Figure 75-3**).[7,8]
- Other symptoms of secondary syphilis include: fever, swollen lymph glands, sore throat, muscle aches, and fatigue.
- Late stage of syphilis occurs 10 to 20 years after the original infection and occurs in about 15 percent of people. During this time the disease will damage internal organs such as the brain, eyes, joints, and bones.

DISTRIBUTION

- Chancres occur on the external genitalia, vagina, anus, and/or the rectum. Chancres may also occur on the lips and the mouth.

LABORATORY TESTING

- Nontreponemal test-nonspecific.
    - These tests include VDRL and RPR. They are inexpensive screening tools but not very specific and can produce false positive results.[7]

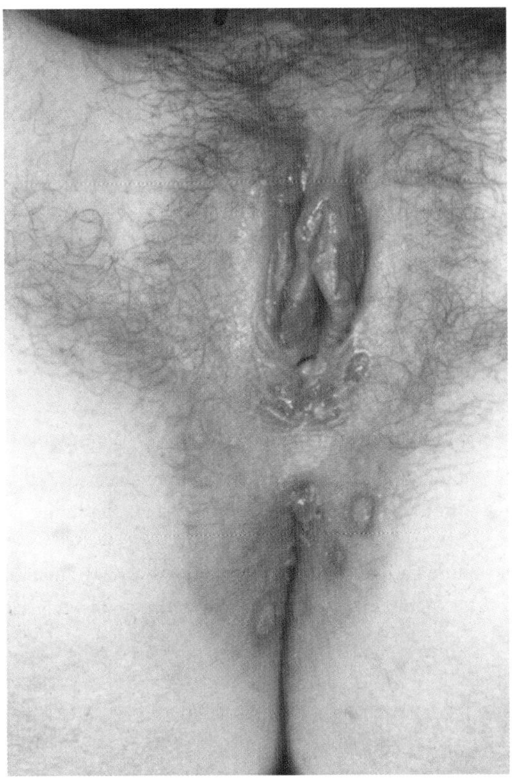

FIGURE 75-3 Condyloma lata lesions involving the vulva and anal region. (*Used with permission from Centers for Disease Control.*)

- Treponemal tests-specific.
  - These tests are necessary to confirm the diagnosis of syphilis.
  - They include Fluorescent treponemal antibody absorbed test (FTA-ABS), *T. pallidum* particle agglutination assey (TP-PA), and treponemal enzyme immunoassay to detect IgG/IgM.[7]

DIFFERENTIAL DIAGNOSIS

- Must differentiate from HSV and chancroid—See these entities in this chapter.
- Lymphogranuloma venereum—Usually manifests with marked inguinal lymphadenopathy. A genital ulcer or papule may occur but often is not seen or missed.
- Granuloma inguinale (Donovanosis)—Very rare in the US. Endemic in some tropical and developing areas, including India; Papua, New Guinea; the Caribbean; central Australia; and southern Africa. Characterized by painless, slowly progressive ulcerative lesions in the genital tract or perineum without regional lymphadenopathy.

MANAGEMENT

MEDICATIONS

- A single intramuscular injection of Benzathine Penicillin G cures a patient with primary, secondary and early latent syphilis.[5] SOR Ⓐ
- Treatment kills the spirochete and prevents further damage.
- Patients who are allergic to penicillin may take doxycycline or tetracycline but the evidence for these treatments is not as firm as for penicillin.

PREVENTION AND SCREENING

- Abstain from intercourse until all the lesions have healed.
- Patients should be tested for other sexually transmitted diseases, especially HIV.
- Patients with syphilis must notify their partners so that they can be tested and treated.
- Consistent use of condoms can reduce the risk of acquiring syphilis.

PROGNOSIS

- Syphilis will not recur but being infected once does not protect one from getting reinfected.

PATIENT EDUCATION

The lesions of syphilis will resolve spontaneously but they must be treated to prevent progression of the infection..

PATIENT RESOURCES

- **www.cdc.gov/std/syphilis/STDFact-Syphilis.htm**.

PROVIDER RESOURCES

- **www.cdc.gov/std/treatment/2010/genital-ulcers.htm#hsv**.

CHANCROID

PATIENT STORY

An 18-year-old female recently returned from a trip to South America and noticed a red bump on her vulva that started one week ago. She is presenting now to her physician as it is quite painful and has an ulcer (**Figure 75-4**). She has had swelling in the inguinal region

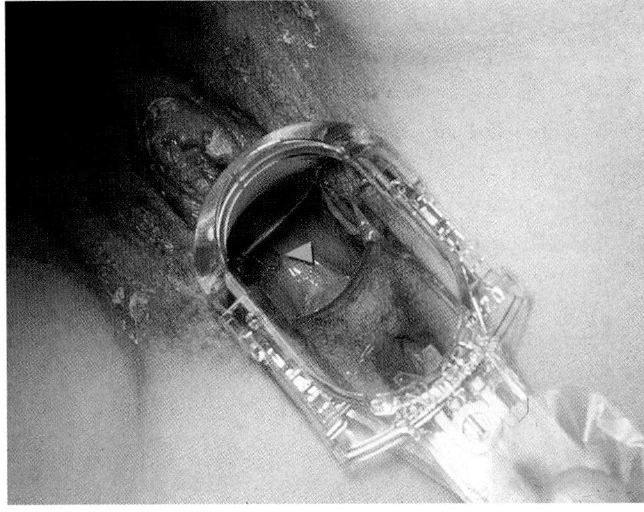

FIGURE 75-4 Chancroid ulcer on the posterior vaginal wall. (*Used with permission from Centers for Disease Control/Susan Lindsley, MD.*)

bilaterally and these areas are painful to her also. She denies any change in her vaginal discharge and states she has been sexually active in the past. A culture of the ulcer is negative for HSV and her syphilis serologies are negative. A diagnosis of probable Chancroid is made and she is treated with one gram of oral azithromycin. The lesions and inguinal lymphadenopathy resolve within 7 days.

INTRODUCTION

Chancroid is an infection caused by *Haemophilus ducreyi*. It presents as genital ulceration that may be associated with regional lymphadenitis and bubo formation.

EPIDEMIOLOGY

- There has been a steady decline in the incidence of chancroid in the US since 1987. Since 2001, only sporadic cases have been reported. In 2010, 24 cases of chancroid were reported.[9]
- It is a major cause of genital ulceration in developing countries.
- Urban outbreaks are occasionally noted more in association with commercial sex work.
- It is more common in Africa, Asia, and Latin America.

ETIOLOGY AND PATHOPHYSIOLOGY

- Caused by *Haemophilus ducreyi*, a gram negative bacteria.[10]
- It is a sexually transmitted infection. Bacteria gain access to tissues from abrasions that occur during sexual intercourse.
- It may spread by auto-inoculation to other anatomical sites
- Its incubation time is 4 to 10 days.
- *H. ducreyi* produces a cytotoxin that causes cell injury and subsequent ulcer formation.

DIAGNOSIS

CLINICAL FEATURES

- The diagnosis is suggested when the combination of painful genital ulcer is seen in conjunction with pustular inguinal lymphadenopathy.
- Lesions are 1 to 2 cm wide with a gray pustular base that bleeds with scraping.
- A definite diagnosis is made when *H. ducreyi* is isolated from the lesion.
- A probable diagnosis is made when:
  - One or more painful genital ulcers exist.
  - No evidence of syphilis 7 days after onset of ulcers (serologies negative).
  - Clinical presentation is typical of chancroid.
  - HSV testing is negative.

LABORATORY TESTING

- Difficult to culture *H. ducreyi*.
- Special culture media necessary to grow *H. ducreyi*.
- No FDA approved PCR test is available in the US.[11]
- Commercial laboratories do have PCR testing available.[12]

DIFFERENTIAL DIAGNOSIS

- HSV and syphilis should always be ruled out when ulcerative genital lesions are present. Note that the RPR is often negative when a syphilitic chancre first appears so repeating the RPR in 2 to 4 weeks may be needed if syphilis is being considered.
- Lymphogranuloma venereum—Usually manifests with marked inguinal lymphadenopathy. A genital ulcer or papule may occur but often is not seen or missed.
- Granuloma inguinale (Donovanosis)—Very rare in the US. Endemic in some tropical and developing areas, including India; Papua, New Guinea; the Caribbean; central Australia; and southern Africa. Characterized by painless, slowly progressive ulcerative lesions in the genital tract or perineum without regional lymphadenopathy.

MANAGEMENT

- Antimicrobial treatment is required to cure the infection, resolve the clinical symptoms, and prevent transmission to others.
- Medications
  - The CDC recommends one of the following regimens:[5]
  - Azithromycin, 1 gram in oral dose in a single dose.
  - Ceftriaxone 250 mg intramuscular dose.
  - Ciprofloxacin 500 mg twice a day for three days, orally (contraindicated in pregnancy).
  - Erythromycin 500 mg three times a day for 7 days.
- Surgery
  - Needle aspiration or incision and drainage of fluctuant slow healing buboes can be considered.[5] SOR Ⓒ
  - Incision and drainage of fluctuant buboes avoids the need for frequent aspirations and possible spontaneous rupture.

PREVENTION AND SCREENING

- All patients should receive health education including information on safe sex.[10]

PROGNOSIS

- Within 3 to 7 days of starting therapy, there should be improvement of ulcerative symptoms.
- The associated lymphadenitis and buboes may respond more slowly.
- If improvement is not seen then the diagnosis should be reconsidered. Co-infection with HIV or another STD such as syphilis should be considered.[11]
- Scarring may occur in advanced cases, despite appropriate therapy.

FOLLOW-UP

- Patients should be offered HIV testing at the time of the diagnosis and then follow-up HIV and serologic syphilis test three months later.

PATIENT RESOURCES

- **www.emedicine.medscape.com/article/214737-overview**.
- **www.nlm.nih.gov/medlineplus/ency/article/000635.htm**.

PROVIDER RESOURCES

- **www.cdc.gov/std/stats10/figures/48.htm**.
- **www.cdc.gov/std/treatment/2010/genital-ulcers.htm#hsv**.

BEHCET DISEASE

PATIENT STORY

A 12-year-old nonsexually active girl presented to the pediatrician with vulvar pain that had begun 4 days prior to presentation. Examination revealed ulcerative lesions on both labia majora (**Figure 75-5**). HSV cultures and syphilis serologies were negative. The lesions resolved over several days. She returned one month later with a similar presentation. Behcet syndrome was suspected and she was referred to pediatric rheumatology.

INTRODUCTION

This is a systemic inflammatory disorder that is characterized by recurrent oral, genital, and cutaneous mucosal lesions, often associated with uveitis.

EPIDEMIOLOGY

- The prevalence of Behcet disease (BD) in North America is 0.12 to 0.33 cases per 100,000 population.[13]
- A higher prevalence is noted from the Far East to the Mediterranean area and the Middle East Countries. Turkey reports the highest prevalence of BD.[14]
- Mean age of presentation is in the third and fourth decade of life. However, it has also been noted in children and adolescents.[15]

ETIOLOGY AND PATHOPHYSIOLOGY

- Pathogenesis of this disease is unknown.[13]
- An interaction of genetic, environmental, and immunologic factors may account for this disease.

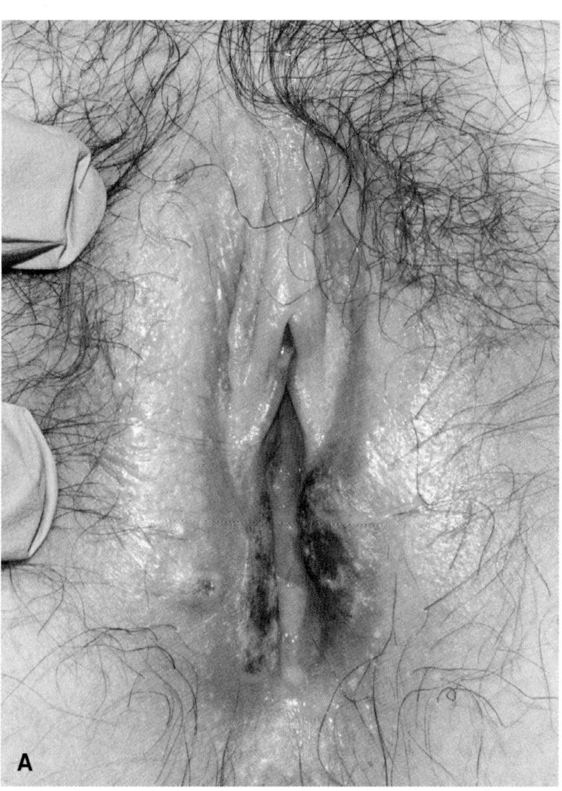

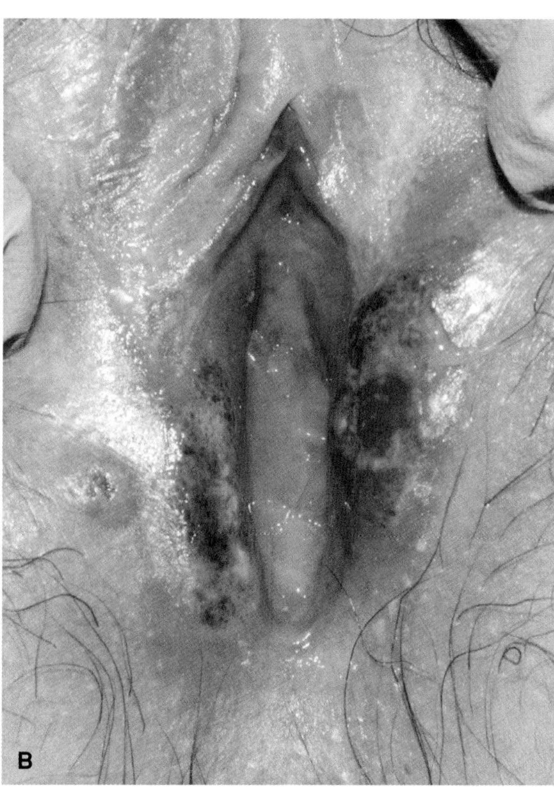

FIGURE 75-5 Bilateral ulcerative lesions in a 12-year-old girl with recurrent vulvar lesions on labia majora (**A**) and close-up view (**B**). The girl was found to have Behcet disease. (*Used with permission from Marjan Attaran, MD.*)

- Genetic abnormalities may explain some cases of BD.[13]
- The most strongly associated genetic factor to BD is HLA-B51. But this accounts for less than 20 percent of the genetic risk.
- There is a possibility that an environmental factor triggers BD in patients with genetic susceptibility. These may be bacterial or viral in origin.
- Neutrophil activity is increased in BD.
- The major lymphocytes implicated in BD pathogenesis are T cells.
- Endothelial cell antibodies have been identified in BD individuals.

RISK FACTORS

- Males are more likely to have BD in the Middle East.
- Females have higher preponderance of BD in Japan.

DIAGNOSIS

The diagnosis depends on the existence of specific clinical features. There is no specific laboratory test. A major or minor aphthous oral ulceration should be noted at least three times in a 12 month period (see Chapter 40, Aphthous Ulcer). In addition the patient should experience two minor criteria, which may include eye lesions, skin lesions, genital lesions, and a positive pathergy test.[14] Pathergy is the appearance or worsening of lesions after trauma to the involved area. A pathergy skin test can be performed with a needle prick and the appearance of a pustule or papule surrounded by erythema 24 to 48 hours after the prick. This is characteristic but not pathognomonic for BD.

CLINICAL FEATURES

- Oral ulcers are usually the initial symptom. They may precede the other manifestations of BD by many years.
- The ulcer is described as a circular aphthous like ulcer with erythematous border and may be located on the buccal mucosa, lips, gingivae, soft palate, and pharynx.
- Genital ulcers are located on the vulva, vagina, cervix in women and prepuce and scrotum in men.
- Eighty percent of patients with BD will have skin lesions. These lesions include erythema nodosum, papulopustular lesions, and pseudofolliculitis.
- Ocular disease is noted in up to 70 percent of BD patients. Uveitis can be detected by an ophthalmologist using a slit lamp. Presenting complaints may be blurry vision and gravelly sensation in the eye.
- Arthritic symptoms may be noted in half of the BD patients.
- Less common associations are thrombophlebitis and gastrointestinal problems. BD can affect arteries and veins and mucosal ulcers can occur anywhere along the gastrointestinal tract.
- The central nervous system may become involved in a small percentage of patients.

LABORATORY TESTING

- Evaluation of the inflammatory cells within a BD lesion usually reveals neutrophils, CD4+ T cells, and cytotoxic cells.

DIFFERENTIAL DIAGNOSIS

- Recurrent aphthous ulcers—Not associated with any systemic manifestations (see Chapter 40, Aphthous Ulcers).
- Recurrent HSV infections—Usually not associated with systemic manifestations except for the primary event, and have classic vesicular lesions (see Chapter 39, Herpes Simplex Gingivostomatitis and Chapter 114, Herpes Simplex).
- Syphilis or chancroid—See discussion in this chapter and Chapter 181, Syphilis.
- Inflammatory bowel disease—May initially present with mucosal ulcerative lesions, but in time develop gastrointestinal symptoms (see Chapter 59, Inflammatory Bowel Disease).
- Reactive arthritis—Usually accompanied by urethritis and conjunctivitis.
- Immunobullous skin disorders—Usually more widespread and have bullous rather than ulcerative lesions (see Chapters 155 to 157).

MANAGEMENT

NONPHARMACOLOGIC

- There are no controlled studies in the pediatric population evaluating treatment of BD.[16,17]
- Sitz baths can help clean the lesions in the external genitalia.

MEDICATIONS

- Mouth washes with sucralfate suspension, or topical and/or corticosteroids may be helpful. SOR C
- A short course of oral corticosteroids is often used for acute ulceration and provides fast relief of symptoms. SOR C
- Long-term colchicine is often used to decrease the frequency of the episodes and the severity of symptoms. SOR C
- Non-steroidal anti-inflammatory medications may be helpful to control the arthritis and arthralgia when used in combination with colchicine. SOR C

REFERRAL

- BD is a multisystem disease that requires a multidisciplinary approach. Referral to rheumatology and ophthalmology should be strongly considered.
- Referral to ophthalmology early is critical to diminishing the morbidity associated with the eye involvement of BD.

PROGNOSIS

- BD is a chronic relapsing disease that will need continued monitoring.
- The ulcerative lesions may continue to recur.

- Patients must be monitored for any systemic manifestations of the disease as this may lead to increased morbidity and mortality.

PATIENT RESOURCES

- **www.behcets.com/site/pp.asp?c=bhJIJSOCJrH&b=262161**.
- **www.medicinenet.com/behcets_syndrome/article.htm**.

PROVIDER RESOURCES

- **www.niams.nih.gov/Health_Info/Behcets_Disease/default.asp**.

REFERENCES

1. Chayavichitsilp P, Buckwalter JV, Krakowski AC, Friedlander SF. Herpes Simplex. *Pediatrics in Review* 2009;30;119.
2. MMWR April 23, 2010/59(15);456-459, NHANES 2005-2008. National Health and Nutrition examination survey.
3. Fleming DT, McQuillan GM, Johnson RE, et al. Herpes simplex virus type 2 in the United States, 1976 to 1994. *N Engl J Med*. 1997;337:1105-1111.
4. Forhan SE, Gottlieb SL, Sternberg MR, et al. Prevalence of sexually transmitted infections among female adolescents aged 14 to 19 in the United States. *Pediatrics*. 2009;124:1505.
5. Centers for Disease Control and Prevention. *2010 Guidelines for Treatment of Sexually Transmitted Diseases*. http://www.cdc.gov/std/treatment/2010/STD-Treatment-2010-RR5912.pdf, accessed December 1, 2011.
6. Centers for Disease Control and Prevention. *Sexually Tansmitted Diseases Guidelines*. http://www.cdc.gov/std, accessed December 1, 2013.
7. Lee V, Kinghorn G. Syphilis and Update. *Clinical Medicine* 2008; 8(3):330-333.
8. Hyman E. Syphilis. *Pediatrics in Review*. 2006; 27(1):37-39.
9. Centers for Disease Control and Prevention. *Sexually Transmitted Diseases, Statistics*. http://www.cdc.gov/std/stats10/figures/48.htm, accessed December 1, 2013.
10. Lewis DA. Chancroid: Clinical manifestations, diagnosis, and management. *Sex Trans Infect*. 2003;79:68-71.
11. Centers for Disease Control and Prevention. *Sexually Transmitted Diseases Guidelines*. http://www.cdc.gov/std/treatment/2010/genital-ulcers.htm#chancroid, accessed December 1, 2013.
12. Orle KA, Gates CA, Martin DH, Body BA, Weiss JB. Simultaneous PCR detection of Haemophilus ducreyi, Treponema pallidum, and herpes simplex virus types 1 and 2 from genital ulcers. *J Clin Microbiol*. 1996;34(1):49.
13. Pineton de Chambrun M, Wechsler B, Geri G, Cacoub P, Saadoun D. New Insights into the pathogenesis of Behcet's disease. *Autoimmunity reviews*. 2012;1:687-698.
14. Yesudian PD, Edirisinghe DN, Mahony CO. Behcet's disease. *International Journal of STD and AIDS*. 2007;18:221-227.
15. Karincaoglu Y, Borlu M, Toker SC, Akman A, Onder M, Gunasti S et al. Demographic and clinical properties of jeuvenile-onset Behcets disease: a controlled multicenter study. *J Am Acad Dermatol*. 2008;58:579-584.
16. Ozen S. Pediatric onset Behcet disease. *Current opinion in Rheumatology*. 2010;22:585-589.
17. Hatemi G, Seyahi E, Fresko I, Hamuryudan V. Behcet's syndrome: a critical digest of the recent literature. *Clinical Experimental Rheumatology*. 2012:30(72):S80-S89.

76 BACTERIAL VAGINOSIS

E.J. Mayeaux, Jr., MD
Richard P. Usatine, MD

PATIENT STORY

A 17-year-old pregnant teen reports some vaginal itching and odor associated with a thin discharge. There is no associated pain. She is unmarried and has had three lifetime sexual partners. On examination, her discharge is visible (**Figure 76-1**). It is thin and off-white. Wet prep examination shows that more than 50 percent of the epithelial cells are clue cells (**Figure 76-2**). Tests for STDs are all negative. The patient is treated with oral metronidazole 500 mg bid for 7 days with good results.

INTRODUCTION

Bacterial vaginosis (BV) is a clinical syndrome resulting from alteration of the vaginal ecosystem. It is called a vaginosis, not a vaginitis, because the tissues themselves are not actually infected, but only have superficial involvement. Women with BV are at increased risk for the acquisition of HIV, *Neisseria gonorrhoeae*, *Chlamydia trachomatis*, and herpes simplex virus (HSV)-2, and they have increased risk of complications after gynecologic surgery.[1]

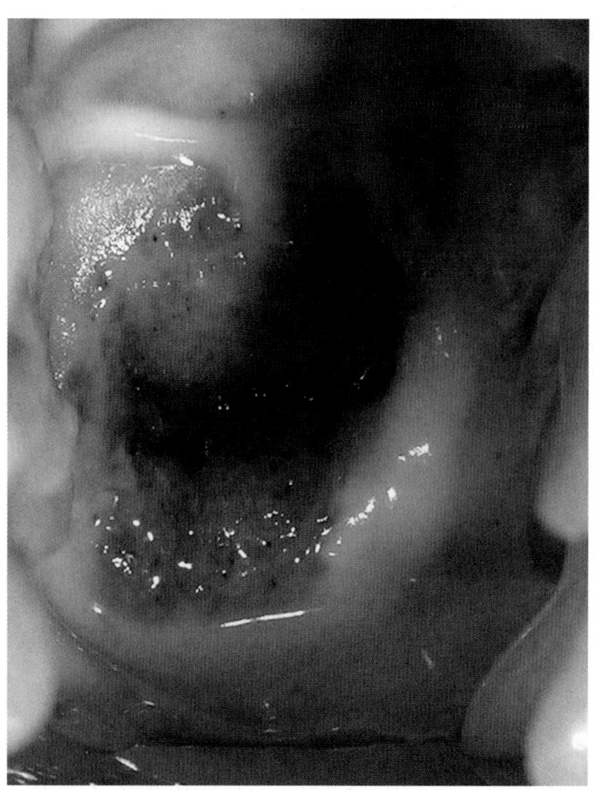

FIGURE 76-1 Bacterial vaginosis in 17-year-old pregnant teen with homogeneous, thin white vaginal discharge. She reports some vaginal itching and odor. *(Used with permission from E.J. Mayeaux, Jr., MD.)*

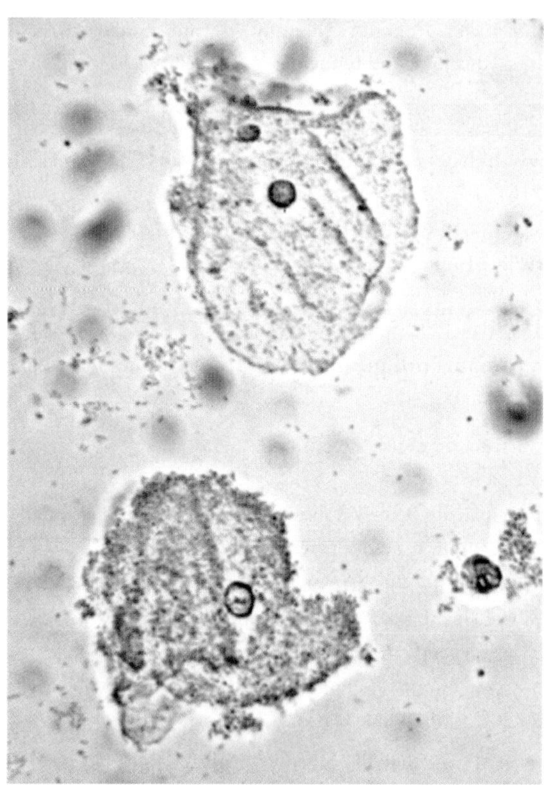

FIGURE 76-2 Clue cell and bacteria seen in bacterial vaginosis. The lower cell is a clue cell covered in bacteria while the upper cell is a normal epithelial cell. Light microscope under high power. *(Used with permission from E.J. Mayeaux, Jr., MD.)*

BV is associated with adverse pregnancy outcomes, including premature rupture of membranes, preterm labor, preterm birth, intraamniotic infection, and postpartum endometritis. However, the only established benefit of BV therapy in pregnant women is the reduction of symptoms and signs of vaginal infection.[1]

SYNONYMS

- Vaginal bacteriosis.
- *Corynebacterium* vaginosis/*vaginalis*/*vaginitis*.
- *Gardnerella vaginalis*/vaginosis.
- *Haemophilus vaginalis*/vaginitis.
- Nonspecific vaginitis.
- Anaerobic vaginosis.

EPIDEMIOLOGY

- BV is estimated to be the most prevalent cause of vaginal discharge or malodor in women presenting for care in the US. However, more than 50 percent of women with BV are asymptomatic.[1] It accounts for more than 10 million outpatient visits per year.[2] The worldwide prevalence is unknown.

ETIOLOGY AND PATHOPHYSIOLOGY

- Hydrogen peroxide-producing *Lactobacillus* is the most common organism composing normal vaginal flora after puberty.[1] In BV, normal vaginal lactobacilli are replaced by high concentrations of anaerobic bacteria such as *Mobiluncus*, *Prevotella*, *Gardnerella*, *Bacteroides*, and *Mycoplasma* species.[1,2]
- The hydrogen peroxide produced by the *Lactobacillus* may help in inhibiting the growth of atypical flora.
- The odor of BV is caused by the aromatic amines produced by the altered bacterial flora in the vagina. These aromatic amines include putrescine and cadaverine—aptly named to describe their foul odor.

RISK FACTORS

- Multiple male or female partners.[1,3]
- A new sex partner.[1]
- Douching.[4]
- Lack of condom use.[1]
- Lack of vaginal lactobacilli.[1]
- Prior BV infection.[1]

DIAGNOSIS

CLINICAL FEATURES

- Symptomatic patients present with an unpleasant, "fishy smelling" discharge that is more noticeable after coitus (the basic pH of seminal fluid is like doing the whiff test with KOH). There may be pruritus but not as often as seen with *Candida* vaginitis. The physical examination should include inspection of the external genitalia for irritation or discharge. Speculum examination is done to determine the amount and character of the discharge. A nucleic acid amplification test for *N. gonorrhoeae*, *Chlamydia*, and/or *C. trachomatis* (or similar test) should be performed on genital specimens (urethral or cervical) or urine.
- BV is usually clinically diagnosed by finding three of the following four signs and symptoms:
  - Homogeneous, thin, white discharge that smoothly coats the vaginal walls (**Figures 76-3** and **76-4**).
  - Presence of clue cells on microscopic examination (**Figure 76-2**).
  - pH of vaginal fluid >4.5.
  - A fishy odor of vaginal discharge before or after addition of 10 percent KOH (i.e., the whiff test).[1]

LABORATORY TESTING

- Vaginal pH testing can be very helpful in the diagnosis of vaginitis. The normal vaginal pH is usually 3.5 to 4.5. A pH above 4.5 is seen with menopausal patients, *Trichomonas* infection, or BV. A small piece of pH paper is touched to the vaginal discharge during the exam or on the speculum. Do not test a wet-prep sample if saline has been added because the saline alters the pH.
- Wet preps are obtained using a cotton-tipped applicator applied to the vaginal sidewall, placing the sample of discharge into normal

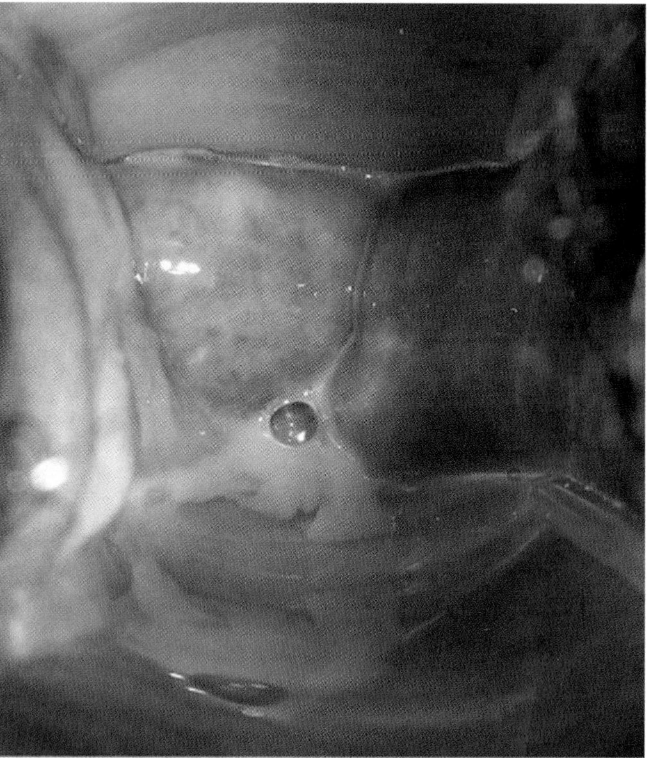

FIGURE 76-3 A homogeneous, off-white creamy malodorous discharge that adheres to the vaginal walls and pools in the vaginal vault in a woman with bacterial vaginosis. (*Used with permission from Richard P. Usatine, MD.*)

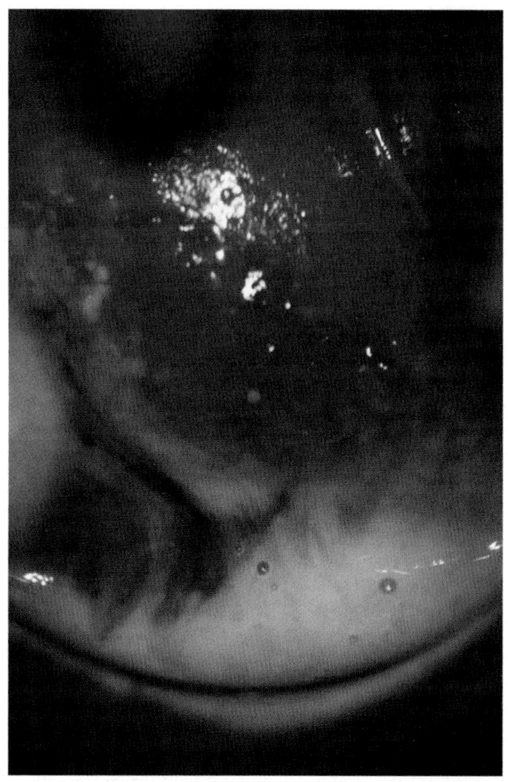

FIGURE 76-4 Bacterial vaginosis seen on the cervix with a white homogeneous discharge. Note the lack of clumping or "cottage-cheese" appearance usually found with *Candida* infections. (*Used with permission from E.J. Mayeaux, Jr., MD.*)

saline (not water). Observe for clue cells, number of white blood cells, trichomonads, and candidal hyphae. Clue cells are squamous epithelial cells whose borders are obscured by attached bacteria. More than 20 to 25 percent of epithelial cells seen in BV should be clue cells (**Figure 76-2**).

- A proline aminopeptidase test card (Pip Activity Test Card), a DNA probe-based test for high concentrations of *G. vaginalis* (Affirm VP III), and the OSOM BVBLUE test have shown acceptable performance characteristics compared with Gram stain (gold standard).[1] However, they are more costly than traditional testing.
- Although a test card is available for the detection of elevated pH and trimethylamine, it has low sensitivity and specificity and is not recommended by the Centers for Disease Control and Prevention (CDC).[1]
- Culture of *G. vaginalis* is not recommended as a diagnostic tool because it is not specific.
- Pap tests are not useful for the diagnosis of BV because of their low sensitivity.[1]

DIFFERENTIAL DIAGNOSIS

- *Trichomonas* also may have the odor of aromatic amines and, therefore, easily confused with BV at first glance. Look for the strawberry cervix on examination and moving trichomonads on the wet prep (Chapter 78, Trichomonas Vaginitis).
- *Candida* vaginitis tends to present with a cottage-cheese-like discharge and vaginal itching (Chapter 77, *Candida* Vulvovaginitis).
- Gonorrhea and chlamydia should not be missed in patients with vaginal discharge. Consider testing for these sexually transmitted diseases (STDs) based on patients' risk factors and the presence of purulence clinically and white blood cells on the wet prep (Chapter 79, Chlamydia Cervicitis).

MANAGEMENT

- Treatment is recommended for women with symptoms.
- Treatment of male sex partners has not been beneficial in preventing the recurrence of BV.[1] SOR Ⓐ

MEDICATIONS

- The established benefits of therapy for BV in nonpregnant women are to (**a**) relieve vaginal symptoms and signs of infection and (**b**) reduce the risk for infectious complications after abortion or hysterectomy.[1] SOR Ⓐ Other potential benefits might include a reduction in risk for other sexually transmitted infections (STIs).[1] SOR Ⓑ **Table 76-1** shows CDC recommended treatments.
- Metronidazole 2 g single-dose therapy has the lowest efficacy for BV and is no longer a recommended or alternative regimen. Clindamycin cream is oil-based and might weaken latex condoms and diaphragms for 5 days after use. Topical clindamycin preparations should not be used in the second half of pregnancy.[1] Multiple studies and meta-analyses have not demonstrated an association between metronidazole use during pregnancy and teratogenic or mutagenic effects in newborns.[1] SOR Ⓐ

TABLE 76-1 CDC Recommended Regimens SOR Ⓐ

Metronidazole 500 mg orally twice a day for 7 days

OR

Metronidazole gel 0.75 percent, 1 full applicator (5 g) intravaginally, once a day for 5 days

OR

Clindamycin cream 2 percent, 1 full applicator (5 g) intravaginally at bedtime for 7 days

CDC Alternative Regimens SOR Ⓐ

Tinidazole 2 g orally once daily for 3 days

OR

Tinidazole 1 g orally once daily for 5 days

OR

Clindamycin 300 mg orally twice a day for 7 days

OR

Clindamycin ovules 100 mg intravaginally once at bedtime for 3 days

OR

Metronidazole 750-mg extended-release tablets once daily for 7 days

CDC Recommended Regimens for Pregnant Women SOR Ⓐ

Metronidazole 500 mg orally twice a day for 7 days

OR

Metronidazole 250 mg orally three times a day for 7 days

OR

Clindamycin 300 mg orally twice a day for 7 days

Data from Centers for Disease Control and Prevention.[1]

- The only established benefit of therapy for BV in pregnant women is to relieve vaginal symptoms and signs of infection.[1] SOR Ⓐ Additional potential benefits of therapy include (**a**) reducing the risk for infectious complications associated with BV during pregnancy and (**b**) reducing the risk for other infections (e.g., other STDs or HIV). Multiple studies and meta-analyses have not demonstrated an association between metronidazole use during pregnancy and teratogenic or mutagenic effects in newborns.[5]
- One randomized trial for persistent BV indicated that metronidazole gel 0.75 percent twice per week for 6 months after completion of a recommended regimen was effective in maintaining a clinical cure for 6 months.[6] SOR Ⓑ
- Limited data suggest that oral nitroimidazole followed by intravaginal boric acid and suppressive metronidazole gel for those women in remission might be an option in women with recurrent BV. SOR Ⓑ[7]
- Intravaginal clindamycin cream has been associated with adverse outcomes if used in the latter half of pregnancy.[1]

COMPLEMENTARY AND ALTERNATIVE THERAPY

- Extended ingestion of live culture, nonpasteurized yogurt may theoretically increase colonization by lactobacilli and decrease the episodes of BV.[8] SOR ⓒ However, health food store lactobacilli are the wrong strain and are not well retained by the vagina.
- The efficacy of exogenous lactobacillus recolonization with probiotic lactobacilli vaginal gelatin capsules has been reported in two small trials.[9,10]

PREVENTION

- Avoidance of risk factors is recommended, although asymptomatic BV is common.
- The evidence is insufficient to assess the impact of screening for BV in pregnant women at high risk for preterm delivery.[1]

FOLLOW-UP

- Follow-up visits are unnecessary in nonpregnant women if symptoms resolve.[1]
- Treatment of BV in asymptomatic pregnant women who are at high risk for preterm delivery might prevent adverse pregnancy outcomes. Therefore, a follow-up evaluation 1 month after comple tion of treatment should be considered to evaluate whether therapy was effective.[1] SOR ⓒ
- If symptoms do recur, consider a treatment regimen different from the original regimen to treat recurrent disease.[1] SOR ⓒ

PATIENT EDUCATION

- Avoid consuming alcohol during treatment with metronidazole and for 24 hours thereafter. Women should be advised to return for additional therapy if symptoms recur because recurrence of BV is not unusual.

PATIENT RESOURCES

- Centers for Disease Control and Prevention. *Bacterial Vaginosis Fact Sheet*—**www.cdc.gov/std/BV/STDFact-Bacterial-Vaginosis.htm**.
- MedicineNet.com—**www.medicinenet.com/bacterial_vaginosis/article.htm**.

PROVIDER RESOURCES

- Centers for Disease Control and Prevention. *2010 Guidelines for Treatment of Sexually Transmitted Diseases*—**www.cdc.gov/std/treatment/2010/STD-Treatment-2010-RR5912.pdf**.

REFERENCES

1. Centers for Disease Control and Prevention. *Guidelines for Treatment of Sexually Transmitted Diseases*. http://www.cdc.gov/std/treatment/2010/STD-Treatment-2010-RR5912.pdf, accessed December 24, 2011.
2. Martius J, Krohn MA, Hillier SL, et al. Relationships of vaginal lactobacillus species, cervical chlamydia trachomatis, and bacterial vaginosis to preterm birth. *Obstet Gynecol.* 1988;71:89-95.
3. Gorgos LM, Marrazzo JM. Sexually transmitted infections among women who have sex with women. *Clin Infect Dis.* 2011;53(3): S84-S91.
4. Klebanoff MA, Nansel TR, Brotman RM, et al. Personal hygienic behaviors and bacterial vaginosis. *Sex Transm Dis.* 2010;37:94.
5. Burtin P, Taddio A, Ariburnu O, et al. Safety of metronidazole in pregnancy: a meta-analysis. *Am J Obstet Gynecol.* 1995;172 (2 Pt 1):525-529.
6. Sobel JD, Ferris D, Schwebke J, et al. Suppressive antibacterial therapy with 0.75% metronidazole vaginal gel to prevent recurrent bacterial vaginosis. *Am J Obstet Gynecol.* 2006;194: 1283-1289.
7. Reichman O, Akins R, Sobel JD. Boric acid addition to suppressive antimicrobial therapy for recurrent bacterial vaginosis. *Sex Transm Dis.* 2009;36:732-734.
8. Baylson FA, Nyirjesy P, Weitz MV. Treatment of recurrent bacterial vaginosis with tinidazole. *Obstet Gynecol.* 2004;104 (5 Pt 1): 931-932.
9. Anukam KC, Osazuwa E, Osemene GI, et al. Clinical study comparing probiotic Lactobacillus GR-1 and RC-14 with metronidazole vaginal gel to treat symptomatic bacterial vaginosis. *Microbes Infect.* 2006;8:2772.
10. Ya W, Reifer C, Miller LE. Efficacy of vaginal probiotic capsules for recurrent bacterial vaginosis: a double-blind, randomized, placebo-controlled study. *Am J Obstet Gynecol.* 2010;203:120.

77 CANDIDA VULVOVAGINITIS

E.J. Mayeaux, Jr., MD
Richard P. Usatine, MD

PATIENT STORY

An 18-year-old woman presents with severe vaginal and vulvar itching and a thick white discharge. **Figure 77-1** shows the appearance of her vulva with redness and excoriations. Note the satellite lesions near the borders of the inflamed areas. Her pelvic examination demonstrated a thick adherent discharge on the vaginal wall and cervix (**Figure 77-2**) that is consistent with an active candida infection. Treatment with a prescription anti-candida drug was successful.

INTRODUCTION

Vulvovaginal candidiasis (VVC) is a common fungal infection in women of childbearing age. Pruritus is accompanied by a thick, odorless, white vaginal discharge. VVC is not a sexually transmitted disease. On the basis of clinical presentation, microbiology, host factors, and response to therapy, VVC can be classified as either uncomplicated or complicated.[1] Uncomplicated VVC is characterized by sporadic or infrequent symptoms, mild-to-moderate symptoms, and the patient is nonimmunocompromised. Complicated VVC is characterized by recurrent (four or more episodes in 1 year) or severe VVC, non-*albicans* candidiasis, or the patient has uncontrolled diabetes, debilitation, or immunosuppression.[1]

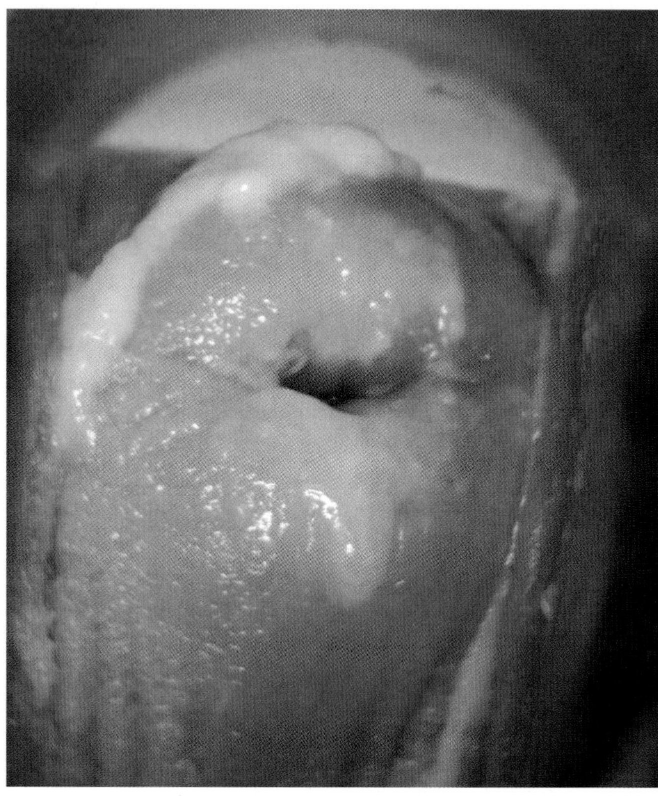

FIGURE 77-2 *Candida* vaginitis. Note the thick white adherent "cottage-cheese-like" discharge. (*Used with permission from E.J. Mayeaux, Jr., MD.*)

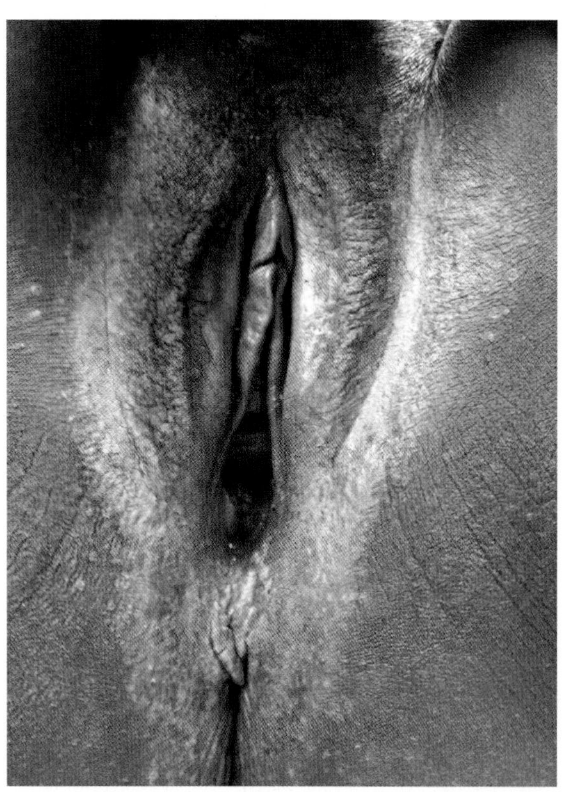

FIGURE 77-1 Candida vulvovaginitis in an 18-year-old who complained of severe vaginal and vulvar itching. She had erythema and excoriations of the vulva. Note the satellite lesions near the borders of the inflamed areas. (*Used with permission from E.J. Mayeaux, Jr., MD.*)

SYNONYMS

Yeast vaginitis, yeast infection, candidiasis, moniliasis.

EPIDEMIOLOGY

- Candida (**Figure 77-3**) is usually not isolated in prepubertal girls except when predisposing factors, such as a recent course of antibiotics, diabetes, or the wearing of diapers are present.[2]
- VVC accounts for approximately 1/3 of vaginitis cases.[1]
- *Candida* species are part of the lower genital tract flora in 20 to 50 percent of healthy asymptomatic women.[3]
- Seventy-five percent of all women in the US will experience at least one episode of VVC. Of these, 40 to 45 percent will have two or more episodes within their lifetime.[4] Approximately 10 to 20 percent of women will have complicated VVC that necessitates diagnostic and therapeutic considerations.
- It is a frequent iatrogenic complication of antibiotic treatment, secondary to altered vaginal flora.

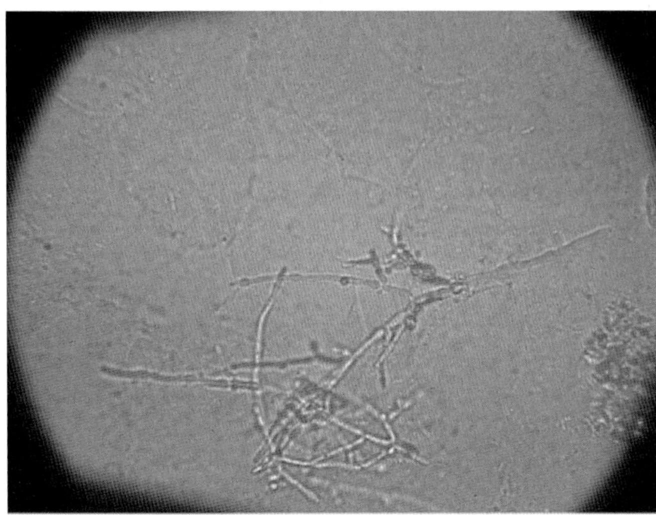

FIGURE 77-3 Wet mount with KOH showing *Candida albicans* in a teen with *Candida* vaginitis. Seen under high power demonstrating branching pseudohyphae and budding yeast. (*Used with permission from Richard P. Usatine, MD.*)

- Approximately half of all women experience multiple episodes, and up to 5 percent experience recurrent disease.[1]
- Recurrent vulvovaginal candidiasis (RVVC) is defined as four or more episodes of symptomatic VVC in 1 year. It affects a small percentage of women (<5%).[5] Recurrent yeast vaginitis is usually caused by relapse, and less often by reinfection. Recurrent infection may be caused by *Candida* recolonization of the vagina from the rectum.[6]

ETIOLOGY AND PATHOPHYSIOLOGY

- Most vulvovaginal Candidiasis is caused by *Candida albicans* (**Figure 77-3**).[1,7] *Candida glabrata* now causes a significant percentage of all *Candida* vulvovaginal infections. This organism is resistant to the nonprescription imidazole creams. It can mutate out of the activity of treatment drugs much faster than *albicans* species.[8]
- The disease is suggested by pruritus in the vulvar area, together with erythema of the vagina and vulva (**Figures 77-1** and **77-2**). The familiar reddening of the vulvar tissues is caused by an ethanol by-product of the *Candida* infection. This ethanol compound also produces pruritic symptoms. A scalloped edge with satellite lesions is characteristic of the erythema on the vulva.
- VVC can occur concomitantly with sexually transmitted diseases (STDs).
- The pathogenesis of recurrent VVC is poorly understood, and most women with these recurrences have no apparent predisposing or underlying conditions.[1]

RISK FACTORS[9,10]

- Diabetes mellitus, especially with higher A1C values.
- Recent antibiotic use.
- Increased estrogen levels.
- Immunosuppression.
- Contraceptive devices (vaginal sponges, diaphragms, and intrauterine devices).
- Genetic susceptibility.
- Behavioral factors—VVC may be linked to orogenital and, less commonly, anogenital sex.
- Wearing diapers.
- Spermicides are **not associated** with *Candida* infection.
- There is no high-quality evidence showing a link between VVC and hygienic habits or wearing tight or synthetic clothing.

DIAGNOSIS

CLINICAL FEATURES

- The diagnosis is usually suspected by characteristic findings (**Figures 77-1** and **77-2**). Typical symptoms include pruritus, vaginal soreness, dyspareunia, and external dysuria. Typical signs include vulvar edema, fissures, excoriations, or thick, curdy vaginal discharge.[1]

LABORATORY TESTING

- Vaginitis solely caused by *Candida* generally has a normal vaginal pH of less than 4.5.
- The wet prep, KOH smear, or Gram stain may demonstrate yeast and/or pseudohyphae (**Figures 77-3** and **77-4**). Wet preps may also demonstrate white blood cells, trichomonads, candidal hyphae, or clue cells.
- The KOH prep is made by adding a drop of KOH solution to a drop of saline suspension of the discharge. The KOH lyses epithelial cells in 5 to 15 minutes (faster if the slide is warmed) and allows easier visualization of candidal hyphae or yeast.[1] Swartz-Lamkins stain (potassium hydroxide, a surfactant, and blue dye) may facilitate diagnosis by staining the yeast organisms a light blue.[11]

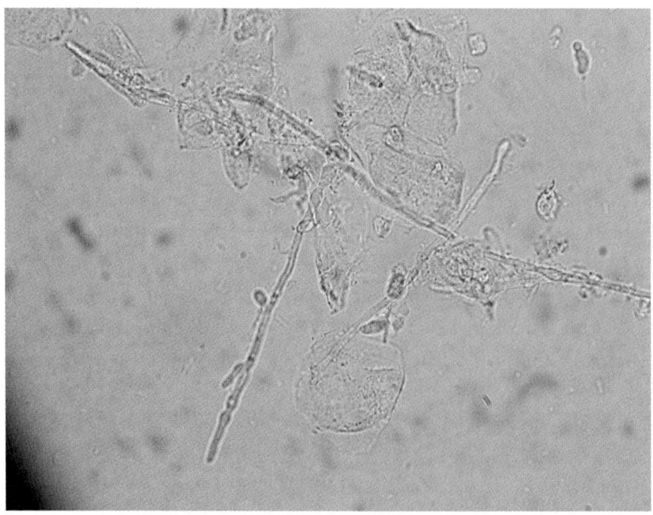

FIGURE 77-4 Wet mount with saline showing *Candida* in a teen with *Candida* vaginitis. Note how the branching pseudohyphae and budding yeast can be seen even though the epithelial cells have not been lysed by KOH. (*Used with permission from Richard P. Usatine, MD.*)

- Rapid antigen testing is also available for *Candida*. The detection of vaginal yeast by rapid antigen testing is feasible for office practice and more sensitive than wet mount. A negative test result, however, was not found to be sensitive enough to rule out yeast and avoid a culture.[7] SOR A
- Fungal culture with Sabouraud agar, Nickerson medium, or Microstix-*Candida* medium should be considered in patients with symptoms and a negative KOH because *C. glabrata* does not form pseudohyphae or hyphae and is not easily recognized on microscopy. If the wet mount is negative and *Candida* cultures cannot be done, empiric treatment can be considered for symptomatic women with any sign of VVC on examination.[1] SOR C Asymptomatic women should not be cultured as 10 to 20 percent of women harbor *Candida* sp. and other yeasts in the vagina.[1] SOR A
- Vaginal cultures should be obtained from patients with RVVC to confirm the clinical diagnosis and to identify unusual species, including non-*albicans* species, particularly *C. glabrata* (*C. glabrata* does not form pseudohyphae or hyphae and is not easily recognized on microscopy).[1] SOR B *C. glabrata* and other non-*albicans Candida* species are observed in 10 to 20 percent of patients with RVVC.[1]
- Given the frequency at which RVVC occurs in the immunocompetent healthy population, the occurrence of RVVC alone should not be considered an indication for HIV testing.[1] SOR C

DIFFERENTIAL DIAGNOSIS

- Trichomoniasis can be confused with candidiasis because patients may report itching and a discharge in both diagnoses. Look for the strawberry cervix on examination and moving trichomonads on the wet prep (Chapter 78, Trichomonas Vaginitis).
- Bacterial vaginosis can be confused with candidiasis because patients may report a discharge and an odor in both diagnoses. The odor is usually much worse in bacterial vaginosis and the quality of the discharge can be different. The wet prep should allow for differentiation between these two infections (Chapter 76, Bacterial Vaginosis).
- Gonorrhea and *Chlamydia* should not be missed in patients with vaginal discharge. Consider testing for these STDs based on patients' risk factors and the presence of purulence clinically and white blood cells on the wet prep (Chapter 79, Chlamydia Cervicitis).
- Cytolytic vaginosis, or Döderlein cytolysis, can be confused with candidiasis. Cytolytic vaginosis is produced by a massive desquamation of epithelial cells related to excess lactobacilli in the vagina. The signs and symptoms are similar to *Candida* vaginitis, except no yeast are found on wet prep. The wet prep will show an overgrowth of lactobacilli. The treatment is to discontinue all antifungals and other agents or procedures that alter the vaginal flora.

MANAGEMENT

NONPHARMACOLOGIC

- VVC is not usually acquired through sexual intercourse; treatment of sex partners is not recommended but may be considered in women who have recurrent infection. Some male sex partners might have balanitis (Chapter 136, Candidiasis) and might benefit from treatment.[1] SOR A
- Any woman whose symptoms persist after using a nonprescription preparation or who has a recurrence of symptoms within 2 months should be evaluated with office-based testing as they are not necessarily more capable of diagnosing themselves even with prior diagnosed episodes of VVC and delay in the treatment of other vulvovaginitis etiologies can result in adverse clinical outcomes.[1] SOR A

MEDICATIONS

- Women with typical symptoms and a positive test result should receive treatment. Short-courses of topical formulations effectively treat uncomplicated VVC (**Table 77-1**).[1] SOR A Topical azole drugs are more effective than nystatin, and result in clinical cure and negative cultures in 80 to 90 percent of patients who complete therapy. The creams and suppositories in **Table 77-1** are oil-based and might weaken latex condoms and diaphragms.[1] SOR A

TABLE 77-1 Centers for Disease Control and Prevention Recommended Treatment Regimens

Intravaginal Agents:

Butoconazole 2 percent cream 5 g intravaginally for 3 days
Butoconazole 2 percent cream 5 g (Butaconazole 1-sustained release), single intravaginal application*
Clotrimazole 1 percent cream 5 g intravaginally for 7 to 14 days
Clotrimazole 2 percent cream 5 g intravaginally for 3 days
Clotrimazole 100 mg vaginal suppositories, one intravaginally for 3 days
Miconazole 2 percent cream 5 g intravaginally for 7 days
Miconazole 100 mg vaginal suppository, 1 suppository for 7 days
Miconazole 200 mg vaginal suppository, 1 suppository for 3 days
Miconazole 1200 mg vaginal suppository, 1 suppository for 1 day
Nystatin 100,000-U vaginal tablet, 1 tablet for 14 days*
Tioconazole 6.5 percent ointment 5 g intravaginally in a single application
Terconazole 0.4 percent cream 5 g intravaginally for 7 days*
Terconazole 0.8 percent cream 5 g intravaginally for 3 days*
Terconazole 80 mg vaginal suppository, 1 suppository for 3 days*

Oral Agent:

Fluconazole 150-mg oral tablet, 1 tablet in single dose*

*Prescription only in the US.
Data from the Centers for Disease Control and Prevention.[1]

- The cure rates with single-dose oral fluconazole and all the intravaginal treatments are equal.[12] Fluconazole (Diflucan) 150-mg single dose has become very popular, but may have clinical cure rates of approximately only 70 percent. Systemic allergic reactions are possible with the oral agents. SOR Ⓐ
- The oral agents fluconazole, ketoconazole, and itraconazole also appear to be effective.[1] SOR Ⓑ
- VVC frequently occurs during pregnancy. Only topical azole therapies, applied for 7 days, are recommended for use among pregnant women.[1] SOR Ⓒ
- The optimal treatment of non-*albicans* VVC remains unknown. Options include longer duration of therapy (7 to 14 days) with topical therapy or a 100-mg, 150-mg, or 200-mg oral dose of fluconazole every third day for a total of 3 doses.[1] SOR Ⓒ
- Severe VVC (i.e., extensive vulvar erythema, edema, excoriation, and fissure formation) is associated with lower clinical response rates in patients treated with short courses of topical or oral therapy. Either 7 to 14 days of topical azole or 150 mg of fluconazole in two sequential doses (second dose 72 hours after initial dose) is recommended.[1] SOR Ⓒ

COMPLEMENTARY AND ALTERNATIVE THERAPY

- If recurrence VVC occurs, 600 mg of boric acid in a gelatin capsule is recommended, administered vaginally once daily for 2 weeks. This regimen has clinical and mycologic eradication rates of approximately 70 percent.[1] SOR Ⓑ
- *Lactobacillus acidophilus* does not adhere well to the vaginal epithelium, and it does not significantly change the incidence of candidal vulvovaginitis.[6,13]
- There is no evidence from randomized trials that other complementary and alternative (CAM) therapies, such as garlic, tea tree oil, yogurt, or douching, are effective for the treatment or prevention of VVC caused by *C. albicans*.[14,15]

PREVENTION

MAINTENANCE REGIMENS

- Oral fluconazole (i.e., 100 mg, 150 mg, or 200 mg dose) weekly for 6 months is the first line of treatment. If this regimen is not feasible, some specialists recommend topical clotrimazole 200 mg twice a week, clotrimazole (500 mg dose vaginal suppositories once weekly), or other topical treatments used intermittently.[1] SOR Ⓒ
- Suppressive maintenance antifungal therapies are effective in reducing RVVC.[1] SOR Ⓐ However, 30 to 50 percent of women will have recurrent disease after maintenance therapy is discontinued. Routine treatment of sex partners is controversial. *C. albicans* azole resistance is rare in vaginal isolates, and susceptibility testing is usually not warranted for individual treatment guidance.

PROGNOSIS

- Women with underlying debilitating medical conditions (e.g., those with uncontrolled diabetes or those receiving corticosteroid treatments) do not respond as well to short-term therapies. Efforts to correct modifiable conditions should be made, and more prolonged (i.e., 7 to 14 days) conventional antimycotic treatment is necessary.[1] SOR Ⓒ
- Symptomatic VVC is more frequent in HIV-seropositive women and correlates with severity of immunodeficiency. In addition, among HIV-infected women, systemic azole exposure is associated with the isolation of non *C. albicans* species from the vagina. According to the available data, therapy for VVC in HIV-infected women should not differ from that for seronegative women.[1] SOR Ⓒ

FOLLOW-UP

- Patients should be instructed to return for follow-up visits only if symptoms persist or recur within 2 months of onset of initial symptoms.[1]

PATIENT EDUCATION

- Studies show that women who were previously diagnosed with VVC are not necessarily more likely to be able to diagnose themselves.[1] Any woman whose symptoms persist after using an nonprescription preparation, or who has a recurrence of symptoms within 2 months, should be evaluated with office-based testing. Explain that unnecessary or inappropriate use of nonprescription preparations can lead to a delay in the treatment of other vulvovaginitis etiologies, which can result in adverse clinical outcomes.[1]

PATIENT RESOURCES

- MedicineNet. *Vaginal Yeast Infection (Yeast Vaginitis)*—**www.medicinenet.com/yeast_vaginitis/article.htm**.
- MedLinePlus. *Yeast Infections*—**www.nlm.nih.gov/medlineplus/yeastinfections.html**.
- eMedicine Health. *Candidiasis*—**www.emedicinehealth.com/candidiasis_yeast_infection/article_em.htm**.

PROVIDER RESOURCES

- Centers for Disease Control and Prevention. *2010 Guidelines for Treatment of Sexually Transmitted Diseases*—**www.cdc.gov/std/treatment/2010/STD-Treatment-2010-RR5912.pdf**.
- American Family Physician. Management of vaginitis. *Am Fam Physician*. 2004;70: 2125-2132.—**www.aafp.org/afp/20041201/2125.html**.
- eMedicine. *Candidiasis*—**www.emedicine.medscape.com/article/213853-overview**.
- eMedicine. *Vulvovaginitis in Emergency Medicine*—**www.emedicine.medscape.com/article/797497-overview**.

REFERENCES

1. Centers for Disease Control and Prevention. *2010 Guidelines for Treatment of Sexually Transmitted Diseases*. http://www.cdc.gov/std/treatment/2010/STD-Treatment-2010-RR5912.pdf, accessed November 2, 2011.
2. Joishy M, Ashtekar CS, Jain A, Gonsalves R. Do we need to treat vulvovaginitis in prepubertal girls? *BMJ*. 2005;330:186.

3. Goldacre MJ, Watt B, Loudon N, et al. Vaginal microbial flora in normal young women. *Br Med J.* 1979;1:1450.
4. Hurley R, De Louvois J. *Candida* vaginitis. *Postgrad Med J.* 1979; 55:645.
5. Sobel JD. Epidemiology and pathogenesis of recurrent vulvovaginal candidiasis. *Am J Obstet Gynecol.* 1985;152:924.
6. Shalev E, Battino S, Weiner E, et al. Ingestion of yogurt containing acidophilus compared with pasteurized yogurt as prophylaxis for recurrent candidal vaginitis and bacterial vaginosis. *Arch Fam Med.* 1996;5:593-596.
7. Cohen DA, Nsuami M, Etame RB, et al. A school-based chlamydia control program using DNA amplification technology. *Pediatrics.* 1998;(1):101.
8. Horowitz BJ, Giaquinta D, Ito S. Evolving pathogens in vulvovaginal candidiasis: implications for patient care. *J Clin Pharmacol.* 1992; 32:248.
9. Foxman B. The epidemiology of vulvovaginal candidiasis: risk factors. *Am J Public Health.* 1990;80:329.
10. Sobel JD. *Candida* vaginitis. *Infect Dis Clin Pract (Baltim Md).* 1994;3:334.
11. Swartz JH, Lamkins BE. A rapid, simple stain for fungi in skin, nail scrapings, and hair. *Arch Dermatol.* 1964 Jan;89:89-94.
12. Sobel JD, Brooker D, Stein GE, et al. Single oral dose fluconazole compared with conventional clotrimazole topical therapy of candida vaginitis. *Am J Obstet Gynecol.* 1995;172:1263-1238.
13. Pirotta M, Gunn J, Chondros P, et al. Effect of lactobacillus in preventing post-antibiotic vulvovaginal candidiasis: a randomised controlled trial. *BMJ.* 2004;329:548.
14. Van Kessel K, Assefi N, Marrazzo J, Eckert L. Common complementary and alternative therapies for yeast vaginitis and bacterial vaginosis: a systematic review. *Obstet Gynecol Surv.* 2003;58(5):351-358.
15. Boskey ER. Alternative therapies for bacterial vaginosis: a literature review and acceptability survey. *Altern Ther Health Med.* 2005;11(5):38-43.

78 *TRICHOMONAS* VAGINITIS

E.J. Mayeaux, Jr., MD
Richard P. Usatine, MD

PATIENT STORY

A 17-year-old teen presents with a vaginal itching, odor, and discharge for several weeks. She has one partner who is asymptomatic. Speculum examination shows a cervix (**Figure 78-1**) with a copious foamy white discharge with a fishy odor. Wet mount shows trichomonads swimming in saline (**Figures 78-2** and **78-3**). The trichomonads are larger than white blood cells (WBCs) and have visible flagella and movement. She is diagnosed with trichomoniasis and treated with 2 g of metronidazole in a single dose. The patient is tested for other sexually transmitted diseases (STDs) and her partner is treated with the same regimen.

INTRODUCTION

Trichomonas vaginitis is a local infection caused by the protozoan *Trichomonas vaginalis* that is associated with vaginal discharge and irritation. The patient often has an itch and an odor along with the discharge but may be asymptomatic.

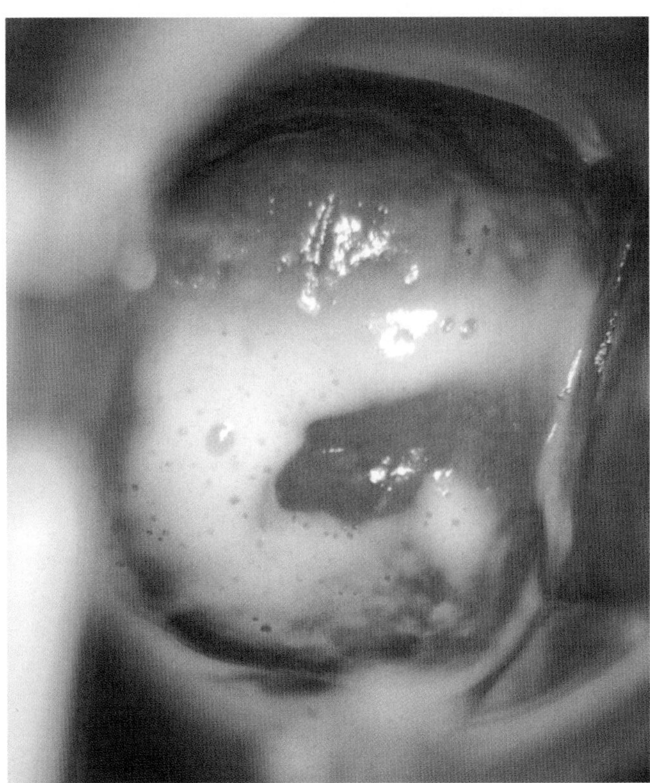

FIGURE 78-1 *Trichomonas* infection seen on the cervix. There is a thick foamy off-white discharge. (*Used with permission from Richard P. Usatine, MD.*)

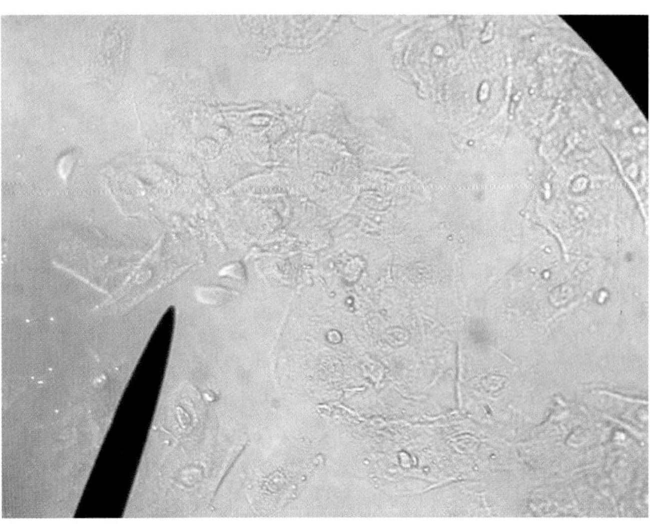

FIGURE 78-2 Wet mount showing *Trichomonas* in saline under low power. There are two visible trichomonads to the right and above the tip of the pointer. The largest cells are vaginal epithelial cells with visible nuclei. (*Used with permission from Richard P. Usatine, MD.*)

SYNONYMS

Trichomoniasis, trich, tricky monkeys.

EPIDEMIOLOGY

- An estimated 3 to 5 million cases of trichomoniasis occur each year in the US.[1]
- The worldwide prevalence of trichomoniasis is estimated to be 180 million cases per year; and these cases account for 10 to 25 percent of all vaginal infections.[2]
- Cross-sectional data from the 2003 to 2004 US National Health and Nutrition Examination Survey (NHANES) shows 3 percent of

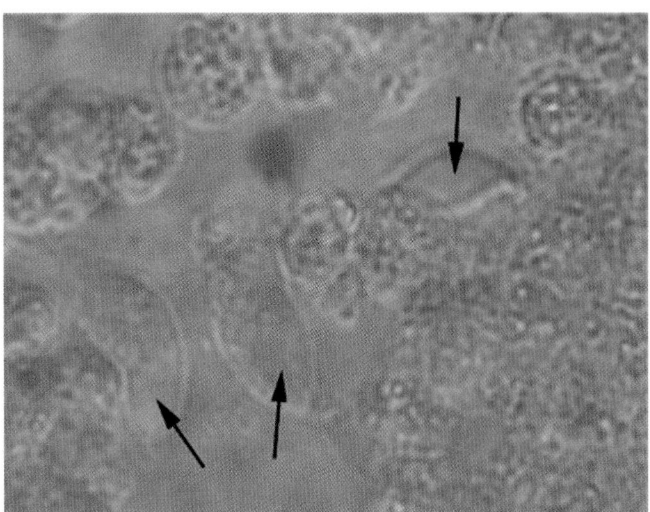

FIGURE 78-3 Wet mount showing *Trichomonas* (*arrows*) in saline under high power. The smaller more granular cells are white blood cells. (*Used with permission from Richard P. Usatine, MD.*)

female adolescents (aged 14 to 19 years) had laboratory evidence of infection with Trichomonas vaginalis.[3]

ETIOLOGY AND PATHOPHYSIOLOGY

- *Trichomonas* infection is caused by the unicellular protozoan *T. vaginalis*.[4]
- The majority of men (90%) infected with *T. vaginalis* are asymptomatic, but many women (50%) report symptoms.[5]
- The infection is predominantly transmitted via sexual contact. The organism can survive up to 48 hours at 10°C (50°F) outside the body, making transmission from shared undergarments or from infected hot spas possible although extremely unlikely.
- *Trichomonas* infection is associated with low-birth-weight infants, premature rupture of membranes, and preterm delivery in pregnant patients.[6]
- In a person coinfected with HIV, the pathology induced by *T. vaginalis* infection can increase HIV shedding. *Trichomonas* infection may also act to expand the portal of entry for HIV in an HIV-negative person. Studies from Africa have suggested that *T. vaginalis* infection may increase the rate of HIV transmission by approximately twofold.[7]

RISK FACTORS[3]

- New or multiple partners.
- A history of STDs.
- Exchanging sex for payment or drugs.
- Injection drug use.

DIAGNOSIS

CLINICAL FEATURES

- The physical examination should include inspection of the external genitalia for irritation or discharge (**Figures 78-1** and **78-5**). Speculum examination is done to determine the amount and character of the discharge and to look for the characteristic strawberry cervix (**Figures 78-4**). This strawberry pattern is caused by inflammation and punctate hemorrhages on the cervix.
- Typically, women with trichomoniasis have a diffuse, malodorous, yellow-green discharge (**Figure 78-5**) with vulvar irritation.[4] Vaginal and vulvar itching and irritation are common.
- It should be determined whether the patient douched recently, because this can lower the yield of diagnostic tests. Patients who have been told not to douche will sometimes start wiping the vagina with soapy washcloths to "keep clean" as an alternative. This greatly irritates the vagina and cervix, lowers test sensitivity, and may cause a discharge.

TYPICAL DISTRIBUTION

- In women, *Trichomonas vaginalis* may be found in the vagina, urethra, and paraurethral glands of infected women. Other sites include the cervix and Bartholin and Skene glands.

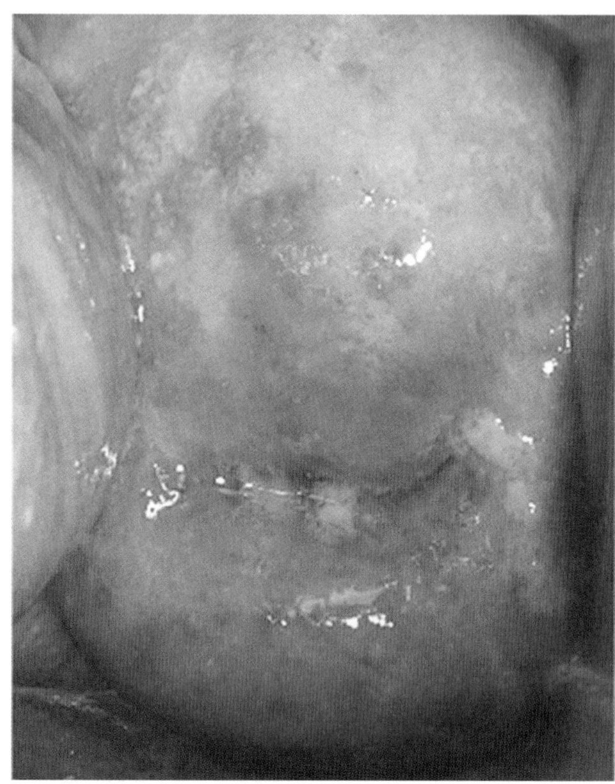

FIGURE 78-4 Close-up of strawberry cervix in a *Trichomonas* infection demonstrating inflammation and punctate hemorrhages. (*Used with permission from Richard P. Usatine, MD.*)

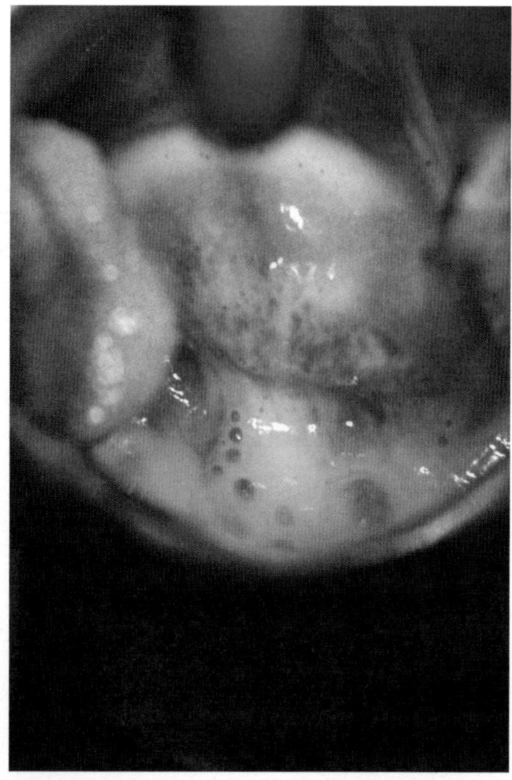

FIGURE 78-5 Speculum examination demonstrating the thick yellow-green discharge that may be seen in *Trichomonas* infection. The discharge can also be frothy white. (*Used with permission from E.J. Mayeaux, Jr., MD.*)

LABORATORY TESTING

- Because of the high prevalence of trichomoniasis, testing should be performed in women seeking care for vaginal discharge. Screening should be considered for women with risk factors.[4]
- Wet preps are obtained using a cotton-tipped applicator applied to the vaginal side-wall, placing the sample of discharge into normal saline (not water). A drop of the suspension is then placed on a slide, covered with a coverslip, and carefully examined with the low-power and high-dry objective lenses. Under the microscope, observe for motile trichomonads, which are often easy to visualize because of their lashing flagella (**Figure 78-2**).
- Wet prep has a sensitivity of only approximately 60 to 70 percent and requires immediate evaluation of wet preparation slide for optimal results.[4] One study found that 20 percent of samples for wet prep became negative by 10 minutes, 35 percent samples by 30 minutes, and 78 percent by two hours. They concluded that in order to maximize the sensitivity of this test, all specimens should be examined immediately after they are taken.[8]
- The OSOM Trichomonas Rapid Test and the Affirm VP III are FDA-cleared for trichomoniasis in women. Both tests are performed on vaginal secretions at the point of care and have a sensitivity greater than 83 percent and a specificity greater than 97 percent. The results of the OSOM Trichomonas Rapid Test are available in approximately 10 minutes, and results of the Affirm VP III are available within 45 minutes. False-positive tests might occur, especially in populations with a low prevalence of disease.[4]
- An FDA-approved polymerase chain reaction (PCR) assay for detection of gonorrhea and chlamydial infection (Amplicor, manufactured by Roche Diagnostic Corp.) has been modified to test for *T. vaginalis* in vaginal or endocervical swabs and in urine from women and men, with sensitivity ranges from 88 to 97 percent and specificity from 98 to 99 percent.[9]
- APTIMA *T. vaginalis* Analyte Specific Reagents (ASR; manufactured by Gen-Probe, Inc.) also can detect *T. vaginalis* RNA using the same instrumentation platforms available for the FDA-cleared APTIMA Combo2 assay for diagnosis of gonorrhea and chlamydial infection. Published validation studies found sensitivity ranging from 74 to 98 percent and specificity from 87 to 98 percent.[10]
- A vaginal pH above 4.5 is seen with menopausal patients, *Trichomonas* infection, or bacterial vaginosis.[5]
- Culture is a sensitive and highly specific method of diagnosis. In women in whom trichomoniasis is suspected but not confirmed by microscopy, vaginal secretions should be cultured for *T. vaginalis*.[4]
- A nucleic acid amplification test for *Neisseria gonorrhoeae*, and/or *Chlamydia trachomatis* should be performed on all patients with *Trichomonas*.
- Although trichomonas may be detected on Pap testing, the sensitivity is low and Pap testing is not indicated in adolescents unless they are HIV infected.[11]

DIFFERENTIAL DIAGNOSIS

- Bacterial vaginosis and *Trichomonas* may have the odor of aromatic amines, and therefore may easily be confused with each other. Look for clue cells and trichomonads on the wet prep to differentiate between the two (Chapter 76, Bacterial Vaginosis).
- *Candida* vaginitis tends to present with a cottage-cheese-like discharge and vaginal itching (Chapter 77, Candida Vaginitis).
- Gonorrhea and *Chlamydia* and should not be missed in patients with vaginal discharge. Consider testing for these STDs based on patients' risk factors and the presence of purulence clinically and WBCs on the wet prep (Chapter 79, Chlamydia Cervicitis).

MANAGEMENT

MEDICATIONS

- **Table 78-1** shows treatments for *T. vaginalis* infections. Metronidazole 2 g orally as a single dose or 500 mg bid for 7 days (including pregnant patients) are the best treatments by Cochrane analysis.[12] SOR Ⓐ
- Tinidazole (Tindamax), a second-generation nitroimidazole, is indicated as a one-time dose of 2 g for the treatment of trichomoniasis (including metronidazole-resistant trichomoniasis).[4] SOR Ⓐ It is effective therapy in nonresistant and resistant *T. vaginalis*.[13,14] The contraindications (including ethyl alcohol [ETOH]) to the use of tinidazole are similar to those for metronidazole.
- Pregnant women may be treated with 2 g of metronidazole in a single dose. Metronidazole is pregnancy category B. Vaginal trichomoniasis is associated with adverse pregnancy outcomes, particularly premature rupture of membranes, preterm delivery, and low birth weight. Unfortunately, data do not suggest that metronidazole treatment results in a reduction in perinatal morbidity and treatment may even increase prematurity or low birth weight.[4] Treatment of *T. vaginalis* might relieve symptoms of vaginal discharge in pregnant women and might prevent respiratory or genital infection of the newborn and further sexual transmission. The Centers for Disease Control and Prevention (CDC) recommends that clinicians counsel patients regarding the potential risks and benefits of treatment during pregnancy.[4]
- Some strains of *T. vaginalis* can have diminished susceptibility to metronidazole. Low-level metronidazole resistance has been identified in 2 to 5 percent of cases of vaginal trichomoniasis. These infections should respond to tinidazole or higher doses or longer durations of metronidazole. High-level resistance is rare.[15]
- Metronidazole gel is 50 percent less efficacious for the treatment of trichomoniasis than oral preparations and is not recommended.[4]

TABLE 78-1 Centers for Disease Control and Prevention Recommended Regimens for Pregnant and Nonpregnant Patients. SOR Ⓐ

Metronidazole 2 g orally in a single dose

OR

Tinidazole 2 g orally in a single dose

CDC Alternative Regimen SOR Ⓐ

Metronidazole 500 mg orally twice a day for 7 days

Data from Centers for Disease Control and Prevention.[2,4]

PREVENTION

- Patients should be instructed to avoid sex until they and their sex partners are cured (i.e., when therapy has been completed and patient and partner[s] are asymptomatic).[4]
- Spermicidal agents such as nonoxynol-9 reduce the rate of transmission of *Trichomonas*.[16]
- The risk of acquiring infection can be reduced by consistent use of condoms and limiting the number of sexual partners.

FOLLOW-UP

- Because of the high rate of reinfection among patients in whom trichomoniasis was diagnosed, rescreening at 3 months following initial infection can be considered for sexually active women.[4]

PATIENT EDUCATION

- Sexual partners of patients with *Trichomonas* should be treated. Patients can be sent home with a dose for a partner when it is believed that the partner will not come in on his own.

PATIENT RESOURCES

- Centers for Disease Control and Prevention information—**www.dpd.cdc.gov/dpdx/HTML/Trichomoniasis.htm**.
- Medline-plus—**www.nlm.nih.gov/medlineplus/ency/article/001331.htm**.
- Centers for Disease Control and Prevention. *STDs: Trichomoniasis*—**www.cdc.gov/std/trichomonas/default.htm**.
- PubMed Health. *Trichomoniasis*—**www.ncbi.nlm.nih.gov/pubmedhealth/PMH0002307/**.
- MedLinePlus. *Trichomoniasis*—**www.nlm.nih.gov/medlineplus/trichomoniasis.html**.
- eMedicine Health. *Trichomoniasis*—**www.emedicinehealth.com/trichomoniasis/article_em.htm**.

PROVIDER RESOURCES

- **www.emedicine.medscape.com/article/230617**.
- Centers for Disease Control and Prevention. *2010 Guidelines for Treatment of Sexually Transmitted Diseases*—**www.cdc.gov/std/treatment/2010/STD-Treatment-2010-RR5912.pdf**.

REFERENCES

1. Sutton M, Sternberg M, Koumans EH, et al. The prevalence of *Trichomonas vaginalis* infection among reproductive-age women in the United States, 2001-2004. *Clin Infect Dis*. 2007;45:1319.
2. Weinstock H, Berman S, Cates W Jr: Sexually transmitted diseases among American youth: incidence and prevalence estimates, 2000. *Perspect Sex Reprod Health*. 2004;36(1):6-10.
3. Forhan SE, Gottlieb SL, Sternberg MR, et al. Prevalence of sexually transmitted infections among female adolescents aged 14 to 19 in the United States. *Pediatrics*. 2009;124:1505.
4. Centers for Disease Control and Prevention. *2010 Guidelines for Treatment of Sexually Transmitted Diseases*. http://www.cdc.gov/std/treatment/2010/STD-Treatment-2010-RR5912.pdf, accessed December 1, 2011.
5. Gjerdngen D, Fontaine P, Bixby M, et al. The impact of regular vaginal pH screening on the diagnosis of bacterial vaginosis in pregnancy. *J Fam Pract*. 2000;49:3-43.
6. Cotch MF, Pastorek JG 2nd, Nugent RP, et al. *Trichomonas vaginalis* associated with low birth weight and preterm delivery: the Vaginal Infections and Prematurity Study Group. *Sex Transm Dis*. 1997;24:353-360.
7. Sorvillo F, Smith L, Kerndt P, Ash L. *Trichomonas vaginalis*, HIV, and African-Americans. *Emerg Infect Dis*. 2001;7(6):927-932.
8. Kingston MA, Bansal D, Carlin EM. 'Shelf life' of Trichomonas vaginalis. *Int J STD AIDS*. 2003 Jan;14(1):28-9.
9. Van Der PB, Kraft CS, Williams JA. Use of an adaptation of a commercially available PCR assay aimed at diagnosis of chlamydia and gonorrhea to detect *Trichomonas vaginalis* in urogenital specimens. *J Clin Microbiol*. 2006;44:366-373.
10. Nye MB, Schwebke JR, Body BA. Comparison of APTIMA *Trichomonas vaginalis* transcription-mediated amplification to wet mount microscopy, culture, and polymerase chain reaction for diagnosis of trichomoniasis in men and women. *Am J Obstet Gynecol*. 2009;200:188-197.
11. Lobo TT, Feijó G, Carvalho SE, Costa PL, Chagas C, Xavier J, Simoes-Barbosa A. A comparative evaluation of the Papanicolaou test for the diagnosis of trichomoniasis. *Sex Transm Dis*. 2003;30(9):694-699.
12. Epling J. What is the best way to treat trichomoniasis in women? (Cochrane review) *Am Fam Physician*. 2001;64:1241-1243.
13. Mammen-Tobin A, Wilson JD. Management of metronidazole-resistant *Trichomonas vaginalis*—a new approach. *Int J STD AIDS*. 2005;16(7):488-490.
14. Hager WD. Treatment of metronidazole-resistant *Trichomonas vaginalis* with tinidazole: case reports of three patients. *Sex Transm Dis*. 2004;31(6):343-345.
15. Kirkcaldy RD, Augostini P, Asbel LE, Bernstein KT, Kerani RP, Mettenbrink CJ, Pathela P, Schwebke JR, Secor WE, Workowski KA, Davis D, Braxton J, Weinstock HS. Trichomonas vaginalis antimicrobial drug resistance in 6 US cities, STD Surveillance Network, 2009-2010. *Emerg Infect Dis*. 2012;18(6):939-943.
16. d'Oro LC, Parazzini F, Naldi L, La Vecchia C. Barrier methods of contraception, spermicides, and sexually transmitted diseases: a review. *Genitourin Med*. 1994;70:410.

79 CHLAMYDIA CERVICITIS

E.J. Mayeaux, Jr., MD
Richard P. Usatine, MD

PATIENT STORY

A 16-year-old girl presents to clinic with a complaint of vaginal discharge. She has only one sexual partner but is unsure if her partner may have had other sexual contacts. On physical examination, there is ectopy and some mucoid discharge (**Figure 79-1**). The cervix bled easily while obtaining discharge and cells for a wet mount and genetic probe test. The wet mount showed many white blood cells (WBCs) but no visible pathogens. The patient was treated with 1 g of azithromycin taken in front of a clinic nurse. She was tested for HIV, syphilis, Trichomonas, GC, and Chlamydia and given a follow-up appointment in 1 week. The genetic probe test was positive for *Chlamydia* and all the other examinations were negative. This information was given to the patient on her return visit and safe sex was discussed.

INTRODUCTION

Chlamydia trachomatis causes genital infections that can result in pelvic inflammatory disease (PID), ectopic pregnancy, and infertility. Asymptomatic infection is common among both men and women so health care providers must rely on screening tests to detect disease.

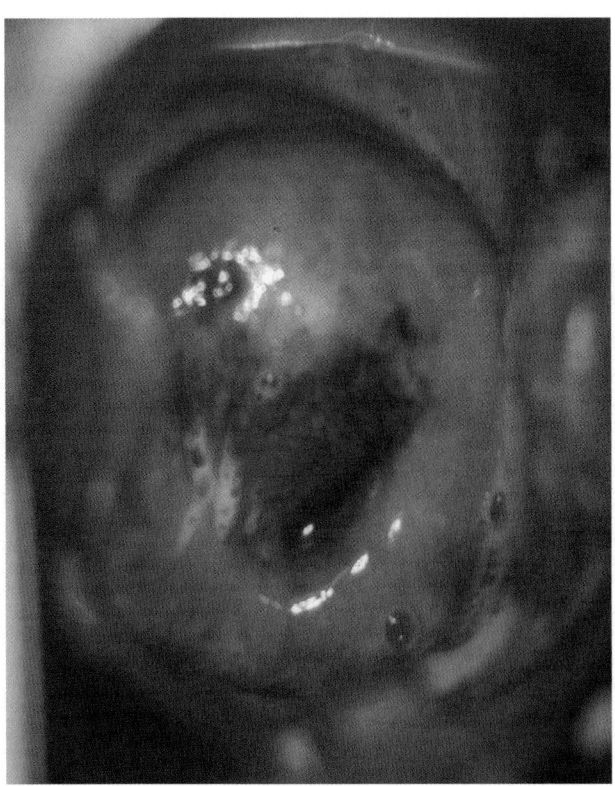

FIGURE 79-1 Chlamydial cervicitis with ectopy, mucoid discharge, and irritation in a 16-year-old girl. The cervix is inflamed and friable. (*Used with permission from E.J. Mayeaux, Jr., MD.*)

The Centers for Disease Control and Prevention (CDC) recommends annual screening of all sexually active women ages 25 years and younger, and of older women with risk factors, such as having a new sex partner or multiple sex partners.[1]

EPIDEMIOLOGY

- A very common STD, *Chlamydia* is the most frequently reported infectious disease in the US (excluding human papillomavirus [HPV]).[1] An estimated 1.2 million cases are reported to the CDC annually in the US.[2]
- The World Health Organization (WHO) estimates there are 140 million cases of Chlamydia trachomatis infection worldwide every year.[3]
- The CDC estimates screening and treatment programs can be conducted at an annual cost of $175 million. Every dollar spent on screening and treatment saves $12 in complications that result from untreated *Chlamydia*.[4]
- It is common among sexually active adolescents and young adults.[5] As many as 1 in 10 adolescent girls tested for *Chlamydia* is infected. Based on reports to the CDC provided by states that collect age-specific data, teenage girls have the highest rates of chlamydial infection. In these states, 15- to 19-year-old girls represent 46 percent of infections and 20- to 24-year-old women represent another 33 percent.[4]
- Cross-sectional data from the 2003-2004 US National Health and Nutrition Examination Survey (NHANES) shows 4 percent of female adolescents (aged 14 to 19 years) had laboratory evidence of infection with Chlamydia trachomatis.[6]

ETIOLOGY AND PATHOPHYSIOLOGY

- *C. trachomatis* is a small Gram-negative bacterium with unique biologic properties among living organisms. *Chlamydia* is an obligate intracellular parasite that has a distinct life-cycle consisting of two major phases: The small elementary bodies attach and penetrate into cells, and the metabolically active reticulate bodies that form large inclusions within cells.
- It has a long growth cycle, which explains why extended courses of treatment are often necessary. Immunity to infection is not long-lived, so reinfection or persistent infection is common.
- The infection may be asymptomatic and the onset often indolent. Symptoms of infection when present in women are most commonly abnormal vaginal discharge, vaginal bleeding (including after intercourse), and dysuria. Only 2 to 4 percent of infected men reported any symptoms.[7]
- It can cause cervicitis, endometritis, PID, infertility, perihepatitis (Fitz-Hugh-Curtis syndrome) urethritis, and epididymitis. It may produce poor neonatal outcomes including premature rupture of membranes, preterm labor, low birth weight, and infant death, conjunctivitis, and pediatric pneumonia.[8] Of exposed babies, 50 percent develop conjunctivitis and 10 to 16 percent develop pneumonia.[1] Perinatal *Chlamydia* is the leading cause of infectious blindness in the world, which is particularly worrisome since adolescents are at increased risk for infection and have more barriers to health care screening.[9]

- *Chlamydia* infections may lead to reactive arthritis, which presents with arthritis, conjunctivitis, and urethritis. Past or ongoing *C. trachomatis* infection may be a risk factor for ovarian cancer.[10,11]
- Up to 40 percent of women with untreated *Chlamydia* will develop PID. Undiagnosed PID caused by *Chlamydia* is common. Of those with PID, 20 percent will become infertile; 18 percent will experience debilitating, chronic pelvic pain; and 9 percent will have a life-threatening tubal pregnancy. Tubal pregnancy is the leading cause of first-trimester, pregnancy-related deaths in American women.[4]

RISK FACTORS[1,2,12]

- Adolescents and young adults.
- Nonwhite populations.
- Multiple and new sexual partners.
- Poor socioeconomic conditions.
- Single marital status.
- Nonbarrier contraceptive use.
- History of prior STD.

DIAGNOSIS

CLINICAL FEATURES

- The cervix is inflamed, friable, and may bleed easily with manipulation. The cervix may show ectopy (columnar cells on the ectocervix). The discharge is usually mucoid or mucopurulent (**Figure 79-1** to **79-3**).[8]

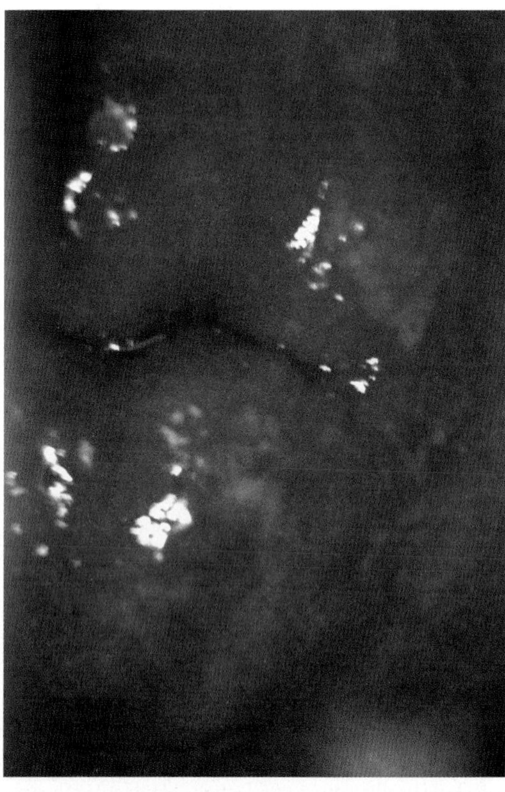

FIGURE 79-2 This patient presented with spotting after intercourse. She has cervicitis with ectopy, friability, and bleeding. NAAT was positive for Chlamydia. (*Used with permission from E.J. Mayeaux, Jr., MD.*)

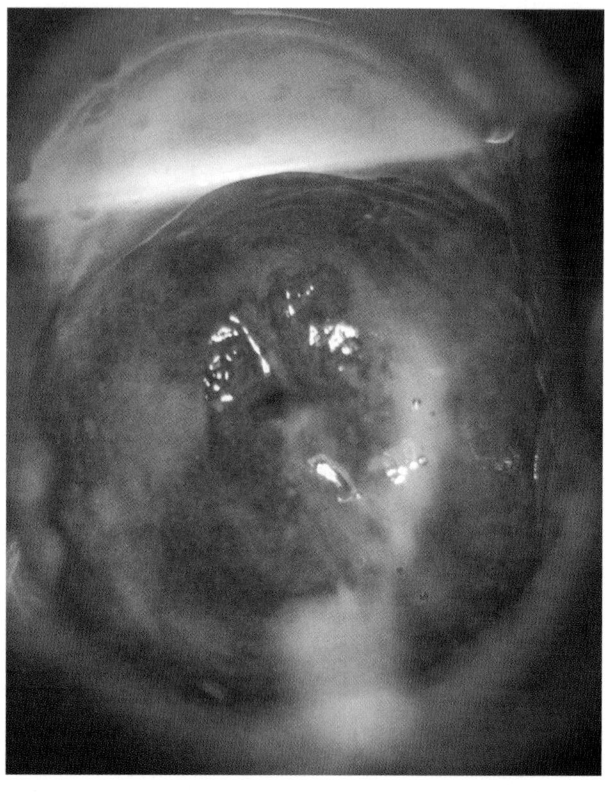

FIGURE 79-3 Chlamydia cervicitis that presented with a mild discharge. A NAAT test was positive for Chlamydia. The rest of her work-up was negative. (*Used with permission from E.J. Mayeaux, Jr., MD.*)

- Persons who have receptive anal intercourse can acquire a rectal infection, which presents as anal pain, discharge, or bleeding. Persons who engage in oral sex can acquire a pharyngeal infection, which may present as an irritated throat.[8]
- Swab test—A white cotton-tip applicator is placed in the endocervical canal and removed to view. A visible mucopurulent discharge constitutes a positive swab test for *Chlamydia* (**Figure 79-4**). This is not specific for *Chlamydia* as other genital infections can cause a mucopurulent discharge, and is not recommended for diagnosis.

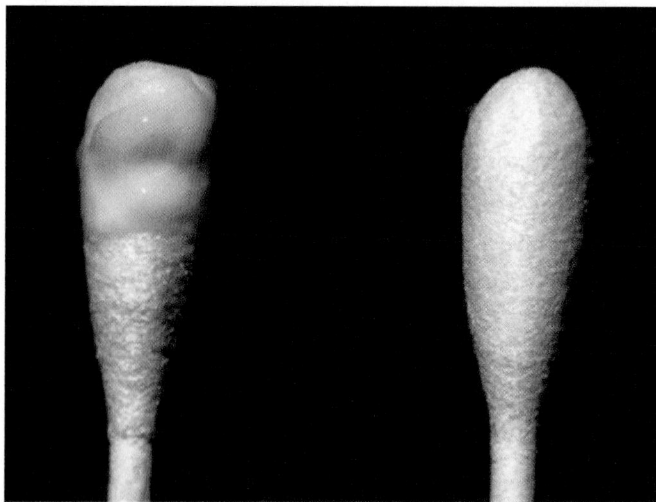

FIGURE 79-4 Mucopurulent discharge on the left swab from a cervix infected with *Chlamydia* (positive swab test). (*Used with permission from Connie Celum and Walter Stamm, Seattle STD/HIV Prevention Training Center, University of Washington.*)

LABORATORY TESTING

- A significant proportion of patients with *Chlamydia* are asymptomatic, providing a reservoir for infection. All pregnant women and sexually active women younger than 25 years of age should be screened with routine examinations. A wet prep is usually negative for other organisms. Only WBCs and normal flora are seen.
- *Chlamydia* cannot be cultured on artificial media because it is an obligate intracellular organism. Tissue culture is required to grow the live organism. When testing for *Chlamydia*, a wood-handled swab must not be used, as substances in wood may inhibit *Chlamydia* organism. Culture has sensitivity of 70 to 100 percent and a specificity of almost 100 percent, which makes it the gold standard.[1]
- The enzyme-linked immunosorbent assay (ELISA) technique (Chlamydiazyme) has a sensitivity of 70 to 100 percent and a specificity of 97 to 99 percent.[5] Fluorescein-conjugated monoclonal antibodies test (MicroTrak) has a sensitivity of 70 to 100 percent and a specificity of 97 to 99 percent.[5]
- *C. trachomatis* can be detected using nucleic acid amplification techniques (NAATs) on swabs or voided urine specimens. These tests are often used for testing to detect gonorrhea and *Chlamydia*. Nucleic acid amplification tests have been used successfully in difficult-to-reach adolescents ("street kids") as well as in pediatric emergency departments and school-based settings.[13,14] Screening in school-based settings was associated with significant reduction in *Chlamydia* rates during a 1-year period. Self-collected vaginal swab specimens perform at least as well as with other approved specimens using NAATs.[15] NAATs can be performed on endocervical, urethral, vaginal, pharyngeal, rectal, or urine samples. The accuracy of NAATs on urine samples has been found to be nearly identical to that of samples obtained directly from the cervix.[16]
- Rectal and oropharyngeal *C. trachomatis* infection in persons engaging in anal or oral intercourse can be diagnosed by testing at the site of exposure. Although not FDA-cleared for this use, NAATs have demonstrated improved sensitivity and specificity compared with culture for the detection at rectal sites,[17] and at oropharyngeal sites in men.[18]
- Certain NAATs have been FDA-cleared for use on liquid-based cytology specimens, although test sensitivity using these specimens might be lower.[19]
- Persons who undergo testing for *Chlamydia* should be tested for other STDs as well.[1]

DIFFERENTIAL DIAGNOSIS

- Gonorrhea frequently coexists with *Chlamydia* and should be tested for when a patient is thought to have *Chlamydia*. The discharge of gonorrhea may be more purulent but this is not always the case.
- Bacterial vaginosis—The aromatic amine odor and clue cells help to distinguish between these infections (Chapter 76, Bacterial Vaginosis).
- Trichomoniasis—Look for the strawberry cervix and *Trichomonas* on the wet prep. There may also be a positive whiff test (see Chapter 78, Trichomonas Vaginitis).

MANAGEMENT

NONPHARMACOLOGIC

- Patients diagnosed with *Chlamydia* cervicitis should be tested for other STDs.[1]

MEDICATIONS

- **Table 79-1** shows CDC recommended treatments for *Chlamydia*. Azithromycin (Zithromax) 1000 mg one-time dose is easy and may be directly observed in the clinic.[1] SOR Ⓐ It is the first-line therapy for *Chlamydia* during pregnancy.
- Other treatments include doxycycline 100 mg PO bid × 7 days.[1] SOR Ⓐ Avoid dairy products around time of dosing.
- Erythromycin might be less efficacious than either azithromycin or doxycycline, mainly because of the frequent occurrence of GI side effects that can lead to nonadherence.

TABLE 79-1 Centers for Disease Control and Prevention Recommended Regimens SOR Ⓐ

Azithromycin 1 g orally in a single dose
OR
Doxycycline 100 mg orally twice a day for 7 days
CDC Alternative Regimens
Erythromycin base 500 mg orally 4 times a day for 7 days
OR
Erythromycin ethylsuccinate 800 mg orally 4 times a day for 7 days
OR
Ofloxacin 300 mg orally twice a day for 7 days
OR
Levofloxacin 500 mg orally once daily for 7 days
CDC Recommended Regimens in Pregnancy
Azithromycin 1 g orally in a single dose
OR
Amoxicillin 500 mg orally 3 times a day for 7 days
Alternative Regimens in Pregnancy
Erythromycin base 500 mg orally 4 times a day for 7 days
OR
Erythromycin base 250 mg orally 4 times a day for 14 days
OR
Erythromycin ethylsuccinate 800 mg orally 4 times a day for 7 days
OR
Erythromycin ethylsuccinate 400 mg orally 4 times a day for 14 days

Data from the Centers for Disease Control and Prevention.[1]

- Ofloxacin (Floxin) 300 mg po bid × 7 days is an alternative that should be taken on an empty stomach.[1] SOR A It is contraindicated in children or pregnant and lactating women, but may also cover *Neisseria gonorrhoeae* infection. Levofloxacin 500 mg orally for 7 days is another fluoroquinolone alternative.[1] SOR A
- A metaanalysis of 12 randomized clinical trials of azithromycin versus doxycycline for the treatment of genital chlamydial infection demonstrated that the treatments were equally efficacious, with microbial cure rates of 97 and 98 percent, respectively.[20]
- Partners need treatment. If concerns exist that sex partners will not seek evaluation and treatment, then delivery of antibiotic therapy (either a prescription or medication) to their partners is an option.[1]
- Medications for chlamydial infections should be dispensed on site and the first dose directly observed to maximize medication adherence.[1]

REFERRAL OR HOSPITALIZATION

- With evidence of complications such as a tuboovarian abscess or severe PID.

PREVENTION

- Individuals who are sexually active should be aware of the risk of STDs and that ways of avoiding infection include mutual monogamy and appropriate barrier protection.

PROGNOSIS

- Treatment failures with full primary therapies are quite rare. Reinfection is very common and is related to nontreatment of sexual partners or acquisition from a new partner.

FOLLOW-UP

- Test-of-cure (repeat testing 3 to 4 weeks after completing therapy) is not recommended for persons treated with the recommended or alterative regimens, unless therapeutic compliance is in question, symptoms persist, or reinfection is suspected. However, test of cure is recommended in pregnant women.[1] If chlamydia is detected during the first trimester, repeat testing for reinfection should also be performed within three to six months, or in the third trimester.[1] Men and nonpregnant women should be retested at three months. If this is not possible, clinicians should retest the patient to screen for reinfection when he or she next presents for medical care within 12 months after treatment.[1]

PATIENT EDUCATION

- To minimize transmission, persons treated for *Chlamydia* should be instructed to abstain from sexual intercourse for 7 days after single-dose therapy or until completion of a 7-day regimen.
- To minimize the risk for reinfection, patients also should be instructed to abstain from sexual intercourse until all of their sex partners are treated.[1]

PATIENT RESOURCES

- eMedicine Health. *Cervicitis*—**www.emedicinehealth.com/cervicitis/article_em.htm**.
- eMedicine Health. *Chlamydia*—**www.emedicinehealth.com/chlamydia/article_em.htm**.
- CDC patient information—**www.cdc.gov/std/Chlamydia/STDFact-Chlamydia.htm**.

PROVIDER RESOURCES

- CDC. *Sexually Transmitted Diseases (STDs) 2010: Diseases Characterized by Urethritis and Cervicitis*—**www.cdc.gov/std/treatment/2010/urethritis-and-cervicitis.htm**.
- *Cervicitis*—**www.emedicine.medscape.com/article/253402**.

REFERENCES

1. Centers for Disease Control and Prevention. *Sexually Transmitted Diseases (STDs) 2010: Diseases Characterized by Urethritis and Cervicitis*. http://www.cdc.gov/std/treatment/2010/urethritis-and-cervicitis.htm, accessed December 23, 2012.
2. Centers for Disease Control and Prevention. *Sexually Transmitted Disease Surveillance, 2009—Chlamydia*. http://www.cdc.gov/std/stats09/default.htm, accessed December 25, 2011.
3. World Health Organization. *Chlamydia Trachomatis. Initiative for Vaccine Research*. http://www.who.int/vaccine_research/diseases/soa_std/en/index.html, accessed December 2, 2011.
4. Centers for Disease Control and Prevention. http://www.cdc.gov/std/Chlamydia/STDFact-Chlamydia.htm, accessed December 23, 2012.
5. Skolnik NS. Screening for *Chlamydia trachomatis* infection. *Am Fam Physician*. 1995;51:821-826.
6. Forhan SE, Gottlieb SL, Sternberg MR, et al. Prevalence of sexually transmitted infections among female adolescents aged 14 to 19 in the United States. *Pediatrics*. 2009;124:1505.
7. Schillinger JA, Dunne EF, Chapin JB, et al. Prevalence of Chlamydia trachomatis infection among men screened in 4 U.S. cities. *Sex Transm Dis*. 2005;32(2):74-77.
8. Mishori R, McClaskey EL, Winkleprins VJ. Chlamydia Trachomatis Infections: Screening, Diagnosis, and Management. *Am Fam Physician*. 2012;86(12):1127-1132.
9. Hu VH, Harding-Esch EM, Burton MJ, Bailey RL, Kadimpeul J, Mabey DC. Epidemiology and control of trachoma: Systematic review. *Trop Med Int Health*. 2010;15(6):673-691.
10. Martius J, Krohn MA, Hillier SL, et al. Relationships of vaginal lactobacillus species, cervical *Chlamydia trachomatis*, and bacterial vaginosis to preterm birth. *Obstet Gynecol*. 1988;71:89-95.
11. Ness RB, Goodman MT, Shen C, Brunham RC. Serologic evidence of past infection with *Chlamydia trachomatis*, in relation to ovarian cancer. *J Infect Dis*. 2003;187:1147-1152.
12. Datta SD, Sternberg M, Johnson RE, et al. Gonorrhea and *Chlamydia* in the United States among persons 14 to 39 years of age, 1999 to 2002. *Ann Intern Med*. 2007;147:89.

13. Monroe KW, Weiss HL, Jones M, Hook EW 3rd: Acceptability of urine screening for *Neisseria gonorrheae* and *Chlamydia trachomatis* in adolescents at an urban emergency department. *Sex Transm Dis.* 2003;30:850.

14. Rietmeijer CA, Bull SS, Ortiz CG, et al. Patterns of general health care and STD services use among high-risk youth in Denver participating in community-based urine *Chlamydia* screening. *Sex Transm Dis.* 1998;25:457.

15. Doshi JS, Power J, Allen E. Acceptability of chlamydia screening using self-taken vaginal swabs. *Int J STD AIDS*. 2008;19:507-509.

16. Cook RL, Hutchison SL, Østergaard L, Braithwaite RS, Ness RB. Systematic review: noninvasive testing for *Chlamydia trachomatis* and *Neisseria gonorrhoeae*. *Ann Intern Med*. 2005; 142(11):914-925.

17. Bachmann LH, Johnson RE, Cheng H, et al. Nucleic acid amplification tests for diagnosis of *Neisseria gonorrhoeae* and *Chlamydia trachomatis* rectal infections. *J Clin Microbiol*. 2010;48:1827-1832.

18. Bachmann LH, Johnson RE, Cheng H, et al. Nucleic acid amplification tests for diagnosis of *Neisseria gonorrhoeae* oropharyngeal infections. *J Clin Microbiol*. 2009;47:902-907.

19. Chernesky M, Freund GG, Hook E, III, et al. Detection of *Chlamydia trachomatis* and *Neisseria gonorrhoeae* infections in North American women by testing SurePath liquid-based Pap specimens in APTIMA assays. *J Clin Microbiol*. 2007;45:2434-2438.

20. Lau C-Y, Qureshi AK. Azithromycin versus doxycycline for genital chlamydial infections: A meta-analysis of randomized clinical trials. *Sex Transm Dis*. 2002;29:497-502.

80 BREAST MASSES IN ADOLESCENTS

Katherine B. Lee, MD

PATIENT STORY

A 13-year-old girl is brought to her pediatrician by her mother because of a left breast mass, which she has noted for the past month. The lump has been very painful and "changed" in color (**Figure 80-1**). Her mother is concerned about the size of the lump, having seen it only three days prior to her visit. The patient reached menarche at age 12 years and is not taking any medications. She has never been pregnant. The diagnosis of giant fibroadenoma was suspected and the girl is referred to a breast surgeon. Given the size of the lesion, and severe asymmetry, it was advised that she have an excision of this mass with reconstruction to achieve a better cosmetic result. She underwent surgical excision of the mass, which confirmed a giant fibroadenoma. After the procedure, her breasts appeared symmetrical and she healed very well. There is concern that her left reconstruction may need to be revised in the future as her other breast will mature appropriately for her age. This will need to be followed into adulthood.

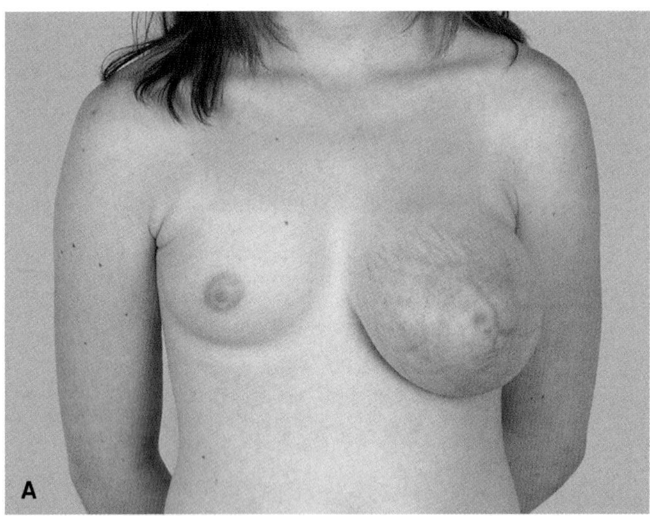

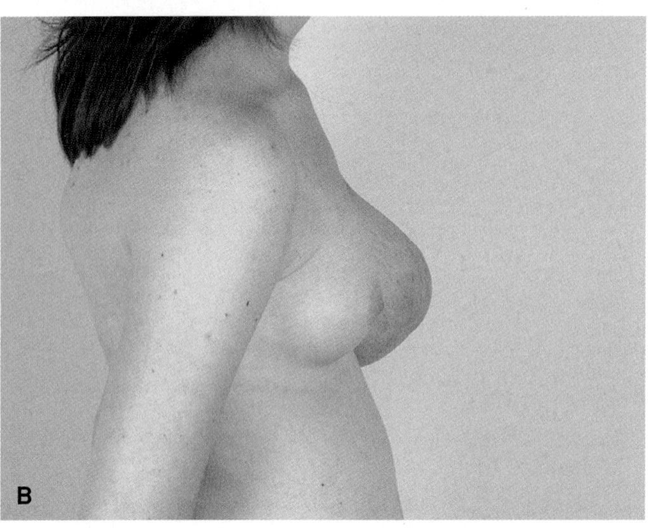

FIGURE 80-1 Giant fibroadenoma in a 13-year-old girl on frontal (**A**) and side view (**B**). (*Used with permission from Katherine B. Lee, MD.*)

INTRODUCTION

Breast masses in female adolescents can range from normal breast tissue to cysts to fibroadenomas to malignancies. The most common cause of breast masses in adolescent girls is a fibroadenoma, which is a benign, well circumscribed lesion composed of abundant stromal and epithelial components. Despite the benign nature of fibroadenomas, accurate diagnosis and management will help alleviate significant fears that are associated with these lesions.

EPIDEMIOLOGY

- Fibroadenomas are the most common breast lesions in adolescent girls.[1,2]
- These occur in about 10 percent of all women, and have a peak incidence in the second and third decades of life.
- Fibrocystic changes of the breast are common in adolescents, although the exact prevalence is not known.[2]

ETIOLOGY AND PATHOPHYSIOLOGY

- Female adolescents usually go through breast development and growth during puberty (**Figure 80-2**). Knowledge of normal development is important in the diagnosis of breast masses in adolescents.
- Pathology of the lesion determines the type of lesion: Cysts are fluid filled masses. Fibroadenomas are fibroepithelial lesions which are filled with numerous cells.
- Fibrocystic changes are thought to result from an imbalance between estrogen and progesterone.
- Women who have fibroadenomas do not appear to have an increased risk of developing breast cancer; however, it is important to note that about 2 percent of carcinomas arise in a fibroadenoma. For this reason, fibroadenomas are usually followed to assure stability over time. Growth beyond 5 cm is consistent with a giant fibroadenoma.
- Fibroadenomas are very responsive to hormonal changes and enlarge during pregnancy or prior to the menses.

RISK FACTORS

- Women in their 20s to 30s are at higher risk, although fibroadenomas are the most common causes of breast lesions in adolescents.
- Hormone exposure such as pregnancy or use of birth control pills.
- Having previous fibroadenomas make women susceptible to having more in the future.
- The role of caffeine as a risk factor for fibroadenomas is not clear.[3–5]

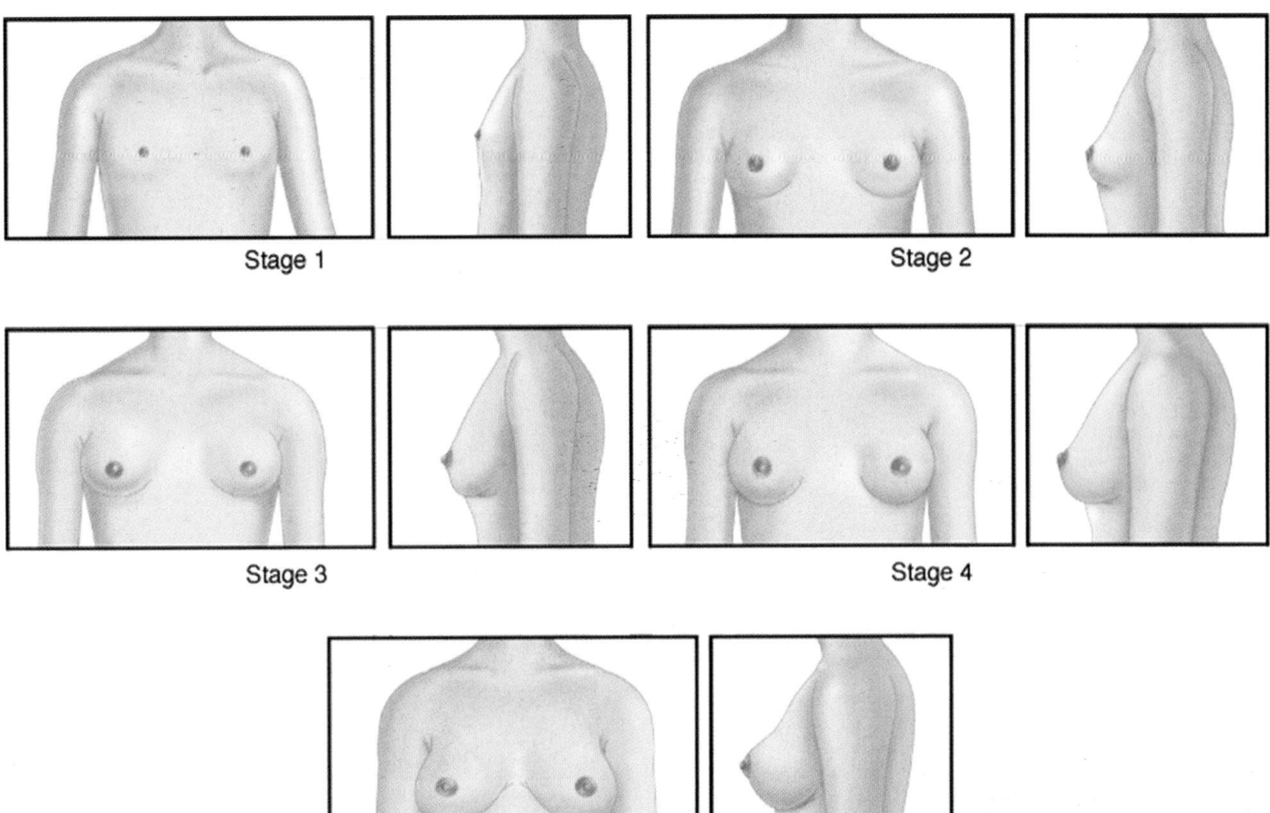

Stage 5

- Stage 1 Preadolescent: juvenile breast with elevated papilla and small flat areola.
- Stage 2 The breast bud forms under the influence of hormonal stimulation. The papilla and areola elevate as a small mound, and the areolar diameter increases.
- Stage 3 Continued enlargement of the breast bud further elevates the papilla. The areola continues to enlarge; no separation of breast contours is noted.
- Stage 4 The areola and papilla separate from the contour of the breast to form a secondary mound.
- Stage 5 Mature: areolar mound recedes into the general contour of the breast; papilla continues to project.

FIGURE 80-2 Tanner staging of breast development. (*Used with permission from Greydanus DE, Pratt HD. Adolescent growth and development, and sport participation. In: Patel DR, Greydanus DE, Baker RJ, eds.* Pediatric Practice: Sports Medicine. *New York, NY: McGraw-Hill; 2009:18. www.accesspediatrics.com*).

DIAGNOSIS

A careful history and physical examination is the first step in the diagnosis of breast lesions in adolescents. Most often, observation of the mass for one to two menstrual cycles will aid in the diagnosis and help rule out more serious causes. In equivocal cases, ultrasonography and/or needle aspiration are helpful.

CLINICAL FEATURES

- Fibroadenomas may be painful but most often are asymptomatic.
- The lesion size can be quite small (1cm) to several centimeters in diameter (as in the patient in the vignette).
- Most fibroadenomas are mobile, have a rubbery consistency, and are well circumscribed.
- Fibroadenomas may affect the contour of the breast (**Figure 80-3**).
- May occur recurrently or found as multiple masses.

DISTRIBUTION

- Can occur in any quadrant, but most frequently found in the upper, outer quadrant of the breast.

LABORATORY TESTING

- If the diagnosis is in question, the most definitive way of making the diagnosis is to sample the lesion via excision or core biopsy.
- Histology reveals proliferating stroma.

IMAGING

- Imaging is usually not necessary, but can help to differentiate cystic from solid masses if the lesion persists for more than two menstrual cycles.
- Ultrasonography of the breast is the modality of choice and will show a well circumscribed hypoechoic mass.[6,7]

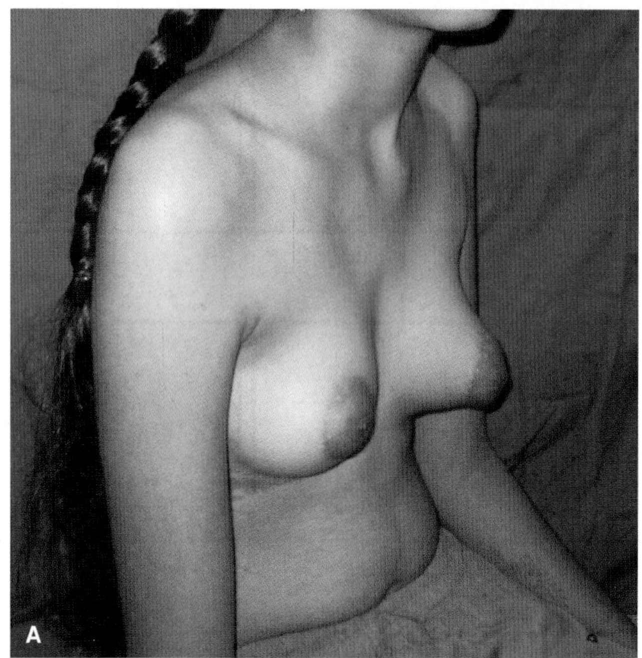

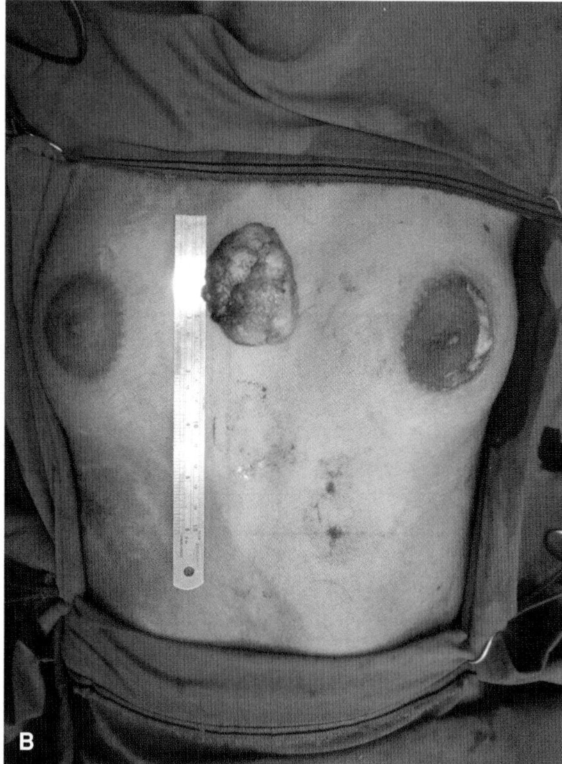

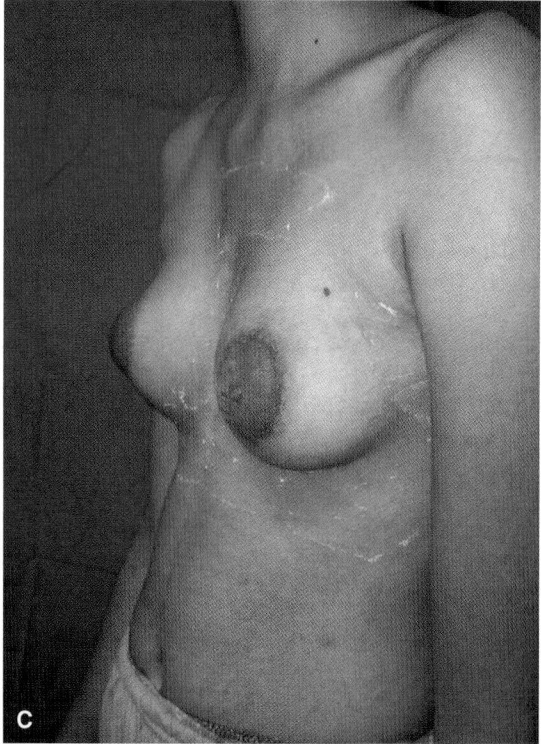

FIGURE 80-3 **A.** Fibroadenoma in a teenage girl presenting with significant change in the left breast contour. **B.** Fibroadenoma removed through a peri-areolar incision. **C.** Healing breast with normal breast contour. (*Used with permission from Dr. N. Jithendran and http://breastsurgeries.blogspot.in/2012/05/fibroadenoma-excision-minimal-scarring.html*)

- Mammography is not helpful in the diagnosis because of the large amount of glandular tissue in adolescents, which makes interpretation of the study difficult.[8]

DIFFERENTIAL DIAGNOSIS

- Breast bud—Breast tissue development can also be confused for an abnormality on examination. It is important to not confuse normal breast bud tissue for an abnormal mass (Figure 80-2).
- Simple cyst—Usually distinguished clinically and disappear over weeks to months.
- Fibroadenoma (Giant)—Greater than 5cm in size and may compress or replace normal breast tissue. Dilated superficial veins often visible (**Figure 80-1**).
- Breast abscess/mastitis—Often associated with overlying mastitis and/or purulent nipple discharge (**Figures 80-4** and **80-5**).
- Phyllodes tumor—A rare primary tumor, which is usually benign, but capable of a wide range of biologic behavior. A biopsy (tissue) is needed to definitely differentiate from fibroadenoma.

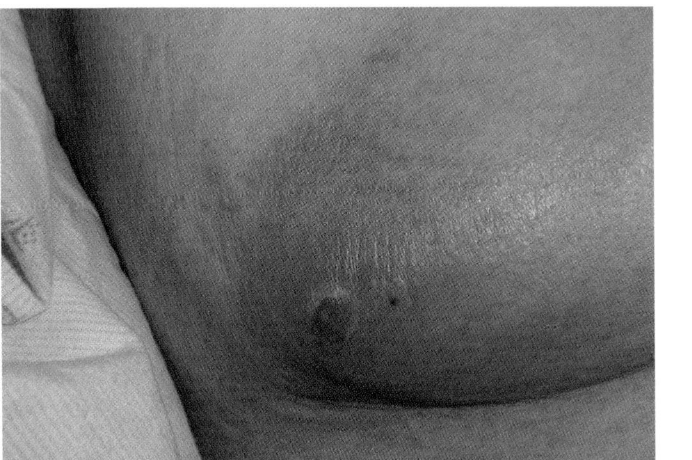

FIGURE 80-4 Breast abscess with surrounding cellulitis. (*Used with permission from Richard P. Usatine, MD.*)

- Breast cancer—Exceedingly rare in the adolescent population. Characterized by a firm, irregular mass.
- Other malignancies such as breast sarcoma—Very rare and characterized by a firm irregular mass that does not change with menstrual cycle.

MANAGEMENT

- The treatment of fibroadenomas in adolescent patients is generally conservative, observing and watching diligently as opposed to surgical excision.[8]
- Observation of the mass for one or two menstrual cycles is the most common approach if the history is typical for fibrocystic changes or a fibroadenoma.
- Asymptomatic solid masses measuring less than 5 cm and consistent with fibroadenomas can be observed.

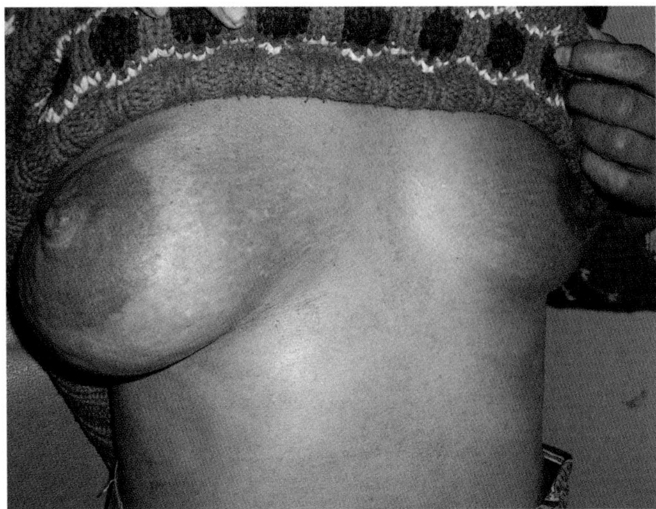

FIGURE 80-5 Postpartum mastitis with massive swelling of the involved breast. (*Used with permission from Richard P. Usatine, MD.*)

- When the mass regresses, observation at 3 to 4 months intervals is appropriate. If the lesion persists over this time period, an ultrasound can be obtained, and if completely consistent with fibroadenoma, can be observed without biopsy unless there are extenuating concerns.[9,10]

SURGERY

- Persistent cystic lesions can be evaluated by needle aspiration, although this is rarely required in adolescents.
- Surgical resection of solid masses may be warranted for nonmobile, hard, enlarging, associated with skin changes, or those associated with significant anxiety for the patients and their parents. SOR Ⓒ
- Giant fibroadenomas should be excised given their large size, severe asymmetry, compression of normal breast tissue and to rule out l tumors.[1,8,11] SOR Ⓒ

REFERRAL

- Removal of the lesion by a breast surgeon along with reconstruction with plastic surgery (**Figure 80-3**).

PREVENTION AND SCREENING

- No known interventions can prevent the development of a fibroadenoma, but a core biopsy is advised if there is question as to the diagnosis or if there is a concern for a phyllodes tumor.
- An ultrasound of the lesion should be performed to aid in the diagnosis.

PROGNOSIS

- Most fibroadenomas in adolescents decrease in size and eventually resolve completely.[12]
- For giant fibroadenomas, the prognosis is good as long as complete excision is achieved.

FOLLOW-UP

- Follow-up and reassurance are paramount in the management of fibroadenomas in adolescents.

PATIENT EDUCATION

- Reassurance as to benign nature of fibroadenomas is very important.
- Reassurance as to the rarity of breast cancer in adolescents is also important.

PATIENT RESOURCES

- **http://www.cancer.org/healthy/findcancerearly/womenshealth/non-cancerousbreastconditions/non-cancerous-breast-conditions-fibroadenomas**.
- **http://emedicine.medscape.com/article/345779-overview**.

REFERENCES

1. Greydanus DE, Matytsina L, Gains M. Breast disorders in children and adolescents. *Prim Care.* 2006;33:455.
2. Templeman C, Hertweck SP. Breast disorders in the pediatric and adolescent patient. *Obstet Gynecol Clin North Am.* 2000;27:19.
3. Schairer C, Brinton LA, Hoover RN. Methylxanthines and benign breast disease. *Am J Epidemiol.* 1986;124:603.
4. Levinson W, Dunn PM. Nonassociation of caffeine and fibrocystic breast disease. *Arch Intern Med.* 1986;146:1773.
5. Jacobson MF, Liebman BF. Caffeine and benign breast disease. *JAMA.* 1986;255:1438.
6. Fornage BD, Lorigan JG, Andry E. Fibroadenoma of the breast: sonographic appearance. *Radiology.* 1989;172:671.
7. Sickles EA, Filly RA, Callen PW. Benign breast lesions: ultrasound detection and diagnosis. *Radiology.* 1984;151:467.
8. De Silva NK, Brandt ML. Disorders of the breast in children and adolescents, Part 2: breast masses. *J Pediatr Adolesc Gynecol.* 2006;19:415.
9. Smith GE, Burrows P. Ultrasound diagnosis of fibroadenoma—is biopsy always necessary? *Clin Radiol.* 2008;63:511.
10. Jayasinghe Y, Simmons PS. Fibroadenomas in adolescence. *Curr Opin Obstet Gynecol.* 2009;21:402.
11. Chao TC, Lo YF, Chen SC, Chen MF. Sonographic features of phyllodes tumors of the breast. *Ultrasound Obstet Gynecol.* 2002;20:64.
12. ACOG Committee on Adolescent Health Care. ACOG Committee Opinion No. 350, November 2006: Breast concerns in the adolescent. *Obstet Gynecol.* 2006;108:1329.

81 COMPLICATIONS OF TATTOOS AND PIERCINGS

Edward A. Jackson, MD
Richard P. Usatine, MD

PATIENT STORY

A teenager presents with itching and swelling along the area of a recent tattoo on the lower leg. She notes that the area has become swollen and is itching and draining (**Figure 81-1**). On examination there is swelling over the areas of red dye usage. The pediatrician recognized this as an allergy to the red dye and noted that there were signs of excoriations and some crusting. This was secondary to the scratching that broke the skin and allowed for a secondary infection to begin. The physician treated the secondary infection with oral cephalexin and referred the patient to dermatology for consideration of intralesional steroid treatment of the red dye allergy.

A teenager presents with a tender red lump around an embedded neck piercing (**Figure 81-2A**). The physician notes that there is a granuloma around the piercing site on the left. The patient requests removal of this piercing which is performed in the office. Four months later a new granuloma forms around the piercing on the right neck (**Figure 81-2B**). The patient requests removal of the second piercing and acknowledges that it is not a good idea for her to get any additional piercings.

INTRODUCTION

Tattoos and piercings in both the adult and adolescent populations have become more commonplace. The complications of both have increased as the popularity of body art grows.

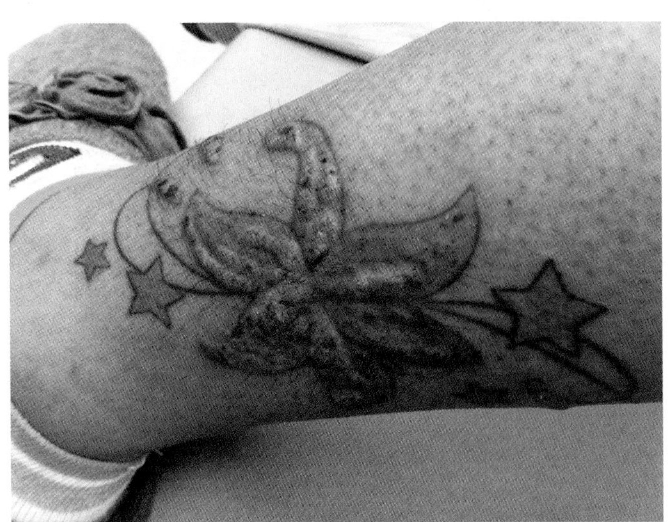

FIGURE 81-1 Allergic reaction to the red pigment in a tattoo on the lower leg of a teenage girl. (*Used with permission from Jonathan Karnes, MD.*)

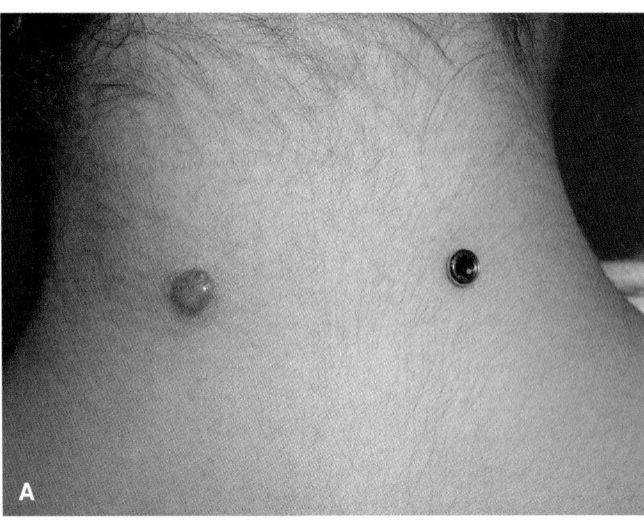

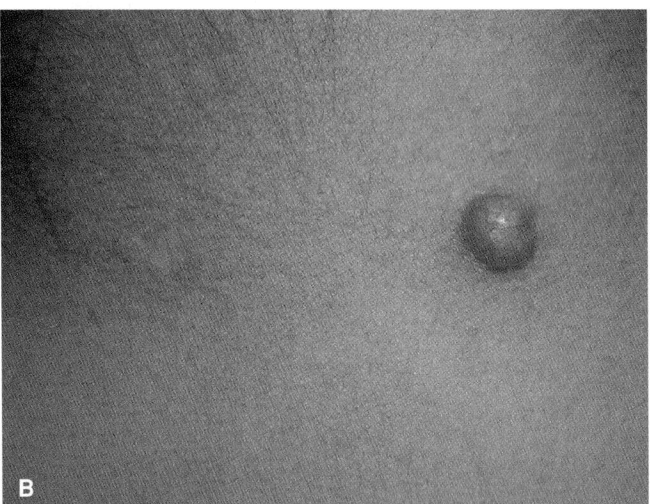

FIGURE 81-2 **A.** Granuloma around the neck piercing on the left. **B.** Five months later a new granuloma has formed around the second neck piercing and the scar from the removal of the first piercing is visible. (*Used with permission from Richard P. Usatine MD.*)

SYNONYMS

Tattoos and piercings are also called body art.

Dye, pigment, and ink are all interchangeable when referring to the color used in tattoos.

EPIDEMIOLOGY

- Body art including tattooing, piercings and scarification have been practiced worldwide since the beginning of history.
- Tattoos are increasingly popular in the US with an estimated percentage of adults with one or more tattoos at about 21 to 25 percent in 2012.[1]
- More adolescent and adults are choosing both tattoos and piercings as an expression of uniqueness.[2]

TABLE 81-1 Common Healing Times for Piercings

Location	Time to Heal
Ear Lobe	6–8 weeks
Ear Cartilage	4 months–1 year
Eyebrow	6–8 weeks
Nostril	2–4 months
Nasal septum	6–8 months
Nasal bridge	8–10 weeks
Tongue	4 weeks
Lip	2–3 months
Nipple	3–6 months
Navel	4 months–1 year
Female genitalia	4–10 weeks
Male genitalia	4 weeks–6 months

ETIOLOGY AND PATHOPHYSIOLOGY

Complications result from permanent tattooing or piercing dependent on the location of the body, the healing time and the type of body art chosen. Because both tattoos and piercings break the protective skin barrier, there are increased risks for infections and bleeding. Further complications for piercings include an increased risk for local trauma, tearing of the skin and mucous membranes, keloid formation, and site-specific piercing complications. Delayed wound healing is also a problem with piercings and may complicate the body art.[4] Healing times for piercings vary by body location and are shown in **Table 81-1**.

RISK FACTORS

- Risk of complications is more common with piercings than with tattoos and reportedly range from 17 to 69 percent.[5] Genital piercings are especially prone to infections (**Figures 81-3** and **81-4**).[7]
- Risks for infection from tattoos is related to contaminated dyes (pigments) and may include bacterial infections such as staph species, mycobacterial,[6–8] viral such as hepatitis B or C, and fungal.[4]
- The most common reported tattoo skin reaction is a hypersensitivity reaction to the pigment. The red pigment is most likely to provoke an allergic reaction (**Figures 81-1** and **81-5**).
- Risks for piercings can be site specific and among these may be delayed healing, allergic reactions to metal of the piercing, (usually to the nickel component in the jewelry), and keloid formation at the piercing site (common in ears) (**Figure 81-6**).

DIAGNOSIS

The following complications are described and illustrated with photographs to help improve early diagnosis and treatment:

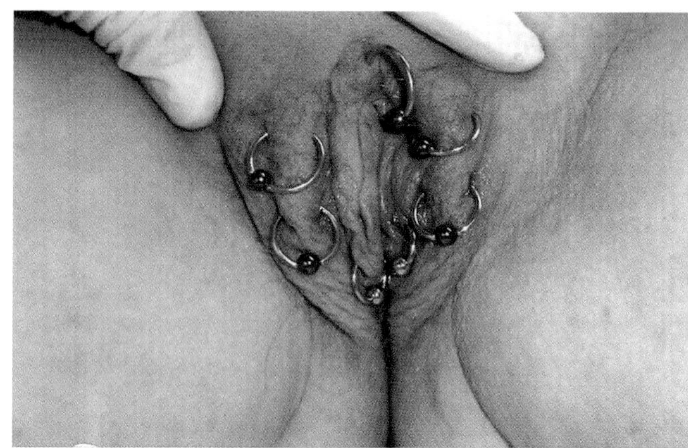

FIGURE 81-3 Clitoral and labial piercing. Piercings in the genital area are at higher risk of developing infections. *(Used with permission from Edward A. Jackson, MD.)*

- Allergic reaction to dye (pigment)—Presents with skin swelling and pruritus. Reactions to red pigment are most common (**Figures 81-1** and **81-5**), but reactions to other colors do occur.
- Contact allergy on skin surface—nickel- or dye- related—presents with erythema, scaling and pruritus (**Figure 81-7**; see Chapter 131, Contact Dermatitis).
- Infection—Has the usual cardinal signs of redness, increased pain at the site, possible purulent drainage, and swelling. Most infections

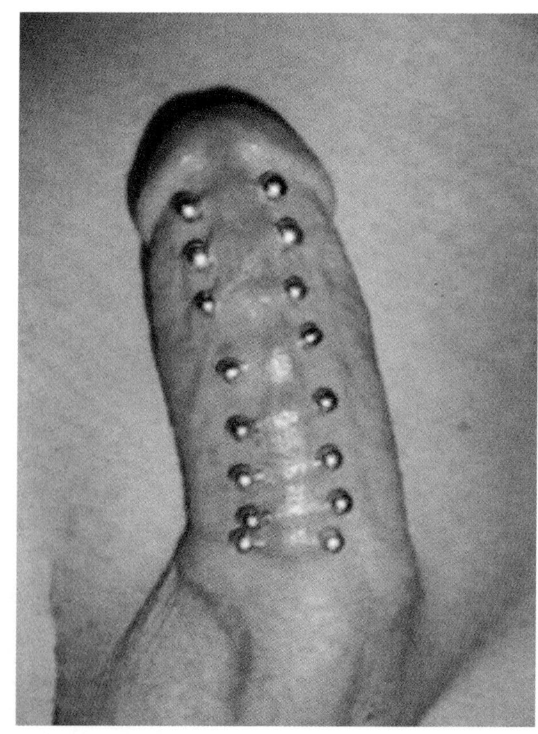

FIGURE 81-4 Penile piercing. While there are no signs of infection there is a higher risk of infections to piercings in the genital region. *(Used with permission from Edward A. Jackson, MD.)*

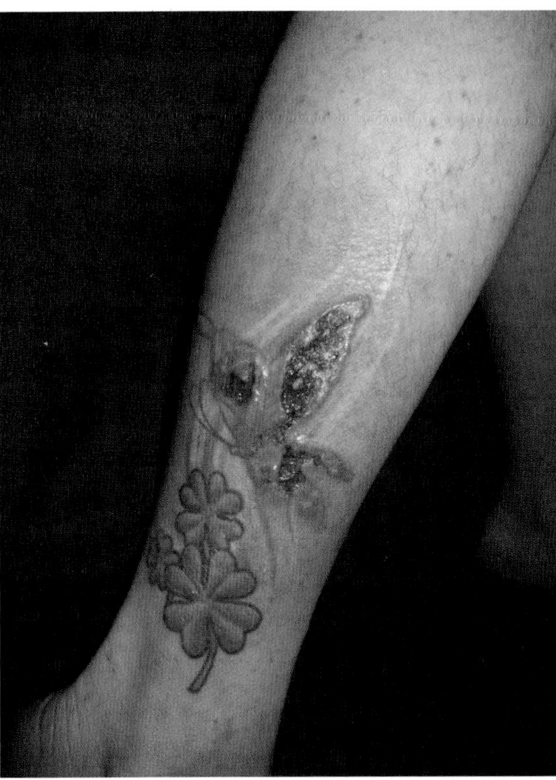

FIGURE 81-5 Allergic reaction to red pigment in a lower leg tattoo. Note that there is granuloma formation as well. (*Used with permission from Jonathan Karnes, MD.*)

around piercings or tattoos are local but systemic symptoms such as fever may occur (**Figure 81-8**).

- Inflammation (granuloma)—Erythema and swelling can occur around piercings and tattoos due to inflammation rather than infection (**Figures 81-2** and **81-5**). Sarcoidosis lesions may develop at sites of tattoos (**Figure 150-7**).
- Photo-aggravated reactions can occur when edema and erythema develop after exposure to sunlight. This occurs most commonly to yellow tattoo pigment.
- Keloids—Benign tumors that arise where skin has been traumatized, cut, or pierced. They are usually the color of the surrounding skin but can also be erythematous or hyperpigmented. The ear is very prone to developing keloids including the earlobe and pinna (**Figure 81-6**; see Chapter 141, Keloids).
- Broken and chipped teeth are most likely to occur with tongue piercings and the piercings (**Figures 81-9** and **81-10**).
- Anatomic distortion—Some piercings are meant to stretch the surrounding skin such as the earlobe (**Figure 81-11**). If the adolescent grows tired of such body art, they are left with anatomic distortions that can only be repaired with plastic surgery.
- Anatomic disruption.
    - Nipple piercings can result in disrupted milk ducts (**Figure 81-12**). While milk production is not a concern of adolescent males, and nipple piercing can be torn from the site resulting in pain and anatomic distortion (**Figure 81-13**).

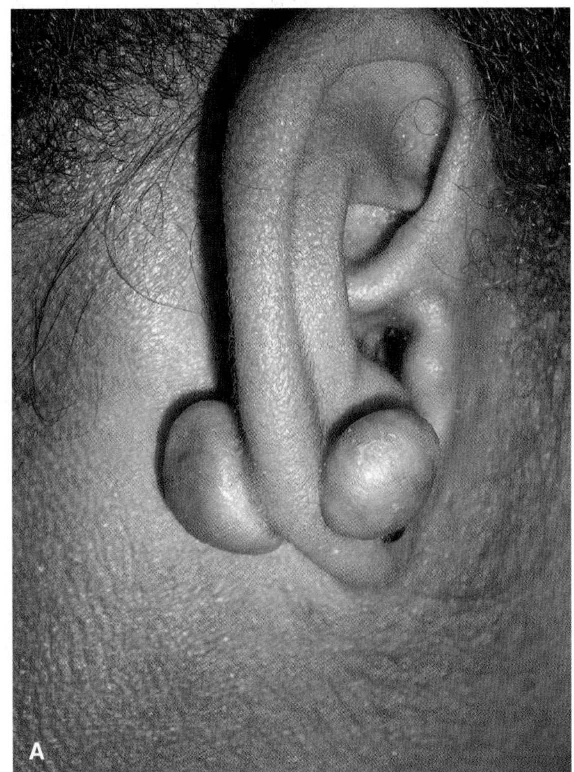

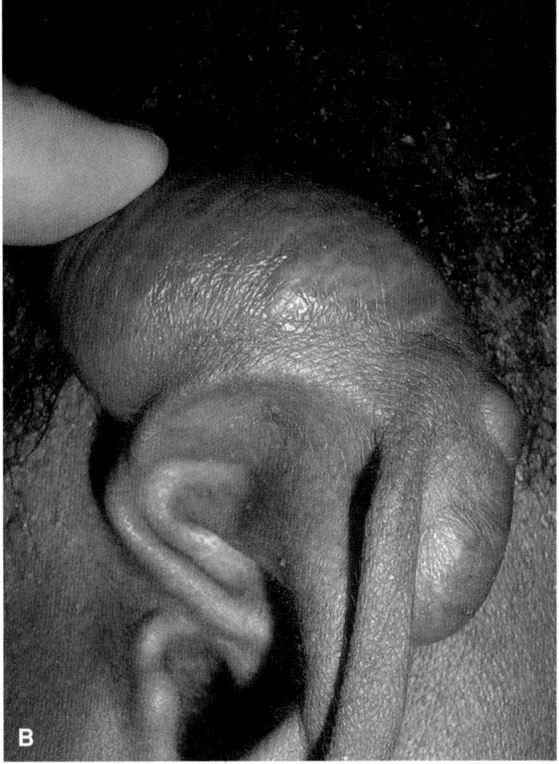

FIGURE 81-6 **A.** Keloids on both sides of the earlobe of this African American teenage female that developed after the piercing of her ears. **B.** Large keloid on the pinna of a young African American female after piercing of the ear cartilage. (*continued*)

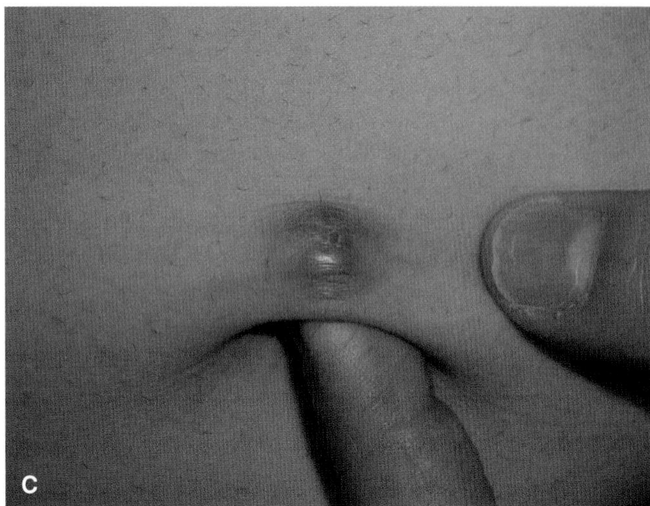

FIGURE 81-6 (*Continued*) **C.** Keloid from a belly-button piercing. (*Used with permission from Richard P. Usatine, MD.*)

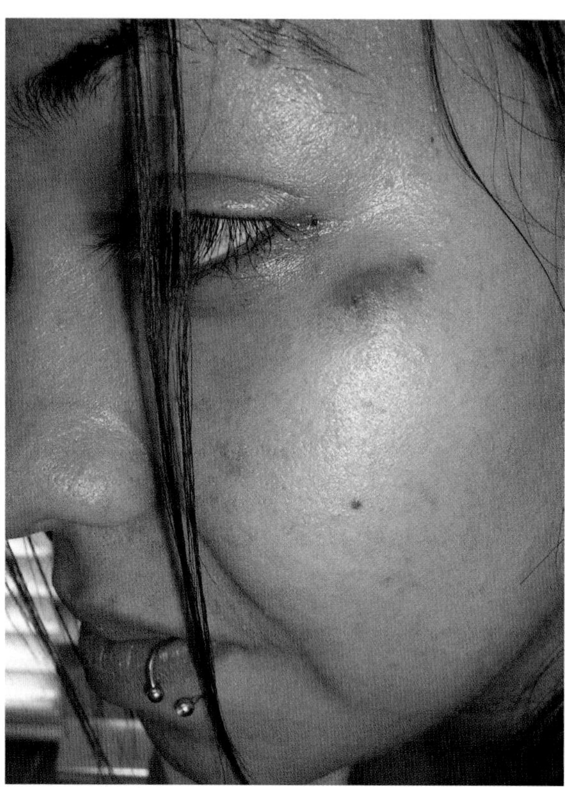

FIGURE 81-8 Infected piercing on the upper cheek of a teenage female secondary to a piercing. Note that her lip has also been pierced. (*Used with permission from Richard P. Usatine, MD.*)

- ◦ Prince Albert piercings go through the urethra of the penis and can lead to a urethral rupture (**Figure 81-14**).
- Piercings can become stuck in the skin so that surgery is needed to remove the piercing (**Figure 81-15**).

LABORATORY TESTING

- Consider bacterial culture of an infected piercing or tattoo if methicillin resistant staphylococcal aureus (MRSA) is suspected.

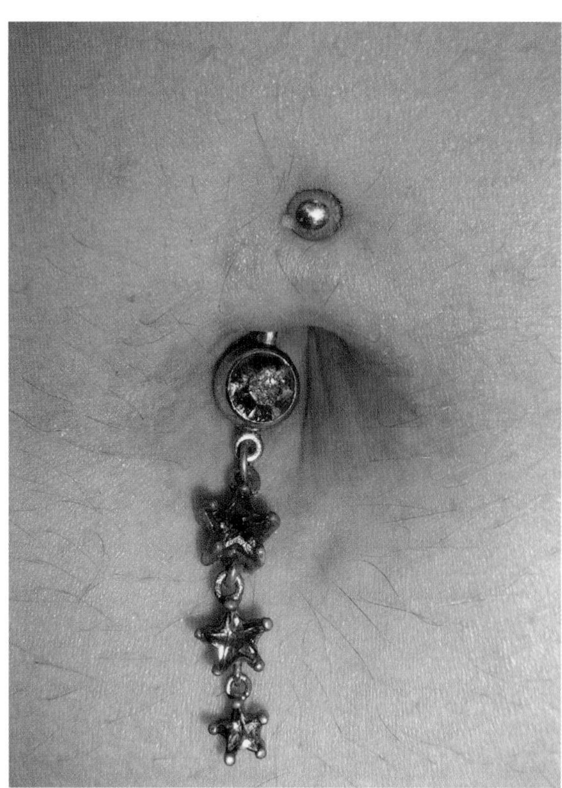

FIGURE 81-7 Nickel contact dermatitis surrounding the jewelry used in a belly button piercing. (*Used with permission from Richard P. Usatine, MD.*)

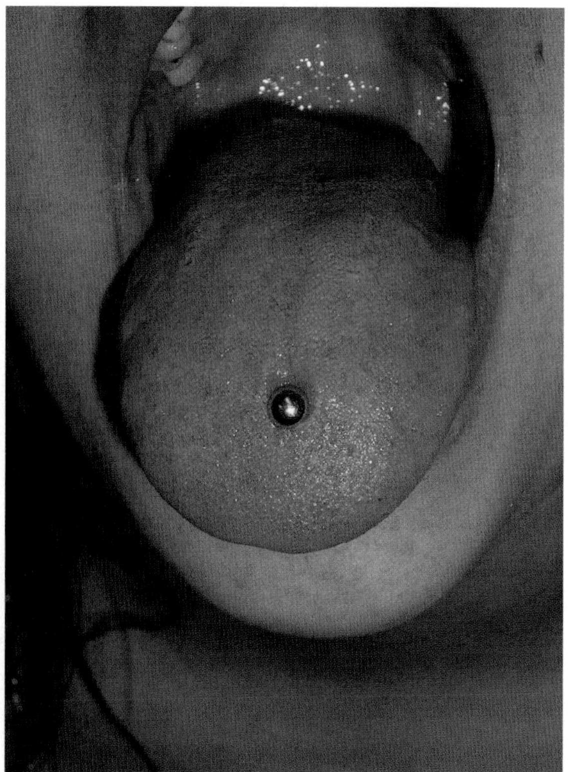

FIGURE 81-9 Tongue piercing putting this patient at risk for cracks and chips to her teeth. (*Used with permission from Richard P. Usatine, MD.*)

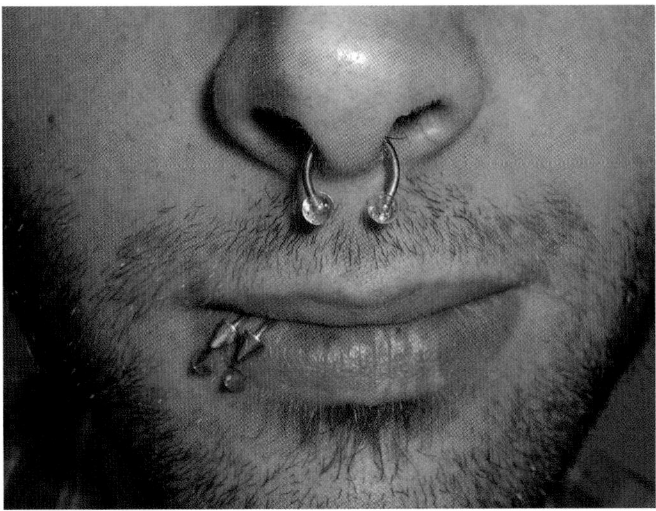

FIGURE 81-10 Facial piercings including a double lip piercing which could result in dental damage. (*Used with permission from Richard P. Usatine, MD.*)

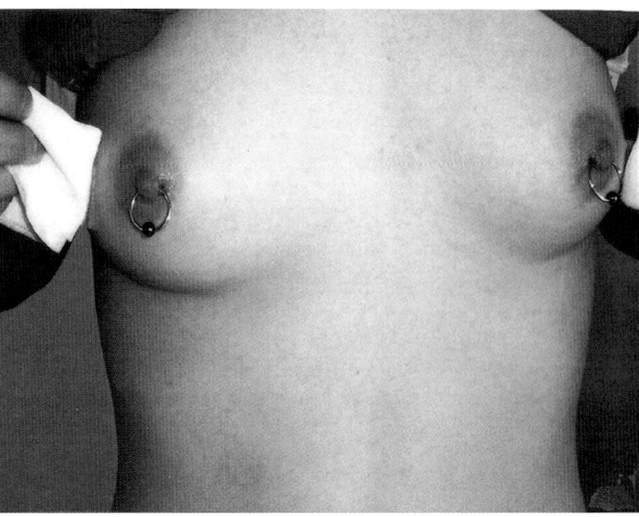

FIGURE 81-12 Bilateral nipple piercings in this teenage female. This type of piercing can result in disruption of the milk ducts that could affect breast-feeding in the future. (*Used with permission from Edward A. Jackson, MD.*)

- Fungal and mycobacterium species have been noted in recent reports to the CDC involving contaminated tattoo inks.[6] Testing for fungus can be performed with a KOH preparation if the suspected fungus is superficial or a punch biopsy sent to the pathologist for a periodic acid Schiff (PAS) stain looking for fungal elements. Mycobacterium species can be detected with an AFB stain from a biopsy of the infected tissue.

DIFFERENTIAL DIAGNOSIS

- Some piercings will continue to ooze fluid after the piercing which may be confused with an infection.[7] A culture may help to differentiate between these two entities.
- Keloid formation may be confused with a hypertrophic scar. A hypertrophic scar will not extend beyond the area of the piercing

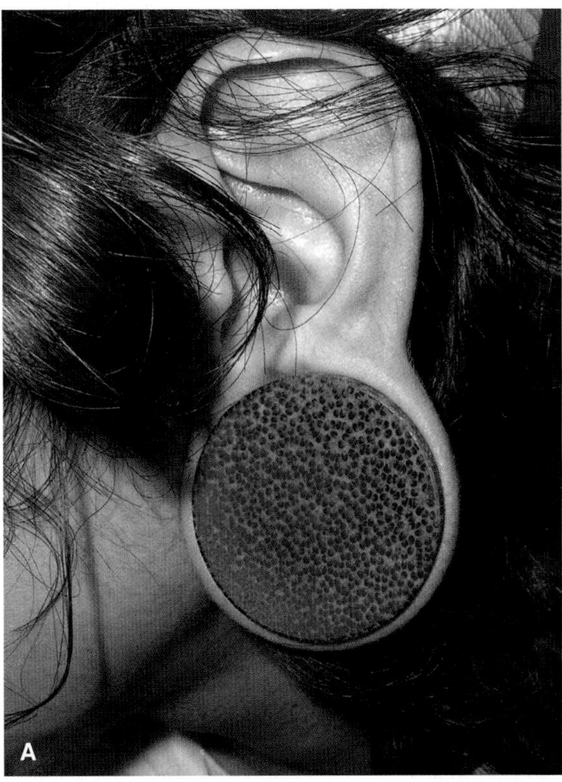

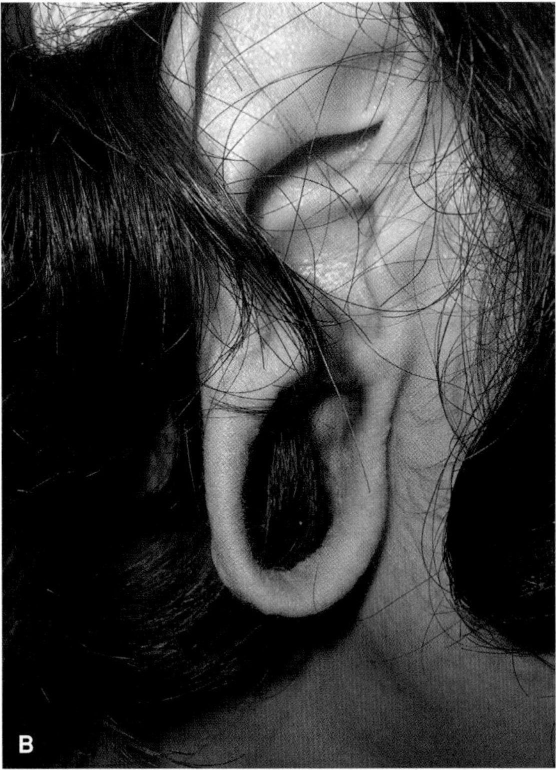

FIGURE 81-11 **A.** Large ear lobe insert used as body art. **B.** Note the anatomic distortion that has occurred to his earlobe when the insert has been removed. If this teenage male decides he no longer wants this body art his earlobe can only be repaired with plastic surgery. (*Used with permission from Richard P. Usatine, MD.*)

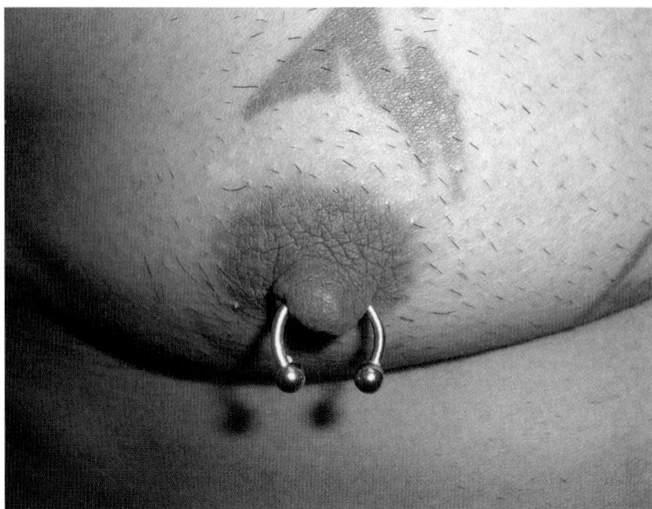

FIGURE 81-13 Nipple piercing in a young man. While breast-feeding is not an issue trauma to this area could pull the ring out and damage the nipple. (*Used with permission from Richard P. Usatine, MD.*)

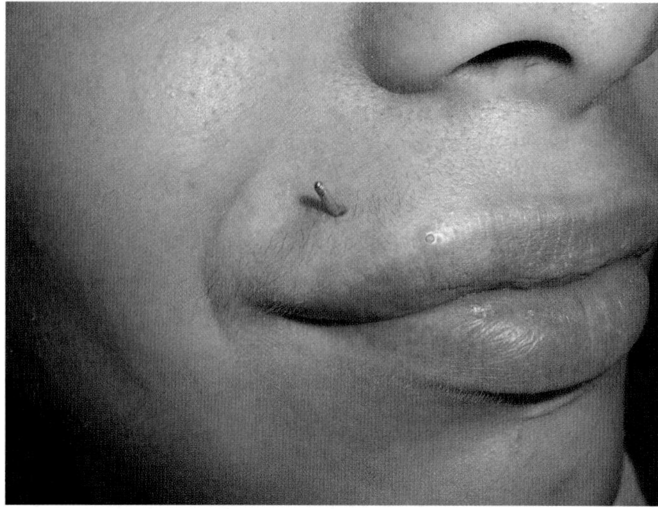

FIGURE 81-15 Lip piercing embedded and stuck in this teenage girl. The lip is somewhat swollen as the area has been anesthetized prior to surgical removal. (*Used with permission from Richard P. Usatine, MD.*)

or trauma.[7] However, hypertrophic scars can be treated the same way that keloids are managed.

MANAGEMENT

- Hypersensitivity reactions to tattoo dyes may be managed with a topical steroid or intralesional injections of 5 mg/mL of triamcinolone. Intralesional injections are more potent and may need to be repeated for adequate results.
- Topical steroids may be used to treat contact dermatitis secondary to nickel or other contact allergens related to piercings or tattoos. Usually a mid-potency topical steroid will be needed for treatment success.
- Hypertrophic scaring and keloids may also be treated with intradermal steroid injections using 10 to 40 mg/mL of triamcinolone.

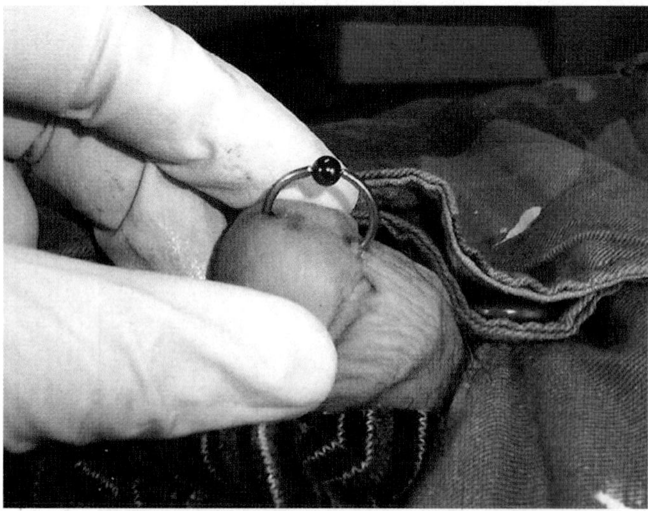

FIGURE 81-14 Prince Albert piercing of the penis, which goes through the urethra and the body of the penis. This can result in damage to the urethra including urethral disruption. (*Used with permission from Edward A. Jackson, MD.*)

- Incision and drainage should be performed to treat an abscess secondary to the piercing (**Figure 81-8**).
- In sites of cellulitis or secondary impetiginization, appropriate selection of antibiotics should cover *Staphylococcus aureus* and *Streptococcus pyogenes*. Consideration for coverage of potential MRSA should be done in those areas that demonstrate high rates of resistance or when the infection is more of an abscess with surrounding cellulitis rather than a superficial impetiginization.
- In the cases with infections that involve piercings, it is recommended to leave the piercing in place during the treatment in order to prevent closure of the site. This may also help in drainage and stop an abscess from forming.[7] A local infection may be managed with good skin cleansers or a topical antibiotic such as mupirocin cream. Avoid ointments as that may delay healing due to their occlusive nature.[8]
- Viral hepatitis is a known complication if clean needles or open vials of pigment were used for tattoos. A viral hepatitis is suspected standard evaluation including liver function tests and hepatitis serologies should be performed.

SURGERY

- When the piercing is stuck in the skin and the patient wants it removed the area may be anesthetized and the piercing may be surgically excised (**Figure 81-15**).
- Piercings which have developed granulomas around them may also need to be excised (**Figure 81-2**).
- In patients with keloids, if intralesional steroids are not successful surgery may be considered.
- For patients that have genital piercings, complications such as urethral rupture may require consultation with urology to repair the damage.
- Removal of tattoos may involve the use of lasers to mechanically disrupt the pigment particles and enable the macrophages to remove the smaller particles. However, this is expensive and may not totally remove the pigment or increase the risk of subsequent

scarring. Since 2007, newer inks have been marketed with micro-encapsulated biocompatible pigments which can be absorbed by the body when the capsule is ruptured by laser treatment.

REFERRALS

- Refer to a dermatologist or surgeon for treatment of keloids or other surgical removals.
- Refer to urology for a urethral rupture.
- For patients wanting laser tattoo removal, refer to a cosmetic dermatologist or another physician trained in the use of cosmetic laser tattoo removal.
- Referral to a hepatologist should be made for any patients newly diagnosed with viral hepatitis.

PREVENTION

- The best method to prevent the complications of tattoos and piercings would to consider not having permanent ones placed in the first place. Many have "buyer remorse" and regret getting a tattoo. Alternatives to permanent tattoos include temporary tattoos, "fake" tattoos or Henna tattoos. There are also "fake" body piercings that may be held in place by a magnet to secure the jewelry.
- Consumers should choose their tattoo or piercing artist with care. Guidelines from the Association of Professional Piercers (AAP) suggest that a good studio should have a certification of recognition by the association. This means that the piercer has had a least 1 year experience, documented training in CPR and blood-borne pathogens, and uses an autoclave with spore testing for sterilization.[8]
- Sterile unused needles and new unopened pigments are essential for safe tattoo technique. Equally important to the use of clean needles is the use of new vials of pigment for each client. The use of an opened bottle of pigment can result in spread of hepatitis from one client to another. Clients should insist on seeing brand-new bottles of pigments opened for their tattoos.
- After a tattoo or piercing, good aftercare may help to prevent the complications of infection.

FOLLOW-UP

Aftercare recommendations for tattoos and piercings include:[8]

- Keep area clean—Wash with antibacterial soap at least twice daily.
- Avoid use of rubbing alcohol, Betadine, or peroxide as these may discolor the jewelry inserted and are not better than soap and water.
- Avoid tight clothing to prevent irritation to the site.
- Avoid hot tubs or pools until healing complete.
- In genital piercings—Condoms or dental dams are recommended during sex to protect the healing wound from the secretions of a sexual partner.
- Oral piercings—Rinse 4 to 5 times daily with an antimicrobial alcohol free rinse.

PATIENT RESOURCES

- Website of association of professional piercers—**www.safepiercing.org**.

PROVIDER RESOURCES

- Tattoo reactions—**www.emedicine.medscape.com/article/1124433**.
- Website of association of professional piercers—**www.safepiercing.org**.

REFERENCES

1. Braverman S. One in five US adults now has a tattoo. New York: Harris Interactive; 2012 (http://www.harrisinteractive.com/vault/Harris%20Poll%2022%20-Tattoos_2.23.12.pdf).
2. Tiggemann M, Hopkins L. Tattoos and piercings: body expression of uniqueness. *Body Image*. 2011;8(3):245-250.
3. Wittman-Price RA, Gittings KK, Collins KM. Nurse and body art: what's your perception? *Nursing*. 2012;42(6):62-64.
4. Desai NA, Smith ML. Body art in adolescents: paint, piercings, and perils. *Adolesc Med*. 2011;022:97-118.
5. Mayers LB, Judelson DA, Moriarty BW et al. Prevalence of body art (body piercing and tattooing) in university undergraduates and incidence of medical complications. *Mayo Clin Proc*. 2002;77:29-34.
6. Center For Disease Control and Prevention. *The Hidden Dangers of Getting Inked*. http://blogs.cdc.gov/publichealthmatters/2012/08/ the-hidden-dangers-of-getting-inked/, accessed March 16, 2014.
7. Braverman PK. Body art: piercing, tattooing, and scarification. *Adolesc MedClin*. 2006;17(3):505-519.
8. Website of association of professional piercers. http://www.safepiercing.org.

PART 13

MUSCULOSKELETAL PROBLEMS

Strength of Recommendation (SOR)	Definition
A	Recommendation based on consistent and good-quality patient-oriented evidence.*
B	Recommendation based on inconsistent or limited-quality patient-oriented evidence.*
C	Recommendation based on consensus, usual practice, opinion, disease-oriented evidence, or case series for studies of diagnosis, treatment, prevention, or screening.*

*See Appendix A on pages 1320–1322 for further information.

82 NURSEMAID'S ELBOW

Paula Sabella, MD

PATIENT STORY

A healthy 2-year-old female is brought to the emergency department because she is not using her left arm. The patient was holding her father's hand while walking when she tripped. To prevent her from falling, her father held onto the patient's left hand and pulled her up as she tripped. The patient cried immediately and then she calmed. She did not seem to be in pain, but she would not move or use her left arm. She held her left arm close to her side with her elbow slightly bent and her palm turned toward her body (**Figure 82-1**). Father denies bruising, swelling, fevers, other injury, or recent illnesses. She was diagnosed with nursemaid's elbow, which was successfully reduced in the emergency department and she regained full use of her arm immediately.

INTRODUCTION

Nursemaid's elbow is a very common injury in preschool aged children. It usually results from a pull to the arm or wrist of a child causing displacement of the annular ligament of the elbow and subluxation of the radial head. This results in pain and refusal to use the arm. The child classically holds the affected elbow close to the body and mildly flexed with pronation of the forearm. The diagnosis is made clinically. The radial head subluxation is usually able to be quickly and easily reduced in the office or emergency department.

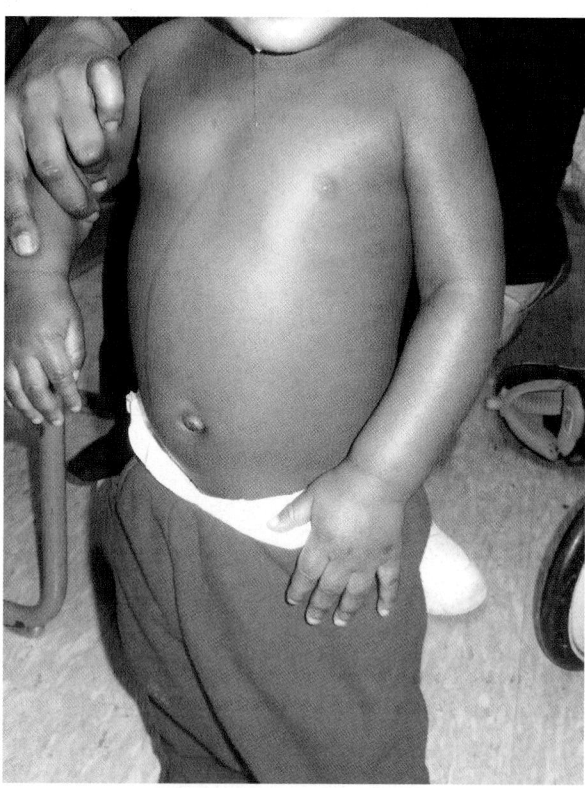

FIGURE 82-1 Typical posture of a child with nursemaid's elbow. Note how the affected left arm is held next to the body with the elbow slightly bent and the forearm pronated. (*Used with permission from Paula Sabella, MD.*)

SYNONYMS

Radial head subluxation; temper tantrum elbow; annular ligament displacement; pulled elbow.

EPIDEMIOLOGY

- Occurs in children aged 6 months to 5 years, with the peak incidence between 2 and 3 years of age.[1-4]
- Left elbow is most commonly affected.[2,4]
- Affects girls more than boys.[1,2,4]

ETIOLOGY AND PATHOPHYSIOLOGY

- The classic mechanism of injury in nursemaid's elbow involves axial traction to a child's pronated forearm or upper extremity.[2] This usually involves a pulling or tugging motion to the upper extremity.
- When the radius is pulled distally, part of the annular ligament shifts proximally over the radial head and becomes caught in the radiohumeral joint (**Figure 82-2**).[2,3] This causes pain and refusal to use the affected arm.
- In many cases of nursemaid's elbow, the typical history of a pulling type of injury is not reported.[5]

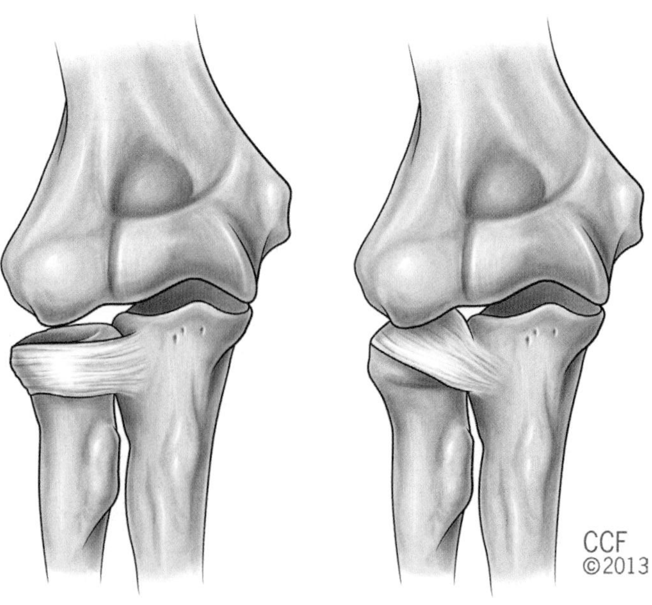

FIGURE 82-2 Drawing of a normal and a displaced annular ligament. Axial traction or tugging to the forearm allows the annular ligament to shift proximally over the radial head and remain caught in the radiohumeral joint. (*Reprinted with permission, Cleveland Clinic Center for Medical Art & Photography © 2013. All Rights Reserved.*)

- Examples of mechanisms reported in patients with nursemaid's elbow include:[1,2,5]
  - Swinging a child while holding the wrists or hands.
  - Lifting a child up by holding the hands or wrists.
  - Catching a child by the hand to prevent a fall.
  - A child holding onto something to prevent a fall.
  - An infant rolling over in bed.
  - Minor trauma to the elbow.

RISK FACTORS

- More common in girls.[1,2,4]
- The left elbow is more commonly affected.[2,4]
- Toddler age group is most affected.[1–4]
- Children with a history of nursemaid's elbow are at an increased risk for recurrence.[2,4]

DIAGNOSIS

- A history of a pull or a traction type of injury to the arm is helpful in making the diagnosis, but is not necessary.[5] A history of brief crying or pain at the time of the injury may also be reported.

CLINICAL FEATURES

- Nursemaid's elbow is a clinical diagnosis, which should be suspected when evaluating a child who refuses to use an upper extremity, and is observed holding the arm in the classic nursemaid's position (**Figure 82-1**).
- The child will typically hold the affected arm next to the body with elbow slightly flexed and the forearm pronated (**Figure 82-1**).
- The child usually does not have severe pain at the time of presentation.[3,5]
- The entire affected upper extremity, including clavicle, should be thoroughly visualized, palpated and evaluated. Children with nursemaid's elbow do not have bruising, swelling, deformity, or other clinical evidence of injury or neurovascular compromise.
- The child may have tenderness with palpation of the radial head.[2,5] There is typically pain with attempts at supination.

DISTRIBUTION

- The elbow is the area involved. Frequently, parents report a concern of wrist or shoulder injury due to the appearance of the child not using the affected arm.

IMAGING

- Radiographs are not indicated to diagnose nursemaid's elbow. Nursemaid's elbow is a clinical diagnosis.[3,6]
- When the history and physical findings are not consistent with nursemaid's elbow, radiographs should be obtained.
- Radiographs are indicated if the child is still not using the arm after failed reduction attempts.[3,6]

DIFFERENTIAL DIAGNOSIS

Fractures (supracondylar, radial, ulnar, clavicular) and dislocations of the arm are usually differentiated from nursemaids elbow by the history of trauma and the presence of pain, distress, point tenderness, swelling, bruising, or deformity on physical examination.

MANAGEMENT

NONPHARMACOLOGIC

- Reduction of the suspected nursemaid's elbow may be carefully attempted when the clinical presentation and physical exam are consistent with nursemaid's elbow.[5] SOR Ⓒ
- The two techniques used for reduction are hyperpronation and supination-flexion.
- Both of the reduction techniques should be performed with the patient seated on the parent's lap facing the examiner. The examiner should be positioned at a similar height to the patient and facing the patient.
- No sedation is required.
- **Reduction Methods**
  - Hyperpronation technique—The examiner holds the affected elbow and applies pressure with a finger over the radial head. The examiner simultaneously holds the patient's distal forearm/wrist with the other hand and hyperpronates the forearm (**Figure 82-3**).[1]
  - Supination/flexion technique—The examiner holds the affected elbow and applies pressure with a finger over the radial head. The examiner simultaneously holds the patient's distal forearm/wrist with the other hand. In one continuous flowing motion, the examiner applies mild traction, full supination of the forearm, and full flexion at the elbow (**Figure 82-4**).[1–3]
- During both methods of reduction, the examiner should feel a click when the annular ligament relocates back into its normal position.[2–4] Most children will cry with the reduction and then calm with family.
- Spontaneous use of the arm usually occurs within 10 to 15 minutes of successful reduction.[1,2,5]
- Toys, books, and family members may be used to entice the child to reach for objects to use the arm (**Figure 82-5**).
- Normal use of the arm after reduction confirms the diagnosis of nursemaid's elbow and of a successful reduction. The patient may immediately resume normal activity.
- If the reduction is unsuccessful, radiographs should be obtained if the child is still not using the arm after several failed reduction attempts.[3,6]
- Reduction may occur spontaneously while waiting for the examiner or en route to the hospital.
- Reduction may also occur after the arm is positioned for radiographs.

REFERRAL

- Referral to an orthopedic specialist is recommended for the child with normal radiographs who is still not using the arm after failed

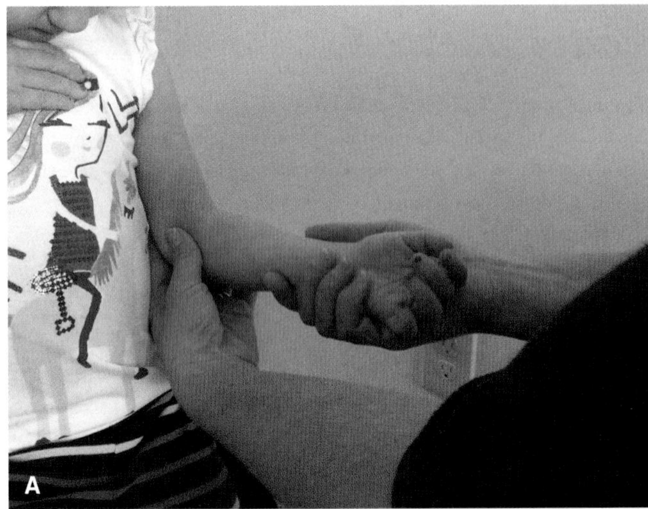

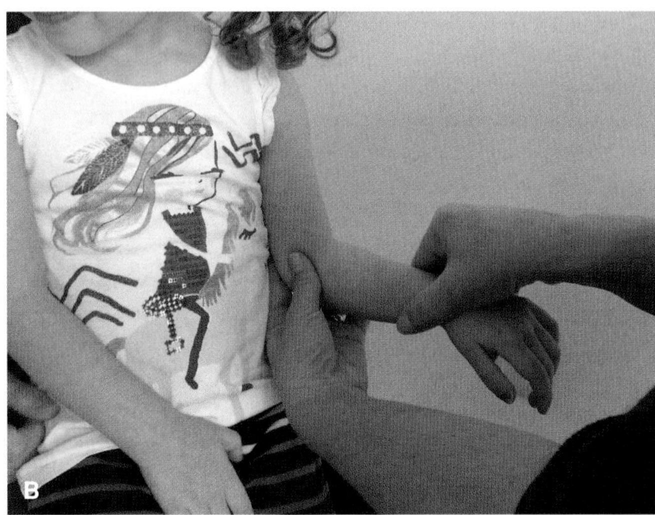

FIGURE 82-3 Hyperpronation Reduction method. (**A**) The examiner firmly holds the affected elbow with one hand and (**B**) hyperpronates the forearm with the other hand. (*Used with permission from Paula Sabella, MD.*)

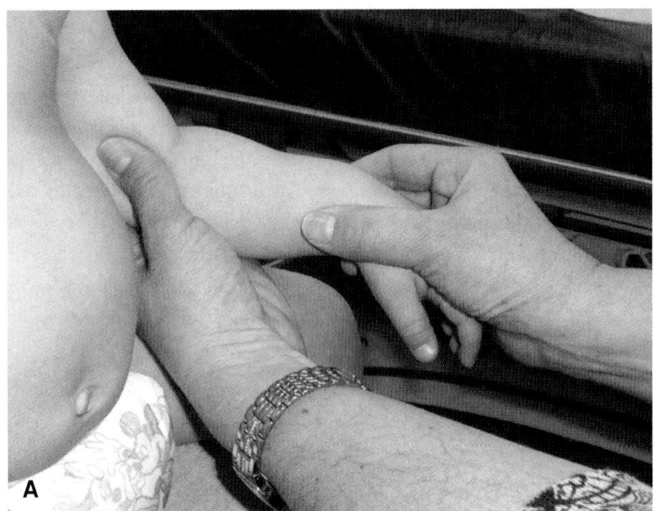

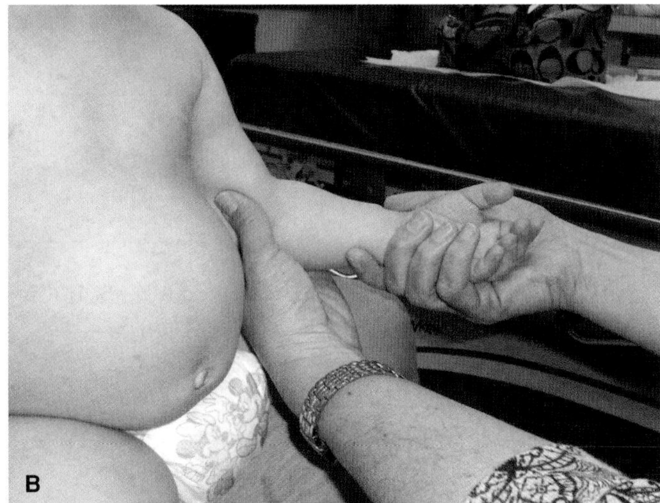

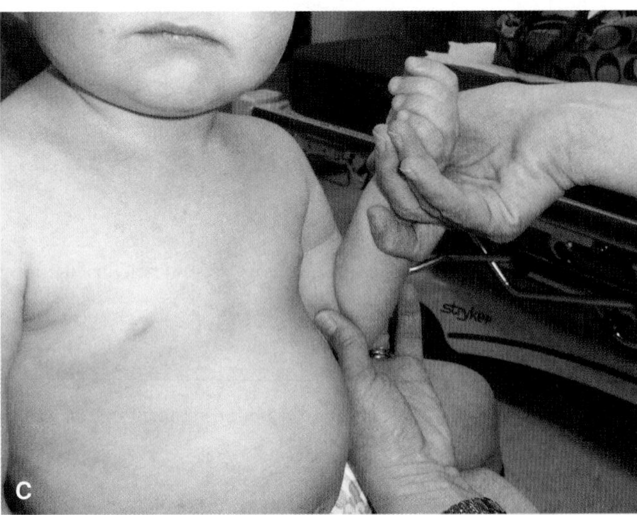

FIGURE 82-4 Supination-Flexion Reduction method. (**A**) The examiner firmly holds the affected elbow with one hand. In one continuous motion, the examiner applies gentle distal traction with the other hand, (**B**) supinates the forearm, and (**C**) then fully flexes the elbow. (*Used with permission from Paula Sabella, MD.*)

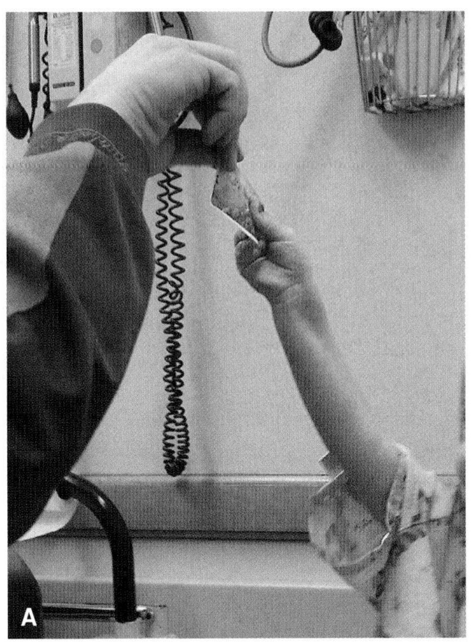
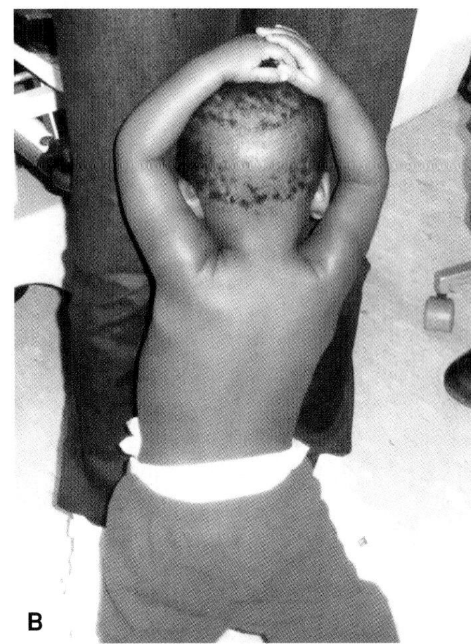

FIGURE 82-5 Successful reduction of nursemaid's elbow results in normal use of the arm (**A**, **B**). *(Used with permission from Paula Sabella, MD.)*

reduction attempts. A sling or splint should be applied to the affected arm.[2,3,6]

PREVENTION AND SCREENING

- Families should be encouraged to lift the child by holding under the axillae.
- Instruct family to avoid tugging, or pulling to the hands, wrists and arms of the child.

PROGNOSIS

- The reduction methods are associated with a very a high rate of success.

FOLLOW-UP

- Follow-up is required for recurrences or if the child is again not using the arm.

PATIENT EDUCATION

- Family should be encouraged to lift the child by holding under the axillae.
- Instruct family to avoid tugging, or pulling to the hands, wrists, and arms of the child.
- Family should be educated regarding the diagnosis and the method of reduction at the time the diagnosis is made.

PATIENT RESOURCES

- **www.nlm.nih.gov/medlineplus/ency/article/000983.htm**.
- **www.healthychildren.org/English/health-issues/conditions/orthopedic/Pages/Nursemaids-Elbow.aspx**.

PROVIDER RESOURCES

- **www.accesspediatrics.com/videoplayer.aspx?aid=8146001**.

REFERENCES

1. Macias CG, Bothner J, Wiebe R. A comparison of supination/flexion to hyperpronation in the reduction of radial head subluxations. *Pediatrics*. 1998;102:e10.
2. Schunk JE. Radial head subluxation: epidemiology and treatment of 87 episodes. *Ann Emerg Med*. 1990;19:1019.
3. Joffe MD, Loiselle JM. *Textbook of Pediatric Emergency Medicine*. Philadelphia: Lippincott Williams.Wilkins; 2006:1695-1696.
4. Quan L, Marcuse EK. The epidemiology and treatment of radial head subluxation. *Am J Dis Child*. 1985;139:1194.
5. Sacchetti A, Ramoska EE, Galcow C. Nonclassic history in children with radial head subluxations. *J Emerg Med*. 1990;8:151.
6. Macias CG, Wiebe R, Bothner J. History and radiographic findings associated with clinically suspected radial head subluxations. *Pediatr Emerg Care*. 2000;16:22.

83 CLAVICULAR FRACTURE

Heidi Chumley, MD
Emily Gale Scott, MD

PATIENT STORY

A 15-year-old girl slipped on the ice and landed directly on her lateral shoulder. She had immediate pain and swelling in the middle of her clavicle. Her parents took her to the emergency room and a radiograph confirmed a displaced mid-clavicular fracture with considerable overlap (**Figure 83-1**). She was placed in a sling and saw her primary care physician the next day. In consultation with a sports medicine expert, she, her family, and her primary care physician decided on conservative treatment. A follow-up radiograph 4 months later demonstrated good healing. The bump on her clavicle is still palpable; but this does not bother her (**Figure 83-2**).

INTRODUCTION

Clavicular fractures are common and are most often caused by accidental trauma. The clavicle most commonly fractures in the midshaft (**Figures 83-3**), but can also fracture distally (**Figure 83-4**). Most fractures can be treated conservatively. Refer patients with significant displacement or distal fractures for surgical evaluation.

EPIDEMIOLOGY

Accounts for 10 to 15 percent of fractures in children; 90 percent are midshaft fractures.[1]

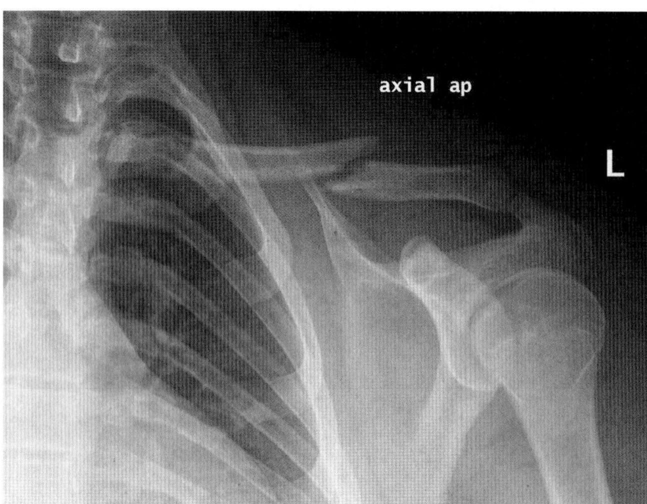

FIGURE 83-1 Midshaft clavicular fracture in a 15-year-old girl who slipped on the ice. (*Used with permission from Emily Scott, MD.*)

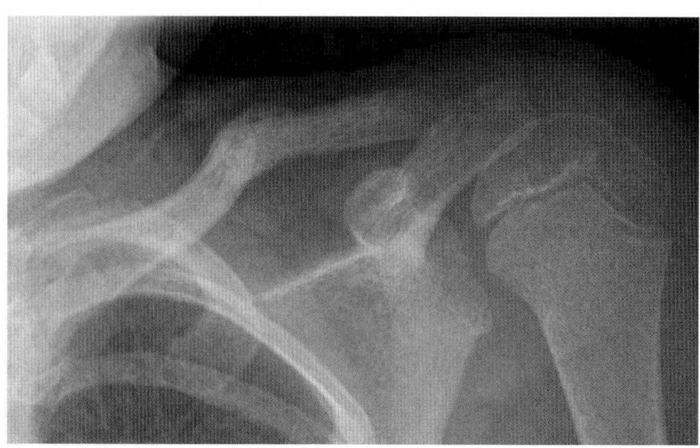

FIGURE 83-2 Healing callous after a midshaft clavicular fracture in the 15-year-old girl in **Figure 83-1**. (*Used with permission from Emily Scott, MD.*)

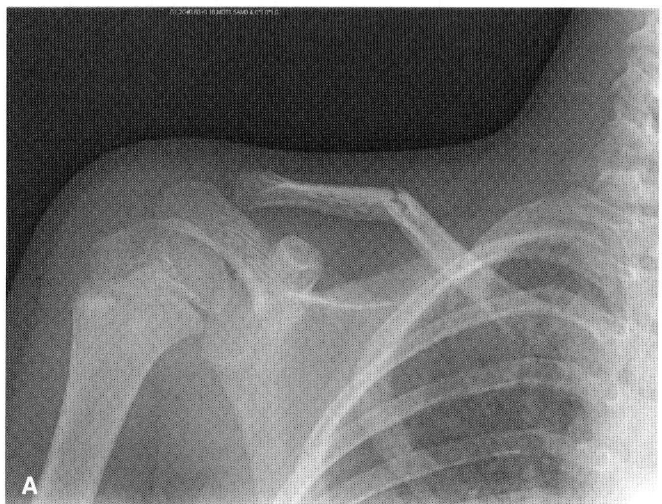

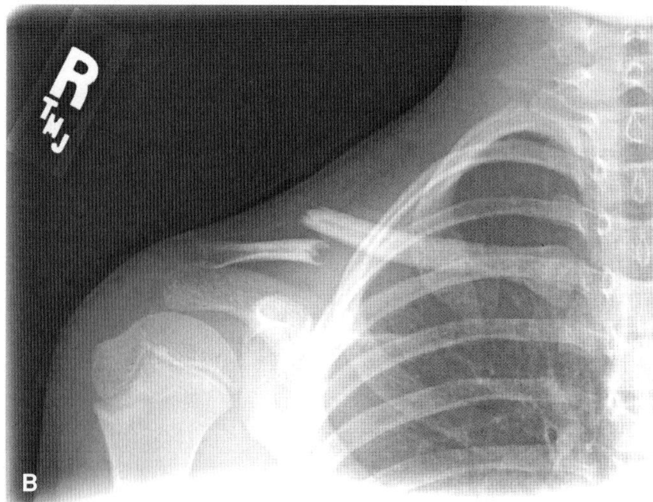

FIGURE 83-3 **A.** Midshaft clavicular fracture with mild angulation but not overriding in 8-year-old child. Midshaft clavicular fracture with overlap in an 11-year-old child. **B.** Usually the proximal fragment is displaced superiorly from the pull of the sternocleidomastoid muscle. (*Used with permission from Emily Scott, MD.*)

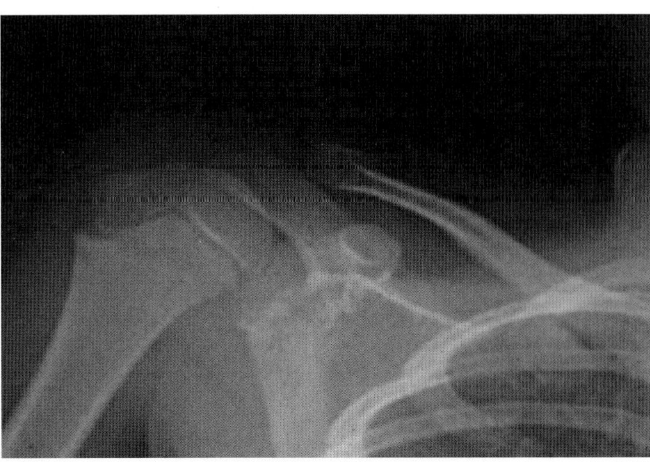

FIGURE 83-4 Right distal clavicular fracture in an 8-year-old boy after he fell off the top bunk. (*Used with permission from Emily Scott, MD.*)

ETIOLOGY AND PATHOPHYSIOLOGY

- Ninety percent of clavicle injuries are caused by accidental trauma from fall against the shoulder as result of a direct blow to the clavicle or can be fall on an outstretched hand.[2] However, stress fractures in gymnasts and divers have been reported.
- Neonatal clavicular injuries are usually from birth trauma, commonly breech presentations.
- In children under 2 years of age, a fall from the bed/crib is most common mechanism.[3]
- Sports injuries are common in the adolescent population.
- Physical assaults and child abuse can cause clavicular fractures and need to be considered (**Figure 83-5**).

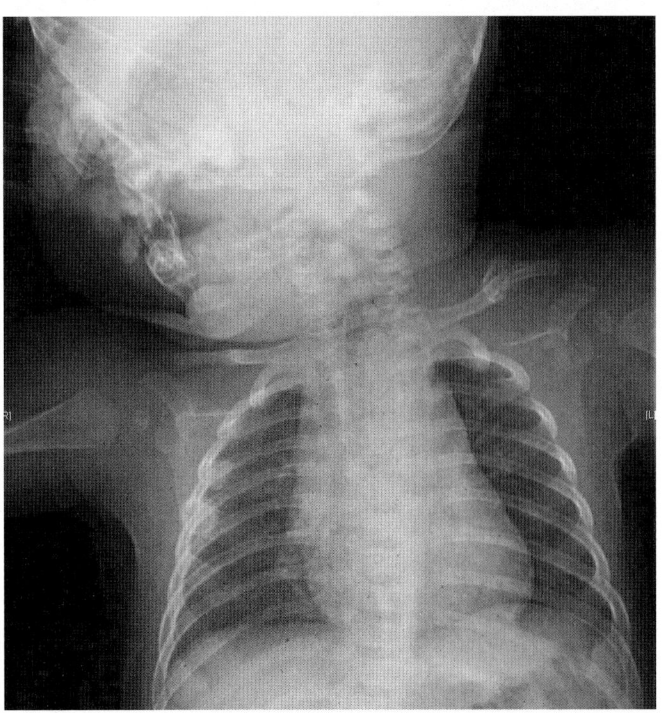

FIGURE 83-5 Healing left clavicular fracture in a 6-month-old infant showing callous formation. This fracture was discovered on radiographic screening for physical abuse. (*Used with permission from Emily Scott, MD.*)

TABLE 83-1 Typical Distribution/Classification

Group (Approx. %)	Fracture Location	Radiographic Appearance
Group I (80%)	Middle third	Upward displacement (**Figure 83-3**)
Group II (15%)	Distal third	Medial side of fragment is displaced upward (**Figure 83-4**)
Type I		Minimal displacement
Type II		Fracture medial to coracoclavicular ligaments; some overlapping of fragments
Type III		Fracture at the articular surface of the acromioclavicular (AC) joint; can look like AC separation
Group III (5%)	Medial third	Medial side of fragment up; distal side down; higher risk of mediastinal injuries

- Pathologic fractures (uncommon) can result from lytic lesions, bony cancers or metastases, or radiation.

TYPICAL DISTRIBUTION

- For the typical distribution and classification of clavicular fractures, see **Table 83-1**.

DIAGNOSIS

CLINICAL FEATURES

- History of trauma with a mechanism known to result in clavicle fractures (i.e., fall on an outstretched hand or lateral shoulder, or direct blow).
- Pain, bruising, and swelling at the fracture site.
- Gross deformity at the site of fracture.
- Young children present with inability to raise their arms above their head and often will present as having trouble getting shirts on and getting into buckled car seats.

IMAGING

- Obtain plain films of the clavicle for radiographic evidence of fracture.

DIFFERENTIAL DIAGNOSIS

- Acromioclavicular (AC) separation—Fall directly on the "point" of the shoulder or a direct blow, pain with overhead movement, tenderness at the AC joint, and AC joint separation on radiographs.

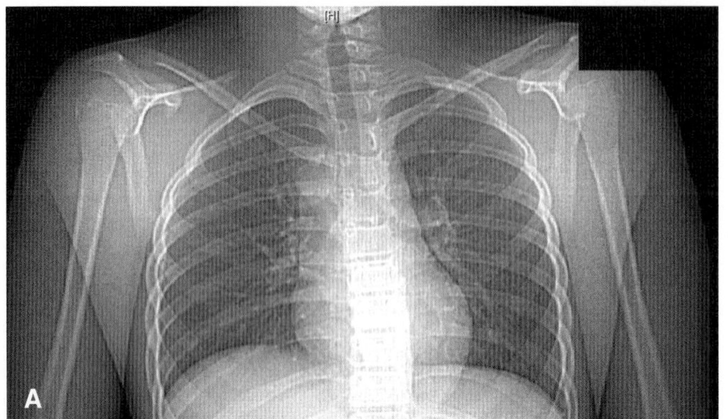

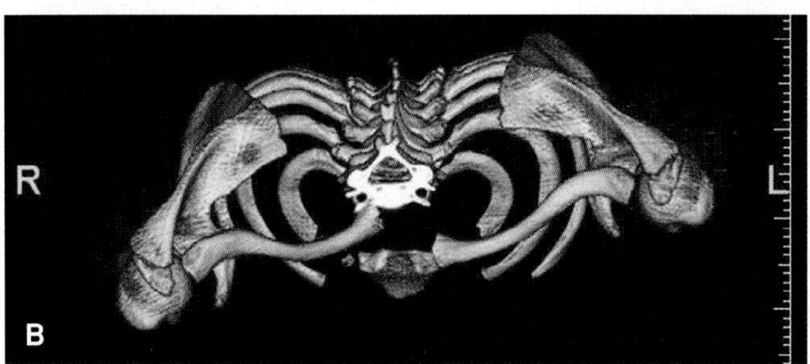

FIGURE 83-6 Sternoclavicular dislocation of right clavicle in a 15-year-old boy who was wrestling and took a knee to the chest. Plain x-ray (**A**) and 3D reconstruction view (**B**). This required surgical repair. (*Used with permission from Emily Scott, MD.*)

- Sternoclavicular dislocation—Fall on the shoulder, chest and shoulder pain exacerbated by arm movement or when lying down, and a prominence from the superomedial displacement of the clavicle (uncommon; **Figure 83-6**).
- Pseudoarthrosis of the clavicle—Painless mass in the middle of the clavicle from failure of the central part of the clavicle to ossify (extremely rare).

MANAGEMENT

- Assess neurovascular status of injured extremity.
- Treat pain as needed with acetaminophen or NSAIDs. Narcotics may be indicated at the time of evaluation and potentially the first few days.
- Assess for damage to lungs (pneumothorax or hemothorax).
- Determine the classification and amount of displacement by radiograph (**Table 83-1**).

TREATMENT

Most clavicular fractures can be treated nonoperatively. Fixation with plates is sometimes required.

- Treat most children with clavicle fracture conservatively, with immobilization figure of eight splints for young children and slings for older patients.[1]
- Children can be treated nonoperatively even with 90-degree displacement and several inches of overlap.[1]
- Operative indications currently are open fractures, comminuted fractures, multitrauma patients and shortened fractures in adolescent population.[4]

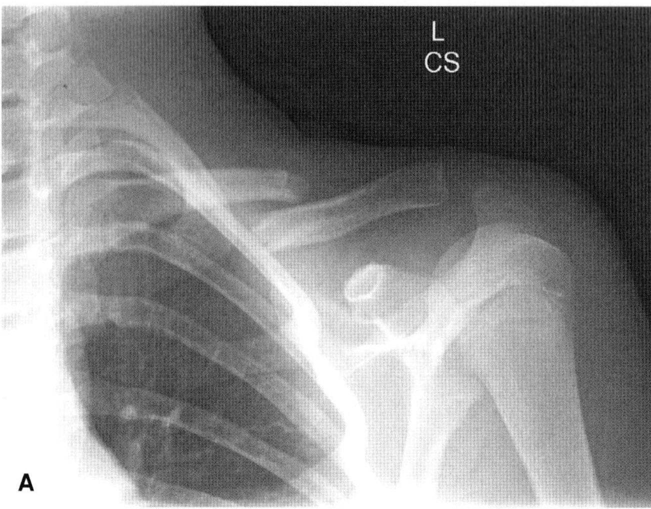

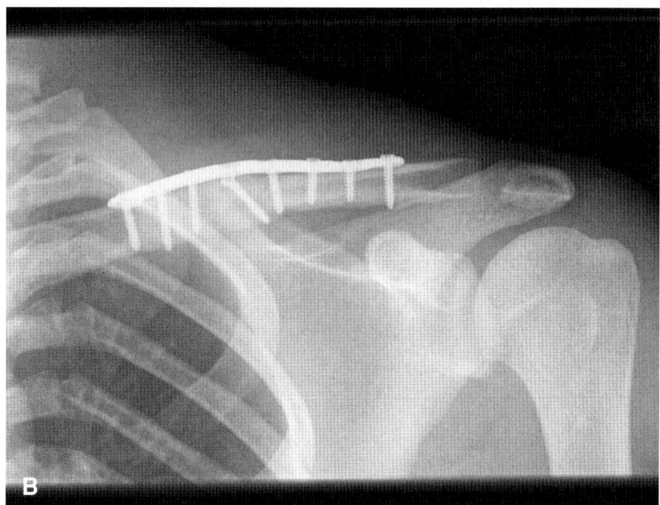

FIGURE 83-7 An overriding clavicular fracture with moderate displacement (**A**), in a 15-year-old hockey player, requiring surgical plating (**B**). (*Used with permission from Emily Scott, MD.*)

- Recent studies have explored earlier operative management in midshaft fractures in the adolescent populations (**Figure 83-7**).[5]

REFERRAL

- Refer for surgical evaluation, children with impingement of soft tissue/muscle, instability of shoulder girdle, displacement with skin perforation/necrosis, or risk to mediastinal structures.[1]
- Consider consulting with a physician skilled in managing clavicular fractures in patients with a distal clavicle fracture. These fractures have a high rate of nonunion; however, only a portion of nonunions are painful or inhibit function. If the patient continues to have a symptomatic nonunion after many months, surgery may be considered.

PROGNOSIS

- Mid-clavicular fractures in newborns and children heal completely without surgery in most cases.
- Mid-clavicular fractures in adolescents heal without surgery in most cases. Return to activities may be shortened from 16 to 12 weeks with operative intervention.[5]

FOLLOW-UP

- Monitor with examination and radiographs until pain has resolved, any lost function has returned, and there is radiographic evidence of healing.
- If the fracture is stable, repeat x-ray every 4 to 6 weeks until the clavicle has healed. If there is no evidence of healing after 2 to 3 months, referral should be considered.

PATIENT EDUCATION

Most clavicle fractures heal without surgery, especially if the fracture is not displaced. Fractures in children take approximately 3 to 4 weeks to heal. Often, there will be a "bump" at the site of the healed fracture, which is underlying bone callous. The callous usually does not does not interfere with any activities but can start forming in the first few days and last for months, which is important to communicate with the families.

PATIENT RESOURCES

- American Academy of Orthopedic Surgeons. Patient information handout under *Broken Collarbone*—**www.orthoinfo.aaos.org/topic.cfm?topic=A00072**.

PROVIDER RESOURCES

- Wheeles' Textbook of Orthopaedics—**www.wheelessonline.com/ortho/clavicular_fractures_in_children**.
- **www.orthobullets.com/pediatrics/4123/medial-clavicle-physeal-fractures**.

REFERENCES

1. Kubiak R, Slongo T. Operative treatment of clavicle fractures in children: a review of 21 years. *J Pediatr Orthop*. 2002;22:736-739.
2. Lenza M, Buchbinder R, Johnston RV, Belloti JC, Faloppa F. Surgical versus conservative interventions for treating fractures of the middle third of the clavicle. *Cochrane Database of Systematic Reviews*. 2013;6.
3. Soto F, Fiesseler F, Morales J, Amato C. Presentation, evaluation, and treatment of clavicle fractures in preschool children presenting to an emergency department. *Pediatr Emerg Care*. 2009;25(11):744-747.
4. Caird MS. Clavicle shaft fractures: are children little adults. *J Pediatr Orthop*. 2012;32(1):S1-4.
5. Vander Have KL, Perdue AM, Caird MS, Farley FA. Operative versus nonoperative treatment of midshaft clavicle fractures in adolescents. *J Pediatr Orthop*. 2010;92(6):811.

84 FOREARM FRACTURES

Emily Gale Scott, MD
Heidi Chumley, MD

PATIENT STORY

A 5-year-old boy fell off his bicycle and had immediate pain and swelling of his right wrist. He continued to complain of pain and could not use his right arm because of severe pain. In the emergency department a radiograph was obtained which showed a Buckle (Torus) right radius fracture (**Figure 84-1**). He was treated by immobilization with a short arm cast for 3 weeks and had an excellent recovery.

INTRODUCTION

Distal radius and forearm fractures are common in children and adolescents. Patients typically present after falling on an outstretched arm. The diagnosis is confirmed by radiographs. Treatment in the pediatric population is usually non-operative with prolonged immobilization but can require operative care depending on the type of fracture, degree of displacement and the age of the patient.

SYNONYMS (TYPES OF FRACTURES)

Physeal fractures (growth plate injuries), Buckle (Torus), Greenstick fractures can occur in the forearm. Galeazzi and Monteggia fractures are more rare forearm fractures, but important to recognize.

EPIDEMIOLOGY

- Radius/ulna fractures are the most common upper extremity fracture (37%) in children under the age of 6 years.[1]
- Distal radial fractures (**Figure 84-2**) accounted for 25 to 30 percent of fractures in children ages 2 to 14.[2,3]
- Incidence is 373/100,000 children.[4]
- Peak incidence is age 11 to 14 in boys and ages 8 to 11 in girls.[4]
- More common in boys across all ages.[2]

ETIOLOGY AND PATHOPHYSIOLOGY

- Classic history is a fall from a height (bed or playground equipment), down stairs, or while running, biking, or skating on an outstretched arm.
- Increase in incidence of fractures during pubertal years is thought to be from increase physical activity concurrent with transient

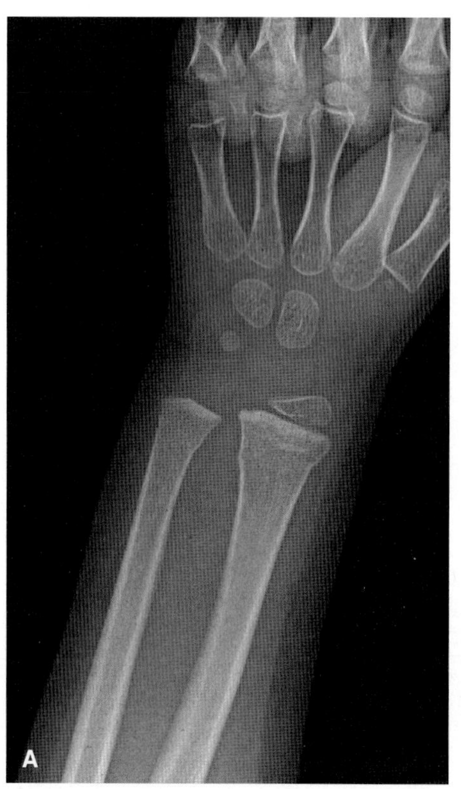

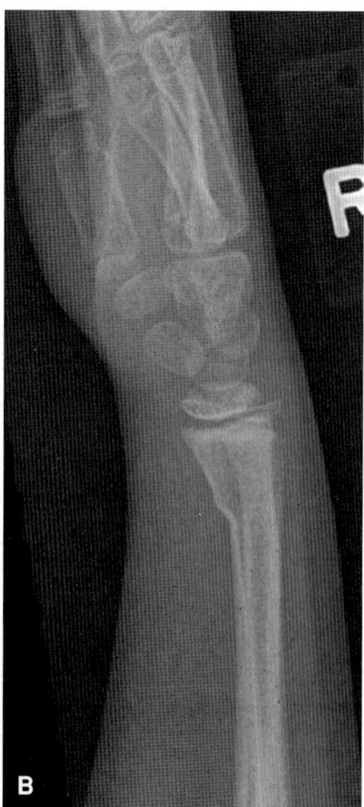

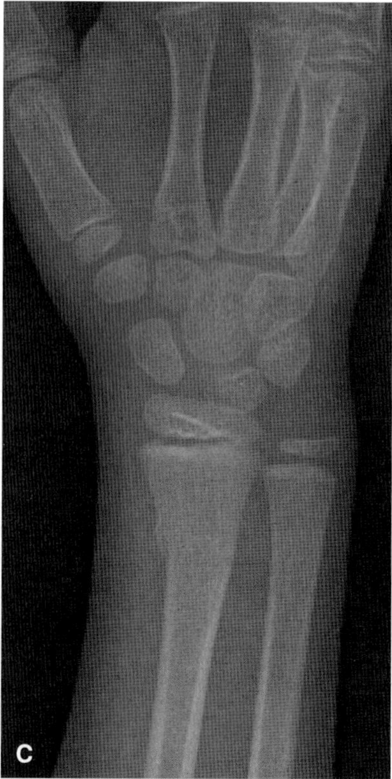

FIGURE 84-1 Buckle fracture (Torus) of the distal radius on AP (**A**), lateral (**B**), and oblique (**C**) forearm x-ray views. This 5-year-old boy fell off his bicycle. (*Used with permission from Emily Scott, MD.*)

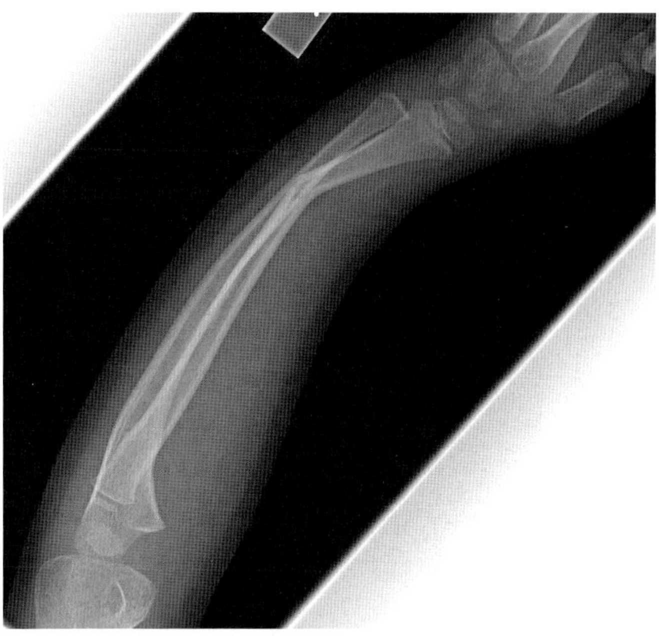

FIGURE 84-2 Distal radius fracture on lateral view in a 7-year-old child. (*Used with permission from Emily Scott, MD.*)

deficit in cortical bone mass and secondary to an increase in height that is not accompanied by an adequately increased accrual of bone mineralization.[4]

- Abuse: in infants (less than one year), should be considered especially if the history of injury is not plausible and inconsistent with injury pattern.[5]

RISK FACTORS

- Male gender.
- Pubertal age.
- Previous history of fracture.

DIAGNOSIS

Diagnosis is suspected by a compatible history such as falling, physical findings of trauma and confirmed by radiographs (two or three views). In regard to radiographs, more than one view is essential to determine the degree of angulation and deformity. Typical radiographs include anterior posterior (AP), lateral and oblique films (**Figure 84-3**). For some specific injuries it is necessary to image the elbow because it can often have dislocation or other injuries associated with forearm fracture.

CLINICAL FEATURES

Pain, obvious swelling, and/or deformity are usually present after accidental injury. External sign of injury and abnormal use of the arm is present in most cases. However, some children under the age of 6 years do not always manifest these signs. Fifteen percent of children will not have an external sign of injury and 16 percent may use a fractured arm normally.[1]

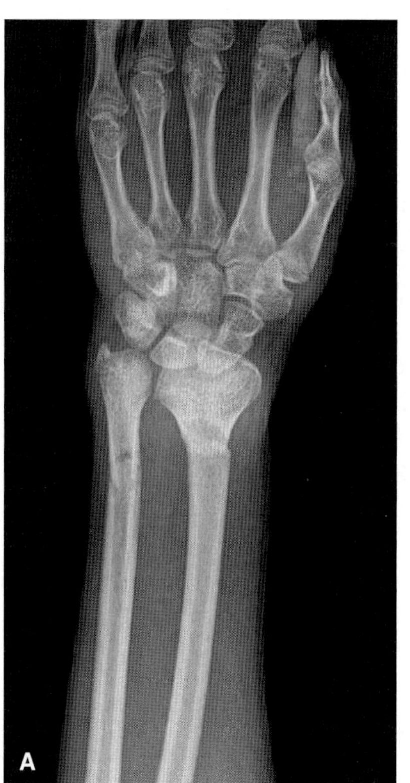

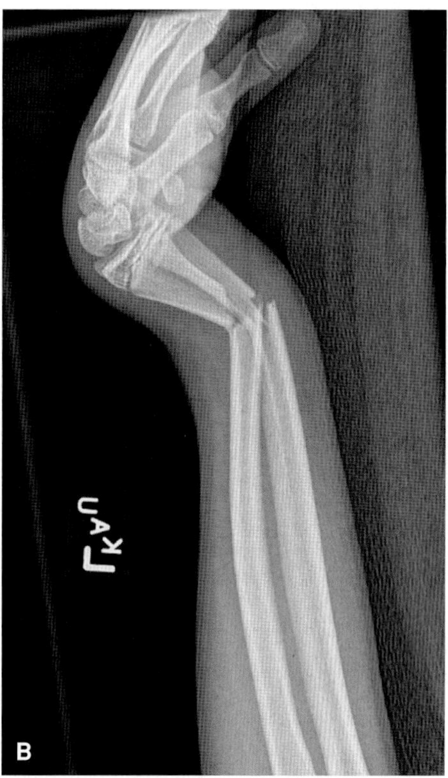

FIGURE 84-3 Midshaft radial fractures in a 10-year-old child. Two x-ray views are essential to determine the degree of injury in forearm fractures. The fracture is seen on the AP (**A**) view, but the lateral (**B**) view clearly demonstrates severe angulation not seen on the AP view. (*Used with permission from Emily Scott, MD.*)

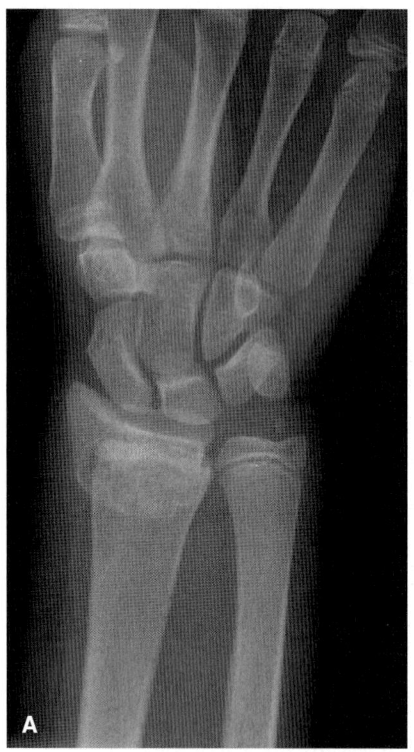

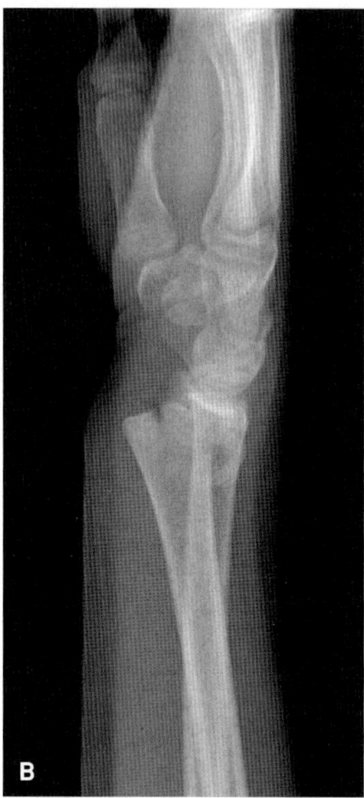

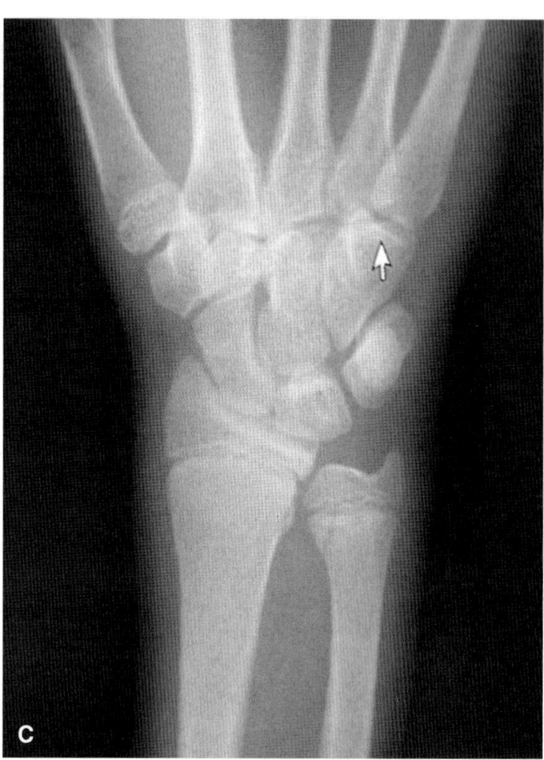

FIGURE 84-4 Salter Harris II physeal radius fracture of the growth plate on AP (**A**), Lateral (**B**) views in a 10-year-old child. (**C**) Classic Salter-Harris II fracture of ulna and buckle fracture of the radius in a 13-year-old boy who fell on an outstretched arm. (*Used with permission from Emily Scott, MD.*)

TYPES OF FRACTURES

Type of forearm fractures in children include:

- Physeal fractures (growth plate injuries)—Most common in children ages 6 to 10 years after falling on an outstretched hand. Most are Salter-Harris type I or II (**Figures 84-4** and **84-5**).

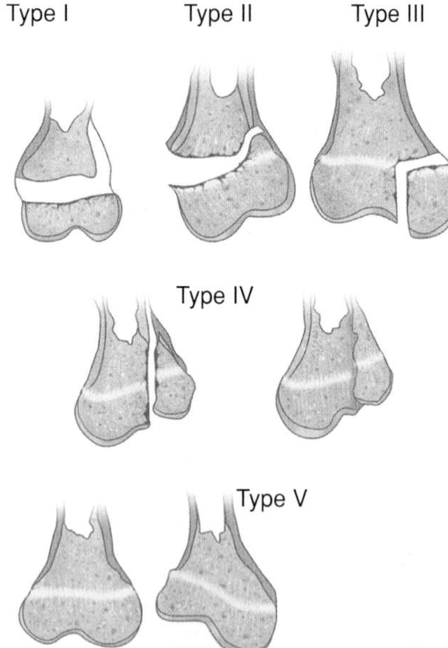

FIGURE 84-5 Salter-Harris classification system of growth plate fractures. Type I, separation of the physis; type II, fracture through the physis and adjacent metaphysis; type III, fracture through the physis and adjacent epiphysis; type IV, fracture through the physis, adjacent metaphysic and epiphysis; type V, crush injury of the physis. (*Used with permission from Patel DR, Greydanus DE, Baker RJ: Pediatric Practice: Sports Medicine: www.accesspediatrics.com.*)

- Torus (Buckle) fractures—Common in young children; fracture through dorsal cortex 2 to 3 cm proximal to the physis with dorsal angulation of distal fragment after falling on an outstretched hand (**Figures 84-6** and **84-7**).
- Greenstick fracture—Incomplete fracture, which may occur on the dorsal or volar side of the radius or ulna or both. Greenstick fracture of one forearm bone can accompany a complete fracture of the other forearm bone (**Figure 84-8**).
- Complex Radius and Ulna fractures—Fractures present in both bones, either complete or incomplete (Greenstick); caused by a fall on an outstretched hand, severe trauma, or intentional injury, especially in infants. These usually occur in the mid-shaft. They often require operative management (**Figure 84-9**).
- Galeazzi fracture—Variant in children is a distal radial fracture with separation of the distal ulnar physis (Salter-Harris type II).
- Monteggia Fracture—A rare specific type of forearm fracture that involves proximal ulna fracture with associated radial head dislocation. If isolated ulna fracture is present, one needs to evaluate the elbow for additional injury (**Figures 84-10** and **84-11**).

DIFFERENTIAL DIAGNOSIS

Other causes of pain at the wrist include:

- Wrist sprains or strains present with tenderness, pain, and swelling but with normal radiographs.

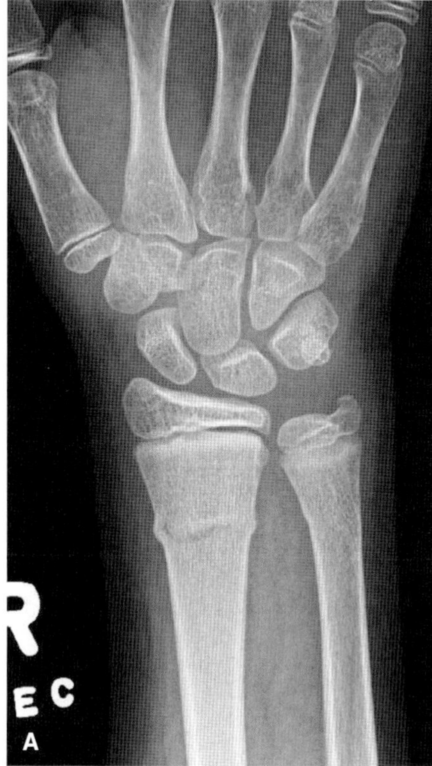

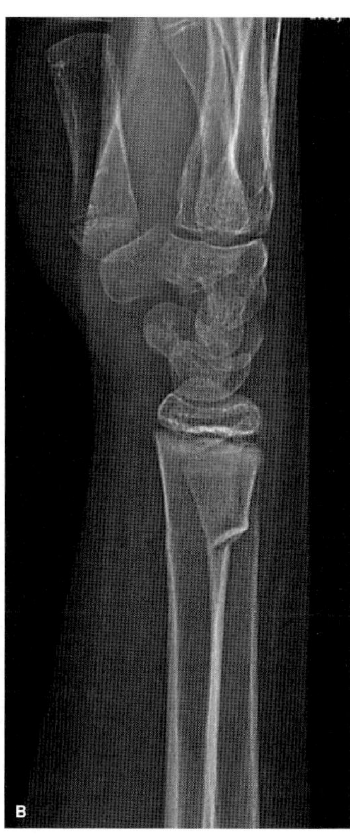

FIGURE 84-6 Distal radius Buckle (Torus) fracture on AP (**A**) and lateral (**B**) views in a 10-year-old child. (*Used with permission from Emily Scott, MD.*)

- Stress or overuse injuries (e.g., in gymnasts) present with less acute onset and include soft-tissue and bony lesions that can be identified on MRI.

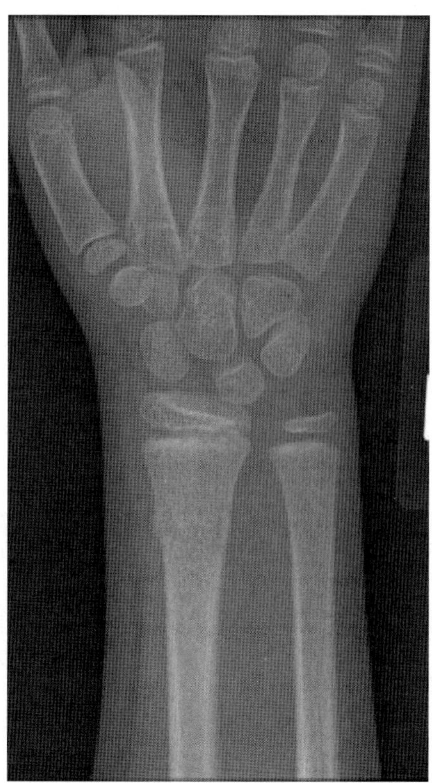

FIGURE 84-7 Buckle (Torus) Fracture in a 13-year-old child. (*Used with permission from Emily Scott, MD.*)

MANAGEMENT

Initial management requires complete exam including neurovascular and motor components, pain management, and radiographs. Type of fracture, amount of displacement, and age of child guide management help guide the management plans for forearm fractures.

PHYSEAL FRACTURES (GROWTH PLATE INJURIES)

- Look for a concomitant distal ulnar fracture and avulsion fracture of ulnar styloid.
- Evaluate for compartment syndrome and acute carpal tunnel and if present, refer immediately.

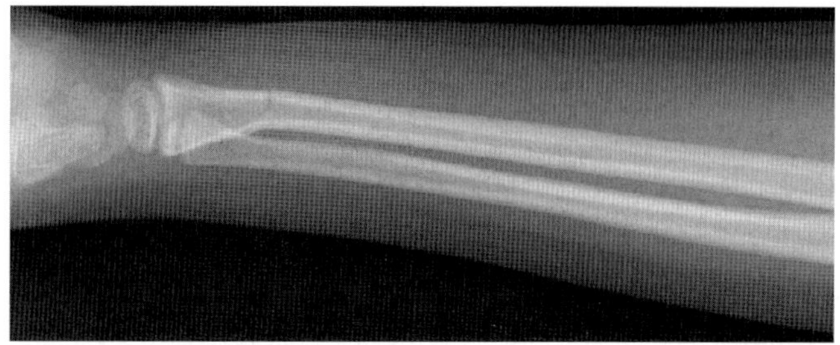

FIGURE 84-8 Greenstick fracture of the radius in an 8-year-old child. (*Used with permission from Emily Scott, MD.*)

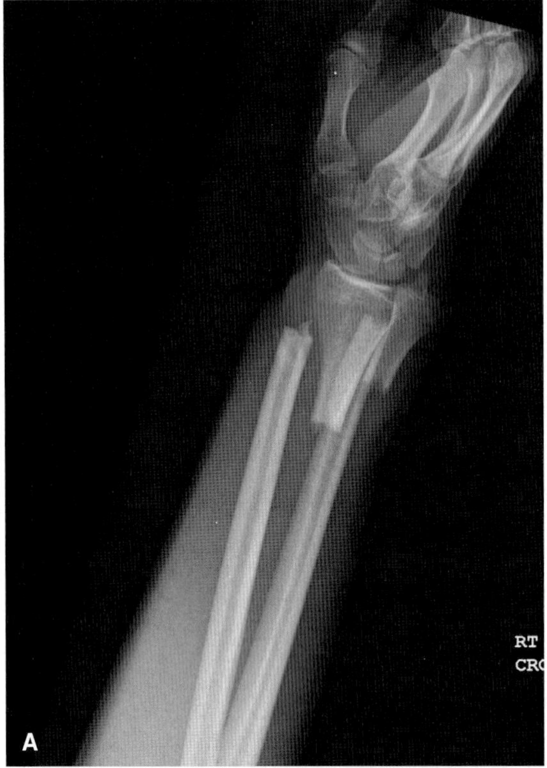

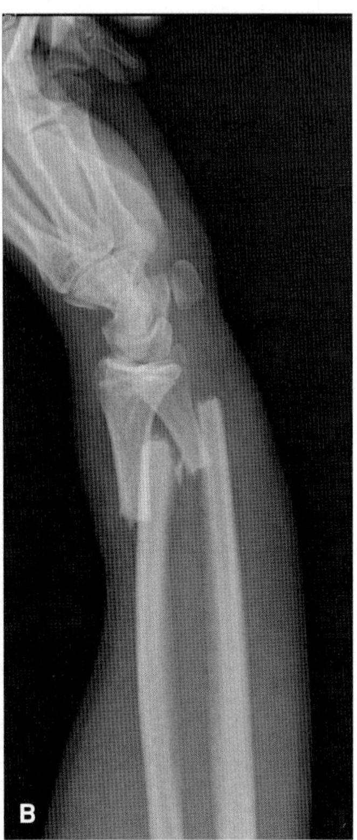

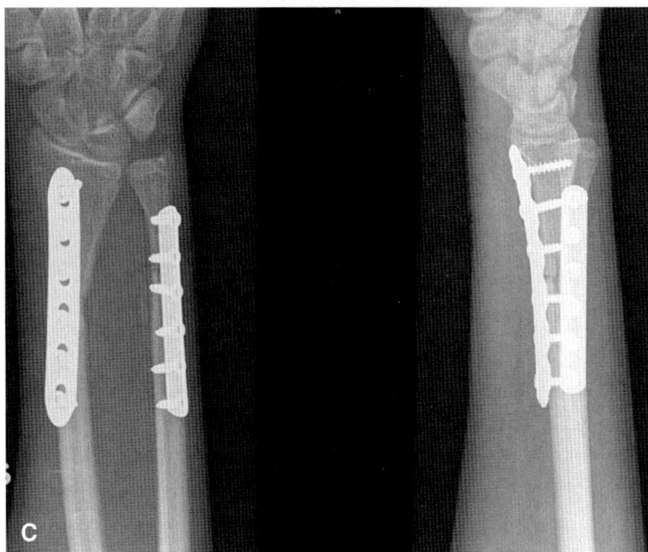

FIGURE 84-9 Complete fracture of the radius and ulna in a 14-year-old child on AP (**A**), lateral (**B**) views. This child required surgical plating (**C**). (*Used with permission from Emily Scott, MD.*)

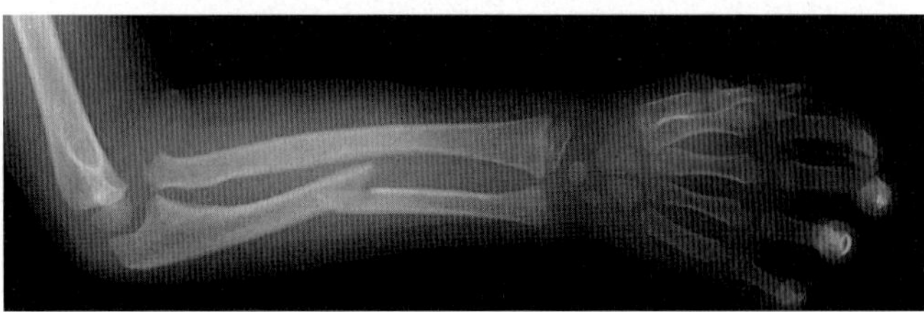

FIGURE 84-10 Monteggia fracture in a 9-year-old child. Lateral view of the elbow and forearm showing the midshaft ulnar fracture with radial head dislocation. (*Used with permission from Emily Scott, MD.*)

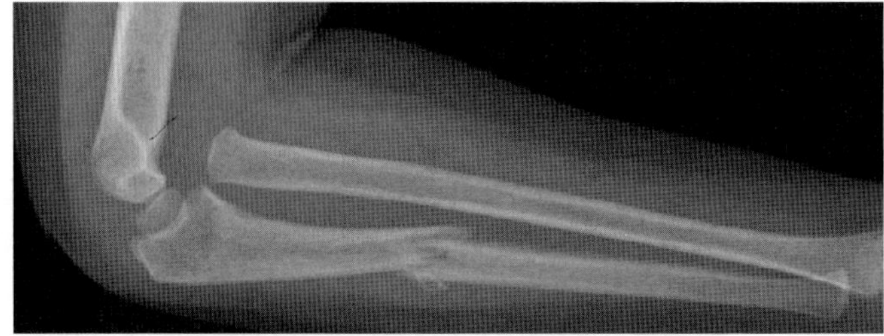

FIGURE 84-11 Monteggia fracture in a 3-year-old child showing a midshaft ulnar fracture with radial head dislocation. (*Used with permission from Emily Scott, MD.*)

TABLE 84-1 Universal Classification of Radial Fractures

Fracture Classification	Management
I Nonarticular, nondisplaced	Immobilization with cast or splint[6] for 4 to 6 weeks
II Nonarticular, displaced	Reduction with cast or splint immobilization; surgical management if irreducible or unstable fracture
III Articular, nondisplaced	Immobilization; pinning if unstable
IV Articular, displaced	Surgical management

- Apply long arm splint with 25 degrees wrist flexion and 15 degrees ulnar deviation.[5]
- Refer to a physician experienced in managing physeal fractures, such as an orthopaedic surgeon
- Described by Salter Harris Classification (**Table 84-1**).

BUCKLE (TORUS) FRACTURES

- Ensure that the fracture is on the compression side and that the tension side is intact.
- Place in a short-arm cast for three weeks.[5]

GREENSTICK FRACTURES

- Minimally angulated (<15 degrees) can be treated with a short arm cast or splint for 4 weeks.[6]
- Consult with a physician experienced in managing Greenstick fractures as they sometimes require completing the fracture to adequately reduce the fracture and minimize the risk of recurrent deformity while in the cast.

COMPLEX RADIUS AND ULNAR FRACTURES

- Evaluate neurovascular status.
- Refer to a physician experienced in managing forearm fractures to determine whether closed or open reduction is most appropriate.

PREVENTION

The Center for Disease Control and Prevention recommends these safety practices to prevent injuries from falls in children.

- Ensure child wears protective gear during sports and recreation including helmets and wrist guards.
- Use window guards, stair gates, and guard rails.
- Ensure the surface under playground equipment is safe and soft (e.g., wood chips instead of dirt).
- Supervise young children at all times when around fall hazards such as staircases and playground equipment.

PROGNOSIS

Most children with distal radial fractures will recover function with appropriate treatment.

FOLLOW-UP

- Management and follow-up often involve a physician with expertise in managing distal radial fractures.[7]

PATIENT EDUCATION

- Most children will recover completely with appropriate management.
- Safe practices can help prevent further injuries.
- Discuss safety tips with parents to prevent future injuries.

PATIENT RESOURCES

- **www.emedicine.medscape.com/article/824949-overview**.
- CDC Fact Sheet: Preventing Falls—**www.cdc.gov/safechild/Falls/index.html**.

PROVIDER RESOURCES

- *Wheeless' Textbook of Orthopaedics* has additional information about the types of distal radius fractures, classification systems, and radiographic findings—**www.wheelessonline.com/ortho/12591**.
- **www.posna.org/education/StudyGuide/fracturesOfShaftOfRadius.asp**.

REFERENCES

1. Farrell C, Rubin DM, Downes K, Dormans J, Christian CW. Symptoms and time to medical care in children with accidental extremity fractures. *Pediatrics*. 2012;129(1):e128-133.
2. Valeria G, Francesca G, Mancusi C, et al. pattern of fractures across pediatric age groups: analysis of individual and lifestyle factors. *BMC Public Health*. 2010;10:656.
3. Nellans KW, Kowalski E, Chung KC. The Epidemiology of Distal Radius Fractures. *Hand Clin*. 2012 28(2):113-125.
4. Khosla S, Melton LJ, Dekutoski MB, Achenback SJ, Oberg AL, Riggs BL. Incidence of childhood distal forearm fractures over 30 years: a population-based study. *JAMA*. 2003;290(11):1479-1485.
5. Wheeless CR. Wheeless' Textbook of Orthopaedics. Pediatric Radial Fractures. http://www.wheelessonline.com/ortho/pediatric_distal_radius_fracture, accessed on Dec 11, 2012.
6. Boutis K, Willan A, Babyn P, Goeree R, Howard A. Cast versus splinting in children with minimally angulated fractures of the distal radius: a randomized controlled trial. *CMAJ*. 2010;182(14):1507-1512.
7. Noonan KJ and Price TP. Forearm and Distal Radius Fractures in Children. *Journ Am Acad Ortho Surg*. 1998;6(3):146-156.

85 METATARSAL FRACTURE

Heidi Chumley, MD

PATIENT STORY

A 13-year-old boy inverted his ankle while playing basketball in his driveway. He felt a pop and had immediate pain. He had tenderness over the base of his fifth metatarsal. Having met the Ottawa ankle rules for radiographs (see Management Section), a radiograph was obtained, which revealed a displaced styloid fracture at the base of the fifth metatarsal (**Figure 85-1**).

INTRODUCTION

Most metatarsal fractures in children over the age of 5 years involve the fifth metatarsal and include avulsion fractures at the base, acute diaphyseal fractures (Jones fracture), and diaphyseal stress fractures (**Figure 85-2**). Fractures of the first through fourth metatarsals are less common but can be associated with a Lisfranc injury. Children under the age of 5 years more commonly fracture the first metatarsal. Diagnosis is based on the mechanism of injury or type of overuse activity and radiographic appearance. Treatment depends on the type of fracture. Most metatarsal fractures have a good prognosis; however, Jones fractures have a high rate of nonunion and Lisfranc injuries can result in chronic symptoms.

SYNONYMS

Avulsion fracture at base of fifth metatarsal: fifth metatarsal tuberosity fracture, dancer fracture, pseudo-Jones fracture.

Jones fracture—Acute diaphyseal fracture of the fifth metatarsal.

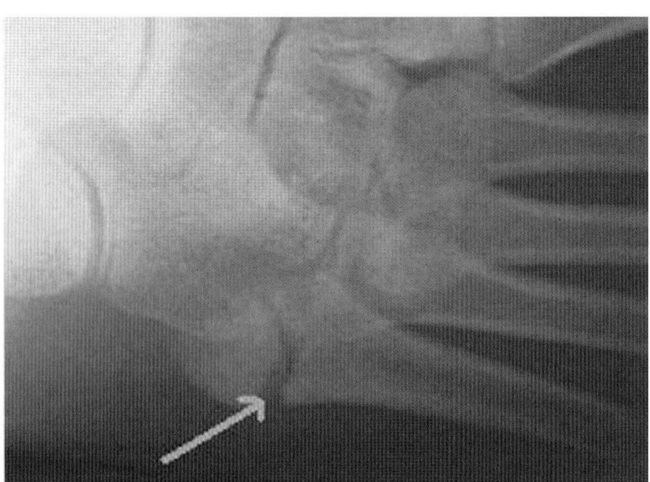

FIGURE 85-1 Displaced styloid fracture at the base of the fifth metatarsal. (*Used with permission from Patel DR, Greydanus DE, Baker RJ: Pediatric Practice: Sports Medicine: www.accesspediatrics.com. Figure 28-26, with permission.*)

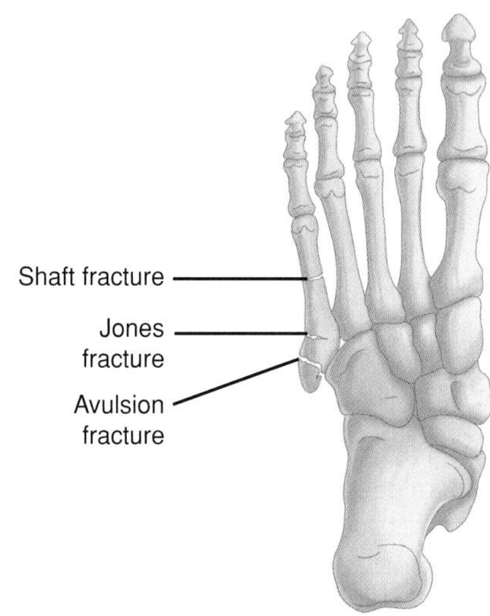

FIGURE 85-2 Fractures of the fifth metatarsal. Avulsions or shaft fractures are most common in pediatrics. The Jones fracture (metaphyseal–diaphyseal junction) is rare in children. (*Used with permission from Strange GR, Ahrens WR, Schafermeyer RW, Wiebe RA: Pediatric emergency Medicine, 3rd edition: http://www.accessemergencymedicine.com. Figure 38-11, with permission.*)

EPIDEMIOLOGY

- Foot fractures are common injuries among recreational and serious athletes; however, incidence and prevalence in most populations is unknown.
- Children under the age of 5 years most frequently fracture the first metatarsal, generally from a fall from a height.[1]
- Children over the age of 5 years most frequently fracture the fifth metatarsal generally from a fall on a level surface.[1]

ETIOLOGY AND PATHOPHYSIOLOGY

- Avulsion fractures result when the peroneus brevis tendon and the lateral plantar fascia pull off the base of the fifth metatarsal, typically during an inversion injury while the foot is in plantar flexion.
- Jones (acute diaphyseal) fracture results from landing on the outside of the foot with the foot plantar flexed.
- Stress fractures at base of second and third metatarsal bones are seen in repetitive trauma in ballet dancing.
- Diaphyseal stress fractures are caused by chronic stress from activities such as jumping and marching.
- Fractures of the first through fourth metatarsals are caused by direct blows or falling forward over a plantar-flexed foot. These fractures may be associated with a Lisfranc injury.

DIAGNOSIS

The diagnosis of avulsion or Jones fractures is made on plain radiographs in a patient with a history of injury and acute lateral foot pain.

Comparative views of the uninjured foot may be helpful. Diaphyseal stress fractures may require CT imaging.

CLINICAL FEATURES

- Avulsion injury—Sudden onset of pain (and tenderness on examination) at the base of the fifth metatarsal after forced inversion with the foot and ankle in plantar flexion.
- Acute Jones fracture—Sudden pain at the base of the fifth metatarsal, with difficulty bearing weight on the foot, after a laterally directed force on the forefoot during plantar flexion of the ankle.
- Stress fracture—History of chronic foot pain with repetitive motion.

IMAGING

- Avulsion fracture—Fracture line at base of fifth metatarsal oriented perpendicularly to the metatarsal shaft (**Figure 85-1**). May extend into joint with cuboid bone, but does not extend into the intermetatarsal joint.
- Acute Jones fractures (**Figure 85-3**) and stress fractures both have a fracture line through the proximal 1.5 cm of the fifth metatarsal shaft. These should be classified into type I, II, or III:[2]
  - Type I fractures have a sharp, narrow fracture line, no intramedullary sclerosis, and minimal cortical hypertrophy.
  - Type II fractures (delayed unions) have a widened fracture line with radiolucency, involve both cortices, and have intramedullary sclerosis.
  - Type III fractures (nonunions) have a wide fracture line, periosteal new bone and radiolucency, and obliteration of the medullary canal by sclerotic bone.
- Early stress fractures may have normal radiographs and can be seen on CT, MRI, or bone scan. Ultrasound may be a less expensive option—sensitivity 83 percent, specificity 76 percent, positive predictive value 59 percent and negative predictive value 92 percent in one small study.[3]

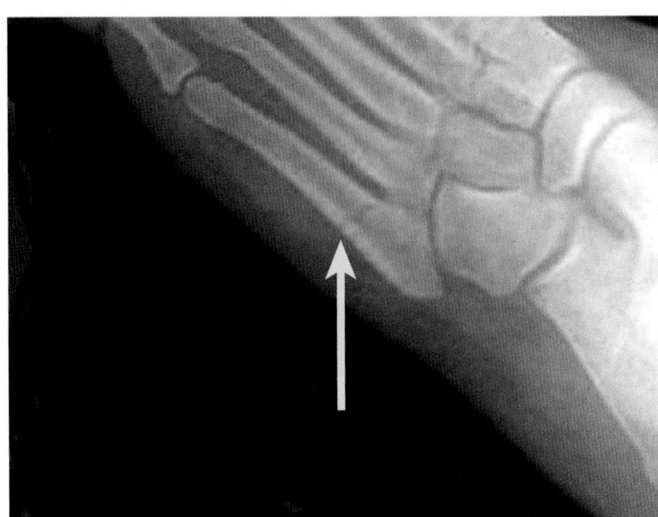

FIGURE 85-3 Jones fracture, a transverse fracture at the junction of the diaphysis and metaphysis. (*Used with permission from Patel DR, Greydanus DE, Baker RJ: Pediatric Practice: Sports Medicine: www.accesspediatrics.com. Figure 28-25, with permission.*)

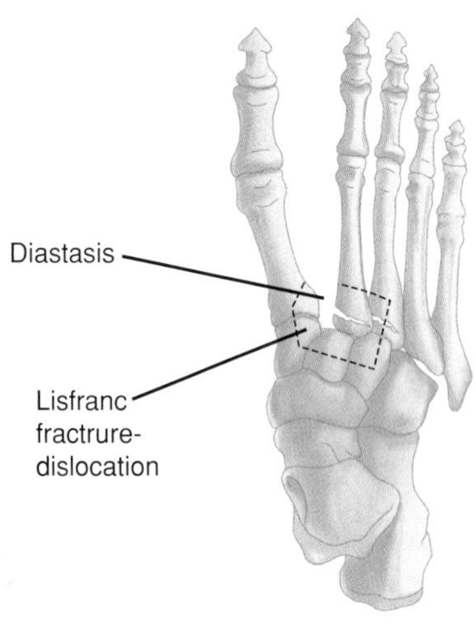

FIGURE 85-4 Illustration of the Lisfranc injury, which is a tarsal–metatarsal dislocation. This is rare in pediatric patients. (*Used with permission from Strange GR, Ahrens WR, Schafermeyer RW, Wiebe RA: Pediatric emergency Medicine, 3rd edition: http://www.accessemergencymedicine.com. Figure 38-12, with permission.*)

DIFFERENTIAL DIAGNOSIS

Pain at the fifth metatarsal can also be caused by:

- Diaphyseal stress fracture—May be radiographically similar to Jones fracture but is often seen more distally in the shaft; occurs in patients with no injury and history of overuse (e.g., ballet dancing, marching).
- Lisfranc injury—Disruption of the tarsal metatarsal joints (**Figure 85-4**). This pain is typically in the midfoot and more commonly medial. May be associated with fractures in the first through fourth metatarsals.

x-ray findings that can be confused with foot fractures include:

- Apophysis, a secondary center of ossification at the proximal end of the fifth metatarsal seen in girls, ages 9 to 11 years, and boys, ages 11 to 14 years. The apophysis is oblique to the metatarsal shaft, whereas avulsion fractures are perpendicular.
- Accessory ossicles (i.e., os peroneum, located at the lateral border of the cuboid) have smooth edges, whereas avulsion fractures have rough edges.

MANAGEMENT

Fractures of fifth metatarsals in children have been found to be similar to those in adults. Management is based on adult literature.[4]

Apply the Ottawa ankle rules in children over the age of 5 years to determine which patients with an injury and ankle/foot pain should have an x-ray.[5,6] SOR Ⓐ Ottawa rules: x-ray patients who cannot walk four steps immediately after the injury or who have localized tenderness at the posterior edge or tip of either malleolus, the navicular, or the base of the fifth metatarsal.[5]

- Treat nondisplaced avulsion fractures with an ankle splint or walking boot with ambulation for 3 to 6 weeks.[7] SOR Ⓑ Refer displaced avulsion fractures.

- Consider referring Jones fractures because of the high rate of nonunion caused by the poor blood supply. Type I or II may be treated with immobilization for at least 6 to 8 weeks. Type II can also be treated with surgery. Type III requires surgical repair. Elite athletes or patients needing a faster recovery are often surgically treated.[8] SOR Ⓑ
- Treat stress fractures with elimination of the causative activity for 4 to 8 weeks. Immobilization is often not required. If walking is painful, partial or non–weight-bearing for 1 to 3 weeks may be necessary.[9]

Refer patients with:[9]

- Neurovascular compromise, compartment syndrome, or open fractures.
- First metatarsal fracture, multiple metatarsal fractures, displaced fracture, intraarticular fracture, or Lisfranc injury.
- Inadequate response to treatment.

PROGNOSIS

Prognosis in children is thought to be excellent. Metatarsal fractures in older adolescents and adults have an excellent outcome, with most patients symptom free at 33 months. Patients with higher body mass index (BMI), diabetes mellitus, women, and a dislocation with the fracture have less-positive outcomes.[10]

FOLLOW-UP

Patients should be followed every 1 to 3 weeks to evaluate for appropriate clinical and radiographic response to treatment.

PATIENT EDUCATION

Patients with nondisplaced avulsion fractures require a splint or boot, but can remain ambulatory. Jones fractures have a poor blood supply and often do not reconnect, even with immobilization. Surgery may result in a faster return to activities in some cases.

PATIENT RESOURCES

- Patient.co.uk has patient information on metatarsal fractures—**www.patient.co.uk/health/Metatarsal-Fractures.htm**.

PROVIDER RESOURCES

- The Ottawa ankle rules are available in several places online including—**www.mdcalc.com/ottawa-ankle-rules**.

REFERENCES

1. Singer G, Cichocki M, Schalamon J, Eberl R, Hollwarth ME. A study of metatarsl fractures in children. *J Bone Joint Surg AM*. 2008;90(4):772-776.
2. Lehman RC, Torg JS, Pavlov H, Delee JC. Fractures of the base of the fifth metatarsal distal to the tuberosity: A review. *Foot Ankle*. 1987;7:245-252.
3. Banal F, Gandjbakhch F, Foltz V, et al. Sensitivity and specificity of ultrasonography in early diagnosis of metatarsal bone stress fractures: a pilot study of 37 patients. *J Rheumatol*. 2009;36(8):1715-1719.
4. Herrera-Soto JA, Scherb M, Duffy MF, Albright JC. Fractures of the fifth metatarsal in children and adolescents. *J Pediatr Orthop*. 2007;27(4):427-431.
5. Stiell IG, Greenberg GH, Mcknight RD, et al. Decision rules for the use of radiography in acute ankle injuries. Refinement and prospective validation. *JAMA*. 1993;269:1127-1132.
6. Dowling S, Spooner CH, Liang Y, et al. Accuracy of Ottawa Ankle Rules to exclude fractures of the ankle and midfoot in children: a meta-analysis. *Acad Emerg Med*. 2009;16(4):277-287.
7. Konkel KF, Menger AG, Retzlaff SA. Nonoperative treatment of fifth metatarsal fractures in an orthopaedic suburban private multi-speciality practice. *Foot Ankle Int*. 2005;26:704-707.
8. Portland G, Kelikian A, Kodros S. Acute surgical management of jones' fractures. *Foot Ankle Int*. 2003;24:829-833.
9. Hatch RL, Alsobrook JA, Clugston JR. Diagnosis and management of metatarsal fractures. *Am Fam Physician*. 2007;76(6):817-826.
10. Cakir H, Van Vliet-Koppert ST, Van Lieshout EM, et al. Demographics and outcome of metatarsal fractures. *Arch Orthop Trauma Surg*. 2011;131(2):241-245.

86 CLUB FEET

David S. Ebenezer, MD
Paul M. Saluan, MD

PATIENT STORY

A 4-day-old baby boy is brought to the pediatrician's office for their first visit after birth. The pregnancy was full-term and uneventful, except for that the baby was a breech birth. The baby's mother has noticed that although both legs and feet appear a little "curved," both feet are almost "sideways" and look abnormal (**Figure 86-1**). On examination of both feet the hindfoot is clearly inverted, the toes point medially, and the foot is plantar flexed. The deformity is somewhat correctible by forcing the foot into a more normal position, but not completely. The baby does not appear to be in pain. He has no other abnormalities, has a normal neurologic exam for his age, and appears to be otherwise healthy. The child is referred to a pediatric orthopaedic surgeon, who begins serial Ponseti casting within one to two weeks. After several weeks of weekly serial casting, the feet have a more normal appearance. The child is then splinted full-time using a special orthosis for approximately three months, after which he is only splinted at night until walking age, at which time splinting is discontinued. He has no residual deformity.

INTRODUCTION

Clubfeet is one of the most common congenital abnormalities of the lower extremities.[1] As with any congenital deformity, it can be very concerning to new parents. However, the current gold standard of early non-operative treatment, with surgery only if needed later in life, has led to generally excellent functional results long-term.[2]

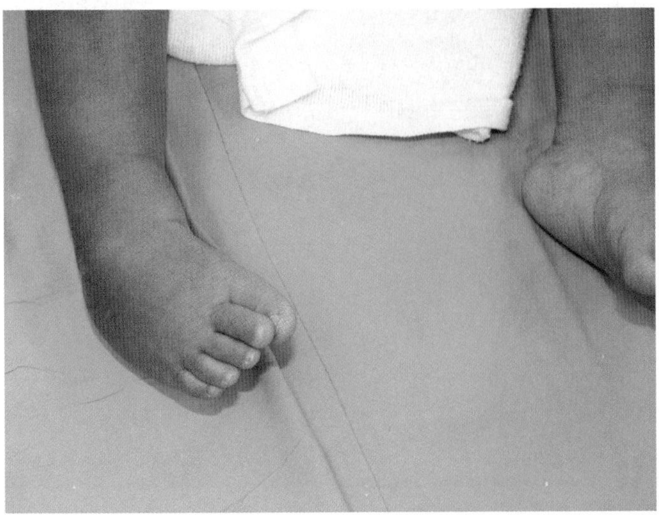

FIGURE 86-1 Bilateral clubfeet in an infant. Note the deepened medial crease (*Used with permission from David Gurd, MD.*)

SYNONYMS

Congenital Talipes Equinovarus.

EPIDEMIOLOGY

- Approximately 1.2 per 1000 live births in Caucasians.[3]
- Varies across cultures, with only 0.39 to 0.5 per 1000 live births in Asian nations to 7 per 1000 live births in the South Pacific.[1,3]
- Two-to-one male predominance across all populations, with 50 percent of cases bilateral.[4]

ETIOLOGY AND PATHOPHYSIOLOGY

- Due to the numerous bones and joints in the foot, a great deal of very descriptive but complicated orthopaedic terminology is associated with understanding the normal and abnormal relationships within the foot. However, this knowledge becomes useful in deciphering and communicating how to correct the deformity.
- The pathophysiology in clubfoot is characterized by four fundamental deformities of the foot, remembered by the mnemonic CAVE:[5]
    - Cavus (a deformity describing a higher or cavitary arch of the foot).
    - Adductus of the forefoot (the rays of the toes abnormally point medially).
    - Varus of the hindfoot (the plantar aspect of the calcaneus points medially if looked at from behind the patient).
    - Equinus (the foot is relatively plantar flexed, usually with a tight Achilles tendon).
- Another useful descriptive term for the forefoot is supination (a combination of inversion and adduction).
- The deformity can vary from mild and very flexible to severe and rigid.[1]
- The etiology is thought to be multifactorial but may include:[1]
    - Genetic factors.
    - Environmental exposure, for example, cigarette smoke.
    - Vascular deficiencies.
    - Abnormal function of the neuromuscular unit.
    - Late-term in utero positioning was historically thought to be a factor, but the evidence appears less likely that it plays a major role in the development of clubfoot.
- May be associated with syndromes such as arthrogryposis, constriction bands (Streeter dysplasia), prune belly, tibial hemimelia, Möbius syndrome, Freeman-Sheldon syndrome, diastrophic dwarfism, Larsen syndrome, Opitz syndrone, and Pierre Robin syndrome.[6]

DIAGNOSIS

CLINICAL FEATURES

- Clubfoot has a very typical appearance.
- After birth clubfoot is primarily a clinical diagnosis based on physical examination showing foot equinus with some degree of cavus, varus, and adductus.[6]

- Frequently the involved calf is smaller in circumference.
- Examination of the skin creases around the foot and ankle can aid in diagnosis.
  - The involved side tends to have a single heel crease, versus multiple on the uninvolved side.[6]
  - The depth of the medial skin crease indicates the severity of the deformity.
- Numerous classification schemes exist, with none entirely prognostic. The system described by Deméglio is most popular to describe severity and track progress of treatment.[5]

IMAGING

- Radiographs can be performed but their role is unclear as the bones of the foot of a newborn are mostly cartilage with ossification centers that are not centered, making the images difficult to interpret.
  - As the bones ossify, classic changes seen include parallelism of the angle made between the long axis of the talus and calcaneus on AP and lateral radiographs when compared to the normal foot (**Figure 86-2**).
  - Clubfoot can be visualized on prenatal ultrasound.
  - Other modalities after birth such as MRI, and CT have been used but are not essential.

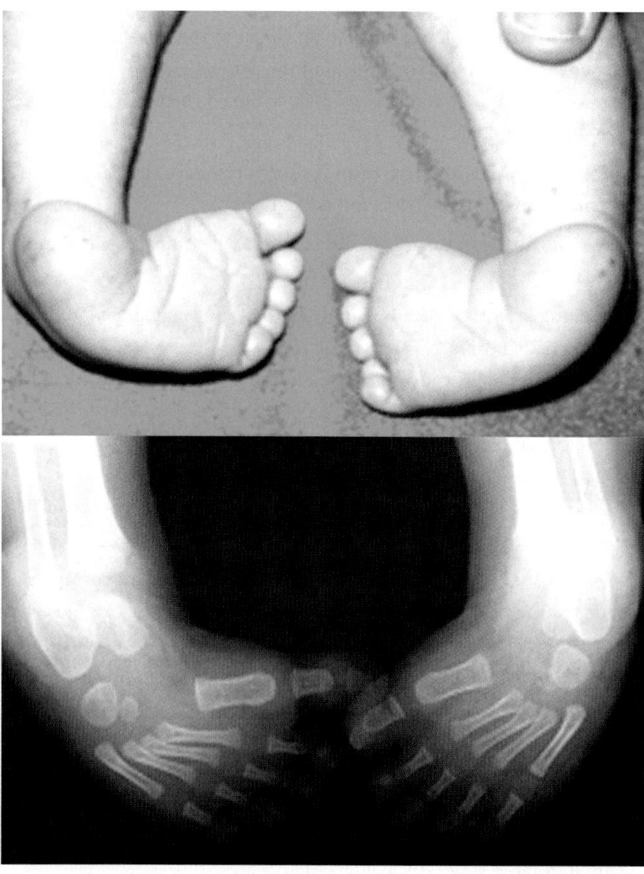

FIGURE 86-2 Bilateral clubfeet with associated radiographic appearance. Note the parallelism of the talus and calcaneus on the radiographs, typical of clubfeet (*Used with permission from Ryan Goodwin, MD.*)

- Radiographs can be useful in cases of tibial hemimelia, or for surgical planning if and when intervention is considered.
- There is a high incidence of associated disorders and syndromes; therefore a full neurologic examination as well as assessment of all joints and the spine is important.[3,6]

DIFFERENTIAL DIAGNOSIS

- Physiologic intrauterine molding/packaging, which results in external rotation of the hips, internal rotation of the tibia, and variable foot position, the combination of which can present with complaints such as "bowed legs" and possibly a foot deformity. These findings are usually mild and usually spontaneously resolve on their own as the child grows.
- Metatarsus Adductus may appear similar to clubfoot, and is one of the component deformities of clubfoot, but can be an isolated entity of its own.[6] In this condition there is no involvement of the hindfoot.
- Congenital vertical talus, characterized by a rocker-bottom foot.[6]

MANAGEMENT

NONSURGICAL

Serial casting has become the preferred choice for initial management of clubfeet among Pediatric Orthopaedic Surgeons over the last decade with dramatic results.[5,7] SOR Ⓐ

- Ideally started within the first month of life.
- Primarily two popular nonsurgical methods utilized today:
  - The Ponseti method of serial casting,
    - Currently the most popular method in the US.[7]
    - Gentle manipulation and casting in a long leg cast (**Figure 86-3**).
    - Casts are changed on a weekly basis.

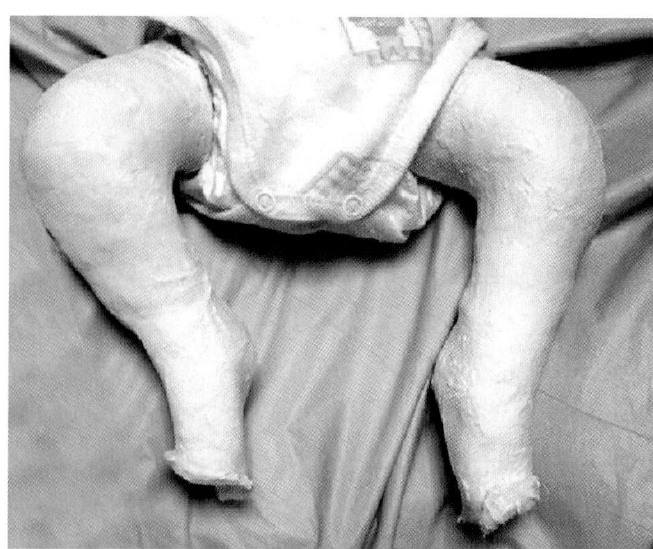

FIGURE 86-3 Bilateral Ponseti casting using plaster casts. The casts must go above the knee as casts below the knee can easily fall off in infants. (*Used with permission from Ryan Goodwin, MD.*)

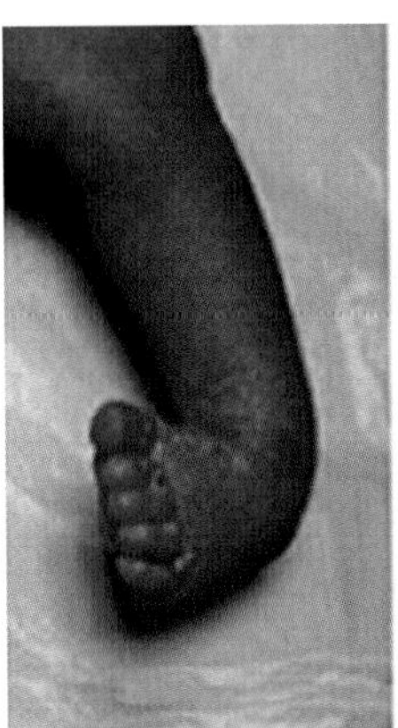
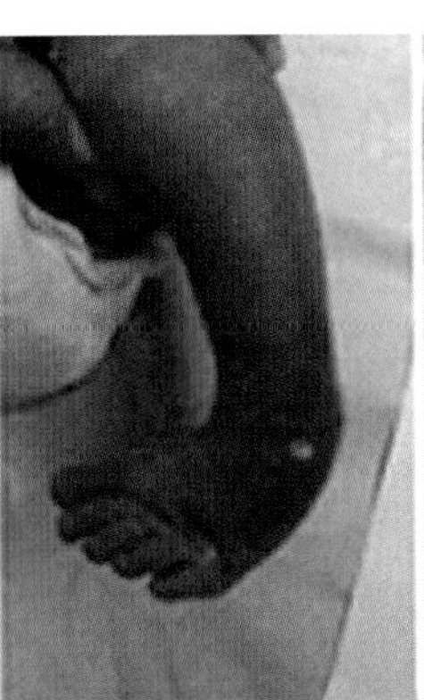
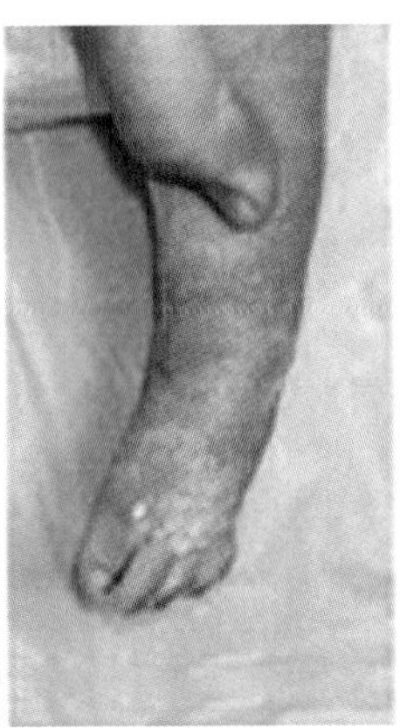
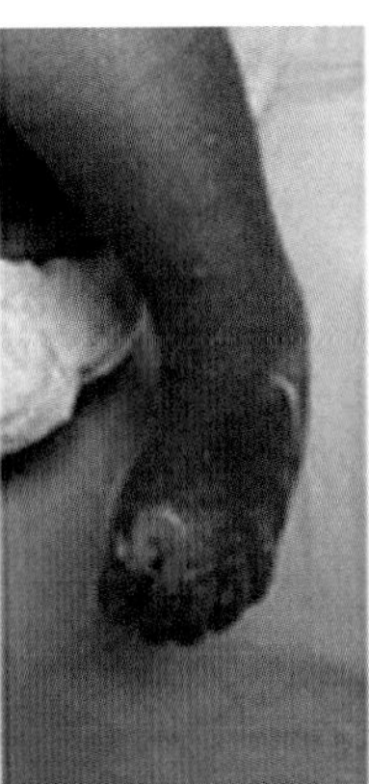
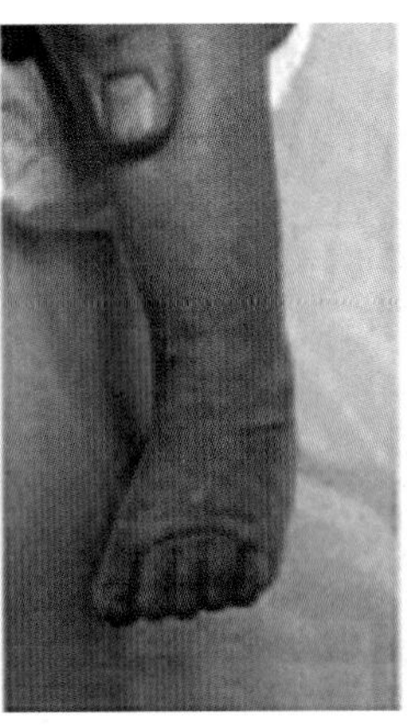
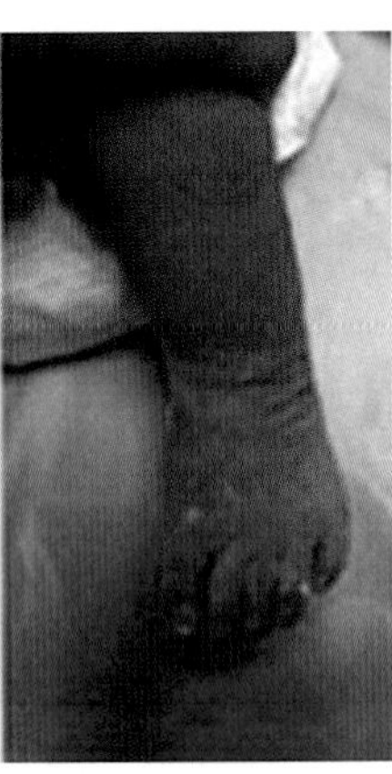

FIGURE 86-4 Time-lapse images of serial Ponseti casting in clubfoot. Note the slow and gradual correction to a normal-appearing foot. (*Used with permission from Ryan Goodwin, MD.*)

        - The mode of deformity correction follows the mnemonic CAVE: first cavus, followed by adductus and then varus; only after all of those are corrected is equinus addressed (**Figure 86-4**).
        - This usually takes between 6 to 8 weeks total.
        - After the fourth or fifth cast, sometimes a percutaneous Achilles tendon tenotomy is performed if there is still an equinus deformity,[1] This usually heals with little to no abnormality of the tendon and no residual weakness,[5] and the foot is casted for 3 to 4 more weeks.
        - Once full correction has been achieved and the final cast is removed, the patient is placed in a foot-abduction brace such as a Denis-Browne bar with the affected foot in approximately 70 degrees of external rotation.[1]
        - This is done 23 hours per day for 3 months, followed by night and nap time wear at least until walking age, although this may be done up to age 4 to prevent recurrence.[1,6]
    - The French method.
        - More dynamic system involving daily manipulations, stretching, and exercises by a trained physical therapist combined with adhesive taping to hold the correction achieved with the therapy.[1,6]
        - Has also incorporated continuous passive motion (CPM) devices into its regimen.[5]
- Compliant patients have been shown to have success with both methods, with minimal difference in success rates between the two, although Ponseti appears to be much more widely used in the US.[8,9]
- Main problem causing recurrence is noncompliance with bracing, which can be treated with recasting and/or subsequent surgery.[9]
- "Successful" nonoperative management often requires an Achilles tendon tenotomy and possibly an anterior tibial tendon transfer to the lateral cuneiform to achieve lasting correction.[1,9]

SURGICAL

- Early operative intervention, with the increased cellularity and collagen response of connective tissues early in life, has been shown to lead to scarring, muscle weakness, pain, recurrence of deformity, damage to neurovascular structures, and overcorrection, and thus should be avoided.[1,3]
- Successful nonoperative treatments have greatly reduced the need for extensive surgical releases and even reduced the overall number of surgeries for clubfoot.[1,6]
- The current trend is toward starting all patients with non-operative management, and approach surgery in a more limited manner, with more selective releases and or tendon transfers as needed to supplement nonoperative management.[1]
- More extensive releases are still required for severe deformity, syndromic clubfoot, neurogenic clubfoot, and refractory recurrent cases.[1,6]
- These can involve release or lengthening of some or all of the soft tissue structures involved, including the Achilles tendon, flexor digitorum longus tendon, flexor hallucis longus tendon, posterior tibial tendon, abductor hallucis, plantar fascia, subtalar and calcaneocuboid capsules, talonavicular capsule, superficial deltoid ligament, talonavicular ("spring") ligament, and the posterior tibiotalar joint capsule.[3]
- Most surgeons prefer to wait until the child is at least 9 months of age to address any of these deformities surgically.[3]
- Many of these extensive releases require reoperation for late loss of correction, or for complications such as wound problems, resultant bony deformity, or overcorrection.
- Some of these late deformities or complications may require osteotomy and bone realignment if the deformity is rigid and cannot be solved by soft tissue releases.
- Very late presentation of severe clubfoot when the child is much older (**Figures 86-5** and **86-6**) may require more heroic efforts, such as treatment with external fixator spatial frames. This presentation is very uncommon in developed countries, however.
- If all other treatments are unsuccessful, eventual joint fusion such as a triple arthrodesis can be performed.

PREVENTION AND SCREENING

- Parents and pediatricians should screen for clubfoot immediately after childbirth and at the first well-child visit.
- Referral to a Pediatric Orthopaedic Surgeon should be made immediately for any suspected clubfoot to allow early treatment and ensure the best possible outcome.

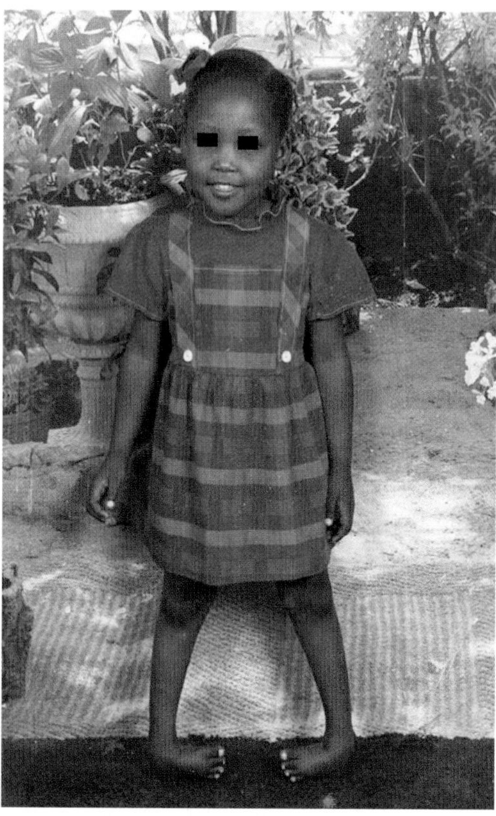

FIGURE 86-5 A young girl with untreated bilateral clubfeet. (*Used with permission from Kaye Wilkins, MD.*)

PROGNOSIS

- With early serial Ponseti casting, compliance with bracing, combined with selective adjunctive surgical procedures (Achilles tenotomy or anterior tibial tendon transfer) in some patients, excellent results have been achieved, reported at 93 to 100 percent.[9]

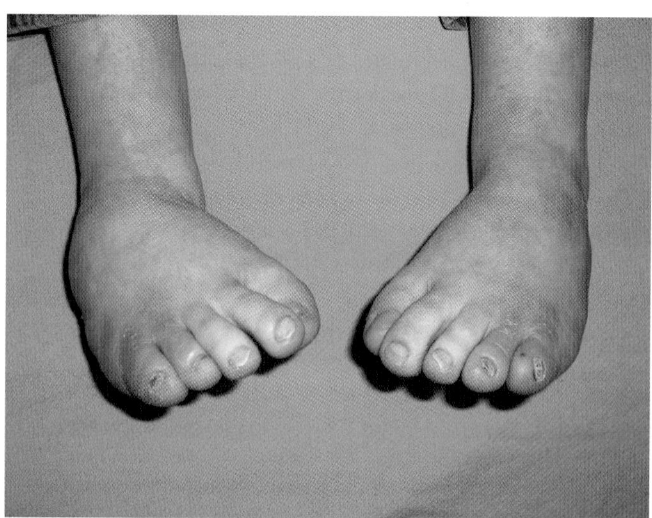

FIGURE 86-6 Late presentation of untreated clubfoot. Note the classic development of calluses along the lateral and dorsal aspect of the foot, reflecting the abnormal areas of the foot the child is forced to walk on due to the deformity. (*Used with permission from Richard Usatine, MD.*)

- Long-term studies have also shown excellent long-term functional results.[2]

FOLLOW-UP

- Children with clubfeet need to be followed very closely while being treated for their serial cast changes, and then for maintenance of correction once they are in the bracing phase.
- These children should continue to be followed periodically into mid-late childhood to monitor for late recurrence.

PATIENT EDUCATION

- Clubfoot has excellent success with nonoperative management and limited surgical intervention as needed.
- It is important to see a pediatrician and have the child seen by an orthopaedic surgeon within the first few weeks of life to start treatment. Late treatment is not as successful.
- Even with successful treatment, brace compliance is critical to long-term success.

PATIENT RESOURCES

- Ponseti International Website—**www.ponseti.info**.
- **www.nlm.nih.gov/medlineplus/ency/article/001228.htm**.
- **www.healthychildren.org/English/health-issues/conditions/developmental-disabilities/Pages/Congenital-Abnormalities.aspx**.
- **www.my.clevelandclinic.org/orthopaedics-rheumatology/diseases-conditions/congenital-clubfoot.aspx**.

PROVIDER RESOURCES

- **www.accesspediatrics.com/content.aspx?aid=7020352#7020390**.
- **www.accesspediatrics.com/content.aspx?aid=56825070#56825073**.

REFERENCES

1. Dobbs MD, Gurnett CA. Update on clubfoot: etiology and treatment. *Clin Orthop Relat Res*. 2009;467(5):1146-53.
2. Cooper DM, Deitz FR. Treatment of idiopathic clubfoot: A thirty-year follow up note. *J Bone Joint Surg Am*. 1995;77:1477-1489.
3. Roye DP Jr, Roye BD. Idiopathic Congenital Talipes Equinovarus. *J Am Acad Orthop Surg*. 2002;10(4):239-48.
4. Wynne-Davies R. Genetic and environmental factors in the etiology of talipes equinovarus. *Clin Orthop Relat Res*. 1972;84: 29-38.
5. Noonan KJ, Richards BS. Nonsurgical Management of idiopathic clubfoot. *J Am Acad Orthop Surg*. 2003;11(6):392-402.

6. Kasser, JR. The Foot, in Lovell and Winter's Pediatric Orthopaedics, edited by Morrissy RT, Weinstein SL. Philadelphia, PA: Lippencott Williams and Wilkins; 2006:1262-1277.

7. Heilig MR, Matern RV, Rosenzweig SD, Bennet JT. Current management of idiopathic clubfoot questionnaire: a multicentric study. *J Pediatr Orthop.* 2003;23(6):780-787.

8. Richards BS, Faulks S, Rathjen KE, Karol LA, Johnston CE, Jones SA. A comparison of two nonoperative methods of idiopathic clubfoot correction: the Ponseti method and the French functional (physiotherapy) method. *J Bone Joint Surg Am.* 2008;90(11): 2313-2321.

9. Abdelgawad AA, Lehman WB, van Bosse HJ, Scher DM, Sala DA. Treatment of idiopathic clubfoot using the Ponseti method: minimum 2-year follow up. *J Pediatr Orthop B.* 2007;16(2): 98-105.

87 DEVELOPMENTAL DYSPLASIA OF THE HIP

Rachel M. Randall
R. Tracy Ballock, MD

PATIENT STORY

A three day old female was brought to her pediatrician for a routine newborn evaluation. Prenatally, the infant was noted by ultrasound to be in the frank breech position, and was born via Cesarean section at 40 weeks of gestation. She is the mother's first child. At this visit, the pediatrician noted that the infant's left thigh segment was shorter than the right, and a palpable "clunk" was felt when pressure was applied to lift the greater trochanter and the left hip was abducted (**Figure 87-1**). The pediatrician ordered an ultrasound of the left hip joint, which revealed a dislocated femoral head. The patient was subsequently placed in a Pavlik harness. After three months, the hip was completely reduced and stable on exam, and the harness was discontinued. Her standing x-ray of the hips at one year was normal.

INTRODUCTION

Developmental Dysplasia of the Hip (DDH) is a disorder of acetabular development leading to a shallow acetabulum (acetabular dysplasia), which may or may not be associated with an unstable or dislocated hip joint.[1]

SYNONYMS

Hip dysplasia, Congenitally dislocated hip.

EPIDEMIOLOGY

- Most common in females, especially those of Native American descent.

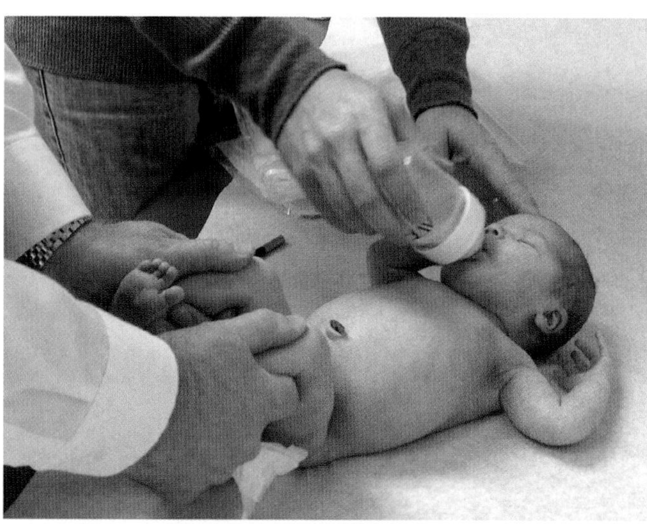

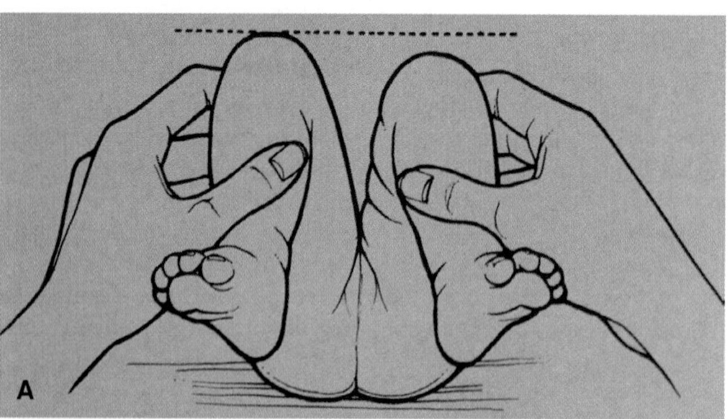

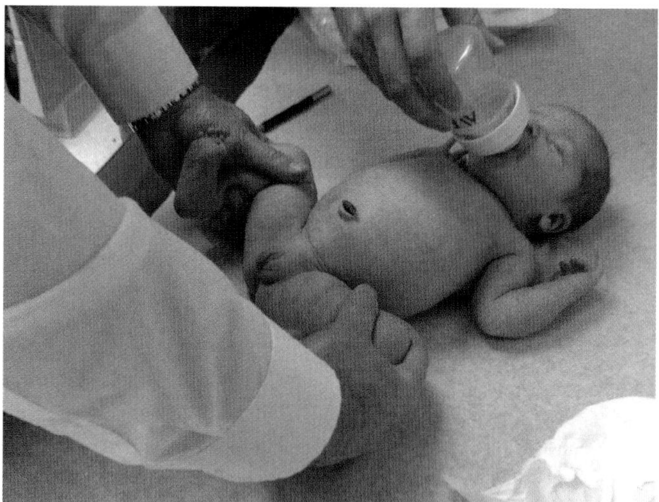

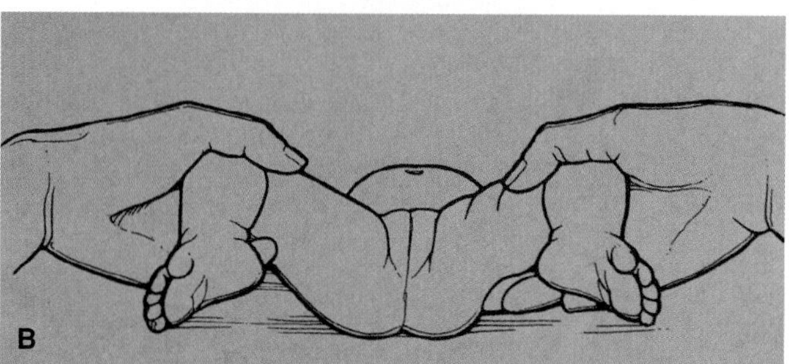

FIGURE 87-1 Physical exam maneuvers for assessment of Developmental Dysplasia of the Hip (DDH). Note that the infant must be calm and relaxed for accurate assessment of these subtle findings. (**A**) Barlow sign (Photo). Gentle posterior pressure over the knee, with hips and knees flexed to 90 degrees, causes subluxation of the femoral head. Galeazzi sign (Sketch). With the hips and knees flexed to 90 degrees, discrepancy of the length of the thigh segment can be evaluated. In DDH, the thigh segment on that side may appear shorter than the unaffected side. (**B**) Ortolani maneuver. Lifting the greater trochanter upwards with the hip maximally abducted causes the dislocated femoral head to reduce back into the acetabulum. (*Sketches Adapted and Reprinted with permission from Ballock and Richards, Contemporary Pediatrics 1997;14:108. Contemporary Pediatrics is a copyrighted publication of Advanstar Communications Inc. All rights reserved.*)

- Incidence of DDH is approximately 1 in 100 live births, but only 1 in 1000 requires treatment.
- Can be discovered in neonates, infancy, or later in childhood.

ETIOLOGY AND PATHOPHYSIOLOGY

- Intrauterine positioning is crucial for proper development of the acetabulum.
- Intrauterine crowding can result in excessive hip flexion and adduction, which leads to acetabular flattening, stretching of the labrum, and ultimately hip joint instability.
- Frank breech positioning and oligohydramnios are the most common causes of intrauterine crowding.

RISK FACTORS

- Breech positioning (especially frank breech, 20 percent risk).
- Positive family history of DDH.
- First born.
- Female (6:1).
- Disorders associated with ligamentous laxity (i.e., Ehlers-Danlos).
- Oligohydramnios.
- Postnatal positioning with hips held in extension.
- Infrequently associated with torticollis and metatarsus adductus.

DIAGNOSIS

CLINICAL FEATURES

- Galeazzi sign—Shortened thigh segment with the hip and knee flexed to 90 degrees compared to the unaffected side (**Figure 87-1A**). One may also see asymmetric skin folds, with excessive folds over the affected side due to superior/posterior dislocation of the femur.
- Barlow sign—Palpable "clunk" with hip adduction and posterior pressure applied on the femur, with the hip and knee flexed to 90 degrees (**Figure 87-1A**). Indicates subluxation of the femoral head out of the acetabulum.
- Ortolani sign—Palpable "clunk" with abduction and anterior pressure applied over the greater trochanter (**Figure 87-1B**). Indicates reduction of a dislocated femoral head.
- In children older than 3 months with DDH, the femur becomes fixed in a dislocated position, and the Barlow and Ortolani tests are no longer helpful. Instead, the prominent physical exam finding is limited abduction on the affected side due to tightening of the adductor muscles (**Figure 87-2**). However, if the DDH is bilateral, the limited abduction is difficult to appreciate. If the child is of walking age, he or she may have a waddling gait, with the unaffected side of the pelvis "dropping" as the child bears weight on the affected side, as well as lumbar hyperlordosis. This is due to weakened abductor muscles on the affected hip.

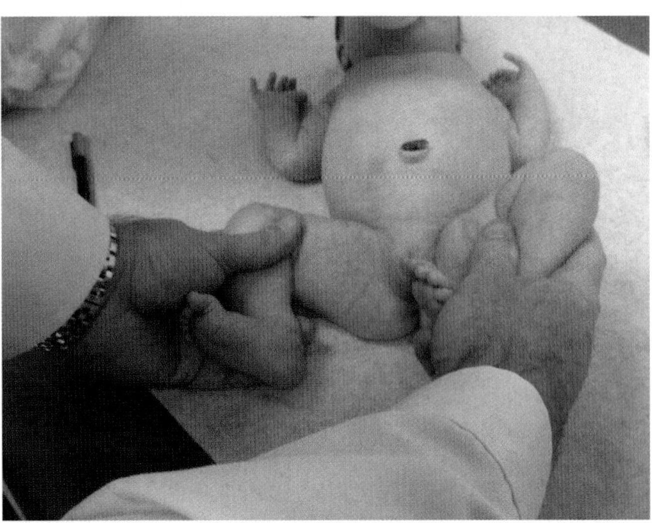

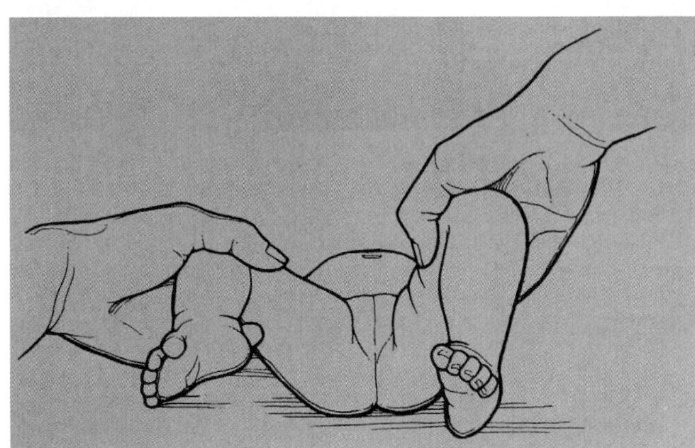

FIGURE 87-2 Limited abduction of the affected left hip. Tight adductor and iliopsoas muscles are often associated with DDH in children older than 3 months, where the femur is in a fixed position out of socket. (*Sketches Adapted and Reprinted with permission from Ballock and Richards, Contemporary Pediatrics 1997;14:108. Contemporary Pediatrics is a copyrighted publication of Advanstar Communications Inc. All rights reserved.*)

DISTRIBUTION

The left hip is disproportionately affected (67 percent of DDH cases) due to the positioning of the left femur against the spinal column in the most common fetal position (left occiput anterior).[1] However, DDH may affect either side or it may be bilateral.

LABORATORY TESTING

- Not usually indicated unless a septic dislocation is suspected.

IMAGING

All infants with breech positioning, a positive family history of DDH, or oligohydramnios should have a screening ultrasound at 6 weeks of age or an AP radiograph at 3 months of age.[2]

- Ultrasound—Best imaging modality before 3 months of age due to the cartilaginous nature of the immature hip joint. Used for evaluation of the degree of hip subluxation or dislocation.
- X-ray—Typically used for diagnosis in children 3 months of age or older at initial presentation. Does not show the anatomic detail or soft tissue structures that ultrasound offers, but can be interpreted

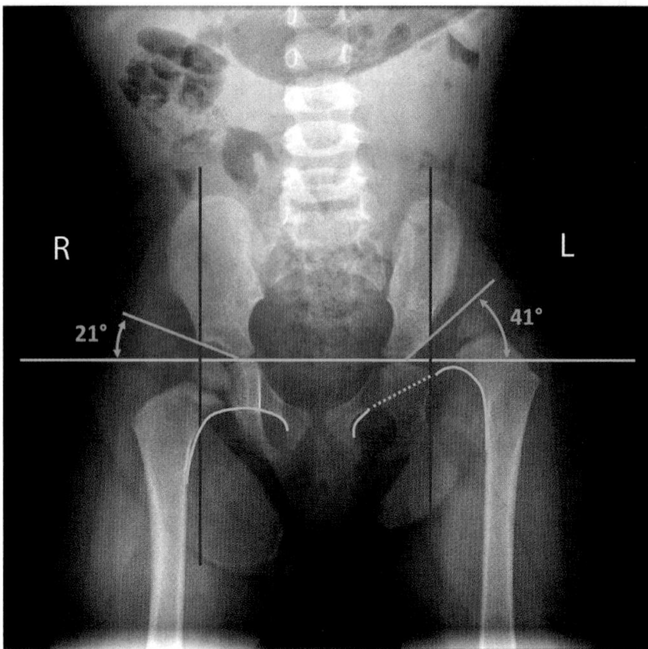

FIGURE 87-3 X-ray of a pelvis with a normal R hip and DDH of the left hip. Hilgenreiner's line (orange), Perkin's line (red), and Shenton's line (green) are shown bilaterally. Note that Shenton's line appears broken on the DDH side. The Acetabular index (blue line and angle) is normal if *less* than 25 to 27 degrees, and decreases with age as the acetabular depth increases. Note how the DDH side has an Acetabular index of 41 degrees. (*Used with permission from R. Tracy Ballock, MD.*)

FIGURE 87-4 Arthrogram of DDH hip. Medial dye pooling, commonly seen in DDH, indicates subluxation of the femoral head (solid arrow). Blunting of the labrum is also seen in this arthrogram (broken arrow). (*Used with permission from R. Tracy Ballock, MD.*)

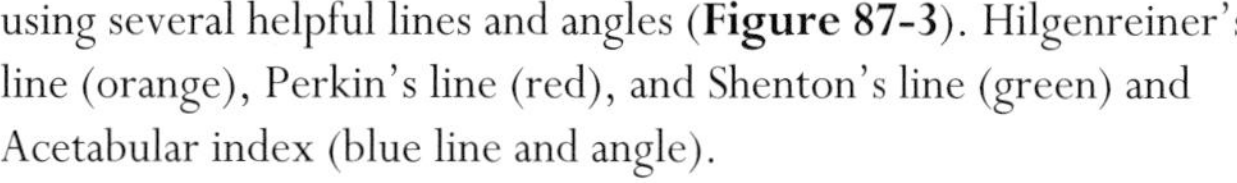

using several helpful lines and angles (**Figure 87-3**). Hilgenreiner's line (orange), Perkin's line (red), and Shenton's line (green) and Acetabular index (blue line and angle).

- Arthrogram—Radio-opaque dye injected directly into the hip joint. Useful for visualizing the cartilaginous femoral head and its relationship to the acetabulum.
  - Medial pooling of dye indicates an abnormal space where the femoral head is normally located (**Figure 87-4**).
  - Shape of the capsule can be distorted by abnormal iliopsoas compression of the capsule (hourglass sign), or an inverted labrum from femoral head subluxation (rose thorn sign).

DIFFERENTIAL DIAGNOSIS

- Septic hip—Usually associated with marked irritability and systemic signs of illness.
- Coxa vara—Varus angulation of the proximal femur.
- Teratologic dislocation of the hip—Associated with neuromuscular conditions, such as arthrogryposis and spina bifida.

MANAGEMENT

NONPHARMACOLOGIC

- Abduction orthosis (such as the Pavlik harness) is most commonly used modality for young infants (**Figure 87-5**).

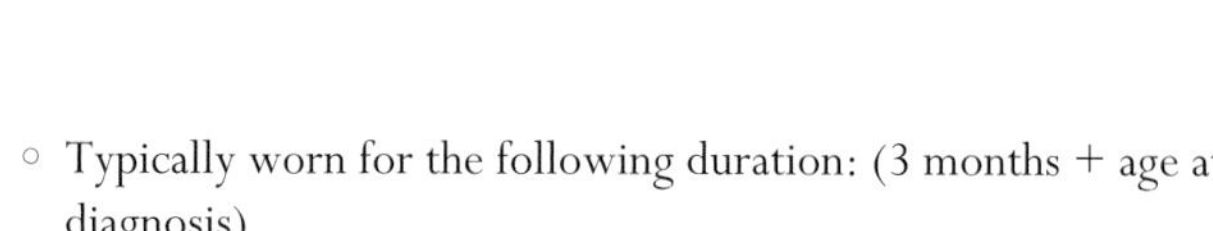

  - Typically worn for the following duration: (3 months + age at diagnosis).
  - Much less effective for infants older than 6 months.
- Observation for stable hips with isolated acetabular dysplasia.

COMPLIMENTARY/ALTERNATIVE THERAPY

- Double- or triple-diapering is not effective as a treatment modality for DDH.[2]

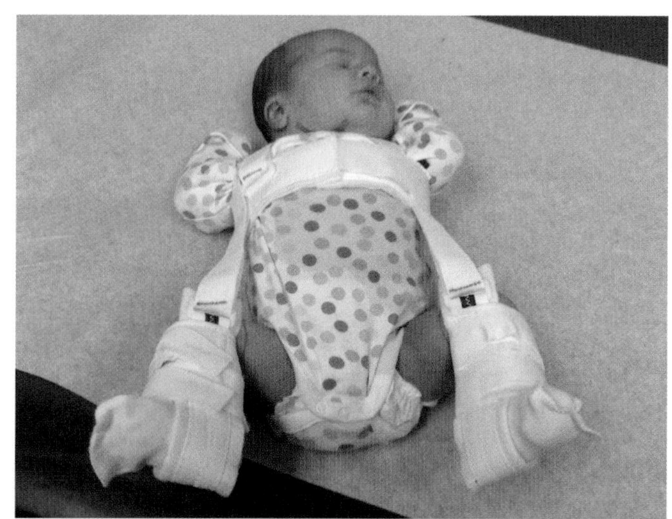

FIGURE 87-5 Pavlik harness for treatment of DDH in infants. The hips are held in 100-120 degrees of flexion and abducted to promote hip stability. (*Used with permission from R. Tracy Ballock, MD.*)

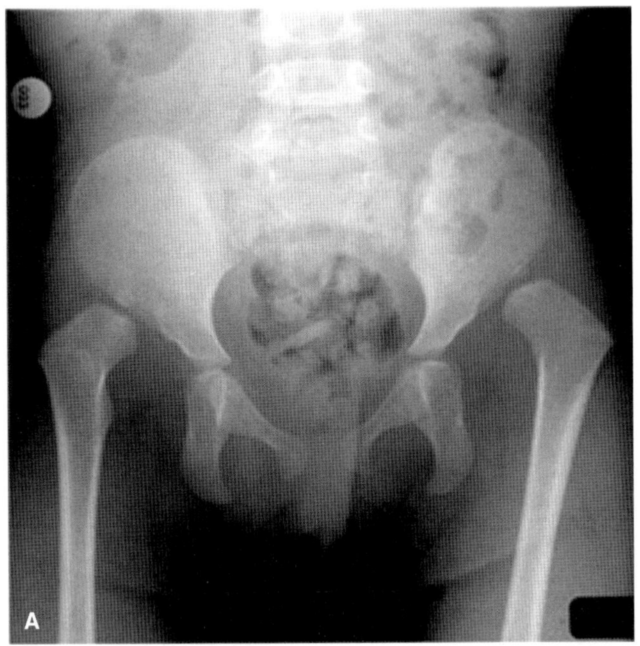

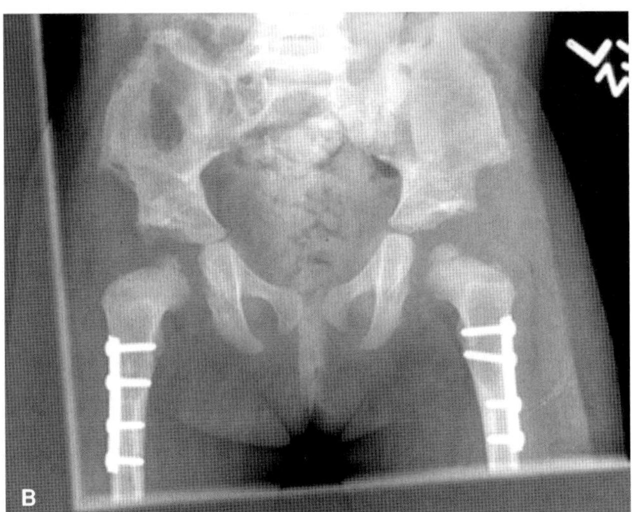

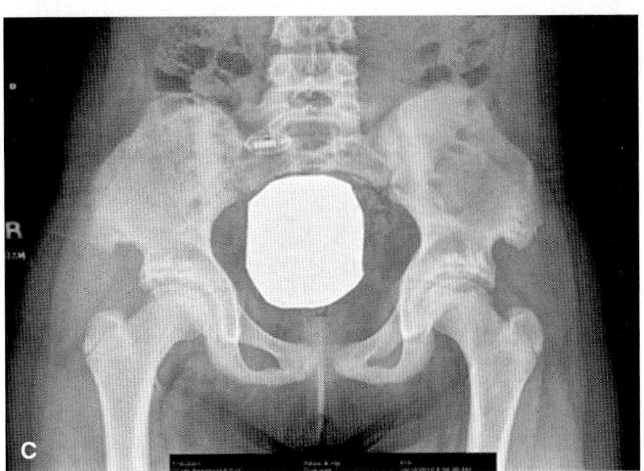

FIGURE 87-6 DDH before and after surgical treatment. X-ray of bilateral DDH before surgery in a 2-year-old female (**A**), postoperatively following Salter innominate osteotomy and femoral shortening osteotomy (**B**), and at long-term follow-up at 11-years of age (**C**). Note the well-formed acetabula following the pelvic osteotomy, and concentric reduction of the femoral heads bilaterally. *(Used with permission from R. Tracy Ballock, MD.)*

SURGERY

- Closed reduction, adductor lengthening tenotomy, spica casting (4 to 6 months of age).
- Open reduction, capsulorrhaphy (>9 months of age).
- Acetabuloplasty (>18 months of age).
  - If triradiate cartilage open—Salter (**Figure 87-6**) or Pemberton osteotomy.
  - If triradiate cartilage closed—Ganz or Steele (Triple) osteotomy.
  - Salvage procedures—Shelf acetabuloplasty, Chiari osteotomy.
- Femoral derotational osteotomy in older children to correct abnormal rotation, and shortening to allow for reduction of the hip joint without excessive stress (**Figure 87-6**).

REFERRAL

Referral to a pediatric orthopedic surgeon is appropriate when clinical signs of DDH are evident on physical examination.

SCREENING

- Every newborn should be screened by physical examination, and subsequently at every well-baby visit until the age of 12 months.[2]
- Children with risk factors including breech presentation in utero or positive family history should be screened with either an ultrasound at 6 weeks or radiograph at 3 months to detect silent acetabular dysplasia.[2]

PROGNOSIS

- Conservative treatment produces excellent results if DDH is diagnosed early.
- Pavlik harness success rate is 95 percent if instituted within the first 6 weeks of life.[1]

FOLLOW-UP

- Serial physical examination for children with risk factors for DDH.
- Pelvic radiographs every 3 to 6 months until age 3 for children with acetabular dysplasia, then every year until age 5, and every 3 years until skeletal maturity for clinical DDH.

PATIENT AND PROVIDER RESOURCES

- **www.orthoinfo.aaos.org/topic.cfm?topic=a00347**.
- **www.aafp.org/afp/2006/1015/p1310.html**.
- **www.tsrhc.org/developmental-hip-dysplasia.htm**.
- **www.emedicine.medscape.com/article/1248135**.

REFERENCES

1. Herring JA. Tachdjian's Pediatric Orthopaedics, 4th edition. Chapter 16: Developmental Dysplasia of the Hip. Saunders-Elsevier, Philadelphia, PA; 2008: 637-770.

2. Committee on Quality Improvement, Subcommittee on Developmental Dysplasia of the Hip: Clinical Practice Guideline: Early Detection of Developmental Dysplasia of the Hip. *American Academy of Pediatrics*. 2000;105(4):896-905.
3. American Academy of Orthopaedic Surgeons: Developmental Dislocation (Dysplasia) of the Hip (DDH). http://orthoinfo.aaos.org/topic.cfm?topic=a00347. Rosemont, IL, 2009.
4. American Academy of Family Physicians: Developmental Dysplasia of the Hip. http://www.aafp.org/afp/2006/1015/p1310.html. Leawood, KS, 2006.
5. Texas Scottish Rite Children's Hospital: Hip Dysplasia and Perthes. http://www.tsrhc.org/developmental-hip-dysplasia.htm. Dallas, TX, 2011.
6. Ballock RT, Richards BS. Hip Dysplasia: Early diagnosis makes a difference. *Contemporary Pediatrics*. 1997;14:108.

88 LEGG-CALVÉ-PERTHES

Keith Bachmann, MD
Ryan C. Goodwin, MD

PATIENT STORY

A 7-year-old boy presents with his parents with a month-long history of "running funny" while playing baseball this season. He does not complain of any pain and has not had any problems like this in the past. The patient and family deny any trauma, fevers, or chills. Radiograph of his pelvis is obtained and shows the early stages of Legg-Calve-Perthes disease (**Figure 88-1**).

INTRODUCTION

Legg-Calvé-Perthes (LCP) disease is a juvenile form of idiopathic osteonecrosis of the femoral head. First described in 1910 as an entity separate from tuberculosis by Legg, Calvé, and Perthes in separate accounts. It still carries unresolved controversy regarding the etiology, pathogenesis, and management.

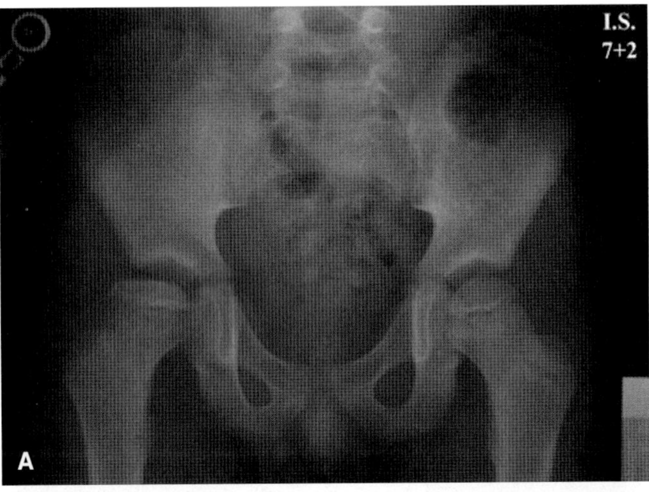

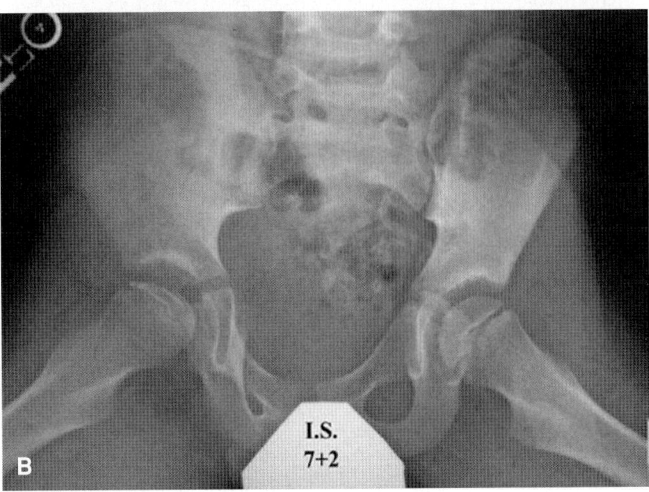

FIGURE 88-1 Initial stage of Perthes disease showing femoral head flattening of the right femoral head in a 7-year-old boy on AP (**A**) and Frog-leg lateral (**B**) radiographs of the pelvis. (*Used with permission from Ryan Goodwin, MD.*)

SYNONYMS

Perthes disease.

EPIDEMIOLOGY

- Can affect a wide age range of children aged 2 to 14 years, but most common at 5 to 8 years of age.
- Male to female ratio 5:1.
- Bilateral in 10 to 15 percent of cases.[1]
- Incidence is 5.1 to 16.9 per 100,000.[2]

ETIOLOGY AND PATHOPHYSIOLOGY[2]

ETIOLOGY

- Probably multifactorial, exact cause still uncertain.
- Possible factors—Trauma, susceptible child, hereditary factors, coagulopathy, hyperactivity, passive smoking, or collagen abnormality.[3]
- Unlikely factors—Endocrinopathy, urban environment, or synovitis.[3]
- Disruption of blood supply to the femoral head and a pathologic repair process cause imbalance of bone resorption and formation.[1]
- Current research focusing on cause of the vascular disruption including a missense mutation in the type II collagen gene in familial cases, thrombophilia also being investigated as possible cause although there are cases of LCP disease without either of these abnormalities.[1]

PATHOPHYSIOLOGY[1]

- Disruption of blood supply affects articular cartilage, bony epiphysis, physis, and metaphysis.
- Cartilage:
  - Necrosis especially in the deep layer, cessation of enchondral ossification, separation from underlying bone followed by revascularization and new accessory ossification.
- Bony Epiphysis:
  - Necrosis of marrow space, compression fractures of trabeculae, fibrovascular granulation tissue invasion, or osteoclastic resorption.
- Physis:
  - Focal areas of growth cartilage columns extending below the endochondral ossification line mostly in the anterior aspect of the femoral head.
- Metaphysis:
  - Physeal cartilage columns as mentioned above, fibrocartilage, fat necrosis, vascular proliferation, and fibrosis all described.

DIAGNOSIS

CLINICAL FEATURES

- Mild pain in groin, anterior hip, or around greater trochanter, knee pain.
- Limp exacerbated by activity that improves with rest.
- Insidious onset but commonly with antecedent trauma.
- Hip irritability (increased pain with motion) due to synovitis.
- Possible Trendelenburg gait (leaning over affected hip).
- Trendelenburg sign—Unaffected side of pelvis drops when standing on affected hip alone and body sways to affected side.
- Possible hip motion limitations depending on stage of disease—Lose abduction and internal rotation first. If in fragmentation stage severe restrictions:
  - Possible limb length discrepancy.
  - Possible thigh and calf muscle atrophy.

LABORATORY TESTING

- No laboratory abnormalities in LCP itself, may reveal an alternate diagnosis through laboratory studies.

IMAGING

- Plain x-rays, AP Pelvis, AP and Lateral views of the hip sufficient.
- Imaging classically involves four radiographic stages: initial (**Figures 88-1**), fragmentation (**Figure 88-2**), reossification, and healed.
- During the initial and fragmentation stages may see flattening of the femoral head that may improve, worsen, or remain unchanged in the reossification stage.
- MRI can show changes in the perfusion of the femoral head potentially helping predict progression but this is still in the early stages of clinical use.

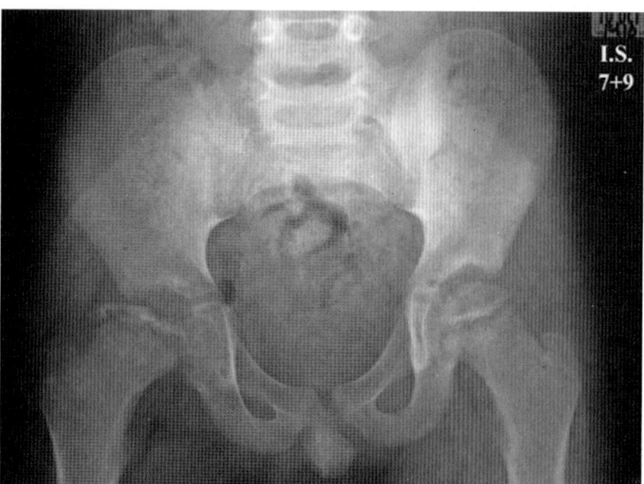

FIGURE 88-2 AP Pelvis radiograph of the same boy as in **Figure 88-1** in the fragmentation stage, demonstrating some lateral subluxation of the right femoral head (*Used with permission from Ryan Goodwin, MD.*)

- X-rays in the healed phase may help classify the patient into the Stulberg classification:
  - Stulberg I: normal hip joint.
  - Stulberg II: Spherical head with enlargement, short neck, or steep acetabulum.
  - Stulberg III: Nonspherical head.
  - Stulberg IV: Flat head.
  - Stulberg V: Flat head with incongruent joint.

DIFFERENTIAL DIAGNOSIS[3,4]

Other causes of a limping child:

- Fracture (Toddler's fracture, Stress Fracture, Physela Fracture)—Can usually be excluded based on history and radiographs.
- Osteomyelitis, Septic Arthritis, Diskitis—Usually accompanied by acute presentation, fever, and systemic symptoms.
- Slipped Capital Femoral Epiphysis—Usually apparent on plain radiographs.
- Arthritis (juvenile rheumatoid, Lyme disease)—Usually diagnosed clinically with the appearance of frank arthritis and evidence of inflammation on laboratory testing.
- Transient synovitis—Preceding upper respiratory tract infection is common.
- Osteochondritis dissecans (knee or ankle)—Knee and ankle pain more prominent.

Other causes of avascular necrosis include:

- Sickle cell disease and hemoglobinopathies—Secondary to vaso-occlusive disease. History of chronic disease usually apparent.
- Steroid use—History of prolonged steroid use usually apparent.
- Traumatic dislocation—History of trauma apparent.
- Iatrogenic—No clear pathogenetic mechanism.
- Epiphyseal Dysplasias including Multiple epiphyseal dysplasia, Spondyloepiphyseal dysplasia, mucopolysaccharidoses, or hypothyroidism—Chronic disorders apparent by history.

MANAGEMENT

NONPHARMACOLOGIC

- Rest followed by abduction exercises (physical therapy).
- Containment Bracing, most frequently studied is a Scottish Rite Orthosis (largely historical).
- Petrie casting (containment).

MEDICATIONS

- No medications to treat or reverse the disease process have been discovered.
- Symptomatic treatment with anti-inflammatory medications may be beneficial. SOR Ⓒ
- Steroids can cause avascular necrosis and would not be recommended.

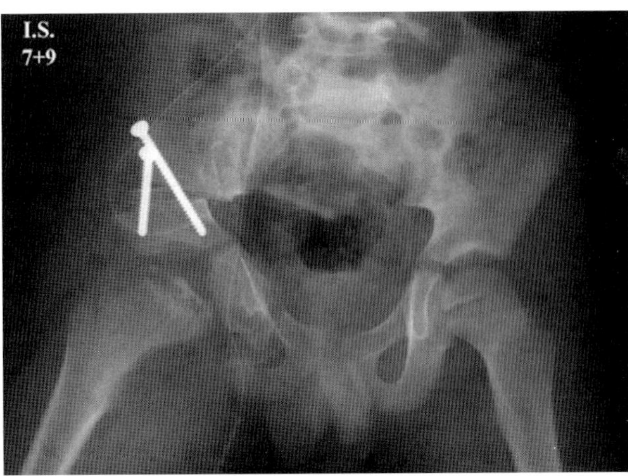

FIGURE 88-3 AP Pelvis radiograph of the same boy as in **Figures 88-1** and **88-2** after undergoing a pelvic osteotomy to obtain better coverage and contain the right femoral head. (*Used with permission from Ryan Goodwin, MD.*)

SURGERY[5]

- Options depend on age at presentation (see the following) and include:
  - Arthrogram.
  - Adductor tenotomy.
  - Petrie casting.
  - Femoral varus osteotomy.
  - Pelvic osteotomy (**Figures 88-3** and **88-4**).
  - Combined procedure.
- Management depends on age at presentation.
  - Less than 6 years of age at onset.
    - Most (80%) achieve good results (Stulberg I/II hips) at maturity with physiotherapy or bracing.
    - This will still leave one to two out of every five patients with a poor outcome, but currently no ability to predict those who will have a poor outcome.
  - Age at onset between 6 and 8 years.
    - Results are mixed in current studies, one showing a significant difference in outcomes with better results obtained with surgical treatment[6] while another showed no difference.[7]
  - Age at onset >8 years.

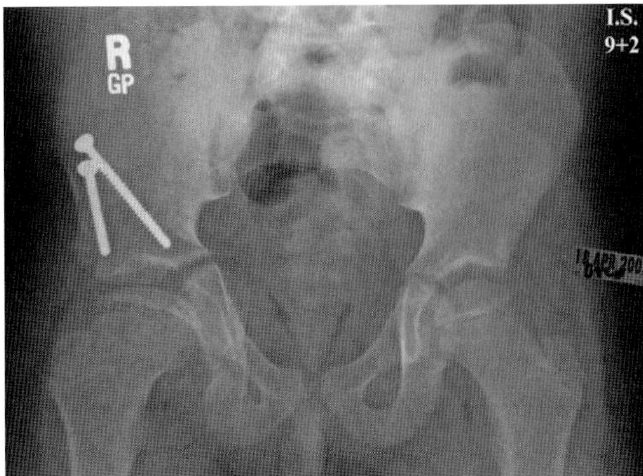

FIGURE 88-4 AP Pelvis radiograph of the same patient as in **Figures 88-1** to **88-3** after healing with a final Stulberg II result. (*Used with permission from Ryan Goodwin, MD.*)

    - Results in follow-up studies favors surgical management although even with this treatment results are still modest with 2/3 achieving Stulberg I/II hips. SOR Ⓒ
- Long term follow-up from Iowa with mean 47.7 years follow up showed only 40 percent of patients with LCP maintained a good level of function, 40 percent underwent total hip arthroplasty (**Figures 88-5** and **88-6**), 10 percent had disabling pain, and 10 percent had poor function.[8]

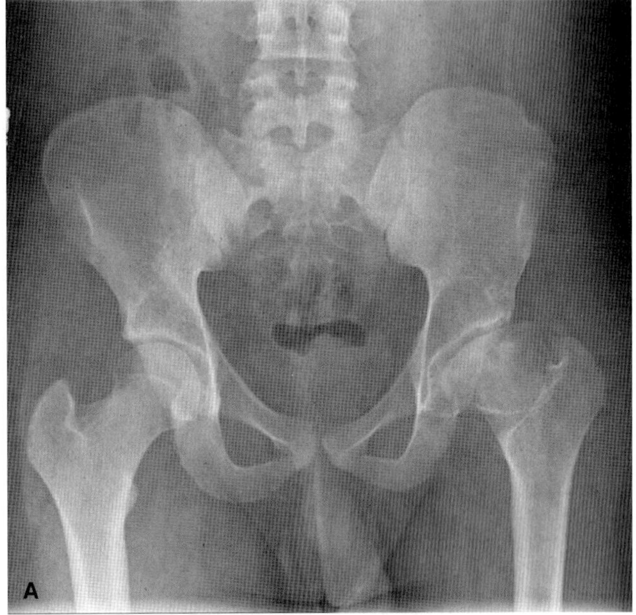

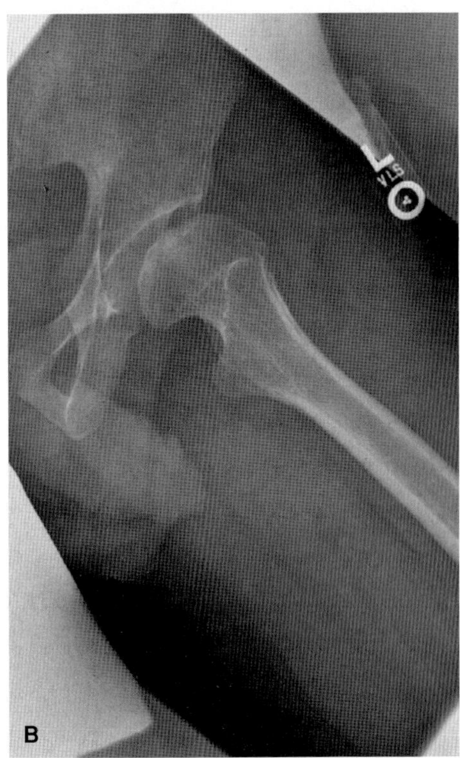

FIGURE 88-5 Legg-Calve-Perthes disease of the left femoral head with a Stulberg IV hip in a 19-year old male. AP (**A**) and lateral (**B**) pelvis radiograph. Note the flattening of the head and uncovering of the lateral aspect on the lateral view. This patient required a total hip replacement. (*Used with permission from Ryan Goodwin, MD.*)

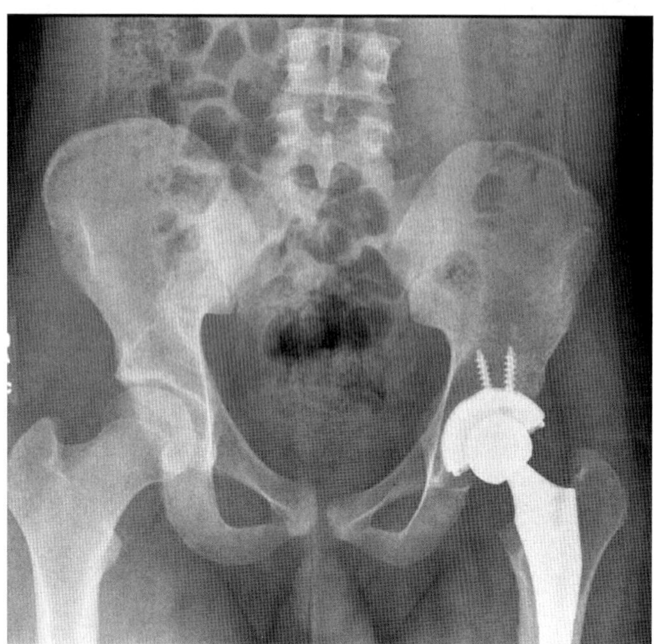

FIGURE 88-6 AP Pelvis radiograph of the patient from **Figure 88-5** after a total hip arthroplasty. (*Used with permission from Ryan Goodwin, MD.*)

REFERRAL

- A Pediatric orthopedic surgeon should be involved in the care of children with LCP to discuss options and institute the preceding therapies.

PREVENTION AND SCREENING

- A high degree of suspicion should be kept in relatives of patients with known LCP disease presenting with a typical story, but there is no routine screening recommended at this time, even in relatives of those with known disease.

FOLLOW-UP

- Should be with a pediatric orthopedic surgeon.
- The radiographic stage at presentation as well as age at presentation will determine treatment and further follow-up.

PATIENT EDUCATION

- Parents should be educated that LCP disease is an evolving clinical entity with multivariable etiology. It is not life-threatening and usually resolves without surgery.

PATIENT RESOURCES

- **www.mayoclinic.com/health/legg-calve-perthes-disease/DS00654.**
- **www.nonf.org/perthesbrochure/perthes-brochure.htm.**

PROVIDER RESOURCES

- **www.mdconsult.com/das/pdxmd/body/389636709-3/0?type=med&eid=9-u1.0-_1_mt_5082301&tab=L.**

REFERENCES

1. Kim HKW. Legg-Calvé-Perthes Disease. *Journal of the American Academy of Orthopaedic Surgeons*. 2010;18(11):676-686.
2. Kim HKW. Pathophysiology and New Strategies for the Treatment of Legg-Calvé-Perthes Disease. *The Journal of Bone and Joint Surgery*. 2012;94-A(7):659-669.
3. Herring JA, Kim HT, Browne R. Legg-Calve-Perthes Disease Part II: Prospective Multicenter Study of the Effect of Treatment on Outcome. *The Journal of Bone and Joint Surgery*. 2004;86(10):2121-2134.
4. Flynn JM, Widmann RF. The Limping Child: Evaluation and Diagnosis. *The Journal of the American Academy of Orthopaedic Surgeons*. 2001;9(2):89-98.
5. Schoenecker PL, Clohisy JC, Millis MB, Wenger DR. Surgical Management of the Problematic Hip in Adolescent and Young Adult Patients. *Journal of the American Academy of Orthopaedic Surgeons*. 2011;19(5):275-286.
6. Wiig O, Terjesen T, Svenningsen S. Prognostic factors and outcome of treatment in Perthes' disease: A prospective study of 368 patients with five-year follow-up. *The Journal of Bone and Joint Surgery [Br]*. 2008;90(10):1362-1371.
7. Herring JA, ed: Legg-Calvé-Perthes Disease. In: *Tachdjian's Pediatric Orthopaedics*. Fourth. Philadelphia, PA: Saunders Elsevier; 2008: 771-826.
8. McAndrew M, Weinstein S. A Long Term Follow-up of Legg-Calve-Perthes Disease. *J Bone Joint Surg [Am]*. 1984;66(6):860-869.

89 SLIPPED CAPITAL FEMORAL EPIPHYSIS (SCFE)

Joel Kolmodin, MD
Paul M. Saluan, MD

PATIENT STORY

A 10-year-old male presents to your office with a 1-month history of left groin pain and intermittent left medial thigh pain as well. His symptoms are typically worse with activity, and his parents have noted that he limps. His parents relate that he has had a similar problems in the past. An x-ray of the left hip shows a slipped capital femoral epiphysis (**Figures 89-1** and **89-2**). The patient is made non-weight bearing, he is immediately admitted to the hospital and Pediatric Orthopedics is consulted for surgical management.

INTRODUCTION

Slipped capital femoral epiphysis (SCFE) is a relatively common disorder of the adolescent hip. "Skiffy" for short, SCFE is failure of the proximal femoral physis during periods of accelerated growth. This failure results in discontinuity arising between the head and neck of the femur. The femoral head stays located in the acetabulum, while the femoral neck migrates superiorly and anteriorly.

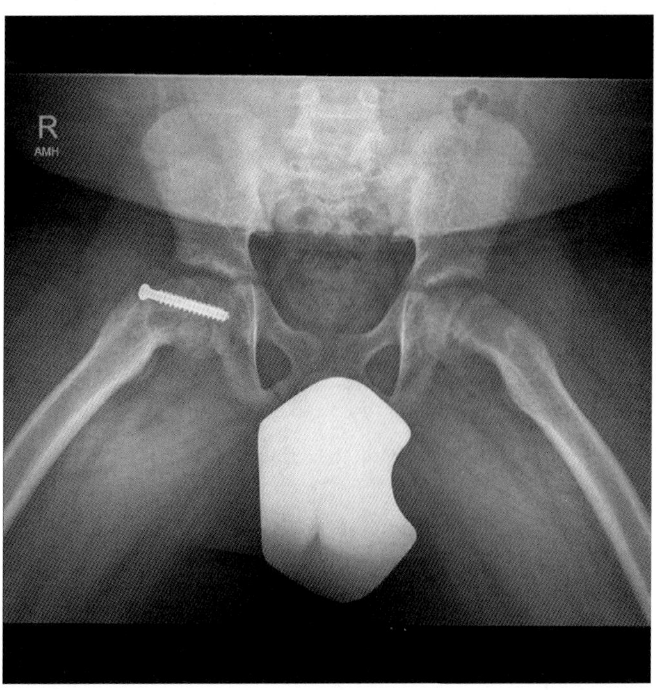

FIGURE 89-1 New slipped capital femoral epiphysis of the left hip in a 10-year-old boy on frog-leg view. Note that the slipped capital femoral epiphysis of the right hip was fixed surgically 18 months prior. (*Used with permission from Thomas Kuivila, MD.*)

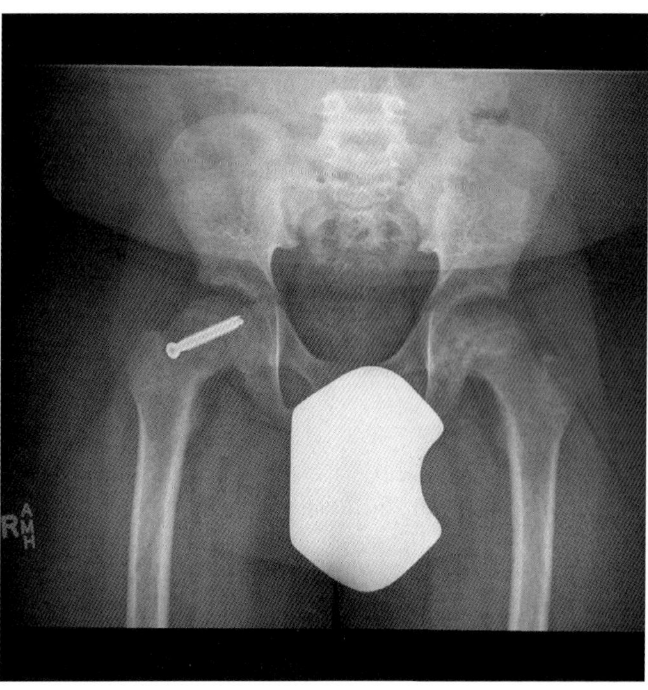

FIGURE 89-2 New slipped capital femoral epiphysis of the left hip on AP view of the same boy as in **Figure 89-1**. (*Used with permission from Thomas Kuivila, MD.*)

SYNONYMS

Slipped upper femoral epiphysis (SUFE).

EPIDEMIOLOGY

- SCFE most commonly occurs in adolescent boys between the ages of 10 and 16 years. It occasionally occurs in girls as well—usually between the ages of 12 and 14 years—but girls are half as likely as boys to have slips.[1]
- Annual incidence is estimated at 8.3 unilateral cases and 0.5 bilateral cases per 100,000 children.[2]
- Slips are more common in obese children[3] and they occur 2 to 4 times more frequently in black and Hispanic children than in white children.[1,4]
- The left hip is involved twice as frequently as the right hip. Bilateral slips occur 20 percent of the time,[1] usually within 12 to 18 months of the first slip.
- Interestingly, SCFE tends to show seasonal and regional variability. Slips tend to occur more frequently in warm months[5], and there is a predilection for slips to occur more frequently in the Northeastern and Western US.[1]

ETIOLOGY AND PATHOPHYSIOLOGY

- Etiological factors for SCFE are thought to be numerous. They include local trauma, mechanical factors (physeal weakness during puberty, stress from obesity),[6,11] endocrine disorders (hypothyroidism, pituitary deficiency),[1] inflammatory conditions, and genetic factors.

- All proposed etiological factors result in a common condition: a weak physis that fails to resist displacement when subjected to sheering stress. Failure occurs in the hypertrophic zone of the physis.[7]

RISK FACTORS

Though the cause of SCFE is has not been fully elucidated, there are a few risk factors that have been identified:

- Male gender.[1]
- Adolescent age.
- Obese children.[3]
- Personal history of hypothyroidism, growth hormone deficiency, and other pituitary axis abnormalities.[8]

DIAGNOSIS

CLINICAL FEATURES

- Patients with a SCFE will typically report hip, thigh (usually medial), or knee pain of a short duration. Medial thigh and knee pain is thought to be referred pain secondary to irritation of the obturator nerve.
- The pain is usually aggravated by activity and relieved with rest.
- Patients often walk with a limp.
- Patients with severe cases of SCFE are completely unable to bear weight, though this is uncommon.
- Often, the affected leg is externally rotated in comparison to the normal leg.
- On exam, there may be obligate external rotation of the affected hip as it is flexed (**Figures 89-3** and **89-4**). There may be a slight leg-length discrepancy. Although prior classification systems (based on duration of symptoms and severity of the slip) have been employed, the most commonly accepted system in use today recognizes slips as stable or unstable. Stable slips are those in which the patient is still able to bear weight; unstable slips are those that prevent any form of ambulation. This classification scheme has implications on prognosis and treatment method.[9]

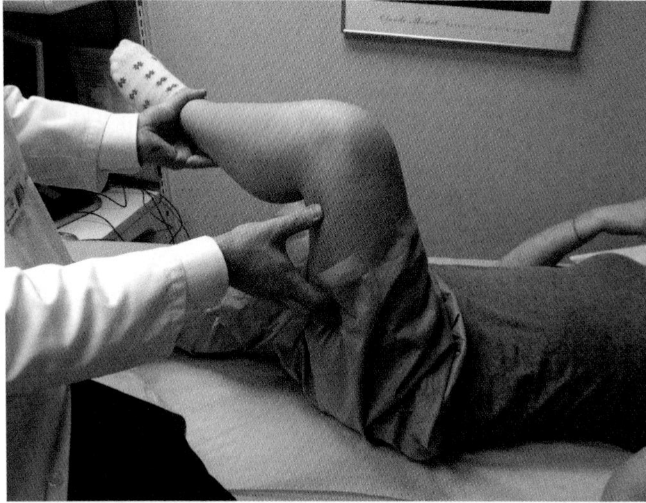

FIGURE 89-3 This patient has been treated for slipped capital femoral epiphysis. Note the obligate external rotation that is seen as the hip is flexed. The examiner is just flexing the hip and the external rotation is occurring spontaneously due to the abnormal anatomy. This is the result of femoral neck impingement on the acetabular rim during hip flexion. (*Used with permission from David Gurd, MD.*)

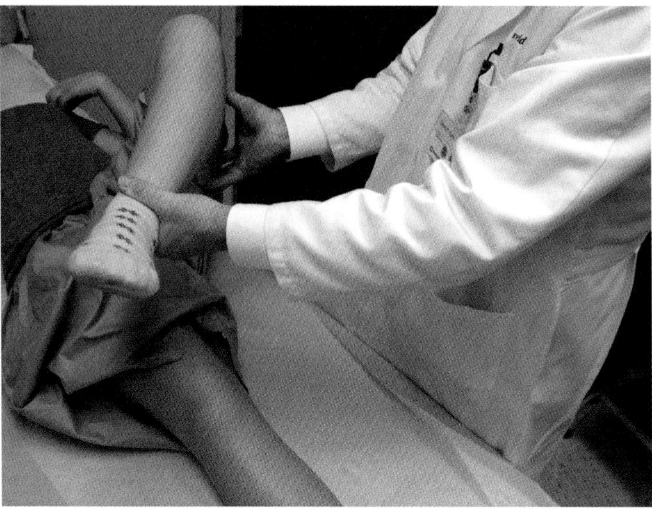

FIGURE 89-4 Obligate external rotation as the hip is flexed from the caudal view in the same boy as in **Figure 89-3**. (*Used with permission from David Gurd, MD.*)

LABORATORY TESTING

- No laboratory tests are necessary to diagnose SCFE.
- However, given the association with endocrine abnormalities, laboratory testing may be indicated if an endocrine etiology is thought possible.
- Pertinent lab tests include thyroid-stimulating hormone (TSH) to evaluate for hypothyroidism, basic metabolic panel to evaluate for renal abnormality, and Growth Hormone levels to evaluate for hypopituitarism, among others.
- Some authors have advocated TSH testing for all patient with SCFE, as well as selective pituitary testing for patients who are short for their age and have hypogonadism.[10]

IMAGING

- SCFE can typically be diagnosed with routine x-rays only. AP and frog-leg lateral views are the most effective ways of observing subtle slips (**Figures 89-1, 89-2**, **89-5**, and **89-6**).
- MRI is used very infrequently to identify slips that are not readily apparent on plain films.
- Ultrasound and CT are not routinely used for the diagnosis of SCFE.

DIFFERENTIAL DIAGNOSIS

- Avascular necrosis of the femoral head (Legg-Calve-Perthes or other etiologies)—Damage to the epiphyseal bone of the femoral head; usually the result of lack of blood supply, often for an

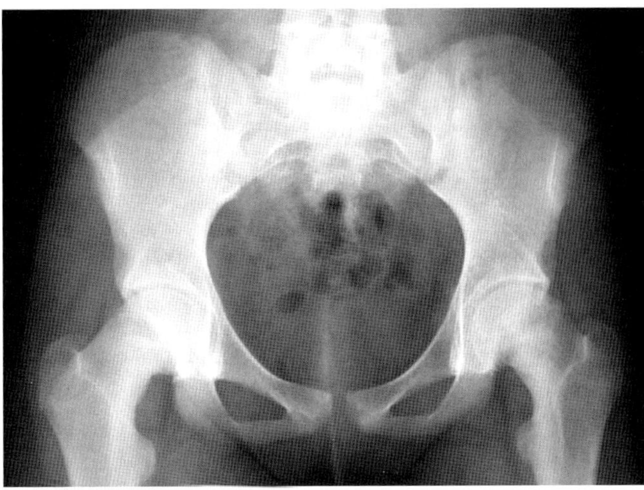

FIGURE 89-5 Bilateral slipped capital femoral epiphysis in a 12-year old boy on AP view. (*Used with permission from Ryan Goodwin, MD.*)

unknown reason. This results in collapse of the overlying articular cartilage, which can lead to premature arthritis if the bone and cartilage are not able to repair and remodel (see Chapter 88, Leg-Calves-Perthes).

- Femoral neck fracture (as well as traumatic proximal femoral physeal fracture)—Fracture through the proximal femoral physis (growth plate fracture), immediately below the femoral head (subcapital femoral neck fracture), or at the base of the neck (basicervical femoral neck fracture). These fractures are almost exclusively traumatic in nature.

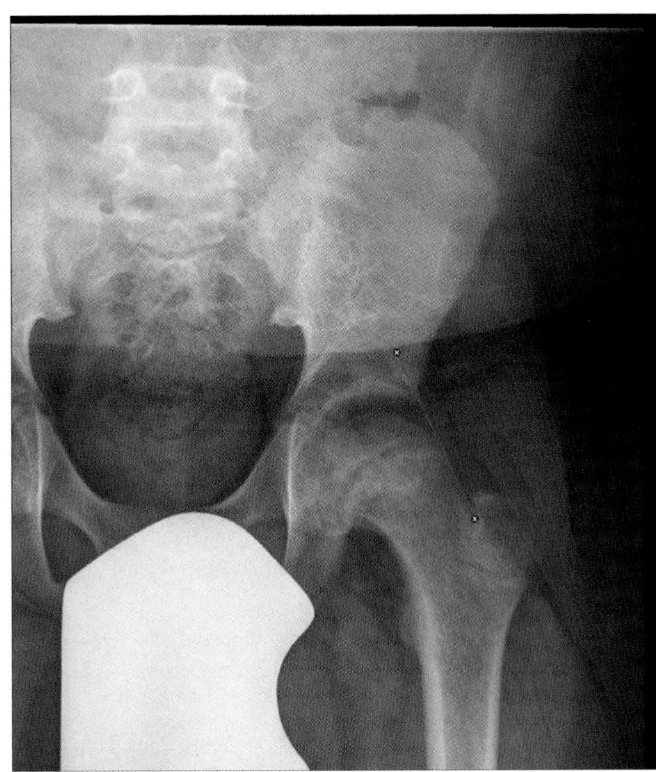

FIGURE 89-6 Klein's line, which runs along the superior aspect of the femoral neck, as seen on AP view of the hip. Slipped capital femoral epiphysis is diagnosed when the line does not intersect any portion of the femoral head. (*Used with permission from Thomas Kuivila, MD.*)

- Femoral neck stress fracture—Fracture through the femoral neck that is a result of overactivity or intense, repetitive activity (military recruits, etc.). Initial radiographs may be negative.
- Adductor strain—Strain of any of the adductor muscles of the thigh, particularly adductor brevis, adductor longus, and adductor magnus. These muscles take their origin from the pubic rami, giving the patient the impression that they have a "pulled groin" when strained.
- Osteitis Pubis—Noninfectious inflammation of the pubic symphysis and the surrounding muscle insertions. It is usually the result of microtrauma to the joint and surrounding muscle insertions during repetitive activities.
- Pelvic apophyseal injury—Avulsion of tendon from bone at the apophysis (a bony process that is the site of ligament or tendon attachment, associated with a growth plate), seen most commonly in the pediatric athlete. In pediatric patients, failure at the apophysis is common, as the growth plate tends to be weaker than its attached tendon or ligament.

MANAGEMENT

NONPHARMACOLOGIC

- Traction or casting has been used successfully in the past, but it is no longer used in current treatment due to its difficulty and complications.
- For obvious reasons, the highly restrictive hip spica cast is tolerated poorly in this demographic, as well as prolonged bedrest for traction.
- Additionally, past studies have shown that the incidence of chondrolysis is far greater in patients treated with casting than with patients treated surgically.[11,12]

MEDICATIONS

- Pain medications are used only for peri-operative pain management in SCFE patients. No medications are used for the treatment of the condition.

SURGERY

Surgical management is the standard of care for the management of SCFE.[11,12] SOR Ⓐ Numerous surgical management options are successfully employed, including percutaneous in situ pinning, open reduction and internal fixation, and osteotomy.

- In general, the slipped epiphysis is not reduced to its original state, as this maneuver causes increased risk of avascular necrosis due to disruption of blood supply.
- Reduction of the slip is only done if the femoral neck and head can be visualized during an open procedure.
- In most cases, the epiphysis is pinned where it lies in situ.
- Percutaneous in situ pinning with a single, large-diameter screw is now the most commonly used treatment option.
- Numerous studies have shown that a single threaded pin is comparable to two or three pins to maintain stability.[13,14] SOR Ⓐ
- For patients with unilateral SCFE, controversy exists over whether or not to pin the unaffected hip prophylactically. In general, it is

recommended that prophylactic pinning of the unaffected hip occur in younger patients (with a low Oxford bone age score)[15] and in patients with a concomitant endocrine abnormality.

REFERRAL

- Diagnosis of SCFE should prompt direct admission to the hospital and strict non–weight-bearing status, followed by a consultation to pediatric orthopedic surgery.
- A patient with SCFE should not be sent home or told to follow up as an outpatient, as further activity and ambulation poses significant risks for further slippage.

PREVENTION AND SCREENING

- Routine screening for SCFE is not employed. However, the astute clinician should suspect SCFE in any adolescent or preadolescent pediatric patient presenting with knee, thigh, or hip pain.
- Indeed, many cases of SCFE have gone undiagnosed when a patient presents with pain outside the hip region.

PROGNOSIS

- The prognosis for stable slips is generally very favorable, with satisfactory results reported to be as high as 96 percent.
- Conversely, the prognosis for unstable slips is poor, with satisfactory results seen in only 1/2 of the patients.[16]
- Complications from SCFE include avascular necrosis of the femoral head and femoro-acetabular impingement (FAI).[3]

FOLLOW-UP

- After diagnosis and surgical management, patients with SCFE must be followed by their surgeon until the physis has become stable, evidenced by a bony bridge across the physis.
- Follow-up with a pediatric specialist may be indicated if a SCFE is found to occur concomitantly with another abnormality (i.e., hypothyroidism).

PATIENT EDUCATION

- Children diagnosed with SCFE need to be educated to not weight-bear between diagnosis and surgery. When the diagnosis is made the child should be evaluated immediately in a hospitalized setting with the parents helping to enforce the no weight-bearing rule.

PATIENT RESOURCES

- The American Academy of Orthopedic Surgery—**www.orthoinfo.aaos.org/topic.cfm?topic=a00052**.
- The US National Library of Medicine—**www.ncbi.nlm.nih.gov/pubmedhealth/PMH0001967**.

PROVIDER RESOURCES

- The Pediatric Orthopedic Society of North America—**www.posna.org/education/StudyGuide/slippedCapitalFemoralEpiphysis.asp**.
- Medscape Reference—**www.emedicine.medscape.com/article/91596**.

REFERENCES

1. Lehmann CL, et al. The epidemiology of slipped capital femoral epiphysis: an update. *J Pediatr Orthop*. 2006;26(3):286-290.
2. Larson AN, et al. Incidence of slipped capital femoral epiphysis: a population-based study. *J Pediatr Orthop B*. 2010;19(1):9-12.
3. Novais EN. Slipped capital femoral epiphysis: prevalence, pathogenesis, and natural history. *Clin Orthop Relat Res*. 2012;9.
4. Kelsey JL. Epidemiology of slipped capital femoral epiphysis: A review of the literature. *Pediatrics*. 1973;51:1042.
5. Brown, D. Seasonal variation of slipped capital femoral epiphysis in the US. *J Pediatr Orthop*. 2004;24(2):139-143.
6. Aronson J, Tursky EA. The torsional basis for slipped capital femoral epiphysis. *Clin Orthop Relat Res*. 1996;322:37.
7. Weiner D. Pathogenesis of slipped capital femoral epiphysis: current concepts. *J Pediatr Orthop B*. 1996;5(2):67-73.
8. Loder RT, et al. Slipped capital femoral epiphysis associated with endocrine disorders. *J Pediatr Orthop*. 1995;15(3):349-356.
9. Mooney JF, et al. Management of unstable/acute slipped capital femoral epiphysis: results of a survey of the POSNA membership. *J Pediatr Orthop*. 2005;25(2):162-166.
10. Wells D. Review of slipped capital femoral epiphysis associated with endocrine disease. *J Pediatr Orthop*. 1993;13(5):610-614.
11. Davidson RS, Weitzel P, Stanton R, et al. Slipped capital femoral epiphysis (SCFE): a multicenter review of the complications by treatment group in 432 hips. Paper presented at the annual meeting of the Pediatric Orthopedic Society of North America, Miami, Fla, April 30, 1995.
12. Betz RR, Steel HH, Emper WD, et al. Treatment of slipped capital femoral epiphysis. *J Bone Joint Surg*. 1990;72A;587.
13. Kibiloski LJ, Doane RM, Karol LA, et al. Biomechanical analysis of single- versus double-screw fixation in slipped capital femoral epiphysis at physiological load levels. *J Pediatr Orthop*. 1994; 14:627.
14. O'Beirne J, McLoughlin R, Dowling F, et al. Slipped upper femoral epiphysis: internal fixation using single central pins. *J Pediatr Orthop*. 1989;9:304.
15. Popejoy D. Prediction of contralateral slipped capital femoral epiphysis using the modified Oxford bone age score. *J Pediatr Orthop*. 2012;32(3):290-294.
16. Loder RT, Richards BS, Shapiro PS, et al. Acute slipped capital femoral epiphysis: the importance of physeal stability. *J Bone Joint Surg*. 1993;75A;1134.

90 OSGOOD-SCHLATTER

Kimberly Giuliano, MD
Ellen Park, MD

PATIENT STORY

An adolescent male presents with unilateral knee pain and swelling (**Figure 90-1**). His pain is worse after athletic participation and with kneeling. On examination, he has point tenderness and edema of the tibial tubercle. He is diagnosed with Osgood-Schlatter disease and treated with rest, ice, and non-steroidal anti-inflammatory medication. His symptoms improve but he continues to have mild flares of pain when he is more active.

INTRODUCTION

Osgood Schlatter disease was described in 1903 by Dr. Osgood and Dr. Schlatter as pain and edema of the anterior tibial tubercle.[1,2] These clinical findings result from traction apophysitis at the patellar tendon insertion site on the proximal tibial tubercle.

SYNONYMS

Osteochondritis of tibial tubercle; tibial tuberosity avulsion.

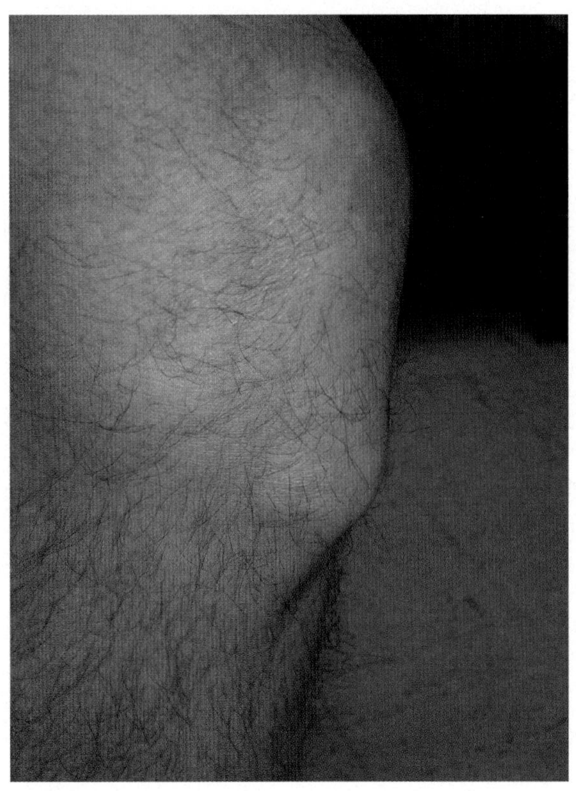

FIGURE 90-1 Prominence of the tibial tuberosity consistent with Osgood-Schlatter disease in an adolescent male. (*Used with permission from Richard P. Usatine, MD.*)

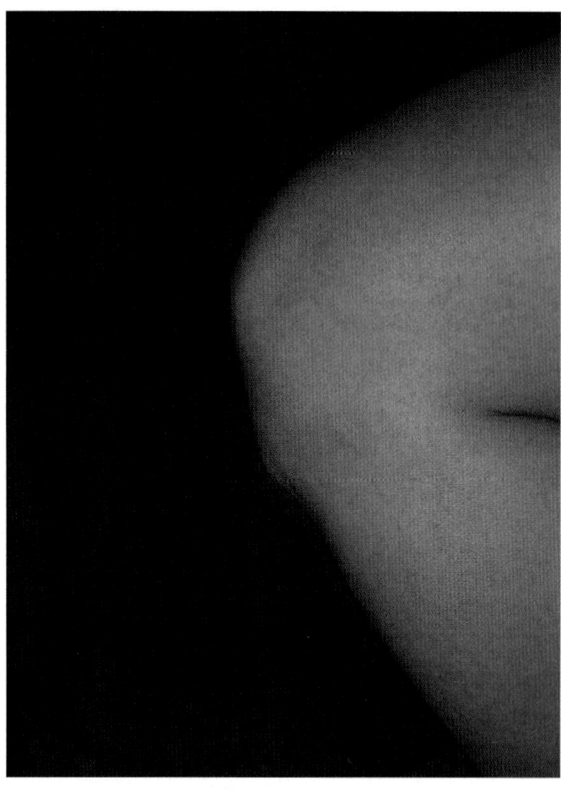

FIGURE 90-2 Prominent tibial tubercle in an adolescent female with Osgood-Schlatter disease. (*Used with permission from Richard P. Usatine, MD.*)

EPIDEMIOLOGY

- Occurs in adolescents after a rapid growth spurt.
- More common in males than females (**Figure 90-2**).[3]
- More common in athletes (21.2%) than nonathletes (4.5%).[4]

ETIOLOGY AND PATHOPHYSIOLOGY

- Overuse injury.
- Repetitive strain leads to chronic avulsion of tibial tubercle apophysis.
- Chronic avulsion results in separation and elevation of the patellar tendon insertion at the tibial tubercle.
- Callous formation during the healing process leads to a pronounced tibial tubercle.

RISK FACTORS

- Participation in athletic activities that involve repetitive running and jumping.
- Pubertal growth spurt.
- More proximal attachment of the patellar tendon.[5]
- Broad patellar tendon attachment at the tibia.[5]
- High riding patella.[6]

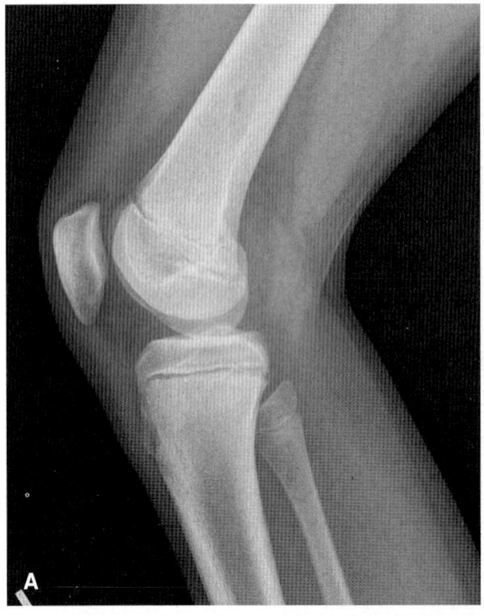

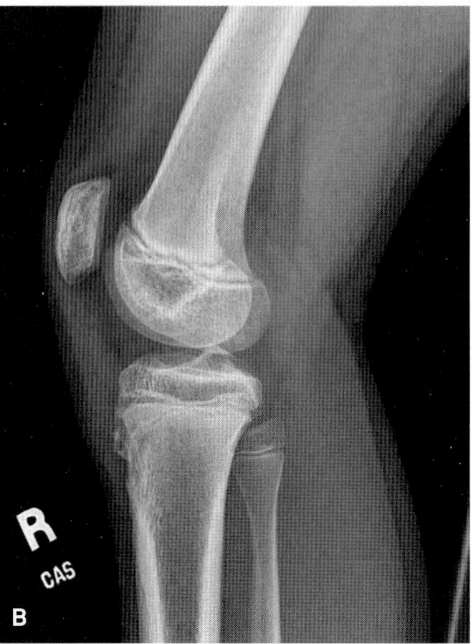

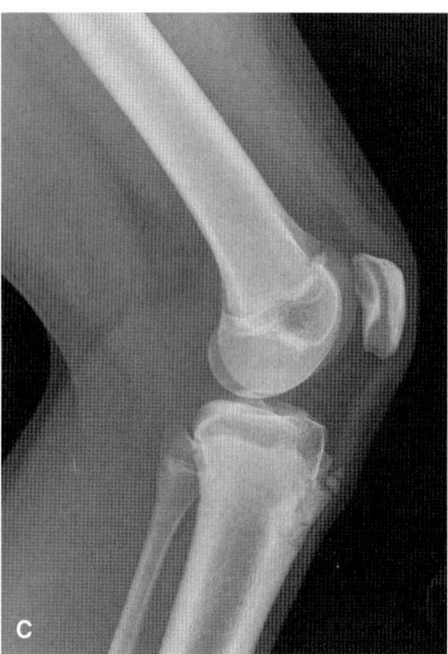

FIGURE 90-3 **A.** Mild changes of Osgood-Schlatter disease in an 11-year-old boy on left knee lateral radiograph. Note mild patellar tendon thickening and edema with slight irregularity of tibial tubercle. **B.** Mild changes of Osgood-Schlatter disease in right knee lateral radiograph with increased patellar tendon thickening, soft tissue edema and irregularity of tibial tubercle. **C.** Fragmentation of the tibial tubercle in Osgood-Schlatter disease. *(Used with permission from Ellen Park, MD.)*

DIAGNOSIS

CLINICAL FEATURES

- Tenderness and prominence of the tibial tubercle.

DISTRIBUTION

- Typically unilateral but can have bilateral involvement.[4]

IMAGING

- Osgood-Schlatter is often a clinical diagnosis. Imaging is not indicated unless unusual features are present to suggest an alternate diagnosis.
- Plain films may demonstrate a spectrum of findings from normal to fragmentation and irregularity of the tibial tubercle, anterior knee soft tissue swelling, and patellar tendon thickening on the lateral knee x-ray (**Figure 90-3**). Plain films may not be helpful if tibial tubercle has not yet ossified (often between the ages of 9 and 11 years).
- Computed tomography and magnetic resonance imaging (MRI) are not typically indicated. MRI is, however, the most sensitive form of imaging and will demonstrate spectrum of findings including soft tissue edema, infrapatellar fat pad edema, patellar tendon thickening, and bony changes (**Figure 90-4**).

DIFFERENTIAL DIAGNOSIS

- Bone tumors—Tumors typically are associated with symptoms that are absent in Osgood-Schlatter (i.e., fever, pain at rest, night awakenings, systemic complaints).
- Osteomyelitis—Overlying erythema, calor and fever should prompt evaluation for infection as these symptoms are not typical for Osgood-Schlatter.
- Avulsion fracture of tibial tubercle—Acute pain with associated injury raises concern for avulsion fracture. Osgood-Schlatter

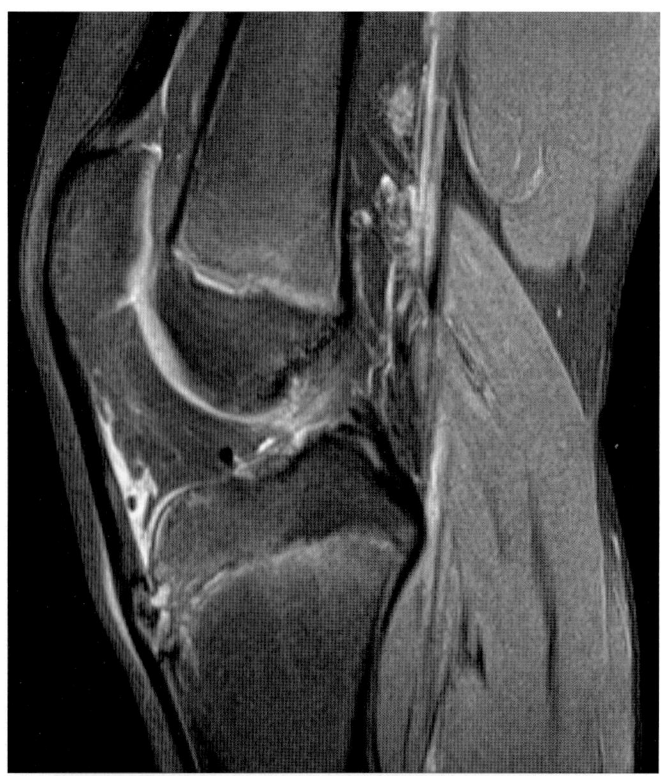

FIGURE 90-4 MRI (T2 weighted imaging) of knee in an 11-year-old with Osgood-Schlatter disease. Bone marrow edema and fragmentation of tibial tubercle is present along with edema of the adjacent soft tissues. *(Used with permission from Ellen Park, MD.)*

typically presents with subacute pain without an identified injury.

- Arthritis—Edema within the knee joint is not consistent with Osgood-Schlatter. Juvenile Idiopathic Arthritis (JIA) and septic arthritis are not isolated to the tibial tubercle and are often associated with systemic symptoms (see Chapter 172, Juvenile Idiopathic Arthritis).
- Tibial stress fracture—Stress fractures generally do not occur within the tibial tubercle.
- Patellar tendonitis—Pain with palpation along the patellar tendon is consistent with tendonitis and is not present in Osgood-Schlatter.
- Sinding-Larsen-Johansson (traction apophysitis of inferior patella)—Pain is located at the inferior patella with traction apophysitis and the tibial tubercle is not involved.
- Plica syndrome (synovial fold inflammation)—Pain is located within the knee joint when the synovial folds are inflamed, but the tibial tubercle is non-tender.
- Hoffa disease (impingement of infrapatellar fat pad)—Fat pad impingement causes pain within the knee joint and does not involve the tibial tubercle.

MANAGEMENT

NONPHARMACOLOGIC

- Rest the involved knee.[7–10] SOR B
- Ice application. SOR C
- Physical load restriction.[11] SOR B
- Wearing a patellar tendon strap may reduce the pain.[12] SOR C
- Wearing a knee pad may help protect the affected area from direct trauma. SOR C
- Stretching the hamstring and quadriceps muscles. SOR C
- Strengthening quadriceps muscles. SOR C

MEDICATIONS

- Non-steroid anti-inflammatory drugs (NSAIDs).[7–10] SOR B
- A small study showed improvement with dextrose injections for refractory cases of Osgood-Schlatter.[13] SOR C

SURGERY

- Surgery is rarely necessary.
- Surgery can be considered for significant refractory Osgood-Schlatter symptoms after the patient reaches skeletal maturity.[14–18] SOR B

REFERRAL

Conservative management by the primary care physician is usually sufficient. Referrals can be considered for refractory or atypical symptoms:

- Physical therapy.
- Sports medicine.
- Orthopedic surgeon.

PREVENTION

- Appropriate stretching of hamstrings and quadriceps prior to sport participation.
- Avoid repetitive jumping on hard surfaces.

PROGNOSIS

- Self-limited course.
- Complete recovery is expected for vast majority of patients upon reaching skeletal maturity.
- Tibial tubercle prominence may persist after symptoms resolve.
- Residual ossicles can result in continued pain after skeletal maturity.

FOLLOW-UP

- Patients should be instructed to follow up with their primary care physician if pain does not decrease with good adherence to conservative treatment measures; however, mild persistent pain is expected.
- Increased pain, night awakenings, overlying erythema, calor, or fevers should prompt further evaluation.

PATIENT EDUCATION

- Patients and parents should be reassured that this is a self-limited process and that adherence to conservative treatment measures is important to recovery from symptoms.

PATIENT RESOURCES

- **www.healthychildren.org/English/health-issues/injuries-emergencies/sports-injuries/Pages/Knee-Pain-and-Osgood-Schlatter-Disease.aspx**.
- **www.orthoinfo.aaos.org/topic.cfm?topic=a00411**.

PROVIDER RESOURCES

- National Athletic Trainers' Association position statement: prevention of pediatric overuse injuries—**www.guideline.gov/content.aspx?id=38462**.

REFERENCES

1. Osgood RB. Lesions of the tibial tubercle occurring during adolescence. *Boston Med Surg J*. 1903;148:114.
2. Schlatter C. Verletzungen des schnabelforminogen fortsatzes der oberen tibiaepiphyse. *Beitre Klin Chir Tubing*. 1903;38:874.
3. Ehrenborg G. The Osgood-Schlatter lesion. A clinical study of 170 cases. *Acta Chir Scand*. 1962;124:89-105.

4. Krause BL, Williams JP, Catterall A. Natural history of Osgood-Schlatter disease. *J Pediatr Orthop.* 1990;10:65-68.
5. Demirag B, Ozturk C, Yazici Z, Sarisozen B. The pathophysiology of Osgood-Schlatter disease: a magnetic resonance investigation. *J Pediatr Orthop B.* 2004;13:379-382.
6. Aparicio G, Abril JC, Calvo E, Alvarez L. Radiologic study of patellar height in Osgood-Schlatter disease. *J Pediatr Orthop.* 1997; 17:63-66.
7. Hussain A, Hagroo GA. Osgood-Schlatter disease. *Sports Exer Injury.* 1996;2:202-206.
8. Mital MA, Matza RA, Cohen J. The so-called unresolved Osgood-Schlatter lesion. *J Bone Joint Surg Am.* 1980;62:732-739.
9. Kujala UM, Kvist M, Heinonen O. Osgood-Schlatter's disease in adolescent athletes. Retrospective study of incidence and duration. *Am J Sports Med.* 1985;13:236-241.
10. Beovich R, Fricker PA. Osgood-Schlatter's disease. A review of the literature and an Australian series. *Aust J Sci Med Sport.* 1988;20:11-13.
11. Gerulis V, Kalesinskas R, Pranckevicius S, Birgeris P. Importance of conservative treatment and load restriction to the course of Osgood-Schaltter's disease. *Medicina.* 2004;40(4):363-369.
12. Levine J, Kashyap S. A new conservative treatment of Osgood-Schlatter disease. *Clin Orthop.* 1981;158:126-128.
13. Topol GA, Podesta LA, Reeves KD, Raya MF, Fullerton BD, Yeh HW. Hyperosmolar dextrose injection for recalcitrant Osgood-Schlatter disease. *Pediatrics.* 2011;128(5):e1121-1128.
14. Orava S, Malinen L, Karpakka JJ, et al. Results of surgical treatment of unresolved Osgood-Schlatter lesion. *Ann Chir Gynaecol.* 2000;89:298-302.
15. Glynn MK, Regan BF. Surgical treatment of Osgood-Schlatter's disease. *J Pediatr Orthop.* 1983;3:216-219.
16. Flowers MJ, Bhadreshwar DR. Tibial tuberosity excision for symptomatic Osgood-Schlatter disease. *J Pediatr Orthop.* 1995;15:292-297.
17. Weiss JM, Jordan SS, Andersen JS, Lee BM, Kocher M. Surgical treatment of unresolved Osgood-Schlatter disease: ossicle resection with tibial tubercleplasty. *J Pediatr Orthop.* 2007;27(7): 844-847.
18. Pihalajamaki HK, Visuri TI. Long-term outcome after surgical treatment of unresolved Osgood-Schlatter disease in young me: surgical technique. *J Bone Joint Surg Am.* 2010;92(1): 258-264.

91 SCOLIOSIS

Joel Kolmodin, MD
David Gurd, MD

PATIENT STORY

A 12-year-old girl presents to the office after a routine school screening. She was told that she has an abnormal curvature of her spine, and she notes an unpleasant hump on the right side of her back. She is found to have a right sided prominence, shoulder height differences, and lateral curvature of her spine on examination (**Figures 91-1** and **91-2**). Neurological examination is normal. PA and lateral x-rays are taken, and the patient is referred to a Pediatric Orthopedic surgeon for evaluation and management.

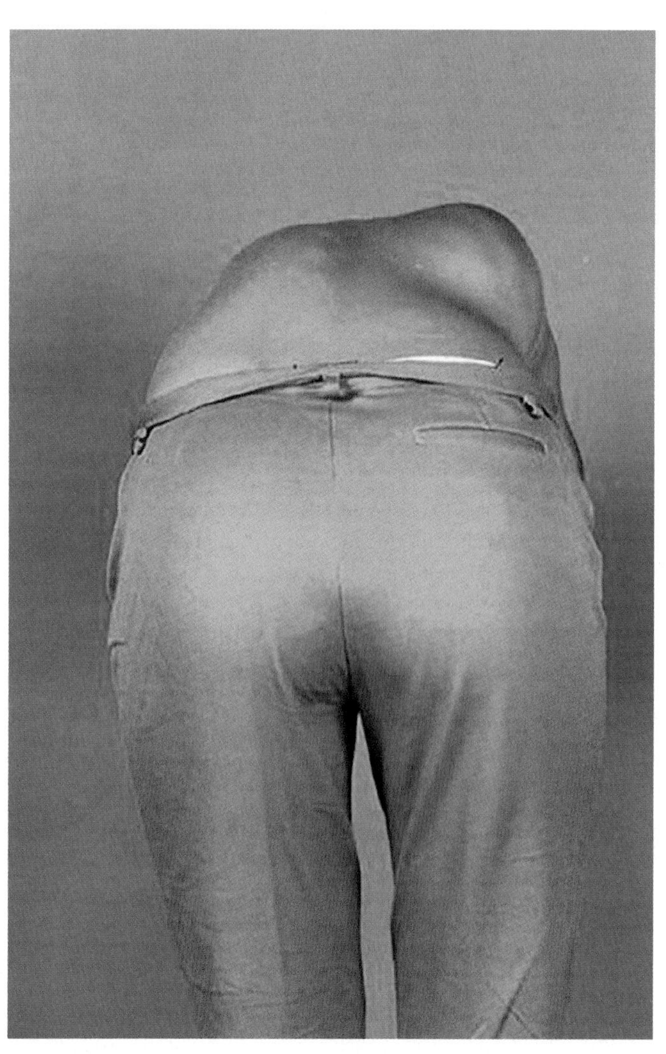

FIGURE 91-1 Typical scoliosis deformities that are seen on forward-bending clinical examination in a 12-year-old girl. Note the thoracic prominence on the right and the sloping angle from the right back to the left. (*Used with permission from David Gurd, MD.*)

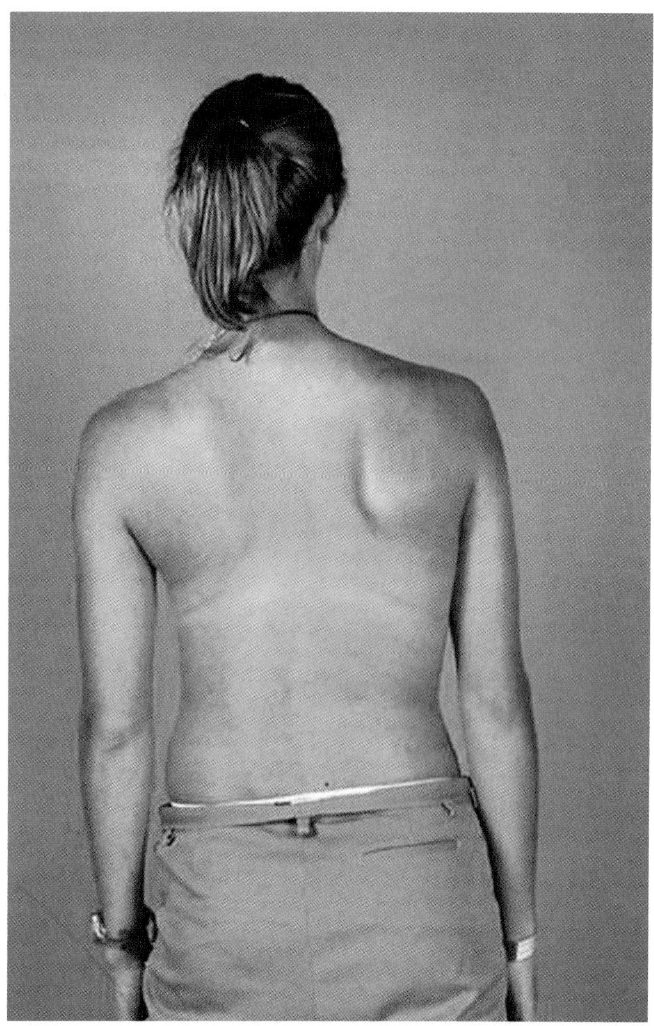

FIGURE 91-2 Typical scoliosis deformities that are seen on posterior clinical examination of the same girl as in Figure 91-1. Note the assymetry of the scapulae and the waist contours. The curvature of the spine is visible along with a slightly higher right shoulder too. (*Used with permission from David Gurd, MD.*)

INTRODUCTION

Scoliosis is a lateral curvature of the spine that is greater than 10 degrees in the coronal plane (**Figure 91-3**). It is often associated with rotational changes and hypokyphotic spinal deformity (flat thoracic spine when viewed from the side).[1]

SYNONYMS

Back curvature; spine deformity; twisted spine.

EPIDEMIOLOGY

- Overall incidence in the population is 2 to 3 percent, with 0.1 to 0.3 percent of the population developing significant curves exceeding 20 degrees.[2]

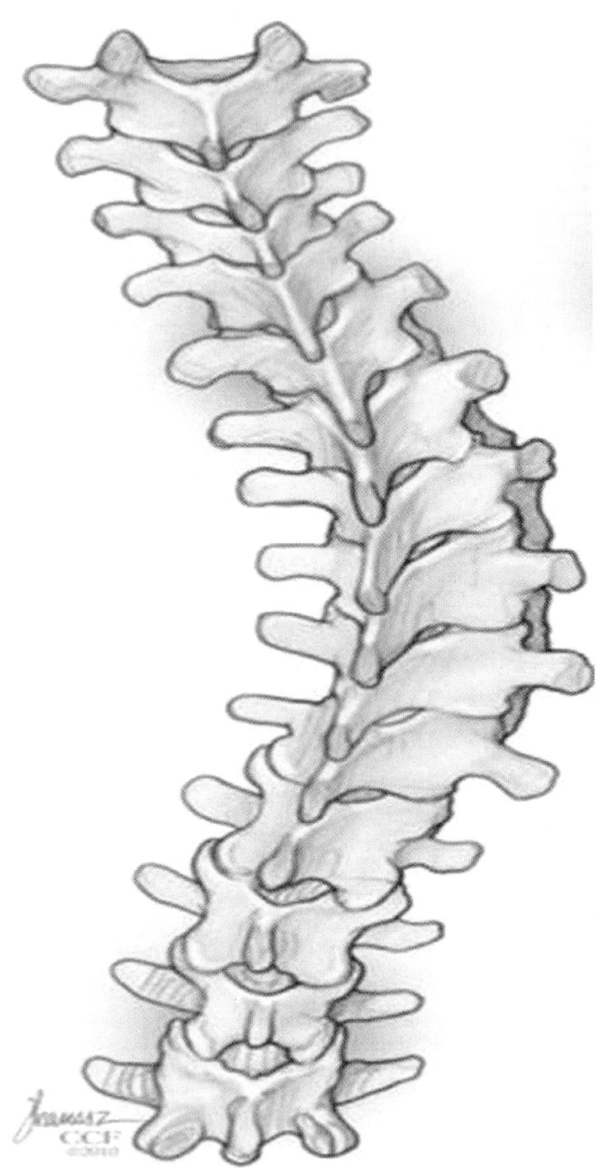

FIGURE 91-3 Example of rotational deformity that occurs with scoliosis. Notice how the vertebral body rotates out toward the apex and convexity of the curve. The majority of the rotation is located nearest to the apex, less away from the apex. (*Reprinted with permission, Cleveland Clinic Center for Medical Art & Photography © 2012. All Rights Reserved.*)

- Scoliosis is classified as:
  - Congenital—Arising from congenital (as an infant) vertebral anomalies such as wedged vertebrae, hemivertebrae, and fused/unsegmented vertebrae.
  - Infantile Idiopathic Scoliosis—Scoliosis which is present between birth and 3 years of age without congenital change. This comprises 4 percent of all idiopathic scoliosis cases.[3]
  - Juvenile Idiopathic Scoliosis—Scoliosis which develops between 4 and 10 years of age. This comprises 10 to 15 percent of all idiopathic scoliosis cases.[4]
  - Adolescent Idiopathic Scoliosis (AIS)—Scoliosis which develops between 10 and 18 years of age. This is by far the most common form of scoliosis.

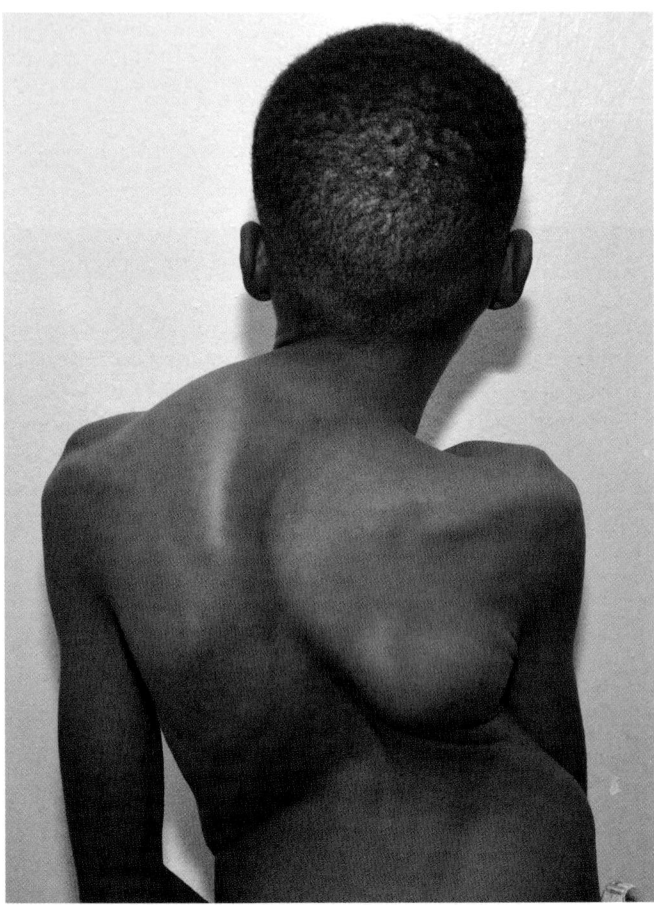

FIGURE 91-4 Severe scoliosis deformity. (*Used with permission from Richard Usatine, MD.*)

ETIOLOGY AND PATHOPHYSIOLOGY

- The vast majority of cases are idiopathic, as is the case with nearly all adolescents presenting with deformity.
- Numerous theories have been proposed for infantile and juvenile cases, including intra-uterine molding, lying infants on their backs, and genetic predisposition.[5]

RISK FACTORS

- There is a positive family history in approximately 30 percent of cases.

DIAGNOSIS

CLINICAL FEATURES

- Patients with scoliosis are typically asymptomatic. They may complain of intermittent back pain, but not more commonly than children without scoliosis. We do not believe that the scoliosis causes back pain unless the deformity is quite severe (**Figures 91-4** and **91-5**).[6] Patients and family members may report a deformity of the spine (curvature), rib cage (hump), shoulders (uneven), or pelvis (waist line asymmetry).

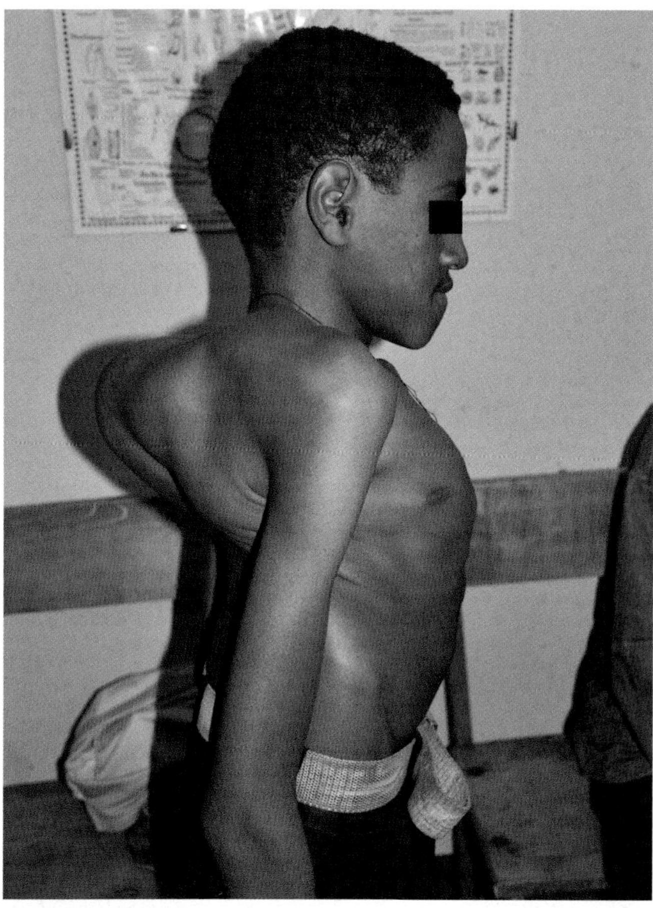

FIGURE 91-5 Severe scoliosis deformity of same patient in Figure 91-4 from lateral view. Note how the upper spine is almost horizontal. (*Used with permission from Richard Usatine, MD.*)

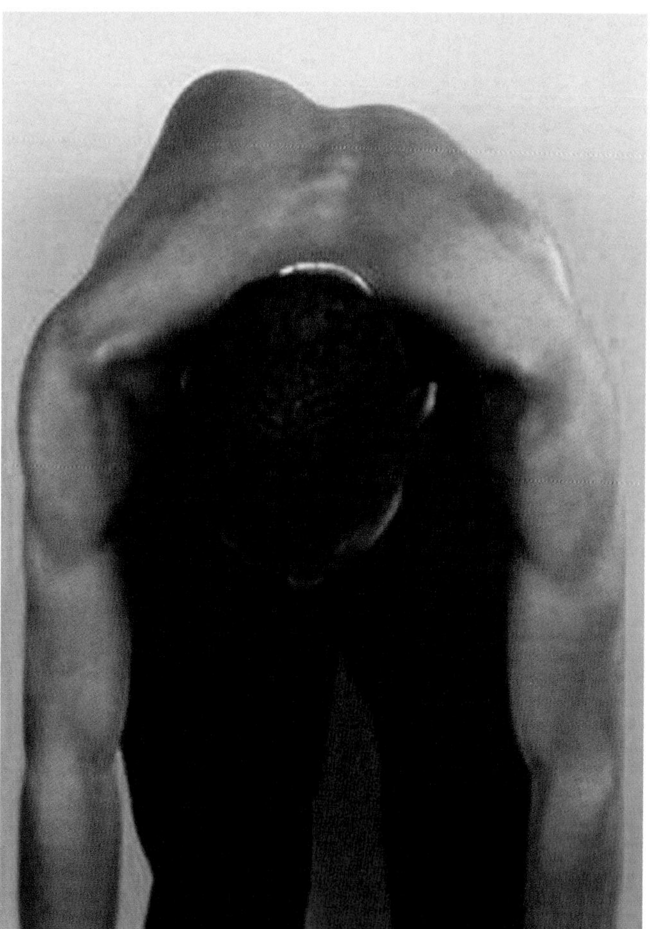

FIGURE 91-6 Typical scoliosis deformities seen on forward-bending clinical exam in a teenage male. (*Used with permission from David Gurd, MD.*)

- The vast majority of curves are right-sided, meaning that the spine curves to the right when the patient is viewed from the back. Often there is a rib prominence noted when the patient bends forward. A curvature of the spine is more evident on forward bending. Patients will often notice unequal shoulder and/or iliac crest (pelvis) heights (**Figure 91-6**).
- Neurologic deficit is uncommon, but it must be checked as scoliosis can be caused by neurological abnormalities. If there is a concern, an MRI can be helpful for assessment.

LABORATORY TESTING

- The SCOLISCORE™ Test is the first clinically validated and highly accurate genetic test for AIS curve progression.[7] It is based on a simple cheek swab. This test gives a numbered score determining likelihood of progression. The lower the score, the less likely for progression. Alternatively, the higher the score, the more likely for progression. There are no other laboratory tests currently available.

IMAGING

- Routine imaging includes PA and lateral x-rays (**Figures 91-7** and **91-8**). Lateral bending x-rays are ordered by an Orthopedic surgeon to assess the flexibility of the patient's curve(s) and are typically only done preoperatively.
- MRI is not routinely ordered. It is ordered by the Orthopedic Surgeon only under specific circumstances to rule out such neurologic abnormalities as syrinx, tethered cord, and Chiari malformation. In a patient with known scoliosis, any abnormality found on neurological exam mandates an MRI.

DIFFERENTIAL DIAGNOSIS

- Kyphosis—Abnormally large forward curvature of the thoracic spine. It is normal to have kyphosis of the thoracic spine, but it is considered abnormal when the kyphosis angle exceeds 50 degrees. As scoliosis can be associated with some degree of abnormal kyphosis, the two diagnosis can mimic one another.
- Postural change—Slouching or hunching over in an asymmetric was can give the appearance of a scoliotic curve. The asymmetry resolves, however, when the patient corrects their incorrect posture.
- Sprengle deformity—Failure of caudal migration (descent) of one scapula during development, resulting in asymmetric scapular heights. This asymmetry can cause a patient to appear to have unequal shoulder heights when viewed from the back (which is also seen in scoliosis), though there is no curvature to the spine.

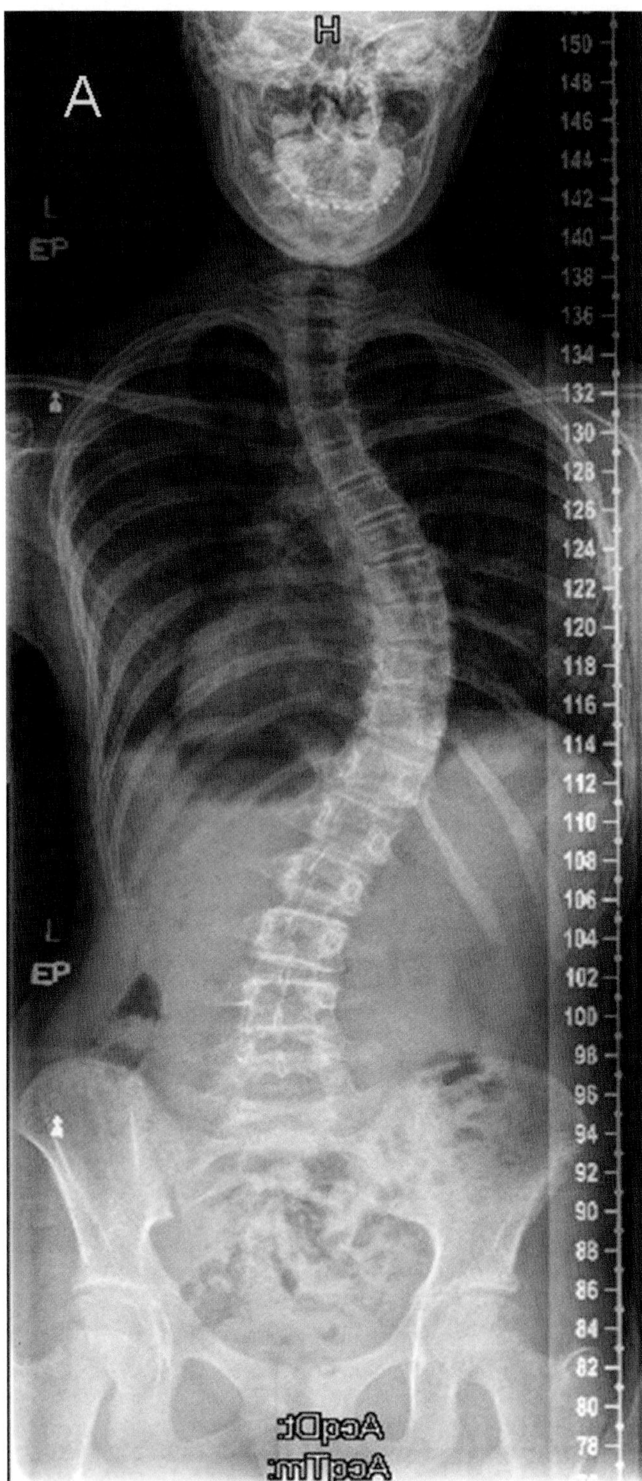

FIGURE 91-7 Scoliosis (mainly right thoracic) with Cobb angle greater than 50 degrees seen on a PA radiograph. (*Used with permission from David Gurd, MD.*)

- Leg length inequality—When one leg is longer than the contralateral side, pelvic obliquity results. This abnormal tilting of the pelvis can cause a compensatory curvature of the spine as the body attempts to keep the keep centered over the sacrum.
- Pectus carinatum and excavatum—Both are common deformities of the anterior chest wall that can occur with or without

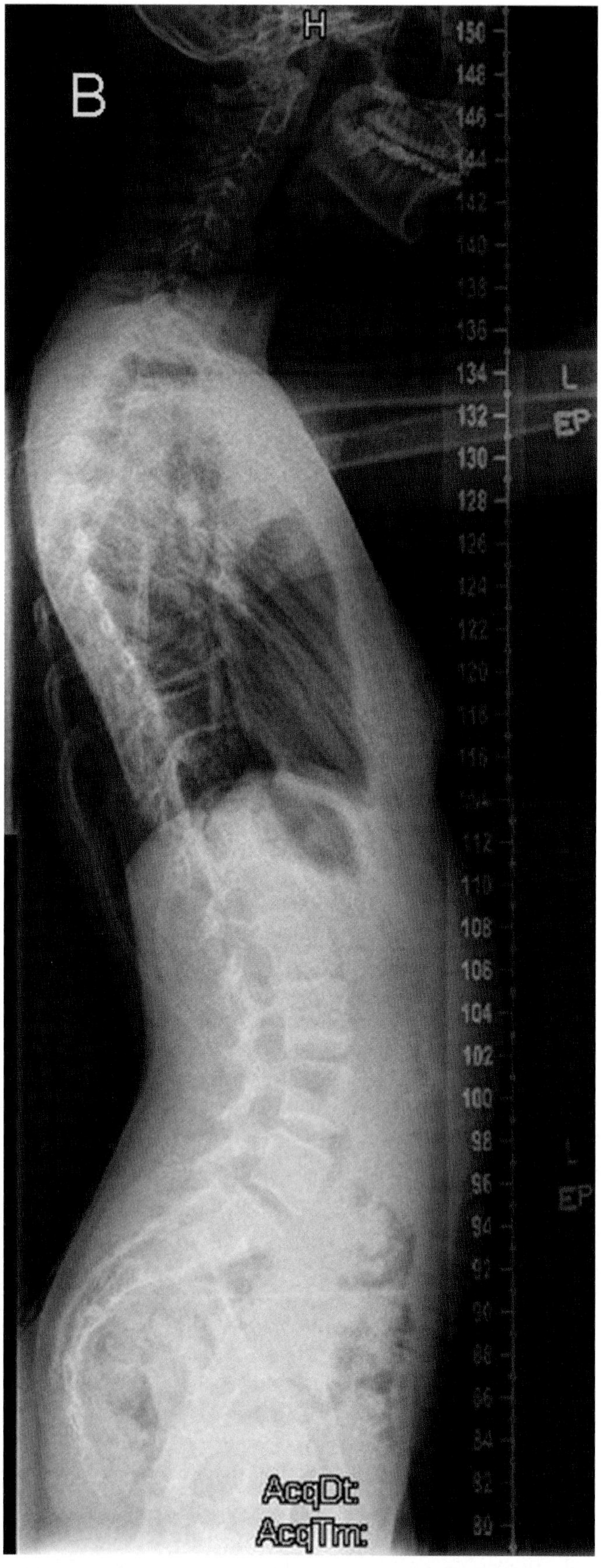

FIGURE 91-8 Hypokyphosis and rib hump deformity seen on lateral radiograph of the same patient as **Figure 91-7**. (*Used with permission from David Gurd, MD.*)

scoliosis. Most often they occur without scoliosis. Pectus carinatum causes a protrusion of the sternum and anterior chest and usually appears during the adolescent growth spurt. It is less common than pectus excavatum in which the anterior chest appears sunken. Both conditions can be asymmetric, giving the appearance of a scoliotic curvature.

MANAGEMENT

NONPHARMACOLOGIC

- Physical therapy has not been shown to prevent the progression of scoliotic curves in any way. It can be helpful, however, in providing the patient some physical benefit in the form of core strengthening to address asymmetry in torso rotation strength,[8] stretching, cardiovascular training, symptom relief, and so on.
- Though its efficacy has been debated in Orthopedic circles, bracing is presently the mainstay of non-operative management of scoliosis.[9] The goal of bracing is to prevent the progression of curves; it is not used to correct curves. Bracing is instituted by an orthopedic surgeon when a patient reaches his/her growth phase and has a curve magnitude of 25 to 40 degrees.[10] SOR B
- The most active growth phase occurs when a patient (1) has not yet begun menstruating, (2) has a low Risser score,[11] and (3) has open triradiate cartilages.
- There are many forms of braces, some of which are worn under clothing for up to 23 hours per day and others of which are only worn at night. Bracing is continued until the active growth phase is completed—usually 2 years after menstruation or when the patient has a Risser score of 4 or 5.[11]
- With early-onset scoliosis, every effort is made to delay surgery until after 10 years of age, a point at which the thoracic cage has adequately developed such that fusion will not confer significant respiratory compromise.
- Surgical management is not medically necessary if the curve can be kept below 45 degrees.[12,13] SOR A

MEDICATIONS

- There are no medications for the treatment of scoliosis.
- Although scoliosis is painless in the cast majority of cases, pain medications (NSAIDs), or anti-spasmotics (cyclobenzaprine, methocarbamol, or diazepam) are infrequently used to treat intermittent symptoms of back pain and/or muscle spasm associated with the diagnosis. SOR C

COMPLIMENTARY/ALTERNATIVE THERAPY

- Generally, alternative therapies are ineffective in managing scoliosis.
- Specifically, studies have shown that chiropractic manipulation, biofeedback, acupuncture, and electrical stimulation[14] do not prevent the progression of scoliosis. SOR B
- They may have a role for these modalities in the treatment of pain or muscle spasm in symptomatic scoliosis.

SURGERY

- Surgery is sometimes employed as a way to manage those patients with early-onset scoliosis where progression is rapid. Growing rods, or metal rods that are attached to the most superior and inferior portions of the curvature, can be lengthened as a child grows. In this way, definitive posterior spinal fusion can be delayed until 10 years of age or later.[15]
- Surgery in the form of posterior spinal fusion is indicated when a curve reaches 45 degrees or more.[12] SOR A The large majority of curves that are 45 to 50 degrees or greater at skeletal maturity will progress as the patient ages, typically at 1 degree per year.[12]
- The goals of surgery are (1) to halt the progression of the deformity, (2) to safely correct the curve, and (3) to address cosmetic deformity such as rib cage prominence. Halting the progression of the curve is the most important goal, as studies have shown that large curves (greater than 90 degrees) can be painful and have a significant impact on respiratory function.[13]
- Surgical treatment utilizes metal implants that are inserted into the spine. These are most often in the form of pedicle screws or hooks and two metal rods that are inserted posteriorly through a midline incision in the back (**Figure 91-9**). Anterior approaches are used as well, though less frequently due to adverse effects on the lungs. This instrumentation is used to correct the coronal curve and any rotational deformity, after which the spine is fused with an allograft and/or autograft. The role of metal instrumentation is to hold the spine in its corrected position until bony fusion occurs. Neuromonitoring is used throughout the case to ensure that there are no changes to neurologic status during the correction.[16] This recent advance has made all corrections more safe and has allowed more aggressive correction of large curves.
- Postoperatively, there are typically no braces or casts used (**Figure 91-10**).
- The patient is encouraged to mobilize the first day after surgery.
- Bending, lifting, and twisting are generally discouraged for up to 6 months, though routine activities are started immediately.

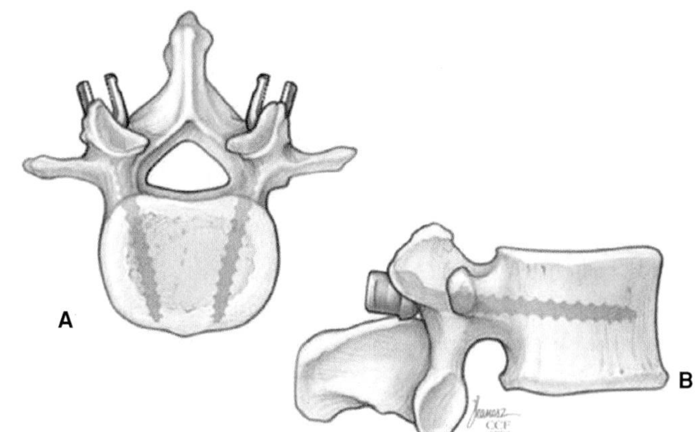

FIGURE 91-9 **A.** Illustration of pedicle screws within the pedicle of a thoracic vertebral body. Just medial to the pedicle is the neural canal and lateral is the rib and pleura. **B.** Same screw from the lateral view. *(Reprinted with permission, Cleveland Clinic Center for Medical Art & Photography © 2012. All Rights Reserved.)*

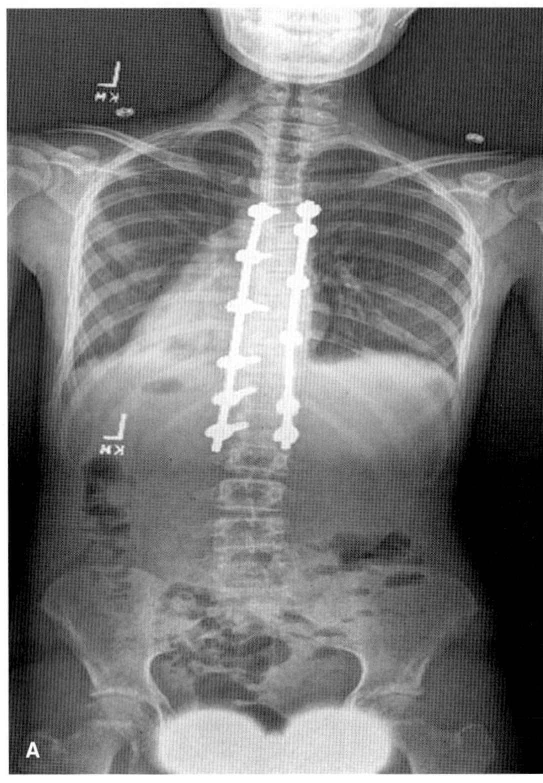
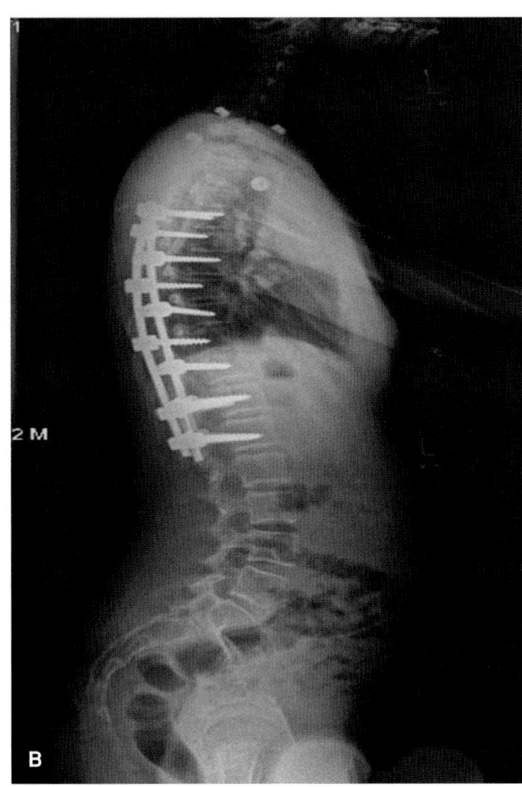

FIGURE 91-10 Postoperative imaging with radiographs of the same 12-year-old girl in **Figure 91-1** and **91-2**. **A.** PA view **B.** Lateral view. (*Used with permission from David Gurd, MD.*)

- It is usually safe to return to noncollision sports 6 months post-operatively.

REFERRAL

- Referral to an Orthopedic surgeon is recommended for any scoliotic curve that is found in infancy or early childhood.
- It is recommended for any child that is found to have a curve greater than 20 degrees and has not yet reached their age of peak growth.

PREVENTION AND SCREENING

- School screening programs are universally in place and they typically start in the elementary school setting, prior to the age at which children reach their peak growth velocity.[17]
- Additionally, scoliosis screening should be performed at yearly well-child check-ups performed by a pediatrician.

PROGNOSIS

- Prognosis is related to the type of scoliosis that the patient has. Infantile scoliosis is known to spontaneously resolve in 20 to 80 percent of cases.[18]
- The prognosis for juvenile and adolescent idiopathic scoliosis is generally favorable if proper screening, conservative management, and definitive treatment are undertaken as they become warranted.
- Curves of all types that are kept below 90 degrees are generally associated with no respiratory compromise, organ dysfunction, or painful sequelae.[13]

FOLLOW-UP

- Once a patient has been found to have scoliosis, regular follow up with a Pediatric Orthopedic surgeon is necessary.
- Children outside their peak growth age can sometimes be followed as infrequently as once per year.
- Patients that are growing rapidly or are treated in a brace are followed as frequently as every 3 to 4 months, but typically every 6 months.

PATIENT RESOURCES

- The Scoliosis Research Society has a helpful site that is easy to navigate and is very informative—**www.srs.org/patient_and_family/scoliosis**.
- The National Institute of Health also has a helpful site, which even gives links to scholarly articles—**www.nlm.nih.gov/medlineplus/scoliosis.html**.
- The Pediatric Orthopedic Society of North America provides a complete patient guide—**www.settingscoliosisstraight.org/education**.

PROVIDER RESOURCES

- The Scoliosis Research Society website has specific links for providers—**www.srs.org/professionals/conditions_and_treatment**.
- The American Academy of Orthopedic Surgery provides up-to-date information and scholarly articles—**www,orthoportal.aaos.org/oko/default**.
- Free patient handouts are provided at the National Institute of Health website—**www.nlm.nih.gov/medlineplus/ency/article/001241.htm**.

REFERENCES

1. Perdriolle R, Vidal J. Thoracic idiopathic scoliosis curve evolution and prognosis. *Spine*. 1985;10:785.
2. Montgomery F, Willner S. The natural history of idiopathic scoliosis: Incidence of treatment in 15 cohorts of children born between 1963 and 1977. *Spine*. 1997;22:772.
3. McMaster MJ. Infantile Idiopathic Scoliosis: Can it be prevented? *J Bone Joint Surg Br*. 1983;65:612.
4. Robinson CM, McMaster MJ. Juvenile idiopathic scoliosis: Curve patterns and prognosis in one hundred and nine patients. *J Bone Joint Surg Am*. 1996;78:1140.
5. Koop SE. Infantile and juvenile idiopathic scoliosis. *Orthop Clin North Am*. 1988;19:331.
6. Ramirez N, Johnston CE, Browne RH. The prevalence of back pain in children who have idiopathic scoliosis. *J Bone Joint Surg Am*. 1997;79:364.
7. Ward K, Ogilvie JW, Singleton, MS, et al. Validation of DNA-based prognostic testing to predict spinal curve progression in Adolescent Idiopathic Scoliosis. *Spine*. 2010;35(25):1455-1464.
8. Mooney V, GulickJ, Pozos R. A preliminary report on the effect of measured strength training in adolescent idiopathic scoliosis. *J Spinal Disord*. 2000;13:102.
9. Nachemson AL, Peterson L-E. Effectiveness of treatment with a brace in girls who have adolescent idiopathic scoliosis. *J Bone Joint Surg (am)*. 1995;77:815-822.
10. Lonstein JE, Carlson JM. The prediction of curve progression in untreated idiopathic scoliosis during growth. *J Bone Joint Surg Am*. 1984;66:1061.
11. Risser JC. The iliac apophysis; an invaluable sign in the management of scoliosis. *Clin Orthop*. 1958;11:111.
12. Weinstein SL, Ponseti IV. Curve progression in idiopathic scoliosis. *J Bone Joint Surg Am*. 1983;65:447.
13. Pehrsson K, Bake B, Larsson S, et al: Lung Function in adult idiopathic scoliosis: A 20 year follow up. *Thorax*. 1991;46:474.
14. Bertrand SL, Drvaric DM, Lange N et al: Electrical stimulation for idiopathic scoliosis. *Clin Orthop Relat Res*. 1992:176.
15. Richards BS. The effects of growth on the scoliotic spine following posterior spinal fusion. In: Buckwalter JA, et al, eds. *Skeletal Growth and Development: Clinical Issues and Basic Science Advances*. Rosemont, IL: American Academy of Orthopedic Surgeons; 1998:577.
16. Cehn ZY, Wong HK, Chan YH. Variability of somatosensory evoked potential monitoring during scoliosis surgery. *J Spinal Disord Tech*. 2004;17:470.
17. American Academy of Orthopedic Surgeons: *School Screening Programs for the Early Detection of Scoliosis*. Rosemont, IL. American Academy of Orthopedic Surgeons; 1992.
18. Lloyd-Roberts GC, Pilcher MF. Structural idiopathic scoliosis in infancy: A study of the natural history of 100 patients: *J Bone Joint Surg Br*. 1965;47;520.

PART 14

DERMATOLOGY

Strength of Recommendation (SOR)	Definition
A	Recommendation based on consistent and good-quality patient-oriented evidence.*
B	Recommendation based on inconsistent or limited-quality patient-oriented evidence.*
C	Recommendation based on consensus, usual practice, opinion, disease-oriented evidence, or case series for studies of diagnosis, treatment, prevention, or screening.*

*See Appendix A on pages 1320–1322 for further information.

SECTION 1 EARLY CHILDHOOD DERMATOLOGY

92 NORMAL SKIN CHANGES OF INFANCY

Mindy Smith, MD, MS
Cristina Fernandez, MD

PATIENT STORY

A 2-week-old infant is brought to the office for her first well-baby check. The parents noticed a rash on the face. You diagnose the white spots on the bridge of the nose as milia and neonatal acne on the cheeks. The parents are happy to hear that the neonatal acne and milia will go away without treatment (**Figures 92-1** and **92-2**).

INTRODUCTION

- Rashes are common in newborns. Physicians will be consulted frequently as they are a common parental concern. Almost all newborn rashes are benign; however, a few are associated with more serious conditions. A newborn's skin shows a variety of changes during the first 2 months of life and most are self-limited. Physicians must be prepared to identify common rashes and provide advice to parents.[1]
- Milia are inclusion cysts that appear as tiny white papules in the skin (**Figure 92-1**) or on the roof of the mouth.
- Neonatal acne is an acneiform eruption appearing as small red papules or whiteheads with surrounding erythema on the skin of newborns (**Figure 92-2**).
- A mongolian spot is a hereditary, congenital macule of bluish-black or bluish-gray pigment usually in the sacral area, back, and buttocks of infants (**Figures 92-3** and **92-4**).
- Erythema toxicum neonatorum (ETN) is a benign, self-limited skin eruption appearing as small yellow-white papules or vesicles with surrounding skin erythema (**Figures 92-5** and **92-6**).

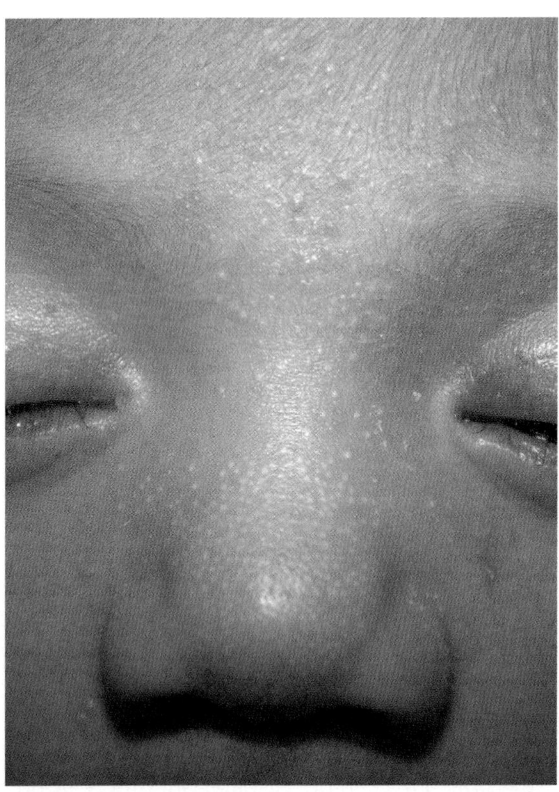

FIGURE 92-1 Milia on the face of a 2-week-old infant with greatest number of milia on the nose. (*Used with permission from Richard P. Usatine, MD.*)

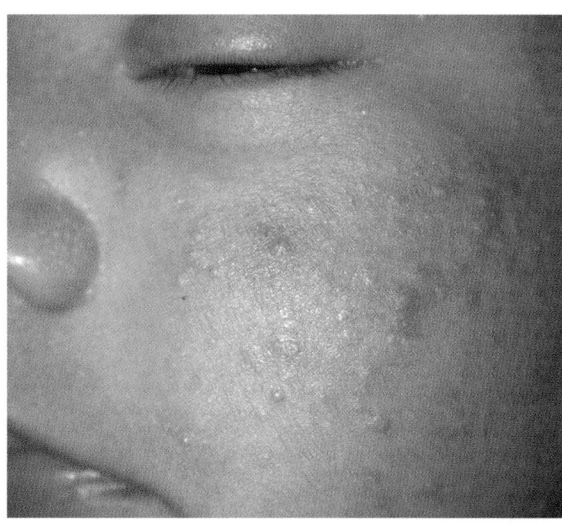

FIGURE 92-2 Neonatal acne on the same infant as in Figure 92-1. (*Used with permission from Richard P. Usatine, MD.*)

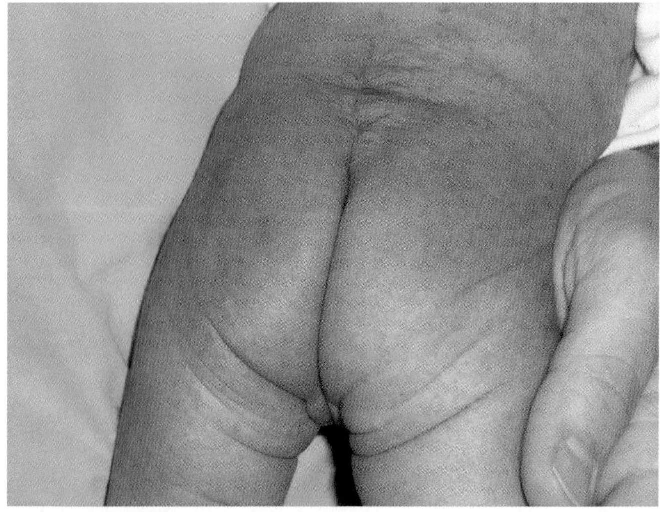

FIGURE 92-3 Large mongolian spots covering the buttocks and back of a Hispanic infant. (*Used with permission from Richard P. Usatine, MD.*)

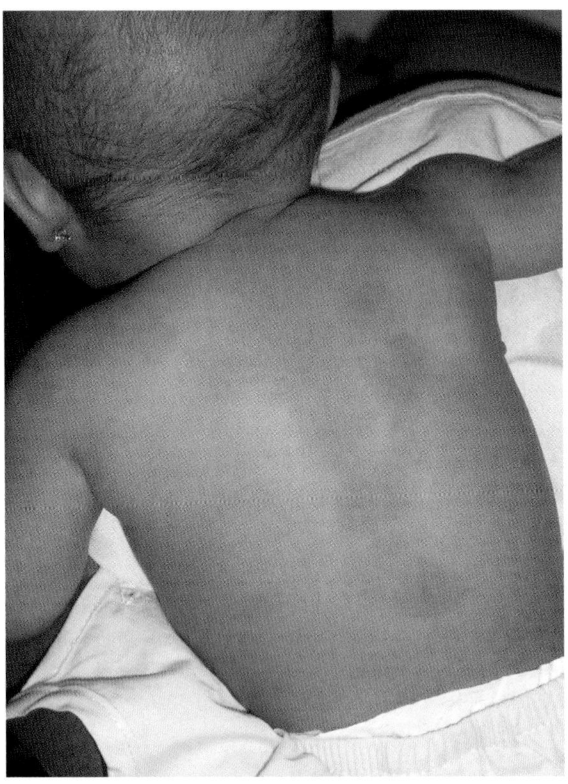

FIGURE 92-4 Prominent mongolian spots on the back of a 1-year-old black child. (*Used with permission from Richard P. Usatine, MD.*)

SYNONYMS

- Milia are also called milk spots or oil seed.
- Neonatal acne is also called acne neonatorum.
- Mongolian spots are also known as mongolian blue spots, congenital dermal melanocytosis, and dermal melanocytosis.

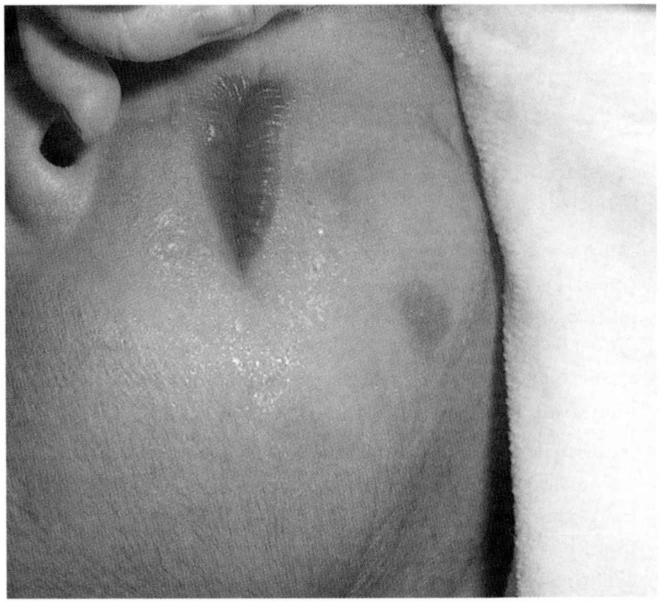

FIGURE 92-5 One small spot of erythema toxicum neonatorum (ETN) on a 2-day-old infant. (*Used with permission from Richard P. Usatine, MD.*)

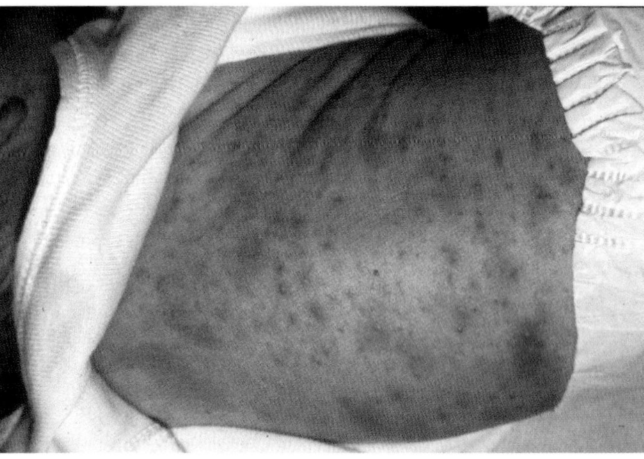

FIGURE 92-6 More widespread case of erythema toxicum neonatorum (ETN) covering the infant. ETN is completely benign and will resolve spontaneously. (*Used with permission from the University of Texas Health Sciences Center, Division of Dermatology.*)

EPIDEMIOLOGY

- Approximately 40 percent of newborn infants in the US develop milia.[2] This condition is mainly associated with newborns carried to full term or near term.
- Neonatal acne occurs in up to 20 percent of the newborns. It typically consists of close comedones of the forehead, nose, and cheeks, although other locations are possible. It is most frequent in boys in the first week of life and is 5 times more common in boys than girls.[3]
- The prevalence of mongolian spots varies among different ethnic groups. They have been reported in approximately 96 percent of black infants, 90 percent of Native American infants, 81 to 90 percent of Asian infants, 46 to 70 percent of Hispanic infants, and 1 to 10 percent of white infants.[2,4,5]
- ETN occurs in 30 to 70 percent of full-term infants and in 5 percent of premature infants. The incidence rises with increasing gestational age and birth weight.[6,7]
- In one case series of infants in the first 48 hours of life in San Diego (N = 594), the incidence of milia was 8 percent and ETN, 7 percent.[8] A prevalence rate of ETN of 16.7 percent was found within the first 72 hours in 1,000 Spanish infants.[9]

ETIOLOGY AND PATHOPHYSIOLOGY

- Milia are inclusion cysts that contain trapped keratinized stratum corneum surrounded by a dense lymphocytic infiltrate. Milia are caused by retention of keratin within the dermis. They may rarely be associated with other abnormalities in syndromes such as epidermolysis bullosa and the orofacial digital syndrome (type 1).[2,10]
- Neonatal acne was thought to be due to maternal androgenic hormones stimulating sebaceous glands; more recently it is theorized that neonatal acne is caused by an increase in dehydroepiandrosterone (DHEA) production causing enlargement and possibly hyperactivity of the fetal adrenal gland.[3]
    - Histologic examination shows hyperplastic sebaceous glands with keratin-plugged orifices.

- The mongolian spot is a hereditary, congenital, developmental condition exclusively involving the skin. It results from entrapment of melanocytes in the dermis during their migration from the neural crest into the epidermis.
  - Mongolian spots are associated with cleft lip, spinal meningeal tumor, melanoma, and phakomatosis pigmentovascularis types 2 and 5.[2,11]
  - A few cases of extensive mongolian spots have been reported with inborn errors of metabolism, the most common being Hurler syndrome, followed by gangliosidosis type 1, Niemann-Pick disease, Hunter syndrome, and mannosidosis. In such cases, they are likely to persist rather than resolve.[2,4]
- The etiology of ETN is not known. ETN is thought to be an immune system reaction; the condition is associated with increased levels of immunologic and inflammatory mediators (e.g., interleukins 1 and 8, eotaxin).[12]
  - The eosinophilic infiltrate of ETN suggests an allergic-related or hypersensitivity-related etiology, but no allergens have been identified. Newborn skin appears to respond to any injury with an eosinophilic infiltrate.
  - Because ETN rarely is seen in premature infants, it is believed that mature newborn skin is required to produce this reaction pattern.

DIAGNOSIS

CLINICAL FEATURES

- Milia are characterized as tiny, pearly white papules (**Figure 92-1**) that are actually small inclusion cysts ranging from 1 to 2 mm in diameter. No visible opening is present.[2]
  - Milia usually appear after 4 to 5 days of life in full-term newborns. Manifestations of milia may be delayed from days to weeks in infants born before term.[11,12]
- Neonatal acne (**Figure 92-2**) includes comedones (i.e., whiteheads), papules, and pustules.
  - Papules and pustules are the most frequent types of lesions (72.7%), followed by comedones only (22.7%).[2]
- A mongolian spot (**Figures 92-3** and **92-4**) is a bluish-black macule or patch typically a few centimeters in diameter, although much larger lesions also can occur. Lesions may be solitary or numerous.
  - Generalized mongolian spots involving large areas covering the entire posterior or anterior trunk and the extremities have been reported.
  - Several variants exist including:[2,4]
    - Persistent mongolian spots—These are larger, have sharper margins, and persist for many years (**Figure 92-4**).
    - Aberrant mongolian spots involve unusual sites such as the face or extremities.
    - Persistent aberrant mongolian spots also are referred to as macular-type blue nevi.
- ETN commonly presents with a blotchy, evanescent, macular erythema (**Figures 92-5** and **92-6**).
  - The macules are irregular, blanchable, and vary in size.
  - In more severe cases (**Figure 92-6**), pale yellow or white wheals or papules on an erythematous base may follow. In approximately 10 percent of patients, 2- to 4-mm pustules develop.[7]
  - ETN occurs within the first 4 days of life in full-term infants, with the peak onset within the first 48 hours following birth. Rare cases have been reported at birth.
  - Delayed onset can rarely occur in full-term and preterm infants up to 14 days of age.
  - Infants with ETN otherwise are healthy and lack systemic symptoms.

TYPICAL DISTRIBUTION

- Milia are found on the forehead, nose, upper lip, cheeks, and scalp. They can, however, occur anywhere and may be present at birth or appear subsequently. The milia on the child in **Figure 92-1** were present at birth.
- Neonatal acne occurs on the face with the cheeks being the most common site (81.8%) (**Figure 92-2**).[2]
- Mongolian spots most commonly involve the lumbosacral area (**Figure 92-3**), but the buttocks, flanks, and shoulders (**Figure 92-4**) may be affected with extensive lesions.
- ETN sites of predilection include the forehead, face, trunk, and proximal extremities, but lesions may occur anywhere, including the genitalia. Involvement of the mucous membranes and palms and soles rarely occurs (**Figures 92-5** and **92-6**).

LABS AND IMAGING

- No laboratory studies are required.
- In extensive mongolian spots involving the back, radiographic studies are needed to rule out a spinal meningeal tumor or anomaly.[4]
- ETN is often diagnosed clinically, based on history and physical examination, but a peripheral smear of intralesional contents can be done to confirm the diagnosis.[2,7]
  - A Tzanck smear or Gram stain shows inflammatory cells with greater than 90 percent eosinophils and variable numbers of neutrophils.
  - A complete blood count (CBC) also shows eosinophilia (up to 18%) in approximately 15 percent of patients. Eosinophilia may be more pronounced when the eruption shows a marked pustular component.

DIFFERENTIAL DIAGNOSIS

Other diagnoses that can be confused with milia, neonatal acne, and ETN include:

- Miliaria—Heat rash (prickly heat) with tiny papules that can be red (miliaria rubra) or clear (miliaria crystallina) or pustular (miliaria pustulosa) (**Figure 92-7**). Miliaria results from sweat retention caused by partial closure of eccrine structures. Both milia and miliaria result from immaturity of the skin structures, but they are clinically distinct entities.
- Neonatal pustular melanosis—This eruption, present at birth, consists of 2- to 4-mm nonerythematous vesicles filled with a milky fluid. This rash occurs in 5 percent of African American newborns and in less than 1 percent of white newborns, and fades in the first 3 to 4 weeks of life (see Chapter 94, Pustular Diseases of Childhood).
- Drug reaction (maternal medication or infant)—History of drug administration and can be more widespread.

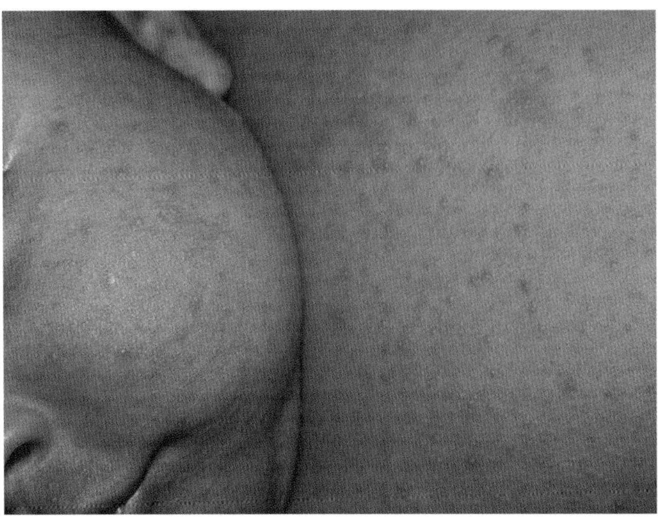

FIGURE 92-7 Miliaria (heat rash) in a 6-month-old infant on a warm summer day. (*Used with permission from Richard P. Usatine, MD.*)

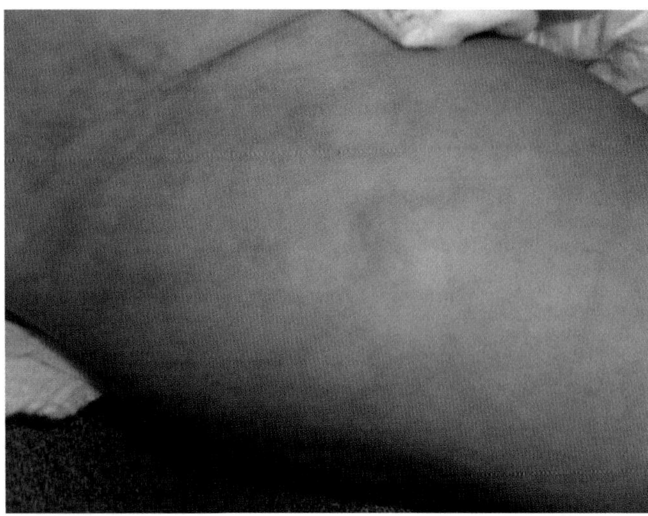

FIGURE 92-8 Cutis marmorata in a 4-month-old infant in a cold exam room. Notice the reticular pattern. This resolved when the infant was warmed. (*Used with permission from Richard P. Usatine, MD.*)

Mongolian spots may be confused with the following lesions also present at birth or shortly after:

- Congenital melanocytic nevi—These lesions are much less common (1 to 2% of newborns). They are of variable color from tan or brown to red or black, often within a single lesion and the pigment may fade off into surrounding skin. The borders are often irregular and the lesion can appear slightly raised over time (although a macular portion is usually found at the edges). Most congenital melanocytic nevi have a darker color and more discrete borders than mongolian spots. A biopsy is only needed if melanoma is suspected (see Chapter 144, Congenital Nevi).
- There are reports of Mongolian spots being confused for the bruising that occurs in child abuse. A good history and a clear knowledge of the pattern of mongolian spots should help to differentiate between these two entities.

ETN can also be confused with the following:

- Miliaria—See preceding information.
- Folliculitis—Primary lesion is a papule or pustule pierced by a central hair, although the hair may not always be visualized. Deeper lesions present as erythematous, often fluctuant, nodules. Folliculitis rarely occurs in the first few days of life when ETN is most commonly seen (see Chapter 100, Folliculitis).
- Herpes simplex virus—A single vesicle or crops of vesicles on an erythematous base are often the first manifestations of neonatal herpes simplex virus infection, which is associated with a high morbidity and mortality. The appearance of these lesions may mimic ETN. Any vesicular rash in the newborn should be evaluated for the possibility of herpes simplex virus infection (see Chapter 187, Congenital Infections).
- Chickenpox—The characteristic rash appears in crops of lesions beginning with red macules and passing through stages of papule, vesicle (on an erythematous base), pustule, and crust. Simultaneous presence of different stages of the rash is a hallmark. Infants are mostly born with adequate maternal antibodies to varicella, so that timing should differentiate between these two conditions (see Chapter 108, Chickenpox).
- Cutis marmorata (**Figure 92-8**) is reticulated mottled skin with symmetric involvement of the trunk and extremities produced by a vascular response to cold; the change resolves with heat. This entity can persist for weeks or months. No treatment is indicated.
- Harlequin color change affects 10 percent of full-term babies and occurs when the newborn lies on one side and erythema develops on one side of the body, while blanching is seen on the contralateral side. The color change fades after 30 seconds to 20 minutes and resolves with increased muscle activity or crying. It begins between the second to fifth days of life and lasts up to 3 weeks.[13]
- Neonatal lupus is a rare syndrome in which maternal autoantibodies are passively transferred to the baby producing well-demarcated, erythematous, scaling patches that are often annular, predominately on the scalp, neck or face (**Figure 92-9**). The condition is self-limited and resolves without scarring by 6 to 7 months of age. It is associated with congenital heart block. Treatment includes photoprotection; mild topical steroids may be helpful.

MANAGEMENT

- Milia, neonatal acne, mongolian spots, and ETN are benign conditions and parents should be reassured that they resolve with time.
- Although acne treatment generally is not indicated, infants can be treated with a topical ketoconazole 2 percent cream twice daily for 1 week.[3] If acne persists more than 4 weeks, infantile acne is likely and 2.5 percent benzoyl peroxide lotion can be used.[3]

PROGNOSIS

- Milia usually disappear within several weeks.
- Neonatal acne may come and go until the baby is between 4 and 6 months of age.
- Mongolian spots may persist for many years but usually disappear within 3 to 5 years and almost always by puberty.

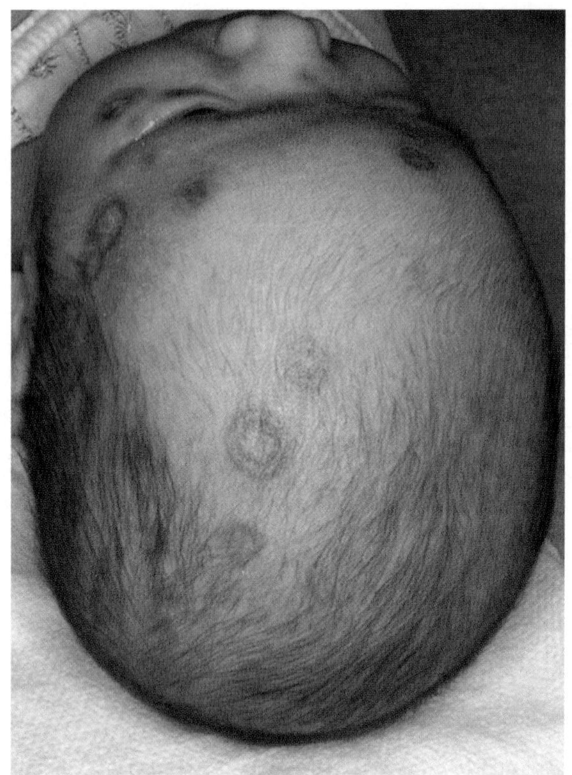

FIGURE 92-9 Neonatal lupus from acquired antibodies through transplacental transmission from the mother with active systemic lupus erythematosus (SLE). Note the annular patterns of scale. (*From Warner AM, Frey KA, Connolly S. Photo rounds: annular rash on a newborn. J Fam Pract. 2006;55(2):127-129. Reproduced with permission from Frontline Medical Communications.*)

- ETN usually lasts for several days but can change rapidly, with lesions appearing and disappearing in different areas over hours.

PATIENT EDUCATION

- Milia is a benign self-limiting rash that disappears within a few months without leaving any scars. No drug therapy is required and use of nonprescription rash medications is not recommended.
- Neonatal acne resolves on its own in weeks. Oils and lotions do not help and may actually aggravate the acne.
- Mongolian spots are likely to fade over time and may disappear by age 7 to 13 years.
- ETN will usually disappear within 2 weeks.

PATIENT RESOURCES

- Milia—**www.ncbi.nlm.nih.gov/pubmedhealth/PMH0002343/**.
- Neonatal acne—**www.womenshealthcaretopics.com/baby_acne.htm**.
- Mongolian spot—**www.nlm.nih.gov/medlineplus/ency/article/001472.htm**.
- ETN—**www.nlm.nih.gov/medlineplus/ency/article/001458.htm**.

PROVIDER RESOURCES

- **www.adhb.govt.nz/newborn/teachingresources/dermatology/BenignLesions.htm**.
- **www.aafp.org/afp/2008/0101/p47.html**.

REFERENCES

1. McLaughlin MR, O'Connor NR, Ham P. Newborn skin: part II. Birthmarks. *Am Fam Physician*. 2008;77(1):56-60.
2. Agrawal R. *Pediatric Milia*. http://emedicine.medscape.com/article/910405-overview, accessed February 2013.
3. Friedlander SF, Baldwin HE, Mancini AJ, et al. The acne continuum: an age-based approach to therapy. *Semin Cutan Med Surg*. 2011;30(3 Suppl):S6-11.
4. Ashrafi MR, Shabanian R, Mohammadi M, Kavusi S. Extensive Mongolian spots: a clinical sign merits special attention. *Pediatr Neurol*. 2006;34(2):143-145.
5. Cordova A. The Mongolian spot: a study of ethnic differences and a literature review. *Clin Pediatr (Phila)*. 1981;20(11):714-719.
6. Clemons RM. Issues in newborn care. *Prim Care*. 2000;27(1):251-267.
7. Liu C, Feng J, Qu R. Epidemiologic study of the predisposing factors in erythema toxicum neonatorum. *Dermatology*. 2005;210(4):269-272.
8. Kanada KN, Merin MR, Munden A, Friedlander SF. A prospective study of cutaneous findings in newborns in the United States: correlation with race, ethnicity, and gestational status using updated classification and nomenclature. *J Pediatr*. 2012;161(2):240-245.
9. Monteagudo B, Labandeira J, Cabanillas M, et al. Prospective study of erythema toxicum neonatorum: epidemiology and predisposing factors. *Pediatr Dermatol*. 2012;29(2):166-168.
10. Johr RH, Schachner LA. Neonatal dermatologic challenges. *Pediatr Rev*. 1997;18(3):86-94.
11. Mallory SB. Neonatal skin disorders. *Pediatr Clin North Am*. 1991;38(4):745-761.
12. Keitel HG, Yadav V. Etiology of toxic erythema. Erythema toxicum neonatorum. *Am J Dis Child*. 1963;106:306-309.
13. Selmogul MA, Dilmen U, Karkelleoglu C, et al. Picture of the month. Harlequin color change. *Arch Pediatr Adolesc Med*. 1995;149(10):1171-1172.

93 CHILDHOOD HEMANGIOMAS AND VASCULAR MALFORMATIONS

Richard P. Usatine, MD
Megha Madhukar, MD

PATIENT STORY

A baby girl is brought to the office because her mother is concerned over the growing strawberry hemangioma on her face. Her mother is reassured that most of these childhood hemangiomas regress over time and that there is no need for immediate treatment (**Figure 93-1**).

INTRODUCTION

Hemangiomas are the most common benign tumors of infancy. They can be problematic if they block vision or interfere with any vital function. Most hemangiomas are small and of cosmetic concern only.

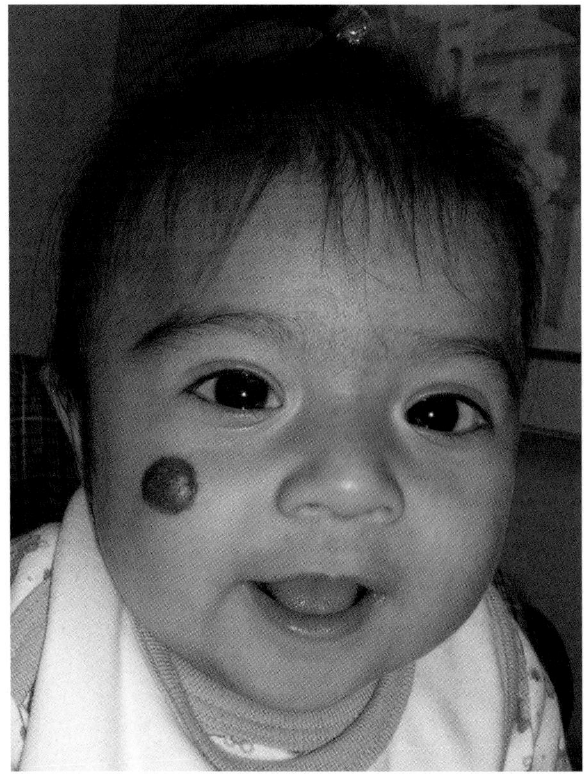

FIGURE 93-1 Strawberry hemangioma on the face causing no functional problems. Treatment is reassurance and watchful waiting. *(Used with permission from Richard P. Usatine, MD.)*

SYNONYMS

Infantile hemangiomas, angiomas. Strawberry hemangiomas are also called superficial hemangiomas of infancy. Cavernous hemangiomas are also called deep hemangiomas of infancy.

EPIDEMIOLOGY

- Approximately 30 percent of hemangiomas are present at birth; the other 70 percent appear within the first few weeks of life.
- Hemangiomas occur more commonly in fair-skinned, premature, female infants. In one study, the mothers of children with hemangiomas are of higher maternal age, have a higher incidence of preeclampsia and placenta previa, and are more likely to have had multiple gestation pregnancies.[1]
- There is an increased incidence of vascular anomalies in the families of children born with hemangiomas.[1]
- The data are mixed as to whether chorionic villus sampling may play a role in the formation of hemangiomas.[1]
- Females are affected more often than males (2.4:1).[1]

ETIOLOGY AND PATHOPHYSIOLOGY

- Hemangiomas consist of an abnormally dense group of dilated blood vessels. Most childhood hemangiomas are thought to occur sporadically.
- Hemangiomas are characterized by an initial phase of rapid proliferation, followed by spontaneous and slow involution, often leading to complete regression. Most childhood hemangiomas are small and innocuous, but some grow to threaten a particular function (**Figure 93-2**) or even life.
- Rapid growth during the first month of life is the historical hallmark of hemangiomas, when rapidly dividing endothelial cells are responsible for the enlargement of these lesions. The hemangiomas become elevated and may take on numerous morphologies (dome-shaped, lobulated, plaque-like, and/or tumoral). The proliferation phase occurs during the first year, with most growth taking place during the first 6 months of life. Proliferation then slows and the hemangioma begins to involute.
- The involutional phase may be rapid or prolonged. No specific feature has been identified in explaining the rate or completeness of involution. However, in one type of hemangioma, the rapidly involuting congenital hemangioma, the proliferation phase occurs entirely in utero such that the lesion is fully developed at birth, followed by complete involution during the second year of life.[1]
- A good rule of thumb is 50 percent of childhood hemangiomas will involute by age 5 years, 70 percent by age 7 years, and the remainder of childhood hemangiomas will take an additional 3 to 5 years to complete the process of involution.[1]
- Of the lesions that have involuted by age 6 years, 38 percent will leave residual evidence of the hemangioma in the form of a scar, telangiectasia, or redundant, "bag-like" skin. The chance of

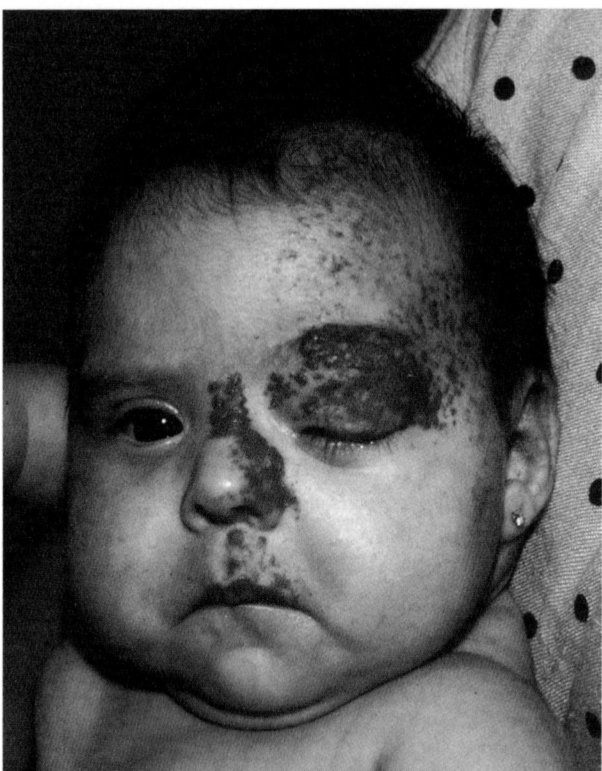

FIGURE 93-2 Large hemangioma on the face needing immediate treatment to prevent amblyopia in the left eye. Although this hemangioma follows the V1 dermatome, this is not a port-wine stain and the patient does not have Sturge-Weber syndrome. (*Used with permission from Richard P. Usatine, MD.*)

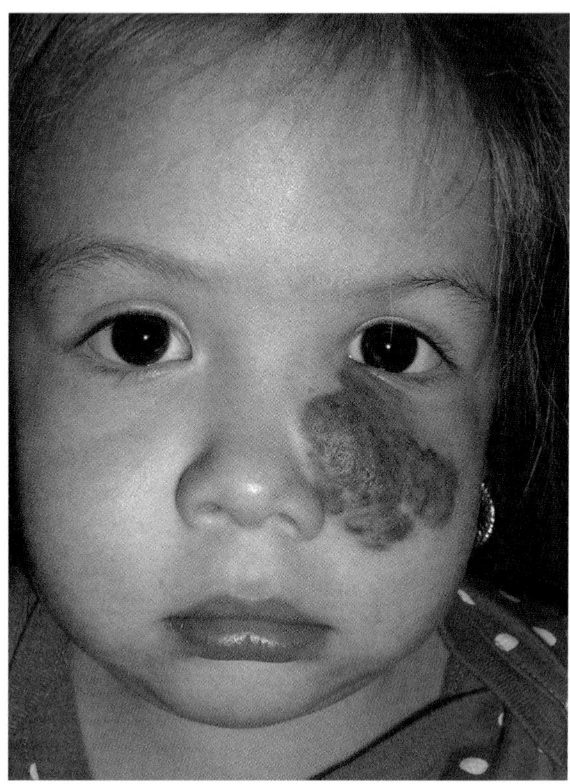

FIGURE 93-3 Strawberry hemangioma present since birth on the face of a 22-month-old girl. Although it is close to her eye, her vision has never been occluded. She has been followed by ophthalmology and no active treatment was recommended. The hemangioma grew larger during the first year of life and is now beginning to involute without treatment. (*Used with permission from Richard P. Usatine, MD.*)

a permanent scar increases the longer it takes to involute. For example, of the lesions that involute after age 6 years, 80 percent may exhibit a cosmetic deformity.[1]

DIAGNOSIS

CLINICAL FEATURES

Early lesions may be subtle, resembling a scratch or bruise, or alternatively may look like a small patch of telangiectasias or an area of hypopigmentation. Hemangiomas can start off as a flat red mark, but as proliferation ensues, it grows to become a spongy mass protruding from the skin. The earliest sign of a hemangioma is blanching of the involved skin with a few fine telangiectasias followed by a red macule. Rarely, a shallow ulceration may be the first sign of an incipient hemangioma.[1] Hemangiomas are typically diagnosed based on appearance, rarely warranting further diagnostic tests.

Hemangiomas may be superficial, deep, or a combination of both. Superficial hemangiomas are well defined, bright red, and appear as nodules or plaques located above clinically normal skin (**Figures 93-1** to **93-3**). Deep hemangiomas are raised flesh-colored nodules, which often have a bluish hue and feel firm and rubbery (**Figure 93-4**).

Most are clinically insignificant unless they impinge on vital structures, ulcerate, bleed, incite a consumptive coagulopathy, or cause high output cardiac failure or structural abnormalities. Blocking vision is a common reason needed for treatment (**Figure 93-2**).

TYPICAL DISTRIBUTION

Anywhere on the body, most often on the face, scalp, back, or chest.

IMAGING

Most hemangiomas of infancy do not need imaging. If the hemangioma is very large, deep or undefined, MRI with and without IV gadolinium helps delineate the location and extent of the hemangioma

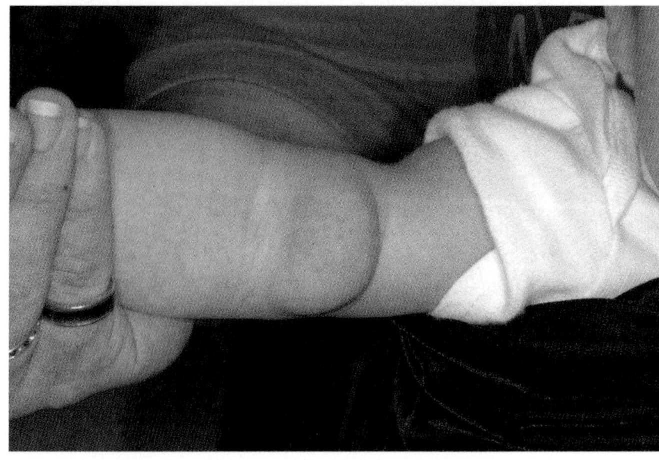

FIGURE 93-4 Deep (cavernous) hemangioma on the arm in a 9-month-old child. Treatment is watchful waiting. (*Used with permission from Richard P. Usatine, MD.*)

while also differentiating them from high flow vascular lesions, like arteriovenous malformations.[1] Ultrasound is a useful tool to differentiate hemangiomas from other subcutaneous structures such as cysts and lymph nodes as well as from other soft-tissue masses.[1]

Plain radiography may be useful for evaluating hemangiomas that impinge on an airway.[1]

BIOPSY

Biopsies are rarely needed and can be risky because vascular lesions may bleed profusely. If a biopsy is being considered, it might be best to refer to a specialist.

DIFFERENTIAL DIAGNOSIS

- Superficial capillary malformations that are frequently seen in infants include those above the eyelids and nape of the neck. These are called *salmon patches* and are not dangerous. The "angel's kisses" on the eyelids usually disappear by age 2 years. The "stork bites" may last into adulthood but are rarely an issue because they often get covered by hair (**Figures 93-5** and **93-6**). These capillary malformations are a variant of nevus flammeus or port-wine stain. They are macular, sharply circumscribed, pink to purple, and varied in size (see Chapter 170, Hereditary and Congenital Vascular Skin Lesions).
- Blue rubber bleb nevus syndrome—Bluish cutaneous vascular malformations that empty with pressure, texture resembles rubbery nodules, similar to deep hemangiomas.[2]
- Maffucci syndrome—Rare congenital nonhereditary mesodermal dysplasia characterized by multiple enchondromata, cutaneous hemangiomas, and more recently spindle cell hemangiomas.[3] It is important to identify Maffucci syndrome early because it is associated with an increased risk of malignancy. May appear as multiple vascular malformations of the skin with a "grape-like" appearance (see Chapter 170, Hereditary and Congenital Vascular Skin Lesions).
- Arteriovenous malformation—Benign, single red papules on head or neck, may be cutaneous or mucosal.[4]

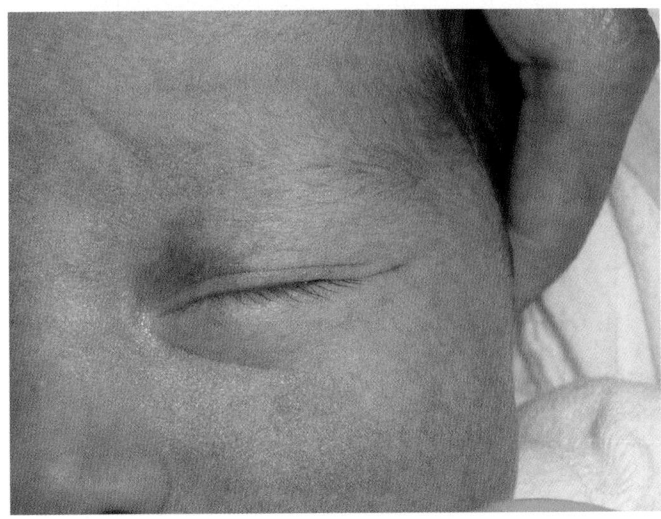

FIGURE 93-5 Salmon patch (a variant of nevus flammeus) on the upper eyelid called an "angel's kiss." These resolve by age 2 years. (*Used with permission from Richard P. Usatine, MD.*)

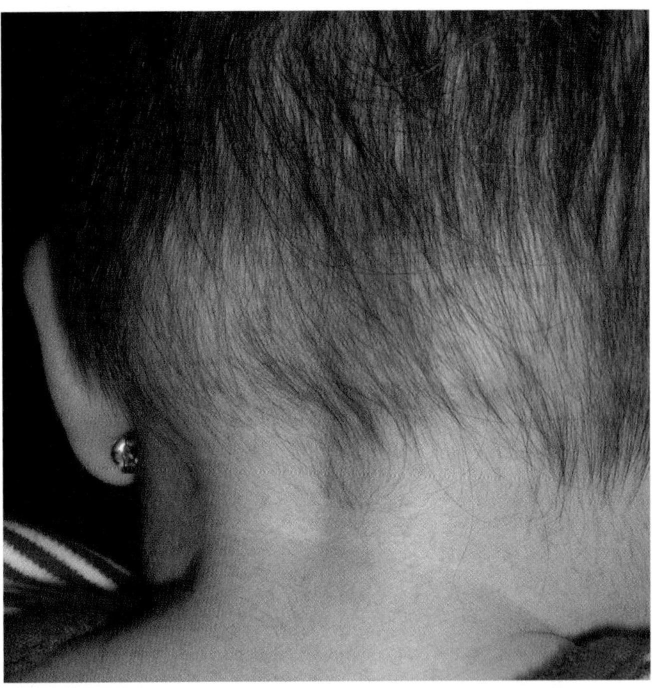

FIGURE 93-6 Salmon patch (a variant of nevus flammeus) on the neck of this young child called a "stork bite." These vascular malformations persist into adulthood. (*Used with permission from Richard P. Usatine, MD.*)

- Infantile fibrosarcoma—A rare and highly malignant tumor of childhood that may take on the form of a highly vascularized mass, resembling a hemangioma, especially after a hemangioma has ulcerated as a result of rapid proliferation.[5]

MANAGEMENT

- The majority of hemangiomas will eventually involute without complications and require no treatment, but approximately 20 percent cause complications like ulcerations, irreversible cutaneous expansion, or threaten vital structures such as the eyes, nose, or airways.[6]
- Any large segmental hemangioma on the face could be part of the PHACE (posterior fossa malformations, hemangiomas, arterial anomalies, coarctation of aorta, cardiac defects, eye abnormalities) syndrome and therefore will need evaluation of the eyes, central nervous system (CNS), and heart (see Chapter 227, PHACE syndrome).
    - **P**osterior fossa—Brain malformations present at birth.
    - **H**emangioma—Segmental hemangioma covers a large area on the head or neck (greater than 5 cm).
    - **A**rterial lesions—Abnormalities of the blood vessels in the neck or head.
    - **C**ardiac abnormalities/aortic coarctation.
    - **E**ye abnormalities.
    - Sternal cleft/pit and supraumbilical raphe may also be present.
- Any lower face or beard hemangioma can be a marker for laryngeal hemangiomatosis. Snoring in such a child can be a bad sign. Refer to a head and neck surgeon.

- Hemangiomas in trauma-prone areas are most likely to ulcerate. These include the diaper area (**Figure 93-7**) and the back of the head. Small ulcerations can be treated with topical mupirocin in morning and metronidazole gel in the evening. SOR Ⓒ
- Propranolol is now the first line of therapy for function-impairing and rapidly proliferating infantile hemangiomas.[2-4] It has been successfully used to treat periorbital infantile hemangiomas and other problematic infantile hemangiomas (**Figure 93-8**).[2-4] SOR Ⓑ
- Propranolol (20 mg/5 mL) is given orally starting with 1 mg/kg per day divided into qid dosing. It is advisable to monitor for hypoglycemia and low blood pressure even though this treatment has been found to be safe in a number of studies.[2-4] If the child is tolerating the treatment well, the dose may be increased to the recommended maintenance dose of 1.5 to 2 mg/kg per day in divided doses.[2,4] Treatment should be maintained until the lesion is completely involuted or the child is 1 year of age.
- Prior to the discovery of the benefits and safety of propranolol as a first-line treatment, prednisone 3 to 5 mg/kg per day had been shown to provide an effective and rapid way of treating hemangiomas.[7] SOR Ⓑ In a study, 68 percent of patients receiving systemic corticosteroid treatment with oral prednisone experienced rapid and virtually complete involution of hemangiomas.[7] Another 25 percent experienced significant regression, and treatment demonstrated no effect in 7 percent of patients. The authors recommended treating with oral prednisone for 6 to 8 weeks, and in more severe cases, for 12 weeks. Side effects include moon facies and irritability, which resolved once therapy was discontinued.[7] Growth may be retarded temporarily.

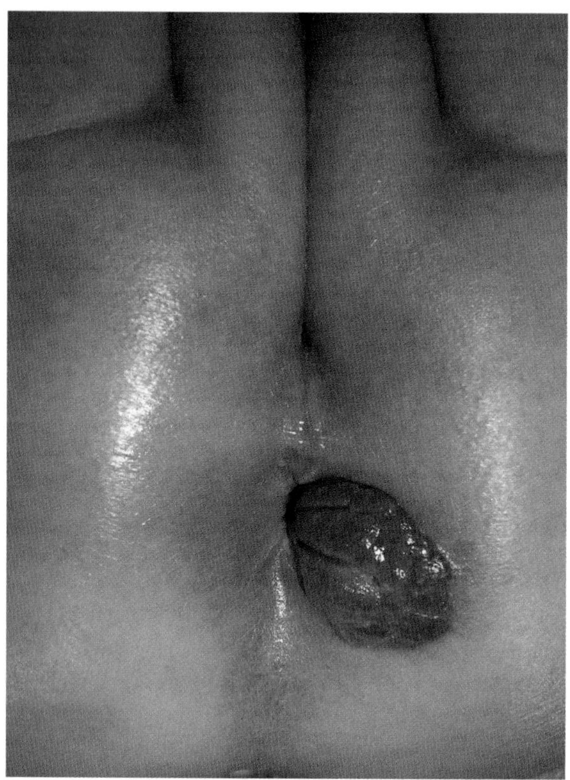

FIGURE 93-7 Strawberry hemangioma in the perianal area of a 5-month-old girl. This is at high risk of ulceration. (*Used with permission from Richard P. Usatine, MD.*)

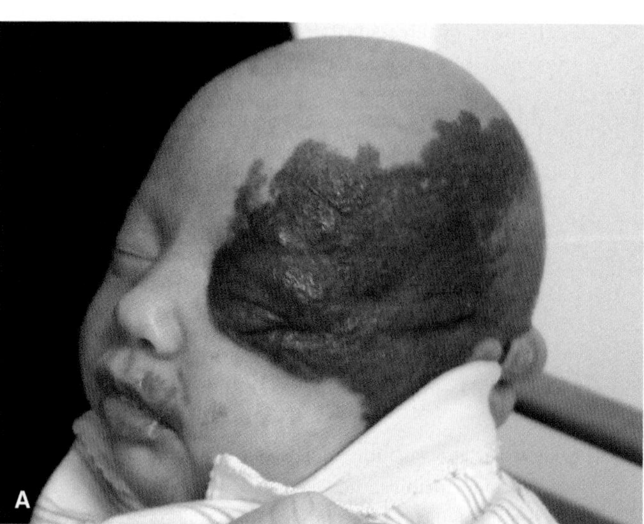

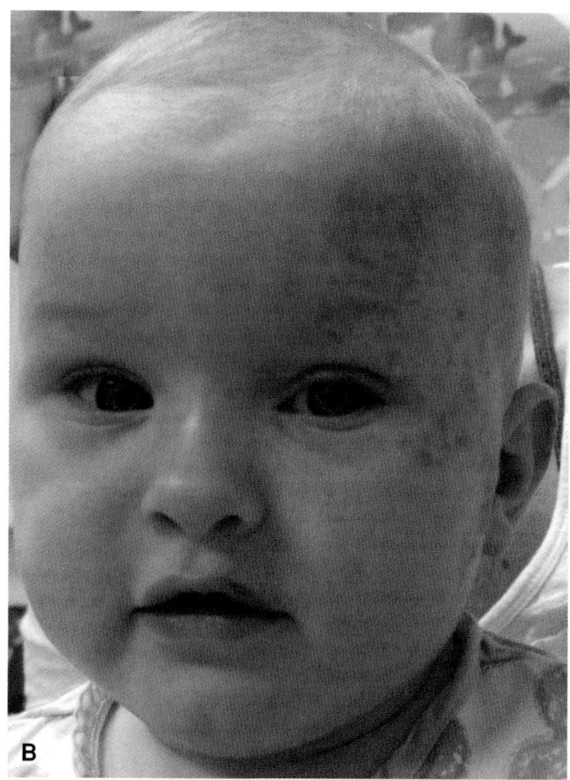

FIGURE 93-8 Large infantile hemangioma in which the child does not have the PHACE syndrome. However, urgent therapy was needed to shrink this hemangioma. **A.** Before propranolol therapy. **B.** After propranolol therapy. (*Used with permission from John Browning, MD.*)

- Ultrapotent topical corticosteroids have been found especially helpful in the treatment of small hemangiomas, especially periocular hemangiomas and those at sites prone to ulceration and disfigurement. Seventy-four percent of patients demonstrated good or at least partial response to treatment with the majority experiencing cessation of growth before what would have been expected for their age. Thinner, more superficial hemangiomas demonstrated better improvement than thicker, deeper lesions.[8] SOR B
- Intralesional corticosteroid injections, composed of a mixture containing triamcinolone acetonide (20 mg average dose) and betamethasone acetate (3 mg average dose) with varying number of injections, have been found to successfully treat head and neck childhood hemangiomas in properly selected infants. In a research study, 13 percent of the hemangiomas treated with intralesional injections almost completely involuted, 32 percent showed greater than 50 percent reduction in volume, 32 percent showed definite but less than 50 percent reduction in volume, and 23 percent showed little to no decrease in size.[9] SOR B Avoid intralesional steroids around eye.
- Treatment with flashlamp-pumped pulsed-dye laser has been found to be an effective treatment method for superficial cutaneous hemangiomas at sites of potential functional impairment and on the face. In a study, 76 percent of patients were found to have excellent or good results with the flashlamp-pumped pulsed-dye laser. Hemangiomas with a deep component do not seem to benefit from flashlamp-pumped pulsed-dye laser therapy to the same degree as a truly superficial hemangioma, as the laser is limited by its depth of vascular injury.[10] SOR B
- Facial hemangiomas causing severe functional disturbance and serious psychological distress are strong reasons to consider surgical excision before the child reaches the expected age of spontaneous regression. SOR C
- Large periocular hemangiomas demand prompt treatment to prevent debilitating consequences such as amblyopia (**Figure 93-2**). Early treatment is also recommended for proliferative labial tumors because not only do they have a tendency to bleed, but they also make eating difficult. Additionally, early treatment with a consideration for surgery is advised for hemangiomas located on the nasal tip as they regress slowly and may ultimately result in distortion of the nasal framework.[11]
- Laser surgery may be considered for selective ablation of vascular tissue, like ulcerated hemangiomas and thin superficial hemangiomas, especially when their locations may result in psychosocial distress for the patient, that is, facial hemangiomas. The pulsed-dye laser seems especially promising with its ability to selectively damage blood vessels with minimal damage to surrounding tissues.[12] This procedure is also associated with decreased pain and increased healing.[12] SOR B
- Surgical excision of involuted hemangiomas is not uncommon to remove the residual tissue that may be causing cosmetic or functional impairment. Excision is performed in late involution to reduce the risk of hemorrhage.
- Depending on the location and how complex the hemangioma is, consultations with pediatric dermatologists, ophthalmologists, otolaryngologists, plastic surgeons, and pediatric neurosurgeons may be necessary to ensure proper care.

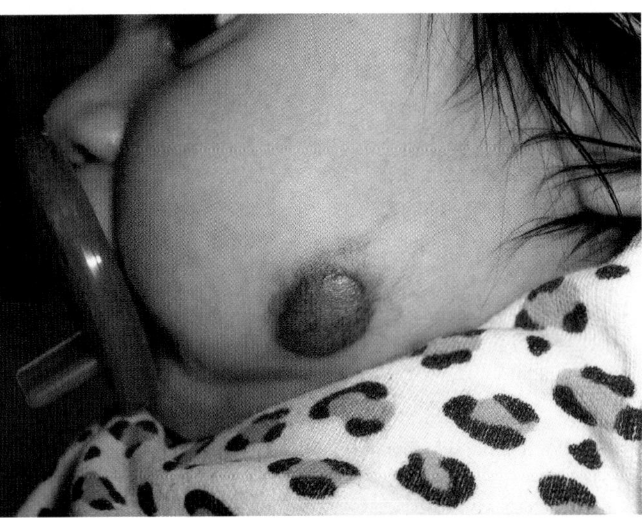

FIGURE 93-9 Strawberry hemangioma on the face causing no functional problems in a 3-month-old girl. The parents requested treatment and a course of topical timolol gel 0.5 percent was initiated. While the hemangioma was in the beard area, the child had no problems with breathing or snoring. A referral to ENT was not needed to investigate for laryngeal hemangiomatosis. *(Used with permission from Richard P. Usatine, MD.)*

NEW TOPICAL THERAPY

- Topical timolol ophthalmic gel or solution has been shown in a number of studies to effectively treat infantile hemangiomas (**Figure 93-9**).[13–15] SOR B One of the studies noted that predictors of better response were superficial type of hemangioma ($p = 0.01$), 0.5 percent timolol concentration ($p = 0.01$), and duration of use longer than 3 months ($p = 0.04$).[14] SOR B Another study using 0.5 percent ophthalmic solution 3 to 4 times daily in patients with small superficial hemangiomas found that treatment was most effective in the early proliferative stage.[13] SOR B

FOLLOW-UP

Watchful waiting and serial observations during well-child examinations are recommended for uncomplicated hemangiomas of infancy. Hemangiomas with complicating factors need close follow-up on an individual basis.

PATIENT EDUCATION

Hemangiomas are benign and not cancer. They are common and up to 1 in 10 white babies will have one. Most hemangiomas will go away spontaneously and not need treatment. For those needing treatments, there are new treatments that are safe and effective (oral propranolol and topical timolol).

PATIENT RESOURCES

- Vascular Birthmarks Foundation—**www.birthmark.org**.

PROVIDER RESOURCES

- National Organization of Vascular Anomalies (NOVA)—**www.novanews.org**.

REFERENCES

1. Antaya R. *Infantile Hemangioma*. http://emedicine.medscape.com/article/1083849, accessed July 16, 2011.
2. Elewski BE, Hughey LC, Parsons ME. *Differential Diagnosis in Dermatology*. St. Louis, MO: Elsevier; 2005:545.
3. McDermott AL, Dutt SN, Shavda SV, Morgan DW. Maffucci's syndrome: clinical and radiological features of a rare condition. *J Laryngol Otol.* 2001;115(10):845-847.
4. Barnhill RL. Vascular tumors. In: Hunt SJ, Santa Cruz DJ, Barnhill RL, eds. *Textbook of Dermatopathology*. New York: McGraw-Hill; 1998:821.
5. Yan AC, Chamlin SL, Liang MG, et al. Fibrosarcoma: a masquerader of ulcerated hemangioma. *Pediatr Dermatol.* 2006;23(4): 330-334.
6. Enjolras O, Wassef M, Mazoyer E, et al. Infants with Kasabach-Merritt syndrome do not have "true" hemangiomas. *J Pediatr.* 1997;130(4):631-640.
7. Sadan N, Wolach B. Treatment of hemangiomas of infants with high doses of prednisone. *J Pediatr.* 1996;128 (1);141-146.
8. Garzon MC, Lucky AW, Hawrot A, Frieden IJ. Ultrapotent topical corticosteroid treatment of hemangiomas of infancy. *J Am Acad Dermatol.* 2005;52:281-286.
9. Sloan G, Reinisch J, Nichter L, et al. Intralesional corticosteroid therapy for infantile hemangiomas. *Plast Reconstr Surg.* 1989;83: 459-466.
10. Poetke M, Phillip C, Berlien HP. Flashlamp-pumped pulsed dye laser for hemangiomas in infancy: treatment of superficial vs. mixed hemangiomas. *Arch Dermatol.* 2000;136(5):628-632.
11. Demiri EC, Pelissier P, Genin-Etcheberry T, et al. Treatment of facial haemangiomas: the present status of surgery. *Br J Plast Surg.* 2001;54(8):665-674.
12. Eedy DJ, Breathnach SM, Walker NPJ. *Surgical Dermatology*. Oxford, UK: Blackwell Science; 1996:245.
13. Oranje AP, Janmohamed SR, Madern GC, de Laat PC. Treatment of small superficial haemangioma with timolol 0.5% ophthalmic solution: a series of 20 cases. *Dermatology*. 2011; 223:330-334.
14. Chakkittakandiyil A, Phillips R, Frieden IJ, et al. Timolol maleate 0.5% or 0.1% gel-forming solution for infantile hemangiomas: a retrospective, multicenter, cohort study. *Pediatr Dermatol.* 2012;29:28-31.
15. Semkova K, Kazandjieva J. Topical timolol maleate for treatment of infantile haemangiomas: preliminary results of a prospective study. *Clin Exp Dermatol.* 2012.

94 PUSTULAR DISEASES OF EARLY CHILDHOOD

Andrew Shedd, MD
Richard P. Usatine, MD
Heidi Chumley, MD

PATIENT STORY

A 1-year-old boy is brought for a second opinion about the recurrent pruritic vesicles and pustules on his hands and feet. This is the third episode, and in both previous episodes, the physicians thought the child had scabies. The child was treated with permethrin both times and within 2 to 3 weeks the skin cleared. No other family members have had lesions or symptoms. **Figures 94-1** to **94-3** demonstrate a typical case of infantile acropustulosis that is often misdiagnosed as scabies. Although the condition can be recurrent, it is ultimately self-limited and will resolve.

INTRODUCTION

Acropustulosis and transient neonatal pustular melanosis (TNPM) are pustular diseases that typically present in infancy. Acropustulosis is a pruritic vesiculopustular disease presenting between 2 and 10 months of age and remitting spontaneously by 36 months of age. TNPM is present at birth and characterized by 2- to 3-mm hyperpigmented macules and pustules. Acropustulosis may require symptomatic treatment of pruritus, but otherwise both illnesses are self-limiting.

EPIDEMIOLOGY

Acropustulosis:

- Rare, intensely pruritic, vesiculopustular disease of young children.[1]

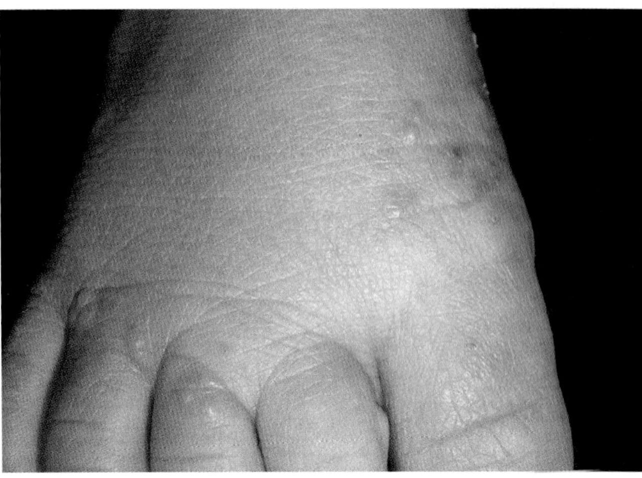

FIGURE 94-2 Acropustulosis with vesiculopustular eruption on the toes of the boy shown in **Figure 94-1**. (*Used with permission from Richard P. Usatine, MD.*)

- Typically begins in the second or third months[1] of life and as late as 10 months of age.[2]
- Occur slightly more often in darker-skinned patients and males.[1]
- Typically spontaneously remits by 6 to 36 months of life.[2]

Transient neonatal pustular melanosis:

- A disease of newborns.[3]
- Equal male-to-female ratio.[3]
- Seen in 4.4 percent of black infants and 0.6 percent of white infants.[4]
- Early, spontaneous remission.[3]

ETIOLOGY AND PATHOPHYSIOLOGY

Acropustulosis:

- The exact cause and mechanism have yet to be determined.[5]

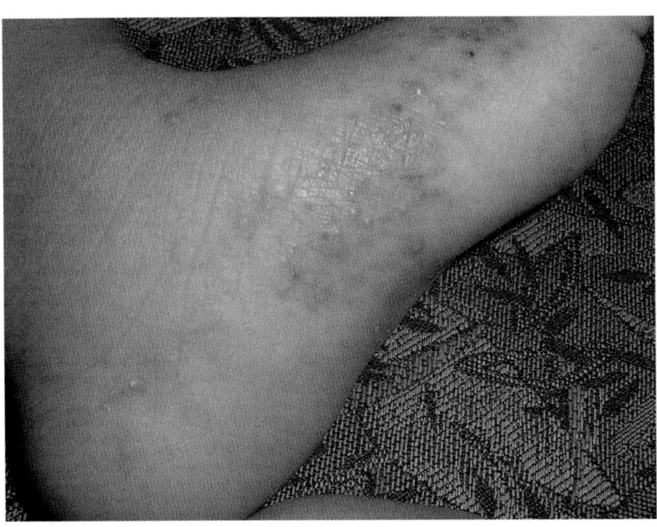

FIGURE 94-1 Infantile acropustulosis (acropustulosis of infancy) on the foot of a 1-year-old boy. (*Used with permission from Richard P. Usatine, MD.*)

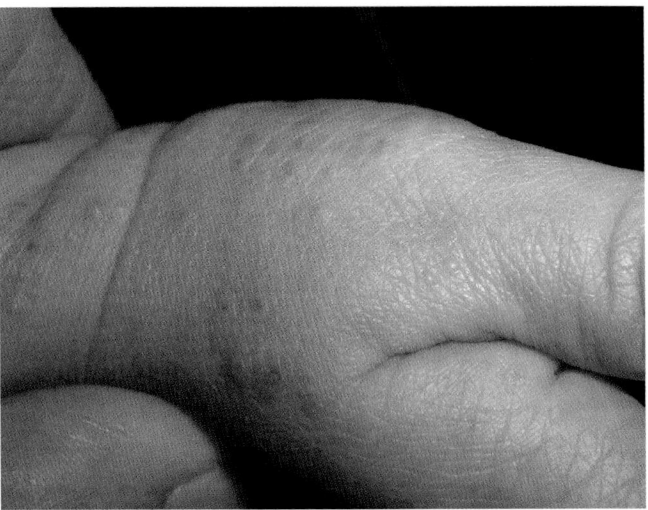

FIGURE 94-3 Acropustulosis with pruritic eruption on the hand and wrist of the boy shown in **Figures 94-1** and **94-2**. (*Used with permission from Richard P. Usatine, MD.*)

- Some physicians speculate that it is a persistent reaction to scabies ("postscabies syndrome"). Suggestive of this infectious etiology, infantile acropustulosis will occasionally be concurrently present among siblings. Also, patients diagnosed with this disorder frequently have received prior treatment for scabies, which may either provide evidence of an infectious etiology or demonstrate the frequent misdiagnosis, as in the previous patient. Odom et al. concludes that in some cases, this disease may represent a hypersensitivity reaction to *Sarcoptes scabiei.*[4]

Transient neonatal pustular melanosis:

- The etiology is uncertain;[6] however, it may result from an obstruction of the pilosebaceous orifice.[3]

DIAGNOSIS

- Acropustulosis—A workup to rule out potentially serious infectious causes should be considered whenever confronted with a new pustular dermatosis early in a child's life. A workup might include a scraping for scabies and KOH preparation as rapid diagnostic tests. If these studies are negative, the diagnosis may be made clinically as described below.
- TNPM—This diagnosis can often be made clinically. However, if performed, a Wright stain of the exudate will reveal a predominance of neutrophils with an occasional eosinophil, and the Gram stain will be negative.[3]

CLINICAL FEATURES

Acropustulosis:

- These vesiculopustular lesions begin around the second or third months of life and are typically concentrated on the hands and feet (**Figures 94-1** to **94-3**).[1]
- They begin acutely as small pink papules and progress within 24 hours to pustules[1] of less than 5 mm in diameter.[2]
- Recurrent episodes of these intensely pruritic lesions typically last 10 days and may recur every 2 to 5 weeks,[1,2] decreasing in frequency and severity[2] until spontaneous remission around 3 years of age.[1]
- There may be a residual scale and postinflammatory hyperpigmentation.[2]

Transient neonatal pustular melanosis:

- This condition is characterized by the presence at birth of 2- to 3-mm macules and pustules[4] on a nonerythematous base (**Figures 94-4** to **94-7**).[7]
- The lesions probably evolve prenatally[7] and subsequently rupture postnatally in 1 to 2 days.
- They heal with hyperpigmented macules that fade by 3 months of age,[3] with lighter-skinned patients experiencing less hyperpigmentation (**Figures 94-6** and **94-7**).[7]
- Sometimes, the only evidence of the disease is the presence of small, brown macules with a rim of scale at birth (**Figure 94-7**).[7]

TYPICAL DISTRIBUTION

- Acropustulosis—Although most commonly found on the palms and soles, the pustules may also be found on the dorsal surfaces of the hands and feet and occasionally the face, scalp, and trunk.[5]
- TNPM—They are most common on the face and chin; however, they may also be present on the neck, chest, sacrum, abdomen, and thighs.[7]

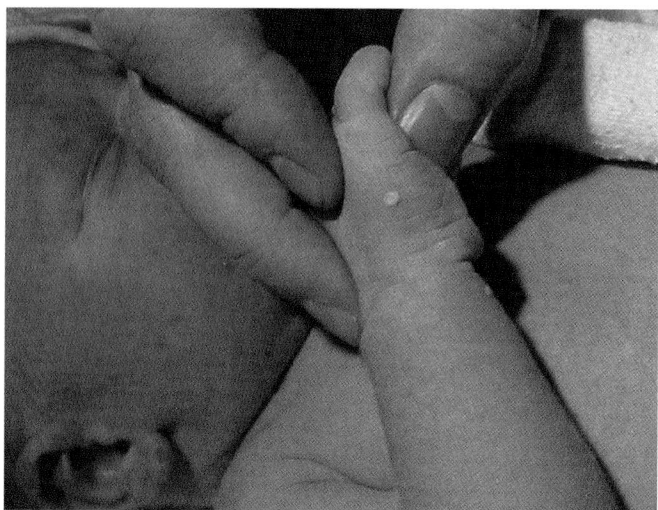

FIGURE 94-4 Transient neonatal pustular melanosis on the hand of a newborn. Note the pustule does not have surrounding erythema. *(Used with permission from Dan Stulberg, MD.)*

LABORATORY TESTING

- Acropustulosis—A blood count is not needed but might reveal a slight leukocytosis and frequently an eosinophilia. Stained smears of the lesions are also not needed but will demonstrate many neutrophils,[1] with some eosinophils possible early in the course.[2]
- TNPM—A Wright stain will reveal numerous neutrophils and some eosinophils, with a negative Gram stain.[3] Blood counts should be normal and no laboratory workup is generally indicated.

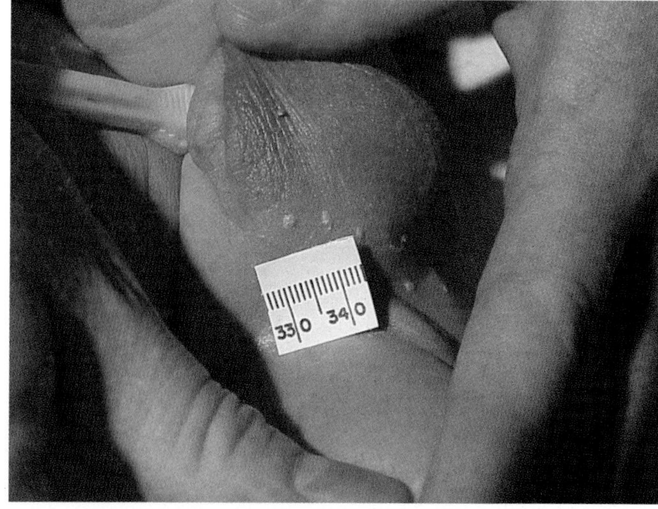

FIGURE 94-5 Transient neonatal pustular melanosis on scrotum of the same newborn with multiple pustules and no erythema. *(Used with permission from Dan Stulberg, MD.)*

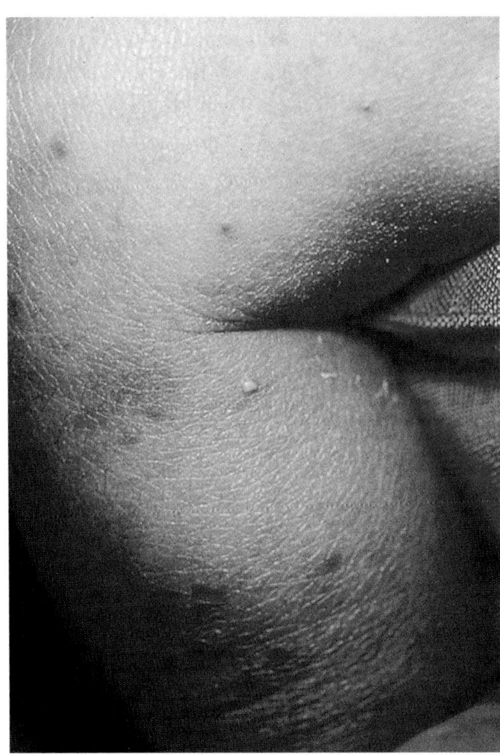

FIGURE 94-6 Transient neonatal pustular melanosis on the leg of a newborn. Note the hyperpigmented macules where the pustules have resolved. (*Used with permission Kane KS, Lio P, Stratigos AJ, Johnson RA. Color Atlas and Synopsis of Pediatric Dermatology, 2nd edition, Figure 1-8, McGraw-Hill, 2009.*)

DIFFERENTIAL DIAGNOSIS

- Scabies infestation—Characterized by pruritic, intraepidermal burrows and vesicles with scale and crust, most commonly found in the web spaces of the digits, wrists, elbow, genitals, and lower extremities. May be present in other family members, and is not present at birth. Microscopic examination of the scrapings of the burrows may reveal mites, feces, eggs, or all of the preceding.[3] Acropustulosis will be refractory to all scabies therapies but scabies therapy may appear to work because each episode of acropustulosis is self-limited (see Chapter 128, Scabies).

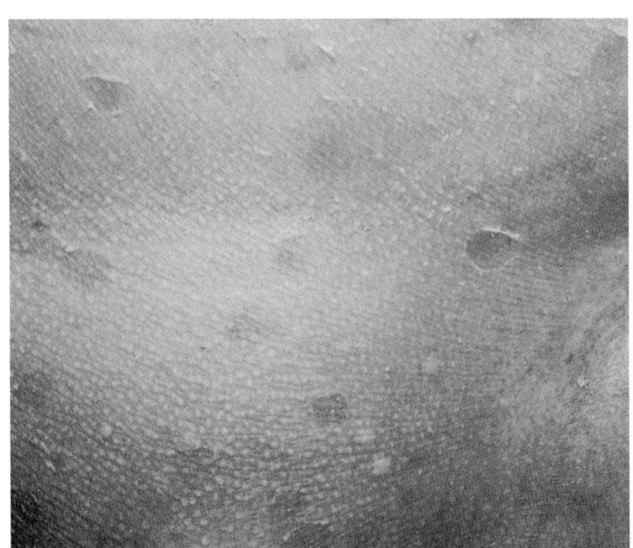

FIGURE 94-7 Transient neonatal pustular melanosis with a number of intact pustules and some hyperpigmented macules with a rim of scale where the previous pustules had ruptured. (*Used with permission from Weinberg SW, Prose NS, Kristal L, Color Atlas of Pediatric Dermatology, 4th edition, Figure 1-3, New York, NY: McGraw-Hill, 2008.*)

- Erythema toxicum neonatorum—Appearing on the neonate 1 to 2 days after birth, this disease of unknown etiology causes 2- to 3-cm diffuse blotchy macules with 1- to 4-mm central vesicles or pustules. The lesions, which spare the palms and soles, contain a predominance of eosinophils and resolve spontaneously by 2 weeks of age (see Chapter 92, Normal Skin Changes).[3]
- Impetigo—A superficial infection of the skin with vesicles, bullae, and honey-colored crusts, caused by group A *Streptococcus*, or *Staphylococcus aureus*. Gram stain and culture should be positive (see Chapter 99, Impetigo).[3]
- Cutaneous candidiasis—Slightly pruritic areas of intensely erythematous papules, pustules, and plaques, possibly with white exudate, found around the genitals and folds of skin. *Candida* yeast forms present on KOH preparation or culture (see Chapter 121, Candidiasis).[3]
- Varicella—Characteristic "dewdrops on a rose petal" that develop in childhood. Uniformly distributed, pruritic, with known contacts likely. Now less common because of immunization (see Chapter 108, Chickenpox).
- Herpes simplex infection—Grouped, painful vesicles on an erythematous base. May occur as gingivostomatitis in young children but rarely seen in the distribution of the pustular diseases of childhood. More likely to be vesicular rather than pustular (see Chapter 114, Herpes Simplex).
- Hand, foot, and mouth disease—This illness is caused by the coxsackievirus and other enteroviruses and produces papules and macules of the hands and feet that progress to flat vesicles before ulceration and eventual resolution. They typically affect the dorsum of the hands and feet and are also accompanied by painful oral lesions (see Chapter 113, Hand, Foot, and Mouth Disease).[3]
- Psoriasis, pustular—This severe form of psoriasis is rare in children and is characterized by the acute appearance of diffuse, painful, pinpoint pustules with high fever, fatigue, and anorexia (see Chapter 136, Psoriasis).[1]

MANAGEMENT

Acropustulosis:

- Corticosteroids (topical and oral) generally are not effective,[1] and not necessary in management.[5] SOR C
- Oral antihistamines may be helpful in controlling pruritus.[1] SOR C
- Pramoxine, lotion or cream, may be used topically for control of itching as it works by a different mechanism than antihistamines.[5] SOR C
- Dapsone (1 to 2 mg/kg per day, maximum dose of 100 mg/day)[5] has been used with good results. However, the risks of complications are generally considered to outweigh the benefits, unless the pruritus is debilitating.[1] SOR C

Transient neonatal pustular melanosis:

- No treatment is necessary. The parents should be reassured that the condition is benign and will resolve spontaneously with eventual normalization of any hyperpigmented macules.[6] SOR B

PROGNOSIS

- Acropustulosis resolves spontaneously by 6 to 36 months of age.
- TNPM resolves spontaneously by 3 months of age.

FOLLOW-UP

Acropustulosis may require initial follow-up for control of symptoms and assurance of a stable disease course. With symptoms controlled, follow-up may be unnecessary as the child ages and the disease decreases in severity and frequency. If dapsone is prescribed, proper monitoring is indicated.

TNPM needs no specific follow-up other than normal well-child care.

PATIENT EDUCATION

Once other conditions have been ruled out, reassurance that these diseases are self-limited is the most important piece of information to communicate to the family.

PATIENT AND PROVIDER RESOURCES

- Medscape. *Acropustulosis of Infancy*—**http://emedicine.medscape.com/article/1109935**.
- Medscape. *Transient Neonatal Pustular Melanosis*—**http://emedicine.medscape.com/article/1112258-overview**.

REFERENCES

1. Ruggero C, Gelmetti C. *Pediatric Dermatology and Dermatopathology: A Concise Atlas*. London, UK: Martin Dunitz; 2002.
2. Weinberg S, Prose NS, Leonard K. *Color Atlas of Pediatric Dermatology*, 3rd ed. New York: McGraw-Hill; 1998.
3. Kane KS, Bissonette J, Baden HP, et al. *Color Atlas and Synopsis of Pediatric Dermatology*. New York: McGraw-Hill; 2002.
4. Odom RB, James WD, Timothy GB. *Andrews' Diseases of the Skin, Clinical Dermatology*, 9th ed. Philadelphia, PA: Saunders; 2000.
5. Pride H. *Acropustulosis of Infancy*. http://www.emedicine.com/derm/topic8.htm, accessed March 30, 2012.
6. Silverman RA. *Neonatal Pustular Melanosis*. http://www.emedicine.com/ped/topic698.htm, accessed March 5, 2012.
7. Cohen BA. *Pediatric Dermatology*, 3rd ed. Philadelphia, PA: Elsevier Mosby; 2005.

95 DIAPER RASH AND PERIANAL DERMATITIS

Bridget Malit, MD
Julie Scott Taylor, MD, MSc
Richard P. Usatine, MD

PATIENT STORY

A 2-month-old baby girl was brought to the office with a severe diaper rash that was not getting better with Desitin. Upon examination, the physician noted a white coating on the tongue and buccal mucosa. The diaper area was red with skin erosions and satellite lesions (**Figure 95-1**). The whole picture is consistent with candidiasis of the mouth (thrush) and the diaper region. The child was treated with oral nystatin suspension and topical clotrimazole cream in the diaper area with good results.

INTRODUCTION

Diaper rash is a general term used to describe any type of red or inflammatory skin rash that is located in the diaper area.

SYNONYMS

Diaper dermatitis, napkin dermatitis.

EPIDEMIOLOGY

- Diaper dermatitis is the most common dermatitis of infancy.
- Variability in prevalence of 4 to 35 percent among children in their first 2 years of life in different studies.[1]
- Diaper rash is thought to be present in 25 percent of children presenting for outpatient visits.[2]

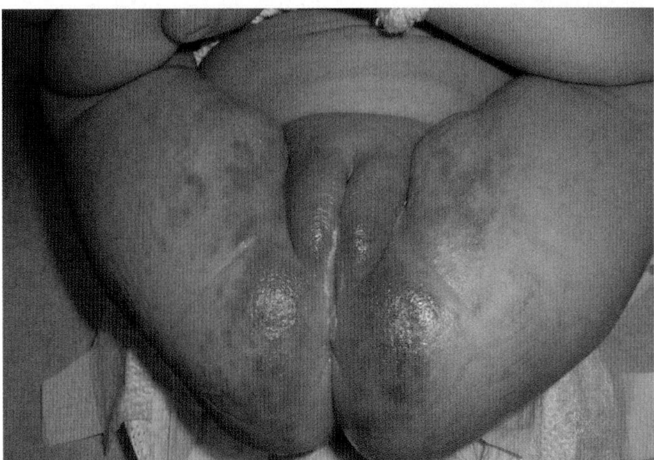

FIGURE 95-1 *Candida* diaper dermatitis in an infant who has oral thrush. (*Used with permission from Richard P. Usatine, MD.*)

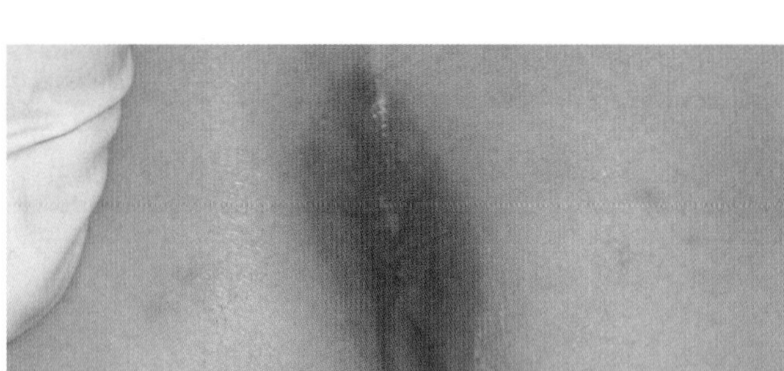

FIGURE 95-2 Perianal dermatitis caused by group A β-hemolytic streptococci. (*From Sheth S, Schechtman AD. Itchy perianal erythema. J Fam Pract. 2007;56(12):1025-1027. Reproduced with permission from Frontline Medical Communications.*)

- No differences in prevalence between genders or among ethnic groups.
- One study showed an incidence of 19.4 percent in children ages 3 to 6 months.[1]
- Higher incidence among formula-fed compared with breastfed infants.[1]
- Condition typically begins around age 3 weeks, peaks at age 9 to 12 months, and then decreases with age until it resolves completely with toilet training.
- Individual episodes last from 1 day to 2 weeks.
- Aggravating factors include poor skin care, diarrhea, recent antibiotic use, and urinary tract abnormalities.
- Perianal streptococcal dermatitis occurs in children between 6 months and 10 years of age (**Figures 95-2** and **95-3**).

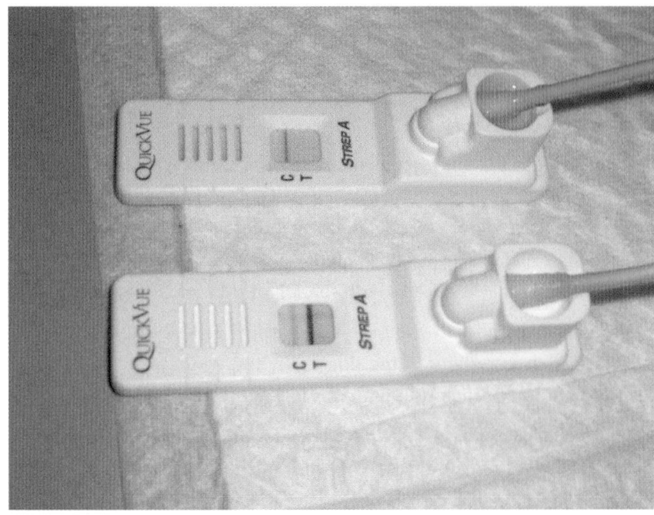

FIGURE 95-3 A positive rapid strep test taken from a swab of the perianal area of the infant in the previous photo. (*From Sheth S, Schechtman AD. Itchy perianal erythema. J Fam Pract. 2007;56(12):1025-1027. Reproduced with permission from Frontline Medical Communications.*)

ETIOLOGY AND PATHOPHYSIOLOGY

- Primary diaper dermatitis—An acute skin inflammation in the diaper area with a multifactorial etiology.[3] The main cause is irritation of thin skin as a result of prolonged contact with moisture including feces and urine. The multiple factors involved are:
  - Occlusion/lack of exposure to air.
  - Friction and mechanical trauma.
  - Local irritants—Fecal proteases and lipases.
  - Increased pH.
  - Maceration of the stratum corneum with loss of the protective barrier function of skin.
- Irritant diaper dermatitis (IDD) is a combination of intertrigo (wet skin damaged from chafing) and miliaria (heat rash) when eccrine glands become obstructed from excessive hydration. It is a noninfectious, nonallergic, often asymptomatic contact dermatitis that typically lasts for less than 3 days after a change in diaper practices.
- Candidal diaper dermatitis—Within 3 days, 45 to 75 percent of diaper rashes are colonized with *Candida albicans* of fecal origin.
- Bacterial diaper dermatitis may be a secondary infection caused by *Staphylococcus aureus* or *Streptococcus pyogenes*. Other common bacterial isolates include *Escherichia coli, Peptostreptococcus*, and *Bacteroides*. Usually occurs during the warm summer months.
- Perianal streptococcal dermatitis is caused by group A β-hemolytic streptococci (**Figures 95-2** and **95-3**).

RISK FACTORS

- Diarrhea.
- Formula-fed infants.
- Recent antibiotic use.
- Urinary tract abnormalities.
- Poor skin care.

DIAGNOSIS

CLINICAL FEATURES

- IDD begins with shiny erythema with or without scale and poorly demarcated margins on the convex skin surfaces in areas covered by diapers. Moderate cases can have papules, plaques, vesicles, and small superficial erosions that can progress to well-demarcated ulcerated nodules typically with sparing of skin folds (**Figure 95-4**).
- Pustules or papules beyond the rash border (called "satellite lesions"), involvement of the skin folds, and white scaling all indicate a fungal infection with *Candida* (**Figure 95-5**).
- Secondary bacterial infections can have redness, honey-colored crusting, swelling, red streaking, and/or purulent discharge. With impetigo in the diaper area, bullae are not usually intact but instead present as superficial erosions.
- Perianal streptococcal dermatitis is a bright red, sharply demarcated rash sometimes associated with blood-streaked stools (**Figure 95-2**).

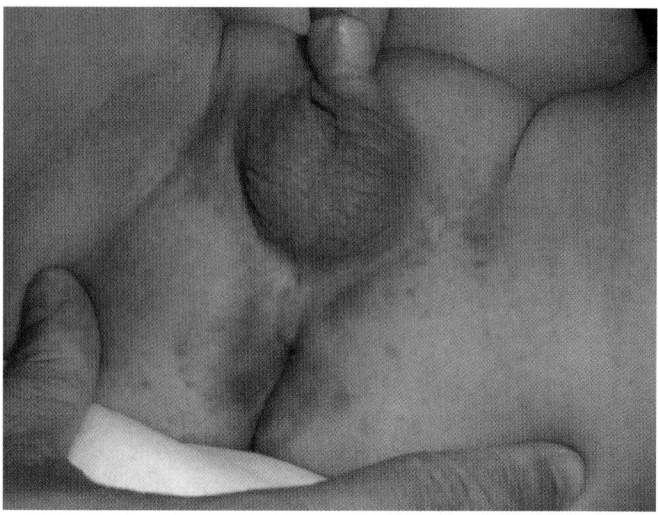

FIGURE 95-4 Irritant diaper dermatitis precipitated by diarrhea secondary to amoxicillin-clavulanate prescribed to treat otitis media. Note the absence of satellite lesions and how it spares the deep folds. (*Used with permission from Richard P. Usatine, MD.*)

TYPICAL DISTRIBUTION

Diaper dermatitis is primarily found on the buttocks, the genitalia, the mons pubis and lower abdomen, and the medial thighs. Be sure to evaluate for rashes outside of the diaper area as well. If *Candida* is suspected, the oropharynx should be inspected for signs of thrush, such as adherent white plaques on the mucosa. If seborrheic dermatitis is suspected, look at the scalp and face.

LABORATORY STUDIES

Clinical diagnosis is based primarily on the physical examination. Rarely indicated tests that are occasionally used in more complicated cases include potassium hydroxide preparation for fungal elements, mineral oil preparation for scabies, complete blood count with differential, zinc level, or skin biopsy (**Figure 95-6**). A rapid strep test can be used to diagnose perianal streptococcal dermatitis (**Figures 95-2** and **95-3**).

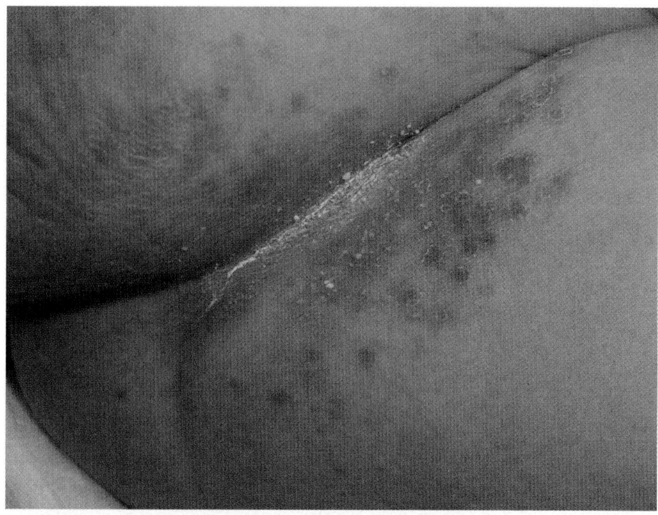

FIGURE 95-5 Close-up of a *Candida* diaper dermatitis in a 5-month-old infant. Note the superficial scaling around the satellite lesions. (*Used with permission from Richard P. Usatine, MD.*)

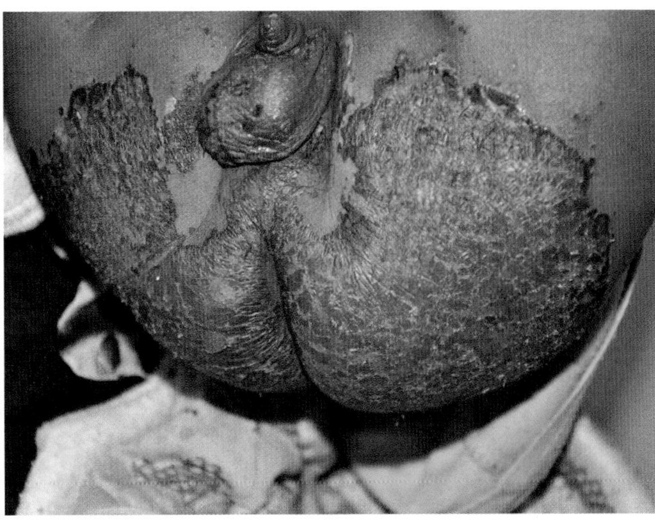

FIGURE 95-6 Acrodermatitis enteropathica caused by zinc deficiency. The child also had perioral dermatitis that appeared similar to the diaper dermatitis. (*Used with permission from Richard P. Usatine, MD.*)

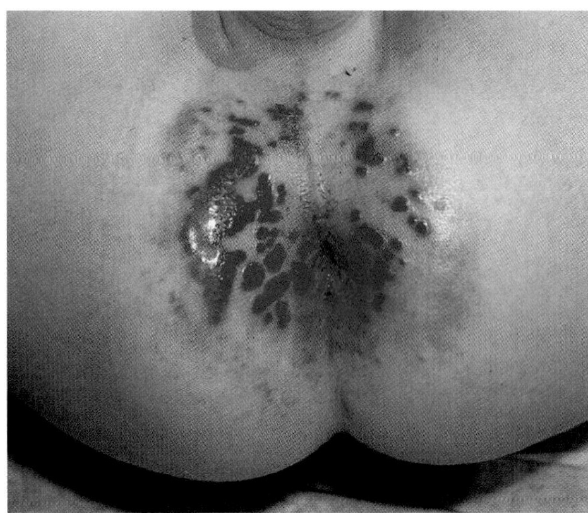

FIGURE 95-8 Erosive diaper dermatitis of Jacquet with bright red erythema, punched-out ulcers and elevated nodules with rolled borders. (*Used with permission from Weinberg SW, Prose NS, Kristal L, Color Atlas of Pediatric Dermatology, 4th edition, Figure 8-42, New York, NY: McGraw-Hill, 2008.*)

DIFFERENTIAL DIAGNOSIS

There are three distinctive severe variants of irritant diaper dermatitis:

1. Erosive diaper dermatitis (dermatitis of Jacquet) is a severe, slow-healing diaper dermatitis in children with persistent diarrhea.[4] The erosions that can lead to nodular lesions with heaped-up borders (**Figures 95-7** and **95-8**).
2. Granuloma gluteale infantum is a rare primary diaper dermatitis that presents with granulomatous nodules that can be large and raised with rolled margins (**Figure 95-9**). Contributing factors are inflammation, candida superinfection and high potency topical steroids. This can resolve over the course of a few months with good diaper care and removal of offending agents. It may leave residual scarring and hyperpigmentation.[5]
3. Pseudoverrucous papules and nodules are shiny, smooth, red, moist, flat-topped perianal lesions that occur with chronic diarrhea. They are commonly confused with the genital warts and can occur with Hirschsprung disease (**Figure 95-10**).

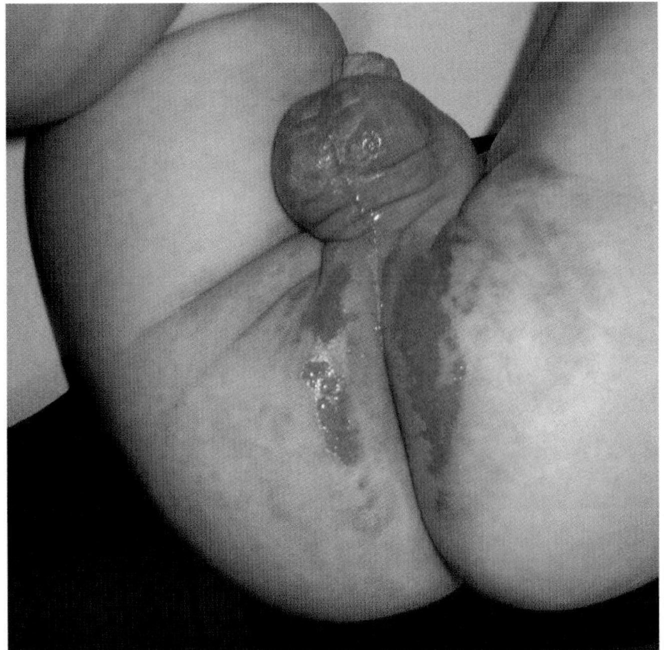

FIGURE 95-7 Erosive diaper dermatitis of Jacquet in an infant with prolonged diarrhea. Note the red erosions and the elevated nodules. (*Used with permission from Richard P. Usatine, MD.*)

Secondary diaper dermatitis is an eruption in the diaper area with a defined etiology. Atopic dermatitis, seborrheic dermatitis, and psoriasis are examples of rashes that can appear anywhere on the body and can be exaggerated in the groin as a result of wearing diapers (**Figure 95-11**). Family history of atopy or psoriasis and rash in other locations besides the groin can be helpful. Look on the scalp for seborrheic dermatitis (cradle-cap) (see Chapter 135, Seborrheic dermatitis).

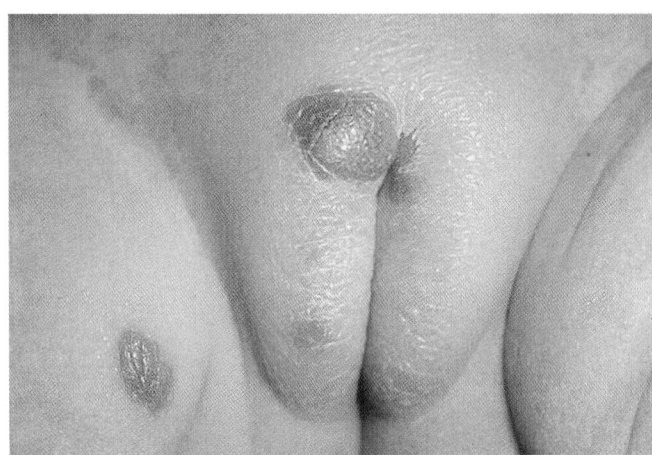

FIGURE 95-9 Granuloma gluteal infantum with two large nodules in the diaper area. While these nodules are brown they can also have a red or purplish hue. In this case, topical steroids were one factor in this nodular granulomatous response. (*Used with permission Kane KS, Lio P, Stratigos AJ, Johnson RA. Color Atlas and Synopsis of Pediatric Dermatology, 2nd edition, Figure 3-5, McGraw-Hill, 2009.*)

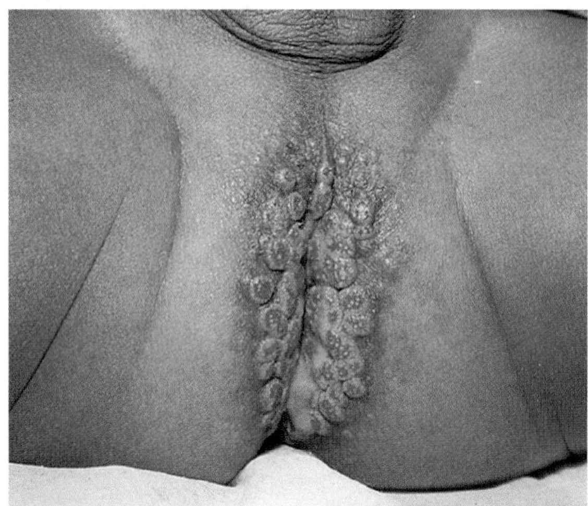

FIGURE 95-10 Pseudoverrucous papules and nodules. The flat-topped or round lesions are shiny, erythematous and moist. This unique diaper dermatitis was originally described in the skin surrounding urostomies, but can occur as a result of chronic diarrhea (sometimes from Hirschsprung's disease), encopresis or urinary incontinence. (*Used with permission from Weinberg SW, Prose NS, Kristal L, Color Atlas of Pediatric Dermatology, 4th edition, Figure 8-45, New York, NY: McGraw-Hill, 2008.*)

Congenital syphilis, scabies, HIV, Langerhans cell histiocytosis (**Figure 95-12**), and acrodermatitis enteropathica (**Figure 95-6**) are examples of rashes in the diaper area unrelated to the diaper. Allergic contact dermatitis as a result of an allergen in the diaper itself is possible but rare. Suspect acrodermatitis enteropathica caused by zinc deficiency when the diaper dermatitis is severe and accompanied by perioral dermatitis (**Figure 95-6**). The serum zinc level will be low and zinc supplementation will be needed.

Intertrigo is an inflammatory condition that occurs in intertriginous areas such as in the inguinal folds (**Figure 95-13**). Other areas involved may be under the neck, in the axillae, or in the gluteal cleft. The term is nonspecific as to the etiology and one should always look for causes such as candida, seborrhea, and psoriasis.

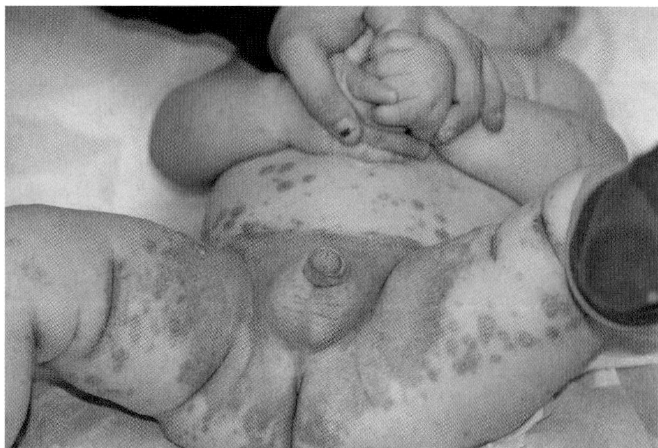

FIGURE 95-11 Severe seborrheic dermatitis in a 1-year-old boy. Note that this condition is not just confined to the diaper area. The whitish-yellow scale is characteristic of seborrhea and the child had involvement on the cheeks and "cradle cap" in the scalp. No satellite pustules of candidiasis are noted. This is not irritant dermatitis as it does not spare the deep folds and the distribution strongly suggests seborrheic dermatitis not candida diaper dermatitis, which would be restricted largely to diaper area or other skin folds. (*Image used with permission from Robert Brodell, MD.*)

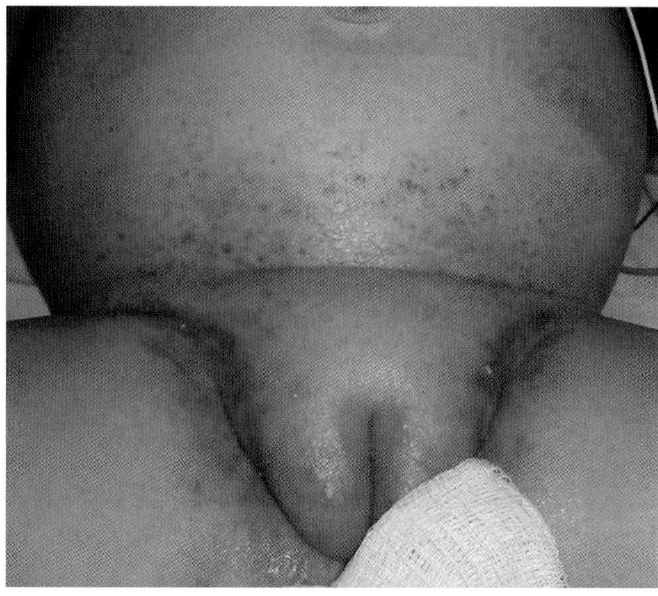

FIGURE 95-12 Langerhans cell histiocytosis in the diaper area. This presented as a refractory diaper rash with scattered erythematous papules and a petechial component. Note the petechiae are particularly prominent on the lower abdomen and the eruption is not only confined to the diaper area. A skin biopsy revealed Langerhans' cells to confirm the diagnosis. (*Used with permission Kane KS, Lio P, Stratigos AJ, Johnson RA. Color Atlas and Synopsis of Pediatric Dermatology, 2nd edition, Figure 3-6, McGraw-Hill, 2009.*)

MANAGEMENT

TREATMENT

- Parental behavior change to keep the skin as exposed and dry as possible. SOR B Frequent diaper changes (as soon as they are wet or soiled and at least every 3 to 4 hours); use disposable diapers. SOR B Frequent gentle cleaning of the affected area with lukewarm tap water instead of commercial wipes containing alcohol

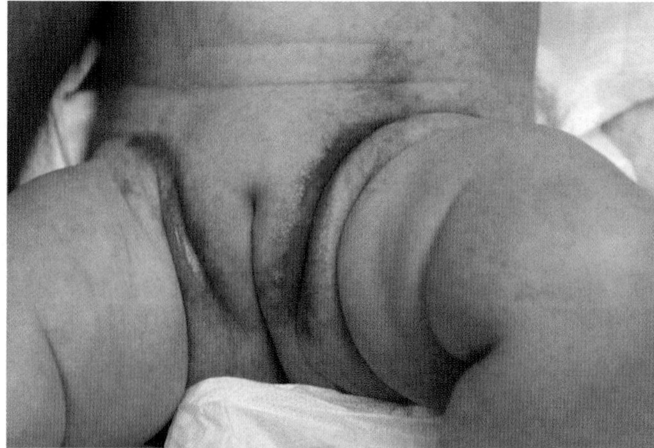

FIGURE 95-13 Intertrigo with bright red erythema in the inguinal folds. One should always look for the contributing factors in any case of intertrigo. Three etiologies to consider are: (1) Irritant dermatitis: This is NOT the classic appearance of an irritant from urine and feces that effects outer skin and spares the deep fold. (2) Candida: Note the papules and papulovesicles on the left abdomen and a few on the thighs (satellite papules and papulovesicles) (3) Seborrheic dermatitis: Look on the scalp and face as this could be a principle cause of this rash. (*Image used with permission from Robert Brodell, MD.*)

and pat dry. A squeeze bottle with lukewarm water can be used to avoid rubbing the delicate skin.

- Superabsorbent diapers that pull moisture away from the skin are helpful.[1] SOR Ⓑ
- Apply barrier preparations, including zinc oxide paste, petroleum jelly, Vitamin A & D ointment, or Burow solution to affected area after each diaper change.[1] SOR Ⓑ Pastes are better than ointments, which, in turn, are better than creams or lotions. Avoid products with fragrances or preservatives to minimize allergic potential. Apply thickly like "icing on a cake." These barrier preparations should be used *on top* of other indicated therapies.
- For moderate to severe inflammation, consider a nonfluorinated, low-potency topical steroid such as 1 percent hydrocortisone ointment (up to 3 times daily) to the affected area until the dermatitis is gone. To avoid skin erosions, atrophy, and striae, it is best to not go beyond 2 weeks of therapy with any topical steroid on a baby's bottom.
- For *Candida*, use topical nonprescription antifungal creams such as clotrimazole, miconazole after every diaper change until the rash resolves. SOR Ⓑ For concomitant oral thrush, treat with oral nystatin swish and swallow 4 times daily.
- Avoid combination antifungal–steroid agents that contain steroids stronger than hydrocortisone (e.g., Lotrisone). Potent topical steroids can cause striae and skin erosions, hypothalamus–pituitary–adrenal axis suppression, and Cushing syndrome.[1]
- For mild bacterial infections, use topical antibiotic ointments such as bacitracin or mupirocin after every diaper change until the rash resolves. SOR Ⓑ
- For more severe bacterial infections, consider a broad-spectrum oral antibiotic such as amoxicillin-clavulanate. Perianal bacterial dermatitis has been reported to be predominantly caused by *S. aureus*.[6] Oral cephalexin is a good choice because it covers *S. aureus* and group A β-hemolytic streptococcus. If methicillin-resistant *S. aureus* (MRSA) is suspected, consider trimethoprim-sulfamethoxazole. SOR Ⓑ
- Ciclopirox 0.77 percent topical suspension (Loprox), a broad-spectrum agent with antifungal, antibacterial, and antiinflammatory properties, was used safely and effectively in 1 trial of 44 children to treat diaper dermatitis caused by *Candida*.[1] SOR Ⓑ
- Recommend dye-free diapers for allergic contact dermatitis. SOR Ⓑ

PREVENTION AND ROUTINE SKIN CARE

- Keep the diaper region as dry and clean as possible.
- Promote the use of barrier preparations daily to maintain skin integrity.
- There is no evidence to suggest that topical vitamin A prevents diaper dermatitis.[7] SOR Ⓑ
- Disposable diapers—Although many individual trials show benefits, a 2006 Cochrane Review found that there is not enough evidence from good quality, randomized, controlled trials to support or refute the use and type of disposable diapers for the prevention of diaper dermatitis in infants.[8] SOR Ⓑ

PROGNOSIS

Diaper dermatitis has an excellent prognosis when treated as previously described.

FOLLOW-UP

No follow-up needed unless the rash worsens or persists. The exception is severe bacterial infection where follow-up is recommended because recurrences are common.

PATIENT EDUCATION

Prevention and early treatment are the best strategies. Keep the child's diaper area as clean, cool, and dry as possible with frequent diaper changes. Do *not* use creams that contain boric acid, camphor, phenol, methyl salicylate, compound of benzoin, or talcum powder or cornstarch. Reassure parents that, although this common condition is sometimes distressing for parents and uncomfortable for children, it is rarely dangerous.

PATIENT RESOURCES

- FamilyDoctor.org. *Diaper Rash*—**www.familydoctor.org/familydoctor/en/diseases-conditions/diaper-rash.html**.
- WebMD. *Diaper Rash–Topic Overview*—**www.children.webmd.com/tc/diaper-rash-topic-overview**.

PROVIDER RESOURCES

- Medscape. *Diaper Rash*—**www.emedicine.medscape.com/article/801222**.

REFERENCES

1. Dib R. *Diaper Rash*. http://emedicine.medscape.com/article/801222-overview#a0199. Updated March 17, 2010.
2. Adalat S, Wall D, Goodyear H. Diaper dermatitis-frequency and contributory factors in hospital attending children. *Pediatr Dermatol.* 2007:24(5):483-488.
3. Adam R. Skin care of the diaper area. *Pediatr Dermatol.* 2008:25(4):427-433.
4. Paradisi A, Capizzi R, Ghitti F, et al. Jacquet erosive diaper dermatitis: a therapeutic challenge. *Clin Exp Dermatol.* 2009:34(7):e385-e386.
5. Al-Faraidy N, Al-Natour S. A forgotten complication of diaper dermatitis: granuloma Gluteale Infantum. *J Family Community Med.* 2010;17(2):107-109.
6. Heath C, Desai N, Silverberg N. Recent microbiological shifts in perianal bacterial dermatitis: *Staphylococcus aureus* predominance. *Pediatr Dermatol.* 2009:26(6):696-700.
7. Davies MW, Dore AJ, Perissinotto KL. Topical vitamin A, or its derivatives, for treating and preventing napkin dermatitis in infants. *Cochrane Database Syst Rev.* 2005 Oct 19;(4):CD004300.
8. Baer EL, Davies MW, Easterbrook KJ. Disposable nappies for preventing napkin dermatitis in infants. *Cochrane Database Syst Rev.* 2006 Jul 19;(3):CD004262.

SECTION 2 ACNEIFORM DISORDERS

96 ACNE VULGARIS

Richard P. Usatine, MD

PATIENT STORY

A 16-year-old boy (**Figure 96-1**) with severe nodulocystic acne and scarring presents for treatment. After trying oral antibiotics, topical retinoids, and topical benzyl peroxide with no significant benefit, the patient and his mother request isotretinoin (Accutane). After 4 months of isotretinoin, the nodules and cysts cleared, and there remained only a few papules (**Figure 96-2**). He is much happier and more confident about his appearance. The skin fully cleared after the last month of isotretinoin.

INTRODUCTION

Acne is an obstructive and inflammatory disease of the pilosebaceous unit predominantly found on the face of adolescents. However, it can occur at any age and often involves the trunk in addition to the face.

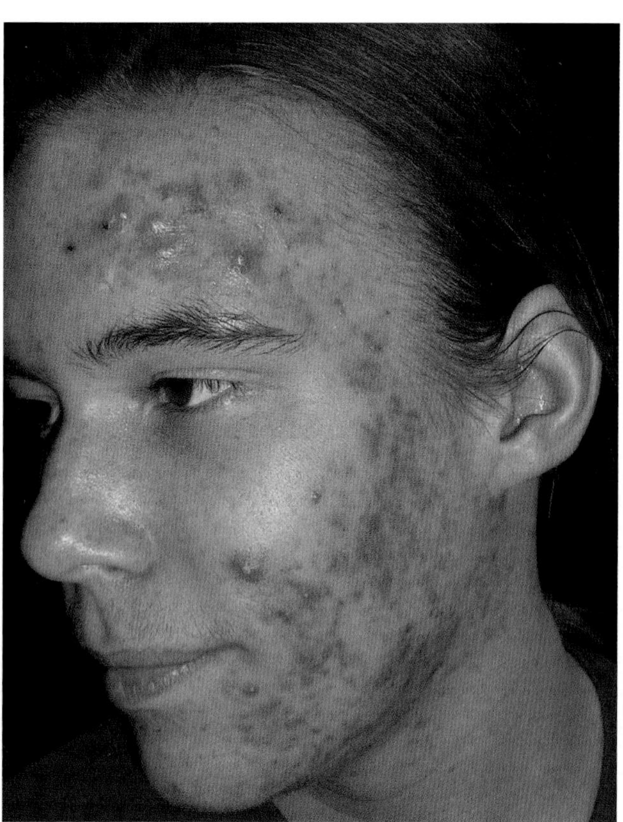

FIGURE 96-1 Severe nodulocystic acne with scarring in a 16-year-old boy. (*Used with permission from Richard P. Usatine, MD.*)

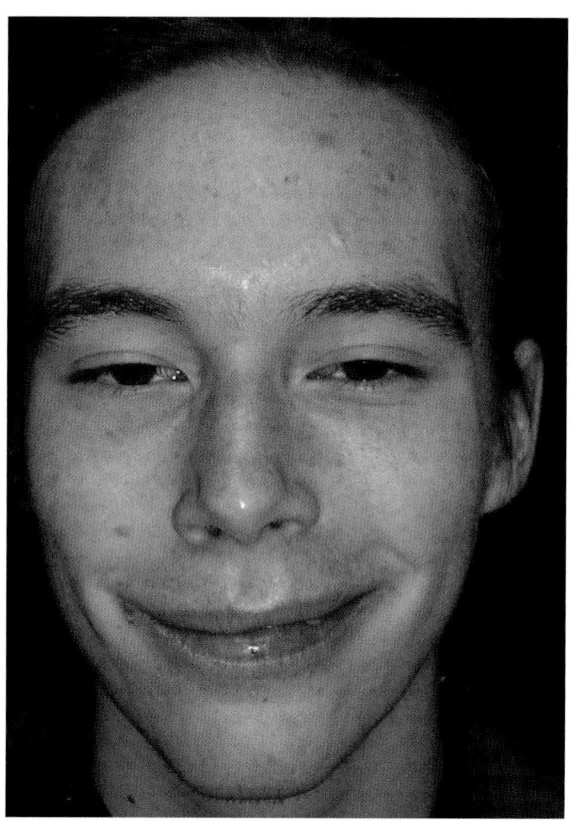

FIGURE 96-2 A happier boy now that his nodules and cysts have cleared at the start of the fifth month of isotretinoin treatment. (*Used with permission from Richard P. Usatine, MD.*)

EPIDEMIOLOGY

Acne vulgaris affects more than 80 percent of teenagers, and persists beyond the age of 25 years in 3 percent of men and 12 percent of women.[1]

ETIOLOGY AND PATHOPHYSIOLOGY

The four most important steps in acne pathogenesis:

1. Sebum overproduction related to androgenic hormones and genetics.
2. Abnormal desquamation of the follicular epithelium (keratin plugging).
3. *Propionibacterium acnes* proliferation.
4. Follicular obstruction, which can lead to inflammation and follicular disruption.

Neonatal acne is thought to be related to maternal hormones and is temporary (**Figure 96-3**).

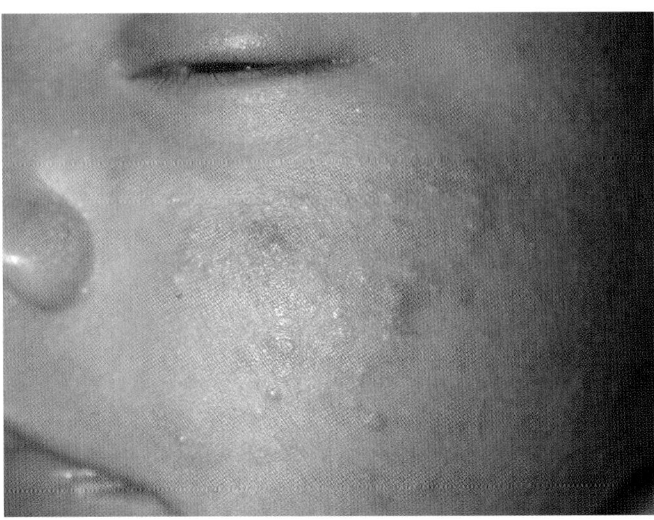

FIGURE 96-3 Neonatal acne in a healthy 2-week-old infant that resolved without treatment. (*Used with permission from Richard P. Usatine, MD.*)

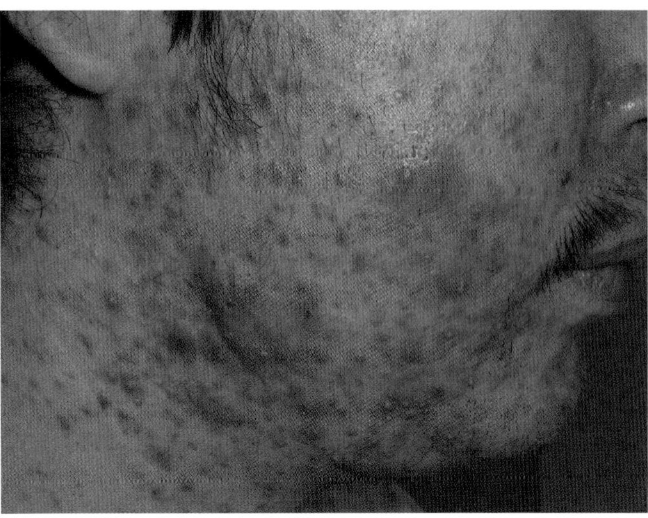

FIGURE 96-5 Severe inflammatory acne in a young adult. His acne worsened when he was started on phenytoin for his seizure disorder. (*Used with permission from Richard P. Usatine, MD.*)

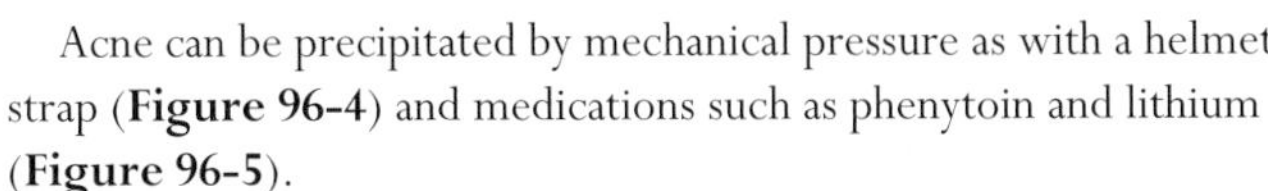

Acne can be precipitated by mechanical pressure as with a helmet strap (**Figure 96-4**) and medications such as phenytoin and lithium (**Figure 96-5**).

There are some studies that suggest that consumption of large quantities of milk (especially skim milk) increase the risk for acne in teenagers.[2]

DIAGNOSIS

CLINICAL FEATURES

Morphology of acne includes comedones, papules, pustules, nodules, and cysts.

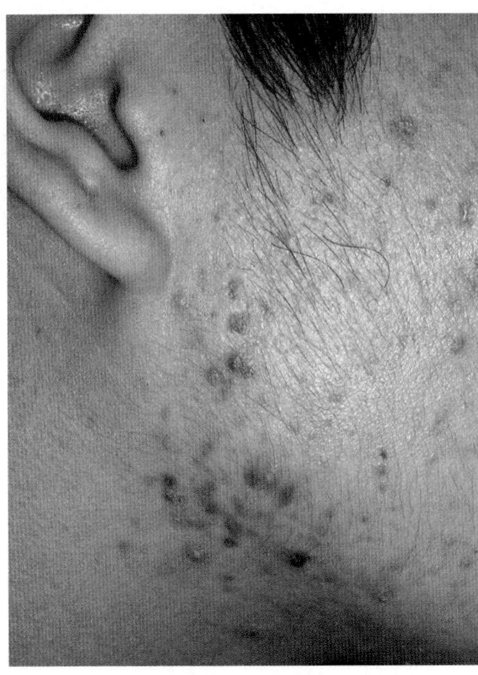

FIGURE 96-4 Inflammatory acne showing pustules and nodules in a 17-year-old boy who uses a helmet while playing football in high school. (*Used with permission from Richard P. Usatine, MD.*)

- Obstructive acne = comedonal acne = noninflammatory acne and consists of only comedones (**Figure 96-6**).
- Open comedones are blackheads (**Figure 96-7**) and closed comedones are called whiteheads and look like small papules.
- Inflammatory acne has papules, pustules, nodules, and cysts in addition to comedones (**Figure 96-5**).

TYPICAL DISTRIBUTION

Face, back, chest, and neck.

LABORATORY STUDIES

None unless you suspect androgen excess and/or polycystic ovarian syndrome (PCOS).[3] SOR A Obtain testosterone and DHEA-S levels if you suspect androgen excess and/or PCOS.

Consider follicle-stimulating hormone (FSH) and luteinizing hormone (LH) levels if you suspect PCOS.

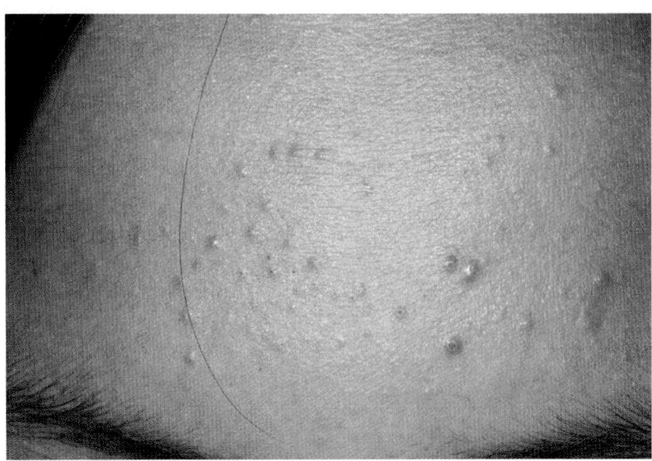

FIGURE 96-6 Comedonal acne in a 15-year-old girl. Open comedones (blackheads) and closed comedones (whiteheads) are visible on her forehead. (*Used with permission from Richard P. Usatine, MD.*)

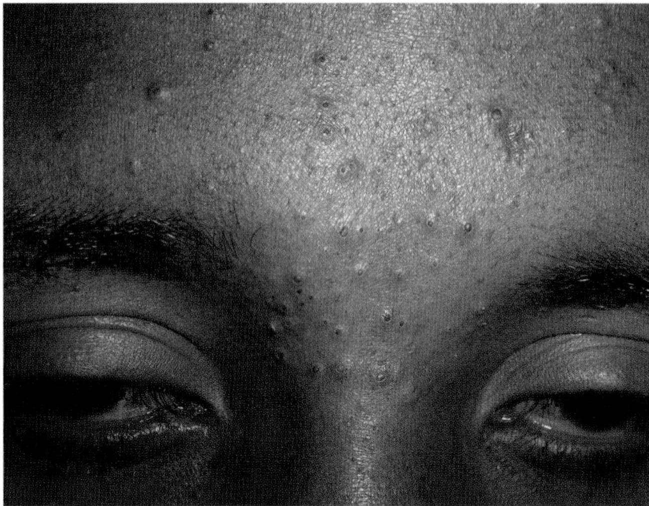

FIGURE 96-7 Comedonal acne in a 17-year-old girl. She has many large open comedones (blackheads). She is a very good candidate for acne surgery along with medical therapy. (*Used with permission from Richard P. Usatine, MD.*)

DIFFERENTIAL DIAGNOSIS (INCLUDING SPECIAL TYPES OF ACNE)

- Acne conglobata is an uncommon and unusually severe form of acne characterized by multiple comedones, cysts, sinus tracks, and abscesses. The inflammatory lesions and scars can lead to significant disfigurement.[4] Sinus tracks can form with multiple openings that drain foul-smelling purulent material (**Figures 96-8** and **96-9**). The comedones and nodules are usually found on the chest, shoulders, back, buttocks, and face. In some cases, acne conglobata is part of a follicular occlusion triad including hidradenitis and dissecting cellulitis of the scalp.
- Acne fulminans is characterized by sudden onset ulcerative crusting cystic acne, mostly on the chest and back (**Figures 96-10** and **96-11**).[5] Fever, malaise, nausea, arthralgia, myalgia, and weight loss are common. Leukocytosis and elevated erythrocyte sedimentation rate are usually found. There may also be focal osteolytic lesions. The term *acne fulminans* may also be used in cases of severe aggravation of acne without systemic features.[5]
- Pomade acne is described as acne that is caused or exacerbate by greasy hair products that get on the skin of the forehead. It is more commonly seen in African Americans (**Figure 96-12**).
- Rosacea can resemble acne by having papules and pustules on the face. It is usually seen in older adults with prominent erythema and telangiectasias. Rosacea does not include comedones and may have ocular or nasal manifestations (Chapter 97, Rosacea).
- Folliculitis on the back may be confused with acne. Look for hairs centrally located in the inflammatory papules of folliculitis to help distinguish it from acne. Acne on the back usually accompanies acne on the face as well (Chapter 100, Folliculitis).
- Acne keloidalis nuchae consists of papules, pustules, nodules, and keloidal tissue found at the posterior hairline. It is most often seen in persons of color after shaving the hair at the nape of the neck (**Figure 96-13**).

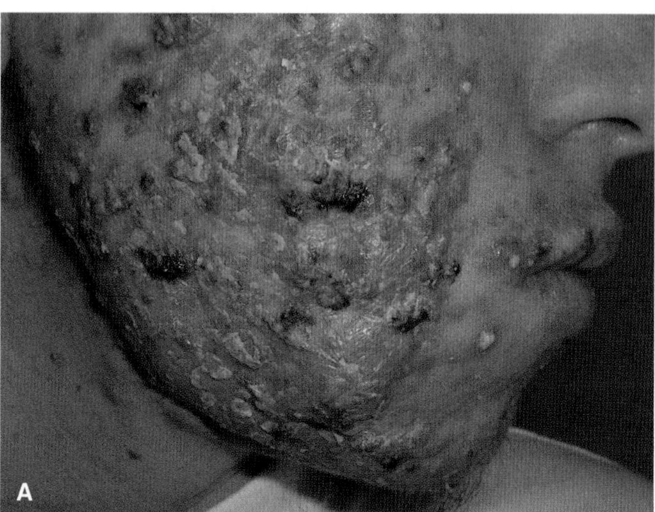

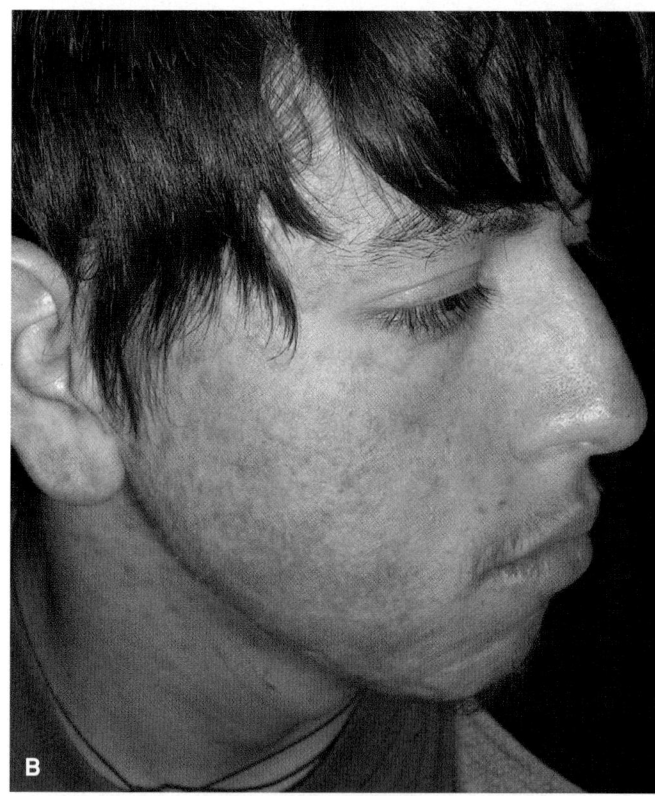

FIGURE 96-8 **A.** Acne conglobata in a 16-year-old boy. He has severe cysts on his face with sinus tracks between them. He required many weeks of oral prednisone before isotretinoin was started. His acne cleared completely with his treatment. **B.** Acne conglobata cleared with minimal scarring after oral prednisone and 5 months of isotretinoin therapy. (*Used with permission from Richard P. Usatine, MD.*)

MANAGEMENT

Treatment is based on type of acne and severity. Categories to choose from are topical retinoids, topical antimicrobials, systemic antimicrobials, hormonal therapy, oral isotretinoin, and injection therapy.

MEDICATIONS FOR ACNE THERAPY

In a review of 250 comparisons, the Agency for Health-care Research and Quality found 14 had evidence of level A.[6] These comparisons

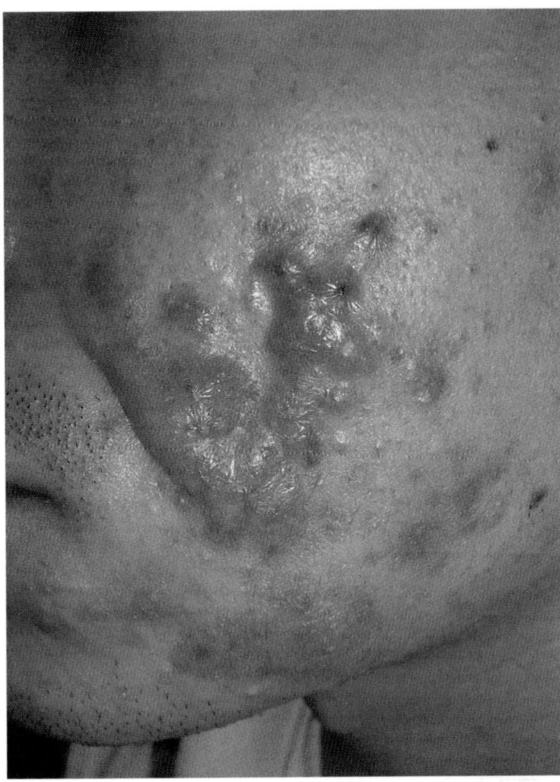

FIGURE 96-9 Acne conglobata on the face with sinus tracts and large cystic lesions in a teenage male. (*Used with permission from Richard P. Usatine, MD.*)

demonstrated the efficacy over vehicle or placebo control of topical clindamycin, topical erythromycin, benzoyl peroxide, topical tretinoin, oral tetracycline, and norgestimate/ethinyl estradiol.[4] Level A conclusions demonstrating equivalence include: Benzoyl peroxide at various strengths was equally efficacious in mild/moderate acne; adapalene and tretinoin were equally efficacious.[6] SOR Ⓐ

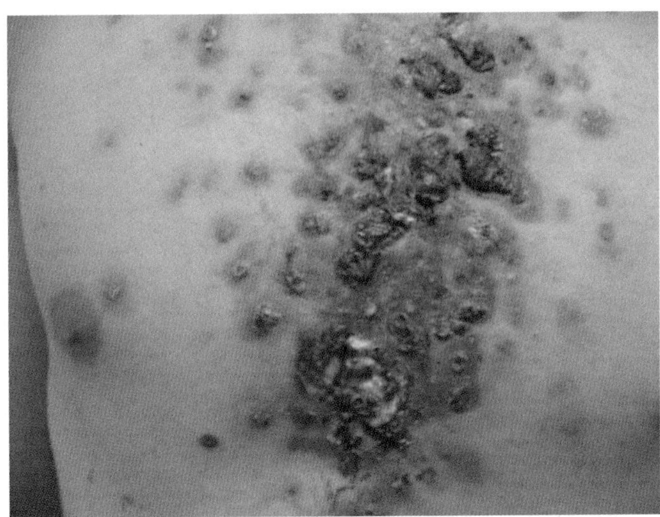

FIGURE 96-10 Acne fulminans in a 17-year-old boy. He was on isotretinoin when he developed worsening of his acne with polymyalgia and arthralgia. He presented with numerous nodules and cysts covered by hemorrhagic crusts on his chest and back. (*From Grunwald MH, Amichai B. Nodulo-cystic eruption with musculoskeletal pain. J Fam Pract. 2007;56:205-206, Reproduced with permission from Frontline Medical Communications.*)

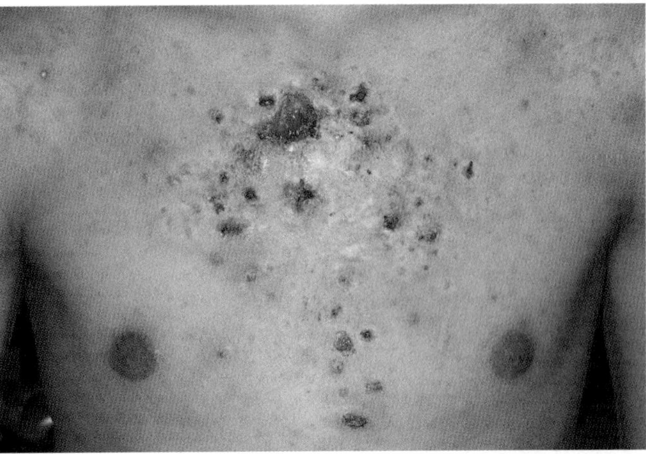

FIGURE 96-11 Acne fulminans with severe rapidly worsening truncal acne in a 15-year-old boy. He did not have fever or bone pain but had a white blood cell count of 17,000. He responded rapidly to prednisone and was started on isotretinoin. The ulcers and granulation tissue worsened initially on isotretinoin but prednisone helped to get this under control. (*Used with permission from Richard P. Usatine, MD.*)

Topical:

- Benzoyl peroxide—Antimicrobial effect (gel, cream, lotion) (2.5%, 5%, 10%) 10 percent causes more irritation and is not more effective.[1] SOR Ⓐ
- Topical antibiotics—Clindamycin and erythromycin are the mainstays of treatment.
- Erythromycin—Solution, gel.[3] SOR Ⓐ
- Clindamycin—Solution, gel, lotion.[3] SOR Ⓐ
- Benzamycin gel—Erythromycin 3 percent, benzoyl peroxide 5 percent.[3] SOR Ⓐ

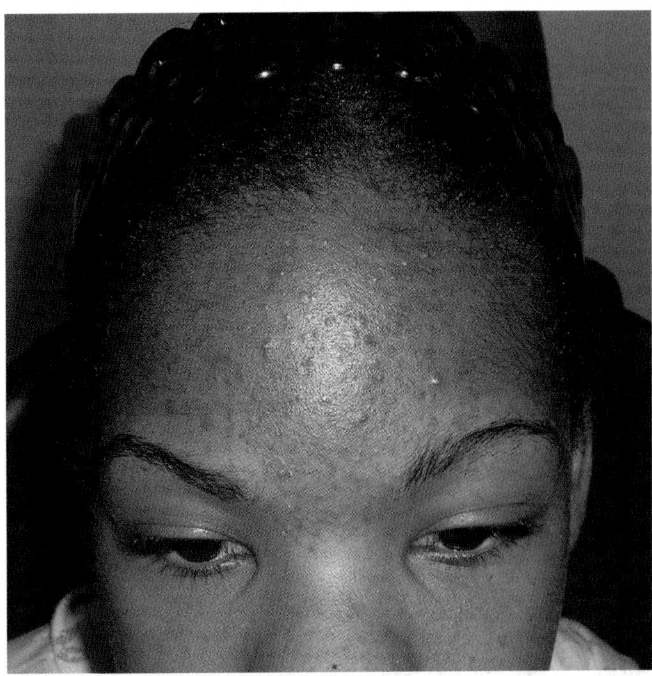

FIGURE 96-12 Pomade acne in a young African American teen that uses oily hair products to style her hair. Note how the acne is predominantly on the forehead. (*Used with permission from Richard P. Usatine, MD.*)

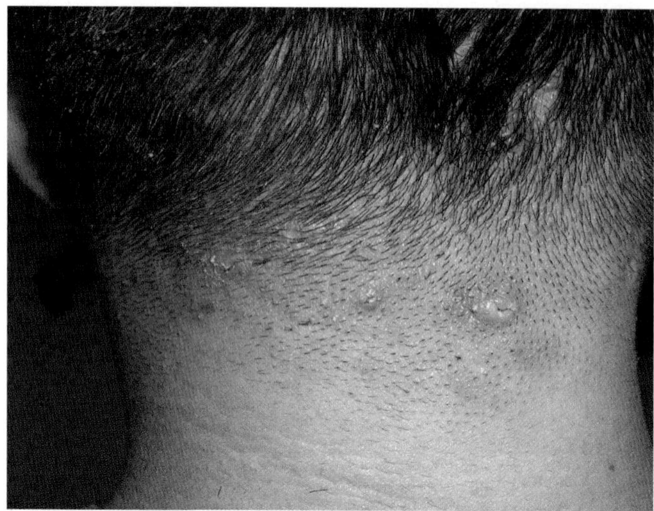

FIGURE 96-13 Acne keloidalis nuchae on the neck of a teen that shaves his hair in the back. The pathophysiology is more related to a folliculitis than actual acne. (*Used with permission from Richard P. Usatine, MD.*)

- BenzaClin gel—Clindamycin 1 percent, benzoyl peroxide 5 percent.[3] SOR Ⓐ
- Dapsone 5 percent gel.[7] SOR Ⓑ

Retinoids:

- Tretinoin (Retin-A) gel, cream, liquid, micronized.[1] SOR Ⓐ
- Adapalene gel—Less irritating than tretinoin.[1] SOR Ⓐ
- Tazarotene—Strongest topical retinoid with greatest risk of irritation.[8] SOR Ⓐ

Topical retinoids will often result in skin irritation during the first 2 to 3 months of treatment, but new systematic reviews do not demonstrate that they worsen acne lesion counts during the initial period of use.[2]

- Azelaic acid—Useful to treat spotty hyperpigmentation and acne (**Figure 96-14**).[3] SOR Ⓑ

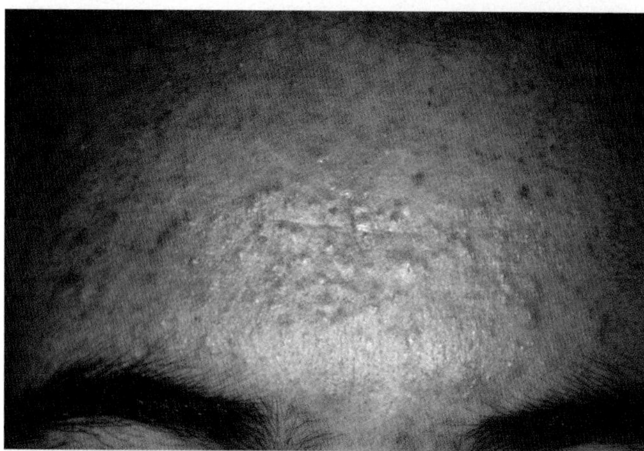

FIGURE 96-14 Obstructive or comedonal acne with spotty hyperpigmentation. Azelaic acid was helpful to treat the acne and the hyperpigmentation. (*Used with permission from Richard P. Usatine, MD.*)

Systemic

- Oral antibiotics.
  - Doxycycline 40 to 100 mg qd to bid—Inexpensive, well tolerated, can take with food and increases sun sensitivity.[3] SOR Ⓐ
  - Minocycline 50 to 100 mg qd to bid—Expensive, not proven to be better than other systemic antibiotics including tetracycline.[3,9] SOR Ⓐ
  - Erythromycin 250 to 500 mg bid—Inexpensive, frequent gastrointestinal (GI) disturbance but can be used in pregnancy.[3] SOR Ⓐ
  - Trimethoprim/sulfamethoxazole DS bid—Effective but risk of Stevens-Johnson syndrome is real. Reserve for short courses in particularly severe and resistant cases.[3] SOR Ⓐ
  - Oral azithromycin has been prescribed in pulse dosing for acne in a number of small poorly done studies and has not been found to be better than oral doxycyline.[10]
- Isotretinoin (Accutane) is the most powerful treatment for acne. It is especially useful for cystic and scarring acne that has not responded to other therapies.[3] SOR Ⓐ Dosed at approximately 1 mg/kg per day for 5 months. Any female of childbearing potential must be abstinent from sexual intercourse or use two forms of contraception. Other risks that are controversial but important to discuss with patients and their parents are depression, suicide, and inflammatory bowel disease.
- The US Food and Drug Administration requires that prescribers of isotretinoin, patients who take isotretinoin, and pharmacists who dispense isotretinoin all must register with the iPLEDGE system (www.ipledgeprogram.com).
- Hormonal treatments are for females only:
  - Oral contraceptives—Choose ones with low androgenic effect.[3] SOR Ⓐ FDA-approved oral contraceptives are Ortho Tri-Cyclen, Yaz, and Estrostep. Other oral contraceptives with similar formulations also help acne in women even though these have not received FDA approval for this indication. Note: Yaz and Yasmin have progestin drospirenone, which is derived from 17α-spirolactone. It shares an antiandrogenic effect with spironolactone.

COMPLEMENTARY/ALTERNATIVE THERAPY

Tea tree oil 5 percent gel.[11] SOR Ⓑ

ACNE PROCEDURES

- Steroid injections for acne are useful for painful nodules and cysts. SOR Ⓒ Patients often report that the lesion flattens and becomes painless by the next day. Follow these directions to avoid producing skin atrophy.
  - Dilute 0.1 mL of 10 mg/mL triamcinolone acetonide (Kenalog) with 0.4 mL of sterile saline in a 0.1 mL syringe to make a 2 mg/mL suspension. Shake the suspension well before injecting.
  - Inject 0.1 mL of this suspension into each nodule or cyst using a 30-gauge needle (**Figure 96-15**).
- Acne surgery is a fancy name for extracting the material from open comedones. It helps to nick the comedone with a needle or #11 blade before expressing the material with a comedone extractor (**Figure 96-16**). The patient in **Figure 96-7** is a very good candidate for this procedure along with medical therapy.

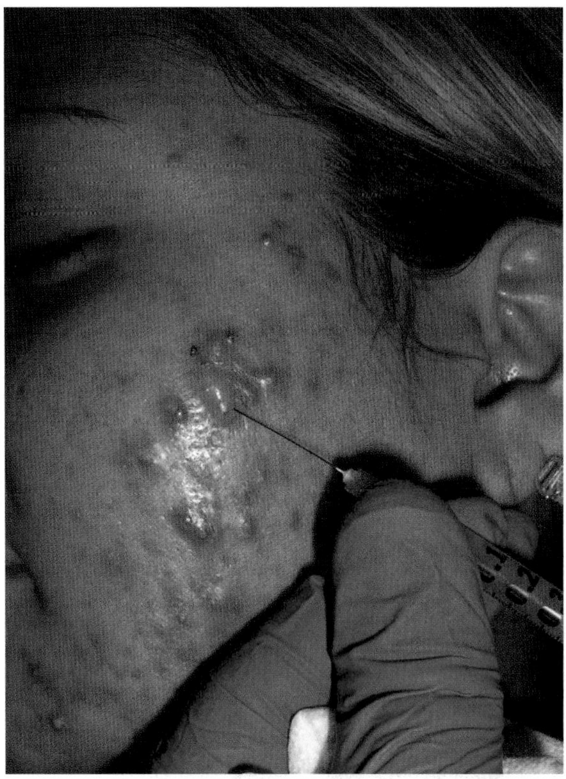

FIGURE 96-15 Injection of acne nodules with 2 mg/cc triamcinolone acetonide. (*Used with permission from Richard P. Usatine, MD.*)

ACNE THERAPY BY SEVERITY

Comedonal acne (Figures 96-6, 96-7, 96-17)

- Topical retinoids or azelaic acid are the most beneficial agents.
- No need for antibiotics—Do not need to kill *P. acnes.*
- Benzoyl peroxide may be beneficial.

Mild papulopustular

- Topical antibiotics and benzoyl peroxide.
- Topical retinoid or azelaic acid.

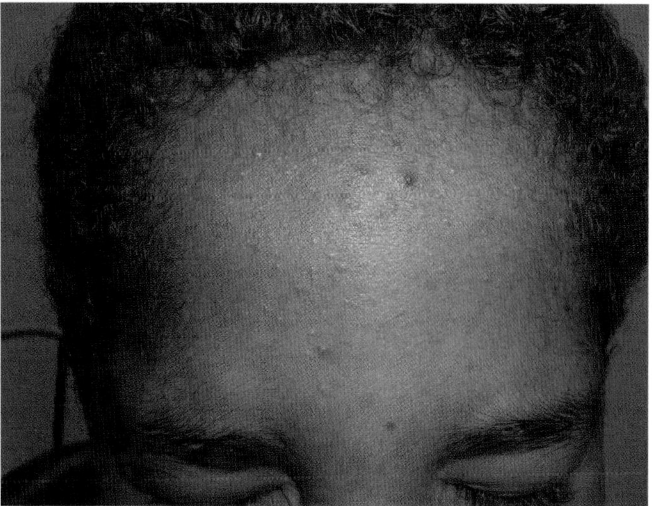

FIGURE 96-17 Comedonal acne beginning on the forehead on 9-year-old boy. (*Used with permission from Richard P. Usatine, MD.*)

- May add oral antibiotics if topical agents are not working (**Figure 96-18**).

Papulopustular or nodulocystic acne—moderate to severe—inflammatory

- Topical antibiotic, benzoyl peroxide, and oral antibiotic.
- Oral antibiotics are often essential at this stage especially if the trunk is involved.
- Topical retinoid or azelaic acid.
- Steroid injection therapy—For painful nodules and cysts.

Severe cystic or scarring acne

- Isotretinoin if there are no contraindications (**Figure 96-19**).
- Steroid injection therapy—For painful nodules and cysts.

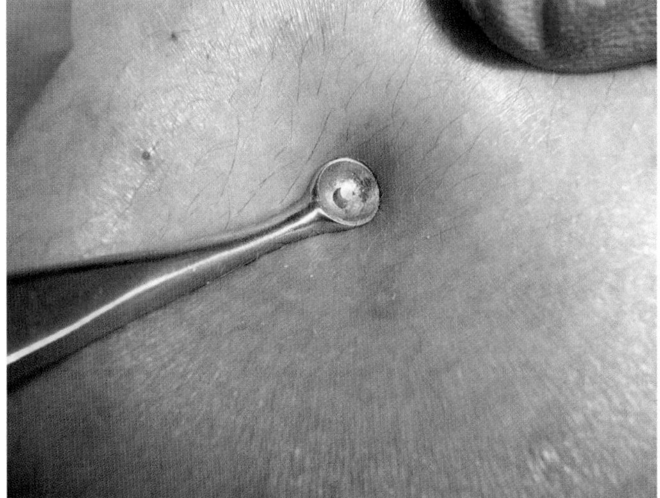

FIGURE 96-16 Acne surgery using a comedone extractor to remove the material from an open comedone after it was nicked with a #11 scalpel blade. (*Used with permission from Richard P. Usatine, MD.*)

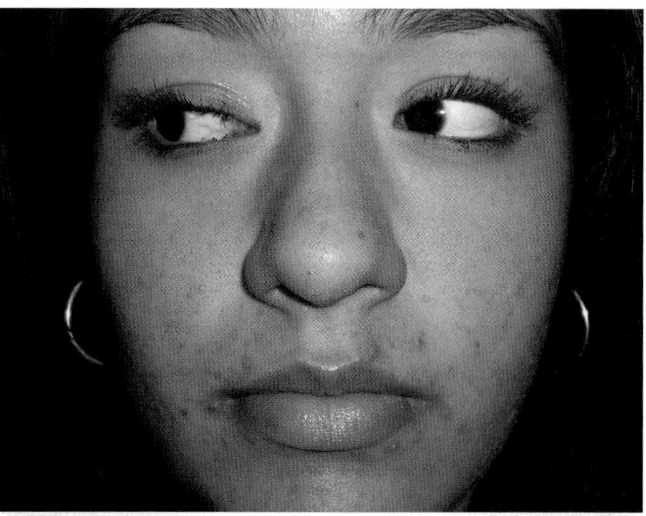

FIGURE 96-18 Mild inflammatory acne failing to fully improve with topical benzyl peroxide and erythromycin. (*Used with permission from Richard P. Usatine, MD.*)

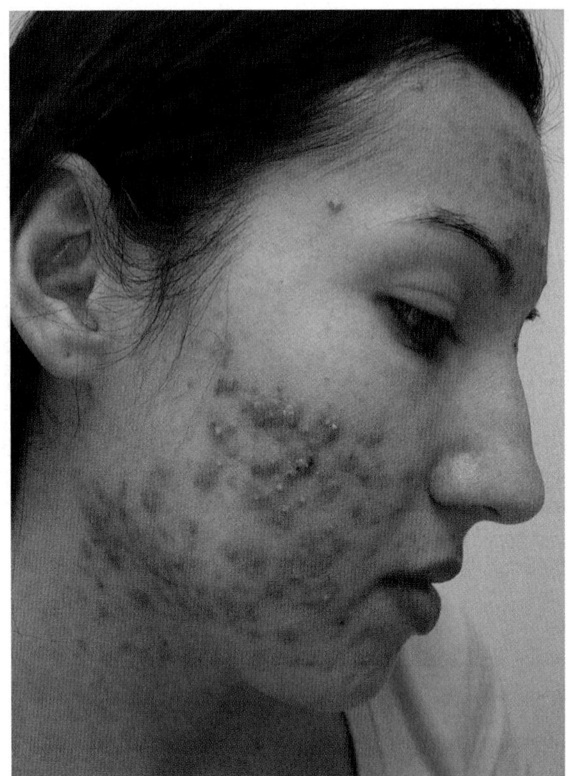

FIGURE 96-19 Severe nodulo-cystic acne in a 17-year-old teen prior to starting oral isotretinoin therapy. (*Used with permission from Richard P. Usatine, MD.*)

Acne fulminans (Figures 96-10 and 96-11)

- Start with systemic steroids (prednisone 40 to 60 mg/day—Approximately 1 mg/kg per day).[12] SOR C
- Systemic steroid treatment rapidly controls the skin lesions and systemic symptoms. The duration of steroid treatment in one Finnish series was 2 to 4 months to avoid relapses.[12] SOR C
- Therapy with isotretinoin, antibiotics, or both was often combined with steroids, but the role of these agents is still uncertain.[12] SOR C
- One British series used oral prednisolone 0.5 to 1 mg/kg daily for 4 to 6 weeks (thereafter slowly reduced to zero).[13] SOR C
- Oral isotretinoin was added to the regimen at the fourth week, initially at 0.5 mg/kg daily and gradually increased to achieve complete clearance.[13] SOR C
- Consider introducing isotretinoin at approximately 4 weeks into the oral prednisone if there are no contraindications. SOR C

Acne conglobata (**Figures 96-8** and **96-9**) may be treated like acne fulminans but the course of oral prednisone does not need to be as long. SOR C

COMBINATION THERAPIES

- Combination therapy with multiple topical agents can be more effective than single agents.[3] SOR B
- Topical retinoids and topical antibiotics are more effective when used in combination than when either are used alone.[3] SOR B
- Benzoyl peroxide and topical antibiotics used in combination are effective treatment for acne by helping to minimize antibiotic resistance.[3] SOR B
- The adjunctive use of clindamycin/benzoyl peroxide gel with tazarotene cream promotes greater efficacy and may also enhance tolerability.[14]
- Combination therapy with topical retinoids and oral antibiotics can be helpful at the start of acne therapy. However, maintenance therapy with combination tazarotene and minocycline therapy showed a trend for greater efficacy but no statistical significance versus tazarotene alone.[15]

MEDICATION COST

The most affordable medications for acne include topical benzoyl peroxide, erythromycin, clindamycin, and oral tetracycline and doxycycline. The most expensive acne medications are the newest brand-name combination products of existing topical medication. These medications are convenient for those with insurance that covers them (Epiduo contains benzoyl peroxide and adapalene; Ziana contains clindamycin and tretinoin).

NEWER EXPENSIVE MODES OF THERAPY

Intense pulsed light and photodynamic therapy (PDT) use lasers, special lights, and topical chemicals to treat acne.[16–18] These therapies are very expensive and the data do not suggest that these should be first-line therapies at this time. Light and laser treatments have been shown to be of short-term benefit if patients can afford therapy and tolerate some discomfort. These therapies have not been shown to be better than simple topical treatments.[2]

One comparative trial demonstrated that PDT was less effective than topical adapalene in the short-term reduction of inflammatory lesions.[2]

FOLLOW-UP

Isotretinoin requires monthly follow-up visits but other therapies can be monitored every few months at first and then once to twice a year. Keep in mind that many treatments for acne take months to work, so quick follow-up visits may be disappointing.

PATIENT EDUCATION

Adherence with medication regimens is crucial to the success of the therapy. Adequate face washing twice a day is sufficient. Do not scrub the face with abrasive physical or chemical agents. If benzoyl peroxide is not being used as a leave-on product, it can be purchased to use for face washing.

PATIENT RESOURCES

- PubMed Health has a good patient education information—**www.ncbi.nlm.nih.gov/pubmedhealth/PMH0001876/**.

PROVIDER RESOURCES

- Usatine R, Pfenninger J, Stulberg D, Small R: *Dermatologic and Cosmetic Procedures in Office Practice*. Philadelphia: Elsevier; 2012—Covers how to do acne surgery, steroid injections for acne, chemical peels, PDT and laser treatment for acne. It is also available as an app: **www.usatinemedia.com**.

REFERENCES

1. Purdy S, de Berker D. Acne vulgaris. *Clin Evid (Online)*. 2011 Jan 5;2011. pii:1714.
2. Smith EV, Grindlay DJ, Williams HC. What's new in acne? An analysis of systematic reviews published in 2009-2010. *Clin Exp Dermatol*. 2011;36:119-122.
3. Strauss JS, Krowchuk DP, Leyden JJ, et al. Guidelines of care for acne vulgaris management. *J Am Acad Dermatol*. 2007;56:651-663.
4. Shirakawa M, Uramoto K, Harada FA. Treatment of acne conglobata with infliximab. *J Am Acad Dermatol*. 2006;55:344-346.
5. Grunwald MH, Amichai B. Nodulo-cystic eruption with musculoskeletal pain. *J Fam Pract*. 2007;56:205-206.
6. AHRQ. *Management of Acne*. http://www ahrq gov/clinic/epcsums/acnesum htm [serial online]. 2001.
7. Draelos ZD, Carter E, Maloney JM, et al. Two randomized studies demonstrate the efficacy and safety of dapsone gel, 5% for the treatment of acne vulgaris. *J Am Acad Dermatol*. 2007;56: 439-410.
8. Webster GF, Guenther L, Poulin YP, et al. A multicenter, double-blind, randomized comparison study of the efficacy and tolerability of once-daily tazarotene 0.1% gel and adapalene 0.1% gel for the treatment of facial acne vulgaris. *Cutis*. 2002;69(2 Suppl):4-11.
9. Garner SE, Eady EA, Popescu C, et al. Minocycline for acne vulgaris: efficacy and safety. *Cochrane Database Syst Rev*. 2003; CD002086.
10. Maleszka R, Turek-Urasinska K, Oremus M, et al. Pulsed azithromycin treatment is as effective and safe as 2-week-longer daily doxycycline treatment of acne vulgaris: a randomized, double-blind, noninferiority study. *Skinmed*. 2011;9:86-94.
11. Enshaieh S, Jooya A, Siadat AH, Iraji F. The efficacy of 5% topical tea tree oil gel in mild to moderate acne vulgaris: a randomized, double-blind placebo-controlled study. *Indian J Dermatol Venereol Leprol*. 2007;73:22-25.
12. Karvonen SL. Acne fulminans: report of clinical findings and treatment of twenty-four patients. *J Am Acad Dermatol*. 1993;28: 572-579.
13. Seukeran DC, Cunliffe WJ. The treatment of acne fulminans: a review of 25 cases. *Br J Dermatol*. 1999;141:307-309.
14. Tanghetti E, Dhawan S, Green L, et al. Randomized comparison of the safety and efficacy of tazarotene 0.1% cream and adapalene 0.3% gel in the treatment of patients with at least moderate facial acne vulgaris. *J Drugs Dermatol*. 2010;9: 549-558.
15. Leyden J, Thiboutot DM, Shalita AR, et al. Comparison of tazarotene and minocycline maintenance therapies in acne vulgaris: a multicenter, double-blind, randomized, parallel-group study. *Arch Dermatol*. 2006;142:605-612.
16. Yeung CK, Shek SY, Bjerring P, et al. A comparative study of intense pulsed light alone and its combination with photodynamic therapy for the treatment of facial acne in Asian skin. *Lasers Surg Med*. 2007;39:1-6.
17. Wiegell SR, Wulf HC. Photodynamic therapy of acne vulgaris using 5-aminolevulinic acid versus methyl aminolevulinate. *J Am Acad Dermatol*. 2006;54:647-651.
18. Horfelt C, Funk J, Frohm-Nilsson M, et al. Topical methyl aminolaevulinate photodynamic therapy for treatment of facial acne vulgaris: results of a randomized, controlled study. *Br J Dermatol*. 2006;155:608-613.

97 ROSACEA

Richard P. Usatine, MD

PATIENT STORY

A 14-year-old girl presents with a red face and a history of easy facial flushing over the last two years (**Figure 97-1**). Her face has become persistently redder and she would like some treatment.

Her mom is in the room and has similar redness in her face. The family is from northern European heritage. The girl also has developed some "pimples." Physical examination reveals some papules and erythema. No comedones are seen. She knows that the sun makes it worse but finds that many sunscreens are irritating to her skin. The patient is started on 0.75 percent metronidazole gel once daily. She agrees to wear a hat and stay out of the sun during the middle of the day. She will continue to look for a sunscreen she can tolerate. She knows that precipitating factors for her include hot and humid weather, alcohol, hot beverages, and spicy foods.

INTRODUCTION

Rosacea is an inflammatory condition of the face and eyes that mostly affects adults but can start in childhood. Most commonly the face becomes reddened over the cheeks and nose and this is often accompanied by telangiectasias and a papulopustular eruption (**Figures 97-2** and **97-3**).

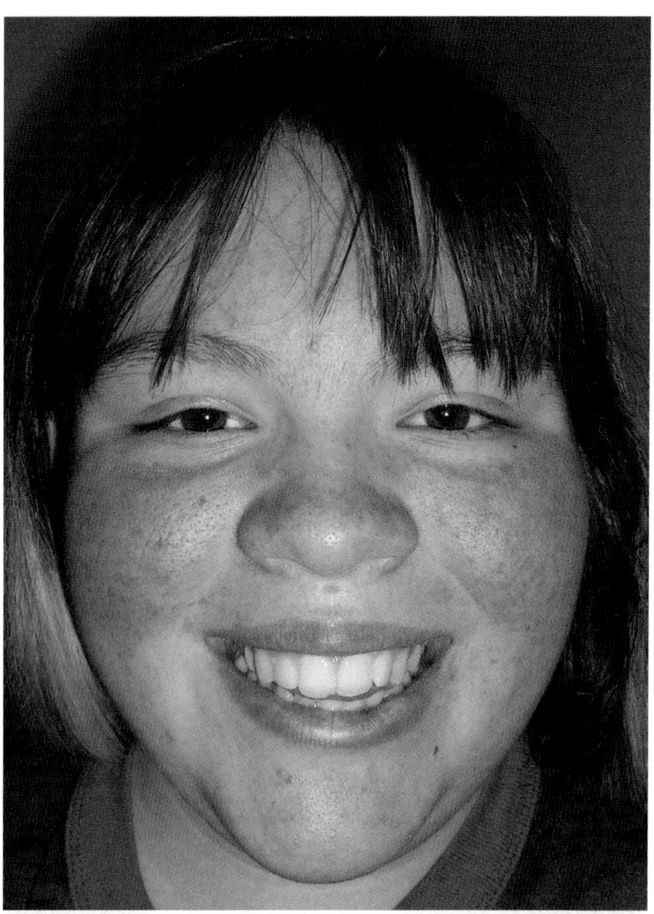

FIGURE 97-1 Rosacea in a 14-year-old girl showing erythema and papules. (*Used with permission from Richard P. Usatine, MD.*)

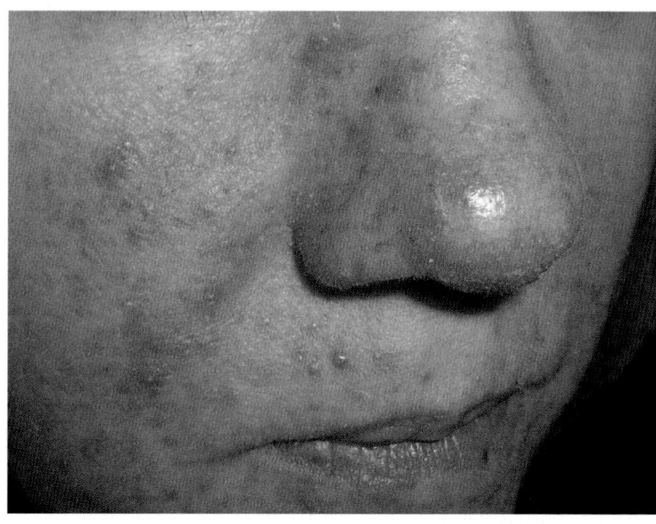

FIGURE 97-2 Close-up of papules and pustules in a young woman with rosacea. Note the absence of comedones. This is not acne. This is papulopustular rosacea. (*Used with permission from Richard P. Usatine, MD.*)

SYNONYMS

Rosacea is also called acne rosacea.

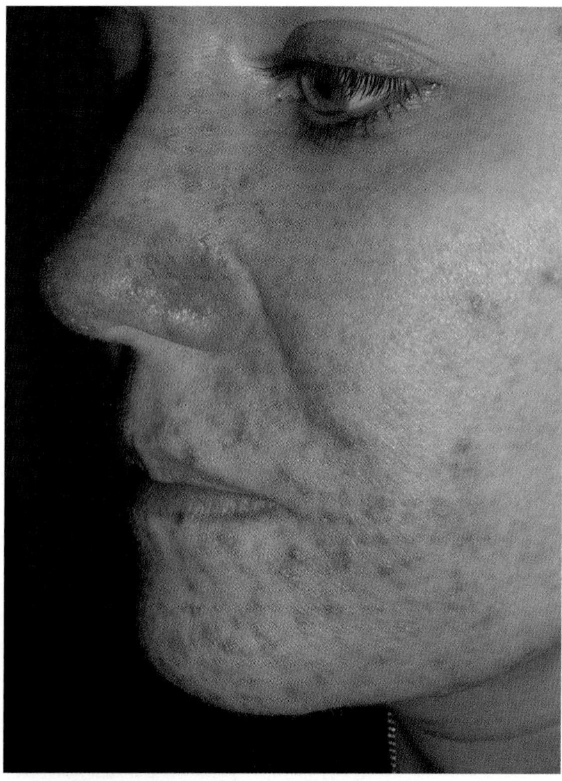

FIGURE 97-3 Close-up showing telangiectasias on the nose and papules around the mouth and chin. (*Used with permission from Richard P. Usatine, MD.*)

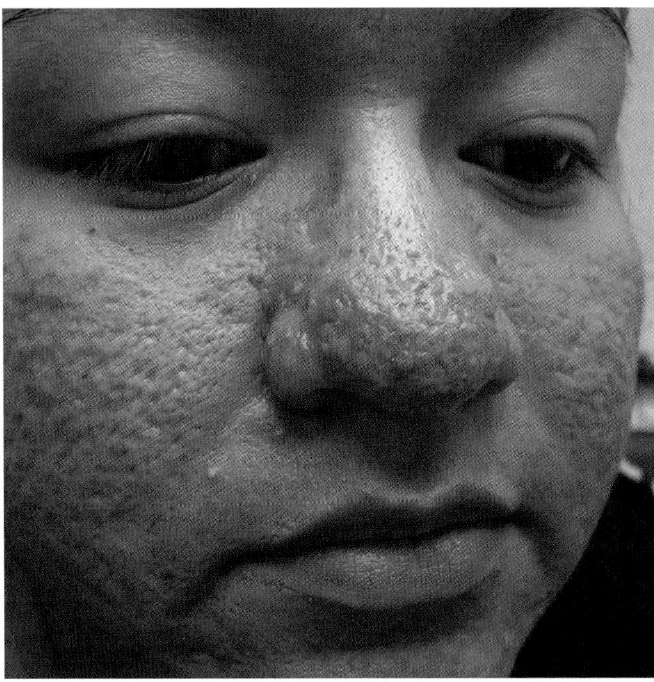

FIGURE 97-4 Rhinophymatous rosacea with hypertrophy of the skin of the nose of a young woman with acne scarring from adolescence. The patient denies heavy alcohol intake. This type of rosacea is very rare in children. (*Used with permission from Richard P. Usatine, MD.*)

EPIDEMIOLOGY

- Common in fair-skinned people of Celtic and northern European heritage.
- Women and girls are more often affected than men and boys.
- Men are more prone to the extreme forms of hyperplasia, which causes rhinophymatous rosacea. However, even young women can have rhinophymatous rosacea. (**Figure 97-4**).

ETIOLOGY AND PATHOPHYSIOLOGY

- Although the exact etiology is unknown, the pathophysiology involves nonspecific inflammation followed by dilation around follicles and hyperreactive capillaries. These dilated capillaries become telangiectasias (**Figures 97-5**).
- As rosacea progresses, diffuse hypertrophy of the connective tissue and sebaceous glands ensues (**Figure 97-4**).
- Alcohol may accentuate erythema, but does not cause the disease. Rosacea runs in families.
- Sun exposure may precipitate an acute rosacea flare, but flare-ups can happen without sun exposure.
- A significant increase in the hair follicle mite *Demodex folliculorum* is sometimes found in rosacea.[1] It is theorized that these mites play a role because they incite an inflammatory or allergic reaction by mechanical blockage of follicles.

RISK FACTORS

Genetics, *Demodex* infestation,[1] sun exposure.

DIAGNOSIS

CLINICAL FEATURES

Rosacea has four stages or subtypes:

1. *Erythematotelangiectatic rosacea* (**Figure 97-5**)—This stage is characterized by frequent mild to severe flushing with persistent central facial erythema.
2. *Papulopustular rosacea* (**Figure 97-6**)—This is a highly vascular stage that involves longer periods of flushing than the first stage, often lasting from days to weeks. Minute telangiectasias and papules start to form by this stage, and some patients begin having

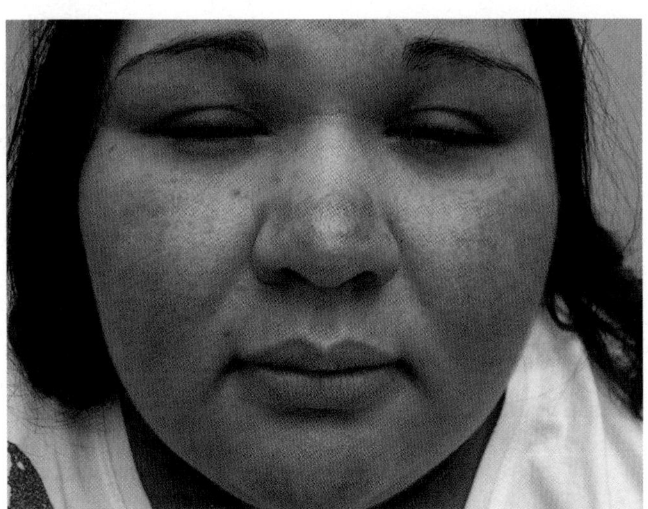

FIGURE 97-5 Erythematotelangiectatic subtype of rosacea in a Hispanic girl. (*Used with permission from Richard P. Usatine, MD.*)

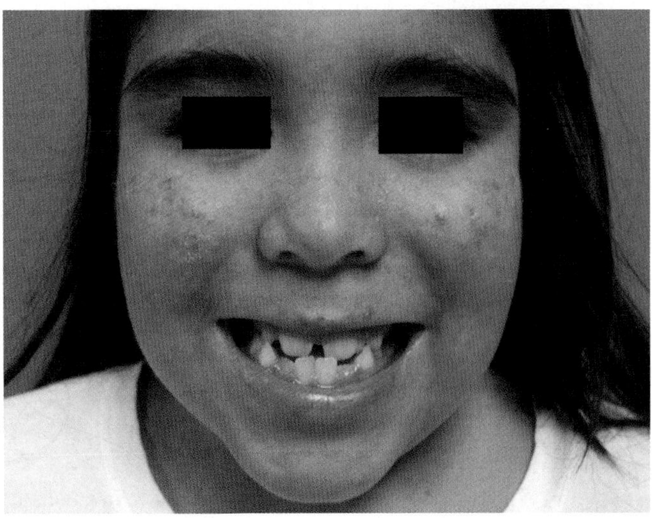

FIGURE 97-6 Papulopustular rosacea in a young girl. (*Used with permission from Jennifer Krejci-Manwaring, MD.*)

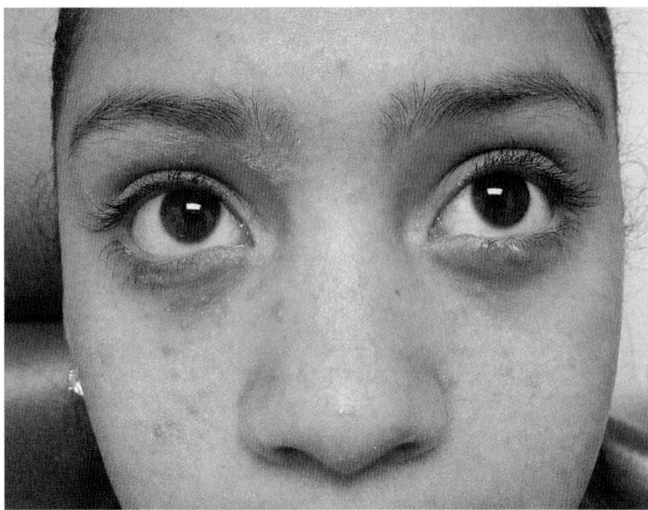

FIGURE 97-7 Ocular rosacea in an 11-year-old girl showing blepharitis, conjunctival hyperemia, and telangiectasias of the lid. (*Used with permission from Lewis Rose, MD.*)

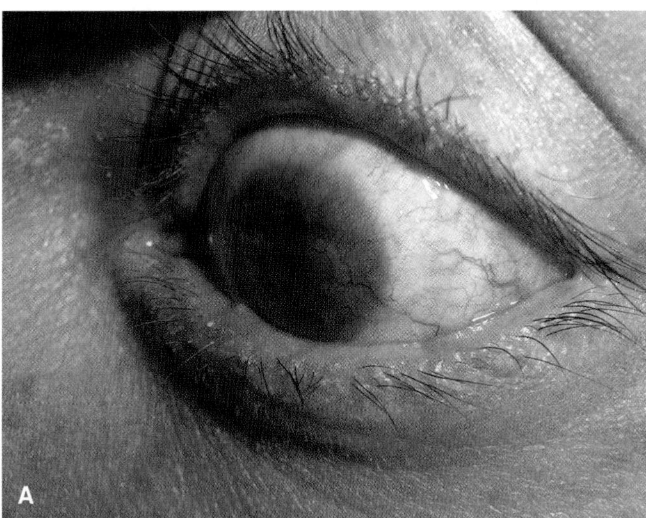

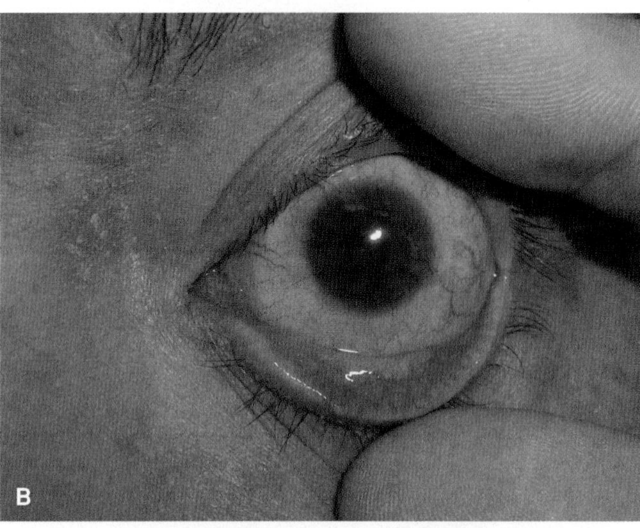

FIGURE 97-8 Neovascularization involving the cornea in a patient with severe ocular rosacea that started in high school. The diagnosis was missed for years and the corneal clouding diminishes her vision. **A.** Side view. **B.** Front view. (*Used with permission from Richard P. Usatine, MD.*)

very mild ocular complaints such as ocular grittiness or conjunctivitis. These patients may have many unsightly pustules with severe facial erythema. They are more prone to develop a hordeolum (stye) (see Chapter 10, Hordeolum and Chalazion).

3. *Phymatous or Rhinophymatous rosacea* (**Figure 97-4**)—Characterized by hyperplasia of the sebaceous glands that form thickened confluent plaques on the nose known as rhinophyma. This hyperplasia can cause significant disfigurement to the forehead, eyelids, chin, and nose. The nasal disfiguration is seen more commonly in men than women. W. C. Fields is famous for his rhinophyma and intake of alcohol. Rhinophyma can occur without any alcohol use.
4. *Ocular rosacea* (**Figures 97-7** and **97-8**)—An advanced subtype of rosacea that is characterized by impressive, severe flushing with persistent telangiectasias, papules, and pustules. The patient may complain of watery eyes, a foreign-body sensation, burning, dryness, vision changes, and lid or periocular erythema. The eyelids are most commonly involved with telangiectasias, blepharitis, and recurrent hordeola and chalazia (**Figure 97-7**). Conjunctivitis may be chronic. Although corneal involvement is least common, it can have the most devastating consequences. Corneal findings may include punctate erosions, corneal infiltrates, and corneal neovascularization. In the most severe cases, blood vessels may grow over the cornea and lead to blindness (**Figure 97-8**).

TYPICAL DISTRIBUTION

Rosacea occurs on the face, especially on the cheeks and nose. However, the forehead, eyelids, and chin can also be involved.

LABORATORY STUDIES

Not needed when the clinical picture is clear. If you are considering lupus or sarcoid, an antinuclear antibody (ANA), chest x-ray, or punch biopsy may be needed (**Figure 97-9**).

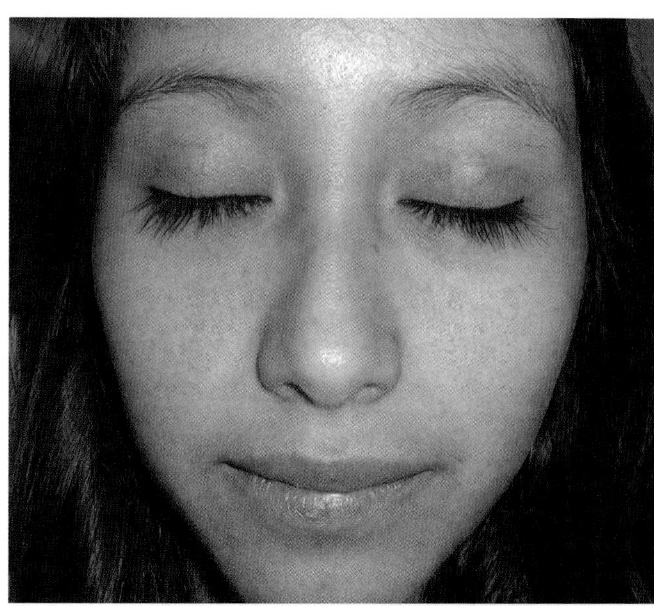

FIGURE 97-9 Biopsy proven rosacea in a 15-year-old girl. The red rash on her cheeks had been present for one year and had not responded to empirical therapy. The butterfly distribution of the rash and the lack of classic rosacea features led the physician to perform a punch biopsy to establish a definitive diagnosis and rule out lupus. (*Used with permission from Richard P. Usatine, MD.*)

DIFFERENTIAL DIAGNOSIS

- Acne—The age of onset for rosacea tends to be 30 to 50 years, much later than the onset for acne vulgaris. Comedones are prominent in most cases of acne and generally absent in rosacea (see Chapter 96, Acne Vulgaris).
- Sarcoidosis on the face is much less common than rosacea, but the inflamed plaques can be red and resemble the inflammation of rosacea (see Chapter 150, Sarcoidosis).
- Seborrheic dermatitis tends to produce scale, whereas rosacea does not. Although both cause central facial erythema, papules and telangiectasias are present in rosacea and are not part of seborrheic dermatitis (see Chapter 135, Seborrheic Dermatitis).
- Systemic lupus erythematosus (SLE) can be scarring, does not usually produce papules or pustules, and it spares the nasolabial folds and nose (see Chapter 173, Lupus: Systemic and Cutaneous). The patient in **Figure 97-9** has a butterfly distribution of her rosacea, but her biopsy clearly demonstrated the histology of rosacea.

The following three diagnoses were once considered variants of rosacea but a recent classification system identified these as separate entities:[2]

- Rosacea fulminans (known as pyoderma faciale) is characterized by the sudden appearance of papules, pustules, and nodules, along with fluctuating and draining sinuses that may be interconnecting. The condition appears primarily in women in their 20s, and intense redness and edema also may be prominent.[2]
- Steroid-induced acneiform eruption is not a variant of rosacea and can occur as an inflammatory response in any patient during or after chronic corticosteroid use. The same inflammatory response may also occur in patients with rosacea.
- Perioral dermatitis without rosacea symptoms should not be classified as a variant of rosacea. Perioral dermatitis is characterized by microvesicles, scaling, and peeling around the mouth (**Figure 97-10**). Perioraficial dermatitis is the same condition but may involve the skin around the nares and eyes (**Figure 97-11**).

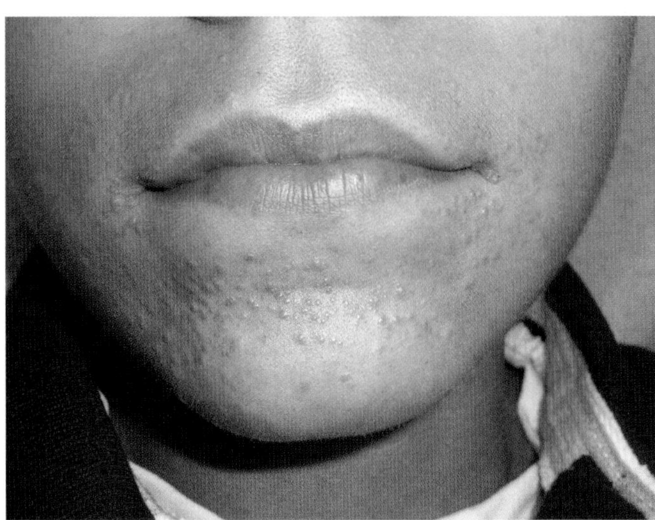

FIGURE 97-10 Perioral dermatitis in this 13-year-old boy with microvesicles, scaling, and peeling around the mouth. (*Used with permission from Richard P. Usatine, MD.*)

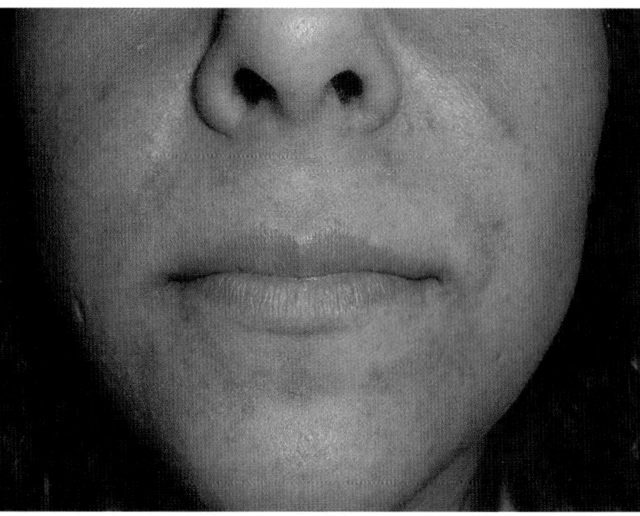

FIGURE 97-11 Perioraficial dermatitis in a teenage girl with papules, scale and erythema around the mouth and nares. Note that there are no comedones as seen with acne. (*Used with permission from Richard P. Usatine, MD.*)

MANAGEMENT

- A Cochrane Database systematic review examined the efficacy of rosacea interventions.[3] Oral doxycycline appeared to be significantly more effective than placebo and there was no statistically significant difference in effectiveness between the 100-mg and 40-mg doses.[3] SOR Ⓐ They found some evidence to support the effectiveness of topical metronidazole (0.75% or 1%), azelaic acid (15% or 20%) for the treatment of moderate to severe rosacea.[3] SOR Ⓐ Cyclosporine ophthalmic emulsion was significantly more effective than artificial tears for treating ocular rosacea (for all outcomes).[3] SOR Ⓐ
- When there are a limited number of papules and pustules, start with topical metronidazole (0.75% or 1%) or topical azelaic acid (15% or 20%).[3]
  - There are no substantial differences between topical metronidazole of 0.75 percent and 1 percent, or between once daily and twice daily regimens.[4] Metronidazole cream, gel, and lotion have similar efficacies as well.[4]
- Azelaic acid in a 15 percent gel applied bid appeared to offer some modest benefits over 0.75 percent metronidazole gel in a manufacturer-sponsored study.[4] Azelaic acid was not as well tolerated, so both medications are reasonable options with the choice depending on patient preference and tolerance.[3] SOR Ⓑ One study found that once-daily azelaic acid 15 percent gel was as effective as twice-daily application, which can translate into a significant cost saving.[5]
- If the skin lesions are more extensive, oral antibiotics, such as doxycycline (40 mg or 100 mg daily) is recommended.[3] SOR Ⓐ When attempting to avoid the photosensitivity side effects of doxycycline it is reasonable to prescribe oral tetracycline (250 mg to 500 mg daily) or oral metronidazole (250 mg to 500 mg daily). SOR Ⓒ
- Patients who are started on oral antibiotics alone and improve may be switched to topical agents such as metronidazole or azelaic acid for maintenance.
- The *Demodex* mite may be one causative agent in rosacea. One study found permethrin 5 percent cream to be as effective as metronidazole

0.75 percent gel and superior to placebo in the treatment of rosacea.[5] SOR B

- Severe papulopustular disease refractory to antibiotics and topical treatments can be treated with oral isotretinoin at a low dose of 0.3 mg/kg per day.[6] SOR B
- Simple electrosurgery or laser without anesthesia can be used to treat the telangiectasias associated with rosacea. SOR C
- Rhinophyma can be excised with radiofrequency electrosurgery or laser. Isotretinoin is also used to treat rhinophyma.[6] SOR B
- Traditional therapies for mild ocular rosacea include oral tetracyclines, lid hygiene, and warm compresses.[1] SOR C Topical ophthalmic cyclosporine 0.05 percent (Restasis) is more effective than artificial tears for the treatment of rosacea-associated lid and corneal changes.[7] SOR B Ocular rosacea that involves the cornea should be immediately referred to an ophthalmologist to prevent blindness (**Figure 97-8**).

FOLLOW-UP

Follow-up can be in 1 to 3 months as needed.

PATIENT EDUCATION

Sun protection, including use of a hat and daily application of sunscreen, should be emphasized. Choose a sunscreen that is nonirritating and protects against UVA and UVB rays. Advise patients to keep a diary to identify and avoid precipitating factors such as hot and humid weather, alcohol, hot beverages, spicy foods, and large hot meals.

PATIENT RESOURCES

- National Rosacea Society. Its mission is to improve the lives of people with rosacea by raising awareness, providing public health information, and supporting medical research—**www.rosacea.org/**.

PROVIDER RESOURCES

- The National Rosacea Society also has an excellent set of materials that are geared for physicians—**www.rosacea.org/**.

REFERENCES

1. Zhao YE, Wu LP, Peng Y, Cheng H. Retrospective analysis of the association between Demodex infestation and rosacea. *Arch Dermatol.* 2010;146:896-902.
2. Wilkin J, Dahl M, Detmar M, et al. Standard classification of rosacea: report of the National Rosacea Society Expert Committee on the Classification and Staging of Rosacea. *J Am Acad Dermatol.* 2002;46:584-587.
3. van Zuuren EJ, Kramer S, Carter B, et al. Interventions for rosacea. *Cochrane Database Syst Rev.* 2011;(3):CD003262.
4. Yoo J, Reid DC, Kimball AB. Metronidazole in the treatment of rosacea: do formulation, dosing, and concentration matter? *J Drugs Dermatol.* 2006;5:317-319.
5. Kocak M, Yagli S, Vahapoglu G, Eksioglu M. Permethrin 5% cream versus metronidazole 0.75% gel for the treatment of papulopustular rosacea. A randomized double-blind placebo-controlled study. *Dermatology.* 2002;205:265-270.
6. Gollnick H, Blume-Peytavi U, Szabo EL, et al. Systemic isotretinoin in the treatment of rosacea—doxycycline- and placebo-controlled, randomized clinical study. *J Dtsch Dermatol Ges.* 2010; 8:505-515.
7. Schechter BA, Katz RS, Friedman LS. Efficacy of topical cyclosporine for the treatment of ocular rosacea. *Adv Ther.* 2009;26:651-659.

98 HIDRADENITIS SUPPURATIVA

Richard P. Usatine, MD

PATIENT STORY

A 17-year-old teenager presents with new tender lesions in her axilla that started during her period 2 weeks ago (**Figure 98-1**). She has had two similar outbreaks in the axilla the year before. The clinician determined that the diagnosis was a mild case of hidradenitis suppurativa with folliculitis as an alternative diagnosis to be considered. The patient was started on doxycycline 100 mg twice daily and the condition cleared within 1 month. The patient was also a one pack per day smoker and she agreed to quit smoking for her health and to decrease her risk of further outbreaks of hidradenitis.

INTRODUCTION

Hidradenitis suppurativa (HS) is an inflammatory disease of the pilosebaceous unit in the apocrine gland-bearing skin. HS is most common in the axilla and inguinal area, but may be found in the inframammary area as well. It produces painful inflammatory nodules, cysts, and sinus tracks with mucopurulent discharge and progressive scarring.

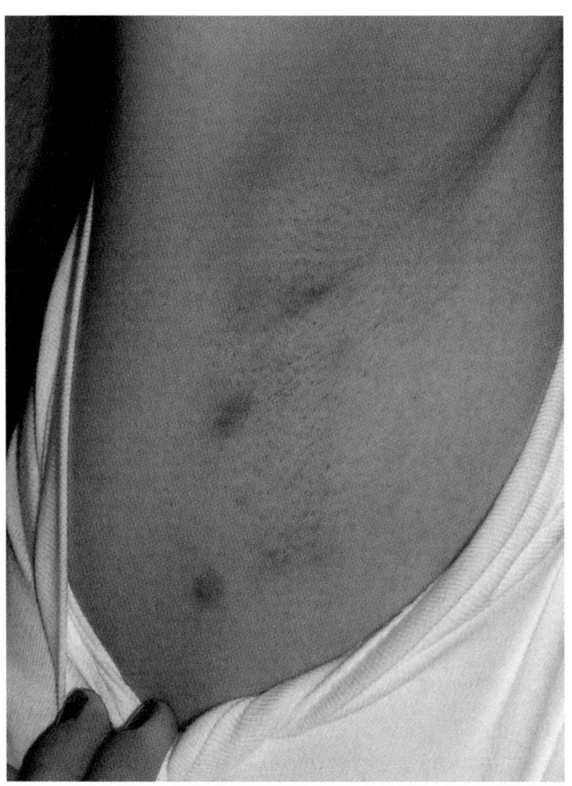

FIGURE 98-1 Mild hidradenitis suppurativa in the axilla. She has a history of recurrent lesions in her axilla. (*Used with permission from Richard P. Usatine, MD.*)

SYNONYMS

It is called acne inversa because it involves intertriginous areas and not the regions affected by acne (similar to inverse psoriasis).

EPIDEMIOLOGY

- Occurs after puberty in approximately 1 percent of the population.[1]
- Incidence is higher in females, in the range of 4:1 to 5:1. Flare-ups may be associated with menses.[1]

ETIOLOGY AND PATHOPHYSIOLOGY

- Disorder of the terminal follicular epithelium in the apocrine gland-bearing skin.[1]
- Starts with occlusion of hair follicles that lead to occlusion of surrounding apocrine glands.
- Chronic relapsing inflammation with mucopurulent discharge.
- Can lead to sinus tracts, draining fistulas and progressive scarring.

RISK FACTORS

Obesity, smoking, and tight-fitting clothing.

DIAGNOSIS

CLINICAL FEATURES

- Most common presentation is painful, tender, firm, nodular lesions in axillae (**Figures 98-1** and **98-2**).
- Nodules may open and drain pus spontaneously and heal slowly, with or without drainage, over 10 to 30 days.[1]

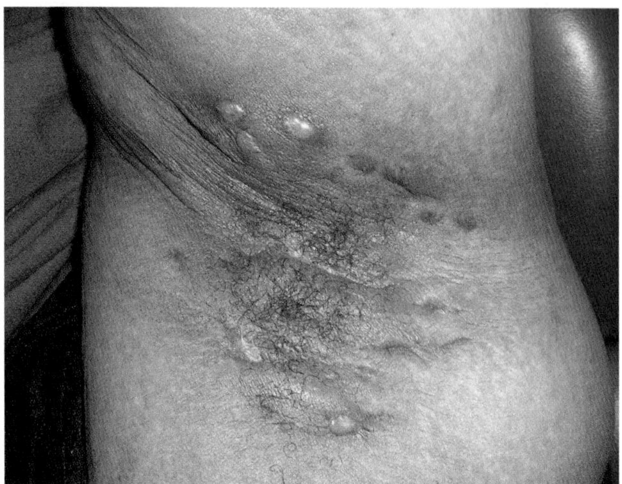

FIGURE 98-2 Hidradenitis in a young woman. The lesions are deeper and there have been some chronic changes with scarring and fibrosis from previous lesions. (*Used with permission from Richard P. Usatine, MD.*)

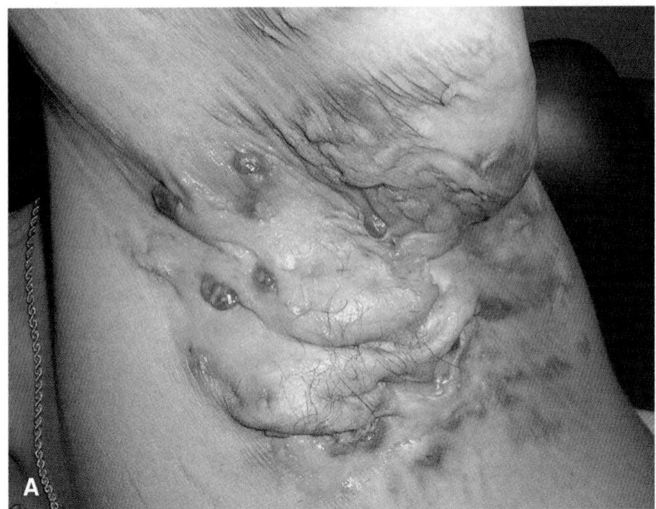

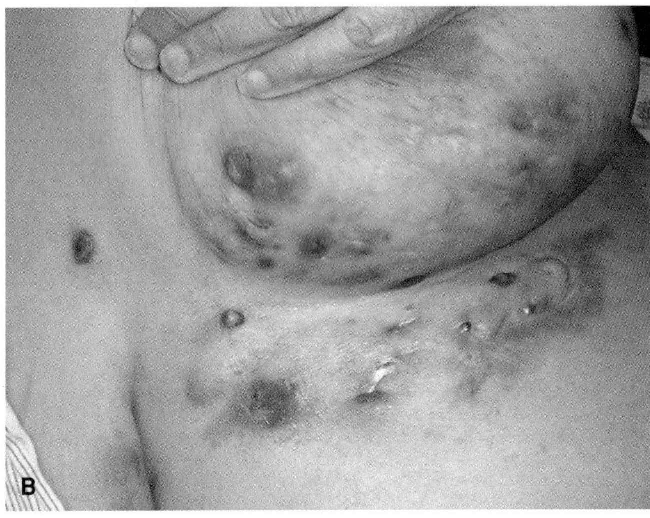

FIGURE 98-3 Severe recalcitrant hidradenitis in this woman with sinus tracts and scarring. **A.** Axillary involvement. **B.** Inframammary involvement. (*Used with permission from Richard P. Usatine, MD.*)

- Nodules may recur several times yearly, or in severe cases new lesions form as old ones heal.
- Surrounding cellulitis may be present and require systemic antibiotic treatment.
- Chronic recurrences result in thickened sinus tracts, which may become draining fistulas (**Figures 98-3**).
- HS can cause disabling pain, diminished range of motion, and social isolation.

TYPICAL DISTRIBUTION

- Axillary, inguinal, periareolar, intermammary (**Figure 98-4**), inframammary, pubic area (**Figure 98-5**), infraumbilical midline, gluteal folds, top of the anterior thighs, and the perianal region.[1]

LABORATORY STUDIES

Culture of purulence is likely to yield staphylococci and streptococci and is usually unnecessary to determine treatment. Culture may be useful if you suspect methicillin-resistant *Staphylococcus aureus.*

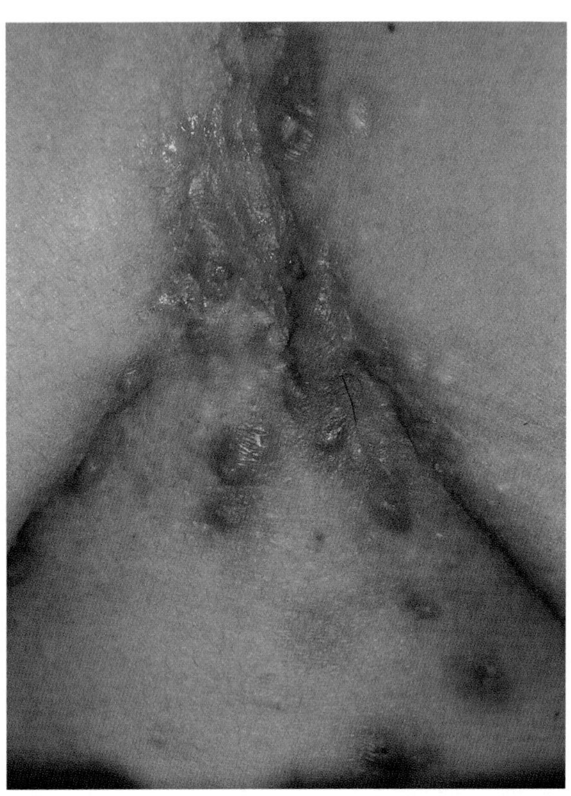

FIGURE 98-4 Long-standing painful severe HS between the breasts of this woman. (*Used with permission from Richard P. Usatine, MD.*)

DIFFERENTIAL DIAGNOSIS

- Bacterial infections, including folliculitis, carbuncles, furuncles, abscess, and cellulitis, may resemble HS but are less likely to be recurrent in the intertriginous areas.
- Epidermal cysts in the intertriginous regions may resemble HS. Theses cysts contain malodorous keratin contents.
- Granuloma inguinale and lymphogranuloma venereum are sexually transmitted infections that can produce inguinal ulcers and adenopathy that could be mistaken for HS.

MANAGEMENT

- Lifestyle changes are recommended, including weight loss if obesity is present. SOR Ⓒ
- Smoking is a risk factor for HS and cessation is highly recommended for many reasons.[1] See SOR Ⓑ for HS and SOR Ⓐ for other health reasons.
- Frequent bathing and wearing loose-fitting clothing may help.

Medical treatment is similar to acne treatment:

- Oral antibiotics are used in acute and chronic treatment. Oral tetracyclines, clindamycin, rifampin, and dapsone have been touted as beneficial. If there is methicillin-resistant *S. aureus* present, trimethoprim/sulfamethoxazole or clindamycin should be used.

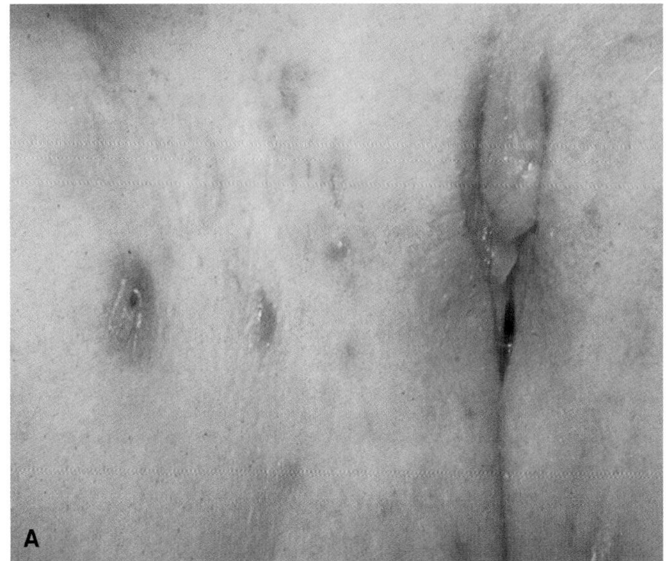

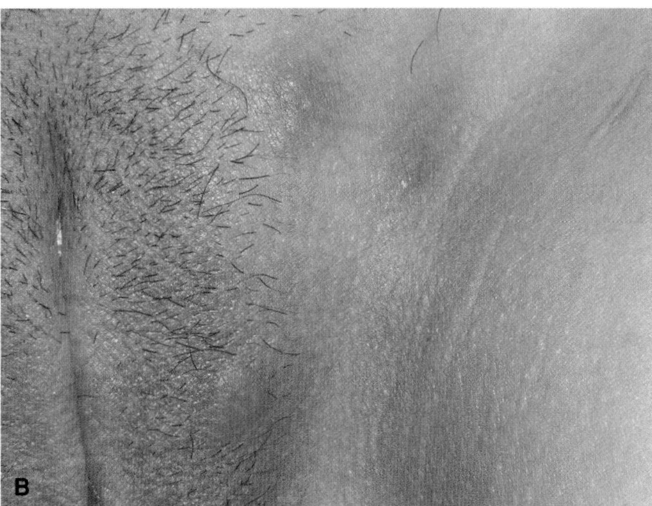

FIGURE 98-5 Hidradenitis of the inguinal area and vulva. **A.** prepubertal. (*Used with permission from Weinberg SW, Prose NS, Kristal L, Color Atlas of Pediatric Dermatology, 4th edition, Figure 2-30, New York, NY: McGraw-Hill, 2008.*) **B.** teenager. (*Used with permission from Richard P. Usatine, MD.*)

- Doxycycline 100 mg bid can be used acutely and to prevent new lesions in the mildest of cases. Many patients do not find these antibiotics to be of great help. SOR Ⓒ
- Topical clindamycin bid may be used in the mildest of cases. In one randomized controlled trial (RCT), systemic therapy with tetracyclines did not show better results than topical therapy with clindamycin.[1] SOR Ⓑ
  - Combination of systemic clindamycin (300 mg twice daily) and rifampin (600 mg daily) is recommended for patients with more severe HS.[2,3] In a series of 116 patients, parameters of severity improved, as did the quality-of-life score.[2] In another study, 28 of 34 patients (82%) experienced at least partial improvement, and 16 (47%) showed a total remission.[3] The maximum effect of treatment appeared within 10 weeks. Following total remission, 8 of 13 (61.5%) patients experienced a relapse after a mean period of 5 months. Nonresponders were predominantly patients with severe disease. The most frequent side effect is diarrhea.[2,3]
  - Oral dapsone may be considered when other therapies fail. However, in one study only 38 percent of patients experienced improvement.[4] SOR Ⓑ Rapid recurrence after stopping treatment suggests that antiinflammatory effects may predominate over antimicrobial effects. The total effect appears to be smaller than that reported with combination therapy using clindamycin and rifampicin. The use of oral dapsone requires frequent monitoring of blood counts because it frequently causes hemolysis. A G6PD level should be checked first to make sure the patient is not at high risk for severe hemolysis.
- Isotretinoin can reduce the severity of attacks in some patients but is not a reliable cure for HS.[5] SOR Ⓒ Also it is a potent teratogen and best avoided for females with this indication.
- Acitretin can be an effective treatment for refractory HS. In one study, all 12 patients achieved remission and experienced a significant decrease in pain. Long-lasting improvement was observed in 9 patients, with no recurrence of lesions after 6 months (n = 1), 1 year (n = 3), more than 2 years (n = 2), more than 3 years (n = 2), and more than 4 years (n = 1).[5] SOR Ⓑ However, acitretin is an oral retinoid that causes birth defects and may remain in the body for 3 years. Therefore, it should be reserved for use in male adolescents only and strictly avoided in females of child-bearing potential.
- Antitumor necrosis factor (TNF) agents are being studied for severe, recalcitrant HS. In one series, infliximab therapy (weight based) was shown to be effective and well tolerated in 6 of 7 patients with HS who were resistant to previous therapy.[6] This was in agreement with preexisting literature showing that 52 of 60 patients (87%) were improved after infliximab therapy.[6] SOR Ⓑ Adalimumab helps in the short-term, but no long-term curative effect was uniformly seen.[7]
- Intense pulsed light (IPL) with laser may be worth considering for patients who can afford the cost and time for treatment. In one study of 18 patients who were randomized to treatment of one axilla, groin, or inframammary area with IPL 2 times per week for 4 weeks, there was a significant improvement in the mean examination score, which was maintained at 12 months. Patients reported high levels of satisfaction with the IPL treatment.[8] SOR Ⓑ

Surgical treatments include the following:

- Intralesional steroids with 5 to 10 mg/mL of triamcinolone may help to decrease inflammation and pain within 24 to 48 hours. SOR Ⓒ
- Incision and drainage of acute lesions are suggested for the large fluctuant abscesses that can occur in HS. Although this may give some relief of the pressure, the surgical treatment and repacking of the wound is painful, and there is no evidence that it speeds healing. SOR Ⓒ
- Lancing small nodules is more painful than helpful and is not recommended.
- Surgical excision of affected area with or without skin grafting is used for recalcitrant disabling disease and should be individualized based on the stage and location of the disease.[9] SOR Ⓑ One surgical group has been using a medial thigh lift for immediate defect closure after radical excision of localized inguinal hidradenitis.[10]

FOLLOW-UP

If there is cellulitis or a large abscess was drained, follow-up should be within days. Chronic relapsing disease can ultimately be managed with appointments every 3 to 6 months depending upon the treatment and its success.

PATIENT EDUCATION

Smoking cessation, weight loss if overweight, and avoidance of tight-fitting clothes.

PATIENT RESOURCES

- Patient education materials at Medline Plus—**www.nlm.nih.gov/medlineplus/hidradenitissuppurativa.html**.

PROVIDER RESOURCES

- **http://emedicine.medscape.com/article/1073117-overview**.

REFERENCES

1. Jemec GB, Wendelboe P. Topical clindamycin versus systemic tetracycline in the treatment of hidradenitis suppurativa. *J Am Acad Dermatol.* 1998;39:971-974.
2. Gener G, Canoui-Poitrine F, Revuz JE, et al. Combination therapy with clindamycin and rifampicin for hidradenitis suppurativa: a series of 116 consecutive patients. *Dermatology.* 2009;219: 148-154.
3. van der Zee HH, Boer J, Prens EP, Jemec GBE. The effect of combined treatment with oral clindamycin and oral rifampicin in patients with hidradenitis suppurativa. *Dermatology.* 2009;219: 143-147.
4. Yazdanyar S, Boer J, Ingvarsson G, et al. Dapsone therapy for hidradenitis suppurativa: a series of 24 patients. *Dermatology.* 2011;222(4):342-346.
5. Boer J, Nazary M. Long-term results of acitretin therapy for hidradenitis suppurativa. Is acne inversa also a misnomer? *Br J Dermatol.* 2011;164:170-175.
6. Delage M, Samimi M, Atlan M, et al. Efficacy of infliximab for hidradenitis suppurativa: assessment of clinical and biological inflammatory markers. *Acta Derm Venereol.* 2011;91:169-171.
7. Miller I, Lynggaard CD, Lophaven S, et al. A double-blind placebo-controlled randomized trial of adalimumab in the treatment of hidradenitis suppurativa. *Br J Dermatol.* 2011;165: 391-398.
8. Highton L, Chan WY, Khwaja N, Laitung JK. Treatment of hidradenitis suppurativa with intense pulsed light: a prospective study. *Plast Reconstr Surg.* 2011;128:459-466.
9. Kagan RJ, Yakuboff KP, Warner P, Warden GD. Surgical treatment of hidradenitis suppurativa: a 10-year experience. *Surgery.* 2005; 138:734-740.
10. Rieger UM, Erba P, Pierer G, Kalbermatten DF. Hidradenitis suppurativa of the groin treated by radical excision and defect closure by medial thigh lift: aesthetic surgery meets reconstructive surgery. *J Plast Reconstr Aesthet Surg.* 2009;62:1355-1360.

SECTION 3 BACTERIAL

99 IMPETIGO

Richard P. Usatine, MD

PATIENT STORIES

A young boy presented to the office with a 3-day history of an untreated skin infection on his ear (**Figure 99-1**). His mother states that he has had white spots on his face for the past year but does not know how the ear infection started. The clinician noted honey crusts and purulent drainage from the lower pinna and pityriasis alba on the face. The child was not febrile and was behaving normally. Oral cephalexin was prescribed for the impetigo and 1 percent hydrocortisone ointment was given for the *p. alba*. Washing and hygiene issues were discussed to avoid spreading the infection within the household. During the 1-week follow-up appointment the impetigo was gone and the *p. alba* was improving.

An 11-year-old-child presented with a 5-day history of a skin lesion that started after a hiking trip (**Figure 99-2**). This episode of bullous impetigo was found to be secondary to methicillin-resistant *Staphylococcus aureus* (MRSA). The lesion was rapidly progressive and was developing a surrounding cellulitis. She was admitted to a hospital and treated with intravenous clindamycin with good results.[1]

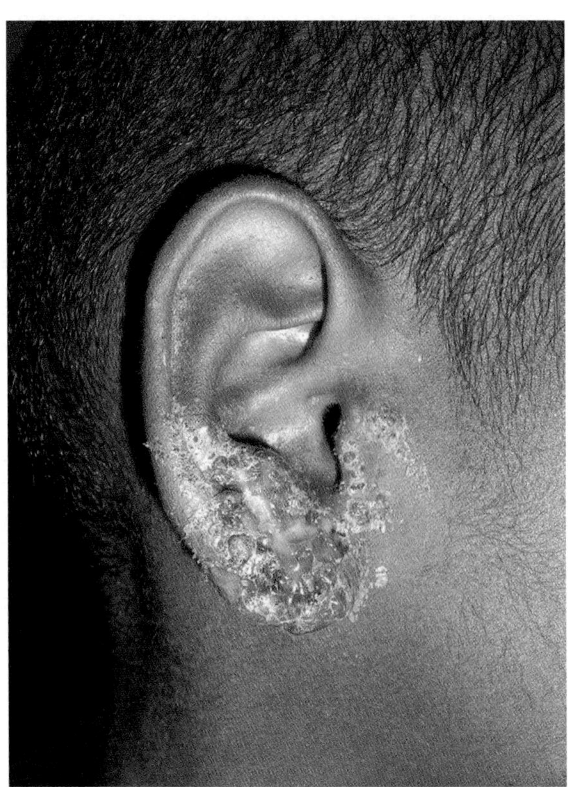

FIGURE 99-1 Typical honey-crusted plaque on the ear of young boy with impetigo. (*Used with permission from Richard P. Usatine, MD.*)

INTRODUCTION

Impetigo is the most superficial of bacterial skin infections. It causes honey crusts, bullae, and erosions.

EPIDEMIOLOGY

- Most frequent in children ages 2 to 6 years, but it can be seen in patients of any age.
- Common among homeless people living on the streets.
  - Seen often in developing countries in persons living without easy access to clean water and soap.
- Contagious and can be spread within a household.

ETIOLOGY AND PATHOPHYSIOLOGY

- Impetigo is caused by *S. aureus* and/or group A β-hemolytic *Streptococcus* (GABHS).
- Bullous impetigo is almost always caused by *S. aureus* and is less common than the typical crusted impetigo.
- Impetigo may occur after minor skin injury, such as an insect bite, abrasion, or dermatitis.

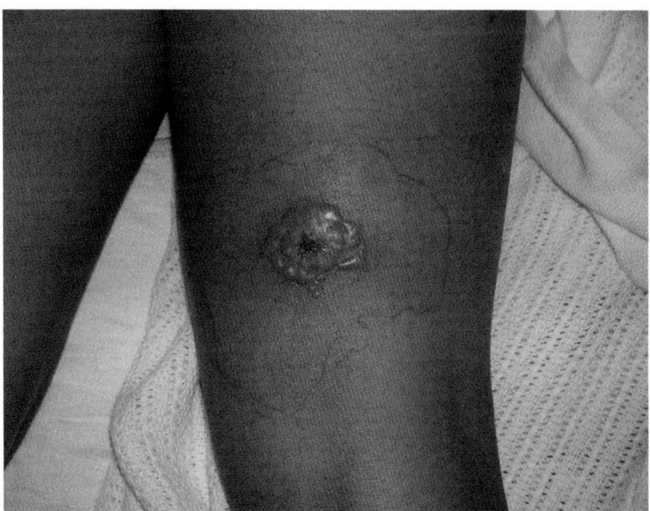

FIGURE 99-2 Bullous impetigo secondary to methicillin-resistant *Staphylococcus aureus* (MRSA) on the leg of an 11-year-old child. Note the surrounding cellulitis. (*With permission from Studdiford J, Stonehouse A. Bullous eruption on the posterior thigh 1. J Fam Pract. 2005;54:1041-1044. Reproduced with permission from Frontline Medical Communications.*)

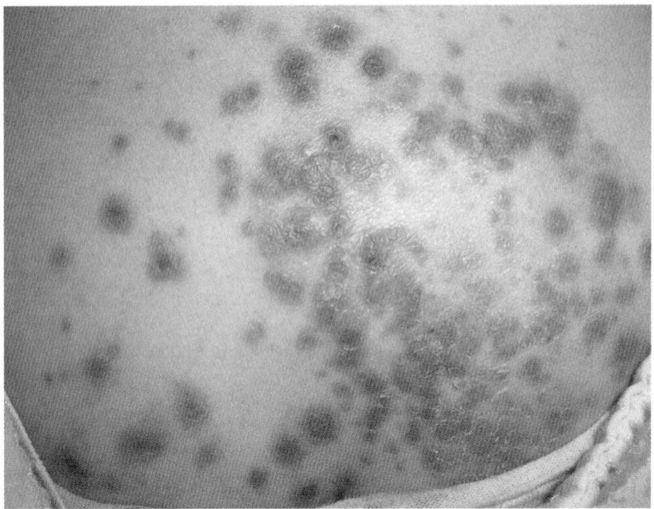

FIGURE 99-3 Widespread impetigo with honey-crusted erythematous lesions on the back of a 7-year-old child. (*Used with permission from Richard P. Usatine, MD.*)

DIAGNOSIS

CLINICAL FEATURES

- Vesicles, pustules, honey-colored (**Figure 99-1**), brown or dark crusts, erythematous erosions (**Figure 99-3**), ulcers in ecthyma (**Figure 99-4**), and bullae in bullous impetigo (**Figures 99-5** to **99-7**).

TYPICAL DISTRIBUTION

- Face (**Figures 99-1, 99-4** to **99-6**, and **99-8**) is most common, followed by hands, legs (**Figures 99-2** and **99-9**), trunk, and buttocks.

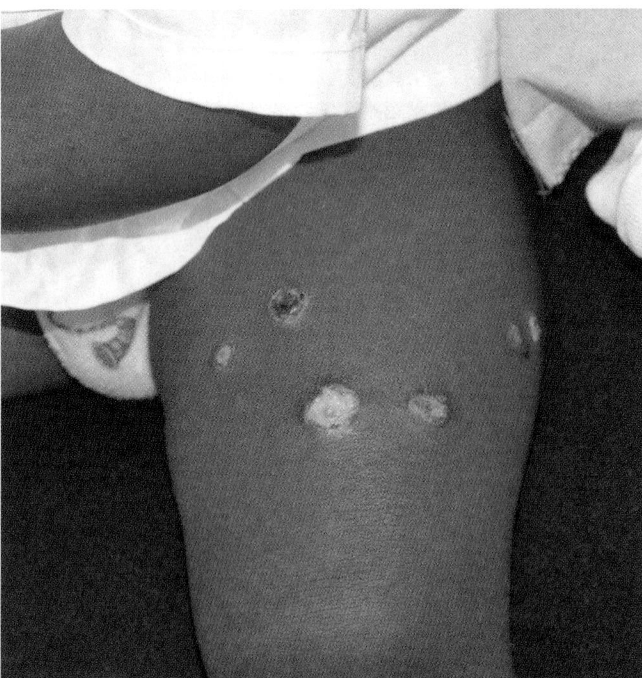

FIGURE 99-4 Impetigo on the leg of a girl in Haiti. Note the ecthyma (ulcerated impetigo) on the mid-thigh. (*Used with permission from Richard P. Usatine, MD.*)

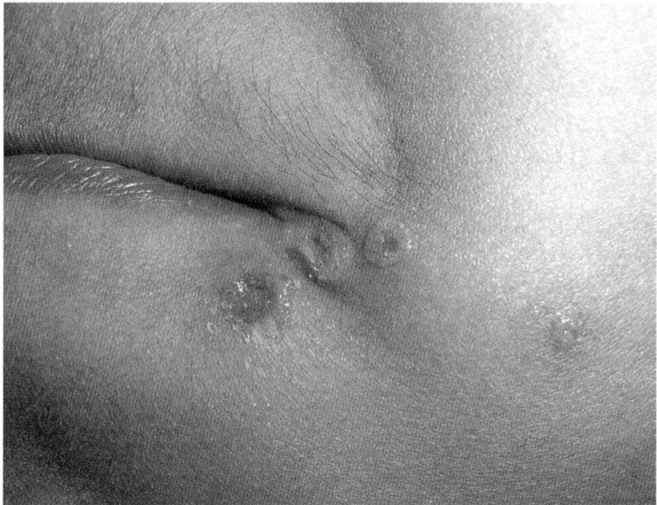

FIGURE 99-5 Bullous impetigo around the mouth of a young boy that progressed to desquamation of the skin on his hands and feet. (*Used with permission from Richard P. Usatine, MD.*)

CULTURE

- Culture should be considered in severe cases because of the rising incidence of MRSA-causing impetigo.

DIFFERENTIAL DIAGNOSIS

Many of the conditions below can become impetigo after being secondarily infected (**Figures 99-10** and **99-11**) with bacteria. This process is called impetiginization.

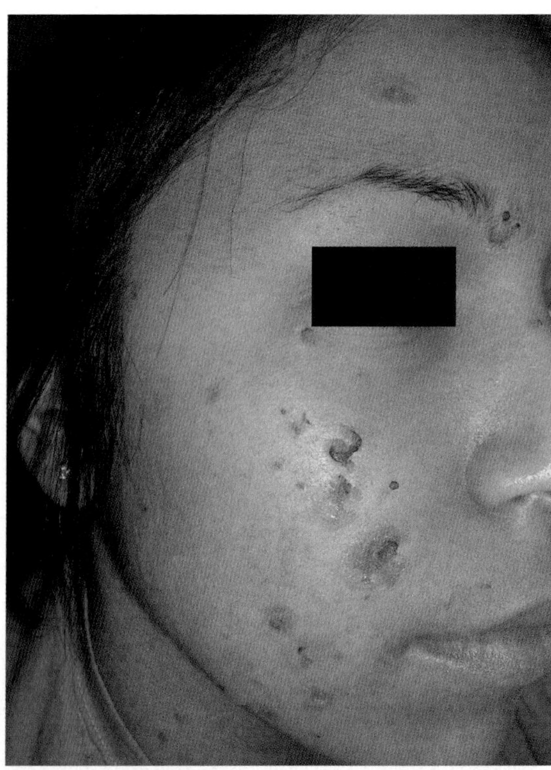

FIGURE 99-6 Bullous impetigo on the face of a 14-year-old girl. Methicillin-resistant *Staphylococcus aureus* was cultured from the impetigo. (*Used with permission from Richard P. Usatine, MD.*)

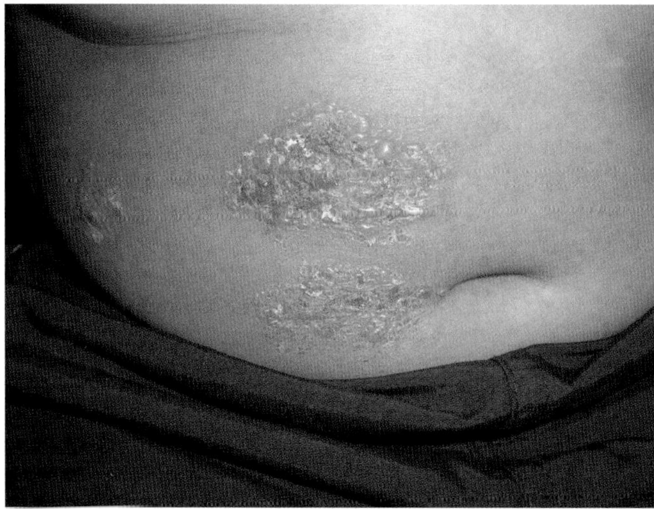

FIGURE 99-7 Bullous impetigo on the abdomen of an 8-year-old boy. (*Used with permission from Richard P. Usatine, MD.*)

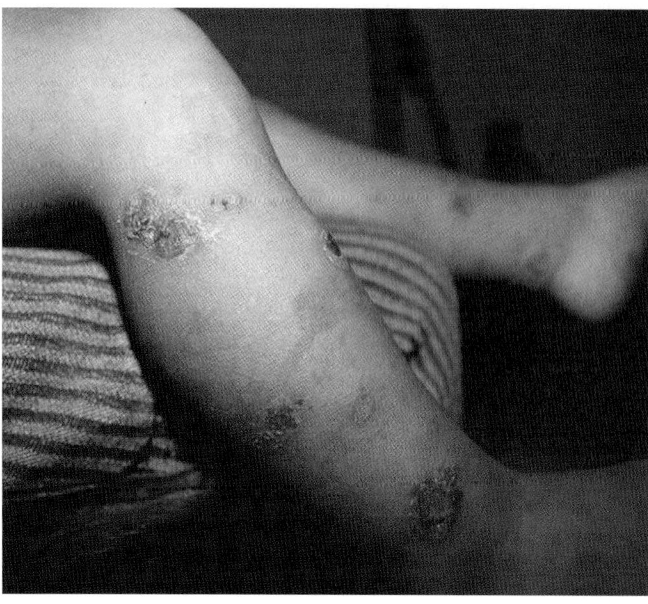

FIGURE 99-9 Impetigo secondary to flea bites on the legs of a young girl. (*Used with permission from Richard P. Usatine, MD. Previously published in the Western Journal of Medicine.*)

- Atopic dermatitis—A common inflammatory skin disorder characterized by itching and inflamed skin. It can become secondarily infected with bacteria (**Figure 99-10**; see Chapter 130, Atopic Dermatitis).
- Herpes simplex virus infection anywhere on the skin or mucous membranes can become secondarily infected (see Chapter 114, Herpes Simplex).
- Eczema herpeticum is eczema superinfected with herpes rather than bacteria (see Chapter 132, Eczema Herpeticum).
- Scabies—Pruritic contagious disease caused by a mite that burrows in skin (see Chapter 128, Scabies).
- Folliculitis—Inflammation and/or infection of hair follicles that may be bacterial (see Chapter 100, Folliculitis).
- Tinea corporis—A cutaneous fungal infection caused by dermatophytes, frequently with ring-like scale (see Chapter 123, Tinea Corporis).

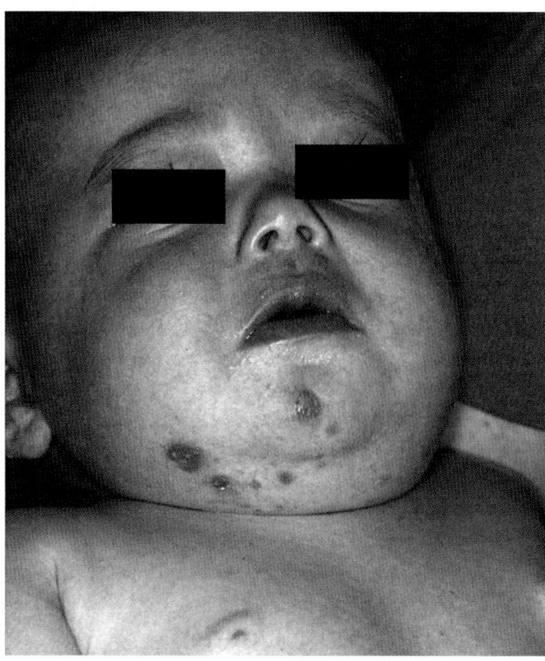

FIGURE 99-8 Impetigo on the face and neck of an infant. (*Used with permission from Richard P. Usatine, MD.*)

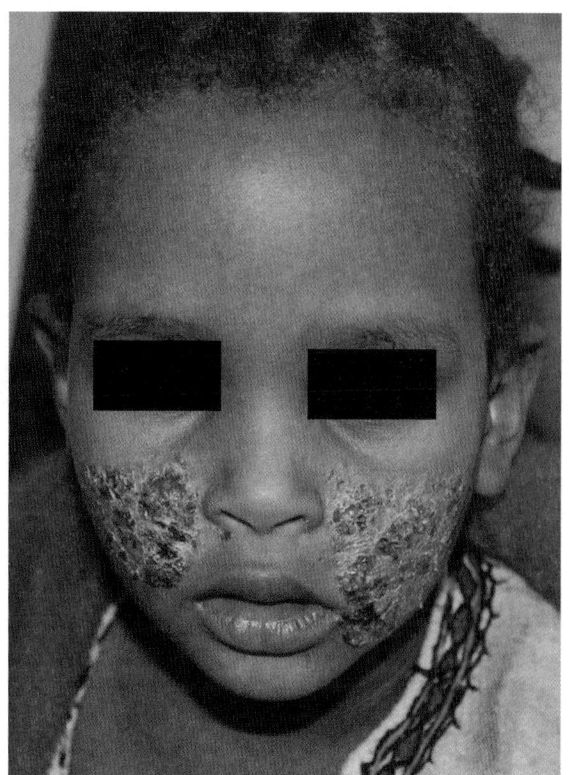

FIGURE 99-10 Atopic dermatitis complicated by secondary impetiginization. (*Used with permission from Richard P. Usatine, MD.*)

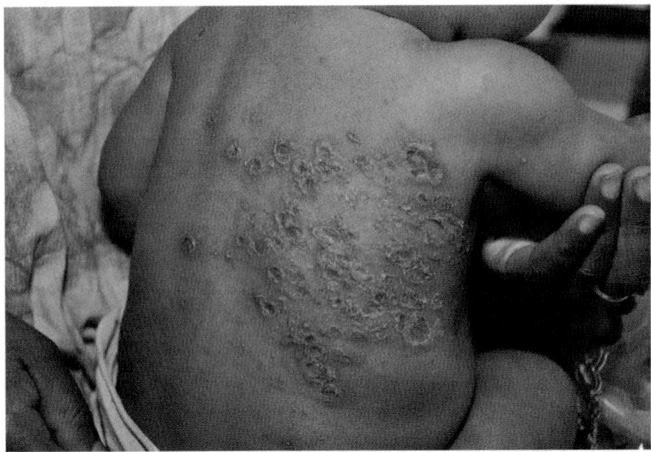

FIGURE 99-11 Bullous impetigo on the trunk of a 6-month-old Ethiopian child that resembles herpes zoster in its distribution and morphology. However, there are lesions on both sides of the back and the child is very young to have had varicella and now zoster. (*Used with permission from Richard P. Usatine, MD.*)

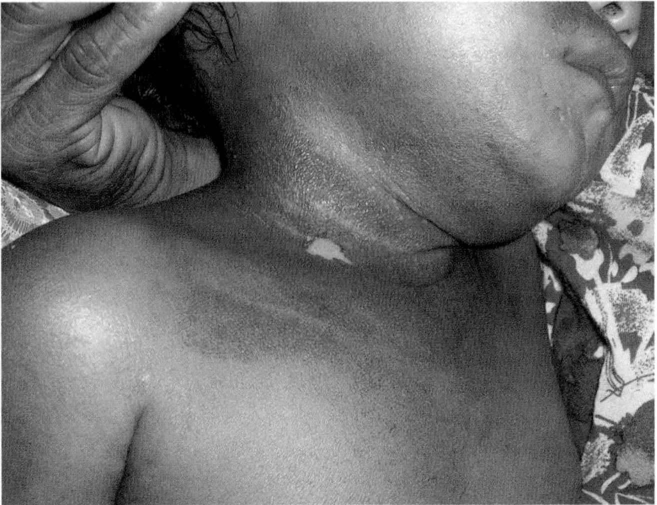

FIGURE 99-12 Staphylococcal scalded skin syndrome in a young child. A severe form of bullous impetigo with large areas of skin exfoliation. Note the prominent involvement of the neck as this condition tends to involve areas with skin folds. (*Used with permission from Richard P. Usatine, MD.*)

- Varicella or Zoster forms vesicles and bullae that can resemble bullous impetigo. See **Figure 99-11** for a case of bullous impetigo that resembles zoster (see Chapters 108 and 109, Chickenpox and Zoster).
- Bullous disease of childhood—An autoimmune condition with multiple tense bullae that can form rosette-like rings (see Chapter 155, Chronic Bullous Disease of Childhood).
- Acute allergic contact dermatitis—Dermatitis from direct cutaneous exposure to allergens such as poison ivy. Acute lesions are erythematous papules and vesicles in a linear pattern (see Chapter 131, Contact Dermatitis).
- Insect bites—Scratched, open lesions can become secondarily infected with bacteria (impetiginized) (**Figure 99-9**).
- Second-degree burn or sunburn—The blisters when opened leave the skin susceptible to secondary infection.
- Staphylococcal scalded skin syndrome—Life-threatening syndrome of acute exfoliation of the skin caused by an exotoxin from a staphylococcal infection. This condition is seen almost entirely in infants and young children (**Figure 99-12**; see Chapter 105, Staphylococcal Scalded Skin Syndrome).

MANAGEMENT

- There is good evidence that topical mupirocin is equally or more effective than oral treatment for people with limited impetigo. SOR Ⓐ Mupirocin also covers MRSA.[2]
- Extensive impetigo could be treated for 7 days with antibiotics that cover GABHS and *S. aureus*, such as cephalexin or dicloxacillin.[3] SOR Ⓐ
- Community-acquired MRSA can present as bullous impetigo in children (**Figures 99-2** and **99-6**) or adults.
- If you suspect MRSA, culture the lesions and start one of the following oral antibiotics: trimethoprim-sulfamethoxazole, clindamycin, or doxycycline (for patients 8 years and older).[4] SOR Ⓐ Trimethoprim-sulfamethoxazole achieved 100 percent clearance in the treatment of impetigo in children cultured with MRSA and GABHS in one small randomized controlled trial (RCT).[6]
- If there are recurrent MRSA infections, one might choose to prescribe intranasal mupirocin ointment and chlorhexidine bathing to decrease MRSA colonization.[5] SOR Ⓑ

PREVENTION

Practice good hygiene with soap and water. Avoid sharing towels and wash clothes.

FOLLOW-UP

Arrange follow-up based on severity of case and the age and immune status of the patient.

PATIENT EDUCATION

Discuss hygiene issues and how to avoid spread within the household or other living situations such as homeless shelters.

REFERENCES

1. Studdiford J, Stonehouse A: Bullous eruption on the posterior thigh 1. *J Fam Pract*. 2005;54:1041-1044.
2. Koning S, Verhagen AP, van-Suijlekom-Smit LWA, et al. Interventions for impetigo. *Cochrane Database Syst Rev*. 2012;CD003261.
3. Stevens DL, Bisno AL, Chambers HF, et al. Practice guidelines for the diagnosis and management of skin and soft-tissue infections. *Clin Infect Dis*. 2005;41:1373-1406.

4. Naimi TS, LeDell KH, Como-Sabetti K, et al. Comparison of community- and health care-associated methicillin-resistant *Staphylococcus aureus* infection. *JAMA.* 2003;290:2976-2984.

5. Wendt C, Schinke S, Württemberger M, et al. Value of whole-body washing with chlorhexidine for the eradication of methicillin-resistant *Staphylococcus aureus:* a randomized, placebo-controlled, double-blind clinical trial. *Infect Control Hosp Epidemiol.* 2007;28(9):1036-1043.

6. Tong SY, Andrews RM, Kearns T, et al. Trimethoprim-sulfamethoxazole compared with benzathine penicillin for treatment of impetigo in aboriginal children: a pilot randomised controlled trial. *J Paediatr Child Health.* 2010;46(3):131-133.

100 FOLLICULITIS

Richard P. Usatine, MD
Khalilah Hunter-Anderson, MD

PATIENT STORY

A young girl is seen for multiple papules and pustules on her lower abdomen (**Figure 100-1**). Further questioning demonstrates that she was in a friend's hot tub twice over the previous weekend. The outbreak started after she went into the hot tub the second time. This is a case of *Pseudomonas* folliculitis or "hot tub" folliculitis. The patient avoided this hot tub and the folliculitis disappeared spontaneously.

INTRODUCTION

Folliculitis is an inflammation of hair follicles usually from an infectious etiology. Multiple species of bacteria have been implicated, as well as fungal organisms.

EPIDEMIOLOGY

- Folliculitis is a cutaneous disorder that affects all age groups and races, and both genders.
- It can be infectious or noninfectious. It is most commonly of bacterial origin (**Figure 100-2**).
- Pseudofolliculitis barbae is most frequently seen in men of color and made worse by shaving (**Figure 100-3**).[1] It is also known as "razor bumps" and can start in the teen years with the onset of shaving.
- Acne keloidalis nuchae or keloidal folliculitis is commonly seen in black patients, but can be seen in patients of any ethnic background (**Figures 100-4** and **100-5**).[2] Like pseudofolliculitis barbae, it is exacerbated by shaving.
- Methicillin-resistant *Staphylococcus aureus* (MRSA) can pose a challenge to the treatment of folliculitis (**Figure 100-6**).

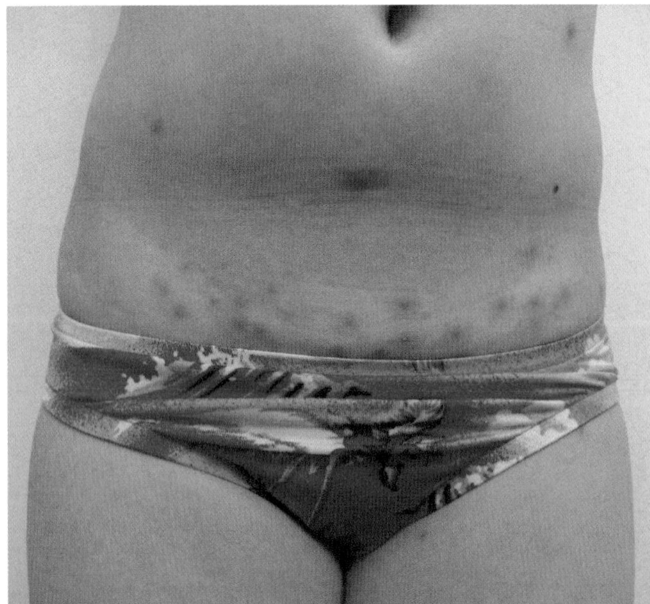

FIGURE 100-1 "Hot-tub" folliculitis from *Pseudomonas aeruginosa* in a hot tub. The folliculitis tends to be distributed under or around the bathing suit. (*Used with permission from Daniel Stulberg, MD.*)

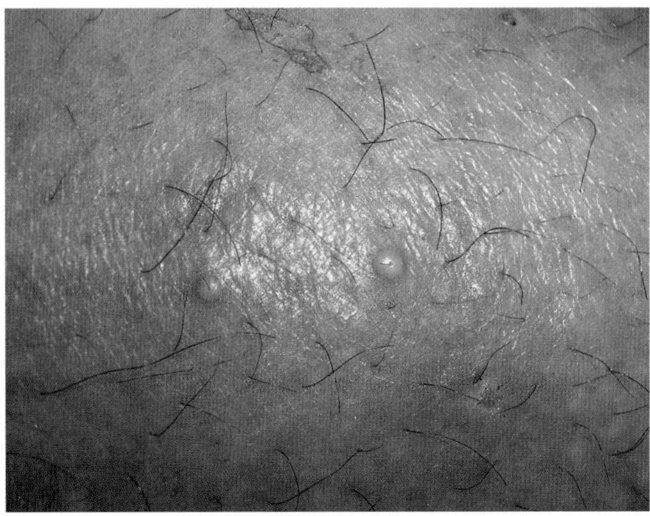

FIGURE 100-2 Close-up of bacterial folliculitis showing hairs coming through pustules. A culture grew out *Staphylococcus aureus*. (*Used with permission from Richard P. Usatine, MD.*)

ETIOLOGY AND PATHOPHYSIOLOGY

- Folliculitis is an infection of the hair follicle and can be superficial, in which it is confined to the upper hair follicle, or deep, in which inflammation spans the entire depth of the follicle.

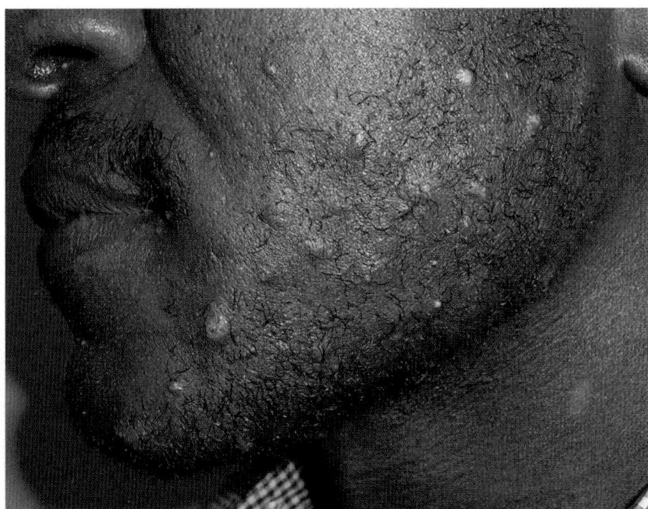

FIGURE 100-3 Pseudofolliculitis barbae in a young black man. Also known as "razor bumps" this started in his teen years with the onset of shaving. (*Used with permission from Richard P. Usatine, MD.*)

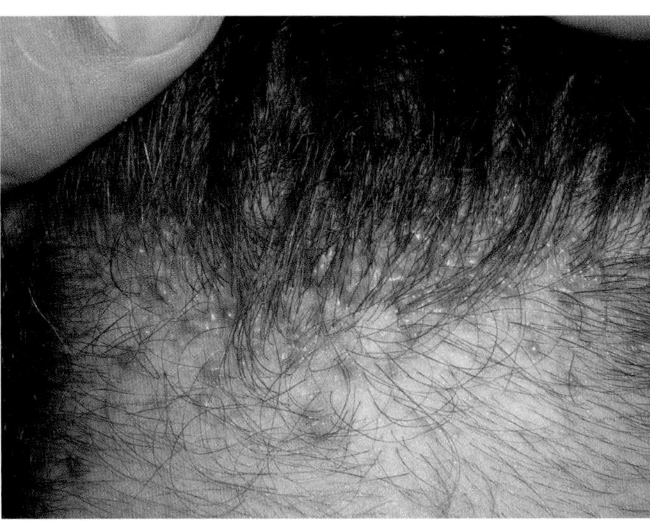

FIGURE 100-4 Acne keloidalis nuchae with inflamed papules and pustules on the neck of a young Hispanic man. (*Used with permission from Richard P. Usatine, MD.*)

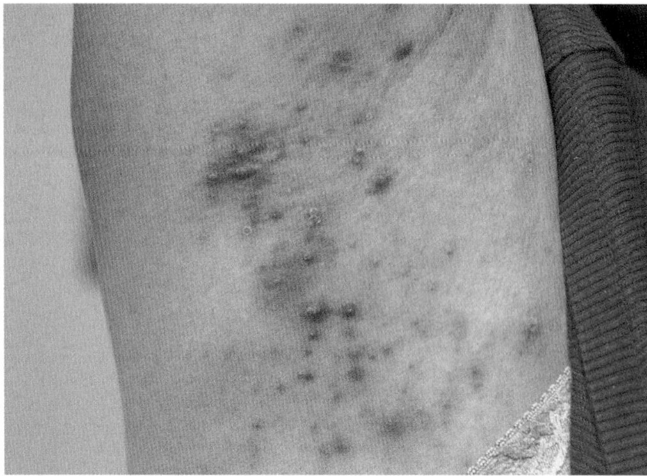

FIGURE 100-6 MRSA folliculitis in the axilla of a young woman. The lesions were present for 4 weeks in the axilla, left forearm, and right thigh. The MRSA was sensitive to tetracyclines and resolved with oral doxycycline. (*Used with permission from Plotner AN, Brodell RT. Bilateral axillary pustules. J Fam Pract. 2008;57(4):253-255.*)

- Infection can be of bacterial, viral, or fungal origin. *S. aureus* is by far the most common bacterial causative agent.
- The noninfectious form of folliculitis is often seen in adolescents and young adults who wear tight-fitting clothes. Folliculitis can also be caused by chemical irritants or physical injury.
- Topical steroid use, ointments, lotions, or makeup can swell the opening to the pilosebaceous unit and cause folliculitis.
- Bacterial folliculitis or *Staphylococcus* folliculitis typically presents as infected pustules most prominent on the face, buttocks, trunk, or extremities. It can progress to a deeper infection with the development of furuncles or boils (**Figure 100-7**). Infection can occur as a result of mechanical injury or via local spread from nearby infected wounds. An area of desquamation is frequently seen surrounding infected pustules in *S. aureus* folliculitis.[1-3]
- Parasitic folliculitis usually occurs as a result of mite infestation (*Demodex*). These are usually seen on the face, nose, and back and typically cause an eosinophilic pustular-like folliculitis.[1]
- Folliculitis decalvans is a chronic form of folliculitis involving the scalp, leading to hair loss or alopecia (**Figure 100-8**). Staphylococci infection is the usual causative agent, but there also has been a suggested genetic component to this condition.[1] It is also called tufted folliculitis because some of the hair follicles will have many hairs growing from them simultaneously (**Figure 100-9**).
- Acne keloidalis nuchae is a chronic form of folliculitis found on the posterior neck that can be extensive and lead to keloidal tissue and alopecia (**Figures 100-4** and **100-5**).[1-3]

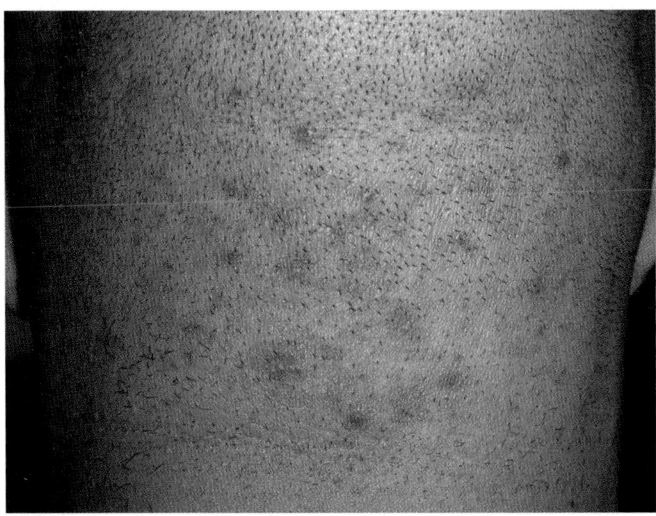

FIGURE 100-5 Acne keloidalis nuchae with inflamed papules and pustules on the posterior neck and scalp of a young African American man who shaves his head. (*Used with permission from Richard P. Usatine, MD.*)

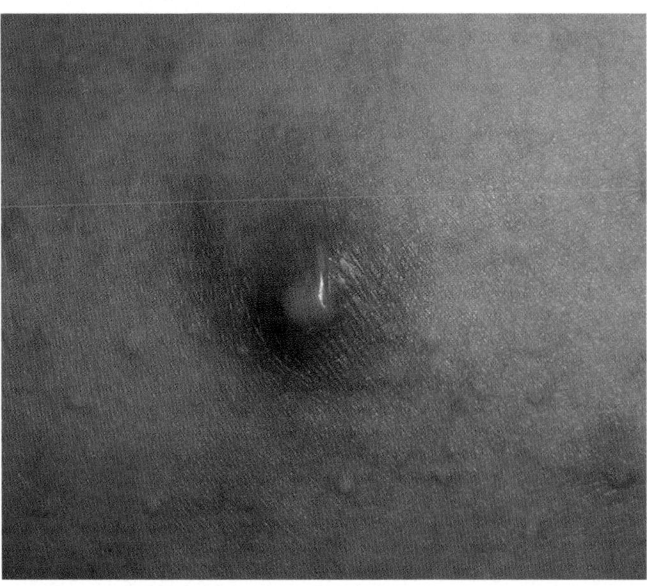

FIGURE 100-7 Isolated single furuncle. (*Used with permission from Richard P. Usatine, MD.*)

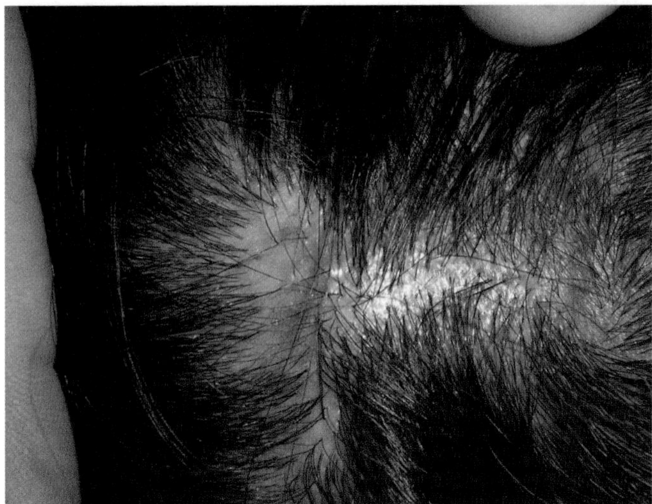

FIGURE 100-8 Early folliculitis decalvans showing scalp inflammation, pustules around hair follicles and scarring alopecia. (*Used with permission from Richard P. Usatine, MD.*)

- Fungal folliculitis is epidermal fungal infections that are seen frequently. Tinea capitis infections are a form of dermatophytic folliculitis (see Chapter 122, Tinea Capitis). *Pityrosporum* folliculitis is caused by yeast infection (*Malassezia* species) and is seen in a similar distribution as bacterial folliculitis on the back, chest, and shoulders (**Figure 100-10**; see Chapter 126, Tinea Versicolor). Candidal infection is less common and is usually seen in individuals who are immunosuppressed, present in hairy areas that are moist, and unlike most cases of folliculitis, may present with systemic signs and symptoms.[1–4]
- *Pseudomonas* folliculitis or "hot tub" folliculitis is usually a self-limited infection that follows exposure to water or objects that are contaminated with *Pseudomonas aeruginosa* (**Figure 100-1**). This occurs when hot tubs are inadequately chlorinated or brominated. This also occurs when loofah sponges or other items used for bathing become a host for pseudomonal growth. Onset of symptoms is usually within 6 to 72 hours after exposure, with the complete resolution of symptoms in a couple of days, provided that the individual avoids further exposure.[4]

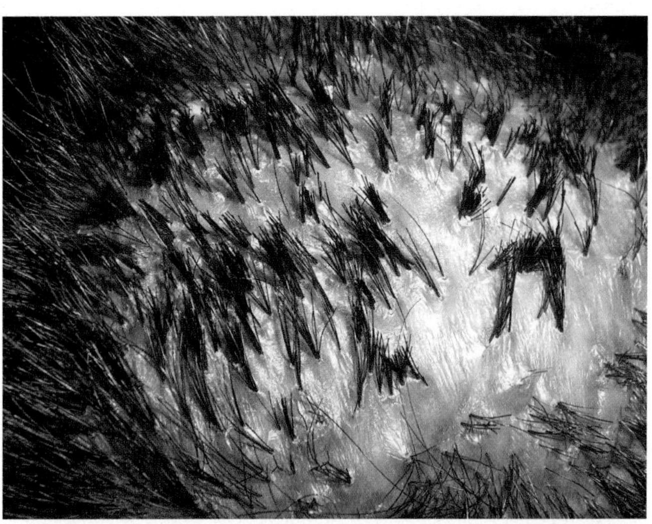

FIGURE 100-9 Tufted folliculitis with visible tufts of hair (multiple hairs from one follicle) growing from a number of abnormal follicles. This is one example of scarring alopecia. (*Used with permission from Richard P. Usatine, MD.*)

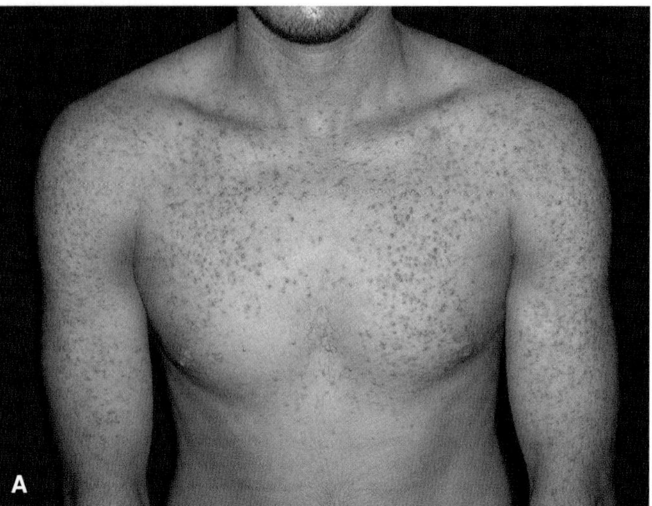

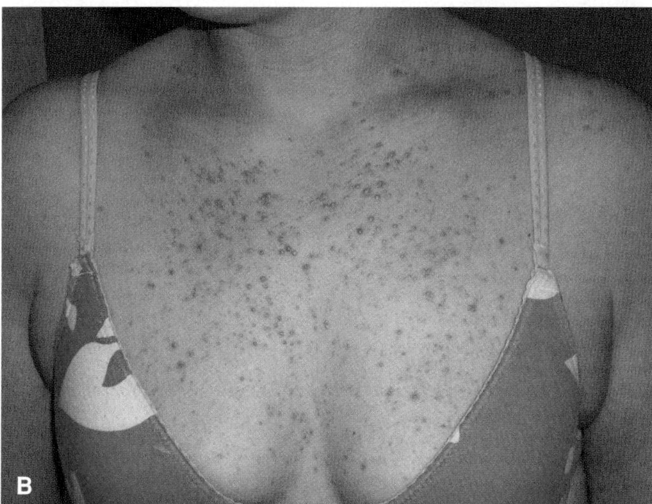

FIGURE 100-10 **A.** *Pityrosporum* folliculitis on the chest, shoulders, and arms of a young man; biopsy proven. **B.** *Pityrosporum* folliculitis on the chest of a young woman. KOH preparation showed *Pityrosporum* looking like ziti and meatballs. (*Used with permission from Richard P. Usatine, MD.*)

- Gram-negative folliculitis is an infection with Gram-negative bacteria that most typically occurs in individuals who have been on long-term antibiotic therapy, usually those taking oral antibiotics for acne. The most frequently encountered infective agents include *Klebsiella*, *Escherichia coli*, *Enterobacter,* and *Proteus*.[5]
- Pseudofolliculitis barbae (razor bumps) is most commonly seen in black males who shave. Papules develop when the sharp edge of the hair shaft reenters the skin (ingrown hairs), and is seen on the cheeks and neck as a result of curled ingrown hair.[2] It can also occur in females with hirsutism who shave or pluck their hairs.
- Viral folliculitis is primarily caused by herpes simplex virus and molluscum contagiosum.[4] Herpetic folliculitis is seen primarily in individuals with a history of herpes simplex infections type I or II. But most notably, it may be a sign of immunosuppression, as is the case with HIV infection.[6] The expression of herpes folliculitis in

HIV infection ranges from simple to necrotizing folliculitis and ulcerative lesions. Molluscum is a pox virus and molluscum contagiosum has been well-documented in similar patient populations (i.e., HIV and AIDS) and in children (see Chapters 114, Herpes Simplex and 115, Molluscum Contagiosum).[6–7]

- Actinic superficial folliculitis is a sterile form of folliculitis seen predominantly in warm climates or during hot or summer months. Pustules occur primarily on the neck, over the shoulders, upper trunk, and upper arms, usually within 6 to 36 hours after sun exposure.[8]

DIAGNOSIS

Often the diagnosis of folliculitis is based on a good history and physical.

CLINICAL FEATURES

Folliculitis has its characteristic presentation as the development of papules or pustules that are thin-walled and surrounded by a margin of erythema or inflammation. Look for a hair at the center of the lesions (**Figure 100-2**). There is usually an absence of systemic signs and patients, symptoms range from mild discomfort and pruritus to severe pain with extensive involvement.

TYPICAL DISTRIBUTION

Any area of the skin may be affected and often location may be related to the pathogen or cause of folliculitis. The face, scalp, neck, trunk, axillae, extremities, and groin are some of the more common areas affected.

LABORATORY TESTS

Laboratory testing may be unnecessary in simple superficial folliculitis and where the history is clear and quick resolution occurs. Clinical diagnosis of herpes and fungal folliculitis may be difficult and diagnosis may be made based on strong clinical suspicion or as a result of failed antimicrobial therapy. KOH preps can be used to look for tinea versicolor or other fungal organisms. Herpes culture or a quick test for herpes can be used when herpes is suspected.[1] SOR Ⓐ

DIFFERENTIAL DIAGNOSIS

- *Miliaria* is blockage of the sweat glands that can resemble the small papules of folliculitis (**Figure 100-11**). The eccrine sweat glands become blocked so that sweat leaks into the dermis and epidermis. Clinically, skin lesions may range from clear vesicles to pustules. These skin lesions primarily occur in times of increased heat and humidity, and are self-limited (see Chapter 92, Normal Skin Changes).[1]
- Impetigo is a bacterial infection of the skin that affects the superficial layers of the epidermis as opposed to hair follicles. It is contagious, unlike folliculitis. It has a bullous and nonbullous form, and honey-crusted lesions frequently predominate as opposed to the usual pustules seen in folliculitis (see Chapter 99, Impetigo).[4]
- Keratosis pilaris consists of papules that occur as a result of a buildup of keratin in the openings of hair follicles, especially on the lateral upper arms and thighs. It is not an infection but can develop into folliculitis if lesions become infected (see Chapter 130, Atopic Dermatitis).[1]

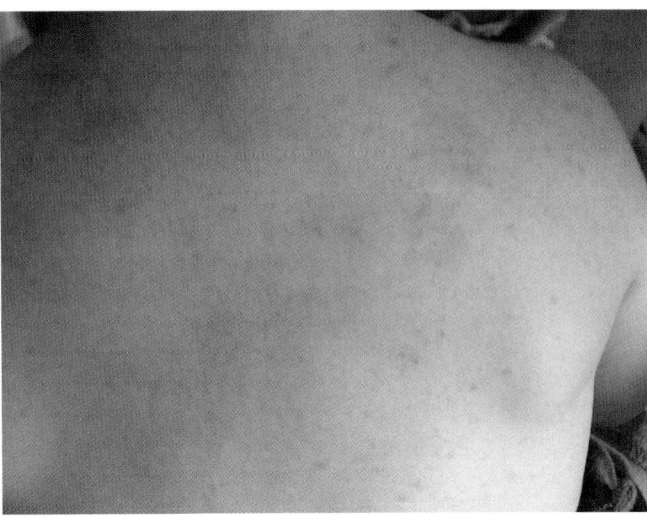

FIGURE 100-11 Miliaria in a 16-month-old child. This is an inflammation and blockage of the eccrine sweat glands and not the pilosebaceous units as seen in folliculitis. (*Used with permission from Richard P. Usatine, MD.*)

- Acne vulgaris is characterized by the presence of comedones, papules, pustules, and nodules that are a result of follicular hyperproliferation and plugging with excessive sebum. Inflammation occurs when *Propionibacterium acnes* and other inflammatory substances get extruded from the blocked pilosebaceous unit. Although acne on the face is rarely confused with folliculitis, acne on the trunk can resemble folliculitis. To distinguish between them look for facial involvement and comedones seen in acne (see Chapter 96, Acne Vulgaris).

MANAGEMENT

- Management of folliculitis varies by causative agent and underlying pathophysiology.
- Antivirals, antibiotics, and antifungals are used as topical and/or systemic agents. Approaches to nonpharmacologic therapy include patient education on the prevention of chemical and mechanical skin irritation. Glycemic control in diabetic patients may help treat folliculitis.[1–3] Good hygiene helps to control symptoms and prevent recurrence.
- With superficial bacterial folliculitis, treatment with topical preparations such as mupirocin (Bactroban) or fusidic acid may be sufficient.[1] SOR Ⓐ Additionally, topical clindamycin may be considered in the mildest cases in which MRSA is involved.[1] SOR Ⓐ
- Deep or extensive bacterial folliculitis warrants oral therapy with first-generation cephalosporins (cephalexin), penicillins (amoxicillin/clavulanate and dicloxacillin), macrolides, or fluoroquinolones.[1,4] SOR Ⓐ
- Pseudomonas or "hot tub" folliculitis usually resolves untreated within a week of onset (**Figure 100-1**). For severe cases, treatment with ciprofloxacin provides adequate antipseudomonal coverage.[1,4] SOR Ⓑ Application of a warm compress to affected areas also provides symptomatic relief.

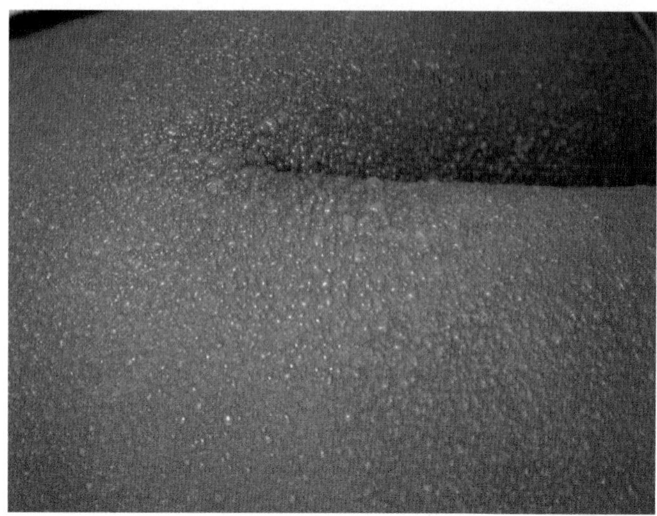

FIGURE 100-12 Miliaria crystallina in which the blockage of the eccrine sweat glands leads to small superficial crystalline vesicles. *(Used with permission from John Browning, MD.)*

- Pityrosporum folliculitis and/or tinea versicolor can be treated with systemic antifungals, topical azoles, and/or with shampoos containing azoles, selenium, or zinc (**Figure 100-12**) (see Chapter 126, Tinea Versicolor).[9]
- Candidal folliculitis in immunosuppressed persons may be treated with oral itraconazole or fluconazole (see Chapter 121, Candidiasis).[1] SOR Ⓑ
- *Demodex* folliculitis can be treated with ivermectin or topically with 5 percent permethrin cream.[4] SOR Ⓑ
- Herpes folliculitis can be treated with acyclovir, valacyclovir, and famciclovir. Regimens may frequently include acyclovir 200 mg five times a day for 5 days (see Chapter 114, Herpes Simplex).[1] SOR Ⓑ

FOLLOW-UP

Most cases of folliculitis are superficial and resolve easily with treatment. Dermatologic and surgical consultation may be required in cases of chronic folliculitis with scarring.

PATIENT EDUCATION

Prevention is most important, and centers on good personal hygiene and proper laundering of clothing. Patients should be encouraged to avoid tight-fitting clothing. Hot tubs should be properly cleaned and the chemicals should be maintained appropriately. Electric razors for shaving can help prevent pseudofolliculitis barbae and should be cleaned regularly with alcohol. Patients with acne keloidalis nuchae should avoid shaving the hair in the involved area.

PATIENT RESOURCE

- **www.ncbi.nlm.nih.gov/pubmedhealth/PMH0001826/**.

PROVIDER RESOURCE

- **http://emedicine.medscape.com/article/1070456**.

REFERENCES

1. Luelmo-Aguilar J, Santandreu MS. Folliculitis recognition and management. *Am J Clin Dermatol.* 2004;5(5):301-310.
2. Habif T. *Clinical Dermatology*, 5th ed. Philadelphia, PA; 2010.
3. Levy AL, Simpson G, Skinner RB Jr: Medical pearl: circle of desquamation, a clue to the diagnosis of folliculitis and furunculosis caused by *Staphylococcus aureus*. *J Am Acad Dermatol.* 2006;55(6):1079-1080.
4. Stulberg DL, Penrod MA, Blatny RA. Common bacterial skin infections. *Am Fam Physician.* 2002;66(1):119-124.
5. Neubert U, Jansen T, Plewig G. Bacteriologic and immunologic aspects of Gram-negative folliculitis: a study of 46 patients. *Int J Dermatol.* 1999;38(4):270-274.
6. Boer A, Herder N, Winter K, Falk T. Herpes folliculitis: clinical histopathological, and molecular pathologic observations. *Br J Dermatol.* 2006;154(4):743-746.
7. Weinberg JM, Mysliwiec A, Turiansky GW, et al. Viral folliculitis. Atypical presentations of herpes simplex, herpes zoster, and molluscum contagiosum. *Arch Dermatol.* 1997;133(8):983-986.
8. Labandeira J, Suarez-Campos A, Toribio J. Actinic superficial folliculitis. *Br J Dermatol.* 1998;138(6):1070-1074.
9. Gupta AK, Batra R, Bluhm R, et al. Skin diseases associated with *Malassezia* species. *J Am Acad Dermatol.* 2004;51(5):785-798.

101 PITTED KERATOLYSIS

Michael Babcock, MD
Richard P. Usatine, MD

PATIENT STORY

A 17-year-old boy comes to the office with a terrible foot odor problem. He is wearing cowboy boots and he says that his feet are always sweaty. He is embarrassed to remove his boots, but when his mother convinces him to do so the odor is unpleasant. The clinician sees the typical pits of pitted keratolysis and notes that the boy's socks are moist. His foot has many crateriform pits on the sole (**Figure 101-1**). He is prescribed topical erythromycin solution for the pitted keratolysis and topical aluminum chloride for the hyperhidrosis. It is suggested that he wear a lighter and more breathable shoe until this problem improves.

INTRODUCTION

Pitted keratolysis is a superficial foot infection caused by Gram-positive bacteria. These bacteria degrade the keratin of the stratum corneum leaving visible pits on the soles of the feet.

EPIDEMIOLOGY

- Seen more commonly in males.
- Often a complication of hyperhidrosis.
- Seen more often in hot and humid climates.
- Prevalence can be as high as 42.5 percent among paddy field workers.[1]
- May be common in athletes with moist, sweaty feet.[2]

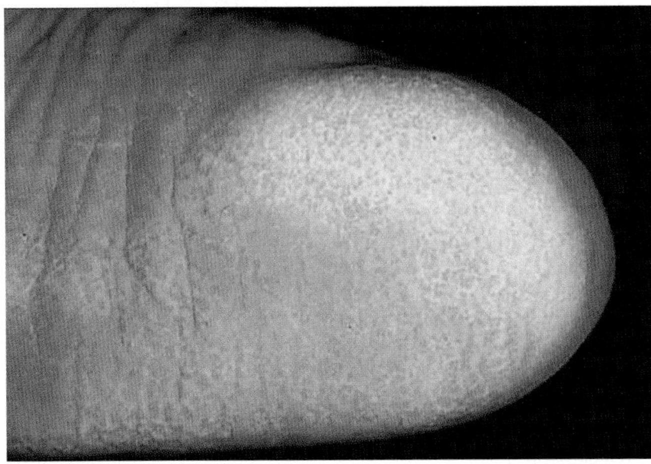

FIGURE 101-1 Many crateriform pits on the heel of the foot with pitted keratolysis and hyperhidrosis. (*Used with permission from Richard P. Usatine, MD.*)

ETIOLOGY AND PATHOPHYSIOLOGY

- *Kytococcus sedentarius* (formerly *Micrococcus* spp.), *Corynebacterium* species, and *Dermatophilus congolensis* have all been shown to cause pitted keratolysis.[3]
- Proteases produced by the bacteria degrade keratins to give the clinical appearance.[4]
- The associated malodor is likely secondary to the production of sulfur byproducts.[3]

DIAGNOSIS

CLINICAL FEATURES

Pitted keratolysis usually presents as painless, malodorous, crateriform pits coalescing into larger superficial erosions of the stratum corneum (**Figures 101-1** to **101-4**). It may be associated with itching and a burning sensation in some patients (**Figure 101-3**).

TYPICAL DISTRIBUTION

Pitted keratolysis usually involves the callused pressure-bearing areas of the foot, such as the heel, ball of the foot, and plantar great toe. It can also be found in friction areas between the toes.[5]

LABORATORY STUDIES

Typically a clinical diagnosis, but biopsy will reveal keratin pits lined by bacteria.

DIFFERENTIAL DIAGNOSIS

Characteristic clinical features make the diagnosis easy, but it is possible to have other diseases causing plantar pits:

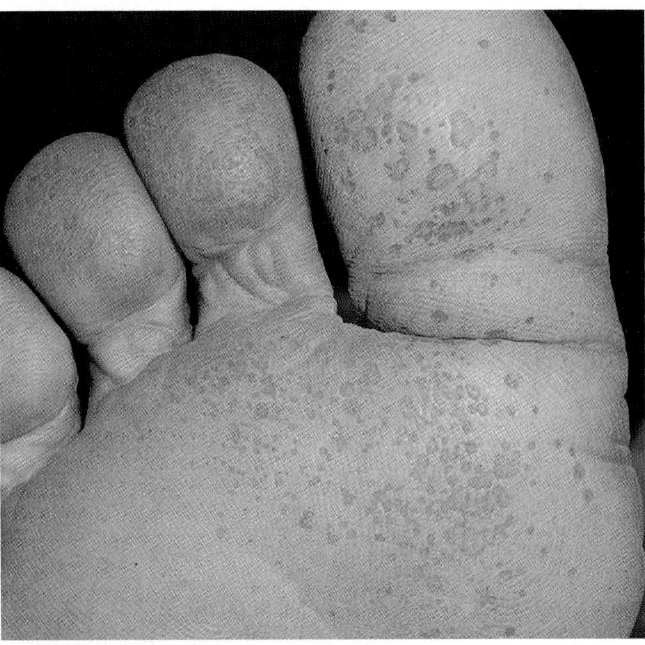

FIGURE 101-2 Pitted keratolysis on the pressure-bearing areas of the toes and the ball of the foot. (*Used with permission from Richard P. Usatine, MD.*)

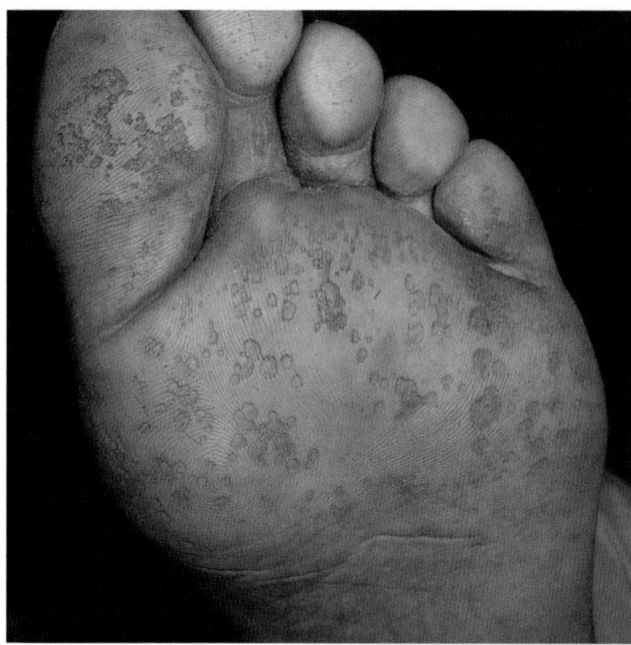

FIGURE 101-3 Pitted keratolysis with hyperpigmented crateriform pits on the pressure-bearing areas of the foot. The patient complained of itching and burning on the feet. (*Used with permission from Richard P. Usatine, MD.*)

- Plantar warts are typically not as numerous. They have a firm callus ring around a soft core with small black dots from thrombosed capillaries (see Chapter 119, Plantar Warts).
- Arsenic toxicity can result in pits on the palms and soles, but it can also have hyperpigmentation, many skin cancers, Mees lines (white lines on the fingernails), or other nail disorders.

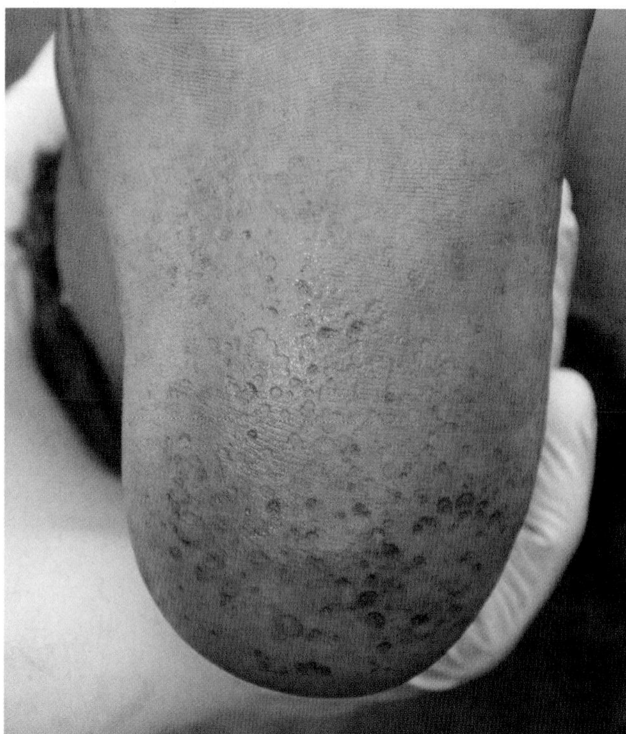

FIGURE 101-4 Pitted keratolysis with many crateriform pits on the heel. (*Used with permission from Richard P. Usatine, MD.*)

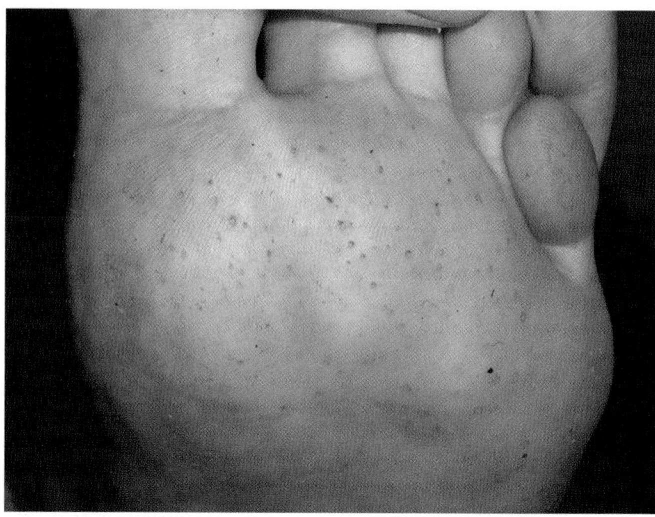

FIGURE 101-5 Pitted keratolysis with small crateriform pits on the ball of the foot. This teen also had hyperhidrosis, which was simultaneously treated with aluminum chloride. Treatment of the hyperhidrosis prevented recurrence of the pitted keratolysis. (*Used with permission from Richard P. Usatine, MD.*)

MANAGEMENT

- Treatment is based on bacterial elimination and reducing the moist environment in which the bacteria thrive. Various topical antibiotics are effective for pitted keratolysis.
- Topical erythromycin or clindamycin solution or gel can be applied twice daily until the condition resolves. SOR C Generic 2 percent erythromycin solution with an applicator top is a very inexpensive and effective preparation. It may take 3 to 4 weeks to clear the odor and skin lesions.
- Topical mupirocin is more expensive but also effective. SOR C
- Oral erythromycin is effective and may be considered if topical therapy fails. SOR C
- Treating underlying hyperhidrosis is also important to prevent recurrence (**Figure 101-5**). This can be done with topical aluminum chloride of varying concentrations. SOR C Drysol is 20 percent aluminum chloride solution and can be prescribed with an applicator top.
- Botulinum toxin injection is an expensive and effective treatment for hyperhidrosis.[6] SOR C It should be reserved for treatment failures because of the cost, the discomfort of the multiple injections, and the need to repeat the treatment every 3 to 4 months.

FOLLOW-UP

Follow-up is needed for treatment failures, recurrences, and the treatment of underlying hyperhidrosis if present. Follow-up can be performed annually for prescription aluminum chloride or approximately every 4 months for botulinum toxin injections.

PATIENT EDUCATION

Patients should be taught about the etiology of this disorder to help avoid recurrence. Helpful preventive strategies include avoiding occlusive footwear and using moisture-wicking socks or changing sweaty socks frequently.

PATIENT RESOURCES

- International Hyperhidrosis Society—**www.sweathelp.org**.

PROVIDER RESOURCES

- Medscape. *Pitted Keratolysis*—**http://emedicine.medscape.com/article/1053078-overview**.

REFERENCES

1. Shenoi SD, Davis SV, Rao S, et al. Dermatoses among paddy field workers—a descriptive, cross-sectional pilot study. *Indian J Dermatol Venereol Leprol.* 2005;71:254-258.
2. Conklin RJ. Common cutaneous disorders in athletes. *Sports Med.* 1990;9:100-119.
3. Bolognia J, Jorizzo J, Rapini R. *Dermatology*, 2nd ed. Philadelphia, PA: Mosby; 2008:1088-1089.
4. Takama H, Tamada Y, Yano K, et al. Pitted keratolysis: clinical manifestations in 53 cases. *Br J Dermatol.* 1997;137(2):282-285.
5. Longshaw C, Wright J, Farrell A, et al. Kytococcus sedentarius, the organism associated with pitted keratolysis, produces two keratin-degrading enzymes. *J Appl Microbiol.* 2002;93(5):810-816.
6. Vadoud-Seyedi J. Treatment of plantar hyperhidrosis with botulinum toxin type A. *Int J Dermatol.* 2004;43(12):969-971.

102 ERYTHRASMA

Anna Allred, MD
Richard P. Usatine, MD
Mindy A. Smith, MD, MS

PATIENT STORY

A 12-year-old Hispanic girl, accompanied by her mother, presents with a 1-year history of a red irritated rash in both axillae (**Figure 102-1**). She has been seen by multiple physicians and has tried many antifungal creams with no results. Even hydrocortisone did not help. She had stopped wearing deodorant for fear that she was allergic to all deodorants. Although the rash barely fluoresced at all, the physical examination and history were most consistent with erythrasma. The patient was given a prescription for oral erythromycin and the erythrasma cleared to the great delight of the patient and her mother.

INTRODUCTION

Erythrasma is a chronic superficial bacterial skin infection that usually occurs in a skin fold.

EPIDEMIOLOGY

- The incidence of erythrasma is approximately 4 percent.[1]
- Both sexes are equally affected.
- The inguinal location is more common in males.

ETIOLOGY AND PATHOPHYSIOLOGY

- *Corynebacterium minutissimum*, a lipophilic Gram-positive non–spore-forming rod-shaped organism, is the causative agent.
- Under favorable conditions, such as heat and humidity, this organism invades and proliferates the upper 1/3 of the stratum corneum.
- The organism produces porphyrins that result in the coral red fluorescence seen under a Wood lamp (**Figure 102-2**).

RISK FACTORS[1]

- Warm climate.
- Diabetes mellitus.
- Immunocompromised states.
- Obesity.
- Hyperhidrosis.
- Poor hygiene.
- Advanced age.

DIAGNOSIS

CLINICAL FEATURES

- Erythrasma is a sharply delineated, dry, red-brown patch with slightly scaling patches. Some lesions appear redder, whereas others have a browner color (**Figures 102-3** and **102-4**).
- The lesions are typically asymptomatic; however, patients sometimes complain of itching and burning when lesions occur in the groin (**Figure 102-3**).

TYPICAL DISTRIBUTION

Erythrasma is characteristically found in the intertriginous areas, especially the axilla and the groin. Patches of erythrasma may also be found in the interspaces of the toes, intergluteal cleft, perianal skin, and inframammary area.

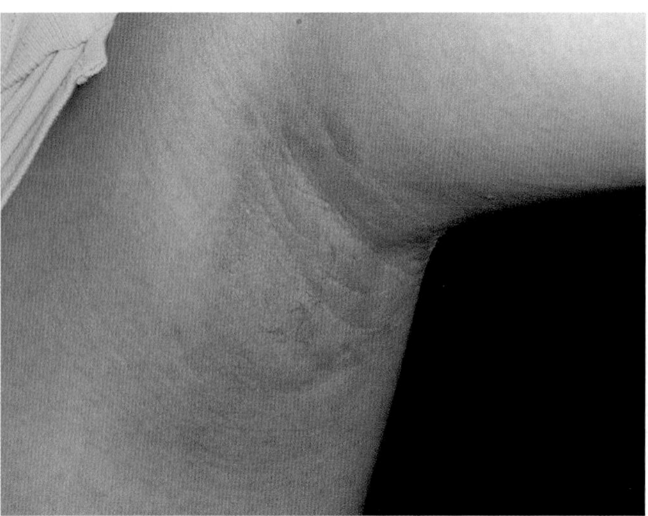

FIGURE 102-1 Erythrasma in the axilla of a 12-year-old Hispanic girl. *(Used with permission from Richard P. Usatine, MD.)*

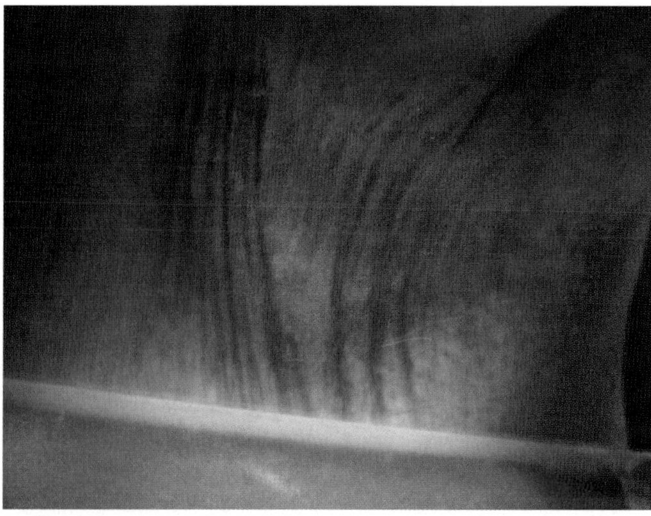

FIGURE 102-2 Coral red fluorescence seen with a Wood lamp held in the axilla of a patient with erythrasma. *(Used with permission from the University of Texas Health Sciences Center, Division of Dermatology.)*

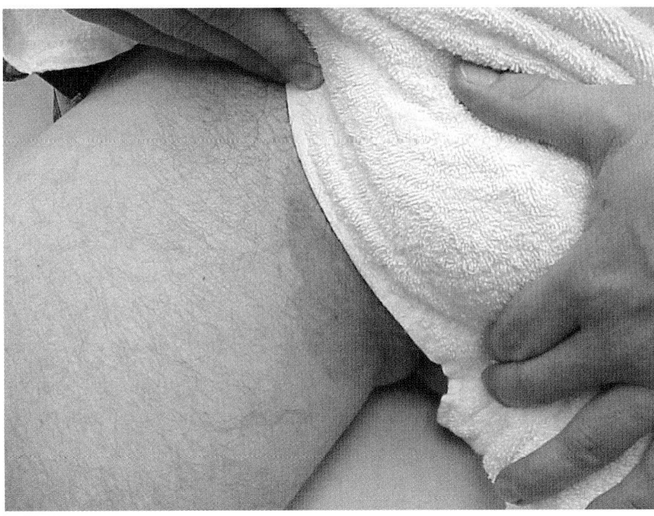

FIGURE 102-3 Light brown erythrasma in the groin of a young man. It does not have the degree of scaling usually seen with tinea cruris. (*Used with permission from Dan Stulberg, MD.*)

LABORATORY STUDIES

- Illumination of the plaque with a Wood lamp reveals coral-red fluorescence. It should be noted that washing the area before examination may eliminate the fluorescence.
- The diagnosis may be confirmed by applying Gram stain or methylene blue stain to scrapings from the skin to reveal Gram-positive rods and dark blue granules, respectively. However, if the presentation is typical and the plaque reveals fluorescence then microscopic examination and cultures are not needed.
- Microscopic examination is useful if erythrasma is suspected but the plaque does not fluoresce.

DIFFERENTIAL DIAGNOSIS

- Psoriasis—Inverse psoriasis occurs in the same areas as erythrasma and also causes pink to red plaques with well-demarcated borders.

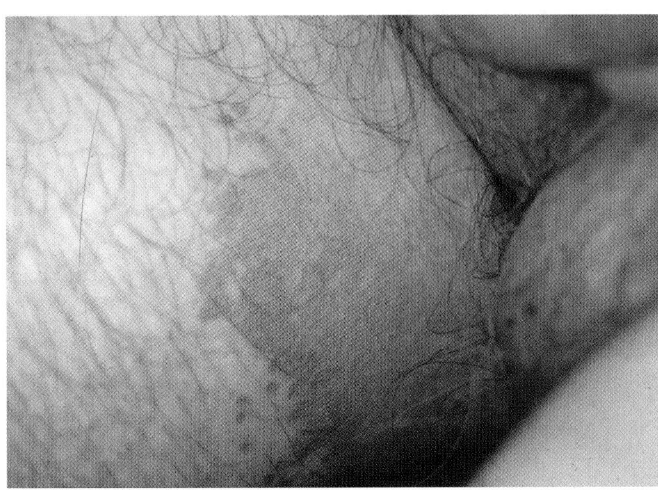

FIGURE 102-4 Brown erythrasma in the groin of a young man with diabetes. (*Used with permission from the University of Texas Health Sciences Center, Division of Dermatology.*)

The best way to distinguish psoriasis from erythrasma is to look for other clues of psoriasis in the patient, including nail pitting or onycholysis and hyperkeratotic plaques on the elbows, knees, or scalp. Also, inverse psoriasis may be seen in the intergluteal cleft as well as below the breasts or pannus in overweight individuals (see Chapter 136, Psoriasis). The Wood lamp may help differentiate between these diagnoses.

- Dermatophytosis—Cutaneous fungal infections also closely resemble erythrasma when they occur in the axillary and inguinal areas. Tinea infections also have well-demarcated borders that can be raised with central clearing. This distinctive ringworm look is more obvious with tinea than erythrasma but a scraping for microscopic examination should be able to distinguish between the two conditions. Examination of the feet will frequently show tinea pedis and onychomycosis when there are tinea infections elsewhere on the body (see Chapters 123, Tinea Corporis and 124, Tinea Cruris).
- Candidiasis—Look for satellite lesions to help distinguish candidiasis from erythrasma. Candidiasis will not fluoresce and a microscopic examination of a *Candida* infection should show branching pseudohyphae (see Chapter 121, Candidiasis).
- Intertrigo—This is a term for inflammation in intertriginous areas (skin folds). It is caused or exacerbated by heat, moisture, maceration, friction, and lack of air circulation. It is frequently made worse by infection with *Candida*, bacteria, or dermatophytes, and therefore overlaps with the erythrasma, *Candida*, and dermatophytosis. Obesity and diabetes especially predispose to this condition. All efforts should be made to find coexisting infections and treat them.
- Contact dermatitis to deodorants can mimic erythrasma. The history and Wood lamp should help to differentiate the two conditions (see Chapter 131, Contact Dermatitis).

MANAGEMENT

NONPHARMACOLOGIC

- It has been advocated that the areas should be vigorously washed with soap and water prior to application of topical antibiotics.[5] SOR C
- Consider loose-fitting cotton undergarments during treatment and to help prevent recurrence.[5] SOR C

MEDICATIONS

- Although the bacteria responds to a variety of antibacterial agents (e.g., penicillins, first-generation cephalosporins), the treatment of choice is oral erythromycin 250 mg four times a day for 14 days. Erythromycin shows cure rates as high as 100 percent.[2–4] SOR B
- However, some advocate that oral erythromycin is only required for the treatment of extensive or resistant cases.[5] SOR C
- Topical therapy (antibacterial, antifungal, benzoic acid 6%) has been recommended in addition to oral therapy in patients with hidden reservoirs of infection (i.e., interdigital involvement). SOR C
- Topical clindamycin may be applied once daily during the course of oral erythromycin therapy and for 2 weeks after physical clearance of the lesions for treatment and prophylaxis.[3,6] SOR C

- Topical erythromycin 2 percent solution applied twice daily.[4,5,7] SOR Ⓒ
- In a Turkish study, topical fusidic acid was more effective than erythromycin or single-dose clarithromycin based on Wood light reflection scores.[8]
- Optimal blood glucose control is recommended in the management of a diabetic patient with erythrasma.[2] SOR Ⓒ

PROGNOSIS

- Usually a benign condition; however, in immunocompromised individuals, *Corynebacterium* can cause abscess formation, bacteremia, endocarditis, pyelonephritis, cellulitis, and meningitis.[1]
- The condition tends to recur if the predisposing condition is not addressed.

FOLLOW-UP

Have the patient follow up in 2 to 4 weeks as needed to determine if erythrasma has resolved.

PATIENT EDUCATION

Reassure the patient that erythrasma is curable with antibiotic treatment.

PATIENT RESOURCES

- PubMed Health. *Erythrasma*—**www.ncbi.nlm.nih.gov/pubmedhealth/PMH0002441/**.
- Dermnet NZ. *Erythrasma*—**www.dermnetnz.org/bacterial/erythrasma.html**.

PROVIDER RESOURCES

- Medscape. *Erythrasma*—**http://emedicine.medscape.com/article/1052532**.

REFERENCES

1. Kibbi AG, Bahhady RF, Saleh Z, Haddad FG. *Erythrasma*. http://emedicine.medscape.com/article/1052532-overview#a0199, accessed April 2, 2012.
2. Ahmed I, Goldstein B. Diabetes mellitus. *Clin Dermatol.* 2006; 24(4):237-246.
3. Holdiness MR. Management of cutaneous erythrasma. *Drugs.* 2002;62(8):1131-1141.
4. James WD, Berger TG, Elston DM. *Andrew's Diseases of the Skin Clinical Dermatology*, 10th ed. London, UK: Saunders/Elsevier; 2006.
5. Karakatsanis G, Vakirlis E, Kastoridou C, Devliotou-Panagiotidou D. Coexistence of pityriasis versicolor and erythrasma. *Mycoses.* 2004;47(7):343-345.
6. Holdiness MR. Erythrasma and common bacterial skin infections. *Am Fam Physician.* 2003;15:67(2):254.
7. Miller SD, David-Bajar K. Images in clinical medicine. A brilliant case of erythrasma. *N Engl J Med.* 2004;14:351(16):1666.
8. Avci O, Tanyildizi T, Kusku E. A comparison between the effectiveness of erythromycin, single-dose clarithromycin and topical fusidic acid in the treatment of erythrasma. *J Dermatolog Treat.* 2011 Sep 18 [Epub ahead of print].

103 CELLULITIS

Richard P. Usatine, MD

PATIENT STORY

A 4-year-old child presents with a fever and a red and swollen foot (**Figure 103-1**). The patient injured her foot 3 days before with a door. On physical examination, the foot was warm, tender, red, and swollen, and the child's temperature was 39.4°C (103°F). This is classic cellulitis and the child was admitted for IV antibiotics.

INTRODUCTION

Cellulitis is an acute infection of the skin that involves the dermis and subcutaneous tissues.

EPIDEMIOLOGY

- In one review of serious skin infections in children admitted to a hospital in New Zealand, the most common types of infection were cellulitis (38%) and subcutaneous abscesses (36%).[1] The most frequent sites of infection were the head, face and neck, (32%) and lower limbs (32%). The most frequently isolated organisms were *Staphylococcus aureus* (48%) and *Streptococcus pyogenes* (20%).[1]
- Facial cellulitis occurs more often in children ages 6 months to 3 years.
- Perianal cellulitis occurs more commonly in young children (see Chapter 95, Diaper Rash and Perianal Dermatitis).

ETIOLOGY AND PATHOPHYSIOLOGY

- Often begins with a break in the skin caused by trauma, a bite, or an underlying dermatosis (e.g., atopic dermatitis) (**Figures 103-1** to **103-4**).
- Is most often caused by group A β-hemolytic *Streptococcus* (GAS) (**Figure 103-3**) or *Staphylococcus aureus*. The most common etiology of cellulitis with intact skin, when it has been determined through needle aspiration and/or punch biopsy, is *S. aureus*, outnumbering GAS by a ratio of nearly 2:1.[2]
- There are increasing concerns about the role of community-acquired methicillin-resistant *S. aureus* (MRSA) in all soft-tissue infections including cellulitis.[3–6]
- After a cat or dog bite, cellulitis is often caused by *Pasteurella multocida* (**Figure 103-4**).
- After saltwater exposure, cellulitis can be secondary to *Vibrio vulnificus* in warm climates. A *Vibrio vulnificus* infection can be especially deadly.
- Erysipelas is a specific type of superficial cellulitis with prominent lymphatic involvement and leading to a sharply defined and elevated border (**Figures 103-5** and **103-6**).
- Risk factors for hospitalization for staphylococcal skin infections in children in California were age less than 3 years, being Black, and lacking private insurance.[7]

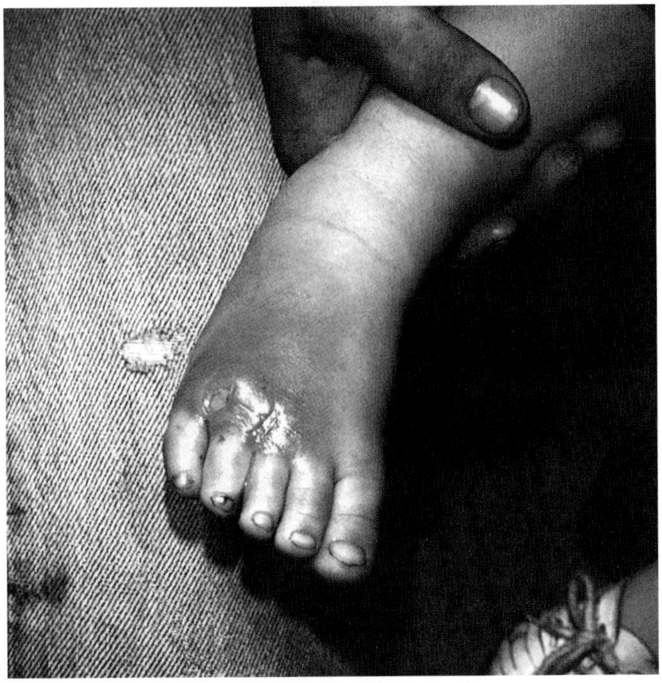

FIGURE 103-1 Cellulitis of the foot after an injury with a door in a 4-year-old girl. (*Used with permission from Richard P. Usatine, MD.*)

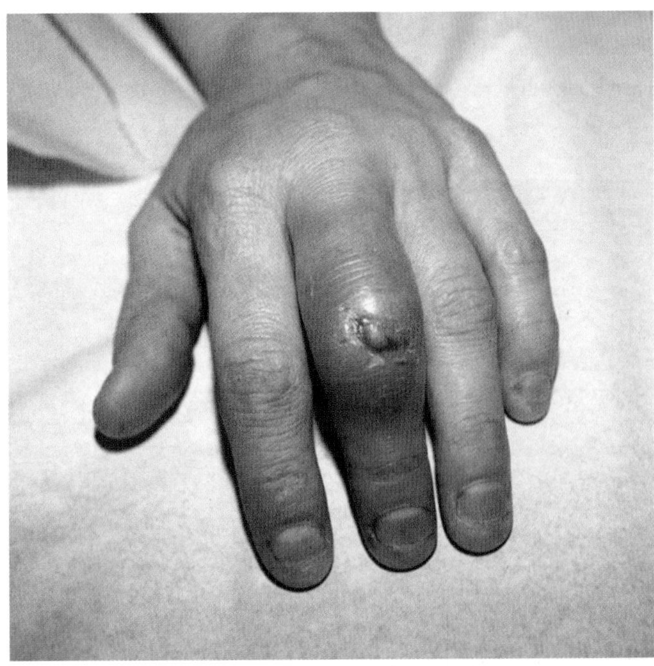

FIGURE 103-2 Cellulitis at the site of a clenched-fist injury when a young man hit another person on the tooth during a fight. This can result in a septic joint as well as a septic tenosynovitis. (*Used with permission from Richard P. Usatine, MD.*)

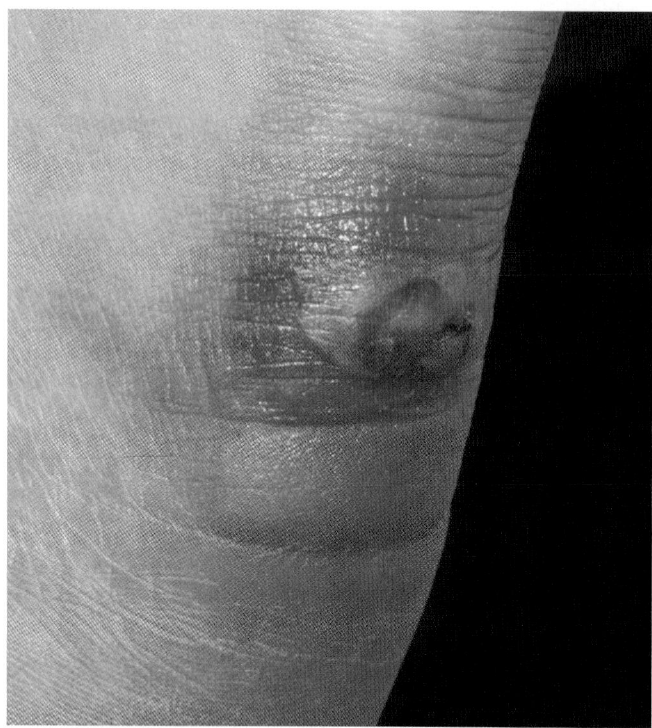

FIGURE 103-3 Group A β-hemolytic *Streptococcus* (GAS) cellulitis of the achilles heel that started as local trauma in a boy. (*Used with permission from Camille Sabella, MD.*)

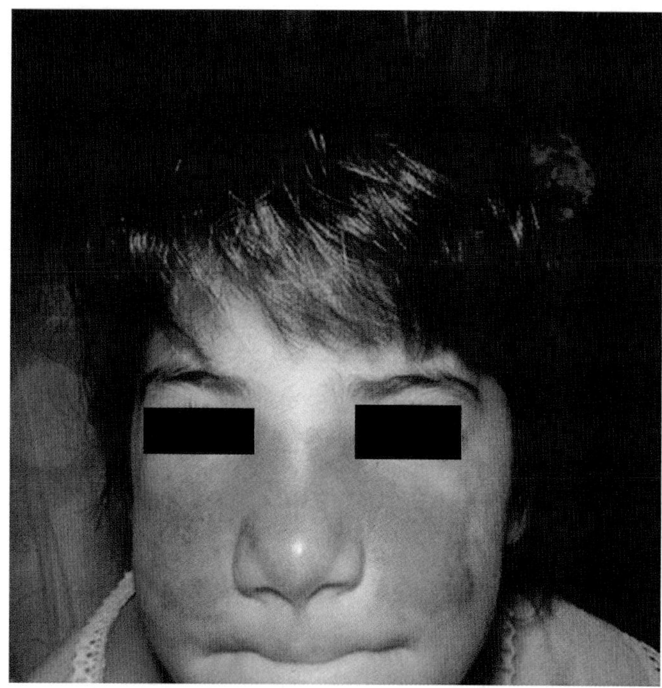

FIGURE 103-5 Butterfly rash of erysipelas. The sharp demarcation between the salmon-red erythema and the normal surrounding skin is evident. (*Reproduced with permission from Shah BR, Lucchesi M: Atlas of Pediatric Emergency Medicine, © 2006, McGraw-Hill, New York.*)

DIAGNOSIS

CLINICAL FEATURES

Rubor (red), calor (warm), tumor (swollen), and dolor (painful).

TYPICAL DISTRIBUTION

Can occur on any part of the body, but is most often seen on the extremities and face (**Figures 103-1** to **103-6**). Periorbital cellulitis

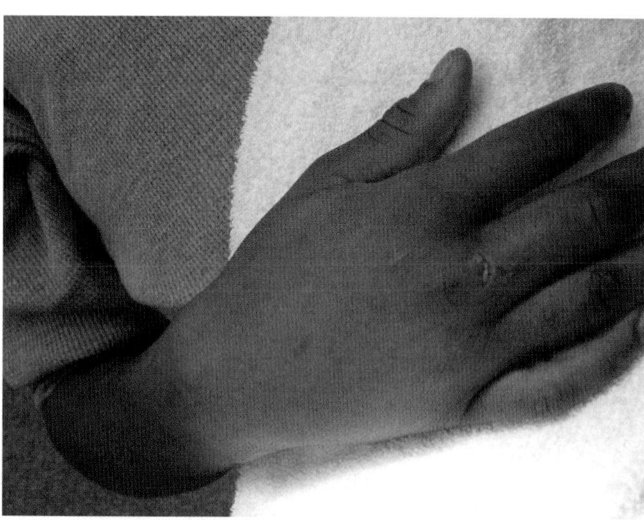

FIGURE 103-4 Cellulitis resulting from a cat bite injury in a child. The most likely organism is *Pasteurella multocida.* (*Used with permission from Emily Scott, MD.*)

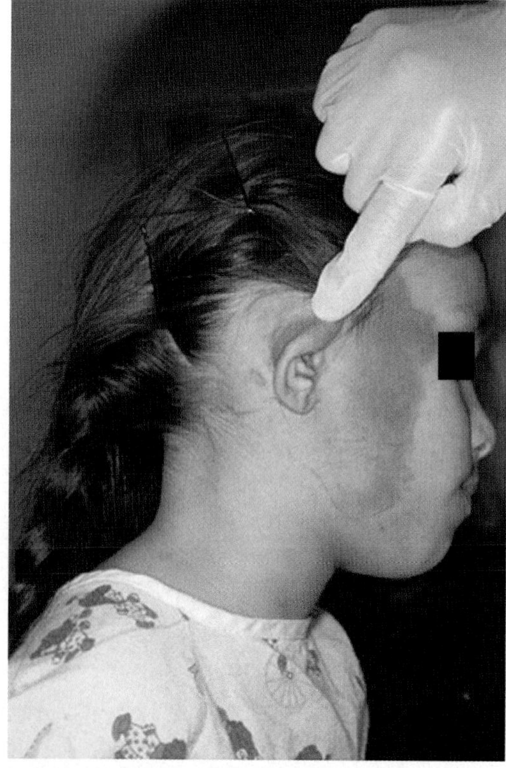

FIGURE 103-6 Erysipelas surrounding the ear of this girl. Note the well-demarcated borders were traced by a pen to monitor treatment progress. (*Reproduced with permission from Shah BR, Lucchesi M: Atlas of Pediatric Emergency Medicine, © 2006, McGraw-Hill, New York.*)

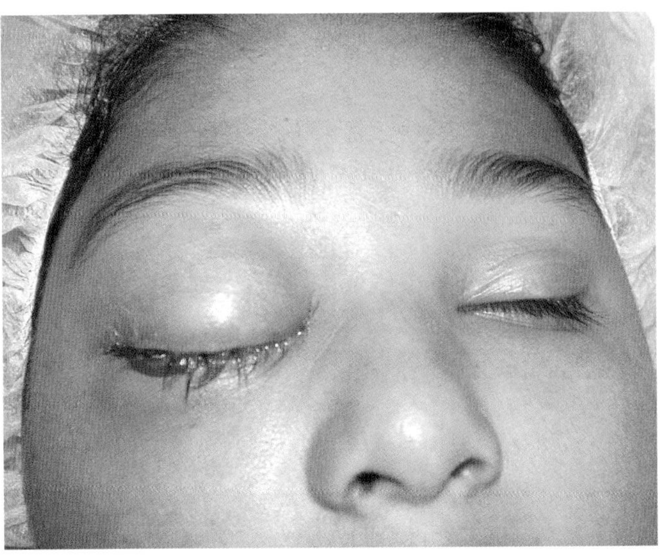

FIGURE 103-7 Life-threatening staphylococcal periorbital cellulitis requiring operative intervention. (*Used with permission from Frank Miller, MD.*)

can be life-threatening (**Figure 103-7**). Infants can develop cellulitis around the umbilicus (omphalitis), which can spread rapidly through the umbilical vessels (**Figure 103-8**).

LABORATORY TESTS

- Aspiration—If there is fluctuance within the area of erythema, a needle aspiration or incision and drainage should be performed (**Figure 103-9**). If pus is aspirated, perform a culture to guide antibiotic use.
- Blood cultures—Results are positive in only 5 percent of cases and the results of culture of needle aspirations of the inflamed skin are variable and not recommended.[5]

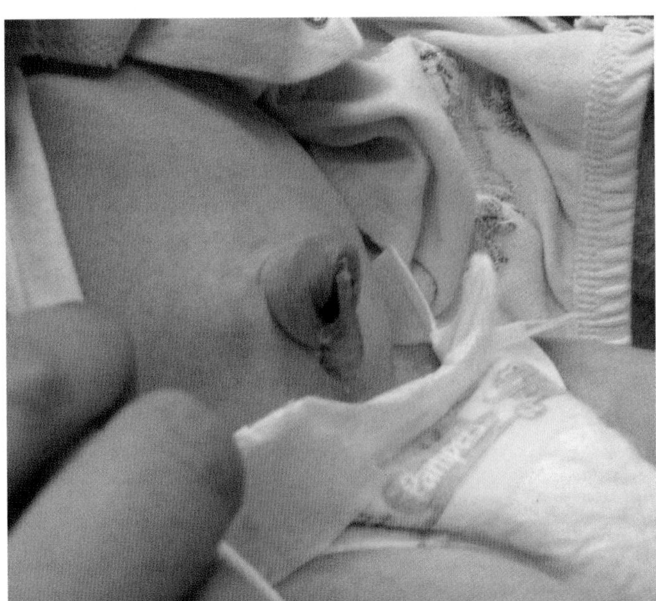

FIGURE 103-8 Omphalitis (cellulitis of the umbilicus) in a newborn. (*Used with permission from Emily Scott, MD.*)

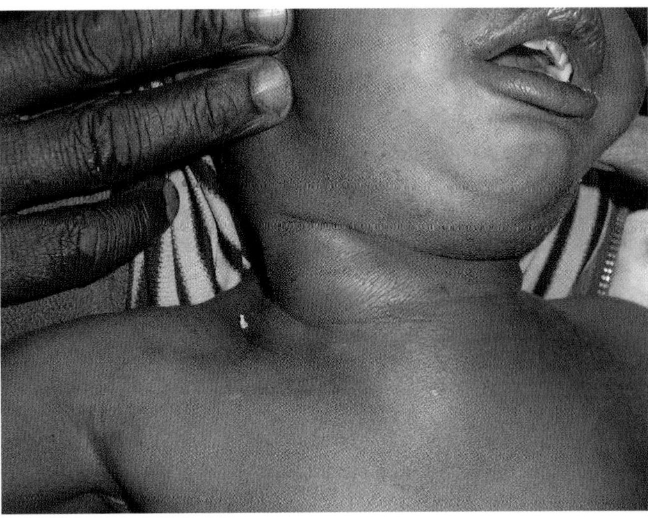

FIGURE 103-9 Cellulitis and abscess of the neck and chest in a 2-year-old girl in Ethiopia. Incision and drainage of the fluctuance over the neck revealed pus. A drain was placed to allow the pus to continue to drain from the incision site. She was treated with IV ceftriaxone and she survived. (*Used with permission from Richard P. Usatine, MD.*)

DIFFERENTIAL DIAGNOSIS

- Abscess can have overlying erythema and appear like cellulitis. If fluctuance can be palpated this is often a sign of an underlying abscess. Sometimes the only way to tell the difference is to aspirate the area with a needle. Of course the two conditions can coexist when an abscess is surrounded by cellulitis (**Figure 103-9**; see Chapter 104, Abscess).
- Staphylococcal scalded skin syndrome (SSSS) is a toxin-mediated illness mediated by exfoliative toxins A and B of *Staphylococcus aureus*. The red skin can appear similar to a cellulitis at first but the exfoliation of skin should be a tip of that this is a toxin mediated illness (**Figure 103-10**; see Chapter 106, Staphylococcal Scalded Skin Syndrome).

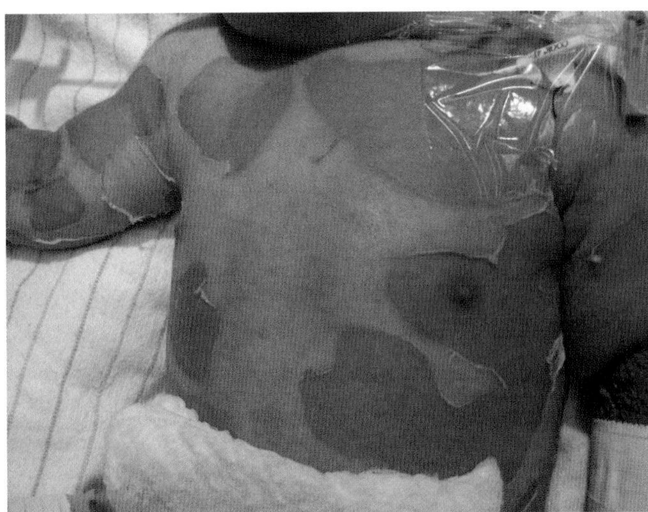

FIGURE 103-10 Erythema and desquamation of the skin in this infant with staphylococcal scalded skin syndrome. (*Used with permission from John C Browning, MD.*)

- Necrotizing fasciitis—Deep infection of the subcutaneous tissues and fascia with diffuse swelling, severe pain, and bullae in a toxic-appearing patient. It is important to recognize the difference between standard cellulitis and necrotizing fasciitis. Imaging procedures can detect gas in the soft tissues. Rapid progression from mild erythema to violaceous or necrotic lesions and/or bullae in a number of hours is a red flag for necrotizing fasciitis. The toxicity of the patient and the other physical findings should encourage rapid surgical consultation (see Chapter 106, Necrotizing Fasciitis).

MANAGEMENT

- The first decision is whether or not the patient needs hospitalization and IV antibiotics. It is often best to hospitalize any immunocompromised patients (e.g., HIV, transplant recipient, chronic renal or liver disease, on prednisone, diabetes out of control) with cellulitis because they may decompensate quickly. SOR C
- Evidence comparing different durations of treatment and oral versus intravenous antibiotics is lacking.[8]
- Standard oral therapy for cellulitis not requiring hospitalization (in the pre-MRSA era) involves covering GAS and *S. aureus* with cephalexin or dicloxacillin.[5] SOR A The typical duration is 7 to 10 days. SOR C
- Penicillin-allergic patients may be treated with clindamycin rather than erythromycin because of macrolide resistance and increasing MRSA prevalence.[5] SOR A
- Parenteral treatment is usually done with penicillinase-resistant penicillins or first-generation cephalosporins such as cefazolin, or, for patients with life-threatening penicillin allergies, clindamycin, or vancomycin.[5] SOR A
- Although MRSA is increasing in its prevalence in skin and soft-tissue infections,[4] the difficulty in obtaining microbiologic cultures for cellulitis still makes it difficult to know how much MRSA is a problem in cellulitis with intact skin. If there is a coexisting abscess or crusting lesion, it is best to obtain a culture to guide therapy and start empiric therapy with trimethoprim-sulfamethoxazole and clindamycin.[3] SOR B
- Do not miss necrotizing fasciitis. Patients with severe pain, bullae, crepitus, skin necrosis, or significant toxicity merit imaging and immediate surgical consultation (see Chapter 106, Necrotizing Fasciitis).
- Treat underlying conditions (e.g., atopic dermatitis, tinea pedis) that predispose the patient to the infection. SOR C

PATIENT EDUCATION

Recommend that the patient rest and elevate the involved extremity. If outpatient therapy is followed, then provide precautions (e.g., vomiting and unable to hold medicine down) for which the patient should seek more immediate follow-up.

FOLLOW-UP

If prescribing oral outpatient therapy, consider follow-up in 1 to 2 days to assess response to the antibiotic and to determine the adequacy of outpatient therapy.

PATIENT RESOURCES

- Medline Plus for patients—**www.nlm.nih.gov/medlineplus/cellulitis.html**.

PROVIDER RESOURCES

- Clinical Practice Guidelines from the Royal Children's Hospital Melbourne—**www.rch.org.au/clinicalguide/guideline_index/Cellulitis_and_Skin_Infections/**.
- **http://emedicine.medscape.com/article/214222**.

REFERENCES

1. O'Sullivan C, Baker MG. Serious skin infections in children: a review of admissions to Gisborne Hospital (2006-2007). *N.Z. Med J.* 2012;55-69.
2. Chira S, Miller LG. *Staphylococcus aureus* is the most common identified cause of cellulitis: a systematic review. *Epidemiol Infect.* 2010;138:313-317.
3. Khawcharoenporn T, Tice A. Empiric outpatient therapy with trimethoprim-sulfamethoxazole, cephalexin, or clindamycin for cellulitis. *Am J Med.* 2010;123:942-950.
4. Moran GJ, Krishnadasan A, Gorwitz RJ, et al. Methicillin-resistant *S. aureus* infections among patients in the emergency department. *N Engl J Med.* 2006;355:666-674.
5. Stevens DL, Bisno AL, Chambers HF, et al. Practice guidelines for the diagnosis and management of skin and soft-tissue infections. *Clin Infect Dis.* 2005;41:1373-1406.
6. Wells RD, Mason P, Roarty J, Dooley M. Comparison of initial antibiotic choice and treatment of cellulitis in the pre- and post-community-acquired methicillin-resistant *Staphylococcus aureus* eras. *Am J Emerg Med.* 2009;27:436-439.
7. Gutierrez K, et al. Staphylococcal infections in children, California, USA, 1985-2009. *Emerg. Infect. Dis.* 2013;10-20.
8. Morris AD. Cellulitis and erysipelas. *Clin Evid (Online).* 2008(2):2008.

104 ABSCESS

Richard P. Usatine, MD

PATIENT STORY

A 2-year-old girl in Ethiopia is brought to see the visiting American doctor for a painful swollen hand. The hand was massively swollen and the child did not want to use it. On examination she had a temperature of 99° F and there was visible pus under the skin (**Figure 104-1**). An incision and drainage was performed and much pus and blood squirted from the abscess. The abscess was packed lightly to stop any bleeding and to prevent it from closing prematurely. Oral antibiotics were given to cover the surrounding cellulitis and any deeper infections. A culture to look for methicillin-resistant *Staphylococcus aureus* (MRSA) was not available in rural Ethiopia, but close follow-up was set for the next day and the patient was doing much better. The medical team performed twice daily home visits and administered the oral trimethoprim-sulfamethoxazole while changing the dressings. Within one week, the child was playing happily, the erythema and swelling were resolving, and she was beginning to use her hand again.

INTRODUCTION

An abscess is a collection of pus in the infected tissues. The abscess represents a walled-off infection in which there is a pocket of purulence. In abscesses of the skin the offending organism is almost always *S. aureus*.

EPIDEMIOLOGY

- MRSA was the most common identifiable cause of skin and soft-tissue infections among patients presenting to emergency departments in 11 US cities. *S. aureus* was isolated from 76 percent of these infections and 59 percent were community-acquired MRSA (CA-MRSA).[1]
- Risk factors for MRSA infection and other abscesses—Intravenous drug abuse, homelessness, dental disease, contact sports, incarceration, and high prevalence in the community.
- In one review of serious skin infections in children admitted to a hospital in New Zealand, the most common types of infection were cellulitis (38%) and subcutaneous abscesses (36%).[2] The most frequent sites of infection were the head, face and neck (32%), and lower limbs (32%). The most frequently isolated organisms were *Staphylococcus aureus* (48%) and *Streptococcus pyogenes* (20%).[2]

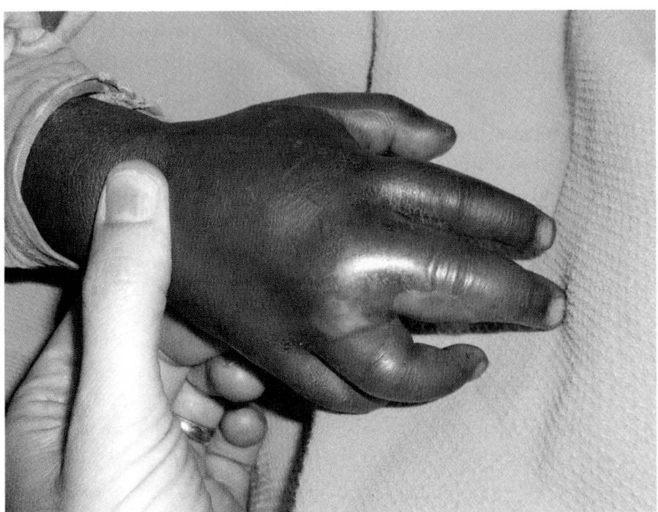

FIGURE 104-1 A large abscess of the hand in a 2-year-old girl in Ethiopia. Incision and drainage was performed and antibiotics were given to cover the surrounding cellulitis and any deeper infections. *(Used with permission from Richard P. Usatine, MD.)*

ETIOLOGY AND PATHOPHYSIOLOGY

- Most cutaneous abscesses are caused by *S. aureus*.
- Risk factors for developing an abscess with MRSA include patients who work or are exposed to a health-care system, intravenous drug use, previous MRSA infection and colonization, recent hospitalization, being homeless, African American, and having used antibiotics within the last 6 months.[3]
- Risk factors for hospitalization for staphylococcal skin infections in children in California were age less than 3 years, being Black, and lacking private insurance.[4]
- CA-MRSA has become prevalent in the US. One study that evaluated management of skin abscesses drained in the emergency department showed that there was no significant association between amount of surrounding cellulitis or abscess size with the likelihood of MRSA-positive cultures.[3]

DIAGNOSIS

CLINICAL FEATURES

Collection of pus in or below the skin. Patients often feel pain and have tenderness at the involved site. There is swelling, erythema, warmth, and fluctuance in most cases (**Figures 104-1** to **104-3**). Determine if the patient is febrile and if there is surrounding cellulitis.

TYPICAL DISTRIBUTION

Skin abscesses can be found anywhere from head to feet. Frequent sites include the hands, feet, extremities (**Figure 104-2**), head, neck, buttocks, and breast.

One type of abscess occurring in the pulp of a distal digit (usually a finger) is called a felon (**Figures 104-4**). This is particularly painful and requires a digital block for incision and drainage.

LABORATORY STUDIES

Clinical cure is often obtained with incision and drainage alone so the benefits of pathogen identification and sensitivities are low in low-risk patients.[3] Most clinical studies have excluded patients who were immunocompromised, diabetic, or had other significant comorbidities.[3] Consequently, it may be reasonable to obtain wound cultures in high-risk patients, those with signs of systemic infection, and in patients with history of high recurrence rates.[3,5]

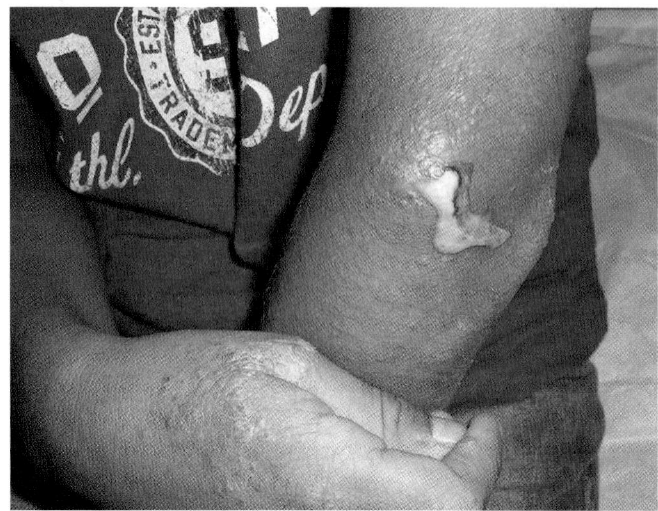

FIGURE 104-2 An atopic boy with bilateral abscesses on the elbows. This abscess drained spontaneously once gentle pressure was applied to the area of fluctuance. The culture revealed *S. aureus* sensitive to methicillin and all the skin infections cleared with oral antibiotics. The atopic dermatitis was treated successfully with 0.1 percent triamcinolone ointment. (*Used with permission from Richard P. Usatine, MD.*)

DIFFERENTIAL DIAGNOSIS

- Epidermal inclusion cyst with inflammation/infection—These cysts (also known as sebaceous cysts) can become inflamed, swollen, and superinfected. Although the initial erythema may be sterile inflammation, these cysts can become infected with *S. aureus*. The treatment consists of incision and drainage and antibiotics if cellulitis is also present. If these are removed before they become inflamed, the cyst may come out intact (**Figure 104-5**).
- Cellulitis with swelling and no pocket of pus—When it is unclear if an area of infected skin has an abscess, needle aspiration with a large-gauge needle may be helpful to determine whether to incise the skin. Cellulitis alone should have no area of fluctuance (see Chapter 103, Cellulitis).

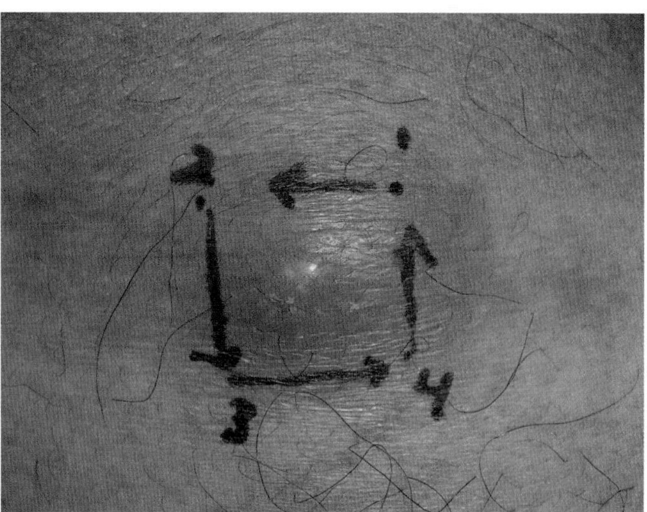

FIGURE 104-3 MRSA abscess on the back of the neck that patient thought was a spider bite. Note that a ring block was drawn around the abscess with a surgical marker to demonstrate how to perform this block. (*Used with permission from Richard P. Usatine, MD.*)

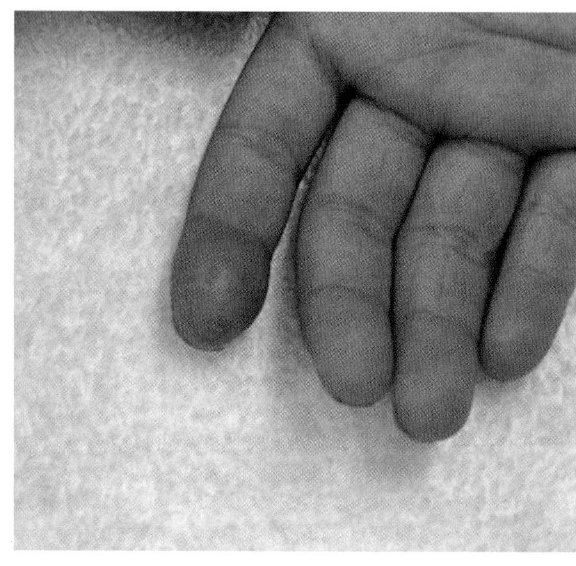

FIGURE 104-4 Felon. An abscess in the pulp of the distal finger. A digital block was required to incise and drain this soft tissue abscess. (*Used with permission from Emily Scott, MD.*)

- Hidradenitis suppurativa—Recurrent inflammation surrounding the apocrine glands of the axilla and inguinal areas (see Chapter 98, Hidradenitis Suppurativa).
- Furuncles and carbuncles—A furuncle or boil is an abscess that starts in hair follicle or sweat gland. A carbuncle occurs when the furuncle extends into the subcutaneous tissue.
- Acne cysts—More sterile inflammation than true abscess, often better to inject with steroid rather than incise and drain (see Chapter 96, Acne Vulgaris).

MANAGEMENT

- The evidence strongly supports the incision and drainage of an abscess.[3,6] SOR Ⓐ Inject 1 percent lidocaine with epinephrine into the skin at the site you plan to open using a 27-gauge needle. A ring block can be helpful rather than injecting into the abscess itself (**Figure 104-3**). Open the abscess with a linear incision using a #11 blade scalpel following skin lines if possible.[7]
- Although many physicians still pack a drained abscess with ribbon gauze, there is limited data on whether or not packing of an abscess cavity improves outcomes. A small study concluded that routine packing of simple cutaneous abscesses is painful and probably unnecessary.[8] SOR Ⓒ The author of this chapter often packs abscesses lightly and has the patient remove the packing in the shower 2 days later, avoiding additional visits and painful repacking of the healing cavity. SOR Ⓒ However, if a large abscess is not packed it can seal over and the pus may reaccumulate.
- Routine use of antibiotics for an initial abscess in addition to incision and drainage is not supported by current evidence.[3,9–11] SOR Ⓐ Three randomized controlled trials (RCTs) performed since the emergence of CA-MRSA have demonstrated that antibiotics do not significantly improve healing rates of superficial skin abscesses, but two of these studies suggest that antibiotics do decrease short-term rates of new lesion development.[9–11]

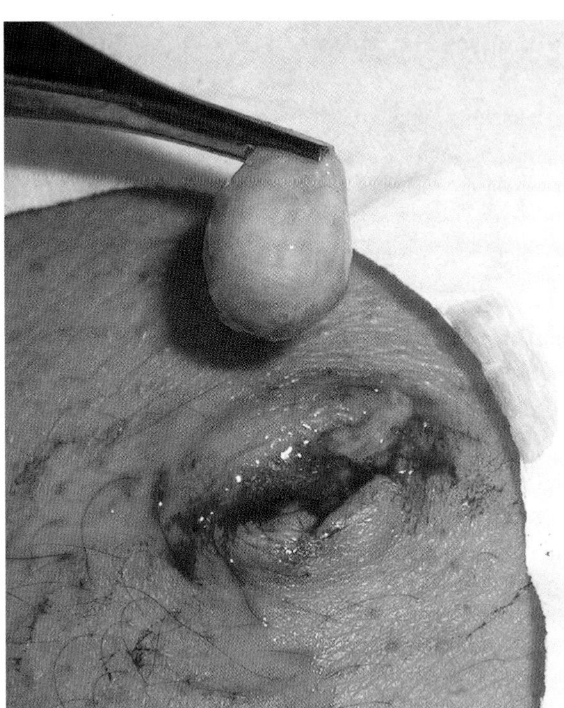

FIGURE 104-5 Epidermal inclusion cyst removed intact. There is no need for antibiotics in this case. (*Used with permission from Richard P. Usatine, MD.*)

- A recent meta-analysis of systemic antibiotics after incision and drainage of simple abscess in children and adults showed that antibiotics did not significantly improve the percentage of patients with complete resolution of their abscesses 7–10 days after treatment.[12]
- Consider the use of oral antibiotics to treat an abscess with suspected CAMRSA in patients who are febrile or have systemic symptoms, have significant surrounding cellulitis, have failed incision and drainage alone, have frequent recurrences, or have a history of close contacts with abscesses.3 SOR Ⓒ
- If an antibiotic is to be used, CA-MRSA is close to 100 percent sensitive to trimethoprim-sulfamethoxazole.3 SOR Ⓑ Alternative antibiotics include oral clindamycin, tetracycline (for children 8 years of age and older), or doxycycline (for children 8 years of age and older). Local sensitivity data should be consulted when available.3 SOR Ⓑ
- There is no current data to support the use of an antimicrobial medication (mupirocin or rifampin) in the eradication of MRSA colonization.[3] SOR Ⓒ

PATIENT EDUCATION

Patients may shower daily 24 to 48 hours after incision and drainage and then reapply dressings. Patients should be given return precautions for worsening of symptoms or continued redness, pain, or pus.

FOLLOW-UP

In patients or wounds at higher risk for complications, follow-up should be scheduled in 24 to 48 hours. If packing was placed, it can be removed by the patient or a family member.

PATIENT RESOURCES

- Skinsight article on abscess—**www.skinsight.com/adult/abscess.htm**.

PROVIDER RESOURCES

- Gillian R: How do you treat an abscess in the era of increased community-associated MRSA (MRSA)? *J Emerg Med*. 2011;41:276-281.
- **www.sciencedirect.com/science/article/pii/S0736467911004252#ref_bib17**.

REFERENCES

1. Moran GJ, Krishnadasan A, Gorwitz RJ, et al. Methicillin-resistant *S. aureus* infections among patients in the emergency department. *N Engl J Med*. 2006;355:666-674.
2. O'Sullivan C. Baker MG. Serious skin infections in children: a review of admissions to Gisborne Hospital (2006-2007). *N.Z. Med J*. 2012;55-69.
3. Gillian R. How do you treat an abscess in the era of increased community-associated methicillin-resistant *Staphylococcus aureus* (MRSA)? *J Emerg Med*. 2011;41:276-281.
4. Gutierrez K, et al. Staphylococcal infections in children, California, USA, 1985-2009. *Emerg. Infect. Dis.* 2013;10-20.
5. Abrahamian FM, Shroff SD. Use of routine wound cultures to evaluate cutaneous abscesses for community-associated methicillin-resistant *Staphylococcus aureus*. *Ann Emerg Med*. 2007;50:66-67.
6. Sorensen C, Hjortrup A, Moesgaard F, Lykkegaard-Nielsen M. Linear incision and curettage vs. deroofing and drainage in subcutaneous abscess. A randomized clinical trial. *Acta Chir Scand*. 1987;153:659-660.
7. Usatine R, Pfenninger J, Stulberg D, Small R. *Dermatologic and Cosmetic Procedures in Office Practice*. Philadelphia: Elsevier; 2012.
8. O'Malley GF, Dominici P, Giraldo P, et al. Routine packing of simple cutaneous abscesses is painful and probably unnecessary. *Acad Emerg Med*. 2009;16:470-473.
9. Duong M, Markwell S, Peter J, Barenkamp S. Randomized, controlled trial of antibiotics in the management of community-acquired skin abscesses in the pediatric patient. *Ann Emerg Med*. 2010;55:401-407.
10. Schmitz GR, Bruner D, Pitotti R, et al. Randomized controlled trial of trimethoprim-sulfamethoxazole for uncomplicated skin abscesses in patients at risk for community-associated methicillin-resistant *Staphylococcus aureus* infection. *Ann Emerg Med*. 2010;56:283-287.
11. Rajendran PM, Young D, Maurer T, et al. Randomized, double-blind, placebo-controlled trial of cephalexin for treatment of uncomplicated skin abscesses in a population at risk for community-acquired methicillin-resistant Staphylococcus aureus infection. *Antimicrob Agents Chemother*. 2007;51:4044-4048.
12. Singer AJ, Thode HC Jr: Systemic antibiotics after incision and drainage of simple abscesses: a meta-analysis. *Emerg. Med. J.* 2013. Published online May 18, 2013.

105 STAPHYLOCOCCAL SCALDED SKIN SYNDROME

Camille Sabella, MD
Charles B. Foster, MD

PATIENT STORY

An 18-month-old girl is admitted to the hospital with fever, irritability, and a tender skin rash on her face. She also has developed facial swelling bilaterally and perioral crusting (**Figure 105-1**). Over the next 24 hours, the rash spreads to her neck and trunk and she develops flaccid blisters on the areas of rash on her neck and trunk. When gentle friction is applied to involved areas of the skin, the skin easily sloughs superficially (Nikolsky sign). She is treated with intravenous anti-staphylococcal antibiotics and recovers completely. A culture taken from her nares grows *Staphylococcal aureus*.

INTRODUCTION

Staphylococcal scalded skin syndrome (SSSS) is a toxin-mediated illness mediated by exfoliative toxins A and B of *Staphylococcus aureus*.

SYNONYMS

Ritter syndrome (SSSS in neonates and young infants).

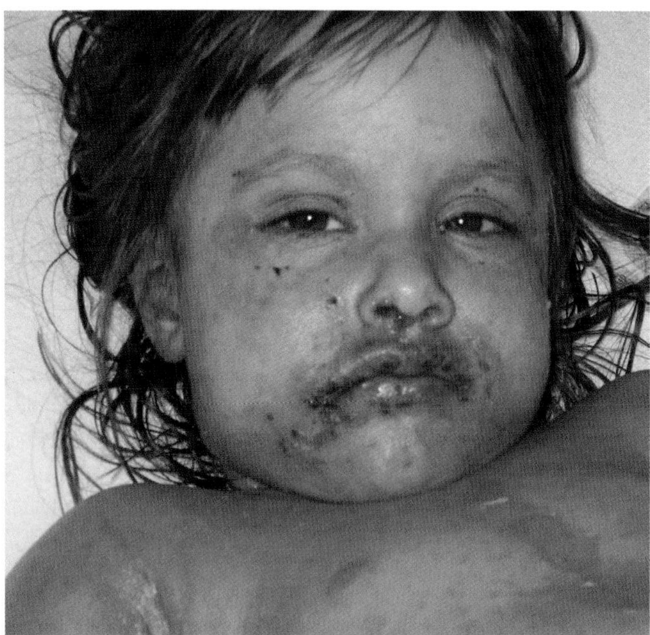

FIGURE 105-1 18-month-old girl with SSSS. Note the edema of the face, perioral crustiness, and extension of the erythema to the neck and trunk. Also note the thin desquamation on the chest and axilla. (*Used with permission from Camille Sabella, MD.*)

EPIDEMIOLOGY

- Occurs mainly in children under 5 years of age.
- May also occur in neonates after becoming colonized or infected with a toxin-producing strain of *S aureus* (Ritter syndrome).

ETIOLOGY AND PATHOPHYSIOLOGY

- Exfoliative toxins A and B of *S aureus* are responsible for the manifestations of the illness.[1,2]
- Mostly caused by *S aureus* belonging to phage group II, types 71 and 55.
- Toxins are hematogenously spread and produce the fever and characteristic rash.
- Toxin targets desmoglein 1, resulting in cleavage of the epidermis in a superficial location.[3,4]

RISK FACTORS

- Primary infection with toxin-producing *S aureus* at sites other than the skin, such as the umbilicus (in neonates), nasopharynx, or conjunctiva.

DIAGNOSIS

CLINICAL FEATURES

- Fever, irritability, and tender erythema of the skin are common.
- Facial edema with perioral and periocular crustiness is typical and may be the primary clinical features (**Figures 105-2** to **105-4**).
- Flaccid blisters and superficial erosions form within 12 to 24 hours, and which progress to become widespread superficial peeling of the skin (**Figure 105-5**).

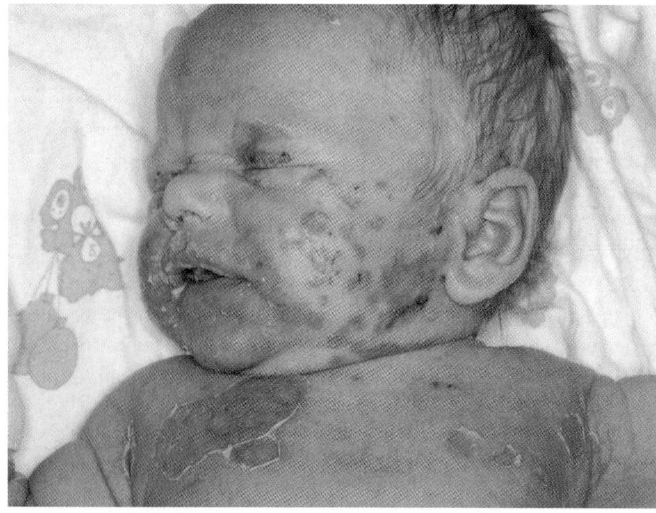

FIGURE 105-2 One-month-old infant with SSSS. Note the crustiness on the face and facial edema. (*Used with permission from Charles B. Foster, MD.*)

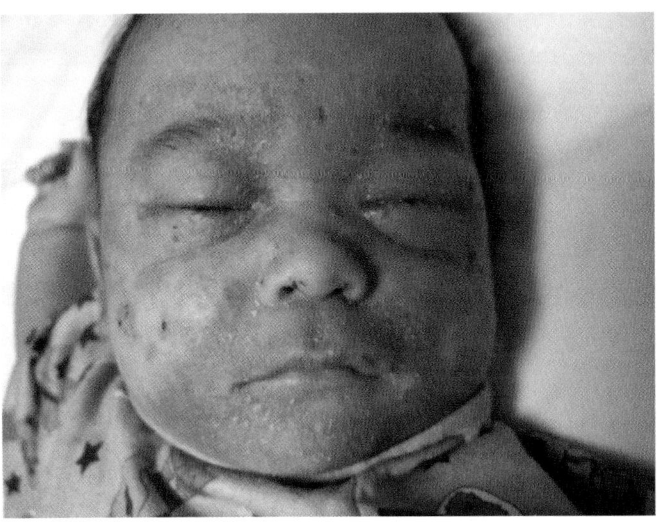

FIGURE 105-3 Infant with edema and crustiness on the face typical for SSSS. (*Used with permission from John C Browning, MD.*)

- Gentle sheering of the skin often results in widespread separation (Nikolsky sign).
- Desquamation of the skin often follows at the involved skin sites (**Figure 105-6**).[5,6]

DISTRIBUTION

- The face, neck, and trunk are most often involved.
- Mucosal surfaces are spared.

LABORATORY TESTING

- The diagnosis is usually made clinically, based on the characteristic features and response to conventional therapy.
- Isolation of *S aureus* from a site distant to the skin—usually the nasopharynx, conjunctiva, site of circumcision, umbilicus (in neonates)—helps to support the diagnosis. Demonstration of toxin production by the isolate provides more definitive diagnosis, but this is rarely performed or required.

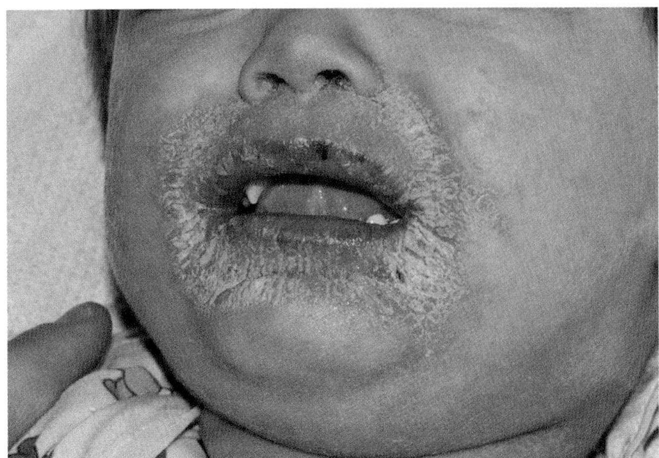

FIGURE 105-4 Toddler with SSSS and marked perioral crustiness, erythema, and edema. (*Used with permission from Camille Sabella, MD.*)

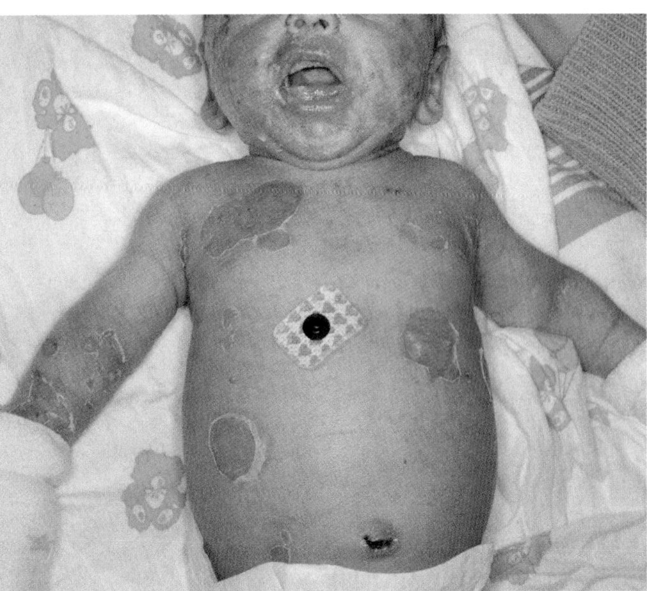

FIGURE 105-5 Same infant as in Figure 105-2, with thin widespread blisters on the trunk. (*Used with permission from Charles B. Foster, MD.*)

- Cultures from the skin lesions and blister fluid are negative for *S aureus*.
- Bacteremia is rare.

SURGERY

- Skin biopsy is usually not necessary for the diagnosis.
- When performed, skin biopsy reveals separation of skin layers at the granular layer within the epidermis.[7]

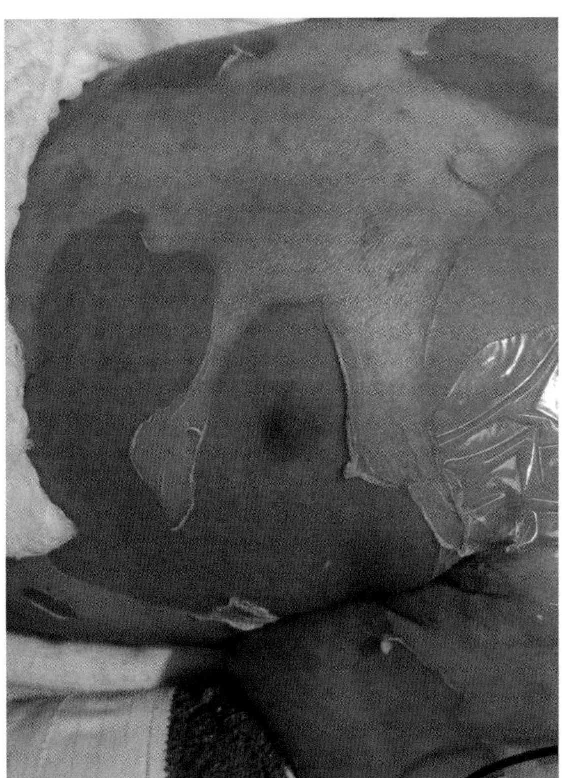

FIGURE 105-6 Desquamation of the skin in this infant with SSSS. (*Used with permission from John C Browning, MD.*)

DIFFERENTIAL DIAGNOSIS

- Drug-induced toxic epidermal necrolysis—Inciting agent often present; mucus membranes usually involved; biopsy shows separation of the skin between the epidermis and the dermis (see Chapter 151, Erythema Multiforme, Stevens-Johnson Syndrome and Toxic Epidermal Necrolysis).[7]
- Scarlet fever—Rash rough, "sandpapery;" pharyngitis and strawberry tongue often present; school aged children are most commonly affected (see Chapter 28, Scarlet Fever and Strawberry Tongue).
- Kawasaki disease—More persistent and higher fever, mucus membrane involvement; rash polymorphous, extremity changes, and lymphadenopathy usually present (see Chapter 177, Kawasaki Disease).
- Toxic Shock Syndrome—Hemodynamic changes present by definition with significant drop in blood pressure (see Chapter 185, Toxic Shock Syndromes).

MANAGEMENT

NONPHARMACOLOGIC

- Supportive—Careful attention to hydration status, electrolyte levels, antipyretics, and anti-analgesics.
- Meticulous attention to wound care and antiseptic measures to prevent superinfection of the skin.
- The skin can be gently moistened and cleansed with isotonic saline or aluminum acetate solution.

MEDICATIONS

- Systemic intravenous anti-staphylococcal antibiotics (such as Nafcillin) is utilized to reduce bacterial burden. This results in prompt clinical improvement. SOR C
- Oral anti-staphylococcal agents are not effective initially.
- Transition from an intravenous to an oral agent can be undertaken after there is clear clinical improvement, to complete a 7- to 10-day course of therapy. SOR C
- Topical antibiotics are not effective and not necessary.
- Application of an emollient, such as petrolatum ointment, can provide lubrication and decreases discomfort.

PROGNOSIS

- The majority of affected children do well and recover without sequelae.
- Healing of the skin occurs without scarring.
- Dehydration and superinfection can occur with major exfoliation.

PATIENT RESOURCES

- **www.nlm.nih.gov/medlineplus/ency/article/001352.htm**.
- **http://emedicine.medscape.com/article/788199-overview**.

PROVIDER RESOURCES

- American Academy of Pediatrics. Staphylococcal infections. In: Pickering LK, Baker CJ, Kimberlin DW, Long SS, eds. *Red Book: 2012 Report of the Committee on Infectious Diseases.* Elk Grove Village, IL: American Academy of Pediatrics; 2012:653-668.
- **http://emedicine.medscape.com/article/1053325**.
- **http://www.accesspediatrics.com/content.aspx?aID=7027999**.

REFERENCES

1. Yamasaki O, et al. Clinical manifestations of staphylococcal scalded-skin syndrome depend on serotypes of exfoliative toxins. *J Clin Microbiol*. 2005;43:1890-1893.
2. Melish ME, Glasgow LA, Turner MD. The staphylococcal scalded-skin syndrome: isolation and partial characterization of the exfoliative toxin. *J Infect Dis*. 1972;125:129-140.
3. Hanakawa Y, Stanley JR. Mechanisms of blister formation by staphylococcal toxins. *J Biochem (Tokyo)*. 2004;136:747-750.
4. Lillibridge CB, Melish ME, Glasgow LA. Site of action of exfoliative toxin in the staphylococcal scaled-skin syndrome. *Pediatrics*. 1972; 50:728-738.
5. Melish ME, Glasgow LA. The staphylococcal scalded-skin syndrome. *N Engl J Med*. 1970;282:1114-1119.
6. Melish ME, Glasgow LA. Staphylococcal scalded skin syndrome: the expanded clinical syndrome. *J Pediatr*.1971;78:958-967.
7. Patel GK, Finlay AY. Staphylococcal scalded skin syndrome: diagnosis and management. *Am J Clin Dermatol*. 2003;4:165-175.

106 NECROTIZING FASCIITIS

Richard P. Usatine, MD
Jeremy A. Franklin, MD
Camille Sabella, MD

PATIENT STORIES

A 9-day-old neonate presented with high fever, moaning, and slightly indurated swelling with bluish discoloration on the back (**Figure 106-1**). Within 12 hours, there was vesiculation and purplish discoloration. The infant was diagnosed with necrotizing fasciitis and surgery was consulted immediately. The first surgical exploration and débridement and shows the underlying muscle and necrotic borders. Both blood and tissue cultures grew *Staphylococcus aureus.* Multiple surgical explorations and débridement were performed followed by skin grafting during recovery. The infant survived with scarring but no other sequelae.

A 16-year-old female presented with necrotizing fasciitis of the left gluteal region following an intramuscular injection received in rural India. She was febrile and in septic shock. The entire left gluteal region had full thickness necrosis and was emitting a foul odor. The skin was violaceous with purple bullae and areas of exfoliation. Previous attempts at incision and drainage were not helpful. She was treated with intravenous fluids, antibiotics and full-thickness extensive surgical debridement in the operating room. She became afebrile and hemodynamically stable. Her subsequent treatment consisted of negative pressure wound therapy followed by skin grafting. She survived with scarring and contour deformities but no other sequelae (**Figure 106-2**).

INTRODUCTION

Necrotizing fasciitis (NF) is a rapidly progressive infection of the deep fascia, with necrosis of the subcutaneous tissues. In children, it usually occurs after surgery, trauma, or varicella infection. Patients have erythema and pain disproportionate to the physical findings. Immediate surgical debridement and antibiotic therapy should be initiated.[1]

SYNONYMS

- Flesh-eating bacteria, necrotizing soft-tissue infection (NSTI), suppurative fasciitis, hospital gangrene, and necrotizing erysipelas. Fournier gangrene is a type of NF or NSTI in the genital and perineal region.[2]

EPIDEMIOLOGY

- Overall incidence of NF in children (<16 years of age) is 2.93 cases per million population per year, according to a recent population-based active surveillance study from Canada; incidence is 0.81 per million for non–Group A Streptococcus-related cases, and 2.12 per million for Group A Streptococcus (GAS)-related cases.[3]
- For non-GAS-related cases, NF typically occurs in children with underlying medical conditions, such as diabetes mellitus, trauma or recent surgery.[3]
- NF caused by *Streptococcus pyogenes* is the most common form of NF in children and adults.[3]
- Non-GAS-related cases are most common in infants less than one-year of age; pre-existing risk factors, such as prematurity, are common, and many of these cases occur in association with omphalitis or circumcision.
- Most cases of GAS-related NF are associated with varicella (**Figure 106-3**).[3,4]

ETIOLOGY AND PATHOPHYSIOLOGY

- Type I NF is a polymicrobial infection with aerobic and anaerobic bacteria:
  - Frequently caused by enteric Gram-negative pathogens including *Enterobacteriaceae* organisms and *Bacteroides*.
  - Can occur with Gram-positive organisms such as non-group A streptococci and *Peptostreptococcus.*[5]
  - Saltwater variant can occur with penetrating trauma or an open wound contaminated with saltwater containing marine vibrios. *Vibrio vulnificus* is the most virulent.[6]
  - Up to 15 pathogens have been isolated in a single wound.
  - Average of five different isolates per wound.[7]
- Type II NF is the most common form in children and is generally a monomicrobial infection caused by GAS:
  - May occur in combination with Staphylococcus aureus.
  - Methicillin-resistant S. aureus is no longer a rare cause of NF.5
  - GAS may produce pyrogenic exotoxins, which act as superantigens to stimulate production of tumor necrosis factor (TNF)-α, TNF-β, interleukin (IL)-1, IL-6, and IL-2.[7]

RISK FACTORS

- Risk factors for type I NF (polymicrobial):
  - Diabetes mellitus.
  - Prematurity.
  - Severe peripheral vascular disease.
  - Obesity.
  - Alcoholism and cirrhosis.
  - Intravenous drug use.
  - Decubitus ulcers.
  - Poor nutritional status.
  - Postoperative patients or those with penetrating trauma.
  - Abscess of the female genital tract.
- Risk factors of type II NF (GAS and *S. aureus*):
  - Varicella.[3,4]
  - Burns.
  - Penetrating trauma.

DIAGNOSIS

Early recognition based on signs and symptoms is potentially life saving. Although lab tests and imaging studies can confirm ones' clinical impression, rapid treatment with antibiotics and surgery are crucial to improving survival.

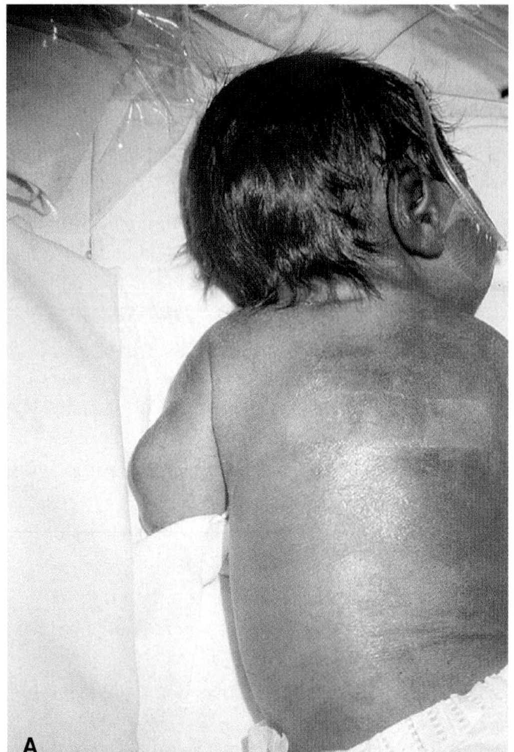

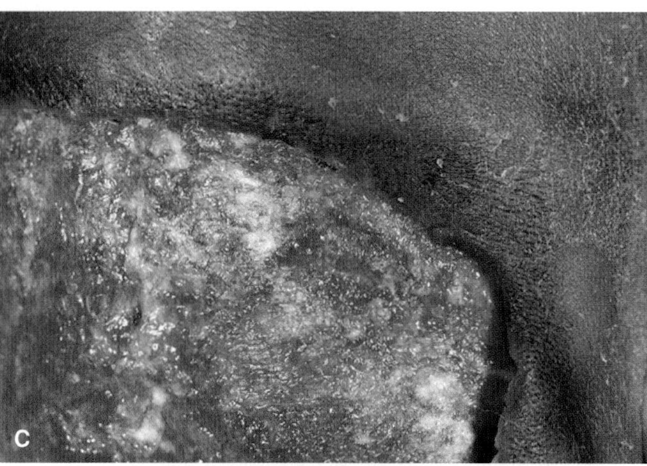

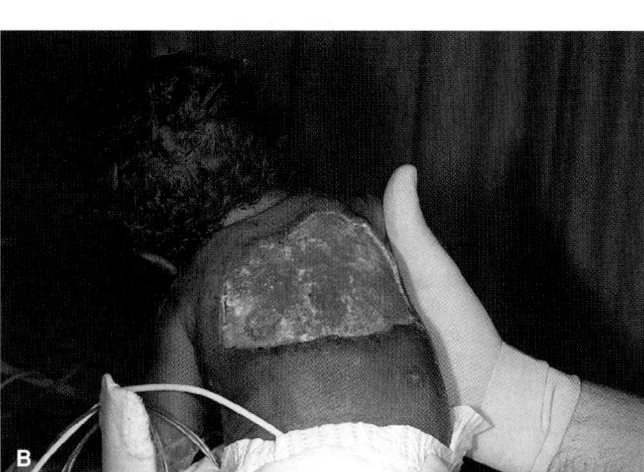

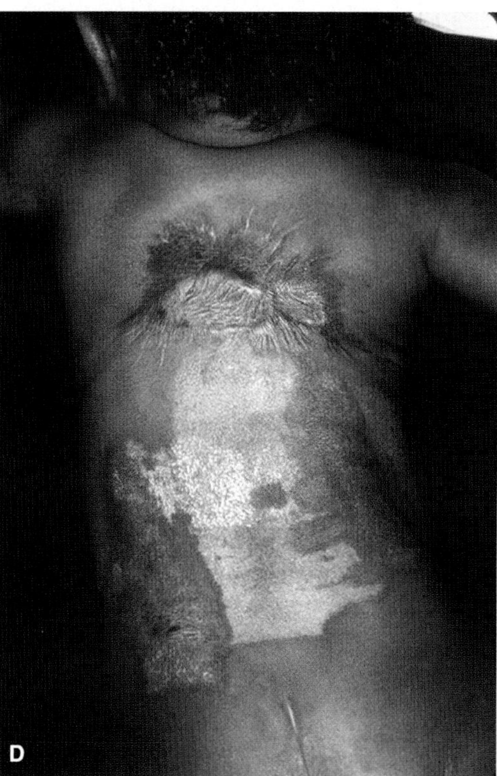

FIGURE 106-1 **A.** A 9-day-old neonate presented with high fever, moaning, and slightly indurated swelling with bluish discoloration on the back. Within 12 hours, there was vesiculation and purplish discoloration. **B.** This photograph was taken 8 hours following the first surgical exploration and débridement and shows the underlying muscle and necrotic borders. **C.** Close-up showing necrotic borders and pus over the underlying muscle. Both blood and tissue cultures grew *Staphylococcus aureus*. **D.** Multiple surgical explorations and débridement were performed followed by skin grafting during recovery. (*Used with permission from Shah BR, Lucchesi M. The Atlas of Pediatric Emergency Medicine, McGraw-Hill, 2006, p. 87.*)

CLINICAL FEATURES

- Soft tissue swelling and pain often appears at the site of trauma or a varicella lesion. This becomes apparent 3 to 4 days after the onset of the exanthem.
- Infants and young children are often irritable and fussy; older children may refuse to bear weight on an involved extremity or refuse to walk.
- Rapid progression of erythema to bullae (**Figure 106-2**), ecchymosis, and necrosis or gangrene.
- The erythematous skin may develop a dusky violaceous discoloration. Vesicular and bullous lesions form over the erythematous skin, with some serosanguineous drainage. The bullae may become violaceous (**Figure 106-2**). The skin can become gangrenous and develop a black eschar.[2]
- Edematous, wooden feel of subcutaneous tissues extending beyond the margin of erythema.
- High fevers and severe systemic toxicity.
- Unrelenting intense pain out of proportion to cutaneous findings.
- Pain progresses to cutaneous anesthesia as disease evolves. Anesthesia of the skin develops as a result of infarction of cutaneous nerves.[2]
- Crepitus occurs when there is gas in the soft tissues.

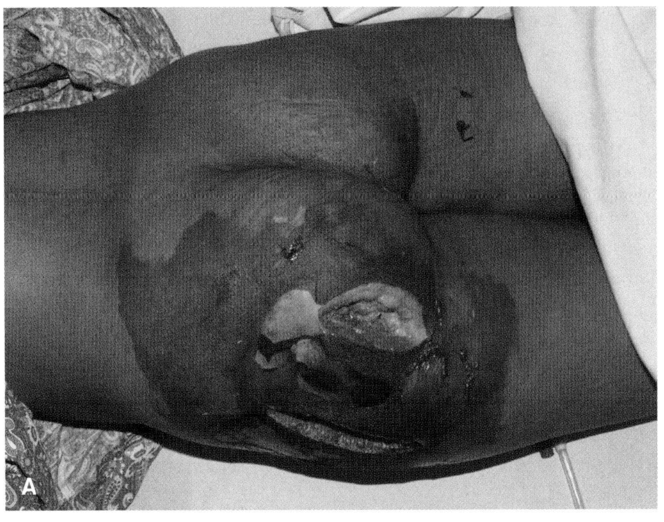

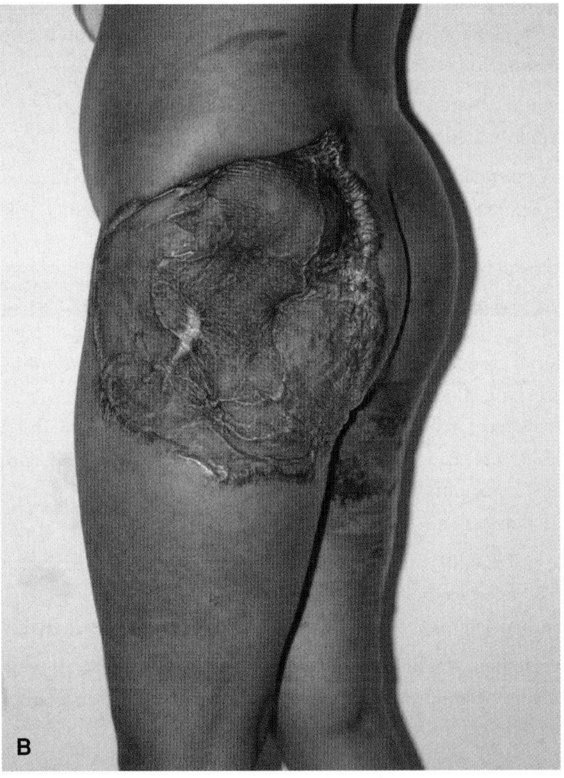

FIGURE 106-2 **A.** Necrotizing fasciitis of the left gluteal region following an intramuscular injection received in rural India. This 16-year-old female was febrile and in septic shock. The entire left gluteal region had full thickness necrosis and was emitting a foul odor. The skin was violaceous with purple bullae and areas of exfoliation. Previous attempts at incision and drainage were not helpful. **B.** Healing with scarring and contour deformities. Treatment consisted of intravenous antibiotics, full-thickness extensive surgical debridement, negative pressure wound therapy followed by skin grafting. (*Used with permission from Dr. N. Jithendran and http://diabeticfootsalvage.blogspot.in/2012/11/post-intramuscular-injection-soft.html.*)

- Unresponsive to empiric antimicrobial therapy.
- May progress to toxic shock syndrome, especially with associated with GAS infection.[5]

TYPICAL DISTRIBUTION

- May occur at any anatomic location.

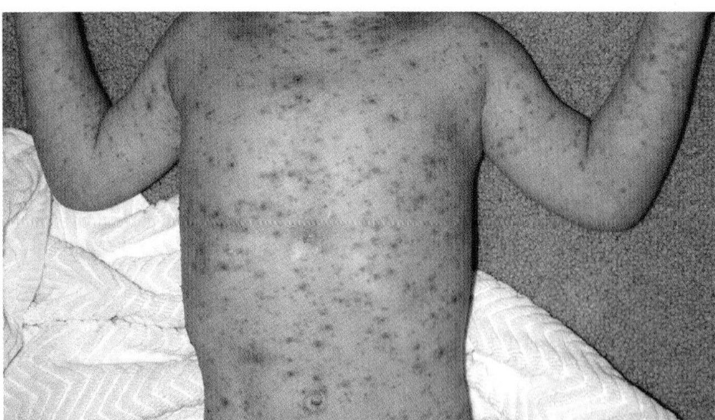

FIGURE 106-3 Varicella in an unimmunized toddler. Although this child did not develop necrotizing fasciitis, bacterial superinfection with *Streptococcus pyogenes* of varicella lesions is one of the most important predisposing factors for necrotizing fasciitis in children. (*Used with permission from Camille Sabella, MD.*)

- Common sites of involvement include the lower extremities (**Figures 106-2**), trunk (**Figure 106-1**), abdomen, gluteal region, upper extremities, and perineum (Fournier gangrene).

LABORATORY AND IMAGING

- Routine laboratory tests are nonspecific but common findings include an elevated white blood cell count (WBC), a predominance of immature neutrophils, a low serum sodium, and a high blood urea nitrogen (BUN).
- Histology and culture of deep tissue biopsy are essential; surface cultures cannot be relied on alone. Gram staining of the exudate may provide clues about the pathogens while awaiting culture results.[2]
- Aerobic and anaerobic blood cultures should be obtained in an attempt to identify the causative organism.
- Standard radiographs are of little value unless air is demonstrated in the tissues.
- CT, ultrasonography, and MRI can be used to assess the level of tissue involvement and to detect gas within soft tissues or muscles.
- Although imaging may help delineate the extent of disease, it should not delay surgical consultation.

BIOPSY

- Gross examination reveals swollen, dull, gray fascia with stringy areas of necrosis.
- Necrosis of superficial fascia and fat produces watery, foul-smelling "dishwater pus."
- Histology demonstrates subcutaneous fat necrosis, vasculitis, and local hemorrhage.

DIFFERENTIAL DIAGNOSIS

- Cellulitis—Acute spreading infection of skin and soft tissues characterized by erythema, edema, pain, and calor. Rapid progression of disease despite antibiotics, systemic toxicity, intense pain, and skin necrosis suggest NF rather than cellulitis (see Chapter 103, Cellulitis).

- Pyomyositis—Suppuration within individual skeletal muscle groups. Synergistic necrotizing cellulitis involves muscle groups in addition to superficial tissues and fascia.[7] Although pyomyositis may occur with NF, it can occur independent of cutaneous and soft-tissue infections. Imaging of the muscle confirms the diagnosis.
- Clostridial myonecrosis—Acute necrotizing infection of muscle tissue caused by clostridial organisms. Surgical exploration and cultures are required to differentiate from NF.
- Streptococcal or staphylococcal toxic shock syndrome—Systemic inflammatory response to a toxin-producing bacteria characterized by fever, hypotension, generalized erythroderma, myalgia, and multisystem organ involvement. NF may occur as part of the toxic shock syndrome.[5]

MANAGEMENT

Start by maintaining a high index of suspicion for NF. If the first debridement occurs within 24 hours from the onset of symptoms, there is a significantly improved chance of survival.[8]

- Surgical debridement is the primary therapeutic modality.[7–10] SOR Ⓐ
  - Extensive, definitive debridement should be the goal with the first surgery. This may require amputation of an extremity to control the disease. Surgical debridement is repeated until all infected devitalized tissue is removed.
- Antibiotics are the main adjunctive therapy to surgery. Broad-spectrum empiric antibiotics should be started immediately when NF is suspected and should include coverage of Gram-positive, Gram-negative, and anaerobic organisms.[7] SOR Ⓐ
  - Antimicrobial therapy must be directed at the known or suspected pathogens and used in appropriate doses until repeated operative procedures are no longer needed, the patient has demonstrated obvious clinical improvement, and fever has been absent for 48 to 72 hours.[7] SOR Ⓐ
  - Clindamycin is useful for coverage of anaerobes and aerobic Gram-positive cocci, including most *S. aureus* serogroups.
  - Clindamycin should be considered in initial coverage for its effects on exotoxin production in group A *Streptococcus* (GAS) infections. NF and/or streptococcal toxic shock syndrome caused by group A streptococci should be treated with clindamycin and penicillin.[7] SOR Ⓐ
    - The rationale for clindamycin is based on in vitro studies demonstrating both toxin suppression and modulation of cytokine (i.e., TNF) production, on animal studies demonstrating superior efficacy versus that of penicillin, and on two observational studies demonstrating greater efficacy for clindamycin than for β-lactam antibiotics.[7] SOR Ⓐ
  - Metronidazole has the greatest anaerobic spectrum against the enteric Gram-negative anaerobes, but it is less effective against the Gram-positive anaerobic cocci. Gentamicin, ticarcillin-clavulanate, or piperacillin-sulbactam is useful for coverage against resistant Gram-negative rods.[7]
  - A common choice of empiric antibiotics for community-acquired mixed infections is a combination of ampicillin-sulbactam or pipercillin-tazobactam plus clindamycin.[7] Aminoglycosides or ciprofloxacin can be used to provide gram-negative coverage for patients who cannot be treated with beta-lactam antibiotics or who are suspected of having multi-drug resistant gram-negative infections. SOR Ⓒ
  - Empiric vancomycin should be considered during pending culture results to cover for the increasing incidence of community-acquired methicillin-resistant *Staphylococcus aureus* (MRSA).[7]
  - For NF due to *V. vulnificus* infection, doxycycline in combination with a third-generation cephalosporin is preferred for children 8 years of age and older, while a combination of trimethorprim sulfamethoxazole and an aminoglycoside is recommended for younger children.[11]
  - Hyperbaric oxygen (HBO_2) may have beneficial effects when used postoperatively in NSTIs. One recent study demonstrated decreased morbidity (amputations 50% versus 0%) and mortality (34% versus 11.9%) with the use of postoperative HBO_2.[12] SOR Ⓑ
- Aggressive fluid resuscitation is often necessary because of massive capillary leak syndrome. Supplemental enteral nutrition is often necessary for patients with NSTIs.
- Vacuum-assisted closure devices may be helpful in secondary wound management after debridement of NSTIs.[10]
- A recommendation to use intravenous gammaglobulin (IVIG) to treat NF or toxic shock syndrome cannot be made with certainty.[7] SOR Ⓑ

PROGNOSIS AND FOLLOW-UP

- Overall case fatality rate in adults remains 20 to 47 percent despite aggressive, modern therapy.[6,7]
  - However, in a retrospective chart review of patients with NSTIs treated at six academic hospitals in Texas between 2004 and 2007 mortality rates varied between hospitals from 9 to 25 percent (n = 296).[13]
- The case fatality rate was 5 percent in the recent pediatric active surveillance study from Canada.[3]
  - Early diagnosis and treatment appears to reduce the case fatality rate.
- Carrying out the first fasciotomy and radical debridement within 24 hours of symptom onset is associated with significantly improved survival.[8]

PATIENT EDUCATION

The serious life-threatening nature of NF should be explained to the patient and family when informed consent is given prior to surgery. The risk of losing life and limb should be explained while giving hope for recovery. For those patients who survive but have lost a limb, counseling should be offered to help them deal with the psychological effects of the amputation.

PATIENT RESOURCES

- **www.cdc.gov/ncidod/dbmd/diseaseinfo/groupastreptococcal_g.htm**.
- **www.pamf.org/health/healthinfo/index.cfm?A=C&hwid=hw140405**.

PROVIDER RESOURCES

- Practice Guidelines for the Diagnosis and Management of Skin and Soft-Tissue Infections—**http://cid.oxfordjournals.org/content/41/10/1373.full#sec-6**.

REFERENCES

1. Usatine RP, Sandy N. Dermatologic emergencies. *Am Fam Physician.* 2010;82:773-780.
2. Koukouras D, Kallidonis P, Panagopoulos C, et al. Fournier's gangrene, a urologic and surgical emergency: presentation of a multi-institutional experience with 45 cases. *Urol Int.* 2011;86: 167-172.
3. Eneli I, Davies HD. Epidemiology and outcome of necrotizing fasciitis in children: an active surveillance study of the Canadian paediatric surveillance program. *J Pediatr.* 2007;151:79-84
4. Zerr DM, Alexander ER, Duchin JS, et al. A case-control study of necrotizing fasciitis during primary varicella. *Pediatrics.* 1999;103:783-790.
5. Stevens DL, Tanner MH, Winship J, et al. Severe group A streptococcal infections associated with a toxic shock-like syndrome and scarlet fever toxin *A. N Engl J Med.* 1989;321:1-7.
6. Horseman MA, Surani S. A comprehensive review of *Vibrio vulnificus*: an important cause of severe sepsis and skin and soft-tissue infection. *Int J Infect Dis.* 2011;15:e157-e166.
7. Stevens DL, Bisno AL, Chambers HF, et al. Practice guidelines for the diagnosis and management of skin and soft-tissue infections. *Clin Infect Dis.* 2005;41:1373-1406.
8. Cheung JP, Fung B, Tang WM, Ip WY. A review of necrotising fasciitis in the extremities. *Hong Kong Med J.* 2009;15:44-52.
9. Angoules AG, Kontakis G, Drakoulakis E, et al. Necrotising fasciitis of upper and lower limb: a systematic review. *Injury.* 2007;38(5):S19-S26.
10. Endorf FW, Cancio LC, Klein MB. Necrotizing soft-tissue infections: clinical guidelines. *J Burn Care Res.* 2009;30:769-775.
11. Centers for Disease Control and Prevention : Management of Vibrio vulnificus wound infections. Available online at http://www.cdc.gov/nczved/divisions/dfbmd/diseases/vibriov/index.html#treatment.
12. Escobar SJ, Slade JB Jr, Hunt TK, Cianci P. Adjuvant hyperbaric oxygen therapy (HBO2) for treatment of necrotizing fasciitis reduces mortality and amputation rate. *Undersea Hyperb Med.* 2005;32:437-443.
13. Kao LS, Lew DF, Arab SN, et al. Local variations in the epidemiology, microbiology, and outcome of necrotizing soft-tissue infections: a multicenter study. *Am J Surg.* 2011;202:139-145.

107 ECTHYMA GANGRENOSUM

Aron Flagg, MD
Camille Sabella, MD

PATIENT STORY

A 13-year-old boy is hospitalized while receiving induction therapy for acute myelogenous leukemia. During a period of profound neutropenia, he develops a fever of 39°C associated with rigors. Blood cultures are taken and he is given broad-spectrum antibiotics. Over the next 48 hours, a tender, erythematous 2 × 2 cm papule develops on his arm, the center of which becomes vesicopustular (**Figure 107-1**). Blood cultures from the initial febrile period are subsequently positive for *Pseudomonas aeruginosa*. He is treated with combination therapy including piperacillin/tazobactam and gentamicin for two weeks until neutrophil recovery.

INTRODUCTION

Ecthyma gangrenosum is an infectious lesion of the skin with a characteristic necrotic center. It is seen predominantly in the immunocompromised patients related to Gram-negative bacteremia, typically *Pseudomonas aeruginosa*.

EPIDEMIOLOGY

- Infrequent condition that is most prevalent in severely immunocompromised hosts with fever.
- The skin lesions may be a presenting feature of acute leukemia.[1]

ETIOLOGY AND PATHOPHYSIOLOGY

- Ecthyma gangrenosum is most commonly associated with disseminated *P aeruginosa* infection; however, it has also been described with other Gram-negative bacilli and fungi, including *Aeromonas hydrophila*, *Enterobacter*, *Escherichia coli*, *Morganella*, *Serratia marcescens*, *Stenotrophomonas maltophilia*, *Aspergillus*, *Candida*, *Fusarium*, and *Mucor*.[1–3]
- Necrotizing, hemorrhagic vasculitis is seen on histopathology.
- Organisms are often seen, particularly within the medial blood vessel layers.[2,4]

RISK FACTORS

- Compromised host immunity, often from malignancy or chemotherapy, is the most significant risk factor. Neutrophil defects may also be seen.[1]

DIAGNOSIS

CLINICAL FEATURES

- Lesions begin as erythematous macules with rapid progression to papules (**Figure 107-2**), then pustules, vesiculopustules (**Figure 107-1**), or bullae. Some lesions may be more nodular in appearance. Central necrosis and ulceration may develop in the later stages of formation (**Figure 107-3**).

DISTRIBUTION

- May appear anywhere on the body; multiple, simultaneous lesions are common.

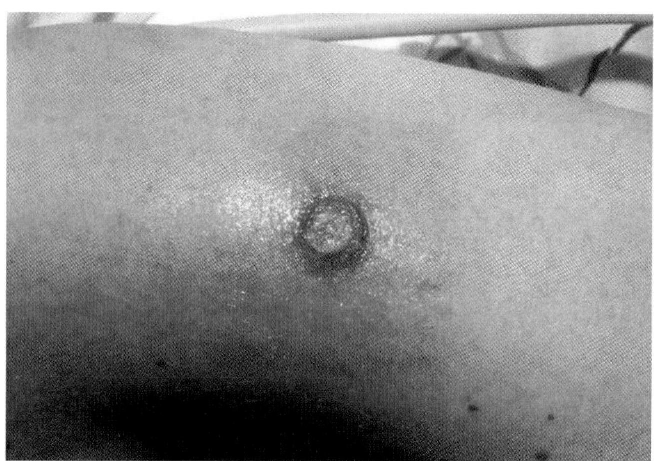

FIGURE 107-1 Ecthyma gangrenosum on the arm of this 13-year-old boy with acute myelogenous leukemia. This lesion is at a vesicopustular stage of formation. Blood cultures grew *Pseudomonas aeruginosa*. (*Used with permission from Johanna Goldfarb, MD.*)

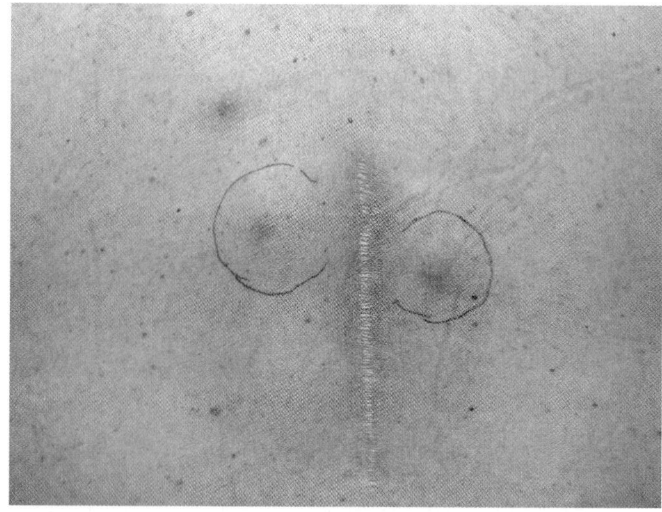

FIGURE 107-2 Ecthyma gangrenosum in the early stage of development. Note the papular lesions surrounding a previous wound in this patient with chemotherapy-induced neutropenia. (*Used with permission from Camille Sabella, MD.*)

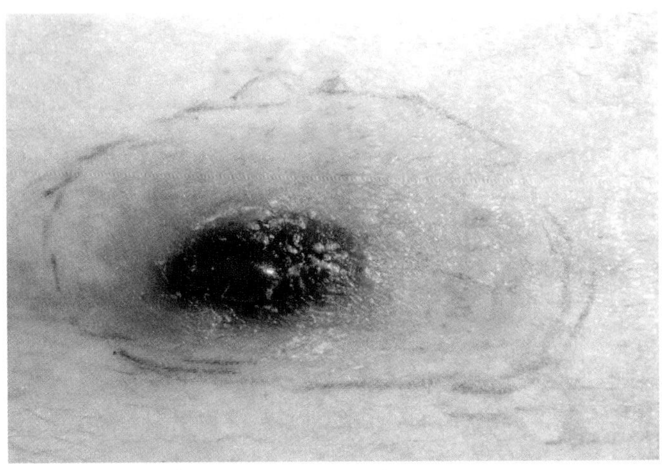

FIGURE 107-3 Ecthyma gangrenosum in a 14-year-old girl with acute myelogenous leukemia. Note the necrotic appearing center of the lesion and surrounding erythema. Blood culture from this patient grew *Pseudomonas aeruginosa*. *(Used with permission from Camille Sabella, MD. From Sabella C, Cunningham RJ III. Intensive Review of Pediatrics, 4th edition. Lippincott Williams Wilkins, p 453.)*

LABORATORY TESTING

- Blood cultures are usually diagnostic of Gram-negative septicemia.
- Biopsy can confirm the diagnosis and tissue culture may also yield a bacteriologic diagnosis.

IMAGING

- Not specifically indicated.

DIFFERENTIAL DIAGNOSIS

- Ecthyma—Community-acquired infection related to *Staphylococcus aureus* or group A streptococcus can be seen in otherwise healthy children, older adults, or diabetics.
- Cutaneous anthrax—Often associated with significant surrounding edema, and with suggestive occupational exposure.[1]
- Sweet syndrome—An acute, febrile, neutrophilic dermatosis not associated with infection usually requiring biopsy diagnosis.
- Leukemia cutis—May be present at leukemia diagnosis or relapse and is not related to infection. Biopsy is required.

MANAGEMENT

MEDICATIONS

- Empiric antibiotic therapy should be directed against *Pseudomonas aeruginosa* and tailored once a bacteriologic diagnosis is made.[1–3] SOR Ⓐ
- Experts recommend double-coverage, at least initially, for serious gram-negative infections in immunocompromised patients to provide synergy and to prevent the development of resistance.[1,2] SOR Ⓐ
- Typical agents used in combination include penicillins (piperacillin, ticarcillin), cephalosporins (ceftazidime, cefepime), carbapenems (imipenem, meropenem), fluoroquinolones (ciprofloxacin), and aminoglycosides (amikacin, gentamicin).[2]

SURGERY

- Rarely, surgical debridement may be necessary in cases of necrosis, abscess formation, or extensive disease.

REFERRAL

- Dermatology consultation may be warranted to confirm the diagnosis or obtain biopsy specimens when required.
- Surgical consultation is warranted when there is extensive necrosis requiring surgical debridement.

PROGNOSIS

- Ecthyma gangrenosum in the immunocompromised host can carry a high mortality, ranging from 30 to 70 percent.[2]

FOLLOW-UP

- Close follow-up is warranted to assure the bacteremia, sepsis, and the ecthymatous lesions have cleared with therapy and recovery of neutropenia.

PATIENT EDUCATION

- As for all patients with chemotherapy-induced neutropenia, fever and/or characteristic lesion or rash warrants immediate medical care.

PATIENT RESOURCES

- **http://en.wikipedia.org/wiki/Ecthyma_gangrenosum**.

PROVIDER RESOURCES

- Weinberg S, Prose NS, Kristal L: Section 15. Cutaneous Manifestations of Systemic Disease. In: Weinberg S, Prose NS, Kristal L, eds. *Color Atlas of Pediatric Dermatology*. 4th ed. New York: McGraw-Hill; 2008. **http://www.accesspediatrics.com/content/6988322**. Accessed March 4, 2013.

REFERENCES

1. Jackson MA. Bacterial skin infections. In: Feigin RD, Cherry JD, Demmler-Harrison GJ, and Kaplan SL, eds. Feigin and Cherry's textbook of pediatric infectious diseases. 6th ed. Philadelphia: Elsevier Saunders; 2009: 784-794.
2. Agger WA, Mardan A. *Pseudomonas aeruginosa* infections of intact skin. *Clin Infect Dis*. 1995;20(2):302-308.
3. Bodey GP. Dermatologic manifestations of infections in neutropenic patients. *Infect Dis Clin North Am*. 1994;8:655-675.
4. Somer T, Finegold SM. Vasculitides associated with infections, immunizations, and antimicrobial drugs. *Clin Infect Dis*. 1995; 20(4):1010-1036.

SECTION 4 VIRAL

108 VARICELLA

E.J. Mayeaux, Jr., MD

PATIENT STORY

A 12-year-old girl presents with a 3-day history of a body-wide pruritic vesicular rash (**Figure 108-1**). The episode started 24 hours before the rash with fever and malaise. The patient is diagnosed with varicella and no antiviral medications are given. Acetaminophen or ibuprofen are recommended for fever and comfort, avoiding aspirin to prevent Reyes syndrome.

INTRODUCTION

Varicella (chickenpox) is a highly contagious viral infection that can become reactivated in the form of zoster.

EPIDEMIOLOGY

- Varicella-zoster virus (VZV) is distributed worldwide.
- The rate of secondary household attack is more than 90 percent in susceptible individuals (**Figure 108-2**).[1]
- Adults and immunocompromised patients generally develop more severe disease than normal children.
- Traditionally, primary infection with VZV occurs during childhood (**Figure 108-3**). In childhood, it is usually a benign, self-limited illness in immunocompetent hosts. It occurs throughout the year in temperate regions, but the incidence peaks in the late spring and summer months.

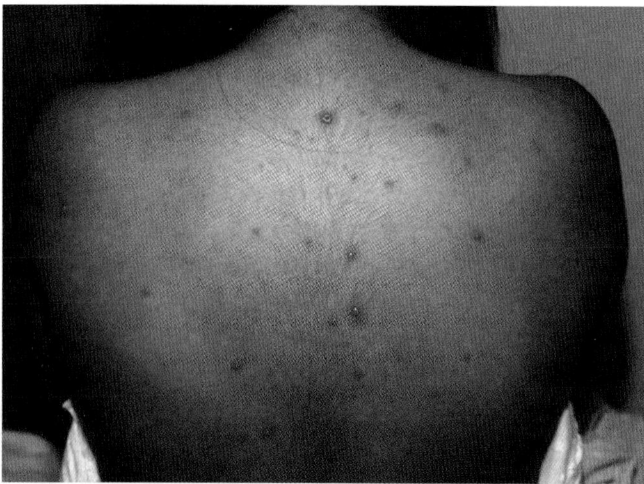

FIGURE 108-1 Chickenpox in a child. Note lesions in various stages (papules, intact vesicles, pustules, and crusted papules) caused by multiple crops of lesions. The vesicles are on a red base. (*Used with permission from Richard P. Usatine, MD.*)

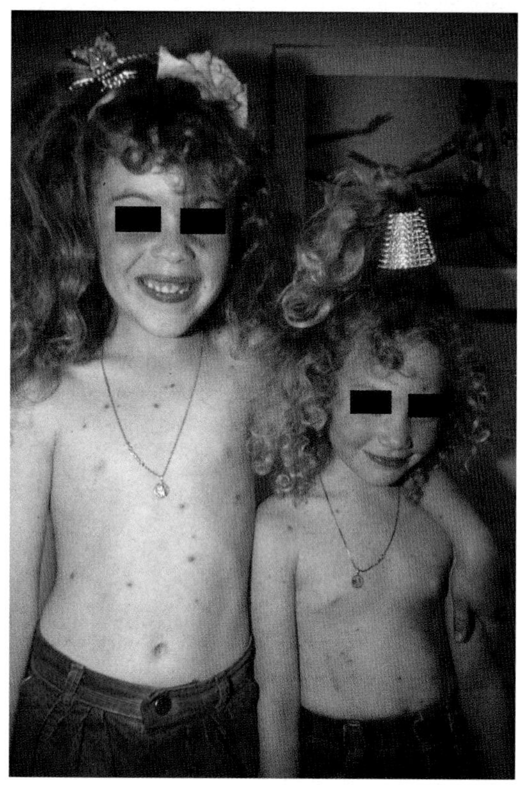

FIGURE 108-2 Chickenpox in sisters seen before the varicella vaccine was available. The girls are feeling better now that the disease is resolving. (*Used with permission from Richard P. Usatine, MD.*)

- Neonatal varicella is a serious illness with a mortality rate up to 30 percent.[2] The risk of infection and the case fatality rate are significantly increased if a mother has symptoms less than five days prior to delivery. The time to delivery allows insufficient time for the development of maternal IgG and passive transfer of protection to the fetus.[3] Postnatally acquired varicella that occurs beyond 10 days after birth usually is mild.[4]
- Prior to the introduction of the varicella vaccine in 1995, the yearly incidence of chickenpox in the US was approximately 4 million cases with approximately 11,000 hospital admissions and 100 deaths.[5]
- As the vaccination rates steadily increased in the US, there has been a corresponding fourfold decrease in the number of cases of chickenpox cases down to disease rates of from 0.3 to 1.0 per 1000 population in 2001.[5]

ETIOLOGY AND PATHOPHYSIOLOGY

- Chickenpox is caused by a primary infection with the VZV, which is a double-stranded, linear DNA herpesvirus.

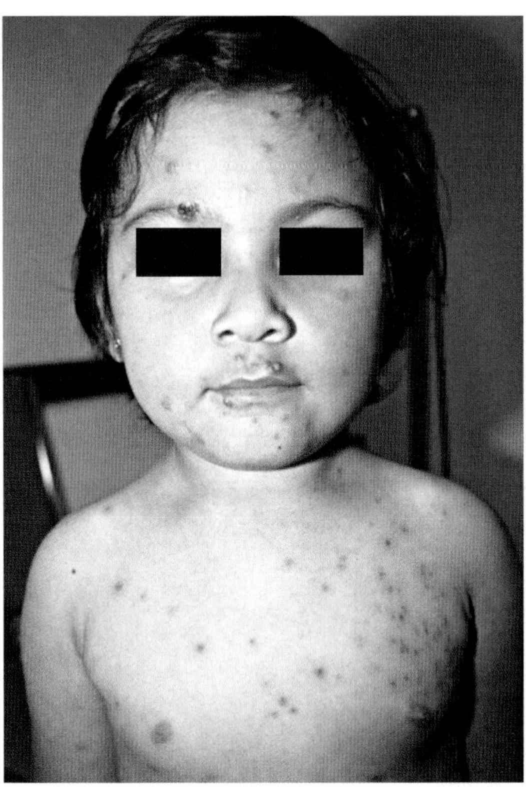

FIGURE 108-3 Chickenpox in a child. Note the widespread distribution of the lesions. The honey-crusted lesion on the eyebrow suggests a secondary bacterial infection (impetigo) has developed. (*Used with permission from Richard P. Usatine, MD.*)

- Transmission occurs via contact with aerosolized droplets from nasopharyngeal secretions or by direct cutaneous contact with vesicle fluid from skin lesions.
- The incubation period for VZV is approximately 15 days, during which the virus undergoes replication in regional lymph nodes, followed by two viremic phases, the second of which persists through the development of skin lesions generally by day 14.[6]

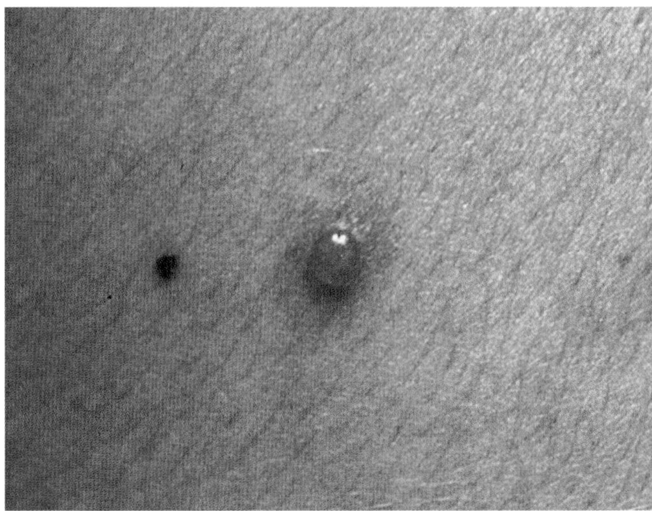

FIGURE 108-4 Dewdrop on a rose petal is the classic description of a varicella vesicle on a red base. (*Used with permission from Richard P. Usatine, MD.*)

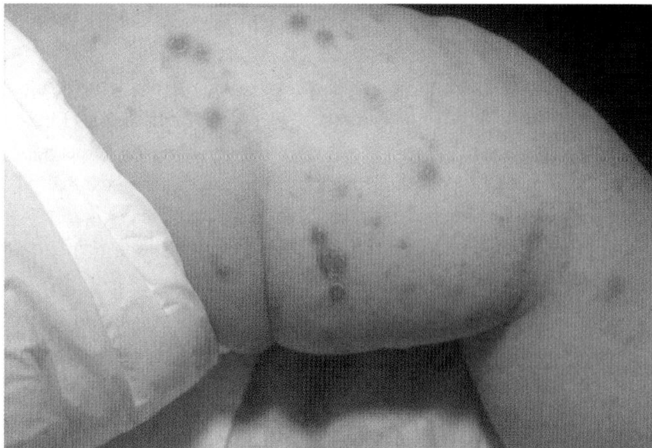

FIGURE 108-5 Varicella on the leg of an infant after the lesions have crusted over. The patient is probably not contagious at this time. (*Used with permission from the University of Texas Health Sciences Center, Division of Dermatology.*)

- The vesicular rash appears in crops for several days. The lesions start as vesicle on a red base, which is classically described as a dewdrop on a rose petal (**Figure 108-4**). The lesions gradually develop a pustular component (**Figure 108-5**) followed by the evolution of crusted papules (**Figure 108-6**). The period of infectivity is generally considered to last from 48 hours prior to the onset of rash until skin lesions have fully crusted.
- The most frequent complication in healthy children is bacterial skin superinfection (**Figure 108-6**). Less common skin complications

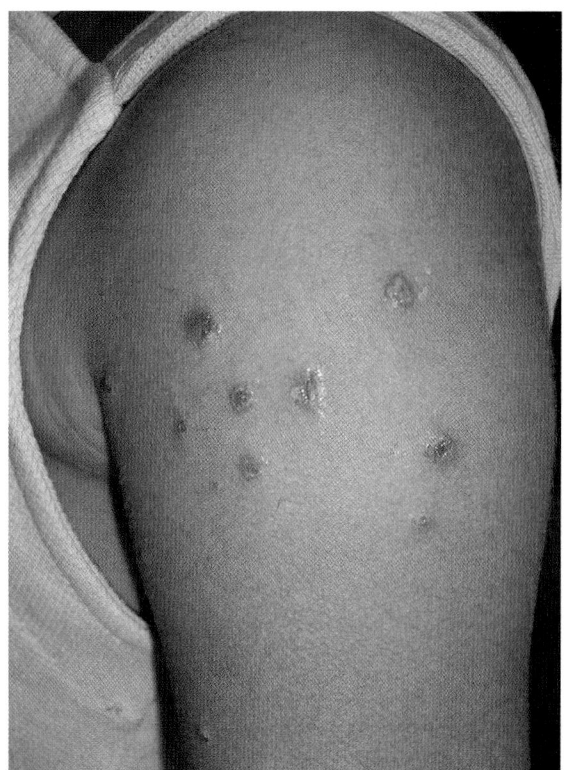

FIGURE 108-6 Honey-crusted lesions of superinfected varicella. This is impetiginized chickenpox caused by a secondary bacterial infection (impetigo). (*Used with permission from Richard P. Usatine, MD.*)

(seen more frequently in immunosuppressed hosts) include bullous varicella, purpura fulminans, and necrotizing fasciitis.

- Encephalitis is a serious potential complication of chickenpox that develops toward the end of the first week of the exanthema. One form, acute cerebellar ataxia, occurs mostly in children and is generally followed by complete recovery. A more diffuse encephalitis most often occurs in adults and may produce delirium, seizures, and focal neurologic signs. It has significant rates of long-term neurologic sequelae and death.
- Pneumonia is rare in healthy children but accounts for the majority of hospitalizations in adults, where it has up to a 30 percent mortality rate.[7] It usually develops insidiously within a few days after the rash has appeared with progressive tachypnea, dyspnea, and dry cough. Chest x-rays reveal diffuse bilateral infiltrates. Treat with prompt administration of intravenous acyclovir. The use of adjunctive steroid therapy is controversial.
- Varicella hepatitis is rare, and typically only occurs in immunosuppressed individuals. It is frequently fatal.
- Reactivation of latent VZV results in herpes zoster or shingles.

DIAGNOSIS

CLINICAL FEATURES

- The typical clinical manifestations of chickenpox include a prodrome of fever, malaise, or pharyngitis, followed in 24 hours by the development of a generalized vesicular rash.
- The lesions are pruritic and appear as successive crops of vesicles more than 3 to 4 days.
- Coexisting lesions in different stages of development on the face, trunk, and extremities are common (**Figure 108-7**).
- New lesions stop forming in approximately 4 days, and most lesions have fully crusted by 7 days.

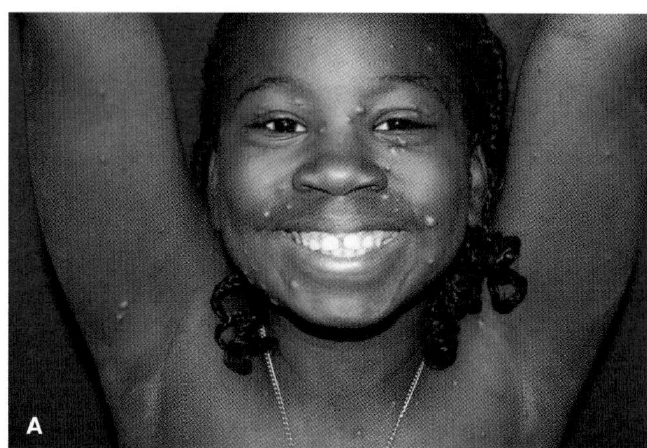

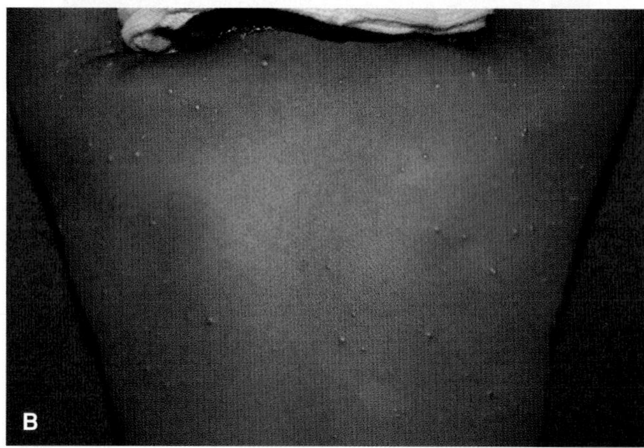

FIGURE 108-7 **A.** Varicella in a young girl that was previously immunized with the varicella vaccine. Note the papules and pustules present. **B.** The back has small evenly distributed pustules. (*Used with permission from Richard P. Usatine, MD.*)

TYPICAL DISTRIBUTION

- Bodywide—No laboratory tests are needed unless the diagnosis is uncertain. For children or adults in which there is uncertainty about previous disease and it is important to establish a quick diagnosis, a direct fluorescent antibody test can be done on a scraping of a lesion. In many laboratories, a result can be obtained within 24 hours (**Figure 108-8**).

LABORATORY TESTING

- Diagnosis is usually based on classic presentation. Culture of vesicular fluid provides a definitive diagnosis, but is positive in less than 40 percent of cases. Direct immunofluorescence has good sensitivity and is more rapid than tissue culture. Latex agglutination blood testing may be used to determine exposure and immunity to VZV.

DIFFERENTIAL DIAGNOSIS

- Pemphigus and bullous pemphigoid are usually seen in adults, whereas varicella is a disease of children.
- Dermatitis herpetiformis is characterized by pruritic papulovesicles over the extremities and on the trunk, and granular immunoglobulin (Ig) A deposits on the basement membrane (see Chapter 155, Chronic Bullous Disease of Childhood).

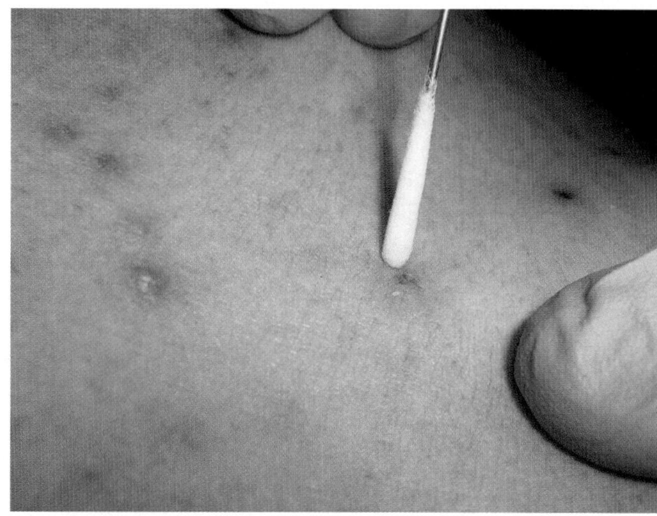

FIGURE 108-8 Direct scraping of a lesion was performed and the varicella virus was identified quickly with a direct fluorescent antibody test. (*Used with permission from Richard P. Usatine, MD.*)

- Herpes simplex infection presents with similar lesions, but is generally restricted to the genital and oral areas. The vesicles of herpes simplex tend to be more clustered in a group rather than the wide distribution of varicella (see Chapter 114, Herpes Simplex).
- Impetigo can have bullous or crusted lesions anywhere on the body. The lesions often have mild erythema and a yellowish color to the crusts (see Chapter 99, Impetigo).
- Insect bites are often suspected by history and can occur on the entire body.

MANAGEMENT

NONPHARMACOLOGIC

- Pruritus can be treated with calamine lotion, pramoxine gel, or powdered oatmeal baths.
- Fingernails should be closely cropped to avoid significant excoriation and secondary bacterial infection.

MEDICATIONS

- Antihistamines are helpful in the symptomatic treatment of pruritus.
- Acetaminophen should be used to treat fever in children, as aspirin use is associated with Reye syndrome in the setting of viral infections.[8] SOR Ⓐ
- Superinfection may be treated with topical or oral antibiotics.
- Prophylactic use of varicella zoster immune globulin (125 U/10 kg, up to 625 U IM) in recently exposed susceptible individuals can prevent or attenuate the disease. However, the immune globulin is extremely hard to obtain at times and is indicated only for those who are at risk for developing severe varicella, such as neonates (see the following section) and immunocompromised individuals.[9]
- Acyclovir (20 mg/kg PO 4 times daily) is US Food and Drug Administration approved for treatment of varicella in healthy children. It should be given during the first 24 hours of rash.[1] However, the Committee on Infectious Disease of the American Academy of Pediatrics issued a statement saying they did not consider the routine administration of acyclovir to all healthy children with varicella to be justified.[10] SOR Ⓒ
- Management of newborns exposed to VZV includes isolation and postexposure prophylaxis with Varicella-zoster immune globulin (VariZIG). The Advisory Committee on Immunization Practices (ACIP) recommends administration within 96 hours to the following newborns:[11] SOR Ⓐ
    - Infants who mothers have signs and symptoms of varicella within five days before or two days after delivery.
    - Premature infants born at >28 weeks of gestation who are exposed during the neonatal period and whose mothers do not have signs of immunity.
    - Premature infants born at <28 weeks of gestation or who weigh <1000 grams at birth and were exposed during the neonatal period, regardless of maternal history of varicella or vaccination.
- Early treatment with intravenous acyclovir may be effective for treatment of varicella hepatitis and pneumonia, and may also be useful in the treatment of immunosuppressed patients. SOR Ⓑ
- Adults who get varicella should be assessed for neurologic and pulmonary disease.

PREVENTION

- Varicella immunization (Varivax) can be used to prevent chickenpox. SOR Ⓐ It is contraindicated in individuals allergic to gelatin or neomycin and in immunosuppressed individuals (it is a live vaccine). In 2006, and again in 2010, the Advisory Committee on Immunization Practices recommended that all children younger than 13 years of age should be routinely administered 2 doses of varicella-containing vaccine, with the first dose administered at 12 to 15 months of age and the second dose at 4 to 6 years of age (i.e., before first grade). The second dose can be administered at an earlier age provided the interval between the first and second dose is at least 3 months.[12]

FOLLOW-UP

- Follow-up is unnecessary for immunocompetent children and adults who are having no complications. All patients or parents should report any respiratory or neurologic problems immediately.

PATIENT EDUCATION

- Avoid scratching the blisters and keep fingernails short. Scratching may lead to superinfection.
- Calamine lotion and oatmeal (Aveeno) baths may help relieve itching.
- Do not use aspirin or aspirin-containing products to relieve fever. The use of aspirin is associated with development of Reye syndrome, which may cause death.

PATIENT RESOURCES

- KidsHealth. *Chickenpox*—**www.kidshealth.org/parent/infections/skin/chicken_pox.html**.
- MedlinePlus. *Chickenpox*—**www.nlm.nih.gov/medlineplus/chickenpox.html**.

PROVIDER RESOURCES

- Centers for Disease Control and Prevention. *Varicella (Chickenpox) Vaccination*—**www.cdc.gov/vaccines/vpd-vac/varicella/default.htm**.
- Centers for Disease Control and Prevention. *Slide Set: Overview of VZV Disease & Vaccination for Health-care Professionals*—**www.cdc.gov/vaccines/vpd-vac/shingles/downloads/VZV_clinical_slideset_Jul2010.ppt**.

REFERENCES

1. Wharton M. The epidemiology of varicella-zoster infections. *Infect Dis Clin North Am.* 1996;10(3):571-581.
2. CDC Chickenpox and Pregnancy. http://www.cdc.gov/pregnancy/infections-chickenpox.html, accessed December 31, 2012.

3. Meyers JD. Congenital varicella in term infants: risk reconsidered. *J Infect Dis*. 1974;129:215.
4. Prober CG, Gershon AA, Grose C, et al. Consensus: varicella-zoster infections in pregnancy and the perinatal period. *Pediatr Infect Dis J*. 1990;9:865.
5. Centers for Disease Control and Prevention (CDC). Decline in annual incidence of varicella—selected states, 1990-2001. *MMWR Morb Mortal Wkly Rep*. 2003;52(37):884-885.
6. Grose C. Variation on a theme by Fenner: the pathogenesis of chickenpox. *Pediatrics*. 1981;68(5):735-737.
7. Schlossberg D, Littman M. Varicella pneumonia. *Arch Intern Med*. 1988;148(7):1630-1632.
8. Belay ED, Bresee JS, Holman RC, et al. Reye's syndrome in the US from 1981 through 1997. *N Engl J Med*. 1999;340(18):1377-1382.
9. Ogilvie MM. Antiviral prophylaxis and treatment in chickenpox. A review prepared for the UK advisory group on chickenpox on behalf of the british society for the study of infection. *J Infect*. 1998;36(1):31-38.
10. Prevention of varicella: recommendations of the Advisory Committee on Immunization Practices (ACIP). Centers for Disease Control and Prevention. *MMWR Morb Mortal Wkly Rep*. 1996;45(RR-11):1-36.
11. Centers for Disease Control and Prevention (CDC). A new product (VariZIG) for postexposure prophylaxis of varicella available under an investigational new drug application expanded access protocol. *MMWR Morb Mortal Wkly Rep*. 2006;55:209.
12. CDC Varicella Vaccination: Information for Health Care Providers-Routine Varicella Vaccination. http://www.cdc.gov/vaccines/vpd-vac/varicella/hcp-routine-vacc.htm, accessed August 5, 2012.

109 HERPES ZOSTER

E.J. Mayeaux, Jr., MD
Richard P. Usatine, MD

PATIENT STORY

A 14-year-old boy presents with deep burning pain and a vesicular eruption in a band starting at the left chest and ending just across the midline of the back (**Figure 109-1**). The varicella-zoster virus (VZV) leaves the dorsal root ganglion to travel down the spinal nerves to the cutaneous nerves of the skin. The vesicles do cross the midline by a few centimeters because the posterior primary ramus of the spinal nerve includes a small cutaneous medial branch that reaches across the midline.[1] The boy was treated with analgesics and an antiviral medication. The zoster healed with scarring.

INTRODUCTION

Herpes zoster (shingles) is a syndrome characterized by a painful, usually unilateral vesicular eruption that develops in a restricted dermatomal distribution (**Figures 109-1** and **109-2**).[2,3]

SYNONYMS

Shingles.

EPIDEMIOLOGY

- According to the Centers for Disease Control and Prevention (CDC), 32 percent of persons in the US will experience zoster during their lifetimes accounting for about 1 million cases annually.[4] Older age groups account for the highest incidence of zoster. Approximately 4 percent of patients will experience a second episode of herpes zoster.[5]
- Herpes zoster is uncommon in healthy children; most cases are seen in immunocompromised patients, including children who have received solid organ and hematologic transplants.

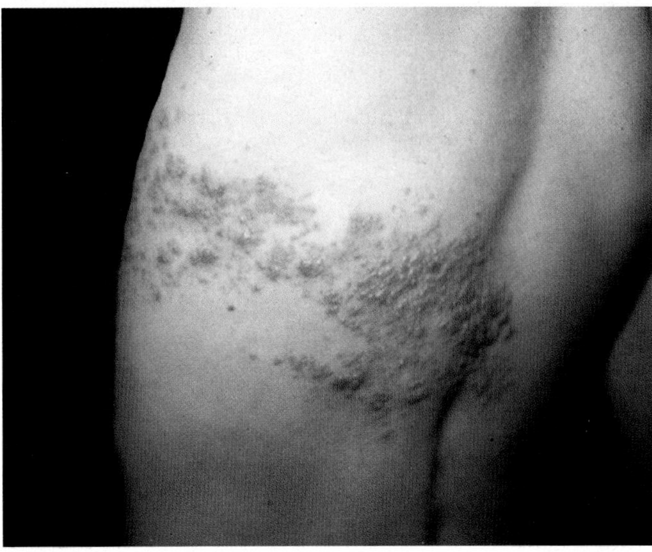

FIGURE 109-1 A 14-year-old boy with severe case of herpes zoster in a thoracic distribution. (*Used with permission from Richard P. Usatine, MD.*)

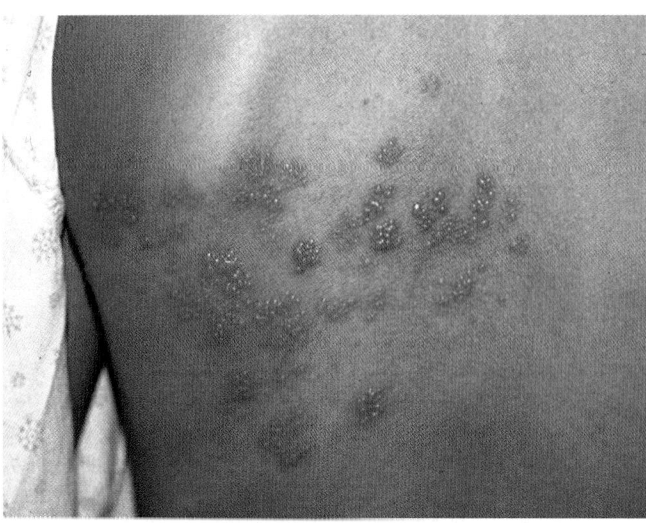

FIGURE 109-2 Close-up of herpes zoster lesions. Note grouped vesicles on a red base. (*Used with permission from Richard P. Usatine, MD.*)

ETIOLOGY AND PATHOPHYSIOLOGY

- After primary infection with either chickenpox or vaccine-type VZV, a latent infection is established in the sensory dorsal root ganglia. Reactivation of this latent VZV infection results in herpes zoster (shingles).
- Both sensory ganglia neurons and satellite cells surrounding the neurons serve as sites of VZV latent infection. During latency, the virus only expresses a small number of viral proteins.
- How the virus emerges from latency is not clearly understood. Once reactivated, virus spreads to other cells within the ganglion. The dermatomal distribution of the rash corresponds to the sensory fields of the infected neurons within the specific ganglion.[3]
- Loss of VZV-specific cell-mediated immune response is responsible for reactivation.[3]
- The pain associated with zoster infections and postherpetic neuralgia (PHN) is thought to result from injury to the peripheral nerves and altered central nervous system processing.
- The most common complication is bacterial superinfection that can delay healing and cause scarring of the zoster lesions.
- Complications may include:[6]
  - PHN—Uncommon in the pediatric population.
  - Ocular complications, including uveitis and keratitis (see Chapter 110, Zoster Ophthalmicus).
  - Bell palsy and other motor nerve plastic.
  - Bacterial skin infection.
  - Meningitis caused by central extension of the infection.
  - Herpes zoster oticus (Ramsay Hunt syndrome; **Figure 109-3**) includes the triad of ipsilateral facial paralysis, ear pain, and vesicles in the auditory canal and auricle.[8] Disturbances in taste

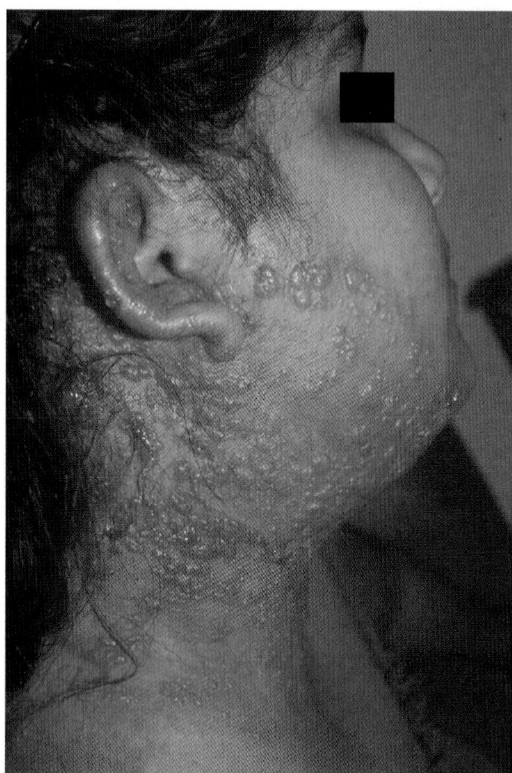

FIGURE 109-3 Herpes zoster oticus (Ramsay Hunt syndrome) with the classic presentation of vesicles on the auricle. (*Used with permission from the University of Texas Health Sciences Center, Division of Dermatology.*)

perception, hearing (tinnitus or hyperacusis), lacrimation, and vestibular function (vertigo) may occur.

- Other rare complications may include acute retinal necrosis, transverse myelitis, encephalitis, leukoencephalitis, contralateral thrombotic stroke syndrome, and granulomatous vasculitis.[7]

- Immunosuppressed patients are at increased risk for complications, including severe complications such as broader dermatomal involvement (**Figure 109-4**), disseminated infection, visceral involvement, pneumonitis, and/or meningoencephalitis.

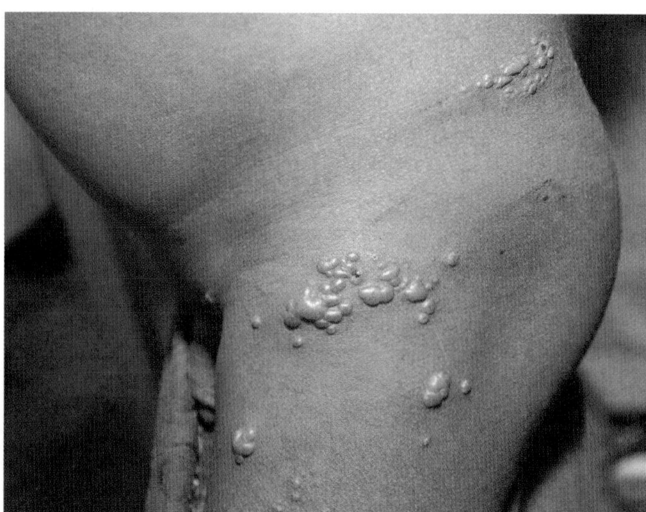

FIGURE 109-4 Herpes zoster in a 4-year-old boy with HIV disease. Note multiple dermatomes are involved. (*Used with permission from Richard P. Usatine, MD.*)

- PHN is the persistence of pain, numbness, and/or dysesthesias precipitated by movement or in response to non-noxious stimuli in the affected dermatome for more than 1 month after the onset of zoster. The incidence of PHN in the general population is 1.38 per 1000 person-years, and it occurs more commonly in individuals older than age 60 years and in immunosuppressed individuals.[3] This is rare in the pediatric population.

RISK FACTORS

ZOSTER[3]

- Older age.
- Underlying malignancy.
- Disorders of cell-mediated immunity, including organ and hematologic transplantation.
- Chronic lung or kidney disease.
- Autoimmune disease.

DIAGNOSIS

CLINICAL FEATURES

- Pediatric patients who develop zoster do not usually experience significant pain or disability.
- Mild tingling or redness in a dermatomal pattern may be the first symptom and can precede the rash.
- A prodrome of fever, dysesthesias, malaise, and headache leads in several days to a dermatomal vesicular eruption. The rash starts as grouped vesicles or bullae, which evolve into pustular or hemorrhagic lesions within 3 to 4 days (**Figures 109-1** to **109-6**). The

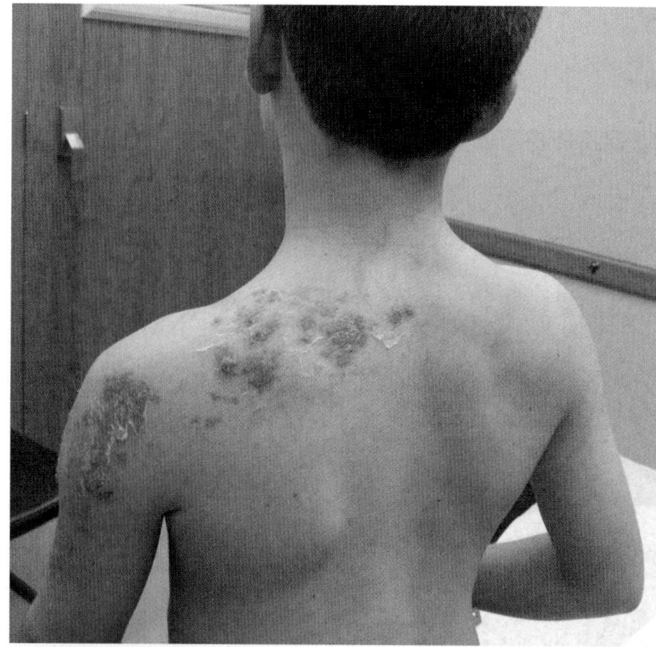

FIGURE 109-5 Herpes zoster following the C6 dermatome in a young otherwise healthy boy. Not all children that have zoster are immunocompromised. (*Used with permission from Emily Scott, MD.*)

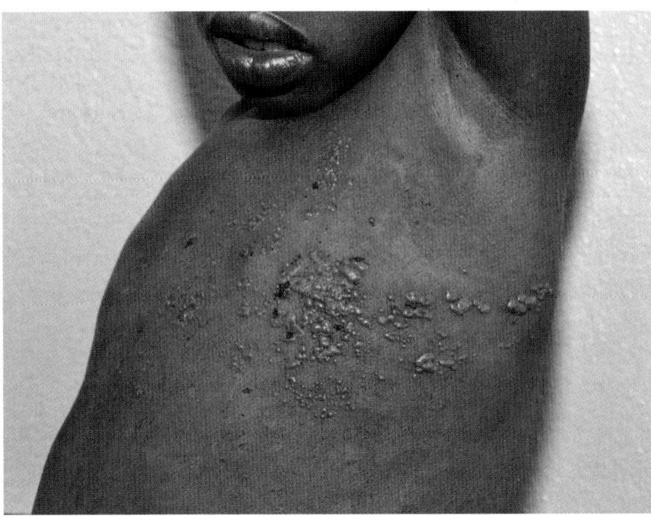

FIGURE 109-6 Herpes zoster in the thoracic distribution in an African child. An HIV serology was ordered because of the various risk factors involved. (*Used with permission from Richard P. Usatine, MD.*)

lesions typically crust in approximately a week, with complete resolution within 3 to 4 weeks.[5]

TYPICAL DISTRIBUTION

- Generally limited to one dermatome in immunocompetent patients, but sometimes affects neighboring dermatomes. Rarely, a few scattered vesicles located away from the involved dermatome as a result of release of VZV from the infected ganglion into the bloodstream.[3] If there are more than 20 lesions distributed outside the dermatome affected, the patient has disseminated zoster. The thoracic and lumbar dermatomes are the most commonly involved. Occasionally zoster will be seen on the extremities (**Figure 109-5**).

LABORATORY TESTING

- Meningitis associated with VZV infection can be diagnosed by cerebrospinal fluid showing pleocytosis.
- If HIV is suspected, serology for HIV antibodies should be ordered (**Figures 109-4** and **109-6**).

DIFFERENTIAL DIAGNOSIS

- Pemphigus and other bullous diseases present with blisters, but not in the classic dermatomal distribution (see Chapter 155, Chronic Bullous Disease of Childhood and Chapter 156, Pemphigus).
- Molluscum contagiosum presents with white or yellow flat-topped papules with central umbilication caused by a pox virus. The lesions are more firm and unless irritated do not have a red base as seen with zoster (see Chapter 115, Molluscum Contagiosum).
- Scabies may present as a pustular rash that is not confined to dermatomes and usually has characteristic lesions in the webs of the fingers (see Chapter 128, Scabies).
- Insect bites are often suspected by history and can occur over the entire body.
- Folliculitis presents with characteristic pustules arising from hair shafts (see Chapter 100, Folliculitis).
- Zoster mimics coronary artery disease when it presents with chest pain before the vesicles are visible.
- Herpes simplex infection presents with similar lesions but is usually restricted to the perioral region, genital area, buttocks, and fingers (see Chapter 114, Herpes Simplex).

MANAGEMENT

NONPHARMACOLOGIC

- Calamine lotion and topically administered lidocaine may be used to reduce pain and itching. SOR Ⓒ

MEDICATIONS

- Healthy children who develop zoster can be treated with analgesics for comfort.
- Acyclovir is not generally recommended in healthy children but may lead to faster resolution of the lesions if started within 48 hours of the onset of the rash. SOR Ⓒ
- Intravenous Acyclovir is indicated for immunocompromised patients to speed recovery and to prevent dissemination. SOR Ⓒ

PREVENTION

- Use of varicella (chickenpox) vaccine has not led to an increase in vaccine-associated herpes zoster in immunized patients or in the general population, and has led to an overall decrease in herpes zoster.[8]

FOLLOW-UP

- Follow-up is based on the severity of the case and the immune status of the patient.

PATIENT EDUCATION

- Herpes zoster in an immunocompetent host is only contagious from contact with open lesions.
- Patients with disseminated zoster or with zoster and are immunocompromised should be isolated from nonimmune individuals with primary varicella infection (in which airborne spread is possible).
- Individuals who have not had varicella and are exposed to a patient with herpes zoster are only at risk of developing primary varicella and not herpes zoster.

PATIENT RESOURCES

- Centers for Disease Control and Prevention. *Vaccine Information Statements*—**www.cdc.gov/vaccines/pubs/vis/**.
- Medinfo UK. *Shingles (Herpes Zoster)*—**www.medinfo.co.uk/conditions/shingles.html**.
- The Skin Site. *Herpes Zoster (Shingles)*—**www.skinsite.com/info_herpes_zoster.htm**.
- MedlinePlus. *Shingles*—**www.nlm.nih.gov/medlineplus/ency/article/000858.htm**.

PROVIDER RESOURCES

- MedlinePlus. *Shingles*—**http://emedicine.medscape.com/article/218683**.
- Stankus SJ, Dlugopolski M, Packer D. Management of herpes zoster (shingles) and PHN. *Am Fam Physician*. 2000;61[8]:2437-2444—**http://www.aafp.org/afp/20000415/2437.html**.
- Varicella-Zoster Infections. *Red Book* 2012:774-789—**http://aapredbook.aappublications.org/content/current.**

REFERENCES

1. Usatine RP, Clemente C. Is herpes zoster unilateral? *West J Med.* 1999;170(5):263.
2. Gnann JW Jr, Whitley RJ. Clinical practice. Herpes zoster. *N Engl J Med.* 2002;347(5):340-346.
3. Oxman MN. Immunization to reduce the frequency and severity of herpes zoster and its complications. *Neurology*. 1995;45(12;8): S41-S46.
4. Harpaz R, Ortega-Sanchez IR, Seward JF; Advisory Committee on Immunization Practices (ACIP) Centers for Disease Control and Prevention (CDC). Prevention of herpes zoster: recommendations of the Advisory Committee on Immunization Practices (ACIP). *MMWR Recomm Rep.* 2008;57(RR-5):1-30.
5. Stankus SJ, Dlugopolski M, Packer D. Management of herpes zoster (shingles) and postherpetic neuralgia. *Am Fam Physician.* 2000;61(18): 2437-2444, 2447-2448.
6. Yawn BP, Saddier P, Wollan PC, et al. A population-based study of the incidence and complication rates of herpes zoster before zoster vaccine introduction. *Mayo Clin Proc.* 2007;82(11): 1341-1349.
7. Arvin AM, Pollard RB, Rasmussen LE, Merigan TC. Cellular and humoral immunity in the pathogenesis of recurrent herpes viral infections in patients with lymphoma. *J Clin Invest.* 1980;65(4): 869-878.
8. Adour KK. Otological complications of herpes zoster. *Ann Neurol.* 1994;35:S62-S64.

110 ZOSTER OPHTHALMICUS

E.J. Mayeaux, Jr., MD
Richard P. Usatine, MD

PATIENT STORY

This 5-year-old girl developed redness and pain on the right side of her forehead. Later a vesicular rash developed (**Figure 110-1**). She was diagnosed with herpes zoster involving the first (ophthalmic) branch of the trigeminal nerve. Note the vesicles and bullae on the forehead and eyelid and the crust on the nasal tip (Hutchinson sign). Fortunately, she did not have ocular complications and her case of zoster fully healed with systemic acyclovir and acyclovir eye ointment.

INTRODUCTION

Herpes zoster is a common infection caused by varicella-zoster virus, the same virus that causes chickenpox. Reactivation of the latent virus in neurosensory ganglia produces the characteristic manifestations of herpes zoster (shingles). Herpes zoster outbreaks may be precipitated by aging, poor nutrition, immunocompromised status (**Figures 110-2** to **110-4**), physical or emotional stress, and excessive fatigue. Although zoster most commonly involves the thoracic and lumbar dermatomes, reactivation of the latent virus in the trigeminal ganglia may result in herpes zoster ophthalmicus (HZO) (**Figures 110-1** to **110-5**).

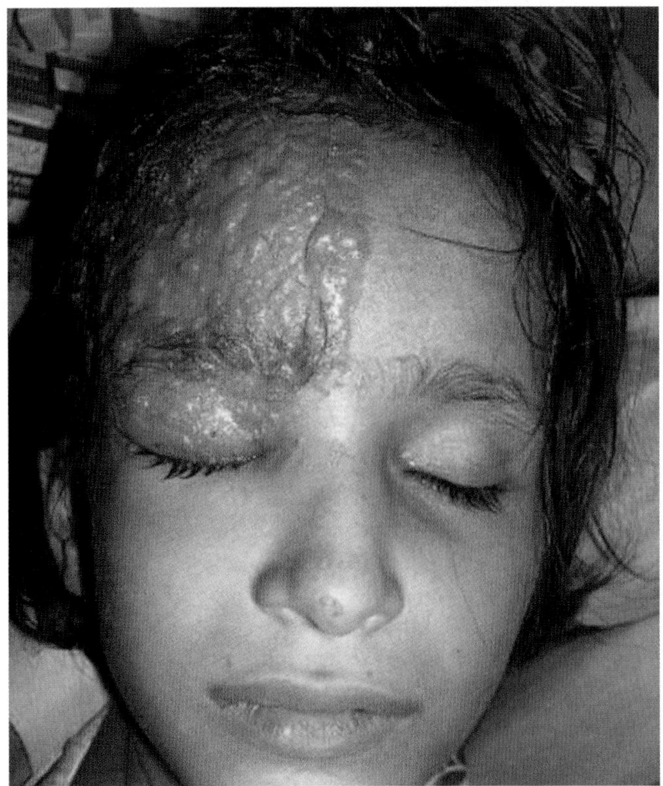

FIGURE 110-1 A 5-year-old girl with herpes zoster involving the ophthalmic branch of the trigeminal nerve. Note the vesicles and bullae on the forehead and eyelid and the crust on the nasal tip (Hutchinson sign). Fortunately, she did not have ocular complications and her case of zoster fully healed with oral acyclovir and acyclovir eye ointment. *(Used with permission from Amor Khachemoune, MD.)*

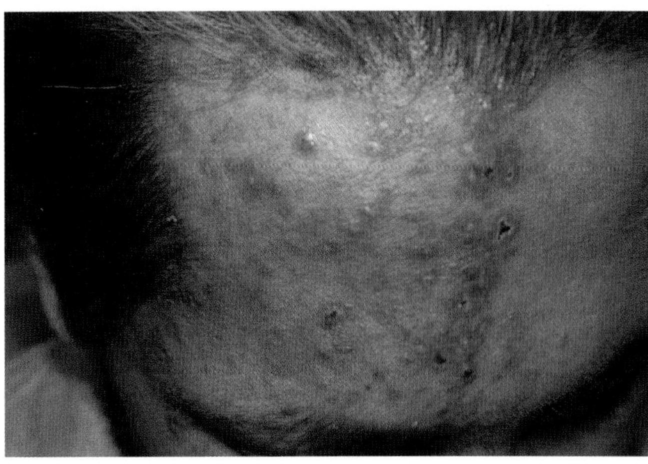

FIGURE 110-2 An HIV-positive Hispanic man with painful herpes zoster of his right forehead. His right eye was red, painful, and very sensitive to light. *(Used with permission from Paul Comeau.)*

SYNONYMS

Ocular herpes zoster.

EPIDEMIOLOGY

- Incidence rates of HZO complicating herpes zoster range from 8 to 56 percent.[1]
- Ocular involvement is not correlated with age, gender, or severity of disease.

ETIOLOGY AND PATHOPHYSIOLOGY

- Serious sequelae may occur including chronic ocular inflammation, vision loss (**Figures 110-2** to **110-4**), and disabling pain. Early

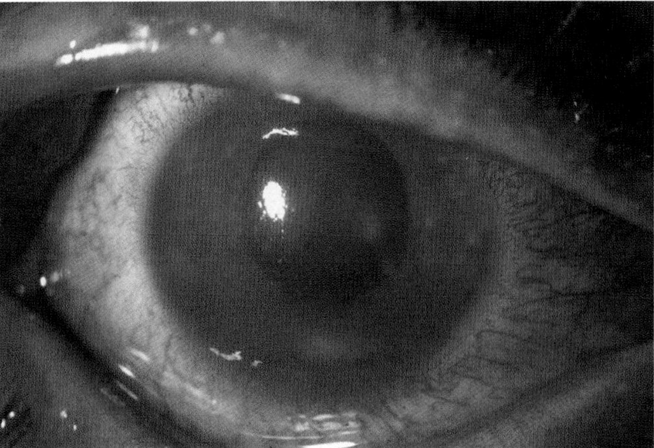

FIGURE 110-3 Acute zoster ophthalmicus of the patient in Figure 110-2. Note the conjunctival injection, corneal punctation (keratitis), and a small layer of blood in the anterior chamber (hyphema). A diagnosis of anterior uveitis was suspected based on the irregularly shaped pupil, the hyphema, and ciliary flush. A slit-lamp examination confirmed the anterior uveitis (iritis). *(Used with permission from Paul Comeau.)*

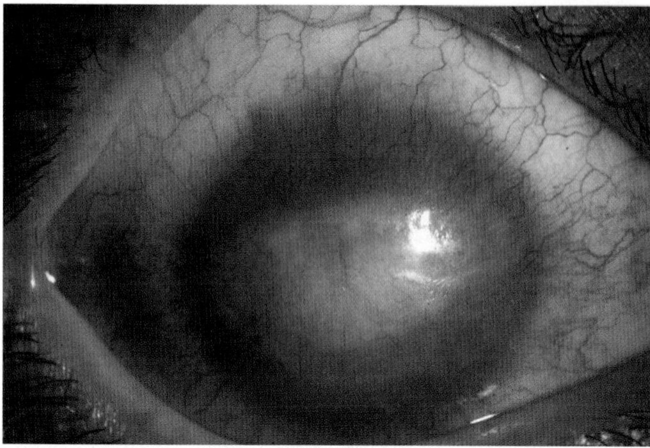

FIGURE 110-4 Corneal scarring and conjunctival injection of the same patient in Figure 110-2 6 months later after being lost to follow-up. *(Used with permission from Paul Comeau.)*

diagnosis is important to prevent progressive corneal involvement and potential loss of vision.[2]

- Because the nasociliary branch of the first (ophthalmic) division of the trigeminal (fifth cranial) nerve innervates the globe (**Figure 110-6**), the most serious ocular involvement develops if this branch is involved.
- Classically, involvement of the side of the tip of the nose (Hutchinson sign) has been thought to be a clinical predictor of ocular involvement via the external nasal nerve (**Figures 110-1** and **110-5**). The Hutchinson sign is a powerful predictor of ocular inflammation and corneal denervation with relative risks of 3.35 and 4.02, respectively. In one study, the manifestation of herpes zoster skin lesions at the dermatomes of both nasociliary branches (at the tip, the side, and the root of the nose) was invariably associated with the development of ocular inflammation.[3]

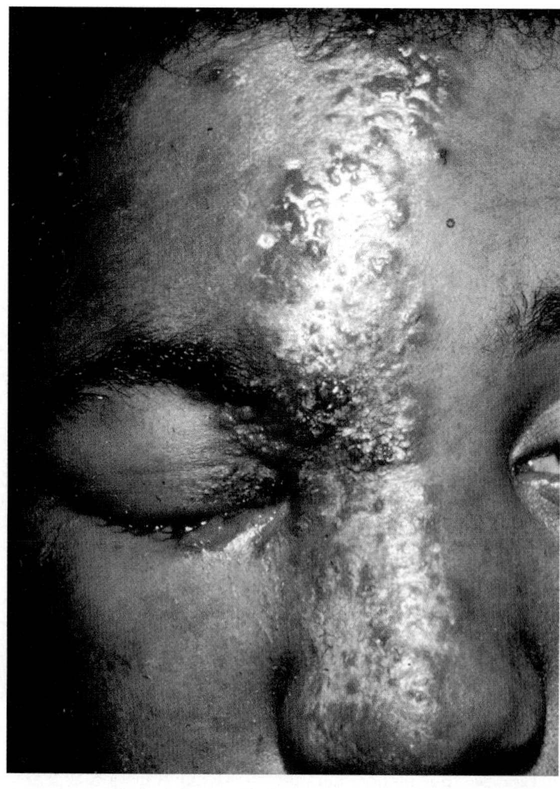

FIGURE 110-5 Herpes zoster ophthalmicus causing eyelid swelling and ptosis. Note the positive Hutchinson sign. *(Used with permission from Richard P. Usatine, MD.)*

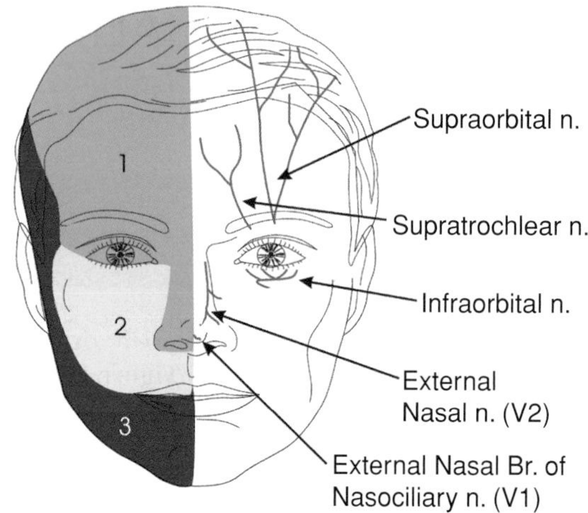

FIGURE 110-6 Diagram demonstrating the sensory distribution of the trigeminal (fifth cranial) nerve, and major peripheral nerves of the first (ophthalmic) division that may be involved with herpes zoster ophthalmicus. The infraorbital nerve from the second division is also shown. *(Used with permission from E.J. Mayeaux, Jr., MD.)*

- Epithelial keratitis is the earliest potential corneal finding (**Figure 110-3**). On slit-lamp examination, it appears as multiple, focal, swollen spots on the cornea that stain with fluorescein dye. They may either resolve or progress to dendrite formation. Herpes zoster virus dendrites form branching or frond-like patterns that have tapered ends and stain with fluorescein dye. These lesions can lead to anterior stromal corneal infiltrates.
- Stromal keratitis occurs in 25 to 30 percent of patients with HZO, and is characterized by multiple fine granular infiltrates in the anterior corneal stroma. The infiltrates probably arise from antigen–antibody reaction and may be prolonged and recurrent.[4]
- Anterior uveitis evolves to inflammation of the iris and ciliary body and occurs frequently with HZO (**Figure 110-3**). The inflammation is usually mild, but may cause a mild intraocular pressure elevation. The course of disease may be prolonged, especially without timely treatment, and may lead to glaucoma and cataract formation.
- Herpes zoster virus is the most common cause of acute retinal necrosis. Symptoms include blurred vision and/or pain in one or both eyes and signs include peripheral patches of retinal necrosis that rapidly coalesce, occlusive vasculitis, and vitreous inflammation. It commonly causes retinal detachment. Bilateral involvement is observed in 1/3 of patients, but may be as high as 70 percent in patients with untreated disease. Treatment includes long courses of oral and intravenous acyclovir, and corticosteroids.[5]
- Varicella-zoster virus is a member of the same family (Herpesviridae) as herpes simplex virus, Epstein-Barr virus, and cytomegalovirus.
- The virus damages the eye and surrounding structures by neural and secondary perineural inflammation of the sensory nerves. This often results in corneal anesthesia.
- Conjunctivitis, usually with *Staphylococcus aureus*, is a common complication of HZO.

RISK FACTORS

- Immunocompromised persons, especially when caused by human immunodeficiency virus infection, have a much higher risk of developing zoster complications, including HZO.

DIAGNOSIS

CLINICAL FEATURES

- The syndrome usually begins with a prodrome of low-grade fever, headache, and malaise that may start up to 1 week before the rash appears.
- Unilateral pain or hypesthesia in the affected eye, forehead, top of the head, and/or nose may precede or follow the prodrome. The rash starts with erythematous macules along the involved dermatome, then rapidly progresses over several days to papules, vesicles and pustules (**Figures 110-5** to **110-5**). The lesions rupture and typically crust over, requiring several weeks to heal completely.
- With the onset of a vesicular rash along the trigeminal dermatome, hyperemic conjunctivitis, episcleritis, and lid droop (ptosis) can occur (**Figure 110-5**).
- Approximately 2/3 of patients with HZO develop corneal involvement (keratitis).[1] The epithelial keratitis may feature punctate or dendritiform lesions (**Figure 110-3**). Complications of corneal involvement can lead to corneal scarring (**Figure 110-4**).[6]
- Iritis (anterior uveitis) occurs in approximately 40 percent of patients and can be associated with hyphema and an irregular pupil (**Figure 110-3**).[1]
- Rarely, zoster can be associated with cranial nerve palsies.

TYPICAL DISTRIBUTION

- The frontal branch of the first division of the trigeminal nerve (which includes the supraorbital, supratrochlear, and external nasal branch of the anterior ethmoidal nerve) is most frequently involved, and 50 to 72 percent of patients experience direct eye involvement (**Figure 110-6**).[1]
- Although HZO most often produces a classic dermatomal rash in the trigeminal distribution, a minority of patients may have only cornea findings.

DIFFERENTIAL DIAGNOSIS

- Bacterial or viral conjunctivitis presents as eye pain and foreign body sensation associated with discharge but no rash (see Chapter 12, Conjunctivitis).
- Trigeminal neuralgia presents with facial pain but without the rash or conjunctival findings.
- Glaucoma that presents as inflammation, pain, and injection, but without the rash or conjunctival findings.
- Traumatic abrasions usually present with a history of trauma and corneal findings but no other zoster findings (see Chapter 11, Corneal Foreign Body and Abrasion).
- Pemphigus and other bullous diseases present with blisters, but not in a dermatomal distribution (see Section 13: Bullous Diseases).

MANAGEMENT

MEDICATIONS

- The standard treatment for HZO is to initiate antiviral therapy with acyclovir (<12 yo: 20 mg/kg/dose IV Q8 hour or >12 yo: 800 mg orally 5 times daily for 7 to 10 days or 10 mg/kg intravenously every 8 hours for 7 to 10 days).[7] SOR Ⓐ
- Topical steroid ophthalmic drops are applied to the involved eye, by the examining ophthalmologist, to reduce the inflammatory response and control immune keratitis and iritis.[1,2] SOR Ⓑ
- The ophthalmologist may prescribe a topical cycloplegic (such as atropine) to treat the ciliary muscle spasm that is painful in iritis. SOR Ⓒ
- Topical ophthalmic antibiotics may also be prescribed to prevent secondary infection of the eye. SOR Ⓒ
- As in all cases of zoster, pain should be treated effectively with oral analgesics.
- Topical anesthetics should never be used with ocular involvement because of their corneal toxicity. SOR Ⓑ
- Secondary infection, usually *S. aureus*, may develop and should be treated with broad-spectrum topical and/or systemic antibiotics.

REFERRAL OR HOSPITALIZATION

- Referral to an ophthalmologist urgently should be initiated when eye involvement is seen or suspected.
- Hospital admission should be considered for patients with loss of vision, severe symptoms, immunosuppression, involvement of multiple dermatomes, or with significant facial bacterial superinfection.

PROGNOSIS

- HZO can become chronic or relapsing. Recurrence is a characteristic feature of HZO.
- Approximately 50 percent of patients with HZO develop complications. Systemic antiviral therapy can lower the emergence of complications.[10,11]

FOLLOW-UP

- Early diagnosis is critical to prevent progressive corneal involvement and potential loss of vision. Patients with herpes zoster should be informed that they should present for medical care with any zoster involving the first (ophthalmic) division of the trigeminal nerve or the eye itself.

PATIENT EDUCATION

- Zoster of the eye is a very serious vision-threatening illness that requires strict adherence to medical therapy and close follow-up.

- Viral transmission to nonimmune individuals from patients with herpes zoster can occur, but it is less frequent than with chickenpox. Virus can be transmitted through contact with secretions.

PATIENT RESOURCES

- American Family Physician. *What You Should Know About HZO*—**www.aafp.org/afp/2002/1101/p1732.html**.
- EyeMDLink.com. *Eye Herpes (Ocular Herpes)*—**www.eyemdlink.com/Condition.asp?ConditionID=223**.

PROVIDER RESOURCES

- Medscape. *Herpes Zoster Ophthalmicus*—**http://emedicine.medscape.com/article/783223**.
- Shaikh S, Ta CN. Evaluation and management of HZO. *Am Fam Physician*. 2002;66[9]:1723-1730—**http://www.aafp.org/afp/20021101/1723.html**.

REFERENCES

1. Pavan-Langston D. Herpes zoster ophthalmicus. *Neurology.* 1995; 45(12;8):S50-S51.
2. Severson EA, Baratz KH, Hodge DO, Burke JP. Herpes zoster ophthalmicus in Olmsted County, Minnesota: Have systemic antivirals made a difference? *Arch Ophthalmol.* 2003;121(3):386-390.
3. Zaal MJ, Völker-Dieben HJ, D'Amaro J. Prognostic value of Hutchinson's sign in acute herpes zoster ophthalmicus. *Graefes Arch Clin Exp Ophthalmol.* 2003;241(3):187-191.
4. Liesegang TJ. Corneal complications from herpes zoster ophthalmicus. *Ophthalmology.* 1985;92(3):316-324.
5. Liesegang TJ. Herpes zoster ophthalmicus natural history, risk factors, clinical presentation, and morbidity. *Ophthalmology.* 2008;115(2 Suppl):S3-S12.
6. Albrecht Ma: *Clinical Features of Varicella-Zoster Virus Infection: Herpes Zoster*. http://www.uptodate.com/contents/clinical-manifestations-of-varicella-zoster-virus-infection-herpes-zoster, accessed September 3, 2012.
7. McGill J, Chapman C, Mahakasingam M. Acyclovir therapy in herpes zoster infection. A practical guide. *Trans Ophthalmol Soc U K.* 1983;103(Pt 1):111-114.
8. Gnann JW Jr, Whitley RJ. Clinical practice. Herpes zoster. *N Engl J Med.* 2002;347(5):340-346.
9. Oxman MN. Immunization to reduce the frequency and severity of herpes zoster and its complications. *Neurology.* 1995;45 (12; 8):S41-S46.
10. Miserocchi E, Waheed NK, Dios E, et al. Visual outcome in herpes simplex virus and varicella zoster virus uveitis: a clinical evaluation and comparison. *Ophthalmology.* 2002;109(8): 1532-1537.
11. Zaal MJ, Volker-Dieben HJ, D'Amaro J. Visual prognosis in immunocompetent patients with herpes zoster ophthalmicus. *Acta Ophthalmol Scand.* 2003;81(3):216-220.

111 MEASLES

E.J. Mayeaux, Jr., MD
Luke Baudoin, MD

PATIENT STORY

An 18-month-old boy, who is visiting family in San Antonio with his parents from Central America, presents with a 3-day history of fever, malaise, conjunctivitis, coryza, and cough. He had been exposed to a child with similar symptoms approximately 2 weeks prior. A day before, he developed a maculopapular rash that blanches under pressure (**Figures 111-1** and **111-2**). His shot records are unavailable but his mother states that his last vaccine was before age 1 year. He is diagnosed with measles and supportive care is provided.

INTRODUCTION

Measles is a highly communicable, acute viral illness that is still one the most serious infectious diseases in human history. Until the introduction of the measles vaccination, it was responsible for millions of deaths worldwide annually. Although the epidemiology of this disease makes eradication a possibility, the ease of transmission and the low percentage of non immunized population that is required for disease survival have made eradication of measles extremely difficult.

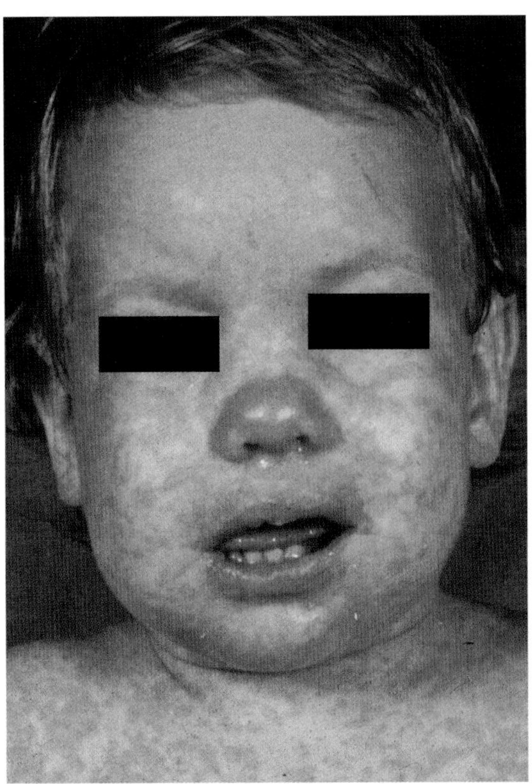

FIGURE 111-1 Typical measles rash that began on the face and became confluent. (*Used with permission from the University of Texas Health Sciences Center, Division of Dermatology.*)

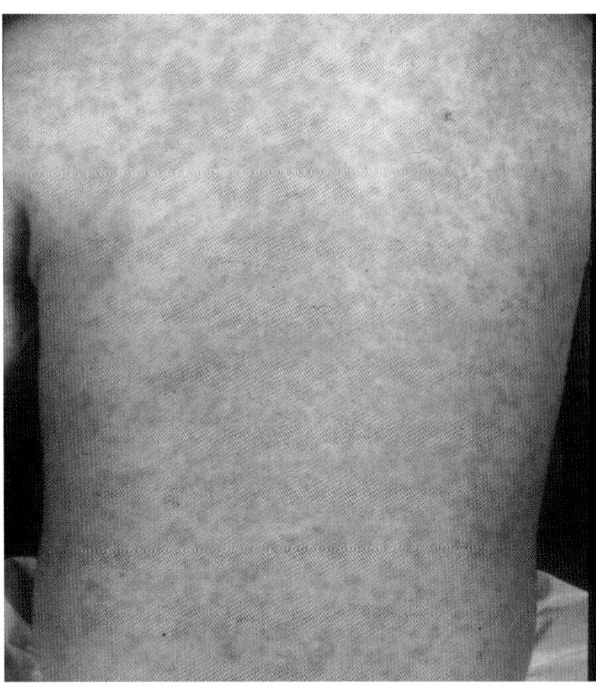

FIGURE 111-2 The typical measles rash on the trunk. (*Used with permission from the University of Texas Health Sciences Center, Division of Dermatology.*)

EPIDEMIOLOGY

- Last major outbreak in the US was during 1989 to 1990 and prompted a change in immunization policy in 1991, so that all children are to have two measles-mumps-rubella (MMR) vaccines before starting kindergarten.
- This practice interrupted the transmission of indigenous measles in the US by 1993 and reduced incidence of measles to an historic low (<0.5 cases per million persons) by 1997 to 1999.[1]
- After an all-time low of 34 cases were reported in 2004 in the US, the annual incidence began to increase with most cases linked to international travel of inadequately vaccinated Americans to endemic areas. Incomplete vaccination rates facilitate the spread once the virus is imported to the US causing clusters of periodic outbreaks.[1]
- The worldwide incidence of death from measles was effectively reduced from an estimated 733,000 deaths in 2000 to an estimated 164,000 deaths in 2008 with mass vaccination campaigns by the member countries of the World Health Assembly.[2] In 2008, about 83 percent of the world's children received one dose of measles vaccine by their first birthday through routine health services—up from 72 percent in 2000.[3]
- Measles elimination is now considered a feasible target. The World Health Organization have renewed their commitment to eliminate measles transmission by 2015. This will require greater than 95 percent of the population receives two doses of the MMR vaccine.[4]

ETIOLOGY AND PATHOPHYSIOLOGY

- Measles is caused by the measles virus, a member of the family paramyxoviridae, genus *Morbillivirus* (hence the name, morbilliform rash).

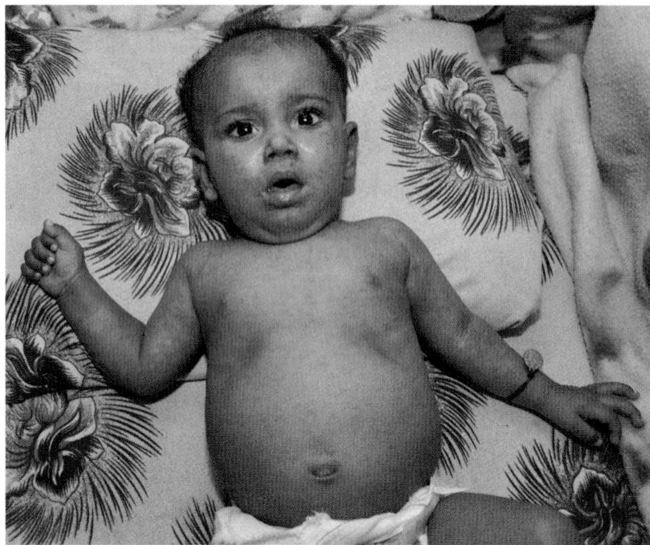

FIGURE 111-3 Measles in an Ethiopian infant during a measles outbreak. The rash is faint but her cough is prominent and subcostal retractions are seen during this cough. She also has rhinorrhea and conjunctivitis. (*Used with permission from Richard P. Usatine, MD.*)

- It is highly contagious, transmitted by airborne droplets, and commonly causes outbreaks.
- Classic measles infection starts with the incubation phase that is usually asymptomatic and lasts for 10 to 14 days. It starts after entry of the virus into the respiratory mucosa with local viral replication. The infection then spreads to regional lymphatic tissues, and then throughout the body through the bloodstream.
- The prodrome phase starts with the appearance of systemic symptoms including fever, malaise, anorexia, conjunctivitis, coryza, and cough (**Figure 111-3**). The respiratory symptoms are caused by mucosal inflammation from viral infection of epithelial cells. Patients may develop Koplik's spots, which are small whitish, grayish, or bluish papules with erythematous bases that develop on the buccal mucosa usually near the molar teeth (**Figure 111-4**). The prodrome usually lasts for 2 to 3 days.
- The classic measles rash (**Figures 111-1**, **111-2**, and **111-5**) is maculopapular and blanches under pressure. Clinical improvement in symptoms typically ensues within 2 days. Three to 4 days after the rash first appears, it begins to fade to a brownish color which is followed by fine flaking. The cough may persist for up to 2 weeks.
- Fever persisting beyond the third day of rash suggests a measles-associated complication.
- Immunity after measles infection is thought to be lifelong in most cases. Measles reinfection occasionally occurs, but it is extremely rare.
- Atypical measles is a measles variant that occurs in previously-vaccinated persons. Patients develop high fever and headache 7 to 14 days after exposure, and often present with a dry cough and pleuritic chest pain. Two to three days later, a rash develops that spreads from the extremities to the trunk. The rash may be vesicular, petechial, purpuric, or urticarial. Patients may develop respiratory distress, peripheral edema, hepatosplenomegaly, paresthesias, or hyperesthesia.
- The measles virus can cause a variety of clinical syndromes including the classic childhood illness and a less intense form in persons with suboptimal levels of anti measles antibodies.

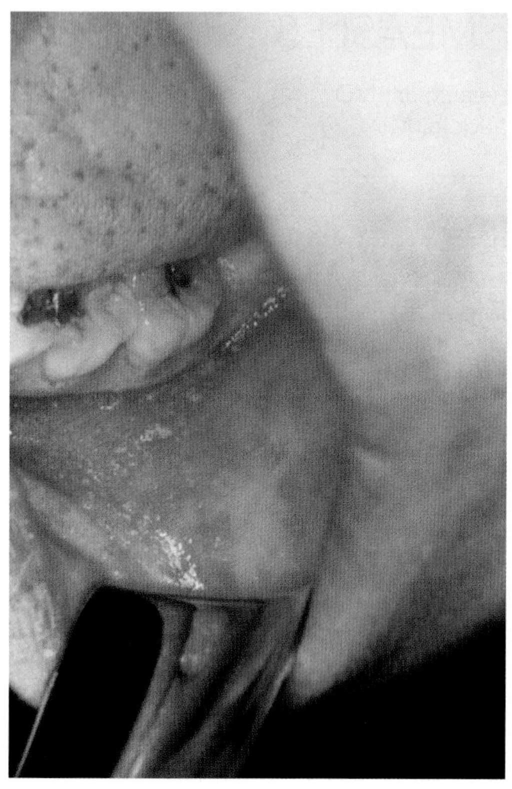

FIGURE 111-4 Koplik's spots occur 1 to 2 days before to 1 to 2 days after the cutaneous rash. Their presence is considered to be pathognomonic for measles, and appear as punctate blue-white spots on the bright red background of the oral buccal (cheek) mucosa. (*Used with permission from the Centers for Disease Control and Prevention.*)

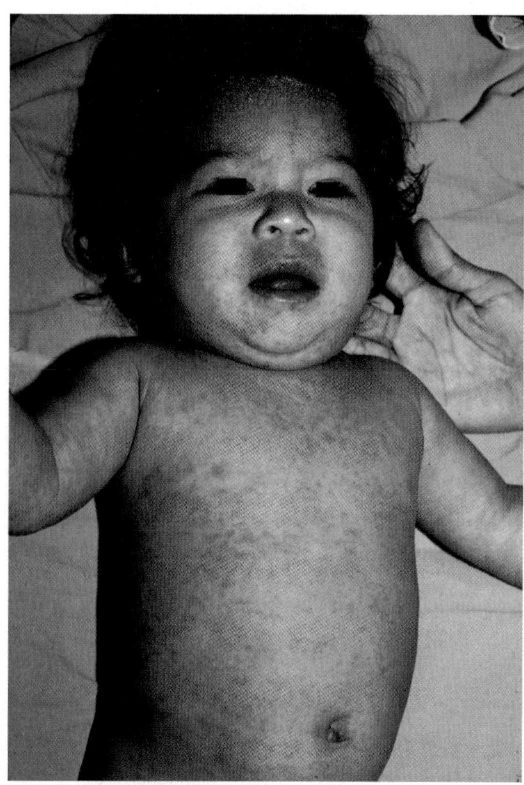

FIGURE 111-5 A South American child with an advanced measles exanthem. (*Used with permission from Eric Kraus.*)

- Measles virus infection can also result in more severe illness, including lymphadenopathy, splenomegaly, laryngotracheobronchitis (croup), giant cell pneumonia, and measles inclusion body encephalitis in immunocompromised patients.[5] This form occurs in the very young, those with vitamin A deficiency, and in pregnant women.
- Postinfection neurologic syndromes can occur. Postinfectious encephalomyelitis is a demyelinating disease that presents during the recovery phase, and is thought to be caused by a postinfectious autoimmune response.[6] The major manifestations include fever, headache, neck stiffness, ataxia, mental status changes, and seizures. CSF analysis demonstrates lymphocytosis and elevated proteins. Postinfectious encephalomyelitis has a 10 to 20 percent mortality rate, and residual neurologic abnormalities are common.[6]
- Subacute sclerosing panencephalitis (SSPE) is a progressive, fatal, neurological degenerative disease that may represent a persistent infection of the central nervous system with a variant of the virus. It usually occurs in patients younger than 20 years of age and 7 to 10 years after natural measles.[7] Patients develop neurologic symptoms, myoclonus, dementia, and eventually flaccidity or decorticate rigidity.
- Measles in pregnancy is a rare entity in areas that practice vaccination. Premature births may be more common in gravid women with measles, but there is no clear evidence of teratogenicity.[8,9]
- When measles occurs during pregnancy, maternal and fetal morbidity is increased. The virus is not responsible for congenital defects but can induce placental damage which may lead to fetal death. Major perinatal risks are also miscarriage and prematurity. When measles occurs in late pregnancy, congenital infection is possible.[8]

RISK FACTORS

For developing measles:

- Failure to receive immunization.
- Failure to receive second immunization dose.
- Travel to endemic areas.
- Exposure to travelers from endemic areas.

For developing severe measles or for developing complications:

- Immunodeficiency.
- Malnutrition.
- Pregnancy.
- Vitamin A deficiency.
- Age younger than 5 years or older than 20 years.

DIAGNOSIS

Measles is a distinct disease characterized by fever, malaise, conjunctivitis, coryza, cough, rash, and Koplik's spots.

CLINICAL FEATURES

Koplik's spots appear during the prodrome phase and are pathognomonic for measles infection and occur approximately 48 hours before the characteristic measles exanthem. The classic blanching rash, along with the prodrome and Koplik spots, is usually adequate to make a tentative diagnosis. The most rapid and accurate test to confirm acute measles is a blood test for measles specific IgM antibodies. By waiting until the third day of the rash, a false-negative IgM result can be avoided.[1]

TYPICAL DISTRIBUTION

The rash begins on the face and spreads centrifugally to involve the neck, trunk, and finally the extremities. The lesions may become confluent, especially on the face. This cranial-to-caudal rash progression is characteristic of measles.

DIFFERENTIAL DIAGNOSIS

- Upper respiratory tract infections—The prodrome stage of measles can be confused with a URI except that significant fever is typically present with measles infection.
- Fordyce spots—Tiny yellow-white granules on the buccal or lip mucosa caused by benign ectopic sebaceous glands, may be mistaken for Koplik's spots. Fordyce spots do not have an erythematous base.
- Alternative diagnoses that may be confused with the measles rash include Rocky Mountain spotted fever, infectious mononucleosis, scarlet fever, Kawasaki disease, toxic shock syndrome, dengue fever, and simple drug eruption (see Chapter 154, Cutaneous Drug Reactions).
- Measles can usually be distinguished clinically from rubella, erythema infectiosum (parvovirus B19 infection), roseola, and enteroviral infection by the intensity of the measles rash, its subsequent brownish coloration, the classic prodrome, and the severe disease course.

MANAGEMENT

NONPHARMACOLOGIC

- The treatment of measles is mostly supportive. Suspected cases of measles should be immediately reported to the local or state department of health.

MEDICATIONS

- Measures to control spread of infection should not be delayed for laboratory confirmation. Vaccine should be promptly administered to all susceptible persons, or they should be removed from the outbreak setting for a minimum of 3 weeks. SOR Ⓒ
- Giving serum immune globulin 0.25 mL/kg of body weight to a maximum dose of 15 mL to a susceptible person within 6 days of exposure to measles, can prevent or modify disease. This is especially important in patients in whom the risk of complications of measles is higher such as pregnant women, children younger than 1 year of age, and immunocompromised patients. SOR Ⓒ
- The World Health Organization recommends vitamin A for all children with acute measles, regardless of their country of residence, to reduce risk of complications. Vitamin A is administered once a day for 2 days at the following doses:

- 50,000 IU for infants aged <6 months.
- 100,000 IU for infants aged 6 to 11 months.
- 200,000 IU for children aged ≥12 months.
- A third, age-specific dose of vitamin A is given 2 to 4 weeks later to patients with clinical signs and symptoms of vitamin A deficiency.[1] SOR Ⓑ

REFERRAL OR HOSPITALIZATION

Consider hospitalization in the following scenarios:

- Difficulty breathing or noisy breathing—Bronchopneumonia occurs in 5 to 10 percent of patients.
- Changes in behavior, confusion—May be a harbinger of acute disseminated encephalomyelitis.
- There is dehydration, which can be the result of diarrhea, vomiting, and poor oral intake.

Refer to ophthalmology if there are changes in vision as measles keratitis can lead to permanent scarring and blindness.

PREVENTION

- Measures to control spread of infection should not be delayed for laboratory confirmation. Vaccine should be promptly administered to all susceptible persons, or they should be removed from the outbreak setting for a minimum of 3 weeks.
- Initial and booster immunization.
- Avoidance of endemic areas without being fully immunized.
- If traveling overseas, the CDC recommends infants 6 to 11 months receive 1 dose of MMR prior to travel (even though the first dose is routinely not recommended until 12 months of age). The MMR given prior to 12 months of age should not be counted as part of the routine vaccination.
- CDC recommends that children over 12 months old traveling overseas should receive the second MMR vaccine at least 28 days apart from the initial vaccination.[1]
- Adequate nutrition including Vitamin A.
- Hand washing.

PROGNOSIS

- The disease is typically self-limited. Measles typically lasts approximately 10 to 14 days from the beginning of the prodrome to the fading of the eruption.
- Approximately 30 percent of measles cases have one or more complications. Complications of measles are more common among patients younger than 5 years of age and adults 20 years of age and older. Centers for Disease Control and Prevention (CDC) reported measles complications include:[6]
  - Diarrhea—8 percent.
  - Otitis media—7 percent.
  - Pneumonia—6 percent.
  - Encephalitis—0.1 percent.
  - Seizures—0.6 to 0.7 percent.
  - Death—0.2 percent.

FOLLOW-UP

- Have patients watched for changes that indicate more severe disease or complications.
- Make sure return appointments for full vaccination is scheduled.

PATIENT EDUCATION

- Avoid exposure to other individuals, particularly unimmunized children and adults, pregnant women, and immunocompromised persons, until at least 4 days after rash onset.
- Avoid contact with potential sources of secondary bacterial pathogens until respiratory symptoms resolve.

PATIENT RESOURCES

- Measles from KidsHealth—**http://kidshealth.org/parent/infections/bacterial_viral/measles.html#cat20028**.
- Centers for Disease Control and Prevention, Two Options for Protecting Your Child Against Measles, Mumps, Rubella, and Varicella—**www.cdc.gov/vaccines/vpd-vac/combo-vaccines/mmrv/vacopt-factsheet-parent.htm**.
- Centers for Disease Control and Prevention, Measles: Make Sure Your Child Is Fully Immunized—**www.cdc.gov/Features/Measles/**.
- Centers for Disease Control and Prevention, Who Should NOT Get Vaccinated with the MMRV (Measles, Mumps, Rubella, and Varicella) vaccine—**www.cdc.gov/vaccines/vpd-vac/should-not-vacc.htm#mmrv**.

PROVIDER RESOURCES

- MedlinePlus-Measles—**www.nlm.nih.gov/medlineplus/measles.html**.
- CDC Measles—http:**//www.cdc.gov/measles/index.html**.
- Centers for Disease Control and Prevention, Manual for the Surveillance of Vaccine-Preventable Diseases (4th edition, 2008). Chapter 7: Measles. **www.cdc.gov/vaccines/pubs/surv-manual/chpt07-measles.html**.
- Centers for Disease Control and Prevention, Epidemiology and Prevention of Vaccine-Preventable Diseases, The Pink Book: Course Textbook, 12th edition (April 2011); Measles. **www.cdc.gov/vaccines/pubs/pinkbook/meas.html**.

REFERENCES

1. Centers for Disease Control and Prevention. *Manual for the Surveillance of Vaccine-Preventable Diseases* (5th edition, 2012). Chapter 7: Measles. http://www.cdc.gov/vaccines/pubs/surv-manual/chpt07-measles.html, accessed December 18, 2012.

2. World Health Organization. *Global eradication of measles: report by the Secretariat*. http://apps.who.int/gb/ebwha/pdf_files/WHA63/A63_18-en.pdf, accessed December 18, 2012.
3. MMWR Morb Mortal Wkly Rep. 2012 Feb 3;61(4):73-8. Progress in global measles control, 2000-2010.Centers for Disease Control and Prevention (CDC). Accessed December 18, 2012
4. Carrillo-Santisteve P, Lopalco PL. Measles still spreads in Europe: who is responsible for the failure to vaccinate? *Clin Microbiol Infect*. 2012;18(5):50-56.
5. Kaplan LJ, Daum RS, Smaron M, McCarthy CA. Severe measles in immunocompromised patients. *JAMA*. 1992;267:1237.
6. Johnson RT, Griffin DE, Hirsch RL, et al. Measles encephalomyelitis—clinical and immunologic studies. *N Engl J Med*. 1984;310:137.
7. Bellini WJ, Rota JS, Lowe LE, et al. Subacute sclerosing panencephalitis: More cases of this fatal disease are prevented by measles immunization than was previously recognized. *J Infect Dis*. 2005;192:1686.
8. Anselem O, Tsatsaris V. Measles and pregnancy. *Presse Med*. 2011; 40(11):1001-1007.
9. Chiba ME, Saito M. Measles infection in pregnancy. *J Infect*. 2003; 47(1):40-44.

112 FIFTH DISEASE

E.J. Mayeaux, Jr., MD
John H. Haynes, Jr., MD
Mathew Prine, MD

PATIENT STORY

A 2-year-old boy presents with mild flu-like symptoms and a rash. He had an erythematous malar rash and a "lace-like" erythematous rash on the trunk and extremities (**Figures 112-1** and **112-2**). The "slapped cheek" appearance made the diagnosis easy for fifth disease. The parents were reassured that this would resolve spontaneously. The child returned to daycare the next day.

INTRODUCTION

Fifth disease is also commonly referred to as erythema infectiosum. The name derives from the fact that it represents the fifth of the 6 common childhood viral exanthems described. Transmission occurs through respiratory secretions, possibly through fomites, and parenterally via vertical transmission from mother to fetus and by transfusion of blood or blood products.

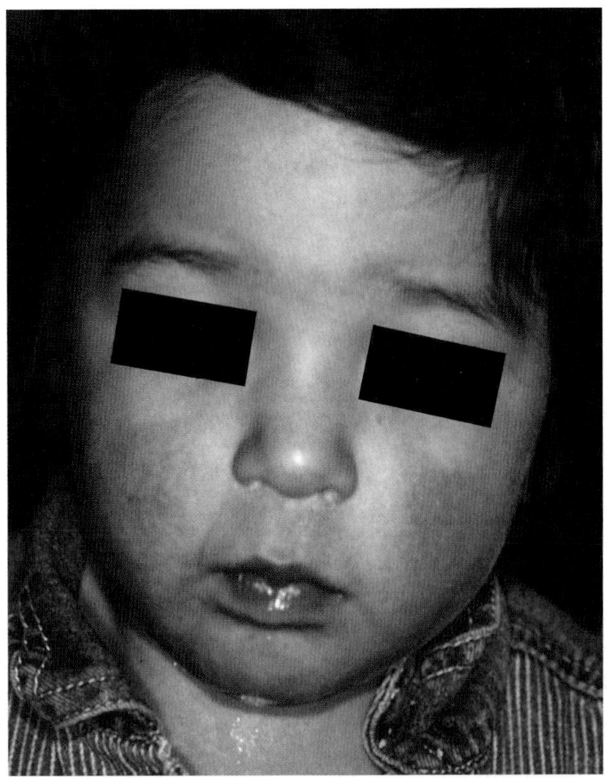

FIGURE 112-1 Classic erythematous malar rash with "slapped cheek" appearance of fifth disease (erythema infectiosum). (*Used with permission from Richard P. Usatine, MD.*)

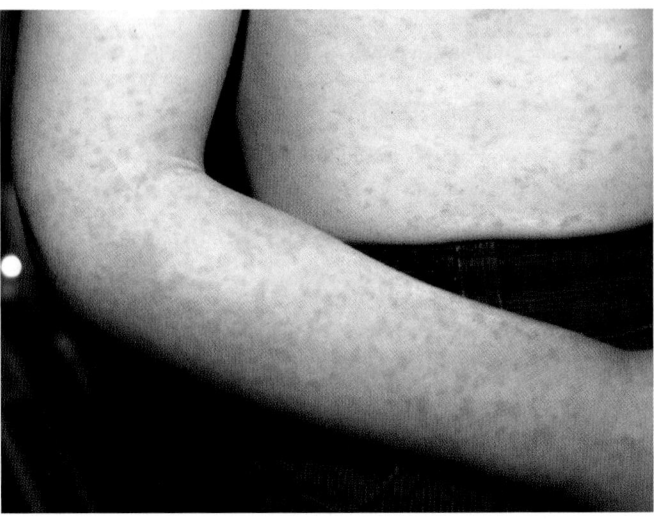

FIGURE 112-2 Classic fifth disease "lace-like" erythematous rash on the trunk and extremities. (*Used with permission from Richard P. Usatine, MD.*)

SYNONYMS

Erythema infectiosum, parvovirus B19 infections, slapped cheek disease.

EPIDEMIOLOGY

- Fifth disease is common throughout the world. Antiparvovirus B19 immunoglobulin (Ig) G is found equally among Americans, Asians, and Europeans.[1] The only known host for B19 is humans.
- Most individuals become infected during their school-age years.
- Fifth disease is very contagious via the respiratory route and occurs more frequently between late winter and early summer. Up to 60 percent of the population is seropositive for antiparvovirus B19 IgG by age 20 years.[2] In some communities, there are cycles of local epidemics every 4 to 10 years.[3]
- Thirty to forty percent of pregnant women lack measurable IgG to the infecting agent and are, therefore, presumed to be susceptible to infection. Infection during pregnancy can in some cases lead to fetal death.

ETIOLOGY AND PATHOPHYSIOLOGY

- Fifth disease is a mild viral febrile illness with an associated rash caused by parvovirus B19 (**Figure 112-3**).
- Most persons with parvovirus B19 infection never develop the clinical picture of fifth disease.
- Parvovirus B19 infects rapidly dividing cells and is cytotoxic for erythroid progenitor cells.
- After initial infection, a viremia occurs with an associated precipitous drop in the reticulocyte count and anemia. The anemia is rarely clinically apparent in healthy patients, but can cause serious anemia if the red blood cell count is already low. Patients with a

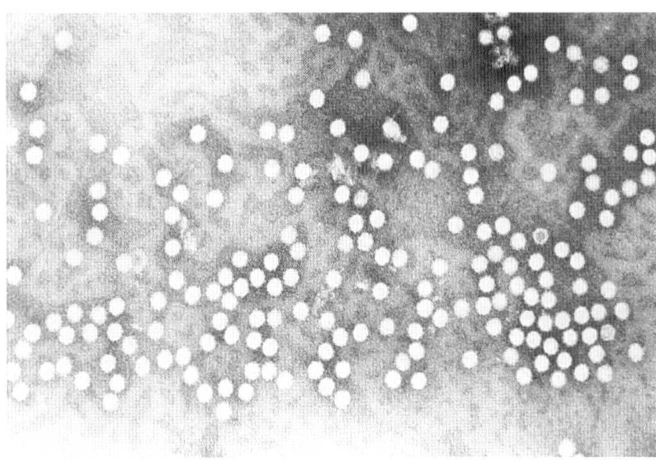

FIGURE 112-3 Transmission electron microscopy of parvovirus B19. *(Used with permission from the Centers for Disease Control and Prevention.)*

chronic anemia such as sickle cell or thalassemia may experience a transient aplastic crisis.[4]

- Vertical transmission can result in congenital infection if a woman becomes infected during her pregnancy.[5] The risk of a fetal loss or hydrops fetalis is greatest (loss rate of 11%) when the infection occurs within the first 20 weeks of gestation.[6]

RISK FACTORS

- Exposure to infected children.
- Reception of blood products.

DIAGNOSIS

CLINICAL FEATURES—HISTORY AND PHYSICAL

- Fifth disease is usually a biphasic illness, starting with upper respiratory tract symptoms that may include headache, fever, sore throat, pruritus, coryza, abdominal pain, diarrhea, and/or arthralgias. These constitutional symptoms coincide with onset of viremia and they usually resolve for about a week before the next stage begins. Associated hematologic abnormalities may be seen with this stage.
- The second stage is characterized by a classic erythematous malar rash with relative circumoral pallor or "slapped cheek" appearance in children (**Figures 112-1** and **112-4**) followed by a "lace-like" erythematous rash on the trunk and extremities (**Figures 112-2** and **112-5**). Arthropathy affecting the hands, wrists, knees, and ankles may precede the development of a rash in adults. The course is usually self-limited.

TYPICAL DISTRIBUTION

- The rash starts with the classic slapped-cheek appearance (**Figures 112-1** and **112-4**). Then an erythematous macular rash occurs on the extremities. After several days, the extremities rash fades into a lacy pattern (**Figures 112-2** and **112-5**). The exanthem may

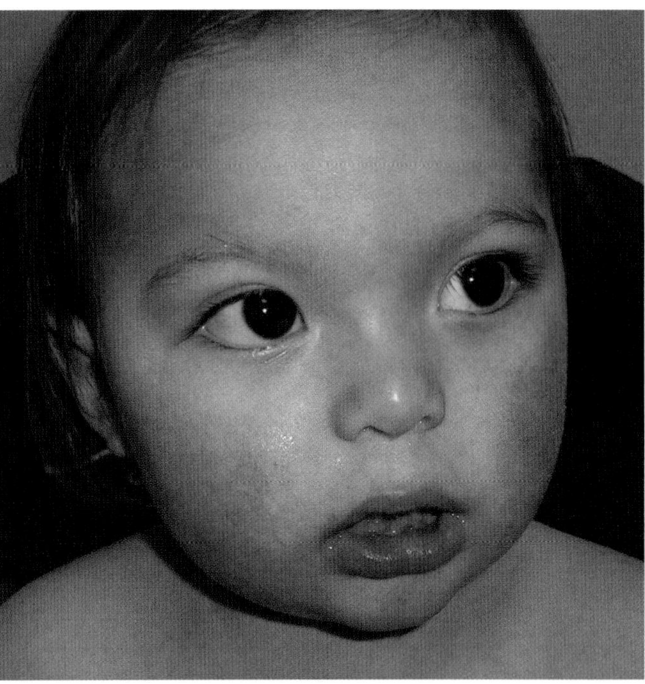

FIGURE 112-4 Classic erythematous malar rash with "slapped cheek" appearance of fifth disease in an 18-month-old child. *(Used with permission from Richard P. Usatine, MD.)*

recur over several weeks in association with exercise, sun exposure, bathing in hot water, or stress.

LABORATORY TESTING

- Laboratory studies are not usually needed as the diagnosis can be made by history and physical exam. Serum B19-specific IgM may be ordered in pregnant women exposed to fifth disease. After 3 weeks, infection is also indicated by a 4-fold or greater rise in serum B19-specific IgG antibody titers.
- Patients with symptoms of anemia, a history of increased red blood cell (RBC) destruction (e.g., sickle cell disease, hereditary

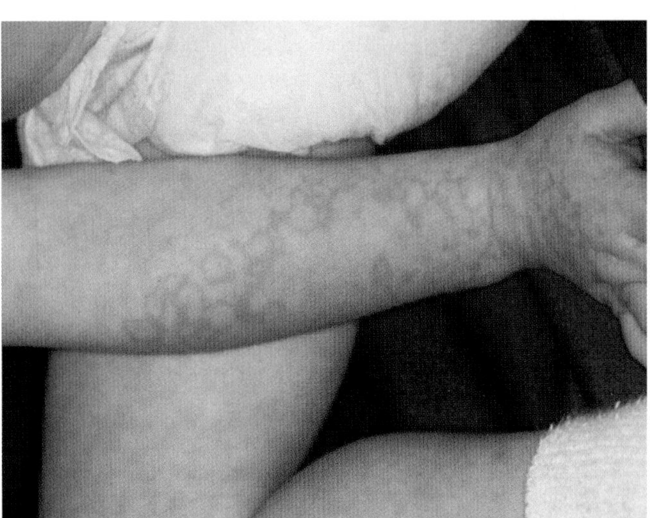

FIGURE 112-5 Classic reticular eruption on the extremities. *(Used with permission from Jeffrey Meffert, MD.)*

spherocytosis), or with decreased RBC production (e.g., iron-deficiency anemia) should be tested to determine the degree of anemia.

- Pregnant women who are exposed to or have symptoms of parvovirus infection should have serologic testing. Prior to 20 weeks' gestation, women testing positive for acute infection (i.e., positive IgM and negative IgG) should be counseled concerning the low risk of fetal loss and congenital anomalies. There are currently no proven associations with congenital abnormalities, but there is low risk of fetal loss.[7]

IMAGING

- If serologic testing in pregnant women is positive, some experts recommend that the patient should receive ultrasounds to look for signs of fetal hydrops. Intrauterine transfusion is currently the only effective treatment to alleviate fetal anemia.[8]

DIFFERENTIAL DIAGNOSIS

- Scarlet fever presents as a fine papular (sandpaper) rash in association with a *Streptococcus* infection (see Chapter 28, Scarlet Fever and Strawberry Tongue).
- Allergic-hypersensitivity reactions (erythema multiforme, erythema nodosum and cutaneous vasculitis) often involve the arms and legs but rarely affect the face (see Section 12: Hypersensitivity Syndromes and Drug Reactions).
- Lyme disease presents with an expanding rash with central clearing (see Chapter 183, Lyme Disease).
- Measles produces a blanching rash that begins on the face and spreads centrifugally to involve the neck, trunk, and finally the extremities. It tends to become more confluent instead of lacy with time (see Chapter 111, Measles).

MANAGEMENT

NONPHARMACOLOGIC

- Fifth disease is usually self-limited and requires no specific therapy.
- See the following "Patient Education" section for further information about parvovirus B19 infections in pregnancy.

MEDICATIONS

- NSAID or acetaminophen therapy may alleviate fevers and arthralgias.
- Transient aplastic anemia occurs in individuals who have baseline anemia and may be severe enough to require transfusion until the patient's red cell production recovers.

PREVENTION

- Because it is spread through respiratory secretions and possibly through fomites, good hand sanitation and infection-control techniques are recommended.
- Infected individuals should avoid excessive heat or sunlight, which can cause rash flare-ups.

PROGNOSIS

- The rash of erythema infectiosum usually is self-limiting, but may last weeks to months with exacerbations.
- Aplastic anemia usually lasts up to 2 weeks but may become chronic. The onset of erythema infectiosum rash usually indicates that reticulocytosis has returned and aplastic crisis will not occur.

PATIENT EDUCATION

- Explain to parents that the disease is usually self-limited. Normal activities may be pursued as tolerated with sun protection or avoidance.
- Children who present with the classic findings of fifth disease are past the infectious state and can attend school and day care.
- During pregnancy, a woman who has an acute infection prior to 20 weeks' gestation should be counseled concerning the low risks of fetal loss and congenital anomalies. Beyond 20 weeks' gestation, some physicians recommend repeated ultrasounds to look for signs of fetal hydrops.

PATIENT RESOURCES

- Centers for Disease Control and Prevention (CDC). *Parvovirus B19 and Fifth Disease*—**www.cdc.gov/parvovirusB19/fifth-disease.html**.
- Centers for Disease Control and Prevention (CDC). *Pregnancy and Fifth Disease*—**www.cdc.gov/parvovirusB19/pregnancy.html**.
- eMedicine health. *Fifth Disease*—**www.emedicinehealth.com/fifth_disease/article_em.htm**.
- PubMed Health. *Fifth Disease*—**www.ncbi.nlm.nih.gov/pubmedhealth/PMH0001972/**.

PROVIDER RESOURCES

- Medscape. *Fifth Disease or Erythema Infectiosum*—**http://emedicine.medscape.com/article/801732**.

REFERENCES

1. Young NS, Brown KE. Parvovirus B19. *N Engl J Med*. 2004;350(6):586-597.
2. American Academy of Pediatrics. *Red Book: 2006 Report on the Committee of Infectious Diseases*. 2006:484-487.
3. Naides SJ. Erythema infectiosum (fifth disease) occurrence in Iowa. *Am J Public Health*. 1988;78(9):1230-1231.
4. Serjeant GR, Serjeant BE, Thomas PW, et al. Human parvovirus infection in homozygous sickle cell disease. *Lancet*. 1993;341(8855):1237-1240.
5. Jordan JA. Identification of human parvovirus B19 infection in idiopathic nonimmune hydrops fetalis. *Am J Obstet Gynecol*. 1996;174(1 Pt 1):37-42.

6. Enders M, Weidner A, Zoellner I, et al. Fetal morbidity and mortality after acute human parvovirus B19 infection in pregnancy: prospective evaluation of 1018 cases. *Prenat Diagn.* 2004; 24(7):513-518.
7. Enders M, Weidner A, Rosenthal T, et al. Improved diagnosis of gestational parvovirus B19 infection at the time of nonimmune fetal hydrops. *J Infect Dis.* 2008;197:58. http://www.ncbi.nlm.nih.gov/pubmed?term=20729141.
8. de Jong EP, de Haan TR, Kroes ACM, et al. Parvovirus B19 infection in pregnancy. *J Clin Virol.* 2006;36(1):1-7.

113 HAND FOOT MOUTH SYNDROME

E.J. Mayeaux, Jr., MD
Steven N. Bienvenu, MD

PATIENT STORY

A 4-year-old boy presents to a free clinic for homeless families with a low-grade fever and lesions on his hands and feet (**Figures 113-1** and **113-2**). The mother notes that two other kids in the transitional living center also have a similar rash. Upon further investigation, mouth lesions are noted (**Figure 113-3**). The mother is reassured that this is nothing more than hand, foot, and mouth disease and will go away on its own. Treatment includes fluids and antipyretics as needed.

INTRODUCTION

Hand, foot, and mouth disease (HFMD) is a viral illness that may affect humans and some animals, and presents with a distinct clinical presentation. The disease occurs worldwide. In 2011 and 2012, an outbreak of a much more severe and atypical form occurred in the US.

EPIDEMIOLOGY

- Epidemics tend to occur every 3 years worldwide. In temperate climates, the peak incidence is in late summer and early fall.
- HFMD generally has a mild course, but it may be more severe in infants and young children.[1,2]
- There is no racial or gender predilection. Most cases affect children younger than 10 years old.[3]

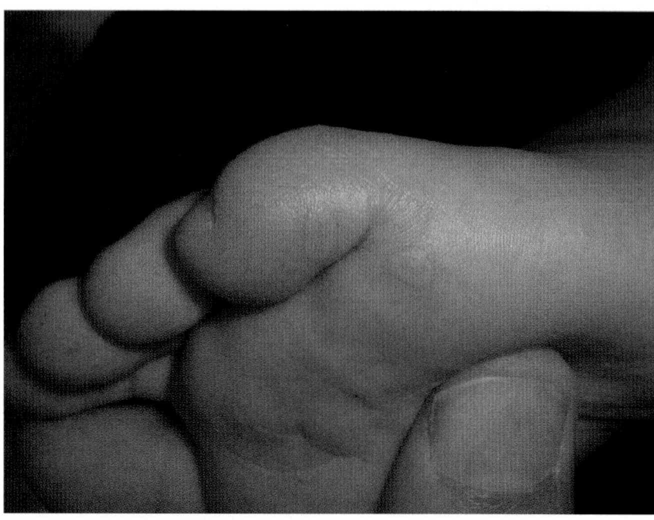

FIGURE 113-2 Foot of the boy in **Figure 113-1**. Lesions tend to be on palms and soles, fingers, and toes. (*Used with permission from Richard P. Usatine, MD.*)

ETIOLOGY AND PATHOPHYSIOLOGY

- HFMD is most commonly caused by members of the enterovirus genus, especially coxsackie viruses. Epidemic infections in the US are usually caused by coxsackievirus A16, and less commonly by other coxsackievirus A strains, coxsackievirus B, or enterovirus 71.[2,3] Sporadic cases occur caused by other coxsackie viruses.
- HFMD is caused by a number of different enteroviruses around the world with different characteristics, but until recently outbreaks of an A6 strain have not been experienced in the US. Most HFMD cases worldwide are due to coxsackievirus A16.[4,5]
- Outbreaks of strains of EV71 enterovirus producing large epidemics of HFMD with significant morbidity and mortality that have occurred recently in east and southeast Asia have not been seen in the US.[5]

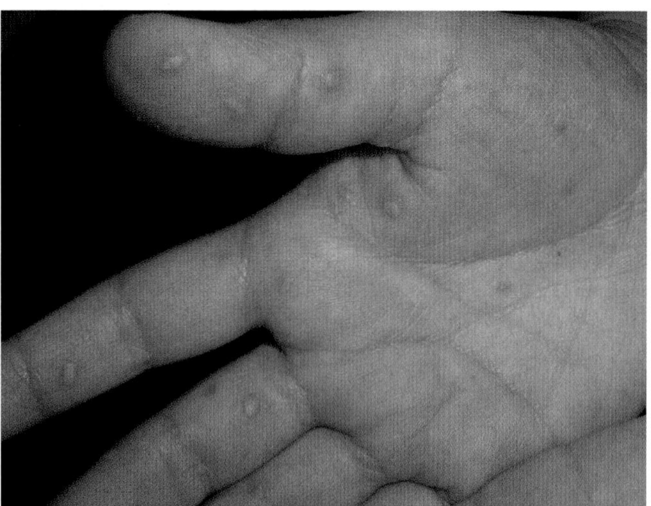

FIGURE 113-1 Typical flat vesicular lesions on the hand of a 4-year-old boy with hand, foot, and mouth disease. (*Used with permission from Richard P. Usatine, MD.*)

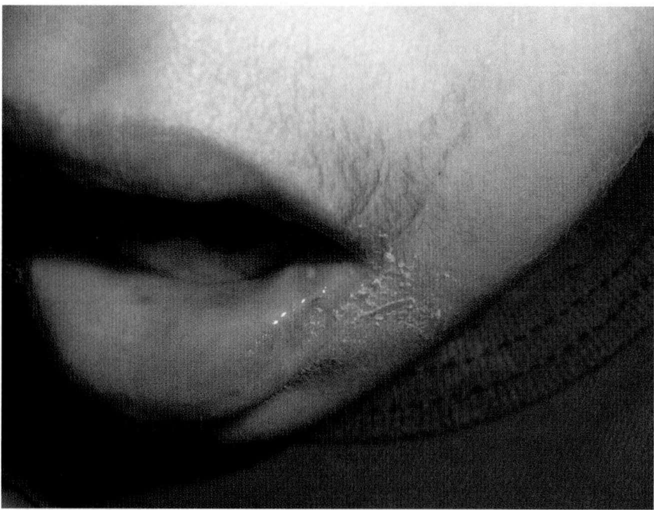

FIGURE 113-3 Mouth lesions in same boy appear as small ulcers on the lips and oral mucosa. (*Used with permission from Richard P. Usatine, MD.*)

- In the fall of 2011 and early winter of 2012, 63 cases of apparent, but more severe HFMD from four US states were reported to the CDC. PCR and gene sequencing detected an A6 strain of coxsackievirus in 74 percent of clinical specimens from 38 cases.[4] Cases of this atypical, severe form of HFMD have now likely been diagnosed throughout much of North America.[4,6,7]
- Coxsackievirus infections are highly contagious. Transmission occurs via aerosolized droplets of nasal and/or oral secretions via the fecal–oral route, or from contact with skin lesions. During epidemics, the virus is spread from child to child and from mother to fetus.
- The incubation period averages 3 to 6 days. Initial viral implantation is in the GI tract mucosa, and it then spreads to lymph nodes within 24 hours. Viremia rapidly ensues, with spread to the oral mucosa and skin. Rarely, aseptic meningitis may occur. Usually by day 7, a neutralizing antibody response develops, and the virus is cleared from the body.
- HFMD may also result in neurologic problems such as a polio-like syndrome, aseptic meningitis, encephalitis, acute cerebellar ataxia, acute transverse myelitis, Guillain-Barré syndrome, and benign intracranial hypertension. Rarely, cardiopulmonary complications such as myocarditis, interstitial pneumonitis, and pulmonary edema may occur.[8,9]
- Infection in the first trimester of pregnancy may lead to spontaneous abortion or intrauterine growth retardation.

RISK FACTORS

- Attendance at child care centers.
- Contact with HFMD.
- Large family.
- Rural residence.

DIAGNOSIS

CLINICAL FEATURES

- A prodrome lasting 12 to 36 hours is usually the first sign of HFMD, and it usually consists of typical general viral infection symptoms with anorexia, abdominal pain, and sore mouth. Lesions are present for 5 to 10 days, and heal spontaneously in 5 to 7 days. Fever is usually mild.
- Atypical, severe HFMD (A6) may be associated with fever as high as 103 to 105 degrees Fahrenheit, produce much more extensive, denser rash in more locations, with greater malaise and likelihood of anorexia, dehydration, and pain.[4]
- Each lesion in typical HFMD begins as a 2- to 10-mm erythematous macule, which develops a gray, oval vesicle that parallels the skin tension lines in its long axis (**Figures 113-1** and **113-2**). The oral lesions (**Figure 113-3**) begin as erythematous macules, evolve into 2- to 3-mm vesicles on an erythematous base, and then rapidly become ulcerated. The vesicles are painful and may interfere with eating. They are not generally pruritic.
- **Atypical** (A6) HFMD may produce lesions that are very protean in their character and evolution. Early lesions are usually maculovesicular as with the milder A16 form, but may coalesce (**Figure 113-4**). Others may be vesiculobullous (**Figure 113-5**) and may drain, or simply papular (**Figure 113-6**), or maculopapular and ulcerative (**Figure 113-7**).[4,6,7]

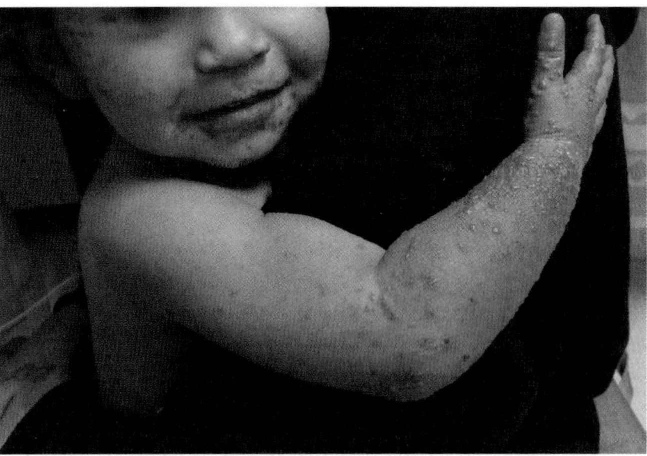

FIGURE 113-4 A one-year-old male with confirmed Coxsackievirus A6 HFMD. His temperature reached 103.8 degrees, and a variety of lesions are visible as well as Koebner phenomenon near the elbow flexure. (*Used with permission from Ann Petru, MD and Julie Kulhanjian, MD.*)

- Cervical or submandibular lymphadenopathy may be present.

TYPICAL DISTRIBUTION

- Skin lesions of the milder form (A16) develop on the hands, feet, and/or buttocks and oral lesions may involve the palate, buccal

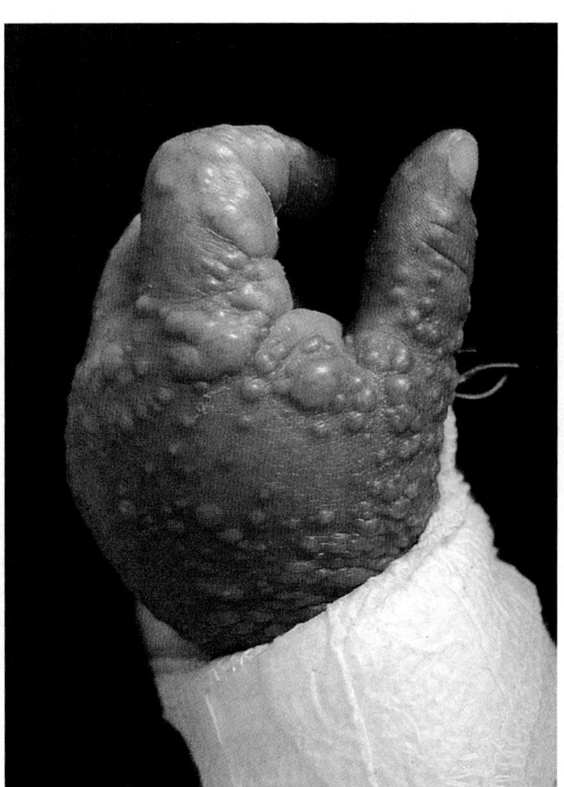

FIGURE 113-5 Vesiculobullous lesions of left hand of child in **Figure 113-4**. Bullous lesions may rupture. (*Used with permission from Ann Petru, MD and Julie Kulhanjian, MD.*)

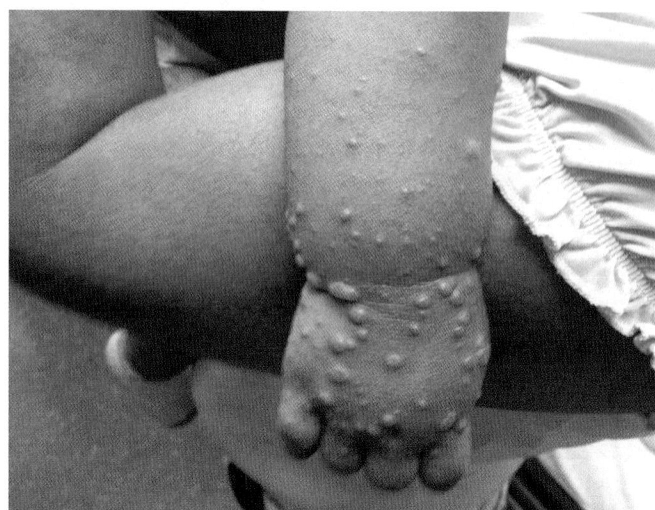

FIGURE 113-6 A 15-month-old female with confirmed A6 infection who demonstrated widespread disease and multiple lesion types. (*Used with permission from Ann Petru, MD.*)

mucosa, gingiva, and/or tongue. Lesions on the hands and feet are largely limited to the palmar and plantar surfaces.

- Atypical, severe HFMD (A6) produces a much more extensive rash, and may include the lips and perioral area of the face (**Figure 113-4** and **113-8**), arms, legs, knees, genitalia, trunk (**Figure 113-7**), buttocks (**Figure 113-9**), perianal area, and distinctively the *dorsal* areas of the hands (**Figures 113-5**, **113-6**, and **113-10**) and feet as well as palmar and plantar surfaces. Distribution can be quite variable, however.[4,7]

LABORATORY TESTING

- Laboratory tests are usually not needed for diagnosis.

BIOPSY

Biopsy is not needed.

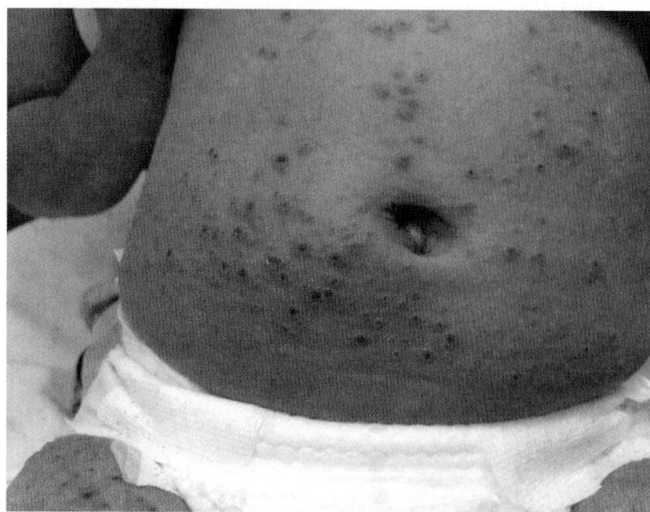

FIGURE 113-7 The abdomen of the child in **Figure 113-5** demonstrating two varieties of lesions in the same patient. (*Used with permission from Ann Petru, MD.*)

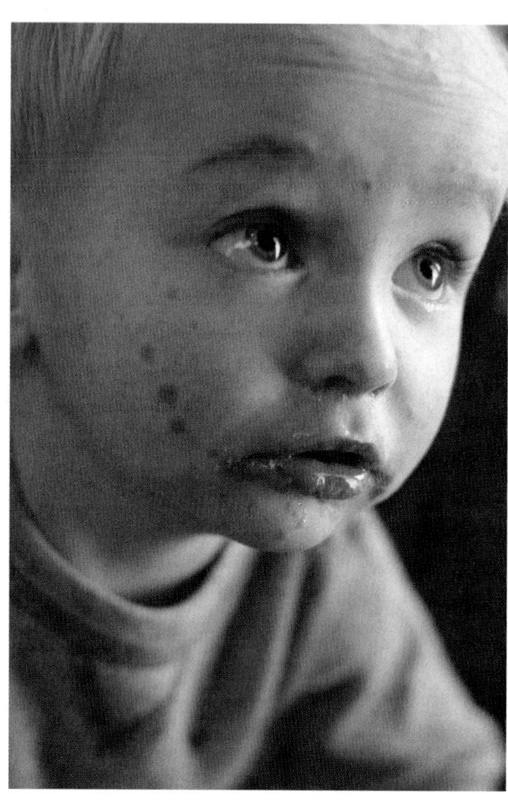

FIGURE 113-8 A 16-month-old male with clinically diagnosed HFMD, likely A6 strain disease. This child had typical perioral / facial, buttocks and leg involvement. (*Used with permission from Storiesofgrandeur.blogspot.com.*)

DIFFERENTIAL DIAGNOSIS

- Aphthous stomatitis presents as single or multiple painful ulcers in the mouth without skin eruptions (see Chapter 40, Aphthous Ulcer).
- Chickenpox presents with body-wide vesicular lesions in multiple crops (see Chapter 108, Chickenpox).
- Erythema multiforme demonstrates body-wide target lesions that also involve the skin of the palms and soles (see Chapter 151,

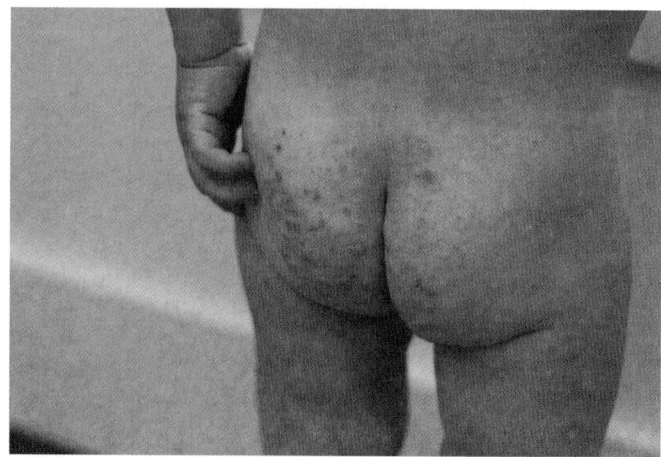

FIGURE 113-9 Buttocks of the child in **Figure 113-8**. (*Used with permission from Storiesofgrandeur.blogspot.com.*)

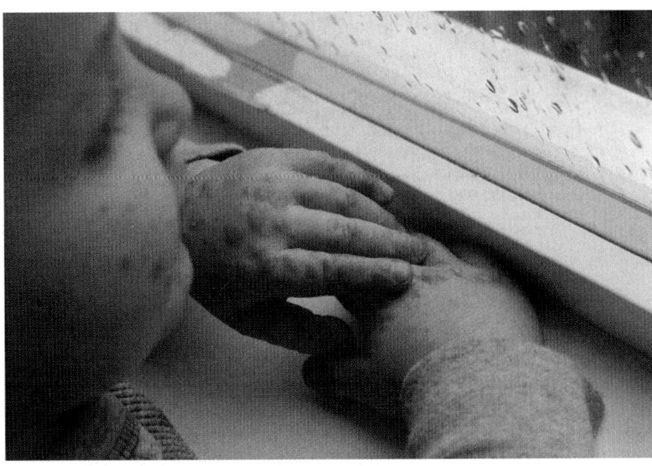

FIGURE 113-10 Dorsal surface papular hand lesions of the child in **Figures 113-8** and **113-9**. (*Used with permission from Storiesofgrandeur. blogspot.com.*)

Erythema Multiforme, Stevens-Johnson Syndrome, and Toxic Epidermal Necrolysis).

- Herpes simplex presents with painful recurrent ulcerations of the lips or genitals without simultaneous hand or foot lesions unless there is a herpetic whitlow on the hand (see Chapter 114, Herpes Simplex).
- Eczema herpeticum lesions may very much resemble those of the atypical (severe) form of HFMD, but careful exam usually reveals the typical perioral/intraoral lesions and concurrent hand and foot distribution of HFMD. This new form of HFMD has also been misdiagnosed as varicella (see Chapter 108, Chickenpox), impetigo (see Chapter 99, Impetigo), poison ivy, and atypical Kawasaki disease. Some cases have not manifested intraoral lesions, or lesions on hands or feet.[6,7]

MANAGEMENT

NONPHARMACOLOGIC

- The treatment of HFMD is usually supportive. Usually the mouth lesions are not as painful as in herpes gingivostomatitis. If there is a lot of mouth pain leading to poor oral intake, the following medications may be considered. Topical oral anesthetics such as 2 percent viscous lidocaine by prescription or 20 percent topical benzocaine (Orabase) nonprescription may be used to treat painful oral ulcers. Benzocaine may not be safe in children under 2 years of age due to the risk of methemoglobinemia.[10] SOR Ⓒ
- A solution combining aluminum and magnesium hydroxide (liquid antacid) and 2 percent viscous lidocaine has been reported as helpful when swished and spit out several times a day as needed for pain. This must be limited to patients old enough to reliably spit out the material and avoid anesthetizing critical swallowing surfaces. SOR Ⓒ

MEDICATIONS

- Acetaminophen or NSAIDs/cyclooxygenase (COX)-2 s may be used to manage fever, and analgesics may be used to treat arthralgias. SOR Ⓒ Aspirin should not be used in viral illnesses in children younger than 12 years of age to prevent Reye syndrome. SOR Ⓒ

REFERRAL OR HOSPITALIZATION

- Patients with central nervous system (CNS) manifestations may require hospitalization.
- Those with the new atypical (A6) form are more likely to require hospitalization due to dehydration, severity of symptoms including pain, and diagnostic uncertainty.[5,8]

PREVENTION

- Good hand-washing is critical to reduce the spread of disease, both at home and at daycare facilities experiencing cases. Virus may be shed in stool for at least several weeks.

PROGNOSIS

- HFMD caused by coxsackie viruses is generally a mild self-limited illness that resolves in around 7 to 10 days. HFMD may rarely recur, persist, or cause serious complications.
- The recent atypical (A6) variety outbreak reported by the CDC resulted in a high rate of hospitalization (about 1 in 5 cases), but of the 63 cases reported to the CDC there were no deaths. Lesions tend to heal completely if not complicated. Beau's lines (Chapter 160, Normal Nail Variants) and onychomadesis (loss of nail) may occur many weeks later, followed by complete healing.[4,7] Illness in both the mild and the "new" atypical form of HFMD is usually followed by complete recovery without scarring. Uncommon CNS involvement has been the cause of most persistent morbidity and deaths associated with HFMD.

PATIENT EDUCATION

- Educate parents of young children to watch for signs of dehydration owing to decreased oral intake secondary to mouth pain.
- To reduce viral spreading, do not rupture blisters.
- The patient may attend school once fever and symptoms subside, no new lesions have appeared, and all lesions have dried or scabbed over.[6]
- The virus that causes hand, foot, and mouth disease may be present in the patient's stool for 1 month.
- Report any neurologic symptoms to health care providers immediately.
- Good hand washing and contact precautions are critical to preventing spread to others.

PATIENT RESOURCES

- Centers for Disease Control and Prevention. *CDC Feature: Hand, Foot, and Mouth Disease*—**www.cdc.gov/Features/HandFootMouthDisease/**.
- Centers for Disease Control and Prevention. *About Hand, Foot, and Mouth Disease (HFMD)*— **www.cdc.gov/hand-foot-mouth/about/**.
- eMedicine. *Hand, Foot and Mouth Disease*—**www.emedicinehealth.com/hand_foot_and_mouth_disease/article_em.htm**.

PROVIDER RESOURCES

- NHS Clinical Knowledge Summaries. *Hand, Foot and Mouth Disease*—**www.cks.nhs.uk/hand_foot_and_mouth_disease/evidence/references#**.
- Frydenberg A, Starr M. Hand, foot and mouth disease. *Aust Fam Physician.* 2003;328:594-595. **http://www.racgp.org.au/afp/200308/20030805starr2.pdf**.
- Centers for Disease Control and Prevention. *Hand, Foot, and Mouth Disease (HFMD)*—**www.cdc.gov/hand-foot-mouth/index.html**.
- A Guide to Clinical Management and Public Health Response for Hand, Foot and Mouth Disease (HFMD).
- **GuidancefortheclinicalmanagementofHFMD.pdf**
- A Quick Reference Sheet for Coxsackievirus A6 Questions—**www.cdph.ca.gov/programs/cder/Documents/CDPH%20-%20Enterovirus%20Quicksheet.doc.pdf**.

REFERENCES

1. Chang LY, King CC, Hsu KH, et al. Risk factors of enterovirus 71 infection and associated hand, foot, and mouth disease/herpangina in children during an epidemic in Taiwan. *Pediatrics.* 2002; 109(6):e88.
2. Chong CY, Chan KP, Shah VA, et al. Hand, foot and mouth disease in Singapore: a comparison of fatal and non-fatal cases. *Acta Paediatr.* 2003;92(10):1163-1169.
3. Frydenberg A, Starr M. Hand, foot and mouth disease. *Aust Fam Physician.* 2003;32(8):594-595.
4. Centers for Disease Control and Prevention (CDC). Notes from the field: severe hand, foot, and mouth disease associated with coxsackievirus A6—Alabama, Connecticut, California, and Nevada, November 2011-February 2012. *MMWR Morb Mortal Wkly Rep.* 2012;61:213-3.
5. World Health Organization Regional Office for the Western Pacific Region. *News Release: Severe hand, foot and mouth disease killed Cambodian children.* http://www.wpro.who.int/mediacentre/releases/2012/20120713/en/index.html, accessed December 8, 2012.
6. Inyo County Health and Human Services, Public Health Division—Inyo County Health Brief http://www.nih.org/docs/ICPHB_hand_foot_7_18_12.pdf. 2012.
7. Flett K, Youngster I, Huang J, McAdam A, Sandora TJ, Rennick M, et al. Hand, foot, and mouth disease caused by coxsackievirus A6 [letter]. Emerg Infect Dis [Internet]. 2012 Oct [date cited]. http://dx.doi.org/10.3201/eid1810.120813.
8. Chan KP, Goh KT, Chong CY, et al. Epidemic hand, foot and mouth disease caused by human enterovirus 71, Singapore. *Emerg Infect Dis.* 2003;9(1):78-85.
9. Chen SC, Chang HL, Yan TR, et al. An eight-year study of epidemiologic features of enterovirus 71 infection in Taiwan. *Am J Trop Med Hyg.* 2007;77(1):188-191.
10. US Food and Drug Administration. Drug Safety Communication: http://www.fda.gov/drugs/drugsafety/ucm250024.htm, accessed December 8, 2012.

114 HERPES SIMPLEX

E.J. Mayeaux, Jr., MD
Richard P. Usatine, MD

PATIENT STORY

A 4-year-old girl is brought to her pediatrician's office because of fever and sores in her mouth for the past 2 days. The child is alert, playful and fully oriented, and her doctor notes that she has crusting on her outer lips (**Figure 114-1A**). The mother pulls back the child's upper lip to show how her daughter's gums are inflamed (**Figure 114-1B**). There are small ulcers on the tip of the tongue (**Figure 114-2A**) and when the lower lip is pulled down there are obvious ulcers on the mucosa (**Figure 114-2B**). The doctor easily diagnoses primary herpes gingivostomatitis and determines that the child is drinking fluids but not eating. Her mucous membranes are moist and there are no signs of dehydration. The doctor recommends giving fluids that are nonacidic and somewhat cold (anything that will be tolerated). Oral acyclovir suspension is prescribed three times daily for 7 days. The following day the child the child became afebrile and was tolerating fluids and food better. Within 1 week, she was fully better and able to go back to preschool.

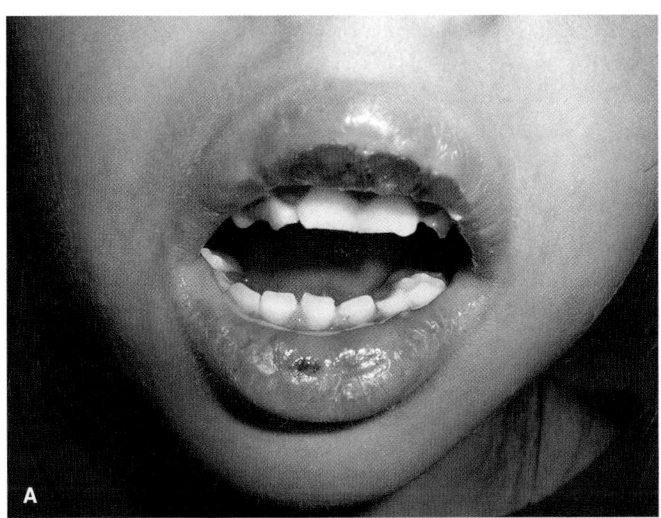

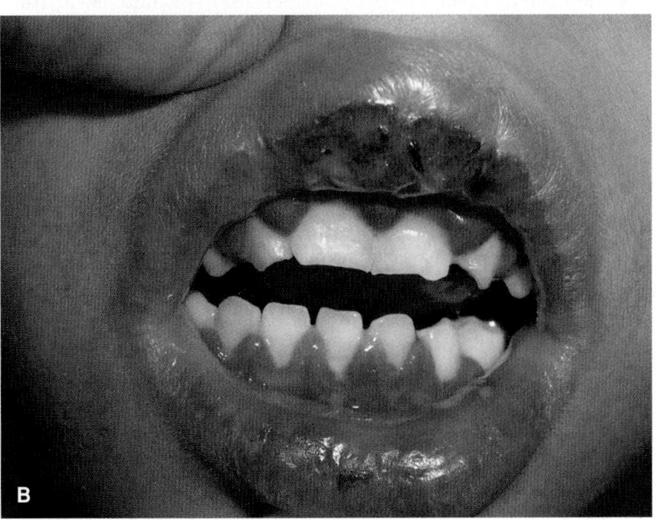

FIGURE 114-1 Primary herpes gingivostomatitis in a 4-year-old girl. **A.** Crusting on the lips. **B.** Gingivitis with significant erythema and swelling of the gums. (*Used with permission from Richard P. Usatine, MD.*)

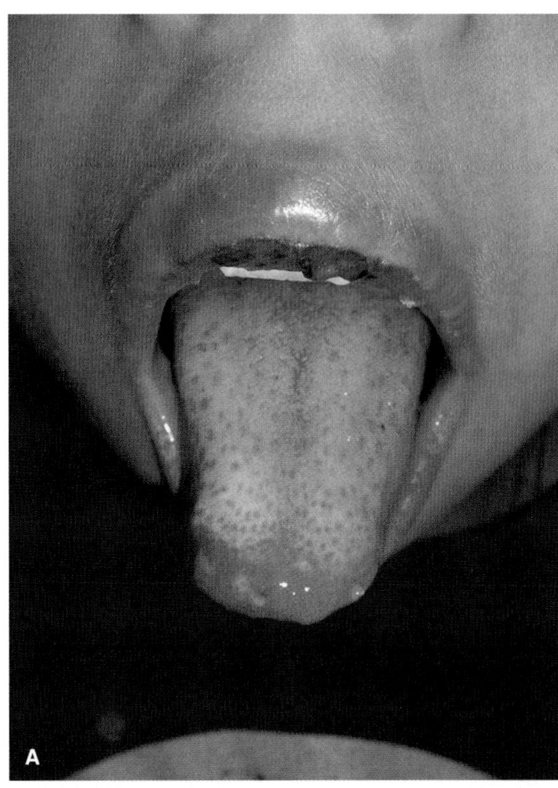

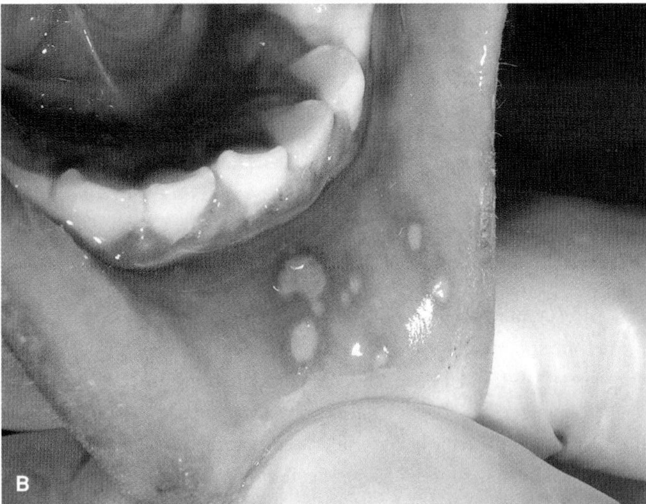

FIGURE 114-2 Primary herpes gingivostomatitis in a 4-year-old girl. **A.** Small ulcers on the tip of the tongue. **B.** HSV ulcers inside the lower lip. (*Used with permission from Richard P. Usatine, MD.*)

INTRODUCTION

Herpes simplex virus (HSV) infection can involve the skin, mucosa, eyes, and central nervous system. HSV establishes a latent state followed by viral reactivation and recurrent local disease. Perinatal

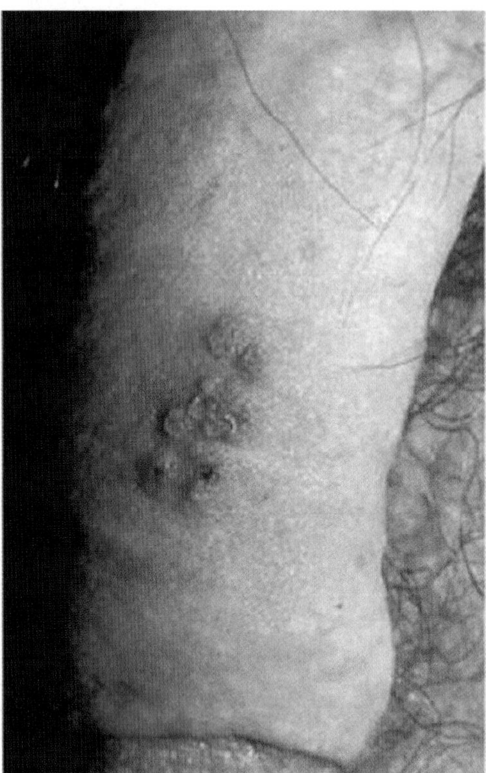

FIGURE 114-3 Herpes simplex on the penis with intact vesicles and visible crusts. (*Used with permission from Jack Rezneck, Sr., MD.*)

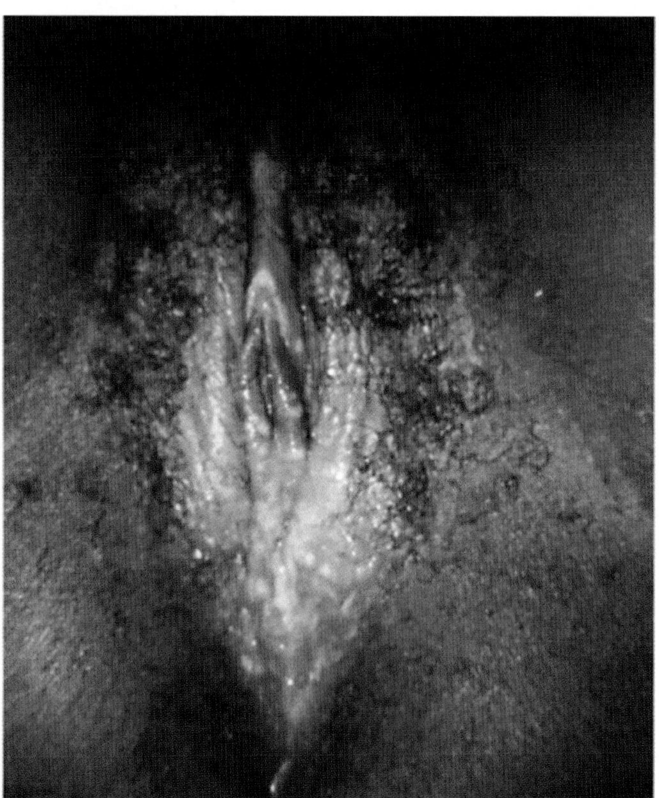

FIGURE 114-4 Vulvar herpes simplex virus at the introitus showing small punched out ulcers. (*Used with permission from the Centers for Disease Control and Prevention and Susan Lindsley.*)

transmission of HSV can lead to significant fetal morbidity and mortality.

EPIDEMIOLOGY

HSV affects more than 1/3 of the world's population, with the 2 most common cutaneous manifestations being orolabial herpes (**Figures 114-1** and **114-2**) and genital (**Figures 114-3** and **114-4**).[1]

HSV-1 infections are transmitted via saliva and are common in children, although primary herpes gingivostomatitis can be observed at any age. Children are most often infected by five years of age with infection rates ranging from 20 to 40 percent depending upon the geographic location and socioeconomic status of the family.[2] Orolabial herpes is the most prevalent form of herpes infection in children and often affects children younger than 5 years of age. The duration of the untreated illness is 2 to 3 weeks, and oral shedding of virus may continue for as long as 23 days.[1]

Acute herpetic gingivostomatitis (**Figures 114-1** and **114-2**) is a manifestation of primary HSV-1 infection that most often occurs in children aged 6 months to 5 years. Adults may also develop acute gingivostomatitis, but it is less severe and is often associated with a posterior pharyngitis. Infected saliva from an adult or another child is the mode of infection. The incubation period is 3 to 6 days.[3]

HSV-2 infections generally affect the genitals but may occur in neonates associated with maternal outbreak at delivery, with an incidence of about 1 in 3000 births.[4] Genital HSV-2 infections most commonly occur once sexual activity begins, often in adolescence. HSV-2 genital infections in children can be an indication of sexual abuse.[5]

The Centers for Disease Control and Prevention (CDC) reports that at least 50 million persons in the US have genital HSV-2 infection (**Figures 114-3** and **114-4**).[6] Over the past decade, the percentage of Americans with genital herpes infection in the US has remained stable. Most persons infected with HSV-2 have not been diagnosed with genital herpes.[6]

Genital HSV-2 infection is more common in women (approximately 1 out of 5 women 14 to 49 years of age) than in men (approximately 1 out of 9 men 14 to 49 years of age). Transmission from an infected male to his female partner is believed to be more likely than from an infected female to her male partner.[6]

Cross-sectional data from the 2003 to 2004 US National Health and Nutrition Examination Survey (NHANES) shows 24 percent of female adolescents (aged 14 to 19 years) had laboratory evidence of infection with human papillomavirus (HPV, 18%), Chlamydia trachomatis (4%), Trichomonas vaginalis (3%), herpes simplex virus type 2 (HSV-2, 2%), or Neisseria gonorrhoeae. Among girls who reported ever having had sex, 40 percent had laboratory evidence of one of the four STDs, most commonly HPV (30%) and chlamydia (7%).[7]

Herpetic whitlow is an intense painful infection of the hand involving the terminal phalanx of one or more digits (**Figures 114-5** and **114-6**). In the US, the estimated annual incidence is 2.4 cases per 100,000 persons.[8]

ETIOLOGY AND PATHOPHYSIOLOGY

- HSV belongs to the family Herpesviridae and is a double-stranded DNA virus.

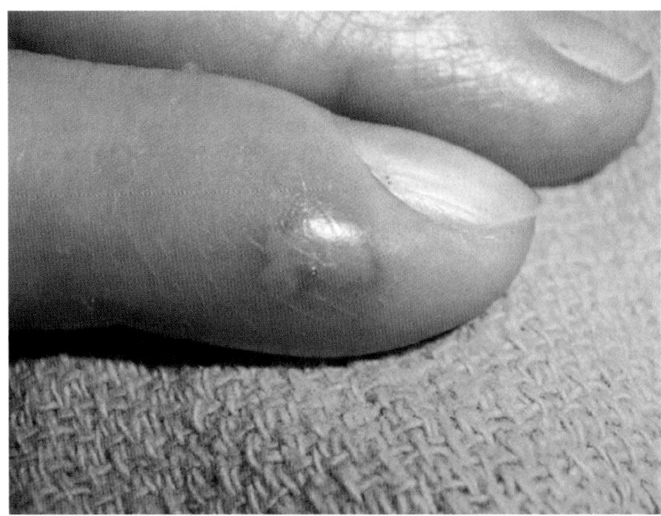

FIGURE 114-5 Herpetic whitlow lesion on distal index finger. (*Used with permission from Richard P. Usatine, MD.*)

- HSV exists as 2 separate types (types 1 and 2), which have affinities for different epithelia.[8] Seventy to ninety percent of HSV-2 infections are genital, whereas 70 to 90 percent of those caused by HSV-1 are oral–labial.
- HSV enters through abraded skin or intact mucous membranes. Once infected, the epithelial cells die, forming vesicles and creating multinucleated giant cells.

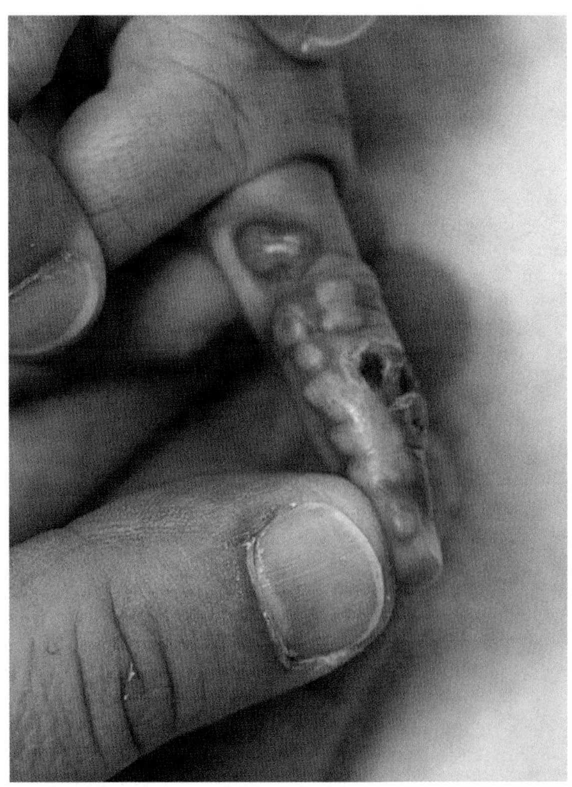

FIGURE 114-6 Herpes whitlow on the left third finger of a 6-month-old child. The mother is demonstrating the lesions on the finger, which are grouped pustules with an erythematous base. The child and mother had a history of recurrent cold sores on the lip and this second primary lesion was most probably from self-inoculation while sucking the finger. A Tzanck prep showed multinucleated giant cells. Viral culture showed HSV1. (*Image used with permission from Robert Brodell, MD.*)

- Retrograde transport into sensory ganglia leads to lifelong latent infection.[1] Reactivation of the virus may be triggered by immunodeficiency, trauma, fever, and UV light.
- Genital HSV infection is usually transmitted through sexual contact. When it occurs in a preadolescent, the possibility of abuse must be considered.
- Evidence indicates that 21.9 percent of all persons in the US, 12 years or older, have serologic evidence of HSV-2 infection, which is more commonly associated with genital infections.[4]
- As many as 90 percent of those infected are unaware that they have herpes infection and may unknowingly shed virus and transmit infection.[9]
- Primary genital herpes has an average incubation period of 4 days, followed by a prodrome of itching, burning, or erythema.
- With both types, systemic symptoms are common in primary disease and include fever, headache, malaise, abdominal pain, and myalgia.[10] Recurrences are usually less severe and shorter in duration than the initial outbreak.[1,10]
- Herpetic whitlow occurs as a complication of oral or genital HSV infection and in medical personnel who have contact with oral secretions (**Figures 114-5** and **114-6**).
- Toddlers and preschool children are susceptible to herpetic whitlow if they have herpes labialis and engage in thumb-sucking or finger-sucking behavior (**Figure 114-6**).
- Like all HSV infections, herpetic whitlow usually has a primary infection, which may be followed by subsequent recurrences. The virus migrates to the peripheral ganglia and Schwann cells where it lies dormant. Recurrences observed in 20 to 50 percent of cases are usually milder and shorter in duration.
- Herpes can remain dormant in nerves, including the trigeminal nerve and recur subsequently (**Figures 114-7** to **114-10**).
- Maternal–fetal transmission of HSV is associated with significant morbidity and mortality. Manifestations of neonatal HSV include

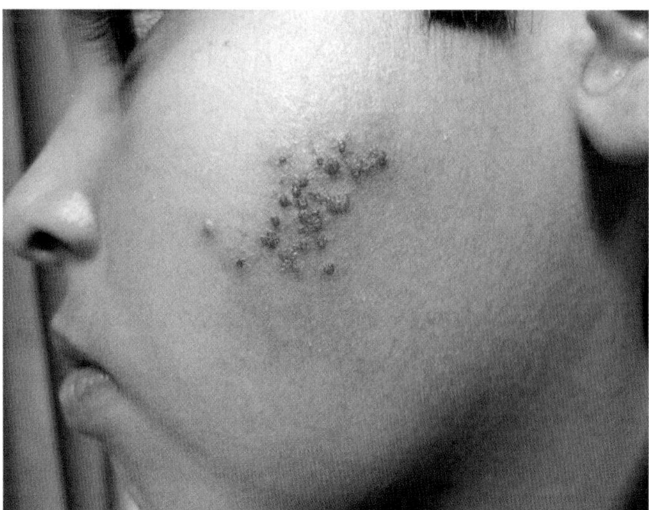

FIGURE 114-7 Recurrent herpes simplex virus on the cheek of a 14-year-old boy. He gets this about once a year since age 8 months. This recurrence started 5 days ago. HSV1 remains dormant in the trigeminal ganglion of V2 between outbreaks. (*Used with permission from Ross Lawler, MD.*)

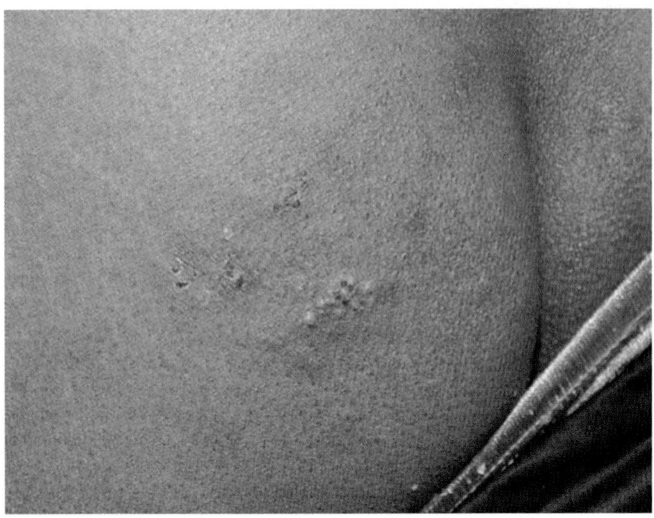

FIGURE 114-8 Recurrent herpes simplex virus on the buttocks of a young woman. Note the vesicles and crusts in a unilateral cluster. (*Used with permission from Richard P. Usatine, MD.*)

localized infection of the skin, eyes, and mouth, central nervous system (CNS) disease, or disseminated multiple organ disease (**Figure 114-11**). The CDC and the American College of Obstetricians and Gynecologists recommend that cesarean delivery should be offered as soon as possible to women who have active HSV lesions or, in those with a history of genital herpes, symptoms of vulvar pain, or burning at the time of delivery.[11]

RISK FACTORS

- Multiple sexual partners.
- Female gender.
- Low socioeconomic status.
- HIV infection.

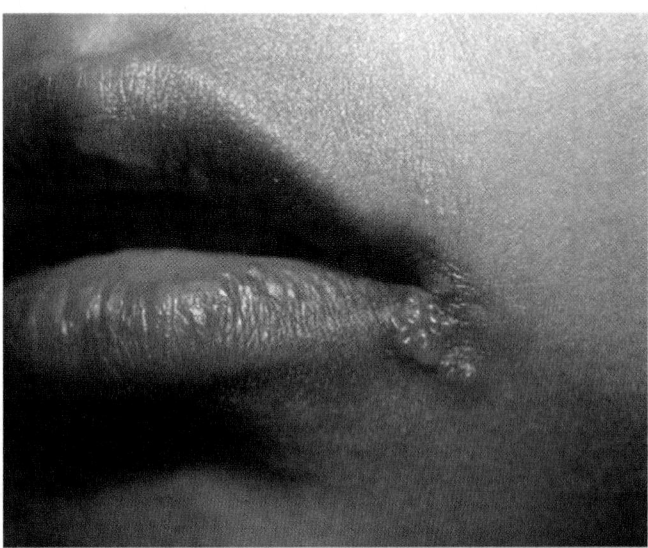

FIGURE 114-9 Close-up of recurrent herpes simplex virus-1 showing vesicles on a red base at the vermillion border in a young girl. (*Used with permission from Richard P. Usatine, MD.*)

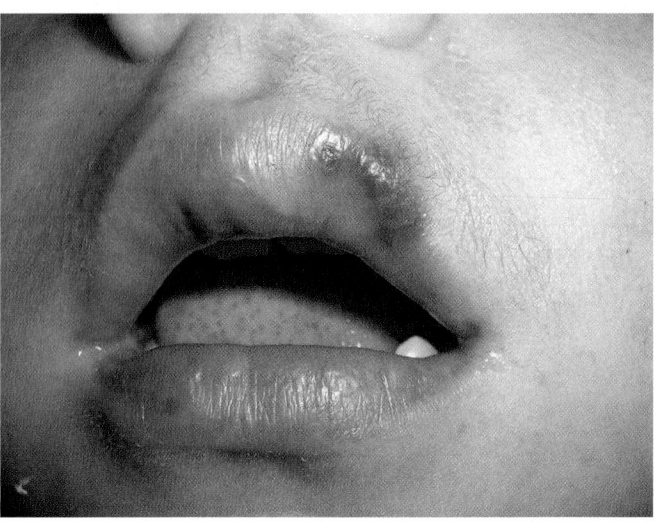

FIGURE 114-10 Orolabial herpes simplex virus in a child showing deroofed blisters (ulcer). (*Used with permission from Richard P. Usatine, MD.*)

DIAGNOSIS

CLINICAL FEATURES

- The diagnosis of HSV infection may be made by clinical appearance. Many patients have systemic symptoms, including fever, headache, malaise, and myalgias.

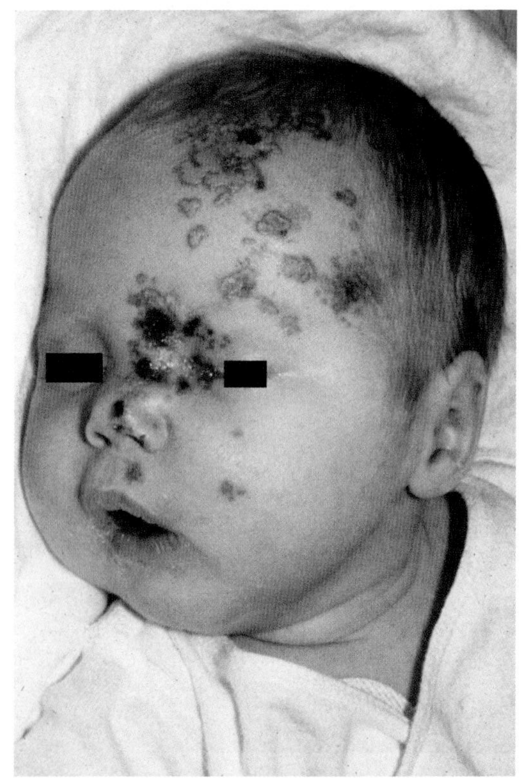

FIGURE 114-11 Neonatal herpes simplex virus-2 infection (culture proven) on the face of an infant most likely acquired during a vaginal birth. The child was hospitalized for intravenous acyclovir and an ophthalmology consult was called due to the skin involvement around the eye. Even though the distribution appears dermatomal this was not a herpes zoster infection. (*Used with permission from Richard P. Usatine, MD.*)

- Primary herpes gingivostomatitis typically takes the form of painful vesicles and ulcerative erosions on the tongue, palate, gingiva, buccal mucosa, and lips (**Figures 114-1** to **114-2**).
- Acute herpetic gingivostomatitis clinical features include an abrupt onset of high fever (102 to 104°F) gingivitis with markedly swollen, erythematous, friable gums, anorexia, listlessness, vesicular lesions, and/or ulcerated plaques of the oral mucosa, tongue, and lips and later rupture and coalesce, tender regional lymphadenopathy, and perioral skin involvement due to contamination with infected saliva.[5]
- Genital herpes presents with multiple transient, painful vesicles that appear on the penis (**Figures 114-3**), vulva (**Figure 114-4**), buttocks (**Figure 114-8**), perineum, vagina or cervix, and tender inguinal lymphadenopathy.[10] The vesicles break down and become ulcers that develop crusts while these are healing.
- Oral and genital herpes infections can recur with variable frequency depending upon many host factors. The duration is shorter and less painful than in primary infections. The lesions are often single and the vesicles heal completely by 8 to 10 days. Recurrent labial herpes is commonly called a "cold sore" because an upper respiratory infection might trigger the outbreak (**Figures 114-9** and **114-10**).
- UV radiation in the form of sunlight may trigger outbreaks. Another reason to use sun protection when outdoors triggers recurrence of orolabial HSV-1, an effect which is not fully suppressed by acyclovir.

LABORATORY STUDIES

- Infants exposed to HSV during birth should be followed carefully in consultation with a pediatric infectious disease specialist (**Figures 114-11**). Surveillance cultures of mucosal surfaces to detect HSV infection might be considered before the development of clinical signs of neonatal herpes.[6]
- The gold standard of diagnosis is viral isolation by tissue culture and polymerase chain reaction (PCR) testing.[6]
    - The culture sensitivity rate is only 70 to 80 percent and depends upon the stage at which the specimen is collected. The sensitivity is highest at first in the vesicular stage and declines with ulceration and crusting. The tissue culture assay can be positive within 48 hours but may take longer.
    - PCR is extremely sensitive (96%) and specific (99%). PCR testing is generally used for cerebrospinal fluid (CSF) testing in suspected HSV encephalitis or meningitis.[6]
- Older type-specific HSV serologic assays that do not accurately distinguish HSV-1 from HSV-2 antibody are still on the market. Both laboratory-based assays and point-of-care tests that provide results for HSV-2 antibodies from capillary blood or serum with sensitivities of 80 to 98 percent are available. Because nearly all HSV-2 infections are sexually acquired, the presence of type-specific HSV-2 antibody implies anogenital infection. Type-specific HSV serologic assays might be useful in patients with recurrent symptoms and negative HSV cultures and an asymptomatic patient with a partner with genital herpes. Screening for HSV-1 and HSV-2 in the general population is not indicated.[6]
- Direct immunofluorescent staining of vesicular lesions (obtained by unroofing a lesion and removing cells from the base of the lesion) is 80 to 90 percent sensitive and very specific. This can provide a rapid diagnosis.
- The Tzanck test has lower sensitivity rates than viral culture and should not be relied on for diagnosis.[6]
- The CDC does not currently recommend routine type 2 HSV testing in someone with no symptoms suggestive of herpes infection (i.e., for the general population).[11]
- If the herpes was acquired by sexual contact, screening should be performed for other sexually transmitted diseases (STDs), such as syphilis and HIV.
- Biopsy is usually unnecessary unless no infectious etiology is found for a genital lesion and a malignancy is suspected.

DIFFERENTIAL DIAGNOSIS

- Syphilis produces a painless or mildly painful, indurated, clean-based ulcer (chancre) at the site of exposure. It is best to investigate for syphilis or coexisting syphilis in any patient presenting for the first time with a genital ulcer of unproven etiology (see Chapter 181, Syphilis).
- Chancroid produces a painful deep, undermined, purulent ulcer that may be associated with painful inguinal lymphadenitis (see Chapter 75, Mucosal Ulcerative Disorders).
- Drug eruptions produce pruritic papules or blisters without associated viral symptoms (see Chapter 154, Cutaneous Drug Reactions).
- Behçet disease produces ulcerative disease around the mouth and genitals, possibly before onset of sexual activity (**Figure 114-12**; see Chapter 75, Mucosal Ulcerative Disorders).
- Acute paronychia which presents as a localized abscess in a nail fold and is the main differential diagnosis in the consideration of herpetic whitlow (see Chapter 164, Paronychia).
- Felon—A red, painful infection, usually bacterial, of the fingertip pulp. It is important to distinguish whitlow from a felon (where the

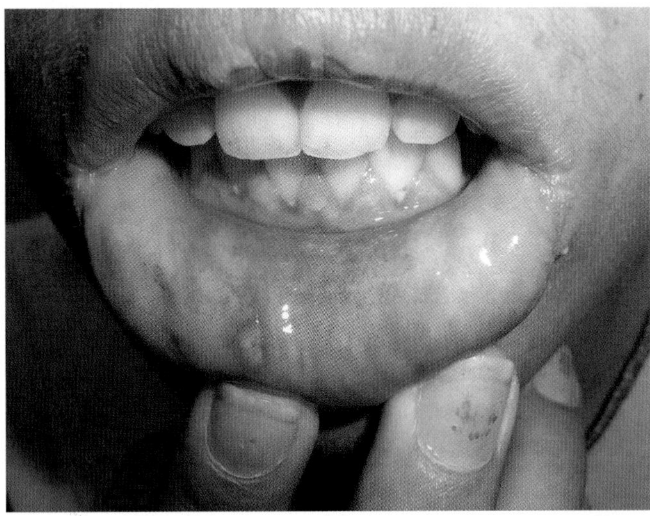

FIGURE 114-12 A 17-year-old girl diagnosed with Behcet's syndrome with recurrent aphthous stomatitis in the mouth and recurrent genital ulcers prior to the onset of sexual activity. (*Used with permission from Richard P. Usatine, MD.*)

pulp space usually is tensely swollen) as incision and drainage of a felon is needed, but should be avoided in herpetic whitlow because it may lead to an unnecessary secondary bacterial infection.

MANAGEMENT

NONPHARMACOLOGIC

- Women with active primary or recurrent genital herpetic lesions at the onset of labor should deliver by cesarean section to lower the chance of neonatal HSV infection.[11] SOR Ⓐ

MEDICATIONS

- Acyclovir is a guanosine analog that acts as a DNA chain terminator which, when incorporated, ends viral DNA replication. It is indicated for use in children for most herpes related indications Valacyclovir is the *l*-valine ester prodrug of acyclovir that has enhanced absorption after oral administration and high oral bioavailability. Famciclovir is the oral form of penciclovir, a purine analog similar to acyclovir. They must be administered early in the outbreak to be effective, but are safe and extremely well-tolerated.[10] SOR Ⓐ Only acyclovir is available as an oral formulation and indicated for young children.
- Treatment for neonatal herpes is intravenous acyclovir and is shown in **Table 114-1**.
- All infants who have neonatal herpes should be promptly evaluated and treated with systemic acyclovir 20 mg/kg IV every 8 hours for 21 days for disseminated and CNS disease or for 14 days for disease limited to the skin and mucous membranes.[6] SOR Ⓑ

Genital herpes:

- Antiviral therapy is recommended for an initial genital herpes outbreak. Although systemic antiviral drugs can partially control the signs and symptoms of herpes episodes, they do not eradicate latent virus.
- Acyclovir, famciclovir, and valacyclovir are equally effective for episodic treatment of genital herpes, but famciclovir appears somewhat less effective for suppression of viral shedding.[6] Only acyclovir is indicated for use in children. SOR Ⓑ
- Effective episodic treatment of herpes requires initiation of therapy during the prodrome period or within 1 day of lesion onset. Providing the patient with a prescription for the medication with instructions to initiate treatment immediately when symptoms begin improves efficacy.[6] SOR Ⓑ
- HSV strains resistant to acyclovir have been detected in immunocompromised patients so that other antivirals (e.g., foscarnet) need to be considered in these patients. SOR Ⓒ
- Topical medication for HSV infection is generally not effective and not recommended. Topical penciclovir applied every 2 hours for 4 days, reduces clinical healing time by approximately 1 day.[1,6]
- All patients with a first episode of genital herpes should receive antiviral therapy as even with mild clinical manifestations initially, they can develop severe or prolonged symptoms.
- Toxicity of these 3 antiviral drugs is rare, but in patients who are dehydrated or who have poor renal function, the drug can crystallize in the renal tubules, leading to a reversible creatinine elevation or, rarely, acute tubular necrosis. Adverse effects, usually mild, include nausea, vomiting, rash, and headache. Lethargy, tremulousness, seizures, and delirium have been reported rarely in studies of renally impaired patients.[12]

Oral herpes:

- Oral acyclovir treatment for primary herpes gingivostomatitis in children, started within the first three days of onset, shortens the duration of all clinical manifestations and the period of infectivity.[13] SOR Ⓑ In this RCT, acyclovir suspension was given (15 mg/kg) five times a day for seven days, or placebo. Children receiving acyclovir (age 1 to 6) had oral lesions for a shorter period than children receiving placebo (median 4 versus 10 days) and earlier disappearance of the following signs and symptoms: fever (1 versus 3 days); extraoral lesions (lesions around the mouth but outside the oral cavity) (0 versus 5.5 days); eating difficulties (4 versus 7 days); and drinking difficulties (3 versus 6 days). Viral shedding was significantly shorter in the group treated with acyclovir (1 versus 5 days).

Dosing of oral acyclovir is based on age and weight:

- 3 months to 2 years old: 15 mg/kg/day IV or oral divided 3 to 5 times per day for 5 to 7 days.

TABLE 114-1 Treatments for Neonatal Herpes

Drug	Dose or Dosage	Evidence Rating†	References
Skin, eyes, and mouth involvement			
Intravenous acyclovir	60 mg/kg/day for 14 days	A	3
Disseminated and central nervous system			
Intravenous acyclovir	60 mg/kg/day for 21 days	A	3
Asymptomatic neonates born to mothers who had primary genital infections			
Intravenous acyclovir	60 mg/kg/day empiric acyclovir therapy pending culture results is recommended by some experts	C	3

†*A*, Consistent, good-quality, patient-oriented evidence; *B*, inconsistent or limited-quality, patient-oriented evidence; *C*, consensus, disease-oriented evidence, usual practice, expert opinion, or case series.
Source: Hollier LM, Wendel GD. Third trimester antiviral prophylaxis for preventing maternal genital herpes simplex virus (HSV) recurrences and neonatal infection. *Cochrane Database Syst Rev.* 2008 Jan 23;(1):CD004946. doi: 10.1002/14651858.CD004946.pub2.

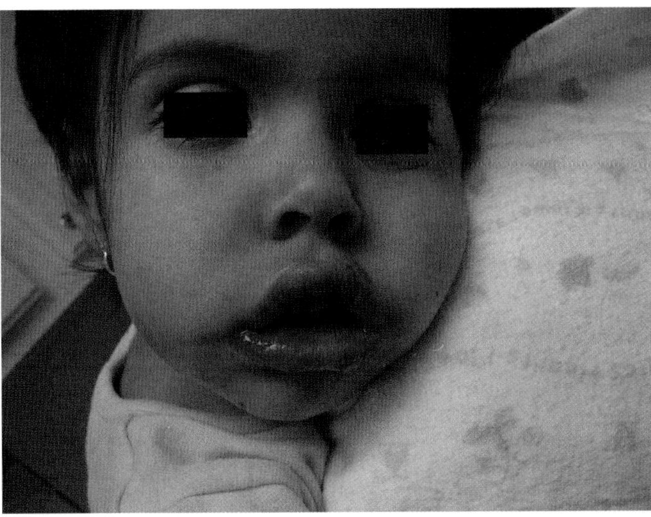

FIGURE 114-13 Primary herpes gingivostomatitis in a toddler. Her lips are swollen and she is drooling because it is painful to swallow. She is febrile and clearly not feeling well at all. (*Used with permission from Richard P. Usatine, MD.*)

- Over 2 years old: 400 mg orally divided q8h for 7 to 10 days (or 15 mg/kg/day).
- The oral lesions in primary herpes gingivostomatitis can lead to poor oral intake especially in children (**Figures 114-13**). To prevent dehydration, the following medications may be considered. Topical oral anesthetics such as 2 percent viscous lidocaine by prescription or 20 percent topical benzocaine OTC may be used to treat painful oral ulcers. SOR Ⓒ A solution combining aluminum and magnesium hydroxide (liquid antacid) and 2 percent viscous lidocaine has been reported as helpful when swished and spit out several times a day as needed for pain. SOR Ⓒ
- Docosanol cream (Abreva) is available without prescription for recurrent oral herpes. One randomized controlled trial (RCT) of 743 patients with herpes labialis showed a faster healing time in patients treated with docosanol 10 percent cream compared with placebo cream (4.1 versus 4.8 days), as well as reduced duration of pain symptoms (2.2 versus 2.7 days).[14] More than 90 percent of patients in both groups healed completely within 10 days.[14] Treatment with docosanol cream, when applied 5 times per day and within 12 hours of episode onset, is safe and somewhat effective.[15]

PREVENTION

- Barrier protection using latex condoms is recommended to minimize exposure to genital HSV infections (see the following section called "Patient Education"). In a large analysis using prospective data, condoms did offer moderate protection against HSV-2 acquisition in men and women.[16] SOR Ⓐ
- Suppressive therapy with antiviral drugs reduces the frequency of genital herpes recurrences by 70 to 80 percent in patients with frequent recurrences.[6] SOR Ⓐ Traditionally this is reserved for use in patients who have more than 4 to 6 outbreaks per year (see **Table 114-1**).
- Short-term prophylactic therapy with acyclovir for orolabial HSV may be used in patients who anticipate intense exposure to UV light.

FOLLOW-UP

- The patient should return for follow-up if pain is uncontrolled or superinfection is suspected. The patient should be periodically evaluated for the need for suppressive therapy based on the number of recurrences per year.
- Acute herpetic gingivostomatitis generally lasts 5 to 7 days, and the symptoms subside in 2 weeks. Viral shedding from the saliva may continue for 3 weeks or more.[5]

PATIENT EDUCATION

Inform women with recurrent genital herpes simplex virus that the risk of neonatal herpes is low. There is insufficient evidence to determine if maternal antiviral prophylaxis reduces the incidence of neonatal herpes. Antenatal antiviral prophylaxis reduces viral shedding and recurrences at delivery and reduces the need for cesarean delivery for genital herpes.[3]

Measures to prevent genital HSV infection:

- Abstain from sexual activity or limit number of sexual partners to prevent exposure to the disease.
- Use condoms to protect against transmission, but this is not foolproof as ulcers can occur on areas not covered by condoms.
- Prevent autoinoculation by patting dry affected areas, not rubbing with towel.
- Studies show that patients may shed virus when they are otherwise asymptomatic.
- A link between HSV genital ulcer disease and sexual transmission of HIV has been established. Safer sex practices should be strongly encouraged to prevent transmission of HSV to others and acquiring HIV by the patient.

PATIENT RESOURCES

- National Institute of Allergy and Infectious Diseases. *Genital Herpes*—**www.niaid.nih.gov/topics/genitalherpes/Pages/default.aspx**.
- Centers for Disease Control and Prevention. *Genital Herpes–CDC Fact Sheet*—**www.cdc.gov/std/Herpes/STDFact-Herpes.htm**.
- Skinsight. *Herpetic Whitlow–Information for Adults*—**www.skinsight.com/adult/herpeticWhitlow.htm**.

PROVIDER RESOURCES

- Medscape. *Herpes Simplex*—**http://emedicine.medscape.com/article/218580**.
- Medscape. *Dermatologic Manifestations of Herpes Simplex*—**http://emedicine.medscape.com/article/1132351**.
- Usatine RP, Tinitigan R. Nongenital HSV. *Am Fam Physician*. 2010;82[9]:1075-1082—**www.aafp.org/afp/2010/1101/p1075.html**.
- Emmert DH. Treatment of common cutaneous HSV infections. *Am Fam Physician*. 2000;61[6]:1697-1704—**www.aafp.org/afp/20000315/1697.html**.

REFERENCES

1. Whitley RJ, Kimberlin DW, Roizman B. Herpes simplex viruses. *Clin Infect Dis.* 1998;26:541-555.
2. Chayavichitsilp P, Buckwalter JV, Krakowski AC, Friedlander SF. Herpes simplex. *Pediatr Rev.* 2009;30(4):119-129.
3. Arduino PG, Porter SR. Oral and perioral herpes simplex virus type 1 (HSV-1) infection: review of its management. *Oral Dis.* 2006;12(3):254-270.
4. Hollier LM, Wendel GD. Third trimester antiviral prophylaxis for preventing maternal genital herpes simplex virus (HSV) recurrences and neonatal infection. *Cochrane Database Syst Rev.* 2008;23(1):CD004946.
5. Fleming DT, McQuillan GM, Johnson RE, et al. Herpes simplex virus type 2 in the United States, 1976 to 1994. *N Engl J Med.* 1997;337:1105-1111.
6. Centers for Disease Control and Prevention. *2010 Guidelines for Treatment of Sexually Transmitted Diseases.* http://www.cdc.gov/std/treatment/2010/STD-Treatment-2010-RR5912.pdf, accessed December 1, 2011.
7. Forhan SE, Gottlieb SL, Sternberg MR, et al. Prevalence of sexually transmitted infections among female adolescents aged 14 to 19 in the United States. *Pediatrics.* 2009;124:1505.
8. Gill MJ, Arlette J, Buchan K. Herpes simplex virus infection of the hand. A profile of 79 cases. *Am J Med.* 1988;84:89-93.
9. Mertz GJ. Epidemiology of genital herpes infections. *Infect Dis Clin North Am.* 1993;7:825-839.
10. Clark JL, Tatum NO, Noble SL. Management of genital herpes. *Am Fam Physician.* 1995;51:175-182, 187-188.
11. Centers for Disease Control and Prevention (CDC). Seroprevalence of herpes simplex virus type 2 among persons aged 14–49 years—United States, 2005–2008. *MMWR Morb Mortal Wkly Rep.* 2010;59(15):456-459.
12. Emmert DH. Treatment of common cutaneous herpes simplex virus infections. *Am Fam Physician.* 2000;61(6):1697-1706, 1708.
13. Amir J, Harel L, Smetana Z, Varsano I. Treatment of herpes simplex gingivostomatitis with aciclovir in children: a randomised double blind placebo controlled study. *BMJ.* 1997;21;314(7097):1800-1803.
14. Sacks SL, Thisted RA, Jones TM, et al. Docosanol 10% Cream Study Group. Clinical efficacy of topical docosanol 10% cream for herpes simplex labialis: a multi-center, randomized, placebo-controlled trial. *J Am Acad Dermatol.* 2001;45(2):222-230.
15. Usatine RP, Tinitigan R. Nongenital herpes simplex virus. *Am Fam Physician.* 2010;82(9):1075-1082.
16. Martin ET, Krantz E, Gottlieb SL, Magaret AS, Langenberg A, Stanberry L, Kamb M, Wald A. A pooled analysis of the effect of condoms in preventing HSV-2 acquisition. *Arch Intern Med.* 2009;169(13):1233-1240.

115 MOLLUSCUM CONTAGIOSUM

E.J. Mayeaux, Jr., MD
Stephen Taylor, MD
Kevin Carlisle, MD

PATIENT STORY

An 8-year-old girl is brought to the office because of an outbreak of bumps on her face for the past 3 months (**Figure 115-1**). Occasionally she scratches them, but she is otherwise asymptomatic. The mother and child are unhappy with the appearance of the molluscum contagiosum and chose to try topical imiquimod 5 percent cream. Fortunately, her health insurance covered this expensive treatment. A topical treatment was chosen to avoid the risk of hypopigmentation that can occur in dark-skinned individuals with cryotherapy.

An 11-year-old girl was also seen with molluscum on her face. The child and her mother decided to try cryotherapy as her treatment. She very bravely tolerated the treatment with liquid nitrogen in a Cryogun (**Figure 115-2**). The molluscum disappeared without scarring or hypopigmentation after 2 treatments.

INTRODUCTION

Molluscum contagiosum is a viral skin infection that produces pearly papules that often have a central umbilication. It is seen most commonly in children, but can also be transmitted sexually among adults.

EPIDEMIOLOGY

- Molluscum contagiosum infection has been reported worldwide. An Australian seroepidemiology study found a seropositivity rate of 23 percent.[1]

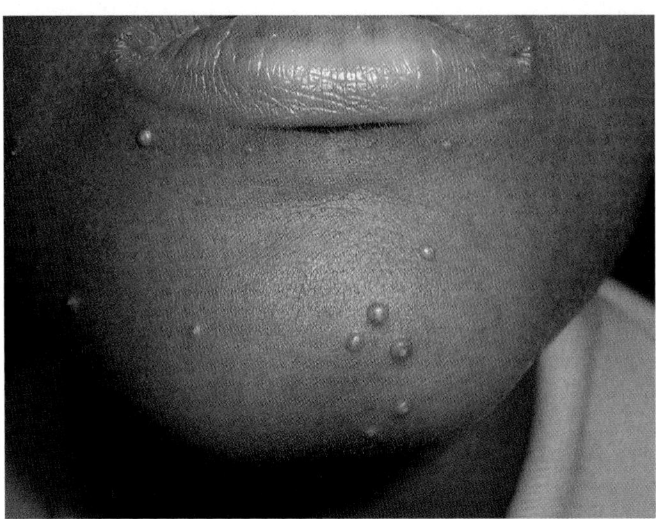

FIGURE 115-1 Molluscum contagiosum on the face of an 8-year-old girl. (*Used with permission from Richard P. Usatine, MD.*)

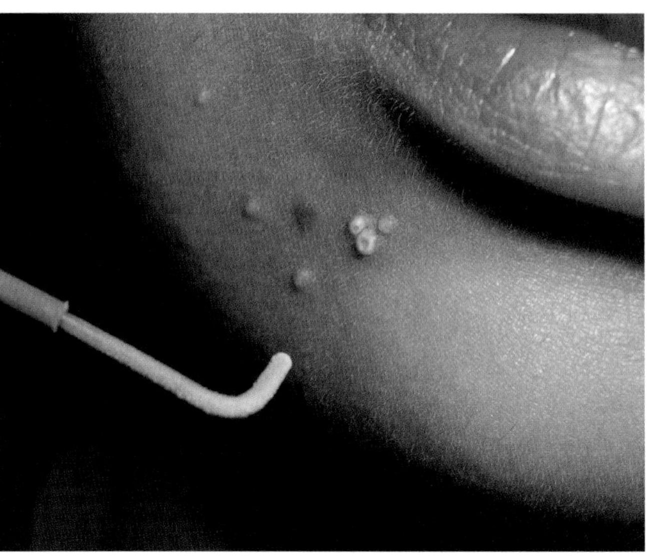

FIGURE 115-2 Cryotherapy of molluscum on the face of an 11-year-old girl. The central umbilication is easily seen in the 2 papules that were just frozen. (*Used with permission from Richard P. Usatine, MD.*)

- Up to 5 percent of children in the US have clinical evidence of molluscum contagiosum infection.[2] It is a common, nonsexually transmitted condition in children (see **Figures 115-1** to **115-4**).
- The number of cases in US adults increased in the 1980s probably as a result of the HIV/AIDS epidemic. Since the introduction of highly active antiretroviral therapy (HAART), the number of molluscum contagiosum cases in HIV/AIDS patients has decreased substantially.[3] However, the prevalence of molluscum contagiosum in patients who are HIV-positive may still be as high as 5 to 18 percent (**Figure 115-5**).[4,5]

ETIOLOGY AND PATHOPHYSIOLOGY

- Molluscum contagiosum is a benign condition that is often transmitted through close contact in children and through sexual contact in adolescents.

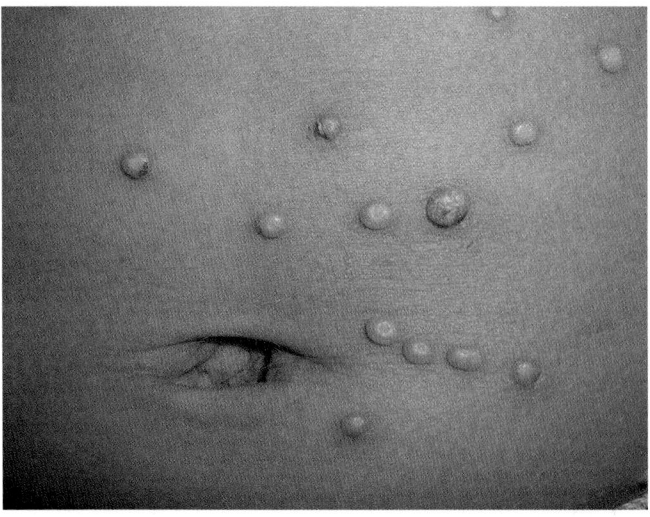

FIGURE 115-3 A group of molluscum contagiosum lesions on the abdomen of a 4-year-old boy. (*Used with permission from Richard P. Usatine, MD.*)

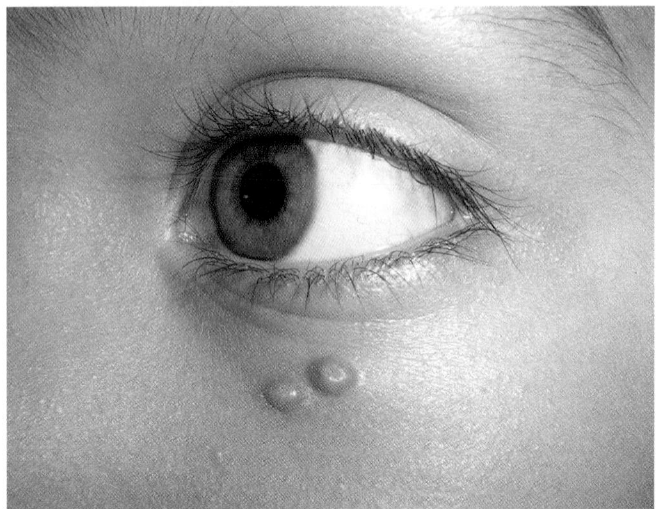

FIGURE 115-4 Molluscum contagiosum under the eye of a young girl with central umbilication. (*Used with permission from Richard P. Usatine, MD.*)

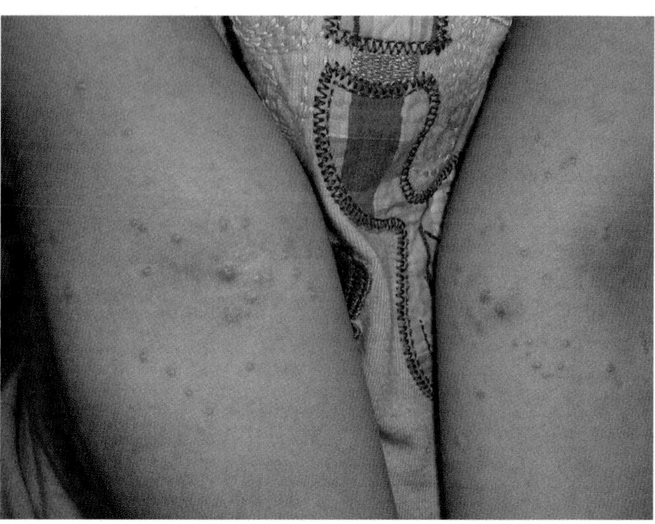

FIGURE 115-6 Molluscum contagiosum in the antecubital fossa of a 6-year-old girl with atopic dermatitis. (*Used with permission from Richard P. Usatine, MD.*)

- It is a large DNA virus of the Poxviridae family of poxvirus. It is related to the orthopoxviruses (variola, vaccinia, smallpox, and monkeypox viruses).
- Molluscum replicates in the cytoplasm of epithelial cells. It causes a chronic localized skin infection consisting of dome-shaped pearly papules on the skin. Like most of the viruses in the poxvirus family, molluscum is spread by direct skin-to-skin contact. It can also spread by autoinoculation when scratching, touching, or treating lesions. Any single lesion is usually present for approximately 2 months, but autoinoculation often causes continuous crops of lesions.

RISK FACTORS

- Common childhood disease.
- Molluscum contagiosum may be more common in patients with atopic dermatitis (**Figure 115-6**).[2]
- The disease also may be spread by participation in contact sports.[2]
- It is also associated with immunodeficient states such as in HIV infection (**Figure 115-5**) and with immunosuppressive drug treatment.

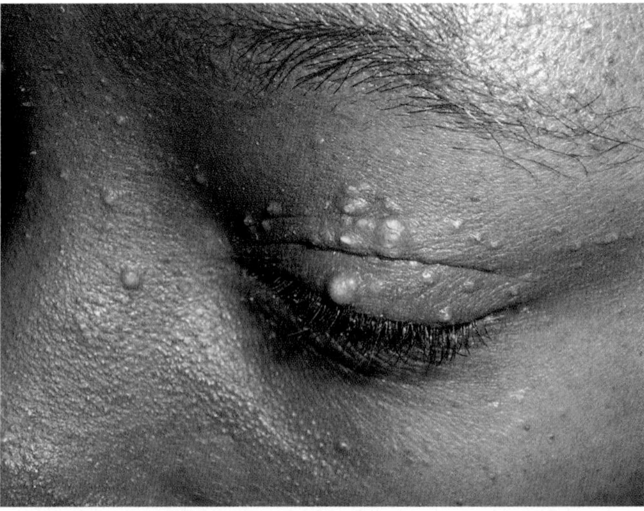

FIGURE 115-5 Extensive molluscum contagiosum on the face of a young girl who has perinatally-acquired HIV infection. (*Used with permission from Richard P. Usatine, MD.*)

DIAGNOSIS

CLINICAL FEATURES

- Firm, multiple, 2- to 5-mm dome-shaped papules with a characteristic shiny surface and umbilicated center (**Figure 115-7**). Not all the papules have a central umbilication, so it helps to take a moment and look for a papule that has this characteristic morphology. If all features point to molluscum and no single lesion has central umbilication, do not rule out molluscum as the diagnosis.

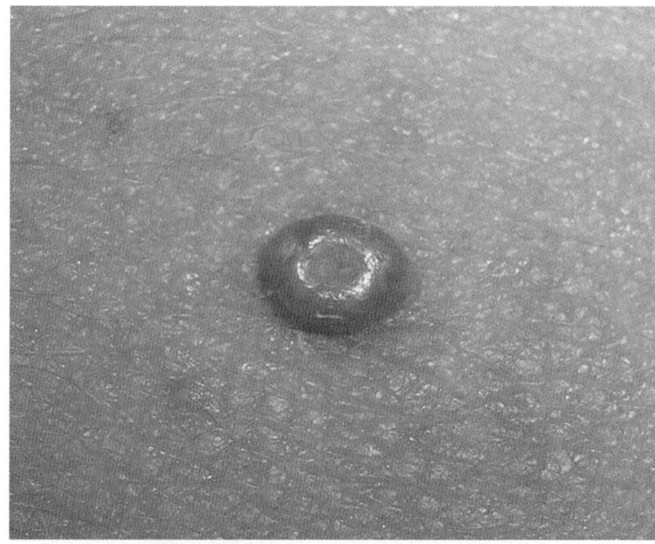

FIGURE 115-7 Close-up of a molluscum lesion on the back of a child showing a dome-shaped pearly papule with a characteristic umbilicated center. (*Used with permission from Richard P. Usatine, MD.*)

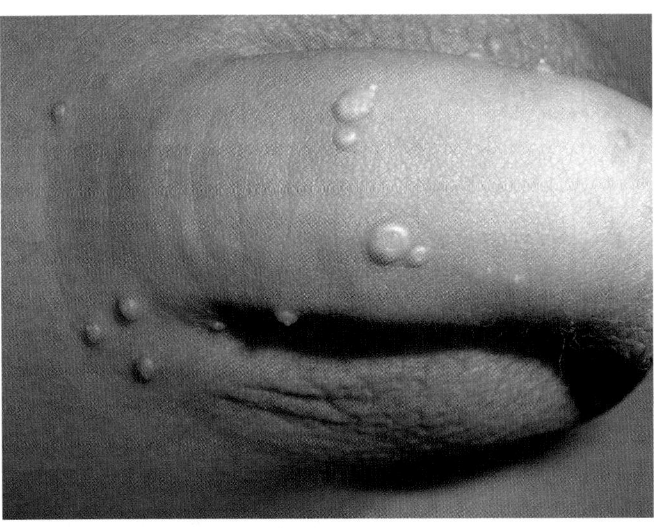

FIGURE 115-8 Molluscum contagiosum on and around the penis of a young boy. There was no evidence for sexual abuse. (*Used with permission from Richard P. Usatine, MD.*)

- The lesions range in color from pearly white to flesh-colored, to pink or yellow.
- Pruritus may be present or absent.

TYPICAL DISTRIBUTION

- The lesions may appear anywhere on the body except the palms and soles. The number of lesions may be greater in an HIV-infected individual. In children, the lesions are often on the trunk or face, but occasionally are found around the genitalia, inguinal area, buttocks, or inner thighs.
- If a child is found to have molluscum contagiosum in the genital area, a history and physical exam should be directed at looking for other clues that might indicate sexual abuse (see Chapter 8, Child Sexual Abuse). Not all cases of molluscum in this area will be secondary to sexual abuse (**Figure 115-8**).

LABORATORY TESTING

- Laboratory testing is not typically indicated.
- Sexually active adolescents with genital lesions should be evaluated for other sexually transmitted diseases, including for HIV infection.

BIOPSY

- If confirmation is needed, smears of the caseous material expressed from the lesions can be examined directly under the microscope looking for molluscum bodies (enlarged keratinocytes that are engorged with viral inclusion bodies). Hematoxylin and eosin (H&E) staining from a shave biopsy usually reveals keratinocytes that contain eosinophilic cytoplasmic inclusion bodies.[5]

DIFFERENTIAL DIAGNOSIS

- Scabies is caused by *Sarcoptes scabiei* mite and can be transmitted through close or sexual contact. Early lesions are flesh-colored to red papules that produce significant itching. The itching and excoriations are greater than seen with molluscum. Scabies lesions also usually appear in the finger webs and ventral wrist fold (see Chapter 128, Scabies).
- Dermatofibromas—Firm to hard nodules ranging in color from flesh to black that typically dimple downward when compressed laterally. Usually not seen in crops as in molluscum. These nodules are deeper in the dermis and do not appear stuck on like molluscum.
- Genital warts may be flat and grossly resemble molluscum but they lack the characteristic shiny surface and central umbilication (see Chapter 118, Genital Warts).

MANAGEMENT

NONPHARMACOLOGIC

- Treatment of nongenital lesions is usually not medically necessary as the infection is usually self-limited and spontaneously resolves after a few months. Treatment may be performed in an attempt to decrease autoinoculation. Patients and parents of children often want treatment for cosmetic reasons and when watchful waiting fails.
- A 2009 Cochrane Database systematic review investigated the efficacy of treatments for nongenital molluscum contagiosum in healthy individuals and found insufficient evidence to conclude that any treatment was definitively effective.[6] SOR Ⓐ
- In the HIV-infected patient, molluscum may resolve after control of HIV disease with HAART.[3] SOR Ⓑ
- Immunocompromised patients should have a full body skin examination to ensure all lesions are identified. Treatment is still optional but should proceed in patients whose parents desire intervention.

MEDICATIONS

- Podophyllotoxin 0.5 percent (Condylox) is an antimitotic agent that is indicated for the treatment of genital warts. The efficacy of podophyllotoxin was established in a randomized trial of patients 10 to 26 years of age who had lesions located on the thighs or genitalia. SOR Ⓑ Local erythema, burning, pruritus, inflammation, and erosions can occur with the use of this agent. The safety and efficacy of this drug has not been established in young children.[7]
- Topical imiquimod 5 percent (Aldara) cream has been shown (not FDA approved) to be better than vehicle alone to treat molluscum.[8,9] SOR Ⓑ It can be well tolerated, although application site irritation can be uncomfortable and lead to discontinuation of therapy. It has been shown not to have systemic or toxic effects in children.[9] In one study, 23 children ranging in age from 1 to 9 years with molluscum contagiosum infection were randomized to either imiquimod cream 5 percent (12 patients) or vehicle (11 patients).
- Parents applied the study drug to the patient's lesions 3 times a week for 12 weeks. Complete clearance at week 12 was noted in 33.3 percent (4/12) of imiquimod patients and in 9.1 percent (1/11) of vehicle patients.[10]
- Tretinoin cream 0.1 percent or gel 0.025 percent applied daily are commonly used but not FDA-approved for this indication.[11] SOR Ⓑ
- Cantharidin was studied in 300 children for molluscum where parents reported 90 percent of children experienced lesion clearing and 8 percent experience lesion improvement (**Figure 115-9**).

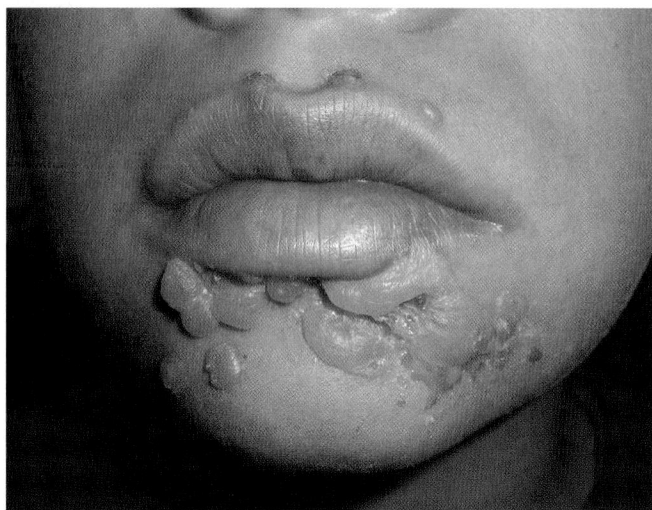

FIGURE 115-9 Blisters that formed the next day after treating molluscum contagiosum with cantharidin. The blisters are not always so large but are supposed to form as the cantharidin is derived from the blister beetle and these blisters help to eradicate the molluscum. (*Used with permission from Richard P. Usatine, MD.*)

Furthermore, 95 percent of parents stated they would use cantharidin therapy again.[12] Local erythema, burning, pruritus, and inflammation were reported side effects.

- Trichloroacetic acid[13] are topical chemicals that can be applied by the physician in the office. SOR B

SURGICAL

- Curettage and cryotherapy are physical methods used to eradicate molluscum.[14,15] SOR B However, many children will fear treatment with a curette or with any form of cryotherapy particularly if multiple lesions are present.

COMPLEMENTARY/ALTERNATIVE THERAPY

- ZymaDermis a nonprescription, topical, homeopathic agent that is marketed for the treatment of molluscum contagiosum, but no published studies have evaluated its efficacy or safety.
- Potassium hydroxide has been used for molluscum but has not proved to be statistically significant when compared to placebo.[16]
- Pulsed dye lasers have shown to be safe and effective in case reports and small uncontrolled studies. One prospective study of 19 children between 2 and 13 concluded that all patients tolerated the 585 nm laser well and 84.3 percent had complete lesion resolution with one treatment.[17]

PREVENTION

- Molluscum contagiosum is a common childhood disease.
- Limiting sexual exposure or number of sexual contact may help prevent exposure.
- Genital lesions should be treated to prevent spread by sexual contact.

PROGNOSIS

- In immunocompetent patients, lesions usually spontaneously resolve within several months. In a minority of cases, disease persists for a few years.[18]

FOLLOW-UP

- Have patients watch for complications that may include irritation, inflammation, and secondary infections. Lesions on eyelids may be associated with follicular or papillary conjunctivitis, so eye irritation should prompt a visit to an eye care specialist.

PATIENT EDUCATION

- Instruct patients to avoid scratching to prevent autoinoculation.

PATIENT RESOURCES

- Centers for Disease Control and Prevention. Molluscum (Molluscum Contagiosum)—**www.cdc.gov/ncidod/dvrd/molluscum**.
- Pubmed Health. Molluscum Contagiosum—**www.ncbi.nlm.nih.gov/pubmedhealth/PMH0001829**.
- American Academy of Dermatology. Molluscum Contagiosum—**www.aad.org/skin-conditions/dermatology-a-to-z/molluscum-contagiosum**.
- eMedicine. Molluscum Contagiosum—**www.emedicinehealth.com/molluscum_contagiosum/article_em.htm**.
- MedlinePlus. Molluscum Contagiosum—**www.nlm.nih.gov/medlineplus/ency/article/000826.htm**.

PROVIDER RESOURCES

- eMedicine. Molluscum Contagiosum—**http://emedicine.medscape.com/article/910570**.
- eMedicine. Molluscum Contagiosum in ED—**http://emedicine.medscape.com/article/762548**.
- Centers for Disease Control and Prevention. Clinical Information: Molluscum Contagiosum—**www.cdc.gov/ncidod/dvrd/molluscum/clinical_overview.htm**.

REFERENCES

1. Konya J, Thompson CH. Molluscum contagiosum virus: antibody responses in persons with clinical lesions and seroepidemiology in a representative Australian population. *J Infect Dis*. 1999; 179(3):701-704.
2. Dohil MA, Lin P, Lee J, et al. The epidemiology of molluscum contagiosum in children. *J Am Acad Dermatol*. 2006;54(1):47-54.
3. Calista D, Boschini A, Landi G. Resolution of disseminated molluscum contagiosum with highly active anti-retroviral therapy (HAART) in patients with AIDS. *Eur J Dermatol*. 1999;9(3):211-213.

4. Schwartz JJ, Myskowski PL. Molluscum contagiosum in patients with human immunodeficiency virus infection. *J Am Acad Dermatol*. 1992;27(4):583-588.

5. Cotell SL, Roholt NS. Images in clinical medicine. Molluscum contagiosum in a patient with the acquired immunodeficiency syndrome. *N Engl J Med*. 1998;338(13):888.

6. van der Wouden JC, van der Sande R, van Suijlekom-Smit LW, et al. Interventions for cutaneous molluscum contagiosum. Cochrane *Database Syst Rev*. 2009;7(4):CD004767.

7. Syed TA, Lundin S, Ahmad M. Topical 0.3% and 0.5% podophyllotoxin cream for self-treatment of molluscum contagiosum in males. A placebo-controlled, double-blind study. *Dermatology*. 1994;189(1):65-68.

8. Hengge UR, Esser S, Schultewolter T, et al. Self-administered topical 5% imiquimod for the treatment of common warts and molluscum contagiosum. *Br J Dermatol*. 2000;143(5):1026-1031.

9. Barba AR, Kapoor S, Berman B. An open label safety study of topical imiquimod 5% cream in the treatment of Molluscum contagiosum in children. *Dermatol Online J*. 2001;7(1):20.

10. Theos AU, Cummins R, Silverberg NB, Paller AS. Effectiveness of imiquimod cream 5% for treating childhood molluscum contagiosum in a double-blind, randomized pilot trial. *Cutis*. 2004;74(2):134-138, 141-142.

11. Papa CM, Berger RS. Venereal herpes-like molluscum contagiosum: treatment with tretinoin. *Cutis*. 1976;18(4):537-540.

12. Silverberg NB, Sidbury R, Mancini AJ. Childhood molluscum contagiosum: experience with cantharidin therapy in 300 patients. *J Am Acad Dermatol*. 2000;43(3):503-507.

13. Yoshinaga IG, Conrado LA, Schainberg SC, Grinblat M. Recalcitrant molluscum contagiosum in a patient with AIDS: combined treatment with CO(2) laser, trichloroacetic acid, and pulsed dye laser. *Lasers Surg Med*. 2000;27(4):291-294.

14. Hanna D, Hatami A, Powell J, et al. A prospective randomized trial comparing the efficacy and adverse effects of four recognized treatments of molluscum contagiosum in children. *Pediatr Dermatol*. 2006;23(6):574-579.

15. Wetmore SJ. Cryosurgery for common skin lesions. Treatment in family physicians' offices. *Can Fam Physician*. 1999;45:964-974.

16. Romiti R, Ribeiro AP, Romiti N. Evaluation of the effectiveness of 5% potassium hydroxide for the treatment of molluscum contagiosum. *Pediatr Dermatol*. 2000;17:495.17.

17. Binder B, Weger W, Komericki P, Kopera D. Treatment of molluscum contagiosum with a pulsed dye laser: Pilot study with 19 children. *J Dtsch Dermatol Ges*. 2008;6:121.

18. Lee R, Schwartz RA. Pediatric molluscum contagiosum: reflections on the last challenging poxvirus infection, part 1. *Cutis*. 2010;86(5):230-236.

116 COMMON WARTS

E.J. Mayeaux, Jr., MD
Anthony Todd Flowers, MD

PATIENT STORY

An 11-year-old girl presents with warts on her fingers that have not responded to nonprescription wart medications (**Figure 116-1**). It causes her and her mother some social embarrassment and they would like to be rid of them. Her mother is also worried that it is affecting her daughter's nails. The girl was able to tolerate the discomfort of liquid nitrogen treatment and wanted all her warts treated. The mother was instructed to purchase 40 percent salicylic acid to continue treatment of any residual warts at home.

INTRODUCTION

Human papillomaviruses (HPVs) are DNA viruses that infect skin and mucous membranes. Infection is usually confined to the epidermis and does not result in disseminated systemic infection. The most common clinical manifestation of these viruses is warts (verrucae). There are more than 100 distinct HPV subtypes based on DNA testing. Some tend to infect specific body sites or types of epithelium. Some HPV types have a potential to cause malignant change but transformation is rare on keratinized skin.

SYNONYMS

Verrucae, verruca vulgaris, common warts.

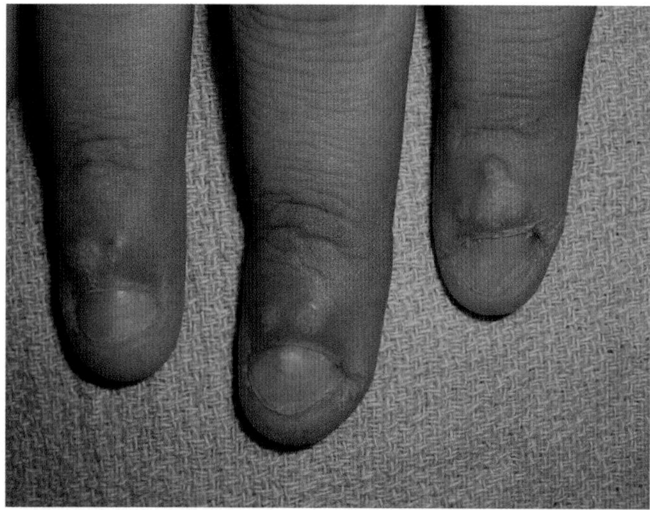

FIGURE 116-1 Common warts on the fingers of an 11-year-old girl. These periungual warts are particularly difficult to eradicate. (*Used with permission from Richard P. Usatine, MD.*)

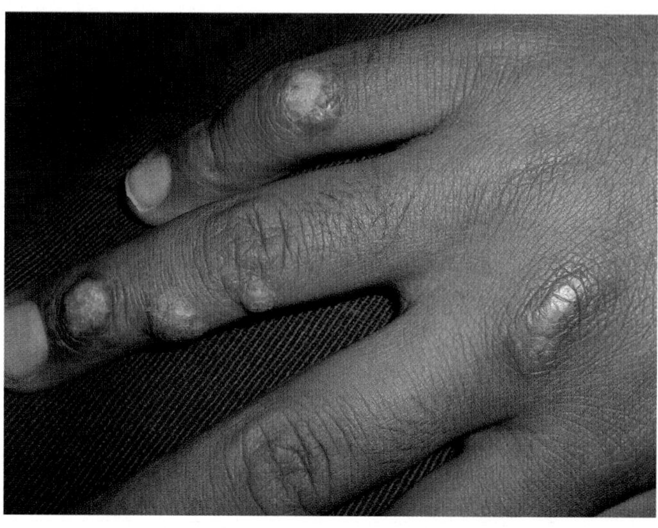

FIGURE 116-2 Common warts on the hand of a 9-year-old boy. (*Used with permission from Richard P. Usatine, MD.*)

EPIDEMIOLOGY

- Nongenital cutaneous warts are widespread worldwide and are more common in children, with a peak incidence in the teenage years and a sharp decline thereafter.[1] Warts are the third most common reason for a pediatric general dermatology clinic visit accounting for about 16 percent of such visits.[2]
- They are most commonly caused by HPV types 1–5, 7, 27, and 29.[1]
- Common warts account for approximately 70 percent of nongenital cutaneous warts.[3]
- Common warts occur most commonly in children and young adults (**Figures 116-1** and **116-2**).[4]

ETIOLOGY AND PATHOPHYSIOLOGY

- Infection with HPV occurs by skin-to-skin contact. It starts with a break in the integrity of the epithelium caused by maceration or trauma that allows the virus to infect the basal layers.
- Warts may infect the skin on opposing digits causing "kissing warts" (**Figure 116-3**).
- Individuals with subclinical infection may serve as a reservoir for HPVs.
- An incubation period following inoculation lasts for approximately 2 to 6 months.

RISK FACTORS[1]

- Young age.
- Disruption to the normal epithelial barrier.
- More common among meat handlers.
- Atopic dermatitis.
- Nail biters more commonly have multiple periungual warts.

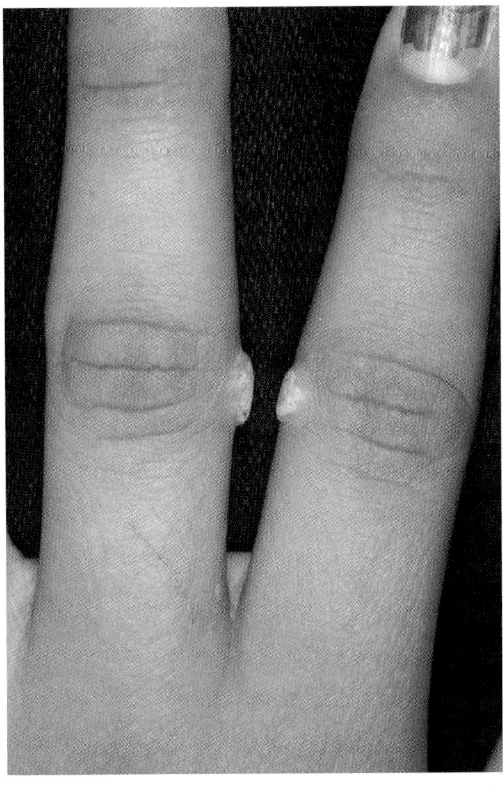

FIGURE 116-3 Warts may infect the skin on opposing digits causing "kissing warts." (*Used with permission from Richard P. Usatine, MD.*)

- Conditions that decrease cell-mediated immunity such as HIV (**Figure 116-4**) and immunosuppressant drugs.

DIAGNOSIS

CLINICAL FEATURES

- The diagnosis of warts is based upon clinical appearance. Warts will obscure normal skin markings (**Figure 116-5**).

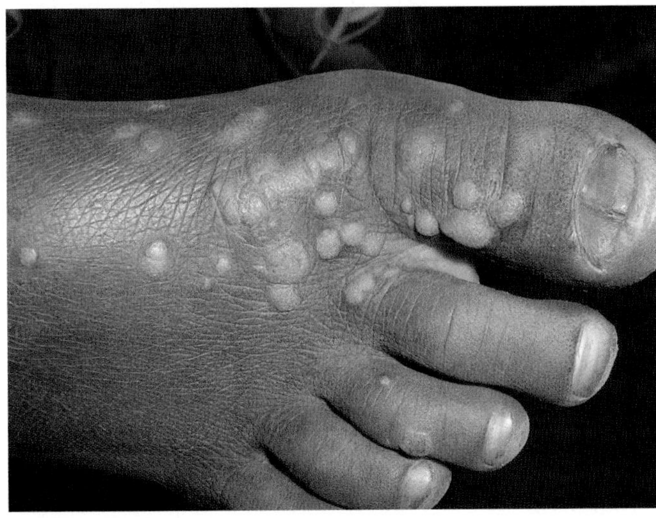

FIGURE 116-4 Large cluster of warts on the foot of a child in Africa suspected of being HIV-positive. (*Used with permission from Richard P. Usatine, MD.*)

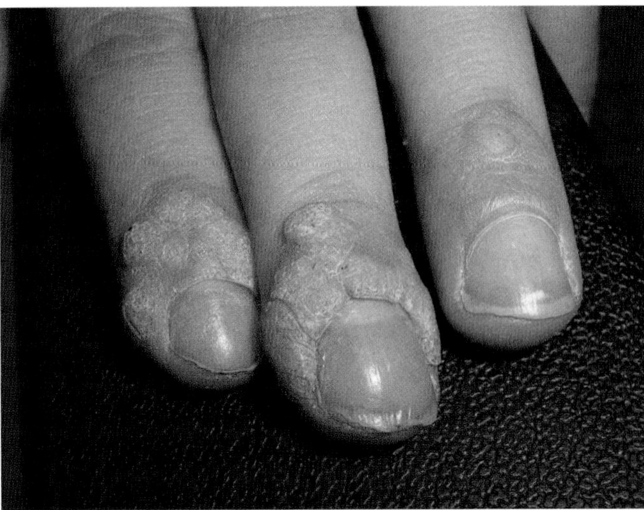

FIGURE 116-5 Periungual warts on the fingers of a child. Warts will obscure normal skin markings. (*Used with permission from Richard P. Usatine, MD.*)

- Common warts are well-demarcated, rough, hard papules with irregular papillary surface. They are usually asymptomatic unless located on a pressure point.
- Warts may form cylindrical of filiform projections (**Figures 116-6** and **116-7**).

TYPICAL DISTRIBUTION

- Common anatomic locations include the dorsum of the hand, between the fingers, flexor surfaces, and adjacent to the nails (periungual; **Figures 116-1**, **116-2**, and **116-5**).

LABORATORY TESTING

- HPV testing is not useful for this condition.[5] In a 2011 study, response to cryotherapy did not correlate HPV type.[6]
- HIV testing may be useful if the warts are severe and there are risk factors present (**Figure 116-4**).

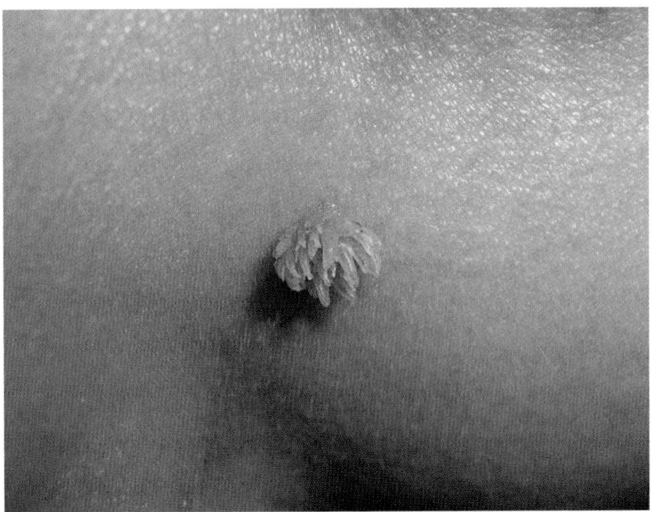

FIGURE 116-6 Filiform warts are identified by their multiple projections as opposed to a unified papule. This wart was on the cheek of a young girl. (*Used with permission from Richard P. Usatine, MD.*)

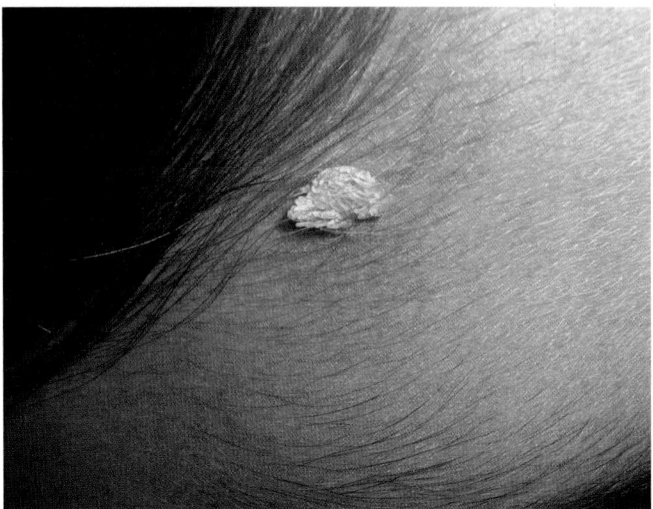

FIGURE 116-7 Filiform wart on the face of a young girl. *(Used with permission from Richard P. Usatine, MD.)*

BIOPSY

- Paring the surface with a surgical blade may expose punctate hemorrhagic capillaries, or black dots, which are thrombosed capillaries. If the diagnosis is in doubt, a shave biopsy is indicated to confirm the diagnosis.

DIFFERENTIAL DIAGNOSIS

- Molluscum contagiosum can appear similar to the common wart when the central umbilication is not easily visible. However, molluscum papules are usually more rounded and appear to be more stuck-on to the top of the skin (see Chapter 115, Molluscum Contagiosum).
- Acrochordon (skin tags) are pedunculated flesh-colored papules that are more common in obese persons. They lack the surface roughness of common warts. Filiform warts also may be pedunculated, but typically have a characteristic filiform appearance.

MANAGEMENT

NONPHARMACOLOGIC

- Because spontaneous regression occurs in 2/3 of warts within 2 years, observation without treatment is always an option. In 17 trials, the average reported cure rate was 30 percent within 10 weeks.[7] Observational studies show that 1/2 of cutaneous warts resolve spontaneously within 1 year, and about 2/3 within 2 years.[8]
- Treatment does not decrease transmissibility of the virus.[9]
- Distraction may help with pediatric acceptance and tolerance of treatment procedures. A 2012 study of patients aged 2 to 6 years who underwent cryotherapy for cutaneous viral warts found that the use of a portable video player significantly reduced preprocedural anxiety levels in patients undergoing cryotherapy for cutaneous viral warts.[10]

MEDICATIONS

- Therapies for common warts do not specifically treat the HPV virus. They work by destruction of virus-containing skin while preserving uninvolved tissue. This usually exposes the blood and its immune cells to the virus, which may promote an immune response against the virus.
- The least-painful methods should be used first in children. SOR Ⓒ
- A Cochrane review found that there is a considerable lack of evidence on which to base the rational use of the local treatments for common warts.[7] The trials are highly variable in method and quality. There is evidence that simple topical treatments containing salicylic acid have a therapeutic effect.[7] SOR Ⓐ There is less evidence for the efficacy of cryotherapy and no convincing evidence that it is any more effective than simple topical treatments. A 2011 meta-analysis of randomized trials for treatments for warts found that salicylic acid was superior to placebo (risk ratio for cure 1.60, 95 percent CI 1.15-2.24) but data were insufficient to draw conclusions on the efficacy of other therapies studied.[11]
- Seventeen percent salicylic acid is a useful first-line agent, especially for thick or multiple warts.[7] SOR Ⓐ It is safe in children. Combined results from five randomized controlled trials (RCTs) showed a 73 percent cure rate with 6 to 12 weeks of salicylic acid treatment, compared with a 48 percent cure rate with placebo (number needed to treat [NNT] = 4).[7] A number of preparations are available without a prescription. Topical 17 percent salicylic acid is applied overnight and is now the most commonly used form for this type of wart. Soak the wart area with warm water for 5 minutes, and then gently file down any thick skin with a pumice stone or emery board. The salicylic acid product should be applied to the wart. Repeat the first 2 steps daily with liquid or gel preparations, or every other day with the patch. Tape may be used to cover the wart after application of salicylic acid liquid. Repeat treatment until the wart has cleared or for up to 12 weeks. Discontinue the treatment if severe redness or pain occurs in the treated area. Do not use salicylic acid on the face because of an increased risk of hypopigmentation.[1]
- Forty percent salicylic acid plasters (Mediplast) are available over the counter for larger and thicker warts. The plasters are cut to fit and then applied a few millimeters beyond the wart for 48 hours. Then the patch is removed, the wart pared down with a nail file, pumice stone, or scalpel, and the process repeated as needed.
- Imiquimod 5 percent is an expensive topical immunomodulator that is indicated for treatment of anogenital warts but is also used on nongenital warts.[12–14] SOR Ⓑ It is nonscarring and painless, although local irritation is common. Debriding heavily keratinized warts may enhance penetration of the medication. The cream is applied in a thin layer to the lesions three times a week (every other night) and covered with a adhesive bandage or tape. The medication is removed with soap and water in the morning. It can also be used as adjunctive therapy. A lower concentration of imiquimod (3.75% cream) is also available, but data for common warts is lacking.
- Intralesional injections with *Candida* antigen induces a localized, cell-mediated and HPV-specific response that may target the injected wart as well as more distant warts (**Figure 116-8**). This method has moderate effectiveness (60% cure rates) for treatment

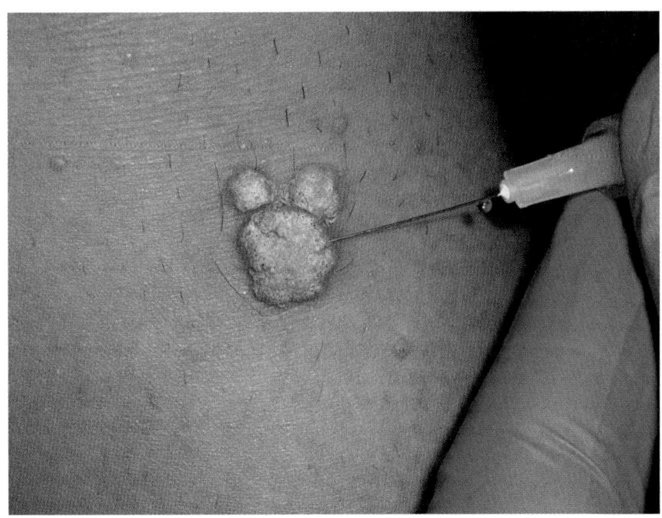

FIGURE 116-8 Candida antigen is being injected into a cluster of warts on the knee of a teenage boy. His warts had not responded to multiple therapies, including topical salicylic acid and cryotherapy. *(Used with permission from Richard P. Usatine, MD.)*

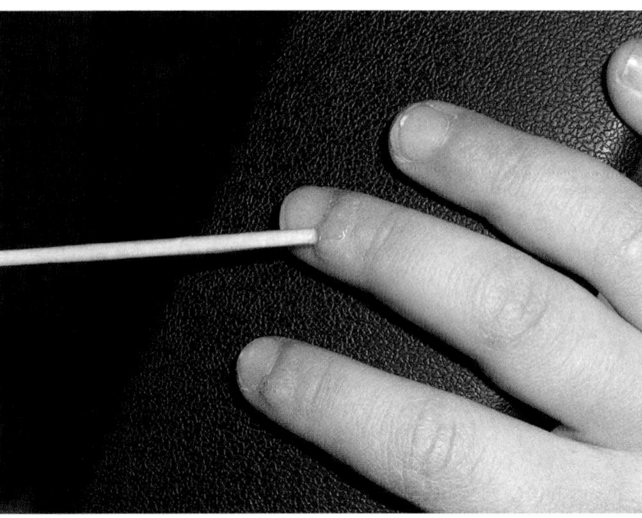

FIGURE 116-9 Cantharidin is being applied to periungual warts on the fingers of a 5-year-old child. Note the use of the wooden stick end of a cotton-tipped applicator. If the cotton tip is used, the cantharidin stays within the cotton and the application is insufficient. *(Used with permission from Richard P. Usatine, MD.)*

of recalcitrant warts in patients with a positive skin antigen pretest.[1] SOR B The *Candida* antigen must be diluted before used (**Table 116-1**). Inject 0.1 to 0.3 mL into the largest warts using a 30-gauge needle and up to 1 mL per treatment. Warn the patient to expect itching in the area, burning, or peeling. Repeat every 4 weeks, up to 3 treatments or until warts are gone.

- Photodynamic therapy with aminolevulinic acid plus topical salicylic acid is a moderately effective option for treatment of recalcitrant warts.[1] SOR B Although it is likely to be beneficial, it is expensive and often requires referral.
- Cantharidin 0.7 percent is an extract of the blister beetle that is applied to the wart, after which blistering occurs on the following day. It may be used in resistant cases. It is also useful in young children because application is painless in the office. However, painful blisters often occur within a day after application. Be careful not to overtreat with cantharidin because the blistering can be quit severe. Carefully apply to multiple lesions using the wooden end of a cotton-tipped applicator (**Figure 116-9**). SOR C
- Contact immunotherapy using dinitrochlorobenzene, squaric acid dibutylester, and diphenylcyclopropenone may be applied to the skin to sensitize the patient and then to the lesion to induce an immune response. SOR C

TABLE 116-1 Candida Dilutions

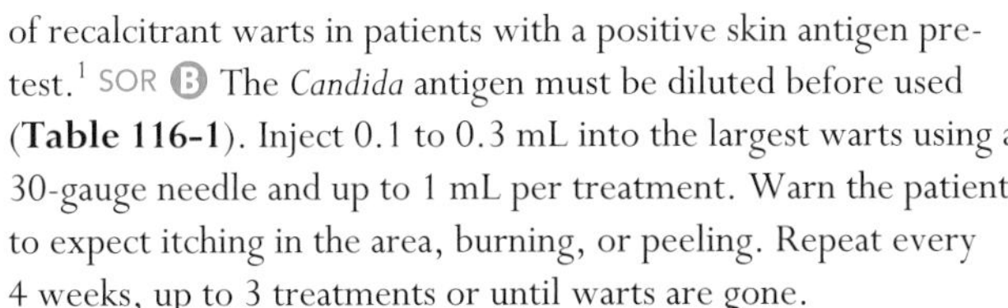

Creating 1.0 mL for Injection	Candida Antigen (mL)	Sterile saline or 2% Lidocaine (no Epi) (mL)
Generic 1:1000	0.25	0.75
Candin 1:500	0.5	0.5

Adapted with permission from: Usatine R, Pfenninger J, Stulberg D, Small R. Dermatologic and Cosmetic Procedures in Office Practice. Elsevier, Inc., Philadelphia. 2012.

- Intralesional injection with bleomycin can be considered for treatment of recalcitrant warts, although the effectiveness is unproven.[1] SOR B
- Early open-label, uncontrolled studies indicate cimetidine might be useful in treating warts. However, three placebo-controlled, double-blind studies and two open-label comparative trials demonstrate that its efficacy is equal to placebo.[15] SOR A

SURGERY

- Cryotherapy, most commonly with liquid nitrogen, is useful but is somewhat painful for younger children.[7] SOR B Chemical cryogens are now available over the counter but are not as cold or effective as liquid nitrogen. Most trials comparing cryotherapy with salicylic acid found similar effectiveness, with overall cure rates of 50 to 70 percent after three or four treatments.[1] Aggressive cryotherapy (10 to 30 seconds) is more effective than less-aggressive cryotherapy, but may increase complications.[1] SOR B Anesthesia is usually unnecessary but may be achieved with 1 percent lidocaine or EMLA (eutectic mixture of local anesthetics) cream. Liquid nitrogen is applied for 10 to 20 seconds via a Cryogun or a cotton swab so that the freeze ball extends 2 mm beyond the lesion (**Figure 116-10**). Two freeze cycles may improve resolution, but it is better to underfreeze than overfreeze as overfreezing may lead to permanent scarring or hypopigmentation. Best results of cryotherapy can be achieved when the patient is treated every 2 or 3 weeks. There is no therapeutic benefit beyond 3 months.[1] SOR B Because HPV can survive in liquid nitrogen, cotton swabs and residual liquid nitrogen should be properly discarded to avoid spreading the virus to other patients or contaminating the liquid nitrogen reservoir.[16] After cryotherapy, the skin shows erythema and may progress to hemorrhagic blistering. Healing occurs in approximately a week and hypopigmentation may occur. Ring warts may result from an inadequate margin of treatment of a common wart (**Figure 116-11**). Common adverse

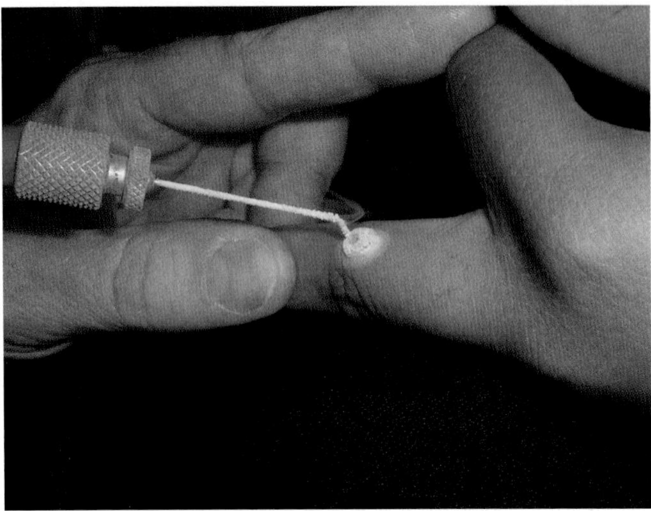

FIGURE 116-10 Cryotherapy showing an adequate free zone (halo) around the wart. (*Used with permission from Richard P. Usatine, MD.*)

effects of cryotherapy include pain, blistering, and hypo- or hyperpigmentation. Cryotherapy must be used cautiously where nerves are located superficially (such as on the fingers) to prevent pain and neuropathy. Overfreezing in the periungual region can result in permanent nail dystrophy.

- Simple excision may be used for small or filiform warts (**Figures 116-6** and **116-7**). The area is injected using lidocaine with epinephrine and the wart is excised with sharp scissors or a scalpel blade. SOR C
- Pulsed-dye laser can be considered for treatment of recalcitrant warts, although the effectiveness is unproven.[1] SOR B

COMPLIMENTARY/ALTERNATIVE THERAPY

- Although preliminary studies were promising, duct tape is of uncertain efficacy for wart treatment.[1] A randomized controlled trial in adults showed it to be no better than moleskin and both groups only had a 21 to 22 percent success rate.[17] SOR B

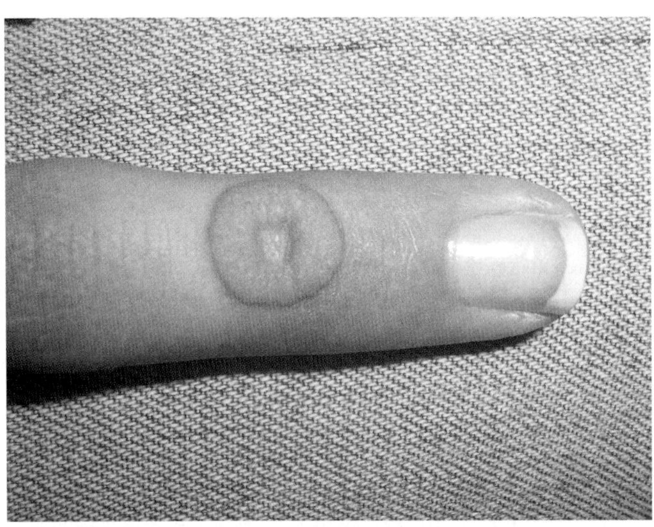

FIGURE 116-11 Ring wart that resulted from inadequate cryotherapy of a common wart. (*Used with permission from Richard P. Usatine, MD.*)

PREVENTION

- Tools used for paring down warts, such as nail files and pumice stones, should not be used on normal skin or by other people.
- Hair-bearing areas with warts should be shaved with depilatories, electric razors, or not at all to help limit spread of warts.

PROGNOSIS

- Sixty to 70 percent of cutaneous warts resolve in 3 to 24 months without treatment.[18,19]
- New warts may appear while others are regressing. This is not a treatment failure but part of the natural disease process with HPV.

FOLLOW-UP

- Schedule patients for return visits after treatment to limit loss of follow-up and to assess therapy.
- Follow-up visits can be left to the patient's discretion when self-applied therapy is being used.

PATIENT EDUCATION

- Therapy often takes weeks to months, so patience and perseverance are essential for successful therapy.

PATIENT RESOURCES

- **www.healthychildren.org/English/health-issues/conditions/skin/Pages/Warts.aspx**.
- **http://kidshealth.org/parent/infections/skin/wart.html**.
- eMedicine Health—**www.emedicinehealth.com/warts/article_em.htm**.
- BUPA. *Warts and verrucas patient information*—**www.bupa.co.uk/individuals/health-information/directory/w/warts-and-verrucas?tab=Resources**.
- **www.webmd.com/skin-problems-and-treatments/features/warts-on-children**.
- MayoClinic.com. Common warts—**www.mayoclinic.com/health/common-warts/DS00370**.

PROVIDER RESOURCES

- eMedicine. *Nongenital Warts*—**http://emedicine.medscape.com/article/1133317**.
- For information on treating warts including how to dilute Candida antigen: Usatine R, Pfenninger J, Stulberg D, Small R. *Dermatologic and Cosmetic Procedures in Office Practice*. Philadelphia, PA: Elsevier; 2012 or may be purchased at purchased as an electronic application at **www.usatinemedia.com**.

- Cutaneous warts: An evidence-based approach to therapy. *Am Fam Physician*. 2005;72:647-652. Available online at **www.aafp.org/afp/20050815/647.html**.
- Medline Plus—**www.nlm.nih.gov/medlineplus/ency/article/000885.htm**.
- Cochrane review. *Topical Treatments for Cutaneous Warts*—**www.cochrane.org/reviews/en/ab001781.html**.

REFERENCES

1. Mulhem E, Pinelis S. Treatment of nongenital cutaneous warts. *Am Fam Physician*. 2011;84(3):288-293.
2. Henderson MD, Abboud J, Cogan CM, Poisson LM, Eide MJ, Shwayder TA, Lim HW. Skin-of-color epidemiology: A report of the most common skin conditions by race. *Pediatr Dermatol*. 2012;29(5):584-589.
3. Micali G, Dall'Oglio F, Nasca MR, et al. Management of cutaneous warts: an evidence-based approach. *Am J Clin Dermatol*. 2004; 5(5):311-317.
4. Kilkenny M, Marks R. The descriptive epidemiology of warts in the community. *Australas J Dermatol*. 1996;37:80-86.
5. Sterling JC, Handfield-Jones S, Hudson PM. British Association of Dermatologists. Guidelines for the management of cutaneous warts. *Br J Dermatol*. 2001;144(1):4-11.
6. Tomson N, Sterling J, Ahmed I, Hague J, Berth-Jones J. Human papillomavirus typing of warts and response to cryotherapy. *J Eur Acad Dermatol Venereol*. 2011;25(9):1108-1111.
7. Gibbs S, Harvey I, Sterling JC, Stark R. Local treatments for cutaneous warts. *Cochrane Database Syst Rev*. 2001;(2):CD001781.
8. Massing AM, Epstein WL. Natural history of warts. A two-year study. *Arch Dermatol*. 1963;87:306-310.
9. Rivera A, Tyring SK. Therapy of cutaneous human papillomavirus infections. *Dermatol Ther*. 2004;17(6):441-448.
10. Tey HL, Tan ES, Tan FG, Tan KL, Lim IS, Tan AS. Reducing anxiety levels in preschool children undergoing cryotherapy for cutaneous viral warts: use of a portable video player. *Arch Dermatol*. 2012;148(9):1001-1004.
11. Kwok CS, Holland R, Gibbs S. Efficacy of topical treatments for cutaneous warts: a meta-analysis and pooled analysis of randomized controlled trials. *Br J Dermatol*. 2011;165:233.
12. Micali G, Dall'Oglio F, Nasca MR. An open label evaluation of the efficacy of imiquimod 5% cream in the treatment of recalcitrant subungual and periungual cutaneous warts. *J Dermatolog Treat*. 2003;14:233-236.
13. Hengge UR, Esser S, Schultewolter T, et al. Self-administered topical 5% imiquimod for the treatment of common warts and molluscum contagiosum. *Br J Dermatol*. 2000;143:1026-1031.
14. Grussendorf-Conen EI, Jacobs S. Efficacy of imiquimod 5% cream in the treatment of recalcitrant warts in children. *Pediatr Dermatol*. 2002;19:263-266.
15. Yilmaz E, Alpsoy E, Basaran E. Cimetidine therapy for warts: a placebo-controlled, double-blind study. *J Am Acad Dermatol*. 1996;34(6):1005-1007.
16. Tabrizi SN, Garland SM. Is cryotherapy treating or infecting? *Med J Aust*. 1996;164(5):263.
17. Wenner R, Askari SK, Cham PM, et al. Duct tape for the treatment of common warts in adults: a double-blind randomized controlled trial. *Arch Dermatol*. 2007;143(3):309-313.
18. Allen AL, Siegfried EC. What's new in human papillomavirus infection. Curr *Opin Pediatr*. 2000;12:365-369.
19. Sterling JC, Handfield-Jones S, Hudson PM. Guidelines for the management of cutaneous warts. *Br J Dermatol*. 2001;144:4-11.

117 FLAT WARTS

E.J. Mayeaux, Jr., MD

PATIENT STORY

A 16-year-old girl presents with multiple flat lesions on her forehead (**Figure 117-1**). It started with just a few lesions but has spread over the past 3 months. She is diagnosed with flat warts and topical imiquimod is prescribed as the initial treatment.

INTRODUCTION

Flat warts are characterized as flat or slightly elevated flesh-colored papules. They may be smooth or slightly hyperkeratotic. They range in size from 1 to 5 mm or more, and numbers range from a few to hundreds of lesions, which may become grouped or confluent. They occur most commonly on the face, hands, and shins. They may appear in a linear distribution as a result of scratching, shaving, or trauma (Koebner phenomenon) (**Figures 117-2** and **117-3**).

SYNONYMS

Plane warts, verruca plana, verruca plana juvenilis, plane warts.

EPIDEMIOLOGY

- Flat warts (verruca plana) are most commonly found in children and young adults (**Figures 117-1** to **117-3**).
- Flat warts are the least common variety of wart, but are generally numerous on an individual.[1]
- Flat warts are usually caused by human papillomavirus (HPV) types 3, 10, 28, and 29.[2]

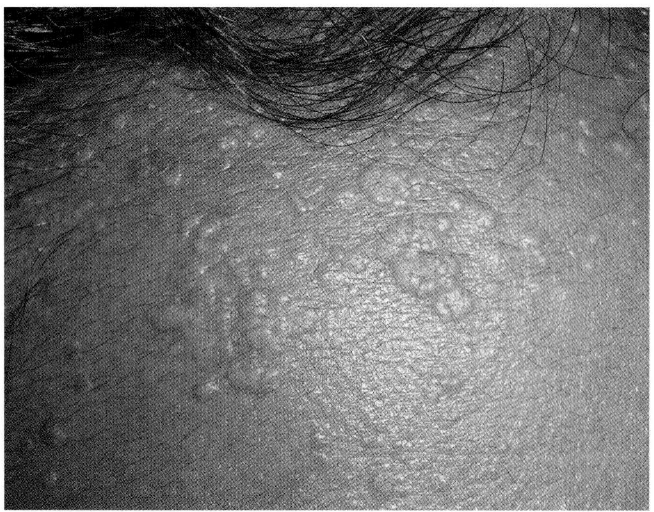

FIGURE 117-1 Flat warts on a patient's forehead. (*Used with permission from Richard P. Usatine, MD.*)

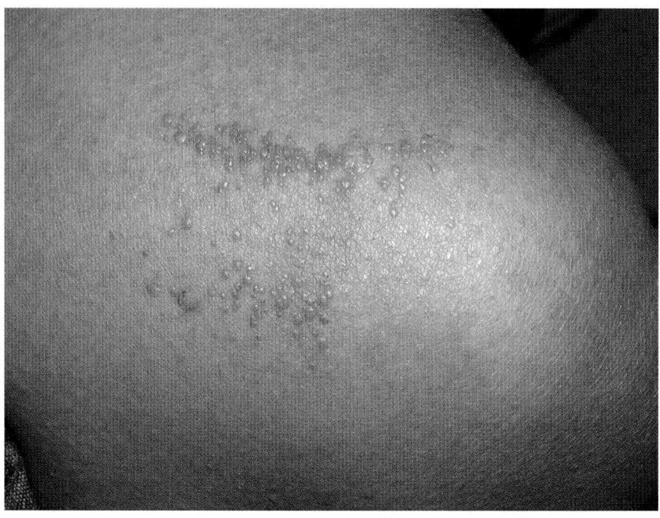

FIGURE 117-2 Flat warts just above the knee of a young woman. Notice the linear distribution probably resulting from spread by shaving (Koebner phenomenon). (*Used with permission from Richard P. Usatine, MD.*)

ETIOLOGY AND PATHOPHYSIOLOGY

- Like all warts, flat warts are caused by HPV.[2]
- Flat warts may spread in a linear pattern secondary to spread by scratching or trauma, such as shaving (**Figure 117-2** and **117-3**).
- Flat warts present a special treatment problem because they persist for a long time, they are generally located in cosmetically important areas, and they are resistant to therapy.

RISK FACTORS

- Shaving next to infected areas (**Figures 117-2** and **117-3**).
- HIV infection or other types of immunosuppression.

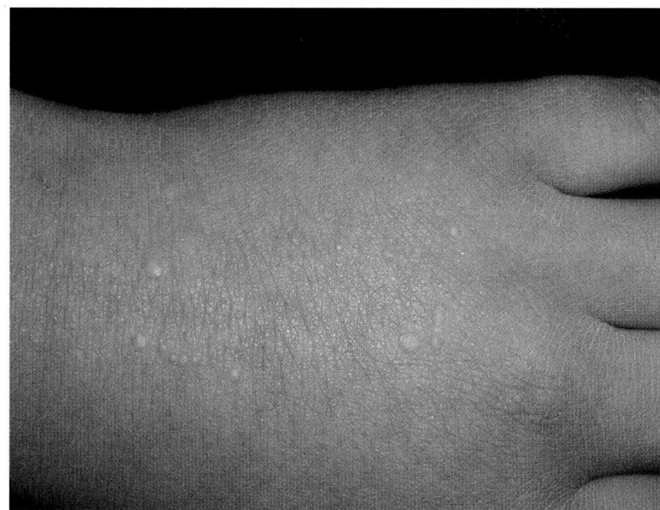

FIGURE 117-3 Flat warts on the hand of a child. Note the linear distribution, which is probably the result of scratching or minor trauma (Koebner phenomenon). (*Used with permission from Richard P. Usatine, MD.*)

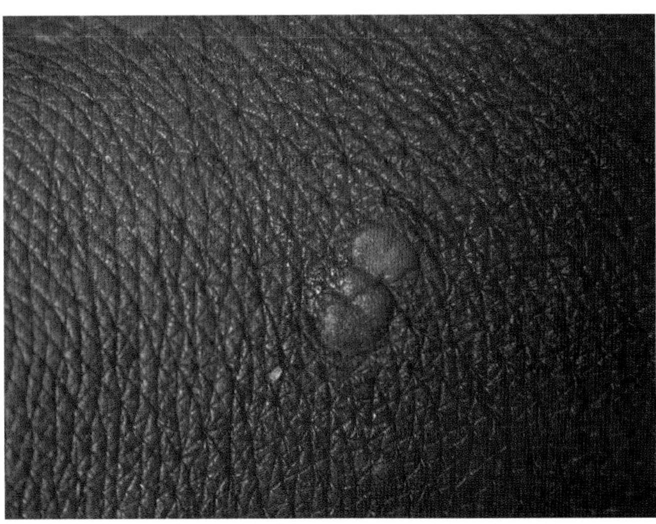

FIGURE 117-4 Close-up of a flat wart. Note typical small, flat-topped papule. (*Used with permission from Richard P. Usatine, MD.*)

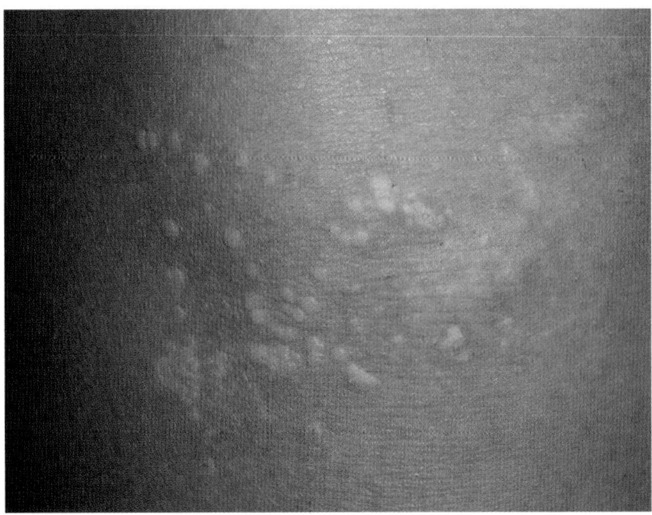

FIGURE 117-6 Flat warts on the leg of a teenager. (*Used with permission from Richard P. Usatine, MD.*)

DIAGNOSIS

CLINICAL FEATURES

- Multiple small, flat-topped papules that may be pink, light brown, or light yellow colored. They may be polygonal in shape (**Figure 117-4**).

TYPICAL DISTRIBUTION

- Flat warts typically appear on the forehead (**Figure 117-1**), around the mouth (**Figure 117-5**), the backs of the hands (**Figure 117-3**), and shaved areas, such as the lower face and neck in men (**Figure 117-3**) and the lower legs in women (**Figures 117-2** and **117-6**).

LABORATORY TESTING

- HPV testing is not useful for this condition.[3]

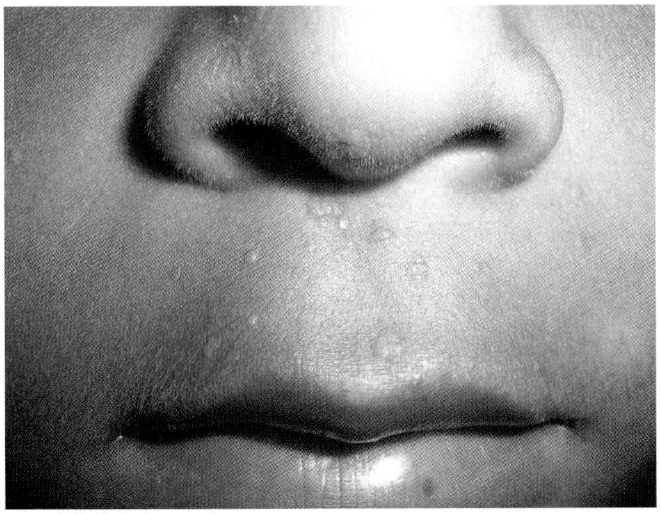

FIGURE 117-5 Flat warts on the upper lip and nose of a young girl. (*Used with permission from Richard P. Usatine, MD.*)

BIOPSY

- Although usually not necessary, a shave biopsy can confirm the diagnosis if the diagnose is in question.

DIFFERENTIAL DIAGNOSIS

- Lichen planus produces flat-topped papules that may be confused with flat warts. Look for characteristic signs of lichen planus such as the symmetric distribution, purplish coloration, and oral lacy lesions. (Wickham striae are white, fine, reticular scale seen on the lesions.) The distribution of lichen planus is different, with the most common sites being the ankles, wrists, and back (see Chapter 138, Lichen Planus). Lichen planus rarely occurs in children.
- Seborrheic keratoses are often more darkly pigmented and have a stuck-on appearance; "horn cysts" may be visible on close examination. These are also rare in children.

MANAGEMENT

NONPHARMACOLOGIC

- Regression of these lesions may occur, which usually is heralded by inflammation.
- There are no current therapies for HPV that are virus specific.
- Distraction may help with pediatric acceptance and tolerance of treatment procedures. A 2012 study of patients aged 2 to 6 years who underwent cryotherapy for cutaneous viral warts found that the use of a portable video player significantly reduced preprocedural anxiety levels i undergoing cryotherapy for cutaneous viral warts.[4]

MEDICATIONS

- Topical salicylic acid treatments by topical liquid or patch are the most effective treatment for all types of warts with a success rate average of 73 percent from five pooled placebo-controlled trials.[5]

Number needed to treat (NNT) = 4. SOR Ⓐ Salicylic acid may be more acceptable on the legs than the face.[2] Often, 17 percent salicylic acid topicals are applied overnight daily until the warts resolve.

- Fluorouracil (Efudex 5% cream, Fluoroplex 1%) may be used to treat flat warts in adults only.[6,7] SOR Ⓑ It is not indicated for use in children.
- Imiquimod 5 percent cream is an expensive topical immunomodulator that has shown some efficacy in treating flat warts.[8,9] It is nonscarring and painless to apply. There are rare reports of systemic side effects. The cream is applied to the lesions 3 times a week (every other day). The cream may be applied to the affected area, not strictly to the lesion itself.[10] It can be used on all external HPV-infected sites, but not on occluded mucous membranes. Therapy can be temporarily halted if symptoms become problematic. Imiquimod has the advantage of having almost no risk of scarring.[8,9] SOR Ⓑ A lower concentration of imiquimod (3.75% cream) is also available, but data for its use with flat or common warts is lacking. It is not indicated for use in children although there are data for its use in adolescents.
- Tretinoin cream, 0.025 percent, 0.05 percent, or 0.1 percent, applied at bedtime over the entire involved area is one accepted treatment. The frequency of application is then adjusted so as to produce a mild, fine scaling and erythema. Sun protection is important. Treatment may be required for weeks or months and may not be effective. No published studies were found to support this treatment. SOR Ⓒ Safety and efficacy in children under age 12 years is not established.
- Intralesional injections with *Candida* antigen induces a localized, cell-mediated, and HPV-specific response that may target the injected wart as well as more distant warts. This method has moderate effectiveness (60% cure rates) for treatment of recalcitrant warts (**Figure 117-3**).[2] The *Candida* antigen must be diluted before used (see **Table 116-1**). Inject 0.1 to 0.3 mL into the largest warts using a 30-gauge needle and up to 1 mL per treatment. Warn the patient to expect itching in the area, burning, or peeling. Repeat every 4 weeks, up to three treatments or until warts are gone.[11] SOR Ⓑ
- Cantharidin 0.7 percent is an extract of the blister beetle that is applied to the wart after which blistering occurs. It may be used in resistant cases.[12] It is also useful in young children because application is painless in the office. However, painful blisters often occur within a day after application. Be careful not to overtreat with cantharidin because the blistering can be quite severe. Carefully apply to multiple lesions using the wooden end of one or two cotton-tipped applicators. SOR Ⓒ

SURGICAL

- Cryotherapy, most commonly with liquid nitrogen, is useful but is somewhat painful for younger children.[7] SOR Ⓑ Chemical cryogens are now available over the counter but are not as cold or effective as liquid nitrogen. Most trials comparing cryotherapy with salicylic acid found similar effectiveness.[2] Liquid nitrogen is applied for 5 to 10 seconds via a Cryogun or a cotton swab so that the freeze ball extends 1 to 2 mm beyond the lesion. Because flat warts are thinner than common warts, the freeze times needed are shorter. Two freeze cycles may improve resolution, but it is better to underfreeze than overfreeze since overfreezing may lead to permanent scarring or hypopigmentation. Best results of cryotherapy can be achieved when the patient is treated every 2 or 3 weeks. There is no therapeutic benefit beyond 3 months.[2] SOR Ⓑ Because HPV can survive in liquid nitrogen, cotton swabs and residual liquid nitrogen should be properly discarded to avoid spreading the virus to other patients or contaminating the liquid nitrogen reservoir.[13] After cryotherapy, the skin shows erythema and may progress to hemorrhagic blistering. Healing occurs in approximately a week and hypopigmentation may occur. Common adverse effects of cryotherapy include pain, blistering, and hypo- or hyperpigmentation.
- Pulsed-dye laser can be considered for treatment of recalcitrant warts, although the effectiveness is unproven.[2] SOR Ⓑ

PREVENTION

- Hair-bearing areas with warts should be shaved with depilatories, electric razors, or not at all to help limit spread of warts.

FOLLOW-UP

- Schedule patients for a return visit in 2 to 3 weeks after therapy to assess efficacy.

PATIENT EDUCATION

- To help avoid spreading warts, patients should avoid touching or scratching the lesions.
- Razors that are used in areas where warts are located should not be used on normal skin or by other people to prevent spread.

PATIENT RESOURCES

- KidsHealth—**www.kidshealth.org/parent/infections/skin/wart.html**.
- American Academy of Dermatology—**www.aad.org/public/Publications/pamphlets/Warts.htm**.
- MedlinePlus. *Warts*—**www.nlm.nih.gov/medlineplus/ency/article/000885.htm**.

PROVIDER RESOURCES

- Bacelieri R, Johnson SM: Cutaneous warts. An evidence-based approach to therapy. *Am Fam Physician*. 2005;72:647-652—**www.aafp.org/afp/20050815/647.html**.
- Cochrane Review. *Topical Treatments for Cutaneous Warts*—**www.cochrane.org/reviews/en/ab001781.html**.
- Treatment of warts is covered extensively in: Usatine R, Pfenninger J, Stulberg D, Small R. *Dermatologic and Cosmetic Procedures in Office Practice*. Elsevier, Inc., Philadelphia. 2012. This can also be purchased as an electronic application at **www.usatinemedia.com**.

REFERENCES

1. Williams H, Pottier A, Strachan D. Are viral warts seen more commonly in children with eczema? *Arch Dermatol.* 1993;129: 717-720.
2. Mulhem E, Pinelis S. Treatment of nongenital cutaneous warts. *Am Fam Physician.* 2011;84(3):288-293.
3. Sterling JC, Handfield-Jones S, Hudson PM. British Association of Dermatologists. Guidelines for the management of cutaneous warts. *Br J Dermatol.* 2001;144(1):4-11.
4. Tey HL, Tan ES, Tan FG, Tan KL, Lim IS, Tan AS. Reducing anxiety levels in preschool children undergoing cryotherapy for cutaneous viral warts: use of a portable video player. *Arch Dermatol.* 2012; 148(9):1001-1004.
5. Gibbs S, Harvey I. Topical treatments for cutaneous warts. *Cochrane Database Syst Rev.* 2006;(3):CD001781.
6. Lockshin NA. Flat facial warts treated with fluorouracil. *Arch Dermatol.* 1979;115:929-1030.
7. Lee S, Kim J-G, Chun SI. Treatment of verruca plana with 5% 5-fluorouracil ointment. *Dermatologica.* 1980;160:383-389.
8. Cutler K, Kagen MH, Don PC, et al. Treatment of facial verrucae with topical imiquimod cream in a patient with human immunodeficiency virus. *Acta Derm Venereol.* 2000;80:134 135.
9. Kim MB. Treatment of flat warts with 5% imiquimod cream. *J Eur Acad Dermatol Venereol.* 2006;20(10):1349-1350.
10. Schwab RA, Elston DM. Topical imiquimod for recalcitrant facial flat warts. *Cutis.* 2000;65:160-162.
11. Ritter SE, Meffert J. Successful treatment of flat warts using intralesional *Candida* antigen. *Arch Dermatol.* 2003;139(4):541-542.
12. Kartal Durmazlar SP, Atacan D, Eskioglu F. Cantharidin treatment for recalcitrant facial flat warts: a preliminary study. *J Dermatolog Treat.* 2009;20(2):114-119.
13. Tabrizi SN, Garland SM. Is cryotherapy treating or infecting? *Med J Aust.* 1996;164(5):263.

118 GENITAL WARTS

E.J. Mayeaux, Jr., MD
Richard P. Usatine, MD

PATIENT STORY

A 16-year-old boy presents with growths in the genital area for about 1 month (**Figure 118-1**). He has never had a sexually transmitted disease (STD) or vaccination against human papillomavirus (HPV) infection. He has had multiple sexual partners. The patient is told that he has genital warts which are an STD caused by HPV. The treatment options are discussed and he chooses to have cryotherapy with liquid nitrogen. A urine test for gonorrhea and *Chlamydia* is performed and the patient is tested for syphilis and HIV. Fortunately, all the additional tests are negative. Further patient education is performed and follow-up is arranged.

INTRODUCTION

More than 100 types of HPV exist, with more than 40 that can infect the human genital area. Most HPV infections are asymptomatic, unrecognized, or subclinical. Low-risk HPV types (e.g., HPV types 6 and 11) cause genital warts, although coinfection with HPV types associated with squamous intraepithelial neoplasia can occur. Asymptomatic genital HPV infection is common in sexually active persons and usually self-limited.[1]

SYNONYMS

Condyloma acuminata.

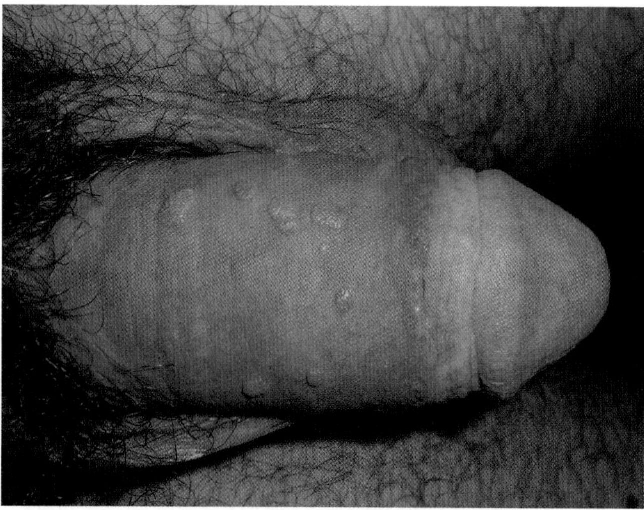

FIGURE 118-1 Condyloma acuminata in 16-year-old circumcised boy not practicing safe sex. He has isolated lesions on the shaft of the penis. He was treated with cryotherapy using liquid nitrogen. (*Used with permission from Richard P. Usatine, MD.*)

EPIDEMIOLOGY

- Anogenital warts are the most common viral STD in the US. There are approximately 1 million new cases of genital warts per year in the US.[2]
- Most infections are transient and cleared within 2 years.[2]
- Some infections persist and recur and cause much distress for the patients.

ETIOLOGY AND PATHOPHYSIOLOGY

- Genital warts are caused by HPV infection in males (**Figure 118-1**) and females (**Figure 118-2**). HPV encompasses a family of primarily sexually transmitted double-stranded DNA viruses. The incubation period after exposure ranges from 3 weeks to 8 months.
- HPV can be transmitted both sexually and non-sexually.[3] Cutaneous HPV types can persist over a long time in healthy skin.[4] HPV DNA detection in amniotic fluid, fetal membranes, cord blood and placental trophoblastic cells all suggest some HPV infection may occur in utero (prenatal transmission).[3]
- The first systematic review on vertical transmission of HPV included 2,113 newborns found the pooled mother-to-child HPV transmission was 6.5 percent. Transmission was higher after vaginal delivery than after caesarean section (18.3% vs 8%) (RR = 1.8; 95% CI 1.3–2.4).[5]

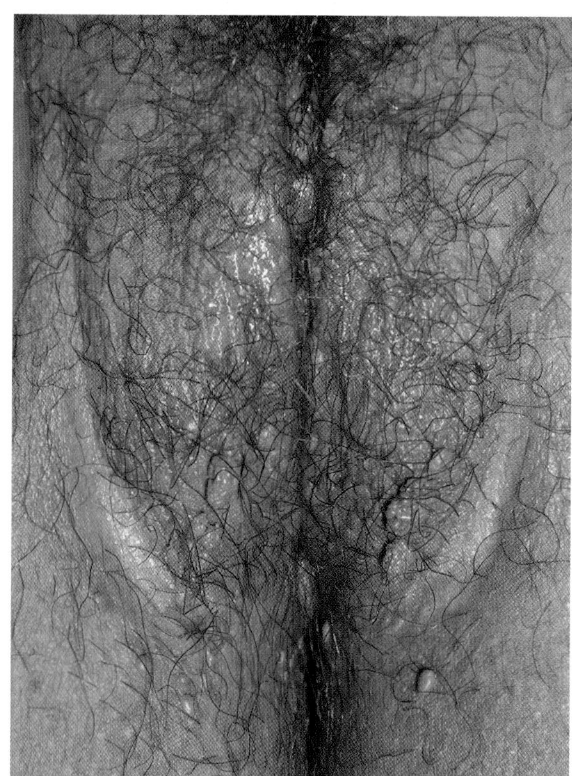

FIGURE 118-2 Multiple vulvar exophytic condyloma in an 18-year-old woman. She had never had a sexually transmitted disease (STD) or vaccination against human papillomavirus (HPV) but admitted to 2 new sexual partners in the prior 6 months. (*Used with permission from Richard P. Usatine, MD.*)

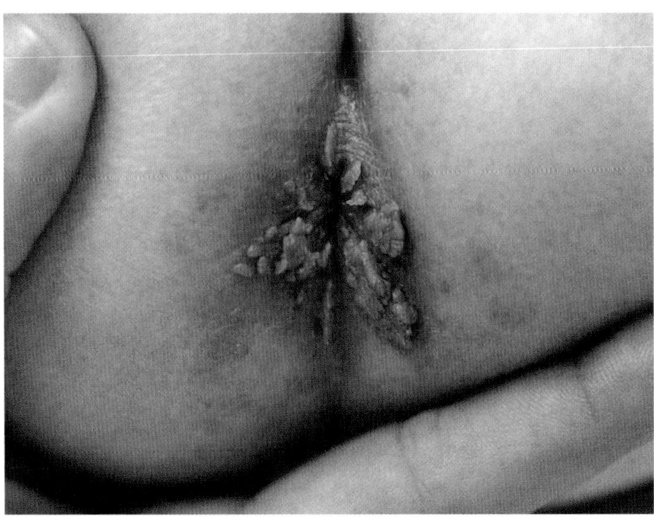

FIGURE 118-3 Perianal condyloma in a 2-year-old girl for 2 months. The child was brought in by her mother who did have warts on her hands. The mother claims that the child is always with her immediate family, never in day care, and no one in the family had genital warts. The clinician did not suspect child abuse, did not file a report and treated the condyloma topically. (*Image used with permission from Robert Brodell, MD.*)

- Most of the mucosal HPV infections in infants are incidental, persistent infections in oral and genital mucosa being found in less than 10 and 2 percent respectively.[3] Condyloma acuminata in children younger than two to three years of age are more likely the result of maternal-child transmission, but may be due to sexual or nonsexual transmission (**Figure 118-3**).
- In one study, 73 children with anogenital warts were examined for sexual abuse during a 2-year period. Approximately 25 percent of these children were younger than age 1 year, and another 50 percent were between the ages of 1 and 3 years. No evidence of sexual abuse was detected in 66 children. The authors concluded that nonsexual transmission is common, particularly in children under 3 years of age.[6]
- HPV testing of mothers does not exclude sexual abuse and is not generally performed.
- Evaluation for potential sexual abuse should be considered, especially in older children, and evaluation by appropriately experienced professionals considered.

RISK FACTORS

- Sexual intercourse and oral sex.
- Other types of sexual activity including digital–anal, oral–anal, and digital–vaginal contact.
- Immunosuppression, especially HIV.

DIAGNOSIS

CLINICAL FEATURES

- Diagnosis of genital warts is usually clinical based on visual inspection.[1]

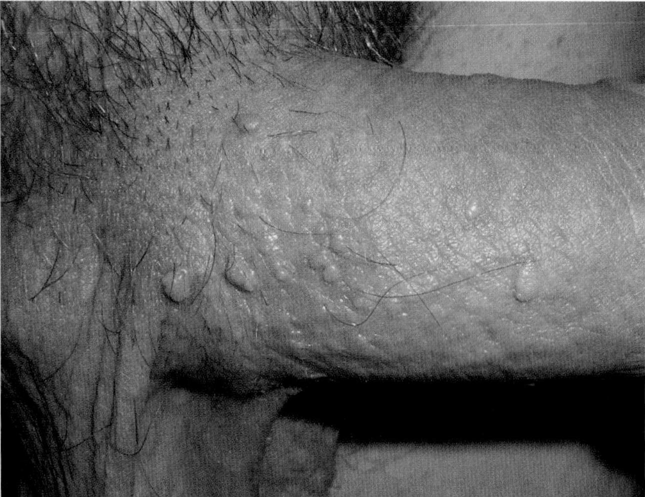

FIGURE 118-4 Smooth-topped condyloma on the well-keratinized skin of a circumcised teen. (*Used with permission from Richard P. Usatine, MD.*)

- Genital warts are usually asymptomatic, and typically present as flesh-colored, exophytic lesions on the genitalia, including the penis, vulva, vagina, scrotum, perineum, and perianal skin.
- External warts can appear as small bumps, or they may be flat, verrucous, or pedunculated (**Figures 118-4** to **188-6**).
- Less commonly, warts can appear as reddish or brown, smooth, raised papules, or as dome-shaped lesions on keratinized skin.

TYPICAL DISTRIBUTION

- In women, the most common sites of infection are the vulva (**Figure 118-2**), perianal area, and the vagina.
- In men, the most common sites of infection are the penis (**Figures 118-1**, and **118-4** to **118-6** and scrotum.
- Perianal warts can occur in men or women who have a history of anal intercourse, and in those who do not have any such history (**Figure 118-7**).[1]

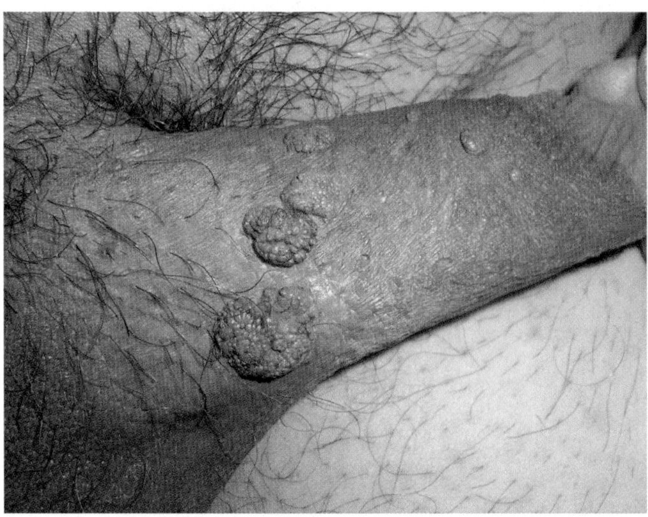

FIGURE 118-5 Condyloma can take on a cauliflower appearance even on the well-keratinized skin of a circumcised male. (*Used with permission from Richard P. Usatine, MD.*)

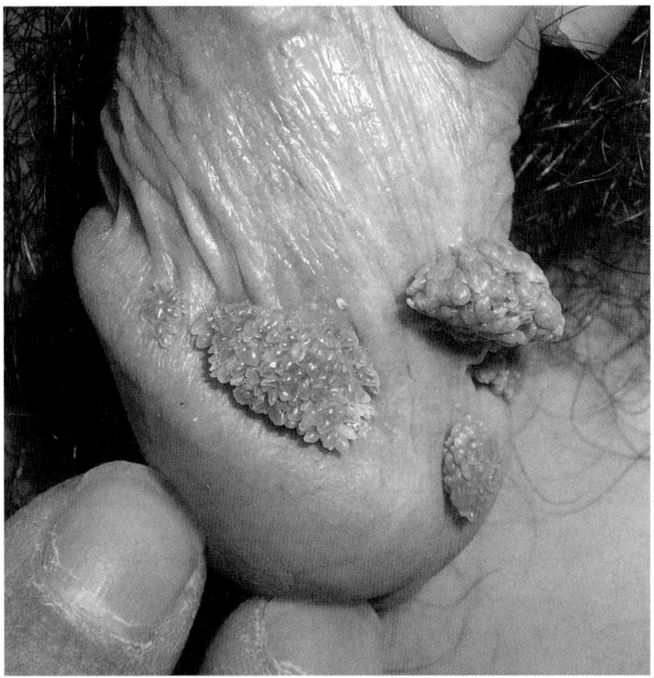

FIGURE 118-6 Condyloma acuminata demonstrating a cauliflower appearance with typical papillary surface seen when the foreskin is retracted in an uncircumcised young man. Note that the top wart is pedunculated with a narrow base. (*Used with permission from Richard P. Usatine, MD.*)

- Condyloma acuminata may be seen on the abdomen or upper thighs in conjunction with genital warts (**Figure 118-8**).

LABORATORY TESTING

- A screen for syphilis and a HIV test should be ordered as well. Genital warts are a sexually transmitted disease and patients who have one STD should be screened for others (**Figure 118-9**).
- HPV viral typing is not recommended because test results would not alter clinical management of the condition. The application of

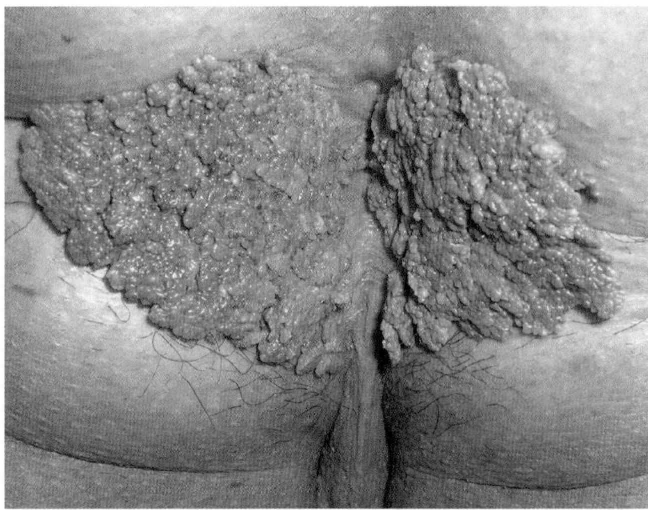

FIGURE 118-7 Extensive perianal warts in a 17-year-old boy who denies sexual abuse and anal intercourse. Patient failed imiquimod therapy and was referred to surgery. (*Used with permission from Richard P. Usatine, MD.*)

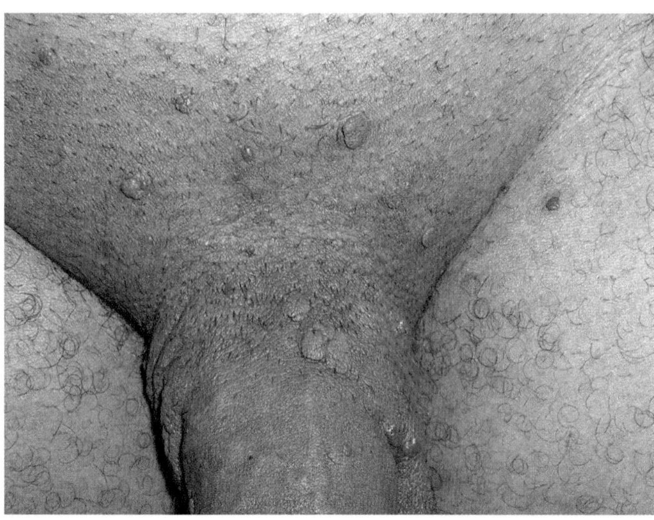

FIGURE 118-8 Condyloma that started on the penis and spread up the abdomen and on to the thighs. Note how these warts are hyperpigmented in this black teenager. (*Used with permission from Richard P. Usatine, MD.*)

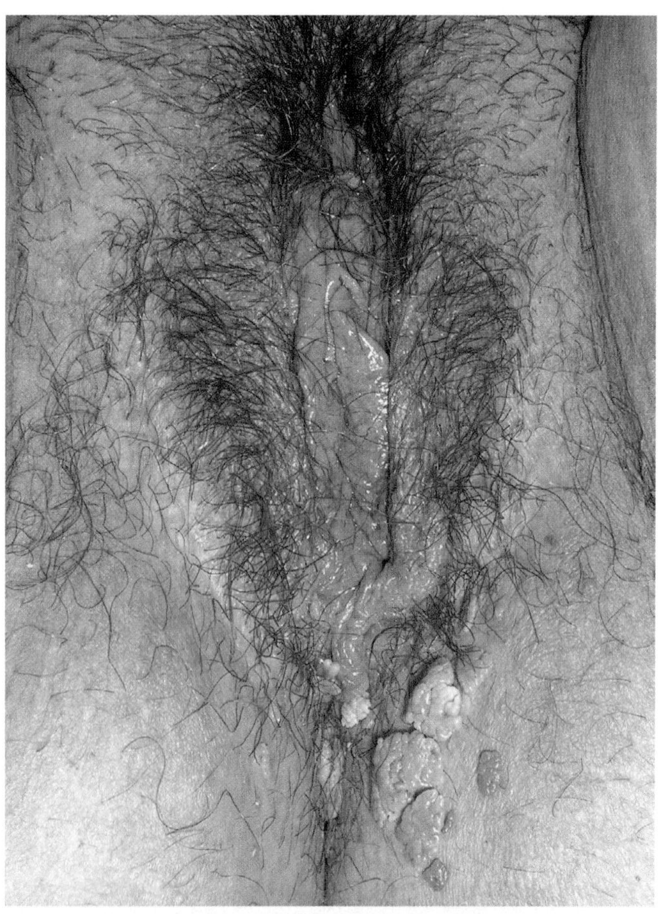

FIGURE 118-9 This teenager tested positive for syphilis at the time she presented with condyloma acuminata. While her RPR was positive these warts were more likely to be HPV related rather than the condyloma lata of secondary syphilis. The patient was treated with IM benzathine penicillin and cryotherapy. (*Used with permission from Richard P. Usatine, MD.*)

3 to 5 percent acetic acid to detect mucosal changes attributed to HPV infection is no longer recommended.[1]

BIOPSY

- Diagnosis may be confirmed by shave or punch biopsy if necessary.[1] Biopsy is indicated if:
  - The diagnosis is uncertain.
  - The patient has a poor response to appropriate therapy.
  - Warts are atypical in appearance (unusually pigmented, indurated, fixed, or ulcerated).
  - The patient has compromised immunity and squamous cell carcinoma is suspected (one type of HPV-related malignancy).

DIFFERENTIAL DIAGNOSIS

- Pearly penile papules, which are small papules around the edge of the glans penis (**Figure 118-10**), may be confused with genital warts.
- Molluscum contagiosum—Waxy umbilicated papules around the genitals and lower abdomen (see Chapter 115, Molluscum Contagiosum).
- Condyloma lata is caused by secondary syphilis infection; lesions appear flat and velvety (see Chapter 181, Syphilis). A full work-up for other STDs, including syphilis, should be done for any patient with genital warts (**Figure 118-9**).
- Micropapillomatosis of the vulva is a normal variant and appears as distinct individual papillary projections from the labia in a symmetrical pattern.

MANAGEMENT

- The primary reason for treating genital warts is the amelioration of symptoms and ultimately removal of the warts.[1]

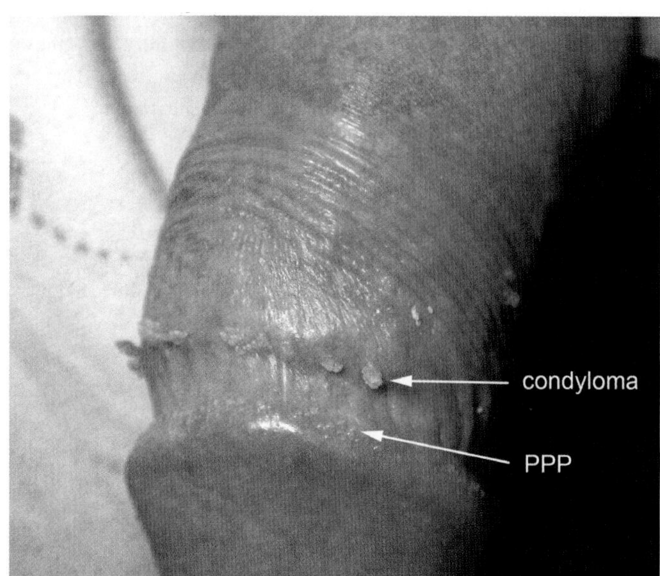

FIGURE 118-10 Condyloma coexisting with pearly penile papules (PPPs), which are a normal variant on the edge of the corona. (*Used with permission from Richard P. Usatine, MD.*)

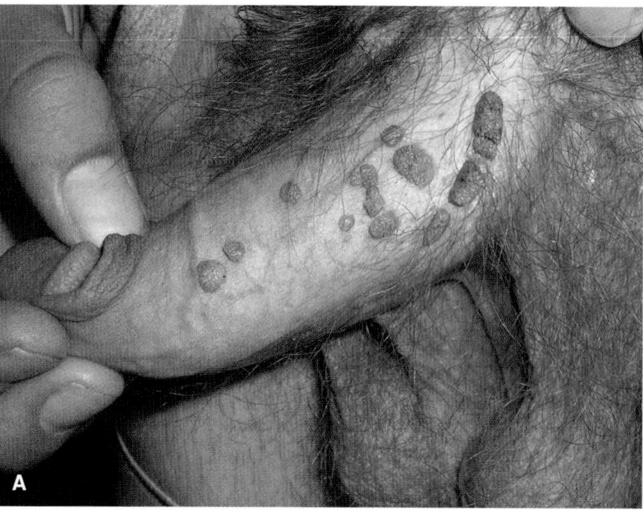

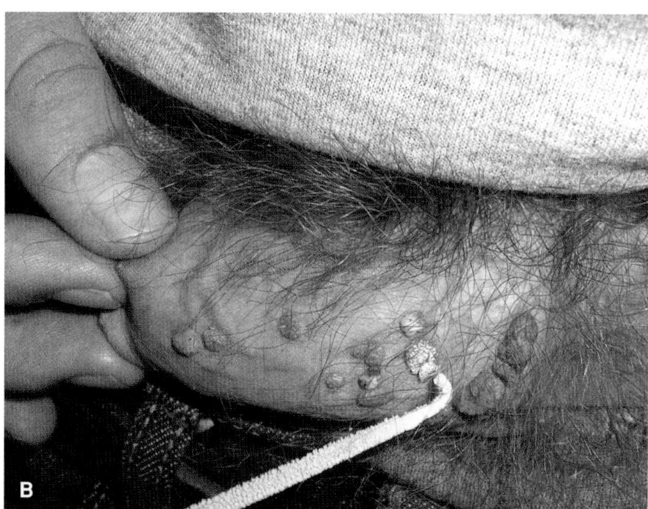

FIGURE 118-11 **A.** Condyloma on the penile shaft of a sexually active teenager not practicing safe sex. **B.** Cryotherapy of the condyloma using a liquid nitrogen spray technique and a bent-tipped applicator. (*Used with permission from Richard P. Usatine, MD.*)

- The choice of therapy is based on the number, size, site, and morphology of lesions, as well as patient preference, treatment cost, convenience, adverse effects, and physician experience.
- Although available therapies for genital warts are likely to reduce HPV infectivity, they probably do not eradicate transmission.[1]

MEDICATIONS AND SURGICAL METHODS

- Treatments for external genital warts include topical medications, cryotherapy (**Figure 118-11**), and surgical methods, and are shown in **Table 118-1**.
- For children under 12 years of age, there are no US Food and Drug Administration-approved treatments for genital warts.[11]
- Cryotherapy is best applied with a bent-tipped spray applicator that allows for precise application with a less painful attenuated flow (**Figure 118-11**).[12] Application may be repeated every 2 weeks if necessary.
- Treatment with 5 percent fluorouracil cream (Efudex) is no longer recommended because of severe local side effects and teratogenicity.[1]

TABLE 118-1 Treatments for External Genital Warts

Treatment	Possible Adverse Effects	Clearance (%)	Recurrence (%)
Patient-Applied Therapy			
Imiquimod (Aldara) is applied at bedtime for 3 days, then rest 4 days; alternatively, apply every other day for 3 applications; may repeat weekly cycles for up to 16 weeks[8] SOR A	Erythema, irritation, ulceration, pain, and pigmentary changes; minimal systemic absorption	30 to 50	15
Sinecatechins 15 percent ointment—Apply a 0.5-cm strand of ointment to each wart 3 times daily[6] SOR A	Erythema, pruritus/burning, pain, ulceration, edema, induration, and vesicular rash	53 to 57	3.7
Podofilox (Condylox) is applied twice daily for 3 days, then rest 4 days; may repeat for 4 cycles[7] SOR A	Burning, pain, inflammation; low risk for systemic toxicity unless applied to occluded membranes	45 to 80	5 to 30
Provider-Applied Therapy			
Cryotherapy performed with liquid nitrogen or a cryoprobe[6] SOR B	Pain or blisters at application site, scarring	60 to 90	20 to 40
Podophyllin resin is applied to each wart and allowed to dry, and is repeated weekly as needed[6,10] SOR A	Local irritation, erythema, burning, and soreness at application site; neurotoxic and oncogenic if absorbed	30 to 80	20 to 65
Surgical treatment for warts involves removal to the dermal–epidermal junction; options include scissor excision, shave excision, laser vaporization, and loop electrosurgical excision procedure (LEEP) excision[9] SOR B	Pain, bleeding, scarring; risk for burning and allergic reaction from local anesthetic; laser and LEEP have risk for spreading HPV in plume	35 to 70	5 to 50
Trichloroacetic acid (TCA) and bichloracetic acid (BCA) are applied to each wart and allowed to dry; repeated weekly[6] SOR B	Local pain and irritation; no systemic side effects	50 to 80	35

- In younger children, cryotherapy is often not well tolerated because of associated pain. Some authors suggest applying topical anesthetics prior to cryotherapy. However, a double-blind, randomized, controlled trial using eutectic lidocaine/prilocaine 5 percent cream for local anesthesia before cryotherapy of nongenital warts in children ages 6 to 18 did not significantly decrease the pain associated with the procedure.[13] SOR A
- Podophyllotoxin 0.5 percent gel and imiquimod 5 percent cream has been safely used in children as young as age 1 year.[14,15] SOR B

REFERRAL OR HOSPITALIZATION

- Consider consultation for patients with very large or recalcitrant lesions.

PREVENTION

- A bivalent vaccine (Cervarix) containing HPV types 16 and 18, and a quadrivalent vaccine (Gardasil) vaccine containing HPV types 6, 11, 16, and 18 are licensed in the US. The quadrivalent HPV vaccine protects against the HPV types that cause 90 percent of genital warts (i.e., types 6 and 11) in males and females when given prophylactically. Both vaccines offer protection against the HPV types that cause 70 percent of cervical cancers (i.e., types 16 and 18). In the US, the quadrivalent (Gardasil) HPV vaccine can also be used in males and females ages 9 to 26 years to prevent genital warts.[7]

PROGNOSIS

- Many genital warts will eventually resolve without treatment. Resolution can usually be hastened with therapy (**Table 118-1**).

FOLLOW-UP

- Patients should be offered a follow-up evaluation 2 to 3 months after treatment to check for new lesions.[1] SOR C

PATIENT EDUCATION

- HPV is transmitted mainly by skin-to-skin contact. Although condoms may decrease the levels of transmission, they are imperfect barriers at best as they can fail, and they do not cover the scrotum or vulva, where infection may reside.

PATIENT RESOURCES

- eMedicineHealth. *Genital Warts (HPV Infection)*—**www.emedicinehealth.com/genital_warts/article_em.htm**.
- PubMed Health. *Genital Warts*—**www.ncbi.nlm.nih.gov/pubmedhealth/PMH0001889/**.
- American Academy of Dermatology. *Genital Warts*—**www.aad.org/skin-conditions/dermatology-a-to-z/genital-warts**.
- MedlinePlus. *Genital Warts*—**www.nlm.nih.gov/medlineplus/ency/article/000886.htm**.

PROVIDER RESOURCES

- Centers for Disease Control and Prevention. *Genital Warts*—**www.cdc.gov/std/treatment/2010/genital-warts.htm**.
- Medscape. *Genital Warts*—**http://emedicine.medscape.com/article/1118201**.
- Medscape. *Genital Warts in Emergency Medicine*—**http://emedicine.medscape.com/article/763014**.

REFERENCES

1. Centers for Disease Control and Prevention. *2010 Guidelines for Treatment of Sexually Transmitted Diseases*. http://www.cdc.gov/std/treatment/2010/STD-Treatment-2010-RR5912.pdf, accessed December 1, 2011.
2. Burk RD, Kelly P, Feldman J, et al. Declining prevalence of cervicovaginal human papillomavirus infection with age is independent of other risk factors. *Sex Transm Dis*. 1996;23:333-341.
3. Syrjänen S. Current concepts on human papillomavirus infections in children. *APMIS*. 2010;118(6-7):494-509.
4. Hsu JYC, Chen ACH, Keleher A, McMillan NAJ, Antonsson A. Shared and persistent asymptomatic cutaneous human papillomavirus infections in healthy skin. *J Med Virol*. 2009;81:1444-1449.
5. Medeiros LR, Ethur AB, Hilgert JB, Zanini RR, Berwanger O, Bozzetti MC, Mylius LC. Vertical transmission of the human papillomavirus: a systematic quantitative review. Cad Saude Publica. 2005;21(4):1006-1015.
6. Cohen BA, Honig P, Androphy E. Anogenital warts in children. Clinical and virologic evaluation for sexual abuse. *Arch Dermatol*. 1990;126(12):1575-1580.
7. Centers for Disease Control and Prevention (CDC). FDA licensure of quadrivalent human papillomavirus vaccine (HPV4, Gardasil) for use in males and guidance from the Advisory Committee on Immunization Practices (ACIP). *MMWR Morb Mortal Wkly Rep*. 2010;59(20):630-632.
8. Gotovtseva EP, Kapadia AS, Smolensky MH, Lairson DR. Optimal frequency of imiquimod (Aldara) 5% cream for the treatment of external genital warts in immunocompetent adults: a meta-analysis. *Sex Transm Dis*. 2008;35(4):346-351.
9. Mayeaux EJ Jr, Dunton C. Modern management of external genital warts. *J Low Genit Tract Dis*. 2008;12:185-192.
10. Langley PC, Tyring SK, Smith MH. The cost effectiveness of patient-applied versus provider-administered intervention strategies for the treatment of external genital warts. *Am J Manag Care*. 1999;5(1):69-77.
11. Thornsberry L, English JC 3rd: Evidence-based treatment and prevention of external genital warts in female pediatric and adolescent patients. J Pediatr Adolesc Gynecol. 2012;25(2):150-154.
12. Usatine R, Stulberg D. Cryosurgery. In: Usatine R, Pfenninger J, Stulberg D, Small R, eds. *Dermatologic and Cosmetic Procedures in Office Practice*. Philadelphia: Elsevier; 2012:182-198.
13. Gupta AK, Koren G, Shear NH. A double-blind, randomized, placebo-controlled trial of eutectic lidocaine/prilocaine cream 5% (EMLA) for analgesia prior to cryotherapy of warts in children and adults. *Pediatr Dermatol*. 1998;15:129e33.
14. Moresi JM, Herbert CR, Cohen BA. Treatment of anogenital warts in children with topical 0.05% podofilox gel and 5% imiquimod cream. *Pediatr Dermatol*. 2001;18:448e50.
15. Leclair E, Black A, Fleming N. Imiquimod 5% cream treatment for rapidly progressive genital condyloma in a 3-year-old girl. *J Pediatr Adolesc Gynecol*. 2012;25 (6):e119-21. doi: 10.1016.

119 PLANTAR WARTS

E.J. Mayeaux, Jr., MD

PATIENT STORY

A 15-year-old boy presents with painful growths on his right heel for approximately 6 months (**Figure 119-1**). It is painful to walk on and he would like it treated. He was diagnosed with multiple large plantar warts called *mosaic warts*. The lesions were treated with gentle paring with a #15 blade scalpel and liquid nitrogen therapy over a number of sessions. He and his mom were instructed on how to use salicylic acid plasters on the remaining warts.

INTRODUCTION

Plantar warts (verruca plantaris) are human papilloma virus (HPV) lesions that occur on the soles of the feet (**Figures 119-1** to **119-5**) and palms of the hands (**Figure 119-6**).

SYNONYMS

Palmoplantar warts, myrmecia.

EPIDEMIOLOGY

- Plantar warts affect mostly adolescents and young adults, affecting up to 10 percent of people in these age groups.[1]
- Prevalence studies demonstrate a wide range of values, from 0.84 percent in the US[2] to 3.3 to 4.7 percent in the United Kingdom,[3] to 24 percent in 16- to 18-year-olds in Australia.[4]

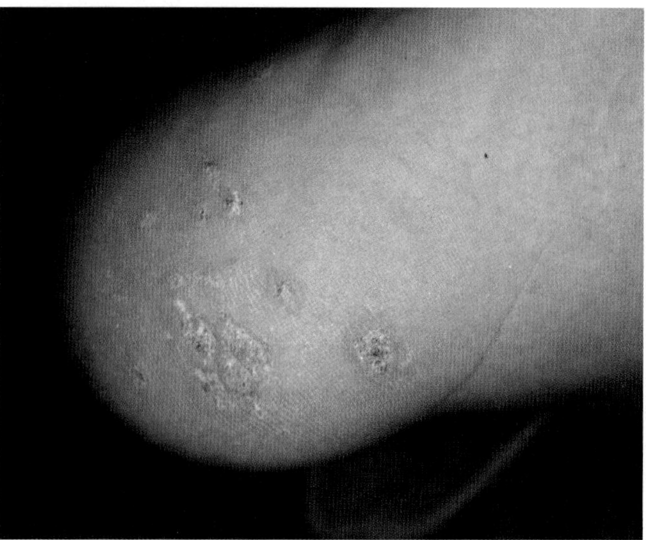

FIGURE 119-1 Plantar warts. Note small black dots in the warts that represent thrombosed vessels. Large plantar warts such as these are called *mosaic warts*. (*Used with permission from Richard P. Usatine, MD.*)

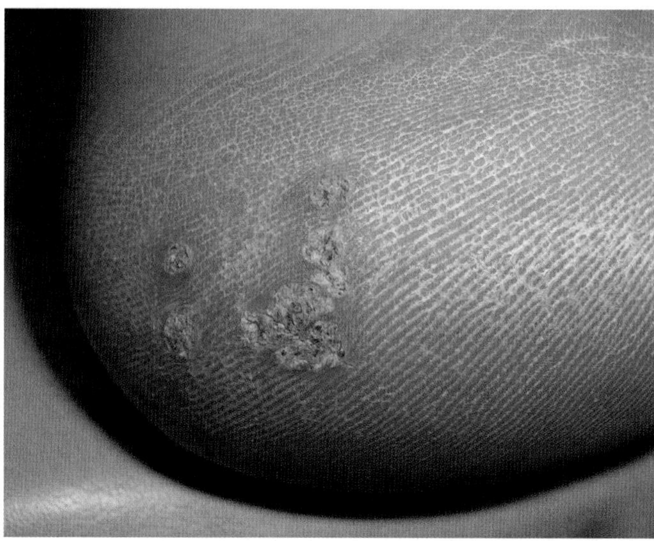

FIGURE 119-2 Close-up of plantar wart on the side of the heel. Note the disruption of skin lines and black dots. (*Used with permission from Richard P. Usatine, MD.*)

ETIOLOGY AND PATHOPHYSIOLOGY

- Plantar warts are caused by HPV.
- They usually occur at points of maximum pressure, such as on the heels (**Figures 119-1** to **119-4**) or over the heads of the metatarsal bones (**Figure 119-5** and **119-6**), but may appear anywhere on the plantar surface including the tips of the fingers (**Figure 119-7**).
- A thick, painful callus forms in response to the pressure that is induced as the size of the lesion increases. Even a minor wart can cause a lot of pain.
- A cluster of many warts that appear to fuse is referred to as a *mosaic wart* (**Figures 119-1** and **119-4**).

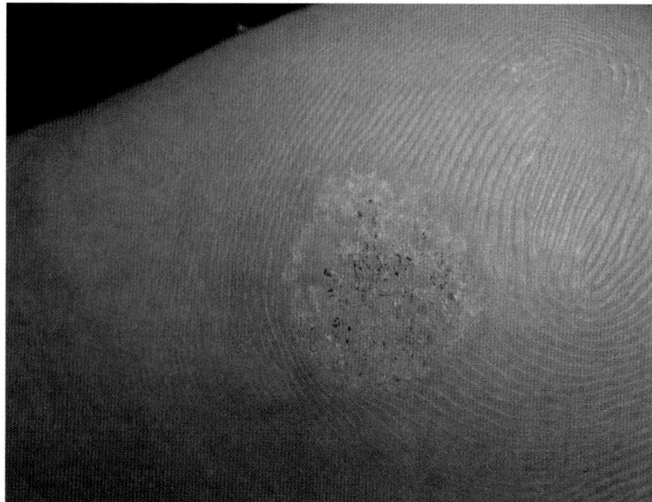

FIGURE 119-3 Close-up of a plantar wart demonstrating disruption of normal skin lines. Corns and callus do not disrupt normal skin lines. The black dots are thrombosed vessels, which are frequently seen in plantar warts. (*Used with permission from Richard P. Usatine, MD.*)

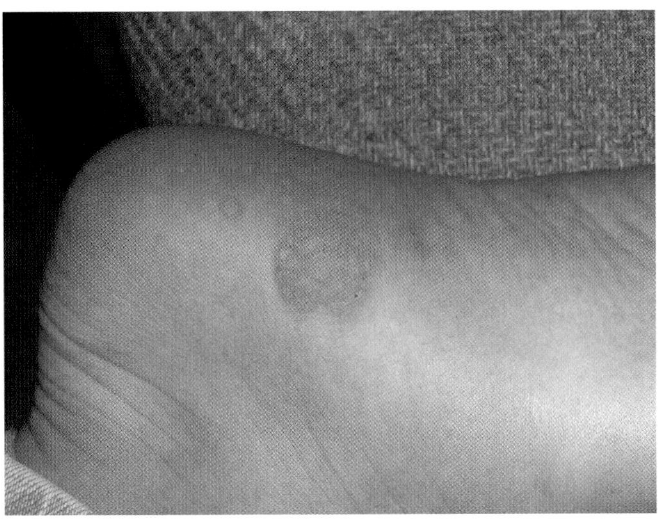

FIGURE 119-4 A mosaic wart is formed when several plantar warts become confluent. (*Used with permission from Richard P. Usatine, MD.*)

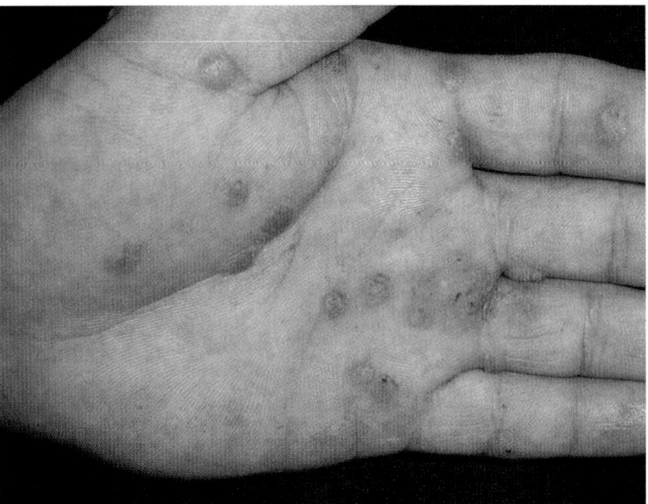

FIGURE 119-6 Multiple plantar warts on the palms of an HIV-positive young man. (*Used with permission from Richard P. Usatine, MD.*)

RISK FACTORS

- Young age.
- Decreased immunity.

DIAGNOSIS

CLINICAL FEATURES

Plantar warts present as thick, painful endophytic plaques located on the soles and/or palms. Warts have the following features:

- Begin as small shiny papules.
- Lack skin lines crossing their surface (**Figure 119-3**).
- Have a highly organized mosaic pattern on the surface when examined with a hand lens.
- Have a rough keratotic surface surrounded by a smooth collar of callused skin
- Painful when compressed laterally.
- May have centrally located black dots (thrombosed vessels) that may bleed with paring (**Figures 119-1** to **119-7**).

TYPICAL DISTRIBUTION

- They occur on the palms of the hands and soles of the feet. They are more commonly found on weight-bearing areas, such as under the metatarsal heads or on the heel.[5]

BIOPSY

- If the diagnosis is doubtful, a shave biopsy is indicated to confirm the diagnosis.[6]

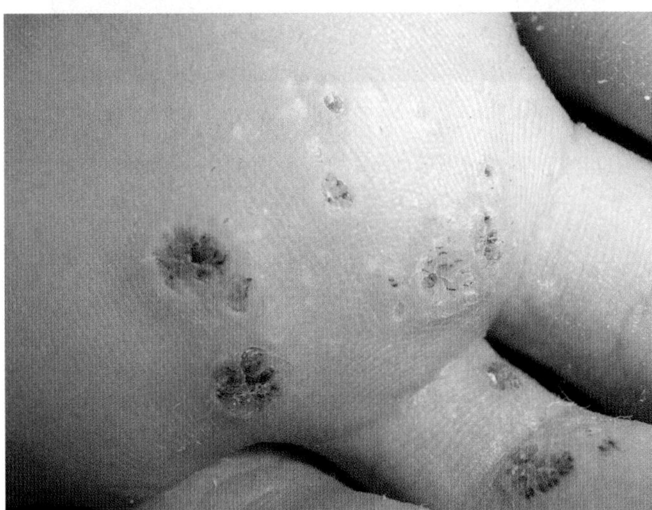

FIGURE 119-5 Multiple plantar warts on the ball of the foot and toes. The thrombosed vessels within the warts appear as black dots. (*Used with permission from Richard P. Usatine, MD.*)

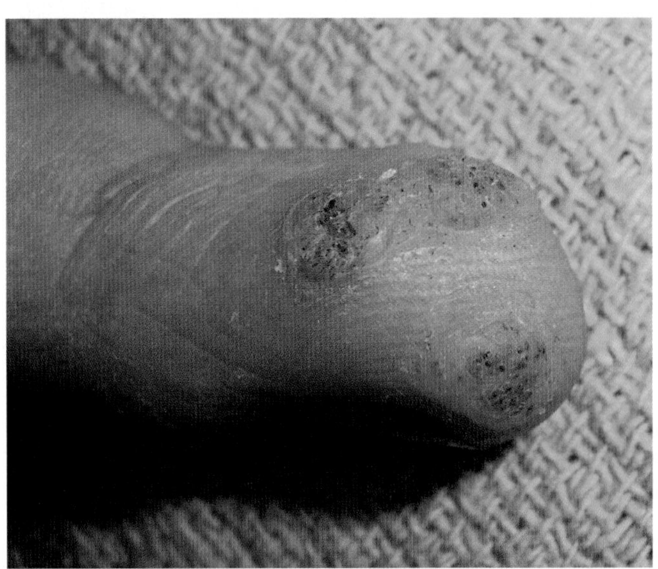

FIGURE 119-7 Close-up of plantar wart on a finger that also shows disruption of skin lines and black dots. (*Used with permission from Richard P. Usatine, MD.*)

DIFFERENTIAL DIAGNOSIS

- Corns and calluses are pressure-induced skin thickenings that occur on the feet and can be mistaken for plantar warts. Calluses are generally found on the sole and corns are usually found on the toes. Calluses and corns have skin lines crossing the surface, and are painless with lateral pressure.
- Black heel presents as a cluster of blue-black dots that result from ruptured capillaries. They appear on the plantar surface of the heel following the shearing trauma of sports that involve sudden stops or position changes. Examination reveals normal skin lines, and paring does not cause additional bleeding. The condition resolves spontaneously in a few weeks.
- Black warts are plantar warts undergoing spontaneous resolution, which may turn black and feel soft when pared with a blade.[7]
- Squamous cell carcinoma should be considered when lesions have irregular growth or pigmentation, ulceration, or resist therapy, particularly in immunosuppressed patients.
- Amelanotic melanoma, although extremely rare, can look similar to HPV lesions. Lesions that are treatment resistant or atypical, particularly on the palms or soles, should be monitored closely. A biopsy is required to establish the diagnosis (see Chapter 147, Melanoma).
- Palmoplantar keratoderma describes a rare heterogeneous group of disorders characterized by thickening of the palms and the soles that can also be an associated feature of different syndromes. They can be classified as having uniform involvement versus focal hyperkeratosis located mainly on pressure points and sites of recurrent friction (**Figure 119-8**). This latter type can be differentiated from plantar warts by the more diffuse locations on the palmoplantar surfaces, the mainly epidermal involvement, and biopsy, if necessary (**Figure 119-9**).

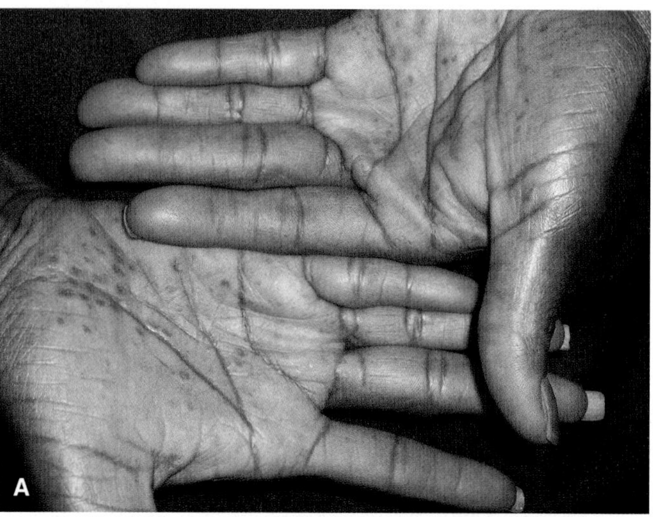

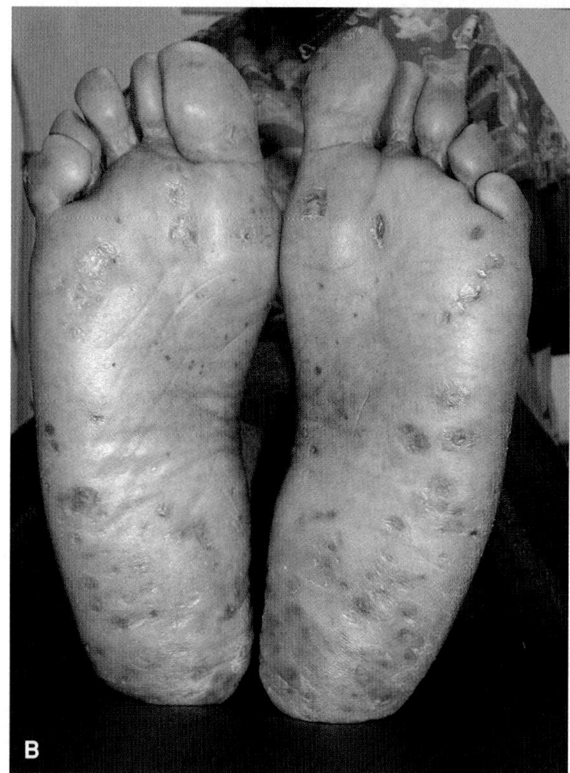

FIGURE 119-8 Focal palmoplantar keratoderma of the palms (**A**) and soles (**B**). This is an inherited genodermatosis. Note lesions are located mainly on higher pressure areas. (*Used with permission from Richard P. Usatine, MD.*)

MANAGEMENT

NONPHARMACOLOGIC

- Painless plantar warts do not require therapy. Minimal discomfort can be relieved by periodically removing the hyperkeratosis with a blade or pumice stone.
- Painful warts should be treated using a technique that causes minimal scarring as scars on the soles of the feet are usually permanent and painful.
- Patients with diabetes must be treated with the utmost care to minimize complications.

MEDICATIONS

- Topical salicylic acid solutions are available in nonprescription form and provide conservative keratolytic therapy. These preparations are nonscarring, minimally painful, and relatively effective, but require persistent application of medication once each day for weeks to months. The wart is first pared with a blade, pumice stone, or emery board, and the area soaked in warm water. The solution is then applied, allowed to dry, reapplied, and occluded with adhesive tape.[8] White, pliable, keratin forms and should be pared away carefully until pink skin is exposed.[9] SOR B
- Seventeen to fifty percent salicylic acid solution and plasters are available in nonprescription and prescription forms. However, the 17 percent solutions are more prevalent and easier to find in nonprescription form. The treatment is similar to the previous process, except that with plasters the salicylic acid has been incorporated into a pad. They are particularly useful in treating mosaic warts covering a large area. Pain is quickly relieved in plantar warts, because a large amount of keratin is removed during the first few days of treatment.[9] SOR B A recent multicenter, open-label, randomized,

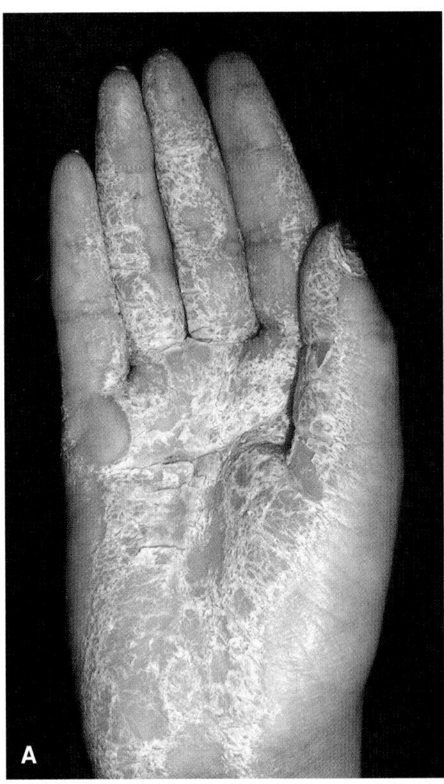

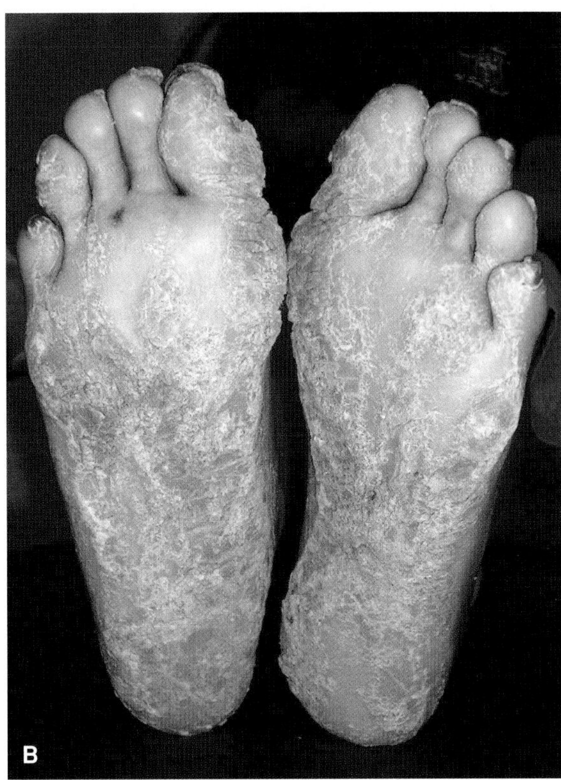

FIGURE 119-9 Diffuse palmoplantar keratoderma of the palms **(A)** and soles **(B)** in an 11-year-old girl. This is an inherited genodermatosis with severe functional consequences. (*Used with permission from Richard P. Usatine, MD.*)

controlled trial found that 50 percent salicylic acid and the cryotherapy were equally effective for clearance of plantar warts.[10] SOR Ⓐ

- Acid chemotherapy with trichloroacetic acid (TCA) or bichloracetic acid (BCA) is commonly employed to treat plantar warts in the office. They are considered safe during pregnancy for external lesions. The excess keratin is first pared with a scalpel, then the entire lesion is coated with acid, and the acid is worked into the wart with a sharp toothpick. The process is repeated every 7 to 10 days. SOR Ⓒ
- Cryotherapy with liquid nitrogen therapy is commonly used, but plantar warts are more resistant than other HPV lesions. The liquid nitrogen is applied to form a freeze ball that covers the lesion and 2 mm of surrounding normal tissue, usually 10 to 20 seconds per freeze. SOR Ⓒ There is no evidence that two freezing episodes are better than one, other than it allows for more freeze time in a way that is more acceptable to the patient. It is always better to underfreeze than to overfreeze in areas where scarring can produce permanent disability.
- Treatments for resistant lesions are often carried out in referral practices that have a high enough volume to use more expensive or specialized therapy. Cantharidin is an extract of the blister beetle that is applied to the wart after which blistering occurs. Intralesional immunotherapy with skin-test antigens (i.e., mumps, *Candida*, or *Trichophyton* antigens) may lead to the resolution both of the injected wart and other warts that were not injected. Contact immunotherapy using dinitrochlorobenzene, squaric acid dibutylester, and diphenylcyclopropenone may be applied to the skin to sensitize the patient and then to the lesion to induce an immune response. Intralesional bleomycin or laser therapy are also useful for recalcitrant warts. SOR Ⓒ

COMPLEMENTARY/ALTERNATIVE THERAPY

- Although many complementary and alternative therapies are promoted for wart therapy, there are no significant data supporting their use in the treatment of plantar warts.

PREVENTION

- Tools used for paring down warts, such as nail files and pumice stones, should not be used on normal skin or by other people.

PROGNOSIS

Most plantar warts will spontaneously disappear without treatment. Treatment often hastens resolution of lesions.

FOLLOW-UP

- Regular follow-up to assess treatment efficacy, adverse reactions, and patient tolerance are recommended to minimize treatment dropouts.

PATIENT EDUCATION

- Because spontaneous regression occurs, observation of painless lesions without treatment is preferable.
- Therapy often takes weeks to months, so patience and perseverance are essential for successful therapy.

PATIENT RESOURCES

- MayoClinic. *Plantar Warts*—**www.mayoclinic.com/health/plantar-warts/DS00509**.
- MedlinePlus. Warts—**www.nlm.nih.gov/medlineplus/warts.html**.
- Fort Drum Medical Activity. *Patient Education Handouts: Warts and Plantar Warts*—**www.drum.amedd.army.mil/pt_info/handouts/warts_Plantar.pdf**.

PROVIDER RESOURCES

- Bacelieri R, Johnson SM: Cutaneous warts: an evidence-based approach to therapy. *Am Fam Physician*. 2005;72[4]:647-652—**www.aafp.org/afp/20050815/647.html**.
- Medscape. *Nongenital Warts*—**http://emedicine.medscape.com/article/1133317**.

REFERENCES

1. Laurent R, Kienzler JL. Epidemiology of HPV infections. *Clin Dermatol*. 1985;3(4):64-70.
2. Johnson ML, Roberts J. Skin conditions and related need for medical care among persons 1-74 years. Rockville, MD. US Department of Health, Education, and Welfare; 1978:1-26.
3. Williams HC, Pottier A, Strachan D. The descriptive epidemiology of warts in British schoolchildren. *Br J Dermatol*. 1993;128:504-511.
4. Kilkenny M, Merlin K, Young R, Marks R. The prevalence of common skin conditions in Australian school students: 1. Common, plane and plantar viral warts. *Br J Dermatol*. 1998;138:840-845.
5. Holland TT, Weber CB, James WD. Tender periungual nodules. Myrmecia (deep palmoplantar warts). *Arch Dermatol*. 1992;128(1):105-106, 108-109.
6. Beutner, KR. Nongenital human papillomavirus infections. *Clin Lab Med*. 2000;20:423-430.
7. Berman A, Domnitz JM, Winkelmann RK. Plantar warts recently turned black. *Arch Dermatol*. 1982;118:47-51.
8. Landsman MJ, Mancuso JE, Abramow SP. Diagnosis, pathophysiology, and treatment of plantar verruca. *Clin Podiatr Med Surg*. 1996;13(1):55-71.
9. Gibbs S, Harvey

Cochrane Summaries. *Topical Treatments for Cutaneous Warts*. http://www.cochrane.org/reviews/en/ab001781.html, accessed April 1, 2008.

10. Cockayne S, Hewitt C, Hicks K, et al. Cryotherapy versus salicylic acid for the treatment of plantar warts (verrucae): a randomized controlled trial. *BMJ*. 2011;342:d3271.

SECTION 5 FUNGAL

120 FUNGAL OVERVIEW

Richard P. Usatine, MD

PATIENT STORY

An otherwise healthy 7-year-old boy is seen in a homeless shelter with a 2-month history of patchy hair loss (**Figure 120-1**). Various anti-dandruff shampoos had not helped. On physical exam, there are moderate areas of patchy alopecia with significant scaling of the scalp. Posterior cervical adenopathy could be seen and palpated on the left side. There was no fluorescence with a Wood's lamp indicating that this fungal infection was most likely *Trichophyton tonsurans*. The pediatrician easily identified this as tinea capitis but decided to confirm the diagnosis with a KOH preparation. Some of the scale was scraped from the scalp using two microscope slides (one to scrape and another to catch the scale). KOH was added and a coverslip placed. Branching hyphae were seen under the microscope. The child was treated with oral griseofulvin at 20 mg per kilogram per day. At the 4-week follow-up there was significant improvement, no reported side effects of the griseofulvin, and the treatment was continued for an additional 4 weeks.

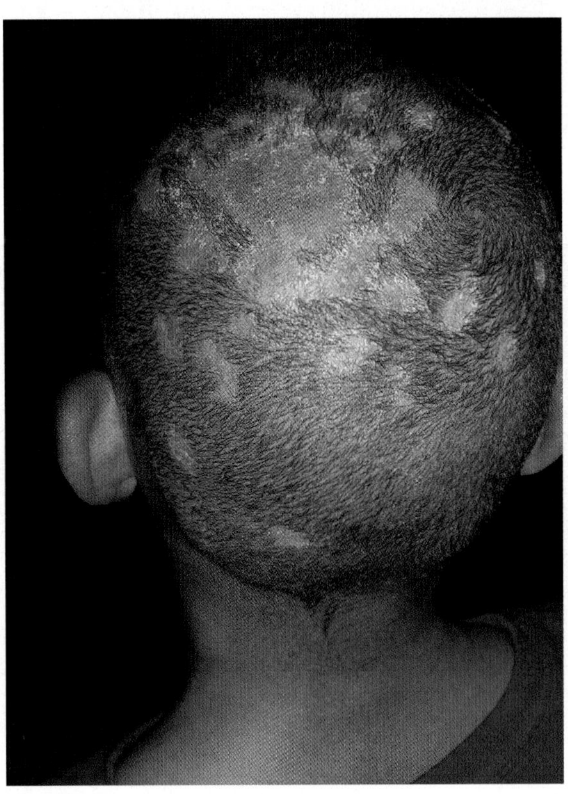

FIGURE 120-1 Tinea capitis in a young African American boy showing patchy alopecia and posterior cervical adenopathy. *(Used with permission from Richard P. Usatine, MD.)*

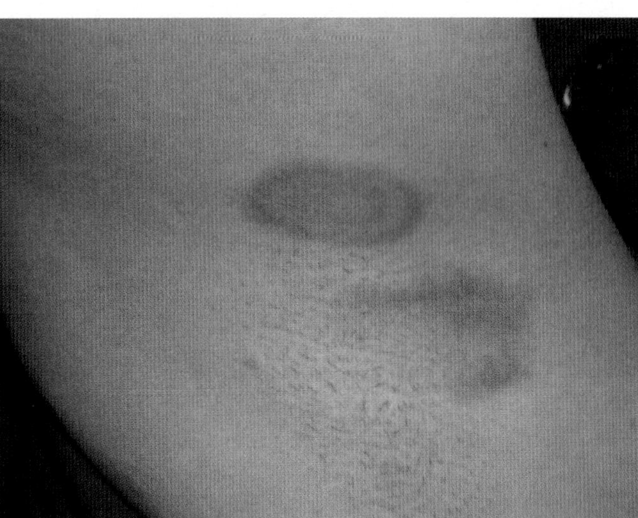

FIGURE 120-2 Annular pruritic lesion with concentric rings in the axilla of a young woman caused by tinea corporis. The concentric rings have a high specificity for tinea infections. *(Used with permission from Richard P. Usatine, MD.)*

INTRODUCTION

Fungal infections of the skin and mucous membranes are ubiquitous and common. There are many types of fungus that grow on humans but they all share a predilection for warm and moist areas. Consequently, hot and humid climates promote fungal infections, but many areas of the skin can get warm and sweaty even in cold climates, such as the feet and groin.

SYNONYMS

Pityriasis versicolor equals tinea versicolor.

PATHOPHYSIOLOGY

Mucocutaneous fungal infections are caused by:

- Dermatophytes in three genera: *Microsporum*, *Epidermophyton,* and *Trichophyton*. There are approximately 40 species in the three genera and these fungi cause tinea pedis and manus, tinea capitis, tinea corporis, tinea cruris, tinea faciei, and onychomycosis (**Figures 120-1** to **120-6**).
- Yeasts in the genera of *Candida* and *Pityrosporum* (*Malassezia*)—There are also multiple types of species and the *Pityrosporum* that cause seborrhea and tinea versicolor (**Figures 120-7** and **120-8**). Although tinea versicolor has the name tinea in it, it is not a true dermatophyte and may be best called pityriasis versicolor.
- There are a number of deep fungal skin infections that can occur in humans. They are all rare and will not be covered in this chapter which focuses on dermatophyte and yeast organisms. One deep

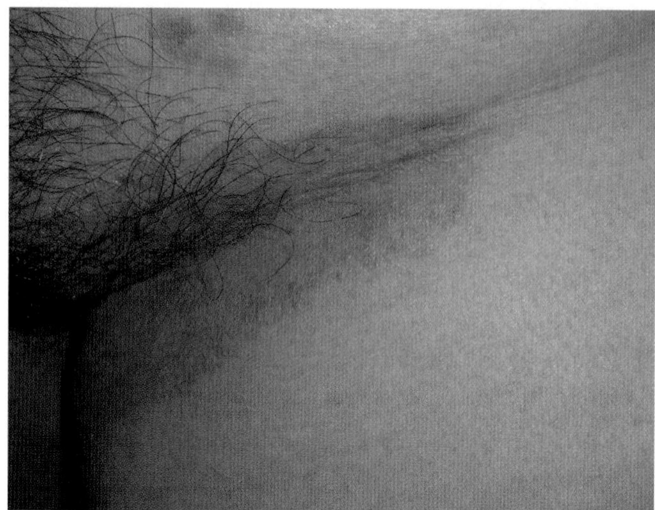

FIGURE 120-3 Tinea cruris with well-demarcated raised border and no central clearing. (*Used with permission from Richard P. Usatine, MD.*)

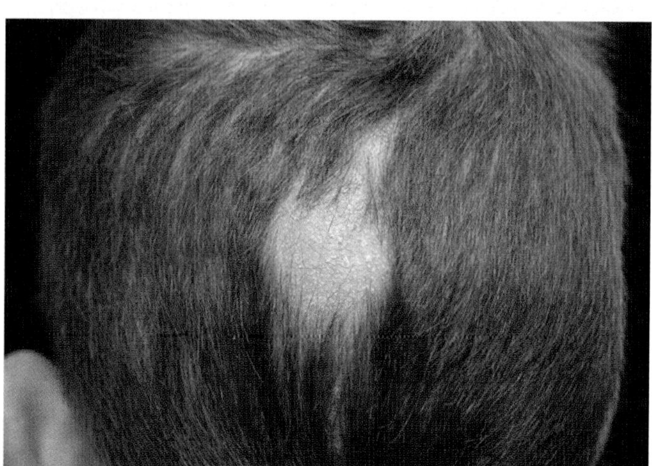

FIGURE 120-4 Tinea capitis in a 6-year-old boy with one major area of alopecia along with scale. (*Photo Credit: Dr. Patrick E. McCleskey, MD.*)

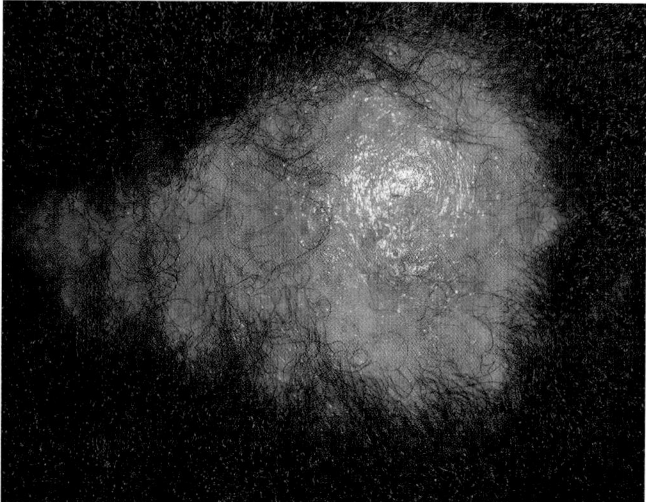

FIGURE 120-5 Tinea capitis in a 5-year-old black girl with hair loss and an inflammatory response. Her kerion is healing after initiating oral griseofulvin. (*Used with permission from Richard P. Usatine, MD.*)

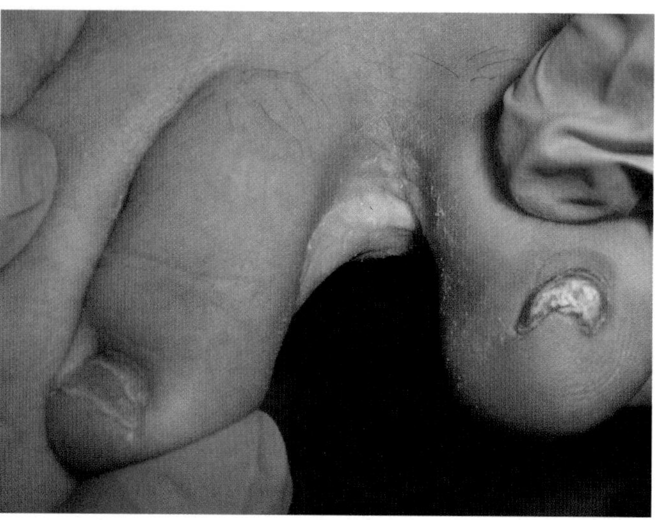

FIGURE 120-6 Tinea pedis with onychomycosis in a 14-year-old boy. (*Used with permission from Richard P. Usatine, MD.*)

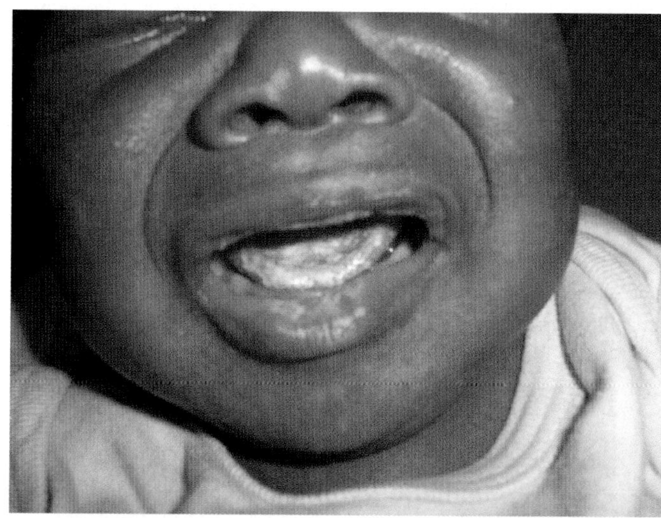

FIGURE 120-7 Thrush in the mouth of an infant caused by *Candida*. (*Used with permission from Richard P. Usatine, MD.*)

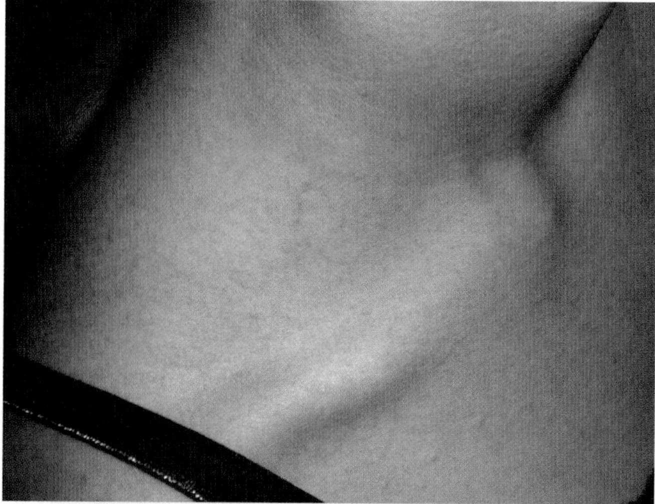

FIGURE 120-8 Tinea versicolor in a 13-year-old girl with an annular pattern on the shoulders. There is some central hypopigmentation and scale. The girl has seborrhea of the scalp also caused by Pityrosporum (Malassezia). The tinea versicolor was proven with a positive KOH. (*Used with permission from Richard P. Usatine, MD.*)

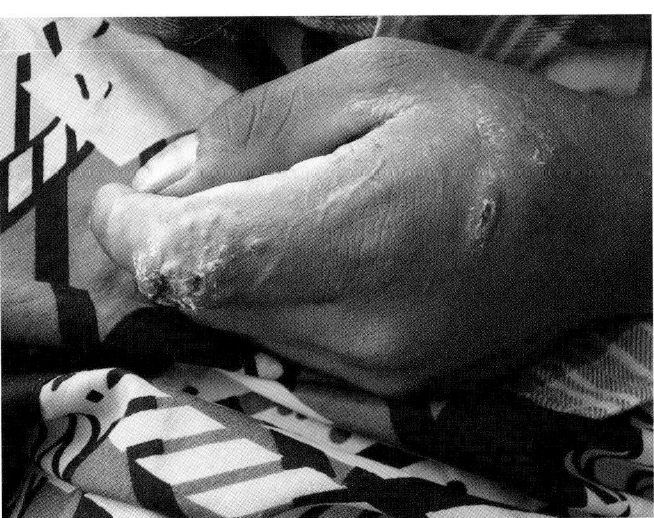

FIGURE 120-9 Sporotrichosis in a teenage boy. This deep fungal infection started with an inoculation to his index finger and spread up his arm. (*Used with permission from Richard P. Usatine, MD.*)

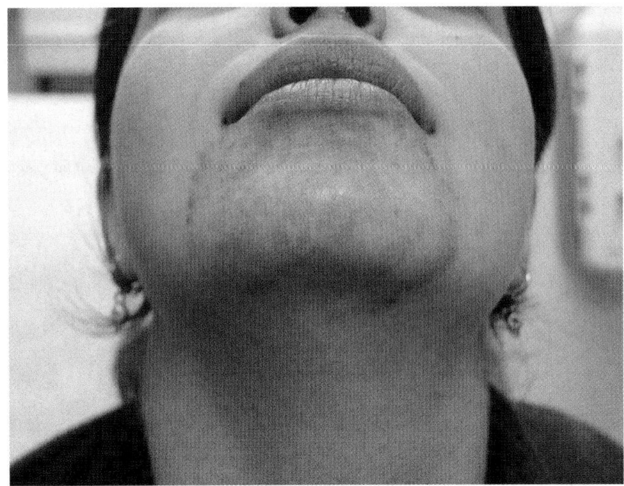

FIGURE 120-10 Tinea faciei on the face of a teenage female with typical scaling and a ring-like pattern (ringworm). Note the well-demarcated raised border and central clearing. (*Photo Credit: Dr. Patrick E. McCleskey, MD.*)

fungal infection that is less rare is Sporotrichosis and can occur from minor trauma with a rosebush thorn **(Figure 120-9)**.

DIAGNOSIS

CLINICAL FEATURES

Clinical features of tinea infections include scaling, erythema, pruritus, central clearing, concentric rings, and maceration (**Table 120-1**). Changes in pigmentation are not uncommon in various types of tinea especially tinea versicolor.

- **Figure 120-2** shows annular pruritic lesion with concentric rings in the axilla of a young woman caused by tinea corporis. The concentric rings have a high specificity (80%) for tinea infections.
- **Figure 120-10** shows tinea faciei on the face with typical scaling and ring-like pattern, hence, the name ringworm. There is also erythema and central clearing. The patient was experiencing pruritus.
- Note that tinea infections will not show central clearing in some cases, as in **Figure 120-3** in which tinea cruris has no central clearing. **Figure 120-11** shows tinea cruris with central clearing.
- Hyperpigmentation secondary to the fungal infection is common in dark-skinned individuals, as seen in **Figure 120-12** on the flank of this young woman. Note the hyperpigmentation is seen in the tinea corporis.
- Hypopigmentation is frequently seen in tinea versicolor (**Figure 120-8**).

TYPICAL DISTRIBUTION

Literally found from head to toes:

- **Figure 120-5** shows tinea capitis in a 5-year-old black girl with hair loss and an inflammatory response. Her kerion is healing after initiating oral griseofulvin.
- **Figure 120-6** shows tinea pedis in a 14-year-old boy with onychomycosis.

TABLE 120-1 Diagnostic Value of Selected Signs and Symptoms in Tinea Infection*

Sign/Symptom	Sensitivity (%)	Specificity (%)	PV+ (%)	PV– (%)	LR+	LR–
Scaling	77	20	17	80	0.96	1.15
Erythema	69	31	18	83	1.00	1.00
Pruritus	54	40	16	80	0.90	1.15
Central clearing	42	65	20	84	1.20	0.89
Concentric rings	27	80	23	84	1.35	0.91
Maceration	27	84	26	84	1.69	0.87

*Signs and symptoms were compiled by 27 general practitioners prior to submission of skin for fungal culture. Specimens were taken from 148 consecutive patients with erythematosquamous lesions of glabrous skin. Culture results were considered the gold standard; level of evidence = 2b.
LR–, Negative likelihood ratio; *LR+*, positive likelihood ratio; *PV–*, negative predictive value; *PV+*, positive predictive value.
Source: From J Fam Pract. 1999;48:611-615. Reproduced with permission from Frontline Medical Communications.

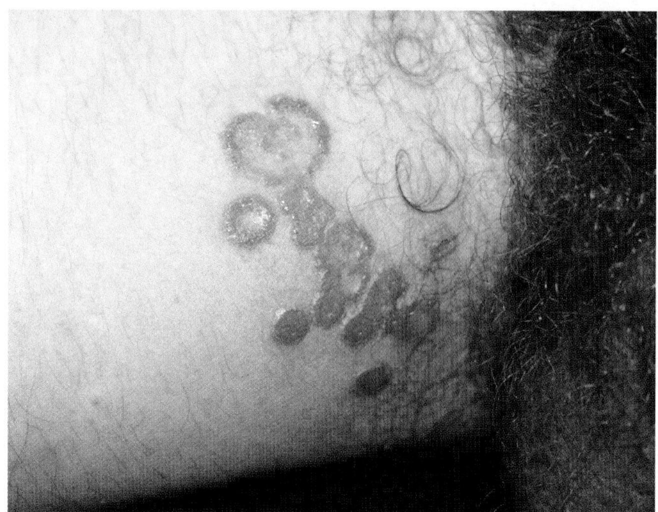

FIGURE 120-11 Inflammatory tinea cruris in a teenage boy on isotretinoin for his acne. The annular eruption is deep red. (*Photo Credit: Dr. Patrick E. McCleskey, MD.*)

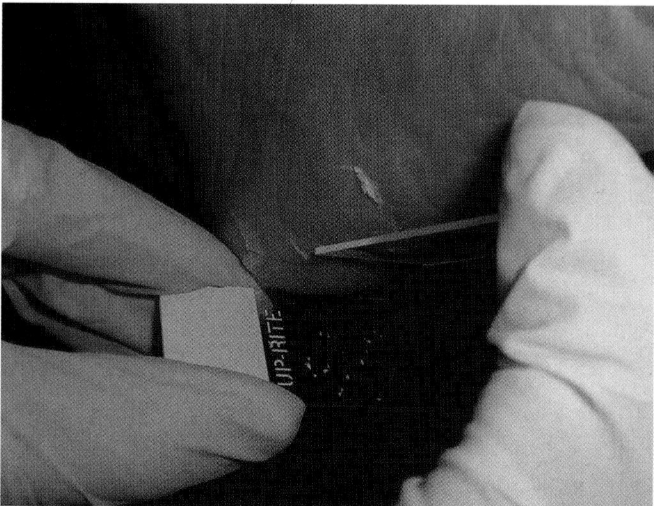

FIGURE 120-13 Making a KOH preparation by scraping in area of scale with two slides. This was a case of tinea pedis. (*Used with permission from Richard P. Usatine, MD.*)

LABORATORY STUDIES

Creating a KOH Prep:

- Scrape the leading edge of the lesion on to a slide using the side of another microscope slide or a #15 scalpel (**Figure 120-13**). For safety reasons with small moving children, it is best to use the 2 slide method and avoid the scalpel.
- Use your coverslip to push the scale into the center of the slide.
- Add two drops of KOH (fungal stain with KOH is preferable) to the slide and place coverslip on top.
- Gently heat with flame from an alcohol lamp or lighter if the pieces of collected skin are large, the sample was from a nail, or if you are using plain KOH without dimethyl sulfoxide (DMSO). Avoid boiling.
- DMSO acts as a surfactant that helps to break up the cell membranes of the epithelial cells without heating. Fungal stains that come with KOH and a surfactant in the solution are very simple to use. These inexpensive stains come conveniently in small plastic squeeze bottles that have a shelf life of 1 to 3 years. Two useful stains that can that make it easier to identify fungus are chlorazol black and Swartz-Lamkins stains. Swartz-Lamkins stain has a longer shelf life.
- Examine with microscope starting with 10 power to look for the cells and hyphae and then switch to 40 power when ready to confirm the findings (**Figures 120-13** to **120-17**). The fungal stain helps the hyphae to stand out among the epithelial cells.
- It helps to start with 10 power to find the clumps of cells and look for groups of cells that appear to have fungal elements within them (**Figure 120-14**).
- Do not be fooled by cell borders that look linear and branching. True fungal morphology at 40 power should confirm the presence of real fungus and rule out artifact. The fungal stains bring out

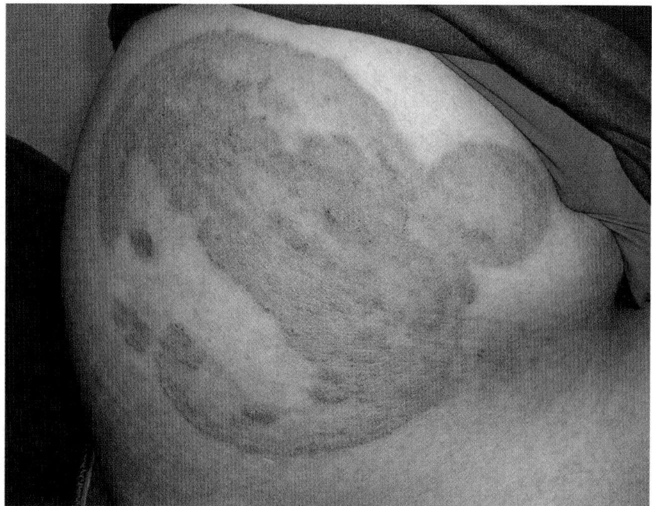

FIGURE 120-12 Tinea corporis on the right flank a young woman bending forward. Note the well-demarcated borders with multiple annular patterns and some postinflammatory hyperpigmentation. (*Used with permission from Richard P. Usatine, MD.*)

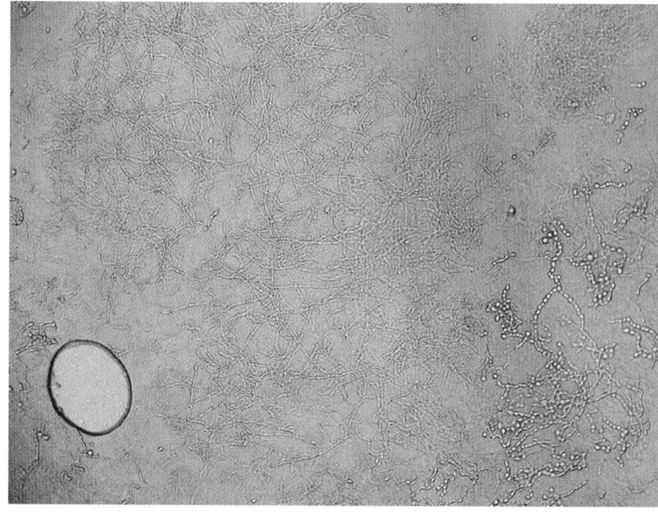

FIGURE 120-14 *Trichophyton rubrum* from tinea cruris visible among skin cells using light microscopy at 10 power and Swartz-Lamkins fungal stain. Start your search on 10 power and move to 40 power to confirm your findings. (*Used with permission from Richard P. Usatine, MD.*)

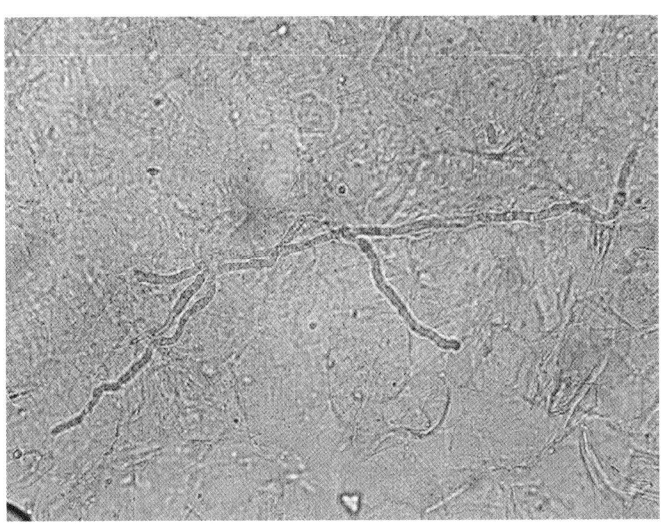

FIGURE 120-15 *Trichophyton rubrum* from tinea cruris using Swartz-Lamkins fungal stain at 40 power. Straight hyphae with visible septae. (*Used with permission from Richard P. Usatine, MD.*)

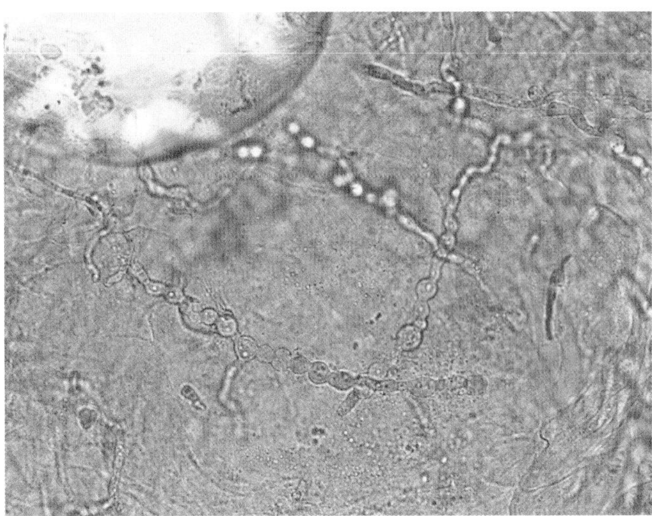

FIGURE 120-16 Arthroconidia visible from tinea cruris using Swartz-Lamkins fungal stain at 40 power. (*Used with permission from Richard P. Usatine, MD.*)

these characteristics including cell walls, nuclei, and Arthroconidia (**Figures 120-15** to **120-17**).

- KOH test characteristics[1] (without fungal stains)—Sensitivity 77 to 88 percent, specificity 62 to 95 percent (**Table 120-2**). The sensitivity and specificity should be higher with fungal stains and increased experience of the person performing the test.

OTHER LABORATORY STUDIES

- Fungal culture—Send skin scrapings, hair, or nail clippings to the laboratory in a sterile container such as a urine cup. These will be plated out on fungal agar and the laboratory can report the species if positive.
- Biopsy specimens and nail clippings can be sent in formalin for periodic acid-Schiff (PAS) staining when KOH and fungal cultures seem to be falsely negative.
- UV light (Woods lamp), looking for fluorescence. The *Microsporum* species are most likely to fluoresce. However, the majority of tinea infections are caused by *Trichophyton* species that do not fluoresce.

MANAGEMENT

There is a wide variety of topical antifungal medications (**Table 120-3**). A Cochrane systematic review of 70 trials of topical antifungals for tinea pedis showed good evidence for efficacy compared to placebo[2] for:

- Allylamines (naftifine, terbinafine, butenafine).
- Azoles (clotrimazole, miconazole, econazole).
- Allylamines cure slightly more infections than azoles but are more expensive.[2]
- No differences in efficacy found between individual topical allylamines or individual azoles.[2] SOR Ⓐ

Evidence for the management onychomycosis by topical treatments is sparse. There is some evidence that ciclopiroxolamine and butenafine are both effective, but they both need to be applied daily for at least 1 year.[3]

Oral antifungals are needed for all tinea capitis infections and for more severe infections of the rest of the body.[4] True dermatophyte

TABLE 120-2 Diagnostic Value of Clinical Diagnosis and KOH Prep in Tinea Infection

Test	Sensitivity (%)	Specificity (%)	PV+ (%)	PV– (%)	LR+	LR–
Clinical diagnosis*	81	45	24	92	1.47	0.42
KOH prep (study one)†	88	95	73	98	17.6	0.13
KOH prep (study two)†	77	62	59	79	2.02	0.37

*The clinical diagnosis set was compiled by 27 general practitioners prior to submission of skin for fungal culture. Specimens were taken from consecutive patients with erythrosquamous lesions. Culture results were considered the gold standard; study quality = 2b.
†Both studies of KOH preps were open analyses of patients with suspicious lesions. Paired fungal culture was initiated simultaneously with KOH prep and was considered the gold standard; study quality = 2b.
LR–, Negative likelihood ratio; *LR+*, positive likelihood ratio; *PV–*, negative predictive value; *PV+*, positive predictive value.
Source: From Thomas B. Clear choices in managing epidermal tinea infections. J Fam Pract. 2003;52(11):850-862. Reproduced with permission from Frontline Medical Communications.

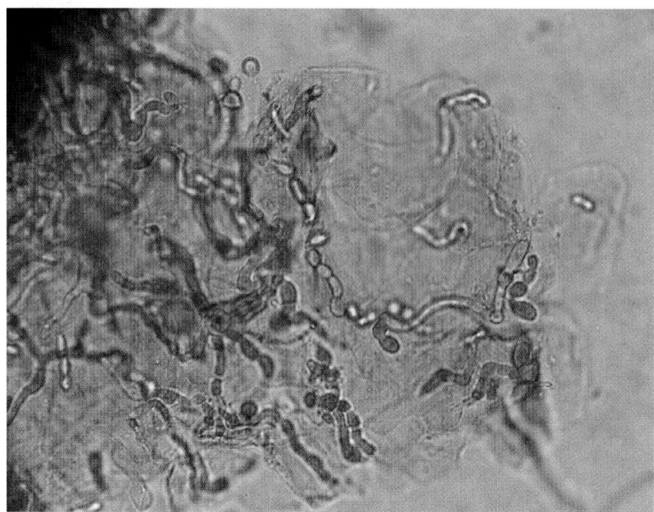

FIGURE 120-17 *Trichophyton rubrum* from tinea cruris using chlorazol black fungal stain at 40 power. (*Used with permission from Richard P. Usatine, MD.*)

infections that do not respond to topical antifungals may need an oral agent.

- A Cochrane systematic review of 12 trials of oral antifungals for tinea pedis showed oral terbinafine for 2 weeks cures 52 percent more patients than oral griseofulvin.[5] SOR Ⓐ

TABLE 120-3 Topical Antifungal Preparations

Generic Name	Brand Name	OTC or R_x	Class
Butenafine	Mentax Lotrimin Ultra	R_x OTC	Allylamine
Ciclopirox	Loprox	R_x	Pyridone
Clotrimazole	Lotrimin AF Cream Lotrimin AF Spray	OTC	Azole
Econazole	Spectazole	R_x	Azole
Ketoconazole	Nizoral	2% R_x	Azole
Miconazole	Micatin Generic	OTC	Azole
Naftifine	Naftin	R_x	Allylamine
Oxiconazole	Oxistat	R_x	Azole
Sertaconazole	Ertaczo	R_x	Azole
Terbinafine	Lamisil AT	OTC	Allylamine
Tolnaftate*	Tinactin cream Lamisil AF defense and Tinactin powder spray Generic cream	OTC	Miscellaneous

*All the above antifungals will treat dermatophytes and *Candida*. Tolnaftate is effective only for dermatophytes and not *Candida*. Nystatin is effective only for *Candida* and not the dermatophytes. *OTC*, over-the-counter.

- Terbinafine is equal to itraconazole in patient outcomes.[5]
- No significant differences in comparisons between a number of other oral agents.[5]

Oral antifungals used for fungal infections of the skin, nails, or mucous membranes:

- Itraconazole (Sporanox).
- Fluconazole (Diflucan).
- Griseofulvin.
- Ketoconazole (Nizoral).
- Terbinafine (Lamisil).

One metaanalysis suggests that terbinafine is more efficacious than griseofulvin in treating tinea capitis caused by *Trichophyton* species, whereas griseofulvin is more efficacious than terbinafine in treating tinea capitis caused by *Microsporum* species.[6] SOR Ⓐ

Details of treatments for multiple types of fungal skin infections are supplied in Chapter 121–126.

PATIENT RESOURCES

- Doctor fungus—**www.doctorfungus.org/**.

PROVIDER RESOURCES

- Fungal skin from New Zealand—**www.dermnetnz.org/fungal/**.
- Doctor fungus from the US—**www.doctorfungus.org/**.
- World of dermatophytes from Canada—**www.provlab.ab.ca/mycol/tutorials/derm/dermhome.htm**.
- Swartz Lamkins fungal stain can be easily purchased online at—**www.delasco.com/pcat/1/Chemicals/Swartz_Lamkins/dlmis023/**.

REFERENCES

1. Thomas B. Clear choices in managing epidermal tinea infections. *J Fam Pract.* 2003;52:850-862.
2. Crawford F, Hart R, Bell-Syer S, et al. Topical treatments for fungal infections of the skin and nails of the foot. *Cochrane Database Syst Rev.* 2000;(2):CD001434.
3. Crawford F, Hollis S. Topical treatments for fungal infections of the skin and nails of the foot. *Cochrane Database Syst Rev.* 2007;(3):CD001434.
4. Gonzalez U, Seaton T, Bergus G, et al. Systemic antifungal therapy for tinea capitis in children. *Cochrane Database Syst Rev.* 2007;(4):CD004685.
5. Bell-Syer SE, Hart R, Crawford F, et al. Oral treatments for fungal infections of the skin of the foot. *Cochrane Database Syst Rev.* 2002;(2):CD003584.
6. Tey HL, Tan AS, Chan YC. Meta-analysis of randomized, controlled trials comparing griseofulvin and terbinafine in the treatment of tinea capitis. *J Am Acad Dermatol.* 2011;64:663-670.

121 CANDIDIASIS

Richard P. Usatine, MD

PATIENT STORY

A 2-month-old infant is being seen for a diaper rash and the pediatrician notes that the tongue and mouth are covered in white (**Figure 121-1**). A diagnosis of thrush and Candida diaper dermatitis is made. The child is treated with oral nystatin for the mouth and topical clotrimazole for the diaper dermatitis.

INTRODUCTION

Cutaneous and mucosal *Candida* infections are seen commonly in infants with thrush and diaper rash (**Figure 121-2**). Also children and teens with obesity, diabetes, and/or immunodeficiency are at higher risk of developing Candida infections.

SYNONYMS

Thrush.

EPIDEMIOLOGY

- *Candida* superinfected diaper dermatitis is highly prevalent in healthy infants (**Figures 121-2** and **121-3**).

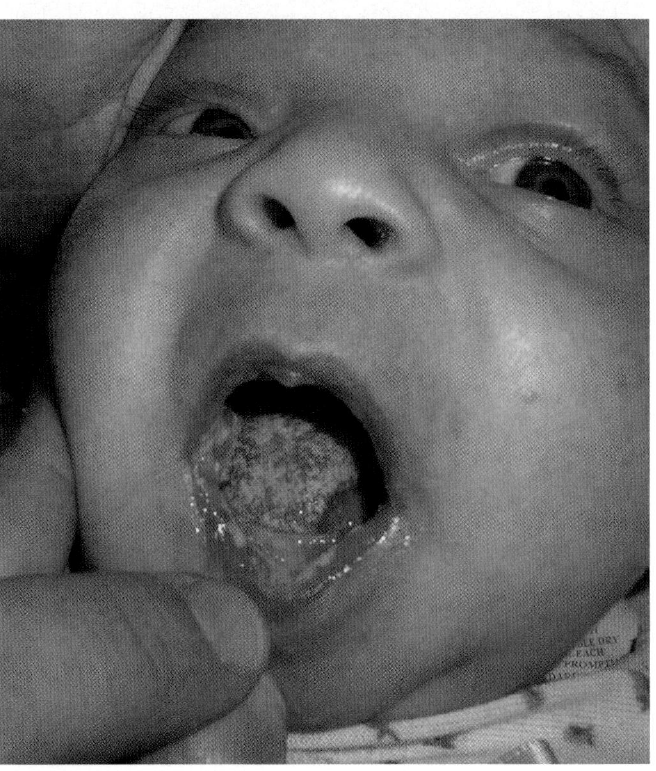

FIGURE 121-1 Thrush in an otherwise healthy infant. (*Used with permission from Richard P. Usatine, MD.*)

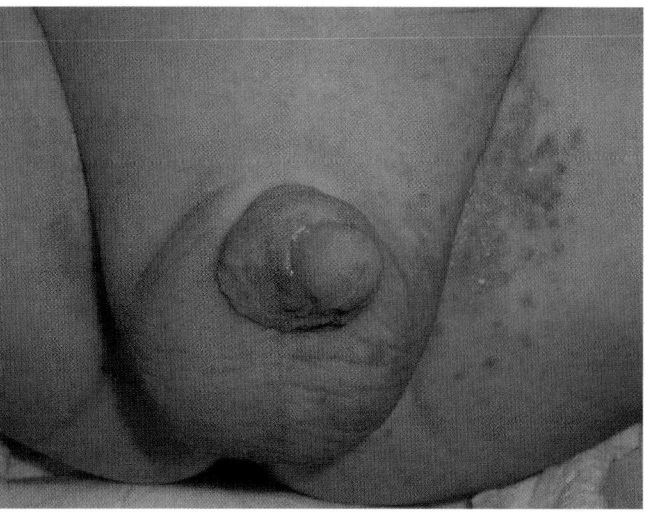

FIGURE 121-2 *Candida* diaper dermatitis in an otherwise healthy infant. Note the satellite lesions and the pink color. (*Used with permission from Richard P. Usatine, MD.*)

- *Candida* thrush is not uncommon in healthy infants (**Figure 121-1**).
- Candidemia is a major source of morbidity and mortality in neonatal intensive care units (NICU).[1] This chapter focuses on cutaneous Candida infections only.

ETIOLOGY AND PATHOPHYSIOLOGY

- Cutaneous infections caused by *Candida* species are primarily *Candida albicans*.
- *C. parapsilosis and C. albicans* infections are the most frequent causes of candidemia in the NICU.[1]
- *C. albicans* has the ability to exist in both hyphal and yeast forms (termed *dimorphism*). If pinched cells do not separate, a chain of cells is produced and is termed *pseudohyphae*.[2]

RISK FACTORS

Infancy, prematurity, hospitalization, being in the NICU, obesity, diabetes, immunodeficiency, HIV, use of oral antibiotics, and use of inhaled or systemic steroids.

DIAGNOSIS

CLINICAL FEATURES

- Ask about recent antibiotic or steroid use in the history.
- Typical distribution—Diaper area (**Figure 121-3**), glans penis, vulva, inframammary (**Figure 121-4**), under abdominal pannus, between fingers, in the creases of the neck, and in the corners of mouth in angular cheilitis.
- Morphology on the skin—Macules, patches, plaques that are pink to bright red with small peripheral satellite lesions (**Figure 121-3**).

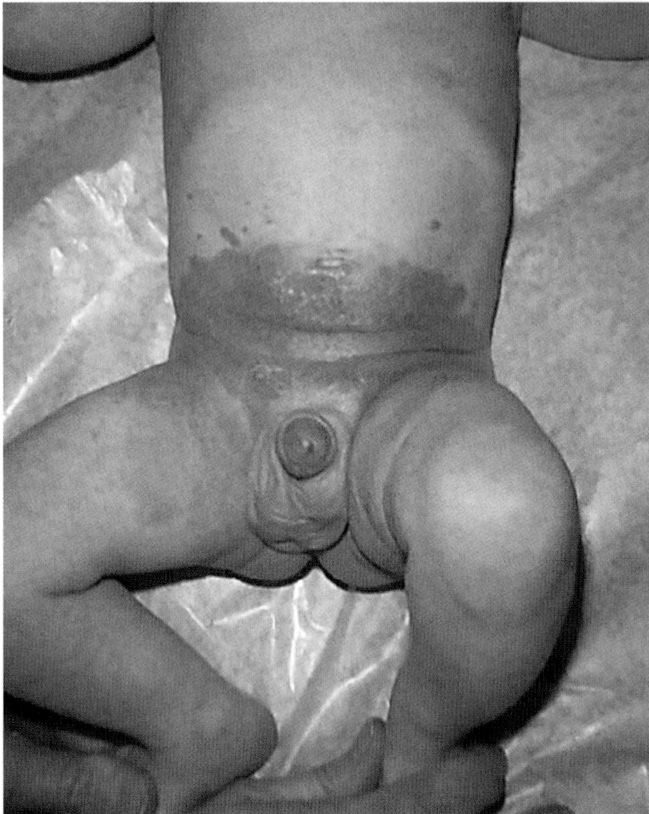

FIGURE 121-3 *Candida* diaper dermatitis after a course of antibiotics for otitis media. Note how the dermatitis has spread up the abdomen but follows the diaper distribution. There are visible satellite lesions. (*Used with permission from the Cleveland Clinic Children's Hospital Photo Files.*)

- Physical exam—Thrush appears as a white coating (velvety or cottage cheese like) on the oral mucosa including the tongue, palate, and buccal mucosa (**Figure 121-1**). Thrush will not be as easy to remove from the buccal mucosa and tongue as breast milk or formula. A gauze-covered finger can be used to test this out. If the white coating does come off and there is red friable tissue below, it is most likely thrush.

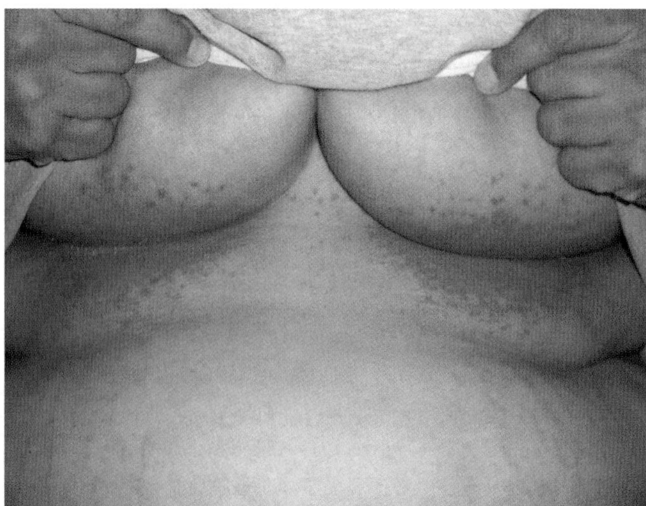

FIGURE 121-4 *Candida* under the breasts of an obese young woman. The border is not well-demarcated and there are satellite lesions. (*Used with permission from Richard P. Usatine, MD.*)

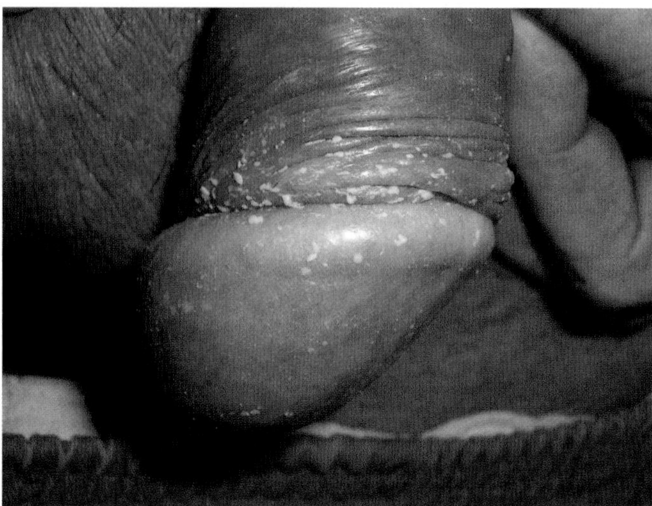

FIGURE 121-5 *Candida* balanitis in an uncircumcised young man. (*Used with permission from Richard P. Usatine, MD.*)

▸ Teens

Candida balanitis is more common in uncircumcised males than in those that have been circumcised (**Figure 121-5**). It presents with penile pruritus and a white discharge under the foreskin.

Candida vaginitis presents with pruritus and a white discharge (**Figure 121-6**). Trichomonas can also present in the same manner so a wet mount is needed to determine the correct diagnosis.

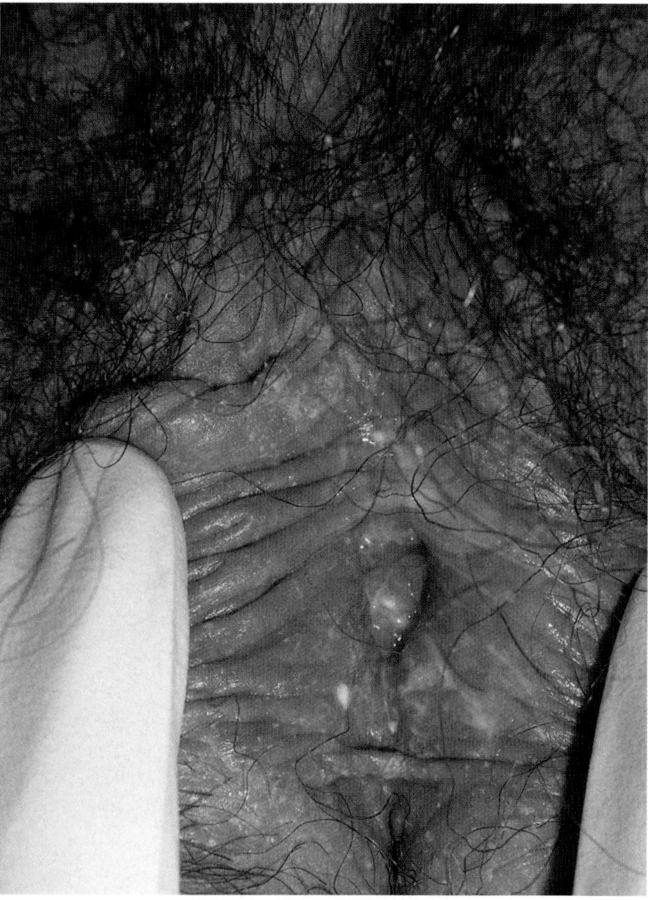

FIGURE 121-6 *Candida* vulvovaginitis in a young woman. (*Used with permission from Richard P. Usatine, MD.*)

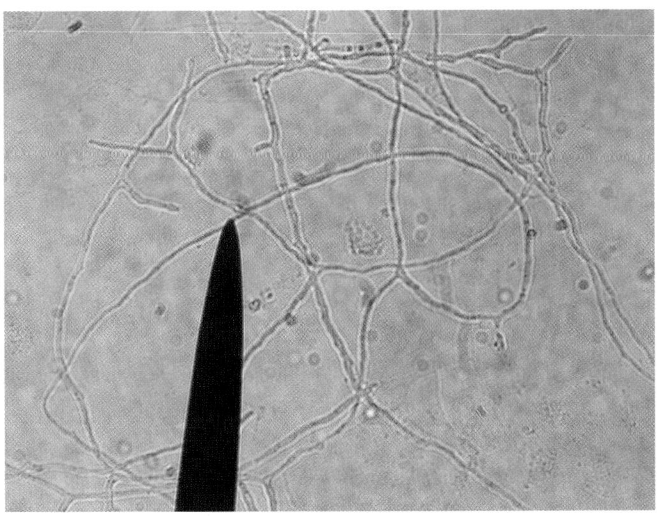

FIGURE 121-7 The branching pseudohyphae and budding yeast of *Candida* under high power. (*Used with permission from Richard P. Usatine, MD.*)

LABORATORY STUDIES

Scrape involved area and add to a slide with KOH (DMSO optional). *C. albicans* exist in both hyphal and yeast forms (dimorphism). Look for pseudohyphae and/or budding yeast (**Figure 121-7**).

DIFFERENTIAL DIAGNOSIS

- Intertrigo is a nonspecific inflammatory condition of the skin folds. It is induced or aggravated by heat, moisture, maceration, and friction. The condition frequently is worsened by infection with *Candida* or dermatophytes (**Figures 121-4**).
- Tinea corporis or cruris—Can be distinguished from *Candida* when you see an annular pattern or concentric circles in the tinea. Typically there is no scrotal involvement in tinea cruris. *Candida* intertrigo may have scrotal involvement (see Chapters 123, Tinea Corporis and 124, Tinea Cruris).
- Erythrasma—Occurs in the inguinal area and axillae. It may be pink or brown and glows a coral red with UV light (see Chapter 102, Erythrasma).
- Seborrhea—Inflammation related to overgrowth of *Pityrosporum*, a yeast-like organism (see Chapter 135, Seborrheic Dermatitis).
- For a full discussion of the differential diagnosis of diaper dermatitis, see Chapter 95, Diaper Rash and Perianal Dermatitis.

MANAGEMENT

PRIMARY CANDIDAL SKIN INFECTIONS

- Topical azoles, including clotrimazole, miconazole, and nystatin (polyenes), are effective.[4] SOR B
- Keeping the infected area of the skin dry is important.[3] SOR C
- For more details of the topical antifungals, see **Table 120-3** in Chapter 120, Fungal Overview.
- In one study, miconazole ointment was well tolerated and significantly more effective than the zinc oxide/petrolatum vehicle control for treatment of diaper dermatitis complicated by candidiasis.[4]
- Do not use tolnaftate, which is active against dermatophytes but not *Candida*.
- If recurrent or recalcitrant, consider oral fluconazole.

OROPHARYNGEAL CANDIDIASIS

- Treat initial episodes with oral nystatin suspension.[3] SOR B
- Oral fluconazole is as effective as—and, in some studies, superior to—topical therapy.[3] SOR A
- Itraconazole solution is as effective as fluconazole.[3] SOR A
- Ketoconazole and itraconazole capsules are less effective than fluconazole, because of variable absorption.[3] SOR A
- HIV/AIDS patients with oral candidiasis may be treated with clotrimazole troches (when old enough to use these safely) or oral fluconazole.[3] SOR A

CHRONIC MUCOCUTANEOUS CANDIDIASIS

- Chronic mucocutaneous candidiasis (**Figure 121-8**) is a spectrum of disorders in which the patients have persistent and/or recurrent candidiasis of the skin, nails and mucous membranes. The patient's T-cells fail to produce cytokines that are essential for expression of cell-mediated immunity to Candida.[5]
- Chronic mucocutaneous candidiasis requires a long-term approach that is analogous to that used in patients with AIDS.[3]
- Systemic therapy is needed, and azole antifungal agents (ketoconazole, fluconazole, and itraconazole) have been used successfully.[3]
- Treatments that restore cellular immunity have produced long term remissions.[5]

PROGNOSIS

Prognosis is based upon the type of Candida infection and the immune status of the host. Healthy infants with thrush and/or

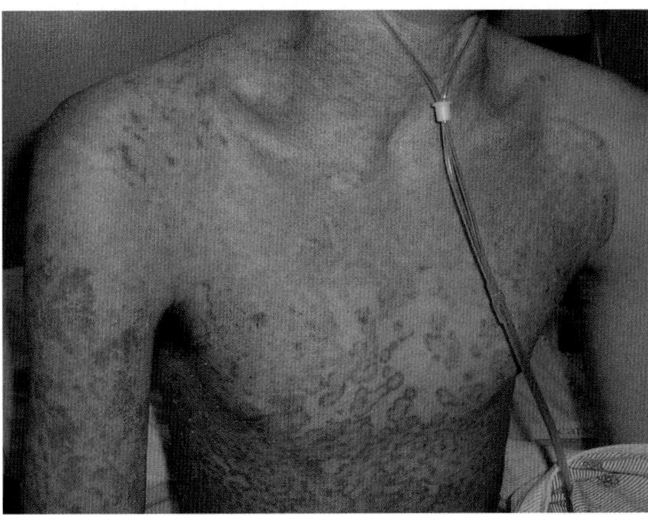

FIGURE 121-8 Chronic mucocutaneous candidiasis. This young man has had persistent candidiasis of his skin, nails and mucous membranes since childhood due to a failure of his T-cell immunity. (*Used with permission from Richard P. Usatine, MD.*)

Candida diaper dermatitis have an excellent prognosis for full recovery.

PATIENT EDUCATION

For skin infections, keep the infected area clean and dry. For thrush in a baby, treat sources of infection such as the mother's breasts and bottle nipples. If the baby is bottle fed, boil the nipples between uses.

PATIENT RESOURCES

- **www.babycenter.com/0_thrush-in-babies_92.bc**.
- **www.nlm.nih.gov/medlineplus/ency/article/000626.htm**.

PROVIDER RESOURCES

- *Pediatric Candidiasis*—**http://emedicine.medscape.com/article/962300**.
- *Cutaneous Candidiasis*—**http://emedicine.medscape.com/article/1090632**.
- *Intertrigo*—**http://emedicine.medscape.com/article/1087691**.

REFERENCES

1. Spiliopoulou A, Dimitriou G, Jelastopulu E, Giannakopoulos I, Anastassiou ED, Christofidou M. Neonatal intensive care unit candidemia: epidemiology, risk factors, outcome, and critical review of published case series. *Mycopathologia*. 2012;173(4):219-228.
2. Scheinfeld N. *Cutaneous Candidiasis*. http://emedicine.medscape.com/article/1090632, accessed May 27, 2013.
3. Pappas PG, Rex JH, Sobel JD, et al. Guidelines for treatment of candidiasis. *Clin Infect Dis*. 2004;38:161-189.
4. Spraker MK, Gisoldi EM, Siegfried EC, et al. Topical miconazole nitrate ointment in the treatment of diaper dermatitis complicated by candidiasis. *Cutis*. 2006;77(2):113-120.
5. Kirkpatrick CH. Chronic mucocutaneous candidiasis. *Pediatr Infect Dis J*. 2001;20(2):197-206.

122 TINEA CAPITIS

Richard P. Usatine, MD
Congjun Yao, MD

PATIENT STORY

An 11-year-old boy has a history of 2 months of progressive patchy hair loss (**Figure 122-1**). He has some itching of the scalp but his mother is worried about his hair loss. Physical examination reveals alopecia with scaling of the scalp and broken hairs looking like black dots in the areas of hair loss. A KOH preparation is created by scraping an area of alopecia onto a slide. A few loose hairs are added to the slide before the KOH and cover slip are placed. Fungal elements are seen under the microscope. After 6 weeks of griseofulvin, the tinea capitis is fully resolved.

INTRODUCTION

Tinea capitis is a fungal infection involving the scalp and hair. It is the most common type of dermatophytoses in children younger than 10 years of age. Common signs include hair loss, scaling, erythema, and impetigo-like plaques.

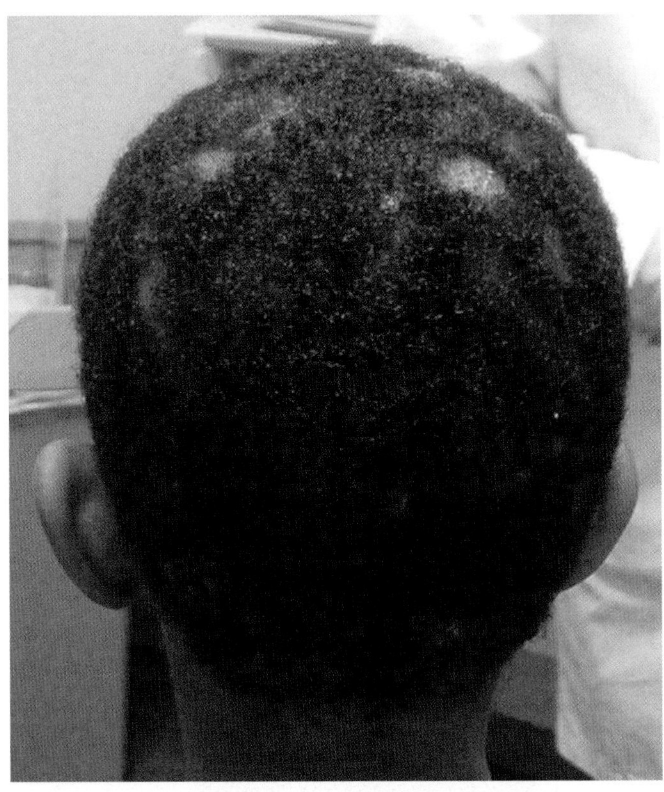

FIGURE 122-1 Tinea capitis in a young black boy. The most likely organism is *Trichophyton tonsurans*. (*Used with permission from Richard P. Usatine, MD.*)

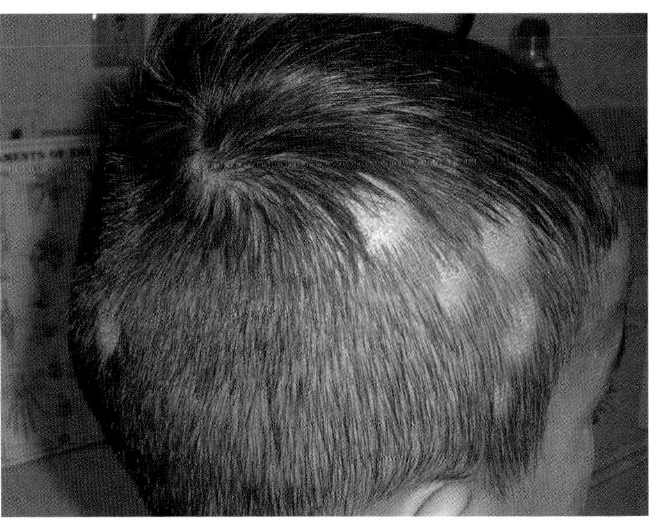

FIGURE 122-2 Tinea capitis with patchy hair loss and scaling of the scalp in a young boy. (*Used with permission from Richard P. Usatine, MD.*)

SYNONYMS

Ringworm of the scalp.

EPIDEMIOLOGY

- Tinea capitis is more common in young, black boys as it has a preference for the follicles of short curly hairs.
- Tinea capitis is the most common type of dermatophytoses in children younger than 10 years (**Figures 122-1** to **122-5**). It rarely occurs after puberty or in adults.[1] The infection has a worldwide distribution.
- Combs, brushes, couches, and sheets may harbor the live dermatophyte for a long period of time.
- Spread from person to person with direct contact or through fomites.
- Occasionally spread from cats and dogs to humans.

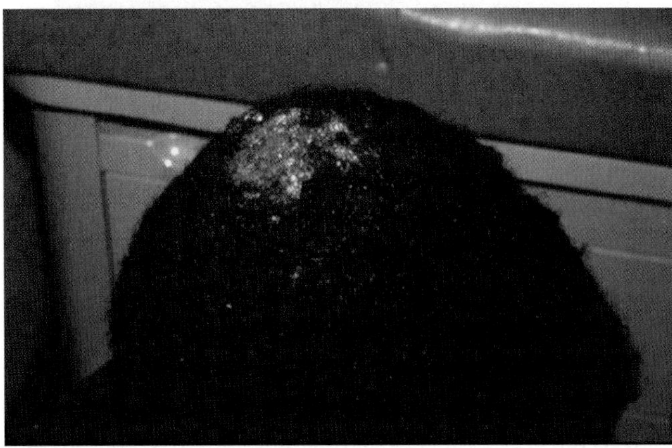

FIGURE 122-3 A kerion resulting from inflammation of the tinea capitis on this young boy. The kerion looks superinfected but it is nothing more than an exuberant inflammatory response to the dermatophyte. (*Used with permission from Richard P. Usatine, MD.*)

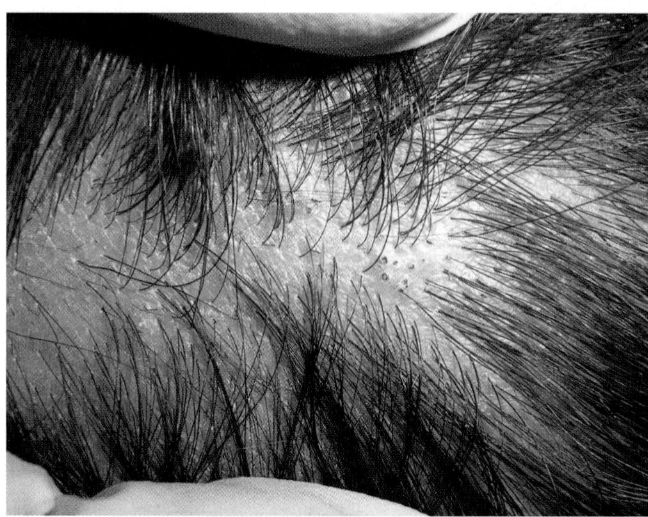

FIGURE 122-4 Close-up of black dot alopecia in a 7-year-old girl showing the black dots where infected hairs have broken off. (*Used with permission from Richard P. Usatine, MD.*)

ETIOLOGY AND PATHOPHYSIOLOGY

- Tinea capitis is a superficial fungal infection affecting hair shafts and follicles on the scalp but could involve the eyebrows and eyelashes.
- Caused by *Trichophyton* and *Microsporum* dermatophytes. The most common organism in the US is *Trichophyton tonsurans,* which is associated with black dot alopecia. *Microsporum canis* is less common now than decades ago. *M. canis* is still highly prevalent in developing countries. The natural reservoir of *M. canis* is dogs and cats.

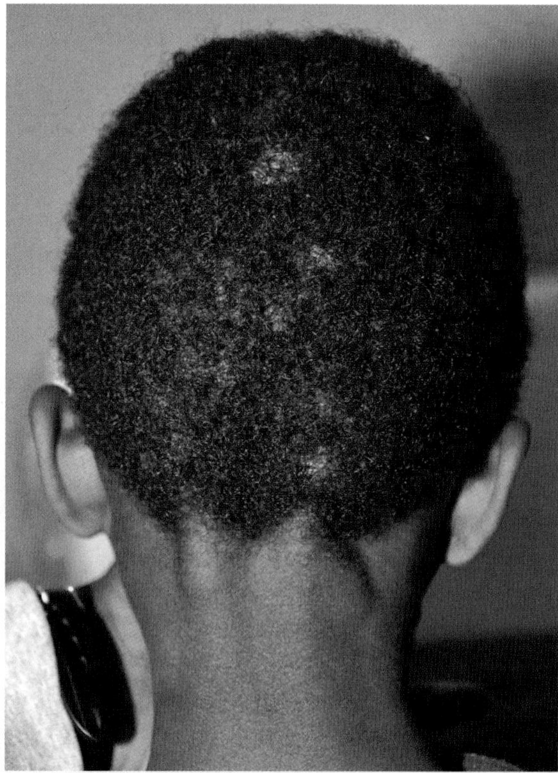

FIGURE 122-5 Lymphadenopathy visible in the neck of this young boy with tinea capitis. The fungal infection shows more scaling and crusting than actual hair loss. The lymphadenopathy is a reaction to the tinea and not a bacterial superinfection. (*Used with permission from Richard P. Usatine, MD.*)

RISK FACTORS

- Lack of access to clean water and soap.
- Poverty and living in rural areas.
- African descent as the dermatophytes grow well in the follicles of short curly hairs.
- Crowded living arrangements in which infected individuals spread the tinea to others.
- Sharing combs, brushes, and hair ornaments.

DIAGNOSIS

- The clinical appearance is often adequate to make the diagnosis.
- Confirm the diagnosis by scraping the scaling areas on the scalp and placing a few loose hairs on a microscope slide with KOH. (DMSO and a fungal stain will help.) Look for hyphae and spores (**Figure 122-6**). Look for endoectothrix invasion of the hair shaft with fungus.

CLINICAL FEATURES

- Alopecia and scaling of the scalp (**Figures 122-1** and **122-2**).
- A kerion occurs when there is an inflammatory response to the tinea. The scalp gets red, swollen, and boggy. There may be serosanguineous discharge and some crusting as this dries (**Figure 122-3**).

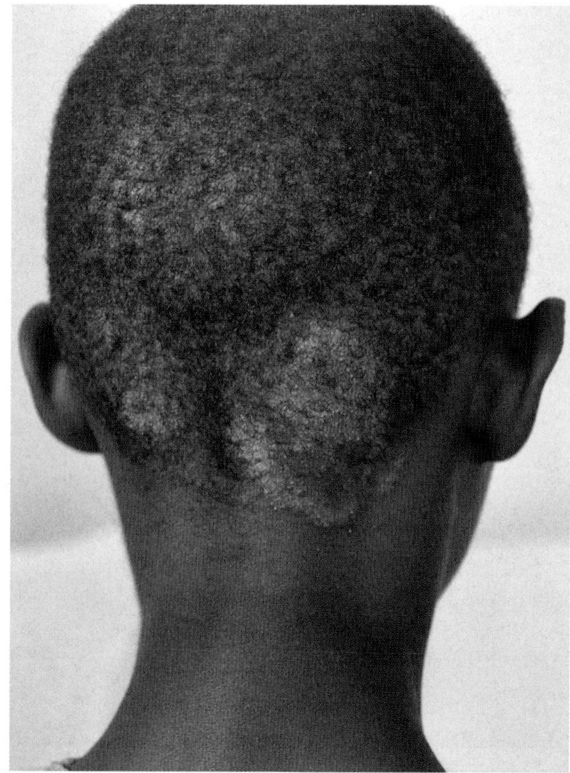

FIGURE 122-6 Tinea capitis with an annular configuration. (*Used with permission from Richard P. Usatine, MD.*)

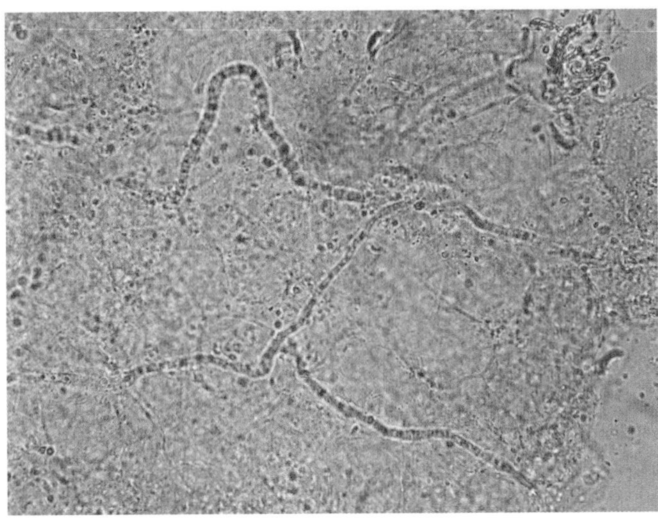

FIGURE 122-7 *Trichophyton tonsurans* from tinea capitis visible among skin cells at 40 power after adding Swartz-Lamkins fungal stain. (*Used with permission from Richard P. Usatine, MD.*)

- There may be broken hairs that look like black dots in the areas of hair loss (**Figure 122-4**).
- Cervical lymphadenopathy is common from the tinea capitis (**Figure 122-5**).
- Tinea capitis can even be annular and have the rings of ringworm (**Figure 122-6**).

TYPICAL DISTRIBUTION

By definition it occurs on the head, but usually is found on the scalp. Rarely involves the eyebrows and eyelashes.

LABORATORY STUDIES

Whenever possible it is very important to confirm or dispel ones' clinical suspicion with mycologic evidence before starting weeks of oral antifungal medicines.

- KOH preparation—Scrape the scale and infected hairs using a #15 blade. Then use KOH or a fungal stain to dissolve the keratin. Use the microscope to look for septate, branching hyphae under 10 and 40 power (**Figure 122-7**). The hyphae of *Microsporum* may also be found on the exterior of the hair (exothrix) while the hyphae of *Trichophyton* is found in the interior of the hair (endothrix) (**Figure 122-8**).
- If the diagnosis is uncertain, send a few loose hairs and a scraping of the scalp scale for a fungal culture.
- You may look at the scalp with a UV light (Woods lamp), looking for fluorescence, but the yield is low. Only the *Microsporum* species will fluoresce (**Figure 122-9**) and this organism is the involved dermatophyte less than 30 percent of the time.

DIFFERENTIAL DIAGNOSIS

- Alopecia areata—Produces areas of hair loss with no scaling, inflammation, or scarring in the underlying scalp. It is an autoimmune process in which the immune system attacks the person's own hair follicles (see Chapter 158, Alopecia Areata).
- Seborrhea of the scalp (dandruff)—is caused by the *Pityrosporum* yeast, resulting in scaling and inflammation but rarely causing hair loss. The scalp involvement tends to be more widespread than patchy and localized as seen in tinea capitis (see Chapter 135, Seborrheic Dermatitis).
- Scalp psoriasis—Rarely causes alopecia. There are mild cases with slight, fine scaling on the scalp, or severe cases with silvery, thick, crusted plaques covering the majority of the scalp. Often psoriatic plaques are seen elsewhere on the body and nail changes are visible.
- Trichotillomania—Self-inflicted alopecia caused when the patient pulls and twists her/his own hair (see Chapter 159, Traction Alopecia and a Trichotillomania).
- Traction alopecia—Alopecia that occurs when the patient or parent pulls the hair to style it into braids or ponytails. There should be no scaling of the scalp (unless there is coexisting seborrhea) and the

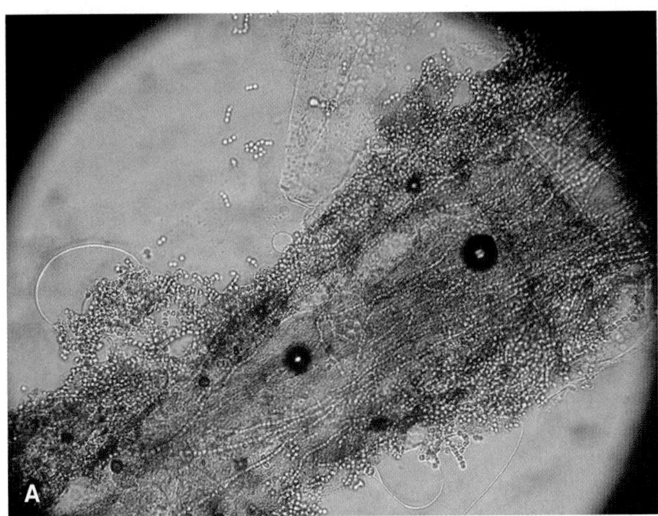

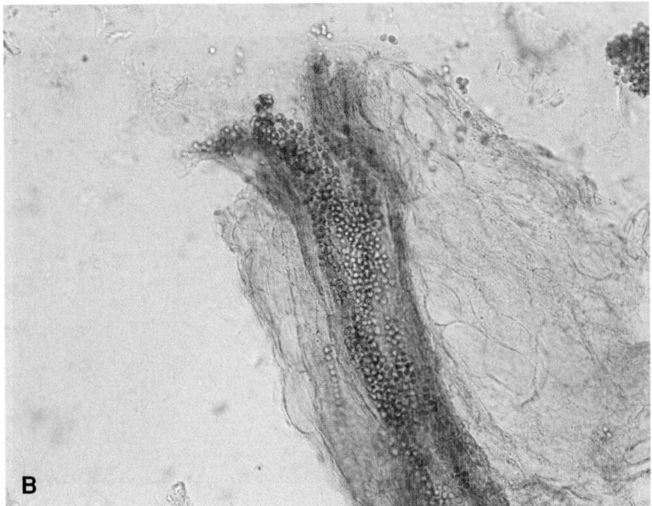

FIGURE 122-8 **A.** *M. canis* showing hyphae on the exterior of the hair (exothrix) at 40 power explaining why this type of tinea fluoresces. (*Used with permission from Eric Kraus, MD.*) **B.** *T. tonsurans* showing hyphae in the interior of the hair (endothrix) at 40 power after adding Swartz-Lamkins fungal stain. This type of tinea capitis does not fluoresce because the fungus is inside the hair. (*Photo Credit: Dr. Patrick E. McCleskey, MD.*)

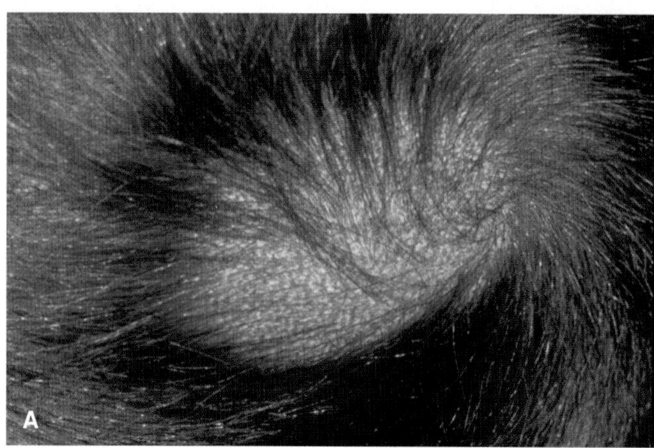

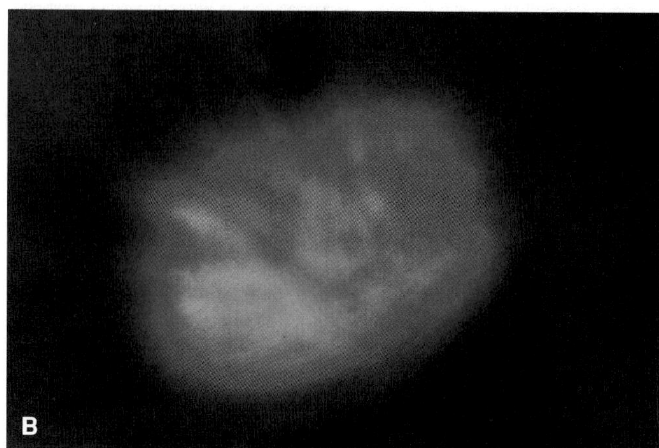

FIGURE 122-9 **A.** Tinea capitis in a young boy. **B.** Fluorescence with an ultraviolet light indicating that this is a *Microsporum* species causing the tinea capitis. (*Used with permission from Jeff Meffert, MD.*)

pattern of hair loss should match the hairstyle (**Figure 122-10**) (see Chapter 159, Traction Alopecia and Trichotillomania).

MANAGEMENT

- Topical antifungal therapy is not adequate and oral treatment is needed.
- Griseofulvin remains the treatment of choice for tinea capitis even if it requires a somewhat longer course than the newer antifungal agents.[2–5] SOR Ⓑ
- Griseofulvin is available in a liquid form for children and often covered by insurance. Prescribe a 6- to 8-week course or longer (12-week course) of griseofulvin for tinea capitis. SOR Ⓒ
- Griseofulvin is available in many forms, including liquid (125 mg microsize/5 cc) for children. Taking the drug with fatty food increases absorption and aids bioavailability. The dose for microsize griseofulvin is 20 mg/kg per day and ultramicrosize griseofulvin tablets is 5 to 15 mg/kg per day. Ultramicrosize preparations are stronger per mg than the microsize, but do not come in liquid form. The tablets are less expensive than the liquids and can be used for children that can swallow a pill. The standard course should be 6 to 12 weeks for tinea capitis to deal with increasing resistance patterns.

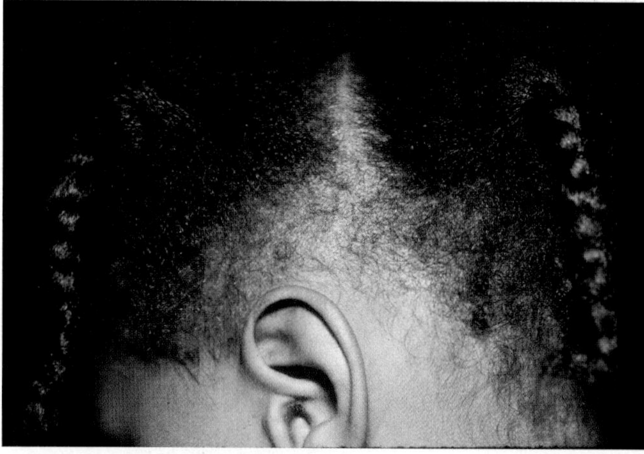

FIGURE 122-10 Traction alopecia that is related to the tight braids that put pressure on the hair follicle. The slight scaling was caused by seborrhea but tinea capitis must be in the differential diagnosis. (*Used with permission from Richard P. Usatine, MD.*)

- Expert opinion in a recent article suggests that griseofulvin microsize should be given at at a dose of 20 to 25 mg/kg per day for 2 to 3 months along with adjunctive shampooing with 2.5 percent selenium sulfide.[6] SOR Ⓒ
- A 2- to 4-week course of terbinafine, fluconazole, and itraconazole are at least as effective as a 6- to 8-week course of griseofulvin for the treatment of *Trichophyton* infections of the scalp.
- A number of RCTs of oral terbinafine (doses ranging from 3 to 8 mg/kg/day and durations of treatment from 2 to 4 weeks) have shown faster and higher cure rates when compared to griseofulvin for treatment of inner city tinea capitis caused by *Trichophyton tonsurans*.[6–10] SOR Ⓐ
- Griseofulvin is likely to be superior to terbinafine for the rare cases caused by *Microsporum* species and inflammatory Trichophyton species.[10,11]
- Terbinafine is effective and offers a shorter course of therapy than griseofulvin. It is not available in liquid form. Recommended dosage for 10- to 20-kg children is 62.5 mg/day; for 20- to 40-kg children, 125 mg daily; and for children who weigh more than 40 kg, 250 mg daily. Treatment duration for *Trichophyton* is 2 to 4 weeks; it is 8 to 12 weeks for *Microsporum* infection.
- Fluconazole is available in liquid form and appears to be effective and safe to treat cutaneous fungal infections. Recommended dosage is 5 to 6 mg/kg per day. Treatment duration for *Trichophyton* is 3 to 6 weeks; 8 to 12 weeks for *Microsporum* infection.
- Itraconazole is also available in liquid form. The recommended dose is 3 mg/kg per day for liquid form. For capsules: 5 mg/kg per day. Treatment duration is 2 to 6 weeks.
- None of these agents require laboratory monitoring at the recommended lengths of treatment for tinea capitis.[1]
- A kerion may resolve with oral antifungal treatment alone. If it is severe and painful, consider a short pulse of oral steroids to speed up resolution (**Figure 122-11**). SOR Ⓒ

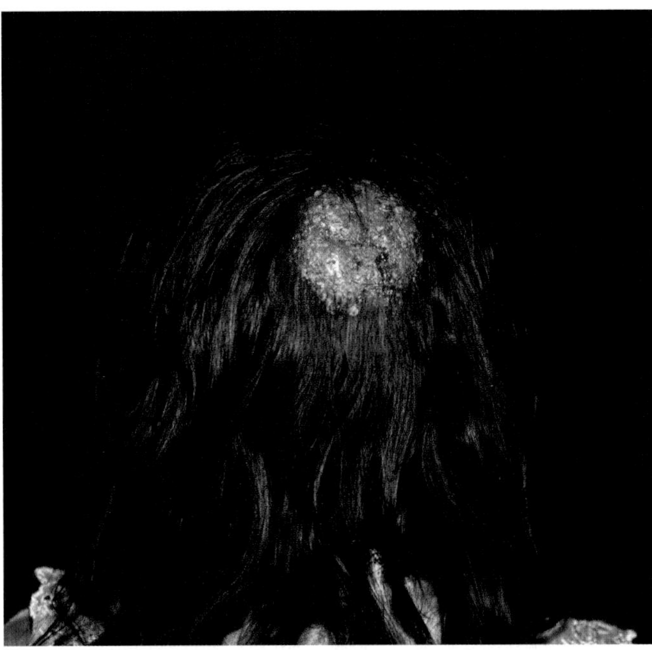

FIGURE 122-11 A kerion in a 5-year-old girl infected with Trichophyton rubrum. (*Used with permission from Eric Kraus, MD.*)

- Although oral therapy is still the recommended treatment for tinea capitis, topical treatment can be used as adjuvant therapy: 1 to 2.5 percent selenium sulfide, 1 percent ciclopirox, or 2 percent ketoconazole shampoo should be applied to the scalp and hair for 5 minutes 2 or 3 times a week for 8 weeks.[12-13] SOR Ⓑ Shampoos with selenium sulfide or ciclopirox have been shown to be of equal efficacy.[13] SOR Ⓑ
- Another use for antifungal shampoo is empirical treatment while waiting for a culture to come back in an equivocal case. Topical antifungal shampoo may decrease the spread of the tinea in crowded living environments while waiting for the oral therapy to work (**Figure 122-12**). SOR Ⓒ

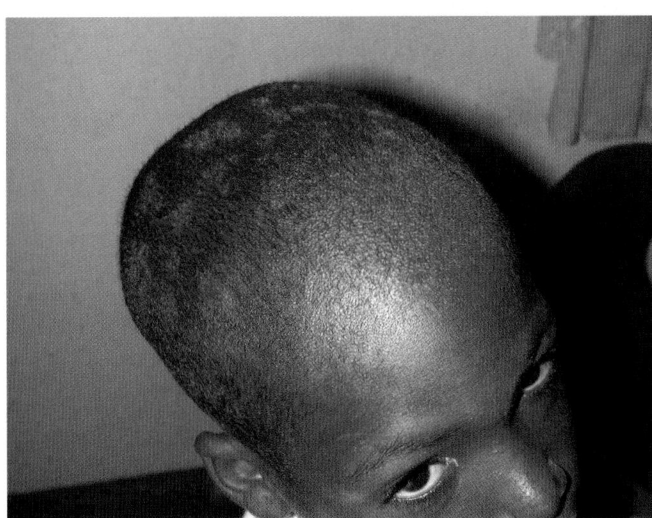

FIGURE 122-12 Tinea capitis in a schoolboy in Panama. Many of his classmates also had tinea capitis. An antifungal shampoo was prescribed for the children while waiting to obtain the needed systemic antifungal agent. (*Used with permission from Richard P. Usatine, MD.*)

PREVENTION

Family members or playmates should be screened and asymptomatic carriers should be treated. Close physical contact and sharing of toys or combs/hairbrushes should be avoided.[14] SOR Ⓑ

PROGNOSIS

Severe hair loss and scarring alopecia can occur if tinea capitis is left untreated.

PATIENT EDUCATION

Patients and parents need to exercise care to avoid spreading the infection to others. Explain the importance of not sharing combs, brushes, and towels.

FOLLOW-UP

Follow-up may be scheduled to check for full resolution of the infection by negative culture or hair regrowth.

PATIENT RESOURCE

- Medline Plus article for patients—**www.nlm.nih.gov/medlineplus/ency/article/000878.htm**.

PROVIDER RESOURCE

- **www.emedicine.com/DERM/topic420.htm**.

REFERENCES

1. Johnston KL, Chambliss ML, DeSpain J. Clinical inquiries. What is the best oral antifungal medication for tinea capitis? *J Fam Pract*. 2001;50:206-207.
2. Tey HL, Tan AS, Chan YC. Meta-analysis of randomized, controlled trials comparing griseofulvin and terbinafine in the treatment of tinea capitis. *J Am Acad Dermatol*. 2011;64(4):663-670.
3. Gupta AK, Cooper EA, Bowen JE. Meta-analysis: griseofulvin efficacy in the treatment of tinea capitis. *J Drugs Dermatol*. 2008;7(4):369-372.
4. González U, Seaton T, Bergus G, et al. Systemic antifungal therapy for tinea capitis in children. *Cochrane Database Syst Rev*. 2007;(4):CD004685.
5. Kakourou T, Uksal U. European Society for Pediatric Dermatology. Guidelines for the management of tinea capitis in children. *Pediatr Dermatol*. 2010;27(3):226-228.
6. Pride HB, Tollefson M, Silverman R. What's new in pediatric dermatology?: Part II. Treatment. *J Am Acad Dermatol*. 2013;68(6):899.e1-899.e11.
7. Elewski BE, Cáceres HW, DeLeon L, El Shimy S, Hunter JA, Korotkiy N, et al. Terbinafine hydrochloride oral granules versus

oral griseofulvin suspension in children with tinea capitis: results of two randomized, investigator-blinded, multicenter, international, controlled trials. *J Am Acad Dermatol*. 2008;59:41-54.

8. Friedlander SF, Aly R, Krafchik B, Blumer J, Honig P, Stewart D, et al. Terbinafine in the treatment of Trichophyton tinea capitis: a randomized, double-blind, parallel-group, duration-finding study. *Pediatrics*. 2002;109:602-607.
9. Deng S, Hu H, Abliz P, Wan Z, Wang A, Cheng W, et al. A random comparative study of terbinafine versus griseofulvin in patients with tinea capitis in western china. *Mycopathologia*. 2011;172:365-372.
10. Gupta AK, Drummond-Main C. Meta-analysis of randomized, controlled trials comparing particular doses of griseofulvin and terbinafine for the treatment of tinea capitis. *Pediatr Dermatol*. 2013;30:1-6.
11. Grover C, Arora P, Manchanda V. Comparative evaluation of griseofulvin, terbinafine and fluconazole in the treatment of tinea capitis. *Int J Dermatol*. 2012;51:455-458.
12. Greer DL. Successful treatment of tinea capitis with 2% ketoconazole shampoo. *Int J Dermatol*. 2000;39(4):302-304.
13. Chen C, Koch LH, Dice JE, et al. A randomized, double-blind study comparing the efficacy of selenium sulfide shampoo 1% and ciclopirox shampoo 1% as adjunctive treatments for tinea capitis in children. *Pediatr Dermatol*. 2010;27(5):459-462.
14. Higgins EM, Fuller LC, Smith CH. Guidelines for the management of tinea capitis. British Association of Dermatologists. *Br J Dermatol*. 2000;143(1):53-58.

123 TINEA CORPORIS

Richard P. Usatine, MD
Adeliza Jimenez, MD

PATIENT STORY

A 6-year-old girl is brought to the office for a round, itchy rash on her body (**Figure 123-1**). It was first noted 2 weeks ago. The family cat does have some patches of hair loss. Note the concentric rings with scaling, erythema, and central sparing. UV light showed green fluorescence (*Microsporum* species) and the KOH is positive for branching and septate hyphae. The child was treated with a topical antifungal cream bid and the tinea resolved in 3 to 4 weeks. The family cat was also taken to the veterinarian for treatment.

INTRODUCTION

Tinea corporis is a common superficial fungal infection of the body, characterized by well-demarcated, annular lesions with central clearing, erythema, and scaling of the periphery.

EPIDEMIOLOGY

Dermatophytes are the most prevalent agents causing fungal infections in the US, with *Trichophyton rubrum* causing the majority of cases of tinea corporis, tinea cruris, tinea manuum, and tinea pedis.

- Excessive heat and humidity make a good environment for fungal growth.

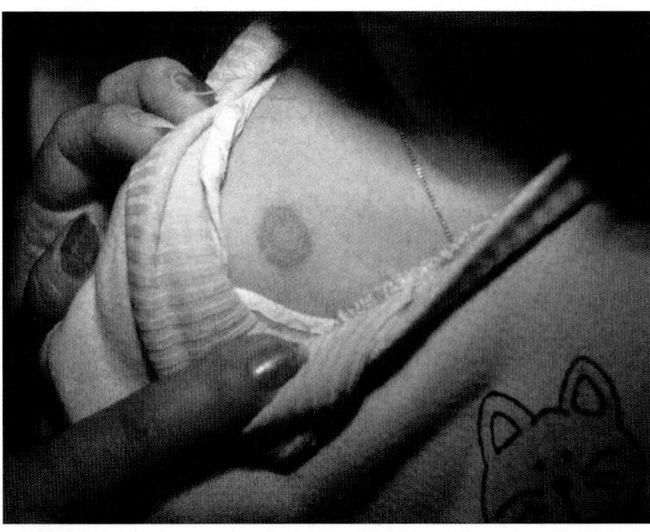

FIGURE 123-1 Tinea corporis on the shoulder of this young girl. This is a very typical annular pattern and the cat on a sweatshirt might be a clue to an infected pet at home spreading a *Microsporum* dermatophyte to the young girl. Note the concentric rings with scaling, erythema, and central sparing. (*Used with permission from Richard P. Usatine, MD.*)

- Dermatophytes are spread by exposure to infected animals or persons and contact with contaminated items.

ETIOLOGY AND PATHOPHYSIOLOGY

Tinea corporis is caused by fungal species from any one of the following three dermatophyte genus': *Trichophyton*, *Microsporum*, and *Epidermophyton*. *T. rubrum* is the most common causative agent of tinea corporis.

- Dermatophytes produce enzymes such as keratinase that penetrate keratinized tissue. Their hyphae invade the stratum corneum and keratin and spread centrifugally outward.

RISK FACTORS

- Participation in daycare centers.
- Poor personal hygiene.
- Living conditions with poor sanitation.
- Warm, humid environments.
- Conditions that cause weakening of the immune system (e.g., AIDS, cancer, organ transplantation, diabetes).

DIAGNOSIS

The diagnosis can be made from history, clinical presentation, culture, and direct microscopic observation of hyphae in infected tissue and hairs after KOH preparation.

CLINICAL FEATURES

- Pruritus of affected area.
- Well-demarcated, annular lesions with central clearing, erythema, and scaling of the periphery. Concentric rings are highly specific (80%) for tinea infections (**Figure 123-1**).
- Central clearing is not always present (**Figure 123-2**).
- Although scale is the most prominent morphologic characteristic, some tinea infections will actually cause pustules from the inflammatory response (**Figure 123-3**).

TYPICAL DISTRIBUTION

- Any part of the body can be involved including the face and extremities (**Figures 123-4**).
- Tinea incognito is a type of tinea infection that was previously not recognized by the physician or patient and topical steroids were used on the site. While applying the steroid, the dermatophyte continues to grow and form concentric rings (**Figures 123-5** and **123-6**).
- Tinea corporis can cover large parts of the body as in **Figure 123-7**.
- In some cases, the infection may cause hyperpigmentation (**Figures 123-5** to **123-7**).

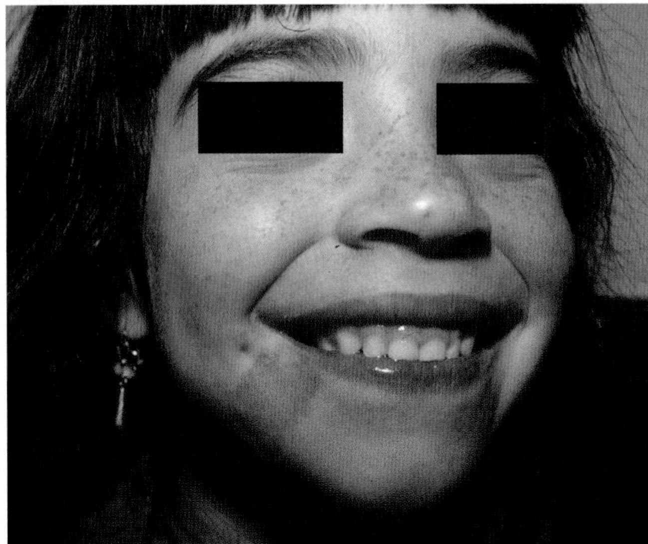

FIGURE 123-2 Tinea faciei in a young girl. There is no central clearing or annular pattern here but the KOH preparation was positive for branching hyphae. It resolved with a topical antifungal medicine. (*Used with permission from Richard P. Usatine, MD.*)

LABORATORY STUDIES

- KOH preparation of skin scraping can be very useful to confirm a clinical impression or when the diagnosis is not certain. Scrape the skin with the side of a slide or scalpel, making sure to scrape the periphery and the erythematous part. Scrape hard enough to get some stratum corneum without causing significant bleeding. False negatives can occur secondary to inadequate scraping, patient using topical antifungals, or an inexperienced microscopist.
- Use KOH (plain, with dimethyl sulfoxide [DMSO], or in a fungal stain) to break up the epithelial cells more rapidly without heating (**Figure 123-8**). It is easy to purchase a small bottle of Swartz-Lamkins fungal stain that includes KOH, a surfactant, and blue ink. The blue ink allows the hyphae to stand out, thereby saving time and decreasing the chance of a false-negative result (**Figure 123-9**). If the epithelial cells are not breaking up sufficiently, use a flame under the slide for approximately 5 seconds to speed up the process.
- Skin scraping and culture—Gold standard, but more costly and may take up to 2 weeks for the culture to grow. Consider culture if

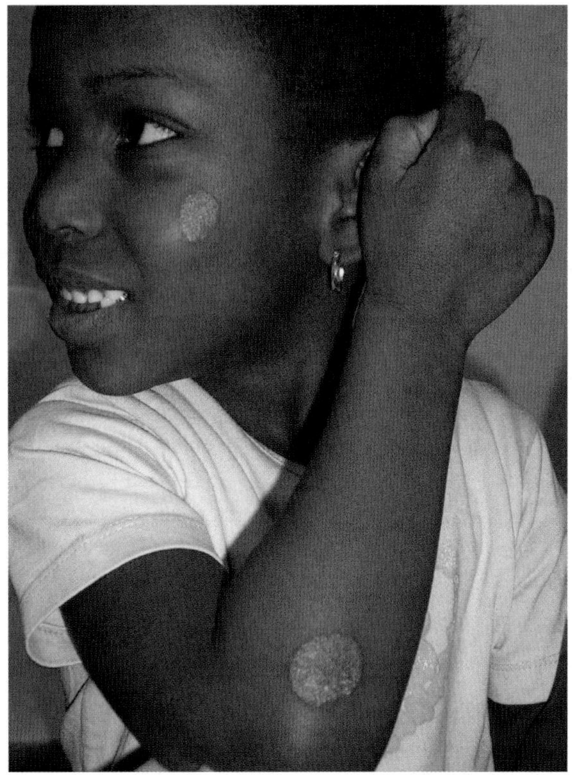

FIGURE 123-4 Tinea corporis with classic scaling rings on the arm and face of this young girl. (*Used with permission from Richard P. Usatine, MD.*)

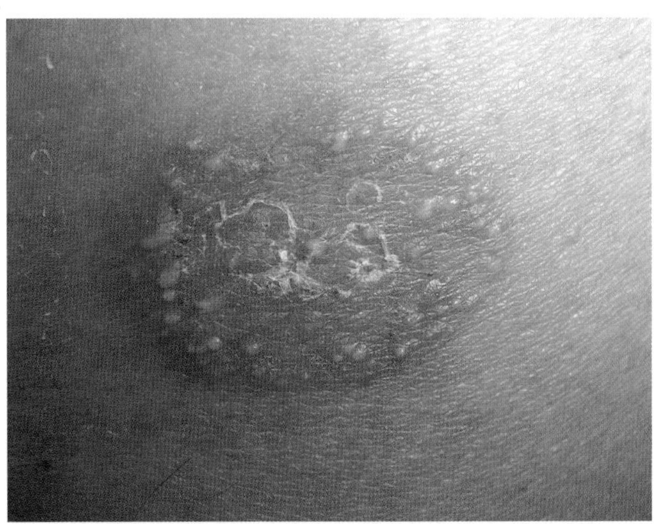

FIGURE 123-3 Tinea corporis with pustules and scale. KOH preparation was positive for branching hyphae. The pustules are a manifestation of an inflammatory response to the dermatophyte infection. (*Used with permission from Richard P. Usatine, MD.*)

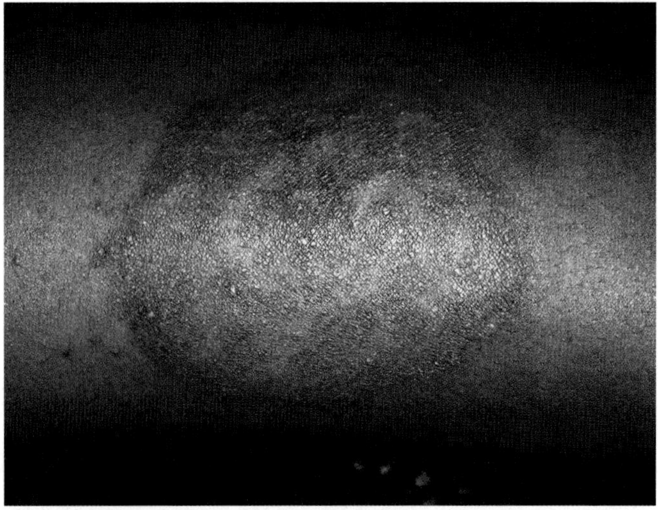

FIGURE 123-5 Tinea incognito on the arm with concentric rings as this dermatophyte infection continued to grow under the influence of the topical steroids mistakenly given to her by her physician. There is an extensive amount of postinflammatory hyperpigmentation. (*Used with permission from Richard P. Usatine, MD.*)

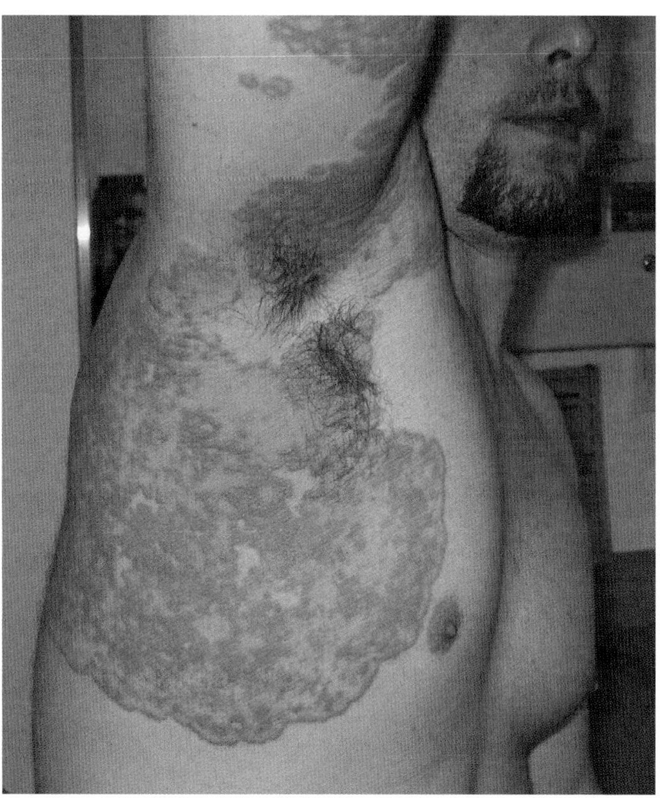

FIGURE 123-6 Tinea incognito in the axillary region of a young man who was prescribed topical steroids. Although there is some hyperpigmentation, erythema is most prominent. (*Used with permission from Chris Wenner, MD.*)

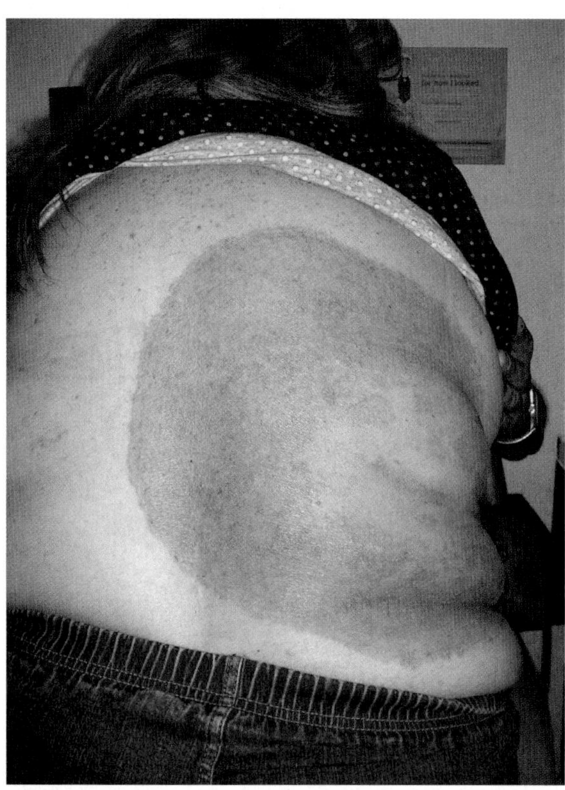

FIGURE 123-7 Tinea corporis covering the back and showing well-demarcated borders. (*Used with permission from Richard P. Usatine, MD.*)

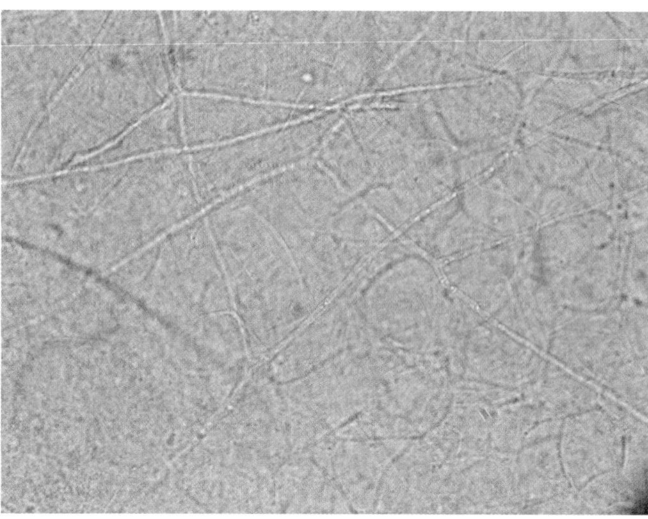

FIGURE 123-8 Branching hyphae at 40× high power from KOH preparation of tinea corporis. (*Used with permission from Richard P. Usatine, MD.*)

the KOH is negative but tinea is still suspected, or when a microscope is not available.

- Skin biopsy sent in formalin for periodic acid-Schiff (PAS) staining when the KOH and culture remain negative but the clinical picture is consistent with a fungal infection.

DIFFERENTIAL DIAGNOSIS

- Granuloma annulare—Inflammatory, benign dermatosis of unknown cause, characterized by both dermal and annular papules (**Figure 123-10**) (see Chapter 148, Granuloma Annulare).
- Psoriasis—Plaque with scale on extensor surfaces and trunk. Occasionally, the plaques can have an annular appearance

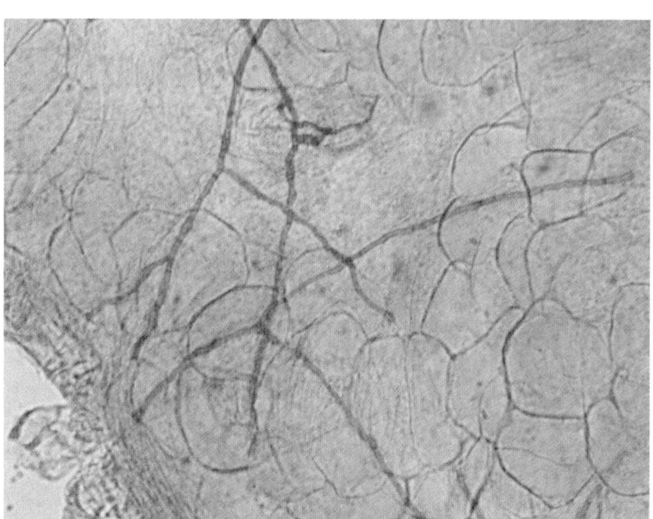

FIGURE 123-9 Branching hyphae easily seen at 40× high power using fungal stain (Swartz-Lamkins) from a scraping of tinea corporis. Note how the hyphae stand out with the blue ink color. (*Used with permission from Richard P. Usatine, MD.*)

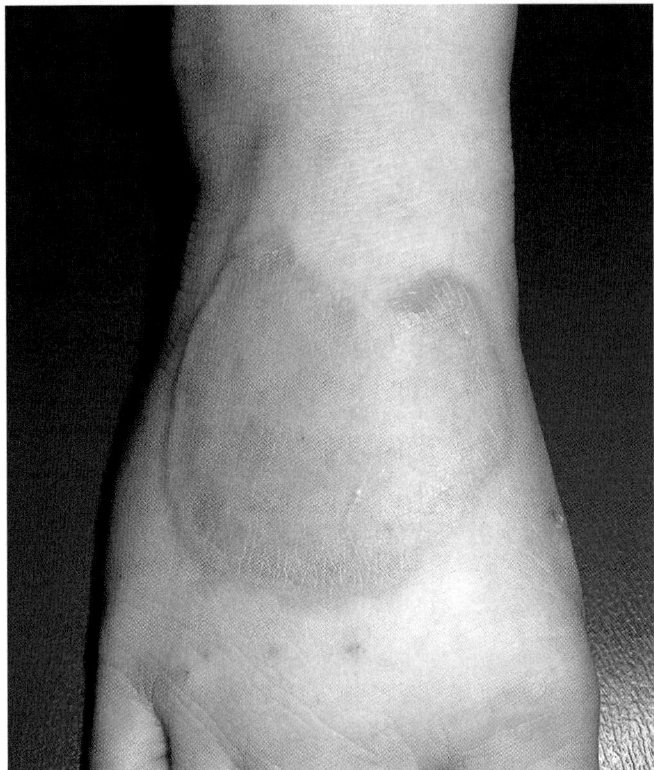

FIGURE 123-10 Granuloma annulare producing an annular lesion on the dorsum of the foot of this 3-year-old boy. No scale is visible. (*Used with permission from Richard P. Usatine, MD.*)

(**Figure 123-11**). Inverse psoriasis in intertriginous areas can also mimic tinea corporis (see Chapter 136, Psoriasis).

- Cutaneous larva migrans has serpiginous burrows made by the hookworm larvae, and these burrows can look annular and be confused with tinea corporis (see Chapter 129, Cutaneous Larva Migrans).
- Nummular eczema—Round coin-like red scaly plaques without central clearing (see Chapter 133, Nummular Eczema).

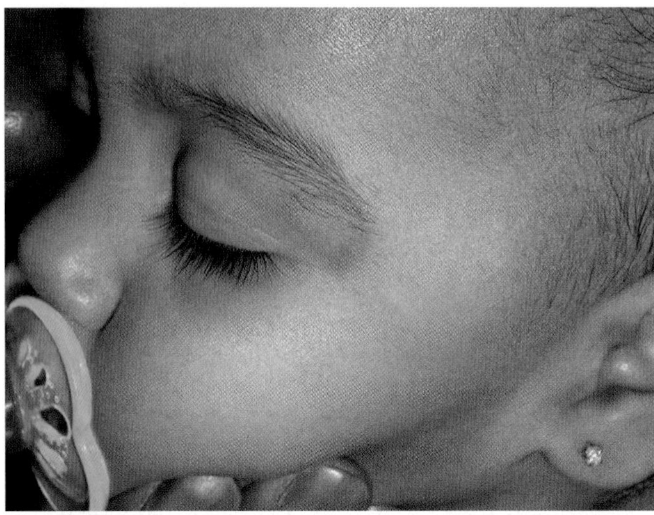

FIGURE 123-12 Tinea faciei near the eyebrow of this infant. (*Used with permission from Richard P. Usatine, MD.*)

MANAGEMENT

- Use topical antifungal medications for tinea corporis that involves small areas of the body as seen in **Figures 123-12** and **123-13**.
- Although all the topical antifungal agents may be effective, the evidence supports the greater effectiveness of the allylamines (terbinafine) over the less-expensive azoles for tinea pedis and corporis. Allylamines cure slightly more infections than azoles and are now available over the counter.[1,2] SOR Ⓐ
- Studies show that terbinafine 1 percent cream or solution applied once daily for 7 days is highly effective for tinea corporis/cruris.[3,4] The 1 percent cream (which is available over the counter as Lamisil AF) produced a mycologic cure of 84.2 percent versus 23.3 percent with placebo. Number needed to treat (NNT) = 1.6.[3] SOR Ⓐ
- Oral antifungal agents should be considered for first-line therapy for tinea corporis covering large areas of the body, as seen in

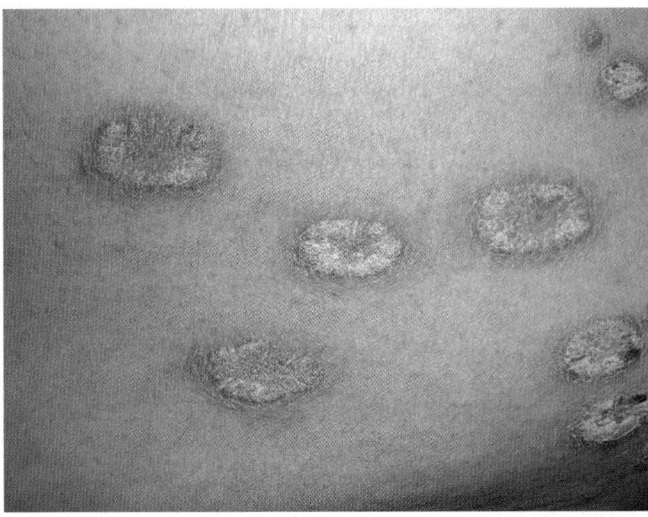

FIGURE 123-11 Annular lesions caused by psoriasis. Not all lesions that are annular with scale are tinea corporis. (*Used with permission from Richard P. Usatine, MD.*)

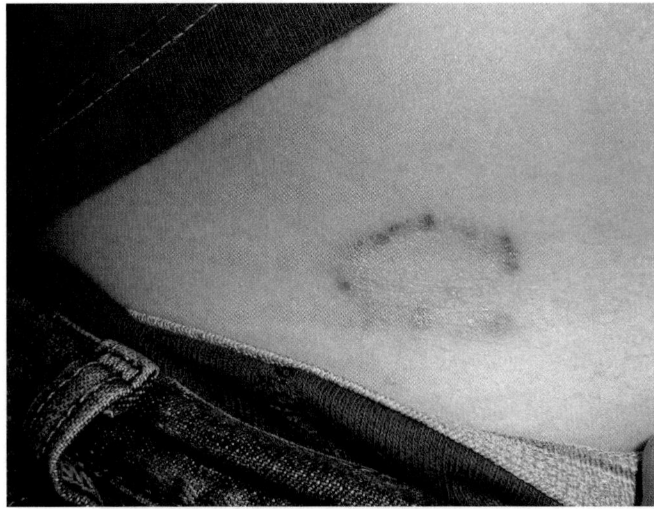

FIGURE 123-13 Tinea corporis producing an open ring near the waist of this 10-year-old boy. Note the erythema and scale along with central clearing. (*Used with permission from Richard P. Usatine, MD.*)

TABLE 123-1 Dosing of Terbinafine By Weight for Tinea Corporis (for Children >2 Years of Age)

Weight in kg	Terbinafine oral dose in mg – give for 2 weeks once daily
<20 kg	62.5 mg (1/4 of 250 mg tablet)
20–40 kg	125 mg (1/2 of 250 mg tablet)
>40 kg	250 mg

Figures 123-6 and **123-7**. However, it is not wrong to attempt topical treatment if the size of the area infected is on the borderline. The patient with tinea incognito in **Figure 123-5** did need oral therapy to resolve her infection. Unfortunately, the postinflammatory hyperpigmentation did not resolve well.

- One randomized controlled trial (RCT) showed that oral itraconazole 200 mg daily for 1 week is similarly effective, equally well tolerated, and at least as safe as itraconazole 100 mg for 2 weeks in the treatment of tinea corporis or cruris.[5] SOR B
- In one study, patients with mycologically diagnosed tinea corporis and tinea cruris were randomly allocated to receive either 250 mg of oral terbinafine once daily or 500 mg of griseofulvin once daily for 2 weeks. The cure rates were higher for terbinafine at 6 weeks.[6] SOR B
- In summary, if an oral agent is needed, the evidence is greatest for the use of:
  - Terbinafine orally daily for 2 weeks.[6] SOR B (Terbinafine is available as an inexpensive generic prescription on the $4 and $5 plans in the US. It also has less drug interactions than itraconazole. For these reasons it is usually the preferred treatment when an oral agent is needed.) See **Table 123-1** for dosing.
  - Itraconazole (10 mg/kg/day) for 1 week or Itraconazole (5 mg/kg/day) daily for 2 weeks.[5] SOR B (More expensive with more drug interactions than terbinafine.)

PREVENTION

Tinea corporis and cruris are dermatophyte infections that are particularly common in areas of excessive heat and moisture. A dry, cool environment may play a role in reducing infection. In addition, avoiding contact with farm animals and other individuals infected with tinea corporis and cruris may help in preventing infection. Preventative measures for tinea infections include practicing good personal hygiene; keeping the skin dry and cool at all times; and avoiding sharing towels, clothing, or hair accessories with infected individuals.[7]

In individuals involved in contact sports such as wrestling, a comprehensive skin disease prevention protocol includes some combination of the following: washing of wrestling mats before and after each practice and competition; showers before and after each practice; use of clean clothing before each practice; and exclusion of infected athletes.[8]

FOLLOW-UP

Consider follow-up appointments in 4 to 6 weeks for difficult and more widespread cases. If there are concerns about bacterial superinfection, follow-up should be sooner.

PATIENT EDUCATION

Keep the skin clean and dry. Infected pets should be treated.

PATIENT RESOURCES

- VisualDxHealth. *Ringworm*—**www.visualdxhealth.com/adult/tineaCorporis.htm**.
- Medline Plus Medical Encyclopedia—**www.nlm.nih.gov/medlineplus/ency/article/000877.htm**.

PROVIDER RESOURCES

- eMedicine topic—**www.emedicine.com/DERM/topic421.htm**.
- Doctor Fungus Web site—**www.doctorfungus.org/**.
- Swartz-Lamkins fungal stain can be easily purchased online at: **www.delasco.com/pcat/1/Chemicals/Swartz_Lamkins/dlmis023/**.

REFERENCES

1. Thomas B. Clear choices in managing epidermal tinea infections. *J Fam Pract*. 2003;52:850-862.
2. Crawford F, Hollis S. Topical treatments for fungal infections of the skin and nails of the foot. *Cochrane Database Syst Rev*. 2007;3:CD001434.
3. Budimulja U, Bramono K, Urip KS, et al. Once daily treatment with terbinafine 1% cream (Lamisil) for one week is effective in the treatment of tinea corporis and cruris. A placebo-controlled study. *Mycoses*. 2001;44:300-306.
4. Lebwohl M, Elewski B, Eisen D, Savin RC. Efficacy and safety of terbinafine 1% solution in the treatment of interdigital tinea pedis and tinea corporis or tinea cruris. *Cutis*. 2001;67:261-266.
5. Boonk W, de Geer D, de Kreek E, et al. Itraconazole in the treatment of tinea corporis and tinea cruris: comparison of two treatment schedules. *Mycoses*. 1998;41:509-514.
6. Voravutinon V. Oral treatment of tinea corporis and tinea cruris with terbinafine and griseofulvin: A randomized double blind comparative study. *J Med Assoc Thai*. 1993;76:388-393.
7. Gupta AK, Chaudhry M, Elewski B. Tinea corporis, tinea cruris, tinea nigra, and piedra. *Dermatol Clin*. 2003;21(3):395-400.
8. Hand JW, Wroble RR. Prevention of tinea corporis in collegiate wrestlers. *J Athl Train*. 1999;34(4):350-352.

124 TINEA CRURIS

Richard P. Usatine, MD
Mindy A. Smith, MD, MS

PATIENT STORY

A 17-year-old girl presents with a rash and itching in the groin (**Figure 124-1**). On examination, she was found to have an expanding scaly erythematous well-demarcated ring in the inguinal area. A skin scraping was treated with Swartz-Lamkins stain and the dermatophyte was highly visible under the microscope (**Figure 124-2**). The clinician diagnosed tinea cruris. She was offered a choice between an oral or topical antifungal medicine and she preferred to have the systemic treatment. She was given 2 weeks of oral terbinafine 250 mg daily and her tinea cruris resolved.

INTRODUCTION

Tinea cruris is an intensely pruritic superficial fungal infection of the groin and adjacent skin.

SYNONYMS

Crotch rot and jock itch.

EPIDEMIOLOGY

- Using data from the National Ambulatory Medical Care Survey and the National Hospital Ambulatory Medical Care Survey (NHAMCS) (1995–2004), there were more than 4 million annual visits for dermatophytoses and 8.4 percent were for tinea cruris.[1]
- Tinea cruris is more common in men than women (three-fold) and rare in children. However, it may be seen in teens after puberty.

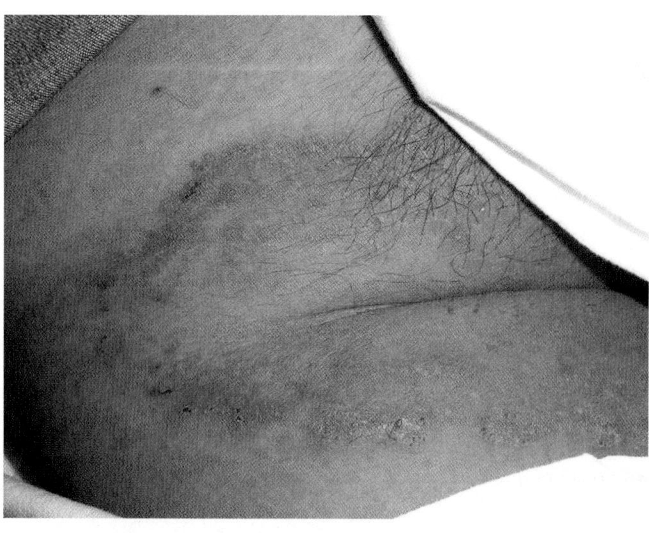

FIGURE 124-1 A 17-year-old woman with tinea cruris showing erythema and scale in an annular pattern. Central clearing is less common in tinea cruris than tinea corporis but can occur. (*Used with permission from Richard P. Usatine, MD.*)

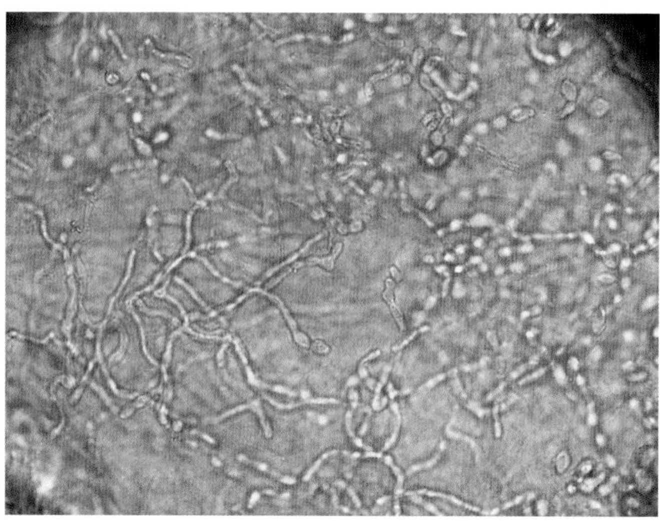

FIGURE 124-2 Microscopic view of the scraping of the groin in a patient with tinea cruris. The hyphae are easy to see under 40-power with Swartz-Lamkins stain. (*Used with permission from Richard P. Usatine, MD.*)

ETIOLOGY AND PATHOPHYSIOLOGY

- Most commonly caused by the dermatophytes: *Trichophyton rubrum, Epidermophyton floccosum, Trichophyton mentagrophytes,* and *Trichophyton verrucosum. T. rubrum* is the most common organism.[2]
- Can be spread by fomites, such as contaminated towels.
- The fungal agents cause keratinases, which allow invasion of the cornified cell layer of the epidermis.[2]
- Autoinoculation can occur from fungus on the feet or hands.

RISK FACTORS

- Wearing tight-fitting or wet clothing or underwear has traditionally been suggested; however, in a study of Italian soldiers, none of the risk factors analyzed (e.g., hyperhidrosis, swimming pool attendance) were significantly associated with any fungal infection.[3]
- Obesity and diabetes mellitus may be risk factors.[4]

DIAGNOSIS

CLINICAL FEATURES

The cardinal features are scale and signs of inflammation. In light-skinned persons, inflammation often appears pink or red and in dark-skinned persons, the inflammation often leads to hyperpigmentation

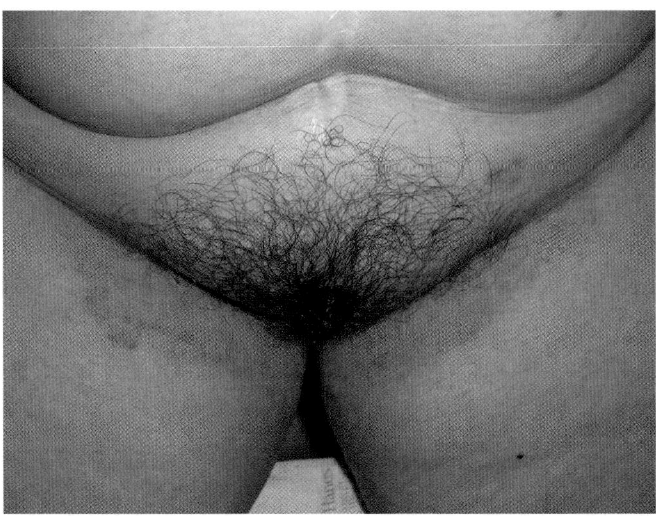

FIGURE 124-3 A woman with tinea cruris showing erythema and scale. This patient had tinea on her feet, face, and under her breasts. (*Used with permission from Richard P. Usatine, MD.*)

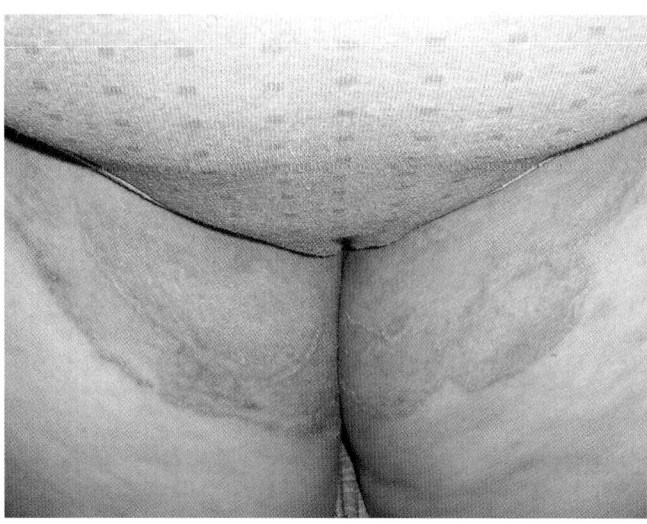

FIGURE 124-5 Tinea incognito with concentric rings within the scaling plaques. The original tinea cruris was misdiagnosed and the patient was given topical steroids for the itching. (*Used with permission from Richard P. Usatine, MD.*)

(see **Figure 124-4**). Occasionally, tinea cruris may show central sparing with an annular pattern as in **Figure 124-1**, but most often is homogeneously distributed as in **Figures 124-3** and **124-4**. If the tinea cruris was missed and the patient was given topical steroids to treat the itching, the tinea cruris can become tinea incognito and the eruption can expand down the thighs (**Figure 124-5**). Tinea incognito often shows concentric rings within the scaling plaques.

TYPICAL DISTRIBUTION

By definition tinea cruris is in the inguinal area. However, the fungus can grow outside of this area to involve the abdomen and thighs (**Figures 124-4** and **124-5**). Tinea may be present in multiple locations simultaneously including the feet.

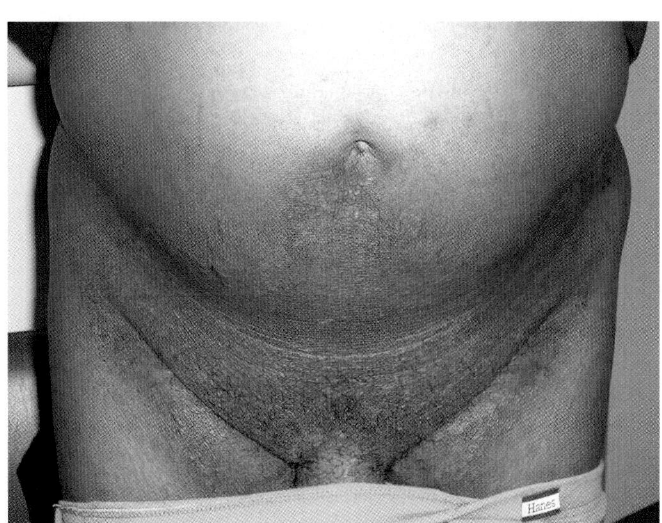

FIGURE 124-4 Tinea cruris that has expanded beyond the inguinal area in this young black man. Postinflammatory hyperpigmentation is visible throughout the infected area. (*Used with permission from Richard P. Usatine, MD.*)

LABORATORY STUDIES

Diagnosis is often made based on clinical presentation, but a skin scraping treated with KOH and a fungal stain analyzed under the microscope can be helpful (**Figure 124-2**). False negatives may occur if scraping is inadequate, patient is using topical antifungals, or the viewer is inexperienced. See Chapter 120, Fungal Overview, for more information on doing a good KOH preparation.

Skin scraping and culture is definitive but expensive, and may take up to 2 weeks for the culture to grow.

UV lamp can be used to look for the coral red fluorescence of erythrasma (see Chapter 102, Erythrasma). Most tinea cruris is caused by *T. rubrum* so will not fluoresce.

DIFFERENTIAL DIAGNOSIS

- Cutaneous *Candida* in the groin can become red and have scaling that extends to the thigh and scrotum. Tinea cruris does not often involve the scrotum. *Candida* often has satellite lesions. However, tinea cruris can also have a few satellite lesions (see Chapter 120, Candidiasis).
- Erythrasma in the groin appears similar to tinea cruris. It is less common than tinea cruris and may show coral red fluorescence with a UV light (**Figure 124-6**) (see Chapter 102, Erythrasma).
- Contact dermatitis can occur anywhere on the body. If the contact is near the groin this can be mistaken for tinea cruris (see Chapter 131, Contact Dermatitis).
- Inverse psoriasis causes inflammation in the intertriginous areas of the body. It does not have the thick plaques of plaque psoriasis. Inverse psoriasis may be misdiagnosed as a fungal infection until an astute clinician recognizes the pattern or does a biopsy (**Figure 124-7**; see Chapter 136, Psoriasis).
- Intertrigo is an inflammatory condition of the skin folds. It induced or aggravated by heat, moisture, maceration, and friction.[5] The

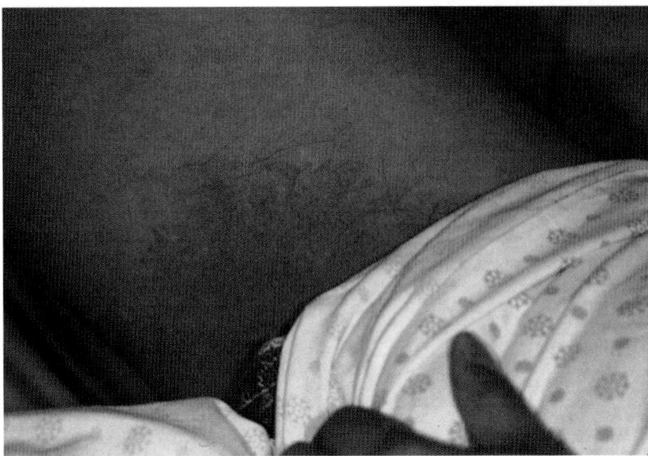

FIGURE 124-6 Erythrasma in the groin can be mistaken for tinea cruris. This erythrasma fluoresced coral red with an ultraviolet light. (*Used with permission from Richard P. Usatine, MD.*)

condition frequently is worsened by infection with *Candida* or dermatophytes so there is some overlap with tinea cruris.

MANAGEMENT

- Tinea cruris (**Figure 124-8**) is best treated with a topical allylamine or an azole antifungal (SOR Ⓐ, based on multiple randomized controlled trials [RCTs]).[6] Differences in current comparison data are insufficient to stratify the two groups of topical antifungals.[7] In one RCT, cure rates were higher at 1 week with butenafine (once daily for 2 weeks) versus clotrimazole (twice daily for 4 weeks) (26.5% vs. 2.9%, respectively), but were not significantly different at 4 or 8 weeks.[8]

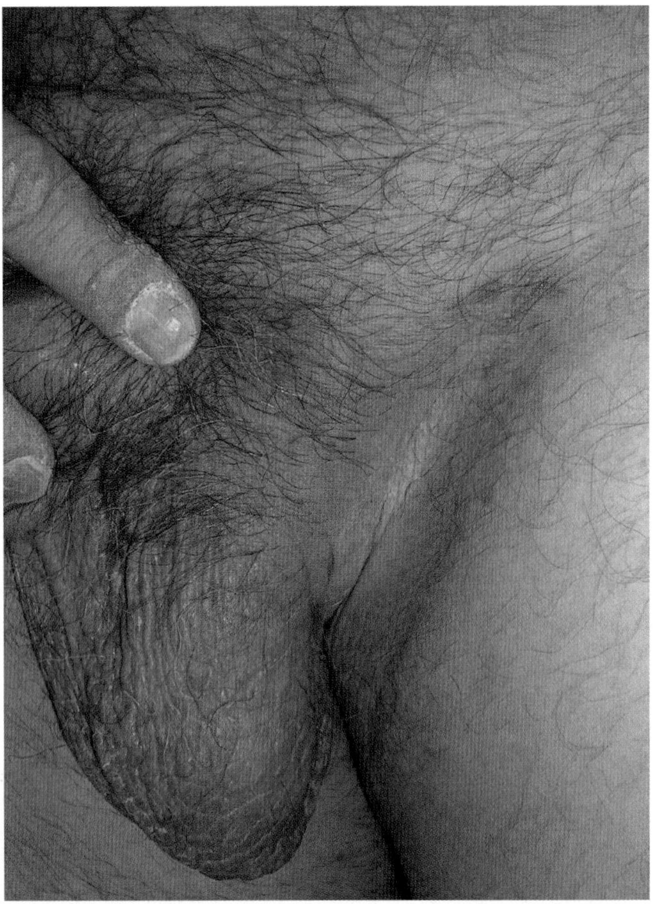

FIGURE 124-7 Inverse psoriasis in a man who also has the nail changes of psoriasis. (*Used with permission from Richard P. Usatine, MD.*)

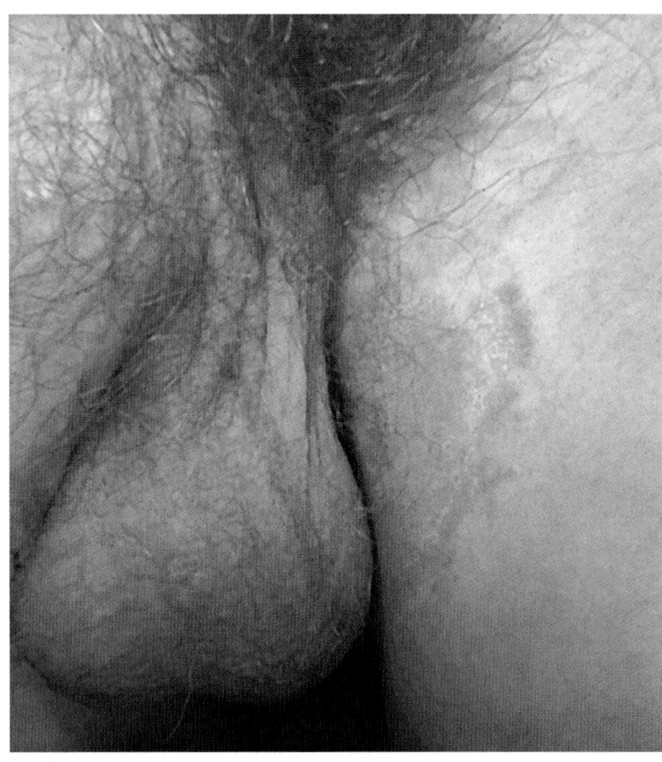

FIGURE 124-8 Tinea cruris in this teenage boy. (*Used with permission from Cleveland Clinic Children's Hospital Photo Files.*)

- The fungicidal allylamines (naftifine and terbinafine) and butenafine (allylamine derivative) are a more costly group of topical tinea treatments, yet they are more convenient as they allow for a shorter duration of treatment compared with fungistatic azoles (clotrimazole, econazole, ketoconazole, oxiconazole, miconazole, and sulconazole).[7]
- Topical azoles should be continued for 4 weeks and topical allylamines for 2 weeks or until clinical cure.[6–8] SOR Ⓐ
- Fluconazole 150 mg once weekly for 2 to 4 weeks appears to be effective in the treatment of tinea cruris in adults.[9] SOR Ⓑ This could be applied to teens as well.
- One RCT showed that itraconazole 200 mg daily for 1 week is similarly effective, equally well tolerated, and at least as safe as itraconazole 100 mg daily for 2 weeks in the treatment of tinea corporis or cruris (clinical response: 73% and 80% at the end of follow-up, respectively).[10] SOR Ⓑ While the study was performed in adults this could be applied to teens.
- Adult patients with mycologically diagnosed tinea corporis and tinea cruris were randomly allocated to receive either 250 mg of oral terbinafine once daily or 500 mg of griseofulvin once daily for 2 weeks. The cure rates were higher for terbinafine at 6 weeks.[11] SOR Ⓑ Oral terbinafine is a good and affordable choice for teenagers if topical treatment fails. SOR Ⓒ

- If there are multiple sites infected with fungus, treat all active areas of infection simultaneously to prevent reinfection of the groin from other body sites. If the tinea is widespread as in the patient in **Figure 124-3**, an oral agent is warranted.

FOLLOW-UP

As needed.

PATIENT EDUCATION

- Advise patients with tinea pedis to put on their socks before their undershorts to reduce the possibility of direct contamination. SOR Ⓒ
- Dry the groin completely after bathing. SOR Ⓒ

PATIENT RESOURCES

- Medscape Family Medicine. *Tinea Cruris in Men: Bothersome But Treatable*—**www.medscape.com/viewarticle/512992**.
- Medline Plus. *Jock Itch*—**www.nlm.nih.gov/medlineplus/ency/article/000876.htm**.

PROVIDER RESOURCES

- DermNet NZ. *Fungal Skin Infections*—**www.dermnetnz.org/fungal/**.
- Doctor Fungus—**www.doctorfungus.org/**.
- Medscape. *Tinea Cruris*—**http://emedicine.medscape.com/article/1091806**.

REFERENCES

1. Panackal AA, Halpern EF, Watson AJ. Cutaneous fungal infections in the United States: analysis of the National Ambulatory Medical Care Survey (NAMCS) and National Hospital Ambulatory Medical Care Survey (NHAMCS), 1995-2004. *Int J Dermatol*. 2009;48(7):704-712.
2. Wiederkehr M, Schwartz RA. *Tinea Cruris*, http://emedicine.medscape.com/article/1091806-overview, accessed April 2, 2012.
3. Ingordo V, Naldi L, Fracchiolla S, Colecchia B. Prevalence and risk factors for superficial fungal infections among Italian Navy cadets. *Dermatology*. 2004;209(3):190-196.
4. Patel GA, Wiederkehr M, Schwartz RA. Tinea cruris in children. *Cutis*. 2009;84(3):133-137.
5. Selden ST. *Intertrigo*, http://emedicine.medscape.com/article/1087691-overview, accessed April 2, 2012.
6. Drake LA, Dinehart SM, Farmer ER, et al. Guidelines of care for superficial mycotic infections of the skin: tinea corporis, tinea cruris, tinea faciei, tinea manuum, and tinea pedis. Guidelines/Outcomes Committee. American Academy of Dermatology. *J Am Acad Dermatol*. 1996;34(2 Pt 1):282-286.
7. Nadalo D, Montoya C, Hunter-Smith D. What is the best way to treat tinea cruris? *J Fam Pract*. 2006;55:256-258.
8. Singal A, Pandhi D, Agrawal S, Das S. Comparative efficacy of topical 1% butenafine and 1% clotrimazole in tinea cruris and tinea corporis: a randomized, double-blind trial. *J Dermatolog Treat*. 2005;16(506):331-335.
9. Nozickova M, Koudelkova V, Kulikova Z, Malina L, Urbanowski S, Silny W. A comparison of the efficacy of oral fluconazole, 150 mg/week versus 50 mg/day, in the treatment of tinea corporis, tinea cruris, tinea pedis, and cutaneous candidosis. *Int J Dermatol*. 1998;37:703-705.
10. Boonk W, de Geer D, de Kreek E, Remme J, van Huystee B. Itraconazole in the treatment of tinea corporis and tinea cruris: comparison of two treatment schedules. *Mycoses*. 1998;41:509-514.
11. Voravutinon V. Oral treatment of tinea corporis and tinea cruris with terbinafine and griseofulvin: a randomized double blind comparative study. *J Med Assoc Thai*. 1993;76:388-393.

125 TINEA PEDIS

Richard P. Usatine, MD
Katie Reppa, MD

PATIENT STORY

An 8-year-old boy presents with itching between his toes for 1 month (**Figure 125-1**). The pediatrician looks between his toes and sees maceration with white material. The patient was diagnosed with tinea pedis and treated successfully with a topical nonprescription antifungal medication.

INTRODUCTION

Tinea pedis is a common cutaneous infection of the feet caused by dermatophyte fungus. The clinical manifestation presents in 1 of 3 major patterns: interdigital, moccasin, and inflammatory. Concurrent fungal infection of the nails (onychomycosis) occurs frequently.

SYNONYMS

Athlete's foot.

EPIDEMIOLOGY

- Tinea pedis is thought to be the world's most common dermatophytosis.[1]
- 70 percent of the population will be infected with tinea pedis at some time.[1]
- More commonly affects males than females.[1]
- Prevalence increases with age and it is rare before adolescence.[1]

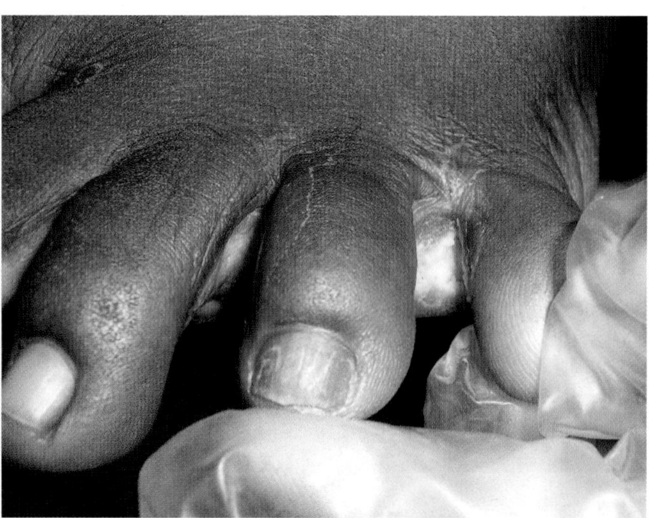

FIGURE 125-1 Tinea pedis seen in the interdigital spaces of an 8-year-old boy. (*Used with permission from Richard P. Usatine, MD.*)

ETIOLOGY AND PATHOPHYSIOLOGY

- A cutaneous fungal infection most commonly caused by *Trichophyton rubrum*.[1]
- *Trichophyton mentagrophytes* and *Epidermophyton floccosum* follow in that order.
- *T. rubrum* causes most tinea pedis and onychomycosis.

RISK FACTORS

- Male gender.
- Use of public showers, baths, or pools.[2]
- Household member with tinea pedis infection.[2]
- Certain occupations (miners, farmers, soldiers, meat factory workers, or marathon runners).[2]
- Use of immunosuppressive drugs.

DIAGNOSIS

TYPICAL DISTRIBUTION AND MORPHOLOGY

Three types of tinea pedis:

- Interdigital type—Most common (**Figure 125-2**).
- Moccasin type (**Figure 125-3**).
- Inflammatory/vesicular type—Least common (**Figure 125-4**).

Some authors describe an ulcerative type (**Figure 125-5**).

CLINICAL FEATURES

- Interdigital—White or green fungal growth between toes with erythema, maceration, cracks, and fissures—especially between fourth and fifth digits (**Figures 125-1** and **125-2**). The dry type has more scale and the moist type becomes macerated.

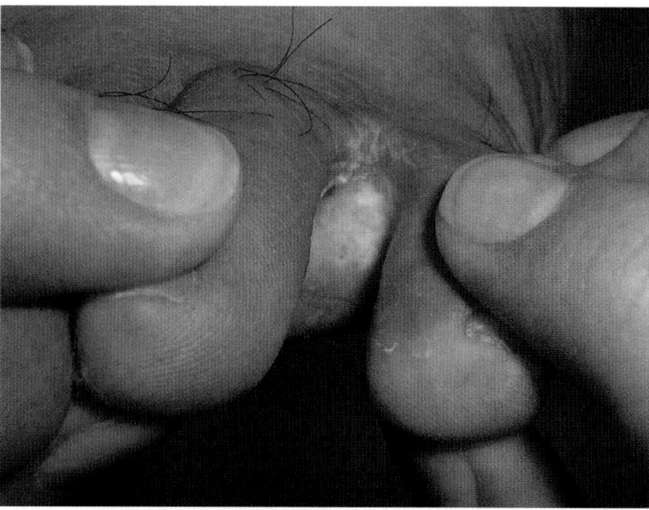

FIGURE 125-2 Tinea pedis seen in the interdigital space between the fourth and fifth digits. This is the most common area to see tinea pedis. (*Used with permission from Richard P. Usatine, MD.*)

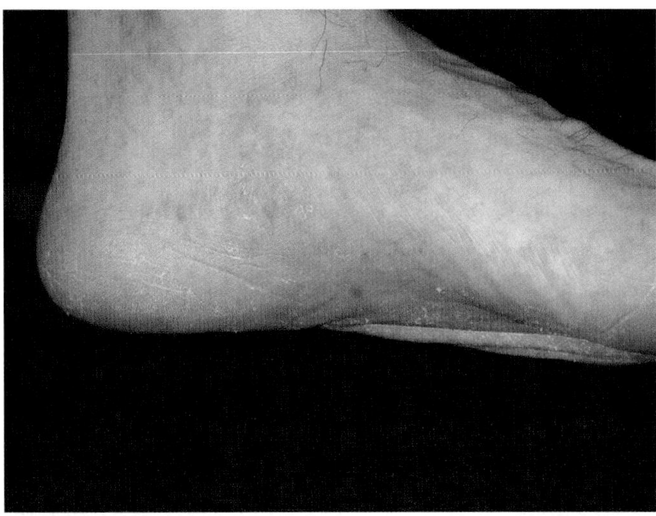

FIGURE 125-3 Tinea pedis in the moccasin distribution. (*Used with permission from Richard P. Usatine, MD.*)

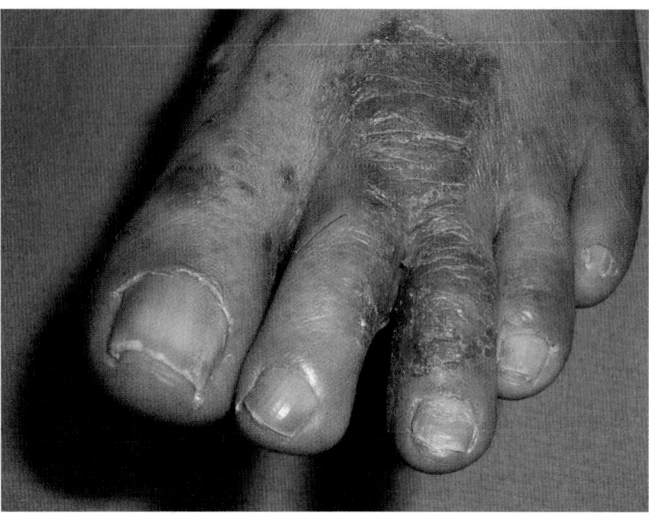

FIGURE 125-5 Ulcerative tinea pedis with spreading vesicles related to a bacterial superinfection. The patient was treated with antifungals and antibiotics. (*Used with permission from Richard P. Usatine, MD.*)

- Moccasin—Scale on sides and soles of feet (**Figure 125-3**).
- Vesicular—Vesicles and bullae on feet especially around the arch (**Figure 125-4**).
- Ulcerative tinea pedis is characterized by rapidly spreading vesiculopustular lesions, ulcers, and erosions, typically in the web spaces (**Figure 125-5**). It is accompanied by a secondary bacterial infection. This can lead to cellulitis or lymphangitis.
- Examine nails for evidence of onychomycosis—Fungal infections of nails may include subungual keratosis, yellow or white discolorations, dysmorphic nails (Chapter 163, Onychomycosis).
- Examine to exclude cellulitis that may show erythema, swelling, tenderness with red streaks tracking up the foot and lower leg (Chapter 103, Cellulitis).

TYPICAL DISTRIBUTION

Between the toes, on the soles, and lateral aspects of the feet.

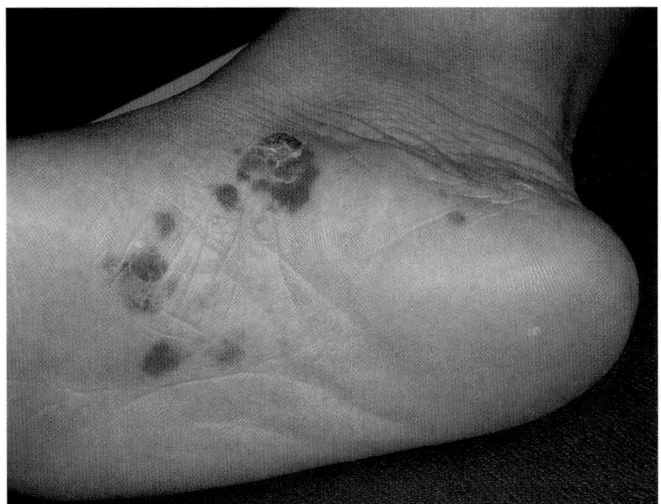

FIGURE 125-4 Vesicular tinea pedis with vesicles and bullae over the arch region of the foot. The arch is a typical location for vesiculobullous tinea pedis. (*Used with permission from Richard P. Usatine, MD.*)

LABORATORY STUDIES

Diagnosis is often made based on clinical presentation but a skin scraping treated with KOH and a fungal stain analyzed under the microscope can be helpful (**Figure 125-6**). The child with the itching foot in **Figure 125-7** could have tinea pedis, dyshidrotic eczema, juvenile plantar dermatosis, or a contact allergy. The positive KOH made the diagnosis easy.

A culture of a skin scraping is helpful if the KOH is negative and there is a fear that it is a false negative. Unfortunately it may take up to 2 weeks for the culture to grow and the cost is higher than a simple KOH.

DIFFERENTIAL DIAGNOSIS

- Juvenile plantar dermatosis causes erythema, scale, cracking and fissures on the weight-bearing surface of the foot in children (**Figure 125-8**). It is also called "sweaty sock syndrome" as these

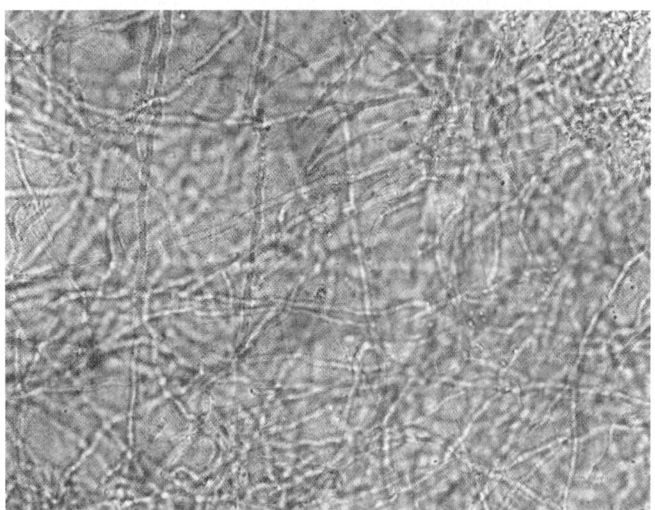

FIGURE 125-6 Microscopic view of the scraping of tinea pedis. The hyphae are easy to see under 40-power with Swartz-Lamkins stain. (*Used with permission from Richard P. Usatine, MD.*)

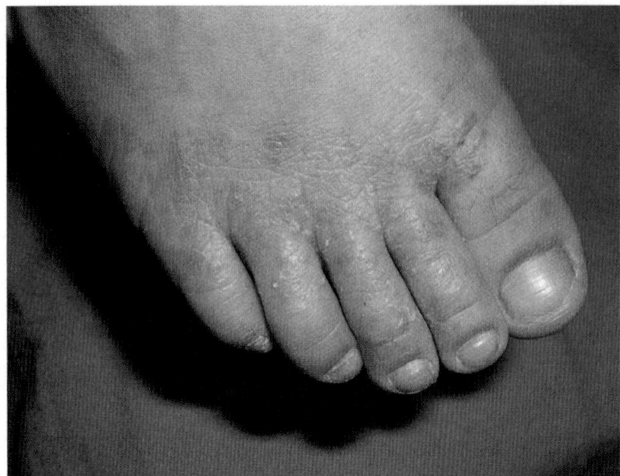

FIGURE 125-7 Tinea pedis around the toes and the forefoot of this child. A KOH preparation was made to confirm the suspicion of tinea pedis as this presentation could be caused by other etiologies. (*Used with permission from Richard P. Usatine, MD.*)

children often have hyperhidrosis and sweaty socks. Another name is "wet-dry foot syndrome" as it is caused by excessive sweating of the feet in occlusive footwear and rapid drying in a low-humidity environment. It tends to be worse in the winter and more common in children with atopic dermatitis. The use of emollient ointments is helpful. A KOH preparation will be negative.

- Pitted keratolysis: well-demarcated pits or erosions in the sole of the foot caused by bacteria (**Figure 125-9**; Chapter 101, Pitted Keratolysis).
- Contact dermatitis: tends to be seen on the dorsum and sides of the foot (**Figure 125-10**) often related to allergens in rubber or leather. It is more common in children with atopic dermatitis (Chapter 131, Contact Dermatitis).
- Dyshidrotic eczema is characterized by scale and tapioca-like vesicles on the hands and feet (**Figure 125-11**). It is also more common in children with atopic dermatitis.

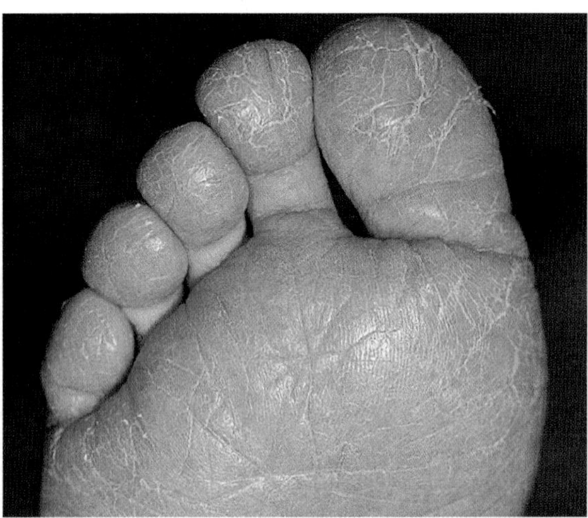

FIGURE 125-8 Juvenile plantar dermatitis causes erythema, scale, cracking and fissures on the weight-bearing surface of the foot. It is also called "sweaty sock syndrome" as these children often have hyperhidrosis and sweaty socks. (*Used with permission from Weinberg SW, Prose NS, Kristal L. Color Atlas of Pediatric Dermatology, 4th ed. Figure 6-13, New York, NY: McGraw-Hill, 2008.*)

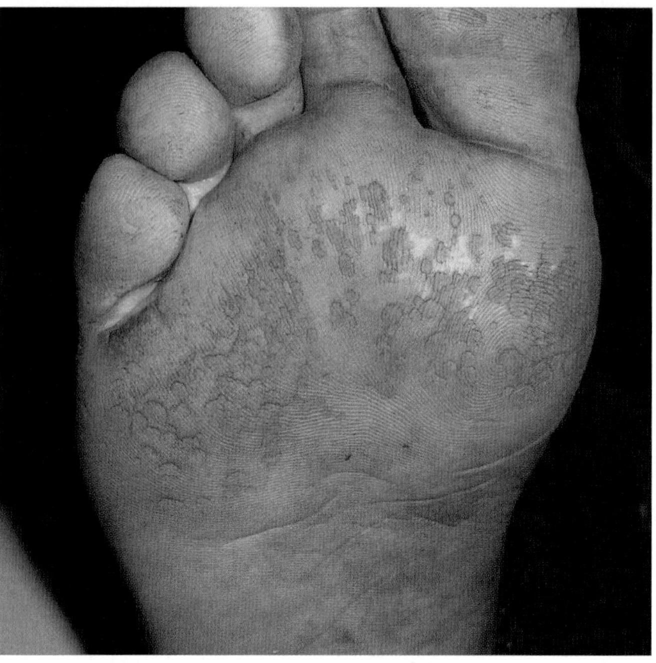

FIGURE 125-9 Pitted keratolysis on the sole of the foot with some interdigital tinea pedis. The pits are caused by bacteria and treatment involves an antibiotic. (*Used with permission from Richard P. Usatine, MD.*)

- Friction blisters—Blisters on the feet of persons leading an active athletic lifestyle.
- Psoriasis—Can mimic tinea pedis but will usually be present in other areas as well (**Figure 125-12**; Chapter 152, Psoriasis).

MANAGEMENT

Table 125-1 discusses management of tinea pedis.

TOPICAL ANTIFUNGALS

- Systematic review of 70 trials of topical antifungals showed good evidence for efficacy compared to placebo for the following:

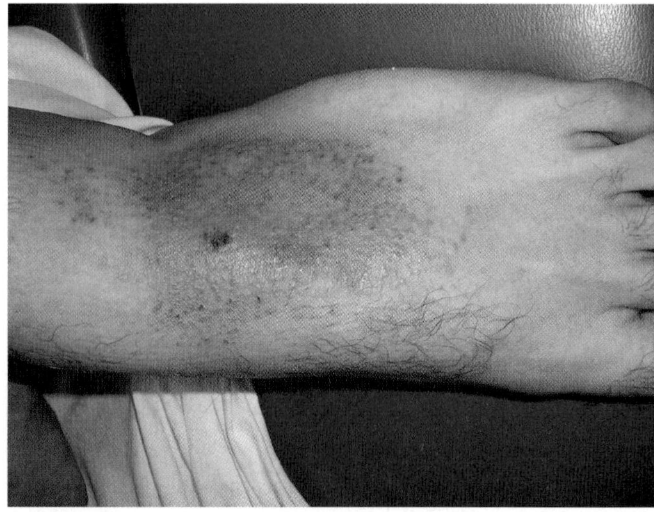

FIGURE 125-10 Contact dermatitis to a chemical in the rubber of the shoes with typical distribution that crosses the dorsum of the foot. (*Used with permission from Richard P. Usatine, MD.*)

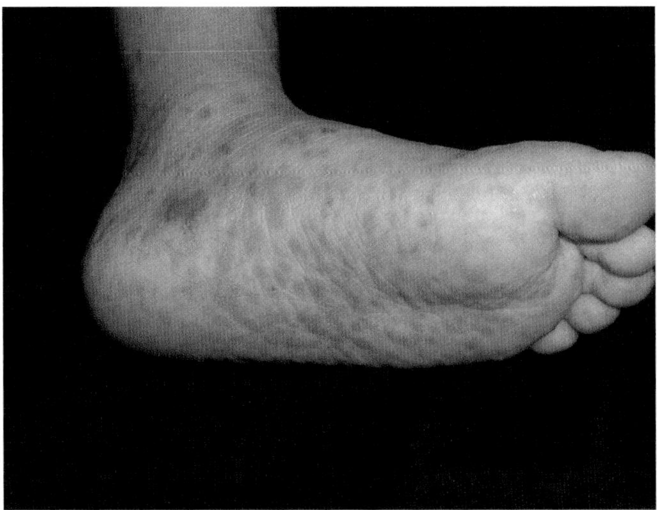

FIGURE 125-11 Dyshidrotic eczema on the foot of a 4-year-old boy showing tapioca vesicles and scaling on the sides and bottom of the foot. This boy also has severe atopic dermatitis. (*Used with permission from Richard P. Usatine, MD.*)

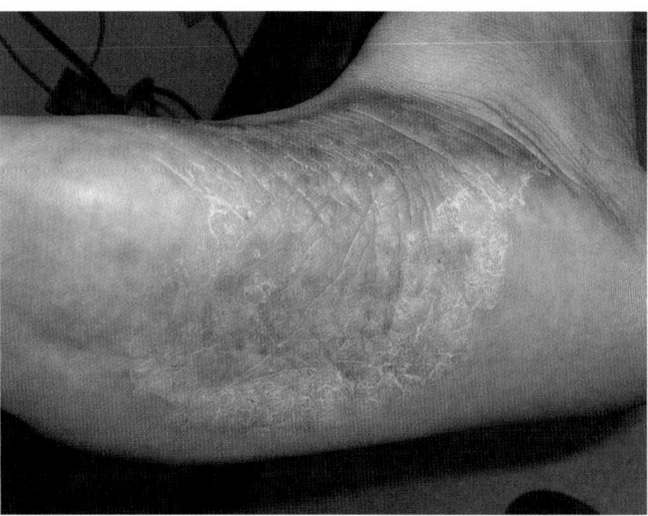

FIGURE 125-12 Plantar psoriasis in a young patient with other areas of psoriasis also present. KOH preparation was negative. (*Used with permission from Richard P. Usatine, MD.*)

- Allylamines (naftifine, terbinafine, butenafine).[3] SOR Ⓐ
- Azoles (clotrimazole, miconazole, econazole).[3] SOR Ⓐ
- Allylamines cure slightly more infections than azoles but are more expensive.[3] SOR Ⓐ
- No differences in efficacy found between individual allylamines or individual azoles (**Table 125-2**). SOR Ⓐ
- In one metaanalysis, topical terbinafine was found to be equally effective as other topical antifungals but the average duration of treatment was shorter (1 week instead of 2 weeks). Additionally, terbinafine is effective as a single-application film-forming solution.[4] SOR Ⓐ

ORAL ANTIFUNGALS

- Systematic review of 12 trials, involving 700 participants: oral terbinafine for 2 weeks cures 52 percent more patients than oral griseofulvin.[5] SOR Ⓐ
- Terbinafine is equal to itraconazole in patient outcomes.[5] SOR Ⓐ
- No significant differences in comparisons between a number of oral agents.[5] SOR Ⓐ

Dosing for tinea pedis needing oral therapy:

- Itraconazole two 100 mg tablets daily for 1 week.[6]
- Terbinafine 250 mg PO daily for 1 to 2 weeks.[6]

Patients with onychomycosis may have recurrences of the skin infection related to the fungus that remains in the nails and, therefore, may need oral treatment for 3 months to achieve better results.

Topical urea (Carmol, Keralac), available in 10 to 40 percent concentrations, may be useful to decrease scaling in patients with hyperkeratotic soles.[5]

ALTERNATIVE THERAPY

One small pilot study with 56 participants showed significant improvement or resolution of symptoms in patients treated by wearing socks containing copper-oxide fibers daily for a minimum of 8 to 10 days.[7] SOR Ⓑ

PATIENT EDUCATION

- Do not go barefoot in public showers and locker rooms. SOR Ⓒ
- Keep feet dry and clean, and use clean socks and shoes that allow the feet to get fresh air. SOR Ⓒ
- Use the topical medication beyond the time in which the feet look clear to prevent relapse.

TABLE 125-1 Management of Tinea Pedis

Tinea Pedis Type	Treatment for Mild Cases	Treatment for Recalcitrant Cases	SOR
Interdigital type	Topical antifungal	Another topical antifungal or an oral antifungal	A
Moccasin type	Topical antifungal	Oral antifungal	A
Inflammatory/vesicular type	Oral antifungal	Oral antifungal	A

Reprinted with permission from Thomas B. Clear choices in managing epidermal tinea infections. *J Fam Pract.* 2003;52(11):857. Reproduced with permission from Frontline Medical Communications.

TABLE 125-2 Topical Antifungal Medications

Agent	Formulation	Frequency*	Duration* (weeks)	NNT†
Imidazoles				
Clotrimazole	1 percent cream 1 percent solution 1 percent swabs	Twice daily	2 to 4	2.9
Econazole	1 percent cream	Twice daily	2 to 4	2.6
Ketoconazole	2 percent cream	Once daily	2 to 4	No data available
Miconazole	2 percent cream 2 percent spray 2 percent powder	Twice daily	2 to 4	2.8 (at 8 weeks)
Oxiconazole	1 percent cream 1 percent lotion	Once to twice daily	2 to 4	2.9
Sulconazole	1 percent cream 1 percent solution	Once to twice daily	2 to 4	2.5
Allylamines				
Naftifine	1 percent cream 1 percent gel	Once to twice daily	1 to 4	1.9
Terbinafine	1 percent cream 1 percent solution	Once to twice daily	1 to 4	1.6 (1.7 for tinea cruris/tinea corporis at 8 weeks)
Benzylamine				
Butenafine	1 percent cream	Once to twice daily	1 to 4	1.9 (1.4 for tinea corporis and 1.5 for tinea cruris)
Other				
Ciclopirox	0.77 percent cream 0.77 percent lotion	Twice daily	2 to 4	2.1
Tolnaftate	1 percent powder 1 percent spray 1 percent swabs	Twice daily	4	3.6 (at 8 weeks)

*Manufacturer guidelines.
†NNT, number needed to treat. NNT is calculated from systematic review of all randomized controlled trials for tinea pedis at 6 weeks after the initiation of treatment except where otherwise noted.
Reprinted with permission from Thomas B. Clear choices in managing epidermal tinea infections. *J Fam Pract.* 2003;52(11):857. Reproduced with permission from Frontline Medical Communications.

PATIENT RESOURCES

- eMedicineHealth. *Athlete's Foot*—**www.emedicinehealth.com/athletes_foot/article_em.htm**.

PROVIDER RESOURCES

- Medscape. *Tinea Pedis*—**http://emedicine.medscape.com/article/1091684**.

REFERENCES

1. Robbins C. *Tinea Pedis*. http://www.emedicine.com/DERM/topic470.htm, accessed June 24, 2007.
2. Seebacher C, Bouchara JP, Mignon B. Updates on the epidemiology of dermatophyte infections. *Mycopathologia*. 2008;166(5-6):335-352.
3. Crawford F, Hart R, Bell-Syer S, Torgerson D, Young P, Russell I. Topical treatments for fungal infections of the skin and nails of the foot. *Cochrane Database Syst Rev*. 2000;CD001434.
4. Kienke P, Korting HC, Nelles S, Rychlik R. Comparable efficacy and safety of various topical formulations of terbinafine in tinea pedis irrespective of the treatment regimen: results of a meta-analysis. *Am J Clin Dermatol*. 2007;8(6):357-364.
5. Bell-Syer SE, Hart R, Crawford F, Torgerson DJ, Tyrrell W, Russell I. Oral treatments for fungal infections of the skin of the foot. *Cochrane Database Syst Rev*. 2002;CD003584.
6. Thomas B. Clear choices in managing epidermal tinea infections. *J Fam Pract*. 2003;52:850-862.
7. Zatcoff RC, Smith MS, Borkow G. Treatment of tinea pedis with socks containing copper-oxide impregnated fibers. *Foot (Edinb)*. 2008;18(3):136-141.

126 TINEA VERSICOLOR

Richard P. Usatine, MD
Melissa M. Chan, MD

PATIENT STORY

A young boy is brought to the office by his parents with a 2-year history of his skin turning white on his trunk (**Figure 126-1**). The boy denies any symptoms. His parents are afraid that he has the same thing that Michael Jackson had (vitiligo). The clinician does a KOH preparation of the white skin and finds the spaghetti and meatball pattern of *Malassezia furfur* under the microscope (**Figure 126-2**). His parents are relieved to receive a prescription for the tinea versicolor and to find out that it is rarely spread to others through contact.

INTRODUCTION

Tinea versicolor is a common superficial skin infection caused by the dimorphic lipophilic yeast *Pityrosporum* (*Malassezia furfur*). The most typical presentation is a set of hypopigmented macules and patches with fine scale over the trunk in a cape-like distribution.

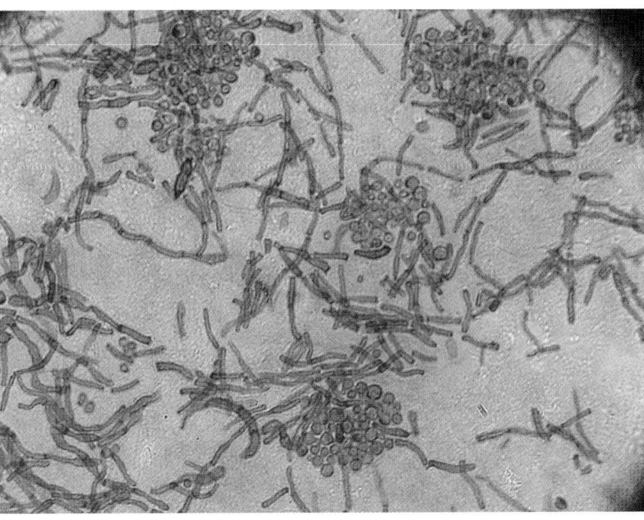

FIGURE 126-2 Positive KOH for tinea versicolor. Microscopic examination of scrapings done from the previous patient showing short mycelial forms and round yeast forms suggestive of spaghetti and meatballs. Swartz-Lamkins stain was used. (*Used with permission from Richard P. Usatine, MD.*)

SYNONYMS

Pityriasis versicolor is actually a more accurate name as "tinea" implies a dermatophyte infection. Tinea versicolor is caused by *Pityrosporum* and not a dermatophyte.

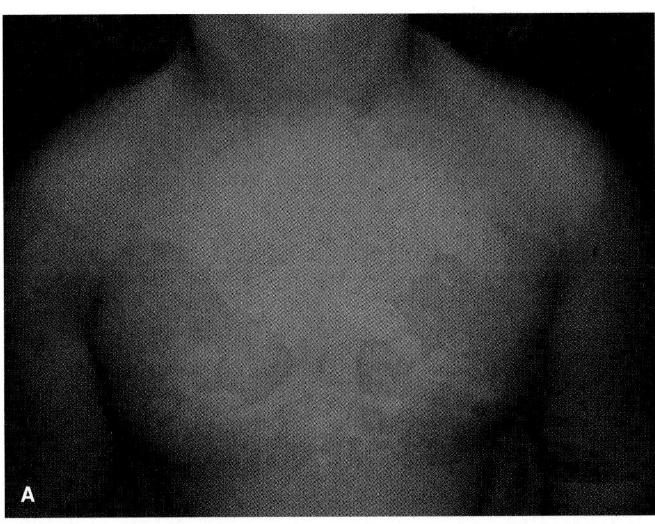

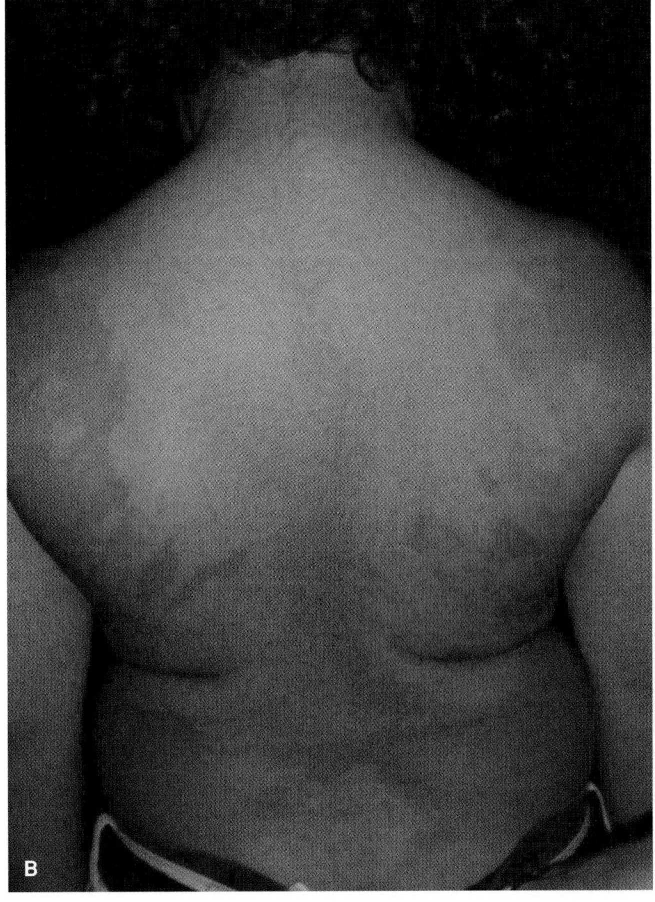

FIGURE 126-1 Tinea versicolor in a young boy showing large areas of hypopigmentation. The darker brown is his normal skin color. The *Malassezia furfur* damages the melanocytes causing the hypopigmentation. The hypopigmentation is reversible with treatment. (*Used with permission from Richard P. Usatine, MD.*)

EPIDEMIOLOGY

- Seen more commonly in men than in women.
- Seen more often during the summer and is especially common in warm and humid climates.

ETIOLOGY AND PATHOPHYSIOLOGY

- Tinea versicolor is caused by *Pityrosporum* (*M. furfur*), which is a lipophilic yeast that can be normal human cutaneous flora.
- *Pityrosporum* exists in two shapes—*Pityrosporum ovale* (oval) and *Pityrosporum orbiculare* (round).
- Tinea versicolor starts when the yeast that normally colonizes the skin changes from the round form to the pathologic mycelial form and then invades the stratum corneum.[1]
- *Pityrosporum* is also associated with seborrhea and *Pityrosporum* folliculitis.
- The white and brown colors are secondary to damage caused by the *Pityrosporum* to the melanocytes, while the pink is an inflammatory reaction to the organism.
- *Pityrosporum* thrive on sebum and moisture; they tend to grow on the skin in areas where there are sebaceous follicles secreting sebum.

DIAGNOSIS

CLINICAL FEATURES

Tinea versicolor consists of hypopigmented, hyperpigmented, or pink macules and patches on the trunk that are finely scaling and well-demarcated. Versicolor means a variety of or variation in colors; tinea versicolor tends to come in white, pink, and brown colors (**Figures 126-1** to **126-5**).

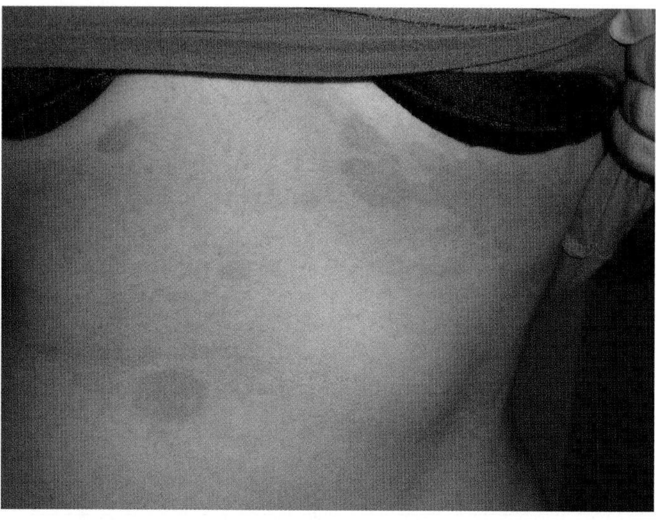

FIGURE 126-4 Brown patches of tinea versicolor on abdomen of this teenage girl. (*Used with permission from Richard P. Usatine, MD.*)

TYPICAL DISTRIBUTION

Tinea versicolor is found on the chest, abdomen, upper arms, and back, whereas seborrhea tends to be seen on the scalp, face, and anterior chest.

LABORATORY STUDIES

A scraping of the scaling portions of the skin may be placed onto a slide using the side of another slide or a scalpel. KOH with DMSO (DMSO helps the KOH dissolve the keratinocytes faster and reduces the need for heating the slide) is placed on the slide and covered with a coverslip. Microscopic examination reveals the typical "spaghetti-and-meatballs" pattern of tinea versicolor. The "spaghetti," or more accurately "ziti," is the short mycelial form and the "meatballs" are the round yeast form (**Figures 126-6** and **126-7**). Fungal stains such as the Swartz-Lamkins stain help make the identification of the fungal elements easier.

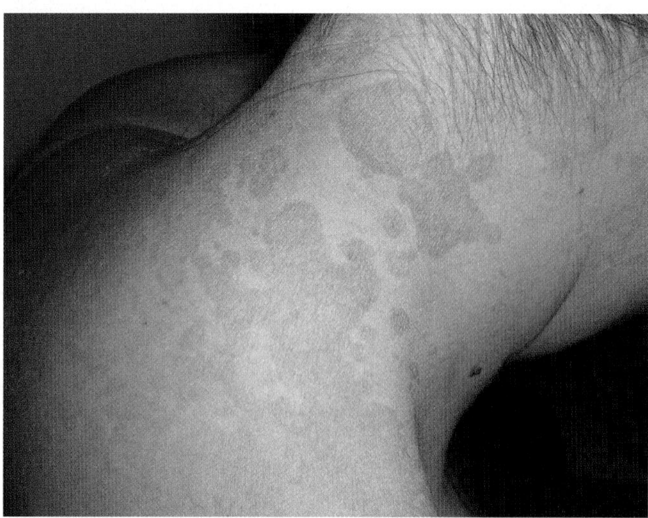

FIGURE 126-3 Pink scaly patches caused by tinea versicolor on the neck of a teenage girl. (*Used with permission from Richard P. Usatine, MD.*)

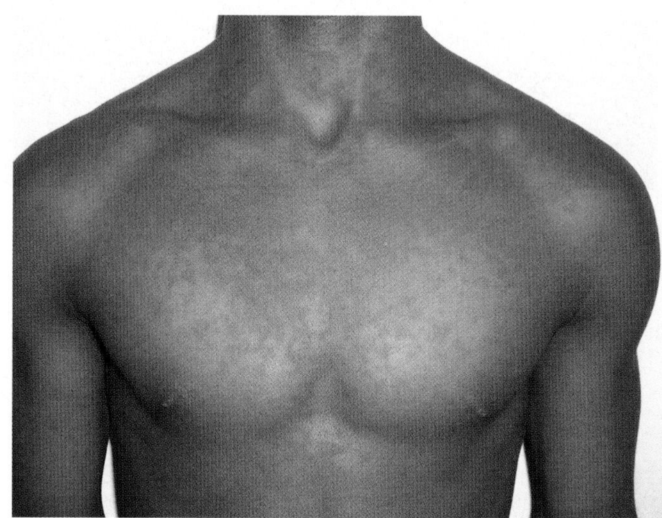

FIGURE 126-5 Hyperpigmented variant of tinea versicolor in a young black man. (*Used with permission from Richard P. Usatine, MD.*)

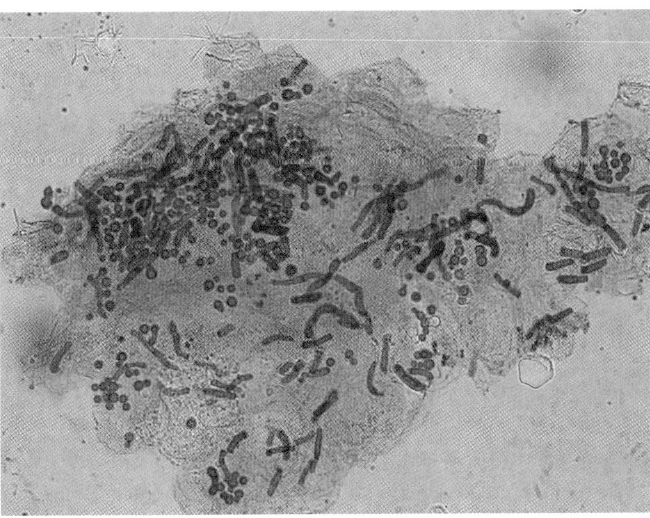

FIGURE 126-6 Positive KOH for tinea versicolor showing short mycelial forms and round yeast forms suggestive of spaghetti (or ziti) and meatballs. Swartz-Lamkins stain was used. (*Used with permission from Richard P. Usatine, MD.*)

DIFFERENTIAL DIAGNOSIS

- Pityriasis rosea has a fine collarette scale around the border of the lesions and is frequently seen with a herald patch. Negative KOH (see Chapter 137, Pityriasis Rosea).
- Secondary syphilis is usually not scaling and tends to have macules on the palms and soles. Negative KOH (see Chapter 181, Syphilis).
- Tinea corporis is rarely as widespread as tinea versicolor and each individual lesion usually has central clearing and a well-defined, raised, scaling border. The KOH preparation in tinea corporis shows hyphae with multiple branch points and not the "ziti-and-meatballs" pattern of tinea versicolor (see Chapter 123, Tinea Corporis).

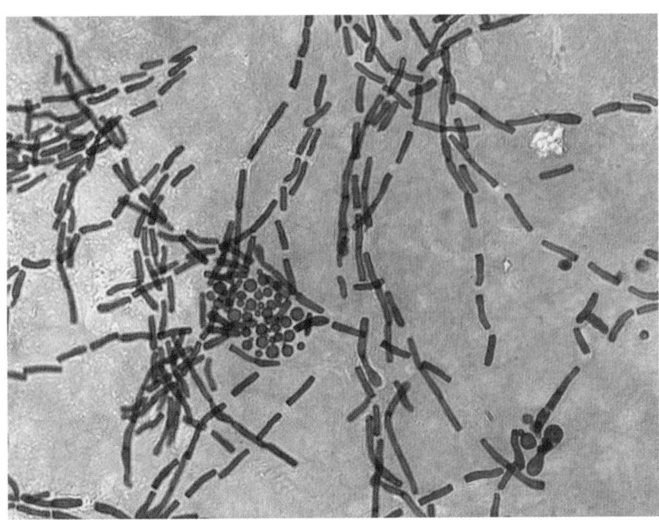

FIGURE 126-7 Close-up of *Malassezia furfur* (*Pityrosporum*) showing the ziti-and-meatball appearance after Swartz-Lamkins stain was applied to the scraping of tinea versicolor. (*Used with permission from Richard P. Usatine, MD.*)

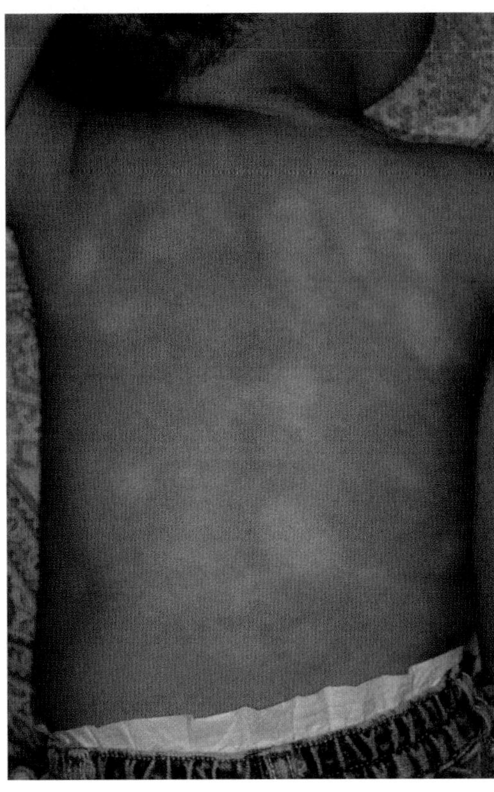

FIGURE 126-8 Pityriasis alba on the back of this young boy that could be mistaken for tinea versicolor. The KOH was negative and the child had other manifestations of atopic dermatitis. (*Used with permission from Richard P. Usatine, MD.*)

- Vitiligo—The degree of hypopigmentation is greater and the distribution is frequently different with vitiligo involving the hands and face (see Chapter 167, Vitiligo and Hypopigmentation).
- Pityriasis alba—Lightly hypopigmented areas with slight scale that tend to be found on the face and trunk of children with atopy. These patches are frequently smaller and rounder than tinea versicolor (**Figures 126-8**; see Chapter 130, Atopic Dermatitis).
- *Pityrosporum* folliculitis is caused by the same organism but presents with pink or brown papules on the back. The patient complains of itchy rough skin and the KOH is positive.

MANAGEMENT

TOPICAL

- Because tinea versicolor is usually asymptomatic, the treatment is mostly for cosmetic reasons.
- The mainstay of treatment has been topical therapy using antidandruff shampoos, because the same *Pityrosporum* species that cause seborrhea and dandruff also cause tinea versicolor.[1,2]
- Patients may apply selenium sulfide 2.5 percent lotion or shampoo, or zinc pyrithione shampoo to the involved areas daily for 1 to 2 weeks. Various amounts of time are suggested to allow the preparations to work, but there are no studies that show a minimum exposure time needed. A typical regimen involves applying the

lotion or shampoo to the involved areas for 10 minutes and then washing it off in the shower. SOR Ⓒ

- One study used ketoconazole 2 percent shampoo (Nizoral) as a single application or daily for 3 days and found it safe and highly effective in treating tinea versicolor.[3] SOR Ⓑ
- Topical antifungal creams for smaller areas of involvement can include ketoconazole and clotrimazole. SOR Ⓒ

ORAL TREATMENT AND PREVENTION

- A single-dose 400-mg oral fluconazole provided the best clinical and mycologic cure rate, with no relapse during 12 months of follow-up.[4] SOR Ⓑ
- A single dose of 300 mg of oral fluconazole repeated weekly for 2 weeks was equal to 400 mg of ketoconazole in a single dose repeated weekly for 2 weeks. No significant differences in efficacy, safety, and tolerability between the two treatment regimens were found.[5] SOR Ⓑ
- A single-dose 400-mg oral ketoconazole to treat tinea versicolor is safe and cost-effective compared to using the newer, more expensive, oral antifungal agents, such as itraconazole.[6,7] SOR Ⓑ
- Oral itraconazole 200 mg given twice a day for 1 day a month has been shown to be safe and effective as a prophylactic treatment for tinea versicolor.[8] SOR Ⓑ
- There is no evidence that establishes the need to sweat after taking oral antifungals to treat tinea versicolor.

FOLLOW-UP

None needed unless it is a stubborn or recurrent case. Recurrent cases can be treated with monthly topical or oral therapy.

PATIENT EDUCATION

Patients should be told that the change in skin color will not reverse immediately. The first sign of successful treatment is the lack of scale. The yeast acts like a sunscreen in the hypopigmented macules. Sun exposure will hasten the normalization of the skin color in patients with hypopigmentation.

PATIENT RESOURCES

- **www.skinsight.com/adult/tineaVersicolor.htm**.

PROVIDER RESOURCES

- **http://emedicine.medscape.com/article/1091575.**

REFERENCES

1. Bolognia J, Jorizzo J, Rapini R. *Dermatology*. St. Louis, MO. Mosby; 2003.
2. Hu SW, Bigby M. Pityriasis versicolor: a systematic review of interventions. *Arch Dermatol.* 2010;146(10):1132-1140.
3. Lange DS, Richards HM, Guarnieri J, et al. Ketoconazole 2% shampoo in the treatment of tinea versicolor: a multicenter, randomized, double-blind, placebo-controlled trial. *J Am Acad Dermatol.* 1998;39(6):944-950.
4. Bhogal CS, Singal A, Baruah MC. Comparative efficacy of ketoconazole and fluconazole in the treatment of pityriasis versicolor: a one year follow-up study. *J Dermatol.* 2001;28(10):535-539.
5. Farschian M, Yaghoobi R, Samadi K. Fluconazole versus ketoconazole in the treatment of tinea versicolor. *J Dermatolog Treat.* 2002;13(2):73-76.
6. Gupta AK, Del Rosso JQ. An evaluation of intermittent therapies used to treat onychomycosis and other dermatomycoses with the oral antifungal agents. *Int J Dermatol.* 2000;39(6):401-411.
7. Wahab MA, Ali ME, Rahman MH, et al. Single dose (400 mg) versus 7 day (200 mg) daily dose itraconazole in the treatment of tinea versicolor: a randomized clinical trial. *Mymensingh Med J.* 2010;19(1):72-76.
8. Faergemann J, Gupta AK, Mofadi AA, et al. Efficacy of itraconazole in the prophylactic treatment of pityriasis (tinea) versicolor. *Arch Dermatol.* 2002;138:69-73.

SECTION 6 INFESTATIONS

127 LICE

E.J. Mayeaux, Jr., MD
Richard P. Usatine, MD

PATIENT STORY

A 12-year-old girl presented to a homeless clinic with her mother for itching on her head. The physical examination revealed multiple nits in her long straight hair (**Figure 127-1**). A live adult louse was also found crawling on the hairs around her neck (**Figure 127-2**). The clinician also examined her mother and found a few nits on the hair behind her ears. There were no other members of the family living at the shelter so both were treated with permethrin now and in one week to kill any remaining live nits before they hatch. The clinician alerted the shelter staff of this infestation and other families were found to be infested. The girl was given permission to return to school if she completed her treatment with the permethrin cream rinse. The clinician recommended that clothes, bed clothes, combs and brushes be washed in hot water.

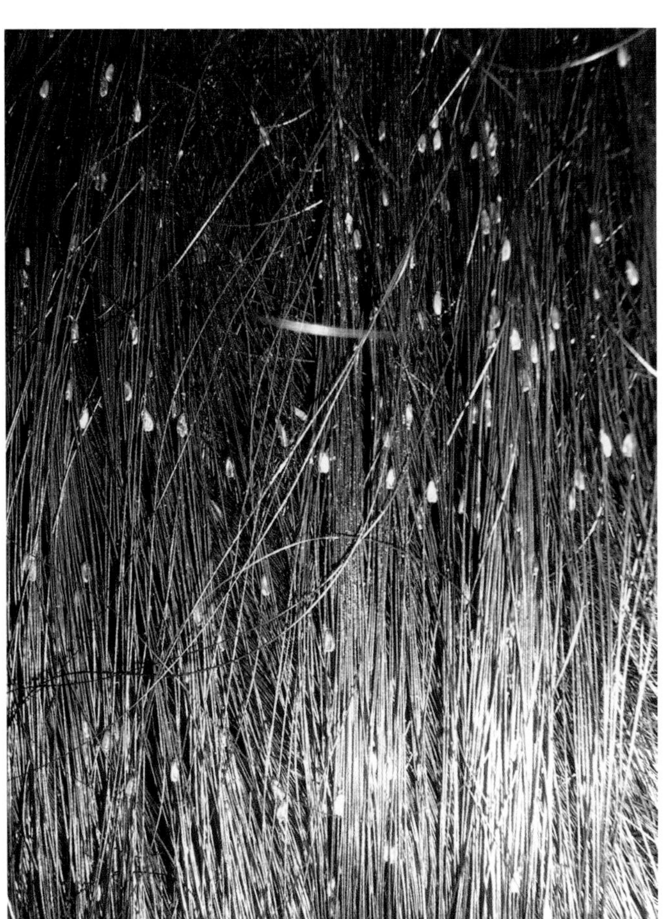

FIGURE 127-1 Pearly nits of the head louse seen in the hair of a 12-year-old girl living in a homeless shelter. (*Used with permission from Richard P. Usatine, MD.*)

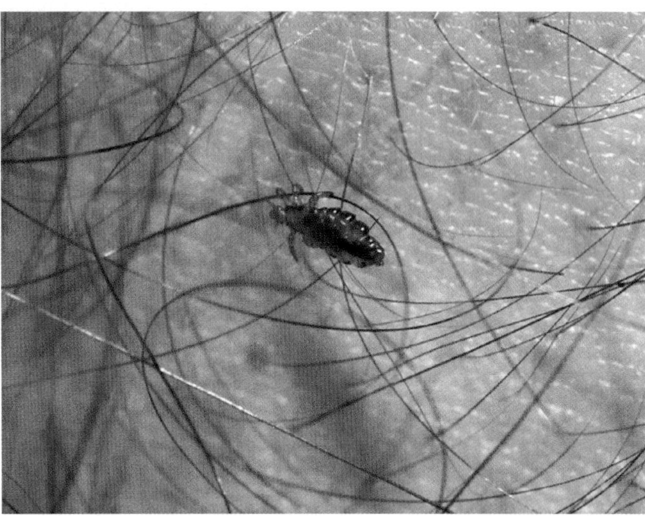

FIGURE 127-2 Adult louse hanging on to the hairs at the nape of the neck. (*Used with permission from Richard P. Usatine, MD.*)

INTRODUCTION

Lice are ectoparasites that live on or near the body.[1] They will die of starvation within 10 days of removal from their human host. Lice have coexisted with humans for at least 10,000 years.[2] Lice are ubiquitous and remain a major problem throughout the world.[3]

SYNONYMS

Pediculosis, crabs (pubic lice).

EPIDEMIOLOGY

- Human lice (pediculosis corporis, pediculosis pubis, and pediculosis capitis) are found in all countries and climates.[3]
- Head lice are most common among school-age children. Each year, approximately 6 to 12 million children, ages 3 to 12 years, are infested.[4]
- Head lice infestation is seen across all socioeconomic groups and is not a sign of poor hygiene.[5]
- In the US, black children are affected less often as a result of their oval-shaped hair shafts that are difficult for lice to grasp.[4]
- Body lice infest the seams of clothing (**Figure 127-3**) and bed linen. Infestations are associated with poor hygiene and conditions of crowding.

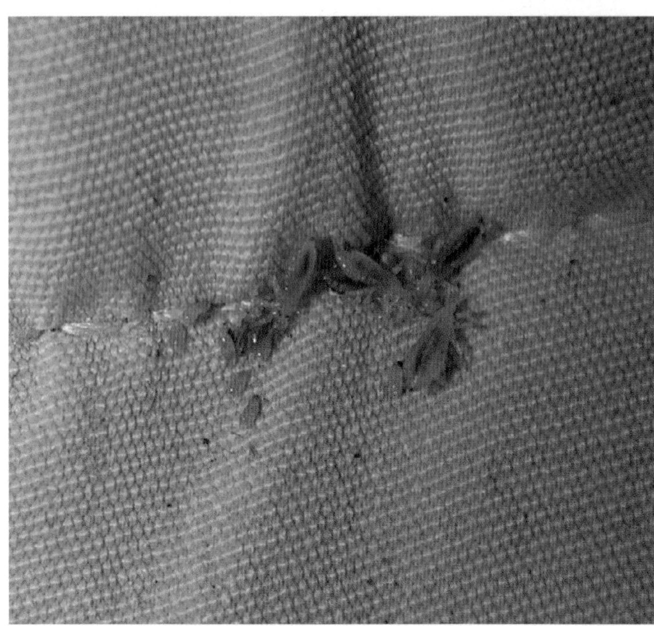

FIGURE 127-3 Adult body lice and nymphs visible along the pant seams of a patient with body lice. (*Used with permission from Richard P. Usatine, MD.*)

- Pubic lice are most common in sexually active adolescents and adults. Young children with pubic lice typically have infestations of the eyelashes. Although infestations in this age group may be an indication of sexual abuse, children generally acquire the crab lice from their parents.[6]

ETIOLOGY AND PATHOPHYSIOLOGY

- Lice are parasites that have six legs with terminal claws that enable them to attach to hair and clothing. There are three types of lice responsible for human infestation. All three kinds of lice must feed daily on human blood and can only survive 1 to 2 days away from the host. The three types of lice are as follows:
    - Head lice (*Pediculus humanus capitis*)—Measure 2 to 4 mm in length (**Figures 127-2** and **127-4**).

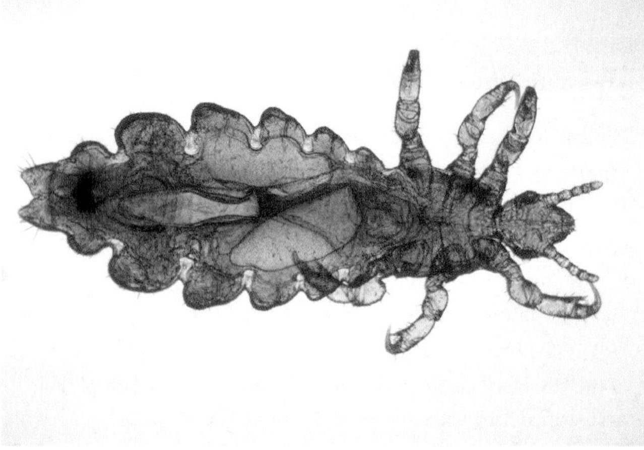

FIGURE 127-4 Adult head louse with elongated body. (*Used with permission from Centers for Disease Control and Prevention and Dennis D. Juranek.*)

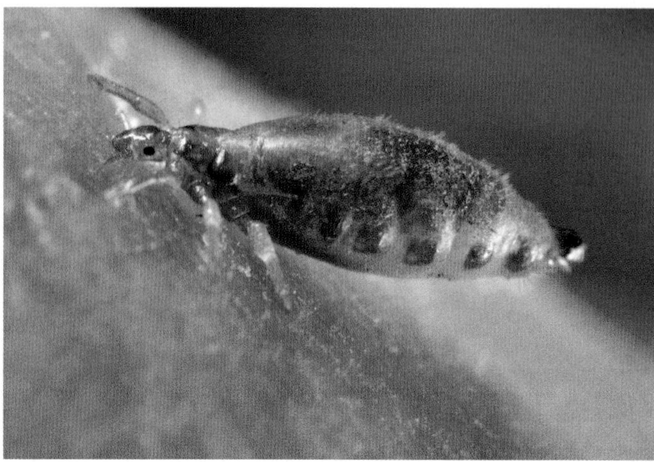

FIGURE 127-5 A body louse feeding on the blood of the photographer. The dark mass inside the abdomen is a previously ingested blood meal. (*Used with permission from Centers for Disease Control and Prevention and Frank Collins, PhD.*)

-
    - Body lice (*Pediculus humanus corporis*)—Body lice similarly measure 2 to 4 mm in length (**Figure 127-5**).
    - Pubic or crab lice (*Phthirus pubis*)—Pubic lice are shorter, with a broader body and have an average length of 1 to 2 mm (**Figure 127-6**).
- Female lice have a lifespan of approximately 30 days and can lay approximately 10 eggs (nits) a day.[4]
- Nits are firmly attached to the hair shaft or clothing seams by a glue-like substance produced by the louse (**Figure 127-7**).
- Nits are incubated by the host's body heat.
- The incubation period from laying eggs to hatching of the first nymph is 7 to 14 days.
- Mature adult lice capable of reproducing appear 2 to 3 weeks later.[5]
- Transmission of head lice occurs through direct contact with the hair of infested individuals. The role of fomites (e.g., hats, combs,

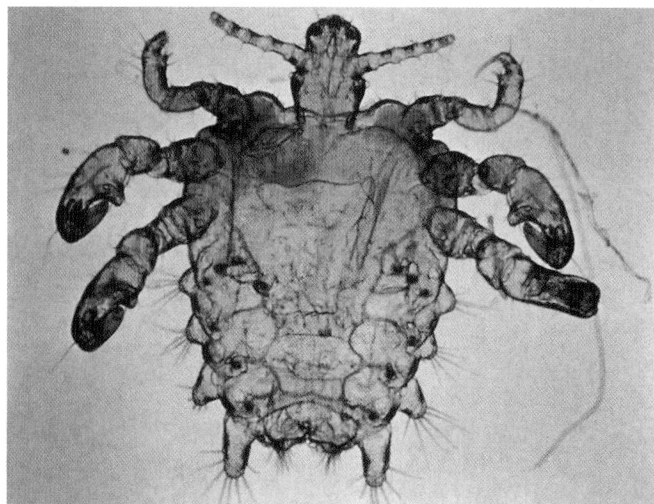

FIGURE 127-6 The crab louse has a short body and its large claws are responsible for the "crab" in its name. (*Used with permission from Centers for Disease Control and Prevention and World Health Organization.*)

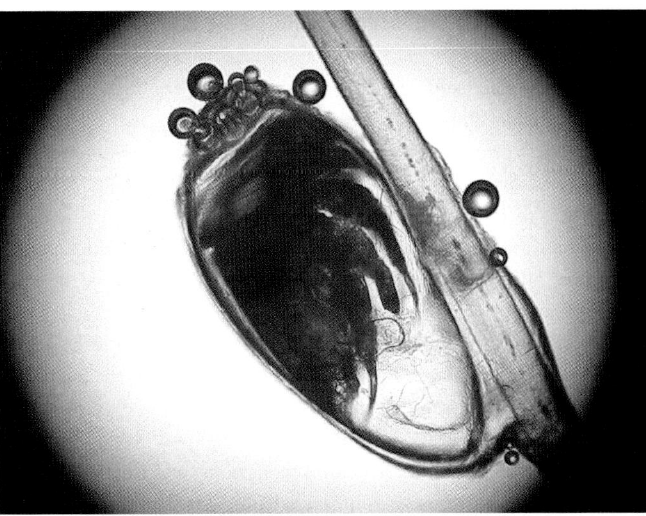

FIGURE 127-7 Microscopic view of a nit cemented to the hair and about to hatch. (*Used with permission from Dan Stulberg, MD.*)

brushes) in transmission is negligible.[6] Head lice do not serve as vectors for transmission of disease among humans.

- Transmission of body lice occurs through direct human contact or contact with infested material. Unlike head lice, body lice are well-recognized vectors for transmission of the pathogens responsible for epidemic typhus, trench fever, and relapsing fever.[5]
- Pubic or crab lice are transmitted primarily through sexual contact. In addition to pubic hair (**Figure 127-8**), infestations of eyelashes, eyebrows, beard, upper thighs, abdominal, and axillary hairs may also occur.

RISK FACTORS

- Contact with an infected individual. This commonly occurs in schools or between siblings at home.
- Living in crowded quarters such as homeless shelters.
- Poor hygiene and mental illness.

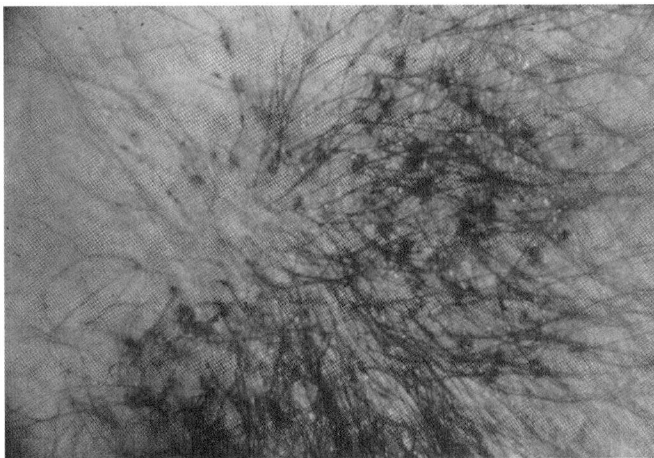

FIGURE 127-8 Crab lice infesting pubic hair. (*Used with permission from the University of Texas Health Sciences Center, Division of Dermatology.*)

DIAGNOSIS

CLINICAL FEATURES

- Nits can be seen in active disease or treated disease. Nits closer to the base of the hairs are generally newer and more likely to be live and unhatched. Unfortunately, nits that were not killed by pediculicides can hatch and start the infestation cycle over again. Note that nits are glued to the hairs and are hard to remove, whereas flakes of dandruff can be easily brushed off.
- Pruritus is the hallmark of lice infestation. It is the result of an allergic response to louse saliva.[7] Head lice are associated with excoriated lesions that appear on the scalp, ears, neck, and back.
- Occipital and cervical adenopathy may develop, especially when lesions become superinfected.
- Body lice result in small maculopapular eruptions that are predominantly found on the trunk and in the seams of the clothing (**Figure 127-3**).
- Chronic infestations often result in hyperpigmented, lichenified plaques known as "vagabond's skin."[8]
- Pubic lice produce bluish-gray spots (macula cerulea) that can be found on the chest, abdomen, and thighs.[8]

TYPICAL DISTRIBUTION

- Head lice—Look for nits and lice in the hair especially above the ears, behind the ears, and at the nape of the neck. There are many more nits present than live adults. Finding nits without an adult louse does not mean that the infestation has resolved (**Figures 127-1** and **127-6**). Systematically combing wet or dry hair with a fine toothed nit comb (teeth of comb are 0.2 mm apart) better detects active louse infestation than visual inspection of the hair and scalp alone.[9]
- Body lice—Look for the lice and larvae in the seams of the clothing (**Figure 127-3**).
- Pubic lice—Look for nits and lice on the pubic hairs (**Figure 127-8**). These lice and their nits may also be seen on the hairs of the upper thighs, abdomen, axilla, beard, eyebrows, and eyelashes. Little specks of dried blood may be seen in the underwear as a clue to the infestation. The diagnosis of pubic lice in a child (under age 18) should prompt the clinician to inquire about sexual abuse.

LABORATORY TESTING

- Direct visualization and identification of live lice or nits are sufficient to make a diagnosis (**Figures 127-1** to **127-9**).
- The use of a magnification lens may aid in the detection or confirmation of lice infestation.
- Under Wood light the head lice nits fluoresce a pale blue.
- If you find an adult louse put it on a slide with a cover slip loosely above it. Look at it under the microscope on the lowest power (**Figures 127-4** and **127-5**). You will see the internal workings of the live organs. If the louse was not found in a typical location, you can use the morphology of the body and legs to determine the type of louse causing the infestation.
- In cases of pubic lice infestations, individuals should be screened for other sexually transmitted diseases.[5]

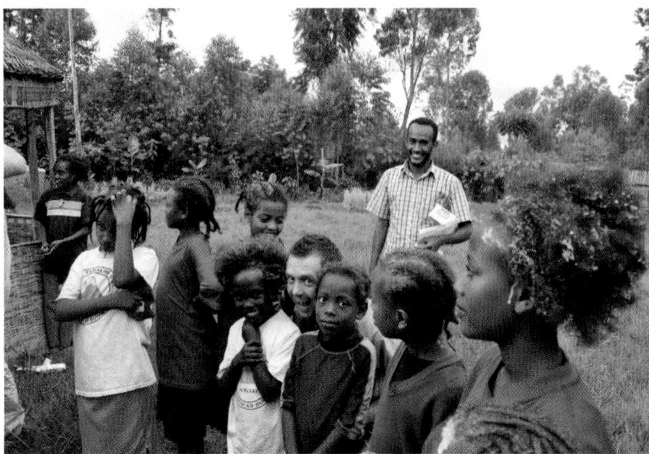

FIGURE 127-9 A group of medical students is helping children in Ethiopia to apply permethrin to their lice infested hair. (*Used with permission from Richard P. Usatine, MD.*)

DIFFERENTIAL DIAGNOSIS

- Dandruff, hair casts, and debris should be ruled out in cases of suspected lice infestations. Unlike nits, these particles are easily removed from the hair shaft. In addition, adult lice are absent.
- Scabies is also characterized by intense pruritus and papular eruptions. Unlike lice infestations, scabies may be associated with vesicles, and the presence of burrows is pathognomonic. Diagnosis is confirmed by microscopic examination of the scrapings from lesions for the presence of mites or eggs (see Chapter 128, Scabies).

MANAGEMENT

NONPHARMACOLOGIC

- In young children or others who wish to avoid topical pediculicides for head lice, mechanical removal of lice by wet combing is an alternative therapy. A 1:1 vinegar: water rinse (left under a conditioning cap or towel for 15 to 20 minutes) or 8 percent formic acid crème rinse may enhance removal of tenacious nits.[8] Combing is performed until no lice are found for 2 weeks. SOR B
  - Nits are also removed with a fine-toothed comb following the application of all treatments. This step is critical in achieving resolution.
  - Combs and hairbrushes should be discarded, soaked in hot water (at a temperature of at least 55°C [130°F]) for 5 minutes, or treated with pediculicides.[10]

MEDICATIONS

- *Pediculus humanus capitis* (head lice):
  - Nonprescription 1 percent permethrin cream rinse (Nix), pyrethrins with piperonyl butoxide (which inhibits pyrethrin catabolism; RID) shampoo, or permethrin 1 percent is applied to the hair and scalp and left on for 10 minutes then rinsed out.[11] SOR A In **Figure 127-9**, a group of medical students is helping children in Ethiopia to apply permethrin to their lice infested hair.
  - Pyrethrins are only pediculicidal, whereas permethrin is both pediculicidal and ovicidal. It is important to note that treatment failure is common with these agents owing to the emergence of resistant strains of lice.
  - After 7 to 10 days repeating the application is optional when permethrin is used, but is a necessary for pyrethrin. Lice persisting after treatment with a pyrethroid may be an indication of resistance.
  - Malathion 0.5 percent (Ovide) is available by prescription only, and is a highly effective pediculicidal and ovicidal agent for resistant lice. Malathion may have greater efficacy than pyrethrins.[12] It is approved for use in children age 6 years and older. The lotion is applied to dry hair for 8 to 12 hours and then washed. Repeat application is recommended after 7 to 10 days if live lice are still present. When used appropriately, malathion is 78 percent to 95 percent effective.[12] SOR A
  - Benzyl alcohol 5 percent lotion (Ulesfia) is a newer treatment option in patients 6 months of age and older. It works by asphyxiating the parasite. It is applied for 10 minutes with saturation of the scalp and hair, and then rinsed off with water. The treatment is repeated after 7 days.[13] SOR A
  - Spinosad (Natroba) is a new topical prescription medication approved by the FDA in 2011 for the treatment of lice. Spinosad is a fermentation product of the soil bacterium *Saccharopolyspora spinosa* that compromises the central nervous system of lice. It is approximately 85 percent effective in lice eradication, usually after one application. It is applied to completely cover the dry scalp and hair, and rinsed off after 10 minutes. Treatment should be repeated if live lice remain 7 days after the initial application.[14] SOR A
  - In February 2012, the US FDA approved ivermectin 0.5 percent lotion for the treatment of head lice for people above 6 months of age. It is applied as a single 10-minute topical application. The safety of ivermectin in infants younger than age 6 months has not been established.[15] SOR A
  - Hair conditioners should not be used prior to the application of pediculicides; these products may result in reduced efficacy.[16]
  - A Cochrane review found no evidence that any one pediculicide was better than another; permethrin, synergized pyrethrin, and malathion were all effective in the treatment of head lice.[17] SOR A
  - Other therapeutic options include permethrin 5 percent cream and lindane 1 percent shampoo. Permethrin 5 percent is conventionally used to treat scabies; however, it is anecdotally recommended for treatment of recalcitrant head lice.[5] SOR C
  - Lindane is considered a second-line treatment option owing to the possibility of central nervous system toxicity, which is most severe in children.
  - Oral therapy options include a 10-day course of trimethoprim-sulfamethoxazole or 2 doses of ivermectin (200 mcg/kg) 7 to 10 days apart. SOR C Trimethoprim-sulfamethoxazole is postulated to kill the symbiotic bacteria in the gut of the louse.[4] Combination therapy with 1 percent permethrin and trimethoprim-sulfamethoxazole is recommended in cases of multiple treatment failure or suspected cases of resistance to therapy.[5,10] SOR C

- *Pediculus humanus corporis* (body lice):
  - Improving hygiene, and laundering clothing and bed linen at temperatures of 65°C (149°F) for 15 to 30 minutes will eliminate body lice.[8]
  - In settings where individuals cannot change clothing (e.g., indigent population), a monthly application of 10 percent lindane powder can be used to dust the lining of all clothing.[8]
  - Additionally, permethrin cream may be applied to the body for 8 to 12 hours to eradicate body lice.
- *Phthirus pubis* (pubic lice):
  - Pubic lice infestations are treated with a 10-minute application of the same topical pediculicides used to treat head lice.
  - Retreatment is recommended 7 to 10 days later.
  - Petroleum ointment applied 2 to 4 times a day for 8 to 10 days will eradicate eyelash infestations.
  - Clothing, towels, and bed linen should also be laundered to eliminate nit-bearing hairs.[8]

PREVENTION

- Washing clothing and linen used by the head or pubic lice-infested person during the 2 days prior to therapy in hot water and/or drying the items on a high-heat dryer cycle (54.5°C [130°F]). Items that cannot be washed may be dry cleaned or stored in a sealed plastic bag for 2 weeks.

FOLLOW-UP

- Patients should be reexamined upon completion of therapy to confirm eradication of lice.

PATIENT EDUCATION

- Patients should be instructed to wash potentially contaminated articles of clothing, bed linen, combs, brushes, and hats.
- Nit removal is important in preventing continued infestation as a result of new progeny. Careful examination of close contacts, with appropriate treatment for infested individuals is important in avoiding recurrence.
- In cases of pubic lice, all sexual contacts should be treated.

PATIENT RESOURCES

- eMedicineHealth. *Lice*—**www.emedicinehealth.com/lice/article_em.htm**.
- Centers for Disease Control and Prevention. *Parasites–Lice*—**www.cdc.gov/parasites/lice/index.html**.

PROVIDER RESOURCES

- Centers for Disease Control and Prevention. *Parasites*—**www.cdc.gov/ncidod/dpd/parasites/lice/default.htm**.
- Medscape. *Pediculosis (Lice)*—**http://emedicine.medscape.com/article/225013**.

REFERENCES

1. Usatine RP, Halem L. A terrible itch: *J Fam Pract*. 2003;52(5): 377-379.
2. Araujo A, Ferreira LF, Guidon N, et al. Ten thousand years of head lice infection. *Parasitol Today*. 2000;16(7):269.
3. Roberts RJ. Clinical practice. Head lice. *N Engl J Med*. 2002;346: 1645.
4. Frankowski BL, Weiner LB. Head Lice. *Pediatrics*. 2002;110(3): 638-643.
5. Pickering LK, Baker CJ, Long SS, McMillan JA. *Red Book: 2006 Report of the Committee on Infectious Diseases*, 27th ed. Elk Grove Village, IL. American Academy of Pediatrics; 2006:488-493.
6. Maguire JH, Pollack RJ, Spielman A. Ectoparasite infestations and arthropod bites and stings. In: Kasper DL, Fauci AS, Longo DL, Braunwald EB, Hauser SL, Jameson JL, eds. *Harrison's Principles of Internal Medicine*, 16th ed. New York, NY: McGraw-Hill; 2005: 2601-2602.
7. Flinders DC, De Schweinitz P. Pediculosis and scabies. *Am Fam Physician*. 2004;69(2):341-348.
8. Darmstadt GL. Arthropod bites and infestations. In: Behrman RE, Kliegman RM, Jenson HB, eds. *Nelson Textbook of Pediatrics*, 16th ed. Philadelphia, PA: Saunders; 2000:2046-2047.
9. Jahnke C, Bauer E, Hengge UR, Feldmeier H. Accuracy of diagnosis of pediculosis capitis: visual inspection vs wet combing. *Arch Dermatol*. 2009;145(3):309-313.
10. Hipolito RB, Mallorca FG, Zuniga-Macaraig ZO, et al. Head lice infestation: single drug versus combination therapy with one percent permethrin and trimethoprim/sulfamethoxazole. *Pediatrics*. 2001;107(3):E30.
11. Meinking TL, Clineschmidt CM, Chen C, et al. An observer-blinded study of 1 percent permethrin creme rinse with and without adjunctive combing in patients with head lice. *J Pediatr*. 2002;141(5):665-670.
12. Meinking TL, Serrano L, Hard B, et al. Comparative in vitro pediculicidal efficacy of treatments in a resistant head lice population in the US. *Arch Dermatol*. 2002;138(2):220-224.
13. Meinking TL, Villar ME, Vicaria M, et al. The clinical trials supporting benzyl alcohol lotion 5 percent (Ulesfia): a safe and effective topical treatment for head lice (pediculosis humanus capitis). *Pediatr Dermatol*. 2010;27(1):19-24.
14. Stough D, Shellabarger S, Quiring J, Gabrielsen AA Jr: Efficacy and safety of spinosad and permethrin creme rinses for pediculosis capitis (head lice). *Pediatrics*. 2009;124(3):e389-e395.
15. *Ivermectin Lotion 0.5% (Sklice) Clinical Review (NDA)*. http://www.fda.gov/downloads/Drugs/DevelopmentApprovalProcess/DevelopmentResources/UCM295584.pdf, accessed April 13, 2012.
16. Lebwohl M, Clark L, Levitt J. Therapy for head lice based on life cycle, resistance, and safety considerations. *Pediatrics*. 2007; 119(5):965-974.
17. Dodd CS. Interventions for treating head lice. *Cochrane Database Syst Rev*. 2006;(4):CD001165.

128 SCABIES

Richard P. Usatine, MD
Pierre Chanoine, MD
Mindy A. Smith, MD, MS

PATIENT STORY

A 2-year-old boy is seen with severe itching and crusting of his hands (**Figures 128-1** and **128-2**). He also has a pruritic rash over the rest of his body. The child has had this problem since 2 months of age and has had a number of treatments for scabies. Other adults and children in the house have itching and rash. Various attempts at treatment have only included topical preparations. A scraping was done and scabies mites and scybala (feces) were seen (**Figures 128-3** and **128-4**). The child and all the family members were put on ivermectin simultaneously and the Norwegian scabies cleared from the child. The family cleared as well and the child was given a repeat dose of ivermectin to avoid relapse.

SYNONYMS

Seven-year itch.

EPIDEMIOLOGY

- Three hundred million cases per year are estimated worldwide.[1] In some tropical countries, scabies is endemic.
- The prevalence of scabies among school children in Nigeria was reported to be 4.7 percent in 2005.[2]
- The prevalence of scabies among boarding school children in Malaysia in 2009 was found to be 8.1 percent.[3]

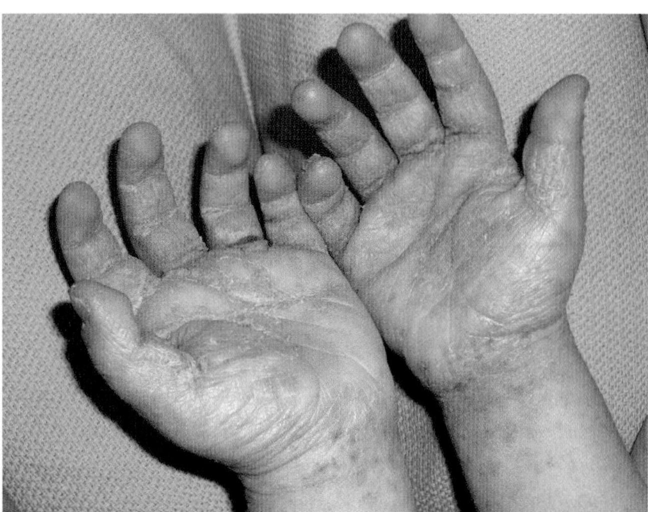

FIGURE 128-1 Crusted scabies (Norwegian scabies) in a 2-year-old boy. (*Used with permission from Richard P. Usatine, MD.*)

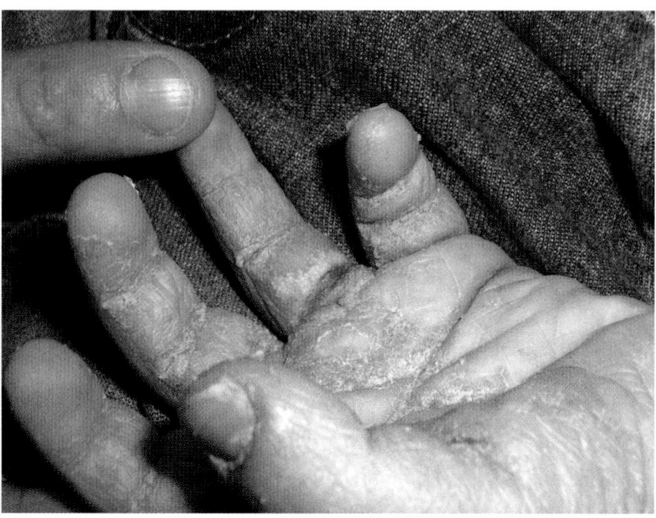

FIGURE 128-2 The boy in **Figure 128-1** with a close-up of his hand showing crusting and a fissure. (*Used with permission from Richard P. Usatine, MD.*)

ETIOLOGY AND PATHOPHYSIOLOGY

- Human scabies is caused by the mite *Sarcoptes scabei*, an obligate human parasite (**Figure 128-3**).[1,4]
- Adult mites spend their entire life cycle, around 30 days, within the epidermis. After copulation the male mite dies and the female mite burrows through the superficial layers of the skin excreting feces (**Figure 128-4**) and laying eggs (**Figure 128-5**).
- Mites move through the superficial layers of skin by secreting proteases that degrade the stratum corneum.
- Infected individuals usually have less than 100 mites. In contrast, immunocompromised hosts can have up to 1 million mites, and are susceptible to crusted scabies also called Norwegian scabies (**Figures 128-1** and **128-2**, and **128-6** to **128-8**).[1]

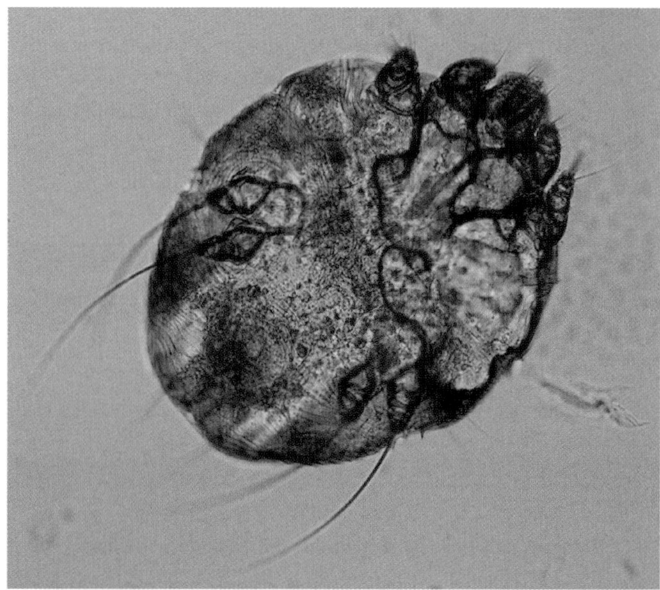

FIGURE 128-3 Microscopic view of the scabies mite from a patient with crusted scabies. (*Used with permission from Richard P. Usatine, MD.*)

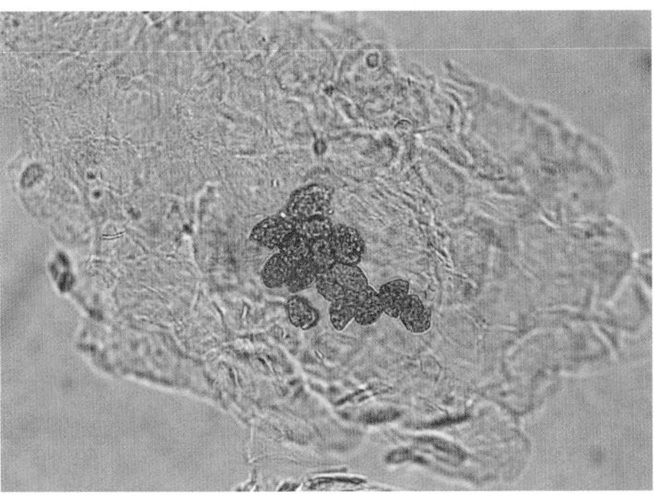

FIGURE 128-4 Scraping of the patient's hand produced a good view of the scybala (the mites' feces). (*Used with permission from Richard P. Usatine, MD.*)

- Transmission usually occurs via direct skin contact (**Figures 128-9**). Scabies in adults is frequently sexually transmitted.[5] Scabies mites can also be transmitted from animals to humans.[1]
- Mites can also survive for 3 days outside of the human epidermis allowing for infrequent transmission through bedding and clothing.
- The incubation period is on average 3 to 4 weeks for an initial infestation. Sensitized individuals can have symptoms within hours of reexposure.

RISK FACTORS

- Scabies is more common in young children, health care workers, homeless and impoverished persons, and individuals who are immunocompromised or suffering from dementia.[1]
- Institutionalized individuals and those living in crowded conditions also have a higher incidence of the infestation.[1]

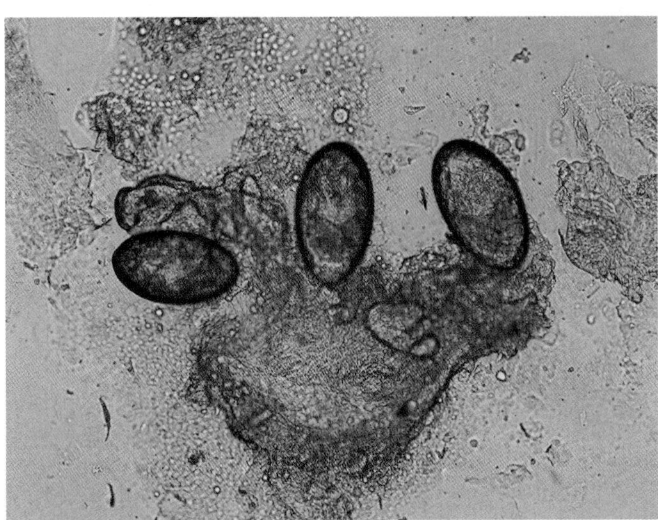

FIGURE 128-5 Scabies eggs from a scraping. (*Used with permission from Richard P. Usatine, MD.*)

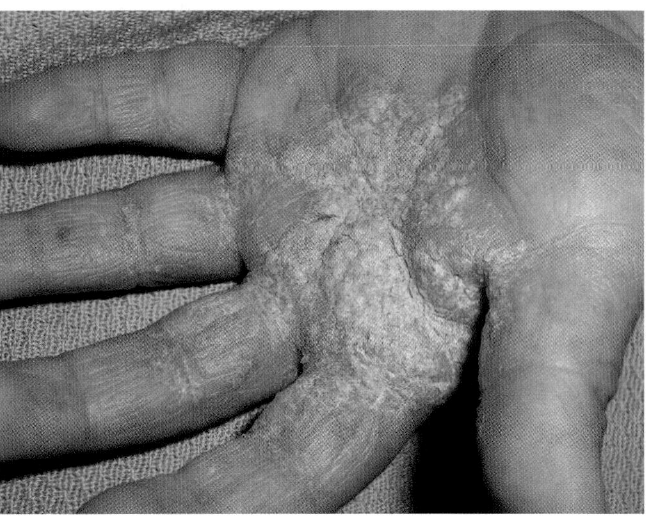

FIGURE 128-6 Norwegian scabies with crusting on the hand of a 3-year-old boy. (*Used with permission from Richard P. Usatine, MD.*)

DIAGNOSIS

CLINICAL FEATURES

- Pruritus is a hallmark of the disease.[1]
- Skin findings include papules (**Figure 128-10**), burrows (**Figures 128-11** and **128-12**) nodules (**Figures 128-13**), and vesiculopustules (**Figure 128-14**).
- Burrows are the classic morphologic finding in scabies and the best location to find the mite (**Figures 128-11** and **128-12**).
- Infants and young children can also exhibit irritability and poor feeding.
- Pruritic papules/nodules around the axillae (**Figure 128-13**), umbilicus, or on the penis (**Figures 128-15** and **128-16**) and scrotum are highly suggestive of scabies.

TYPICAL DISTRIBUTION

- Classic distribution in scabies includes the interdigital spaces (**Figure 128-17**), wrists (**Figure 128-18**), ankles (**Figure 128-19**),

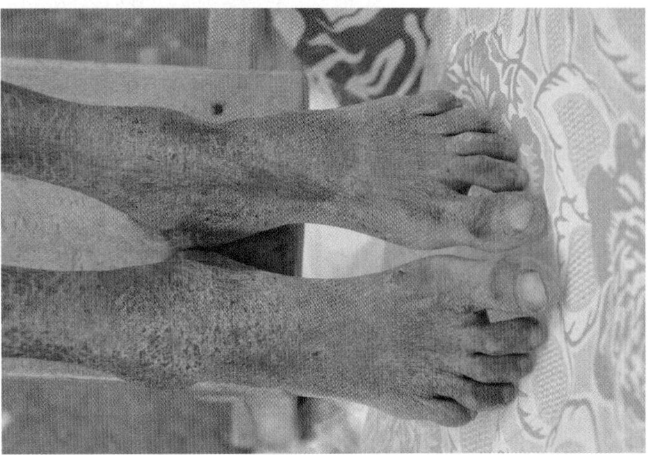

FIGURE 128-7 Crusted scabies on the feet of a malnourished girl in Haiti. (*Used with permission from Richard P. Usatine, MD.*)

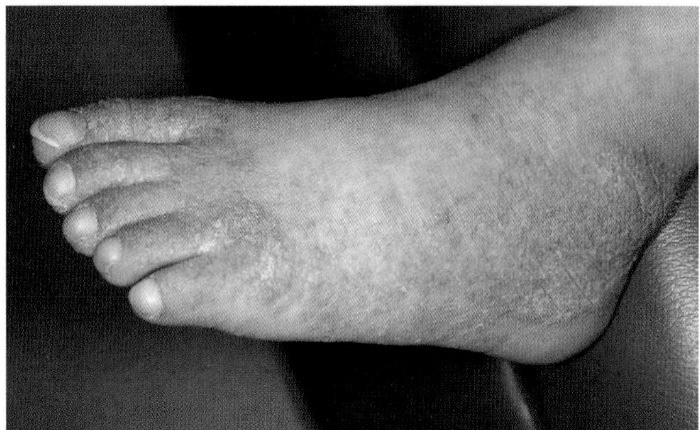

FIGURE 128-8 Crusted scabies on the foot of a 5-year-old boy with Down syndrome. (*Used with permission from Richard P. Usatine, MD.*)

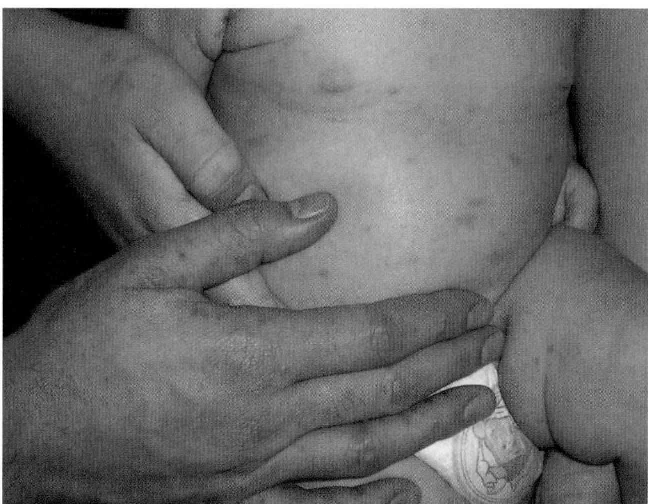

FIGURE 128-9 Scabies has been transmitted by skin to skin contact in this family. The photograph shows the active infection on the skin of the infant and the hands of the mother and father. (*Used with permission from Richard P. Usatine, MD.*)

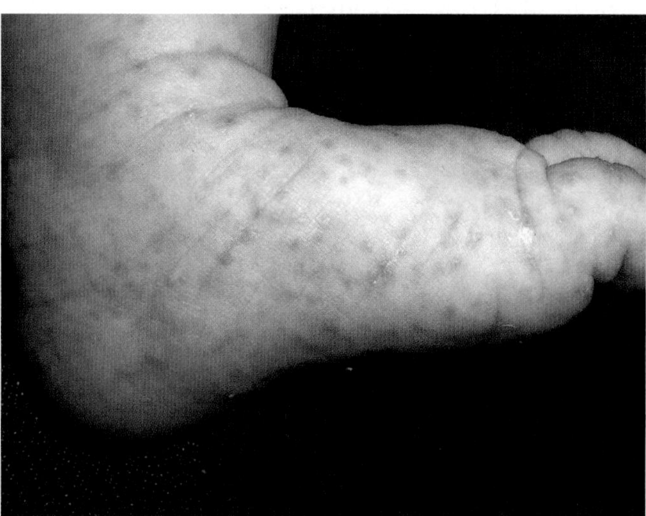

FIGURE 128-10 Scabies papules on the foot of a 3-month-old child. (*Used with permission from Richard P. Usatine, MD.*)

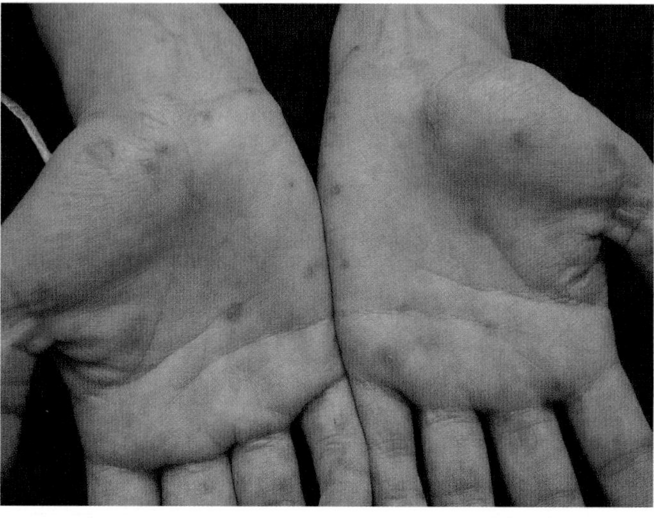

FIGURE 128-11 Scabies infestation on the hand of a 17-year-old teenager with visible burrows and papules. Dermoscopy revealed scabies mites within burrows. (*Used with permission from Richard P. Usatine, MD.*)

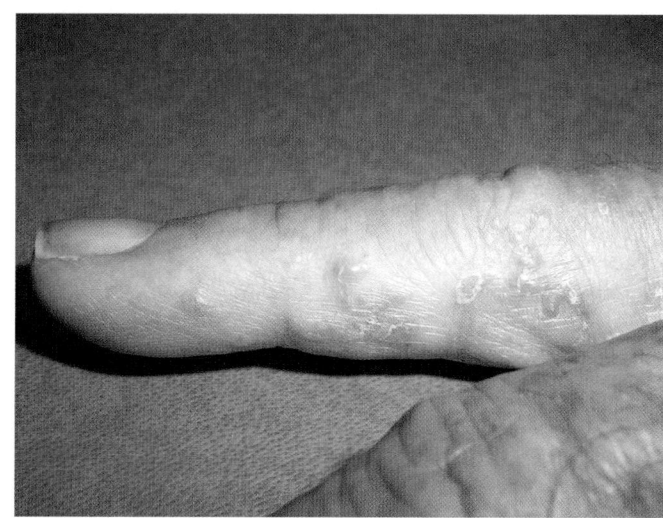

FIGURE 128-12 Burrows prominently visible between the fingers. Burrows are a classic manifestation of scabies. (*Used with permission from Richard P. Usatine, MD.*)

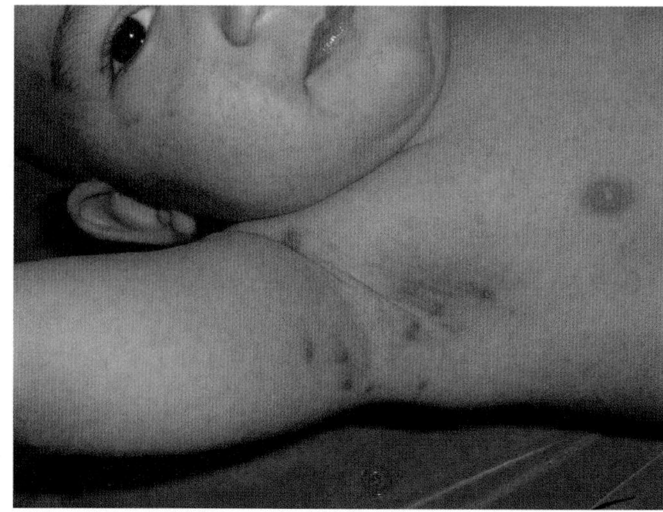

FIGURE 128-13 Scabetic nodules in the axilla of a toddler with scabies. (*Used with permission from Richard P. Usatine, MD.*)

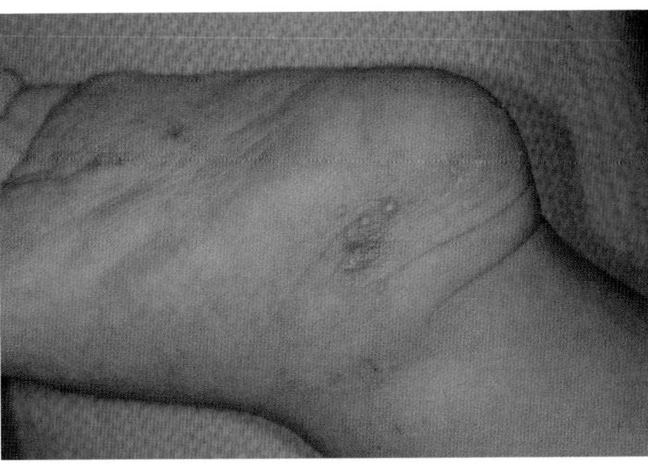

FIGURE 128-14 Scabies on the foot of a 9-month-old infant with pustules. Although this also looks like acropustulosis, the mother also had scabies. (*Used with permission from Richard P. Usatine, MD.*)

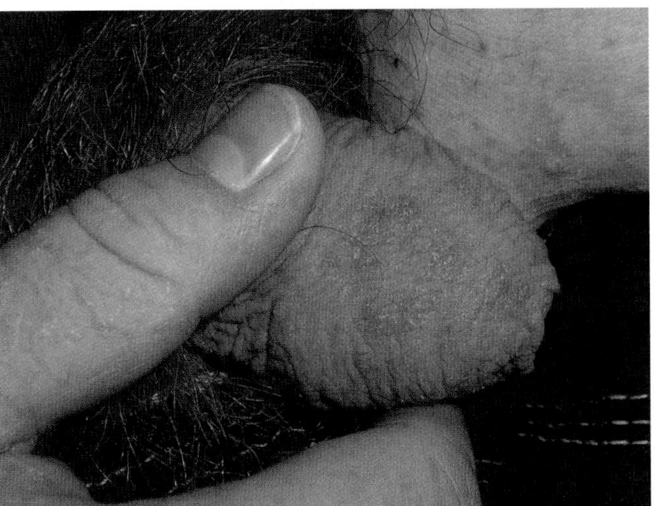

FIGURE 128-15 Pruritic papules of scabies on the foreskin of the penis, hands, and groin acquired as a sexually transmitted disease. (*Used with permission from Richard P. Usatine, MD.*)

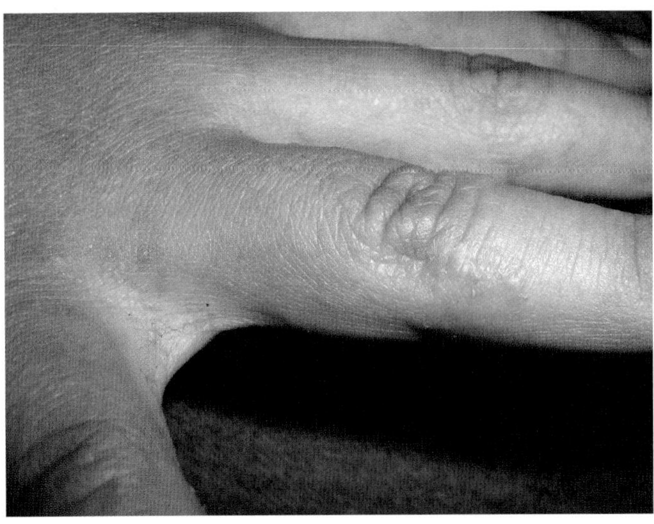

FIGURE 128-17 Scabies found in the classic location between the fingers in this interdigital webspace. (*Used with permission from Richard P. Usatine, MD.*)

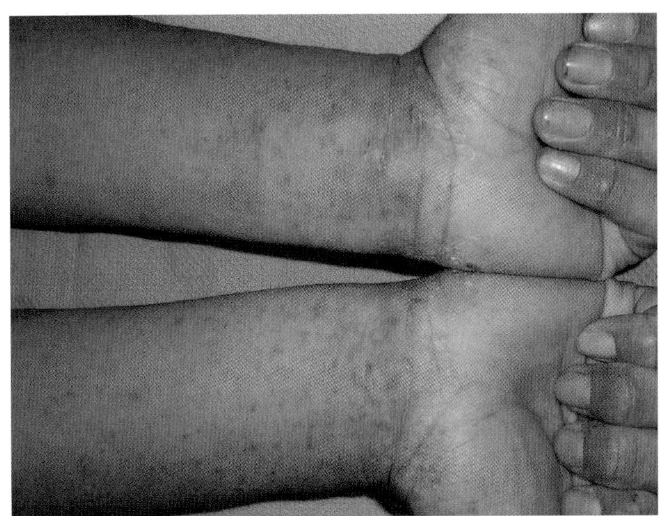

FIGURE 128-18 Scabies papules found prominently around the wrists of this 15-year-old boy. (*Used with permission from Richard P. Usatine, MD.*)

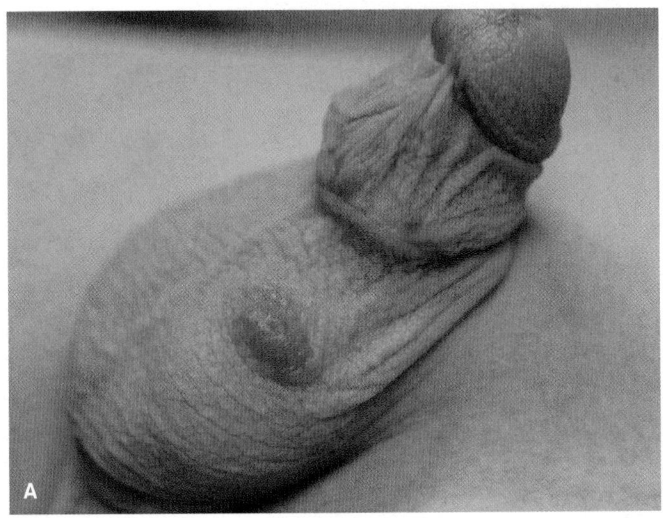

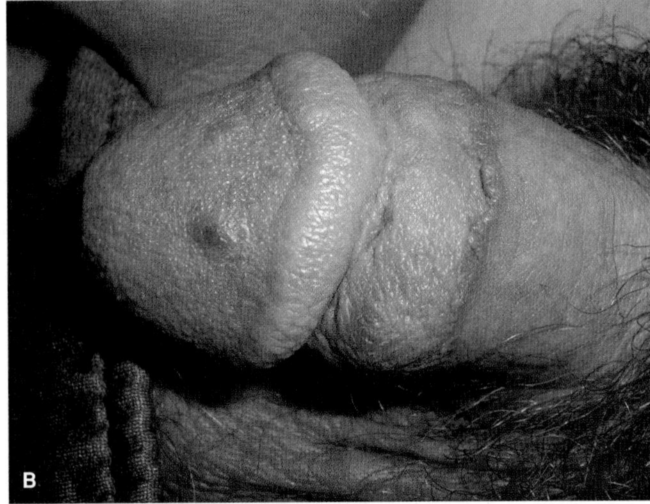

FIGURE 128-16 Papules and nodules on the glans penis, penile shaft and scrotum are typical of scabies. **A.** Nodular scabies in a 6-year-old boy. (*Used with permission from Robert Brodell, MD.*) **B.** Pruritic papules of scabies on the glans of this teenager. (*Used with permission from Richard P. Usatine, MD.*)

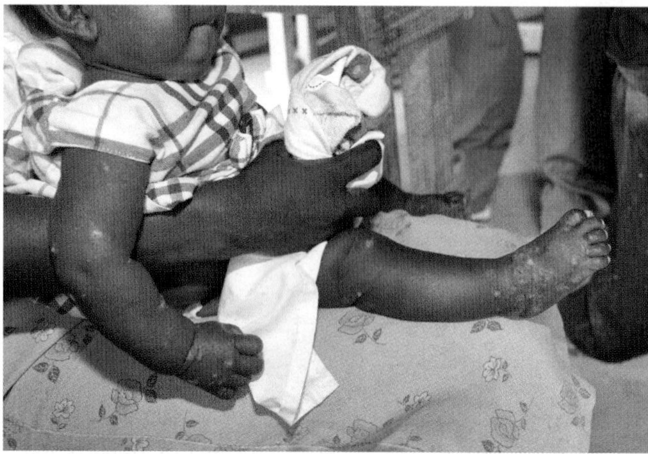

FIGURE 128-19 Ethiopian child with widely distributed scabies seen prominently on the wrists and ankles. (*Used with permission from Richard P. Usatine, MD.*)

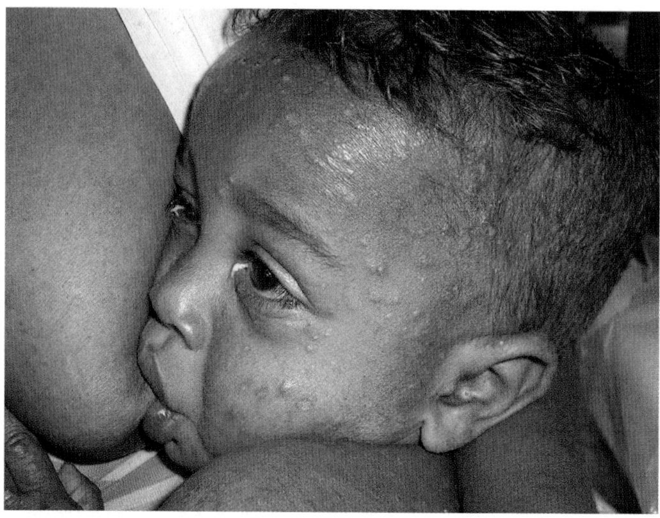

FIGURE 128-21 Scabies on the head and face of a young breastfeeding boy. (*Used with permission from Richard P. Usatine, MD.*)

waist (**Figure 128-20**), groin, axillae (**Figure 128-13**), palms, and soles (**Figures 128-1, 128-2, 128-6,** and **128-7**).

- Genital involvement can also occur (**Figures 128-15** and **128-16**).
- In children, the head can also be involved (**Figure 128-21**).

LABORATORY STUDIES AND IMAGING

- Light microscopy of skin scrapings provides a definitive diagnosis when mites, eggs, or feces are identified (**Figures 128-3** to **128-5**). This can be challenging and time-consuming, even when mites, eggs, or feces are present. Packing tape stripping of skin has also been used instead of a scalpel to find mites for examination under the microscope.[6] The inability to find these items should not be used to rule out scabies in a clinically suspicious case. In what is believed to be a recurrent case, it is helpful to find definitive evidence that your diagnosis is correct.
- Dermoscopy is a useful and rapid technique for identifying a scabies mite at the end of a burrow (see Appendix 3: Dermoscopy).[7] The mite has been described as an arrowhead or a jet plane in its appearance (**Figure 128-22**). The advantage of the dermoscope is that multiple burrows can be examined quickly without causing any pain to the patient. Children are more likely to stay still for this than scraping with a scalpel or skin stripping with tape.
- If a dermoscope is available, start with this noninvasive examination. If the findings are typical, then a microscopic examination is not needed. If the findings are not convincing, or a dermoscope is not available, perform a scraping. It is best to scrape the skin at the end of a burrow. Use a #15 scalpel that has been dipped into mineral oil or microscope immersion oil. Scrape holding the blade perpendicular to the skin until the burrow (or papule) is opened (some

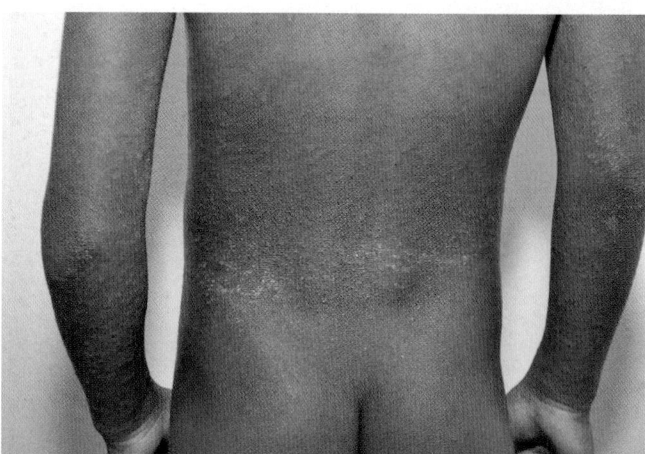

FIGURE 128-20 Scabies around the waist showing postinflammatory hyperpigmentation along with multiple papules and some crusting. (*Used with permission from Richard P. Usatine, MD.*)

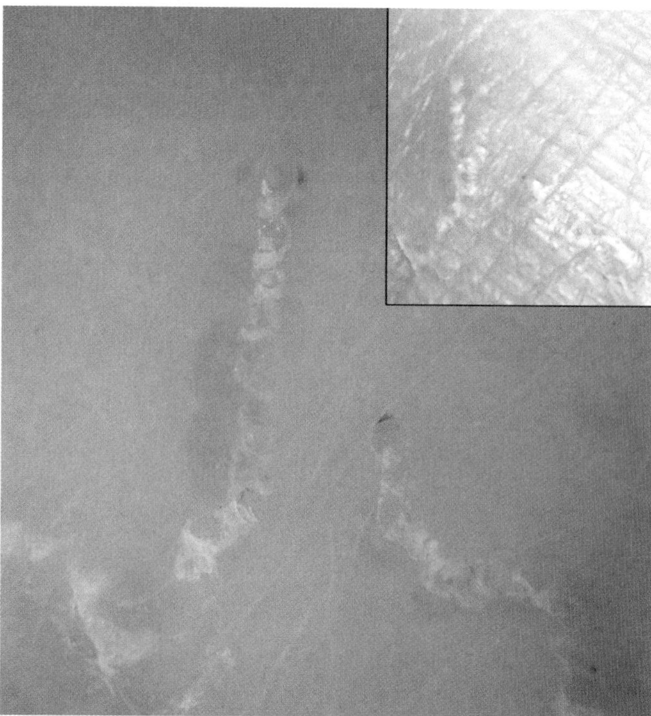

FIGURE 128-22 Two scabies mites visible with dermoscopy. Note how the darkest most visible aspect of the mite looks like an arrowhead or jet plane. In this case the oval bodies of the mites are also visible. The *upper right inset* shows the same burrows without dermoscopy. (*Used with permission from Richard P. Usatine, MD.*)

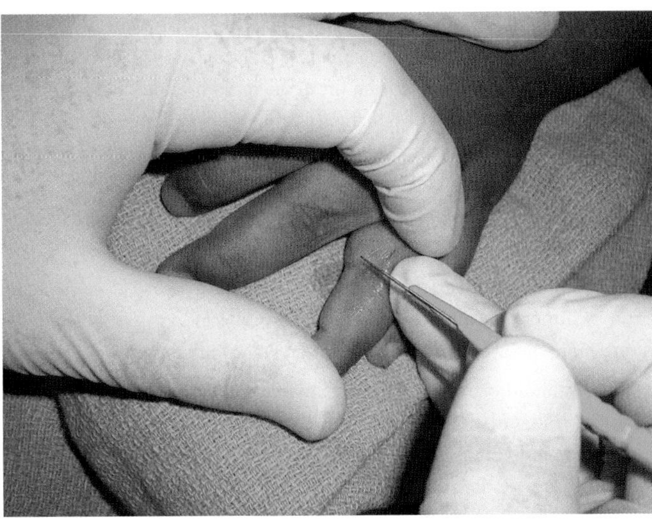

FIGURE 128-23 Using a #15 scalpel held perpendicular to the skin to scrape a suspicious burrow for scabies. Some mineral oil was applied to the scalpel and the scraping must be deep enough to get some tissue. (*Used with permission from Richard P. Usatine, MD.*)

slight bleeding is usual; **Figure 128-23**). Transfer the material to a slide and add a cover slip.

- Tips for microscopic examination—Start by examining the slide with the lowest power available as mites may be seen under 4 power and the slide can be scanned most quickly with the lowest power. If no mites are seen, switch to 10 power and scan the slide again looking for mites, eggs, and feces. Forty power may be used to confirm findings under 10 power.
- In one study comparing dermoscopic mite identification with microscopic examination of skin scrapings, found the former technique to be of comparable sensitivity (91% and 90%, respectively) with specificity of 86 percent (versus 100% by definition), even in inexperienced hands.[8] Another study reported sensitivity of dermoscopy at 83 percent (95% confidence interval, 0.70 to 0.94).[9] In this study, the negative predictive value was identical for dermoscopy and the adhesive tape test (0.85), making the latter a good screening test in resource-poor areas.
- Videodermatoscopy can also be used to diagnose scabies.[10] Videodermatoscopy allows for skin magnification with incidental lighting at high magnifications for viewing mites and eggs. The technique is noninvasive and does not cause pain.
- *S. scabiei* recombinant antigens have diagnostic potential and are under investigation for identifying antibodies in individuals with active scabies.[11]

BIOPSY

Rarely necessary unless there are reasons to suspect another diagnosis.

DIFFERENTIAL DIAGNOSIS

- Atopic dermatitis—Itching is a prominent symptom in atopic dermatitis and scabies. The distribution of involved skin can help to differentiate the 2 diagnoses. Look for burrows in scabies and a history of involved family members. In children, atopic dermatitis is often confined to the flexural and extensor surfaces of the body. In adults, the hands are a primary site of involvement (see Chapter 130, Atopic Dermatitis).
- Contact dermatitis—Characterized by vesicles and papules on bright red skin, which are rare in scabies. Chronic contact dermatitis often leads to scaling and lichenification and may not be as pruritic as scabies (see Chapter 131, Contact Dermatitis).
- Seborrheic dermatitis—A papulosquamous eruption with scales and crusts that is limited to the sebum rich areas of the body; namely, the scalp, the face the postauricular areas, and the intertriginous areas. Pruritus is usually mild or absent (see Chapter 135, Seborrheic Dermatitis).
- Impetigo—Honey-crusted plaques are a hallmark of impetigo. Scabies can become secondarily infected, so consider that both diagnoses can occur concomitantly with papules and pustules present (**Figure 128-24**) (see Chapter 99, Impetigo).

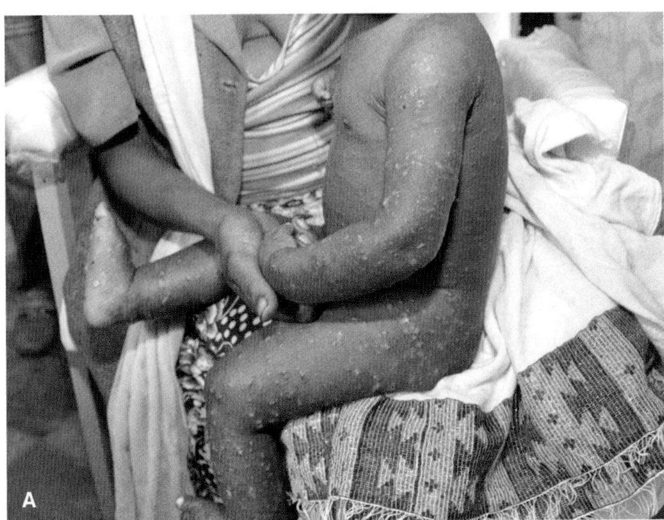

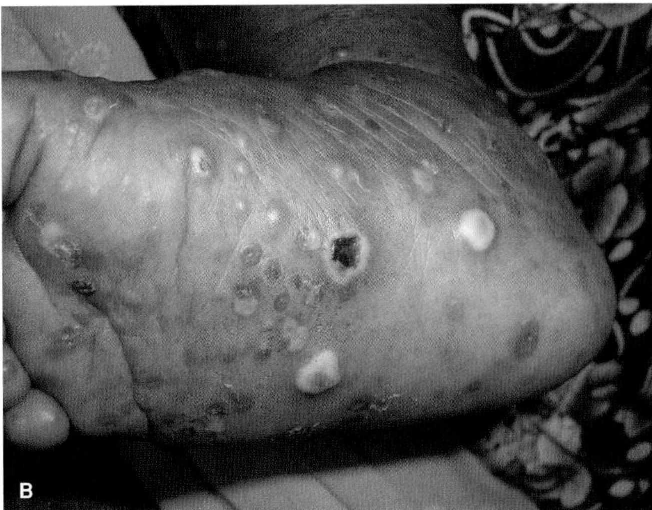

FIGURE 128-24 **A.** Superinfected scabies from head to toe in this young boy. **B.** Note the large pustules on the foot of this boy demonstrating the bacterial superinfection. (*Used with permission from Richard P. Usatine, MD.*)

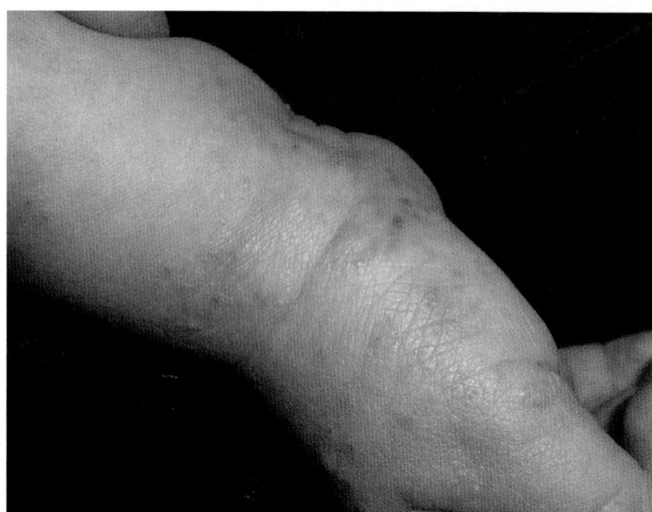

FIGURE 128-25 Infantile acropustulosis in a 9-month-old child that was mistakenly treated for scabies. No one else in the household had lesions and the scabies treatment did not lead to resolution of the pustules and vesicles. (*Used with permission from Richard P. Usatine, MD.*)

- Arthropod bites—Bites may exhibit puncta that allow for differentiation from scabies.
- Acropustulosis of infancy (**Figure 128-25**)—A vesicopustular recurrent eruption limited to the hands, wrists, feet, and ankles. It is rare after 2 years of age (see Chapter 94, Pustular Diseases of Childhood).

MANAGEMENT

NONPHARMACOLOGIC

- Environmental decontamination is a standard component of all therapies. SOR B Clothing, bed linens, and towels should be machine washed in hot water. Clothing or other items (e.g., stuffed animals) that cannot be washed may be dry cleaned or stored in sealed bags for at least 72 hours.[12]

MEDICATIONS

Treatment includes administration of an antiscabicide and an antipruritic.[1,13]

- Permethrin 5 percent cream (Elimite, Acticin) is the most effective treatment based upon a systematic review in the Cochrane Database.[13] SOR A The cream is applied from the neck down (include the head when it is involved) and rinsed off 8 to 14 hours later. Usually, this is done overnight. Repeating the treatment in 1 to 2 weeks may be more effective. SOR C In patients with crusted scabies, use of a keratolytic cream may facilitate the breakdown of skin crusts and improve penetration of the cream.[14] Unfortunately, scabies resistance to permethrin is increasing.
- Ivermectin is an oral treatment for resistant or crusted scabies. Studies have demonstrated its safety and efficacy. Most studies used a single dose of ivermectin at 200 mcg/kg.[13] SOR A Taking the drug with food may enhance drug penetration into the epidermis.[14] Some experts advocate repeating a dose 1 week later. It is worth noting that the FDA has not labeled this drug for use in children weighing less than 15 kg. Ivermectin is currently available only in 3- and 6-mg tablets, so dosing often needs to be rounded up to accommodate the use of whichever tablets are available. As there is no oral suspension available, tablets may need to be cut and given with food for use in children.
- Diphenhydramine, hydroxyzine, and mid-potency steroid creams can be used for symptomatic relief of itching. SOR C. It is important to note that pruritus may persist for 1 to 2 weeks after successful treatment because the dead scabies mites and eggs still have antigenic qualities that may cause persistent inflammation.
- All household or family members living in the infested home and sexual contacts should be treated. SOR C Failure to treat all involved individuals often results in recurrences within the family. Use of insecticide sprays and fumigants is not recommended.
- Other less-effective medications include topical benzyl benzoate, crotamiton, lindane (no longer used in the US because of concerns regarding neurotoxicity), and synergized natural pyrethrins.[9] SOR A Topical agents used more commonly in other countries include 5 to 10 percent sulfur in paraffin (widely in Africa and South America), 10 to 25 percent benzyl benzoate (often used in Europe and Australia), and malathion.[14] In infants younger than 2 months of age, crotamiton or a sulfur preparation is recommended by one author instead of permethrin because of theoretical concerns of systemic absorption of permethrin.[14]
- Antibiotics are needed if there is evidence of a bacterial superinfection (**Figure 128-23**). SOR C

COMPLEMENTARY/ALTERNATIVE THERAPY

- Tea tree oil contains oxygenetic terpenoids, found to have rapid scabicidal activity.[15]

PREVENTION

- Avoid direct skin-to-skin contact with an infested person or with items such as clothing or bedding used by an infested person.
- Treat members of the same household and other potentially exposed persons at the same time as the infested person to prevent possible reexposure and reinfestation.

PROGNOSIS

- The prognosis with proper diagnosis and treatment is excellent unless the patient is immunocompromised; reinfestation, however, often occurs if environmental risk factors continue.[1]
- Postinflammatory hyper- or hypopigmentation can occur.[1]

FOLLOW-UP

- Routine follow-up is indicated when symptoms do not resolve.
- Consider an immunologic work-up for individuals with crusted scabies.

PATIENT EDUCATION

- Patients should avoid direct contact including sleeping with others until they have completed the first application of the medicine.
- Patients may return to school and work 24 hours after first treatment.
- Patients should be warned that itching may persist for 1 to 2 weeks after successful treatment but that if symptoms are still present by the third week, the patient should return for further evaluation.

PATIENT RESOURCES

- **www.cdc.gov/parasites/scabies/**.
- **www.ncbi.nlm.nih.gov/pubmedhealth/PMH0001833/**.

PROVIDER RESOURCES

- **http://emedicine.medscape.com/article/1109204**.
- **http://dermnetnz.org/arthropods/scabies.html**.

REFERENCES

1. Hengge UR, Currie B, Jäger G, et al. Scabies: a ubiquitous neglected skin disease. *Lancet Infect Dis.* 2006;6(12):769-779.
2. Ogunbiyi AO, Owoaje E, Ndahi A. Prevalence of skin disorders in school children in Ibadan, Nigeria. *Pediatr Dermatol.* 2005;22:6-10.
3. Yap FB-B, Elena E, Pabalan M. Prevalence of scabies and head lice among students of secondary boarding schools in Kuching, Sarawak, Malaysia. *Pediatr Infect Dis J.* 2010; 29:682-683.
4. Paller AS, Mancini AJ. Scabies. In: Paller AS, Mancini AJ, eds. *Hurwitz Clinical Pediatric Dermatology: A Textbook of Skin Disorders of Childhood and Adolescence*. Philadelphia, PA: Saunders; 2006: 479-488.
5. Centers for Disease Control and Prevention. *Scabies: Epidemiology and Risk Factors*. http://www.cdc.gov/parasites/scabies/epi.html, accessed April 2012.
6. Albrecht J, Bigby M. Testing a test. Critical appraisal of tests for diagnosing scabies. *Arch Dermatol.* 2011;147(4):494-497.
7. Fox GN, Usatine RP. Itching and rash in a boy and his grandmother. *J Fam Pract.* 2006;55(8):679-684.
8. Dupuy A, Dehen L, Bourrat E, et al. Accuracy of standard dermoscopy for diagnosing scabies. *J Am Acad Dermatol.* 2007; 56(1):53-62.
9. Walter B, Heukelbach J, Fengler G, et al. Comparison of dermoscopy, skin scraping, and the adhesive tape test for the diagnosis of scabies in a resource-poor setting. *Arch Dermatol.* 2011;147(4): 468-473.
10. Lacarrubba F, Musumeci ML, Caltabiano R, et al. High-magnification videodermatoscopy: a new noninvasive diagnostic tool for scabies in children. *Pediatr Dermatol.* 2001;18(5):439-441.
11. Walton SF, Currie BJ. Problems in diagnosing scabies, a global disease in human and animal populations. *Clin Microbiol Rev.* 2007; 20(2):268-279.
12. Centers for Disease Control and Prevention. *Scabies: Treatment*. http://www.cdc.gov/parasites/scabies/treatment.html, accessed April 2012.
13. Strong M, Johnstone PW. Interventions for treating scabies. *Cochrane Database Syst Rev.* 2007;3:CD000320.
14. Currie BJ, McCarthy JS. Permethrin and ivermectin for scabies. *N Engl J Med.* 2010;362(8):717-725.
15. Carson CF, Hammer KA, Riley TV. *Melaleuca alternifolia* (Tea Tree) oil: a review of antimicrobial and other medicinal properties. *Clin Microbiol Rev.* 2006;19(1):50-62.

129 CUTANEOUS LARVA MIGRANS

Jennifer A. Keehbauch, MD

PATIENT STORY

A mother brought her 18-month-old son to the physician's office for an itchy rash on his feet and buttocks (**Figures 129-1** and **129-2**).[1] The first physician examined the child and made the incorrect diagnosis of tinea corporis. The topical clotrimazole cream failed. The child was unable to sleep because of the intense itching and was losing weight secondary to his poor appetite. He was taken to an urgent care clinic where the physician learned that the family had returned from a trip to the Caribbean prior to the visit to the first physician. The child had played on beaches that were frequented by local dogs. The physician recognized the serpiginous pattern of cutaneous larva migrans (CLM) and successfully treated the child with oral ivermectin. The child was 15 kg so the dose was 3 mg (0.2 mg/kg), and the tablet was ground up and placed in applesauce.

SYNONYMS

Creeping eruption, Plumber's itch.

EPIDEMIOLOGY

- Endemic in developing countries, particularly Brazil, India, South Africa, Somalia, Malaysia, Indonesia, and Thailand.[2,3]
- Peak incidence in the rainy seasons.[3]
- During peak rainy seasons, the prevalence in children is as high as 15 percent in resource poor areas, but much less common in affluent communities in these same countries with only 1 to 2 per 10,000 individuals per year.[4]
- In the US, it is found predominantly in Florida, southeastern Atlantic states, and the Gulf Coast.[2]
- Children are more frequently affected than adults.[4]

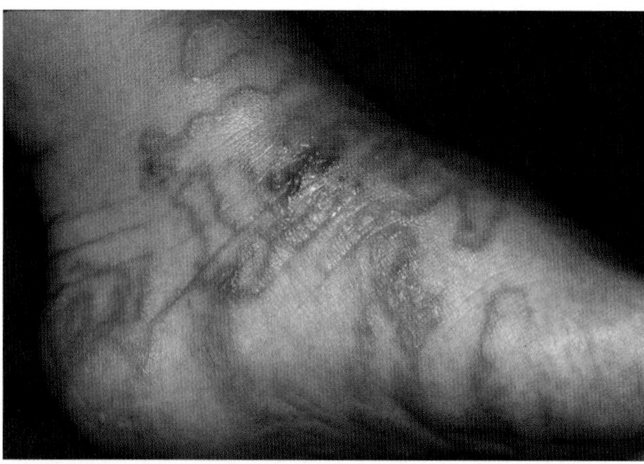

FIGURE 129-1 The serpiginous rash of cutaneous larva migrans on the foot of an 18-month-old boy after a family trip to the beaches of the Caribbean. (*Used with permission from Richard P. Usatine, MD. Usatine RP. A rash on the feet and buttocks. West J Med. 1999;170(6): 344-335.*)

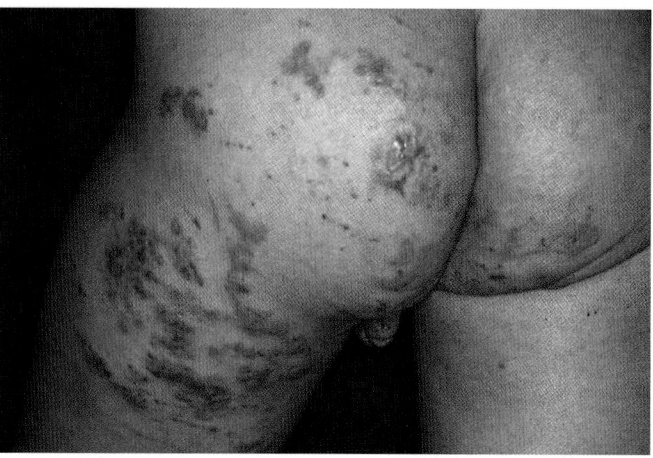

FIGURE 129-2 Cutaneous larva migrans on the buttocks and thigh of the same boy showing significant excoriations. (*Used with permission from Richard P. Usatine, MD. Usatine RP. A rash on the feet and buttocks. West J Med. 1999;170(6):344-335.*)

ETIOLOGY AND PATHOPHYSIOLOGY

- Caused most commonly by dog and cat hookworms (i.e., *Ancylostoma braziliense*, *Ancylostoma caninum*, or *Uncinaria stenocephala*).[4]
- Eggs are passed in cat or dog feces.[2]
- Larvae are hatched in moist, warm sand or soil.[2]
- Infective stage larvae penetrate the skin.[2]

DIAGNOSIS

The diagnosis is based on history and clinical findings.

CLINICAL FEATURES

- Elevated, serpiginous, or linear reddish-brown tracks 1 to 5 cm long (**Figures 129-1** to **129-3**).[2,5]
- Intense pruritus, which often disrupts sleep.[3]
- Symptoms last for weeks to months, and, rarely, years. Most cases are self-limiting.[5]

TYPICAL DISTRIBUTION

- Feet and lower extremities (73%), buttocks (13% to 18%), and abdomen (16%) (**Figure 129-4**).[6,7]
- Areas that come in contact with contaminated sand or soil.
  - Most commonly the feet, buttocks, and thigh.[3]

LABORATORY AND IMAGING

- Not indicated, but rarely blood tests shows Eosinophilia or elevated immunoglobulin E levels.[5]

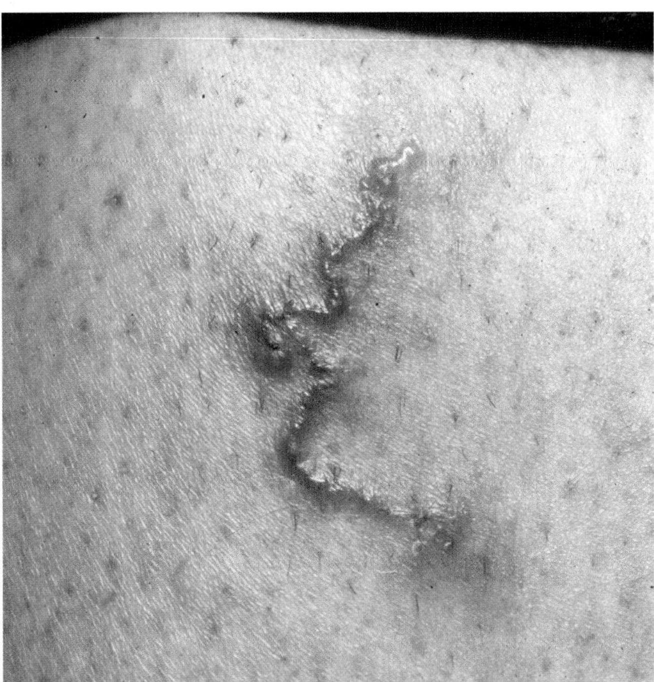

FIGURE 129-3 Close-up of a serpiginous burrow from cutaneous larva migrans on the leg. The actual larva is 2 to 3 cm beyond the visible tracks. (*Used with permission from John Gonzalez, MD.*)

DIFFERENTIAL DIAGNOSIS

May be confused with the following conditions:

- Cutaneous fungal infections—Lesions are typically scaling plaques and annular macules with central clearing. If the serpiginous track of CLM is circular, this can lead to the incorrect diagnosis of "ringworm." The irony is that ringworm is a dermatophyte fungus whereas CLM really is a worm (see Chapter 123, Tinea Corporis).
- Contact dermatitis—Differentiate by distribution of lesions, presence of vesicles, and absence of classical serpiginous tracks (see Chapter 131, Contact Dermatitis).
- Erythema migrans of Lyme disease—Lesions are usually annular macules or patches and are not raised and serpiginous (see Chapter 183, Lyme Disease).
- Phytophotodermatitis—The acute phase of phytophotodermatitis is erythematous with vesicles; this later develops into postinflammatory hyperpigmented lesions. This may be acquired while preparing drinks with lime on the beach and not from the sandy beach infested with larvae.

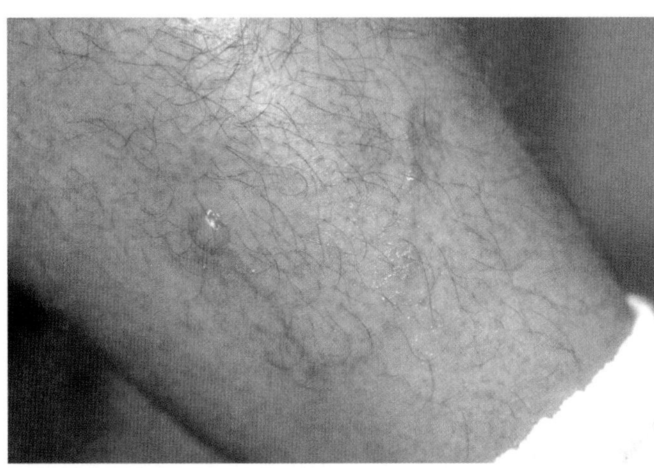

FIGURE 129-4 Cutaneous larva migrans on the leg of a teenager. He developed this pruritic serpiginous rash several days after returning from the beach. It extended several mm in length each day and a blister developed at the distal point of the burrow in the past 24 hours. (*Used with permission from Robert T. Brodell, MD.*)

MANAGEMENT

- Oral thiabendazole was the first proven therapy with FDA approval. It was removed from the market in 2010.
- Albendazole has been successfully prescribed for more than 25 years, and is the Centers for Disease Control and Prevention (CDC) drug of choice.[3,5] Albendazole lacks FDA approval for this indication.
  - The recommended dose is 400 mg daily for 3 days.[3,5] SOR B
  - Cure rates with albendazole exceed 92 percent, but are less with single dosage.[3]
- Ivermectin (Stromectol) has been well studied and is an appropriate alternative as per the CDC with dosing of 0.2 mg/kg daily for 1 to 2 days.[3,5] It also lacks FDA approval for this indication.
  - A single dose of ivermectin 0.2 mg/kg is also recommended.[3] SOR B
  - Cure rates of 77 to 100 percent with a single dose.[3]
  - Ivermectin has been used worldwide on millions with an excellent safety profile.[3]
  - Ivermectin is contraindicated in pregnancy, breastfeeding mothers, and in children weighing less than 15 kg.[3]
  - Studies on compounded ivermectin and albendazole for topical use are limited, but promising for use in children.[3]
- Cryotherapy is ineffective and harmful and should be avoided.[3] SOR B

ADJUNCT THERAPY

- Antihistamines may relieve itching.
- Antibiotics may be used if secondary infection occurs.

FOLLOW-UP

- Follow-up if lesions persist.

PATIENT EDUCATION

- Wear shoes on beaches where animals are allowed.
- Keep covers on sand boxes.
- Pet owners should keep pets off the beaches, deworm pets, and dispose of feces properly.

PATIENT AND PROVIDER RESOURCES

- eMedicine. *Dermatology*—**http://emedicine.medscape.com/article/1108784**.
- eMedicine. *Pediatrics*—**http://emedicine.medscape.com/article/998709**.
- CDC—**http://www.cdc.gov/parasites/zoonotichookworm/health_professionals/index.html**.

REFERENCES

1. Usatine RP. A rash on the feet and buttocks. *West J Med*. 1999;170(6):334-335.
2. Bowman D, Montgomery S, Zajac A, et al. Hookworms of dogs and cats as agents of cutaneous larva migrans *Trends Parasitol*. 2010;26(4):162-167.
3. Heukelbach J, Feldmeier H. Epidemiological and clinical characteristics of hookworm-related cutaneous larva migrans. *Lancet Infect Dis*. 2008;8(5):302-309.
4. Feldmeier H, Heukelbach J. Epidermal parasitic skin diseases: a neglected category of poverty-associated plagues. *Bull World Health Organ*. 2009;87(2):152-159.
5. Montgomery S. Cutaneous larva migrans. In: *Infectious Disease Related to Travel. CDC Yellow Book*. 2012. http://wwwnc.cdc.gov/travel/yellowbook/2012/chapter-3-infectious-diseases-related-to-travel/cutaneous-larva-migrans.htm, accessed October 26, 2012.
6. Hotez P, Brooker S, Bethony J, et al. Hookworm infection. *N Engl J Med*. 2004;351(8):799-807.
7. Jelinek T, Maiwald H, Nothdurft H, Loscher T. Cutaneous larva migrans in travelers: Synopsis of histories, symptoms and treating 98 patients. *Clin Infect Dis*. 1994;19:1062-1066.

SECTION 7 DERMATITIS/ALLERGIC

130 ATOPIC DERMATITIS

Richard P. Usatine, MD
Lindsey B. Finklea, MD

PATIENT STORYX

A 1-year-old Asian American girl is brought to her family physician for a new rash on her face and legs (**Figures 130-1** and **130-2**). The child is scratching both areas but is otherwise healthy. There is a family history of asthma, allergic rhinitis, and atopic dermatitis (AD) on the father's side. The child responded well to low-dose topical corticosteroids and emollients.

INTRODUCTION

AD is a chronic and relapsing inflammatory skin disorder characterized by itching and inflamed skin that is triggered by the interplay of genetic, immunologic, and environmental factors.

SYNONYMS

Eczema, atopic eczema.

EPIDEMIOLOGY

- AD is the most frequent inflammatory skin disorder in the US and the most common skin condition in children.[1]

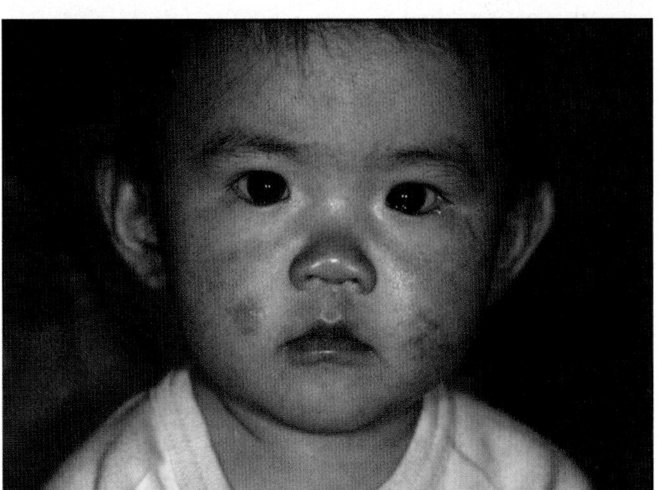

FIGURE 130-1 Atopic dermatitis on the cheeks of an infant. (*Used with permission from Milgrom EC, Usatine RP, Tan RA, Spector SL. Practical Allergy. Philadelphia, PA: Elsevier; 2004.*)

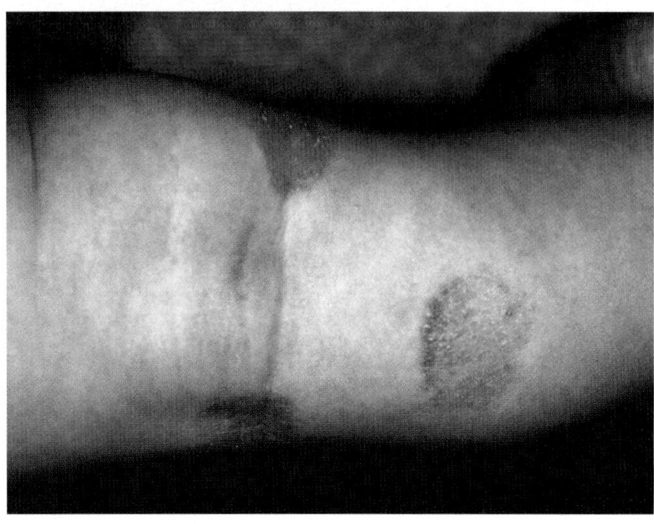

FIGURE 130-2 Atopic dermatitis on the leg of the infant in **Figure 130-1**. The coin-like pattern is that of nummular eczema. (*Used with permission from Milgrom EC, Usatine RP, Tan RA, Spector SL. Practical Allergy. Philadelphia, PA: Elsevier; 2004.*)

- Worldwide prevalence in children is 15 to 20 percent and is increasing in industrialized nations.[2]
- Sixty percent of cases begin during the first year of life and 90 percent by 5 years of age.[1] 1/3 will persist into adulthood.[2]
- Sixty percent of adults with AD have children with AD (**Figure 130-3**).[1]

ETIOLOGY AND PATHOPHYSIOLOGY

- Strong familial tendency, especially if atopy is inherited from the maternal side.

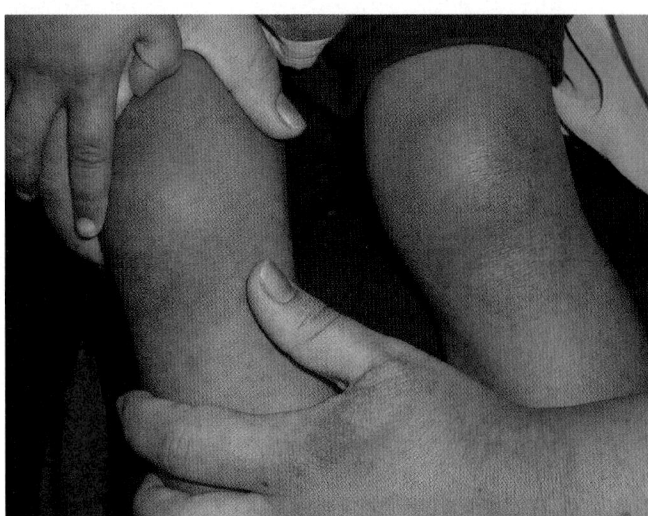

FIGURE 130-3 The child and his mother both have atopic dermatitis but not in the most typical distribution. (*Used with permission from Richard P. Usatine, MD.*)

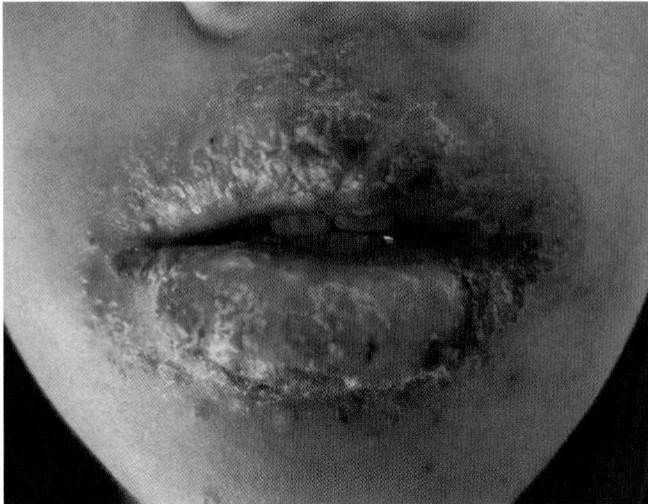

FIGURE 130-4 A teenager with atopic dermatitis superinfected by herpes (eczema herpeticum). (*Used with permission from Richard P. Usatine, MD.*)

- Associated with elevated T-helper (Th) 2 cytokine response, elevated serum immunoglobulin (Ig) E, hyperstimulatory Langerhans cells, defective cell-mediated immunity, and loss of function mutation in filaggrin, an epidermal barrier protein.
- Exotoxins of *Staphylococcus aureus* act as superantigens and stimulate activation of T-cells and macrophages, worsening AD without actually showing signs of superinfection.
- Patients may have a primary T-cell defect. This may be why they can get more severe skin infections caused by herpes simplex virus (eczema herpeticum as seen in **Figure 130-4**) or bacteria (widespread impetigo). They are also at risk of a bad reaction to the smallpox vaccine with dissemination of the attenuated virus beyond the vaccination site. Eczema vaccinatum is a potentially deadly complication of smallpox vaccination (**Figure 130-5**).

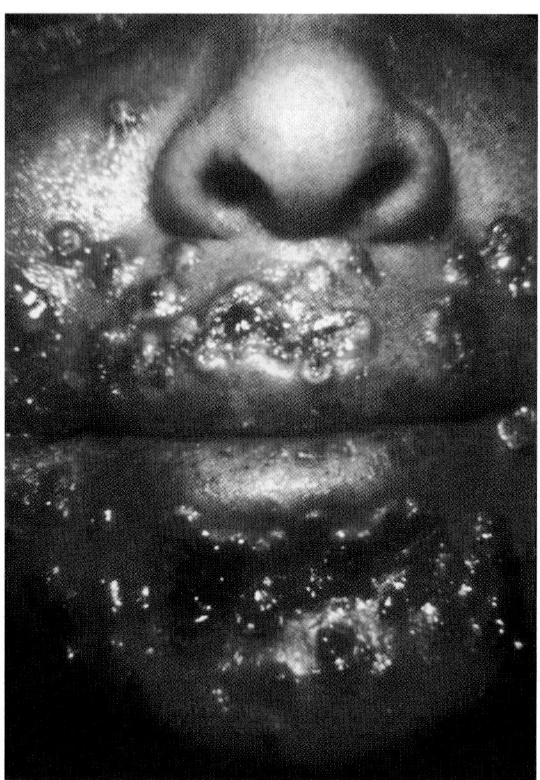

FIGURE 130-5 Eczema vaccinatum in a 17-year-old woman with atopic dermatitis who was given the smallpox vaccine. This eruption became this severe 8 days after her vaccination. (*Used with permission from CDC and Arthur E. Kaye.*)

TYPICAL DISTRIBUTION

- AD often starts on the face in infancy and childhood (**Figures 130-1** and **130-7**) and then appears in the flexural folds, especially the antecubital and popliteal fossa (**Figures 130-8** to **130-10**).
- Involvement of the neck, wrists, and ankles also may occur (**Figures 130-11** and **130-12**).

DIAGNOSIS

- History—Pruritus is the hallmark symptom of AD. It is referred to as "the itch that rashes" as patients will often feel the need to scratch before a primary lesion appears. If it does not itch, it is not AD. Persons with AD often have a personal or family history of other allergic conditions, namely asthma and allergic rhinitis.
- The atopic triad is AD, allergic rhinitis, and asthma. Atopic persons have an exaggerated inflammatory response to factors that irritate the skin.
- Physical examination—Primary lesions include vesicles, scale, papules, and plaques.
- Secondary (or sequential) lesions include linear excoriations from scratching or rubbing, which may result in lichenification (thickened skin with accentuation of skin lines), fissuring, and prurigo nodularis. Crust may indicate that a secondary infection has occurred. Postinflammatory hyperpigmentation and follicular hyperaccentuation (more prominent hyperkeratotic follicles; **Figure 130-6**) may also be identified.

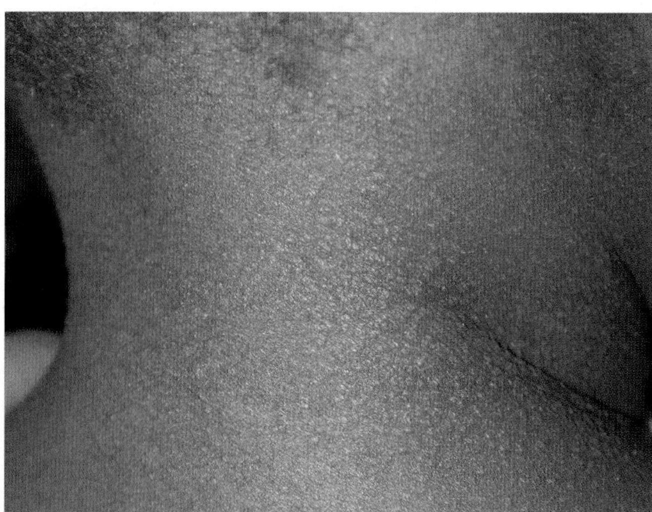

FIGURE 130-6 A young black girl with atopic dermatitis showing follicular hyperaccentuation on the neck. This pattern of atopic dermatitis is more common in persons of color. (*Used with permission from Richard P. Usatine, MD.*)

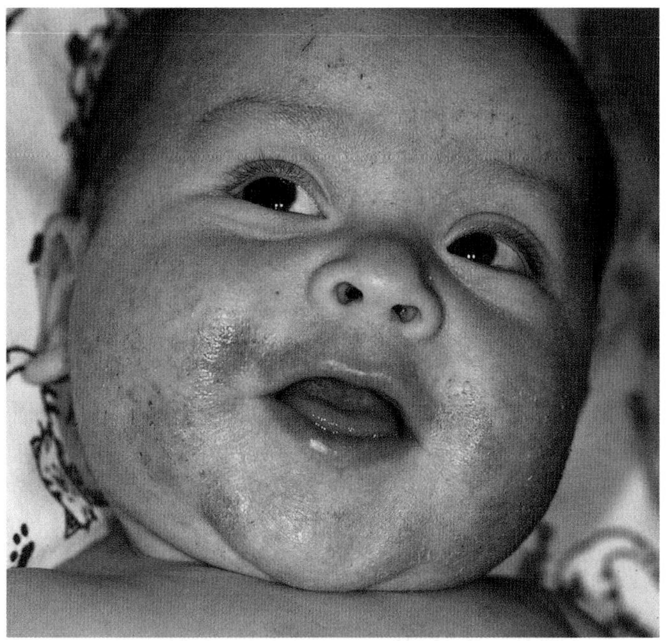

FIGURE 130-7 An infant with atopic dermatitis on the face that has become superinfected. (*Used with permission from Milgrom EC, Usatine RP, Tan RA, Spector SL. Practical Allergy. Philadelphia, PA: Elsevier; 2004.*)

- AD in adults can occur on the hands, around the mouth, or eyelids as well as all the other areas (**Figures 130-13** and **130-14**).
- In one series, the prevalence of hand involvement in patients with active AD was 58.9 percent. There was a significant trend toward an increasing prevalence of hand involvement with increasing age.[3]

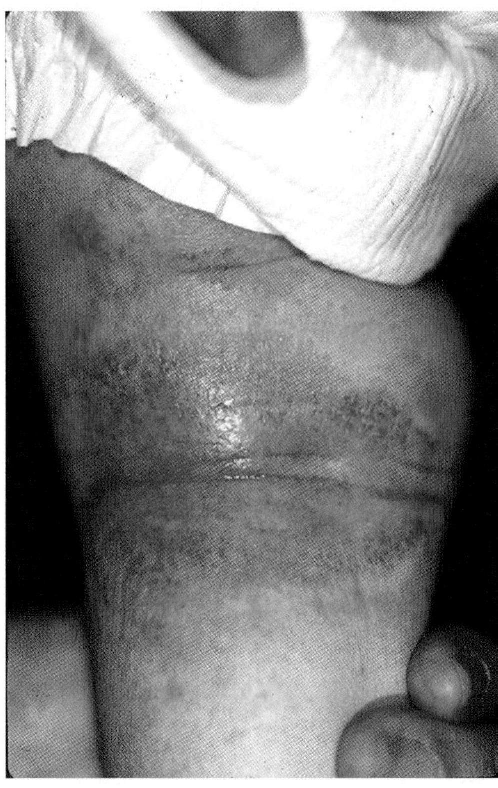

FIGURE 130-8 The same infant with superinfected atopic dermatitis of the popliteal fossa. (*Used with permission from Milgrom EC, Usatine RP, Tan RA, Spector SL. Practical Allergy. Philadelphia, PA: Elsevier; 2004.*)

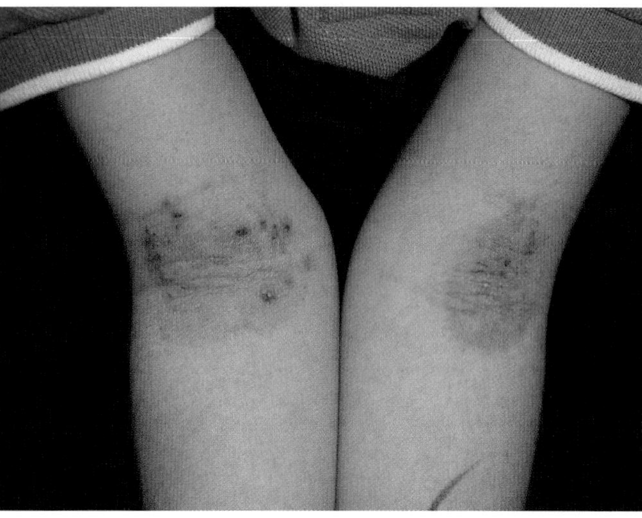

FIGURE 130-9 Atopic dermatitis in the antecubital fossae of a 6-year-old boy. Note the erythematous plaques with excoriations. (*Used with permission from Richard P. Usatine, MD.*)

OTHER FEATURES OR CONDITIONS ASSOCIATED WITH ATOPIC DERMATITIS

- Keratosis pilaris (**Figure 130-15**).
- Ichthyosis (**Figure 130-16**).
- Pityriasis alba (**Figures 130-17** and **130-18**).
- Palmar or plantar hyperlinearity.
- Angular Cheilitis (**Figure 130-13**).
- Dennie-Morgan lines (infraorbital fold) (**Figure 130-14**).
- Hand or foot dermatitis
- Susceptibility to cutaneous infections (**Figures 130-4** and **130-5**).
- Xerosis (dry skin) (**Figure 130-19**).

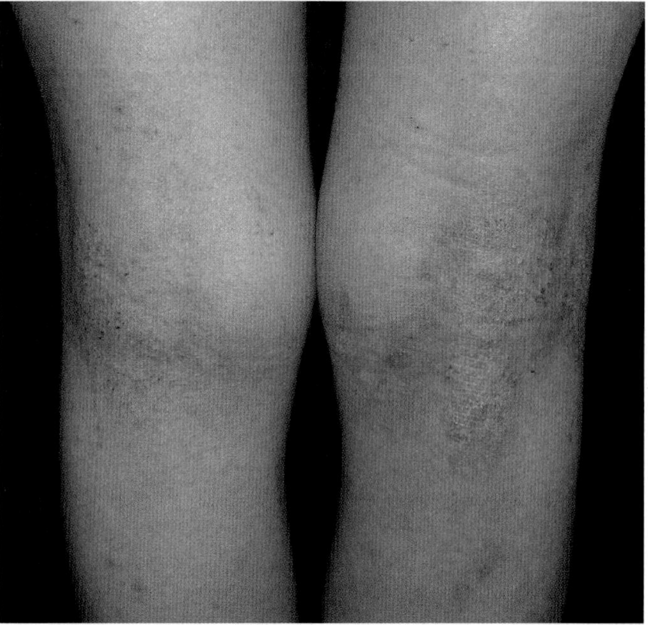

FIGURE 130-10 A 20-year-old young woman with severe chronic atopic dermatitis showing lichenification and hyperpigmentation in the popliteal fossa. (*Used with permission from Richard P. Usatine, MD.*)

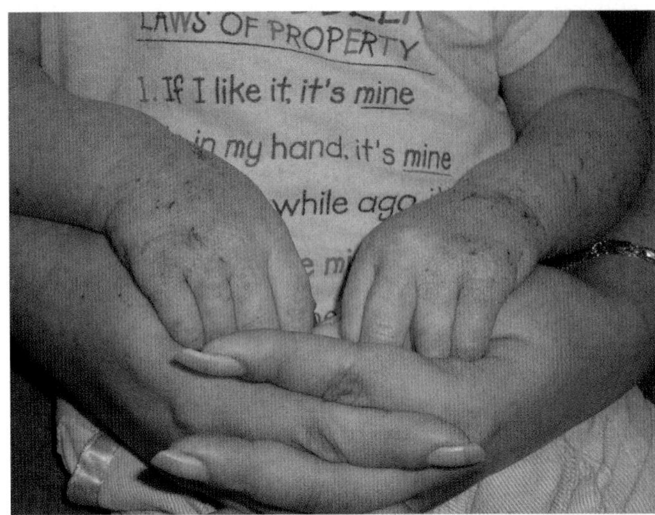

FIGURE 130-11 A 2-year-old girl with atopic dermatitis visible on her hands, wrists, and arms. (*Used with permission from Richard P. Usatine, MD.*)

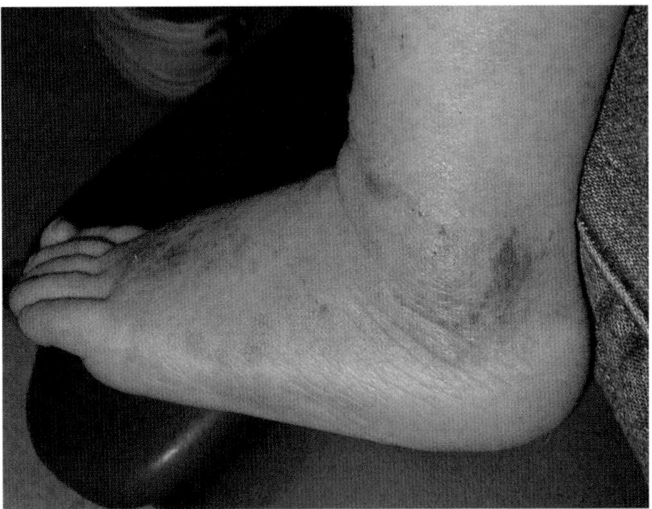

FIGURE 130-12 The girl in Figure 130-11 with an exacerbation of her atopic dermatitis on the ankle showing many excoriations. (*Used with permission from Richard P. Usatine, MD.*)

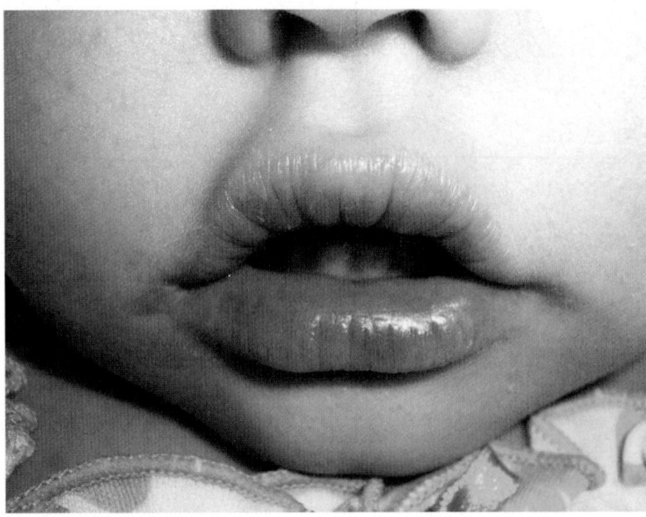

FIGURE 130-13 Angular cheilitis in an infant with atopic dermatitis. (*Used with permission from Richard P. Usatine, MD.*)

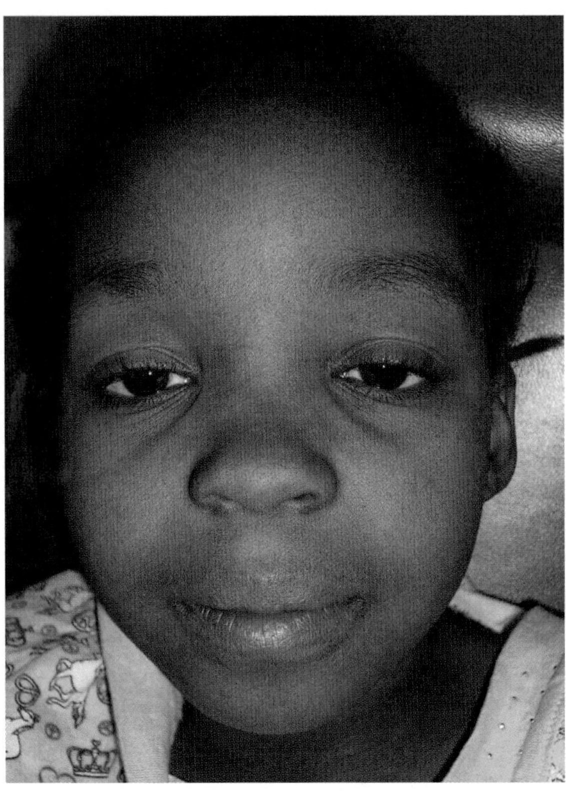

FIGURE 130-14 A young girl with the atopic triad. The patient has Denny Morgan lines visible on the lower eyelids. She was observed doing the allergic salute many times during her office visit. (*Used with permission from Richard P. Usatine, MD.*)

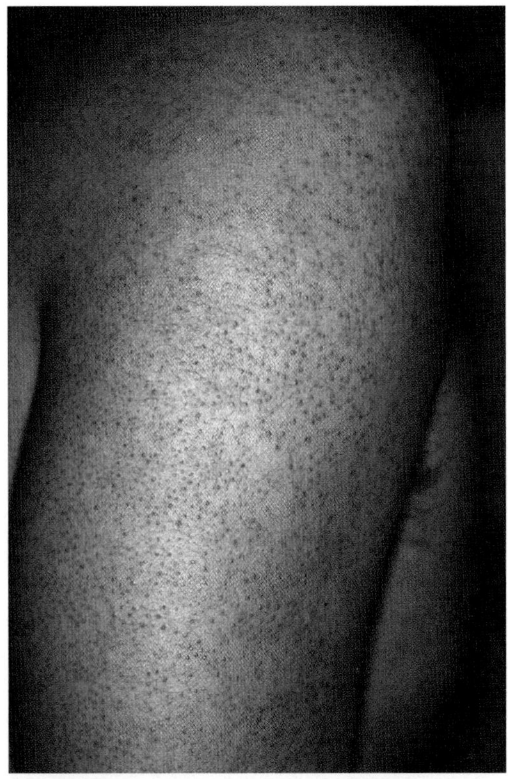

FIGURE 130-15 Keratosis pilaris on the lateral upper arm. The papules can vary in color from pink to brown to white depending upon the skin color of the person. (*Used with permission from Richard P. Usatine, MD.*)

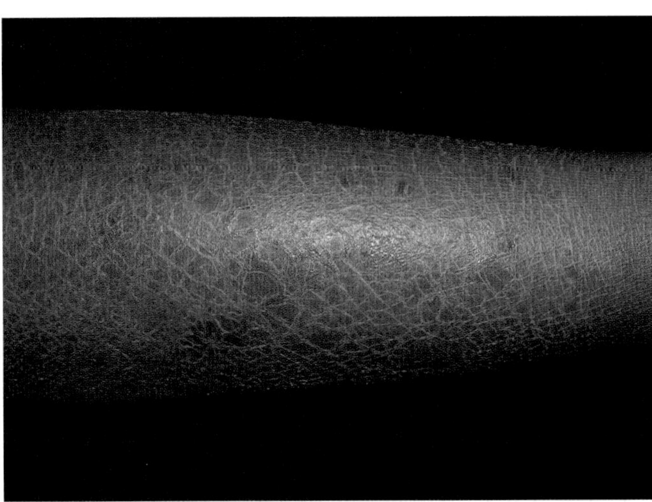

FIGURE 130-16 Acquired ichthyosis on the leg of a 9-year-old boy with atopic dermatitis. Note the fish-scale appearance along with the dry skin. (*Used with permission from Richard P. Usatine, MD.*)

- Eye findings—Recurrent conjunctivitis, keratoconus (**Figure 130-20**), cataracts, and orbital darkening.
- A horizontal nasal crease may be seen over the bridge of the nose in a patient with allergic rhinitis prone to performing the allergic salute. In some patients, this crease may become hyperpigmented (**Figure 130-21**).

LABORATORY STUDIES

Labs are rarely needed if the history and physical examination support the diagnosis. Occasionally, a KOH preparation may be needed to rule out tinea or a skin scraping to rule out scabies. Of course, both of these conditions can occur on top of AD. A Radioallergosorbent test (RAST) for food allergies and serum IgE levels are not of proven benefit.

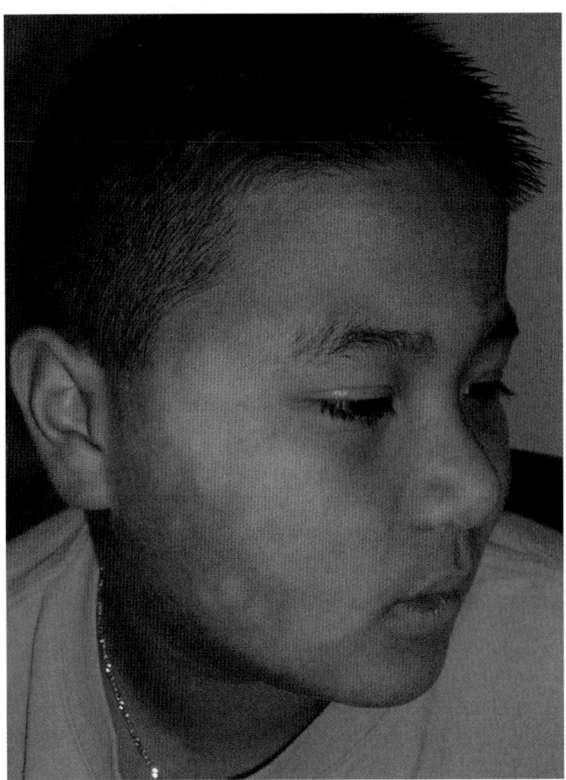

FIGURE 130-17 Pityriasis alba on the face of a young boy. (*Used with permission from Richard P. Usatine, MD.*)

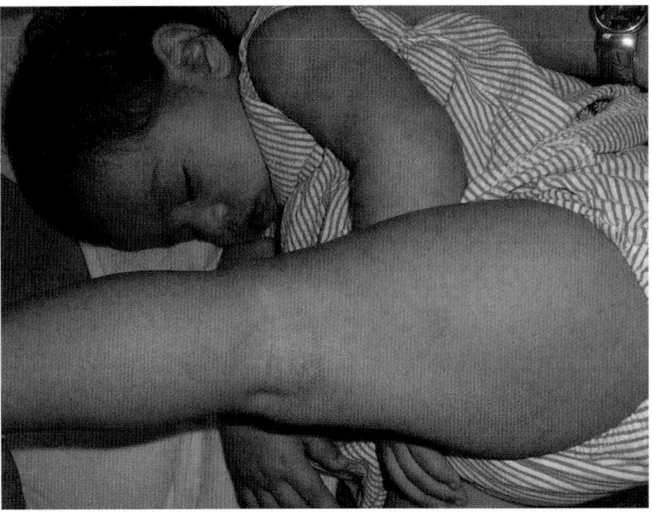

FIGURE 130-18 An 18-month-old girl with atopic dermatitis visible in her popliteal fossa and pityriasis alba on her arm (*Used with permission from Richard P. Usatine, MD.*)

DIFFERENTIAL DIAGNOSIS

- Dyshidrotic eczema—Dry inflamed scaling skin on the hands and feet with tapioca-like vesicles, especially seen between the fingers.
- Seborrheic dermatitis—Greasy, scaly lesions on scalp, face, and chest (see Chapter 135, Seborrheic Dermatitis).
- Psoriasis—Thickened plaques on extensor surfaces, scalp, and buttocks; pitted nails (see Chapter 136, Psoriasis).

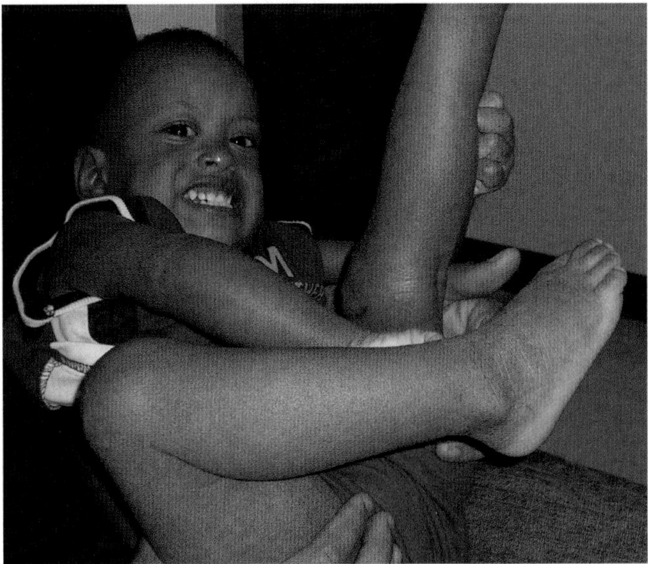

FIGURE 130-19 Severe atopic dermatitis in a 2-year-old black boy with very dry (xerotic) skin. He is spontaneously scratching and crying out in discomfort. (*Used with permission from Richard P. Usatine, MD.*)

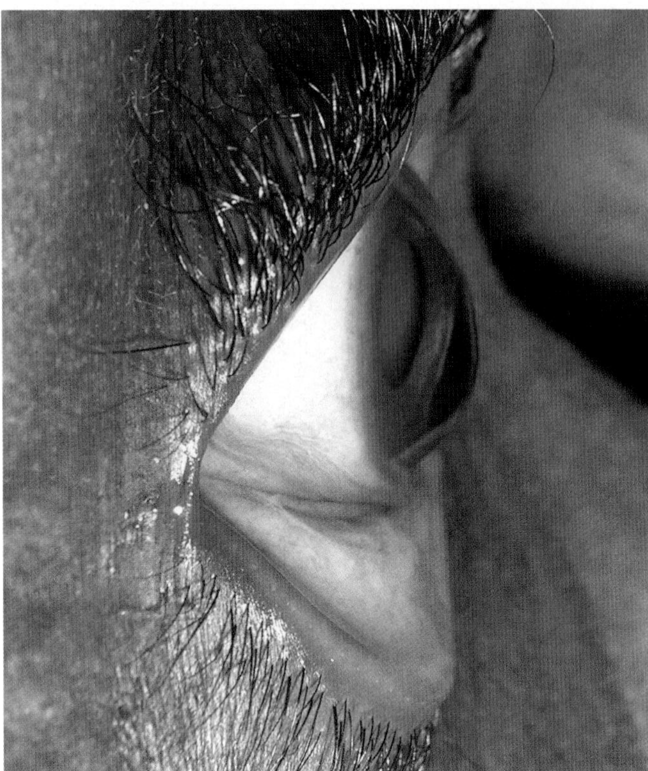

FIGURE 130-20 Keratoconus in a young woman with severe atopic dermatitis. She admits to rubbing her eyes frequently. In keratoconus the cornea bulges out in the middle like a cone and can adversely affect the health of the eye. (*Used with permission from Richard P. Usatine, MD.*)

- Lichen simplex chronicus (sometimes called neurodermatitis)—Usually, a single patch in an area accessible to scratching such as the ankle, wrist, and neck.
- Contact dermatitis—Positive exposure history, rash in area of exposure; absence of family history. Patch testing may be helpful in distinguishing from AD (see Chapter 131, Contact Dermatitis).

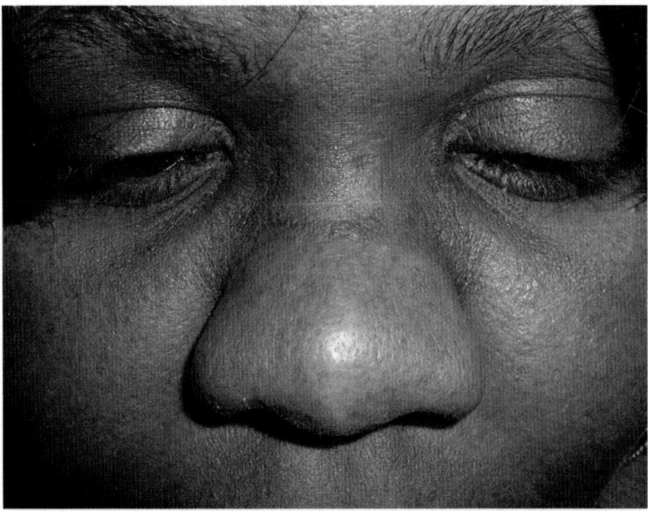

FIGURE 130-21 Hyperpigmented horizontal nasal crease in a patient with the atopic triad who repeatedly performs the allergic salute when her nose is feeling itchy. (*Used with permission from Richard P. Usatine, MD.*)

- Scabies—Papules, burrows, finger web involvement, positive skin scraping (see Chapter 128, Scabies).
- Dermatophyte infection—On the hands or feet can look just like hand or foot dermatitis; a positive KOH preparation for hyphae can help make the diagnosis (see Chapter 125, Tinea Pedis).

MANAGEMENT

- There is some evidence suggesting that controlling house dust mites reduces severity of symptoms in patients with the atopic triad. Bedding covers were found to be the most effective method to control dust mites and AD symptoms in this subgroup of AD patients. Unfortunately, dust mite interventions are not proven to be effective for patients with AD that do not have the full atopic triad.[1] SOR B
- Dietary restriction is controversial but may be useful for infants with proven egg allergies. SOR B There is insufficient evidence that dietary manipulation in children or adults reduces symptom severity and may cause iatrogenic malnourishment.
- Patient education, avoidance of possible triggers (enzyme-rich detergents, wool clothing), and dry skin care should be optimized.
- Dilute bleach baths (0.5 cup of 6 percent bleach in tub of bath water) lower the *S. aureus* burden on the skin, decreasing severity of AD.[4] SOR B
- There is some evidence suggesting probiotic treatment of pregnant mother and prolonged nursing of child may delay onset of AD.[1] SOR B

TOPICAL THERAPIES

- Topical steroids and emollients have been proven to work for AD and are the mainstay of treatment.[1] SOR A
- Vehicle selection and steroid strength area based on age, body location, and lesion morphology. The ointments are best for dry and cracked skin and are more potent. Creams are easier to apply and are better tolerated by some patients.
- Use stronger steroids for thicker skin, severe outbreaks, or lesions that have not responded to weaker steroids. Avoid strong steroids on face, genitals, and armpits and in infants and small children.
- To avoid adverse effects, the highest potency steroids (e.g., clobetasol) should not be used for longer than 2 weeks continuously. However, they can be used intermittently for recurring AD in a pulse-therapy mode (e.g., apply every weekend, with no application on weekdays).
- Topical calcineurin inhibitors (immunomodulators, such as pimecrolimus and tacrolimus) reduce the rash severity and symptoms in children and adults.[1] SOR A These work by suppressing antigen-specific T-cell activation and inhibiting inflammatory cytokine release. These are steroid-sparing medications that are helpful for eyelid eczema and in other areas when steroids may thin the skin (**Figure 130-22**). These agents are now only approved for persons older than 2 years of age and the FDA states that they

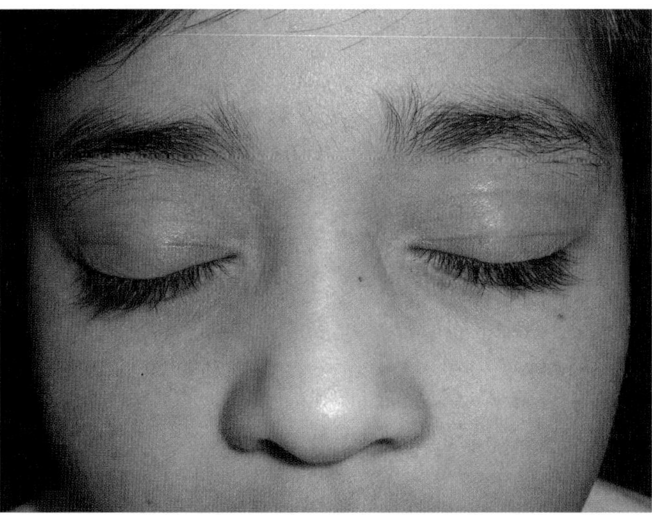

FIGURE 130-22 Atopic dermatitis involving the eyelids in this 8-year-old girl with atopic dermatitis since infancy. A topical calcineurin inhibitor helped to get the eyelid eczema under control. (*Used with permission from Richard P. Usatine, MD.*)

should not be used as first-line agents because of a possible risk of causing cancer. The American Academy of Dermatology (AAD) has released a statement that the "data does not prove that the proper topical use of pimecrolimus and tacrolimus is dangerous."

- Short-term adjunctive use of topical doxepin may aid in the reduction of pruritus.[1] SOR Ⓐ
- Topical and systemic antibiotics are used for AD that has become secondarily infected with bacteria. The most common infecting organism is *S. aureus*. Weeping fluid and crusting during an exacerbation should prompt consideration of antibiotic use[1] (**Figures 130-7**, **130-8**, and **130-23**). SOR Ⓐ

ORAL/SYSTEMIC THERAPIES

- For extensive flares, consider oral prednisone or an IM shot of triamcinolone (40 mg in 1 mL of 40 mg/mL suspension for adults).[1] SOR Ⓒ

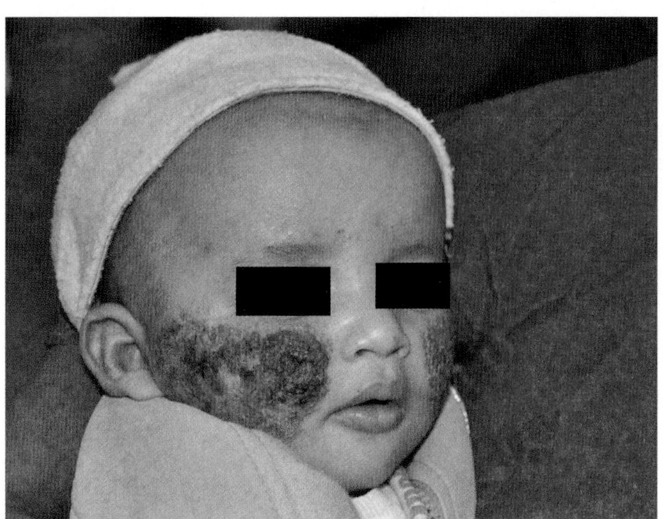

FIGURE 130-23 Superinfected atopic dermatitis on the cheeks. The crusting is a sign of secondary infection usually caused by Staph. aureus or Strep. pyogenes. (*Used with permission from Richard P. Usatine, MD.*)

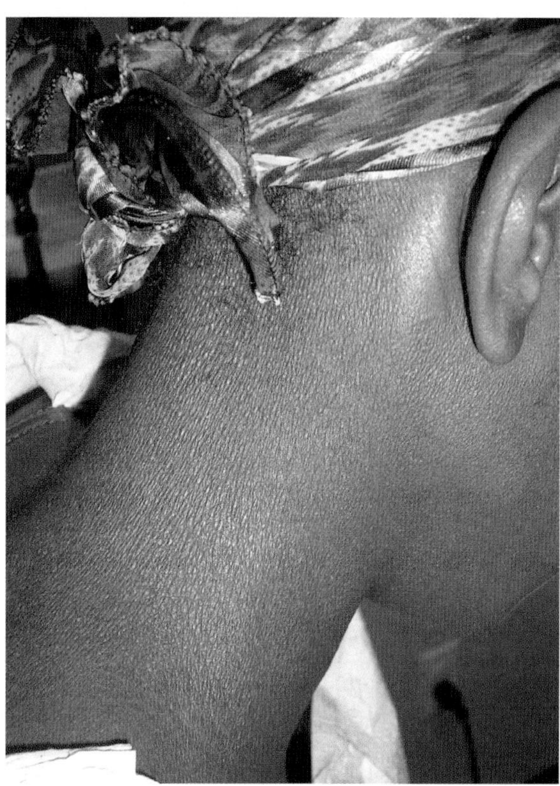

FIGURE 130-24 Atopic dermatitis so flared up from head to ankles that this 17-year-old teen was started on oral cyclosporine. Her response to cyclosporine over the next 2 months was so excellent that she was able to go off the cyclosporine and keep her skin clear with emollients and occasional topical steroids. (*Used with permission from Richard P. Usatine, MD.*)

- The value of antihistamines in AD is controversial. If antihistamines are to be used, the sedating agents are most effective and can be given at night.[1] SOR Ⓑ
- Cyclosporine for severe refractory AD can be used in long-term maintenance therapy to treat and avoid relapse.[1] SOR Ⓐ Cyclosporine is approved for 1 year of lifetime therapy for skin diseases in the US and 2 years in Europe (**Figure 130-24**). A short course with careful monitoring can be very helpful.
- UV phototherapy may also be used in severe refractory AD with some success.[1] SOR Ⓐ
- Azathioprine, methotrexate, and mycophenolate mofetil are of possible benefit, but there is less evidence for their effectiveness.[1] SOR Ⓒ

FOLLOW-UP

Regular follow-up should be given to patients with chronic and difficult-to-control AD. Establishing a good regimen is crucial to good control and then visits may be adjusted to longer intervals between visits.

PATIENT EDUCATION

Patients need to know that scratching their AD makes it worse. Behavior modification is especially challenging in young children

TABLE 130-1 Written Action Plan to Be Given to Patients (or Their Parents)

No skin lesions or dry skin	Prevention: Emollients, dry skin care, fragrance-free detergent, no drier sheets, once weekly bleach bath
Mild flare	Prevention plus low-mid potency topical steroid and/or calcineurin inhibitors (e.g., hydrocortisone 2.5 percent or tacrolimus 0.1 percent to face, axillae, genitals; desonide 0.1 percent or triamcinolone 0.1 percent to body)
Moderate flare	Prevention plus mid-high potency topical steroids and/or calcineurin inhibitor (e.g., triamcinolone under wet pajamas bid to clobetasol for short course)
Severe flare	Systemic therapy

Adapted from Rance F, Boguniewicz M, and Lau S,[2] and from Chisolm SS, Taylor SL, Balkrishnan R, et al.[5]

and may involve cutting fingernails short and occluding hands/body at night with cotton gloves or clothing. Because of its chronicity and cyclic nature, AD patients may have poor adherence. In one recent study, overall adherence was 32 percent. A written action plan may be employed to improve adherence (**Table 130-1**).

REFERENCES

1. Hanifin JM, Cooper KD, Ho VC, et al. Guidelines of care for atopic dermatitis. *J Am Acad Dermatol.* 2004;50:391-404.
2. Rance F, Boguniewicz M, Lau S. New visions for atopic eczema: an iPAC summary and future trends. *Pediatr Allergy Immunol.* 2008;19(19):17-25.
3. Simpson EL. Prevalence and morphology of hand eczema in patients with atopic dermatitis. *Dermatitis.* 2006;17:123-127.
4. Huang JT, Abrams M, Tlougan B, et al. Dilute bleach baths for *Staphylococcus aureus* colonization in atopic dermatitis to decrease disease severity. *Pediatrics.* 2009;123(5):e808-e814.
5. Chisolm SS, Taylor SL, Balkrishnan R, et al. Written action plans: potential for improving outcomes in children with atopic dermatitis. *J Am Acad Dermatol.* 2008;59:677-683.

131 CONTACT DERMATITIS

Richard P. Usatine, MD

PATIENT STORY

An 11-year-old girl presents with a rash on her abdomen for the past month (**Figure 131-1**).

She denies other skin problems but her mother states that she had atopic dermatitis as a baby. The clinician readily identifies the problem as a nickel allergy to the nickel found in her belt buckle and jeans. He prescribes avoidance of nickel contact to the skin and prescribes 0.1 percent triamcinolone ointment to be applied twice daily until the contact dermatitis resolves. He describes various methods to cover medal snaps intense including sewing and fabric or painting clear nail polish over the metal. Neither method works 100 percent but it is hard to find jeans without metal snaps. The patient responded rapidly to treatment.[1,2]

INTRODUCTION

Contact dermatitis (CD) is a common inflammatory skin condition characterized by erythematous and pruritic skin lesions resulting from the contact of skin with a foreign substance. Irritant contact dermatitis (ICD) is caused by the non–immune-modulated irritation of the skin by a substance, resulting in a skin changes. Allergic contact dermatitis (ACD) is a delayed-type hypersensitivity reaction in which a foreign substance comes into contact with the skin, and upon reexposure, skin changes occur.[3]

EPIDEMIOLOGY

- Some of the most common types of CD are secondary to exposures to poison ivy, nickel, and fragrances.[4]

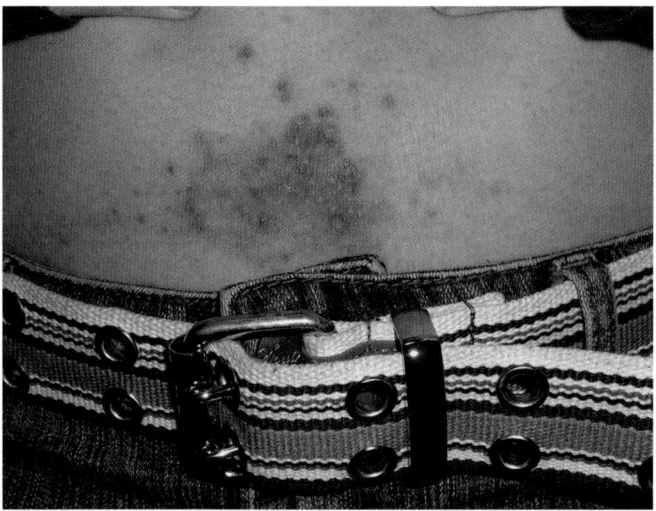

FIGURE 131-1 Allergic contact dermatitis to the nickel in the jeans' fastener and the belt buckle causing erythema, scaling, and hyperpigmentation. (*Used with permission from Richard P. Usatine, MD.*)

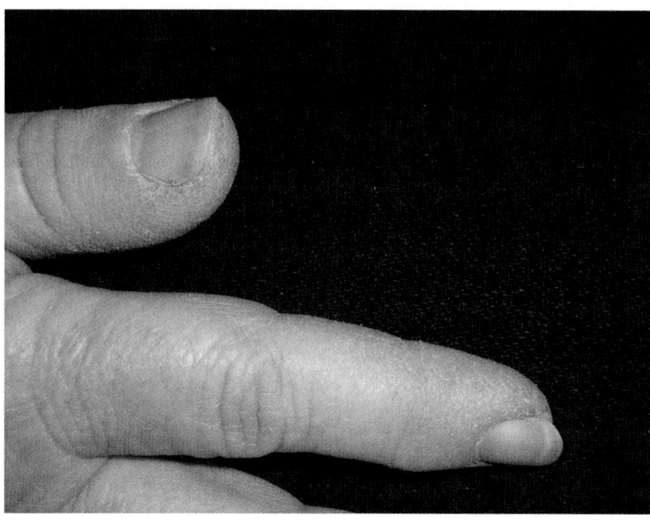

FIGURE 131-2 Occupational irritant contact dermatitis in a woman whose hands are exposed to chemicals while making cowboy hats in Texas. Occupational exposures might affect teens as they begin to enter the work force. (*Used with permission from Richard P. Usatine, MD.*)

- Patch testing data indicate that the five most prevalent contact allergens out of more than 3700 known contact allergens are nickel (14.3% of patients tested), fragrance mix (14%), neomycin (11.6%), balsam of Peru (10.4%), and thimerosal (10.4%).[5]
- Occupational skin diseases (chiefly CD) rank second only to traumatic injuries as the most common type of occupational disease. Chemical irritants such as solvents and cutting fluids account for most ICD cases. Sixty percent were ACD and 32 percent were ICD. Hands were primarily affected in 64 percent of ACD and 80 percent of ICD[4] (**Figure 131-2**).

ETIOLOGY AND PATHOPHYSIOLOGY

- CD is a common inflammatory skin condition characterized by erythematous and pruritic skin lesions resulting from the contact of skin with a foreign substance.
- ICD is caused by the non–immune-modulated irritation of the skin by a substance, resulting in a skin rash.
- ACD is a delayed-type hypersensitivity reaction in which a foreign substance comes into contact with the skin, and is linked to skin protein forming an antigen complex that leads to sensitization. Upon reexposure of the epidermis to the antigen, the sensitized T cells initiate an inflammatory cascade, leading to the skin changes seen in ACD.

DIAGNOSIS

HISTORY

Ask about contact with known allergens (i.e., nickel, fragrances, neomycin, and poison ivy/oak).

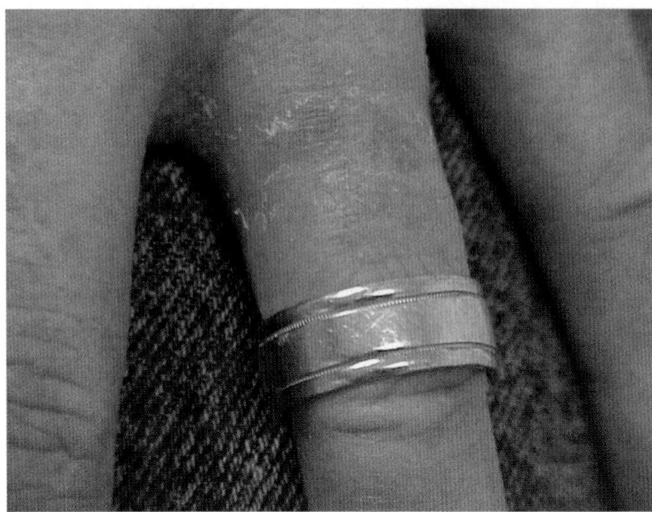

FIGURE 131-3 Patient moved up his ring to show the allergic contact dermatitis secondary to a nickel allergy to the ring. (*Used with permission from Milgrom EC, Usatine RP, Tan RA, Spector SL. Practical Allergy. Philadelphia, PA: Elsevier, Inc; 2004.*)

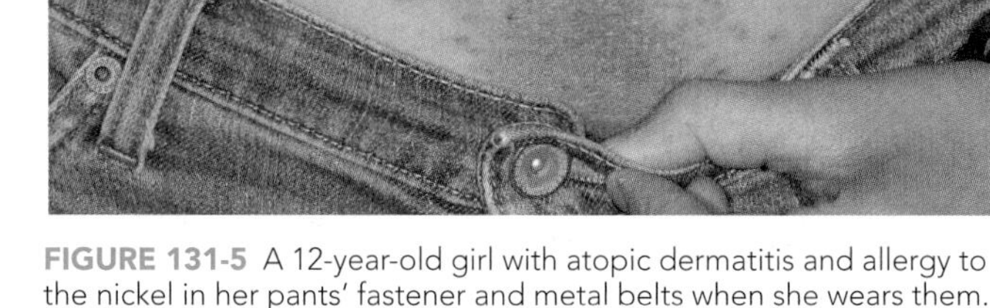

FIGURE 131-5 A 12-year-old girl with atopic dermatitis and allergy to the nickel in her pants' fastener and metal belts when she wears them. (*Used with permission from Richard P. Usatine, MD.*)

- Nickel exposure is often related to the wearing of rings, jewelry, and metal belt buckles (**Figures 131-3** to **131-5**).
- Lip licking—Saliva can cause an irritant contact dermatitis (**Figure 131-6**).
- Fragrances in the forms of deodorants and perfumes (**Figure 131-7**).
- Neomycin applied as a triple antibiotic ointment by patients (**Figures 131-8** and **131-9**).

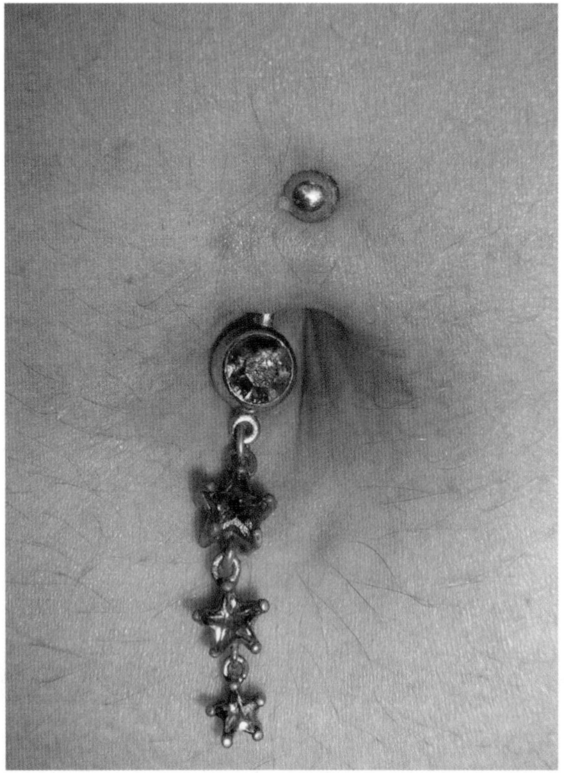

FIGURE 131-4 Allergic contact dermatitis to the metal in the bellybutton ring of a teenage girl. (*Used with permission from Richard P. Usatine, MD.*)

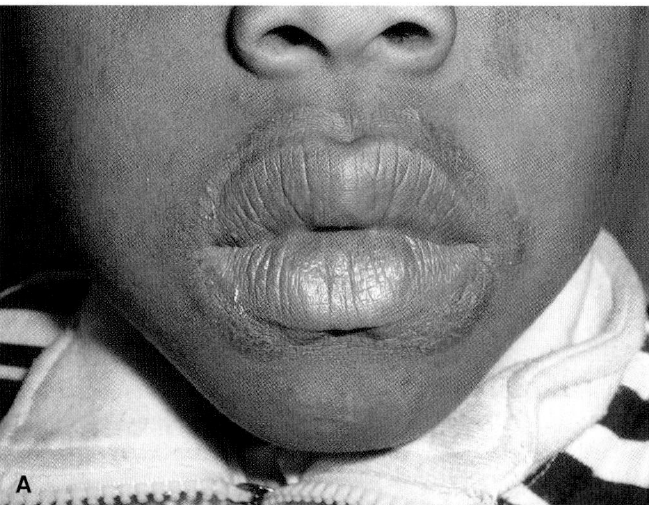

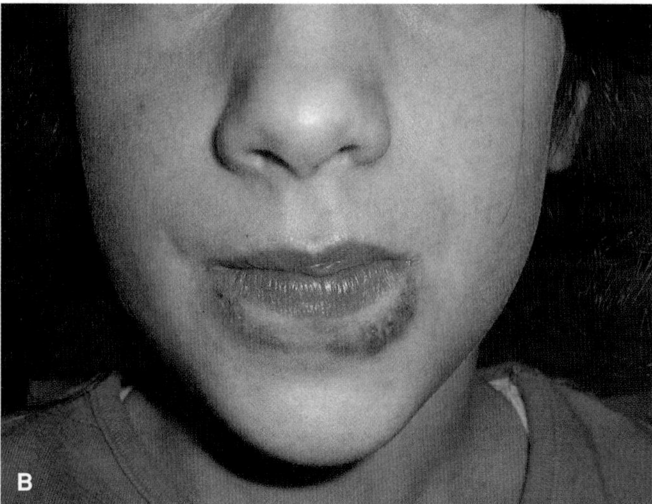

FIGURE 131-6 Two children with lip licking irritant contact dermatitis. **A.** Note the postinflammatory hyperpigmentation. **B.** Note the pink color and crusting. (*Used with permission from Richard P. Usatine, MD.*)

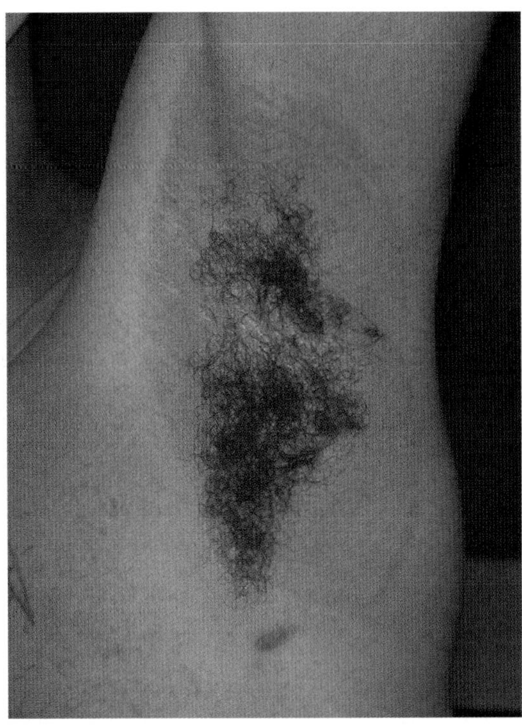

FIGURE 131-7 Allergic contact dermatitis to the fragrance in a new deodorant. (*Used with permission from Milgrom EC, Usatine RP, Tan RA, Spector SL. Practical Allergy. Philadelphia, PA: Elsevier, Inc; 2004.*)

- Poison ivy/oak in outdoor settings. Especially ask when the distribution of the reaction is linear (**Figures 131-10** and **131-11**).
- Ask about occupational exposures, especially solvents. For example, chemicals used in hat making can cause ICD on the hands (**Figure 131-2**).
- Tapes applied to skin after cuts or surgery are frequent causes of CD (**Figure 131-12**).
- If the CD is on the feet, ask about new shoes (**Figures 131-13** and **131-14**).

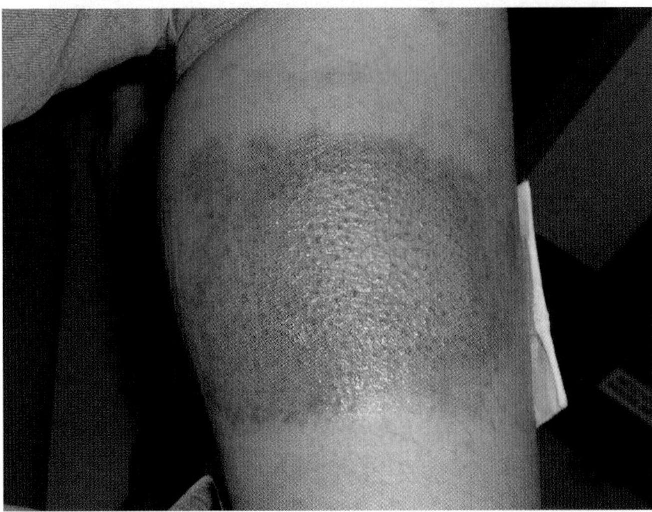

FIGURE 131-8 Allergic contact dermatitis to neomycin applied to the leg of a young woman. Her mom gave her triple antibiotic ointment to place over a bug bite with a large nonstick pad. The contact allergy follows the exact size of the pad and only occurs where the antibiotic was applied. (*Used with permission from Richard P. Usatine, MD.*)

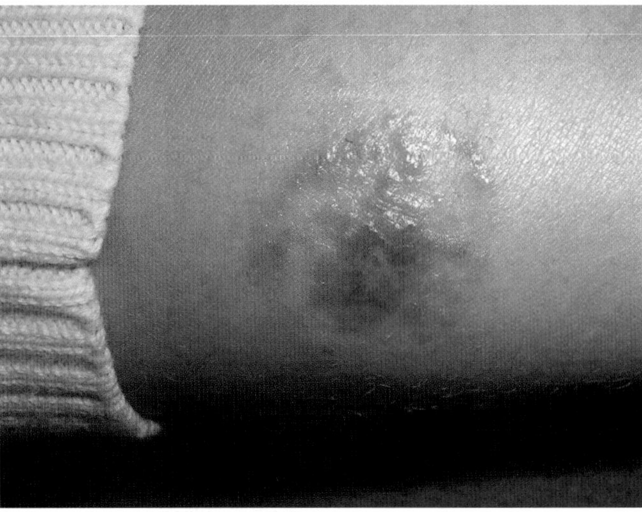

FIGURE 131-9 Allergic contact dermatitis to a neomycin containing topical antibiotic. (*Used with permission from Richard P. Usatine, MD.*)

A detailed history of products used on the skin may reveal a suspected allergen. Sometimes patch testing results will lead to the answer when the history is only suggestive. For example, an 8-year-old girl with mild atopic dermatitis was found to be allergic to a chemical in an over-the-counter product used to moisturize her skin. The history that her mother gave about the child developing a rash to a particular soap was a clue that the new hand dermatitis may have been secondary to contact dermatitis. Patch testing was used to identify the chemical (**Figures 131-15** to **131-17**).

CLINICAL FEATURES

All types of CD have erythema. Although it is not always possible to distinguish between ICD and ACD, here are some features that might help:

- ICD:
  - Location—Usually the hands.
  - Symptoms—Burning, pruritus, pain.
  - Dry and fissured skin (**Figure 131-2**).
  - Indistinct borders.

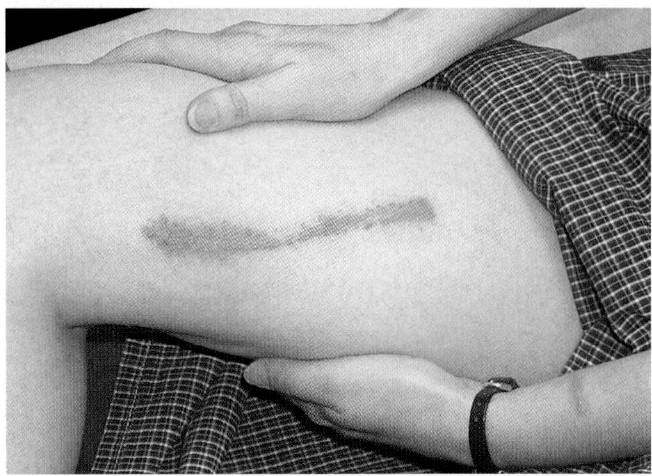

FIGURE 131-10 A linear pattern of allergic contact dermatitis from poison ivy. (*Used with permission from Jack Resneck, Sr., MD.*)

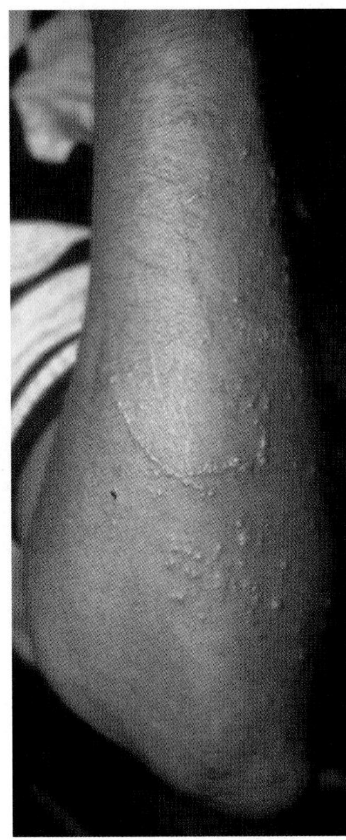

FIGURE 131-11 Multiple lines of vesicles from poison oak on the arm of this teen boy. (*Used with permission from Milgrom EC, Usatine RP, Tan RA, Spector SL. Practical Allergy. Philadelphia, PA: Elsevier, Inc; 2004.*)

- ACD:
  - Location—Usually exposed area of skin, often the hands.
  - Pruritus is the dominant symptom.
  - Vesicles and bulla (**Figures 131-1** and **131-8**).
  - Distinct angles, lines, and borders (**Figures 131-8** to **131-12**).

Both ICD and ACD may be complicated by bacterial superinfection showing signs of exudate, weeping, and crusts.

Toxicodendron (Rhus) dermatitis (poison ivy, poison oak, and poison sumac) is caused by urushiol, which is found in the saps of this plant family. Clinically, a line of vesicles can occur from brushing against one of the plants. Also, the linear pattern occurs from scratching oneself and dragging the oleoresin across the skin with the fingernails (**Figures 131-10** and **131-11**).

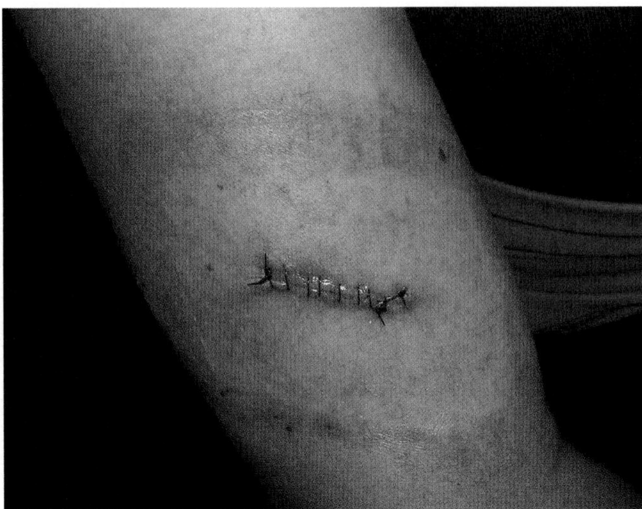

FIGURE 131-12 Contact dermatitis to tape. (*Used with permission from Richard P. Usatine, MD.*)

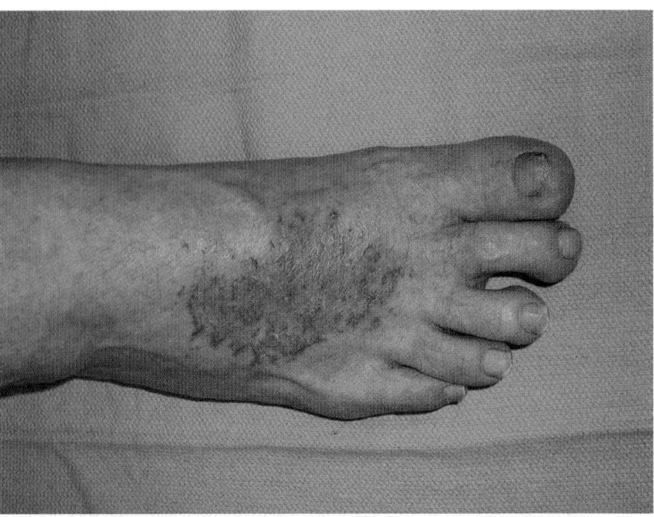

FIGURE 131-13 Allergic contact dermatitis from new shoes. This is the typical distribution found on the dorsum of the feet. Patch testing revealed that the allergy was to thiurams found in rubber. (*Used with permission from Richard P. Usatine, MD.*)

Systemic CD is a rare form of CD seen after the systemic administration of a substance, usually a drug, to which topical sensitization has previously occurred.[6]

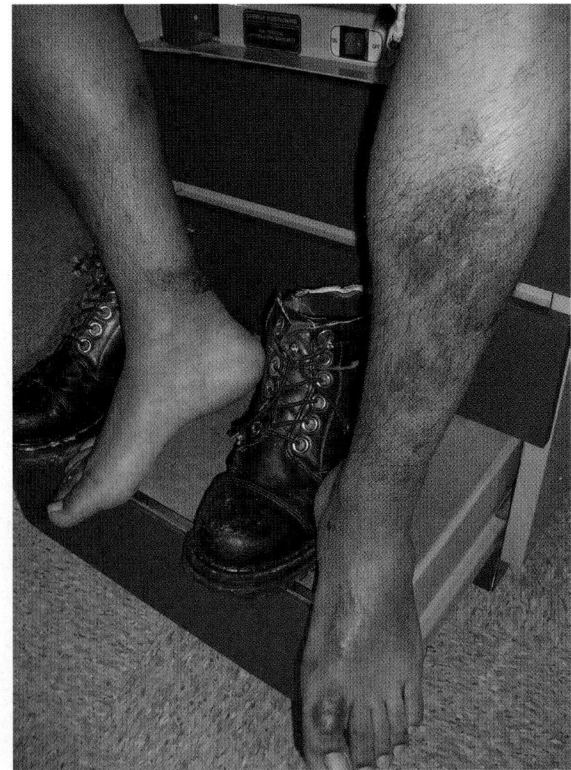

FIGURE 131-14 A young man with allergic contact dermatitis to a chemical in his boots. His boots were higher but he cut them down to try to alleviate the discomfort coming from the boots higher on his leg. (*Used with permission from Milgrom EC, Usatine RP, Tan RA, Spector SL. Practical Allergy. Philadelphia, PA: Elsevier, Inc; 2004.*)

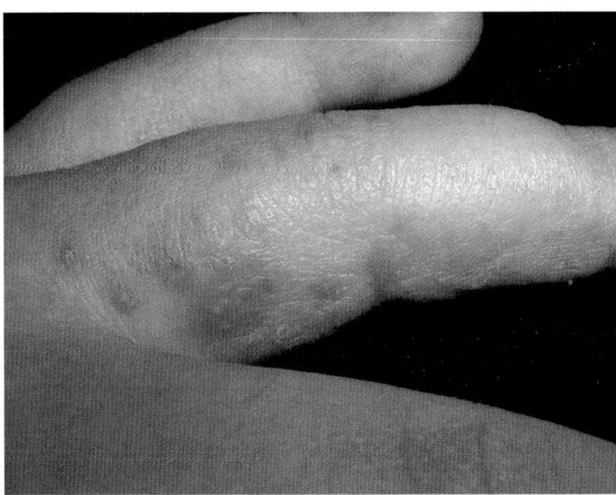

FIGURE 131-15 Allergic contact dermatitis on the hands of an 8-year-old girl with history of mild atopic dermatitis. Patch testing ultimately revealed that she was allergic to $Cl^+ Me^-$ isothiazolinone. Her mother discovered this was one of the ingredients in a moisturizer they were using on her skin. Her allergic contact dermatitis resolved once exposure to $Cl^+ Me^-$ isothiazolinone was eliminated. (*Used with permission from Richard P. Usatine, MD.*)

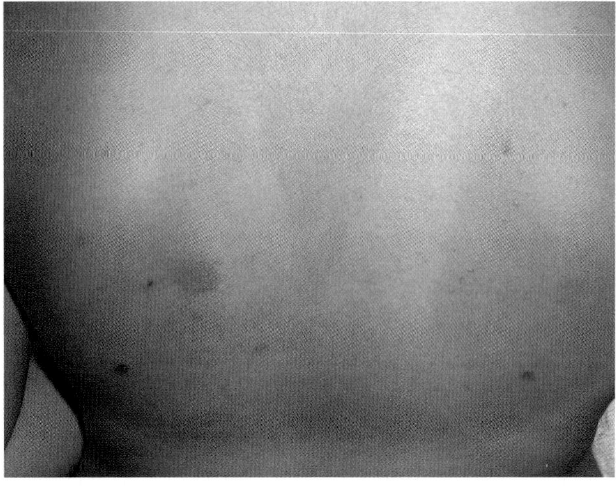

FIGURE 131-17 This positive patch test result for $Cl^+ Me^-$ isothiazolinone shows small vesicles on an erythematous base. The T.R.U.E. Test reading strip is held against the skin using the skin markings to identify the positive antigen. This is the same 8-year-old girl in **Figures 131-15** and **131-16**. (*Used with permission from Richard P. Usatine, MD.*)

LABORATORY STUDIES

The diagnosis is most often made by history and physical examination. Consider culture if there are signs of superinfection and there is a concern for methicillin-resistant *Staphylococcus aureus* (MRSA). The following tests may be considered when the diagnosis is not clear.

- KOH preparation and/or fungal culture if tinea is suspected.
- Microscopy for scabies mites and eggs.
- Latex allergy testing—This type of reaction is neither ICD (nonimmunologic) nor ACD. The latex allergy type of reaction is a type I, or immunoglobulin (Ig)E-mediated response to the latex allergen.
- Patch testing—Common antigens are placed on the skin of a patient. The T.R.U.E. Test comes in three tape strips that are easy to apply to the back (**Figure 131-16**). There is no preparation needed to test for the 35 common allergens embedded into these strips (**Table 131-1** for a list of the 35 allergens). The strips are removed in 2 days and read at that time and again in two more days (**Figure 131-17**). The T.R.U.E. Test website provides detailed information on how to perform the testing and how to counsel patients about the meaning of their results. Any clinician with an interest in patch testing can easily perform this service in the office.
    - A meta-analysis of the T.R.U.E. Test shows that nickel (14.7% of tested patients), thimerosal (5.0%), cobalt (4.8%), fragrance mix (3.4%), and balsam of Peru (3.0%) are the most prevalent allergens detected using this system.[5]
    - Critics of the T.R.U.E. Test state that it misses other important antigens. There are a number of dermatologists who create their own more extensive panels in their office. If the suspected allergen is not in the T.R.U.E. Test, refer to a specialist who will customize the patch testing. Also, personal products, such as cosmetics and lotions, can be diluted for special patch testing.
    - A meta-analysis of children patch tested for ACD showed the top five allergens to be nickel, ammonium persulfate, gold sodium thiosulfate, thimerosal, and toluene-2,5-diamine (*p*-toluenediamine).[7] Only two of these five allergens are in the T.R.U.E. Test, so it may be best to not use this standardized patch testing for children.
    - Once the patch test results are known, it is important to determine if the result is "relevant" to the patient's dermatitis. One method for classifying clinical relevance of a positive patch test reaction is:
        - current relevance—the patient has been exposed to allergen during the current episode of dermatitis and improves when the exposure ceases;
        - past relevance—past episode of dermatitis from exposure to allergen;
        - relevance not known—not sure if exposure is current or old;
        - cross-reaction—the positive test is a result of cross-reaction with another allergen; and
        - exposed—a history of exposure but not resulting in dermatitis from that exposure, or no history of exposure but a definite positive allergic patch test.[6]

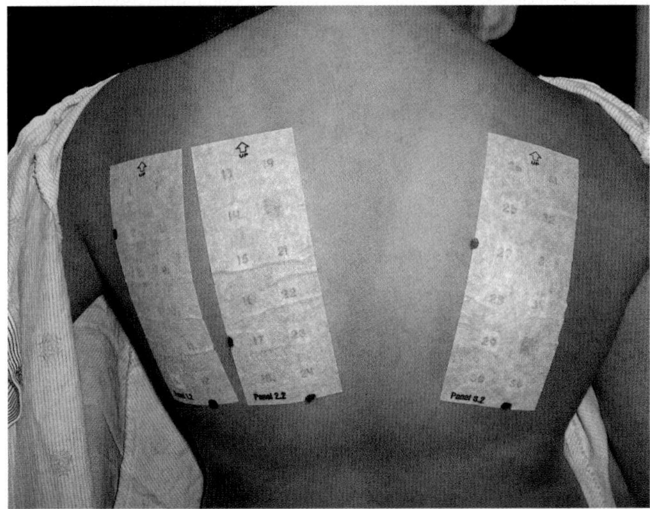

FIGURE 131-16 The T.R.U.E. Test is an easy-to-use standardized patch test that is applied to the back using 3 tape strips to test for 35 common allergens. This 8-year-old girl is starting the process of patch testing to determine the cause of her hand dermatitis. Hypoallergenic tape is about to be applied to keep the strips from peeling off for 2 days. (*Used with permission from Richard P. Usatine, MD.*)

TABLE 131-1 Allergens in T.R.U.E. Test (Patch Test for Contact Dermatitis)

Panel 1.2	Panel 2.2	Panel 3.2
1. Nickel Sulfate	13. *p*-tert-Butylphenol Formaldehyde Resin	25. Diazolidinyl urea
2. Wool Alcohols	14. Epoxy Resin	26. Quinoline mix
3. Neomycin Sulfate	15. Carba Mix	27. Tixocortol-21-pivalate
4. Potassium Dichromate	16. Black Rubber Mix	28. Gold sodium thiosulfate
5. Caine Mix	17. Cl^{+} Me^{-} Isothiazolinone (MCI/MI)	29. Imidazolidinyl urea
6. Fragrance Mix	18. Quaternium-15	30. Budesonide
7. Colophony	19. Methyldibromo glutaronitrile	31. Hydrocortizone-17-butyrate
8. Paraben Mix	20. *p*-Phenylenediamine	32. Mercaptobenzothiazole
9. Negative Control	21. Formaldehyde	33. Bacitracin
10. Balsam of Peru	22. Mercapto Mix	34. Parthenolide
11. Ethylenediamine Dihydrochloride	23. Thimerosal	35. Disperse blue 106
12. Cobalt Dichloride	24. Thiuram Mix	36. 2-Bromo-2-nitropropane-1,3-diol (Bronopol)

There are 35 allergens and one negative control at number 9.

- Punch biopsy—When another underlying disorder is suspected that is best diagnosed with histology (e.g., psoriasis).

DIFFERENTIAL DIAGNOSIS

- Atopic dermatitis is usually more widespread than CD. There is often a history of other atopic conditions, such as allergic rhinitis and asthma. There may be family history of allergies. However, persons with atopic dermatitis are more prone to CD (**Figure 131-6**; Chapter 130, Atopic Dermatitis).
- Dyshidrotic eczema—Seen on the hands and feet with tapioca vesicles, erythema, and scale. Although this is not primarily caused by contact to allergens, various irritating substances can make it worse.
- Immediate IgE contact reaction (e.g., latex glove allergy)—Immediate erythema, itching, and possibly systemic reaction after contact with a known (or suspected) allergen.
- Fungal infections—A dermatophyte infection that can closely resemble CD when it occurs on the hands and feet. Tinea pedis is usually seen between the toes, on the soles or on the sides of the feet. CD of the feet is often on the dorsum of the foot and related to rubber or other chemicals in the shoes (**Figures 131-13** and **131-14**; Chapter 125, Tinea Pedis).
- Scabies on the hands can be mistaken for CD. Look for burrows and for the typical distribution of the scabies infestation to distinguish this from CD (see Chapter 128, Scabies).
- Allergies to the dyes used in tattoos can occur. Although this is not strictly a CD because the dye is injected below the skin, the allergic process is similar (**Figure 131-18**).

MANAGEMENT

- Identify and avoid the offending agent(s).[4] SOR Ⓐ
  - Be aware that some patients are actually allergic to topical steroids. This unfortunate situation can be diagnosed with patch testing.
  - In cases of nickel ACD, we recommend the patient cover the metal tab of their jeans with an iron-on patch or a few coats of clear nail polish.
- Cool compresses can soothe the symptoms of acute cases of CD.[4] SOR Ⓒ

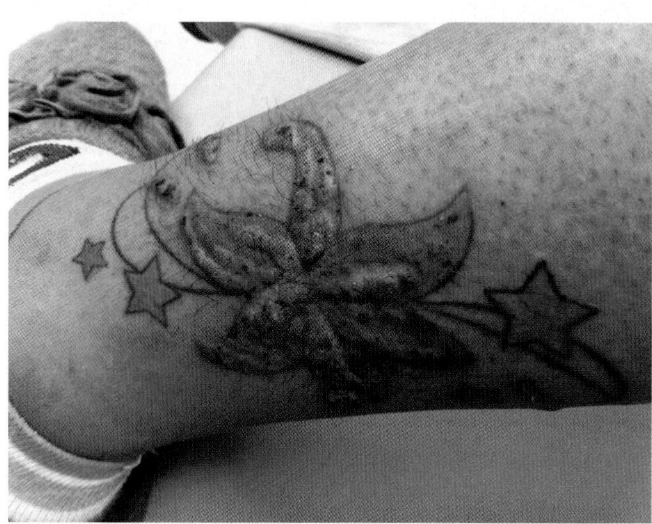

FIGURE 131-18 Allergic dermatitis to the red dye in a new tattoo. *(Used with permission from Jonathan Karnes, MD.)*

- Calamine and colloidal oatmeal baths may help to dry and soothe acute, oozing lesions.[3,4] SOR C
- Localized acute ACD lesions respond best with mid-potency to high-potency topical steroids such as 0.1 percent triamcinolone to 0.05 percent clobetasol, respectively.[4] SOR A
- On areas of thinner skin (e.g., flexural surfaces, eyelids, face, or anogenital region) lower-potency steroids such as desonide ointment can minimize the risk of skin atrophy.[3,4] SOR B
- There is insufficient data to support the use of topical steroids for ICD, but because it is difficult to distinguish clinically between ACD and ICD, these agents are frequently tried. SOR C
- If ACD involves extensive skin areas (>20%), systemic steroid therapy is often required and offers relief within 12 to 24 hours. The recommended dose is 0.5 to 1 mg/kg daily for 5 to 7 days, and if the patient is comfortable at that time, the dose may be reduced by 50 percent for the next 5 to 7 days. The rate of reduction of steroid dosage depends on factors such as severity, duration of ACD, and how effectively the allergen can be avoided.[4] SOR B
- Oral steroids should be tapered over 2 weeks because rapid discontinuance of steroids can result in rebound dermatitis. Severe poison ivy/oak is often treated with oral prednisone for 2 to 3 weeks. Avoid using a Medrol dose-pack, which has insufficient dosing and duration.[4] SOR B
- The efficacy of topical immunomodulators (tacrolimus and pimecrolimus) in ACD or ICD has not been well established.[4] However, one randomized controlled trial (RCT) did demonstrate that tacrolimus ointment is more effective than vehicle in treating chronically exposed, nickel-induced ACD.[8] SOR B
- Although antihistamines are generally not effective for pruritus associated with ACD, they are commonly used. Sedation from more soporific antihistamines may offer some degree of palliation (diphenhydramine, hydroxyzine).[4] SOR C
- Bacterial superinfection should be treated with an appropriate antibiotic that will cover *Streptococcus pyogenes* and *S. aureus*. Treat for MRSA if suspected.
- Once the diagnosis of any CD is established, emollients and moisturizers may help soothe irritated skin.[4] SOR C

For ICD and occupational CD of the hands:

- Wear protective gloves when working with known allergens or potentially irritating substances such as solvents, soaps, and detergents.[6,9] SOR A
- Use cotton liners under the gloves for both comfort and the absorption of sweat. Wearing cotton glove liners can prevent the development of an impaired skin barrier function caused by prolonged wearing of occlusive gloves.[9] SOR B
  - There is insufficient evidence to promote the use of barrier creams to protect against contact with irritants.[6,9] SOR A
  - After work, conditioning creams can improve skin condition in workers with damaged skin.[9] SOR A
- Keep hands clean, dry, and well-moisturized whenever possible.
- Petrolatum applied twice a day is a great way to moisturize dry and cracked skin without exposing the patient to new irritants.

If the CD is severe enough, the patient may need to change activities to completely avoid the offending irritant or antigen.

FOLLOW-UP

May need frequent follow-up if the offending substance is not found, the rash does not resolve and if patch testing will be needed.

PATIENT EDUCATION

Avoid the offending agent and take the medications as prescribed to relieve symptoms.

PATIENT RESOURCES

- PubMed Health. *Contact Dermatitis*—**www.ncbi.nlm.nih.gov/pubmedhealth/PMH0001872/**.
- The T.R.U.E. Test website has a wealth of information on reading labels, common allergens and patch testing for patients—**www.truetest.com/**.

PROVIDER RESOURCES

- American Family Physician. *Diagnosis and Management of Contact Dermatitis*—**www.aafp.org/afp/2010/0801/p249.html**.
- The T.R.U.E. Test website has a wealth of information on patch testing for health care professionals—**www.truetest.com/**.

REFERENCES

1. Usatine RP. A red twisted ankle. *West J Med.* 1999;171:361-362.
2. Halstater B, Usatine RP. Contact dermatitis. In: Milgrom E, Usatine RP, Tan R, Spector S, eds. *Practical Allergy*. Philadelphia, PA: Elsevier; 2004.
3. Usatine RP, Riojas M. Diagnosis and management of contact dermatitis. *Am Fam Physician.* 2010;82:249-255.
4. Beltrani VS, Bernstein IL, Cohen DE, Fonacier L. Contact dermatitis: a practice parameter. *Ann Allergy Asthma Immunol.* 2006;97:S1-S38.
5. Krob HA, Fleischer AB Jr, D'Agostino R Jr, Haverstock CL, Feldman S. Prevalence and relevance of contact dermatitis allergens: a meta-analysis of 15 years of published T.R.U.E. test data. *J Am Acad Dermatol.* 2004;51:349-353.
6. Bourke J, Coulson I, English J. Guidelines for the management of contact dermatitis: an update. *Br J Dermatol.* 2009;160:946-954.
7. Bonitsis NG, Tatsioni A, Bassioukas K, Ioannidis JP. Allergens responsible for allergic contact dermatitis among children: a systematic review and meta-analysis. *Contact Dermatitis.* 2011;64:245-257.
8. Belsito D, Wilson DC, Warshaw E, et al. A prospective randomized clinical trial of 0.1% tacrolimus ointment in a model of chronic allergic contact dermatitis. *J Am Acad Dermatol.* 2006;55:40-46.
9. Nicholson PJ, Llewellyn D, English JS. Evidence-based guidelines for the prevention, identification and management of occupational contact dermatitis and urticaria. *Contact Dermatitis.* 2010;63:177-186.

132 ECZEMA HERPETICUM

Carla Torres-Zegarra, MD
Camille Sabella, MD

PATIENT STORY

A 16-year-old-boy with a past medical history significant for atopic dermatitis presented to the Emergency Department with a 1-day history of sudden onset of tender blistering lesions on the face and neck associated with a burning sensation. Associated symptoms included lethargy, headache, and four episodes of vomiting since onset of symptoms. On exam, the boy was noted to be ill-appearing, moderately dehydrated, and febrile to 39°C. He was tachycardic but normotensive, warm, and well perfused. The skin exam revealed pustules, vesicles and crusts over his face, neck, elbows, both hands and both knees (**Figure 132-1**). He was admitted and treated with intravenous (IV) fluids, IV antibiotics, and IV acyclovir. Viral culture taken from an unroofed vesicular lesion revealed herpes simplex virus type 1. Bacterial cultures taken from the impetiginized lesions grew *Staphylococcus aureus*.

INTRODUCTION

Eczema herpeticum is an acutely disseminated herpes simplex virus (HSV) infection associated with systemic symptoms that develops in the setting of underlying skin conditions or epidermal barrier disruption, such as atopic dermatitis. HSV type 1 is most commonly involved, but cases of HSV type 2 infection and other viruses have rarely been implicated.

SYNONYMS

Kaposi varicelliform eruption.

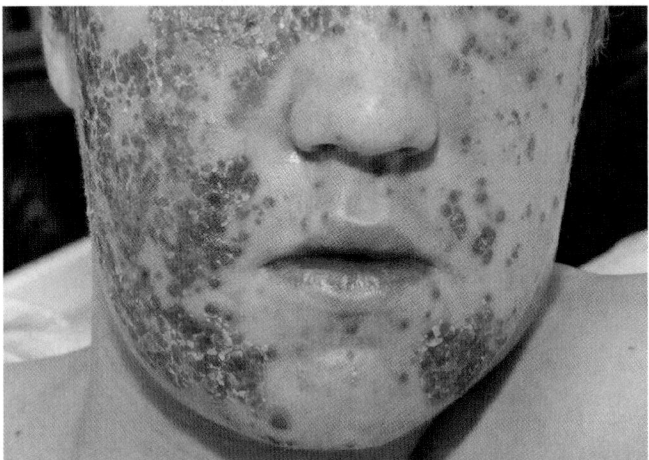

FIGURE 132-1 Eczema herpeticum in a 16-year-old-boy with a history of severe atopic dermatitis. Eczema herpeticum is a severe HSV infection in a patient with atopic dermatitis. *(Used with permission from Camille Sabella, MD.)*

EPIDEMIOLOGY

- Infants and children with atopic dermatitis are at highest risk.[1]

ETIOLOGY AND PATHOPHYSIOLOGY

- Diverse immune mechanisms have been proposed to explain the development of eczema herpeticum in patients with atopic dermatitis:
  - A disruption of the immune response against herpes simplex mediated by T cells.
  - A defect in antibody production against the virus.
  - A decrease in natural killer cells and IL-2 receptors.
  - Inhibition of TH-1 response due to increase in IL-4.
  - Decrease in dendritic cells that produce IL-1.[2]
- Another possibility is that viral dissemination is directly favored by the disruption of the skin barrier that exists in atopic dermatitis.[3]

RISK FACTORS

- Early onset of atopic dermatitis and high levels of IgE in atopic patients, based on a retrospective study involving 100 patients with eczema herpeticum.[4]
- The use of topical corticosteroids is not a predisposing factor.
- Patients with chronic skin pathology like Darier disease, cutaneous T cell lymphoma, pityriasis rubra pilaris, benign familial pemphigus, seborrheic dermatitis, Wiskott-Aldrich syndrome, psoriasis, and systemic lupus erythematosis are susceptible to eczema herpeticum. Severe infections may develop even when the dermatitis is inactive.[2]
- Other risk factors include conditions where the epidermal barrier has been disrupted, like burns, contact dermatitis, skin grafts, and dermabrasion.

DIAGNOSIS

CLINICAL FEATURES

- The diagnosis is primarily clinical, supported by isolation of HSV in culture.
- Eczema herpeticum is characterized by cutaneous pain and multiple clusters of monomorphic papules, vesicles, pustules and crusts in areas of preexisting atopic dermatitis (**Figure 132-2**).
- These lesions can spread rapidly leading to severe morbidity and mortality.[5]
- The eruption of eczema herpeticum may sometimes be difficult to distinguish from the patient's baseline eczema if the latter is poorly controlled.
- Impetigo secondary to bacterial infection can be difficult to differentiate from eczema herpeticum, and can complicate the diagnosis.
- The lesions can appear pustular or hemorrhagic (**Figure 132-3**) and can be associated with systemic symptoms like fever and

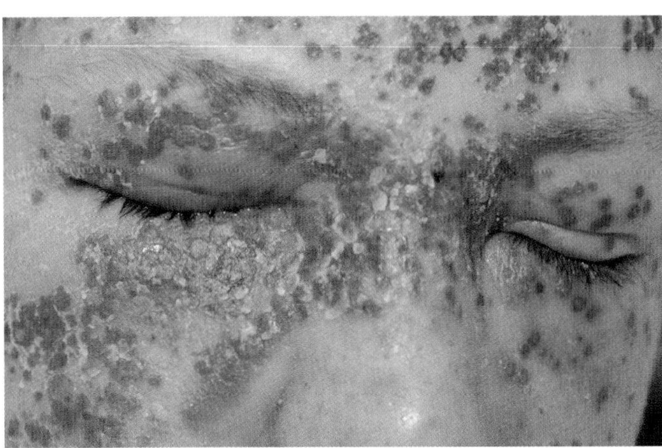

FIGURE 132-2 Close up of the eczema herpeticum lesions in the atopic patient in **Figure 132-1** showing clusters of papules, vesicles and crusted lesions secondary to HSV. Some of the crusting is secondary to impetiginized lesions from a *S. aureus* bacterial superinfection. (*Used with permission from Camille Sabella, MD.*)

general malaise. Such a presentation is also consistent with bacterial superinfection, which is one of the key considerations in the differential diagnosis.

- Erythema and swelling of the periorbital area may be marked and may represent the primary process or a secondary bacterial cellulitis (**Figure 132-4**).
- Duration of illness is 16 days on average, but ranges from 2 to 6 weeks. About 13 to 16 percent of patients can develop recurrent episodes, which tend to be milder, with limited skin involvement and are less commonly associated with systemic symptoms.[2]
- The most common complication is secondary bacterial infection of the skin; *S aureus* is the most common pathogen isolated.
- Rarely, eczema herpeticum may present as a fulminating disease with widespread lesions, multiorgan involvement, bone marrow suppression, and disseminated intravascular coagulation.

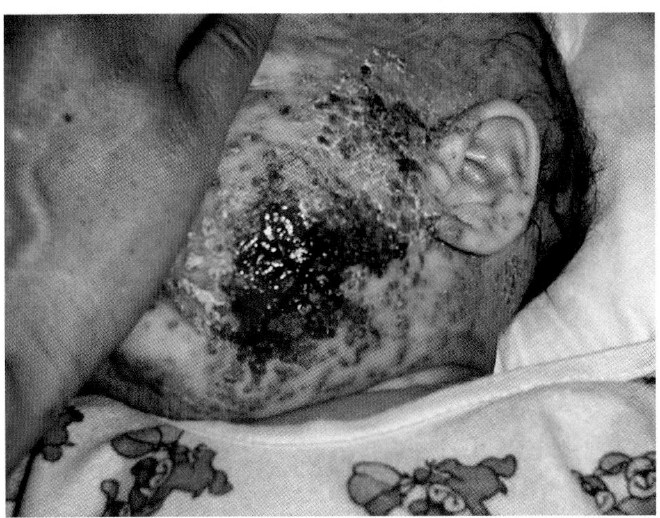

FIGURE 132-3 Eczema herpeticum in a 5-month-old infant with severe atopic dermatitis presenting with ulcerated and hemorrhagic lesions along with vesicles, papules and crusts. Viral culture from an unroofed vesicle yielded HSV. (*Used with permission from Camille Sabella, MD.*)

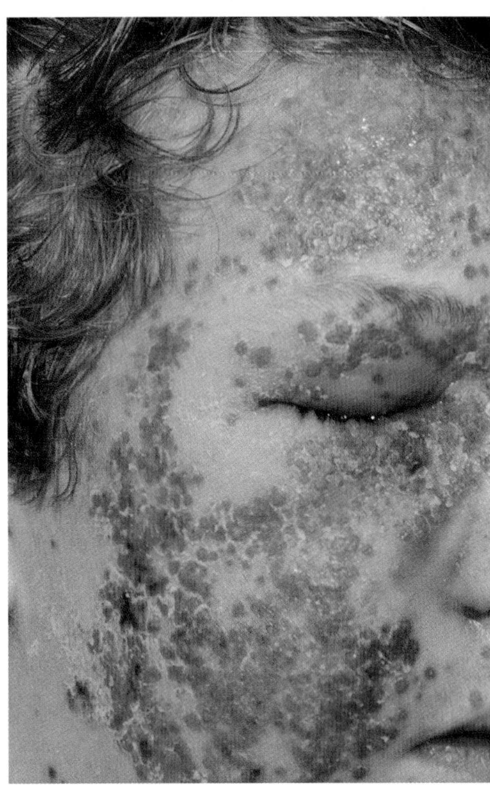

FIGURE 132-4 Periorbital erythema and induration associated with eczema herpeticum in the same patient as **Figure 132-1**. (*Used with permission from Camille Sabella, MD.*)

LABORATORY TESTING

- Culture of HSV from skin lesions is the most sensitive and specific method of diagnosing an active HSV infection.[6]
- Direct fluorescent antibody (DFA) staining of infected cells is 80 to 90 percent sensitive and very specific. DFA can provide a rapid diagnosis within 24 hours.[7,8] Many labs will do the DFA staining and then set up a culture if this is negative.
- Cells for culture and DFA are best obtained by unroofing an intact vesicle and removing cells from the base of the lesion. When an intact vesicle is not available, new lesions are better than old lesions and ulcers are better than crusts.
- Tzank smear of material from the floor of an intact vesicle may reveal multinucleated giant cells, which supports the diagnosis. Although this provides a rapid and inexpensive method of diagnosis, it is no longer recommended, given the availability of culture and DFA, which are more sensitive and specific.
- Bacterial cultures from the skin lesions and blood cultures should be obtained if secondary bacterial infection is suspected.

DIFFERENTIAL DIAGNOSIS

- Coxsackie virus A16, which causes hand-foot-and-mouth disease. The lesions are usually flat-topped vesicles on the palms, soles and oral mucosa. These lesions do not have the same degree of crusting seen in eczema herpeticum (see Chapter 113, Hand, Foot, and Mouth Disease).

- Impetigo that presents with honey-crusted lesions usually has slower evolution and fewer systemic symptoms. Discrete vesicular lesions are not usually present (see Chapter 99, Impetigo).
- Varicella (Chickenpox) is characterized by crops of polymorphic lesions in various stages of development. It often has a more widespread distribution (see Chapter 108, Varicella).
- Other uncommon causes of vesicobullous virus infections include Coxsackie virus A5, 9, and 10; Echovirus 4, 9, 11, 17, and 25; and variola and vaccinia (cowpox).

MANAGEMENT

MEDICATIONS

- Prompt intravenous antiviral therapy with acyclovir is indicated while awaiting diagnostic testing for HSV. Patients should be hospitalized and the route should be intravenous if systemic symptoms are present.[9,10] SOR B
- Delay of acyclovir initiation is associated with increased length of stay (LOS) in hospitalized children with eczema herpeticum.[11] SOR B
- Use of topical corticosteroids on admission is not associated with increased LOS.[11] SOR B
- Emollients may be used to treat the underlying eczema.
- If bacterial superinfection is suspected, intravenous or oral systemic antibiotics active against *S aureus* and *Streptococcus pyogenes* should be given. SOR C
- There is no evidence to support the use of topical antibiotics.[2] SOR B
- Topical ophthalmic acyclovir may be added if there is evidence of periocular involvement, to prevent herpetic keratitis.

REFERRAL

- Dermatology consultation should be obtained on admission.
- Ophthalmology consultation should be obtained if periocular involvement is present.

PREVENTION AND SCREENING

- Good control of atopic dermatitis may be important in helping to control the severity of involvement and decrease risk of bacterial superinfection.

PROGNOSIS

- Prompt use of acyclovir has decreased mortality from 50 to 10 percent.[10,11]
- If left untreated, skin loss may lead to all complications usually associated with severe burns: hypovolemia, hypothermia, hypoalbuminemia, hypokalemia, disseminated intravascular coagulation, and superadded bacterial infections.
- With periocular involvement, herpetic keratitis and conjunctivitis can occur.

FOLLOW-UP

- Dermatology and ophthalmology follow-up may be indicated depending on the initial presentation and course.
- If the original atopic dermatitis was not controlled, then dermatology follow-up is needed for that reason alone.

PATIENT EDUCATION

- With early recognition, eczema herpeticum can be effectively treated. Any patient with history of atopic dermatitis, who develops acute blistering should be evaluated and treated empirically for eczema herpeticum.
- Consider advising patients to discard previously used emollients or creams (especially if it is stored in tubs) if contamination is suspected.
- It is important to keep atopic dermatitis well treated and under control to preserve the important barrier function of the skin.

PATIENT RESOURCES

- **http://emedicine.medscape.com/article/1132622-overview**.
- **www.nationaleczema.org/living-with-eczema/tips/ask-the-experts/eczema-herpeticum**.

PROVIDER RESOURCES

- Varicelliform eruption—**www.emedicine.com/derm/topic 204.htm**.

REFERENCES

1. Knoell K, Greer K. Atopic dermatitis. Pediatrics in review 1999:20(2):46-52.
2. Schroeder HF, Elgueta NA, Martínez GMJ. Eczema herpeticum caused by herpes simplex virus type 2. Review of the literature about one case. *Rev Chilena Infectol.* 2009;26(4):356-359.
3. Kramer S, Thomas C, Tyler W, Elston D. Kaposi's varicelliform eruption: A case report and review of the literature. *Cutis.* 2004;73:115-122.
4. Wollenberg A, Zoch C, Wetzel S, Plewig G, Przybilla B. Predisposing factors and clinical features of eczema herpeticum: a retrospective analysis of 100 cases. *J Am Acad Dermatol.* 2003;49: 198-205.
5. Sanderson IR, L A Brueton L, Savage M, and Harper J. Eczema herpeticum: a potentially fatal disease. *Br Med J (Clin Res Ed).* 1987;294(6573):693-694.
6. Moseley RC, Corey L, Benjamin D, et al. Comparison of viral isolation, direct immunofluorescence, and indirect immunoperoxidase techniques for detection of genital herpes simplex virus infection. *J Clin Microbiol.* 1981;13:913.

7. Goldstein LC, Corey L, McDougall JK, et al. Monoclonal antibodies to herpes simplex viruses: Use in antigenic typing and rapid diagnosis. *J Infect Dis*. 1983;147:829.
8. Pouletty P, Chomel JJ, Thouvenot D, et al. Detection of herpes simplex virus in direct specimens by immunofluorescence assay using a monoclonal antibody. *J Clin Microbiol*. 1987;25:958.
9. Nikkels AF, Pièrard GE. Treatment of mucocutaneous presentations of herpes simplex virus infections. *Am J Clin Dermatol*. 2002;3(7):475.
10. Wetzel S, Wollenberg A. Eczema herpeticatum. Hautarzt. 2006;57 (7):586-591.
11. Aronson P, Yan A C, Mittal M, Mohamad Z, Shah S. Delayed Acyclovir and Outcomes of Children Hospitalized With Eczema Herpeticum. *Pediatrics*. 2011:128(6):1161-1167.

133 NUMMULAR ECZEMA

Yu Wah, MD
Richard P. Usatine, MD

PATIENT STORY

A 2-year-old Hispanic male presents to the clinic with erythematous, round, moist, crusted lesions on the left thigh (**Figure 133-1**) and right arm. His mother noted several small bumps initially, which developed into coin-shaped lesions over the next few weeks. The child is scratching them but is otherwise healthy. A KOH preparation of the scraping from the lesions did not show fungal structures. The child responds well to treatment with topical mid-potency corticosteroids, emollients, and dressing in long-sleeve clothes to prevent scratching the lesions. His nummular eczema resolved in 6 weeks.

INTRODUCTION

Nummular eczema (NE) is a type of eczema characterized by circular or oval-shaped scaling plaques with well-defined borders. The term *nummular* refers to the shape of a coin (Latin for coin is *nummus*). The lesions are typically multiple and most commonly found on the dorsa of the hands, arms, and legs. It often overlaps with other clinical types of eczema: atopic dermatitis, stasis dermatitis, and asteatotic eczema.[1,2]

SYNONYMS

Nummular dermatitis, discoid eczema, microbial eczema, and orbicular eczema.

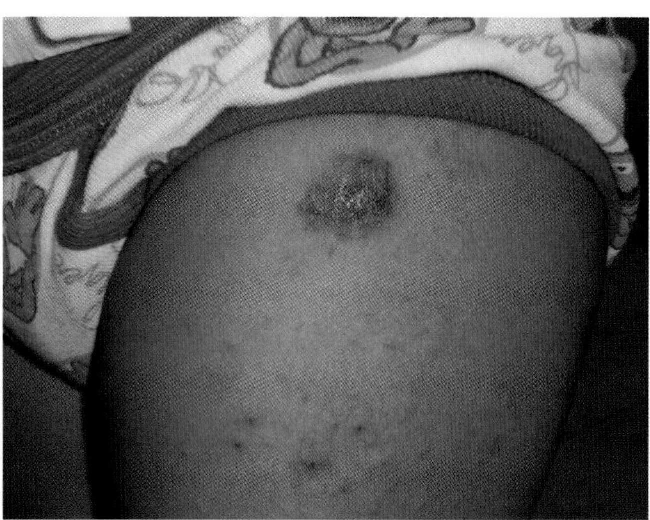

FIGURE 133-1 A 2-year-old child with nummular eczema on the left thigh. The lesion shows abrasions and excoriations from scratching. He has another similar lesion on the right arm. (*Used with permission from Yu Wah, MD.*)

EPIDEMIOLOGY

- Prevalence is reported to range widely from 0.1 to 9.1 percent.[1]
- It is slightly more common in males than in females.[1]
- Males are also affected at a later age (peak older than age 50 years) than females (peak younger than age 30 years).[1]
- It is less common in children.

ETIOLOGY AND PATHOPHYSIOLOGY

Many factors have been reported in association with NE but their role in the etiology and pathogenesis is not well established:

- NE has been viewed as microbial in origin, either secondary to bacterial colonization or hematogenous spread of bacterial toxins,[1,3] but an infectious source is not identified in most cases of NE.
- NE is reported to be associated with xerosis of the skin that subsequently weakens the skin barrier function and sensitizes it to environmental allergens.[4]
- NE is frequently reported in association with contact sensitization to various agents, including nickel, chromate, balsam of Peru, and fragrances. Allergic or chronic contact dermatitis has been frequently reported to manifest as NE on the dorsa of the hands.[1,5]
- Onset of NE has been reported in association with various medications, including interferon and ribavirin therapy for hepatitis C[6,7] and isotretinoin.[8] Most of these reports are based on single or limited number of cases.
- Mercury in the dental amalgam was reported to induce NE in two cases with relapsing NE.[9]

DIAGNOSIS

HISTORY

- Onset is reported to be within days to week. Simultaneous or subsequent development of multiple lesions is often reported.
- Intense pruritus or burning is common.
- Lesions may last months to years without treatment and may be recurrent.
- History of medications, atopy, and exposure to allergens may be helpful to tailor the management of NE.

PHYSICAL EXAMINATION

- Primary morphology includes small papules and vesicles that coalesce to form circular to oval shape patches and plaques (**Figures 133-2** and **133-3**).
- Secondary morphology includes abrasion and excoriations from scratching (**Figure 133-1**), weeping and crusting after the vesicles leak (**Figures 133-2** to **133-4**), and scaling and lichenification in more chronic lesions (**Figures 133-5** and **133-6**). Excessive weeping and crusting may indicate secondary bacterial infection.

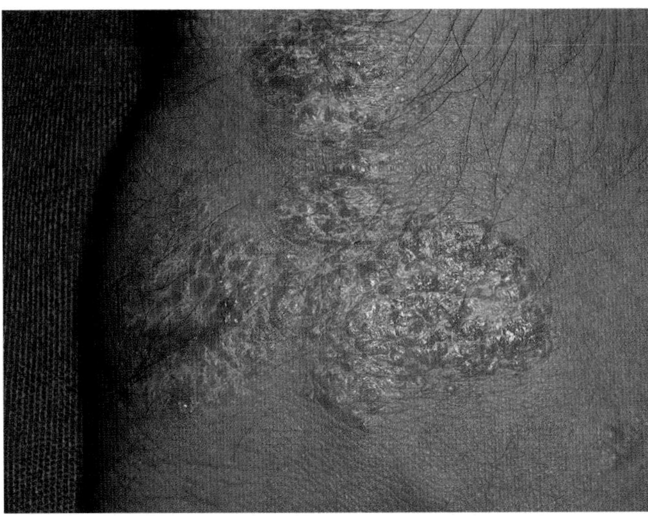

FIGURE 133-2 Multiple nummular lesions on the dorsum of the hand, a common site of nummular eczema. The lesions show multiple papules and vesicles that coalesce to form coin-shaped plaques; oozing and crusting can be seen from ruptured vesicles. (*Used with permission from Richard P. Usatine, MD.*)

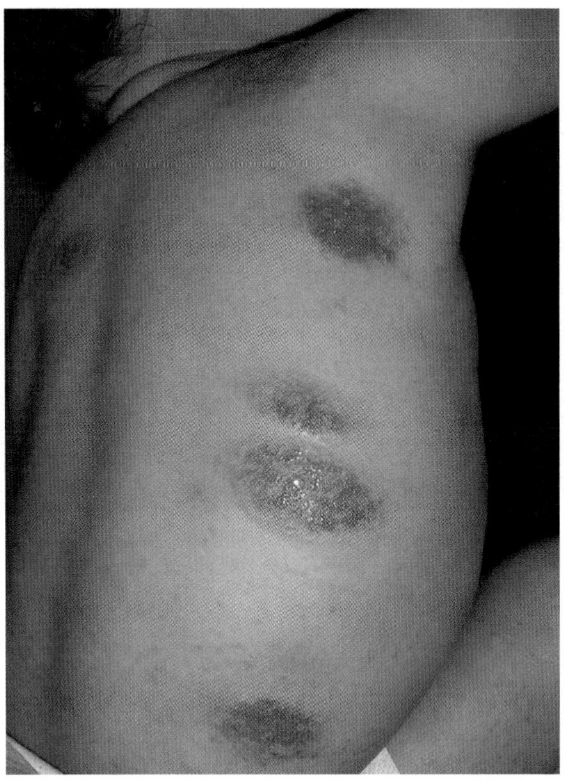

FIGURE 133-4 Superinfected nummular eczema healing on the trunk of a 2-year-old girl receiving topical triamcinolone ointment and oral cephalexin. (*Used with permission from Richard P. Usatine, MD.*)

TYPICAL DISTRIBUTION

- Dorsal hand is most commonly affected (**Figures 133-2** and **133-7**). The extensor aspects of the forearm (**Figures 133-3** and **133-6**) and the lower leg (**Figure 133-5**), the thighs (**Figure 133-1**), and the flanks are frequently involved, but NE may be seen in any part of the body (**Figures 133-4**, **133-8**, and **133-9**).

LABORATORY TESTING

- Diagnosis in most cases is made from clinical features.
- KOH preparation is helpful to investigate for tinea corporis.
- Patch testing may be considered if contact allergy is suspected.

BIOPSY

- Biopsy is rarely needed, but should be performed if there is suspicion of other serious clinical entities (e.g., mycosis fungoides, psoriasis) or if the diagnosis is uncertain.

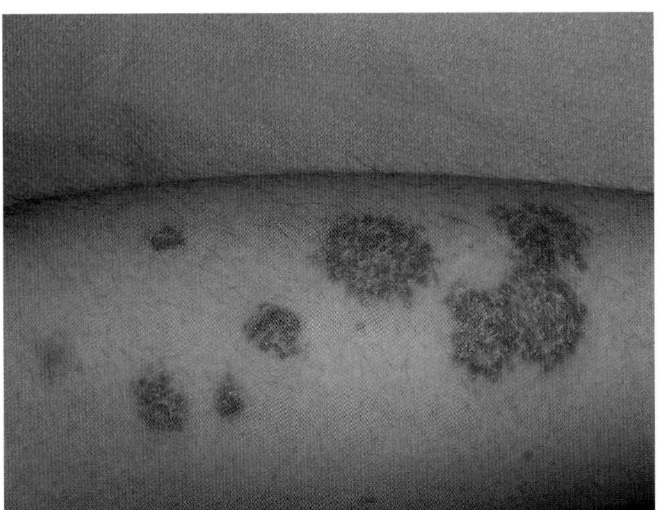

FIGURE 133-3 Nummular eczema on the forearm of a young man. The lesions show multiple papules and vesicles that coalesce to form coin-shaped plaques; oozing and crusting can be seen from ruptured vesicles. (*Used with permission from Richard P. Usatine, MD.*)

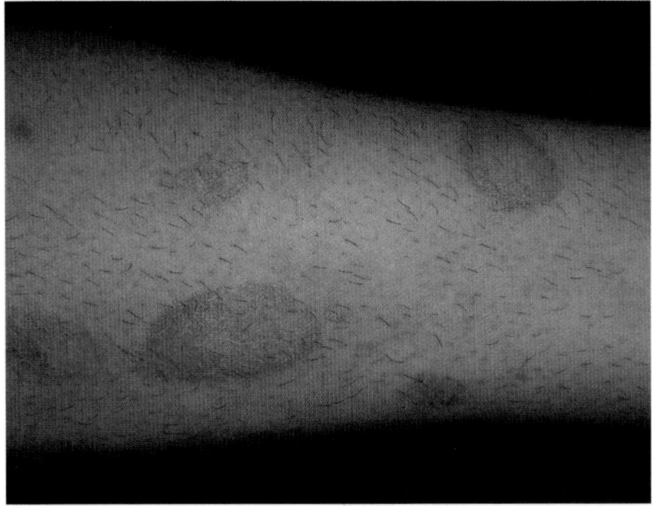

FIGURE 133-5 Multiple nummular lesions on the lower leg of a 15-year-old girl. Lesions of nummular eczema can be dry and scaly. The lesions prevented the patient from shaving her legs. (*Used with permission from Richard P. Usatine, MD.*)

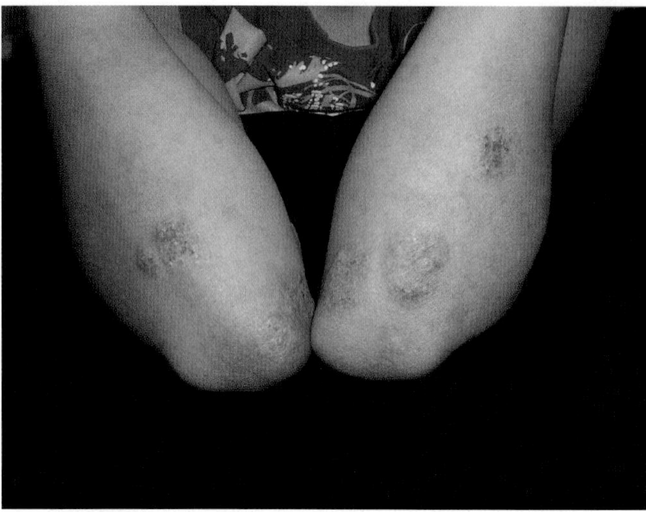

FIGURE 133-6 Nummular eczema on the extensor surface of the forearms and elbows. Thickened, scaly lesions resemble psoriatic plaques. A biopsy was performed to confirm the diagnosis of nummular eczema. (*Used with permission from Richard P. Usatine, MD.*)

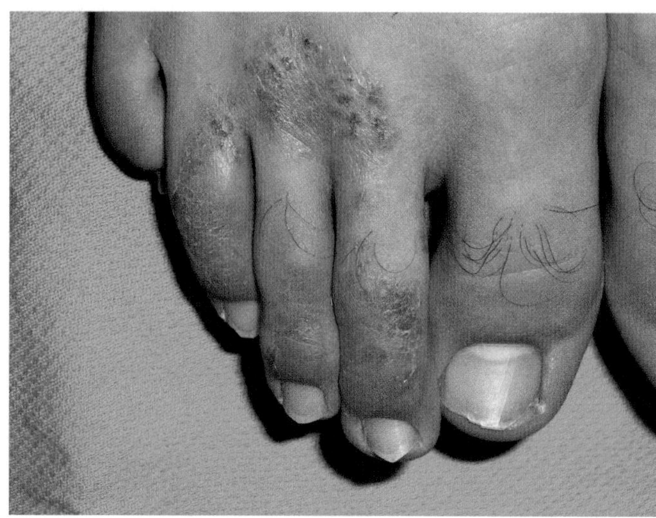

FIGURE 133-8 Nummular eczema on the dorsum of the foot. Contact dermatitis and tinea pedis are also in the differential diagnosis. KOH preparation was negative and the lesions did resolve with a topical steroid. (*Used with permission from Richard P. Usatine, MD.*)

DIFFERENTIAL DIAGNOSIS

- Tinea corporis may present as pruritic annular lesions with scales and vesicles. Vesicles are typically at the periphery of the lesion compared to NE, where they are also seen in the center. A positive KOH preparation for hyphae can help with the diagnosis (see Chapter 123, Tinea Corporis).
- Psoriasis typically presents with thickened plaques on the extensor surfaces of arms and legs, scalp and sacral areas. Nail changes may be present (see Chapter 136, Psoriasis).
- Lichen simplex chronicus usually presents as a single plaque in an area easily accessible to scratching such as the ankle, wrist, and neck (**Figures 133-10** to **133-12**).
- Nummular lesions of atopic dermatitis may have features similar to NE. Presence of other lesions typically on flexural surfaces, and a history of atopy, asthma, or seasonal allergies may help make the diagnosis (see Chapter 130, Atopic Dermatitis).
- Contact dermatitis (CD) may present with nummular lesions. History of exposure to contact allergens at the affected areas can raise the suspicion for CD. Patch testing may be used to confirm the clinical suspicion (see Chapter 131, Contact Dermatitis).

MANAGEMENT

- Emollients are beneficial to help restore and maintain normal skin barrier function. SOR Ⓒ
- Hydration by bathing before bedtime followed by ointment application to wet skin is reported as an effective method of skin care in patients with eczema.[10] SOR Ⓑ

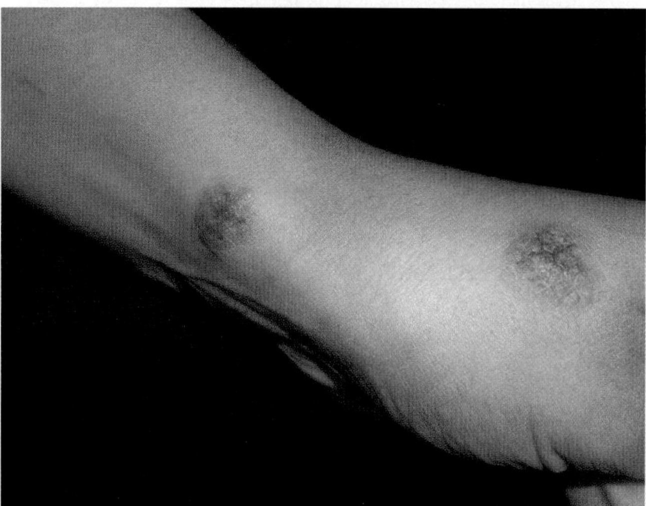

FIGURE 133-7 Nummular eczema on the dorsum of the hand and wrist. (*Used with permission from Richard P. Usatine, MD.*)

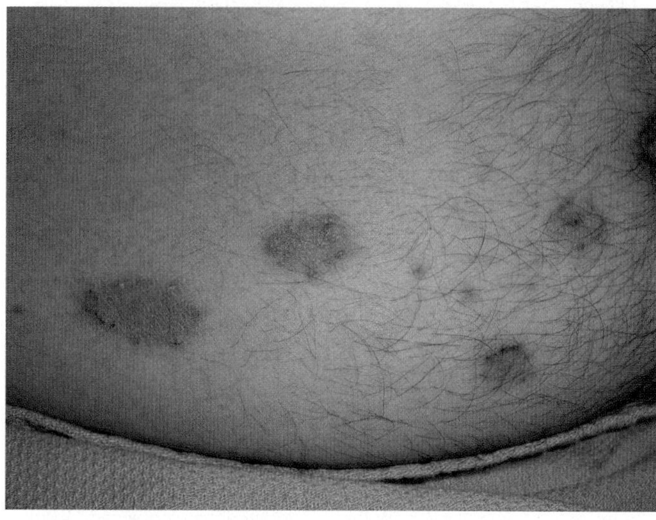

FIGURE 133-9 Nummular eczema on the abdomen of a young man. (*Used with permission from Richard P. Usatine, MD.*)

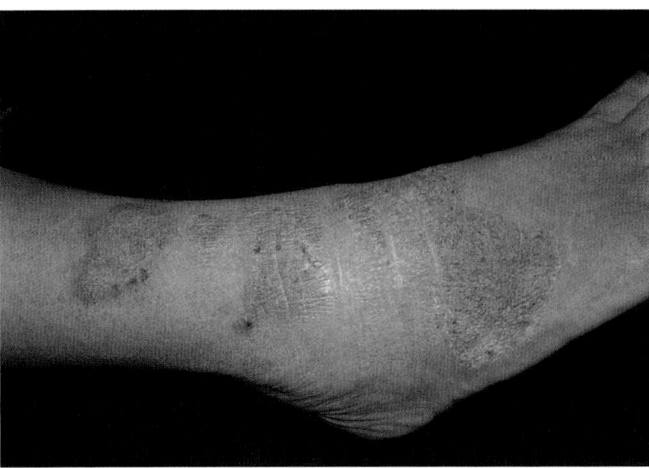

FIGURE 133-10 Lichen simplex chronicus on the ankle. Note the lichenification of the involved skin which has become thickened with accentuated skin lines. There is also postinflammatory hyperpigmentation. (*Used with permission from Richard P. Usatine, MD.*)

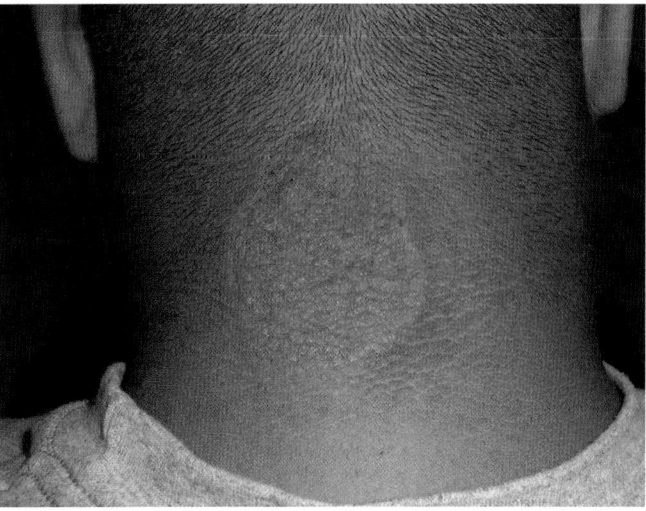

FIGURE 133-12 Lichen simplex chronicus on the neck of a 15-year-old boy. (*Used with permission from Richard P. Usatine, MD.*)

- A medium- to high-potency topical corticosteroid ointment is the first line of treatment. A cream preparation may be used if patient compliance is a concern with ointments. SOR Ⓒ
- Topical calcineurin inhibitors such as topical tacrolimus and pimecrolimus have the benefit of not causing skin atrophy and have been shown to be effective in many types of eczema.[1] SOR Ⓑ They have a higher cost compared to topical corticosteroids and have a black box warning because of a reported risk of malignancies.

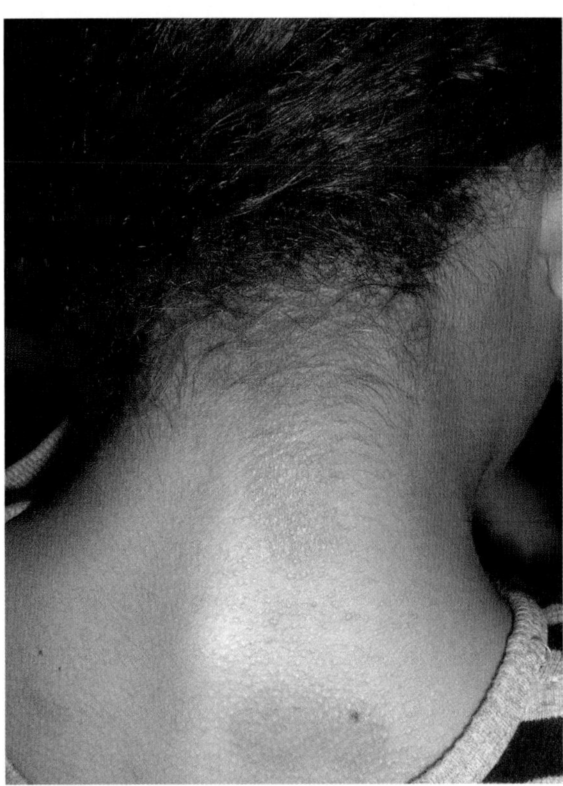

FIGURE 133-11 Lichen simplex chronicus on the neck of a 13-year-old girl. Lichen simplex chronicus is frequently found on the neck. (*Used with permission from Richard P. Usatine, MD.*)

- Short courses of systemic corticosteroids may be necessary in severe or acute cases. SOR Ⓒ
- Methotrexate is reported to be safe, effective, and well-tolerated in treatment of moderate to severe childhood NE.[11] This was reported in a case series of 25 pediatric patients with refractory NE treated with 5 or 10 mg of methotrexate per week. Sixty-four percent had total clearance after an average of 10.5 months. No serious adverse events were observed in this study.[11] SOR Ⓑ
- Phototherapy may be used in generalized, severe, or refractory cases.[1,2] Narrow-band UVB is commonly used and psoralen UVA has been used in more severe cases.[2] SOR Ⓒ
- Topical and oral antihistamines are often needed to treat pruritus. Topical doxepin is reported to be effective in treatment of pruritus associated with eczematous conditions and has a favorable safety profile.[12] SOR Ⓑ
- Topical and systemic antibiotics may be needed to treat secondary or associated bacterial infection. SOR Ⓒ
- Complementary therapy with probiotics is not effective in treatment of eczema and carries a small risk of adverse events.[13] SOR Ⓐ

FOLLOW-UP

Regular follow-up is needed for the patient with chronic, refractory, or relapsing nummular dermatitis until remission or resolution is achieved.

PATIENT EDUCATION

Hydration and protection of skin form irritants is important. Apply moisturizer or topical medications immediately after bathing while the skin is still moist. Avoid strong soaps and use mild fragrance-free soap, or soap alternatives. Avoid tight clothing and fabrics that irritate the skin.

PATIENT RESOURCES

- American Academy of Dermatology. *Nummular Dermatitis*—**www.aad.org/skin-conditions/dermatology-a-to-z/nummular-dermatitis**.
- British Association of Dermatologists. *Discoid Eczema*—**www.bad.org.uk/site/811/Default.aspx**.

PROVIDER RESOURCES

- Medscape. *Nummular Dermatitis*—**http://emedicine.medscape.com/article/1123605**.

REFERENCES

1. Bolognia J. *Dermatology*. St. Louis, MO: Mosby/Elsevier; 2008.
2. Miller J. *Nummular Dermatitis*, http://emedicine.medscape.com/article/1123605, updated May 20, 2011, accessed November 12, 2011.
3. Tanaka T, Satoh T, Yokozeki H. Dental infection associated with nummular eczema as an overlooked focal infection. *J Dermatol.* 2009;36(8):462-465.
4. Aoyama H, Tanaka M, Hara M, Tabata N, Tagami H. Nummular eczema: an addition of senile xerosis and unique cutaneous reactivities to environmental aeroallergens. *Dermatology*. 1999;199(2):135-139.
5. Wilkinson DS. Discoid eczema as a consequence of contact with irritants. *Contact Dermatitis.* 1979;5(2):118-119.
6. Moore MM, Elpern DJ, Carter DJ. Severe, generalized nummular eczema secondary to interferon alfa-2b plus ribavirin combination therapy in a patient with chronic hepatitis C virus infection. *Arch Dermatol.* 2004;140(2):215-217.
7. Shen Y, Pielop J, Hsu S. Generalized nummular eczema secondary to peginterferon Alfa-2b and ribavirin combination therapy for hepatitis C infection. *Arch Dermatol.* 2005;141(1):102-103.
8. Bettoli V, Tosti A, Varotti C. Nummular eczema during isotretinoin treatment. *J Am Acad Dermatol.* 1987;16(3 Pt 1):617.
9. Adachi A, Horikawa T, Takashima T, Ichihashi M. Mercury-induced nummular dermatitis. *J Am Acad Dermatol.* 2000;43(2):383-385.
10. Gutman AB, Kligman AM, Sciacca J, James WD. Soak and smear: a standard technique revisited. *Arch Dermatol.* 2005;141(12):1556-1569.
11. Roberts H, Orchard D. Methotrexate is a safe and effective treatment for paediatric discoid (nummular) eczema: a case series of 25 children. *Australas J Dermatol.* 2010;51(2):128-130.
12. Drake LA, Millikan LE. The antipruritic effect of 5% doxepin cream in patients with eczematous dermatitis. Doxepin Study Group. *Arch Dermatol.* 1995;131(12):1403-1408.
13. Boyle RJ, Bath-Hextall FJ, Leonardi-Bee J, Murrell DF, Tang ML. Probiotics for treating eczema. *Cochrane Database Syst Rev.* 2008;(4):CD006135.

134 URTICARIA AND ANGIOEDEMA

Richard P. Usatine, MD

PATIENT STORY

A penicillin allergic young boy was given trimethoprim-sulfamethoxazole for otitis media and broke out in hives one week later. The hives were on his trunk and arms (**Figure 134-1**). He had no airway symptoms and had only urticaria without angioedema. His fever was gone, his ear pain was resolved, and his tympanic membranes were not bulging, so his parents were told to stop the antibiotic. The pediatrician prescribed an H_1-blocker that gave him relief of symptoms and the wheals disappeared over the next 2 days.

INTRODUCTION

Urticaria and angioedema are a heterogeneous group of diseases that cause swelling of the skin and other soft tissues. They both result from a large variety of underlying causes, are elicited by a great diversity of factors, and present clinically in a highly variable way.[1] Standard hives with transient wheals is the most common manifestation of urticaria.

FIGURE 134-1 A young boy with acute urticaria due to trimethoprim-sulfamethoxazole. (*Used with permission from Richard P. Usatine, MD.*)

SYNONYMS

Hives.

EPIDEMIOLOGY

- It is estimated that 15 to 25 percent of the population may have urticaria sometime during their lifetime.[2]
- Urticaria affects 6 to 7 percent of preschool children and 17 percent of children with atopic dermatitis.[2]
- Among all age groups, approximately 50 percent have both urticaria and angioedema, 40 percent have isolated urticaria, and 10 percent have angioedema alone.[2]
- Acute urticaria is defined as less than 6 weeks' duration. A specific cause is more likely to be identified in acute urticaria.[2]
- The cause of chronic urticaria (>6 weeks' duration) is determined in less than 20 percent of cases.[2]
- Chronic urticaria predominantly affects adults.[3]
- Up to 40 percent of patients with chronic urticaria of more than 6 months' duration still have urticaria 10 years later.[3]

ETIOLOGY AND PATHOPHYSIOLOGY

- The pathophysiology of angioedema and urticaria can be immunoglobulin (Ig) E mediated, complement mediated, related to physical stimuli, autoantibody mediated, or idiopathic.
- These mechanisms lead to mast cell degranulation resulting in the release of histamine. The histamine and other inflammatory mediators produce the wheals, edema, and pruritus.
- Urticaria is a dynamic process in which new wheals evolve as old ones resolve. These wheals result from localized capillary vasodilation, followed by transudation of protein-rich fluid into the surrounding skin. The wheals resolve when the fluid is slowly reabsorbed.
- Angioedema is an edematous area that involves transudation of fluid into the dermis and subcutaneous tissue (**Figures 134-2** and **134-3**).

The following etiologic types exist:

- Immunologic—IgE mediated, complement mediated. Occurs more often in patients with an atopic background. Antigens are most commonly foods or medications. The most common foods are milk, nuts, wheat, and shellfish.
- Physical urticaria—Dermatographism, cold, cholinergic, solar, pressure, and vibratory urticaria (**Figures 134-4** to **134-6**).
- Urticaria caused by mast cell-releasing agents—Mastocytosis and urticaria pigmentosa (**Figures 134-7** and **134-8**).
- Urticaria associated with vascular/connective tissue autoimmune disease.
- Hereditary angioedema is a potentially life-threatening disorder that is inherited in an autosomal dominant manner. In this disease, angioedema occurs without urticaria.

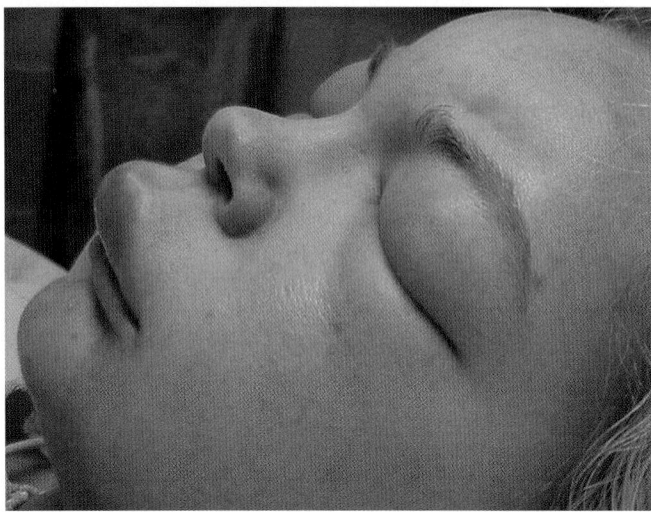

FIGURE 134-2 Severe angioedema around the eyes and mouth in a high school girl. (*Used with permission from Daniel Stulberg, MD.*)

DIAGNOSIS

CLINICAL FEATURES

- Symptoms include itching, burning, and stinging.
- Wheals vary in size from small, 2-mm papules of cholinergic urticaria (**Figure 134-6**) to giant hives where a single wheal may cover a large portion of the trunk.
- The wheal may be all red or white, or the border may be red with the remainder of the surface white.
- Wheals may be annular (**Figures 134-9** to **134-11**).
- If dermatographism is present, one can write on the skin and be able to see the resulting words or shapes (**Figure 134-5**).
- If you suspect urticaria pigmentosa, stroke a lesion with the wooden end of a cotton-tipped applicator. This induces erythema of the plaque and the wheal is confined to the stroke site. This is called Darier sign (**Figures 134-12** and **134-13**).

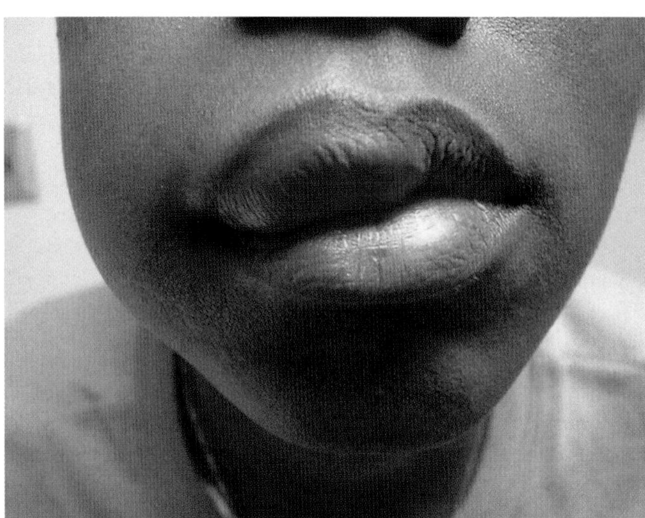

FIGURE 134-3 Young black woman with angioedema after being started on an angiotensin-converting enzyme (ACE) inhibitor for essential hypertension. (*Used with permission from Adrian Casillas, MD.*)

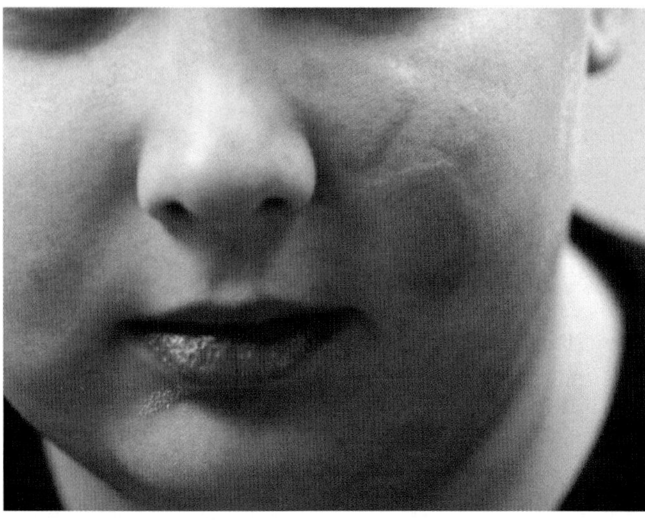

FIGURE 134-4 Cold urticaria demonstrated on the face of a young boy using a 2-minute application of an ice cube to the face. This "ice cube test" is diagnostic as the reaction mirrored the shape of the cube held against the skin. Avoiding cold and the use of antihistamines are the mainstay of treatment. Jumping into a pool can lead to hypotension and drowning in these children. Prescribe an Epi Pen for safety. (*Image used with permission from Robert Brodell, MD.*)

TYPICAL DISTRIBUTION

- Angioedema is seen more often on the face and is especially found around the mouth and eyes (**Figures 134-2** and **134-3**). Sometimes angioedema can occur on the genitals or the trunk.
- Urticaria can be found anywhere on the body and is often on the trunk and extremities (**Figures 134-14** and **134-15**).

LABORATORY STUDIES

Consider tests that might help reveal the cause of the urticaria and/or angioedema.

- Order complement studies to investigate for hereditary or acquired C1 esterase inhibitor deficiency when angioedema occurs repeatedly without urticaria.

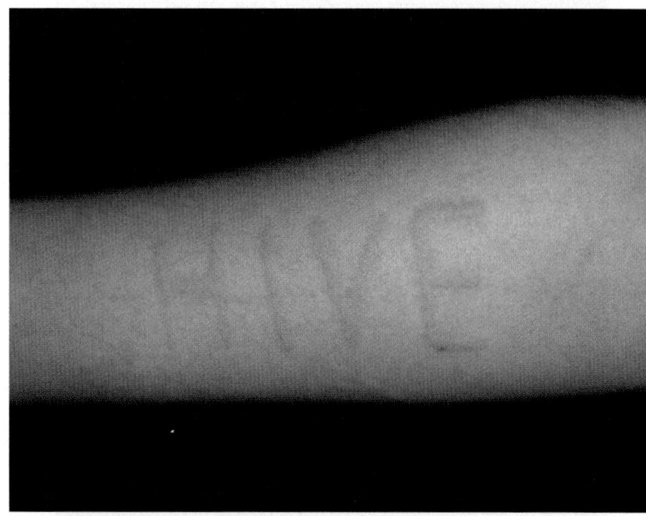

FIGURE 134-5 Dermatographism in a 15-year-old girl with chronic urticaria. Note the exaggerated triple reaction. (*Used with permission from Richard P. Usatine, MD.*)

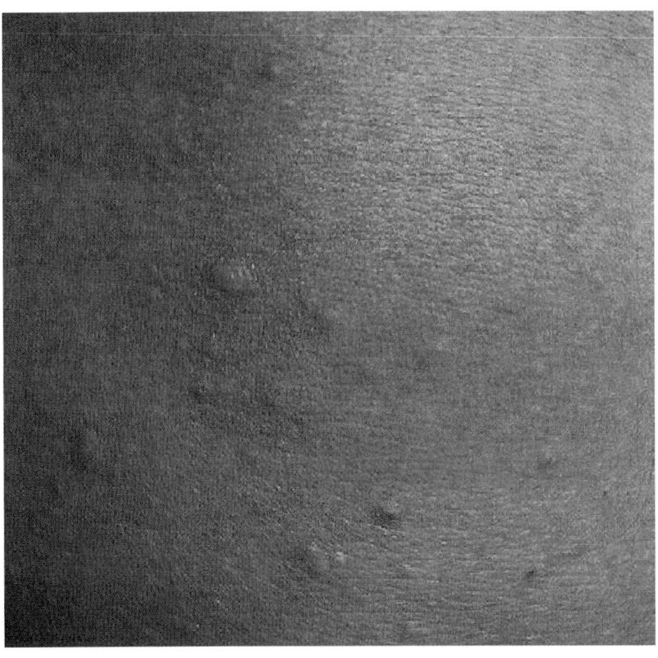

FIGURE 134-6 Cholinergic urticaria showing small wheals. The patient would get this urticaria after exercising. (*Used with permission from Philip C. Anderson, MD.*)

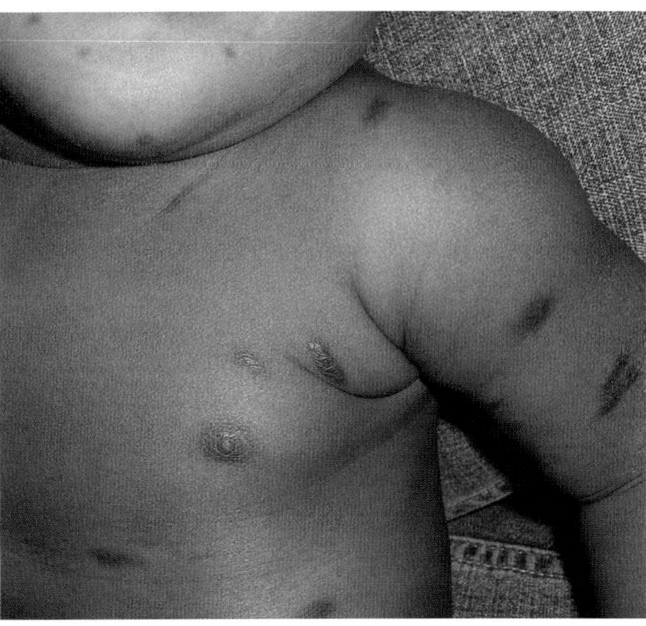

FIGURE 134-8 Urticaria pigmentosa in a 4-month-old black boy. His lesions started on day 2 of life and have proliferated. (*Used with permission from Richard P. Usatine, MD.*)

- Consider allergen skin testing and/or in vitro tests for when the history reveals that urticaria/angioedema occurs after direct contact with a suspected allergen.
- Punch biopsy of the involved area may be used to diagnose urticarial vasculitis or mastocytosis.

DIFFERENTIAL DIAGNOSIS

- Insect bites—A good history and physical examination should help to distinguish between insect bites and urticaria.
- Erythema multiforme like urticaria can occur in response to an allergic/immunologic reaction to medications, infections, and neoplasms. The classic lesion of erythema multiforme is the target lesion in which there is disruption of the epithelium in the center. This disruption may be a vesicle, bulla, or erosion. Do not confuse annular lesions or concentric rings with erythema multiforme if the epidermis is intact (**Figure 134-11** is *not* erythema multiforme) (see Chapter 151, Erythema Multiforme, Stevens-Johnson Syndrome, and Toxic Epidermal Necrolysis).
- Urticarial vasculitis typically has lesions that last longer than 24 hours. The lesions are found more commonly on the lower extremities, and when they heal, they often leave hyperpigmented areas. Causes range from a hypersensitivity vasculitis, such as

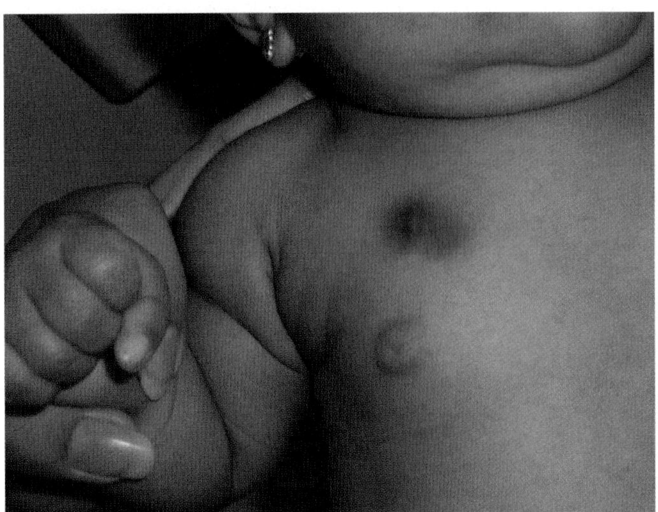

FIGURE 134-7 Urticaria pigmentosa on the chest of this 9-month-old girl. She has a positive Darier sign in which stroking the lesion results in edema. (*Used with permission from Richard P. Usatine, MD.*)

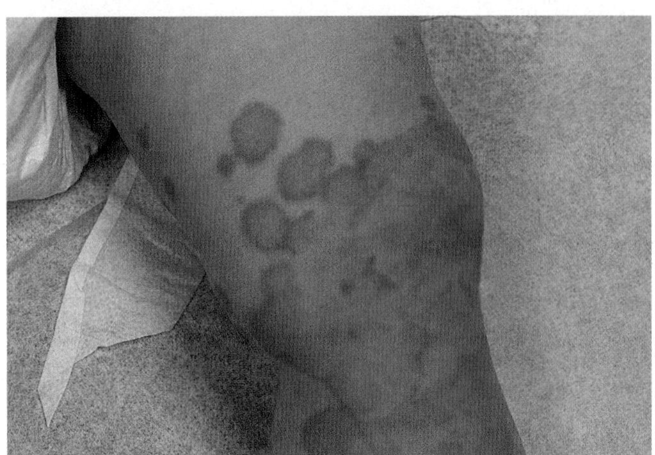

FIGURE 134-9 Giant urticaria on the left thigh of a 1-year-old boy with some areas that are annular (urticaria multiforme). No underlying cause identified. (*Image used with permission from Robert Brodell, MD.*)

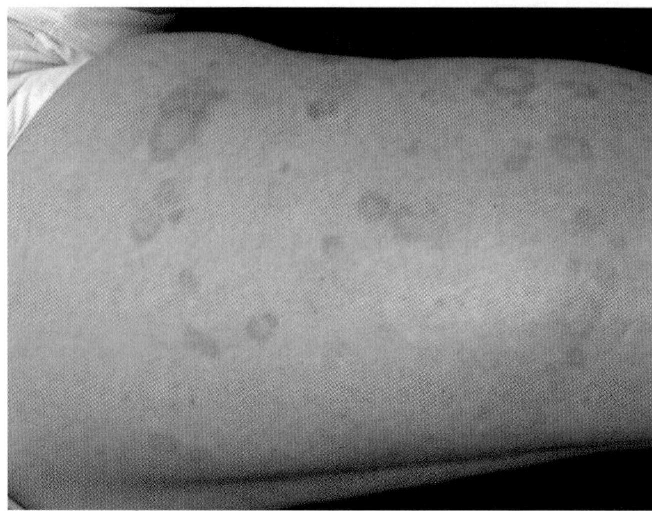

FIGURE 134-10 Chronic urticaria with annular urticarial wheals. (*Used with permission from Richard P. Usatine, MD.*)

Henoch-Schönlein purpura, to underlying connective tissue disease (**Figure 134-14**).[2]

- Mast cell releasability syndromes are syndromes in which there are too many mast cells in the skin or other organs of the body. These include cutaneous mastocytosis and urticaria pigmentosa (**Figures 134-5**, **134-6**, **134-11**, and **134-12**).
- Asymmetric periflexural exanthem of childhood. This condition resolves on its own over weeks or months. It is often misdiagnosed as a contact dermatitis, eczema, or urticaria. These children are healthy and asymptomatic unless they have mild pruritus.

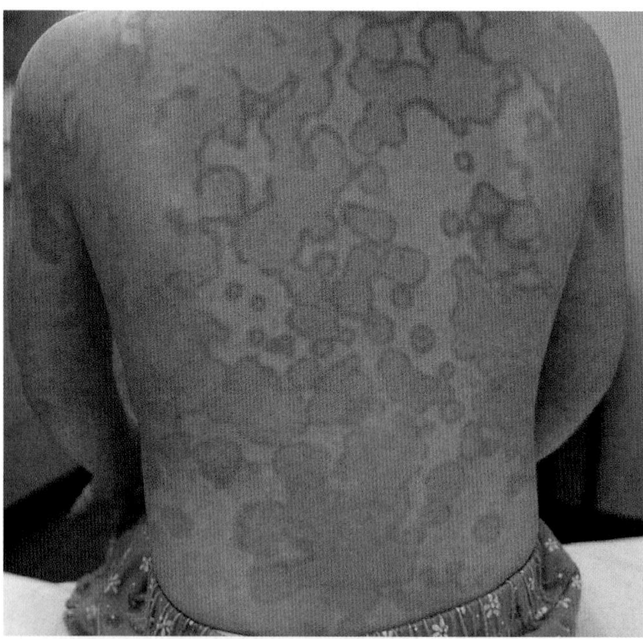

FIGURE 134-11 Giant urticaria (urticaria multiforme). Although this appears to have targets the real target lesions of erythema multiforme have a central lesion with a scaling or bullous component affecting the epidermis. The history suggests that this may have been a serum sickness type reaction. (*Used with permission from Milgrom EC, Usatine RP, Tan RA, Spector SL. Practical Allergy. Philadelphia, PA: Elsevier; 2003; and Daniel Stulberg, MD.*)

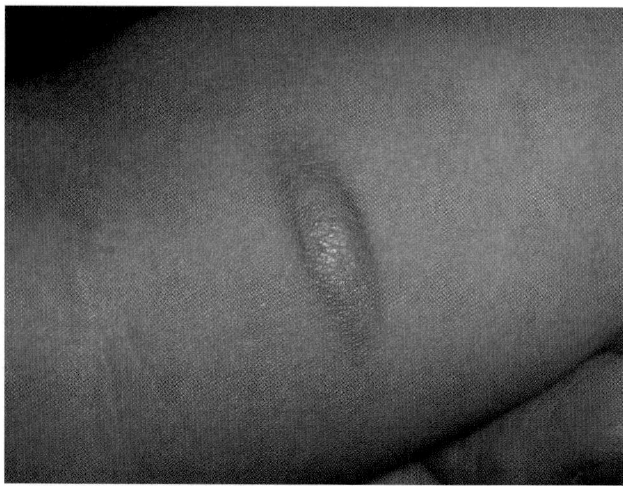

FIGURE 134-12 Positive Darier sign in which stroking the lesion of urticaria pigmentosum results in edema. (*Used with permission from Richard P. Usatine, MD.*)

The cause is unknown and serologic studies are generally negative (**Figure 134-16**).

MANAGEMENT

NONPHARMACOLOGIC

- Avoid any causative agent, medication, stimulus, or antigen if found. SOR Ⓑ
- Angiotensin-converting enzyme inhibitors (ACEIs) are especially prone to causing angioedema so should be stopped as soon as possible when suspected to be causative of angioedema or urticaria (**Figure 134-3**).[1] SOR Ⓐ Even an angiotensin receptor blocker (ARB) can cause angioedema and should be suspected in a patient on this class of medication (**Figure 134-16**).
- In chronic urticaria, patients may benefit from avoidance of potential urticarial precipitants such as aspirin, NSAIDs (**Figure 134-17**), opiates, and alcohol.[1] SOR Ⓑ

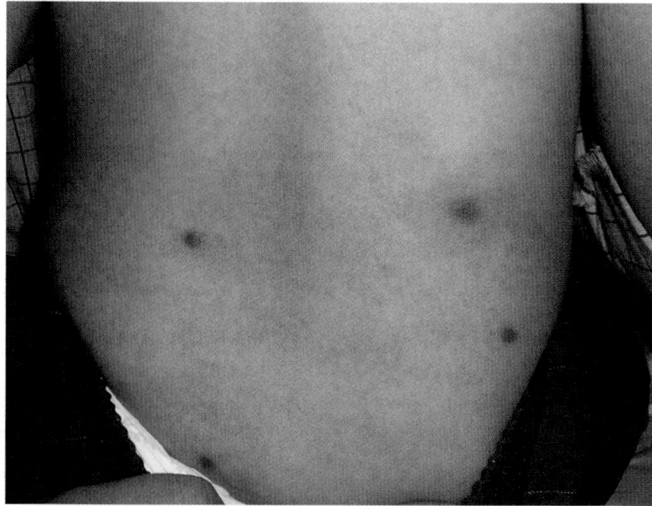

FIGURE 134-13 Positive Darier sign in which stroking the lesions of urticaria pigmentosum on the back resulted in erythema and edema at the site of the stroke. (*Used with permission from Richard P. Usatine, MD.*)

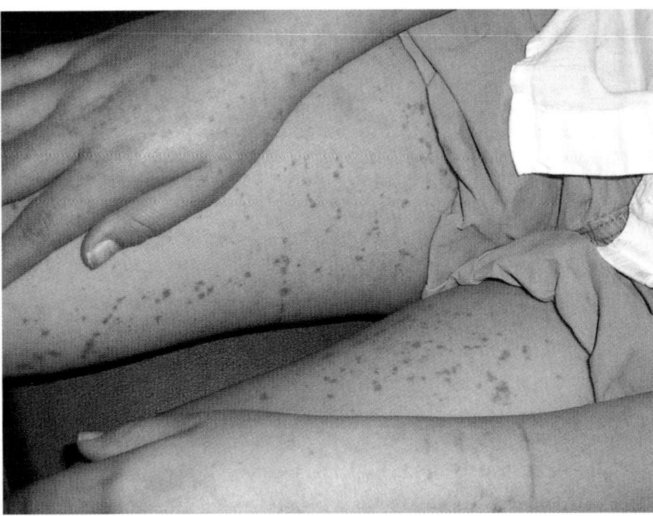

FIGURE 134-14 Henoch-Schönlein purpura on the leg of an 11-year-old girl. This is a type of urticarial vasculitis. (*Used with permission from Richard P. Usatine, MD.*)

- Infections may be a cause, an aggravating factor, or an unassociated bystander.[1] Look for sources of chronic infections such as parasitic infections, dental infections, GI infections, respiratory infections, and tinea pedis. Treat these, as it is possible, but unproven, that they can contribute to the chronic urticaria. SOR C
- Stop all unnecessary nonprescription medications, supplements, and vitamins in chronic urticaria. SOR C
- Avoidance of physical stimuli for the treatment of physical urticaria is desirable, but not always possible (observational studies only).[1] SOR B

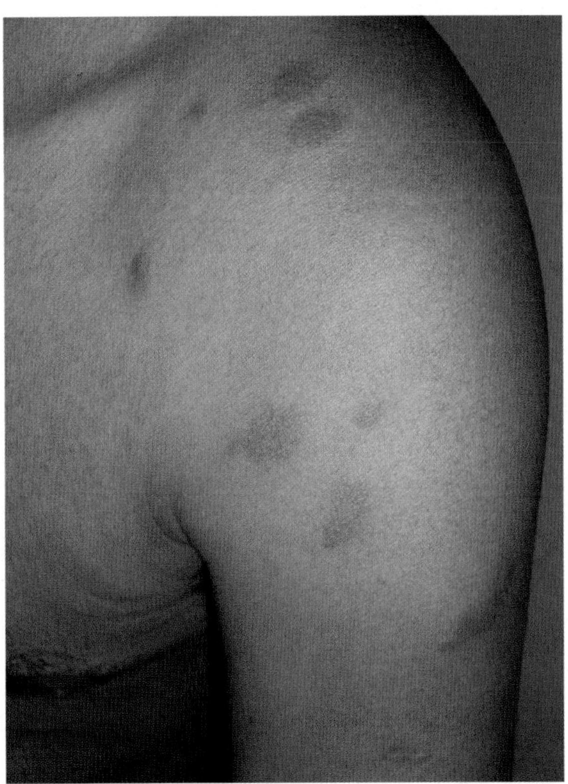

FIGURE 134-15 Urticaria in a young man that was acute and idiopathic. (*Used with permission from Richard P. Usatine, MD.*)

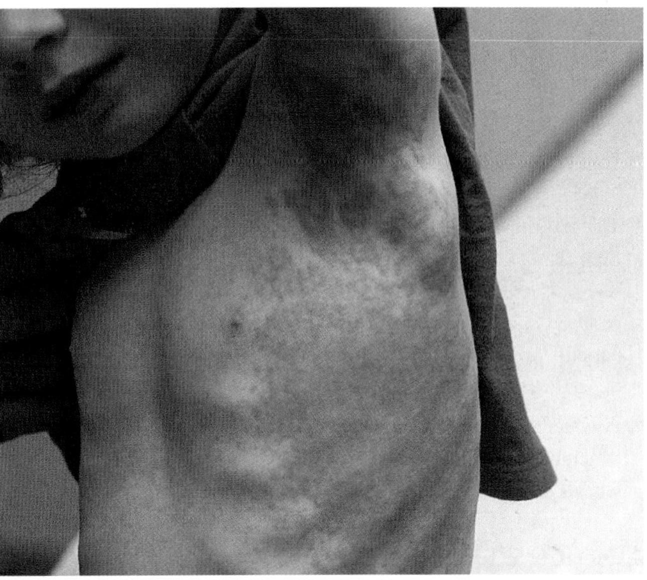

FIGURE 134-16 Asymmetric periflexural exanthem of childhood on the left flank of a 9-year-old girl. This resolves on its own over weeks or months and is often misdiagnosed as a contact dermatitis or eczema. These kids are healthy and asymptomatic unless they have mild pruritus. The cause is unknown. (*Image used with permission from Robert Brodell, MD.*)

- Stress reduction techniques may help in chronic urticaria but this is unproven. SOR C

ANTIHISTAMINES

- Low-sedating, second-generation antihistamines should be prescribed as a first-line treatment for chronic urticaria.[4–6] SOR A
- Increasing the dose of cetirizine from 10 mg to 20 mg daily produced a significant improvement in the severity of wheal and itching in urticaria refractory to the standard doses of antihistamines.[7] SOR B
- The British guidelines even suggest using antihistamines at up to quadruple the manufacturers' recommended dosages before changing to an alternative therapy. They also recommend waiting up to 4 weeks to allow full effectiveness of the antihistamines before considering referral to a specialist.[1] SOR C

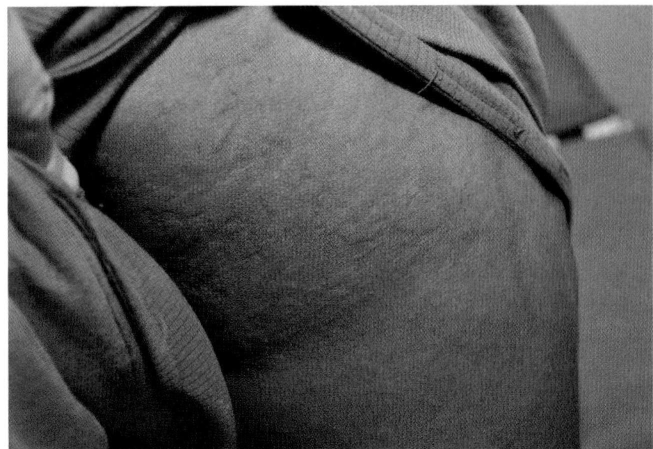

FIGURE 134-17 Urticaria that occurred within an hour after a boy was given ibuprofen to treat a high fever. (*Used with permission from Richard P. Usatine, MD.*)

- All patients should be offered the choice of at least two low-sedating H_1 antagonists because responses and tolerance vary between individuals.[8] SOR Ⓐ
- Addition of a sedating antihistamine at night may help patients sleep better, although they probably add little to existing H_1 receptor blockade.[8]
- The addition of an H_2 antagonist may give better control of urticaria than H_1 antagonists alone, although a benefit is not always seen.[8] SOR Ⓑ In one study, adding H_2 blockers to H_1 antagonists resulted in improvement of certain cutaneous outcomes for patients presenting with acute allergic syndromes to an emergency department.[9] SOR Ⓑ
- Low-sedating antihistamines seem to be effective in the treatment of acquired cold urticaria by significantly reducing the presence of wheals and pruritus after cold exposure.[10] SOR Ⓐ

CORTICOSTEROIDS

- Oral corticosteroids should be restricted to short courses for severe acute urticaria or angioedema affecting the mouth (e.g., prednisone 1–2 mg/kg/day for 3 to 4 days).[8,11] SOR Ⓑ
- Short tapering courses of oral steroids over 3 to 4 weeks may be necessary for urticarial vasculitis and severe delayed pressure urticaria.
- Long-term oral corticosteroids should not be used in chronic urticaria. It is better to use oral cyclosporine if needed as it has a far better risk-to-benefit ratio compared with steroids.[1,8]
- A randomized controlled trial showed that clobetasol 0.05 percent in a foam formulation was safe and effective in the short-term treatment of patients with delayed pressure urticaria.[12] SOR Ⓑ

OTHERS

- Epinephrine is valuable in severe acute urticaria or angioedema, especially if there is a suspicion of airway compromise or anaphylaxis.
- The evidence for leukotriene modifiers in the treatment of urticaria is poor. SOR Ⓒ
- Ecallantide is a new plasma kallikrein inhibitor for the subcutaneous treatment of acute attacks of hereditary angioedema.[13] SOR Ⓑ
- Anti-inflammatory drugs, such as colchicine, dapsone and sulfasalazine, have been reported as helpful in uncontrolled trials or case series.[1]

FOLLOW-UP

Follow-up is especially needed when the urticaria/angioedema persist or recur.

PATIENT EDUCATION

In most cases, it is not possible to find the cause of urticaria. This is especially true for chronic urticaria. Fortunately, most chronic urticaria will subside over time and there are medicines to treat the condition until it runs its course. If one medication doesn't work keep your follow-up visits to try other medications. Carefully observe for causative agents.

PATIENT RESOURCES

- eMedicineHealth.com is a consumer health site with information and support groups—**www.emedicinehealth.com/hives_and_angioedema/article_em.htm**.

PROVIDER RESOURCES

- Well-written guidelines based upon a joint initiative of a number of European dermatology, allergy, and immunology organizations—**http://onlinelibrary.wiley.com/doi/10.1111/j.1398-9995.2009.02178.x/full**.

REFERENCES

1. Zuberbier T, Asero R, Bindslev-Jensen C, et al. EAACI/GA(2) LEN/EDF/WAO guideline: management of urticaria. *Allergy*. 2009;64:1427-1443.
2. Baxi S, Dinakar C. Urticaria and angioedema. *Immunol Allergy Clin North Am*. 2005;25:353-367, vii.
3. Usatine RP. Urticaria and agioedema. In: Milgrom E, Usatine RP, Tan R, Spector S, eds. *Practical Allergy*. Philadelphia, PA: Elsevier; 2003:78-96.
4. Finn AF Jr, Kaplan AP, Fretwell R, et al. A double-blind, placebo-controlled trial of fexofenadine HCl in the treatment of chronic idiopathic urticaria. *J Allergy Clin Immunol*. 1999;104:1071-1078.
5. Ortonne JP, Grob JJ, Auquier P, Dreyfus I. Efficacy and safety of desloratadine in adults with chronic idiopathic urticaria: a randomized, double-blind, placebo-controlled, multicenter trial. *Am J Clin Dermatol*. 2007;8:37-42.
6. Ortonne JP. Chronic urticaria: a comparison of management guidelines. *Expert Opin Pharmacother*. 2011;12(17):2683-2693.
7. Okubo Y, Shigoka Y, Yamazaki M, Tsuboi R. Double dose of cetirizine hydrochloride is effective for patients with urticaria resistant: a prospective, randomized, non-blinded, comparative clinical study and assessment of quality of life. *J Dermatolog Treat*. 2011. [Epub ahead of print]
8. Grattan C, Powell S, Humphreys F. Management and diagnostic guidelines for urticaria and angio-oedema. *Br J Dermatol*. 2001; 144:708-714.
9. Lin RY, Curry A, Pesola GR, et al. Improved outcomes in patients with acute allergic syndromes who are treated with combined H1 and H2 antagonists. *Ann Emerg Med*. 2000;36:462-468.
10. Weinstein ME, Wolff AH, Bielory L. Efficacy and tolerability of second- and third-generation antihistamines in the treatment of acquired cold urticaria: a meta-analysis. *Ann Allergy Asthma Immunol*. 2010;104:518-522.
11. Pollack CV Jr, Romano TJ. Outpatient management of acute urticaria: the role of prednisone. *Ann Emerg Med*. 1995;26:547-551.
12. Vena GA, Cassano N, D'Argento V, Milani M. Clobetasol propionate 0.05% in a novel foam formulation is safe and effective in the short-term treatment of patients with delayed pressure urticaria: a randomized, double-blind, placebo-controlled trial. *Br J Dermatol*. 2006;154:353-356.
13. Stolz LE, Horn PT. Ecallantide: a plasma kallikrein inhibitor for the treatment of acute attacks of hereditary angioedema. *Drugs Today (Barc)*. 2010;46:547-555.

SECTION 8 PAPULOSQUAMOUS CONDITIONS

135 SEBORRHEIC DERMATITIS

Meredith Hancock, MD
Yoon-Soo Cindy Bae-Harboe, MD
Richard P. Usatine, MD

PATIENT STORY

A 3-month-old African American boy is brought to the clinic with white spots on his face for one month (**Figure 135-1**). The child is otherwise in great health, eating well and gaining weight. The mother was negative for HIV during pregnancy. On physical exam, there are hypopigmented patches on the face especially at the hair line and under the eyebrows. There is visible scale in each of these patches. The hypopigmentation occurs secondary to the toxic effect of the Malassezia (Pityrosporum) on the melanocytes (as seen in tinea versicolor). The diagnosis of seborrheic dermatitis is made and treatment is begun with appropriate topical agents to treat the inflammation and the Malassezia. The mother is told to shampoo the infant's hair with a selenium-based shampoo every 1 to 2 days and to apply 1 percent hydrocortisone cream to the hypopigmented areas twice daily for the next 2 weeks. At a 2-week follow-up, the scale is gone and the hypopigmentation is resolving.

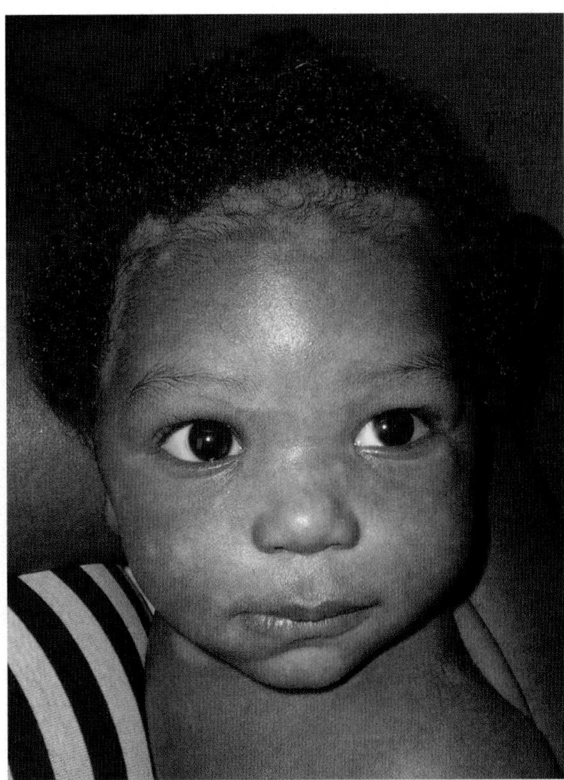

FIGURE 135-1 Seborrheic dermatitis on the scalp and face with visible hypopigmentation. Note how the hypopigmentation is particularly visible around the hairline and under the eyebrows. (*Used with permission from Richard P. Usatine, MD.*)

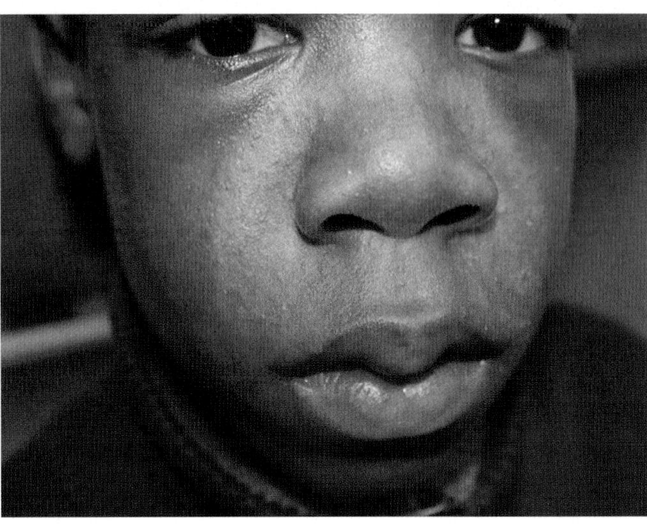

FIGURE 135-2 Seborrheic dermatitis in a 13-year-old boy demonstrating confluent scaling and erythema along with areas of hypopigmentation. Patients with more pigmentation often show a raised lateral margin reminiscent of the advancing border of dermatophyte infections and subsequent post-inflammatory hypopigmentation that can be temporarily disfiguring. (*Image used with permission from Robert Brodell, MD.*)

PATIENT STORY

A 13-year-old African American boy presented to clinic with a mildly pruritic central facial rash and scalp dandruff that had persisted for two years (**Figure 135-2**). There was no history to suggest an allergic contact dermatitis or drug allergy. On physical exam, confluent scaling and erythema with areas of hypopigmentation were noted in the nasomesial folds and over the eyebrows. Additionally, diffuse scaling and erythema were noted throughout the scalp. The patient was diagnosed with seborrheic dermatitis. Patients with more pigmentation often show a raised lateral margin reminiscent of the advancing border of dermatophyte infections and subsequent postinflammatory hypopigmentation that can be temporarily disfiguring. This patient responded to ketoconazole 2 percent cream applied twice daily to the face and other non-hair-bearing areas and ketoconazole 2 percent shampoo twice weekly for his scalp. His hypopigmentation improved over time.

INTRODUCTION

Seborrheic dermatitis is a common, chronic, relapsing dermatitis affecting sebum-rich areas of the body. Children and adults, males and females may be affected. Presentation may vary from mild erythema to greasy scales, and rarelyas erythroderma. Treatment is targeted to reduce inflammation and irritation, as well as to eliminate Malassezia fungus, whose exact role is not completely understood.

SYNONYMS

Seborrhea, seborrheic eczema, dandruff, and cradle cap (pityriasis capitis).

EPIDEMIOLOGY

- The prevalence of seborrheic dermatitis was 10 percent in children from infancy to 5 years of age in a skin survey of over 1,000 children in Australia. The highest rate was in the first 3 months of life, decreasing rapidly by the age of 1 year, after which it slowly decreased over the next 4 years. Most (72%) had disease classified as minimal to mild. Cradle cap occurred in 42 percent of the children examined, with 86 percent categorized as minimal to mild only.[1]
- Prevalence of scalp seborrheic dermatitis in a survey of male adolescents in Brazil was 11 percent. The prevalence was higher in persons with white skin and a higher body fat content.[2]
- Seborrheic dermatitis affects 1 to 3 percent of the general population, 3 to 5 percent of young adults, and 20 to 83 percent of patients with AIDS.[3]

ETIOLOGY AND PATHOPHYSIOLOGY

- Seborrheic dermatitis is a chronic, superficial, localized inflammatory dermatitis that is found in sebum-producing areas of the body.
- The actual cause of seborrheic dermatitis is not well understood. It appears to be related to the interplay between host susceptibility, environmental factors, and local immune response to antigens.[4–6]
- Patients with seborrheic dermatitis may be colonized with certain species of lipophilic yeast of the genus *Malassezia*; however, *Malassezia* is considered normal skin flora and unaffected persons also may be colonized.
- Recent evidence suggests that *Malassezia* may produce different irritants or metabolites on affected skin.[6]

RISK FACTORS

- Infancy.
- Male gender.
- Immunocompromise (HIV/AIDS, Parkinson disease, or malignancy).
- Stress.
- Environmental factors (cold, dry weather).

DIAGNOSIS

The clinical diagnosis is made by history and physical examination. **Figures 135-3** and **135-4** reveal erythema and scale across the eyebrows, forehead, central face, and scalp. Biopsy is not generally indicated unless ruling out other possibilities (see the following section "Differential Diagnosis").

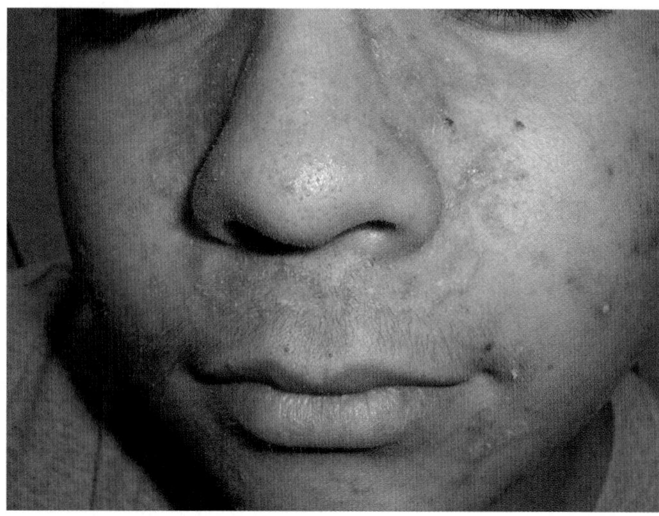

FIGURE 135-3 Seborrheic dermatitis on the face of a 14-year-old boy. Note the erythema and scale especially concentrated around the central face. He also had seborrhea of the scalp and acne. (*Used with permission from Richard P. Usatine, MD.*)

CLINICAL FEATURES

- Chronic skin condition characterized by remissions and exacerbations.
- Poorly demarcated, erythematous plaques of greasy, yellow scale (**Figure 135-3**), in the characteristic seborrheic distribution (see the following description).
- Common precipitating factors are stress, immunosuppression, and cold weather.
- Face, scalp, and ears may be very pruritic.
- May be the presenting sign of HIV seropositivity.

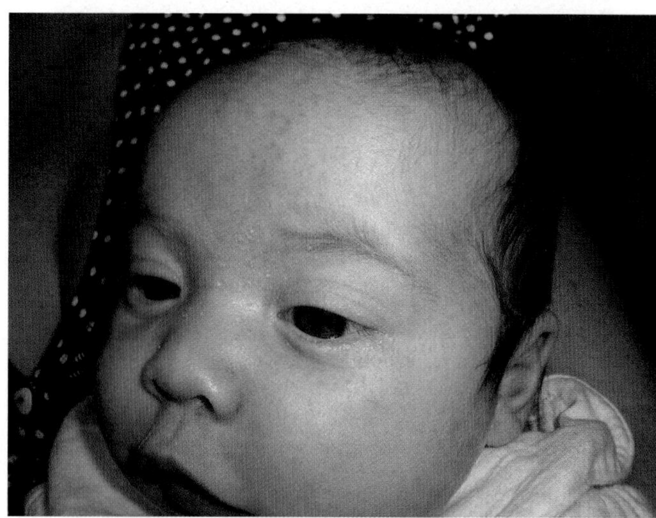

FIGURE 135-4 Mild seborrheic dermatitis with subtle flaking around the eyebrows of a 2-month-old girl who also has cradle cap. (*Used with permission from Richard P. Usatine, MD.*)

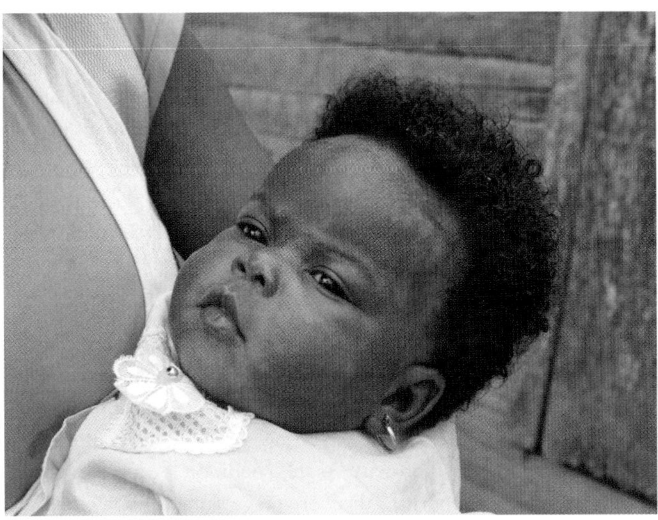

FIGURE 135-5 Seborrheic dermatitis on the face of an infant with hypopigmentation around the scalp and over the eyebrows. Hypopigmentation is secondary to postinflammatory changes. (*Used with permission from Richard P. Usatine, MD.*)

- In dark-skinned individuals, the involved skin and scale may become hyperpigmented or hypopigmented (**Figures 135-2, 135-3**, and **135-5**).

TYPICAL DISTRIBUTION

Scalp (i.e., dandruff), eyebrows (**Figures 135-4** and **135-5**), nasolabial creases, forehead, cheeks, around the nose, behind the ears (**Figure 135-6**), external auditory meatus, and under facial hair. Seborrhea can also occur over the sternum and in the axillae, submammary folds, umbilicus, groin, and gluteal creases.

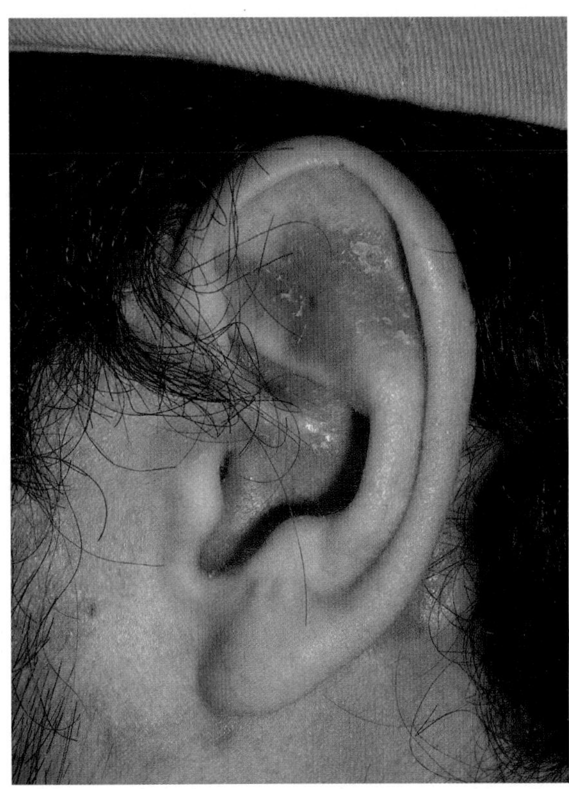

FIGURE 135-6 Seborrheic dermatitis in and around the ear of a teenager. (*Used with permission from Richard P. Usatine, MD.*)

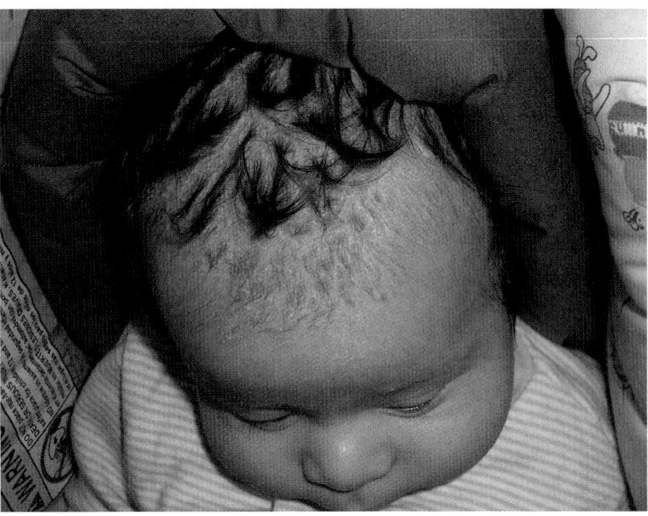

FIGURE 135-7 Cradle cap in a healthy infant showing brown adherent scale over the central scalp. (*Used with permission from Richard P. Usatine, MD.*)

Infants may develop scales on the scalp, known as cradle cap (**Figures 135-7** and **135-8**). The eyebrows may also be affected (**Figure 135-5**). Some infants have a wider distribution involving the neck creases, armpits, leg creases, and groin (**Figure 135-9**).

LABORATORY STUDIES

- Test for HIV if patient has risk factors.
- Consider KOH preparation to look for the spaghetti and meatballs pattern of Malassezia furfur (Pityrosporum yeast).
- Consider zinc level or alkaline phosphatase to rule out nutritional/zinc deficiency.

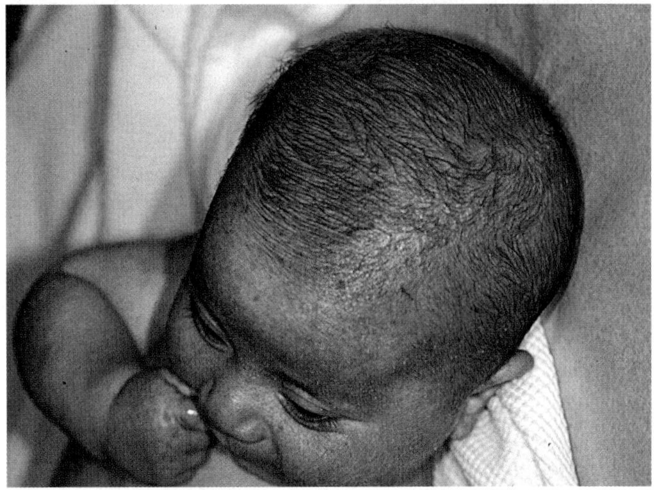

FIGURE 135-8 Widespread severe seborrheic dermatitis with cradle cap in an infant that also has atopic dermatitis. (*Used with permission from Richard P. Usatine, MD.*)

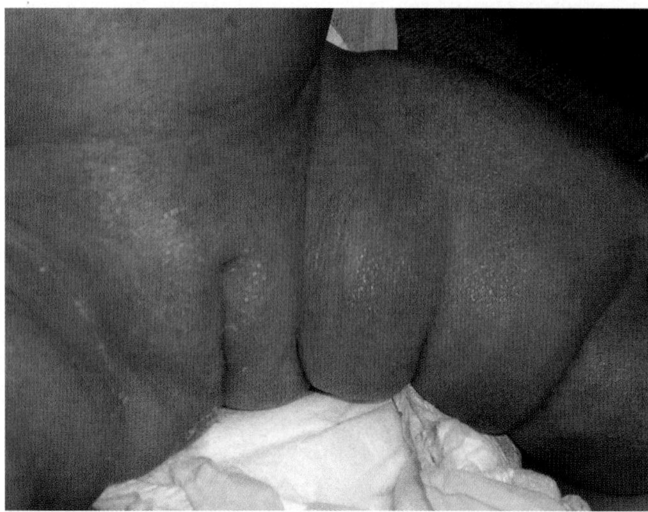

FIGURE 135-9 Seborrheic dermatitis in the diaper area and skin folds of the thighs in an otherwise healthy infant. (*Used with permission from Richard P. Usatine, MD.*)

DIFFERENTIAL DIAGNOSIS

- Langerhans cell histiocytosis is a group of disorders characterized by proliferation of Langerhans cells. The proliferation leads to lesions in the skin, bone marrow, endocrine system, or lungs. It may present with a severe refractory diaper rash that has scattered erythematous papules and a petechial component (**Figure 135-10**). A skin biopsy is needed to make the diagnosis (see Chapter 214, Langerhans cell Histiocytosis).
- Psoriasis—The scale of psoriasis tends to be thicker, on well-demarcated plaques distributed over extensor surfaces along with the scalp. Look for signs of nail involvement that may support the diagnosis of psoriasis (see Chapter 136, Psoriasis).

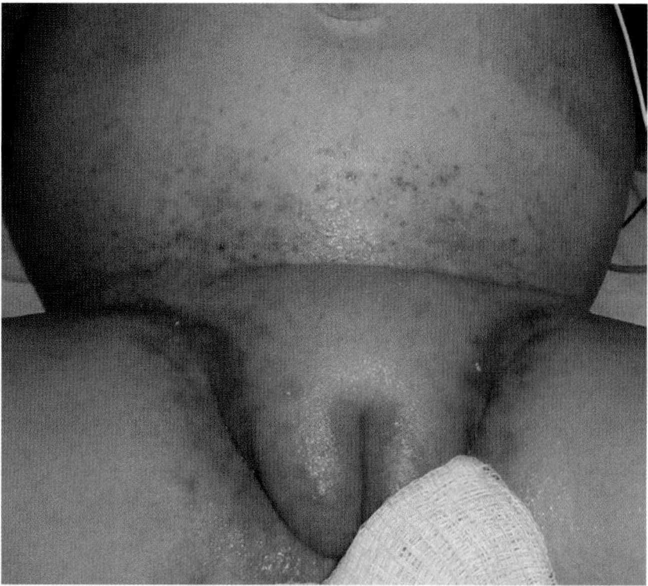

FIGURE 135-10 Langerhans cell histiocytosis in the diaper area presented as a diaper rash, which did not respond to treatment. This refractory diaper rash has scattered erythematous papules and a petechial component. A skin biopsy revealed Langerhans' cells. (*Used with permission from Kane KS, Lio P, Stratigos AJ, Johnson RA. Color Atlas and Synopsis of Pediatric Dermatology, 2nd edition, Figure 3-6, New York, NY: McGraw-Hill, 2009.*)

- Rosacea—The erythema on the face is often associated with papules, pustules, telangiectasia, and an absence of scales. May also present with chalazia or hordeola (see Chapter 97, Rosacea).
- Tinea capitis—Scale and erythema commonly with associated hair loss. KOH and/or culture can help make the distinction (see Chapter 122, Tinea Capitis).
- Perioral dermatitis—Usually restricted around the mouth with minimal scale.
- Tinea versicolor (trunk and neck)—The scale of tinea versicolor is fine and white and scales with scraping. The *Malassezia* infection affects the melanocytes leading to changes in color of the affected areas (white, pink and brown). As this condition is caused by the same organism as seborrhea there are many similarities in clinical appearance and treatment (see Chapter 126, Tinea Versicolor).
- Allergic or irritant contact dermatitis—May present with a well demarcated lesion with fine white scale, secondarily impetiginized lesions may have associated yellow colored crust, not scale.
- Candidiasis—May be found in intertriginous areas, but presents with significant erythema and satellite lesions.
- Nutritional deficiency (i.e., zinc)—May present with facial lesions and acral rash as seen in acrodermatitis enteropathica (see Chapter 7, Global Health).

MANAGEMENT

As seborrheic dermatitis is a recurrent, chronic condition, repeated and/or maintenance therapy is often required.

- Mainstay of treatment is topical antifungals.
- For seborrheic dermatitis of the scalp, patients should wash their hair with antifungal shampoos (containing selenium sulfide, ketoconazole, or ciclopirox) several times per week, each time leaving the lather on the affected areas for several minutes until remission is attained. Patients may continue to use antifungal shampoo as maintenance therapy.[5]
- Shampoos containing ketoconazole, selenium sulfide or zinc pyrithione (ZPT) are active against the *Malassezia* and are effective in the treatment of moderate to severe dandruff.[7,8] SOR Ⓐ
- Ketoconazole 2 percent shampoo was found to be superior to ZPT 1 percent shampoo when used twice weekly. Ketoconazole led to a 73 percent improvement in the total dandruff severity score compared with 67 percent for ZPT 1 percent at 4 weeks.[8] SOR Ⓑ
- Ciclopirox shampoo 1 percent is effective and safe in the treatment of seborrheic dermatitis of the scalp.[9,10] SOR Ⓐ It is by prescription only and is expensive.
- Ketoconazole 2 percent cream, gel, or emulsion is safe and effective for facial seborrheic dermatitis.[11–13] SOR Ⓑ
- Ciclopirox 1 percent cream is also safe and effective for facial seborrheic dermatitis and is equivalent to ketoconazole 2 percent cream.[11,14] SOR Ⓑ
- Oral terbinafine 250 mg daily for 4 weeks was found to be effective for moderate to severe seborrhea in adults.[15,16] SOR Ⓑ However,

because of the potential for harmful side effects of oral antifungals and the limited study of their efficacy, they are not first-line treatments.[5] Oral terbinafine may be considered to treat erythroderma caused by seborrhea in an adolescent.

Topical corticosteroids are useful in treating associated erythema and pruritis.[5] Long-term use may lead to skin atrophy[5] and should be used with caution.

- Lotion or solution is preferable on hair-covered area for patient comfort and usability.
- Hydrocortisone 1 to 2.5 percent cream or lotion can be used bid on the face, scalp, and other affected areas.[13,17] SOR B
- Desonide 0.05 percent lotion is safe and effective for short-term treatment of seborrheic dermatitis of the face.[15] SOR B It is a nonfluorinated low to midpotency steroid that is higher in potency than hydrocortisone 1 percent.
- For moderate to severe seborrheic dermatitis on the scalp of a teenager:
  - Fluocinonide 0.05 percent solution once daily is affordable and beneficial. SOR C

OTHER TREATMENTS

- Pimecrolimus cream 1 percent is an effective and well-tolerated treatment for facial seborrheic dermatitis.[17,19,20] SOR B In one study, there was more burning noted with the pimecrolimus than with the betamethasone 17-valerate 0.1 percent cream.[19]
- Metronidazole gel—Two small studies have found different results in the treatment of seborrheic dermatitis on the face. One suggests it works better than the vehicle alone and the other found no statistically significant difference from placebo.[21,22] SOR B

COMPLEMENTARY/ALTERNATIVE THERAPY

- Tea tree oil 5 percent shampoo showed a 41 percent improvement in the quadrant-area-severity score compared with 11 percent in the placebo. Statistically significant improvements were also observed in the total area of involvement score, the total severity score, and the itchiness and greasiness components of the patients' self-assessments.[23] SOR B
- One small randomized controlled trial using homeopathic medication consisting of potassium bromide, sodium bromide, nickel sulfate, and sodium chloride for 10 weeks showed significant improvement over placebo.[24] SOR B

FOLLOW-UP

Patients with longstanding and severe seborrhea will appreciate a follow-up visit in most cases. Milder cases can be followed as needed.

PATIENT EDUCATION

For improved treatment results, encourage patients (or the parents of younger children) to wash the hair and scalp daily with an antifungal shampoo. Some patients (or their parents) fear that washing their hair too often will cause a "dry" scalp and need to understand that the scaling and flaking will improve rather than worsen with more frequent hair washing. It is helpful to explain that the flaking is not because the scalp is dry but secondary to the overgrowth of the fungus that needs to be washed off the scalp.

PATIENT RESOURCES

- PubMed Health. Seborrheic Dermatitis—**www.ncbi.nlm.nih.gov/pubmedhealth/PMH0001959/**.

PROVIDER RESOURCES

- Medscape. Seborrheic Dermatitis—**http://emedicine.medscape.com/article/1108312**.

REFERENCES

1. Foley P, Zuo Y, Plunkett A, Merlin K, Marks R. The frequency of common skin conditions in preschool-aged children in Australia: seborrheic dermatitis and pityriasis capitis (cradle cap). *Arch Dermatol.* 2003;139(3):318-322.
2. Breunig Jde A, de Almeida HL Jr, Duquia RP, Souza PR, Staub HL. Scalp seborrheic dermatitis: prevalence and associated factors in male adolescents. *Int J Dermatol.* 2012;51(1):46-49.
3. Schechtman RC, Midgley G, Hay RJ. HIV disease and Malassezia yeasts: a quantitative study of patients presenting with seborrhoeic dermatitis. *Br J Dermatol.* 1995;133(5):694-698.
4. Gaitanis G, Magiatis P, Hantschke M, Bassukas ID, Velegraki A. The Malassezia genus in skin and systemic diseases. *Clin Microbiol Rev.* 2012;25(1):106-141.
5. Naldi L, Alfredo Rebora A. Seborrheic dermatitis. *N Engl J Med.* 2009;360;4:387-396.
6. Hay RJ. Malassezia, dandruff and seborrheic dermatitis: an overview. *Br J Dermatol.* 2011;165 (2):2-8.
7. Danby FW, Maddin WS, Margesson LJ, Rosenthal D. A randomized, double-blind, placebo-controlled trial of ketoconazole 2% shampoo versus selenium sulfide 2.5% shampoo in the treatment of moderate to severe dandruff. *J Am Acad Dermatol.* 1993;29: 1008-1012.
8. Pierard-Franchimont C. A multicenter randomized trial of ketoconazole 2% and zinc pyrithione 1% shampoos in severe dandruff and seborrheic dermatitis. *Skin Pharmacol Appl Skin Physiol.* 2002;15(6):434-441.
9. Aly R. Ciclopirox gel for seborrheic dermatitis of the scalp. *Int J Dermatol.* 2003;42(1):19-22.
10. Lebwohl M, Plott T. Safety and efficacy of ciclopirox 1% shampoo for the treatment of seborrheic dermatitis of the scalp in the US population: results of a double-blind, vehicle-controlled trial. *Int J Dermatol.* 2004;43(1):17-20.
11. Chosidow O, Maurette C, Dupuy P. Randomized, open-labeled, non-inferiority study between ciclopiroxolamine 1% cream and ketoconazole 2% foaming gel in mild to moderate facial seborrheic dermatitis. *Dermatology.* 2003;206:233-240.
12. Pierard GE, Pierard-Franchimont C, Van CJ, Rurangirwa A, Hoppenbrouwers ML, Schrooten P. Ketoconazole 2% emulsion in the

treatment of seborrheic dermatitis. *Int J Dermatol.* 1991;30: 806-809.

13. Katsambas A, Antoniou C, Frangouli E, Avgerinou G, Michailidis D, Stratigos J. A double-blind trial of treatment of seborrheic dermatitis with 2% ketoconazole cream compared with 1% hydrocortisone cream. *Br J Dermatol.* 1989;121:353-357.
14. Dupuy P, Maurette C, Amoric JC, Chosidow O. Randomized, placebo-controlled, double-blind study on clinical efficacy of ciclopiroxolamine 1% cream in facial seborrheic dermatitis. *Br J Dermatol.* 2001;135:1033-1037.
15. Vena GA, Micali G, Santoianni P, Cassano N, Peruzzi E. Oral terbinafine in the treatment of multi-site seborrheic dermatitis: a multicenter, double-blind placebo-controlled study. *Int J Immunopathol Pharmacol.* 2005;18:745-753.
16. Scaparro E, Quadri G, Virno G, Orifici C, Milani M. Evaluation of the efficacy and tolerability of oral terbinafine (Daskil) in patients with seborrheic dermatitis. A multicentre, randomized, investigator-blinded, placebo-controlled trial. *Br J Dermatol.* 2001;135(4): 854-857.
17. Firooz A, Solhpour A, Gorouhi F, et al. Pimecrolimus cream, 1%, vs hydrocortisone acetate cream, 1%, in the treatment of facial seborrheic dermatitis: a randomized, investigator-blind, clinical trial. *Arch Dermatol.* 2006;142:1066-1067.
18. Freeman SH. Efficacy, cutaneous tolerance and cosmetic acceptability of desonide 0.05% lotion (Desowen) versus vehicle in the short-term treatment of facial atopic or seborrheic dermatitis. *Australas J Dermatol.* 2002;43(3):186-189.
19. Rigopoulos D, Ioannides D, Kalogeromitros D, Gregoriou S, Katsambas A. Pimecrolimus cream 1% vs. betamethasone 17-valerate 0.1% cream in the treatment of seborrheic dermatitis. A randomized open-label clinical trial. *Br J Dermatol.* 2004;135:1071-1075.
20. Warshaw EM, Wohlhuter RJ, Liu A, et al. Results of a randomized, double-blind, vehicle-controlled efficacy trial of pimecrolimus cream 1% for the treatment of moderate to severe facial seborrheic dermatitis. *J Am Acad Dermatol.* 2007;57(2): 257-264.
21. Parsad D, Pandhi R, Negi KS, Kumar B. Topical metronidazole in seborrheic dermatitis—a double-blind study. *Dermatology.* 2001; 202:35-37.
22. Koca R. Is topical metronidazole effective in seborrheic dermatitis? A double-blind study. *Int J Dermatol.* 2003;42(8):632-635.
23. Satchell AC, Saurajen A, Bell C, Barnetson RS. Treatment of dandruff with 5% tea tree oil shampoo. *J Am Acad Dermatol.* 2002; 47(6):852-855.
24. Smith SA, Baker AE, Williams JH. Effective treatment of seborrheic dermatitis using a low dose, oral homeopathic medication consisting of potassium bromide, sodium bromide, nickel sulfate, and sodium chloride in a double-blind, placebo-controlled study. *Altern Med Rev.* 2002;7(1):59-67.

136 PSORIASIS

Richard P. Usatine, MD

PATIENT STORY

A 5-year-old boy presents to his pediatrician with a new onset rash 2 weeks after being treated for strep pharyngitis. He had been treated with a10-day course of amoxicillin after a positive rapid strep test in the office. The mother states that her son is otherwise feeling well with a good appetite and no change in his activities. The pediatrician notes small plaques on the child's face, arms and trunk and sees the resemblance to drops of water (**Figure 136-1**). The vital signs are normal as is the rest of the physical examination. A diagnosis of guttate psoriasis is made without any laboratory tests or biopsies. The child is started on 0.1 percent triamcinolone ointment to be applied twice daily. A referral to dermatology is also made.

INTRODUCTION

Psoriasis is a chronic inflammatory papulosquamous and immune-mediated skin disorder. It is also associated with joint and cardiovascular comorbidities. Psoriasis can present in many different patterns, from the scalp to the feet, and cause psychiatric distress and physical disabilities. It is crucial to be able to identify psoriasis in all its myriad presentations so that patients receive the best possible treatments to improve their quality of life and avoid comorbidities.

EPIDEMIOLOGY

- Psoriasis affects approximately 2 percent of the world population.[1]
- The prevalence of psoriasis was 2.5 percent in white patients and was 1.3 percent in African American patients in one population study in the US.[2]
- Sex—No gender preference.
- Age—Psoriasis can begin at any age. In one population study of the age of onset of psoriasis two peaks was revealed, one occurring at the age of 16 years (female) or 22 years (males) and a second peak at the age of 60 years (female) or 57 years (males).[3]
- The prevalence rates for pediatric psoriasis increased in a linear way from 0.2 percent at the age of one year to 1.2 percent at the age of 18 years in a German study.[4]
- Psoriasis begins before the age of 20 in about 1/3 of patients.[5]
- Psoriatic arthritis affects about 20 percent of all psoriasis patients.[5]

ETIOLOGY AND PATHOPHYSIOLOGY

- Immune-mediated skin disease, where the T cell plays a pivotal role in the pathogenesis of the disease.

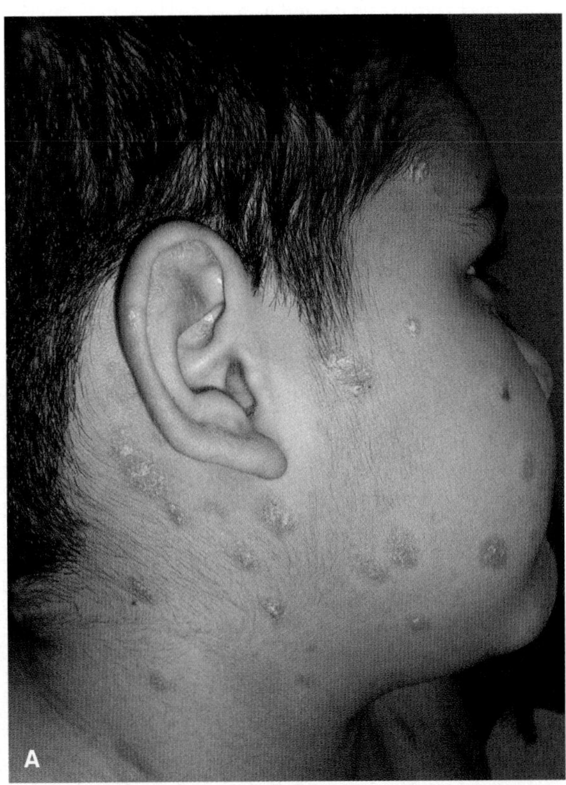

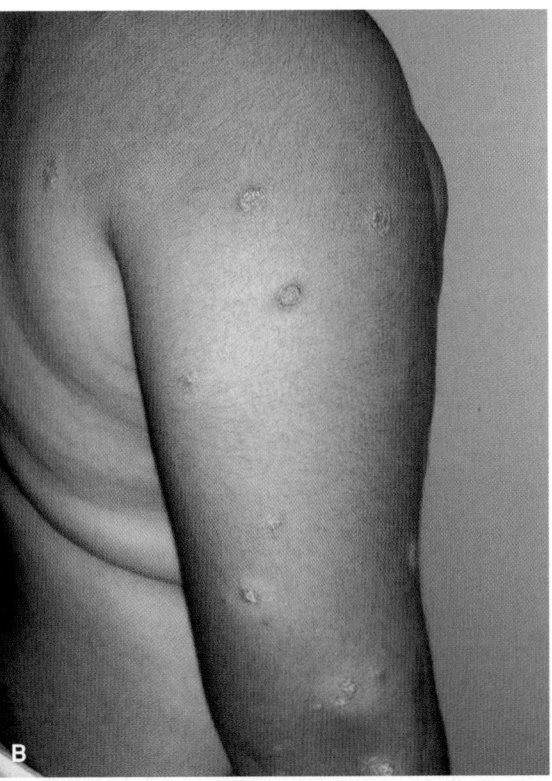

FIGURE 136-1 This 5-year-old boy developed guttate psoriasis 2 weeks after a strep throat. **A.** Note the drop-like pink plaques on the face and neck. **B.** Drop-like plaques on the arms and trunk. (*Used with permission from Richard P. Usatine, MD.*)

TABLE 136-1 Factors that Trigger and Exacerbate Psoriasis

• Stress • Physical trauma to the skin (Koebner phenomenon) • Cold, dry weather • Sun exposure and hot weather • Infections (eg, strep throat, HIV) • Medications (eg, ACE inhibitors, antimalarial agents, beta-blockers, lithium, NSAIDs)

- Langerhans cell (antigen-presenting cells in the skin) migrate from the skin to regional lymph nodes, where they activate T cells that migrate to the skin and release cytokines.
- Cytokines are responsible for epidermal and vascular hyperproliferation and proinflammatory effects.

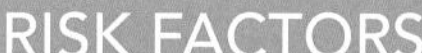

RISK FACTORS

- Family history.
- Obesity.
- Smoking and environmental smoke.
- Heavy alcohol use.

Table 136-1 lists the factors that trigger and exacerbate psoriasis.[6]

The risk of psoriasis is higher with:[7]

- Family history of psoriasis (odds ratio [OR] = 33.96; 95 percent confidence interval [CI] 14.14 to 81.57).
- Urban dwellers (OR = 3.61; 95% CI = 0.99 to 13.18).
- Alcohol consumption (OR = 2.55; 95% CI = 1.26 to 5.17).
- Environmental tobacco smoke at home (OR = 2.29; 95% CI = 1.12 to 4.67).

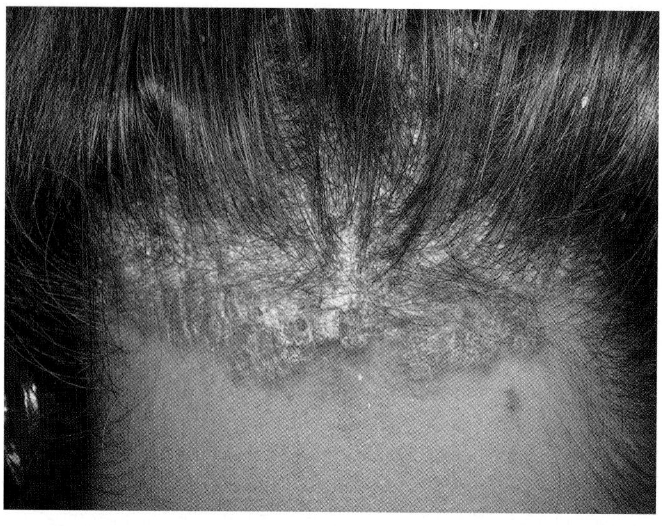

FIGURE 136-3 Scalp psoriasis visible at the posterior hairline in a teenage girl. (*Used with permission from Richard P. Usatine, MD.*)

In a multicenter case-control study of environmental risk factors in pediatric psoriasis the most important risk factors were:

- Environmental tobacco smoke at home or smoking—Odds ratio 2.90 (95% confidence interval [CI] = 2.27–3.78).
- Stressful life events—Odds ratio 2.94 (95% CI = 2.28–3.79).
- Higher BMI (>26)—odds ratio 2.52 (95% CI = 1.42–4.49).[8]

DIAGNOSIS

Psoriasis has many forms and locations. These nine categories were used to describe psoriasis in a consensus statement of the American Academy of Dermatology (AAD):[9]

1. Plaque psoriasis (**Figure 136-2**).
2. Scalp psoriasis (**Figure 136-3**).
3. Guttate psoriasis (**Figures 136-4** and **136-5**).

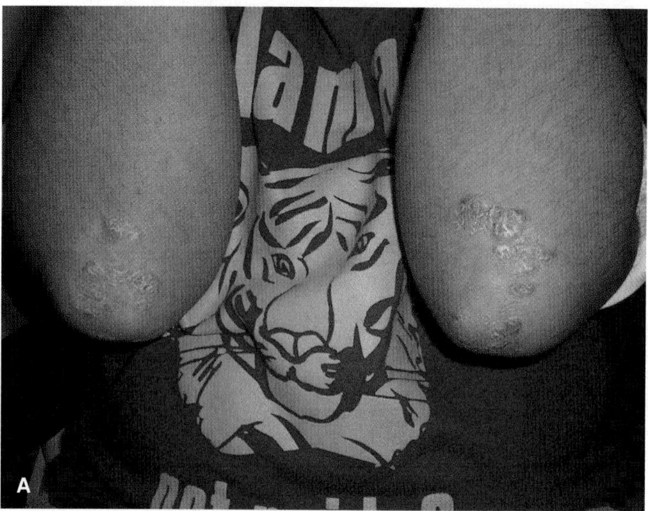

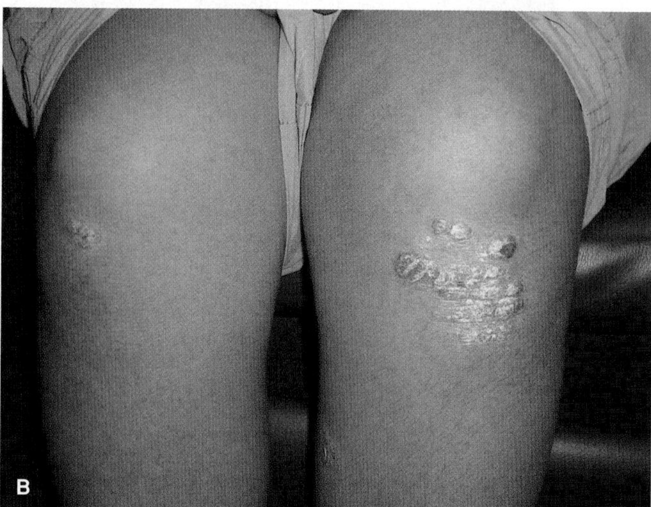

FIGURE 136-2 Typical plaque psoriasis in a 9-year-old child on the **A.** elbows and **B.** knees. (*Used with permission from Richard P. Usatine, MD.*)

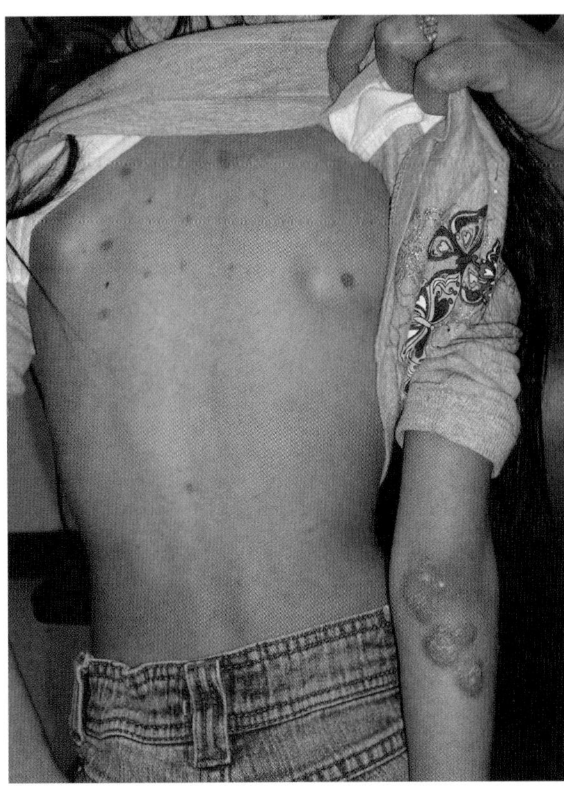

FIGURE 136-4 Guttate psoriasis in a 6-year-old girl seen 2 weeks after strep pharyngitis. Note the small drop-like plaques on her back along with larger plaques over her elbow. (*Used with permission from Richard P. Usatine, MD.*)

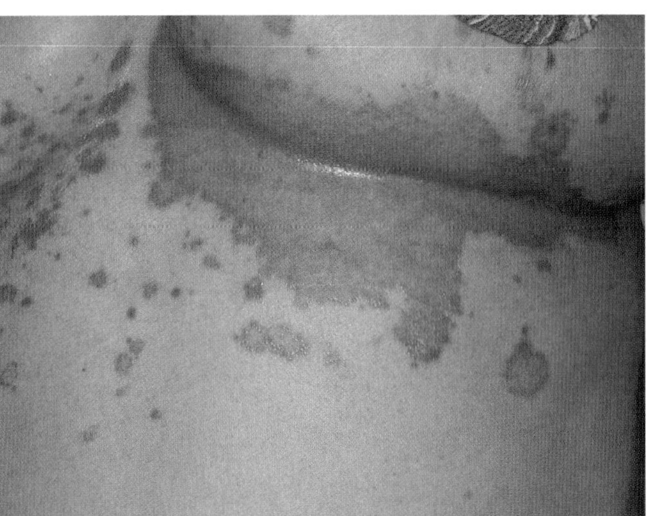

FIGURE 136-6 Inverse psoriasis in the inframammary folds of this obese teenage patient. This is not a *Candida* infection. (*Used with permission from Richard P. Usatine, MD.*)

4. Inverse psoriasis (**Figure 136-6**).
5. Palmar-plantar psoriasis (**Figure 136-7**); also known as palmoplantar psoriasis.
6. Erythrodermic psoriasis (**Figure 136-8**).
7. Pustular psoriasis—Localized and generalized (**Figure 136-9**).
8. Nail psoriasis (**Figure 136-10**; see Chapter 165, Psoriatic Nails).
9. Psoriatic arthritis (**Figure 136-11**).

Typical distribution involves: elbows, knees, extremities, trunk, scalp, face, ears, hands, feet, genitalia, and intertriginous areas, and nails.

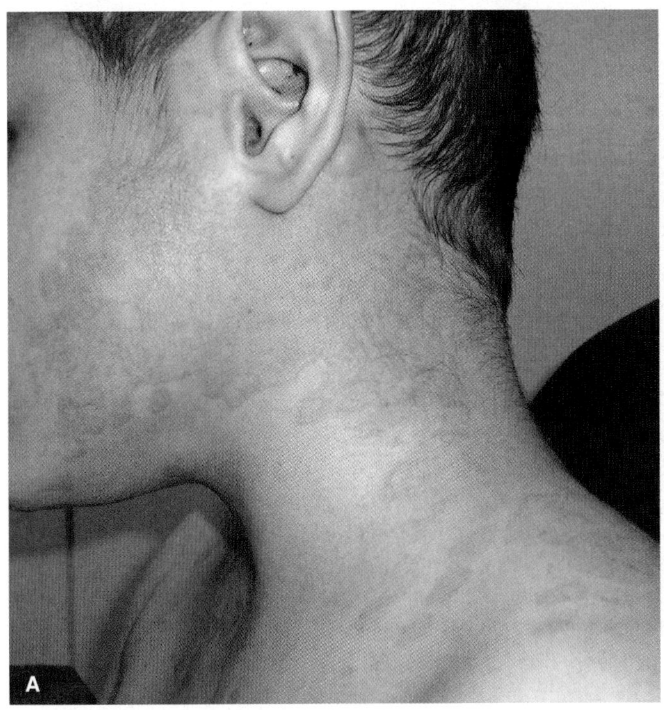

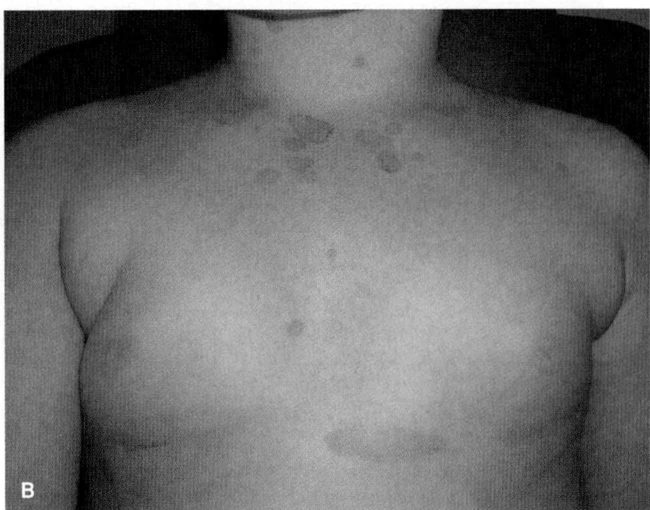

FIGURE 136-5 **A.** Guttate psoriasis that started 2 weeks after strep pharyngitis in this 7-year-old boy. The salmon patches of guttate psoriasis are prominent over the neck, ear, face and scalp. **B.** Other guttate plaques are visible on the chest. (*Used with permission from Richard P. Usatine, MD.*)

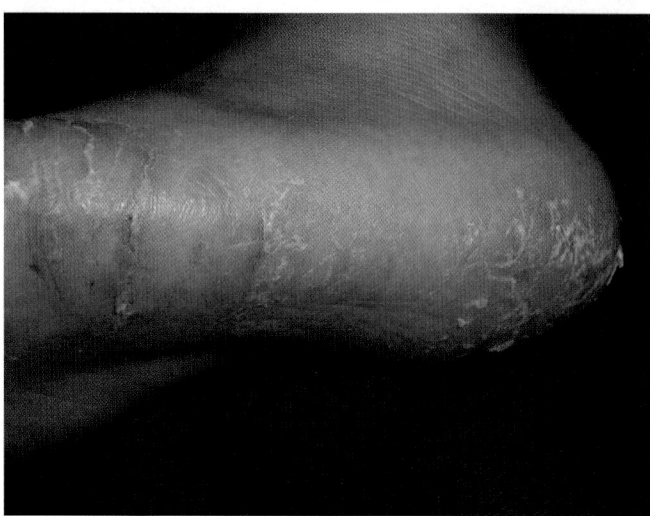

FIGURE 136-7 Plantar psoriasis in a 3-year-old girl who also has psoriasis on her hands and in her nails. Note that the widespread erythema and scale could be mistaken for tinea pedis. (*Used with permission from Richard P. Usatine, MD.*)

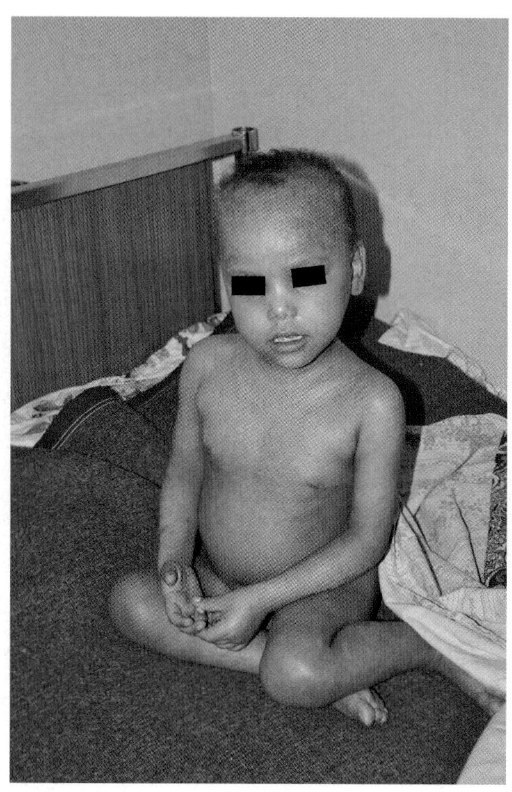

FIGURE 136-8 Erythrodermic psoriasis being treated in a young girl. This young girl was covered with erythematous psoriasis from head to toe prior to being started on systemic treatment in the hospital. (*Used with permission from Richard P. Usatine, MD.*)

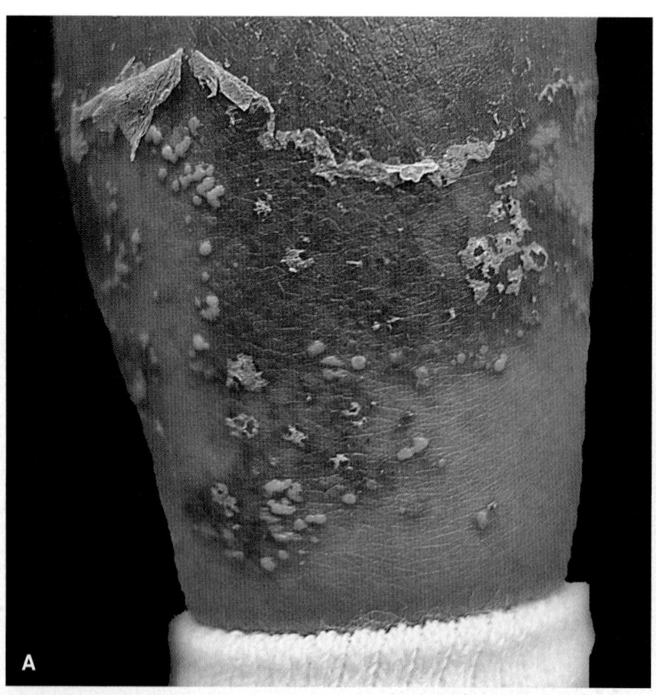

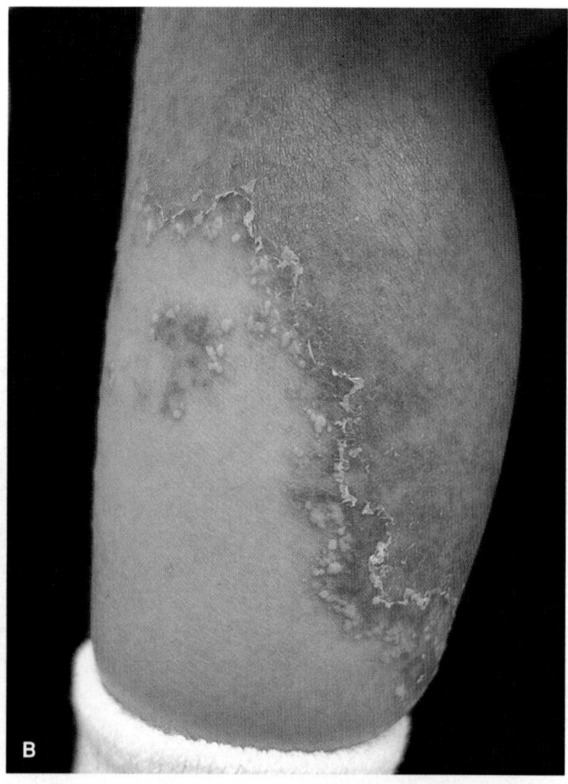

FIGURE 136-9 Pustular psoriasis in a 3-year-old boy. He presented with fever, erythroderma and no history of psoriasis. He was admitted for a presumed infection and then developed pustules. He was started on cyclosporine as an inpatient and then transitioned to acitretin as an outpatient. Note the clusters of pustules and the exfoliation of skin at the borders of the involved areas. **A.** Many pustules are visible on the lower leg. **B.** Pustules on the other leg are on the edge of an area of erythema. (*Used with permission from Emily Becker, MD.*)

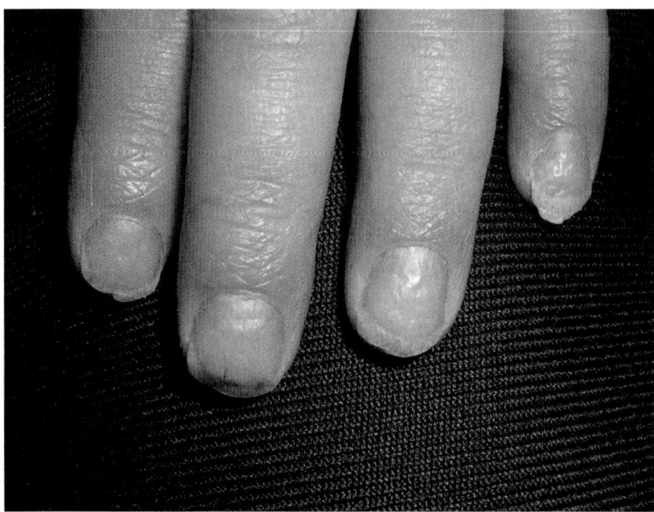

FIGURE 136-10 Nail pitting from psoriasis in a 3-year-old girl. This is the same girl with plantar psoriasis in **Figure 136-7**. (*Used with permission from Richard P. Usatine, MD.*)

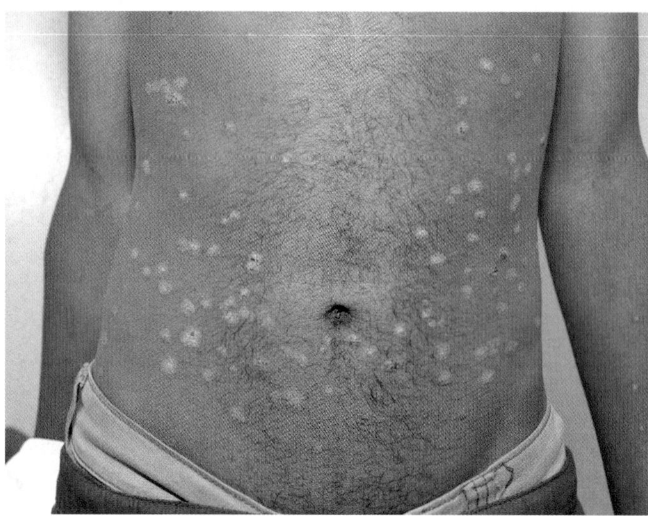

FIGURE 136-12 Guttate psoriasis in a 17-year-old young African teen following an episode of strep pharyngitis. Note how the small plaques are a silvery gray color rather than the erythema seen in lighter pigmented individuals. (*Used with permission from Richard P. Usatine, MD.*)

Plaque psoriasis

- White scale on an erythematous raised base with well-demarcated borders (**Figures 136-2**).
- Plaques can appear in different colors including silvery gray (**Figure 136-12**) and hypopigmented (**Figure 136-13**).
- Positive Auspitz sign in which the peeling of the scale produces pinpoint bleeding on the plaque below.
- Typical distribution includes the elbows and knees and other extensor surfaces. The plaques can be found from head to toe including the umbilicus, vulva, and penis. In children, plaques are more likely to be seen on the face than in adults (**Figure 136-14**).
- Plaques tend to be symmetrically distributed.
- Plaques can be annular with central clearing (**Figure 136-15**).
- When plaques occur at a site of injury, it is known as the Koebner phenomenon.

Scalp psoriasis

- Plaque on the scalp that may be seen at the hairline and around the ears (**Figure 136-3**).
- The thickness and extent of the plaques are variable as seen in plaque psoriasis.

Guttate psoriasis

- Small round plaques that resemble water drops (guttate means like a water drop; **Figure 136-16**).

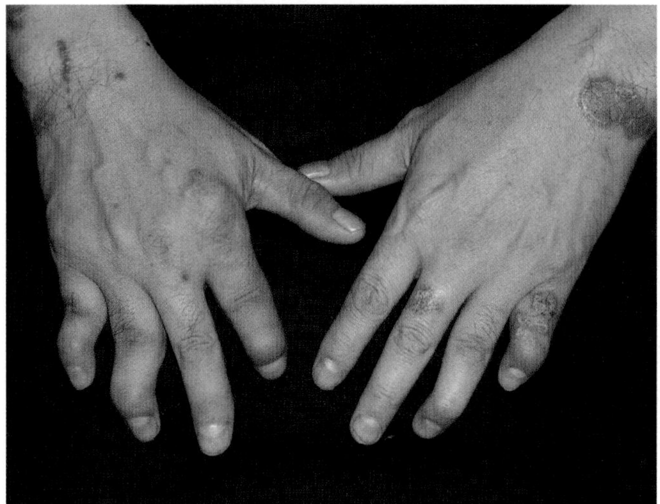

FIGURE 136-11 Psoriatic arthritis that has become crippling to this patient. Note the swan-neck deformities. Psoriatic arthritis should be diagnosed and treated before it gets to this stage. (*Used with permission from Richard P. Usatine, MD.*)

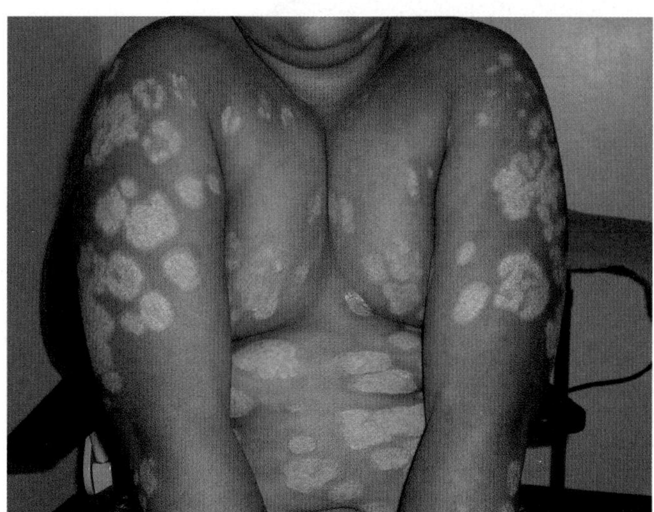

FIGURE 136-13 Plaque psoriasis with hypopigmentation in this 12-year-old obese boy. (*Used with permission from Richard P. Usatine, MD.*)

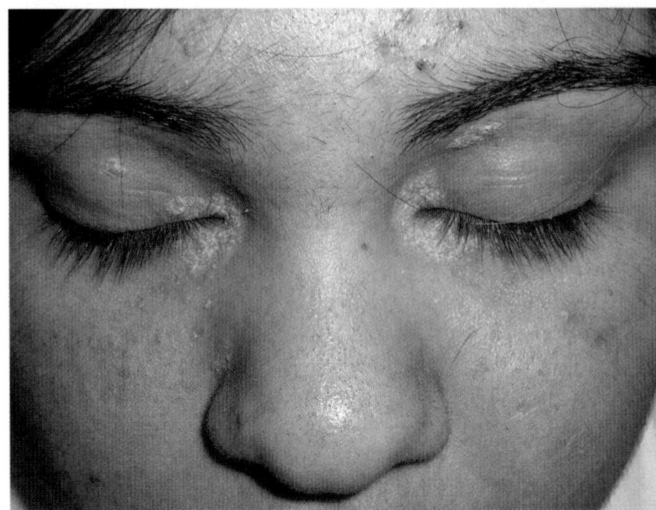

FIGURE 136-14 Plaque psoriasis on the face of a 15-year-old girl. She also has scalp psoriasis. (*Used with permission from Richard P. Usatine, MD.*)

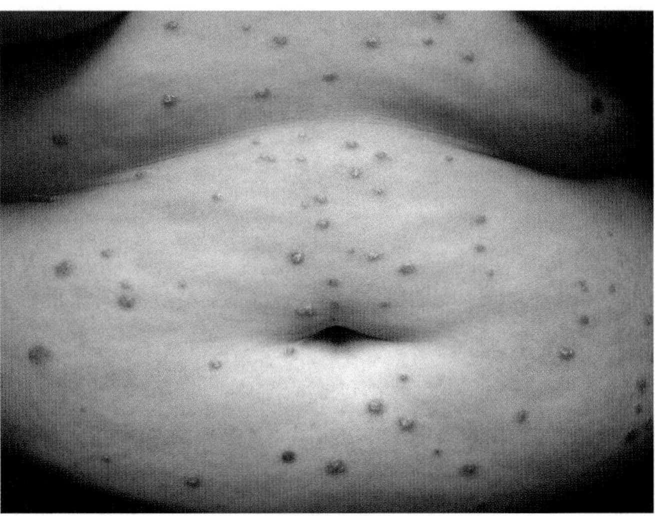

FIGURE 136-16 Guttate psoriasis in an obese 8-year-old girl. After many attempts to treat this with topical corticosteroids and ultraviolet light therapy she finally cleared with etanercept. (*Used with permission from Richard P. Usatine, MD.*)

- Classically described as occurring after strep pharyngitis or another bacterial infection. This is one type of psoriasis that occurs in childhood.
- Typical distribution—The trunk and extremities but may include the face and neck (**Figures 136-1** and **136-5**).

Inverse psoriasis

- Found in the intertriginous areas of the axilla, groin, inframammary folds, and intergluteal fold (**Figure 136-6**). It can also be seen within adipose folds in obese individuals.
- The term *inverse* refers to the fact that the distribution is not on extensor surfaces but in areas of body folds.
- Morphologically the lesions have little to no visible scale.
- Color is generally pink to red but can be hyperpigmented in dark-skinned individuals.

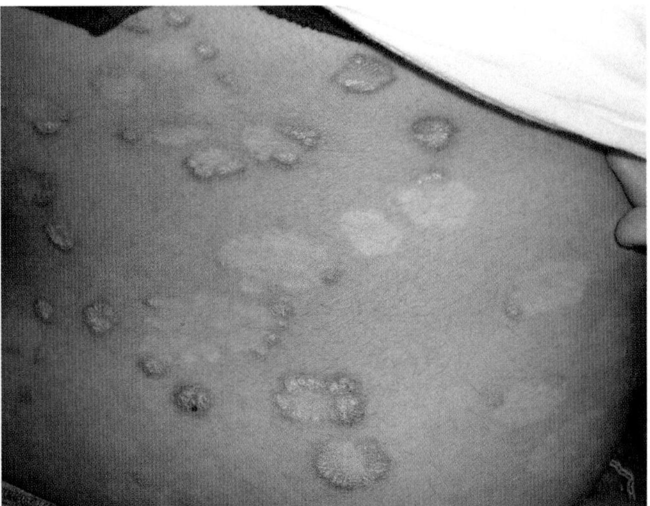

FIGURE 136-15 Plaque psoriasis with annular patterns on the trunk of a 15-year-old girl. Some of the healed plaques have left postinflammatory hypopigmentation. (*Used with permission from Richard P. Usatine, MD.*)

Palmar-plantar (palmoplantar) psoriasis

- Psoriasis that occurs on the plantar aspects of the hands and feet (palms and soles) (**Figure 136-7**). The psoriasis can also be seen on other parts of the hands and feet.
- Patients with this type of psoriasis often experience severe foot and hand pain that can impair walking and other daily activities of living. Hand involvement can result in pain with many types of work.
- Morphologically this can be plaque-like, vesicular, or pustular. Brown spots may be present as macules or flat papules. These are called mahogany spots and although they are not always present, they are characteristic of palmar-plantar psoriasis. Exfoliation of the skin can occur on the palms and soles.

Erythrodermic psoriasis

- Erythrodermic psoriasis is widespread and erythematosus covering most of the skin (**Figure 136-8**).
- Morphologically, it can have plaques and erythema or the erythroderma can appear with the desquamation of pustular psoriasis.
- Widespread distribution can impair the important functions of the skin and this can be a dermatologic urgency requiring hospitalization and IV fluids. Chills, fever, tachycardia, and orthostatic hypotension are all signs that the patient may need hospitalization.

Pustular psoriasis

- Pustular psoriasis comes in localized and generalized types. **Figure 136-9** is an example of localized pustular psoriasis on the lower legs.
- In the generalized type (**Figure 136-17**), the skin initially becomes fiery red and tender, and the patient experiences constitutional signs and symptoms such as headache, fever, chills, arthralgia, malaise, anorexia, and nausea. The desquamation that occurs in the generalized form can impair the important functions of the skin predisposing to dehydration and sepsis. This is a dermatologic emergency requiring hospitalization and IV fluids, preferably in a monitored bed with good nursing care.

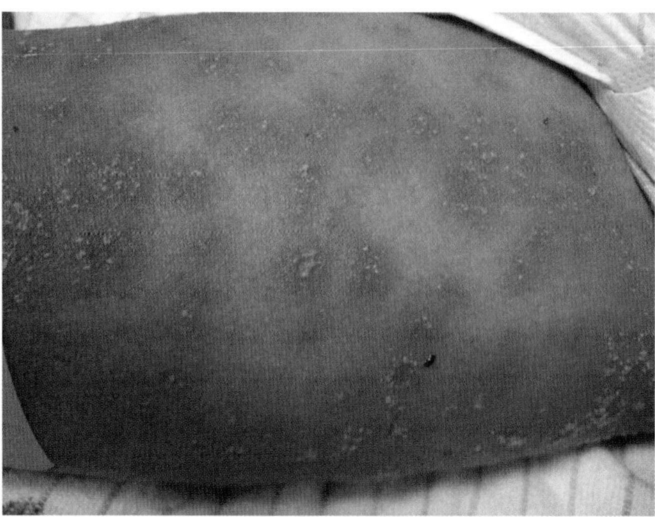

FIGURE 136-17 Generalized pustular psoriasis in a 2-year-old boy not known to have psoriasis before this presentation. The child had fever and was hospitalized for diagnosis and treatment. Note the large areas of erythema and the many pustules present. In some areas, the pustules are beginning to coalesce into lakes of pus and there is desquamation starting to occur. (*Used with permission from John C. Browning, MD.*)

- Typical distribution—Flexural and anogenital. Less often, facial lesions occur. Pustules may occur on the tongue and subungually, resulting in dysphagia and nail shedding, respectively.
- Time course—Within hours, clusters of nonfollicular, superficial 2- to 3-mm pustules may appear in a generalized pattern. These pustules coalesce within 1 day to form lakes of pus that dry and desquamate in sheets, leaving behind a smooth erythematous surface on which new crops of pustules may appear. These episodes of pustulation may occur for days to weeks causing the patient severe discomfort and exhaustion. Upon remission of the pustular component, most systemic symptoms disappear; however, the patient may be in an erythrodermic state or may have residual lesions.[1]

Nail psoriasis

- Nail involvement in psoriasis can lead to pitting, onycholysis, subungual keratosis, splinter hemorrhages, oil spots, and nail loss (**Figure 136-10**; see Chapter 165, Psoriatic Nails).

Psoriatic arthritis

- Asymmetric oligoarthritis typically involving the hands, feet, and knees. The arthritis can also be symmetric and in children is a form of juvenile idiopathic arthritis (see Chapter 172, Juvenile Idiopathic Arthritis). Distal interphalangeal joint (DIP) involvement is a classic finding, but DIP predominance is present in the minority of cases. The fingers may be swollen like sausages, which is called dactylitis.
- Hand involvement can become disabling (**Figure 136-11**). X-rays should be ordered when a patient with psoriasis has joint pains suggesting psoriatic arthritis. At first, the x-rays will be negative other than soft-tissue swelling. Over time, untreated psoriatic arthritis will demonstrate juxtaarticular erosions and pencil-cup deformities seen with the interphalangeal joints.
- There may be inflammation at the insertion of tendons onto bone (enthesopathy). This may occur at the Achilles tendon.
- Patients with psoriatic arthritis need to be treated with systemic agents (methotrexate or biologics) to prevent advancement of the disease.

DISEASE SEVERITY

- Moderate-to-severe disease is defined by psoriasis of the palms, soles, head and neck, or genitalia, and in patients with more than 5 percent body surface area (BSA) involvement. A person's palm is approximately 1 percent BSA and can be used to estimate BSA.
- Another grading system for severity uses the following numbers:
  - Mild—Up to 3 percent BSA.
  - Moderate—3 to 10 percent BSA.
  - Severe—>10 percent BSA (**Figure 136-18**).
- Patients with psoriatic arthritis may have limited skin disease but require more aggressive systemic therapies.
- Note that palmoplantar psoriasis is considered moderate-to-severe even if the BSA involved is not above 3 or 5 percent because of its disabling effect on the patient.

LABORATORY STUDIES

Laboratory studies are rarely needed. A punch biopsy or deep shave is used for evaluating atypical cases. For pustular psoriasis, a 4-mm punch around an intact pustule is preferred.

IMAGING

Plain films should be ordered when a person with psoriasis has joint pains suggesting psoriatic arthritis. Early psoriatic arthritis often has

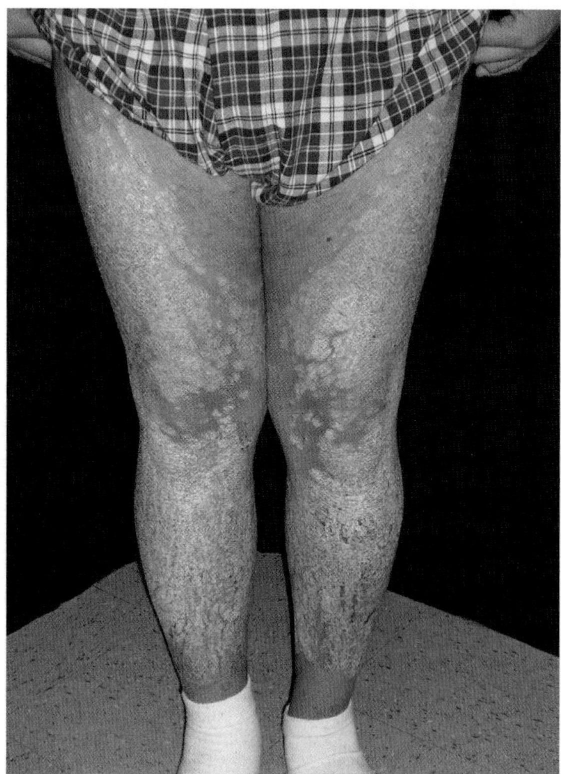

FIGURE 136-18 Widespread plaque psoriasis in the initial presentation of psoriasis in a teenage male. He also had severe pain in his feet and ankles from psoriatic arthritis. His disease was ultimately controlled with a biologic agent. (*Used with permission from Richard P. Usatine, MD.*)

no bone findings on plain films, but if history and physical exam suggest the diagnosis, one should not wait for irreversible visible joint damage to initiate therapy.

DIFFERENTIAL DIAGNOSIS

- Tinea corporis or cruris can resemble inverse psoriasis in the intertriginous areas as both conditions tend to have erythema and thinner plaques without central clearing in these regions. Tinea corporis in nonintertriginous areas typically presents with annular plaques with central clearing. Tinea corporis usually does not have as many plaques as psoriasis but a KOH preparation can be used to look for fungal elements to distinguish between these two conditions (see Chapter 123, Tinea Corporis).
- Lichen planus is a papulosquamous disease similar to psoriasis. Its distribution is more on flexor surfaces and around the wrists and ankles than the elbows and knees (see Chapter 138, Lichen Planus). It is very uncommon in children.
- Lichen simplex chronicus is a hyperkeratotic plaque with lichenification. It usually presents with fewer plaques than psoriasis and is typically found on the posterior neck, ankle, wrist, or lower leg. There is usually more lichenification than thick scale and it is always pruritic (**Figure 136-19**).
- Nummular eczema presents with coin-like plaques. These are most commonly found on the legs and are usually not as thick as the plaques of psoriasis. Nummular eczema may also have vesicles and bullae. Psoriasis has a different distribution and often includes nail changes (see Chapter 133, Nummular Eczema).

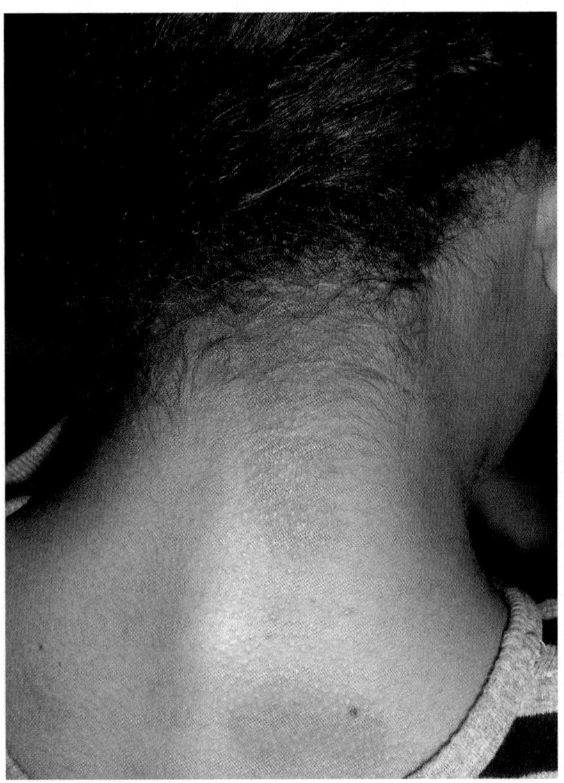

FIGURE 136-19 Lichen simplex chronicus on the neck of a 13-year-old Hispanic female. (*Used with permission from Richard P. Usatine, MD.*)

- Pityriasis rosea is a self-limited process that has papulosquamous plaques. These plaques are less keratotic and have a collarette scale. Pityriasis rosea frequently has a herald patch (see Chapter 137, Pityriasis Rosea).
- Seborrheic dermatitis of the scalp can closely resemble psoriasis of the scalp, especially when it is severe. Psoriasis generally has thicker plaques on the scalp and the plaques often cross the hairline. Seborrhea and psoriasis can both involve the ear. Both conditions respond to topical steroids (see Chapter 135, Seborrheic Dermatitis).
- Syphilis is the great imitator and secondary syphilis can have a papulosquamous eruption similar to psoriasis. Secondary syphilis often involves the palms and soles and the rapid plasma reagin (RPR) will be positive (see Chapter 181, Syphilis).
- Cutaneous candidiasis appears similar to inverse psoriasis when found in intertriginous areas (see Chapter 121, Candidiasis). A KOH prep should be positive and satellite lesions may be visible.

MANAGEMENT

Treat precipitating and underlying factors when these are known. Encourage smoking cessation to all who smoke. Avoid alcohol use. Stress management techniques can be suggested in children and teens who admit that stress is an important factor in worsening their condition. Use preventive techniques as much as possible by avoiding known precipitants.

Patient perception of their disease and expectations for therapy are as important as the evidence and recommendations that follow. Some patients and their parents are willing to live with some skin changes rather than go on systemic treatment, whereas others want everything done with a goal of 100 percent clearance. Consequently, therapeutic choices are made in conjunction with patient and the parent's values and their life situation (economics and time issues surrounding treatment options).

▶ Choice of topical vehicles

- An ointment has a petrolatum base and will penetrate thick scale best.
- An emollient cream has some of the advantages of an ointment but is cosmetically more appealing to patients who find a basic ointment to be too greasy.
- Some patients prefer cream to avoid the oily feel of ointment even though it is less effective in general than an ointment. However, in most cases the most effective vehicle is the one the patient will use as directed.
- Lotions and foams are good for hair-bearing areas when some moisturizing is desired.
- Steroid solutions work well for psoriasis of the scalp.
- New foam preparations have rapid absorption and are cosmetically appealing. These tend to be more expensive and are less likely to be covered by insurance.

▶ Topical treatments

- **Table 136-2** summarizes the strength of recommendations for the treatment of psoriasis using topical therapies. Most studies have

TABLE 136-2 Strength of Recommendations for the Treatment of Psoriasis Using Topical Therapies[1]

Agent	Strength of Recommendation	Level of Evidence
Class I corticosteroids (highest potency)	A	I
Class II corticosteroids	B	II
Classes III/IV corticosteroids (medium potency)	A	I
Classes V/VI/VII corticosteroids (lowest potency)	A	I
Vitamin D analogs	A	I
Tazarotene	A	I
Tacrolimus and pimecrolimus	B	II
Anthralin	C	III
Coal tar	B	II
Combination corticosteroid and salicylic acid	B	II
Combination corticosteroid and vitamin D analog	A	I
Combination corticosteroid and tazarotene	A	I
Combination tacrolimus and salicylic acid	B	II

Adapted from Menter A, Korman NJ, Elmets CA, et al; American Academy of Dermatology. Guidelines of care for the management of psoriasis and psoriatic arthritis. Section 3. Guidelines of care for the management and treatment of psoriasis with topical therapies. J Am Acad Dermatol. 2009;60(4):643-659.

been performed in adults, so evidence is extrapolated to children when adult data is all that is available.

- Research supports potent topical steroids as first-line therapy.[10] SOR A Clobetasol is an ultrahigh-potency steroid that is generic and comes in many vehicles for use on the body and scalp. Clobetasol has FDA approval for children greater than 12 years of age. A meta-analysis of the studies with clobetasol demonstrated 68 to 89 percent of patients had clear improvement or complete healing.[11] SOR A
- In one study, clobetasol foam was found to be safe and effective for treatment of mild-to-moderate plaque-type psoriasis in patients aged 12 years or older.[12] SOR B Reversible hypothalamic-pituitary-adrenal axis suppression secondary to topical clobetasol was observed in 47 percent of participants aged 6 to 12 years.[12]
- Topical 0.1 percent triamcinolone is a moderate strength corticosteroid and can be used on children of any age.
- There are two vitamin D analogs available for topical use: calcipotriene (Dovonex and generic) and calcitriol (Vectical). These vitamin D preparations are recommended as first-line therapy with or without topical corticosteroids for the treatment of childhood psoriasis.[13] SOR A
- Comparable efficacy has been shown for topical calcipotriene (vitamin D analog) and tazarotene (retinoid) with a slight increase in adverse effects for tazarotene.[10] SOR A
- Using topical steroids and calcipotriene or tazarotene is an effective regimen. It has increased efficacy and fewer side effects.[10–11] SOR A However, in monotherapy studies of topical agents in psoriasis, steroids caused fewer adverse reactions compared to vitamin D analogs and tazarotene.[14] SOR A
- Clobetasol in the morning and tazarotene in the evening is a good combination to reduce irritation and increase efficacy.[10] SOR A
- Two trials randomized potent steroid treatment responders to either an intermittent maintenance regime (three applications each weekend) or to no maintenance. The results of more than 6 months indicate that patients receiving maintenance therapy were more than three times as likely to stay in remission.[15] SOR B
- Older treatments still in use include topical coal tar.[11] Evidence does not support the use of coal tar alone or in combination at this time.[11] SOR A
- Topical calcineurin inhibitors previously approved for eczema are being studied for use in psoriasis. Tacrolimus ointment seems most effective in treating psoriasis of the face and intertriginous areas where the skin is thin. Clinical trials suggest that tacrolimus (0.1%) ointment twice a day produces a good response in a majority of patients with facial and intertriginous (inverse) psoriasis (**Figures 136-6** to **136-14**). SOR B
- Emollients and keratolytics are safe and probably beneficial as adjunctive treatment. SOR C
- Intralesional steroids may help small plaques resolve in older children if they will allow these injections. Use triamcinolone acetonide 5 to 10 mg/mL injected with a 27-gauge needle into the plaque. SOR C

Phototherapy

- Is indicated in the presence of extensive and widespread disease (practically defined as more lesions than can be easily counted) and psoriasis not responding to topical therapy.
- Phototherapy is only safe in children old enough and mature enough to sit in a small light box alone with protective eyewear for a number of minutes. They have to understand that the eyewear must be worn the whole time to protect their vision from the damage of the intense ultraviolet light.
- Narrowband UVB is more effective than broadband UVB and approaches psoralen and UVA (PUVA) in efficacy for the treatment of psoriasis in patients with skin types I to III (lighter skin).[19] SOR A
- At present, there are no predictors of the type(s) of psoriasis most responsive to narrowband UVB.[19]
- Of adult patients with psoriasis, 63 to 80 percent will clear with a course of narrowband UVB with equivalent relapse rates compared with PUVA.[19]

- Methotrexate pretreatment (15 mg per week × 3) allowed physicians to clear psoriasis in fewer phototherapy sessions than when phototherapy was administered alone in one study.[20] SOR B
- According to one consensus conference, acitretin combined with UV therapy is safe and effective and limits treatment frequency, duration, and cumulative doses of both agents. They state this combination is better tolerated, more convenient, less costly, and, perhaps, safer during long-term treatment than phototherapy alone.[21] SOR C
- Avoid use of cyclosporine with UV therapy because of an increased risk of skin cancer.[22]

Systemic

- When topical agents (and/or phototherapy fail), systemic agents (including biologic agents) are the next step. **Table 136-3** summarizes the systemic drugs used in treatment of psoriasis.[23]
- Methotrexate and biologic agents are especially valuable in patients with psoriatic arthritis and may be started early in the course of treatment to prevent permanent joint damage.
- Do not use systemic corticosteroid therapy for psoriasis. Pustular flares of disease may be provoked and these flares can be fatal.
- Methotrexate and oral retinoids can cause birth defects so appropriate counseling, contraception, and testing should accompany therapy with these agents.
- In one systematic literature review of the efficacy and safety of treatments for childhood psoriasis, methotrexate was considered to be the systemic treatment of choice.[24] In a consensus statement of pediatric rheumatologists in Germany, the primary treatment of choice for psoriasis and psoriatic arthritis in childhood was methotrexate followed by etanercept.[5] SOR C
- Methotrexate (MTX) is given as a weekly dose titrated to response and side effects.[25] SOR A Tuberculosis screening with purified protein derivative (PPD) or QuantiFERON-TB Gold blood test should precede treatment (if positive results, then the tuberculosis [TB] needs treatment before starting this therapy). Pretreatment laboratories should include a complete blood count (CBC), differential, liver function tests (LFTs), a chemistry profile, and hepatitides B and C serologies. A CBC and LFTs should be followed regularly. Patients should take folic acid daily to prevent some of the possible adverse effects of MTX. For MTX, reliable contraceptive methods should be used during and for at least 3 months after therapy in both males and females.[24]
- The major risk of MTX is liver damage. Type 2 diabetes and obesity appear to be significant risk factors for hepatic fibrosis.[23] The question of whether or when to do a liver biopsy and/or stop MTX is controversial. The National Psoriasis Foundation has published that liver "biopsies are now advocated after a cumulative dose of 3.5 g in low-risk patients and 1.5 g in high-risk patients." The same recommendations are cited in the 2009 National Psoriasis Foundation Consensus Conference on MTX and psoriasis.[26] SOR C
- Cyclosporine (oral) is a T-cell inhibitor and is very effective in rapidly treating psoriasis. The recommended starting dose is 2.5 to 6 mg/kg per day (actual body weight) divided twice a day.[22] SOR C Serum creatinine and blood pressure should be monitored monthly. Also CBC, uric acid, potassium, lipids, LFTs, and magnesium should be monitored monthly. Cyclosporine can be used for long-term therapy in patients with severe psoriasis for up to 2 years life-time maximum based on European guidelines and 1 year maximum based upon the US guidelines.[11,22] SOR C Cyclosporine is pregnancy category C, with several studies

TABLE 136-3 Systemic Drugs Used in Treatment of Psoriasis.[29]

Drug Name	Classification/ Mechanism of Action	Comments
Acitretin	Oral retinoid	Systemic drug for chronic palmoplantar or pustular psoriasis in boys. Avoid in girls as it is teratogenic and has a long half-life.
Cyclosporine	Oral calcineurin inhibitor	Fast-acting systemic drug that is used first-line for pustular psoriasis or erythrodermic psoriasis. For intermittent use in periods up to 12 wk as a short-term agent to control a flare of psoriasis. Is FDA approved to prevent transplant rejections in children but has been used in children off label for atopic dermatitis and psoriasis.
Methotrexate	Inhibitor of folate biosynthesis	May be used as a first-line systemic drug for psoriatic arthritis in all ages with careful monitoring. It has FDA approval for juvenile idiopathic arthritis (JIA) over age 2 but not for cutaneous psoriasis alone.
Adalimumab	TNF inhibitor	FDA approved for juvenile idiopathic arthritis (JIA) over age 4 but not for cutaneous psoriasis alone.
Etanercept	TNF inhibitor	FDA approved for juvenile idiopathic arthritis (JIA) over age 2 but not for cutaneous psoriasis alone. Commonly used as a first-line systemic drug for chronic plaque psoriasis and psoriatic arthritis. Approved in Europe for children aged 8 years and over for the treatment of severe plaque psoriasis.

None FDA approved in children for cutaneous psoriasis but some approved for juvenile idiopathic arthritis (JIA) of which psoriatic arthritis is one type.

indicating an increased risk of premature birth but no major malformations.[22]

- Oral retinoids—Acitretin is a potent systemic retinoid used for psoriasis.[27] SOR Ⓐ Acitretin appears to provide better efficacy in pustular psoriasis (including palmoplantar psoriasis) than in plaque-type psoriasis as a single agent treatment.[28] SOR Ⓐ Acitretin is known to cause fetal malformations just like isotretinoin so it is best to avoid use in women capable of pregnancy, especially as it may remain in the body for up to 3 years after stopping therapy.

▶ Biologic agents

There are 4 biologic agents available and FDA approved for treating psoriasis in adults. See **Table 136-3** for the 2 biologic agents that have been FDA approved for treating children with JIA of which psoriatic arthritis is one type. In Europe, etanercept was approved for children aged 8 years and over for the treatment of severe plaque psoriasis.[29]

- Before starting therapy, obtain a PPD or QuantiFERON-TB *Gold* blood test. These agents can reactivate dormant TB. Screening for TB should continue yearly during biologic therapy.[30]
- The TNF inhibitors (adalimumab, etanercept) share a common mechanism of action that leads to safety concerns. Safety concerns include serious infections (e.g., sepsis, tuberculosis, and viral infections), autoimmune conditions (lupus and demyelinating disorders), and lymphoma.[31]
- Etanercept was studied in 211 children (4 to 17 years of age) in a 48-week study and found to significantly reduce disease severity in children and adolescents with moderate-to-severe plaque psoriasis.[32] The children were given once-weekly subcutaneous injections of placebo or 0.8 mg of etanercept per kilogram of body weight (to a maximum of 50 mg). A subgroup analysis of the original study concluded that etanercept provided significant, sustained improvement in disease severity and was well tolerated in children > or = 8 years with severe plaque psoriasis.[33]
- While the biologic agents are all very expensive, insurance may cover them and there are patient assistance programs for uninsured patients with limited resources.

▶ Methotrexate versus biologic agents[25]

- MTX is a very inexpensive medication with more than a 40-year track record, but with known potential for hepatotoxicity. It is very effective, but requires monitoring of the LFTs and the blood count on a regular basis.
- The biologic agents are engineered proteins with a potentially safer profile than MTX. However, they are very expensive and require parenteral administration. Biologics have the advantage of requiring less monitoring with blood tests. The biologic agents are not side-effect free and some of the potential side effects, while rare, are quite dangerous, and include the risks of sepsis, malignancy, and demyelinating disease.

THERAPY BY TYPE OF PSORIASIS

▶ Plaque type

Mild-to-moderate plaque psoriasis: Start with triamcinolone ointment twice daily for 2 to 4 weeks. Consider topical clobetasol, a stronger topical steroid, if needed. Then decrease use of topical steroid when possible and consider adding a steroid-sparing topical agent such as a vitamin D topical product.

Severe plaque form psoriasis: One systematic review found 665 studies dealing with the treatment of severe plaque psoriasis.[20] Photochemotherapy showed the highest average proportion of patients with clearance (70% [6947/9925]) and good response (83% [8238/9925]), followed by UVB (67.9% [620/913]) and cyclosporine (64% [1030/ 1609]) therapy.[34] SOR Ⓐ Expert consensus in a meeting following data analysis supported the following sequence for the treatments: UVB, photochemotherapy, MTX, acitretin, and cyclosporine.[34] SOR Ⓒ

The Consensus guidelines for the management of plaque psoriasis published in 2012 is based on US National Psoriasis Foundation review and update of the Canadian Guidelines for the Management of Plaque Psoriasis.[29] **Table 136-3** summarizes the systemic treatments for plaque type psoriasis.

▶ Scalp

One head-to-head trial (no pun intended) in scalp psoriasis demonstrated no therapeutic difference between a topical vitamin D derivative and a topical potent steroid.[15] Generic fluocinonide solution daily to the scalp is effective. Derma-smooth is another affordable scalp product that combines a high-potency steroid with a peanut oil. Calcipotriene daily to scalp also helps but is more expensive. Mineral oil may be used to moisturize and remove scale. Shampoos with tar and/or salicylic acid (T-Gel and T-Sal) can help to dissolve and wash away some of the scale. Of course, systemic therapies for more severe psoriasis will help clear scalp psoriasis.

▶ Guttate psoriasis

Phototherapy works particularly well for guttate psoriasis in patients old enough to be able to use phototherapy safely.[9] SOR Ⓒ Narrow-band UVB therapy may produce clearing in less than one month. Topical therapies are a reasonable option when phototherapy is not available.[9] SOR Ⓒ Although both antibiotics and tonsillectomy have frequently been advocated for patients with guttate psoriasis, there is no good evidence that either intervention is beneficial.[35]

▶ Inverse psoriasis

Mid- to high-potency topical steroids can be used for inverse psoriasis even though the disease occurs in skinfolds (**Figure 136-6**). A number of studies have shown that tacrolimus works well to treat inverse psoriasis when applied twice daily.[16–18] SOR Ⓑ Some patients did report a warm sensation or pruritus upon application so patients should be warned of this and told not to stop using the tacrolimus as this may improve over time.[13–15]

▶ Palmar-plantar psoriasis

For mild disease, start with topical treatments as in plaque psoriasis. For moderate to severe cases, systemic therapy such as oral acitretin, MTX, or one of the biologics may be needed.

▶ Erythrodermic/generalized psoriasis

Treatment considerations include hospitalization for dehydration and close monitoring, cyclosporine, MTX, oral retinoids, or phototherapy.[9] SOR Ⓒ Cyclosporine is very effective in rapidly treating the most severe erythrodermic psoriasis.

▸ Pustular psoriasis

Options include oral retinoids such as isotretinoin or acitretin (depends on sex and age of the patient), MTX, cyclosporine, phototherapy, and hospitalization as needed.[9] SOR Ⓒ Cyclosporine is very effective in rapidly treating pustular psoriasis.[22]

REFERRAL

Children with psoriasis that is more than mild and/or requiring more than topical therapy should be referred to a dermatologist. Children with psoriatic arthritis should be referred to a pediatric rheumatologist and/or a pediatric dermatologist.

PROGNOSIS

In one study, the first signs of psoriasis occurred before the age of 18 in 37 percent of patients. The type of childhood onset psoriasis often remained the same from childhood to adulthood. They found no evidence that getting psoriasis before the age of 18 years influences disease severity in later life. The authors concluded that the age of onset of psoriasis essentially does not influence the subsequent course of the disease.[36]

FOLLOW-UP

- Follow-up may need to be frequent for various therapies including cytotoxic drugs, the biologics, and light therapy.
- While there are many safety concerns with the biologic agents a recent integrated safety analysis of short- and long-term safety profiles of etanercept in patients with psoriasis concluded that rates of noninfectious and infectious adverse events were comparable between placebo and etanercept groups.[37] Also, there was no increase in overall malignancies with etanercept therapy compared with the psoriasis population.[37]
- Well-controlled psoriasis on topical agents does not require frequent follow-up.

PATIENT EDUCATION

This is a chronic disease that cannot be cured. There are many methods to control psoriasis. Patients and their families need to develop a relationship with the dermatologist to control the psoriasis for maximum quality of life. **Table 136-4** lists discussion points.

PATIENT RESOURCES

- The National Psoriasis Foundation—**www.psoriasis.org/**.
- About psoriasis in children—**www.psoriasis.org/learn_children**.
- Psoriasis Association—**www.psoriasis-association.org.uk/pages/view/about-psoriasis/children-and-psoriasis**.

TABLE 136-4 Discussion Points for Health care Provider and Patient/Parents at Initial Visits

- Hereditary aspects
- Systemic manifestations
- Exacerbating and ameliorating factors
- Past treatment responses
- Range of therapeutic options
- Chronic long-term disease
- Psychological issues
- Optimism for tomorrow based on rapid research developments
- Support/services available from the National Psoriasis Foundation

PROVIDER RESOURCES

- Hsu S, Papp KA, Lebwohl MG, et al. Consensus guidelines for the management of plaque psoriasis. *Arch Dermatol*. 2012;148(1):95-102. **http://archderm.ama-assn.org/cgi/content/short/148/1/95**.
- National Guideline Clearinghouse. Guidelines of Care for the Management of Psoriasis and Psoriatic Arthritis. Section 3. Guidelines of Care for the Management and Treatment of Psoriasis with Topical Therapies—**www.guidelines.gov/content.aspx?id =14572&search=psoriasis**.
- The National Psoriasis Foundation—**www.psoriasis.org/health-care-providers/treating-psoriasis**.
- Medscape. *Psoriasis*—**http//emedicine.medscape.com/article/1943419**.
- Medscape. *Guttate Psoriasis*—**http//emedicine.medscape.com/article/1107850**.

REFERENCES

1. Menter A, Korman NJ, Elmets CA, et al. Guidelines of care for the management of psoriasis and psoriatic arthritis. Section 3. Guidelines of care for the management and treatment of psoriasis with topical therapies. *J Am Acad Dermatol*. 2009;60:643-659.
2. Gelfand JM, Stern RS, Nijsten T, et al. The prevalence of psoriasis in African Americans: results from a population-based study. *J Am Acad Dermatol*. 2005;52:23-26.
3. Henseler T, Christophers E. Psoriasis of early and late onset: characterization of two types of psoriasis vulgaris. *J Am Acad Dermatol*. 1985;13:450-456.
4. Radtke MA, Folster-Holst R, Beikert F, Herberger K, Augustin M. Juvenile psoriasis: rewarding endeavours in contemporary dermatology and pediatrics. *G Ital Dermatol Venereol*. 2011;146:31-45.
5. Sticherling M, Minden K, Kuster RM, Krause A, Borte M. [Psoriasis und Psoriasis arthritis in childhood and adolescence. Overview and consensus statement of the 9th Worlitz Expert Round Table Discussion 2006 for the Society for Child and Adolescent Rheumatology]. *Z Rheumatol*. 2007;66:349-354.

6. Menter A, Weinstein GD. An overview of psoriasis. In: Koo YM, Lebwohl MD, Lee CS, eds. *Therapy of Moderate-to-Severe Psoriasis*. London, UK: Informa Healthcare; 2008:1-26.
7. Jankovic S, Raznatovic M, Marinkovic J, et al. Risk factors for psoriasis: a case-control study. *J Dermatol.* 2009;36:328-334.
8. Ozden MG, Tekin NS, Gurer MA et al. Environmental risk factors in pediatric psoriasis: a multicenter case-control study. *Pediatr Dermatol.* 2011;28:306-312.
9. Callen JP, Krueger GG, Lebwohl M, et al. AAD consensus statement on psoriasis therapies. *J Am Acad Dermatol.* 2003;49:897-899.
10. Afifi T, de Gannes G, Huang C, Zhou Y. Topical therapies for psoriasis: evidence-based review. *Can Fam Physician.* 2005;51:519-525.
11. Nast A, Kopp I, Augustin M, et al. German evidence-based guidelines for the treatment of Psoriasis vulgaris (short version). *Arch Dermatol Res.* 2007;299:111-138.
12. Kimball AB, Gold MH, Zib B, Davis MW. Clobetasol propionate emulsion formulation foam 0.05%: review of phase II open-label and phase III randomized controlled trials in steroid-responsive dermatoses in adults and adolescents. *J Am Acad Dermatol.* 2008; 59:448-54, 454.
13. de Jager ME, de Jong EM, van de Kerkhof PC, Seyger MM. Efficacy and safety of treatments for childhood psoriasis: a systematic literature review. *J Am Acad Dermatol.* 2010;62:1013-1030.
14. Bruner CR, Feldman SR, Ventrapragada M, Fleischer AB Jr: A systematic review of adverse effects associated with topical treatments for psoriasis. *Dermatol Online J.* 2003;9:2.
15. Mason J, Mason AR, Cork MJ. Topical preparations for the treatment of psoriasis: a systematic review. *Br J Dermatol.* 2002;146: 351-364.
16. Brune A, Miller DW, Lin P, et al. Tacrolimus ointment is effective for psoriasis on the face and intertriginous areas in pediatric patients. *Pediatr Dermatol.* 2007;24:76-80.
17. Lebwohl M, Freeman AK, Chapman MS, et al. Tacrolimus ointment is effective for facial and intertriginous psoriasis. *J Am Acad Dermatol.* 2004;51:723-730.
18. Martin EG, Sanchez RM, Herrera AE, Umbert MP. Topical tacrolimus for the treatment of psoriasis on the face, genitalia, intertriginous areas and corporal plaques. *J Drugs Dermatol.* 2006;5:334-336.
19. Ibbotson SH, Bilsland D, Cox NH, et al. An update and guidance on narrowband ultraviolet B phototherapy: a British Photodermatology Group Workshop Report. *Br J Dermatol.* 2004;151: 283-297.
20. Asawanonda P, Nateetongrungsak Y. Methotrexate plus narrowband UVB phototherapy versus narrowband UVB phototherapy alone in the treatment of plaque-type psoriasis: a randomized, placebo-controlled study. *J Am Acad Dermatol.* 2006;54:1013-1018.
21. Lebwohl M, Drake L, Menter A, et al. Consensus conference: acitretin in combination with UVB or PUVA in the treatment of psoriasis. *J Am Acad Dermatol.* 2001;45:544-553.
22. Rosmarin DM, Lebwohl M, Elewski BE, Gottlieb AB. Cyclosporine and psoriasis: 2008 National Psoriasis Foundation Consensus Conference. *J Am Acad Dermatol.* 2010;62:838-853.
23. Montaudie H, Sbidian E, Paul C, et al. Methotrexate in psoriasis: a systematic review of treatment modalities, incidence, risk factors and monitoring of liver toxicity. *J Eur Acad Dermatol Venereol.* 2011;25 Suppl 2:12-18.
24. de Jager ME, de Jong EM, van de Kerkhof PC, Seyger MM. Efficacy and safety of treatments for childhood psoriasis: a systematic literature review. *J Am Acad Dermatol* 2010;62: 1013-1030.
25. Saporito FC, Menter MA. Methotrexate and psoriasis in the era of new biologic agents. *J Am Acad Dermatol.* 2004;50:301-309.
26. Kalb RE, Strober B, Weinstein G, Lebwohl M. Methotrexate and psoriasis: 2009 National Psoriasis Foundation Consensus Conference. *J Am Acad Dermatol.* 2009;60:824-837.
27. Pearce DJ, Klinger S, Ziel KK, et al. Low-dose acitretin is associated with fewer adverse events than high-dose acitretin in the treatment of psoriasis. *Arch Dermatol.* 2006;142:1000-1004.
28. Sbidian E, Maza A, Montaudie H, et al. Efficacy and safety of oral retinoids in different psoriasis subtypes: a systematic literature review. *J Eur Acad Dermatol Venereol.* 2011;25 Suppl 2:28-33.
29. Hsu S, Papp KA, Lebwohl MG, et al. Consensus guidelines for the management of plaque psoriasis. *Arch Dermatol.* 2012;148: 95-102.
30. Sivamani RK, Goodarzi H, Garcia MS, et al. Biologic therapies in the treatment of psoriasis: a comprehensive evidence-based basic science and clinical review and a practical guide to tuberculosis monitoring. *Clin Rev Allergy Immunol.* 2012 Feb 5. [Epub ahead of print.]
31. Gottlieb A, Korman NJ, Gordon KB, et al. Guidelines of care for the management of psoriasis and psoriatic arthritis: section 2. Psoriatic arthritis: overview and guidelines of care for treatment with an emphasis on the biologics. *J Am Acad Dermatol.* 2008;58:851-864.
32. Paller AS, Siegfried EC, Langley RG et al. Etanercept treatment for children and adolescents with plaque psoriasis. *N Engl J Med.* 2008;358:241-251.
33. Landells I, Paller AS, Pariser D et al. Efficacy and safety of etanercept in children and adolescents aged > or = 8 years with severe plaque psoriasis. *Eur J Dermatol.* 2010;20:323-328.
34. Spuls PI, Bossuyt PM, van Everdingen JJ, et al. The development of practice guidelines for the treatment of severe plaque form psoriasis. *Arch Dermatol.* 1998;134:1591-1596.
35. Owen CM, Chalmers RJ, O'Sullivan T, Griffiths CE. A systematic review of antistreptococcal interventions for guttate and chronic plaque psoriasis. *Br J Dermatol.* 2001;145:886-890.
36. de Jager ME, de Jong EM, Meeuwis KA, van de Kerkhof PC, Seyger MM. No evidence found that childhood onset of psoriasis influences disease severity, future body mass index or type of treatments used. *J Eur Acad Dermatol Venereol.* 2010;24: 1333-1339.
37. Pariser DM, Leonardi CL, Gordon K, Gottlieb AB, Tyring S, Papp KA, Li J, Baumgartner SW. Integrated safety analysis: Short- and long-term safety profiles of etanercept in patients with psoriasis. *J Am Acad Dermatol.* 2012;67(2):245-256.

137 PITYRIASIS ROSEA

David Henderson, MD
Richard P. Usatine, MD

PATIENT STORY

A 17-year-old is brought to the office by her mom because of a rash that appeared 3 weeks ago for no apparent reason (**Figures 137-1** to **137-3**). She was feeling well and the rash is only occasionally pruritic. With and without mom in the room, the patient denied sexual activity. The diagnosis of pityriasis rosea was made by the clinical appearance even though there was no obvious herald patch. The collarette scale was visible and the distribution was consistent with pityriasis rosea. The patient and her mom were reassured that this would resolve spontaneously. At a subsequent visit for a college physical, the skin was found to be completely clear with no scarring.

INTRODUCTION

Pityriasis rosea is a common, self-limited, papulosquamous skin condition originally described in the 19th century. It is seen in children and adults. Despite the long history, its etiology remains elusive. A number of infectious etiologies have been proposed, but at present, supporting evidence is inconclusive. Pityriasis rosea has unique features including a herald patch in many cases and collarette scale that are useful in distinguishing it from other papulosquamous eruptions.

EPIDEMIOLOGY

- Pityriasis rosea is a papulosquamous eruption of unknown etiology.[1]
- It occurs throughout the life cycle. It is most commonly seen between the ages of 10 and 35 years.[3]

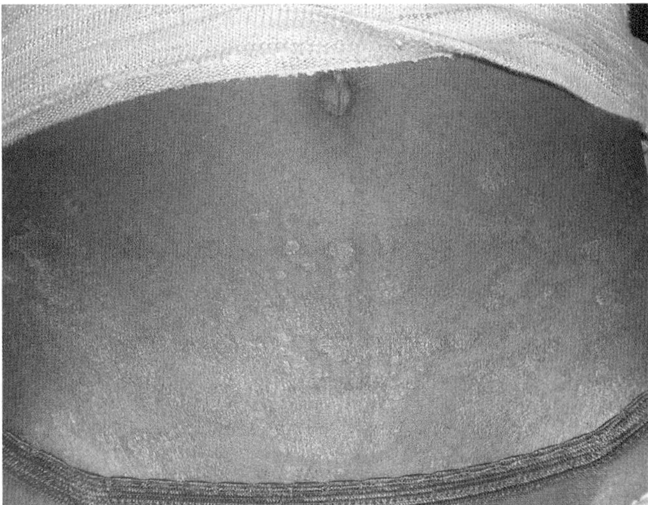

FIGURE 137-1 Pityriasis rosea in a 17-year-old. Lesions are often concentrated in the lower abdominal area. (*Used with permission from Richard P. Usatine, MD.*)

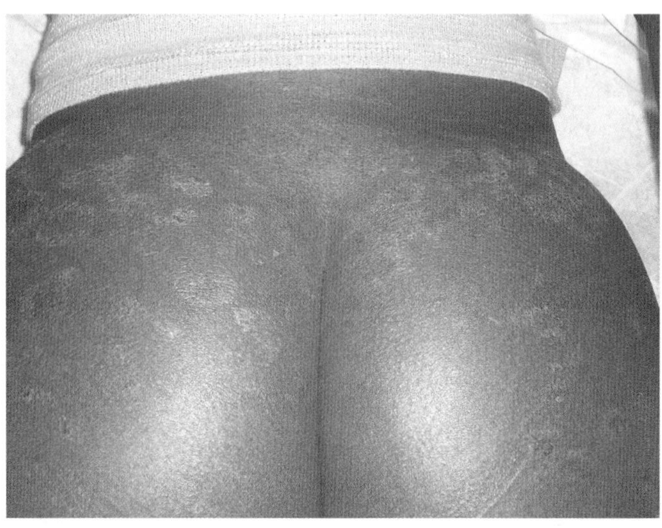

FIGURE 137-2 Scaling lesions seen on the buttocks of the same teen as in **Figure 137-1**. Note how some of the lesions are annular. (*Used with permission from Richard P. Usatine, MD.*)

- The peak incidence is between 20 and 29 years of age.[1]
- The gender distribution is essentially equal.[1]
- The rash is most prevalent in winter months.[4]

ETIOLOGY AND PATHOPHYSIOLOGY

- The cause of pityriasis rosea is unknown, although numerous causes have been proposed.
- It has long been suspected that it may have a viral etiology because a viral-like prodrome often occurs prior to the onset of the rash. Human herpesviruses 6 and 7 have been proposed as causes, but numerous studies have failed to demonstrate conclusive supportive evidence.[1,2]
- *Chlamydophila pneumoniae, Mycoplasma pneumoniae, and Legionella pneumophila* have been proposed as potential etiologic agents, but studies have not demonstrated any significant rise in antibody levels against any of these pathogens in patients with pityriasis rosea.[1]

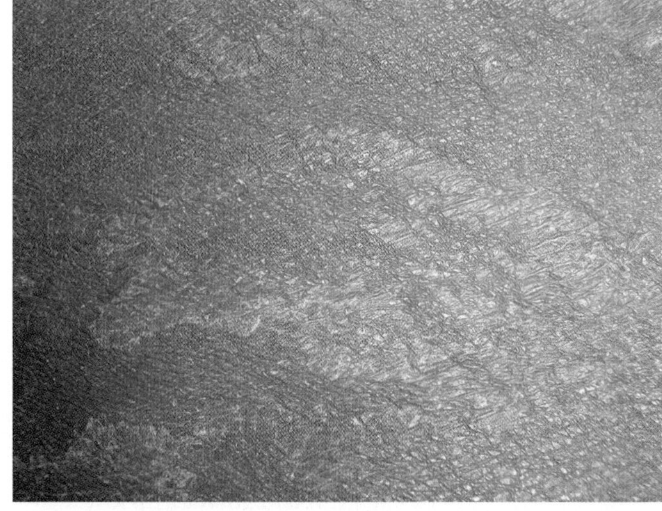

FIGURE 137-3 Close-up of lesion showing collarette scale. Note how the lesions can be annular with some central clearing. (*Used with permission from Richard P. Usatine, MD.*)

- Pityriasis rosea has also been associated with negative pregnancy outcomes, particularly premature birth. The risk seems to be greatest when the condition occurs in the first 15 weeks of gestation.[2]
- Pityriasis rosea may rarely occur as the result of a drug reaction. Documented drug reactions that have produced a pityriasis rosea-like eruption include barbiturates, captopril, clonidine, interferon, bismuth, gold, and the hepatitis B vaccine.[1,2]

DIAGNOSIS

CLINICAL FEATURES

- In approximately 20 to 50 percent of cases, the rash of pityriasis rosea is preceded by a viral-like illness consisting of upper respiratory or GI symptoms.
- This is followed by the appearance of a *herald patch* in 17 percent of cases (**Figures 137-4** to **137-6**).[4]
- The herald patch is a solitary, oval, flesh-colored to salmon-colored lesion with scaling at the border. It often occurs on the trunk, and is generally 2 to 10 cm in diameter (**Figures 137-4** and **137-5**).
- One to two weeks after the appearance of the herald patch, other papulosquamous lesions appear on the trunk and sometimes on the extremities.
- These lesions vary from oval macules to slightly raised plaques, 0.5 to 2 cm in size. They are salmon colored (or hyperpigmented in individuals with dark skin), and typically have a collarette of scaling at the border (**Figure 137-3**). It is common for some of the lesions to appear annular with central clearing.
- In many cases, the herald patch has resolved by the time the rest of the exanthem erupts which can make the diagnosis more difficult.
- There are no systemic symptoms.
- Itching occurs in approximately 25 percent of patients.
- The exanthem resolves in 8 weeks in 80 percent of patients.[1] However, it can last up to 3 to 5 months.[3]

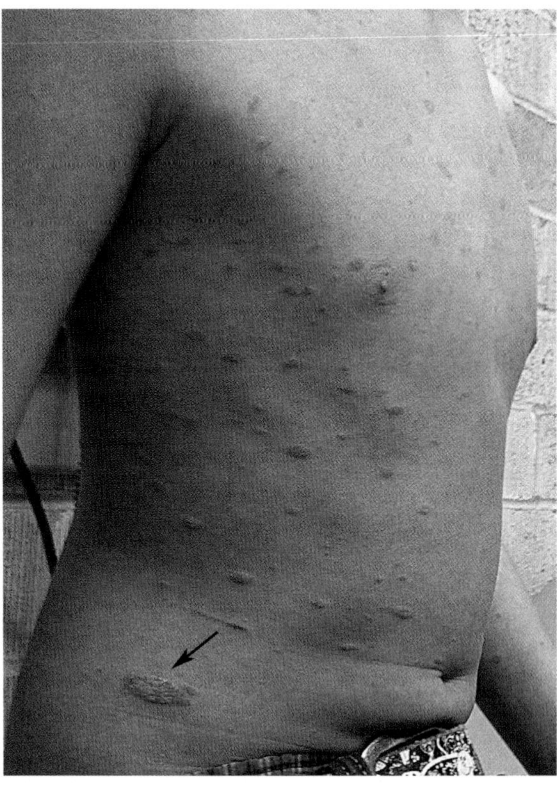

FIGURE 137-5 Pityriasis rosea in a 13-year-old boy. *Arrow* points to herald patch. (*Used with permission from Richard P. Usatine, MD.*)

TYPICAL DISTRIBUTION

- The rash is bilaterally symmetrical, generally most dense on the trunk, but also involves the upper and lower extremities.
- The lesions follow the cleavage, or Langer lines, and may create the typical *fir* or *Christmas tree* pattern over the back (**Figure 137-7**). Do not expect to always see a Christmas tree pattern.
- Over the chest, the lesions create a V-shaped pattern, and run transversely over the abdomen (**Figures 137-8** and **137-9**).

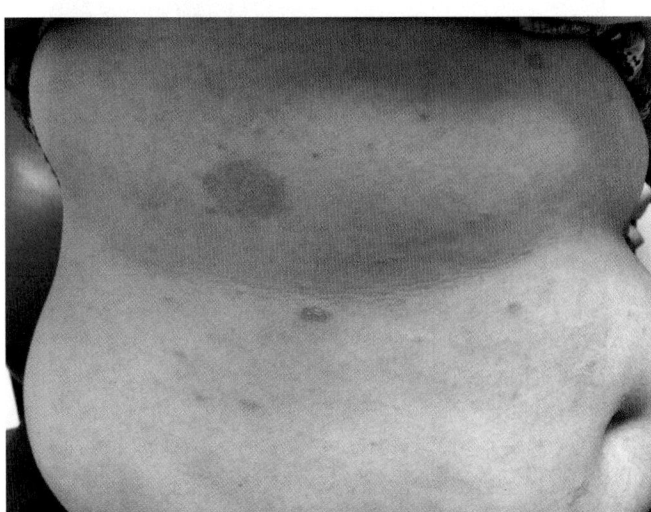

FIGURE 137-4 Pityriasis rosea with prominent pink herald patch on the abdomen of this overweight teenager. (*Used with permission from Richard P. Usatine, MD.*)

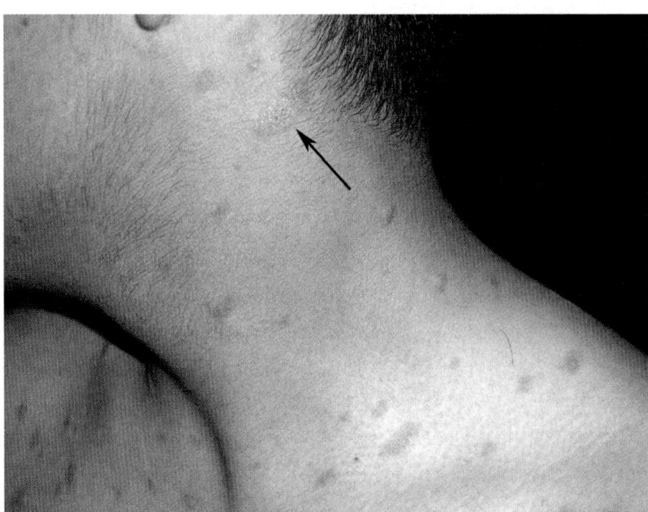

FIGURE 137-6 Pityriasis rosea in a 15-year-old boy with the herald patch on the neck near the hairline. (*Used with permission from Richard P. Usatine, MD.*)

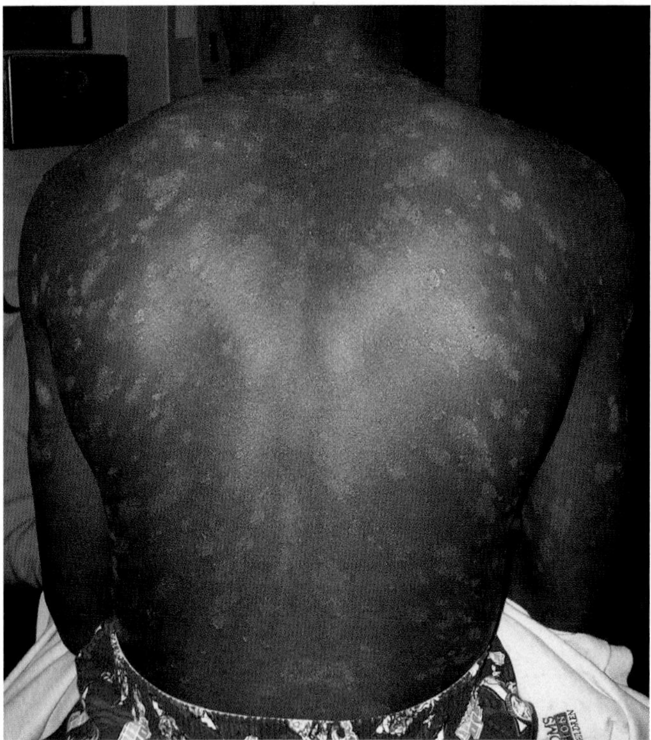

FIGURE 137-7 Pityriasis rosea in a 16-year-old boy. The scaling lesions follow skin lines and resemble a Christmas tree. (*Used with permission from E.J. Mayeaux, Jr., MD.*)

- An inverse form has been described, characterized by more intense involvement of the extremities and relative sparing of the trunk (**Figures 137-10** and **137-11**).

LABORATORY STUDIES

Pityriasis rosea is a clinical diagnosis. There are no laboratory tests that aid in the diagnosis. Biopsy of lesions typically reveals only non-specific inflammatory changes. Because secondary syphilis is also a papulosquamous eruption and can be difficult to distinguish from pityriasis rosea on clinical grounds, taking a sexual history is important when a diagnosis of pityriasis rosea is being considered. In patients

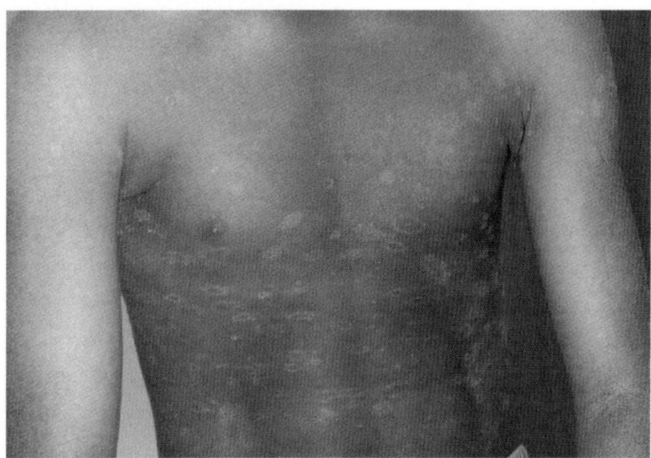

FIGURE 137-8 Pityriasis rosea in a 12-year-old boy showing classic scaling lesions across the chest and abdomen. Small annular lesions are visible. (*Used with permission from Jeffrey Meffert, MD.*)

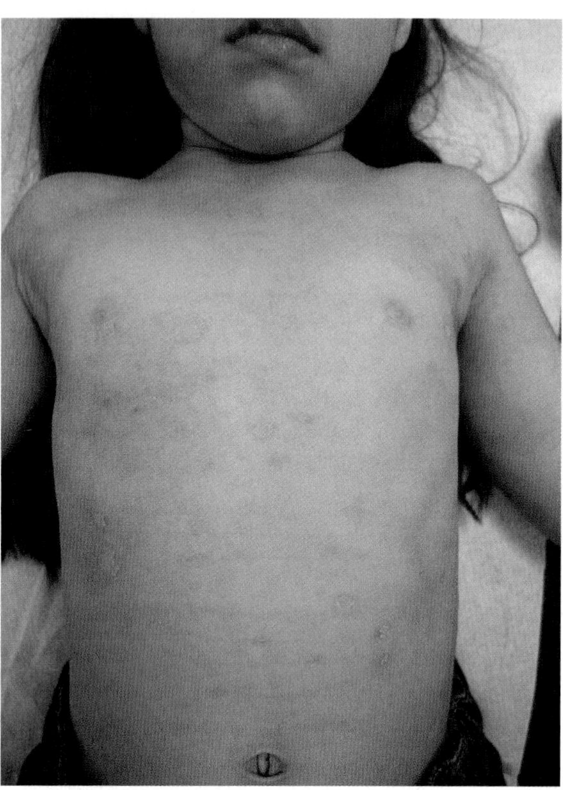

FIGURE 137-9 Pityriasis rosea on the chest and abdomen of this young girl. While the lesions are subtle, close-up examination reveals a trailing scale pattern. (*Used with permission from Emily Becker, MD.*)

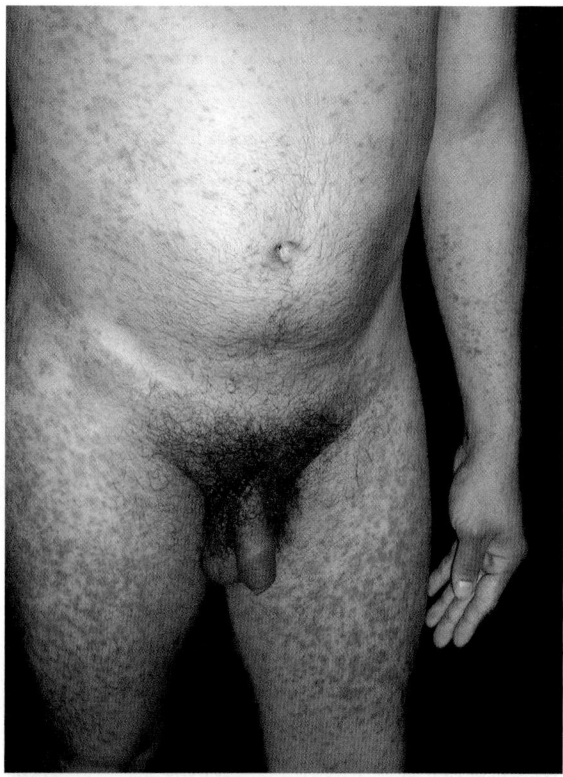

FIGURE 137-10 Pityriasis rosea with an inverse pattern. Note how there is a higher density of lesions on the legs. Rapid plasma reagin (RPR) was negative and the diagnosis was confirmed with a punch biopsy. (*Used with permission from Richard P. Usatine, MD.*)

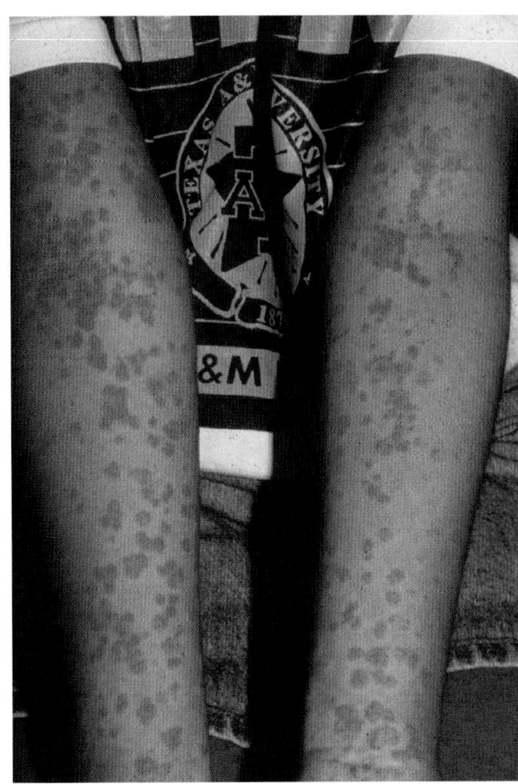

FIGURE 137-11 Pityriasis rosea with an inverse pattern on the arms with prominent erythematous lesions. (*Used with permission from the University of Texas Health Sciences Center, Division of Dermatology.*)

with a history of sexually transmitted diseases, or sexual practices that place them at risk, a blood test for syphilis should be considered (**Figures 137-10**) (see Chapter 181, Syphilis).

DIFFERENTIAL DIAGNOSIS

- Tinea corporis is usually more localized than pityriasis rosea. However, the annular patterns, scale, and central clearing of some lesions in pityriasis rosea can mislead the clinician to misdiagnose tinea corporis. Tinea corporis tends to have fewer annular lesions and may have concentric circles rather than a single ring. Microscopy with KOH usually demonstrates branching hyphae (see Chapter 123, Tinea Corporis).
- Tinea versicolor has a distribution similar to pityriasis rosea, but is not associated with a herald patch. The pattern of scaling noted is generally more diffuse and not annular. Microscopy with KOH demonstrates the *spaghetti-and-meatball* pattern typical of *Pityrosporum* (see Chapter 126, Tinea Versicolor).
- Secondary syphilis is also a papulosquamous eruption. Lesions are often found on the palms and soles, which is not the case in pityriasis rosea; however, because the two conditions cannot always be accurately distinguished on clinical grounds, a blood test for syphilis is indicated if there is a significant doubt in the diagnosis (see Chapter 181, Syphilis).
- Nummular eczema has coin-like areas of scale that can resemble pityriasis rosea. The scale is not collarette and nummular eczema has a predilection for the legs, an area that is less often involved with pityriasis rosea (see Chapter 130, Atopic Dermatitis).
- Guttate psoriasis generally presents as oval to round, scaly macules on the trunk, and so can be confused with pityriasis rosea. However, the scaling is generally thicker and more adherent than in pityriasis rosea (see Chapter 136, Psoriasis).

MANAGEMENT

- Pityriasis rosea often requires no treatment at all other than reassurance.
- Topical steroids and oral diphenhydramine may be used to relieve itching when there is pruritus involved. SOR Ⓒ
- One study found oral erythromycin to be effective in treating patients with pityriasis rosea,[5] although a subsequent study did not find erythromycin to be better than placebo.[6] SOR Ⓑ
- Azithromycin did not cure pityriasis rosea in a study of children with this condition.[7]
- A Cochrane systematic review found inadequate evidence for efficacy for most treatments for pityriasis rosea.[8] Based on one small randomized controlled trial (RCT), the review authors noted that oral erythromycin may be effective in treating the rash and decreasing the itch.[5,8] The authors stated that this result should be treated with caution as it comes from only one small RCT.[5,8] SOR Ⓑ

FOLLOW-UP

- Patients should be instructed to follow up if the rash persists for longer than 3 months as reevaluation and consideration of an alternate diagnosis may be prudent.

PATIENT EDUCATION

- Patients are often concerned about the duration of the rash and whether they are contagious. They should be reassured that pityriasis rosea is self-limited and not truly contagious. Although there have been reported clusters of pityriasis rosea in settings where people are living in close quarters (e.g., dormitories), it is not considered to be contagious. It has a reported recurrence rate of only 2 percent.[5]

PATIENT RESOURCES

- Mayo Clinic. *Pityriasis Rosea*—**www.mayoclinic.com/health/pityriasis-rosea/DS00720**.
- WebMD. *Pityriasis Rosea: Topic Overview*—**www.webmd.com/skin-problems-and-treatments/tc/pityriasis-rosea-topic-overview**.

PROVIDER RESOURCES

- Medscape. *Pityriasis Rosea in Emergency Medicine*—**http://emedicine.medscape.com/article/762725**.
- American Academy of Dermatology. *Pityriasis Rosea*—**www.aad.org/skin-conditions/dermatology-a-to-z/pityriasis-rosea**.

REFERENCES

1. Stulberg DH, Wolfrey J. Pityriasis rosea. *Am Fam Physician.* 2004;69: 87-92, 94.

2. Browning JC. An update on pityriasis rosea and other similar childhood exanthems. *Curr Opin Pediatr.* 2009;21(4):481-485.

3. Youngquist S, Usatine R. It's beginning to look a lot like Christmas. *West J Med.* 2001;175(4):227-228.

4. Habif TP. *Clinical Dermatology*, 5th ed. St Louis, MO. Mosby; 2009:316-319.

5. Sharma PK, Yadav TP, Gautam RK, et al. Erythromycin in pityriasis rosea: a double-blind, placebo-controlled clinical trial. *J Am Acad Dermatol.* 2000;42(2 Pt 1):241-244.

6. Rasi A, Tajziehchi L, Savabi-Nasab S. Oral erythromycin is ineffective in the treatment of pityriasis rosea. *J Drugs Dermatol.* 2008;7(1):35-38.

7. Amer H, Fischer H. Azithromycin does not cure pityriasis rosea. *Pediatrics.* 2006;117(4):1702-1705.

8. Chuh AA, Dofitas BL, Comisel GG, et al. Interventions for pityriasis rosea. *Cochrane Database Syst Rev.* 2007;(2):CD005068.

138 LICHEN PLANUS

Robert Kraft, MD
Richard P. Usatine, MD

PATIENT STORY

A 12-year-old boy presents with a rash on his wrists, forearms and ankle for one month (**Figure 138-1**). The rash itches and he does not know where it comes from. The father states that there are no other members of the family with such a rash now or in the past. The pediatrician recognized the morphology and distribution as that of lichen planus. The papules and plaques on the wrist were pink and purple, planar, pruritic and polygonal. The pediatrician looked inside the mouth and the mucosa was clear with no Wickham's striae. The boy was started on a mid-potency topical steroid ointment and a follow up appointment was scheduled.

INTRODUCTION

Lichen planus (LP) is a self-limited, recurrent, or chronic autoimmune disease affecting the skin, oral mucosa, and genitalia. LP is generally diagnosed clinically with lesions classically described using the six Ps (planar, purple, polygonal, pruritic, papules, and plaques).

EPIDEMIOLOGY

- LP is an inflammatory dermatosis of skin or mucous membranes that occurs in approximately 1 percent of all new patients seen at health care clinics.[1]

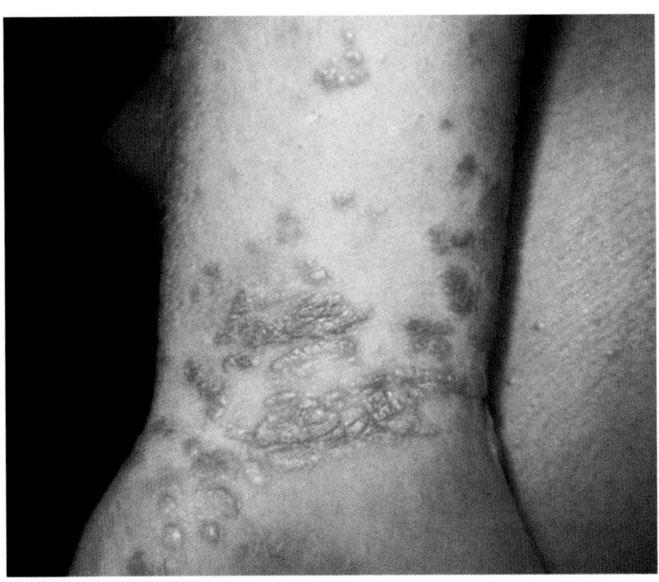

FIGURE 138-1 Lichen planus on the flexor surface of the wrist of a 12-year-old boy. *(Used with permission from Weinberg SW, Prose NS, Kristal L, Color Atlas of Pediatric Dermatology, 4th edition, Figure 9-40, New York, NY: McGraw-Hill, 2008.)*

- Although most cases occur between ages 30 and 60 years, LP can occur at any age with fewer than 4 percent of cases in patients under age 20.[1–4]
- There may be a slight female predominance.[2,5–7]

ETIOLOGY AND PATHOPHYSIOLOGY

- Usually idiopathic, thought to be a cell-mediated immune response to an unknown antigen.[2,5,8]
- Possible human leukocyte antigen (HLA)-associated genetic predisposition.[2]
- Lichenoid-type reactions may be associated with medications (e.g., angiotensin-converting enzyme inhibitors [ACEIs], thiazide-type diuretics, tetracycline, and chloroquine), metals (e.g., gold and mercury), or infections (e.g., secondary syphilis).[2,8]
- Associated with liver disease, especially related to hepatitis C virus.[2,8,9]
- A few cases of LP after hepatitis B vaccination have been reported.[10]
- LP may be found with other diseases of altered immunity (e.g., ulcerative colitis, alopecia areata, myasthenia gravis).[1]
- Malignant transformation has been reported in ulcerative oral lesions in men.[1]

RISK FACTORS

- Possible HLA-associated genetic predisposition; however, a positive family history is not consistently found.[11]
- Hepatitis C virus infection, and possibly hepatitis B vaccination, although causal relationship is not established.[6,12]
- Certain drugs (see the previous section "Etiology and Pathophysiology").

DIAGNOSIS

CLINICAL FEATURES[2,8]

- Classically, the six Ps of LP are planar, purple, polygonal, pruritic, papules, and plaques (**Figure 138-2**). These well-demarcated flat-topped violaceous lesions are often covered by lacy, reticular white lines (called Wickham striae or Wickham lines; **Figure 138-3**).
- An initial lesion is usually located on the flexor surface of the limbs, such as the wrists, followed by a generalized eruption with maximal spreading within 2 to 16 weeks.[1]
- Lesions may demonstrate the Koebner phenomenon (linear distribution) from scratching (**Figure 138-4**).
- Lesions are often hyperpigmented rather than purple or pink in dark-skinned persons, and skin may remain hyperpigmented after lesions resolve (**Figure 138-5**).
- Lesions can also be annular (**Figure 138-5**).
- Skin variants:
  - Hypertrophic (**Figure 138-6**)—Typical papules develop into thicker reddish-brown to purple plaques most commonly on the foot and shins.

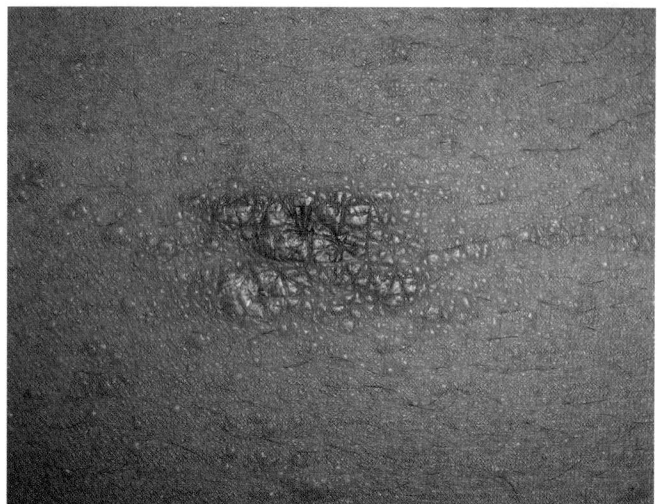

FIGURE 138-2 Lichen planus on the back with all the 6 Ps (planar, purple, polygonal, pruritic, papules, and plaques). Some of the papules are also pink and follow a linear pattern. (*Used with permission from Richard P. Usatine, MD.*)

- Follicular—Pinpoint hyperkeratotic projections often on scalp, may lead to cicatricial alopecia (**Figure 138-7**).
- Vesicular—Vesicles or bullae occur alongside the more typical LP lesions (**Figure 138-8**).
- Actinic—Typical lesions in sun-exposed areas, such as the face, back of hands and arms.
- Atrophic—The lesions are atrophic rather than standard plaques.
- Ulcerative—Ulcers develop within typical lesions or start as waxy semitranslucent plaques on palms and soles; may require skin grafting.

- Mucous membrane variants:
  - May be reticular (net-like; **Figure 138-9**), atrophic, erosive, or bullous. It is almost always bilateral.
  - Oral lesions may be asymptomatic or have a burning sensation; pain occurs with ulceration.[1,6,9]
  - Found in up to 40 percent of pediatric patients.[13]
  - Oral LP is often associated with extraoral LP.[4,14,15]

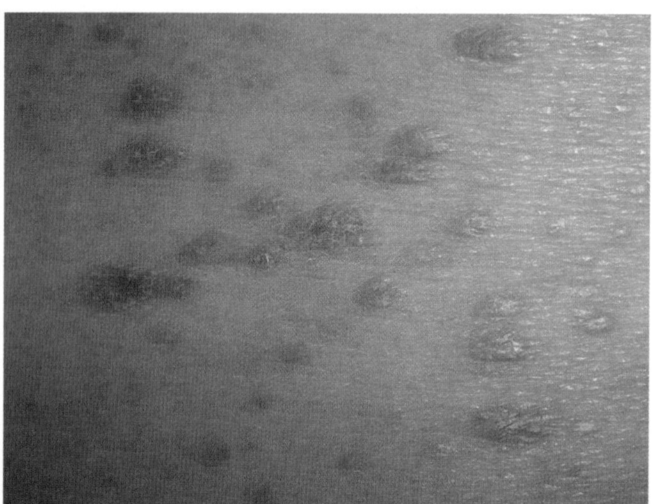

FIGURE 138-3 Close-up of lesions on the back showing Wickham striae crossing the flat papules of lichen planus. These lines are white and reticular like a net. (*Used with permission from Richard P. Usatine, MD.*)

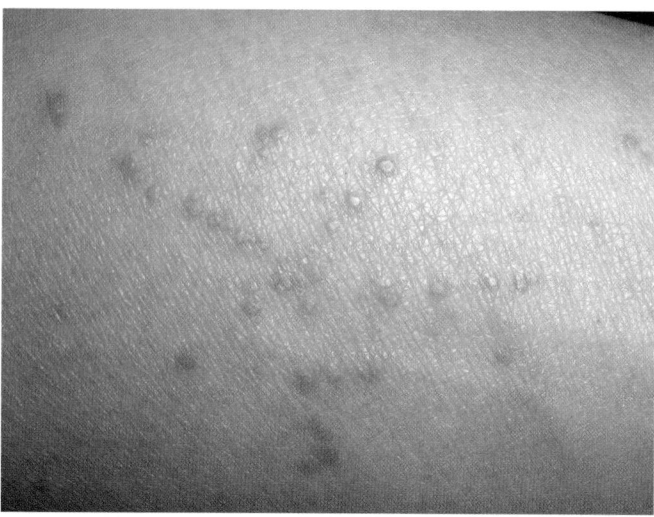

FIGURE 138-4 Close-up of wrist showing linearity of the lesions on the flexor surface secondary to the Koebner phenomenon. Lesions may be pink rather than purple. (*Used with permission from Richard P. Usatine, MD.*)

- Genitalia variants:
  - Reticular, annular, papular, or erosive lesions on penis, scrotum, labia, or vagina.
  - Vulvar/vaginal lesions may be associated with dyspareunia, a burning sensation, and/or pruritus.[1,14]
  - Vulvar and urethral stenosis can also be present.[1,14]
- Hair and nail variants (**Figure 138-10**); the latter present in 10 percent of adult patients, but less commonly in pediatric patients:[1,11,13]
  - Violaceous, scaly, pruritic papules on the scalp can progress to scarring alopecia. Lichen planopilaris (LP of the scalp) can cause widespread hair loss.[16]
  - Nail plate thinning results in longitudinal grooving and ridging; rarely destruction of nailfold and nail bed with splintering (**Figure 138-9**).
  - Hyperpigmentation, subungual hyperkeratosis, onycholysis, and longitudinal melanonychia can result from LP.[1]

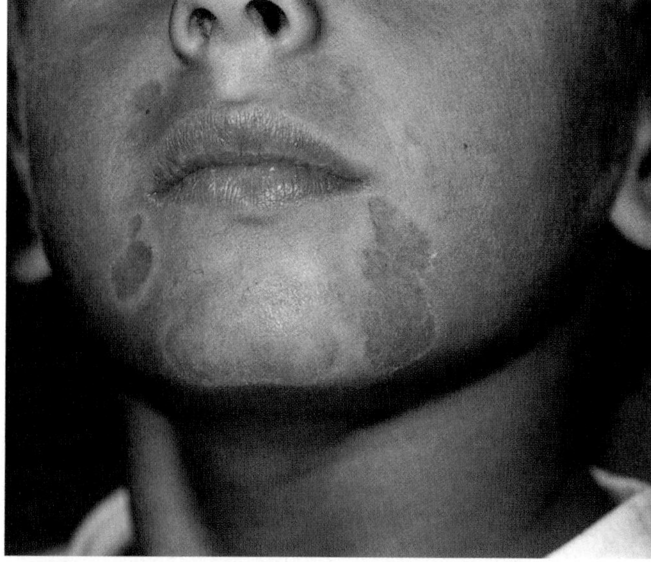

FIGURE 138-5 Annular lichen planus on the face of a young boy. Note how the lesion is hyperpigmented rather than purple or pink. (*Used with permission from Weinberg SW, Prose NS, Kristal L, Color Atlas of Pediatric Dermatology, 4th edition, Figure 9-47, New York, NY: McGraw-Hill, 2008.*)

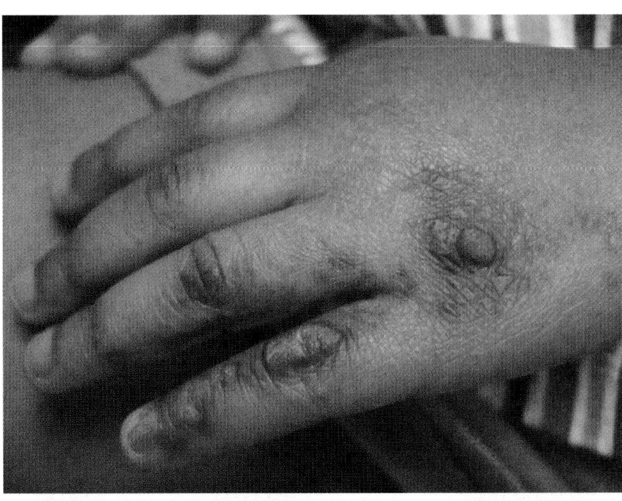

FIGURE 138-6 Hypertrophic lichen planus on the hand of a child. As this also resembles verruca vulgaris a shave biopsy was performed to determine the diagnosis. (*Used with permission from John C. Browning, MD.*)

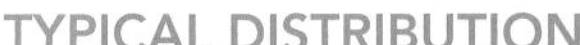

TYPICAL DISTRIBUTION

Wrists (**Figure 138-1**), ankles, lower back, eyelids, shins, scalp, penis, or mouth (i.e., buccal mucosa, lateral tongue, and gingiva).[2,8] Lesions can also appear on the dorsum of the hand (**Figures 138-6** and **138-11**) and on the legs (**Figure 138-12**).

LABORATORY STUDIES

- Wickham striae can be accentuated by a drop of oil on the skin plaque and magnification.[8] Not all LP has visible Wickham striae. This study is rarely needed. If the diagnosis is uncertain, a punch biopsy should be performed.

BIOPSY

- A punch biopsy is a valuable method to make as initial diagnosis if the clinical picture is not certain. A biopsy is rarely needed to evaluate for malignant transformation.[8,17]

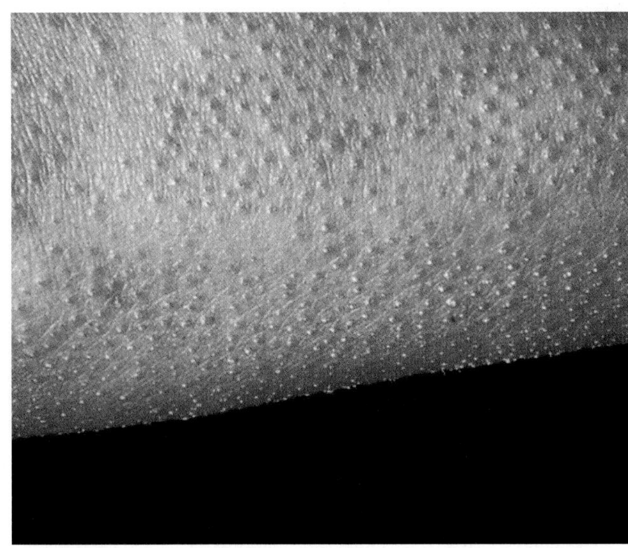

FIGURE 138-7 Lichen planopilaris (follicular lichen planus) primary involvement is around hair follicles and this is more common in females. When it involves the scalp it can cause scarring alopecia. (*Used with permission from Weinberg SW, Prose NS, Kristal L, Color Atlas of Pediatric Dermatology, 4th edition, Figure 9-48, New York, NY: McGraw-Hill, 2008.*)

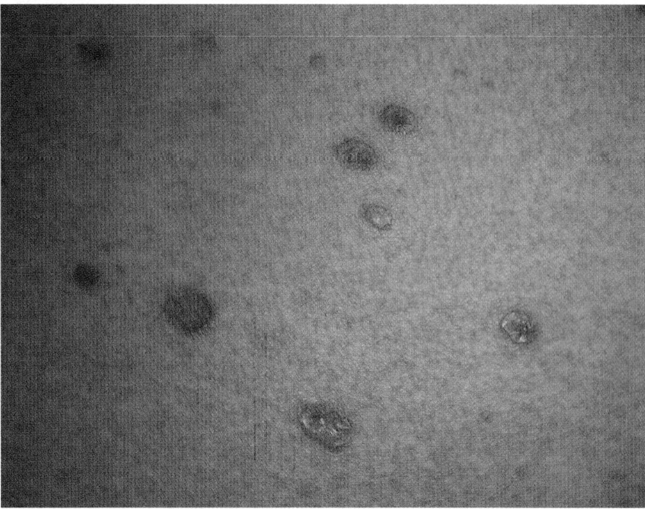

FIGURE 138-8 Bullous lichen planus on the lower back. (*Used with permission from Richard P. Usatine, MD.*)

- Mainly lymphocytic immunoinflammatory infiltrate with hyperkeratosis, increased granular layer and liquefaction of basal cell layer.[2,8]
- Linear fibrin and fibrinogen deposits along basement membrane.[2,8]
- Direct immunofluorescence on biopsy specimen reveals globular deposits of immunoglobulin (Ig) G, IgM, IgA, and complement at dermal–epidermal junction.[8]

DIFFERENTIAL DIAGNOSIS

Skin lesions that may be confused with LP:

- Eczematous dermatitis—"The itch that rashes": dry skin, itching, often excoriations and lichenification of skin with predilection for flexor surfaces (see Chapter 130, Atopic Dermatitis).

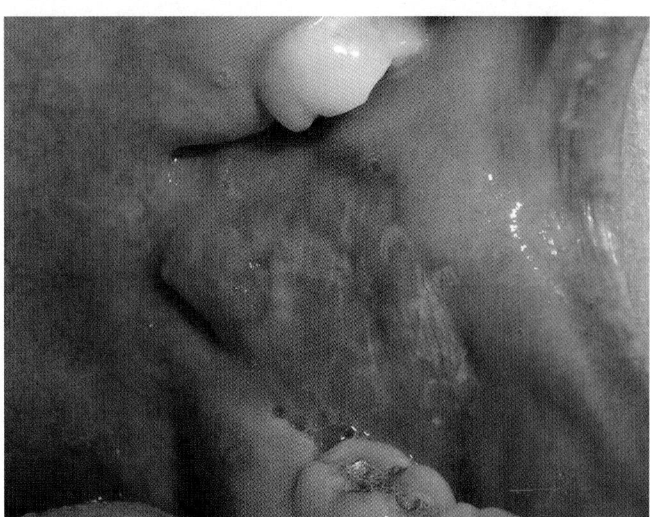

FIGURE 138-9 Asymptomatic white keratotic striae of lichen planus on left buccal mucosa. The patient had similar involvement of the right buccal mucosa and gingivae. Lichen planus in the mouth is bilateral. (*Used with permission from Richard P. Usatine, MD.*)

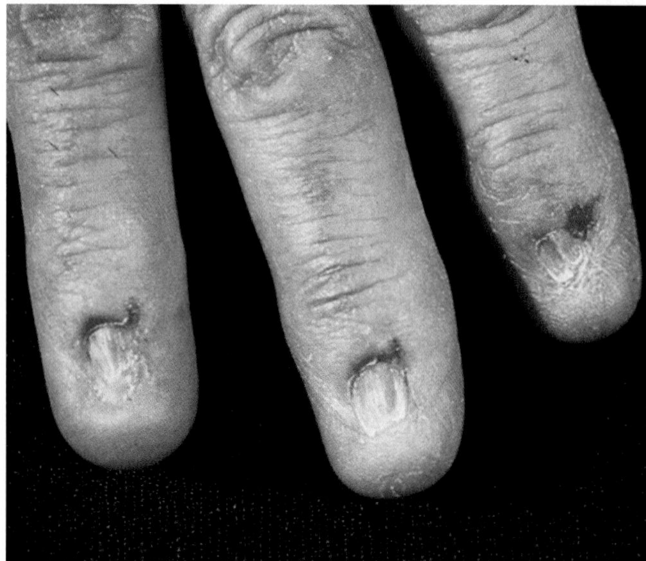

FIGURE 138-10 Lichen planus of the nails with pterygium formation and permanent nail loss. (*Used with permission from Weinberg SW, Prose NS, Kristal L, Color Atlas of Pediatric Dermatology, 4th edition, Figure 9-46, New York, NY: McGraw-Hill, 2008.*)

- Psoriasis has more prominent silvery scale and is generally located on extensor surfaces.[8] A punch biopsy can be used to distinguish between these two when the clinical picture is not clear (see Chapter 136, Psoriasis).
- Pityriasis rosea—Herald patch and subsequent pink papules and plaques with long axes along skin lines (Christmas tree pattern) (see Chapter 137, Pityriasis Rosea).
- Chronic cutaneous lupus erythematosus—Bright red sharply demarcated papules with adherent scale. Tend to regress centrally and can be light induced. Generally located on face, scalp, or forearms, and hands. Biopsy may be necessary to differentiate (see Chapter 173, Lupus: Systemic and Cutaneous).[8]

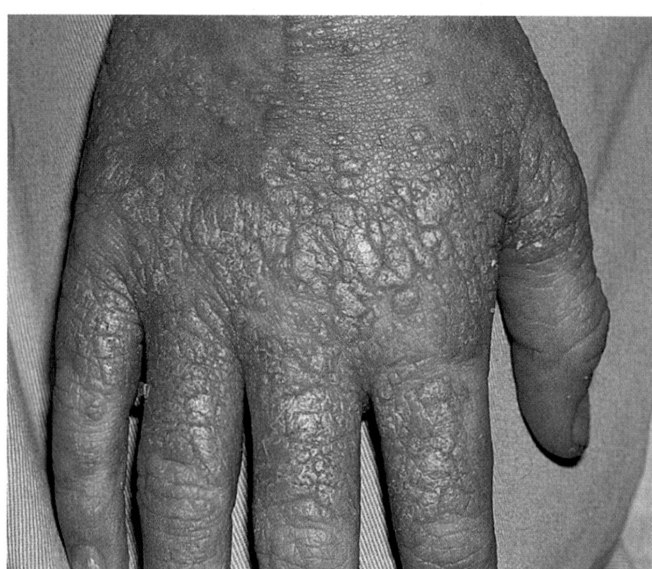

FIGURE 138-11 Lichen planus on the dorsum of the hand and fingers of a child. (*Used with permission from Weinberg SW, Prose NS, Kristal L, Color Atlas of Pediatric Dermatology, 4th edition, Figure 9-39, New York, NY: McGraw-Hill, 2008.*)

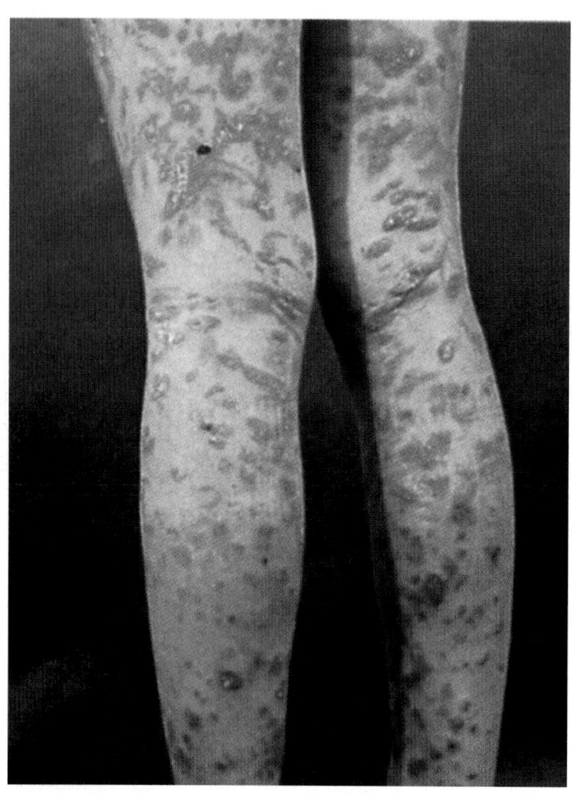

FIGURE 138-12 Severe lichen planus on the legs of a child. (*Used with permission from Weinberg SW, Prose NS, Kristal L, Color Atlas of Pediatric Dermatology, 4th edition, Figure 9-41, New York, NY: McGraw-Hill, 2008.*)

Other mucous membrane lesions that may appear similar:[8]

- Thrush—Removable whitish plaques over an erythematous mucosal surface caused by *Candida* infection, confirmed by KOH preparation (see Chapter 121, Candidiasis).
- Bite trauma in the mouth—May result in white areas of the lip or buccal mucosa. Persons may have a white bite line where the upper and lower molars occlude and this can be confused with oral LP. If in doubt, a biopsy may be needed.

Genital lesions that may be differentiated from LP:[8]

- Psoriasis on the penis can look like LP on the penis. A shave biopsy can be used to differentiate between these two diagnoses (see Chapter 136, Psoriasis).

MANAGEMENT

LP may persist for months to years. Hypertrophic LP and oral LP can last for decades.[2] Any type of LP can recur. Antihistamines can be used for symptomatic pruritus.[8] SOR C Symptomatic and severe cases can be treated as follows:

- Localized/topical treatment.
  - Topical corticosteroids twice a day.[18–20] SOR B Mid- to high-potency steroids are usually needed. Clobetasol cream or ointment

may be used on the skin and clobetasol ointment or gel may be used in the mouth.
  - Topical aloe vera gel has demonstrated efficacy against oral LP.[21,22] SOR B
  - Intralesional triamcinolone (3 to 5 mg/mL) for hypertrophic or mucous membrane lesions, may repeat every 3 to 4 weeks.[2,8,17,18,23] SOR B
  - Tacrolimus, pimecrolimus, retinoids, or cyclosporine in mouthwash or adhesive base for oral disease unresponsive to topical corticosteroids.[5,6,17,19,24–27] SOR B
  - Topical corticosteroids, tacrolimus, and aloe vera gel have demonstrated efficacy for vulvar LP.[28,29] SOR B
- Systemic treatment can be considered for resistant, widespread, or severe cases.
  - Oral steroids may be used starting with a 3-week tapered course of oral prednisone.[2,17,18,30,31] SOR B
  - Systemic retinoids, that is, acitretin 25 mg/day. Monitor serum creatinine, liver function tests (LFTs), and fasting lipids.[5,8,31] SOR B Contraindicated in women of childbearing potential.
  - Cyclosporine (5 mg/kg per day). Monitor complete blood count, serum creatinine, LFTs, and blood pressure.[2] SOR B
  - Azathioprine may be used as a steroid-sparing agent. Monitor complete blood count and LFTs.[8,17] SOR C
  - Psoralen UVA (PUVA) phototherapy may be effective but can cause phototoxic reactions and has long-term risks, including the development of squamous cell carcinoma.[32] SOR C
  - Carbon dioxide laser and low-level laser therapy have reports of treatment success against oral LP.[33,34] SOR C

PROGNOSIS

- Generally self-limiting and spontaneous resolution may occur in 12 to 18 months.
- Recurrences are common.
- Mucosal LP is generally more persistent than cutaneous forms.
- Malignant transformation of LP is rare.

FOLLOW-UP

- Follow-up depends on severity and treatment course.
- Oral and vaginal disease may be most challenging to treat.
- Follow oral or vaginal lesions for possible malignant transformation. Because of low risk of transformation even with oral LP (best estimate: 0.2% per year), routine screening and biopsy is not recommended.[17] Biopsy if suspecting malignancy; lesion becomes larger, ulcerated, nodular, or lose reticular pattern.

PATIENT EDUCATION

- Patients should understand that LP is often self-limiting and may resolve in 12 to 18 months.
- There is a significant chance of recurrence.

PATIENT RESOURCES

- Handout available—**http://familydoctor.org/600.xml**.
- Online support group for LP—**www.mdjunction.com/lichen-planus**.
- Online support group for oral LP—**http://bcdwp.web.tamhsc.edu/iolpdallas/**.

PROVIDER RESOURCES

- Usatine RP, Tinitigan M. Diagnosis and treatment of LP. *Am Fam Physician.* 2011;84(1):53-60. Available online—**www.aafp.org/afp/2011/0701/p53.html# afp20110701p53-b14**.

REFERENCES

1. Chuang T-Y, Stitle L. http://emedicine.medscape.com/article/1123213-overview, accessed September 20, 2011.
2. Wolff K, Johnson RA. *Fitzpatrick's Color Atlas and Synopsis of Clinical Dermatology*, 6th ed. New York, NY: McGraw-Hill; 2009;128-133.
3. Jue MS, Lee JW, Ko JY, et al. Childhood lichen planus with palmoplantar involvement. *Ann Dermatol.* 2010;22(1):51-53.
4. Handa S, Sahoo B. Childhood lichen planus: a study of 87 cases. *Int J Dermatol.* 2002;41(7):423-427.
5. Zakrzewska JM, Chan ES-Y, Thornhill MH. A systematic review of placebo-controlled randomized clinical trials of treatments used in oral lichen planus. *Br J Dermatol.* 2005;153:336-341.
6. Laeijendecker R, Tank B, Dekker SK, Neumann HA. A comparison of treatment of oral lichen planus with topical tacrolimus and triamcinolone acetonide ointment. *Acta Derm Venereol.* 2006;86(3):227-229.
7. Walton KE, Bowers EV, Drolet BA, Holland KE. Choldhood lichen planus: demographics of a U.S. population. *Pediatr Dermatol.* 2010;27(1):34 38.
8. Habif TP. *Clinical Dermatology: A Color Guide to Diagnosis and Therapy*, 5th ed. Philadelphia, PA: Mosby; 2010.
9. Shengyuan L, Songpo Y, Wen W, et al. Hepatitis C virus and lichen planus: a reciprocal association determined by a meta-analysis. *Arch Dermatol.* 2009;145(9):1040-1047.
10. Limas C, Limas CJ. Lichen planus in children: a possible complication of hepatitis B vaccines. *Pediatr Dermatol.* 2002; 19(3):204-209.
11. Luis-Montoya P, Domínguez-Soto L, Vega-Memije E. Lichen planus in 24 children with review of the literature. *Pediatr Dermatol.* 2005;22(4):295-298.
12. Mérigou D, Léauté-Labrèze C, Louvet S, et al. Lichen planus in children: role of the campaign for hepatitis B vaccination. *Ann Dermatol Venereol.* 1998;125(6-7):399-403.
13. Paller AS, Mancini AJ. *Hurwitz Clinical Pediatric Dermatology: A Textbook of Skin Disorders of Childhood and Adolescence,* 3rd ed. Philadelphia, PA: Elsevier Saunders; 2006.
14. Di Fede O, Belfiore P, Cabibi D, et al. Unexpectedly high frequency of genital involvement in women with clinical and histological features of oral lichen planus. *Acta Derm Venereol.* 2006;86(5):433-438.

15. Imail SB, Kumar SK, Zain RB. Oral lichen planus and lichenoid reactions: etiopathogenesis, diagnosis, management and malignant transformation. *J Oral Sci.* 2007;49(2):89-106.

16. Cevacso NC, Bergfeld WF, Remzi BK, de Knott HR. A case-series of 29 patients with lichen planopilaris: the Cleveland Clinic Foundation experience on evaluation, diagnosis, and treatment. *J Am Acad Dermatol.* 2007;57(1):47-53.

17. Lodi G, Scully C, Carrozzo M, et al. Current controversies in oral lichen planus: report of an international consensus meeting, part 2. Clinical management and malignant transformation. *Oral Surg Oral Med Oral Pathol Oral Radiol Endod.* 2005;100:164-178.

18. Cribier B, Frances C, Chosidow O. Treatment of lichen planus. An evidence-based medicine analysis of efficacy. *Arch Dermatol.* 1998;134(12):1521-1530.

19. Corrocher G, Di Lorenzo G, Martinelli N, et al. Comparative effect of tacrolimus 0.1% ointment and clobetasol 0.05% ointment in patients with oral lichen planus. *J Clin Periodontol.* 2008;35(3):244-249.

20. Carbone M, Arduino PG, Carrozzo M, et al. Topical clobetasol in the treatment of atrophic-erosive oral lichen planus: a randomized controlled trial to compare two preparations with different concentrations. *J Oral Pathol Med.* 2009;38(2):227-233.

21. Choonhakarn C, Busaracome P, Sripanidkulchai B, Sarakam P. The efficacy of aloe vera gel in the treatment of oral lichen planus: a randomized controlled trial. *Br J Dermatol.* 2008;158(3):573-577.

22. Salazar SN. Efficacy of topical Aloe vera in patients with oral lichen planus: a randomized double-blind study. *J Oral Pathol Med.* 2010;39(10):735-740.

23. De Moraes PC, Teixeira RG, Tacchelli DP, et al. Atypical case of oral lichen planus in a pediatric patient: clinical presentation and management. *Pediatr Dent.* 2011; 33(5):445-447.

24. Conrotto D, Carbone M, Carrozzo M, et al. Ciclosporine vs. clobetasol in the topical management of atrophic and erosive oral lichen planus: a double-blind, randomized controlled trial. *Br J Dermatol.* 2006;138(1):139-145.

25. Swift JC, Rees TD, Plemons JM, et al. The effectiveness of 1% pimecrolimus cream in the treatment of oral erosive lichen planus. *J Periodontol.* 2005;76(4):627-635.

26. Volz T, Caroli U, Ludtke H, et al. Pimecrolimus cream 1% in erosive oral lichen planus—a prospective randomized double-blind vehicle-controlled study. *Br J Dermatol.* 2008;159(4):936-941.

27. Thongprasom K, Carrozzo M, Furness S, Lodi G. Interventions for treating oral lichen planus. *Cochrane Database Syst Rev.* 2011;(7):CD001168.

28. Rajar UD, Majeed R, Parveen N, et al. Efficacy of aloe vera gel in the treatment of vulval lichen planus. *J Coll Physicians Surg Pak.* 2008;18(10):612-614.

29. McPherson T, Cooper S. Vulval lichen sclerosis and lichen planus. *Dermatol Ther.* 2010;23(5):523-532.

30. Thongprasom K, Dhanuthai K. Steroids in the treatment of lichen planus: a review. *J Oral Sci.* 2008;50(4):377-385.

31. Asch S, Goldenberg G. Systemic treatment of cutaneous lichen planus: an update. *Cutis.* 2011;87(3):129-134.

32. Wackernagel A, Legat FJ, Hofer A, et al. Psoralen plus UVA vs. UVB-311 nm for the treatment of lichen planus. *Photodermatol Photoimmunol Photomed.* 2007;23(1):15-19.

33. van der Hem PS, Egges M, van der Wal JE, Roodenburg JL. CO_2 laser evaporation of oral lichen planus. *Int J Oral Maxillofac Surg.* 2008;37(7):630-633.

34. Cafaro A, Albanese G, Arduino PG, et al. Effect of low-level laser irradiation on unresponsive oral lichen planus: early preliminary results in 13 patients. *Photomed Laser Surg.* 2010;28 Suppl 2:S99-S103.

139 LICHEN NITIDUS AND LICHEN STRIATUS

Michaela R. Marek, MD
Catherine Kowalewski, DO

PATIENT STORY

An 8-year-old Hispanic boy presents for evaluation of mildly itchy, pinpoint bumps that have been present for 2 to 3 months. The "rash" is primarily involving the patient's trunk. Patient is otherwise healthy, and no one else at home has a similar eruption. The mother of the patient has tried some over-the-counter hydrocortisone, which has helped some with the mild itching, but the lesions persist. The pediatrician noted the linear pattern of the pinpoint papules and made the clinical diagnosis of lichen nitidus (**Figure 139-1**). These lines represent the Koebner phenomenon caused by scratching done by the child in areas that are reachable.

INTRODUCTION

Lichen nitidus and lichen striatus are two distinct entities under the umbrella of lichenoid dermatoses, a grouping that is based on clinical findings resembling lichen planus, the prototypical lichenoid dermatosis, and the characteristic histologic findings of a band-like inflammatory infiltrate with or without vacuolar alteration of the dermoepidermal junction. Both conditions can present in a linear array; lichen nitidus because it exhibits the Koebner phenomenon (**Figure 139-1**) and lichen striatus (**Figure 139-2**) because it follows the lines of Blaschko. We will further discuss some of the similarities and distinguishing features of these two entities.

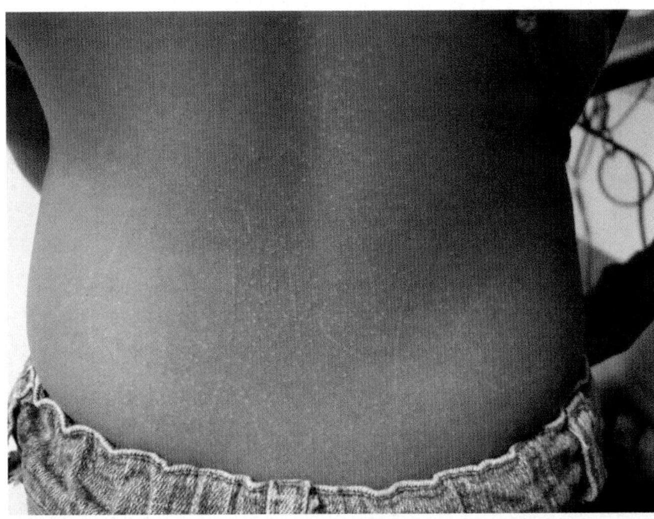

FIGURE 139-1 Lichen nitidus with several linearly arranged groups of tiny, skin-colored papules amidst a background of scattered pinpoint papules on the trunk of a child. The linearly arranged groups of papules are secondary to scratching (Koebner phenomenon). *(Used with permission from John Browning, MD.)*

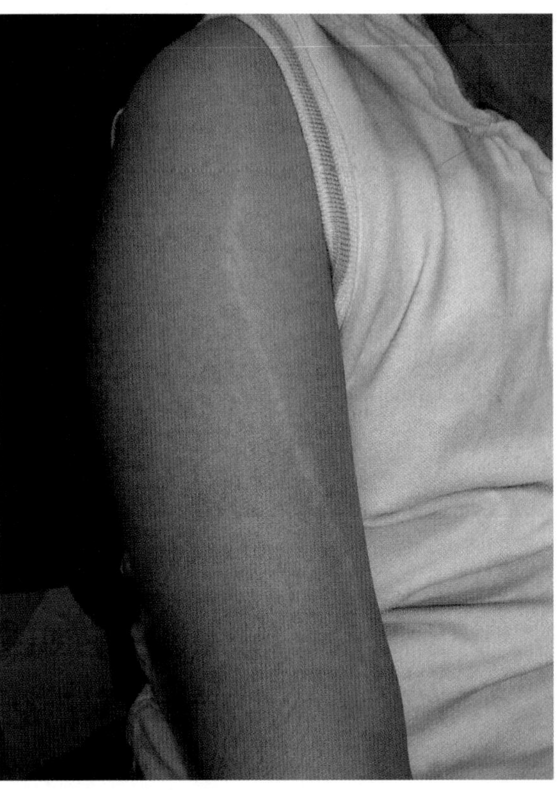

FIGURE 139-2 Lichen striatus with a curvilinear configuration of pink, slightly scaly, flat-topped papules on the upper extremity of a young girl. *(Used with permission from Richard P. Usatine, MD.)*

SYNONYMS

Lichen striatus—Linear lichenoid dermatosis, *B*laschko *l*inear *a*cquired *i*nflammatory *s*kin *e*ruption (BLAISE).

EPIDEMIOLOGY

LICHEN NITIDUS

- Lichen nitidus is a relatively rare disorder, more common in children and young adults.
- Lichen nitidus often presents in preschool and school-aged children.
- There does not seem to be a race or sex predilection.

LICHEN STRIATUS

- Lichen striatus is seen primarily in children 5 to 15 years of age.[1]
- Females are more often affected than males, with some reports of a female to male ratio as great as 2-3:1 (**Figure 139-3**).

ETIOLOGY AND PATHOPHYSIOLOGY

LICHEN NITIDUS

- Lichen nitidus was once thought to be a tuberculous reaction because of its distinctive histologic findings of a lymphohistiocytic infiltrate, but no infectious agents have ever been elucidated.

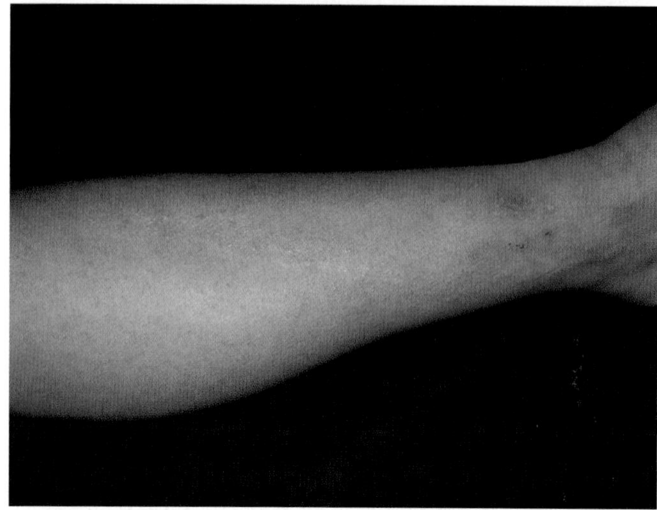

FIGURE 139-3 Lichen striatus with a Blaschkoid distribution of pink, slightly scaly papules on the leg of an 11-year-old girl. (*Used with permission from Richard P. Usatine, MD.*)

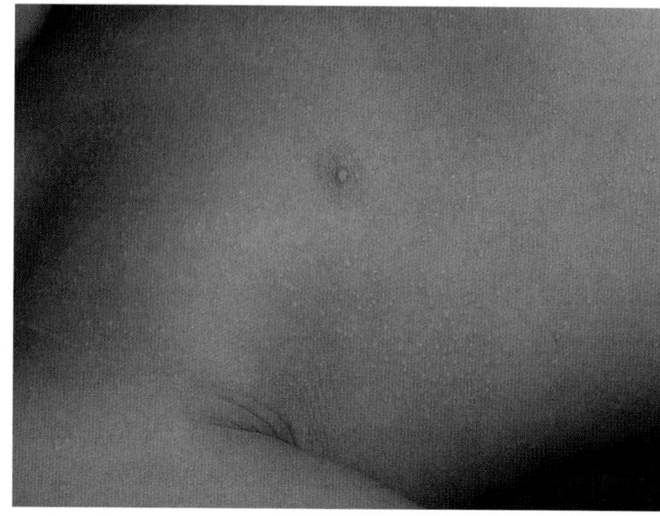

FIGURE 139-4 Lichen nitidus with scattered 1 to 2mm shiny, skin-colored, flat-topped papules of the trunk of a 7-year-old Hispanic boy. (*Used with permission from Richard P. Usatine, MD.*)

LICHEN STRIATUS

- Lichen striatus is also thought to be related to infectious agents, viruses in particular. This postulation is based on the predominance of lichen striatus in children and its tendency to appear more commonly in the spring and summer.
- The Blaschkoid distribution of lesions in lichen striatus point to a somatic mutation as another potential cause, but no gene association has been established.
- Some hypothesize that a combination of the two previously mentioned processes may be required for development of lichen striatus.
- Still, lichen striatus may be related to atopy.

RISK FACTORS

LICHEN NITIDUS

There are no proven risk factors, but some authors do believe that lichen nitidus is a cutaneous manifestation of Crohn's disease.[2]

LICHEN STRIATUS

Atopy may be a predisposing factor for lichen striatus, but it is suspected that an infectious agent is still a necessary trigger.

DIAGNOSIS

LICHEN NITIDUS

CLINICAL FEATURES

Lichen nitidus is characterized by numerous, discrete, skin-colored, shiny, flat-topped 1 to 2mm papules, clustered in groups (**Figures 139-4** and **139-5**). If inflammatory, the papules may appear more red.

Sometimes the pinhead-sized papules are more yellow or red-brown.

In dark-skinned persons, the papules are most often hypopigmented, but can also be hyperpigmented.

Tiny grey-white papules can be seen on the buccal mucosa, along with grey-white plaques involving the tongue and hard palate.

Nail changes are seen in approximately 10 percent of patients, more often in adults, and consist of pitting, longitudinal ridging, and rippling.

Often seen in a linear pattern, secondary to koebnerization (**Figure 139-6**).

Lesions can be pruritic, with pruritus more common in the generalized form.

SALE (summertime actinic lichenoid eruption) or lichen nitidus actinicus has similar clinical appearance as lichen nitidus, but is seen in type IV and V skin, and is pruritic and photodistributed.

FIGURE 139-5 Close-up view of lichen nitidus with scattered skin-colored, flat-topped papules on the trunk. (*Used with permission from Richard P. Usatine, MD.*)

FIGURE 139-6 Lichen nitidus showing skin-colored, flat-topped papules in a linear array across mid-back of an adolescent. This is an example of Koebnerization. (*Used with permission from Richard P. Usatine, MD.*)

DISTRIBUTION

Flexor aspects of the upper extremities, dorsal hands, anterior trunk, and genitalia are sites most often involved.

Lichen nitidus has also been reported to occur on the palms of pediatric patients, albeit rarely.[3]

LABORATORY TESTING AND IMAGING

Other than skin biopsy, labs and imaging studies are typically not useful in the diagnosis of lichen nitidus. Biopsy shows a distinctive pattern of "ball in claw" consisting of lymphs, histiocytes, and epitheloid cells clutched in hyperplastic rete.

LICHEN STRIATUS

CLINICAL FEATURES

Clinically lichen striatus presents as a band of clustered, skin-colored to pink, slightly scaly, flat-topped papules (**Figure 139-7**).

The individual papules are usually larger than that seen in lichen nitidus, ranging from 2 to 4 mm in size. They can be smooth or scaly.

Occasionally vesicles may be present.

Nail changes may be the only clinical finding and present as thickened nails with ridges and/or longitudinal split. The nail changes can occur before, after, or simultaneous with appearance of skin lesions.[4]

Lichen striatus can also be intensely pruritic.

DISTRIBUTION

Lichen striatus usually presents as a single, unilateral streak along Blaschko's lines (**Figures 139-8** and **Figure 139-9**).

The eruption tends to affect a single extremity (**Figure 139-10**), but can be seen bilaterally and involving the face1 or the trunk (**Figure 139-11**).

LABORATORY TESTING AND IMAGING

Usually a clinical diagnosis, labs do not play a significant role in diagnosing lichen striatus except for possible conformational skin biopsy. Imaging studies are not indicated.

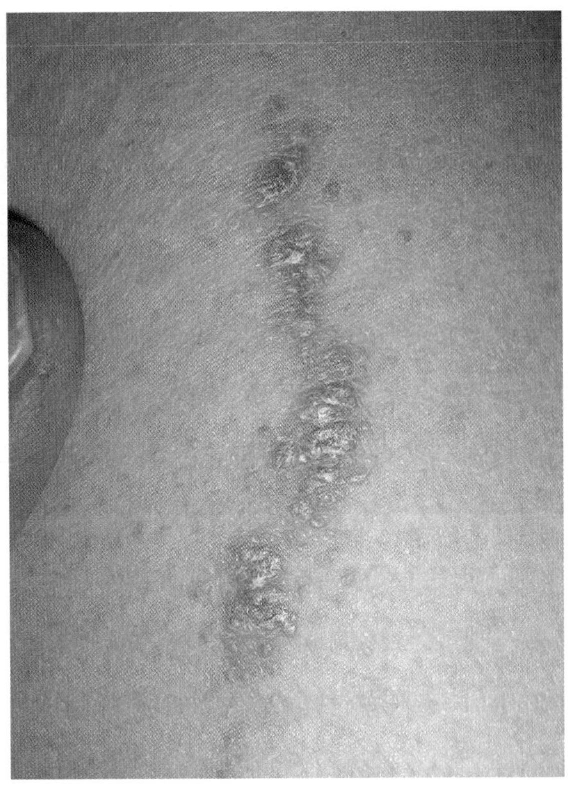

FIGURE 139-7 Lichen striatus close-up showing a linear band of pink, scaly papules. (*Used with permission from Richard P. Usatine, MD.*)

DIFFERENTIAL DIAGNOSIS

LICHEN NITIDUS

- Lichen planus—Purple, polygonal, planar papules, more pruritic and larger than papules of lichen nitidus (see Chapter 138, Lichen Planus).
- Molluscum contagiosum—Smooth, skin-colored to pink, dome-shaped papules with central umbilication (see Chapter 115, Molluscum Contagiosum).

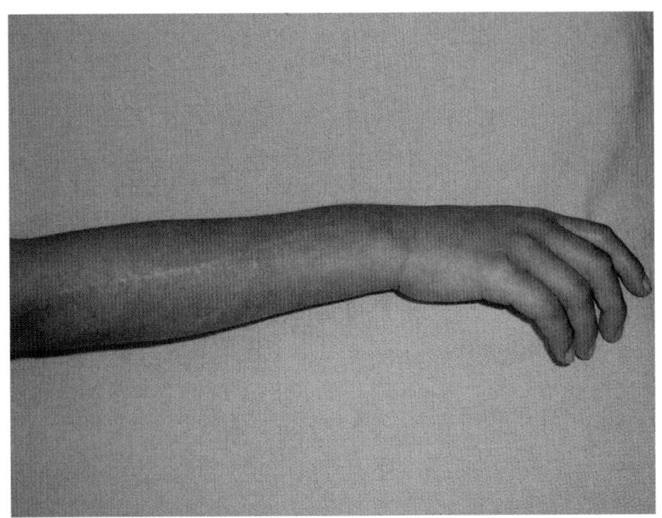

FIGURE 139-8 Lichen striatus with skin-colored to pink, slightly scaly papules coalescing into a linear plaque on the upper extremity of a young girl. (*Used with permission from Richard P. Usatine, MD.*)

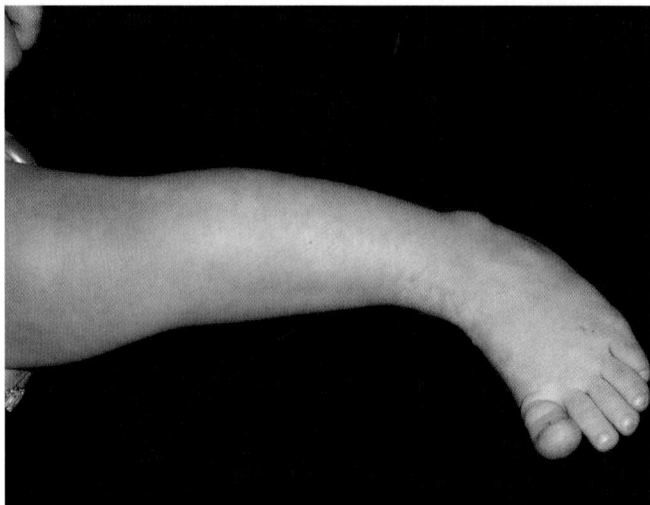

FIGURE 139-9 Lichen striatus with hypopigmented to pink, flat-topped papules in a Blaschkoid distribution on the leg of an infant. (*Used with permission from Richard P. Usatine, MD.*)

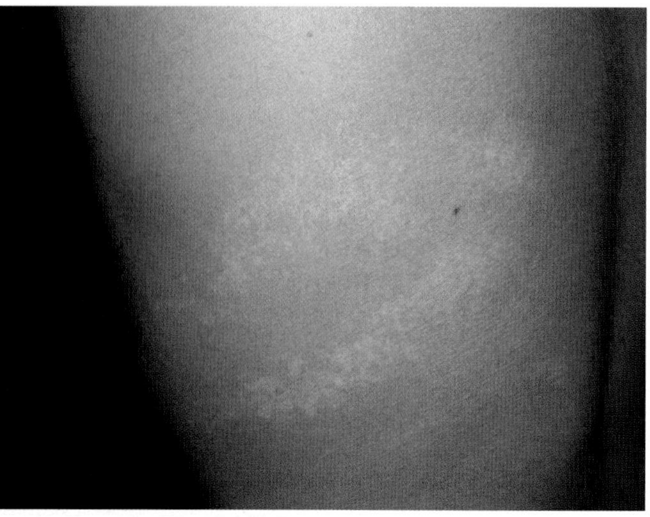

FIGURE 139-11 Lichen striatus with hypopigmented to pink, flat-topped papules in a Blaschkoid distribution on the trunk of a 13-year-old boy. (*Used with permission from Richard P. Usatine, MD.*)

- Atopic dermatitis (popular form)—Scattered pin-head sized erythematous papules, frequently in the flexures (see Chapter 130, Atopic Dermatitis).
- Lichen spinulosus—Multiple discrete, follicular-based, skin-colored papules with central keratin spine, coalescing into circumscribed plaques, usually bilateral and symmetric.
- Keratosis pilaris—Monomorphic, roughly 1mm folliculocentric papules, most often affecting the extensor arms and thighs (**Figures 139-12** and **139-13**).
- Pearly penile papules—Skin-colored to pink, regular papules arranged in rows on the coronal ring or at the frenulum, usually presenting after puberty.

LICHEN STRIATUS

- Linear lichen planus—Purple, polygonal, planar papules in a linear distribution.

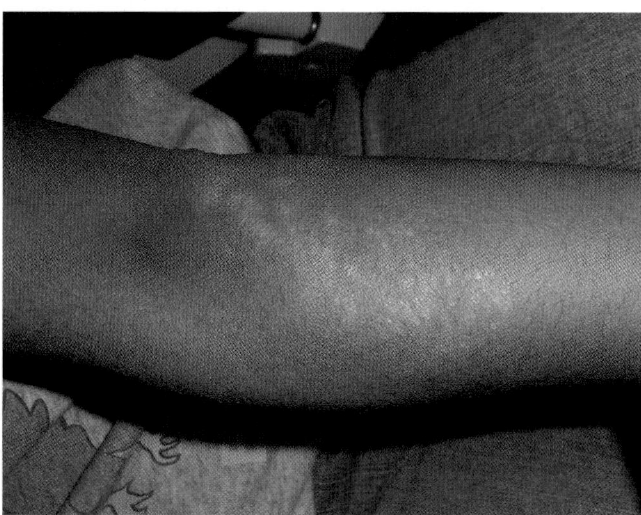

FIGURE 139-10 Lichen striatus on one arm with hypopigmented to pink, flat-topped papules in a Blaschkoid distribution. (*Used with permission from Richard P. Usatine, MD.*)

- Linear epidermal nevus—Flesh-colored to tan to brown verrucous papules coalescing into linear plaques.
- Blaschkitis—Relapsing papulovesicular eruption in a Blaschkoid distribution.
- Inflammatory linear verrucous epidermal nevus—Erythematous, verrucous papules grouped together in a linear distribution.
- Linear Darier's disease—Autosomal dominantly inherited linear grouping of yellow-brown, greasy, hyperkeratotic papules.
- Incontinentia pigmenti—X-linked recessive found almost exclusively in females, usually presenting within a few weeks

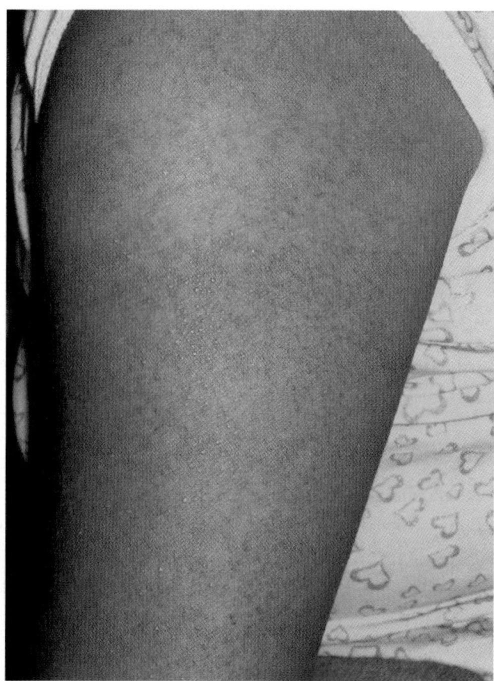

FIGURE 139-12 Keratosis pilaris on the upper arm of this young girl. Keratosis pilaris most often affects the extensor surface of the extremities, unlike lichen nitidus, which has a predilection for the flexural surfaces of the arms. (*Used with permission from Richard P. Usatine, MD.*)

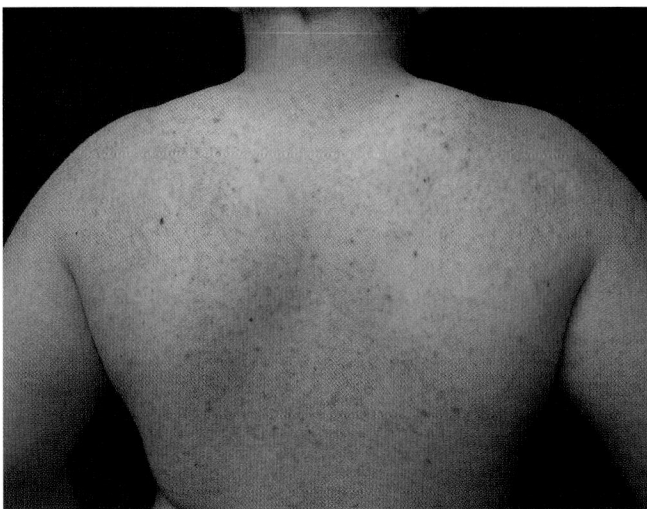

FIGURE 139-13 Keratosis pilaris on the back of this 17-year-old boy. The folliculocentric skin-colored to pink papules of keratosis pilaris can also be seen on the back. Lichen nitidus is more likely to occur on the anterior trunk although it too can occur on the back. (*Used with permission from Richard P. Usatine, MD.*)

of birth. Four stages including vesicular, verrucous, hyperpigmented and hypopigmented (see Chapter 228, Incontinentia Pigmenti).

MANAGEMENT

Both lichen nitidus and lichen striatus are self-limited conditions so treatment is usually indicated for symptomatic cases only. Although more common in lichen nitidus, both entities can cause significant pruritus that generally responds well to topical corticosteroids. Aggressive measures such as surgery should be avoided as the natural history of both conditions is for spontaneous regression.

LICHEN NITIDUS

MEDICATIONS

Topical corticosteroids are usually first line in the treatment of significant pruritus. In children, it is important to use a low potency corticosteroid and avoid use to face and intertriginous areas as much as possible to avoid the potential side effects of atrophy, striae and telangiectasia.

Topical calcineurin inhibitors (TCI), such as tacrolimus and pimecrolimus, have also been shown to be effective. TCI affect the cutaneous immune response by preventing the transcription of proinflammatory cytokines, which may explain its effectiveness in lichen nitidus.[4]

- Oral antihistamines may help to abate intense itching. Children's dosing of a sedating antihistamine can be used at bedtime, but a non-sedating antihistamine would be preferred during the day.
- Generalized lichen nitidus not responding to topical corticosteroids may do well with narrowband UVB or PUVA.
- Acitretin, isotretinoin, and other retinoids have been used rarely.
- Immunomodulatory treatments that have been reported in severe cases include cyclosporine, dinitrochlorobenzene, itraconazole, and isoniazid.[5]

REFERRAL

- Referral may be indicated for confirmation of diagnosis. One may also seek dermatology referral for generalized pruritus that has not responded to topical medications and/or oral antihistamines. In that scenario, narrowband UVB or PUVA or other systemic therapy may be necessary, and this therapy should be facilitated and monitored by a dermatologist.

LICHEN STRIATUS

MEDICATIONS

- Topical corticosteroids are also the mainstay of treatment for lichen striatus. They have been used under occlusion to accelerate its spontaneous resolution. As per the preceding, precautions must be taken to avoid unwanted side effects.
- Topical calcineurin inhibitors have been reported to be effective as well.

REFERRAL

- As with lichen nitidus or any other cutaneous eruption, dermatology consult may be appropriate to confirm a diagnosis. In lichen striatus in particular, it would be of benefit to rule out some of the other entities in the differential, such as incontinentia pigmenti and linear epidermal nevus, which can present with or develop additional findings, including systemic findings.

PREVENTION AND SCREENING

- As the exact etiology and pathogenesis of both conditions remains theoretical at best, prevention and screening measures are not practical at this time.

PROGNOSIS

Lichen nitidus and lichen striatus purport excellent prognoses as an eventual spontaneous resolution is the natural progression of both conditions, usually within a few years.

FOLLOW-UP

Follow-up should be made on an as needed basis for symptomatic patients to ensure that their pruritus is adequately controlled.

PATIENT EDUCATION

- Reassure patients and parents that lichen nitidus and lichen striatus are self-limited.
- Offer low potency topical steroids if pruritus is a problem.

PATIENT RESOURCES

- Lichen nitidus—**http://us.cnn.com/HEALTH/library/lichen-nitidus/DS00721.html**.
- Lichen striatus—**http://www.dermnetnz.org/dermatitis/lichen-striatus.html**.

PROVIDER RESOURCES

- Lichen nitidus—**http://emedicine.medscape.com/article/1123127**.
- Lichen striatus—**emedicine.medscape.com/article/1111723**.

REFERENCES

1. Mu EW, Abuav R, Cohen BA. Facial Lichen Striatus in Children: Retracing the Lines of Blaschko. *Pediatric Dermatology*. 2013; 30(3):364-366.
2. Wanat KA, Elenitsas R, Chachkin S, Lubinski S, Rosenbach M. Extensive lichen nitidus as a clue to underlying Crohn's disease. *Journal of the American Academy of Dermatology*. 2012;67(5):e218-220.
3. Cakmak SK, Unal E, Gonul M, Yayla D, Ozhamam E. Lichen Nitidus with Involvement of the Palms. *Pediatric Dermatology*. 2013: 1-2.
4. Vozza A, Baroni A, Nacca L, Piccolo V, Falleti J, Vozza G. Lichen striatus with nail involvement in an 8-year-old child. *The Journal of Dermatology*. 201;38(8):821-823.
5. Lee WJ, Park OJ, Won CH, Chang SE, Lee MW, Choi JH, Moon KC. Penile lichen nitidus successfully treated with topical pimecrolimus 1% cream. *The Journal of Dermatology*. 2013;40:1-2.

SECTION 9 BENIGN NEOPLASMS

140 JUVENILE XANTHOGRANULOMA

Olvia Revelo, MD
Richard P. Usatine, MD

PATIENT STORY

A 2-year-old healthy Caucasian male is brought in by his mother for evaluation of a solitary mass-like lesion that developed on his scalp over the past couple of months. The nodule was asymptomatic. His mother denies other symptoms or medical problems. Physical examination was normal except for a 1cm yellow, dome-shaped, smooth nodule on scalp apex (**Figure 140-1**). Clinical diagnosis of juvenile xanthogranuloma was made and mother was given reassurance that lesion would regress spontaneously over the next months.

INTRODUCTION

- Juvenile Xanthogranuloma (JXG) is considered a benign, non-Langerhan cell, histiocyte proliferation disorder.
- It usually presents as a solitary or few dome shaped red to yellow papules involving the upper body, although many variants are known to exist.
- Juvenile Xanthogranuloma usually only involves the skin. These lesions generally resolve spontaneously within months to years.
- Rarely JXG may be associated with systemic findings such as involvement of the central nervous system, liver, spleen, lungs, eyes, oropharynx, and muscle.[1] Only 5 patients (3.9%) of 129 patients were found to have systemic involvement in a retrospective review of a German pediatric tumor registry.[2]

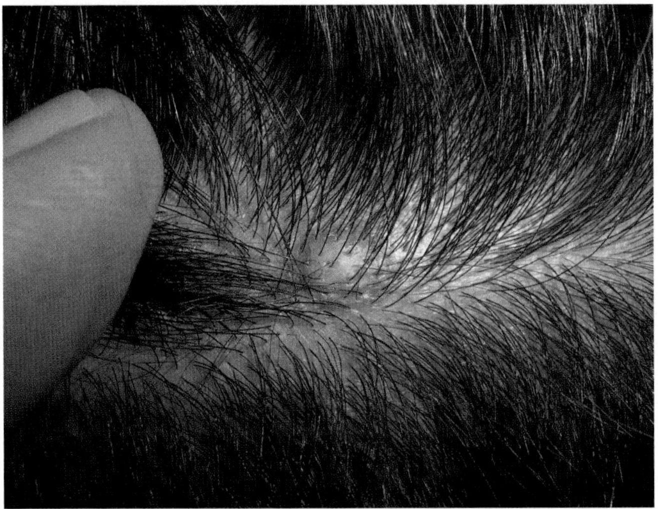

FIGURE 140-1 Juvenile xanthogranuloma on the scalp of a 2-year-old boy. Note the yellow color. *(Used with permission from Richard P. Usatine, MD.)*

- There is a 0.3–0.5 percent incidence of ocular JXG. Children at maximum risk are 2 years of age or younger, have multiple skin lesions, and are newly diagnosed JXG.[3] Two percent of JXG involving the eye are complicated by blindness usually from hyphema or glaucoma.[4]
- Juvenile Xanthogranuloma may also be associated with other disorders including neurofibromatosis 1, juvenile chronic myelogenous leukemia (CML), urticaria pigmentosa, insulin-dependent diabetes mellitus, aquagenic pruritis, and possibly cytomegalovirus infection. Children with JXG associated with NF1 have a 20 time increased risk of developing CML.[1]
- The xanthomas of JXG are not associated with primary hyperlipidemia.[4]

SYNONYMS

Nevoxanthoendothelioma, xanthoma multiplex, juvenile xanthoma, congenital xanthoma tuberosum, xanthoma neviforme, and juvenile giant-cell granuloma.

EPIDEMIOLOGY

- Disease incidence is unknown. JXG may be under recognized and under reported. The relative incidence from a retrospective review of 26,400 patients was 0.52 percent.[2,5]
- It commonly affects children 2 years or younger with 75 percent of cases diagnosed by age 1, and 15 percent of cases presenting at birth.[4]
- There may be a slight male predilection in children. Estimates run between 1.5 to 4: 1 male to female ratio.[1]
- It may rarely present in adults.

ETIOLOGY AND PATHOPHYSIOLOGY

- The pathogenesis is unknown.
- There is still controversy about the origin of the cell involved and histiologic criteria since there is a mixed pattern among the non-Langerhans cell histiocyte proliferation disorders with many authorities considering them all a spectrum of the same disorder.[2,4]

DIAGNOSIS

CLINICAL FEATURES

- There are two distinct variants in presentation. First there is a small nodular form with multiple pink, 2 to 5mm, dome-shaped papules that become red-brown and later turn yellow. They mainly affect the upper trunk (**Figure 140-2**).

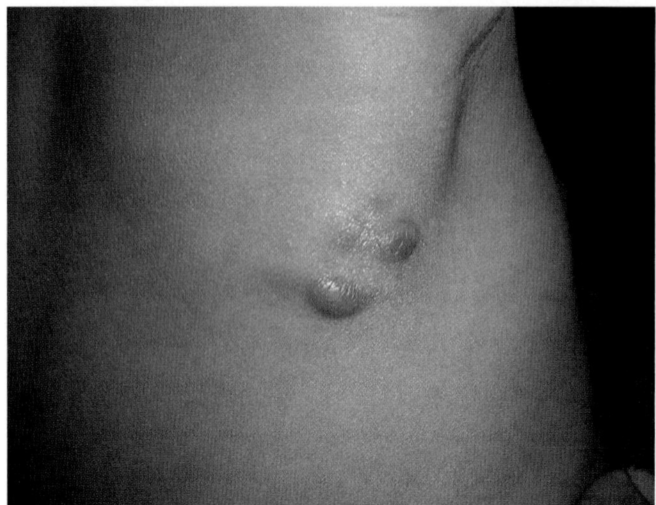

FIGURE 140-2 Multiple nodular juvenile xanthogranuloma on the trunk of a 20-month-old African American boy. Note the pink coloration at an early stage of development. (*Used with permission from Richard P. Usatine, MD.*)

- The second variant is the large nodular form in which a solitary or a couple of 1 to 2 cm nodules develop (**Figure 140-3**).
- Both variants may coexist at the same time.

DISTRIBUTION

- Areas most commonly involved include head, face (**Figure 140-4**), neck, upper torso, upper and lower extremities, and rarely in the oral mucosa.[2,4–7]

LABORATORY TESTING

- Clinical diagnosis can be supplemented by biopsy (**Figures 140-5** and **140-6**) and histologic examination for definitive diagnosis.

IMAGING

- Consider imaging if systemic involvement is suspected by clinical symptoms.

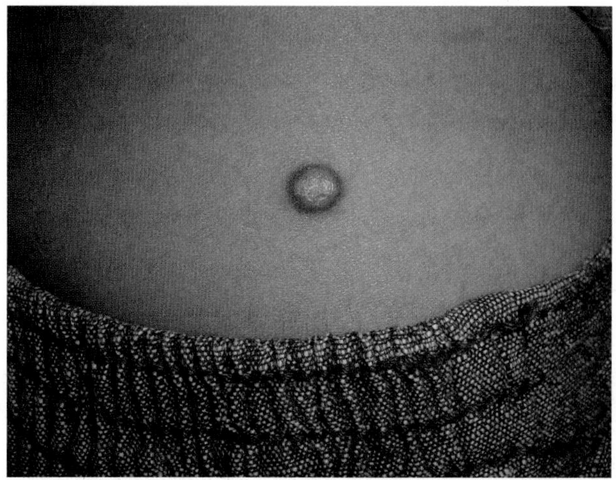

FIGURE 140-3 Solitary juvenile xanthogranuloma on the trunk with overlying scale and a red-brown color. Dermatofibroma is on the differential diagnosis. (Used with permission from Weinberg SW, Prose NS, Kristal L, Color Atlas of Pediatric Dermatology, 4th Edition, Figure 15-29, McGraw-Hill, 2008.)

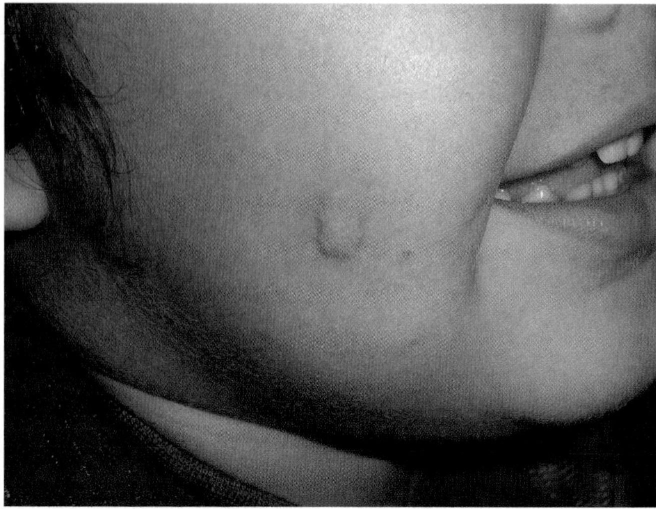

FIGURE 140-4 Solitary juvenile xanthogranuloma on the face of a 2.5 year old boy with obvious yellow coloration. (*Used with permission from Richard P. Usatine, MD.*)

DIFFERENTIAL DIAGNOSIS

- Juvenile Xanthogranuloma may be confused with other histiocytic proliferating disorders such as
  - Langerhan Cell Histiocytosis—These infants typically present with refractive scalp seborrheic-like dermatitis associated with diaper dermatitis and cutaneous xanthomatous papules. It is frequently associated with systemic symptoms such as bone lesions, hepatosplenomegaly, and diabetes insipidus (see Chapter 214, Langerhans Cell Histiocytosis).[5,8,9]
  - Generalized Eruptive Histiocytosis—This disorder usually involves older children and even adults and present as recurrent, multiple, red to brown papules over upper trunk, face, and proximal extremities. These lesions may leave a hyperpigmented scar behind.[4,5]

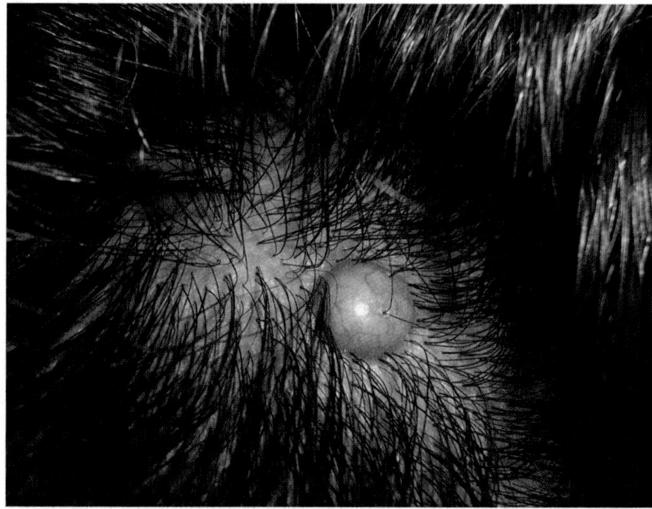

FIGURE 140-5 Juvenile xanthogranuloma on the scalp of a 2-year-old boy. Note the yellow color and the telangiectasias. This was biopsy proven. (*Used with permission from Richard P. Usatine, MD.*)

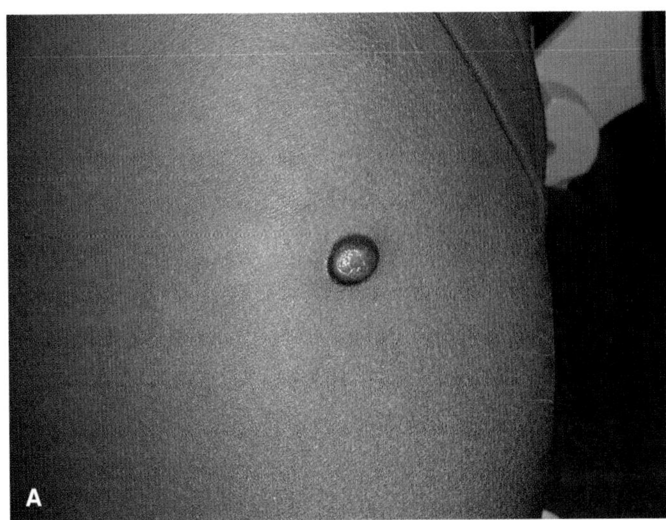

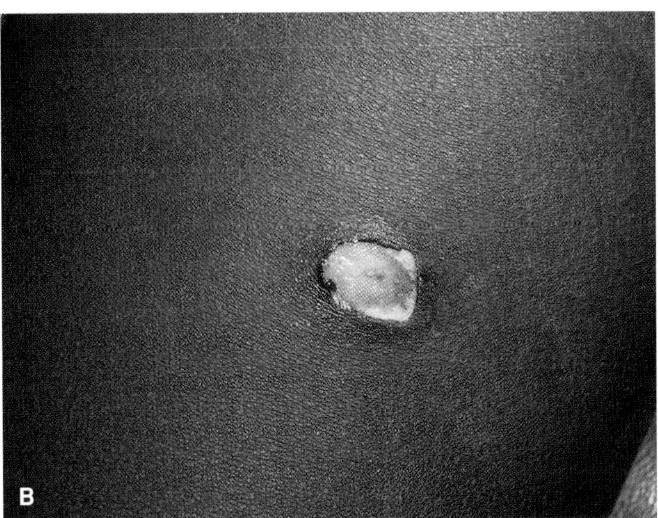

FIGURE 140-6 **A.** Six-month-old girl presented with growing tumor on her trunk. No yellow color was visible within the dark skin of the tumor. **B.** Yellow color of juvenile xanthogranuloma visible after shave biopsy using local anesthesia. (*Used with permission from Richard P. Usatine, MD.*)

  - Benign Cephalic Histiocytosis—This entity typically involves erythematous macules/papules on the face, and may also appear on the ears, neck, trunk and upper extremities (**Figure 140-7**).[4,5]
  - Xanthoma disseminatum—Rare condition including triad of cutaneous and mucous membrane xanthomas along with diabetes insipidus. Xanthomas are usually numerous, symmetric and involve the face along with flexural and intertriginous skin.[4,5]
- It can also look similar to molluscum contagiosum, Spitz nevus, dermatofibroma (**Figure 140-3**), keloid, and pyogenic granuloma.[4] Histologic examination may be the only way to differentiate between entities.

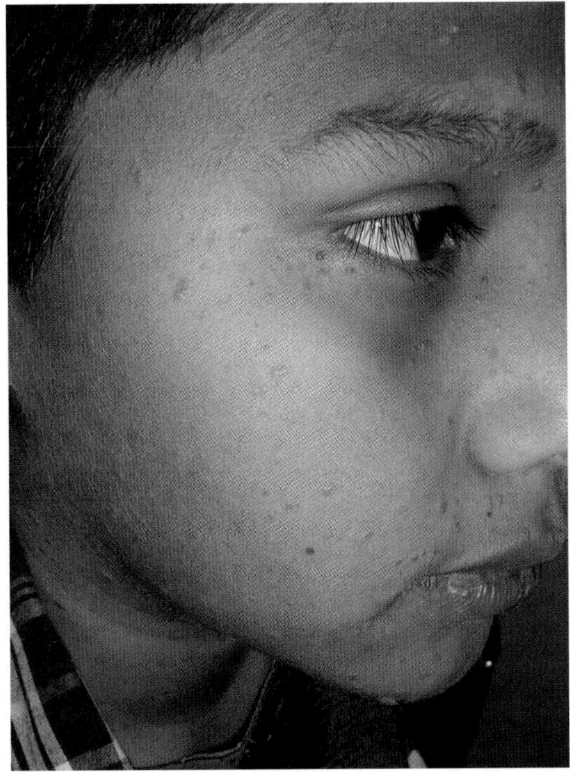

FIGURE 140-7 Benign cephalic histiocytosis on the face of 8-year-old boy, biopsy proven. (*Used with permission from Richard P. Usatine, MD.*)

MANAGEMENT

- Juvenile Xanthogranuloma, when only involving the skin, is usually a self-limited proliferation and requires no therapy. Look for systemic involvement or other systemic disorders. If no other organ is involved and there is no other risk associated with other disorders, then patient is given reassurance with good prognosis. Granulomas usually regress in 3 months to 6 years.[2,4–7] SOR Ⓐ
- If systemic involvement is found, then referral to appropriate specialist for monitoring, resection or other ablative therapy is indicated.[1,5,10] SOR Ⓐ
- Isolated cases have reported use of various chemotherapy agents (i.e., Cladribine), high dose prednisone, and cyclosporine or radiation therapy for systemic cases.[4,8] SOR Ⓒ
- Surgical excision may be pursued for cosmetic or compressive indications. SOR Ⓑ
- Routine referral for asymptomatic patients to an ophthalmologist is not recommended. Referral to ophthalmology for eye examination may be consider in patients 2 years old or younger, at time of diagnoses, or in patients that have multiple lesions because they may be at increased risk.[3,5] SOR Ⓐ

PROGNOSIS

Prognosis for cutaneous JXG is good, with high likelihood of spontaneous resolution of lesions without scarring. When there is systemic involvement prognosis is variable depending on degree of disease and organs involved.

FOLLOW-UP

Follow-up for resolution of lesion and development of new systemic or ocular symptoms as needed.

PATIENT EDUCATION

Reassure patient that if this is only confined to the skin there is a good prognosis and only rarely affects other organ systems. Reassure that lesions will resolve with little to no scar. At times nodules may develop superficial scaling or crusting which can be ameliorated with emollients (**Figure 140-3**). Lesions are usually asymptomatic.

PATIENT RESOURCES

- Juvenile Xanthogranuloma (JXG) Online Support—**www.jxgonlinesupport.org/p/home.html**.
- Histiocytosis Association—**www.histio.org/page.aspx?pid=391**.

PROVIDER RESOURCES

- eMedicine—**http://emedicine.medscape.com/article/1111629-overview**.
- DermNet NZ—**www.dermnetnz.org/lesions/xanthogranuloma.html**.

REFERENCES

1. Freyer, D et al. Juvenile Xanthogranuloma: Forms of Systemic Disease and their Clinical Implications. *Journal of Pediatrics*. 1996;129(2):227-237.
2. Janssen, D and Harms, D. Juvenile Xanthogranuloma in Childhood and Adolescence: A Clinicopathologic Study of 129 Patients From the Kiel Pediatric Tumor Registry. *American Journal of Surgical Pathology*. 2005; 29(1):21-28.
3. Chang, MW et al. The Risk of Intraocular Juvenile Xanthogranuloma: Survey of Current Practices and Assessment of Risk. *Journal of American Academy of Dermatology*. 1996;34(3):445-449.
4. Bologna, J et al. Dermatology volume 2. Juvenile Xanthogranuloma. 2003; Mosby;Spain: 1436-1438.
5. Puttgen, KB. Juvenile xanthogranuloma. UpToDate. http://www.uptodate.com/contents/juvenile-xanthogranuloma-jxg. Accessed on March 29, 2014.
6. Hernandez-Martin, A et al. Juvenile Xanthogranuloma. *Journal of American Academy of Dermatology*. 1997;36(3):355-367.
7. Wagner, A. Lumps and Bumps in Childhood. *Current Problems in Dermatology*. 1996 Jul-Aug;8(4):137-188.
8. Patrizi, A et al. Langerhan cell hystiocytosis and juvenile xanthogranuloma. Two case reports. *Dermatology*. 2004;209(1):57-61.
9. Yu, H et al. A Child with Coexistent Juvenile Xanthogranuloma and Langerhan Cell Histiocytosis. *Journal of American Academy of Dermatology*. 2010;62(2):329-332.
10. Chang, MW et al. Update on Juvenile Xanthogranuloma: Unusual Cutaneous and Systemic Variants. *Seminars in Cutaneous Medicine and Surgery*. 1999;18(3):195-205.

141 KELOIDS

Richard P. Usatine, MD
E.J. Mayeaux, Jr., MD

PATIENT STORY

A large keloid (**Figure 141-1A**) has been present on the upper ear of this 14-year-old boy for more than 2 years, since he experienced trauma to this area. The keloid was excised in the office with local anesthetic and the defect sutured using 5-0 Prolene (**Figure 141-1B**). The cosmetic result was excellent and the patient was happy.

INTRODUCTION

Keloids are benign dermal fibroproliferative tumors that form in scar because of altered wound healing. They form as a result of overproduction of extracellular matrix and dermal fibroblasts that have a high mitotic rate.

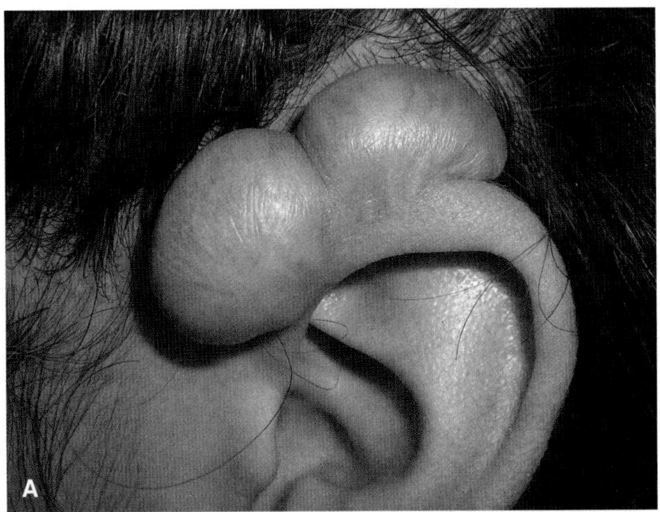

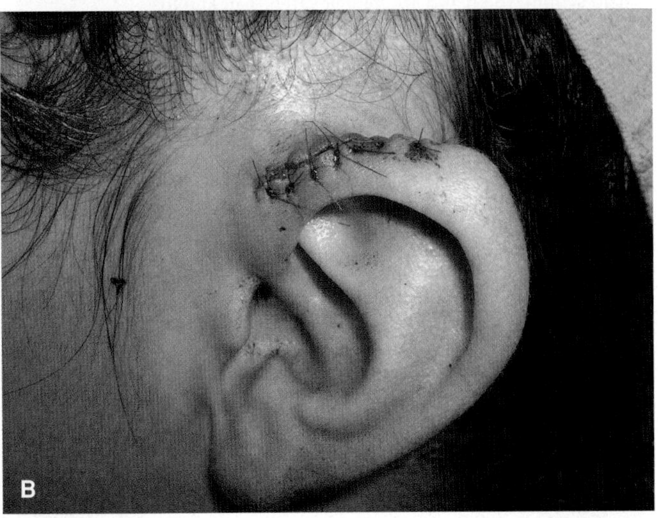

FIGURE 141-1 **A.** A large keloid has been present on the upper ear of this 14-year-old boy for more than 2 years, since he experienced trauma to this area. **B.** The keloid was excised in the office with local anesthetic and the defect sutured using 5-0 Prolene. The cosmetic result was excellent. *(Used with permission from Richard P. Usatine, MD.)*

SYNONYMS

Cheloid.

EPIDEMIOLOGY

- Individuals with darker pigmentation are more likely to develop keloids. Sixteen percent of black persons reported having keloids in a random sampling.[1]
- Men and women are generally affected equally except that keloids are more common in young adult women—probably secondary to a higher rate of piercing the ears (**Figure 141-2**).[2]
- Highest incidence is in individuals ages 10 to 20 years.[2,3]

ETIOLOGY AND PATHOPHYSIOLOGY

- Keloids are dermal fibrotic lesions that are a variation of the normal wound-healing process in the spectrum of fibroproliferative disorders.
- Keloids are more likely to develop in areas of the body that are subjected to high skin tension such as over the sternum.

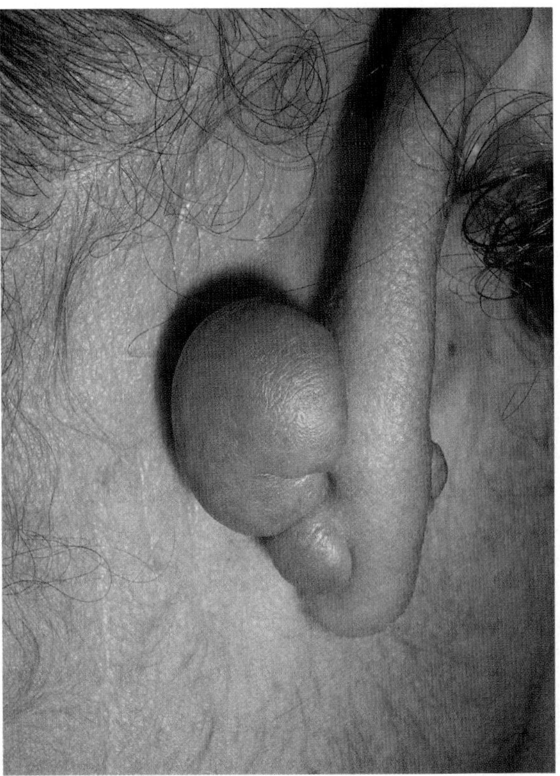

FIGURE 141-2 A keloid on the earlobe that started from piercing the ear. *(Used with permission from Richard P. Usatine, MD.)*

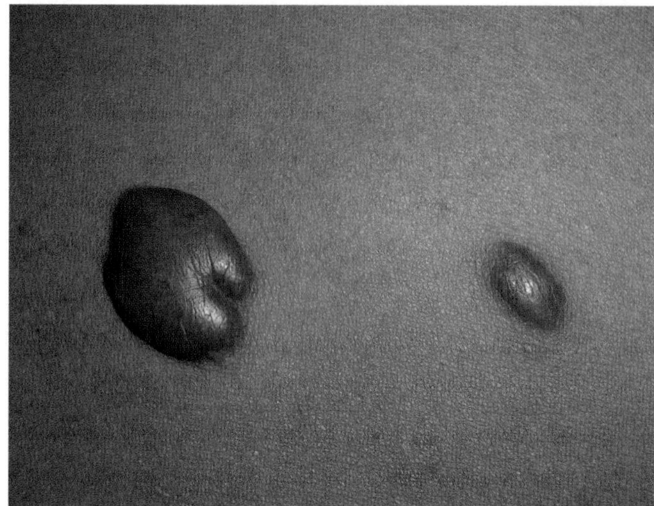

FIGURE 141-3 Two keloids on the back of this young African American woman. (*Used with permission from Richard P. Usatine, MD.*)

- These can occur even up to a year after the injury and will enlarge beyond the scar margin. Burns and other injuries can heal with a keloid in just one portion of the area injured.
- Wounds subjected to prolonged inflammation (acne cysts) are more likely to develop keloids.

RISK FACTORS[3]

- Darker skin pigmentation (African, Hispanic, or Asian ethnicity) (**Figure 141-3**).
- A family history of keloids.
- Wound healing by secondary intention.
- Wounds subjected to prolonged inflammation.
- Sites of repeated trauma.
- Pregnancy.
- Body piercings (**Figure 141-4**).

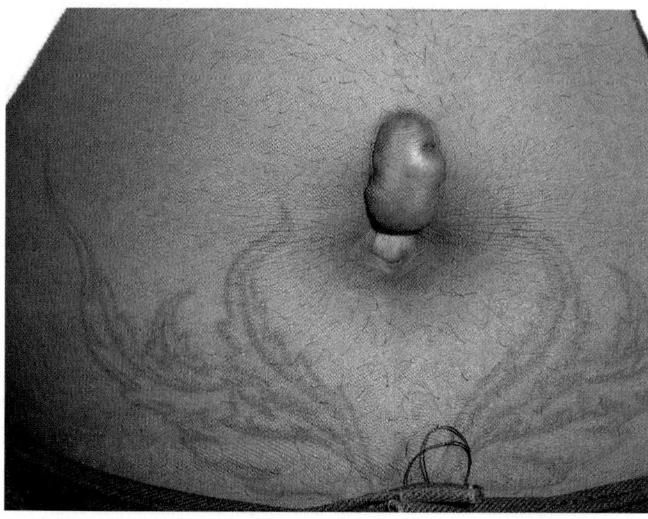

FIGURE 141-4 This keloid formed at the site of a belly button piercing. (*Used with permission from Richard P. Usatine, MD.*)

DIAGNOSIS

CLINICAL FEATURES

- Some keloids present with pruritic pain or a burning sensation around the scar.
- Initially manifest as erythematous lesions devoid of hair follicles or other glandular tissue.
- Papules to nodules to large tuberous lesions.
- Range in consistency from soft and doughy to rubbery and hard. Most often, the lesions are the color of normal skin but can become brownish red or bluish and then pale as they age.[4]
- May extend in a claw-like fashion far beyond any slight injury.
- Lesions on neck, ears, and abdomen tend to become pedunculated.

TYPICAL DISTRIBUTION

- Anterior chest, shoulders, flexor surfaces of extremities, anterior neck, earlobes, and wounds that cross skin tension lines.

LABORATORY TESTING

- Biopsy is rarely needed to make a diagnosis because the clinical appearance is usually distinctive and clear.

DIFFERENTIAL DIAGNOSIS

- Hypertrophic scars can appear similar to keloids but are confined to the site of original injury.
- Acne keloidalis nuchae is an inflammatory disorder around hair follicles of the posterior neck that results in keloidal scarring (**Figure 141-5**). Although the scarring is similar to keloids the location and pathophysiology are unique. This process can also cause alopecia.
- Dermatofibromas are common button-like dermal nodules usually found on the legs or arms. They may umbilicate when the surrounding skin is pinched. These often have a hyperpigmented halo around them and are less elevated than keloids.

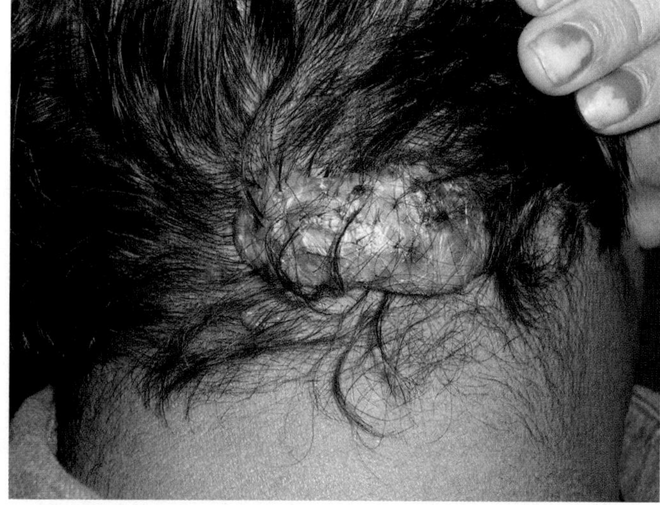

FIGURE 141-5 Acne keloidalis nuchae on the posterior neck of this young Hispanic man. (*Used with permission from Richard P. Usatine, MD.*)

MANAGEMENT

- Patients frequently want keloids treated because of symptoms (pain and pruritus) and concerns about appearance.
- A 2006 systematic review of 396 studies and an accompanying meta-analysis of 36 articles concluded that no optimal evidence-based therapy exists and recommended choosing treatment based on cost and adverse effect profile.[5]

NONPHARMACOLOGIC

- Silicone gel sheeting as a treatment for hypertrophic and keloid scarring is supported by poor-quality trials susceptible to bias. There is only weak evidence of a benefit of silicone gel sheeting as prevention for abnormal scarring in high-risk individuals.[6,7] SOR B

MEDICATIONS

- Intralesional steroid injections—Intralesional injection of triamcinolone acetonide (10 to 40 mg/mL) may decrease pruritus, as well as decreasing size and flattening of keloids (**Figure 141-6**). SOR C This may be repeated monthly as needed.[5,8]
- Earlobe keloids can be treated with imiquimod 5 percent cream following tangential shave excision on both sides of the earlobe.[9,10] SOR B Patients were instructed to administer imiquimod 5 percent cream to the excision sites the night of the surgery and daily for 6 to 8 weeks postsurgery. Imiquimod 5 percent cream only temporarily prevented the recurrence of presternal keloids after excision.[11] SOR C

COMPLEMENTARY/ALTERNATIVE THERAPY

- No available evidence supports using nonprescription products such as Mederma and other creams, gels, and oils, to treat scars.[7] Limited clinical trials have failed to demonstrate lasting improvement of established keloids and hypertrophic scars with onion extract topical gel (e.g., Mederma) or topical vitamin E.[3] SOR B

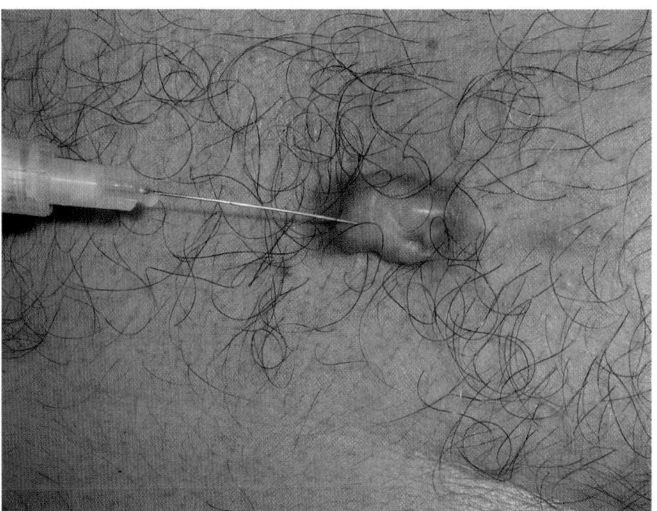

FIGURE 141-6 Triamcinolone injected into this symptomatic keloid on the chest. Note how the keloid is blanching white, demonstrating that the steroid is properly injected into the body of the keloid. A Luer lock syringe is used to avoid the needle popping off during the injection under pressure and a 27-gauge needle is used to minimize patient discomfort. (*Used with permission from Richard P. Usatine, MD.*)

SURGICAL

- Cryosurgery and intralesional triamcinolone have been used to treat smaller keloids (e.g., secondary to acne) with similar success to other therapies.[3,12] SOR B
- Combined cryosurgery and intralesional triamcinolone—The lesion is initially frozen with liquid nitrogen spray and allowed to thaw. Then it is injected with triamcinolone acetate (10 to 40 mg/mL). SOR C
- Earlobe keloids can be surgically excised with a shave or excisional technique and then injected with triamcinolone acetate (10 to 40 mg/mL) after hemostasis is obtained. The triamcinolone injection can be repeated in 1 month to decrease the chance of recurrence.[8] SOR B
- Keloids on the upper ear can be excised and the skin closed with sutures (**Figure 141-1**). SOR C
- Pulsed-dye laser treatment can be beneficial for keloids.[13] Combination treatment with pulsed-dye laser plus intralesional therapy with corticosteroids and/or fluorouracil 50 mg/mL 2 to 3 times per week may be superior to either approach alone.[14] SOR C
- Keloids can be treated with cryosurgery alone or in combination with intralesional steroids. In one, small, controlled study, 10 patients with keloids were treated with intralesional steroid and cryosurgery vs. intralesional steroid or cryosurgery alone.[15] SOR B Patients were treated at least 3 times 4 weeks apart. Based upon keloid thickness, the keloids responded significantly better to combined cryosurgery and triamcinolone versus triamcinolone alone or cryotherapy alone. Pain intensity was significantly lowered with all treatment modalities. Pruritus was lowered only with the combined treatment and intralesional corticosteroid alone.[15]
- In another study, 20 patients with hypertrophic and keloidal scars received two 15-second cycles (total 30 seconds) of cryosurgery treatments once monthly for 12 months with intralesional injections of 10 to 40 mg/mL triamcinolone once monthly for 3 months.[16] SOR B Topical application of silicone gel was added 3 times daily for 12 months. The control group included 10 patients who received treatment with silicone sheeting only. After 1 year there was improvement in all the parameters, especially in terms of symptoms, cosmetic appearance, and associated signs, compared to baseline and compared to the control group.[16] SOR B
- Layton et al. reported that the intralesional injection of a steroid is helpful but cryotherapy is more effective (85% improvement in terms of flattening) for recent acne keloids located on the back.[17] Treatment with intralesional triamcinolone was beneficial, but the response to cryosurgery was significantly better in early, vascular lesions.[17] SOR B
- If the keloid is older and/or firmer, it may not respond to injection therapy as well as softer and newer lesions. It may help to pretreat the keloid with cryotherapy. It is not necessary to freeze a margin of normal tissue. After liquid nitrogen or another freezing modality is applied to the keloid, it is allowed to thaw and develop edema. This generally takes 1 to 2 minutes, which allows an easier introduction of intralesional steroids into the lesions. SOR C

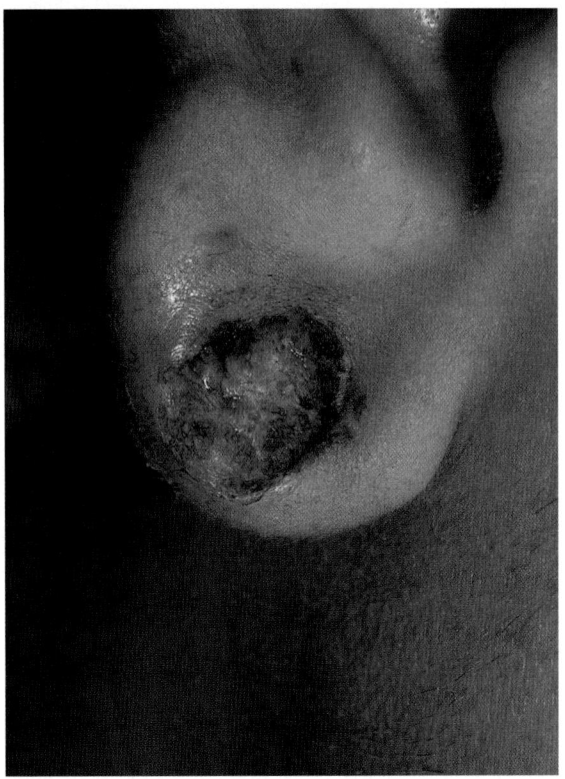

FIGURE 141-7 Ear lobe keloid was shaved off with a DermaBlade and the base was treated with electrosurgery to stop the bleeding. Then 0.1 mL of 40 mg/mL triamcinolone was injected into the base of the remaining keloid. *(Used with permission from Richard P. Usatine, MD.)*

- In one double-blind, clinical trial, 40 patients were randomized to receive intralesional triamcinolone (TAC) or a combination of TAC and 5-fluorouracil (5-FU).[18] Both groups received injections at weekly intervals for 8 weeks and lesions were assessed for erythema, pruritus, pliability, height, length, and width. Both groups showed an acceptable improvement in nearly all parameters, but these were more significant in the TAC plus 5-FU group ($P < 0.05$ for all except pruritus and percentage of itch reduction). Good-to-excellent improvement was reported by 20 percent of the patients receiving TAC alone and by 55 percent of the patients in the group receiving TAC plus 5-FU.[18] SOR Ⓑ
- Earlobe keloids may be excised with a shave excision and injection of the base with steroid (**Figure 141-7**). It is hard to get much volume of steroid into the base of these keloids, so 40 mg/mL triamcinolone is preferred as the concentration for injection. SOR Ⓒ Another option is to use radiofrequency electrosurgery technique with a pure cutting setting (and using steroid in the anesthetic).
- According to one article, simple excision of earlobe keloids can result in recurrence rates approaching 80 percent.[19] A randomized, prospective trial comparing steroid injections versus radiation therapy found that 2 of 16 keloids (12.5%) recurred after surgery and radiation therapy, whereas 4 of 12 (33%) recurred after surgery and steroid injections. These results did not produce a statistically significant difference. No alteration of skin pigmentation, wound dehiscence, or chronic dermatitis was observed in any patient in either group.[19] Although radiation therapy was considered easy to obtain in this study, it is reasonable to use steroid injections in office practice.

PREVENTION

- Avoiding trauma, including surgical trauma, whenever possible may decrease keloids in susceptible individuals.

PROGNOSIS

- A 2006 systematic review of 396 studies and an accompanying meta-analysis of 36 articles concluded that any treatment gave patients an overall 70 percent (95% confidence interval, 49% to 91%) chance of improvement.[5]

FOLLOW-UP

- Follow-up is based on the chosen treatment. Follow-up for intralesional steroid injections is usually in 1 month.

PATIENT EDUCATION

- Advise patients to avoid local skin trauma, for example, ear piercing, body piercing, and tattoos, and to control inflammatory acne.

PATIENT RESOURCES

- MedlinePlus. *Keloids*—**www.nlm.nih.gov/medlineplus/ency/article/000849.htm**.
- Skinsight. *Keloid Information for Adults*—**www.skinsight.com/adult/keloid.htm**.

PROVIDER RESOURCES

- Medscape. *Keloid and Hypertrophic Scar* (Dermatology)—**http://emedicine.medscape.com/article/1057599**.
- Medscape. *Keloids* (Plastic Surgery)—**http://emedicine.medscape.com/article/1298013**.
- Usatine R, Pfenninger J, Stulberg D, Small R: Dermatologic and Cosmetic Procedures in Office Practice. Philadelphia, PA: Elsevier; 2012. Available as a text with DVD or electronic application. Contains details, photographs and videos on how to use cryosurgery and intralesional injections to treat keloids—**http://usatinemedia.com/Usatine_Media_LLC/DermProcedures_Overview.html**.

REFERENCES

1. Chike-Obi CJ, Cole PD, Brissett AE. Keloids: pathogenesis, clinical features, and management. *Semin Plast Surg*. 2009;23:178-184.
2. Alhady SM, Sivanantharajah K. Keloids in various races. A review of 175 cases. *Plast Reconstr Surg*. 1969;44(6):564-566.
3. Juckett G, Hartman-Adams H. Management of keloids and hypertrophic scars. *Am Fam Physician*. 2009;80(3):253-260.

4. Urioste SS, Arndt KA, Dover JS. Keloids and hypertrophic scars: review and treatment strategies. *Semin Cutan Med Surg*. 1999;18: 159-171.

5. Leventhal D, Furr M, Reiter D. Treatment of keloids and hypertrophic scars: a meta-analysis and review of the literature. *Arch Facial Plast Surg*. 2006;8:362-368.

6. O'Brien L, Pandit A. Silicon gel sheeting for preventing and treating hypertrophic and keloid scars. *Cochrane Database Syst Rev*. 2006;(1):CD003826.

7. Williams CC, De Groote S. Clinical inquiry: what treatment is best for hypertrophic scars and keloids? *J Fam Pract*. 2011;60(12):757-758.

8. Shaffer JJ, Taylor SC, Cook-Bolden F. Keloidal scars: a review with a critical look at therapeutic options. *J Am Acad Dermatol*. 2002;46:S63.

9. Patel PJ, Skinner RB Jr: Experience with keloids after excision and application of 5% imiquimod cream. *Dermatol Surg*. 2006;32:462.

10. Stashower ME. Successful treatment of earlobe keloids with imiquimod after tangential shave excision. *Dermatol Surg*. 2006;32:380-386.

11. Malhotra AK, Gupta S, Khaitan BK, Sharma VK. Imiquimod 5% cream for the prevention of recurrence after excision of presternal keloids. *Dermatology*. 2007;215:63-65.

12. Layton AM, Yip J, Cunliffe WJ. A comparison of intralesional triamcinolone and cryosurgery in the treatment of acne keloids. *Br J Dermatol*. 1994;130:498-501.

13. Alster TS, Williams CM. Treatment of keloid sternotomy scars with 585 nm flashlamp-pumped pulsed-dye laser. *Lancet*. 1995;345:1198.

14. Asilian A, Darougheh A, Shariati F. New combination of triamcinolone, 5-fluorouracil, and pulsed-dye laser for treatment of keloid and hypertrophic scars. *Dermatol Surg*. 2006;32:907-915.

15. Yosipovitch G, Widijanti SM, Goon A, Chan YH, Goh CL. A comparison of the combined effect of cryotherapy and corticosteroid injections versus corticosteroids and cryotherapy alone on keloids: a controlled study. *J Dermatolog Treat*. 2001;12:87-89.

16. Boutli-Kasapidou F, Tsakiri A, Anagnostou E, Mourellou O. Hypertrophic and keloidal scars: an approach to polytherapy. *Int J Dermatol*. 2005;44:324-327.

17. Layton AM, Yip J, Cunliffe WJ. A comparison of intralesional triamcinolone and cryosurgery in the treatment of acne keloids. *Br J Dermatol*. 1994;130:498-501.

18. Darougheh A, Asilian A, Shariati F. Intralesional triamcinolone alone or in combination with 5-fluorouracil for the treatment of keloid and hypertrophic scars. *Clin Exp Dermatol*. 2009;34: 219-223.

19. Sclafani AP, Gordon L, Chadha M, Romo T, III. Prevention of earlobe keloid recurrence with postoperative corticosteroid injections versus radiation therapy: a randomized, prospective study and review of the literature. *Dermatol Surg*. 1996;22:569-574.

142 PYOGENIC GRANULOMA

Mindy A. Smith, MD, MS
Richard P. Usatine, MD

PATIENT STORY

A young girl is brought in by her mother to see their pediatrician for a red growth on the face that has been there for two months (**Figure 142-1**). The red growth bleeds easily if traumatized. The pediatrician recognizes the typical features of a pyogenic granuloma and presents various treatment options to the mother including excision with biopsy. It is clear that the child will not stay still for local anesthetic with the needle but is willing to allow the physician to use a Cryo Tweezer to freeze the pyogenic granuloma. The pediatrician places the Cryo Tweezer in liquid nitrogen and applies the device to the pyogenic granuloma. As the child is cooperative with the procedure a second freeze is performed in the same manner. On follow-up visit in 3 weeks, the pyogenic granuloma is gone. The mother is warned if there is regrowth to return for further evaluation and treatment.

INTRODUCTION

Pyogenic granuloma (PG) is the name for a common, benign, acquired, vascular neoplasm of the skin and mucous membranes.

SYNONYMS

- The term "lobular capillary hemangioma" is an accepted and preferred term because PG is neither pyogenic (purulent bacterial infection) nor a granuloma.[1] We continue to use "pyogenic granuloma" as this is still the most recognized term.

EPIDEMIOLOGY

- Most often seen in children and young adults (0.5% of children's skin lesions); 42 percent of cases occur by 5 years of age and about 1 percent are present at birth.[1]
- Oral lesions occur most often in the second and third decade, more commonly in women (2:1).[1] In a case series from Israel of pediatric gingival lesions (N = 233), one-quarter were PGs.
- Also common during pregnancy.
- PG has also been reported in the gastrointestinal tract, the larynx, and on the nasal mucosa, conjunctiva, and cornea.

ETIOLOGY AND PATHOPHYSIOLOGY

- Etiology is unknown but may be the result of trauma, infection, or preceding dermatoses.
- Consists of dense proliferation of capillaries and fibroblastic stroma that is infiltrated with polymorphonuclear leukocytes.
- Multiple PGs have been reported at burn sites and following use of oral contraceptives, protease inhibitors, and topical application of tretinoin for acne.[2]
- PGs are known to regress following pregnancy. Vascular endothelial growth factor (VEGF) was found in one study to be high in the granulomas in pregnancy and was almost undetectable after parturition and associated with apoptosis of endothelial cells and regression of granuloma.[3]

RISK FACTORS

- Trauma (up to 50%), including nose piercing,[4] or chronic irritation (e.g., orthodontic appliance).[1,5]
- Multiple lesions can follow manipulation of a primary lesion.[6]

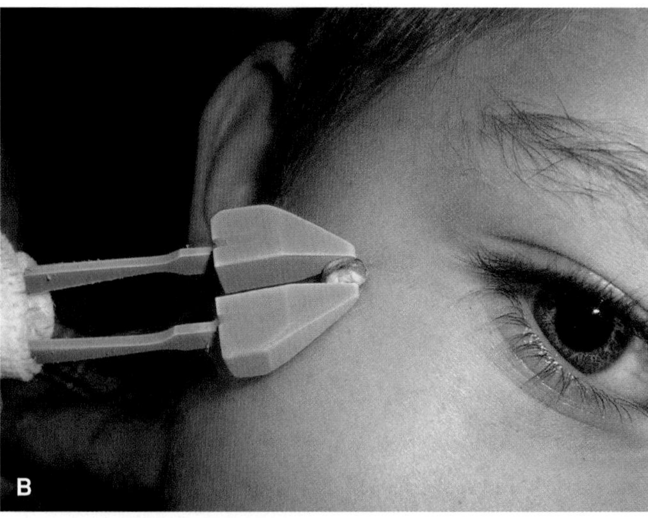

FIGURE 142-1 **A.** Pyogenic granuloma on the cheek of a young girl. **B.** Cryotherapy of the pyogenic granuloma using a cryo tweezer. This method was chosen because the girl was afraid of the needle needed for local anesthesia and surgical excision. She tolerated the cryotherapy well. (*Used with permission from Richard P. Usatine, MD.*)

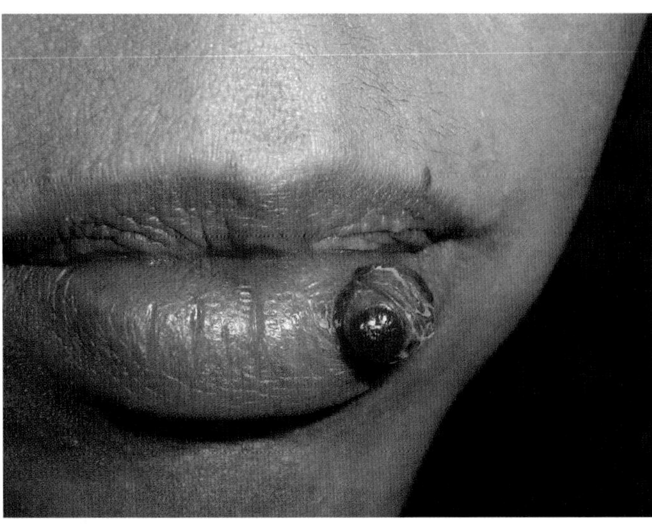

FIGURE 142-2 Pyogenic granuloma on the lip. This was surgically excised. (*Used with permission from Richard P. Usatine, MD.*)

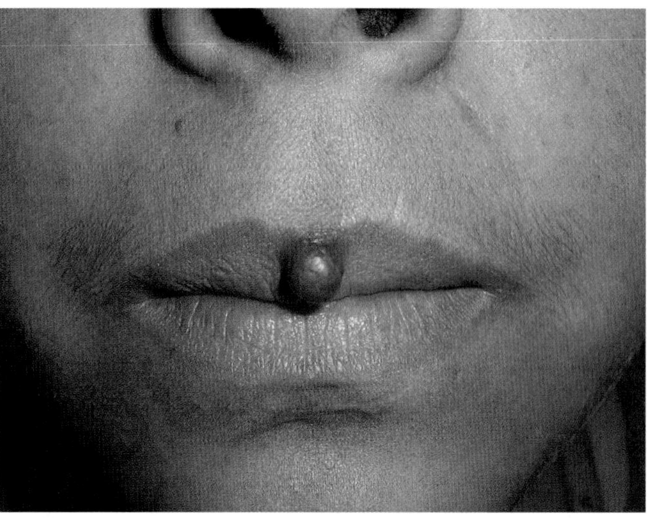

FIGURE 142-4 Pyogenic granuloma on the upper lip. (*Used with permission from Richard P. Usatine, MD.*)

- Pregnancy or use of oral contraceptives for oral PGs; postulated due to imbalance between angiogenesis enhancers and inhibitors.[1]
- Infection with *Bartonella*.[1]

DIAGNOSIS

CLINICAL FEATURES

- Usually solitary, erythematous, dome-shaped papule or nodule that bleeds easily (**Figures 142-1** to **142-6**); rarely causes anemia. Satellite lesions may rarely occur.
- Prone to ulceration, erosion, and crusting.
- Size ranges from a few millimeters to several centimeters (average size is 6.5 mm).[1]
- Rapid growth over a period of weeks to maximum size.
- Variants include cutaneous, oral mucosal (granuloma gravidarum), satellite, subcutaneous, intravenous, and congenital types.[1]
- PG can also arrive within port-wine stains (PWS); in one case series (N = 31 with nodules arising within PWS), 14 biopsy specimens were PGs.[7] Most PGs and arteriovenous malformations (10 specimens) occurred in the area innervated by the second branch of the trigeminal nerve. In one case series, PGs arising with PWS were seen as a complication of 595 nm tunable pulsed dye laser treatment of the original lesion.[8]

TYPICAL DISTRIBUTION

- Cutaneous PG most often found on the head and neck (62.5%) (specifically the gingiva, lips as in **Figure 142-2** to **142-4**), nose, face (**Figure 142-5**), neck (**Figure 142-6**), trunk (20%), and extremities (18%; **Figure 142-7**).[1] The fingers and hands are very commonly involved (**Figure 142-7**). PGs have also been reported on the glans penis in association with phimosis.[9]
- Pregnancy PG occurs most commonly along the maxillary intraoral mucosal surface.

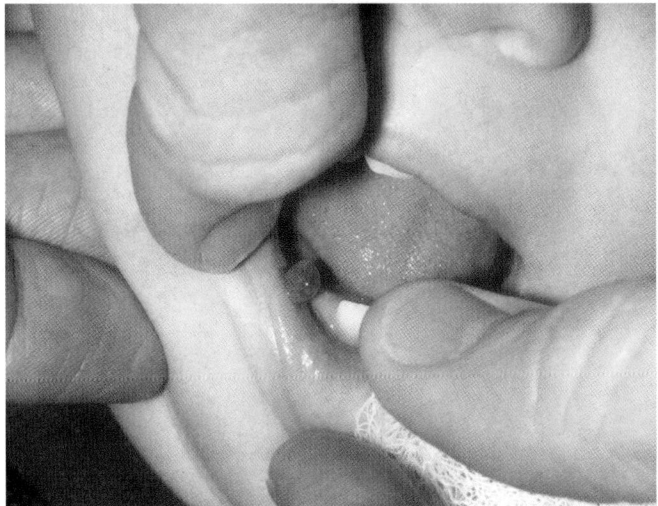

FIGURE 142-3 Pyogenic granuloma on the lip of an infant. (*Used with permission from Richard P. Usatine, MD.*)

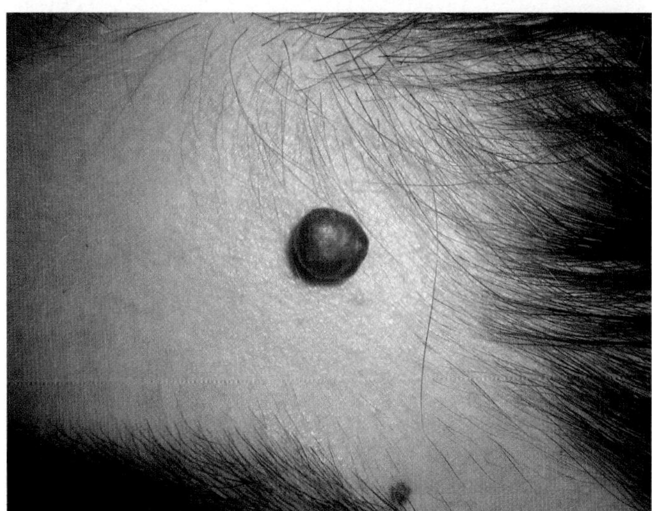

FIGURE 142-5 Pyogenic granuloma on the forehead and a 14-year-old girl. (*Used with permission from Richard P. Usatine, MD.*)

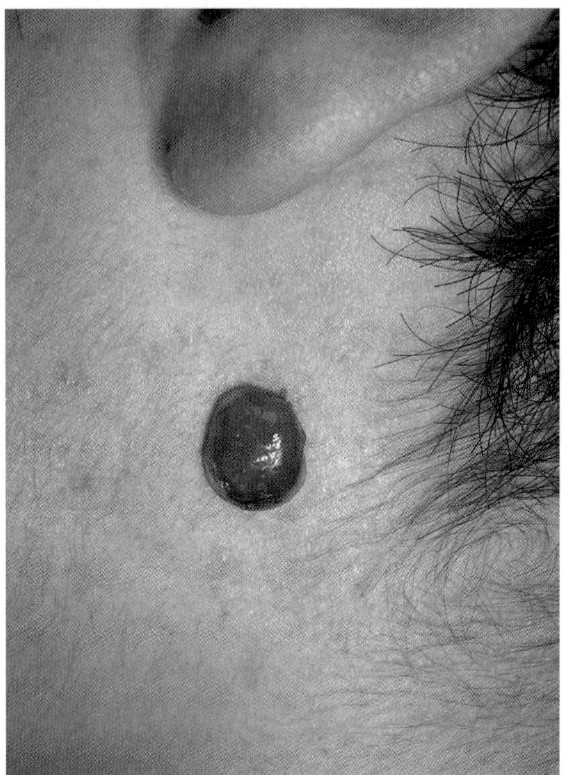

FIGURE 142-6 Pyogenic granuloma on the neck 12-year-old boy. (*Used with permission from Richard P. Usatine, MD.*)

- In one retrospective study (N = 58 cases) and literature review, causes of PG included drugs, local trauma, and peripheral nerve injury.[10] The authors suggested that histological examination might be needed to rule out malignant melanoma.

IMAGING

- Reddish homogeneous area surrounded by a white collarette is the most frequent dermoscopic pattern in pyogenic granulomas (85%).[11] In more advanced lesions, white lines that intersect the central areas may be seen that are likely fibrous septa. Slight pressure can obscure vascular structures within a PG so care should be taken as the visualization of vascular structures within a red tumor requires assessment for melanoma.[12]
- In vivo reflectance confocal microscopy is under investigation for differentiation of acquired vascular lesions.[13]

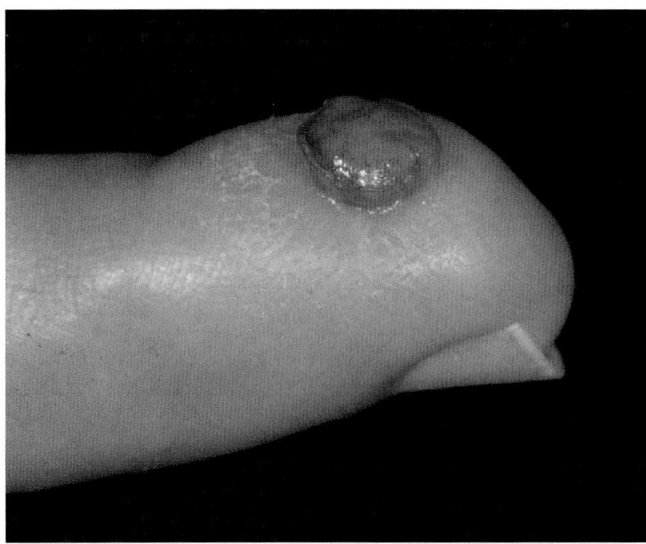

FIGURE 142-7 Small pyogenic granuloma on the finger of a 17-year-old boy for 2 months. It started with a small injury to the finger. (*Used with permission from Richard P. Usatine, MD.*)

BIOPSY

- If treatment involves excision, than the tissue should be sent to pathology to confirm the diagnosis and exclude malignancy.
- Early lesions resemble granulation tissue (numerous capillaries and venules with endothelial cells arrayed radially toward the skin surface; stroma is edematous).[1]
- The mature PG exhibits a fibromyxoid stroma separating the lesion into lobules. Proliferation of capillaries is present, with prominent endothelial cells. The epidermis exhibits inward growth at the lesion base.[1]

DIFFERENTIAL DIAGNOSIS

Although cutaneous malignancies are rare in children, PG may be confused with lesions including atypical fibroxanthoma, basal cell carcinoma, Kaposi carcoma, metastatic cutaneous lesions, squamous cell carcinoma, and amelanotic melanoma (**Figure 142-8**). It is especially important to send the excised lesion that appears to be a PG for pathology to make sure that a malignancy is not missed.

Benign tumors that may be confused with PG include:

- Cherry hemangioma—Small, bright-red, dome-shaped papules that represent benign proliferation of capillaries (**Figure 142-9**). These tend to be flatter and do not bleed as easily as a PG. Many cherry

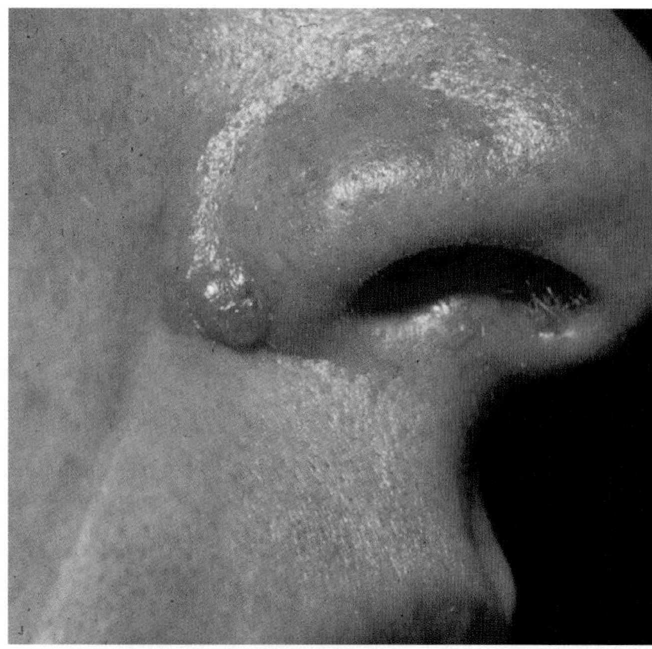

FIGURE 142-8 Amelanotic melanoma on the nose that could be confused with a pyogenic granuloma. Always send what you suspect to be a PG to the pathologist. (*Used with permission from UTHSCSA Division of Dermatology.*)

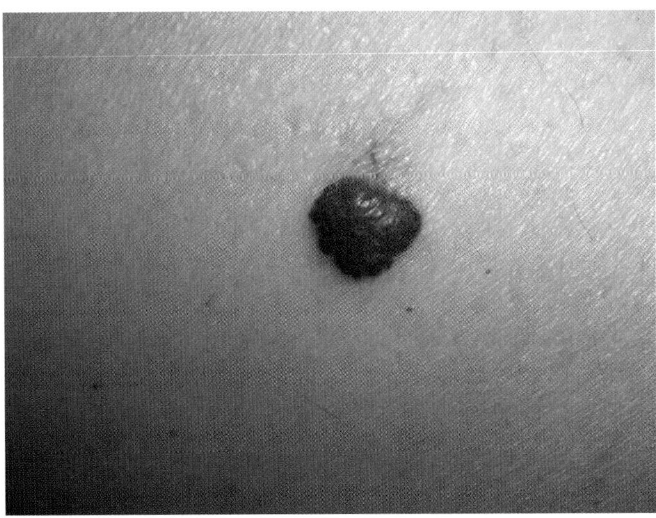

FIGURE 142-9 Cherry hemangioma on the arm. (*Used with permission from Richard P. Usatine, MD.*)

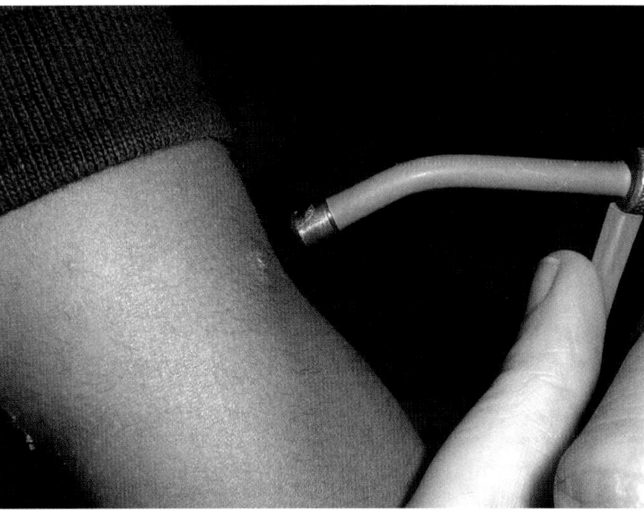

FIGURE 142-10 Pyogenic granuloma on the arm of a 7-year-old boy being treated with cryotherapy using a probe delivery device to allow for compression of the lesion at the same time that the cold is being delivered to the site. (*Used with permission from Richard P. Usatine, MD.*)

angiomas are acquired as part of normal aging so are seen more frequently in older adults.

- Fibrous papule of the nose is a benign tumor of the nose. Most are skin colored and not confused with PG. A benign clear cell variant of a fibrous papule can closely resemble a PG.

MANAGEMENT

Removal of the lesion is indicated to alleviate any bleeding or discomfort, for cosmetic reasons or when the diagnosis is uncertain.

NONPHARMACOLOGIC

- Untreated PGs eventually atrophy, become fibromatous, and slowly regress, especially if the causative agent is removed.

MEDICATIONS

- A case of successful treatment of a recurrent pyogenic granuloma was reported using a 14-week course of twice-weekly imiquimod 5 percent topical application.[14] SOR Ⓒ
- Topical 98 percent phenol (3 applications, 1 minute each consecutively followed by silver sulfadine, and 10 percent povidone iodine) has also been successfully used without scarring for periungual PGs, but required weekly treatment over 2 to 14 weeks in one case series.[15]

PROCEDURES

A number of procedures have been used for elimination of PGs; data are limited to case series reports.[16]

- Cryotherapy is more likely to be tolerated by young children rather than an excision, which requires a needle injection with a local anesthetic. A Cryo Tweezer (**Figure 142-1**) or cryoprobe (**Figure 142-10**) is likely to be more effective as both devices can compress the vascular structures for more effective cryodestruction. Also, both devices may be less frightening and painful than a spray application (author experience).
- Simple surgical excision has a low recurrence rate (<4%) but is associated with scarring (55%).[16] SOR Ⓒ
- Removal can be accomplished with shave excision and electrodesiccation—The latter reduces recurrence (about 10%); scarring appears less than with simple excision (31%) or cauterization alone (43.5%).[1,16] PGs bleed extensively when manipulated or cut. It is important to use lidocaine with epinephrine, wait 10 minutes for the epinephrine to work and have an electrosurgery device to control bleeding. Cut the PG off with a blade and send to pathology. Curetting the base will also help stop the bleeding and prevent recurrence. The base is curetted and electrodesiccated until the bleeding can be stopped. A pressure dressing should be applied before the patient leaves the office. SOR Ⓒ
- Both cryosurgery and laser surgery often require more than one treatment and scarring may be high (12% to 42% and 44%, respectively).[1,16] SOR Ⓒ In one case series, 19 of 20 patients had recurrence-free healing after one to four treatments using a 1,064-nm neodymium-doped yttrium aluminum garnet (Nd:YAG) laser.[17]
- Sclerotherapy in one case series was reported to leave no scarring or recurrence.[16] SOR Ⓒ

PROGNOSIS

- PG develops over weeks, and growth typically stabilizes over several months.[1] Eventually, it shrinks to become a fibrotic angioma. Some nodules spontaneously infarct and involute. In one pediatric retrospective case series with telephone follow-up, four untreated patients had spontaneous resolution within 6 to 18 months with no recurrences.[18]
- Congenital PG is an uncommon disseminated variant that presents with multiple lesions, similar in appearance to the cutaneous form, present at birth. The condition appears to follow a benign course, with spontaneous resolution over 6 to 12 months.[1]

FOLLOW-UP

- As needed.

PATIENT EDUCATION

- Explain to patients that lesions may resolve spontaneously and that multiple treatments are available.
- Once treated, if the lesion begins to recur, patients should follow-up quickly before the lesion gets larger and harder to treat.

PATIENT RESOURCES

- **www.nlm.nih.gov/medlineplus/ency/article/001464.htm**.
- **www.ncbi.nlm.nih.gov/pubmedhealth/PMH0002435/**.

PROVIDER RESOURCES

- **http://emedicine.medscape.com/article/910112**.

REFERENCES

1. Lin RL, Janniger CK. Pyogenic granuloma. *Cutis*. 2004;74(4): 229-233.
2. Teknetzis A, Tonannides D, Vakali G, et al. Pyogenic granulomas following topical application of tretinoin. *J Eur Acad Dermatol Venereol*. 2004;18(3):337-339.
3. Yuan K, Lin MT. The roles of vascular endothelial growth factor and angiopoietin-2 in the regression of pregnancy pyogenic granuloma. *Oral Dis*. 2004;10(3):179-185.
4 Kumar GS, Bandyopadhyay D. Granuloma pyogenicum as a complication of decorative nose piercing: report of eight cases from eastern India. *J Cutan Med Surg*. 2012;16(3):197-200.
5. Acharya PN, Gill D, Lloyd T. Pyogenic granuloma: a rare side complication from an orthodontic appliance. *J Orthod*. 2011; 38(4):290-293.
6. Blickenstaff RD, Roenigk RK, Peters MS, et al. Recurrent pyogenic granuloma with satellitosis. *J Am Acad Dermatol*. 1989;21: 1241-1244.
7. Chen D, Hu XJ, Lin XX, et al. Nodules arising within port-wine stains: a clinicopathologic study of 31 cases. *Am J Dermatopathol*. 2011;33(2):144-151.
8. Liu S, Yang C, Xu S, et al. Pyogenic granuloma arising as a complication of 595 nm tunable pulsed dye laser treatment of port-wine stains: report of four cases. *Dermatol Surg*. 2010;36(8):1341-1343.
9. Eickhorst KM, Nurzia MJ, Barone JG. Pediatric pyogenic granuloma of the glans penis. *Urology*. 2003;61(3):644.
10. Piraccini BM, Bellavista S, Misciali C, et al. Periungual and subungual pyogenic granuloma. *Br J Dermatol*. 2010;163(5):941-953.
11. Zaballos P, Llambrich A, Cuellar F, et al. Dermoscopic findings in pyogenic granuloma. *Br J Dermatol. 2006;154(6):1108-11.*
12. Oiso N, Kawada A. Dermoscopy of pyogenic granuloma on the lip: the differing appearances of vascular structures with and without pressure. *Eur J Dermatol*. 2011;21(3):441.
13. Astner S, González S, Cuevas J, et al. Preliminary evaluation of benign vascular lesions using in vivo relectance confocal microscopy. *Dermatol Surg*. 2010;36(7):1099-1110.
14. Goldenberg G, Krowchuk DP, Jorizzo JL. Successful treatment of a therapy-resistant pyogenic granuloma with topical imiquimod 5% cream. *J Dermatolog Treat*. 2006;17(2):121-123.
15. Losa Iglesias ME, Becerro de Bengoa Vallejo R. Topical phenol as a conservative treatment for periungual pyogenic granuloma. *Dermatol Surg*. 2010;36(5):675-678.
16. Gilmore A, Kelsberg G, Safranek S. Clinical inquiries. What's the best treatment for pyogenic granuloma? *J Fam Pract*. 2010;59(1): 40-42.
17. Hammes S, Kaiser K, Pohl L, et al. Pyogenic granuloma: treatment with the 1,064-nm long-pulsed neodymium-doped yttrium aluminum garnet laser in 20 patients. *Dermatol Surg*. 2012;38(6): 918-923.
18. Pagliai KA, Cohen BA. Pyogenic granuloma in children. *Pediatr Dermatol*. 2004;21:10-13.

SECTION 10 NEVI AND MELANOMA

143 BENIGN NEVI

Mindy A. Smith, MD, MS
Richard P. Usatine, MD

PATIENT STORY

A teenager is brought to the office by her mother who has noted that the moles on her daughter's back are changing (**Figure 143-1**). A few have white halos around the brown pigmentation and some have lost their pigment completely, with a light area remaining. The teenager has no symptoms but wants to make sure these are not skin cancers. Halo nevi are an uncommon variation of common nevi. These appear benign and the patient and her mother are reassured.

INTRODUCTION

Most nevi are benign tumors caused by the aggregation of melanocytic cells in the skin. However, nevi can occur on the conjunctiva, sclera and other structures of the eye. There are also nonmelanocytic nevi that are produced by other cells as seen in Becker nevi and comedonal nevi. Although most nevi are acquired, many nevi are present at birth.

SYNONYMS

Moles.

EPIDEMIOLOGY

- Acquired nevi are common lesions, forming during early childhood; few adults have none.
- Prevalence appears to be lower in dark-skinned individuals.
- Present in 1 percent of neonates, increasing through childhood, and peaking at puberty; new ones may continue to appear in adulthood. In a convenience sample of children in Colorado, non-Hispanic white children had the highest number of nevi compared to other racial/ethnic groups. Beginning at age 6 years, non-Hispanic white boys had significantly more nevi than non-Hispanic white girls (median, 21 versus 17), Hispanic white children (median 11), black children (median 7), and Asian/Pacific Islander children (median 6).[1] This number is similar to a study of children (N = 180, ages 1 to 15 years) in Barcelona where the mean number of nevi was 17.5.[2]
- In the Colorado study previously cited, non-Hispanic white children developed an average of 4 to 6 new nevi per year from 3 to 8 years of age. Development of new nevi leveled off in chronically exposed body sites at 7 years of age and at a higher level for boys than girls.[1]
- Adults typically have 10 to 40 nevi scattered over the body.
- The peak incidence of melanocytic nevi (MN) is in the fourth to fifth decades of life; the incidence decreases with each successive decade.[3]

ETIOLOGY AND PATHOPHYSIOLOGY

- Benign tumors composed of nevus cells derived from melanocytes, pigment-producing cells that colonize the epidermis.
- MN represent proliferations of melanocytes that are in contact with each other, forming small collections of cells known as nests. Genetic mutations present in common nevi as well as in melanomas include BRAF, NRAS, and *c*-kit.[4]
- Sun (UV) exposure, skin-blistering events (e.g., sunburn), and genetics play a role in the formation of new nevi.[3]

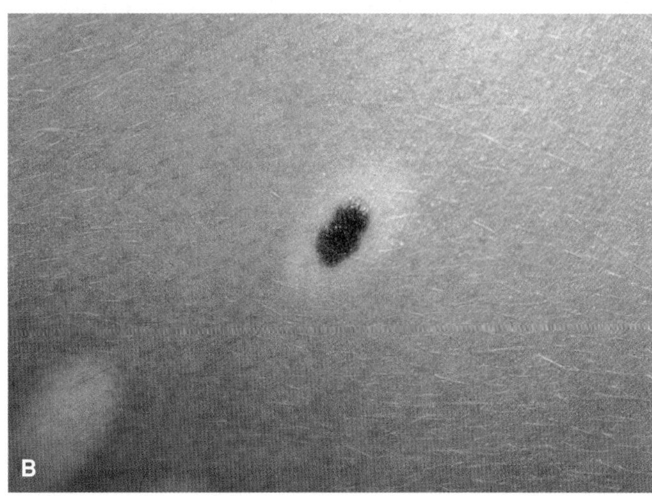

FIGURE 143-1 **A.** Multiple halo nevi on the back. **B.** Close-up of a halo nevus in transition. (*Used with permission from Richard P. Usatine, MD.*)

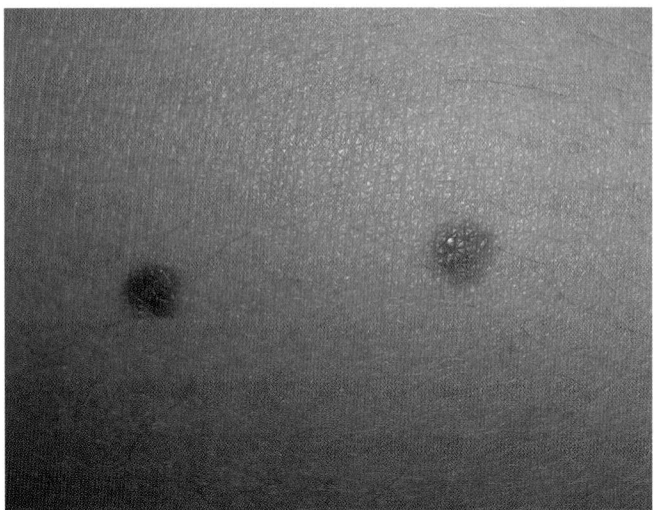

FIGURE 143-2 Two benign junctional nevi on the arm of a teenage girl. Note how these are flat macules. (*Used with permission from Richard P. Usatine, MD.*)

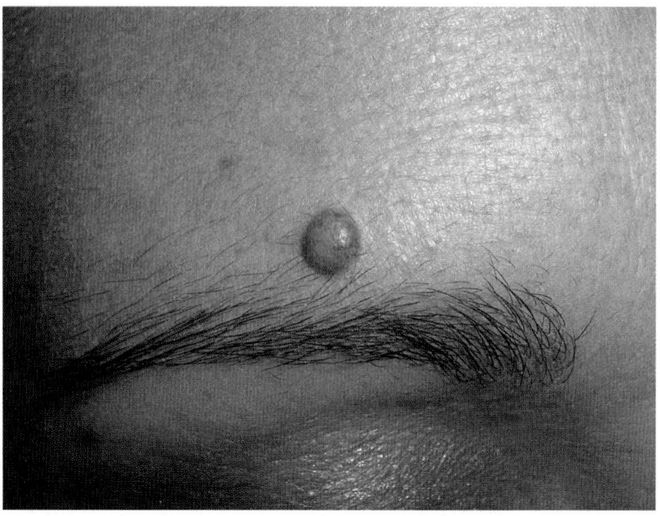

FIGURE 143-4 Dermal nevus (intradermal melanocytic nevus)—dome shaped with some scattered pigmentation. (*Used with permission from Richard P. Usatine, MD.*)

- Three broad categories of MN are based on location of nevus cells:[5]
  - Junctional nevi—Composed of nevus cells located in the dermoepidermal junction; may change into compound nevi after childhood (except when located on the palms, soles, or genitalia; **Figure 143-2**).
  - Compound nevi—A nevus in which a portion of nevus cells have migrated into the dermis (**Figure 143-3**).
  - Dermal nevi—Composed of nevus cells located within the dermis (usually found only in adults). These are usually raised and have little to no visible hyperpigmentation (**Figures 143-4** and **143-5**).
- Special categories of nevi:
  - Halo nevus—Compound or dermal nevus that develops a symmetric, sharply demarcated, depigmented border (**Figure 143-1**). Most commonly occurs on the trunk and develops during adolescence. Repigmentation may occur.
  - Blue nevus—A dermal nevus that contains large amounts of pigment so that the brown pigment absorbs the longer wavelengths of light and scatters blue light (Tyndall effect; **Figure 143-6**). Blue nevi are not always blue and color varies from tan to blue, black, and gray. The nodules are firm because of associated stromal sclerosis. Usually appears in childhood on the extremities, dorsum of the hands and face. A rare variant, the cellular blue nevus is large (>1 cm), frequently located on the buttocks, and may undergo malignant degeneration.
  - Nevus spilus—Hairless, oval, or irregularly shaped brown lesion with darker brown to black dots containing nevus cells (**Figure 143-7**). May appear at any age or be present at birth; unrelated to sun exposure.

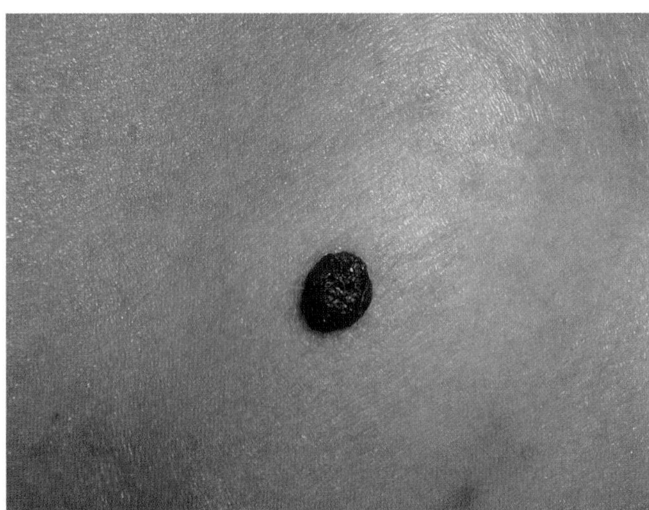

FIGURE 143-3 Benign compound nevus on the chest of a 14-year-old girl proven by biopsy. Note the brown pigmentation and the fact that the nevus is raised. (*Used with permission from Richard P. Usatine, MD.*)

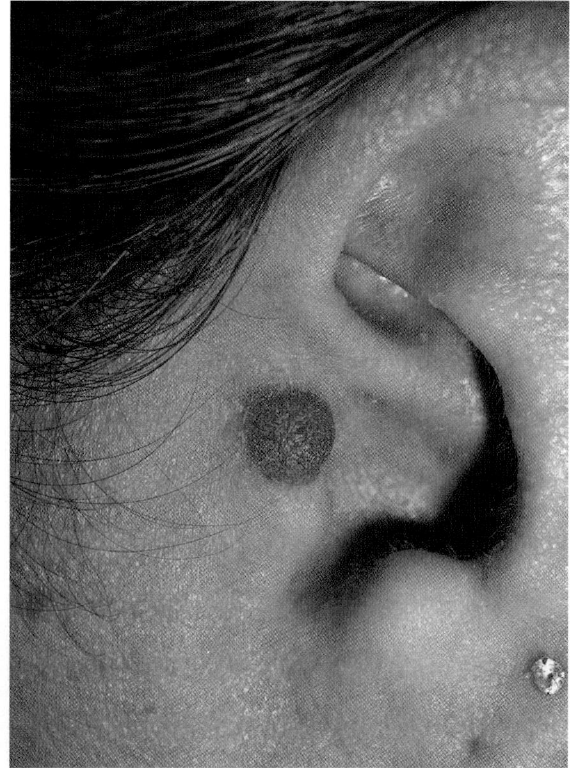

FIGURE 143-5 Dermal nevus over the tragus. This biopsy proven dermal nevus was uniformly pigmented. (*Used with permission from Richard P. Usatine, MD.*)

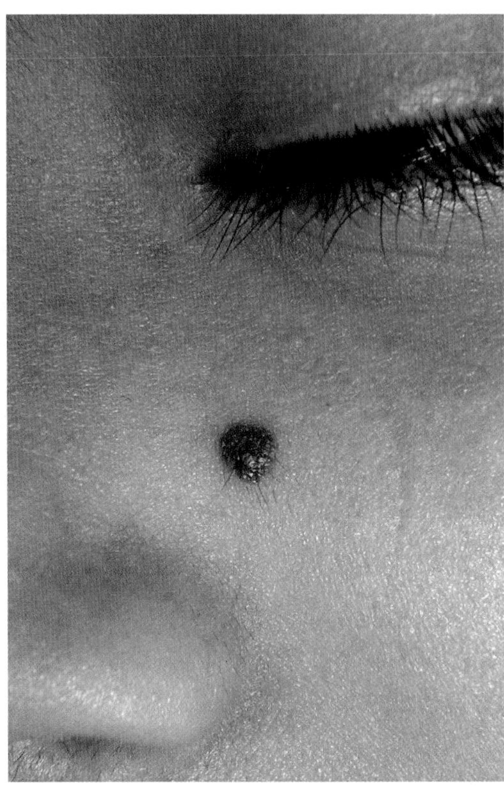

FIGURE 143-6 Blue nevus on the left cheek that could resemble a melanoma with its dark color. In this case it was fully excised with a 5-mm punch with a good cosmetic result. Blue nevi are benign and do not need to be excised unless there are suspicious changes. (*Used with permission from Richard P. Usatine, MD.*)

- Spitz nevus (formerly called benign juvenile melanoma because of its clinical and histologic similarity to melanoma)—Hairless, red, or reddish brown dome-shaped papules generally appearing suddenly in children, sometimes following trauma (**Figures 143-8** and **143-9**). The pink color is caused by increased vascularity. Most importantly, these should be fully excised with clear margins.
- Nevus of Ota—Dark brown nevus that occurs most commonly around the eye and can involve the sclera (**Figure 143-10**).

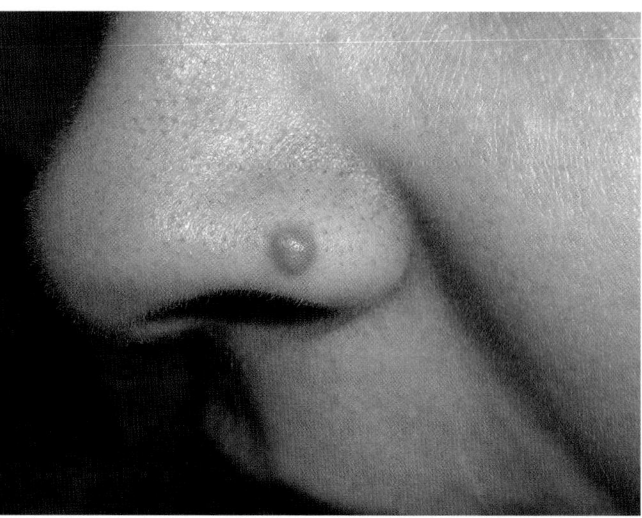

FIGURE 143-8 Spitz nevus that grew over the past year on the nose of this 18-year-old female. It was fully excised with no complications. (*Used with permission from Richard P. Usatine, MD.*)

- Both acquired and congenital MN hold some risk for the development of melanoma; the number of MN, especially more than 100, is an important independent risk factor for cutaneous melanoma.[6]

NONMELANOCYTIC NEVI

- Becker nevus—A brown patch often with hair located on the shoulder, back or submammary area, most often in adolescent boys (**Figures 143-11** and **143-12**). The lesion may enlarge to cover an entire shoulder or upper arm. Although it is called a nevus, it does not actually have nevus cells and has no malignant potential. It is a type of hamartoma, an abnormal mixture of cells and tissues normally found in the area of the body where the growth occurs.
- Nevus depigmentosus is usually present at birth or starts in early childhood. There is a decrease number of melanosomes within a normal number of melanocytes. It typically has a serrated or jagged edge (**Figure 143-13**).

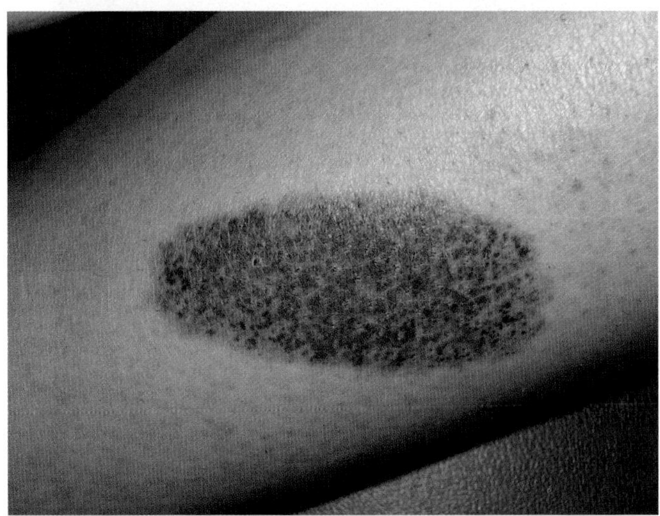

FIGURE 143-7 Nevus spilus on the leg of a young woman from birth. It appears benign and needs no intervention. (*Used with permission from Richard P. Usatine, MD.*)

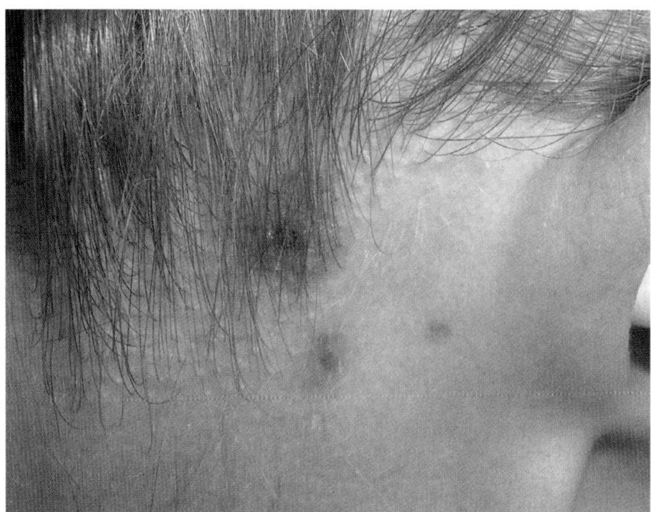

FIGURE 143-9 Spitz nevus on face of this 9-year-old boy. He very bravely allowed us to excise it with local anesthesia. (*Used with permission from Richard P. Usatine, MD.*)

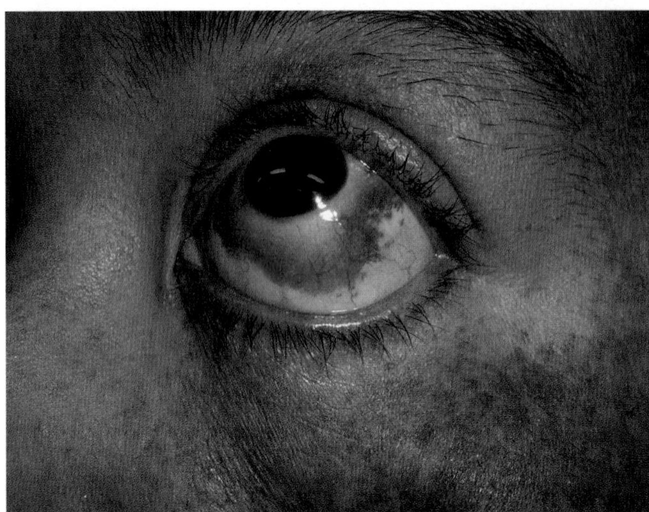

FIGURE 143-10 Nevus of Ota on the face of this young woman since early childhood. It involved both eyes and the skin around both eyes. The scleral pigmentation looks blue. (*Used with permission from Richard P. Usatine, MD.*)

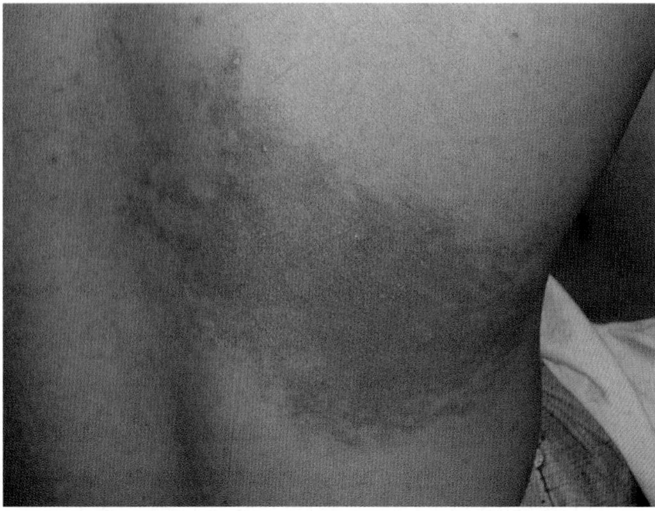

FIGURE 143-12 Becker nevus on the back of a 16-year-old Hispanic boy for 2 years. While this nevus did not have hair, it did have increased acne within the area—another feature of the Becker nevus. (*Used with permission from Richard P. Usatine, MD.*)

- Nevus anemicus—A congenital hypopigmented macule or patch that is stable in relative size and distribution. It occurs as a result of localized hypersensitivity to catecholamines and not a decrease in melanocytes. On diascopy (pressure with a glass slide) the skin is indistinguishable from the surrounding skin (**Figure 143-14**).
- Nevus comedonicus (comedonal nevus) is a rare congenital hamartoma characterized by an aggregation of comedones in one region of the skin (**Figure 143-15**).
- Epidermal nevi are congenital hamartomas of ectodermal origin classified on the basis of their main component: sebaceous, apocrine, eccrine, follicular, or keratinocytic. See Chapter 144, Congenital Nevi for a full discussion of this type of nevus.

Note that nevus comedonicus and epidermal nevi tend to follow Blaschko lines, which come from embryologic development.

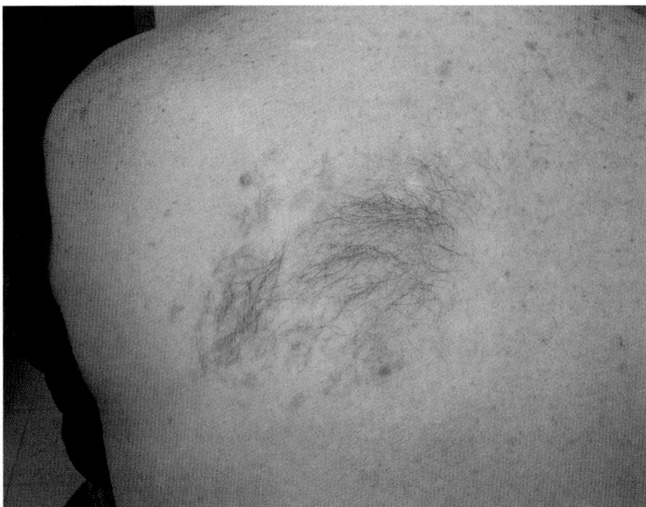

FIGURE 143-11 Becker nevus that developed during adolescence. Hair is frequently seen on this type of nonmelanocytic nevus. (*Used with permission from Richard P. Usatine, MD.*)

RISK FACTORS

- In the Barcelona study of children, male gender, past history of sunburns, facial freckling, and family history of breast cancer were independent risk factors for having a higher number of nevi.[2]
- In one study among very light-skinned (and not darker skinned) children without red hair, children who develop tans have greater numbers of nevi.[7]

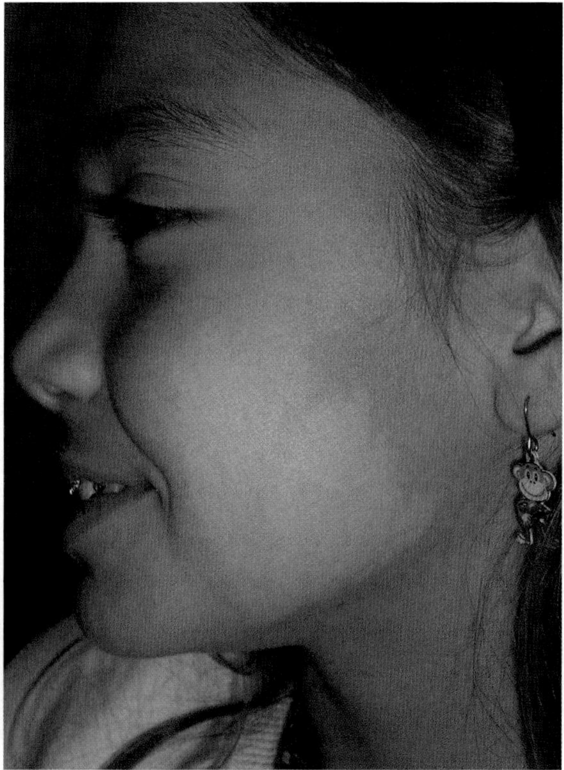

FIGURE 143-13 Nevus depigmentosus on the face of this young girl since birth. (*Used with permission from Richard P. Usatine, MD.*)

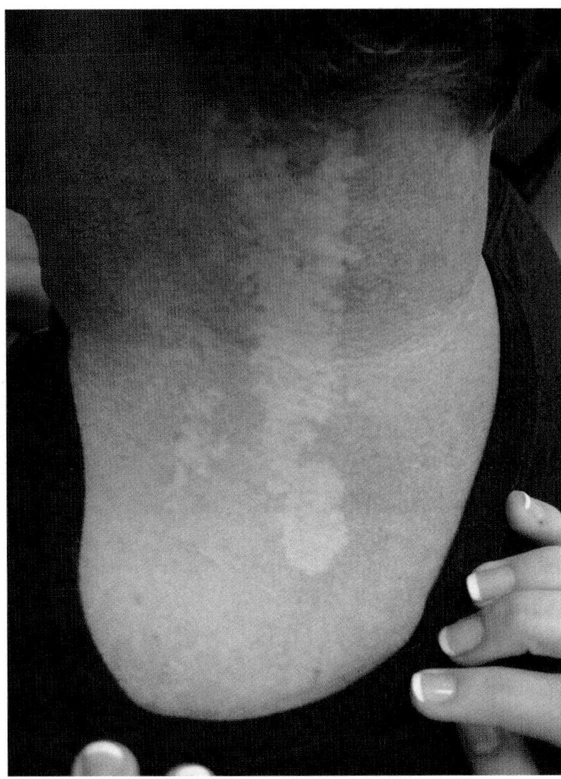

FIGURE 143-14 Nevus anemicus on the posterior neck. The localized hypersensitivity to catecholamines causes the area to stay lighter than the surrounding skin. (*Used with permission from the University of Texas Health Sciences Center, Division of Dermatology.*)

- Engaging in outdoor sports increases the number of nevi.[8]
- Although neonatal blue-light phototherapy (NBLP) was not related to nevus count at age 9 years in one study,[9] investigators of a twin study (N = 59 sets) in which one of the pair received NBLP found a higher prevalence of both cutaneous and uveal melanocytic lesions in exposed twins.[10]

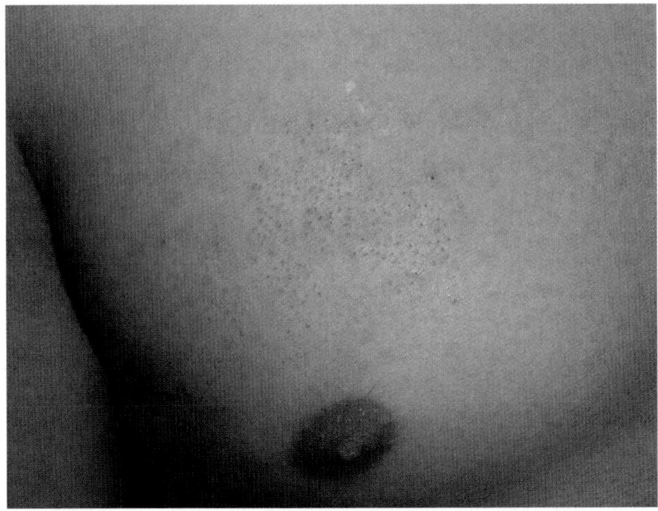

FIGURE 143-15 Nevus comedonicus on the chest of this 15-year-old boy since birth. This is a congenital hamartoma with open comedones. It is not acne. (*Used with permission from Richard P. Usatine, MD.*)

DIAGNOSIS

CLINICAL FEATURES

Most benign MN are tan to brown, usually less than 6 mm, with round shape and sharp borders.

- Junctional nevi—Macular or slightly elevated mole of uniform brown to black pigmentation, smooth surface, and a round or oval border (**Figure 143-2**). Most are hairless and vary from 1 to 6 mm.
- Compound nevi—Slightly elevated, symmetric, flesh colored or brown with a round or oval border, often becoming more elevated with age (**Figure 143-3**). Hair may be present and a white halo may form.
- Dermal nevi (same as intradermal nevi)—Skin color or brown color that may fade with age; dome shaped is most common, but shapes vary, including polypoid, warty, and pedunculated. Often found on the face (**Figures 143-4** and **143-5**) with the size ranging from 2 to 10 mm.

TYPICAL DISTRIBUTION

- Most often above the waist on sun-exposed areas but may appear anywhere on the cutaneous surface; less commonly found on the scalp, breasts, or buttocks.
- Among children in the Barcelona study, 61.1 percent had nevi on the face and neck, 17.2 percent on the buttocks, and 11.7 percent on the scalp; approximately 1/3 had congenital nevi (Chapter 144, Congenital Nevi).[2]
- In an Australian study of white children, MN of all sizes were highest on the outer forearms, followed by the outer upper arms, neck, and face.[11] Boys had higher densities of MN of all sizes on the neck than girls, and girls had higher densities of MN of 2 mm or greater on the lower legs and thighs than boys. Habitually sun-exposed body sites had higher densities of small MN and highest prevalence of larger MN.

IMAGING

- Dermoscopy can be a useful technique for diagnosing benign nevi. For MN, dermoscopic diagnosis relies on color; pattern (i.e., globular, reticular, starburst, and homogeneous blue pattern); pigment distribution (i.e., multifocal, central, eccentric, and uniform); and special sites (e.g., face, acral areas, nail, and mucosa), in conjunction with patient factors (e.g., history, pregnancy).[12]
- Authors of a review of dermoscopy in the pediatric population reported that acquired MNs in children show peripheral globules and nevo-melanocytic junctional nests at the perimeter.[13] Lesions tend to grow in a symmetric, centrifugal fashion with peripheral globules becoming sparser and eventually disappearing as the lesions mature; mature MNs manifest a reticular or homogeneous pattern. Investigators in one study found change in 16.2 percent of 2497 benign melanocytic lesions with minor suspicion of melanoma undergoing short term dermoscopy.[14] Change was more often seen in younger (0 to 18 years and 19 to 35 years) and older patients.
- In the Barcelona study, the most frequent dominant dermoscopic pattern in children was the globular type (**Figure 143-16**) with the homogeneous pattern predominating in the youngest children and the reticular pattern predominating in adolescents.[2]

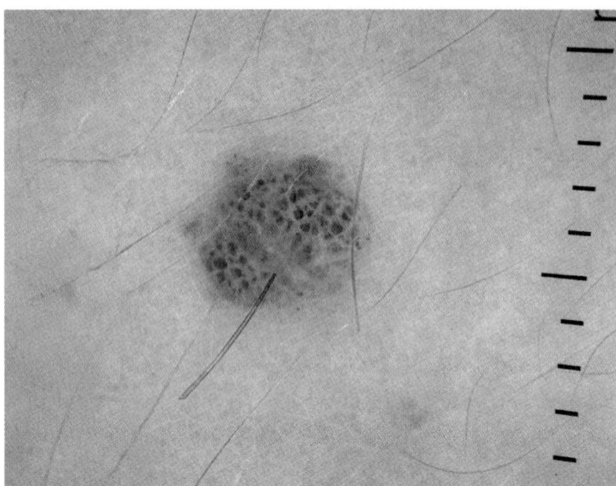

FIGURE 143-16 Dermoscopy of a benign melanocytic nevus in a teenage girl showing a globular pattern often seen in the nevi of children. (*Used with permission from Richard P. Usatine, MD.*)

BIOPSY

Biopsy is necessary if you suspect melanoma or a Spitz nevus (**Figure 143-9**). A biopsy that cuts below the pigmented area is preferred if there is a reasonable suspicion for melanoma. This can be done with a scoop shave, a punch that gets the whole lesion, or an elliptical excision. If the patient wants a raised benign appearing nevus excised for cosmetic reasons, a shave excision may be adequate. Send all lesions (except skin tags) to the pathologist for examination, even when they appear benign, to avoid missing a melanoma.

- Immunostaining is performed by the pathologist as a valuable adjunct to histopathologic evaluation in differentiating benign from malignant melanocytic tumors.[15]

DIFFERENTIAL DIAGNOSIS

Benign nevi may develop atypia or become melanoma. This should be suspected if a lesion has atypical features including asymmetry, border irregularity, color variability, diameter greater than 6 mm, and evolving (called the ABCDE approach [asymmetry, border irregularity, color irregularity, diameter >6 mm, evolution]). Any lesion that becomes symptomatic (e.g., itchy, painful, irritated, or bleeding), or develops a loss or increase in pigmentation, should be evaluated and biopsied if needed. Dermoscopy can be used to increase one's accuracy in distinguishing between benign and malignant lesions.

- Melanomas are skin cancers that can develop from a preexisting nevus. Distinguishing a benign nevus from a nevus that might be malignant melanoma is an important skill to develop. However, because clinical appearance can be misleading, a biopsy is necessary when there is a reasonable suspicion for cancer (Chapter 147, Melanoma).
- Dysplastic or atypical nevi are variants that are relatively flat, thinly papular, and relatively broad. Often, the lesions exhibit target-like or fried egg-like morphology, with a central papular zone and a macular surrounding area with differing pigmentation (Chapter 146, Dysplastic Nevus).
- Labial melanotic macules are benign dark macules on the lip that are not nevi and not melanomas (**Figure 143-17**). They can be removed for cosmetic purposes.

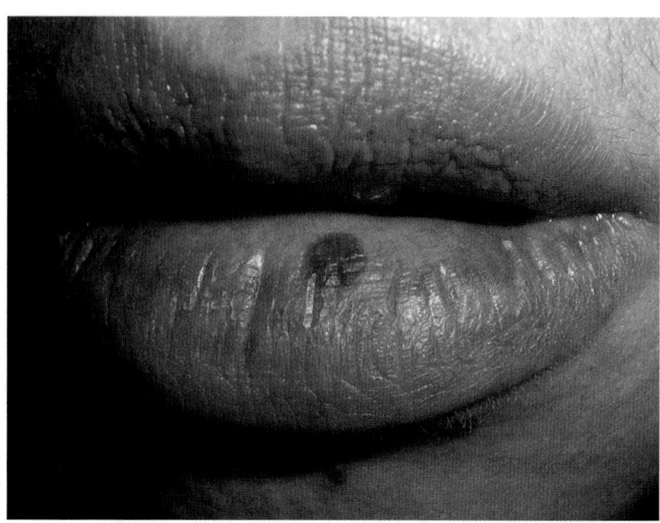

FIGURE 143-17 Labial melanotic macule. These are benign but are not nevi. (*Used with permission from Richard P. Usatine, MD.*)

MANAGEMENT

Nevi are generally only removed for cosmetic reasons or because of concern over changes in the lesion suggestive of dysplasia or melanoma.

- A full excisional biopsy with a sutured closure is usually the best means to diagnose a lesion if concern exists regarding the possibility of melanoma. If the lesion is found to be benign, no further treatment is usually required.
- Punch excision can be used to excise smaller lesions.
- Scoop shave—Unfortunately, if a punch biopsy is used to sample a larger lesion it may miss a melanoma in another part of the lesion. A broad scoop shave is better than a punch biopsy when a full elliptical excision is not possible or desirable (e.g., a large flat pigmented lesion on the face).
- Nevi removed for cosmesis are often removed by shave excision.[3]

If a Spitz nevus is suspected, either biopsy it now or schedule the patient for a full excision. The histopathology is too close to a melanoma to just watch it.

- Becker nevi and comedonal nevi do not become melanoma because they lack melanocytes. Therefore, there is no reason to excise them. Generally, these are large and the risks of excision for cosmetic reasons outweigh the benefits.

PREVENTION

- Sun protection to limit sunburn may help reduce the appearance of nevi. In a trial of 209 white children, children randomized to the sunscreen group, especially those with freckles, had significantly fewer new nevi on the trunk than did children in the control group at 3-year follow-up.[16]
- In another study, a partially tailored mailed intervention on child sun protection behaviors was effective in increasing parental reported use of sunscreen, protective clothing and hats, shade-seeking, and midday sun avoidance, and resulted in fewer reported sunburns and fewer nevi ≥2 mm at 1 year.[17]

PROGNOSIS

- Degeneration of common nevi into melanoma is very rare.
- Patients with multiple or large MN appear to have an increased risk of melanoma.[3]
- Nevi may recur or persist following removal; in one study, dysplastic MN were the most likely to persist.[18] In another study, of 61 benign nevi biopsy sites reexamined, two (3.3%) recurred.[19]

FOLLOW-UP

- Patients with multiple or sizable MN should be followed by an experienced clinician because they appear to have an increased lifetime risk of melanoma, with the risk increasing in rough proportion to the size and/or number of lesions.[3]
- As noted in the section on imaging, MN in children often undergo change. Change may be more common for scalp nevi; in a follow-up study of 44 scalp nevi in children (30% of total population), most (77%) showed clinical signs of change during mean follow-up of 2.8 years; about half (53%) became more atypical and the other half (47%) became less atypical since the initial examination.[20] Scalp MN may require closer monitoring.

PATIENT EDUCATION

- Patients and their parents should be encouraged to use sunscreen to prevent skin cancer as well as to reduce the development of new nevi.
- Patients with multiple or sizable MN and their parents should be taught to look for and report asymmetry, border irregularity, new symptoms, and color and size changes.

PATIENT RESOURCES

- VisualDxHealth. Good information for parents with excellent photographs—**www.skinsight.com/child/commonAcquiredNevusMole.htm**.
- MedlinePlus—**www.nlm.nih.gov/medlineplus/moles.html**.
- American Osteopathic College of Dermatology—**www.aocd.org/skin/dermatologic_diseases/moles.html**.

PROVIDER RESOURCES

- **http://emedicine.medscape.com/article/1058445-overview**.

REFERENCES

1. Crane LA, Mokrohisky ST, Dellavalle RP, et al. Melanocytic nevus development in Colorado children born in 1998: a longitudinal study. *Arch Dermatol*. 2009;145(2):148-156.
2. Aguilera P, Puig S, Guilabert A, et al. Prevalence study of nevi in children from Barcelona. Dermoscopy, constitutional and environmental factors. *Dermatology*. 2009;18(3):203-214.
3. McCalmont T. *Melanocytic Nevi*. http://emedicine.medscape.com/article/1058445-overview#a0199, Aaccessed April 2013.
4. Zembowicz A, Phadke PA. Blue nevi and variants: an update. *Arch Pathol Lab Med*. 2011;135(3):327-336.
5. Schafer T, Merkl J, Klemm E, et al. The Epidemiology of nevi and signs of skin aging in the adult general population: Results of the KORA-Survey 2000. *J Invest Dermatol*. 2006;126(7):1490-1496.
6. Gandini S, Sera F, Cattaruzza MS, et al. Meta-analysis of risk factors for cutaneous melanoma: I. Common and atypical nevi. *Eur J Cancer*. 2005;41(1):28-44.
7. Aalborg J, Morelli JG, Mokrohisky ST, et al. Tanning and increased nevus development in very-light-skinned children without red hair. *Arch Dermatol*. 2009;145(9):989-996.
8. Mahé E, Beauchet A, de Paula Corrêa M, et al. Outdoor sports and risk of ultraviolet radiation-related skin lesions in children: evaluation of risks and prevention. *Br J Dermatol*. 2011;165(2):360-367.
9. Mahé E, Beauchet A, Aegerter P, Saiag P. Neonatal blue-light phototherapy does not increase nevus count in 9-year-old children. *Pediatrics*. 2009;123(5):e896-e900.
10. Csoma Z, Tóth-Molnár E, Balogh K, et al. Neonatal blue light phototherapy and melanocytic nevi: a twin study. *Pediatrics*. 2011; 128(4):e856-64.
11. Harrison SL, Buettner PG, MacLennan R. Body-site distribution of MN in young Australian children. *Arch Dermatol*. 1999; 135(1):47-52.
12. Zalaudek I, Docimo G, Argenziano G. Using dermoscopic criteria and patient-related factors for the management of pigmented melanocytic nevi. *Arch Dermatol*. 2009;145(7):816-826.
13. Haliasos HC, Zalaudek I, Malvehy J, et al. Dermoscopy of benign and malignant neoplasms in the pediatric population. *Semin Cutan Med Surg*. 2010; 29(4):218-231.
14. Menzies SW, Stevenson ML, Altamura D, Byth K. Variables predicting change in benign melanocytic nevi undergoing short-term dermoscopic imaging. *Arch Dermatol*. 2011:147(6):655-659.
15. Jakobiec FA, Bhat P, Colby KA. Immunohistochemical studies of conjunctival nevi and melanomas. *Arch Ophthalmol*. 2010;128(2):174-183.
16. Lee TK, Rivers JK, Gallagher RP. Site-specific protective effect of broad-spectrum sunscreen on nevus development among white schoolchildren in a randomized trial. *J Am Acad Dermatol*. 2005;52(5):786-792.
17. Crane LA, Asdigian NL, Barón AE, et al. Mailed intervention to promote sun protection of children: a randomized controlled trial. *Am J Prev Med*. 2012;43(4):399-410.
18. Sommer LL, Barcia SM, Clarke LE, Helm KF. Persistent melanocytic nevi: a review and analysis of 205 cases. *J Cutan Pathol*. 2011;38(6):503-507.
19. Goodson AG, Florell SR, Boucher KM, Grossman D. Low rates of clinical recurrence after biopsy of benign to moderately dysplastic melanocytic nevi. *J Am Acad Dermatol*. 2010;62(4):591-596.
20. Gupta M, Berk DR, Gray C, et al. Morphologic features and natural history of scalp nevi in children. *Arch Dermatol*. 2010;146(5):506-511.

144 CONGENITAL NEVI

Mindy A. Smith, MD, MS
Richard P. Usatine, MD

PATIENT STORY

A small congenital nevus (**Figure 144-1**) was noted on this 6-month-old child by his new family physician during a routine exam. The parents acknowledged that it was present from birth and asked if it needed to be removed. They were reassured that nothing needs to be done about it and unless there were suspicious changes in the future it could remain there for the remainder of their child's life.

INTRODUCTION

Congenital melanocytic nevi (CMN) are benign pigmented lesions that have a wide variation in size and presentation and are composed of melanocytes, the pigment-forming cells in the skin.

SYNONYMS

- Garment nevus, bathing trunk nevus (**Figure 144-2**), giant hairy nevus, giant pigmented nevus, pigmented hairy nevus, nevus pigmentosus, nevus pigmentosus et pilosus (pigmented nevus with hair).[1]
- Tardive congenital nevus refers to a nevus with similar features to congenital nevi, but appears at age 1 to 3 years.

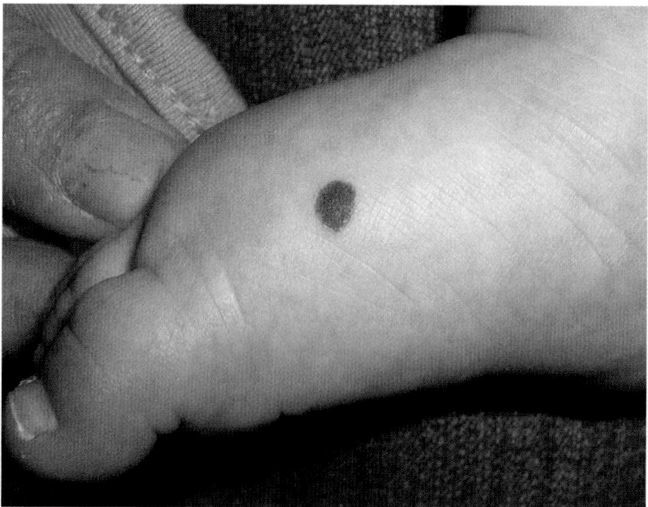

FIGURE 144-1 Small congenital nevus found on the foot of a 6-month-old child. The parents were counseled to not get it excised at this time. *(Used with permission from Richard P. Usatine, MD.)*

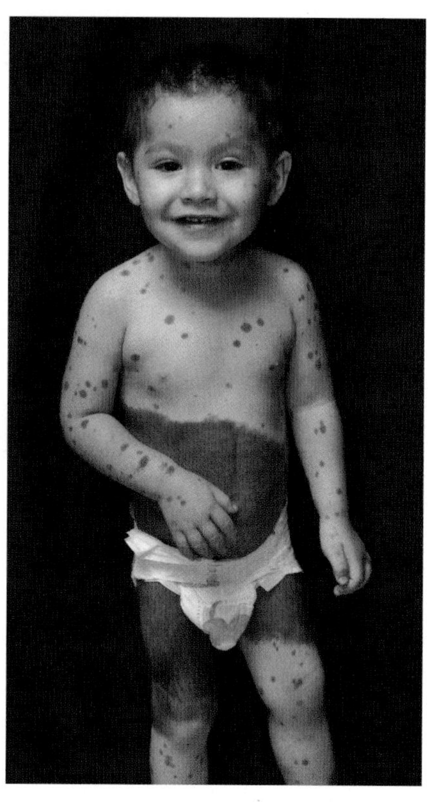

FIGURE 144-2 Large bathing trunk nevus with multiple satellite nevi on this happy 2-year old boy. The mother has opted for no surgical intervention. *(Used with permission from Richard P. Usatine, MD.)*

EPIDEMIOLOGY

- CMN develop in 1 to 6 percent of newborns and are present at birth or occasionally develop during the first year of life.[1] In a recent case series in California (N = 594), 2.4 percent of the infants had CMN.[2]
- In an Italian prevalence study of over 3000 children aged 12–17 years, congenital melanocytic nevi or congenital nevus-like nevi were found in 17.5 percent; most (92%) were small (<1.5 cm).[3]
- Congenital nevi are also seen in neurocutaneous melanosis, a rare syndrome characterized by the presence of congenital melanocytic nevi and melanotic neoplasms of the central nervous system.
- The development of melanoma within CMN (**Figure 144-8**) is believed to occur at a higher rate than in normal skin. Estimates range from 4 to 10 percent with smaller lesions having lowest risk.[1]
  - In a systematic review, 46 of 651 patients with CMN (0.7%) followed for 3.4 to 23.7 years developed melanomas, representing a 465-fold increased relative risk of developing melanoma during childhood and adolescence.[4] The mean age at diagnosis of melanoma was 15.5 years (median 7 years).
  - Patients with giant CMN (larger than 20 cm; **Figures 144-2** to **144-5**) appear to be at highest risk where subsequent melanoma has been reported in 5 to 7 percent by age 60 years.[5] In one study, 70 percent of patients who had a large CMN diagnosed with melanoma were diagnosed within the first 10 years of life.[6]

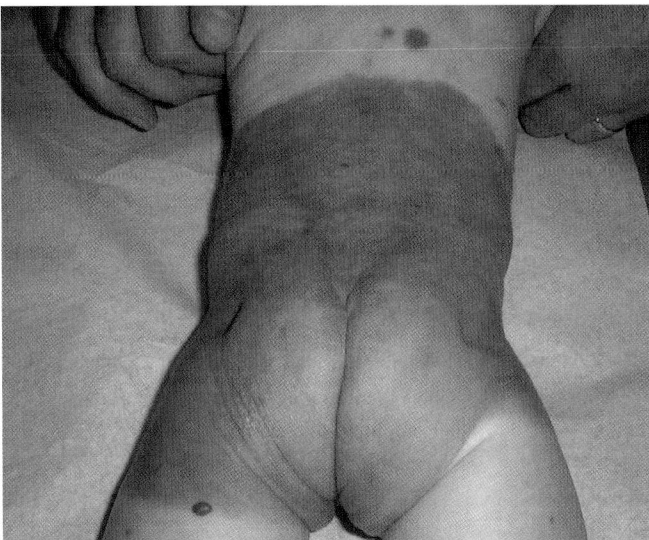

FIGURE 144-3 Bathing trunk congenital melanocytic nevus has fine velus hairs on the surface. In time, these hairs become terminal hairs and the lesion could then be termed congenital hairy nevus. It has a significant premalignant potential. Staged excisions are often performed to debulk the lesion even if it cannot all be removed. Careful clinical follow-up is required on at least an annual basis at the physician's office and monthly at home looking for any changes that would prompt biopsy to exclude malignant degeneration. (*Image used with permission from Robert Brodell, MD.*)

- However, in a prospective study of 230 medium-sized congenital nevi (1.5 to 19.9 cm; (**Figures 144-6** to **144-7**) in 227 patients from 1955 to 1996, no melanomas occurred. The average follow-up period was 6.7 years to an average age of 25.5 years.[7]
- Other risk factors for melanoma include personal or family history of melanoma or other skin cancer, presence of multiple nevi, red hair, blue eyes, freckling, and history of radiation (see Chapter 147, Melanoma).[1]

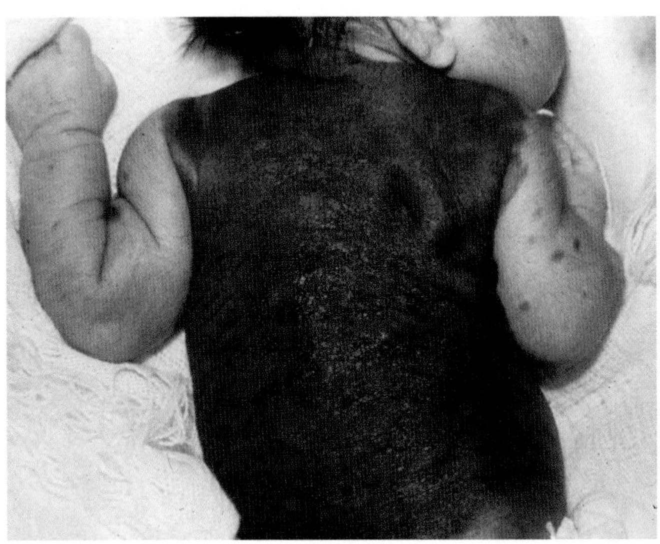

FIGURE 144-4 Infant born with large bathing trunk nevus covering most of the back and chest. (*Used with permission from UTHSCSA Division of Dermatology.*)

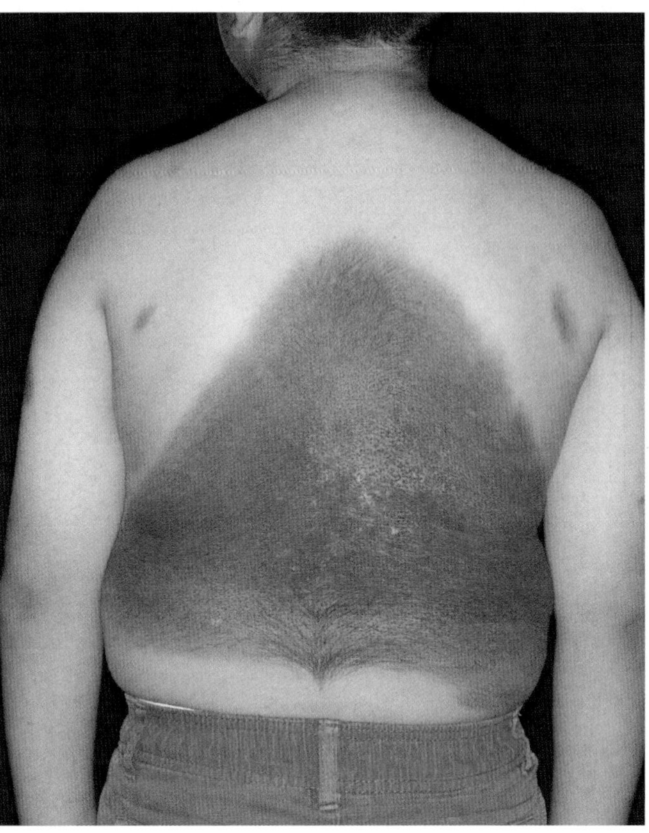

FIGURE 144-5 Giant congenital bathing trunk nevus surrounded by satellite nevi in a 7-year-old Hispanic boy. The patient was referred for consideration of staged removal of this potentially dangerous lesion. (*Used with permission from Richard P. Usatine, MD.*)

ETIOLOGY AND PATHOPHYSIOLOGY

- The etiology of CMN is unknown.
- Congenital nevi result from a proliferation of benign melanocytes in the dermis, epidermis, or both. Melanocytes of the skin originate

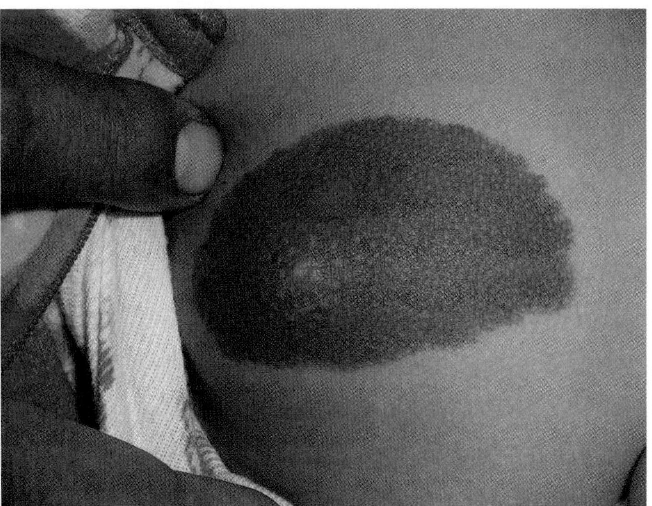

FIGURE 144-6 Congenital nevus on around the areola of a 4-month-old girl. It was recommended to not excise this nevus as it would likely cause damage to breast development in the future. As there are no malignant features this nevus will be followed with yearly clinical exams. (*Used with permission from Richard P. Usatine, MD.*)

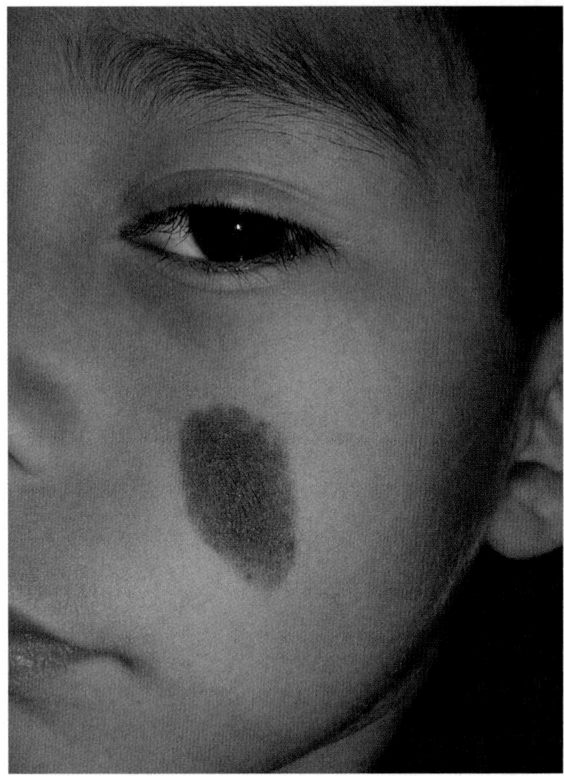

FIGURE 144-7 Medium-sized congenital nevus on the face of this 4-year-old boy. (*Used with permission from Richard P. Usatine, MD.*)

in the neuroectoderm and migrate vertically to the skin and other locations such as the central nervous system and eye.[1] Defects in migration or maturation are hypothesized as causal.

MAKING THE DIAGNOSIS

Diagnosis is usually made based on clinical features.

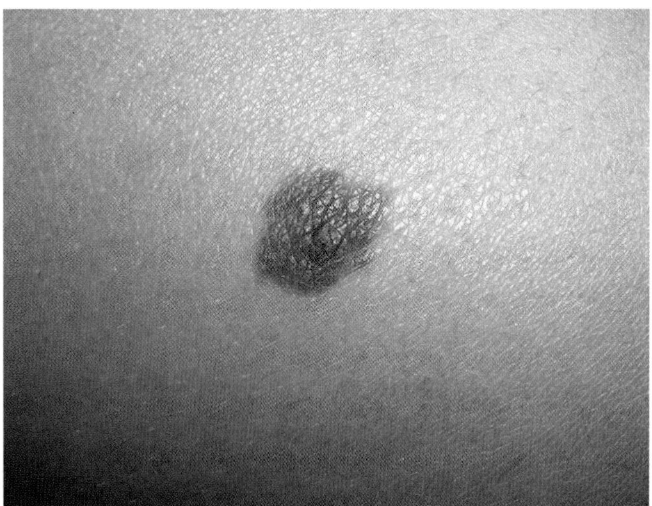

FIGURE 144-8 Congenital nevus on the shoulder of this 10-year-old girl that was biopsied to confirm that it was benign. Note the small area of raised pigmentation in the middle of the nevus that prompted the parent's request for a biopsy. (*Used with permission from Richard P. Usatine, MD.*)

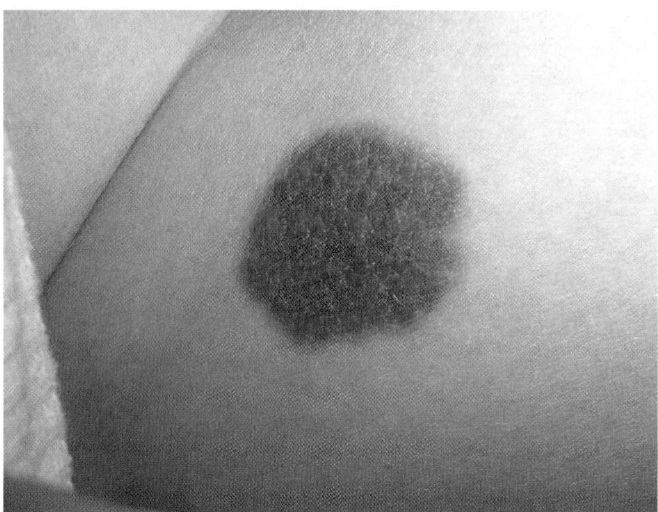

FIGURE 144-9 Congenital nevus on a 7-year-old boy with a pebbly surface. (*Used with permission from Richard P. Usatine, MD.*)

CLINICAL FEATURES[1]

- Variable mixtures of color including pink-red (primarily at birth), tan, brown, black, or multiple shades within a single lesion; color usual remains constant over time but the nevus will grow as the child grows.
- Shapes are also highly variable including oval, round, linear, and random; lesions have irregular but well demarcated borders. The pigment may fade off into surrounding skin.
- Nevi may become raised over time or a portion may become raised (**Figure 144-8**). The skin surface ranges from smooth to pebbly (**Figure 144-9**) to hyperkeratotic.
- Macular portion usually found at edges.
- Frequently exhibit hypertrichosis (**Figures 144-10** and **144-11**).
- Heavily pigmented large congenital melanocytic nevi over a limb may be associated with underdevelopment of the limb.[1]

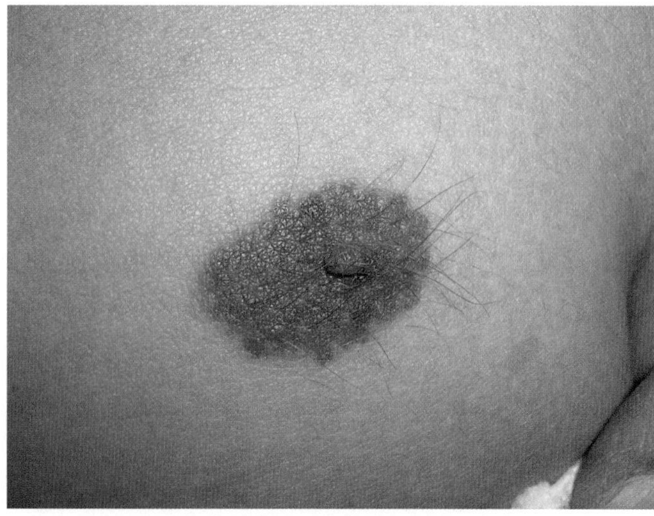

FIGURE 144-10 A benign hairy congenital nevus on the upper buttocks of a 7-year-old boy. (*Used with permission from Richard P. Usatine, MD.*)

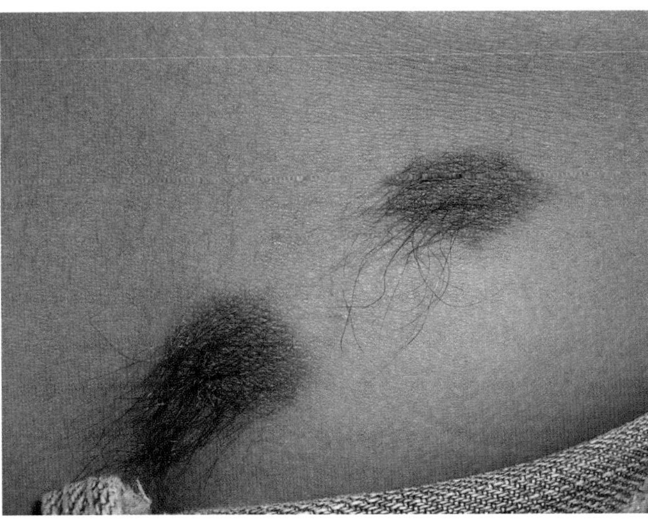

FIGURE 144-11 Two satellite nevi with hypertrichosis in a child with one larger congenital nevus not shown in this photograph. (*Used with permission from Richard P. Usatine, MD.*)

- Lesions are classified by size in adulthood as:[1]
  - Small (<1.5 cm; **Figure 144-1**).
  - Medium (1.5 cm-19.9 cm; **Figures 144-6** and **144-10**).
  - Large (>20 cm; **Figures 144-2** through **144-5**). Giant nevi are often surrounded by several smaller satellite nevi (**Figures 144-2** through **144-5** and **144-11**).
  - Lesions on a child's head of >9 cm are considered large based on likely eventual growth.[1]

IMAGING

- Dermoscopy findings depend on the age and location. In one study, the globular pattern (**Figure 144-12**) was most common in children under age 11 years and on the trunk.[8] The majority of reticular lesions were located on the limbs and the variegated pattern was the most specific for congenital nevi. In one Japanese follow-up study of children with acral CMN (N=24 lesions), changes in dermoscopic features were observed in 4 lesions on patients younger than age 14 years.[9]
- Magnetic resonance imaging (MRI) of the central nervous system can be a useful diagnostic tool in patients suspected of having neurocutaneous melanosis; one author recommended a screening MRI for patients with giant congenital melanocytic nevi.[10]

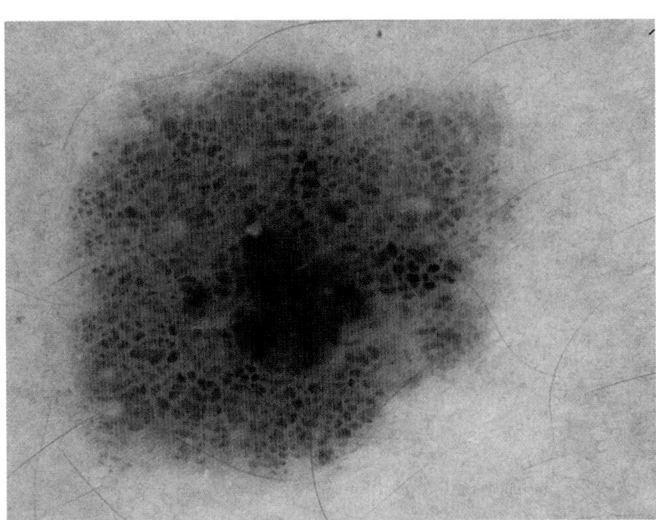

FIGURE 144-12 Dermoscopy of a congenital nevus in a child showing a globular pattern. This is the congenital nevus on the 10-year-old girl in **Figure 144-8**. (*Used with permission from Richard P. Usatine, MD.*)

TYPICAL DISTRIBUTION

- Congenital nevi may be found anywhere on the body.

BIOPSY

- Although there are many histological subtypes, distinguishing histologic features of CMN include:[1]
  - Involvement by nevus cells of deep dermal appendages and neurovascular structures (e.g., hair follicles, sebaceous glands, arrector pili muscles, and within walls of blood vessels).
  - Infiltration of nevus cells between collagen bundles.

DIFFERENTIAL DIAGNOSIS

- Acral nevi—Congenital nevi that appear on the palms and soles are one type of acral nevus (**Figure 144-13**). Other acral nevi may be acquired. If acral nevi appear benign we do not need to be biopsied. The most benign easily recognizable benign pattern of an acral

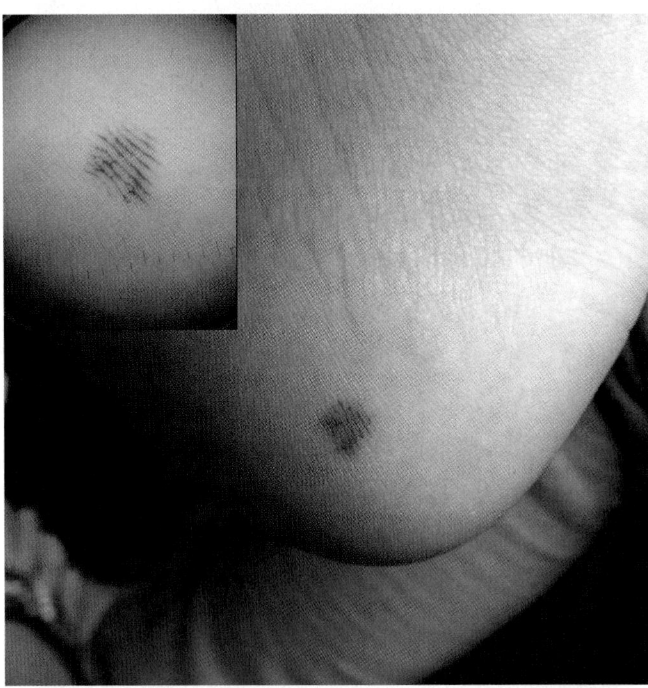

FIGURE 144-13 Acral congenital nevus close to the sole of the foot of an 8-year-old girl. The dermascopic image in the upper left corner shows parallel pigmented lines running in the valleys of the acral skin reassuring the physician that this is a benign nevus. (*Used with permission from Richard P. Usatine, MD.*)

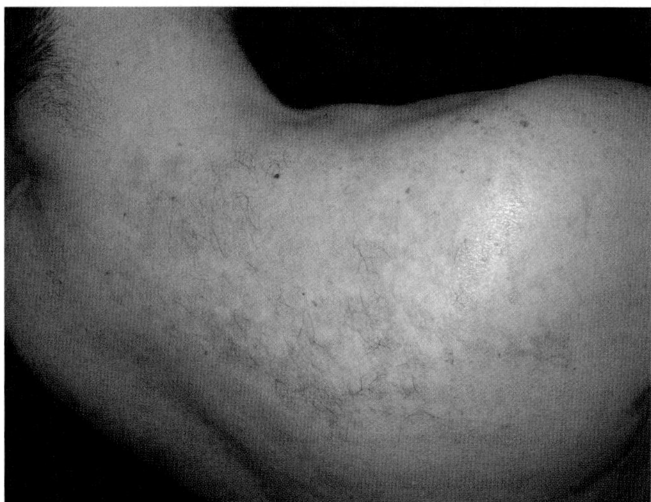

FIGURE 144-14 A congenital Becker's nevus presenting with hyperpigmentation and hair growth on the right shoulder of this teenage boy. (*Used with permission from Richard P. Usatine, MD.*)

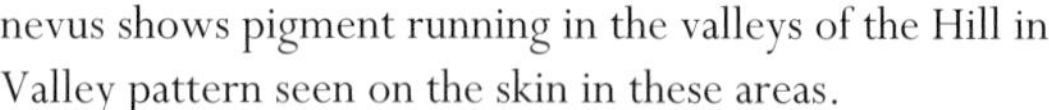

nevus shows pigment running in the valleys of the Hill in Valley pattern seen on the skin in these areas.

- Becker nevus—A brown macule, patch of hair, or both on the shoulder, back, or submammary area that most often develops in adolescence. The border is irregular and the lesion may enlarge to cover an entire shoulder or upper arm. It is a type of hamartoma and is not a melanocytic nevus (see Chapter 143, Nevus). A

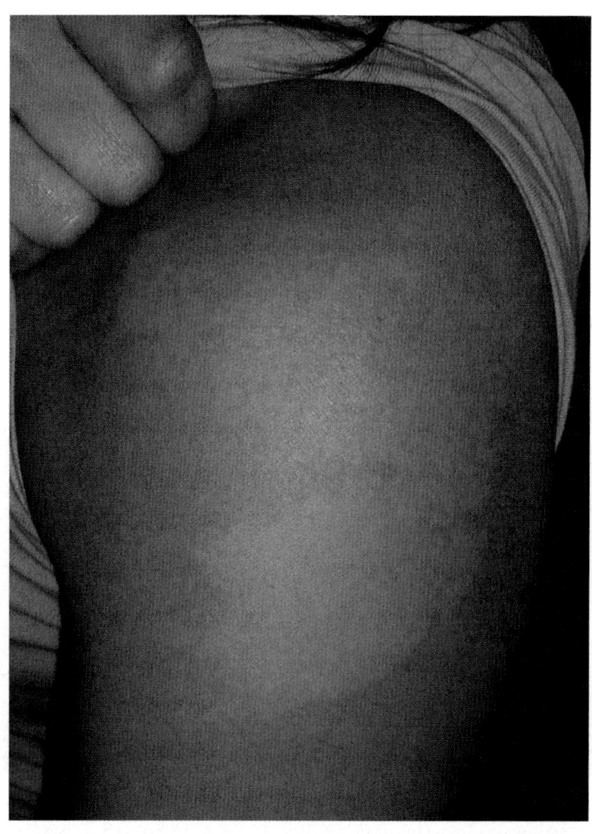

FIGURE 144-15 Congenital nevus depigmentosus on the shoulder of a 17-year-old girl since birth. (*Used with permission from Richard P. Usatine, MD.*)

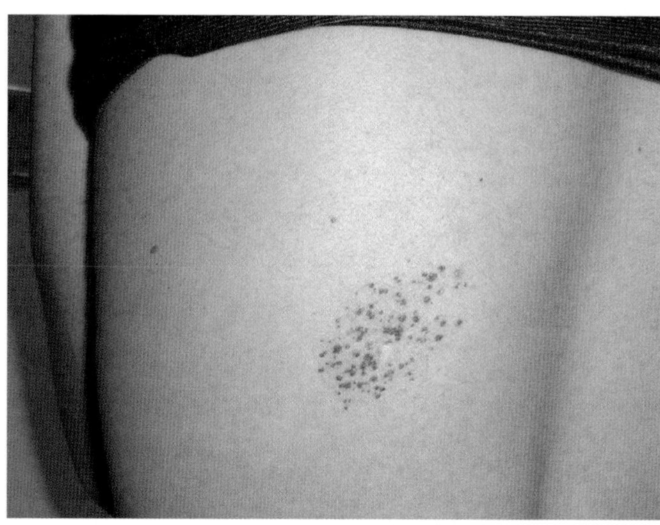

FIGURE 144-16 A speckled congenital nevus (nevus spilus) on the back. (*Used with permission from Richard P. Usatine, MD.*)

Becker's nevus can appear at birth and enlarge during adolescence (**Figure 144-14**).

- Café-au-lait spots—Coffee-and-milk-colored patch that can be present at birth or develop during early childhood. Although a number of large café-au-lait spots are associated with neurofibromatosis, a few of them can occur in completely unaffected children. These light-brown patches have increased melanin but are not nevi (see Chapter 206, Neurofibromatosis).
- Dermal Melanocytosis (Mongolian Spot)—Blue-gray hyperpigmented patch present at birth with less well-defined borders than a congenital nevus. They are seen most often on the buttocks and back and can be quite large (see Chapter 168, Hyperpigmentation).
- Nevus depigmentosus—A benign nonmelanocytic nevus with hypopigmentation that may have jagged edges resembling a continent. These are often congenital but can also be acquired (**Figure 144-15**).
- Nevus spilus (speckled nevus)—Hairless, oval or irregularly shaped brown lesion with darker brown to black dots containing nevus cells. These may appear at birth or any age (**Figure 144-16**; see Chapter 143, Benign Nevus).
- Changes that can occur to a congenital nevus may include the development of a halo (**Figure 144-17**) or pigment incontinence (**Figure 144-18**). It is best to biopsy any suspicious changes.

MANAGEMENT

The management of CMN depends on size and location of the lesion (difficulty in monitoring), associated symptoms, the age of patient, the effect on cosmesis, and the potential for malignant transformation.

- For small and medium-sized CMN, the risk of malignant transformation is small and prophylactic removal is not recommended. For cosmesis, treatments include dermabrasion, curettage, laser therapy, and surgical excision.

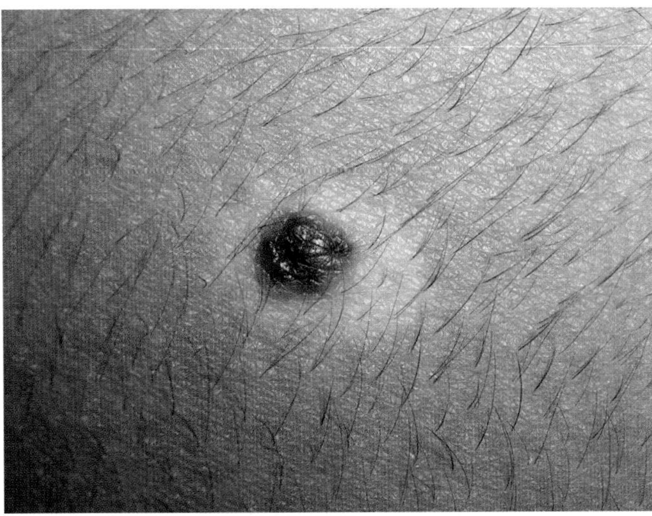

FIGURE 144-17 This congenital nevus on a 12-year-old girl became darker and developed a halo around it. Upon excision it was determined that it was an inflamed congenital intradermal nevus with no malignant features. (*Used with permission from Richard P. Usatine, MD.*)

- Larger CMN can be surgically removed but may require tissue expanders, tissue grafts, and tissue flaps to close large defects. Because the melanocytes may extend deep into underlying tissues (including muscle, bone, and central nervous system), removing the cutaneous component may not eliminate the risk of malignancy.
  - There is also concern that surgical intervention may adversely affect CMN cells.[11]
- Laser treatment of the lesions has been performed with a number of different types of lasers.[12] Because of the lack of penetrance to deeper tissue levels, long-term recurrence or malignant transformation is also an issue with these techniques.
  - In a case series of patients with CMN (N-52) at a mean of 8 years follow-up, most (87%) were satisfied with their treatment and about three quarters had minimal visible pigmentation after treatment completion.[13] Treatment failure occurred in 5 patients and recurrence developed in 5; a few patients had hypertrophic scarring or hyperpigmentation and 1 patient developed an intracranial melanoma.

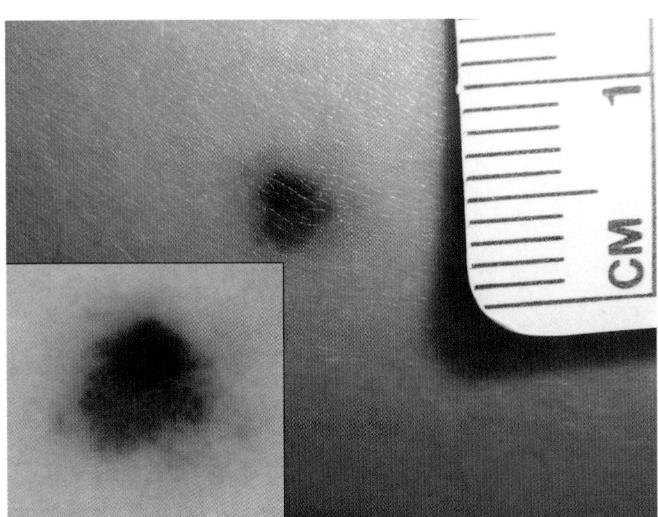

FIGURE 144-18 Color changes appearing in a congenital nevus. The dermoscopic image in the bottom left corner was not reassuring and a biopsy revealed pigment incontinence but no signs of malignancy. (*Used with permission from Richard P. Usatine, MD.*)

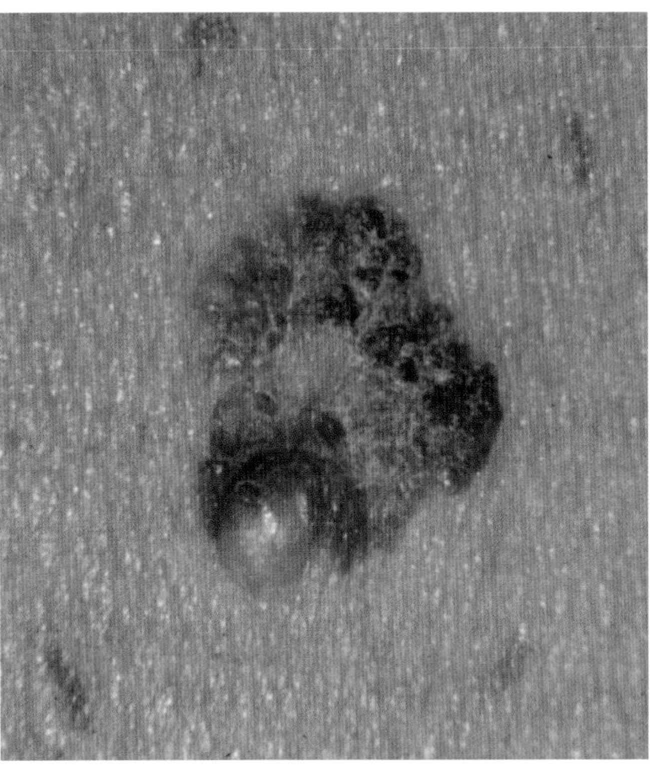

FIGURE 144-19 Melanoma arising in an acquired nevus showing features of central regression and a new elevated nodule. These are the same features that would make a congenital nevus suspicious for melanoma. (*Used with permission from UTHSCSA Division of Dermatology.*)

- Careful life-long follow-up with photographs is an acceptable approach, especially with the affordability of digital cameras.
- Garment or bathing trunk nevi (**Figures 144-2** through **144-5**).
  - About half of the melanomas that develop in bathing trunk nevi do so before age 5 years.[14] These melanomas can be missed by observation because they can have non-epidermal origins.
- Surgical excision is recommended by some experts to prevent melanoma.[14] SOR C
- Changes to watch for that call for a biopsy include:
  - Partial regression (depressed white areas).
  - Inflammation.
  - Rapid growth or color change.
  - Development of a firm nodule (**Figure 144-19**).

FOLLOW-UP

- Patients with giant CMN or multiple CMN may benefit from consultation with a neurologist, pediatrician, or both because of the risk of neurocutaneous melanosis and its neurologic manifestations or obstructive hydrocephalus.
- Bathing trunk nevi can also be associated with spina bifida, meningocele, and neurofibromatosis.[14]

- Because patients with all forms of CMN, especially giant CMN, have an increased risk of developing melanoma, physicians should consider baseline photography and regular follow-up with an experienced clinician for these patients.

PATIENT EDUCATION

- All patients should be told about the importance of protection from ultraviolet light exposure. This is especially important in people with giant CMN, because they at a significantly increased risk of melanoma.
- Patients (or their parents) should be taught to look for signs of melanoma (ABCDE: asymmetry, border irregularity, color irregularity, diameter >5 mm, evolution).

PATIENT RESOURCES

- **www.nevus.org/faqs-about-cmn_id555.html**.
- **www.nevusnetwork.org**.

PROVIDER RESOURCES

- **http://emedicine.medscape.com/article/1118659-overview**.
- **www.dermatlas.org**.

REFERENCES

1. Lyon VB. Congenital melanocytic nevi. *Pediatr Clin N Am*. 2010; 57:1155-1176.
2. Kanada KN, Merin MR, Munden A, Friedlander: A prospective study of cutaneous findings in newborns in the United States: correlation with race, ethnicity, and gestational status using updated classification and nomenclature. *J Pediatr*. 2012;161(2): 240-245.
3. Gallus S, Naldi L. Oncology Study Group of the Italian Group for Epidemiologic Research in Dermatology. Distribution of congenital melanocytic naevi and congenital naevus-like naevi in a survey of 3406 Italian schoolchildren. *Br J Dermatol*. 2008; 159(2):433-438.
4. Krengel S, Hauschild A, Schafer T. Melanoma risk in congenital melanocytic naevi: a systematic review. *Br J Dermatol*. 2006 Jul; 155(1):1-8.
5. Bett BJ. Large or multiple congenital melanocytic nevi: occurrence of cutaneous melanoma in 1008 persons. *J Am Acad Dermatol*. 2005; 52(5): 793-797.
6. Marghoob AA, Agero AL, Benvenuto-Andrade C, et al. Large congenital melanocytic nevi, risk of cutaneous melanoma, and prophylactic surgery. *J Am Acad Dermatol*. 2006;54(5):868-870.
7. Sahin S, Levin L, Kopf AW, Rao BK, Triola M, Koenig K, Huang C, Bart R. Risk of melanoma in medium-sized congenital melanocytic nevi: A follow-up study. *J Am Acad Dermatol*. 1998;39:428-433.
8. Seidenari S, Pellacani G, Martella A, et al. Instrument-, age- and site-dependent variations of dermoscopic patterns of congenital melanocytic naevi: a multicentre study. *Br J Dermatol*. 2006; 155(1):56-61.
9. Minagawa A, Koga H, Saida T. Dermoscopic characteristics of congenital melanocytic nevi affecting acral volar skin. *Arch Dermatol*. 2011;147(7):809-913.
10. Arneia JS, Gosain AK. Giant congenital melanocytic nevi. *Plast Reconstr Surg*. 2009;124(1):1e-13e.
11. Kinsler V, Bulstrode N. The role of surgery in the management of congenital melanocytic naevi in children: a perspective from Great Ormond Street Hospital. *J Plast Reconstr Aesthet Surg*. 2009; 62(5):595-601.
12. Ferguson RE Jr, Vasconez HC. Laser treatment of congenital nevi. *J Craniofac Surg*. 2005;16(5):908-914.
13. Al-Hadithy N, Al-Nakib K, Quaba A. Outcomes of 52 patients with congenital melanocytic naevi treated with UltraPulse Carbon Dioxide and Frequency Doubled Q-Switched Nd-Yag laser. *J Plast Reconstr Aesthet Surg*. 2012;65(8):1019-1028.
14. Habif T. Clinical Dermatology: A Color Guide to Diagnosis and Therapy. Fourth Edition. Mosby, 2003.

145 EPIDERMAL NEVI AND NEVUS SEBACEOUS

Mindy A. Smith, MD, MS
Richard P. Usatine, MD

PATIENT STORY

A 15-year-old boy is brought in by his mother with a concern about growth of his birthmark. It has become somewhat more raised and bumpy in the past year (**Figure 145-1**). The adolescent reports no symptoms and is not worried about the appearance. He is otherwise healthy with no neurologic symptoms. The joint decision of the family and the doctor was to not excise the epidermal nevus at this time. He may choose to have this removed by a plastic surgeon in the future.

INTRODUCTION

- Epidermal nevi (EN) are congenital hamartomas of ectodermal origin classified on the basis of their main component: sebaceous, apocrine, eccrine, follicular, or keratinocytic.
- Nevus sebaceous (NS) is a hamartoma of the epidermis, hair follicles, and sebaceous and apocrine glands. A hamartoma is the disordered overgrowth of benign tissue in its area of origin.

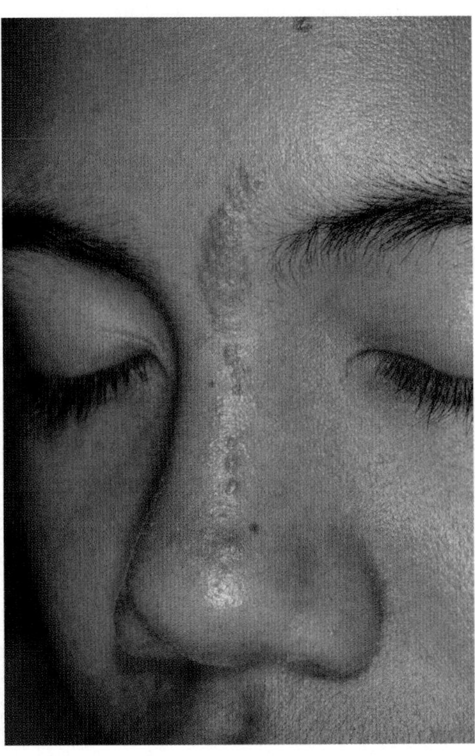

FIGURE 145-1 Epidermal nevus on the face of a teenager. This nevus has been present since birth, and the patient is otherwise healthy. *(Used with permission from Richard P. Usatine, MD.)*

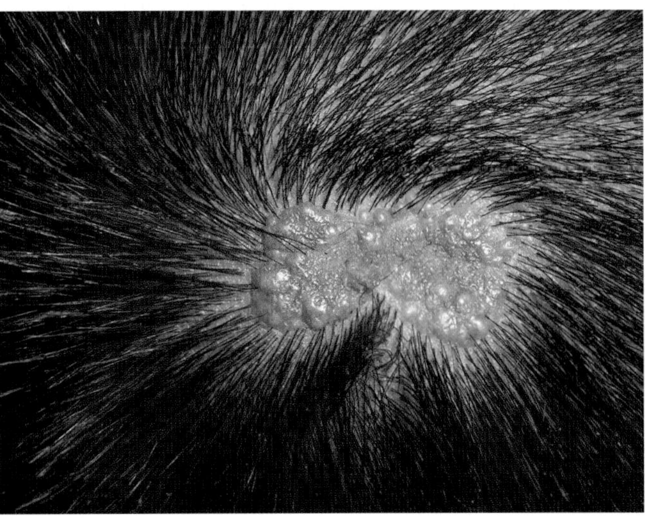

FIGURE 145-2 Nevus sebaceous on the scalp of a 14-year-old boy. *(Used with permission from Richard P. Usatine, MD.)*

SYNONYMS

- EN syndrome is also called Solomon syndrome and is a neurocutaneous disorder characterized by EN and an assortment of neurologic and visceral manifestations.
- NS is also called sebaceous nevus and nevus sebaceous of Jadassohn (**Figure 145-2**).
- An inflammatory linear verrucous epidermal nevus (ILVEN; **Figure 145-3**) can be part of an epidermal nevus syndrome but some affected persons only have the cutaneous EN.

EPIDEMIOLOGY

- EN are uncommon (approximately 1 to 3 percent of newborns and children), sporadic, and usually present at birth, although they can appear in early childhood.

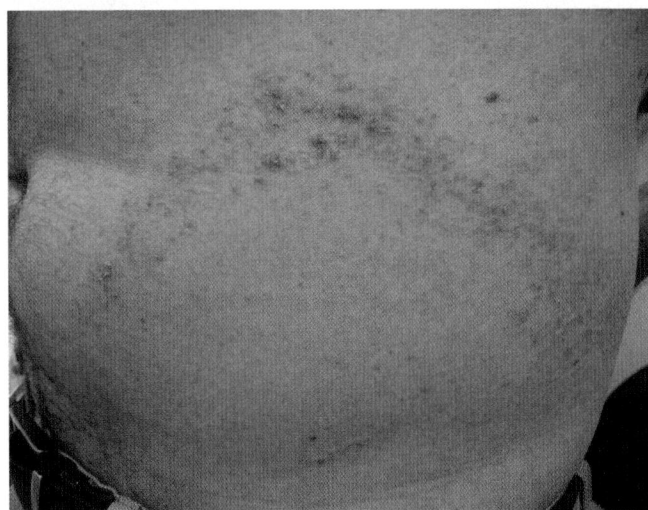

FIGURE 145-3 Inflammatory linear verrucous epidermal nevus (ILVEN) on the trunk. Topical steroids were not helpful in diminishing his pruritus. *(Used with permission from Robert T. Gilson, MD.)*

- EN are associated with disorders of the eye, nervous, and musculoskeletal systems in 10 to 30 percent of patients; in one study, 7.9 percent of patients with EN had one of the nine syndromes—an estimated one per 11,928 pediatric patients.[1]
- In another review of 131 cases of EN, most (60%) had noninflammatory EN, 1/3 had NS, and 6 percent had inflammatory linear verrucous EN.[2]
- NS are usually present at birth or noted in early childhood.[3] Most cases are sporadic but familial cases have been reported.
- Linear NS is estimated to occur in 1 per 1000 live births.[4]
- Linear NS syndrome includes a range of abnormalities including in the central nervous system (CNS). Patients with CNS involvement typically have cognitive impairment and seizures.[4] The cardiovascular, skeletal, ophthalmologic, and urogenital systems may also be involved.

ETIOLOGY AND PATHOPHYSIOLOGY

- EN histologically displays hyperkeratosis and papillomatosis, similar microscopically to seborrheic keratosis.[3] Also similar to seborrheic keratosis, some ENs of keratinocyte differentiation (about one third) have been found to have a mutation in the fibroblast growth factor receptor 3 (FGFR3) gene.[3]
- Nine EN syndromes have been reported and are described in the referenced article.[5]
- ENs frequently have a linear pattern that follows Blaschko lines (**Figures 145-1**, **145-3**, and **145-4**), which are believed to represent epidermal migration during embryogenesis.

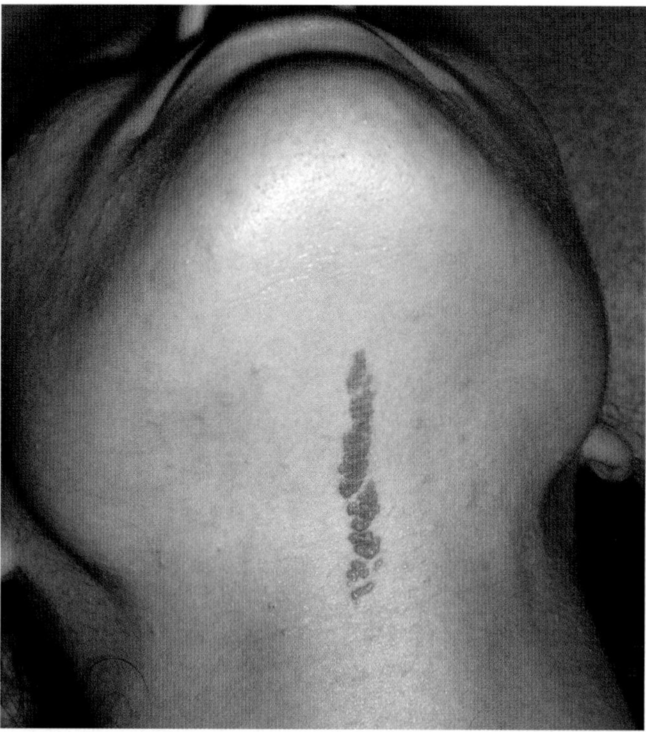

FIGURE 145-4 Linear epidermal nevus on the neck that appeared in early childhood. The patient had no neurologic, musculoskeletal, or vision problems. (*Used with permission from Richard P. Usatine, MD.*)

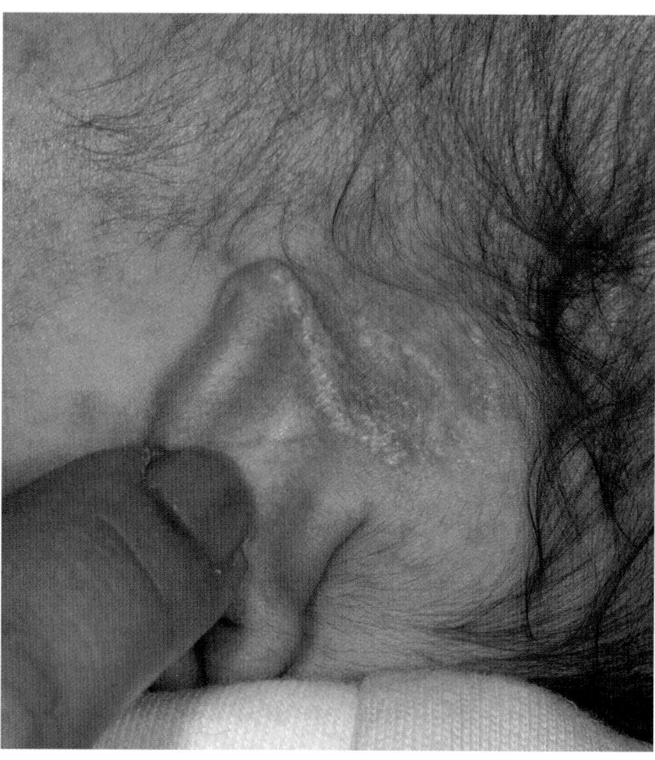

FIGURE 145-5 Nevus sebaceous behind the ear of an infant. Note the light color and the subtle presentation. (*Used with permission from Richard P. Usatine, MD.*)

- EN tend to become thicker, verrucous (**Figure 145-4**), and hyperpigmented at puberty.[3]
- Similarly, NS demonstrate stages of evolution paralleling the histologic differentiation of normal sebaceous glands:[6]
  - Infancy and young children—Smooth to slightly papillated, waxy, hairless thickening (**Figure 145-5**).
  - Puberty—Epidermal hyperplasia resulting in verrucous irregularity of the surface covered with numerous closely aggregated yellow-to-brown papules (**Figure 145-6**).

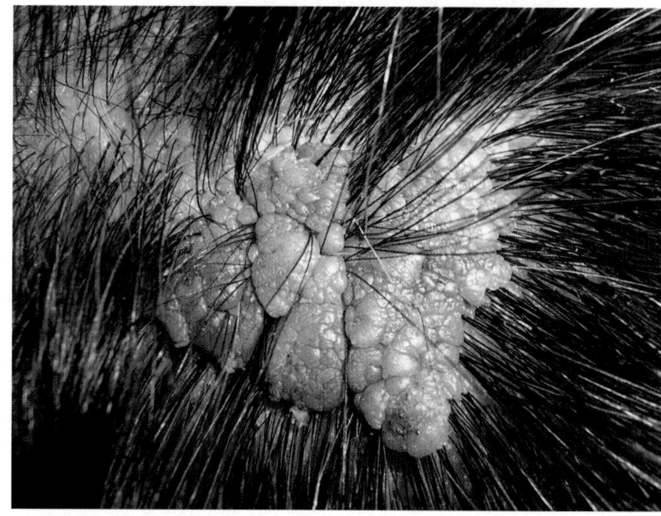

FIGURE 145-6 Nevus sebaceous on the scalp of a teenage female that is verrucous and brown. (*Used with permission from Richard P. Usatine, MD.*)

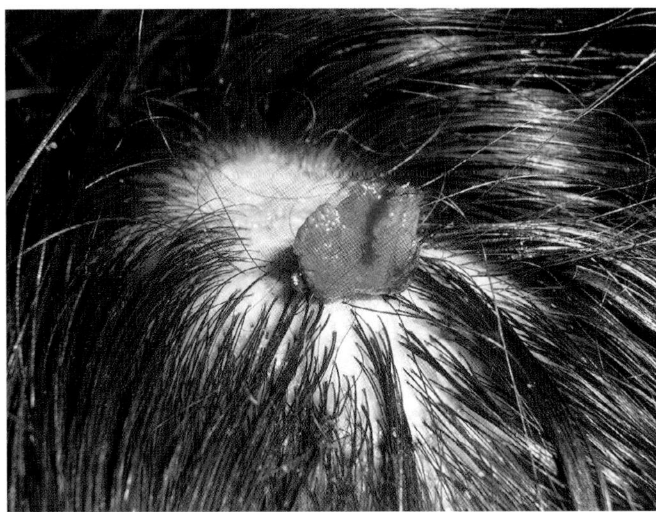

FIGURE 145-7 Nevus sebaceous with a benign tumor identified as a syringocystadenoma papilliferum by shave biopsy. Patient was referred for full removal of the nevus sebaceous. (*Used with permission from Richard P. Usatine, MD.*)

  - Development of secondary appendageal tumors (**Figures 145-7**) occurs in 20 to 30 percent of patients, most are benign (most commonly basal cell epithelioma or trichoblastoma), but single (most commonly basal cell carcinoma) or multiple malignant tumors of both epidermal and adnexal origins may be seen and metastases have been reported. Rarely, these malignancies are seen in childhood.
- NS were shown to have a high prevalence of human papillomavirus DNA and authors postulate that HPV infection of fetal epidermal stem cells could play a role in the pathogenesis.[7]

MAKING THE DIAGNOSIS

CLINICAL FEATURES OF EPIDERMAL NEVI

- EN are linear, round or oblong, well circumscribed, elevated, and flat-topped (**Figures 145-8** and **145-9**).

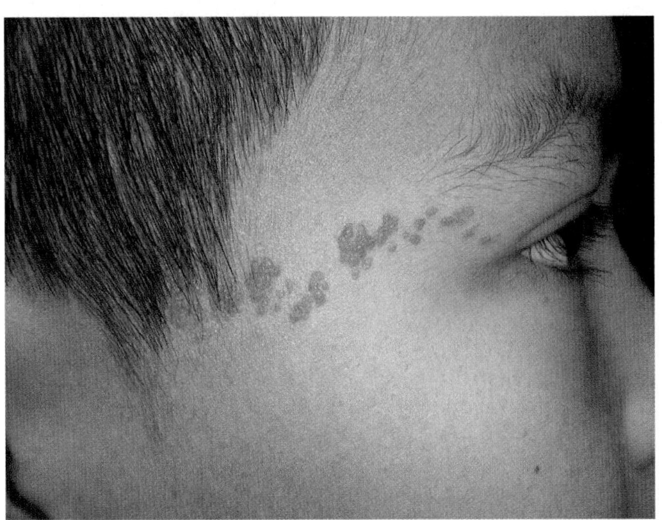

FIGURE 145-8 Epidermal nevus that is linear on the side of this young boy's face. (*Used with permission from Richard P. Usatine, MD.*)

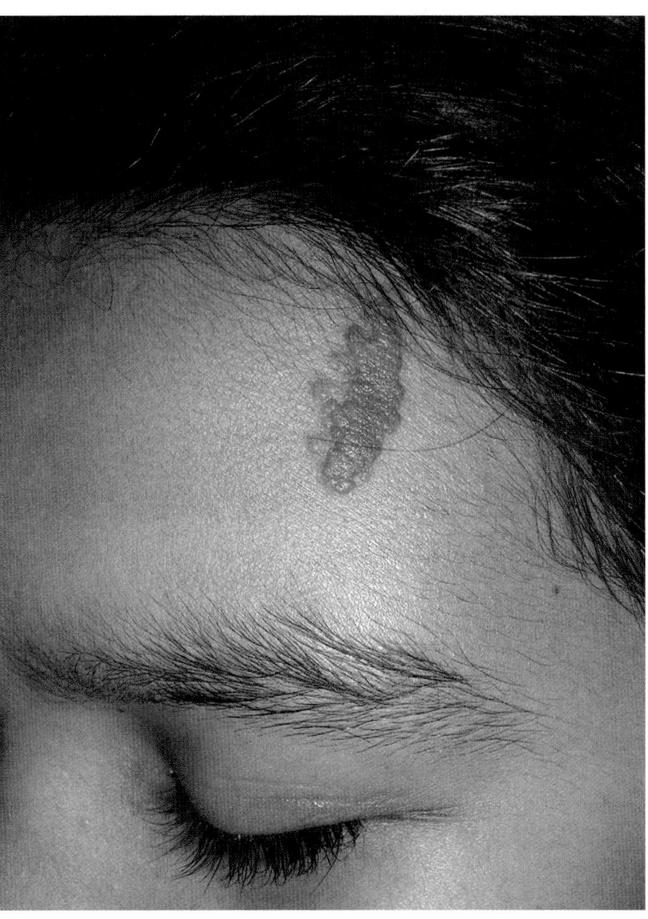

FIGURE 145-9 Epidermal nevus with some hyperpigmentation on the forehead of this young girl. (*Used with permission from Richard P. Usatine, MD.*)

- Color is yellow-tan to dark brown.
- Surface is uniform velvety or warty (**Figures 145-8** and **145-9**).
- ILVEN, a less common type of EN, is pruritic and erythematous (**Figure 145-3**).

CLINICAL FEATURES OF NEVUS SEBACEOUS

- NS has an oval to linear shape ranging from 0.5 × 1 cm to 7 × 9 cm.
- NS is usually solitary, smooth, waxy, hairless thickening noted on the scalp at birth or in early childhood (**Figures 145-6**, **145-6**, and **145-10**). [PE: Repeated '6'. Pls. check.]
- Early NS may be pink, orange, yellow or tan; later lesions can appear verrucous and nodular (**Figure 145-10**).

TYPICAL DISTRIBUTION

- EN occur most commonly on the head and neck followed by the trunk and proximal extremities; only 13 percent have wide spread lesions (**Figure 145-11**). Lesions may spread beyond their original distribution with age. Inflammatory verrucous EN is found on the limbs.
- NS are commonly found on the scalp followed by forehead and retroauricular region (**Figures 145-10** and **145-5**) and rarely involves the neck, trunk, or other areas.

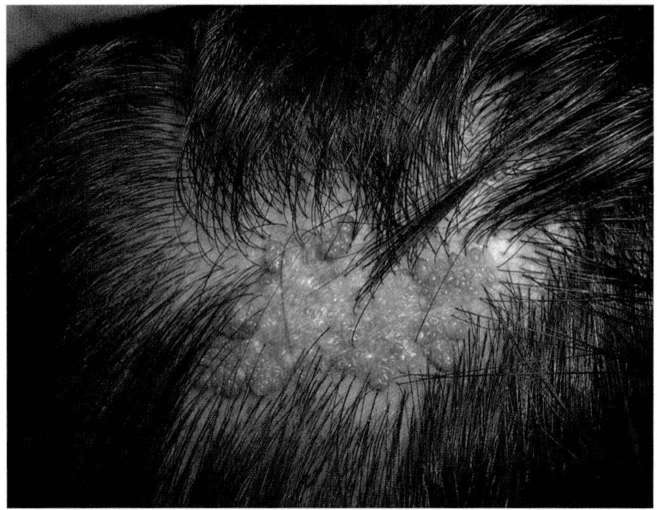

FIGURE 145-10 Nevus sebaceous on the scalp appearing verrucous with pink and brown coloration. (*Used with permission from Richard P. Usatine, MD.*)

BIOPSY

- Biopsy is the most definitive method for diagnosing these nevi. A biopsy is not needed if the clinical picture is clear and no operative intervention is planned. A shave biopsy should provide adequate tissue for diagnosis because the pathology is epidermal and in the upper dermis.

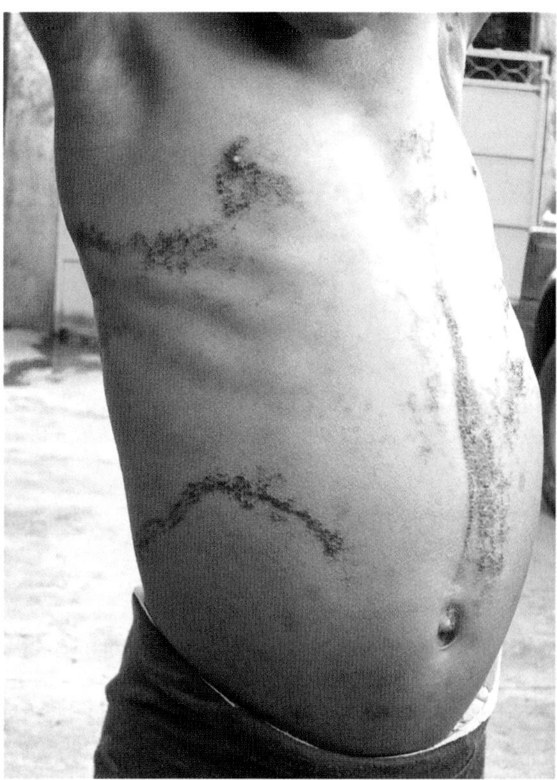

FIGURE 145-11 Extensive epidermal nevus following Blaschko lines on the trunk of this boy. Note how the lines are similar to the patient with inflammatory linear verrucous epidermal nevus (ILVEN) in **Figure 145-2**. (*Used with permission from Rick Hodes, MD.*)

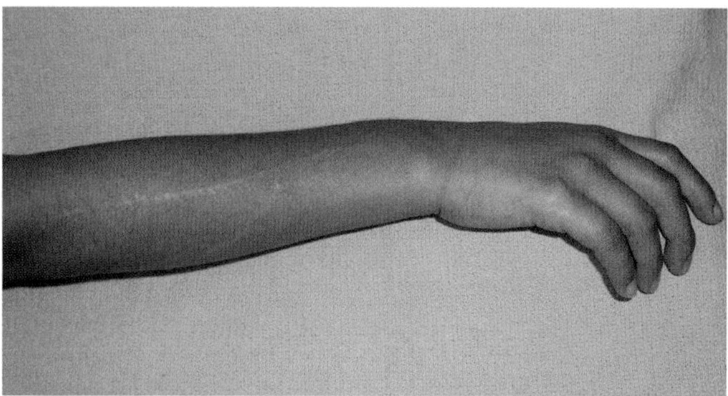

FIGURE 145-12 Lichen striatus that appeared suddenly on the arm of a young boy. (*Used with permission from Richard P. Usatine, MD.*)

 - Histologic features of epidermolytic hyperkeratosis within an EN are associated with mutations in the keratin gene that may be transmitted to offspring; widespread cutaneous involvement may be seen.[3]

DIFFERENTIAL DIAGNOSIS

- Lichen striatus—Discrete pink, tan, or skin-colored asymptomatic papules in a linear band that suddenly appear. The papules may be smooth, scaly, or flat topped. It is mostly seen in children. While it is most commonly seen on an extremity, it can appear on the trunk (**Figure 145-12**). It can resemble a linear EN but lichen striatus will spontaneously regress within one year.
- Syringoma (**Figure 145-13**)—Benign adnexal tumor derived from sweat gland ducts. Autosomal dominant transmission, soft, small, skin-colored to brown papules develop during childhood and adolescence, especially around the eyes but may be found on the face, neck, and trunk.

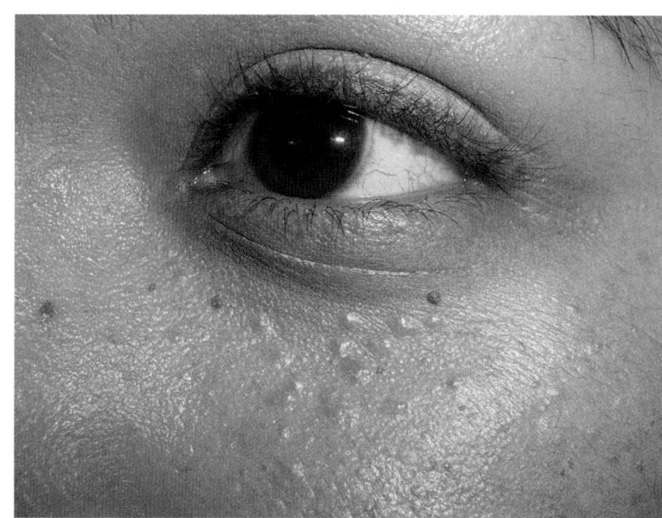

FIGURE 145-13 Syringoma on the lower eyelid of a teenage girl. (*Used with permission from Richard P. Usatine, MD.*)

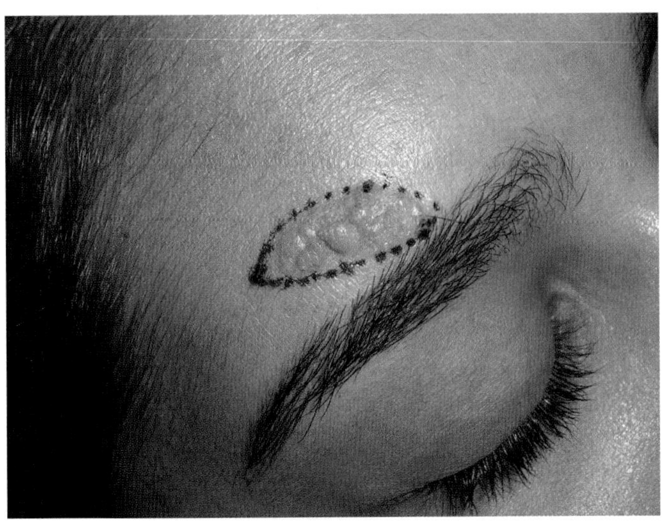

FIGURE 145-14 Nevus sebaceous about to be elliptically excised from the forehead of a 15-year-old girl. Careful surgery by an experienced surgeon produced an excellent cosmetic result. The girl and her parents requested the surgery for cosmetic and psychologic reasons as there were no signs of malignant degeneration. The girl and her parents were delighted with the results. *(Used with permission from Richard P. Usatine, MD.)*

MANAGEMENT

MEDICATIONS

- There are no proven topical methods for treatment of these lesions. Topical retinoids may improve lesion appearance but recurrence is common.[3]

PROCEDURES

- Destructive modalities for EN such as electrodessication or cryotherapy may temporally improve the appearance of the lesion, but recurrence is frequent.[3]
- Carbon dioxide laser is an alternative option for EN; however, scarring and pigment changes are potential permanent complications, especially in patients with darker skin types.[8] This treatment does not completely remove NS and there is recurrence risk.
- Surgical excision is an option, but may be complicated by scarring.
- Because of the potential for malignant transformation particularly following puberty, many authors recommend early complete plastic surgical excision for NS (**Figure 145-14**); reconstructive surgery may be needed. SOR Ⓒ
- Excision of large lesions may require reconstructive surgery with a rotation flap to close.[9]

PROGNOSIS

- There are reports of spontaneous improvement in patients with widespread involvement of EN.
- Malignant potential is low in EN.[3]
- Malignant potential in NS is uncertain. Reports range from 0 to 2.7 percent.[3]
  - Early reports suggested a high rate of developing basal cell carcinomas while more recent studies identified trichoblastoma and syringocystadenoma papilliferum in NS, usually in adulthood.
  - In a retrospective analysis of 757 cases of NS from 1996 to 2002 in children ≤ age 16 years, investigators found no malignancies and question the need for prophylactic surgical removal.[10] In a study using data pooled from six large retrospective studies of giant NS (N = 2520), the cumulative incidence of malignant tumors was 0.5 percent.[11]
  - Squamous cell carcinoma has also been described in a NS.[12]

FOLLOW-UP

- Patients with NS should be examined for other associated findings. Consider a consultation with a neurologist and/or ophthalmologist.
  - In a study of 196 subjects with NS examined for clinical neurologic abnormalities, only 7 percent had abnormalities.[13] Abnormal exams were more frequent in individuals with extensive nevi (21% versus 5%) and a centrofacial location (21% versus 2%). The patients in **Figures 145-1** through **145-3** had no neurological abnormalities.

PATIENT RESOURCES

- Support group—**www.nevus.org/other-kinds-of-nevi_id559.html**.
- **http://ghr.nlm.nih.gov/condition/epidermal-nevus**.

PROVIDER RESOURCES

- Nevus sebaceous—**http://emedicine.medscape.com/article/1058733-overview**.
- Epidermal nevus syndrome—**http://emedicine.medscape.com/article/1117506-overview**.

REFERENCES

1. Vidaurri-de la Cruz H, Tamayo-Sanchez L, Duran-McKinster C, et al. Epidermal nevus syndromes: clinical findings in 35 patients. *Pediatr Dermatol*. 2004;21(4):432-439.
2. Rogers M, McCrossin I, Commens C. Epidermal nevi and the epidermal nevus syndrome. A review of 131 cases. *J Am Acad Dermatol*. 1989;20(3):476-488.
3. Brandling-Bennett HA, Morel KD. Epidermal Nevi. *Pediatr Clin N Am*. 2010;57:1177-1198.
4. Menascu S, Donner EJ. Linear nevus sebaceous syndrome: case reports and review of the literature. *Pediatr Neurol*. 2008;38(3):207-210.
5. Happle R. The group of epidermal nevous syndromes. Part I. Well defined phenotypes. *J Am Acad Dermatol*. 2010;63:1-22.
6. Hammadi AA. *Nevus sebaceous*. Emedicine. Last updated May 29, 2012. http://emedicine.medscape.com/article/1058733-overview, accessed November 2012.
7. Carlson JA, Cribier B, Nuovo G, et al. Epidermodysplasia verruciformis-associated and genital-mucosal high-risk human

papillomavirus DNA are prevalent in nevus sebaceus of Jadassohn. *J Am Acad Dermatol*. 2008;59(2):279–294.

8. Boyce S, Alster TS. CO2 laser treatment of epidermal nevi: long-term success. *Dermatol Surg*. 2002;28(7):611–614.
9. Davison SP, Khachemoune A, Yu D, Kauffman LC. Nevus sebaceus of Jadassohn revisited with reconstruction options. *Int J Dermatol*. 2005;44(2):145-150.
10. Santibanez-Gallerani A, Marshall D, Duarte AM, et al. Should nevus sebaceus of Jadassohn in children be excised? A study of 757 cases, and literature review. *J Craniofac Surg*. 2003;14(5):658-660.
11. Chepla KJ, Gosain AK. Giant nevus sebaceous: definition, surgical techniques, and rationale for treatment. *Plast Reconstr Surg*. 2012; 130(2):296e-304e.
12. Aguayo R, Pallarés J, Casanova JM, et al. Squamous cell carcinoma developing in Jadassohn's sebaceous nevus: case report and review of the literature. *Dermatol Surg*. 2010;36(11): 1763-1768.
13. Davies D. Rogers M. Review of neurological manifestations in 196 patients with sebaceous naevi. *Australas J Dermatol*. 2002;43(1):20-23.

146 DYSPLASTIC NEVUS

Mindy A. Smith, MD, MS
Richard P. Usatine, MD

PATIENT STORY

A teenage boy presents with concern over a mole on his back that his mother says is growing larger and more variable in color. His mother, who is present with him, reports that his father had a melanoma that was caught early and successfully treated. The edges are irregular and the color almost appears to be "leaking" into the surrounding skin. He reports no symptoms related to this lesion. On physical exam, the nevus is 9 mm in diameter with asymmetry, variations in color and an irregular border (**Figure 146-1**). A full-body skin exam did not demonstrate any other suspicious lesions. Dermoscopy showed an irregular network with multiple asymmetrically placed dots off the network (**Figure 146-2**). A scoop saucerization was performed with a DermaBlade taking 2-mm margins of clinically normal skin (**Figure 146-3**). The pathology showed a completely excised compound dysplastic nevus with no signs of malignancy. No further treatment was needed except yearly skin exams to monitor for melanoma.

INTRODUCTION

Dysplastic nevi (DN)/atypical moles are acquired melanocytic lesions of the skin whose clinical and histologic definitions are controversial and still evolving. These lesions have some small potential for malignant transformation and patients with multiple DN have an increased risk for melanoma.[1]

The presence of multiple DN is a marker for increased melanoma risk, similar to red hair, and, analogously, cutting off the red hair or cutting out all the DN does not change melanoma risk. The problem with DN is that any one lesion suspicious for melanoma must be biopsied to avoid missing melanoma, not to prevent melanoma from occurring in that nevus in the future.

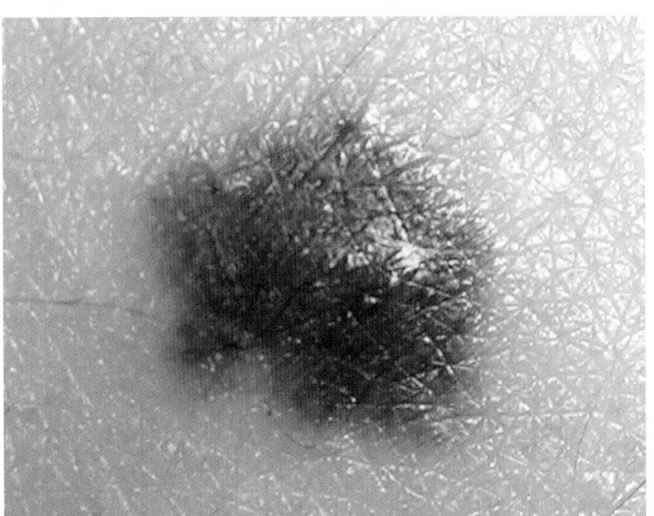

FIGURE 146-1 Growing 9-mm pigmented lesion on the back with asymmetry, variations in color and an irregular border. Pathology after excision revealed this to be a compound dysplastic nevus. (*Used with permission from Richard P. Usatine, MD.*)

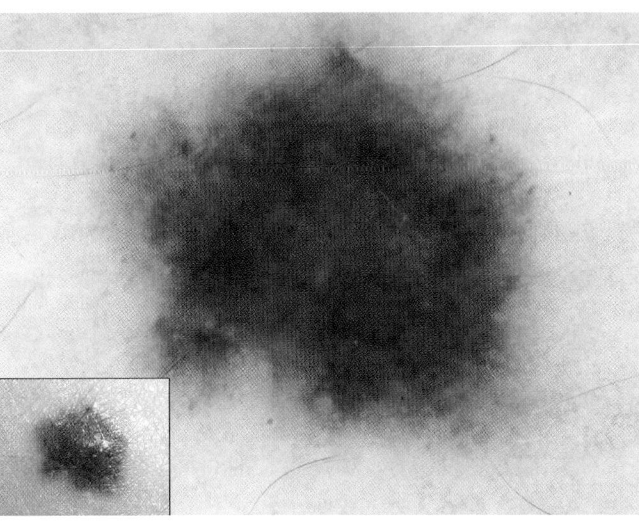

FIGURE 146-2 Dermoscopy of this compound dysplastic nevus shows an irregular network with multiple asymmetrically placed dots off the network. (*Used with permission from Richard P. Usatine, MD.*)

SYNONYMS

Atypical nevus, atypical mole, Clark nevus, nevus with architectural disorder, and melanocytic atypia.[1]

EPIDEMIOLOGY

- DN are uncommon in children; in a study of Swedish children (N = 524), none had DN.[2] In another study of pathology reports

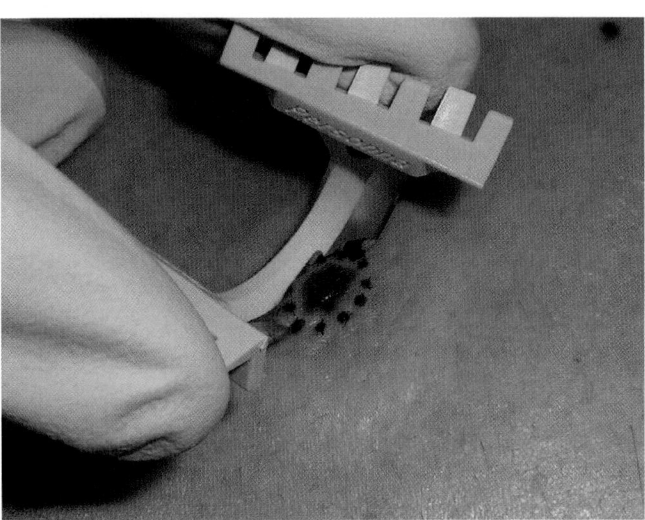

FIGURE 146-3 A scoop saucerization was performed with a DermaBlade taking 2-mm margins of clinically normal skin. Although this could have been an early thin melanoma, the pathology showed a completely excised compound dysplastic nevus with no signs of malignancy. (*Used with permission from Richard P. Usatine, MD.*)

from nevi removed from patients younger than 18 years, 3 of 199 nevi submitted for histologic analysis met the histologic criteria for DN.[3]

- Two percent to 9 percent of the population has atypical moles (AMs).[4,5] Among patients with melanoma, the rate of DN ranges from 34 to 59 percent.[4]
- Individuals with fair skin types are at higher risk of DN.[4]
- The sudden eruption of benign and atypical melanocytic nevi has been reported and is associated with blistering skin conditions and a number of disease states, including immunosuppression. Subsets of patients with immunosuppression have increased numbers of nevi on the palms and soles.[6]
- The National Institute of Health Consensus Conference on the diagnosis and treatment of early melanoma defined a syndrome of familial atypical mole and melanoma (FAMM). The criteria of FAMM syndrome are[7]:
  - The occurrence of malignant melanoma in one or more first- or second-degree relatives.
  - The presence of numerous (often >50) melanocytic nevi, some of which are clinically atypical.
  - Many of the associated nevi show certain histologic features (see the following section "Biopsy").

ETIOLOGY AND PATHOPHYSIOLOGY

- Most DN are compound nevi (**Figure 146-1**) possessing a junctional and intradermal component (see Chapter 143, Benign Nevi).[1] The junctional component is highly cellular and consists of an irregular distribution of melanocytes arranged in nests and lentiginous patterns along the dermoepidermal junction. The dermal component, located at the center, consists of nests and strands of melanocytes with distinct sclerotic changes.[1]
- DN exhibit a host response consisting of irregular rete ridge elongation, subepidermal sclerosis, proliferation of dermal capillaries, and a perivascular, lymphohistiocytic inflammatory infiltrate.[1]
- Individuals with DN may have deficient DNA repair, and DN lesions are associated with overexpression of pheomelanin (pigment produced by melanocytes), which may lead to increased oxidative DNA damage and tumor progression.[8]

DIAGNOSIS

CLINICAL FEATURES

- Variable mixtures of color including tan, brown, black, and red within a single lesion (**Figures 146-4** and **146-5**).
- Irregular, notched borders; pigment may fade off into surrounding skin.
- Flat or slightly raised (**Figures 146-4** to **146-6**) with the macular portion at edge. Not verrucous or pendulous.
- Lesions frequently surrounded by a reddish hue from reactive hyperemia making them appear target-like.

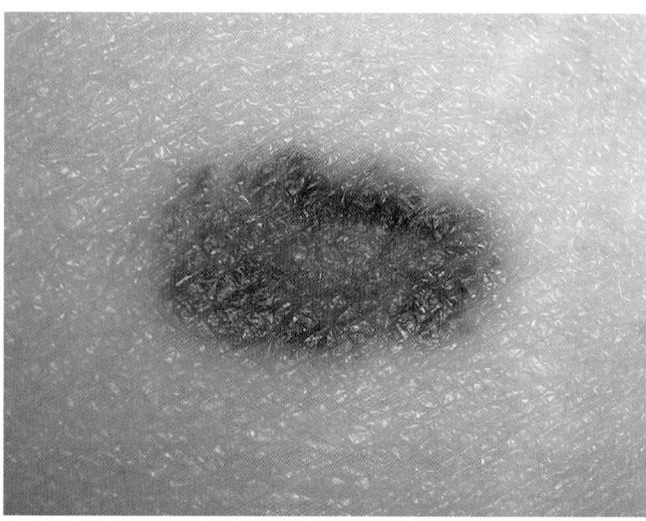

FIGURE 146-4 Dysplastic nevus in a young woman with malignant melanoma in a different region of her body. The size was greater than 6 mm and there was variation in color. This was fully excised to make sure there was no melanoma present. *(Used with permission from Richard P. Usatine, MD.)*

- Usually larger than 6 mm; may be larger than 10 mm (**Figures 146-1** and **146-4**).
- Patients with FAMM syndrome may have more than 100 lesions, far greater than the average number of common moles (<50) in most individuals.

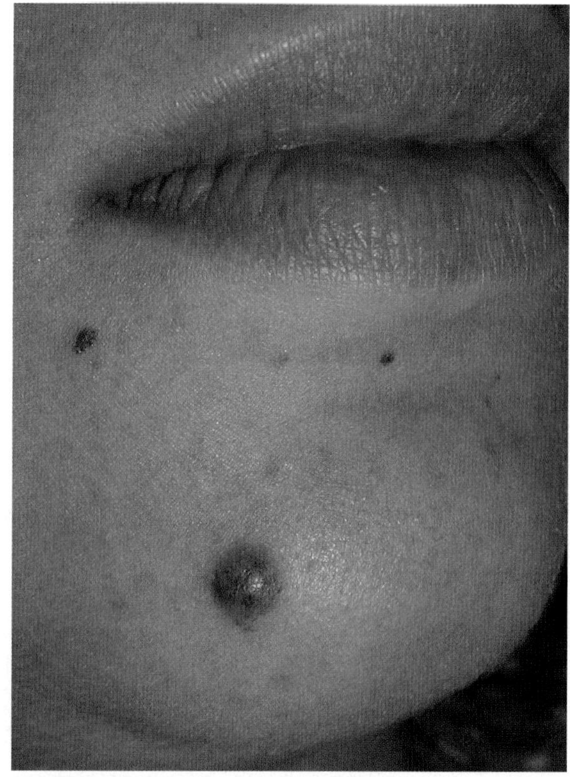

FIGURE 146-5 Dysplastic nevus on the chin of a teenage girl. A punch biopsy successfully removed the whole lesion and confirmed that it was not melanoma. *(Used with permission from Richard P. Usatine, MD.)*

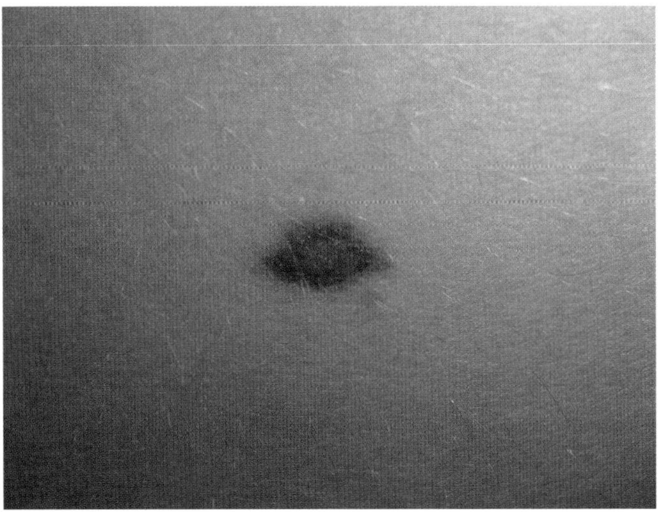

FIGURE 146-6 Dysplastic nevus on the back proven by biopsy. Note the fried egg appearance of this atypical mole. (*Used with permission from Richard P. Usatine, MD.*)

TYPICAL DISTRIBUTION

- Usually on sun-exposed areas, especially the back (**Figures 146-1** and **146-6**); may be found on sites where nevi are usually absent or rare such as the scalp, breasts, genital skin, buttocks, palm, and dorsa of feet.

IMAGING

- Although eccentric peripheral hyperpigmented and multifocal hyper- or hypopigmented types are more commonly seen in melanoma, no digital dermatoscopic criteria have been identified that can clearly distinguish DN from in situ melanomas.[9] However, dermoscopy increases diagnostic sensitivity and specificity of cutaneous melanoma from 60 to greater than 90 percent, especially using pattern recognition.[4]
- Investigators in one study found change in 16.2 percent of 2497 benign melanocytic lesions with minor suspicion of melanoma undergoing short-term dermoscopy.[10] Change was more often seen in younger (0 to 18 years and 19 to 35 years) and older patients.

BIOPSY

- The importance of histology is to distinguish DN from melanoma. Although not universally accepted, the World Health Organization Melanoma Program proposed a list of characteristics/criteria with individual lesions requiring two major and two minor criteria to be classified as a DN:[4]
    - Major criteria are basilar proliferation of atypical nevomelanocytes and organization of this proliferation in a lentiginous or epithelioid cell pattern.
    - Minor criteria are: (a) the presence of lamellar fibrosis or concentric eosinophilic fibrosis, (b) neovascularization, (c) inflammatory response, and (d) fusion of rete ridges. These established criteria yielded 92 percent mean concordance overall by panel members.

DIFFERENTIAL DIAGNOSIS

- Melanocytic nevi—Most common moles are tan to brown, smaller than 6 mm, round in shape, and with sharp borders (see Chapter 143, Benign Nevi).
- Melanoma—Skin cancer is often asymmetric, with irregular border and varied colors. It is usually larger than 6 mm in diameter (see Chapter 147, Melanoma).

MANAGEMENT

NONPHARMACOLOGIC

- Obtain a family history of DN and melanoma for patients presenting with DN.
- Because of the low risk of any one DN developing malignant transformation, the prophylactic removal of all DN is not recommended. SOR Ⓒ

MEDICATIONS

- Of the medications tested, including topical 5-fluorouracil, systemic isotretinoin, topical tretinoin with or without hydrocortisone, and topical imiquimod, none completely destroy DN.[4]

PROCEDURES

- Removal of at least one lesion is reasonable to histologically confirm the diagnosis and rule out melanoma. This should be accomplished with excisional biopsy and histologic confirmation of DN versus melanoma. DN is usually removed with conservative surgical margins (about 2 mm) to provide adequate tissue for the pathologist.[3] SOR Ⓒ
- Scoop saucerizations (deep shave biopsy with a DermaBlade or razor blade) including at least a 2-mm margin of clinically normal skin surrounding the pigmented lesion is a rapid and acceptable method of excision for pathology (**Figure 146-7**).

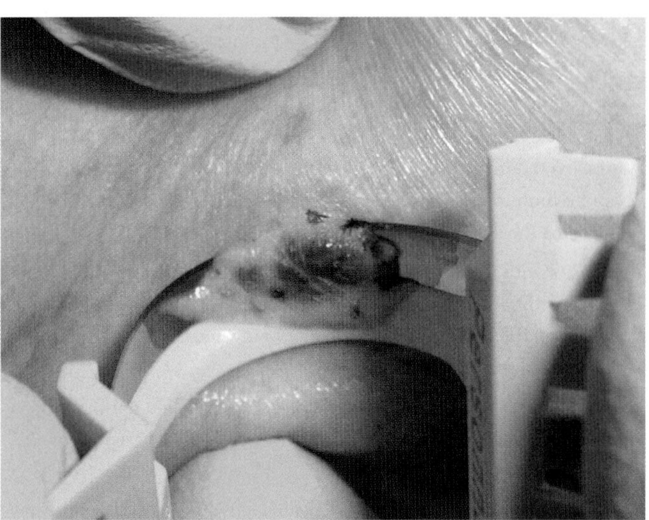

FIGURE 146-7 Scoop saucerization of a suspicious pigmented lesion that turned out to be a dysplastic junctional nevus with moderate atypia. The whole lesion was successfully excised with this deep shave. (*Used with permission from Richard P. Usatine, MD.*)

PREVENTION

- Avoid direct sunlight.
- Sun protection to limit sunburn may also help reduce the appearance of nevi. In one trial (N = 209 white children), children randomized to the sunscreen group, especially those with freckles, had significantly fewer new nevi on the trunk than did children in the control group at 3-year follow-up.[11]

PROGNOSIS

- The risk of a melanoma arising within a DN is estimated at 1:3000 per year.[1] However, there is also an increased risk of melanoma arising elsewhere on the skin in patients with DN; the actual incidence rate is uncertain and ranges from 0.5 to 46 percent.[4] There is also a substantially increased risk of melanoma associated with the number of atypical nevi (relative risk [RR] = 6.36; 95% confidence interval [CI]: 3.80, 10.33; for 5 versus 0).[12]
- In one case-control study, the estimated 10-year cumulative risk for developing melanoma in patients with AM syndrome was 10.7 percent (versus 0.62% in a control population).[13]
- DNs appear to be dynamic throughout adulthood. In a study of the natural history of DN, investigators found that 51 percent of all evaluated nevi (297 of 593) showed clinical signs of change during an average follow-up of 89 months.[14] New nevi were common in adulthood, continuing to form in more than 20 percent of patients older than age 50 years, and some nevi disappeared. Less is known about DN in children but change is common in other nevi (see Chapter 143, Benign Nevi).

FOLLOW-UP

- Patents with DN should have regular skin examinations with biopsy performed of any suspicious lesions (**Figure 146-7**).[4]
- Consider total-body photographs for monitoring (**Figures 146-8** and **146-9**).[4] In a study of 50 patients with 5 or more DN, the use of baseline digital photographs improved the diagnostic accuracy of skin self-examination on the back, chest, and abdomen, and improved detection of changing and new moles.[15] Individual DN can be monitored more precisely with digital dermoscopic photos added to the skin photographs (**Figure 146-9**).
- Patients with numerous DN and who have a family history of melanoma are at a higher risk of developing melanoma and should be encouraged to have regular follow-up with a provider skilled in detecting melanoma.
- Patients with FAMM should also consider a baseline ophthalmologic examination because of a possible association between uveal melanoma and FAMM syndrome.[4]
- First-degree relatives of patients diagnosed with FAMM syndrome should be encouraged to be examined for DN and melanoma.

In a cohort study of 115 patients with dysplastic nevi an average follow-up of 17.4 years (range: 0.0 to 29.9) was achieved.[16] During these long-term follow-up periods, no patient developed melanoma at the site of an incompletely or narrowly removed histological dysplastic nevus. The authors concluded that this provides evidence that routine re-excision of mildly or moderately dysplastic nevi may not be necessary.[16]

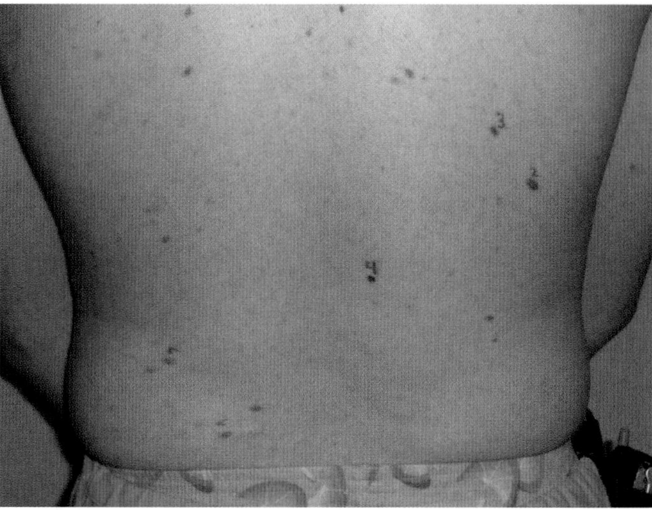

FIGURE 146-8 Multiple dysplastic nevi on the back of a young man. Multiple biopsies have all been negative, so patient is being followed by serial digital photography with numbering of the dysplastic nevi. (*Used with permission from Richard P. Usatine, MD.*)

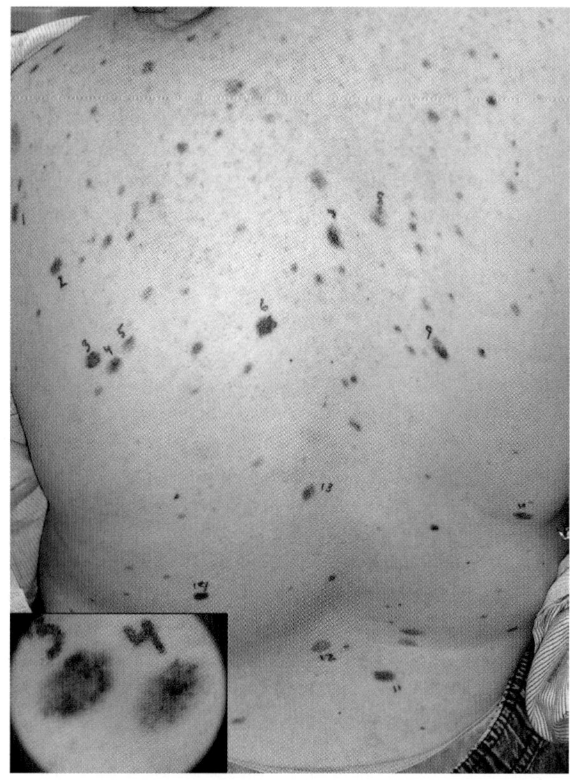

FIGURE 146-9 More than 14 dysplastic nevi are seen on the back of this young woman. She has never had a melanoma and has no family history of melanoma. Multiple biopsies so far have only shown dysplastic nevi, so she is being followed with serial digital photography of her nevi along with corresponding dermoscopic photographs. Note the dermoscopic images of nevi 3 and 4 in the bottom left corner. (*Used with permission from Richard P. Usatine, MD.*)

PATIENT EDUCATION

- Patients with DN should avoid excessive exposure to natural or artificial UV light and routinely use a broad-spectrum sunscreen with a sun protective factor of 30 or greater and/or sun-protective clothing.
- Patients and their parents should be taught self-examination to detect changes in existing moles and to recognize clinical features of melanomas. Patients should be taught to look for and report asymmetry, border irregularity, new symptoms (e.g., pain, pruritus, bleeding, or ulceration), and color and size changes.

PATIENT RESOURCES

- **www.nlm.nih.gov/medlineplus/moles.html.**
- **www.cancer.gov/cancertopics/wyntk/moles-and-dysplastic-nevi.**

PROVIDER RESOURCES

- **www.dermatlas.com.**
- **http://emedicine.medscape.com/article/1056283-overview.**
- **www.ncbi.nlm.nih.gov/books/NBK7030/.**

REFERENCES

1. Clarke LE. Dysplastic nevus. *Clin Lab Med*. 2011;31:255-265.
2. Synnerstad I, Nilsson L, Fredrikson M, Rosdahl I. Frequency and distribution pattern of melanocytic naevi in Swedish 8-9-year-old children. *Acta Derm Venereol*. 2004;84(4):271-276.
3. Haley JC, Hood AF, Chuang TY, Rasmussen J. The frequency of histologically dysplastic nevi in 199 pediatric patients. *Pediatr Dermatol.* 2000;17(4):266-269.
4. Friedman RJ, Farber MJ, Warycha MA, et al. The "dysplastic" nevus. *Clin Dermatol*. 2009;27:103-115.
5. Mooi WJ. The dysplastic naevus. *J Clin Pathol*. 1997;50: 711-715.
6. Woodhouse J, Maytin EV. Eruptive nevi of the palms and soles. *J Am Acad Dermatol*. 2005;52(5:1):S96-S100.
7. Friedman RJ, Farber MJ, Warycha MA, et al. The "dysplastic" nevus. *Clin Dermatol*. 2009;27:103-115.
8. Elder DE. Dysplastic naevi: an update. *Histopathology*. 2010; 56(1):112-120.
9. Burroni M, Sbano P, Cevenini G, et al. Dysplastic naevus vs. in situ melanoma: digital dermoscopy analysis. *Br J Dermatol*. 2005; 152(4):679-684.
10. Menzies SW, Stevenson ML, Altamura D, Byth K. Variables predicting change in benign melanocytic nevi undergoing short-term dermoscopic imaging. *Arch Dermatol*. 2011:147(6): 655-659.
11. Lee TK, Rivers JK, Gallagher RP. Site-specific protective effect of broad-spectrum sunscreen on nevus development among white schoolchildren in a randomized trial. *J Am Acad Dermatol.* 2005; 52(5):786-792.
12. Gandini S, Sera F, Cattaruzza MS, et al. Meta-analysis of risk factors for cutaneous melanoma: I. Common and atypical naevi. *Eur J Cancer*. 2005;41(1):28-44.
13. Marghoob AA, Kopf AW, Rigel DS, et al. Risk of cutaneous malignant melanoma in patients with "classic" atypical-mole syndrome. A case-control study. *Arch Dermatol*. 1994;130:993-998.
14. Trock B, Synnestvedt M, Humphreys T. Natural history of dysplastic nevi. *J Am Acad Dermatol*. 1993;29(1):51-57.
15. Oliveria SA, Chau D, Christos PJ, et al. Diagnostic accuracy of patients in performing skin self-examination and the impact of photography. *Arch Dermatol*. 2004;140(1):57-62.
16. Hocker TL, Alikhan A, Comfere NI, Peters MS. Favorable long-term outcomes in patients with histologically dysplastic nevi that approach a specimen border. *J* Am Acad Dermatol. 2013; 68(4):545-51.

147 PEDIATRIC MELANOMA

Jonathan B. Karnes, MD
Richard P. Usatine, MD

PATIENT STORY

A 13-year-old red-haired female with a family history of melanoma in her father and multiple moles presents for a routine physical and is found to have a thin 8 mm pink papule on the right neck that has appeared in the last 6 months and occasionally bleeds when it rubs on a shirt (**Figure 147-1**). A narrow margin excisional biopsy was performed which revealed invasive melanoma 0.7 mm in depth with 2 mitoses per high power field. She was referred to pediatric surgery where she underwent wide local excision and sentinel lymph node biopsy of the neck, which revealed micrometastasis in one node. After PET scan showed no distant metastasis, she underwent lymph node dissection and was enrolled in a clinical trial through a major referral hospital in the region. Her prognosis is guarded, but similar to adults with the same cancer stage.

EPIDEMIOLOGY

- Although extremely rare, malignant melanoma is the most common skin cancer in children and represents 1 percent of all new cases of melanoma.[1]
- Between 1973 and 2009, 1230 children in the US were diagnosed with melanoma at a rate of 6 per million overall. Children aged 0 to 9 had the lowest rate at 1.1 per million while children aged 15 to 19 were diagnosed at the highest rate of 18 cases per million.[1]

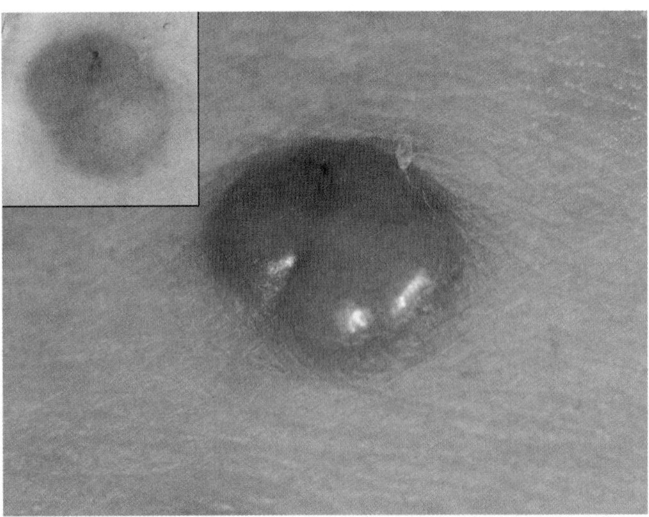

FIGURE 147-1 Amelanotic nodular melanoma with atypical vascular structures seen on dermoscopy (see inset in upper left corner). (*Used with permission from Ashfaq A.Marghoob, MD.*)

- Melanoma incidence is on the rise in adults and children with the incidence increasing in children by 2 percent per year and 4 to 8 percent per year in adults.[1]
- In the US, the death rate is decreasing among persons younger than 65.[2]
- The lifetime risk of developing melanoma is 1 in 55 for men and 1 in 36 for women.[3]

RISK FACTORS

Risk factors can be broadly thought of as genetic risks, environmental risks, and phenotypic risks—arising from a combination of genetic and environmental risks. For example, a fair skinned child (genetic risk) who gets a sunburn (environmental) is much more likely to develop freckles (phenotypic) and melanoma. Childhood sun exposure is a significant risk factor for developing melanoma as an adult.[4]

ENVIRONMENTAL RISKS

- Exposure to sunlight.
- History of sunburn doubles the risk of melanoma and is worse at a young age.
- Artificial tanning.
- History of immunosuppression.
- Higher socioeconomic status (likely associated with more frequent opportunity for sunburns).

GENETIC RISKS

- Fair skin, blue or green eyes, red or blonde hair.
- In children, female sex is higher risk, in adulthood, male sex is higher risk.
- Melanoma in a first-degree relative.
- History of xeroderma pigmentosa or familial atypical mole melanoma syndrome.
- Personal history of a BRCA2 mutation confers a high risk of uveal melanoma.[5]

PHENOTYPIC RISKS

- Many nevi.
- Congenital nevi (**Figure 147-2**).
- Multiple dysplastic nevi.
- Increased age.
- Personal history of skin cancer.

DIAGNOSIS

CLINICAL FEATURES

Melanoma in children may deviate significantly from the traditional ABCDE criteria used to assess risk of melanoma.[6] The traditional

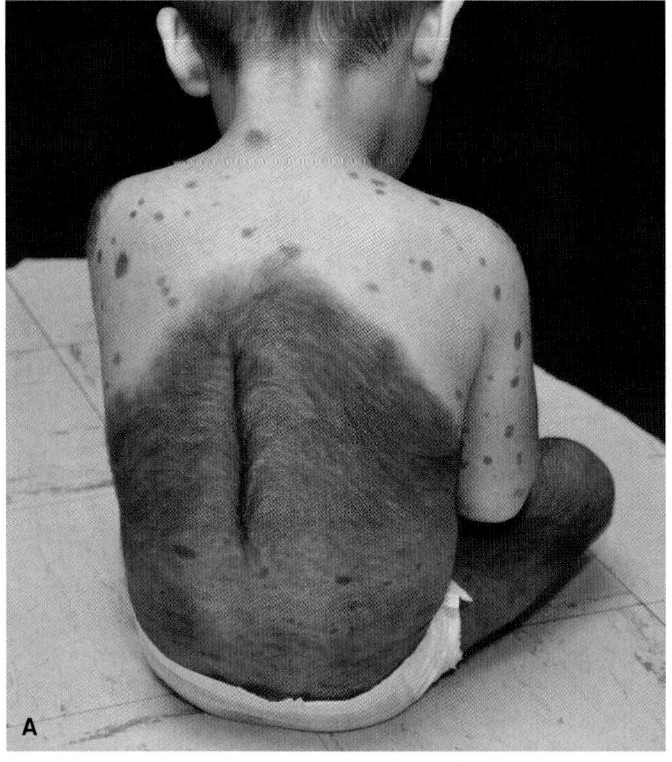

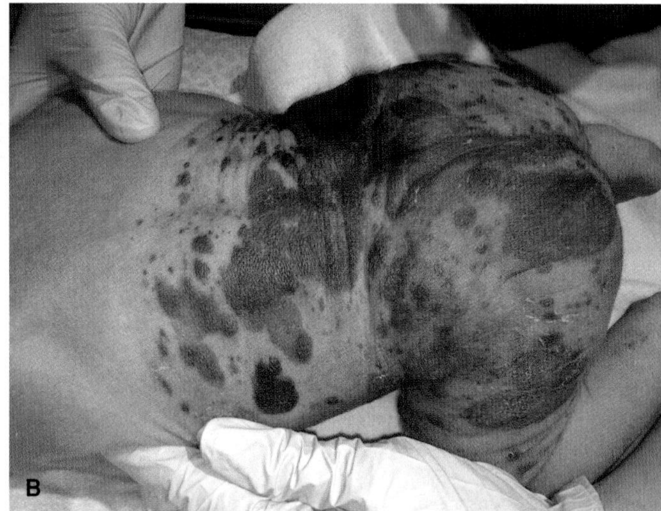

FIGURE 147-2 **A.** A 2-year-old boy with a bathing trunk nevus and numerous satellite congenital nevi. He benefits from regular skin screening and mole monitoring. (*Used with permission from Richard P. Usatine, MD.*) **B.** A giant bathing trunk nevus noted at birth. The dark black colors and variations in color make this a very concerning congenital nevus. Again, regular skin screening and mole monitoring will be a regular part of his care. (*Used with permission from Carrie Griffin, MD.*)

ABCDE guidelines are listed below followed by newly proposed guidelines to increase the sensitivity of detecting melanoma in children.

TRADITIONAL ABCDE GUIDELINES

ABCDE guidelines for diagnosing melanoma (**Figure 147-3**).[7]

A = *Asymmetry*. Most early melanomas are asymmetrical—A line through the middle will not create matching halves. Benign nevi are usually round and symmetrical (**Figure 147-4**).

B = *Border*. The borders of early melanomas are often uneven and may have scalloped or notched edges. Benign nevi have smoother, more even borders (**Figure 147-4**).

C = *Color* variation. Benign nevi are usually a single shade of brown. Melanomas are often in varied shades of brown, tan, or black, but may also exhibit red, white, or blue (**Figures 147-4** and **147-5**).

D = *Diameter* greater than or equal to 6 mm. Melanomas tend to grow larger than most nevi. Note that melanomas in children or adults can present less than 6 mm in diameter (**Figure 147-5**).

E = *Evolving* could be in size, shape, symptoms (itching, tenderness), surface (especially bleeding), and shades of color.

Modified ABCD criteria in children were developed and proposed by Cordoro, et al. in a recent large cohort study.[6] The criteria were developed from the data presented in **Figure 147-6** that compared conventional ABCDE criteria with other presenting features of melanoma in children.

In children, particularly those younger than 13, new ABCD detection criteria are needed as many childhood melanomas present as pink or skin colored uniform bumps. The modified ABCD detection criteria are listed below:

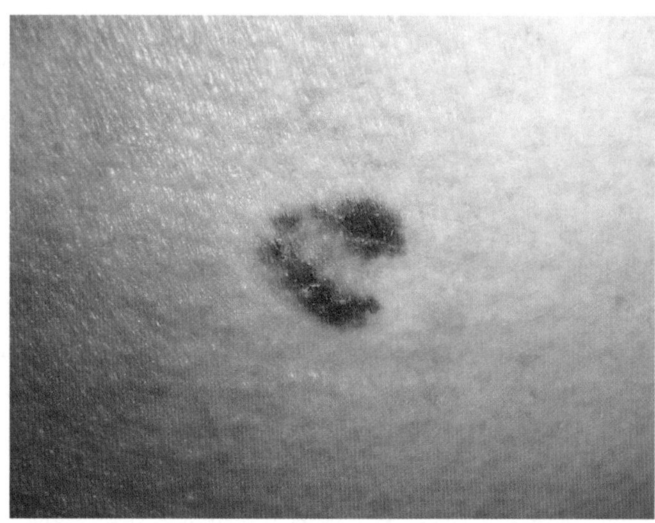

FIGURE 147-3 Superficial spreading melanoma on the neck demonstrates many traditional ABCDE features of melanoma. (*Used with permission from Richard P. Usatine, MD.*)

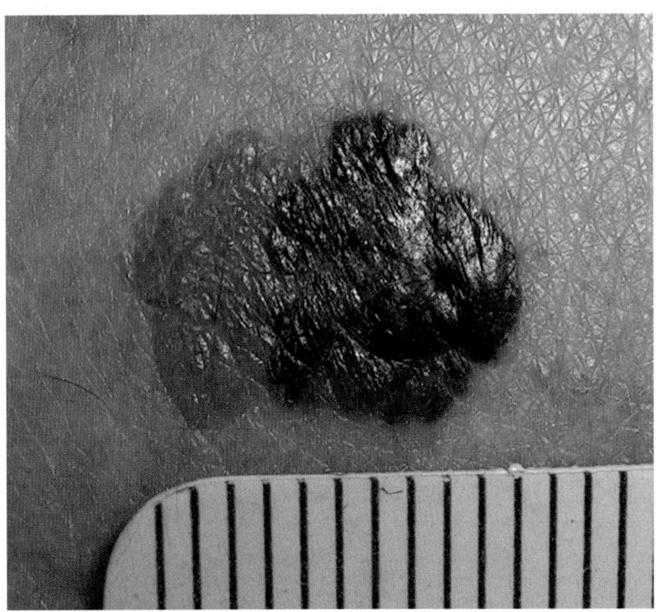

FIGURE 147-4 Marked asymmetry, border irregularity, color variation, and increased diameter characterize this thin melanoma. (*Used with permission from Richard P. Usatine, MD.*)

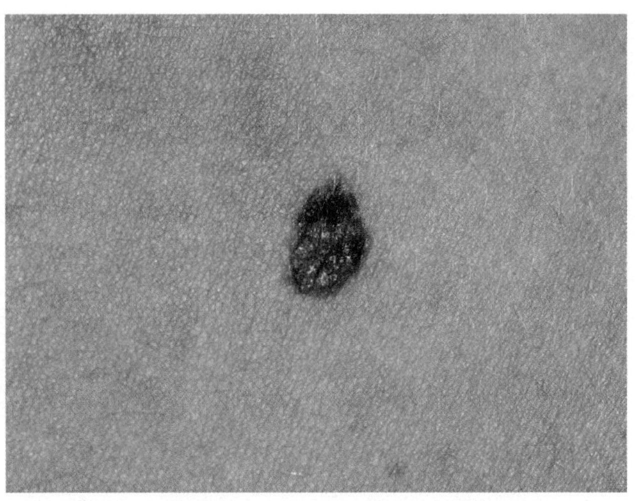

FIGURE 147-5 Small 4 × 5 mm melanoma that developed on the back of an 11-year-old boy. This melanoma demonstrated asymmetry and variation in color only. (*Used with permission from Kelly M. Cordoro, MD.*)

A = *Amelanotic* lesions are more common in children than adults (**Figures 147-1**, **147-6**, and **147-7**).

B = *Bleeding, Bump*. Suspect any new bleeding papule or macule.

C = *Color uniformity* may be present in childhood melanoma rather than the color variation that is traditionally associated with melanoma (**Figure 147-8**).

D = *De Novo, any diameter*. Any lesion arising out of the blue is suspicious in children.

Conventional subtypes of adult melanomas—superficial spreading, nodular, lentigo maligna melanoma, and acral lentiginous melanoma—are not as relevant in diagnosing childhood melanoma. In contrast, most childhood melanoma—especially in children under 10—is more clinically and histologically ambiguous and defies these classifications.[6] Any subtype may be classified as amelanotic when pigment is absent to a degree that the lesion is pink in color. In adults, this is rare, representing less than 5 percent of all melanoma. In children, however, up to 70 percent of melanoma may be amelanotic (**Table 147-1**).[6]

- Other rare melanoma variants include (**1**) nevoid melanomas, (**2**) malignant blue nevus, (**3**) Desmoplastic/Spindled/Neurotropic Melanoma, (**4**) Clear Cell Sarcoma (in fact a melanoma), (**5**) Animal-Type Melanoma, (**6**) Ocular Melanoma (**7**) and mucosal (lentiginous) melanoma.[8]

TYPICAL DISTRIBUTION

In children, the most common sites of melanoma are the trunk and lower limbs in females and the head and neck in males.[1]

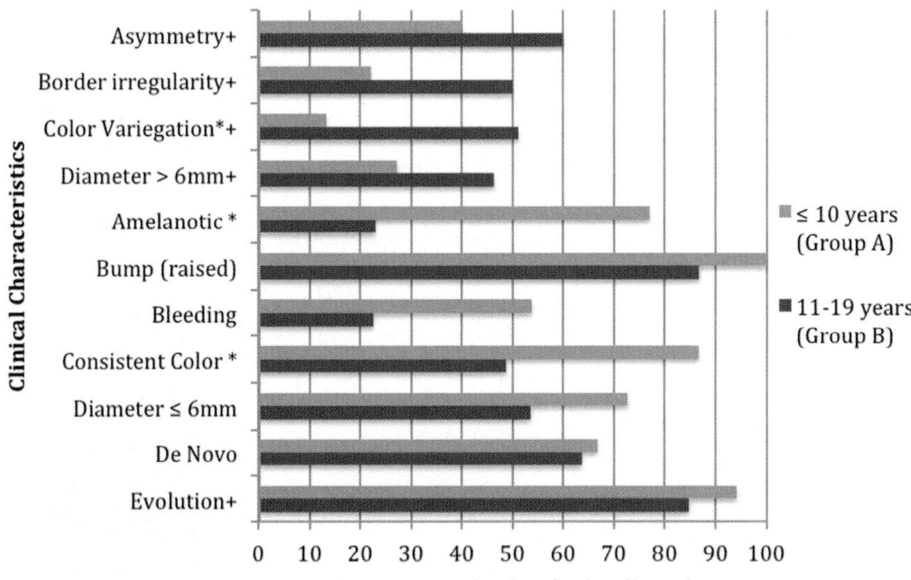

FIGURE 147-6 Comparison of conventional ABCDE criteria with other presenting features of melanoma in children. (*Used with permission from and copyright Cordoro KM, et al. Pediatric melanoma: Results of a large cohort study and proposal for modified ABCD detection criteria for children. J Am Acad Dermatol. 2013.*)

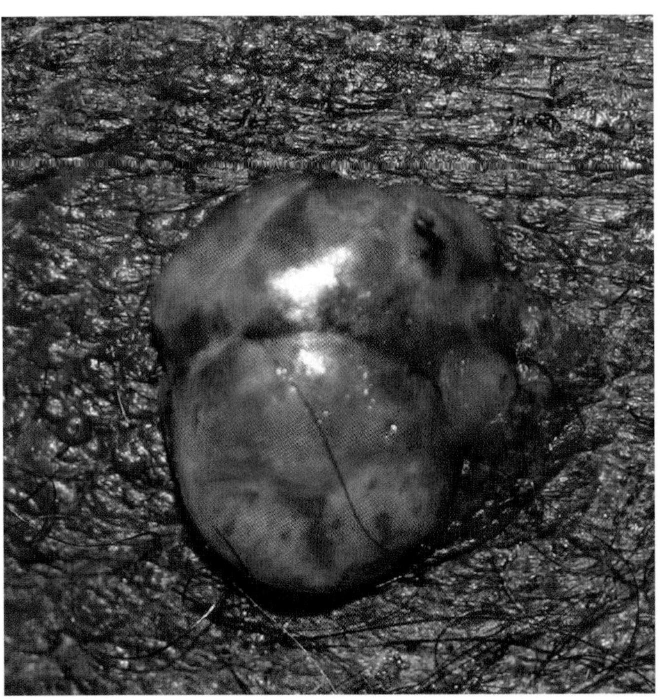

FIGURE 147-7 Amelanotic melanoma that developed in a large congenital melanocytic nevus. The boy was only 16-years old. (*Used with permission from Kelly M. Cordoro, MD.*)

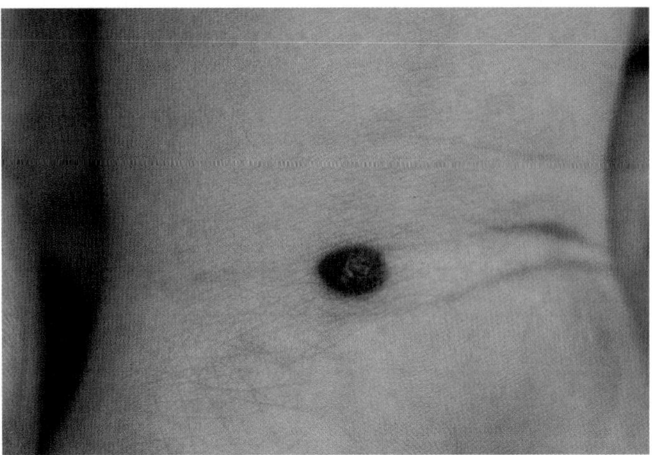

FIGURE 147-8 Spitzoid melanoma on the wrist of a 4-year-old girl. (*Used with permission from John L. Pfenninger, MD.*)

DERMOSCOPY

Dermoscopy is a useful tool in pigmented lesions in adults and in children, though it is less well characterized in children. Dermoscopy is painless, adds information, and can assist in the decision to biopsy.[9] In a prospective study of 401 lesions evaluated for melanoma by experts in dermoscopy, the sensitivity of 66.6 percent with ABCDE criteria

TABLE 147-1 Melanoma Subtypes Versus Melanoma Subtypes in Children

Melanoma Subtypes in Adults	Melanoma Subtypes in Children
From most frequent to least frequent	From most frequent to least frequent.
1. Superficial spreading melanoma	1. *Unclassified or ambiguous melanoma* represents a large majority of those found in children. Childhood melanoma often defies traditional histologic classification.
2. Nodular melanoma	2. *Nodular melanoma* is the most common subtype of melanoma in children and is represented by an enlarging papule or nodule. A flat macule that is atypical may be monitored over a short period, but a papule or raised lesion should be biopsied rather than monitored if clinically suspicious.
3. Lentigo maligna melanoma	3. *Superficial spreading* melanoma has a radial growth pattern prior to vertical invasion. The first sign is the appearance of a flat macule or slightly raised and discolored papule or plaque. Colors may vary and include tan, brown, black, red, blue, or white. These lesions may arise at the edge of an older nevus and can arise anywhere on the body.
4. Acral lentiginous melanoma	4. *Spitzoid melanoma* presents with features similar to a Spitz nevus with a smooth dome shaped papule or nodule that is hairless and brown or red-brown in color (**Figure 147-8**).
5. Amelanotic melanoma represents less than 5 percent of adult melanomas and present as pink to flesh colored macules or papules that may be easily mistaken for an inflammatory papule or non-melanoma skin cancer. In children, up to 70 percent of melanoma may be amelanotic.[6]	5. *Acral lentiginous melanoma* of the hands and feet is rare in children.

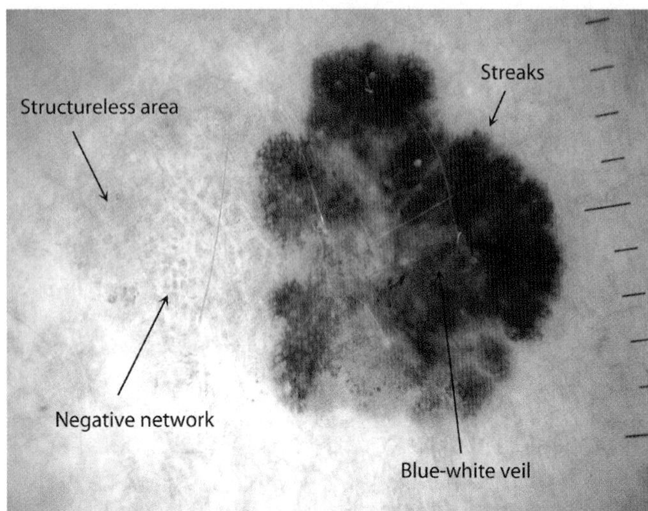

FIGURE 147-9 Observe many dermoscopic features of melanoma in this superficial spreading melanoma. This is the dermoscopic view of the melanoma in **Figure 147-4**. (*Used with permission from Richard P. Usatine, MD.*)

improved to 80 percent, and specificity rose from 79.3 to 89.1 percent (**Figure 147-9**).[9]

In a study of dermoscopy done by 60 physicians (35 general practitioners, 10 dermatologists, and 16 dermatology trainees) on unaided photos of 40 lesions using the ABCD rule, the Menzies method, a 7-point checklist, and pattern analysis, the sensitivity rose over the unaided eye.[10] In children, melanoma will deviate from the benign dermoscopic patterns and have at least one melanoma specific criteria, most commonly atypical vascular structure and crystalline structure (**Figure 147-1**).[11]

Accepted dermoscopic local features of melanoma include:

- Atypical network (includes branched-streaks).
- Streaks—Pseudopods and radial streaming.
- Atypical dots and globules.
- Negative pigment network.
- Blotch (off center).
- Blue-white veil/peppering over macular areas (regression).
- Blue-white veil over raised areas.
- Vascular structures.
- Peripheral tan/brown structureless areas.
- Crystalline structures

Figure 147-8 demonstrates a number of these features.

BIOPSY

In children, melanoma diagnosis is often delayed because of the rarity of the diagnosis and a natural tendency to avoid biopsy. Still, a full thickness skin biopsy remains the gold standard for diagnosing melanoma. Complete excisional biopsy with close margins (2 mm) is ideal for histologic diagnosis and tumor staging. Although there is evidence that an incisional biopsy of a portion of a melanoma does not worsen the prognosis, this should only be the rare case when a lesion is too large to excise in the office. When the clinical impression differs markedly from the pathology report, discuss the case with the reading pathologist and share clinical photos if you haven't done so already. You may need to have the pathologist prepare "deeper sections" or "step sections"—meaning more slices from the same "loaf of bread." Additionally, if the diagnosis of melanoma was expected and the result of an incisional biopsy does not meet the expectation, go forward with a complete excision or refer to a surgeon who can.

The National Comprehensive Cancer Network (NCCN) Melanoma Guidelines on the Principles of Biopsy state:[12]

- Excisional biopsy (elliptical, punch [when whole lesion is small], or saucerization) with 1- to 3-mm margins is preferred. Avoid wider margins to permit accurate subsequent lymphatic mapping.
- The orientation of the biopsy should be planned with definitive wide excision in mind.
- Full-thickness incisional or punch biopsy of clinically thickest portion of the lesion is acceptable in certain anatomic areas (e.g., palm/sole, digit, face, and ear) or for very large lesions.
- Shave biopsy (not saucerization or deep shave) may compromise pathologic diagnosis and complete assessment of Breslow thickness, but is acceptable when the index of suspicion is low.[13]

Despite strong opinions about biopsy technique, there is evidence that a scoop shave biopsy leads to an accurate diagnosis and staging 97 percent of the time.[13] Still, a shallow shave biopsy may miss important staging information and may cause "upstaging" and unnecessary lymph node biopsy.

DIFFERENTIAL DIAGNOSIS

Nevi of all types may mimic melanoma. In children, because of the high percentage of melanomas that are melanocytic, broaden the differential to include many inflammatory and vascular papules. Nevi of all types can mimic melanoma. Congenital nevi can be especially large and asymmetrical. Therefore, it is important to ask the patient if the pigmented area has been there from birth and consider how it has changed over time.

- Atypical nevi, also called dysplastic nevi, often mimic melanoma (**Figure 147-10**). When an atypical nevus is suspicious for

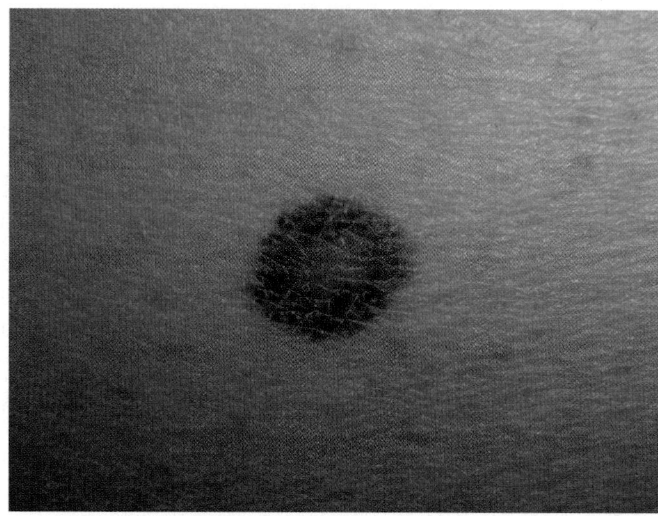

FIGURE 147-10 This benign compound dysplastic nevus has several features of melanoma including color variation and size greater than 6 mm. (*Used with permission from Richard P. Usatine, MD.*)

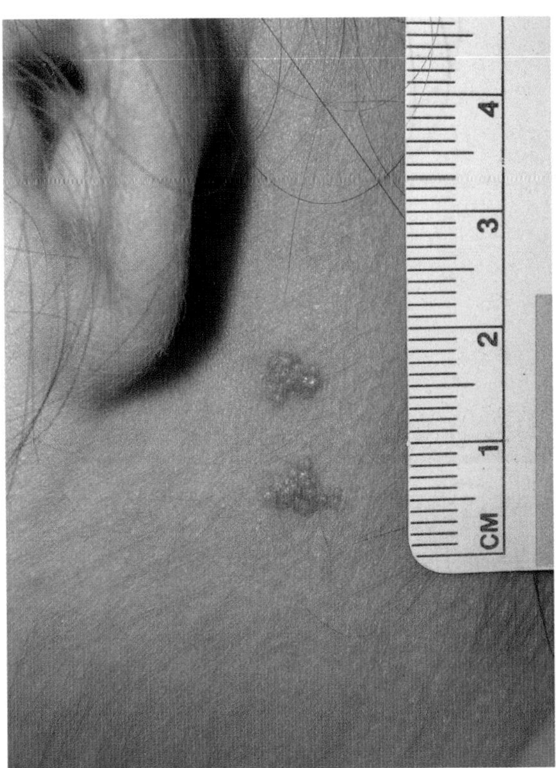

FIGURE 147-11 These epidermal nevi were increasing in size, but are not melanocytic in origin and have no potential to become melanoma. (*Used with permission from Richard P. Usatine, MD.*)

melanoma, perform a full thickness biopsy or a broad scoop shave for histology. Only the less suspicious dysplastic nevi should be followed with photography or serial exams.

- Epidermal nevi are warty in appearance and may fall along embryonic cleavage lines. These are benign and not precancerous but may grow rapidly especially during puberty (**Figure 147-11**).
- Pyogenic granulomas are benign vascular neoplasms that grow rapidly and are often friable. They are frequently associated with pregnancy, but can occur without a clear cause and mimic an amelanotic nodular melanoma (**Figures 147-12** and **147-13**).
- Pseudolymphoma presents as a pink papule or plaque without significant scaling that persists for weeks to months and may be associated with a history of an insect or spider bite (**Figure 147-14**).
- Dermatofibromas are fibrotic nodules that occur most frequently on the legs and arms. They can be any color from skin color to black and often have a brown halo surrounding them. A pinch test will produce a dimpling of the skin in most cases.
- Warts in children may mimic melanocytic lesions including Spitz nevi and melanoma (**Figures 147-15** and **147-16**).
- Benign adnexal tumors such as pilomatricomas may appear similar to a nodular melanoma and can occur on the head and neck (**Figure 147-17**).

MANAGEMENT

- Cutaneous melanoma is surgically treated with complete full skin depth excision using margins determined by the Breslow depth.

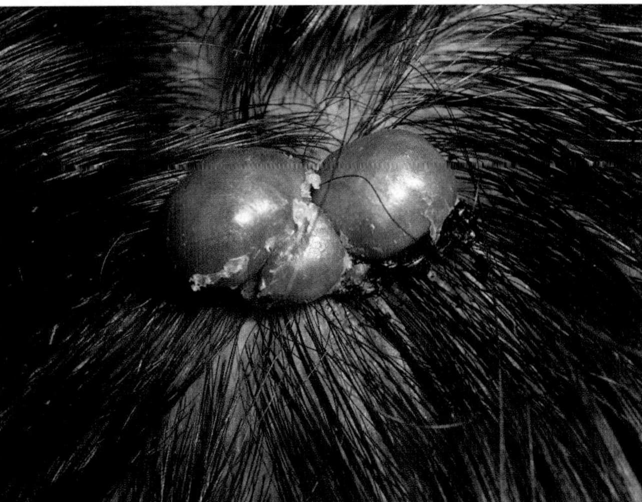

FIGURE 147-12 This pyogenic granuloma formed rapidly and bled easily on the scalp of this teenager. It was excised and sent for pathology to make sure it was not an amelanotic melanoma. (*Used with permission from Richard P. Usatine, MD.*)

This depth is a measure of tumor thickness from the granular layer of the epidermis to the point of deepest invasion using an ocular micrometer.

- Current recommendations for excision margins range from 5 mm for in situ lesions to 1 to 2 cm for invasive lesions. A recent study showed significant benefit with a 9 mm margin on Mohs excision of melanoma in situ compared with 6 mm margins at a referral center.[14]
- Sentinel lymph node biopsies are recommended for tumors of greater than or equal to 1 mm in depth (**Figure 147-18**) and should be considered for thinner lesions with ulceration or more than 1 mitosis per mm^2. Even in patients with thin melanoma with mitoses above 1 per mm^2 sentinel lymph node biopsy should be considered according to the most recent guidelines.[15] In these guidelines, mitoses per mm^2 has replaced Clark's levels to distinguish T1a from T1b tumors.[15]

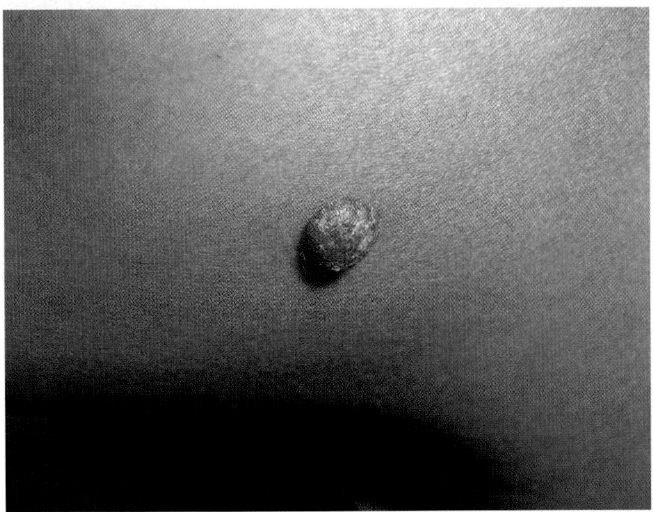

FIGURE 147-13 A pyogenic granuloma on the arm of a young boy mimics an amelanotic melanoma. (*Used with permission from Richard P. Usatine, MD.*)

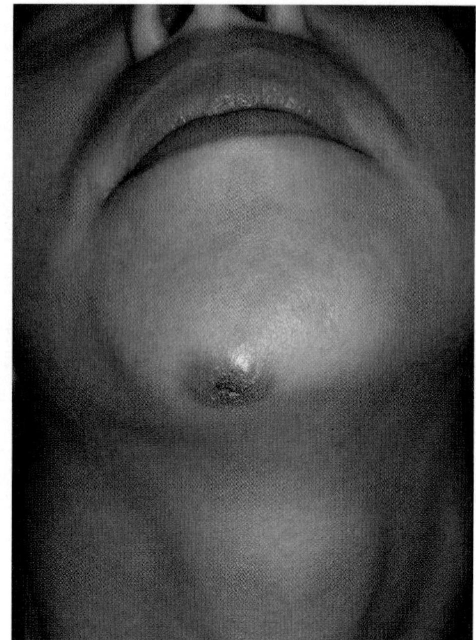

FIGURE 147-14 This pink nodule developed rapidly on the chin of a 11-year-old girl and did not resolve after several months. Pathology was consistent with pseudolymphoma. (*Used with permission from Richard P. Usatine, MD.*)

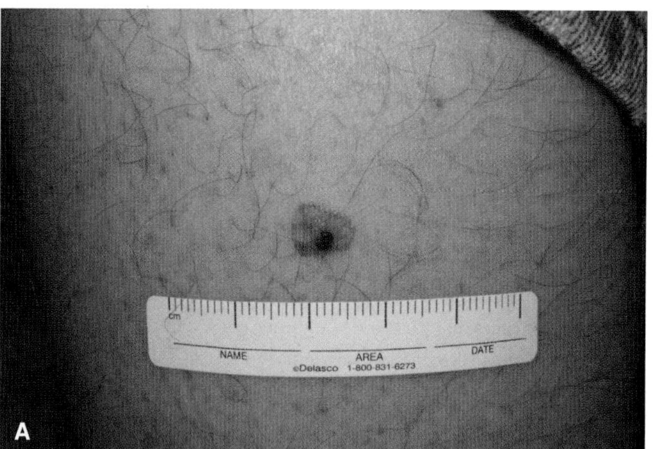

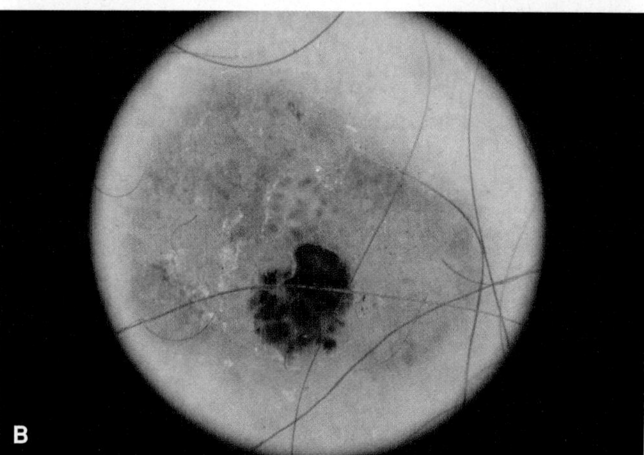

FIGURE 147-15 This pink and black wart with dotted vessels appeared suddenly on the leg of a teenage boy and shares some features of melanoma. (**A**) Clinical (**B**) Dermoscopy. (*Used with permission from Jonathan B. Karnes, MD.*)

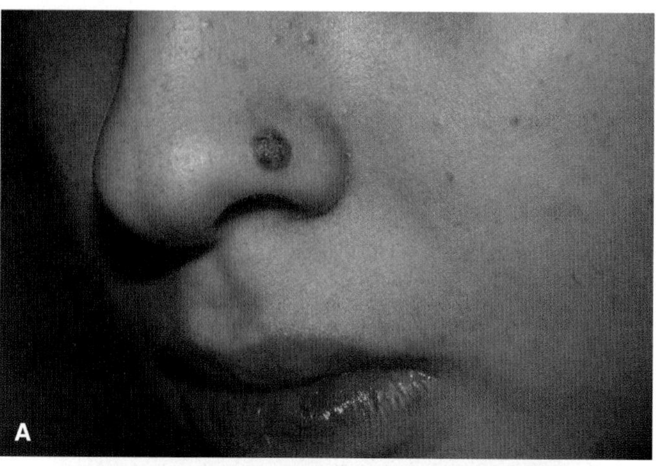

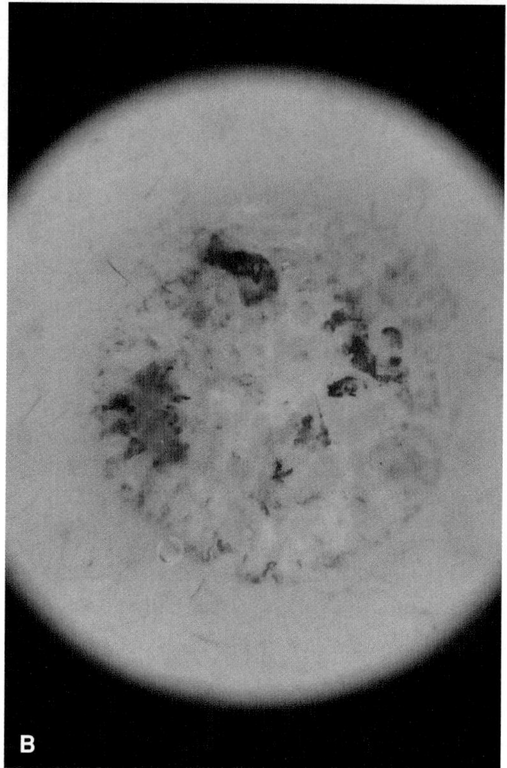

FIGURE 147-16 **A** and **B**. This papule appeared most consistent with a Spitz nevus, but histology revealed a wart with unusual pseudoepitheliomatous hyperplasia. (*Used with permission from Jonathan B. Karnes, MD.*)

- Melanoma staging takes into account tumor thickness and metastasis and prognosis worsens statistically with each increasing stage from 0 to IV. A patient with an in situ melanoma and no nodal metastasis is considered stage 0. Thicker tumors that remain localized to the skin may be staged as high as stage IIC and subcategories are based on tumor thickness and presence of ulceration. Any lymph node metastasis is considered stage III or higher and any distant metastasis beyond lymph nodes is categorized as stage IV.[16]
- Patients with advanced melanoma should be referred to medical oncology and may receive combination therapy with multiple chemotherapeutic agents and immunotherapy. Many trials are ongoing and three new drugs including interferon 2-alpha, vemurafenib,

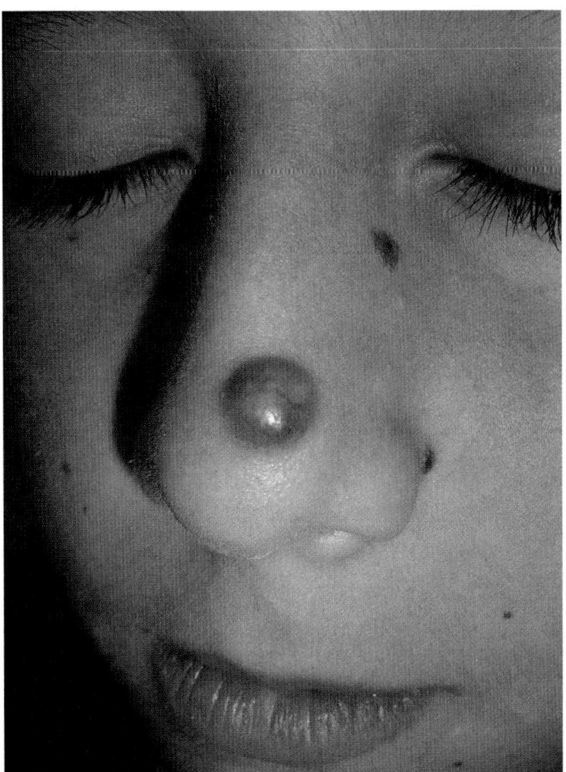

FIGURE 147-17 A pink and purple nodule on the nose that had grown over several months. This was excised and turned out to be a benign pilomatricoma. This is clinically suspected when rock hard calcifications are palpable within the tumor. (*Used with permission from Richard P. Usatine, MD.*)

and ipilimumab have been approved for use in advanced melanoma. Treatment regimens in children are similar to regimens in adults.

- Recently two new chemotherapeutic agents have been FDA approved for the treatment of metastatic melanoma. One, vemurafenib is a monoclonal antibody targeting the BRAF mutation

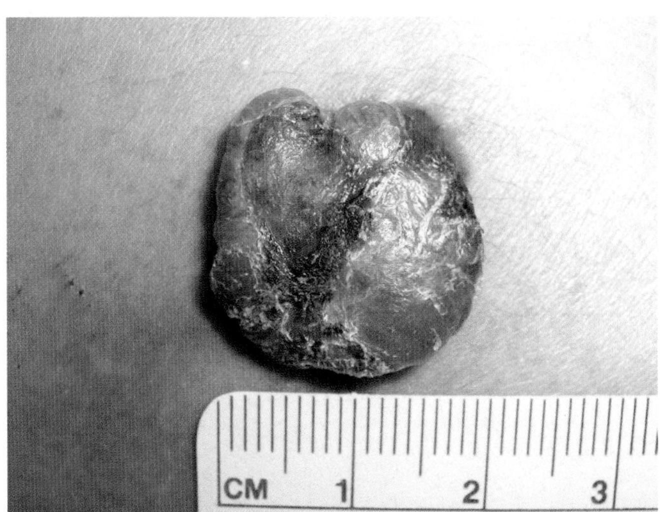

FIGURE 147-18 Thick ulcerated nodular melanoma on the back was mostly amelanotic in appearance. The melanoma depth was greater than 1 mm and the patient was sent for a complete excision with a sentinel node biopsy. (*Used with permission from Richard P. Usatine, MD.*)

expressed on many melanomas. Ipilimumaub prevents dampening of the immune system by blocking a regulatory molecule CTLA-4. Both of these medications used in combination with dacarbazine have shown a small but significant increase in progression free survival in adults and are in ongoing trials in children.[17]

FOLLOW-UP

The need for follow-up is largely determined by the stage of the disease. Updates to the staging criteria are published by the American Joint Committee. As previously mentioned, the prognosis is worsened by increasing depth, mitotic rate, ulceration, positive lymph nodes, and metastases.

The follow-up for stage 0 and 1 cutaneous melanoma includes regular skin examinations by a physician trained in skin screening. Total body photography is available in limited areas, but may be of benefit in monitoring patients with multiple nevi. The rate of subsequent cutaneous melanomas among persons with a history of melanoma was found to be more than 10 times the rate of a first cutaneous melanoma and the highest incidence of recurrence was in the first 3 to 5 years after initial diagnosis.[18,19]

PATIENT EDUCATION

Advise patients to avoid future sun exposure and monitor their skin for new and changing moles. Advise avoidance of artificial tanning. Recommend a complete skin examination yearly by a physician trained to detect early melanoma. A large portion of adult melanoma is caused from childhood exposure.[4]

REFERENCES

1. Wong JR, Harris JK, Rodriguez-Galindo C, Johnson KJ. Incidence of childhood and adolescent melanoma in the United States: 1973-2009. *Pediatrics*. 2013;131(5):846-854.
2. Jemal A, Saraiya M, Patel P, et al. Recent trends in cutaneous melanoma incidence and death rates in the United States, 1992-2006. *J Am Acad Dermatol*. 2011;65(5:1):S17-25.e1–3.
3. Siegel R, Naishadham D, Jemal A. Cancer statistics, 2012. *CA Cancer J Clin*. 2012;62(1):10-29.
4. Whiteman DC, Whiteman CA, Green AC. Childhood sun exposure as a risk factor for melanoma: a systematic review of epidemiologic studies. *Cancer Causes Control*. 2001;12(1):69-82.
5. Moran A, O'Hara C, Khan S, et al. Risk of cancer other than breast or ovarian in individuals with BRCA1 and BRCA2 mutations. *Familial Cancer*. 2011;11(2):235-242.
6. Cordoro KM, Gupta D, Frieden IJ, McCalmont T, Kashani-Sabet M. Pediatric melanoma: Results of a large cohort study and proposal for modified ABCD detection criteria for children. *J Am Acad Dermatol*. 2013.
7. Thomas L, Tranchand P, Berard F, Secchi T, Colin C, Moulin G. Semiological value of ABCDE criteria in the diagnosis of cutaneous pigmented tumors. *Dermatology (Basel)*. 1998;197(1):11-17.

8. MD JLB, MD JLJ, MD RPR. *Dermatology e-dition: Text with Continually Updated Online Reference, 2-Volume Set, 2e*. 2nd ed. Mosby; 2007.

9. Benelli C, Roscetti E, Pozzo VD, Gasparini G, Cavicchini S. The dermoscopic versus the clinical diagnosis of melanoma. *Eur J Dermatol*. 1999;9(6):470-476.

10. Dolianitis C, Kelly J, Wolfe R, Simpson P. Comparative performance of 4 dermoscopic algorithms by nonexperts for the diagnosis of melanocytic lesions. *Archives of Dermatology*. 2005;141(8):1008-1014.

11. Haliasos EC, Kerner M, Jaimes N, et al. Dermoscopy for the Pediatric Dermatologist Part III: Dermoscopy of Melanocytic Lesions. *Pediatr Dermatol*. 2013;30(3):281-293.

12. Coit DG, Andtbacka R, Bichakjian CK, et al. NCCN Melanoma Panel. Melanoma. *J Natl Compr Canc Netw*. 2009;7(3):250-275.

13. Zager JS, Hochwald SN, Marzban SS, et al. Shave biopsy is a safe and accurate method for the initial evaluation of melanoma. *J. Am. Coll. Surg*. 2011;212(4):454-460.

14. Kunishige JH, Brodland DG, Zitelli JA. Surgical margins for melanoma in situ. *J Am Acad Dermatol*. 2012;66(3):438-444.

15. Lens MB, Dawes M, Goodacre T, Bishop JAN. Excision margins in the treatment of primary cutaneous melanoma: a systematic review of randomized controlled trials comparing narrow vs wide excision. *Arch Surg*. 2002;137(10):1101-1105.

16. Balch CM, Gershenwald JE, Soong S-J, et al. Final version of 2009 AJCC melanoma staging and classification. *J. Clin. Oncol*. 2009;27(36):6199-6206.

17. Lee B, Mukhi N, Liu D. Current management and novel agents for malignant melanoma. *J Hematol Oncol*. 2012;5(1):3-3.

18. Tsao H, Atkins MB, Sober AJ. Management of cutaneous melanoma. *N. Engl. J. Med*. 2004;351(10):998-1012.

19. Levi F, Randimbison L, Te V-C, La Vecchia C. High constant incidence rates of second cutaneous melanomas. *Int. J. Cancer*. 2005;117(5):877-879.

SECTION 11 INFILTRATIVE IMMUNOLOGIC

148 GRANULOMA ANNULARE

Melissa Muszynski, MD
Richard P. Usatine, MD

PATIENT STORY

A 3-year-old boy presents with an annular eruption on the dorsum of his foot for 6 months. Prior to this visit the child was treated with multiple topical antifungal creams prescribed by other health care providers for presumed tinea corporis. The absence of significant scaling and the failure to respond to topical antifungals point to the diagnosis of granuloma annulare (GA). Also, this is a common location for GA. A KOH preparation was also negative for hyphae. The diagnosis was discussed with the parents and the decision was made to try a mid-potency corticosteroid topically for treatment. While intralesional steroids are more effective this is not a viable option for 3-year-old child.

INTRODUCTION

GA is a common dermatologic condition that presents as small, light-red, dermal papules coalescing into annular plaques without scale. As the previous vignette describes, it is often mistaken as nummular eczema or tinea corporis. Distribution, pattern, and lack of scale are important diagnostic clues.

EPIDEMIOLOGY

- GA affects twice as many females than males.[1]
- The four presentations of GA are localized, disseminated/generalized, perforating, and subcutaneous.
- Of the four variations, the localized form is seen most often.[1]

ETIOLOGY AND PATHOPHYSIOLOGY

- Benign cutaneous, inflammatory disorder of unknown origin.[1]
- Disease may be self-limiting, but may persist for many years.
- There is a reported association between type 1 diabetes and subcutaneous granuloma annulare in children. One retrospective study looked at 34 children less than 10 years of age with subcutaneous granuloma annulare and found 2 of these children (5.9%) had type 1 diabetes.[2,3] While this is much higher than the prevalence of childhood type 1 diabetes, this does not prove causality.
- Reported associations include viral infections (including HIV), *Borrelia* and streptococcal infections, insect bites, lymphoma, tuberculosis, and trauma.[4,5]
- One proposed mechanism for GA is a delayed-type hypersensitivity reaction as a result of T-helper–type cell (Th)-1 lymphocytic differentiation of macrophages. These macrophages become effector cells that express tumor necrosis factor (TNF)-α and matrix metalloproteinases. The activated macrophages are responsible for dermal collagen matrix degradation.[6]
- An association between high expression of gil-1 oncogene and granulomatous lesions of the skin, including GA, has been established.[7]

RISK FACTORS

The only identifiable risk factor is being a female. There are several associations, but nothing has been shown to be causative.

DIAGNOSIS

CLINICAL FEATURES

Annular lesions have raised borders that are skin-colored to erythematous (**Figures 148-1** and **148-2**). The rings may become

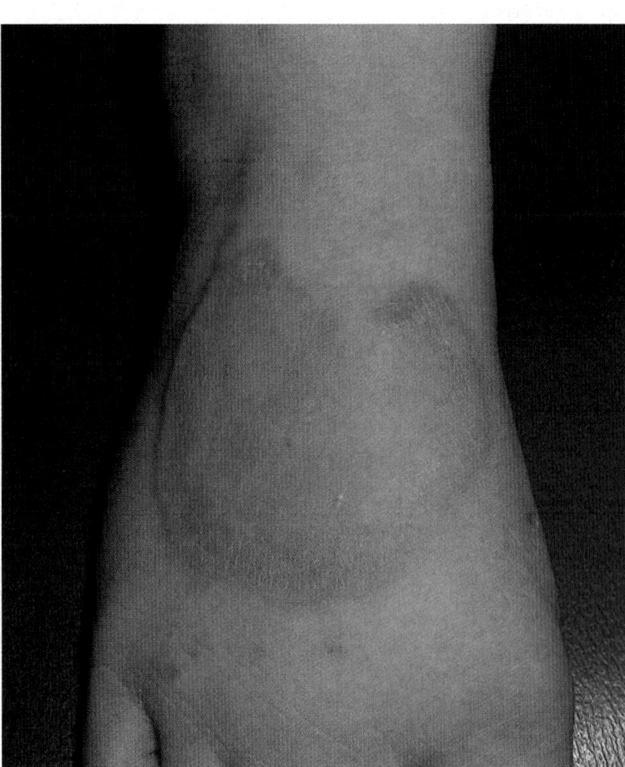

FIGURE 148-1 Granuloma annulare on the dorsum of the foot of a 3-year-old boy for 6 months. (*Used with permission from Richard P. Usatine, MD.*)

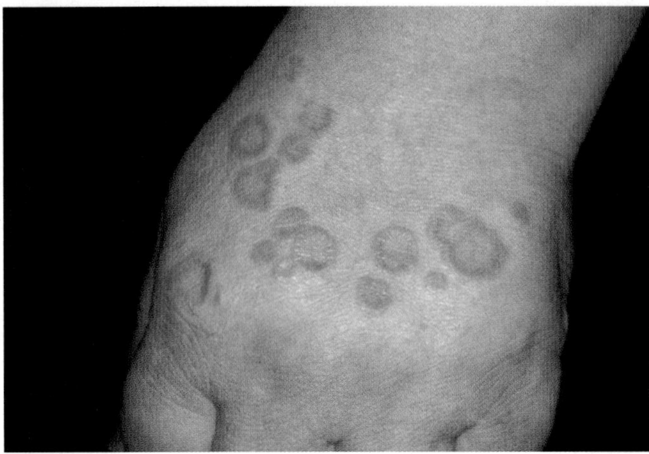

FIGURE 148-2 Disseminated granuloma annulare on the dorsum of the hand. (*Used with permission from Richard P. Usatine, MD.*)

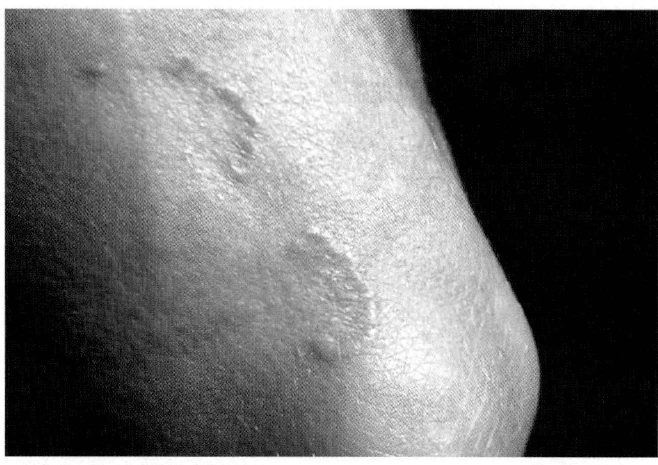

FIGURE 148-4 Granuloma annulare on the elbow showing how the rings may not be complete. (*Used with permission from Richard P. Usatine, MD.*)

hyperpigmented or violaceous (**Figure 148-3**). There is often a central depression within the ring. These lesions range from 2 mm to 5 cm. Although the classical appearance of GA is annular, the lesions may be arcuate instead of forming a complete ring (**Figure 148-4**). Most importantly, there should be no scaling as seen in tinea corporis (ringworm).

TYPICAL DISTRIBUTION

Each of the four types of GA has a different distribution. Localized and disseminated GA differ only in that disseminated lesions can spread to the trunk and neck and may be more pronounced in sun-exposed areas.[8]

1. Localized—This is the most common form of GA affecting 75 percent of GA patients.[1] It typically presents as solitary lesions on the dorsal surfaces of extremities, especially of hands and feet (**Figures 148-1** to **148-3**).
2. Disseminated or generalized—Adults are most affected by this form, which begins in the extremities and can spread to the trunk and neck (**Figures 148-2** and **148-3**).
3. Perforating—Children and young adults present with 1 to hundreds of 1- to 4-mm pinpoint to annular papules (**Figure 148-5**). They may coalesce to form a typical annular plaque. Although this form can appear anywhere on the body, it has an affinity for extremities, especially the hands and fingers.[9] The papules may exude a thick and creamy or clear and viscous fluid.
4. Subcutaneous—These lesions present as rapidly growing, nonpainful, subcutaneous or dermal nodules on the feet, fingers, hands, scalp, and forehead. Subcutaneous GA most commonly affects children, with a mean age of 3.9 years (**Figure 148-6**).[8,10] These lesions are often ill-defined and less discrete (**Figure 148-7**). They can erupt as a single lesion or crops of lesions.

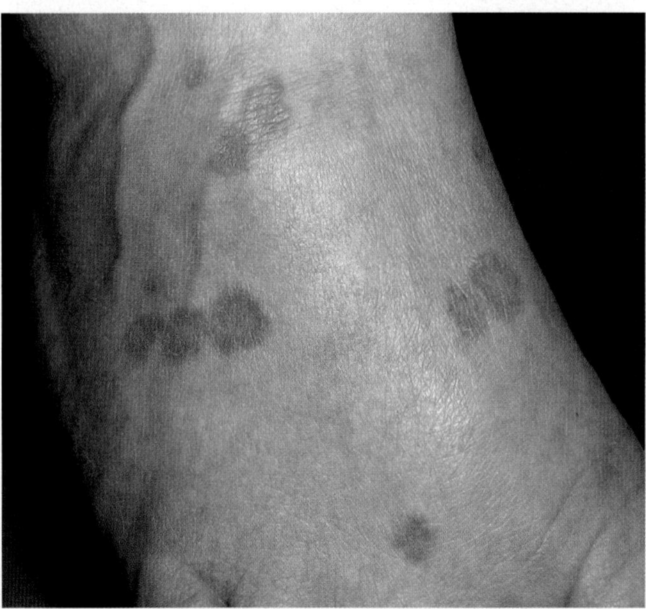

FIGURE 148-3 Disseminated granuloma annulare on the dorsum of the foot. The rings are flatter and many are conjoined. Note the hyperpigmentation. (*Used with permission from Richard P. Usatine, MD.*)

LABORATORY STUDIES

Often a diagnosis of GA is made on clinical presentation alone, without the need for biopsy. Subcutaneous GA may be an exception, as the unusual appearance may be mistaken for a rheumatoid nodule. Histologic examination reveals an increase of mucin, which is a hallmark of GA. There is also a dense infiltrate of histiocytes in the mid-dermis and sparse perivascular lymphocytic infiltrate. The histiocytes are either organized as palisading cells lining a collection of mucin or as a diffuse interstitial pattern. There are no signs of epidermal change.[5]

DIFFERENTIAL DIAGNOSIS

- Tinea corporis has a raised, scaling border and can present on any body surface. KOH preparation reveals hyphae with multiple branches (see Chapter 123, Tinea Corporis).
- Erythema annulare centrifugum has an affinity for thighs and legs. The diameter of these lesions can expand at a rate of 2 to 5 mm/day

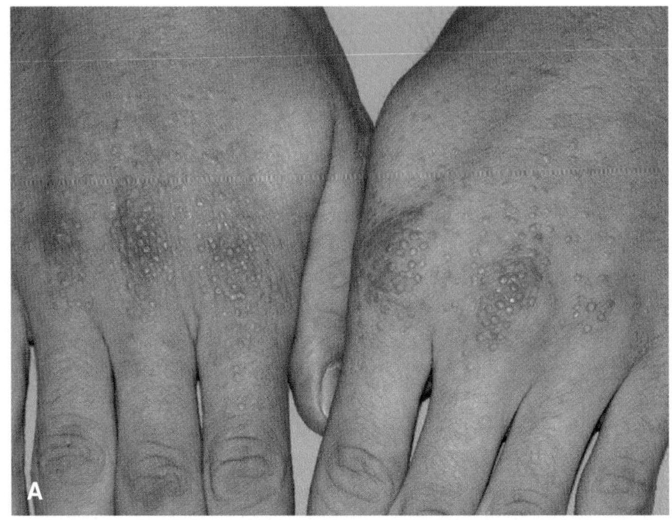

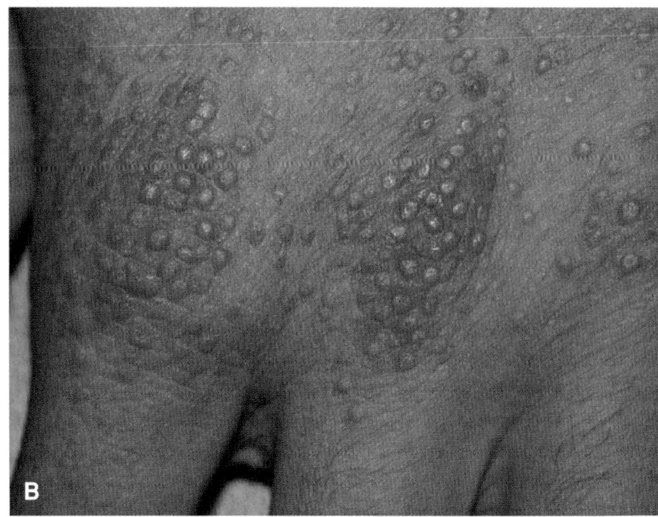

FIGURE 148-5 **A.** Perforating granuloma annulare in a 17-year-old boy with asymptomatic dorsal hand lesions since 9 months of age. Within the previous six months lesions began to appear on both elbows. This was previously misdiagnosed as molluscum contagiosum. **B.** This rare perforating subset of granuloma annulare affects the dorsum of the hands and extensor surfaces in children and young adults. (*Used with permission from Eric Kraus, MD.*)

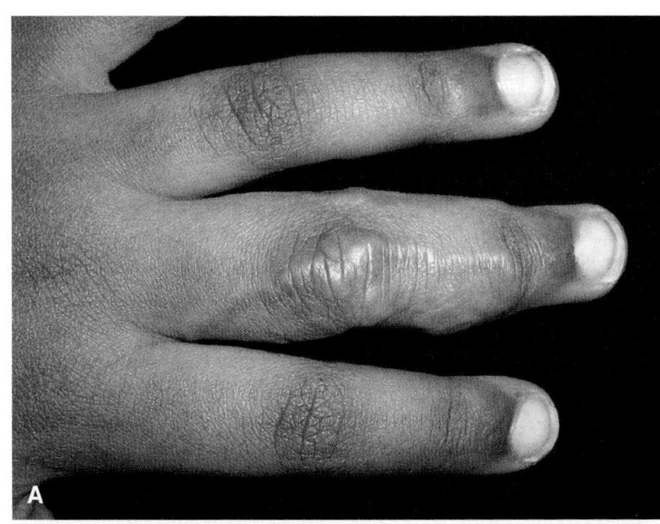

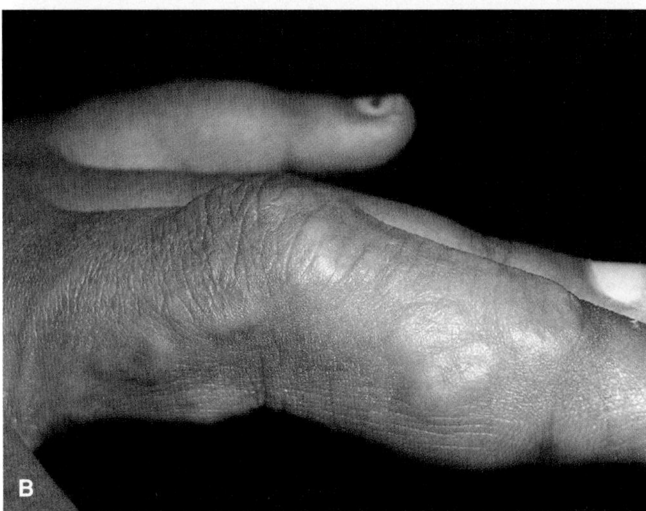

FIGURE 148-6 **A.** Subcutaneous granuloma annulare in a 7-year-old girl showing one large ring on the dorsum of the finger with soft-tissue infiltration. **B.** Subcutaneous GA in a 7-year-old girl showing thickening of the involved finger along with the small annular patterns. Note the soft-tissue infiltration that has distorted the finger anatomy. (*Used with permission from Richard P. Usatine, MD.*)

and may present with a trailing scale inside the advancing border.[2] Biopsy is helpful to differentiate this condition from GA.

- Nummular eczema presents commonly on extremities, but is almost always associated with scaling plaques and intense itching (see Chapter 133, Nummular Eczema).
- Pityriasis rosea often has oval lesions with a trailing collarette of scale. The lesions are minimally raised and have scale that is absent in GA (see Chapter 137, Pityriasis Rosea).
- Rheumatoid nodules may mimic appearance of subcutaneous GA. These nodules are often seen over the elbows, fingers, and other joints in a patient with joint pains and other clinical signs of arthritis (see Chapter 172, Juvenile Rheumatoid Arthritis). Rheumatoid nodules have fibrin deposition on histologic examination, in contrast to mucin in GA.

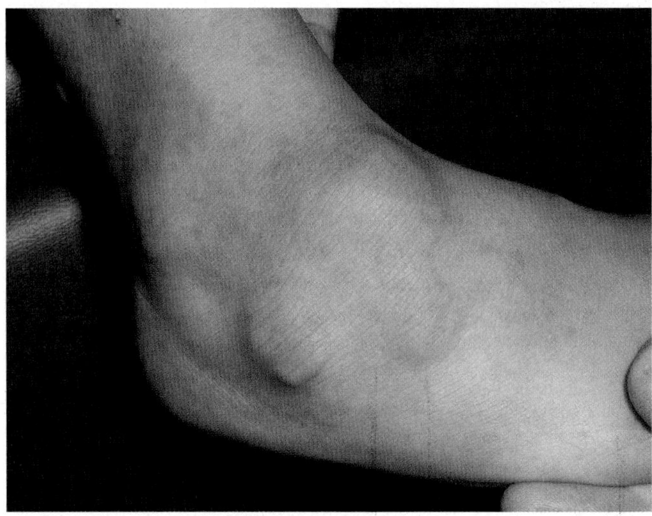

FIGURE 148-7 Subcutaneous granuloma annulare in a 4-year-old boy over the lateral foot with soft-tissue infiltration. The rings are less discrete than localized granuloma annulare. (*Used with permission from Richard P. Usatine, MD.*)

MANAGEMENT

The evidence for various treatments is at best small series of cases that are not randomized controlled trials. This disease is asymptomatic, and treatments only improve cosmetic appearance. Many patients may want intervention as diffuse lesions can cause psychological distress. Although GA will eventually resolve, some treatments may cause pigment change or atrophy that might be permanent. Several of the treatments below have shown promise, but these treatments may appear to work when in fact the resolution was natural.

LOCALIZED GA

- In a retrospective study of children with localized GA (mean age: 8.6 years), 39 of 42 presented with complete clearance within 2 years. The average duration was 1 year. Researchers of this study consider most treatments unnecessary because of the self-limiting nature of this variation.[9] One treatment option is watchful waiting, and may be the most appropriate in children with this condition after discussing other options with the parents.[10,11] SOR B
- Intralesional corticosteroids can be injected into GA lesions with resolution of the area injected. Inject directly into the ring itself with 3 to 5 mg/mL triamcinolone acetonide (Kenalog) using a 27-gauge needle. SOR C A large completed ring may take 4 injections to reach 360 degrees of the circle. The major complications include hypopigmentation and skin atrophy at the injected sites.
- Cryotherapy was studied using nitrous oxide for 9 patients and liquid nitrogen for 22 patients. The results showed 80 percent clearing after a single freeze; however, 4 of 19 patients treated with liquid nitrogen developed atrophic scars when lesions were larger than 4 cm. All patients developed blisters.[12] Cryoatrophy may possibly be prevented by avoiding freeze thaw cycles greater than 10 seconds and not overlapping treatment areas.[13] SOR C

GENERALIZED/DISSEMINATED GA

- This variant is more difficult to treat, and often has a longer duration than localized GA. It is very rare in children and all the studies have been performed in adults only. Even these studies involved small sample sizes and were not randomized. The studies often involved the use of antibiotics with some reported benefits (rifampin, ofloxacin, minocycline and dapsone).[14,15] SOR C
- UVA1 phototherapy provided good or excellent results in 10 of 20 patients with disseminated GA. In patients with only a satisfactory treatment response, the disease reappeared soon after phototherapy was discontinued.[16] SOR C
- Topical 5 percent imiquimod cream and 0.1 percent tacrolimus ointment were also touted as beneficial in small studies of adults.[17,18] SOR C
- Three adults were treated with vitamin E 400 IU daily and zileuton 2400 mg daily. All responded within 3 months with complete clinical clearing.[20] SOR C

PERFORATING, SUBCUTANEOUS

- Although we could find no specific data to inform the treatment of these less-common types of GA, treatments for both localized and disseminated GA could be applied based on clinical judgment along with patient's severity and preferences.

PROGNOSIS

In 50 percent of cases, there is spontaneous resolution within 2 years; however, recurrence rate is as high as 40 percent.[21] In the study of 34 children with SGA, local recurrence occurred in 38 percent within 1 month to 7 years and recurrences at other locations were documented in 15 percent. Three patients with skin of color may have postinflammatory hyperpigmentation once the papules and plaques resolve.

FOLLOW-UP

Follow-up visits should be offered to patients who want active treatment.

PATIENT EDUCATION

It is important to reassure patients and parents that this disease is self-limiting. Despite a displeasing appearance, the best treatment may be to let lesions resolve naturally. Numerous individual case studies and treatments have been attempted without consistent success. Treatments may produce side effects that are equally as unwanted, but more permanent, than the GA.

PATIENT RESOURCES

- Skinsight. Granuloma Annulare: Information for Adults—**www.skinsight.com/adult/granulomaAnnulare.htm**.

PROVIDER RESOURCES

- Medscape. *Granuloma Annulare*—**http://emedicine.medscape.com/article/1123031**.

REFERENCES

1. Cyr PR. Diagnosis and management of granuloma annulare. *Am Fam Physician*. 2006;74(10):1729-1484.
2. Agrawal, AK, Kammen, BF, Guo H, et al. An unusual presentation of subcutaneous granuloma annulare in associateion with juvenile-onset diabetes: case report and literature review. *Pediatr Dermatolo*. 2012;29(2):202-205.
3. Grogg KL, Nascimento AG. Subcutaneous granuloma annulare in childhood: clinicopathologic features in 34 cases. *Pediatrics* 2001; 107:e42
4. Ghadially R, Garg A. *Granuloma Annulare*. http://emedicine.medscape.com/article/1123031-overview, accessed May 10, 2012.
5. Ko CJ, Glusac EJ, Shapiro PE. Noninfectious granulomas. In: Elder DE, ed. *Lever's Histopathology of the Skin*, 10th ed. Philadelphia, PA: Lippincott Williams & Wilkins; 2009:361-364.

6. Fayyazi A, Schweyer S, Eichmeyer B, et al. Expression of IFN-gamma, coexpression of TNF-alpha and matrix metalloproteinases and apoptosis of T lymphocytes and macrophages in granuloma annulare. *Arch Dermatol Res.* 2000;292:384-390.
7. Macaron NC, Cohen C, Chen SC, Arbiser JL. gli-1 Oncogene is highly expressed in granulomatous skin disorders, including sarcoidosis, granuloma annulare, and necrobiosis lipoidica diabeticorum. *Arch Dermatol.* 2005;141:259-262.
8. Habif TP. *Clinical Dermatology*, 4th ed. St Louis, MO. Mosby; 2004.
9. Smith MD, Downie JB, DiCostanzo D. Granuloma annulare. *Int J Dermatol.* 1997;36:326-333.
10. Martinón-Torres F, Martinón-Sánchez JM, Martinón-Sánchez F. Localized granuloma annulare in children: a review of 42 cases. *Eur J Pediatr.* 1999;158(10):866.
11 Paller AS and Mancini AJ. *Hurwitz Clinical Pediatric Dermatology*, 4th Edition, Philadelphia, PA: Elsevier; 2011.
12. Blume-Peytavi U, Zouboulis CC, Jacobi H, et al. Successful outcome of cryosurgery in patients with granuloma annulare. *Br J Dermatol.* 1994;130(4):494-497.
13. Lebwohl MG, Berth-Jones M, Coulson I. *Treatment of Skin Disease, Comprehensive Therapeutic Strategies*, 2nd ed. St. Louis, MO: Mosby; 2006:251.
14. Marcus DV, Mahmoud BH, Hamzavi IH. Granuloma annulare treated with rifampin, ofloxacin, and minocycline combination therapy. *Arch Dermatol.* 2009;145(7):787-789.
15. Czarnecki DB, Gin D. The response of generalized granuloma annulare to Dapsone. *Acta Derm Venereol (Stockh).* 1986;66;82-84.
16. Schnopp C, Tzaneva S, Mempel M, et al. UVA1 phototherapy for disseminated granuloma annulare. *Photodermatol Photoimmunol Photomed.* 2005;21(2):68-71.
17. Badavanis G, Monastirli A, Pasmatzi E, Tsambaos D. Successful treatment of granuloma annulare with imiquimod cream 5%: a report of four cases. *Acta Derm Venereol.* 2005;85(6):547-548.
18. Jain S, Stephens CJM. Successful treatment of disseminated granuloma annulare with topical tacrolimus. *Br J Dermatol.* 2004; 150:1042-1043.
19. Looney M. Isotretinoin in the treatment of granuloma annulare. *Ann Pharmacother.* 2004;38(3):494-497.
20. Smith KJ, Norwood C, Skelton H. Treatment of disseminated granuloma annulare with a 5-lipoxygenase inhibitor and vitamin E. *Br J Dermatol.* 2002;146(4):667-670.
21. Reisenauer A, White KP, Korcheva V, White CR. Non-infectious granulomas. In: Bolognia JL, Jorizzo JL, Schaffer JV, eds. *Dermatology*, 2nd ed. Philadelphia, PA: Elsevier; 2012.

149 PYODERMA GANGRENOSUM

E.J. Mayeaux, Jr., MD
Richard P. Usatine, MD

PATIENT STORY

During a medical mission trip to Africa a child was seen with pyoderma gangrenosum on the dermatology ward of a hospital. She has had a long history of pyoderma gangrenosum with ulcerations on her face, neck, and chest (**Figure 149-1**). The scarring has caused adhesions between the face, neck, and chest.

INTRODUCTION

Pyoderma gangrenosum (PG) is an uncommon ulcerative disease of the skin of unknown origin that affects both children and adults. It is a type of neutrophilic dermatosis.

EPIDEMIOLOGY

- PG occurs in approximately 1 person per 100,000 people of all ages each year.[1]
- Children account for only 3 to 4 percent of the total number of cases. There is nothing clinically distinctive about pyoderma gangrenosum in children and adolescents other than the age of the patients.[2]
- No racial predilection is apparent.
- A slight female predominance may exist.
- Predominately occurs in fourth and fifth decade, but all ages may be affected.

ETIOLOGY AND PATHOPHYSIOLOGY

- Etiology is poorly understood.
- Pathergy (initiation at the site of trauma or injury) is a common process and it is estimated that 30 percent of patients with PG experienced pathergy.[1]
- Up to 50 percent of all cases are idiopathic.[3]
- At least 50 percent of cases are associated with systemic diseases such as inflammatory bowel disease, hematologic malignancy, and arthritis.[3]
- It occurs in up to 5 percent of patients with ulcerative colitis and 2 percent of those with Crohn disease (**Figure 149-2**).[4,5]
- In one study of 46 patients 18 years of age or younger with pyoderma gangrenosum, an underlying systemic disease was present in 74 percent of the older children, and as in adults it was most commonly ulcerative colitis.[2]
- The lesions tend to affect the lower extremities (**Figure 149-3**), but infants tend to have ulcers more commonly than adults in the genital and perianal distribution,[6] the head and face (**Figure 149-1**), and the buttocks (**Figure 149-4**).[7]

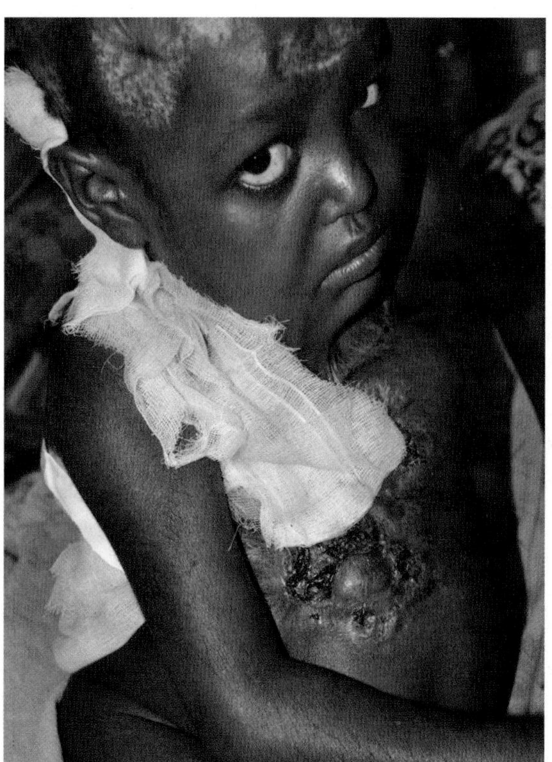

FIGURE 149-1 Pyoderma gangrenosum on the face, neck, and chest of a child in Africa. The scarring has caused adhesions between the face, neck, and chest. *(Used with permission from Richard P. Usatine, MD.)*

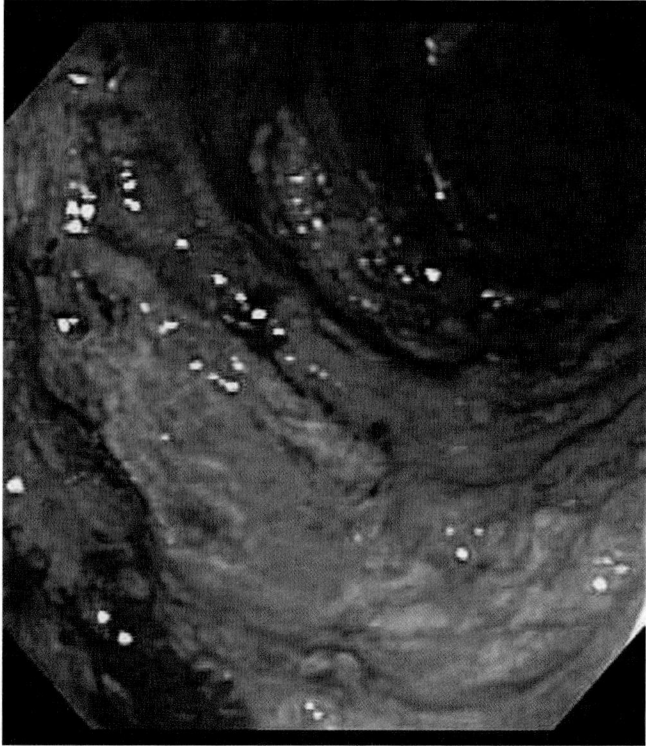

FIGURE 149-2 Friable inflamed mucosa of the colon in Crohn disease. *(Used with permission from Shashi Mittal, MD.)*

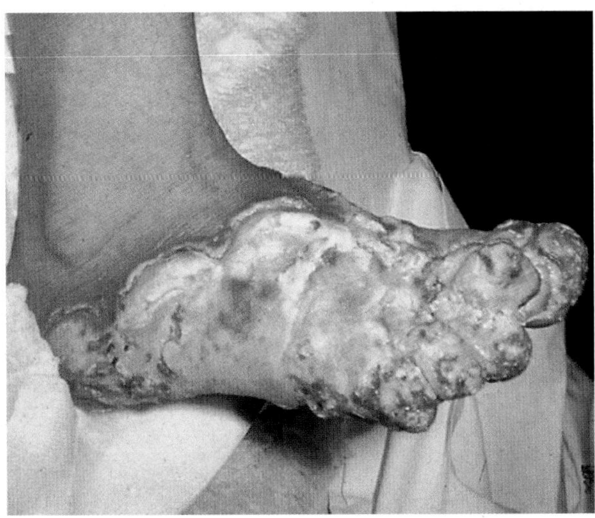

FIGURE 149-3 Pyoderma gangrenosum on the foot of a child. The lower extremity is the most common location for this rare disease in children. (*Used with permission from Weinberg SW, Prose NS, Kristal L, Color Atlas of Pediatric Dermatology, 4th edition, Figure 15-29, New York, NY: McGraw-Hill, 2008.*)

- Biopsies usually show a polymorphonuclear cell infiltrate with features of ulceration, infarction, and abscess formation.

RISK FACTORS

- Ulcerative colitis.
- Crohn disease.[3,8]

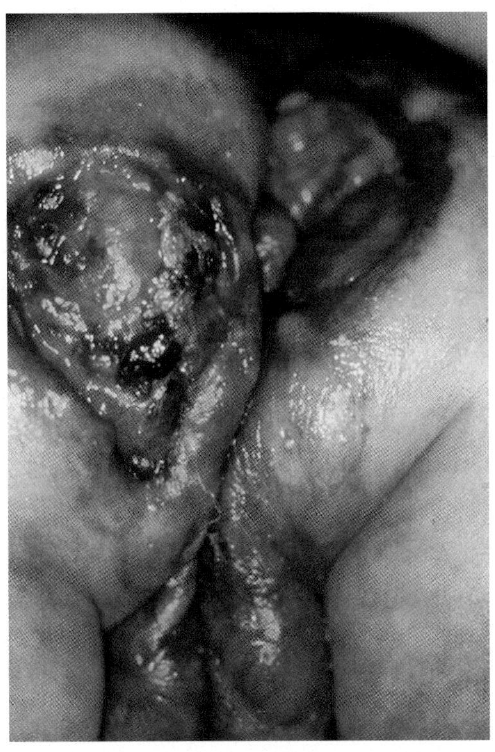

FIGURE 149-4 Pyoderma gangrenosum on the buttocks of an infant. Note the necrotic ulcers with undermined borders. (*Used with permission Kane KS, Lio P, Stratigos AJ, Johnson RA. Color Atlas and Synopsis of Pediatric Dermatology, 2nd edition, Figure 15-17, New York, NY: McGraw-Hill, 2009.*)

- Polyarthritis (seronegative or seropositive).
- Hematologic diseases/disorders such as leukemia (predominantly myelocytic).
- Monoclonal gammopathies (primarily immunoglobulin A).
- Psoriatic arthritis and rheumatoid arthritis.
- Hepatic diseases (hepatitis and primary biliary cirrhosis).
- Immunologic diseases (lupus erythematosus and Sjögren syndrome).

DIAGNOSIS

CLINICAL FEATURES

- Typically PG presents with deep painful ulcer with a well-defined border, which is usually violet or blue (**Figures 149-3** and **149-4**). The color has also been described as the color of gun metal. The ulcer edge is often undermined and the surrounding skin is erythematous and indurated. It usually starts as a pustule with an inflammatory base, an erythematous nodule, or a hemorrhagic bulla on a violaceous base. The central area then undergoes necrosis to form a single ulcer.[8]
- The lesions are painful and the pain can be severe.[3] Patients may have malaise, arthralgia, and myalgia.
- Two main variants of PG exist: classic and atypical.[3]
  - Classic PG is characterized by a deep ulceration with a violaceous border that overhangs the ulcer bed.[3] These lesions of PG most commonly occur on the legs (**Figure 149-3**).[3]
  - Atypical PG has a vesiculopustular wet component. This is usually only at the border, is erosive or superficially ulcerated, and most often occurs on the dorsal surface of the hands, the extensor parts of the forearms, or the face.[3]
- Other variants:
  - Peristomal PG may occur around stoma sites. This form is often mistaken for a wound infection or irritation from the appliance.[9]
  - Vulvar or penile PG occurs on the genitalia and must be differentiated from ulcerative sexually transmitted diseases (STDs) in adolescents such as chancroid and syphilis.[3]
  - Intraoral PG is known as pyostomatitis vegetans. It occurs primarily in patients with inflammatory bowel disease.[3]

TYPICAL DISTRIBUTION

- Most commonly seen on the legs and hands, but can occur on any skin surface including the genitalia, buttocks, head and around a stoma. PG can be seen on the scalp, head, and neck (**Figure 149-1**).

LABORATORY TESTING

- Complete blood count (CBC), urinalysis (UA), and liver function tests (LFTs) should be obtained. Order a hepatitis profile to rule out hepatitis.[3] Systemic disease markers may be elevated if associated conditions exist, that is, erythrocyte sedimentation rate (ESR), antinuclear antibody (ANA), and rheumatoid factor. Obtain rapid plasma reagin (RPR), protein electrophoresis, and skin cultures as indicated. Consider culturing the ulcer/erosion for bacteria, fungi, atypical *Mycobacteria*, and viruses.[3]
- If GI symptoms exist, perform or refer for colonoscopy to look for inflammatory bowel disease.

BIOPSY

- Although there are no specific pathologic signs of PG, a biopsy of an active area of disease along with the border, can be used to rule out other causes of ulcerative skin lesions.
- The pathologist may be able to confirm your clinical impression. Biopsy of the earliest lesions reveal a neutrophilic vascular reaction. Fully developed lesions exhibit dense neutrophilic infiltrate, and some lymphocytes and macrophages surrounding marked tissue necrosis. Ulceration, infarction of tissue, and abscess formation with fibrosing inflammation at the edge of the ulcer may be seen.[10]

DIFFERENTIAL DIAGNOSIS

- PG is sometimes a diagnosis of exclusion diagnosed with successful wound healing following immunosuppressant therapy.[11] When misdiagnosed it is often confused for vascular occlusive or venous disease, vasculitis, cancer, primary infection, drug-induced or exogenous tissue injury, and other inflammatory disorders.[12] Biopsy of a questionable lesion may be the only way to ultimately distinguish PG as the cause of ulcerative skin lesions.
- Ulcerative STDs, such as chancroid and syphilis, can resemble vulvar or penile PG. These STDs are more common than PG and should be diagnosed with appropriate tests, including RPR and bacterial culture for *Haemophilus ducreyi*. If these tests are negative, then PG should be considered. RPR should also be repeated in 2 weeks if it is initially negative at the start of a chancre—it takes some weeks to become positive and syphilis is easily treatable (see Chapter 75, Ulcerative Mucosal Disorders and Chapter 181, Syphilis).
- Acute febrile neutrophilic dermatosis (Sweet syndrome) is a neutrophilic dermatosis like PG, but the patients are generally febrile with systemic symptoms (**Figure 149-5**). The diagnosis of Sweet syndrome is made when the patient fulfills 2 of 2 major criteria and 2 of 4 minor criteria. The 2 major criteria are (a) an abrupt onset of tender or painful erythematous plaques or nodules occasionally with vesicles, pustules, or bullae, and (b) predominantly neutrophilic infiltration in the dermis without leukocytoclastic vasculitis. Minor criteria include specific preceding or concurrent medical conditions, fever, abnormal lab values, including leukocytosis and an elevated sedimentation rate, and a rapid response to systemic steroids.

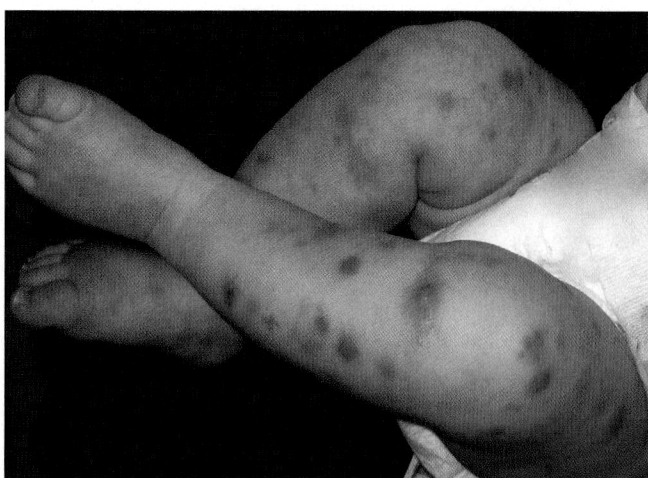

FIGURE 149-5 Sweet's syndrome in an infant. Erythematous plaques and nodules with central bullous changes are present on the legs. *(Used with permission Kane KS, Lio P, Stratigos AJ, Johnson RA. Color Atlas and Synopsis of Pediatric Dermatology, 2nd edition, Figure 15-16, New York, NY: McGraw-Hill, 2009.)*

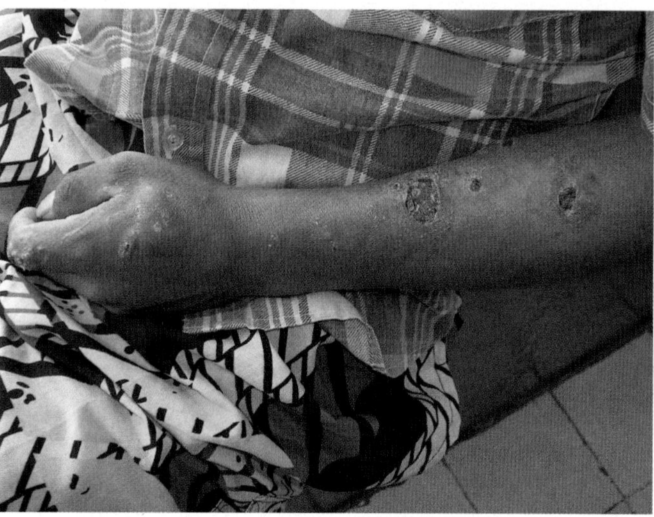

FIGURE 149-6 Sporotrichosis (fungal infection) with the typical sporotrichoid spread up the arm from an inoculation of the hand. Note the ulcers that resemble pyoderma gangrenosum on the arm of this Panamanian child. *(Used with permission from Richard P. Usatine, MD.)*

- Systemic vasculitis is perhaps the most difficult to differentiate, but history of minor trauma in the area preceding lesion formation (pathergy) and undermining of the violaceous border should lead one toward the diagnosis of PG.[12]
- Ecthyma is a type of impetigo in which ulcers form. Bacterial cultures will be positive and this disease should respond to cephalexin or other oral antibiotics (see Chapter 99, Impetigo).
- Spider bites from the black recluse spider can easily resemble PG when they ulcerate. The history of a spider bite can help differentiate this from PG.
- Sporotrichosis is a fungal infection that often starts from an injury while gardening with roses. It is usually on the arm or hand and can resemble PG (**Figure 149-6**). Use fungal culture to diagnose this when the history suggests this as the diagnosis. Oral antifungal medications can treat this.
- Venous insufficiency ulcers are typically seen around the medial malleolus and the most severe of these ulcers resembles PG, although they are rare in children and usually associated with other severe vaso-occlusive problems. The presence of signs and symptoms of venous insufficiency should help differentiate this from PG.

MANAGEMENT

NONPHARMACOLOGIC

- At each visit, measure and document the lesion's depth, length, and width to track treatment progression.[13]
- Surgical debridement is contraindicated as pathergy occurs in 25 to 50 percent of cases and surgery will make the lesions worse. SOR Ⓑ

MEDICATIONS

- Patients frequently are in pain from the lesions, so treatment is aimed at pain relief as well as healing the skin lesions.
- Therapy directed at the underlying inflammatory bowel disease (IBD), when present, usually results in healing, although treatment with steroids is often necessary.[13] SOR B
- Topical medications are first-line therapy in cases of localized PG that are not severe. Start with potent corticosteroid ointments or tacrolimus ointment (over age 2 years).[13–16] SOR B
- Small ulcers can be managed with topical steroid creams, silver sulfadiazine, or potassium iodide solution. SOR C
- Intralesional injections with corticosteroids are also an option.[13, 14] SOR B
- Systemic treatment with oral corticosteroids, such as methylprednisolone (0.5–1.7 mg/kg/day divided q12hr IV for 3 days), prednisone (0.5–1 mg/kg/day PO qDay or divided BID; not to exceed 80 mg/day), or oral cyclosporine (e.g., 5 mg/kg per day) alone or together appears to be effective (in the absence of controlled trials) in many cases and should be considered first-line therapy.[9,14] SOR B Response is usually rapid, with stabilization of the PG within 24 hours.[17]
- In steroid-refractory PG associated with IBD, infliximab 5 mg/kg IV at 0, 2 and 6 weeks then every 8wk was effective in case series and a small placebo-controlled trial.[18,19] SOR B Other biologic therapies reported to improve symptoms include etanercept and adalimumab.[13] SOR C
- To date, case reports have been published that show therapeutic efficacy of oral dapsone, azathioprine, mycophenolate mofetil, cyclophosphamide, and tacrolimus.[14,20] SOR C

REFERRAL

In most cases, referral to a dermatologist is needed.

PROGNOSIS

- The prognosis of PG is generally good, but residual scarring is common (**Figure 149-1**) and recurrences may occur.
- Although many patients improve with initial immunosuppressive therapy, patients may follow a refractory course and require multiple therapies.

FOLLOW-UP

- All patients suspected of having PG need close and frequent follow-up to obtain a definitive diagnosis and treat this challenging condition.

PATIENT EDUCATION

- PG is a rare ulcerative skin condition that is poorly understood.
- A skin biopsy is needed to rule out other diagnoses.
- Most treatments are empirical and based on small studies.
- The risks and benefits of steroids and/or other immunosuppressive medications need to be explained.
- Surgical treatments are contraindicated because they increase the ulcer size.

PATIENT RESOURCES

- American Autoimmune Related Diseases Association, Inc. Tel: 800-598-4668—**www.aarda.org/**.
- Crohn's and Colitis Foundation of America. Tel: 800-932-2423—**www.ccfa.org**.

PROVIDER RESOURCES

- Medscape. *Pyoderma Gangrenosum*—**http://emedicine.medscape.com/article/1123821**.
- MayoClinic. *Pyoderma Gangrenosum*—**www.mayoclinic.com/health/pyoderma-gangrenosum/DS00723**.
- Wollina U. PG–a review. *Orphanet J Rare Dis.* 2007;2:19—**www.ncbi.nlm.nih.gov/pmc/articles/PMC1857704/**.

REFERENCES

1. Brooklyn T, Brooklyn T, Dunnill G, Probert C. Diagnosis and treatment of pyoderma gangrenosum. *BMJ*. 2006;333(7560):181-184.
2. Graham JA, Hansen KK, Rabinowitz LG, Esterly NB. Pyoderma gangrenosum in infants and children. Pediatr Dermatol. 1994;11(1):10-17.
3. Jackson JM, Callen JP. *Pyoderma Gangrenosum*. http://emedicine.medscape.com/article/1123821-overview, accessed on March 30, 2012.
4. Mir-Madjlessi SH, Taylor JS, Farmer RG. Clinical course and evolution of erythema nodosum and pyoderma gangrenosum in chronic ulcerative colitis: a study of 42 patients. *Am J Gastroenterol.* 1985;80(8):615-620.
5. McCallum DI, Kinmont PD. Dermatological manifestations of Crohn's disease. *Br J Dermatol.* 1968;80(1):1-8.
6. Burgess NA. Pyoderma gangrenosum with large circumferential perianal skin loss in a child. *Br J Clin Pract* 1991;45:223-224.
7. Prystowsky JH, Kahn SN, Lazarus GS. Present status of pyoderma gangrenosum. *Arch Dermatol.* 1989;125:57-64.
8. Habif T. *Clinical Dermatology*, 4th ed. Philadelphia, PA: Mosby; 2004:653-654.
9. Keltz M, Lebwohl M, Bishop S. Peristomal pyoderma gangrenosum. *J Am Acad Dermatol.* 1992;27(2):360-364.
10. Su WP, Schroeter AL, Perry HO, Powell FC. Histopathologic and immunopathologic study of pyoderma gangrenosum. *J Cutan Pathol.* 1986;13(5):323-330.
11. Banga F, Schuitemaker N, Meijer P. Pyoderma gangrenosum after caesarean section: a case report. *Reprod Health*. 2006;3:9.
12. Weenig RH, Davis MD, Dahl PR, Su WP. Skin ulcers misdiagnosed as pyoderma gangrenosum. *N Engl J Med*. 2002;347(18):1412-1418.

13. Miller J, Yentzer BA, Clark A, et al. Pyoderma gangrenosum: a review and update on new therapies. *J Am Acad Dermatol.* 2010;62(4):646-654.

14. Reichrath J, Bens G, Bonowitz A, Tilgen W. Treatment recommendations for pyoderma gangrenosum: an evidence-based review of the literature based on more than 350 patients. *J Am Acad Dermatol.* 2005;53(2):273-283.

15. Nybaek H, Olsen AG, Karlsmark T, Jemec GB. Topical therapy for peristomal pyoderma gangrenosum. *J Cutan Med Surg*. 2004;8(4): 220-223.

16. Jackson JM. TNF- alpha inhibitors. *Dermatol Ther*. 2007;20(4): 251-264.

17. Chow RK, Ho VC. Treatment of pyoderma gangrenosum. *J Am Acad Dermatol*. 1996;34(6):1047-1060.

18. De la Morena F, Martín L, Gisbert JP, et al. Refractory and infected pyoderma gangrenosum in a patient with ulcerative colitis: response to infliximab. *Inflamm Bowel Dis.* 2007;13(4):509-510.

19. Brooklyn TN, Dunnill MG, Shetty A, et al. Infliximab for the treatment of pyoderma gangrenosum: a randomised, double blind, placebo controlled trial. *Gut.* 2006;55(4):505-509.

20. Eaton PA, Callen JP. Mycophenolate mofetil as therapy for pyoderma gangrenosum. *Arch Dermatol.* 2009;145(7):781-785.

150 PEDIATRIC SARCOIDOSIS

Yoon-Soo Cindy Bae-Harboe, MD
Khashayar Sarabi, MD
Amor Khachemoune, MD

PATIENT STORY

A 4-year-old boy presents with "multiple bumps" that have been growing on his face (**Figure 150-1**). The differential diagnosis of these lesions included cutaneous sarcoidosis and granuloma annulare. A punch biopsy was performed and the diagnosis of sarcoidosis was made.

INTRODUCTION

Sarcoidosis is a multisystem granulomatous disease most commonly involving the skin, lungs, lymph nodes, liver, and eyes. There is no clear gender predominance in childhood sarcoidosis.[1] Of interest, outside the US sarcoidosis mainly occurs in the predominant race of the country.[2] Higher incidences of cases occur in certain parts of the world, including Sweden in Europe and the South Atlantic and Gulf States in the US.[3–5]

In the pediatric population, sarcoidosis is divided into early and late onset. Early onset involves children in their first four years of life, presenting with a triad of arthritis, rash, and uveitis.[4] In this patient population, typical pulmonary disease occurs in about 22 percent of children in this age group.[6] Early onset sarcoidosis is seen mostly in Caucasian patients and these patients may have a protracted course with severe morbidity and residual impairments.[7,8]

Late onset sarcoidosis in children presents as a multisystem disorder, with lung involvement most common.[6] Up to 60 percent of children have an abnormal chest x-ray at initial presentation, with the predominant symptom being a mild, dry, chronic cough.[6] The eyes are also affected in older children (20 to 30%).[3,9] Symptoms include eye redness, blurred vision, photophobia, and ocular pain. Ophthalmic sarcoidosis manifests as uveitis with anterior segment involvement (84% of cases).[9] Other complications include optic neuritis, band keratopathy, cataracts, glaucoma, and retinal vasculitis. Other organ systems may be involved including the reticuloendothelial system (enlargement of lymph nodes),[1] cutaneous (erythema nodosum),[2] musculoskeletal (joint effusions, arthralgias, myositis),[2] renal (nephrocalcinosis, abnormal urinalysis),[3,10] cardiovascular (arrhythmias, sudden death),[11] central nervous system (seizures, cranial neuropathies, diabetes insipidus, growth hormone deficiency),[6,12,13] and hepatic (abnormal liver function tests) systems.[14]

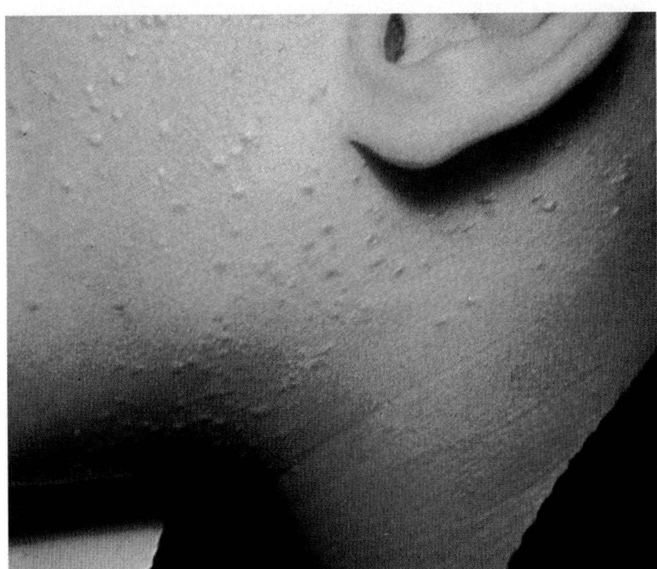

FIGURE 150-1 Papular lesions of sarcoidosis on the face of a 4-year-old boy. *(Used with permission from Weinberg SW, Prose NS, Kristal L. Color Atlas of Pediatric Dermatology, 4th edition, Figure 15-23, New York, NY: McGraw-Hill, 2008.)*

SYNONYMS

- Juvenile early onset sarcoidosis.
- Juvenile late onset sarcoidosis.
- Juvenile systemic granulomatosis.
- Childhood sarcoidosis.
- Lupus pernio (sarcoidosis of the face that resembles cutaneous lupus).

EPIDEMIOLOGY

- Rare in pediatric age group; more common in adolescents and young adults.
- Male/female ratio = 1.
- Two distinct forms of juvenile sarcoidosis—Early onset and late onset.
    - Early:
        - Presents within the first four years of life.
        - Triad of arthritis/rash/uveitis.
        - Predominantly Caucasian patients.
        - Progressive and debilitating course
    - Late:
        - Older children, adolescence.
        - Multi organ involvement.
        - Predominantly African American patients.
- Common types are maculopapular, lupus pernio, cutaneous, or subcutaneous nodules, and infiltrative scars.
- Erythema nodosum (EN) occurs in 31 percent of patients with sarcoidosis and is the most common associated skin finding (see Chapter 152, Erythema Nodosum).

ETIOLOGY AND PATHOPHYSIOLOGY

- Studies reveal that siblings of patients with sarcoidosis exhibit an increased risk of involvement thus implying a genetic component.[15]
- Sarcoidosis is a granulomatous disease with involvement of multiple organ systems with an unknown etiology.

- The typical findings in sarcoid lesions are characterized by the presence of circumscribed granulomas of epithelioid cells with little or no caseating necrosis, although fibrinoid necrosis is not uncommon.
- Granulomas are usually in the superficial dermis but may involve the thickness of dermis and extend to the subcutaneous tissue. These granulomas are referred to as "naked" because they only have a sparse lymphocytic infiltrate at their margins.

RISK FACTORS

- Positive family history.
- African descent, as familial clustering is more commonly observed in this population.

DIAGNOSIS

CLINICAL FORMS OF DISEASE

Cutaneous involvement is either *specific* or *nonspecific*.

- Specific:
  - Typical noncaseating granulomas, no evidence of infection, foreign body, or other causes.
  - May be disfiguring, but almost always nontender and rarely ulcerate.
  - Papules, plaques or nodules is most common, red-brown or purplish, usually smaller than 1 cm, and found mostly on face, neck, upper back, and limbs (**Figure 150-2**).
  - Lupus pernio type sarcoidosis (**Figures 150-3** to **150-5**) presents as purplish lesions resembling frostbites with shiny skin covering them, typically affecting nose, cheeks, ears, and lips.
  - Plaque sarcoidosis is typically chronic, occurring over the forehead, extremities, and shoulders, but may heal without scarring.
  - Nodular cutaneous and subcutaneous plaques that are skin-colored or violaceous without epidermal involvement are typically seen in advanced systemic sarcoidosis.
  - Areas of old scars that are damaged by trauma, radiation, surgery, or tattoo may also be infiltrated with sarcoid granulomas (**Figures 150-6** and **150-7**). Lesions may be tender and appear indurated with red or purple discoloration.
- Nonspecific:
  - Erythema nodosum (EN) lesions usually are not disfiguring, but tender to touch, especially when they occur with fever, polyarthralgias, and sometimes arthritis and acute iritis.
  - EN appears abruptly with warm, tender, reddish nodules on the lower extremities, most commonly the anterior tibial surfaces, ankles, and knees.
  - EN nodules are 1 to 5 cm, usually bilateral, and evolve through color stages: first bright red, then purplish, and lastly a bruise-like yellow or green appearance.
  - EN is seen in the setting of Löfgren syndrome, appearing in conjunction with hilar lymphadenopathy (bilateral most often), and occasionally anterior uveitis and/or polyarthritis.
  - Ulceration is typically not observed in EN, which heals without scarring.
  - Early-onset childhood sarcoidosis may present with enchondromatosis.[16]

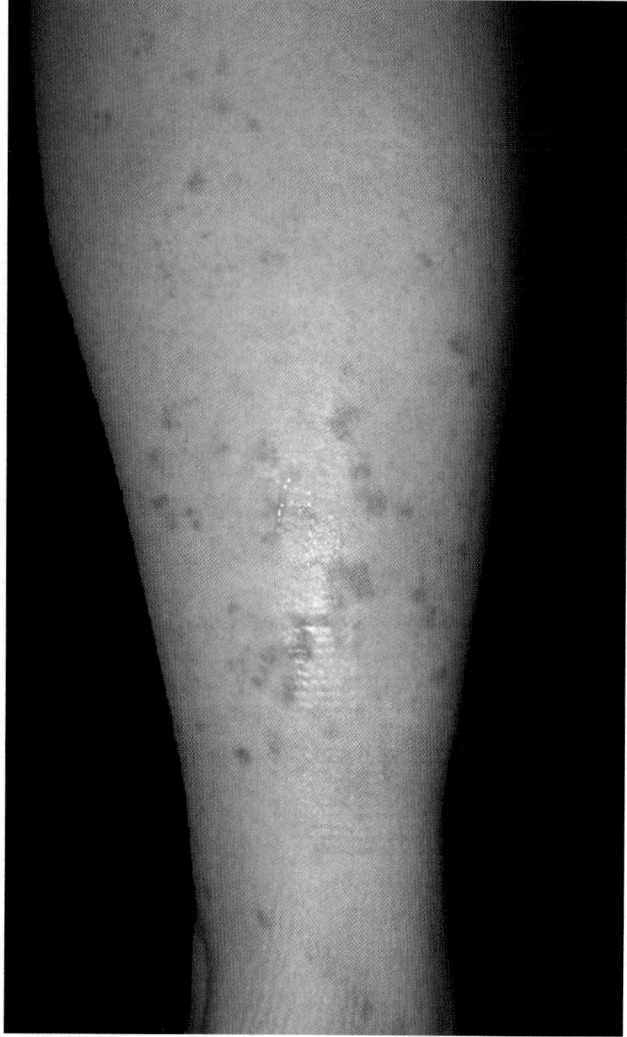

FIGURE 150-2 Maculopapular sarcoidosis on the leg. (*Used with permission from Amor Khachemoune, MD.*)

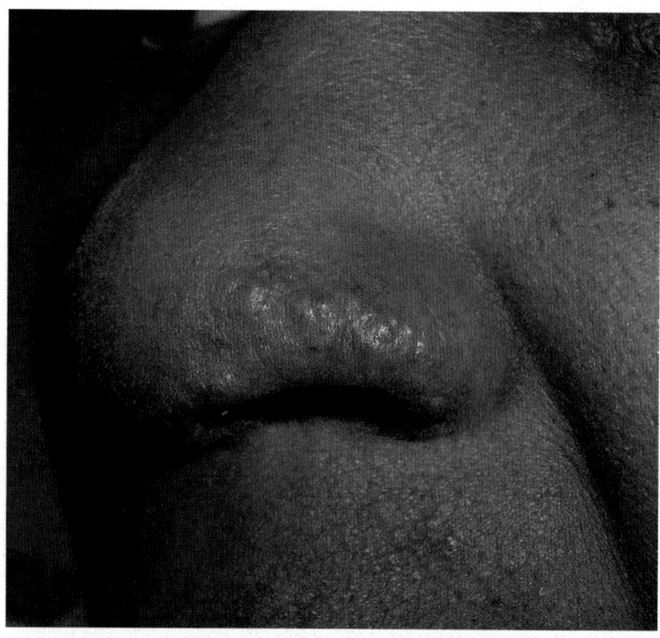

FIGURE 150-3 Lupus pernio type sarcoidosis involving the nasal rim. (*Used with permission from Richard P. Usatine, MD.*)

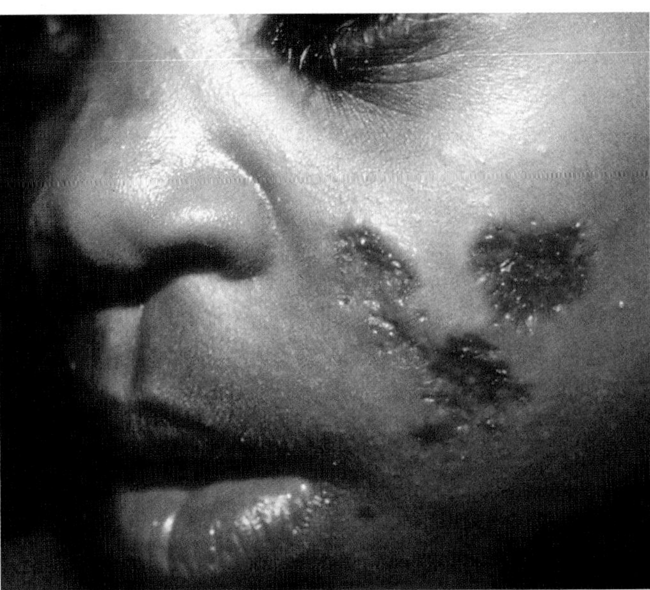

FIGURE 150-4 Lupus pernio type sarcoidosis with violaceous scarred plaques on cheek of a child. (*Used with permission from Kane K, Lio PA, Stratigos AJ, Johnson RA. Color Atlas & Synopsis of Pediatric Dermatology, 2nd edition, Figure 15-18, New York, NY: McGraw-Hill, 2009.*)

LABORATORY STUDIES

- Complete blood count (CBC) count with differential:
  - Leukopenia, eosinophilia, and anemia may be seen.
- Serum calcium and 24-hour urine calcium levels:
  - Hypercalciuria has been found in 49 percent of patients in some studies, whereas 13 percent of patients had hypercalcemia.
  - Hypercalcemia occurs in sarcoidosis because of increased intestinal absorption of calcium that results from overproduction of a metabolite of vitamin D by pulmonary macrophages.
- Serum angiotensin-converting enzyme (ACE) level is elevated:

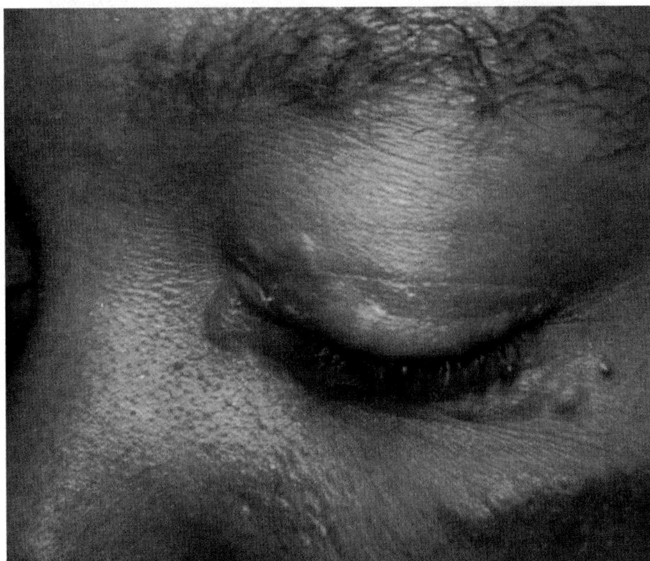

FIGURE 150-5 Lupus pernio (sarcoidosis) with violaceous papules and plaques around the eye and on the cheek of a child. (*Used with permission from Weinberg S, Prose NS, Kristal L. Color Atlas of Pediatric Dermatology, 4th edition, Fig. 15-25, McGraw-Hill, 2008.*)

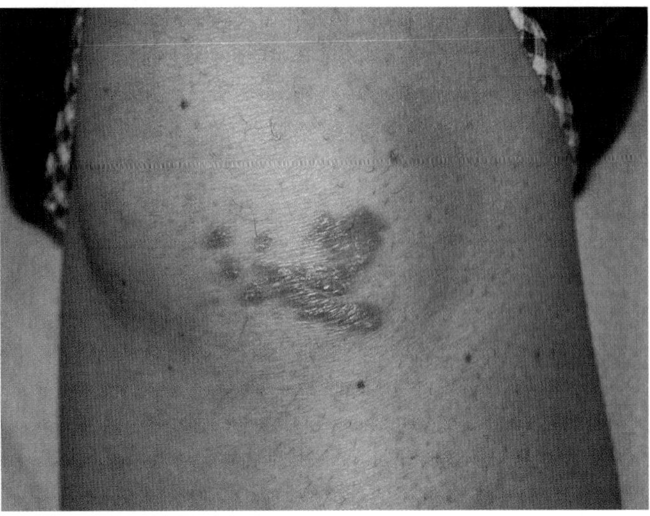

FIGURE 150-6 Sarcoidal plaque of the knee, which appeared after a trauma to the knee. (*Used with permission from Amor Khachemoune, MD.*)

  - Age related variations in normal serum ACE levels should be taken into account as values of 40 to 50 percent higher than in adults have been observed in children younger than 15 years.[11,17]
- Chitotriosidase involved in the defense against pathogens containing chitin may be a potential marker for disease activity:
  - Chitotriosidase activity was found to be correlated with SACE and lung CT scores for sarcoidosis.[18]
- Serum chemistries, such as alanine aminotransferase, aspartate aminotransferase, alkaline phosphatase, blood urea nitrogen (BUN), and creatinine levels. In addition, urinalysis may reveal proteinuria, hematuria, leucocyturia and concentration defect. These levels may be elevated with hepatic and renal involvement.
- Other—Elevated erythrocyte sedimentation rate, diabetes insipidus, and renal failure may be noted.

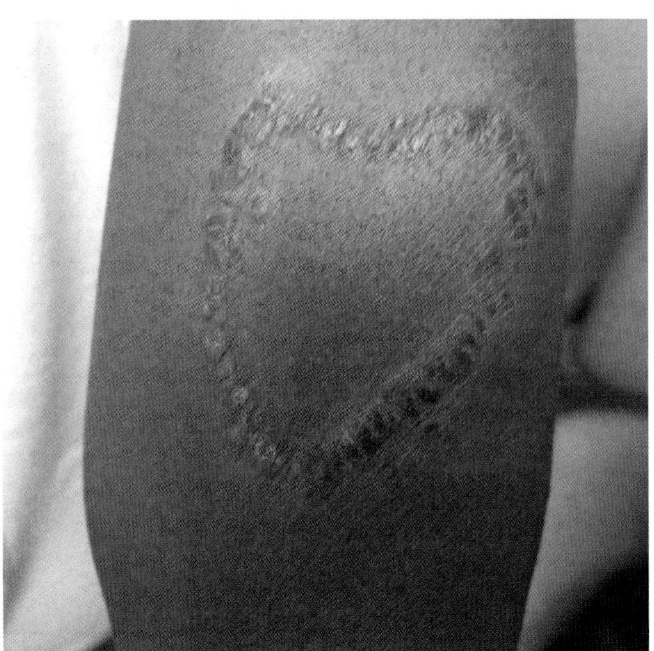

FIGURE 150-7 Sarcoid on a heart-shaped homemade tattoo over the knee. (*Used with permission from Amor Khachemoune, MD.*)

IMAGING STUDIES

- Chest x-ray (CXR):
  - Intrathoracic lymphadenopathy involving the right paratracheal area and both hila are detected in 95 percent of cases.[19]
  - Stage I disease shows bilateral hilar lymphadenopathy (BHL). Stage II disease shows BHL plus pulmonary infiltrates. Stage III disease shows pulmonary infiltrates without BHL. Stage IV disease shows pulmonary fibrosis.
- CT of the thorax may demonstrate lymphadenopathy or granulomatous infiltration. Other findings may include small nodules with a bronchovascular and subpleural distribution, thickened interlobular septae, honeycombing, bronchiectasis, and alveolar consolidation.
- Pulmonary function tests—Evidence of both restrictive abnormalities and obstructive abnormalities may be found.

BIOPSY

- Punch biopsy is adequate to obtain a sample of skin that includes dermis.
- If EN nodules are deep, a biopsy should also include subcutaneous tissue.
- Biopsy specimens are sent for histologic examination, as well as stains and cultures to rule out infectious causes.

DIFFERENTIAL DIAGNOSIS

- Granulomatous sarcoidosis of the skin (**Figure 150-8**).
  - Granuloma annulare (GA) is also a granulomatous skin disease, which appears in single or multiple rings in adults and children (see Chapter 148, Granuloma Annulare).
  - Rheumatoid nodules—These usually appear in the context of a diagnosed rheumatoid arthritis with joint disease present (see Chapter 172, Juvenile Rheumatoid Arthritis).
  - Granulomatous mycosis fungoides—This is a type of cutaneous lymphoma with many clinical forms including granuloma formation.

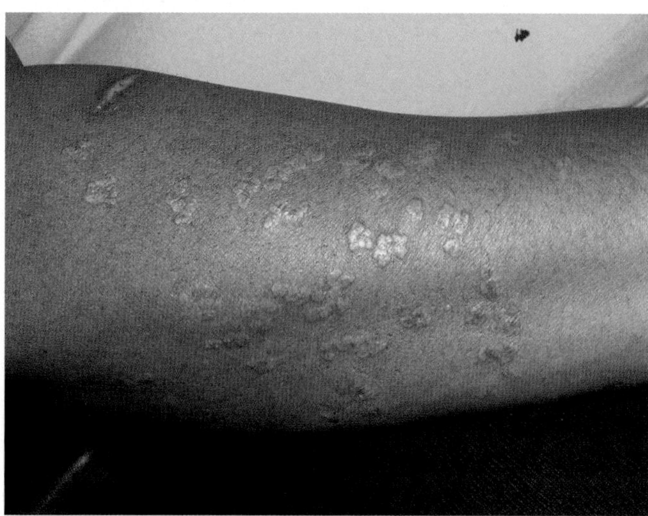

FIGURE 150-8 Granulomatous plaques of biopsy proven sarcoidosis on the arm of a woman. She also has sarcoidosis of the lung. (*Used with permission from Richard P. Usatine, MD.*)

  - Granulomatous periorificial dermatitis—Also known as facial Afro-Caribbean childhood eruption (FACE), GPD occurs in prepubertal children and is usually self limited.[20]
- Maculopapular type:
  - Lupus vulgaris—This is a type of cutaneous involvement with *Mycobacterium tuberculosis*.
  - Syringoma—These are small firm benign adnexal tumors usually appearing around the upper cheeks and lower eyelids.
  - Xanthelasma—These are the most common type of xanthomas. They are benign yellow macules, papules, or plaques often appearing on the eyelids. Approximately one half of the patients with xanthelasma have a lipid disorder (see Chapter 193, Hyperlipidemia and Xanthomas).
  - Lichen planus—This is a very pruritic skin eruption with pink to violaceous papules and plaques. It may present in different body locations but the most common areas are the wrists and ankles (see Chapter 138, Lichen Planus).
  - Granulomatous rosacea—This is a variant of rosacea made of uniform papules involving the face.
  - Acne keloidalis nuchae—This is commonly seen in dark-skinned patients. It presents with multiple perifollicular papules and nodules. The most common location is the back of the neck at the hairline.
  - Pseudofolliculitis barbae—This is most commonly seen in patients with darker skin color, triggered by ingrown hair involving the beard area.
- Annular or circinate type of sarcoidosis (**Figure 150-9**):
  - Granuloma annulare—Annular type (described previously, see also Chapter 148, Granuloma Annulare).

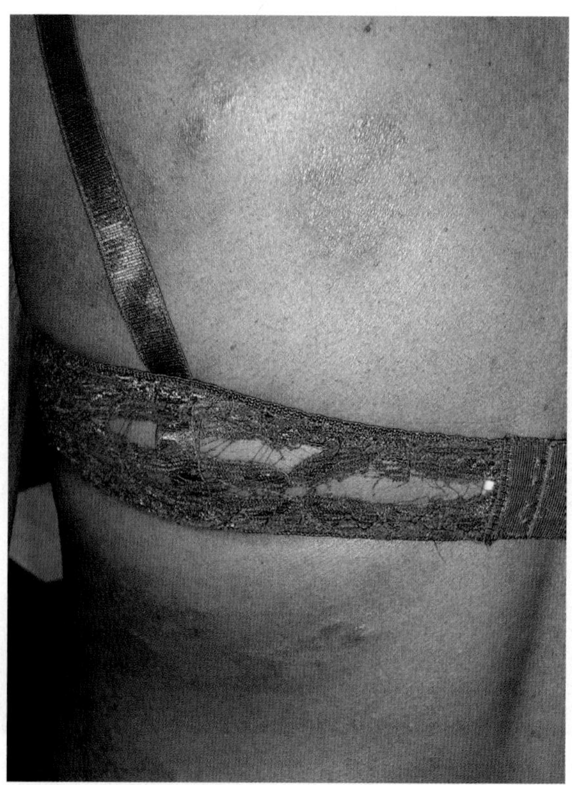

FIGURE 150-9 Violaceous sarcoidal papules coalescing into annular plaques on the back. (*Used with permission from Richard P. Usatine, MD.*)

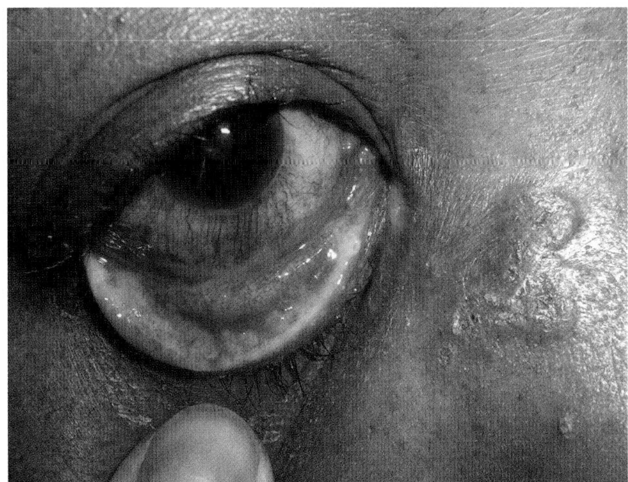

FIGURE 150-10 Sarcoidosis of the eye with involvement of the conjunctiva and infiltration of the inner lower eyelid. (*Used with permission from Richard P. Usatine, MD.*)

MANAGEMENT

- Cutaneous involvement of sarcoidosis is typically not life-threatening and, therefore, the major rationale for treatment is to prevent or minimize disfigurement. Cosmetic issues are particularly important on the face. Also, the lesions can be painful.
- Corticosteroids (oral and topical) are the mainstay of treatment.[3] SOR B
- Steroid sparing agents used to treat sarcoidosis include methotrexate, azathioprine cyclophosphamide and cyclosporin.[21,22] SOR C

REFERRAL

- A multidisciplinary approach is imperative in patients with systemic sarcoidosis.
- Patients with eye symptoms should be referred to an ophthalmologist (**Figure 150-10**).
- Patients with lung involvement should be referred to a pulmonologist.
- Sarcoidosis may affect the following organ systems: pulmonary, reticuloendothelial, musculoskeletal, renal, cardiovascular, neurologic, hepatic; thus, thorough review of systems and results from laboratory work-up should dictate appropriate referral.

PREVENTION AND SCREENING

As the cause remains to be elucidated, no preventative measures have been established. Patients presenting with cutaneous sarcoidosis should be screened as clinically indicated.

PROGNOSIS

- The prognosis of sarcoidosis in children is unclear as the disease is rare and the number of the reported cases is small.
- Generally the prognosis is poorer in the African-American adult population.

In early onset disease, 80 to 100 percent of patients suffer from chronic debilitating sequelae.[7,8]

- Hilar lymphadenopathy in combination with acute or subacute onset (fever, arthralgia, erythema nodosum) is associated with a remission rate of 80 to 90 percent.[23]
- Hypercalcemia, cutaneous sarcoid lesions, and generalized lymphadenopathy are associated with poorer prognosis.[11]
- Mortality rate has been estimated to be about 1 to 5 percent.[24]

FOLLOW-UP

Patients with cutaneous sarcoidosis should be worked up for systemic sarcoidosis. Regular follow-up is necessary.

PATIENT EDUCATION

Inform patients about the risk that systemic sarcoidosis can occur even if the skin is the only area currently involved.

PATIENT RESOURCES

- National Heart, Lung, and Blood Institute. *What Is Sarcoidosis?*—**www.nhlbi.nih.gov/health/dci/Diseases/sarc/sar_whatis.html**.

PROVIDER RESOURCE

- Medscape. *Dermatologic Manifestations of Sarcoidosis*—**http://emedicine.medscape.com/article/1123970**.

REFERENCES

1. Fretzayas A, Moustaki M, Vougiouka O. The puzzling clinical spectrum and course of juvenile sarcoidosis. *World J Pediatr*. 2011;7(2):103-110.
2. Shetty AK, Gedalia A. Childhood sarcoidosis: a rare but fascinating disorder. *Pediatr Rheumatol Online*. 2008;6:6.
3. Shetty AK, Gedalia A. Sarcoidosis: a pediatric perspective. *Clin Pediatr (Phila)*, 1998;37:707-717.
4. Cimaz R, Ansell BM. Sarcoidosis in the pediatric age. *Clin Exp Rheumatol*. 2002;20:231-237.
5. Pattishall EN, Kendig EL Jr: Sarcoidosis in children. *Pediatr Pulmonol*. 1996;22:195-203.
6. Pattishall EN, Strope GL, Spinola SM, Denny FW. Childhood sarcoidosis. *J Pediatr*. 1986;108:169-177.
7. Hetherington S. Sarcoidosis in young children. *Am J Dis Child*. 1982; 136:13-15.
8. Fink CW, Cimaz R. Early onset sarcoidosis: not a benign disease. *J Rheumatol*. 1997;24:174-177.
9. Kataria S, Trevathan GE, Holland JE, Kataria YP. Ocular presentation of sarcoidosis in children. *Clin Pediatr (Phila)*. 1983;22:793-797.
10. Blau EB. Familial granulomatous arthritis, iritis, and rash. *J Pediatr*. 1985;107:689-693.

11. Milman N, Hoffmann AL, Byg KE. Sarcoidosis in children. Epidemiology in Danes, clinical features, diagnosis, treatment and prognosis. *Acta Paediatr*. 1998;87:871-878.
12. Koné-Paut I, Portas M, Wechsler B, Girard N, Raybaud C. The pitfall of silent neurosarcoidosis. *Pediatr Neurol*. 1999;20:215-218.
13. Basdemir D, Clarke W, Rogol AD. Growth hormone deficiency in a child with sarcoidosis. *Clin Pediatr (Phila)*. 1999;38:315-316.
14. Bean MJ, Horton KM, Fishman EK. Concurrent focal hepatic and splenic lesions: a pictorial guide to differential diagnosis. *J Comput Assist Tomogr*. 2004;28:605-612.
15. Rybicki BA, Iannuzzi MC, Frederick MM, Thompson BW, Rossman MD, Bresnitz EA, et al. Familial aggregation of sarcoidosis. A case-control etiologic study of sarcoidosis (ACCESS). *Am J Respir Crit Care Med*. 2001;164:2085-2091.
16. Lee JH, Lim YJ, Lee S, Joo KB, Choi YY, Park CK, Lee YH. Early-onset childhood sarcoidosis with incidental multiple enchondromatosis. *J Korean Med Sci*. 2012 Jan;27(1):96-100.
17. Bénéteau-Burnat B, Baudin B, Morgant G, Baumann FC, Giboudeau J. Serum angiotensin-converting enzyme in healthy and sarcoidotic children: comparison with the reference interval for adults. *Clin Chem*. 1990;36:344-346.
18. Rust M, Bergmann L, Kühn T, Tuengerthal S, Bartmann K, Mitrou PS, et al. Prognostic value of chest radiograph, serumangiotensin-converting enzyme and T helper cell count in blood and in bronchoalveolar lavage of patients with pulmonary sarcoidosis. *Respiration*. 1985;48:231-236.
19. Park HJ, Jung JI, Chung MH, Song SW, Kim HL, Baik JH, et al. Typical and atypical manifestations of intrathoracic sarcoidosis. *Korean J Radiol*. 2009;10:623-631.
20. Lucas CR, Korman NJ, Gilliam AC. Granulomatous periorificial dermatitis: a variant of granulomatous rosacea in children? *J Cutan Med Surg*. 2009;13(2):115-118.
21. Cron RQ, Sharma S, Sherry DD. Current treatment by United States and Canadian pediatric rheumatologists. *J Rheumatol*. 1999; 26:2036-2038.
22. Yasui K, Yashiro M, Tsuge M, Manki A, Takemoto K, Yamamoto M, et al. Thalidomide dramatically improves the symptoms of early-onset sarcoidosis/Blau syndrome: its possible action and mechanism. *Arthritis Rheum*. 2010;62:250-257.
23. Tsagris VA, Liapi-Adamidou G. Sarcoidosis in infancy: a case with pulmonary involvement as a cardinal manifestation. *Eur J Pediatr*. 1999;158:258-260.
24. Statement on sarcoidosis. Joint Statement of the American Thoracic Society (ATS), the European Respiratory Society (ERS) and the World Association of Sarcoidosis and Other Granulomatous Disorders (WASOG) adopted by the ATS Board of Directors and by the ERS Executive Committee, February 1999. *Am J Respir Crit Care Med*. 1999;160:736-755.

SECTION 12 HYPERSENSITIVITY SYNDROMES AND DRUG REACTIONS

151 ERYTHEMA MULTIFORME, STEVENS-JOHNSON SYNDROME, AND TOXIC EPIDERMAL NECROLYSIS

Carolyn Milana, MD
Mindy A. Smith, MD, MS

PATIENT STORY

A 14-year-old boy presents to the emergency department with a 1-day history of fever associated with lip swelling and peeling (**Figure 151-1A**). Within 48 hours, he developed involvement of his ocular (**Figure 151-1B**) and urethral mucosa along with an erythematous papular rash on his trunk that spread to his extremities. In **Figure 151-1C**, target lesions can be seen on the back. He was diagnosed with Stevens-Johnson syndrome and admitted to the hospital.

INTRODUCTION

Erythema multiforme (EM), Stevens-Johnson syndrome (SJS), and toxic epidermal necrolysis (TEN) are skin disorders thought to be types of hypersensitivity reactions (undesirable reactions produced by a normal immune system in a presensitized host) that occur in response to medication, infection, or illness. Both SJS and TEN are severe cutaneous reactions thought to describe the same disorder, only differing in severity (TEN, more severe); however, there is debate as to whether these three fall into a spectrum of disease that includes EM.

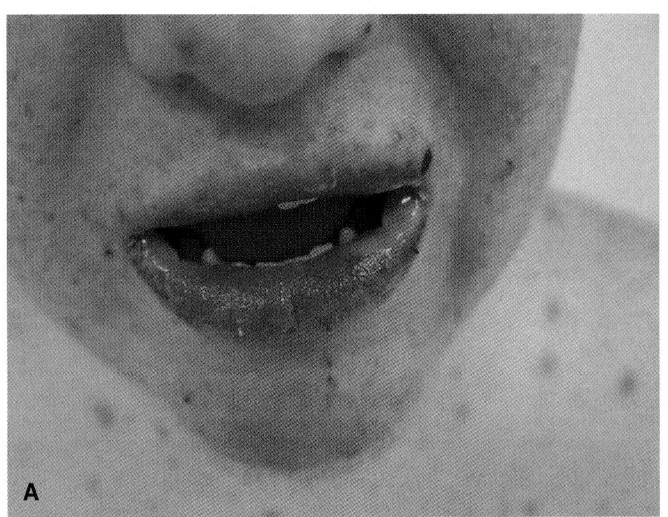

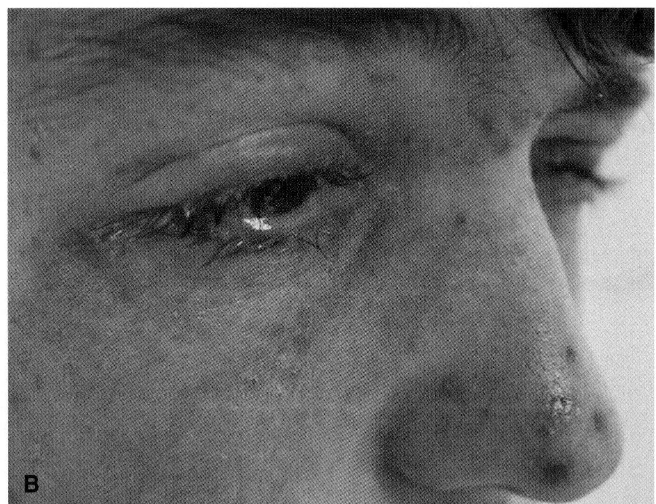

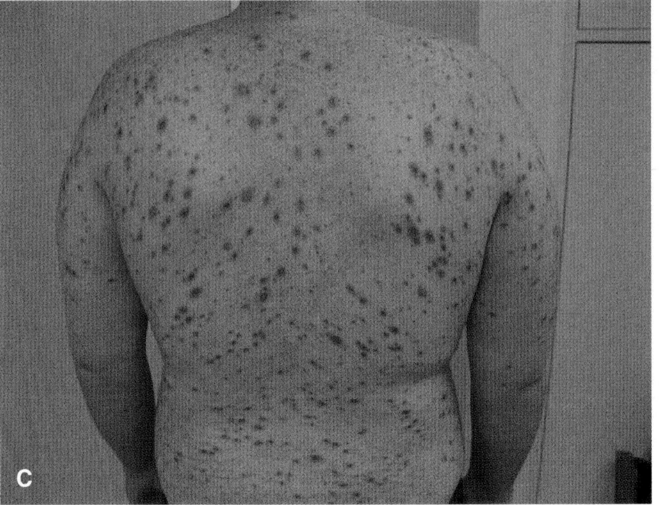

FIGURE 151-1 Stevens-Johnson syndrome in a 14-year-old boy who received penicillin for pneumonia. **A.** Lips and mouth are involved. **B.** Eye involvement. **C.** Target lesions on his back. (*Used with permission from Dan Stulberg, MD.*)

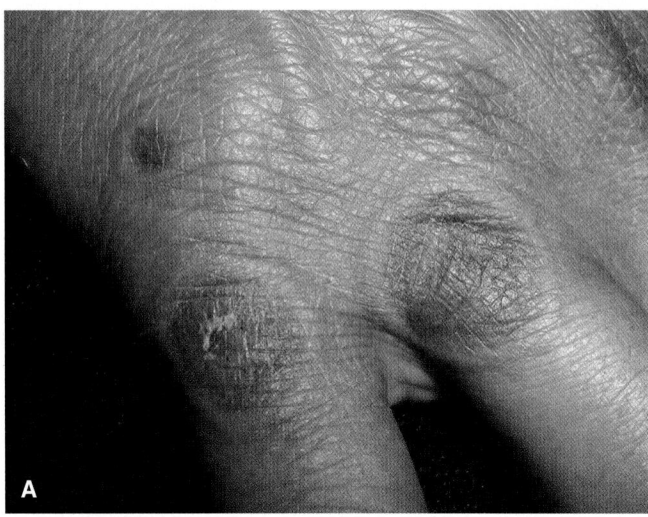

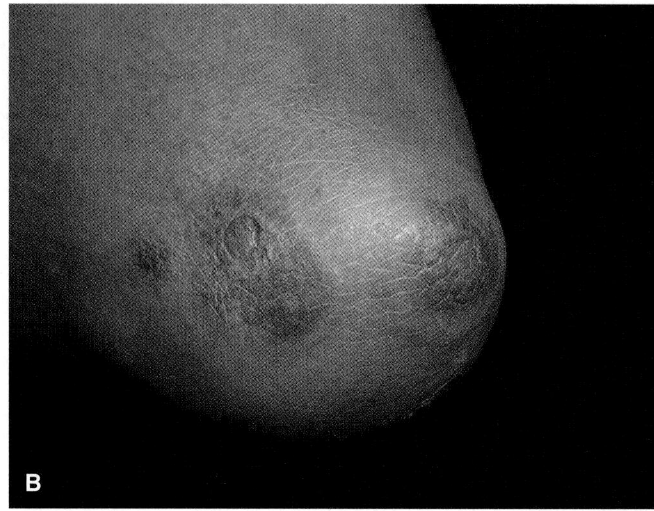

FIGURE 151-2 Erythema multiforme in a woman that recurs every time she breaks out with genital herpes. **A.** Target lesions on hand. **B.** Target lesions on elbow. (*Used with permission from Richard P. Usatine, MD.*)

SYNONYMS

- EM has also been called EM minor.
- SJS has been called EM major in the past but it is now thought to be a distinct entity different from all types of EM.
- TEN is also known as Lyell syndrome.

EPIDEMIOLOGY

- The incidence of EM has been estimated to range from 1 in 1000 persons to 1 in 10,000 persons.[1] The true incidence of the disease is unknown.[1]
- SJS and TEN are rare severe cutaneous reactions often caused by drugs. Reports of incidence vary from 1.2 to 6 per 1 million for SJS and from 0.4 to 1.2 per 1 million for TEN.[2–4]
- EM most commonly occurs between the ages of 10 and 30 years, with 20 percent of cases occurring in children and adolescents.[5]
- With respect to EM, males are affected slightly more often than females.[5]

ETIOLOGY AND PATHOPHYSIOLOGY

Numerous factors have been identified as causative agents for EM:

- Herpes simplex virus (HSV) I and HSV II are the most common causative agents, having been implicated in at least 60 percent of the cases (**Figure 151-2**).[6,7] The virus has been found in circulating blood,[8] as well as on skin biopsy of patients with EM minor.[6]
- For SJS and TEN, the majority of cases are drug induced. Drugs most commonly known to cause SJS and TEN in children are the anticonvulsants phenytoin, carbamazepine, and lamotrigine followed by sulfonamide antibiotics.[3]
- *Mycoplasma pneumoniae* has been identified as the most common infectious cause for SJS (**Figure 151-3**).[7]

Other less-common causative agents for EM, SJS, and TEN include:

- Infectious agents such as *Mycobacterium tuberculosis*, group A streptococci, hepatitis B, Epstein Barr virus, *Francisella tularensis*, *Yersinia*, enteroviruses, *Histoplasma*, and *Coccidioides*.[1]
- Neoplastic processes, such as leukemia and lymphoma.[1]
- Drugs including antibiotics (e.g., penicillin, isoniazid, tetracyclines, cephalosporins, and quinolones), other anticonvulsants (e.g., phenobarbital and valproic acid),[1,7] and NSAIDS.
- Immunizations, such as diphtheria-tetanus toxoid, hepatitis B, measles-mumps-rubella, poliomyelitis, and Calmette-Guérin bacillus.[6]
- Other agents or triggers, including radiation therapy, sunlight, pregnancy, connective tissue disease, and menstruation.[1]

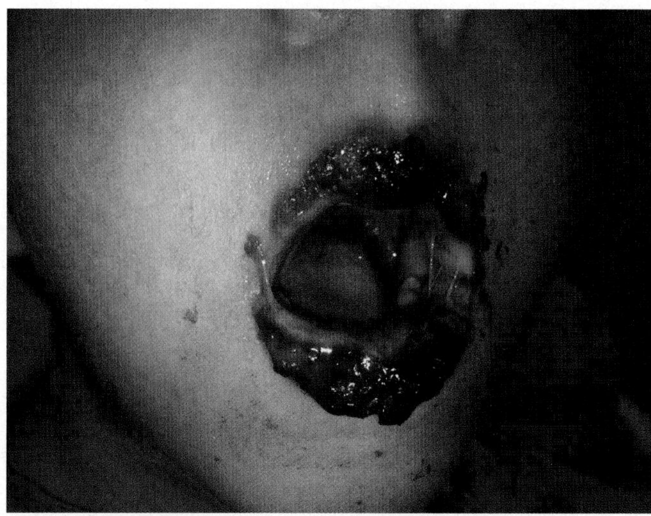

FIGURE 151-3 Stevens-Johnson syndrome with typical appearing oral mucosa showing hemorrhagic ulcerations and crusting in this young child. The child was diagnosed with a respiratory *Mycoplasma* infection. (*Used with permission from Camille Sabella, MD.*)

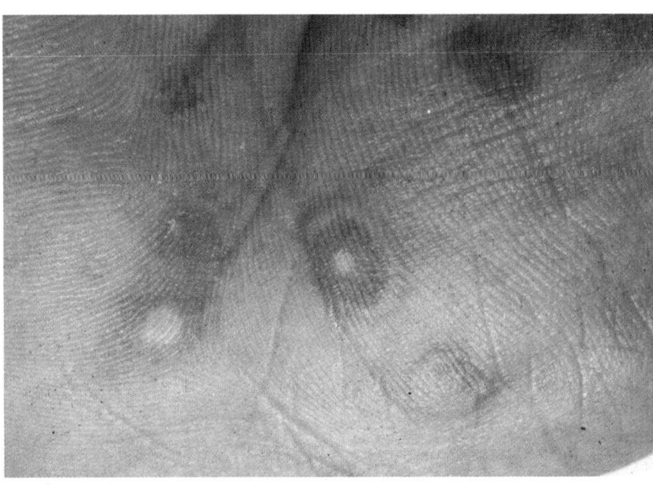

FIGURE 151-4 Erythema multiforme on the palm with target lesions that have a dusky red and white center. (*Used with permission from the University of Texas Health Sciences Center, Division of Dermatology.*)

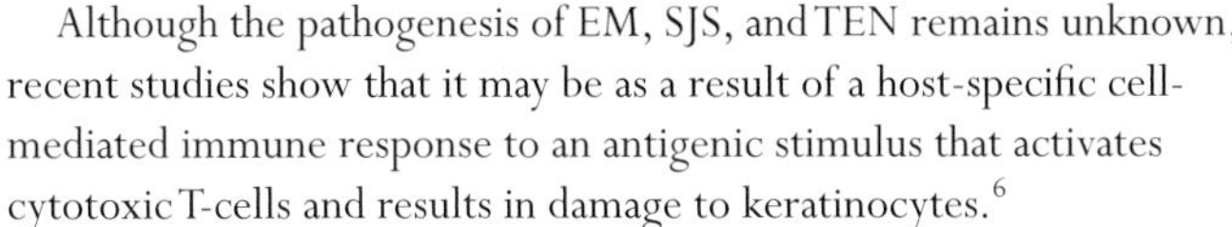

Although the pathogenesis of EM, SJS, and TEN remains unknown, recent studies show that it may be as a result of a host-specific cell-mediated immune response to an antigenic stimulus that activates cytotoxic T-cells and results in damage to keratinocytes.[6]

- The epidermal detachment (skin peeling) seen in SJS and TEN appears to result from epidermal necrosis in the absence of substantial dermal inflammation.

RISK FACTORS

- Recent evidence shows individuals with certain human leukocyte antigen (HLA) alleles may be predisposed to developing SJS/TEN when taking certain drugs.[2]
- Certain diseases, such as HIV/AIDS, malignancy, or autoimmune disease, also predispose individuals to SJS/TEN.[2,9]

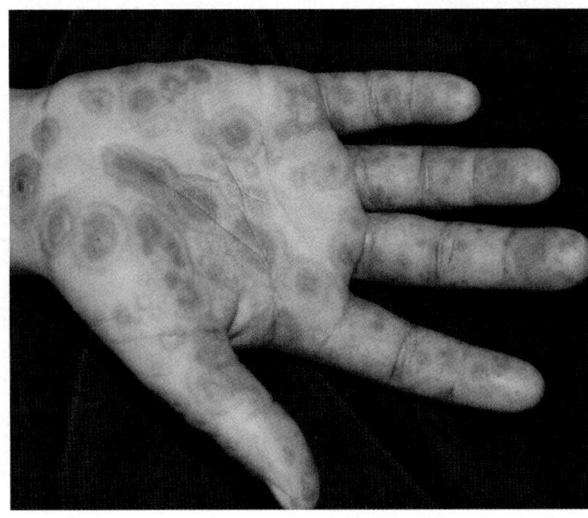

FIGURE 151-5 Erythema multiforme with target lesions on the palms. Note that there are some central bulla and crusts. (*Used with permission from Weinberg SW, Prose NS, Kristal L. Color Atlas of Pediatric Dermatology, 4th edition, Figure 13-8, 2008, New York: McGraw-Hill.*)

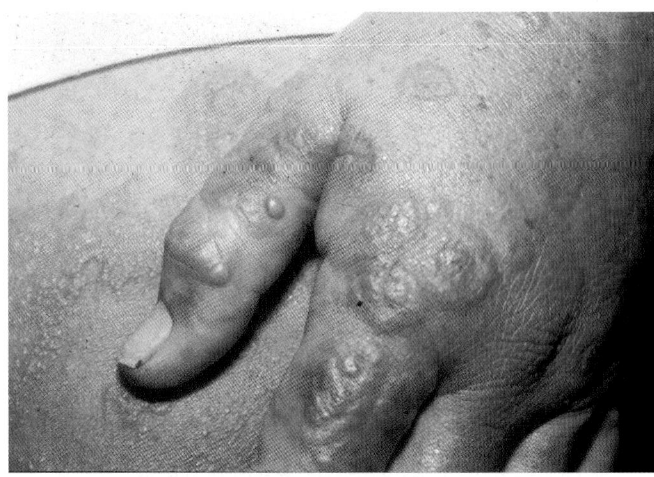

FIGURE 151-6 Erythema multiforme with vesicles and blistering of the target lesions on the hand. (*Used with permission from the University of Texas Health Sciences Center, Division of Dermatology.*)

DIAGNOSIS

CLINICAL FEATURES

In all of these conditions, there is a rapid onset of skin lesions. EM is a disease in which patients present with the following lesions:

- Classic lesions begin as red macules and expand centrifugally to become target-like papules or plaques with an erythematous outer border and central clearing (iris or bull's-eye lesions) (**Figures 151-4 to 151-7**). Target lesions, although characteristic, are not necessary to make the diagnosis. The center of the lesions should have some epidermal disruption, such as vesicles or erosions.
- Lesions can coalesce and form larger lesions up to 2 cm in diameter with centers that can become dusky purple or necrotic.
- Unlike urticarial lesions, the lesions of EM do not appear and fade; once they appear they remain fixed in place until healing occurs many days to weeks later.
- Patients are usually asymptomatic, although a burning sensation or pruritus may be present.

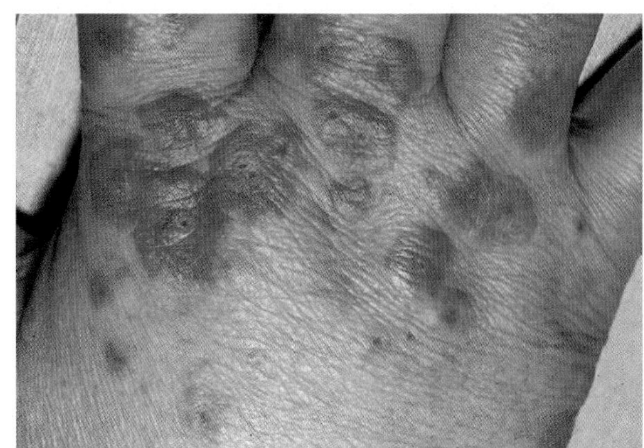

FIGURE 151-7 Erythema multiforme on the dorsum of the hand showing targets with small, eroded centers. There should be some epidermal erosion to diagnose erythema multiforme. (*Used with permission from the University of Texas Health Sciences Center, Division of Dermatology.*)

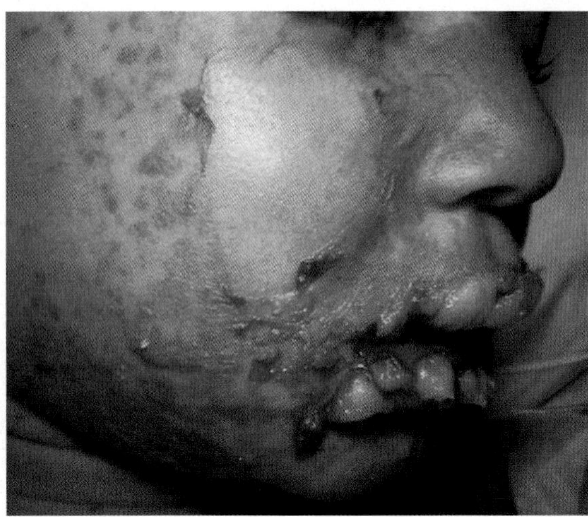

FIGURE 151-8 Toxic epidermal necrolysis with extensive desquamation of the skin on the face and lips of a young child. (*Used with permission from Weinberg SW, Prose NS, Kristal L. Color Atlas of Pediatric Dermatology, 4th edition, Figure 13-13, 2008, New York: McGraw-Hill.*)

- Lesions typically resolve without any permanent sequelae within 2 weeks.
- Recurrent outbreaks are often associated with HSV infection (**Figure 151-2**).[6,7]

In both SJS and TEN, patients may have blisters that develop on dusky or purpuric macules. SJS is diagnosed when less than 10 percent of the body surface area is involved, SJS/TEN overlap when 10 to 30 percent is involved, and TEN when greater than 30 percent is involved.

- Lesions can become more widespread and rapidly progress to form areas of central necrosis, bullae, and areas of denudation (**Figure 151-8**).
- Fever higher than 39°C (102.2°F) is often present.
- In addition to skin involvement, there is involvement of at least 2 mucosal surfaces, such as the eyes, oral cavity, upper airway, esophagus, GI tract, or the anogenital mucosa (**Figures 151-1**, **151-3**, and **151-9**).
- New lesions occur in crops and may take 4 to 6 weeks to heal.
- Large areas of epidermal detachment occur (**Figure 151-10**).
- Nikolsky's sign (denuding of skin when rubbed) may be seen when the child is handled.
- Severe pain can occur from mucosal ulcerations, but skin tenderness is minimal.
- Skin erosions lead to increased insensible blood and fluid losses as well as an increased risk of bacterial superinfection and sepsis.
- These patients are at high risk for ocular complications that can lead to blindness. Additional sequelae include bronchitis, pneumonitis, myocarditis, hepatitis, enterocolitis, polyarthritis, hematuria, and acute tubular necrosis.

TYPICAL DISTRIBUTION

- The distribution of the rash in EM can be widespread.
- The distal extremities, including the palms and soles, are most commonly involved.

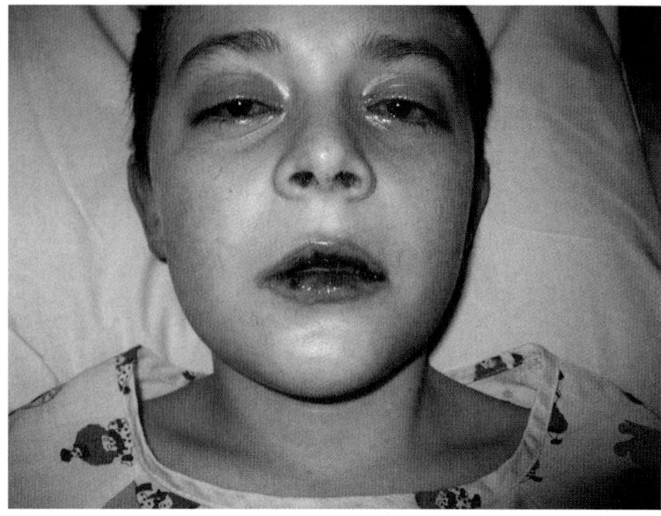

FIGURE 151-9 Stevens-Johnson syndrome with debilitating mucosal involvement of the eyes and mouth. Note the hemorrhagic ulcerations and crusting. This young boy required hospital admission for IV fluids and supportive care. (*Used with permission from Kane KS, Lio P, Stratigos AJ, Johnson RA. Color Atlas and Synopsis of Pediatric Dermatology, 2nd edition, Figure 15-7, 2009, New York: McGraw-Hill.*)

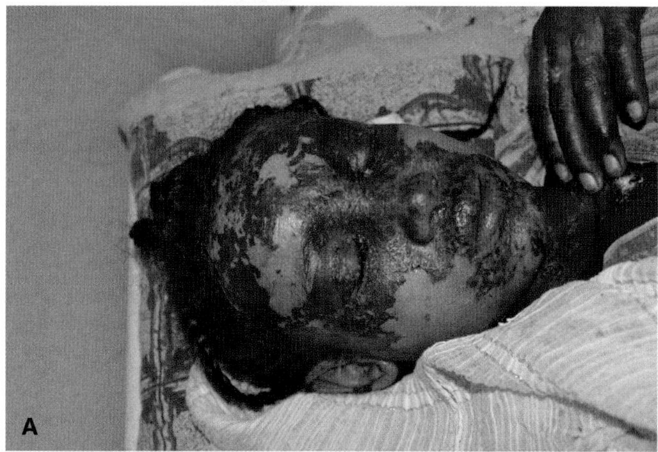

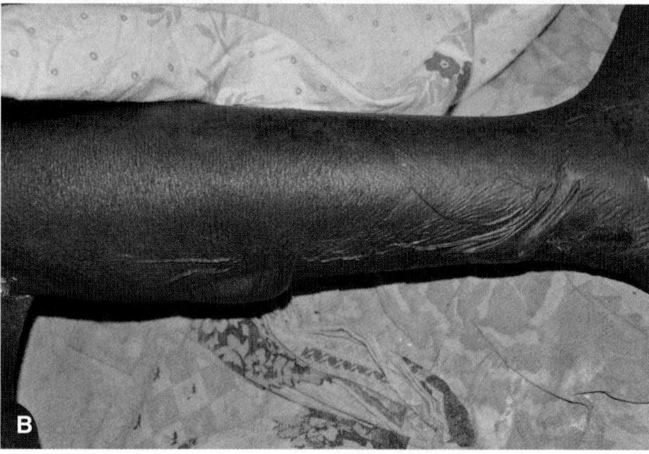

FIGURE 151-10 Toxic epidermal necrolysis secondary to amoxicillin. **A.** Face with large areas of desquamation and loss of pigmentation. **B.** Skin detaching from leg in large sheets and bullae. (*Used with permission from Richard P. Usatine, MD.*)

- Extensor surfaces are favored.
- Oral lesions may be present, especially in SJS (**Figures 151-1, 151-3**, and **151-9**).
- Severe lesions with exfoliation and extensive mucosal lesions occur in SJS and TEN (**Figures 151-8** and **151-10**).

LABORATORY AND IMAGING

- There are no consistent laboratory findings with these conditions. The diagnosis is usually made based on clinical findings.
- Routine blood work may show leukocytosis, elevated liver transaminases, and an elevated erythrocyte sedimentation rate.
- In TEN, leukopenia may occur.

BIOPSY

- A cutaneous punch biopsy can be performed to confirm the diagnosis or to rule out other diseases.
- Histologic findings of EM will show a lymphocytic infiltrate at the dermal–epidermal junction. There is a characteristic vacuolization of the epidermal cells and necrotic keratinocytes within the epidermis.[1]

DIFFERENTIAL DIAGNOSIS

- Urticaria—A skin reaction characterized by red wheals that are usually pruritic. Unlike EM, individual lesions rarely last more than 24 hours (Chapter 134, Urticaria and Angioedema). Giant urticaria (urticaria multiforme) can have targetoid patterns and be confused with EM (**Figure 151-11**).
- Kawasaki disease (see Chapter 177, Kawasaki disease)—Fever persists at least 5 days and there must be at least four of the following features[10]:
  - Changes in extremities—*Acute:* erythema of palms, soles; edema of hands and feet; or *subacute:* periungual peeling of fingers and toes in weeks 2 and 3.
  - Polymorphous exanthem.
  - Bilateral bulbar conjunctival injection without exudate.
  - Changes in lips and oral cavity—Erythema, lips cracking, strawberry tongue (see Chapter 28, Scarlet Fever and Strawberry Tongue), diffuse injection of oral and pharyngeal mucosae.
  - Cervical lymphadenopathy (>1.5 cm diameter), usually unilateral.
- Cutaneous vasculitis (see Chapter 153, Vasculitis)—Also caused by a hypersensitivity reaction, lesions are palpable papules or purpura. Blisters, hives, and necrotic ulcers can occur on the skin. In Henoch-Schönlein Purpura (see Chapter 175, Henoch Schönlein Purpura), the most common cutaneous vasculitis of childhood, lesions are usually located on the legs, trunk, and buttocks.
- Staphylococcal scalded skin syndrome (see Chapter 105, Staphylococcal Scalded Skin Syndrome)—Rash may also follow a prodrome of malaise and fever but is macular, brightly erythematous, and initially involves the face, neck, axilla, and groin. Skin is markedly tender. Like SJS and TEN, large areas of the epidermis peel away. Unlike TEN, the site of the staphylococcal infection is usually extracutaneous (e.g., otitis media, pharyngitis) and not the skin lesions themselves (Chapter 99, Impetigo).

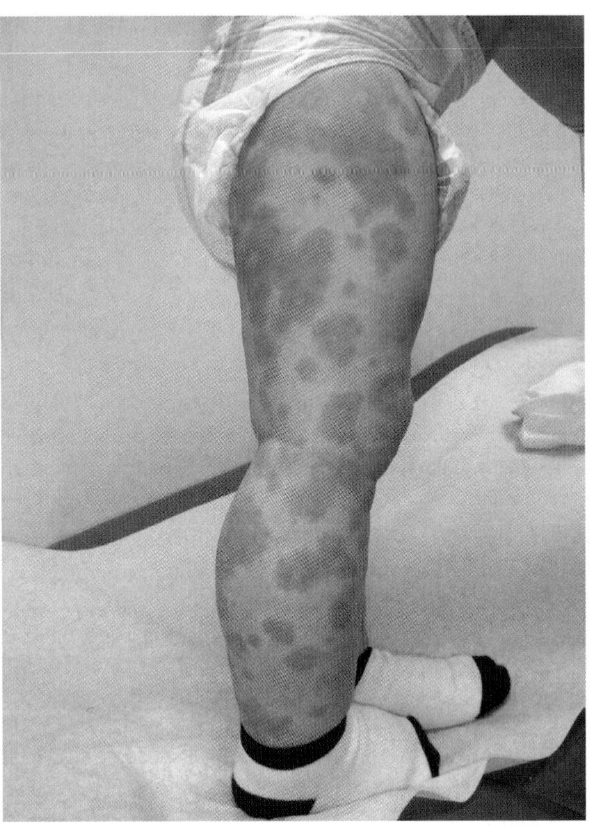

FIGURE 151-11 Well-appearing child with clinical pattern that could support a diagnosis of urticaria multiforme (UM) or erythema multiforme (EM). Some of the targetoid lesions have a dusky center (supporting EM) but there is no disruption of the epithelium and no palmar involvement (supporting UM). Clinically, if individual lesions last less than 24 hours, respond to antihistamines and they itch that supports UM. If they persist, burn more than itch, involve palms and soles and don't respond to antihistamines it is more likely to be EM.

MANAGEMENT

EM

- The treatment is mainly supportive. Symptomatic relief may be provided with topical emollients, systemic antihistamines, and acetaminophen. These do not, however, alter the course of the illness.
- The use of corticosteroids has not been well studied, but is thought to prolong the course or increase the frequency of recurrences in HSV-associated cases.[7]
- Prophylactic acyclovir has been used to control recurrent HSV-associated EM with some success.[7]

SJS AND TEN

- Treatment again, is mainly supportive and may require intensive care or placement in a burn unit. Early diagnosis is imperative so that triggering agents can be discontinued.
- Oral lesions can be managed with mouthwashes and glycerin swabs.
- Skin lesions should be cleansed with saline or Burow solution (aluminum acetate in water).
- IV fluids should be given to replace insensible losses.
- Daily examinations for secondary infections should occur and systemic antibiotics should be started as needed.

- Consultation with an ophthalmologist is important because of the high risk of ocular sequelae.
- Pharmacologic therapy is widely debated in the literature and not well studied in children. Evidence suggests that intravenous immunoglobulin (IVIG) can help shorten the course and improve outcome if started early in the course of the disease in adults; however, there is an association between IVIG use and increased ocular complications in children.[3,11]
- Systemic corticosteroids have been the mainstay of treatment for SJS/TEN. Recent evidence, however, suggests there may be an increase in morbidity and mortality when used for TEN.[11]
- Although still debated, the use of these pharmacologic therapies (IVIG, corticosteroids or a combination of both) has been shown to alter severity and improve overall outcome better than supportive therapy alone.[4]
- Other agents that have been tried with limited success include thalidomide, tumor necrosis factor (TNF)-α inhibitors, cyclophosphamide, cyclosporine, and plasmapheresis.

PREVENTION

Screening populations known to carry HLA alleles prior to starting medications with higher risks for SJS/TEN has been suggested by some researchers.[2]

PROGNOSIS

- EM usually resolves spontaneously within 1 to 2 weeks.
- Recurrence of EM is common, especially when preceded by HSV infection.
- Prognosis is poorer for patients with SJS and TEN if they are older, have a large percentage of body surface area involved, or have intestinal or pulmonary involvement.
- Mortality for SJS/TEN can be predicted based on the severity of illness score for TEN.[12] This scoring system, however, was based on adult literature and many of the criteria cannot be applied to children.
- Predictors for poor outcomes in children are unknown. Evidence suggests that approximately half of children with SJS/TEN develop long term sequelae, the most common involving the skin (hypopigmentation and scaring) and eye (uveitis, keratitis, corneal defects, and chronic conjunctivitis).[4]

FOLLOW-UP

- For uncomplicated cases, no specific follow-up is needed.
- For patients with EM major and any of the complications previously listed, follow-up should be arranged with the appropriate specialist.

PATIENT EDUCATION

- If an offending drug is found to be the cause, it should be discontinued immediately.
- Patients with HSV-associated EM should be made aware of the risk of recurrence.

PATIENT RESOURCES

- Erythema multiforme—**www.nlm.nih.gov/medlineplus/ency/article/000851.htm**.

PROVIDER RESOURCES

- Medscape. *Erythema Multiforme*—**http://emedicine.medscape.com/article/1122915**.
- Medscape. *Stevens-Johnson Syndrome*—**http://emedicine.medscape.com/article/1197450**.

REFERENCES

1. Shaw JC. Erythema multiforme. In: Noble J, Green H, Levinson W, et al, eds. *Textbook of Primary Care Medicine*, 3rd ed. St. Louis, MO: Mosby; 2001:815-816.
2. Tan SK, Tay YK. Profile and Pattern of Stevens-Johnson syndrome and toxic epidermal necrolysis in a general hospital in Singapore: treatment outcomes. *Acta Derm Venereol.* 2012;92(1):62-66.
3. Finkelstein Y, Soon GS, Acuna P, et al. Recurrence and outcomes of Stevens-Johnson syndrome and toxic epidermal necrolysis in children. *Pediatrics.* 2011;128(4):723-728.
4. Del Pozzo-Magana BR, Lazo-Langner A, Carleton B. A systematic review of treatment of drug-induced Stevens-Johnson syndrome and toxic epidermal necrolysis in children. *J Popul Ther Clin Pharmacol.* 2011;18:e121-e133.
5. Plaza JA. *Erythema Multiforme*. Updated July 29, 2011. http://emedicine.medscape.com/article/1122915-overview, accessed January 2012.
6. Darmstadt GL. Erythema multiforme. In: Long S, Pickering L, Prober C, eds. *Principles and Practice of Pediatric Infectious Diseases*, 2nd ed. New York, NY: Churchill Livingstone; 2003:442-444.
7. Morelli JG. Vesiculobullous disorders. In: Behrman R, Kliegman RM, Jenson HB, eds. *Nelson Textbook of Pediatrics*, 19th ed. Philadelphia, PA: Saunders; 2011:2241-2249.
8. Weston WL. Herpes associated erythema multiforme. *J Invest Dermatol.* 2005;124(6):xv-xvi.
9. Sanmarkan AD, Tukaram S, Thappa DM, et al. Retrospective analysis of Stevens-Johnson syndrome and toxic epidermal necrolysis over a period of 10 years. *Indian J Dermatol.* 2011;56(1):25-29.
10. Newburger JW, Takahashi M, Gerber MA, et al. Diagnosis, treatment, and long-term management of Kawasaki disease: a statement for health professionals from the Committee on Rheumatic Fever, Endocarditis and Kawasaki Disease, Council on Cardiovascular Disease in the Young, American Heart Association. *Circulation* 2004;110(17):2747-2771.
11. Worswick S, Cotliar J. Stevens-Johnson syndrome and toxic epidermal necrolysis: a review of treatment options. *Dermatol Ther.* 2011;24(2):207-218.
12. Bastuji-Garin S, Fouchard N, Bertocchi M, et al. SCORTEN: a severity of illness score for toxic epidermal necrolysis. *J Invest Dermatol.* 2000;115(2):149-153.

152 ERYTHEMA NODOSUM

E.J. Mayeaux, Jr., MD

PATIENT STORY

A 9-year-old boy presented to the office with a 2-day history of fever and sore throat. At the time of presentation, he and his mother noted some painful bumps on his lower legs, and denied trauma (**Figure 152-1**). No history of recent cough or change in bowel habits was reported. The patient had no chronic medical problems, took no medications and had no known drug allergies. On examination, his oropharynx revealed tonsillar erythema and exudates. Bilateral lower extremities were spotted with multiple slightly-raised, tender, erythematous nodules that varied in size from 2 to 6 cm. Rapid strep test was positive and he was diagnosed clinically with erythema nodosum (EN) secondary to group A β-hemolytic *Streptococcus*. He was treated with penicillin and NSAIDs. He experienced complete resolution of the EN within 6 weeks.

INTRODUCTION

EN is a common inflammatory panniculitis characterized by ill-defined, erythematous patches with underlying tender, subcutaneous nodules. It is a reactive process caused by chronic inflammatory states, infections, medications, malignancies, and unknown factors.

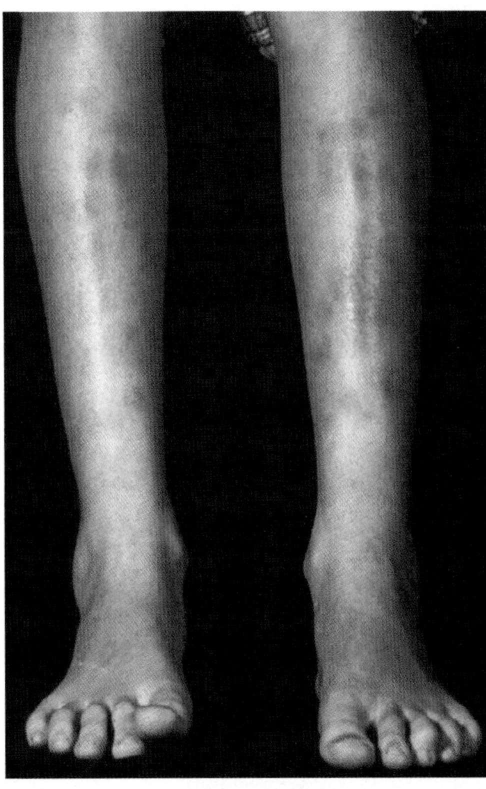

FIGURE 152-1 Erythema nodosum on the leg of a boy secondary to group A β-hemolytic *Streptococcus*. (*Used with permission from Cleveland Clinic Children's Hospital Photo Files.*)

SYNONYMS

Lofgren syndrome (with hilar adenopathy).

EPIDEMIOLOGY

- Erythema nodosum occurs in approximately 1 to 5 per 100,000 persons.[1] It is the most frequent type of septal panniculitis (inflammation of the septa of fat lobules in the subcutaneous tissue).[2]
- In the childhood form, the sexes are equally represented. In adults EN tends to occur more often in women, with a male-to-female ratio of 1:4.5.[3]
- In 1 study, an overall incidence of 54 million people worldwide was cited in patients older than 14 years of age.[4]

ETIOLOGY AND PATHOPHYSIOLOGY

- Most EN is idiopathic (**Figures 152-2**). Although the exact percentage is unknown, 1 study estimated that 55 percent of EN is idiopathic.[5] This may be influenced by the fact that EN may precede the underlying illness. The distribution of etiologic causes may be seasonal.[6] Identifiable causes can be infectious, reactive, pharmacologic, or neoplastic.
- Histologic examination is most useful in defining EN. Defining characteristics of EN are a septal panniculitis without presence of vasculitis. That this pattern develops in certain areas of skin may be linked to local variations in temperature and efficient blood drainage.
- Septal panniculitis begins with polymorphonuclear cells infiltrating the septa of fat lobules in the subcutaneous tissue. It is thought that this is in response to existing immune complex deposition in these

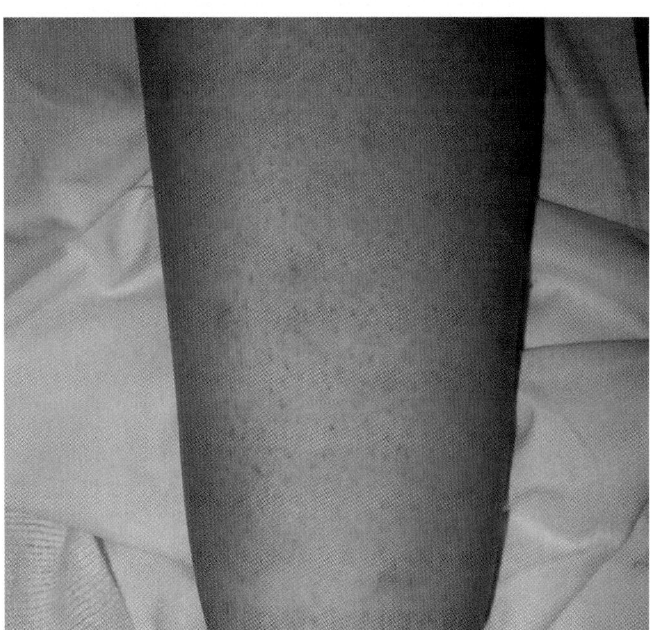

FIGURE 152-2 Erythema nodosum presenting with tender nodules on the pretibial area of an adolescent. (*Used with permission Kane KS, Lio P, Stratigos AJ, Johnson RA. Color Atlas and Synopsis of Pediatric Dermatology, 2nd edition, Figure 15-4, McGraw-Hill, 2009.*)

areas.[7] This inflammatory change consists of edema and hemorrhage which is responsible for the nodularity, warmth, and erythema.

- The infiltrate progresses from predominantly polymorphonuclear cells, to lymphocytes, and then histiocytes where fibrosis occurs around the lobules. There may be some necrosis though minimal as complete resolution without scarring is the typical course.
- The histopathologic hallmark of EN is the Miescher radial granuloma. This is a small, well-defined nodular aggregate of small histiocytes around a central stellate or banana-shaped cleft.

RISK FACTORS

- Group A β-hemolytic streptococcal pharyngitis has been linked to EN (**Figure 152-1**). A retrospective study of 129 cases of EN over several decades reports 28 percent had streptococcal infection.[5]
- Nonstreptococcal upper respiratory tract infections may also play a role.[1]
- Historically, tuberculosis (TB) was a common underlying illness with EN, but TB is now a rare cause of EN in developed countries. There are reports of EN occurring in patients receiving the bacille Calmette-Guérin vaccination.[8]
- EN is less frequently associated with other infections agents, including *Yersinia* gastroenteritis, *Salmonella*, *Campylobacter*, toxoplasmosis, syphilis, amebiasis, giardiasis, brucellosis, leprosy, *Chlamydia*, *Mycoplasma*, *Brucella*, hepatitis B (infection and vaccine), Epstein-Barr virus, and *Bartonella*.[4,9,10]
- The literature reports that EN is seen in patients with inflammatory bowel diseases. It is usually prominent around the time of GI flare-ups, but may occur before a flare (**Figure 152-3**). Most sources report a greater association between Crohn disease and EN than between ulcerative colitis and EN. Other chronic diseases associated with EN include Behçet disease, sarcoidosis, and Sweet syndrome.[10,11]
- EN may be seen as a hypersensitivity reaction to a fungal infection, such as Histoplasmosis and Coccidioidomycosis.[12]
- Some debate exists over causality from pregnancy and oral contraceptives in the occurrence of EN.
- Besides oral contraceptives, medications implicated as causing EN are antibiotics including sulfonamides, penicillins, and bromides. However, the antibiotics may have been prescribed for the underlying infection that had caused EN.[10]
- Lymphomas, acute myelogenous leukemia, carcinoid tumor, and pancreatic carcinoma are associated with EN and should be considered in cases of persistent or recurrent EN.[10,13]

DIAGNOSIS

CLINICAL FEATURES

- The diagnosis is usually clinical.
- The lesions of EN are deep-seated nodules that may be more easily palpated than visualized (**Figure 152-2**).
- Lesions are initially firm, round or oval, and are poorly demarcated.
- Lesions may be bright red, warm, and painful (**Figure 152-2**).

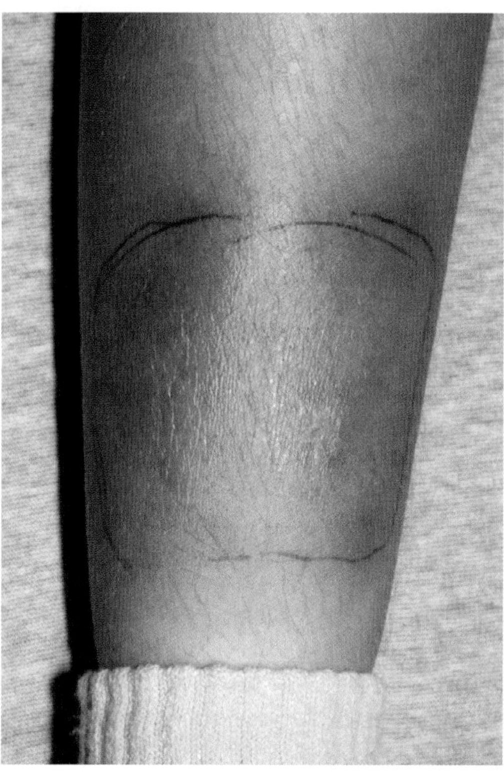

FIGURE 152-3 Erythema nodosum in a 14-year old who was diagnosed with inflammatory bowel disease. Erythema nodosum was the presenting manifestation in this child, prior to the development of gastrointestinal symptoms. (*Used with permission from Camille Sabella, MD.*)

- Lesions number from 1 to more than 10.5 and vary in size from 1 to 15 cm.
- Over their course, the lesions begin to flatten and change to a purplish color before eventually taking on the yellowish hue of a bruise.
- A characteristic of EN is the complete resolution of lesions with no ulceration or scarring.
- EN is associated with systemic occurrence of fever, malaise, and polyarthralgia sometime near eruption.

TYPICAL DISTRIBUTION

- Lesions appear on the anterior/lateral aspect of both lower extremities (**Figures 152-1** and **152-2**).

LABORATORY TESTING

- Blood tests may help to identify the underlying cause. Typical tests include complete blood count, chemistries, liver function tests, and erythrocyte sedimentation rate. Erythrocyte sedimentation rate may be elevated.
- For suspected *Streptococcus* cases, rapid strep test or throat cultures are best during acute illness, whereas antistreptolysin O titers may be used in the convalescent phase.[4]
- In sarcoid, angiotensin-converting enzyme levels may be helpful but are neither sensitive nor specific.[2] A chest x-ray and/or skin biopsy of a suspected sarcoid lesion can help make this diagnosis (see Chapter 150, Pediatric Sarcoidosis).
- Tuberculin skin test (PPD) or Interferon gamma release assay may be obtained when tuberculosis is a consideration.

BIOPSY

- The diagnosis of EN is mostly made on physical examination. When the diagnosis is uncertain, a biopsy that includes subcutaneous fat is performed. This can be a deep punch biopsy or a deep incisional biopsy sent for standard histology. If a biopsy is needed, this can be done by choosing a lesion not over a joint or vital structure and burying a 4-mm punch biopsy instrument to the hilt.

DIFFERENTIAL DIAGNOSIS

- Cellulitis should be considered and not missed. These patients tend to be sicker and have more fever and systemic symptoms. EN tends to appear in multiple locations while cellulitis is usually in one localized area (see Chapter 103, Cellulitis).
- Nodular cutaneous and subcutaneous sarcoid is skin-colored or violaceous without epidermal involvement. The lack of surface involvement makes this resemble EN. Subcutaneous sarcoid may be seen in advanced systemic sarcoidosis that can also be the cause of EN. Skin biopsy is the best method to distinguish between these two conditions. Either way, treatment is directed toward the sarcoidosis (see Chapter 150, Pediatric Sarcoidosis).
- Erythema induratum of Bazin is a lobular panniculitis that occurs on the posterior lower extremity of women with tendency of lesions to ulcerate with residual scarring.[7] This condition is typically caused by TB and is more chronic in nature than EN.[2]
- Erythema nodosum leprosum may occur in patients with leprosy and probably represent an immune complex or hypersensitivity reaction (**Figure 152-4**). Erythema nodosum leprosum is typically seen as a type 2 reaction to standard leprosy therapy.[14] It is more common in multibacillary lepromatous leprosy. Although the lesions often look like standard EN, the lesions may also ulcerate.
- An infectious panniculitis should also be considered in the differential, especially in immunocompromised patients. These lesions are often asymmetric and the patient may be febrile. If suspected, a punch biopsy of a lesion should be sent for tissue culture (bacteria, fungus, and *Mycobacteria*).

MANAGEMENT

- Look for and treat the underlying cause. There is limited evidence to guide treatment unless an underlying cause is found.

NONPHARMACOLOGIC

- Cool, wet compresses, elevation of the involved extremities, bedrest, gradient support stockings, or pressure bandages may help alleviate the pain.[10] SOR C

MEDICATIONS

- Treat the pain and discomfort of the nodules with NSAIDs and/or other analgesics.[15] SOR C
- The value of oral prednisone is controversial and should be avoided unless it is being used to treat the underlying cause (such as sarcoidosis) and if underlying infection, risk of bacterial dissemination or sepsis, and malignancy have been excluded.[1] SOR C
- Oral potassium iodide, which is contraindicated in pregnancy, led to resolution of EN in several small studies.[6,7] SOR B
- Colchicine, hydroxychloroquine, and dapsone have been used as well.[2,7] SOR C

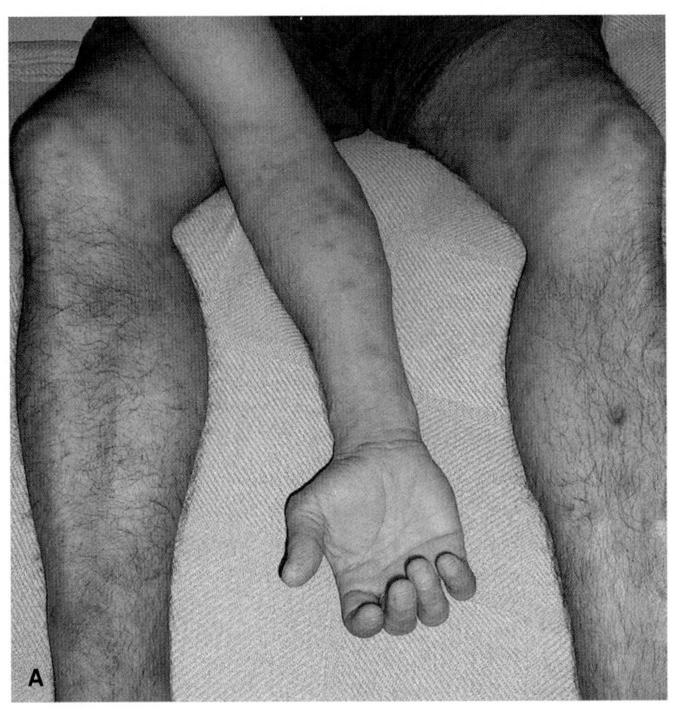

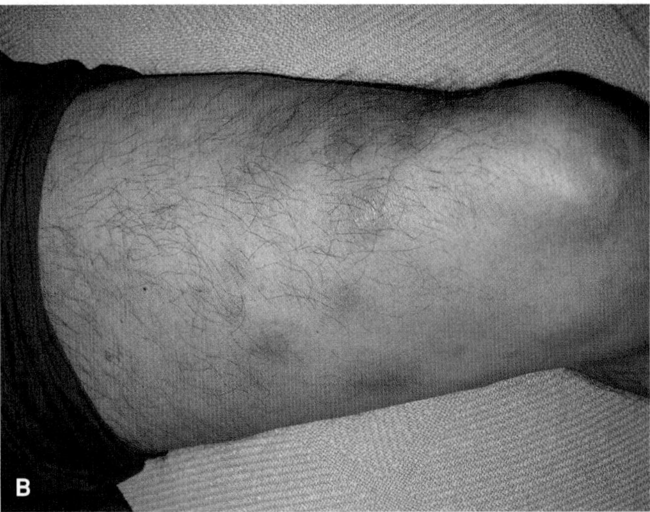

FIGURE 152-4 Erythema nodosum leprosum (ENL) in a patient who acquired multibacillary leprosy from handling and eating armadillos. His ENL started when he started the antibacterial treatment. **A.** Note the many subcutaneous nodules on his arms and legs. **B.** Close-up of the ENL lesions. *(Used with permission from Richard P. Usatine, MD.)*

- There are a few case reports of EN treated with penicillin, erythromycin, adalimumab, etanercept, infliximab, mycophenolate mofetil, cyclosporine, thalidomide, and extracorporeal monocyte granulocytapheresis.[1,16,17] SOR C
- There is one case report of minocycline and tetracycline leading to EN improvement.[18] SOR C

PREVENTION

- Good hand washing and general health measures may prevent respiratory infections that may predispose to EN.

PROGNOSIS

- EN is usually self-limited or resolves with treatment of the underlying disorder.
- Patients may continue to develop nodules for a few weeks.
- The course depends on the etiology, but usually lasts only 6 weeks.
- Lesions completely resolve with no ulceration or scarring.
- Recurrences occur in 33 to 41 percent of cases, usually when the etiology is unknown.[17]

FOLLOW-UP

- Follow-up is needed to complete the work-up for an underlying cause and to make sure that the patient is responding to symptomatic treatment.

PATIENT EDUCATION

Reassure the patient that there is complete resolution in most cases within 3 to 6 weeks. Inform the patient that some EN outbreaks may persist for up to 12 weeks, and some cases are recurrent.[6]

PATIENT RESOURCES

- NYU Department of Pediatrics Division of Pediatric Rheumatology. *Erythema Nodosum*—**http://pediatrics.med.nyu.edu/rheumatology/conditions-we-treat/conditions/erythema-nodosum**.
- MedicineNet. *Erythema Nodosum*—**www.medicinenet.com/erythema_nodosum/article.htm**.

PROVIDER RESOURCES

- Medscape. *Erythema Nodosum*—**http://emedicine.medscape.com/article/1081633-overview**.
- Schwartz RA, Nervi SJ. Erythema nodosum: a sign of systemic disease. *Am Fam Physician*. 20071;75(5):695-700. Available at **http://www.aafp.org/afp/2007/0301/p695.html**.
- Consultant for Pediatricians: *Erythema Nodosum*—**www.pediatricsconsultant360.com/content/erythema-nodosum**.

REFERENCES

1. Schwartz RA, Nervi SJ. Erythema nodosum: a sign of systemic disease. *Am Fam Physician*. 2007;75(5):695-700.
2. Atzeni F, Carrabba M, Davin JC, et al. Skin manifestations in vasculitis and erythema nodosum. *Clin Exp Rheumatol*. 2006;24(1:40):S60-S66.
3. Garcia-Porrua C, González-Gay MA, Vázquez-Caruncho M, et al. Erythema nodosum: etiologic and predictive factors erythema nodosum and erythema induratum in a defined population. *Arthritis Rheum*. 2000:43:584-592.
4. Gonzalez-Gay MA, Garcia-Porrua C, Pujol RM, Salvarani C. Erythema nodosum: a clinical approach. *Clin Exp Rheumatol*. 2001;19(4):365-368.
5. Cribier B, Caille A, Heid E, Grosshans E. Erythema nodosum and associated diseases. A study of 129 cases. *Int J Dermatol*. 1998;37(9):667-672.
6. Hannuksela M. Erythema nodosum. *Clin Dermatol*. 1986;4(4):88-95.
7. Requena L, Requena C. Erythema nodosum. *Dermatol Online J*. 2002;8(1):4.
8. Fox MD, Schwartz RA. Erythema nodosum. *Am Fam Physician*. 1992;46(3):818-822.
9. Shimizu M, Hamaguchi Y, Matsushita T, Sakakibara Y, Yachie A. Sequentially appearing erythema nodosum, erythema multiforme and Henoch-Schönlein purpura in a patient with Mycoplasma pneumoniae infection: a case report. *J Med Case Rep*. 2012 Nov 23;6(1):398.
10. Day AS, Ledder O, Leach ST, Lemberg DA. Crohn's and colitis in children and adolescents. World J Gastroenterol. 2012;18(41):5862-5869.
11. Gilchrist H, Patterson JW. Erythema nodosum and erythema induratum (nodular vasculitis): diagnosis and management. *Dermatol Ther*. 2010;23(4):320-327.
12. Body BA. Cutaneous manifestations of systemic mycoses. *Dermatol Clin*. 1996;14(1):125-135.
13. Cho KH, Kim YG, Yang SG, et al. Inflammatory nodules of the lower legs: a clinical and histological analysis of 134 cases in Korea. *J Dermatol*. 1997;24:522-529.
14. Van Brakel WH, Khawas IB, Lucas SB. Reactions in leprosy: an epidemiological study of 386 patients in west Nepal. *Lepr Rev*. 1994;65(3):190-203.
15. Ubogy Z, Persellin RH. Suppression of erythema nodosum by indomethacin. *Acta Derm Venereol*. 1982;62:265.
16. Allen RA, Spielvogel RL. Erythema nodosum. In: Lebwohl MG, Heymann WR, Berth-Jones J, Coulson I, eds. *Treatment of Skin Disease*, 3rd ed. Philadelphia, PA: Saunders; 2010:223-225.
17. Gilchrist H, Patterson JW. Erythema nodosum and erythema induratum (nodular vasculitis): diagnosis and management. *Dermatol Ther*. 2010;23(4):320-327.
18. Davis MD. Response of recalcitrant erythema nodosum to tetracyclines. *J Am Acad Dermatol*. 2011;64(6):1211-1212.

153 VASCULITIS

E.J. Mayeaux, Jr., MD
Nathan Scott Martin, MD
Richard P. Usatine, MD

PATIENT STORY

A previously healthy 11-year-old girl presents to her pediatrician with a rash on her legs and knee pain. She admits to having abdominal pain the day before but her stomach is feeling better today. She denies fever, nausea, vomiting, and diarrhea. The right knee hurts sufficiently that she has been limping since she woke up. Upon exam the child is afebrile and does not appear to be in distress. She has an impressive rash on her legs with right knee swelling (**Figure 153-1**). The rash is petechial and purpuric and slightly palpable. The linear pattern running down the thigh matches the seams of her pants. A urinalysis performed in the office reveals blood in the urine but no protein. The pediatrician diagnoses Henoch Schonlein purpura (a type of vasculitis) and discusses the treatment plan with the girl and her mother.

INTRODUCTION

Vasculitis refers to a group of disorders characterized by inflammation and damage in blood vessel walls. They may be limited to skin or may be a multisystem disorder. Cutaneous vasculitic diseases are classified according to the size (small versus medium to large vessel) and type of blood vessel involved (venule, arteriole, artery, or vein). Small and medium-size vessels are found in the dermis and deep reticular dermis, respectively. The clinical presentation varies with the intensity of the inflammation, and the size and type of blood vessel involved.[1] Hypersensitivity vasculitis (HSP) is also known as leukocytoclastic vasculitis. HSP is a type of leukocytoclastic vasculitis.

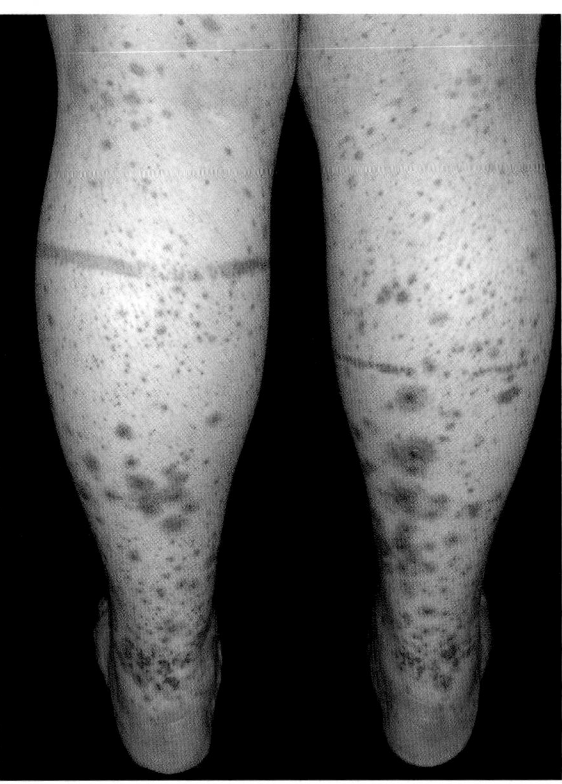

FIGURE 153-2 Henoch-Schönlein purpura presenting as palpable purpura on the lower extremity. The visible sock lines are from lesions that formed where the socks exerted pressure on the legs. (*Used with permission from Richard P. Usatine, MD.*)

EPIDEMIOLOGY

- HSP (**Figures 153-1** to **153-3**) occurs mainly in children with an incidence of approximately 1 in 5000 children annually.[2] It is the most common vasculitis in the pediatric population.[3]

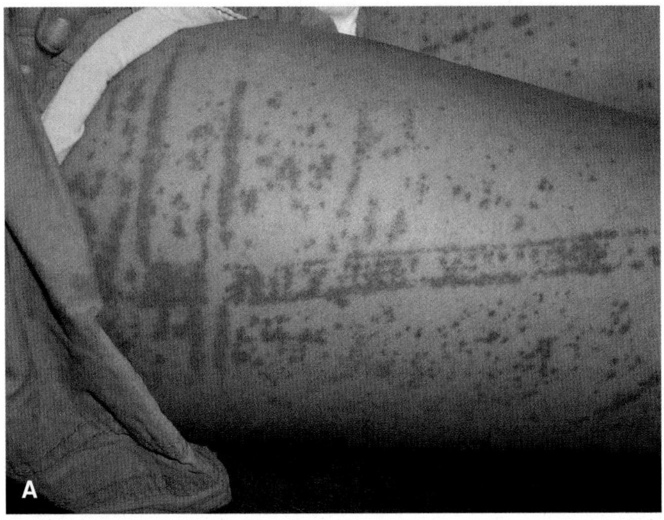

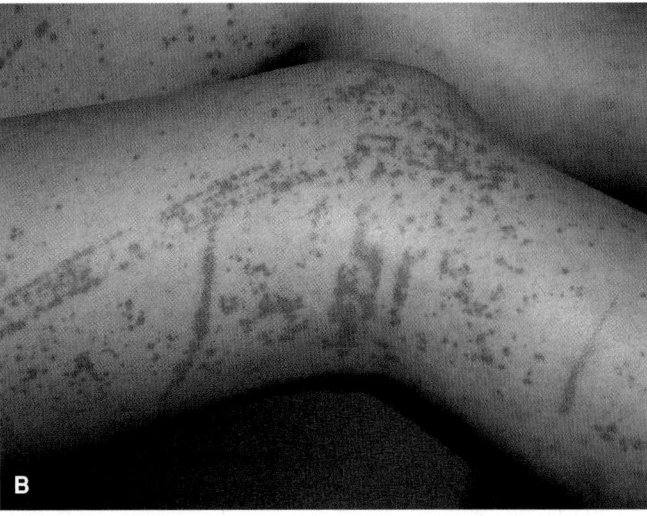

FIGURE 153-1 Henoch-Schönlein purpura in an 11-year-old girl. **A.** In addition to the palpable purpura, this patient also had abdominal pain. Note how the seam of her jeans is visible in the purpuric pattern. **B.** She also had knee pain and swelling and was walking with a limp. (*Used with permission from Richard P. Usatine, MD.*)

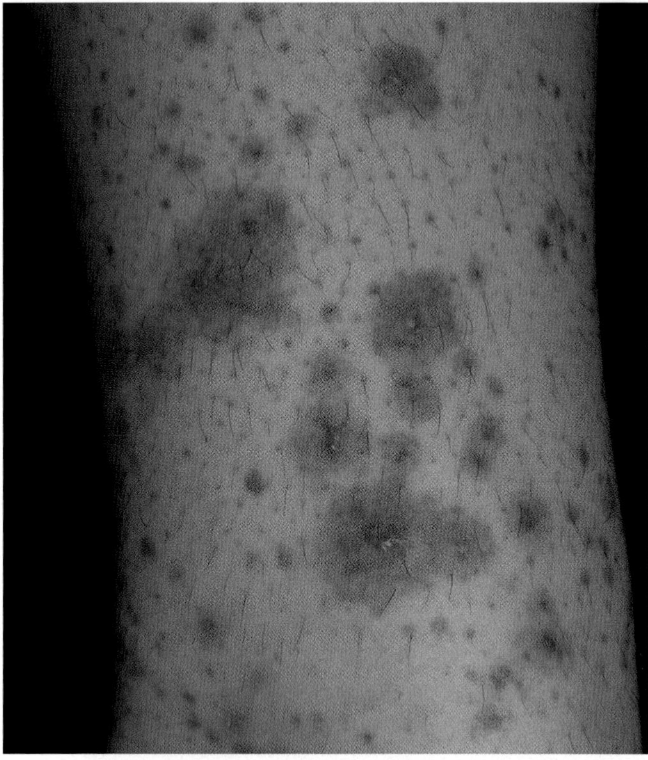

FIGURE 153-3 Close-up of palpable purpura from the patient in **Figure 153-2**. Some lesions look like target lesions but this is Henoch-Schönlein purpura and not erythema multiforme. (*Used with permission from Richard P. Usatine, MD.*)

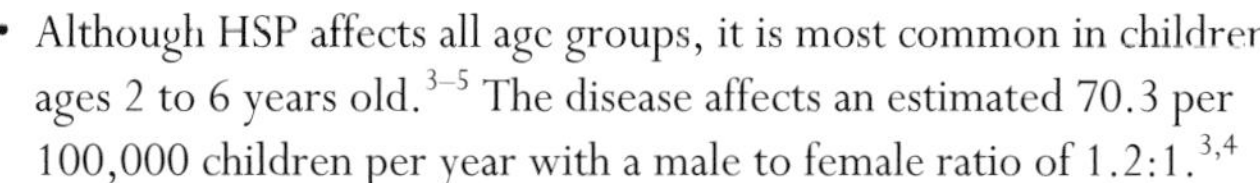

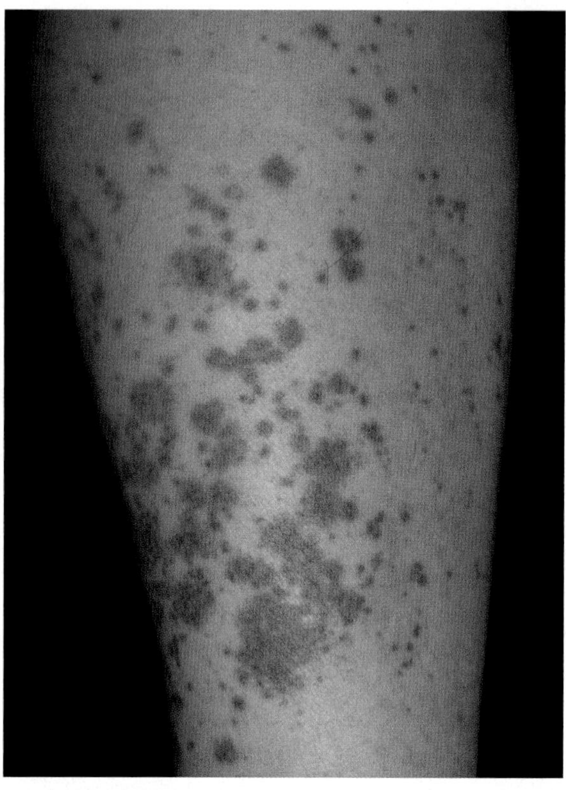

FIGURE 153-4 Leukocytoclastic vasculitis on the leg of a young woman. (*Used with permission from Richard P. Usatine, MD.*)

- Although HSP affects all age groups, it is most common in children ages 2 to 6 years old.[3–5] The disease affects an estimated 70.3 per 100,000 children per year with a male to female ratio of 1.2:1.[3,4]
- White children have a much higher incidence of HSP compared to black children.[3,4]
- Although the incidence in children has been reported to be about 100 times greater than adults, HSP is typically less severe in the pediatric population.[6]

ETIOLOGY AND PATHOPHYSIOLOGY

- HSP is usually benign and self-limiting, and tends to occur in the springtime. It results from immunoglobulin (Ig) A-containing immune complexes in blood vessel walls in the skin, kidney, and GI tract. A streptococcal or viral upper respiratory infection often precedes the disease by 1 to 3 weeks. Prodromal symptoms include anorexia and fever. Most children with HSP also have joint pain and swelling with the knees and ankles being most commonly involved (**Figure 153-1**). In half of the cases there are recurrences, typically in the first 3 months. Recurrences are more common in patients with nephritis and are milder than the original episode. To make the diagnosis of HSP, the patient should have palpable purpura or petechiae more in lower limbs and one or more of the following:[7,8]
- Bowel angina (pain).
- Arthritis or arthralgia.
- GI bleeding.
- Hematuria (renal involvement).
- Leukocytoclastic vasculitis (**Figures 153-4** and **153-5**) is the most commonly seen form of small vessel vasculitis. Prodromal symptoms include fever, malaise, myalgia, and joint pain. The palpable purpura begins as asymptomatic localized areas of cutaneous hemorrhage that become palpable. Few or many discrete lesions are most commonly seen on the lower extremities but may occur on any dependent area. Small lesions itch and are painful, but nodules, ulcers, and bullae may be very painful. Lesions appear in crops, last for 1 to 4 weeks, and may heal with residual scarring and hyperpigmentation. Patients may experience 1 episode (drug reaction or viral infection) or multiple episodes (RA or SLE). The disease is usually self-limited and confined to the skin. To make the diagnosis, look for presence of 3 or more of the following:[9]
- Age older than 16 years (not for HSP).
- Use of a possible offending drug in temporal relation to the symptoms.
- Palpable purpura.
- Maculopapular rash.
- Biopsy of a skin lesion showing neutrophils around an arteriole or venule. Systemic manifestations of leukocytoclastic vasculitis may include kidney disease, heart, nervous system, GI tract, lungs, and joint involvement.
- Vasculitis is defined as inflammation of the blood vessel wall. The mechanisms of vascular damage consist of a humoral response, immune complex deposition, or cell-mediated T-lymphocyte response with granuloma formation.[10]

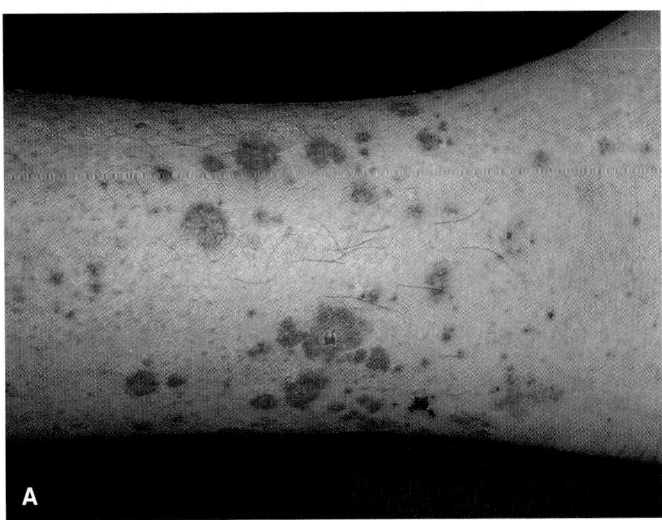

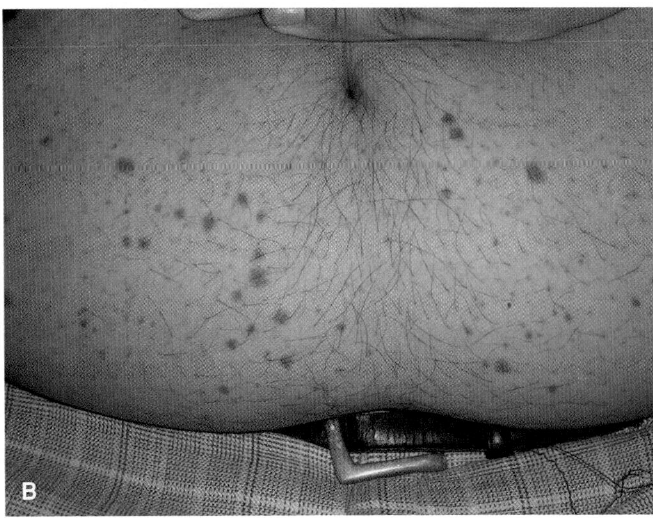

FIGURE 153-5 Leukocytoclastic vasculitis in a young man. **A.** Palpable purpura on the lower leg. **B.** Involvement of the lower abdomen. *(Used with permission from Richard P. Usatine, MD.)*

- Vasculitis induced injury to blood vessels may lead to increased vascular permeability, vessel weakening, aneurysm formation, hemorrhage, intimal proliferation, and thrombosis that result in obstruction and local ischemia.[10]
- Small-vessel vasculitis is initiated by hypersensitivity to various antigens (drugs, chemicals, microorganisms, and endogenous antigens), with formation of circulating immune complexes that are deposited in walls of postcapillary venules. The vessel-bound immune complexes activate complement, which attracts polymorphonuclear leukocytes. They damage the walls of small veins by release of lysosomal enzymes. This causes vessel necrosis and local hemorrhage.
- Small-vessel vasculitis most commonly affects the skin and rarely causes serious internal organ dysfunction, except when the kidney is involved. Small-vessel vasculitis is associated with leukocytoclastic vasculitis, HSP, essential mixed cryoglobulinemia, connective tissue diseases or malignancies, serum sickness, and serum sickness-like reactions, chronic urticaria, and acute hepatitis B or C infection.
- Hypersensitivity (leukocytoclastic) vasculitis causes acute inflammation and necrosis of venules in the dermis. The term *leukocytoclastic vasculitis* describes the histologic pattern produced when leukocytes fragment.
- Some patients with systemic lupus erythematosus (SLE; **Figure 153-6**) and other connective tissue disorders develop an associated necrotizing vasculitis. It most frequently involves the small muscular arteries, arterioles, and venules. The blood vessels can become blocked leading to tissue necrosis (**Figure 153-6**). The skin and internal organs may be involved.

RISK FACTORS

- Viral infections.
- Autoimmune disorders.
- Drug hypersensitivity.
- Cocaine (adulterated with levamisole; **Figure 153-7**).

DIAGNOSIS

- Initially, determining the extent of visceral organ involvement is more important than identifying the type of vasculitis, so that organs at risk of damage are not jeopardized by delayed or inadequate treatment. It is critical to distinguish vasculitis occurring as a primary autoimmune disorder from vasculitis secondary to infection, drugs, malignancy, or connective tissue disease such as SLE.[10]

CLINICAL FEATURES

- The clinical features of HSP include nonthrombocytopenic palpable purpura mainly on the lower extremities and buttocks (**Figures 153-1** to **153-3**), GI symptoms, arthralgia, and nephritis.

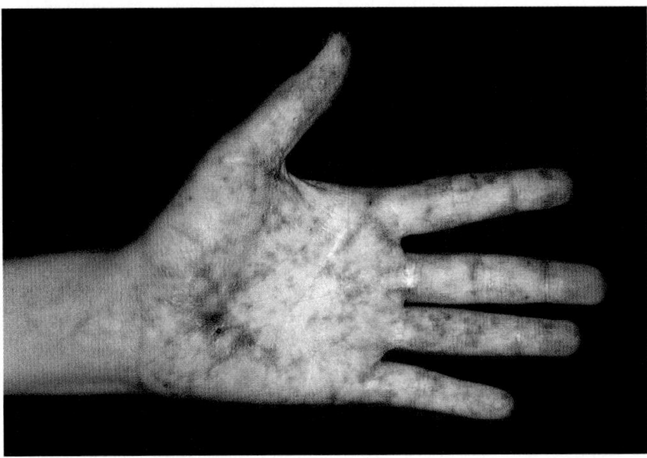

FIGURE 153-6 Necrotizing vasculitis in a young Asian woman with systemic lupus erythematosus. The circulation to the fingertips was compromised and the woman was treated with high-dose intravenous steroids and intravenous immunoglobulins to prevent tissue loss. *(Used with permission from Richard P. Usatine, MD.)*

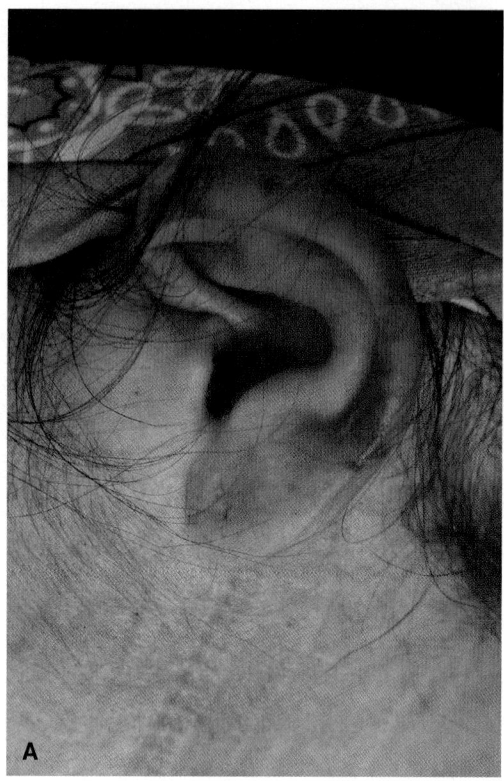

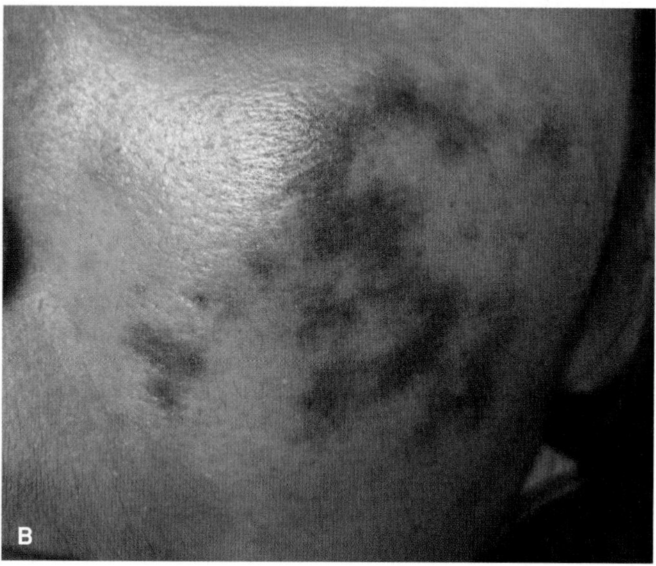

FIGURE 153-7 **A.** Cutaneous vasculitis of the ear caused by levamisole-adulterated cocaine. (*Used with permission from Jonathan Karnes, MD.*) **B.** Cutaneous vasculitis in a retiform (net-like) pattern caused by the use of levamisole-adulterated cocaine. This is called *retiform purpura*. (*Used with permission from John M. Martin IV, MD.*)

- Small-vessel vasculitis is characterized by necrotizing inflammation of small blood vessels, and may be identified by the finding of "palpable purpura." The lower extremities typically demonstrate "palpable purpura," varying in size from a few millimeters to several centimeters (**Figures 153-1** to **153-5**). In its early stages, leukocytoclastic vasculitis may not be palpable.

TYPICAL DISTRIBUTION

- Cutaneous vasculitis is found most commonly on the legs, but may be seen on the hands and abdomen (**Figures 153-1 to 153-5**).

LABORATORY TESTING

- Laboratory evaluation is geared to finding the antigenic source of the immunologic reaction. Consider throat culture, antistreptolysin-*O* titer, erythrocyte sedimentation rate, platelets, complete blood count (CBC), serum creatinine, urinalysis, antinuclear antibody, serum protein electrophoresis, circulating immune complexes, hepatitis B surface antigen, hepatitis C antibody, cryoglobulins, and rheumatoid factor. The erythrocyte sedimentation rate is almost always elevated during active vasculitis. Immunofluorescent studies are best done within the first 24 hours after a lesion forms. The most common immunoreactants present in and around blood vessels are IgM, C3, and fibrin. The presence of IgA in blood vessels of a child with vasculitis suggests the diagnosis of HSP.
- Basic laboratory analysis to assess the degree and types of organs affected should include serum creatinine, creatinine kinase, liver function studies, hepatitis serologies, urinalysis, and possibly chest x-ray and ECG.

BIOPSY

- The clinical presentation is so characteristic that a biopsy is generally unnecessary. In doubtful cases, a punch biopsy should be taken from an early active (nonulcerated) lesion or, if necessary, from the edge of an ulcer.
- Renal biopsy is not usually required but may be considered In patients with nephritic/nephrotic presentation, raised creatinine, hypertension, oliguria, heavy proteinuria (urine albumin/urine creatinine Ratio persistently >100 mg/mmol), persistent proteinuria (>4 weeks), or GFR <80.[11]

DIFFERENTIAL DIAGNOSIS

- Lichen aureus is a localized pigmented purpuric dermatosis seen in younger persons that may occur on the leg or in other parts of the body (**Figures 153-8** to **153-10**). The color may be yellow brown or golden brown.
- There is also a pigmented purpuric dermatosis of the Majocchi type that has an annular appearance with prominent elevated erythematous borders that may have telangiectasias (**Figure 153-11**). A dermatoscope can help to visualize the red or pink dots that represent inflamed capillaries in these conditions.

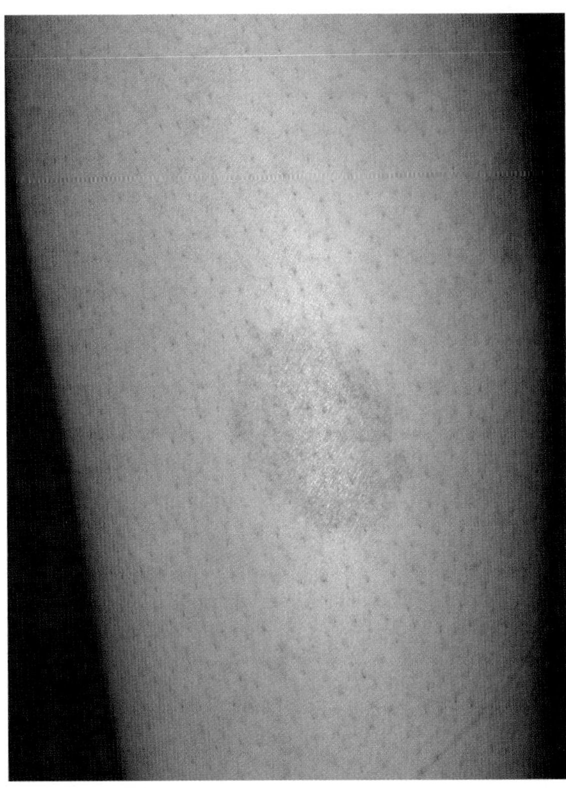

FIGURE 153-8 Lichen aureus on the leg of a 16-year-old girl. The light pink color is typical and it often is somewhat round or annular. Dermoscopy or magnification shows pinpoint capillaries with light hemosiderin deposits. (*Used with permission from Richard P. Usatine, MD.*)

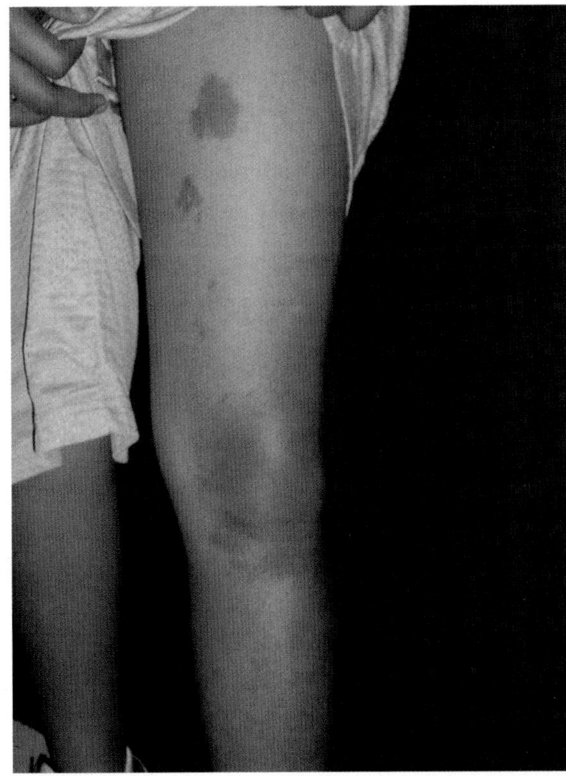

FIGURE 153-9 Lichen aureus (pigmented purpuric dermatosis) on the leg of an 8-year-old boy showing hemosiderin deposits and a cayenne pepper capillaritis. Note that this condition is hyperpigmented and not palpable. (*Used with permission from Richard P. Usatine, MD.*)

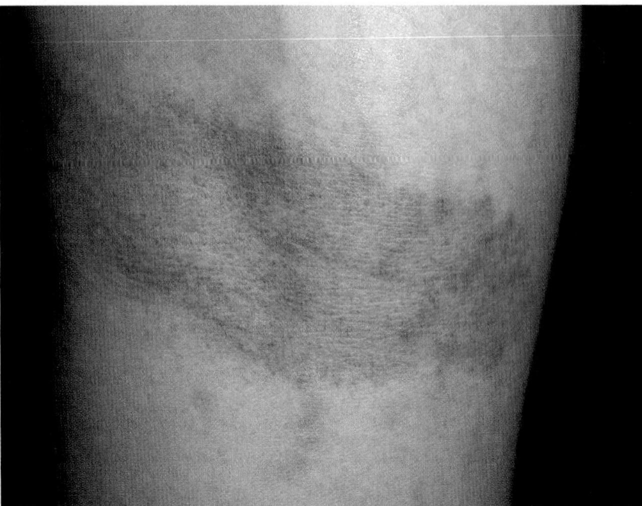

FIGURE 153-10 Lichen aureus (pigmented purpuric dermatosis) of the popliteal fossa in a teenage girl showing hemosiderin deposits and a cayenne pepper capillaritis. Note that this condition is not palpable but the cosmetic appearance is distressing to this teen. (*Used with permission from Richard P. Usatine, MD.*)

- Meningococcemia that presents with purpura in severely ill patients with or without central nervous system symptoms (**Figure 153-12**).
- Rocky Mountain spotted fever is a rickettsial infection that presents with pink to bright red, discrete 1- to 5-mm macules that blanch with pressure and may be pruritic. The lesions start distally and spread to the soles and palms (see **Figure 175-5**).
- Stevens-Johnson syndrome and toxic epidermal necrolysis (see Chapter 151, Erythema Multiforme, Stevens-Johnson Syndrome, and Toxic Epidermal Necrolysis).
- Idiopathic thrombocytopenia purpura can be easily distinguished from vasculitis by measuring the platelet count. Also, the purpura is usually not palpable and the petechiae can be scattered all over the body (**Figure 153-13**).

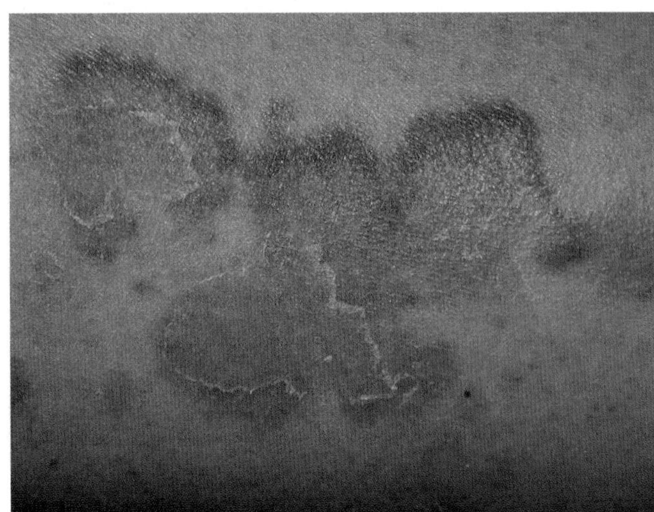

FIGURE 153-11 Pigmented purpuric dermatosis of the Majocchi type. Note the annular appearance and the prominent elevated erythematous borders. (*Used with permission from Suraj Reddy, MD.*)

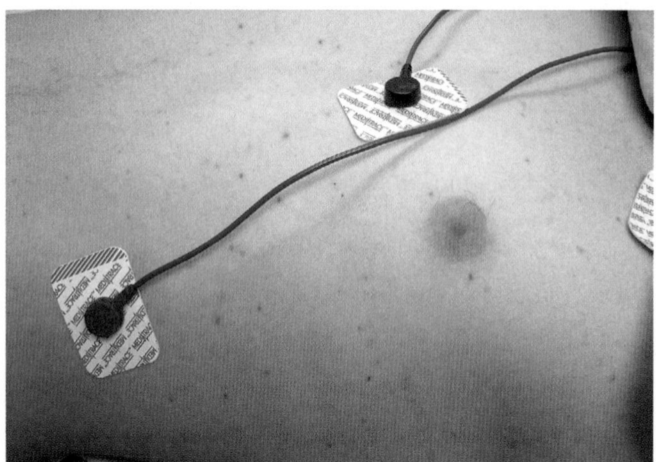

FIGURE 153-12 Petechiae of meningococcemia on the trunk of a hospitalized adolescent. (*Used with permission from Tom Moore, MD.*)

- Wegener granulomatosis is an unusual multisystem disease characterized by necrotizing granulomatous inflammation and vasculitis of the respiratory tract, kidneys, and skin.
- Churg-Strauss syndrome (allergic granulomatosis) that presents with a systemic vasculitis associated with asthma, transient pulmonary infiltrates, and hypereosinophilia.
- Cutaneous manifestations of cholesterol embolism, which are leg pain, livedo reticularis (blue-red mottling of the skin in a net-like pattern), and/or blue toes in the presence of good peripheral pulses.

MANAGEMENT

NONPHARMACOLOGIC

- The offending antigen should be identified and removed whenever possible. With a mild hypersensitivity vasculitis is due to a drug, discontinuing the offending drug may be all the treatment that is necessary. SOR C

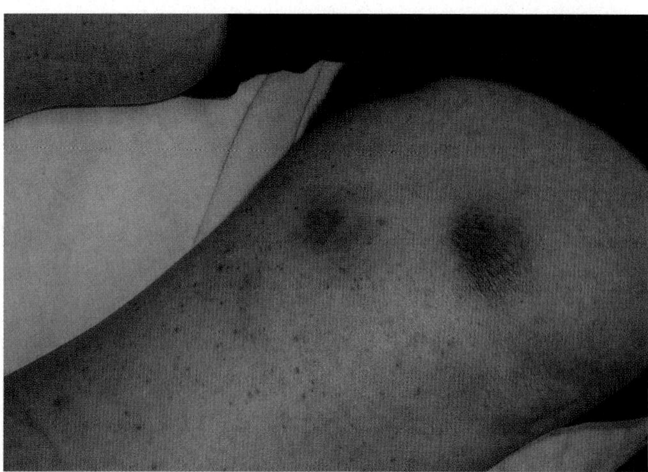

FIGURE 153-13 Petechiae and purpura in a patient with idiopathic thrombocytopenic purpura and a platelet count of 3000. Note that this purpura is not palpable. (*Used with permission from Richard P. Usatine, MD.*)

MEDICATIONS

- In HSP and prolonged hypersensitivity vasculitis, treatment with nonsteroidal antiinflammatory drugs is usually preferred. Treatment with corticosteroids may be of more benefit in patients with more severe disease such as more pronounced abdominal pain and renal involvement.[14] SOR B Adding cyclophosphamide to the steroids may also be effective. SOR C Azathioprine also may be used.[15]
- An antihistamine might be used for itching. SOR C
- Oral prednisone is used to treat visceral involvement and more severe cases of vasculitis of the skin. Short courses of prednisone (1 mg/kg/day) are effective and should be tapered slowly over 2 weeks.[12,13] SOR B
- Colchicine and dapsone inhibit neutrophil chemotaxis and have been used in adults but data is limited on their effectiveness in pediatric patients. SOR B
- There may be a role for the use of Ace inhibitors in patients with proteinuria related to vasculitis but data is still inconclusive on long-term benefit to preserving renal function.[17]

PROGNOSIS

- In leukocytoclastic (hypersensitivity) vasculitis, the cutaneous lesions usually resolve without sequelae. Visceral involvement (such as kidney and lung) most commonly occurs in HSP, cryoglobulinemia and vasculitis associated with SLE.[16] Extensive internal organ involvement should prompt an investigation for coexistent medium-size vessel disease and referral to a rheumatologist.

FOLLOW-UP

- Relapses may occur, especially when the precipitating factor is an autoimmune disease. Regular monitoring is necessary.

PATIENT EDUCATION

- Reassure patients and parents that most cases of acute cutaneous vasculitis resolve spontaneously.

PATIENT RESOURCES

- MedicineNet. *Vasculitis (Arteritis, Angiitis)*—**www.medicinenet.com/vasculitis/article.htm**.
- National Kidney and Urologic Diseases Information Clearinghouse. *Henoch-Schönlein Purpura*—**http://kidney.niddk.nih.gov/kudiseases/pubs/HSP/**.
- National Heart Blood and Lung Institute. *What Is Vasculitis?*—**www.nhlbi.nih.gov/health/dci/Diseases/vas/vas_whatis.html**.

PROVIDER RESOURCES

- Roane DW, Griger DR: An approach to diagnosis and initial management of systemic vasculitis. *Am Fam Physician* 1999:60: 1421-1430—**www.aafp.org/afp/991001ap/1421.html**.
- Sharma P, Sharma S, Baltaro R, Hurley J: Systemic vasculitis. *Am Family Physician* 2011;83(5):556-565—**www.aafp.org/afp/2011/0301/p556.html**.

REFERENCES

1. Stone JH, Nousari HC. "Essential" cutaneous vasculitis: what every rheumatologist should know about vasculitis of the skin. *Curr Opin Rheumatol* 2001;13(1):23-34.
2. Gardner-Medwin JM, Dolezalova P, Cummins C, Southwood TR. Incidence of Henoch-Schönlein purpura, Kawasaki disease, and rare vasculitides in children of different ethnic origins. *Lancet* 2002;360(9341):1197-1202.
3. McCarthy HJ, Tizard EJ. Clinical practice: Diagnosis and management of Henoch-Schonlein purpura. *Eur J Pediatr*. 2010;169: 643-650.
4. Gardner-Medwin JM, Dolezalova P, Cummins C, Southwood TR. Incidence of Henoch–Schönlein purpura, Kawasaki disease, and rare vasculitides in children of different ethnic origins. *Lancet*. 2002; 360(9341):1197-1202.
5. Aalberse J, Dolman K, Ramnath G, et al. Henoch Schönlein purpura in children: an epidemiological study among Dutch paediatricians on incidence and diagnostic criteria. *Ann Rheum Dis*. 2007; 66(12):1648-1650.
6. Ozen S. The spectrum of vasculitis in children. *Best Pract Res Clin Rheumatol*. 2002; 16:411-425.
7. Michel BA, Hunder GG, Bloch DA, Calabrese LH. Hypersensitivity vasculitis and Henoch-Schönlein purpura: a comparison between the 2 disorders. *J Rheumatol.* 1992;19:721.
8. Ozen S, Pistorio A, Iusan SM, et al. EULAR/PRINTO/PRES criteria for Henoch-Schönlein purpura, childhood polyarteritis nodosa, childhood Wegener granulomatosis and childhood Takayasu arteritis: Ankara 2008. Part II: Final classification criteria. Ann *Rheum Dis*. 2010; 69:798.
9. Calabrese LH, Michel BA, Bloch DA, et al. The American College of Rheumatology 1990 criteria for the classification of hypersensitivity vasculitis. *Arthritis Rheum* 1990;33:1108.
10. Sharma P, Sharma S, Baltaro R, Hurley J. Systemic vasculitis. *Am Fam Physician* 2011;83(5):556-565.
11. Brogan P, Eleftheriou D, Dillon M. Small vessel vasculitis. *Pediatric Nephrology*. 2010; 25:1025-1035.
12. Martinez-Taboada VM, Blanco R, Garcia-Fuentes M, Rodriguez-Valverde V. Clinical features and outcome of 95 patients with hypersensitivity vasculitis. *Am J Med.* 1997;102:186-191.
13. Sais G, Vidaller A, Jucgla A, et al. Colchicine in the treatment of cutaneous leukocytoclastic vasculitis. Results of a prospective, randomized controlled trial. *Arch Dermatol.* 1995;131: 1399-1402.
14. Weiss PF, Feinstein JA, Luan X, et al. Effects of corticosteroid on Henoch-Schonlein purpura: A systematic review. *Pediatrics.* 2007; 120:1079-1087.
15. Saulsbury FT. Henoch-Schönlein purpura. *Curr Opin Rheumatol* 2001;13:35-40.
16. Roane DW, Griger DR. An approach to diagnosis and initial management of systemic vasculitis. *Am Fam Physician.* 1999;60: 1421-1430.
17. Zaffanello, M. & Fanos, V. 2009. Treatment-based literature of Henoch-Schonlein purpura nephritis in childhood. *Pediatric Nephrology*. 2009; 24:1901-1911.

154 CUTANEOUS DRUG REACTIONS

Richard P. Usatine, MD
Anna Allred, MD
Mindy A. Smith, MD, MS

PATIENT STORY

A young college student was seen for fatigue and an upper respiratory infection and started on amoxicillin for a sore throat. Six days later, she broke out with a red rash all over her body (**Figure 154-1**). She went to see her family physician back home with the rash and lymphadenopathy. A monospot was drawn and found to be positive. This morbilliform rash (like measles) is typical of an amoxicillin drug eruption in a person with mononucleosis. Amoxicillin was stopped, and diphenhydramine was used for the itching.

INTRODUCTION

Cutaneous drug reactions are skin manifestations of drug hypersensitivity. Drug hypersensitivity may be defined as symptoms or signs initiated by a drug exposure at a dose normally tolerated by non-hypersensitive persons.[1] Drug-induced adverse reactions are often classified as type A and type B. Type A reactions are common (80%) predictable side effects caused by a pharmacologic action of the drug, and type B reactions are uncommon (10% to 15%) and considered idiosyncratic, a result of individual predisposition (e.g., an enzyme defect).[2] Cutaneous drug reactions range from mild skin eruptions (e.g., exanthem, urticaria, and angioedema) to severe cutaneous drug reactions (SCARs), the latter category including Stevens-Johnson syndrome (SJS), toxic epidermal necrolysis (TEN), and drug reaction with eosinophilia and systemic symptoms (DRESS) syndrome.[3]

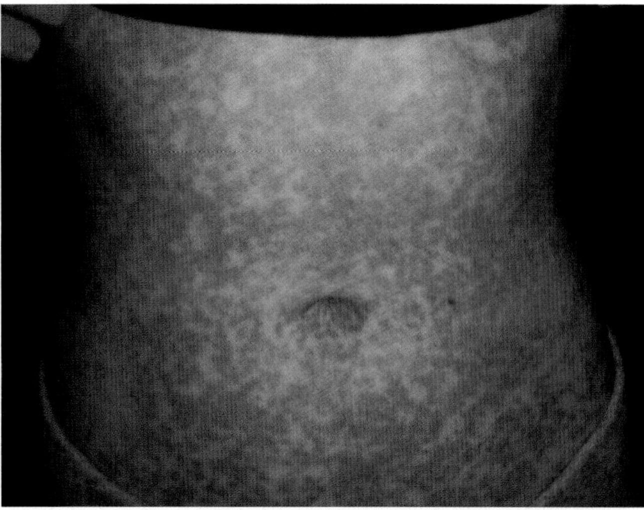

FIGURE 154-1 Amoxicillin rash in a teenage girl with mononucleosis. This is a morbilliform eruption. (*Used with permission from Richard P. Usatine, MD.*)

SYNONYMS

Cutaneous adverse reactions, drug reactions, medication reactions, adverse effects to drugs, or hypersensitivity reactions. DRESS syndrome is also called drug-induced hypersensitivity syndrome.

EPIDEMIOLOGY

- Cutaneous drug reactions are common complications of drug therapy occurring in 2 to 3 percent of hospitalized patients.[4]
- One study found that 45 percent of all adverse drug reactions were manifested in the skin.[4]
- Approximately 1 in 6 adverse drug reactions represents drug hypersensitivity, and are allergic or non–immune-mediated (pseudoallergic) reactions.[2]
- Maculopapular eruptions, also known as exanthematous drug eruptions, are the most frequent of all cutaneous drug reactions, representing 95 percent of skin reactions.[5] They are often confused with viral exanthems. This occurs most commonly with β-lactams such as amoxicillin, but also with barbiturates, gentamicin, isoniazid, phenytoin, sulfonamides, thiazides, and trimethoprim-sulfamethoxazole (**Figures 154-1** and **154-2**).

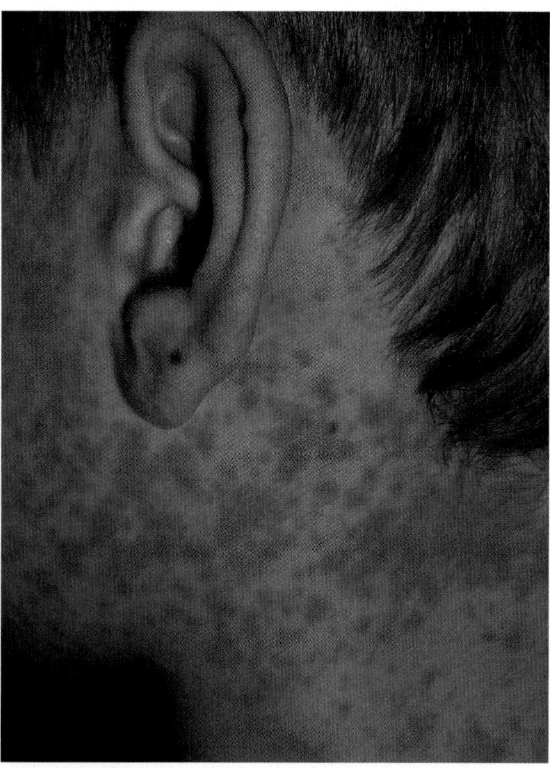

FIGURE 154-2 Maculopapular drug eruption in a 5-year-old boy with an upper respiratory infection started on amoxicillin for a questionable otitis media. Four days later he broke out with a red rash all over his face and body. This morbilliform rash (like measles) is typical of an amoxicillin drug eruption. (*Used with permission from Robert Tunks, MD.*)

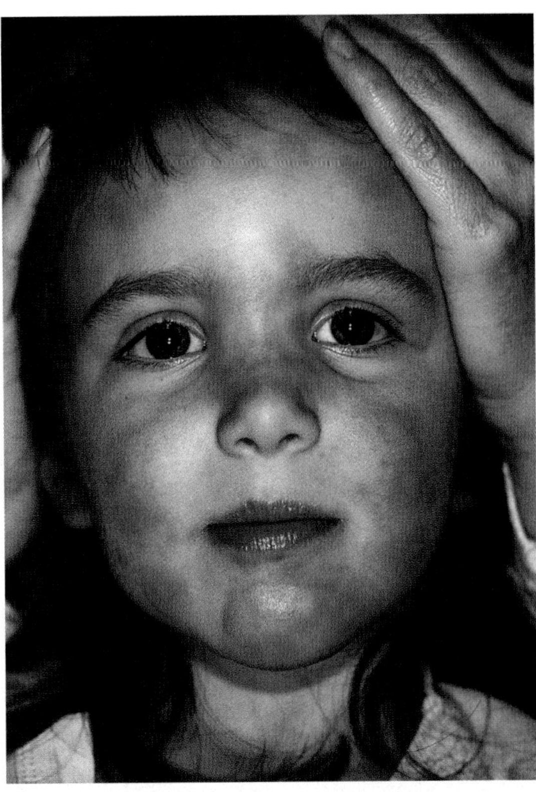

FIGURE 154-3 Urticarial drug eruption secondary to trimethoprim/sulfamethoxazole. (*Used with permission from Richard P. Usatine, MD.*)

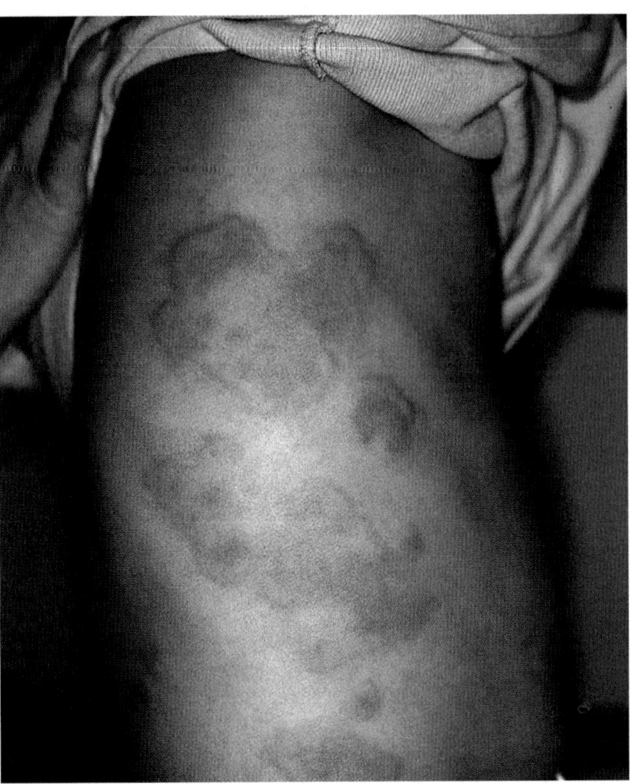

FIGURE 154-4 Giant urticarial eruption (urticaria multiforme) in the patient in **Figure 154-3** with drug reaction to sulfa. (*Used with permission from Richard P. Usatine, MD.*)

- Urticarial drug reactions are the second most common skin eruptions, representing approximately 5 percent of cutaneous drug reactions.[5] This reaction can result from any drug but commonly occurs with aspirin, penicillin, sulfa, angiotensin-converting enzyme (ACE) inhibitors, aminoglycosides, and blood products. Urticaria results from immunoglobulin (Ig) E reactions within minutes to hours of drug administration (**Figures 154-3** and **154-4**).
- Drug-induced hyperpigmentation occurs with antiarrhythmics (amiodarone), antibiotics (minocycline), NSAIDs, and chemotherapy agents (Adriamycin).
- Fixed drug eruptions (FDEs) can occur with many medications, including phenolphthalein, doxycycline, ibuprofen, sulfonamide antibiotics, and barbiturates (**Figures 154-5** to **154-8**). FDEs are more commonly observed in males.
- Erythema multiforme (EM) and SJS can occur secondary to drug reactions (**Figure 154-9**). Incidence of SJS is estimated at 1.2 per 6 million people.[3]
- DRESS (drug reaction with eosinophilia and systemic symptoms) syndrome is also a severe adverse drug-induced reaction characterized by eosinophilia with liver involvement, fever, and lymphadenopathy. In a case series (N = 172), 44 drugs were associated with DRESS.[6] DRESS syndrome is estimated to occur in 1 per 1000 to 1 per 10,000 exposures to antiepileptic drugs.[7]
- **Tables 154-1** lists the most common medications associated with allergic cutaneous drug reactions and the rates of reactions found.[8]
- **Table 154-2** lists the frequency of various classes of drugs associated with an eruption (in cases with <4 suspected drugs) based on a 5-year study.[9]

ETIOLOGY AND PATHOPHYSIOLOGY

- Two mechanisms are responsible for cutaneous drug reactions—Immunologic, including all four types of hypersensitivity reactions,

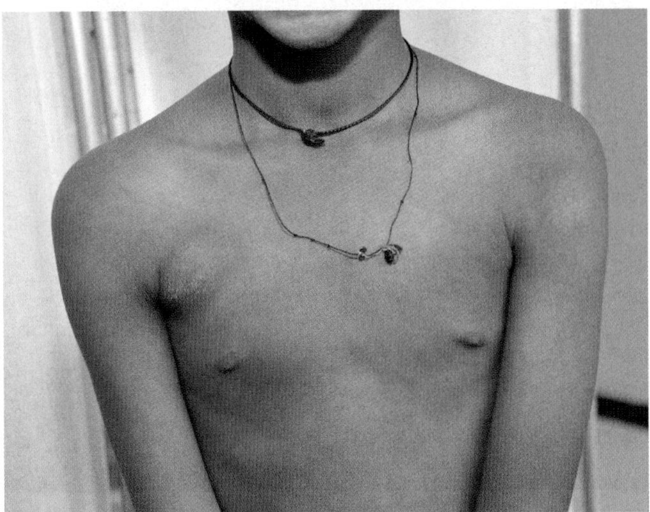

FIGURE 154-5 Fixed drug eruption to trimethoprim/sulfamethoxazole with hyperpigmented plaques in a 10-year-old boy. (*Used with permission from Richard P. Usatine, MD.*)

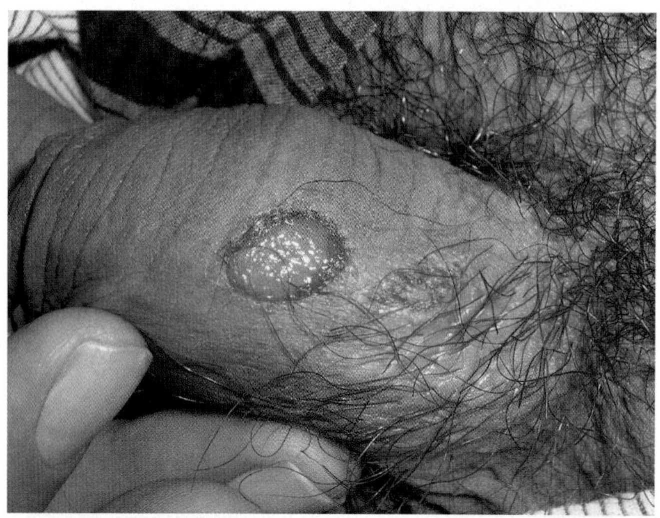

FIGURE 154-6 Fixed drug eruption to ibuprofen with violaceous and hyperpigmented macules and erosions on the penis. (*Used with permission from Richard P. Usatine, MD.*)

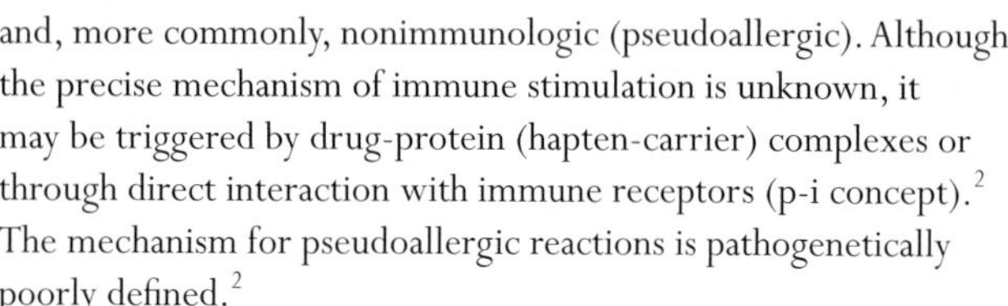

and, more commonly, nonimmunologic (pseudoallergic). Although the precise mechanism of immune stimulation is unknown, it may be triggered by drug-protein (hapten-carrier) complexes or through direct interaction with immune receptors (p-i concept).[2] The mechanism for pseudoallergic reactions is pathogenetically poorly defined.[2]

- Hypersensitivity to NSAIDs is a nonimmunologic reaction that can be immediate (within hours after exposure) or delayed (more than 24 hours after administration).[1]
- SJS/TEN is most commonly associated with penicillins and sulfonamide antibiotics but can also occur with anticonvulsants, NSAIDs, allopurinol, and corticosteroids. It is hypothesized that a specific human leukocyte antigen (HLA)-B molecule may present the drug

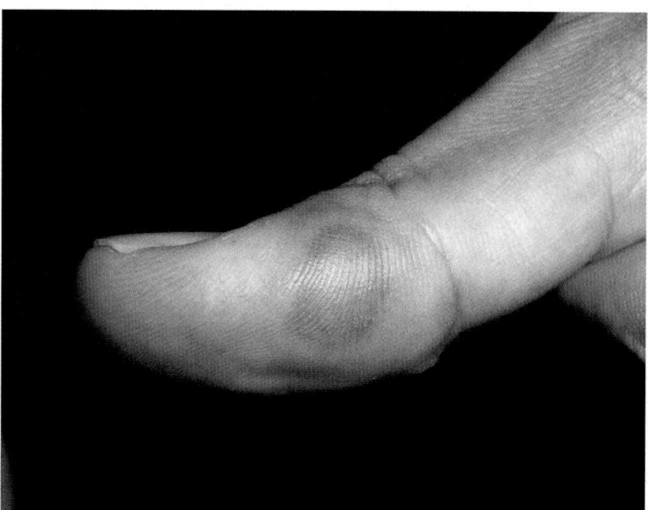

FIGURE 154-7 Third episode of fixed drug eruption to doxycycline. Note how the finger lesion is similar to a target lesion in erythema multiforme. However, there is no central epithelial disruption in this target lesion. (*Used with permission from Richard P. Usatine, MD.*)

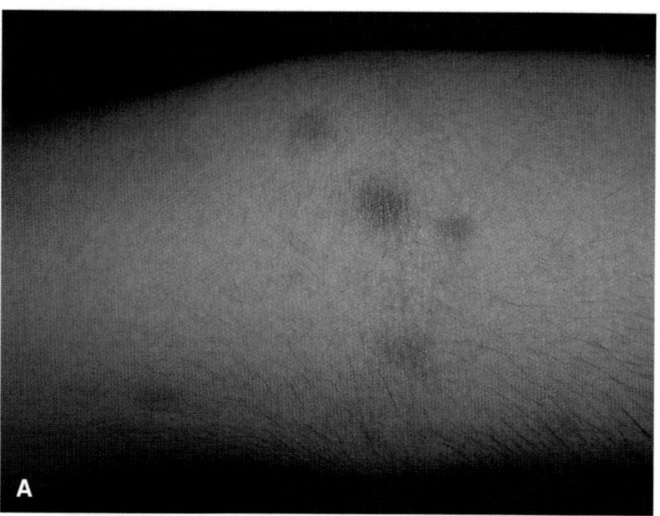

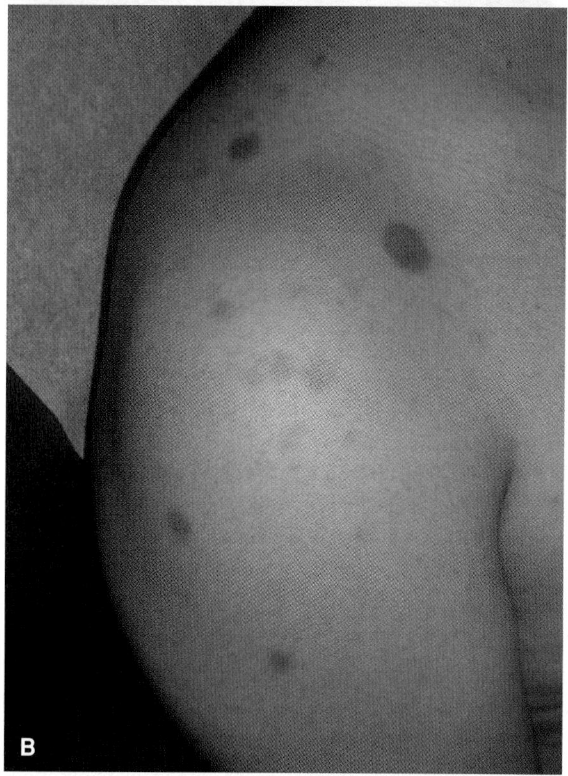

FIGURE 154-8 Fixed drug eruption to hydrocodone on the **A.** arm and **B.** shoulder. (*Used with permission from Richard P. Usatine, MD.*)

or its metabolites to naïve CD8 cells resulting in clonal expansion of CD8 cytotoxic lymphocytes and induction of cytotoxic effector responses, resulting in apoptosis of keratinocytes.[10] This pathway is not likely to be specific to SJS.

RISK FACTORS

- Drug hypersensitivity reactions increase with the drug dose, duration, route of administration (topical > subcutaneous > intramuscular > oral > intravenous),[11] immune activation of the individual, and

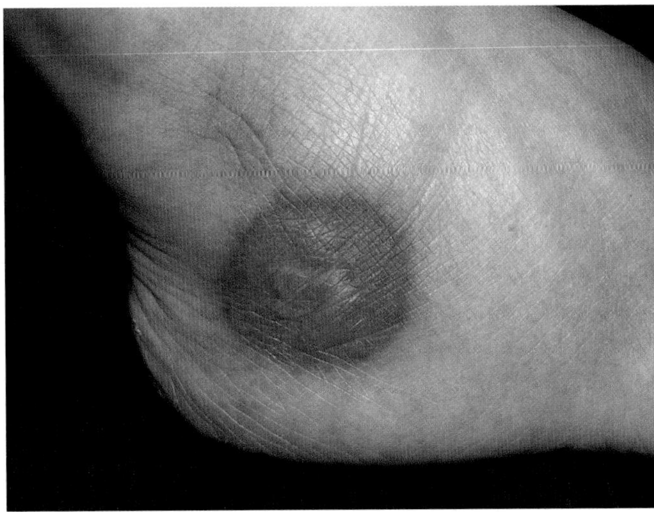

FIGURE 154-9 Bullous fixed drug eruption with a dusky color and an annular pink border on the ankle. (*Used with permission from Richard P. Usatine, MD.*)

immunogenetic predisposition; they are also more frequent in women.[2] Multiple drug therapy may also increase risk.[11]

- Patients with the following HLAs are at higher risk for cutaneous drug reactions: HLA-B*1502 (confers a very high risk of carbamazepine-induced and other antiepileptic drug-induced SJS among people of southeastern Asian ethnicity); HLA-B*5801 (higher risk of allopurinol-induced severe cutaneous reactions); HLA-B*5701 (higher risk of abacavir [an antiretroviral drug] hypersensitivity reactions); HLA-B*3501, HLA-B*3505, HLA-B*1402, and HLA-Cw8 (nevirapine [an antiretroviral drug] sensitivity with rash; the latter two found in a Sardinian population); HLA-DRB1*0101 (nevirapine hypersensitivity rash with hepatitis).[2,6]
- Prior drug reaction may result in a faster recurrence on reexposure.[11]
- Concomitant illness, especially viral infections and autoimmune disorders.[11]

TABLE 154-2 Frequency of Various Classes of Drugs Associated with an Eruption (in cases with <4 suspected drugs)

Class of Drug	No. of Cases (N = 82)
Antibiotic	37
Antiepileptic	12
Phenytoin	9
Antiarrhythmic	6
Calcium ion inhibitors	3
Anticoagulant	5
Enoxaparin	2
Clopidogrel	2
Warfarin	1
Antifungal	4
Antigout	4
Proton pump inhibitors	4
ACE[1] inhibitors	3
Contrast	3
Diuretics	3
Anti-inflammatory	2
Antiretroviral (HIV)	2
Antiviral	2
Beta blockers	2
Chemotherapeutic	2
Other	11

[1]ACE, Angiotensin-converting enzyme.
Used with permission from: Gerson D, Sriganeshan V, Alexis JB. Cutaneous drug eruptions: a 5-year experience. *J Am Acad Dermatol.* 2008 Dec;59(6):995-999.

TABLE 154-1 Allergic Cutaneous Reactions to Drugs Received by at Least 1000 Patients

Drug	Reactions, No.	Recipients, No.	Rate, Percent	95 Percent Confidence Interval
Fluoroquinolones	16	1015	1.6	0.8 to 2.3
Amoxicillin	40	3233	1.2	0.9 to 1.6
Augmentin	12	1000	1.2	0.5 to 1.9
Penicillins	63	5914	1.1	0.8 to 1.3
Nitrofurantoin	7	1085	0.6	0.2 to 1.1
Tetracycline	23	4981	0.5	0.3 to 0.7
Macrolides	5	1435	0.3	0.0 to 0.7

Source: Reprinted from: van der Linden PD, van der Lei J, Vlug AE, Stricker BH: Skin reactions to antibacterial agents in general practice. *J Clin Epidemiol.* 1998;(51)703-708. Copyright 1998, with permission from Elsevier.

DIAGNOSIS

CLINICAL FEATURES AND TYPICAL DISTRIBUTION (THE MOST COMMON AND IMPORTANT DRUG ERUPTIONS)

- Maculopapular—These eruptions, red macules with papules, can occur any time after drug therapy is initiated (often 7 to 10 days) and last 1 to 2 weeks. The reaction usually starts on the upper trunk or head and neck then spreads symmetrically downward to limbs. The eruptions may become confluent in a symmetric, generalized distribution that spares the face (**Figure 154-1**). Mild desquamation is normal as the exanthematous eruption resolves.
- Urticaria and angioedema—Urticaria reactions present as circumscribed areas of blanching-raised erythema and edema of the superficial dermis (**Figures 154-3** and **154-4**). They may occur on any skin area and are usually transient, migratory, and pruritic. Angioedema represents a deeper reaction, with swelling usually around the lips and eyes (see Chapter 150, Urticaria and Angioedema).
- Hyperpigmentation—Drug-induced hyperpigmentation presents in many ways. Amiodarone causes a dusky red coloration that turns blue-gray with time in photo-exposed areas. Minocycline can cause a blue-gray color in acne lesions, on the gingiva and on the teeth. Phenytoin (Dilantin) and other hydantoins may cause melasma-like brown pigmentation on the face.
- NSAIDs—The cutaneous reactions to NSAID-associated drug hypersensitivity are urticaria, angioedema, or anaphylaxis.[1] These reactions can be caused by a single NSAID or multiple NSAIDs. There is also an NSAID-exacerbated urticaria and angioedema that occurs in patients with chronic idiopathic urticaria.
- Fixed drug eruption (FDE)—Presents with single or multiple sharply demarcated circular, violaceous or hyperpigmented plaques that may include a central blister (**Figures 154-3** to **154-9**). The lesion(s) appear after drug exposure and reappear exactly at the same site each time the drug is taken. The site resolves, leaving an area of macular hyperpigmentation (**Figures 154-5** and **154-8**). Lesions can occur anywhere including the hands and feet, but are commonly found on the penis (**Figure 154-6**). The eruption presents 30 minutes to 8 hours after drug administration. Bullous *fixed drug eruptions* occur when the lesion blisters and erodes, followed by desquamation and crusting (**Figure 154-9**).
- EM—It presents with typical target or raised edematous papules distributed acrally. Most importantly, there should be some type of epidermal disruption with bullae or erosions within the target lesions (**Figure 154-10**). Severe EM becomes and more widespread epidermal detachment may occur involving less than 10 percent of total body surface area (see Chapter 151, Erythema Multiforme, Stevens-Johnson Syndrome, and Toxic Epidermal Necrolysis).
- SJS—It presents with erythematous or pruritic macules, widespread blisters on the trunk and face, and erosions of one or more mucous membranes (**Figure 154-11**). Atypical target lesions or widespread erythema, particularly in the upper chest and back, are potential early signs of both SJS and TEN.[11] Burning or painful skin can be a sign of increased severity. Epidermal detachment occurs and involves less than 30 percent of total body surface area.

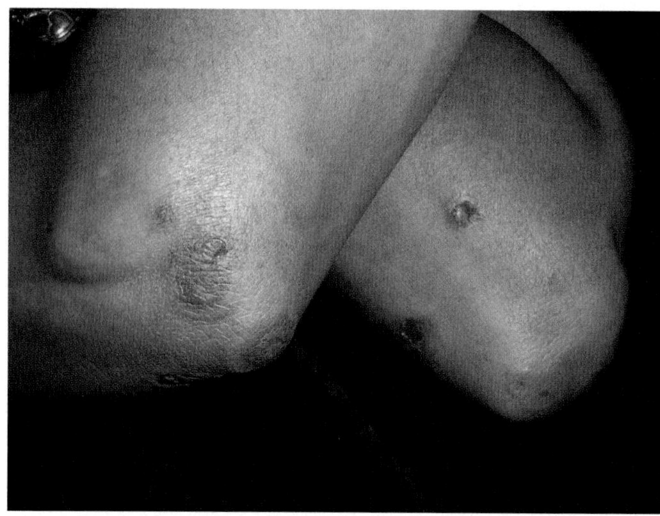

FIGURE 154-10 Erythema multiforme on the elbows. Note the epithelial disruption in the center of each target lesion. (*Used with permission from Richard P. Usatine, MD.*)

- Toxic epidermal necrolysis (TEN)—It is on the most severe side of the SJS spectrum. EM is diagnosed when less than 10 percent of the body surface area is involved, SJS/TEN when 10 to 30 percent is involved, and toxic epidermal necrolysis when more than 30 percent is involved (see Chapter 151, Erythema Multiforme, Stevens-Johnson Syndrome and Toxic Epidermal Necrolysis).
- Drug reaction with eosinophilia and systemic symptoms (DRESS) or drug-induced hypersensitivity syndrome (DIHS)—Infiltrated,

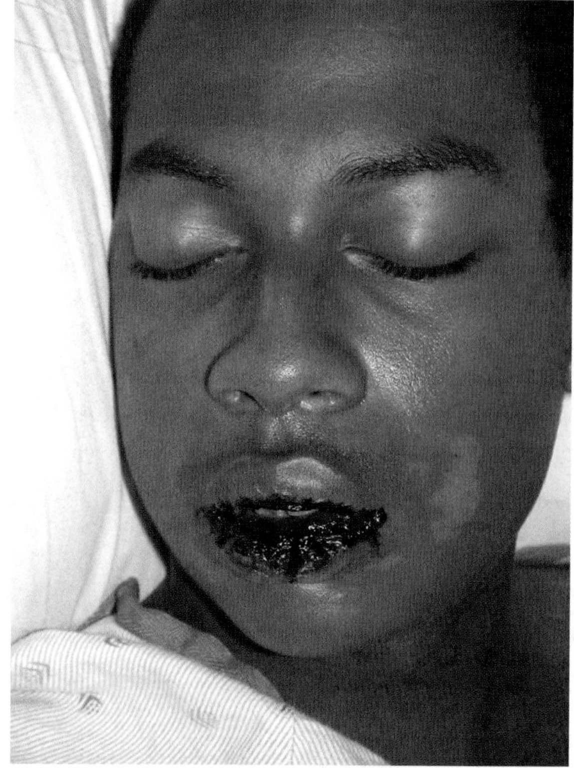

FIGURE 154-11 Stevens-Johnson syndrome secondary to a sulfa antibiotic. (*Used with permission from Eric Kraus, MD.*)

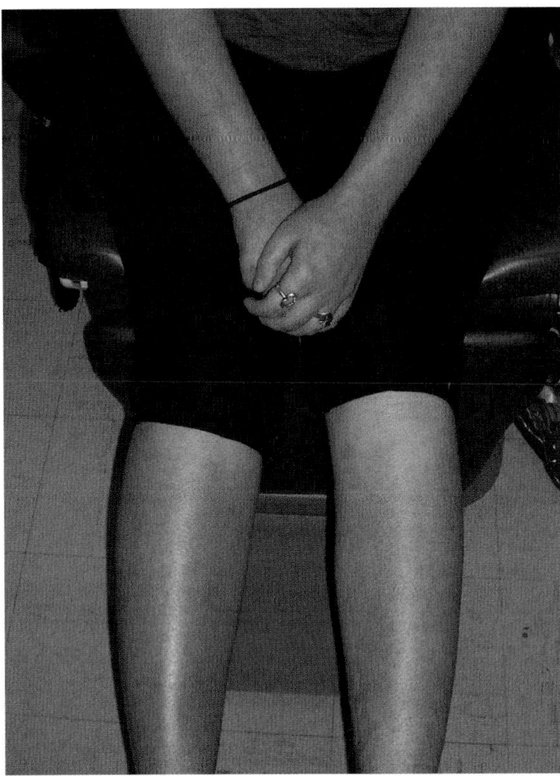

FIGURE 154-12 Drug reaction with eosinophilia and systemic symptoms syndrome (drug reaction, eosinophilia, systemic symptoms) in a teenage girl. Erythroderma has persisted but the patient is feeling better after treatment and discharge from the hospital. (*Used with permission from Richard P. Usatine, MD.*)

palpable lesions are potential heralds of this disorder.[11] Central facial edema and erythema and a maculopapular rash are seen along with high fever, generalized lymphadenopathy, and arthralgias. Drug reaction with eosinophilia and systemic symptoms can also cause an erythroderma (**Figure 154-12**). Latency between starting a drug and first signs of drug reaction with eosinophilia and systemic symptoms can be up to 12 weeks.[11]

- Drugs most commonly known to cause SJS and TEN are sulfonamide antibiotics, allopurinol, nonsteroidal antiinflammatory agents, amine antiepileptic drugs (phenytoin and carbamazepine), and lamotrigine (see Chapter 151, Erythema Multiforme, Stevens-Johnson Syndrome, and Toxic Epidermal Necrolysis).[12] Fifty percent of SJS/TEN cases have no identifiable cause.
- Acute generalized exanthematous pustulosis (AGEP)—is a type of drug eruption that results in clusters of small pustules along with erythematous skin (**Figure 154-13**). The patients are often febrile and the pustules are primarily nonfollicular and sterile.

LABORATORY STUDIES

The diagnosis of drug eruptions is usually made based on history and physical examination.

- An FDE may be diagnosed by "provoking" the appearance of the lesion with an oral rechallenge with the suspected drug; however, this can be dangerous in bullous cases.

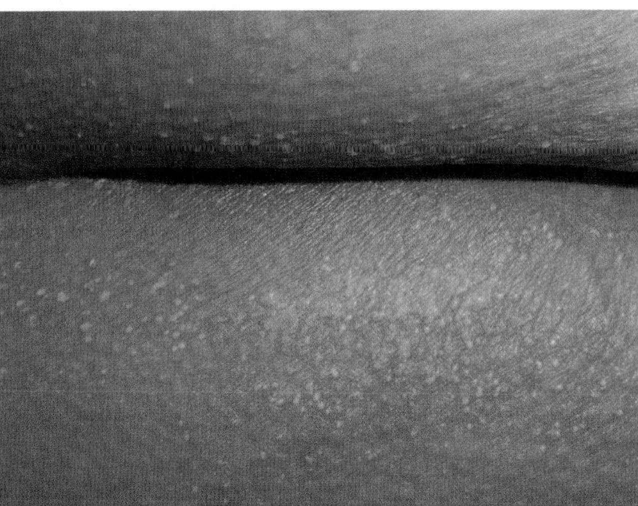

FIGURE 154-13 Acute generalized exanthematous pustulosis (AGEP) caused by a drug eruption. The clusters of small pustules with erythematous skin are seen on the buttocks. In this case, the pustules and erythema covered major portions of the back and buttocks. (*Used with permission from Robert T. Gilson, MD.*)

- Severe reactions may need a complete blood count (CBC) with differential and comprehensive serum chemistry panel to look for systemic involvement and check hydration status.
- In more challenging cases, a skin biopsy may be helpful to confirm the diagnosis.
- Intradermal skin testing may be hazardous to patients, and patch tests are not useful.
- Skin biopsies are usually not required for diagnosis of WISN, but may aid in the diagnosis.
- Testing for thrombophilia (high platelet count) may also be done in WISN.
- Laboratory tests in patients with DRESS/DIHS may show atypical lymphocytes, eosinophilia, lymphocytopenia, and thrombocytopenia; liver abnormalities are often seen.

DIFFERENTIAL DIAGNOSIS

- Viral exanthems look just like generalized maculopapular drug eruptions. Sometimes when a patient is given an antibiotic for an upper respiratory infection, the rash that ensues may be the viral exanthem rather than a drug eruption. The best way to avoid this confusion is only to use antibiotics when the evidence for bacterial infection is sufficient to justify the risks of a drug reaction (see Chapters 108 to 115 for more information on viral exanthems).
- Urticarial reactions present as transient migratory circumscribed areas of blanching-raised erythema and edema of the superficial dermis. Patients experience itching. Identifying urticaria is easy compared with finding the precipitating factors. If there is a temporal association with starting a new drug, it is best to stop the drug (in most cases) and see if the urticaria resolves (see Chapter 134, Urticaria and Angioedema).

- EM presents with sudden onset of rapidly progressive, symmetrical, and cutaneus lesions with centripetal spread. The patient may have a burning sensation in affected areas but usually has no pruritus. EM is most often caused by a reaction to an infection such as herpes simplex virus (HSV) or mycoplasma but may be caused by a drug reaction. Careful history and physical examination can help differentiate between the possible causes (see Chapter 151, Erythema Multiforme, Stevens-Johnson Syndrome, and Toxic Epidermal Necrolysis).
- SJS and TEN present with generalized cutaneous lesion with blisters, fever, malaise, arthralgias, headache, sore throat, nausea, vomiting, and diarrhea. The patient may also have difficulty in eating, drinking, or opening his or her mouth secondary to erosion of oral mucous membranes (**Figure 154-11**). Not all SJS or TEN is secondary to drug exposure, but it is the job of the clinician to investigate this cause and stop any suspicious medications. SJS and TEN can be life-threatening (see Chapter 151, Erythema Multiforme, Stevens-Johnson Syndrome, and Toxic Epidermal Necrolysis).
- DRESS syndrome can be distinguished by involvement of organs other than skin including liver (hepatitis in 50% to 70%), kidney (nephritis in 10%), and, more rarely, pneumonitis, colitis, myocarditis, parotitis, meningitis, encephalitis, and pancreatitis; the pattern of organ involvement appears to depend on the drug trigger.[7,13] Some of the sequelae from DRESS syndrome are strongly related to herpes virus reactivation.[7] A recurrence of symptoms at the third week is common. Diagnostic criteria have been proposed to include all of the following: maculopapular rash developing more than 3 weeks after drug exposure, prolonged clinical symptoms after drug discontinuation, fever (>38°C [100.4°F]), liver abnormalities or other organ involvement, leukocyte abnormalities (atypical lymphocytosis, leukocytosis, eosinophilia), lymphadenopathy, and human herpesvirus-6 reactivation.[13]
- Pityriasis rosea (PR) is a mysterious eruption of unknown etiology that could easily mimic a maculopapular drug eruption. Look and ask for the herald patch to help make the diagnosis of PR. In PR, look for the collarette scale and observe whether the eruption follows the skin lines (causing a Christmas tree pattern on the back). These features should help positively identify PR because there are no laboratory tests that are specific to PR or most drug eruptions (see Chapter 137, Pityriasis Rosea).
- Syphilis is the great imitator. Any generalized rash without a known etiology may be caused by secondary syphilis. A rapid plasma reagin (RPR) will always be positive in secondary syphilis and is easy to run (see Chapter 181, Syphilis).
- Chronic bullous disease of childhood and pemphigus vulgaris can resemble a bullous drug eruption. Biopsies are the best way to diagnose these bullous diseases. Their clinical pictures are described in detail in Chapters 155, Chronic Bullous Disease of Childhood, and Chapter 156, Pemphigus.

MANAGEMENT

NONPHARMACOLOGIC

- Discontinue the offending medication for all types of drug reactions whenever possible. Older patients with drug eruptions may be on multiple medications and may be very ill; however, efforts should be made to discontinue all nonessential medications.[5] SOR Ⓒ
- Patients with maculopapular reactions may continue to be treated with the offending agent if it is essential for treating a serious underlying condition.[5]
- Maculopapular drug eruptions are not a precursor to severe reactions such as TEN.[5]
- Local wound care, debridement, and skin grafting may need to be performed to repair resultant disfigurement from necrosis.[15]

MEDICATIONS

- Maculopapular- and urticarial/angioedema-type drug reactions are treated with antihistamines. If the angioedema is causing airway compromise, epinephrine (10 mcg/kg intramuscular) and other treatments will be necessary.[5,13] SOR Ⓒ Usually an H_1-blocker is started. In some cases of urticaria/angioedema, an H_2-blocker is added on for broader antihistamine effects (see Chapter 134, Urticaria and Angioedema).
- Diphenhydramine (Benadryl)—Orally every 4 to 6 hours (nonprescription).
- Hydroxyzine (Atarax)—Pediatric dose 0.5 to 1.0 mg/kg per day orally 4 times daily.[5]
- Loratadine (Claritin)—Once daily[5] (nonprescription).
- H_2-blockers can be used by prescription or nonprescription.
- Topical steroids such as triamcinolone or desonide may be used for symptomatic relief of pruritus.[5] SOR Ⓒ
- Oral steroids have been used, but little benefit has been shown in most drug reactions.[5] SOR Ⓒ
- Systemic steroids are recommended for treatment of DRESS syndrome.[13,14] SOR Ⓒ
- FDEs are treated by discontinuing the drug and applying topical corticosteroids to the affected area.[4] SOR Ⓒ

REFERRAL OR HOSPITALIZATION

Patients with SJS, TEN, and DRESS syndrome are usually hospitalized.

- SJS, TEN, DRESS/DIHS—Start with early diagnosis, rapid discontinuing of offending agent, intravenous fluid replacement, and placement in an intensive care unit (ICU) or burn unit (see Chapter 151, Erythema Multiforme, Steven-Johnson Syndrome, and Toxic Epidermal Necrolysis).[4,5] Liver transplant has been used in patients with DRESS.[13]
- Most experts and studies now agree that systemic corticosteroids should not be used except in DRESS syndrome.[4] SOR Ⓑ
- Nutritional support, careful wound care, temperature control, and anticoagulation are recommended.[4] SOR Ⓒ
- Daily skin samples should be sent for bacterial Gram stain and culture to monitor for developing infection.[4] SOR Ⓒ

PREVENTION

- In the future, prevention may occur through screening for HLA associations and drug avoidance.[1]
- Avoid reexposure to the drug.

- Screening for HLA-B*1502 is advised by the US FDA and Health Canada for patients of southeastern Asian ethnicity before carbamazepine therapy.[1]

PROGNOSIS

- Most cutaneous drug reactions resolve with discontinuation of the causative agent.
- Mortality, however, is high at 10 percent for SJS and DRESS and 30 to 50 percent for TEN.[5,15] In a case series of patients with possible or probably DRESS, case fatality rate was 5 percent (9/172).[6]
- Some studies show the occurrence of autoimmune diseases, including type 1 diabetes mellitus, autoimmune thyroid disease, sclerodermoid graft-versus-host disease (GVHD)-like lesions, and lupus erythematosus months to years after resolution of DRESS syndrome.[7] Because of the long symptom-free interval in some patients, this relationship is questioned.

FOLLOW-UP

- Follow-up is most important when the case is severe or the diagnosis is uncertain. Clear-cut mild drug reactions may not need scheduled follow-up.
- Continued surveillance for autoimmune disorders may be warranted in patients following DRESS syndrome.

PATIENT EDUCATION

- Most patients with drug eruptions recover fully without any complications. The patient should be warned that even after the responsible medication is stopped the eruptions may clear slowly or even worsen at first; the patient should be advised that the reaction may not resolve for 1 to 2 weeks.
- The patient should also be counseled that mild desquamation is normal as the exanthematous eruption resolves. Confirming the diagnosis of an FDE, especially lesions presenting on the glans, with a drug challenge may allay the patient anxiety about the venereal origin of the disease.
- The family should be counseled as to the genetic predisposition of some drug-induced eruptions.
- The patient should be advised to enroll in a medic alert program and to wear a bracelet detailing the allergy.

PATIENT RESOURCES

- MedlinePlus. *Drug Allergies*—**www.nlm.nih.gov/medlineplus/ency/article/000819.htm**.
- Mayo Clinic. *Stevens-Johnson Syndrome*—**www.mayoclinic.com/print/stevens-johnson-syndrome/DS00940/DSECTION=all&METHOD=print**.

PROVIDER RESOURCES

- **www.patient.co.uk/doctor/Drug-Eruptions.htm**.
- **http://dermnetnz.org/reactions/drug-eruptions.html**.
- Medscape. *Drug Eruptions*—**http://emedicine.medscape.com/article/1049474-overview**.

If the skin eruption is rare, serious, or unexpected, the drug reaction should be reported to the manufacturer and FDA.

REFERENCES

1. Sánchez-Borges M. NSAID hypersensitivity (respiratory, cutaneous, and generalized anaphylactic symptoms). *Med Clin North Am.* 2010;94(4):853-864.
2. Pichler WJ, Adam J, Daubner B, et al. Drug hypersensitivity reactions: pathomechanism and clinical symptoms. *Med Clin North Am.* 2010;94(4):645-664.
3. Phillips EJ, Chung WH, Mockenhaupt M, et al. Drug hypersensitivity: pharmacogenetics and clinical syndromes. *J Allergy Clin Immunol.* 2011;127(3):S60-S66.
4. Nigen S, Knowles SR, Shear NH. Drug eruptions: approaching the diagnosis of drug-induced skin diseases. *J Drugs Dermatol.* 2003;2(3):278-299.
5. Habif T. *Skin Disease Diagnosis and Treatment*, 2nd ed. Philadelphia, PA: Mosby; 2005.
6. Cacoub P, Musette P, Descamps V, et al. The DRESS syndrome: a literature review. *Am J Med.* 2011;124(7):588-597.
7. Kano Y, Ishida T, Kazuhisa K, Shiohara T. Visceral involvements and long-term sequelae in drug-induced hypersensitivity syndrome. *Med Clin North Am.* 2010;94(4):743-759.
8. van der Linden PD, van der Lei J, Vlug AE, Stricker BH. Skin reactions to antibacterial agents in general practice. *J Clin Epidemiol.* 1998;(51)703-708.
9. Gerson D, Sriganeshan V, Alexis JB. Cutaneous drug eruptions: a 5-year experience. *J Am Acad Dermatol.* 2008 Dec;59(6):995-999.
10. Fernando SL, Broadfoot J. Prevention of severe cutaneous adverse drug reactions: the emerging value of pharmacogenetic screening. *CMAJ.* 2010;182(5):476-480.
11. Scherer K, Bircher AJ. Danger signs in drug hypersensitivity. *Med Clin North Am.* 2010;94(4):681-689.
12. Chosidow OM, Stern RS, Wintroub BU. Cutaneous drug reactions. In: Kasper DL, Fauci AS, Longo DL, Braunwald EB, Hauser SL, Jameson JL, eds. *Harrison's Principles of Internal Medicine*, 16th ed. New York, NY: McGraw-Hill; 2005:318-324.
13. Schnyder B. Approach to the patient with drug allergy. *Med Clin North Am.* 2010;94(4):665-679.
14. Husain Z, Reddy BY, Schwartz RA. DRESS syndrome: Part II. Management and therapeutics. *J Am Acad Dermatol.* 2013;(68):709.e1-709.e9.
15. Mockenhaupt M, Norgauer J. Cutaneous adverse drug reactions: Stevens-Johnson syndrome and toxic epidermal necrolysis. *Allergy Clin Immunol Int.* 2002;14:143-150.

SECTION 13 BULLOUS DISEASE

155 CHRONIC BULLOUS DISEASE OF CHILDHOOD

Holly H. Volz, MD
Richard P. Usatine, MD

PATIENT STORY

An 8 year-old girl presented with a two-day history of blisters on her face, trunk, and extremities (**Figure 155-1**). She complained of moderate discomfort from the blisters, but denied itching, burning, fever, and recent illness. She was not taking any medications. Biopsy demonstrated subepidermal vesicles and a rich neutrophilic infiltrate in the dermal papillary tips. Direct immunofluorescence revealed a linear deposition of IgA along the basement membrane confirming the diagnosis of chronic bullous disease of childhood.The patient was started on systemic therapy with dapsone and her lesions quickly resolved.

INTRODUCTION

Chronic bullous disease of childhood (CBDC) is the most common autoimmune bullous disorder in children.[1] This subepidermal vesiculo-bullous disorder is characterized by linear IgA deposits at the dermal-epidermal junction. It shares the same immunopathologic mechanism with its adult counterpart, adult linear IgA dermatosis. Although there is a great deal of overlap between the adult and childhood forms of linear IgA dermatosis, CBDC classically appears before the age of 5 years old, whereas adult linear IgA disease appears after age 60 years old. CBDC is considered a benign condition because it does not increase mortality; however, it may carry significant morbidity and, therefore, warrants treatment aimed at controlling the disease. Treatment with dapsone or sulfapyridine usually results in rapid resolution of the lesions. No correlation between the severity of blistering and the chronicity of disease exists. Most patients undergo spontaneous remission within months to years of initial presentation.

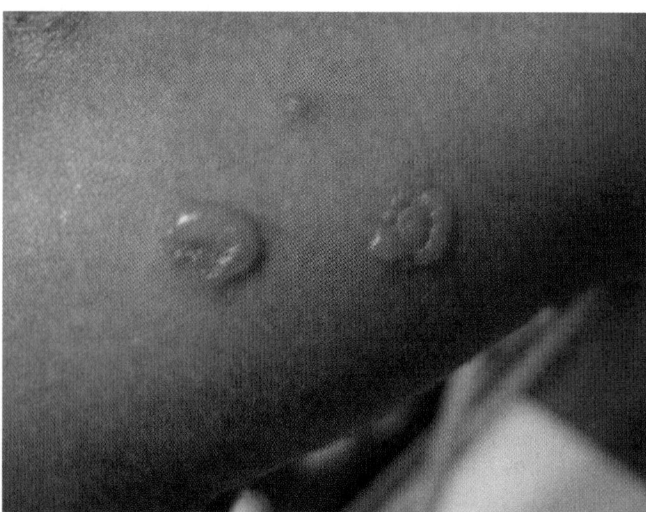

FIGURE 155-1 Chronic bullous disease of childhood in an 8-year-old girl. She had blisters on her face, trunk, and extremities. Note the annular and arcuate patterns of the bullae. (*Used with permission from John Browning, MD.*)

SYNONYMS

IgA bullous dermatosis of childhood, Linear IgA dermatosis, bullous disease of childhood, or chronic bullous dermatosis of childhood.

EPIDEMIOLOGY

- CBDC is a rare disorder with an incidence of 1:500,000.[2]
- It is the most common autoimmune bullous disorder in children.[1]
- Age of onset generally ranges from 1 to 11 years old with a mean of 3.5 to 4.5 years;[2] however, some case reports have documented neonatal onset of disease.[3,4]
- All races may be affected, although the disease appears to be more common in developing countries.[2]
- Data on the sex predilection of CBDC is heterogeneous and appears to vary with location.[5] Both sexes are affected, and some of the literature notes a slight female predominance.[2,6]

ETIOLOGY AND PATHOPHYSIOLOGY

- The etiology and exact pathophysiology of CBDC has not yet been defined, although both humoral and cellular immune responses are implicated in the disease process. The characteristic blister formation occurs as a result of IgA antibody formation against a heterogenous group of antigens located in the basement membrane zone of the epidermis. Over the last few decades, studies have identified a significant number of these targeted antigens, most commonly the 120-kDa and 97-kDa protein fragments of collagen XVII. Collagen XVII, also known as the 180-kDa bullous pemphigoid antigen (BP180), is a hemidesmosomal transmembrane protein that helps maintain the structural integrity of the dermal-epidermal junction.[4]
- Most cases of CBDC are idiopathic, and the inciting event that induces the production of autoantibodies remains unknown; however, a thorough history is imperative as numerous precipitating factors have been identified. These include:
    - Infection—Recent upper respiratory tract infection, gastroenteritis, varicella, and other viral or bacterial infections.[2,7]
    - Drugs—Vancomycin is most commonly associated; others include nonsteroidal antiinflammatory drugs such as diclofenac and naproxen, antibiotics such as amoxicillin, amoxicillin-clavulanate,

ampicillin, ceftriaxone-metronidazole, and penicillin, as well as amiodarone, captopril, and phenytoin.[5,6,8]
    - Skin trauma—Local skin injury, burns, UV light exposure[5–7]
- The literature highlights a notable association between the development of CBDC and the presence of certain human leukocyte antigen (HLA) genotypes, including HLA-B8, CW7, DR3, and DQW2.[2,4,9,10] The presence of these haplotypes has been associated with an early onset of disease,[6] particularly in homozygous individuals.[2]

DIAGNOSIS

CLINICAL FEATURES

- A non-specific prodromal illness may precede development of the skin lesions.
- Onset of blisters is abrupt; systemic symptoms such as fever may or may not be present.
- Disease presentation is variable with respect to both the distribution and morphology of the skin lesions.
- Classically, the primary lesions of CBDC are tense, clear or hemorrhagic vesicles or bullae. The vesicobullous lesions may develop on normal-appearing skin or the skin may appear erythematous or urticated. The blister size is variable, and lesions frequently assume annular or arcuate patterns (**Figures 155-2** to **155-4**).
- The development of new lesions around resolving lesions creates the pathognomonic "string of pearls" or "rosette" appearance of CBDC (**Figures 155-2** to **155-4**).
- Mucous membrane involvement is present in the majority of patients with variable presentation. Possible manifestations include oral ulceration, desquamative gingivitis, erosive cheilitis, nasal congestion, and bleeding. Ocular involvement may present as a conjunctivitis associated with photosensitivity, dryness, and irritation. Importantly, eye involvement can progress to serious sequelae including scarring and blindness.
- Patients may be asymptomatic or may experience a variety of symptoms ranging from mild pruritus to severe pruritus or burning.
- Skin lesions are usually most severe at initial presentation. Subsequent attacks, if they occur, are less severe.
- Healed lesions may cause transient skin hypopigmentation or hyperpigmentation known as "postinflammatory dyspigmentation." Permanent scarring is not typical.

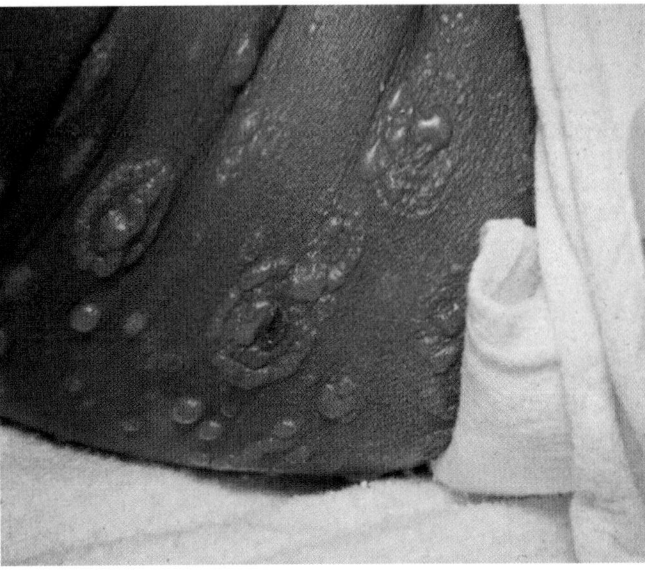

FIGURE 155-3 Chronic bullous disease of childhood with annular lesions and a "string of pearls" appearance. (*Used with permission from Weinberg SW, Prose NS, Kristal L. Color Atlas of Pediatric Dermatology, 4th edition, Figure 14-28, New York, NY: McGraw-Hill, 2008.*)

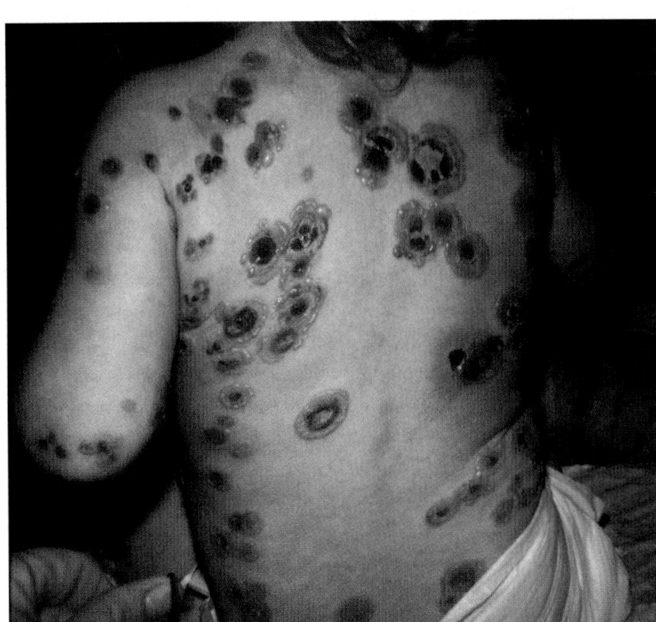

FIGURE 155-2 Bullae in a ring-like pattern in a young girl with chronic bullous disease of childhood. Note the pathognomonic "rosette" or "string of pearls" appearance. (*Used with permission from Jack Resneck, Sr., MD.*)

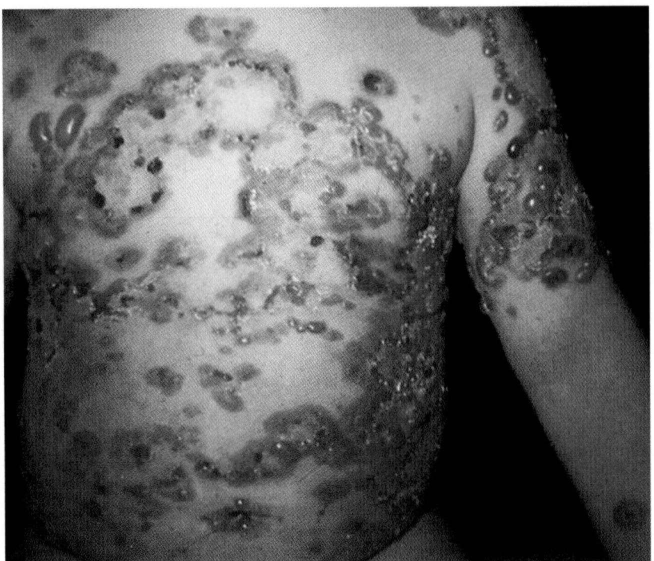

FIGURE 155-4 Chronic bullous disease of childhood with extensive annular lesions on the trunk and arm. Note the 'string of pearls" appearance. (*Used with permission from Weinberg SW, Prose NS, Kristal L. Color Atlas of Pediatric Dermatology, 4th edition, Figure 14-30, New York, NY: McGraw-Hill, 2008.*)

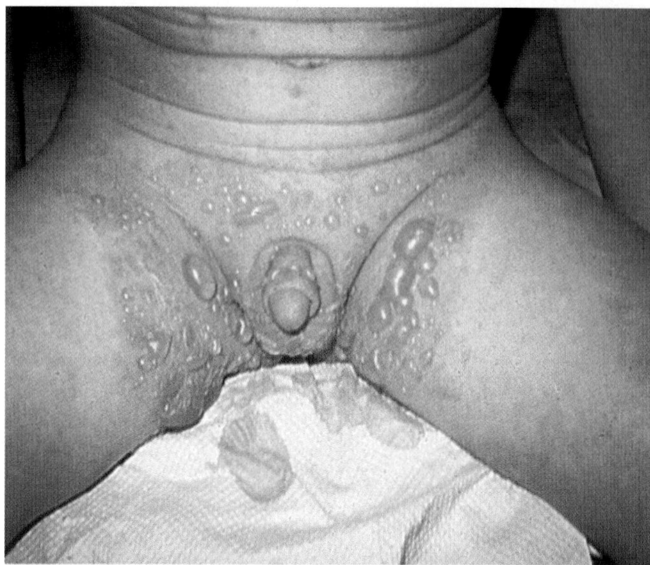

FIGURE 155-5 Chronic bullous disease of childhood involving the penis, groin and upper thighs. (*Used with permission from Weinberg SW, Prose NS, Kristal L. Color Atlas of Pediatric Dermatology, 4th edition, Figure 14-29, New York, NY: McGraw-Hill 2008.*)

TYPICAL DISTRIBUTION

- Lesions may be localized or widespread.
- The most commonly affected areas include the face, trunk, perineum, external genitalia, and thighs (**Figures 155-4** and **155-5**).
  - Lesions on the face typically occur in a perioral distribution (**Figure 155-6**) or around the eyes, including the eyelids.
  - Eruptions that initially manifest in the perineum have been mistaken for sexual abuse.[4]
- Other sites of involvement include the hands and feet (**Figure 155-7**).
- Younger children frequently demonstrate the classic distribution of both facial and perineal lesions. Older children more commonly present with a more generalized distribution.[4]

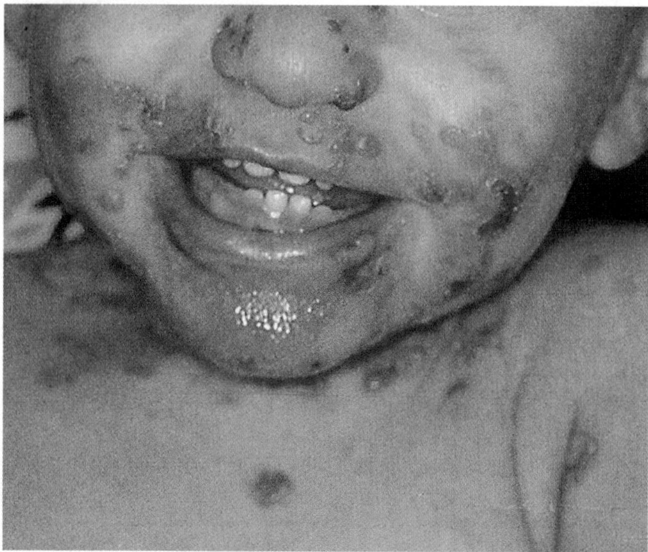

FIGURE 155-6 Chronic bullous diseases of childhood on the face of a 13-month-old infant. (*Used with permission from Kane KS, Lio P, Stratigos AJ, Johnson RA. Color Atlas and Synopsis of Pediatric Dermatology, 2nd edition, Figure 5-4b, 2009, New York: McGraw-Hill.*)

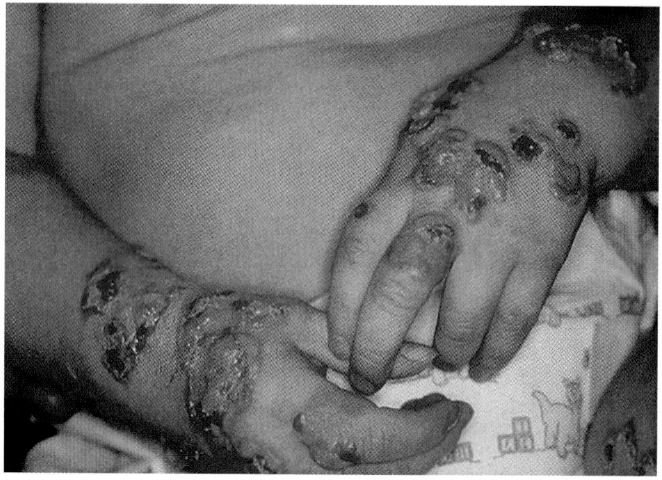

FIGURE 155-7 Chronic bullous disease of childhood on the hands and arms of this 13-month-old infant. Note the rosette appearance of some of the lesions. (*Used with permission from Kane KS, Lio P, Stratigos AJ, Johnson RA. Color Atlas and Synopsis of Pediatric Dermatology, 2nd edition, Figure 5-4c, New York, NY: McGraw-Hill, 2009.*)

LABORATORY STUDIES

- If detected, circulating antibodies are of the IgA1 subclass. In general, indirect immunofluorescence has a variable rate of positivity; low titers of autoantibody are detected in greater than 90 percent of patients.[4] Notably, the detection of circulating IgA occurs at a higher frequency in CBDC compared to the adult form of the disease.[6] Detection of circulating antibody is not necessary for diagnosis.
- All patients should be screened for glucose-6-phosphate dehydrogenase deficiency before initiating therapy with dapsone. Individuals with this deficiency are at risk for the development of severe hemolysis. Other initial laboratory tests include a complete blood count with differential, liver function tests, renal function tests, and urinalysis. A CBC should be monitored regularly during the first three months of therapy with dapsone with periodic blood work thereafter.
- If corticosteroids or immunosuppressive agents are required for treatment, a baseline complete blood count and a comprehensive metabolic profile should be obtained to allow for proper surveillance.

BIOPSY

- CBDC is diagnosed by the combination of clinical features along with hematoxylin-eosin–stained biopsy and direct immunofluorescence testing. Although histopathology can support the diagnosis, it does not distinguish CBDC from other important diseases in the differential diagnosis, including bullous pemphigoid and dermatitis herpetiformis; therefore, immunopathologic examination is required. Histologically, CBDC is characterized by subepidermal blisters and a rich inflammatory infiltrate along the basement membrane and in the dermal papillary tips. The gold standard for diagnosis is the immunohistochemical demonstration of linear IgA deposits along the dermal-epidermal junction.
- Direct immunofluorescence (DIF) testing should be performed on perilesional, uninvolved skin. Biopsy the perilesional skin and send the specimen in special Michel media or sterile saline and let the lab know to transfer it to Michel media when it arrives. The easiest way to do this is to take a shave biopsy that includes the bulla and

the perilesional skin. Then cut the specimen in half and send the perilesional skin for DIF and the blister for standard pathology. Biopsy from the skin of the forearm appears to be less sensitive,[6] and false-negative results may be seen early in the disease and necessitate repeat biopsy.

DIFFERENTIAL DIAGNOSIS

- Bullous impetigo is the most common bullous disease seen in children. Vesicles and bullae on normal appearing skin secondary to a superficial bacterial skin infection (usually *Staphylococcus aureus*). It commonly occurs on the face and in the intertriginous areas, and surrounding erythema may or may not be present (**Figure 155-8**; see Chapter 99, Impetigo).
- Bullous pemphigoid is much more common in older adults than children. Bullae are tense because they occur in the deeper subepidermal layer. In childhood, bullous pemphigoid has a predilection to involve the palms, soles and face but can also be generalized.[11] Biopsy (including DIF) is needed to make the diagnosis.
- Pemphigus is a rare group of autoimmune bullous diseases of skin and mucous membranes characterized by flaccid bulla and erosions. While it is more commonly seen in adults, it can occur in childhood. It often affects the oral mucosa in the form of pemphigus vulgaris. Biopsy (including DIF) is needed to make the diagnosis.
- Dermatitis herpetiformis is rare in children with typical onset in the second to fourth decades of life. Herpes-like lesions in the form of grouped vesicles and erosions occur especially on the elbows and extensor surfaces. It is associated with gluten-induced enteropathy. Blood tests for antigliadin and antiendomysial antibodies can help diagnose the gluten-induced enteropathy and a skin biopsy is helpful to diagnose the associated skin disease.

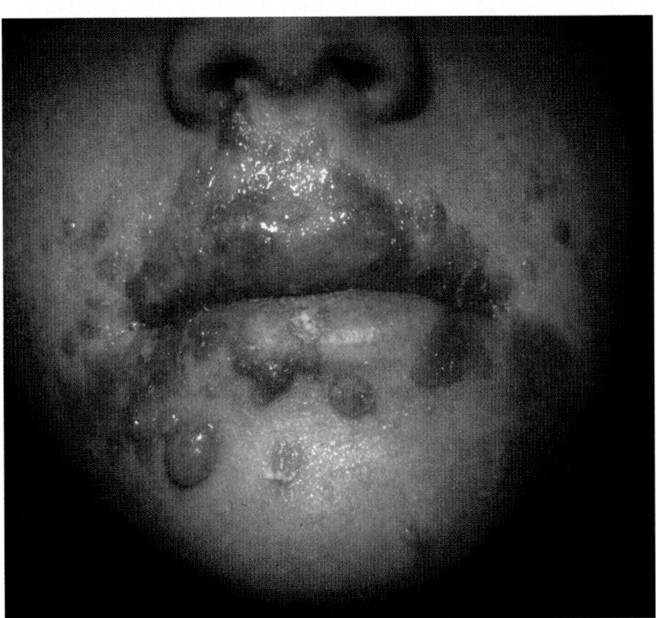

FIGURE 155-8 Bullous impetigo on the face of a child. Note the honey crusts, vesicles and bulla. (*Used with permission from Jack Resneck, Sr., MD.*)

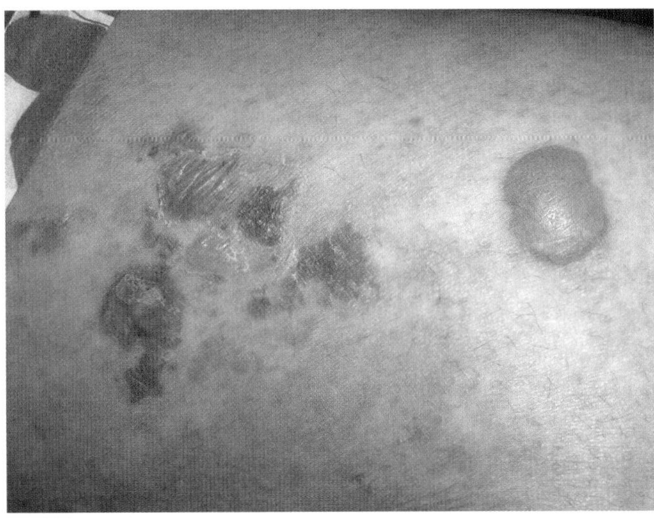

FIGURE 155-9 Epidermolysis bullosa simplex with trauma induced bullae on the leg of 15-year-old girl. (*Used with permission from Richard P. Usatine, MD.*)

- Epidermolysis bullosa is a rare group of inherited bullous diseases in which bullae form in response to even minor mechanical trauma. These diseases can manifest in infancy with most cases being epidermolysis bullosa simplex (**Figure 155-9**).
    - Severe cases can be fatal in infancy. Biopsy (including DIF) is needed to make the diagnosis (see Chapter 157, Other Bullous Diseases).
- Erythema multiforme—Erythematous papular and vesiculobullous lesions that typically involve the extremities and mucous membranes. Most cases are related to herpes simplex virus infection. The typical lesion is targetoid and may have a vesiculobullous component (see Chapter 151, Erythema Multiforme, Stevens-Johnson Syndrome, and Toxic Epidermal Necrolysis).

MANAGEMENT

Treatment of CBDC is directed by the extent of cutaneous and mucosal involvement and may require a multidisciplinary approach. As a rare disease, large, randomized, double-blind, controlled trials on the treatment of CBDC are lacking. In general, referral to a dermatologist is necessary and involvement of an ophthalmologist, otolaryngologist, or gastroenterologist should be considered when appropriate. Treatment is initially aimed at achieving control of the blistering while avoiding side effects. The majority of patients rapidly respond to treatment with sulfones or sulfonamides, anti-inflammatory antibiotics, and topical steroids. If drug-induced CBDC is suspected, discontinuation of the medication may lead to resolution of the disease. Complete clinical remission is expected, and patients should subsequently be tapered from medications. A maintenance dosage of medications may be required and should be scheduled based on clinical judgment.

SYSTEMIC THERAPY

Sulfones: dapsone

Dapsone is considered the first line agent for treatment of CBDC. SOR C It is effective as both an anti-inflammatory and immunomodulatory drug.

- Begin treatment at a low dose and slowly titrate upward until adequate symptom control has been achieved. A good starting point for initial therapy is less than 0.5 mg/kg of body weight per day. Most patients maintain symptom control at doses around 2 mg/kg per day.[12] Unfortunately, mucous membrane involvement may be refractory to monotherapy with dapsone[13] and an additional agent will be required.
- All patients should be screened for glucose-6-phosphate dehydrogenase (G6PD) deficiency before initiating therapy with dapsone. Patients with this deficiency are at an increased risk of hemolytic anemia.
- All patients receiving dapsone will have some hemolysis so it is important to monitor a CBC weekly at first and then less often when the dose and blood count are stable.
- Other adverse effects associated with dapsone therapy include methemoglobinemia, bone marrow suppression including agranulocytosis, hepatitis, peripheral neuropathy, and dapsone hypersensitivity syndrome.[12,13]

Sulfonamide drugs

Sulfonamide drugs, often considered first or second-line therapy in the treatment of CBDC, are an effective alternative treatment option with a side effect profile similar but less severe than that of dapsone. This class of drugs can be used as monotherapy or in combination with dapsone without an increased risk of adverse effects.

- Sulfapyridine and sulfasalazine are the most commonly used drugs in this class; however, the therapeutic dosages in children are not well established.[12] Because sulfapyridine is not readily available in the US, its prodrug, sulfasalazine, is being used in its place.[12] SOR C
- Other sulfonamides, such as trimethoprim-sulfamethoxazole, may be effective.[5] SOR C
- The potential side effects of sulfonamides include hemolysis, granulocytopenia, aplastic anemia, pancreatitis, and hepatotoxicity.[5]

Corticosteroids and other immunosuppressive agents

Widespread or poorly controlled disease may necessitate the use of systemic corticosteroids. Corticosteroids should also be considered when patients have contraindications to dapsone or sulfonamide drugs such as G6PD deficiency. Ideally, corticosteroids are used for short term control of symptoms, tapered, and then discontinued.

- The recommended dose of corticosteroid is 0.05 to 2.0 mg/kg/day of oral prednisone[5] or 1.0 mg/kg/day of oral prednisolone.[10] SOR C Short-term treatment for 1 to 3 weeks followed by a taper over 3 to 6 weeks is recommended in order to avoid the adverse side effects of prolonged steroid use.[10]
- Other immunosuppressive agents have been used with some success. These include colchicine, azathioprine, and cyclosporine.[2,5,12,13] SOR C

Antibiotic therapy

Non-sulfa antibiotics are another potential therapeutic option for the treatment of CBDC. The successful use of various antibiotics, including amoxicillin, dicloxacillin, oxacillin, erythromycin, and tetracyclines, have been reported in the literature.[5,8,12–14,16] SOR C Consider these drugs in patients who are not candidates for therapy with dapsone or sulfonamides, patients who cannot comply with regular blood monitoring, or as adjuncts to treatment.

Adjuvant agents

- The use of alternative therapeutic strategies, including intravenous immunoglobulin and immunoadsorption, have been successfully documented in adults with refractory linear IgA disease.[5] The use of these therapies in children has not been thoroughly evaluated; however, there are case reports documenting successful treatment of CBDC with intravenous immunoglobulin.[16] SOR C

LOCAL THERAPY

- Mild cases of CBDC may resolve with treatment with a topical steroid alone.[13] SOR C Higher potency ointments are more likely to be beneficial than low potency creams. SOR C
- Alternatively, topical steroids can be used in combination with systemic therapy.

PROGNOSIS

Most cases of CBDC carry a good prognosis; however, a select number of patients suffer from severe mucosal disease with ocular and pharyngeal involvement that may progress to blindness or dysphagia.[4] In most cases, however, the disease remits after months to years and lesions heal without scarring.[6] Although most cases resolve before puberty, some patients may continue to suffer from the disease into adulthood.[6] Notably, the severity of blistering has not been shown to correlate with disease chronicity.

FOLLOW-UP

Patients should be regularly followed by their physician to allow for assessment of disease severity, medication adjustments, and monitoring of blood work.

PATIENT EDUCATION

- Education is an important aspect of patient care. Patients and family members should be informed regarding the disease, possible complications, prognosis, and therapeutic options.

PATIENT RESOURCES

- Great Ormond Street Hospital in the United Kingdom—**http://www.gosh.nhs.uk/medical-conditions/search-for-medical-conditions/chronic-bullous-disease-of-childhood/**.

PROVIDER RESOURCES

- Medscape—**http://emedicine.medscape.com/article/1063590**. Linear IgA Dermatosis.
- Information on how to perform the appropriate biopsy can be found in Usatine R, Pfenninger J, Stulberg D, Small R. *Dermatologic and Cosmetic Procedures in Office Practice*. Philadelphia, PA: Elsevier; 2012. The text and the accompanying videos can also be purchased as an electronic application at: **www.usatinemedia.com**.

REFERENCES

1. Mihai S, Sitaru C. Immunopathology and molecular diagnosis of autoimmune bullous diseases. *J Cell Mol Med*. 2007;11(3):462-481.
2. Brenner S, Mashiah J. Autoimmune blistering diseases in children: signposts in the process of evaluation. *Clin Dermatol*. 2000;18(6): 711-724.
3. Kishida Y, Kameyama J, Nei M, Hashimoto T, Baba K. Linear IgA bullous dermatosis of neonatal onset: case report and review of the literature. *Acta Paediatr*. 2004;93(6):850-852.
4. Mintz EM, Morel KD. Clinical features, diagnosis, and pathogenesis of chronic bullous disease of childhood. *Dermatol Clin*. 2011;29 (3):459-462, ix.
5. Fortuna G, Marinkovich MP. Linear immunoglobulin A bullous dermatosis. *Clin Dermatol*. 2012;30(1):38-50.
6. Venning VA. Linear IgA disease: clinical presentation, diagnosis, and pathogenesis. *Dermatol Clin*. 2011;29(3):453-8, ix.
7. Ljubojevic S, Lipozencic J. Autoimmune bullous diseases associations. *Clin Dermatol*. 2012;30(1):17-33.
8. Sansaricq F, Stein SL, Petronic-Rosic V. Autoimmune bullous diseases in childhood. *Clin Dermatol*. 2012;30(1):114-127.
9. Patricio P, Ferreira C, Gomes MM, Filipe P. Autoimmune bullous dermatoses: a review. *Ann NY Acad Sci*. 2009;1173:203-210.
10. Lara-Corrales I, Pope E. Autoimmune blistering diseases in children. *Semin Cutan Med Surg*. 2010;29(2):85-91.
11. Bickle K, Roark TR, Hsu S. Autoimmune bullous dermatoses: a review. *Am Fam Physician*. 2002;65:1861-1870.
12. Mintz EM, Morel KD. Treatment of chronic bullous disease of childhood. *Dermatol Clin*. 2011;29(4):699-700.
13. Ng SY, Venning VV. Management of linear IgA disease. *Dermatol Clin*. 2011;29(4):629-630.
14. Kharfi M, Khaled A, Karaa A, Zaraa I, Fazaa B, Kamoun MR. Linear IgA bullous dermatosis: the more frequent bullous dermatosis of children. *Dermatol Online J*. 2010;16(1):2.
15. Jablonska S, Chorzelski TP, Rosinska D, Maciejowska E. Linear IgA bullous dermatosis of childhood (chronic bullous dermatosis of childhood). *Clin Dermatol*. 1991;9(3):393-401.
16. Nanda A, Khawaja F, Nanda M, Al-Sabah H, Selim MK, Dvorak R, et al. Linear immunoglobulin a bullous disease of childhood responsive to intravenous immunoglobulin monotherapy. Pediatr Dermatol 2012;29(4):529-532.

156 PEMPHIGUS

Richard P. Usatine, MD
Shashi Mittal, MD

PATIENT STORY

A teenage boy presented with painful blisters on his face and mouth (**Figure 156-1**). The patient was referred to dermatology that day. The dermatologist recognized likely pemphigus vulgaris (PV) and did shave biopsies for histopathology and direct immunofluorescence of facial vesicles/bullae to confirm the presumed diagnosis. The patient was started on 60 mg of prednisone daily until the pathology confirmed PV. Steroid-sparing therapy was then discussed and started in 2 weeks from presentation.

INTRODUCTION

Pemphigus is a rare group of autoimmune bullous diseases of skin and mucous membranes characterized by flaccid bulla and erosions. The three main types of pemphigus are PV (with the pemphigus vegetans variant), pemphigus foliaceous (with the pemphigus erythematosus variant), and paraneoplastic pemphigus. All types of pemphigus cause significant morbidity and mortality. Although pemphigus is not curable, it can be controlled with systemic steroids and immunosuppressive medications. These medications can be lifesaving, but also place pemphigus patients at risk for a number of complications. The word *pemphigus* is derived from the Greek word *pemphix*, which means bubble or blister.

EPIDEMIOLOGY

Epidemiology of the three major types of pemphigus:

- PV (**Figures 156-1** to **156-4**):

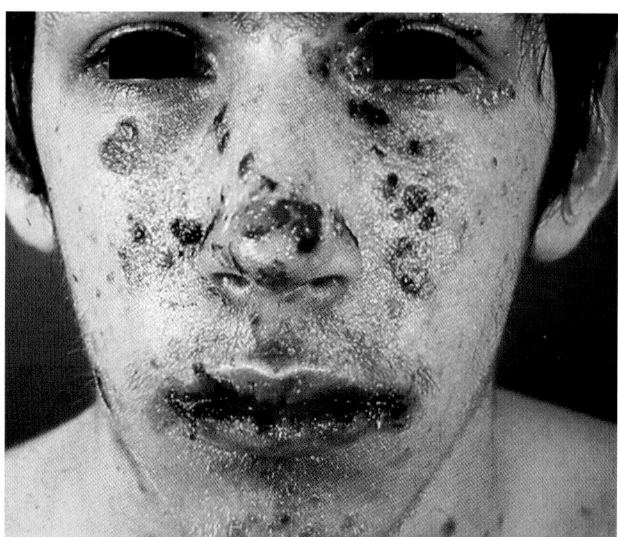

FIGURE 156-1 Pemphigus vulgaris on the face of a teenage boy with mouth involvement. Note the crusting that appears when the bullae erode. (*Used with permission from Weinberg SW, Prose NS, Kristal L. Color Atlas of Pediatric Dermatology, 4th edition, Figure 14-2, New York, NY: McGraw-Hill, 2008.*)

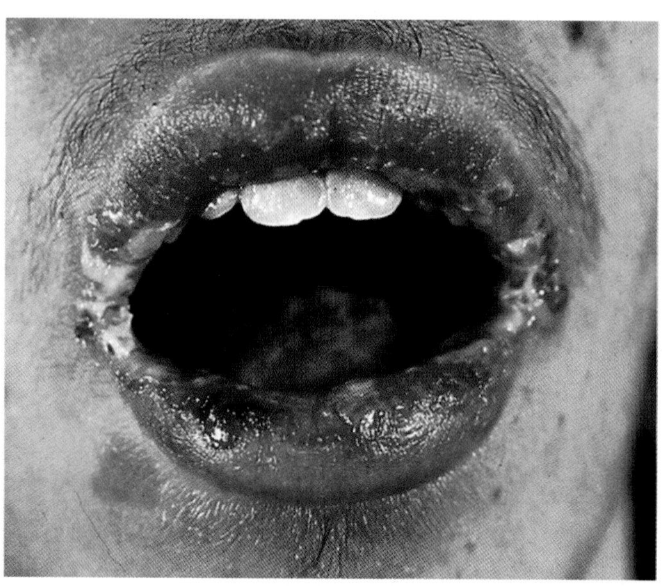

FIGURE 156-2 Pemphigus vulgaris with erosions of the lips and tongue. There are also erosions of the gums and palate that are not visible. This patient was in severe pain when attempting to eat or drink fluids. (*Used with permission from Weinberg SW, Prose NS, Kristal L. Color Atlas of Pediatric Dermatology, 4th edition, Figure 14-1, New York, NY: McGraw-Hill 2008.*)

  - Most common form of pemphigus is in the US.
  - Annual incidence is 0.75 to 5 cases per 1 million population.[1]
  - Usually occurs between 30 and 50 years of age, but can occur in childhood.[2]
  - Increased incidence in Ashkenazi Jews and persons of Mediterranean origin.[2]
  - Pemphigus vegetans is a variant form of PV (**Figures 156-5** and **156-6**).
- Pemphigus foliaceus (PF): Superficial form of pemphigus (**Figure 156-7**).

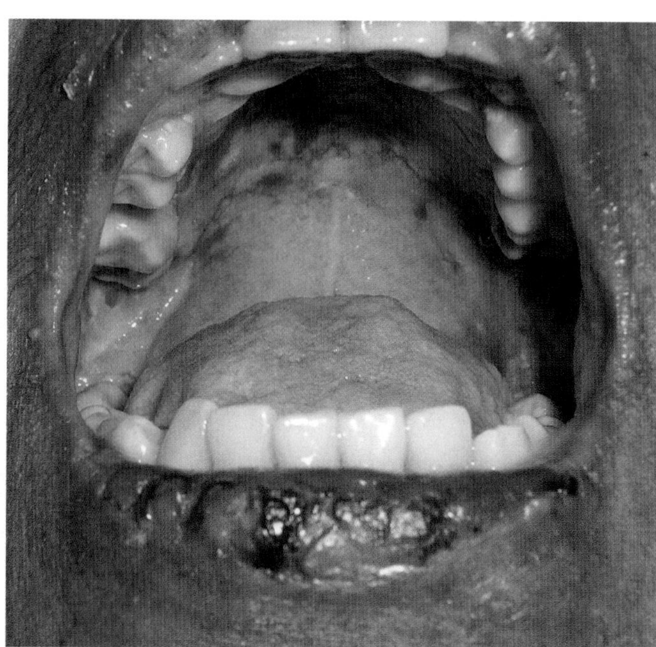

FIGURE 156-3 Pemphigus vulgaris involving the lips and palate. This is severely painful, making it difficult to eat or drink. (*Used with permission from Dan Shaked, MD.*)

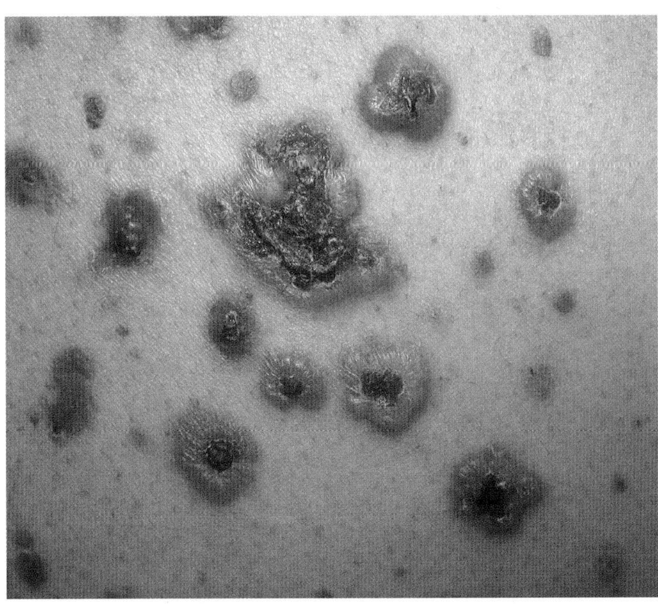

FIGURE 156-4 Pemphigus vulgaris on the back with crusted and intact bullae. (*Used with permission from of Eric Kraus, MD.*)

- Variant forms include pemphigus erythematosus (resembles the malar rash of lupus erythematosus) and fogo selvagem.
- Fogo selvagem is an endemic form of PF seen in Brazil and affects teenagers and individuals in their 20.[1]

- Paraneoplastic pemphigus (PNP):
  - Onset at age 60 years and older.
  - Associated with occult neoplasms commonly lymphoreticular.

ETIOLOGY AND PATHOPHYSIOLOGY

- The basic abnormality in all three types of pemphigus is acantholysis, a process of separating keratinocytes from one another. This occurs as a result of autoantibody formation against desmoglein (the adhesive molecule that holds epidermal cells together). Separation of epidermal cells leads to formation of intraepidermal clefts, which enlarge to form bullae.[1]

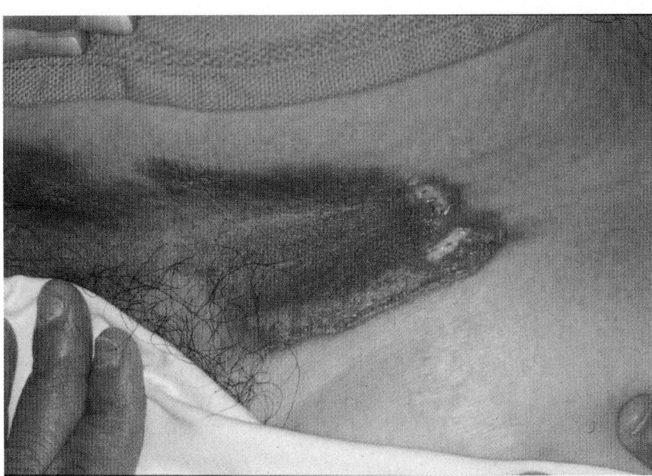

FIGURE 156-5 Pemphigus vegetans in the groin. (*Used with permission from Eric Kraus, MD.*)

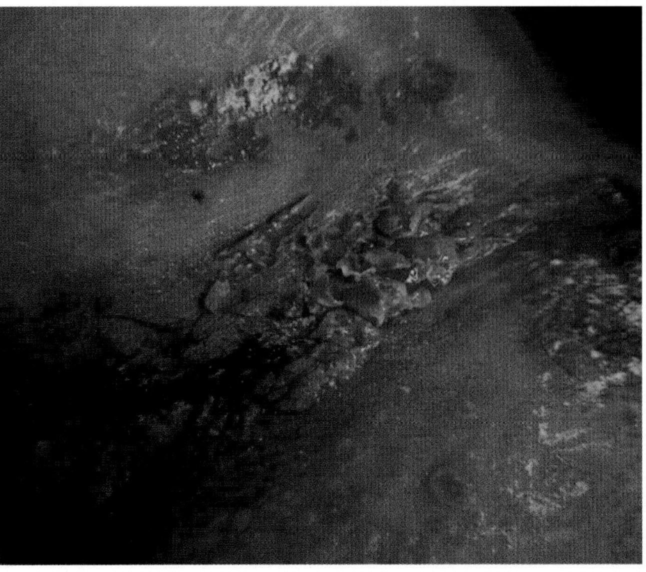

FIGURE 156-6 Pemphigus vegetans in the groin with boggy inflammation and tumid granulation. (*Used with permission from Weinberg SW, Prose NS, Kristal L. Color Atlas of Pediatric Dermatology, 4th edition, Figure 14-4, New York, NY: McGraw-Hill, 2008.*)

- The mechanism that induces the production of these autoantibodies in most individuals is unknown. Yet PF may be triggered by drugs, most commonly thiol compounds like penicillamine, captopril, piroxicam, and others, like penicillin and imiquimod.[3] An environmental trigger in the presence of susceptible human leukocyte antigen (HLA) gene is suggested to induce autoantibodies in fogo selvagum.[1]
- The autoantibodies in pemphigus are usually directed against desmoglein 1 and 3 molecules (Dsg1 and Dsg3). Dsg1 is present predominantly in the superficial layers of the epidermis, whereas Dsg3 is expressed in deeper epidermal layers and in mucous membranes. As a result, clinical presentation depends on the antibody profile. In PV, a limited mucosal disease occurs when only anti-Dsg3 antibody

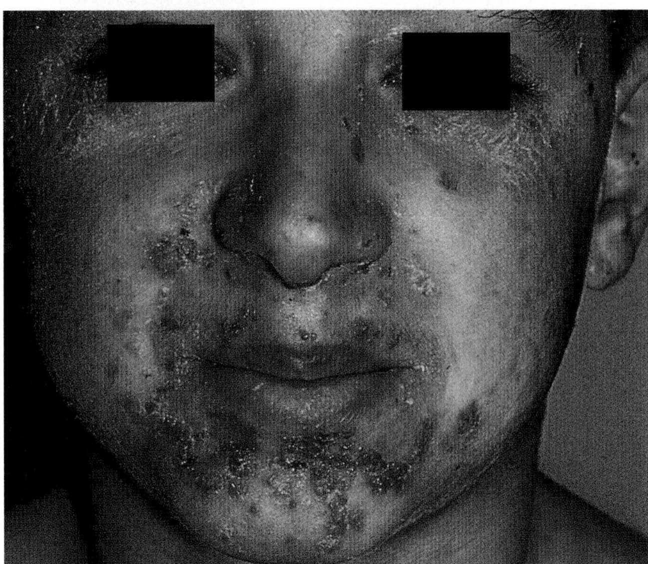

FIGURE 156-7 Pemphigus foliaceous in the perioral area without oral mucosal involvement. This can be mistaken for impetigo as impetigo is much more common than pemphigus. (*Used with permission from Weinberg SW, Prose NS, Kristal L. Color Atlas of Pediatric Dermatology, 4th edition, Figure 14-8, New York, NY: McGraw-Hill, 2008.*)

is present, but extensive mucosal and cutaneous disease occurs when both anti-Dsg1 and Dsg3 antibodies are present. In PF, mucosal lesions are absent and the cutaneous lesions are superficial because of isolated anti-Dsg1 antibody.

- Patients with PNP demonstrate both anti-Dsg1 and Dsg3 antibodies. However, unlike PV, autoantibodies against plakin proteins (another adhesive molecule) are also observed in patients with PNP and these autoantibodies form a reliable marker for this type of pemphigus.

DIAGNOSIS

CLINICAL FEATURES

- Pemphigus vulgaris (**Figures 156-1** to **156-4**)—Classical lesions are flaccid bullae that rupture easily, creating erosions. Since bullae are short-lived, erosions are the more common presenting physical finding (**Figure 156-4**). Lesions are typically tender and heal with postinflammatory hyperpigmentation that resolves without scarring. A positive Asboe-Hansen or Nikolsky sign may be present, but neither sign is diagnostic. A positive Asboe-Hansen sign occurs when a bulla extends to surrounding skin while pressure is applied directly to the bulla. The Nikolsky sign is positive when skin shears off while lateral pressure is applied to unblistered skin during active disease. Sometimes the Asboe-Hansen sign is also attributed to Nikolsky and called a Nikolsky sign, too.
- Pemphigus vegetans is a variant of PV where healing is associated with vegetating proliferation of the epidermis (**Figures 156-5** and **156-6**). Tumid granulation occurs with boggy inflammation (**Figure 156-6**).
- Pemphigus foliaceous: Multiple red, scaling, crusted, and pruritic lesions described as "corn flakes" are seen. Shallow erosions arise when crusts are removed, but intact blisters are rare as the disease is superficial (**Figures 156-7** to **156-10**).

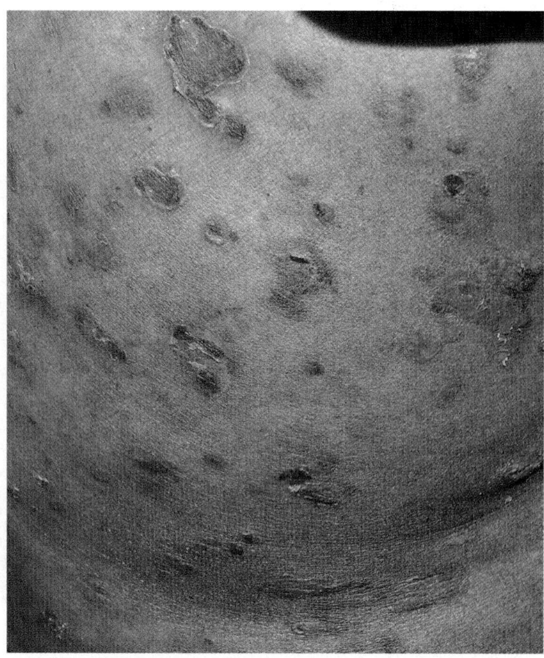

FIGURE 156-8 Pemphigus foliaceous on the back with superficial blisters and erosions. (*Used with permission from Richard P. Usatine, MD.*)

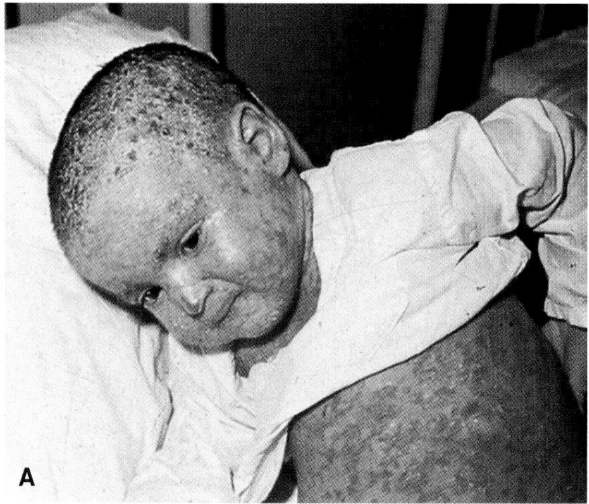

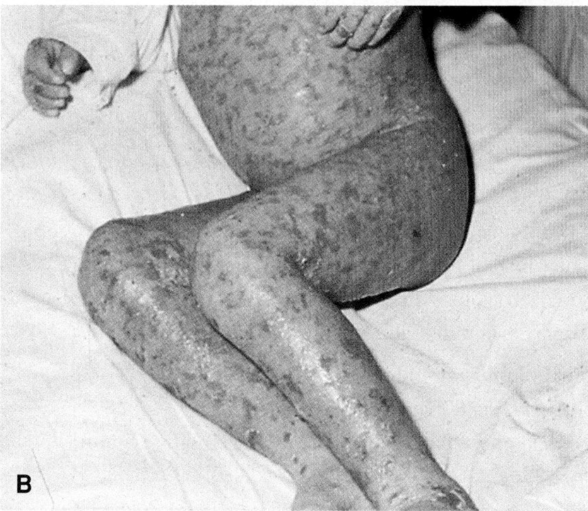

FIGURE 156-9 **A** and **B.** Pemphigus foliaceous from head to toe in this young child. The blister formation occurs high in the epidermis and is not unusual to only see "corn flake" crusting of the skin with no intact blisters. (*Used with permission from Weinberg SW, Prose NS, Kristal L. Color Atlas of Pediatric Dermatology, 4th edition, Figure 14-6 (for part A), Figure 14-7 (for part B), New York, NY: McGraw-Hill, 2008.*)

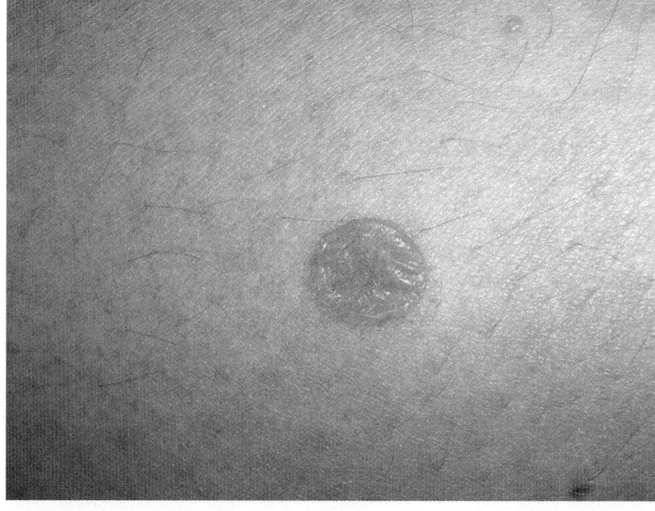

FIGURE 156-10 An intact flacid bullae that just appeared on the leg of a person with pemphigus foliaceous. (*Used with permission from Richard P. Usatine, MD.*)

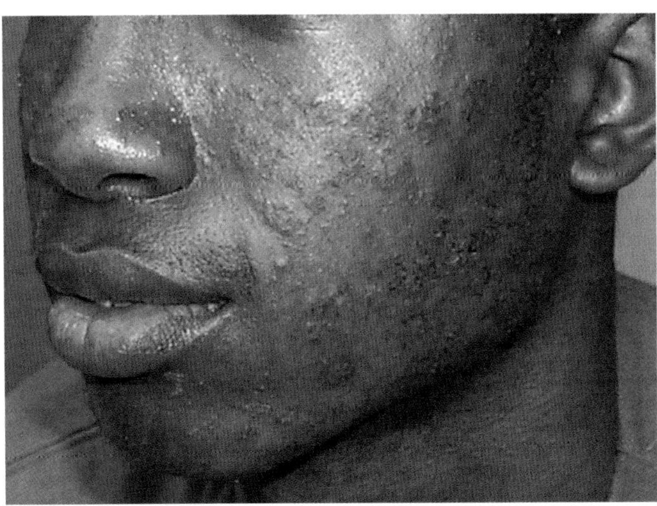

FIGURE 156-11 Pemphigus foliaceous (erythematosus) on the face. Note how the lesions have a butterfly pattern on the cheek. (*Used with permission from Jack Resneck, Sr., MD.*)

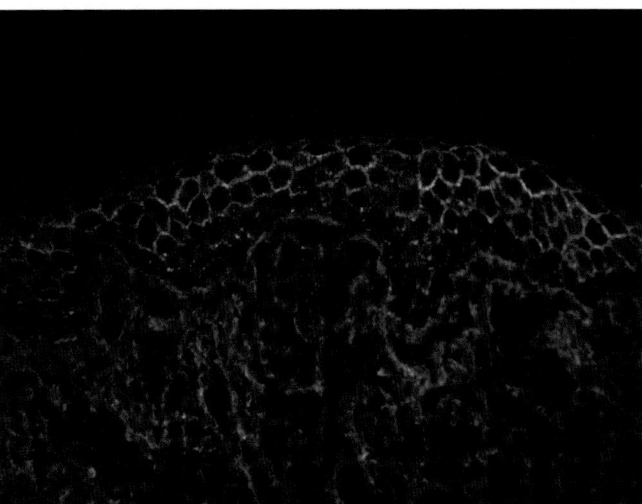

FIGURE 156-12 Direct immunofluorescence against immunoglobulin (Ig) G antibodies surrounding cells of the epidermis in a patient with pemphigus vulgaris. Note the chicken-wire appearance. (*Used with permission from Martin Fernandez, MD, and Richard P. Usatine, MD.*)

TYPICAL DISTRIBUTION

- PV—Common mucosal site is oral mucosa, although any stratified squamous epithelium may be involved. Mucosal lesions may be followed by skin lesions after weeks to months usually on scalp, face, and upper torso. PV should be suspected if an oral ulcer persists beyond a month (**Figures 156-2** and **156-3**).
- Pemphigus vegetans—Usually seen in intertriginous areas like the axilla, groin, and genital region (**Figures 156-5** and **156-6**).
- PF—Initially affects face and scalp, though may progress to involve chest and back (**Figures 156-7** to **156-10**). When the facial involvement in PF is in a lupus-like pattern, this is called pemphigus erythematosus (**Figure 156-11**).

LABORATORY STUDIES

- Circulating desmoglein antibodies levels may be measured in the blood using indirect immunofluorescence. This is usually not necessary unless the diagnosis is in question and further data are needed.
- Complete blood count and a comprehensive metabolic profile including liver function tests, creatinine, and glucose will be needed as a baseline, as all the systemic therapies have significant toxicities.
- Patients at risk for steroid-induced osteoporosis should have a dual-energy x-ray absorptiometry (DEXA) scan performed.

BIOPSY

- Skin biopsy is essential for accurate diagnosis. The depth of acantholysis and site of deposition of antibody complexes help differentiate pemphigus from other bullous diseases. Two specimens should be sent. Perform a shave of the edge of the bulla to include the surrounding normal appearing epidermis. This biopsy should be of the freshest lesion with an intact bulla, if possible. Cut the specimen in half and send the portion with the bulla in formalin for routine histopathology. The second half should be perilesional adjacent normal skin. This is sent on a gauze pad soaked in normal saline or Michel solution for direct immunofluorescence (DIF). Routine histopathology demonstrates suprabasal acantholysis and DIF shows antibody deposition in the intercellular spaces of the epidermis. The pattern of the DIF fluorescence is described as chicken wire (**Figure 156-12**).

DIFFERENTIAL DIAGNOSIS

- Chronic bullous disease of childhood (CBDC) is the most common autoimmune bullous disorder in children. This subepidermal vesiculo-bullous disorder is characterized by linear IgA deposits at the dermal-epidermal junction. Typical lesions are described as "string of pearls," which is an urticarial plaque surrounded by vesicles and bullae (see Chapter 155, Chronic Bullous Disease of Childhood).
- Hailey-Hailey disease (benign familial pemphigus)—A genodermatosis with crusted erosions and flaccid vesicles distributed in the intertriginous areas (**Figure 156-13**). It most closely resembles

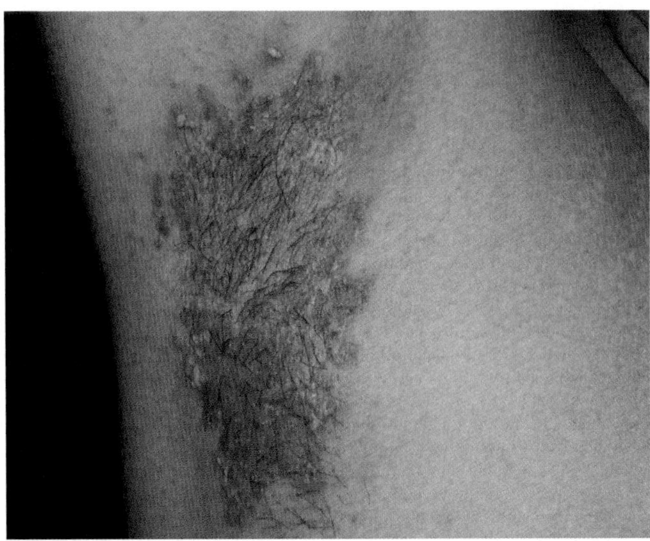

FIGURE 156-13 Hailey-Hailey disease (benign familial pemphigus) with erythema and pustules in the axilla. This is not true pemphigus but resembles pemphigus vegetans. (*Used with permission from Jonathan B. Karnes, MD.*)

pemphigus vegetans clinically but has a completely different pathophysiology than true pemphigus. It is called benign because it is not life-threatening. A 4-mm punch biopsy is adequate to make this diagnosis as the histology is different than pemphigus.

- Bullous pemphigoid—Bullae are tense because they occur in the deeper subepidermal layer. Mucous membrane involvement is rare. Biopsy illustrates subepidermal acantholysis and immunoglobulin deposition along the basement membrane.[3]
- Dermatitis herpetiformis—Herpes-like lesions in the form of grouped vesicles and erosions occur especially on the elbows and extensor surfaces. It is associated with gluten-induced enteropathy. Biopsy reveals neutrophilic microabscesses at the tips of dermal papillae with deposition of immunoglobulin (Ig) A antibody complexes. Blood tests for antigliadin and antiendomysial antibodies can help diagnose the gluten-induced enteropathy (Chapter 157, Other Bullous Diseases).

MANAGEMENT

Treatment of pemphigus should be undertaken in consultation with a dermatologist. Treatment is directed initially at disease control and remission followed by disease suppression. The goal is to eventually discontinue all medications and achieve complete remission. Unfortunately, this goal is hard to achieve. Most studies of the treatment of pemphigus have been performed in adults so the following recommendations are based on a combination of adult studies and pediatric case reports and expert reviews.

SYSTEMIC THERAPY

▶ Corticosteroids

Oral steroids with a steroid-sparing adjuvant agent is the most effective treatment for all forms of pemphigus (two randomized controlled trials [RCTs]).[4,5] SOR B

- Treatment should begin with the corticosteroid.[4–6] SOR B Mild disease may be controlled with prednisone (or prednisolone) 1 mg/kg/day but for rapidly progressive and extensive disease, a higher dose prednisone 2 mg/kg/day may be initiated. SOR C In most cases, the prednisone daily will need to be continued for at least 1 month. Once remission is induced, the dose is tapered by 25 percent every 1 to 2 weeks to the lowest dose needed to suppress recurrence of new lesions.[1]
- High-dose and prolonged treatment with steroids can have serious side effects. Consequently, it is advisable to start adjuvant steroid-sparing therapy within 2 to 4 weeks of treatment. Adjuvant agents have a lag period of 4 to 6 weeks before they become effective, so starting them sooner allows for earlier steroid taper. They may be used alone to maintain remission after steroid withdrawal.

▶ Adjuvant agents

- Adjuvant agents include azathioprine, methotrexate, mycophenolate, cyclophosphamide, dapsone, and intravenous immunoglobulin.[6–10] The efficacy of steroids have been shown to be enhanced when combined with a cytotoxic drug.[5]
- In one RCT open-label trial of four treatment regimens for adult PV, the most efficacious cytotoxic drug to reduce steroid was found to be azathioprine, followed by cyclophosphamide (IV pulse therapy), and mycophenolate mofetil.[5] SOR B
- Azathioprine and methotrexate are often the preferred adjuvants for childhood pemphigus.[10] SOR C
- Dapsone is an alternative adjuvant for pemphigus.[6] SOR C In one small study of adults with pemphigus vulgaris, 8 (73%) of 11 patients receiving dapsone versus 3 (30%) of 10 receiving placebo reached the primary outcome of a prednisone dosage of 7.5 mg/day or less. This was not statistically significant and only showed a trend to efficacy of dapsone as a steroid-sparing drug in maintenance-phase PV.[11]
- Intravenous immunoglobulin (IVIG) may be used as adjuvant therapy in refractory cases of pemphigus.[6,12–14] SOR B In one RCT of adult patients, it was used as a 5-day cycle to treat pemphigus that was relatively resistant to systemic steroids. In this multicenter study of 61 adult patients with PV or foliaceous, there was a decrease in disease activity subsequent to the cycle of IVIG.[14] SOR B
- Rituximab is a chimeric monoclonal antibody against CD20 on B lymphocytes. It leads to depletion of pathogenic B cells for up to 12 months, resulting in a reduction of plasma cells secreting pathogenic autoantibodies. Rituximab is infused weekly for 4 consecutive weeks in addition to the standard immunosuppressive treatment. It has shown promise in several case reports and cohort studies in the treatment of refractory cases of PV and foliaceus.[15–18] SOR B

▶ Treating and preventing complications of therapy

- Growth retardation has been reported in 50 percent of patients receiving oral corticosteroids.[19]
- Obesity and steroid-induced diabetes may also occur. Good diet, exercise, and monitoring of blood sugars and hemoglobin A_{1c} can be helpful.

LOCAL THERAPY

- Solitary lesions may be treated with topical high-potency steroids, such as clobetasol, or with intralesional steroid injections; for example, 20 mg/mL triamcinolone acetonide. Isolated oral lesions may be treated with steroid paste, sprays, or lozenges.
- Normal saline compresses or bacteriostatic solutions such as potassium permanganate are useful in keeping lesions clean. Oral hygiene is crucial. Mouthwashes such as chlorhexidine 0.2 percent or 1:4 hydrogen peroxide may be used. Topical anesthetics may be used for pain.[6]

PROGNOSIS

Pemphigus is a chronic group of diseases that are potentially life-threatening. There is no cure and the long-term use of steroids and immunosuppressive drugs places the patients at risk for a number of complications including infections, sepsis, steroid-induced diabetes, and steroid-induced osteoporosis. Some patients will be lucky and go into remission while others will need systemic therapy for life. Complications of treatment have become the greatest source of morbidity and mortality in pemphigus.

FOLLOW-UP

Prolonged follow-up is needed for medication adjustment and to monitor disease activity and drug side effects.

PATIENT EDUCATION

- Educate patients regarding disease, complications, and side effects of medications.
- Advise patients on avoiding trauma to skin such as with contact sports. Similarly, oral lesions may be aggravated by nuts, spicy foods, chips, and dental plates and bridges.
- Instruct patients on wound care to prevent infections and relieve local discomfort.
- Provide information on support groups such as the International Pemphigus Pemphigoid Foundation.

PATIENT RESOURCES

- MedlinePlus. *Pemphigus*—**www.nlm.nih.gov/medlineplus/pemphigus.html**.
- Mayo Clinic. *Pemphigus*—**www.mayoclinic.com/health/pemphigus/DS00749**.
- International Pemphigus Pemphigoid Foundation—**www.pemphigus.org/**.

PROVIDER RESOURCES

- Medscape. *Pemphigus Vulgaris*—**http://emedicine.medscape.com/article/1064187**.
- Information on how to perform the appropriate biopsy can be found in Usatine R, Pfenninger J, Stulberg D, Small R: *Dermatologic and Cosmetic Procedures in Office Practice*. Philadelphia, PA: Elsevier; 2012. The text and the accompanying videos can also be purchased as an electronic application at: **www.usatinemedia.com**.

REFERENCES

1. Bystryn JC, Rudolph JL. Pemphigus. *Lancet*. 2005;366:61-73.
2. Ettlin DA. Pemphigus: *Dent Clin North Am*. 2005;49:107-1ix.
3. Bickle K, Roark TR, Hsu S. Autoimmune bullous dermatoses: a review. *Am Fam Physician*. 2002;65:1861-1870.
4. Beissert S, Mimouni D, Kanwar AJ, Solomons N, Kalia V, Anhalt GJ. Treating pemphigus vulgaris with prednisone and mycophenolate mofetil: a multicenter, randomized, placebo-controlled trial. *J Invest Dermatol*. 2010;130:2041-2048.
5. Chams-Davatchi C, Esmaili N, Daneshpazhooh M, et al. Randomized controlled open-label trial of four treatment regimens for pemphigus vulgaris. *J Am Acad Dermatol*. 2007; 57:622-628.
6. Harman KE, Albert S, Black MM. Guidelines for the management of pemphigus vulgaris. *Br J Dermatol*. 2003;149:926-937.
7. Frew JW, Martin LK, Murrell DF. Evidence-based treatments in pemphigus vulgaris and pemphigus foliaceus. *Dermatol Clin*. 2011; 29:599-606.
8. Martin LK, Werth VP, Villaneuva EV, Murrell DF. A systematic review of randomized controlled trials for pemphigus vulgaris and pemphigus foliaceus. *J Am Acad Dermatol*. 2011;64:903-908.
9. Singh S. Evidence-based treatments for pemphigus vulgaris, pemphigus foliaceus, and bullous pemphigoid: a systematic review. *Indian J Dermatol Venereol Leprol*. 2011;77:456-469.
10. Wananukul S, Pongprasit P. Childhood pemphigus. Int *J Dermatol*. 1999;38(1):29-35.
11. Werth VP, Fivenson D, Pandya AG, et al. Multicenter randomized, double-blind, placebo-controlled, clinical trial of dapsone as a glucocorticoid-sparing agent in maintenance-phase pemphigus vulgaris. *Arch Dermatol*. 2008;144:25-32.
12. Sami N, Qureshi A, Ruocco E, Ahmed AR. Corticosteroid-sparing effect of intravenous immunoglobulin therapy in patients with pemphigus vulgaris. *Arch Dermatol*. 2002;138:1158-1162.
13. Gurcan HM, Jeph S, Ahmed AR. Intravenous immunoglobulin therapy in autoimmune mucocutaneous blistering diseases: a review of the evidence for its efficacy and safety. *Am J Clin Dermatol*. 2010; 11:315-326.
14. Amagai M, Ikeda S, Shimizu H, et al. A randomized double-blind trial of intravenous immunoglobulin for pemphigus. *J Am Acad Dermatol*. 2009;60:595-603.
15. Fuertes I, Guilabert A, Mascaró JM Jr, Iranzo P. Rituximab in childhood pemphigus vulgaris: a long-term follow-up case and review of the literature. *Dermatology*. 2010;221(1):13-16.
16. Kanwar AJ, Sawatkar GU, Vinay K, Hashimoto T. Childhood pemphigus vulgaris successfully treated with rituximab. *Indian J Dermatol Venereol Leprol*. 2012;78(5):632-634.
17. Mamelak AJ, Eid MP, Cohen BA, Anhalt GJ. Rituximab therapy in severe juvenile pemphigus vulgaris. *Cutis*. 2007;80(4):335-340.
18. Connelly EA, Aber C, Kleiner G, Nousari C, Charles C, Schachner LA. Generalized erythrodermic pemphigus foliaceus in a child and its successful response to rituximab treatment. *Pediatr Dermatol*. 2007;24(2):172-176.
19. Gürcan H, Mabrouk D, Razzaque Ahmed A. Management of pemphigus in pediatric patients. *Minerva Pediatr*. 2011;63(4): 279-291.

157 OTHER BULLOUS DISEASES

Jimmy H. Hara, MD
Richard P. Usatine, MD

INTRODUCTION

There are a number of bullous diseases other than pemphigus and bullous pemphigoid that are important to recognize. Epidermolysis bullosa belongs to a family of inherited diseases where blister formation can be caused by even minor skin trauma. PLEVA (pityriasis lichenoides et varioliformis acuta) is a minor cutaneous lymphoid dyscrasia that can appear suddenly and persist for weeks to months. Dermatitis herpetiformis is a recurrent eruption that is usually associated with gluten and diet-related enteropathies. These diseases will be discussed in succession.

EPIDERMOLYSIS BULLOSA

PATIENT STORY

A 12-year-old girl with the Dowling-Meara type of epidermolysis bullosa (EB) simplex presents to her pediatrician for a URI. While examining her respiratory tract, the pediatrician notes the extensive, severe blistering over many areas of the body including, the (A) trunk, (B) extremities, and (C) the hands (**Figure 157-1**). She has been followed by a dermatologist since early childhood when the EB simplex was first diagnosed. It turns out that she only has a viral URI so no antibiotics are needed and standard treatment with fluids and analgesics is recommended. Her mom states that the girl has an appointment with her dermatologist next month.

EPIDEMIOLOGY

- Epidermolysis bullosa (EB) is a family of inherited diseases characterized by skin fragility and blister formation caused by minor skin trauma.[1]
- There are autosomal recessive and autosomal dominant types; the severity of this disease may vary widely.
- Onset is in childhood and in later years severe dystrophic deformities of hands and feet are characteristic (**Figure 157-2**).

ETIOLOGY AND PATHOPHYSIOLOGY

Blistering occurs at different levels for these 3 types of EB:

1. Epidermolysis bullosa simplex (**Figure 157-1**) blisters within the epidermis (most superficial).[2,3]
2. Dystrophic epidermolysis bullosa (dominant and recessive) has vesiculobullous skin separation occurring at the sub-basal lamina level of the dermis (deepest layer of all 3 types; **Figures 157-2** to **157-4**).

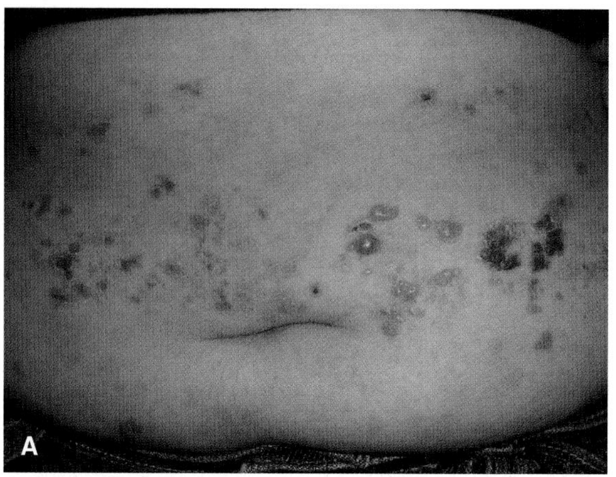

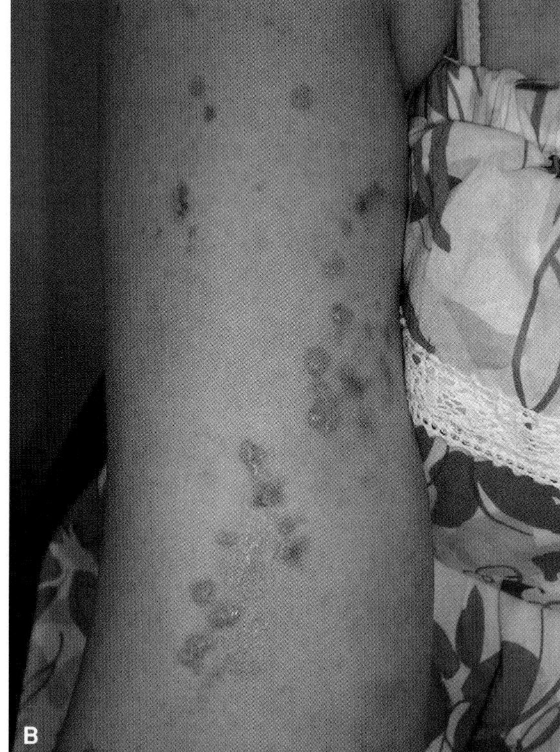

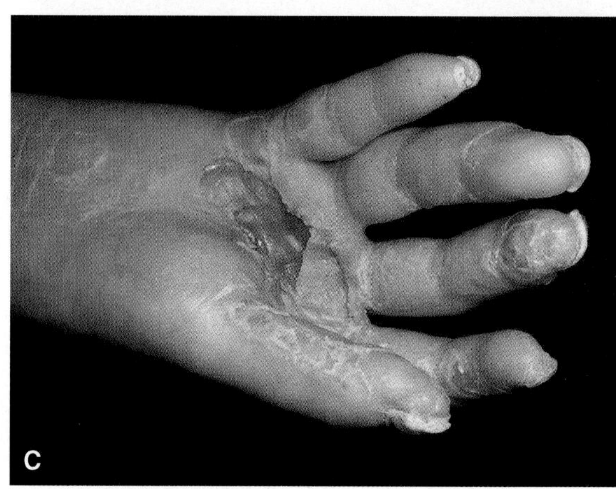

FIGURE 157-1 A 12-year-old girl with the Dowling-Meara type of epidermolysis bullosa simplex. It is the most severe form with extensive, severe blistering over many areas of the body including, the (**A**) trunk, (**B**) extremities, and (**C**) the hands. (*Used with permission from Richard P, Usatine, MD.*)

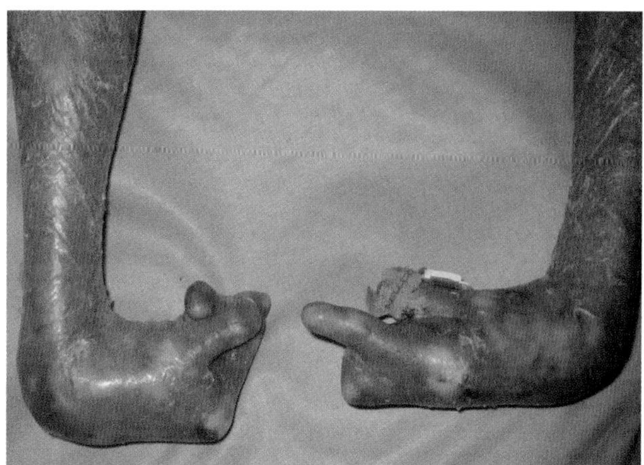

FIGURE 157-2 Recessive dystrophic epidermolysis bullosa in an adolescent with a mitten deformity and flexion contractures at the wrists. (*Used with permission from Kane KS, Lio PA, Stratigos AJ, Johnson RA. Color Atlas & Synopsis of Pediatric Dermatology, 2nd edition, Figure 5-3b, New York, NY: McGraw-Hill, 2009.*)

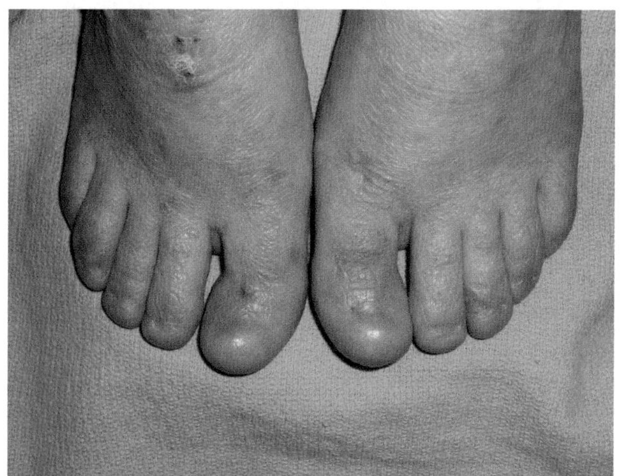

FIGURE 157-3 Recessive dystrophic epidermolysis bullosa with loss of all her toenails starting as a young child. (*Used with permission from Richard P. Usatine, MD.*)

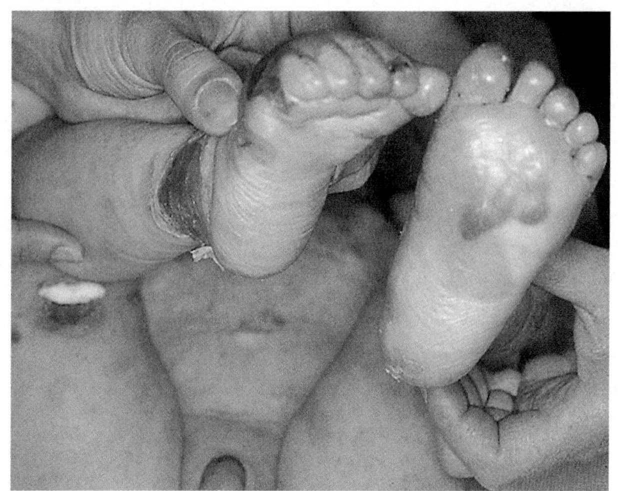

FIGURE 157-4 Recessive dystrophic epidermolysis bullosa in a newborn. Bullae occur at areas of minimal trauma at or near birth. (*Used with permission from Kane KS, Lio P, Stratigos AJ, Johnson RA. Color Atlas and Synopsis of Pediatric Dermatology, 2nd edition, Figure 5-3a, New York, NY: McGraw-Hill, 2009.*)

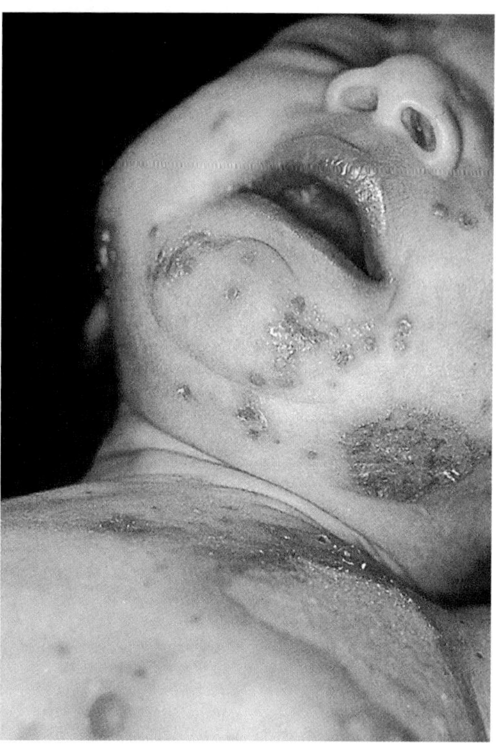

FIGURE 157-5 Junctional epidermolysis bullosa in a newborn with severe perioral, oral and GI involvement. This infant was subsequently hospitalized and despite burn unit supportive measures eventually passed away because of sepsis. (*Used with permission from Kane KS, Lio P, Stratigos AJ, Johnson RA. Color Atlas and Synopsis of Pediatric Dermatology, 2nd edition, Figure 5-2c, New York, NY: McGraw-Hill, 2009.*)

3. Junctional epidermolysis bullosa blisters at the dermal-epidermal junction (**Figure 157-5**).

DIAGNOSIS

CLINICAL FEATURES

Acral skin fragility and blistering are the hallmark in childhood. Minor trauma can induce severe blistering. As the disease progresses initially, painful and ultimately debilitating dystrophic deformities are typical. Repeated blistering of the hands can lead to fusion of the fingers and the "mitten" deformity (**Figure 157-2**).

TYPICAL DISTRIBUTION

The typical distribution is acral (hands and feet), although blistering may extend proximally secondary to trauma.

LABORATORY STUDIES AND BIOPSY

There are no laboratory tests to confirm the diagnosis. A punch biopsy can provide adequate tissue for the dermatopathologist to differentiate between the different forms of epidermolysis bullosa: simplex, junctional, and dystrophic.

DIFFERENTIAL DIAGNOSIS

- Erythema multiforme bullosum may have a similar appearance, but the distribution is less apt to be limited to the distal extremities.

- The first appearance of the condition may be confused, with staphylococcal scalded skin syndrome (see Chapter 105, Staphylococcal Scalded Skin Syndrome).[4]

MANAGEMENT

Management is primarily prevention of trauma, careful wound care, and treatment of complicating infections. Other supportive measures such as pain management and nutritional support are often necessary. Screening the skin for squamous cell carcinoma is important in adulthood for the dystrophic form.[2]

FOLLOW-UP

Periodic skin examinations should be done to help manage symptoms and screen for malignancy.

PATIENT EDUCATION

Avoid trauma and come in early if there are any signs of infection or malignancy.

PITYRIASIS LICHENOIDES ET VARIOLIFORMIS ACUTA

PATIENT STORY

A young man presented with a varicelliform eruption that he has had for 6 weeks (**Figure 157-6**). Initially, he was diagnosed with varicella and given a course of acyclovir. Then he was misdiagnosed with scabies and treated with permethrin. A correct diagnosis of PLEVA was made by clinical appearance and confirmed with biopsy. His skin lesions cleared with oral doxycycline.

EPIDEMIOLOGY

- PLEVA or Mucha-Habermann disease and pityriasis lichenoides chronica are maculopapular erythematous eruptions that can occur in crops of vesicles that can become hemorrhagic over a course of weeks to months (**Figures 157-7**).[5]
- There is a predilection for males in the second and third decades.
- PLEVA occurs in preschool and preadolescent children as well.[6]

ETIOLOGY AND PATHOPHYSIOLOGY

- PLEVA has traditionally been classified as a benign papulosquamous disease. However, there is increasing evidence that suggests that PLEVA should be considered a form of cutaneous lymphoid dyscrasia.[7] It may even represent an indolent form of mycosis fungoides.

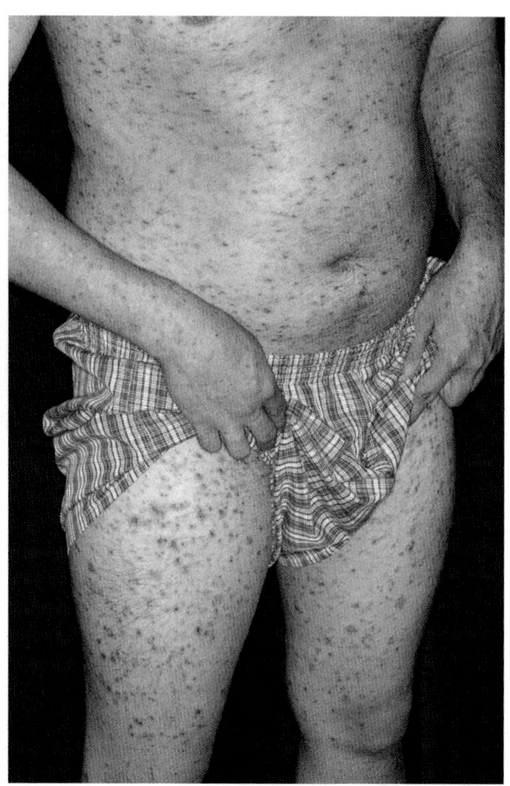

FIGURE 157-6 A college student with pityriasis lichenoides et varioliformis acuta. His skin lesions cleared with oral doxycycline. (*Used with permission from Richard P, Usatine, MD.*)

DIAGNOSIS

CLINICAL FEATURES

PLEVA occurs with crops of maculopapular and papulosquamous lesions that can vesiculate and form hemorrhagic vesicles (**Figures 157-6** and **157-7**). Although it resembles varicella, new crops of

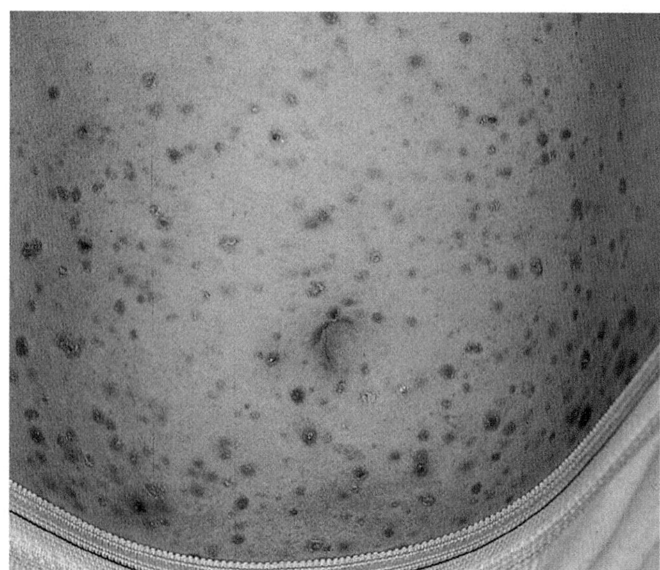

FIGURE 157-7 A teenager with pityriasis lichenoides et varioliformis acuta (PLEVA, Mucha-Habermann disease). (*Used with permission from Weinberg SW, Prose NS, Kristal L. Color Atlas of Pediatric Dermatology, 4th edition, Figure 9-35, New York, NY: McGraw-Hill, 2008.*)

lesions continue to appear over weeks and months. It can be thought of as "chickenpox that lasts for weeks to months."

TYPICAL DISTRIBUTION

Lesions typically occur over the anterior trunk and flexural aspects of the proximal extremities. The face is spared.

LABORATORY STUDIES

There are no specific laboratory tests for PLEVA except biopsy.

BIOPSY

A punch biopsy is helpful in making the diagnosis. It may be necessary to differentiate PLEVA from lymphomatoid papulosis (see the following section "Differential Diagnosis").

DIFFERENTIAL DIAGNOSIS

- Varicella—A varicella direct fluorescent antibody test can confirm acute varicella. If no viral testing was done and what appeared to be varicella persists, PLEVA should be considered (Chapter 108, Chickenpox).
- Pityriasis lichenoides chronica is the chronic form of PLEVA and can be distinguished from PLEVA by length of time and biopsy (**Figure 157-8**). It has a more low-grade clinical course than PLEVA and the lesions appear over a longer course of time.
- Erythema multiforme is a hypersensitivity syndrome in which target lesions are seen. The target lesions have epidermal disruption in the center with vesicles and/or erosions. Look for the target lesions to help differentiate this from PLEVA (see Section 12, Hypersensitivity Syndromes and Drug Reactions).

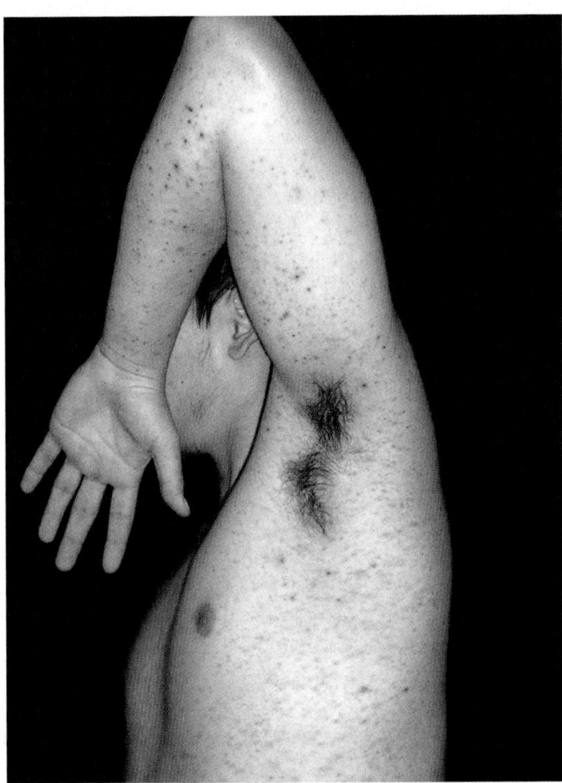

FIGURE 157-8 Pityriasis lichenoides chronica is the chronic form of pityriasis lichenoides et varioliformis acuta that may persist for months to years. *(Used with permission from Richard P. Usatine, MD.)*

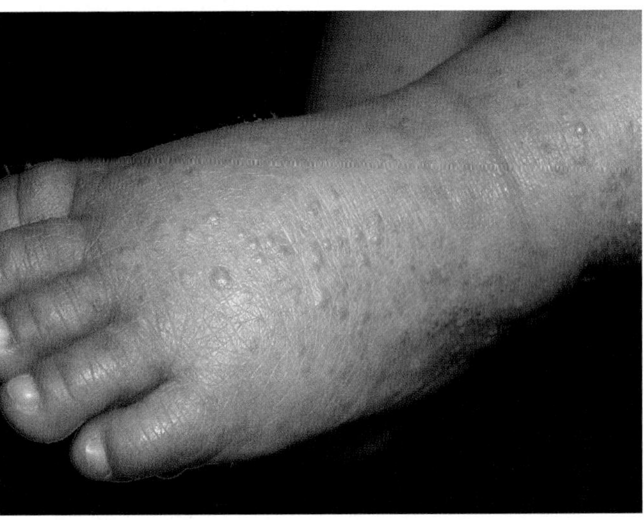

FIGURE 157-9 Gianotti-Crosti syndrome, "papular acrodermatitis of childhood," in a 7-month-old child. The acral eruption started just after a viral upper respiratory infection and involved the feet, lower legs, and buttocks. *(Used with permission from Richard P. Usatine, MD.)*

- Lymphomatoid papulosis presents in a manner similar to PLEVA with recurrent crops of pruritic papules at different stages of development that appear on the trunk and extremities. Although it has histologic features that suggest lymphoma, lymphomatoid papulosis alone is not fatal. It is important to differentiate this from PLEVA because these patients need to be worked up for coexisting malignancy. These patients tend to be older and a punch biopsy can make the diagnosis.
- Gianotti-Crosti syndrome (papular acrodermatitis of childhood) may resemble PLEVA but the lesions are usually acral in distribution (**Figure 157-9**).[3] The erythematous papules and vesicles are found on the extremities and sometimes on the face. It is a benign syndrome associated with many childhood viruses that may last 2 to 8 weeks.

MANAGEMENT

- UV A1 phototherapy has been deployed with some success.[8] Various reports suggest the efficacy of macrolides and tetracyclines, probably more for their antiinflammatory properties than for their antibacterial effects.

FOLLOW-UP

Needed only if the disease does not resolve.

PATIENT EDUCATION

This is usually a temporary disease but if it becomes chronic there are treatments that could help such as oral macrolides or doxycycline.

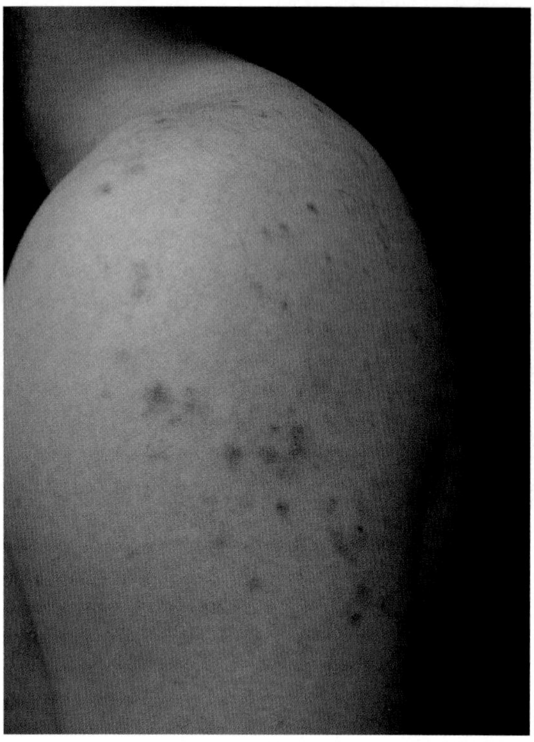

FIGURE 157-10 A young man with dermatitis herpetiformis and gluten-induced enteropathy. The daily vesicles that form are fragile and rapidly become small erosions. (*Used with permission from Richard P. Usatine, MD.*)

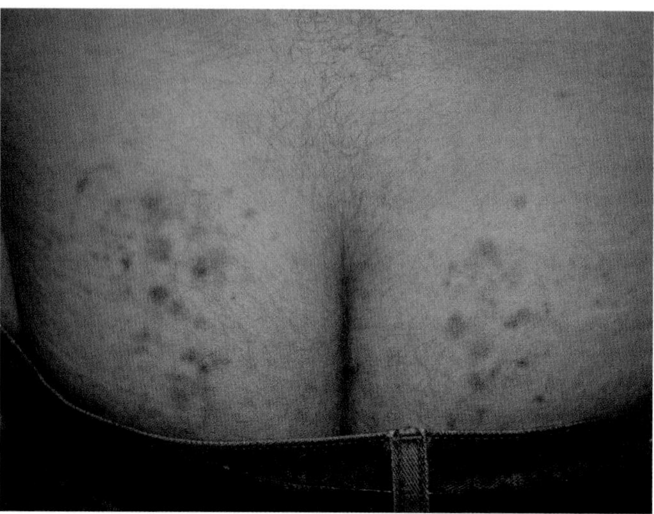

FIGURE 157-11 Dermatitis herpetiformis that has persisted even though he is on a strict gluten-free diet. The buttocks is a commonly involved area. His gastrointestinal symptoms have resolved on the gluten-free diet but his eruption has only diminished. His skin lesions resolved with oral dapsone. (*Used with permission from Richard P. Usatine, MD.*)

DERMATITIS HERPETIFORMIS

PATIENT STORY

A young man with a past history of diarrhea and malabsorption carries a past diagnosis of gluten-induced enteropathy. Despite a gluten-free diet he continues to have a pruritic eruption on his shoulders, back, extremities and buttocks (**Figures 157-10** and **157-11**). While the most likely diagnosis is dermatitis herpetiformis, a punch biopsy was performed to confirm this before starting the patient on oral dapsone.

EPIDEMIOLOGY

- Dermatitis herpetiformis is a chronic recurrent symmetric vesicular eruption that is usually associated with diet-related enteropathy.[9] It most commonly occurs in the 20 to 40 years of age group. Men are affected more often than women.

ETIOLOGY AND PATHOPHYSIOLOGY

- The disease is related to gluten and other diet-related antigens that cause the development of circulating immune complexes and their subsequent deposition in the skin. The term *herpetiformis* refers to the grouped vesicles that appear on extensor aspects of the extremities and trunk and is not a viral infection or related to the herpes viruses. The disease is characterized by the deposition of immunoglobulin (Ig) A along the tips of the dermal papillae. The majority of patients will also have blunting and flattening of jejunal villi, which leads to diarrhea even to the point of steatorrhea and malabsorption.

DIAGNOSIS

CLINICAL FEATURES

The clinical eruption is characterized by severe itching, burning, or stinging in the characteristic extensor distribution. Herpetiform vesicles and urticarial plaques may be seen. Because of the intense pruritus, characteristic lesions may be excoriated beyond recognition (**Figures 157-10** to **157-12**).

TYPICAL DISTRIBUTION

Classically, the lesions (or excoriations) are seen in the extensor aspects of the extremities, shoulders (**Figure 157-10**), lower back, and buttocks (**Figures 157-11** and **157-12**).

LABORATORY STUDIES

If the patient has gluten-induced enteropathy, antigliadin and antiendomysial antibodies may be present. A blood test for antigliadin antibody is a sensitive test for gluten-induced enteropathy.

BIOPSY

Diagnosis is confirmed by a punch biopsy. It is best to biopsy new crops of lesions. A standard histologic examination will show eosinophils and microabscesses of neutrophils in the dermal papillae and subepidermal vesicles. Direct immunofluorescence reveals deposits of IgA and complement within the dermal papillae.

DIFFERENTIAL DIAGNOSIS

- Scabies may have a similar appearance with pruritus, papules, and vesicles. If the lesions and distribution suggest scabies, it should be

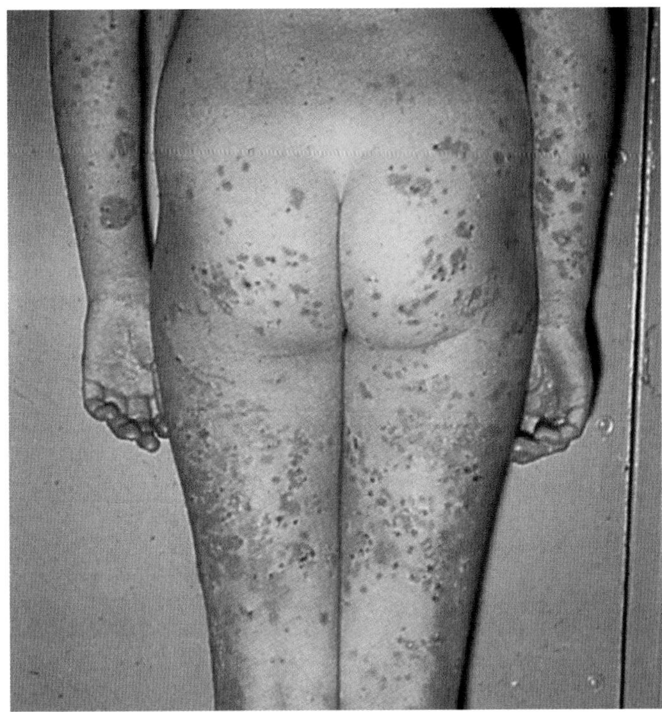

FIGURE 157-12 Dermatitis herpetiformis showing erosions from vesicles and bullae on the buttocks, legs and arms in a young girl with gluten-induced enteropathy. (*Used with permission from Weinberg SW, Prose NS, Kristal L. Color Atlas of Pediatric Dermatology, 4th edition, Figure 14-32, New York, NY: McGraw-Hill, 2008.*)

ruled out with skin scraping looking for the mite, feces, and eggs. If the scraping is negative, but the clinical appearance suggests scabies, empiric treatment with permethrin should be considered as well. If the lesions persist, consider a punch biopsy to look for dermatitis herpetiformis (Chapter 128, Scabies).
- Nummular and dyshidrotic eczema may also be diagnostic considerations, but response to steroids in eczema may be helpful in differentiation (Chapter 130, Atopic Dermatitis).

MANAGEMENT

- With a gluten-free diet, 80 percent of patients will show improvement in the skin lesions. The degree of benefit is dependent upon the strictness of the diet.[9]
- A gluten-free diet may help the enteropathy and decrease the subsequent development of small bowel lymphoma.
- Dapsone may be necessary indefinitely.[10]

FOLLOW-UP

Follow-up is needed to control the disease and monitor nutritional status.

PATIENT EDUCATION

Nutritional counseling is important for all patients with gluten-induced enteropathy. Persons with dermatitis herpetiformis and gluten-induced, enteropathy should not eat wheat and barley but can eat rice, oats, and corn.

PATIENT RESOURCES

- Genetics Home Reference. Epidermolysis Bullosa Simplex—**http://ghr.nlm.nih.gov/condition=epidermolysisbullosasimplex**.
- National Institute of Arthritis and Musculoskeletal and Skin Diseases. Epidermolysis Bullosa—**www.niams.nih.gov/Health_Info/Epidermolysis_Bullosa/default.asp**.
- DermNet NZ. Pityriasis Lichenoides—**http://dermnetnz.org/scaly/pityriasis-lichenoides.html**.
- PubMed Health. Dermatitis Herpetiformis—**www.ncbi.nlm.nih.gov/pubmedhealth/PMH0002451/**.

PROVIDER RESOURCES

- Medscape. *Epidermolysis Bullosa*—**http://emedicine.medscape.com/article/1062939**.
- Medscape. *Pityriasis Lichenoides*—**http://emedicine.medscape.com/article/1099078**.
- Medscape. *Dermatitis Herpetiformis*—**http://emedicine.medscape.com/article/1062640**.

REFERENCES

1. Horn HM, Tidman MJ. The clinical spectrum of epidermolysis bullosa. *Br J Dermatol*. 2002;146(2):267-274.
2. Fine JD, Johnson LB, Weiner M, et al. Epidermolysis bullosa and the risk of life-threatening cancers: the National EB Registry experience, 1986-2006. *J Am Acad Dermatol*. 2009;60(2):203-211.
3. Paller AS, Mancini AJ. Bullous diseases in children. In: Paller AS, Mancini AJ, eds. *Hurwitz's Clinical Pediatric Dermatology*, 3rd ed. Philadelphia, PA: Elsevier; 2006:345.
4. Patel GK, Finlay AY. Staphylococcal scalded skin syndrome: diagnosis and management. *Am J Clin Dermatol*. 2003;4(3):165-175.
5. Bowers S, Warshaw EM. Pityriasis lichenoides and its subtypes. *J Am Acad Dermatol*. 2006;55(4):557-572.
6. Ersoy-Evans S, Greco MF, Mancini AJ, et al. Pityriasis lichenoides in childhood: a retrospective review of 124 patients. *J Am Acad Dermatol*. 2007;56(2):205-210.
7. Magro C, Crowson AN, Kovatich A, Burns F. Pityriasis lichenoides: a clonal T-cell lymphoproliferative disorder. *Hum Pathol*. 2002;33(8):788-795.
8. Pinton PC, Capezzera R, Zane C, De Panfilis G. Medium-dose ultraviolet A1 therapy for pityriasis lichenoides et varioliformis acuta and pityriasis lichenoides chronica. *J Am Acad Dermatol*. 2002;47(3):410-414.
9. Patient.co.uk. *Dermatitis Herpetiformis*. http://www.patient.co.uk/showdoc/40001007/. Accessed October 7, 2007.
10. AGA Institute: AGA Institute Medical Position Statement on the Diagnosis and Management of Celiac Disease. *Gastroenterology*. 2006;131(6):1977-1980.

SECTION 14 HAIR AND NAIL CONDITIONS

158 ALOPECIA AREATA

Richard P. Usatine, MD

PATIENT STORY

An 8-year-old Hispanic girl was brought to her physician by her mother, who noticed two bald spots on the back of her daughter's scalp while brushing her hair. The child had no itching or pain. The mother was more worried that her beautiful girl would become bald. The girl was pleased that the bald spots could be completely covered with her long hair, as she did not want anyone to see them. The child was otherwise healthy. When the mother lifted the hair in the back, two round areas of hair loss were evident (**Figure 158-1**). On close inspection, there was no scaling or scarring. The mother and child were reassured that alopecia areata (AA) is a condition in which the hair is likely to regrow without treatment. Neither of them wanted intralesional injections or topical therapies. During a well-child examination 1 year later, it was noted that the girl's hair had fully regrown.[1]

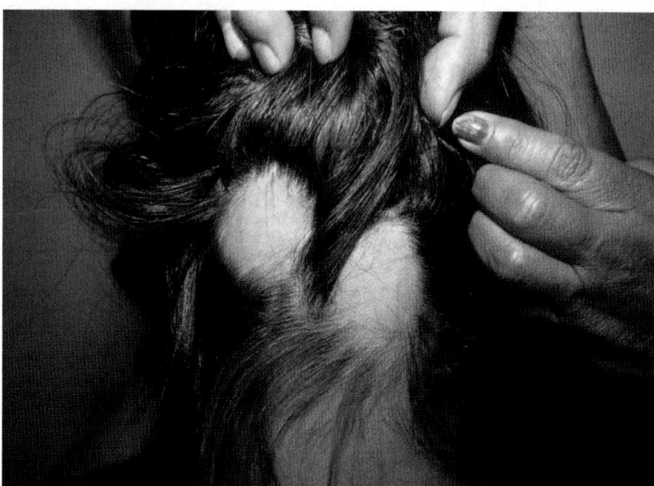

FIGURE 158-1 Alopecia areata in an 8-year-old girl. (*From Usatine R. Bald spots on a young girl. J Fam Pract. 2004;53(1):33-36. Reproduced with permission from Frontline Medical Communications.*)

INTRODUCTION

AA is a common disorder that causes patches of hair loss without inflammation or scarring. The areas of hair loss are often round and the scalp is often very smooth at the site of hair loss.

SYNONYMS

Alopecia totalis involves the whole scalp. Alopecia universalis (AU) involves the whole scalp, head, and body (**Figure 158-2**). Limited alopecia areata on the scalp is called "patchy" alopecia areata or patch AA.

EPIDEMIOLOGY

- Alopecia areata affects approximately 0.2 percent of the population at any given time with approximately 1.7 percent of the population experiencing an episode during their lifetime.[2,3]
- Males and females are equally affected.
- Patients with alopecia totalis and/or universalis were younger at the age of onset than those with patchy AA, were more likely to have atopic dermatitis, thyroid disease, and had a greater number of relatives affected by AA.[4]

ETIOLOGY AND PATHOPHYSIOLOGY

- The etiology is unknown but experts presume that the AA spectrum of disorders is secondary to an autoimmune phenomenon involving antibodies, T cells, and cytokines.

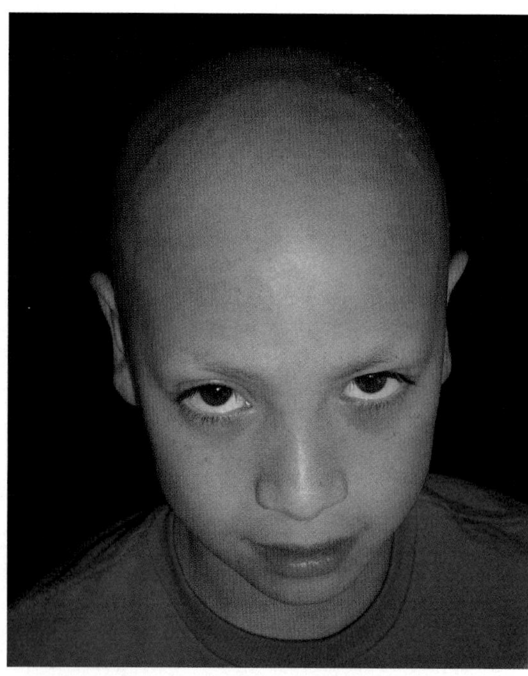

FIGURE 158-2 Alopecia universalis in a 10-year-old boy that started when he was 3 years old. The hyperpigmentation and peeling on his scalp is from repeated sun burns. He does have eyelashes and the medial sides of his eyebrows. Many children with alopecia universalis lose their eyebrows and eyelashes along with all their body hair. (*Used with permission from Richard P. Usatine, MD.*)

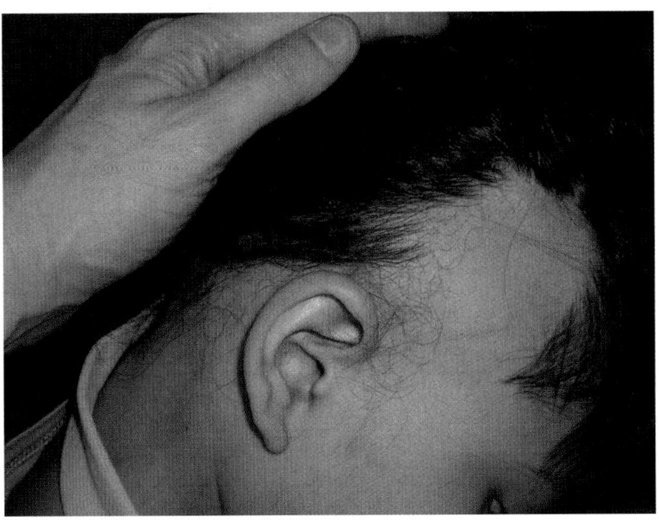

FIGURE 158-3 Alopecia areata for 2 years in a young girl. (*Used with permission from Richard P. Usatine, MD.*)

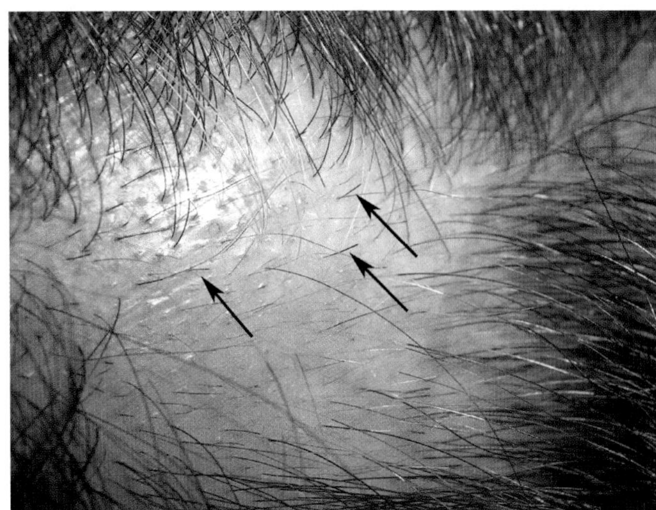

FIGURE 158-5 Exclamation point hairs (*arrows*) can be seen in this case of alopecia areata. The hair is narrow at the base, short and wide at the end. (*Used with permission from Richard P. Usatine, MD.*)

RISK FACTORS

- Previous episode of AA.
- Family history of AA—In one study, the estimated lifetime risks were 7.1 percent in siblings, 7.8 percent in parents, and 5.7 percent in offspring of patients with AA.[5]

DIAGNOSIS

CLINICAL FEATURES

- Sudden onset of 1 or more 1- to 4-cm areas of hair loss on the scalp (**Figures 158-1** and **158-3**). This can occur in the eyebrows or other areas of hair (**Figure 158-4**).
- The affected skin is smooth and may have short stubble hair growth.
- "Exclamation point" hairs are often noted (**Figure 158-5**). These hairs are characterized by proximal thinning while the distal portion remains of normal caliber.
- When hair begins to regrow, it often comes in as fine white hair (**Figure 158-6**).
- Nail dystrophy can occur and might suggest a worse prognosis for hair regrowth.

TYPICAL DISTRIBUTION

- Scalp and eyebrows but can involve any area with hair.
- Ophiasis is the term used to describe the distribution of alopecia areata when the hair loss follows a serpent-like distribution on the scalp (**Figures 158-7** and **158-8**). It is said to have a worse prognosis but studies to prove this are lacking. This pattern can also be seen with traction alopecia so hair care practices should be queried.

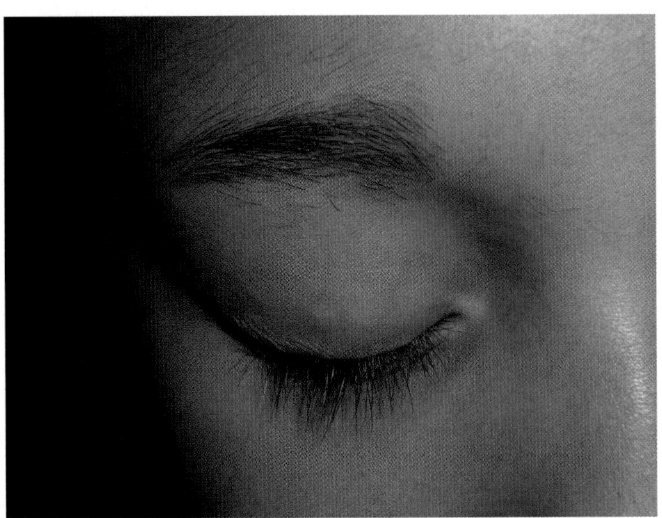

FIGURE 158-4 Alopecia areata in the medial eyebrow a 7-year-old girl. (*Used with permission from Richard P. Usatine, MD.*)

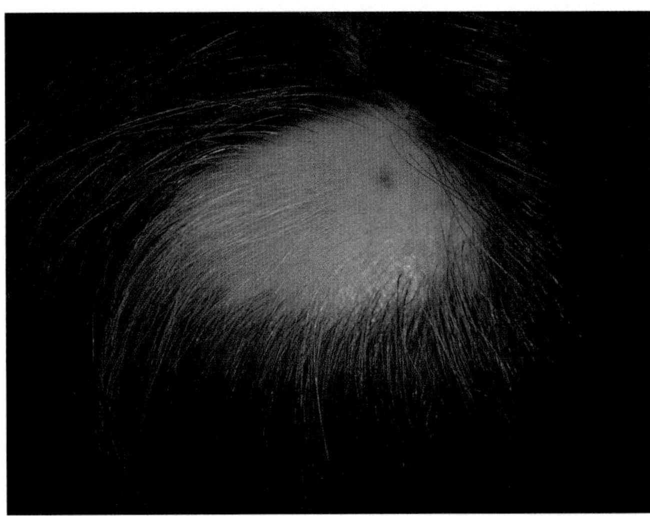

FIGURE 158-6 New growth of white hair after 7 months of alopecia areata. (*Used with permission from Richard P. Usatine, MD.*)

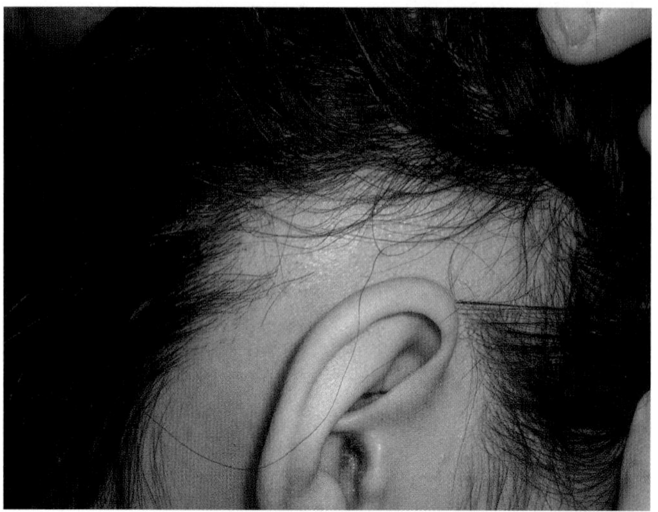

FIGURE 158-7 Ophiasis pattern of alopecia areata in a 12-year-old girl with atopic dermatitis. Ophiasis means "serpent-like." (*Used with permission from Richard P. Usatine, MD.*)

LABORATORY STUDIES

- Typically, the diagnosis can be made with history and physical examination alone (**Figure 158-9**).
- Thyroid abnormalities, vitiligo, and pernicious anemia often accompany AA. Consequently, screening laboratory tests (e.g., thyroid-stimulating hormone, complete blood count [CBC]) may be helpful to look for thyroid disorders and anemia.

BIOPSY

Not needed unless the diagnosis is uncertain. Histology examination shows peribulbar lymphocytic infiltration, frequently including eosinophils and the previously mentioned (see "Clinical Features") "exclamation point" hairs.

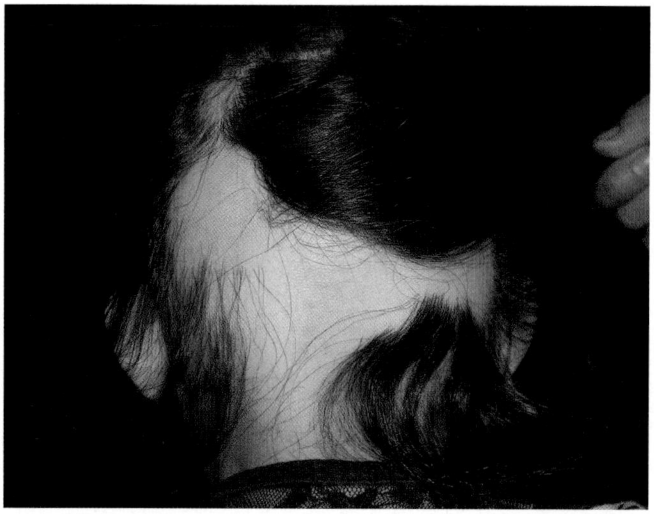

FIGURE 158-8 Ophiasis pattern of extensive alopecia areata in a 6-year-old girl. (*Used with permission from Richard P. Usatine, MD.*)

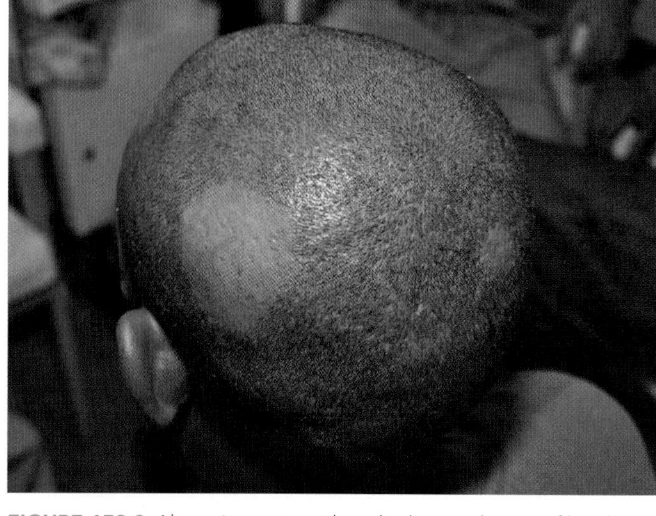

FIGURE 158-9 Alopecia areata with multiple round areas of hair loss in this young African boy. Note how the skin of the affected area appears smooth and there is no scale. (*Used with permission from Richard P. Usatine, MD.*)

DIFFERENTIAL DIAGNOSIS

- Trichotillomania—History of hair pulling; short, "broken" hairs are seen (see Chapter 159, Traction Alopecia and Trichotillomania).
- Telogen effluvium—Even distribution of hair loss; may be drug-induced (e.g., warfarin, β blockers, or lithium) or occur after pregnancy.
- Anagen effluvium—History of drug use (e.g., chemotherapy); even distribution of hair loss.
- Tinea capitis—Skin scaling and inflammation; KOH prep or fungal culture, if necessary (see Chapter 122, Tinea Capitis).
- Secondary syphilis—"Moth-eaten" appearance in beard or scalp; risk factors and rapid plasma reagin (RPR) will help distinguish (see Chapter 181, Syphilis).
- Lupus erythematosus—Skin scarring; antinuclear antibody (ANA) if clinical presentation compatible with this diagnosis (see Chapter 173, Lupus: Systemic and Cutaneous).

MANAGEMENT

- Alopecia areata can lead to significant psychological distress for the child and family. Counseling the child and parents about the nature and course of the condition as well as the available treatments is critical to management.[6]
- Treatment for AA includes immune-modulating agents (e.g., corticosteroids or anthralin), and biologic response modifiers (e.g., minoxidil).[6,7] SOR C
  - A commonly used treatment in patients older than 10 years of age with less than 50 percent scalp involvement is intralesional steroids (**Figure 158-10**). SOR B
    - In one randomized controlled trial (RCT), intralesional triamcinolone acetonide (10 mg/mL every 3 weeks) was better than

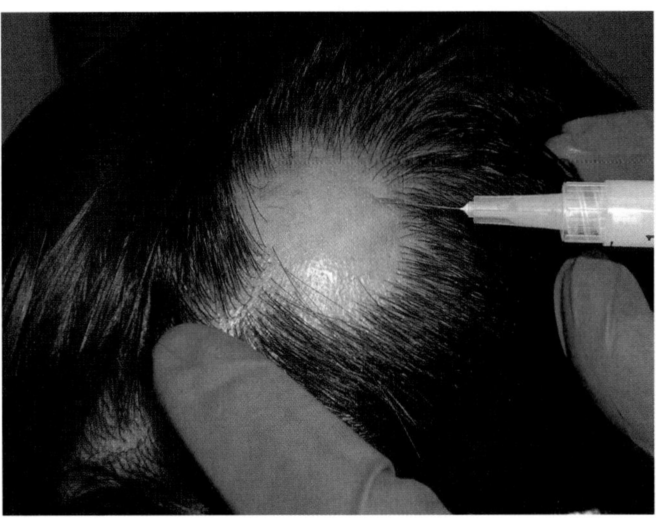

FIGURE 158-10 Injecting alopecia areata with triamcinolone acetonide 5 mg/mL. (*Used with permission from Richard P. Usatine, MD.*)

betamethasone valerate foam and topical tacrolimus in the management of localized AA.[8] There was no satisfactory hair regrowth in the tacrolimus group.[8] Although 10 mg/mL triamcinolone is often used as treatment, there is a higher rate of scalp atrophy than with 5 mg/mL. Start with 5 mg/mL and consider 10 mg/mL in subsequent injections if there is acceptance of a higher risk of scalp atrophy.

- Triamcinolone acetonide (Kenalog)—Dilute with sterile saline to 5 mg/mL. Inject with a 3-mL or 5-mL syringe and a 27- or 30-gauge needle. Inject into the dermis of the involved areas but not to exceed 4 mL per visit. Use 2.5 mg/mL for involved areas of the eyebrows or beard. SOR C
- Skin atrophy can be reduced by injecting intradermally and limiting both the volume per site and the frequency of injections (4 to 6 weeks between injections). Do not reinject areas that show atrophy and in most cases, the atrophy will resolve spontaneously. SOR C
- Spontaneous regrowth may still occur, so steroid injections should be discontinued after 6 months.

- For patients younger than age 10 years, a mid-potency topical steroid such as triamcinolone 0.1 percent cream applied twice daily is one option. SOR C

A Cochrane review in 2008 concluded that most trials have been reported poorly and are so small that any important clinical benefits are inconclusive.[9] They stated that considering the possibility of spontaneous remission (especially for those in the early stages of the disease) the options of not treating or wearing a wig are reasonable alternatives.[9]

- Hairpieces and hair transplantation may be used for those patients with unresponsive, recalcitrant disease.

COMPLEMENTARY/ALTERNATIVE THERAPY

- One RCT showed aromatherapy with topical essential oils to be a safe and effective treatment for AA.[10] The active group massaged essential oils (thyme, rosemary, lavender, and cedarwood) in a mixture of carrier oils (jojoba and grapeseed) into their scalp daily. This is a good option for families that want to do something but want to avoid the use of steroids. SOR B

PATIENT EDUCATION AND PROGNOSIS

- Although spontaneous recovery usually occurs, the course of AA is unpredictable and often characterized by recurrent periods of hair loss and regrowth.
- Spontaneous long-term regrowth in alopecia totalis and AU is poor.
- Prognosis is worse if the alopecia persists longer than 1 year.
- Alopecia areata, totalis and universalis can actually resolve spontaneously at any time as the hair follicle retains its ability to regrow even years after the initial loss of hair.
- Patients with a family history of AA, younger age at onset, coexisting immune disorders, nail dystrophy, atopy, and widespread hair loss have a poorer prognosis.[5]

FOLLOW-UP

- Spontaneous recovery usually occurs within 6 to 12 months and the prognosis for total permanent regrowth with limited involvement (AA) is excellent.
- The regrown hair is usually of the same texture and color but may be fine and white at first (**Figure 158-5**).
- Ten percent of patients never regrow hair and advance to chronic disease. Clinicians should provide contact information to the National Alopecia Areata Foundation and offer follow-up in the office as necessary.

PATIENT RESOURCES

- The National Alopecia Areata Foundation (**http://www.naaf.org/**) publishes a newsletter and can provide information regarding these support groups as well as hairpiece information.
- **www.niams.nih.gov/hi/topics/alopecia/ff_alopecia_areata.htm**.

PROVIDER RESOURCES

- British Association of Dermatologists' guidelines for the management of alopecia areata 2012—**http://www.alopeciaonline.org.uk/viewNews.asp?news_id=121**.

REFERENCES

1. Usatine RP. Bald spots on a young girl. *J Fam Pract*. 2004;53:33-36.
2. Firooz A, Firoozabadi MR, Ghazisaidi B, Dowlati Y. Concepts of patients with alopecia areata about their disease. *BMC Dermatol*. 2005;5:1.
3. Springer K, Brown M, Stulberg DL. Common hair loss disorders. *Am Fam Physician*. 2003;68:93-102.

4. Goh C, Finkel M, Christos PJ, Sinha AA. Profile of 513 patients with alopecia areata: associations of disease subtypes with atopy, autoimmune disease and positive family history. *J Eur. Acad Dermatol Venereol*. 2006:20(9);1055-1060.

5. Blaumeiser B, van der Goot I, Fimmers R, et al. Familial aggregation of alopecia areata. *J Am Acad Dermatol*. 2006;54: 627-632.

6. Garg, S and Messenger, AG. Alopecia areata: evidence-based treatments. *Semin. Cutan. Med. Surg*. 2009:28(1);15-18.

7. Price VH. Treatment of hair loss. *N Engl J Med*. 1999;341:964-973.

8. Kuldeep C, Singhal H, Khare AK, et al. Randomized comparison of topical betamethasone valerate foam, intralesional triamcinolone acetonide and tacrolimus ointment in management of localized alopecia areata. *Int J Trichology*. 2011;3:20-24.

9. Delamere FM, Sladden MM, Dobbins HM, Leonardi-Bee J. Interventions for alopecia areata. *Cochrane Database Syst Rev*. 2008:16(2):CD004413.

10. Hay IC, Jamieson M, Ormerod AD. Randomized trial of aromatherapy. Successful treatment for alopecia areata. *Arch Dermatol*. 1998;134:1349-1352.

159 TRACTION ALOPECIA AND TRICHOTILLOMANIA

E.J. Mayeaux, Jr., MD

PATIENT STORY

A 17-year-old Hispanic girl is brought to the office by her mother who is worried about the hair loss that has been going on for the past 3 months. The physician recognized the pattern of trichotillomania (**Figure 159-1**) and asked the girl if she was pulling on her hair. She told the doctor that this has been a very stressful year for her as she is currently taking four Advanced-Placement courses simultaneously. She admitted to playing with her hair while studying and sometimes that involved pulling on the hairs. The physician explained to the girl and her mother that this was a case of trichotillomania. He asked if the girl would be willing to stop pulling on her hairs and if she would like further counseling. She promised the doctor and her mother that she would stop pulling her hair and preferred to not enter counseling at this time. A follow-up appointment for one month was set.

INTRODUCTION

Traction alopecia is hair loss caused by damage to the dermal papilla and hair follicle by constant pulling or tension over a long period. It often occurs in persons who wear tight braids, especially "cornrows" that lead to high tension, pulling, and breakage of hair. Trichotillomania (Greek for "hair-pulling madness") is a traction alopecia related to a compulsive disorder caused when patients pull on and pluck hairs, often creating bizarre patterns of hair loss.

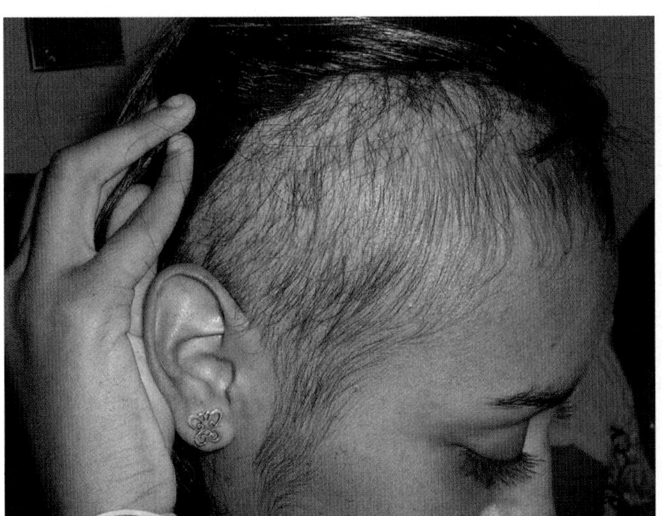

FIGURE 159-1 Trichotillomania in his 17-year-old honors student who is currently taking four Advanced Placement courses simultaneously. *(Used with permission from Richard P. Usatine, MD.)*

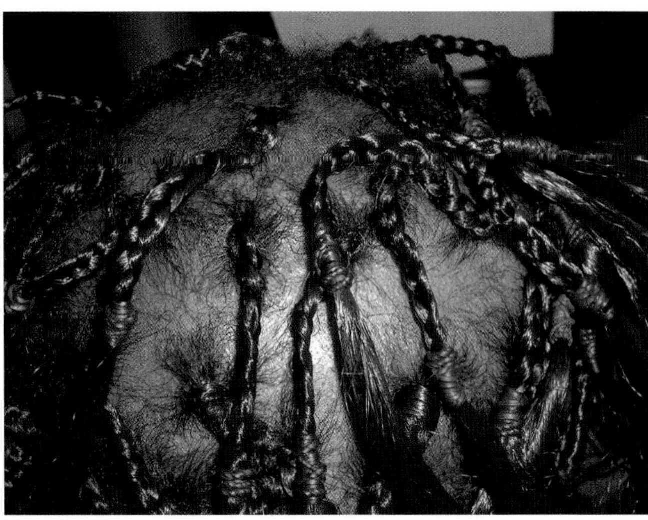

FIGURE 159-2 Traction alopecia in a young African American girl whose mom braids her hair tightly. *(Used with permission from Richard P. Usatine, MD.)*

EPIDEMIOLOGY

- The prevalence of traction alopecia (**Figures 159-1** and **159-2**) is unknown and varies by cultural hairstyle practices. It is most commonly seen in females and children.[1]
- The prevalence of trichotillomania (**Figures 159-3** to **159-6**) is also difficult to determine, but is estimated to be approximately 1.5 percent of males and 3.4 percent of females in the US. The mean age of onset of trichotillomania is 8 years in boys and 12 years in girls, and it is the most common cause of childhood alopecia.[2]

ETIOLOGY AND PATHOPHYSIOLOGY

- Traction alopecia is seen in individuals who place chronic tension on the hair shafts with tight braids, heavy natural hair, use of hair

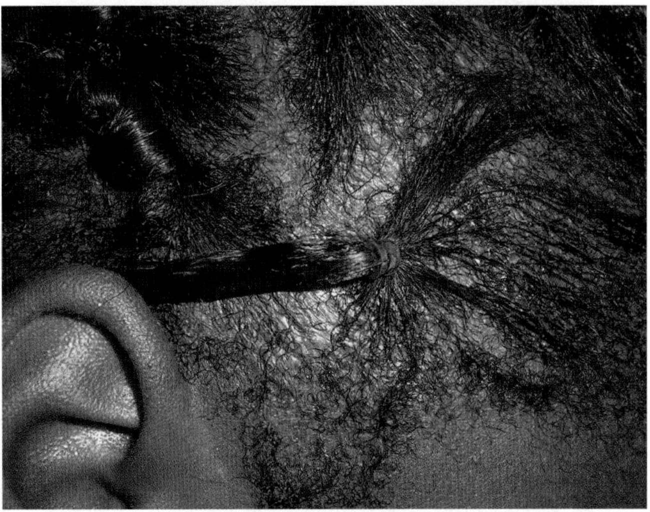

FIGURE 159-3 Traction alopecia on the lateral aspect of the scalp of a young girl due to pulling the hair tightly with rubber bands. *(Used with permission from Richard P. Usatine, MD.)*

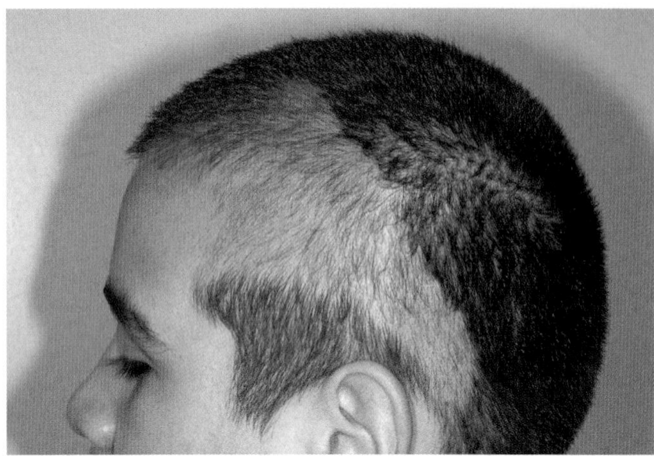

FIGURE 159-4 Trichotillomania in an 11-year-old boy. Note the incomplete hair loss and unusual geometric pattern. He was receiving help and the hair is now growing in. (*Used with permission from Richard P. Usatine, MD.*)

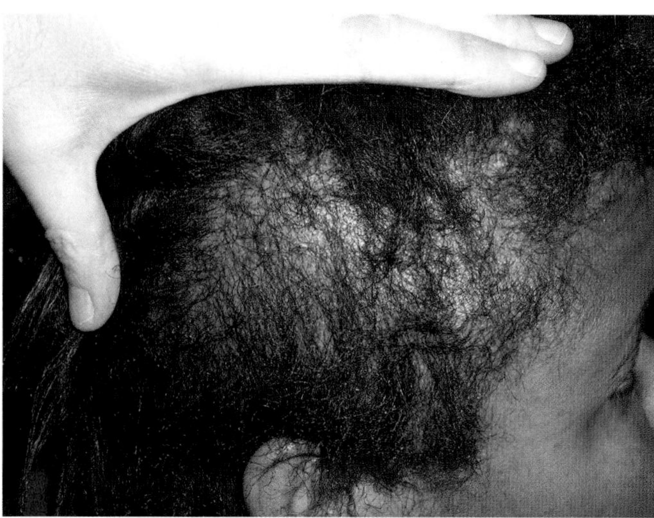

FIGURE 159-5 Trichotillomania in a 12-year-old black girl. The lateral right scalp was most involved. (*Used with permission from Richard P. Usatine, MD.*)

prostheses, or chronic pulling (**Figures 159-1** and **159-2**).[1] It also occurs commonly in female athletes who pull their hair into tight ponytails.

- Chronic tension on the hair shaft seems to create inflammation within the hair follicle that eventually leads to cessation of hair growth. Because hair loss from traction alopecia may become permanent, prevention and early treatment are important.
- It is seen most frequently in black women who tightly braid or pull the hair into a hairstyle during youth and on into adulthood. May also be seen in individuals who wear hair prostheses or extensions for a prolonged period of time. It is also seen in Sikh men of India and Japanese women whose traditional hairstyles may pull and damage hair.
- Trichotillomania is a subtype of traction alopecia manifested by chronic hair pulling (**Figures 159-3** to **159-6**) and sometimes

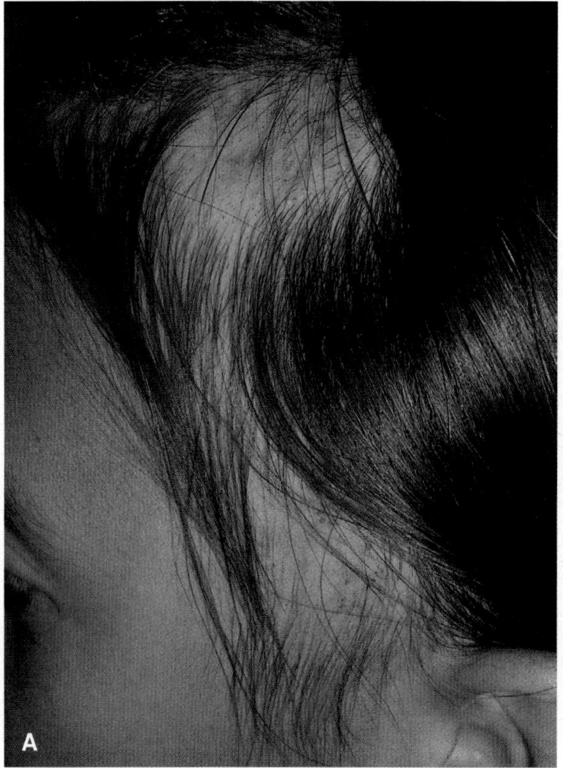

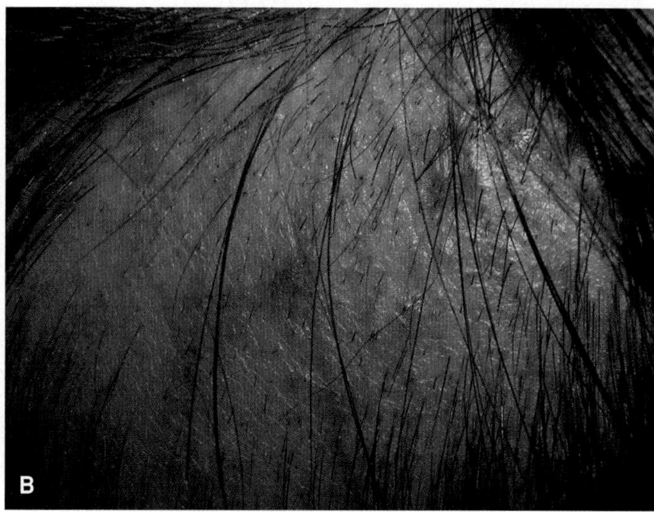

FIGURE 159-6 **A.** Trichotillomania in a 12-year-old girl undergoing much stress because of conflict in her family. **B.** Close-up of trichotillomania showing broken hairs, black dots, and excoriations. (*Used with permission from Richard P. Usatine, MD.*)

hair eating (trichophagy), which can lead to a trichobezoar. It is classified as a psychiatric impulse-control disorder.[3]

- Trichotillomania may be a manifestation of the inability to cope with stress rather than more severe mental disorders.
- Children who exhibit trichotillomania may discontinue the hair pulling with parental support and maturity. Adults who exhibit trichotillomania, even though they are aware of the problem, may require psychiatric intervention to limit the behavior. The hair loss is initially reversible but may become permanent if the habits persist.

DIAGNOSIS

CLINICAL FEATURES

In patients with traction alopecia, there are decreased follicular ostia in the affected area coupled with decreased hair density. The hair loss usually occurs in the frontal and temporal areas but depends on the precipitating hairstyle (**Figures 159-1** and **159-2**). No scalp inflammation or scaling is typically visible. No pain or other discomfort is associated with the condition. Patients with trichotillomania often demonstrate short, broken hairs (**Figure 159-6**) without the presence of inflammation or skin scale early in the disease. The affected areas are not bald, but rather possess hairs of varying length. There may be telltale stubble of hairs too short to pull. The hair loss often follows bizarre patterns with incomplete areas of clearing. The scalp may appear normal or have areas of erythema and pustule formation. With chronic pulling, the hair loss becomes permanent (**Figure 159-4**). The patient may be observed pulling or twisting the hair by friends or family members.

TYPICAL DISTRIBUTION

Trichotillomania most commonly occurs on the scalp and can involve any area of the body that can be reached by the patient.[1] Traction alopecia can occur anywhere on the scalp, but is most commonly seen at the anterior hairline. This is the site where the hair is pulled back from the face into braids or a bun.

LABORATORY STUDIES

Laboratory tests are not needed to make the diagnosis. A hand lens can be used to examine the affected scalp for decreased follicular ostia, if desired. A scalp biopsy (4-mm punch biopsy) may be necessary to make the diagnosis and rule out other etiologies, especially in trichotillomania, because patients may not acknowledge the habit.

Hypothyroidism or hyperthyroidism may be associated with telogen effluvium or alopecia areata. It may be worth ordering a thyroid-stimulating hormone (TSH) if the history and physical exam are not completely convincing for self-induced hair loss.

DIFFERENTIAL DIAGNOSIS[1]

- Alopecia areata is characterized by the total absence of hair in an area and the presence of exclamation point hairs. These hairs are thinner in diameter closer to the scalp and thicker in diameter away from the scalp, creating the appearance of an exclamation point. Hairs are often white when they start to regrow (see Chapter 158, Alopecia Areata).
- Tinea capitis exhibits hairs broken off at the skin surface and the presence of scale and/or inflammation. Some varieties fluoresce when examined with a Wood light (UV light). Microscopy of a KOH preparation may detect the dermatophyte. Sometimes it is necessary to culture some hairs and scale to make this diagnosis (see Chapter 122, Tinea Capitis).

MANAGEMENT

NONPHARMACOLOGIC

- Stop hairstyling practices that led to the traction alopecia. No tight braiding or buns should be worn.[1] SOR Ⓒ
- For trichotillomania, open discussions with the patient, and the family, if appropriate, are important to understand the reason for the behavior. Many times there are secondary social or emotional issues that must be resolved before the trichotillomania ceases.
    - Cognitive behavioral treatment is the most effective treatment for trichotillomania.[1,3] SOR Ⓑ
    - Cognitive-behavioral therapy usually is successful if the patient is recalcitrant to simple education.[5] SOR Ⓒ

MEDICATIONS

- Topical corticosteroids can be used to decrease scalp inflammation if erythema or itching is present. SOR Ⓒ
- Topical minoxidil is sometimes used to speed hair regrowth in the area. SOR Ⓒ
- Fluoxetine hydrochloride (Prozac) 20 to 40 mg/day in adults or clomipramine (Anafranil) 25 to 250 mg/day in adults or a maximum of 3 mg/kg per day in children has had some success for alleviating compulsive hair pulling.[4–6] SOR Ⓑ
- Olanzapine (Zyprexa) has been studied for the treatment of trichotillomania in a 12-week, randomized, double-blind, placebo-controlled trial. A dose of 10 mg/day showed a significant decrease in the CGI-Severity of Illness scale in 85 percent of subjects.[7] SOR Ⓑ
- Methylphenidate also has showed limited efficacy in trichotillomania patients with comorbid attention deficit hyperactivity disorder (ADHD) in a 12-week study.[8] SOR Ⓑ

FOLLOW-UP

Specific follow-up is not required for traction alopecia but psychiatric/behavioral counseling follow-up is indicated for trichotillomania.

PATIENT EDUCATION

Explain that in traction alopecia, current grooming practices are responsible for the hair loss and a new hairstyle must be selected. It is important to tell the patient that some of the hair loss may be permanent and no guarantee can be given regarding the amount of expected hair regrowth. Similar hair grooming practices should be avoided in the patient's children to prevent traction alopecia from occurring. Prevention is definitely the best treatment.

Explain that trichotillomania is a self-induced disease that can often resolve if the hair pulling or twisting is discontinued. Patients may exhibit hair pulling or twisting unconsciously when stressed or use it as a calming activity when relaxing or going to sleep. The underlying reasons for the behavior should be explored and discussed. Sometimes trichotillomania can be substituted with another behavior, such as playing with beads or rubbing a stone.

PATIENT RESOURCES

- Trichotillomania Support and Therapy Site. *Emphasis on Growth*—**www.trichotillomania.co.uk/**.
- WebMD. *Mental Health and Trichotillomania*—**www.webmd.com/anxiety-panic/guide/trichotillomania**.
- *Traction Alopecia: Causes and Treatment Options*—**www.traction-alopecia.com/**.
- MedlinePlus. *Trichotillomania*—**http://www.nlm.nih.gov/medlineplus/ency/article/001517.htm**.
- Mental Health America. *Trichotillomania*—**www.nmha.org/go/information/get-info/trichotillomania**.

PROVIDER RESOURCES

- *Trichotillomania*—**http://emedicine.medscape.com/article/1071854-overview**.
- *Traction Alopecia*—**www.emedicine.com/derm/topic895.htm**.

REFERENCES

1. Springer K, Brown M, Stulberg DL: Common hair loss disorders. *Am Fam Physician.* 2003;68:93-102, 107-108.
2. Messinger ML, Cheng TL: Trichotillomania. *Pediatr Rev.* 1999;20: 249-250.
3. Bloch MH, Landeros-Weisenberger A, Dombrowski P, et al. Systematic review: pharmacological and behavioral treatment for trichotillomania. *Biol Psychiatry.* 2007;62(8):839-846.
4. Christenson GA, Crow SJ: The characterization and treatment of trichotillomania. *J Clin Psychiatry.* 1996;57(8):42-47.
5. Streichenwein SM, Thornby JI: A long-term, double-blind, placebo-controlled crossover trial of the efficacy of fluoxetine for trichotillomania. *Am J Psychiatry.* 1995;152:1192-1196.
6. Ninan PT, Rothbaum BO, Marsteller FA, et al. A placebo-controlled trial of cognitive-behavioral therapy and clomipramine in trichotillomania. *J Clin Psychiatry.* 2000;61:47-50.
7. Van Ameringen M, Mancini C, Patterson B, et al. A randomized, double-blind, placebo-controlled trial of olanzapine in the treatment of trichotillomania. *J Clin Psychiatry.* 2010;71(10): 1336-1343.
8. Golubchik P, Sever J, Weizman A, Zalsman G: Methylphenidate treatment in pediatric patients with attention-deficit/hyperactivity disorder and comorbid trichotillomania: a preliminary report. *Clin Neuropharmacol.* 2011;34(3):108-110.

160 NORMAL NAIL VARIANTS

E.J. Mayeaux, Jr., MD

PATIENT STORY

A 14-year-old boy was brought into the office for a well-child visit and his mother pointed out white streaks in his fingernail (**Figure 160-1**). He has had them for about a year and his mother is concerned that he may have a vitamin deficiency. They were reassured that this is a normal nail finding often associated with minor trauma.

INTRODUCTION

The anatomy of the nail unit is shown in **Figure 160-2**. The nail unit includes the nail matrix, nail plate, nail bed, cuticle, proximal and lateral folds, and fibrocollagenous supportive tissues. The proximal matrix produces the superficial aspects of the plate, and the distal matrix the deeper portions. The nail plate is composed of hard and soft keratins, is formed via onychokeratinization, which is similar to hair sheath keratinization.[1] Most normal nail variants occur as a result of accentuation or disruption of normal nail formation.

SYNONYMS

- Leukonychia.
  - Transverse striate leukonychia.

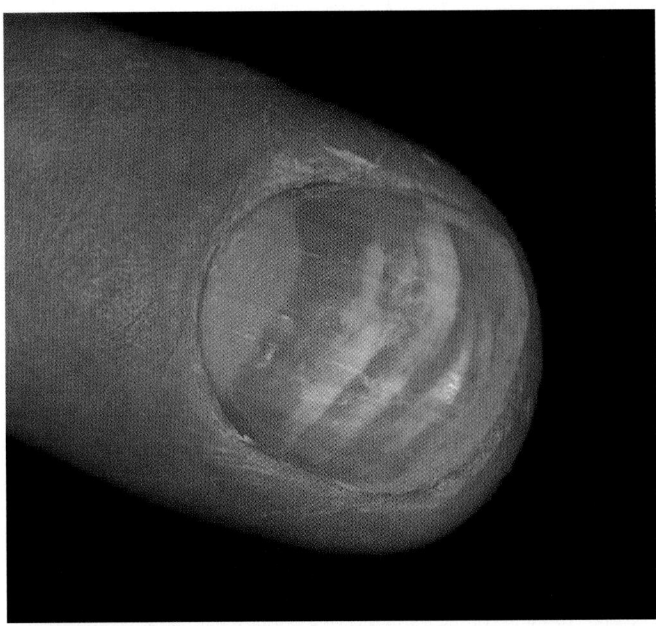

FIGURE 160-1 Transverse striate leukonychia (transverse white streaks) in a healthy patient. Note that the lines do not extend all of the way to the lateral folds, which indicates a probable benign process. (*Used with permission from Richard P. Usatine, MD.*)

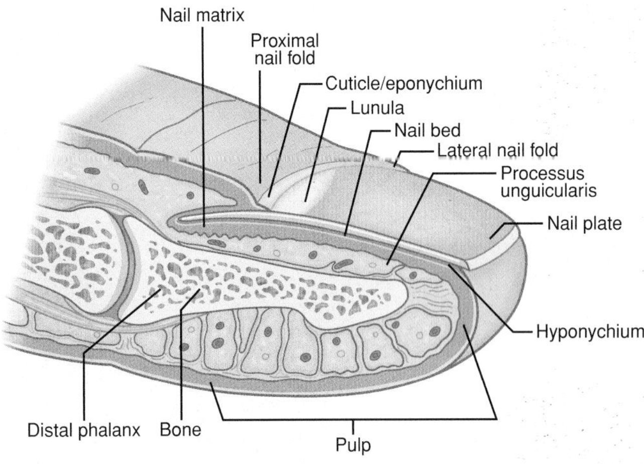

FIGURE 160-2 The anatomy of the nail unit. (*Used with permission from Usatine R, Pfenninger J, Stulberg D, Small R. Dermatologic and Cosmetic Procedures in Office Practice. Elsevier, Inc., Philadelphia. 2012.*)

  - Leukonychia punctata.
  - White nails.
- Longitudinal melanonychia (LM).
  - Racial melanonychia in African Americans.
- Nail hypertrophy.
  - Oyster-like deformity.
  - Lateral nail hypertrophy.
  - Thickened toenail.

EPIDEMIOLOGY

Melanonychia often involves several nails and is a more common occurrence in those patients with darker skin types. Among African Americans, benign melanonychia affects up to 77 percent of young adults and nearly 100 percent of those age 50 years or older. In the Japanese, LM affects 10 to 20 percent of adults.[1] Nail matrix nevi have been reported to represent approximately 12 percent of LM in adults and 48 percent in children.[2] The incidences of most other benign nail findings are not well established.

ETIOLOGY AND PATHOPHYSIOLOGY

- *Leukonychia* represents benign, single or multiple, white spots or lines in the nails. Patchy patterns of partial, transverse white streaks (transverse striate leukonychia, **Figure 160-1**) or spots (leukonychia punctata, **Figure 160-3**) are the most common patterns of leukonychia.[3] Leukonychia is common in children and becomes less frequent with age. Parents may fear that it represents a dietary deficiency, in particular a lack of calcium, but this concern is almost always unfounded.
- Most commonly, no specific cause for leukonychia can be found. It is usually the result of minor trauma to the nail cuticle or matrix and is the most commonly found nail condition in children.[4] When the lesions are caused by overly aggressive manicuring or nervous habit, behavior modification often is helpful. Leukonychia can also be

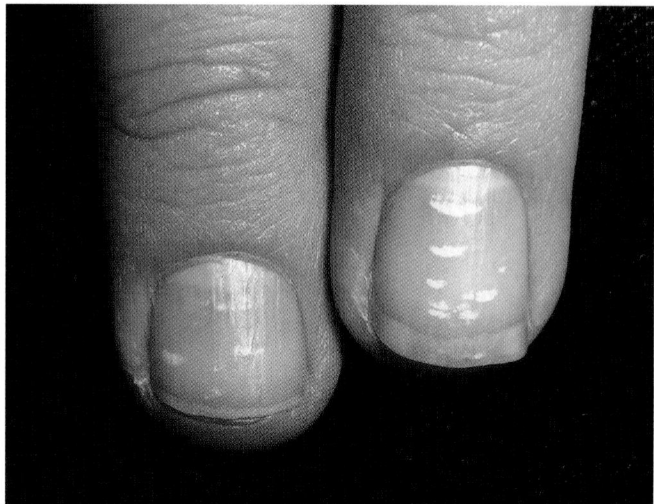

FIGURE 160-3 Leukonychia punctata showing distinct punctate white spots and lines on the fingernails. (*Used with permission from Richard P. Usatine, MD.*)

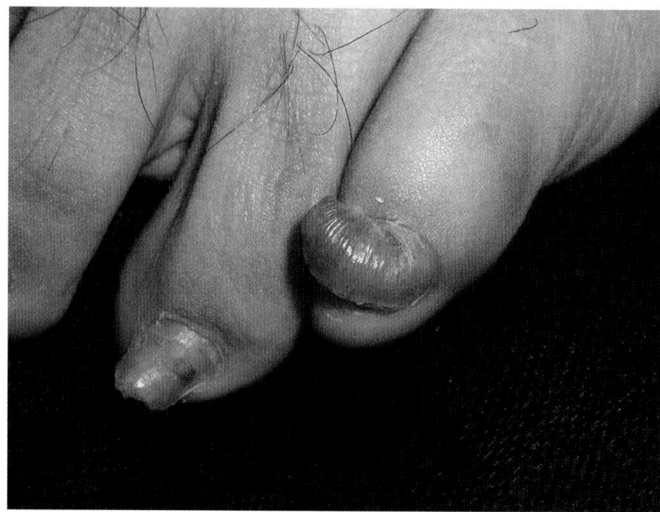

FIGURE 160-5 Onychogryphosis (ram's horn nail) is a type of lateral nail hypertrophy most frequently found in the toenails and often associated with onychomycosis. (*Used with permission from Richard P. Usatine, MD.*)

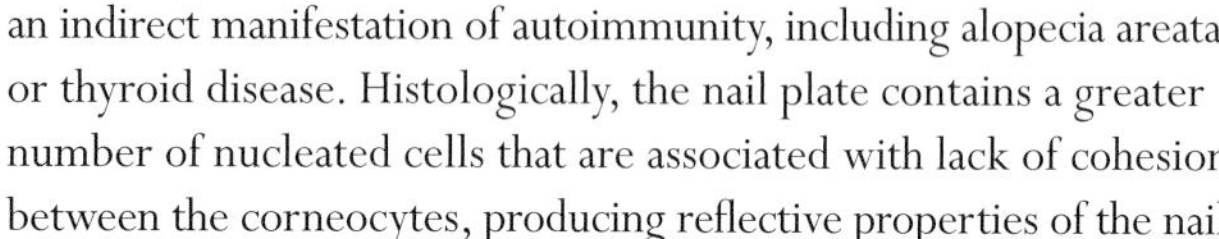

an indirect manifestation of autoimmunity, including alopecia areata or thyroid disease. Histologically, the nail plate contains a greater number of nucleated cells that are associated with lack of cohesion between the corneocytes, producing reflective properties of the nail.

- Longitudinal melanonychia (**Figure 160-4**) represents a longitudinal pigmented band in the nail plate. Melanonychia is ultimately caused by melanocyte activation. Causes of nongenetic nail matrix melanocyte activation include drugs, inflammatory processes, trauma, mycosis, systemic diseases, and neoplasms (melanomas).[1] LM is often caused by lentigines, benign melanocytic hyperplasia, or nevus of the nail matrix. However, it must be differentiated from subungual melanoma (see Chapter 161, Pigmented Nail Disorders). Benign causes of LM produce melanocytic activation with bands that usually measure 3 to 5 mm or less in width, whereas melanoma tends to produce wider bands. Most lentigines and nevi display a band with a tan-to-brown hue. A benign nail band is generally relatively homogeneous with respect to color and color intensity and if it expands, tends to expand slowly.[1]
- *Nail hypertrophy* (Figure **160-5**) is the development of opaque thickened nails with exaggerated upward, or lateral growth. It may be associated with age, fungal infections and trauma. It can cause pain with pressure.
- *Habit-tic deformity* (**Figures 160-6** and **160-7**) is caused by habitual picking of the proximal nail fold. The resulting inflammation induces the nail plate to be wavy and ridged, while its substance remains intact and hard.

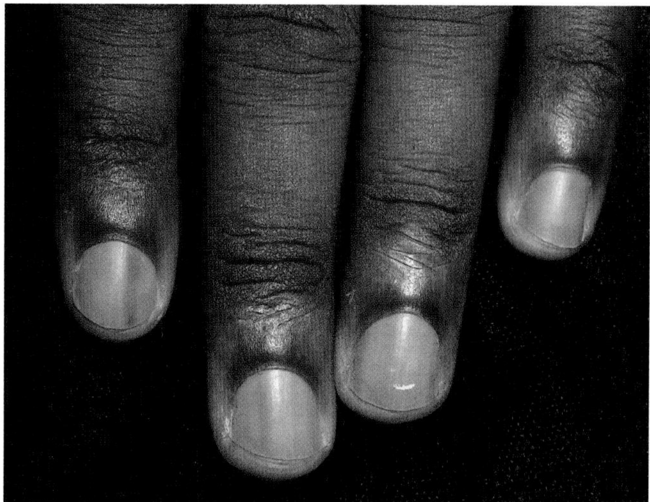

FIGURE 160-4 Longitudinal melanonychia in multiple fingers. These bands of translucent nail pigmentation in multiple fingers are typical of racial longitudinal melanonychia and not suspicious for melanoma. Note the dark pigment on the proximal nail folds represents a pseudo-Hutchinson sign. (*Used with permission from Richard P. Usatine, MD.*)

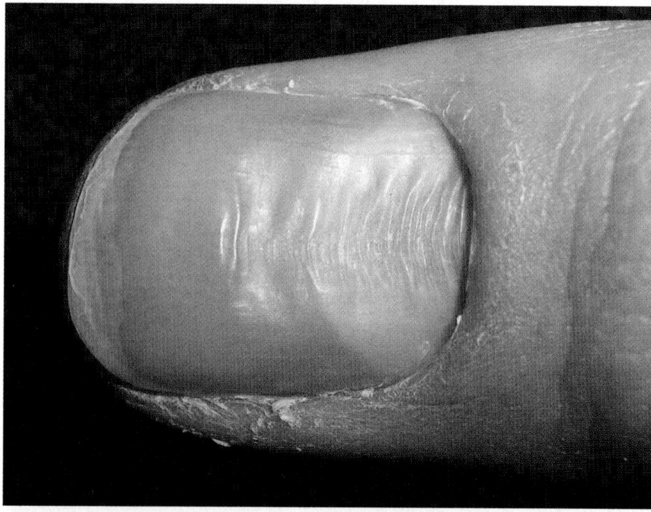

FIGURE 160-6 Habit-tic deformity of the thumbnail caused by a conscious or unconscious rubbing or picking of the proximal nails and nail folds. Horizontal grooves are formed proximally and move distally with fingernail growth. The thumbnails are most often affected. This was found in a high-school girl. (*Used with permission from Richard P. Usatine, MD.*)

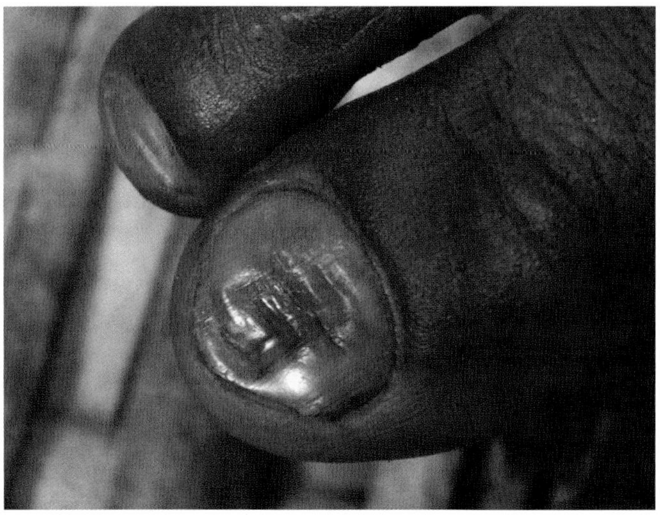

FIGURE 160-7 Habit-tic deformity of the large toenail in a teen that walks barefoot often. He acknowledged that he picks at the nail and cuticle. (*Used with permission from Richard P. Usatine, MD.*)

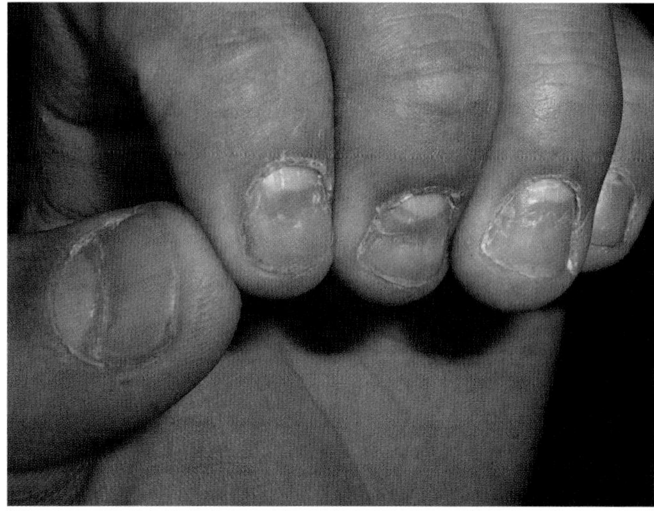

FIGURE 160-9 Beau lines in the fingernails of a young girl who was hospitalized with pneumonia 4 months prior to this visit. (*Used with permission from Richard P. Usatine, MD.*)

- *Beau lines* are transverse linear depressions in the nail plate (**Figures 160-8** and **160-9**). They are thought to result from suppressed nail growth secondary to local trauma or severe illness.[5] They most commonly appear symmetrically in several or all nails and may have associated white lines. They usually grow out over several months. One may estimate the time since onset of systemic illness by measuring the distance from the Beau line to the proximal nail fold and applying the conversion factor of 6 to 10 days per millimeter of growth.[4]

RISK FACTORS

- Leukonychia.
  - Use of nail enamels, nail hardeners, or artificial nails as a result of trauma and allergic reactions.
  - Repetitive trauma from work, sports, or leisure activities.

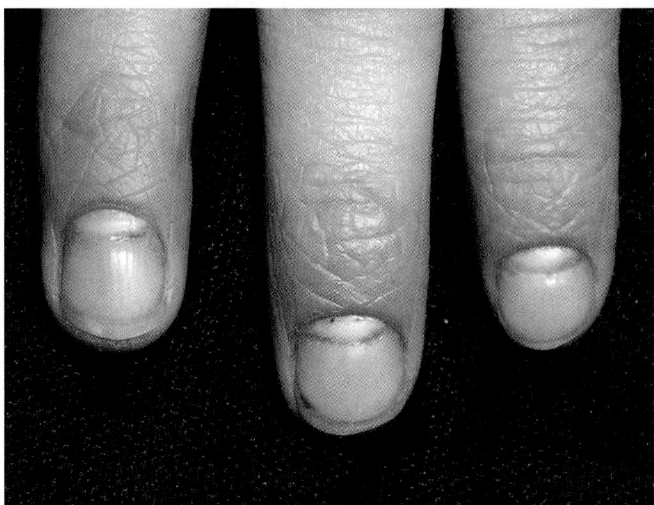

FIGURE 160-8 Beau lines in the fingernails of a young boy that had erythema multiforme and exfoliation approximately 2 months prior to this visit. (*Used with permission from Richard P. Usatine, MD.*)

- LM.
  - Race.
  - Age.
- Nail hypertrophy and onychogryphosis.
  - Age.
  - Fungal Infection.
- Habit-tic deformity.
  - Psychological dysfunctions.
- Beau lines.
  - Severe illness.
  - High fever.

DIAGNOSIS

CLINICAL FEATURES

- All diagnoses of nail disorders should begin with a focused history and physical exam. It is especially important to ask about trauma and recent illnesses.

LABORATORY TESTING

- If renal disease is suspected, order a urinalysis and a serum creatinine.

IMAGING

- The use of nail plate or matrix dermoscopy has been proposed as a way to further define areas to biopsy in LM, but their accuracy in the diagnosis of subungual melanoma has not been established.[2] SOR Ⓒ

BIOPSY

- Definitive diagnosis of a nail discoloration may be made with a biopsy of the nail or matrix. Patients with darker skin tones and multiple digits with translucent LM often need only be observed. A new dark line in a single nail should be biopsied. A 3-mm punch biopsy can be performed at the origin of the darkest part of a dark band. This usually involves reflecting the skin of the proximal nail fold back while performing a punch biopsy of the distal matrix. Histologic diagnosis of atypical melanocytic hyperplasia necessitates the complete removal of the lesion.[1] SOR Ⓒ

DIFFERENTIAL DIAGNOSIS

- Pigmented lesions in the nail bed do not cause LM, only nail matrix lesions do. Nail bed lesions make spots under the nails but do not grow out as stripes. These are viewed through the nail as a grayish to brown or black spot.[6]
- The diagnosis of subungual melanoma must always be considered in patients with LM. A biopsy should be performed in an adult if the cause of LM is not apparent. Extension of pigmentation to the skin adjacent to the nail plate involving the nail folds or the fingertip is called Hutchinson sign, which is an important indicator of nail melanoma (see Chapter 147, Pediatric Melanoma).
- Hematoma may be confused with LM, but the color grows out with the nail plate, exhibiting a proximal border that reproduces the shape of the lunula. A hole punched in the nail plate allows for the visualization of the underlying nail bed and confirmation of the nature of the coloration (see Chapter 166, Subungual Hematoma).
- Mees and Muehrcke lines may be confused with leukonychia or Beau lines. Mees lines are multiple white transverse lines that begin in the nail matrix and extend completely across the nail plate (**Figure 160-10**). They are caused by heavy-metal poisoning or severe systemic insults. Muehrcke lines are white transverse lines that represent an abnormality of the nail vascular bed and may occur with chronic hypoalbuminemia or renal disease

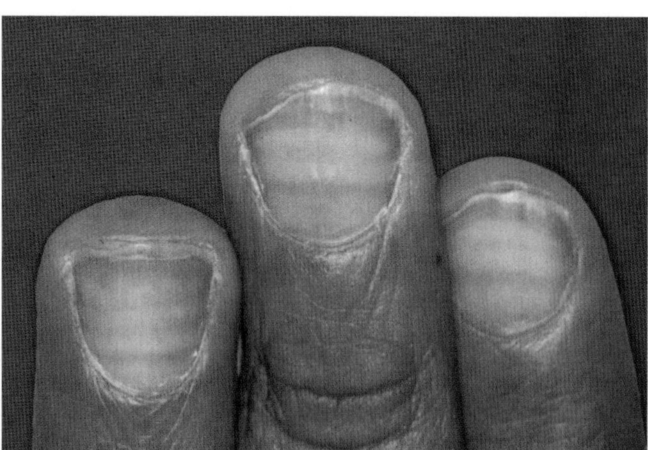

FIGURE 160-10 Mee lines that spread transversely across the entire breadth of the nail and are somewhat rounded with a contour similar to the distal lunula. (*Used with permission from Jeffrey Meffert, MD.*)

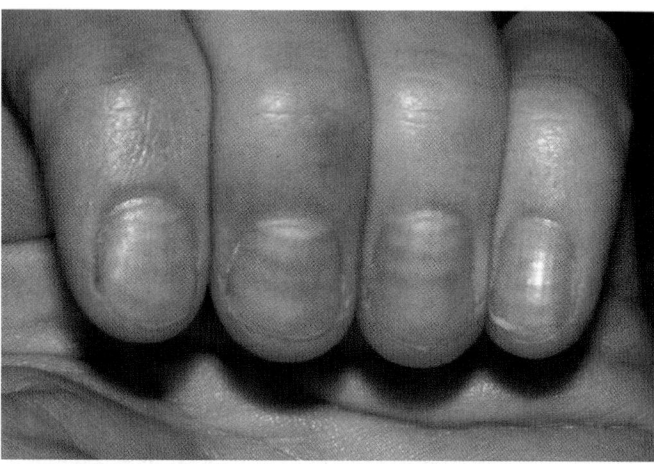

FIGURE 160-11 Muehrcke lines in a patient with chronic hypoalbuminemia from nephrotic syndrome. The white transverse lines extend across the full nail bed and represent an abnormality of the nail vascular bed.

(**Figure 160-11**). In contrast to Beau lines, they are not grooved and they do not move with nail growth. **Table 160-1** lists the clinical signs that help differentiate local trauma-induced lesions from those associated with systemic disease.

- Leukonychia must also be differentiated from localized white onychomycosis, half-and-half nails, which are white proximal nails and pink or brown distal nails seen in renal failure (**Figure 160-12**), and Terry nails, which are white proximal nails and reddened distal nails that are seen in liver cirrhosis.
- The differential diagnosis of habit-tic deformity includes several nail dystrophies. In median nail, dystrophy produces a distinctive longitudinal split in the center of the nail plate with several cracks projecting laterally. Chronic paronychia is a *Candida* induced inflammation of the proximal nail folds that may induce ripples that can mimic the habit-tic deformity. Chronic eczematous inflammation may produce similar changes. Onychomycosis, Beau lines, and psoriatic nail lesions may also appear similar to habit-tic deformity.[7]
- Twenty-nail dystrophy (**Figure 160-13**) is an idiopathic nail dystrophy that starts in childhood and resolves slowly with age. The nails lose their luster and develop longitudinal striations. It often starts with the fingernails and then affects the toenails.

MANAGEMENT

NONPHARMACOLOGIC

Most normal variants do not require treatment. Cosmetic concerns may often be addressed with nail buffing, polish, or false nail application.

MEDICATIONS

- Fluoxetine has been reported as being helpful in the treatment of habit-tic deformity.[8] SOR Ⓒ

TABLE 160-1 Signs that Help Differentiate Local Trauma-Induced Nail Changes from Those Associated with Systemic Disease

Characteristic	Mees Lines (Figure 160-10)	Muehrcke Lines (Figure 160-11)	Beau lines (Figures 160-8 and 160-9)	Leukonychia (Figures 160-1 and 160-3)
Number of Nails involved	Tend to be single but may occur on several nails at once	Tend to occur on several nails at once	Appear symmetrically in several or all nails	Usually on one or two nails
Nail coverage	Spread transversely across the entire breadth of the nail	Spread across the entire breadth of the nail bed or plate, often disappear with nail plate pressure	Spread transversely across the entire breadth of the nail	Often do not span the entire breadth of the nail plate
Line shape	Tend to have contour similar to the distal lunula, with a rounded distal edge	White transverse lines that have contour similar to the distal lunula, with a rounded distal edge	Tend to have contour similar to the distal lunula, with a rounded distal edge	More linear and resemble the contour of the proximal nail fold
Nail surface changes	Absent	Absent	Usually depressed	Absent
Etiology	Fragmented nail plate structure as a result of a compromised nail matrix	Abnormality of the nail vascular bed	Suppressed nail growth	Disruption of nail plate formation
Associated conditions	History of a systemic insult correlated with the onset of the lines such as chemotherapy, heart failure, and heavy-metal poisoning	Chronic hypoalbuminemia (hepatic and renal disease)	History of a physiologic stressor such as surgery or a severe illness	History of physical trauma (often not identified)

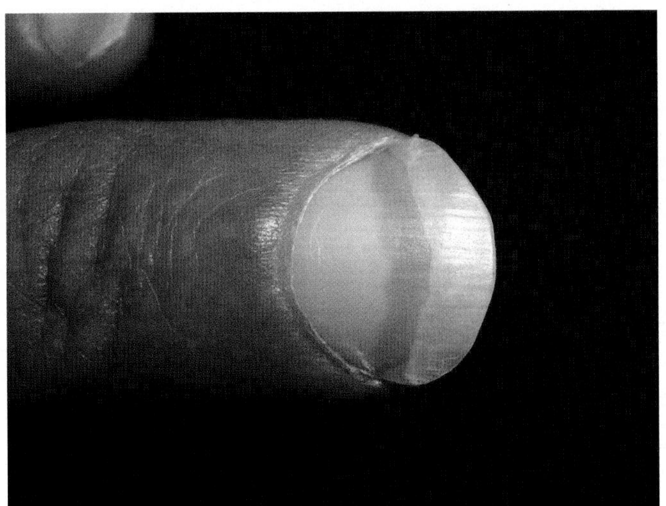

FIGURE 160-12 Half-and-half nail ("Lindsay nails") with the proximal portion of the nail being white and the distal portion pink. Note the sharp line of demarcation between the two halves. This patient has cirrhosis. *(Used with permission from Richard P. Usatine, MD.)*

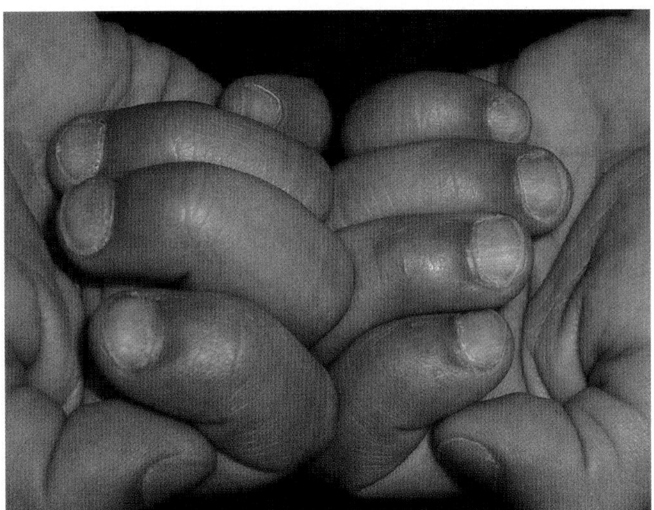

FIGURE 160-13 Twenty-nail dystrophy in a healthy 8-year-old girl. Note how all the fingernails are uniformly affected with longitudinal striations and loss of nail luster. Her skin is otherwise normal. *(Used with permission from Richard P. Usatine, MD.)*

PATIENT RESOURCES

- *Melanonychia*—**www.diseasesatoz.com/melanonychia.htm**.

PROVIDER RESOURCES

- Emedicine. *Nail Surgery*—**www.emedicine.com/derm/topic818.htm**.
- Color pictures at Dermatlas.org—**www.dermatlas.com/derm/** and select body site: *nails (all)*.
- Medscape. *Melanonychia*—**http://emedicine.medscape.com/article/1375850-overview#showall**.
- Medscape Education. *Examining the Fingernails*—**http://www.medscape.org/viewarticle/571916_2**.
- DermnetNZ. *"Nail Diseases"*—**http://dermnetnz.org/hair-nails-sweat/nails.html**.

REFERENCES

1. Ruben B: Pigmented lesions of the nail unit: clinical and histopathologic features. *Semin Cutan Med Surg*. 2010;29:148-158.
2. Tosti A, Piraccini BM, de Farias DC: Dealing with melanonychia. *Semin Cutan Med Surg*. 2009;28:49-54.
3. Grossman M, Scher RK: Leukonychia. Review and classification. *Int J Dermatol*. 1990;29:535-541.
4. Baran R, Kechijian P: Diagnosis and management. *J Am Acad Dermatol*. 1989;21:1165-1175.
5. Daniel CR, Zaias N: Pigmentary abnormalities of the nails with emphasis on systemic diseases. *Dermatol Clin*. 1988;6:305-313.
6. Noronha PA, Zubkov B: Nails and nail disorders in children and adults. *Am Fam Physician*. 1997;55:2129-2140.
7. Farnell EA 4th: Bilateral thumbnail deformity. *J Fam Pract*. 2008; 57(11):743-745.
8. Vittorio CC, Phillips KA: Treatment of habit-tic deformity with fluoxetine. *Arch Dermatol*. 1997;133(10):1203-1204.

161 PIGMENTED NAIL DISORDERS

E.J. Mayeaux, Jr., MD
Richard P. Usatine, MD

PATIENT STORY

A four-year-old boy presents with a newly pigmented line on his right thumb for 6 months. He already had one pigmented line on that same thumb since age one. His parents want to know if this pigmentation is dangerous. The child is otherwise healthy. On examination there are two longitudinal pigmented lines easily visible on the right thumbnail (**Figure 161-1A**). The boy is referred to a pediatric dermatologist. Examination with a dermatoscope shows the details of the many lines and confirms his concern for melanoma (**Figure 161-1B**). The concerns are expressed to the parents and the child is set up for a nail matrix biopsy with sedation. The differential diagnosis also includes a congenital melanocytic nevus that is growing.

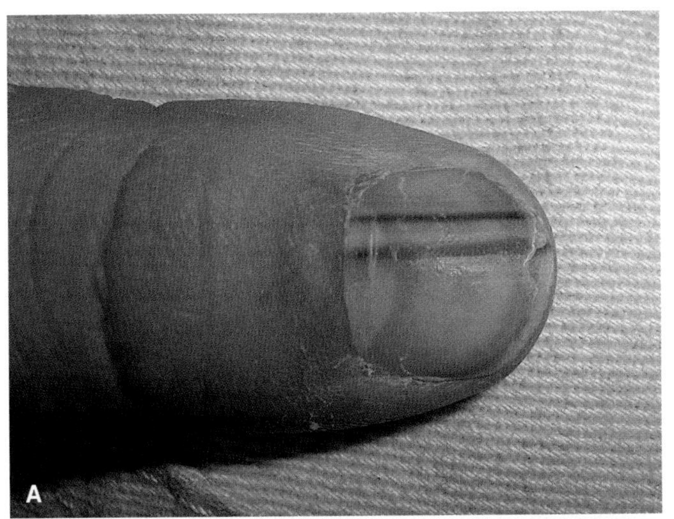

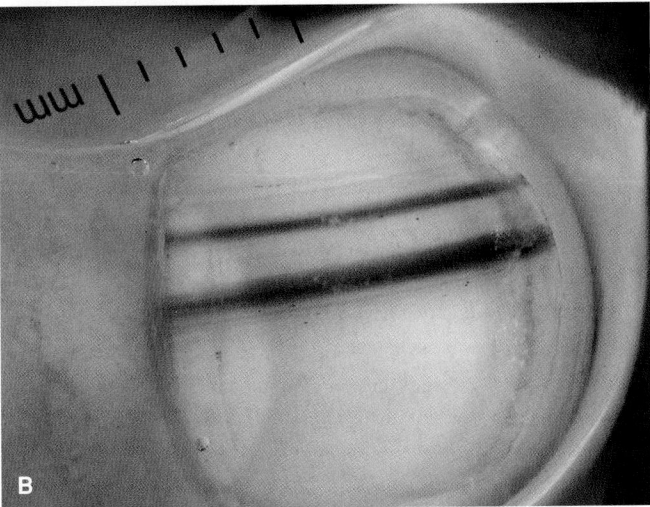

FIGURE 161-1 **A.** Longitudinal melanonychia on the right thumb of four-year-old boy with two prominent pigmented lines. One of the two lines is new. **B.** Dermoscopic examination of the nail shows the complex pigment pattern with many lines and melanocytic dots. This is suspicious for melanoma but could also be a congenital nevus that is growing. (*Used with permission from Richard P. Usatine, MD.*)

INTRODUCTION

Atypical pigmentation of the nail plate may result from many nonmalignant causes, such as fungal infections, benign melanocytic hyperplasia, nevi and medications. It may also result from development of subungual melanoma. The challenge for the clinician is separating the malignant from the nonmalignant sources.

Longitudinal melanonychia (LM) is a clinically descriptive term that represents a longitudinal pigmented band in the nail plate (**Figures 161-1** to **161-3**). It may be caused by any of the conditions listed above but is often due to normal ethnic hyperpigmentation (**Figure 161-3**). It may involve 1 or several digits, vary in color

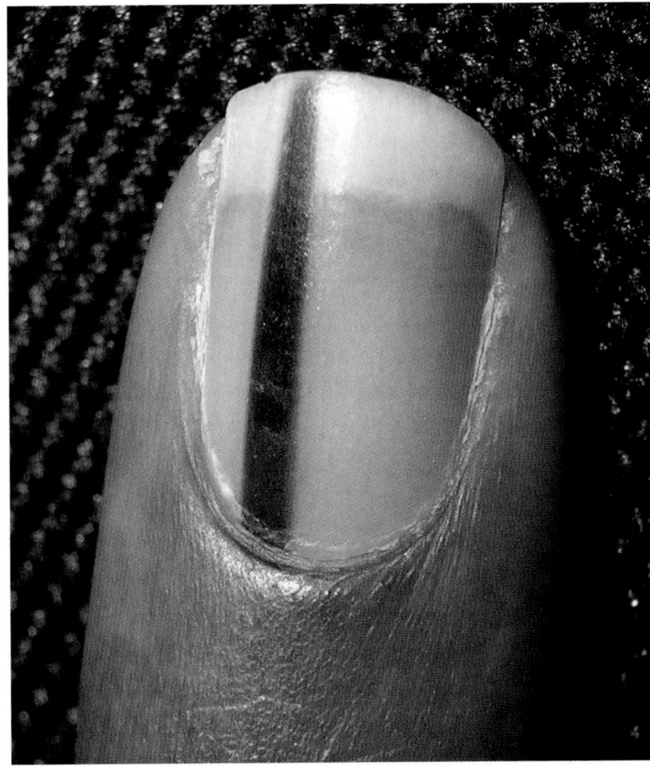

FIGURE 161-2 Longitudinal melanonychia—a single dark band of nail pigment appearing in the matrix region and extended to the tip of the nail. This is concerning for melanoma. The widening of the band in the proximal nail shows that the melanocytic lesion in the matrix is growing. A biopsy showed this to be a benign nevus. (*Used with permission from Richard P. Usatine, MD.*)

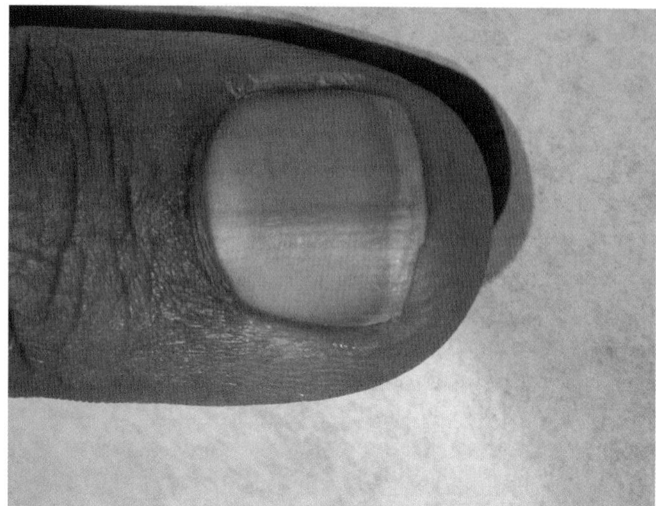

FIGURE 161-3 During a routine sports physical for a black adolescent boy, a translucent darker stipe was discovered in the nail plate of one of his thumbs. The line was faint and uniform in width. He was reassured it was most likely benign but the lesion was noted in his medical record so it could be rechecked in the future and he was instructed to return to clinic if it rapidly changed. (*Used with permission from E.J. Mayeaux, Jr., MD.*)

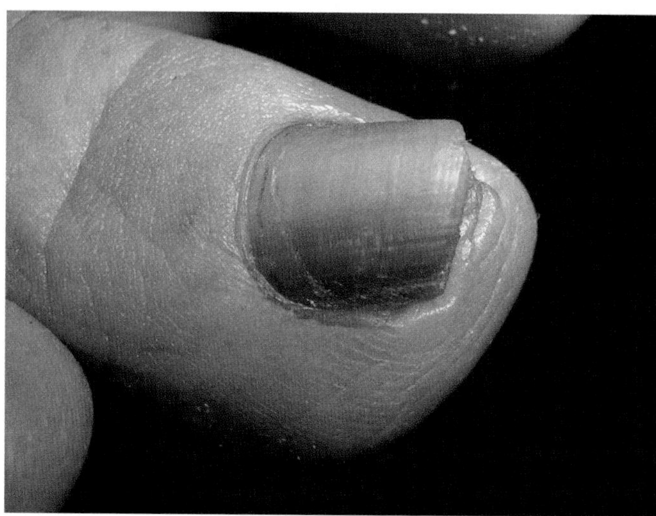

FIGURE 161-4 Longitudinal melanonychia of the toenail of a young person. Biopsy demonstrated benign melanocytosis. (*Used with permission from Richard P. Usatine, MD.*)

from light brown to black, vary in width (most range from 2 to 4 mm), and have sharp or blurred borders.

SYNONYMS

Acrolentiginous melanoma = acral lentiginous melanoma, subungual melanoma is one type of acral lentiginous melanoma involving the nail unit.

EPIDEMIOLOGY

- LM is more common in more darkly pigmented persons. It occurs in 77 percent of African Americans older than age 20 years and in almost 100 percent of those older than age 50 years.[1,2] It also occurs in 10 to 20 percent of persons of Japanese descent. LM is common in Hispanic and other dark-skinned groups. LM is unusual in whites, occurring in only approximately 1 percent of the population.[1]
- Melanoma is the seventh most common cause of cancer in patients in the US. Subungual melanoma is a relatively rare tumor with reported incidences between 0.7 percent and 3.5 percent of all melanoma cases in the general population.[3]

ETIOLOGY AND PATHOPHYSIOLOGY

- LM originates in the nail matrix and results from increased deposition of melanin within the nail plate. This deposition may result from greater melanin synthesis or from an increase in the total number of melanocytes (**Figure 161-4**). Pigment clinically localized within the dorsal half of the nail plate indicates a proximal matrix origin, and pigment localized within the ventral nail plate indicates a distal matrix origin. Look at the distal edge of the nail in a cross-sectional view to see whether the pigment is dorsal or ventral (a dermatoscope may help).
- LM may also be caused by chronic trauma, especially in the great toes.
- Inflammatory changes accompanying skin diseases located in the nail unit, such as psoriasis, lichen planus, amyloidosis, and localized scleroderma, rarely may result in LM.
- Benign melanocytic hyperplasia (lentigo) is observed in 30 percent of the pediatric cases of single-biopsied LM.[4]
- Nevi represent almost 50 percent of cases in children. A brown-black coloration is observed in two thirds of the cases and periungual pigmentation (benign pseudo-Hutchinson sign) in 1/3.
- Certain drugs may also cause LM, especially chemotherapeutic agents, and antimalarial drugs (mepacrine, amodiaquine, and chloroquine).
- Endocrine disorders, such as Addison disease, Cushing syndrome, hyperthyroidism, and acromegaly, can be responsible for LM.
- The diagnosis of subungual melanoma must always be considered in patients with LM (**Figures 161-5** to **161-7**). Separating benign from malignant lesions is often difficult. Both arise most often in the thumb or index fingers, and both are more common in dark-skinned persons.[5] A biopsy should be performed if the cause of LM is suspicious for melanoma. **Table 161-1** lists diagnostic clues for subungual melanomas. Many subungual melanomas have a history of trauma preceding the diagnosis so it is important to not be fooled by this history (**Figure 161-7**).
- Hutchinson sign is the extension of pigmentation to the skin adjacent to the nail plate involving the nail folds or the fingertip. It is an important indicator for nail melanoma (**Figures 161-5** to **161-6**).[6]
- Pseudo-Hutchinson sign is the presence of dark pigment around the proximal nail fold secondary to benign conditions such as racial melanosis and not melanoma (**Figure 161-8**). Another cause of pseudo-Hutchinson sign is a translucent cuticle below which the pigment of LM is visible. Trauma and drug-induced pigmentation can also produce a pseudo-Hutchinson sign.

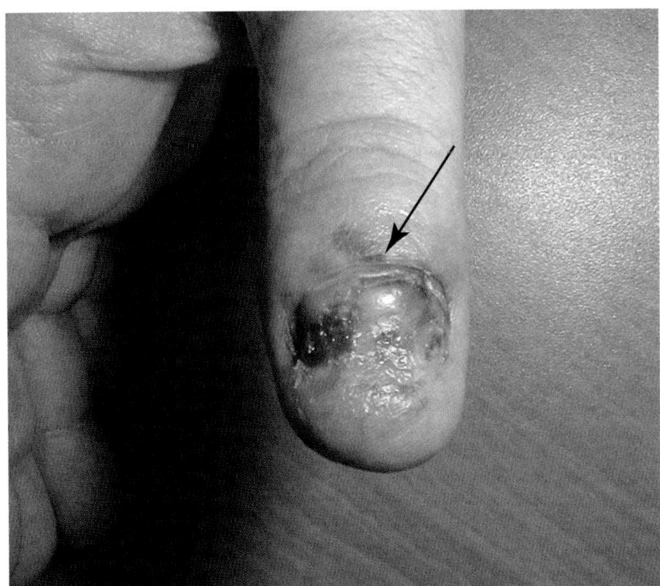

FIGURE 161-5 Advanced acral lentiginous melanoma of the thumb with destruction of the nail plate and ulceration. Note the hyperpigmentation of the proximal nail fold (Hutchinson sign), which is strongly indicative of melanoma. (*Used with permission from Dr. Dubin at http://www.skinatlas.com.*)

- Subungual melanoma arises on the hand in 45 to 60 percent of cases, and most of those occur in the thumb (**Figures 161-5** to **161-6**).[4] On the foot, subungual melanoma usually occurs in the great toe.[5] The median age at which subungual melanoma is usually diagnosed is in the sixth and seventh decades. It appears with equal frequency in males and females.[5]

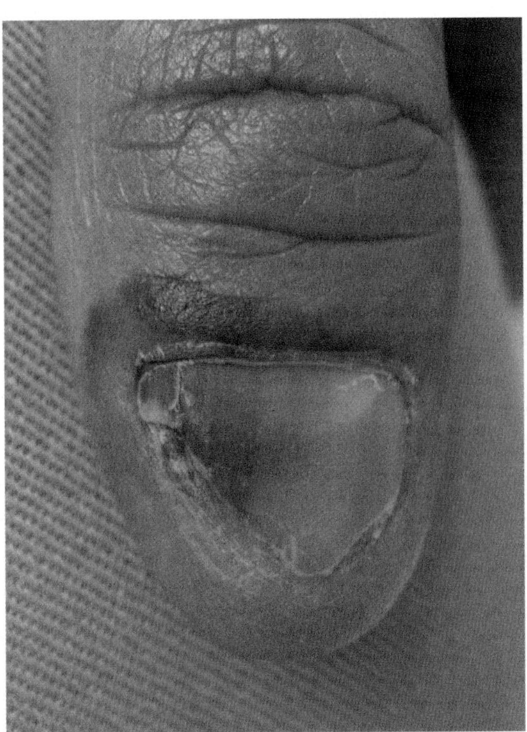

FIGURE 161-6 Acral lentiginous melanoma of the thumb with a very positive Hutchinson sign. Note how the pigmented band on the nail is greater than 3 mm in width. (*Used with permission from Robert T. Gilson, MD.*)

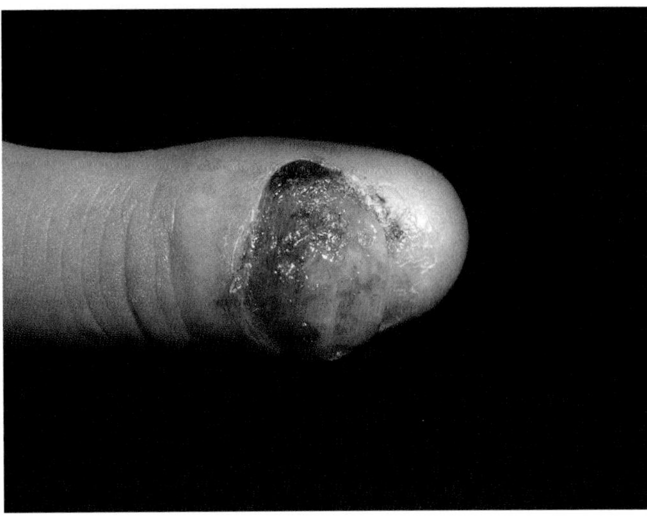

FIGURE 161-7 Nodular melanoma growing within the pinkie nail (not the thumb) of a young woman. The patient claims that it started with a dark spot under the nail of this fifth digit after she caught it in a dresser drawer. When it did not heal she pursued medical care and was treated for a presumed nail fungus and then a paronychia until she was finally seen by a physician who recognized the gravity of this situation. A biopsy was performed immediately and it showed a thick nodular melanoma greater than 3 mm in depth with a high mitotic index and ulceration. The patient will undergo an amputation of the finger at the PIP joint along with a sentinel node biopsy. (*Used with permission from Richard P. Usatine, MD.*)

RISK FACTORS

Table 161-1 lists diagnostic clues that indicate an increased risk for the presence of subungual melanoma.

TABLE 161-1 Diagnostic Clues that Indicate Longitudinal Melanonychia is Suspicious for Subungual Melanoma

Hutchinson sign (melanoma until proven otherwise)
In a single digit
Sixth decade of life or later
Develops abruptly in a previously normal nail plate
Suddenly darkens or widens (change in the LM morphology)
Occurs in either the thumb, index finger, or great toe
History of digital trauma
Dark-skinned patient, particularly if the thumb or great toe is affected
Blurred, rather than sharp, lateral borders
Personal history of malignant melanoma
Increased risk for melanoma (e.g., familial atypical mole and melanoma [FAMM] syndrome)
Nail dystrophy, such as partial nail destruction or disappearance

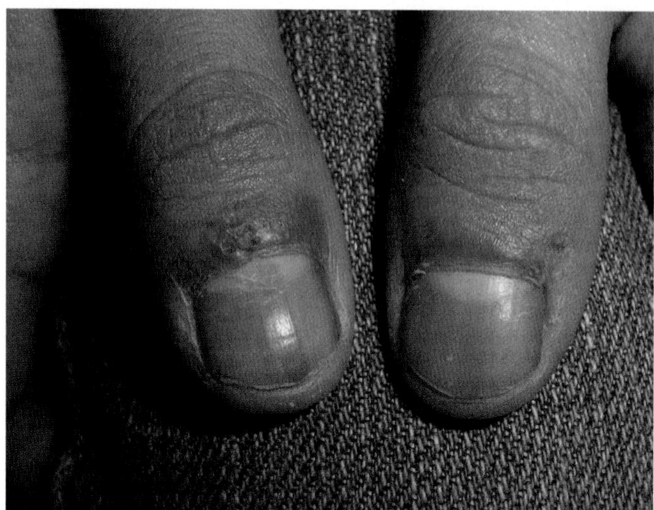

FIGURE 161-8 The fingers of this child demonstrate longitudinal melanonychia with pseudo-Hutchinson sign that was found to be due to racial melanosis. The small bruise on the proximal nail fold of the right thumb was due to recent trauma and not melanoma. *(Used with permission from Richard P. Usatine, MD.)*

DIAGNOSIS

CLINICAL FEATURES

There is an ABCDEF mnemonic system that applies to subungual melanoma:

- In this system "A" stands for age (peak incidence being between the fifth to seventh decades) and African Americans, Asians, and Native Americans in whom subungual melanoma accounts for 1/3 of melanoma cases.
- "B" stands for "brown to black" and with "breadth" of 3 mm or more.
- "C" stands for change in the nail band coloration or lack of change after adequate treatment.
- "D" stands for the digit most commonly involved.
- "E" stands for extension of the pigment onto the proximal and/or lateral nailfold (Hutchinson sign).
- "F" stands for family or personal history of dysplastic nevus or melanoma.

TYPICAL DISTRIBUTION

The digits used for grasping (thumb, index finger, and middle finger) are the most commonly involved in LM and melanoma, but either may be found in any finger or toe.

BIOPSY

Definitive diagnosis of a nail discoloration may be made with a biopsy of the nail matrix. Patients with darker skin color and multiple digits with translucent LM often need only be observed. Single dark lines in whites should always be biopsied. A 3-mm punch biopsy can be performed at the origin of the darkest part of a dark band within the nail matrix (**Figure 161-9**). Histologic diagnosis of atypical melanocytic hyperplasia necessitates the complete removal of the lesion.

DIFFERENTIAL DIAGNOSIS

- Pigmented lesions in the nail bed usually do not cause LM and are viewed through the nail as a grayish to brown or black spot.[7]

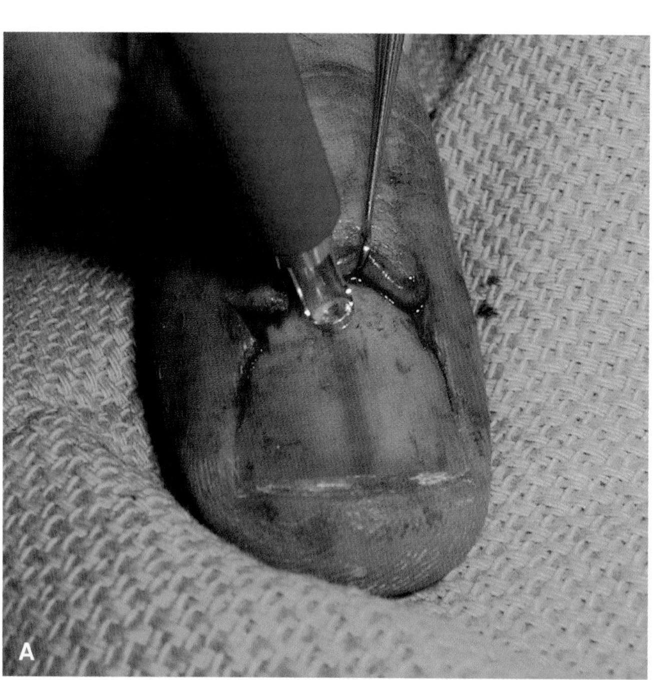

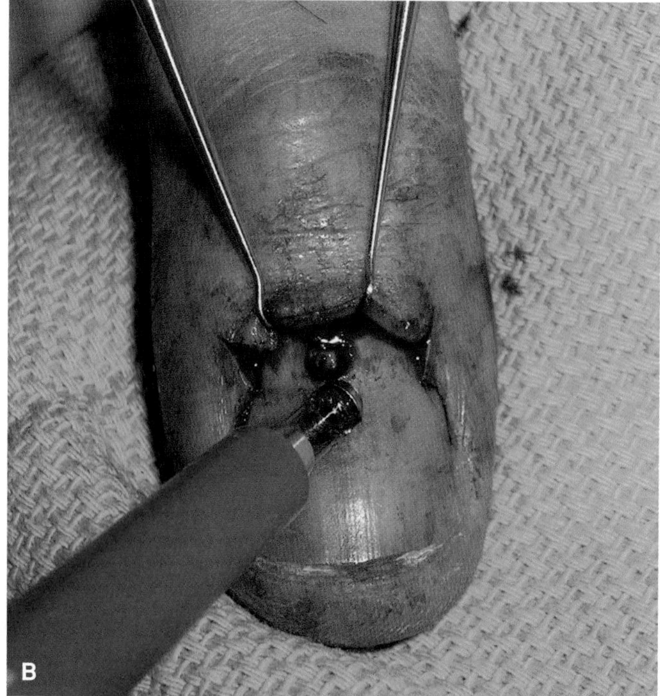

FIGURE 161-9 **A.** The proximal nail fold is reflected back to perform a nail matrix biopsy in a young man with new onset of longitudinal melanonychia. The 3-mm punch is placed over the origin of the dark band at the distal matrix. **B.** The 3-mm punch now contains the specimen for pathology. The longitudinal melanonychia was caused by melanocytic hyperplasia. *(Used with permission from Richard P. Usatine, MD.)*

- Subungual hematoma may be confused with LM, but the color grows out with the nail plate, exhibiting a proximal border that reproduces the shape of the lunula. A hole punched in the nail plate allows for the visualization of the underlying nail bed and confirmation of the nature of the coloration (see Chapter 166, Subungual Hematoma).

MANAGEMENT

NONPHARMACOLOGIC

No treatment is required for benign LM.

REFERRAL OR HOSPITALIZATION

Treatment of primary subungual melanomas includes amputation at the level of the interphalangeal joint for thumb lesions, SOR Ⓑ the distal or proximal interphalangeal joint for fingers, SOR Ⓒ and the metatarsophalangeal joint for toes.[8] For melanoma in situ, it may be possible to remove the full nail apparatus and save the digit. Sentinel lymph node biopsy is often indicated to establish the disease stage. Chemotherapy is recommended for nodal or visceral metastases.

PROGNOSIS

The 5-year survival is approximately 74 percent for patients with stage I subungual melanoma and 40 percent for patients with stage II disease. Prognostic variables negatively affecting survival include stage at diagnosis, deeper Clark level of invasion, African American race, and ulceration.[9]

FOLLOW-UP

Because LM may indicate an undiagnosed melanoma of the nail unit, biopsy, or regular monitoring is extremely important. If there is any doubt about the diagnosis of melanoma, biopsy immediately or refer to someone who can. Have the patient report any changes in pigmentation of the nail plate or nail folds, and strongly consider biopsy in these individuals.

PATIENT RESOURCES

- Medscape. *Nail Diseases In Childhood*—**www.medscape.com/viewarticle/585158_8**.
- DermNet NZ. *Subungual Melanoma*—**http://dermnetnz.org/hair-nails-sweat/melanoma-nailunit.html**.

PROVIDER RESOURCES

- DermNet NZ. *Nail Diseases*—**http://dermnetnz.org/hair-nails-sweat/nails.html**.
- eMedicine. *Nail Surgery*—**www.emedicine.com/derm/topic818.htm**.
- Braun RP, Baran R, Le Gal FA, et al. Diagnosis and management of nail pigmentation. *J Am Acad Dermatol*. 2007;56:[5] 835-847.
- Jellinek N. Nail matrix biopsy of longitudinal melanonychia: diagnostic algorithm including the matrix shave biopsy. *J Am Acad Dermatol*. 2007;56:[5] 803-810.
- Usatine R. Nail procedures. In: Usatine R, Pfenninger J, Stulberg D, Small R, eds. *Dermatologic and Cosmetic Procedures in Office Practice*. Philadelphia, PA: Elsevier; 2012:216-228. The whole procedure depicted in **Figure 161-9** is described in detail.

REFERENCES

1. Baran R, Kechjijian P: Longitudinal melanonychia (melanonychia striata): diagnosis and management. *J Am Acad Dermatol*. 1989;21:1165-1175.
2. Ruben B: Pigmented lesions of the nail unit: clinical and histopathologic features. *Semin Cutan Med Surg*. 2010;29:148-158.
3. Finley RK, Driscoll DL, Blumenson LE, Karakousis CP: Subungual melanoma: an eighteen year review. *Surgery*. 1994;116:96-100.
4. Goettmann-Bonvallot S, André J, Belaich S: Longitudinal melanonychia in children: a clinical and histopathologic study of 40 cases. *J Am Acad Dermatol*. 1999;41:17-22.
5. Papachristou DN, Fortner JG: Melanoma arising under the nail. *J Surg Oncol*. 1982;21:219-222.
6. Mikhail GR: Hutchinson's sign. *J Dermatol Surg Oncol*. 1986;12:519-521.
7. Baran R, Perrin C: Linear melanonychia due to subungual keratosis of the nail bed: report of two cases. *Br J Dermatol*. 1999;140:730-733.
8. Moehrle M, Metzger S, Schippert W, et al. "Functional" surgery in subungual melanoma. *Dermatol Surg*. 2003;29(4):366-374.
9. O'Leary JA, Berend KR, Johnson JL, et al. Subungual melanoma: a review of 93 cases with identification of prognostic variables. *Clin Orthop Relat Res*. 2000;378:206-212.

162 INGROWN TOENAIL

E.J. Mayeaux, Jr., MD
Heather M. Guillot, MD

PATIENT STORY

A 13-year-old boy presents with recurrent ingrown toenails. He presents to the clinic with another episode (**Figure 162-1**). He was treated with partial nail avulsion and a lateral matrixectomy was performed using topical phenol to ablate the matrix. This treatment produced long-term remission of his condition.

INTRODUCTION

Onychocryptosis (ingrown toenails) is a common childhood and adult problem. Patients often seek treatment because of the significant levels of discomfort and disability associated with the condition.

SYNONYMS

Onychocryptosis, unguis incarnatus.

EPIDEMIOLOGY

- The prevalence of onychocryptosis is unknown as many patients do not seek medical care and it is not a reportable disease. The toenails, especially the great toenail, are most commonly affected. Ingrown toenails at birth and in early childhood do occur, but are very rare.

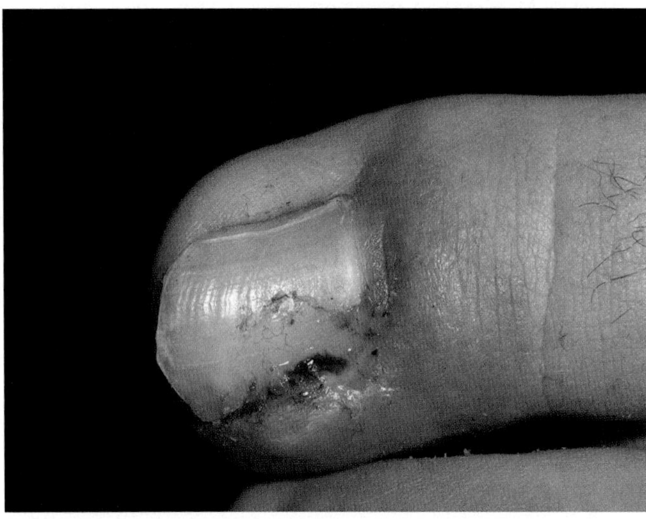

FIGURE 162-1 Recurrent ingrown toenail in a 13-year-old boy. Note the local redness and swelling. (*Used with permission from Richard P. Usatine, MD.*)

ETIOLOGY AND PATHOPHYSIOLOGY

Onychocryptosis occurs when the lateral nail plate damages the lateral nail fold. The laterally edge of the nail plate penetrates and perforates the adjacent nail fold skin. Perforation of the lateral fold skin results in painful inflammation that manifests clinically as mild edema, erythema, and pain. In advanced stages, drainage, infection, and ulceration may be present. Hypertrophy of the lateral nail wall occurs, and granulation tissue forms over the nail plate and the nail fold during healing of the ulcerated skin.[1] It is a common affliction that can result from a variety of conditions that cause improper fit of the nail plate in the lateral nail grove (**Figure 162-1**).

RISK FACTORS[1]

- Genetic predisposition.
- Poor-fitting footwear.
- Excessive trimming of the lateral nail plate.
- Pincer nail deformity (**Figure 162-2**).
- Trauma.
- Sports in which kicking or running is important.
- Hyperhidrosis.
- Anatomic features such as nail fold width.
- Congenital malalignment of the digit.
- Overcurvature of the nail plate.
- Onychomycosis and other diseases that result in abnormal changes in the nail plate.
- Obesity causing deepening of the nail groove.

DIAGNOSIS

CLINICAL FEATURES—HISTORY AND PHYSICAL

- The diagnosis is based upon clinical appearance and rarely is difficult. Characteristic signs and symptoms include pain, edema, exudate, and granulation tissue (**Figure 162-1**).

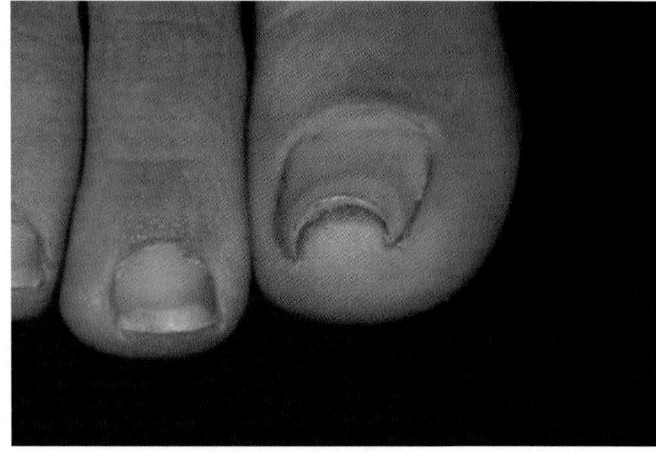

FIGURE 162-2 The curved infolding of the lateral edges of the nail plate indicates this patient has a pincer nail, which predisposes to onychocryptosis. (*Used with permission from Richard P. Usatine, MD.*)

TYPICAL DISTRIBUTION

- The great toe is most commonly affected; fingers are rarely involved except when nail biting is present.

LABORATORY TESTING

- Since the diagnosis is made clinically, laboratory testing is usually not necessary.

DIFFERENTIAL DIAGNOSIS

- Cellulitis—Presents with redness, pain, and swelling beyond the nail fold (see Chapter 103, Cellulitis).
- Paronychia—Presents with redness and abscess formation (pus) in a nail fold (see Chapter 164, Paronychia).
- Pseudo-ingrown toenails—Presents in infants 0 to 12 months of age; common and transient deformity, which usually self-corrects.
- Osteomyelitis—Presents with redness, pain, and swelling of the toe and fever.

MANAGEMENT

- The treatment of ingrown toenails depends upon the age of the patient and the severity of the lesion.

NONPHARMACOLOGIC

- Lesions characterized by minimal to moderate pain and no discharge can be treated conservatively with soaking the affected foot in warm water for 20 minutes, 3 times per day, and pushing the lateral nailfold away from the nail plate.[2] SOR Ⓒ
- Other palliative measures include cotton wedging underneath the lateral nail plate and trimming the lateral part of the nail plate below the area of nail fold irritation.
- Numerous alternative methods of conservative treatment have been described, including splints and commercially available devices. Devices that have shown promise include shape memory alloys (SMAs), either of a Cu-Al-Mn base or a Ni-Ti base.[3–5]

MEDICATIONS

- Although many elect to treat apparent infections with oral antibiotics, studies show the use of antibiotics does not decrease healing time or postprocedure morbidity in otherwise normal patients.[6] SOR Ⓐ
- A medium- to high-potency topical corticosteroid can be applied after soaking to decrease inflammation, but is often unnecessary.
- If nail avulsion and/or matrix ablation is used, pain relievers for mild to moderate pain may be necessary.
- When placing digital blocks for surgical procedures, the best evidence indicates the use of lidocaine with epinephrine is equally safe and efficacious for anesthesia.[7]

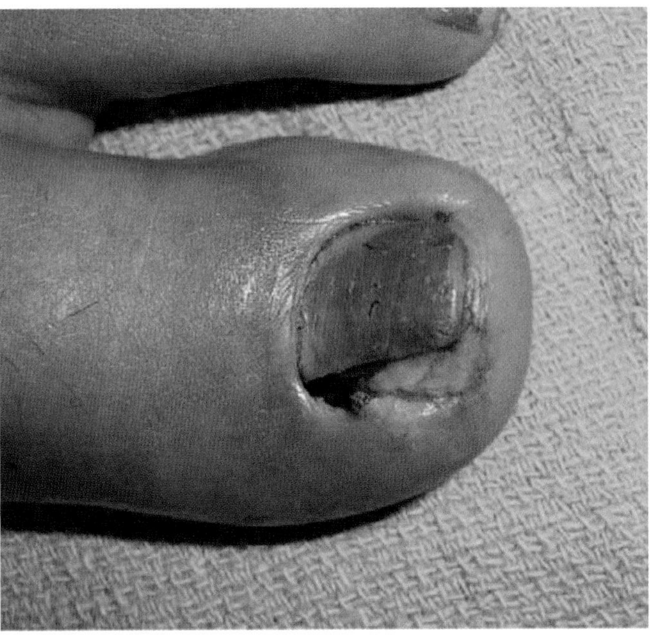

FIGURE 162-3 Status post partial nail avulsion procedure for an ingrown toenail. (*Used with permission from Richard P. Usatine, MD.*)

SURGICAL

- Nonresponders to conservative therapy and patients with more severe lesions (substantial erythema, granulation tissue and pus) need surgical therapy.[8,9] SOR Ⓒ
- Surgical interventions are more effective at preventing the recurrence of an ingrowing toenail when compared to non-surgical interventions.[10]
- Surgical intervention involves partial or full nail plate avulsion. Usually it is only necessary to remove the part of the nail that is placing pressure on the lateral nail fold (**Figure 162-3**). SOR Ⓒ
- Patients who develop recurrent ingrown toenails benefit from permanent nail ablation of the lateral nail matrix. This may be achieved with the combination of partial nail plate avulsion plus phenol matrixectomy, which can cut recurrence rates by 90 percent (**Figure 162-4**).[8,9,11,12] SOR Ⓐ

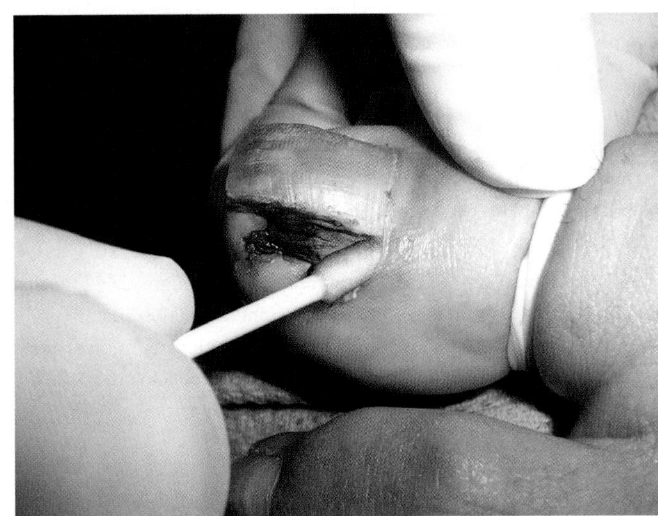

FIGURE 162-4 Phenol matrixectomy to destroy a portion of the nail matrix to prevent a recurrent ingrown toenail. Note the phenol is applied with a twisting motion. (*Used with permission from Richard P. Usatine, MD.*)

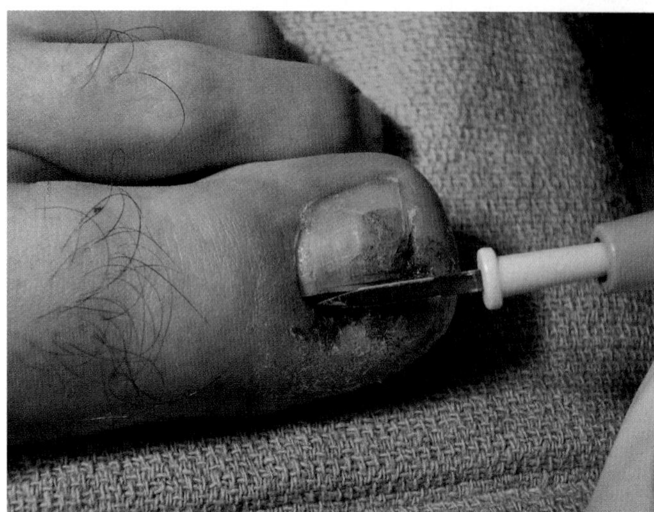

FIGURE 162-5 Use of electrosurgery to ablate the lateral nail matrix. This results in a narrower nail and a decreased likelihood of onychocryptosis recurrence. (*Used with permission from Richard P. Usatine, MD.*)

- In a Cochrane Systematic Review of surgical treatments for ingrowing toenails nail avulsion with the use of phenol is more effective at preventing symptomatic recurrence than nail avulsion without the use of phenol.[11] Unfortunately the use of phenol does increase the risk of postoperative infection (by 5 times) compared with simple nail avulsion.[11,13] SOR A
- Chemical matrixectomy is performed mainly by phenol (full-strength 88%), but 10 percent sodium hydroxide is another alternative. In a comparison study of the use of chemical matrixectomy for the treatment of ingrown toenails, the overall success rates were 95 percent for both phenol and sodium hydroxide.[14] SOR A
- One study found that partial nail avulsion with phenolization gave better results than partial avulsion with matrix excision. Local antibiotics applied to the surgical site did not reduce signs of infection or recurrence. The use of phenol did not produce more signs of infection than matrix excision.[15] SOR B
- Electrosurgical ablation can be performed with electrosurgery units on the fulguration setting or using a special matrixectomy electrode with a high-frequency electrosurgical unit (**Figure 162-5**). SOR C
- A surgical alternative to nail plate avulsion with or without matrixectomy is soft tissue nail fold excision consisting of excision of the offending nail fold, leaving a soft tissue defect that heals by secondary intention (Vandenbos procedure). No portion of the nail or matrix is excised using this procedure. One case series report found no recurrence of ingrown toenail after a median 14-month follow-up.[16]
- A Cochrane Systematic Review of treatments for ingrowing toenails found that no postoperative intervention including postoperative antibiotics, manuka honey, povidone-iodine with paraffin, hydrogel with paraffin, or paraffin gauze was effective in reducing the risk of postoperative infection or pain or reducing healing time.[10]

PREVENTION

There are several things that the patient may do to decrease the likelihood of getting an ingrown toenail.

- Trim nails straight across the top, not in a rounded shape.
- Wear shoes that fit properly. Shoes that place excessive pressure on the toes or pinch the toes.
- Switch to longer shoes with a bigger toe box.
- Wear protective footwear, especially if there is a risk of injuring the toes.

FOLLOW-UP

- After surgical intervention, consider follow-up in 3 to 4 days to assess treatment and exclude cellulitis.

PATIENT EDUCATION

- Patients should be educated about proper nail trimming so as to minimize trauma to the lateral nail fold. The lateral nail plate should be allowed to grow well beyond the lateral nail fold before trimming horizontally.
- Patients should also be educated about the importance of avoiding shoes that are too tight over the toes to help minimize recurrences.

PATIENT RESOURCES

- Ingrown Toenails information at the familydoctor.org—**http://familydoctor.org/online/famdocen/home/common/skin/disorders/208.html**.
- NYU Department of Pediatrics: Ingrown Toenail—**www.mch.com/page/EN/4317/Skin-And-Rashes/Ingrown-toenail.aspx**.

PROVIDER RESOURCES

- Medscape Emedicine Article "Ingrown Nails"—**http://emedicine.medscape.com/article/909807-overview#showall**.

REFERENCES

1. Siegle RJ, Swanson NA. Nail surgery: a review. *J Dermatol Surg Oncol*. 1982;8(8):659-666.
2. Connolly B, Fitzgerald RJ. Pledgets in ingrowing toenails. *Arch Dis Child*. 1988;63:71.
3. Nazari S. A simple and practical method in treatment of ingrown nails: splinting by flexible tube. *J Eur Acad Dermatol Venereol*. 2006;20(10):1302-1306.
4. Arai H. Formable acrylic treatment for ingrowing nail with gutter splint and sculptured nail. *Int J Dermatol*. 2004;43(10):759-765.
5. Ishibashi M, Tabata N, Suetake T, et al. A simple method to treat an ingrowing toenail with a shape-memory alloy device. *J Dermatolog Treat*. 2008;19(5):291-292.
6. Reyzelman AM, Trombello KA, Vayser DJ, et al. Are antibiotics necessary in the treatment of locally infected ingrown toenails? *Arch Fam Med*. 2000;9:930.

7. Altinyazar HC, Demirel CB, Koca R, Hosnuter M. Digital block with and without epinephrine during chemical matricectomy with phenol. *Dermatol Surg*. 2010;36(10):1568-1571.

8. Grieg JD, Anderson JH, Ireland AJ, Anderson JR. The surgical treatment of ingrowing toenails. *J Bone Joint Surg Br*. 1991; 73:131.

9. Vaccari S, Dika E, Balestri R, et al. Partial excision of matrix and phenolic ablation for the treatment of ingrowing toenail: a 36-month follow-up of 197 treated patients. *Dermatol Surg*. 2010; 36(8):1288-1293.

10. Eekhof JAH, Van Wijk B, Knuistingh Neven A, van der Wouden JC. Interventions for ingrowing toenails. Cochrane Database of Systematic Reviews 2012, Issue 4. Art. No.: CD001541. DOI: 10.1002/14651858.CD001541.pub3

11. Rounding C, Bloomfield S. Surgical treatments for ingrowing toe-nails. *Cochrane Database Syst Rev*. 2005;(2):CD001541.

12. Islam S, Lin EM, Drongowski R, et al. The effect of phenol on ingrown toenail excision in children. *J Pediatr Surg*. 2005;40: 290-292.

13. Kaleel SS, Iqbal S, Arbuthnot J, et al. Surgical options in the management of ingrown toenails in paediatric age group. *The Foot*. 2007;17:214-217.

14. Bostanci S, Kocyigit P, Gurgey E. Comparison of phenol and sodium hydroxide chemical matricectomies for the treatment of ingrowing toenails. *Dermatol Surg*. 2007;33:680-685.

15. Bos AM, van Tilburg MW, van Sorge AA, Klinkenbijl JH. Randomized clinical trial of surgical technique and local antibiotics for ingrowing toenail. *Br J Surg*. 2007;94:292-296.

16. Haricharan RN, Masquijo J, Bettolli M. Nail-fold excision for the treatment of ingrown toenail in children. *J Pediatr*. 2012.

163 ONYCHOMYCOSIS

E.J. Mayeaux, Jr., MD

PATIENT STORY

A 12-year-old boy was brought in by his mother with discoloration and some pain in his toenails (**Figure 163-1**). The clinical diagnosis of onychomycosis was confirmed with microscopic examination of a potassium hydroxide preparation. The onychomycosis resolved after a 3 month course of oral terbinafine.

INTRODUCTION

Onychomycosis is a term used to denote nail infections caused by any fungus, including dermatophytes, yeasts, and nondermatophyte molds. One, some, and occasionally all of the toenails and/or fingernails may be involved. Although most toenail onychomycosis is caused by dermatophytes, many cases of fingernail onychomycosis are caused by yeast. Onychomycosis may involve the nail plate and other parts of the nail unit, including the nail matrix.

SYNONYMS

Toenail fungus, tinea unguium, dermatophytosis of nails.

EPIDEMIOLOGY

- The incidence of onychomycosis has been reported to be 2 to 13 percent in North America.[1]

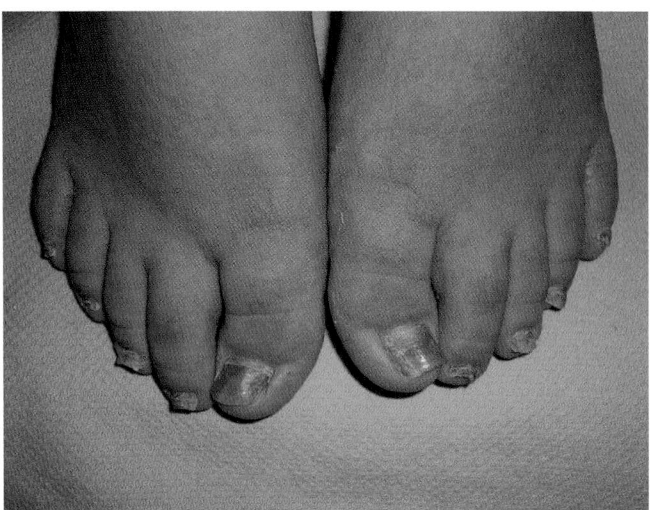

FIGURE 163-1 Onychomycosis in a child. Note the discoloration in the nail plate of the great toes, and the onycholysis and hyperkeratotic debris under the nail plate visible in the other toes. The diagnosis was confirmed with a positive nail culture. (*Used with permission from Richard P. Usatine, MD.*)

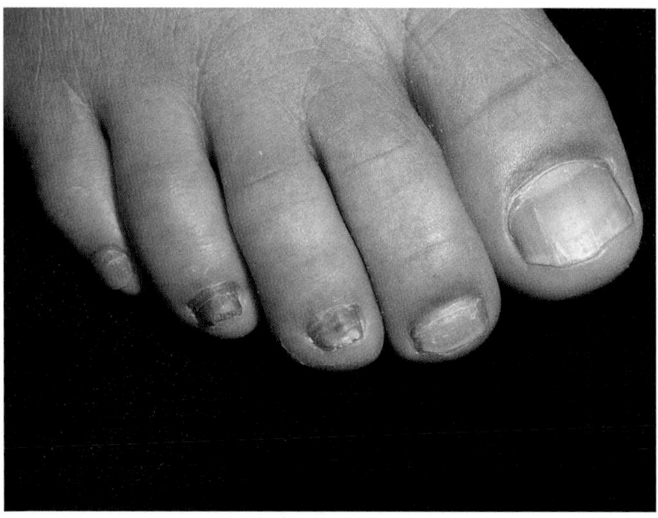

FIGURE 163-2 Onychomycosis in the toe nails of a 8-year-old boy proven by the visualization of hyphae under the microscope with a KOH preparation from a nail scraping. (*Used with permission from Richard P. Usatine, MD.*)

- Most patients (7.6%) only have toenail involvement and only 0.15 percent have fingernail involvement alone.[2]
- The prevalence of onychomycosis varies from 4 to 18 percent.[3,4]
- The disease is very common in adults, but may also occur in children.

ETIOLOGY AND PATHOPHYSIOLOGY

- Dermatophytes are responsible for most toenail (**Figures 163-1** to **163-3**) and finger infections (**Figures 163-4** and **163-5**).
- Nonpathogenic fungi and *Candida* (including the rare syndrome of chronic mucocutaneous candidiasis) also can infect the nail plate (**Figure 163-6**).

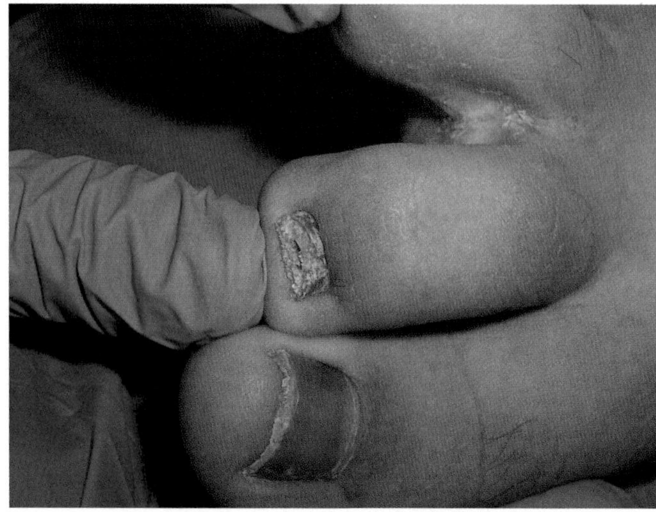

FIGURE 163-3 Onychomycosis in a 14-year-old Hispanic male. Note the coexisting tinea pedis between his toes. (*Used with permission from Richard P. Usatine, MD.*)

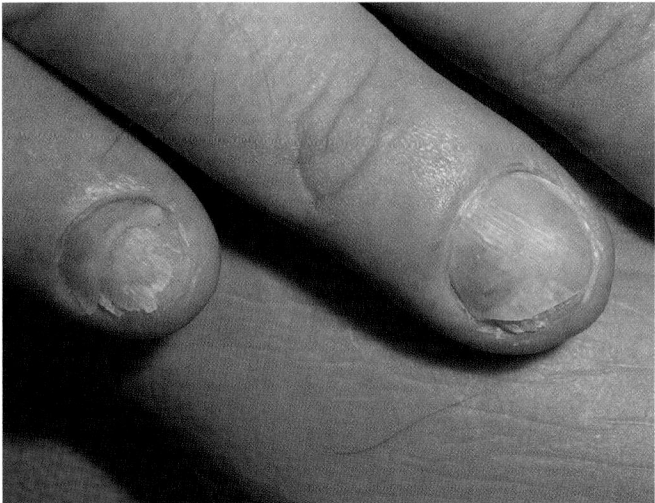

FIGURE 163-4 Fingernail onychomycosis demonstrating onycholysis and degeneration of the nail plane. (*Used with permission from Richard P. Usatine, MD.*)

- Dermatophytic onychomycosis (tinea unguium) occurs in three distinct forms: distal subungual, proximal subungual, and white superficial.
- The vast majority of distal and proximal subungual onychomycosis results from *Trichophyton rubrum*.
- White superficial onychomycosis is usually caused by *Trichophyton mentagrophytes*, although cases caused by *T. rubrum* have also been reported.
- Yeast onychomycosis is most common in the fingers caused by *Candida albicans* (**Figure 163-6**).

RISK FACTORS

- Tinea pedis.[5]
- Trauma predisposes to infection but can also cause a dysmorphic nail that can be confused for onychomycosis.[5]

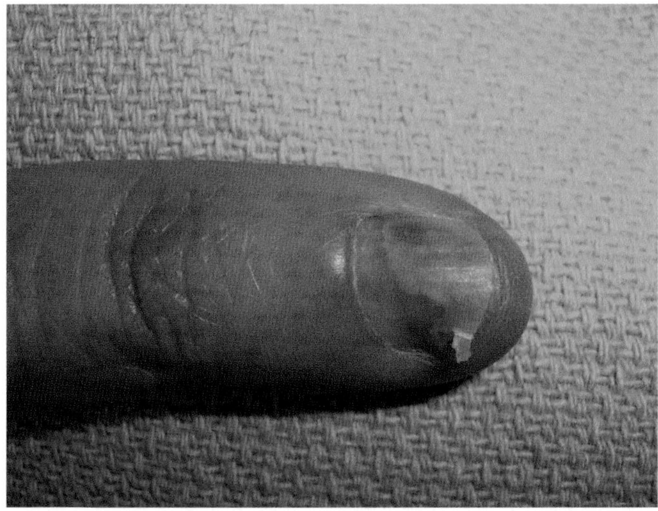

FIGURE 163-5 Onychomycosis in the finger nail proven by the visualization of hyphae under the microscope with a KOH preparation from a nail scraping. (*Used with permission from Richard P. Usatine, MD.*)

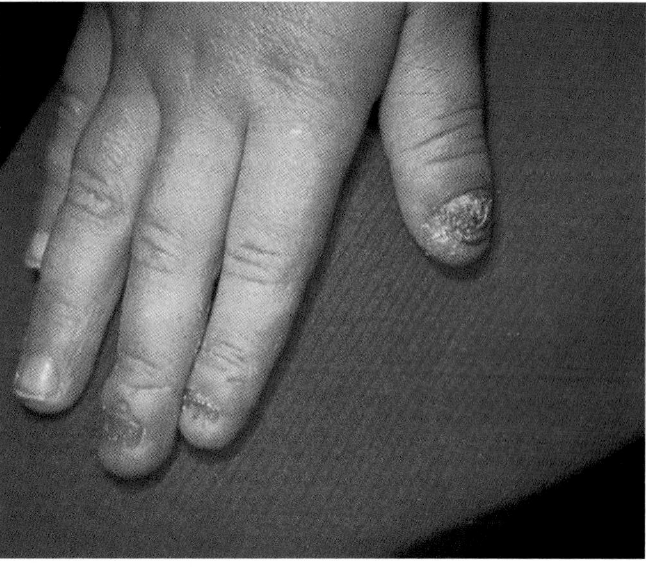

FIGURE 163-6 Mucocutaneous candidiasis in a child, which often associated with severe zinc or iron deficiency. (*Used with permission from Weinberg S, Prose NS, Kristal. Color Atlas of Pediatric Dermatology, 4th edition, New York: McGraw-Hill, 2008, Figure 6-47.*)

- Older age.[5]
- Swimming.[5]
- Diabetes.[5]
- Living with family members who have onychomycosis.[5]
- Immunosuppression.[6]

DIAGNOSIS

CLINICAL FEATURES

- Distal subungual onychomycosis is the most common presentation.
- Distal subungual onychomycosis begins with a whitish, yellowish, or brownish discoloration of a distal corner of the nail, which gradually spreads to involve the entire width of the nail plate and extends slowly toward the cuticle. Keratin debris collecting between the nail plate and its bed is the cause of the discoloration (**Figures 63-1** to **163-3**).
- Proximal subungual onychomycosis progresses in a manner similar to distal subungual onychomycosis but affects the nail in the vicinity of the cuticle first and extends distally. It usually occurs in individuals with a severely compromised immune system.
- White superficial onychomycosis appears as dull white spots on the surface of the nail plate. Eventually the whole nail plate may be involved. The white areas may be soft and can be lightly scraped to yield a chalky scale that may be examined or cultured.

TYPICAL DISTRIBUTION

- Nail infection may occur in a single digit but most often occurs simultaneously in multiple digits of the foot (**Figure 163-1** to **163-3**). Toenails and fingernails may be affected at the same time especially in patients that are immunocompromised.

LABORATORY TESTING

- KOH and culture—Clippings of nail plate and scrapings of subungual keratosis can be examined with KOH and microscopy and/or sent to the laboratory in a sterile container to be inoculated onto Sabouraud medium to culture.
- Dermatophyte test medium (DTM) culture is an alternative to Sabouraud medium culture. DTM is less expensive and can be performed in the physician's office, with results becoming available within 3 to 7 days. Dermatophyte growth is indicated by a change in the medium's color from yellow to red. It is important that DTM cultures be read in a timely fashion, as saprophytic organisms may grow over several weeks and cause a false-positive result. DTM does not identify the specific causative organism, but such identification is unnecessary as all dermatophyte infections are treated the same way. DTM cultures had good positive and negative correlation with culture on Sabouraud medium.[7]
- Clippings—Nail clippings may be sent to pathology in formalin to be examined with periodic acid-Schiff (PAS) stain for fungal elements. This can be more sensitive than KOH and culture.[8]
- Comparison of diagnostic methods:
  - In a 2003 study by Weinberg et al, the sensitivities for onychomycosis detection were KOH 80 percent, Bx/PAS 92 percent, and culture 59 percent. The specificities were KOH 72 percent, Bx/PAS 72 percent, and culture 82 percent. The positive predictive values were KOH 88 percent, Bx/PAS 89.7 percent, and culture 90 percent. The negative predictive values were KOH 58 percent, Bx/PAS 77 percent, and culture 43 percent.[8]
  - In a 2007 study of the diagnosis of onychomycosis by Hsiao et al, the sensitivities of KOH, PAS, and culture were 87 percent, 81 percent, and 67 percent, respectively, and the negative predictive values of KOH, PAS, and culture were 50 percent, 40 percent, and 28 percent, respectively. One reason that the KOH may have done so well is that the nail specimen was immersed in 20 percent KOH in a test tube for 30 minutes or longer before looking under the microscope.[9]
  - KOH may be equivalent to PAS if done and read properly. It is less expensive and the results are available while the patient is in the office. PAS is a good second line if the KOH is negative and the suspicion for onychomycosis is still present.

DIFFERENTIAL DIAGNOSIS

- Nail trauma can cause a dysmorphic nail that is discolored and thickened. It is especially seen in the big toenail in runners. Ask about nail trauma before diagnosing onychomycosis. Although onychomycosis often starts in the big toenail, it usually spreads to other nails. Traumatic changes often present with only one nail involved.
- Psoriatic and lichen planus nail changes may easily be confused with onychomycosis, especially when the nail becomes thickened and discolored. Pitting of the nail plate surface, which is common in psoriasis, is not a feature of fungal infection. It is possible for a patient with psoriasis to get onychomycosis. Fungal studies can help determine if the changes are truly secondary to onychomycosis (see Chapter 165, Psoriatic Nails).

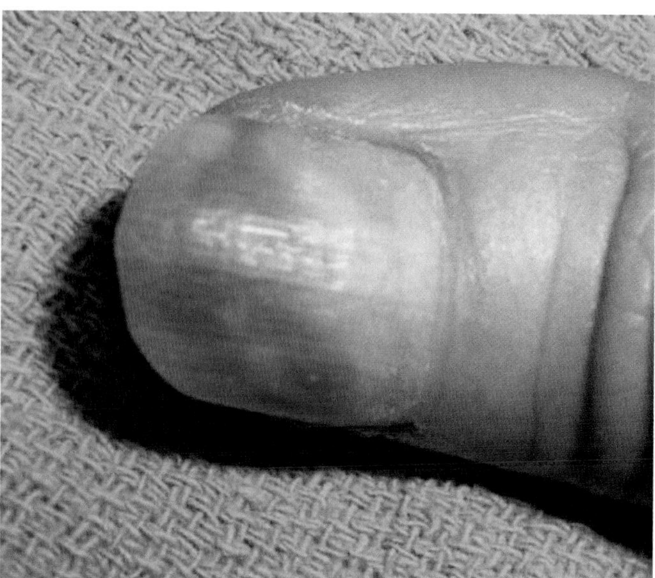

FIGURE 163-7 *Pseudomonas* of the nail showing a blue-green discoloration. (*Used with permission from Richard P. Usatine, MD.*)

- Pseudomonal nail infection—Produces a blue-green tint to the nail plate (**Figure 163-7**).
- Leukonychia—White spots or bands that appear proximally and proceed out with the nail may be confused with white superficial onychomycosis (see Chapter 160, Normal Nail Variants).
- Habitual picking of the proximal nail fold—induces the nail plate to be wavy and ridged, although its substance remains intact and hard (see Chapter 160, Normal Nail Variants).

MANAGEMENT

- Treating onychomycosis can be discouraging. Most topical creams and lotions do not penetrate the nail plate well and are of little value except in controlling inflammation at the nail folds.
- Surgical avulsion may be used to decrease pain caused by pressure on an elevated nail plate because of a dermatophytoma (a collection of dermatophytes and cellular debris under the nail plate). Recurrences are common in the absence of additional systemic or topical therapy with ciclopirox, as the infection typically involves the nail matrix and bed. SOR Ⓒ
- There has been a resurgence of interest in phototherapy modalities for the treatment of onychomycosis. UV light therapy, near-infrared photoinactivation therapy, photodynamic therapy, and photothermal ablative therapy are being studied for treatment of onychomycosis.[10] Further studies are required to determine the clinical role of laser and light therapy in the treatment of onychomycosis. The Pinpointe FootLaser was approved for use to treat onychomycosis in February 2011. SOR Ⓒ

TABLE 163-1 Common Treatments for Onychomycosis

Drug	Pediatric Dose	Adult Dose	Course	Toenail Cure Rate
Griseofulvin (Grifulvin V)	Microsize 15 to 20 mg/kg per day	500 mg po qd	4 to 9 months (f), 6 to 12 months (t)	60 ± 6 percent
Terbinafine (Lamisil)	10 to 20 kg: 62.5 mg/day 20 to 40 kg: 125 mg/day	250 mg po qd	6 weeks (f), 12 weeks (t)	76 ± 3 percent
Terbinafine (Lamisil) pulse*	—	250 mg bid 1 wk/mo	2 months (f), 3 months (t)	NR
Itraconazole (Sporanox)	—	200 mg daily	6 weeks (f), 12 weeks (t)	59 ± 5 percent
Itraconazole (Sporanox) pulse	<20 kg: 5 mg/kg per day for 1 wk/mo 20 to 40 kg: 100 mg daily for 1 wk/mo	200 mg bid or 5 mg/kg per day capsules for 1 wk/mo	2 months (f), 3 months (t)	63 ± 7 percent
Fluconazole (Diflucan)	3 to 6 mg/kg once a wk	150 mg once a wk	12 to 16 weeks (f), 18 to 26 weeks (t)	48 ± 5 percent
Ciclopirox 8 percent nail lacquer (Penlac)	—	Apply daily to nail and surrounding 5-mm skin	Up to 48 weeks	Approximately 7 percent

NR, Not recorded.
*Not indicated for treating onychomycosis by the FDA.
From: Harrell TK, Necomb WW, Replogle WH, et al. Onychomycosis: improved cure rates with itraconazole and terbinafine. *J Am Board Fam Pract.* 2000;13(4):268-273; Bell-Syer S, Porthouse J, Bigby M. Oral treatments for toenail onychomycosis. *Cochrane Database Syst Rev.* 2004;(2):CD004766. DOI: 10.1002/14651858. CD004766; Crawford F, Hart R, Bell-Syer S, et al. Topical treatments for fungal infections of the skin and nails of the foot. *Cochrane Database Syst Rev.* 1999;(3):CD001434. DOI: 10.1002/14651858. CD001434; Havu V, Heikkila H, Kuokkanen K, et al. A double-blind, randomized study to compare the efficacy and safety of terbinafine (Lamisil) with fluconazole (Diflucan) in the treatment of onychomycosis. *Br J Dermatol.* 2000;142(1):97-102.

MEDICATIONS

- Oral therapy (**Table 163-1**) is no longer expensive now that terbinafine is generic and on many discounted drug lists.
- A Cochrane review found that the evidence suggests that terbinafine is more effective than griseofulvin and that terbinafine and itraconazole are more effective than no treatment.[11] SOR Ⓐ
- Terbinafine is used daily for 3 months for toenail onychomycosis and daily for 2 months to treat fingernail involvement.[11] SOR Ⓐ
- Another Cochrane review found two trials of nail infections that did not provide any evidence of benefit for topical treatments (ciclopirox not included) compared with placebo.[12] SOR Ⓐ
- Terbinafine has a preferable drug interaction profile, may have better long-term cure rates, and daily dosing may be the most effective treatment.[6,11] SOR Ⓐ
- Itraconazole (Sporanox) has more drug interactions. Pulse dosing is as effective as daily dosing, but even with pulse dosing, therapy is more costly than terbinafine. Consider itraconazole if terbinafine does not effectively treat onychomycosis caused by fungus other than dermatophytes. SOR Ⓒ
- Fluconazole (Diflucan) is not currently FDA approved for nail therapy and is not as effective as other oral therapies.[6,13] SOR Ⓑ
- Ciclopirox 8 percent nail lacquer (Penlac) used daily (with weekly nail cleaning and filing) is an FDA-approved topical treatment for ages 12 years and above for mild to moderate onychomycosis. A metaanalysis of 2 randomized controlled trials showed a clinical cure rate of 8 percent versus 1 percent for vehicle alone.[14] Such a low cure rate is disappointing, but a larger group of patients had some improvement without cure. This is one option for persons able to afford this topical treatment but who are not able to take oral antifungals.
- Amorolfine is a topical antifungal agent with activity against dermatophytes, yeasts, and fungi that is available over the counter in Australia and the United Kingdom, but is not approved for use in the US. Amorolfine 5 percent nail lacquer has been used as monotherapy for the treatment of onychomycosis. It is applied once weekly after the surface of the nail is filed with a disposable file and wiped with alcohol. Once weekly application of amorolfine 5 percent nail lacquer for 6 months led to both clinical and mycologic cure in 38 percent and 46 percent of patients. It may also be used to increase cure rates when used in combination with oral antifungals.[15]

COMPLEMENTARY/ALTERNATIVE THERAPY

- There are numerous complementary and alternative medicine (CAM) therapies described on the Internet, most of which have minimal or no evidence of clinical efficacy.
- Mentholated chest rub—There is minimal data on the efficacy of a mentholated chest rub (Vicks VapoRub) in the treatment of onychomycosis. In a series of 18 patients who applied the medication to affected nails daily for 48 weeks, 4 patients (22%) achieved both clinical and mycologic cure.[16] Although these products are unlikely to be harmful, additional studies that support their efficacy in onychomycosis are necessary before widespread use can be recommended.

PREVENTION

Patients should be educated about the use of appropriate footwear, especially in high-exposure areas such as communal bathing facilities and health clubs.

PROGNOSIS

The condition may persist indefinitely if left untreated.

In patients with diabetes or other immunocompromised states, onychomycosis may increase the risk of secondary bacterial infections.[17]

FOLLOW-UP

Routine monitoring of liver function tests during therapy is probably not necessary in patients without underlying liver disease. However, because the manufacturer of terbinafine recommends checking pretreatment serum aminotransferases and monitoring for potential symptoms of hepatotoxicity during treatment, many clinicians routinely obtain pretreatment and mid-therapy values.

PATIENT EDUCATION

Patients should be advised that with treatment, nails may not appear normal for up to 1 year. The normal nail must grow out as treatment progresses. The appearance of normal appearing nails at the proximal edge of the nail is an encouraging sign at the completion of therapy.

PATIENT RESOURCES

- eMedicineHealth. *Onychomycosis*—**http://www.emedicinehealth.com/onychomycosis/article_em.htm**.
- Familydoctor.org website. *Fungal Infections of Fingernails and Toenails*—**http://familydoctor.org/online/famdocen/home/common/infections/common/fungal/663.html**.
- MedicineNet. *Fungal Nails (Onychomycosis, Tinea Unguium)*—**http://www.medicinenet.com/fungal_nails/article.htm**.

PROVIDER RESOURCES

- Tosti A. *Onychomycosis*—**http://emedicine.medscape.com/article/1105828-overview.** Accessed November 25,2011.
- Roger P, Bassler M; American Family Physician. *Treating Onychomycosis*—**http://www.aafp.org/afp/20010215/663.html.** Accessed November 25,2011.
- Elewski BE. Onychomycosis: pathogenesis, diagnosis, and management. *Clin Microbiol Rev*. 1998;11[3]:415-429. **http://www.ncbi.nlm.nih.gov/pmc/articles/PMC88888/**. Accessed November 25,2011.
- DermNetNZ. *Fungal Nail Infections*—**http://dermnetnz.org/fungal/onychomycosis.html.** Accessed November 25,2011.
- Roberts DT, Taylor WD, Boyle J. Guidelines for treatment of onychomycosis. *Br J Dermatol*. 2003;148:402-410. **http://www.bad.org.uk/for-the-public/patient-information-leaflets/fungal-infections-of-the-nails?q=Fungal infections of the nails**. Accessed November 25,2011.

REFERENCES

1. Kemna ME, Elewski BE. A U.S. epidemiologic survey of superficial fungal diseases. *J Am Acad Dermatol.* 1996;35(4):539-542.
2. Gupta AK. Prevalence and epidemiology of onychomycosis in patients visiting physicians' offices: A multicenter Canadian survey of 15,000 patients. *J Am Acad Dermatol*. 2000;43:244.
3. Erbagci Z, Tuncel A, Zer Y, Balci I. A prospective epidemiologic survey on the prevalence of onychomycosis and dermatophytosis in male boarding school residents. *Mycopathologia*. 2005;159: 347.
4. Sahin I, Kaya D, Parlak AH, et al. Dermatophytoses in forestry workers and farmers. *Mycoses*. 2005;48:260.
5. Sigurgeirsson B, Steingrímsson O. Risk factors associated with onychomycosis. *J Eur Acad Dermatol Venereol.* 2004;18:48.
6. Harrell TK, Necomb WW, Replogle WH, et al. Onychomycosis: improved cure rates with itraconazole and terbinafine. *J Am Board Fam Pract*. 2000;13(4):268-273.
7. Elewski BE, Leyden J, Rinaldi MG, Atillasoy E. Office practice-based confirmation of onychomycosis: a US nationwide prospective survey. *Arch Intern Med.* 2002;162:2133.
8. Weinberg JM, Koestenblatt EK, Tutrone WD, et al. Comparison of diagnostic methods in the evaluation of onychomycosis. *J Am Acad Dermatol*. 2003;49(2):193-197.
9. Hsiao YP, Lin HS, Wu TW, et al. A comparative study of KOH test, PAS staining and fungal culture in diagnosis of onychomycosis in Taiwan. *J Dermatol Sci*. 2007;45(2):138-140.
10. Bornstein E. A review of current research in light-based technologies for treatment of podiatric infectious disease states. *J Am Podiatr Med Assoc*. 2009;99(4):348-352.
11. Bell-Syer S, Porthouse J, Bigby M. Oral treatments for toenail onychomycosis. *Cochrane Database Syst Rev*. 2004;(2):CD004766. DOI: 10.1002/14651858. CD004766.

12. Crawford F, Hart R, Bell-Syer S, et al. Topical treatments for fungal infections of the skin and nails of the foot. *Cochrane Database Syst Rev*. 1999;(3):CD001434. DOI: 10.1002/14651858. CD001434.

13. Havu V, Heikkila H, Kuokkanen K, et al. A double-blind, randomized study to compare the efficacy and safety of terbinafine (Lamisil) with fluconazole (Diflucan) in the treatment of onychomycosis. *Br J Dermatol*. 2000;142(1):97-102.

14. Gupta AK, Joseph WS. Ciclopirox 8% nail lacquer in the treatment of onychomycosis of the toenails in the United States. *J Am Podiatr Med Assoc*. 2000;90(10):495-501.

15. Baran R, Kaoukhov A. Topical antifungal drugs for the treatment of onychomycosis: An overview of current strategies for monotherapy and combination therapy. *J Eur Acad Dermatol Venereol*. 2005;19:21.

16. Derby R, Rohal P, Jackson C, et al. Novel treatment of onychomycosis using over-the-counter mentholated ointment: a clinical case series. *J Am Board Fam Med*. 2011;24:69.

17. Bristow IR, Spruce MC. Fungal foot infection, cellulitis and diabetes: a review. *Diabet Med*. 2009;26:548.

164 PARONYCHIA

Brian Elkins, MD
E.J. Mayeaux, Jr., MD

PATIENT STORY

A teenage girl presents with mild itching and redness in her finger nail folds (**Figure 164-1**). The pediatrician diagnosed her with chronic paronychia, probably due to chronically pushing back her cuticles for cosmetic reasons. Behavior modification resulted in resolution of symptoms.

INTRODUCTION

Paronychia is a localized, superficial infection or abscess of the nail folds. Paronychia can be acute or chronic. Acute paronychia usually presents as an acutely painful abscess in the nail fold. It is most commonly treated with incision and drainage (**Figure 164-2**). Chronic paronychia is defined as bring present for longer then 6 weeks duration. It is a generalized red, tender, swelling of the proximal or lateral nail folds. It is usually nonsuppurative and is more difficult to treat.

EPIDEMIOLOGY

Paronychia is the most common infection of the hand representing 35 percent of all hand infections in the US.[1]

ETIOLOGY AND PATHOPHYSIOLOGY

- Paronychial infections develop when a disruption occurs between the seal of the nail fold and the nail plate or the skin of a nail fold is disrupted and allows a portal of entry for invading organisms.[2]

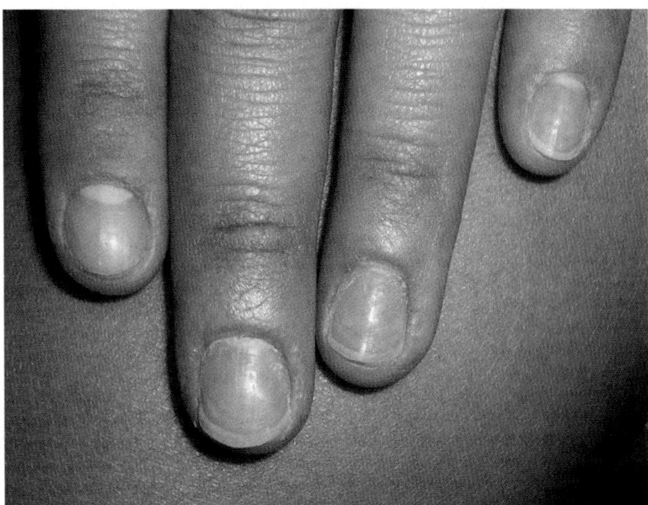

FIGURE 164-1 Chronic paronychia in a teenage girl probably due to chronically pushing back her cuticles for cosmetic reasons. Note the redness in the finger nail folds. (*Used with permission from Richard P. Usatine, MD.*)

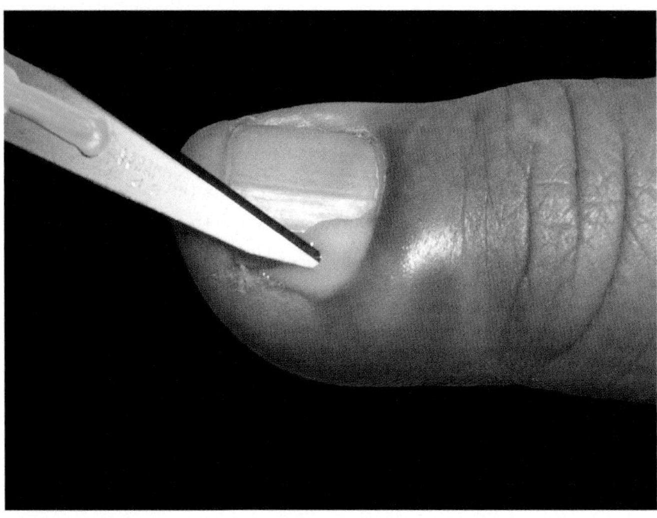

FIGURE 164-2 Incision and drainage of the acute paronychia with a #11 scalpel. Note the exuberant pus draining from the incision. (*Used with permission from Richard P. Usatine, MD.*)

- Acute paronychia is most commonly caused by *S. aureus*, followed by *Streptococcus pyogenes*, *Pseudomonas pyocyanea*, and *Proteus vulgaris*.[3]
- Chronic paronychia is thought to be a multifactorial inflammatory and/or allergic phenomenon in which a variety of microorganisms, including bacteria and fungi, may be secondarily present.[4]
- Untreated persistent chronic paronychia may cause horizontal ridging, undulations and other changes to the nail plate (**Figures 164-3** and **164-4**).

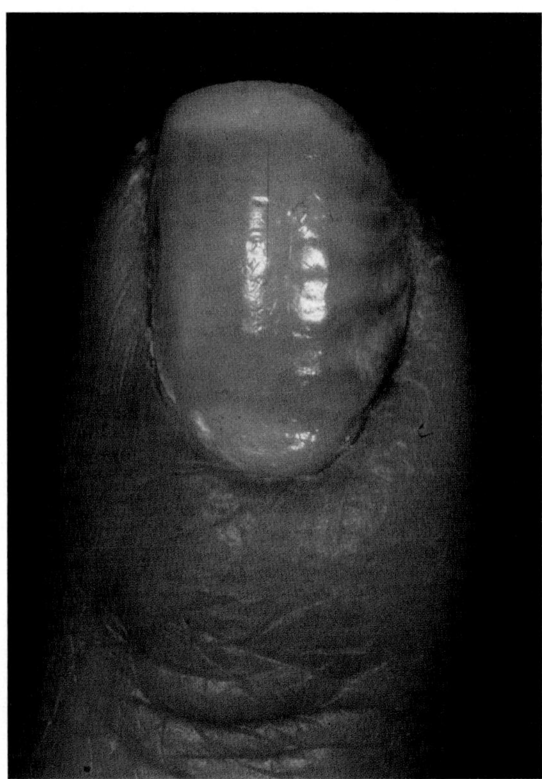

FIGURE 164-3 Chronic paronychia. Note horizontal ridges on one side of the nail plate as a result of chronic inflammation. (*Used with permission from Richard P. Usatine, MD.*)

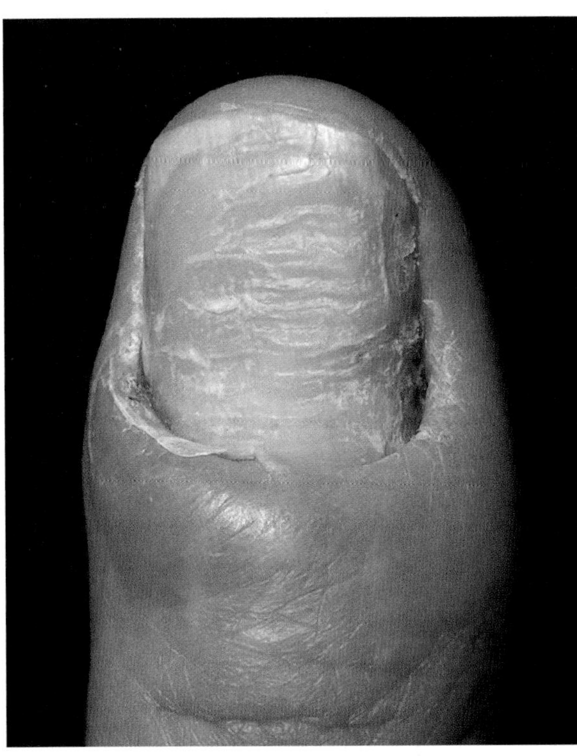

FIGURE 164-4 Chronic *Candida* paronychia causing a dysmorphic fingernail with horizontal ridging. (*Used with permission from Richard P. Usatine, MD.*)

RISK FACTORS

- Acute paronychia commonly results from nail biting (**Figure 164-5**), finger sucking, aggressive manicuring (**Figure 164-6**), hang nails (**Figure 164-7**), trauma, and artificial nails.[2]
- Children are prone to acute paronychia through direct infection of fingers with mouth flora from finger sucking and nail biting.
- Patients with diabetes mellitus, compromised immune systems, or a history of oral steroid use are at increased risk for paronychia, as well as children with chronic pulmonary disease.[5]

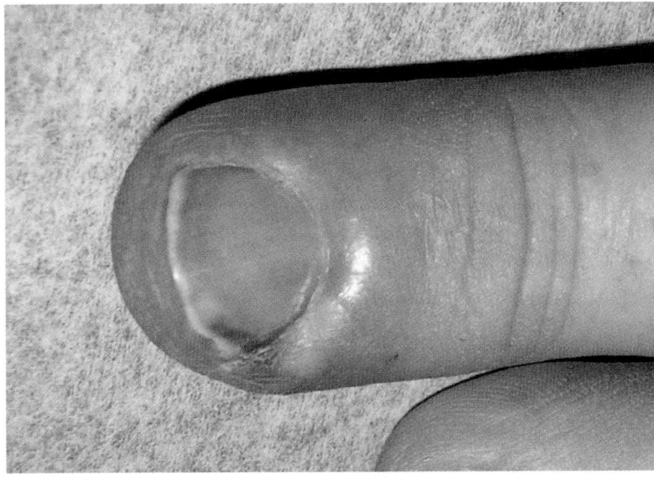

FIGURE 164-5 Acute paronychia from nail biting. Note abscess formation in the lateral nail fold that is extending into the proximal fold. (*Used with permission from E.J. Mayeaux, Jr., MD.*)

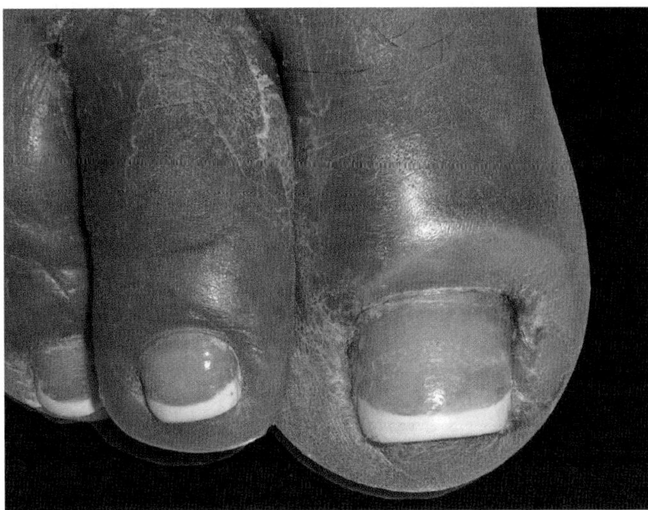

FIGURE 164-6 Acute paronychia of the great toe. Note extensive manicure of the nails, which may predispose to paronychia if the cuticle or nail folds are disrupted. (*Used with permission from Jennifer P. Pierce, MD.*)

- Paronychia may in some cases be a manifestation of zinc deficiency.[6]
- Retroviral therapy use, especially indinavir and lamivudine, may be associated with an increased incidence of paronychia.[7] Several cancer chemotherapeutic drugs, especially taxanes/anthracyclines and epidermal growth factor receptor (EGFR) inhibitors, have also been implicated.[8,9]

DIAGNOSIS

CLINICAL FEATURES

- Acute paronychia presents with localized pain and tenderness. The nail fold appears erythematous and inflamed, and a collection of pus usually develops (**Figures 164-1, 164-2, 161-5,** and **161-6**).

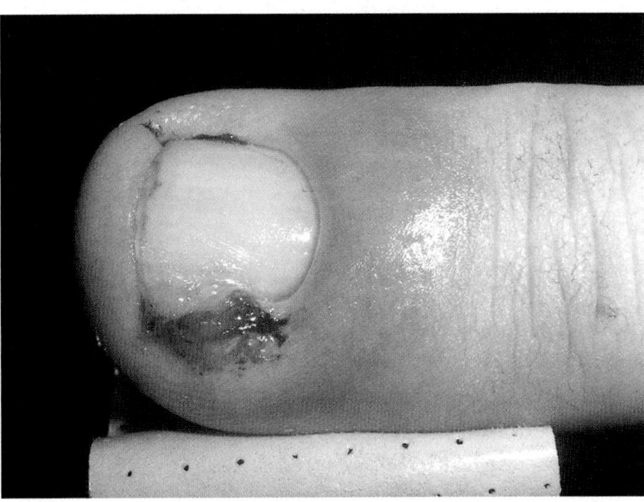

FIGURE 164-7 Paronychia with cellulitis of the skin of the fingertip and granulation tissue formation. This all started when the patient began manipulating a hang nail. (*Used with permission from Richard P. Usatine, MD.*)

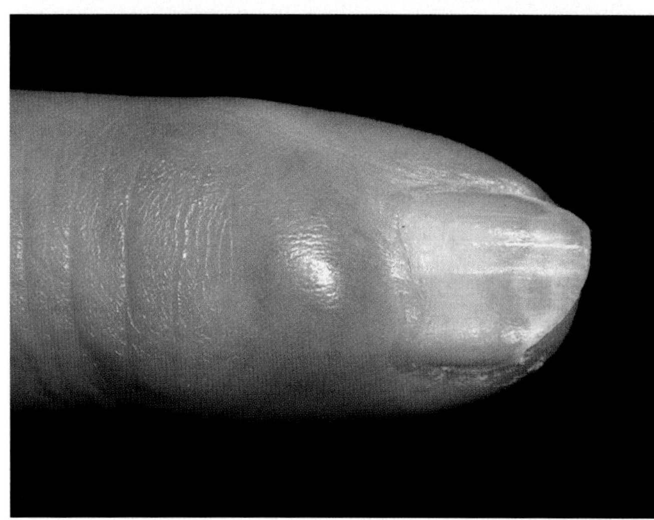

FIGURE 164-8 Digital mucus cyst presenting as a painless swelling of the nail fold in a young woman. Note the indented area of the nail caused by the pressure of the mucus cyst on the nail matrix. (*Used with permission from Richard P. Usatine, MD.*)

Granulation tissue may develop along the nail fold and cellulitis may develop (**Figure 164-7**).

- Chronic paronychia is a red, tender, painful swelling of the proximal or lateral nail folds. A small collection of pus or abscess may form but typically only redness and swelling are present. Eventually, the nail plates may become thickened and discolored, with pronounced horizontal ridges (see **Figures 164-3** and **164-4**).[10]

DIFFERENTIAL DIAGNOSIS

- Mucus cyst, which presents as a painless swelling lateral and proximal to the nail plate (**Figure 164-8**). This can also cause changes in the nail morphology.
- Ingrown nail (onychocryptosis) is a condition in which the nail plate is too large for the nail bed. The pressure applied to the lateral nail fold causes a painful inflammation. Although this is sometimes called paronychia, it is different from the type of paronychia caused by an infection of the nail fold (see Chapter 162, Ingrown Toenail).
- Glomus tumor, which presents with constant severe pain, nail plate elevation, bluish-discoloration of the nail plate, and blurring of the lunula.
- Herpetic whitlow, which results from herpes simplex virus (HSV) infection presents with acute onset of vesicles or pustules, severe edema, erythema, and pain. Tzanck staining of vesicles will demonstrate multinucleated giant cells and viral culture will grow HSV (see Chapter 114, Herpes Simplex).
- Felon—Paronychia must be distinguished from a felon, which is an infection of the digital pulp. It is characterized by severe pain, swelling, and erythema in the pad of the fingertip.
- Benign and malignant neoplasms, which may present early with redness and swelling should always be ruled out when chronic paronychia does not respond to conventional treatment.

MANAGEMENT

NONPHARMACOLOGIC

- Milder cases of acute paronychia without abscess formation may be treated with warm soaks for 20 minutes 3 to 4 times a day.[2] SOR Ⓒ
- When an abscess or fluctuance is present, drainage is necessary.[11] SOR Ⓒ It is performed with digital block anesthesia. The affected nail fold is incised with a scalpel with the blade parallel to the edge of the nail plate and the pus expressed (see **Figure 164-2**). Warm soaks 4 times a day are initiated to keep the incision from sealing until all of the pus is gone.[12] Between soakings, an adhesive bandage can protect the nail fold. Antibiotic therapy is usually not necessary unless there is accompanying cellulitis. SOR Ⓒ

MEDICATIONS

- Acute cases with more inflammation but no abscess formation may be treated with a topical antibiotic cream (e.g., mupirocin [Bactroban], bacitracin) combined with a topical corticosteroid such as betamethasone.[13]
- Lesions that persist after drainage, or which are associated with surrounding cellulitis, should be treated with antistaphylococcal antibiotics (e.g., cephalexin 25 to 50 mg/kg/day divided q6-8hr or dicloxacillin 12.5to 25 mg/kg/day divided q6hr), and cultures should be obtained in severe cases to guide antimicrobial therapy.[13] Clindamycin (20 to 40 mg/kg/day divided q6-8hr) or trimethoprim/sulfamethoxazole (8 to 12 mg TMP/kg/day divided q12hr) may be preferred in communities with a high incidence of community-acquired methicillin-resistant *S. aureus* (CA-MRSA).
- Both children who suck their fingers and patients who bite their nails and who require antibiotics should be covered against anaerobes. Clindamycin and amoxicillin-clavulanate potassium are effective against most pathogens isolated from infections originating in the mouth.[14]
- Long-term treatment of chronic paronychia primarily involves avoiding predisposing factors such as prolonged exposure to water, nail trauma, and finger sucking. Treatment with topical antifungals (topical miconazole or ketoconazole) or a combination of topical steroids and an antifungal agent has been shown to be successful.[2,7] SOR Ⓑ Oral antifungal therapy is usually not necessary.[2]

SURGICAL

- The most common treatment for acute paronychia is incision and drainage. The basic procedures involves obtaining informed consent then performing a digital block on the affected digit. A #11 scalpel blade is places against the nail plate and the abscess is incised where the nail fold meets the nail plate (see **Figure 164-2**). Express the pus and lightly bandage. Have the patient soak the digit several times daily. Antibiotics are usually not necessary unless there is coexisting cellulitis. [15]

PREVENTION

- Trim hangnails to a semilunar smooth edge with a clean sharp nail plate trimmer. Trim toenails flush with the toe tip.

- Avoid nail biting, picking, manipulation, and finger sucking.
- Avoid prolonged hand exposure to moisture. If hand washing must be frequent, use antibacterial soap, thoroughly dry hands with a clean towel, and apply an antibacterial moisturizer. Use cotton glove liners under waterproof gloves to keep hands dry from sweat and condensation.
- Wear rubber or latex-free gloves when there is potential exposure to pathogens.
- Control diabetes mellitus.
- Keep fingernails clean.
- Moisturize the skin, don't let it become chafed and cracked.

PROGNOSIS

Although the nail fold should improve with treatment, some chronic nail plate changes may not resolve. Paronychia has rarely been associated with distant, necrotizing soft-tissue infections,[15] so it may be prudent to advise caregivers to observe for signs of remote infection.

FOLLOW-UP

Patients can perform warm soaks 3 to 4 times per day and should have a follow-up examination several days after incision and drainage to assure the infection is resolving appropriately.

PATIENT EDUCATION

Educate patients on measures that may prevent or improve paronychia.

PATIENT RESOURCES

- Paronychia @ FamilyDoctor.org—**http://familydoctor.org/familydoctor/en/diseases-conditions/paronychia.html**.
- Paronychia (nail fold infection) @ DermNet NZ—**http://dermnetnz.org/fungal/paronychia.html**.

PROVIDER RESOURCES

- Rigopoulos D. Acute and chronic paronychia. *Am Fam Physician*. 2008;77(3):339-346. **http://www.aafp.org/afp/2008/0201/p339.html**.
- eMedicine Paronychia—**http://www.emedicine.com/emerg/topic357.htm**.

REFERENCES

1. Rockwell PG. Acute and chronic paronychia. *Am Fam Physician*. 2001;63(6):1113-1116.
2. Hochman LG. Paronychia: more than just an abscess. *Int J Dermatol*. 1995;34:385-386.
3. Ritting AW. Acute paronychia. *J Hand Surg Am*. 2012;37(5): 1068-1070.
4. Tully AS. Evaluation of Nail Abnormalities. *Am Fam Physician*. 2012;85(8):779-787.
5. Shah KN. Nail disorders as signs of pediatric systemic disease. *Curr Probl Pediatr Adolesc Health Care*. 2012; 42(8):204-211.
6. Yan AC. Skin signs of pediatric nutritional disorders. *Curr Probl Pediatr Adolesc Health Care*. 2012; 42(8):212-217.
7. Tosti A, Piraccini BM, D'Antuono A, et al. Paronychia associated with antiretroviral therapy. *Br J Dermatol*. 1999;140(6):1165-1168.
8. Belloni B. Cutaneous drug eruptions associated with the use of new oncological drugs. *Chem Immunol Allergy*. 2012;97:191-202.
9. Gilbar P. Nail toxicity induced by cancer chemotherapy. *J Oncol Pharm Pract*. 2009;15(3):143-155.
10. Canales FL, Newmeyer WL 3d, Kilgore ES. The treatment of felons and paronychias. *Hand Clin*. 1989;5:515-523.
11. Keyser JJ, Littler JW, Eaton RG. Surgical treatment of infections and lesions of the perionychium. *Hand Clin*. 1990;6(1):137-153.
12. Zuber T, Mayeaux EJ Jr: Atlas of Primary Care Procedures. Philadelphia, PA: Lippincott, Williams, & Wilkins; 2003:233-238.
13. Rigopoulos D. Acute and chronic paronychia. *Am Fam Physician*. 2008;77(3):339-346.
14. Brook I. Aerobic and anaerobic microbiology of paronychia. *Ann Emerg Med*. 1990;19:994-996.
15. Mayeaux EJ Jr: Paronychia Surgery. In: Mayeaux EJ Jr. *The Essential Guide to Primary Care Procedures*. Philadelphia: Wolters Kluwer: Lippincott, Williams, & Wilkins. 2009.
16. Losanoff JE. Can paronychia cause a remote necrotizing soft tissue infection? *Emerg Med*. 2011;40(1):e11-e13.

165 PSORIATIC NAILS

E.J. Mayeaux, Jr., MD
Joshua Rai Clark, MD

PATIENT STORY

A 3-year-old girl presents with one year of rashes from head to toe that are not responding to topical steroids. The girl's mother and her chart reflect a diagnosis of severe atopic dermatitis. The physician meticulously examines the girl's skin and nails and finds splinter hemorrhages, pitting, longitudinal ridging and onycholysis in the fingernails with splinter hemorrhages and nail thickening of the toenails (**Figure 165-1**). With this new information in mind, the physician notes other skin findings that are more suggestive of psoriasis than atopic dermatitis. This careful examination of the nails leads the clinician to the correct diagnosis and more effective treatment of the psoriasis.

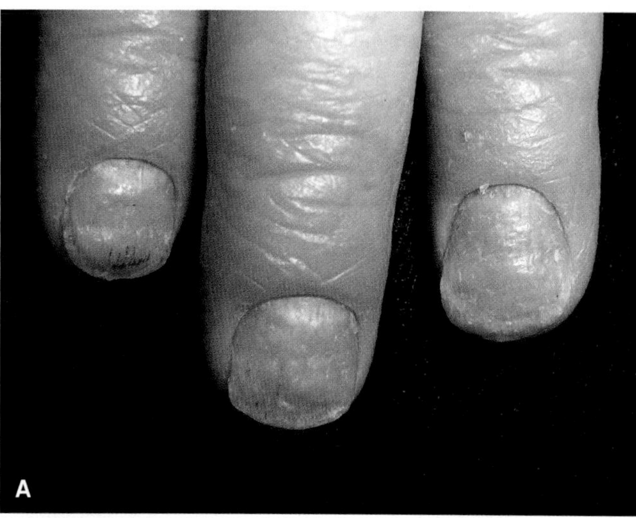

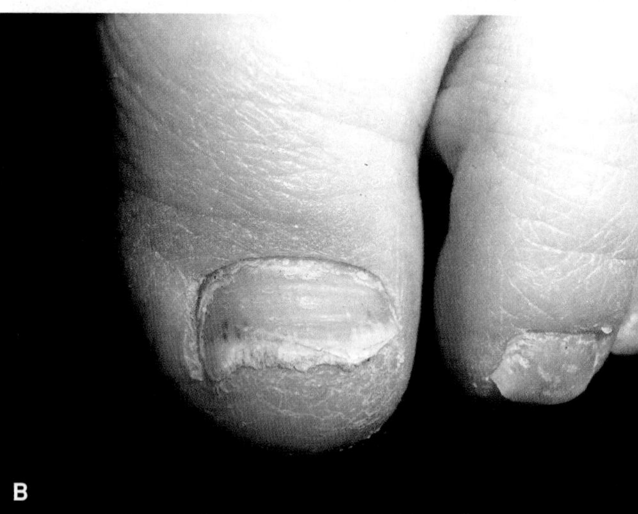

FIGURE 165-1 Nail psoriasis in a 3-year-old girl that helped to correctly diagnose her skin rash as psoriasis and not atopic dermatitis. **A.** Note the nail pitting, onycholysis, oil drop sign, longitudinal ridging and splinter hemorrhages in the fingernails. **B.** Note the splinter hemorrhages and nail thickening in the toenails. (*Used with permission from Richard P. Usatine, MD.*)

INTRODUCTION

Psoriasis is a hereditary disorder of skin with numerous clinical expressions. It affects millions of people throughout the world.[1] Nail involvement is common and can have a significant cosmetic impact.

EPIDEMIOLOGY

- Nails are involved in 30 to 50 percent of psoriasis patients at any given time, and up to 90 percent develop nail changes over their lifetime.[1] In most cases, nail involvement coexists with cutaneous psoriasis, although the skin surrounding the affected nails need not be involved. Psoriatic nail disease without overt cutaneous disease occurs in 1 to 5 percent of psoriasis. Patients with nail involvement are thought to have a higher incidence of associated arthritis.[2]
- The most common nail change seen with psoriasis is nail plate pitting (**Figures 165-1** and **165-2**).

ETIOLOGY AND PATHOPHYSIOLOGY

- In psoriasis, parakeratotic cells within the stratum corneum of the nail matrix alters normal keratinization.[3] The proximal nail matrix forms the superficial portion of the nail plate, so that involvement in this part of the matrix results in pitting of the nail plate (**Figures 165-1** and **165-2**.) The pits may range in size from pinpoint depressions to large punched-out lesions. People without psoriasis can have nail pitting.
- Longitudinal matrix involvement produces longitudinal nail ridging or splitting (**Figure 165-3**). When transverse matrix involvement occurs, solitary or multiple "growth arrest" lines (Beau lines) may occur (see Chapter 160, Normal Nail Variants). Psoriatic

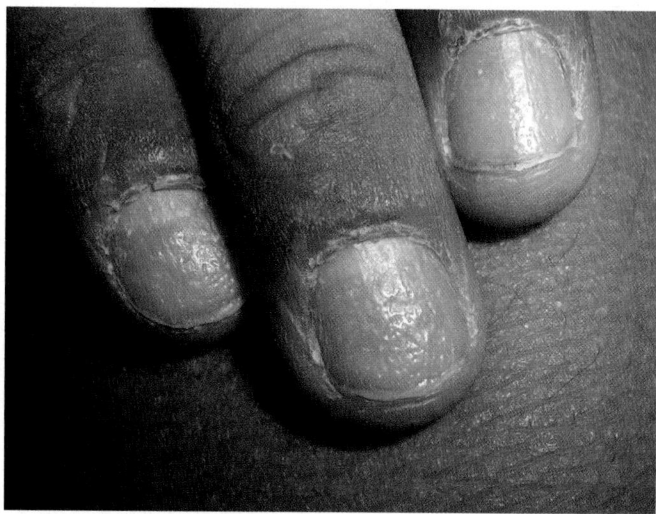

FIGURE 165-2 Nail pitting in a young boy with psoriasis. (*Used with permission from Richard P. Usatine, MD.*)

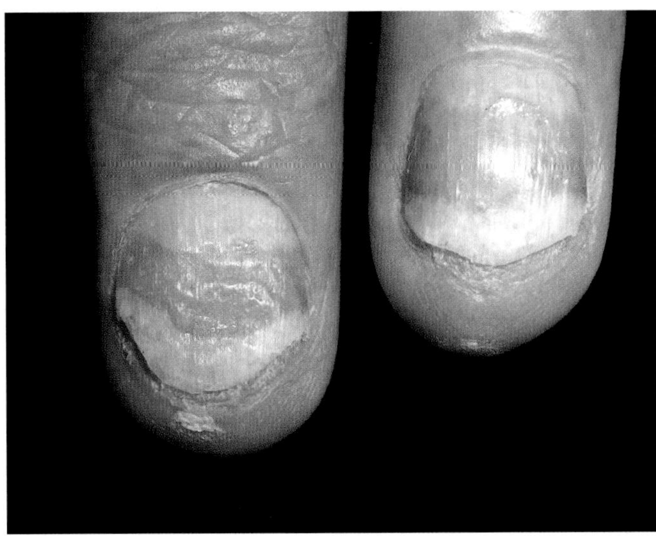

FIGURE 165-3 Nail psoriasis demonstrating onycholysis, pits, and transverse and longitudinal ridging. (*Used with permission from Richard P. Usatine, MD.*)

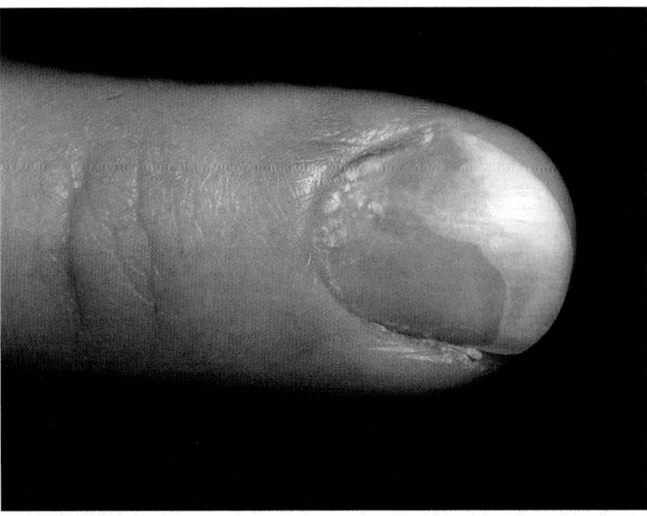

FIGURE 165-5 Nail psoriasis with the oil drop sign proximal to the lighter onycholysis at the distal nail. (*Used with permission from Richard P. Usatine, MD.*)

involvement of the intermediate portion of the nail matrix leads to leukonychia and diminished nail plate integrity.

- Parakeratosis of the nail bed with thickening of the stratum corneum causes discoloration of the nail bed, producing the "salmon spot" or "oil drop" signs (**Figure 165-4**).[3]
- Desquamation of parakeratotic cells at the hyponychium leads to onycholysis, which may allow for bacteria and fungi infection (**Figure 165-5**).[4]

RISK FACTORS

- Psoriasis of the skin.
- Psoriatic arthritis.
- Nail unit trauma.
- Generalized psoriasis flair.

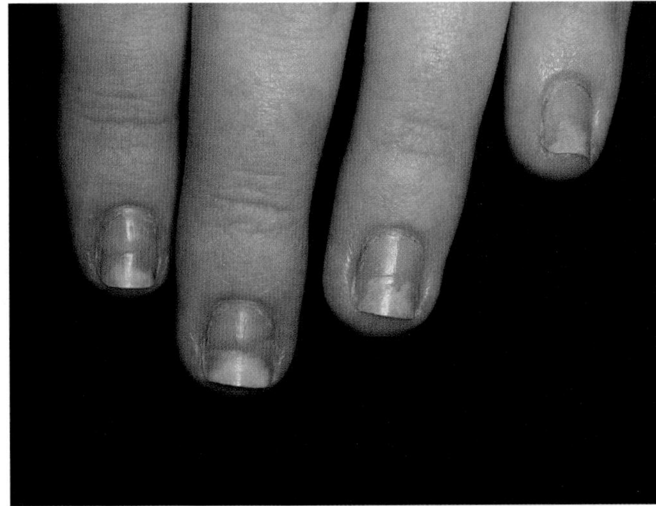

FIGURE 165-4 Nail psoriasis with onycholysis and oil drop sign in a teenage female. Note that end of the nail plates are no longer attached to the nail bed and there is a light brown discoloration where the nail loses its attachment. (*Used with permission from Richard P. Usatine, MD.*)

DIAGNOSIS

CLINICAL FEATURES

- The diagnosis of nail psoriasis is usually straightforward when characteristic nail findings coexist with cutaneous psoriasis. Nail pitting and onycholysis are the most common findings (**Figures 165-1** to **165-5**).
- Nail psoriasis and onychomycosis are often indistinguishable by clinical examination alone. Psoriasis at the hyponychium produces subungual hyperkeratosis and distal onycholysis (**Figures 165-4** and **165-5**). Trauma may accentuate this process. Secondary microbial colonization by *Candida* or *Pseudomonas* organisms may occur (**Figure 165-6**).
- Nail bed psoriasis produces localized onycholysis which often appears like a drop of oil on a piece of paper (oil drop sign; see **Figures 165-4**, and **165-5**). This same condition is also called the salmon patch sign.
- Extensive germinal matrix involvement may result in loss of nail integrity and transverse (horizontal) ridging (**Figure 165-3**).
- Psoriasis causes dermal vascular dilation and tortuosity, and in the nails is associated with splinter hemorrhages of the nail bed caused by foci of capillary bleeding. Extravasated blood becomes trapped between the longitudinal troughs of the nail bed and the overlying nail plate grows out distally along with the plate (**Figures 165-1** and **165-7**). The splinter hemorrhages of the psoriatic nail are analogous to the cutaneous Auspitz sign.

LABORATORY TESTING

- KOH preparation and fungal culture will usually provide an answer. However, it may be necessary to clip a portion of the nail plate and send it for fungal staining (periodic acid-Schiff [PAS]

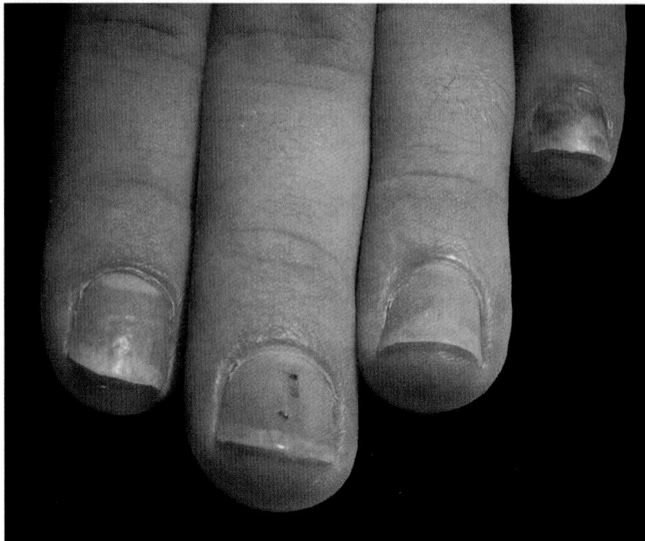

FIGURE 165-6 Patient with nail psoriasis demonstrating the oil drop sign (second digit), nail pitting (second and third digit), onycholysis (second, fourth and fifth digit), and secondary pseudomonas infection (fifth digit). (*Used with permission from E.J. Mayeaux, Jr., MD.*)

stain) if the first test results are not consistent with the clinical picture.[5] Psoriasis and onychomycosis can occur concomitantly.

BIOPSY

- Biopsy of the nail unit is rarely necessary unless a malignancy is suspected.

DIFFERENTIAL DIAGNOSIS

- Onychomycosis produces distal onycholysis and hyperkeratosis that appear identical to psoriasis and may coexist with it (see Chapter 163, Onychomycosis).

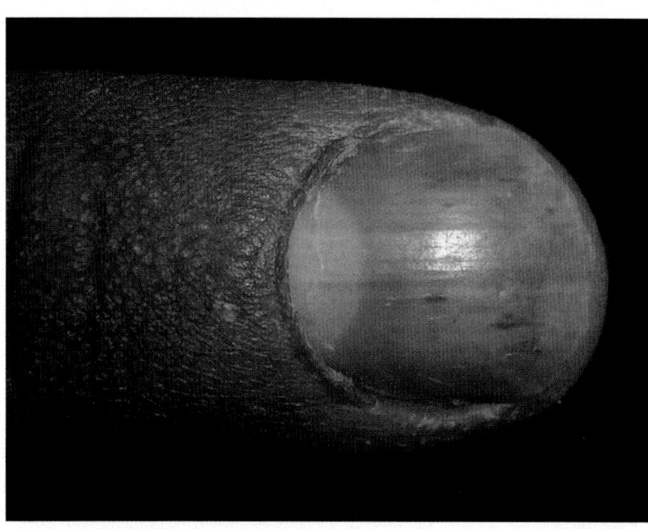

FIGURE 165-7 Prominent splinter hemorrhages and onycholysis in the nail of a person with psoriasis. (*Used with permission from Richard P. Usatine, MD.*)

- Alopecia areata also can produce pitting of the nails. As a general rule, pitting in psoriasis is more irregular and broader based; pitting in alopecia areata is more regular, shallow, and geometric and produces fine pits (see Chapter 158, Alopecia Areata).
- Neoplastic and dysplastic diseases may produce psoriasiform nail changes in a single nail. Bowen disease, squamous cell carcinoma, and verruca vulgaris may appear as an isolated subungual or periungual plaque, possibly with accompanying nail plate destruction. A biopsy can establish a definitive diagnosis.

MANAGEMENT

NONPHARMACOLOGIC

- Psoriatic nail disease is often persistent and refractory to treatment. There is insufficient evidence to recommend a standard treatment.
- The nails should be kept short, to avoid traumatic exacerbation of onycholysis and to avoid the accumulation of exogenous material under the nail.[3] SOR C
- Nail polish may be very helpful in concealing a range of nail unit changes.[6] SOR C
- Nail plate buffing may diminish surface imperfections.[6] SOR C

MEDICATIONS

- Unfortunately, specific evidence for systemic therapy in nail psoriasis is generally lacking. It should be considered in those with significant cutaneous involvement in addition to nail disease.
- One treatment option for nail psoriasis, especially with matrix involvement, is intralesional corticosteroid injection. Triamcinolone acetonide (0.4 mL, 10 mg/mL) is injected into the nail bed, matrix, or proximal fold following digital block, and then at 3-month intervals.[3,7] SOR A Subungual hyperkeratosis, ridging, and thickening respond better than pitting and onycholysis, with benefit sustained for at least 9 months.[7] Pain, periungual hypopigmentation, subungual hemorrhage and atrophy have been reported.[3]
- Nail bed disease, including subungual hyperkeratosis, distal onycholysis, and "oil drop" changes may also need the lateral nail folds injected close to the nail bed. Direct injection into the nail bed is prevented by the nail plate and extreme pain sensitivity of the hyponychial region. Atrophy and subungual hematoma formation are potential complications.
- Topical tazarotene improves onycholysis and nail pitting (if applied under occlusion) in those treated for 24 weeks.[3] SOR A
- Narrow-band UVB and psoralen UVA (PUVA) phototherapy for 3 to 6 months is effective for cutaneous psoriasis but it's efficacy for nail psoriasis is poorly defined.[3]
- Systemic retinoid therapy is often effective for pustular psoriasis, and early intervention is most likely to prevent chronic nail-associated scarring.
- However, in a single uncontrolled retrospective study in patients ranging in ages from 15 to 81 years old found that Infliximab (5mg/kg) given at 0, 2, 6 and every 8 weeks up to 38 weeks showed a decrease in psoriatic nail lesions. This study suggests

that the psoriatic nail should be treated early as its presence may correlate with an increased chance of developing psoriatic arthritis. This study is limited by sample size and lack of long term follow up.[8] SOR B

PREVENTION[9]

- Wearing gloves during wet work and during exposure to harsh materials may minimize trauma to the skin and nail unit.
- Trimming the nail short to minimize leverage at the free edge and resulting trauma.
- If dry skin or scaling develop, application of emollients may be helpful.
- Cosmetic manipulations of the nail risk exacerbating the disease due to minor trauma. Discretion and care should be exercised when trimming the cuticle and clearing subungual debris.

PROGNOSIS

- Psoriatic nail changes may be reversible because scarring typically does not occur. An exception to this may develop in severe cases of generalized pustular psoriasis.

FOLLOW-UP

- Follow-up can be combined with regular follow-ups for cutaneous psoriasis.

PATIENT EDUCATION

- Nail psoriasis is mainly a cosmetic problem. Nail polish or artificial nails can be used in some patients to conceal psoriatic pitting and onycholysis. When subungual hyperkeratosis becomes uncomfortable because of pressure exerted by footwear, the nail can be pared down to relieve the pressure.
- Patients should be instructed to trim nails back to the point of firm attachment with the nail bed to minimize further nail-bed and nail-plate disassociation. Wearing gloves while working may minimize trauma to the nails. Tell patients to avoid vigorous cleaning and scraping under the nails as this may break the skin where the nail is attached and lead to an infection.

PATIENT RESOURCES

- National Psoriasis Foundation. *Hands, Feet and Nails*—**www.psoriasis.org/page.aspx?pid=445**.
- eMedicineHealth. *Nail Psoriasis*—**www.emedicinehealth.com/nail_psoriasis/article_em.htm**.

PROVIDER RESOURCES

- Medscape. *Nail Psoriasis: Overview of Nail Psoriasis*—**http://emedicine.medscape.com/article/1107949**.
- DermNet NZ. *Nail Psoriasis*—**http://dermnetnz.org/scaly/nail-psoriasis.html**.

REFERENCES

1. Jiaravuthisan MM, Sasseville D, Vender RB, et al. Psoriasis of the nail. Anatomy, pathology, clinical presentation, and a review of the literature on thereapy. *J Am Acad Dermatol*. 2007;57(1):1-27.
2. Noronha PA, Zubkov B: Nails and nail disorders in children and adults. *Am Fam Physician*. 1997;55(6):2129-2140.
3. Edwards F, de Berker D: Nail psoriasis: clinical presentation and best practice recommendations. *Drugs*. 2009;69(17):2351-2361.
4. Jiaravuthisan MM, Sasseville D, Vender RB, et al. Psoriasis of the nail: anatomy, pathology, clinical presentation, and a review of the literature on therapy. *J Am Acad Dermatol*. 2007;57(1):1-27.
5. Grammer-West NY, Corvette DM, Giandoni MB, Fitzpatrick JE: Clinical pearl: nail plate biopsy for the diagnosis of psoriatic nails. *J Am Acad Dermatol*. 1998;38(2:1):260-262.
6. de Berker D: Management of psoriatic nail disease. *Semin Cutan Med Surg*. 2009;28(1):39-43.
7. de Berker DA, Lawrence CM: A simplified protocol of steroid injection for psoriatic nail dystrophy. *Br J Dermatol*. 1998;138(1):90-95.
8. Fabroni C, Gori A, Troiano M, Prignano F, Lotti T: Infliximab efficacy in nail psoriasis. A retrospective study in 48 patients. *J European Academy of Dermatology and Venereology*. 2011;25:549-553.
9. André J: Artificial nails and psoriasis. *J Cosmet Dermatol*. 2005;4(2):103-106.

166 SUBUNGUAL HEMATOMA

E.J. Mayeaux, Jr., MD

PATIENT STORY

A 14-year-old boy presented to the office 1 week after slamming his finger in a car door. He was seen at an urgent care clinic after the acute event and told to follow-up in 1 week. A healing subungual hematoma was evident (**Figure 166-1**). He has full range-of-motion and no pain. Since there is no pain, there is no indication for nail perforation and drainage.

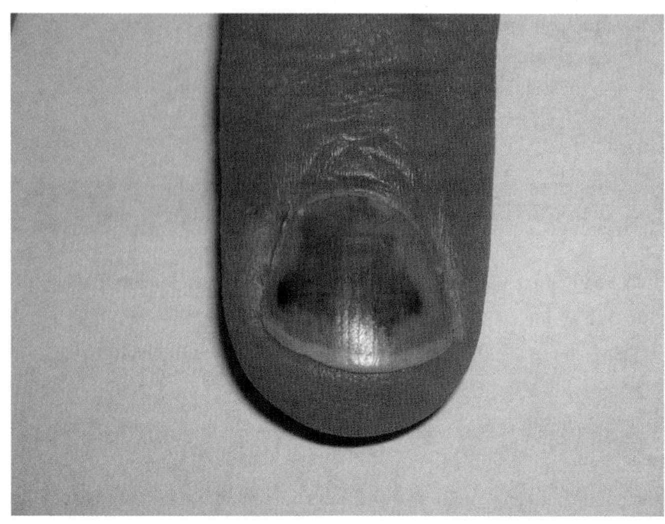

FIGURE 166-1 Subungual hematoma healing in a 14-year-old boy one week after slamming his finger in a car door. (*Used with permission from E.J. Mayeaux, Jr., MD.*)

INTRODUCTION

Subungual hematoma (blood under the fingernail or toenail) is a common injury. It is typically caused by a blow to the distal phalanx (e.g., smashing with a tool, crush in a door jamb, stubbing one's toe). The blow causes bleeding of the nail matrix or bed with resultant subungual hematoma formation. Patients usually present because of throbbing pain associated with blue-black discoloration under the nail plate. Subungual hematomas may be simple (i.e., the nail and nail fold are intact) or accompanied by significant injuries to the nail fold and digit.[1] The patient may not be aware of the precipitating trauma, because it may have been minor and/or chronic (e.g., rubbing in a tight shoe).

EPIDEMIOLOGY

Subungual hematoma is a common childhood injury.

ETIOLOGY AND PATHOPHYSIOLOGY

- The injury causes bleeding of the nail matrix and nail bed, which results in subungual hematoma formation. Pain is produced by the pressure in the contained space under the nail plate pressing against nerve receptors, although soft tissue or bony injury may also contribute to the pain when present (**Figures 166-1** to **166-5**).
- In most cases the discoloration grows out with the nail plate, exhibiting a proximal border that reproduces the shape of the lunula. Occasionally, a hematoma does not migrate because of repeated daily trauma. An extended, nonmigrating "hematoma" should be considered suspicious. Nail plate punch biopsy can be performed if melanoma is a worry. If the dark area was only a hematoma the dark color lifts off with nail plate.
- Potential complications of subungual hematoma include onycholysis, nail deformity (usually splitting as in **Figure 166-6**), and infection. Complications are more likely to occur when presentation is delayed or there is an underlying fracture.[2]

DIAGNOSIS

CLINICAL FEATURES

- Patients experience throbbing pain and blue-black discoloration under the nail as the hematoma progresses. Pain is relieved immediately in most patients with simple nail trephination (**Figure 166-3**).

IMAGING

- If the mechanism of injury and clinical picture suggest a possible distal phalanx or distal interphalangeal (DIP) fracture, obtain a radiograph. SOR Ⓒ

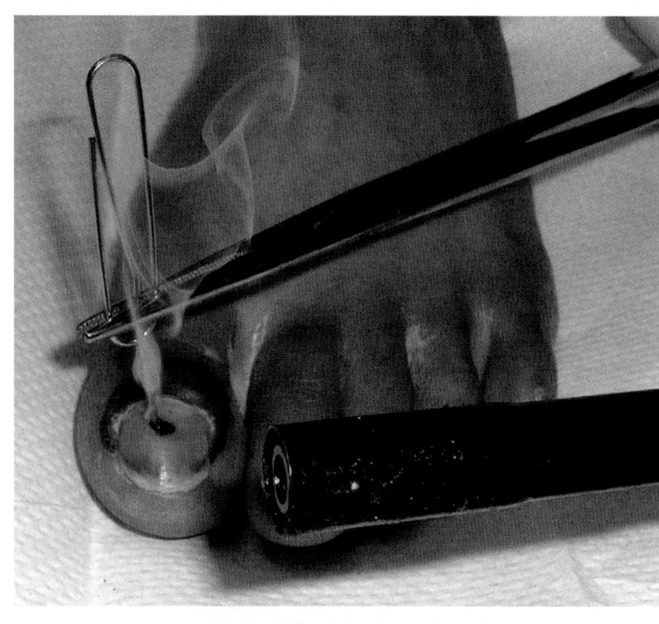

FIGURE 166-2 A subungual hematoma occurred when an iron fell on the toe of this young woman. A paperclip was held in a hemostat and heated with a torch to pierce the patient's nail plate in order to relieve the subungual hematoma. (*Used with permission from Richard P. Usatine, MD.*)

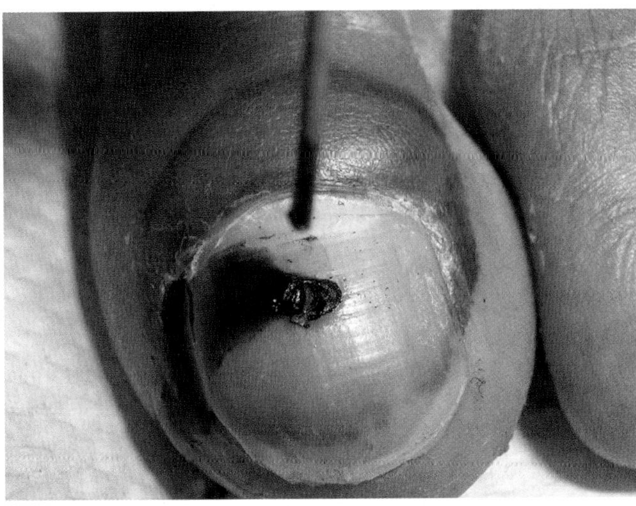

FIGURE 166-3 The hot paper clip formed a nice hole in the nail plate and the blood drained out spontaneously. This relieved the pressure and gave the patient immediate pain relief. (*Used with permission from Richard P. Usatine, MD.*)

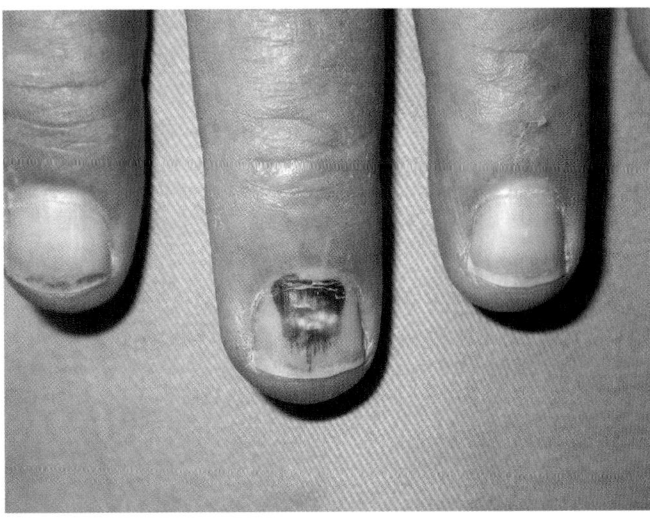

FIGURE 166-5 This persistent discoloration of the nail in this adolescent was correctly diagnosed as a subungual hematoma by history and physical exam so a nail plate biopsy was not needed. (*Used with permission from Richard P. Usatine, MD.*)

DIFFERENTIAL DIAGNOSIS

- Nail bed nevus—Appears as a stable or slowly growing painless dark spot in the nail bed or matrix.
- Longitudinal melanonychia—Appears as painless pigmented bands that start in the matrix and extend the length of the nail (see Chapter 161, Pigmented Nail Disorders).
- Subungual melanoma—May start as a painless darkly pigmented band in the matrix and extend the length of the nail. It may be associated with pigment deposition in the proximal nail fold (Hutchinson sign; see Chapter 161, Pigmented Nail Disorders).
- Splinter hemorrhages—Appears as reddish streaks in the nail bed and are seen in psoriasis more commonly than endocarditis (see Chapter 165, Psoriatic Nails).
- The diagnosis of child abuse must be considered in cases of chronic or frequently recurrent subungual hematomas in children.[3]

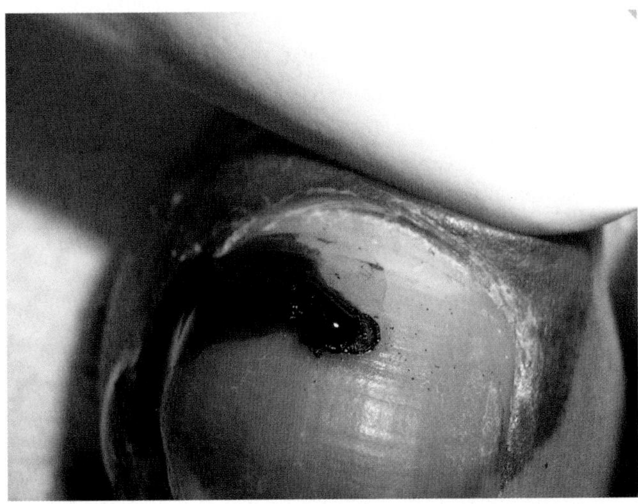

FIGURE 166-4 After the nail plate is pierced, the blood drains easily with a little pressure on the proximal nail fold. (*Used with permission from Richard P. Usatine, MD.*)

MANAGEMENT

NONPHARMACOLOGIC

- Subungual hematomas are treated with nail trephination, which removes the extravasated blood and relieves the pressure and resulting pain. Beyond 48 hours, most subungual hematomas have clotted and pain has decreased, so trephination is ineffective. SOR C

SURGERY

- Nail perforation is a painless procedure because there are no nerve endings in the nail plate that is perforated. The nail is perforated with a steel paper clip (**Figures 166-2** to **166-4**) or an electrocautery device. This allows the collected blood to drain out (**Figures 166-3** and **166-4**). The hole must be large enough for continued drainage, which can continue for 24 to 36 hours. The puncture site should be

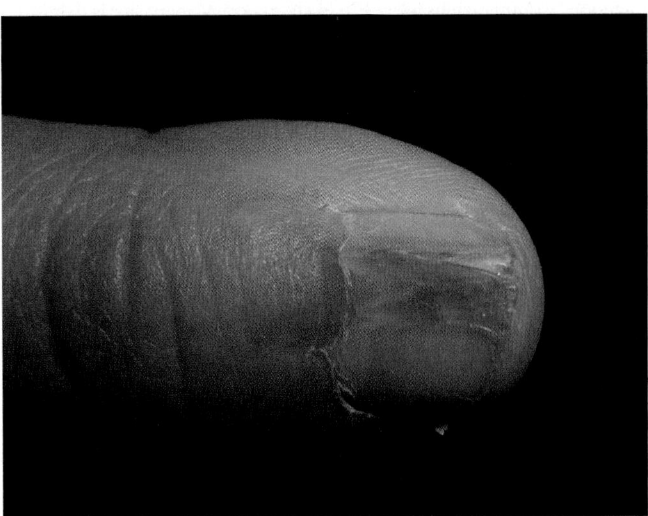

FIGURE 166-6 Split-nail deformity in a 6-year-old girl 1 year after her finger was closed in a car door and sutured in the emergency department. The matrix did not come together well and the nail will remain split (onychoschizia). (*Used with permission from Richard P. Usatine, MD.*)

kept covered with sterile gauze dressing while the wound drains, and the gauze should be changed daily. Extreme caution should be used with open flame in a medical (and especially pediatric) setting.

- The bevel of a large-bore needle may be twisted against the nail plate like a mechanical spade bit to produce a hole to drain the hematoma.[4] This method causes compression of the nail against the hematoma and nail bed during the procedure and may temporarily increase pain.
- Insulin syringe needle (29 gauge) may also be used for aspiration of distal nail subungual hematomas.[5]
- Mesoscission device (e.g., PathFormer) may be used to bore multiple holes in the nail over the hematoma. It monitors electrical resistance to determine depth of mechanical boring, thus avoiding inadvertent puncture of the nail bed.[6]

MEDICATIONS

- The use of prophylactic antibiotics does not appear to improve outcomes in patients with subungual hematomas and intact nail folds.[7] SOR B If a prophylactic antibiotic is used, a first generation cephalosporin (e.g., cephalexin 25–50 mg/kg/day divided every 6 to 8 hours for 10 days) would be the drug of choice.[8,9]
- Oral analgesia such as ibuprofen 10 mg/kg (maximum dose: 800 mg) every 6 to 8 hours may be used with more painful digits. SOR C

REFERRAL

- Some authors recommend removal of the nail with inspection instead of nail trephination when the hematoma involves more than 25 to 50 percent of the nail because of the increased likelihood of significant nail bed injury and fracture of the distal phalanx.[10,11] SOR C
- When deeper injuries are involved, nail plate removal after a digital block allows for nail bed repair.[12] SOR C

PROGNOSIS

The potential complications of a subungual hematoma include onycholysis (separation of the nail plate from the nail bed), nail deformity, nail loss, and infection. Complications are more likely to occur when care is delayed.

A retrospective analysis of 123 patients treated with simple trephination found that 85 percent of patients reported an excellent or very good outcome, 2 percent reported a poor outcome (nail splitting), and no correlation was found between outcome and size of the hematoma or the presence of fracture or infection.[2]

FOLLOW-UP

After drainage, instruct the patient to soak the affected digit in warm water several times per day for 2 days, and to keep the area dressed between soaks. Have the patient return if there are any signs of reaccumulation of blood or infection.

PATIENT EDUCATION

- Potential complications of subungual hematoma and nail trephination should be discussed with the patient and/or the patient's parents or guardian.
- Inform the patient that residual discoloration usually slowly grows out with the nail.

PATIENT RESOURCES

- eMedicineHealth. *Subungual Hematoma*—**www.emedicinehealth.com/subungual_hematoma_bleeding_under_nail/article_em.htm**.
- HealthSquare. *Subungual Hematoma*—**www.healthcentral.com/symptoms/guide-154582–75.html**.
- WebMD. *Subungual Hematoma*—**www.webmd.com/skin-problems-and-treatments/bleeding-under-nail**.

PROVIDER RESOURCES

- American Family Physician. *Fingertip Injuries*—**http://www.aafp.org/afp/20010515/1961.html**.
- InteliHealth. *Nail Trauma*—**www.intelihealth.com/IH/ihtIH/WSIHW000/9339/25971.html**.

REFERENCES

1. Roser SE, Gellman H. Comparison of nail bed repair versus nail trephination for subungual hematomas in children. *J Hand Surg Am*. 1999;24:1166-1170.
2. Meek S, White M. Subungual haematomas: is simple trephining enough? *J Accid Emerg Med*. 1998;15:269-271.
3. Gavin LA, Lanz MJ, Leung DY, Roesler TA. Chronic subungual hematomas: a presumed immunologic puzzle resolved with a diagnosis of child abuse. *Arch Pediatr Adolesc Med*. 1997;151:103-105.
4. Bonisteel PS. Practice tips. Trephining subungual hematomas. Can Fam Physician 2008; 54:693.
5. Kaya TI, Tursen U, Baz K, Ikizoglu G. Extra-fine insulin syringe needle: an excellent instrument for the evacuation of subungual hematoma. *Dermatol Surg*. 2003;29:1141.
6. Salter SA, Ciocon DH, Gowrishankar TR, Kimball AB. Controlled nail trephination for subungual hematoma. *Am J Emerg Med*. 2006;24:875
7. Seaberg DC, Angelos WJ, Paris PM. Treatment of subungual hematomas with nail trephination: a prospective study. *Am J Emerg Med*. 1991;9:209-210.
8. Kensinger DR, Guille JT, Horn BD, Herman MJ. The stubbed great toe: importance of early recognition and treatment of open fractures of the distal phalanx. *J Pediatr Orthop* 2001; 21:31.
9. Fox IM. Osteomyelitis of the distal phalanx following trauma to the nail. A case report. *J Am Podiatr Med Assoc*. 1992; 82:542.
10. Zook EG, Guy RJ, Russell RC. A study of nail bed injuries: causes, treatment, and prognosis. *J Hand Surg Am*. 1984;9:247-252.
11. Zacher JB. Management of injuries of the distal phalanx. *Surg Clin North Am*. 1984;64:747-760.
12. Hart RG, Kleinert HE. Fingertip and nail bed injuries. *Emerg Med Clin North Am*. 1993;11:755-765.

SECTION 15 PIGMENTARY CONDITIONS

167 VITILIGO AND HYPOPIGMENTATION

Richard P. Usatine, MD
Karen A. Hughes, MD
Mindy A. Smith, MD, MS

PATIENT STORY

An 8-year-old Hispanic boy is brought in to the clinic by his mother, who is concerned about his pigment loss (**Figure 167-1**). He is starting to develop this vitiligo around the mouth and his mother wants him to be treated. The child was started on a topical steroid and the use of narrow band UVB was discussed if the steroid does not prove helpful. Realistic expectations of the treatments were provided to the mother and her son.

INTRODUCTION

Vitiligo is an acquired, progressive loss of pigmentation of the epidermis. The Vitiligo European Task Force defines nonsegmental vitiligo as "an acquired chronic pigmentation disorder characterized by white patches, often symmetrical, which usually increase in size with time, corresponding to a substantial loss of functioning epidermal and sometimes hair follicle melanocytes."[1] Segmental vitiligo is defined similarly except for a unilateral distribution that may totally or partially match a dermatome; occasionally more than one segment is involved.[1]

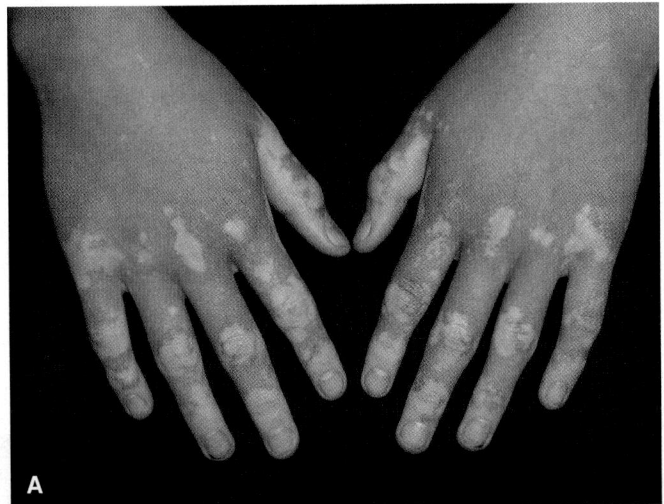

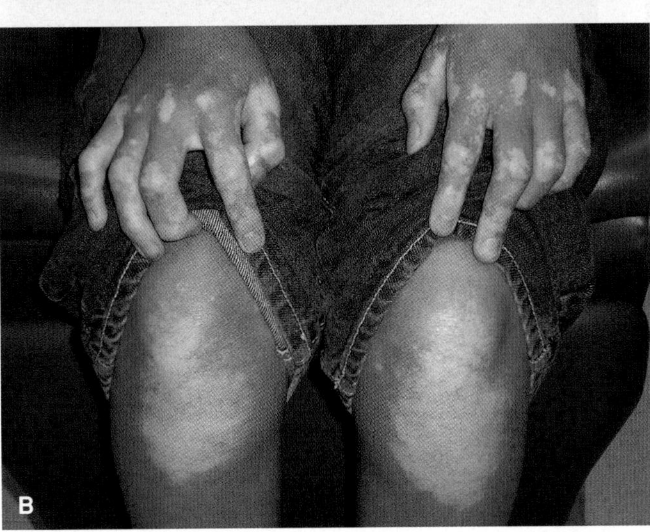

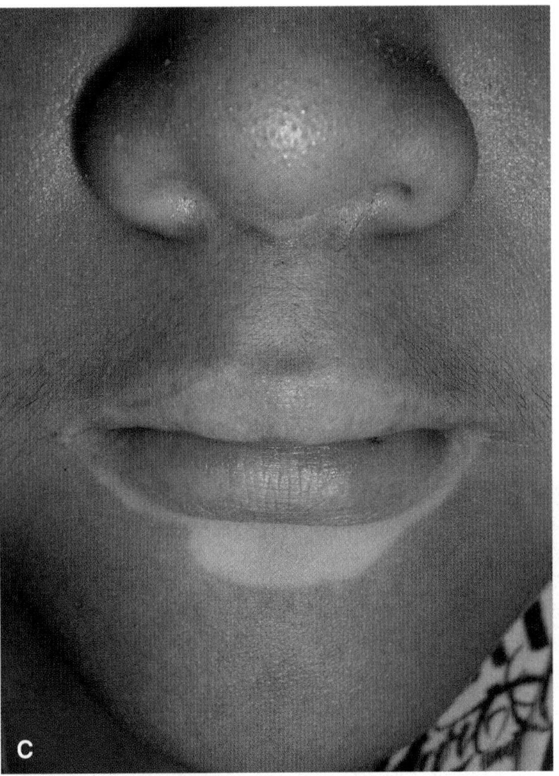

FIGURE 167-1 Vitiligo in an 8-year-old Hispanic boy. **A.** Hands. **B.** Knees and hands. **C.** Perioral. (*Used with permission from Richard P. Usatine, MD.*)

SYNONYMS

Vitiligo vulgaris.

EPIDEMIOLOGY

- Vitiligo occurs in approximately 0.5 to 2 percent of the worldwide population.[2,3]
- It can occur at any age but typically develops between the ages of 10 and 30 years.[2]
- Vitiligo has equal rates in males and females.[2]
- It occurs in all races but is more prominent in those with darker skin.

ETIOLOGY AND PATHOPHYSIOLOGY

- Autoimmune disease with destruction of melanocytes.
- Genetic component in approximately 30 percent of cases. Toll-like receptor genes were found to be associated with vitiligo in a population of Turkish patients.[4]
- Can trigger or worsen with illness, emotional stress, and/or skin trauma (Koebner phenomenon).

DIAGNOSIS

CLINICAL FEATURES

- Macular regions of depigmentation with scalloped, well-defined borders (**Figures 167-1** to **167-3**).
- Depigmented areas often coalesce over time to form larger areas (**Figure 167-4**).
- Depigmented areas are more susceptible to sunburn. Tanning of the normal surrounding skin makes the depigmented areas more obvious.

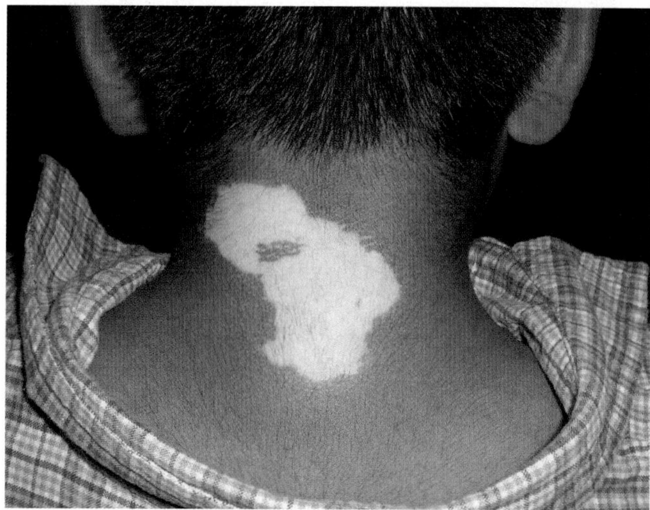

FIGURE 167-2 Vitiligo on the neck of a Hispanic boy. (*Used with permission from Richard P. Usatine, MD.*)

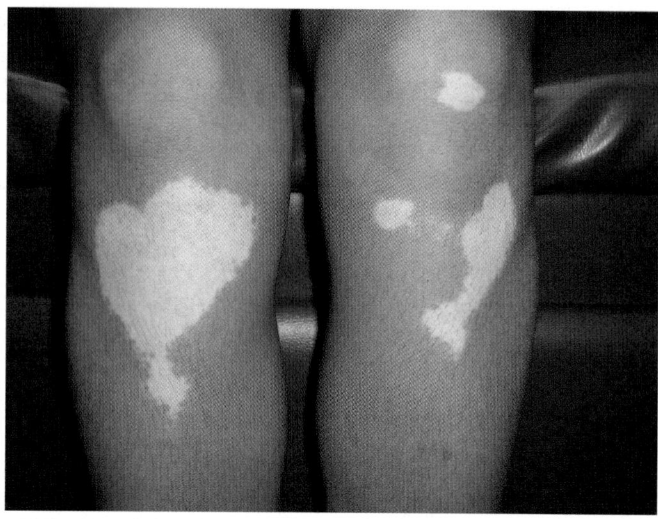

FIGURE 167-3 Vitiligo on the knees with the typical jagged edges. (*Used with permission from Richard P. Usatine, MD.*)

- There is no standardized method for assessing vitiligo; strategies include subjective clinical assessment, semiobjective assessment (e.g., Vitiligo Area Scoring Index [VASI] and point-counting methods), macroscopic morphologic assessment (e.g., visual, photographic in natural or UV light, or computerized image analysis), micromorphologic assessment (e.g., confocal laser microscopy), and objective assessment (e.g., software-based image analysis or spectrophotometry).[5] Authors of a literature review concluded that the VASI, the rule of 9, and Wood's lamp were the best techniques for assessing the degree of pigmentary lesions and measuring the extent and progression of vitiligo.[5]
- Conditions associated with vitiligo include thyroid disease and the presence of thyroid antibodies,[6,7] congenital nevi (in one study, 6.2 percent versus 2.8 percent in those without vitiligo),[4] and halo nevi,[1] and possibly primary open-angle glaucoma (57% of patients in one case series).[8]

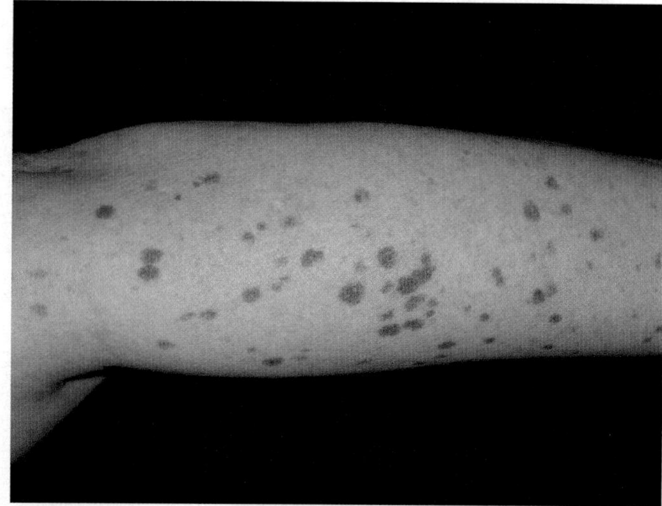

FIGURE 167-4 This previously dark-skinned patient has only a few spots of pigment remaining on her arm because of the extensive vitiligo. Her father has the same condition. (*Used with permission from Richard P. Usatine, MD.*)

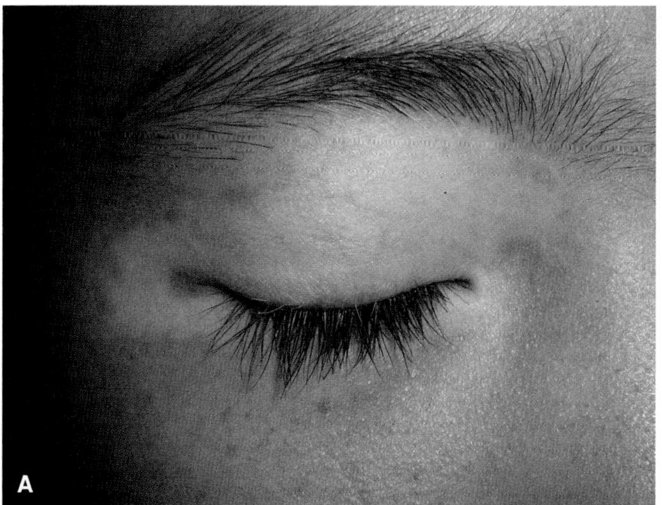

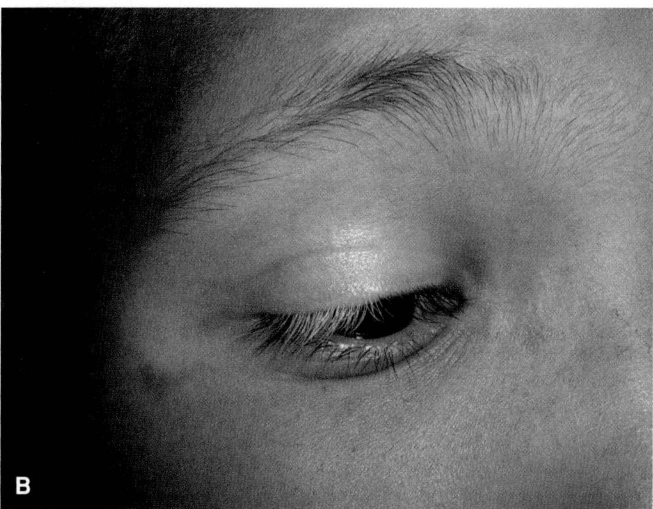

FIGURE 167-5 Vitiligo occurs commonly around the eye. **A.** Vitiligo with normal eyelashes. **B.** Vitiligo with leukotrichia. The loss of melanocytes has turned some of the eyelashes white. (*Used with permission from Richard P. Usatine, MD.*)

TYPICAL DISTRIBUTION

- Widespread, but generally seen first on the face, hands, arms, and genitalia.
- Depigmentation around body openings such as eyes, mouth, umbilicus, and anus is common (**Figure 167-5**). When the eyelashes are involved it is called *leukotrichia*. When other hair is involved it is called *poliosis*.
- Vitiligo can be unilateral or bilateral; in one study, patients with unilateral vitiligo were younger, and had an earlier age at onset while those with bilateral vitiligo were more likely to have light skin types and more commonly had associated autoimmune disease.[9]

LABORATORY AND IMAGING

- Evaluation for endocrine disorders such as hyper- or hypothyroidism (e.g., thyroid-stimulating hormone [TSH]) and diabetes mellitus (e.g., fasting blood sugar) should be considered, as vitiligo can be associated with these disorders.[10]

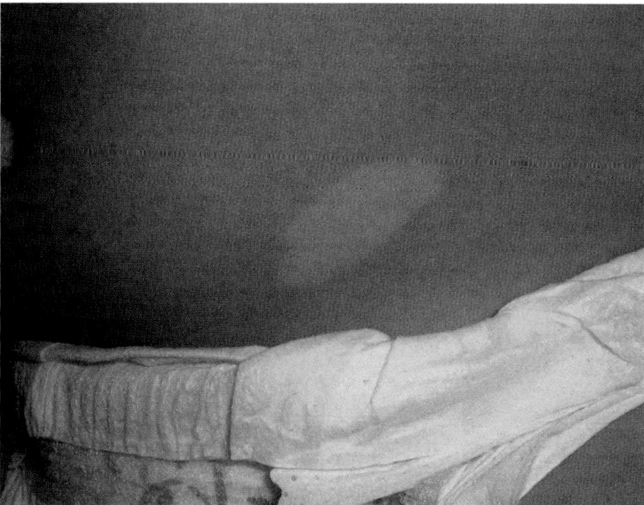

FIGURE 167-6 A hypopigmented patch on the abdomen of an infant in a shape that suggests an ash leaf. The child is otherwise healthy with no seizures or developmental delay but should be monitored for signs of tuberous sclerosis. This may be nothing more than nevus depigmentosus. (*Used with permission from Richard P. Usatine, MD.*)

BIOPSY

Not indicated unless the diagnosis is not clear and then a 4-mm punch biopsy will suffice.

DIFFERENTIAL DIAGNOSIS

- Pityriasis alba—Areas of decreased pigmentation with scaling and mild itching. Seen in young children and usually associated with eczema and improves with age (see Chapter 130, Atopic Dermatitis).
- Ash leaf spots—Lance-shaped macules of hypopigmentation, which remain stable in size and shape over time (**Figure 167-6**). Often the earliest sign of tuberous sclerosis. More concerning if there are 3 or more present in one child (see Chapter 205, Tuberous Sclerosis).
- Halo nevus—Hypopigmentation confined to areas surrounding pigmented nevi that typically appear in adolescents and young adults (see Chapter 143, Benign Nevi).
- Hypomelanosis of Ito is a rare syndrome with hypopigmented whorls of skin present at birth along the Blaschko lines of development. This pattern may be accompanied by congenital abnormalities involving the eyes, or neurologic or renal systems. Its presence at birth helps distinguish it from vitiligo (**Figures 167-7** and **167-8**).
- Nevus anemicus—A congenital hypopigmented macule or patch that is stable in relative size and distribution. It occurs as a result of localized hypersensitivity to catecholamines and not a decrease in melanocytes. On diascopy (pressure with a glass slide) the skin is indistinguishable from the surrounding skin. Its presence from birth helps distinguish it from vitiligo (**Figure 167-9**).
- Nevus depigmentosus is usually present at birth or starts in early childhood. There is a decreased number of melanosomes within a normal number of melanocytes. It typically has a serrated or jagged edge. Its presence at birth or early in childhood helps to differentiate it from vitiligo (**Figure 167-10**).

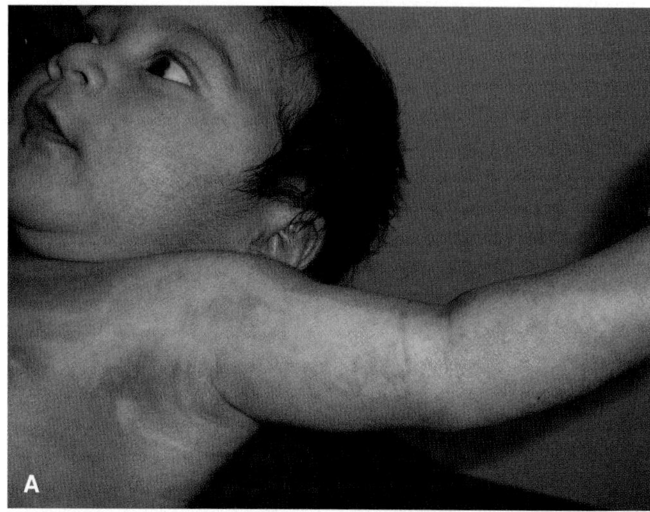

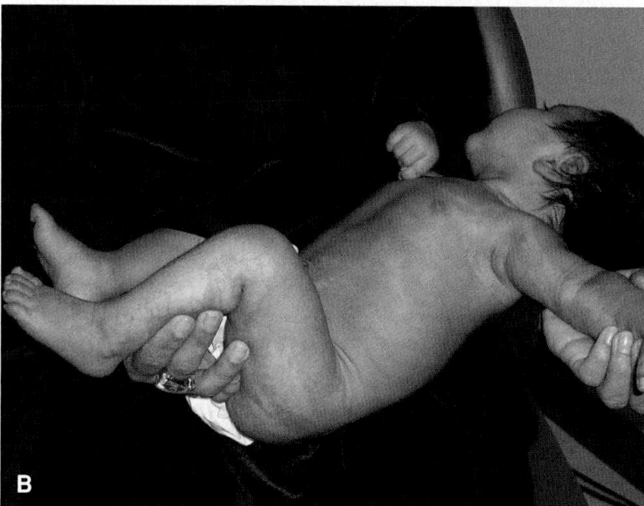

FIGURE 167-7 **A.** Hypomelanosis of Ito in a 2-month-old girl. It is a rare syndrome with hypopigmented whorls of skin present at birth along the Blaschko lines of development. It is typically unilateral and extends down an extremity. **B.** Note the whorls on the chest and upper arm. (*Used with permission from Richard P. Usatine, MD.*)

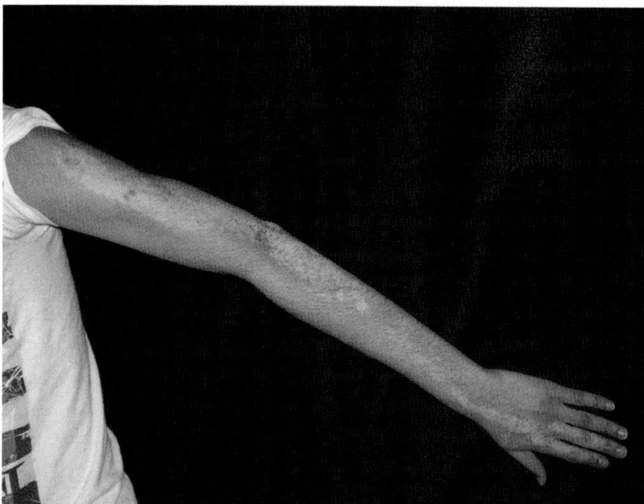

FIGURE 167-8 Hypomelanosis of Ito extending down the arm of this 17-year-old boy since birth. This was unilateral and could be mistaken for segmental vitiligo if it had not been present since birth. (*Used with permission from Richard P. Usatine, MD.*)

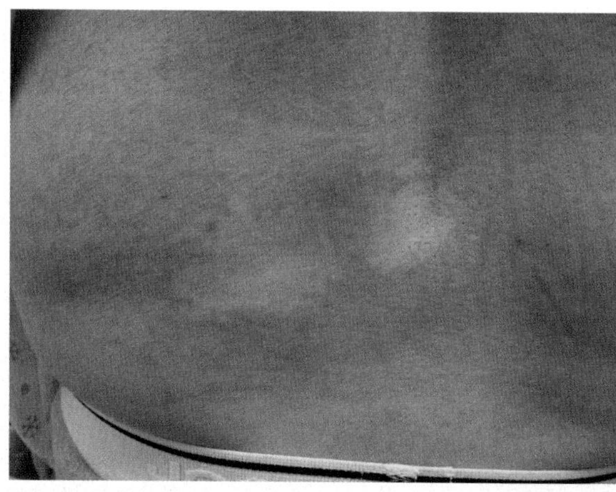

FIGURE 167-9 Nevus anemicus on the back of this patient since birth. This is a congenital hypersensitivity to localized catecholamines. On diascopy the skin was indistinguishable from the surrounding skin. The irregular broken-up outline is seen in nevus anemicus and nevus depigmentosus. (*Used with permission from Ryan O'Quinn, MD.*)

MANAGEMENT

For assessing outcomes to treatment, the Vitiligo European Task Force suggests a system combining analysis of extent using percentage of body area involved (rule of 9), stage of disease based on cutaneous and hair pigmentation in vitiligo patches and staged 0 to 4 (with 0 representing normal pigment and 4 complete hair whitening) on the largest macule in each body region except hands and feet, and disease progression (spreading) assessed with Wood's lamp examination of the same largest macule in each body area.[1] An evaluation sheet can be found in the citation.[1]

NONPHARMACOLOGIC

- Addressing the psychological distress that this disfiguring skin disorder causes should be a primary focus as the clinical course is unpredictable and, in some cases, little can be done to modify the condition itself.

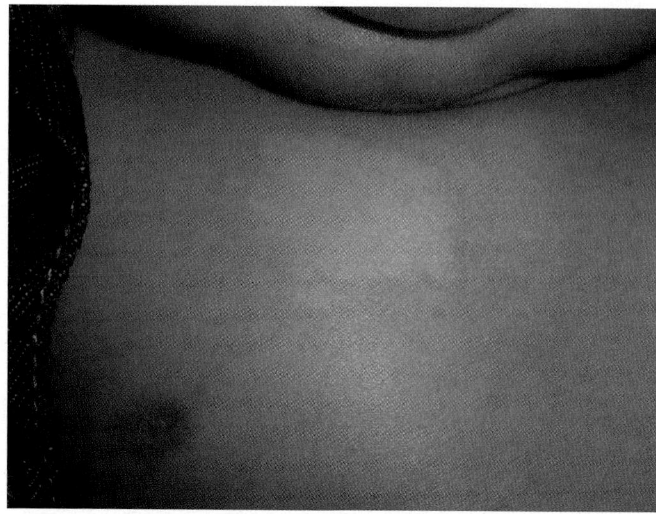

FIGURE 167-10 Nevus depigmentosus, present since birth, on the chest of this 4-month-old infant. Note the serrated or jagged edge. Vitiligo is not present at birth. (*Used with permission from Richard P. Usatine, MD.*)

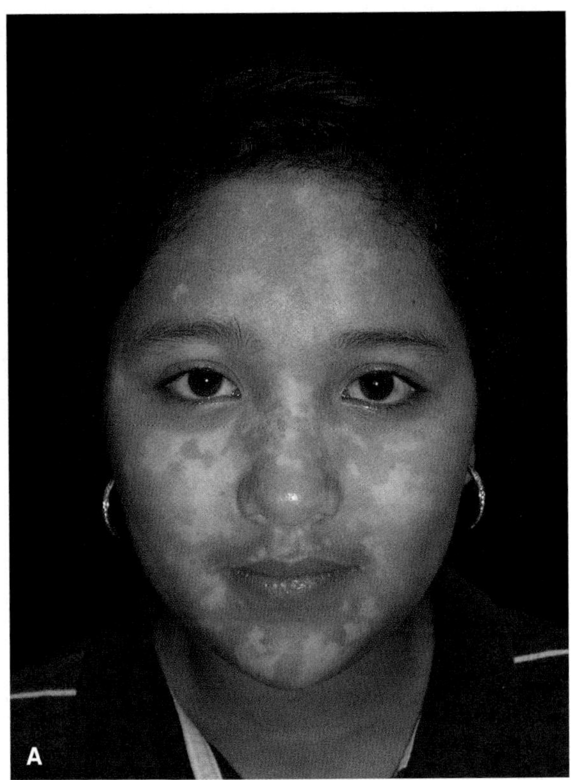

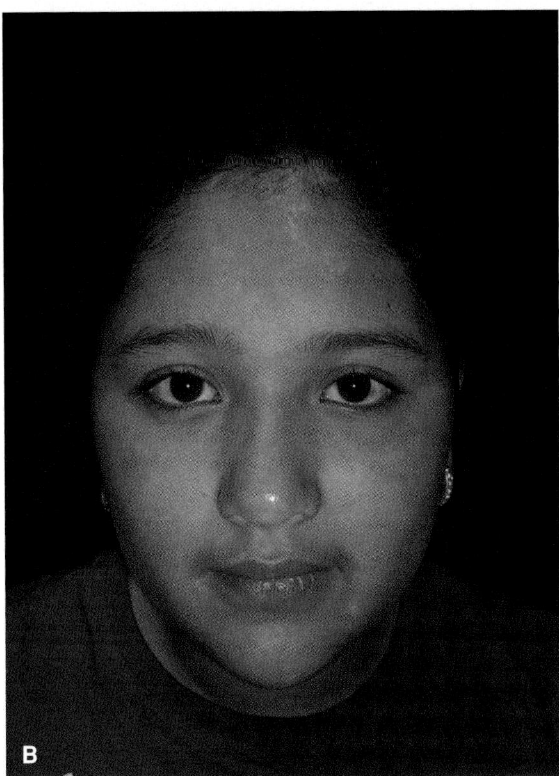

FIGURE 167-11 **A.** Vitiligo on the face of an 11-year-old girl. **B.** Significant resolution of the vitiligo 2 months later after using 0.1 percent triamcinolone cream once to twice daily. The patient and the mother were so happy with the results. There were no signs of skin atrophy or steroid side effects. *(Used with permission from Richard P. Usatine, MD.)*

- Management of inciting factors such as illness, stress, and skin trauma may be useful. SOR Ⓒ

MEDICATIONS

Topical treatments used for vitiligo include corticosteroids, immunomodulators, vitamin D analogs, and psoralens; these treatments had mixed outcomes based on a systematic review, with topical steroids having the highest rate of adverse events.[11] SOR Ⓑ Ineffective topical agents include melagenina, topical phenylalanine, topical L-DOPA (levodopa), coal tar, anacarcin forte oil, and minoxidil.[12]

- In a retrospective study of 101 children with vitiligo treated with moderate- to high-potency topical corticosteroids 64 percent (45/70) had repigmentation of the lesions, 24 percent (17/70) showed no change, and 11 percent (8/70) were worse than at the initial presentation.[13] SOR Ⓑ (**Figure 167-11**). Local steroid side effects were noted in 26 percent of patients at 81.7 ± 44 days of follow-up. Two children were given the diagnosis of steroid-induced adrenal suppression. Children with head and/or neck affected areas were eight times more likely to have an abnormal cortisol level compared with children who were affected in other body areas.[13] Therefore, a trial of topical steroids may be useful for patients with localized vitiligo that does not predominantly involve the head and neck. SOR Ⓒ
- Based on several reviews, topical corticosteroids (potent or very potent) are the preferred drugs for localized vitiligo (<20% of skin area);[11,12] a less-than-2-month trial is recommended.[12] SOR Ⓑ
- Topical immunomodulators (tacrolimus, pimecrolimus) are an alternative for localized vitiligo and display comparable effectiveness with fewer side effects.[14] SOR Ⓑ
- In a small case series (N = 6), various antitumor necrosis factor α agents (infliximab, etanercept, and adalimumab given according to treatment regimens used for psoriasis) were not effective for widespread nonsegmental vitiligo.[15]

COMPLEMENTARY/ALTERNATIVE THERAPY

- Antioxidants may be useful adjunctive therapy.[11]

OTHER TREATMENT

- Use sunscreen to prevent burns to the depigmented areas and further trauma to unaffected skin, and to minimize contrast between these areas.[14] SOR Ⓐ
- Bleaching the unaffected skin in patients with widespread depigmentation to reduce contrast with depigmented areas can improve cosmetic appearance.[14] SOR Ⓑ A monobenzylether of hydroquinone 20 percent cream (Benoquin) is available by prescription to produce a permanent bleaching of the skin around the vitiligo. It is irreversible and makes the skin at higher risk for sunburn.

PROCEDURES

- Combination therapies are likely to be more effective than monotherapy, and most combinations include a form of phototherapy; narrow-band UVB appears to be the most effective with the fewest adverse effects (**Figure 167-12**).[11,14] SOR Ⓑ Psoralen UVA (PUVA) is the second-best choice. Authors of a Cochrane review

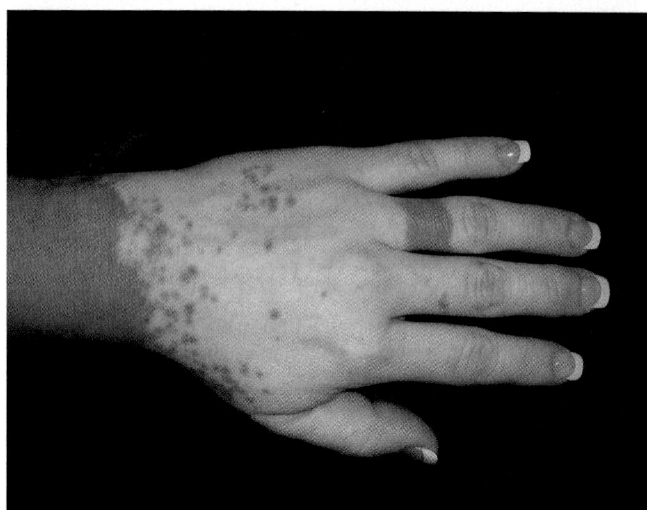

FIGURE 167-12 Vitiligo, which spared the area under a ring; the patient has spotty return of pigment on hand with narrowband UVB treatment. (*Used with permission from Richard P. Usatine, MD.*)

concurred that majority of analyses showing statistically significant differences in treatment outcomes were from studies that assessed combination interventions including some form of light treatment.[16]

- Excimer laser is an alternative to UVB therapy, achieving good responses especially in localized vitiligo of the face, where the excimer laser may be superior to UVB therapy. By combining with topical immunomodulators, treatment response can be accelerated.[14] SOR Ⓑ In one prospective study of 14 patients, repigmentation rates for once, twice, and thrice weekly treatment approached each other (60%, 79%, and 82%, respectively) at 12 weeks.[17] Although repigmentation occurred fastest with thrice weekly treatment, the final repigmentation depends on the total number of treatments, not their frequency. SOR Ⓑ
- No single therapy for vitiligo can be regarded as the most effective as the success of each treatment modality depends on the type and location of vitiligo. SOR Ⓑ

PROGNOSIS

The course of vitiligo varies, but is usually progressive with periods of activity interspersed with times of inactivity.[18] Spontaneous repigmentation can occur but is rare.

- The face and neck respond best to all therapeutic approaches, while the acral areas are least responsive.[14] SOR Ⓑ
- Vitiligo does not appear to be associated with adverse outcomes in pregnancy.[19]

FOLLOW-UP

- Counseling and emotional support are a mainstay of follow-up treatment.
- Trials of various combination therapies may be needed.

PATIENT EDUCATION

- Reassurance that this is a benign condition while acknowledging any psychological distress.
- Advise patients about the highly variable course of vitiligo with usually progressive periods of activity interspersed with times of inactivity.
- Inform patients about the multiple treatment options and possible need for prolonged or repeat treatment.

PATIENT RESOURCES

- National Institutes of Health. *Vitiligo*—**http://health.nih.gov/topic/Vitiligo**.
- National Organization for Albinism and Hypopigmentation—**http://www.healthfinder.gov/orgs/HR2242.htm**.
- National Vitiligo Foundation—**http://nvfi.org/index.php**.
- MedLine Plus. *Vitiligo*—**http://www.nlm.nih.gov/medlineplus/ency/article/003224.htm**.

PROVIDER RESOURCES

- Medscape. *Vitiligo*—**http: //emedicine.medscape.com/article/1068962**.
- National *Vitiligo* Foundation. A Handbook for Physicians—**http://nvfi.org/pages/info_physician_handbook.php**.

REFERENCES

1. Taïeb A, Picardo M; VETF Members: The definition and assessment of vitiligo: a consensus report of the Vitiligo European Task Force. *Pigment Cell Res*. 2007;20(1):27-35.
2. Njoo MD, Westerhof W. Vitiligo: pathogenesis and treatment. *Am J Clin Dermatol*. 2001;2(3):167-181.
3. Krüger C, Schallreuter KU. A review of the worldwide prevalence of vitiligo in children/adolescents and adults. *Int J Dermatol*. 2012 Mar 27. doi: 10.1111/j.1365-4632.2011.05377.x. [Epub ahead of print].
4. Karaca N, Ozturk G, Gerceker BT, et al. TLR2 and TLR4 gene polymorphisms in Turkish vitiligo patients. *J Eur Acad Dermatol Venereol*. 2012 Mar 16. doi: 10.1111/j.1468-3083.2012.04514.x. [Epub ahead of print].
5. Alghamdi KM, Kumar A, Taïeb A, Ezzedine K. Assessment methods for the evaluation of vitiligo. *J Eur Acad Dermatol Venereol*. 2012 Mar 15. doi: 10.1111/j.1468-3083.2012.04505.x. [Epub ahead of print].
6. Schallreuter KU, Lemke R, Brandt O, et al. Vitiligo and other diseases: coexistence or true association? Hamburg study on 321 patients. *Dermatology*. 1994;188(4):269-275.
7. Hegedüs L, Heidenheim M, Gervil M, et al. High frequency of thyroid dysfunction in patients with vitiligo. *Acta Derm Venereol*. 1994;74(2):120-123.
8. Rogosić V, Bojić L, Puizina-Ivić N, et al. Vitiligo and glaucoma – an association or a coincidence? A pilot study. *Acta Dermatovenerol Croat*. 2010;18(1):21-26.

9. Barona MI, Arrunátegui A, Falabella R, Alzate A. An epidemiologic case-control study in a population with vitiligo. *J Am Acad Dermatol*. 1995;33(4):621-625.

10. Hacker SM. Common disorders of pigmentation: When are more than cosmetic cover-ups required? *Postgrad Med*. 1996;99(6):177-186.

11. Bacigalupi RM, Postolova A, Davis RS. Evidence-based, non-surgical treatments for vitiligo: a review. *Am J Clin Dermatol*. 2012 Mar 16. doi: 10.2165/11630540–000000000-00000. [Epub ahead of print].

12. Hossani-Madani AR, Halder RM. Topical treatment and combination approaches for vitiligo: new insights, new developments. *G Ital Dermatol Venereol*. 2010;145(1):57-78.

13. Kwinter J, Pelletier J, Khambalia A, Pope E. High-potency steroid use in children with vitiligo: a retrospective study. *J Am Acad Dermatol*. 2007;56(2):236-241.

14. Forschner T, Buchholtz S, Stockfleth E. Current state of vitiligo therapy—evidence-based analysis of the literature. *J Dtsch Dermatol Ges*. 2007;5(6):467-475.

15. Alghamdi KM, Khurrum H, Taieb A, Ezzedine K. Treatment of generalized vitiligo with anti-TNF-α agents. *J Drugs Dermatol*. 2012;11(4):534-539.

16. Whitton ME, Pinart M, Batchelor J, et al. Interventions for vitiligo. *Cochrane Database Syst Rev*. 2010;(1):CD003263.

17. Hofer A, Hassan AS, Legat FJ, et al. Optimal weekly frequency of 308-nm excimer laser treatment in vitiligo patients. *Br J Dermatol*. 2005;152(5):981-985.

18. Viles J, Monte D, Gawkrodger DJ. Vitiligo. *BMJ*. 2010;341:c3780.

19. Horev A, Weintraub AY, Sergienko R, et al. Pregnancy outcome in women with vitiligo. *Int J Dermatol*. 2011;50(9):1083-1085.

168 DISORDERS OF HYPERPIGMENTATION

Sigrid M Collier, MD
Jennifer Krejci-Mannwaring, MD
Richard P. Usatine, MD

PATIENT STORY

A 7-year-old African American girl was brought to her pediatrician by her mom who was worried that she was itching and that her skin was getting darker. The pediatrician knew the girl well as a patient with asthma and allergic rhinitis. In fact, the girl performed the allergic salute more than once in the office as she rubbed her itchy nose. Morgan-Dennie lines were seen under her eyes (**Figure 168-1A**). The mom undressed the girl to show the dark patches of skin around her knees (**Figure 168-1B**). Atopic dermatitis is common in the popliteal fossae and this girl clearly demonstrated the atopic triad: atopic dermatitis, asthma, and allergic rhinitis. The darkening of the skin around the knees and also seen on the neck is related to the scratching and rubbing of the skin secondary to the pruritus of atopic dermatitis. The pediatrician explained to the mom and child about the need to more aggressively treat the atopic dermatitis with emollients and topical steroids. No promises were made about the reversibility of the hyperpigmentation as each patient will respond differently to treatment.

INTRODUCTION

Postinflammatory hyperpigmentation (PIH) is an accumulation of melanin in response to chronic inflammation that usually appears as brown, black, or grey macules or patches in the pattern of an underlying inflammatory condition. Postinflammatory hyperpigmentation can result from any kind of irritant to the skin, but is more common in conditions resulting in chronic irritation and inflammation, and is more common in individuals with darker Fitzpatrick Skin Types IV, V, and VI. It is more severe and longer lasting if the underlying inflammatory condition goes untreated though most PIH will fade within 6 to 12 months of treating the underlying inflammatory condition. For the girl in the preceding case, the PIH may resolve without treatment after her atopic dermatitis clears up, but if the atopic dermatitis persists then the PIH will continue until the resolution of the underlying condition.

EPIDEMIOLOGY

- The prevalence of disorders of hyperpigmentation including post-inflammatory hyperpigmentation in the general population ranges from 0.42 percent in Kuwait to 55.9 percent in a sample population from Michigan.[1]
- The prevalence in children in the US is around 22 percent based on a sample of hospitalized children in Kentucky.[2]

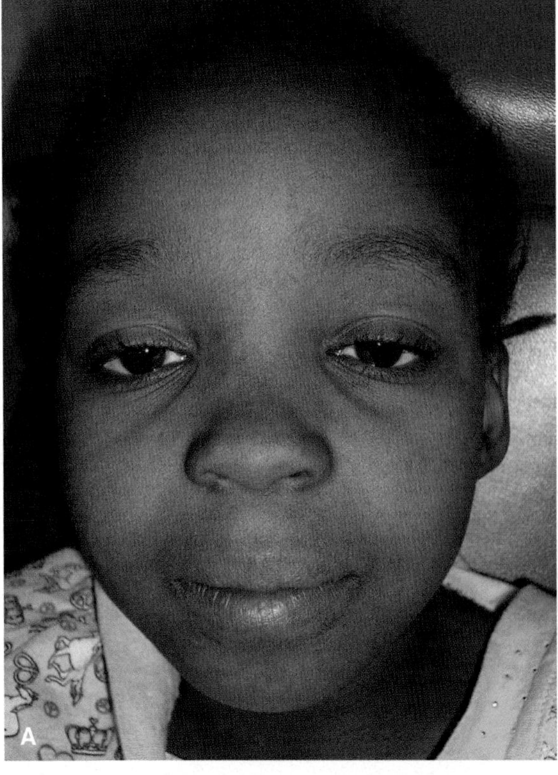

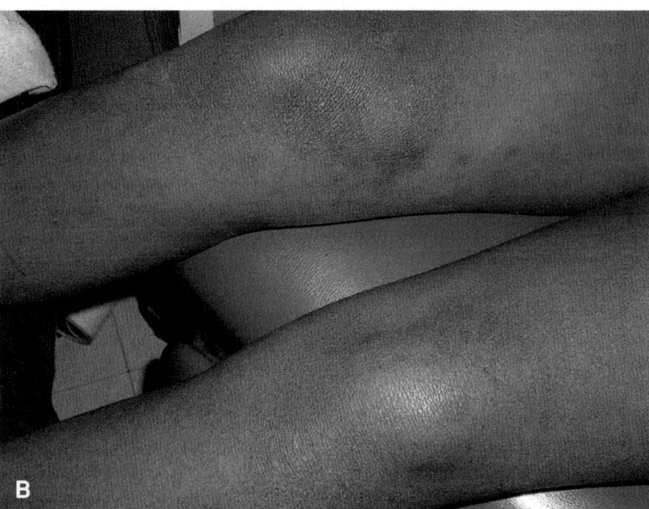

FIGURE 168-1 **A.** Atopic triad in a 7-year-old girl with Dennie-Morgan lines and a nasal crease. **B.** Postinflammatory hyperpigmentation around the knees in the same girl. (*Used with permission from Richard P. Usatine, MD.*)

- Postinflammatory hyperpigmentation (PIH) is one of the most common types of cutaneous hyperpigmentation, and although there are no good estimates of its prevalence in the children of the US, studies in Nigeria estimate PIH to represent 49.5 percent of skin lesions present in hospitalized children.[3] In studies of adults, "dyschromia" is often used to combine disorders of hyperpigmentation, which would include melasma, lentigines, and PIH so true prevalence is difficult to obtain. In one study dyschromia was the second most common diagnosis among African American patients, but failed to make it into the top 10 for Caucasian patients.[4]
- The distribution of PIH is equal among males and females of all ages.[5]
- PIH is more common in dark-skinned individuals (Fitzpatrick skin types IV, V, and VI), and therefore is frequently found in individuals from Asia, Africa (**Figure 168-2**), South America, and Native Americans.[6]
- The age at which a child could present with a hyperpigmented lesion varies, and PIH, erythema ab igne, and confluent and reticulated papillomatosis (CARP) are more common in older children and young adults versus young children (**Figure 168-3**).[7]
- Other hyperpigmented lesions such as "linear and whorled hypermelanosis," nevus of Ota, and Café au Lait spots are linked to embryologic mosaicism or genetic abnormalities, and may be seen at birth or within a few weeks after birth (**Figures 168-4** and **168-5**). Mongolian spots are nearly always present at birth (**Figure 168-6**).[7]
- Just as PIH is most common in darker-skinned individuals, Nevus of Ota, Mongolian spot, Café au Lait macules, and CARP are more common in Asians and Blacks.[7] Conversely, linear and whorled hypermelanosis shows no racial predilection.[8]

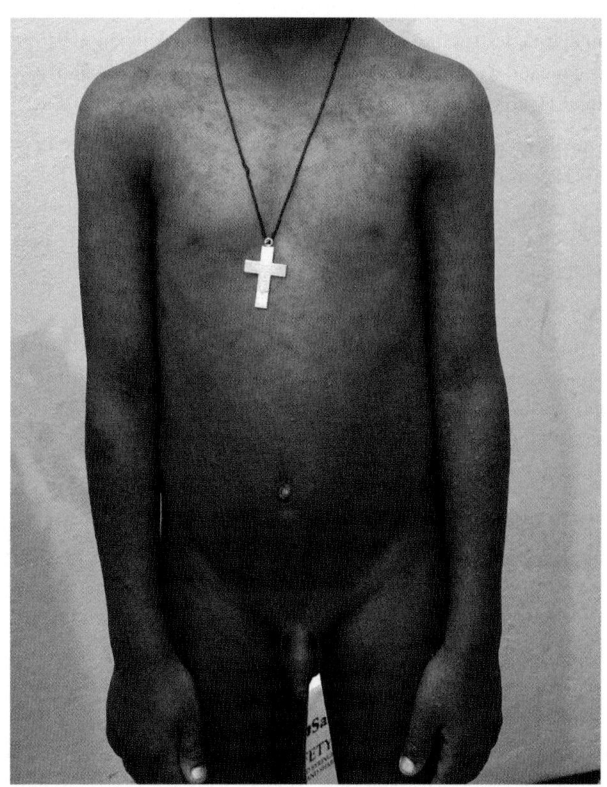

FIGURE 168-2 An African boy with a long history of atopic dermatitis and newly diagnosed scabies. Note how the postinflammatory hyperpigmentation is concentrated around the waist and forearms. (*Used with permission from Richard P. Usatine, MD.*)

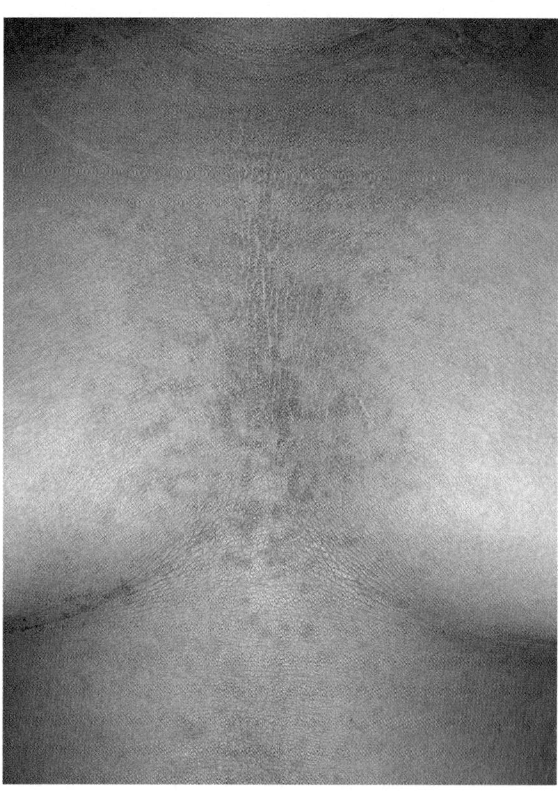

FIGURE 168-3 Confluent and reticulated papillomatosis (CARP) in an obese 15-year-old boy with gynecomastia. (*Used with permission from Richard P. Usatine, MD.*)

ETIOLOGY AND PATHOPHYSIOLOGY

- The most common causes of postinflammatory hyperpigmentation are acne vulgaris, atopic dermatitis (**Figure 168-7**), and impetigo, but any insult to the skin from bug bites and minor burns to drug reactions and other rashes can result in postinflammatory hyperpigmentation.[1,5]
- Postinflammatory hyperpigmentation may be divided based on whether the pigment accumulates in the epidermis or in the dermis.

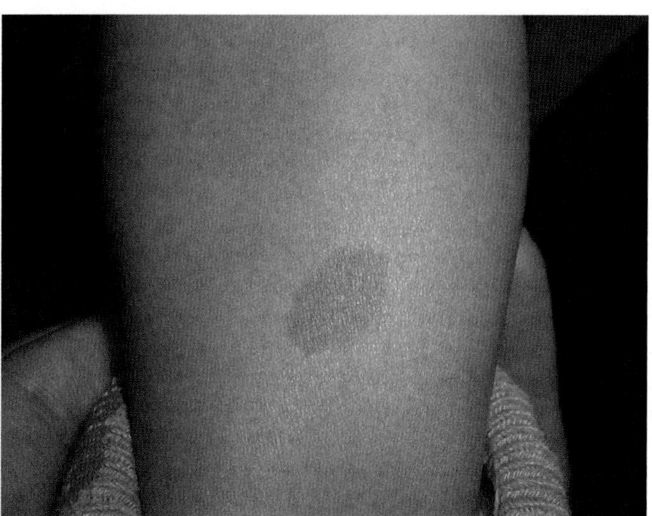

FIGURE 168-4 Café au lait macule in a girl found to have tuberous sclerosis. (*Used with permission from Richard P. Usatine, MD.*)

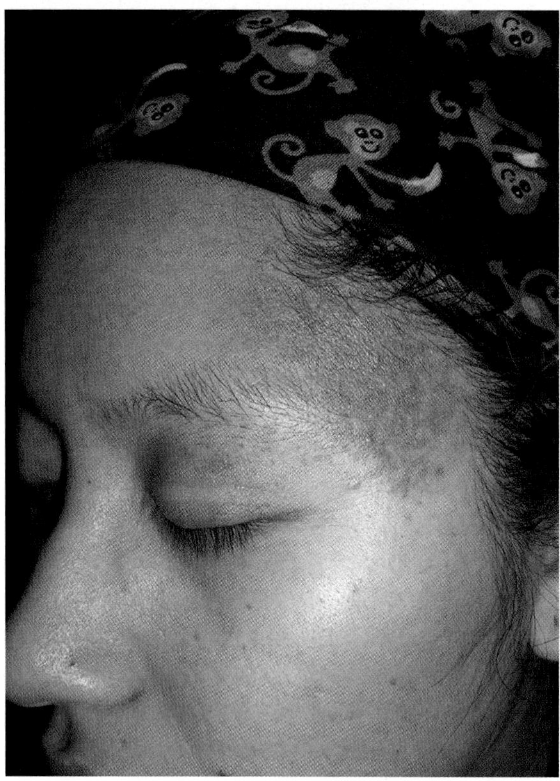

FIGURE 168-5 Nevus of the Ota with a blue-gray coloration around the eye. (*Used with permission from Richard P. Usatine, MD.*)

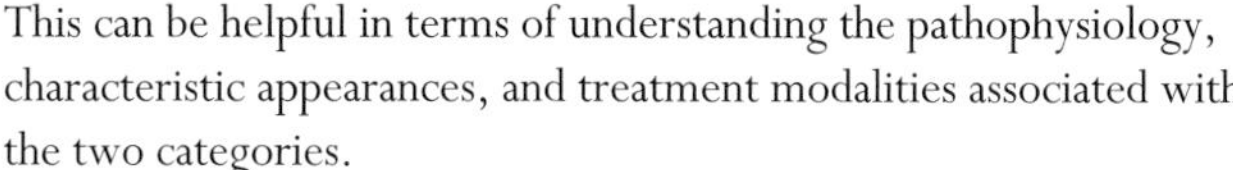

This can be helpful in terms of understanding the pathophysiology, characteristic appearances, and treatment modalities associated with the two categories.

- Epidermal hyperpigmentation is thought to be in part caused by the release of inflammatory molecules such as prostanoids, cytokines, chemokines, and other products of arachidonic acid which leads to increased melanocyte activity, increased melanin production and release, and accumulation of melanin in adjacent keratinocytes.[1,5,9,10]

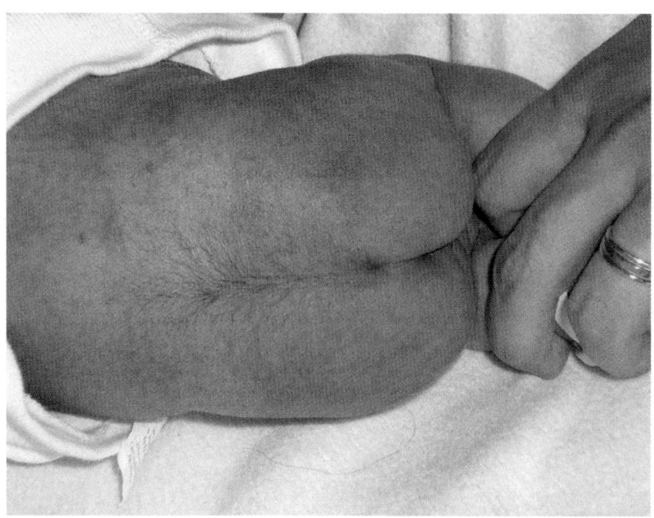

FIGURE 168-6 Dermal melanocytosis (Mongolian spot) over the buttocks of a newborn. (*Used with permission from Richard P. Usatine, MD.*)

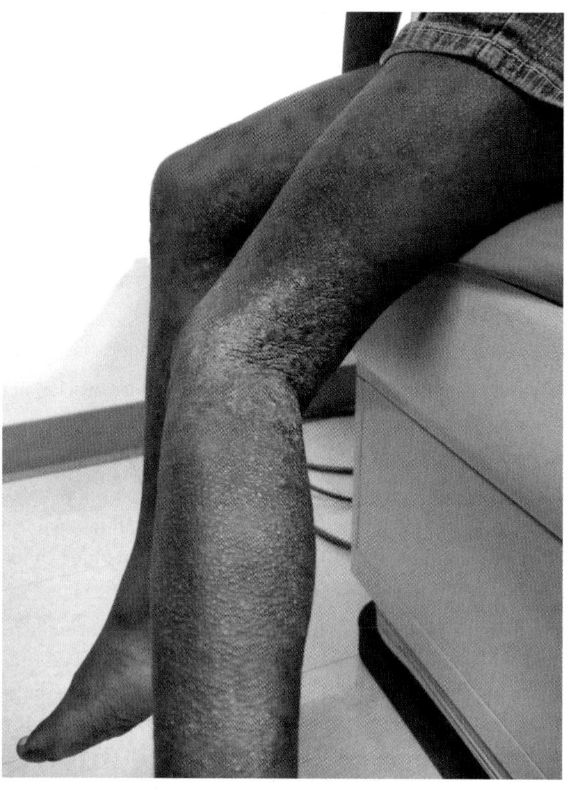

FIGURE 168-7 Postinflammatory hyperpigmentation over the legs in a black child with severe atopic dermatitis. (*Used with permission from John Browning, MD.*)

- Dermal hyperpigmentation is thought to result from inflammatory mediated destruction of keratinocytes, which results in melanin release and its accumulation within macrophages in the upper dermis.[1] Histologically this is described as "pigment incontinence."
- The distinction between accumulation of pigment in the epidermis and accumulation of pigment in the dermis is reflected in the appearance of the lesion on the skin. Dermal lesions tend to be a blue-gray color with indistinct boundaries and epidermal lesions tend to be tan, brown, or dark brown and with more sharply demarcated borders.[1,11]
- In other disorders of hyperpigmentation the connection between the pathophysiology and the cutaneous appearance also exists; the color and shape of the pigment generally reflects both the location of melanin and the degree of melanocytic hyperplasia or release of melanin.[7]

DIAGNOSIS

CLINICAL FEATURES

- The degree of pigmentation is strongly correlated with the total duration of the inflammatory process, where chronic or relapsing inflammatory processes cause darker and longer lasting hyperpigmentation.[1]
- Darker-skinned individuals have larger and more densely distributed melanin pigment in their skin. In turn, they tend to react to inflammation with more accumulation of pigment, and therefore PIH tends to present with darker lesions that last longer.[1,12]

- UV exposure is also associated with darkening and persistence of hyperpigmented lesions.[13]
- The location of the pigmentation in the skin also effects the persistence of PIH, and dermal hyperpigmentation tends to last longer since the dermis does not continuously turnover like the epidermis.[13]

TYPICAL DISTRIBUTION

- Postinflammatory hyperpigmentation typically follows the pattern of the initial inflammatory process and consists of macules or patches.[12]

LABORATORY AND IMAGING

- A Wood's lamp examination can be used to distinguish between epidermal and dermal hyperpigmentation, where epidermal lesions will have distinct margins and a prominent border whereas dermal lesions will have fluffy, indistinct margins.[5]

BIOPSY

In general, skin biopsies are unnecessary, but if the etiology is uncertain a 4-mm punch biopsy can help determine the underlying cause of PIH. The Fontana-Masson stain is used to identify melanin in the skin and is useful in distinguishing between epidermal and dermal hyperpigmentation.[5]

DIFFERENTIAL DIAGNOSIS

- CARP is characterized by hyperkeratotic or verrucous scaly brown papules that coalesce into plaques, with peripheral reticular pattern with or without pruritus (**Figure 168-8**). It is generally first seen in inframammary region or interscapular region, and often spreads to the chest or abdomen (**Figure 168-3**). It can be found on the face, neck, extremities, flanks, or gluteal cleft. The etiology is unknown, but potential causes include a keratinization disorder, a reaction to a fungal or bacterial infection, photosensitivity, amyloidosis, and genetic factors.[14,15]

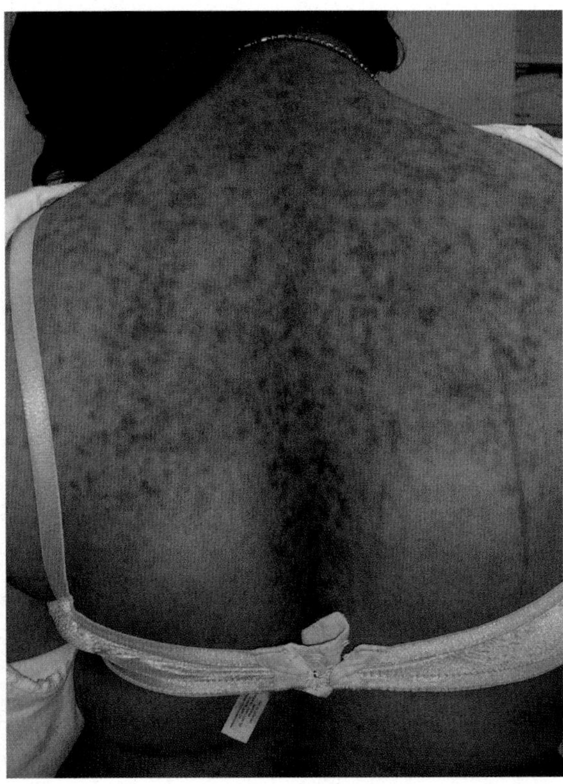

FIGURE 168-8 Confluent and reticulated papillomatosis (CARP) on the back of an African American girl. (*Used with permission from Richard P. Usatine, MD.*)

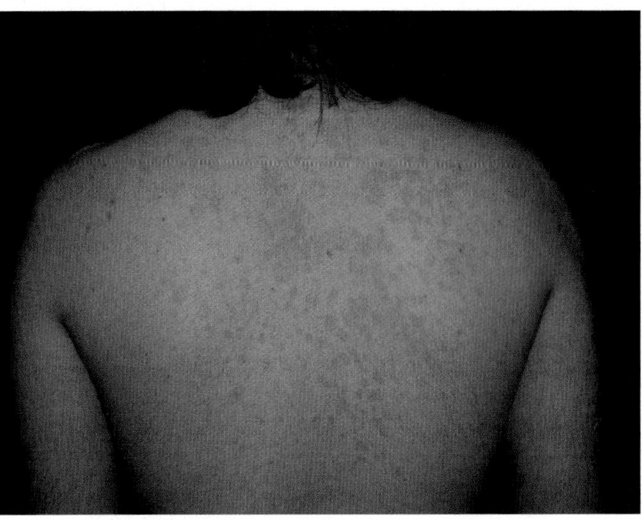

FIGURE 168-9 Tinea versicolor on the back of a 16-year-old boy. Note the pinkish brown coloration. (*Used with permission from Richard P. Usatine, MD.*)

CARP can be distinguished from PIH both clinically and by its unique histology. CARP is raised and keratotic papules and plaques on the torso while PIH is typically flat macules or patches where there were previous lesions. Tinea versicolor occurs in a similar distribution to CARP (on the torso) but tinea versicolor is scaly patches and responds to oral or topical antifungal therapy (**Figures 168-9** and **168-10**).

CARP is a rare disorder, but it is most commonly seen in young adults (ages 18 to 21), and people with skin of color. In the US, it is more common in females than in males, but the gender distribution varies in different parts of the world. Minocycline is

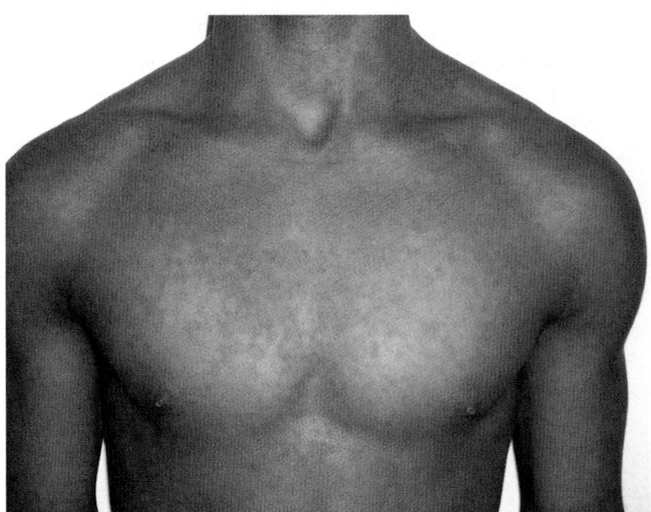

FIGURE 168-10 Tinea versicolor with a cape-like distribution over the chest in a black teenage boy. Note how the Malassezia furfur has caused a brown hyperpigmentation. (*Used with permission from Richard P. Usatine, MD.*)

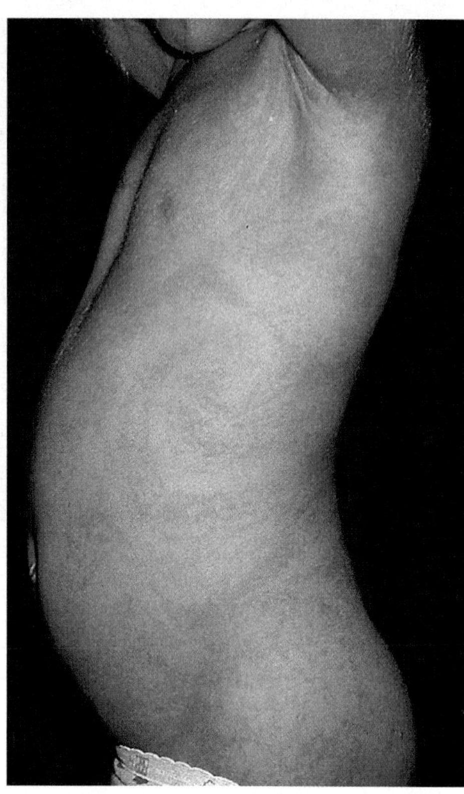

FIGURE 168-11 Linear and whorled hypermelanosis has been present since birth in this otherwise healthy child. (*Used with permission from Kane KS, Lio P, Stratigos AJ, Johnson RA. Color Atlas and Synopsis of Pediatric Dermatology, 2nd edition, Figure 12-8, New York, NY: McGraw-Hill, 2009.*)

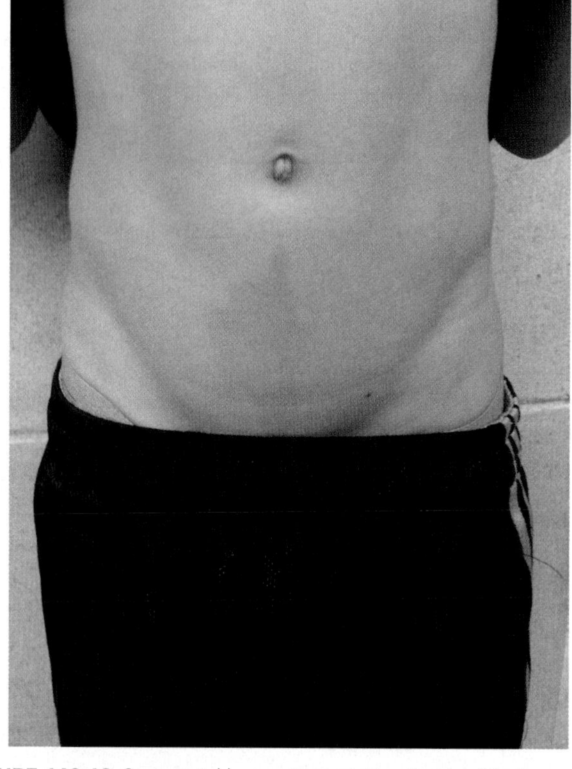

FIGURE 168-12 Segmental hyperpigmentation in a healthy 8-year-old boy. Lesion appeared shortly after birth as a faint patch and became more apparent in early childhood. (*Used with permission from Jennifer Krejci-Mannwaring, MD.*)

considered the first line treatment, but azithromycin, clarithromycin, fusidic acid, and retinoic acid have also been effective in case reports and case studies.[14]

- Linear and Whorled Hypermelanosis (LAWH; **Figure 168-11**) is characterized by linear and whorled patches that occur along the lines of Blaschko (lines of embryological development).[16] The lesions can occur anywhere on the body, but typically spare the mucous membranes, palms, soles, and eyes.[16] LAWH appears within a few weeks of birth and will progressively expand and darken until the child is 1 to 2 years of age. The exact cause of LAWH is unknown, but it may be associated with underlying genetic mosaicism.[8] There have been a few cases where LAWH was associated with neurologic abnormalities, but the association is very rare.[16,17] In general, there is no need to do neurologic testing or brain imaging if the child seems normal and healthy.[8]
- Segmental Hyperpigmentation presents at birth or in early childhood as a hyperpigmented patch on the truck with a characteristic delineation at midline, usually ventral giving them a dermatomal appearance (**Figure 168-12**). They are typically not Blaschkoid like LAWH and are more geometric than CALMs. There are no known associated abnormalities and is thought to be due to a somatic mosaicism.[18]
- Erythema ab igne is reticular tan-brown pigmented patch (**Figure 168-13**). It is most commonly caused by prolonged exposure to heat or infrared.[19] Although it is rare in children, it has been reported in children who use laptop computers directly on their

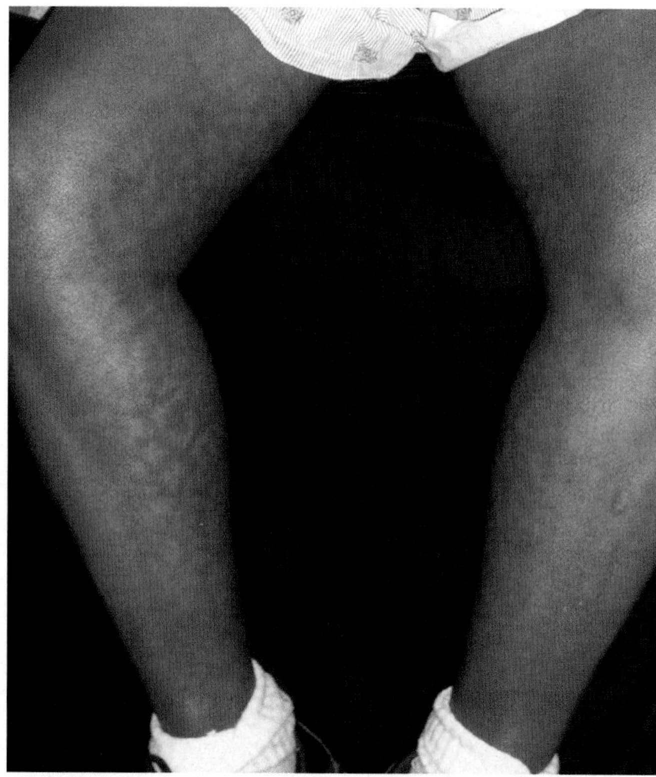

FIGURE 168-13 Erythema ab igne caused by repeated straddling of a place heater in an attempt to keep warm in a home without central heating. (*Used with permission from Richard P. Usatine, MD.*)

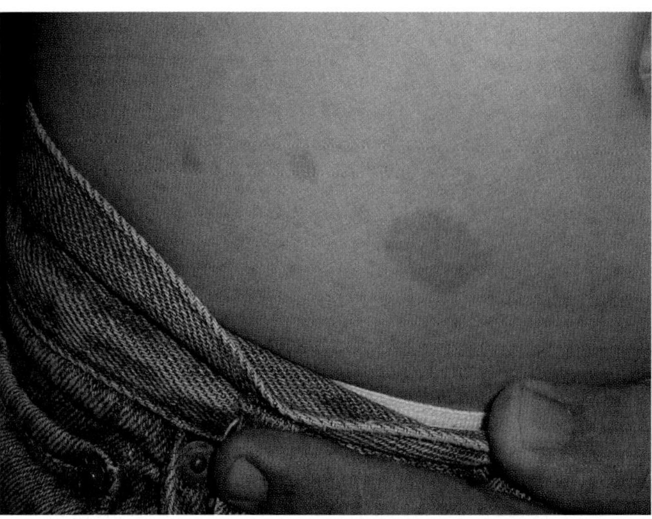

FIGURE 168-14 Café au lait macule in a child with neurofibromatosis. (*Used with permission from Richard P. Usatine, MD.*)

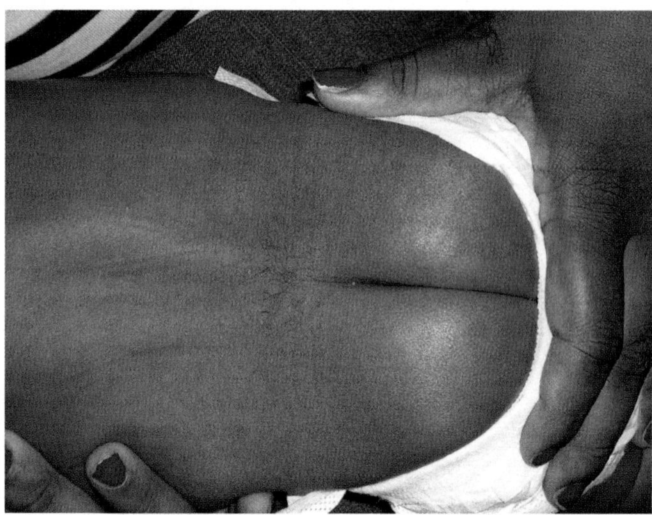

FIGURE 168-15 Dermal melanocytosis (Mongolian spot) in a black infant. (*Used with permission from Richard P. Usatine, MD.*)

laps.[19] Other common causes include hot-water bottles, heating pads, and heated blankets. It is generally a self-limited condition, but prolonged exposure and recurrence of the lesions may predispose to squamous cell carcinoma or Merkel cell carcinoma.[19]

- Café au Lait Macules (CALMs) are evenly pigmented light brown macules or patches (**Figure 168-14**). They are commonly solitary and present at birth though they can appear any time in the first few years of life.[20] CALMs are also more common in blacks than whites. If CALMs continue to appear into adulthood or are multiple this warrants further investigation as these characteristics increase the likelihood of a coexisting condition like neurofibromatosis, tuberous sclerosis, McCune-Albright, or Noonan syndrome (**Figures 168-4** and **168-14**).[20] There is no medical reason to treat CALMs. These lesions are caused by epidermal melanin, giant melanosomes, and increased melanocyte density. Skin lightening creams are not effective, but several lasers have been used with variable responses including Pulsed Dye, Erbium:YAG, Q-Switched Nd:YAG, QS Ruby, and QS Alexandrite. The risks of laser surgery include hypo/hyperpigmentation, scarring, incomplete removal, and recurrence.[21]
- Dermal Melanocytosis (Mongolian Spot) is a blue-gray hyperpigmented patch that can vary in size, but is most commonly found on the gluteal region of newborns and infants (**Figure 168-15**).[22] It is most prevalent in individuals of Asian and African ancestry, but it can occur in individuals of any race. The lesion is benign, has no known association with other congenital abnormalities, and will disappear in most children by the age of 4 but sometimes persists.[22] Given the likelihood of spontaneous regression, there is no need for treatment.
- Ashy Dermatosis (Erythema Dyschromicum Perstans [EDP]) is characterized by blue-gray macules that may have a raised erythematous border.[23] They are most often found on the trunk, extremities, and neck (**Figures 168-16** and **168-17**). These lesions of unknown etiology are chronic and may grow larger and multiply over time. The prevalence is highest among Latin Americans though other races can be affected. EDP most commonly presents between the ages of 10 and 30, but can occur at any age.[23] The treatment of EDP is limited and lesions are often permanent. Many therapies have been attempted but none are very effective.[24]
- Nevus of Ota (oculodermal melanocytosis) is a speckled blue-gray or brown macular lesion that follows a dermatomal distribution usually unilaterally within the distribution of the ophthalmic and maxillary branches of the trigeminal nerve. In addition to skin, it may involve ocular and oral mucosal surfaces (**Figure 168-18**).[25] These lesions represent a hamartoma of dermal melanocytes. Nevus Of Ito is the same process on the body and usually found on the shoulder. These lesions are often present at birth and tend to darken and expand with age. It is more commonly seen in Asian children, but can occur in any race and shows no gender predilection. The risk of malignant transformation in Nevus of Ota/Ito is extremely rare but there is up to 10 percent risk of glaucoma if the eye is involved. Nevus of Ota have also been associated with Sturge-Weber, Klippel-Trenaunay-Weber, and neurodevelopmental abnormalities.[25] These risks make close follow-up important in pediatric patients. This

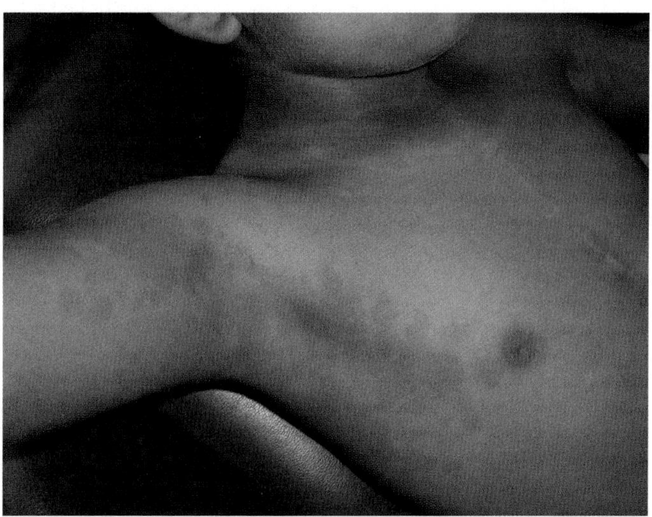

FIGURE 168-16 Ashy dermatosis (erythema dyschromicum perstans) in an 8-year-old boy that was confirmed by a punch biopsy. (*Used with permission from Richard P. Usatine, MD.*)

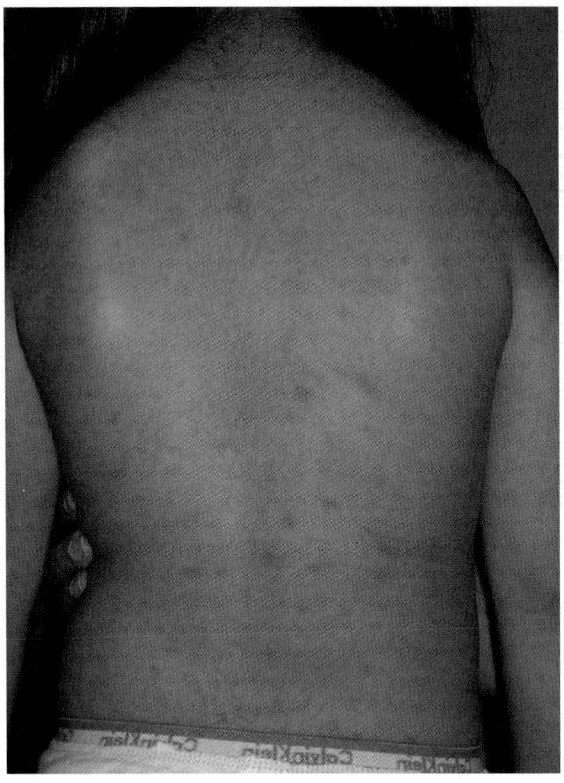

FIGURE 168-17 Ashy dermatosis (erythema dyschromicum perstans) in a 4-year-old girl. (*Used with permission from Richard P. Usatine, MD.*)

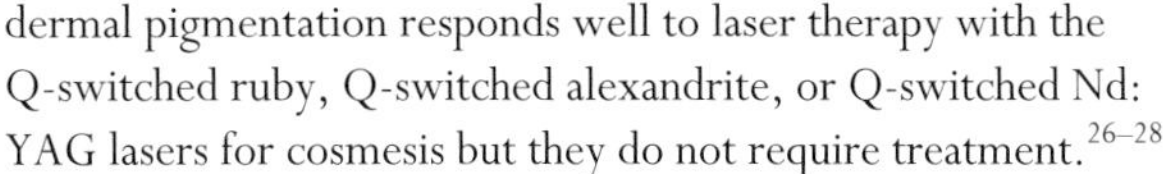

dermal pigmentation responds well to laser therapy with the Q-switched ruby, Q-switched alexandrite, or Q-switched Nd: YAG lasers for cosmesis but they do not require treatment.[26–28]

- In children with pigmented lesions, it is especially important to consider and rule out child abuse as a possibly cause.[12] Bruising or PIH that is linear or geometric in nature should raise concern for abuse. Also, lesions of abuse on the back or buttocks in a child can mimic EDP or dermal melanocytosis (**Figure 168-19**); however, traumatic lesions will fade quickly compared to the latter.

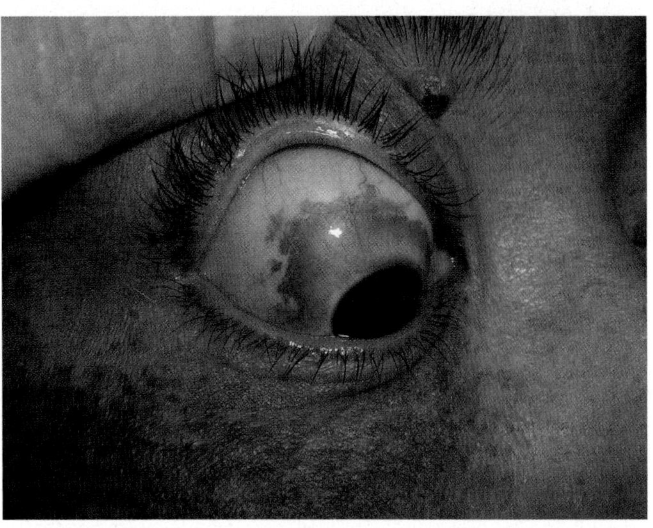

FIGURE 168-18 Nevus of Ota around the eye with blue-gray scleral hyperpigmentation. (*Used with permission from Richard P. Usatine, MD.*)

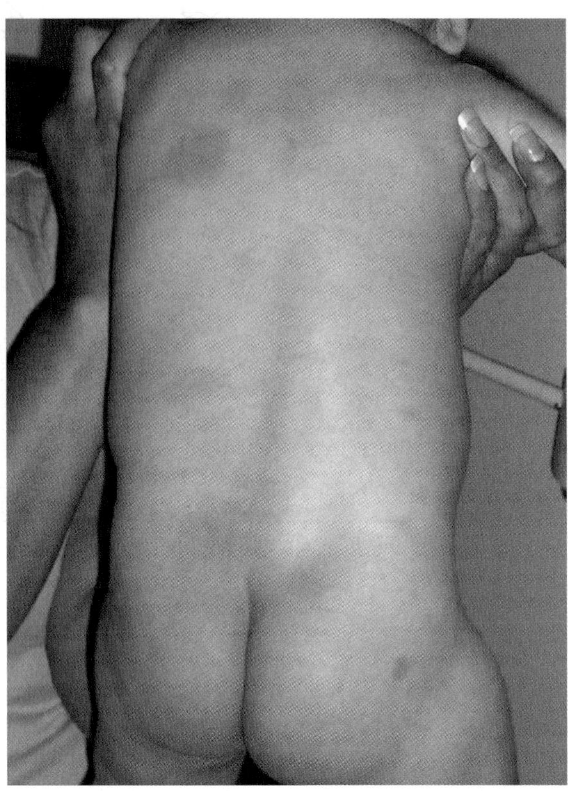

FIGURE 168-19 Multiple patches of dermal melanocytosis (Mongolian spots) on the back and buttocks of a young black child. (*Used with permission from Richard P. Usatine, MD.*)

MANAGEMENT

The first step in the management of PIH is to ascertain the underlying cause of cutaneous inflammation or trauma and rule out other causes of pigmented lesions.

The shape and distribution of the lesions should mirror the pattern of the underlying disorder and most patients with PIH will have a history of chronic skin disease or trauma. When there is no history of a chronic skin condition it is important to consider congenital diseases or other causes of hyperpigmentation, see differential diagnoses, which was previously discussed.

If the underlying cause is a treatable condition then prompt treatment is essential. Decreasing the development of additional PIH requires controlling the source of cutaneous inflammation.[12]

NONPHARMACOLOGIC

- The first line of therapy for PIH is *daily* sunscreen use. Daily use of sunscreen with an SPF of 30 or greater has been shown to decrease the duration of postinflammatory hyperpigmentation and to prevent darkening of existing lesions.[1] Any gains made with topical or other therapies can quickly be undone by short exposures to ultraviolet light. Behavior modification often requires additional patient/parent education. While darker skin types are more prone to pigmentary disorder they may not be as familiar sun protection behaviors given that they have a lower propensity for sunburn. “Physical sunscreens” (ones that are zinc or titanium based) are preferred, however, on darkly pigmented skin they may leave a gray or violaceous hue when applied and therefore an aesthetically acceptable product may be tricky. Sun protection should also include avoidance of peak sun hours (10 am to 4 pm), the use of wide brimmed hats, and long sleeves or pants depending on the body part affected.

TOPICAL TREATMENTS

- Various topical skin-lightening agents have been used to treat PIH and other disorders of hyperpigmentation. The treatments include topical medication such as hydroquinone, retinoids, mequinol, azelaic acid, kojic acid, and licorice extract, ascorbic acid, niacinamide, N-acetyl glucosamine, and soy.[1,12,29] In general, topical skin-lightening agents are most effective on epidermal pigmentation and less effective for dermal hyperpigmentation.[12]
- The first line in topical treatment for PIH is hydroquinone, which can be used at various concentrations though there is no increase in efficacy at concentrations higher than 5 percent.[13,30] Controlled trials have shown a decrease in skin hyperpigmentation as compared to baseline by 4 weeks after beginning therapy.[31] The potential side effects include allergic dermatitis (most common), the development of a ring of hypopigmentation around the lesions, and rarely paradoxical darkening of the lesions (exogenous ochronosis).[32]
- Combination therapies with hydroquinone show additional efficacy. Small trials of 4 percent hydroquinone and 0.15 percent retinol have shown significant improvement in the degree of pigmentation and the lesion size.[31] Triple therapies combining 4 percent hydroquinone, 0.1 percent tretinoin, or 0.5 percent ascorbic acid, and topical steroids (dexamethasone or fluocinolone acetonide) resulted in higher rates of complete skin clearing of melasma than either hydroquinone monotherapy or dual therapy, but there is no such trial on the use of triple therapy in PIH.[33]
- There is some evidence for the efficacy of tretinoin (retinoic acid) as monotherapy in the treatment of PIH. In one randomized control trial, 91 percent of the participants in the treatment group had significant lightening of their lesions compared to 57 percent in the control group based on clinical evaluation.[34]
- There is some limited clinical evidence for the efficacy of such compounds as kojic acid, arbutin, niacinamide, n-acetyl glucosamine, ascorbic acid, licorice extract, and soy in treating hyperpigmentation. Most of the evidence for the efficacy of these naturally occurring chemicals is from trials for the treatment of melasma.[29] Of the agents listed, topical soy extract is the only agent with significant evidence in PIH.[13] Many of these compounds are marketed in over-the-counter products and may also contain derivatives of retinoic acid such as retinol or retinyl.

PROCEDURES

- The most common procedures used in the treatment of hyperpigmented lesions are chemical peels and laser therapy. Both have been shown to be efficacious in randomized controlled trials, but they remain second-line treatments and are generally only indicated in combination with or after treatment with topical agents have failed.[21]
- Chemical peels are used to treat hyperpigmentation.[13] The chemical agents used for these procedures include glycolic acid (GA), salicylic acid, and trichloracetic acid.[35,36] In general, superficial peels are recommended for people with skin of color to decrease the risk of additional postinflammatory hyperpigmentation. Side effects of chemical peels include erythema, burning/stinging, hypo/hyperpigmentation, ulceration, scarring, reactivation of HSV, and superficial desquamation. Repeated peels (5 or more) are often needed to achieve results.
- A few randomized controlled trials have indicated that the use of GA chemical peels in addition to hydroquinone therapy was as effective in PIH as hydroquinone therapy and tended to work more quickly with more dramatic results.[37] There is little data in the current literature assessing the safety of these therapies in children, though there are a few case reports of good outcomes in children with xeroderma pigmentosum and congenital melanocytic nevi.[38,39]
- Lasers are used in the treatment of hyperpigmentation. Q-switch alexandrite, Q-switch ruby, Q-switch Nd:YAG, and nonablative fractional protolysis laser treatments have been effective in treatment of many hyperpigmented lesions including PIH, Mongolian Spots, Nevus of Ota, and Café Au Lait Macules.[21,40,41] The wavelength of the system should be correctly matched to the depth of the lesion, and epidermal hyperpigmentation tends to respond best to shorter wavelengths, whereas dermal hyperpigmentation tends to respond best to longer wavelengths.[41] Great care must also be taken to avoid increasing the pigmentation of the lesion or inducing postinflammatory hyperpigmentation, as both of these are known potential side effects of laser therapy.[40] A review of laser use in children concluded that laser therapies are safe in children and in some cases are more efficacious than in adults.[41]

PROGNOSIS

- The course of postinflammatory hyperpigmentation is strongly dependent on controlling the underlying inflammatory disease. Once the underlying disease is treated most epidermal hyperpigmentation will resolve in 6 to 12 months, and with treatment the lesions may resolve as quickly as 4 weeks.[5,31] Dermal hyperpigmentation has a comparatively prolonged course, and lesions can persist for years or be permanent despite treatment.[5]

FOLLOW-UP

- The first step for children with PIH is to treat the underlying cause. Once the cause is treated simple reassurance and regular follow-up may be sufficient. More aggressive treatment should be considered for lesions in aesthetically sensitive areas such as the face, or, if the child experiences significant psychological distress.
- In children with congenital hyperpigmented lesions that may lead to psychological distress, consider initiating treatment early but to give parents realistic expectations. Most congenital or persistent lesions, if responsive, will do so to more invasive treatments such as laser therapy.

PATIENT EDUCATION

- PIH will generally resolve spontaneously over time, and the primary objective is to identify and eliminate the cause of inflammation in the skin.

- Strict sun protection may prevent worsening of PIH and can help it fade more quickly.
- If PIH persists, there are other treatment options but they have variable effectiveness and side effects and should be reserved for cases that have not resolved with watchful waiting.

PATIENT RESOURCES

- **www.nlm.nih.gov/medlineplus/ency/article/003242.htm.**
- **www.skinsight.com/infant/cafeauLaitMacule.htm.**
- **www.dermnetnz.org/colour/pigmentation.html.**

PROVIDER RESOURCES

- **http://emedicine.medscape.com/article/1069191-overview.**

REFERENCES

1. Davis EC, Callender VD. Postinflammatory hyperpigmentation: a review of the epidemiology, clinical features, and treatment options in skin of color. *J Clin Aesthet Dermatol.* 2010;3(7):20-31.
2. Hubert JN, Callen JP, Kasteler JS. Prevalence of cutaneous findings in hospitalized pediatric patients. *Pediatr Dermatol.* 1997; 14(6):426-429.
3. Okafor OO, Akinbami FO, Orimadegun AE, Okafor CM, Ogunbiyi AO. Prevalence of dermatological lesions in hospitalized children at the University College Hospital, Ibadan, Nigeria. *Niger J Clin Pract.* 2011;14(3):287-292.
4. Alexis AF, Sergay AB, Taylor SC. Common dermatologic disorders in skin of color: a comparative practice survey. *Cutis.* 2007;80(5): 387-394.
5. Lacz NL, Vafaie J, Kihiczak NI, Schwartz RA. Postinflammatory hyperpigmentation: a common but troubling condition. *Int J Dermatol.* 2004;43(5):362-365.
6. Epstein JH. Postinflammatory hyperpigmentation. *Clin Dermatol.* 1989;7(2):55-65.
7. Taieb A, Boralevi F. Hypermelanoses of the newborn and of the infant. *Dermatol Clin.* 2007;25(3):327-336, viii.
8. Loomis CA. Linear hypopigmentation and hyperpigmentation, including mosaicism. *Semin Cutan Med Surg.* 1997;16(1):44-53.
9. Tomita Y, Maeda K, Tagami H. Melanocyte-stimulating properties of arachidonic acid metabolites: possible role in postinflammatory pigmentation. *Pigment Cell Res.* 1992;5(5 Pt 2):357-361.
10. Ortonne JP. Retinoic acid and pigment cells: a review of in-vitro and in-vivo studies. *Br J Dermatol.* 1992;127(41):43-47.
11. Pandya AG, Guevara IL. Disorders of hyperpigmentation. *Dermatol Clin.* 2000;18(1):91-98, ix.
12. Ruiz-Maldonado R, Orozco-Covarrubias ML. Postinflammatory hypopigmentation and hyperpigmentation. *Semin Cutan Med Surg.* 1997;16(1):36-43.
13. Callender VD, St Surin-Lord S, Davis EC, Maclin M. Postinflammatory hyperpigmentation: etiologic and therapeutic considerations. *Am J Clin Dermatol.* 2011;12(2):87-99.
14. Jang HS, Oh CK, Cha JH, Cho SH, Kwon KS. Six cases of confluent and reticulated papillomatosis alleviated by various antibiotics. *J Am Acad Dermatol.* 2001;44(4):652-655.
15. Scheinfeld N. Confluent and reticulated papillomatosis: a review of the literature. *Am J Clin Dermatol.* 2006;7(5):305-313.
16. Di Lernia V. Linear and whorled hypermelanosis. *Pediatr Dermatol.* 2007;24(3):205-210.
17. Nehal KS, PeBenito R, Orlow SJ. Analysis of 54 cases of hypopigmentation and hyperpigmentation along the lines of Blaschko. *Arch Dermatol.* 1996;132(10):1167-1170.
18. Hogeling M, Frieden IJ. Segmental pigmentation disorder. *Br J Dermatol.* 2010;162(6):1337-1341.
19. Arnold AW, Itin PH. Laptop computer-induced erythema ab igne in a child and review of the literature. *Pediatrics.* 2010;126(5):e1227-1230.
20. Shah KN. The diagnostic and clinical significance of cafe-au-lait macules. *Pediatr Clin North Am.* 2010;57(5):1131-1153.
21. Polder KD, Landau JM, Vergilis-Kalner IJ, Goldberg LH, Friedman PM, Bruce S. Laser eradication of pigmented lesions: a review. *Dermatol Surg.* 2011;37(5):572-595.
22. Cordova A. The Mongolian spot: a study of ethnic differences and a literature review. *Clin Pediatr (Phila).* 1981;20(11):714-719.
23. Osswald SS, Proffer LH, Sartori CR. Erythema dyschromicum perstans: a case report and review. *Cutis.* 2001;68(1):25-28.
24. Torrelo A, Zaballos P, Colmenero I, Mediero IG, de Prada I, Zambrano A. Erythema dyschromicum perstans in children: a report of 14 cases. *J Eur Acad Dermatol Venereol.* 2005;19(4):422-426.
25. Sinha S, Cohen PJ, Schwartz RA. Nevus of Ota in children. *Cutis.* 2008;82(1):25-29.
26. Chang CJ, Kou CS. Comparing the effectiveness of Q-switched Ruby laser treatment with that of Q-switched Nd:YAG laser for oculodermal melanosis (Nevus of Ota). *J Plast Reconstr Aesthet Surg.* 2011;64(3):339-345.
27. Liu J, Ma YP, Ma XG, et al. A retrospective study of q-switched alexandrite laser in treating nevus of ota. *Dermatol Surg.* 2011;37(10):1480-1485.
28. Fusade T, Lafaye S, Laubach HJ. Nevus of Ota in dark skin–an uncommon but treatable entity. *Lasers Surg Med.* 2011;43(10): 960-964.
29. Leyden JJ, Shergill B, Micali G, Downie J, Wallo W. Natural options for the management of hyperpigmentation. *J Eur Acad Dermatol Venereol.* 2011;25(10):1140-1145.
30. Perez-Bernal A, Munoz-Perez MA, Camacho F. Management of facial hyperpigmentation. *Am J Clin Dermatol.* 2000;1(5):261-268.
31. Cook-Bolden FE, Hamilton SF. An open-label study of the efficacy and tolerability of microencapsulated hydroquinone 4% and retinol 0.15% with antioxidants for the treatment of hyperpigmentation. *Cutis.* 2008;81(4):365-371.
32. Lynde CB, Kraft JN, Lynde CW. Topical treatments for melasma and postinflammatory hyperpigmentation. *Skin Therapy Lett.* 2006;11(9):1-6.
33. Taylor SC, Torok H, Jones T, et al. Efficacy and safety of a new triple-combination agent for the treatment of facial melasma. *Cutis.* 2003;72(1):67-72.

34. Bulengo-Ransby SM, Griffiths CE, Kimbrough-Green CK, et al. Topical tretinoin (retinoic acid) therapy for hyperpigmented lesions caused by inflammation of the skin in black patients. *N Engl J Med.* 1993;328(20):1438-1443.

35. Grimes PE. The safety and efficacy of salicylic acid chemical peels in darker racial-ethnic groups. *Dermatol Surg.* 1999;25(1):18-22.

36. Grover C, Reddu BS. The therapeutic value of glycolic acid peels in dermatology. *Indian J Dermatol Venereol Leprol.* 2003;69 (2):148-150.

37. Burns RL, Prevost-Blank PL, Lawry MA, Lawry TB, Faria DT, Fivenson DP. Glycolic acid peels for postinflammatory hyperpigmentation in black patients. A comparative study. *Dermatol Surg.* 1997;23(3):171-174; discussion 175.

38. Nelson BR, Fader DJ, Gillard M, Baker SR, Johnson TM. The role of dermabrasion and chemical peels in the treatment of patients with xeroderma pigmentosum. *J Am Acad Dermatol.* 1995;32(4):623-626.

39. O'Neill TB, Rawlins J, Rea S, Wood F. Treatment of a large congenital melanocytic nevus with dermabrasion and autologous cell suspension (ReCELL(R)): a case report. *J Plast Reconstr Aesthet Surg.* 2011;64(12):1672-1676.

40. Tierney EP, Hanke CW. Review of the literature: Treatment of dyspigmentation with fractionated resurfacing. *Dermatol Surg.* 2010;36(10):1499-1508.

41. Cordisco MR. An update on lasers in children. *Curr Opin Pediatr.* 2009;21(4):499-504.

SECTION 16 GENETIC SKIN DISORDERS

169 GENODERMATOSES

Olvia Revelo, MD
Michael Babcock, MD
Richard P. Usatine, MD

INTRODUCTION

There are more than 100 genetic syndromes with cutaneous manifestations that are referred to as genodermatoses. There are disorders of: pigmentation (e.g., albinism), cornification (e.g., the ichthyoses and Darier disease), vascularization (e.g., Sturge-Weber syndrome), connective tissue (e.g., Ehlers-Danlos syndrome), metabolism (e.g., phenylketonuria), immune system (e.g., Wiskott-Aldrich syndrome), and DNA repair (e.g., xeroderma pigmentosa). Some textbooks are dedicated to the topic of genodermatoses alone.[1] This chapter introduces the topic and illustrates several genodermatoses. We will focus our discussion on Darier disease and pachyonychia congenita as an introduction to the genodermatoses.

DARIER DISEASE

PATIENT STORY

A 12-year-old girl presents to her pediatrician with a scaling rash around her neck. A family history reveals that her mother, maternal grandmother, maternal aunt, and uncle all have Darier's disease. Because this genodermatosis is inherited as an autosomal dominant trait, the pediatrician states that this is likely to be the onset of her Darier disease. The pediatrician prescribes a low potency steroid cream to help the occasional itching that occurs with this new rash. She suggests that the patient also see a local dermatologist. Years later, the young woman returns and her rash is much worse. Upon examination she had red greasy scale around the neck and over the anterior chest (**Figures 169-1** to **169-3**). The patient states that she was given the diagnosis of Darier disease by the dermatologist but was unable to get an appointment during this acute flare-up. She asked the pediatrician if she could prescribe some 0.1 percent triamcinolone cream because that is what has helped her in the past and she ran out of it 1 month ago. The pediatrician agrees to give her a prescription but encourages her to make an appointment with her dermatologist to see what else can be done. She also notes that the nails have the distinctive red-and-white striping seen in Darier disease (**Figure 169-4**).

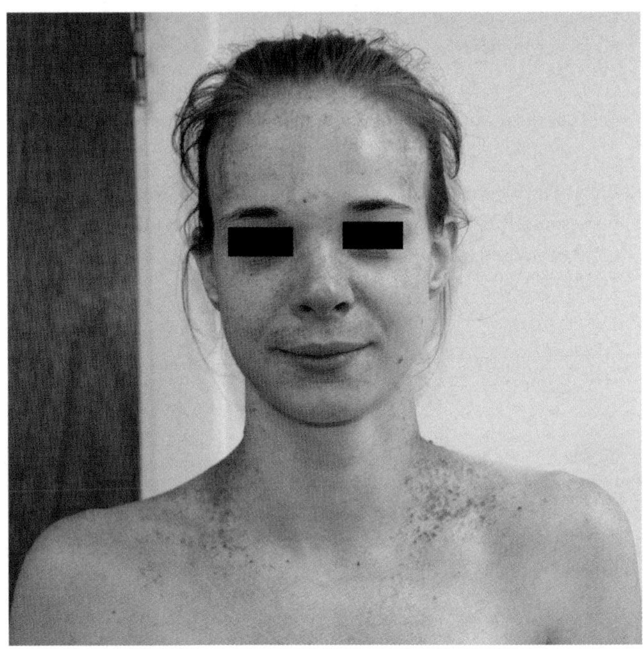

FIGURE 169-1 Darier disease with greasy hyperkeratotic scale in a seborrheic distribution involving the face, neck, and chest. As this is an autosomal dominant genodermatosis, many members of her mother's family have this condition. (*Used with permission from Yoon Cohen, MD.*)

EPIDEMIOLOGY

- Darier disease, also known as keratosis follicularis, has been reported in approximately 1:30,000 to 1:100,000 people.
- Males and females are equally affected as this occurs through autosomal dominant inheritance.
- Clinically it becomes apparent near puberty.

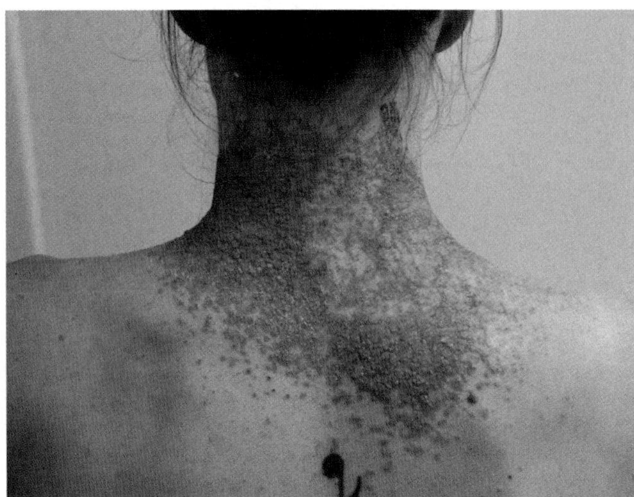

FIGURE 169-2 Darier disease flared up on the posterior neck and upper back in the same patient from **Figure 169-1**. Note the erythema and greasy yellow hyperkeratotic scale in the seborrheic area. (*Used with permission from Yoon Cohen, MD.*)

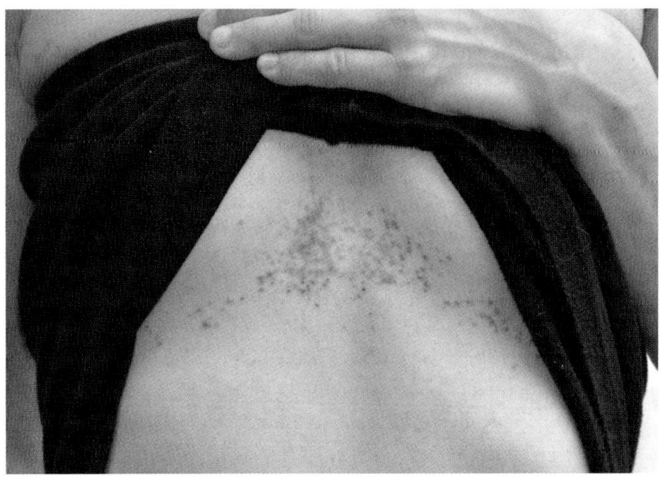

FIGURE 169-3 Darier disease on the chest in any seborrheic distribution over the sternum and around the breasts in the same patient from **Figure 169-1**. (*Used with permission from Yoon Cohen, MD.*)

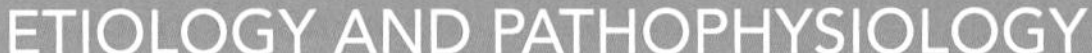

ETIOLOGY AND PATHOPHYSIOLOGY

- In Darier disease, a gene mutation in the ATP2A2 gene in chromosome 12q23-24.1 results in production of an abnormal calcium pump in the sarcoendoplasmic reticulum, SERCA2. How this mutation affects the way the cells interact together is still unknown, but it results in abnormal epidermal differentiation.[2] It is inherited in an autosomal-dominant fashion.

DIAGNOSIS

- Clinical features—Greasy, hyperkeratotic, yellowish-brown papules and plaques with scale in a seborrheic distribution (**Figures 169-1** to **169-3**). The feet can be covered with hyperkeratotic plaques. The palms may have pits or keratotic papules, and the nails can have V-shaped nicking and alternating longitudinal red and white bands (**Figures 169-4** and **169-5**). The keratotic papules can be intensely malodorous such that it can interfere with normal social situations (**Figure 169-6**).
- Typical distribution—The clinical lesions involve skin in the seborrheic distribution (face, ears, scalp, upper chest, upper back, and groin; **Figures 169-1** to **169-3** and **169-6**). The axilla and inframammary areas may be involved (**Figure 169-3**). In early, mild, or partially treated disease, only the skin behind the ears may be affected.[3] The nails are characteristically involved (**Figures 169-4** and **169-5**).
- Laboratories—Skin biopsy reveals the characteristic histopathology. A test for the ATP2A2 gene mutation can be performed.

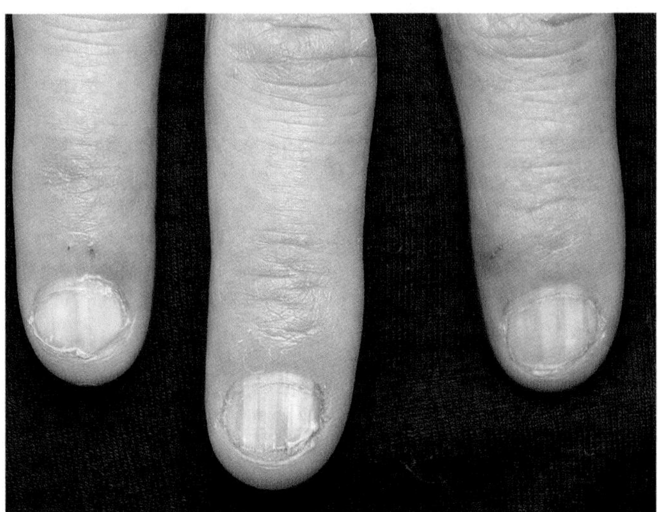

FIGURE 169-4 Darier disease of the fingernails with the typical red and white striping in the same patient from **Figure 169-1**. (*Used with permission from Yoon Cohen, MD.*)

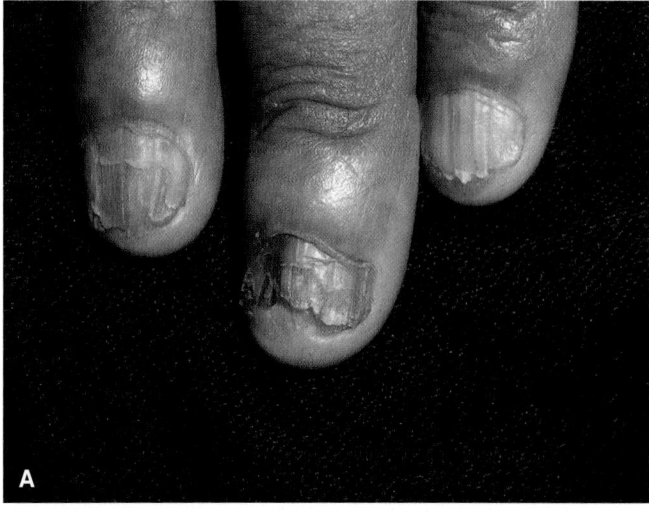

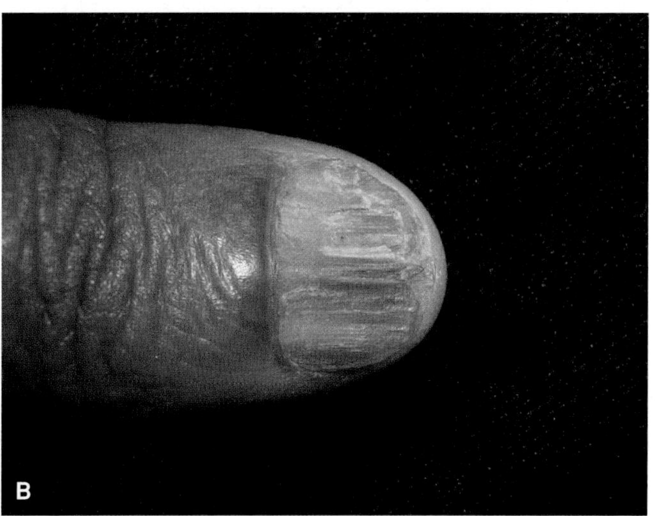

FIGURE 169-5 **A.** Typical nail findings in Darier disease showing longitudinal bands and longitudinal splitting. **B.** V-shaped nick at the free margin of the fingernail—the most pathognomonic nail finding in Darier disease. (*Used with permission from Richard P. Usatine, MD.*)

DIFFERENTIAL DIAGNOSIS

- Hailey-Hailey disease (aka benign familial pemphigus)—Another genodermatosis with crusted erosions and flaccid vesicles distributed

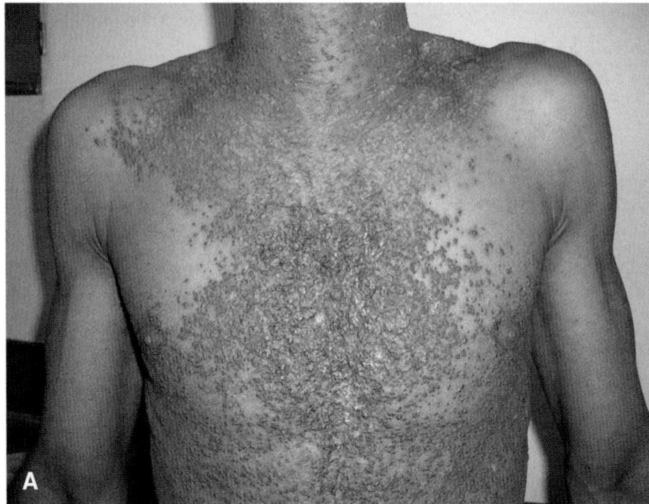

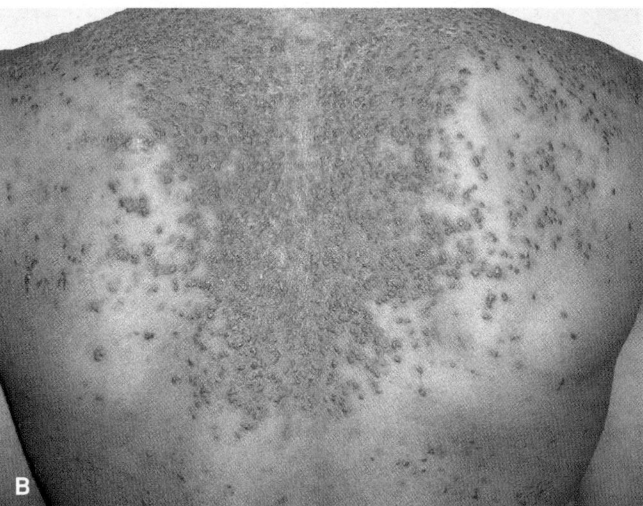

FIGURE 169-6 Darier disease in a more advanced stage. **A.** Central chest and neck are completely covered with hyperkeratotic greasy scale. **B.** The central back is also covered with hyperpigmented hyperkeratotic greasy scale. The patient states that warm weather worsens the rash and causes increased itching and an unpleasant odor. (*Used with permission from Richard P. Usatine, MD.*)

in the intertriginous areas as opposed to the greasy keratotic papules in the seborrheic distribution. A 4-mm punch biopsy is adequate to make this diagnosis.

- Seborrheic dermatitis—Erythematous patches and thin plaques with yellow greasy scale on the scalp, central face, and chest. This is rarely as severe as Darier disease (see Chapter 135, Seborrheic Dermatitis).

MANAGEMENT

- Darier disease is so rare that there are no randomized controlled trials to guide treatment.
- Mild-to-moderate disease can be treated by avoiding exacerbating factors (sunlight, heat, and occlusion) and with topical medications, SOR C but severe disease is best treated with oral retinoids. SOR C
- Frequent application of emollients, humectants, and keratolytics are the mainstay of therapy. SOR C There are many effective nonprescription and prescription products that contain propylene glycol, urea, or lactic acid. Ammonium lactate can be obtained in a 6 percent lotion OTC and can be prescribed in a 12 percent lotion.
- Topical retinoids (adapalene, tretinoin, or tazarotene) are effective in some patients, but their main limitation is irritation. Adapalene use may be effective in localized variants.[4] SOR C All retinoids are contraindicated in pregnancy.
- Topical corticosteroids may be of some help. Lower-potency topical corticosteroids should be used on the face, groin, and axillae to minimize side effects in these areas. SOR C
- Topical calcineurin inhibitors (pimecrolimus and tacrolimus) may also be helpful as noted in some case reports.[5,6] SOR C These do not have a risk of skin atrophy like steroids, but are generally more expensive and have the controversial black box warning related to the rare risk of skin malignancy and lymphoma.
- Systemic retinoids (acitretin initial 10 to 20 mg/day or isotretinoin 0.5 to 1mg/kg/day) are the most potent treatment and treatment of choice for severe disease.[2] SOR C They should only be prescribed by physicians who have experience with these medications. Patients on systemic retinoids require close monitoring and careful selection, as they are teratogenic (category X) and can cause hyperlipidemia, hypertriglyceridemia, mucous membrane dryness, alopecia, hepatotoxicity, and possible mood disturbances. Females must not get pregnant for at least 1 month after stopping isotretinoin and at least 3 years after stopping acitretin.
- Topical or oral antibiotics may be necessary for flares as they often are secondarily infected with bacteria. SOR C
- Laser, radiation, photodynamic, and gene therapy are newer treatment modalities that are being investigated.
- Refer to an urologist or ophthalmologist if testicular abnormality or corneal opacities are detected. SOR C
- Gene therapy has also been studied but has not yet become a viable treatment option.
- The malodor that accompanies the disease, as well as the facial involvement, often adversely affects the patient's quality of life; thus, treatment is often warranted.

FOLLOW-UP

- Follow-up is needed if patients are on oral retinoids to monitor patients' lipid panel and liver function tests approximately every 3 months. Patients should also be monitored for signs of secondary bacterial infection.

PATIENT EDUCATION

- Avoid direct sunlight, heat, occlusion, and people acutely infected with herpes simplex virus (HSV) or varicella-zoster virus.
- Watch for signs of secondary cutaneous bacterial or viral infections.

PATIENT RESOURCES

- There are patient advocacy groups for several genetic skin conditions. A quick search online can obtain their websites and contact information.
- The American Academy of Dermatology has a summer camp that is free of charge for children with skin conditions called Camp Discovery—**www.campdiscovery.org/**.

PROVIDER RESOURCES

- A helpful free online resource for the genodermatoses, or any genetic disease, is the Online Mendelian Inheritance of Man website—**www.omim.org**.
- For information on laboratories that perform rare genetic tests and clinics that perform prenatal diagnostic testing for certain conditions—**www.genetests.org**.
- Skin Advocate is a free application for mobile devices that is provided by the Society of Investigative Dermatology. Patient advocacy groups—**www.skinadvocateapp.com**.

PACHYONYCHIA CONGENITA (PC)

PATIENT STORY

A college student comes to the pediatrician's office for a school physical exam and his influenza vaccine. He is aware that he was born with pachyonychia congenita (type-1) and has been dealing with the ramifications of this condition since he was 9 years old. He has come to accept the nail abnormalities (**Figure 169-7**) but finds that the hyperkeratotic lesions on his hands, feet, and elbows can be painful (**Figures 169-8** to **169-10**). The thick calluses on his feet cause him the most pain and he describes this problem to be like walking with pebbles in your shoes. His dermatologist has given him 12 percent ammonium lactate to help dissolve some of the thickened hyperkeratoses. He also uses a pumice stone after bathing to sand down the callus on the feet and the papules on the hands and elbows. He wonders if there is anything else that can be done to help him. As this is a rare genodermatosis, the pediatrician refers the young student to his dermatologist.

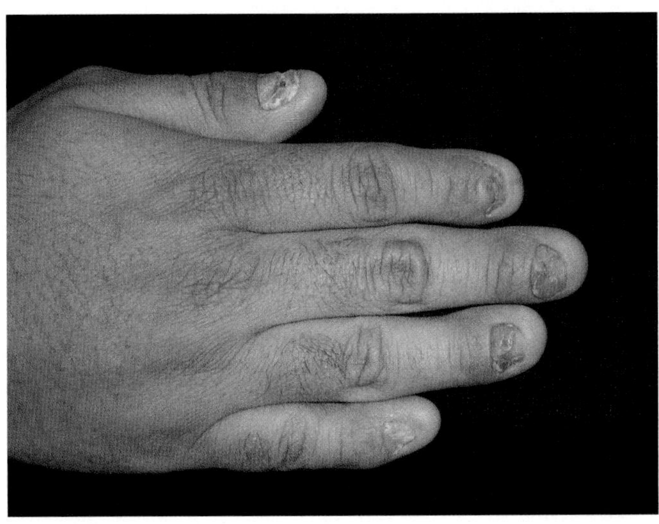

FIGURE 169-7 Pachyonychia congenita (type 1) showing the hyperkeratotic nail dystrophy. (*Used with permission from Richard P. Usatine, MD.*)

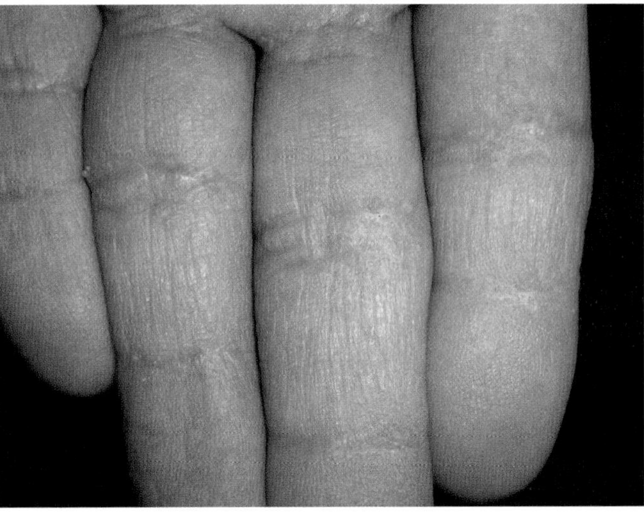

FIGURE 169-8 Pachyonychia congenita showing the small keratotic papules on the palmar side of the fingers. (*Used with permission from Richard P. Usatine, MD.*)

EPIDEMIOLOGY

- Rare disorder with unknown prevalence. Mutations in individuals from at least 227 families have been published.[7] Increasing data is currently being analyzed since the initiation of the International Pachyonychia Research Registry.
- Increased in Slavic and Jewish populations. Increased incidence in males that in females.[1]

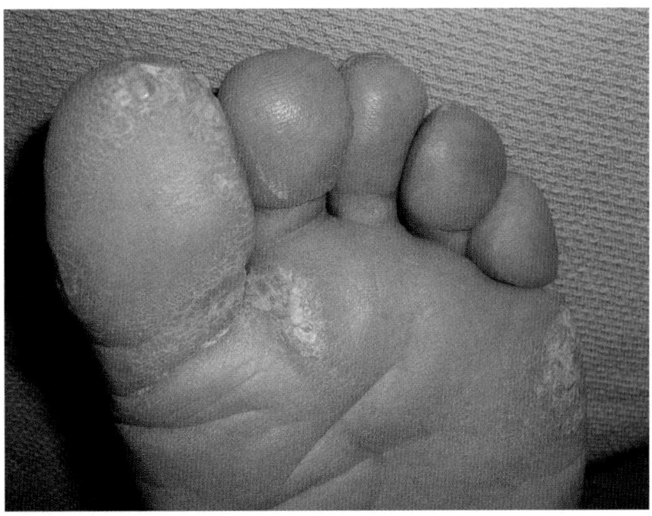

FIGURE 169-9 Pachyonychia congenita demonstrating the hypertrophic callus found on the soles of the feet. This patient religiously uses keratolytic topical medications to keep the callus under control. At one time he was using a wheelchair because it was too painful to walk on his feet. (*Used with permission from Richard P. Usatine, MD.*)

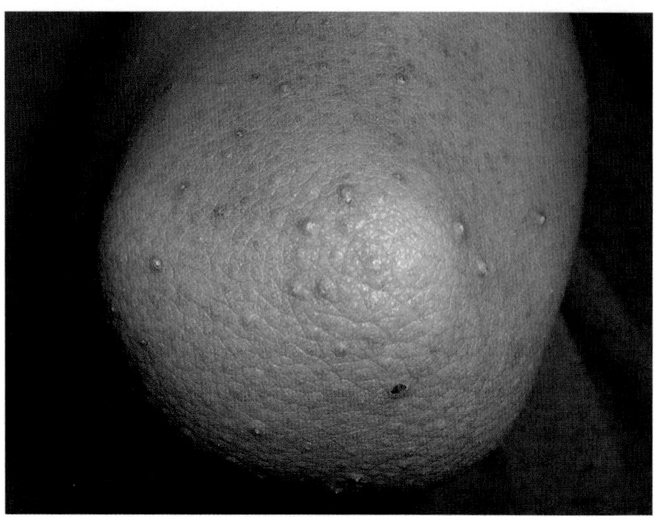

FIGURE 169-10 Pachyonychia congenita showing hyperkeratotic papules on the elbows. This patient also gets these on the buttocks, which can make it painful to sit. (*Used with permission from Richard P. Usatine, MD.*)

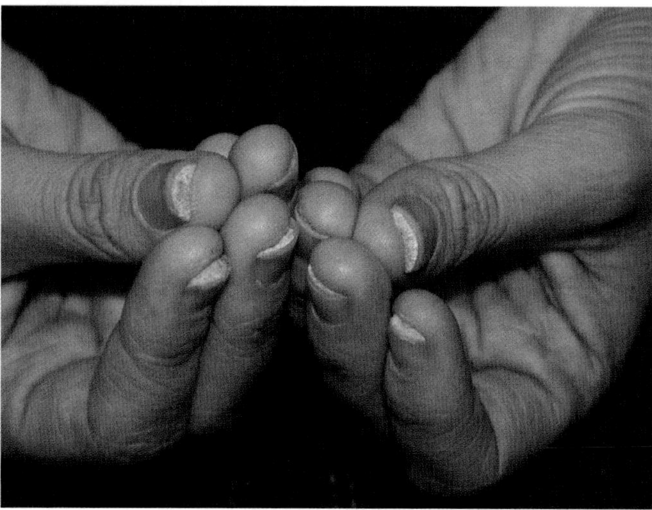

FIGURE 169-11 Pachyonychia congenita involving all 10 fingernails with subungual hyperkeratosis elevating the distal nail plate and causing some pincer-like deformities. (*Used with permission from Eric Kraus, MD.*)

ETIOLOGY AND PATHOPHYSIOLOGY

- Pachyonychia congenita is considered a spectrum of clinical manifestations of ectodermal dysplasia associated with abnormal keratin proteins involved in normal intermediate filament assembly.[7] This defect disrupts the integrity of epithelial cells especially when frictional stressors are applied.
- About half of all cases are inherited in an autosomal dominant manner, the rest arise from spontaneous mutations.[1,2]
- Historically, the disorder had 2 variants called Jadassohn-Lewandsowsky (PC Type-1) and Jackson-Lawler (PC Type-2) based on clinical presentation. There has been an international effort in data collection registry that has led to a new classification system proposed at the 2010 International Pachyonychia Congenita Symposium based on the link between 4 genetic mutations and clinical presentation.[7]
- The four genetic mutations carry the name of the protein and the chromosome number associated with the keratin gene abnormality: KRT6A, KRT6B, KRT16, KRT17. Therefore the new nomenclature used to classify PC is as follows: PC-K6a, PC-K6b, PC-K16, PC-K17, and PC-U when the genetic mutation is unknown.[7]

DIAGNOSIS

- Diagnosis is made by clinical findings and molecular genetic testing of the four known keratin genes. The most common clinical finding is hypertrophic nail dystrophy (**Figure 169-7**). It is associated with painful focal keratoderma typically found on palms and soles or on pressure points or areas under recurrent friction stress (**Figures 169-8** to **169-10**).[2,7]
- First sign that may be appreciated during infancy is erythema of the nail bed prior to typical nail changes.
- Nails—Subungual hyperkeratosis with increased transverse curvature, "pincer nail effect," and elevation of distal nail plate (**Figure 169-11**). Typically involves all 20 nails, with fingernails being affected more often than toenails. Nail plates may also be darkened, thickened and friable with increased risk of shedding the entire nail plate. May be associated with paronychial infection with Staphylococcus or Candida.
- Skin—Focal symmetric palmoplantar keratoderma, follicular hyperkeratosis of elbows, knees, extensor extremities. May be associated with hyperhydrosis, steatocystoma multiplex, or epidermoid cysts. Steatocystoma multiplex is a condition in which there are many superficial cutaneous cysts filled with a fatty substance. It is frequently located on the back and chest (**Figure 169-12**). Hair may be coarse and brittle (pili torti).
- Oropharynx—May be associated with oral leukokeratosis, angular cheilitis, and hoarseness. Natal teeth have most frequently been associated with KRT17 mutation.
- Eyes/Ears—Rarely associated with corneal dystrophy, cataracts, and excessive cerumen accumulation.
- Phenotypes associated with genetic mutations are as follows:
    - KRT6A and KRT6B exist as the classic painful nail dystrophy and palmoplantar keratoderma typically not associated with other phenotypes.[2]
    - KRT16 is a focal nonepidermolytic palmoplantar keratoderma, defined as keratoderma of varying severity that may occur on the palms and soles with absent or mild nail dystrophy.[2]
    - KRT17 is associated with steatocystoma multiplex (**Figure 169-12**), and can have absent or only mild nail dystrophy and palmoplantar keratoderma.[2]

DIFFERENTIAL DIAGNOSIS

- Dyskeratosis congenita—May be difficult to differentiate from PC since both may show nail dystrophy, palmoplantar keratoderma, hyperhidrosis, and oral leukoplakia. However, reticulate hyperpigmentation, skin tumors, and hematologic manifestations are more specific to dyskeratosis congenita.

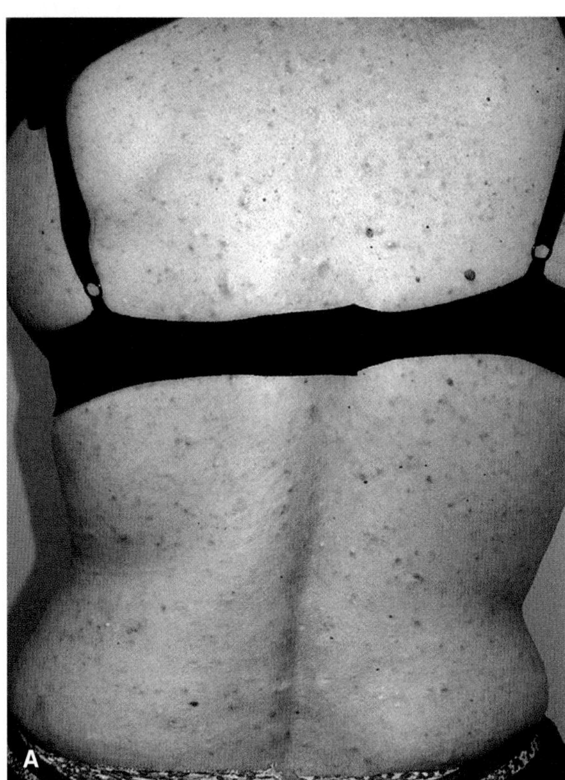

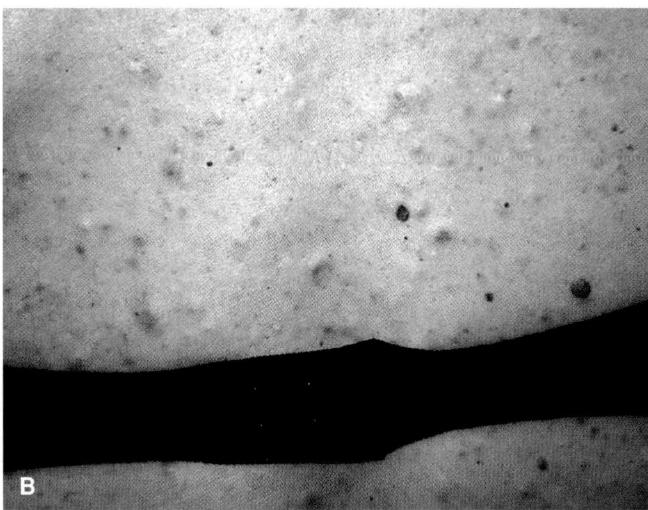

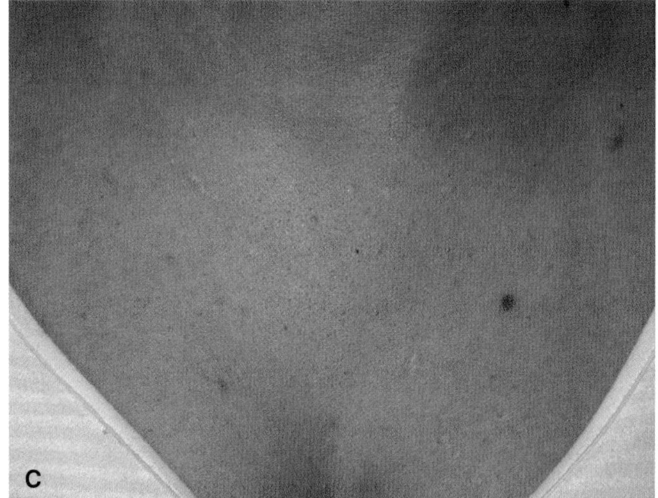

FIGURE 169-12 **A.** pachyonychia congenita type 2 with extensive steatocystoma multiplex on the back. **B.** Close-up of steatocystoma multiplex. **C.** The daughter is beginning to develop steatocystoma multiplex on the chest. (*Used with permission from Eric Kraus, MD.*)

- Onychomycosis—Typically does not involve all 20 nails and is not associated with painful palmoplantar keratoderma or other PC findings. May perform a KOH preparation or culture the affected nail plate.
- Twenty nail dystrophy—May occur without keratoderma or other findings associated with PC. Genetic testing may be necessary to differentiate these entities.
- Palmoplantar psoriasis—Psoriasis is usually associated with mahogany (red-brown) spots and pustules. Also look for other signs of psoriasis such as plaques elsewhere or nail findings such as nail pitting or oil spots. Punch biopsy of plaque shows typical histopathologic changes.
- Other palmoplantar keratodermas—May present similarly and require syndromic phenotype clues or genetic testing to differentiate.

MANAGEMENT

- Treatment is mainly supportive and tailored to each patient according to age and severity of symptoms. Often there is need to treat overlying skin infection. Education about grooming practices is imperative.
- Topical therapies useful for ameliorating hyperkeratosis include lactic acid and urea based creams and lotions. Ammonium lactate can be obtained in a 6 percent lotion OTC and can be prescribed in a 12 percent lotion. SOR C
- Mechanical nail paring with electric file, dental drill, or blade can be attempted. Avulsion of the nail plate with matrix destruction can be used in severe, symptomatic cases. SOR C
- Systemic antibiotics or antifungals may be needed to treat underlying infection. SOR C
- Pain can be reduced by limiting friction and trauma to the feet. Attempting to minimize prolonged walking or standing may be helpful. Patients should select comfortable, ventilated footwear and attempt to maintain an ideal body weight. SOR C
- Routine grooming of the feet is essential and includes paring down the hyperkeratotic areas to avoid painful buildup that can add further friction and trauma to the foot. Soaking the feet in warm water prior to the paring is helpful when plaques are hard. The surface of the skin and the instruments used should be clean to avoid infection. If blisters develop, they can be drained with a sterile needle. SOR C

- Treatments currently under investigation include use of genetic modulators, rapamycin, simvastatin, anti-TNF biologics, and even botulinum toxin.[1]

FOLLOW UP

- Referral to dermatology and podiatry as needed for management and supportive treatment of complications from skin excess. Genetic referral should be considered for reproductive counseling and assessment of at-risk family members.

PATIENT EDUCATION

- Lesions persist throughout life. Reduction of trauma, friction, and sheer forces to the skin and nails improves the condition. Heat or perspiration may worsen the condition and should be avoided.
- Molecular genetic testing of at-risk relatives in a family with PC is not indicated because the phenotype is readily observed from a young age and no interventions can prevent the development of manifestations or reduce their severity.
- It is rarely associated with blindness secondary to corneal dystrophy. There are no other known associated systemic risks or conditions.

Additional Examples

XERODERMA PIGMENTOSA

- Xeroderma pigmentosa (XP) is an autosomal recessive genetic repair disorder resulting in early predisposition to malignancy mainly secondary to UV-light damage (**Figure 169-13**). The condition affects approximately 1 in 1 million people in the US, but there seems to be an increased incidence in Japan.[8] The earliest sign is increased sun sensitivity with easy sun burning in infancy. Dyschromic macules and telangiectasias start to develop in a sun-exposed distribution within the first few years of life. After some time actinic keratosis followed by various forms of skin cancer start to appear depending on the amount of sun exposure. Ophthalmologic and neurologic manifestations are associated. Treatment includes extreme sun avoidance (only out early morning and evening) as well as protective barriers, cancer screening, excision of skin cancers, and referral to dermatology, ophthalmology, or neurology accordingly.

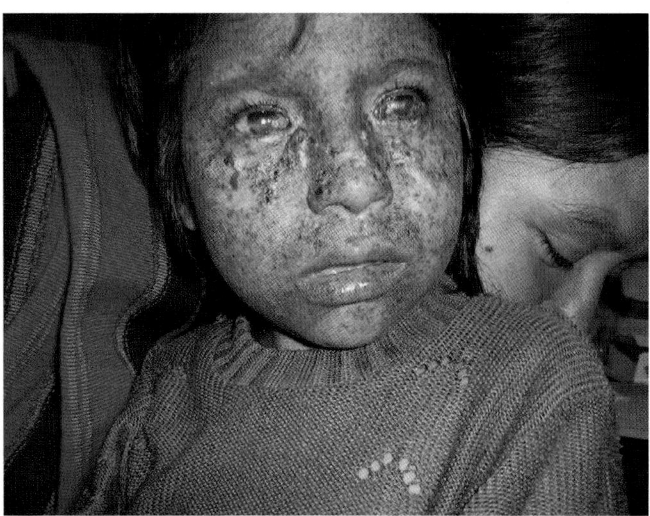

FIGURE 169-13 Xeroderma pigmentosum in an 8-year-old girl from Guatemala showing large hyperkeratotic lesions with some induration suspicious of actinic keratosis and early squamous cell carcinoma. There are also numerous hyperpigmented solar lentigines. Marked corneal scarring and conjunctival injection is present. (*Used with permission from James Halpern, Bryan Hopping, Joshua M Brostoff and Wikimedia Commons.*)

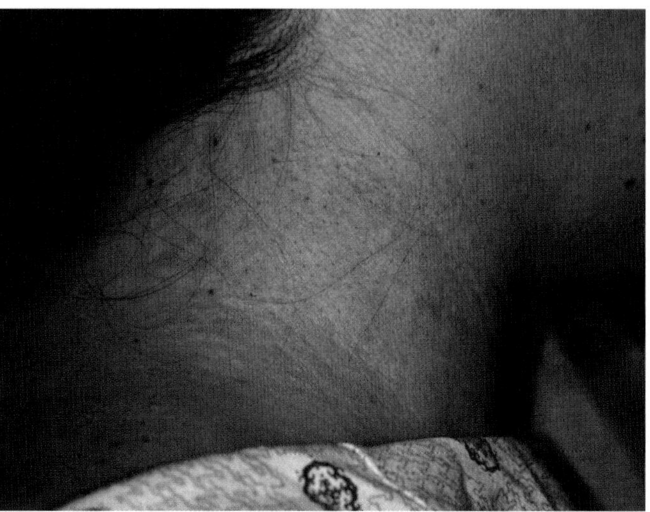

FIGURE 169-14 Pseudoxanthoma elasticum with a typical patch of soft thickened pink skin on the neck. This young woman went on to have early coronary artery disease. (*Used with permission from Richard P. Usatine, MD.*)

PSEUDOXANTHOMA ELASTICUM

- Pseudoxanthoma elasticum (PXE) is considered a genetic disorder of connective tissue. There is a rare mutation in a transmembrane transporter gene that in some way leads to the clinical manifestations observed. Incidence is approximately 1 in 100,000, affecting both sexes equally.[9] Some key clinical features include yellow papules/plaques over redundant, lax, soft skin folds on the sides of neck (**Figure 169-14**), axillae, antecubital fossae, abdomen, groin, and thighs as well as mucous membranes. Eyes exhibit angioid streaks, retinal pigmentation alteration, and may be associated with macular degeneration and retinal hemorrhages causing blindness. Other systems involved are the cardiovascular system (gastric artery hemorrhage) and reproductive system (first trimester miscarriage). Diagnosis is clinical or with biopsy if needed. Treatment is supportive with appropriate referrals as complications arise.

PATIENT RESOURCES

- Genetics Home Reference—**http://ghr.nlm.nih.gov/condition/pachyonychia-congenita**.
- Pachyonychia Congenita Project—**www.pachyonychia.org**.
- International Pachyonychia Congenita Research Registry (IPCRR)—**www.pachyonychia.org**.

PROVIDER RESOURCES

- A helpful free online resource for the genodermatoses, or any genetic disease for that matter, is the Online Mendelian Inheritance of Man website—**www.omim.org**.
- For information on laboratories that perform rare genetic tests and clinics that perform prenatal diagnostic testing for certain conditions—**www.genetests.org**.
- Skin Advocate is a free application for mobile devices that is provided by the Society of Investigative Dermatology. It lists contact information for various patient advocacy groups.

REFERENCES

1. Spitz J: *Genodermatoses: A Clinical Guide to Genetic Skin Disorders*, 2nd ed. Philadelphia, PA: Lippincott Williams & Wilkins; 2005.
2. Bolognia J, Jorizzo J, Rapini R: *Dermatology*. London, UK: Mosby; 2003.
3. James W, Berger T, Elston D: *Andrews' Diseases of the Skin: Clinical Dermatology*, 11th ed. Amsterdam, The Netherlands: Elsevier; 2011.
4. Casals M, Campoy A, Aspiolea F, et al. Successful treatment of linear Darier disease with topical adapalene. *J Eur Acad Dermatol Venerol*. 2009;23(2):237-238.
5. Pérez-Carmona L, Fleta-Asín B, Moreno-García-Del-Real C, et al. Successful treatment of Darier disease with topical pimecrolimus. *Eur J Dermatol*. 2011;21(2):301-302.
6. Rubegni P, Poggiali S, Sbano P, et al. A case of Darier disease successfully treated with topical tacrolimus. *J Eur Acad Dermatol Venereol*. 2006;20(1):84-87.
7. Smith, F et al. Pachyonychia Congenita. *Gene Reviews*. 2006; U of WA, Seattle; http://www.ncbi.nlm.nih.gov/books/NBK1280/#_ncbi_dlg_citbx_NBK1280.
8. Lehmann AR, McGibbon D, Stefanini M: Xeroderma pigmentosum. *Orphanet Journal of Rare Diseases*. 2011;6:70. http://www.ncbi.nlm.nih.gov/pubmed/22044 607.
9. Sharon TF and Bercovitch L: Pseudoxanthoma elasticum. *Gene Reviews*. 2001; U of WA, Seattle; http://www.ncbi.nlm.nih.gov/books/NBK1113/#_ncbi_dlg_citbx_NBK1113.

170 VASCULAR AND LYMPHATIC MALFORMATIONS

Richard P. Usatine, MD
Nathan Hitzeman, MD

PATIENT STORY

A 6-month-old African American boy is brought to his pediatrician for his six-month well-baby exam and immunizations. The mother asks whether the red mark on the forehead and right eyebrow from birth will ever go away (**Figure 170-1**). The pediatrician refers the child to a dermatologist that explains that this is a capillary malformation called a port-wine stain and that it will remain there for the rest of the child's life. He also notes that it is less likely but still possible for this to be a salmon patch that could resolve spontaneously (although most salmon patches are lighter and midline). He states that it is not necessary to perform a biopsy because either way it is a capillary malformation that will not cause the child any physical harm. As it only involves part of V1 and none of V2, it is extremely unlikely to be part of the neurocutaneous syndrome known as Sturge-Weber syndrome. The pediatrician decides to not even bring up Sturge-Weber to avoid making the mother anxious but will continue to follow the child's development over time. The dermatologist also explained that the child may choose to have laser treatment in the future if the capillary malformation is causing psychological distress.

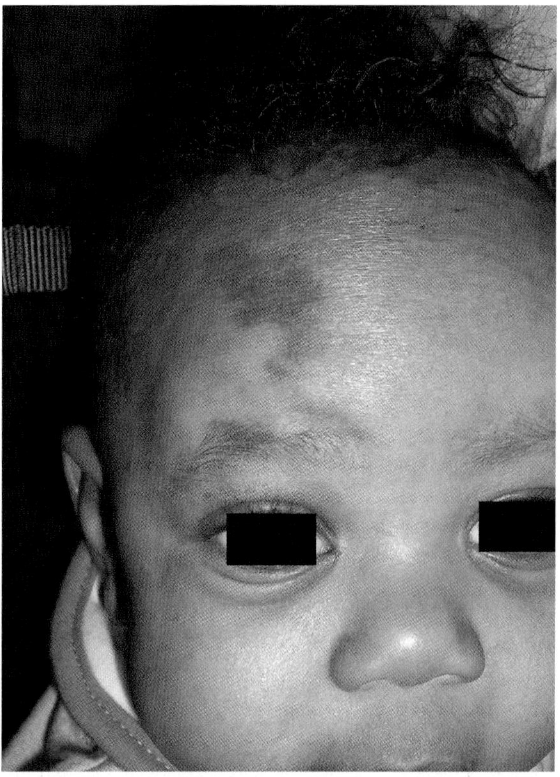

FIGURE 170-1 Capillary malformation since birth on the forehead and right eyebrow of this 6-month-old infant. This is likely to be a port-wine stain since it is not midline and it is darker than most salmon patches. As it only involves part of V1 and none of V2 it is extremely unlikely to be part of the Sturge-Weber syndrome. (*Used with permission from Richard P. Usatine, MD.*)

INTRODUCTION

Vascular malformations at birth range from the very common and benign salmon patch to rare but serious neurocutaneous syndromes (Sturge-Weber syndrome). Cutaneous lymphatic malformations are seen in a relatively rare condition called lymphangioma circumscripta. Osler-Weber-Rendu syndrome (hereditary hemorrhagic telangiectasia) is a rare vascular disorder that is inherited an autosomal dominant manner. Childhood hemangiomas are covered separately in Chapter 93, Childhood Hemangiomas.

SYNONYMS

There are two major types of capillary malformations present at birth:

- Salmon patch (stork bite, angel kiss, capillary stain, nuchal nevus, nevus simplex, telangiectatic nevus, and nevus flammeus nuchae) is a superficial capillary malformation and is likely to resolve spontaneously (**Figure 170-2**). Using the term capillary stain is one-way to denote how superficial it is.
- Port-wine stain (nevus flammeus) is deeper capillary malformation in the dermis and does not involute over time (**Figure 170-3**). In fact, it may increase in size, thickness, and become more nodular over time. It is this type of capillary malformation that may be associated with Sturge-Weber syndrome or Klippel-Trenaunay syndrome.
- Microcystic lymphatic malformations are called lymphangioma circumscriptum or cutaneous lymphangioma circumscriptum (**Figure 170-4**).

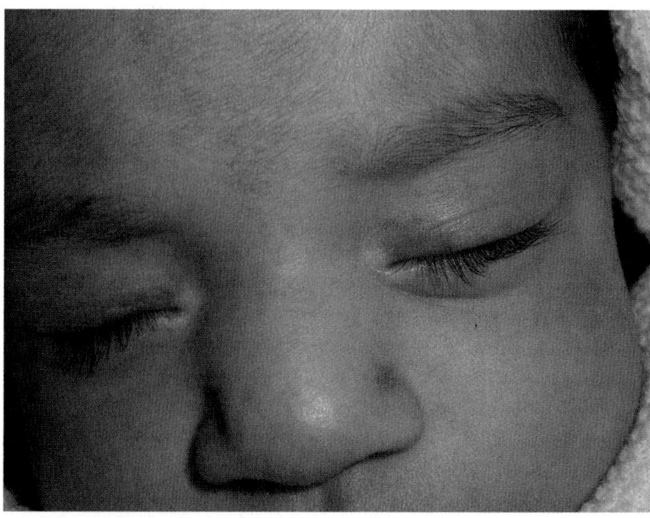

FIGURE 170-2 Salmon patches on the eyelids (angel kisses), glabella, forehead and nose in this healthy 2-month-old infant. Note how the pink color is faint and the forehead involvement is midline. (*Used with permission from Richard P. Usatine, MD.*)

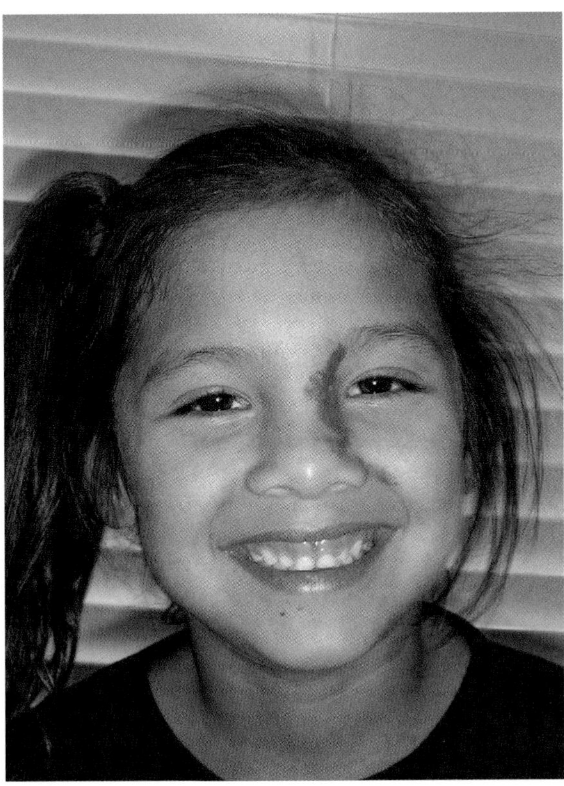

FIGURE 170-3 Port-wine stain on the face of this 6-year-old happy and healthy girl. While her mother would like to see the port-wine stain removed she understands that her daughter is too young for laser therapy. (*Used with permission from Richard P. Usatine, MD.*)

EPIDEMIOLOGY

- Salmon patches, also known as "stork bites" or "angel kisses" are present in 26 to 64 percent of newborns.[1–4] The angel kisses over the face tend to fade with time but the stork bites on the nape of the neck often persist (**Figure 170-2**).

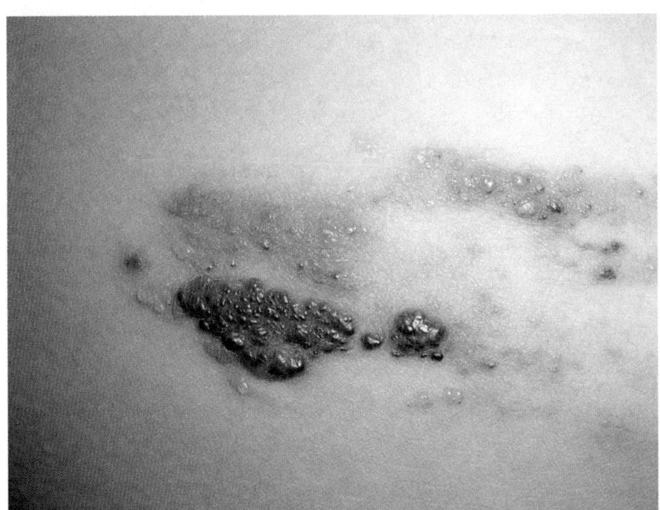

FIGURE 170-4 Close-up of lymphangioma circumscriptum present from birth on the trunk of this 7-year-old girl. The vesicles vary in color from yellow to pink and red. The red color is due to blood within the dilated lymphatic vessels. Note how this pattern resembles frog spawn. (*Used with permission from Richard P. Usatine, MD.*)

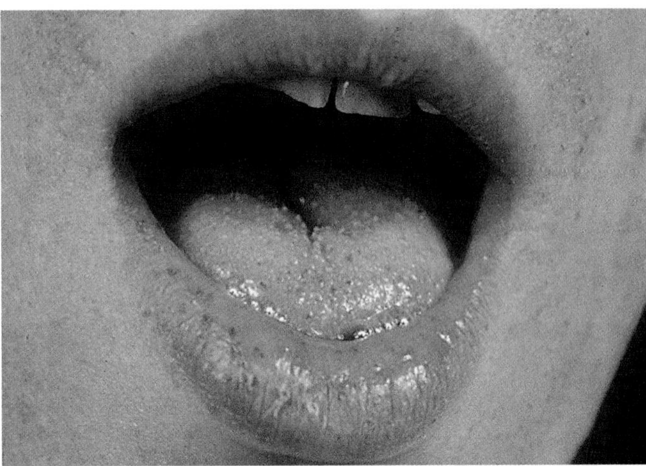

FIGURE 170-5 Hereditary hemorrhagic telangiectasias (Osler-Weber-Rendu syndrome) in a teen with recurrent nosebleeds and visible telangiectasias on the lips and tongue. (*Used with permission from Kane KS, Lio P, Stratigos AJ, Johnson RA. Color Atlas and Synopsis of Pediatric Dermatology, 2nd edition, Figure 8-10b, New York, NY: McGraw-Hill, 2009.*)

- Port-wine stains are congenital vascular malformations that occur in 0.6 to 2.8 percent of infants as developmental anomalies.[3,4] They persist into adulthood. They may be associated with rare syndromes such as Klippel-Trenaunay and Sturge-Weber syndromes (see Chapter 207, Sturge-Weber Syndrome).
- Hereditary hemorrhagic telangiectasia (HHT) is an autosomal-dominant vascular disorder that affects one in several thousands of people (**Figure 170-5**). Certain populations in Europe and the US have a higher prevalence of this disease.[5]
- Lymphangioma circumscriptum consists of dilated cutaneous lymphatic tissue and is rare.

ETIOLOGY AND PATHOPHYSIOLOGY

- Port-wine stains are vascular ectasias or dilations thought to arise from a deficiency of sympathetic nervous innervation to the blood vessels. Dilated capillaries are present throughout the dermis layer of the skin.
- HHT is associated with mutations in two genes: endoglin on chromosome 9 (HHT type 1) and activin receptor-like kinase-1 on chromosome 12 (HHT type 2). These genes are involved in vascular development and repair. With the mutations, arterioles become dilated and connect directly with venules without a capillary in between. Although manifestations are not present at birth, telangiectasias later develop on the skin, mucous membranes, and GI tract. In addition, AVMs often develop in the hepatic (up to 70% of patients), pulmonary (5% to 300%), and cerebral circulations (10% to 15%). Any of these lesions may become fragile and prone to bleeding.[5]
- Congenital malformations of the lymphatic system may involve the skin, subcutaneous tissues and intestines.[6] These lymphangiomas are hamartomatous in nature with the most superficial version being lymphangioma circumscriptum. Deeper versions are called cavernous lymphangiomas and cystic hygromas. The dilated ectopic lymph vessels protrude from the skin forming vesicles.

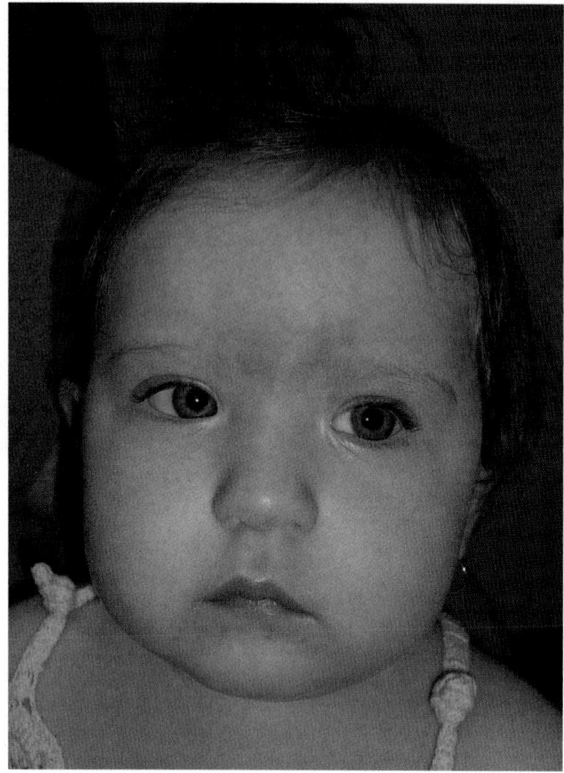

FIGURE 170-6 Salmon patch on the forehead and glabella of this otherwise healthy infant. This will spontaneously fade over time. Note how the pink color is faint and the forehead involvement is midline. (*Used with permission from Richard P. Usatine, MD.*)

DIAGNOSIS

CLINICAL FEATURES

- Salmon patches present with fine pink to salmon-colored dilated superficial capillaries over the eyelids, glabella, forehead and posterior neck (**Figures 170-2** and **170-6**). These may be so faint that they are only visible when the baby is crying. Most salmon patches on the forehead are midline.
- Port-wine stains are irregular red-to-purple patches that start out smooth in infancy but may hypertrophy and develop a cobblestone texture with age (**Figures 170-1** and **170-3**).
- Klippel-Trenaunay syndrome is characterized by vascular malformations, venous varicosities, and soft-tissue hyperplasia over an entire limb or another part of the body. This may cause hemihypertrophy of a single extremity such as the leg (**Figure 170-7**).
- Patients with Sturge-Weber syndrome often have developmental delays, epilepsy, and ophthalmology problems (see Chapter 207, Sturge-Weber Syndrome).
- HHT is diagnosed if three of the following four Curaçao criteria are met (and suspected if two are present):
  1. Recurrent spontaneous nosebleeds (the presenting sign in more than 90 percent of patients, often during childhood);
  2. Mucocutaneous telangiectasia (**Figure 170-5**; typically develops in the third decade of life);
  3. Visceral involvement (lungs, brain, liver, and colon); and/or
  4. An affected first-degree relative.[7]
- Lymphangioma circumscriptum appears as fluid-filled vesicles in groups are clusters on the skin. These can be clear, pink or red depending upon the amount of blood within them (**Figures 170-8** and **170-9**). These vesicles can resemble frog spawn (**Figure 170-10**).

TYPICAL DISTRIBUTION

- Salmon patches are presents over the eyelids, glabella, forehead and posterior neck (**Figures 170-2** and **170-6**). Most salmon patches on the forehead are midline.
- Port-wine stains tend to affect the face and neck, although lesions may affect any body surface, including mucous membranes (**Figures 170-1** and **170-3**). Lesions of Klippel-Trenaunay syndrome tend to affect the lower extremities (**Figure 170-7**). A diagnosis of

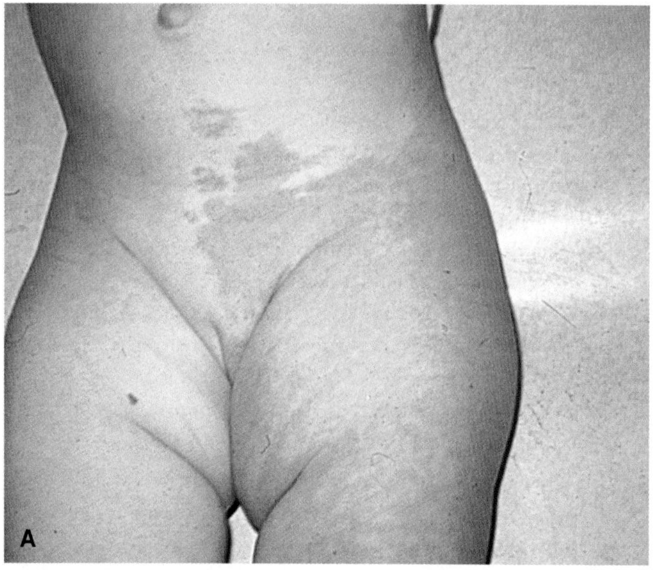

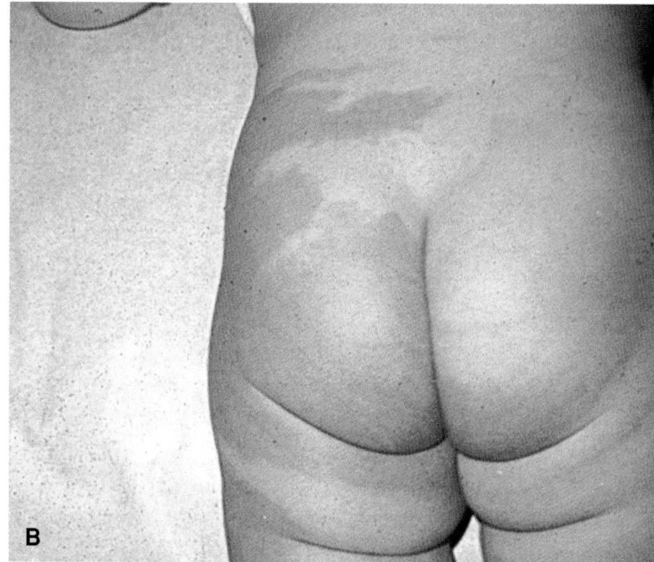

FIGURE 170-7 Klippel-Trenaunay syndrome with a port-wine stain over the left thigh. Over time, more massive vascularization and enlargement of the limb will develop. **A.** Anterior left thigh. **B.** Buttocks and posterior thigh. (*Used with permission from Weinberg SW, Prose NS, Kristal L. Color Atlas of Pediatric Dermatology, 4th edition, Figures 20-35 and 20-36, New York, NY: McGraw-Hill, 2008.*)

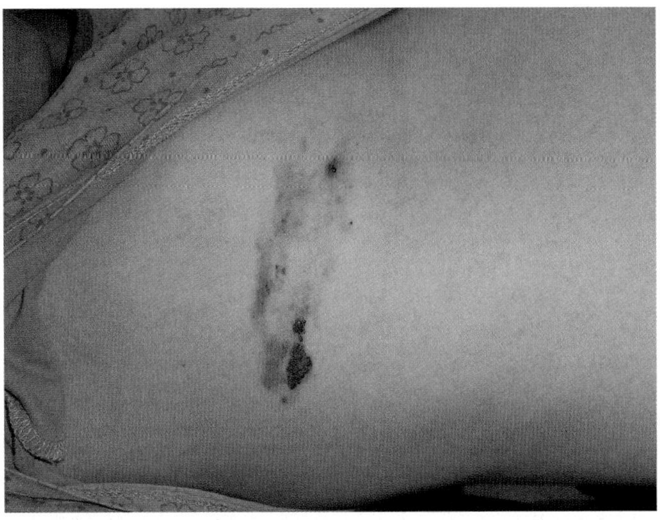

FIGURE 170-8 Lymphangioma circumscriptum since birth on the trunk of this 7-year-old girl. It is asymptomatic but the parents would like to know if it can be removed. (*Used with permission from Richard P. Usatine, MD.*)

Sturge-Weber syndrome requires that a port-wine stain be present in the trigeminal nerve distribution (see Chapter 207, Sturge-Weber Syndrome).

- HHT skin manifestations are few to numerous lesions on the tongue, lips, nasal mucosa, hands, and feet (**Figure 170-5**). However, any skin area or internal organ may be involved.
- Common locations for lymphangioma circumscriptum include the trunk (**Figures 170-8** to **170-10**), extremities, tongue, vulva, and genitalia.

LABORATORY STUDIES

- Patients with benign-appearing salmon patches, port-wine stains, lymphangiomas who lack other concerning symptoms, do not require laboratory testing.

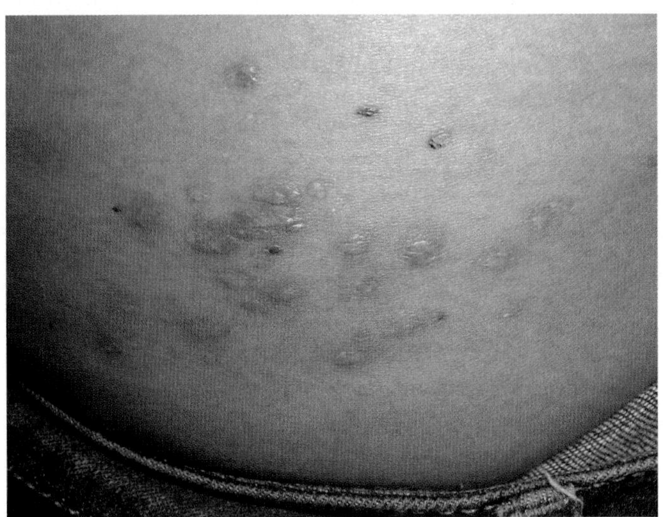

FIGURE 170-9 Lymphangioma circumscriptum near the waist of this 18-year-old female after sclerotherapy was partially effective. She is hoping that additional therapy will remove this from her skin. (*Used with permission from Richard P. Usatine, MD.*)

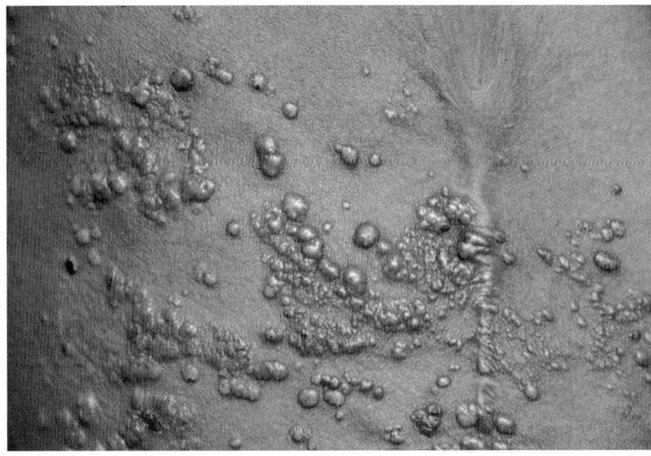

FIGURE 170-10 Lymphangioma circumscriptum on the trunk of teenager that occurred after surgery. Not all lymphangioma circumscriptum is congenital. Note how this pattern resembles frog spawn. (*Used with permission from Richard P. Usatine, MD.*)

- Check an annual complete blood count (CBC) and fecal occult blood in patients with HHT. They are at higher risk for iron-deficiency anemia because of recurrent nosebleeds and/or GI bleeding.
- If Sturge-Weber syndrome is suspected, perform neuroimaging and glaucoma testing. Neuroimaging may reveal leptomeningeal malformations ipsilateral to the port-wine stain. An electroencephalogram may reveal epilepsy. Elevated ocular pressures or visual field deficits may indicate glaucoma (see Chapter 207, Sturge-Weber Syndrome).

DIFFERENTIAL DIAGNOSIS

- Childhood hemangiomas are most likely to be confused with capillary malformations, especially if they are relatively flat. These are very different pathophysiologically as these hemangiomas are actually benign vascular tumors rather than malformations. Hemangiomas are usually raised and will involute over time (see Chapter 93, Childhood Hemangiomas).
- Childhood hemangiomas on the face may be part of the PHACES syndrome (see Chapter 227, PHACES Syndrome). As these may be segmental, they can be confused with the port-wine stain following a dermatomal distribution of the trigeminal nerve (**Figures 170-11** and **170-12**).
- Cutis marmorata is found in infants and presents with a reticulated mottling of the skin with a pink, red or bluish coloration when the infant is exposed to cold temperatures. It usually occurs on the lower extremities and is evanescent (**Figure 170-13**).
- Acquired capillary malformations seen in pyogenic granulomas (lobulated capillary hemangioma) could be mistaken for a congenital capillary or lymphatic malformation but a good history should prevent this confusion. Pyogenic granulomas are not present at birth and often follow local trauma to the area. They are often friable and bleed easily (see Chapter 142, Pyogenic Granuloma).
- CREST (calcinosis, Raynaud phenomenon, esophageal involvement, sclerodactyly, and telangiectasia) syndrome and scleroderma usually have multiple telangiectasias as in HHT. Other clinical

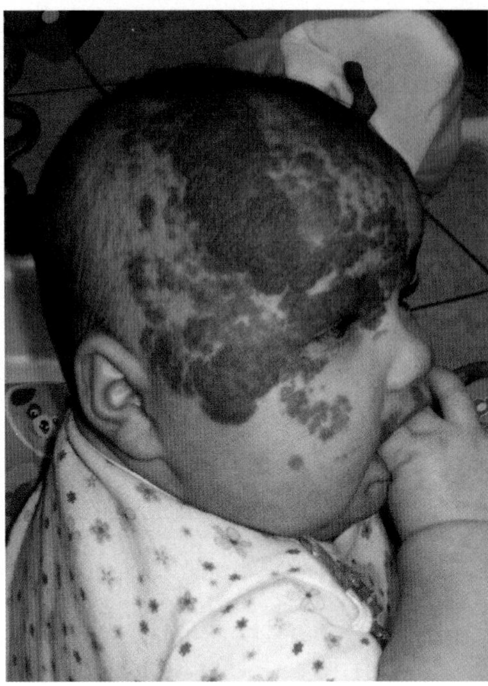

FIGURE 170-11 Infant with PHACE syndrome and a large segmental hemangioma over the face. The child also has a congenital coloboma of the right eye. (*Used with permission from angel face.com.*)

features and laboratory tests such as the antinuclear antibody (ANA) can differentiate between these rheumatologic conditions and HHT (see Chapter 178, Scleroderma and Morphea).

MANAGEMENT

- Port-wine stains may be treated with makeup (see the "Patient Resources" section at the end of this chapter). Pulsed-dye laser treatment is another cosmetic option available to teens and adults able to tolerate this procedure. Laser treatments blanch

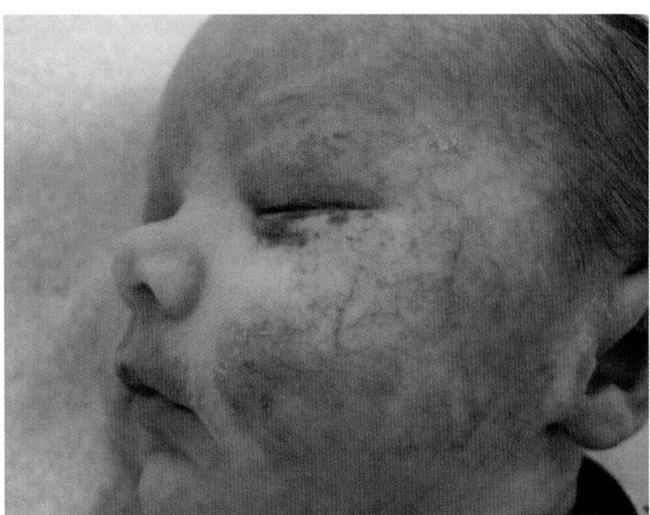

FIGURE 170-12 Infant with PHACE syndrome. In this case the hemangioma is flat with many telangiectasias and resembles a port-wine stain. (*Used with permission from John Browning, MD.*)

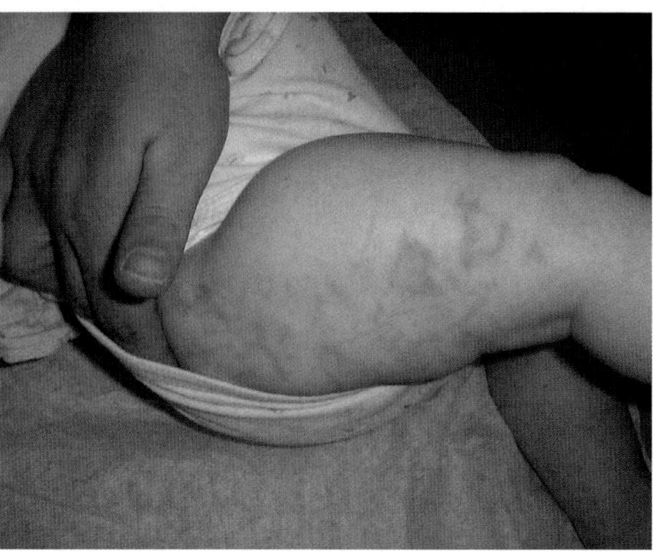

FIGURE 170-13 Infant with cutis marmorata showing a reticular pink network that occurs when the child is cold. (*Image used with permission from Robert Brodell, MD.*)

most port-wine lesions to some degree, but complete resolution is difficult to achieve and the recurrence rate is high.[8] SOR B In a Cochrane systematic review of the literature, pulse dye laser resulted in a 25 percent reduction in redness over 1 to 3 treatments.[9]
- HHT has no cure. Oral iron supplementation and transfusions are sometimes needed as a result of bleeding. Few randomized controlled trials exist regarding treatment of bleeding. Estrogen/progesterone supplementation for heavily transfusion-dependent female patients decreases recurrent bleeding.[10] SOR B Case reports and uncontrolled studies regarding epistaxis treatment show some benefit from laser treatment, surgery, embolization, and topical therapy. SOR C Cauterization is not recommended because of complications from local tissue damage. Embolization procedures have been described for AVMs in the liver, lungs, and brain. Surgical resection of AVMs is sometimes done as a last resort when other measures fail.[5] In short, it is often best to do as little intervention as possible with HHT and, if any intervention is done, it is done by specialists experienced with this disease, as complications and recurrence are frequently encountered.
- There are many treatments that have been tried for lymphangioma circumscriptum including surgery, electrosurgery, cryosurgery, sclerotherapy, topical imiquimod, and carbon dioxide laser.[11–15] In a systematic review of carbon dioxide laser for lymphangioma circumscriptum, 11 case reports and 5 case series with a total of 28 separate patients were identified. Eight patients remained disease free from 4 months to 3 years, 10 experienced partial recurrence, and two experienced complete recurrence.[16]
- In a case report of a 16-year-old female with a life-long history of a weeping, hemorrhagic, and painful lymphangioma on her right buttock, the authors attempted therapeutic treatment with pulsed dye laser.[15] The lesion appeared unchanged after two trials and so three sessions of electrodessication were applied to the aberrant lymphatic vessels. The lesion largely resolved without complications and was no longer causing pain or emotional distress.[15]

- In one series, 10 patients were treated with the combination technique of radiofrequency ablation (RFA) and sclerotherapy for their lymphangioma circumscriptum.[11] The sessions were repeated at monthly intervals until complete clearance. Nine of 10 patients who were treated with the combination technique achieved near-complete clearance. RFA ablates the lesions and achieves hemostasis while the sclerosant injected in and around the lesion reaches the deeper vascular lesions, preventing recurrence.[11]

FOLLOW-UP

- The need for follow-up varies from not at all to regular follow-up for patients with HHT and Sturge-Weber syndrome.
- Patients with Sturge-Weber syndrome should have yearly eye examinations that include testing of intraocular pressures SOR Ⓒ (see Chapter 207, Sturge-Weber Syndrome).

PATIENT EDUCATION

- Whatever the vascular condition is, patients can benefit from reliable information about the current and future outlook for their condition.

PATIENT RESOURCES

- Stork Bite—**www.nlm.nih.gov/medlineplus/ency/article/001388.htm**.
- HHT Foundation International. Excellent patient information on HHT can be found at the Foundation's website—**www.hht.org**.
- Covermark. Port-wine stains are often psychologically distressing. Cosmetic makeup may be purchased through Covermark—**www.covermark.com**.
- Dermablend is another effective cosmetic product for port-wine stains—**www.dermablend.com**.

PROVIDER RESOURCES

- Capillary malformation—**http://emedicine.medscape.com/article/1084479**.
- Medscape. *Laser Treatment of Acquired and Congenital Vascular Lesions*—**http://emedicine.medscape.com/article/1120509**.

REFERENCES

1. Monteagudo B, Labandeira J, Leon-Muinos E et al. Prevalence of birthmarks and transient skin lesions in 1,000 Spanish newborns. *Actas Dermosifiliogr* 2011;102:264-269.
2. Moosavi Z, Hosseini T. One-year survey of cutaneous lesions in 1000 consecutive Iranian newborns. *Pediatr Dermatol.* 2006;23:61-63.
3. Lorenz S, Maier C, Segerer H, Landthaler M, Hohenleutner U. Skin changes in newborn infants in the first 5 days of life. *Hautarzt* 2000;51:396-400.
4. Shih IH, Lin JY, Chen CH, Hong HS. A birthmark survey in 500 newborns: clinical observation in two northern Taiwan medical center nurseries. *Chang Gung Med J.* 2007;30:220-225.
5. Grand'Maison A. Hereditary hemorrhagic telangiectasia. *CMAJ* 2009;180:833-835.
6. Patel GA, Schwartz RA. Cutaneous lymphangioma circumscriptum: frog spawn on the skin. *Int J Dermatol.* 2009;48:1290-1295.
7. Shovlin CL, Guttmacher AE, Buscarini E et al. Diagnostic criteria for hereditary hemorrhagic telangiectasia (Rendu-Osler-Weber syndrome). *Am J Med Genet.* 2000;91:66-67.
8. Lanigan SW, Taibjee SM. Recent advances in laser treatment of port-wine stains. *Br J Dermatol.* 2004;151:527-533.
9. Faurschou A, Olesen AB, Leonardi-Bee J, Haedersdal M. Lasers or light sources for treating port-wine stains. *Cochrane Database Syst Rev.* 2011;CD007152.
10. van CE, Rutgeerts P, Vantrappen G. Treatment of bleeding gastrointestinal vascular malformations with oestrogen-progesterone. *Lancet.* 1990;335:953-955.
11. Niti K, Manish P. Microcystic lymphatic malformation (lymphangioma circumscriptum) treated using a minimally invasive technique of radiofrequency ablation and sclerotherapy. *Dermatol Surg.* 2010;36:1711-1717.
12. Ikeda M, Muramatsu T, Shida M et al. Surgical management of vulvar lymphangioma circumscriptum: two case reports. *Tokai J Exp Clin Med.* 2011;36:17-20.
13. AlGhamdi KM, Mubki TF. Treatment of lymphangioma circumscriptum with sclerotherapy: an ignored effective remedy. *J Cosmet Dermatol.* 2011;10:156-158.
14. Wang JY, Liu LF, Mao XH. Treatment of lymphangioma circumscriptum with topical imiquimod 5% cream. *Dermatol Surg.* 2012;38:1566-1569.
15. Emer J, Gropper J, Gallitano S, Levitt J. A case of lymphangioma circumscriptum successfully treated with electrodessication following failure of pulsed dye laser. *Dermatol Online J.* 2013;19:2.
16. Savas JA, Ledon J, Franca K, Chacon A, Zaiac M, Nouri K. Carbon dioxide laser for the treatment of microcystic lymphatic malformations (lymphangioma circumscriptum): a systematic review. *Dermatol Surg.* 2013;39:1147-1157.

171 ICHTHYOSIS

William A. Miller, MD, MPH, MSc
Richard P. Usatine, MD

PATIENT STORY

Two brothers are seen during a medical mission in Africa for their dry skin. The clinician recognizes the pattern of X-linked ichthyosis sparing the antecubital fossae of the arms amidst the heavy scales (**Figure 171-1**). With the help of a translator, the condition is explained to the mother and her boys. It turns out the mother's father also had the same condition but never received a diagnosis or had any medical care. The suggested treatment is daily emollients and keratolytics.

INTRODUCTION

Ichthyoses were recently reclassified by consensus with respect to nomenclature and whether they involved organs in addition to the skin (syndromic).[1] This chapter addresses four relatively more common ichthyoses pediatricians may encounter: ichthyosis vulgaris, X-linked recessive ichthyosis, epidermolytic ichthyosis, and lamellar ichthyosis. Common features of the ichthyoses include thick, dry skin, various forms and degrees of scaling, cutaneous inflammation, hypohidrosis, and skin fragility. Management is typically symptomatic, attempting to reduce morbidity, and often involves coordinated care with a dermatologist.

SYNONYMS

Epidermolytic ichthyosis (EI)—Formerly known as epidermolytic hyperkeratosis (EHK) or bullous ichthyosiform erythroderma (BIE), nonbullous congenital ichthyosiform erythroderma (NBIE) or congenital ichthyosiform erythroderma (CIE).

Lamellar ichthyosis—Also known as nonbullous congenital ichthyosis, one of the autosomal recessive congenital ichthyoses (ARCI).

EPIDEMIOLOGY

- Ichthyosis vulgaris—A common ichthyosis (**Figure 171-2**), with approximately 1 in 250 individuals affected.[2] Males and females are affected equally.
- X-linked recessive ichthyosis—Occurs in approximately 1 in 2000 to 6000 males.[3] Because of its frequent occurrence, steroid sulfatase deficiency accounts for most cases of X-linked ichthyosis, but a normal steroid sulfatase level in a male with ichthyosis does not rule out an X-linked pattern of inheritance.[4]
- Epidermolytic ichthyosis (bullous ichthyosiform erythroderma)—Prevalence of approximately 1 in 200,000 to 300,000 persons.[5]

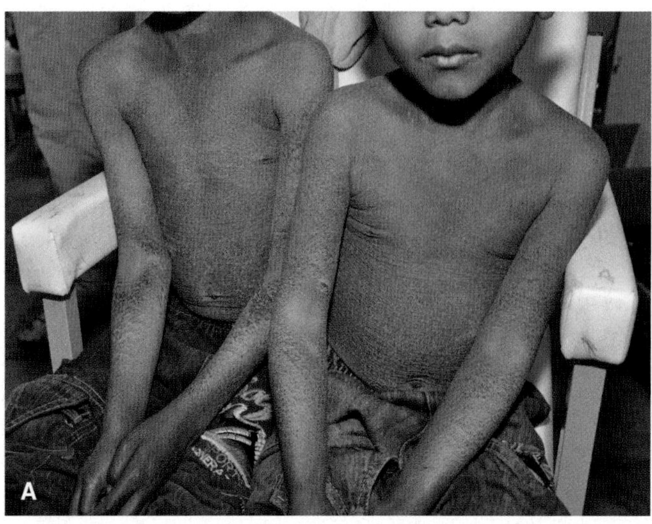

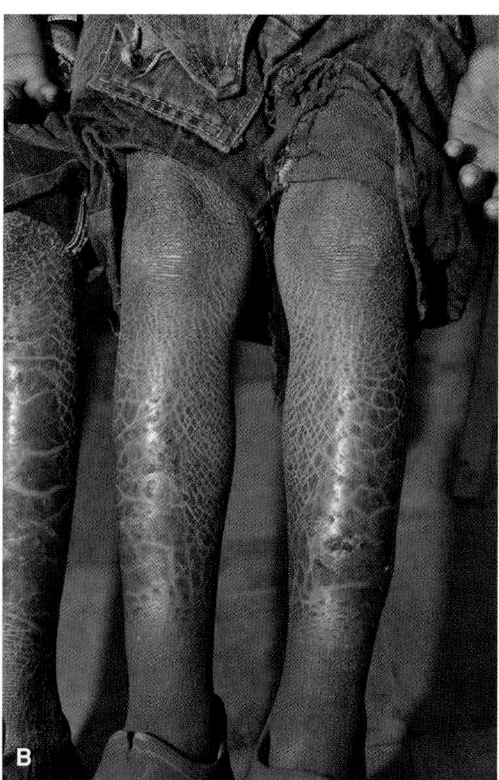

FIGURE 171-1 **A.** X-linked ichthyosis in two brothers showing sparing of the antecubital fossae of the arms amid the heavy scales. **B.** Heavy fish scale of X-linked ichthyosis on the legs of the same two affected brothers. (*Used with permission from Richard P. Usatine, MD.*)

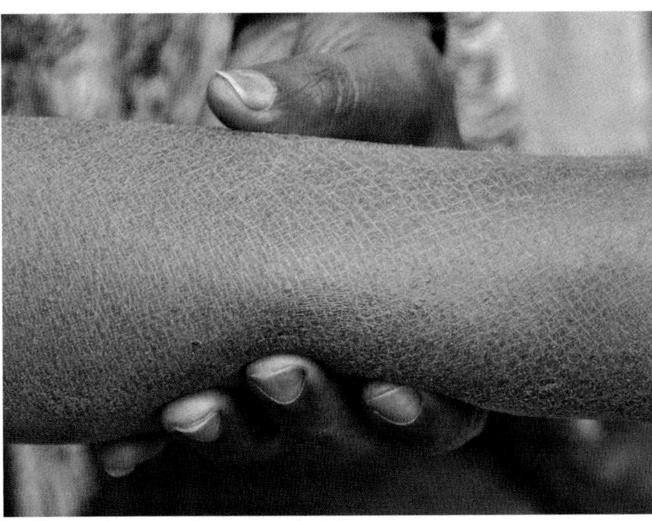

FIGURE 171-2 Ichthyosis vulgaris starts in childhood and has a fine scale. (*Used with permission from Richard P. Usatine, MD.*)

- Lamellar ichthyosis (non-bullous ichthyosiform erythroderma)—The most common form of autosomal recessive congenital ichthyosis (**Figure 171-3**).[6,7]

ETIOLOGY AND PATHOPHYSIOLOGY

- Ichthyosis vulgaris—A relatively common condition caused by loss of function mutations in the filaggrin gene.[2,8] It is inherited in an autosomal dominant manner and presents in childhood with a fine adherent scale in similar distribution to X-linked ichthyosis (**Figure 171-2**). Patients frequently have hyperlinear palms, keratosis pilaris, and atopic dermatitis, which are not commonly associated with X-linked ichthyosis.
- X-linked ichthyosis—A deletion of the steroid sulfatase gene results in keratinocyte retention by inhibiting desmosome degradation.[9] It is inherited in an X-linked recessive manner (**Figure 171-4**).
- Epidermolytic ichthyosis—Inherited in an autosomal dominant manner and is due mutations leading to production of faulty keratin proteins that function poorly.[10]
- Lamellar ichthyosis—A more severe and rare disorder resulting from mutations in the transglutaminase 1 gene.[11] Manifests with plate-like scales involving most of the body, including the face and flexures (**Figure 171-3**). Patients are typically born as a collodion baby (a thin translucent membrane that surrounds the baby at birth).[12]

DIAGNOSIS

ICHTHYOSIS VULGARIS

- Clinical features—Onset is usually between ages 3 and 12 months, presenting with fine scale, sometimes centrally tacked-down with superficial fissuring, varying degrees of dry skin, and hyperlinear palms and soles.[2] Some patients improve with age and especially

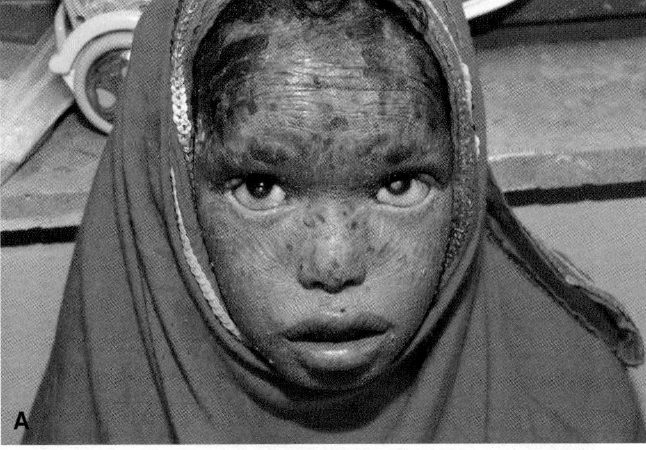

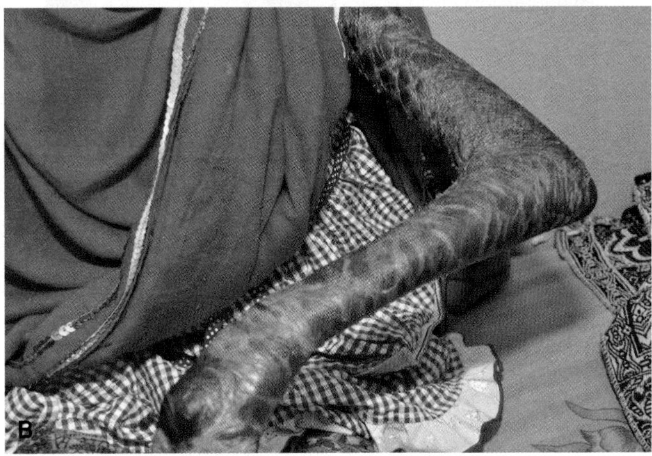

FIGURE 171-3 Lamellar ichthyosis is more rare and severe than X-linked ichthyosis. **A.** Note the deep lines and severe dryness of the skin on the face of this girl with lamellar ichthyosis. **B.** Her arm is severely affected so that she cannot extend her elbow fully. (*Used with permission from Richard P. Usatine, MD.*)

with warm weather. However, it typically does not clear completely.

- Typical distribution—Scaling is most prominent on legs, buttocks, abdomen, and trunk, while flexural areas are typically spared.
- Other findings—Can be associated with atopic eczema and keratosis pilaris.
- Laboratories—Appropriate genetic testing.

X-LINKED ICHTHYOSIS

- Clinical features—Firm, adherent, fish-like brown scale noted early in the life of young affected boys whose mothers were carriers of the gene on their X chromosome (**Figures 171-1** and **171-4**). Extracutaneous involvement may include ocular and testicular manifestations. Patients have an increased incidence of cryptorchidism and are at an increased risk of testicular cancer, independent of the risk from cryptorchidism alone.[2,3] These patients may have corneal opacities which do not affect their vision.[9,13] Often, they are delivered by caesarean section because a placental sulfatase deficiency results in failure of labor progression.[14,15]

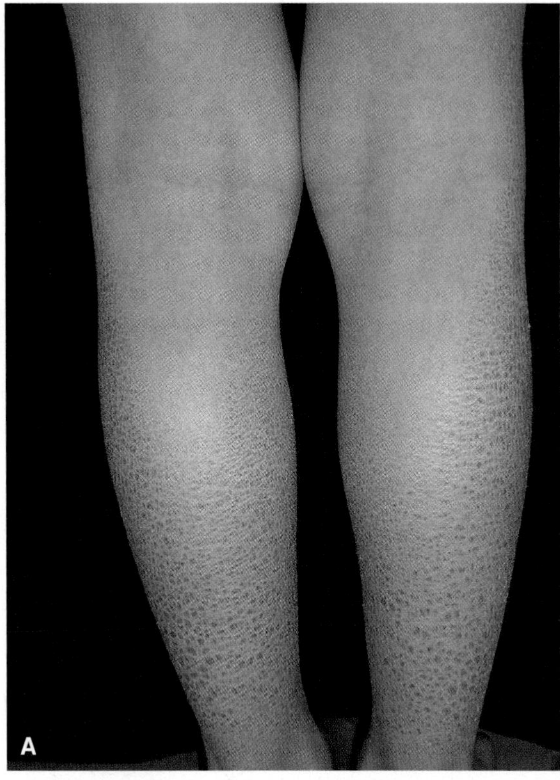

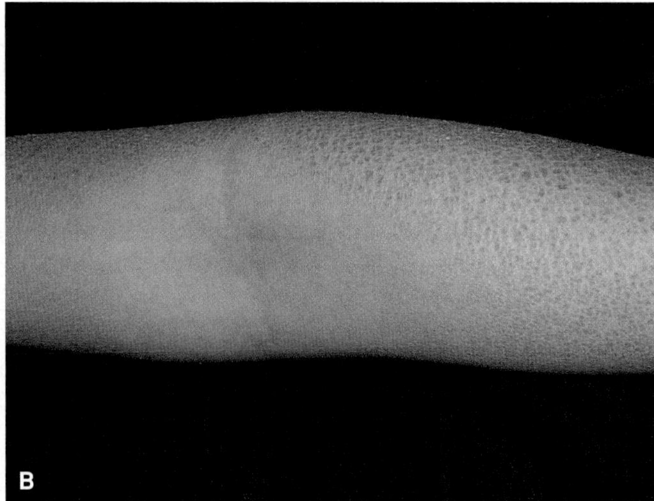

FIGURE 171-4 X-linked ichthyosis in a 9-year-old boy whose maternal uncle is also affected. **A.** Ichthyosis showing sparing of the popliteal fossa. **B.** Ichthyosis sparing antecubital fossa. (*Used with permission from Richard P. Usatine, MD.*)

- Typical distribution—Most of the body is involved, except for the typical sparing of the flexures, face, palms, and soles. The antecubital fossae are notably spared (**Figures 171-1** and **171-4**). There is an accentuation noted on the neck, giving these patients a characteristic "dirty neck" appearance (**Figure 171-5**).

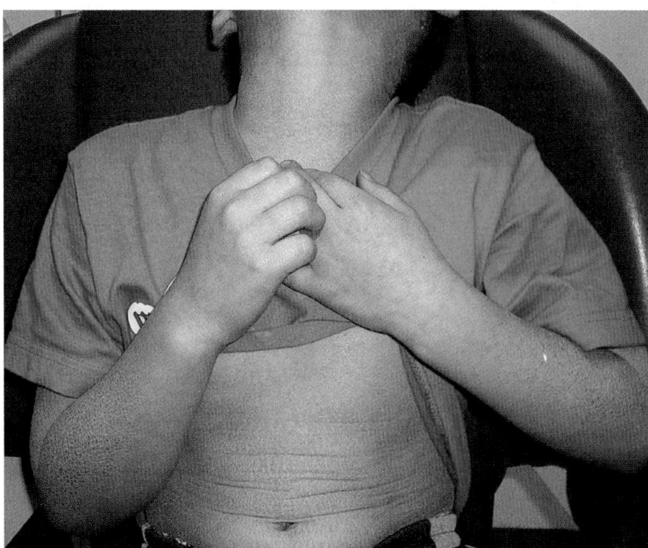

FIGURE 171-5 X-linked ichthyosis in a 9-year-old boy. His mother states that she could never get his neck clean. This is the "dirty neck appearance" of X-linked ichthyosis. Of course the neck is not dirty—this is the scale of ichthyosis which is also readily seen on the arms and abdomen. (*Used with permission from Richard P. Usatine, MD.*)

- Laboratories—Increased levels of serum cholesterol sulfate levels (steroid sulfatase hydrolyses cholesterol sulfate). Steroid sulfatase activity can also be measured directly. Appropriate genetic testing.

EPIDERMOLYTIC ICHTHYOSIS

- Clinical features—Patients present with fragile skin that eventually progresses to ichthyosis. Within hours after birth, minor trauma may cause blisters, superficial erosions, and peeling.[16]
- Typical distribution—Presents as a bullous disease shortly after birth with blistering resulting from even minor trauma. Only focal areas of hyperkeratosis and signs of skin weakness at sites of minor trauma may hint toward the diagnosis. Later in childhood, hyperkeratosis is noticeable on flexures, the abdominal wall, and scalp.
- Other findings—Skin colonization by staphylococcus, other bacteria, and possibly yeast creates an unwanted body odor.
- Laboratories—Appropriate genetic testing.

LAMELLAR ICHTHYOSIS

- Clinical features—Usually seen at birth presenting with collodion membrane (**Figure 171-6**).[12] After shedding membrane, patients demonstrate flushing and large, rough, dark-brown scales.[17]
- Typical distribution—Typically the whole body is affected, however some patients may experience partial resolution resulting in a bathing suit-pattern ichthyosis.
- Other findings—Ectropion improves during growth, but may persist into adulthood in many patients. Nail findings may include

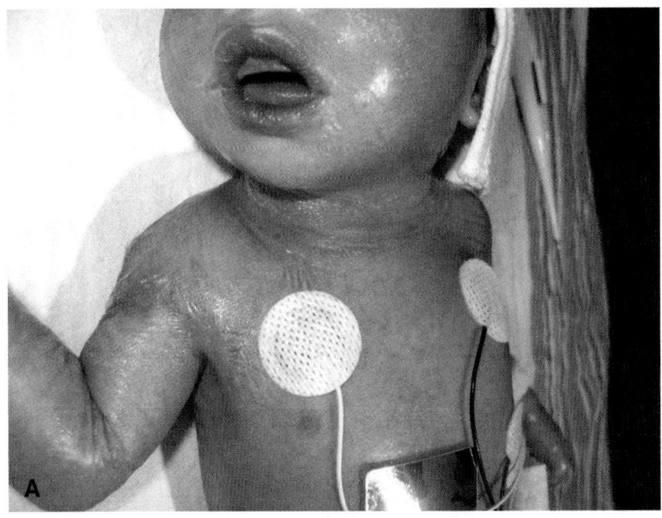

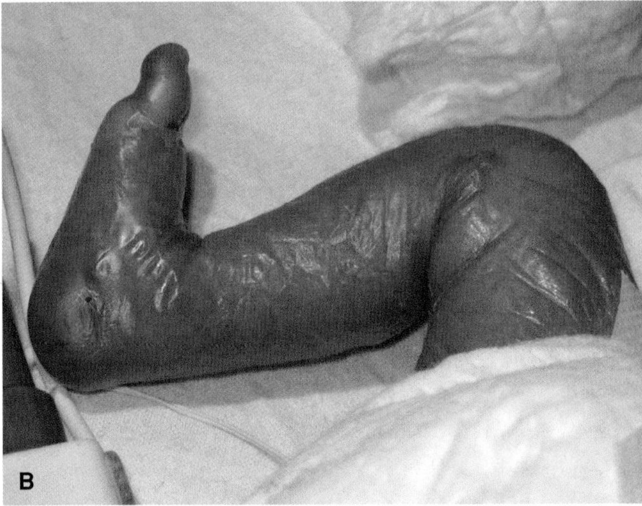

FIGURE 171-6 **A.** Collodion baby just after birth. Note the shiny skin covered with a thin membrane and the turning out of the lips (eclabium). This baby also had eversion of the eyelids (ectropion). **B.** The shiny skin is very prominent on the foot. (*Used with permission from Jeffrey Meffert, MD.*)

ridging, subungual hyperkeratosis, or hypoplasia. Patients typically cope with decreased sweat gland function. Bacterial and viral cutaneous infections are rare, however, fungal infections are common. Severe lamellar ichthyosis may affect growth and nutritional deficiencies may be present, including vitamin D deficiency. Possible vitamin D deficiency imparts an increased risk of rickets.[18-20]

- Laboratories—Vitamin D levels and appropriate genetic testing.

DIFFERENTIAL DIAGNOSIS

- Atopic dermatitis (eczema)—Much more common than the ichthyoses and typically presents with generalized dry skin (xerosis) resulting in pruritus that manifests the infamous itch-scratch cycle of atopic dermatitis. Repetitive scratching leads to skin thickening (lichenification) and accentuation in skin markings. Notably, atopic dermatitis is frequently the first condition to present in the "atopic march" of atopic dermatitis, food allergy, asthma, and allergic rhinitis (Chapter 130, Atopic Dermatitis).[21]

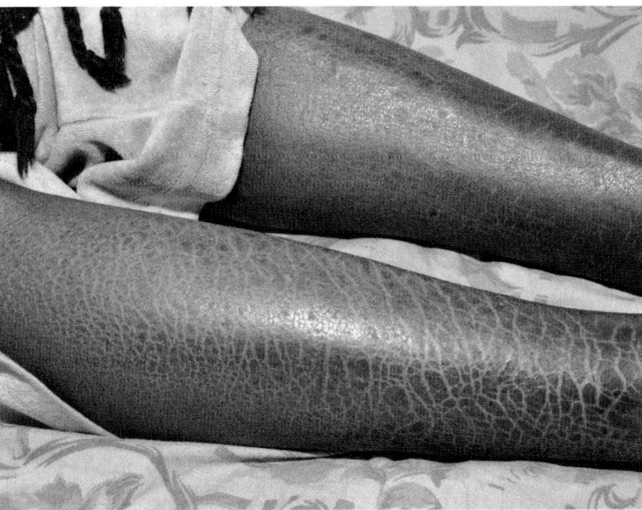

FIGURE 171-7 Acquired ichthyosis starts in adulthood and is especially prominent on the legs. (*Used with permission from Richard P. Usatine, MD.*)

- Acquired ichthyosis—Does not occur until adulthood. It is not inherited and may be associated with some systemic disease. The time of onset is the key to diagnosis. The legs are often are most involved and the skin appears similar to fish-scales (**Figure 171-7**).

MANAGEMENT

- Generally, frequent application of emollients and keratolytics are the mainstay of therapy.[22] There are many effective nonprescription and prescription products that contain petrolatum, propylene glycol, urea, or lactic acid.[22] Good choices for emollients include petrolatum, Aquaphor, and Eucerin. Ammonium lactate is an effective keratolytic available as a 6 percent OTC product or a 12 percent prescription. SOR Ⓒ
- Topical salicylic acid products used for their keratolytic properties to remove scale should be applied only on a limited area, as systemic absorption has led to salicylate toxicity in some patients.
- Epidermolytic ichthyosis tends to improve with age. If manifested in newborns as denuded skin, it may necessitate treatment in an intensive care unit due to increased risk of electrolyte irregularities and infectious complications. Further, patients should be handled carefully to avoid new trauma. Symptomatic care for blistering and use of emollients are particularly helpful in newborns. Moisturization and topical emollients continue to be the foundation of management as children age. Keratolytics may be avoided if they irritate the skin. Special diet and activity restrictions are not necessary.
- Systemic retinoids such as acitretin may be used in boys for severe lamellar ichthyosis by physicians experienced in their use (**Figure 171-8**). These agents are strong teratogens and should be avoided in any female of childbearing potential (including up to 3 years before menarche). SOR Ⓒ
- Gene therapy is an active area of research but is not yet a viable treatment option.

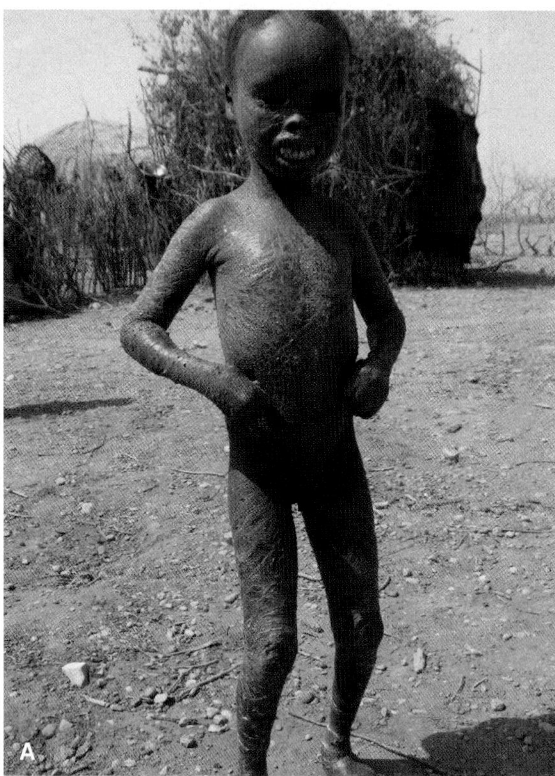

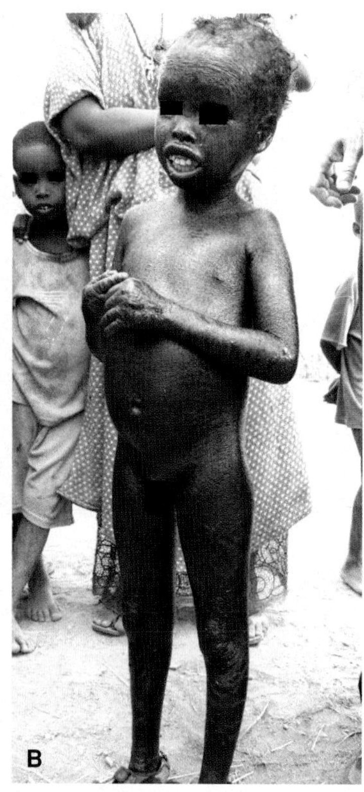

FIGURE 171-8 **A.** Lamellar ichthyosis in a young boy in Ethiopia. **B.** Great improvement in the ichthyosis after systemic retinoids (acitretin). (*Used with permission from Rick Hodes, MD and Richard Lord.*)

REFERRAL

- Refer to a urologist or ophthalmologist if testicular abnormality or corneal opacities are detected.

FOLLOW-UP

- Ichthyosis vulgaris—The prognosis is excellent, however, infection can result from fissured skin that has been refractory to management.
- X-linked ichthyosis—Adolescent males may experience cosmetic morbidity. Further, regular physical exams monitoring for corneal opacities and for testicular cancer in males should be performed at follow-up visits.
- Epidermolytic ichthyosis—Requires lifelong management but symptoms may improve with age.
- Lamellar ichthyosis—Specialist care by a dermatologist is recommended for skin assessment and treatment. Patients with ectropion should be referred to an ophthalmologist.

PATIENT EDUCATION

- Consider genetic counseling for all families that have a child with a hereditary ichthyosis.
- Ichthyosis vulgaris—For most patients, emphasis on regular and consistent treatment is important in achieving satisfactory management.
- X-linked ichthyosis—Use daily moisturizers, especially in dry climates and in the winter. Patients should understand the need for and should regularly conduct self-examination for testicular carcinoma.
- Lamellar ichthyosis—Patients should be informed of a higher risk of heat stroke.

PATIENT RESOURCES

- Foundation for Ichthyosis and Related Skin Types—**www.firstskinfoundation.org**.
- **www.ichthyosis.com** and **www.ichthyosis.org.uk** have support groups and information for patients and their parents.
- The American Academy of Dermatology has a summer camp that is free of charge for children with chronic skin conditions called Camp Discovery—**www.campdiscovery.org**.

PROVIDER RESOURCES

- **http://emedicine.medscape.com/article/1198130**.
- A helpful free online resource for the genodermatoses, or any genetic disease for that matter, is the Online Mendelian Inheritance of Man website—**www.omim.org**.
- For information on laboratories that perform rare genetic tests and clinics that perform prenatal diagnostic testing for certain conditions—**www.genetests.org**.
- Skin Advocate is a free application for mobile devices that is provided by the Society of Investigative Dermatology. It lists contact information for various patient advocacy groups—**https://itunes.apple.com/us/app/skin-advocate/id465525999?mt=8**.

REFERENCES

1. Oji V et al. Revised nomenclature and classification of inherited ichthyoses: results of the First Ichthyosis Consensus Conference in Soreze 2009. *J Am Acad Dermatol*. 2010;63(4):607-641.
2. Thyssen JP, Godoy-Gijon, E and Elias, PM. Ichthyosis vulgaris: the filaggrin mutation disease. *Br J Dermatol*. 2013;168(6): 1155-1166.
3. Ingordo V, et al. X-linked ichthyosis in southern Italy. *J Am Acad Dermatol*. 2003;49(5):962-963.
4. Craig WY, et al. Prevalence of steroid sulfatase deficiency in California according to race and ethnicity. *Prenat Diagn*. 2010; 30(9):893-898.
5. DiGiovanna JJ and Bale SJ. Clinical heterogeneity in epidermolytic hyperkeratosis. *Arch Dermatol*. 1994;130(8):1026-1035.
6. Bale, SJ and Doyle, SZ. The genetics of ichthyosis: a primer for epidemiologists. *J Invest Dermatol*. 1994;102(6):49S-50S.
7. Bale, SJ and Richard, G. *Autosomal recessive congenital ichthyosis. GeneReviews [Sitio en Internet]*. Seattle, WA. University of Washington, Seattle; 2001.
8. Harding CR, Aho S, and Bosko, CA. Filaggrin—revisited. *Int J Cosmet Sci*. 2013.
9. Fernandes NF, Janniger, CK and Schwartz, RA. *X-linked ichthyosis: an oculocutaneous genodermatosis. J Am Acad Dermatol*. 2010;62(3): 480-485.
10. Oji, V and Traupe, H. Ichthyosis: clinical manifestations and practical treatment options. *Am J Clin Dermatol*. 2009;10(6):351-364.
11. Oji, V and Traupe, H. Ichthyoses: differential diagnosis and molecular genetics. *Eur J Dermatol*. 2006;16(4):349-359.
12. Prado R et al. Collodion baby: an update with a focus on practical management. *J Am Acad Dermatol*. 2012;67(6):1362-1374.
13. Haritoglou C et al. Corneal manifestations of X-linked ichthyosis in two brothers. *Cornea*. 2000;19(6);861-863.
14. Bradshaw KD and Carr, BR. Placental sulfatase deficiency: maternal and fetal expression of steroid sulfatase deficiency and X-linked ichthyosis. *Obstet Gynecol Surv*. 1986;41(7):401-413.
15. Rizk DE and Johansen, KA. Placental sulfatase deficiency and congenital ichthyosis with intrauterine fetal death: case report. *Am J Obstet Gynecol*. 1993;168(2):570-571.
16. Lacz NL, Schwartz RA, and Kihiczak G. Epidermolytic hyperkeratosis: a keratin 1 or 10 mutational event. *Int J Dermatol*. 2005; 44(1):1-6.
17. Rodriguez-Pazos L et al. Autosomal recessive congenital ichthyosis. *Actas Dermosifiliogr*. 2013;104(4):270-284.
18. Kothari D et al. Ichthyosis associated with rickets in two Indian children. *Indian J Dermatol*. 2013;58(3):244.
19. Sathish Kumar T et al. Vitamin D deficiency rickets with Lamellar ichthyosis. *J Postgrad Med*. 2007;53(3):215-217.
20. Thacher TD et al. *Nutritional rickets in ichthyosis and response to calcipotriene. Pediatrics*. 2004;114(1):e119-123.
21. Carlsten C. et al. Atopic dermatitis in a high-risk cohort: natural history, associated allergic outcomes, and risk factors. *Ann Allergy Asthma Immunol*. 2013;110(1):24-28.
22. Hernandez-Martin A et al. A systematic review of clinical trials of treatments for the congenital ichthyoses, excluding ichthyosis vulgaris. *J Am Acad Dermatol*. 2013;69(4):544-549 e8.

PART 15

RHEUMATOLOGY

Strength of Recommendation (SOR)	Definition
A	Recommendation based on consistent and good-quality patient-oriented evidence.*
B	Recommendation based on inconsistent or limited-quality patient-oriented evidence.*
C	Recommendation based on consensus, usual practice, opinion, disease-oriented evidence, or case series for studies of diagnosis, treatment, prevention, or screening.*

*See Appendix A on pages 1320–1322 for further information.

172 JUVENILE IDIOPATHIC ATHRITIS

Shoghik Akoghlanian, MD
Andrew Zeft, MD MPH

PATIENT STORY

A 2-year-old Caucasian girl has had left knee swelling for 2 months (**Figure 172-1**). On physical examination, she has a warm left knee with limited range of motion and an effusion. Her left leg is longer than her right, and she walks with an antalgic gait. She has no other systemic signs and symptoms. Her antinuclear antigen (ANA) test is positive (1:160, speckled pattern) and her erythrocyte sedimentation rate is normal. She is diagnosed with oligoarticular juvenile idiopathic arthritis (oligoJIA). After initially taking nonsteroidal antiinflammatory medication around the clock, she is given an intra-articular steroid injection to treat her synovitis followed by physical therapy. Six weeks later, her knee exhibits full range of motion and is free of swelling. Six months later, she is found to have anterior uveitis (**Figure 172-2**) on routine screening slit lamp ophthalmology exam. Her uveitis is treated with ocular steroid drops, but her eye disease remains active, and requires the disease modifying antirheumatic drug, methotrexate.

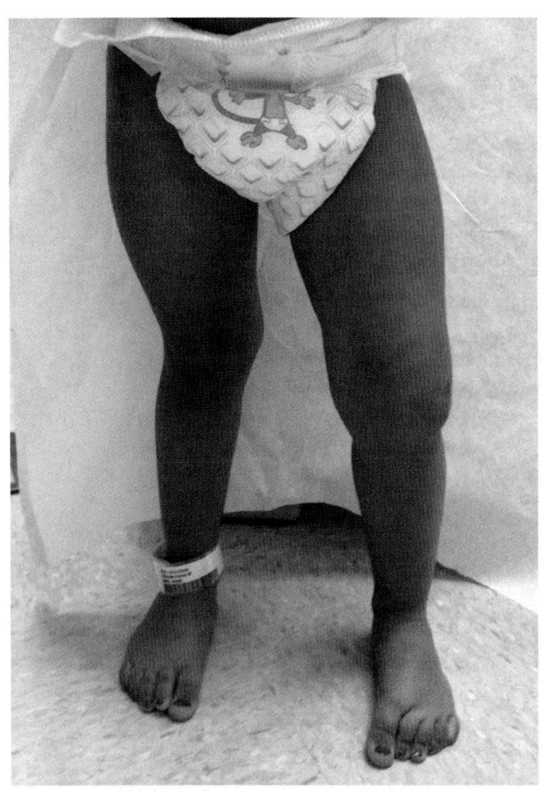

FIGURE 172-1 Swelling of the left knee in a 2-year-old girl with oligoarticular JIA. (*Used with permission from Vidya Raman, MD.*)

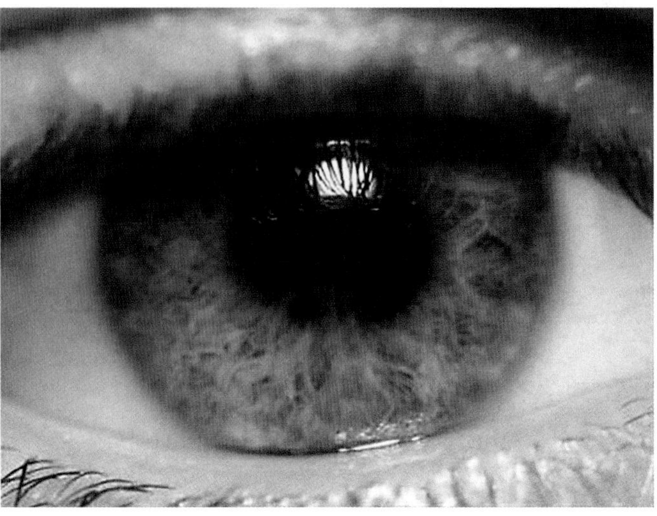

FIGURE 172-2 Synechiae complicating anterior nongranulomatous uveitis in a child with juvenile idiopathic arthritis. (*Used with permission from Carol A. Wallace, MD.*)

INTRODUCTION

Juvenile Idiopathic Arthritis (JIA), the most common chronic rheumatologic disease of childhood,[1] is defined by arthritis lasting greater than 6 weeks clinically beginning in a child before their 16th birthday after infection or other systemic etiologies have been ruled out. JIA is divided into 7 phenotypic subtypes which include: oligoarticular (persistent, extended), polyarticular (rheumatoid factor [RF] positive), polyarticular (RF negative), systemic onset, psoriatic, enthesitis related, and undifferentiated.[2]

SYNONYMS

Juvenile chronic arthritis (JCA) and juvenile rheumatoid arthritis (JRA).

EPIDEMIOLOGY

- JIA occurs worldwide.
- The prevalence is ~1 per 1,000 children, and the incidence is ~12 new cases per 100,000 children.[3]
- JIA appears to occur more commonly in children of Northern European ancestry.
- A striking age of onset peak in the oligoarticular type is noted between 1 to 2 years of age, in contrast to polyarticular JIA, which has a biphasic clinical onset with one peak between 1 to 3 years of age and another late in school age and into adolescence. Systemic onset JIA is more common in toddler-aged children, but otherwise onset is rather equally distributed amongst ages.
- In general, girls are affected more often than boys, but gender distribution varies with disease subtypes. The most common subtype, oligoJIA, occurs most commonly in toddler-aged girls (F: M, 3:1) and accounts for close to half of JIA diagnoses.

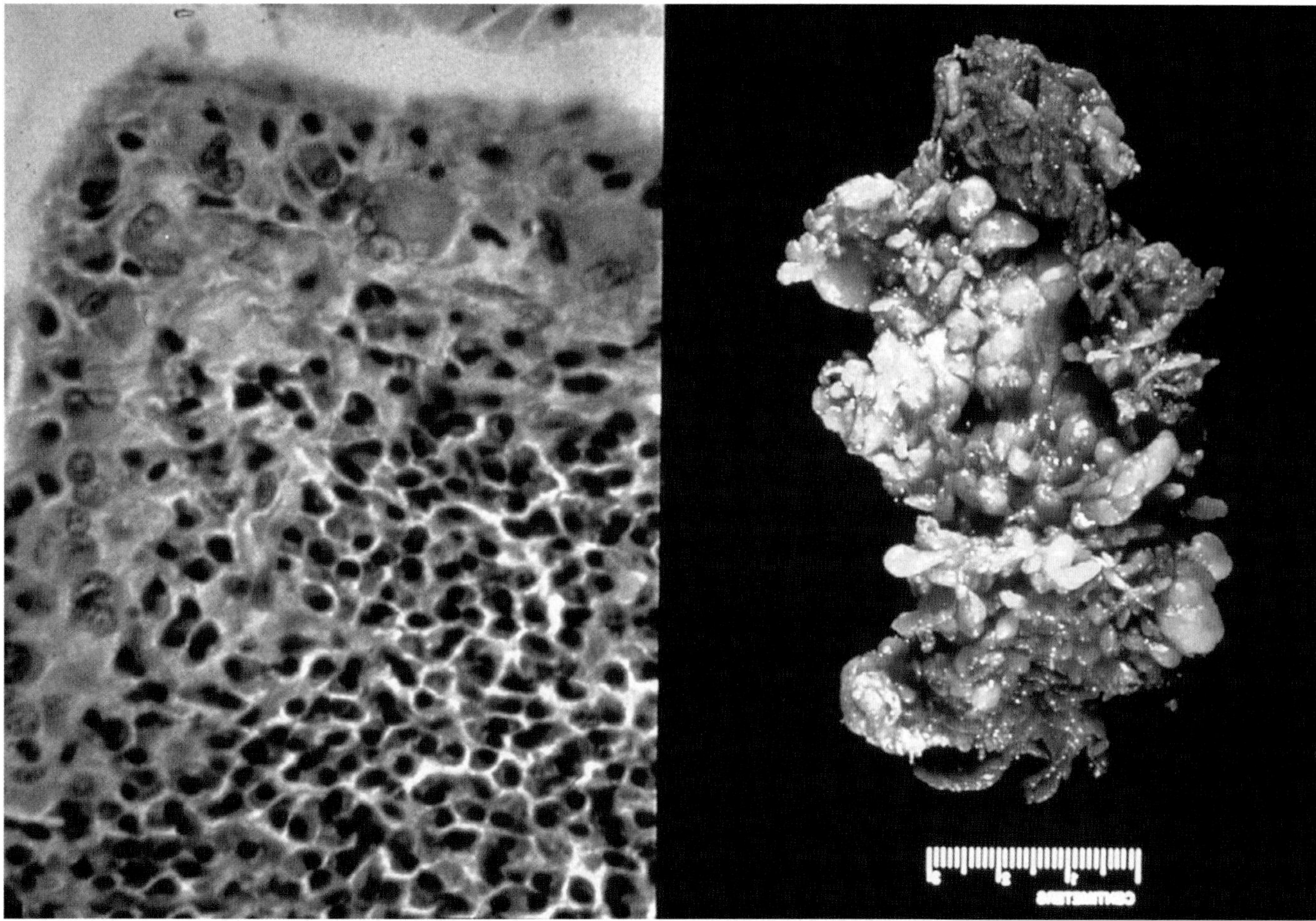

FIGURE 172-3 Pannus, composed of mixed lymphocytes and macrophages (left), seen after gross removal (right) from a joint of a patient with active juvenile idiopathic arthritis. (*Used with permission from Carol A. Wallace, MD.*)

- Anterior nongranulomatous uveitis occurs in ~15 percent of ANA-positive patients with either the oligoJIA or RF-negative polyarticular subtype (**Figure 172-2**).

ETIOLOGY AND PATHOPHYSIOLOGY

- The etiology of JIA is related to both genetic and environment factors.
- Synovitis describes synovial hypertrophy and a proliferation of inflammatory pannus (abnormal fibrovascular tissue). The presence of synovitis is diagnostic in children with JIA. Pannus is composed partially of T and B-lymphocytes as well as macrophages and is accompanied by angiogenesis (**Figure 172-3**).
- Contiguous cartilage and bone may be invaded and damaged.
- Cytokines released primarily by proinflammatory macrophages precipitate pannus formation and cartilage/osseus damage.

RISK FACTORS

- Genetic factors, aberrant immune responses, and putative environmental triggers play roles in JIA pathogenesis.
- Associations of HLA class I and II alleles with JIA are well established, further suggesting the involvement of T cells and antigen presentation in the pathogenesis of JIA.
- Hormonal influences may affect pathogenesis given the predominance of females with both oligoJIA and RF-positive polyJIA.

DIAGNOSIS

CLINICAL FEATURES[2]

- Arthritis is defined as:
  - Persistent joint swelling or effusion.
  - Presence of two or more of the following signs in one or more joints:
    - Limitation of range of motion.
    - Tenderness or pain on motion.
    - Increase in tactile heat.
- Enthesitis defined as inflammation where tendon, ligament, joint capsule, or fascia attach to bone.
- Specific JIA Subgroups and Definitions.
  - Systemic onset JIA (soJIA)—Presents with systemic symptoms such as fever, evanescent salmon-colored rash (typically truncal and nonpruritic; **Figure 172-4**), lymphadenopathy, and

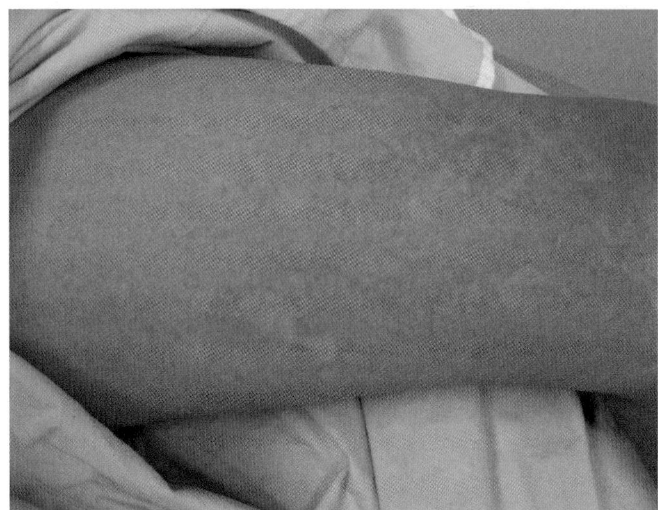

FIGURE 172-4 Salmon-colored, evanescent, macular eruption in a child diagnosed with systemic-onset juvenile idiopathic arthritis. (*Used with permission from Steven Spalding, MD.*)

hepatosplenomegaly with or followed by arthritis. Macrophage activation syndrome can be a life-threatening presentation of undertreated soJIA.

- OligoJIA—Arthritis involving 4 or fewer joints in the first 6 months of disease (**Figures 172-1** and **172-5**). OligoJIA is described as persistent (or extended) if the joint involvement persists beyond 6 months. Disease in children with persistent oligoJIA often remits with therapy, but risk for flares remain.
- Polyarticular JIA (polyJIA)—Arthritis involving five or more joints, further divided by JIA International League Against Rheumatism criteria into seropositive and seronegative polyarticular subgroups based on the presence or absence of IgM RF (**Figure 172-6**). Children with seropositive polyJIA share clinical and immunologic features of adult patients with rheumatoid arthritis, including symmetric arthritis disease involving wrists and small joints of the hands and feet, with or without subcutaneous rheumatoid nodules and articular erosions. Unfortunately, many patients with polyJIA enter adulthood with active disease and require continued treatment on disease modifying or biologic therapy.

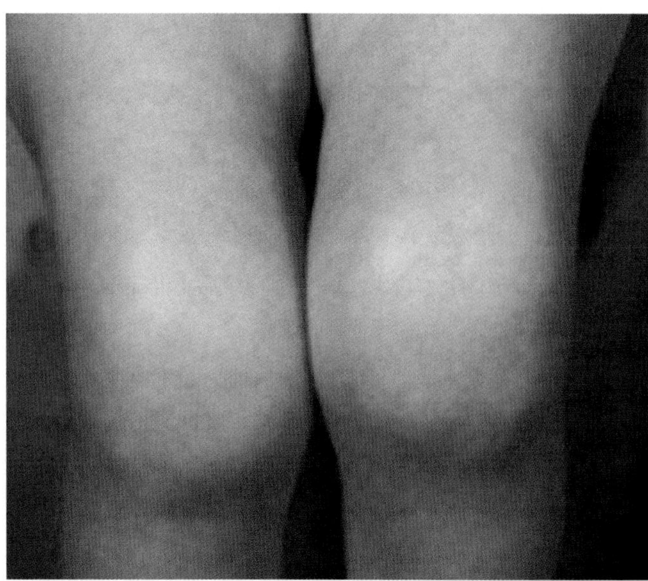

FIGURE 172-5 Left knee swelling in a young child with oligoarticular juvenile idiopathic arthritis. (*Used with permission from the Cleveland Clinic Children's Hospital Photo files.*)

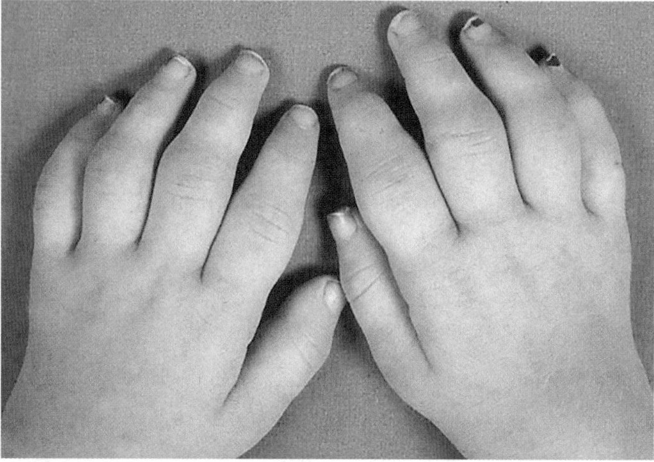

FIGURE 172-6 Small joint arthritis in a young child with polyarticular juvenile idiopathic arthritis. (*Used with permission from the Cleveland Clinic Children's Hospital Photo files.*)

- Psoriatic JIA (psJIA)—Either the presence of:
  - Arthritis and psoriasis.
  - Arthritis and 2 of 3 features including: dactylitis, nail changes ranging from mild nail pitting to onycholysis, and family history of a first degree relative having psoriasis or psoriatic arthritis.
- Enthesitis related arthritis (ERA)—The presence of arthritis and enthesitis *or* arthritis or enthesitis with greater than or equal to 2 of the following: history of sacroiliac joint tenderness and/or inflammatory lumbosacral pain, HLA-B27+, onset in a male >8 years of age, acute (symptomatic) anterior uveitis, or family history in at least one first- or second-degree relative of medically confirmed HLA-B27 associated disease. Typically enthesitis involves the lower extremities at tendon insertions at the posterior and anterior iliac crest, femoral greater trochanter, patella, tibial tuberosity, Achilles tendon, and/or planter fascia.
- Undifferentiated JIA—The patient's features of arthritis and other associated symptoms do not fit any other JIA category *or* fit more than one category.

LABORATORY TESTING

- No specific laboratory result is diagnostic for JIA.
- Hematological abnormalities may reflect the state of systemic inflammation (anemia of chronic disease, thrombocytosis, elevated ESR, as well as thrombocytopenia and dampened ESR in soJIA).
- ANA is associated with increased risk for chronic anterior uveitis in oligoJIA and seronegative polyJIA patients.
- Anticyclic citrullinated peptide (CCP) antibody is a specific but insensitive test for seropositive polyarticular arthritis.[4]
- Variable levels of synovial fluid cellularity, often (but not characteristically) <50,000 white blood cells per high power field.

DIFFERENTIAL DIAGNOSIS

- Infection—Lyme disease, bacterial (streptococcal or staphylococcus), brucella, and viral (influenza or parvovirus); mycoplasma, usually more acute in onset than JIA and have specific epidemiologic clues.
- Reactive arthritis in response to bacterial gastroenteritis (Yersinia, E. coli, salmonella, Shigella, or campylobacter) or genitourinary tract infection (gonococcal)—Preceding infection or specific symptoms help to differentiate these entities.
- Malignancy—Acute lymphoblastic leukemia (pre-B cell most common), metastatic bone, primary bone, cartilage, synovium, or soft tissue tumors can be distinguished from JIA by characteristic laboratory and radiographic features.
- Other pediatric autoimmune diseases involving arthritis, such as systemic lupus erythematosis and inflammatory bowel disease—Should be suspected when other organ systems are involved such as the renal and gastrointestinal systems (see Chapter 173, Lupus, Systemic and Cutaneous and Chapter 59, Inflammatory Bowel Disease).
- Metabolic.
    - Hurler's Syndrome—Bone and joint symptoms often occur in conjunction with other manifestations, such as growth delays, deafness, facial features, and heart valve abnormalities.

MANAGEMENT

NONPHARMACOLOGIC

- Physical and occupational therapy are recommended to restore and maintain function and prevent disability.
- Ophthalmology consultation in oligoarticular and polyarticular JIA patients to screen for intraocular signs of anterior uveitis and in psJIA or ERA patients, primarily for treatment of symptomatic scleritis, episcleritis.

MEDICATIONS

- Intra-articular glucocorticoid injection is first line therapy for oligo-JIA and utilized for other JIA patients with persistent disease activity despite systemic therapy.[6,7] SOR Ⓑ
- Non-steroidal anti-inflammatory drugs.[8–12] Provide symptomatic pain relief, but do not modify disease. SOR Ⓐ
- Systemic corticosteroids.[5] Induction treatment or may be kept at a low daily dose. Limiting daily systemic steroids is essential to avoid unwarranted side effects in children. SOR Ⓒ
- Disease-modifying antirheumatic drugs: methotrexate (most commonly), leflunomide, or sulfasalazine.[5,13] SOR Ⓑ
- Biologic agents[14]—Inhibit the action of proinflammatory cytokines:
    - Tumor necrosis factor-α (TNF-α; etanercept, adalimumab, and infliximab).[15,16] SOR Ⓐ for polyJIA
    - IL-1 (anakinra, canakinumab, or rilonacept).
    - IL-6 (tocilizumab).
    - Other medications target T-cell (abatacept) and B-cell (rituximab) function.
- Side effects of immune modulatory and biologic medications include increased risk of infection (tuberculosis dissemination with anti-TNF therapy). Screening for latent tuberculosis should be performed prior to treatment.
- Avoid administering live vaccines (MMR or varicella) while the patient is receiving chronic steroids, methotrexate, or biologic therapy.

SURGERY

- Synovectomy—Arthroscopic approach to remove chronic, persistent hypertrophic synovial tissue.
- Reconstructive surgeries and joint replacement for dysfunctional joints with long standing erosive arthritis, advanced secondary osteoarthritic changes, or to correct pronounced leg length discrepancy due to long-standing, unilateral disease.

PROGNOSIS

- Long-term functional limitations are common and often persist into adulthood.[17–19]
- Recent advances in therapy, especially the use of biologic agents, have improved the short- and medium-term outcomes.[15,16,20]

PATIENT RESOURCES

- **http://my.clevelandclinic.org/childrens-hospital/health-info/diseases-conditions/rheumatology/hic-Juvenile-Idiopathic-Arthritis.aspx.**
- **www.healthychildren.org/English/health-issues/conditions/orthopedic/pages/Juvenile-Idiopathic-Arthritis.aspx?nfstatus=401&nftoken=00000000-0000-0000-0000-000000000000&nfstatusdescription=ERROR%3a+No+local+token.**
- Arthritis Foundation—**www.arthritis.org**.
- American College of Rheumatology—**www.rheumatology.org**.
- Pediatric Rheumatology International Trials Organization—**www.printo.it/pediatric-rheumatology/index.htm**.

PROVIDER RESOURCES

- **www.rheumatology.org/Practice/Clinical/Guidelines/Juvenile_Idiopathic_Arthritis/**.
- **http://emedicine.medscape.com/article/1007276**.

REFERENCES

1. Gowdie, PJ and Tse, SM. Juvenile idiopathic arthritis. *Pediatr Clin North Am*. 2012;59(2):301-327.
2. Petty, RE et al. International League of Associations for Rheumatology classification of juvenile idiopathic arthritis: second revision, Edmonton. 2001. *J Rheumatol*. 2004;31(2):390-392.
3. Gabriel SE, Michaud K. Epidemiological studies in incidence, prevalence, mortality, and comorbidity of the rheumatic diseases. *Arthritis Res Ther*. 2009;11(3):1-16.

4. Tebo A, et al. Profiling anti-cyclic citrillinated peptide anibodies in patients with juvenile idiopathic arthritis. *Pediatric Rheumatology Online Journal*. 2012;10(1):29.

5. Beukelman, T., et al. 2011 American College of Rheumatology recommendations for the treatment of juvenile idiopathic arthritis: initiation and safety monitoring of therapeutic agents for the treatment of arthritis and systemic features. *Arthritis Care Res.* 2011;63(4): 465-482.

6. Zulian F, Martini G, Gobber D, Plebani M, Zacchello F, Manners P. Triamcinolone acetonide and hexacetonide intra-articular treatment of symmetrical joints in juvenile idiopathic arthritis: a double-blind trial. *Rheumatology*. 2004;43:1288-1291.

7. Sherry DD, Stein LD, Reed AM, Schanberg LE, Kredich DW. Prevention of leg length discrepancy in young children with pauciarticular juvenile rheumatoid arthritis by treatment with intraarticular steroids. *Arthritis Rheum*. 1999;42:2330-2334.

8. Giannini EH, Brewer EJ, Miller ML, Gibbas D, Passo MH, Hoyeraal HM, et al. for the Pediatric Rheumatology Collaborative Study Group. Ibuprofen suspension in the treatment of juvenile rheumatoid arthritis. *J Pediatr*. 1990;117:645-652.

9. Bhettay E. Double-blind study of sulindac and aspirin in juvenile chronic arthritis. *S Afr Med J*. 1986;70:724-726.

10. Kvien TK, Hoyeraal HM, Sandstad B. Naproxen and acetylsalicylic acid in the treatment of pauciarticular and polyarticular juvenile rheumatoid arthritis: assessment of tolerance and efficacy in a single-centre 24-week double-blind parallel study. *Scand J Rheumatol*. 1984;13:342-350.

11. Haapasaari J, Wuolijoki E, Ylijoki H. Treatment of juvenile rheumatoid arthritis with diclofenac sodium. *Scand J Rheumatol*. 1983;12:325-330.

12. Brewer EJ, Giannini EH, Baum J, Bernstein B, Fink CW, Emery HM, et al. Aspirin and fenoprofen (Nalfon) in the treatment of juvenile rheumatoid arthritis results of the double blind-trial: a segment II study. *J Rheumatol*. 1982;9:123-138.

13. Wallace CA, Giannini EH, Spalding SJ, Hashkes PJ, et al. and for the Childhood Arthritis and Rheumatology Research Alliance. Trial of early aggressive therapy in polyarticular juvenile idiopathic arthritis. *Arthritis & Rheumatism*. 2012;64: 2012-2021.

14. Ringold S, Weiss Pamela F, Beukelman T, DeWitt EM, IlowiteNT, Kimura Y, Laxer RM, Lovell DJ, Nigrovic PA, Robinson AB, Vehe RK. Update of the 2011 American College of Rheumatology Recommendations for the Treatment of Juvenile Idiopathic Arthritis: Recommendations for the Medical Therapy of Children With Systemic Juvenile Idiopathic Arthritis and Tuberculosis Screening Among Children Receiving Biologic Medications. *Arthritis & Rheumatism*. 2013;65(10):2499-2512.

15. Lovell DJ, Giannini EH, Reiff A, Cawkwell GD, Silverman ED, Nocton JJ, et al. for the Pediatric Rheumatology Collaborative Study Group. Etanercept in children with polyarticular juvenile rheumatoid arthritis. *N Engl J Med*. 2000;342:763-769.

16. Lovell DJ, Ruperto N, Goodman S, Reiff A, Jung L, Jarosova K, et al. Adalimumab with or without methotrexate in juvenile rheumatoid arthritis. *N Engl J Med*. 2008;359:810-820.

17. Zak M, Pedersen FK. Juvenile chronic arthritis into adulthood: a long-term follow-up study. *Rheumatology*. 2000;39:198-204.

18. Minden K, Niewerth M, Listing J, Biedermann T, Bollow M, Schontube M, et al. Long-term outcome in patients with juvenile idiopathic arthritis. *Arthritis Rheum*. 2002;46:2392-2401.

19. Bowyer SL, Roettcher PA, Higgins GC, Adams B, Myers LK, Wallace C, et al. Health status of patients with juvenile rheumatoid arthritis at 1 and 5 years after diagnosis. *J Rheumatol.* 2003;30:394-400.

20. Lovell DJ, Reiff A, Ilowite NT, Wallace CA, Chon Y, Lin SL, et al. for the Pediatric Rheumatology Collaborative Study Group. Safety and efficacy of up to eight years of continuous etanercept therapy in patients with juvenile rheumatoid arthritis. *Arthritis Rheum*. 2008;58:1496-1504.

173 LUPUS—SYSTEMIC AND CUTANEOUS

Vidya Raman, MD
E.J. Mayeaux, Jr., MD

PATIENT STORY

A previously healthy 16-year-old African American girl presented to the clinic with alopecia and rash over her face and arms for 6 months (**Figures 173-1** and **173-2**). She reported pain in her knees and ankles for a year and an oral ulcer 3 months ago, which had healed. Laboratory evaluation was remarkable for a low white blood cell count at 2.4 × 1000/uL (normal 5.0–13.0 × 100/uL), hemoglobin of 10.8 g/dL (normal 11.8–16.0 g/dL), and platelet count of 109 × 1000/uL (normal 142–424 × 1000/uL). Erythrocyte sedimentation rate was elevated at 45 mm/hr (normal 0–15 mm/hr). Antinuclear antibody was positive at 1:640 with a strongly positive antidouble stranded DNA antibody confirming a diagnosis of systemic lupus erythematosus (SLE). Urinalysis did not show proteinuria to suggest renal involvement. She was treated with prednisone and hydroxychloroquine resulting in improvement in her problems.

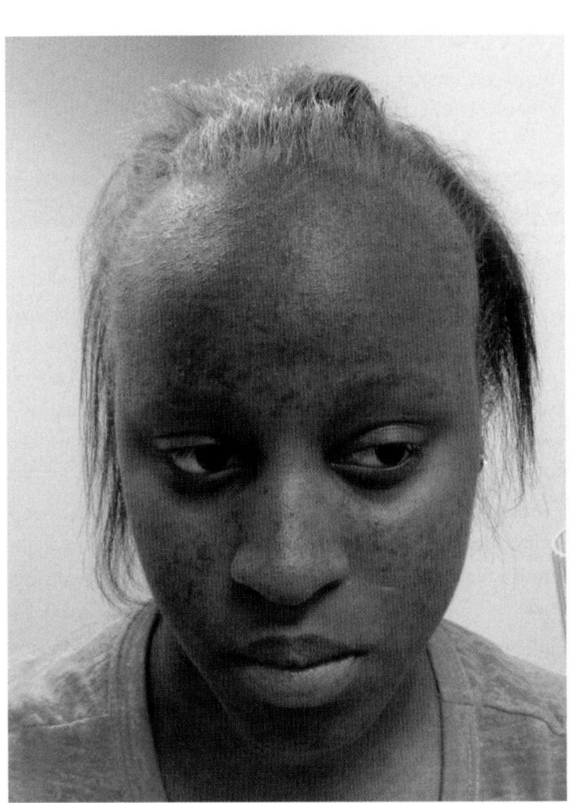

FIGURE 173-1 New onset systemic lupus erythematosus (SLE) presenting with 6 months of a facial rash and alopecia in a 16-year-old African American girl. She also had pain in her knees and oral ulcers. (*Used with permission from Vidya Raman, MD.*)

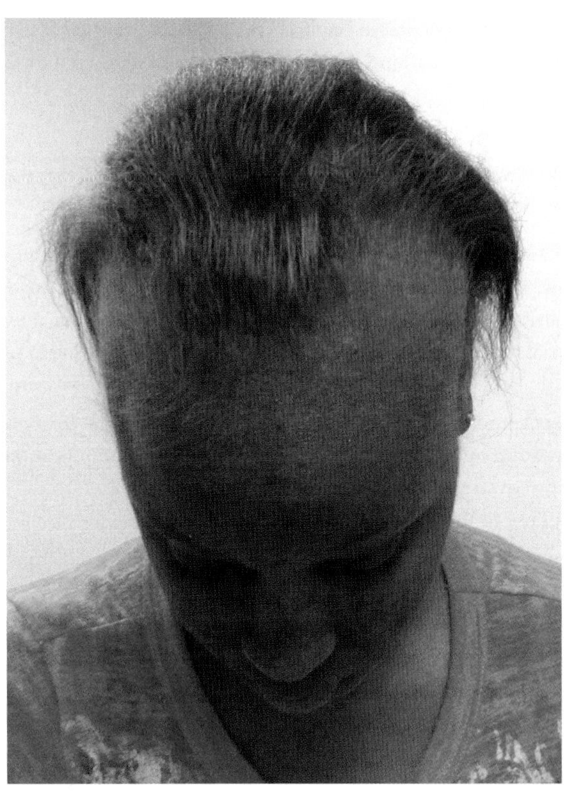

FIGURE 173-2 New onset SLE in a 16-year-old girl (as seen in **Figure 173-1**) demonstrating her alopecia. Her ANA was 1:640. (*Used with permission from Vidya Raman, MD.*)

INTRODUCTION

Systemic lupus erythematosus (SLE) is a chronic inflammatory disease that can affect many organs of the body including the skin, joints, kidneys, lungs, nervous system, and mucus membranes.

SYNONYMS

- Chronic cutaneous lupus erythematosus = discoid lupus = DLE.
- Lupus profundus = lupus panniculitis.

EPIDEMIOLOGY

- The true incidence of pediatric SLE is difficult to estimate since there are very few studies in the pediatric population. It is believed that approximately 15 percent of patients with SLE have onset of disease in childhood. Childhood SLE occurs in 6 to 18.9 cases per 100,000 white females, with higher prevalence in African Americans and Hispanics.[1]
- The mean age of presentation of SLE in children is 12 to 13 years.
- Discoid lupus erythematosus (DLE), which develops in up to 25 percent of adults with SLE, is less common in children.[3] Patients with only DLE have a 5 to 10 percent risk of eventually developing SLE, which tends to follow a mild course.[4] DLE lesions usually slowly expand with active inflammation at the periphery, and then

to heal, leaving depressed central scars, atrophy, telangiectasias, and hypopigmentation.[5] The female–male ratio of discoid lupus erythematosus (DLE) is 2:1.

ETIOLOGY AND PATHOPHYSIOLOGY

- SLE is a multisystem autoimmune disease with variable presentations. Based on current understanding, an environmental exposure, occurring in a genetically susceptible individual, results in activation of the innate and adaptive immune response resulting in production of auto-antibodies and loss of tolerance to self antigens.
- Recent studies in children have revealed a central role for type I interferon in the disease pathogenesis through an amplification loop activating T and B cells and may be useful in monitoring response to therapy.[6]
- Many of the signs and symptoms of SLE are caused by the circulating immune complexes or by the direct effects of antibodies to cells.
- A genetic predisposition for SLE exists. The concordance rate in monozygotic twins is between 25 percent and 70 percent. If a mother has SLE, her daughter's risk of developing the disease is 1:40 and her son's risk is 1:250.
- The course of SLE is one of intermittent remissions punctuated by disease flares. Organ damage often progresses over time.
- Rarely, neonates may develop a lupus rash and can have complete heart block from acquired antibodies through transplacental transmission from mother if she has active SLE (**Figures 173-3** and **173-4**).

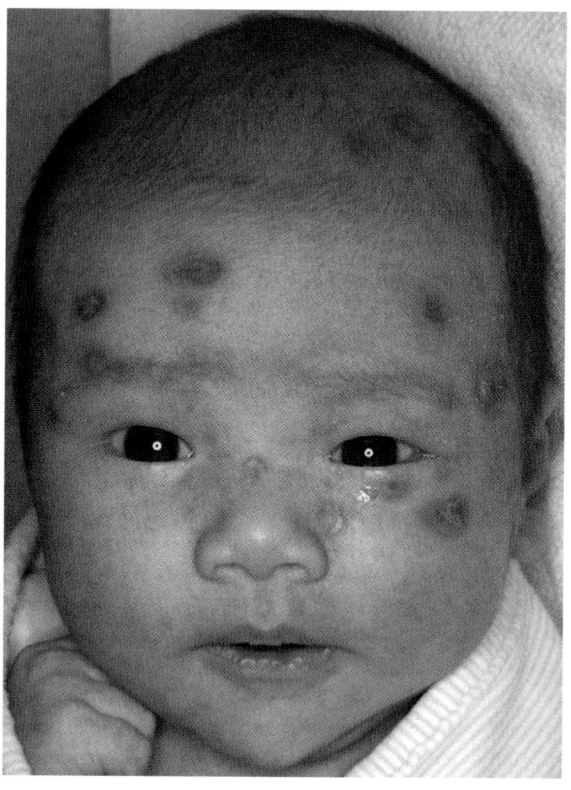

FIGURE 173-4 Neonatal lupus from acquired antibodies through transplacental transmission from the mother with active SLE. (*Used with permission from Warner AM, Frey KA, Connolly S. Annular rash on a newborn. J Fam Pract. 2006;55(2):127-129. Reproduced with permission from Frontline Medical Communications.*)

RISK FACTORS

- Precipitating factors for SLE include:
  - Exposure to the sunlight (ultraviolet light, especially UVB).
  - Infections.
  - Stress.
  - Trauma or surgery.
  - Pregnancy (especially in the postpartum period).

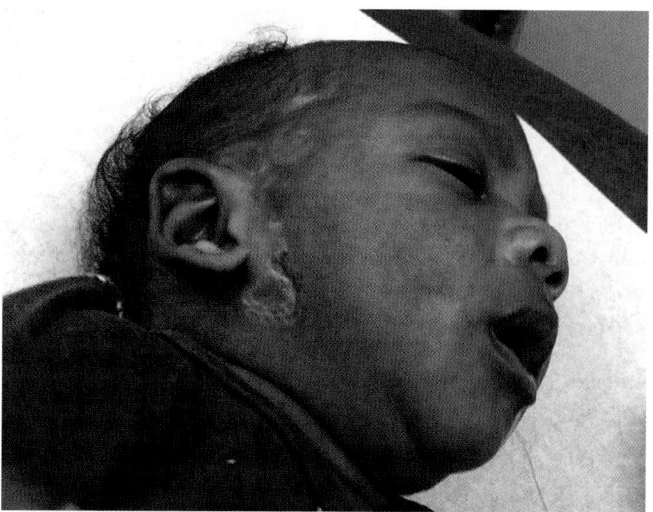

FIGURE 173-3 Neonatal lupus from acquired antibodies through transplacental transmission from the mother with positive SSA (Ro) and SSB (La) antibodies. (*Used with permission from Vidya Raman, MD.*)

DIAGNOSIS

CLINICAL FEATURES

- SLE is a chronic, recurrent, potentially fatal inflammatory disorder that can be difficult to diagnose. It is an autoimmune disease involving multiple organ systems that is defined clinically with associated autoantibodies directed against cell nuclei. The disease has no single diagnostic sign or marker (**Table 173-1**). Accurate diagnosis is important because treatment can reduce morbidity and mortality.[7]
- SLE most often presents with a mixture of constitutional symptoms including fatigue, fever, myalgia, anorexia, nausea, and weight loss. The mean length of time between onset of symptoms and diagnosis is 5 years.
- The disease is characterized by exacerbations and remissions as well as symptoms. The diagnosis of SLE is made if four or more of the manifestations mentioned in the following are either present, serially or simultaneously, in the patient at the time of presentation or were present in the past. Arthralgias, which are often the initial complaint, are usually out of proportion to physical findings. The polyarthritis is symmetric, nonerosive, and usually nondeforming. In longstanding disease, rheumatoid-like deformities with swan-neck fingers are commonly seen.

TABLE 173-1 American College of Rheumatology Criteria for Diagnosis of Systemic Lupus Erythematosus[1,2]

Criterion	Definition
Malar rash	Fixed erythema, flat or raised, over the malar eminences, tending to spare the nasolabial folds.
Discoid rash	Erythematosus raised patches with adherent keratotic scaling and follicular plugging and later atrophic scarring.
Photosensitivity	Skin rash as a result of unusual reaction to sunlight, by history or physician observation.
Oral ulcers	Oral or nasopharyngeal ulceration, usually painless, observed by a physician.
Arthritis	Nonerosive arthritis involving 2 or more peripheral joints, characterized by tenderness, swelling, or effusion.
Serositis	Pleuritis—Convincing history of pleuritic pain or rub heard by a physician or evidence of pleural effusion **OR** pericarditis documented by EKG, rub, or evidence of pericardial effusion.
Renal disorder	Persistent proteinuria greater than 0.5 grams per day or greater than 3+ if quantitation not performed **OR** red cell, hemoglobin, granular, tubular, or mixed cellular casts.
Neurologic disorder	Seizures **OR** psychosis—In the absence of offending drugs or known metabolic derangements (uremia, ketoacidosis, or electrolyte imbalance).
Hematologic disorder	Hemolytic anemia with reticulocytosis **OR** leukopenia (<4,000/mm^3 on two or more occasions) **OR** lymphopenia (<1,500/mm^3 on two or more occasions) **OR** thrombocytopenia (<100,000/mm^3) in the absence of offending drugs.
Immunologic disorders	Positive antiphospholipid antibody **OR** anti-DNA—Antibody to native DNA in abnormal titer **OR** anti-Sm—Presence of antibody to Sm nuclear antigen **OR** false positive serologic test for syphilis known to be positive for at least six months and confirmed by Treponema pallidum immobilization or fluorescent treponemal antibody absorption test.
Antinuclear antibody	An abnormal titer of antinuclear antibody by immunofluorescence or an equivalent assay at any point in time and in the absence of drugs known to be associated with "drug-induced lupus" syndrome.

[1]Four of the criterion are required to make the diagnosis.
[2]*Modified with permission from Callahan LF, Pincus T. Mortality in the rheumatic diseases. Arthritis Care Res. 1995;8:229.*

- A malar or butterfly rash is fixed erythema over the cheeks and bridge of the nose sparing the nasolabial folds (**Figures 173-5** and **173-6**). It may also involve the chin and ears. More severe malar rashes may cause severe atrophy, scarring, and hypopigmentation.
- The rash is often associated with photosensitivity to ultraviolet (UV) light.
- A discoid rash consisting of erythematosus raised patches with adherent keratotic scaling and follicular plugging. Atrophic scarring may occur in older lesions.
- Ulcers (usually painless) in the nose, mouth, or vagina are frequent complaints.
- Pleuritis as evidenced by a convincing history of pleuritic pain or rub or evidence of pleural effusion.
- Pericarditis as documented by EKG, rub, or evidence of pericardial effusion.
- Renal disorder such as cellular casts or persistent proteinuria >0.5 g/d or >3+ if quantitation not performed.
- Central nervous system (CNS) symptoms ranging from mild cognitive dysfunction to psychosis or seizures. Any region of CNS can be involved. Intractable headaches and difficulties with memory and reasoning are the most common features of neurologic disease in lupus patients.
- Hematologic disorders such as hemolytic anemia, leukopenia (<4000/mm^3 total on two or more occasions), lymphopenia (<1500/mm^3 on two or more occasions), or thrombocytopenia (<100,000/mm^3 in the absence of precipitating drugs).
- GI symptoms may include abdominal pain, diarrhea, and vomiting. Intestinal perforation and vasculitis are important diagnoses to exclude.
- Vasculitis (**Figures 173-6** and **173-7**) can be severe and can include retinal vasculitis.
- Immunologic disorders such as a positive antiphospholipid antibody, anti-DNA, anti-Sm, or a false positive serologic test for syphilis (known to be positive for at least 6 months and confirmed by a negative treponema specific test).
- An abnormal titer of antinuclear antibody at any point in time and in the absence of drugs associated with "drug-induced lupus."
- DLE (cutaneous lupus) lesions are characterized by discrete, erythematous, slightly infiltrated papule or plaques covered by a

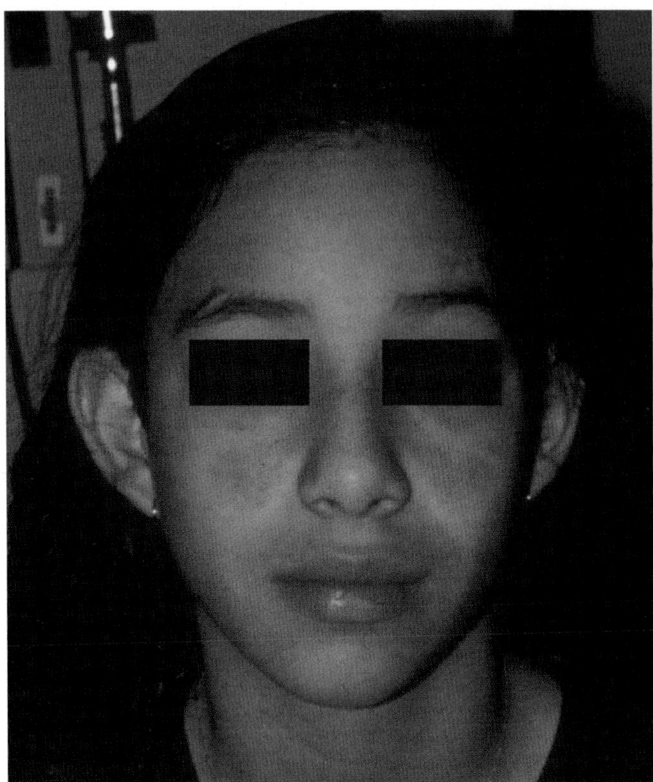

FIGURE 173-5 Malar rash in adolescent Hispanic girl with SLE. Note the relative sparing of the nasolabial fold. (*Used with permission from the University of Texas Health Sciences Center, Division of Dermatology.*)

well-formed adherent scale (**Figures 173-8** to **173-11**). As the lesion progresses, the scale often thickens and becomes adherent. Hypopigmentation develops in the central area and hyperpigmentation develops at the active border. Resolution of the active lesion results in atrophy and scarring. When they occur in the scalp, scarring alopecia often results (**Figure 173-12**). If the scale on the scalp is removed, it may leave a "carpet tack sign" from follicular plugging.

TYPICAL DISTRIBUTION

- SLE is known for its typical malar rash across the face like a butterfly (**Figures 173-5** and **173-13**).

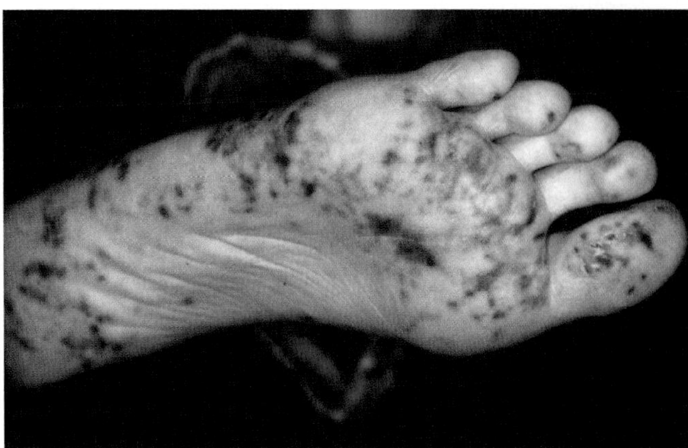

FIGURE 173-6 Necrotizing angiitis in a Japanese American patient with a severe lupus flare. Palpable purpura was evident on both feet and hands. (*Used with permission from Richard P. Usatine, MD.*)

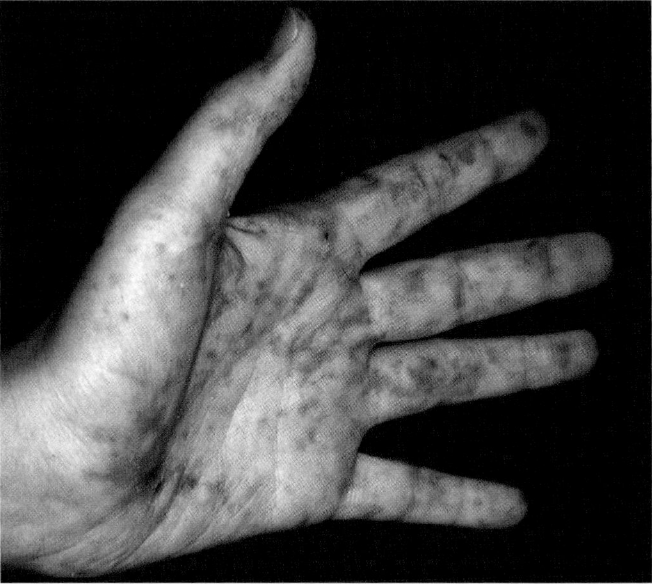

FIGURE 173-7 Necrotizing angiitis on the hand of the patient in **Figure 173-6** with lupus. (*Used with permission from Richard P. Usatine, MD.*)

- Discoid lesions are most often seen on the face, neck, and scalp, but also occur on the ears, and infrequently on the upper torso.
- DLE lesions may be localized or widespread. Localized DLE occurs only in the head and neck area, while widespread DLE occurs anywhere. Patients with widespread involvement are more likely to develop SLE.
- Lupus panniculitis, or lupus profundus, is a variant of LE that primarily affects subcutaneous fat. It usually involves the proximal extremities, trunk, breasts, buttocks, and face (**Figure 173-14**).

LABORATORY TESTING

- The American College of Rheumatology recommends ANA testing in patients who have two or more unexplained signs or symptoms

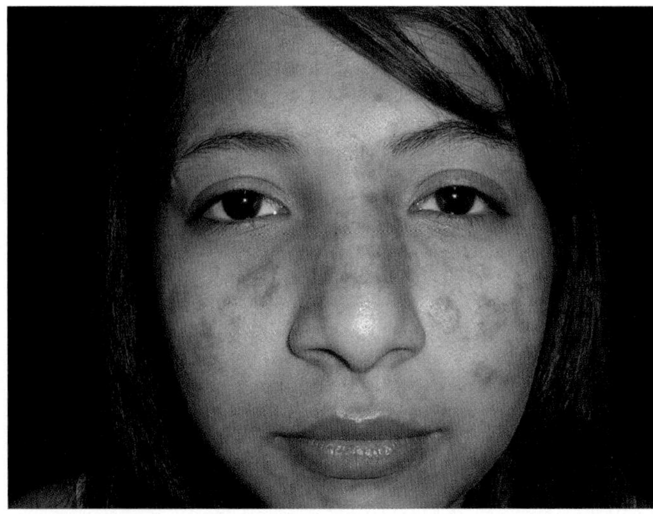

FIGURE 173-8 Cutaneous lupus (discoid lupus) on the face of this teenage Hispanic girl. (*Used with permission from Richard P. Usatine, MD.*)

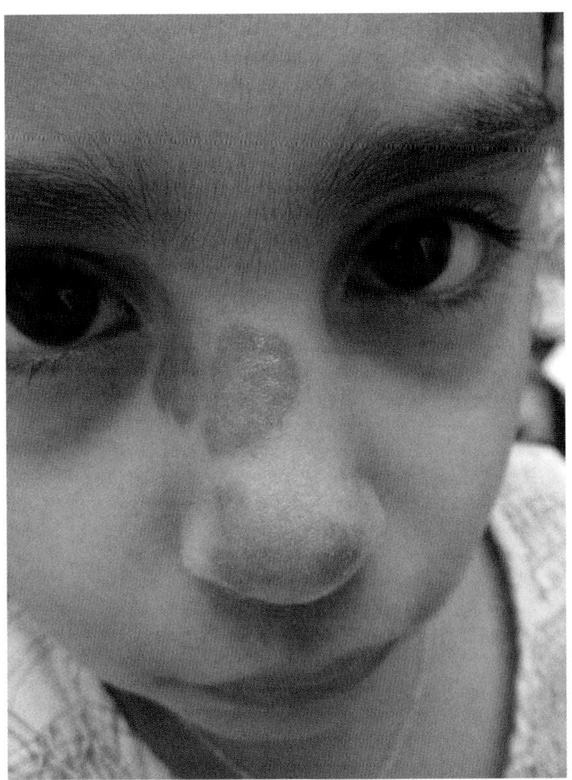

FIGURE 173-9 Cutaneous lupus on the face of a 5-year-old girl. She is responding to hydroxychloroquine with improvement in the facial lesions. (*Used with permission from Lewis Rose, MD.*)

that could be lupus. Elevation of the ANA titer to or above 1:80 is the most sensitive of the American College of Rheumatology diagnostic criteria. Although many patients may have a negative ANA titer early in the disease, more than 99 percent of SLE patients will eventually have an elevated ANA titer.[9] The ANA test is not specific for lupus, and the most common reason for a positive ANA test without SLE (usually at titers <1:80) is the presence of another connective tissue disease. ANA titer is useful in screening and

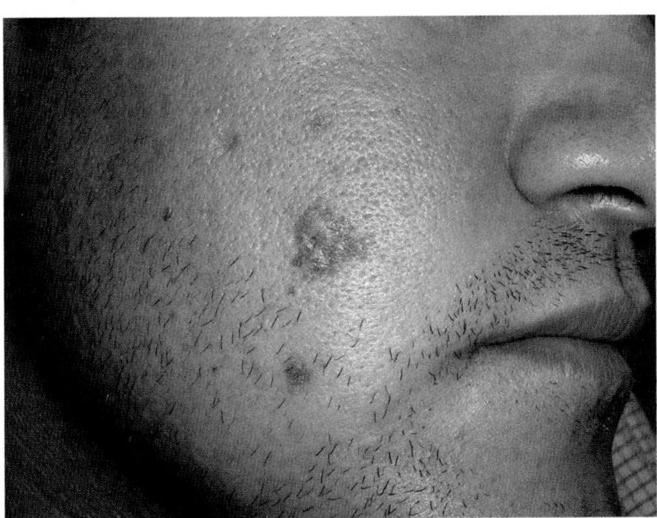

FIGURE 173-10 Discoid lupus with hyperpigmentation and scarring on the face of this young man.

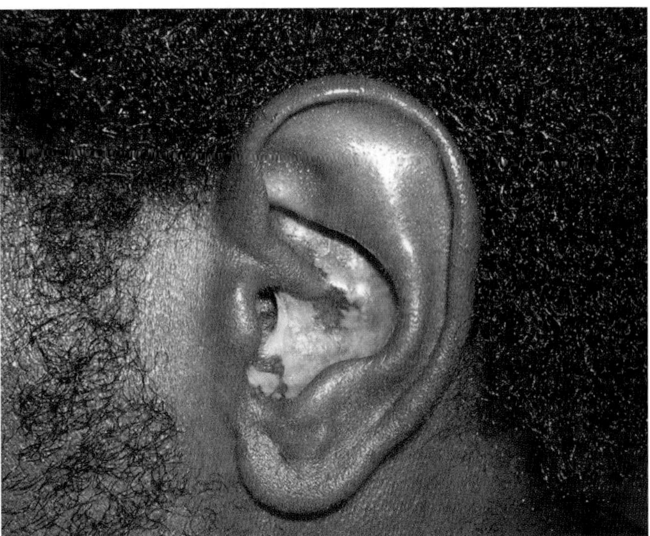

FIGURE 173-11 Discoid lupus with hypopigmentation and scarring inside the pinna. (*Used with permission from E.J. Mayeaux, Jr., MD.*)

diagnosis but not in monitoring disease activity. Specific antibodies used in confirming the diagnosis include anti-double stranded DNA (anti-DS DNA) and anti-Smith antibodies.

- Active SLE is often heralded by a rise in IgG anti-double-stranded DNA titers and/or a fall in complement levels.[10]
- Patients with only DLE generally have negative or low-titer ANA titers, and rarely have low titers of anti-Ro antibodies.[11]

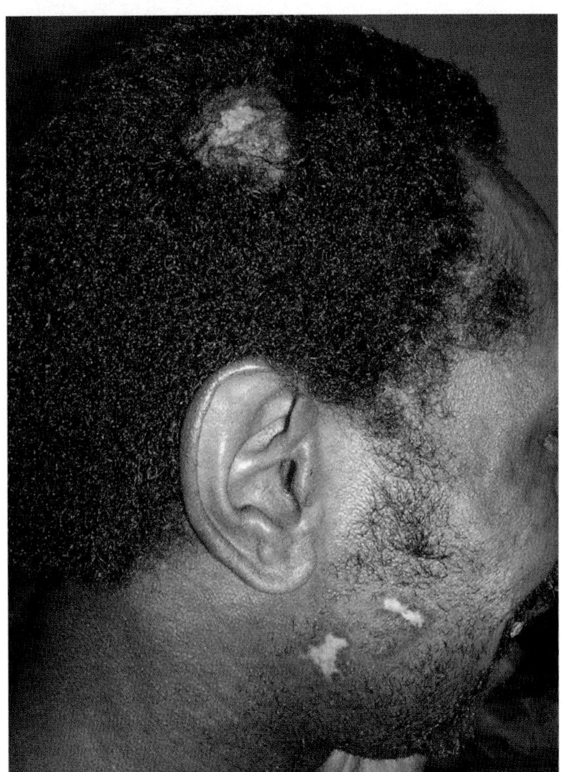

FIGURE 173-12 Discoid lupus with scarring alopecia and hypopigmentation on the scalp and face. (*Used with permission from E.J. Mayeaux, Jr., MD.*)

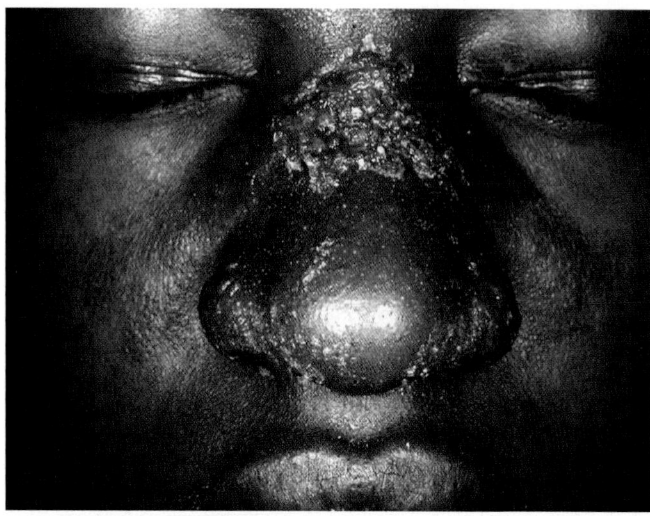

FIGURE 173-13 An 18-year-old girl presenting with crusted sores on her nose and malar rash. This was impetigo over the malar rash from new onset SLE. Months later she developed a severe lupus cerebritis. (*Used with permission from Richard P. Usatine, MD.*)

DIFFERENTIAL DIAGNOSIS

- Drug-induced lupus is a lupus-like syndrome most strongly associated with procainamide, hydralazine, isoniazid, chlorpromazine, methyldopa, and quinidine.
- Scleroderma presents with thickening of the skin and multi-system sclerosis (see Chapter 178, Scleroderma and Morphea).

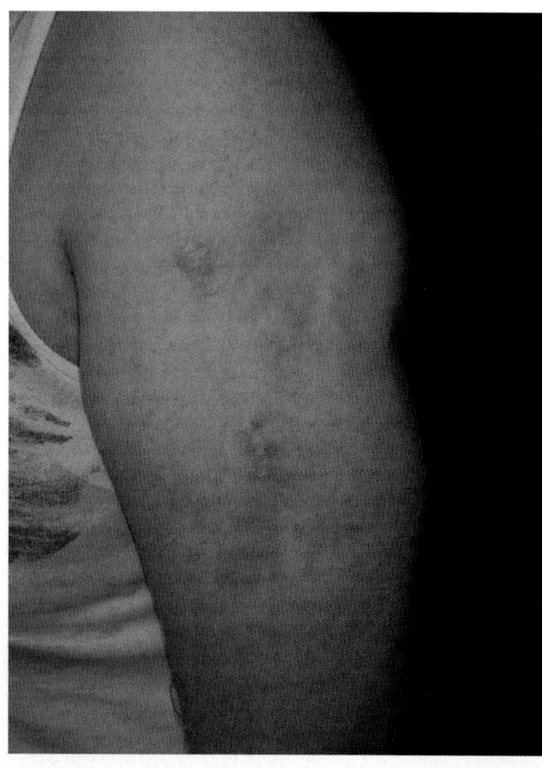

FIGURE 173-14 Lupus profundus showing localized atrophic changes of the arm secondary to the panniculitis. This teenager also has the lupus profundus on the face and other arm. The atrophy has been present for more than 1 year despite treatment. (*Used with permission from Richard P. Usatine, MD.*)

- Dermatomyositis presents with facial swelling, "heliotrope" rash around the eyes, Gottron's papules, and periungual erythema in the hands, and proximal muscular limb girdle weakness (see Chapter 174, Juvenile Dermatomyositis).
- Psoriasis demonstrates silver-white plaques that cover the elbows, knees, scalp, back, or vulva. There may also be nail and scalp involvement (see Chapter 136, Psoriasis).
- Rosacea is associated with mid-facial skin erythema, papules, and pustules without the systemic symptoms of LE, and usually involves the nasolabial folds (see Chapter 97, Rosacea).
- Sarcoidosis may produce skin plaques but without the central clearing and atrophy of LE (see Chapter 150, Pediatric Sarcoidosis).
- Syphilis may produce a plaque like rash that can be confused with DLE. The short course of the disease and serologic testing can distinguish the diseases. However, lupus autoantibodies may produce a false-positive screening test for syphilis (see Chapter 181, Syphilis).

MANAGEMENT

NONPHARMACOLOGIC

- Since UV light can flare SLE, use of sunscreen, preferably those that block both UV-A and UV-B, should be encouraged. SOR C

MEDICATIONS

- Conservative management for SLE with nonsteroidal anti-inflammatory drugs or cyclooxygenase-2 selective inhibitors are recommended for arthritis, arthralgias, and myalgias.[12] SOR B
- Antimalarial drugs (hydroxychloroquine (Plaquenil) maximum 6.5 mg/kg/d) most commonly for skin manifestations and for musculoskeletal complaints that do not adequately respond to nonsteroidal anti-inflammatory drugs. They may also prevent major damage to the kidneys and CNS and reduce the risk of disease flares.[13] SOR B
- Systemic glucocorticoids (1–2 mg/kg/d of prednisone or equivalent) alone or with immunosuppressive agents for patients with significant renal and CNS disease or any other organ threatening manifestation.[14] SOR B Lower doses of glucocorticoids for symptomatic relief of severe or unresponsive musculoskeletal symptoms. In severe, life-threatening situations, high-dose methylprednisolone can be given for three consecutive days.
- Immunosuppressive medications (e.g., methotrexate, cyclophosphamide, azathioprine, mycophenolate, or rituximab) are generally reserved for patients with significant organ involvement, or who have had an inadequate response to glucocorticoids.[15] SOR B
- Belimumab, a monoclonal antibody against B cell activating factor, was recently approved for therapy of mild to moderate SLE in adults but is not yet approved in children.[16]
- Patients with thrombosis, usually associated to the presence of antiphospholipid antibodies, require anticoagulation with warfarin for a target international normalized ratio of 3:3.5 for arterial thrombosis and 2:3 for venous thrombosis.[17]
- DLE therapy includes corticosteroids (topical or intralesional) and antimalarials. SOR C Alternative therapies include auranofin, oral or topical retinoids, and immunosuppressive agents.

PREVENTION

- Avoiding precipitating factors may decrease exacerbations.

PROGNOSIS

- SLE can have a varied clinical course, ranging from a relatively benign illness to a rapidly progressive disease with organ failure and death. Children have a higher risk of renal and neurologic involvement and a higher mortality than adults.
- Poor prognostic factors for survival in SLE include:[18]
  - Renal disease (especially diffuse proliferative glomerulonephritis).
  - Hypertension.
  - Male sex.
  - Young age.
  - Older age at presentation.
  - Poor socioeconomic status.
  - African American and Hispanic race, which may primarily reflect low socioeconomic status.
  - Presence of antiphospholipid antibodies.
  - Antiphospholipid syndrome.
  - High overall disease activity.

FOLLOW-UP

- The patient should have regular follow-up appointments to monitor for and attempt to prevent end organ damage. Regular follow-up visits are needed to monitor medication benefits and side effects and to coordinate care of the whole person.

PATIENT EDUCATION

- Educate the patient on the necessity of protection from the sun, since UV exposure can cause lupus flares. They should use sunscreen, preferably those that block both UV-A and UV-B, with a minimum skin protection factor of 30.
- Since cigarette smoking may increase the risk of developing SLE and smokers generally have more active disease, children and adolescents with SLE should be counseled to avoid smoking. Have patients report any signs of secondary infection in their rash, since this requires antibiotic therapy (**Figure 173-13**).
- If possible, avoid sulfa drugs, which have been related to lupus flares.

PATIENT RESOURCES

- Arthritis Foundation—**www.arthritis.org/conditions-treatments/disease-center/systemic-lupus-erythematosus-lupus-sle/**.
- PubMed Health: Systemic lupus erythematosus—**www.ncbi.nlm.nih.gov/pubmedhealth/PMH0001471/**.
- Mayo Clinic: Lupus—**www.mayoclinic.com/health/lupus/DS00115**.
- Womenshealth.gov: Lupus fact sheet—**http://www.womenshealth.gov/publications/our-publications/fact-sheet/lupus.pdf**.

PROVIDER RESOURCES

- Medscape: Systemic Lupus Erythematosus (SLE)—**http://emedicine.medscape.com/article/332244-overview**.
- Medscape: Discoid Lupus Erythematosus—**http://emedicine.medscape.com/article/1065529-overview**.

REFERENCES

1. Malleson PN, Fung MY, et al. The incidence of pediatric rheumatic diseases: results from the Canadian Pediatric Rheumatology Association Disease Registry. *J Rheumatol*. 1996;23:1981-1987.
2. Danchenko N, Satia JA, Anthony MS. Epidemiology of systemic lupus erythematosus: a comparison of worldwide disease burden. *Lupus*. 2006;15(5):308-318.
3. Pistiner M, Wallace DJ, Nessim S, et al. Lupus erythematosus in the 1980s: A survey of 570 patients. *Semin Arthritis Rheum*. 1991;21:55.
4. Healy E, Kieran E, Rogers S. Cutaneous lupus erythematosus—a study of clinical and laboratory prognostic factors in 65 patients. *Ir J Med Sci*. 1995;164:113.
5. Rowell NR. Laboratory abnormalities in the diagnosis and management of lupus erythematosus. *Br J Dermatol*. 1971;84:210.
6. Liu Z, Davidson A. Taming lupus—a new understanding of pathogenesis is leading to clinical advances. *Nature Medicine*. 18;6:871-882.
7. Gill JM, Quisel AM, Rocca PV, Walters DT. Diagnosis of systemic lupus erythematosus. *Am Fam Physician*. 2003;68:2179-2186.
8. Hochberg MC. Updating the American College of Rheumatology revised criteria for the classification of SLE [letter]. *Arthritis Rheum*. 1997;40:1725.
9. Tan EM, Cohen AS, Fries JF, et al. The 1982 revised criteria for the classification of systemic lupus erythematosus. *Arthritis Rheum*. 1982;25:1271-1277.
10. Kao AH, Navratil JS, Ruffing MJ, et al. Erythrocyte C3d and C4d for monitoring disease activity in systemic lupus erythematosus. *Arthritis Rheum*. 2010;62:837.
11. Provost TT. The relationship between discoid and systemic lupus erythematosus. *Arch Dermatol*. 1994;130:1308.
12. Lander SA, Wallace DJ, Weisman MH. Celecoxib for systemic lupus erythematosus: case series and literature review of the use of NSAIDs in SLE. *Lupus*. 2002;11:340.
13. Fessler BJ, Alarcon GS, McGwin G Jr., et al. Systemic lupus erythematosus in three ethnic groups: XVI. Association of hydroxychloroquine use with reduced risk of damage accrual. *Arthritis Rheum*. 2005;52:1473-1480.
14. Parker BJ, Bruce IN. High dose methylprednisolone therapy for the treatment of severe systemic lupus erythematosus. *Lupus*. 2007;16:387-393.

15. Fortin PR, Abrahamowicz M, Ferland D, et al. Steroid-sparing effects of methotrexate in systemic lupus erythematosus: a double-blind, randomized, placebo-controlled trial. *Arthritis Rheum*. 2008;59:1796.

16. FDA news release. FDA approves Benlysta to treat lupus. www.fda.gov/NewsEvents/Newsroom/PressAnnouncements/ucm246489.htm, accessed February 18, 2012.

17. Erkan D, Lockshin MD. New treatments for antiphospholipid syndrome. *Rheum Dis Clin N Am*. 2006;32:129-148.

18. Cervera R, Khamashta MA, Font J, et al. Morbidity and mortality in systemic lupus erythematosus during a 10-year period: a comparison of early and late manifestations in a cohort of 1,000 patients. *Medicine*. 2003;82:299.

174 JUVENILE DERMATOMYOSITIS

Margaret L. Burks, MD
Richard P. Usatine, MD

PATIENT STORY

A teenage girl presents with a new rash on her face and hands for the past few months. In addition to going to school she works as a waitress and has noted that it is harder to carry heavy trays. She also has gum inflammation and is wondering if this could be related to everything else. The physician notes the heliotrope rash around her eyes (**Figure 174-1**) and the Gottron papules on the dorsum of her knuckles (**Figure 174-2**). He considers that this may be dermatomyositis and tests for proximal muscle weakness. The proximal muscles are not found to be weak on physical exam although a subsequent blood test showed a mildly elevated CK and AST. The physician uses his dermatoscope to look at the nail folds and sees many dilated capillary loops (**Figure 174-3**). On the oral examination, there is a marginal gingivitis and the dermatoscope shows a similar dilated capillary pattern around the tooth. A diagnosis of dermatomyositis is made. The patient was treated with prednisone and hydroxychloroquine and improves greatly. The patient was then tapered off the prednisone fully with no relapse.

INTRODUCTION

Juvenile dermatomyositis is a rare, idiopathic inflammatory disease involving the striated muscles and the skin. Similar to adult cases of dermatomyositis, the disease is primarily characterized by

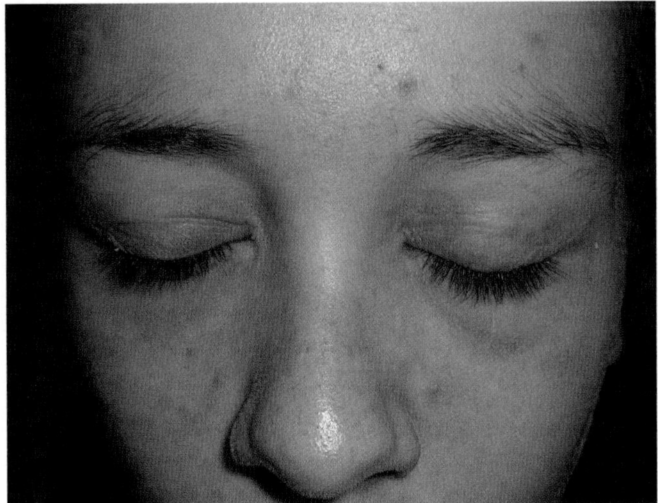

FIGURE 174-1 Classic heliotrope rash around the eyes of this teenager newly diagnosed with dermatomyositis. The color "heliotrope" is a pink-purple tint named after the color of the heliotrope flower. As expected, her heliotrope rash is bilaterally symmetrical. This rash resolved with prednisone and hydroxychloroquine. *(Used with permission from Richard P. Usatine, MD.)*

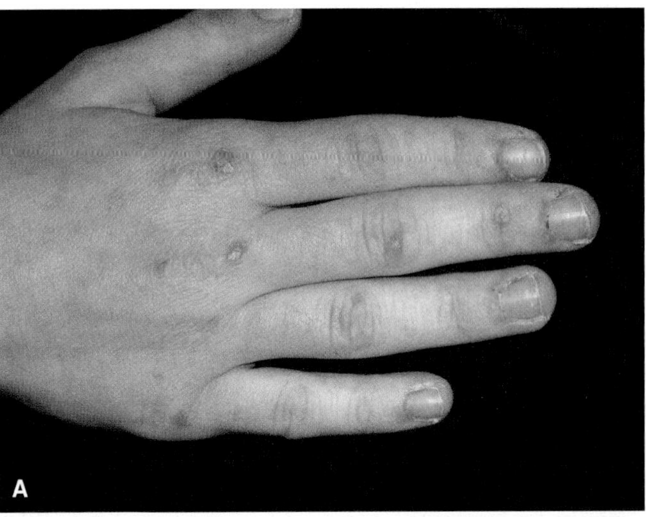

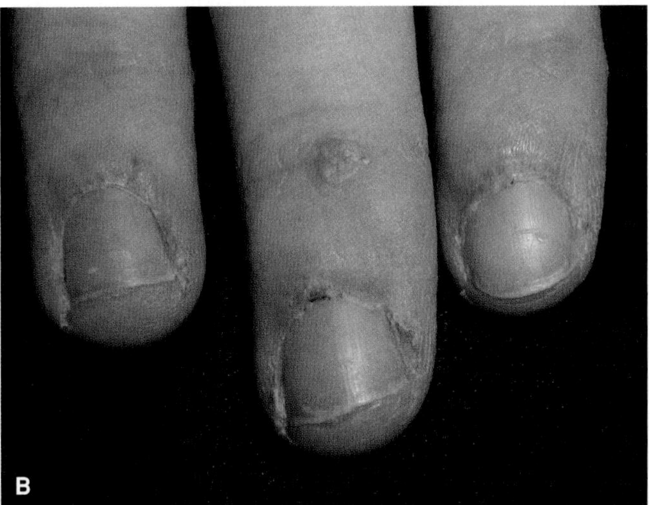

FIGURE 174-2 Hand involvement in the teenager in **Figure 174-1** with Gottron papules over the finger joints. She has nailfold erythema and ragged cuticles (Samitz sign). *(Used with permission from Richard P. Usatine, MD.)*

progressive, symmetrical, proximal muscle weakness. Dermatologic manifestations may occur with or without muscular disease and include the heliotrope rash (**Figures 174-1**, **174-4**, and **174-5**), "shawl sign," and Gottron papules over the finger joints (**Figures 174-4** to **174-7**). Although primarily a disease of muscle and skin, juvenile dermatomyositis has a clear association with myocarditis, vasculitis, calcinosis and interstitial lung disease.[1] Unlike adult dermatomyositis, juvenile cases are much less likely to be associated with an underlying malignancy.

EPIDEMIOLOGY

- Annual incidence of 3.2 cases per 1 million population.[2]
- More common in females.[1,2]
- Children tend to have better long-term prognosis and survival compared to adults with dermatomyositis.[1]
- Mortality rate in children with dermatomyositis is lower than that of adults (less than 5.0% versus 20.8%).[1,3,4]

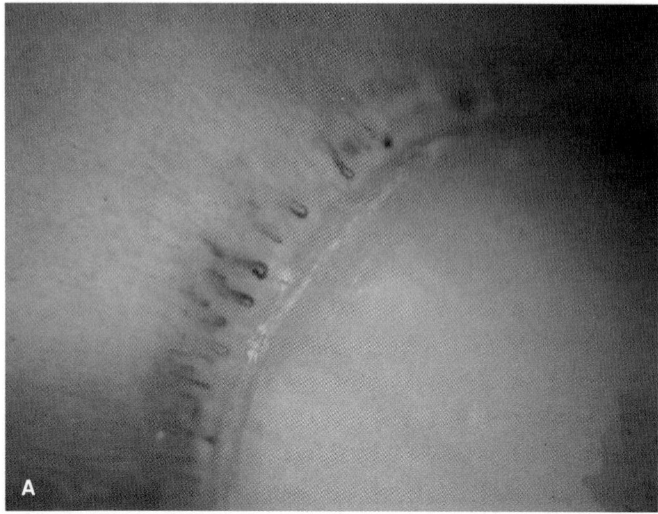
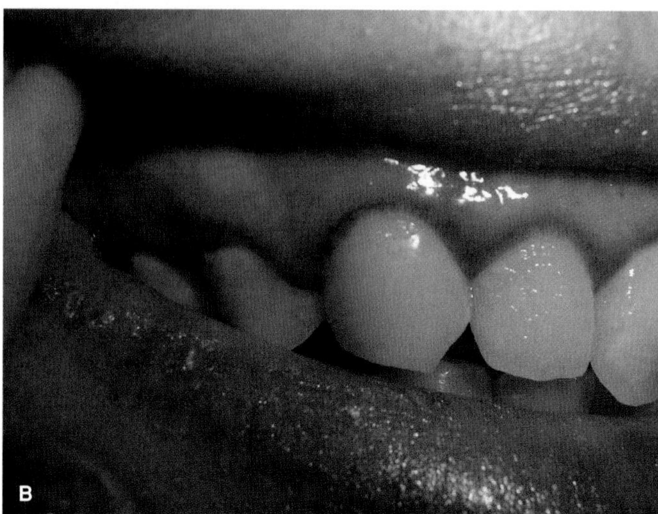
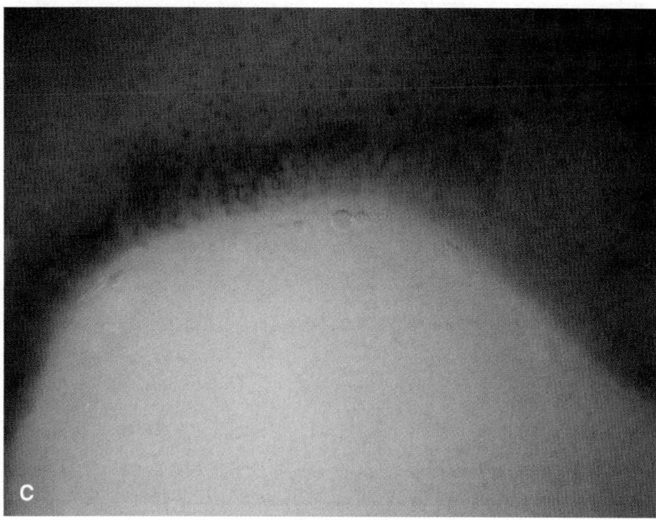

FIGURE 174-3 **A.** Dilated nailfold capillary loops visible with dermoscopy in a teenager with newly diagnosed dermatomyositis. **B.** Marginal gingivitis in the same teen with newly diagnosed dermatomyositis. **C.** She also had dilated capillary loops on the gingival borders of her teeth seen with dermoscopy. The nailfold findings and gingival findings both resolved with treatment. (*Used with permission from Richard P. Usatine, MD.*)

- Peak age of disease onset is 7 years old.[5–7]
- In contrast to adult patients with dermatomyositis, juvenile cases are much less likely to have concomitant interstitial lung disease (14% of juvenile cases versus 35% to 40% of adult cases).[8,9]
- Though linked to malignancy in 12 to 32 percent of adults, malignancy is not typically seen in children with dermatomyositis (approximately 1% of cases).[1,3,10,11,12]

ETIOLOGY AND PATHOPHYSIOLOGY

- Dermatomyositis is considered an autoimmune disease of unknown etiology. Environmental exposure and infectious agents may play a role in disease pathogenesis.[1]
- In children, some studies have shown a high incidence of infectious symptoms in the months prior to disease onset, although no specific pathogen has been linked to the disease.[6]
- Dermatomyositis is a microangiopathy that affects the skin and muscle. The muscle weakness and skin manifestations are likely a result of inflammatory cell infiltrate and activation and deposition of complement, causing lysis of endomysial capillaries and muscle ischemia.[13]
- Muscle biopsy reveals perivascular and perifascicular inflammation, focal muscle necrosis, vasculopathy, and inflammatory cell infiltrate (particularly CD4 cells, B cells, and macrophages).[1,13]

DIAGNOSIS

- Diagnosis includes five criteria: "definite" (typical skin findings plus any three of criteria 1 to 4 that indicate muscle inflammation), "probable" (skin findings plus two of any criteria 1 to 4), or "possible" (skin findings plus any one of criteria 1 to 4).[1,14,15]
  - Proximal symmetric muscle weakness that progresses over weeks to months.
  - Elevated serum levels of muscle enzymes (CK, AST, lactate dehydrogenase [LDH] and aldolase).
  - Abnormal electromyogram (EMG) demonstrating muscle irritability.
  - Abnormal muscle biopsy with muscle necrosis or inflammatory infiltrate.
  - Skin findings—Presence of cutaneous disease characteristic of dermatomyositis. The heliotrope rash (**Figures 174-1**, **174-4**, and **174-5**) and Gottron papules (**Figures 174-4** to **174-7**) are

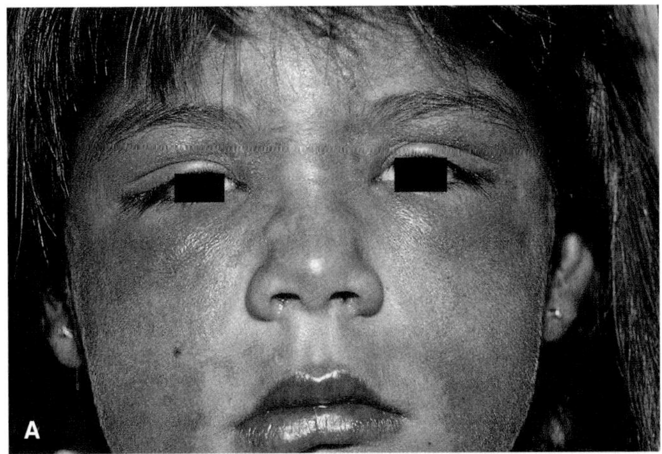

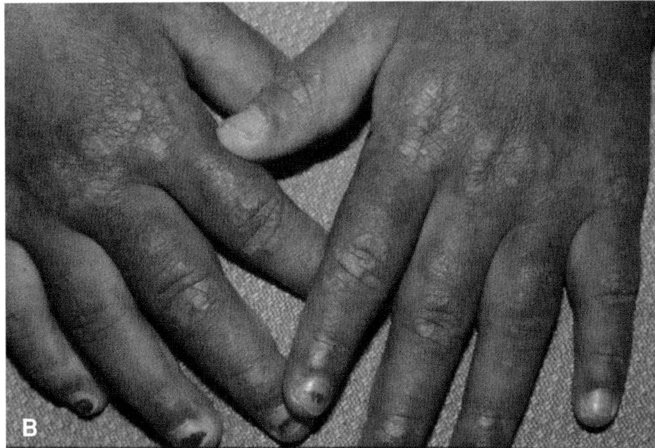

FIGURE 174-4 **A.** Juvenile dermatomyositis in a young girl with the characteristic heliotrope rash that is periorbital and violaceous. The periorbital edema and facial swelling are also commonly seen in juvenile dermatomyositis. **B.** Gottron papules on the dorsa of the knuckles. *(Used with permission from Eric Kraus, MD.)*

considered pathognomonic. Nonpathognomonic manifestations include malar erythema, and periungual and cuticular changes (**Figures 174-2** and **174-3**).

- These criteria are still considered the "gold standard," although they are old (1975) and currently under critical review because of several limitations. The criteria do not include specific autoantibodies or MRI findings.[5]
- Dilated nailfold capillary loops (**Figure 174-3**) have shown promise in juvenile dermatomyositis as a marker for both skin and muscle disease activity to guide treatment. Some authors propose adding this finding to criteria for diagnosis.[16,17]

CLINICAL FEATURES

- Bilateral periorbital heliotrope erythema (pathognomonic; **Figures 174-1**, **174-4**, and **174-5**) and scaling violaceous papular dermatitis in a patient complaining of proximal muscle weakness points to dermatomyositis.
- A psoriasiform scalp dermatitis may be seen in up to 25 percent and pruritus in up to 38 percent of new cases of juvenile dermatomyositis.[18]

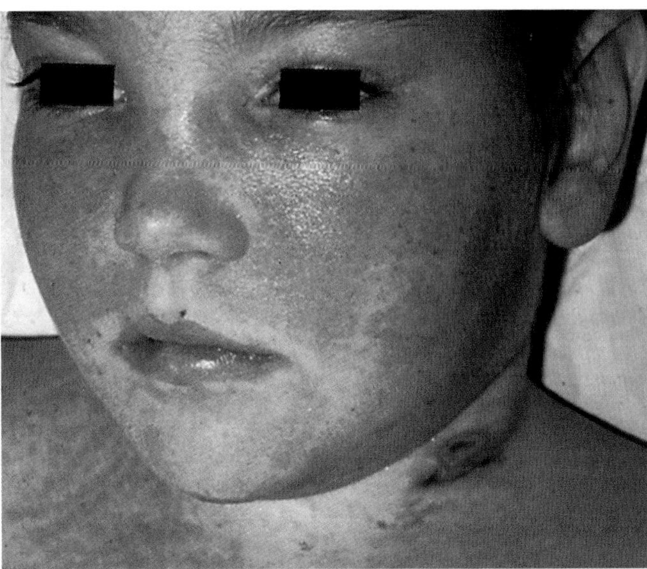

FIGURE 174-5 Heliotrope rash of juvenile dermatomyositis around the eyes of this young boy. Note the periorbital and facial edema. The erythema covers the cheeks, chin and shoulders. He also has a skin ulcer on the neck. Skin ulcerations are found in juvenile dermatomyositis. *(Used with permission from Weinberg S, Prose NS, Kristal L. Color Atlas of Pediatric Dermatology, 4th edition, New York: McGraw-Hill, 2008.)*

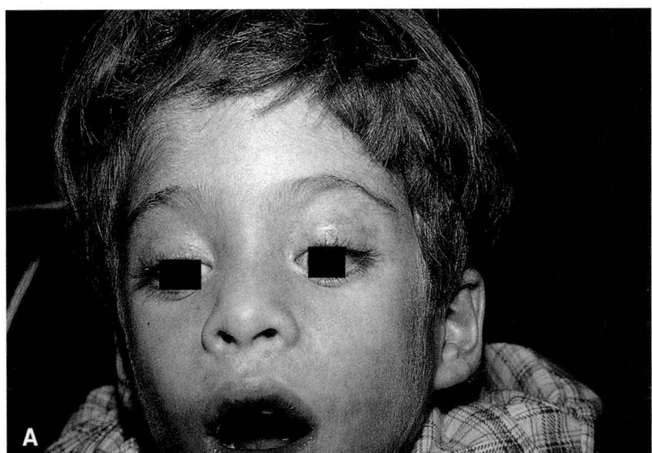

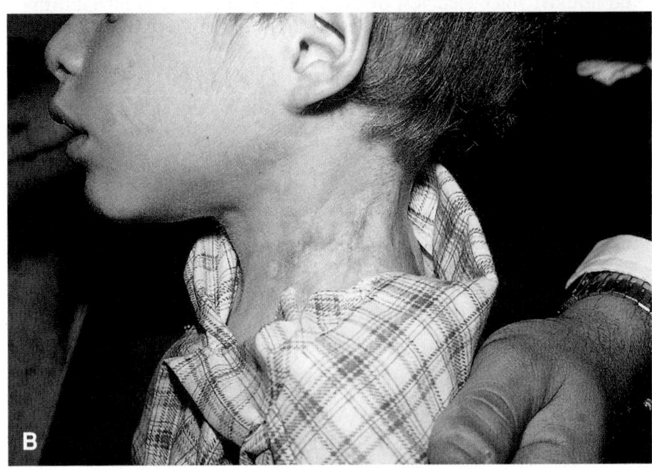

FIGURE 174-6 Juvenile dermatomyositis in a 5-year-old boy demonstrating **A**. heliotrope rash around the eyes. **B.** Calcinosis in the skin of the neck. *(Used with permission from Eric Kraus, MD.)*

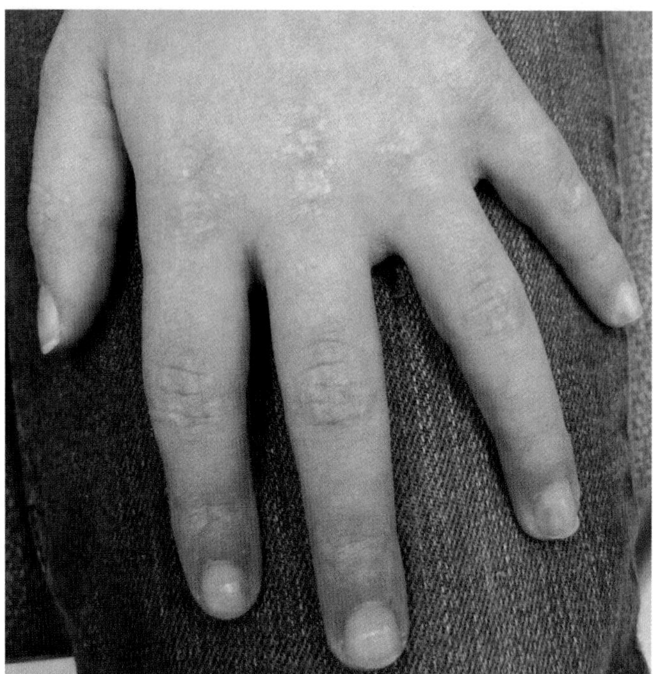

FIGURE 174-7 Child with juvenile dermatomyositis and Gottron plaques on the dorsum of the knuckles. (*Used with permission from John Browning, MD.*)

- An older child may complain of difficulty climbing stairs, rising from a seat, or combing their hair. Notably the skin manifestations may precede, follow, or present simultaneously with muscle involvement.
- In younger children, proximal muscle weakness is often difficult for the clinician to evaluate. Signs to look for include a child not wanting to walk or who insists on being carried, hesitancy to stand up off of the floor, difficulty keeping the head up after infancy, or the "Gower sign."[1] The "Gower sign" is typically associated with muscular dystrophy but can be seen in the proximal myopathy of dermatomyositis (see **Figure 208-1**).
- Severe muscular disease may include difficulty swallowing, choking on liquids, voice changes, or even acute respiratory failure if muscles of respiration are affected.[1,19]
- Hand involvement includes abnormal nailfolds and Gottron papules. "Moth-eaten" cuticles, also called the Samitz sign, are evidenced by periungual erythema and telangiectasias (**Figures 174-2** and **174-3**).
- Juvenile dermatomyositis is more often associated with vascular disease compared to adult cases. Telangiectasias (periungual and gingival) are more common in the pediatric population (**Figure 174-3**).[1]
- Severe vascular disease in juvenile dermatomyositis can lead to skin ulceration in up to 24 percent of pediatric cases (**Figure 174-5**).[20] Similarly, vascular disease may lead to abdominal pain, pneumatosis intestinalis, and GI hemorrhage with risk of perforation. Persistent or severe abdominal pain in a child with juvenile dermatomyositis should prompt immediate evaluation.[21]
- Gottron papules, smooth, purple-to-red papules and plaques, are classically located over the knuckles and on the sides of fingers (**Figures 174-2**, **174-4**, **174-7**, and **174-8**). Plaques may be present over the knuckles instead of or in addition to papules (**Figure 174-7**). The papules are much more evident upon presentation of juvenile-onset dermatomyositis.
- Calcinosis of tissues is present in up to 30 percent of cases (**Figure 174-6**). Calcinosis is due to precipitation of calcium and phosphate in inflamed tissues, which can lead to functional disability.[5,21–23] Typically, the deposits are on the extensor surfaces of joints and pressure points of the extremities, although they may be present anywhere.[22] The presence of calcinosis may be decreased if patients are treated early and aggressively.[21,24] Calcinosis can lead to ulceration, pain from nerve entrapment, and joint contractures.[21]
- Lipodystrophy has been associated with up to 10 to 40 percent of cases of juvenile dermatomyositis. This disease complication presents with loss of visceral and subcutaneous fat accompanied by increased insulin resistance and glucose intolerance.[1,21,25]

TYPICAL DISTRIBUTION

- Face—The characteristic heliotrope rash occurs around the eyes. The color "heliotrope" is a pink-purple tint named after the color of the heliotrope flower. This color is best seen in **Figure 174-1**. The heliotrope rash can also be a dusky-red color as seen in **Figures 174-4** and **174-6**. This heliotrope rash is bilaterally symmetrical.
- Hands—There is usually hand involvement with Gottron papules (and plaques) and abnormal nailfolds and cuticles (**Figures 174-2** and **174-4**, **174-7**, and **174-8**).
- Neck and upper trunk—A red or poikiloderma-type rash can be seen in a V-neck or in a shawl distribution. Poikiloderma refers to hyperpigmentation of the skin demonstrating a variety of shades and associated with telangiectasias. The rash here can be scaling and look psoriasiform.
- Extremities may have erythematous plaques and papules with scale.
- Scalp is often involved with erythema and scale and appears similar to seborrhea or psoriasis.
- Sun-exposed areas are often involved and worsen with sun exposure. This is why so many of the skin findings are on the face and upper chest. However, patients rarely complain of sun sensitivity.

LABORATORY STUDIES AND DIAGNOSTIC TESTS

- Elevated muscle enzymes, evidence of inflammation on electromyography (EMG), and inflammatory infiltrates on muscle biopsy confirm the diagnosis of dermatomyositis. The following serum muscle enzymes can be drawn during the acute active phase and may be found to be elevated: CK, LDH, alanine aminotransferase, aspartate aminotransferase, and aldolase. Of note, it is necessary to measure all of the aforementioned enzymes as only one of them may be elevated.
- The diagnosis may be made with confidence in a patient with characteristic skin findings and elevated muscle enzymes. If the presentation is not straightforward, then muscle biopsy should be performed.[5]
- T2-weighted MRI may be useful in unclear diagnoses and to assess disease activity. This imaging can show edema in the muscle and subcutaneous tissue.[5,26]

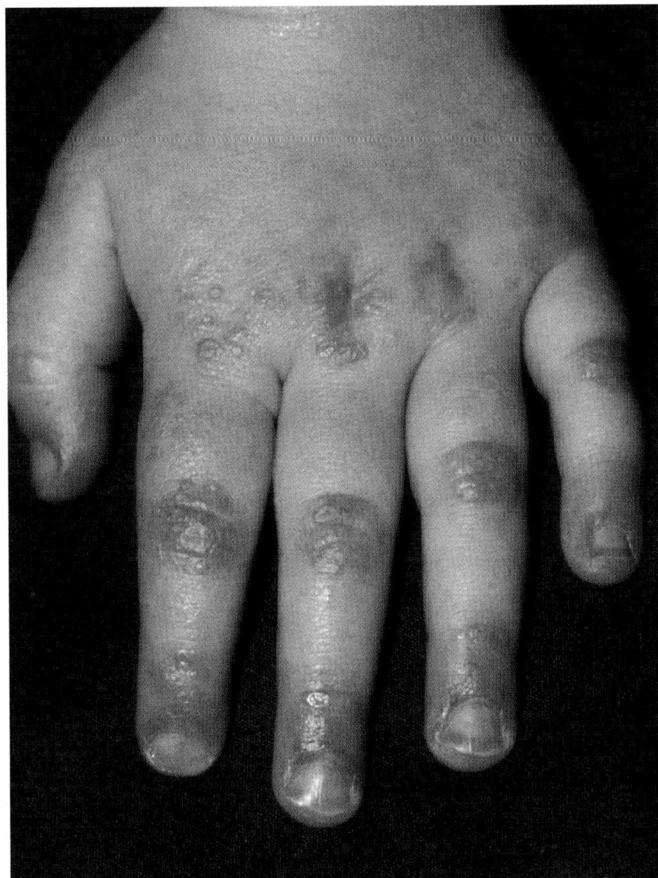

FIGURE 174-8 Prominent Gottron papules in this boy with juvenile dermatomyositis. in a young boy. Note how the erythematous papules and plaques are most prominent over the finger joints and spare the space between joints. *(Used with permission from Richard P. Usatine, MD, and from Goodall J, Usatine RP. Skin rash and muscle weakness. J Fam Pract. 2005;54(10):864-868. Reproduced with permission from Frontline Medical Communications.)*

- The diagnosis can be supported with positive antibodies such as antinuclear antibody (ANA), anti-Mi-2, and anti-Jo-1. It is not necessary to order these antibodies to make the diagnosis of dermatomyositis. Antinuclear antibody can be present in >70 percent of juvenile dermatomyositis cases.[27] Anti-Jo and anti-Mi-2 are considered myositis-specific antibodies; however, they are positive in approximately 5 percent of Caucasian patients with juvenile dermatomyositis. This percentage is higher in African Americans.[13,28]
- Other papulosquamous diseases, such as lichen planus and psoriasis, may be differentiated from dermatomyositis with a punch biopsy.
- Seven to 19 percent of juvenile dermatomyositis cases have been associated with interstitial lung disease.[9,29–31] Though their use is not clearly defined, pulmonary function tests (PFTs), chest radiograph, and high-resolution CT have been used to identify patients with interstitial lung disease.[32] Many children with restrictive lung disease or ILD features seen on imaging may not report symptoms of dyspnea.[9,33] Some experts thus recommend the use of imaging and PFTs for evaluating all children diagnosed with juvenile dermatomyositis for lung involvement, regardless of the presence or absence of symptoms.[33]
- PFTs demonstrate a restrictive pattern with interstitial lung disease. Abnormal results must be confirmed by CT scan as PFT results may also reflect coexisting respiratory muscle weakness. High resolution CT abnormalities may correlate with a child's reported health status and cumulative organ damage.[9]

BIOPSY

Muscle biopsy is typically recommended when the diagnosis is not clear or the patient presents with varying signs and symptoms. Muscle biopsy of dermatomyositis will show inflammatory cells around intramuscular blood vessels. Atrophic muscle fibers are seen around the periphery of muscle fascicles ("perifascicular atrophy"). Biopsy of juvenile dermatomyositis cases reveals increased destruction of capillaries compared to adult cases.[1] Muscle biopsy can also help determine disease severity and may help with predicting the long term impact of the disease.[34,35]

DIFFERENTIAL DIAGNOSIS

- Polymyositis is another form of inflammatory myopathy. It is distinguished from dermatomyositis by its lack of cutaneous involvement. Dermatomyositis can also occur without muscle involvement. This is called *dermatomyositis sine myositis* or *amyopathic dermatomyositis*. In children, it is unknown whether this represents a very mild muscle inflammation and whether or not these cases will eventually progress if left untreated.[1]
- Polymorphous light eruption or other photosensitivity reactions may be mistaken for the dermatologic findings of dermatomyositis as the cutaneous findings may be predominantly in light-exposed areas. Therefore, it is essential in the management and follow-up with patients with suspected photosensitivity reactions to inquire about muscle weakness and to look for other signs of dermatomyositis. Examination of the hands and tests for muscle enzyme elevations might help to distinguish dermatomyositis from photosensitivity reactions.
- Juvenile idiopathic arthritis (JIA) is a cause of pain and rash in the pediatric population, although the pain in JIA is typically localized to joints. The rash in the systemic subtype of JIA is classically described as a salmon colored, macular rash that can accompany fever in children with JIA. This rash is characteristically distinct from those previously described in dermatomyositis (see Chapter 172, Juvenile Idiopathic Arthritis).
- Viral myositis can cause muscle aches and pains in pediatric patients, similar to dermatomyositis. However, viral myositis will not present with the classic cutaneous findings seen in juvenile dermatomyositis.
- Hypothyroidism can cause a proximal myopathy just like polymyositis and dermatomyositis. Although hypothyroidism can cause a dermopathy, it does not resemble the skin findings of dermatomyositis. All patients with proximal muscle weakness should have a screening thyroid-stimulating hormone (TSH) to rule out hypothyroidism regardless of their skin findings (see Chapter 191, Hypothyroidism).
- In children, eczema causes an erythematous rash on the face, as is often seen in dermatomyositis. Of course eczema does not cause muscle weakness and the erythema of eczema is classically confined

to the flexor surfaces of the extremities (see Chapter 130, Atopic Dermatitis).

- Steroid myopathy may develop as a side effect of systemic steroid therapy. The symptoms develop 4 to 6 weeks after starting oral steroids for dermatomyositis and other autoimmune diseases. Therefore if muscle weakness recurs after improving, it could be from the steroids not the disease.
- Dermatomyositis-like reaction rarely may present with similar skin findings with initiation of the following medications and improvement with their discontinuation: penicillamine, NSAIDs, and carbamazepine.
- Overlap syndrome—The term *overlap* denotes that certain signs are seen in both dermatomyositis and other connective tissue diseases, such as scleroderma, rheumatoid arthritis, and lupus erythematosus. Scleroderma and dermatomyositis are the most commonly associated conditions and have been termed sclerodermatomyositis or mixed connective disease. In mixed connective tissue disease, features of systemic lupus erythematosus (SLE), scleroderma, and polymyositis are evident, such as malar rash, alopecia, Raynaud phenomenon, waxy-appearing skin, and proximal muscle weakness.

MANAGEMENT

Given the autoimmune mechanism likely central to the disease process, treatment is geared toward the proximal muscle weakness and skin changes using immunosuppressive or immunomodulatory therapy. Treatment is nonspecific as the target antigen remains elusive.[1] Cutaneous manifestations do not always parallel muscle disease in response to therapy. Clinical improvement and physician judgment should guide treatment regimens.[36] Enzyme levels should not be used as a sole guide for gauging responsiveness to therapy because they frequently become normal during treatment even if active disease is present.[5] Effective therapies for the myopathy are oral corticosteroids, immunosuppressants, biologic agents, and/or intravenous immunoglobulin. Effective therapies for the skin disease are sun protection, topical corticosteroids, antimalarials, methotrexate, and/or immunoglobulin. Drug therapy for dermatomyositis continues to be based on empirical rather than evidence-based practice because of lack of controlled trials.[36]

NONPHARMACOLOGIC

- Physical and/or occupational therapy has been shown to preserve and increase muscle function and strength.[37]
- Photoprotective measures, which could consist of a broad-spectrum sunscreen, protective outerwear, and limitation of sun exposure.[13] SOR B

TOPICAL TREATMENT

- Topical corticosteroids may be used for refractory skin disease and may improve redness and itching; however resistant skin disease should clue the clinician to potentially increasing systemic disease activity.[1] SOR B
- Topical pimecrolimus also is also an adjunctive therapy used to decrease redness and itching in the treatment of refractory skin manifestations.[1]

ORAL TREATMENT

- Corticosteroids are the mainstay for treatment of juvenile dermatomyositis. First-line therapy for muscle disease is high-dose (2 mg/kg oral single daily dose with a maximum daily dose of 60 mg) systemic corticosteroids, usually prednisone, with or without an immunosuppressive ("steroid-sparing") agent. Typically in children this agent is methotrexate (oral or subcutaneous).[13,36]
- Experts typically agree that steroid taper should be initiated based on: improved or normal muscle strength, enzymes improved or normal, rash stable or improved, and physician judgment after about 4 weeks on high-dose steroid treatment.[36]
- High dose oral steroid taper should be slow, typically over a minimum of 1 to 2 years.[24,36,38]
- If no response, based on clinician judgment, to initial four weeks of treatment with high-dose steroids, addition of an immune modulators (intravenous immunoglobulin, cyclosporine, mycophenolate mofetil, azathioprine, or biologic agent), or IV methylprednisolone should be considered.[36] SOR B
- Lack of response after 2 to 3 months of treatment should lead to a reexamination of the diagnosis and perhaps another muscle biopsy.[39]
- Methotrexate is effective in treating the muscular symptoms of juvenile dermatomyositis as a steroid-sparing agent. Methotrexate, when added to prednisone in initial therapy, has been shown to result in good disease control and limit the cumulative dose of steroid.[38] SOR B
- Oral or subcutaneous methotrexate dosing starts at 1mg/kg once weekly or 15 mg/m^2 weekly (maximum dose of 40 mg).[1,36]
- Using methotrexate safely requires a number of precautions. All patients should have a complete blood count with differential, liver and renal function panels, hepatitis, and VZV serology, a urinalysis, C-reactive protein, and erythrocyte sedimentation rate. A purified protein derivative (PPD) should be placed or a QuantiFERON-TB Gold assay performed to rule out latent tuberculosis. Patients with active liver disease, including hepatitis C and alcoholic cirrhosis, should receive alternative forms of therapy. Female patients should avoid becoming pregnant during therapy. Folic acid supplementation while on methotrexate of 1 mg of folic acid daily is important to prevent side effects.[40]
- While taking methotrexate, the patient should be followed with regular laboratory tests including: complete blood count with differential, liver and renal function panels, and a urinalysis. This should typically be performed after 4 weeks of treatment then every 8 to 12 weeks.[40] Methotrexate should only be prescribed by doctors familiar with its risks and benefits.
- Cyclosporine is a steroid sparing agent that is typically considered a second line agent in the treatment of juvenile dermatomyositis but has shown to be beneficial in the treatment of refractory disease.[1,39] SOR B Cyclosporine should be used cautiously with monitoring of blood pressure, renal function, liver function, and hematologic parameters. Side effects may include headache, tremor, and gastrointestinal symptoms.[39]
- Cyclosporine has also been shown to be efficacious in steroid-resistant interstitial lung disease associated with juvenile dermato-

myositis. Initiation of cyclosporine has been recommended for rapidly progressive interstitial lung disease.[33,39]

- Azathioprine is also considered a second line agent in the treatment of juvenile dermatomyositis.[1] It is commonly used in chronic inflammatory diseases as a steroid-sparing agent. Like all of the other immunosuppressive agents, azathioprine must be used cautiously by physicians familiar with its risks.
- Tacrolimus, a calcineurin inhibitor, is second line therapy and has adverse effects similar to cyclosporine; however, tacrolimus has greater potency. It is effective in refractory juvenile dermatomyositis.[1,39]
- Mycophenolate mofetil, an inhibitor of T-cell and B-cell proliferation, is a corticosteroid-sparing agent that affects both refractory cutaneous and muscular disease. It is considered a second line therapy for juvenile dermatomyositis.[1]
- Hydroxychloroquine is used as a steroid-sparing agent in mild disease. It has been shown to be particularly beneficial for the rash of juvenile dermatomyositis.[41,42] One report, however, note worsening of the rash and another found a higher incidence of cutaneous drug reactions in patients taking hydroxychloroquine with dermatomyositis.[43,44] SOR Ⓒ
- Biologics, including tumor necrosis factor (TNF)-α inhibitors, are currently being tested for use in juvenile dermatomyositis. Conflicting and discouraging initial results prompt the need for further clinical trials. The TNF-α inhibitor, infliximab, has been used with good effect in the treatment of calcinosis in juvenile dermatomysositis.[1,45]
- Other agents used in the treatment of calcinosis include bisphosphonates and calcium channel blockers. Some patients may require surgical excision in areas causing chronic pain, recurrent infection, or debilitating functional status.[1]
- It is important to look at these medications' side-effect profiles and monitor the patient accordingly during treatment. Patients must not get pregnant while on these medications and various labs need to be followed.

INTRAVENOUS TREATMENT

- Pulsed intravenous methylprednisolone has been advocated for severe disease in juvenile dermatomyositis.[41] SOR Ⓒ
- The safest and most efficacious route of steroid administration in juvenile dermatomyositis is unclear. IV methylprednisolone has not been shown to be superior to oral corticosteroids in the early treatment of moderate cases of juvenile dermatomyositis; however, it may improve cost effectiveness by decreasing the duration of disease.[46,47]
- Studies investigating the efficacy of intravenous immunoglobulin (IVIG) in children are lacking.[1] IVIG may be beneficial as a steroid-sparing agent.[48] Risks associated with the use of IVIG include infusion reactions (nausea, vomiting, fever, or lethargy) and exposure to blood product. In children, this may be associated with the presence of IgA in the infusion.[49] SOR Ⓒ
- Rituximab is a monoclonal antibody directed primarily against proteins present on B-cells. Adult studies have shown potential efficacy in the treatment of myositis. Currently, placebo-controlled trials are underway to determine its potential benefit in the treatment of juvenile dermatomyositis.[1,39]

MALIGNANCY WORK-UP

- The association between adult cases of dermatomyositis and malignancy has been well documented. Adult patients with dermatomyositis, regardless of age, should undergo an age- and gender-relevant malignancy work-up beginning at the time of diagnosis. In contrast, malignancy is very rare in cases of juvenile dermatomyositis, often consisting of isolated case reports.[3,50]
- Extensive evaluation for an underlying malignancy at diagnosis is not recommended.[5,50]
- Cases of juvenile dermatomyositis that are associated with an underlying malignancy typically have additional features noted on physical exam, including extensive lymphadenopathy, splenomegaly, or an atypical rash. The finding of these additional features on exam indicates the need for further evaluation of malignancy in these patients before the initiation of immunosuppressive therapy.[50]
- The most common malignancies noted on review of patients with juvenile dermatomyositis were leukemias and lymphomas.[50]
- The link between malignancy and juvenile dermatomyositis remains unclear, though it is possible that dermatomyositis represents a paraneoplastic syndrome. Underlying changes in the immune system along with the effects of immunosuppressive agents used in treatment may play a role.[50]
- Patients with juvenile dermatomyositis should be continually monitored for malignancy during treatment with immunosuppressive therapy, even if malignancy is not suspected at diagnosis or on initiation of treatment.[50]

PROGNOSIS

The mortality rate of juvenile dermatomyositis is less than 5 percent, which is notably lower than that seen in adult cases.[1,3,4] Despite this, over half of patients have a chronic disease course, with continued disease activity and need for medications two to three years after diagnosis.[16,23] Eight percent of patients may have continued moderate to severe disability.[23] The median time to remission (absence of rash, no active myositis, and no need for immunosuppressive agents for 6 months) has been reported to be approximately 4.67 years.[16] Poor outcome has been linked to delay in treatment and the initiation of low-dose treatment.[24] The presence of lipodystrophy and calcinosis, both complications of dermatomyositis, is associated with a longer duration of active disease.[4] Similarly, the presence of Gottron papules 3 months after diagnosis and Gottron papules plus abnormal nailfold capillaries at 6 months after diagnosis may predict a longer time to remission.[16]

FOLLOW-UP

These patients need very close and frequent follow-up to manage their medications and overall care. High doses of steroids and steroid-sparing agents, such as methotrexate, have numerous potential side effects. These patients need to be closely followed with laboratory tests and careful titration of the toxic medicines used for treatment. Patients need physical therapy, periodic eye exams for cataracts, and weight monitoring. Specific supplements including calcium, vitamin D and folic acid may be added to prevent some of the side effects of the strong medications being prescribed. Children on long-term corticosteroids should also be monitored for decelerated growth, one of the side effects of long-term corticosteroid use.

PATIENT EDUCATION

Discuss the importance of sun protection as sun exposure does make the cutaneous manifestations worse. Counseling about the serious nature of the disease and prognosis is important as many patients may develop substantial weakness and decline in physical functioning. Patients need to understand that the medications being used have many risks along with their benefits and need to report side effects to their physicians. Pregnancy prevention is needed for females of childbearing potential while on a number of the medications used to treat this disease.

PATIENT RESOURCES

- The Myositis Association—**www.myositis.org**.
- American College of Rheumatology—**www.rheumatology.org/practice/clinical/patients/diseases_and_conditions/dermatomyositis.asp**.
- National Institute of Neurological Disorders and Stroke. *NINDS Dermatomyositis Information Page*—**www.ninds.nih.gov/disorders/dermatomyositis/dermatomyositis.htm**.

PROVIDER RESOURCES

- Medscape. *Juvenile Dermatomyositis*—**http://emedicine.medscape.com/article/1417215**.

REFERENCES

1. Robinson AB, Reed AM. Clinical features, pathogenesis and treatment of juvenile and adult dermatomyositis. *Nat Rev Rheumatol.* 2011;7(11):664-675.
2. Mendez EP. et al. US incidence of juvenile dermatomyositis, 1995–1998: results from the National Institute of Arthritis and Musculoskeletal and Skin Diseases Registry. *Arthritis Care Res.* 2003;49:300-305.
3. Na SJ, Kim SM, Sunwoo IN, Choi YC. Clinical characteristics and outcomes of juvenile and adult dermatomyositis. *J. Korean Med. Sci.* 2009;24:715-721.
4. Ravelli A, et al. Long-term outcome and prognostic factors of juvenile dermatomyositis: a multinational, multicenter study of 490 patients. *Arthritis Care Res.* 2010;62:63-72.
5. Feldman BM, Rider LG, Reed AM, Pachman LM. Juvenile dermatomyositis and other idiopathic inflammatory myopathies of childhood. *Lancet.* 2008;371:2201-2212.
6. Pachman, LM, et al. History of infection before the onset of juvenile dermatomyositis: results from the National Institute of Arthritis and Musculoskeletal and Skin Diseases Research Registry. *Arthritis Rheum.* 2005;53:166-172.
7. Rider LG, Miller FW. Deciphering the clinical presentations, pathogenesis, and treatment of the idiopathic inflammatory myopathies. *JAMA.* 2011;305:183-190.
8. Connors GR, Christopher-Stine L, Oddis CV, Danoff SK. Interstitial lung disease associated with the idiopathic inflammatory myopathies: what progress has been made in the past 35 years? *Chest.* 2010;138;1464-1474.
9. Sanner H, et al. Pulmonary outcome in juvenile dermatomyositis: a case-control study. *Ann. Rheum. Dis.* 2011;70:86-91.
10. Hill CL Zhang Y, Sigurgeirsson B, Pukkala E, et al. Frequency of specific cancer types in dermatomyositis and polymyositis: a population-based study. *Lancet.* 2001;357:96-100.
11. Huang YL, Chen YJ, Lin MW, Wu CY, et al. Malignancies associated with dermatomyositis and polymyositis in Taiwan: a nationwide population-based study. *British Journal of Dermatology.* 2009:161:854-860.
12. Sigurgeirsson B, Lindelof B, Edhag O, et al. Risk of cancer in patients with dermatomyositis or polymyositis. A population-based study. *N Engl J Med.* 1992;326:363-367.
13. Wedderburn LR, Rider, LG. Juvenile dermatomyositis: new developments in pathogenesis, assessment and treatment. *Best Pract. Res. Clin. Rheumatol.* 2009;23:665-678.
14. Bohan A, Peter JB. Polymyositis and dermatomyositis (first of two parts). *N Engl J Med.* 1975;292(7):344-347.
15. Bohan A, Peter JB. Polymyositis and dermatomyositis (second of two parts). *N Engl J Med.* 1975;292(8):403-407.
16. Stringer E, Singh-Grewal D, Feldman BM. Predicting the course of juvenile dermatomyositis: significance of early clinical and laboratory features. *Arthritis Rheum.* 2008;58:3585-3592.
17. Schmeling H, Stephens S, Goia C. et al. Nailfold capillary density is importantly associated over time with muscle and skin disease activity in juvenile dermatomyositis. *Rheumatology.* 2011;50:885-893.
18. Peloro TM, Miller OF, Hahn TF, and Newman ED. Juvenile dermatomyositis: a retrospective review of a 30-year experience. *J Am Acad Dermatol.* 2001;43(1):28-34.
19. Fathi M, Lundberg IE, and Tomling, G. Pulmonary complications of polymyositis and dermatomyositis. *Semin. Respir. Crit. Care Med.* 2007;28:451-458.
20. Rider LG, Lachenbruch PA, Monroe JB, et al. Damage extent and predictors in adult and juvenile dermatomyositis and polymyositis as determined with the myositis damage index. *Arthritis & Rhematism.* 2007;60(11);3425-3435.
21. Lowry CA, Pilkington CA. Juvenile dermatomyositis: extramuscular manifestations and their management. *Curr. Opin. Rheumatol.* 2009:21:575-580.
22. Eidelman N et al. Microstructure and mineral composition of dystrophic calcification associated with the idiopathic inflammatory myopathies. *Arthritis Res. Ther.* 2009;11:R159.
23. Huber AM, et al. Medium- and long-term functional outcomes in a multicenter cohort of children with juvenile dermatomyositis. *Arthritis Rheum.* 2000;43:541-549.
24. Bowyer SL, Blane CE, Sullivan, DB, Cassidy JT. Childhood dermatomyositis: factors predicting functional outcome and development of dystrophic calcification. *J. Pediatr.* 1983;103:882-888.

25. Huemer C, et al. Lipodystrophy in patients with juvenile dermatomyositis—evaluation of clinical and metabolic abnormalities. *J. Rheumatol.* 2001;28:610-615.

26. Kimball AB, Summers RM, Turner M, et al. Magnetic resonance imaging detection of occult skin and subcutaneous abnormalities in juvenile dermatomyositis. Implications for diagnosis and therapy. *Arthritis Rheum* 2000;43:1866-1873.

27. Wedderburn LR, et al. HLA class II haplotype and autoantibody associations in children with juvenile dermatomyositis and juvenile dermatomyositis-scleroderma overlap. *Rheumatology.* 2007;46:1786-1791.

28. O'Hanlon TP, et al. HLA polymorphisms in African Americans with idiopathic inflammatory myopathy: allelic profiles distinguish patients with different clinical phenotypes and myositis autoantibodies. *Arthritis Rheum.* 2006;54:3670-3681.

29. Chiu SK, Yang YH, Wang LC, et al. Ten-year experience of juvenile dermatomyositis: a retrospective study. *J Microbiol Immunol Infect.* 2007;40:68-73.

30. Morinishi Y, Oh-Ishi T, Kabuki T, et al. Juvenile dermatomyositis: clinical characteristics and the relatively high risk of interstitial lung disease. *Mod Rheumatol.* 2007;17:413-417.

31. Constantin T, Ponyi A, Orban I, et al. National registry of patients with juvenile idiopathic infl ammatory myopathies in Hungary: clinical characteristics and disease course of 44 patients with juvenile dermatomyositis. *Autoimmunity.* 2006;39:223-232.

32. Fathi M, Dastmalchi M, Rasmussen E, et al. Interstitial lung disease, a common manifestation of newly diagnosed polymyositis and dermatomyositis. *Ann Rheum Dis.* 2004;63:297-301.

33. Kobayashi I, Yamada M, Takahashi Y, et al. Interstitial lung disease associated with juvenile dermatomyositis: clinical features and efficacy of cyclosporin A. *Rheumatology (Oxford).* 2003;42: 371-374.

34. Lopez de Padilla CM, et al. Plasmacytoid dendritic cells in inflamed muscle of patients with juvenile dermatomyositis. *Arthritis Rheum.* 2007;56:1658-1668.

35. Miles L, et al. Predictability of the clinical course of juvenile dermatomyositis based on initial muscle biopsy: a retrospective study of 72 patients. *Arthritis Rheum.* 2007;17:725-730.

36. Huber AM, Robinson AB, Reed AM, et al. Consensus treatments for moderate juvenile dermatomyositis: beyond the first two months. Results of the Second Childhood Arthritis and Rheumatology Research Alliance Consensus Conference. *Arthritis Care and Research.* 2012;64(4):546-553.

37. Omori CH, Silva CA, Sallum AM, et al. Exercise training in juvenile dermatomyositis. *Arthritis Care and Research.* 2012;54(8):1186-1194.

38. Ramanan AV, et al. The effectiveness of treating juvenile dermatomyositis with methotrexate and aggressively tapered corticosteroids. *Arthritis Rheum.* 2005;52:3570-3578.

39. Aggarwal R, Oddis CV. Therapeutic approaches in myositis. *Curr Rheumatol Rep.* 2011;13(3):182-191.

40. Niehues T, Horneff G, Michels H, Höck MS, and Schuchmann L. Evidence-based use of methotrexate in children with rheumatic diseases: a consensus statement of the Working Groups Pediatric Rheumatology Germany (AGKJR) and Pediatric Rheumatology Austria. *Rheumatol Int.* 2005;25:160-178.

41. Stringer E, et al. Treatment approaches to juvenile dermatomyositis (JDM) across North America: The Childhood Arthritis and Rheumatology Research Alliance (CARRA) JDM Treatment Survey. *J. Rheum.* 2010;37:1953-1961.

42. Woo TY, Callen JP, Voorhees JJ, Bickers DR, Hanno R, Hawkins C. Cutaneous lesions of dermatomyositis are improved by hydroxychloroquine. *J Am Acad Dermatol.* 1984;10:592-600.

43. Bloom BJ, Tucker LB, Klein-Gitelman M, Miller LC, Schaller JG. Worsening of the rash of juvenile dermatomyositis with hydroxychloroquine therapy. *J Rheumatol.* 1994;21:2171-2172.

44. Pelle MT, Callen JP. Adverse cutaneous reactions to hydroxychloroquine are more common in patients with dermatomyositis than in patients with cutaneous lupus erythematosus. *Arch Dermatol.* 2002;138:1231-1233.

45. Riley P. et al. Effectiveness of infliximab in the treatment of refractory juvenile dermatomyositis with calcinosis. *Rheumatology (Oxford).* 2008;47:877-880.

46. Seshadri R, Feldman BM, Ilowite N, Cawkwell G, Pachman LM. The role of aggressive corticosteroid therapy in patients with juvenile dermatomyositis: a propensity score analysis. *Arthritis Rheum.* 2008;59:989-995.

47. Klein-Gitelman MS, Waters T, Pachman LM. The economic impact of intermittent high-dose intravenous versus oral corticosteroid treatment of juvenile dermatomyositis. *Arthritis Care Res.* 2000;13:360-368.

48. Lang BA, Laxer RM, Murphy G, Silverman ED, Roifman CM. Treatment of dermatomyositis with intravenous gammaglobulin. *Am J Med.* 1991;91:169-172.

49. Manlhiot C, et al. Safety of intravenous immunoglobulin in the treatment of juvenile dermatomyositis: adverse reactions are a ssociated with immunoglobulin A content. *Pediatrics.* 2008;121:e626-e630.

50. Morris P, Dare J. Juvenile dermatomyositis as a paraneoplastic phenomenon: an update. *J. Pediatr. Hematol. Oncol.* 2010;32: 189-191.

51. Huber AM, et al. Medium- and long-term functional outcomes in a multicenter cohort of children with juvenile dermatomyositis. *Arthritis Rheum.* 2000;43:541-549.

175 HENOCH SCHONLEIN PURPURA

Margaret L. Burks, MD
Richard P. Usatine, MD

PATIENT STORY

A previously healthy 8-year-old boy presented with 2 days of knee and ankle pain with no known cause. His parents denied that he had any trauma or fever. On physical examination, he was afebrile in no apparent distress. His left knee was swollen and tender (**Figure 175-1**). He admitted to other joint pains but there was no swelling or tenderness in the other joints. The pediatrician noted a petechial and purpuric eruption from his buttocks down to his ankles (**Figure 175-1**). It was non-blanching but only barely palpable. There were prominent circumferential petechiae around the left sock area. Upon further questioning, the mother admitted that her son had a viral upper respiratory infection 2 weeks ago. A urinalysis showed mild hematuria but no proteinuria. He never developed abdominal pain. Therapy was supportive and systemic corticosteroids were not used.

INTRODUCTION

Henoch-Schonlein Purpura (HSP) is a small vessel vasculitis characterized in children by a classic, palpable, purpuric rash over the lower extremities. In addition to the rash, children may also exhibit arthralgias, hematuria, and abdominal pain. The exact disease trigger is unknown; however, the symptoms of HSP are attributed to IgA deposition in the systemic vasculature. Though a minority of patients may develop long-term renal complications, the majority of cases are self-limited.

SYNONYMS

- In the early 20th century, HSP was thought to be due to anaphylaxis. Consequently, the disease was named "anaphylactoid purpura." Occasionally, this term may still be used in reference to HSP.[1]

EPIDEMIOLOGY

- HSP is the most common vasculitis in the pediatric population.[2]
- Although HSP may affect all age groups, it is most common between children ages 2 to 6 years old.[2–4]

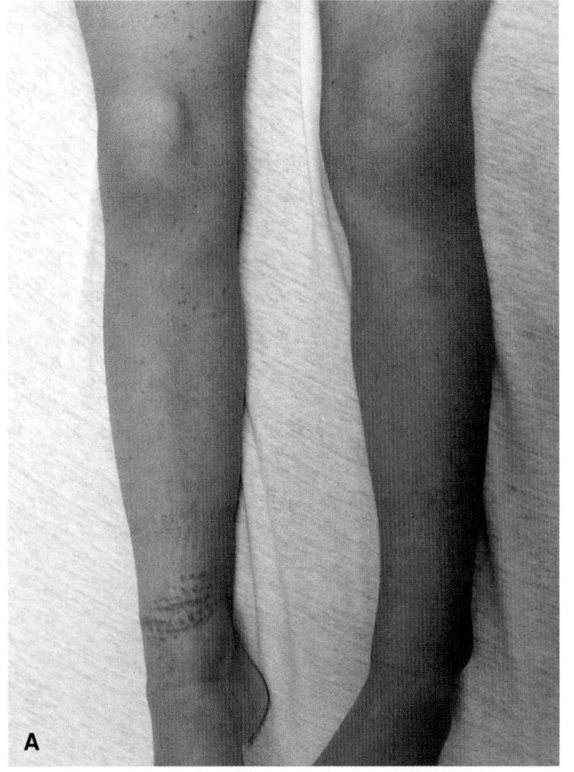

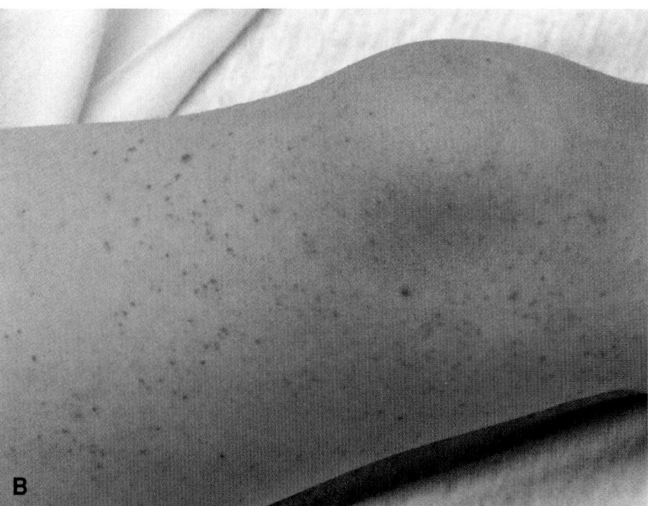

FIGURE 175-1 Henoch-Schönlein purpura (HSP) in an 8-year-old boy presenting with 2 days of knee and ankle pain 2 weeks after a viral upper respiratory infection. **A.** petechiae are visible on both legs with a prominent sock mark on the right ankle. Note the left knee is somewhat swollen. **B.** A close-up of the petechiae that are slightly palpable. There is no obvious purpura at this time. (*Used with permission from Camille Sabella, MD.*)

- The disease affects an estimated 70.3 per 100,000 children per year.[2,3]
- A very slight male predominance exists with a 1.2:1 male to female ratio.[2,3]
- White children have a much higher incidence compared to black children.[2,3]
- Though the incidence has been reported to be about 100 times greater in children than adults, HSP is typically less severe in the pediatric population.[5]
- The peak disease occurrence is in the fall and winter months.[1]

ETIOLOGY AND PATHOPHYSIOLOGY

- HSP is an immune complex-mediated disease.[2]
- Clinical symptoms are due to widespread IgA deposits in the small vessels of the GI tract, renal glomeruli, and skin.[1,4] IgA activates a local inflammatory response which leads to necrosis of the blood vessels.[2]
- IgA may bind to endothelial cells of the vasculature and lead to the destruction of these cells by activation of complement or PMNs with the subsequent release of reactive oxygen species. The exact pathogenic mechanism, however, remains unknown.[6]

RISK FACTORS

- HSP is preceded by an upper respiratory tract infection in up to 90 percent of patients (**Figure 175-1**).[7] Many different respiratory pathogens have been linked to HSP, including group A β-hemolytic streptococcus.[1,5,7,8]
- Although many studies have speculated that a potential relationship exists between respiratory pathogens and the development of HSP, no single pathogen has shown to be the definitive causal agent.[1]
- Risk factors for renal disease in HSP remain unclear. Older age at onset, persistent purpura, and severe abdominal pain have been cited by some studies as risk factors for the development of renal disease.[9–11]
- Some experts hypothesize a genetic susceptibility towards the development of HSP as well as toward renal involvement; however, no definitive genetic polymorphism has been linked to the disease.[2,6,12]
- HSP is more common in children with a history of familial Mediterranean fever.[2,13]

DIAGNOSIS

- HSP is a clinical diagnosis.[5]
- Diagnostic criteria include—The presence of nonthrombocytopenic palpable purpura (considered a mandatory criteria) plus at least one of the following four clinical features:[5,14]
  - Diffuse abdominal pain.
  - Any biopsy showing predominantly IgA deposition.
  - Arthritis or arthralgia.
  - Renal involvement (proteinuria and/or hematuria).
- The majority of children do not require renal or skin biopsy to confirm diagnosis unless severe renal involvement is suspected or skin findings appear atypical.[15]
- Biopsy of the purpura, as well as of nonaffected areas, will reveal IgA deposition under immunofluorescence.[15]
- Renal biopsy will demonstrate mesangial proliferation and focal necrosis, classically described as a "focal and segmental proliferative glomerulonephritis." Cresecent formation is evident in cases of rapidly progressive disease.[2,15]

CLINICAL FEATURES

- The classic palpable, purpuric rash is essential for diagnosis.[2] It is the presenting symptom in over half of the cases of HSP; however, it may not always be seen at initial presentation.[2,16,17]
- Both joint pain and abdominal pain may precede the classic rash in up to 43 percent of patients by up to two weeks.[1,2]
- The purpura are typically 2 to 10 mm in diameter and accompanied by scattered pinpoint petechiae and ecchymoses (**Figure 175-2**).[1]
- The rash may appear urticarial or macular-papular for the first 24 hours.[1]
- Bullous lesions may develop in some children.[1]
- Fatigue and low-grade fever are common.[18]
- Joint pain is present in up to 82 percent of patients. It most often involves the lower extremities, including the feet, ankles, and knees; however, up to 37 percent of patients may have additional pain in the hands, wrists and elbows.[1,2]
- Abdominal pain is present in 50 percent to 75 percent of cases of HSP (**Figure 175-3**). It is described as "colicky," or a "bowel angina," and may be accompanied by vomiting.[1,2,6]
- The abdominal pain is often considered mild, however severely debilitating pain may occur in some individuals.[2]
- Gastrointestinal bleeding, either gross or occult, is noted in approximately half of children with abdominal pain related to HSP.[1]
- Renal involvement is present in approximately 50 percent of cases.[5,19,20]
- While rarely severe, renal manifestations can range from mild and benign to a rapidly progressive glomerulonephritis with crescent formation and renal failure.[20,21]
- Nephritis is typically evidenced by microscopic hematuria with or without proteinuria; however, macroscopic hematuria may also be present.[2,21]
- Some children with renal involvement may also have hypertension.[2]
- A less common clinical feature includes testicular involvement in male children. This may present as epididymitis or orchitis with swelling and pain.[1,2,16] Testicular involvement may be the presenting symptom in some male children.[16]
- CNS involvement is rare, but may occur. Headache, seizures, intracranial hemorrhage and cerebral vasculitis may be present in about 2 percent of patients.[2,22]
- Most CNS manifestations are mild and resolve without permanent consequences. Severe or fatal neurologic complications are very rare.[22]

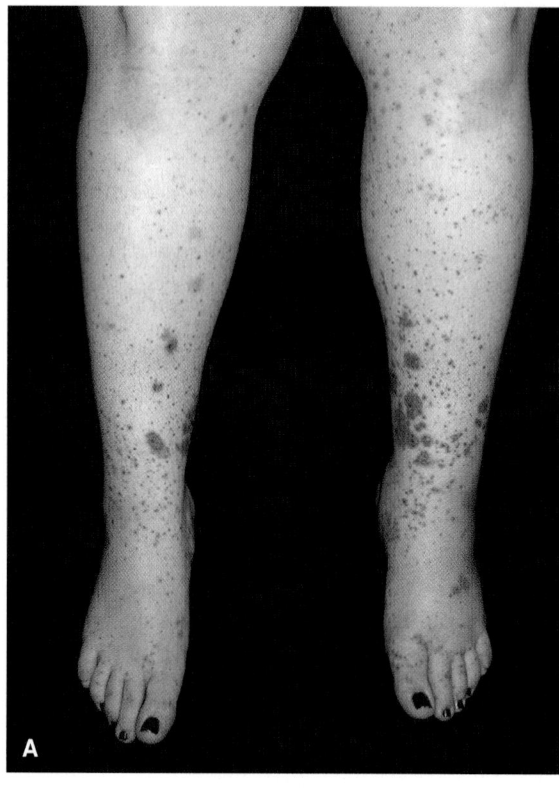

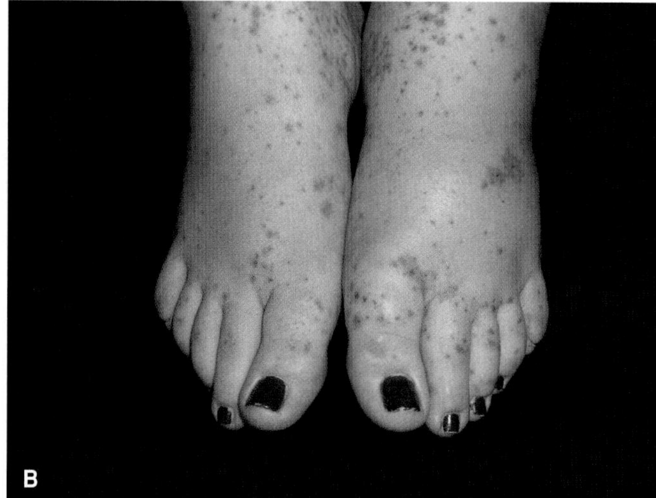

FIGURE 175-2 Henoch-Schönlein purpura (HSP) in an overweight teenage girl presenting with a rash, ankle pain and swelling. **A.** Note the palpable purpura on both legs and the ankle swelling. **B.** Note the soft tissue swelling of the feet along with the petechial eruption. *(Used with permission from Richard P. Usatine, MD.)*

DISTRIBUTION

- The classic palpable, purpuric rash is symmetrical and distributed predominantly over the extensor surfaces of the lower extremities (**Figures 175-1** to **175-4**) and buttocks; however, it may be present in other areas as well.[1,2]
- In some cases, the purpuric lesions may spread to the child's trunk and face.[2]

LABORATORY TESTING

- No single laboratory test is diagnostic for HSP.[2]
- Experts recommend the following for initial investigation of HSP:[2]
  - CBC (anemia due to GI bleeding and a leukocytosis may be present).
  - ESR (may be elevated).
  - Clotting profile (normal in HSP).

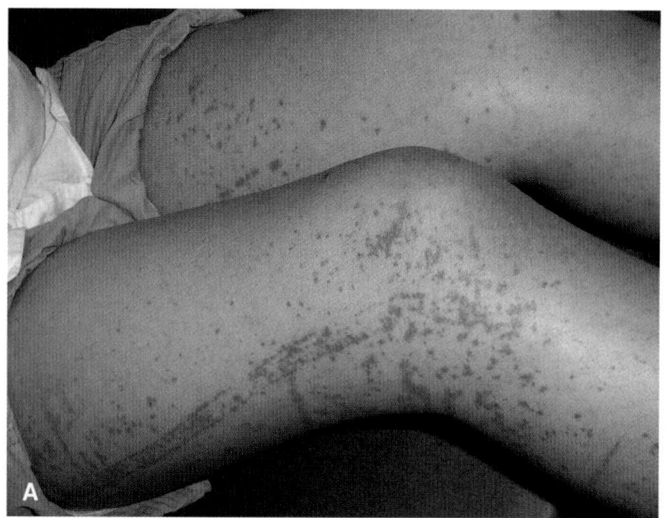

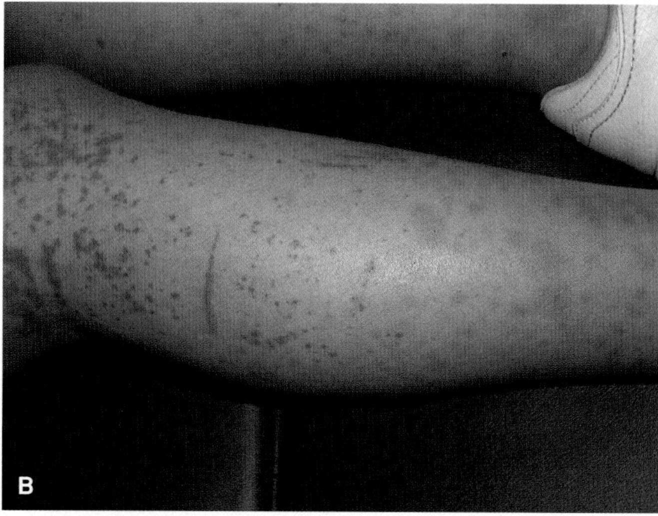

FIGURE 175-3 Henoch-Schönlein purpura (HSP) in an 11-year-old girl. She presented with a rash, knee pain and abdominal pain that was already resolving. **A.** Petechial eruption is particularly evident under the area where the seams of her jeans pressed on the leg. **B.** Petechiae and purpura on the lower leg. *(Used with permission from Richard P. Usatine, MD.)*

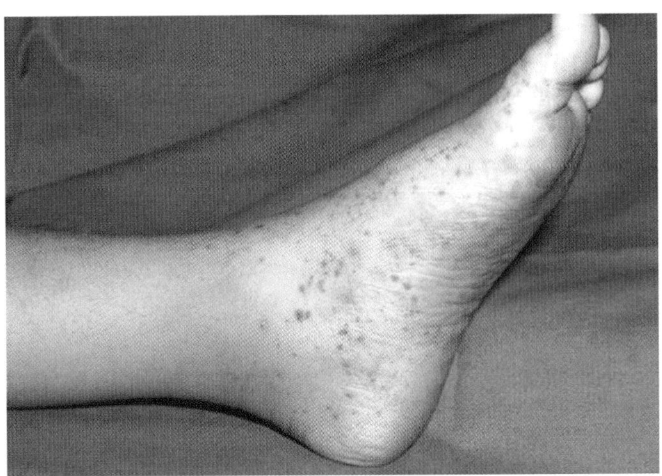

FIGURE 175-4 Henoch-Schönlein purpura (HSP) with prominent involvement of the foot of this child. (*Used with permission from Camille Sabella, MD.*)

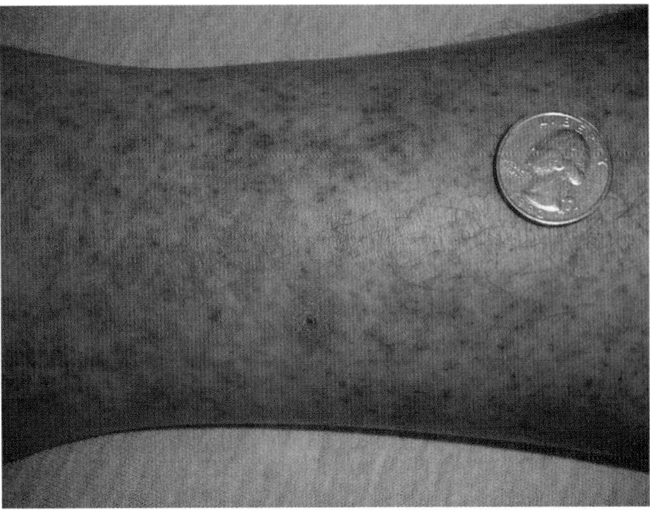

FIGURE 175-5 Rocky Mountain spotted fever with many petechiae visible around the original tick bite. This rickettsial disease looks similar to vasculitis. (*Used with permission from Tom Moore, MD.*)

 - Serum chemistry (to monitor renal function).
 - Albumin (may be low due to GI or renal involvement).
 - ASO titer and anti-DNase B (for possible preceding streptococcal infection).
 - Urine dipstick (evaluate for proteinuria and hematuria).
 - If purpura are present and the diagnosis is unclear, a full sepsis work-up may be warranted.
- Increased levels of serum IgA are often present, especially during the acute phase of the disease.[6,7]
- Complement levels in HSP are typically normal.[23]

IMAGING

- Imaging is not routinely performed in the evaluation of HSP.[18]
- Intussusception is a rare complication of HSP in the pediatric population.[2,12] Ultrasound or CT may be used to look for a suspected intussusception in a child with abdominal pain.[24]
- MRI may be used for the diagnosis of suspected cerebral vasculitis.[22]

DIFFERENTIAL DIAGNOSIS

- IgA nephropathy (Berger's disease) has similar renal manifestations and histologic findings on renal biopsy, including hypercellularity and mesangial proliferation.[2] HSP and IgA nephropathy are both attributed to IgA deposition.[4] Some experts even suggest that HSP and IgA nephropathy actually represent different manifestations of the same disease process.[23,25]
- Septic meningococcal infection may present with purpura on the extremities, similar to HSP.[15] However, in meningococcal infection, the patient likely has additional symptoms of fever and meningitis (see **Figure 153-12**).
- Wegner's granulomatosis may mimic the renal effects of HSP with proteinuria and hematuria;[15] however, Wegner's will typically also affect the upper respiratory tract. In contrast to HSP, patients with Wegner's classically test positive for c-ANCA antibodies.[15,18]
- Rocky Mountain spotted fever may present with palpable purpura, similar in appearance to HSP.[18] The rash, however, has a characteristic spreading pattern and will begin on the palms and soles and spread to the trunk and extremities (see **Figures 175-5** and **188-1**).
- Cutaneous leukocytoclastic vasculitis can present with palpable purpura and arthralgia; however, cutaneous leukocytoclastic vasculitis will not have renal involvement (see Chapter 153, Vasculitis).[15,18]
- Purpura due to thrombocytopenia of many causes (including leukemia in children) may mimic the characteristic rash of HSP with the appearance of purpura and petechiae; however, HSP will show a normal platelet count and coagulation profile.[15,18]

MANAGEMENT

- There is not a consensus among experts about optimal treatment regimens for children diagnosed with HSP.[2]
- Not all patients with HSP require treatment with steroids. In general, patients with mild disease require only symptomatic treatment.[15,23]
- Some experts recommend that steroid treatment be specifically used in patients with a high risk of renal involvement or severe extrarenal symptoms.[9]

NONPHARMACOLOGIC

- Supportive therapy with hydration is adequate in mild cases.[18]
- Arthralgias may be lessened with rest and elevation.[15,18]

MEDICATIONS

- For skin lesions, most patients will not need treatment, as these lesions are typically self-resolving. However, bullous lesions may respond to corticosteroid treatment.[2]
- NSAIDS have been used with good effect in arthritis associated with HSP; however, caution must be exercised due to the detrimental effects of NSAIDS on renal function.[2]
- Prednisone has proven to be effective in the treatment of extrarenal symptoms such as joint pain and abdominal pain.[2,9,12,18] The early

use of prednisone has been recommended for severe extrarenal symptoms, typically at 1mg/kg/day for 2 weeks with weaning over the following 2 weeks.[9,15] SOR Ⓒ

- There is a lack of evidence and controlled trials to guide treatment of HSP nephritis.[12] It is controversial whether early treatment with corticosteroids is effective preventing the progression of renal disease.[9,26]
- For children with >6 months of proteinuria, use of an ACE inhibitor may help reduce glomerular injury.[15,20]
- Though very little data exists about the treatment of rapidly progressive glomerulonephritis due to HSP, uncontrolled data has shown that treatment options include aggressive therapy with corticosteroids, cyclophosphamide, and, potentially, plasma exchange.[15,20]
- Cyclosporine A, azathioprine, and cyclophosphamide may also be effective in rapidly progressive disease.[15,20]

- Plasma exchange has been reported for use in rapidly progressive glomerulonephritis, though it is not recommended currently due to scarcity of data.[20]

SURGERY

- Contrast enema was shown in one recent study to be safe, though typically unsuccessful, in the reduction of intussusceptions due to HSP.[18,24]
- Intussusception in HSP is typically ileocolic or ileoileal and contrast enemas are often unable to reach these locations. The patient may subsequently require surgical reduction and resection.[24]

REFERRAL

- Immediate referral to a nephrologist should be made if the patient displays hypertension, abnormal renal function, acute nephritis, nephrotic syndrome, persistent proteinuria, or macroscopic hematuria for longer than 5 days.[2]

PREVENTION AND SCREENING

- Despite HSP being the most common vasculitis in children, definitive data on preventative measures is lacking in the literature.[5]
- Corticosteroid treatment at presentation has not been shown to prevent the development of nephritis in newly diagnosed cases of HSP.[9,12,20,27]
- Similarly, corticosteroids have not been shown to prevent recurrence of disease.[1]

PROGNOSIS

- In general, the prognosis of HSP is very good. The majority of children will not develop long term renal complications.[21]
- The mortality rate of HSP is <1 percent.[28]
- Most of the features of HSP are self-resolving, lasting an average of 4 weeks.[12]
- Chronic renal impairment is seen in only 1.1 to 5.0 percent of patients with HSP.[10,23,28]
- Long term prognosis is linked to the severity of renal disease.[2,12] Poor long-term outcome is associated with severe renal disease at diagnosis, while patents with hematuria and mild or absent proteinuria typically have a very benign course with full recovery.[23,29]
- No single prognostic factor (proteinuria, hematuria, renal function) can reliably predict outcomes of glomerulonephritis due to HSP in children; however, symptoms and severity of nephritis at onset of disease have been shown to be more predictive of long term morbidity than renal biopsy.[29–31]
- One study suggests that severity of renal symptoms at diagnosis should be regarded as equally important in making treatment decisions as biopsy results.[29]
- Patients with nephrotic syndrome have a worse prognosis, with 20 to 50 percent of these patients experiencing long-term renal impairment.[12,19,21]
- If no renal symptoms develop within one month of the onset of HSP, there is likely a very favorable prognosis for long term renal function.[9,29]
- Adult women with a history of HSP in childhood are at increased risk of hypertension and proteinuria during pregnancy and require frequent monitoring for these complications.[2] This risk exists even if the patient had only mild renal disease at diagnosis.[4,29]

FOLLOW-UP

- Up to 1/3 of patients will have a recurrence of their disease 6 months after the initial diagnosis.[18] Recurrence is more common in patients with renal disease and is usually is less severe and of shorter duration than the initial episode.[1,2,18]
- It is recommended by some experts that children diagnosed with HSP should be evaluated monthly for at least 6 months following their diagnosis, even if urinalysis is normal at diagnosis.[2,21]
- Follow-up should include monitoring of blood pressure as well as a urinalysis to evaluate for proteinuria and hematuria.[2,18] If proteinuria or hematuria is present, BUN and creatinine should be evaluated.[18,21]
- It is suggested that no follow up is needed after 6 months if the patient's urinalysis remains normal; however, patients diagnosed with nephritis due to HSP should be followed for longer than 6 months.[19,21]

PATIENT EDUCATION

- Reassure parents that most children with HSP have no long lasting effects.
- Renal disease is the most common long term complication so urine testing will be needed for some time.

PATIENT RESOURCES

- Kids Health: *Henoch-Schönlein Purpura*—**http://kidshealth.org/parent/medical/heart/hsp.html**.
- Mayo Clinic: *Henoch-Schonlein Purpura*—**www.mayoclinic.com/health/henoch-schonlein-purpura/DS00838**.

PROVIDER RESOURCES

- The Johns Hopkins Vasculitis Center. *Henoch Schonlein Purpura*—**www.hopkinsvasculitis.org/types-vasculitis/henochschnlein-purpura**.
- Medscape. *Henoch-Schonlein Purpura*—**www.emedicine.medscape.com/article/984105**.

REFERENCES

1. Saulsbury, FT. Henoch-Schönlein purpura in children. Report of 100 patients and review of the literature. *Medicine* (Baltimore). 1999;78(6):395-409.
2. McCarthy HJ, Tizard EJ. Clinical practice: Diagnosis and management of Henoch-Schonlein purpura. *Eur J Pediatr*. 2010;169:643-650.
3. Gardner-Medwin JM, Dolezalova P, Cummins C, Southwood TR. Incidence of Henoch–Schönlein purpura, Kawasaki disease, and rare vasculitides in children of different ethnic origins. *Lancet*. 2002;360(9341):1197-1202.
4. Aalberse J, Dolman K, Ramnath G, et al. Henoch Schönlein purpura in children: an epidemiological study among Dutch paediatricians on incidence and diagnostic criteria. *Ann Rheum Dis*. 2007; 66(12):1648-1650.
5. Ozen S. The spectrum of vasculitis in children. *Best Pract Res Clin Rheumatol*. 2002;16:411–425.
6. Yang YH, Chuang YH, Wang LC, et al. The immunobiology of Henoch-Schonlein Purpura. *Autoimmun Rev*. 2008;7:179-184.
7. Ozaltin F, Bakkaloglu A, Ozen S, et al. The significance of IgA class of antineutrophil cytoplasmic antibodies (ANCA) in childhood Henoch–Schönlein purpura. *Clin Rheumatol*. 2004; 23(5):426-429.
8. Al Shayyeb M, Batieha A, El-Shanti H, et al. Henoch-Schonlein purpura and streptococcal infection: a prospective case-control study. *Annals of Tropical Paediatrics*. 1999;19:253-255.
9. Ronkainen J, Koskimies O, Ala-Houhala M, et al. Early prednisone therapy in Henoch–Schönlein purpura: a randomized, double-blind, placebo-controlled trial. *J Pediatr*. 2006;149(2):241-247.
10. Kaku Y, Nohara K, Honda S. Renal involvement in Henoch-Schönlein purpura: a multivariate analysis of prognostic factors. *Kidney Int*. 1998;53:1755-1759.
11. Sano H, Izumida M, Shimizu H, Ogawa Y. Risk factors of renal involvement and significant proteinuria in Henoch-Schönlein purpura. *Eur J Pediatr*. 2002;161:196-201.
12. Saulsbury FT. Henoch-Schonlein purpura. *Current Opinion in Rheumatology*. 2010;22:598-602.
13. Ozçakar ZB, Yalçinkaya F, Cakar N, et al. MEFV mutations modify the clinical presentation of Henoch–Schönlein purpura. *J Rheumatol*. 2008;35(12):2427–2429.
14. Ozen S, Ruperto N, Dillon MJ, et al. EULAR/PReS endorsed consensus criteria for the classification of childhood vasculitides. *Ann Rheum Dis*. 2006;65(7):936–941.
15. Brogan P, Eleftheriou D, Dillon M. Small vessel vasculitis. *Pediatr Nephrol*. 2010;25:1025-1035.
16. Ha TS, Lee JS. Scrotal involvement in childhood Henoch–Schönlein purpura. *Acta Paediatr*. 2007;96(4):552–555.
17. Robson WL, Leung AK. Henoch-Schonlein purpura. *Adv Pediatr*. 1994;41:163-194.
18. Reamy BV, Williams PM, Lindsay TJ. Henoch-Schonlein purpura. *Am Fam Physician*. 2009;80(7):697-704.
19. Jauhola O, Ronkainen J, Koskimies O, et al. Renal manifestations of Henoch-Schonlein purpura in a 6-month prospective study of 223 children. *Arch Dis Child*. 2010;95:877-882.
20. Zaffanello M, Fanos V. Treatment-based literature of Henoch-Schonlein purpura nephritis in childhood. *Pediatr Nephrol*. 2009;24:1901-1911.
21. Narchi H. Risk of long term renal impairment and duration of follow up recommended for Henoch–Schönlein purpura with normal or minimal urinary findings: a systematic review. *Arch Dis Child*. 2005;90(9):916-920.
22. Wen YK, Yang Y, Chang CC. Cerebral vasculitis and intracerebral hemorrhage in Henoch–Schönlein purpura treated with plasmapheresis. *Pediatr Nephrol*. 2005;20(2):223-225.
23. Roberti I, Reisman L, Churg J. Vasculitis in childhood. *Pediatr Nephrol*. 1993;7:479-489.
24. Schwab J, Benya E, Lin R, Majd K. Contrast enema in children with Henoch-Schönlein purpura. *J Pediatr Surg*. 2005;40(8):1221-1223.
25. Meadow SR, Scott DG. Berger disease: Henoch-Schonlein syndrome without the rash. *J Pediatr*. 1985;106:27-32.
26. Huber AM, King J, McLaine P, Klassen T, Pothos M. A randomized, placebo-controlled trial of prednisone in early Henoch-Schönlein purpura. *BMC Med*. 2004;2:7.
27. Chartapisak W, Opastiraku S, Willis NS, et al. Prevention and treatment of renal disease in Henoch-Schonlein purpura: a systematic review. *Arch Dis Child*. 2009;94:132-137.
28. Stewart M, Savage JM, Bell B, McCord B. Long term renal prognosis of Henoch–Schönlein purpura in an unselected childhood population. *Eur J Pediatr*. 1988;147:113-115.
29. Ronkainen J, Nuutinen M, Koskimies O. The adult kidney 24 years after childhood Henoch–Schonlein purpura: a retrospective cohort study. *Lancet*. 2002;360:666-670.
30. Coppo R, Mazzucco G, Cagnoli L, Lupo A, Schena FP. Long-term prognosis of Henoch-Schönlein nephritis in adults and children. *Nephrol Dial Transplant*. 1997;12:2277-2283.
31. Mir S, Yavascan O, Mutlubas F, et al. Clinical outcome in children with Henoch- Schönlein nephritis. *Pediatr Nephrol*. 2007;22:64-70.

176 PERIODIC FEVER SYNDROMES

Shoghik Akoghlanian, MD
Andrew Zeft, MD MPH

PATIENT STORY

A 6-year-old Caucasian boy is seen by his pediatrician for a 14-month history of fever episodes lasting up to 10 days. During these episodes, he develops a red rash, nonspecific joint pains, and abdominal pain variably accompanied by diarrhea. Between episodes he is asymptomatic. He has had serial evaluations in the primary care clinic and has been admitted to a children's hospital for work up to rule out potential infectious, gastrointestinal, and oncologic etiologies. The work-up is only positive for nonspecific elevations in inflammatory markers and a mild leukocytosis. The pediatrician suspects a periodic fever syndrome and refers the child to a pediatric rheumatologist. During an episode of fever, the child is evaluated by the pediatric rheumatologist. The only clinical finding is a rash on the back and trunk (**Figure 176-1**). Work-up for a periodic fever syndrome reveals a heterozygous missense mutation in the gene encoding the cell surface receptor for tumor necrosis factor (TNF) TNFRSF1A, and the diagnosis of tumor necrosis factor receptor-associated periodic syndrome (TRAPS) is made. The boy is treated with etanercept, a soluble TNF-α receptor fusion protein, after which the frequency and severity of his episodes lessen.

INTRODUCTION

Periodic fever syndromes refer to a class of auto-inflammatory (AI) disorders characterized by spells of fever with other associated symptoms, typically occurring with three or more episodes of unexplained fever in a six-month period at least seven days apart. As in the case presented, a recurrent fever syndrome diagnosis may have a monogenetic etiology; however, many cases are characterized phenotypically,[1] There is an expanding spectrum of genetic AI diseases including but not limited to: TRAPS, familial Mediterranean fever (FMF), mevalonate kinase deficiency (MVK), otherwise known as hyperimmunoglobulin D syndrome (HIDS), and cryopyrin associated periodic syndromes (CAPS), which includes three overlapping phenotypes (familial cold auto-inflammatory syndrome, Muckle-Wells syndrome, or neonatal onset multisystem inflammatory disease). The disorder termed periodic fever, aphthous stomatitis, pharyngitis, cervical adenitis syndrome (PFAPA or Marshall Syndrome), is a benign condition with regular intervals of high fever which last approximately 5 days (**Table 176-1**).[2]

SYNONYMS

Periodic fever syndrome, recurrent fever syndrome, or auto-inflammatory disorder.

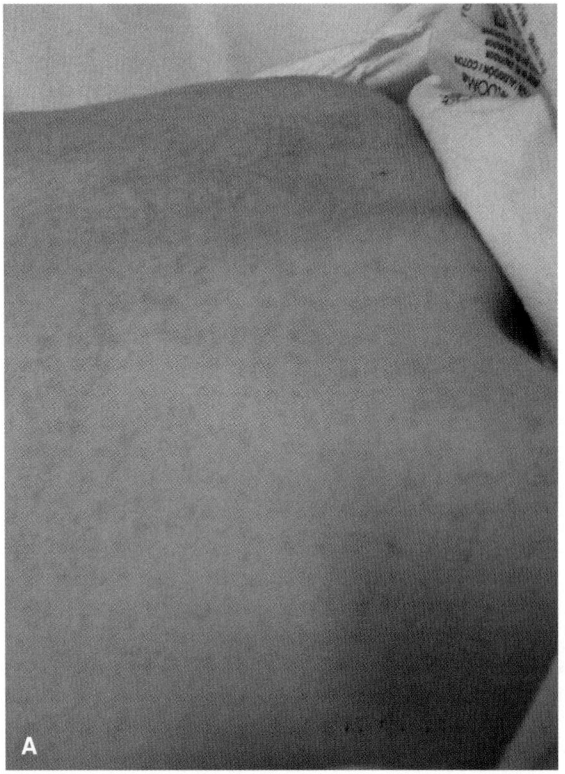

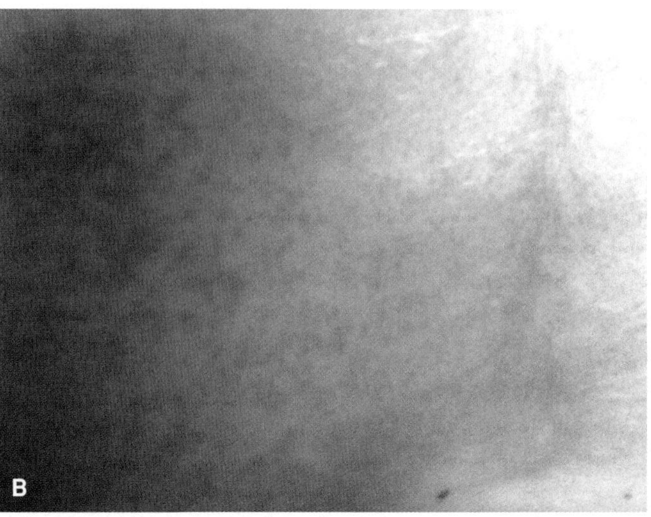

FIGURE 176-1 **A.** Erythematous eruption on the back of a child (a) with periodic fever who was confirmed to have tumor necrosis factor receptor associated periodic syndrome (TRAPS). **B.** A close-up view reveals speckled patches with some areas of confluence, which is characteristic of this syndrome. This resembles a viral exanthem. (*Used with permission from Andrew Zeft, MD.*)

TABLE 176-1 Summary of Autoinflammatory Syndromes and Their Acronyms

- TRAPS—Tumor necrosis factor receptor-associated periodic syndrome.
- FMF—Familial Mediterranean fever.
- MVK—Mevalonate kinase deficiency = HIDS-hyperimmunoglobulin globulin D syndrome.
- CAPS—Cold auto inflammatory syndromes. Includes Familial cold autoinflammatory syndrome (FCAS), Muckle-Wells syndrome (MWS), and Neonatal-onset multisystem inflammatory disorder (NOMID).
- PFAPA—Periodic fever, aphthous stomatitis, pharyngitis, or cervical adenitis syndrome.

EPIDEMIOLOGY

- Of the periodic fever syndromes, PFAPA is perceived to be the most prevalent.
- TRAPS may present from infancy into adulthood, but most commonly presents in toddlers. TRAPS patients characteristically have an Irish ancestral pattern.
- FMF is more common in those with Sephardic Jewish, Armenian, or Turkish ancestry. Clinical signs of FMF typically develop by 10 years of age.
- The first HIDS episode typically occurs prior to 12 months. HIDS was first described in patients from the Netherlands and is believed more common in those from Western Europe.
- In France, the prevalence of CAPS with NLRP-3 (pyrin domain) mutations has been estimated 1/360,000.[3]

ETIOLOGY AND PATHOPHYSIOLOGY

- Unlike classic rheumatic diseases with autoimmune pathogenesis, autoinflammatory diseases do not rely on autoreactive T lymphocytes or pathogenic autoantibodies.
- To date, nearly all mutations linked to AI syndromes disrupt inflammatory signaling within the innate immune system. This disruption generates a pro-inflammatory state, often leading to a final common pathway ending with activation of the inflammasome, a complex of distinct proteins, which serve to convert inactive pro-IL-1β to active pro-IL-1β (**Figure 176-2**).
- Stress or infection may trigger episodes by stimulating an inflammatory process through the inflammasome.
- TRAPS is an autosomal dominantly inherited disease with incomplete penetrance.
- CAPS' inheritance is autosomal dominant, while FMF and HIDS inheritance is autosomal recessive.

RISK FACTORS

- Family history of unexplained recurrent fever symptoms, hearing loss (Muckle-Wells), renal failure, recurrent abdominal pain, amyloidosis with or without renal failure.[4]
- Although no associated genetic mutation has been identified in PFAPA, close to half of patients have a positive family history of a parent or sibling with symptoms suggestive of the disorder.[5]

DIAGNOSIS

- A symptom log documenting fever duration and associated triggers and symptoms is very important in the diagnostic evaluation.

CLINICAL FEATURES

- Fever, rash, serositis, lymphadenopathy, GI disturbance, and musculoskeletal involvement are the most common clinical signs and symptoms of AI syndromes.
    - Familial Mediterranean Fever is characterized by symptomatic episodes of short duration (12 to 72 hours), fever (~90%), and severe abdominal pain (peritonitis) which may mimic appendicitis. Acute monoarthritis (typically knee or ankle) occurs in over half although chronic arthritis may be present. Headaches may be due to aseptic meningitis.
    - Tumor necrosis factor receptor-associated periodic syndrome is characterized by longer episodes (often >7 days) of fever, abdominal pain, erythematous rash (typically travels proximal to distal), regions of myopathy (**Figure 172-1**), with or without periocular swelling. Deep tissue biopsy often demonstrates a neutrophilic fasciitis sparing the underlying musculature.
    - Hyper Immunoglobulin D syndrome is characterized by cervical lymphadenopathy (90%) and polymorphic erythematous rash (80%, typically palms and soles; **Figure 176-3**). Attacks may be triggered by vaccination or infection; they typically last 3 to 7 days and may reoccur every 3 to 6 weeks.
    - Periodic fever, aphthous stomatitis, pharyngitis, cervical adenitis syndrome is classically characterized by periodic fevers, aphthous stomatitis, pharyngitis, and cervical lymphadenopathy. However, all the features are rarely present at once during the fever episodes, making the diagnosis difficult.

LABORATORY TESTING

- Elevated acute phase reactants (ESR, CRP) are typical of AI disorders. These may normalize between the attacks.
- FMF is primarily a clinical diagnosis supported by a response to colchicine, but sequencing a mutation within the Mediterranean fever (MEFV) gene is confirmative.
- TRAPS is confirmed by a mutation in the TNFRSF1A gene. Unlike other AI disorders, acute inflammatory markers (ESR, CRP) may remain elevated during subclinical periods.
- Urine mevalonic acid is usually elevated during HIDS attacks. A mevalonic kinase gene mutation is diagnostic. Elevated immunoglobulin D (IgD) is not specific for the diagnosis, but is commonly elevated in HIDS patients.

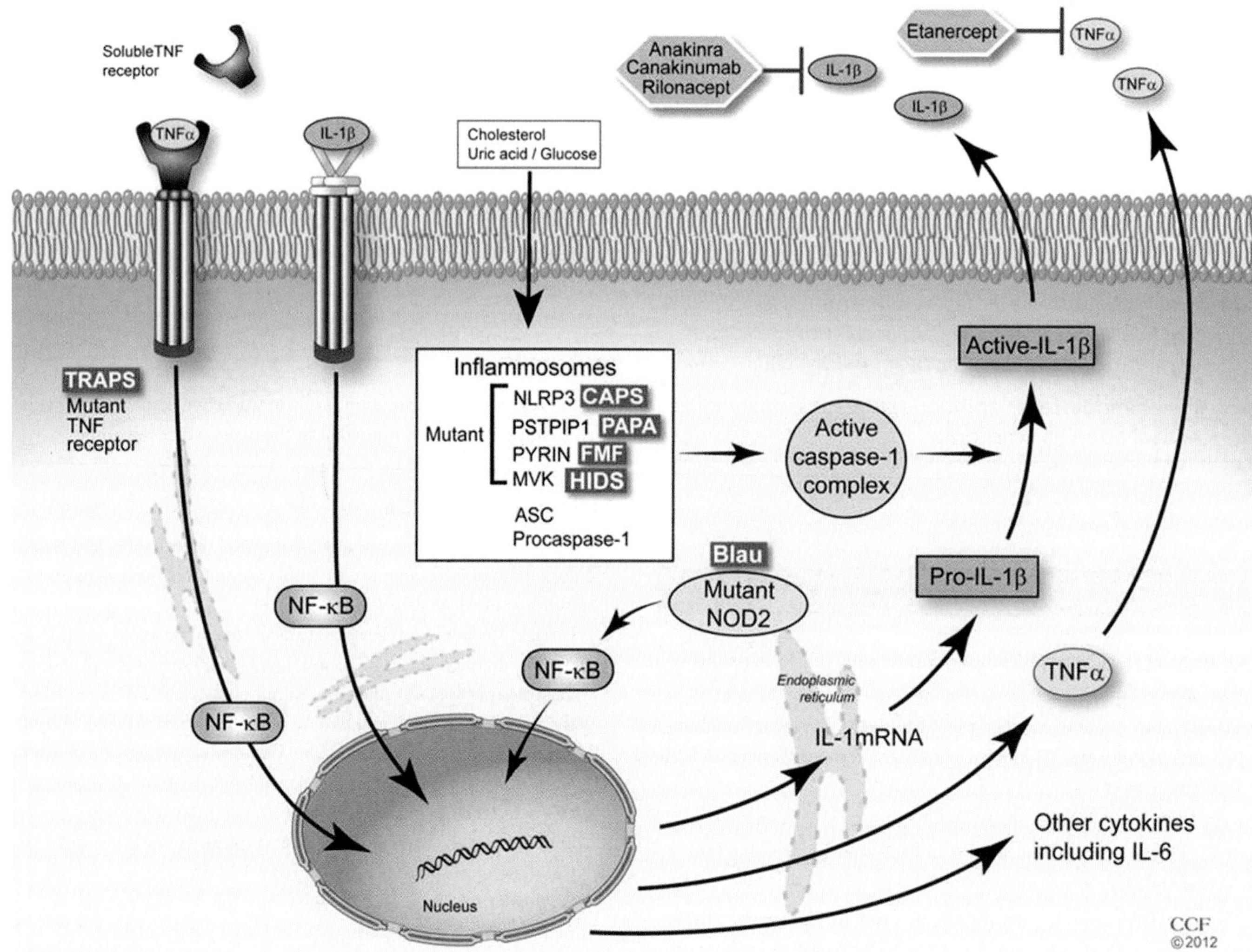

FIGURE 176-2 The inflammasome, is a complex of distinct proteins that when brought together, serve to convert inactive pro-IL 1beta to active IL-1 beta. In CAPS, FMF, and HIDS, mutations stimulate the inflammasome, resulting in activation of Interleukin-1β. In TRAPS, mutant tumor necrosis factor receptor is sequestered, leading to the transcription of pro-inflammatory markers, including Interleukin-1β.
Abbreviations key:

- TRAPS—Tumor necrosis factor receptor-associated periodic syndrome.
- FMF—Familial Mediterranean fever.
- MVK—Mevalonate kinase deficiency.
- HIDS—Hyperimmunoglobulin globulin D syndrome.
- CAPS—Cold auto inflammatory syndrome.
- PFAPA—Periodic fever, aphthous stomatitis, pharyngitis, cervical adenitis syndrome.
- NF—Nuclear factor.
- ASC—Apoptosis-associated speck-like protein containing a casepase activation and recruitment domain.
- TNF—Tumor necrosis factor.
- IL—Interleukin.

(*Reprinted with permission, Cleveland Clinic Center for Medical Art & Photography © 2012-2013. All Rights Reserved.*)

DIFFERENTIAL DIAGNOSIS

- Recurrent viral or bacterial infections are the most common cause of fever in the pediatric population and should primarily be ruled out.
- *Mycobacteria tuberculosis* and tick-borne relapsing fever may present with prolonged fever and rash. History of recent travel to an endemic area is critical when considering these diagnoses.
- Hematologic disorders such as cyclic neutropenia, leukemia, lymphoma, and inflammatory myofibroblastic tumor ("inflammatory pseudotumor") should be considered, and prompt referral to a hematologist/oncologist may be necessary.
- Systemic onset Juvenile Idiopathic Arthritis (sJIA) is characterized by prolonged quotidian fever (typically at symptom onset) for >2 weeks, differentiating this condition from true periodic fever syndromes. Arthritis in one or more joint, evanescent erythematosus rash, lymphadenopathy, and hepatosplenomegaly are features of sJIA (see Chapter 172, Juvenile Idiopathic Arthritis).

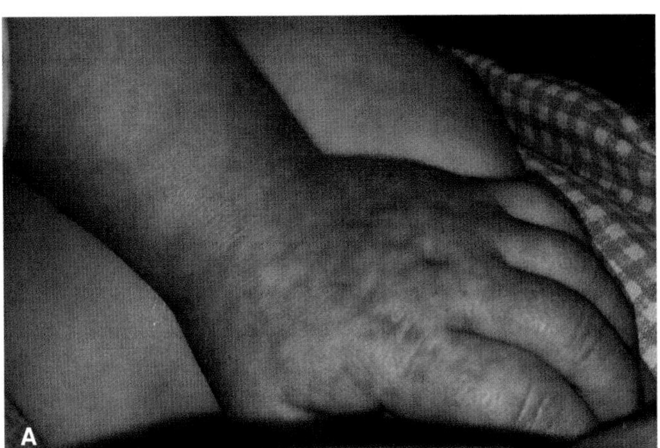

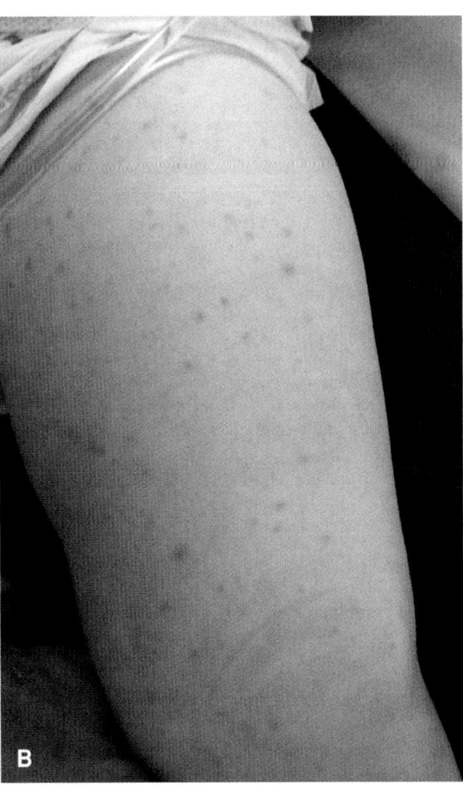

FIGURE 176-3 Polymorphic eruption in a child with hyperimmunoglobulin D syndrome (HIDS). **A.** Reticular pattern on hand and forearm. **B.** Diffuse petechial pattern on the leg. (*Used with permission from Sivia Lapidus, MD.*)

- Inflammatory bowel disease should be considered in patients with fever and associated abdominal pain, bloody stool, weight loss, joint or eye manifestations (see Chapter 59, Inflammatory Bowel Disease).

MANAGEMENT

- Supportive care with antipyretics and antianalgesics during the acute episodes are often helpful.

MEDICATIONS

- Systemic corticosteroids may be effective in treating flares of AI syndromes.[6] SOR Ⓒ However, the adverse effects of recurrent steroid use is a significant concern.
- Etanercept, a fusion protein linked to the Tumor necrosis factor (TNF) receptor, has variable efficacy in treating TRAPS.[7] SOR Ⓑ
- In cases not responding adequately to etanercept, an interleukin 1 (IL-1) inhibitor (anakinra, rilonacept) may be efficacious. SOR Ⓒ
- Colchicine is profoundly effective in minimizing the frequency and severity of FMF attacks and in preventing long-term complications (amyloidosis).[6] SOR Ⓐ IL-1 inhibitors may be efficacious in those not tolerating colchicine due to gastrointestinal-related side effects.[7] SOR Ⓑ
- In HIDS, a nonsteroidal anti-inflammatory agent may provide symptomatic relief; otherwise, systemic corticosteroids, colchicine, or biologic TNF or IL-1 inhibitors may be effective.[8] SOR Ⓑ Fortunately, the frequency of HIDS attacks typically decreases with age.[9]

SURGERY

Tonsillectomy leads to complete resolution of PFAPA related symptoms in approximately 2/3 of cases.[10]

REFERRAL

- A referral to a pediatric rheumatologist and/or a pediatric infectious diseases physician should be considered when the diagnosis of a periodic fever syndrome is suspected.
- A referral to an otolaryngologist should be considered for possible tonsillectomy for patients with PFAPA.

PROGNOSIS

- Prognosis depends on the specific periodic fever syndrome. The spectrum of complications is evolving for many of the more recently characterized disorders.
- PFAPA is a benign process that often resolves over time. The time to resolution however, is variable.
- The long-term complications of FMF (amyloidosis) can usually be prevented with appropriate therapy (colchicine).

FOLLOW-UP

- Close follow-up to assess the frequency of episodes and associated symptoms and the response to therapy is essential.

- Pediatric rheumatologists and/or pediatric infectious diseases specialists are often involved in the follow-up of these patients.

PATIENT EDUCATION

- A thorough log diary of the frequency of the episodes and associated features are very important.
- Parents should be told that a precise etiology for the periodic fevers is often not ascertained.

PATIENT AND PROVIDER RESOURCES

- **http://my.clevelandclinic.org/orthopaedics-rheumatology/diseases-conditions/periodic-fever-syndrome.aspx**.
- **www.rheumatology.org/practice/clinical/patients/diseases_and_conditions/pfapa.asp**.
- NOMID alliance—**http://www.nomidalliance.org/index.php**.
- Pediatric Rheumatology International Trials Organization—**www.printo.it/pediatric-rheumatology/information/UK/index.htm**.
- **http://pedsinreview.aappublications.org/content/30/5/e34.full.pdf+html**.

REFERENCES

1. Zeft AS, Spalding SJ. Autoinflammatory syndromes: fever is not always a sign of infection. *Cleve Clin J Med*. 2012;79(8):569-581.
2. Marshall SJ, Edwards KM, and Lawton AR. PFAPA syndrome. *Pediatr Infect Dis J*. 1989;8(9):658-659.
3. Cuisset L, et al. Mutations in the autoinflammatory cryopyrin-associated periodic syndrome gene: epidemiological study and lessons from eight years of genetic analysis in France. *Ann Rheum Dis*. 2011;70(3):495-499.
4. Shinar Y, et al. Guidelines for the genetic diagnosis of hereditary recurrent fevers. *Ann Rheum Dis*. 2012;71(10):1599-1605.
5. Cochard M, et al. PFAPA syndrome is not a sporadic disease. *Rheumatology (Oxford)*. 2010;49(10):1984-1987.
6. Ter Haar N, et al. Treatment of autoinflammatory diseases: results from the Eurofever Registry and a literature review. *Ann Rheum Dis*. 2013;72(5):678-685.
7. Bulua AC, et al. *Efficacy of etanercept in the tumor necrosis factor receptor-associated periodic syndrome: a prospective, open-label, dose-escalation study. Arthritis Rheum*. 2012;64(3):908-913.
8. Bodar et al. On-demand anakinra treatment is effective in mevalonate kinase deficiency. *Ann Rheum Dis*. 2011;70(12):2155-2158.
9. Zemer D, et al. Colchicine in the prevention and treatment of the amyloidosis of familial Mediterranean fever. *N Engl J Med*. 1986;314(16):1001-1005.
10. Hashkes PJ, et al. Rilonacept for colchicine-resistant or -intolerant familial Mediterranean fever: a randomized trial. *Ann Intern Med*. 2012;157(8):533-541.
11. van der Hilst, JC, et al. Long-term follow-up, clinical features, and quality of life in a series of 103 patients with hyperimmunoglobulinemia D syndrome. *Medicine (Baltimore)*. 2008.87(6):301-310.
12. Licameli G ,et al. Long-term surgical outcomes of adenotonsillectomy for PFAPA syndrome. *Arch Otolaryngol Head Neck Surg*. 2012;138(10):902-906.

177 KAWASAKI DISEASE

Camille Sabella, MD
Athar M. Qureshi, MD

PATIENT STORY

A 13-month-old previously healthy boy was admitted to the hospital with a 7-day history of high fever and marked irritability. Over the past 3 days, his parents noted that he had developed a red rash over his face, trunk, and extremities, as well as redness and cracking of his lips. He was also noted to have swelling in his hands and feet. He was admitted because of concern of Kawasaki disease. On physical examination, he was irritable and ill-appearing, had a diffuse pleomorphic rash on his face, trunk, and extremities (**Figure 177-1**), nonpurulent conjunctivitis, cracked fissured lips (**Figure 177-2**), a tender 2 cm-diameter lymph node in his posterior cervical area, and swelling in his extremities (**Figure 177-3**). He was treated with intravenous immune globulin and high-dose aspirin and recovered completely. Baseline echocardiography did not reveal any coronary artery abnormalities. Follow-up echocardiograms 2 weeks and 8 weeks after his presentation were normal.

INTRODUCTION

Kawasaki disease is an acute vasculitis that has emerged as the most common cause of acquired heart disease in children in the developed world. Based on the epidemiology and clinical features of this disorder, an infectious etiology is considered likely, although the precise etiology remains elusive. It is important to recognize the clinical manifestations of KD because the diagnosis is based on clinical criteria, and because timely treatment significantly reduces the risk of coronary artery disease, the most feared consequence of this disease.

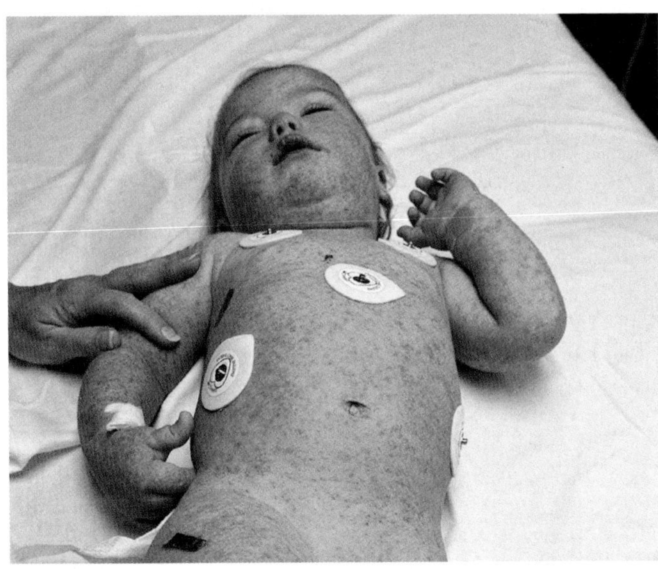

FIGURE 177-1 Pleomorphic rash in a 13-month-old with Kawasaki disease. (*Used with permission from Camille Sabella, MD.*)

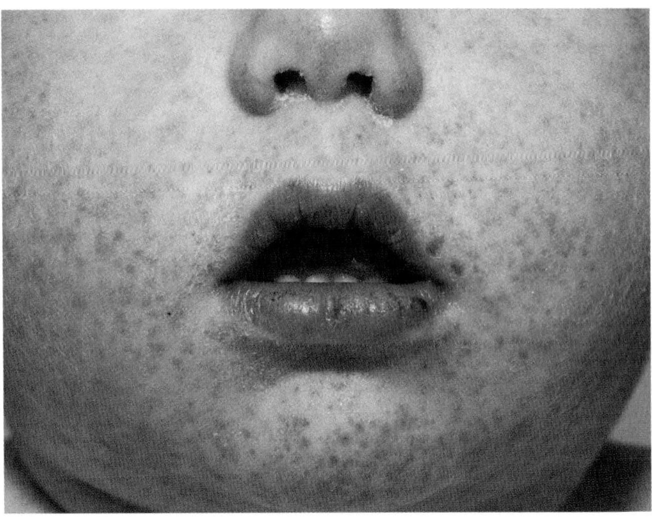

FIGURE 177-2 Cracked, fissured, and erythematous lips in the 13 month old with Kawasaki disease. (*Used with permission from Camille Sabella, MD.*)

SYNONYMS

Mucocutaneous Lymph Node Syndrome or Kawasaki Syndrome.

EPIDEMIOLOGY

- Eighty percent of children are under 5 years of age; rare in infants less than 3 months of age and children older than 8 years of age.[1]
- Male: Female ratio is 3:2.
- Predominance of cases in winter-spring in temperate climates.
- Incidence highest among Asian children, even in those living in non-Asian countries.[2]
- Epidemics of disease can occur in all ethnic groups.
- Recurrence of disease occurs rarely.
- No person-to-person spread of disease.

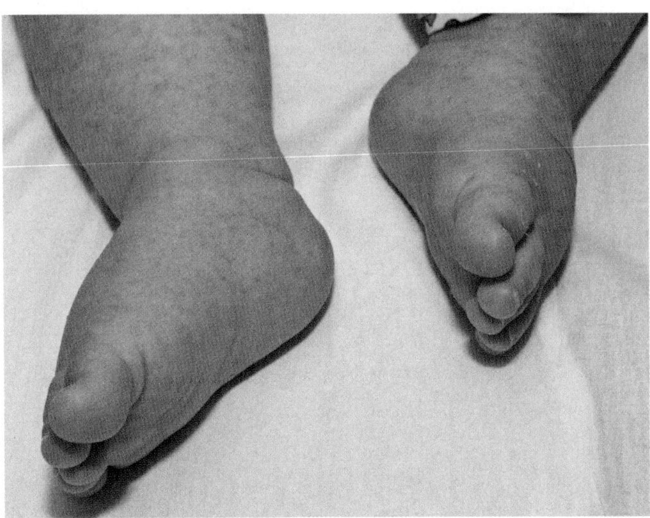

FIGURE 177-3 Extremity swelling in the 13-month-old with Kawasaki disease. (*Used with permission from Camille Sabella, MD.*)

ETIOLOGY AND PATHOPHYSIOLOGY

- Precise etiology is not known, but epidemiologic features (age group affected, seasonal predilection, occurrence of epidemics) point to an infectious etiology.
- Marked immunological activation in affected patients leads to inflammatory cell infiltration of blood vessels, particularly involving the coronary arteries.

RISK FACTORS

- Occurs in previously healthy infants and children.
- Infants and young children less than 5 years of age are most commonly affected.
- Annual incidence in Japanese children is 215 per 100,000 children younger than 5 year of age.[2]
- The attack rate in Caucasian children is 10-fold lower than in Asians; African- Americans have an intermediate incidence.
- Risk factors for the development of coronary artery disease on those affected include:
  - Age younger than 1 year.
  - Duration of fever longer than 16 days.
  - Recurrence of fever after an afebrile period of at least 48 hours.
  - Anemia.
  - Thrombocytopenia.
  - Hypoalbuminemia.

DIAGNOSIS

CLINICAL FEATURES

- Three phases of KD are classically described:
  - The acute phase, which lasts 7 to 14 days and is characterized by the classic clinical diagnostic criteria (see the following section).
  - The subacute phase occurs from about day 10 to day 25 of the illness, characterized by periungual desquamation, arthritis, and thrombocytosis.
  - The convalescent phase occurs from when all the clinical signs of illness have resolved until 6 to 8 weeks after the onset of the illness.
- The diagnosis of classic acute KD relies on clinical criteria, which include the presence of fever persisting for at least 5 days, along with four or the following five clinical findings:
  - Bilateral bulbar conjunctival injection without exudate (**Figure 177-4**).
  - Erythematous mouth and pharynx, red, cracked, fissured lips, and "strawberry tongue" (**Figure 177-5**).
  - Polymorphous, generalized, erythematous rash (may be maculopapular, morbilliform, scarlatiniform, or erythema multiforme-like; **Figure 177-6**).
  - Erythema and swelling of the hands and feet, with subsequent periungual desquamation (**Figures 177-7** to **177-9**)
  - Cervical lymph node enlargement (usually unilateral) with at least one lymph node measuring 1.5 cm in diameter (**Figure 177-10**).
- Other findings that may be present include:
  - Irritability, which is often marked.
  - Abdominal pain.

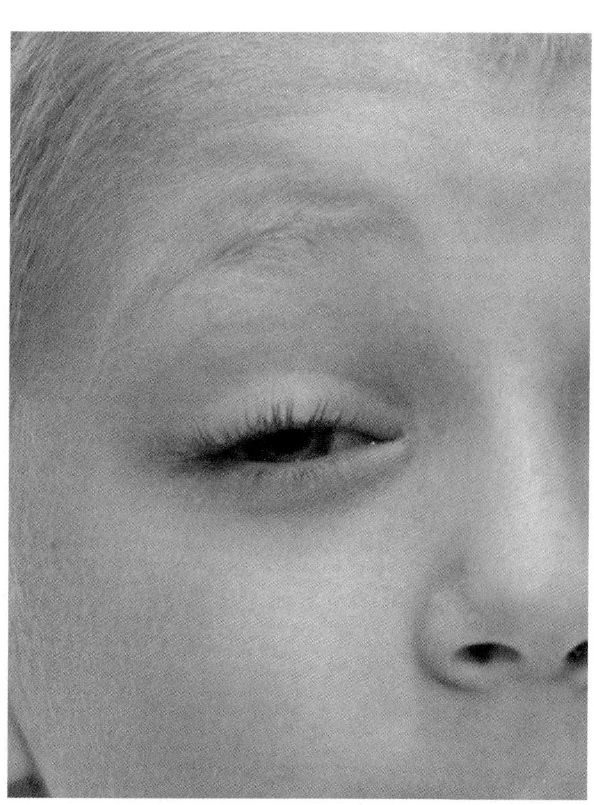

FIGURE 177-4 Nonpurulent conjunctivitis in a 5-year-old boy with Kawasaki disease (*Used with permission from Camille Sabella, MD.*)

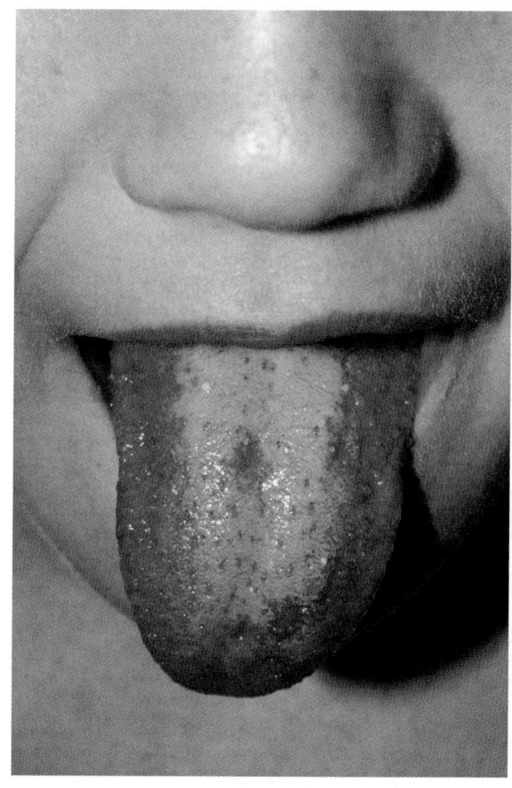

FIGURE 177-5 "Strawberry" tongue in a young boy with Kawasaki disease. (*Used with permission from Johanna Goldfarb, MD.*)

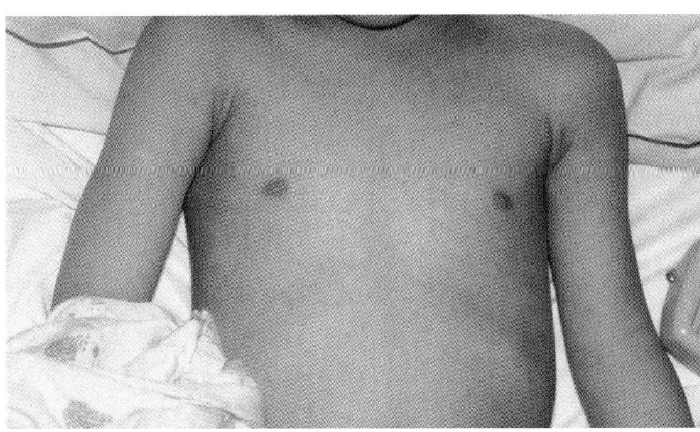

FIGURE 177-6 Diffuse maculopapular rash in a 5-year-old boy with Kawasaki disease. (*Used with permission from Johanna Goldfarb, MD.*)

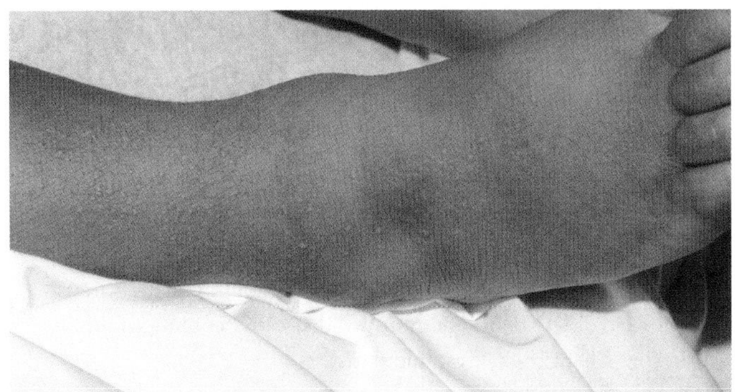

FIGURE 177-7 Extremity swelling, including the ankle joint, in a 2-year-old boy with Kawasaki disease. (*Used with permission from Camille Sabella, MD.*)

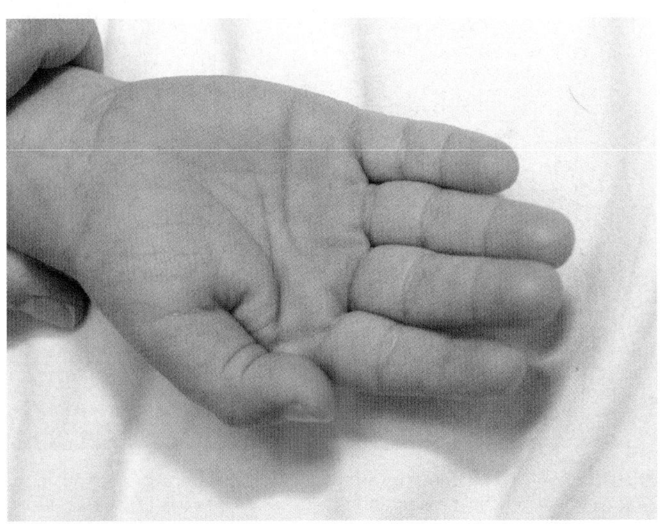

FIGURE 177-8 Palmar swelling and erythema in a 5-year-old boy with Kawasaki disease. (*Used with permission from Camille Sabella, MD.*)

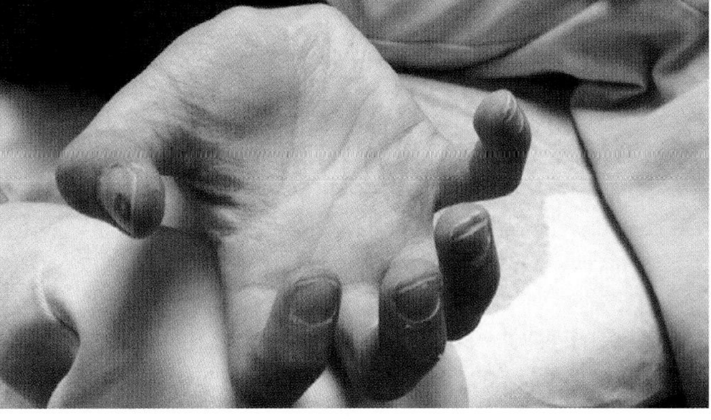

FIGURE 177-9 Periungual desquamation on day 10 of illness in this 9-year-old child with incomplete Kawasaki disease. (*Used with permission from Blanca Gonzalez, MD.*)

  - Diarrhea and vomiting.
  - Arthritis or arthralgia.
  - Meningismus.
- Coronary artery aneurysms, myocarditis, and pericarditis are well-known complications.
- Incomplete cases of KD can occur, particularly in young infants, usually heralded by the presence of fever and fewer than 4 of the 5 clinical features of the illness; these can be challenging to diagnose.[3,4]
- Periungual desquamation occurs during the subacute phase of the illness, usually occurring from day 10 to day 25 of the illness (**Figure 177-9**).

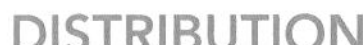

DISTRIBUTION

- Although the rash associated with KD is generalized, perineal involvement and accentuation is common.[5]
- Mild anterior uveitis may occur in 25 to 50 percent of patients.[6]

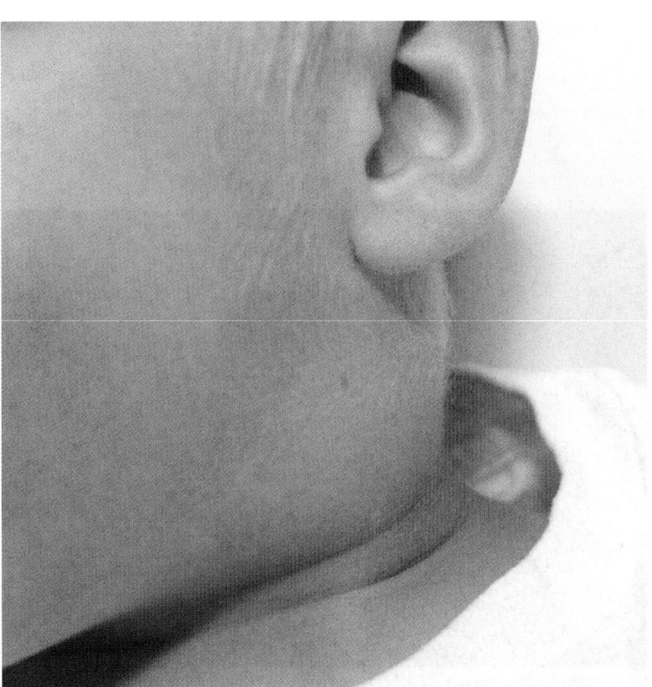

FIGURE 177-10 Posterior cervical adenopathy in a child with Kawasaki disease. (*Used with permission from Camille Sabella, MD.*)

LABORATORY TESTING

- Common laboratory findings include:
  - Leukocytosis.
  - Anemia.
  - Markedly elevated acute phase reactants.
  - Sterile pyuria (secondary to urethritis).
  - Hepatitis (elevated serum transaminases with or without elevated serum bilirubin).
  - Hypoalbuminemia.
  - Cerebrospinal fluid pleocytosis.
  - Thrombocytosis (seen during the subacute phase of the illness).
- Although laboratory parameters are characteristic and helpful in making the diagnosis, none are diagnostic.
- Thrombocytosis is not present during the acute phase of the illness, the period during which the diagnosis should be made.

IMAGING

- A baseline 2D-echocardiographic study should be obtained at diagnosis and repeated during the subacute phase of the illness (1 to 2 weeks after diagnosis).[7]
- If the initial and second echocardiographic studies are normal, a follow-up echocardiogram should be obtained 6 to 8 weeks after diagnosis to assure that abnormalities have not developed during the subacute or convalescent phase of the illness.
- If abnormalities are detected at any time, such as saccular or fusiform aneurysms (**Figures 177-11** and **177-12**), additional studies are necessary.
- Angiography may be necessary in cases of unusual coronary artery abnormalities (**Figure 177-13**) or for long-term follow-up of large aneurysms (**Figure 177-14**). Cardiac Computed tomographs or magnetic resonance imaging may be performed as well; however, they have limitations particularly in small children.
- Hydrops of the gallbladder can be detected in about 10 percent of children with KD (**Figure 177-15**).[8]

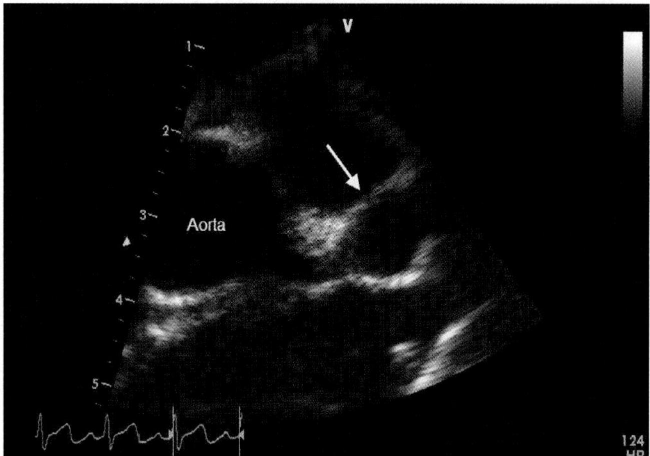

FIGURE 177-11 Transthoracic two-dimensional echocardiogram short axis view showing a saccular aneurysm (arrow) of the left anterior descending coronary artery. (*Used with permission from Athar M. Qureshi, MD.*)

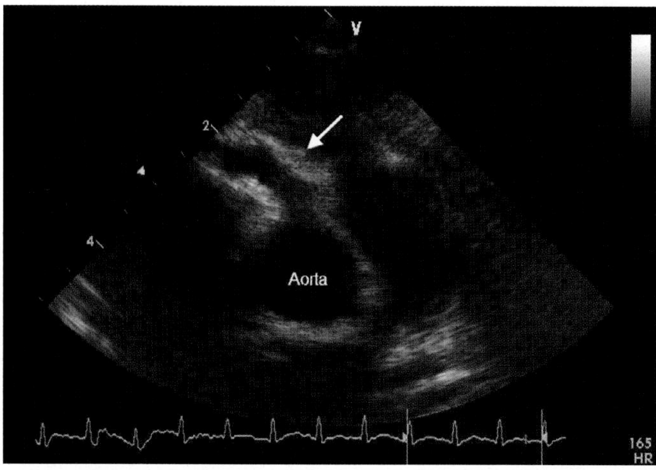

FIGURE 177-12 Transthoracic two-dimensional echocardiogram short axis view showing a fusiform aneurysm (arrow) of the right coronary artery. (*Used with permission from Athar M. Qureshi, MD.*)

DIFFERENTIAL DIAGNOSIS

- KD is difficult to differentiate from many other febrile illnesses of childhood.
- Perineal accentuation of the rash without accentuation in other skin folds (as in scarlet fever) is characteristic of KD (see Chapter 28, Strawberry Tongue and Scarlet Fever).
- The presence of a bulbar conjunctivitis without exudate is more suggestive of KD than other entities that cause conjunctival injection (see Chapter 12, Conjunctivitis).

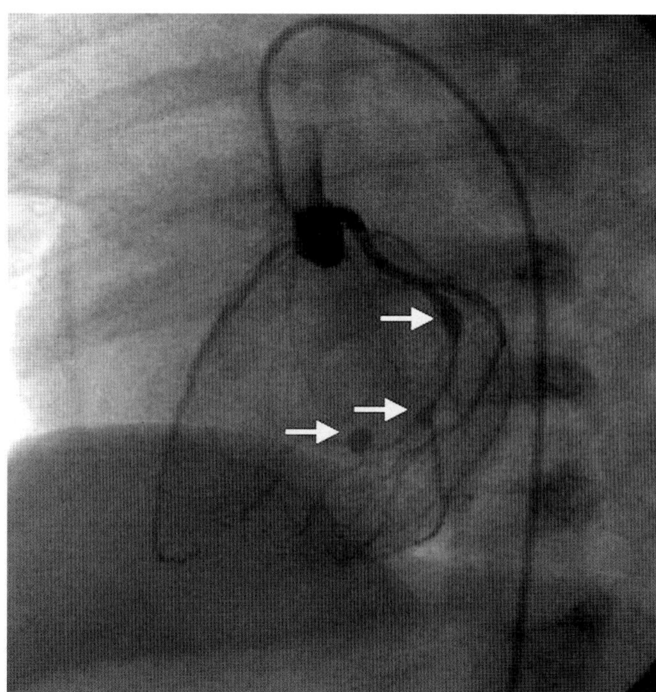

FIGURE 177-13 Left coronary artery angiogram (lateral projection) in an infant with an unusual presentation of Kawasaki disease. The circumflex coronary artery is seen with three aneurysms—one fusiform aneurysm (superior arrow) and two saccular aneurysms (inferior arrows). (*Used with permission from Athar M. Qureshi, MD.*)

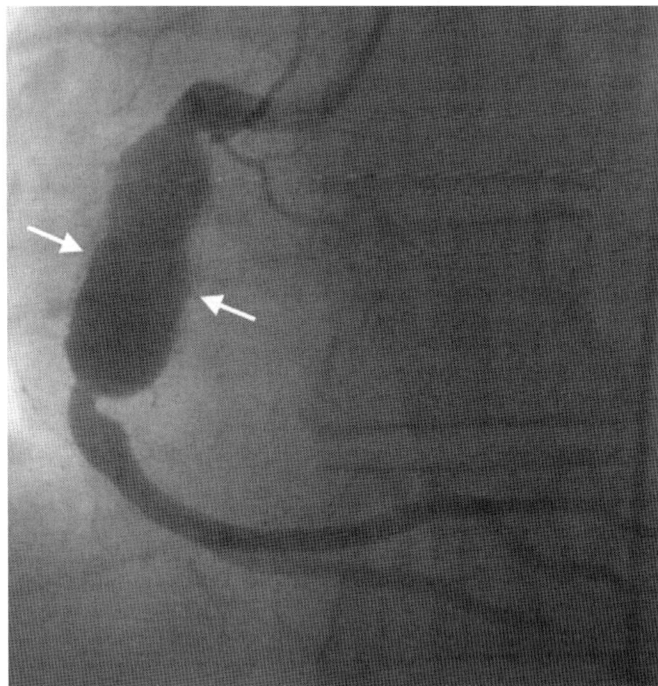

FIGURE 177-14 This right coronary artery angiogram was performed in an 18-year-old who had been followed for a giant right coronary artery aneurysm (arrow) since he was 3 years old. Note the rim of calcification surrounding the aneurysm and stenosis proximal and distal to the aneurysm. (*Used with permission from Athar M. Qureshi, MD.*)

- In general, children with KD are ill-appearing throughout the illness; this can help to distinguish KD from viral illnesses and scarlet fever.
- Although the rash of KD is polymorphous, vesicular and bullous lesions are not characteristic.
- Measles and Streptococcus pyogenes (Group A) are the illnesses that most commonly resemble KD (see Chapter 111, Measles).
- Measles should be considered in the ill-appearing child whose immunization history suggests susceptibility to measles; serum IgM testing can confirm the diagnosis of measles.

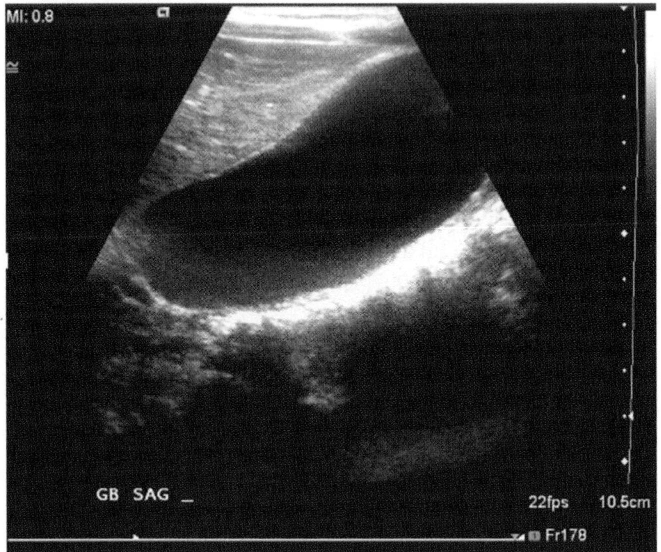

FIGURE 177-15 Hydrops of the gallbladder visualized on ultrasound of the liver and gallbladder. This occurs in about 10 percent of patients with Kawasaki disease. (*Used with permission from Camille Sabella, MD.*)

- The clinical features and positive throat culture or rapid antigen test for GAS can help distinguish KD from GAS infection.
- Other entities in the differential diagnosis of KD include a viral illness/exanthem (especially adenovirus), toxic shock syndrome, erythema multiforme/Erythema multiforme, and juvenile rheumatoid arthritis (see Chapter 185, Toxic Shock Syndromes, Chapter 151, Erythema Multiforme/Stevens Johnson Syndrome, and Toxic Epidermal Necrolysis, and Chapter 172, Juvenile Rheumatoid Arthritis).

MANAGEMENT

- KD is a self-limited vasculitis. However, 20 to 25 percent of untreated children will develop coronary artery abnormalities.[9] The goal of therapy is to reduce the clinical symptoms and prevent the development of coronary artery abnormalities by reducing inflammation.

MEDICATIONS

- The combination of intravenous immune globulin (IVIG) and high dose aspirin given within the first 10 days of illness has been demonstrated to reduce the prevalence of coronary artery abnormalities from about 20 to 25 percent (in aspirin-treated patients) to about 5 percent.[9,10] SOR Ⓐ
  - IVIG is given as a single infusion of 2g/kg over 12 hours, which results in a dramatic response in 90 percent of patients.
  - Aspirin should be given in anti-inflammatory doses (80 to 100 mg/kg/day divided every 6 hours) until the acute phase of the illness has subsided; the dose can then be reduced to anti-thrombotic effects (3 to 5 mg/kg/day); aspirin is discontinued 6 to 8 weeks after the onset of therapy provided coronary artery abnormalities have not developed during the course of the illness and if the echocardiogram at that time does not show any abnormalities.
- About 10 percent of children with KD do not respond to IVIG and remain afebrile 48 hours after completing the IVIG infusion; most of these children respond to a second dose of IVIG.[11–13] SOR Ⓐ
- Optimal treatment of children who are refractory to 2 doses of IVIG is not clear; these children are often treated with corticosteroids or infliximab. SOR Ⓒ
- The addition of corticosteroids to high-dose aspirin and IVIG as primary therapy does not appear to be effective and is not indicated.[14] SOR Ⓐ
- If abnormalities of the coronary arteries are detected, low-dose aspirin therapy is continued; large aneurysm may require the use of additional anticoagulant therapy, such as warfarin, low-molecular weight heparin, or acute thrombolytic therapy, to prevent thrombosis.[7] SOR Ⓒ

INTERVENTIONAL CARDIOLOGY TREATMENT/SURGERY

- Rarely, patients with significant coronary artery abnormalities will require interventions such as transluminal coronary angioplasty, coronary atherectomy, stent implantation, coronary artery bypass surgery, or heart transplantation.

REFERRAL

- A pediatric cardiologist with expertise in the interpretation of echocardiographic studies of coronary arteries in children is mandatory.

- The care of patients with significant cardiac abnormalities should involve a pediatric cardiologist with experience in the management of children with KD.

PROGNOSIS

- Without treatment, 20 to 25 percent of children with KD will develop coronary artery abnormalities; the risk is reduced to less than 5 percent with appropriate treatment.
- Long-term prognosis depends on the severity of coronary artery disease; those with giant aneurysms are more likely to require surgical intervention and their prognosis is more guarded.

FOLLOW-UP

- Acute follow-up after the initial hospitalization is important in assuring a good clinical response to the initial therapy.
- Repeat echocardiographic studies during the subacute and convalescent phase is recommended as previously outlined.
- Long-term management of children with KD should be based on the extent of coronary artery abnormalities.
- Even in the absence of coronary artery disease, periodic cardiovascular risk assessment should be performed as some patients may develop premature atherosclerotic changes.

PATIENT EDUCATION

- Children with prolonged fever or fever associated with irritability or any of the other features of KD should receive medical attention.
- Once the diagnosis of KD is made, close follow-up will be required depending on the course and complications.

PATIENT RESOURCES

- **www.nhlbi.nih.gov/health/health-topics/topics/kd/treatment.html**.
- **www.healthychildren.org/English/health-issues/conditions/heart/pages/Kawasaki-Disease.aspx?**.
- **www.ncbi.nlm.nih.gov/pubmedhealth/PMH0001984/**.
- **www.kdfoundation.org/**.

PROVIDER RESOURCES

- **www.cdc.gov/kawasaki/**.
- Holman RC, Curns AT, Belay ED, Steiner CA, Schonberger LB: Kawasaki syndrome hospitalizations in the United States, 1997 and 2000. *Pediatrics*. 2003;112:495-501.
- Newburger JW, Takahashi M, Gerber MA: Diagnosis, treatment, and long-term management of Kawasaki disease: a statement for health professionals from the Committee on Rheumatic Fever, Endocarditis and Kawasaki Disease, Council on Cardiovascular Disease in the Young, American Heart Association. *Circulation* 110 (2004):2747-2771.

REFERENCES

1. Holman RC, Belay ED, Christensen KY. Hospitalizations for Kawasaki syndrome among children in the United States, 1997–2007. *Pediatr Infect Dis J*. 2010;29:483-488.
2. Nakamura Y, Yashiro M, Uehara R. Epidemiologic features of Kawasaki disease in Japan: results of the 2007–2008 nationwide survey. *J Epidemiol*. 2010;20:302-307.
3. Rosenfeld EA, CorydonKE, Shulman ST. Kawasaki disease in infants less than one year of age. *J Pediatr*. 1995;126:524-529.
4. Rowley AH, Gonzalez-Crussi F, Gidding SS, Duffy CE, Shulman ST. Incomplete Kawasaki disease with coronary artery involvement. *J Pediatr*. 1987;110:409-413.
5. Friter BS, Lucky AW. The perineal eruption of Kawasaki syndrome. *Arch Dermatol*. 1988;124:1805-1810.
6. Burke MJ, Rennebohm RM. Eye involvement in Kawasaki disease. *J Pediatr Ophthalmol Strabismus*. 1981;18:7-12.
7. Newburger JW, Takahashi M, Gerber MA. Diagnosis, treatment, and long-term management of Kawasaki disease: a statement for health professionals from the Committee on Rheumatic Fever, Endocarditis and Kawasaki Disease, Council on Cardiovascular Disease in the Young, American Heart Association. *Circulation*. 2004;110:2747-2771.
8. Tizard EJ, Suzuki A, Levin M, Dillon MJ. Clinical aspects of 100 patients with Kawasaki disease. *Arch Dis Child*. 1991;66:185-188.
9. Newburger JW, Takahashi M, Burns JC. The treatment of Kawasaki syndrome with intravenous gamma globulin. *N Engl J Med*. 1986; 315:341-347.
10. Newburger JW, Takahashi M, Beiser AS. A single intravenous infusion of gamma globulin as compared with four infusions in the treatment of acute Kawasaki syndrome. *N Engl J Med*. 1991; 324:1633-1639.
11. Sundel RP, Burns JC, Baker A. Gamma globulin re-treatment in Kawasaki disease. *J Pediatr*. 1993;123:657-659.
12. Burns JC, Capparelli EV, Brown JA. Intravenous gamma-globulin treatment and retreatment in Kawasaki disease. US/Canadian Kawasaki Syndrome Study Group *Pediatr Infect Dis J*. 1998;17:1144-1148.
13. Han RK, Silverman ED, Newman A, McCrindle BW. Management and outcome of persistent or recurrent fever after initial intravenous gamma globulin therapy in acute Kawasaki disease. *Arch Pediatr Adolesc Med*. 2000;154:694-699.
14. Newburger JW, Sleeper LA, McCrindle BW. Randomized trial of pulsed corticosteroid therapy for primary treatment of Kawasaki disease *N Engl J Med*. 2007;356:663-675.

178 SCLERODERMA AND MORPHEA

E.J. Mayeaux, Jr., MD
Vidya Raman, MD

PATIENT STORY

A 4-year-old boy presented with a one-year history of skin redness and tightening over the right upper extremity. His mother had initially noticed the lesion after applying a temporary tattoo. He complained of occasional itching and pain over the area. His mother was concerned that his arm appeared to be "shrinking." He had no prior medical problems or preceding infections and his immunizations were up-to-date. He had difficulty grasping a crayon due to involvement of his fingers. On exam, he had a large area of skin tightening extending from the right scapular region and upper arm down to the forearm, index finger and thumb (**Figure 178-1**). He was referred to a dermatologist who performed a punch biopsy confirming a diagnosis of morphea (localized scleroderma). He was treated with topical fluticasone without benefit and referred to a pediatric rheumatologist for systemic therapy with methotrexate. Serologic testing showed a negative ANA and scleroderma antibody and he has had no features of systemic scleroderma.

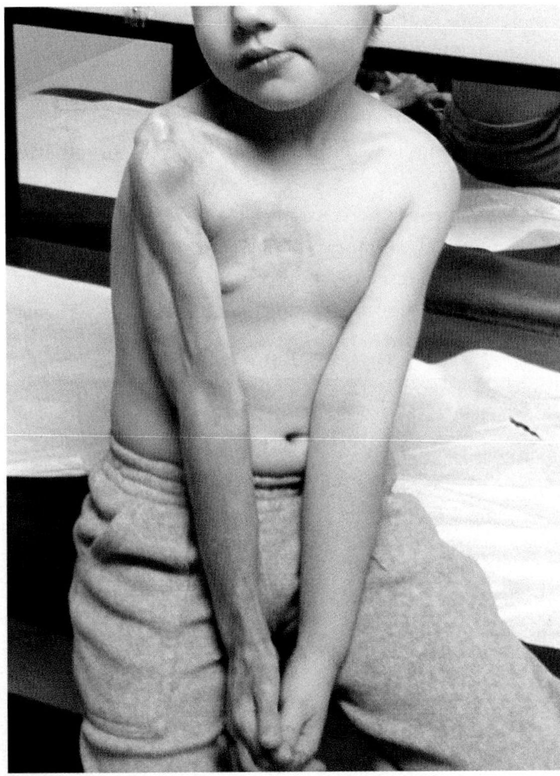

FIGURE 178-1 Morphea on the arm of a 4-year-old boy. He had a large area of skin tightening extending from the right scapular region and upper arm down to the index finger and thumb. (*Used with permission from Vidya Raman, MD.*)

INTRODUCTION

Scleroderma (from the Greek *scleros*, to harden) is a term that describes the presence of thickened, hardened skin. It may affect only limited areas of the skin (morphea), most or all of the skin (scleroderma), or also involve internal organs (systemic sclerosis).

EPIDEMIOLOGY

- Scleroderma is a spectrum of disorders that can be occur at any stage of life, but the clinical patterns seen in childhood differ somewhat from that seen in adults.
- The prevalence rates of diseases that share scleroderma as a clinical feature are reported ranging from 4 to 253 cases per 1 million individuals of all ages.[1]
- The most common form of childhood scleroderma is morphea (localized scleroderma or LSc) which principally involves the skin, subcutaneous fascia, muscle, and bone. It is 10 times more common than systemic sclerosis and may include circumscribed or generalized morphea, bullous morphea, deep morphea, and linear morphea (including the en coup de sabre subtype, characterized by a vertical scar on the forehead resembling a stroke from a sword).[2]
- In a retrospective multicenter review of 750 children with LSc, the most common subtype was linear morphea (65%), followed by circumscribed morphea (26%), mixed subtype (15%), generalized morphea (7%), and deep morphea (2%). Overall, the mean age of presentation was 7.3 years (range 0 to 16 years, median age 6.1 years).[3]
- In the US, the incidence of morphea has been estimated at 25 cases per 1 million individuals (of any age) per year.[1] Although data are scarce, it is estimated that childhood LSc occurs only in 1 per 1 million.[2] LSc infrequently progresses into a systemic form and can sometimes merge or overlap with eosinophilic fasciitis.[4]
- Juvenile systemic sclerosis (JSSc) is a chronic multisystem connective tissue disorder characterized by sclerodermic skin changes and abnormalities of the visceral organs. Systemic sclerosis has an annual incidence of 1 to 2 per 100,000 adults and children in the US.[1] Onset of JSSc in childhood is very uncommon and accounts for only 3 percent of all cases of systemic sclerosis.[6]
- The risk of JSSc is similar in both sexes in younger children, but it occurs three times more often in girls than in boys aged eight years or more.[7]
- The incidence of JSSc in the United Kingdom and Ireland was estimated to be 0.27 cases per million children/year in a 2005 to 2007 survey.[8] The incidence of JSSc in other populations is unknown.
- Worldwide, there are higher rates of scleroderma in the US and Australia than in Japan or Europe.[9]
- Pulmonary, cardiac, and renal disease are the leading causes of death as a consequence of these diseases.[10]

ETIOLOGY AND PATHOPHYSIOLOGY

- The etiology and pathogenesis of scleroderma remains uncertain. Two theorized contributing pathogenic processes include vasculopathy, abnormal fibroblast function, and autoimmune dysfunction.

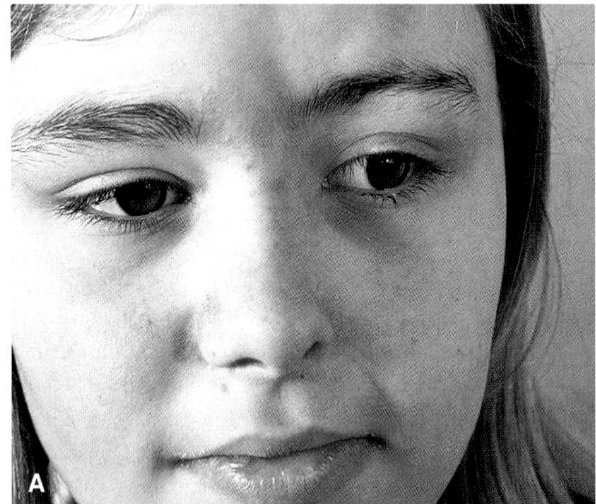

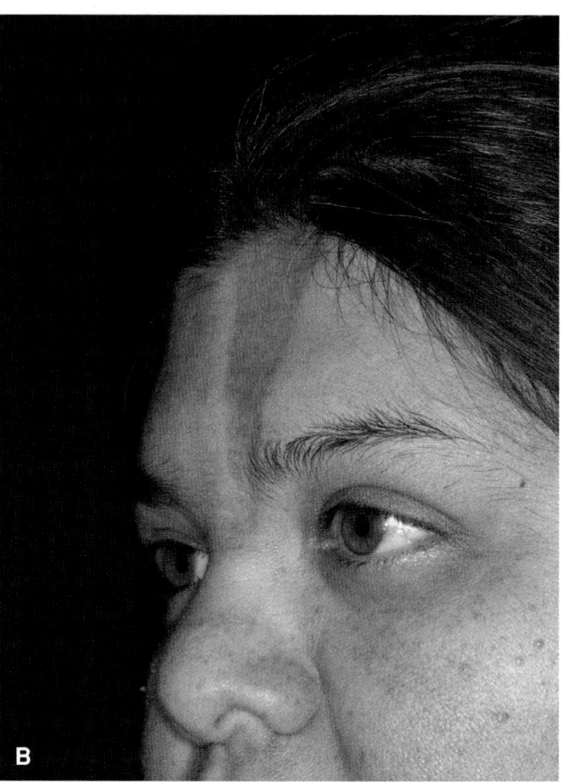

FIGURE 178-2 **A.** Linear morphea on one side of the brow on the forehead, commonly known as an "en coup de sabre" lesion, meaning the blow of a sword. (*Used with permission from Weinberg SW, Prose NS, Kristal L. Color Atlas of Pediatric Dermatology, 4th edition, Figure 17-4, New York, NY: McGraw-Hill, 2008.*) **B.** Another "en coup de sabre" lesion on the forehead with significant atrophy and hyperpigmentation. (*Used with permission from Richard P. Usatine, MD.*)

- Scleroderma disorders can be subdivided into three groups: localized scleroderma (morphea; **Figures 178-1** to **178-3**), systemic sclerosis (**Figures 178-4** to **178-7**), and other scleroderma-like disorders that are marked by the presence of thickened, sclerotic skin lesions.
- A multicenter European study of 750 children with LSc defined the prevalence and the clinical features of extracutaneous findings in patients with LSc.[11] There was one or more extracutaneous manifestations in 22 percent of children. In 92 percent of the cases, the skin lesion was the presenting sign of disease. The overall distribution of extracutaneous manifestations included:
    - Arthritis—19 percent.
    - Neurologic findings—4 percent.
    - Raynaud's phenomenon—3 percent.
    - Vascular findings (vasculitic rash and deep vein thrombosis)—2 percent.
    - Ocular findings—3 percent.
    - Gastrointestinal symptoms (GERD)—2 percent.
    - Restrictive lung disease—1 percent.
    - Two patients had cardiac findings (pericarditis and arrhythmia) and one patient had nephritis.

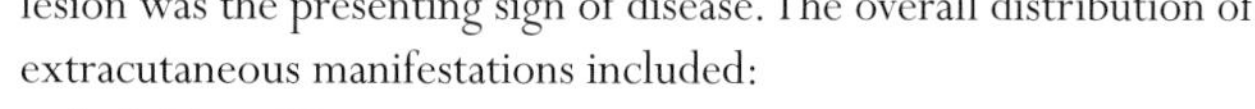

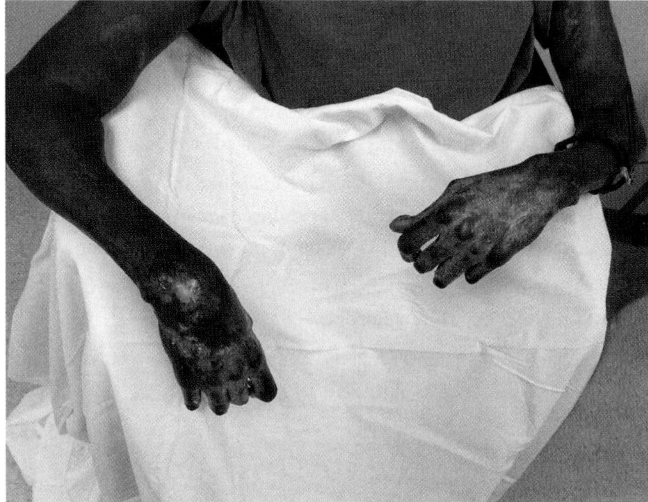

FIGURE 178-3 Pansclerotic morphea, a rare variant of localized scleroderma, in a 13-year-old African American male. Note the "bound-down" skin with hypopigmentation and hyperpigmentation that occurs with this disease. (*Used with permission from Vidya Raman, MD.*)

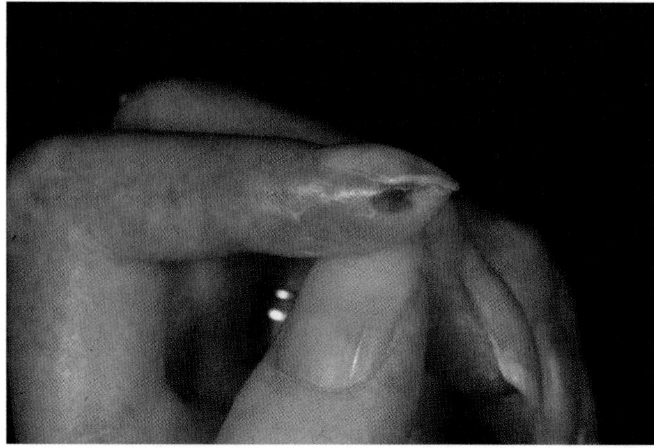

FIGURE 178-4 Sclerodactyly with tapering of the fingers and mottled hyperpigmentation. (*Used with permission from Jeffrey Meffert, MD.*)

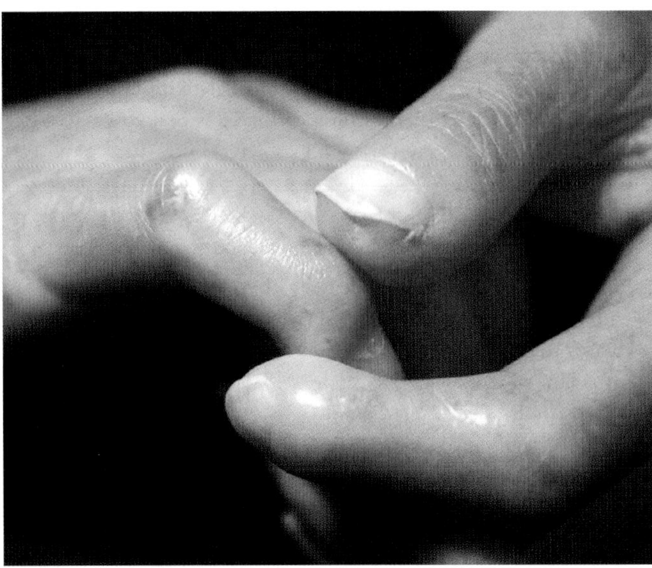

FIGURE 178-5 Scleroderma showing sclerodactyly with tight shiny skin over the fingers. (*Used with permission from Everett Allen, MD.*)

- Systemic sclerosis is used to describe a systemic disease characterized by skin induration and thickening accompanied by variable tissue fibrosis and inflammatory infiltration in numerous visceral organs. Systemic sclerosis can be diffuse (DcSSc) or limited to the skin and adjacent tissues (limited cutaneous systemic sclerosis [LcSSc]).
- The majority of children with JSSc present with Raynaud phenomenon and/or skin changes (tightening, thinning, and atrophy) of the hands and face. In a multicenter retrospective study of 153 children with JSSc, the median age of onset was 8.1 years and the mean duration of symptoms prior to diagnosis was 1.9 years.[7] Eleven percent had a family history of autoimmune disease. Findings at diagnosis included:
    - Raynaud phenomenon—70 percent.
    - Skin induration proximal to the MCP and MTP joints—63 percent.
    - Musculoskeletal symptoms (arthralgia, muscle weakness, and arthritis)—33 percent.
    - Weight loss—18 percent.

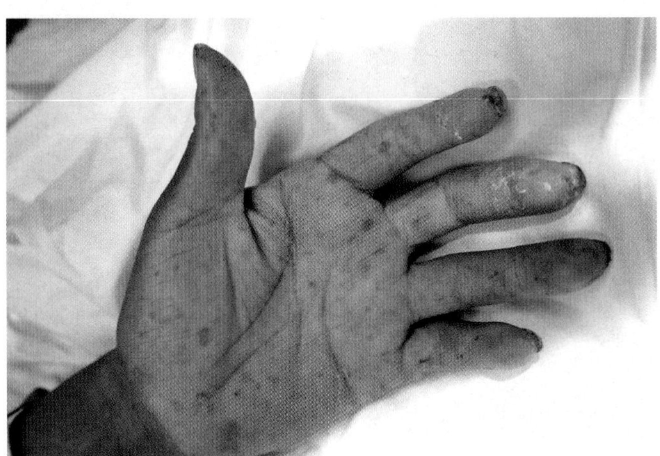

FIGURE 178-6 Scleroderma with telangiectasias and digital necrosis of the hands. (*Used with permission from Everett Allen, MD.*)

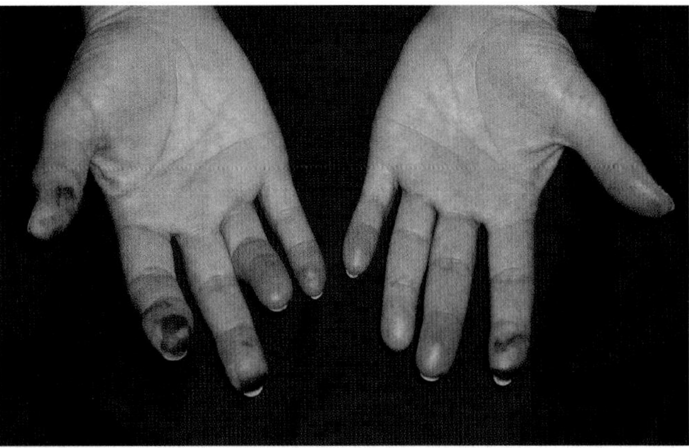

FIGURE 178-7 Raynaud phenomenon with severe ischemia leading to the necrosis of the fingertips. (*Used with permission from Ricardo Zuniga-Montes, MD.*)

    - Dyspnea—10 percent.
    - Dysphagia—10 percent.
- The most common vascular dysfunction associated with scleroderma is Raynaud phenomenon (**Figure 178-7**). Raynaud phenomenon is produced by arterial constriction in the digits. The characteristic color changes progress from white (pallor), to blue (acrocyanosis), to finally red (reperfusion hyperemia). Raynaud phenomenon generally precedes other disease manifestations, sometimes by years. Many patients develop progressive structural changes in their small blood vessels, which permanently impair blood flow, and can result in digital ulceration or infarction. Other forms of vascular injury include pulmonary artery hypertension, renal crisis, and gastric antral vascular ectasia.
- Patients with limited cutaneous scleroderma (LcSSc) usually have skin sclerosis restricted to the hands and, to a lesser extent, the face and neck. With time, some patients develop scleroderma of the distal forearm. They often eventually display the CREST syndrome, which presents with Raynaud phenomenon (**Figure 178-7**), esophageal dysmotility, sclerodactyly (**Figures 178-4** and **178-5**), telangiectasias (**Figure 178-6**), and calcinosis cutis (**Figure 178-8**). This variant is rare in children.

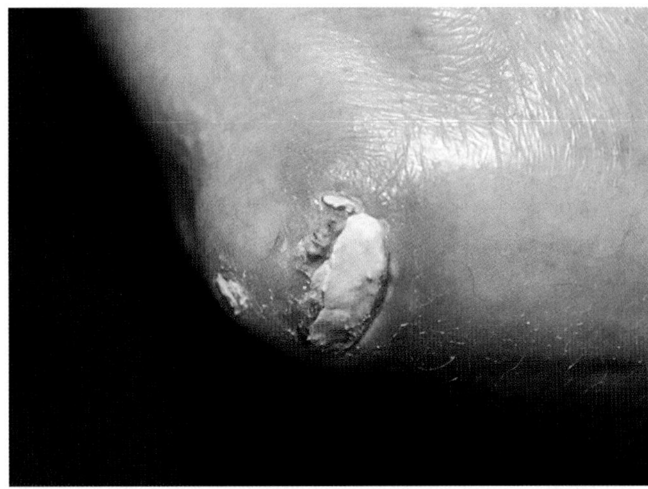

FIGURE 178-8 Calcinosis over the elbow in a patient with CREST syndrome. (*Used with permission from Everett Allen, MD.*)

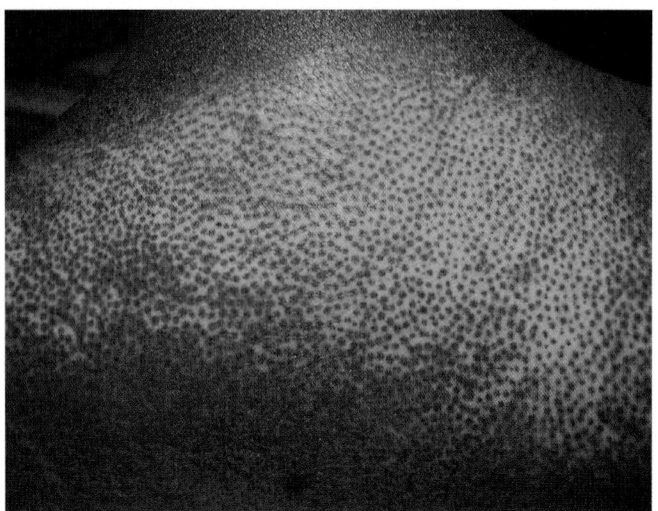

FIGURE 178-9 Scleroderma with mottled hypopigmentation. The skin may have a salt-and-pepper appearance as shown here. (*Used with permission from Ricardo Zuniga-Montes, MD.*)

- Patients with diffuse cutaneous scleroderma (DcSSc) often present with sclerotic skin on the chest, abdomen, or upper arms and shoulders. The skin may take on a "salt-and-pepper" look (**Figure 178-9**). They are more likely to develop internal organ damage caused by ischemic injury and fibrosis than those with LcSSc or morphea.
- Arthralgias are the presenting symptom in about 15 percent of children and are usually mild and transient. Joint contractures are most common at the proximal intraphalangeal joints and elbows. Arthritis and myositis may occur in up to 30 percent of children, and may precede the diagnosis of JSSc.[7] Myositis leads to muscle weakness and myalgia, and is associated with elevated levels of creatinine kinase (CPK).
- GI involvement is seen in 30 to 74 percent of children with systemic sclerosis,[7,12] although half of these patients may be asymptomatic. Any part of the GI tract may be involved. Potential signs and symptoms include dysphagia, choking, heartburn, cough after swallowing, bloating, constipation, and/or diarrhea, pseudoobstruction, malabsorption, and fecal incontinency. Chronic gastroesophageal reflux is more common in children and recurrent episodes of aspiration may contribute to the development of interstitial lung disease. Vascular ectasia in the stomach (often referred to as "water-melon stomach" on endoscopy) is a common late finding, and may lead to GI bleeding and anemia.
- Pulmonary involvement is seen in more than 70 percent of patients, usually presenting as dyspnea on exertion and a nonproductive cough. Fine "Velcro" rales may be heard at the lung bases with lung auscultation. Pulmonary vascular disease occurs in 10 to 40 percent of patients with systemic sclerosis, and is more common in patients with limited cutaneous disease. The risk of lung cancer is increased approximately 5-fold in patients with scleroderma.
- Autopsy data suggest that 60 to 80 percent of patients with DcSSc have evidence of kidney damage.[13] Some degree of proteinuria, a mild elevation in the plasma creatinine concentration, and/or hypertension are observed in as many as 50 percent of patients.[14] Severe renal disease develops in 10 to 15 percent of patients, most commonly in patients with DcSSc.
- Symptomatic pericarditis occurs in 7 to 20 percent of patients, which has a 5-year mortality rate of 75 percent.[15] Primary cardiac involvement includes pericarditis, pericardial effusion, myocardial fibrosis, heart failure, myocarditis associated with myositis, conduction disturbances, and arrhythmias.[16] Patchy myocardial fibrosis is characteristic of systemic sclerosis, and is thought to result from recurrent vasospasm of small vessels. Arrhythmias are common and are most caused by fibrosis of the conduction system.
- Pulmonary vascular disease occurs in 10 to 40 percent of patients with scleroderma, and is more common in patients with limited cutaneous disease. It may occur in the absence of significant interstitial lung disease, generally a late complication in adults, and is usually progressive. Severe pulmonary arterial hypertension, sometimes with pulmonale and right-sided heart failure or thrombosis of the pulmonary vessels may develop.
- Contractures may develop, with contractures of the fingers being most common. Neuropathies and central nervous system involvement, including headache, seizures, stroke, vascular disease, radiculopathy, and myelopathy, occur.

DIAGNOSIS

CLINICAL FEATURES

- The diagnosis of systemic sclerosis and related disorders is based primarily upon the presence of characteristic clinical findings. Skin involvement is characterized by variable thickening and hardening of the skin with possible involvement of the underlying tissues. Skin pigmentary changes may occur, especially a salt-and-pepper appearance from patchy hypopigmentation (**Figure 178-9**). Other prominent skin manifestations include:
  - Pruritus and edema in the early stages.
  - Sclerodactyly (**Figures 178-3** and **178-4**).
  - Digital ulcers and pitting at the fingertips (**Figures 178-6** and **178-10**).
  - Telangiectasia (**Figures 178-6** and **178-11**).
  - Calcinosis cutis (**Figure 178-8**).

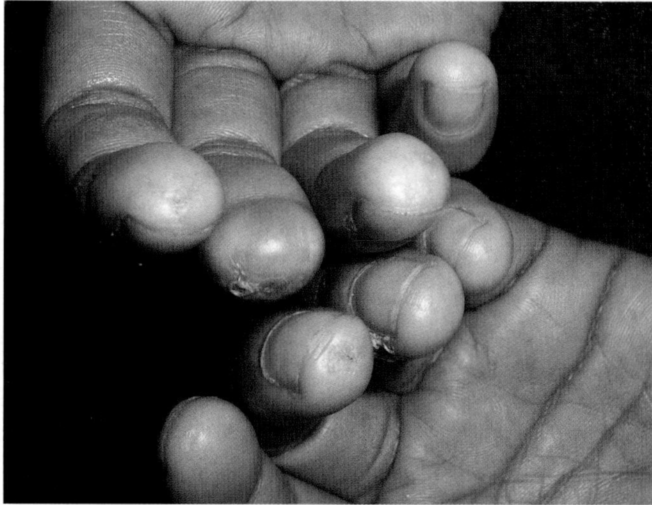

FIGURE 178-10 Digital pitting scars and loss of substance from finger pads in this patient with scleroderma and sclerodactyly. (*Used with permission from Richard P. Usatine, MD.*)

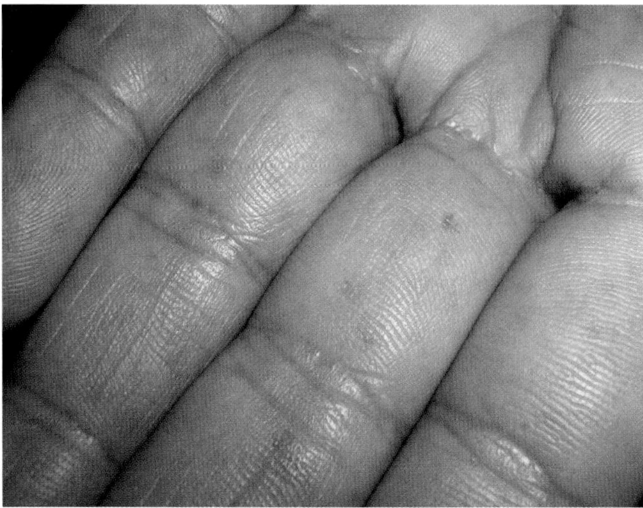

FIGURE 178-11 Telangiectasias on the hands of this patient with CREST syndrome. (*Used with permission from Richard P. Usatine, MD.*)

- The diagnosis of localized scleroderma (morphea) is suggested by the presence of typical skin thickening and hardening confined to one area, with absence of internal organ involvement (**Figures 178-1** and **178-2**). The diagnosis of systemic sclerosis is suggested by the presence of typical skin thickening and hardening (sclerosis) that is not confined to one area (i.e., not localized scleroderma) and occuring proximal to the metacarpophalangeal (MCP) and metatarsophalangeal (MTP) joints. The combination of skin signs plus one or more of the typical systemic features supports the diagnosis of systemic sclerosis.
- Linear scleroderma is the most common type of LSc in children. The fibrotic lesion is elongated, and the direction is usually transverse when on the trunk and longitudinal on the limbs. When the lesion involves the face or scalp, it is referred to as "en coup de sabre." Patients may develop contractures and defects of the limb with associated unequal growth and disabilities.
- The American College of Rheumatology, the Pediatric Rheumatology European Society, and European League Against Rheumatism defined criteria for the diagnosis and classification of JSSc.[17] In a patient less than 16 years of age, JSSc is diagnosed if the major criterion and at least 2 of the minor criteria are present:
  - Major criterion (required)—Sclerosis/induration of the skin proximal to the MCP and MTP joints.
- Minor criteria—Two of the following criteria are required:
  - Skin—Sclerodactyly.
  - Vascular—Raynaud phenomenon, nailfold capillary abnormalities, or digital tip ulcers.
  - Gastrointestinal—Dysphagia or gastroesophageal reflux.
  - Renal—Renal crisis or new onset arterial hypertension.
  - Cardiac—Arrhythmias or heart failure.
  - Respiratory—Evidence of pulmonary fibrosis, abnormality of diffusion capacity, or pulmonary hypertension.
  - Musculoskeletal—Tendon friction rubs, arthritis, or myositis.
  - Neurological—Neuropathy or carpal tunnel syndrome.
  - Serological testing—Presence of antinuclear antibodies or SSc selective autoantibodies.

LABORATORY TESTING

- A positive ANA with a speckled, homogenous, or nucleolar staining pattern is common in systemic scleroderma and is seen in 81 to 97 percent of children with JSSc.[7] A positive ANA was found in 42 percent of a large series of children with localized scleroderma, however, there was no correlation between the presence of ANA and disease course in this patient population.[3] Anticentromere antibodies are often associated with LcSSc. Anti-DNA topoisomerase I (Scl-70) antibodies are highly specific for both systemic sclerosis, and related interstitial lung and renal disease.[18] Although not very sensitive, anti-RNA polymerases I and III antibodies are specific for systemic sclerosis. Other testing for specific organ dysfunction is routinely done.
- The presence of characteristic autoantibodies, such as anticentromere, antitopoisomerase I (Scl-70), anti-RNA polymerase, or U3-RNP antibodies is supportive of the diagnosis of systemic sclerosis.
- Consider checking a CPK in children with myositis or any cardiac symptom. Children with significantly elevated CPK should be appropriately evaluated for cardiac disease.[7]

IMAGING

All patients with systemic sclerosis should have a chest x-ray (CXR) and pulmonary function tests (PFTs) screening for pulmonary involvement. The most common types of pulmonary involvement are interstitial lung disease and pulmonary hypertension. The diffusing capacity, DLCO, (as part of PFTs) is the most sensitive test for pulmonary disease in systemic sclerosis. High-resolution chest CT may be indicated for further evaluation of active pulmonary disease.

BIOPSY

- A punch biopsy can be used to diagnose morphea and scleroderma when the clinical diagnosis is not clear and to rule out other conditions such as eosinophilic fasciitis.

DIFFERENTIAL DIAGNOSIS

- Idiopathic occurrence of systemic sclerosis associated diseases such as Raynaud phenomenon, renal failure, and gastroesophageal reflux disease.
- Systemic lupus erythematosus (SLE) presents with systemic symptoms and a typical rash that may be scarring. ANA testing with lupus-specific antibodies usually helps establish the diagnosis (see Chapter 173, Lupus—Systemic and Cutaneous).
- Discoid lupus erythematosus (DLE) presents as localized plaque lesion that eventually scar. Biopsy usually makes the diagnosis (see Chapter 173, Lupus—Systemic and Cutaneous).
- Myxedema is associated with hypothyroidism and is characterized by thickening and coarseness of the skin. Thyroid testing usually makes the diagnosis (see Chapter 191, Hypothyroidism).
- Lichen sclerosus when it occurs away from the genital area can resemble morphea. Although it most commonly affects the genital (**Figure 178-12**) and perianal area, it can occur on the upper trunk, breasts, and upper arms. The plaques appear atrophic but a thin cigarette-paper crinkling appearance may help to differentiate it from morphea. A punch biopsy will lead to the correct diagnosis.

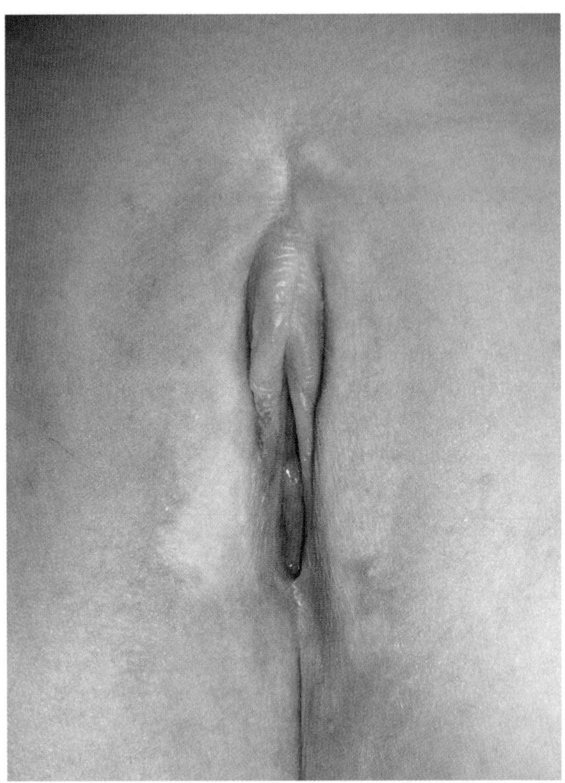

FIGURE 178-12 Lichen sclerosus of the vulva of a 4-year-old girl, which can be confused with morphea or a chronic candida infection. Affected girls may complain of vulvar itching, soreness, or painful urination. However, the degree of discomfort may not be proportional to the amount of disease present. (*Used with permission from Richard P. Usatine, MD.*)

- Amyloidosis of the skin may result in thickening and stiffness of the skin. Skin biopsy reveals amyloid infiltration. Biopsy usually makes the diagnosis.
- Juvenile idiopathic arthritis (juvenile rheumatoid arthritis) may produce joint symptoms and contractures similar to JSc (see Chapter 172, Juvenile Idiopathic Arthritis).

MANAGEMENT

NONPHARMACOLOGIC

- Localized scleroderma, including morphea, appears to soften with UVA light therapy.[19] SOR B
- Physical therapy and massage is recommended in many children with LSc. SOR C Regular physical therapy maintains functional ability, muscle strength, and joint movement while preventing flexion contractures. Deep connective tissue massage may be taught to parents to improve dermal elasticity. Attention to positive joint alignment and muscle development is important in linear scleroderma. SOR C
- Telangiectasias may be covered with foundation make-up or treated with laser therapy.
- Small localized lesions of morphea can be removed surgically, but only after the active phase of the disease has abated and the child's growth is complete.[20] SOR C
- The use of corrective or functional splints may be necessary to treat or prevent contractures. Splints may be required for an extended period of time.

MEDICATIONS

- For symptomatic therapy, skin lubrication, histamine 1 (H_1) and histamine 2 (H_2) blockers, oral doxepin, and low-dose oral glucocorticoids may be used to treat pruritus. SOR C
- Treatment options for morphea include topical steroids such as clobetasol and topical calcipotriol.[21,22] SOR B
- Methotrexate has been used successfully in children and adults with LSc (15 mg/m^2 as a single oral or subcutaneous dose per week for at least one year—maximum dose 25 mg per week).[23] SOR B Addition of glucocorticoids (prednisone 1 mg/kg/day (maximum dose to 50 mg/day) orally or methylprednisolone 20 to 30 mg/kg/day (maximum dose to 1000 mg/kg/day) intravenously for three consecutive days monthly) during the first two to three months of therapy may be helpful for those with rapidly progressive disease.
- The combination of high-dose oral prednisone and low-dose oral methotrexate has been used successfully in adults and larger adolescents for localized scleroderma.[24] SOR B Methotrexate can be started at 7.5 mg PO weekly and titrated up as needed. Of course the long-term goal is to taper the prednisone while using the oral methotrexate as a steroid-sparing agent.
- Calcium channel blockers (nifedipine at a dose of 0.2–0.3 mg/kg every eight hours—maximum 10 mg/dose), dipyridamole, aspirin, and topical nitrates may help symptoms of Raynaud phenomenon.[25,26] SOR B Patients should be advised to avoid cold, stress, nicotine, caffeine, and sympathomimetic decongestant medications. Acid-reducing agents may be used empirically for gastroesophageal reflux disease. Prokinetic agents, such as erythromycin, may be useful for patients with esophageal hypomotility. SOR C
- The mainstay of treatment of renal disease is control of blood pressure, with angiotensin-converting enzyme (ACE) inhibitors being the first-line agent. SOR C Hemodialysis or peritoneal dialysis may be used as needed.
- Treatments of pulmonary hypertension associated with the systemic sclerosis being tested include the endothelin receptor antagonist bosentan (62.5 mg PO bid for 4 weeks, then increase to 125 mg PO bid), the phosphodiesterase-5 inhibitor sildenafil, and various prostacyclin analogs (e.g., epoprostenol, treprostinil, and iloprost). Pulmonary fibrosing alveolitis may be treated with cyclophosphamide.[27] SOR B
- Myositis may be treated with oral prednisone 0.3 to 0.5 mg/kg per day. However, several studies have suggested that use of steroids in scleroderma is associated with a higher risk of scleroderma renal crisis and therefore, patients on steroids should have close monitoring of blood pressure and renal function. SOR B Arthralgias can be treated with acetaminophen and NSAIDs. SOR C

REFERRAL

Patients with systemic sclerosis should be referred to a rheumatologist as this is a complicated disease that requires the use of toxic medications. Depending upon the complications, patients with scleroderma may also need referral to pulmonology, cardiology, and nephrology.

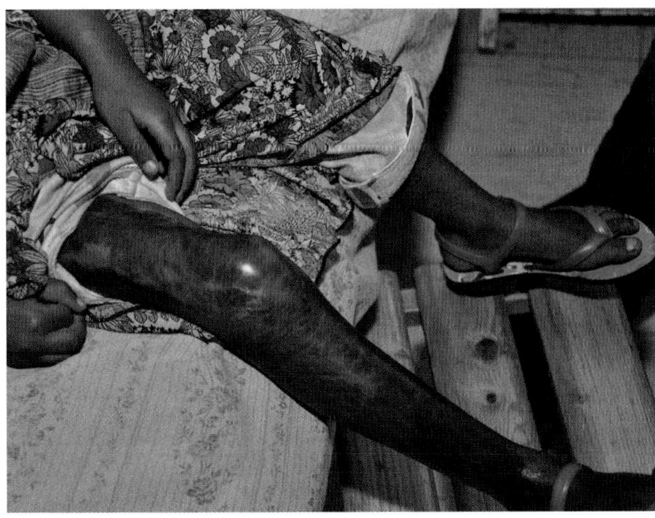

FIGURE 178-13 Localized morphea of the leg in this young girl. Although her disease is not systemic, the tightening of the skin around the knee does cause problems with knee movement and ambulation. (*Used with permission from Richard P. Usatine, MD.*)

PROGNOSIS

- In general, the prognosis of SSc in children is better than in adults. The commonest causes of death in children are related to the involvement of cardiac, renal, and pulmonary systems. Cardiomyopathy is a leading cause of early death, especially in children.[28]
- The prognosis for morphea is excellent as it only affects the skin. Although the appearance may be disturbing to the patient it is not life-threatening. If the morphea is extensive and over an extremity, it can affect function (**Figure 178-13**).

FOLLOW-UP

- The patient with systemic sclerosis needs to be evaluated at least every 3 to 6 months to monitor disease activity and progression.

PATIENT EDUCATION

- Instruct the patient and parents to avoid skin trauma (especially the fingers), cold exposure, and smoking. Make patients aware of potential complications and have them watch for signs of systemic disease occurrence or progression.
- Encourage the child to be as physically active as possible. Physical therapy will help maintain functional ability, muscle strength, and joint movement while preventing flexion contractures. It should be performed consistently since irregular regimens will be less effective.
- Avoid exposures that irritate or dry the skin. Daily application of lanolin or water-soluble cream as an emollient may minimize this effect.
- Patients and parents should be told to avoid cold, trauma, heat, and sun exposure. Cold and trauma can exacerbate symptoms. These children are also susceptible to hyperpigmentation from sunlight and have difficulty in dissipating heat through sclerotic skin.

PATIENT RESOURCES

- American College of Rheumatology. *Handout on Localized Scleroderma*—**www.niams.nih.gov/Health_Info/Scleroderma/default.asp**.
- Arthritis Foundation. Handout on scleroderma—**www.afstore.org/Products-By-Topic/Other-Diseases/SCLERODERMA-FREE-PDF**.
- The John Hopkins Scleroderma Center: Living with Scleroderma—**www.hopkinsscleroderma.org/patients/living-scleroderma/**.
- Cleveland Clinic: Pediatric Scleroderma—**http://www.cchs.net/health/health-info/docs/1600/1679.asp?index=4910**.

PROVIDER RESOURCES

- National Institute of Arthritis and Musculoskeletal and Skin Diseases. *Handout on Health: Scleroderma*—**www.niams.nih.gov/Health_Info/Scleroderma/default.asp**.
- The John Hopkins Scleroderma Center—**http://emedicine.medscape.com/article/331864**.

REFERENCES

1. Lawrence RC, Helmick CG, Arnett FC, et al. Estimates of the prevalence of arthritis and selected musculoskeletal disorders in the United States. *Arthritis Rheum*. 1998;41(5):778-799.
2. Peterson LS, Nelson AM, Su WP. Classification of morphea (localized scleroderma). *Mayo Clin Proc*. 1995;70:1068.
3. Zulian F, Athreya BH, Laxer R, et al. Juvenile localized scleroderma: clinical and epidemiological features in 750 children. An international study. *Rheumatology (Oxford)*. 2006;45:614.
4. Rossi P, Fossaluzza V, Gonano L. Localized scleroderma evolving into systemic sclerosis. *J Rheumatol*. 1985;12:629.
5. Kornreich HK, King KK, Bernstein BH, et al. Scleroderma in childhood. *Arthritis Rheum*. 1977;20:343.
6. Cassidy JT, Sullivan DB, Dabich L, Petty RE. Scleroderma in children. *Arthritis Rheum*. 1977;20:351.
7. Martini G, Foeldvari I, Russo R, et al. Systemic sclerosis in childhood: clinical and immunologic features of 153 patients in an international database. *Arthritis Rheum*. 2006;54:3971.
8. Herrick AL, Ennis H, Bhushan M, et al. Incidence of childhood linear scleroderma and systemic sclerosis in the UK and Ireland. *Arthritis Care Res (Hoboken)*. 2010;62:213.
9. Chifflot H, Fautrel B, Sordet C, et al. Incidence and prevalence of systemic sclerosis: a systematic literature review. *Semin Arthritis Rheum*. 2008;37(4):223-235.
10. Steen VD, Lucas M, Fertig N, Medsger TA Jr: Pulmonary arterial hypertension and severe pulmonary fibrosis in systemic sclerosis patients with a nucleolar antibody. *J Rheumatol*. 2007;34(11):2230-2235.
11. Zulian F, Vallongo C, Woo P, et al. Localized scleroderma in childhood is not just a skin disease. *Arthritis Rheum*. 2005;52:2873.

12. Akesson A, Wollheim FA. Organ manifestations in 100 patients with progressive systemic sclerosis: a comparison between the CREST syndrome and diffuse scleroderma. *Br J Rheumatol.* 1989; 28(4):281-286.

13. Medsger TA Jr, Masi AT. Survival with scleroderma. II. A life-table analysis of clinical and demographic factors in 358 male U.S. veteran patients. *J Chronic Dis.* 1973;26(10):647-660.

14. Tuffanelli DL, Winkelmann RK. Systemic scleroderma, a clinical study of 727 cases. *Arch Dermatol.* 1961;84:359-371.

15. Janosik DL, Osborn TG, Moore TL, et al. Heart disease in systemic sclerosis. *Semin Arthritis Rheum.* 1989;19(3):191-200.

16. Byers RJ, Marshall DA, Freemont AJ. Pericardial involvement in systemic sclerosis. *Ann Rheum Dis.* 1997;56(6):393-394.

17. Zulian F, Woo P, Athreya BH, et al. The Pediatric Rheumatology European Society/American College of Rheumatology/European League against Rheumatism provisional classification criteria for juvenile systemic sclerosis. *Arthritis Rheum.* 2007;57:203.

18. Reveille JD, Solomon DH. Evidence-based guidelines for the use of immunologic tests: Anticentromere, Scl-70, and nucleolar antibodies. *Arthritis Rheum.* 2003;49(3):399-412.

19. Kreuter A, Breuckmann F, Uhle A, et al. Low-dose UVA1 phototherapy in systemic sclerosis: effects on acrosclerosis. *J Am Acad Dermatol.* 2004;50(5):740-747.

20. Lapiere JC, Aasi S, Cook B, Montalvo A. Successful correction of depressed scars of the forehead secondary to trauma and morphea en coup de sabre by en bloc autologous dermal fat graft. *Dermatol Surg.* 2000;26:793.

21. Seyger MM, van den Hoogen FH, de Boo T, de Jong EM. Low-dose methotrexate in the treatment of widespread morphea. *J Am Acad Dermatol.* 1998;39(2;1):220-225.

22. Cunningham BB, Landells ID, Langman C, et al. Topical calcipotriene for morphea/linear scleroderma. *J Am Acad Dermatol.* 1998; 39:211.

23. Zulian F, Martini G, Vallongo C, et al. Methotrexate treatment in juvenile localized scleroderma: a randomized, double-blind, placebo-controlled trial. *Arthritis Rheum.* 2011;63:1998.

24. Kreuter A, Gambichler T, Breuckmann F, et al. Pulsed high-dose corticosteroids combined with low-dose methotrexate in severe localized scleroderma. *Arch Dermatol.* 2005;141(7):847-852.

25. Thompson AE, Shea B, Welch V, et al. Calcium-channel blockers for Raynaud's phenomenon in systemic sclerosis. *Arthritis Rheum.* 2001;44(8):1841-1847.

26. Clifford PC, Martin MF, Sheddon EJ, et al. Treatment of vasospastic disease with prostaglandin E1. *Br Med J.* 1980;281(6247): 1031-1034.

27. Tashkin DP, Elashoff R, Clements PJ, et al. Cyclophosphamide versus placebo in scleroderma lung disease. *N Engl J Med.* 2006; 354(25):2655-2666.

28. Quartier P, Bonnet D, Fournet JC, et al. Severe cardiac involvement in children with systemic sclerosis and myositis. *J Rheumatol.* 2002;29:1767.

PART 16

INFECTIOUS DISEASES

Strength of Recommendation (SOR)	Definition
A	Recommendation based on consistent and good-quality patient-oriented evidence.*
B	Recommendation based on inconsistent or limited-quality patient-oriented evidence.*
C	Recommendation based on consensus, usual practice, opinion, disease-oriented evidence, or case series for studies of diagnosis, treatment, prevention, or screening.*

*See Appendix A on pages 1320–1322 for further information.

179 GASTROINTESTINAL INECTIONS (INCLUDING DIARRHEA)

Heidi Chumley, MD
Camille Sabella, MD

Gastrointestinal infections can be caused by a wide variety of infectious agents, including bacteria, viruses, and parasites. In this chapter, common viral and bacterial causes of diarrhea will be discussed, followed by a discussion of the most important parasitic infections.

BACTERIAL AND VIRAL GASTROENTERITIS

PATIENT STORY

A 3-year-old boy who attends a child care center presents to his pediatrician with a 2-day history of bloody diarrhea with mucus. On physical examination, he is well hydrated and has mild abdominal tenderness. The pediatrician orders a stool culture for enteric pathogens and recommends supportive care including appropriate hydration and close follow-up. Forty-eight hours later, the stool culture is reported as positive for *Shigella sonnei* (**Figure 179-1**). Because the boy continued to have bloody diarrhea, the pediatrician treated the boy with a 5-day course of azithromycin and he recovered completely. Two stool cultures obtained after the completion of therapy were negative and the boy was able to resume child care.

INTRODUCTION

Gastrointestinal infections frequently manifest as diarrhea (loose, watery stools), frequently with fever, vomiting, and abdominal pain. Although many of these infections are self-limited, these infections can be associated with intestinal and extra-intestinal manifestations and can lead to significant morbidity.

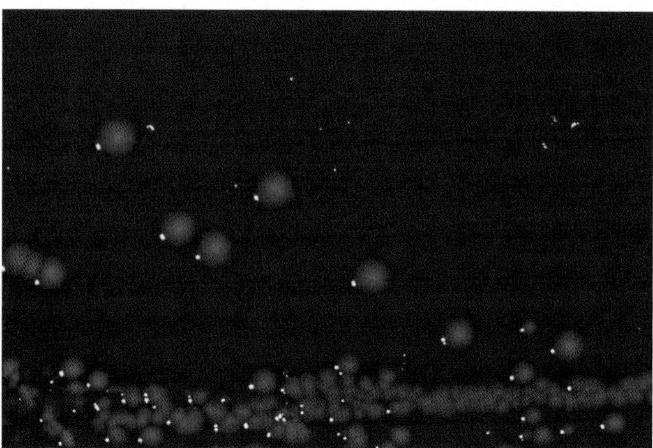

FIGURE 179-1 *Shigella* colonies on a blood agar plate. (*Used with permission from CDC Public Health Image Library.*)

EPIDEMIOLOGY

- Worldwide, diarrheal illness is a leading cause of morbidity and mortality.
- Diarrhea accounts for 2 to 4 million health care visits, 220,000 hospitalizations, and 300 to 400 deaths annually in the US.[1]
- Diarrhea is the most common illness encountered by international travelers to developing countries.[2]
- Acquisition of intestinal pathogens occurs through the fecal-oral route, from person-to-person contact or from contaminated food and water. Many pathogens can be spread by either person-to-person contact or from contaminated food and water.
- Pathogens that are spread through person-to-person contact include *Shigella spp*, *Escherichia coli* O157:H7, and most viral causes of diarrhea. These agents are commonly implicated in outbreaks in childcare centers.
- Pathogens that are spread through contaminated food and water include *Salmonella spp*, *Campylobacter spp*, enterotoxigenic *E coli*, and many viruses.
- Enterotoxigenic *E coli*, *Salmonella*, *Campylobacter*, and *Shigella* are the most common causes of traveler's diarrhea.
- Pet reptiles are common sources of *Salmonella* infection. Transmission of this organism to household members, especially young infants, can occur in the absence of direct contact in household. Salmonella bacteremia and meningitis has occurred from transmission from pet lizards.

ETIOLOGY AND PATHOPHYSIOLOGY

- Common bacterial causes of gastroenteritis include *Campylobacter* spp, *Salmonella* spp, diarrheal-producing strains of *E coli*, *Shigella* spp, and *Yersinia* spp.
- Virulent traits of these agents include enterotoxins and cytotoxins that promote aggregation and invasiveness that result in clinical symptoms.
- Antibiotic-associated colitis is due to toxin-producing strains of *Clostridium difficile.*
- Common viral causes of diarrhea include rotavirus, enteric adenovirus, norovirus, and astrovirus.
- Universal immunization of infants in the US with rotavirus vaccine has resulted in a dramatic decline in rotavirus illness requiring hospitalization.[3]
- Viruses exert their diarrheal effect through selective destruction of absorptive cells in the mucosa, reduction of brush border enzymes, and alteration of the absorptive fluid balance in the gut.
- Host factors also influence susceptibility to infection and colonization. Children with underlying immunodeficiencies and premature infants are more at risk for severe episodes of diarrhea and complications of diarrhea, leading to increased morbidity and mortality.
- Extraintestinal manifestations of enteric pathogens result from direct local or remote spread of infection or are the result of immune-mediated mechanisms.

RISK FACTORS

- Child care attendance.
- Immunodeficiency.
- Prematurity.
- Ingestion of undercooked food.
- Exposure to animals and pets that may harbor infectious organisms like *Salmonella*.
- Travel to developing countries.

DIAGNOSIS

CLINICAL FEATURES

- Watery diarrhea is characteristic of infection with enteric viruses and enterotoxin-producing bacteria.
- Dysentery—Stools containing blood and mucus can result from bacterial causes that invade the large intestine, such as *Shigella* infection.
- Vomiting with minimal or no diarrhea—Can occur with viral causes as well as toxin-producing bacteria.
- Mesenteric adenitis is often a feature of bacterial gastroenteritis. This can simulate appendicitis if the pain is in the right lower quadrant.
- Disseminated infection and meningitis is a complication of *Salmonella* gastroenteritis and occurs mostly in young infants.
- Disseminated disease can occur with any bacterial cause of gastroenteritis in immunocompromised hosts.
- Extraintestinal immune mediated manifestations and the related pathogens include:
  - Erythema nodosum—Related to *Salmonella* spp, *Campylobacter* spp, and *Yersinia* spp.
  - Guillain Barre Syndrome—May follow *Campylobacter jejuni* infection.
  - Reactive arthritis—Related to *Shigella*, *Salmonella*, *Yersinia*, and *Campylobacter* infections.
  - Hemolytic uremic syndrome (HUS)—Most commonly related to Shiga-toxin producing *E coli*.
  - Seizures—Can be a feature of *Shigella* infection and may occur prior to the onset of diarrhea. These are benign and self-limited.

LABORATORY TESTING

- Most episodes of diarrhea are self-limited and testing is not warranted for most cases.
- Stool should be examined for the presence of blood and mucus, which may serve as a clue as to the pathogen. In general, pathogens causing invasion, such as shiga-toxin producing *E coli* and some serotypes of *Shigella*, produce bloody diarrhea.
- In general, stool cultures are indicated when stools contain blood or fecal leukocytes, when hemolytic uremic syndrome is suspected, during outbreaks, and in immunocompromised children.
- Routine stool cultures in most laboratories test for *Campylobacter*, *Salmonella*, *Shigella*, and *Yersinia* species. Identification of *E coli* O157:H7 requires special assays, which should be used for cases of suspected hemolytic uremic syndrome.
- Identification of toxin producing strains of *C. difficile* can be done using enzyme immunoassays or polymerase chain reaction techniques.
- Stool antigen tests can be used to detect rotavirus infection.
- When HUS is suspected, a renal panel and CBC are indicated. The finding of a microangiopathic hemolytic anemia, thrombocytopenia and renal dysfunction is consistent with HUS (see Chapter 69, Hemolytic Uremic Syndrome).

DIFFERENTIAL DIAGNOSIS

- Other causes of diarrhea such as irritable bowel disease, toddler's diarrhea, and inflammatory bowel disease need to be considered in the differential diagnosis. A thorough history and associated findings such as fever are helpful clinically. Stool studies help to rule out infectious etiologies when the diagnosis is not clear.
- Toddler's diarrhea (chronic nonspecific diarrhea of childhood) affects children from 6 months to 5 years of age. Children with toddler's diarrhea will have 3 to 10 loose stools per day but continue to grow and gain weight normally. These children will grow out of this on their own without treatment.
- Bacterial causes of gastroenteritis can cause an intense mesenteric adenitis and can mimic appendicitis. This is classically attributed to *Yersinia* infection, but can occur with other bacteria that cause gastroenteritis.

MANAGEMENT

NONPHARMACOLOGIC

- Careful attention to fluid and electrolyte status is of the utmost importance in all cases of diarrhea.
- Oral rehydration therapy is preferred modality for the management of diarrhea in otherwise healthy children who have mild or moderate dehydration.[4]
- Current oral rehydration therapies in the US, such as Pedialyte, Rehydralyte, Enfalyte, and CeraLyte-50 are glucose-electrolyte solutions that can be used in infants and children with mild to moderate dehydration.
- Multiple studies, both in the US and in developing countries, have shown that early feeding of age-appropriate foods, including milk, to children with diarrhea after rehydration is associated with decreased stool output and reduction in duration of diarrhea.

MEDICATIONS

- Antimotility agents have not been shown to be effective in t reating acute diarrhea in infants and children, and are associated with systemic toxic effects that may be exaggerated in infants and children; thus, their use is not recommended.
- Probiotics, especially *Lactobacillus rhamnosus* GG, used early in the course of acute viral gastroenteritis, may reduce the duration of diarrhea by 1 day.[5,6] SOR B
- Probiotics may also prevent antibiotic-associated diarrhea.
- There is no evidence to support probiotics in the prevention of infectious diarrhea or in the treatment of antibiotic-associated diarrhea.

- Definite recommendations regarding the use of specific probiotics are lacking and await further clinical trials in infants and children.
- Antimicrobial therapy for most cases of acute gastroenteritis is generally not of benefit. Antimicrobial therapy for acute gastroenteritis may be of benefit in specific cases:
    - *Shigella* infections—Therapy may be effective in shortening duration of diarrhea and hastening eradication of the organism and is recommended for patients with severe disease, dysentery, or underlying immunosuppressive conditions. Azithromycin, ciprofloxacin, or a parenteral third-generation cephalosporin may be used for treatment when required.[7] SOR Ⓑ
    - *Campylobacter jejuni*—Azithromycin and erythromycin shorten the duration of illness and excretion of organisms and prevent relapse when given early in gastrointestinal tract infection.[8] SOR Ⓑ
    - Non-typhi *Salmonella* infections in infants less than 3 months—Antimicrobial therapy is used in young infants to prevent dissemination of the organism, although the benefit of this practice is unproven. Treatment of Salmonella gastroenteritis in otherwise healthy children 3 months of age and older is not beneficial and not recommended.[9] SOR Ⓒ
    - Traveler's diarrhea—Azithromycin is preferred for children who develop a diarrheal illness in a developing country.
    - *C difficile* infections—Metronidazole administered orally or parenterally is the first line treatment. Oral vancomycin is reserved for refractory cases.
    - *Salmonella typhi*—See Chapter 7, Global Health.
    - Cholera—See Chapter 7, Global Health.

REFERRAL

- Children with severe dehydration, complications of gastroenteritis, or with extra-intestinal manifestations may require hospitalization and/or referral with a pediatric gastroenterologist or infectious disease specialist.

PREVENTION AND SCREENING

- Careful attention to public and personal hygienic practices is important in decreasing diarrheal illnesses.
- Assuring clean water, food, and sanitation is essential in preventing diarrheal illness.
- Careful hand hygienic practices are the most important personal measures that can be used to prevent transmission of diarrheal agents.
- Breastfeeding decreases morbidity and mortality associated with diarrheal illness.
- Proper food preparation is important in preventing contamination and transmission of infectious agents.
- Pet reptiles should not be avoided in households where young children and immunocompromised individuals reside.[9]
- A rotavirus vaccine should be given to all infants starting at 2 months of age; two vaccines are currently available for infants, and are safe and effective.[10]
- Two *S typhi* vaccines are licensed for children traveling to countries where *S typhi* is endemic; a polysaccharide vaccine parenteral vaccine is available for children 2 years and older, and a live oral typhoid vaccine is available for children 6 years of age and older.[9]

PROGNOSIS

- Morbidity and mortality associated with diarrheal illness is related to adequacy of treatment of dehydration.
- Meticulous supportive management of complications of diarrheal illness, such as HUS, is important in limiting morbidity and mortality.

FOLLOW-UP

- Close follow-up for patients with dehydration secondary to diarrheal illness is required.
- Documentation of negative stool cultures are required for *Shigella* and shiga-toxin producing *E coli* infections prior to the return to child care.

PATIENT EDUCATION

- The importance of adequate hydration should be stressed to parents of children with diarrhea.
- Travelers should be educated about appropriate food and water precautions.
- Parents of young infants and children should be educated as to the importance of proper food preparation.

PATIENT RESOURCES

- **wwwnc.cdc.gov/travel**.
- **http://patiented.aap.org/content.aspx?aid=5473**.
- **www.healthychildren.org/english/tips-tools/symptom-checker/pages/Diarrhea.aspx**.

PROVIDER RESOURCES

- American Academy of Pediatrics. *Red Book: 2012 Report of the Committee on Infectious Diseases*. Pickering LK, ed. 29th ed. Elk Grove Village, IL: American Academy of Pediatrics; 2012.
- **http://pedsinreview.aappublications.org/content/33/11/487.extract**.

PARASITIC INFECTIONS

PATIENT STORY

A parent brings in a 4-year-old boy suffering with anal itching. On examination the physician finds several excoriations around the anus and suspects pinworms. The physician then applies scotch tape to the perianal area and places the tape on a glass slide. Review of the slide demonstrates adult worms and ova of *Enterobius vermicularis* (pinworms; **Figure 179-2**). The boy is treated with a single dose of chewable mebendazole and his symptoms resolve. The parent is told

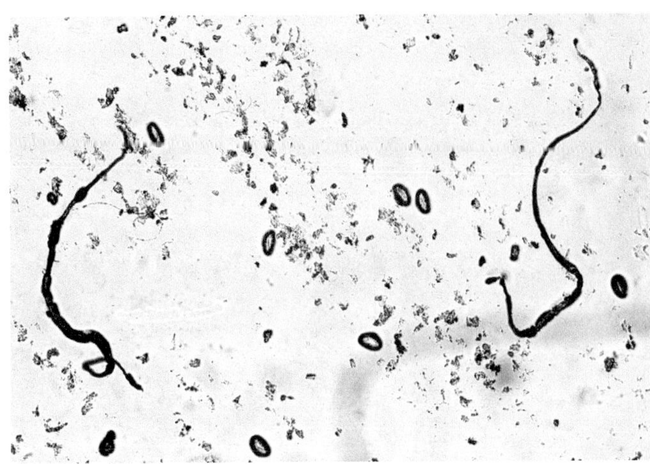

FIGURE 179-2 *Enterobius vermicularis* (pinworms and ova) seen under the microscope from a scotch tape specimen taken of the perianal region of a 4-year-old boy with anal itching. (*Used with permission from James L. Fishback, MD.*)

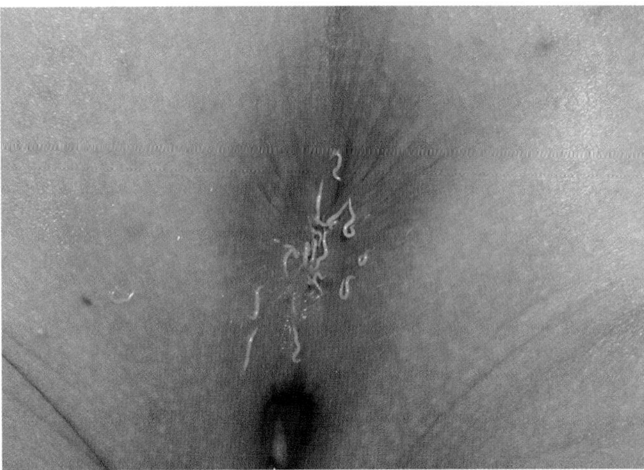

FIGURE 179-3 *Enterobius vermicularis* (pinworms) seen on the perianal and perineal regions of a young girl with anal itching. (*Used with permission from the Atlas of Emergency Medicine and Lawrence E. Heiskell, MD.*)

to repeat the mebendazole dose in 2 weeks to increase the long-term cure rate. If the scotch tape test were negative, the physician could choose to treat empirically as mebendazole is a very safe medication. Another option is to test again having the parent apply the scotch tape to the boy's perianal area first thing in the morning and bring that back to the office (the yield is higher in the morning).

INTRODUCTION

Intestinal parasites are most common in places with warmer temperatures and high humidity, poor sanitation and unclean water, and a large number of individuals (especially children) living in close proximity. In general, the parasites are either asymptomatic or cause symptoms related to their presence in the GI tract. Several migrate through the lungs and can also cause pulmonary symptoms during the migration. Diagnoses are made by history of worms being seen by the patient or parents or by laboratory examination for ova and parasites in the stool.

EPIDEMIOLOGY

- Nematoda is the phylum that contains pinworms, hookworms, *Ascaris*, *Strongyloides*, and whipworms.
  - *E. vermicularis* (pinworm) is the most prevalent nematode in the US. Populations at risk include preschool and school aged children, institutionalized persons, and household members of persons with pinworm infection (**Figure 179-3**).[11]
  - *Necator americanus* (hookworm) is found predominately in the Americas and Australia, and is the second most common nematode identified in stool studies in the US (**Figures 179-4** and **179-5**).[11] *Ancylostoma duodenale* (hookworm) is found mostly in southern Europe, North Africa, the Middle East, and Asia.[11]
  - *Ascaris lumbricoides* is the largest and most common roundworm found in humans in the world; although less common in the US, it is seen mostly in the rural southeast. It is found in tropical and subtropical areas, including the southeastern rural US (**Figures 179-6** and **179-7**).[11]
  - *Strongyloides stercoralis* is seen mostly in tropical and subtropical areas, but can be found in temperate areas, including the southern US (**Figure 179-8**). It is more frequently found in rural areas, institutional settings, and lower socioeconomic groups.[11]
  - *Trichuris trichiura* (whipworm) is the third most common roundworm found in humans worldwide. Infections are more frequent in areas with tropical weather and poor sanitation practices, and among children (**Figure 179-9**). It is estimated that 800 million people are infected worldwide. Trichuriasis occurs in the southern US.[11]
- Cestodes (tapeworm) are a class in the phylum Platyhelminthes that contains *Taenia solium* (pork tapeworm).
  - *T. solium* is found worldwide where pigs and humans live in close proximity.
- Protozoa is the kingdom of one-celled organisms that includes *Giardia lamblia, Cryptosporidium species*, and *Entamoeba histolytica*.

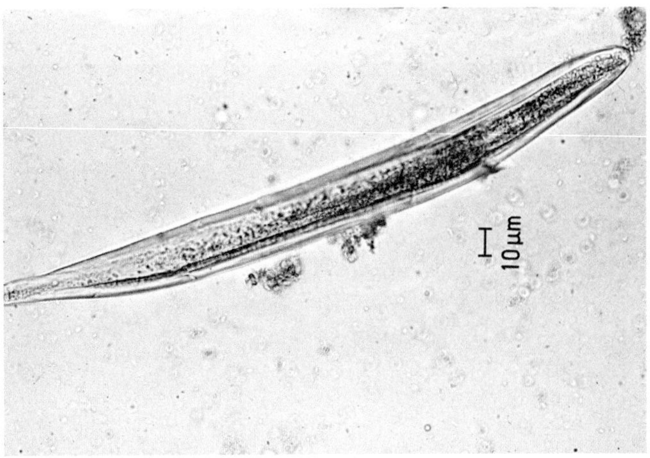

FIGURE 179-4 *Necator americanus* (hookworm) larvae can penetrate the skin, travel through veins to the heart then lungs, climb the bronchial tree to the pharynx, are swallowed, and attach to intestine walls. (*Used with permission from James L. Fishback, MD.*)

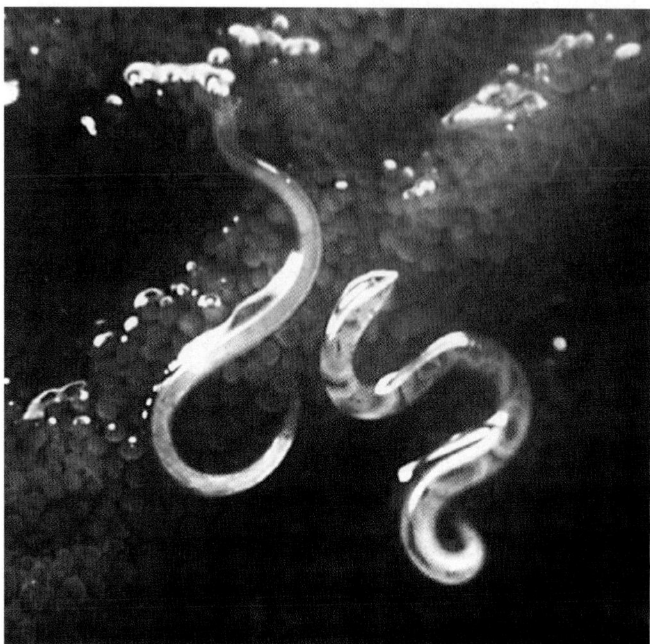

FIGURE 179-5 Adult hookworm attached to the intestinal wall. (*Used with permission from Centers for Disease Control and Prevention.*)

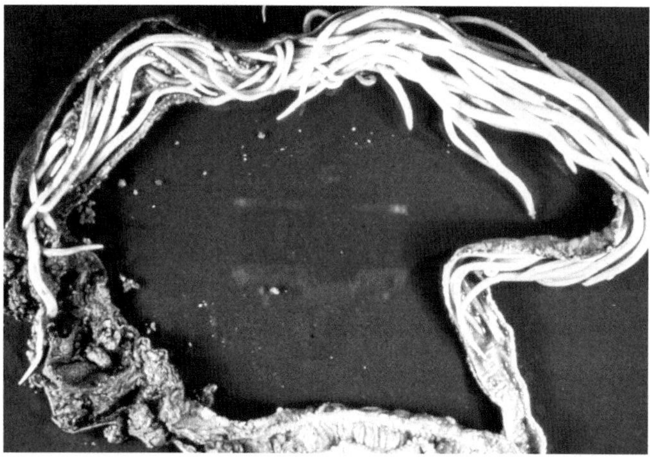

FIGURE 179-6 *Ascaris lumbricoides* in the resected bowel of a patient with bowel obstruction. (*Used with permission from James L. Fishback, MD.*)

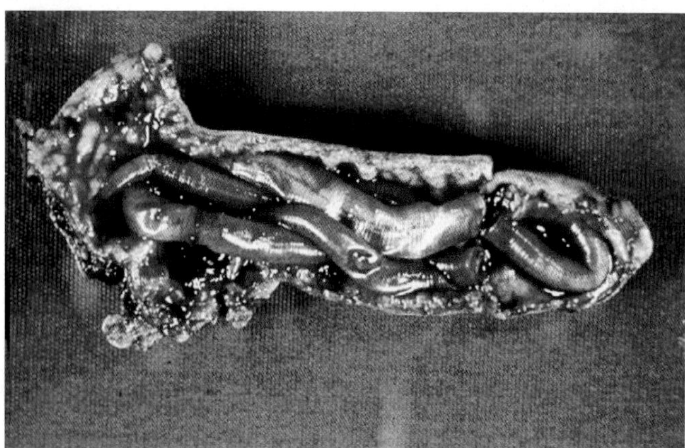

FIGURE 179-7 *Ascaris lumbricoides* in the appendix after being removed with an appendectomy for acute appendicitis. (*Used with permission from James L. Fishback, MD.*)

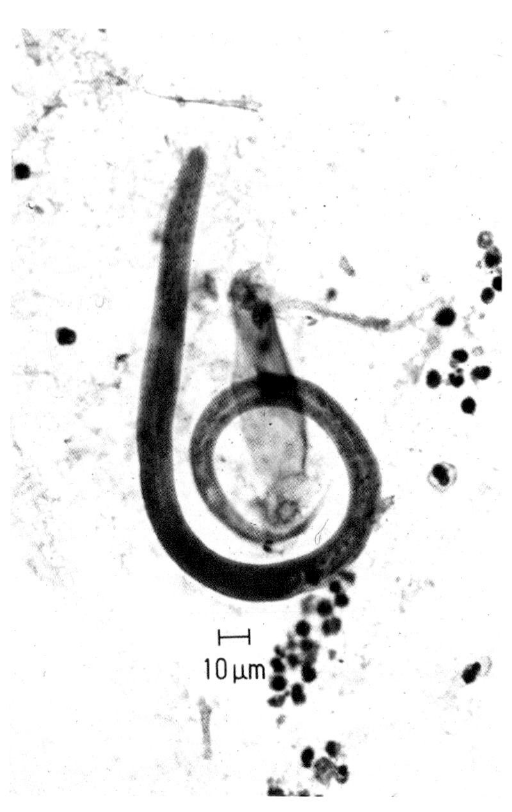

FIGURE 179-8 *Strongyloides stercoralis* ova and parasite in stool. (*Used with permission from James L. Fishback, MD.*)

- *G. lamblia (Giardia intestinalis)* is the most common parasite infection worldwide and the second most common in the US (after pinworm), causing 2.5 million infections annually (**Figure 179-10**).[11]
- *Cryptosporidium hominis* and *C parvum* causes diarrheal illness in normal and immunocompromised hosts. Large community

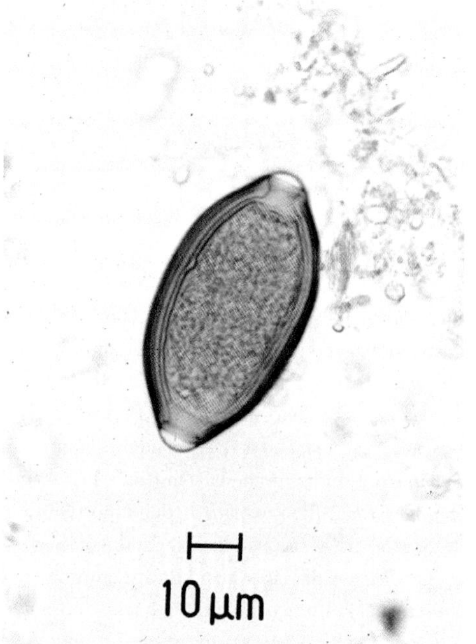

FIGURE 179-9 *Trichuris trichiura* (whipworm) egg in stool. (*Used with permission from James L. Fishback, MD.*)

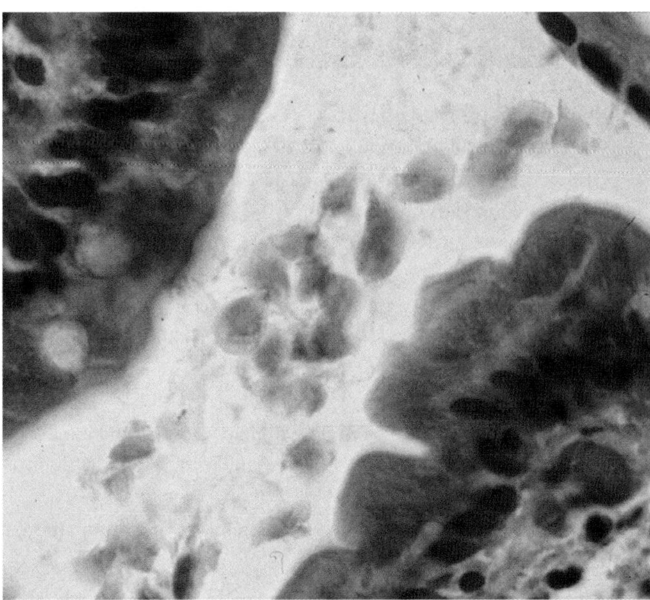

FIGURE 179-10 *Giardia lamblia* in a duodenal biopsy obtained by esophagogastroduodenoscopy in a patient with typical symptoms of chronic giardiasis (excessive flatulence and sulfurous belching) that failed to improve on metronidazole. (*Used with permission from Tom Moore, MD.*)

outbreaks have occurred from contaminated municipal water supplies and swimming pools, and smaller outbreaks have occurred in child care centers.
  - *E. histolytica* is seen worldwide, with higher incidence in developing countries. In the US, risk groups include men who have sex with men, travelers and recent immigrants, and institutionalized populations.[11]

ETIOLOGY AND PATHOPHYSIOLOGY

- Nematodes (roundworms).
  - *E. vermicularis* (pinworm; **Figures 179-2** and **179-3**) is acquired through an oral route when hands that have contacted contaminated objects are placed in the mouth. Larvae hatch in the small intestine. Adults live in the cecum. The pregnant female goes to the perianal region at night to lay eggs.
  - *N. americanus* (hookworm; **Figure 179-4**) larvae penetrate the skin, travel through veins to the heart and then to the lungs, climb the bronchial tree to the pharynx, and then are swallowed and attach to intestine walls (**Figure 179-5**).
  - When fertilized eggs of *A. lumbricoides* (**Figure 179-6**) are ingested, they hatch and the larvae enter the circulation through intestinal mucosa, travel to the lungs, climb to the pharynx, then are swallowed, and finally the adult *Ascaris* worms live in the small intestine.
  - *S. stercoralis* have both a free-living and parasitic cycle. In the parasitic cycle, larvae penetrate the skin, travel through the circulation to the lungs and are swallowed, and travel to the small intestine (**Figure 179-8**) to become adults. Adult females lay eggs, which become rhabditiform larvae, which can either become free living or can cause autoinfection by reentering the parasitic cycle or disseminating widely in the body.
  - *T. trichiura* (whipworm; **Figure 179-9**) eggs are ingested and hatch in the small intestine; worms live in the cecum or colon.
  - Cestodes (tapeworms)—*T. solium* is acquired by ingesting undercooked contaminated pork. *Diphyllobothrium latum* is the fish tapeworm that is acquired by ingesting uncooked contaminated fresh-water fish.
- Protozoa.
  - *G. lamblia* cysts are ingested from contaminated water, food, or fomites and travel to the small intestine (**Figure 179-10**).
  - Cryptosporidium species can be acquired and spread from person-to-person or from ingestion of contaminated water.
  - *E. histolytica* cysts or trophozoites are ingested from fecally contaminated food, water, or hands or from fecal contact during sexual practices; these then travel to the large intestine, where these either remain or travel through the bloodstream to the brain, liver, or lungs.

RISK FACTORS

- Endemic in developing countries with limited access to clean water.
- Living in an environment conducive to parasites (warm, humid climate) and parasitic transfer (crowded conditions, contaminated water supply, or poor hygiene) dramatically raises the risk of parasitic infection.
- Household contacts or caretakers of persons with intestinal parasites are at risk for contracting the parasites.
- Children or others with poor hygiene are also at high risk.
- Immunocompromised patients, once infected, may have a more serious course.

DIAGNOSIS

CLINICAL FEATURES

- Nematodes.
  - *E. vermicularis* (pinworm)—Perianal pruritus is the most common; female genital tract irritation also reported; rarely abdominal pain or appendicitis; infants show irritability, but can be asymptomatic.[11]
  - *N. americanus* (hookworm)—Most commonly presents with iron-deficiency anemia.[11]
  - *A. lumbricoides*—Frequently asymptomatic; high numbers of worms can cause abdominal pain or intestinal obstruction. Cough, dyspnea, hemoptysis, or eosinophilic pneumonitis when in the lungs. Patients may cough up visible worms.
  - *S. stercoralis*—Frequently asymptomatic; eosinophilia; may cause abdominal pain or diarrhea, cough, shortness of breath, or hemoptysis when in the lungs; can disseminate in immunocompromised patients causing abdominal pain, distention, septicemia, shock, or death.
  - *T. trichiura* (whipworm)—Frequently asymptomatic; high number of worms can cause abdominal pain or intestinal obstruction, especially in children.

- Cestodes.
  - *T. solium*—Frequently asymptomatic; risk of developing cysticercosis with symptoms based on location of cysts in brain (e.g., seizures, focal neurologic signs, and death), eyes, heart, or spine.
- Protozoa.
  - *G. lamblia*—Diarrhea, nausea, emesis, abdominal bloating occurs 1 to 14 days after ingestion for up to 3 weeks and can be asymptomatic.
  - Cryptosporidiosis in otherwise healthy children often results in asymptomatic infection. Some children may develop a self-limited watery diarrhea associated with vomiting, abdominal pain, and fever. Immunodeficient individuals, particularly those with human immunodeficiency virus infection and other T-cell deficiencies, may develop a severe protracted diarrheal illness with malabsorption and weight loss, or may develop disseminated infection and cholangitis.
  - *E. histolytica*—Asymptomatic, intestinal symptoms (e.g., colitis and appendicitis), or extraintestinal (e.g., abscess in the liver or lungs, peritonitis, and skin or genital lesions).

LABORATORY TESTING

- Nematodes.
  - *E. vermicularis* (pinworm)—Microscopic identification of eggs (**Figure 179-2**) collected from perianal area; apply transparent adhesive tape to the unwashed perianal area at the time of presentation or in the morning and then place tape on slide.
  - *N. americanus* (hookworm)—Microscopic identification of eggs in the stool.
  - *A. lumbricoides*—Microscopic identification of eggs in the stool.
  - *S. stercoralis*—Microscopic identification of larvae in stool (**Figure 179-8**) or duodenal fluid; often requires several samples. Immunologic tests are useful when infection is suspected, but larvae are not seen in several samples. Immunologic tests do not differentiate from past or present infections.
  - *T. trichiura* (whipworm)—Microscopic identification of eggs in stool (**Figure 179-9**).
- Cestodes.
  - *T. solium*—Microscopic identification of eggs or proglottids in stool indicates taeniasis; presumed neurocysticercus diagnosed from Centers for Disease Control and Prevention (CDC)'s immunoblot assay.[11]
- Protozoa.
  - *G. lamblia*—Microscopic identification of cysts or trophozoites in stool or trophozoites in duodenal fluid or biopsy (**Figure 179-10**). Antigen tests and immunofluorescence are available.
  - Cryptosporidium species—Microscopic identification of oocytes in stool using a modified acid-fast stain. Antigen assays are available and used commonly.
  - *E. histolytica*—Microscopic identification of cysts or trophozoites in stool (difficult to distinguish from nonpathogens); antibody detection for extraintestinal disease; antigen detection can distinguish pathogenic and nonpathogenic infections.[11]

IMAGING

- Cestodes.
  - *T. solium*—MRI is typically used to identify brain cysts.

DIFFERENTIAL DIAGNOSIS

- Abdominal symptoms seen with several intestinal parasites can also be caused by the following:
  - Viral or bacterial infections—May present with acute onset of emesis and diarrhea often with fever (see the preceding).
  - Irritable bowel disease—Chronic symptoms of abdominal cramping with diarrhea or loose stools and/or constipation; usually no bloody stools, weight loss, or anemia.
  - Inflammatory bowel disease—Intermittent abdominal pain and bloody stools; diagnosis confirmed by colonoscopy with biopsy.
  - Iron-deficiency anemia seen with hookworms can be seen with blood loss from any site from one of many causes. Of course, iron deficiency can be seen with a diet deficient in iron without having hookworms.
  - GI blood loss can be seen with other infections or inflammation, polyps, or masses.

MANAGEMENT

MEDICATIONS

All medication doses are from *The Medical Letter*.[12]

- Nematodes.
  - *E. vermicularis* (pinworm)—Pyrantel pamoate 11 mg/kg once (maximum 1 g), repeat in 2 weeks; or mebendazole 100 mg once, repeat in 2 weeks.
  - *N. americanus* (hookworm)—Albendazole 400 mg once; or mebendazole 100 mg twice a day for 3 days 500 mg once or pyrantel pamoate 11 mg/kg (maximum 1 g) for 3 days.
  - *A. lumbricoides*—Albendazole 400 mg once; alternate therapy mebendazole 500 mg once or ivermectin 150 to 200 mcg/kg po once.
  - *S. stercoralis*—Ivermectin 200 mcg/kg per day for 2 days; alternate therapy albendazole 400 mg bid for 7 days.
  - *T. trichiura* (whipworm)—Mebendazole 100 mg twice a day for 3 days or 500 mg once; alternate therapy albendazole 400 mg once a day for 3 days or ivermectin 0.2 mg/kg daily for 3 days.
- Cestodes.
  - *T. solium*—Praziquantel 5 to 10 mg/kg once for intestinal stage; cysticercosis require seizure prophylaxis and steroids in conjunction with albendazole 15 mg/kg per day up to 400 mg bid for 8 to 30 days; ophthalmologic examination for eye cysts is recommended.
- Protozoa.
  - *G. lamblia*—Metronidazole 15 mg/kg per day, up to 750 mg, divided tid for 5 to 7 days; or tinidazole 50 mg/kg (maximum 2 g) once; or nitazoxanide 500 mg bid for 3 days (age >12 years), 100 mg bid for 3 days (age 1 to 3 years), 200 mg po bid for 3 days (age 4 to 11 years).
  - Cryptosporidiosis—Nitazoxanide 500 mg bid for 3 days (age >12 years), 100 mg bid for 3 days (age 1 to 3 years), 200 mg bid for 3 days (age 4 to 11 years).
  - *E. histolytica*—Metronidazole 35 to 50 mg/kg per day, up to 1500 mg, divided in 3 doses for 7 to 10 days or 50 mg/kg per

day in 3 doses up to 2 g for 3 days. Then iodoquinol 30 to 40 mg/kg per day up to 2 g in 3 doses for 20 days; or paromomycin 25 to 35 mg/kg per day in 3 doses for 7 days.

REFERRAL OR HOSPITALIZATION

Refer or hospitalize patients:

- Who do not respond to initial therapy or have recurrent infections.
- Suspected of having cysticercosis.
- Experiencing severe abdominal symptoms suggesting obstruction or an acute abdomen.

PREVENTION

- Clean uncontaminated water for drinking and cooking—Use bottled water, chemically treated water, or boiled water in endemic areas.
- Good hygiene, especially hand washing.
- When travelling to endemic areas, drink bottled water when possible. Water can also be treated with chlorine, iodine, or boiled if bottled water is not available. Clean water should be used for brushing teeth. Avoid eating fresh salads washed in local water.
- Children in developing countries who are drinking contaminated water (and lack access to clean water) should be considered for deworming with albendazole every 3 to 6 months (see Chapter 7, Global Health).

PROGNOSIS

Prognosis is excellent for most infections if adequate therapy and clean water is available.

FOLLOW-UP

Follow-up at completion of therapy.

PATIENT EDUCATION

Most intestinal parasites are asymptomatic and easily treatable. Avoid infecting others by practicing good hygiene, including hand washing.

PATIENT RESOURCES

- The Centers for Disease Control and Prevention division of parasitic diseases has information on many parasitic diseases—**www.cdc.gov/parasites**.

PROVIDER RESOURCES

- Centers for Disease Control and Prevention (CDC)—**www.cdc.gov/parasites**.
- The Medical Letter's "Drugs for Parasitic Infections" is available online at **www.medletter.com** for individual and institutional subscribers.

REFERENCES

1. Centers for Disease Control and Prevention. Prevention of rotavirus gastroenteritis among infants and children. Recommendations of the Advisory Committee on Immunization Practices. *MMWR*. 2006;55:1-53.
2. http://wwwnc.cdc.gov/travel/page/travelers-diarrhea.
3. http://www.cdc.gov/vaccines/pubs/surv-manual/chpt13-rotavirus.html.
4. Hartling L, Bellemar S, Wiebe N, et al. Oral versus intravenous rehydration for treating dehydration due to gastroenteritis in children. *Cochrane Database Syst Rev*. 2006;3CD004390.
5. Allen SJ, Okoko B, Martinez E, Gregorio G, Dans LF. Probiotics for treating infectious diarrhoea. *Cochrane Database Syst Rev*. 2004;(2):CD003048.
6. Thomas DW, Greer FR. Committee on Nutrition. Clinical report—probiotics and prebiotics in pediatrics. *Pediatrics*. 2010;126:1217-1222.
7. American Academy of Pediatrics: Shigella infections. *Red Book: 2012 Report of the Committee on Infectious Diseases.* Pickering LK, ed. 29th ed. Elk Grove Village, IL: American Academy of Pediatrics; 2012:645-647.
8. American Academy of Pediatrics. Campylobacter infections. *Red Book: 2012 Report of the Committee on Infectious Diseases.* Pickering LK, ed. 29th ed. Elk Grove Village, IL: American Academy of Pediatrics; 2012:262-264.
9. American Academy of Pediatrics. Salmonella Infections. *Red Book: 2012 Report of the Committee on Infectious Diseases.* Pickering LK, ed. 29th ed. Elk Grove Village, IL: American Academy of Pediatrics; 2012:635-640.
10. American Academy of Pediatrics. Rotavirus infections. *Red Book: 2012 Report of the Committee on Infectious Diseases.* Pickering LK, ed. 29th ed. Elk Grove Village, IL: *American Academy of Pediatrics*. 2012:626-629.
11. Centers for Disease Control and Prevention. *Parasites*. http://www.cdc.gov/parasites, accessed September 11, 2011.
12. The Medical Letter. Drugs for parasitic infections. Treatment guidelines. 2nd ed, 2010. http://secure.medicalletter.org/system/files/private/parasitic.pdf, accessed September 11, 2011.

180 GONOCOCCAL INFECTIONS

Heidi Chumley, MD
Richard P. Usatine, MD

PATIENT STORY

A 17-year-old male presents to his pediatrician with 3 days of dysuria and penile discharge. A heavy purulent urethral discharge is seen (**Figure 180-1**). He has been sexually active with four female partners. He was diagnosed with gonococcal urethritis by clinical appearance and a urine specimen was sent for testing to confirm the gonorrhea and test for *Chlamydia*. He was treated with Ceftriaxone 250 mg IM for gonorrhea and 1 g of oral azithromycin for possible coexisting *Chlamydia*. He was offered and agreed to testing for other sexually transmitted diseases. He was told to inform his partners of the diagnosis. He was counseled about safe sex. On his 1-week follow-up visit, his symptoms were gone and he had no further discharge. His gonorrhea nucleic acid amplification test was positive and his *Chlamydia*, rapid plasma reagin (RPR), and HIV tests were negative. His case was reported to the Health Department for contact tracing.

INTRODUCTION

Infections with *Neisseria gonorrhoeae* are the second most commonly reported sexually transmitted disease in the US. Gonorrhea can cause cervicitis, urethritis, proctitis, and conjunctivitis. Untreated infections can lead to pelvic inflammatory disease, increasing the risk for infertility, ectopic pregnancy and chronic pelvic pain. Exposed newborns can develop ophthalmia neonatorum. Diagnosis is suspected clinically and confirmed by a urine nucleic acid amplification test. Treat for both gonorrhea and *Chlamydia* until one or both are ruled out by laboratory testing.

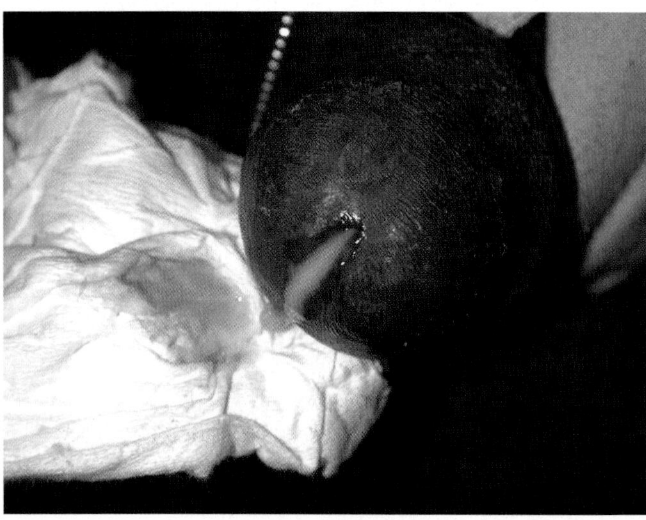

FIGURE 180-1 A 17-year-old with gonococcal urethritis and a heavy purulent urethral discharge. (*Used with permission from Richard P. Usatine, MD.*)

EPIDEMIOLOGY

- The prevalence of gonorrhea in boys and girls ages 15 to 19 was 248.6 and 556.5 per 100,000 persons in the US in 2011. In 2011, gonorrhea rates remained highest among black men and women (427.3), which was 17 times the rate among whites (25.2 per 100,000 population). The rates among Hispanics (53.8) was 2.1 times those of whites.[1]

ETIOLOGY AND PATHOPHYSIOLOGY

- *Neisseria gonorrhoeae* is a gram-negative cocci.
- Urethritis is most common infection in males, with an incubation period of 2 to 7 days.
- Cervicitis is the most common infection in females, with symptoms typically developing within 10 days of exposure.
- Vaginitis is rare in adolescents but can be seen in prepubertal girls due to lack of estrogen effect on the vaginal mucosa.
- May also cause anorectal or pharyngeal infections.
- Ophthalmia neonatorum presents 2 to 5 days after birth (see Chapter 72, Neonatal Conjunctivitis).
- Gonococcal bacteremia can cause a polyarthritis often accompanied by skin lesions.

DIAGNOSIS

CLINICAL FEATURES

Male patients with urethritis can be asymptomatic or present with urethral discharge, dysuria, or urethral pruritus.

Urethritis is diagnosed when one of the following is present:[2]

- Mucopurulent or purulent urethral discharge (**Figures 180-1** and **180-2**).

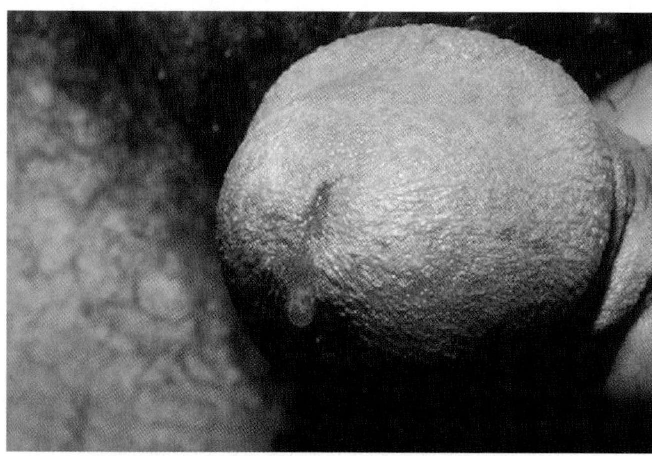

FIGURE 180-2 Nongonococcal urethritis caused by *Chlamydia*. Note the discharge is clearer and less purulent than seen with gonorrhea. (*Used with permission from Seattle STD/HIV Prevention Training Center, University of Washington.*)

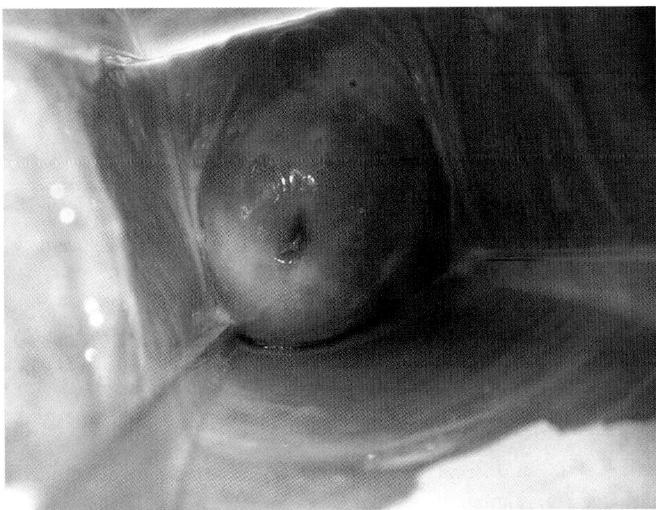

FIGURE 180-3 Normal appearing cervix in a patient with a mild white vaginal discharge and proven gonorrhea and Chlamydia. During this visit when the liquid-based Pap test was performed the specimen was also sent for gonorrhea and chlamydia and found to be positive. She was enrolled in a residential drug rehabilitation program and had a history of unprotected sex with multiple partners. (*Used with permission from Richard P. Usatine, MD.*)

- First-void urine positive leukocyte esterase test ≥10 white blood cells (WBCs) per high-power field. (This can also be seen with a urinary tract infection [UTI]; however, the incidence of UTI in men younger than 50 years of age is approximately 50 per 100,000 per year, much lower than the incidence of gonococcal or chlamydial urethritis in this age group.)
- Female patients can be asymptomatic, present with mild symptoms such as scant discharge or dysuria, or present with mucopurulent vaginal discharge (**Figures 180-3** and **180-4**).

LABORATORY TESTING

- Nucleic acid amplification test (NAAT) is the recommended test for screening asymptomatic at-risk adolescent boys and testing symptomatic adolescent boys.[2] Urine is a better specimen than urethral swab and does not hurt.[2,3]
- Self collected vulvovaginal swabs, in women age 16 or older, are equivalent to clinician collected endocervical swabs.[4]
- Gram stain of urethral secretions with ≥5 WBC per oil immersion field. (If Gram-negative intracellular diplococci are seen, gonococcal urethritis is present.) Gram stain will identify most cases; ≥5 WBCs are seen in 82 percent of *Chlamydia* and 94 percent of gonococcal infections.[5] Government regulations concerning in-office laboratory testing have severely curtailed the use of Gram stains in the office.
- In males, leukocyte esterase test on urine has a good negative predictive value (NPV) but poor positive predictive value (PPV) in a low-prevalence population (NPV 96.4% and PPV 35.4%).[6] Urethral culture is less commonly necessary when NAAT is available.
- Consider culture when tests for gonorrhea and *Chlamydia* are negative, or symptoms persist despite adequate treatment in a patient who is unlikely to have been reinfected by an untreated partner.

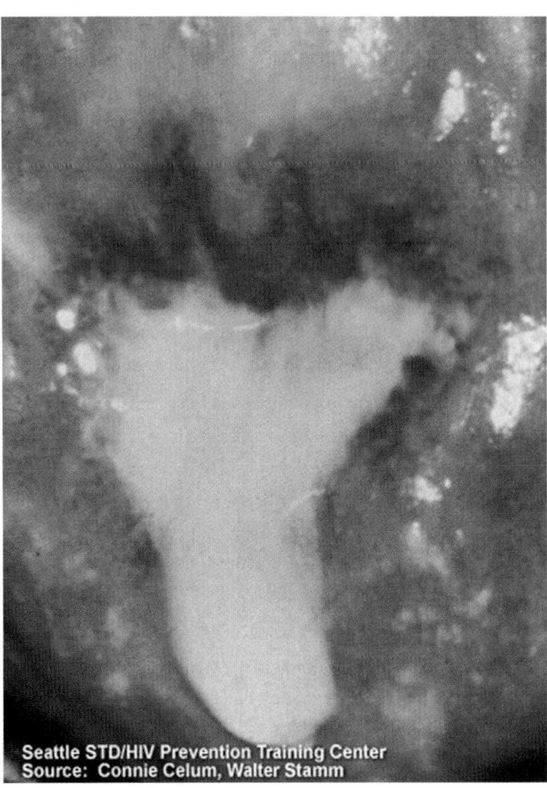

FIGURE 180-4 Thick mucopurulent discharge from the cervix infected with gonorrhea. (*Used with permission from Seattle STD/HIV Prevention Training Center, University of Washington. http://depts.washington.edu/handbook/gallery/index.html image 7-6.*)

DIFFERENTIAL DIAGNOSIS

Dysuria in males can be caused by the following:[7]

- Infections in other sites or the urogenital tract—Cystitis, prostatitis with perineal pain or prostate tenderness, or epididymitis with scrotal pain.
- Penile lesions—Vesicles of herpes simplex, ulcers of syphilis, chancroid, or lymphogranuloma venereum, and glans irritation from balanitis.
- Mechanical causes—Obstruction from benign prostatic hyperplasia (BPH) causing inflammation without infection, trauma including catheterization, urethral strictures, or genitourinary cancers.
- Inflammatory conditions—Spondyloarthropathies, drug reactions, or autoimmune diseases.

Vaginal discharge is also commonly caused by Chlamydia, Trichomonas, or candidiasis. Co-infection with gonorrhea should be ruled out with any sexually transmitted infection causing vaginal discharge.

MANAGEMENT

When clinical suspicion is high, treat male and female patients empirically for both *N. gonorrhoeae* and *C. trachomatis* until results are available. In males, treat patients who meet criteria for urethritis. Test patients with dysuria who do not meet criteria for urethritis, for

N. gonorrhoeae and *C. trachomatis*, and treat if positive. Advise sex partners to be evaluated and treated.[1]

MEDICATIONS

- The 2010 CDC STD treatment guidelines recommend treating uncomplicated gonococcal urethritis or cervicitis with ceftriaxone 250 mg IM in a single dose plus treatment for *Chlamydia* with azithromycin or doxycycline. Most gonococci in the US are susceptible to doxycycline and azithromycin, so that routine co-treatment might also hinder the development of antimicrobial-resistant *N. gonorrhoeae*.[8] Avoid fluoroquinolones and oral cefixime as drug resistance is too high.[8,9] SOR A
- The 2010 CDC STD treatment guidelines recommend treating *Chlamydia* urethritis or cervicitis with azithromycin 1 g orally in a single dose or doxycycline 100 mg orally twice a day for 7 days.[10] SOR A Acceptable alternate regimens include:
  - Erythromycin base 500 mg 4 times a day for 7 days or erythromycin ethylsuccinate 800 mg 4 times a day for 7 days or ofloxacin 300 mg orally twice a day for 7 days or levofloxacin 500 mg orally once daily for 7 days.[10]
- For persistent urethritis or cervicitis, consider *Trichomonas vaginalis* as a possible cause—Culture and treat with a single dose of metronidazole 2 g.
- Consider expedited partner therapy (EPT). EPT is the delivery of medications or prescriptions by persons infected with a sexually transmitted disease (STD) to their sex partners without clinical assessment of the partners. Legal status by state is available at www.cdc.gov/std/ept/legal/default.htm.

PREVENTION

- Encourage safe-sex practices.
- From the US Preventive Services Task Force:
  - Screen asymptomatic sexually active adolescent females for gonorrhea. SOR B
  - There is insufficient evidence to recommend screening asymptomatic sexually active adolescent males for gonorrhea. SOR A
- Offer STI testing, including testing for gonorrhea, in patients with an STI.
- Use prophylactic ocular topical medicine in all newborns. SOR A

PROGNOSIS

Gonococcal and chlamydial urethritis and cervicitis respond well to appropriate antibiotic therapy. Partners must be treated to avoid reinfection.

FOLLOW-UP

- Reevaluate patients with persistent or recurrent symptoms after treatment. Reexamine for evidence of urethral or cervical inflammation and retest for gonorrhea and *Chlamydia*.
- Routine test-of-cure laboratory examination is not recommended by the CDC for gonorrhea infections unless therapeutic compliance is in question, symptoms persist, or reinfection is suspected.[8,10]
- However, patients who have symptoms that persist after treatment of gonorrhea should be evaluated by culture for *N. gonorrhoeae*, and any gonococci isolated should be tested for antimicrobial susceptibility.[8]

PATIENT EDUCATION

The Centers for Disease Control and Prevention (CDC) recommends the following for patients diagnosed with gonorrhea:[1]

- Return for evaluation if the symptoms persist or return after therapy is completed.
- Abstain from sexual intercourse until 7 days after starting therapy, symptoms have resolved, and sexual partners have been adequately treated.
- Undergo testing for other STDs, including HIV and syphilis.
- Advise sexual partners of the need for treatment and/or take medications directly to them using EPT.

PATIENT RESOURCES

- Centers for Disease Control and Prevention—**www.cdc.gov/std/Gonorrhea/STDFact-gonorrhea.htm**.

PROVIDER RESOURCES

- The Centers for Disease Control and Prevention (CDC) website has the latest epidemiologic data and management recommendations—**www.cdc.gov/std/default.htm**.
- The newest CDC Treatment Guidelines—**www.cdc.gov/std/treatment**.
- The Practitioners Handbook for the Management of Sexually Transmitted Diseases. From the Seattle STD/HIV Prevention Training Center. Includes an image gallery—**http://depts.washington.edu/handbook/index.html**.

REFERENCES

1. U.S. Centers for Disease Control and Prevention. http://www.cdc.gov/std/stats10/chlamydia.htm, accessed September 2, 2012.
2. Brill JR. Diagnosis and treatment of urethritis in men. *Am Fam Physician*. 2010;81(7):873-878.
3. Sugunendran H, Birley HD, Mallinson H, et al. Comparison of urine, first and second endourethral swabs for PCR based detection of genital *Chlamydia trachomatis* infection in male patients. *Sex Transm Infect*. 2001;77(6):423-426.
4. Stewart CM, Schoeman SA, Booth RA, et al. Assessment of self taken swabs versus clinician taken swab cultures for diagnosing gonorrhea in women: single centre, diagnostic accuracy study. *BMJ*. 2012;345:e8107.

5. Geisler WM, Yu S, Hook EW III. Chlamydial and gonococcal infection in men without polymorphonuclear leukocytes on Gram stain: implications for diagnostic approach and management. *Sex Transm Dis.* 2005;32(10):630-634.

6. Bowden FJ. Reappraising the value of urine leukocyte esterase testing in the age of nucleic acid amplification. *Sex Transm Dis.* 1998;25(6):322-326.

7. Bremnor J, Sadovsky R. Evaluation of dysuria in adults. *Am Fam Physician.* 2002;65(8):1589-1596.

8. Centers for Disease Control and Prevention (CDC). *Sexually Transmitted Diseases Treatment Guidelines, 2010: Gonococcal-infections.* http://www.cdc.gov/std/treatment/2010/gonococcal-infections.htm, accessed September 2, 2012.

9. Update to CDC's Sexually Transmitted Diseases Treatment Guidelines, 2010: Oral Cephalosporins No Longer a Recommended Treatment for Gonococcal Infections. *MMWR.* 2012; 61(31):590-594. http://www.cdc.gov/mmwr/preview/mmwrhtml/mm6131a3.htm?s_cid=mm6131a3_w, accessed September 2, 2012.

10. Centers for Disease Control and Prevention (CDC). *Sexually Transmitted Diseases Treatment Guidelines, 2010: Chlamydial Infections.* http://www.cdc.gov/std/treatment/2010/chlamydial-infections.htm, accessed September 2, 2012.

181 SYPHILIS

Richard P. Usatine, MD
Heidi Chumley, MD

PATIENT STORY

A young woman presents to the office with a total body rash for one week (**Figure 181-1**). She denies other symptoms and the rash does not itch. Upon examination, tattoos on her hands are visible and she does admit to experimenting with crack and IV heroine. The physician suspects that she may have secondary syphilis and she admits to many sexual partners especially while using drugs. She is given a shot of 2.4 million units of benzathine penicillin IM in the office and her blood is drawn for an RPR and an HIV test. The RPR and HIV tests come back positive along with a treponemal specific confirmatory test. The patient is called to return to the office for some serious counseling and a referral to an infectious disease specialist. The ID specialist is called on the phone to see if he wants to admit her for a lumbar puncture or if he will do this as an outpatient. She needs investigation for neurosyphilis due to her positive HIV status.

INTRODUCTION

Syphilis, caused by *Treponema pallidum*, is a systemic disease characterized by multiple overlapping stages: primary syphilis (ulcer), secondary syphilis (skin rash, mucocutaneous lesions, or lymphadenopathy), tertiary syphilis (cardiac or gummatous lesions), and early or late latent syphilis (positive serology without clinical manifestations). Neurosyphilis can occur at any stage. Diagnosis is made using treponemal and nontreponemal tests. Treatment is penicillin; the dose and duration depend on the stage.

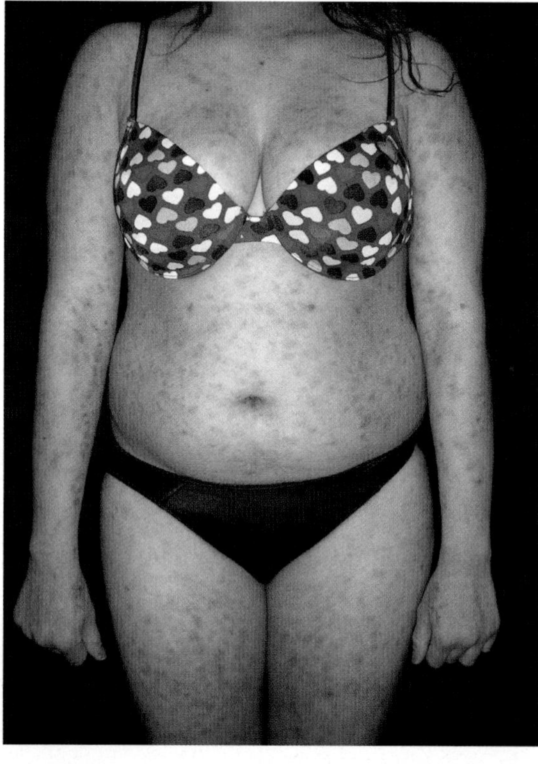

FIGURE 181-1 Secondary syphilis in a young woman with a history of injection drug use and multiple sexual partners. Her HIV test was also positive so she was worked up for neurosyphilis. (*Used with permission from Richard P. Usatine, MD.*)

SYNONYMS AND ACRONYMS

Lues is another word for syphilis.

NONTREPONEMAL TESTS

- VDRL—Venereal Disease Research Laboratory.
- RPR—Rapid Plasma Reagin.

TREPONEMAL TESTS

- EIA—Enzyme immunoassay.
- TPPA—*T. pallidum* particle agglutination.
- FTA-ABS—Fluorescent treponemal antibody absorption.
- MHA-TP—Microhemagglutination assay for *T. pallidum*.

EPIDEMIOLOGY

- Primary and secondary (P&S) syphilis cases reported to CDC increased from 11,466 in 2007 to 13,970 in 2011, an increase of 22 percent.[1] The rate of P&S syphilis in the US in 2011 (4.5 cases per 100,000 population) was 2.2 percent lower than the rate in 2009 (4.6 cases). This is the first overall decrease in P&S syphilis in 10 years.[1]
- The prevalence of P&S syphilis per 100,000 population is extremely low in ages 0 to 4 (0.0), 5 to 9 (0.0), and 10 to 14 (0.1) year olds, with only 25 reported cases in 2011.[1]
- The prevalence of P&S syphilis per 100,000 between the ages of 15 and 19 is 3.9, and is higher in males (5.4) than females (2.4).[1]
- Syphilis in persons ages 15 to 19 differs by races/ethnicities. In 2011, prevalence per 100,000 was 16.7 in black, 2.5 in Hispanic, and 0.9 in white persons.[1]
- In 2008, 63 percent of the reported cases of P&S (adolescents and adults combined) were in men who have sex with men (MSM).[2]
- HIV-infected patients were found to have syphilis rates of 62.3 per 1000 compared to 0.8 per 1000 in HIV-uninfected patients in a population study of adults in California.[3]
- In 2011, there were 362 reported cases of congenital syphilis, 8.4 per 100,000 live births.[1]

ETIOLOGY AND PATHOPHYSIOLOGY

- Syphilis is caused by the spirochete *T. pallidum* and contracted through direct sexual contact with primary or secondary lesions.
- Congenital syphilis can be contracted across the placenta. Seventy-five percent to 95 percent of fetuses are infected when untreated maternal syphilis was contracted within 2 years. Thirty-five percent

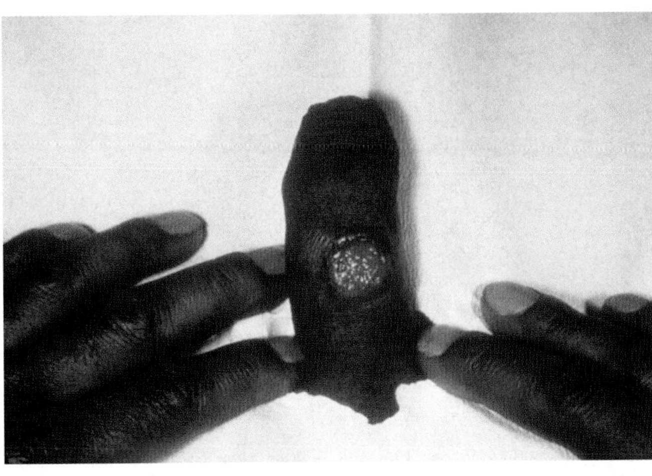

FIGURE 181-2 A painless chancre at the location of treponemal entry. *(Used with permission from the Public Health Image Library, Centers for Disease Control and Prevention.)*

of fetuses are infected when maternal syphilis was contracted more than 2 years before pregnancy.

RISK FACTORS

- Sexual contact with a person with primary or secondary syphilis.
- Gay males.
- Prostitution.
- Sex for drugs.
- HIV/AIDS.

DIAGNOSIS

CLINICAL FEATURES

- Primary syphilis is associated with a chancre—Usually a nonpainful ulcer (**Figures 181-2** and **181-4**). The presence of pain does not

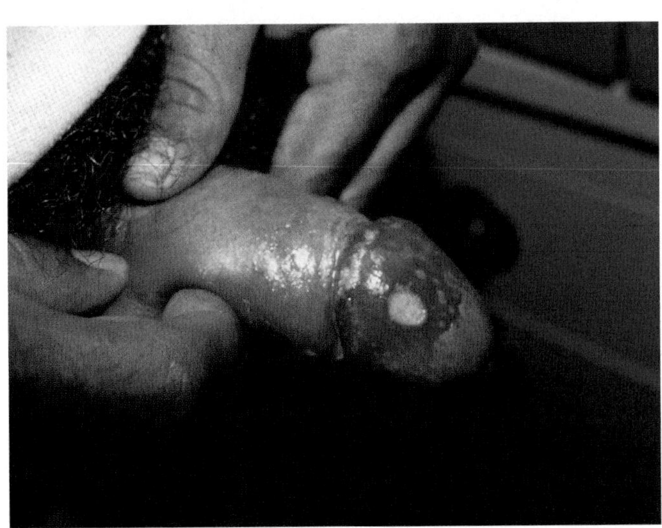

FIGURE 181-3 Primary syphilis with a large chancre on the glands of the penis. The multiple small surrounding ulcers are part of the syphilis and not herpes. *(Used with permission from Richard P. Usatine, MD.)*

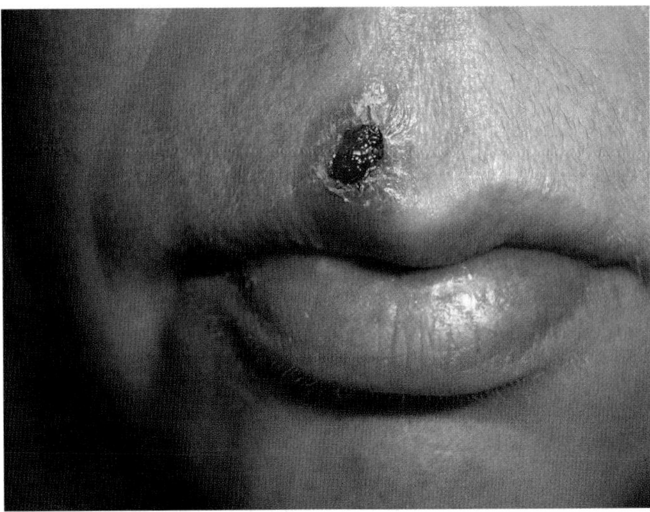

FIGURE 181-4 Primary syphilis with a chancre over the lip of a young woman. *(Used with permission from Richard P. Usatine, MD.)*

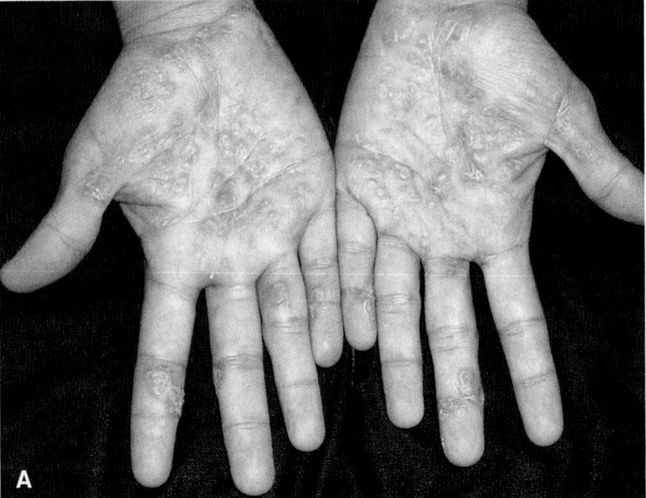

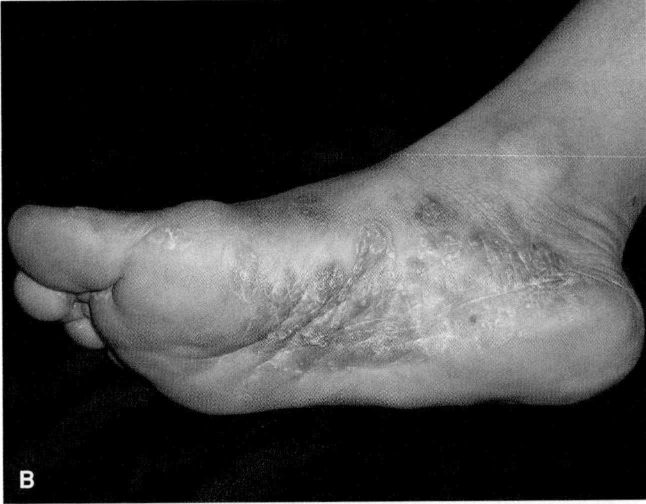

FIGURE 181-5 Secondary syphilis in a pregnant patient. **A.** Typical palmar lesions. **B.** Typical lesions on the sole. **C.** Mucous patches on the labia. *(Used with permission from Richard P. Usatine, MD.)* *(continued)*

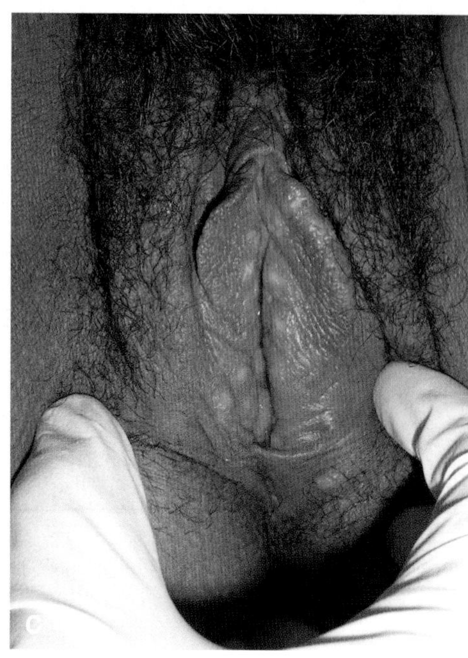

FIGURE 181-5 *(Continued)*

rule out syphilis, and the patient with a painful genital ulcer should be tested for both syphilis and herpes.

- Secondary syphilis occurs when the spirochetes become systemic and may present as a rash with protean morphologies, condyloma lata, and/or mucous patches (**Figures 181-5** to **181-7**).
- Tertiary syphilis may be visualized with gummas on the skin, but many of the manifestations are internal such as the cardiac and neurologic diseases that occur (e.g., aortitis, tabes dorsalis, and iritis). As tertiary syphilis takes years to develop and penicillin treatment is readily available, it is unlikely to ever see this in a child.
- Neurosyphilis can occur at any stage. Clinical symptoms include cognitive dysfunction, vision or hearing loss, uveitis or iritis, motor or sensory abnormalities, cranial nerve palsies, or symptoms of meningitis.
- Congenital syphilis.

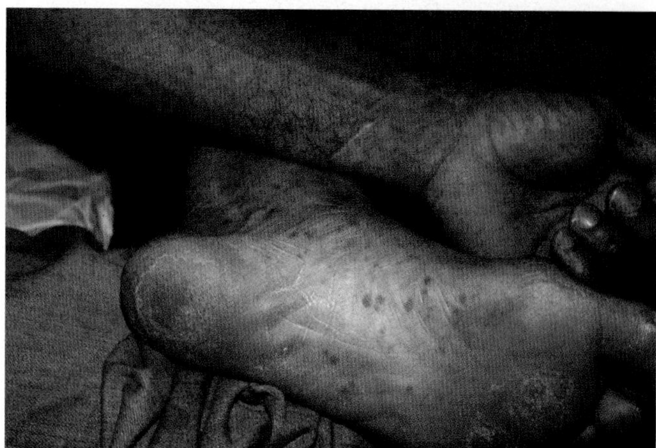

FIGURE 181-6 Pink macules on the feet and wrists of a patient with secondary syphilis. (*Used with permission from Richard P. Usatine, MD.*)

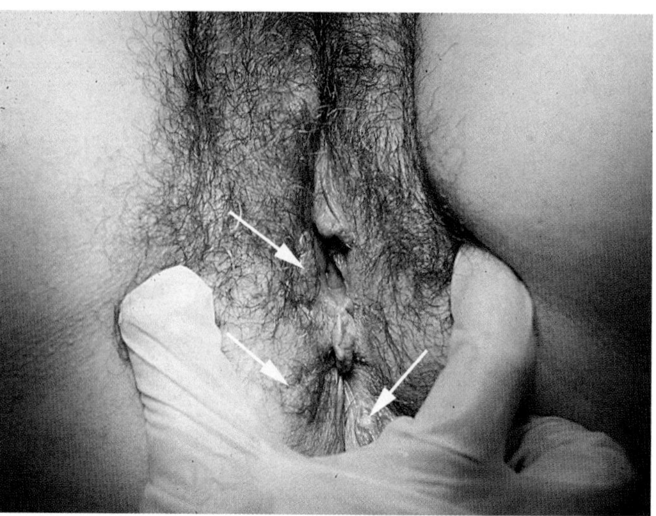

FIGURE 181-7 Condylomata lata (*arrows*) on the vulva of a patient with secondary syphilis. (*Used with permission from Richard P. Usatine, MD.*)

  - Early manifestations (within 2 years, typically by 2 to 3 months) include rhinitis, mucocutaneous lesions, bone changes, hepatosplenomegaly, lymphadenopathy, anemia and jaundice (**Figures 181-8** and **181-9**).
  - Late manifestations (after 2 years of age, without treatment) include interstitial keratitis, eight-nerve deafness, recurrent arthropathy, saber shins, saddle nose, tooth abnormalities, and neurosyphilis (**Figures 181-10** to **181-12**).

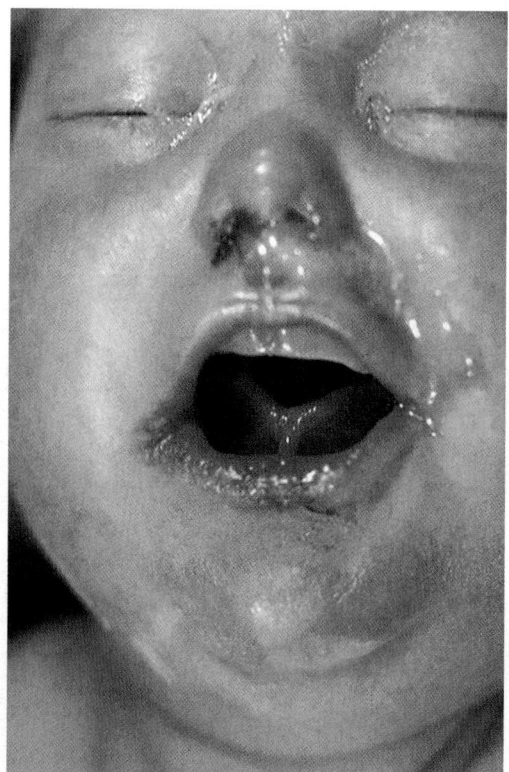

FIGURE 181-8 Congenital syphilis in a newborn infant with snuffles (mucous discharge from the nose). (*Used with permission from the CDC/Dr. Norman Cole.*)

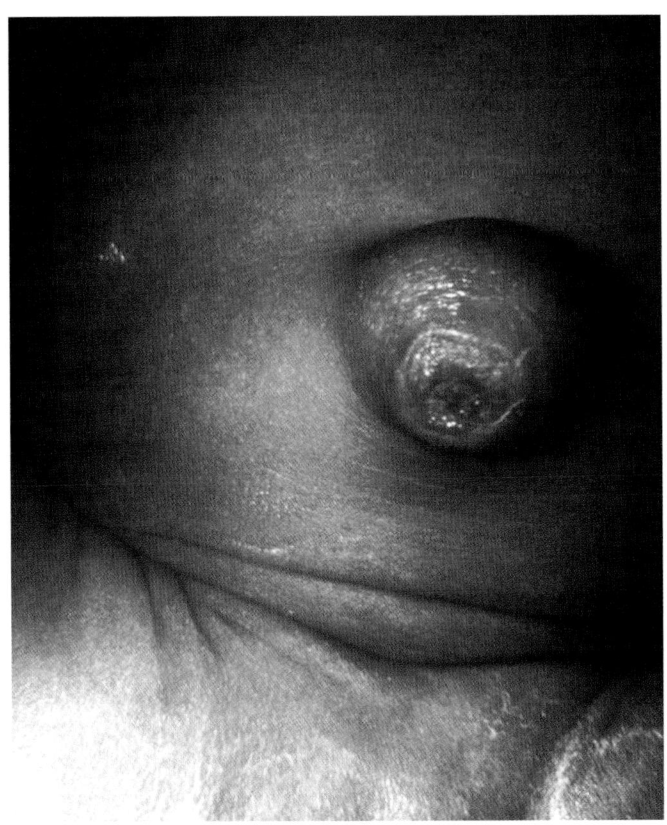

FIGURE 181-9 Congenital syphilis presenting with an inflamed lesion on the umbilicus. Dark field examination revealed the presence of Treponema pallidum spirochetes. (*Used with permission from the Public Health Image Library, Centers for Disease Control and Prevention.*)

TYPICAL DISTRIBUTION

- Primary syphilis is usually a single ulcer (chancre) that is not painful in the genital region (**Figures 181-2** and **181-3**). A chancre can be seen on the lip (**Figure 181-4**).
- Secondary syphilis may present with various eruptions on the trunk, palms, and soles (**Figures 181-5** to **181-7**).
- Mucous patches of secondary syphilis are found on the genitals or in the mouth (**Figure 181-5C**).

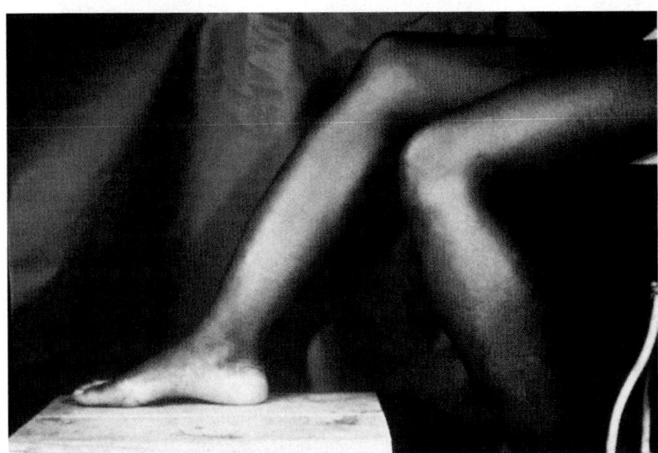

FIGURE 181-10 Saber shins or osteoperiostitis of the tibia is a result of untreated congenital syphilis. (*Used with permission from the CDC/ Robert E. Sumpter.*)

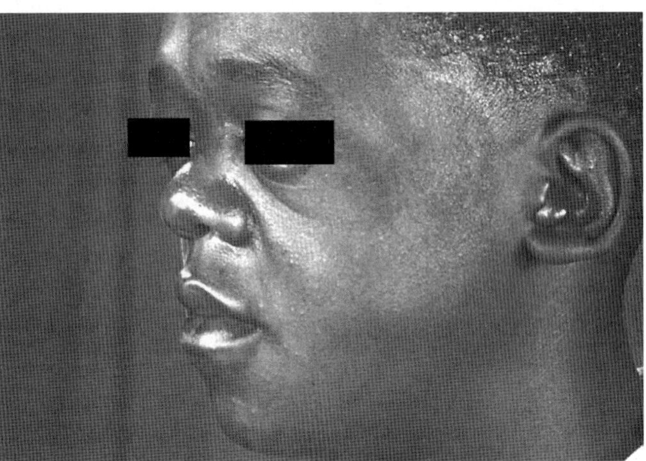

FIGURE 181-11 Saddle nose deformity in a 16-year-old patient due to congenital syphilis. (*Used with permission from the Public Health Image Library, Centers for Disease Control and Prevention.*)

LABORATORY TESTING

- Serologic tests are either nontreponemal (RPR or VDRL), which measure anticardiolipin antibodies, or treponemal (EIA, TPPA, FTA-ABS, or MHA-TP), which measure antibodies to *T. pallidum.*
- There are two algorithms for laboratory testing currently in use around the world:
  1. Start with a low-cost nontreponemal test and confirm a positive result with a treponemal test.
  2. Start with the EIA treponemal test, followed by a nontreponemal test for confirmation.
- In 2008, the Centers for Disease Control and Prevention (CDC) recommended a treponemal EIA initially, with positive results followed by a nontreponemal test for confirmation, a strategy that detected an additional 3 percent of positive samples not identified in the nontreponemal–treponemal sequence.[4]
- A nontreponemal test is required for confirmation, as a treponemal EIA indicates exposure but not active infection.

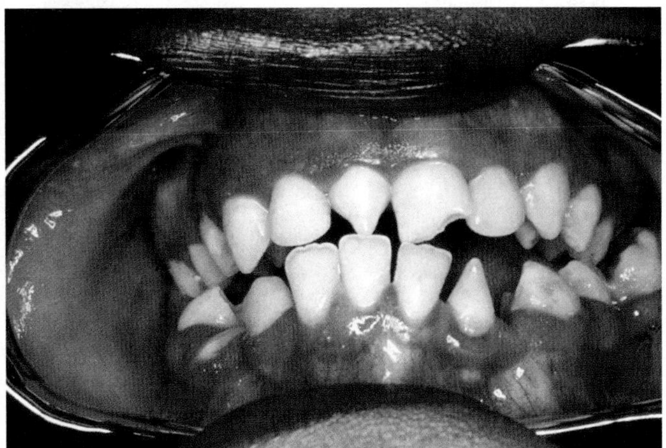

FIGURE 181-12 Hutchinson incisors caused by a congenital syphilis infection. Triangular appearing teeth are Hutchinson incisors, a known manifestation of congenital syphilis. (*Used with permission from the CDC/ Robert E. Sumpter.*)

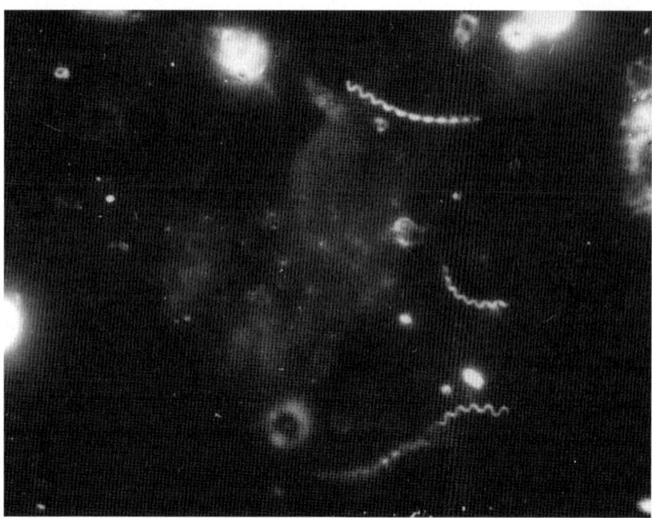

FIGURE 181-13 Live spirochetes of *T. pallidum* seen in a darkfield preparation. (*Used with permission from the Public Health Image Library, Centers for Disease Control and Prevention.*)

- A positive EIA with a negative RPR can be a previous treated or untreated infection, a false positive, or early primary syphilis. In this case, retest with a second treponemal test.
- Dark-field microscopy is useful in evaluating moist cutaneous lesions, such as chancre, mucous patches, and condyloma lata (**Figure 181-13**).
- Test all patients with syphilis for HIV (**Figure 181-14**).
- Patients with syphilis who have any signs or symptoms suggesting neurologic disease including vision or hearing need a cerebrospinal fluid (CSF) exam, a slit-lamp ophthalmologic examination, and an otologic examination to determine if neurosyphilis is present.

DIFFERENTIAL DIAGNOSIS

- Herpes simplex—Most common cause of genital ulcers in the US. These ulcers are painful and often start as vesicles (see Chapter 114, Herpes Simplex).
- Chancroid—Painful beefy red ulcers on the penis or vulva (**Figure 181-15**). It is less common than syphilis but in the early stage of the ulceration can resemble primary syphilis. If the RPR in a patient with a presumed syphilis chancre is negative and remains negative, bacterial cultures of the ulcer for *Haemophilus ducreyi* should be submitted. Chancroid is also known to cause large painful inguinal adenopathy (bubo; **Figure 181-16**).(See Chapter 75, Mucosal Ulcerative Disorders.)
- Drug eruptions—Can be on the genital area such as seen in a fixed drug eruption. Also whole-body drug eruptions can appear similar to secondary syphilis (see Chapter 154, Cutaneous Drug Reactions).
- Erythema multiforme—Can look like the rash of secondary syphilis but may have target lesions (see Chapter 151, Erythema Multiforme, Stevens-Johnson Syndrome, and Toxic Epidermal Necrolysis).

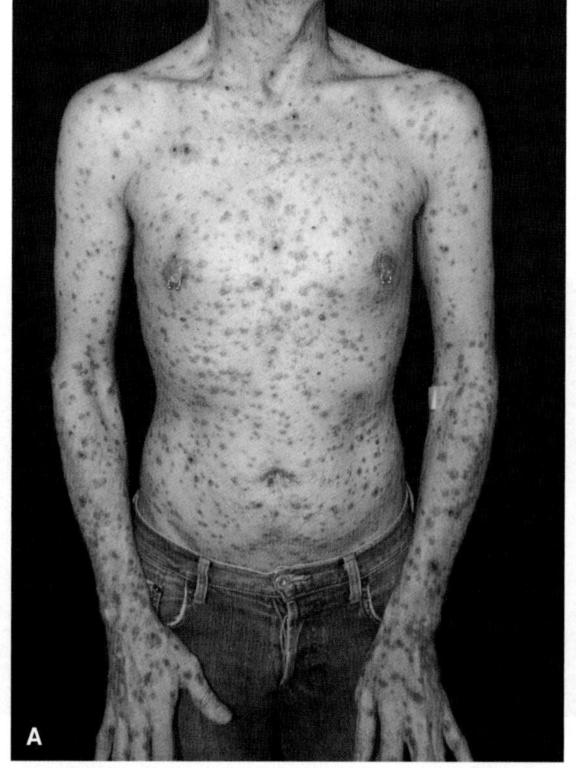

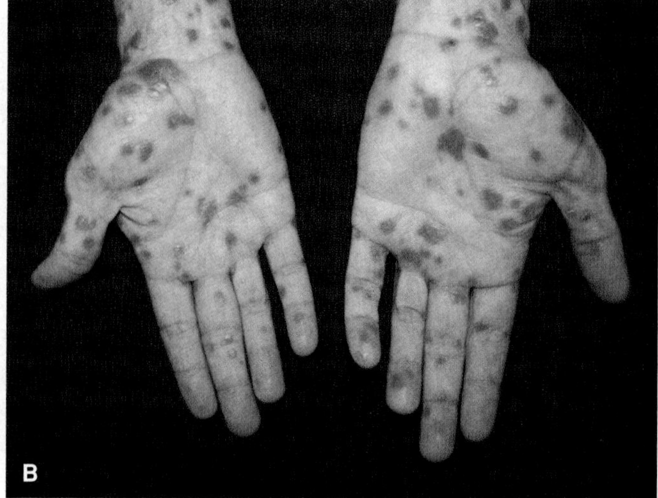

FIGURE 181-14 Secondary syphilis in a young man with known HIV/AIDS **A.** Impressive red papulosquamous eruption from head to toe is present. **B.** Close-up showing the palmar patches and plaques. (*Used with permission from Jonathan B. Karnes, MD.*)

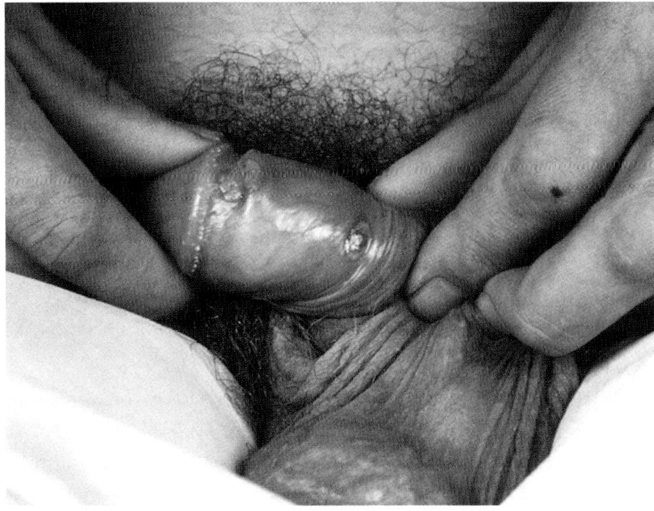

FIGURE 181-15 Chancroid ulcers caused by the bacterium, *Haemophilus ducreyi*. The patient was originally thought to have syphilis. Chancroidal ulcers are classically painful and beefy but chancroid should be considered on the differential diagnosis of any sexually acquired genital ulcer. (*Used with permission from CDC/ Dr. Pirozzi.*)

- Pityriasis rosea—A self-limited cutaneous eruption that often begins with a herald patch and may have a Christmas tree distribution on the back (see Chapter 137, Pityriasis Rosea).
- The differential diagnosis for congenital syphilis includes other congenital infections such as rubella, cytomegalovirus, herpes simplex virus, and toxoplasmosis (see Chapter 187, Congenital Infections). Erythroblastosis fetalis is also on the differential diagnosis for congenital syphilis.

MANAGEMENT

MEDICATIONS

Benzathine penicillin is the treatment of choice for all stages of syphilis. Dose and duration depend on stage. The following treatment information is from the CDC.[5]

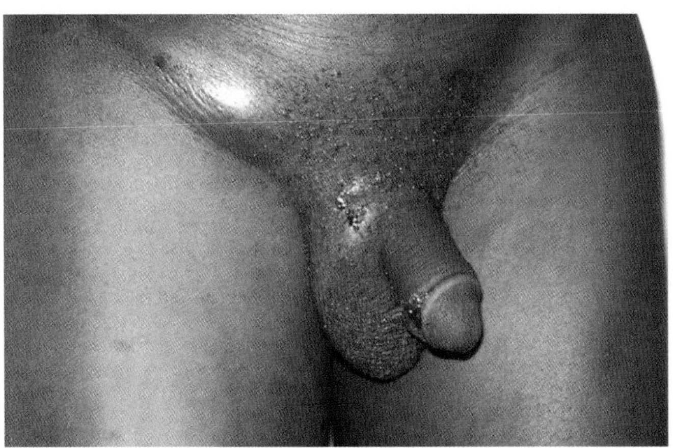

FIGURE 181-16 Chancroid lesions of the groin and penis affecting the ipsilateral inguinal lymph nodes. (*Used with permission from CDC/J. Pledger.*)

- Primary, secondary, and early latent (immunocompetent and nonpregnant):
  - Children older than 1 month with acquired primary or secondary—Benzathine penicillin 50,000 U/kg IM up to 2.4 million U one time.
- Penicillin allergy:
  - Doxycycline 100 mg twice daily × 14 days (For children 8 years of age and older) or
  - Ceftriaxone 1 g IM/IV daily × 10 to 14 days (limited studies) or
  - Azithromycin 2 g single oral dose; however, azithromycin resistance has been documented in several areas of the US. Use only when penicillin or doxycycline cannot be used. Do not use in gay males.
- Late latent syphilis or syphilis of unknown duration.
  - Children—Benzathine penicillin 50,000 U/kg IM (up to 2.4 million U) every week for 3 weeks.
- Penicillin allergy—Doxycycline is the only acceptable alternative available (for children 8 years of age and older).
- For the management of congenital, tertiary, and neurosyphilis, see the *Sexually Transmitted Diseases Treatment Guidelines* published by the CDC in 2010—www.cdc.gov/std/treatment/2010/genital-ulcers.htm#syphilis.

REFERRAL OR HOSPITALIZATION

- Refer patients when the stage of syphilis is unclear. Consider referral to an infectious disease specialist in children younger than 1 month of age, pregnant women with a penicillin allergy, patients with tertiary or neurosyphilis, or patients who have failed treatment.

PREVENTION

PRIMARY PREVENTION

Safe sex practices—Sexual transmission occurs when mucocutaneous syphilitic lesions are present.

SECONDARY PREVENTION

- Treat presumptively (regardless of serology) sexual partners who were exposed within 90 days of the partner's diagnosis of primary, secondary, or early latent syphilis.
- Consider presumptive treatment when exposure was greater than 90 days before partner's diagnosis if serology is unavailable or follow-up is uncertain.[5]

Primary prevention of congenital syphilis: Screen all pregnant patients and treat as soon as possible when positive. Treatment before the 16th week of pregnancy prevents fetal damage in most cases.

PROGNOSIS

When syphilis is recognized and appropriately treated, the prognosis is excellent.

FOLLOW-UP

- Reexamine clinically and serologically at 6 and 12 months. Consider treatment failure if signs and/or symptoms persist or the nontreponemal test titer does not decline by 2 dilutions after 6 to 12 months of therapy. Fifteen percent will not achieve this decline in titer after 1 year.[5]

- For treatment failures—Retest for HIV and perform a lumbar puncture for CSF analysis and treat for neurosyphilis if positive.

PATIENT EDUCATION

Condoms can prevent the spread of syphilis. Patients should be advised to get HIV testing and need to know that syphilis is a risk factor for the spread of HIV. HIV/AIDS is also a risk factor for acquiring syphilis (**Figure 181-14**). Patients should be advised of the importance of completing treatment and follow-up to prevent complications.

PATIENT RESOURCES

- Centers for Disease Control and Prevention (CDC). *Sexually Transmitted Diseases (STDs): Syphilis–CDC Fact Sheet*—**www.cdc.gov/std/syphilis/stdfact-syphilis.htm**.

PROVIDER RESOURCES

- **http://emedicine.medscape.com/article/229461**.
- The Centers for Disease Control and Prevention. *Sexually Transmitted Diseases Treatment Guidelines*—**www.cdc.gov/std/treatment/2010/toc.htm**. (Also available to download as an ebook for Apple iPad, iPhone, or iPod Touch—**www.cdc.gov/std/2010-ebook.htm**.)

REFERENCES

1. Centers for Disease Control and Prevention (CDC). *Sexually Transmitted Diseases Surveillance.* Syphilis. http://www.cdc.gov/std/stats10/Syphilis.htm, accessed February 21, 2013.
2. Centers for Disease Control and Prevention (CDC). *Sexually Transmitted Diseases.* Syphilis. http://www.cdc.gov/std/syphilis/, accessed April 8, 2014.
3. Horberg MA, Ranatunga DK, Quesenberry CP, et al. Syphilis epidemiology and clinical outcomes in HIV-infected and HIV-uninfected patients in Kaiser Permanente Northern California. *Sex Transm Dis.* 2010;37(1):53-58.
4. Centers for Disease Control and Prevention (CDC): Syphilis testing algorithms using treponemal tests for initial screening—four laboratories, New York City, 2005-2006. *MMWR Morb Mortal Wkly Rep.* 2008;57(32):872-875.
5. Centers for Disease Control and Prevention (CDC): *Sexually Transmitted Diseases Treatment Guidelines, 2010: Diseases Characterized by Genital, Anal, or Perianal Ulcers.* http://www.cdc.gov/std/treatment/2010/genital-ulcers.htm#syphilis, accessed April 8, 2014.

182 PEDIATRIC HUMAN IMMUNODEFICIENCY VIRUS (HIV) INFECTION

Rebecca Schein, MD

PATIENT STORIES

A 6-month-old girl is seen by her pediatrician for because her mother is concerned about a white coating on the infant's tongue and poor feeding. On exam, the child appears cachectic and has thrush visible throughout her oropharynx (**Figure 182-1**). Palpable cervical and axillary lymph nodes are noted as well. A human immunodeficiency virus (HIV) antibody test is obtained and is positive. Diagnosis is confirmed with a HIV DNA polymerase chain reaction (PCR). The mother of the baby also tests positive for HIV. The child is treated with antiretroviral (ARV) therapy and improves with treatment.

A 15-year-old male presents to a community clinic with penile discharge and anal itching due to anal warts (**Figure 182-2**). On further questioning, he admits to being homeless. He supports himself through commercial sex work, mainly with male partners. A urine nucleic acid test is positive for chlamydia and the oral rapid HIV antibody test is positive as well. Diagnosis of HIV is confirmed via Western Blot testing.

INTRODUCTION

HIV is a retrovirus that causes disseminated infection resulting in suppression of T-cell mediated immunity and development of opportunistic infections.

SYNONYMS

Acquired Immunodeficiency Syndrome (AIDS) refers to clinical syndrome seen with advanced disease.[1]

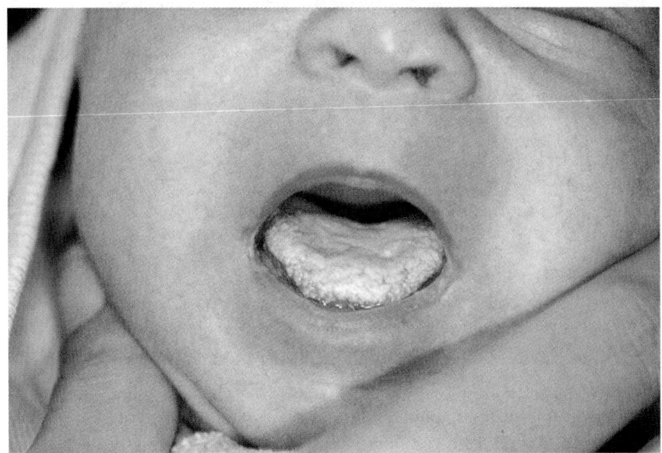

FIGURE 182-1 Oral thrush in an infant with human immunodeficiency virus (HIV) infection. (*Used with permission from David Effron, MD.*)

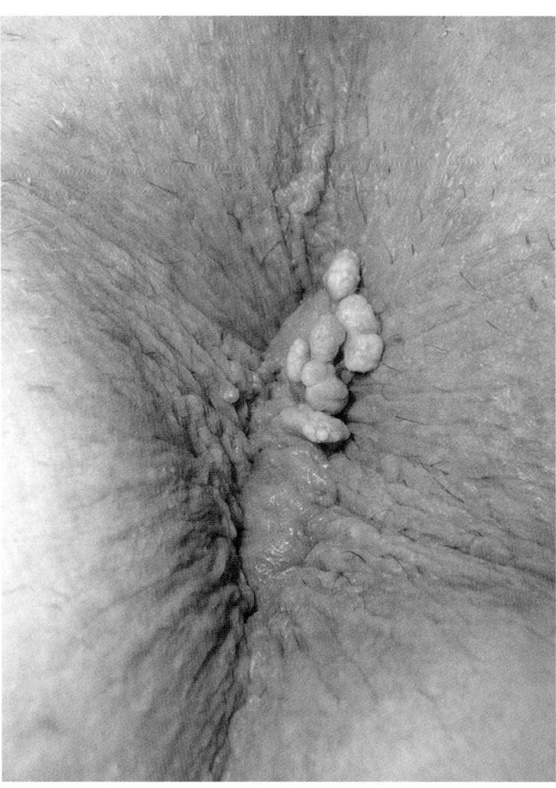

FIGURE 182-2 Anal warts (condyloma) caused by Human Papilloma Virus in an adolescent male with HIV infection and a history of anal receptive intercourse. (*Used with permission from Richard P. Usatine, MD.*)

EPIDEMIOLOGY

- Humans are the only known reservoir for HIV-1 and HIV-2.
- HIV lives in peripheral blood mononuclear cells, brain cells, bone marrow, and genital tract cells.
- Transmission occurs via sexual contact, blood exposure, mucous membrane exposure to blood or breast milk, and mother to child transmission.[2]
- Risk of mother to child transmission at birth without intervention is approximately 30 percent;[2] with current therapy this risk is now 1 to 2 percent in the US. High maternal HIV viral load at delivery, primary maternal infection during pregnancy, and breast feeding all increase transmission risk.[3]
- Risk of sexual transmission varies from 0.1 to 30 percent per encounter with highest risk from receptive anal sex.[4]

ETIOLOGY AND PATHOPHYSIOLOGY

- Lentivirus of the family *Retroviridae*.
- Two forms—HIV-1 and HIV-2. HIV-2 causes a milder form of disease and is found predominantly in West Africa.
- RNA virus that requires conversion of viral RNA to DNA to incorporate into host cell genome.[2]
- Major enzymes and regulatory genes required for replication, assembly, and release viral particles are encoded in the viral

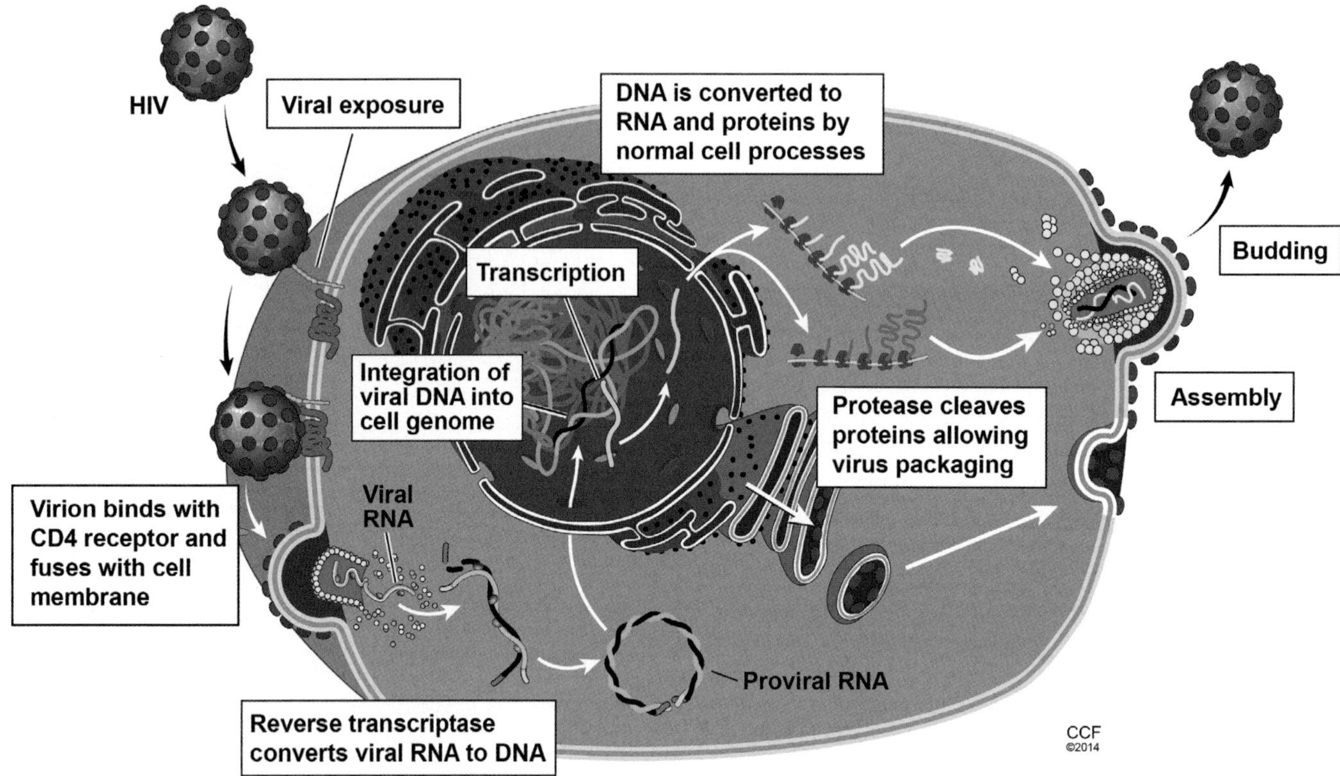

FIGURE 182-3 Model of HIV viral replication. (*Used with permission from Cleveland Clinic Center for Medical Art & Photography © 2014. All Rights Reserved.*)

genome including Reverse Transcriptase, Integrase, and Protease enzymes (**Figure 182-3**). See Diagram.

RISK FACTORS

- Unprotected sexual intercourse particularly receptive anal sex, genital ulcers or concomitant sexually transmitted diseases, intravenous drug use, maternal HIV, contaminated blood transfusion, and rarely needle stick injury.[2]

DIAGNOSIS

CLINICAL FEATURES

- Fevers, generalized lymphadenopathy, hepatosplenomegaly, failure to thrive, recurrent oral thrush, persistent diarrhea, interstitial pneumonia, invasive bacterial infection, and/or other opportunistic infection (OI).[2]
- OIs include respiratory or esophageal candidiasis, cryptococcosis (**Figure 182-4**), disseminated endemic fungal infection, cytomegalovirus (**Figure 182-5**), chronic herpes simplex (**Figure 182-6**), progressive multifocal leukoencephalopathy caused by JC virus (**Figure 182-7**), Kaposi's sarcoma caused by HHV 8 (**Figure 182-8**), *Mycobacterium avium-intracellulare*, other mycobacterial disease, cryptosporidium, *Pneumocystic jirovecii* (**Figure 182-9**), and toxoplasmosis.[5]
- Children may also present with more severe presentations of common childhood infections (**Figures 182-10** and **182-11**).
- Cervical lymphadenopathy not resolving should prompt the clinician to check for generalized lymphadenopathy and to consider HIV on the differential diagnosis (**Figure 182-12**).

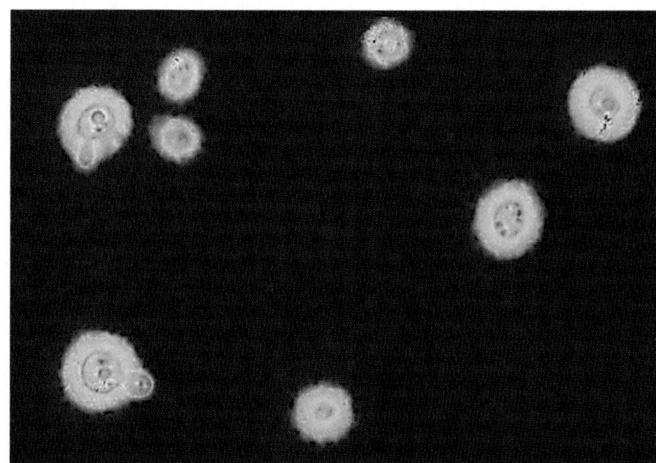

FIGURE 182-4 *Cryptococcus neoformans* in cerebral spinal fluid as seen on India ink stain, in a patient infected with HIV. (*Used with permission from Rebecca Schein, MD.*)

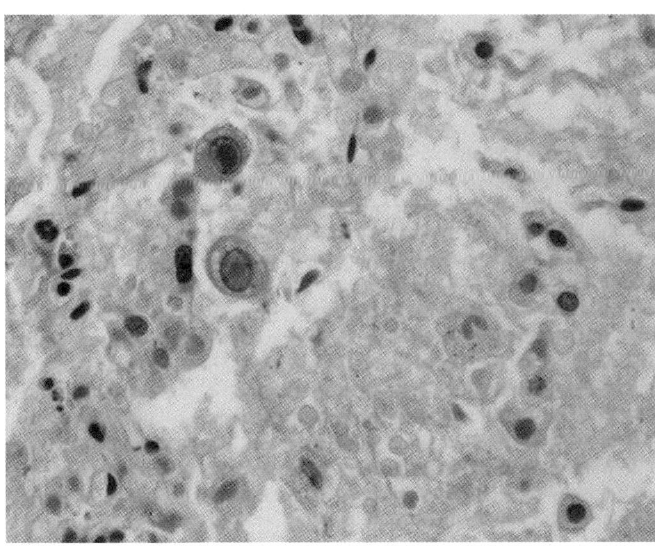

FIGURE 182-5 Cytomegalovirus infection of lung resulting in nucleated giant cells seen on microscopic view of a patient with HIV infection. *(Used with permission from Rebecca Schein, MD.)*

LABORATORY TESTING

- Neonates.
  - Diagnosis in this age group is via HIV DNA PCR because passively acquired maternal antibodies can persist until 18 months of age. Two negative PCR tests after 2 weeks of age effectively rules out infection.[6]
- Adolescents and children >18 months of age.
  - Initial screen is an HIV antibody test via enzyme immunoassay. Rapid testing is available and may be performed on blood or saliva. Confirmation of positive antibody testing is via Western blot.[1]
  - US Preventative Services Task Force recommends one time screening for HIV of all persons 15 to 65 years of age.

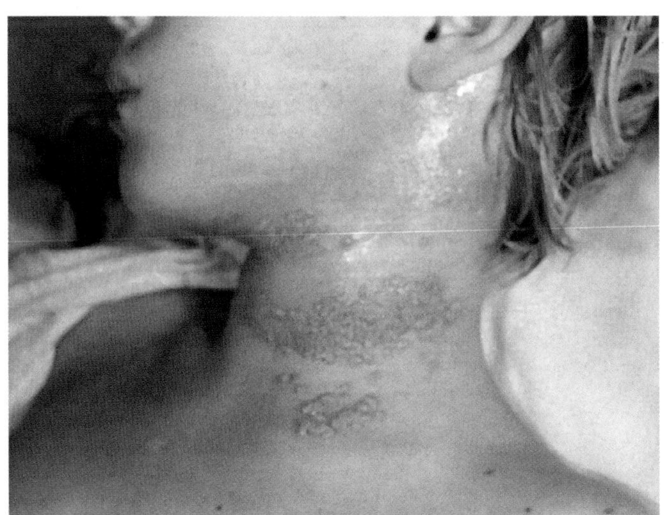

FIGURE 182-6 Herpes simplex skin infection in an immunocompromised child with HIV. *(Used with permission from Bernard Portnoy, MD.)*

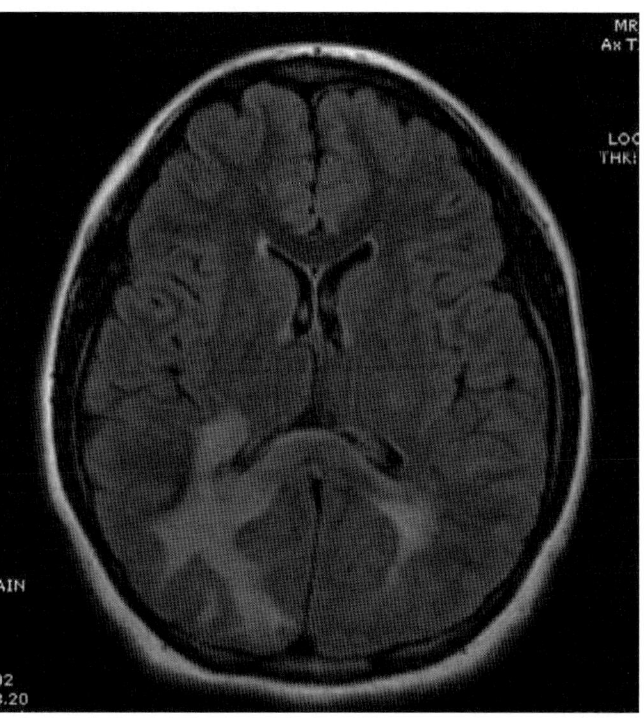

FIGURE 182-7 Progressive multifocal leukoencephalopathy (PML) on MRI image of the brain of a teenage girl with perinatal HIV infection who did not take her medications. She passed away soon after this MRI was taken. *(Used with permission from James Homans, MD.)*

MANAGEMENT

- Current therapy consists of a combination of ARV agents and current recommendations can be found on the National Institutes of Health AIDSinfo website—http://aidsinfo.nih.gov/.
- HIV therapy is based on frequently revised guidelines, viral resistance patterns, and adverse effects of medications. Management in collaboration with experts in pediatric and adolescent HIV care is recommended.
- Treatment is currently recommended for all persons with HIV regardless of CD4 count. Therapy requires a multidisciplinary

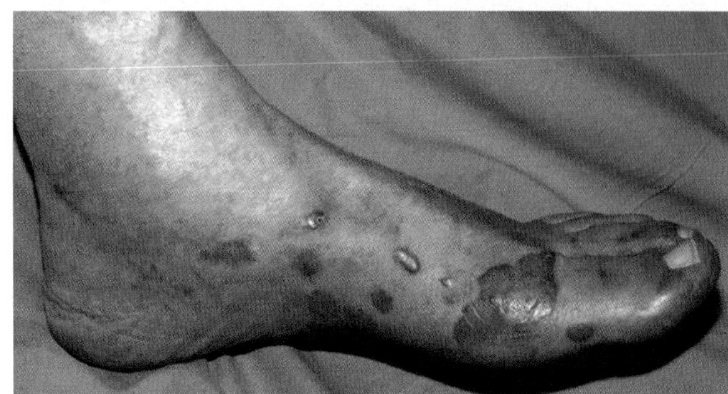

FIGURE 182-8 Kaposi sarcoma in a young adult with HIV infection. *(Used with permission from David Effron, MD.)*

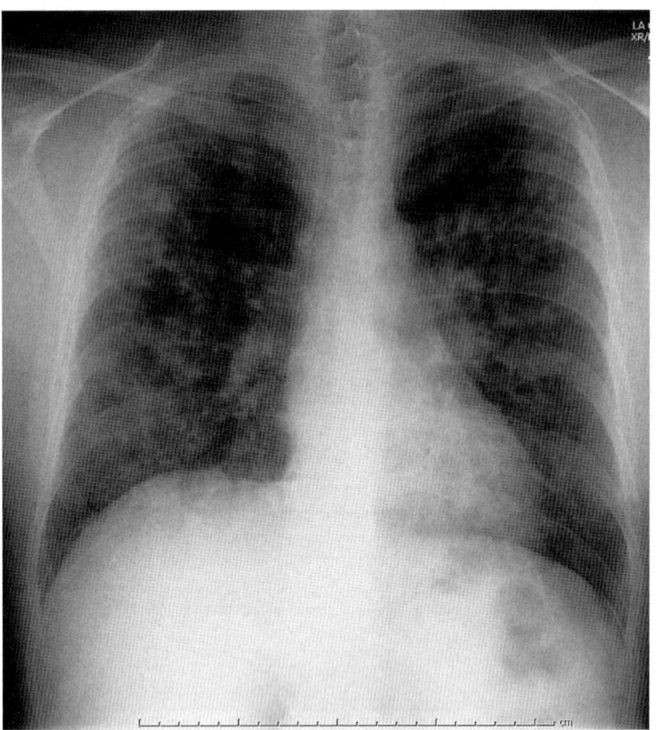

FIGURE 182-9 *Pneumocystis jirovecii* Pneumonia on chest x-ray. (*Used with permission from Rebecca Schein, MD.*)

approach that includes medical care, mental health care, and social support programs.[7]

MEDICATIONS

- Highly Active Anti-Retroviral Therapy or HAART is defined as 3 or more drugs in 2 or more classes.
- ARV agents are directed at blocking viral infection and/or replication and are characterized by their mechanism of action. See **Table 182-1** for further information.[7]

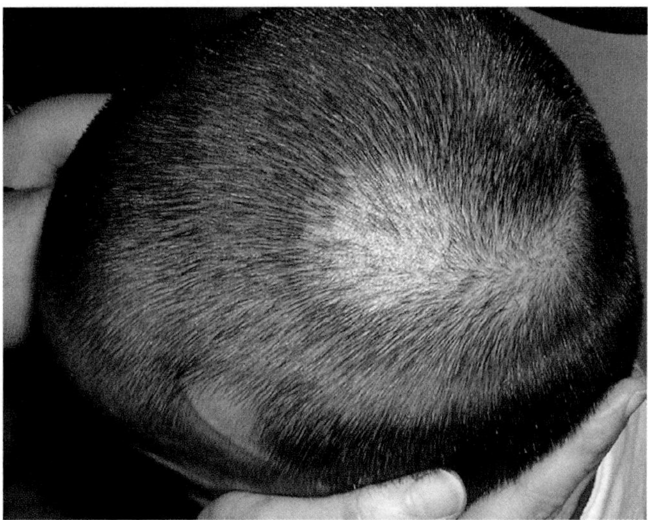

FIGURE 182-10 Tinea capitis in a child with human immunodeficiency virus infection. (*Used with permission from Ann Petru, MD.*)

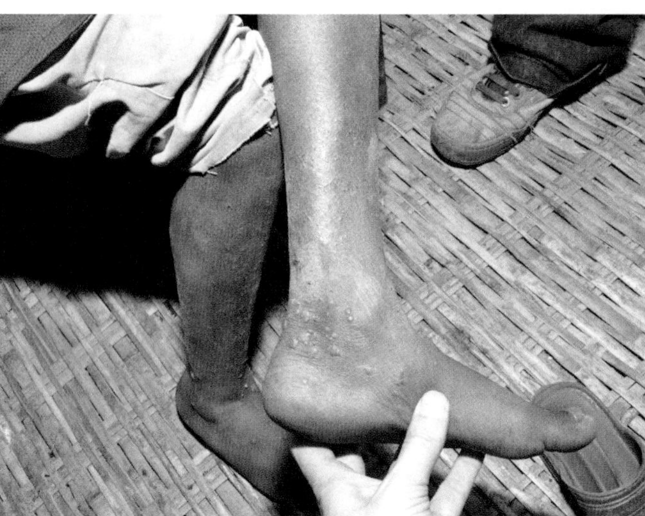

FIGURE 182-11 The cluster of warts on the foot of this African boy prompted an HIV test, which was positive. While warts alone are very common in children, the large cluster of warts was a stimulus to ask about HIV in the family. The mother knew that she was positive for HIV but had resisted having her son tested until this time. (*Used with permission from Richard P. Usatine, MD.*)

PREVENTION AND SCREENING

- Maternal-Child transmission.
  - All pregnant women should be tested for HIV in the first trimester and women with high-risk behaviors should be retested in the third trimester or at delivery.[3] HIV positive women are treated with HAART. Newborn infants are treated with a minimum of six weeks of oral zidovudine (AZT). SOR Ⓐ Additional therapy is recommended on a case by case basis.[8]
- Sexual transmission.
  - Limit numbers of sexual partners, encourage condom use, treat sexually transmitted infections, and encourage partner notification.

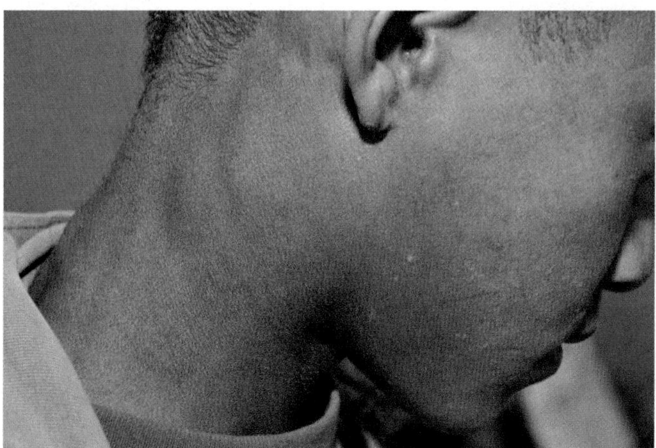

FIGURE 182-12 Cervical lymphadenopathy in an 12-year-old African boy with perinatal HIV infection. (*Used with permission from Richard P. Usatine, MD.*)

TABLE 182-1 Anti-Retroviral Agents

Class	Mechanism of Action	Examples	Additional Information
Entry inhibitors	Either block CCR5 or inhibit membrane fusion	Maraviroc Enfuvirtide	Maraviroc requires trophism testing Enfuvirtide is only injectable
NRTI[1]	Nucleotide analog prevents DNA elongation	Zidovudine Lamivudine Tenofovir	Abacavir causes hypersensitivity reaction Zidovudine (AZT) may result in anemia, lactic acidosis, and GI upset
NNRTI[2]	Bind and inhibit Reverswe Transcriptase	Nevirapine Efavirenz Etravirine	Resistance develops rapidly Very long half-life Efavirenz has CNS side effects and is contra-indicated in 1st trimester of pregnancy
Integrase inhibitor	Block integration into cell genome	Raltegravir Elvitegravir	
Protease inhibitor	Bind and inhibit Protease	Lopinavir Atazanavir Darunavir	Associated with lipodystrophy Ritonavir is used to boost effect of other protease inhibitors

[1]NRTI = Nucleotide Reverse Transcriptase Inhibitor.
[2]NNRTI = Non-nucleotide Reverse Transcriptase Inhibitor.

    - Combination tenofovir plus emtricitabine has been shown to decrease transmission in discordant couples and may be used for preexposure prophylaxis or PrEP.[9] SOR B
- Injection drug use transmission.
    - Encourage use of clean needle programs and avoid needle sharing, methadone maintenance programs, and bleach to disinfect drug paraphernalia.
- Postexposure prophylaxis.
    - If exposure occurs despite interventions then combination anti-retroviral therapy may be used in high-risk cases to prevent infection. Typically treatment should be initiated within 72 hours of exposure and is continued for 28 days.[4] SOR B

PROGNOSIS

- With early and appropriate treatment HIV has become a chronic disease. Further studies are in progress on the long-term effects of the various ARVs. In general, patients are expected to lead full lives.

FOLLOW-UP

- Patients are typically followed at 3- to 4-month intervals. CD4 counts and HIV viral loads are followed to determine response to therapy and additional testing is tailored to evaluate for medication toxicity.[7]

PATIENT EDUCATION

- Counsel patients and their parents regarding the importance of adherence to medication and the risk of resistance of medications.
- Counsel adolescent patients regarding the need and methods to prevent transmission, as previously outlined.

PATIENT RESOURCES

- The Body: the Complete HIV/AIDS Resource—**www.thebody.com**.
- AIDS Alliance for Children, Youth, & Families—**www.aids-alliance.org**.
- Project Inform—**www.projectinform.org**.

PROVIDER RESOURCES

- NIH website: AIDSinfo Offering information on HIV/AIDS treatment, prevention and research—**www.aidsinfo.nih.gov/**.
- CDC website: Act Against AIDS—**www.cdc.gov/actagainstaids/index.html**.
- WHO guidelines on HIV/AIDS—**www.who.int/publications/guidelines/hiv_aids/en/index.html**.

REFERENCES

1. Schneider E, Whitmore S, Glynn MK, et al. Revised Surveillance Case Definitions for HIV Infection Among Adults, Adolescents, and Children Aged <18 Months and for HIV Infection and AIDS Among Children Aged 18 Months to <13 Years—United States, 2008. *MMWR Reccommendations and Reports*. 2008;57(RR10): 1-8.
2. American Academy of Pediatrics: Human Immunodeficiency Virus Infection. In *Red Book: 2012 Report of the Committee on Infectious Disease,* edited by LK Pickering, CJ Baker, DW Kimberlin, SS Long. Elk Grove Village, IL: American Academy of Pediatrics; 2012:418-438.

3. Chou, R, Cantor AG, Zakher B, Bougatsos C: Screening for HIV in Pregnant Women: Systematic Review to Update the 2005 U.S. Preventive Services Task Force Recommendation. *Annals of Internal Medicine.* 2012;157(10):719-728.

4. Landovitz, RJ, Currier, JS: Postexposure Prophylaxis for HIV Infection. *The New England Journal of Medicine.* 2009;361(18):1768-1775.

5. Recommendations from CDC, the National Institutes of Health,the HIV Medicine Association of the Infectious Diseases Society, and the American Academy of Pediatrics: Guidelines for the Prevention and Treatment of Opportunistic Infections Among HIV-Exposed and HIV-Infected Children. *MMWR Reccommendations and Reports.* 2009;58(RR-11):1-165.

6. Read, JS: From the American Academy of Pediatrics: Diagnosis of HIV-1 Infection in Children Younger Than 18 Months in the United States. *Pediatrics.* 2007;120(6):e1547-e1562.

7. HHS Panel on Antiretroviral Therapy and Medical Mangement of HIV-infected Children: Guidelines for the Use of Antiretroviral Agents in Pediatric HIV Infection. http://aidsinfo.nih.gov/contentfiles/PediatricGuidelines.pdf.

8. Nielsen-Saines, K, Watts, H and Veloso, VG, et al. Three postpartum Antiretroviral regimens to prevent intrapatum infection. *The New England Journal of Medicine.* 2012;366(25):2368-2379.

9. Smith, DK, Thigpen, M and Nesheim, S, et al. Interim Guidance for Clinicians Considering the Use of Preexposure Prophylaxis for the Prevention of HIV Infection in Heterosexually Active Adults. *MMWR.* 2012;61(31):586-589.

183 LYME DISEASE

Thomas J. Corson, DO
Richard P. Usatine, MD
Camille Sabella, MD

PATIENT STORY

On a warm, summer afternoon an 11-year-old girl presents having had low-grade fevers for 4 days and a rash. On physical examination, the pediatrician notes annular eruptions with erythema on her shoulder and legs (**Figure 183-1**). The mother states that the rash has gotten progressively larger during the last 3 days and her daughter complains of intermittent joint pain. She does not recall being bitten by an insect. She denies taking medications within the last month and has no known allergies. When asked about recent travel, the mother admits to taking the family on a camping trip in eastern Massachusetts with a return of 5 days ago. The patient was diagnosed with Lyme borreliosis (acute Lyme disease) and started on doxycycline 100 mg twice daily for 14 days. She responded quickly to the antibiotics and never developed the late stage of Lyme disease.

INTRODUCTION

Lyme disease is an infection caused by the spirochete *Borrelia burgdorferi*, transmitted via tick bite. Most cases of Lyme disease occur in the northeast between April and November. Patients experience flu-like symptoms and may develop the pathognomonic rash, erythema migrans. Lyme disease is prevented by avoiding exposure to the tick vector using insect repellent and protective clothing.

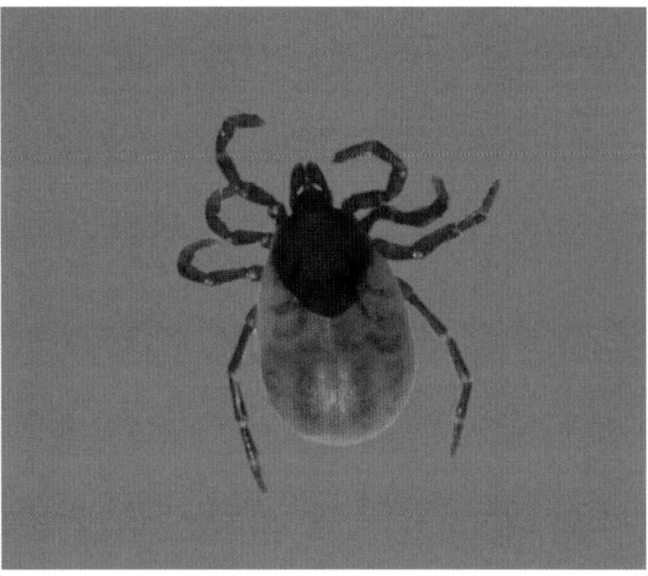

FIGURE 183-2 The deer tick transmits the *Borrelia* spirochete. This is an unengorged female black-legged deer tick. The tick is tiny and can be undetected in its unengorged state. (*Used with permission from Thomas Corson, MD.*)

EPIDEMIOLOGY

- In 1977, clusters of patients in Old Lyme, Connecticut, began reporting symptoms originally thought to be juvenile rheumatoid arthritis.[1]
- In 1981, American entomologist, Dr. Willy Burgdorfer, isolated the infectious pathogen responsible for Lyme disease from the midgut of *Ixodes scapularis* (a.k.a., black-legged deer ticks; **Figure 183-2**), which serve as the primary transmission vector in the US.[1]
- It was identified as a bacterial spirochete and named *B. burgdorferi* in honor of its founder.

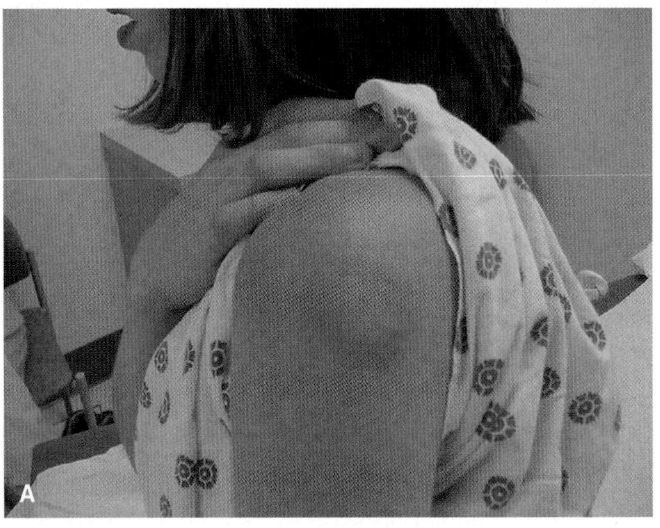

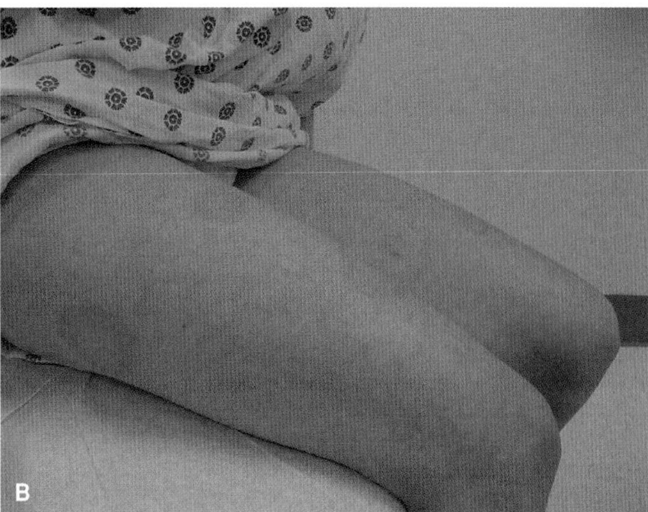

FIGURE 183-1 An 11-year-old girl with early disseminated Lyme disease presenting with multiple erythema migrans (EM) lesions, low grade fever and some intermittent joint pain. **A.** EM with its annular configuration on her shoulder. **B.** Multiple rings of EM on her legs. (*Used with permission from Jeremy Golding, MD.*)

- Based on Centers for Disease Control and Prevention (CDC) data reported in 2007, Lyme disease (or Lyme borreliosis) is the most common tickborne illness in the US, with an overall incidence of 7.9 per 100,000 persons.[2]
- In 2010, 94 percent of Lyme disease cases were reported from 12 states: Connecticut, Delaware, Maine, Maryland, Massachusetts, Minnesota, New Jersey, New Hampshire, New York, Pennsylvania, Virginia, and Wisconsin.[3]
- Patients living between Maryland and Maine accounted for 93 percent of all reported cases in the US in 2005, with an overall incidence of 31.6 cases for every 100,000 persons.[2]
- The incidence is highest among children 5 to 14 years of age, and more than 90 percent of cases report onset between April and November.[2]

ETIOLOGY AND PATHOPHYSIOLOGY

- *B. burgdorferi* begins to multiply in the midgut of *I. scapularis* ticks upon attaching to humans.
- Migration from midgut to salivary glands of ticks requires 24 to 48 hours.
- Prior to this migration, host infection rarely occurs.
- Common hosts include field mice, white-tailed deer, and household pets.
- Ticks must feed on infested hosts in order to infect humans.
- Thirty percent of infected patients do not recall being bitten.[4]
- Once a human is infected, disease progression is categorized into three clinical stages: early localized, early disseminated, and late disseminated.

DIAGNOSIS

CLINICAL FEATURES

Early Localized (3 to 32 days after tick bite)

- Erythema migrans (formerly known as erythema chronicum migrans)—This pathognomonic finding occurs in roughly 68 percent of Lyme disease cases.[4] Described as a "bull's-eye" eruption (**Figures 183-1** and **183-3**), this nonpruritic, maculopapular lesion typically occurs near the site of infection. The erythematous perimeter migrates outward over several days while the central area clears. Erythema migrans can persist for 2 to 3 weeks if left untreated.
- Flu-like symptoms—Roughly 67 percent of patients will develop flu-like symptoms that can include fever, myalgias, headache, malaise, and lymphadenopathy. Symptoms usually subside within 7 to 10 days.

Early Disseminated (3 to 10 weeks after tick bite)

- *Erythema migrans*—Multiple lesions (**Figure 183-4**).
    - May develop as a consequence of bacteremic dissemination to multiple sites.
    - About 25 percent of children are first diagnosed with Lyme disease based on these lesions.
    - Lesions are usually smaller than primary lesions and often accompanied by flu-like symptoms.

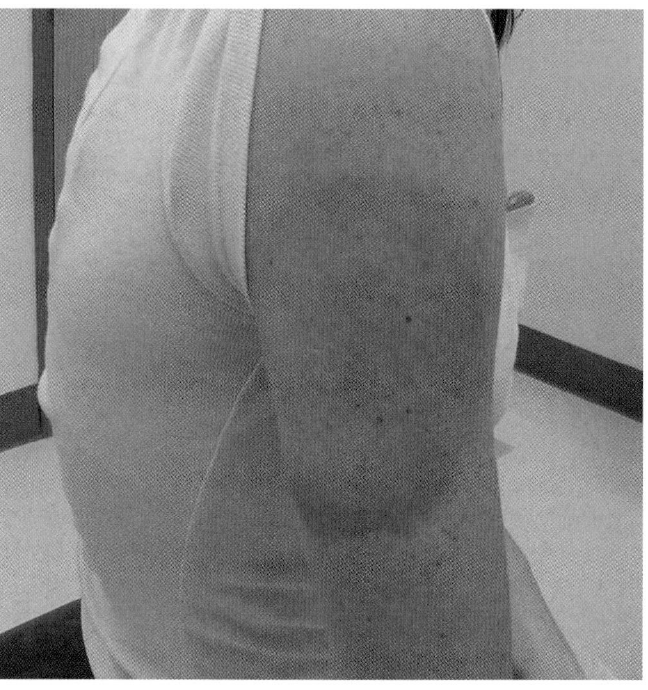

FIGURE 183-3 A 12-year-old girl with erythema migrans eruption on her right arm. The annular border is somewhat raised and there is central clearing. (*Used with permission from Jeremy Golding, MD.*)

- Cranial nerve palsy—Bell's palsy (seventh cranial nerve) is the most common neurologic manifestation of Lyme disease, occurring in 3 to 5 percent of children with Lyme disease. However, nearly every cranial nerve has been reported to be involved. Facial nerve palsy is a lower motor neuron lesion that results in weakness of both the lower face and the forehead. Lasting up to 8 weeks, the resolution of symptoms is gradual, begins shortly after initial onset, and does not appear to be influenced by antimicrobial therapy (see Chapter 202, Bell's Palsy).
- Aseptic meningitis—Patients may present with complaints similar to bacterial meningitis (photophobia, nuchal rigidity, and

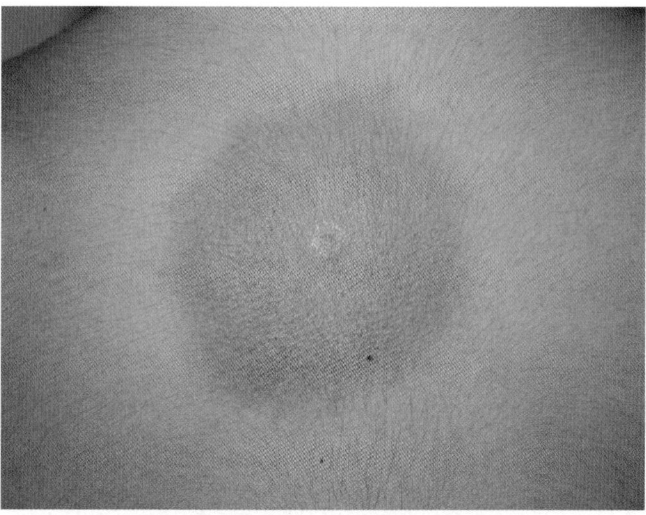

FIGURE 183-4 Erythema migrans on the back of an 11-year-old boy who was camping in Western Pennsylvania. The central papule/excoriated lesion is the site of the bite and some central clearing is visible. (*Used with permission from Charles B. Foster, MD.*)

headache), but symptoms are generally less severe in nature. This can also occur with or without concomitant cranial nerve palsy.[4]

- Atrioventricular blockade—This is a very uncommon finding in children with Lyme disease. When it does occur, syncope, lightheadedness, and dyspnea are classic symptoms consistent with atrioventricular (AV) dysfunction.[3] However, patients can be completely asymptomatic. The degree of Lyme-associated blockade varies so that symptoms are generally episodic. Most cases resolve spontaneously within 1 week.[4]
- All of the following can be accompanied by nonspecific signs and symptoms as fatigue, myalgia, headache, fever, and lymphadenopathy.

Late Disseminated Disease (2 to 12 months after tick bite)

- Arthritis—This is generally a monoarticular arthritis involving the knee (90%), although other sites such as the shoulder, ankle, elbow, or wrist may be involved. Approximately 7 percent of children with Lyme disease will have this as their presenting manifestation.[4] Swelling and tenderness of the joint, along with an effusion is most common. With treatment, the arthritis resolves over days to weeks, although recurrence occurs in 5 to 10 percent of treated patients and usually resolves with retreatment. An immune mediated chronic arthritis has been rarely associated in adults with Lyme disease but is extremely rare in children.[5]
- Children who are adequately treated for Lyme disease in the early stages almost never develop late manifestations.

LABORATORY TESTING

Diagnosing Lyme disease is generally based on pertinent history findings and/or the presence of an erythema migrans lesion, especially in endemic areas. In cases where an erythema migrans lesion is absent, serologic testing may be warranted utilizing the following tests:

- Enzyme-linked immunosorbent assay (ELISA; sensitivity: 94%, specificity: 97%)[6]—Used as a *screening* test in patients lacking physical signs of erythema migrans. Up to 50 percent of patients with early infection can have a false-negative result. Thus, serologic testing is generally not recommended in the first 4 weeks of the illness. If strong suspicion remains, convalescent titers should be obtained in 6 weeks.[6] Prior infection does not indicate immunity. Lyme titers may be falsely positive in patients with mononucleosis, periodontal disease, connective tissue disease, and other less common conditions.[7]
- Western blot (immunoglobulin [Ig] M and IgG for *B. burgdorferi*)—If ELISA test yields a positive result, Western blot test is used as a *confirmatory* test. IgM antibodies are detectable between 2 weeks and 6 months after inoculation. IgG may be present indefinitely after 6 weeks, despite appropriate antibiotic therapy. Once it is determined that a person is seropositive for Lyme disease, antibiotic therapy should be initiated promptly. Repeat testing to assess for success of therapy should not be performed, as positive serologic tests may persist indefinitely.
- Because of the frequency of false positive serologic results of Lyme testing, the American Academy of Pediatrics state that, "The widespread practice of ordering serologic tests for patients with nonspecific symptoms, such as fatigue or arthralgia, who have a low probability of having Lyme disease or because of parental pressure, is discouraged. Almost all positive serologic test results in these patients are false-positive results. In areas with endemic infection, subclinical infection and seroconversion also can occur, and the patient's symptoms merely are coincidental. Patients with acute Lyme disease almost always have objective signs of infection (e.g., erythema migrans, facial nerve palsy, arthritis). Nonspecific symptoms commonly accompany these specific signs but almost never are the only evidence of Lyme disease."[8]

Empiric antibiotic therapy (no test necessary) should be considered in any of the following clinical presentations: presence of EM rash, flu-like symptoms (in absence of upper respiratory infection [URI] or GI symptoms) after known tick bite, Bell's palsy in endemic areas, especially between June and September, and tick bites occurring during pregnancy.

CHARACTERISTIC LABORATORY FINDINGS

- Complete blood count (CBC)—Leukocytosis (11,000 to 18,000/μL). Anemia and thrombocytopenia are rare.
- Elevated erythrocyte sedimentation rate (ESR) (>20 mm/h).
- Elevated γ-glutamyltransferase (GGT) and aspartate aminotransferase (AST).
- Cerebrospinal fluid—Pleocytosis and elevated protein levels if central nervous system (CNS) is involved. Spirochete antibodies may be detectable.
- Blood culture—Low yield; not recommended.
- Nerve conduction studies and EM—Useful in patients with paresthesias or radicular pain.

DIFFERENTIAL DIAGNOSIS[9]

- Cellulitis—Spreads more rapidly than Lyme disease. Induration and tenderness are more common (see Chapter 103, Cellulitis).
- Urticaria—Can resemble erythema migrans when the urticarial lesions are annular. Urticaria is generally more widespread and the wheals come and go over time whereas the lesion of EM is more fixed (see Chapter 134, Urticaria and Angioedema).
- Rocky Mountain spotted fever—Associated with *Dermacentor variabilis* (American dog) tick; rash is petechial and the spots are widely distributed over the body (see Chapter 175, Henoch Schonlein Purpura, **Figure 175-5**). Patients often appear toxic.
- Cutaneous fungal infections—Usually pruritic and may be annular; associated with scaling, which is not characteristic of erythema migrans; and spreads slowly if at all. The similarity is that the annular appearance of tinea corporis can mimic EM (see Chapter 123, Tinea Corporis).
- Local reaction to tick bites—Tick bites may cause a local reaction in skin and do not expand with time; generally less than 2 cm in diameter, and are usually papular.
- Febrile viral illnesses (particularly enteroviruses during summer)—Rash, myalgias, arthralgias, and headache; GI symptoms; sore throat and/or cough.
- Facial nerve palsy—May be bilateral in Lyme disease. This is uncommon in facial nerve palsy not associated with Lyme disease (see Chapter 202, Bell's Palsy).

- Viral meningitis—Lymphocytic (aseptic) meningitis caused by viral infection generally results in transient illness that resolves within several days, usually after a monophasic course.
- Juvenile idiopathic arthritis may be indistinguishable from acute arthritis associated with Lyme disease. Serologic testing and clinical history can help to discriminate (see Chapter 172, Juvenile Idiopathic Arthritis).

MANAGEMENT

MEDICATIONS

▶ Early localized disease

- Eight years of age and older—Doxycycline 4 mg/kg divided twice a day up to 100 mg/dose for 14 to 21 days.[5] SOR Ⓐ
- Younger than 8 years of age or for those who can't tolerate Doxycycline—Amoxicillin 50 mg/kg divided 3 times a day up to 500 mg per dose or cefuroxime 30 mg/kg divided twice a day up to 1000 mg per dose for 14 to 21 days.

▶ Early disseminated disease and late disease

- Multiple erythema migrans—Same oral regimen as for early localized disease, but for 21 days.
- Isolated facial palsy—Same oral regimen as for early localized disease, but for 14 to 21 days.
- Arthritis—Same oral regimen as for early localized disease, but for 28 days.
- Persistent or recurrent arthritis—Ceftriaxone sodium, 50 to 75 mg/kg, IV, once a day (maximum 2 g/day) for 14 to 28 days.
    - Alternatives: Penicillin, 200 000 to 400 000 U/kg per day, IV, given in divided doses every 4 h (maximum 18 to 24 million U/day) for 14 to 28 days.
    - Cefotaxime 150 to 200 mg/kg per day, IV, divided into 3 or 4 doses (maximum 6 g/day) for 14 to 28 days.
    - Same oral regimen as for early disease (retreatment) but for 28 days.

▶ Atrioventricular heart block or carditis

- Oral regimen as for early disease if asymptomatic but for 14 to 21 days. Ceftriaxone or penicillin IV for symptomatic: see persistent or recurrent arthritis for dosing, but for 14 to 21 days.

▶ Meningitis

- Ceftriaxone 50 to 75 mg/kg IV up to a maximum of 2 g/day for 14 days; alternative therapy cefotaxime 150 to 200 mg/kg per day up to a maximum of 6 g/day, divided into 3 to 4 doses per day.[5] SOR Ⓑ
- Doxycycline (oral) 100 to 200 mg twice a day for 14 days.[5] SOR Ⓑ

REFERRAL OR HOSPITALIZATION

- Consider referring patients in whom the diagnosis is unclear, have severe clinical manifestations, or who do not respond to initial therapy.

PREVENTION

- Avoid exposure to ticks by using protective clothing and tick repellant. If hiking in tick-infested areas check body daily for ticks and promptly remove any attached ticks.
- Prophylactic doxycycline (1 dose of 200 mg) is recommended only if the tick is identified as an adult or nymphal *I. scapularis* tick that has been attached for at least 36 hours; medication can be started within 72 hours of tick removal; local rate of infection of ticks with *B. burgdorferi* is at least 20 percent; and doxycycline is not contraindicated.[5]

PROGNOSIS

- The outcome for children who receive conventional appropriate antimicrobial therapy is excellent.
- Non-specific symptoms such as fatigue, arthralgia or myalgia may continue after appropriate treatment, but will resolve over weeks to months. This is not due to persistence of the organism and repeated courses of antibiotics are not effective in hastening resolution of these symptoms.[3]
- True treatment failures are uncommon and prolonged oral or parenteral antibiotic courses are emphatically discouraged. In patients who continue to present with residual subjective symptoms, providers should seek alternate diagnoses and/or referral to an appropriate specialist.

FOLLOW-UP

Follow patients during antibiotic therapy through recovery.

PATIENT EDUCATION

Prevention is accomplished by reducing exposure to ticks. If you live in an area that has Lyme disease then use protective clothing, tick repellent, tick checks, and other simple measures to prevent tick bites. This is especially important during the high-risk months of April through November. Patients should know the early signs of Lyme disease so that they can get care early when it is most curable.

If a tick is found on the skin, remove it early using fine-tipped tweezers. See the following patient resources.

PATIENT RESOURCES

- Centers for Disease Control and Prevention (CDC). *Lyme Disease*—**www.cdc.gov/lyme/**.
- Centers for Disease Control and Prevention (CDC). *Tick Removal*—**www.cdc.gov/lyme/removal/index.html**.

PROVIDER RESOURCE

- Centers for Disease Control and Prevention (CDC). *Lyme Disease*—**www.cdc.gov/lyme/**.

REFERENCES

1. Sternbach G, Dibble CL. Willy Burgdorfer: Lyme disease. *J Emerg Med.* 1996;14(5):631-634.
2. Centers for Disease Control and Prevention. Lyme disease—United States, 2003 2005. *MMWR Morb Mortal Wkly Rep.* 2007; 56(23):573-576.
3. Centers for Disease Control and Prevention. *Lyme Disease.* http://www.cdc.gov/lyme, accessed December 7, 2013.
4. Meyerhoff JO. *Lyme Disease.* http://emedicine.medscape.com/article/330178, accessed December 7, 2013.
5. Wormser GP, Dattwyler RJ, Shapiro ED, et al. The clinical assessment, treatment, and prevention of lyme disease, human granulocytic anaplasmosis, and babesiosis: clinical practice guidelines by the Infectious Diseases Society of America. *Clin Infect Dis.* 2006; 43(9):1089-1134.
6. *Lyme Disease Executive Summary.* http://www.harp.org/eng/kaiserslymesummary.htm, accessed December 7, 2013.
7. Columbia University Medical Center Lyme and Tick-Borne Diseases Research Center. http://www.columbia-lyme.org/, accessed December 7, 2013.
8. American Academy of Pediatrics. Lyme disease. *Red Book: 2012 Report of the Committee on Infectious Diseases.* Pickering LK, ed. 29th ed. Elk Grove Village, IL: American Academy of Pediatrics; 2012: 474, 479.
9. American College of Physicians. *Differential Diagnosis of Lyme Disease.* http://www.acponline.org/journals/news/jun07/critters.pdf, accessed December 7, 2013.

184 EPSTEIN BARR VIRUS INFECTIONS (INFECTIOUS MONONUCLEOSIS)

Blanca E. Gonzalez, MD

PATIENT STORY

A 16-year-old boy comes to see his pediatrician because of a 7-day history of intense sore throat, fever, malaise, and abdominal pain. He also complains of bilateral neck swelling and tenderness. On examination, he has markedly enlarged tonsils with bilateral whitish exudates, and very large lymph nodes palpable in the posterior neck bilaterally (**Figure 184-1**). In addition, his spleen is palpable at 1 cm below the left costal margin. A heterophile antibody test (monospot) is positive and he is offered symptomatic treatment. His symptoms persist for about 10 days, after which he recovers completely.

INTRODUCTION

Epstein Barr virus (EBV) is a DNA virus that belongs to the Herpes virus family. It is the most common etiological agent of infectious mononucleosis, a clinical syndrome characterized by fever, pharyngitis and cervical lymphadenopathy. Rarely, encephalitis, myocarditis, and hemolytic anemia can develop as a consequence of EBV infections.[1] In the immunocompromised host, this virus can cause life-threatening infections.[2]

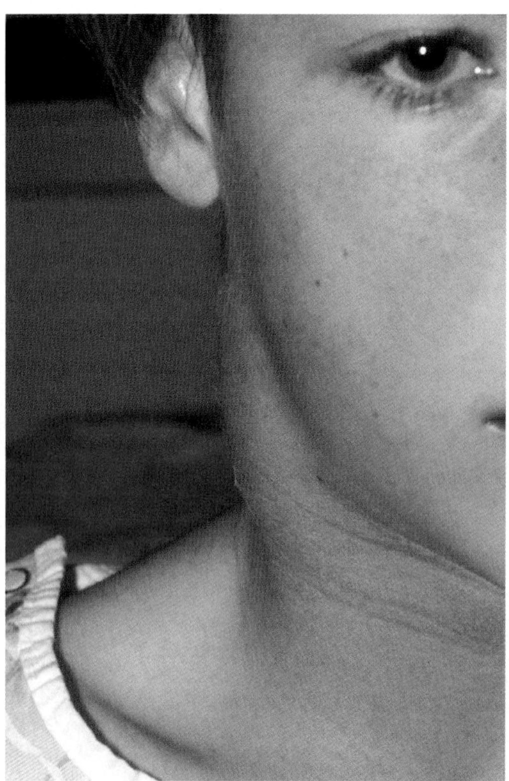

FIGURE 184-1 Posterior cervical lymphadenopathy in an adolescent with infectious mononucleosis. (*Used with permission from Johanna Goldfarb, MD.*)

SYNONYMS

EBV infection is synonymous with infectious mononucleosis although infectious mononucleosis can be caused by other viruses such as cytomegalovirus (CMV). Other terms associated with EBV are glandular syndrome and human herpes virus 4. It is referred to as "the kissing disease" in the popular vernacular.

EPIDEMIOLOGY

- Ubiquitous in the environment.
- In developed countries, EBV infections are not common in infants and young children. In contrast, in developing nations, 90 percent of children less than 6 years of age have been exposed to the virus.[1,3,4]
- The majority of primary infections occur in adolescents and young adults.
- By adulthood, greater than 90 percent have serological evidence of previous EBV exposure.
- The virus has no defined seasonal variations and occurs year round with slightly higher incidence during summer months.[5–7]
- Oral secretions are the main source of transmission; that is, deep kissing, toddlers sharing toys.[8]
- In childhood, EBV infections may be asymptomatic.
- EBV infection results in infectious mononucleosis in 30 to 40 percent of adolescents.
- Incubation 30 to 50 days.

ETIOLOGY AND PATHOPHYSIOLOGY

- The virus infects epithelial cells in the tonsillar crypts and B lymphocytes.[2]
- The virus is disseminated throughout the reticuloendothelial system (tonsils, spleen, and lymph nodes) by the infected B cells.
- CD4 and CD8 T cell responses are activated.
- The virus establishes permanent latent infections in the host.
- Disease severity may be related to high numbers of NK and $CD8^+$ T cells and elevated blood viral loads.[8]

RISK FACTORS

- In developed countries, teenagers and college students are the highest risk group. Behaviors such as "deep kissing"[8] and sexual activity are risk factors for primary EBV infections.
- Immunocompromised hosts, including patients with diabetes, HIV, transplant patients, and patients on immunomodulators are at risk of developing severe manifestations of EBV infections.

DIAGNOSIS

- Infectious Mononucleosis—The classical presentation consists of the triad of fever, exudative pharyngitis and lymphadenopathy.
- Younger children may present with mild symptoms, or may present with fever as their only sign of infection.
- Constitutional symptoms such as fever, myalgias, malaise, and headache may precede the lymphadenopathy and pharyngitis by 3 to 5 days.
- Cervical lymphadenopathy can be significant and give the neck the appearance of "bull's neck." The posterior cervical chains are commonly involved. Epitrochlear nodes can also be enlarged (**Figure 184-1**).[9,10] Splenomegaly occurs in 80 percent of the patients and may lead to splenic rupture after mild trauma.[11,12]
- Hepatomegaly is less common.
- Fatigue is a common feature and often persists throughout the course of illness.

OCULAR MANIFESTATIONS

- Periorbital edema may be the presenting sign of infectious mononucleosis and can be confused with cellulitis.[13,14]
- Oculo-glandular syndromes (eyelid swelling with non-tender pre-auricular lymphadenopathy).[15,16]
- Less commonly keratitis, uveitis and acute retinal necrosis.[17,18]

DERMATOLOGICAL MANIFESTATIONS

- A rash may be present in 10 percent of the patients. The rash is morbilliform and usually is present over the trunk and arms (**Figure 184-2**). Occasionally the rash may be urticarial or petechial.[19–21]
- Over 90 percent will develop a rash if exposed to ampicillin.[20]
- Papular acrodermatitis, also known as Gianotti-Crosti syndrome, has been associated with EBV.[21] It tends to occur in infancy and early childhood (**Figure 184-3**).
- Erythema nodosum (**Figure 184-4**).

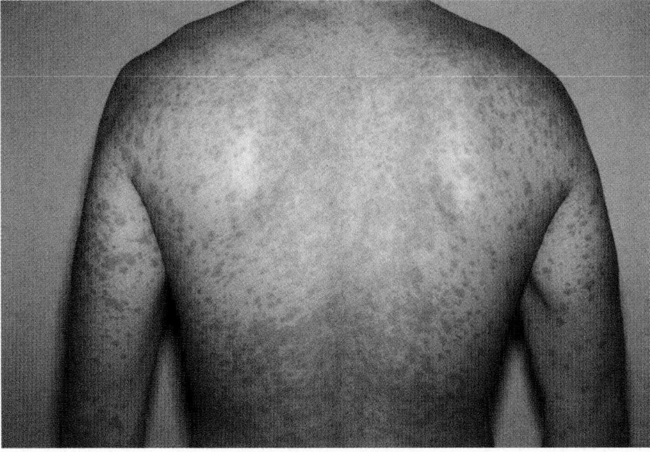

FIGURE 184-2 Morbilliform rash in an adolescent with infectious mononucleosis. (*Used with permission from Johanna Goldfarb, MD.*)

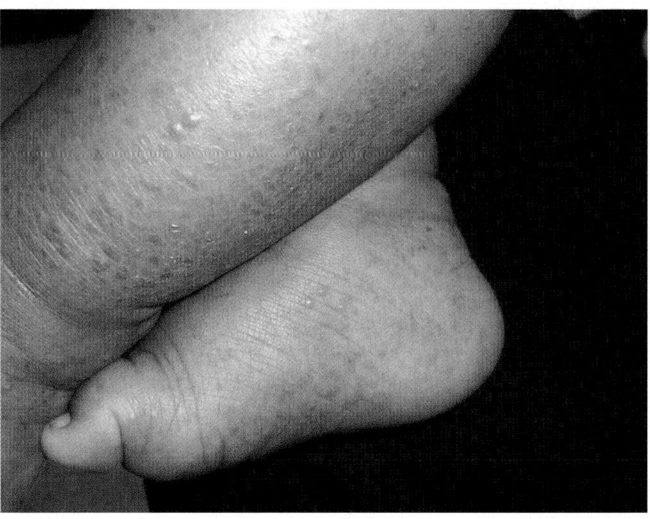

FIGURE 184-3 Papular acrodermatitis (also known as Gianotti-Crosti syndrome) in an infant. (*Used with permission from Richard P. Usatine, MD.*)

- Genital ulcerations in adolescent girls can be seen in conjunction with EBV infections (Ulcus Vulvae Acutum). They can be single or multiple and very painful.[22,23]

CENTRAL NERVOUS SYSTEM MANIFESTATIONS

- The virus may affect central and peripheral and nervous system and has been associated with encephalitis, meningitis, encephalomyelitis, and radiculitis.[24]

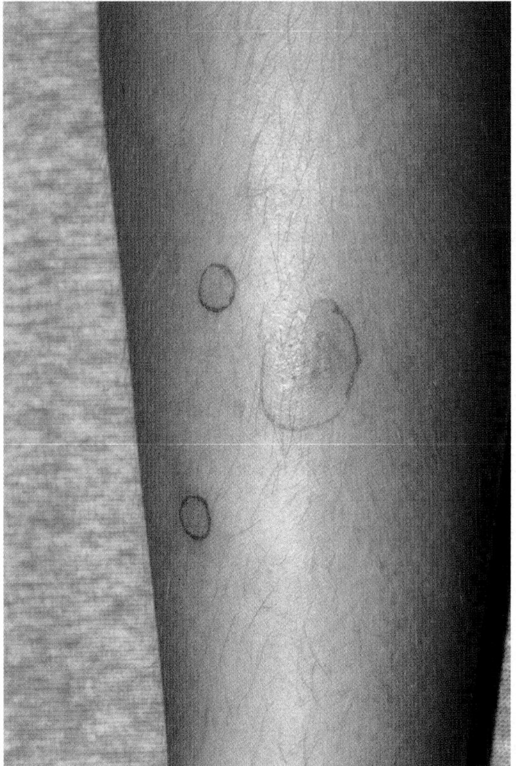

FIGURE 184-4 Erythema nodosum distributed over the shins of this adolescent. These are painful nodules and are associated with many infections, including EBV infection. (*Used with permission from Camille Sabella, MD.*)

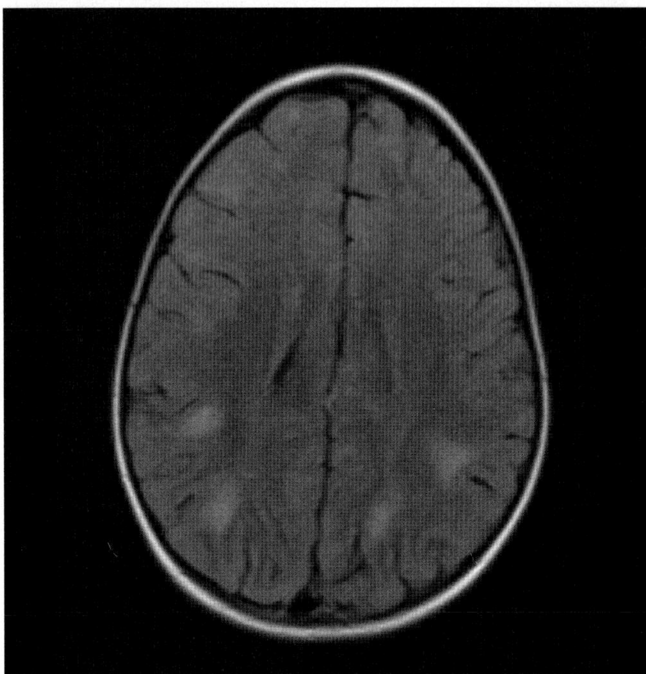

FIGURE 184-5 Acute disseminated encephalomyelitis. Note the hypodense areas in the occipital and parietal areas. Many different etiologic agents have been associated with ADEM, including EBV infections. (*Used with permission from Neil Friedman, MD.*)

- Acute disseminated encephalomyelitis (ADEM; **Figure 184-5**).[25]
- Alice in Wonderland syndrome—Associated with EBV and consists of abnormal perceptions where patients experience distortions of forms, size, or colors. Children will say objects look long, or small or different. This condition usually transient and improves with the improvement of the infectious mononucleosis.[26]

OTHER MANIFESTATIONS OF EBV INFECTIONS[1,2]

- Carditis, pericarditis.
- Pneumonia.
- Hemolytic anemia.
- Transient thrombocytopenic purpura.
- Interstitial nephritis.

ASSOCIATED MALIGNANT PROCESSES WITH EBV IN CHILDREN[2]

- Burkitt's lymphoma.
- Hodgkin's disease (**Figure 184-6**).
- X-linked lymphoproliferative syndrome (XLPS).
- Leiomyosarcoma in children with Human Immunodeficiency virus (HIV) or immunodeficiencies (i.e., transplant) and post-transplant lymphoproliferative disorder (PTLD) after organ transplantation.

LABORATORY TESTING

- Atypical lymphocytes—Reactive lymphocytes that are larger and with dents in the cytoplasm (**Figure 184-7**). They are also present

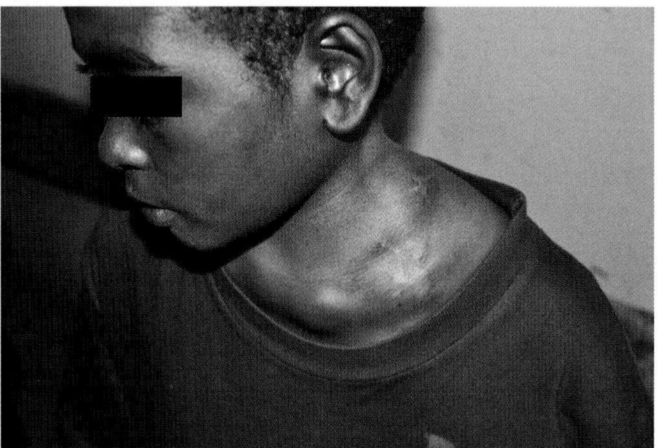

FIGURE 184-6 Cervical and supraclavicular lymphadenopathy in a boy with Hodgkin's disease. (*Used with permission from Richard P. Usatine, MD.*)

with CMV infections. Less commonly present in other viral illnesses.[27]

- Heterophile antibody—These are nonspecific antibodies that cross react with many antigens. The monospot detects these antibodies using slide tests with horse or sheep red blood cells. These antibodies are most elevated between 2 to 5 weeks of illness and may be negative in the first weeks of the disease process. The test is usually negative in 10 to 50 percent of children under the age of 4 years. Overall sensitivity of the test is around 80 percent and the specificity is around 89 to 100 percent. Therefore, a negative monospot does not exclude EBV.[1,28]
- Cytomegalovirus associated infectious mononucleosis is monospot negative.[29]
- Serologies—Four specific EBV antibodies are used to establish the diagnosis: Early antigen, viral capsid antibody (VCA) IgM, VCA IgG, and Epstein Barr nuclear antigen (EBNA) IgG (**Figure 184-8**).[30] These are used to make the diagnosis in younger children in whom

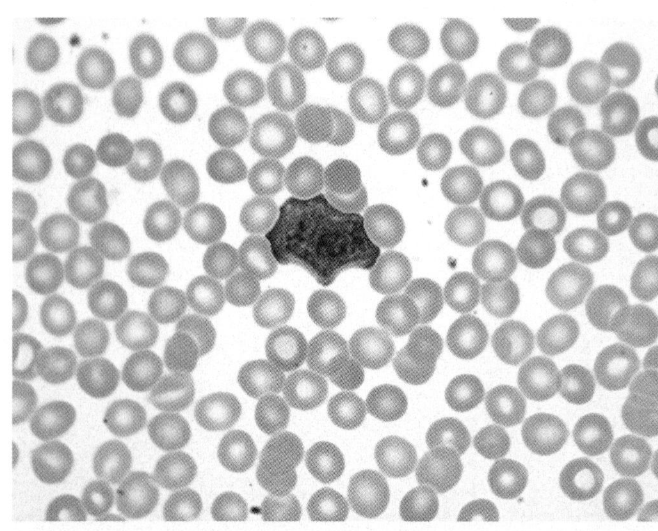

FIGURE 184-7 Atypical lymphocyte with indentation of the nuclei on a peripheral blood smear, characteristic of infectious mononucleosis. (*Used with permission from Eric Hsi, MD.*)

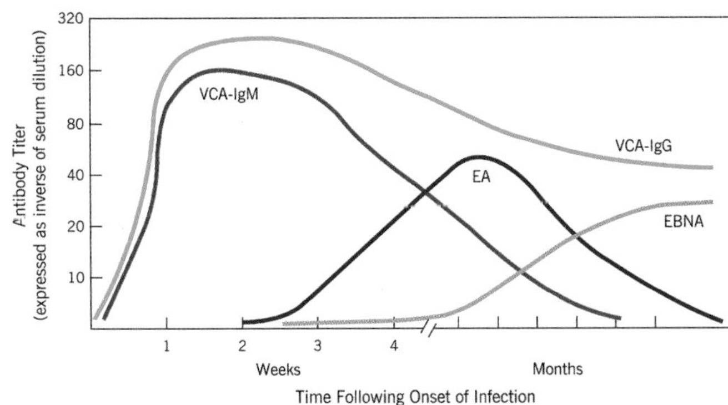

FIGURE 184-8 EBV antibodies during infectious mononucleosis. The first antibodies to appear are IgM and IgG against the viral capside antigen (IgM VCA and IGG VCA). The IgM VCA rises quickly and remains positive for approximately 4 months. The IgG VCA remains positive for life after the infection. The early antigen (EA) antibody follows the VCA antibodies and may remain positive for more than 6 months and in some patients may be positive lifelong. The Epstein Barr nuclear antigen (EBNA) is the last antibody to appear 1 to 3 months after the infection and usually remains positive for life.[1,30]

the heterophile antibody test may negative or when the heterophile antibody test is negative and infectious mononucleosis remains suspected.

- Polymerase chain reaction (PCR) is utilized to detect the virus in CSF when central nervous system complications are suspected or to measure the viral load in blood of immunocompromised patients.[31,32]

DIFFERENTIAL DIAGNOSIS[33]

- CMV—Causes a heterophile-negative infectious mononucleosis syndrome and can be indistinguishable from EBV infection. Diagnosis usually made with serology.
- Toxoplasmosis—May present with similar features to EBV infection. The pharyngitis features and less pronounced and splenomegaly often absent.
- Acute retroviral syndrome (acute HIV)—Should be suspected as a cause of heterophile-negative infectious mononucleosis syndrome, especially if there is a history of possible epidemiological exposure.
- Hepatitis A—Commonly causes fever, nausea and jaundice, but not often with pharyngitis and lymphadenopathy.
- Adenovirus—Usually more acute presentation and not associated with splenomegaly.
- Enterovirus—Common cause of fever in infants and young children and may present similarly to EBV infection at these ages. Often have herpangina or hand-foot-mouth disease (see Chapter 113, Hand Foot Mouth Syndrome).
- HHV6—Very common cause of fever with/without rash in infants and thus in the differential diagnosis of EBV infection in young infants.
- Mycoplasma—Common in adolescents, who usually have respiratory manifestations as the primary focus of infection.
- Group A streptococcal infection—Common cause of pharyngitis and lymphadenopathy and can occur concurrently with EBV infection. It can be excluded with appropriate microbiologic testing of the pharynx (see Chapter 29, URI Including Pharyngitis).
- Hodgkin's lymphoma (Hodgkin's disease)—Can present with lymphadenopathy, fever, night sweats, and fatigue similar to mononucleosis. These children may have larger more tender lymph nodes but any systemic illness with these features should prompt consideration of Hodgkin's disease as well as mononucleosis (**Figure 184-6**). Hodgkin's disease may even follow an episode of mononucleosis.

MANAGEMENT

- Mainly supportive: hydration, rest.
- Antibiotics have no role and may cause rash (amoxicillin). If there is coexisting strep pharyngitis use penicillin (not amoxicillin) as treatment to avoid the common amoxicillin mononucleosis exanthem (see Chapter 154, Cutaneous Drug Reactions).
- Routine therapy with corticosteroids is not indicated. They may offer benefit in reducing edema when there is airway compromise.[34] SOR Ⓒ
- Contact sports should be avoided until the spleen is no longer palpable because of risk of splenic rupture.
- Acyclovir and ganciclovir are active against the virus in vitro by means of inhibition of the lytic phase but there is limited or no evidence that they improve symptoms of infectious mononucleosis. Antiviral treatment is reserved for immunocompromised patients.[35]

RADIOLOGY

- Ultrasound technique may be used to assess the size of the spleen and help determine when a child can go back to participate in contact sports; however, there are no well-defined norms related to a normal spleen size are available (**Figure 184-9**).[36–39]

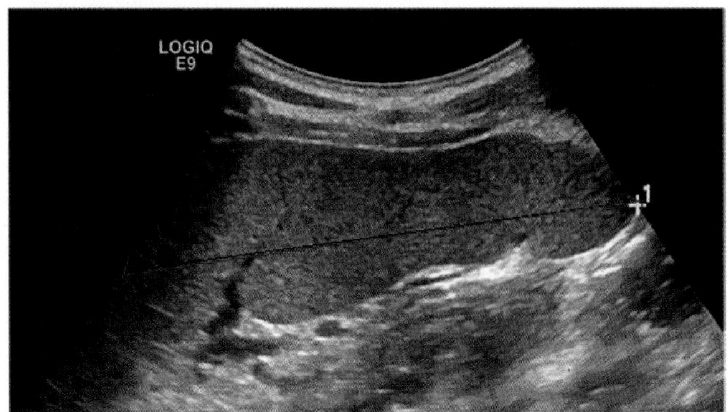

FIGURE 184-9 Splenomegaly on ultrasound of the spleen in a 16 year-old- patient with infectious mononucleosis. The spleen measures 17cm. Even though there are no clearly defined norms of splenic size in adolescents, measurement closer to 12 to 13 are considered normal for this age group.[37,38] The disruption in the splenic perimeter at the bottom left portion of this enlarged spleen is due to a splenic vessel and not a splenic rupture. (*Used with permission from Blanca Gonzalez, MD.*)

SURGERY

- Surgery may be indicated in splenic rupture, although conservative approaches have also been successful in treating splenic rupture associated with EBV infectious mononucleosis.[40]
- Spontaneous splenic rupture, though rare, can occur most frequently within the first 2 weeks of illness.[39]
- Late ruptures are associated with trauma.

PREVENTION

- Because the virus may persist in saliva for a long time and patients may be infectious prior to the onset of symptoms, prevention strategies are difficult; nevertheless, patients should avoid deep kissing and sharing food or utensils during the acute phase of the disease.

PROGNOSIS

- The fatigue that patients experience may persist for up to 6 months.[41] Fatigue and non-specific symptoms persisting longer than this cannot be attributed to active viral infection and other diseases such as Hodgkin's lymphoma should be considered.
- Chronic EBV infections are a very rare occurrence and manifest as persistent symptoms of infectious mononucleosis for more than 6 months with evidence of other organ involvement (i.e., Hepatitis, hemolytic anemia).[42]
- EBV infection confers lifelong immunity to re-infection.
- Even though reactivations may occur, they tend to be asymptomatic in the immune competent host.
- Lymphomas and epithelial malignancies may develop in some patients.[2]
- In the transplant patient, EBV reactivation may lead to the development of PTLD.[43]

FOLLOW-UP

- Follow-up with primary physician for clearance for participation in sports.
- Generally, once the acute manifestations and splenomegaly on physical exam have resolved, the patient may return to sports participation. A 6-week period from the onset of symptoms is often used as a guideline.

PATIENT EDUCATION

- The expected course of illness should be discussed with the patient and the family.
- After an initial period of rest, a return to school and noncontact activities is important to re-establish a normal routine.

PATIENT RESOURCES

- **http://my.clevelandclinic.org/disorders/mononucleosis/hic_overview.aspx**.
- **www.healthychildren.org/English/health-issues/conditions/infections/Pages/Infectious-Mononucleosis**.
- **www.emedicinehealth.com/epstein-barr_virus_infection/article_em.htm**.

PROVIDER RESOURCES

- **http://www.cdc.gov/epstein-barr/about-mono.html**.
- **http://pedsinreview.aappublications.org/content/32/9/375.short**.

REFERENCES

1. Bravender T. Epstein-Barr virus, cytomegalovirus, and infectious mononucleosis. *Adolesc Med State Art Rev*. 2010;21(2):251-264.
2. Macsween KF, Crawford DH. *Epstein-Barr virus-recent advances. Lancet Infect Dis*. 2003;3(3):131-140.
3. Gonzalez Saldana N, et al. Clinical and laboratory characteristics of infectious mononucleosis by Epstein-Barr virus in Mexican children. *BMC Res Notes*. 2012;5:361.
4. Pereira MS, Blake JM, and Macrae AD. EB virus antibody at different ages. *Br Med J*. 1969;4(5682):526-527.
5. Grotto I, et al. Clinical and laboratory presentation of EBV positive infectious mononucleosis in young adults. *Epidemiol Infect*. 2003;131(1):683-689.
6. Levine H et al. Secular and seasonal trends of infectious mononucleosis among young adults in Israel: 1978-2009. *Eur J Clin Microbiol Infect Dis*. 2012;31(5):757-760.
7. Son, KH, Shin MY. Clinical features of Epstein-Barr virus-associated infectious mononucleosis in hospitalized Korean children. *Korean J Pediatr*. 2011;54(10):409-413.
8. Balfour HH, Jr, et al. Behavioral, virologic, and immunologic factors associated with acquisition and severity of primary epstein-barr virus infection in university students. *J Infect Dis*. 2013;207(1):80-88.
9. Abdel-Aziz M, et al. Epstein-Barr virus infection as a cause of cervical lymphadenopathy in children. *Int J Pediatr Otorhinolaryngol*. 2011;75(4):564-567.
10. Selby CD, Marcus HS, and Toghill PJ. Enlarged epitrochlear lymph nodes: an old physical sign revisited. *J R Coll Physicians Lond*. 1992;26(2):159-161.
11. Konvolinka CW, Wyatt DB. Splenic rupture and infectious mononucleosis. *J Emerg Med*. 1989;7(5):471-475.
12. Aldrete JS. Spontaneous rupture of the spleen in patients with infectious mononucleosis. *Mayo Clin Proc*. 1992;67(9):910-912.
13. van Hasselt W, Schreuder RM, and Houwerzijl EJ. Periorbital oedema. *Neth J Med*. 2009;67(8):338-339.
14. Bass MH. Periorbital edema as the initial sign of infectious mononucleosis. *J Pediatr*. 1954;45(2):204-205.

15. Charbel Issa P, et al. Oculoglandular syndrome associated with reactivated Epstein-Barr-virus infection. *Br J Ophthalmol*. 2008; 92(6):740,855.

16. Meisler DM, Bosworth, DE and Krachmer, JH. Ocular infectious mononucleosis manifested as Parinaud's oculoglandular syndrome. *Am J Ophthalmol*. 1981;92(5):722-726.

17. Matoba AY. Ocular disease associated with Epstein-Barr virus infection. *Surv Ophthalmol*. 1990;35(2):145-150.

18. Lau CH, et al. Acute retinal necrosis features, management, and outcomes. *Ophthalmology* 2007;114(4):756-762.

19. de Moraes JC et al. Etiologies of rash and fever illnesses in Campinas, Brazil. *J Infect Dis*. 2011;204(2):S627-S636.

20. Jappe U. Amoxicillin-induced exanthema in patients with infectious mononucleosis: allergy or transient immunostimulation? *Allergy*. 2007;62(12):1474-1475.

21. Mendoza N, et al. Mucocutaneous manifestations of Epstein-Barr virus infection. *Am J Clin Dermatol*. 2008;9(5):295-305.

22. DeKlotz CM and Frieden, IJ. Picture of the month quiz case. Vulvar ulcerations resulting from acute Epstein-Barr virus infection. *Arch Pediatr Adolesc Med*. 2008;162(1):86-87.

23. Sardy M, et al. Genital ulcers associated with Epstein-Barr virus infection (ulcus vulvae acutum). *Acta Derm Venereol*. 2011;91(1): 55-59.

24. Bathoorn E, et al. Primary Epstein-Barr virus infection with neurological complications. *Scand J Infect Dis*. 2011;43(2):136-144.

25. Dale RC. Acute disseminated encephalomyelitis. *Semin Pediatr Infect Dis*. 2003;14(2):90-95.

26. Hausler M, et al. Neurological complications of acute and persistent Epstein-Barr virus infection in paediatric patients. *J Med Virol*. 2002;68(2):253-263.

27. Brigden ML, et al. Infectious mononucleosis in an outpatient population: diagnostic utility of 2 automated hematology analyzers and the sensitivity and specificity of Hoagland's criteria in heterophile-positive patients. *Arch Pathol Lab Med*. 1999;123(10):875-881.

28. Ventura KC and Hudnall, SD. Hematologic differences in heterophile-positive and heterophile-negative infectious mononucleosis. *Am J Hematol*. 2004;76(4):315-318.

29. Klemola E, et al. Infectious-mononucleosis-like disease with negative heterophil agglutination test. Clinical features in relation to Epstein-Barr virus and cytomegalovirus antibodies. *J Infect Dis*. 1970;121(6):608-614.

30. Klutts JS, et al. Evidence-based approach for interpretation of Epstein-Barr virus serological patterns. *J Clin Microbiol*. 2009; 47(10):3204-3210.

31. Weinberg A, et al. Quantitative CSF PCR in Epstein-Barr virus infections of the central nervous system. *Ann Neurol*. 2002;52(5): 543-548.

32. Schonberger S, et al. Prospective, comprehensive, and effective viral monitoring in children undergoing allogeneic hematopoietic stem cell transplantation. *Biol Blood Marrow Transplant*. 2010;16(10):1428-1435.

33. Horwitz CA, et al. Heterophil-negative infectious mononucleosis and mononucleosis-like illnesses. Laboratory confirmation of 43 cases. *Am J Med*. 1977;63(6):947-957.

34. Candy B, Hotopf M. Steroids for symptom control in infectious mononucleosis. *Cochrane Database Syst Rev*. 2006(3):CD004402.

35. Gershburg E, Pagano JS. Epstein-Barr virus infections: prospects for treatment. *J Antimicrob Chemother*. 2005;56(2):277-281.

36. Hosey RG, et al. Ultrasonographic evaluation of splenic enlargement in athletes with acute infectious mononucleosis. *Br J Sports Med*. 2008;42(12):974-977.

37. McCorkle R, et al. Normative spleen size in tall healthy athletes: implications for safe return to contact sports after infectious mononucleosis. *Clin J Sport Med*. 2010;20(6):413-415.

38. O'Connor TE, et al. Return to contact sports following infectious mononucleosis: the role of serial ultrasonography. *Ear Nose Throat J*. 2011;90(8):E21-E24.

39. Rinderknecht AS, Pomerantz, WJ. Spontaneous splenic rupture in infectious mononucleosis: case report and review of the literature. *Pediatr Emerg Care*. 2012;28(12):1377-1379.

40. Stephenson JT, DuBois, JJ. Nonoperative management of spontaneous splenic rupture in infectious mononucleosis: a case report and review of the literature. *Pediatrics*. 2007;120(2):e432-e435.

41. Katz BZ, et al. Exercise tolerance testing in a prospective cohort of adolescents with chronic fatigue syndrome and recovered controls following infectious mononucleosis. *J Pediatr*. 2010;157(3): 468-472.

42. Kimura H. Pathogenesis of chronic active Epstein-Barr virus infection: is this an infectious disease, lymphoproliferative disorder, or immunodeficiency? *Rev Med Virol*. 2006;16(4):251-261.

43. Hatton O, Martinez OM, and Esquivel CO. Emerging therapeutic strategies for Epstein-Barr virus+ post-transplant lymphoproliferative disorder. *Pediatr Transplant*. 2012;16(3):220-229.

185 TOXIC SHOCK SYNDROMES

Camille Sabella, MD

PATIENT STORY

An 11-year-old boy presented to the emergency department with a 12-hour history of fever, rash over his trunk, vomiting, and diarrhea. In the emergency department, he had a fever to 39.3°C., pulse 140/minute, respiratory rate 40/minute, and blood pressure 90/60 mm Hg. He had conjunctival injection and inflamed oral mucus membranes, and intense erythroderma (red skin) on his trunk and back (**Figure 185-1**). Laboratory tests revealed thrombocytopenia, transaminitis, and an elevated creatinine level that was twice normal for his age. He was given fluid resuscitation and was admitted to the pediatric intensive care unit, where he required several fluid boluses and inotropic support to maintain adequate blood pressure and perfusion. He was treated with vancomycin and clindamycin. *Staphylococcus aureus* was isolated from an infected wound on his lower extremity that he sustained from a sports injury a few days prior to his presentation.

INTRODUCTION

Toxic shock syndrome (TSS) is an acute illness characterized by fever, rash, hypotension, and multi-organ system involvement that can progress to shock, renal failure, myocardial dysfunction, and adult respiratory distress syndrome. TSS was originally described in 1978 in children who had infection caused by *Staphylococcus aureus*, and has been well described in menstruating females using tampons.[1,2] A similar toxic shock-like syndrome has been described in association with group A streptococcal (GAS) infection.[3,4]

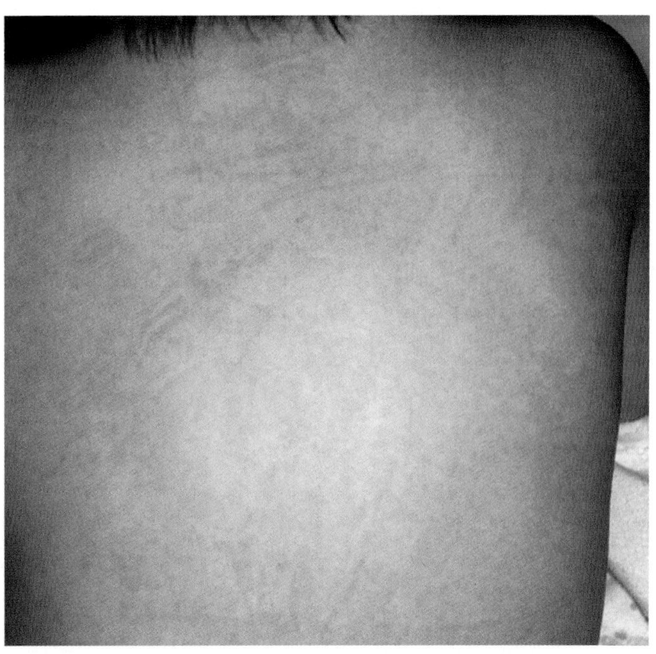

FIGURE 185-1 Erythroderma in a child with toxic shock syndrome. *(Used with permission from Johanna Goldfarb, MD.)*

EPIDEMIOLOGY

STAPHYLOCOCCAL TOXIC SHOCK

- There is a strong correlation between menstruation, use of high absorbency tampons, and the development of TSS.[5]
- Sixty percent of TSS cases occur in menstruating women while 40 percent occur in males and nonmenstruating females.[6]
- More likely to occur in younger individuals who have not had previous exposure to TSS toxins and lack neutralizing antibody.[7]
- Young women who have vaginal colonization with toxin-producing strains of *S aureus* and who have no antibody to TSS toxin 1 (TSST-1) are at highest risk of developing TSS during menstruation, especially with tampon use.
- Children who have focal infection caused by *S aureus* can develop TSS. These infections may be clinically apparent, such as wound infections, skin abscesses, cellulitis, tracheitis, or may be occult, such as with sinusitis.

STREPTOCOCCAL TOXIC SHOCK-LIKE SYNDROME

- Usually related to GAS bacteremia, and in many cases often associated with cellulitis and necrotizing fasciitis.[3,4]
- Associated with varicella infections in which GAS secondarily infects skin lesions.

ETIOLOGY AND PATHOPHYSIOLOGY

- TSS is caused by *S aureus* strains that produce TSS toxin 1 or possibly other Staphylococcal enterotoxins.[8]
- TSS toxins are thought to act as superantigens that stimulate the production of inflammatory mediators such as tumor necrosis factor and interleukin 1. These mediators cause capillary leakage that lead to hypotension and multisystem organ dysfunction.[9–11]
- The degree of hypotension predicts the extent of multisystem organ dysfunction.
- Current clones of community-associated strains of methicillin-resistant *S aureus* (MRSA) rarely produce TSS toxin.[12]
- Most cases of GAS toxic shock-like syndrome are due to strains of M types 1 and 3.

RISK FACTORS

- TSS is most common in young menstruating women using high absorbency tampons.
- The lack of antibody to TSS-toxin 1 is a risk factor for infection.
- Varicella infection is an important risk factor for Streptococcal toxic shock-like syndrome (**Figure 185-2**).

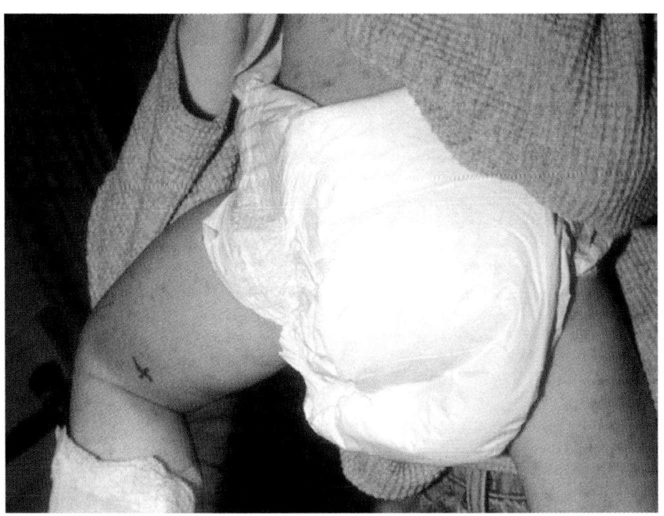

FIGURE 185-2 Child with varicella who developed a secondary bacterial cellulitis caused by group A streptococcus. (*Used with permission from Camille Sabella, MD.*)

DIAGNOSIS

CLINICAL FEATURES

- Formal case definitions for TSS and Streptococcal toxic shock-like syndrome have been published (**Tables 185-1** and **185-2**).
- Acute onset of fever, sore throat and myalgia are the first symptoms.
- Gastrointestinal manifestations, especially profuse diarrhea, are common.
- Rash is erythrodermal or scarlatiniform in nature (**Figures 185-1** and **185-3**).
- Symptoms of hypotension are often present (dizziness or fainting).
- "Strawberry tongue" (**Figure 185-4**), nonpurulent conjunctival injection (**Figure 185-5**), and pharyngeal inflammation are common features on physical examination.
- Altered consciousness is a sign of hypotension.
- Desquamation of the skin occurs 7 to 21 days after the onset of illness; this commonly occurs in a full-thickness, sheet like manner (**Figure 185-6**).

TABLE 185-1 Clinical Case Definition for Staphylococcal Toxic Shock Syndrome[1]

Clinical Manifestations

Fever—Temperature greater than or equal to 38.9 C (102 F).
Rash—Diffuse macular erythroderma.
Desquamation—1 to 2 weeks after onset of illness, particularly palms and soles.
Hypotension—Systolic blood pressure less than or equal to 90 mm Hg for adults or less than fifth percentile by age for children <16 years of age; orthostatic drop in diastolic blood pressure greater than or equal to 15 mm Hg from lying to sitting, orthostatic syncope, or orthostatic dizziness.

Multisystem Involvement

Three or more of the following:

- Gastrointestina—Vomiting or diarrhea at onset of illness.
- Muscular—Severe myalgia or creatine phosphokinase level at least twice the upper limit of normal for laboratory.
- Mucous membrane—Vaginal, oropharyngeal, or conjunctival hyperemia.
- Renal—Blood urea nitrogen or creatinine at least twice the upper limit of normal for laboratory or urinary sediment with pyuria (greater than or equal to 5 leukocytes per high-power field) in the absence of urinary tract infection.
- Hepatic—Total bilirubin, serum glutamic-oxaloacetic transa- minase (SGOT), or serum glutamic-pyruvic transaminase (SGPT) at least twice the upper limit of normal for laboratory.
- Hematologic—Platelets <100,000/mm superscript 3.
- Central nervous system—Disorientation or alterations in consciousness without focal neurologic signs when fever and hypotension are absent.

Negative results on the following tests, if obtained:

- Blood, throat, or cerebrospinal fluid cultures (blood culture may be positive for Staphylococcus aureus).
- Rise in titer to Rocky Mountain spotted fever, leptospirosis, or measles.

Case Classification

Probable—A case with five of the six clinical findings described previously.
Confirmed—A case with all six of the clinical findings described above, including desquamation, unless the patient dies before desquamation could occur.

[1]*Adapted from Wharton M, Chorba TL, Vogt RL, Morse DL, Buehler JW. Case definitions for public health surveillance. MMWR Recomm Rep. 1990;39(RR-13):1-43.*

TABLE 185-2 Clinical Case Definition of Streptococcal Toxic Shock Syndrome[1]

I. Isolation of Group A Streptococcus *(Streptococcus pyogenes).*
   A. From a normally sterile site (e.g., blood, cerebrospinal fluid, peritoneal fluid, or tissue biopsy specimen)—Definite case if combined with IIA and IIB in the following.
   B. From a nonsterile site (e.g., throat, sputum, vagina, open surgical wound, or superficial skin lesion)—Probable case if combined with IIA and IIB below if no other cause of the illness is identified.

II. Clinical Signs of Severity.
   A. Hypotension—Systolic pressure 90 mm Hg or less in adults or lower than the fifth percentile for age in children.

   AND

   B. Two or more of the following signs:
      Renal impairment—Creatinine concentration 177 µmol/L (2 mg/dL) or greater for adults or at least 2 times the upper limit of normal for age.
      Coagulopathy—Platelet count 100 000/mm^3 or less or disseminated intravascular coagulation.
      Hepatic involvement—Elevated alanine transaminase, aspartate transaminase, or total bilirubin concentrations at least 2 times the upper limit of normal for age.
      Adult respiratory distress syndrome.
      A generalized erythematous macular rash that may desquamate.
      Soft tissue necrosis, including necrotizing fasciitis or myositis, or gangrene.

[1]*Adapted from National Notifiable Diseases Surveillance System (NNDSS), 2010 Case Definition; Centers for Disease Control and Prevention. Found at: http://wwwn.cdc.gov/nndss/script/casedef.aspx?CondYrID=858&DatePub=1/1/2010.*

- The clinical features of GAS toxic shock-like syndrome are similar to that of Staphylococcal toxic shock; however, GAS toxic shock is more often preceded by wound infection, cellulitis or pneumonia (**Figure 185-7**).

DISTRIBUTION

- Rash is more prominent on the trunk than on the extremities, except in the presence of severe hypotension.
- Desquamation of the digits, palms, and soles is most common.

LABORATORY TESTING

- Leukocytosis with a predominance of neutrophils and premature forms are common.
- Hepatic dysfunction is common and usually heralded by mildly elevated serum transaminases and disproportionately elevated conjugated bilirubin levels.
- Renal function is often compromised.
- Consumption coagulopathy may occur.

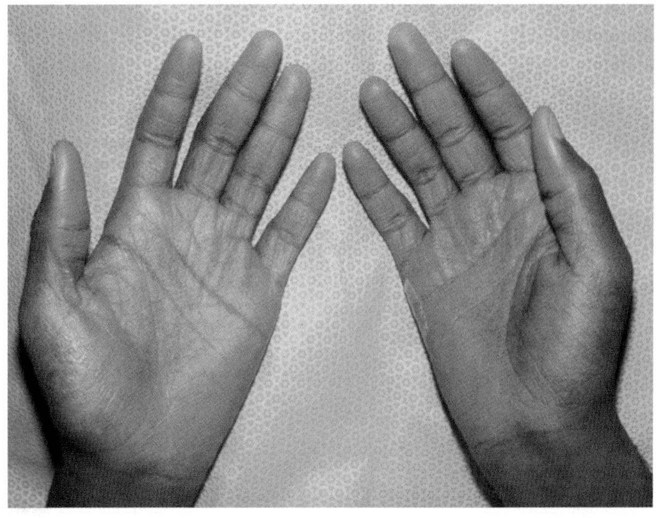

FIGURE 185-3 Child with palmar erythema characteristic of early toxic shock syndrome. *(Used with permission from Camille Sabella, MD.)*

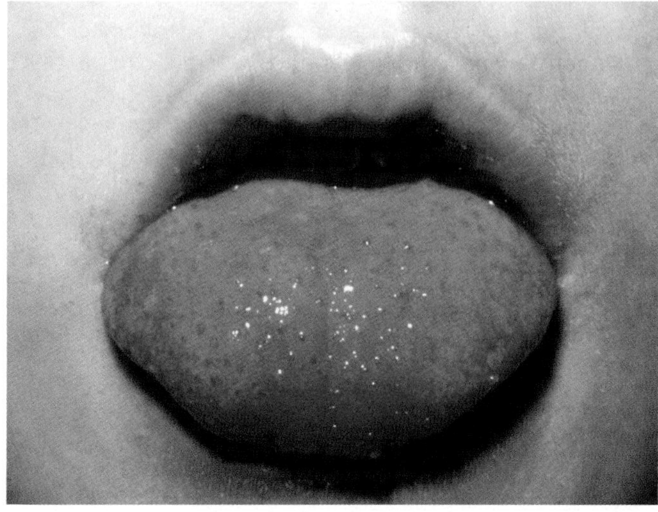

FIGURE 185-4 Strawberry tongue, which is one of the features of toxic shock syndrome. *(Used with permission from Johanna Goldfarb, MD.)*

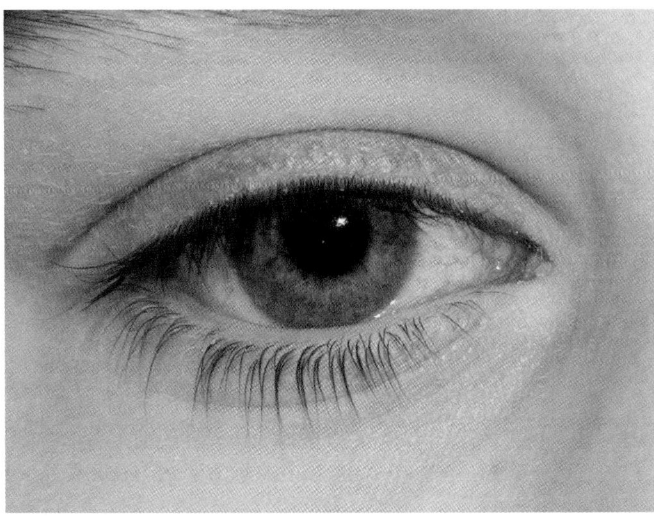

FIGURE 185-5 Conjunctival hyperemia in a child with toxic shock syndrome. (*Used with permission from Camille Sabella, MD.*)

- Isolation of *S aureus* is not required to make the diagnosis of TSS, but every effort should be made to identify and drain any focus of infection.
- A definitive diagnosis of GAS toxic shock-like syndrome requires meeting the clinical case definition plus isolation of GAS from the blood or other sterile body site (probable case if GAS isolated from nonsterile body site).

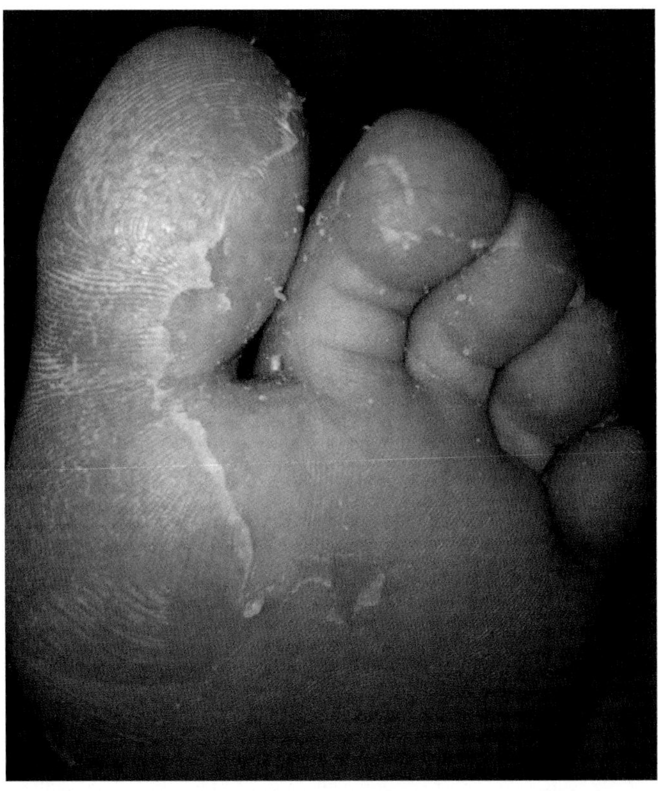

FIGURE 185-6 Sheet-like desquamation, which occurs 7 to 10 days after the onset of toxic shock syndrome. (*Used with permission from Camille Sabella, MD.*)

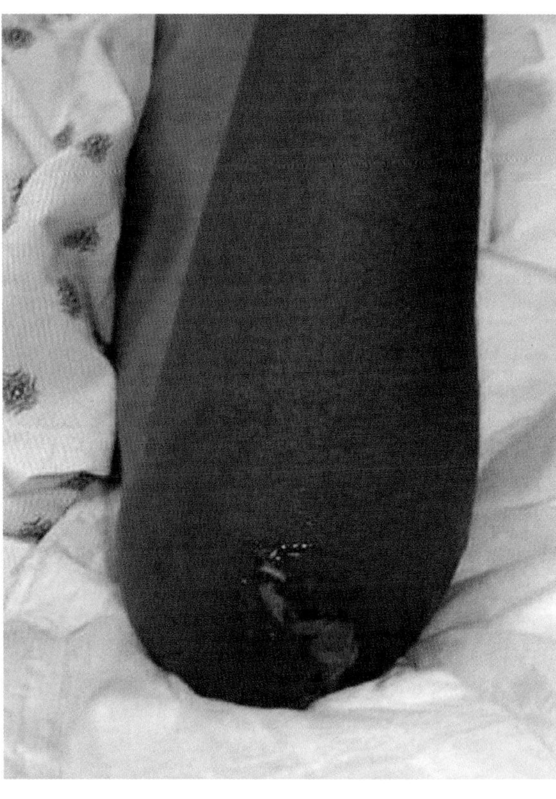

FIGURE 185-7 Wound infection caused by group A streptococcus as a risk factor for streptococcal toxic shock-like syndrome. (*Used with permission from Camille Sabella, MD.*)

DIFFERENTIAL DIAGNOSIS

- TSS should be considered in the differential of fever, rash (erythroderma), and hypotension.
- Kawasaki disease has many similar findings as TSS but the prolonged fever, absence of gastrointestinal symptoms, and lack of hypotension in most cases of Kawasaki disease helps to differentiate these entities.
- Septic shock caused by organisms other than *S. aureus* can usually be differentiated on the basis of positive blood cultures, purpuric rather than an erythrodermal rash, and lack of conjunctivitis and mucositis.
- Other toxin-mediated illnesses such as Staphylococcal scalded skin syndrome and scarlet fever are not usually associated with the toxicity and hypotension of TSS.

MANAGEMENT

NONPHARMACOLOGIC

- Vigorous administration of intravenous fluids to correct the hemodynamic compromise is critical.
- Inotropic support may be necessary depending on the degree of hemodynamic compromise and myocardial dysfunction.
- Drainage of any foci of infection is important in limiting the amount of toxin produced by the organism.

- Any foreign material that may be contributing to the infection, such as a tampon or other vaginal foreign body, should be removed.

MEDICATIONS

- Empiric therapy for TSS is recommended to eradicate the organism and prevent relapses and should include coverage against *S. aureus* and GAS. SOR Ⓒ
- The combination of vancomycin and clindamycin is an appropriate empiric choice to cover *S. aureus*, including MRSA and GAS. SOR Ⓒ
- Clindamycin is useful as an adjunctive agent because of its ability to inhibit toxin production. SOR Ⓒ
- For cases caused by GAS, treatment with a penicillin and clindamycin are often used once the organisms is isolated; clindamycin in these situations is advantageous because of its superior activity against high inoculum, low-replication setting of GAS skin and soft tissue infection, as well as its anti-toxin effects.[13,14]
- Corticosteroids and intravenous immunoglobulin (IVIG) may be considered in severe cases of staphylococcal toxic shock, although data from clinical trials showing clear benefit are lacking.[15,16] SOR Ⓒ
- IVIG may be useful for severe refractory GAS toxic shock.[17,18] SOR Ⓑ

SURGERY

- Drainage of purulent foci of infection and removal of any infected foreign material should be undertaken.
- Early surgical exploration and debridement of infected skin and soft tissues is especially critical in cases of GAS toxic-shock like syndrome that involve severe cellulitis and necrotizing fasciitis.

REFERRAL

- Children who manifest signs of TSS or who are suspected of having TSS should be admitted to the hospital and managed in a pediatric intensive care unit.

PREVENTION AND SCREENING

- The routine use of age-appropriate varicella vaccination for all children decreases the risk of varicella and bacterial superinfection, which is an important risk factor for TSS.
- Women who develop menses-associated TSS should be counseled to not use tampons for several menstrual cycles and to use pads instead of tampons at night.[19]
- Routine screening for *S aureus* carriage in patients who have recovered from TSS is controversial and not routinely recommended.

PROGNOSIS

- Most patients improve with aggressive fluid resuscitation, drainage of any purulent material, and appropriate antimicrobial therapy.[15]
- The case fatality rate for TSS is lower in children than in adults.
- Causes of fatalities in patients with TSS include myocardial dysfunction, refractory shock, and adult respiratory distress syndrome.

FOLLOW-UP

- Recurrence of TSS can occur especially in women who continue to use tampons. Close follow-up of these patients is warranted.

PATIENT EDUCATION

Parents should be advised to seek care for high fever and rash in any child who has a wound or skin infection.

PATIENT RESOURCES

- **www.ncbi.nlm.nih.gov/pubmedhealth/PMH0001676**.
- **www.toxicshock.com**.
- **www.nlm.nih.gov/medlineplus/ency/article/000653.htm**.

PROVIDER RESOURCES

- Wiesenthal AM, Todd JK. Toxic shock syndrome in children aged 10 years or less. *Pediatrics*. 1984;74:112-117.
- American Academy of Pediatrics. Committee on Infectious Diseases. Severe invasive group A streptococcal infections: a subject review. *Pediatrics*. 1998;101:136-140.

REFERENCES

1. Todd J, Fishaut M, Kapral F, et al. Toxic shock syndrome associated with phagegroup I staphylococci. *Lancet*. 1978;2:116-118.
2. Shands KN, Schmid GP, Dan BB, et al. Toxic shock syndrome in menstruating women: association with tampon use and *Staphylococcus aureus* and clinical features in 52 cases. *N Engl J Med*. 1980; 303:1436-1442.
3. Stevens DL. Invasive group A streptococcus infections. *Clin Infect Dis*. 1992;14:2-11.
4. Wheeler MC, Roe MH, Kaplan EL, et al. Clinical, epidemiological, and microbiological correlates of an outbreak of group A streptococcal septicemia in children. *JAMA*. 1991;266:533-537.
5. Schlech WF, Shands KN, Reingold AL, et al. Risk factors for development of toxic shock syndrome: association with a tampon brand. *JAMA*. 1982;248:835-839.
6. Todd JK, Weisenthal AM, Ressman M, et al. Toxic shock syndrome. II. Estimated occurrence in Colorado as influenced by case ascertainment methods. *Am J Epidemiol*. 1985;122:857-867.
7. Todd JK. Toxic shock syndrome. *Clin Microbiol Rev*. 1988;1:432-446.
8. Marples RR, Wieneke AA. Enterotoxins and toxic-shock syndrome toxin-1 in nonenteric staphylococcal disease. *Epidemiol Infect*. 1993;110:477-488.
9. Akatusuka H, Imanishi K, Inada K, et al. Production of tumour necrosis factors by human T cells stimulated by a superantigen, toxic shock syndrome toxin-1. *Clin Exp Immunol*. 1994;96: 422-426.

10. Hackett SP, Stevens DL. Superantigens associated with staphylococcal and streptococcal toxic shock syndrome are potent inducers of tumor necrosis factorbeta synthesis. *J Infect Dis*. 1993;168: 232-235.

11. Schlievert PM. Role of superantigens in human disease. *J Infect Dis*. 1993;167:997-1002.

12. American Academy of Pediatrics. Staphylococcal infections. In: Pickering LK, Baker CJ, Kimberlin DW, Long SS, eds. *Red Book: 2012 Report of the Committee on Infectious Diseases*. Elk Grove Village, IL: American Academy of Pediatrics; 2012:653-668.

13. Stevens DI, Gibbons AE, Bergstrom R, et al. The Eagle effect revisited: efficacy of clindamycin, erythromycin, and penicillin in the treatment of streptococcal myositis. *J Infect Dis*. 1988;158:23-28.

14. Zimbelman J, Palmer A, Todd J. Improved outcome of clindamycin compared with beta-lactam antibiotic treatment of invasive *Streptococcus pyogenes* infection. *Pediatr Infect Dis J*. 1999;18:1096-1100.

15. Todd JK, Ressman M, Caston SA, et al. Corticosteroid therapy for patients with toxic shock syndrome. *JAMA*. 1984;252:3399-3402.

16. Barry W, Hudgins L, Donta ST, et al. Intravenous immunoglobulin therapy for toxic shock syndrome. *JAMA*. 1992;267:3315-3316.

17. Kaul R, McGeer A, et al. Intravenous immunoglobulin therapy for streptococcal toxic shock syndrome: a comparative observational study. The Canadian Streptococcal Study Group. *Clin Infect Dis*. 1999;28:800-807.

18. Norrby-Teglund A, Muller MP, McGeer A, et al. Successful management of severe group A streptococcal soft tissue infections using an aggressive medical regimen including intravenous polyspecific immunoglobulin together with a conservative surgical approach. *Scand J Infect Dis*. 2005;37:166-172.

19. Todd, JK. Toxic shock syndrome. In: Long SS, Pickering LK, Prober CG, eds. Priciples and practice of pediatric infectious diseases. 3rd edition. Philadelphia, PA: Elsevier; 2008:110-113.

186 PEDIATRIC TUBERCULOSIS

Nazha Abughali, MD
Jessie Maxwell, MD
Frits van der Kuyp, MD

PATIENT STORY

A 17-month-old Hispanic boy presented to the emergency department with a 2-week history of cough, wheezing, fever, and weight loss. The child was born in the US and lives with his dad and uncle, both employed as migrant farm workers. He was admitted to the hospital with the diagnosis of bacterial pneumonia and asthma exacerbation. His initial chest radiograph (CXR) showed right upper and lower lobe infiltrates (**Figure 186-1**). He continued to have high grade fever despite intravenous antibiotics. After further history revealed that his mother recently died of tuberculosis (TB), he was immediately placed in respiratory isolation. A tuberculin skin test (TST) was positive with a 17 mm of induration, and a computed tomography (CT) of the chest showed a large lymph node compressing the trachea and the right main bronchus (**Figure 186-2**). Gastric aspirates for acid fast bacilli (AFB) stain and culture were obtained and he was started on anti-TB medications. The culture was positive for *Mycobacterium tuberculosis*. His father, sister and uncle all had a positive TST and evidence of active pulmonary TB. They were referred expeditiously for evaluation and treatment.

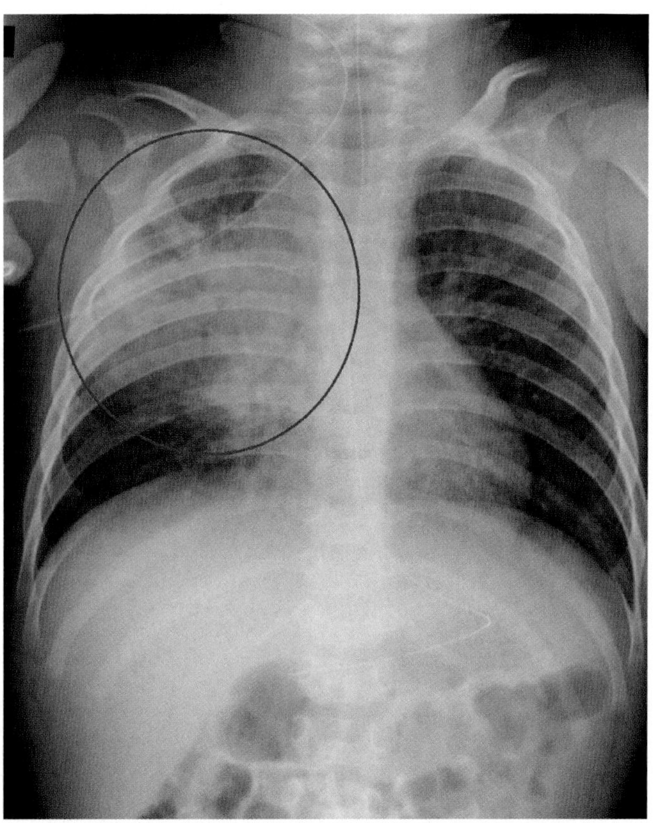

FIGURE 186-1 Right, upper, and middle lobe infiltrates (circled) due to primary pulmonary tuberculosis on chest x-ray of a 17-month-old boy. (*Used with permission from Nazha Abughali, MD.*)

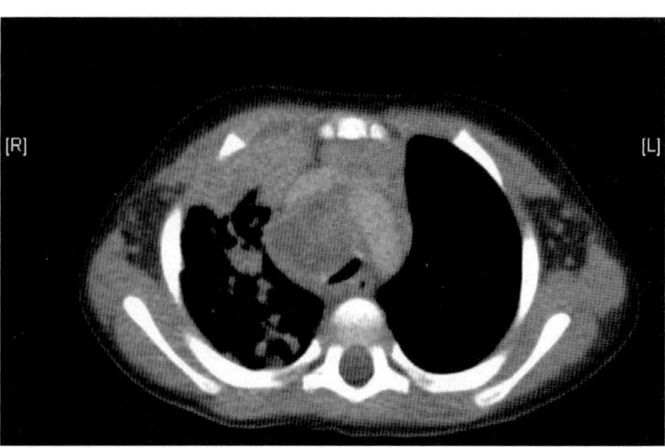

FIGURE 186-2 Compression of the trachea and right main stem bronchus due to an enlarged and necrotic lymph node on chest CT of the boy in **Figure 186-1** with primary pulmonary tuberculosis. (*Used with permission from Nazha Abughali, MD.*)

INTRODUCTION

Despite the significant decrease in TB rates in the US and other developed countries, tuberculosis continues to be a major cause of morbidity in developing countries. It is estimated that one third of the world's population is currently infected with TB, with 90 percent occurring in developing countries. Diagnosis of TB in children can be very challenging due to its non-specific clinical presentation and its paucibacillary nature coupled with the decrease in TB expertise among practitioners in developed countries. Without timely diagnosis and prompt institution of appropriate antituberculous therapy, TB in children can be associated with significant morbidity as well as mortality.

SYNONYMS

Tuberculosis: Phthisis, Consumption, Wasting disease, White plague.

Scrofula: TB adenitis, usually affecting the cervical lymph nodes.

Pott's disease: Tuberculosis of the spine.

EPIDEMIOLOGY

- Worldwide, around 9 million new cases of tuberculosis and approximately 1.5 million deaths are annually reported by the world health organization (WHO), with an estimated 500,000 cases and 64,000 deaths occurring among children <15 years of age.[1]
- In spite of the steady decrease in TB rates in the US among adults and children, tuberculosis continues to occur especially among certain ethnic and racial groups as well as among foreign-born individuals.
- Currently, more than 60 percent of the total TB cases occur among the foreign born persons in the US.[2]

- In children, specific groups with greater TB infection and disease rates include immigrants, international adoptees, and refugees from or travelers to high-prevalence regions.

ETIOLOGY AND PATHOPHYSIOLOGY

- Tuberculosis is caused by aerobic, fastidious, acid fast bacilli belonging to the *M. tuberculosis* complex group, which is composed of multiple species.
- The most important species include *Mycobacterium tuberculosis* (M.tb) that causes the majority of human tuberculosis and *Mycobacterium bovis* that could causes disease in humans by consumption of unpasteurized milk.[3]

TRANSMISSION

- Mainly airborne with inhalation of droplet nuclei containing tubercle bacilli.
- Transmission to a pediatric patient occurs from an adult or adolescent with active TB disease.
- Occurs during coughing, sneezing, and singing.
- Young children are rarely contagious.
- Infection is usually transmitted from a close adult contact.

PATHOPHYSIOLOGY

- Tubercle bacilli are deposited in the alveoli where they multiply forming the initial pulmonary focus or the "Ghon focus." Infection is spread to the regional lymph nodes (hilar, mediastinal, paratracheal, or subcarinal). The initial pulmonary focus and the draining regional nodes forms what is known as the "primary complex" that is more likely to be seen radiographically in children compared to adults.
- Occult mycobacterial lymphohematogenous spread could occur at this initial phase of infection with possible dissemination throughout the body, including the lymph nodes, kidneys, bones, brain, and the lungs. This provides a nidus for subsequent progressive disease or reactivation disease.
- The incubation period from the initial infection to the development of tuberculin hypersensitivity is around 2 to 10 weeks and can be demonstrated by either a positive tuberculin skin test (TST) or interferon γ release assay (IGRA) blood test.

RISK FACTORS

RISK FACTORS FOR TB INFECTION

- The ultimate risk for TB infection in a child is contact with an adult with untreated or inadequately treated pulmonary TB.
- Epidemiologic risk factors—Foreign birth, history of travel to high TB prevalent areas or history of incarceration. Also, history of exposure to adults with the following risk factors: foreign birth, abuse of intravenous drugs, dwellers of homeless shelters, and migrant farm workers.

RISK FACTORS FOR PROGRESSION FROM TB INFECTION TO DISEASE (TUBERCULOSIS)

- Recent infection—Risk for progression to TB in immunocompetent individuals is 5 to 10 percent during their whole life spans with 50 percent of this risk occurring within the first two years after infection.
- Age—Young infants and adolescents are especially at risk for TB progression. Children <1 year of age with TB infection have 40 percent risk of progression to disease.
- Immunosuppressive conditions—HIV infection, prolonged use of high dose steroids, and use of tumor necrosis factor-alpha (TNF-alpha) antagonists.
- Chronic conditions—Diabetes, renal failure, malnutrition, lymphoma.

DIAGNOSIS

DEFINITIONS

- Tuberculosis Exposure—Patient with history of exposure to suspected contagious TB case, with negative IGRA and negative TST, with no clinical, physical or radiological findings that are consistent with TB.
- Latent TB infection (LTBI)—Patient with a positive IGRA and/or TST, with no clinical, physical or radiological findings that are consistent with TB. These patients are non-contagious. The onset of the hypersensitivity reaction could be associated with erythema nodosum (**Figure 186-3**) or phlyctenular keratoconjunctivitis.

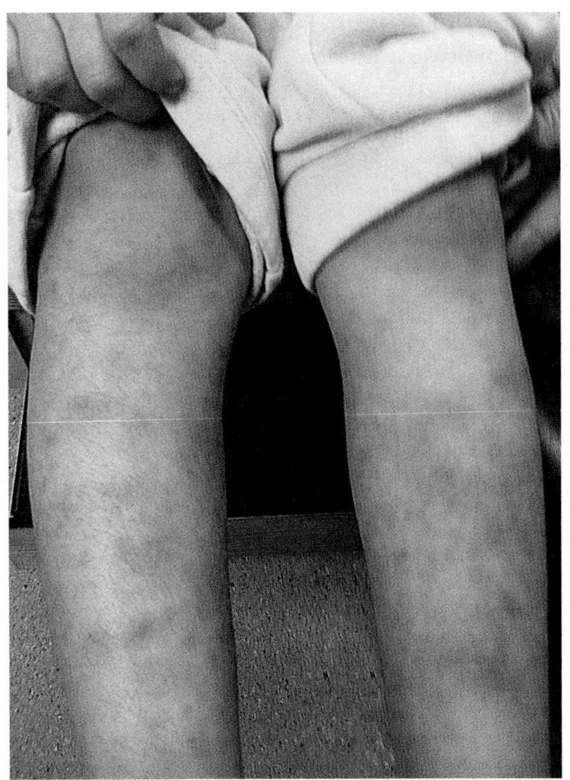

FIGURE 186-3 Erythema nodosum seen in a young patient diagnosed with TB infection. (*Used with permission from Nazha Abughali, MD.*)

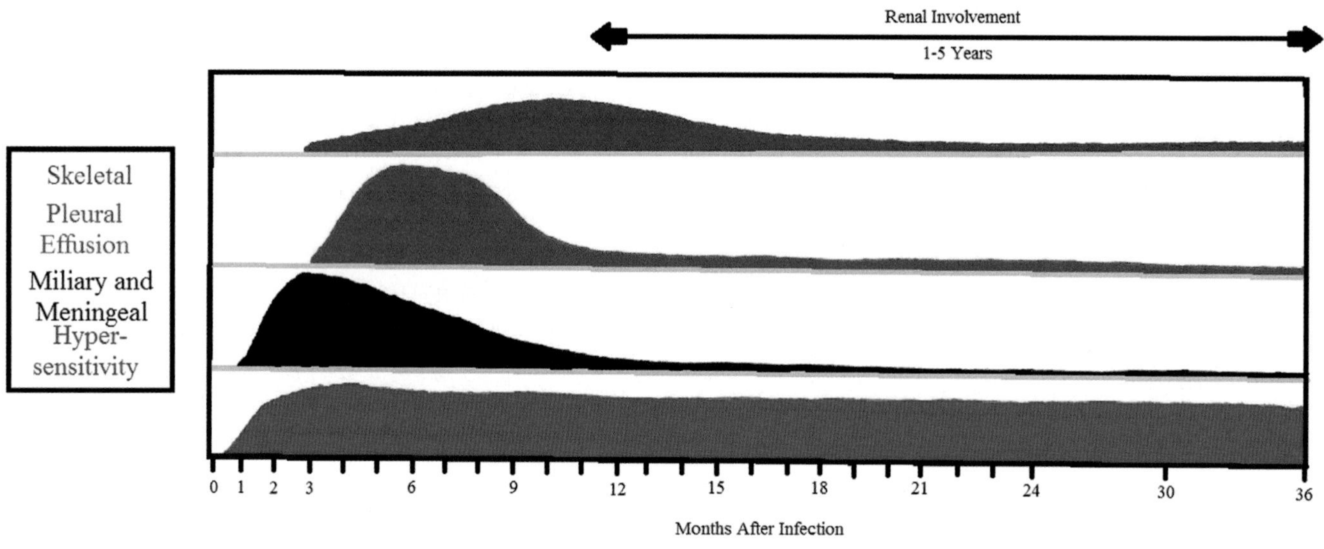

FIGURE 186-4 The clinical manifestations of tuberculosis occur at different times in the disease course in children. Renal involvement is the last manifestation to occur typically. *(Adapted from Marais, BJ, Gie, RP, Schaaf, HS, et al. The natural history of childhood intra-thoracic tuberculosis: A critical review of the pre-chemotherapy literature. Int. J. Tuberc. Lung Dis. 8:392-402, 2004. "Reprinted with permission of the International Union Against Tuberculosis and Lung Disease. Copyright © The Union.")*

- Tuberculosis disease (Tuberculosis)—Patient with a positive TST and/or IGRA with clinical symptoms or signs (physical, radiological, bacteriologic, or histological examination) that are consistent with tuberculosis.

CLINICAL FEATURES

- In general, pulmonary disease predominates in both adults and children.
- TB can develop in any organ system; however, both the frequency and severity of extrapulmonary TB are increased among children. Different manifestations of TB disease tend to occur after different periods of latency in children (**Figure 186-4**).[4]
- Signs and symptoms of TB in children depend on the organ of involvement.

DISTRIBUTION

▶ Pulmonary disease

Primary tuberculosis

- The most common type of TB in children.
- Children are mostly asymptomatic, but could present with fever, persistent cough, and weight loss.
- Typically diagnosed in an asymptomatic child who has a positive TST/IGRA and an abnormal CXR, which shows intrathoracic lymph node enlargement especially of the hilar or mediastinal nodes (**Figures 186-1**, **186-2**, and **186-5**).
- Bronchial compression and Endobronchial disease—Enlarged nodes may cause compression or obstruction of adjoining airways (**Figure 186-2**). In addition, bronchial obstruction may be caused by severe tuberculous disease secondary to invasion by an infected node into the bronchus (**Figure 186-6**). Children may present with persistent cough, wheezing or recurrent localized bacterial pneumonia.
- Diagnosis—Mainly clinical and epidemiological based on history of exposure to TB. AFB smear and culture are best obtained from early morning gastric aspirates.

Progressive primary tuberculosis

- The primary parenchymal focus may enlarge and caseate. This may drain into adjacent bronchi, resulting in local cavitation and spread into other areas of the lung (**Figure 186-7**).

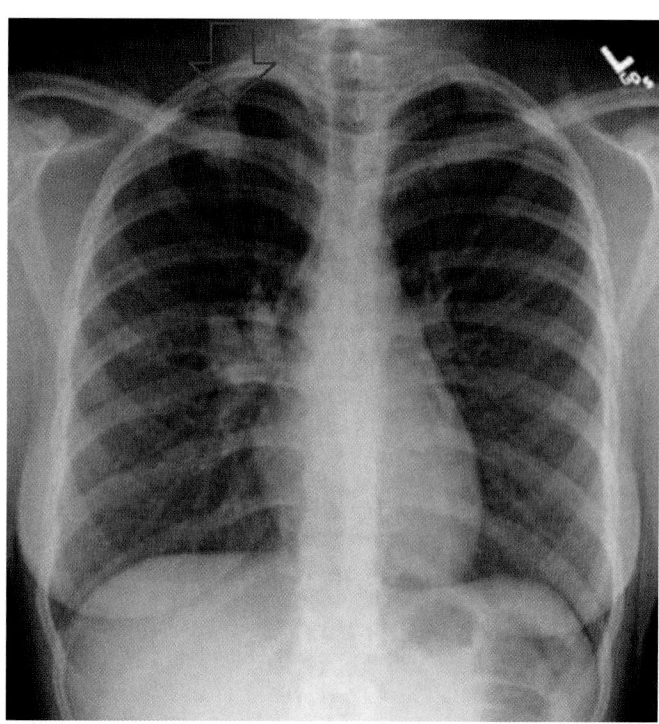

FIGURE 186-5 Right hilar lymphadenopathy with infiltrates in the right middle and upper lobes (arrow) on chest x-ray (CXR) of an 18-year-old female with primary tuberculosis. *(Used with permission from Nazha Abughali, MD.)*

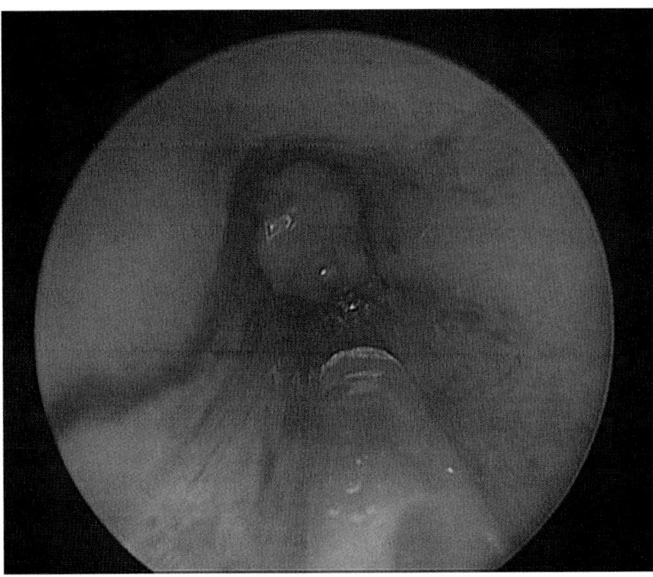

FIGURE 186-6 Bronchial obstruction caused by endobronchial disease. (*Used with permission from Nazha Abughali, MD.*)

- Children are quite ill with productive cough, weight loss, fever, and malaise.
- Progressive primary TB develops more frequently in infants and immunosuppressed patients.
- AFB cultures can be obtained from sputum, gastric aspirates, or bronchoalveolar lavage.

Tuberculous pleural effusion

- Pleural effusions are more often seen in older children and appear within 6 to 9 months after the primary infection (**Figure 186-8**).

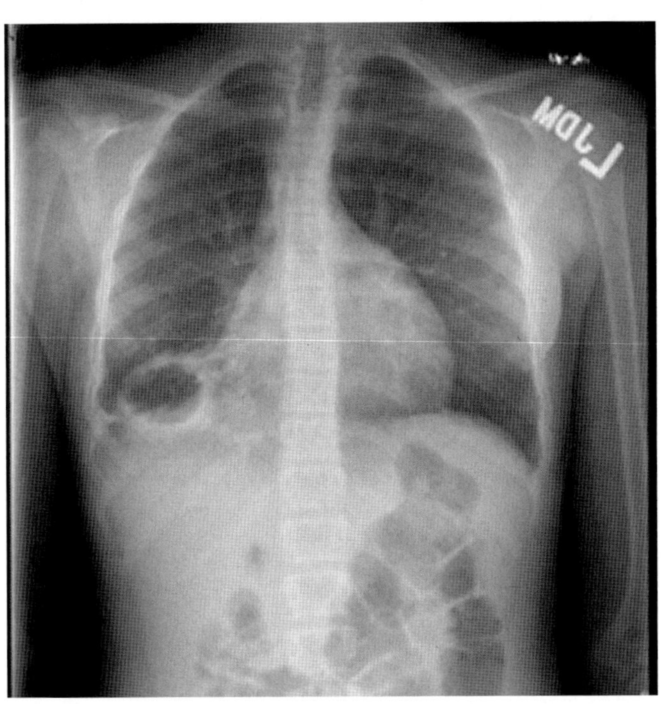

FIGURE 186-7 Right lower lobe tuberculous cavity on chest x-ray of a 12-year-old female immigrant from Uganda. (*Used with permission from Richard Blinkhorn, MD.*)

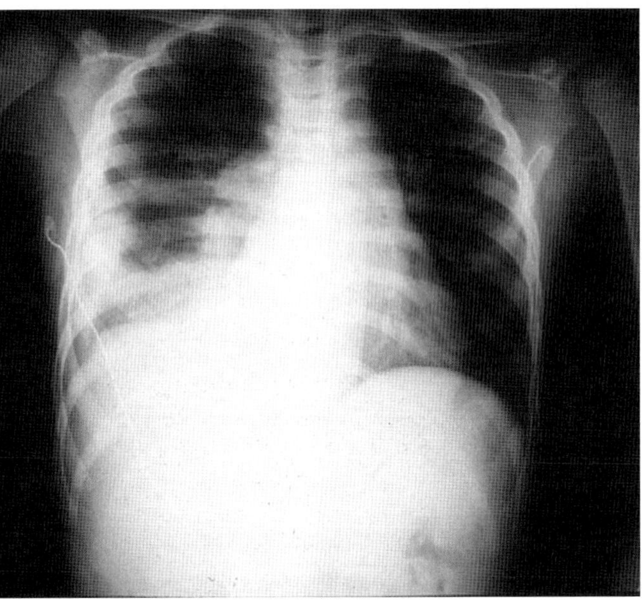

FIGURE 186-8 Right-sided pleural effusion following primary tuberculous infection. (*Used with permission from Nazha Abughali, MD.*)

- Presentation is sudden onset of fever, cough, chest pain, and shortness of breath.
- The majority of pleural effusions are believed to be secondary to hypersensitivity reaction to mycobacterial antigens in the pleural space.
- Pleurocentesis shows pleocytosis with lymphocytic predominance. AFB stain is usually negative. Pleural biopsy may show caseating granulomas with positive AFB culture.

Adult type pulmonary tuberculosis

- Similar to adult type TB disease, representing reactivation of TB in a previously healed focus. Commonly seen in adolescents (**Figures 186-9** and **186-10**).

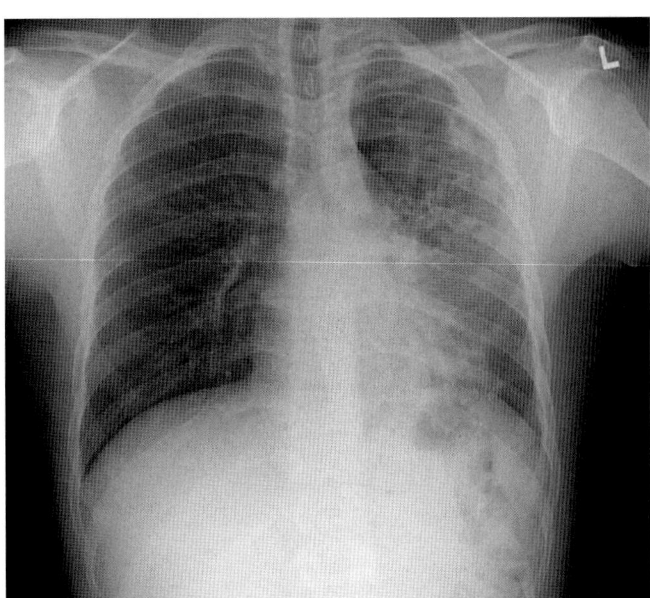

FIGURE 186-9 Significant left upper and left lower lobe infiltrates on chest x-ray of a 16-year-old male with TB pneumonia. (*Used with permission from Nazha Abughali, MD.*)

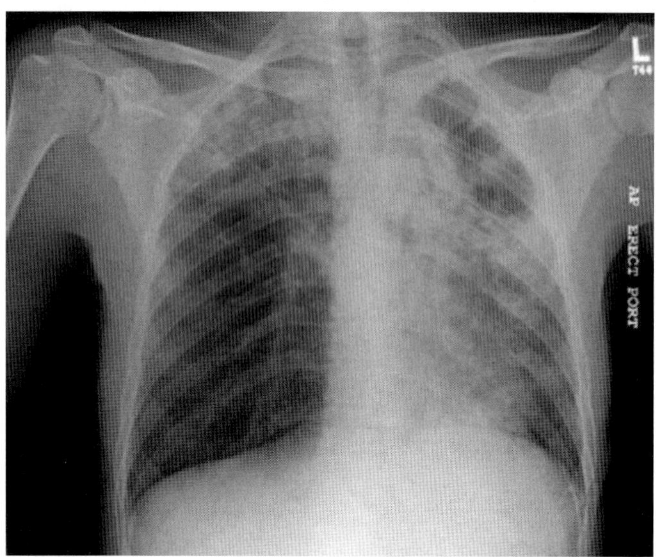

FIGURE 186-10 Nodular infiltrates predominantly in the right upper lobe and entire left lung with cavitary disease in the left upper lobe in a young adult male with tuberculosis. (*Used with permission from Nazha Abughali, MD.*)

- Presents with fever, night sweats, weight loss, cough, malaise, and occasionally hemoptysis.
- CXR shows pulmonary infiltrates with cavitary formation (**Figure 186-7**).
- Patients could be highly contagious and should be placed in respiratory isolation.
- Sputum samples should be obtained for AFB smear, culture, and sensitivity.

▶ Extrapulmonary tuberculosis

Miliary tuberculosis

- A caseous focus may erode into a blood vessel, causing widespread dissemination, usually involving multiple organs.
- More common in infants and young children.
- It occurs early, within 2 to 6 months after the initial infection.
- The patient usually presents with acute onset of high fever, weakness, anorexia, and lethargy. Close to 1/2 of children with miliary TB have evidence of meningitis at the time of diagnosis.
- Physical examination may show evidence of hepatomegaly, splenomegaly, and generalized lymphadenopathy.
- The CXR shows a typical diffuse bilateral miliary pattern throughout the lung fields (**Figure 186-11**).
- AFB stains, cultures, and polymerase chain reaction (PCR) may be obtained from gastric aspirates, tracheal aspirates, and bone marrow and liver biopsies.
- Without prompt recognition and treatment, miliary TB has a very high morbidity mortality rate.

Tuberculous meningitis

- The most severe complication of tuberculous disease.
- It occurs most frequently in children less than 6 years within 3 to 6 months after the primary infection.

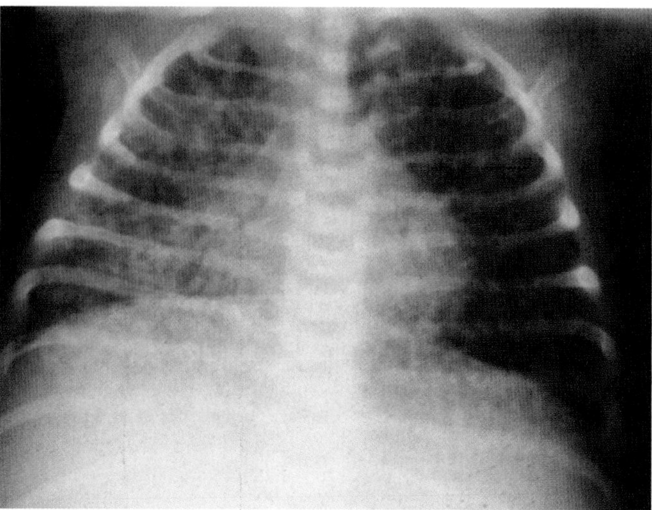

FIGURE 186-11 Miliary tuberculosis in an infant with congenital tuberculosis. (*Used with permission from Nazha Abughali, MD.*)

- The base of the brain is mostly affected with frequent involvement of the cranial nerves II, VI, and VII.
- There are clinically three stages of the disease:
  - Stage I
    - Typically lasts 1 to 2 weeks.
    - Nonspecific symptoms such as fever, headache, irritability, and drowsiness are common.
  - Stage II
    - Begins abruptly.
    - Lethargy, nuchal rigidity, seizures, vomiting, cranial nerve abnormalities, focal neurologic signs, encephalitis, disorientation, and speech impairment are manifestations.
  - Stage III
    - Symptoms include coma, hemiplegia or paraplegia, hypertension, decerebrate or decorticate posturing, and death.
- Prognosis of tuberculous meningitis correlates with the clinical stage of illness and early initiation of therapy.
- Diagnosis is challenging—Up to 40 percent have negative TST and 50 percent have negative CXR.
- Magnetic resonance imaging (MRI) and CT typically show basilar meningitis, communicating hydrocephalus or cranial nerve involvement (**Figures 186-12** and **186-13**).
- CSF studies typically show elevated protein, low glucose, and leukocytosis with lymphocytic predominance. CSF samples should be sent for AFB stain, cultures, and PCR.
- TB brain tuberculomas occur in 5 percent of children with central nervous system (CNS) TB. They usually appear as a ring-enhancing lesion on MRI or CT (**Figure 186-14**). They are more common in developing countries, accounting for 10 to 20 percent of pediatric brain occupying lesions.

Tuberculous lymphadenitis

- TB lymphadenitis involving superficial lymph nodes is the most frequent extrapulmonary manifestation of TB.
- It arises from either a localized extension of a primary lesion or from lymphohematogenous spread of bacilli during the primary infection.

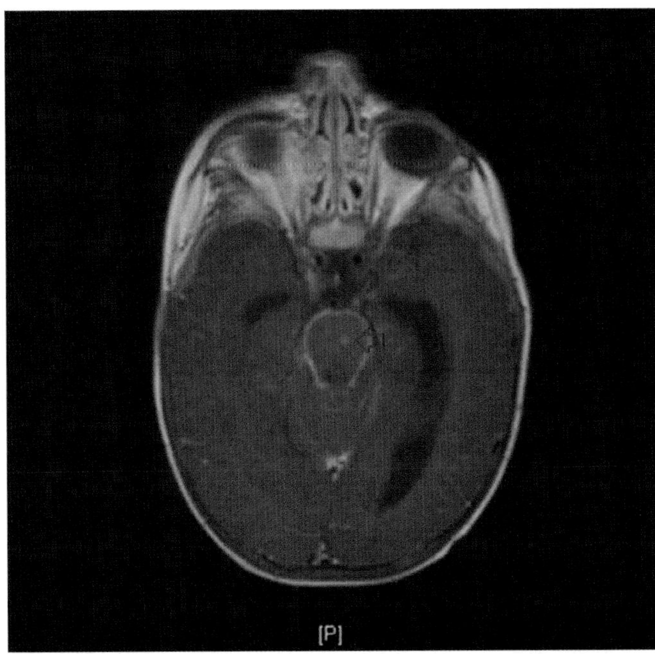

FIGURE 186-12 Tuberuculous meningitis in a 10-month-old girl. Note the leptomeningeal enhancement involving the basal pia-arachnoid and intraparenchymal enhancement (arrow) on MRI. The enlargement of the temporal horn supports the presence of hydrocephalus. (*Used with permission from Nazha Abughali, MD.*)

- It occurs mostly in the neck (known as scrofula). Lymph nodes involved in terms of frequency are anterior cervical, posterior cervical, supraclavicular, submandibular, and submental. The nodes are usually firm and nontender, but may later become matted, indurated, and fluctuant (**Figure 186-15**).

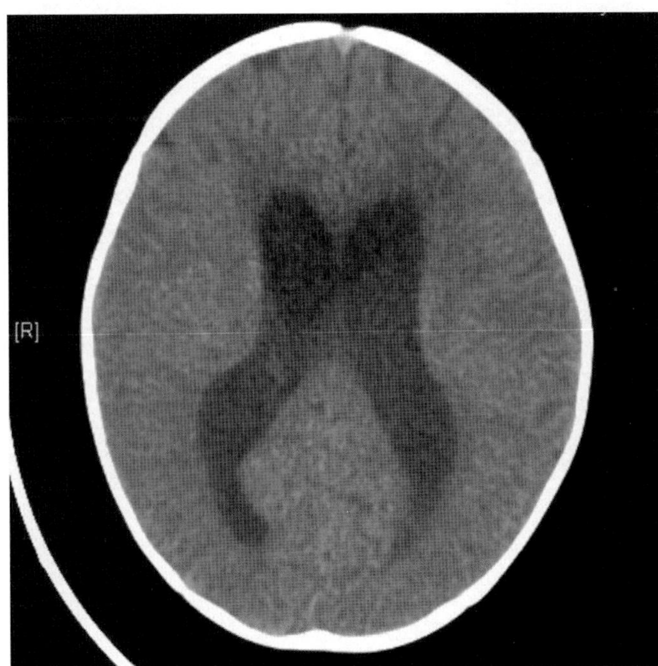

FIGURE 186-13 Communicating hydrocephalus secondary to tuberculous meningitis seen on the head CT of the infant in **Figure 186-11**. (*Used with permission from Nazha Abughali, MD.*)

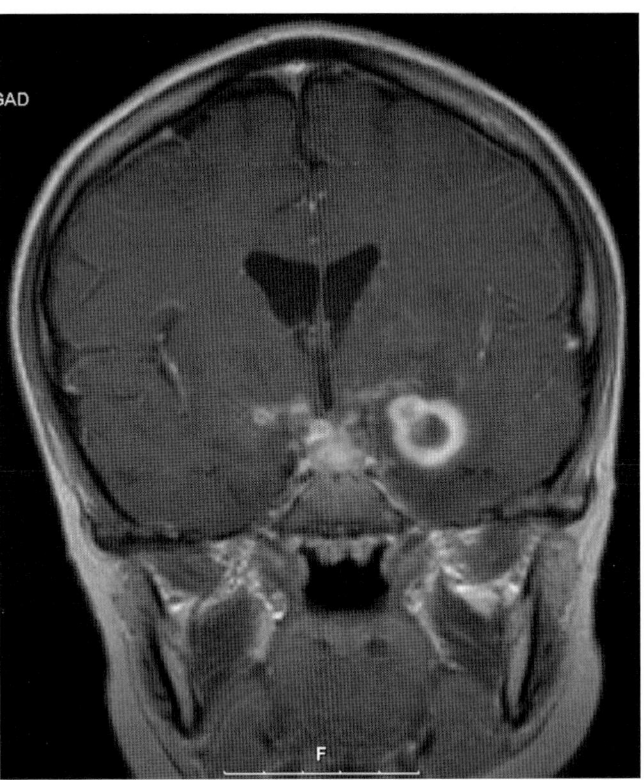

FIGURE 186-14 A tuberculoma shown with an MRI of the brain using gadolinium in an 11-year-old Hispanic child with TB meningitis. The tuberculoma is visualized as a ring enhancing lesion in the left medial and temporal lobe with surrounding edema. Leptomeningeal enhancement is also present. (*Used with permission from Nazha Abughali, MD.*)

- It is important to differentiate between TB lymphadenitis (caused by M.tb) and adenitis caused by non-tuberculous mycobacteria (NTM or MOTT—Mycobacteria other than TB). The TST may be positive in both forms; positive IGRA favors M.tb (**Table 186-1**).
- Biopsy is usually not indicated. If obtained, specimens should be sent for AFB and culture and sensitivity studies.

Skeletal tuberculosis

- Approximately 1/2 of cases of skeletal TB involve the spine. Other areas are the hip, knee, shoulders, and elbow (**Figure 186-16**). Involvement of the smaller bones in the hands and feet (tuberculous dactylitis) may be seen in young children.
- Pathogenesis is mainly secondary to lymphohematogenous dissemination to the bone or synovium at the time of the initial infection, with reactivation occurring 12 to 18 months after the initial infection in children. The presence of a primary focus on CXR strongly supports the diagnosis.
- The clinical presentation depends on the location and may consist of localized pain, swelling, and warmth of the affected joint.
- TST is usually positive.
- Diagnosis—MRI or x-ray. AFB stains and cultures from synovial aspirate and bone biopsy.

Abdominal tuberculosis

- Uncommon, this occurs secondary to ingestion or lymphohematogenous spread of TB.

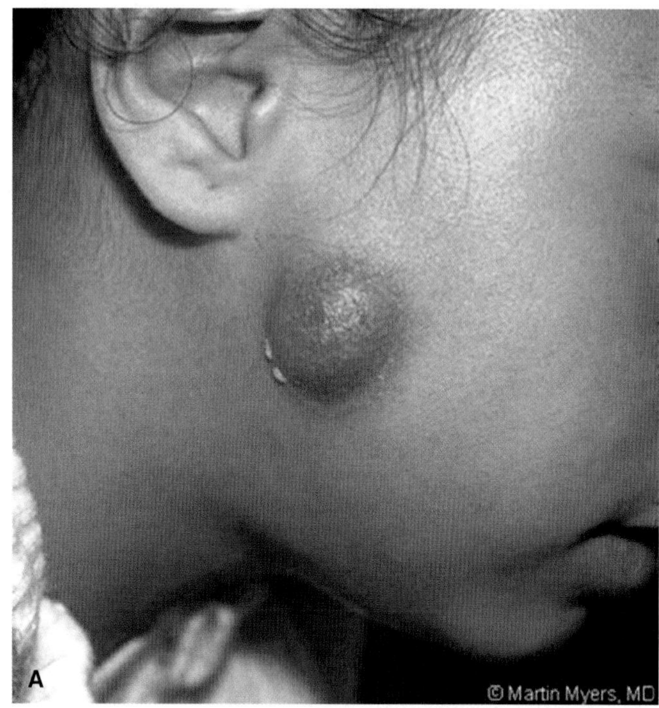

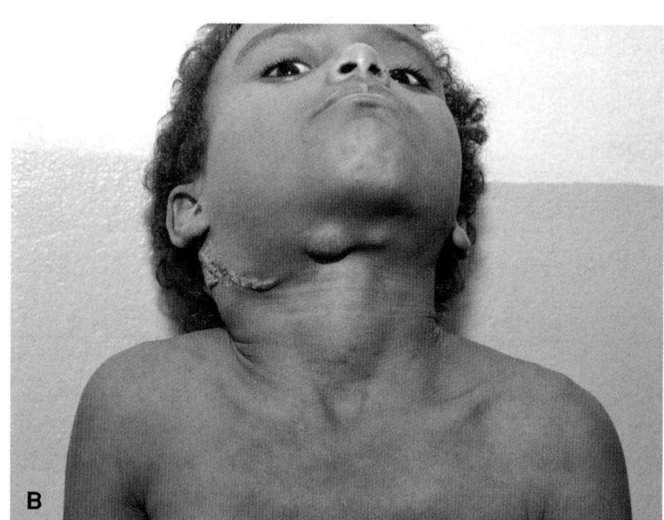

FIGURE 186-15 **A.** *Mycobacterium tuberculosis* scrofula in a young female. (*Used with permission from Martin G. Myers, MD.*) **B.** *Mycobacterium tuberculosis* scrofula in a young boy in Africa. Note the crusting around the areas of drainage in the lateral neck region. (*Used with permission from Richard P. Usatine, MD.*)

- TB enteritis may present with abdominal pain, diarrhea, bloody stools, and weight loss. The ileocecal area is the most commonly involved with the formation of shallow ulcers.
- TB mesenteric lymphadenitis can present as colicky abdominal pain, especially after exercise due to adhesions.

TABLE 186-1 Comparison of Tuberculin Skin Test (TST) with Interferon γ Release Assay (IGRA) Blood Test

TST	IGRA
Intradermal injection	Blood draw
Result is observer dependent	Standardized laboratory results
Requires laboratory expertise and special laboratory equipment	No laboratory equipment or laboratory expertise required
Cannot differentiate disease and infection	Cannot differentiate disease and infection
Requires 2 visits	Requires 1 visit
Booster effect with repeated testing	No booster effect
Less specific, can be positive after BCG vaccination and NTM infection	More specific for M.tb
Can be used for all ages	Recommended for children >4 years of age[1]

[1]Limited data for children under 4 years of age.

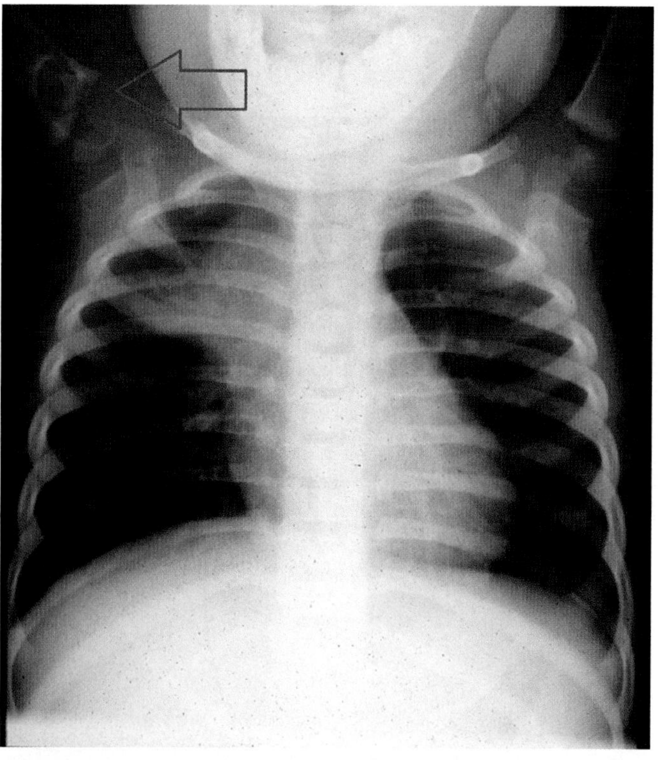

FIGURE 186-16 *Mycobacterium tuberculosis* infection in an 18-month-old with a right upper lobe infiltrate and TB osteomyelitis in the metaphysis of the right humerus (arrow). (*Used with permission from Nazha Abughali, MD.*)

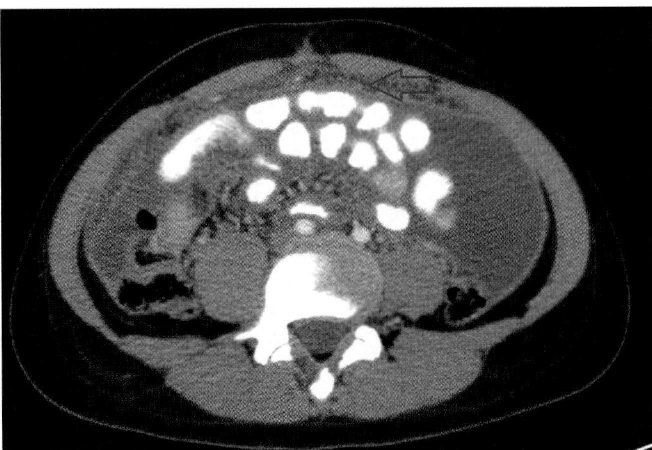

FIGURE 186-17 CT abdomen showing somewhat loculated collection of mesenteric ascites with peripheral enhancement and soft tissue thickening of the omentum. This thickening is known as "caking" (arrow). (*Used with permission from Nazha Abughali, MD.*)

- TB peritonitis could be either plastic or serous type. Plastic peritonitis presents with tender "doughy abdomen." Serous peritonitis might have an insidious presentation with ascites, or could present with fever as bacterial peritonitis.
- Diagnosis—CT of the abdomen could show calcification and nodules in the liver and spleen or mesenteric lymph node enlargement. In TB peritonitis, CT could also show the typical omental caking (**Figure 186-17**). Biopsies of involved organs such as liver, lymph node or omentum and peritoneal fluid could be sent for AFB culture as well as PCR.

LABORATORY TESTING

Currently there are two tests available for the diagnosis of TB infection: TST and IGRA.[5]

- TST is the most common method for diagnosing LTBI. Purified protein derivative (PPD) of tuberculin is injected intradermally into the forearm; the induration is then measured to determine the presence of TB infection (**Table 186-2**).

TABLE 186-2 Risk Factors Associated with a Positive Tuberculin Skin Test (TST)

Induration Size	Risk Factors Associated with a Positive TST
≥5 mm	Immunocompromised Individual Known contact with a TB case Chest radiograph of patient consistent with TB
≥10 mm	Young age (<4 years old) Chronic medical conditions Health care provider Residence/birth in country with high prevalence
≥15 mm	All considered positive

TABLE 186-3 Recommended Uses of Tuberculin Skin Test (TST) and Interferon γ Release Assay (IGRA) Blood Test

Recommended Uses of TST
- Children <5 years of age

Recommended Uses of IGRA
- Persons who have previously received BCG (vaccine)
- Person unlikely to return for TST reading
- Persons with possible exposure due to occupation

Recommended Uses of TST and IGRA
- When initial testing is indeterminate
- If initial testing is negative, but clinical suspicion is high or the outcome is poor
- If initial testing is positive, but there is a history of BCG, confirmatory testing is needed, or if nontuberculous mycobacterial disease is suspected

- Interferon Gamma Release Assays (IGRA) were recently developed and approved for the diagnosis of TB infection. Two tests are currently licensed in the US. The first is the QuantiFERON-TB (Cellestix, Carnegie, Australia) that measures whole-blood interferon γ production. The second test is the enzyme-linked immunospot (ELISPOT, T-SPOT.TB, Oxford Immunotec, Oxford, UK), which measures the number of lymphocytes that produce interferon γ (**Tables 186-1** and **186-3**). Both employ incubation of blood lymphocytes with M.tb specific antigens.

LABORATORY DIAGNOSIS OF TB DISEASE

- The most commonly used AFB stains are the Ziehl-Neelsen and the Fluorochrome stains. The AFB smear cannot differentiate M. tuberculosis from mycobacteria other than TB (MOTT).
- Specimens for AFB stain and culture can be obtained from gastric aspirates, sputum, bronchial washings, pleural fluid, CSF, urine, or tissue biopsies. Early morning gastric lavage in young children and induced sputum in older children have the highest yield. Drug susceptibility testing should be performed on all positive cultures.
- *M. tuberculosis* is a very slow growing organism. Cultures may take 3 to 6 weeks to grow on solid media, with drug susceptibility testing requiring an additional 4 weeks (**Figure 186-18**). Use of solid media allows examination of colony morphology and quantification of growth. Growth can be detected in 1 to 3 weeks by utilizing a liquid media; drug susceptibilities results in an additional 3 to 5 days.
- The presence of *M. tuberculosis* in clinical specimens sometimes can be detected directly within hours using nucleic acid amplification (NAA) tests (including PCR); studies in children are limited.
- Mycobacterial TB cultures are positive in less than 50 percent of children with clinical diagnosis of pulmonary TB.
- Histological examination of all specimens from lymph nodes, liver, pleura, and peritoneal mesentery with demonstration of AFB and granulomas can be very supportive of TB diagnosis (**Figures 186-19** and **186-20**).

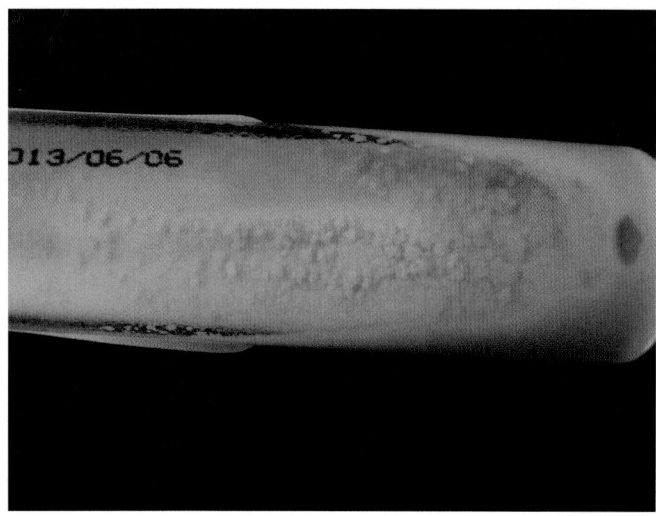

FIGURE 186-18 Tan crumb-like colonies of *M. tuberculosis* on Lowenstein-Jense agar. (*Used with permission from Joseph Tomashefksi, MD.*)

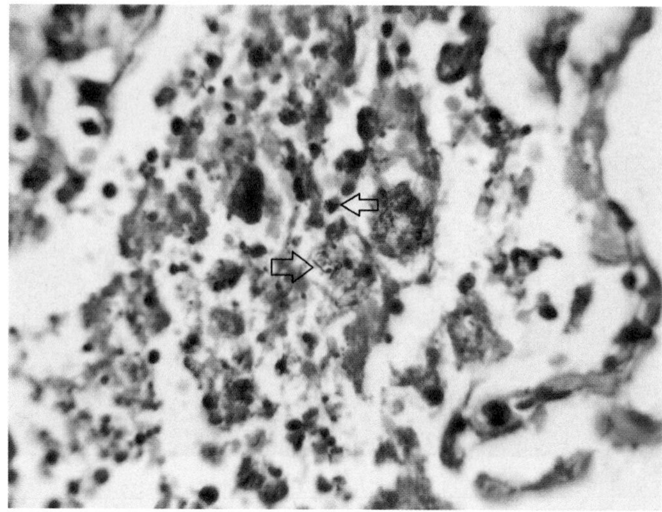

FIGURE 186-20 Acid fast bacilli (arrows) associated with caseous necrosis shown on Ziehl-Neelsen staining. (*Used with permission from Joseph Tomashefski, MD.*)

IMAGING

- CXR is recommended for all patients with a positive TST and/or IGRA.
- Depending on the extent of infection, patients may need skeletal radiograph, MRI, CT of the chest, and/or CT of the head as well as other specialized radiographic studies.

DIFFERENTIAL DIAGNOSIS

The presenting differential diagnosis of TB is elucidated in **Table 186-4**.

MANAGEMENT[6–9]

- Young children with TB are usually not contagious and do not require respiratory isolation when hospitalized. However, pulmonary TB needs to be ruled out in the caregivers before they are allowed on the pediatric ward.

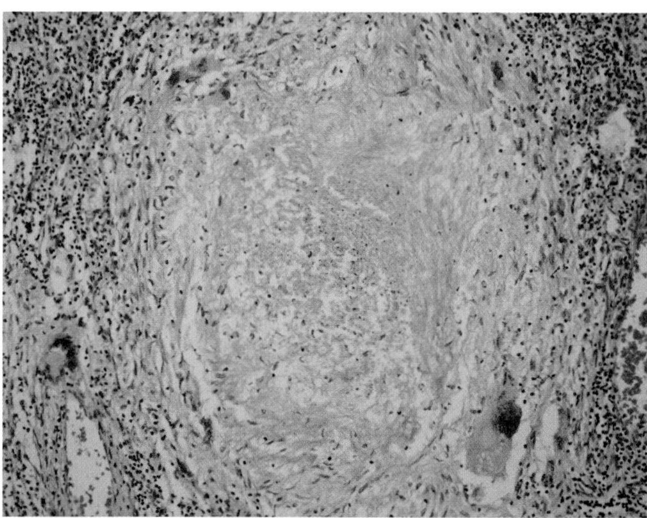

FIGURE 186-19 A caseating granuloma with central caseous necrosis, peripheral epithelioid cells, Langhans giant cells, and a lymphocyte cuff. (*Used with permission from Joseph Tomashefski, MD.*)

- Older children and adolescents require respiratory isolation when they have a cough.
- Whenever possible, AFB cultures and susceptibilities should be obtained in every child with suspected TB especially in the presence of:
  - Extrapulmonary TB.
  - Possible exposure to a source case with multiple drug resistant TB (MDR-TB).
  - HIV infection.
  - Child is suspected to have MDR-TB based on a history of travel or birth in areas with high TB prevalence.
- It is important to be aware of the TB resistance pattern in different areas of the world, especially in foreign-born children. All TB cases should be reported to the local TB program, and contact investigation of all family members and close contacts should be performed.
- Ideally all children with TB should have directly observed therapy to ensure compliance with treatment.

PHARMACOLOGIC

- The choice of the initial TB regimen in a child usually depends on:
  - The type of TB disease.
  - Susceptibility pattern in the child and/or the source case (if available).
  - The countries TB resistance pattern.
- See **Table 186-5** for a summary of treatment recommendations.
- Corticosteroids are indicated as an adjunct therapy in tuberculosis meningitis and may be considered in endobronchial disease, or pleural/pericardial effusions and abdominal TB. SOR Ⓒ
- Vitamin B6 is recommended for breastfed infants, and HIV infected and/or malnourished children. SOR Ⓒ

TABLE 186-4 Presenting Differential Diagnosis of TB

Presenting Diagnosis	
Pneumonia	• Infectious: Bacterial: *Streptococcus pneumoniae, Streptococcus pyogenes, Staphylococcus aureus, Nocardia* Fungal: Blastomycosis, Histoplasmosis, Actinomycosis, Nontuberculous mycobacteria • Malignancy: Squamous cell carcinoma
Meningitis	• Infectious: Bacterial: *Streptococcus pneumoniae, Neisseria meningitides*, Brucellosis Fungal: Cryptococcosis, Deep-seated granulomatous fungal infections
Brain Tuberculoma	• Abscess (Bacterial or Fungal) • Tumor
Lymphadenopathy	Intrathoracic: • Infectious: Fungal (Histoplasmosis), HIV, Nontuberculous mycobacteria • Malignancy: Hodgkin Lymphoma and Non-Hodgkin Lymphoma • Other: Sarcoidosis Peripheral: • Infectious: Nontuberculous mycobacteria, *Bartonella henselae, Staphylococcus aureus, Streptococcus pyogenes*, CMV, EBV, HIV, *Toxoplasma gondii* • Malignancy: Lymphoma
Peritonitis	• Bacterial peritonitis • Peritoneal Carcinomatosis
TB Enteritis	• Inflammatory bowel disease
Osteoarthritis	• Infectious: Group A *Streptococcus, Staphylococcus aureus* • Fungal
Miliary	• Malignancy: Disseminated neuroblastoma, Thyroid carcinoma • Fungal: Histoplasmosis • Lymphocytic interstitial pneumonia

TABLE 186-5 Treatment Recommendations for Tuberculosis

	Primary Treatment	Recommendations for Drug Resistance
TB Exposure	• Child <4 years of age and those with HIV infection should receive isoniazid or rifampin therapy until second testing.	• Consult specialist for any additional resistance[1]
Latent Tuberculosis Infection	• Isoniazid once daily for 9 months	• Rifampin for 6 months • Consult specialist for any additional resistance[1]
Pulmonary and Extrapulmonary Disease Excluding Meningitis	• Isoniazid, rifampin, pyrazinamide, ethambutol for 2 months followed by isoniazid and rifampin for 4 months[2]	• If hilar adenopathy only is present, treat with 6 months of isoniazid and rifampin • Consult specialist for any additional resistance[1]
Meningitis	• Isoniazid, Rifampin, pyrazinamide, and an aminoglycoside or ethambutol or ethionamide for 2 months followed by 7 to 10 months of isoniazid and rifampin	• If resistance to streptomycin is present, use kanamycin, amikacin, or capreomycin • Consult specialist for any additional resistance[1]

[1]Duration of therapy is longer for HIV infected patients, and additional drugs may be indicated.
[2]In the initial CXR shows cavitary lesions, and sputum remains positive after 2 months of therapy, the duration of therapy is extended to 9 months.

SURGERY

- Surgical intervention includes obtaining a biopsy or aspiration sample when needed for diagnosis.
- Some patients will develop hydrocephalus and require a cerebral shunt to be placed.

REFERRAL

- Patients should be referred to the local tuberculosis program and/or infectious disease specialist.
- Ophthalmology referrals may be required for infants on ethambutol to rule out optic neuritis.
- Patients that require surgical intervention will need referred to the appropriate surgical specialist.

PREVENTION AND SCREENING

- TB prevention and control is a collaborative responsibility between health care workers and public health officials. Health care workers are required to report all suspected TB cases to their local TB program. In turn, it is the responsibility of the TB program to:
- Complete contact investigation of all TB exposed individuals.
- Prescribe TB preventive therapy to all exposed children under the age of 4 years until the second TB test results are available.
- Prescribe treatment to all LTBI cases, especially in individuals that are young, newly converted, or immunocompromised.

The American Association of Pediatrics (AAP) has recommendations for screening children who are at risk for TB (2):

Immediate Testing

- If a contact person of the child has TB disease.
- If the child was born in a high risk country.
- Any child with radiographic findings that suggest TB infection.

Non-Urgent Testing

- If a family member of the child has a positive TST.
- If the child has traveled to a high risk country and stayed for more than 1 week or immigrated from a high risk country.

Annual Testing

- Yearly TST screening should be done in all children with HIV or adolescents that are incarcerated.
- The only vaccine currently available is the BCG vaccine. It is used worldwide except in the US and the Netherlands. In general it has low efficacy, with the primary value of the vaccine being in the prevention of miliary TB and tuberculous meningitis in young infants.

PROGNOSIS

- In children, isoniazid treatment of LTBI is close to 100 percent effective in preventing future TB disease.
- Prognosis for children with drug susceptible TB who are compliant with antituberculous therapy is usually excellent, with cure rates of 95 to 100 percent.
- Without early diagnosis and prompt initiation of appropriate therapy, TB meningitis and miliary TB could be associated with high morbidity and mortality.

FOLLOW-UP

- A CXR, CT, or additional imaging should be completed as clinically indicated for patients with pulmonary tuberculosis.
- Follow-up with neurology and neurosurgery is needed in any patient with central nervous system involvement. Ophthalmology will need to follow up patients with ocular involvement.
- Liver function tests are not routinely recommended unless the child has history of hepatitis or has signs or symptoms such as jaundice, vomiting and abdominal pain.

PATIENT RESOURCES[8]

- CDC website has fact sheets available for patients—**www.cdc.gov/tb/publications/factsheets/general/tb.htm**.

PROVIDER RESOURCES[9]

- TB program information is also available at the CDC website—**www.cdc.gov/tb/programs/Evaluation/Default.htm**.
- CDC website has fact sheets available for providers—**www.cdc.gov/tb/publications/factsheets/general/tb.htm**.

REFERENCES

1. World Health Organization. *Tuberculosis*. http://www.who.int/topics/tuberculosis/en/, accessed 2012.
2. Red Book Online. *Tuberculosis*. http://aapredbook.aappublications.org/content/1/SEC131/SEC283.body, accessed 2012.
3. Centers for Disease Control. *Tuberculosis*. http://www.cdc.gov/tb/statistics/default.htm, accessed 2012.
4. Marais, BJ, Gie, RP, Schaaf, HS, et al: The natural history of childhood intra-thoracic tuberculosis: A critical review of the pre-chemotherapy literature. *Int. J. Tuberc. Lung Dis*. 2004;8:392-402.
5. Center for Disease Control: Updated Guidelines for Using Interferon Gamma Release Assays to Detect Mycobacterium tuberculosis Infection—United States, 2010. www.cdc.gov/mmwr/pdf/rr/rr5905.pdf.
6. Fitzgerald, DW, Sterling, TR, Haas, DW: Mandell: Mandell, Douglas, and Bennett's Principles and Practice of Infectious Diseases. In: *Mycobacterium Tuberculosis*, 7th ed. Philadelphia, PA: Churchill Livingstone, Elsevier; 2009:3129-3163.
7. Starke JR, Feigin RD, Cherry J, Demmler-Harrison GJ, Kaplan SL, eds. *Tuberculosis*. St. Louis, MO: Saunders Elsevier; 2009: 771-786.
8. Newton SM, Brent AJ, Aderson S, et al. Pediatric Tuberculosis. *Lancet Infect Dis*. 2008;8:498-510. http://www.cdc.gov/mmwr/preview/mmwrhtml/rr5905a1.htm?s_cid=rr5905a1_e. Mazurek, GH, Jereb, J, Vernon, A, et al. 2010.
9. Cruz, AT, Starke, JR: Pediatric Tuberculosis. *Pediatrics in Review*. 2010;31:13-26.

187 CONGENITAL AND PERINATAL INFECTIONS

Camille Sabella, MD

PATIENT STORY

A 7-day-old infant is seen in the emergency department because of a rash that was noted on the infant's trunk and back. The rash consisted of crops of vesicular lesions on an erythematous base (**Figure 187-1**). The infant was born at term gestation to an 18-year-old mother who had poor prenatal care. The mother denied a history of herpes simplex infection or other sexually transmitted infections. A direct fluorescent antibody test for herpes simplex virus (HSV) was positive and an HSV culture from the lesion was positive. A lumbar puncture was normal, and blood and CSF tests for HSV DNA were negative. The infant was admitted and treated with intravenous acyclovir for 14 days and recovered without sequelae.

INTRODUCTION

Many microbiological agents can cause infection in the newborn infant. These infections may be acquired *in utero*, at the time of delivery, or in the immediate newborn period. Although the majority of congenital infections result in inapparent infection, it is imperative to recognize infections that manifest symptomatically. Although the clinical manifestations of these infections may be similar regardless of the pathogen, specific clinical findings and patterns may serve as important clues for specific microorganisms.

EPIDEMIOLOGY

- The epidemiology varies depending on the organism responsible for the infection:

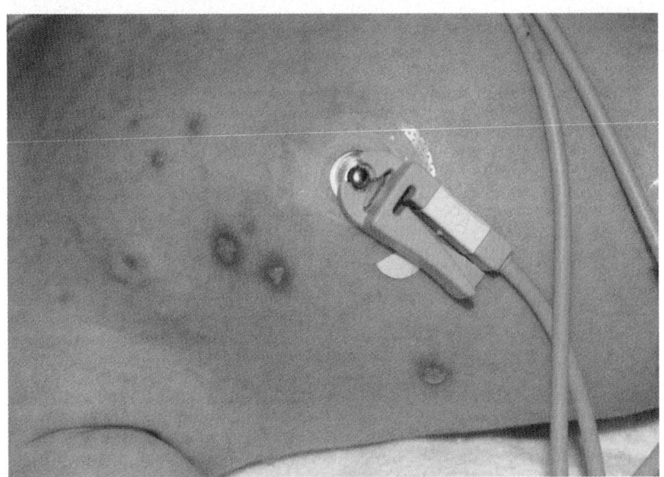

FIGURE 187-1 Vesicular lesions of HSV in an infant. (*Used with permission from Johanna Goldfarb, MD.*)

Streptococcus agalactiae (Group B Streptococci)

- Incidence of early onset disease (presentation in the first week of life) is 0.3/1000 live births.[1,2]
- Early-onset disease is related to perinatal transmission of the organism.
- Fifteen to forty percent of pregnant women are colonized with the organism in the genital and/or gastrointestinal tract.
- Fifty to seventy percent of colonized mothers transmit the organism to their infants; 1 to 2 percent of colonized infants develop early-onset sepsis (if intrapartum antimicrobial prophylaxis is not provided); risk higher if risk factors are present (see the following section "Risk Factors").
- Incidence of early-onset GBS infection has decreased significantly since the implementation of maternal intrapartum antibiotic prophylaxis.[3]

Herpes Simplex Virus (HSV)

- Incidence is estimated to be 1 per 3200 deliveries.[4]
- Most neonates acquire the virus from an infected maternal genital tract at the time of delivery.[5]
- HSV-2 accounts for 70 percent of neonatal cases while HSV-1 accounts from 30 percent of cases.
- Because most maternal genital infections are asymptomatic, 60 to 80 percent of neonates who have HSV infection are born to mothers who have no history of current or past genital HSV infection.[5]
- The transmission rate from mother to infant during maternal primary infection is 35 to 50 percent, while the transmission rate during a recurrence of HSV is 2 to 5 percent.

Enteroviruses

- Newborns who become infected most commonly acquire these viruses at the time of delivery.
- In temperate climates, these viruses most commonly cause infections in late summer and early autumn.
- Recent maternal febrile illness and abdominal pain, lack of obstetrical complications, and summertime or autumn illness may serve as clues to the diagnosis.[6]

Cytomegalovirus (CMV)

- Most common congenital infection, affecting approximately 1 percent of all newborns in the US.[7]
- Can be acquired in utero, perinatally, or postnatally, through breastfeeding or blood transfusion.
- Can be acquired as a result of maternal primary or recurrent infection; risk considerably higher if infection is a result of a primary maternal infection.

Toxoplasma infection

- Incidence in the US is 1 per 1,000 to 8,000 live births.[8]
- Maternal acquisition of the organism occurs via the ingestion of food containing cysts or by exposure to oocytes excreted by cats.

- Congenital infection can occur when a pregnant mother has a primary infection.
- Risk of transmission to the fetus increases with advancing gestational age; however, neonatal manifestations are more severe when the fetus is infected early in pregnancy (i.e., first trimester).[9]

Rubella

- The incidence of congenital rubella in the US today is very low because of widespread immunization against the virus.
- All congenital cases are due to maternal primary infection during pregnancy.
- Overall risk of infection of the fetus is 80 to 100 percent if maternal infection occurs during the first trimester. Risk is significantly lower if maternal infection occurs in the second or third trimester.[10]

Syphilis

- The incidence of congenital syphilis had declined to the lowest reported levels in 2000. Since that time, the rate of primary and secondary syphilis has increased among women, with a concomitant increase in cases of congenital syphilis since 2005.[11]

ETIOLOGY AND PATHOPHYSIOLOGY

- Bacterial causes of perinatal infections include *Streptococcus agalactiae* (Group B), *Escherichia coli*, and *Listeria monocytogenes.*
- Bacterial pathogens that cause early-onset infection are most commonly transmitted to the infant at the time of delivery.
- HSV is most commonly acquired by the neonate at the time of delivery; infection of the neonate may occur *in utero* (very rare) or may occur after postnatal acquisition from an oro-labial HSV infection.
- CMV infection in the neonate may follow a primary or recurrent maternal infection and may be acquired *in utero*, at the time of delivery or postnatally, through breastfeeding or blood transfusion.
- *Toxoplasma gondii* and Rubella congenital infections are a result of maternal primary infection.
- Transplacental transmission of *Treponema pallidum* may result in congenital syphilis; because the fetus acquires the infection from hematogenous spread, the clinical manifestations in the newborn are similar to those of secondary syphilis.

RISK FACTORS

- Risk factors for Group B Streptococcal sepsis include:
  - Maternal colonization at the time of delivery.
  - Prematurity (less than 37 weeks gestation).
  - Prolonged rupture of membranes (>18 hours).
  - Chorioamnionitis/maternal fever.
  - Group B Streptococcal bacteriuria.
- A risk factor for neonatal enteroviral infection is exposure of a pregnant mother to a contact who is shedding enterovirus.
- Prolonged contact with young children, especially among parents, is a risk factor for primary CMV infection during pregnancy.[12]
- Ingestion of undercooked pork, beef, and lamb during pregnancy serve as an important source of primary *Toxoplasma* maternal infection.
- Non-immunity to rubella during pregnancy—either from lack of vaccination or incomplete vaccination—is a risk factor for maternal rubella infection.
- Untreated syphilis in a pregnant mother may result in congenital syphilis.

DIAGNOSIS

CLINICAL FEATURES

▶ Perinatally acquired infections

- The clinical manifestations of infections acquired around the time of delivery usually become apparent soon after birth but may occur anytime in the neonatal period. Examples of these infections include *S. agalactiae* (Group B), *E. coli*, *L. monocytogenes*, herpes simplex virus, and enteroviruses.
- Pneumonia, septic shock, and meningitis are manifestations of perinatally acquired infections; brain abscess may complicate meningitis caused by neonatal pathogens, especially gram negative organisms (**Figure 187-2**).
- The clinical manifestations of infection in the neonatal period may be subtle and are similar regardless of etiology; meningitis is clinically indistinguishable from sepsis in this age group.
- Common manifestations include temperature instability, respiratory distress, apnea, feeding intolerance, lethargy, and jaundice.

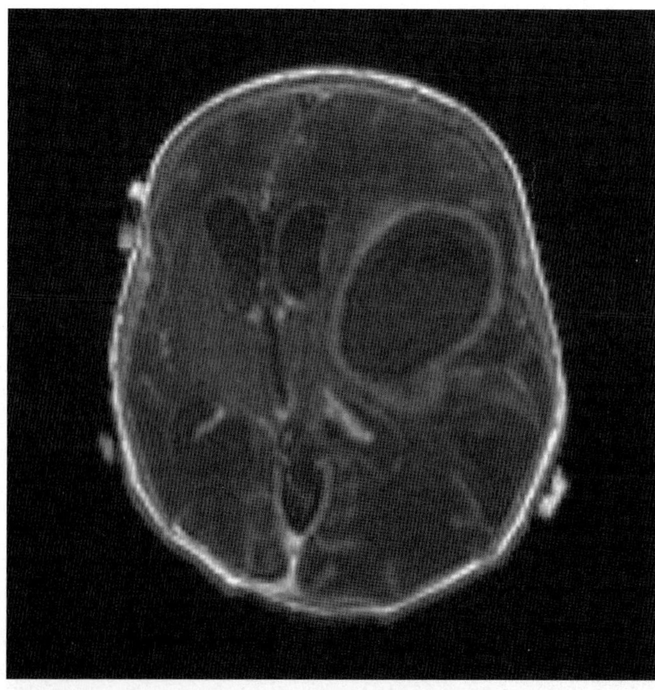

FIGURE 187-2 Multiple brain abscesses seen on MRI in a 3-week-old infant. Brain abscess is a complication of meningitis in neonates, and most commonly is caused by gram-negative organisms like *Citrobacter koseri, Serratia marcescens,* and *E. coli.* (*Used with permission from Camille Sabella, MD.*)

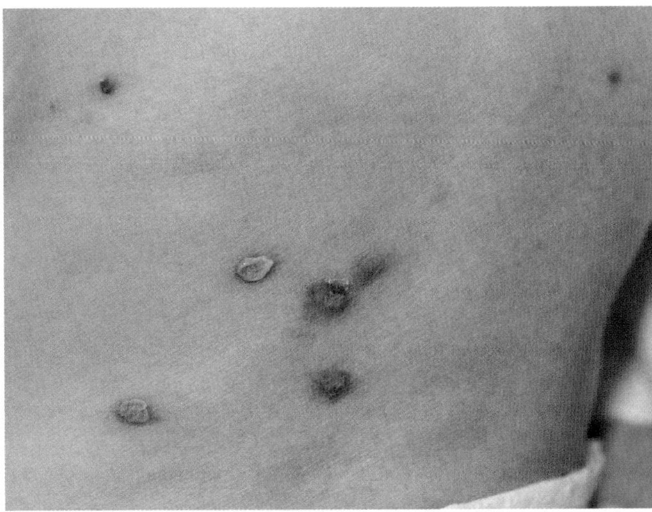

FIGURE 187-3 Crops of vesicular lesions on an erythematous base, characteristic of HSV infections in a 10-day-old infant. (*Used with permission from Blanca E. Gonzalez, MD.*)

- Herpes simplex virus infection in the newborn may manifest with localized disease (confined to the skin, eyes, or mucous membranes), disseminated infection, or infection confined to the central nervous system.[13]
- Vesicular lesions, forming singly, or in clusters, on an erythematous base (**Figure 187-3**) are the hallmark features of localized HSV infection in the newborn.
- Enteroviral infections in the newborn may be mild and nonspecific, or may be severe and life-threatening; a macular, maculopapular, vesicular, or petechial rash may be present in these infants (**Figure 187-4**).[6]

Intrauterine infections

- The manifestations of intrauterine infections may be apparent at or shortly after birth, or they may become apparent months to years later.
- Clinical features of congenital infections are similar regardless of the etiology and are listed in **Table 187-1**.

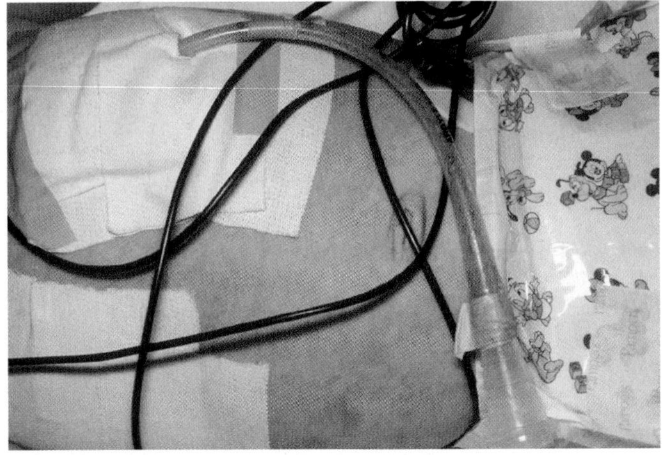

FIGURE 187-4 Enteroviral infection in a critically ill infant. Note the subtle maculopapular rash which can serve as a clue to the diagnosis. (*Used with permission from Camille Sabella, MD.*)

TABLE 187-1 Common Clinical Manifestations of Intrauterine Infection

Hepatosplenomegaly
Jaundice
Rash
Microcephaly
Intracranial calcifications
Meningoencephalitis
Chorioretinitis
Cataracts
Microphthalmia
Bone lesions
Adenopathy
Cardiac abnormalities
Pneumonitis
Thrombocytopenia
Anemia
Sensorineural hearing loss

- Infections with certain pathogens may result in more specific congenital abnormalities:
  - Infants with CMV infection may manifest with cytomegalic inclusion disease consisting of intrauterine growth retardation, hepatosplenomegaly, jaundice, thrombocytopenia, lymphadenopathy, petechial/purpuric rash, and microcephaly (**Figure 187-5**).[14]
  - Common manifestations of rubella infection include hepatosplenomegaly, jaundice, cataracts (**Figure 187-6**), blueberry

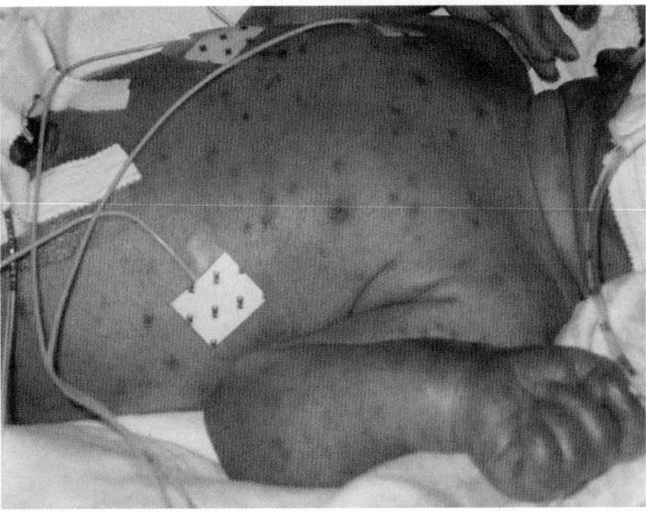

FIGURE 187-5 Infant with the "blueberry muffin" rash representing extramedullary hematopoiesis. This is classically described for congenital rubella but can be seen with congenital CMV as well. (*Used with permission from Shah SS. Pediatric Practice: Infectious Diseases. Figure 50-1. www.accesspediatrics.com.*)

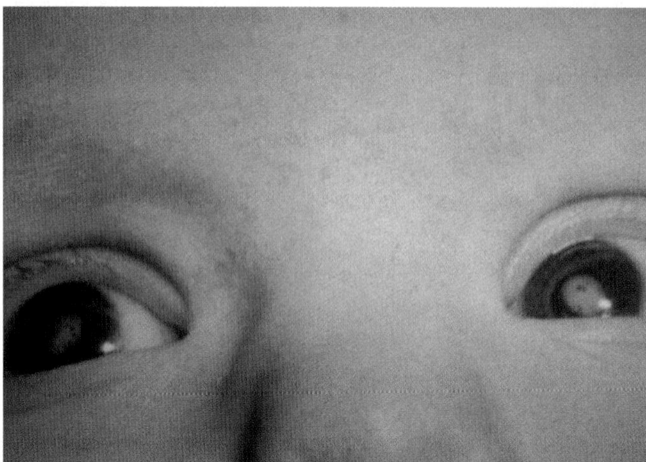

FIGURE 187-6 Bilateral cataracts in an infant with congenital rubella syndrome. (*Used with permission from CDC.*)

muffin lesions (dermal erythropoiesis; **Figure 187-7**), and congenital heart disease.
- The classic triad of congenital toxoplasma infection include chorioretinitis, hydrocephalus, and cerebral calcifications.[15]
- Early features (first 3 months of age) of congenital syphilis include syphilitic rhinitis (snuffles), maculopapular, or vesicobullous rash on the palms, soles, mouth or anus, and long bone periostitis (**Figures 187-8** and **187-9**; see Chapter 181, Syphilis).[16]

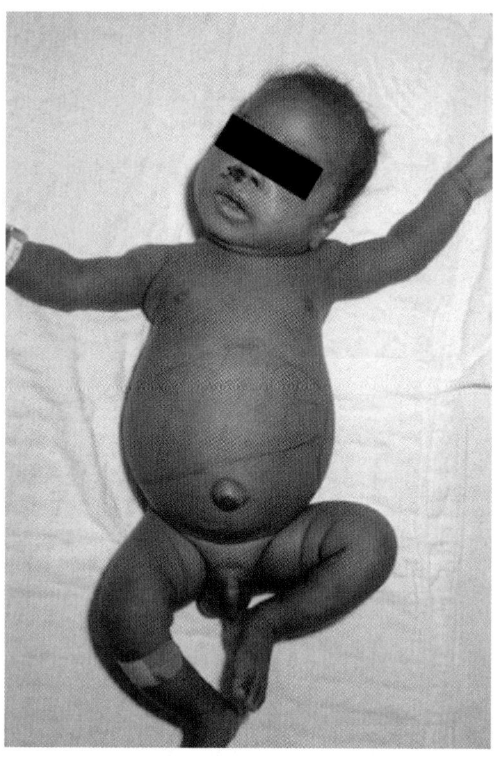

FIGURE 187-8 A newborn infant with congenital syphilis. Note the hepatosplenomegaly as outlined, right sided axillary adenopathy, and the bloody, mucousy nasal discharge (snuffles). (*Used with permission from Camille Sabella, MD.*)

LABORATORY TESTING

- The diagnosis of bacterial sepsis and meningitis relies on isolating an organism from the blood or cerebrospinal fluid.
- Hematologic abnormalities and inflammatory markers are neither sensitive nor specific for the diagnosis of neonatal sepsis.
- Viral culture from a vesicular lesion is the most reliable method of diagnosing localized HSV infection in the newborn; direct fluorescent antibody testing of cells from a skin lesion can also be utilized to provide a rapid diagnosis.[17,18]
- Viral culture for HSV from sites such as the nasopharynx, conjunctivae, and rectum is used to diagnose disseminated HSV infection.
- Polymerase chain reaction testing for HSV DNA in blood mononuclear cells is recommended for diagnosing disseminated infection.[19]

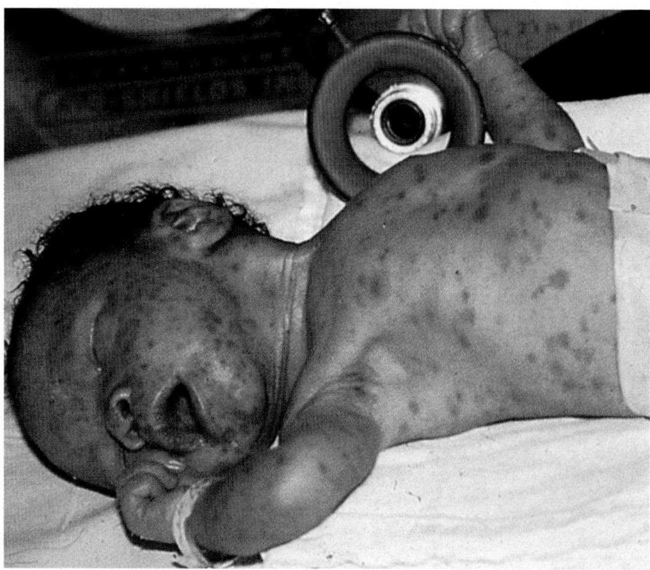

FIGURE 187-7 A neonate with congenital rubella syndrome. Note the "blueberry muffin" rash, which represents sites of extramedullary hematopoiesis. Also note the microcephaly. (*Used with permission from Weinberg SW, Prose NS, Kristal L. Color Atlas of Pediatric Dermatology, 4th edition, Figure 5-51, New York, NY: McGraw-Hill, 2008.*)

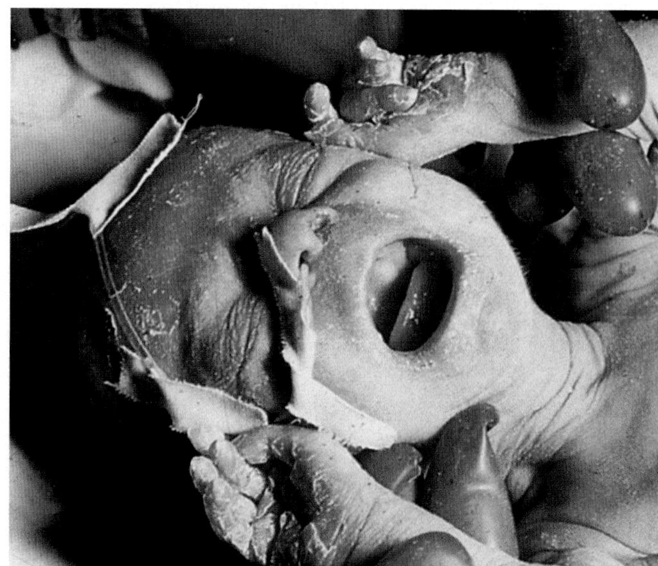

FIGURE 187-9 Infant with congenital syphilis. Note the scaly, bullous rash on the rash and extremities, including the palms in this infant. (*Used with permission from Weinberg SW, Prose NS, Kristal L. Color Atlas of Pediatric Dermatology, 4th edition, Figure 4-1, New York, NY: McGraw-Hill, 2008.*)

- Polymerase chain reaction testing for HSV DNA in the cerebrospinal fluid is the diagnostic test of choice for diagnosing central nervous system infection.[20]
- Viral culture for enterovirus from the nasopharynx and/or rectum is helpful in diagnosing neonatal enteroviral infection; Polymerase chain reaction for enterovirus RNA from cerebrospinal fluid is more sensitive than viral culture for the diagnosis of enteroviral meningoencephalitis.[21]
- A positive urine culture for CMV in the first 2 to 3 weeks of life confirms congenital infection.
- Rubella virus can be isolated in cell culture from sites such as the urine, cerebrospinal fluid or nasopharynx in suspected cases; Rubella specific IgG and IgM titers may also be helpful in establishing the diagnosis.
- The diagnosis of congenital toxoplasmosis is difficult and usually relies on serologic assays on the infant and mother; persistent or rising IgG titers in the infant, or positive specific IgM or IgA assays help establish the diagnosis; nucleic acid assays, histopathology of the placenta or infected tissues and mouse inoculation assays on the infant's blood or placenta may also be helpful.
- Definitive diagnosis of congenital syphilis is difficult; positive nontreponemal and treponemal antibody testing in the mother and the infant is recommended; A positive result of a nontreponemal antibody test in an infant that does not disappear by 6 months of age, a rising titer after birth, or a titer in an infant that is fourfold higher than the mother's titer are highly suggestive of congenital infection.[22]

IMAGING

- Neonatal pneumonia, such as that caused by Group B Streptococcus, is indistinguishable from respiratory distress syndrome of the newborn (**Figure 187-10**).

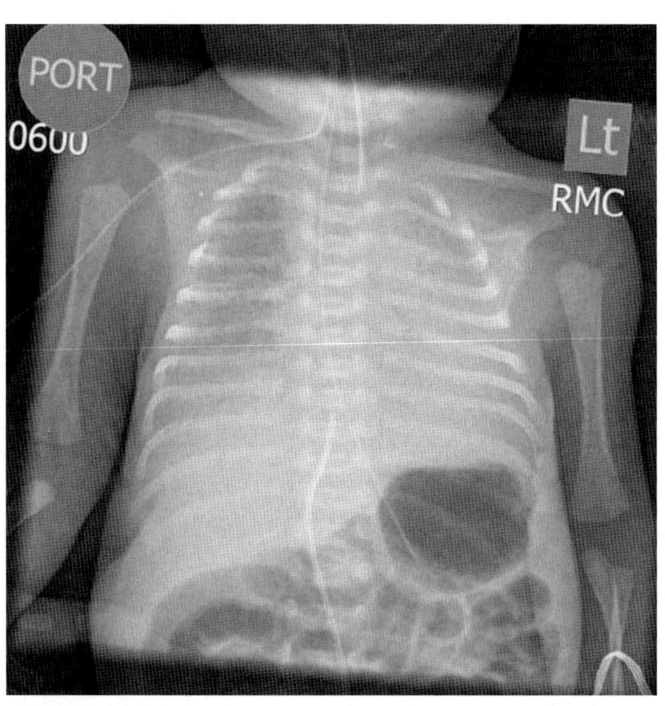

FIGURE 187-10 X-ray of neonatal pneumonia. (*Used with permission from Camille Sabella, MD.*)

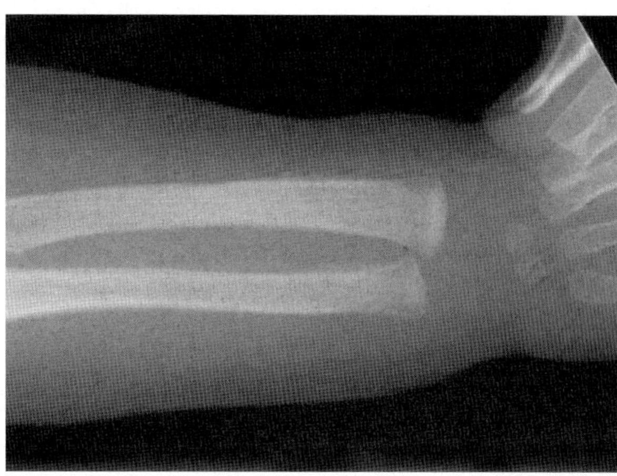

FIGURE 187-11 X-ray of the arm of an infant with congenital syphilis. There are transverse metaphyseal lucent bands seen involving the distal radius and ulna and smooth organized lamellated periosteal new bone seen involving the ulnar diaphysis and metaphysis. (*Used with permission from Camille Sabella, MD.*)

- Brain abscess is a well-known complication of neonatal meningitis, and is a relatively common complication of gram negative meningitis (**Figure 187-2**).
- Periostitis or osteochondritis of long bones may be features of congenital infection, and is a common finding in infants with congenital syphilis (**Figure 187-11**).
- Intracranial calcifications can occur with congenital infection caused by CMV and *Toxoplasma*; calcifications caused by CMV are often periventricular in distribution (**Figure 187-12**) while those caused by *Toxoplasma* are commonly intraparenchymal (**Figure 187-13**).

DIFFERENTIAL DIAGNOSIS

- The clinical manifestation of newborn sepsis and meningitis are often indistinguishable for other newborn illnesses, such as respiratory distress syndrome, congenital heart disease, and metabolic disorders.

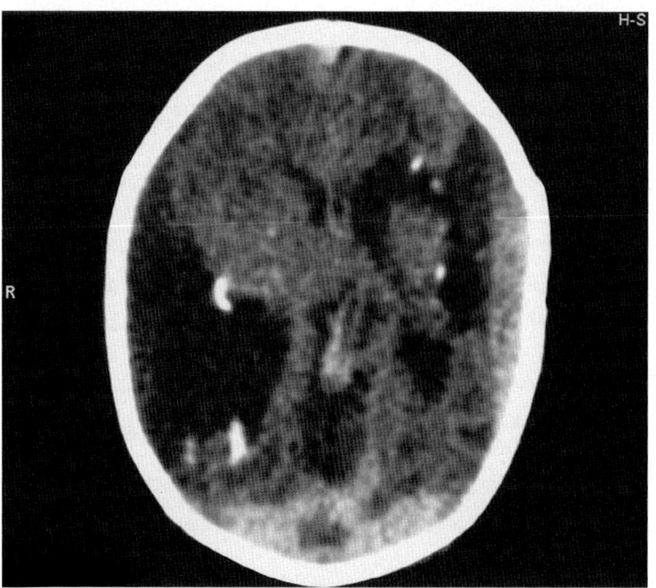

FIGURE 187-12 Periventricular calcifications in an infant with congenital CMV. (*Used with permission from Camille Sabella, MD.*)

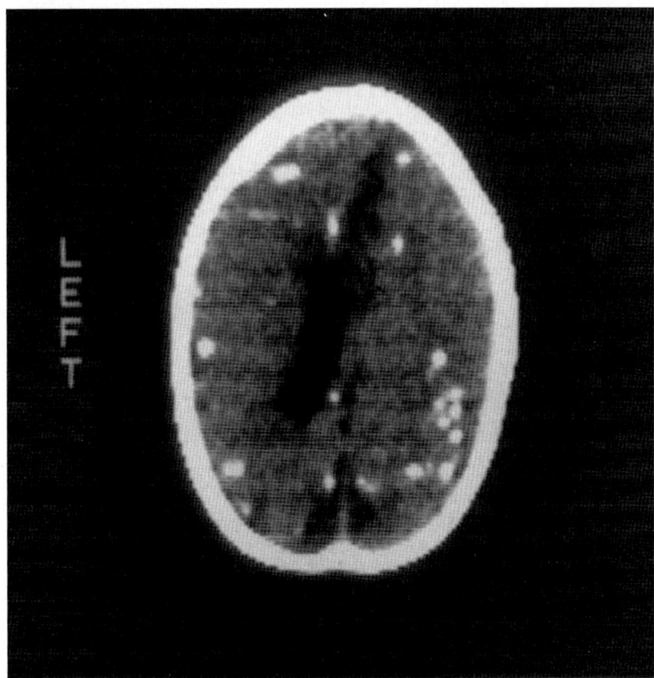

FIGURE 187-13 Parenchymal calcifications seen on CT in the brain an infant with congenital toxoplasmosis. (*Used with permission from Camille Sabella, MD.*)

MANAGEMENT

NONPHARMACOLOGIC

- Appropriate respiratory and hemodynamic support should be provided for every newborn suspected of having or proven to have an infection.

MEDICATIONS

- Antimicrobial therapy for newborns suspected of having bacterial sepsis should be initiated empirically and must include coverage for Group B Streptococci, *E. coli*, and *L. monocytogenes*.
- Ampicillin and gentamicin is appropriate therapy for such infants; more specific therapy directed against a particular pathogen can be undertaken once a pathogen is identified. SOR Ⓒ
- Parenteral acyclovir is the treatment of choice for infants with HSV infection.[23,24] SOR Ⓐ
- The benefit of antiviral therapy for congenital CMV infection is currently under study; antiviral therapy for infants with congenital CMV infection is not routinely recommended at this time.[25] SOR Ⓒ
- Early institution of pyrimethamine and sulfadiazine for infants with congenital T*oxoplasma* infection decreases the severity of disease and the frequency of sequelae.[26] SOR Ⓑ
- Parenteral Penicillin G therapy is recommended for infants with proven or suspected congenital syphilis.[27,28] SOR Ⓐ

PREVENTION AND SCREENING

- Vaginal and rectal cultures for Group B Streptococcal carriage should be performed in all pregnant women at 35 to 37 weeks' gestation.[29,30]
- Intrapartum antibiotic prophylaxis (penicillin is preferred agent) is recommended for mothers who have:
  - A positive screening test for Group B streptococcus.
  - Group B streptococcal bacteriuria during current pregnancy.
  - Previous infant with group B streptococcal disease.
- If the group B streptococcal status of the mother is unknown at the time of delivery, maternal intrapartum prophylaxis is indicated if any of the following are present:
  - Delivery at less than 37 weeks gestation.
  - Membranes ruptured for 18 hours or longer.
  - Intrapartum fever (temperature ≥38°C [100.4°F]).
  - Positive intrapartum nucleic acid amplification test for group B streptococcus.
- All women should be screened serologically for syphilis early in pregnancy and preferably again at delivery; no newborn should be discharged from the hospital without determination of the mothers syphilis serologic status at least once during pregnancy.[27,31]

PROGNOSIS

- The case fatality rate of perinatally acquired bacterial sepsis and meningitis is 10 to 25 percent.
- Long-term neurologic sequelae develop in 25 to 50 percent of survivors of neonatal bacterial meningitis.
- Despite antiviral therapy, there is a 30 percent mortality rate among neonates with disseminated HSV infection; those with localized infections that are appropriately treated with antiviral therapy all survive.[24]
- Long-term neurologic sequelae are common in survivors of disseminated and central nervous system HSV infection.[13,24]
- Ten to 15 percent of infants with localized HSV infection have long-term neurologic sequelae, despite appropriate treatment.[24]
- The prognosis of infants with congenital infection is highly variable and dependent upon the agent, the extent of involvement, and the organ systems affected.
- The mortality rate of infants with cytomegalic inclusion disease is 30 percent, whereas the overall mortality of symptomatic CMV congenital infection is 10 to 15 percent.[14]
- Long-term neurologic sequelae, especially hearing loss and intellectual deficits, occur in approximately 5 to 10 percent of infants who have asymptomatic congenital CMV infection.[32–34]

FOLLOW-UP

- Close follow-up of all infants born with perinatally acquired or congenital infection is mandatory, with particular attention to neurodevelopment, hearing, and vision.

PATIENT EDUCATION

- Pregnant women should receive good prenatal care to lower the risk of transmission of infection to their infants.

PATIENT RESOURCES

- **www.congenitalcmv.org/public.htm.**
- **www.cmvfoundation.org.**
- **www.bcm.edu/pediatrics/cmvregistry.**
- **www.cdc.gov/features/pregnancy.**
- **www.cdc.gov/Features/PrenatalInfections.**

PROVIDER RESOURCES

- American Academy of Pediatrics. Pickering LK, Baker CJ, Kimberlin DW, Long SS, eds. *Red Book: 2012 Report of the Committee on Infectious Diseases*. Elk Grove Village, IL: American Academy of Pediatrics; 2012.
- Corey L, Wald A. Maternal and neonatal herpes simplex virus infections. *N Engl J Med*. 2009;361:1376-1385.
- James SH, Kimberlin DW, Whitley RJ. Antiviral therapy for herpesvirus central nervous system infections: Neonatal herpes simplex virus infection, herpes simplex encephalitis, and congenital cytomegalovirus infection. *Antiviral Res*. 2009;83:207-213.

REFERENCES

1. Centers for Disease Control and Prevention. 2011 Active Bacterial Core Surveillance Report, Emerging Infections Program Network, Group B Streptococcus. http://www.cdc.gov/abcs/reports-findings/survreports/gbs10.pdf.
2. Bizzarro MJ, Raskind C, Baltimore RS. Seventy-five years of neonatal sepsis at Yale: 1928–2003. *Pediatrics* 2005;116:595-602.
3. Schrag SJ, Zywicki S, Farley MM, Reingold AL, Harrison LH, Lefkowitz LB et al. Group B streptococcal disease in the era of intrapartum antibiotic prophylaxis. *N Engl J Med*. 2000;342(1):15-20.
4. Brown ZA, Wald A, Morrow RA, SElke S, Zeh J, Corey L. Effect of serologic status and cesarean delivery on transmission rates of herpes simplex virus from mother to infant. *JAMA*. 2003;289:203-209.
5. Brown ZA, Selke SA, Zeh J, et al. The acquisition of herpes simplex virus during pregnancy. *N Engl J Med*. 1997;337:509-515.
6. Lake AM, Lauer BA, Clark JC, Wesenberg RL, McIntosh K. Enterovirus infections in neonates. *J Pediatr*. 1976;89:787-791.
7. Gaytant MA, Steegers EAP, Semmekrot BA, Merkus HMMW, Galama JMD. Congenital cytomegalovirus infection: review of the epidemiology and outcome. *Obstet Gynecol Surv*. 2002;57:245-256.
8. Remington JS, McLeod R, Thuilliez P, and Desmonts G. *Toxoplasmosis*. In: JS Remington, JO Klein, CB Wilson, eds. Infectious Diseases of the Fetus and Newborn Infant, 7th ed. St. Louis, MO: Elsevier Saunders, Philadelphia; 2011.
9. Dunn, M Wallon, Peyron F. Mother-to-child transmission of toxoplasmosis: risk estimates for clinical counseling. *Lancet*. 1999;353:1829-1833.
10. Miller E, Cradock-Watson JE, Pollock JE. Consequences of confirmed maternal rubella at successive stages of pregnancy. *Lancet* 1982; 8302:782-784.
11. Centers for Disease Control and Prevention. Congenital syphilis–United States, 2003-2008. *MMWR*. 2010;59:413-417.
12. Kenneson A, Cannon MJ. Review and meta-analysis of the epidemiology of congenital cytomegalovirus (CMV) infection. *Rev Med Virol*. 2007;17(4)253-276.
13. Kimberlin DW, Lin CY, Jacobs RF, et al. Natural history of neonatal herpes simplex virus infections in the acyclovir era. *Pediatrics*. 2001;108:223-229.
14. Boppana SB, Pass RF, Britt WJ, Stagno S, Alford CA. Symptomatic congenital cytomegalovirus infection: neonatal morbidity and mortality. *Pediatr Infect Dis J*. 1992;11:93-99.
15. Brown ED, Chau JK, Atashband S, et al. A systematic review of neonatal toxoplasmosis exposure and sensorineural hearing loss. *Int J Pediatr Otorhinolaryngol*. 2009;73:707-711.
16. Brion LP, Manuli M, Rai B, et al. Longbone radiographic abnormalities as a sign of active congenital syphilis in asymptomatic newborns. Pediatrics. 1991;88:1037-1040.
17. Goldstein LC, Corey L, McDougall JK, et al. Monoclonal antibodies to herpes simplex viruses: Use in antigenic typing and rapid diagnosis. *J Infect Dis*. 1983;147:829.
18. Pouletty P, Chomel JJ, Thouvenot D, et al. Detection of herpes simplex virus in direct specimens by immunofluorescence assay using a monoclonal antibody. *J Clin Microbiol*. 1987;25:958.
19. American Academy of Pediatrics. Herpes simplex. In: Pickering LK, Baker CJ, Kimberlin DW, Long SS, eds. *Red Book: 2012 Report of the Committee on Infectious Diseases*. Elk Grove Village, IL; 2012: 398-408.
20. Lakeman FD, Whitley RJ. Diagnosis of herpes simplex encephalitis: application of polymerase chain reaction to cerebrospinal fluid from brainbiopsied patients and correlation with disease. *J Infect Dis*. 1995;171:857.
21. Sawyer M, Holland D, Aintablian N, et al. Diagnosis of enteroviral central nervous system infection by polymerase chain reaction during a large community outbreak. *Pediatr Infect Dis J*. 1994;13:177-182.
22. American Academy of Pediatrics. Syphilis. In: Pickering LK, Baker CJ, Kimberlin DW, Long SS, eds. *Red Book: 2012 Report of the Committee on Infectious Diseases*. Elk Grove Village, IL; 2012: 690-703.
23. Whitley R, Arvin A, Prober C, et al, and the NIAID Collaborative Antiviral Study Group. A controlled trial comparing vidarabine with acyclovir in neonatal herpes simplex virus infection. *N Engl J Med*. 1991;324:444-449.
24. Kimberlin DW, Lin CY, Jacobs RF, et al, and the NIAID Collaborative Antiviral Study Group. Safety and efficacy of high-dose intravenous acyclovir in the management of neonatal herpes simplex virus infections. *Pediatrics*. 2001;108:230-238.
25. American Academy of Pediatrics. Cytomegalovirus infection. In: Pickering LK, Baker CJ, Kimberlin DW, Long SS, eds. *Red Book: 2012 Report of the Committee on Infectious Diseases*. Elk Grove Village, IL; 2012:300-305.
26. McLeod R, Boyer K, Karrison T, et al. Outcome of treatment for congenital toxoplasmosis, 1981–2004: the National Collaborative

Chicago-Based, Congenital Toxoplasmosis Study. *Clin Infect Dis*. 2006;42:1383-1394.

27. American Academy of Pediatrics. Syphilis. In: Pickering LK, Baker CJ, Kimberlin DW, Long SS, eds. *Red Book: 2012 Report of the Committee on Infectious Diseases*. Elk Grove Village, IL; 2012:690-703.
28. Centers for Disease Control and Prevention. Sexually transmitted infection treatment guidelines—United States, 2010. *MMWR Recomm Rep*. 2010;59:1-110.
29. Centers for Disease Control and Prevention. Prevention of perinatal group B streptococcal disease. Revised guidelines from CDC, 2010. *MMWR Recomm Rep*. 2010;59:1-36.
30. American Academy of Pediatrics, Committee on Infectious Diseases. Recommendations for the prevention of perinatal group B streptococcal (GBS) disease. Pediatrics. 2011;128(3):611-616.
31. Wolff T, Shelton E, Sessions C, Miller T. Screening for syphilis infection in pregnant women: evidence for the US Preventive Services Task Force reaffirmation recommendation statement. *Ann Intern Med*. 2009;150(10):710-716.
32. Kumar ML, Nankervis GM, Jacobs IB, et al. Congenital and postnatally acquired cytomegalovirus infections: long term follow-up. *J Pediatr*. 1984;104:674-679.
33. Saigal S, Luynk O, Larke B, et al. The outcome in children with congenital cytomegalovirus infection: a longitudinal follow-up study. *Am J Dis Children*. 1982;136:896-901.
34. Pass RF, Fowler KB, Boppana S. Clinical importance of cytomegalovirus infection: an overview. In: Landini MP, ed. *Progress in Cytomegalovirus Research*. New York, NY: Elsevier Science Publishers; 1991:3-10.

188 ZOONOSES

Lara Danziger-Isakov, MD, MPH
Camille Sabella, MD

PATIENT STORY

A 12-year-old boy developed fever to 38.9°C and felt ill. Over the next 2 days, he developed a red spots on his hands and arms, which became petechial (**Figure 188-1**) and spread to involve his entire upper extremities and trunk. He also developed abdominal pain and a headache. History was significant for a recent camping trip with his family to the Southeastern coast of the US. The parents report that he did sustain several tick bites while camping. He was treated presumptively for Rocky Mountain Spotted Fever (RMSF) with doxycycline, and his symptoms resolved over several days.

INTRODUCTION

Zoonoses are infectious agents spread to humans by animals. Infection may occur through direct contact with the animal or via vectors such as ticks (**Table 188-1**). Examples of zoonotic diseases include RMSF, Ehrlichiosis, Tularemia, Cat-scratch disease, and Rat-bite fever.

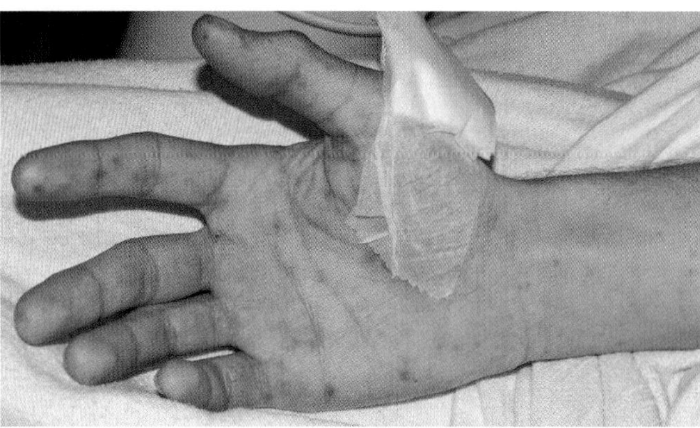

FIGURE 188-1 Petechial rash characteristic of late Rocky Mountain Spotted Fever (RMSF). *(Used with permission from Johanna Goldfarb, MD.)*

EPIDEMIOLOGY

- RMSF
    - Incidence is highest (19 to 77 cases/1 million people in 2008) in Southeastern (Virginia, Carolinas) and Central (Tennessee, Missouri, Arkansas and Oklahoma) US (**Figure 188-2**).[1]
    - Approximately 2,000 cases are reported annually in the US.
    - 1/3 of all cases are in the pediatric age group.[2,3]
- Ehrlichiosis
    - Incidence is highest (14 to 33 cases/1 million people in 2008) in Central States (Missouri, Arkansas and Oklahoma) with moderate

TABLE 188-1 Epidemiologic Characteristics of Selected Zoonoses

Disease	Infectious Agent	Seasonality	Reservoir	Vector/Exposure	Risk Area
RMSF	*Rickettsia rickettsia*	Late spring through early fall	Wild mammals, such as squirrels, opossums, rabbits, dogs, and mice	Ticks: *Dermacentor andersoni*, in western US; *Dermacentor variabilis* in the eastern US; *Rhipicephalus sanguineus* in Arizona and Mexico	Southeastern US
Ehrlichiosis/ Anaplasmosis	*E. chaffeensis; E. ewingii; Anaplasma phagocytophila*	Late spring through early fall	Deer	Ticks: *Ixodes scapularis* and *Amblyomma americanum*	Eastern seaboard, South Central, Midwest and Northern California
Tularemia	*Francisella tularensis*	Late spring through early fall	Rabbits, hares and small rodents	Direct exposure or Ticks	Central US
Rat-bite Fever	*Streptobacillus moniliformis* in the US *Spirillum minus*	None	Rats, mice, squirrels	Direct exposure/bite	
Cat-scratch disease	*Bartonella henselae*		Cats	Direct exposure	

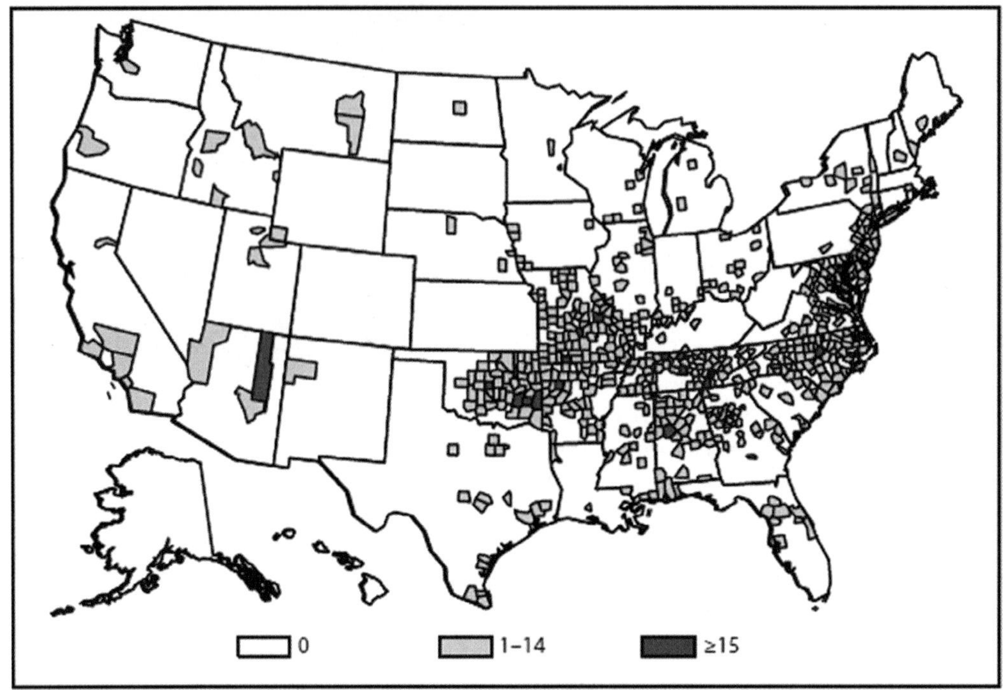

FIGURE 188-2 Rocky Mountain Spotted Fever. Number of reported cases, by county, US, 2010. (*Used with permission from the National Notifiable Disease Surveillance System, Centers for Disease Control and Prevention. MMWR Morb Mortal Wkly Rep. 2012 Jun 1;59(53):1-111.*)

incidence (1.7 to 14 cases/1 million people in 2008) in Upper Midwest and Southeastern states (**Figure 188-3**).[1]
  - Approximately 2500 cases were reported in 2010.
  - Number of reported cases as well as size of endemic regions appears to be growing with spread of tick vectors.
- Tularemia
  - Rare; only 124 cases were reported in the US in 2010.[1]
- Cat-scratch
  - Uncommon, although not routinely reported through National Notifiable Disease Surveillance System (NNDSS) at the Centers of Disease Control and Prevention (CDC).
- Rat-bite fever.
  - Rare, but not routinely reported to NNDSS.

ETIOLOGY AND PATHOPHYSIOLOGY

- RMSF.
  - Etiologic agent is *Rickettsia rickettsii*, which produces endothelial cell infection resulting in a systemic small-vessel vasculitis.
  - Ticks are the natural hosts, reservoirs and vectors. Rocky Mountain wood ticks (Dermacentor andersoni) are the most common vector for RMSF in Western North America (**Figure 188-4**). There are 3 other ticks that have been identified as vectors of *Rickettsia rickettsii* in North America.
- Ehrlichiosis.
  - Etiologic agents are obligate intracellular gram-negative bacteria *Ehrlichia chaffeensis, E. ewingii,* and *Anaplasma phagocytophilum*, which have tropisms for different white blood cells.
- Tularemia.
  - *Francisella tularensis* is the etiologic agent.
- Cat scratch disease.
  - *Bartonella henselae* is the etiologic agent.
- Rat-bite fever.
  - In the US, *Streptobacillus moniliformis* is the etiologic agent, whereas *Spirillum minus* is found in Asia.

RISK FACTORS

- RMSF/Ehrlichiosis.
  - Tick exposure in endemic areas and younger age are risk factors for infection.
- Tularemia.
  - Exposure to infected rabbits, including skinning, is a risk factor for infection.
  - Tick bite in endemic area is common mode of spread.
- Cat-scratch disease.
  - Exposure to cats, particularly kittens, is the main risk factor.
  - Can occur following a recent scratch or bite.
  - About 20 to 30 percent of patients who have cat scratch disease have no cat or kitten exposure.
- Rat-bite fever
  - Infected rodents serve as vectors.
  - May also be acquired from ingestion of unpasteurized milk, water or other food contaminated with *S. moniliformis* (Haverhill fever).

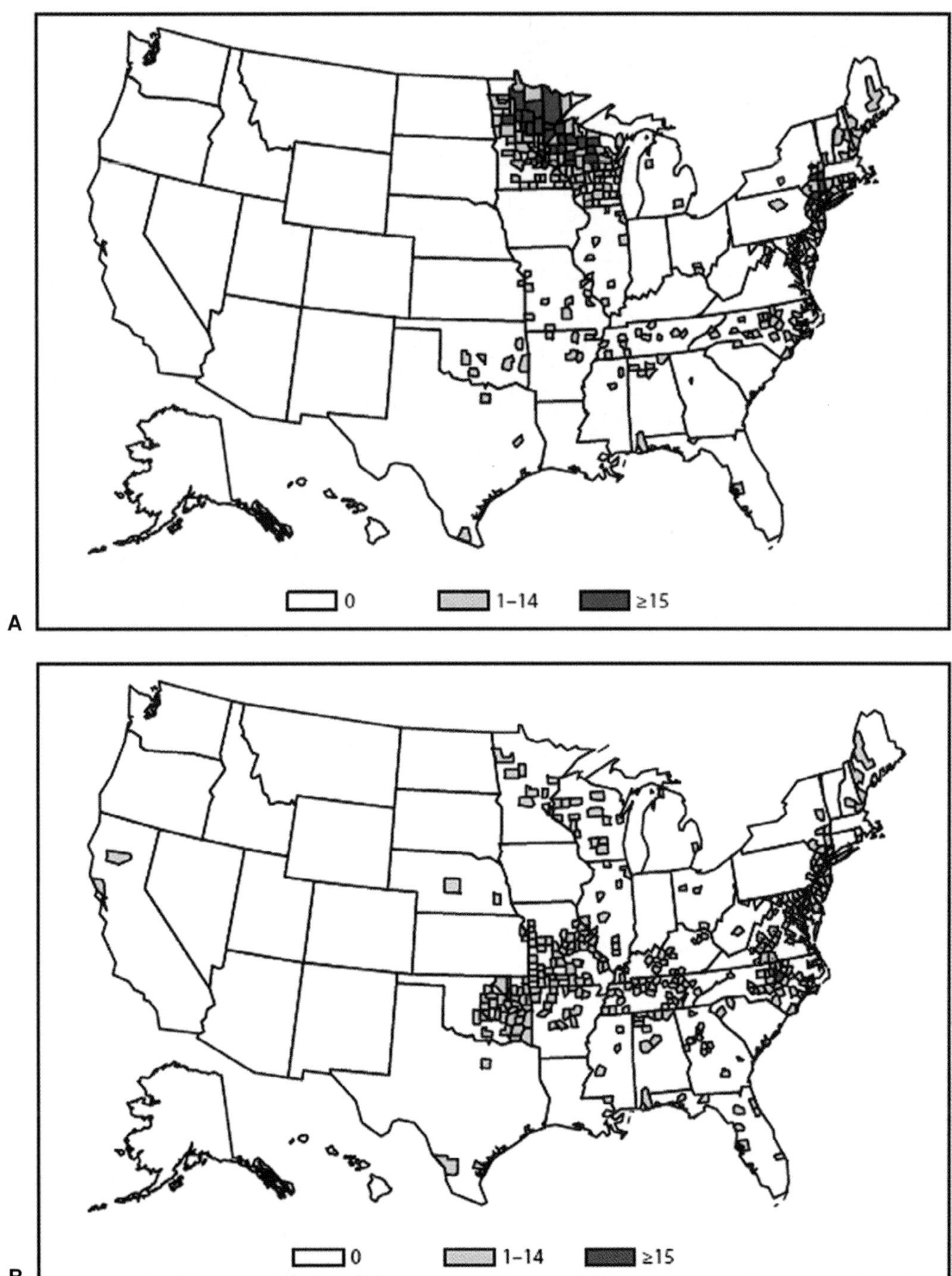

FIGURE 188-3 **A.** Ehrlichiosis. Number of reported cases, by county, US, 2010. *Anaplasma phagocytophilia* and **B.** *Ehrlichia chaggeensis (Used with permission from the National Notifiable Disease Surveillance System, Centers for Disease Control and Prevention. MMWR Morb Mortal Wkly Rep. 2012;59(53):1-111.)*

DIAGNOSIS

- RMSF.
  - Definitive diagnosis is difficult, as there are no widely available sensitive laboratory assays to confirm the diagnosis.
  - Treatment should be presumptive, pending testing results, as a delay in therapy is associated with a poor outcome.[4]
  - A confirmed case, as defined by the CDC,[4] includes the appropriate clinical symptoms and:
    - Serological evidence of a fourfold change in immunoglobulin G (IgG)-specific antibody titer reactive with *R. rickettsii* or other spotted fever group antigen by indirect immunofluorescence assay (IFA) between paired serum specimens (one taken in the first week of illness and a second 2 to 4 weeks later)., OR
    - Detection of *R. rickettsii* or other spotted fever group DNA in a clinical specimen (skin biopsy) via amplification of a specific target by polymerase chain reaction (PCR) assay, or demonstration of

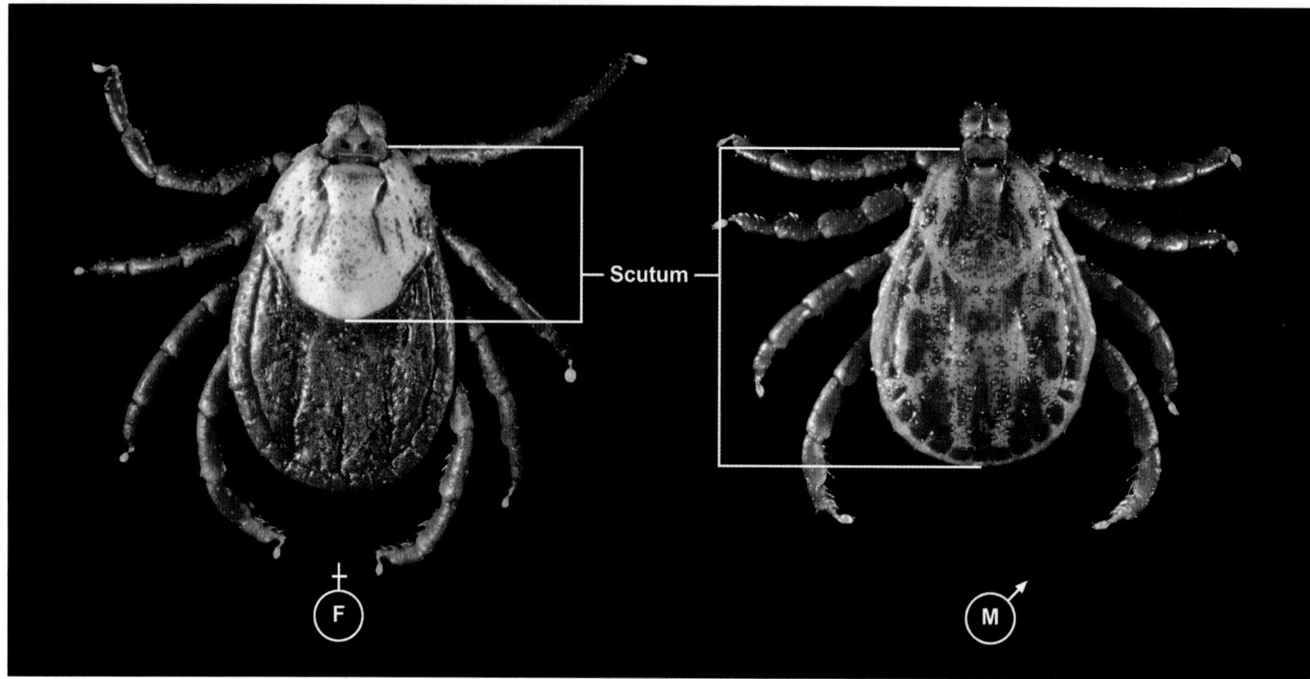

FIGURE 188-4 Rocky Mountain wood ticks (Dermacentor andersoni). A North American vector of Rickettsia rickettsii, the etiologic agent of Rocky Mountain spotted fever. Note the smaller size of the female's scutum (shield) compared to the male's larger scutum. The dorsal shield covers only a small part of the female's dorsal surface enabling her abdomen to expand and becoming engorged during feeding. (*Used with permission from CDC/ Dr. Christopher Paddock.*)

spotted fever group antigen in a biopsy or autopsy specimen by Immunohistochemical staining, OR
  - Isolation of *R. rickettsii* or other spotted fever group rickettsia from a clinical specimen in cell culture.
- Ehrlichiosis.
  - A confirmed case, as defined by the CDC,[4] includes the appropriate clinical symptoms and:
    - Serological diagnosis with a fourfold change in specific antibody titers between acute (at illness onset) and convalescent sera (4 weeks after illness), OR
    - Detection of *Ehrlichia* or *Anaplasma* DNA in a clinical specimen via PCR assay, OR
    - Demonstration of Ehrlichia antigen in a biopsy or autopsy sample by immunohistochemical methods, OR
    - Isolation of *E. chaffeensis* from a clinical specimen in cell culture.
  - A probable case, as defined by the CDC,[4] includes:
    - Presence of morulae (clusters of phagocytized ehrlichial organisms in vacuoles) in cytoplasm of peripheral blood granulocytes, monocytes, or macrophages (**Figure 188-5**), OR
    - Serologic evidence of IgG or IgM reactive to *Ehrlichia* antigen by IFA, enzyme-linked immunosorbent assay (ELISA), dot-ELISA, or assays in other formats.
- Tularemia.
  - Growth of the organism in culture is definitive.
    - Appropriate specimens include swabs or scrapping of skin lesions, lymph node aspirates or biopsies, pharyngeal washings, sputum specimens, or gastric aspirates, depending on the form of illness.
    - Paradoxically, blood cultures are often negative.
  - Serological diagnosis with a fourfold change in specific antibody titers between acute (at illness onset) and convalescent sera (4 weeks after illness) can confirm the diagnosis. However, this is not helpful in acute clinical management because of the delay in diagnosis.
  - A presumptive diagnosis of tularemia can be made when there is:
    - Evidence of an elevated serum antibody titer to *F. tularensis* antigen without evidence of a four-fold increase,[5] OR
    - A positive result using direct fluorescent antibody, immunohistochemical staining, or PCR.
- Cat-scratch disease.
  - The diagnosis is usually confirmed by demonstrating serological evidence of antibodies to *Bartonella* antigens using an indirect immunofluorescent antibody (IFA) assay.[6]
  - PCR of body fluids is available at CDC or reference laboratories.

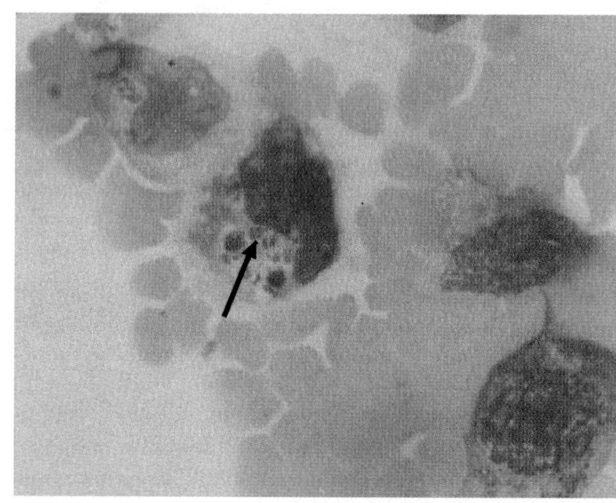

FIGURE 188-5 Peripheral blood smear showing intraleukocytic morulae in granulocytic cell. This is supportive evidence of the diagnosis of Ehrlichiosis. (*Used with permission from Camille Sabella, MD.*)

- Histopathologic evidence of organisms on Warthin-Starry silver staining is not specific for *B. henselae* infection.

- Rat-bite fever.
  - The diagnosis of *S. moniliformis* infection is made via culture of blood, synovial fluid, or other body fluids using specific media; cultures should be held for 3 weeks because of the slow growth of this agent.
  - The diagnosis of *S. minus* infection is made with darkfield microscopy of blood or infected body fluids.

CLINICAL FEATURES

- RMSF.
  - Fever, headache, malaise, myalgias, nausea, and vomiting are the initial symptoms.
  - These symptoms are followed several days later by a maculopapular rash that evolves into petechial rash (late finding), spreading from the extremities (wrists/ankles) centrally (**Figure 188-1**).
  - If untreated, RMSF progresses to involve the central nervous, renal, cardiac, pulmonary, and gastrointestinal systems, and often includes disseminated intravascular coagulation and shock.
  - Delays in therapy are associated with increased risk of death.
- Ehrlichiosis.
  - Fever, headache, malaise, and myalgia are the most common features.
  - Vomiting, abdominal pain, and arthralgia are less common.
  - Rash occurs less frequently than with RMSF, but is more common in children than adults.
- Tularemia.
  - There are multiple syndrome profiles depending on the site of inoculation:
    - Ulceroglandular (ulceration at inoculation site followed by healing and localized regional lymphadenopathy; **Figure 188-6**).
    - Glandular (without ulceration).
    - Oculoglandular.

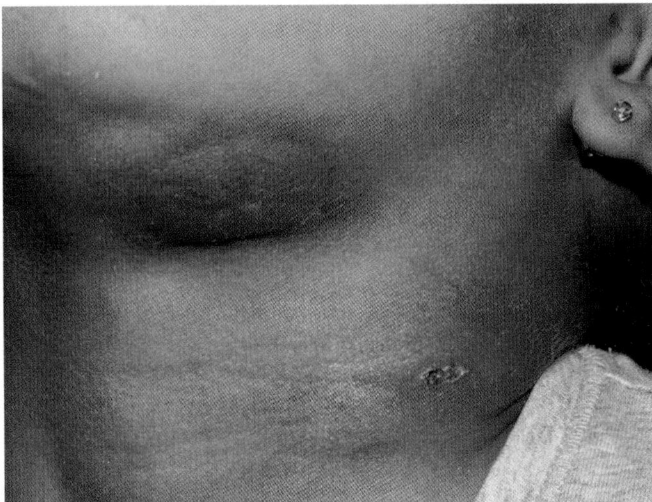

FIGURE 188-6 Ulceration with eschar at the site of inoculation with regional lymphadenopathy. This is characteristic of the ulceroglandular presentation of tularemia or cat scratch adenitis. (*Used with permission from Charles B. Foster, MD.*)

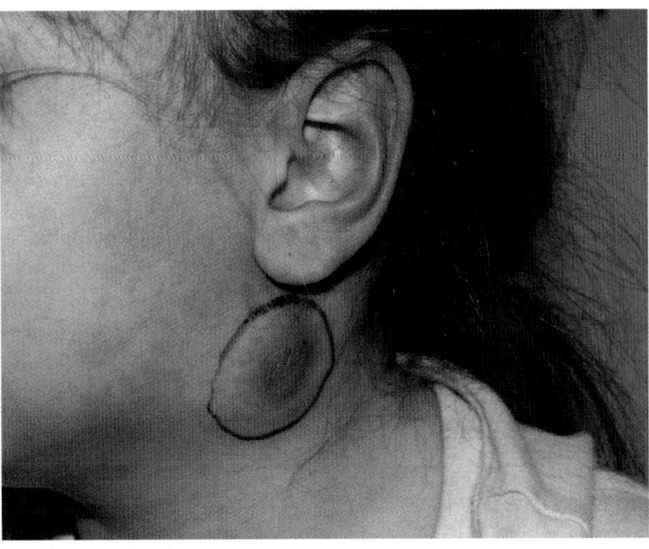

FIGURE 188-7 Cat-scratch adenitis with central fluctuance. (*Used with permission from Camille Sabella, MD.*)

    - Oropharyngeal.
    - Intestinal.
    - Pneumonic.
- Cat-scratch disease.
  - Regional lymphadenopathy with overlying erythema, tenderness, warmth, and induration is the most common presentation (**Figure 188-7**).
  - A primary papule at the inoculation site may be present at diagnosis (**Figure 188-8**).
  - Less common presentations including fever of unknown origin, hepatitis, splenic calcifications, neuroretinitis, and aseptic meningitis.[7,8]
  - Parinaud oculoglandular syndrome with conjunctivitis and ipsilateral preauricular lymphadenopathy is a distinctive manifestation (**Figure 188-9**).
- Rat-bite fever.
  - Abrupt onset of fever, malaise, myalgia with swelling, erythema, and purulence from the inoculation site are common manifestations.

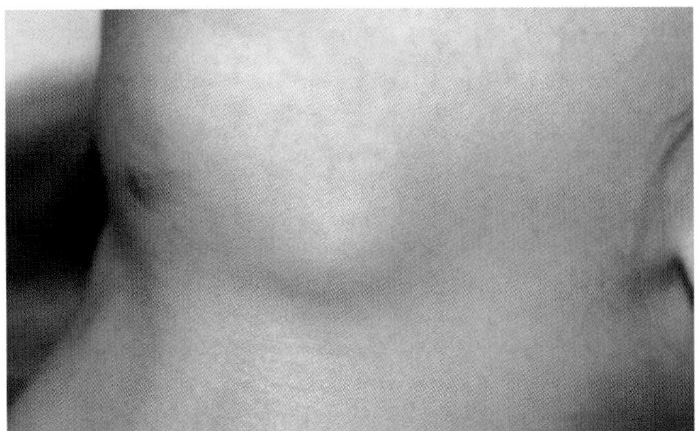

FIGURE 188-8 Cat-scratch adenitis. Note the primary papule at the inoculation site with adjacent adenitis. (*Used with permission from Johanna Goldfarb, MD.*)

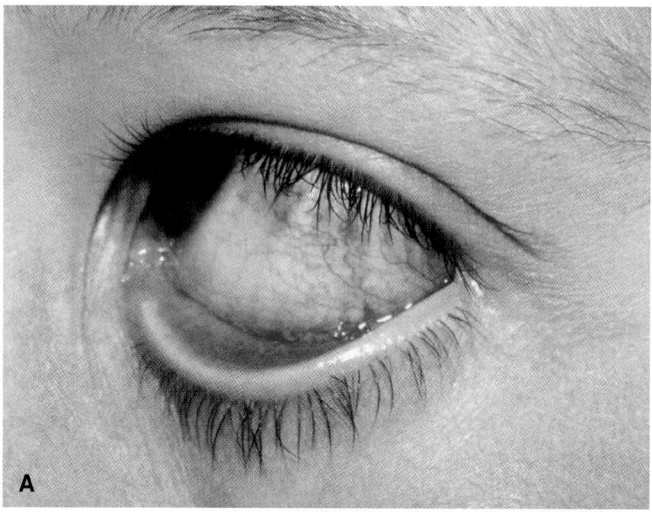

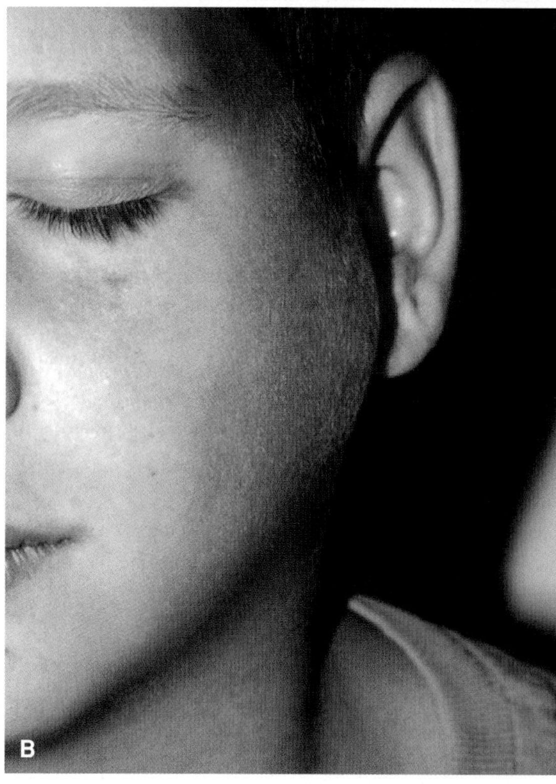

FIGURE 188-9 Parinaud oculoglandular syndrome with (**A**) conjunctivitis and (**B**) pre-auricular lymphadenitis. This child had cat scratch disease, proven by serology, but the differential diagnosis includes tularemia, adenovirus and *H influenzae* infection. (*Used with permission from Camille Sabella, MD. From Sabella C, Cunningham RJ III. Intensive Review of Pediatrics, 4th edition. Lippincott Williams Wilkins, p 448, Figure 53-2, 53-3.*)

- A maculopapular or petechial rash spreading from extremities (palms/soles) centrally is most common (**Figure 188-10**).
- Fifty percent of patients develop migratory polyarthritis after the rash has appeared when due to *S. moniliformis* infection; arthritis is uncommon in *S. minus* infections.
- A relapsing course over several weeks can occur in untreated patients.
- Complications include septic arthritis, endocarditis, meningitis and abscesses.[9]

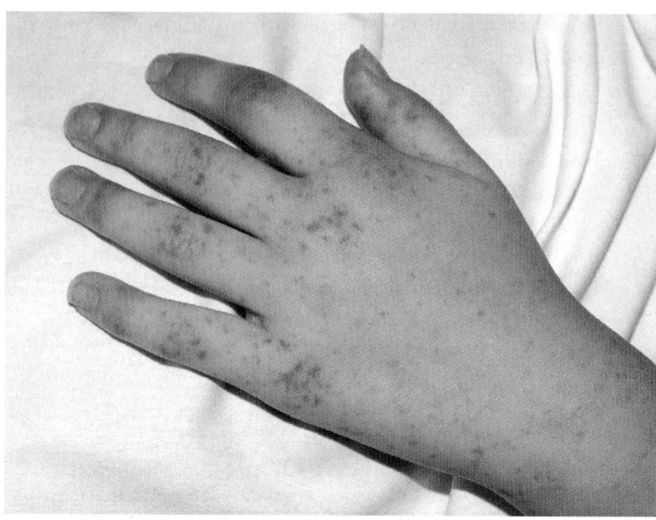

FIGURE 188-10 Maculopapular and petechial rash in 9-year old girl who developed rat-bite fever after being bitten by her pet rat. Inoculation site with swelling and erythema seen on the index finger. (*Used with permission from Camille Sabella, MD.*)

ADDITIONAL LABORATORY FINDINGS

- Thrombocytopenia, neutropenia, hyponatremia, and increased hepatic transaminases are common laboratory findings in RMSF, but may not be apparent until later in the course of the illness.
- Leukopenia or lymphopenia, thrombocytopenia, and increased hepatic transaminases are common findings in Ehrlichiosis.

IMAGING

- Cat-scratch disease.
  - Ultrasound is often utilized to assess for suppuration of lymph nodes in patients who are suspected of having cat scratch disease.
  - Ultrasound or Computed Tomography of the liver and spleen may demonstrate granulomatous lesions in patients with cat scratch disease. These patients may present with fever of unknown origin.[8]

DIFFERENTIAL DIAGNOSIS

- The rash that is associated with many of the infections previously discussed may mimic the rash of Meningococcemia, Kawasaki, Rubeola (measles), and Henoch Schonlein Purpura (see Chapters 177, Kawasaki Disease, Chapter 111, Measles, and Chapter 175, Henoch Schonlein Purpura). The epidemiology and route of acquisition of the zoonoses serve as important clues in differentiating these entities.
- The lymphadenitis of cat scratch disease and tularemia is sometimes difficult to differentiate from other causes of lymphadenitis, such as pyogenic (Staphylococcal and streptococcal), mycobacterial, and toxoplasma infections. A thorough history of exposures and the finding of an inoculation site can be helpful in the diagnosis of cat scratch disease and tularemia.
- The differential diagnosis of Parinaud Oculoglandular syndrome (named after Henri Parinaud) includes tularemia, cat-scratch disease, adenovirus, and *H. influenzae* infection. A thorough exposure history and appropriate diagnostic cultures for adenovirus and *H influenzae* can help to differentiate these infections.

MANAGEMENT

NONPHARMACOLOGICAL

- Supportive care for critically ill patients with any of these zoonoses is essential.
- Cat-scratch disease lymphadenopathy is usually self-limited and management is aimed at symptom relief.
- Remove ticks found on people carefully to avoid having the tick expel its contents into the patient during removal.

MEDICATIONS

- RMSF/Ehrlichiosis.
  - Doxycycline is the drug of choice for all patient with these infections, including those who are less than 8 years of age.[10] SOR Ⓐ
- Tularemia.
  - Gentamicin or streptomycin for 10 days is the recommended treatment of choice for tularemia.[11] SOR Ⓐ
  - Alternatively, doxycycline for 14 days can be given for patients 8 years of age and older who do not have severe illness.
- Cat-scratch disease.
  - Azithromycin may decrease the size of lymphadenopathy in the first month of therapy, but does not impact the overall outcome.[12] SOR Ⓑ
  - Antimicrobial therapy may hasten recovery of systemic manifestations, such as hepatic or splenic granulomas, and in immunocompromised hosts,[13] although the role of such therapy in these patients is not clear. SOR Ⓒ
  - Azithromycin, gentamicin, ciprofloxacin, trimethoprim-sulfamethoxazole, and rifampin are possible treatment options for these patients. SOR Ⓒ
- Rat-bite fever.
  - Penicillin G for 7 to 10 days is the treatment of choice.[14] SOR Ⓐ
  - Four weeks of penicillin G recommended for endocarditis.[14]
  - Doxycycline, gentamicin, or streptomycin recommended for those with severe penicillin allergy.

SURGERY

- Cat-scratch disease.
  - Needle aspiration of the involved lymph node(s) can be performed for symptom relief. SOR Ⓒ
  - Incision and drainage of the involved lymph node(s) may result in the development of a draining sinus, and is not recommended. SOR Ⓒ
  - Surgical excision is rarely necessary for enlarged lymph nodes but if performed, should be undertaken prior to the development of spontaneous drainage, if possible. SOR Ⓒ

REFERRAL

- Referral to infectious diseases may be helpful for the diagnosis and management of zoonoses, depending on the specific infection and the severity of the manifestations.
- Referral to surgery for aspiration of an infected lymph node or drainage of a pyogenic focus of infection may be required.

PREVENTION AND SCREENING

- Avoidance of direct animal contact will decrease the risk of some zoonoses such as rat bite fever, cat scratch disease, and tularemia.
- Periodic evaluation for tick-bites and prompt tick removal when in at-risk areas will help prevent tick-borne infections.
- Treatment of domestic animals for ticks as directed by veterinarian is recommended.
- Prompt and thorough cleansing of any scratches or bites from animal contacts is important in decreasing the risk of infection.

PROGNOSIS

- RMSF.
  - A delay of disease suspicion and treatment after the fifth day of illness is association with an increased risk of death.[15,16]
- Ehrlichiosis.
  - The case fatality rate is reported to be from 1 to 3 percent (*E. chaffeensis*) to <1 percent (*A. phagocytophilum*), although this may be overestimated because many individuals who are infected are asymptomatic.[17]
- Tularemia.
  - Suppuration of lymph nodes may occur despite adequate therapy.
- Cat-scratch disease.
  - Lymphadenopathy is usually self-limited and resolves over 1 to 2 months.
  - Suppuration of lymph nodes may occur in up to 25 percent of cases.
- Rat-bite fever.
  - The course of rat bite fever can be rapid and fatal.

PATIENT EDUCATION

Parents should seek medical attention if symptoms of infection develop after zoonotic exposures.

PATIENT RESOURCES

- Centers for Disease Control and Prevention—**www.cdc.gov**. Offers many resources on zoonoses including the following:
  - Rocky Mountain spotted fever (RMSF)—**www.cdc.gov/rmsf/**.
  - Cat scratch disease—**http://www.cdc.gov/healthypets/**.

PROVIDER RESOURCES

- Centers for Disease Control and Prevention—**www.cdc.gov**.
- Morbidity and Mortality Weekly from the Centers for Disease Control and Prevention—**www.cdc.gov/mmwr**.
- National Notifiable Disease Surveillance System (NNDSS)—**wwwn.cdc.gov/nndss**.
- American Academy of Pediatrics. Pickering LK, Baker CJ, Kimberlin DW, Long SS, eds. *Red Book: 2012 Report of the Committee on Infectious Diseases*. Elk Grove Village, IL: American Academy of Pediatrics; 2012.

REFERENCES

1. Centers for Disease Control and Prevention (CDC). *MMWR Morb Mortal Wkly Rep*. 2012;59(53):1-111.
2. Treadwell TA, Holman RC, Clarke MJ, et al. Rocky Mountain spotted fever in the United States 1993-1996. *Am J Trop Med Hyg*. 2000;63:21-26.
3. Chapman AS, Murphy SM, Demma LJ, et al. Rocky Mountain spotted fever in the United States, 1997-2002. *Vector Borne Zoonotic Dis*. 2006;6:170-178.
4. Centers for Disease Control and Prevention. Diagnosis and management of tickborne rickettsial diseases: Rocky Mountain spotted fever, ehrlichiosis, and anaplasmosis—United States. A practical guide for physicians and other health care and public health professionals. *MMWR Morb Mortal Wkly Rep*. 2006; 55(RR-4):1-29.
5. Chu MC, Weyant RS. Francisella and Brucella. In: Murray PR, Baron EJ, Pfaller MA, et al., eds. *Manual of Clinical Microbiology, 8th ed*. Washington, DC; American Society for Microbiology; 2003:789-808.
6. Murakami K, Tsukahara M, Tsuneoka H, et al. Cat scratch disease: analysis of 130 seropositive cases. *J Infect Chemother*. 2002;8:686-691.
7. Arisoy ES, Correa AG, Wagner ML, et al. Hepatosplenic cat-scratch disease in children: selected clinical features and treatment. *Clin Infect Dis*. 1999;28:778-784.
8. Jacobs RF, Schutze GE. *Bartonella henselae* as a cause of prolonged fever and fever of unknown origin in children. *Clin Infect Dis*. 1998;26:80-84.
9. Hagelskjaer L, Sorensen I, Randers E. *Streptobacillus moniliformis* infection: 2 cases and a literature review. *Scand J Infect Dis*. 1998;30:309.
10. American Academy of Pediatrics. Rocky Mountain Spotted Fever. In: Pickering LK, Baker CJ, Kimberlin DW, Long SS, eds. *Red Book: 2012 Report of the Committee on Infectious Diseases*. Elk Grove Village, IL: American Academy of Pediatrics; 2012:623-625.
11. American Academy of Pediatrics. Tularemia. In: Pickering LK, Baker CJ, Kimberlin DW, Long SS, eds. *Red Book: 2012 Report of the Committee on Infectious Diseases*. Elk Grove Village, IL: American Academy of Pediatrics; 2012:768-769.
12. Bass JW, Freitas BC, Freitas AD, et al. Prospective randomized double blind placebo-controlled evaluation of azithromycin for treatment of cat-scratch disease. *Pediatr Infect Dis J*. 1998;17: 147-152.
13. American Academy of Pediatrics. Cat Scratch Disease (Bartonella henselae). In: Pickering LK, Baker CJ, Kimberlin DW, Long SS, eds. *Red Book: 2012 Report of the Committee on Infectious Diseases*. Elk Grove Village, IL: American Academy of Pediatrics; 2012: 269-271.
14. American Academy of Pediatrics. Rat-Bite Fever. In: Pickering LK, Baker CJ, Kimberlin DW, Long SS, eds. *Red Book: 2012 Report of the Committee on Infectious Diseases*. Elk Grove Village, IL: American Academy of Pediatrics; 2012:608-609.
15. Kirkland KB, Wilkiinson WE, Sexton DJ. Therapeutic dealy and mortality in cases of rocky mountain spotted fever. *Clin Infect Dis*. 1995;20(5):1118.
16. Buckingham SC, Marshall GS, Schutze GE, et al. Clinical and laboratory features, hospital course, and outcome of rocky mountain spotted fever in children. *J Pediatr*. 2007;150(2):180.
17. Bakken JS, Dumler JS. Human granulocytic ehrlichiosis. *Clin Infect Dis*. 2000;31(2):554.

PART 17

ENDOCRINOLOGY

Strength of Recommendation (SOR)	Definition
A	Recommendation based on consistent and good-quality patient-oriented evidence.*
B	Recommendation based on inconsistent or limited-quality patient-oriented evidence.*
C	Recommendation based on consensus, usual practice, opinion, disease-oriented evidence, or case series for studies of diagnosis, treatment, prevention, or screening.*

*See Appendix A on pages 1320–1322 for further information.

189 DIABETES OVERVIEW

Todd D. Nebesio, MD

PATIENT STORY

A 7-year-old girl presents with increased thirst and urination over the last 2 weeks. Despite previously being dry at night, she has wet the bed a few times over the past week. She has not been ill and has had a good appetite. She has had no abdominal pain or vomiting. Physical examination is remarkable for dry, tacky oral mucous membranes. Her weight is down 3 kg since her last well-child visit. A blood sugar is checked (**Figure 189-1**) on a meter and is "high" or too elevated to be read by the meter. A urinalysis shows positive glucose and ketones in his urine. A basic metabolic profile reveals sodium of 131 mEq/L, bicarbonate of 20 mEq/L, and plasma glucose of 652 mg/dL. Hemoglobin A1c is 10.8 percent. She is admitted to the hospital with the diagnosis of new onset diabetes. She is treated with intravenous fluids and insulin. While in the hospital, she is started on SQ insulin injections and she and her family receive diabetes education. With her age, the patient most likely has type 1 diabetes mellitus (T1DM).

INTRODUCTION

The classic symptoms of new onset diabetes are polydipsia, polyuria, and unexpected weight loss.

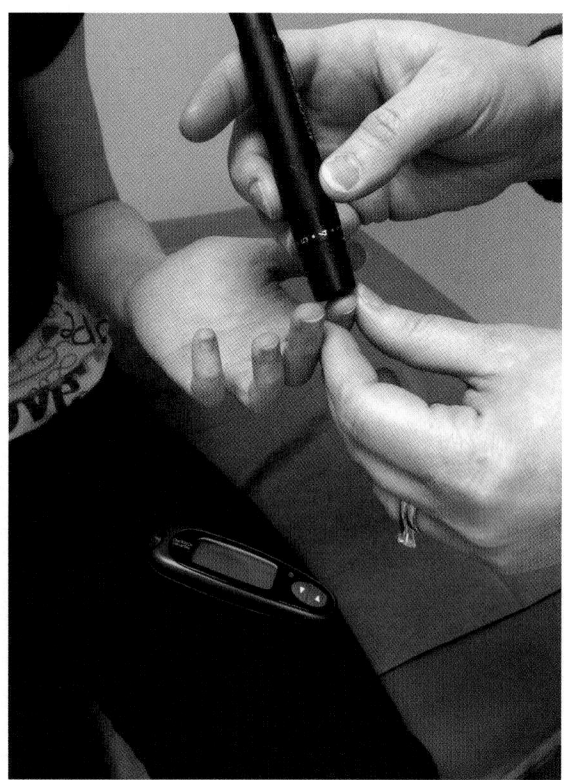

FIGURE 189-1 Blood sugar testing in a girl with suspected diabetes. *(Used with permission from Todd D. Nebesio, MD.)*

SYNONYMS

T1DM has also been called insulin-dependent diabetes, juvenile-onset diabetes, and immune-mediated diabetes.

EPIDEMIOLOGY

- The incidence of T1DM is increasing by about 3 percent per year for unknown reasons.
- Less common forms of diabetes in children and adolescents include type 2 diabetes (T2DM), cystic fibrosis related diabetes (CFRD), steroid-induced diabetes, and rare genetic forms of diabetes.[1]
- The prevalence of T1DM in the US at 18 years of age is about 2 to 3 per 1,000 individuals.[2]
- Males and females are equally affected.
- There are two peaks in incidence of T1DM in children: as they start school (4 to 6 years) and early adolescence (10 to 14 years).
- The incidence of T2DM has also increased associated with the rise in childhood obesity. T2DM most often occurs in pubertal adolescents.

ETIOLOGY AND PATHOPHYSIOLOGY

- T1DM is due to autoimmune beta cell destruction in the pancreas resulting in absolute insulin deficiency.
- T2DM is due to insulin resistance and relative insulin deficiency.

RISK FACTORS

- There is an increased risk of developing T1DM if there is an already affected relative: 6 percent risk in a sibling; <50 percent chance in an identical twin; higher risk if the father has T1DM compared to a mother with T1DM.[2]
- Obesity, positive family history, ethnic minority, and evidence of insulin resistance are common risk factors for T2DM.

DIAGNOSIS

CLINICAL FEATURES

- Polyuria, polydipsia, polyphagia, and weight loss are the classic features of new onset diabetes.
- When presenting in diabetic ketoacidosis (DKA), additional features include nausea, vomiting, abdominal pain, mental status changes, and Kussmaul breathing.
- Acanthosis nigricans on the neck, axilla, or other skin folds is a sign of insulin resistance seen in T2DM and obese individuals (**Figure 189-2**; see Chapter 190, Acanthosis Nigricans). Genetic defects in insulin action can result in extreme insulin resistance (**Figure 189-3**).

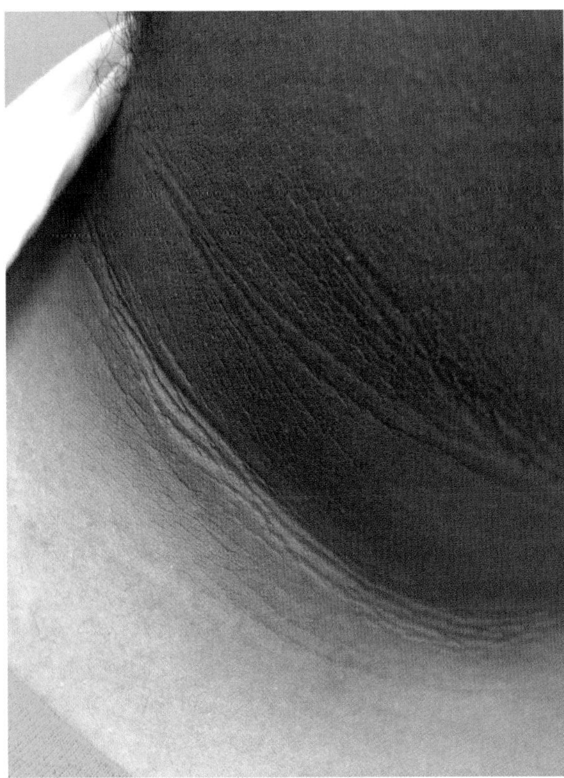

FIGURE 189-2 Acanthosis nigricans on the neck of an obese African American teenager with insulin resistance. (*Used with permission from Todd D. Nebesio, MD.*)

- Necrobiosis lipoidica diabeticorum (NLD) is a rare skin condition occurring in <0.5 percent of diabetics and seldom seen in children (**Figure 189-4**).

LABORATORY TESTING

- Criteria for the diagnosis of diabetes mellitus include symptoms of diabetes and a random plasma glucose ≥200 mg/dL, a fasting plasma glucose ≥126 mg/dL, a 2-hour plasma glucose ≥200 mg/dL during an oral glucose tolerance test (OGTT), or hemoglobin A1c ≥6.5 percent (3). If there are no classic symptoms of hyperglycemia, testing needs to be repeated on a second day.

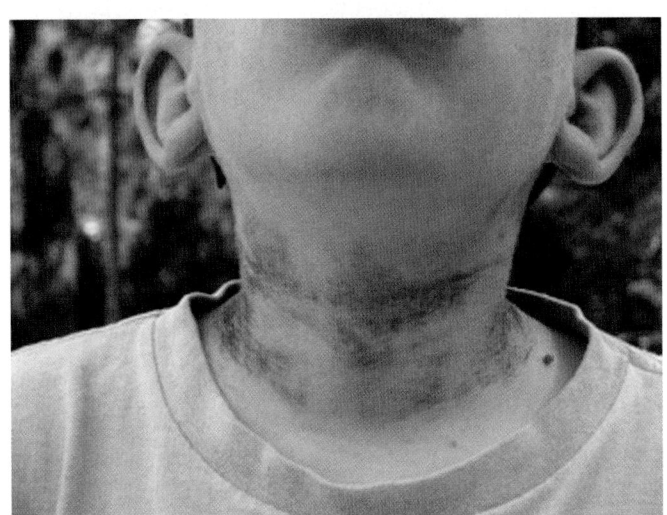

FIGURE 189-3 Severe insulin resistance and acanthosis nigricans in a child with Rabson-Mendenhall syndrome, which is due to defects in the insulin receptor gene. (*Used with permission from Todd D. Nebesio, MD.*)

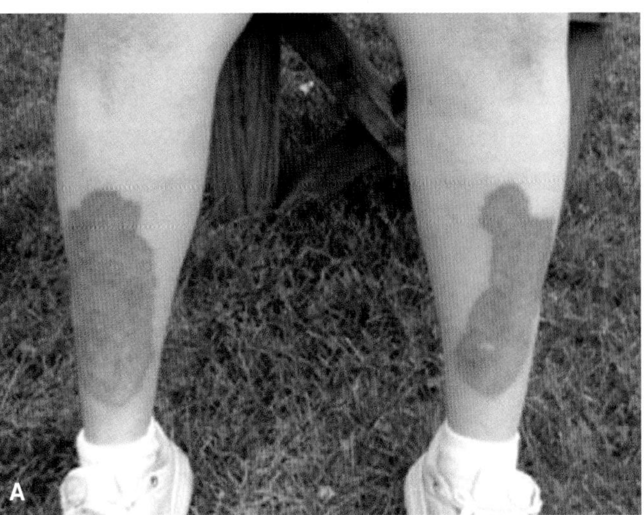

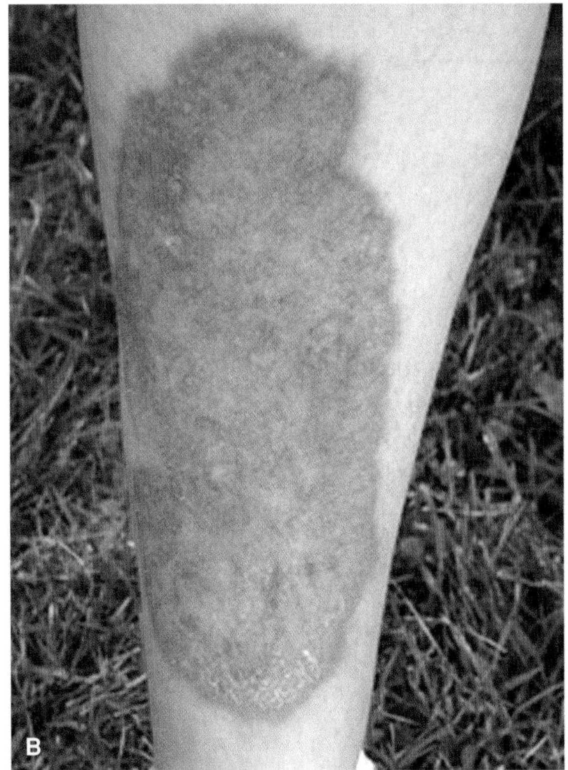

FIGURE 189-4 **A.** Necrobiosis lipoidica diabeticorum (NLD) in an adolescent girl with type 1 diabetes. Although rare, it commonly occurs along the pretibial region of the lower legs. **B.** Closer view of NLD on her right leg. (*Used with permission from Todd D. Nebesio, MD.*)

- Fasting plasma glucose between 100 to 125 mg/dL indicates impaired fasting glucose (IFG) and 2-hour plasma glucose during an OGTT between 140 to 199 mg/dL indicates impaired glucose tolerance (IGT). IFG and IGT are pre-diabetic states and indicate a higher risk of developing diabetes in the future.
- Diabetes autoantibodies are commonly positive in T1DM but can also be seen in a small percentage of T2DM. Up to 25 percent of

new onset patients with T1DM can be obese, which confuses the diagnosis between T1DM versus T2DM.[4,5]

- Glucosuria is present if the plasma glucose level is >180 mg/dL.
- Positive urine or blood ketones indicate insulin deficiency.
- Hyperglycemia causes pseudohyponatremia; for every 100 mg/dL increase in the plasma glucose above 100 mg/dL, a 1.6 mEq/L decrease occurs in the measured serum sodium level.
- Acidosis with a bicarbonate level <15 mEq/L indicates DKA, which is the most common cause of death in children with T1DM.

DIFFERENTIAL DIAGNOSIS

- In the setting of hyperglycemia and positive symptoms, the diagnosis is typically straightforward. However, differentiating the type of diabetes can sometimes be difficult.
- Differential for polyuria and polydipsia: diabetes mellitus, diabetes insipidus, psychogenic, hypercalcemia, hypokalemia, and hyperthyroidism.

MANAGEMENT

NONPHARMACOLOGIC

- Nutrition and meal planning is important in diabetics to maintain normal weight and growth.
- Physical fitness and regular exercise potentiates the action of insulin.
- Blood sugar testing is typically performed at least 4 times per day, specifically before meals and at bedtime (**Figure 189-5**).
- Blood or urine ketones are checked if the blood sugar is repeatedly elevated or the patient is sick, feels nauseated, or is vomiting, or has abdominal pain.

MEDICATIONS

- Insulin is the initial management in children with diabetes. Injection sites, including the arms, thighs, abdomen, hips, and buttocks, need to be rotated to avoid localized areas of hypertrophy (**Figure 189-6**).
- Rapid-acting insulin is given at meal times for food coverage and correction of the blood sugar to a certain goal level.
- Long-acting or basal insulin is given once or twice a day and suppresses ketone body production.
- Metformin is an oral medication used in patients with T2DM.

COMPLIMENTARY THERAPY

- Insulin pumps continuously deliver rapid short-acting insulin through a pump site that is changed every 2 to 3 days (**Figure 189-7**).

PREVENTION AND SCREENING

- Prevention of T1DM at this time is not possible.
- In overweight and obese children with signs of insulin resistance and a positive family history of T2DM, lifestyle intervention can prevent the development of T2DM.

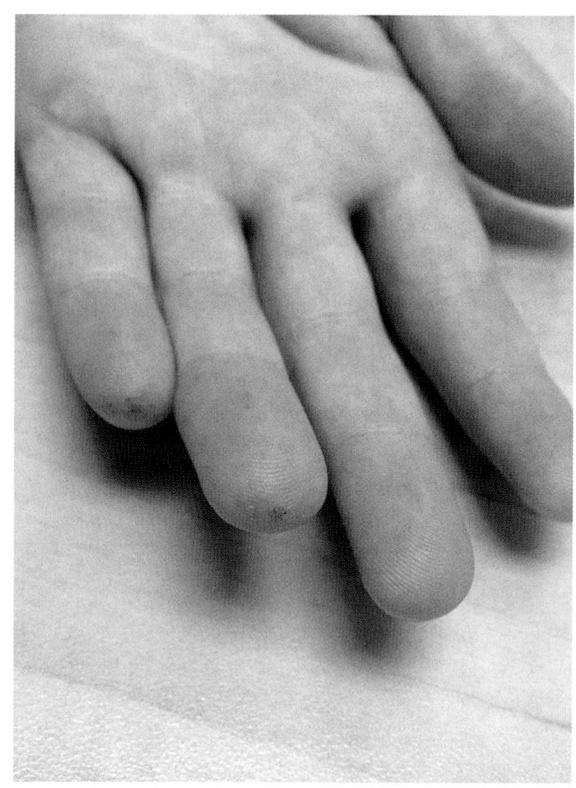

FIGURE 189-5 Evidence of blood sugar testing at the ends of the fingers in a teen with type 1 diabetes. (*Used with permission from Todd D. Nebesio, MD.*)

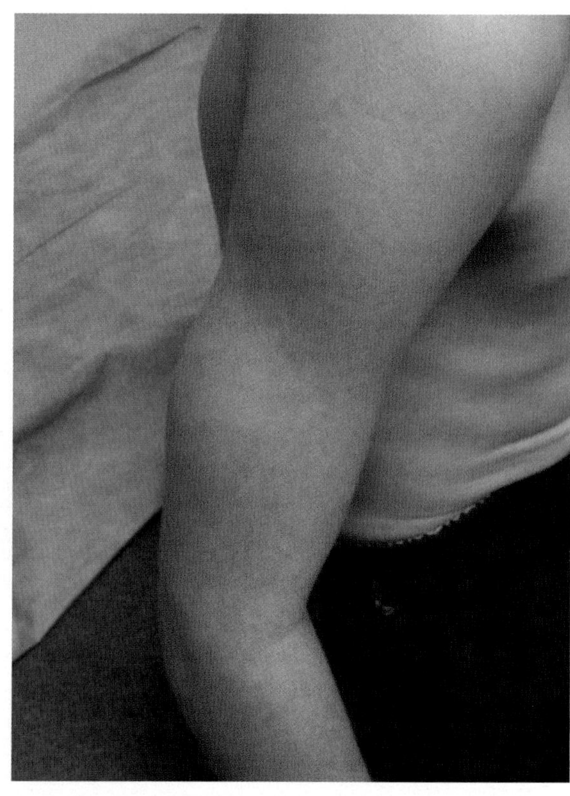

FIGURE 189-6 Repeated insulin injections in the same location on the arm can cause hypertrophy, which results in slow and erratic insulin absorption. (*Used with permission from Todd D. Nebesio, MD.*)

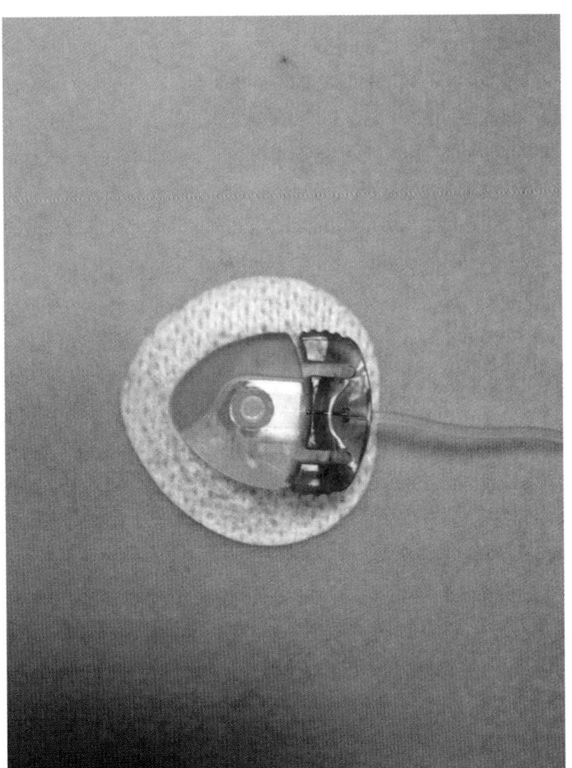

FIGURE 189-7 An insulin pump site. At the top is where a previous pump site was placed. (*Used with permission from Todd D. Nebesio, MD.*)

- Screening in asymptomatic children with positive risk factors of developing T2DM should begin at 10 years or at the onset of puberty and then every 3 years.[6]

PROGNOSIS

- Blood sugar ranges and hemoglobin A1c targets vary with age.[6,7]
- In very young children with T1DM, significant hypoglycemia can potentially lead to neuropsychological impairment.[7]
- The most common cause of a known diabetic presenting in DKA is from not taking their insulin injections.
- Chronic complications from hyperglycemia include growth problems, nephropathy, retinopathy, and neuropathy.[2,5,7] Diabetes complications are decreased with intensive therapy and improved blood sugar control.[8]
- In T1DM, there is an increased risk of other autoimmune diseases, most commonly thyroid disease and celiac disease.

FOLLOW-UP

- Hemoglobin A1c, height, weight, and blood pressure are checked every 3 months at clinic visits.
- Dilated eye exam should be done yearly after having T1DM for 5 years or after the age of 10 years; an eye exam should be done shortly after diagnosis of T2DM.
- Periodic screening for other conditions and co-morbidities: hypertension, dyslipidemia, microalbuminuria, psychiatric disorders (e.g., depression and eating disorders), hepatic steatosis (in T2DM), and hypothyroidism and celiac disease (in T1DM).

PATIENT EDUCATION

- Lifestyle interventions such as dietary measures and exercise can prevent and control the onset and course of T2DM.
- New onset diabetics and their families need education regarding nutrition, exercise, and blood sugar testing.

PATIENT RESOURCES

- **www.childrenwithdiabetes.com**.
- **www.jdrf.org**.
- **www.diabetes.org**.

PROVIDER RESOURCES

- **www.cdc.gov/diabetes/projects/cda2.htm**.
- Fagot-Campagna A, Pettitt DJ, Engelgau MM, Burrows NR, Geiss LS, Valdez R, et al. Type 2 diabetes among North American children and adolescents: An epidemiologic review and a public health perspective. *J Pediatr* 2000;136(5):664-672.

REFERENCES

1. Steck AK, Winter WE. Review of monogenic diabetes. *Curr Opin Endocrinol Diabetes Obes.* 2011;18:252-258.
2. Cooke DW, Plotnick L. Type 1 diabetes mellitus in pediatrics. *Pediatr Rev.* 2008;29:374-385.
3. American Diabetes Association. Diagnosis and classification of diabetes mellitus. *Diabetes Care.* 2013;36(1):S67-79.
4. Jones KL. Role of obesity in complicating and confusing the diagnosis and treatment of diabetes in children. *Pediatrics.* 2008; 12:361-368.
5. Rosenbloom AL, Silverstein JH, Amemiya S, Zeitler P, Klingensmith GJ. Type 2 diabetes in children and adolescents. *Pediatr Diabetes.* 2009;10(12):17-32.
6. American Diabetes Association. Standards of medical care in diabetes—2013. *Diabetes Care.* 2013;36(1):S11-66.
7. Silverstein J, Klingensmith G, Copeland K, et al. Care of children and adolescents with type 1 diabetes. *Diabetes Care.* 2005;28:186-212.
8. The Diabetes Control and Complications Trial (DCCT) Research Group. The effect of intensive treatment of diabetes on the development and progression of long-term complications in insulin-dependent diabetes mellitus. *N Engl J Med.* 1993;329:977-986.

190 ACANTHOSIS NIGRICANS

Mindy A. Smith, MD, MS

PATIENT STORY

A 10-year-old girl with obesity and recently diagnosed type II diabetes mellitus (DM) presents to her pediatrician with concerns about a "dirty area" under her arms and on her neck that "couldn't be cleaned" (**Figure 190-1**). The pediatrician makes the diagnosis of acanthosis nigricans and explains to the mother the importance of weight loss, good diet, and exercise. She uses this as a teachable moment to explain how the obesity and diabetes are adversely affecting the daughter and how this is visible on the skin. The role of genetics is discussed too but there is emphasis on the risk factors that can be altered.

INTRODUCTION

- Acanthosis nigricans (AN) is a localized form of hyperpigmentation that involves epidermal alteration. AN is associated with insulin resistance and usually seen in patients with endocrine disorders (e.g., type 2 DM, Cushing syndrome, acromegaly), obesity, and polycystic ovary syndrome.

EPIDEMIOLOGY

- In a cross-sectional study conducted in a southwestern practice-based research network (N = 1133), AN was found in 17 percent of children and 21 percent of adults.[1]

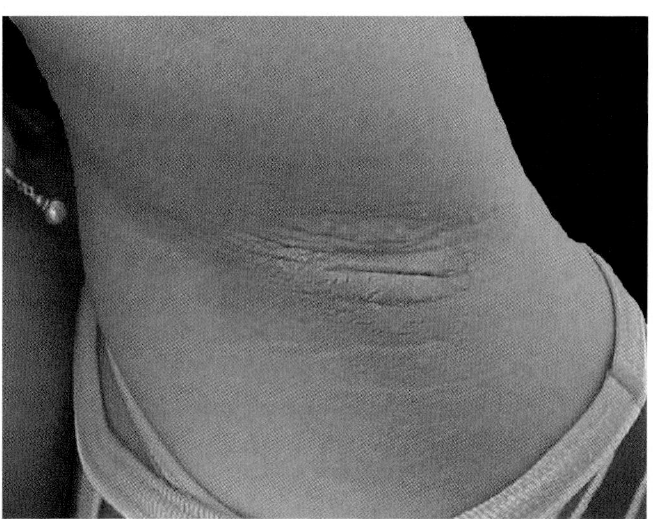

FIGURE 190-1 Acanthosis nigricans in the left axilla of an overweight Hispanic 10-year-old girl. Note areas of dark velvety discoloration and pink filiform hypertrophy. (*Used with permission from Richard P. Usatine, MD.*)

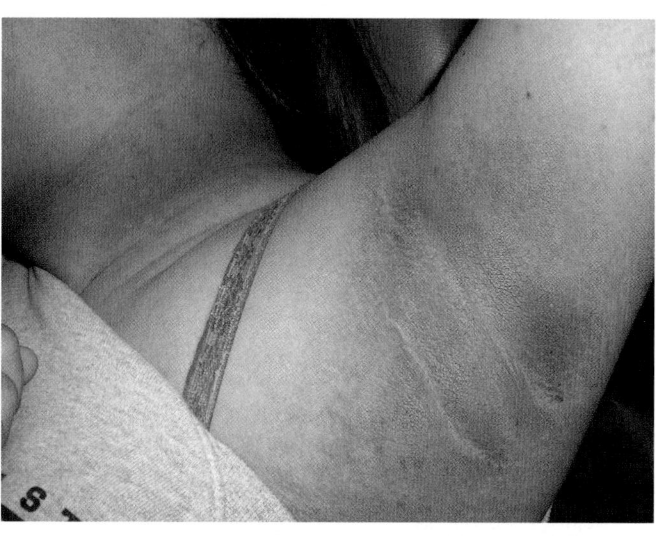

FIGURE 190-2 Acanthosis nigricans on the neck and in the axilla of an overweight 13-year-old Hispanic female with insulin resistance, hirsutism, and secondary amenorrhea. She was diagnosed with HAIR-AN syndrome and treated accordingly. (*Used with permission from Richard P. Usatine, MD.*)

- In two studies, AN was present in 36 percent of patients with newly diagnosed DM and 39 percent of children with obesity.[2,3] AN prevalence rates have been reported to be as high as 60 to 92 percent of black and Hispanic children with diabetes.[4]
- AN has been reported in children with Wilms' tumor and osteogenic sarcoma.[4]
- A condition of hyperandrogenism (HA), insulin resistance (IR), and acanthosis nigricans (AN) called HAIR-AN syndrome is a subphenotype of the polycystic ovary syndrome (**Figure 190-2**).[5–7] It is one of the most common causes of menstrual problems, hyperandrogenic symptoms, and insulin resistance among adolescent patients.[6] In one series of patients with HAIR-AN in an adolescent clinic, the mean age of affected patients was 15.5, initial mean weight at diagnosis was 94.5 kg, and the mean BMI was 33 kg/2.6 m.
- AN can be an adverse effect from hormonal therapies.[8]

ETIOLOGY AND PATHOPHYSIOLOGY

- AN results from long-term exposure of keratinocytes to insulin and is an indicator of insulin sensitivity independent of body mass index (BMI).[4]
- Type A IR appears responsible for producing AN in patients who are obese and Type B resistance, mediated by antibody formation against insulin receptors, appears to cause AN in patients with other autoimmune diseases.[4]
- Keratinocytes have insulin and insulin-like growth receptors on their surface and the pathogenesis of this condition is linked to insulin binding to insulin-like growth receptors in the epidermis.
- Fibroblast growth factor receptor 3 (FGFR3) gene mutations should be considered in patients with coexistent AN and skeletal dysplasia (e.g., thanatophoric dysplasia, severe achondroplasia with developmental delay and AN [SADDAN syndrome], and Crouzon

syndrome with AN);[9,10] in these patients, IR does not appear to be the mechanism in producing AN.[10] Insulin receptor mutations have also been described.[4]

- Malignant AN likely occurs as a result of tumor cell expression of peptides that enhance proliferation of transforming growth factor-a and epidermal growth factor.[4]

DIAGNOSIS

The diagnosis of AN is made clinically in a patient with or at risk for IR who has the characteristic lesions.

CLINICAL FEATURES

- AN ranges in appearance from diffuse streaky thickened brown velvety lesions to leathery verrucous papillomatous lesions (**Figures 190-1** to **190-6**).
- Women with HAIR-AN syndrome have evidence of virilization (e.g., increased body hair in male distribution, enlarged clitoris) in addition to AN.[6]
- There is a significant correlation between AN and obesity (**Figures 190-3** and **190-4**) and hypertension.[11]

TYPICAL DISTRIBUTION

- Commonly located on the neck (**Figures 190-4** to **190-6**) or skin folds (i.e., axillae [**Figures 190-1** to **190-3**], inframammary folds, groin, and perineum).
- Less often AN is seen on the nipples or areolae, perineum, groin, and extensor surfaces of the legs.[6]
- Verrucous AN can affect the eyelids, lips, and buccal mucosa.[6]
- In patients with malignancy, the onset of AN can be abrupt and the distribution of lesions is more widespread and may include the periorbital skin and the palms and soles.[12]

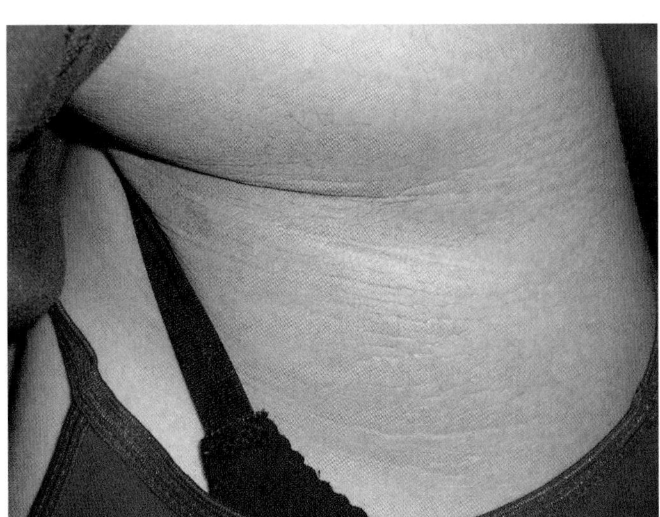

FIGURE 190-3 Acanthosis nigricans in the axilla of an 11-year-old obese Hispanic girl. (*Used with permission from Richard P. Usatine, MD.*)

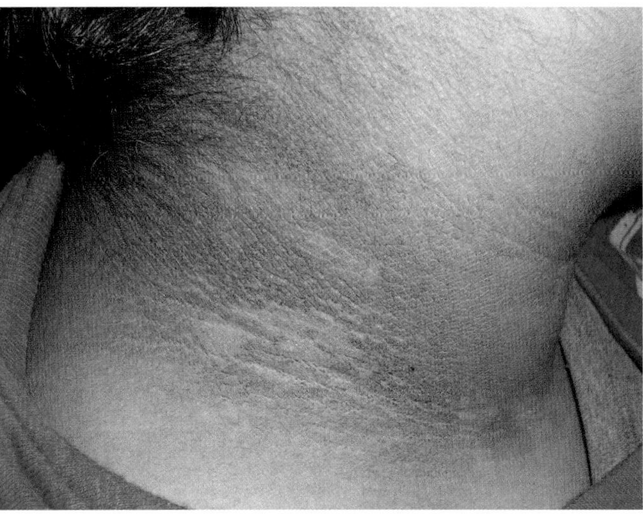

FIGURE 190-4 Acanthosis nigricans on the neck of a 15-year-old obese Hispanic male. (*Used with permission from Richard P. Usatine, MD.*)

BIOPSY

- Biopsy is rarely needed in unusual cases.
- Histologic examination reveals hyperkeratosis and papillary hypertrophy, although the epidermis is only mildly thickened.[13]

DIFFERENTIAL DIAGNOSIS

Other hyperpigmented lesions that may be confused with AN include:

- On the neck, AN can be confused with tinea corporis (see Chapter 123, Tinea Corporis) or atopic dermatitis (see Chapter 130, Atopic Dermatitis).
- Ichthyosis hystrix, a rare form of ichthyosis, can cause massive hyperkeratosis that can resemble AN; distinguishing features are

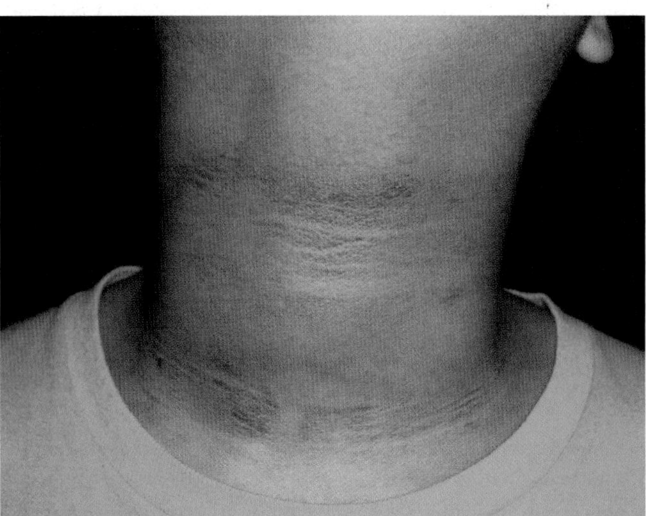

FIGURE 190-5 Acanthosis nigricans on neck of a 12-year-old African American boy with a strong family history of diabetes. Note that this child is not overweight and currently does not have diabetes. The acanthosis nigricans makes the neck appear dirty but this child has very good hygiene. (*Used with permission from Richard P. Usatine, MD.*)

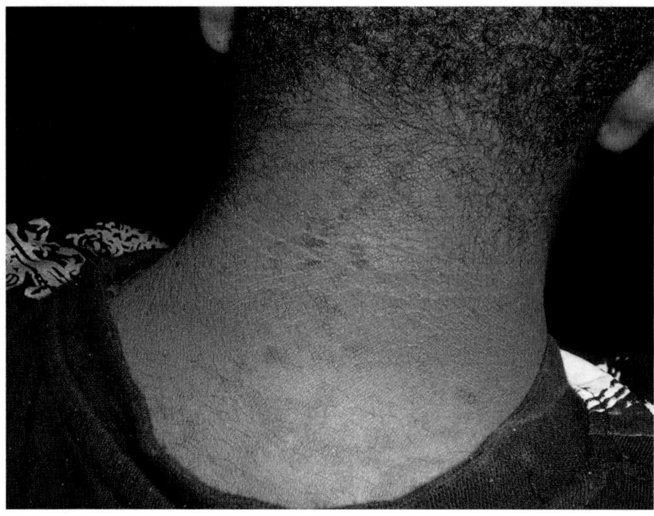

FIGURE 190-6 Acanthosis nigricans on the neck of a 15-year-old boy with no obesity or diabetes. His mother has very prominent acanthosis nigricans. (*Used with permission from Richard P. Usatine, MD.*)

greater body distribution including palmar and plantar keratoderma and resolution in the summer months.[4]

- There is also a rare AN form of epidermal nevus that shows histopathological evidence of both lesions (see Chapter 145, Epidermal Nevus and Nevus Sebaceous for additional information on epidermal nevi).[14]

MANAGEMENT

NONPHARMACOLOGIC

- Children with AN are at higher risk of metabolic syndrome, and lipid screening should be considered along with consideration of testing for DM. There is controversy about whether children should be screened for AN as marker for early detection of diabetes mellitus. In a cohort of Native American youth (N = 161), BMI was a more sensitive marker for insulin resistance although less specific than AN,[15] and the Centers for Disease Control and Prevention do not recommend screening for AN. The American Academy of Pediatrics recommends screening children with obesity for hyperlipidemia and hyperglycemia.[16]
- Treat the underlying cause, if identified. Weight loss through diet and exercise helps reverse both IR and compensatory hyperinsulinemia and can improve the condition in obese patients.
- Resolution of AN also occurs with removal of the associated malignancy or associated drug in drug-induced AN.[4]

MEDICATIONS

- Keratolytic agents (e.g., salicylic acid) can improve the cosmetic appearance. Other topical therapies, including 0.1 percent tretinoin cream (to lighten the lesion), combination tretinoin cream with 12 percent ammonium lactate cream, or topical vitamin D ointments,[17] may be useful.[6] SOR Ⓒ
- Metformin[18] and octreotide have also been used to manage AN. SOR Ⓒ
- Adolescent girls with HAIR-AN were treated with a diet, exercise, oral contraceptive pills, and metformin (in most cases) in one large series.[6] All the girls who took their oral contraceptive pills began to have regular menstrual periods and their acne and/or hirsutism improved or remained unchanged. Only 20 percent of the adolescents had improvement in their acanthosis nigricans with treatment.[6]

COMPLEMENTARY AND ALTERNATIVE THERAPY

- The use of omega-3-fatty acid and dietary fish oil supplementation has also been reported to improve AN.[19] SOR Ⓒ

PROGNOSIS

- AN may regress when the underlying condition (e.g., diabetes, HAIR-AN syndrome, malignancy) is treated.[6] However, in one series of girls with HAIR-AN syndrome, only 20 percent of the adolescents had improvement in their acanthosis nigricans with treatment.[6]

PATIENT EDUCATION

- Patients who are overweight should be encouraged to lose weight through diet and exercise because weight loss may help diminish this condition.

PATIENT RESOURCES

- **www.ncbi.nlm.nih.gov/pubmedhealth/PMH0001855/**.
- **www.nlm.nih.gov/medlineplus/ency/article/000852.htm**.

PROVIDER RESOURCES

- Diabetes Public Health Resource, National Center for Chronic Disease Prevention and Health Promotion of the Centers for Disease Control and Prevention—**www.cdc.gov/diabetes/news/docs/an.htm**.

REFERENCES

1. Kong AS, Williams RL, Smith M, et al. Acanthosis nigricans and diabetes risk factors: prevalence in young persons seen in southwestern US primary care practices. *Ann Fam Med.* 2007;5:202-208.
2. Litonjua P, Pinero-Pilona A, Aviles-Santa L, et al. Prevalence of acanthosis nigricans in newly-diagnosed type 2 diabetes. *Endocr Pract.* 2004;10:101-106.
3. Miura N, Ikezaki A, Iwama S, et al. Genetic factors and clinical significance of acanthosis nigricans in obese Japanese children and adolescents. *Acta Paediatr.* 2006;95:170-175.
4. Sinha S, Schwartz RA. Juvenile acanthosis nigricans. *J Am Acad Dermatol.* 2007;57:502-508.
5. McClanahan KK, Omar HA. Navigating adolescence with a chronic health condition: a perspective on the psychological

effects of HAIR-AN syndrome on adolescent girls. Scientific-WorldJournal. 2006;6:1350-1358.

6. Omar HA, Logsdon S, Richards J. Clinical profiles, occurrence, and management of adolescent patients with HAIR-AN syndrome. *ScientificWorldJournal*. 2004;4:507-511.
7. Esperanza LE, Fenske NA. Hyperandrogenism, insulin resistance, and acanthosis nigricans (HAIR-AN) syndrome: spontaneous remission in a 15-year-old girl. *J Am Acad Dermatol*. 1996;34(5): 892-897.
8. Downs AM, Kennedy CT. Somatotrophin-induced acanthosis nigricans. *Br J Dermatol*. 1999;141:390-391.
9. Blomberg M, Jeppesen EM, Skovby F, Benfeldt E. FGFR3 mutations and the skin: report of a patient with a FGFR3 gene mutation, acanthosis nigricans, hypochondroplasia and hyperinsulinemia and review of the literature. *Dermatology*. 2010;220(4):297-305.
10. Alatzoglou KS, Hindmarsh PC, Brain C, et al. Acanthosis nigricans and insulin sensitivity in patients with achondroplasia and hypochondroplasia due to FGFR3 mutations. *J Clin Endocrinol Metab*. 2009;94(10):3959-3963.
11. Otto DE, Wang X, Tijerina SL, et al. A comparison of blood pressure, body mass index and acanthosis nigricans in school-age children. *J Sch Nurs*. 2010;26(3):223-229.
12. Stulberg DL, Clark N. Hyperpigmented disorders in adults: part II. *Am Fam Physician*. 2003;68:1963-1968.
13. Sibbald RG, Landolt SJ, Toth D. Skin and diabetes. *Endocrinol Metab Clin North Am*. 1996;25(2):463-472.
14. de Waal AC, van Rossum MM, Bovenschen HJ. Extensive segmental acanthosis nirgricans form of epidermal nevus. *Dermatol Online J*. 2010;16(6):7.
15. Nsiah-Kumi PA, Beals J, Lasley S, et al. Body mass index percentile more sensitive than acanthosis nigricans for screening Native American children for diabetes risk. *J Natl Med Assoc*. 2010; 102(10):944-949.
16. Barlow SE. Expert committee recommendations regarding the prevention, assessment, and treatment of child and adolescent overweight and obesity: summary report. *Pediatrics*. 2007; 120(4):S164-S192.
17. Hermanns-Le T, Scheen A, Pierard GE. Acanthosis nigricans associated with insulin resistance: pathophysiology and management. *Am J Clin Dermatol*. 2004;5(3):199-203.
18. Wasniewska M, Arrigo T, Crisafulli G, et al. Recovery of acanthosis nigricans under prolonged metformin treatment in an adolescent with normal weight. *J Endocrinol Invest*. 2009;32:939-940.
19. Sheretz EF. Improved acanthosis nigricans with lipodystrophic diabetes during dietary fish oil supplementation. *Arch Dermatol*. 1988;124:1094-1096.
19. Rosenbach A, Ram R. Treatment of acanthosis nigricans of the axillae using a long-pulsed (5-msec) alexandrite laser. *Dermatol Surg*. 2004;30(8):1158-1160.

191 HYPOTHYROIDISM

Mindy A. Smith, MD, MS

PATIENT STORY

A 6-week-old girl, who was born at home and was not screened at birth for congenital hypothyroidism, presented to her pediatrician with signs of jaundice and was found to be hypothyroid with an elevated TSH (**Figure 191-1**). She was started on levothyroxine and her dose was titrated until her TSH was normal. At her 1 year old visit she was a normal healthy child with a normal developmental exam.

INTRODUCTION

- Hypothyroidism is a condition caused by lack of thyroid hormone and usually develops as a result of thyroid failure from intrinsic thyroid disease. The most common cause of nonendemic goitrous hypothyroidism in both children and adults is chronic lymphocytic (Hashimoto) thyroiditis, also called autoimmune thyroiditis.[1]
- Congenital hypothyroidism (CH) is decreased or absent thyroid function and thyroid hormone production that is present at birth. Historically this was due to lack of iodine. In iodine-replete countries, most cases of CH are caused by defects in embryonic development (e.g., congenitally absent, underdeveloped, or ectopic thyroid gland). Other causes include inherited enzymatic defects in the synthesis of thyroxine (T_4), prematurity, and anti-thyroid drugs taken during pregnancy.
- Goiter is a spectrum of changes in the thyroid gland ranging from diffuse enlargement to nodular enlargement depending on the cause. In the US, the most common cause of goiter with normal thyroid function or transient dysfunction is thyroiditis.
- Subclinical thyroid disease refers to a patient with no or minimal thyroid-related symptoms but abnormal laboratory values (elevated TSH and thyroxine level within the normal range).

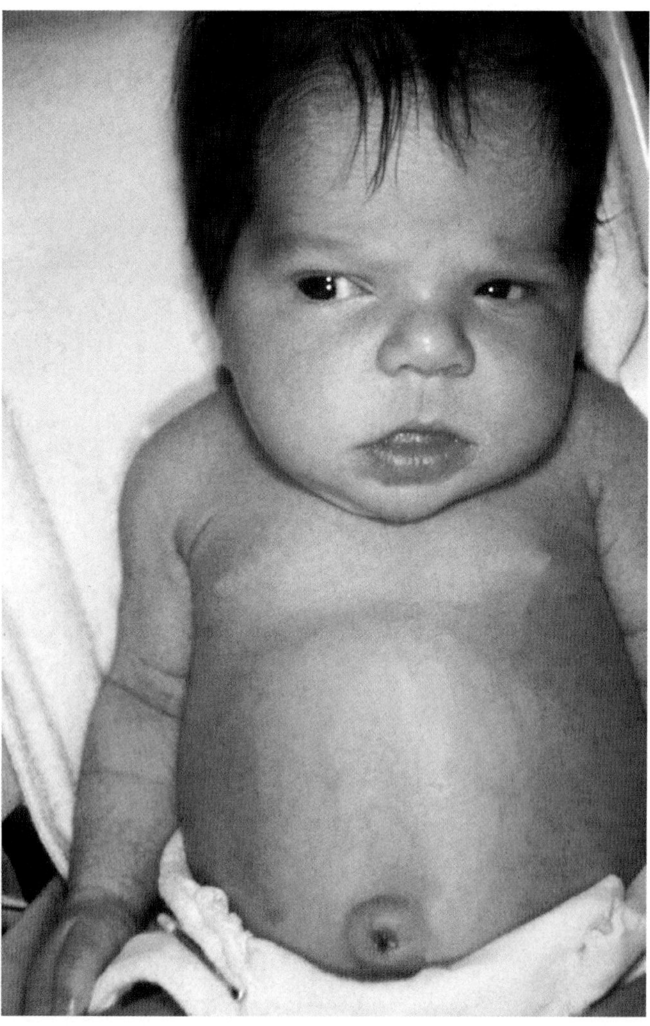

FIGURE 191-1 Congenital hypothyroidism in a 6-week-old girl with signs of jaundice and an elevated TSH. *(Used with permission from the CDC/ Dr. Hudson.)*

EPIDEMIOLOGY

- Based on a population study in Scotland, the prevalence of hypothyroidism in children (<22 years of age) is 0.135 percent; the prevalence is 0.113 percent in children aged 11 to 18 years.[2] These values are twice those of previous estimates. The most common cause of acquired hypothyroidism was autoimmune disease.
- CH occurs in about 1 per 3000 to 4000 births in the US with a female to male ratio of 2: 1. It is the most preventable cause of cognitive impairment in children.[3] There is a higher incidence of CH in some ethnic groups such as Greek Cypriots (1 per 1800) and Asians (1 per 918 in Northern England).[4,5]
- In a New Zealand population study, the overall incidence of CH rose from 2.6 to 3.6 per 10,000 live births over an 18-year period thought to be due to a shift in population with proportionately more Asian and Pacific Island births.[6]
- Worldwide, goiter is the most common endocrine disorder with rates of 4 to 15 percent in areas of adequate iodine intake and more than 90 percent where there is iodine deficiency.[7] Endemic goiter is defined as goiter that affects more than 5 percent of the population (**Figure 191-1**).
- Most goiters are not associated with thyroid dysfunction.
- The prevalence of goitrous hypothyroidism varies from 0.7 to 4 percent of the population. Among adolescents, the incidence of Hashimoto thyroiditis during adolescence is approximately 1 to 2 percent.[3]
- Subclinical hypothyroidism is present in 3 to 10 percent of population groups.[8,9]
- Prevalence rates of hypothyroidism and subclinical hypothyroidism are higher for children with certain conditions including Down syndrome (10.8% of children with Down syndrome in one 11-year population study filled a new prescription for thyroid medication),[10] Turner syndrome, type 1 diabetes mellitus (7.2% of children in one study had subclinical hypothyroidism),[11] celiac disease, and cystic fibrosis (CF) (108/129 children with CF in one study were iodine deficient and 11.6 percent had subclinical hypothyroidism).[12] Autoimmune thyroid disease is also more common in

individuals with vitiligo. In a recent report of 104 Iranian children age 5 to 15 years referred with migraine headache, 24 percent had subclinical hypothyroidism.[13]

ETIOLOGY AND PATHOPHYSIOLOGY

Hypothyroidism can be caused by disease of the thyroid gland itself (e.g., Hashimoto thyroiditis or thyroid dysgenesis), treatment of hyperthyroidism (e.g., anti-thyroid medication or radioiodine thyroid ablation in the patient or mother during pregnancy, or thyroidectomy), high-dose head and neck radiation therapy, medications (e.g., lithium or alpha-interferon) or, rarely, by pituitary or hypothalamic disorders (e.g., tumors, inflammatory conditions, infiltrative diseases, infections, pituitary surgery, pituitary radiation therapy, and head trauma).[8]

Hashimoto thyroiditis is caused by thyroid peroxidase (TPO) antibodies.

- There is marked lymphocytic infiltration of the thyroid in Hashimoto thyroiditis; the infiltrate is composed of activated CD4+ and CD8+ T cells, as well as B cells.
- Thyroid destruction in Hashimoto thyroiditis is believed to be primarily mediated by CD8+ cytotoxic T cells.

CH can be either permanent or temporary.

- Permanent causes include defective embryonic development resulting in congenitally absent, underdeveloped, or ectopic thyroid gland (85%); inherited enzymatic defect in the synthesis of thyroxine (T4) caused by an autosomal recessive gene (10%); abnormal function of hypothalamus or pituitary, or thyroid hormone resistance (<5%). In the New Zealand study previously cited, of 330 new cases of CH over an 18-year period, 86 percent of cases had a scintiscan of which 67 percent showed thyroid dysgenesis (female to male ratio 5:1), and 33 percent demonstrated dyshormonogenesis (female to male ratio 0.9:1.0).[6]
- About 2 percent of thyroid dysgenesis is familial. In one case series, TSHR was found to be the main causative locus in autosomal recessively inherited thyroid dysgenesis.[14]
- Among cases of temporary hypothyroidism, causes include antithyroid drugs taken during pregnancy, prematurity, and iodine deficiency or excess.

Contributing factors for goiter are:

- Iodine deficiency or excess (**Figures 191-2** and **191-3**).
- TSH stimulation.
- Drugs, including lithium, amiodarone, anticonvulsants, and α-interferon.
- Autoimmunity/heredity.

RISK FACTORS

Other risk factors for hypothyroidism include[2]:

- Symptoms of thyroid hormone deficiency.
- Goiter.

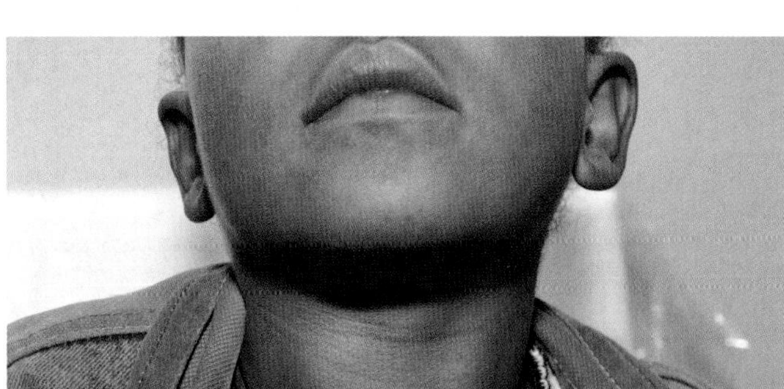

FIGURE 191-2 Goiter developing in a 12-year-old girl in an endemic area for goiters. (*Used with permission from Richard P. Usatine, MD.*)

- Personal or family history of thyroid disease.
- Personal treatment of thyroid disease.
- History of an autoimmune disease, especially diabetes mellitus.

DIAGNOSIS

CLINICAL FEATURES

Many children with autoimmune thyroiditis are asymptomatic at diagnosis.[15] Classic signs and symptoms of hypothyroidism are[3]:

- A decrease in linear growth.
- Fatigue and/or weakness.
- Dry and cool skin (**Figure 191-4**).

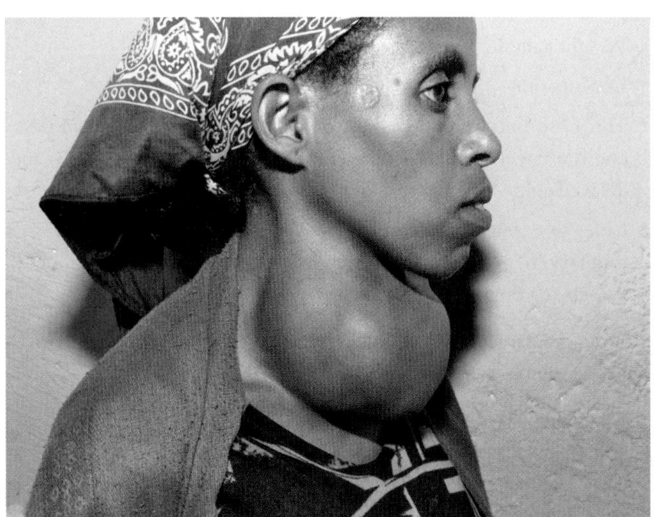

FIGURE 191-3 Massive goiter in an Ethiopian woman who lives in an endemic area for goiters. Many adults have large goiters in Ethiopia where there is little iodine in their diets. (*Used with permission from Richard P. Usatine, MD.*)

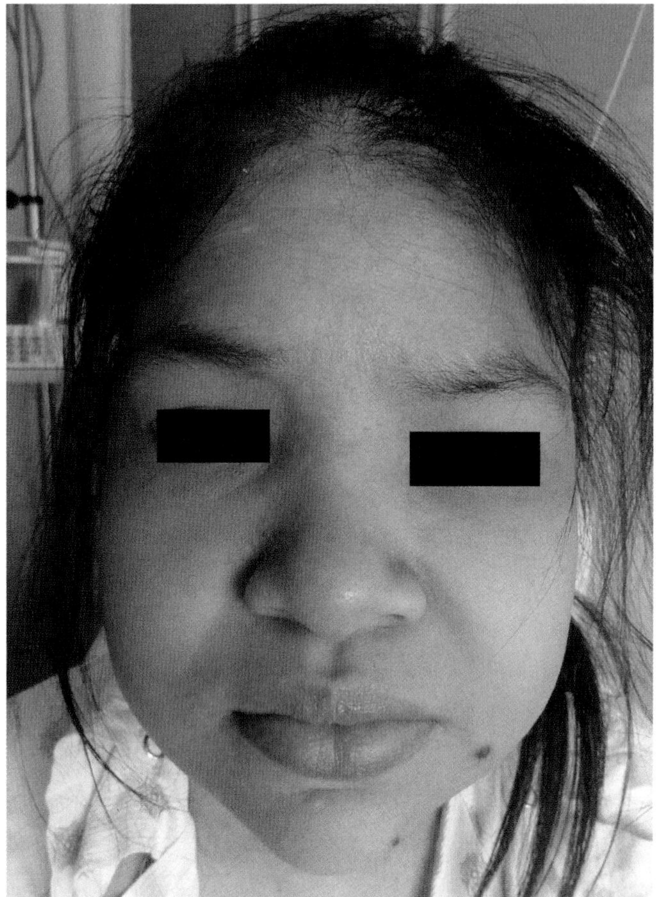

FIGURE 191-4 Myxedema with puffiness of the face, dry skin, some hair loss of the scalp, and eyebrows. (*Used with permission from the University of Texas Health Sciences Center, Division of Dermatology.*)

- Increased body hair.
- Difficulty concentrating with poor school performance.
- Bradycardia.
- Delayed deep tendon reflex relaxation.
- Weight gain despite poor appetite.
- Constipation.
- The most useful signs in adults for diagnosing hypothyroidism in one study were puffiness (likelihood ratio positive [LR+] 16.2) and delayed ankle reflex (LR+ 11.8).[16]
- Clues to a central cause of hypothyroidism include a history of pituitary/hypothalamic surgery or radiation, headache, visual field defects, or ophthalmoplegia.[8]

Among infants with CH, the vast majority (95%) has few clinical manifestations.[3] Features suggestive of CH include:[3]

- An open posterior fontanelle in a term baby.
- Lethargy or hypotonia.
- Hoarse cry.
- Feeding problems or macroglossia.
- Constipation.
- Umbilical hernia (**Figure 191-5**).

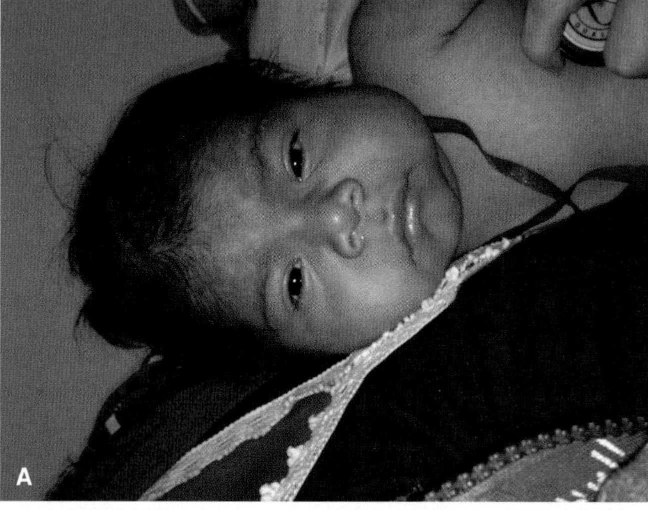

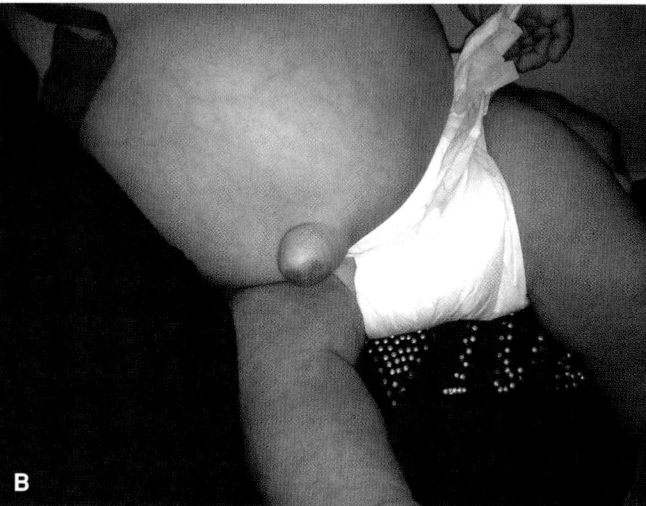

FIGURE 191-5 Congenital hypothyroidism in a 3-year-old child in Peru. The child was developmentally delayed and was not diagnosed until a medical mission team provided access to health care for this child. **A.** Note the puffiness of the cheeks and the increased facial hair on the forehead. **B.** Note the persistent umbilical hernia and the fact that the child is still in diapers. (*Used with permission from Sangeeta Krishna, MD.*)

- Dry skin.
- Hypothermia.
- Prolonged jaundice.

Features of goiter are:

- A painful neck mass is usually a form of thyroiditis.
- Large goiters are easily visible before palpating the neck (**Figures 191-2** and **191-3**). In a case series of children with autoimmune thyroiditis (N = 61), the vast majority of patients had a goiter; approximately half were euthyroid (N = 29), nine had hypothyroidism and seven had hyperthyroidism.[17]
- Physical examination maneuvers that help detect goiter are neck extension (**Figure 191-6**), observation from the side, palpation by locating the isthmus first, and having the patient swallow.[18]
- Asymmetric goiters can shift the trachea away from the midline.

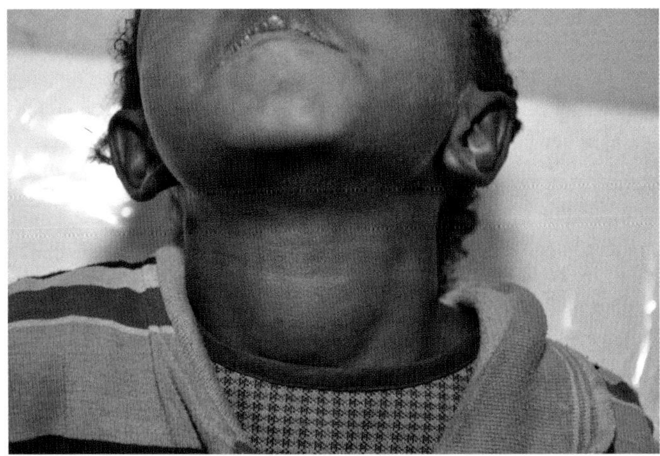

FIGURE 191-6 Child with goiter and kwashiorkor (protein malnutrition) in Africa. Note how the goiter is easily visible when she extends her neck. (*Used with permission from Richard P. Usatine, MD.*)

LABORATORY AND IMAGING STUDIES

Laboratory tests include an erythrocyte sedimentation rate (ESR) if thyroiditis is suspected, and TSH (elevated in hypothyroidism and subclinical disease) and FT_4 levels (low in hypothyroidism).

- In acute granulomatous thyroiditis, ESR is >50 (LR+ 95) and the TSH and FT_4 are usually normal.
- In primary hypothyroidism, the TSH is >10 mU/L (LR+ 16) and FT_4 is <8 (LR+ 11).
- Based on several case series, about half of children with autoimmune thyroiditis are euthyroid at diagnosis.[15,17]
- The presence of antibodies to TPO and thyroglobulin help establish the diagnosis of Hashimoto thyroiditis but is unnecessary for treatment. TPO antibodies will be positive in 90 to 95 percent of adult patients and the majority of children.[3,15]
- Confirming a positive neonatal screening result with formal thyroid function testing is a matter of urgency.[19] SOR Ⓐ
- Thyroid imaging with radionuclide scan for children with CH along with ultrasound will identify thyroid dysgenesis (accounts for 85% of cases). Radionuclide scintigraphy is considered the 'gold standard' for visualizing ectopic thyroid tissue. In one study (N = 174 screening-referred infants),151 had normally located thyroid on scintigraphy, ultrasound was found to be 95.8 percent sensitive (95% CI, 76.8 to 99.7), and 99.3 percent specific (95.8 to 100) for absence of normal thyroid.[20]
- In pituitary causes of hypothyroidism (central hypothyroidism), the TSH may be normal or elevated but FT_4 will be low.[8]
- In the future, reference limits may need to change as TSH distribution and reference limits have been shown to shift to higher concentrations with age and are unique for different racial/ethnic groups.[21]

DIFFERENTIAL DIAGNOSIS

Goiter presenting as a painful neck mass is most commonly caused by subacute granulomatous (de Quervain) thyroiditis (likely viral) or hemorrhage into a thyroid cyst or adenoma. Other causes include the following:

- Painful Hashimoto thyroiditis—Hypothyroidism with the presence of antibodies helps to confirm this diagnosis.
- Infected thyroglossal duct or branchial cleft cyst—Mass palpates as cystic and may be fluctuant; focal (e.g., erythema and warmth) and systemic symptoms of infection (e.g., fever) may be present. Even a noninfected thyroglossal duct cyst can be confused for an enlarged thyroid.
- Acute suppurative thyroiditis (microbial)—Focal (e.g., erythema and warmth) and systemic symptoms of infection (e.g., fever) are usually present.

Painless goiter and hypothyroidism are most often caused by Hashimoto thyroiditis, but may also be caused by the following:

- Environmental goitrogens (e.g., excess iodine, foods such as cassava, cabbage, and soybeans).
- Iodine deficiency.
- Pharmacologic inhibition (rare)—Drugs include lithium, amiodarone, and interferon-α.

Painless goiter and hyperthyroidism may be caused by the following:

- Graves disease—Symptoms of nervousness, fatigue, weight loss, heat intolerance, palpitations, and exophthalmus (Chapter 192, Hyperthyroidism).
- Postpartum thyroiditis (2% to 16% within 3 to 6 months of delivery)—Recent delivery.

MANAGEMENT

NONPHARMACOLOGIC

- For nonendemic goiter, identify and remove goitrogens.

MEDICATIONS

- Patients with endemic goiter should be provided with iodine. SOR Ⓒ
- The goal for children with acquired hypothyroidism treatment is euthyroidism by treating with levothyroxine.[3] SOR Ⓐ Dose ranges for children are 5 to 8 mcg/kg for children aged 6 to 12 months, 4 to 6 mcg/kg for children aged 1 to 3 years, 3 to 5 mcg/kg for children aged 3 to 10 years, and 2 to 4 mcg/kg for children aged 10 to 18 years.[3] Dosing should be titrated to achieve the treatment goal of a normal TSH.
- The goal of treatment for children with CH is to rapidly achieve euthyroidism. SOR Ⓐ In the first year of life, target serum T_4 level should be 10 to 16 mcg/dL (128.7 to 205.9 nmol/L), serum free T_4 should be 1.4 to 2.3 ng/dL (18.0 to 29.6 pmol/L), and TSH concentration <5 mU/L.[3] Oral levothyroxine is administered daily at 10 to 15 mcg/kg (usually 37.5 to 50 mcg/day); one author suggests a dose of 50 mcg/day in term infants for optimal preservation of cognitive abilities.[3] Authors of a Cochrane review, however, found only a single randomized clinical trial and therefor insufficient evidence to support high versus low dose initial thyroid replacement.[22] Parents can crush and mix tables with a small volume of human milk, formula, or water; soy formulas or preparations containing concentrated iron or calcium should be avoided as they can reduce thyroxine absorption.

- There is controversy over whether brand-name levothyroxine (Synthroid) performs better than generic medication in normalizing TSH in children with severe CH.[23,24]
- There is also controversy over whether children with subclinical hypothyroidism should be treated with levothyroxine. Based on a systematic literature review, overt hypothyroidism is more likely to develop in children with goiter and elevated thyroglobulin antibodies, children with celiac disease, and children demonstrating a progressive increase in thyroperoxidase antibodies and TSH value (see Prognosis);[25] in adults, a TSH >10 mIU/L is also likely to predict subsequent hypothyroidism.
  - It is reasonable to treat children at high likelihood of progression or if they have symptoms of thyroid deficiency or are pregnant.[8,26] SOR Ⓒ
  - In children with subclinical hypothyroidism, an increased growth velocity with treatment was observed in two studies and reduced thyroid volume was seen in 25 to 100 percent of children with subclinical hypothyroidism and autoimmune thyroiditis in two studies.[25] There were no observed effects on neuropsychological functions (one study) or posttreatment evolution of hypothyroidism (one study).[25]
  - Authors of a Cochrane review of 12 small randomized controlled trials (RCTs) determined that treatment of subclinical hypothyroidism did not improve survival or decrease cardiovascular morbidity.[27]
- Levothyroxine treatment is effective in reducing thyroid volume in children and can be considered for the treatment of goiter caused by autoimmune thyroiditis, even in children who are euthyroid.[28]
- Patients with acute microbial thyroiditis are treated with antibiotics (e.g., amoxicillin/clavulanate, first- or second-generation cephalosporin) for 7 to 10 days against the most common pathogens (i.e., *Staphylococcus aureus, Streptococcus pyogenes,* and *Streptococcus pneumoniae*). In patients with subacute thyroiditis, oral corticosteroids can reduce pain and swelling. SOR Ⓒ Symptoms of hyperthyroidism can be treated with β-blockers. SOR Ⓑ

COMPLICATIONS AND REFERRAL

- Large goiters that impinge upon the trachea or do not respond to medications can be treated with surgery.
- Children with hypothyroidism should be referred to a pediatric endocrinologist.
- Patients with myxedema coma should be hospitalized in an intensive care unit; without treatment, mortality approaches 100 percent.
- Hashimoto's encephalopathy (HE) is a rare complication. In a case series of patients (all girls) with HE (N = 8), all had high levels of antithyroid peroxidase (TPO) antibodies at onset (4043.3 ± 2969.8 IU/mL) despite normal T4 and TSH levels in six of them. Relapses were observed in five children despite steroid therapy and four subsequently developed hypothyroidism.[29]
- Severe hypothyroidism is associated with pseudoprecocious puberty (24% of 33 children in one case series).[30]

PREVENTION AND SCREENING

- The US Preventive Services Task Force recommends screening for CH in newborns. SOR Ⓐ Screening is done with TSH with backup serum T_4, primary T_4 with backup TSH, or both tests in initial screening, optimally at 2 to 4 days of age.
- Periodic screening may also be justified in high-risk populations; in an observational study of children with Down syndrome, early administration of levothyroxine for hypothyroidism appeared to improve growth.[31]
- There is insufficient evidence to support screening for hypothyroidism in pregnant and nonpregnant patients;[32] however, pregnant patients with subclinical hypothyroidism are more likely to have placental abruption (three-fold increase) and preterm delivery (two-fold increase) and their infants are at higher risk for intraventricular hemorrhage and respiratory distress syndrome.[33] Authors of a literature review found a single intervention trial demonstrating a decrease in preterm delivery among thyroid antibody-positive women treated with levothyroxine.[34]

PROGNOSIS

- Suppression of TSH with levothyroxine effectively reduces the goiter of Hashimoto thyroiditis and should be continued indefinitely. In one study of adults, withdrawal of medication after 1 year resulted in only 11.4 percent remaining euthyroid.[35]
- Children with CH, especially severe CH, are at risk for motor and cognitive problems.[36] In a survey of 10-year-old patients with CH, reported health-related quality of life and self-worth were lower than general population ratings, independent of disease factors, IQ and motor skills.[37]
- In the most extensive community survey on goiter (Whickham, England), goiter was present in 15.5 percent of the population.[38] At the 20-year follow-up, 20 percent of women and 5 percent of men no longer had goiter and 4 percent of women and no men had acquired a goiter.
- In patients with subclinical hypothyroidism, progression to clinically overt hypothyroidism is 2.6 percent each year if TPO antibodies are absent and 4.3 percent if they are present.[39] In a review of pediatric patients with subclinical hypothyroidism, most children reverted to euthyroidism or remained with subclinical hypothyroidism; overt hypothyroidism occurred in between 0 and 28.8 percent.[25] In a 2-year follow-up study of 92 children with subclinical hypothyroidism, TSH normalized or remained unchanged in 88 percent and increased above 10 mU/L in 11 children; none developed overt hypothyroidism.[40]

FOLLOW-UP

- Children with CH should be followed with serum T_4 or free T_4 and TSH concentrations at 2 and 4 weeks after the initiation of treatment, every 1 to 2 months during the first 6 postnatal months, and every 3 to 4 months between 6 months and 3 years of age.[3] If hypothyroidism is permanent (expected in about 80%), serum tests should continue every 6 to 12 months until growth is complete or more frequently if adherence is questioned or abnormal results are obtained. If the medication dose is altered, test in 2 weeks.

- Serum free T^4 and TSH should be rechecked in children approximately 6 to 8 weeks after initiation of levothyroxine therapy and again in 4 to 6 months, with dosing adjustments made as needed. If normal, testing should continue every 3 to 6 months thereafter until growth is complete unless otherwise clinically indicated, then annually.[3,20] SOR C
- Although the need for thyroid replacement is lifelong, dose requirements can change over time. For example, the thyroxine dose may need to be increased during pregnancy (20% to 40%), with use of estrogens, or in situations of weight gain, malabsorption, *Helicobacter pylori*-related gastritis and atrophic gastritis and with use of some medications. Requirements may decrease with increased age, androgen use, reactivation of Graves' disease, or the development of autonomous thyroid nodules.[8]
- The frequency of other autoimmune disease is increased in patients with Hashimoto thyroiditis (14.3% in one study), including rheumatoid arthritis, pernicious anemia, systemic lupus erythematosus, Addison disease, celiac disease, and vitiligo, and increased monitoring should be considered.[41]

PATIENT RESOURCES

- Booklets from the American Thyroid Association—**www.thyroid.org/patients/brochures.html**.
- National Library of Medicine—**www.nlm.nih.gov/medlineplus/thyroiddiseases.html**.

PROVIDER RESOURCE

- **http://reference.medscape.com/article/922777**.
- Counts D, Varma SK. Hypothyroidism in children. *Pediatr Rev.* 2009;30(7):251-257.

REFERENCES

1. Wasniewska M, Vigone MC, Cappa M, et al. Study Group for Thyroid diseases of Italian Society for Pediatric Endocrinology. Acute suppurative thyroiditis in childhood: relative frequency among thyroid inflammatory diseases. *J Endocrinol Invest.* 2007;30:346-347.
2. Hunter I, Greene SA, MacDonald TM, Morris AD. Prevalence and aetiology of hypothyroidism in the young. *Arch Dis Child.* 2000;83:207-210.
3. Counts D, Varma SK. Hypothyroidism in children. *Pediatr Rev.* 2009;30(7):251-257.
4. Skordis N, Toumba M, Savva SC, et al. High prevalence of congenital hypothyroidism in the Greek Cypriot population: results of the neonatal screening program 1990-2000. *J Pediatr Endocrinol Metab.* 2005;18:453-461.
5. Rosenthal M, Addison GM, Price DA. Congenital hypothyroidism: increased incidence in Asian families. *Arch Dis Child* 1988;63:790-793.
6. Albert BB, Cutfield WS, Webster D, et al. Etiology of increasing incidence of congenital hypothyroidism in New Zealand from 1993-2010. *J Clin Endocrinol Metab.* 2012;3155-3160.
7. Wang C, Crapo LM. The epidemiology of thyroid disease and implications for screening. *Endocrinol Metab Clin North Am.* 1997; 26(1):189-218.
8. McDermott MT. In the clinic. Hypothyroidism. *Ann Intern Med.* 2009;151(11):ITC61.
9. Fatourechi V. Subclinical hypothyroidism: an update for primary care physicians. *Mayo Clin Proc.* 2009;84(1):65-71.
10. Carroll KN, Arbogast PG, Dudley JA, Cooper WO. Increase in incidence of medically treated thyroid disease in children with Down syndrome after rerelease of American Academy of Pediatrics Health Supervision guidelines. *Pediatrics.* 2008; 122(2):e493-498.
11. Denzer C, Karges B, Näke A, et al. Subclinical hypothyroidism and dyslipidemia in children and adolescents with type 1 diabetes mellitus. *Eur J Endocrinol.* 2013 Feb 5. [Epub ahead of print].
12. Naehrlich L, Dörr HG, Bagheri-Behrouzi A, Rauh M. Iodine deficiency and subclinical hypothyroidism are common in cystic fibrosis patients. *J Trace Elem Med Biol.* 2012 Oct 26. [Epub ahead of print].
13. Fallah R, Mirouliaei M, Bashardoost N, Partovee M. Frequency of subclinical hypothyroidism in 5- to 15-year-old children with migraine headache. *J Pediatr Endocrinol Metab.* 2012;25(9-10): 859-862.
14. Cangul H, Aycan Z, Saglam H, et al. TSHR is the main causative locus in autosomal recessively inherited thyroid dysgenesis. *J Pediatr Endocrinol Metab.* 2012;25(5-6):419-426.
15. Skarpa V, Kappaousta E, Tertipi A, et al. Epidemiological characteristics of children with autoimmune thyroid disease. *Hormones (Athens).* 2011;10(3):207-214.
16. Zulewski H, Müller B, Exer P, et al. Estimation of tissue hypothyroidism by a new clinical score: Evaluation of patients with various grades of hypothyroidism and controls. *J Clin Endocrinol Metab.* 1997;82:771-776.
17. Roth C, Scortea M, Stubbe P, et al. Autoimmune thyroiditis in childhood-epidemiology, clinical and laboratory findings in 61 patients. *Exp Clin Endocrinol Diabetes.* 1997;105(4):66-69.
18. Siminoski K. Does this patient have a goiter? *JAMA.* 1995; 273(10):813-819.
19. American Academy of Pediatrics, Rose SR; Section on Endocrinology and Committee on Genetics, American Thyroid Association, Brown RS; Public Health Committee, Lawson Wilkins Pediatric Endocrine Society, Foley T, Kaplowitz PB, Kaye CI, Sundararajan S, Varma SK. Update of newborn screening and therapy for congenital hypothyroidism. *Pediatrics.* 2006;117: 2290-2303.
20. Ohnishi H, Inomata H, Watanabe T. Clinical utility of thyroid ultrasonography in the diagnosis of congenital hypothyroidism. *Endocr J.* 2002;49:293-297.
21. Surks MI, Boucai L. Age- and race-based serum thyrotropin reference limits. *J Clin Endocrinol Metab.* 2010;95(2):496-502.

22. Ng SM, Anand D, Weindling AM. High versus low dose of initial thyroid hormonr replacement for congenital hypothyroidism. *Cochrane Database Syst Rev*. 2009;(1):CD006972.

23. Carswell JM, Gordon JH, Popovsky E, et al. Generic and brand-name L-thyroxine are not bioequivalent for children with severe congenital hypothyroidism. *J Clin Endocrinol Metab*. 2013;98(2): 610-607.

24. Lomenick JP, Wang L, Ampah SB, et al. Generic levothyroxine compared with Synthroid in young children with congenital hypothyroidism. *J Clin Endocrinol Metab*. 2013;98(2):653-658.

25. Monzani A, Prodam F, Rapa A, et al. Endocrine disorders in childhood and adolescence. Natural history of subclinical hypothyroidism in children and adolescents and potential effects of replacement therapy: a review. *Eur J Endocrinol*. 2012;168(1):R1-R11.

26. Fatourechi V. Subclinical hypothyroidism: an update for primary care physicians. *Mayo Clin Proc*. 2009;84(1):65-71.

27. Villar HCCE, Saconato H, Valente O, Atallah ÁN. Thyroid hormone replacement for subclinical hypothyroidism. *Cochrane Database Syst Rev*. 2007;(3):CD003419.

28. Svensson J, Ericsson US, Nilsson P, et al. Levothyroxine treatment reduces thyroid size in children and adolescents with chronic autoimmune thyroiditis. *J Clin Endocrinol Metab*. 2006;91(5): 1729-1734.

29. Mamoudjy N, Korff C, Maurey H, et al. Hashimoto's encephalopathy: identification and long-term outcome in children. *Eur J Paediatr Neurol*. 2012 Dec 3. [Epub ahead of print]

30. Cabrera SM, Dimeglio LA, Eugster EA. Incidence and characteristics of pseudoprecocious because of severe primary hypothyroidism. *J Pediatr*. 2013;162(3):637-639.

31. Kowalczyk K, Pukajło K, Malczewska A, et al. L-thyroxine therapy and growth processes in children with Down syndrome. *Adv Clin Exp Med*. 2013;22(1):85-92.

32. United States Preventive Services Task Force. *Screening for Thyroid Disease*. http://www.uspreventiveservicestaskforce.org/uspstf/uspsthyr.htm, accessed November 2011.

33. Casey BM, Dashe JS, Spong CY, et al. Perinatal significance of isolated maternal hypothyroxinemia identified in the first half of pregnancy. *Obstet Gynecol*. 2007;109:1129-1135.

34. Stagnaro-Green A. Material thyroid disease and preterm delivery. *J Clin Endocrinol Metab*. 2009;94(1):21-25.

35. Comtois R, Faucher L, Lafleche L. Outcome of hypothyroidism cause by Hashimoto's thyroiditis. *Arch Intern Med*. 1995;155(13): 1404-1408.

36. van der Sluijs Veer L, Kempers MJ, Wiedijk BM, et al. Evaluation of cognitive and motor development in toddlers with congenital hypothyroidism diagnosed by neonatal screening. *J Dev Bahv Pediatr*. 2012;33(8):633-640.

37. van der Sluijs Veer L, Kempers MJ, Maurice-Stam H, et al. Health-related quality of life and self-worth in 10-year old children with congenital hypothyroidism diagnosed by neonatal screening. *Child Adolesc Psychiatry Ment Health*. 2012;6(1):32.

38. Wang C, Crapo LM. The epidemiology of thyroid disease and implications for screening. *Endocrinol Metab Clin North Am*. 1997; 26(1):189-218.

39. Vanderpump MP, Tunbridge WM, French JM, et al. The incidence of thyroid disorders in the community: a twenty-year follow-up of the Whickham Survey. *Clin Endocrinol (Oxf)*. 1995;43(1):55-68.

40. Wasniewska M, Salerno M, Cassio A, et al. Prospective evaluation of the natural course of idiopathic subclinical hypothyroidism in childhood and adolescence. *Eur J Endocrinol*. 2009;160(3):417-421.

41. Boelaert K, Newby PR, Simmonds MJ, et al. Prevalence and relative risk of other autoimmune diseases in subjects with autoimmune thyroid disease. *Am J Med*. 2010;123(2): 183.e1-183.e9.

192 HYPERTHYROIDISM

Mindy A. Smith, MD, MS

PATIENT STORY

A 12-year-old girl presents with fatigue, palpitations, and inability to sleep. She has been an excellent student in school but has had increasing difficulty concentrating in class and difficulty focusing her eyes. Family history was significant for thyroid disease in her mother (hypothyroid) and maternal aunt (Graves' disease [GD]). On examination, her pulse is 105 beats per minute, blood pressure 112/60 mm Hg, and she is mildly underweight with a BMI of 15. She has a mild resting tremor, proptosis (R >L), and her thyroid exam reveals a slightly enlarged but symmetric gland (**Figure 192-1**). You obtain blood work that reveals a low thyroid-stimulating hormone (TSH) and an elevated free thyroxin level (T_4). A thyroid scan and uptake shows a diffusely increased intake of 54 percent with no nodules (**Figure 192-2**). The patient was diagnosed with GD and the therapeutic options are presented to the family.

INTRODUCTION

GD is an autoimmune thyroid disorder characterized by circulating antibodies that stimulate the thyroid-stimulating hormone (TSH) receptor and resulting in hyperthyroidism.[1]

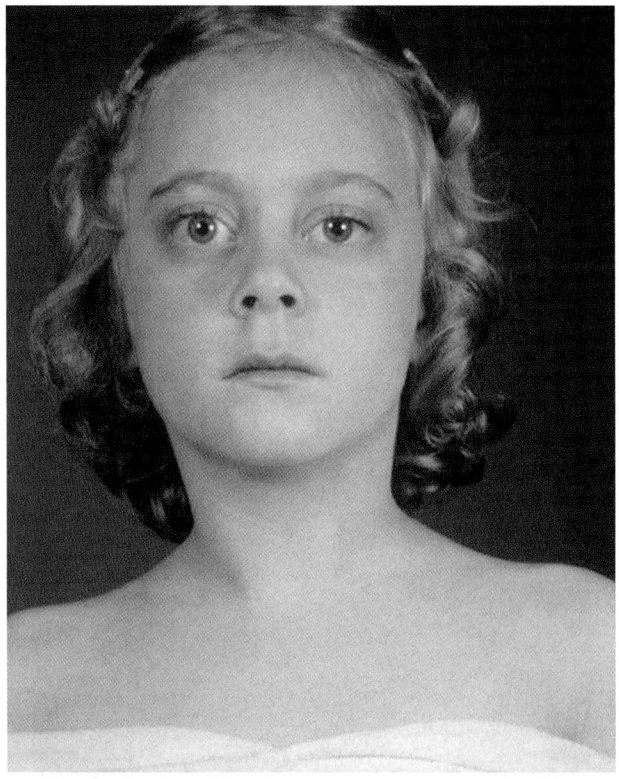

FIGURE 192-1 Graves disease presenting in a 12-year-old girl. Note the lid retraction and proptosis (exophthalmos), particularly evident on the right eye. (*Used with permission from Cleveland Clinic Children's Hospital Photo Files.*)

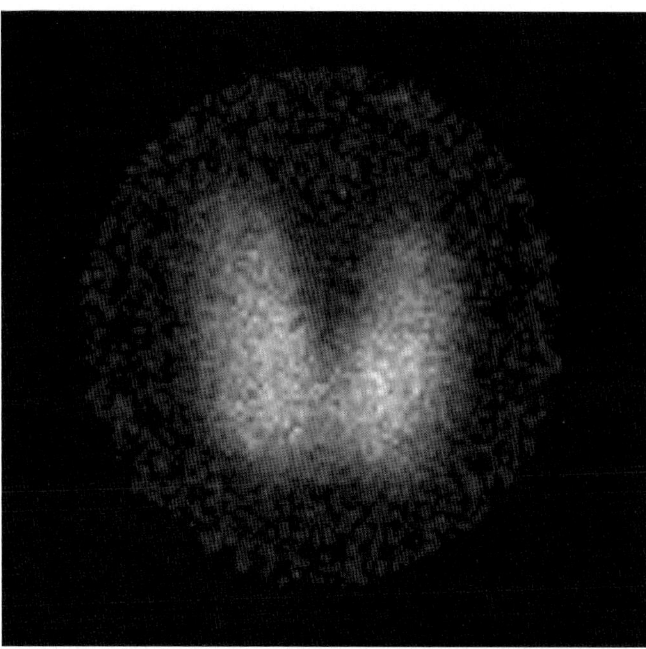

FIGURE 192-2 Nuclear scan of the thyroid in Graves disease showing increased uptake (54%) in a diffusely enlarged thyroid gland (with a homogeneous pattern). (*Used with permission from Richard P. Usatine, MD.*)

SYNONYMS

Thyrotoxicosis (clinical state resulting from inappropriately high thyroid hormone levels); hyperthyroidism (thyrotoxicosis caused by elevated synthesis and secretion of thyroid hormone), autoimmune hyperthyroidism, von Basedow's disease (in Europe).

EPIDEMIOLOGY

- GD is the most common cause of thyrotoxicosis in children (up to 95 percent of cases), with a prevalence in children and adolescents of between 1:2000 and 1:10,000 and an incidence between 0.1 and 3 per 100,000.[2,3] The incidence peaks in adolescence; only 1 to 5 percent of cases of childhood hyperthyroidism begin before the age of 16 years.[4]
- Similar to adults, there is a female predominance of between 3:1 to 5:1.[4]
- Autoimmune hyperthyroidism can occurs in about 2 percent of infants born to mothers with GD, but is usually transient (resolving in 3 to 12 weeks).[4,5] Cases of persistent congenital hyperthyroidism and non-autoimmune familial hyperthyroidism due to mutations in the TSH-receptor gene have been reported.[4]
- Rare forms of hyperthyroidism in children include pituitary adenomas, functioning thyroid nodules, pituitary resistance to thyroid hormones, and ingestion thyroid hormone or iodine.[4] Thyrotoxicosis of variable duration can also occur as part of Hashimoto thyroiditis (see Chapter 191, Hypothyroidism). Authors of one small case series (N = 14) reported resolution of hyperthyroidism by 8.3 ± 6.3 months after diagnosis (range 3 to 23 months); duration was positively correlated with thyroid peroxidase autoantibody level at presentation.[6]

- Graves' ophthalmopathy (see the following section "Clinical Features") occurs in more than 80 percent of patients within 18 months of diagnosis of GD. The ophthalmopathy is clinically apparent in 30 to 50 percent of patients, including children.[4,7]
- Untreated hyperthyroidism can lead to osteoporosis, atrial fibrillation, cardiomyopathy, and congestive heart failure; thyrotoxicosis (thyroid storm) has an associated mortality rate of 20 to 50 percent.[8] In newborns, untreated hyperthyroidism can cause irreversible nervous system damage and developmental delay.[4]

ETIOLOGY AND PATHOPHYSIOLOGY

- The hyperthyroidism of GD results from circulating immunoglobulin (Ig) G antibodies that stimulate the TSH receptor.[7] These antibodies are synthesized in the thyroid gland, bone marrow, and lymph nodes. Activation of the TSH receptor stimulates follicular hypertrophy and hyperplasia causing thyroid enlargement (goiter) and an increase in thyroid hormone production with an increased fraction of triiodothyronine (T_3) relative to T_4 (from approximately 20 to up to 30 percent).[7]
- The etiology is seen as a combination of genetic (polygenetic, including human leukocyte antigen-D related [HLA-DR] and cytotoxic (T-lymphocyte antigen 4 [CTLA-4] polymorphisms) and environmental factors, including physical and emotional stress (e.g., infection, childbirth, life events).[4,7] In addition, insulin-like growth factor-1 receptor (IGF-1R)-bearing fibroblasts and B-cells exhibiting the IGF-1R(+) phenotype may be involved in the connective tissue manifestations.[9] Siblings have a higher incidence of both GD and Hashimoto thyroiditis (Chapter 191, Hypothyroidism).
- The ophthalmopathy is believed to result from an autoimmune response directed toward an antigen shared by the thyroid and the eye's orbit. There is infiltration of the extraocular muscles by activated T cells, which release cytokines, activating fibroblasts (fibrosis can lead to diplopia) and increasing the synthesis of glycosaminoglycans (water trapping causes swelling).[7]

RISK FACTORS

- Family history of thyroid disease, especially in maternal relatives.
- Smoking (a strong risk factor for Graves ophthalmopathy).
- Children with McCune-Albright syndrome are at higher risk of hyperthyroidism and nodular goiter.[10]
- Type 1 diabetes mellitus does not appear to confer an increased risk of GD.[3]

DIAGNOSIS

CLINICAL FEATURES

Symptoms depend on the severity of thyrotoxicosis, duration of disease (initial symptoms can be nonspecific), and age. Children with congenital hyperthyroidism may be born prematurely and postnatally can display restlessness, irritability, failure to thrive, and tachycardia; premature craniosynostosis can occur if diagnosis is delayed.[4] Common symptoms of Graves' disease are:[4,7]

- Nervousness.
- Fatigue.
- Weight loss.
- Increased appetite.
- Diarrhea.
- Behavioral changes including poor school performance, insomnia, restlessness and irritability, and nocturia.

Signs of disease include:

- Tachycardia.
- Goiter—Listening over the goiter with a stethoscope may reveal a thyroid bruit (**Figures 192-3 to 192-5**).
- Resting tremor.
- Hyperreflexia
- Skin changes include:
  - Warm, erythematous, moist skin (from increased peripheral circulation).
  - Palmer erythema.
- Eye involvement can occur before hyperthyroidism (in 20% of patients) and gradually progresses with only mild discomfort (a gritty sensation with increased tearing is the earliest manifestation). The eye findings in GD are less severe in children and include:[4,7,11]
  - Lid retraction (drawing back of the eyelid allowing more sclera to be visible; **Figures 192-1** and **192-5**).

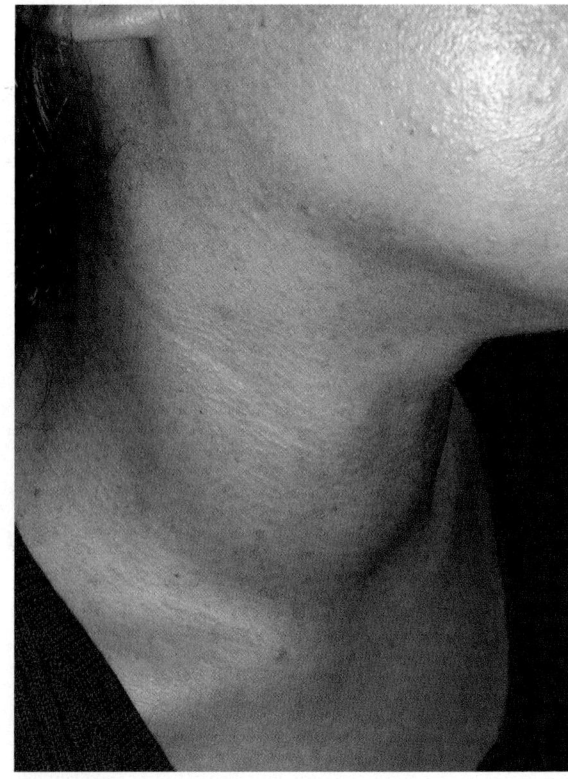

FIGURE 192-3 This young woman has Graves disease and a loud bruit over her enlarged hyperactive thyroid gland. She was thyrotoxic at this time. (*Used with permission from Richard P. Usatine, MD.*)

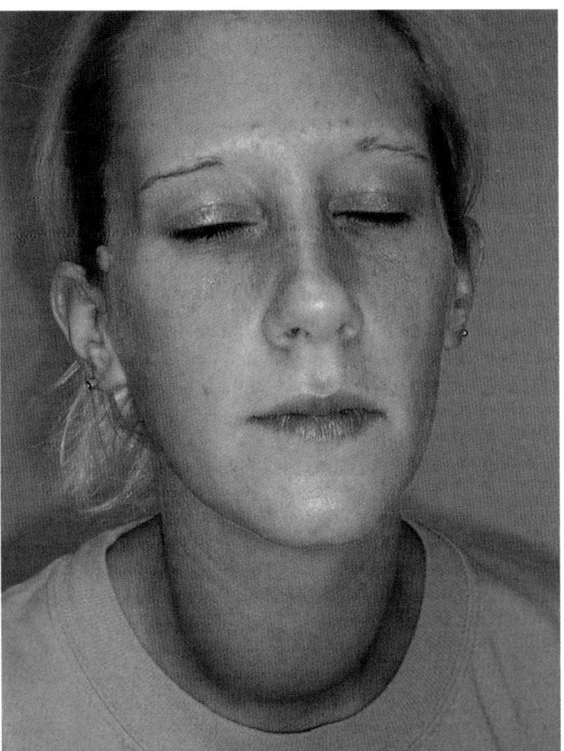

FIGURE 192-4 Flushed skin and temporal wasting in this thyrotoxic young woman with new-onset Graves disease. Her thyroid gland was diffusely enlarged. (*Used with permission from Richard P. Usatine, MD.*)

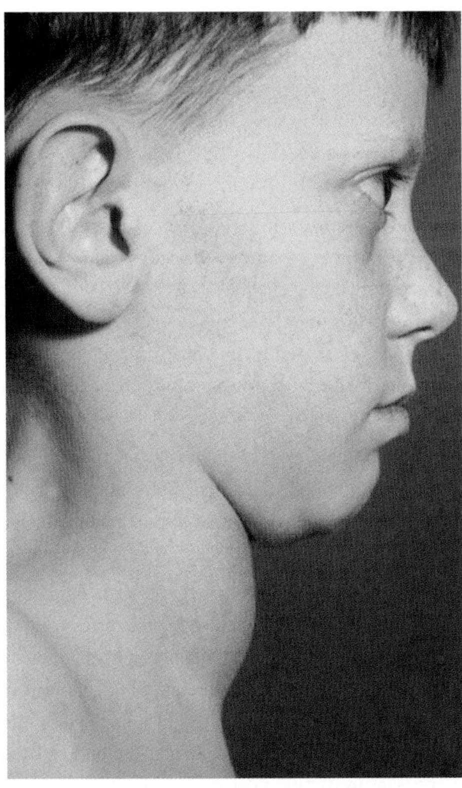

FIGURE 192-5 Graves disease presenting in a young boy with a diffusely enlarged thyroid gland and proptosis (exophthalmos). (*Used with permission from Cleveland Clinic Children's Hospital Photo Files.*)

- Frank proptosis (displacement of the eye in the anterior direction; **Figures 192-1** and **192-5**).
- It is possible to have unilateral or asymmetric eye involvement with Graves ophthalmopathy (**Figure 192-1**).
- Extraocular muscle dysfunction (e.g., diplopia), severe strabismus, and optic neuropathy are rare in children.

LABORATORY TESTING AND IMAGING

- With typical symptoms, you can confirm the diagnosis of GD with a low or undetectable sensitive assay for TSH and an elevated free T_4 level or T_3 level (T3 thyrotoxicosis is more common in children, especially prepubertal children).[4]
- The presence of TSH-receptor antibodies (present in 70% to 100% of adult patients at diagnosis) has a positive and negative likelihood ratio of 247 and 0.01, respectively.[12] TSH-receptor antibodies have been reported to be higher in younger (age 5 years or younger) compared to older children.[13] These antibodies are not usually required for diagnosis.
- For children with suspected congenital hyperthyroidism, one author recommends measurements of iodothyronines and antibodies at birth (in cord blood), after one week when the effects of maternal antithyroid drugs have disappeared, and after 6 to 8 weeks of life because TSH-stimulating immunoglobulins persist.[4]
- A thyroid ultrasound can be obtained to document gland enlargement or to detect nodules in an asymmetric or irregular gland. Consider a RAI scan and uptake if there is thyroid nodularity or if the diagnosis is uncertain in the face of a suppressed TSH to rule out toxic multinodular goiter, thyroiditis, or autonomous functioning nodules.[2,4] Distinguishing between the toxicosis that can occur with Hashimoto thyroiditis and GD can be difficult (see Chapter 191, Hypothyroidism).
- Needle biopsy of an isolated thyroid nodule should be considered as differentiated thyroid cancer can be seen in children and adolescents with GD.[2]

DIFFERENTIAL DIAGNOSIS

Other causes of hyperthyroidism:

- Autonomous functioning nodule—This is an uncommon cause of thyrotoxicosis and most nodules do not cause hyperthyroidism. These present as a discrete swelling in an otherwise normal thyroid gland, and thyroid scan would show a discrete nodule.
- Thyrotropin-secreting pituitary adenoma (rare)—Adenomas can cause visual disturbance (in the absence of exophthalmos), and other hormonal stimulation may occur (e.g., elevated serum prolactin).
- Thyroiditis—May be painless or painful, short duration, low update on RAI scan.
- Exogenous thyroid hormone ingestion—History of overdosage of prescribed or acquired thyroid medication.

The differential diagnoses for the eye findings include the following:

- Metastatic disease to the extraocular muscles.
- Pseudotumor—This condition's rapid onset and pain differentiate it from Graves ophthalmopathy.

MANAGEMENT

- Three options are available to treat the hyperthyroidism: antithyroid drugs (ATD), RAI therapy, and surgery, as discussed in the following section.[4,7]

NONPHARMACOLOGIC

- Supportive measures for eye symptoms include dark glasses, artificial tears, propping up the head and taping the eyelids closed at night.

MEDICATIONS

- Symptoms of hyperthyroidism can be controlled with β-adrenergic blockers (e.g., propranolol, 1 to 2 mg/kg divided twice daily).[2] SOR B
- The antithyroid drug methimazole (0.5 to 1 mg/kg once daily) is considered the first-line agent for children in the US.[1,2,4,7] SOR A Potential side effects include rash, joint pain, liver inflammation, and, rarely, agranulocytosis.[7] Propylthiouracil (PTU; 5 to 10 mg/kg divided every 8 hours) can be considered for children allergic or intolerant to methimazole; however, PTU causes more severe liver injury.[1,14] Baseline liver enzymes and complete blood count (CBC) (including white blood cells [WBCs] and differential) is recommended.[15]
- The ATD dose can be reduced after the patient is euthyroid (typically by one third or one half to maintain a normal serum thyroxine level). Alternatively, the initial dosage can be continued to induce hypothyroidism and initiating L-thyroxine therapy.[4] This approach may reduce frequency of monitoring for development of hypothyroidism.
- PTU is preferred just before and during the first trimester of pregnancy as congenital malformations have been reported approximately three times more often with prenatal exposure to methimazole.[14]
- Pretreatment with methimazole prior to RAI is suggested for patients with GD who are at high risk for complications of extreme hyperthyroidism.[15]
- The optimal duration of titrated antithyroid drug therapy is 12 to 18 months to minimize relapse (see the "Follow-Up" section).[15] SOR A If remission (defined as normal thyroid function off ATDs) is not seen, other treatments are considered.[1]
- In one study, predictors of with higher relapse rates following ATD were non-Caucasian race, young patients, and patients with severe disease at diagnosis (high serum TSH-receptor antibodies and free T_4 levels).[16]
- Children have been reported to have less severe ophthalmopathy than adults, perhaps related to less smoking exposure. Graves' ophthalmopathy can be treated with a course of prednisone (2 to 20 g daily) depending on severity; side effects of prolonged treatment can include weight gain, immune suppression and growth failure.[17] Somatostatin-analogs have been investigated in adults with limited success.

RADIOTHERAPY

- Radioiodine therapy (RAI) is the most commonly prescribed treatment in the US, but is contraindicated in pregnancy or with breastfeeding. A dose of >150 μCi/g of thyroid tissue is recommended by one author for children.[1] Another author recommended doses of between 220 and 275 μCi/g, increased to 300 μCi/g for larger goiters or less elevated radioiodine uptake.[2]
- RAI can also be used after initial treatment with antithyroid drugs; these drugs should be discontinued for 3 to 7 days before treatment.[7]
- The long-term safety of RAI in children is unknown. Because of concerns about subsequent thyroid cancer, treatment is generally avoided in children under age 5 years,[2,4] although several long-term follow-up studies (up to 36 years) did not find adverse effects on fertility, congenital abnormalities or miscarriage, or increased cancer above the general population.[2]
- RAI can cause painful thyroid inflammation for a few weeks in approximately 1 percent of patients; this condition can be treated with nonsteroidal antiinflammatory agents, β-blockers, and possibly steroids.[8]
- In addition, radiation-induced thyroiditis can aggravate ophthalmopathy. This side effect can be minimized by an oral glucocorticoid starting on or 1 day after RAI treatment and tapering over the next 1 to 3 months).[2]

SURGICAL TREATMENT

- Near-total to total thyroidectomy by a high-volume thyroid surgeon is recommended as one treatment option for patients with GD.[15]
- Indications for surgery are very large goiters, presence of suspicious nodules, pregnant women requiring high doses of ATDs, and allergy or failure of other therapies.
- Children who fail an ATD are candidates for surgery if a high volume surgeon practicing in a hospital capable of providing pediatric anesthesia and post-operative care is available.[2] One author prefers surgery over RAI for children under age 10 years, those with severe ophthalmopathy or large thyroids (more than two times normal), adolescents considering pregnancy, and in cases where adherence with RAI and follow-up are questionable.[2]
- In most cases for patients with GD, pretreatment with methimazole until euthyroid is recommended prior to surgery and levothyroxine is started following surgery.[15] A 7- to 10-d course of concentrated iodine solution (three to five drops [50 to 150 mg/dose] three times daily), given the week before surgery can help to decrease thyroid hormone production with the added benefit of decreasing thyroid vascularity.[2]
- Following surgery, small remnants of thyroid tissue (<4 g) result in rates of hypothyroidism of greater than 50 percent; large remnants (>8 g) have higher rates of recurrent hyperthyroidism (15%).
- Complications following surgery, reported for adults, include hypocalcemia (40%), hematoma (2%), recurrent laryngeal nerve injury (2%), and hypoparathyroidism (1%).[1] Complication rates may be higher for young children; Rivkees reported postoperative complication rates for children aged 0 to 6 years of 22 percent using a national database, which was twice the rate for older children.[1] Postoperative rapid PTH testing, drawn at the end of the procedure, is helpful in predicting postoperative hypocalcemia.[2]
- With respect to the eye findings, most symptoms except for proptosis improve with control of the hyperthyroidism.

REFERRAL

- Children who have or are suspected of having hyperthyroidism should be referred to a pediatric endocrinologist for diagnosis and management.
- Patients with significant eye symptoms or clinical findings should be referred to a pediatric ophthalmologist.

PROGNOSIS

- With use of ATDs, symptoms improve in 3 to 4 weeks; weight gain (about 4.5 kg) often occurs as metabolism normalizes.[7] Cortical bone density has also been shown to normalize by 2 years in children rendered euthyroid on ATDs.[18] Remission rates following ATDs vary from 37 to 70 percent and remission usually occurs within 6 to 8 weeks.
- Following RAI, 50 to 75 percent of patients become euthyroid after 5 to 8 weeks, but 50 to 90 percent of patients with GD eventually become hypothyroid (10% to 20% in year 1 and 5% per year afterward).[8] Transient hypocalcemia has been reported following RAI for GD.[19] Retreatment with radioiodine may be needed in 14 percent of patients with GD, 10 to 30 percent of patients with toxic adenoma, and 6 to 18 percent of patients with toxic nodular goiter.[8] In one large Chinese case series (N=1,874 children with GD), the cure rate for RAI was half with an incidence of hypothyroidism of 37.8 percent.[20] The relapse rate was 6.3 percent and adverse effects were reported in less than 2 percent.
- Delayed diagnosis in prepubertal children can lead to increased height, advanced bone age, and lower weight; with appropriate treatment, pubertal progression can be maintained and final predicted height preserved.[2]

FOLLOW-UP

- The goals of therapy are to resolve hyperthyroid symptoms and to restore the euthyroid state. Close follow-up is needed in the initial treatment period; medications for symptoms of hyperthyroidism can be withdrawn slowly following treatment.
- ATD dosages can be reduced after the patient becomes euthyroid, but drugs should be continued for 12 to 18 months to minimize relapse. SOR Ⓐ Follow-up blood tests (T_4 or T_3, because prolonged suppression of TSH is common) are recommended at 4 to 6 weeks after initial treatment and every 2 to 3 months after the appropriate dose is determined.[2] Despite initial remission, relapse rates are high (50% to 70%).[5] Longer duration of treatment reduces relapse rates, but about half of children require additional treatment.[5]
- There is an association between GD, antithyroid medications, and myeloperoxidase-antineutrophil cytoplasmic antibody (MPO-ANCA) vasculitis potentially involving the kidneys, respiratory tract, joints, eyes, gastrointestinal tract, and brain.[2] An MPO-ANCA level can be obtained if this condition is suspected (normal range, <20 EU/mL).
- Following treatment with RAI, most patients eventually become hypothyroid (20% within the first year) and so periodic monitoring of thyroid function is important. Follow-up blood testing within the first 1 to 2 months (free T_4 and T_3) is recommended and then at 4 to 6 weeks if hyperthyroidism continues; consider retreatment with RAI if there is minimal response at 3 months or hyperthyroidism persists at 6 months.[7]
- Following surgery, patients may become hypothyroid or have a recurrence of hyperthyroidism, depending on the size of the remnant remaining; patients should be monitored with periodic blood tests and for symptoms. For those with GD following surgery and levothyroxine, a TSH is recommended at 6 to 8 weeks postoperation.[15] In cases where hyperthyroidism recurs after surgery, RAI is considered as repeat surgery is associated with increased complications.[13]
- An in-office exophthalmometer can be used to track changes in eye prominence over time.
- Patients with GD are at high risk for development of other autoimmune disease; in one cross-sectional study in the United Kingdom of patients attending a thyroid clinic, the frequency of another autoimmune disorder (e.g., rheumatoid arthritis [3.15%], pernicious anemia, systemic lupus erythematosus, Addison disease, celiac disease, and vitiligo) was 9.67 percent in patients with GD.[21]

PATIENT EDUCATION

- Patients should be told that the goals of therapy are to resolve the symptoms of thyroid excess and to restore the thyroid function to normal.
- The treatment choices should be discussed, as each has advantages and disadvantages; treatment should be individualized.
- Regardless of the therapy chosen, long-term follow-up is needed to monitor thyroid status; there is a high risk of becoming hypothyroid in the future or to relapse again into hyperthyroidism. Patients should be made aware of symptoms to watch for and to report any recurrent symptoms.
- Following RAI, patients should avoid intimate contact (including kissing) and contact with other children for 5 days; avoid contact with pregnant women for 10 days (maintain distance of approximately 6 feet); limit close contact with other adults to 2 hours for 5 days; sit while voiding and flush twice with the lid closed; not share toothbrushes, utensils, dishes, towels, or clothes, and wash these separately.[8]
- Ophthalmopathy usually runs its own course independent of the thyroid function. Additional treatment may be needed in consultation with an ophthalmologist.
- Smoking cessation can have a beneficial effect on the course of ophthalmopathy.
- Siblings and children should be made aware of their increased risk of developing thyroid disease or associated disorders and should monitor themselves for symptoms.

PATIENT RESOURCES

- Booklets from the American Thyroid Association—**www.thyroid.org/patients/brochures.html**.
- National Library of Medicine—**www.nlm.nih.gov/medlineplus/thyroiddiseases.html**.
- National Graves' Disease Foundation—**www.ngdf.org**.

PROVIDER RESOURCES

- Bahn RS, Burch HB, Cooper DS, et al. Hyperthyroidism and other causes of thyrotoxicosis: management guidelines of the American Thyroid Association and the American Association of Clinical Endocrinologists. *Thyroid*. 2011;21(6):593-641.
- Bauer AJ. Approach to the pediatric patient with Graves' disease: when is definitive therapy warranted? *J Clin Endocrinol Metab*. 2011;96(3):580-588.

REFERENCES

1. Rivkees SA. Pediatric Graves disease: controversies in management. *Horm Res Paediatr*. 2010;74:305-311.
2. Bauer AJ. Approach to the pediatric patient with Graves' disease: when is definitive therapy warranted? *J Clin Endocrinol Metab*. 2011;96(3):580-588.
3. Lombardo F, Messina MF, Salzano G, et al. Prevalence, presentation and clinical evolution of Graves' disease in children and adolescents with type 1 diabetes mellitus. *Horm Res Pediatr*. 2011; 76(4):221-225.
4. Bettendorf M. Thyroid disorders in children from birth to adolescence. *Eur J Nucl Med*. 2002;29(2):S439-S446.
5. Léger J, Carel JC. Hyperthyroidism in childhood: causes, when and how to treat. *J Clin Res Pediatr Endocrinol*. 2012 Nov 15. [Epub ahead of print]
6. Wasniewska M, Corrias A, Salerno M, et al. Outcomes of children with hashitoxicosis. *Horm Res Paediatr*. 2012;77(1):36-40.
7. Brent GA. Graves' disease. *N Engl J Med*. 2008;358(24):2594-2605.
8. Ross DS. Radioiodine therapy for hyperthyroidism. *N Engl J Med*. 2011;364:542-550.
9. Douglas RS, Naik V, Hwang CJ, et al. B cells from patients with Graves' disease aberrantly express the IGF-1 receptor: implications for disease pathogenesis. *J Immunol*. 2008;181(8):5768-5774.
10. Tessaris D, Corrias A, Matarazzo P, et al. Thyroid abnormalities in children and adolescents with McCune-Albright syndrome. *Horm Res Paediatr*. 2012;78(3):151-157.
11. Gogakos AI, Boboridis K, Krassas GE. Pediatric aspects in Graves' orbitopathy. *Pediatr Endocrinol Rev*. 2010;7(2):234-244.
12. Costagliola S, Marganthaler NG, Hoermann R, et al. Second generation assay for thyrotropin receptor antibodies has superior diagnostic sensitivity for Graves' disease. *J Clin Endocrinol Metab*. 1999;84:90-97.
13. Kaguelidou F, Carel JC, Léger J. Graves' disease in childhood: advances in management with antithyroid drug therapy. *Horm Res*. 2009;71:310-317.
14. Krassas S, Tzotzas T, Krassas GE. Toxicological considerations for antithyroid drugs in children. *Expert Opin Drug Metab Toxicol*. 2011;7(4):399-410.
15. Bahn RS, Burch HB, Cooper DS, et al. Hyperthyroidism and other causes of thyrotoxicosis: management guidelines of the American Thyroid Association and the American Association of Clinical Endocrinologists. *Thyroid*. 2011;21(6):593-641.
16. Kaguelidou F, Alberti C, Castanet M, et al. Predictors of autoimmune hyperthyroidism relapse in children after discontinuation of antithyroid drug treatment. *J Clin Endocrinol Metab*. 2008; 93:3817-3826.
17. Krassas GE, Gogakos A. Thyroid-associated ophthalmopathy in juvenile Graves' disease—clinical, endocrine and therapeutic aspects. *J Pediatr Endpcrinol Metab*. 2006;19(10):1190-1206.
18. Numbenjapon N, Costin G, Pitukcheewanont P. Normalization of cortical bone density in children and adolescents with hyperthyroidism treated with antithyroid medication. *Osteoporos Int*. 2012;23(9):2277-2282.
19. Komarovskiy K, Raghavan S. Hypocalcemia following treatment with radioiodine in a child with Graves' disease. *Thyroid*. 2012; 22(2):218-222.
20. Chao M, Jiawei X, Guoming W, et al. Radioiodine treatment for pediatric hyperthyroid Graves' disease. *Eur J Pediatr*. 2009; 168(10):1165-1169.
21. Boelaert K, Newby PR, Simmonds MJ, et al. Prevalence and relative risk of other autoimmune diseases in subjects with autoimmune thyroid disease. *Am J Med*. 2010;123(2):183.e1-183.e9.

193 HYPERLIPIDEMIA AND XANTHOMAS

Alia Chauhan, MD, FAAP
Mindy A. Smith, MD, MS

PATIENT STORY

A 5-year-old boy is undergoing a complete physical exam prior to starting kindergarten and the pediatrician notes some papules over the right Achilles tendon (**Figure 193-1A**). She also notes rings around the peripheral corneas of both eyes that could be arcus juvenilis (**Figure 193-1B**). The mom noticed the papules near the foot about 2 months ago but had not noticed anything unusual about the eyes. The pediatrician suspects that these findings could be secondary to elevated lipids and discovers that the mother has type 2 diabetes along with high cholesterol. The child is sent for a fasting lipid panel and blood sugar. The results confirm familial hypercholesterolemia (total cholesterol of 810 mg/dL and a low density lipoprotein of 507 mg/dL). The papules over the Achilles tendon are tendinous xanthomas and the eyes do show arcus juvenilis secondary to the elevated lipids. The child is referred to endocrinologist and the mother is told that all the family should be tested and everyone should be eating a low fat diet.

INTRODUCTION

Hyperlipidemia refers to an elevated concentration of one or more of the measured serum lipid components (total cholesterol [TC], low-density lipid [LDL], high-density lipoprotein [HDL], and triglycerides [TGs]). Xanthomas are a skin manifestation of familial or severe secondary hyperlipidemia, although they can occur in patients with normal lipid levels. Hyperlipidemia is a major modifiable risk factor for cardiovascular disease.

EPIDEMIOLOGY

- Among young adults, ages 12 to 19 years, 20.3 percent have abnormal lipids; boys are more likely than girls to have at least 1 lipid abnormality (24.3% versus 15.9%, respectively).[1]
- Patients with homozygous familial hypercholesterolemia (FH) (1 in 1 million persons worldwide) present in childhood with cutaneous xanthomas on the hands, wrists, elbows, knees, heels, or buttocks.[2]
- In one population study, children of parents with coronary artery disease were more likely to be overweight and have dyslipidemia in childhood.[3]
- Large epidemiological studies indicate that children's lipid levels correlate with their adult family members levels.[4]

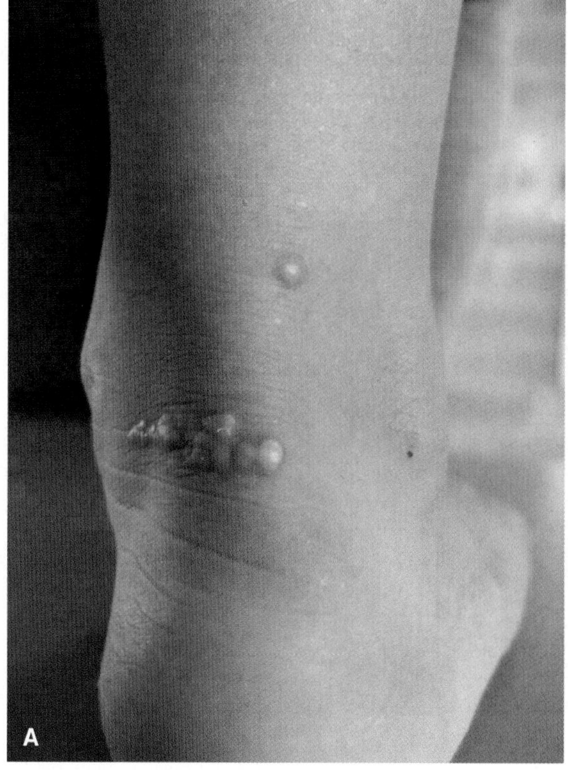

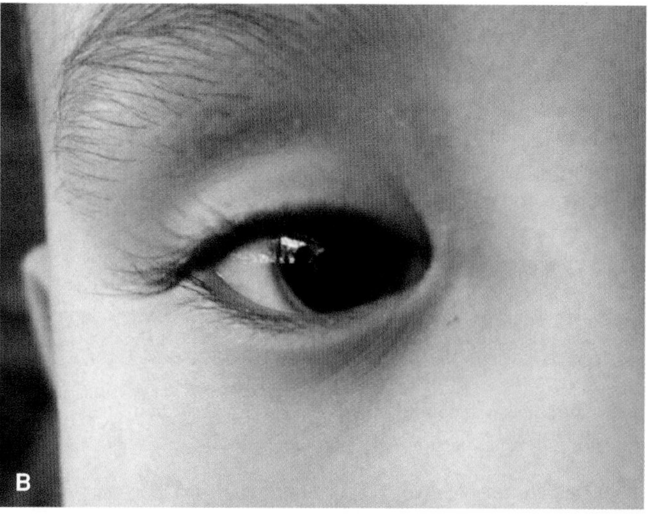

FIGURE 193-1 **A.** Tendinous xanthomas over the Achilles tendon of a 5-year-old boy with familial hypercholesterolemia. **B.** Arcus juvenilis secondary to elevated lipids in the same boy with familial hypercholesterolemia. The white ring is due to lipid infiltration of the corneal stroma and leaves some normal cornea at the limbus. (*Used with permission from John Browning, MD.*)

ETIOLOGY AND PATHOPHYSIOLOGY

- Causes of primary lipid disorders most common seen in children and adolescents are familial combined hyperlipidemia and FH (heterozygous; **Figure 193-1**). Secondary causes include obesity, metabolic syndrome, hypothyroidism, hypopituitarism, diabetes mellitus (type 1 and type 2), polycystic ovary syndrome, juvenile rheumatoid arthritis, chronic renal disease including nephrotic syndrome, Kawasaki disease, and hepatitis.
- Lipoproteins are complexes of lipids and proteins essential for transporting cholesterol, TGs, and fat-soluble vitamins.
- Elevated levels can result from genetically based derangement of lipid metabolism and/or transport or from secondary causes (listed above), cigarette smoking, obesity, or drugs (e.g., corticosteroids, estrogens, retinoids, and high-dose β-blockers).
- Increased circulating LDL becomes incorporation into atherosclerotic plaques. These plaques can grow to block blood supply and oxygen delivery resulting in ischemia to vital organs. In addition, if the plaque ruptures, it can precipitate a clot, causing for example myocardial infarction.
- Elevated TG is an independent risk factor for CHD and increases the risk of hepatomegaly, splenomegaly, hepatic steatosis, and pancreatitis. Contributing factors include obesity, physical inactivity, cigarette smoking, excess alcohol intake, medical diseases (e.g., type 2 DM, chronic renal failure, nephrotic syndrome), drugs (as previously discussed), and genetic disorders (e.g., familial combined hyperlipidemia).[5]
- Autopsy studies show a correlation between lipid levels and arterial fat disposition in young adults and children.[6,7]
- Xanthomas are deposits of lipid in the skin or subcutaneous tissue, usually occurring as a consequence of primary or secondary hyperlipidemia. Xanthomas can also be seen in association with monoclonal gammopathy.[8] There are five basic types of xanthomas:
  - Eruptive xanthomas (also called tuberoeruptive) are the most common form. These appear as crops of yellow or hyperpigmented papules with erythematous halos in white persons (**Figure 193-2**), appearing hyperpigmented in black persons.
  - Tendon xanthomas are frequently seen on the Achilles (**Figure 193-1**) and extensor finger tendons.
  - Plane xanthomas are flat and commonly seen on the palmar creases, face, upper trunk, and on scars.
  - Tuberous xanthomas are found most frequently on the hand or over large joints.
  - Xanthelasma are yellow papules found on the eyelids (**Figure 193-3**). Fifty percent of individuals with xanthelasmas have normal lipid profiles.

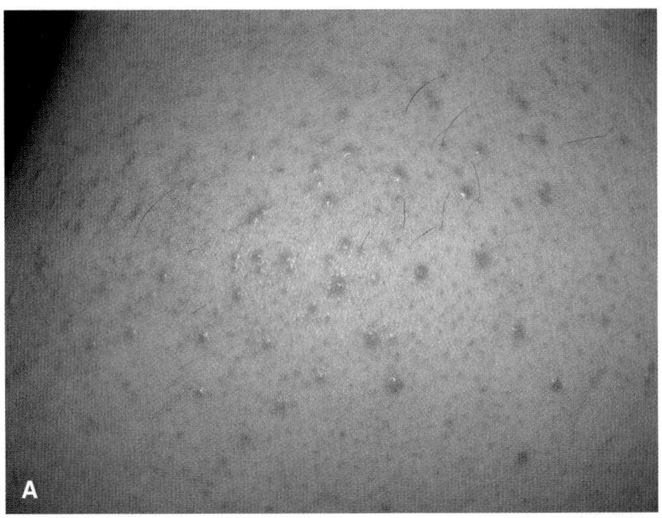

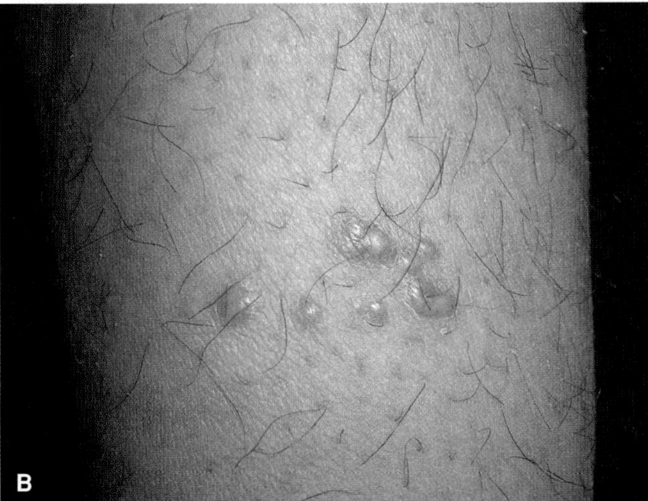

FIGURE 193-2 **A.** Eruptive xanthomas on the back of young man with uncontrolled diabetes (BS = 350) and elevated lipids (triglycerides >9000 mg/dL, total cholesterol >800 mg/dL) **B.** Eruptive xanthomas on the arm of the same patient. (*Used with permission from Richard P. Usatine, MD.*)

RISK FACTORS/CONDITIONS

Risk factors and high-risk conditions to consider for treatment decisions in children with hyperlipidemia include:[9]

- Positive family history of myocardial infarction; angina; coronary artery bypass graft/stent/angioplasty; sudden cardiac death in parent, grandparent, aunt, or uncle (if male at age <55 years and female at age <65 years).

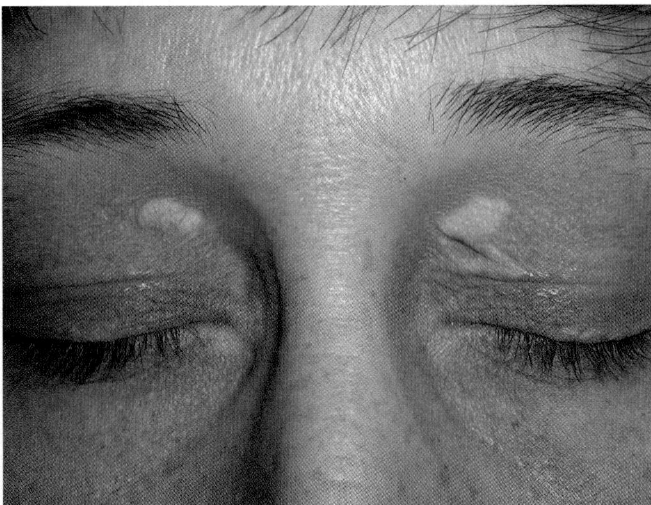

FIGURE 193-3 Xanthelasma around the eyes (xanthoma palpebrarum); most often seen on the medial aspect of the eyelids, with upper lids being more commonly involved than lower lids. This patient has a total cholesterol of over 300 mg/dL. (*Used with permission from Richard P. Usatine, MD.*)

- High-level risk factors including hypertension requiring drug therapy, BMI ≥97th percentile, and current cigarette smoker.
- Moderate level risk factors including hypertension not requiring drug therapy, BMI ≥95th but <97th percentile, and HDL-C <40 mg/dL.
- The presence of high risk conditions including diabetes mellitus, chronic kidney disease/end-stage renal disease/post renal transplant, post orthotopic heart transplant, and Kawasaki disease with current aneurysms.
- The presence of moderate risk conditions including Kawasaki disease with regressed coronary aneurysms, chronic inflammatory disease (e.g., systemic lupus erythematosus, juvenile rheumatoid arthritis), nephrotic syndrome, and human immunodeficiency virus infection.

DIAGNOSIS

CLINICAL FEATURES

- Most patients with hyperlipidemia are asymptomatic.
- A very high TC level (>2000 mg/dL) can result in eruptive xanthomas or lipemia retinalis (white appearance of the retina; also seen with isolated high TG). Very high LDL can lead to the formation of tendinous xanthomas.
- Xanthomas manifest clinically as yellowish papules, nodules, or tumors (**Figure 193-1**).
- Eruptive xanthomas (**Figures 193-4** to **193-5**) begin as clusters of small papules on the elbows, knees, and buttocks that can grow to the size of grapes.

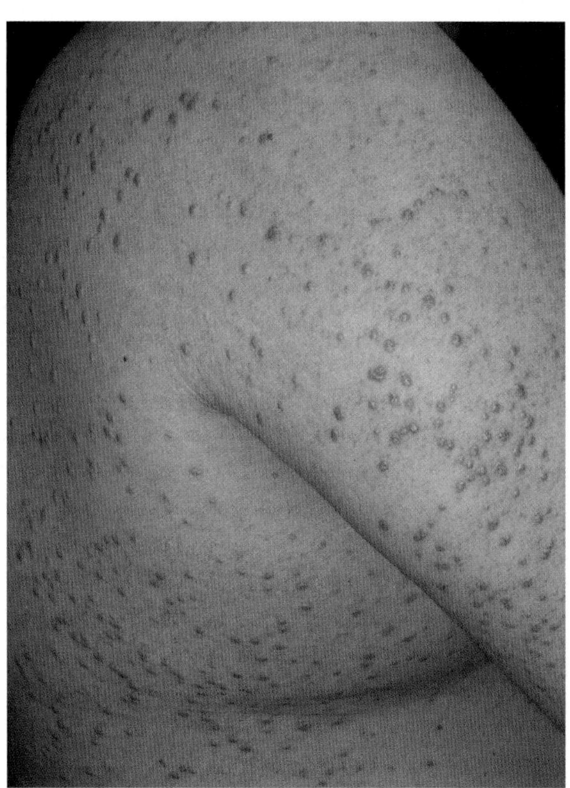

FIGURE 193-4 Eruptive xanthomas on the arm and trunk in an obese patient with untreated hyperlipidemia and diabetes. (*Used with permission from Richard P. Usatine, MD.*)

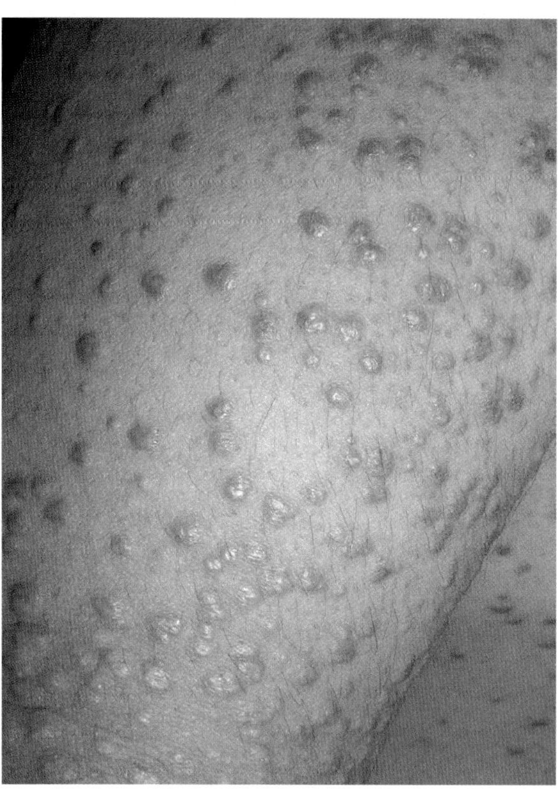

FIGURE 193-5 Close-up of eruptive xanthomas in a patient with untreated hyperlipidemia and diabetes. (*Used with permission from Richard P. Usatine, MD.*)

TYPICAL DISTRIBUTION

Xanthomas are most commonly found in superficial soft tissues, such as skin and subcutis, or on tendon sheaths.

LABORATORY TESTING

- Acceptable, borderline, and high values for plasma lipid and lipoprotein levels based on the National Cholesterol Education Program (NCEP) Expert Panel on Cholesterol Levels in Children are shown in **Table 193-1**.[10] The cut points for high and borderline represent approximately the 95th and 75th percentiles, respectively.[11,12] Low cut points for HDL-C represent approximately the 10th percentile.[13]
- If thyroid dysfunction is suspected, obtain a thyroid-stimulating hormone level to determine whether thyroid dysfunction is contributing to the lipid abnormalities.

BIOPSY

Biopsy is rarely needed and shows collections of lipid-filled macrophages.

DIFFERENTIAL DIAGNOSIS

Other skin papules that can be mistaken for xanthomas include the following:

- Molluscum contagiosum—Caused by a virus; lesions can be papular and widespread but generally have a central depression (see Chapter 115, Molluscum Contagiosum).

TABLE 193-1 Acceptable, Borderline, and High Plasma Lipid, Lipoprotein Concentrations (mg/dL) for Children and Adolescents[1,2,3]

Category	Acceptable	Borderline High	High+
TC	<170	170–199	≥200
LDL-C	<110	110–129	≥130
Non–HDL-C	<120	120–144	≥145
Apo B	<90	90–109	≥110
TG			
0 to 9 years	<75	75–99	≥100
10 to 19 years	<90	90–129	≥130
HDL-C	>45	40–45	<40
ApoA-1	>120	115–120	<115

[1]Values for plasma lipid and lipoproteins levels are from the National Cholesterol Education Program (NCEP) Expert Panel on Cholesterol Levels in Children. Non–HDL-C values from the Bogalusa Heart Study are equivalent to the NCEP Pediatric Panel cut points for LDL-C. Values for plasma ApoB and ApoA-1 are from the National Health and Nutrition Examination Survey III.
[2]Abbreviations: TC, total cholesterol; LDL-C, low density lipid cholesterol; HDL-C, high density lipid cholesterol; TG, triglycerides.
[3]From: Expert Panel on Integrated Guidelines for Cardiovascular Health and Risk Reduction in Children and Adolescents Summary Report. National Heart Lung and Blood Institute. NIH publication No. 12-7486A. October 2012 (reference 33).

- Pseudoxanthoma elasticum—A disorder caused by abnormal deposits of calcium on the elastic fibers of the skin and eye (see Chapter 169, Genodermatoses).

MANAGEMENT

For children with elevated lipids, diet is recommended as first-line treatment. Referral to a pediatric endocrinologist or dietician may be beneficial.

NONPHARMACOLOGIC

- Smoking cessation should be encouraged and attempts actively supported; cessation lowers both cardiovascular risk and lipid levels. SOR Ⓐ
- AAP recommends that all children engage in moderate-to-vigorous physical activity for 1 hour/day and <2 hours/day of sedentary screen time.
- The Expert Panel accepts the 2010 *Dietary Guidelines for Americans* (2010 *DGA*) as appropriate recommendations for diet and nutrition in children 2 years of age and older. Consider referral to a registered dietician.
  - CHILD 1—The Cardiovascular Health Integrated Lifestyle Diet (CHILD 1) is the first stage in dietary change for children with identified dyslipidemia, overweight and obesity, children with a risk factor/ high-risk medical condition, and children with a positive family history of early cardiovascular disease. Dietary components: Primary beverage: fat-free unflavored milk; limit/avoid sugar sweetened beverages, encourage water; fat content: Total fat 25 to 30 percent of daily kcal/EER; saturated fat 8 to 10 percent of daily kcal/EER; avoid trans fat as much as possible; monounsaturated and polyunsaturated fat up to 20 percent of daily kcal/EER; cholesterol <300 mg/d; encourage high dietary fiber intake from foods.
  - CHILD 2-LDL (for high LDL). Dietary Components: 25 to 30 percent of calories from fat, ≤7 percent from saturated fat, 10 percent from monounsaturated fat, <200 mg/day of cholesterol and avoid trans fat as much as possible, plant sterol esters and/or plant stanol esters up to 2 g/day as replacement for usual fat sources can be used after age 2 years in children with FH. Water-soluble fiber psyllium can be added to a low-fat, low saturated fat diet as cereal enriched with psyllium at a dose of 6 g/day for children 2-12 years, and 12 g/day for those ≥12 years.
  - CHILD 2-TG (for high triglycerides [average fasting levels of TG ≥500 mg/dL or any single measurement ≥1,000 mg/dL related to a primary hypertriglyceridemia]). Dietary components: 25 to 30 percent of calories from fat, ≤7 percent from saturated fat, 10 percent from monounsaturated fat; <200 mg/d of cholesterol, avoid trans fat, decrease sugar intake (e.g., no sugar-sweetened beverages), increase dietary fish to increase omega-3 fatty acids. These children should be treated in conjunction with a lipid specialist.
- Elevated TG levels are very responsive to weight loss, diet composition, and exercise. Most importantly, in overweight and obese children and adolescents with elevated TG levels, even small amounts of weight loss are associated with significant decreases in TG levels and increases in HDL-C levels.[14–16]
- Initial treatment of xanthomas should target the underlying hyperlipidemia (when present).

MEDICATIONS

Decisions regarding the need for medication therapy should be based on the average of results from at least two fasting lipid profiles obtained at least 2 weeks but no more than 12 weeks apart. SOR Ⓒ The cut points used to define the level at which drug therapy should be considered come from the 1992 *NCEP Pediatric Guidelines* which have been used as the basis for multiple drug safety and efficacy trials in dyslipidemic children.[10] The goal of LDL-lowering therapy in childhood and adolescence is a LDL-C below the 95th percentile (≤130 mg/dL).

- The following are indications for drug therapy in children with elevated LDL:[10]
  - Children Younger Than Age 10 Years—In this age group, medication should only be used if LDL-C is ≥400 mg/dL (homozygous hypercholesterolemia), TG is ≥500 mg/dL (primary hypertriglyceridemia), or the child has a high-risk condition that is associated with serious medical morbidity. SOR Ⓒ
  - Children 10 to 20 years—Children with an average LDL-C ≥250 mg/dL should be referred to a lipid specialist for treatment. If, after a 6-month trial of lifestyle/diet changes, the LDL-C remains ≥190 mg/dL, statin therapy should be considered.[10] SOR Ⓐ

    - If LDL-C remains between 130 mg/dL and 190 mg/dL in a child with a negative family history of premature CVD in first-degree relatives and no high-level or moderate-level risk factor or risk condition, management should continue to focus on diet changes plus weight management if BMI ≥85th percentile. Treatment with bile acid sequestrants can be considered in consultation with a lipid specialist.[10] SOR B
    - If LDL-C remains between 160 to 189 mg/dL after a trial of lifestyle/diet management in children with a positive family history of premature CVD/events in first-degree relatives or at least one high-level risk factor or risk condition or at least two moderate-level risk factors or risk conditions, statin therapy should be considered.[10] SOR B
    - If LDL-C remains between 130 to 159 mg/dL after a trial of lifestyle/diet management in a child with at least two high-level risk factors or risk conditions or at least one high-level risk factor or risk condition together with at least two moderate-level risk factors or risk conditions, statin therapy should be considered.[10] SOR C
    - For children ages 8 and 9 years with LDL-C persistently ≥190 mg/dL after a trial of lifestyle/diet management together with multiple first-degree family members with premature CVD/events or the presence of at least one high-level risk factor or risk condition or the presence of at least two moderate-level risk factors or risk conditions, statin therapy might be considered.[10] SOR B
- The following are indications for drug therapy in children with elevated triglycerides (TG; average fasting levels of TG ≥ 500 mg/dL or any single measurement ≥1,000 mg/dL related to a primary hypertriglyceridemia) or elevated non-HDL-C:[10]
    - In conjunction with a lipid specialist, the child should be placed on a CHILD 2-TG diet and should consider use of fish oil, fibrate, or niacin to prevent pancreatitis.[10] SOR C
    - Children with fasting levels of TG between 200 to 499 mg/dL after a trial of lifestyle/diet management, should have non-HDL recalculated and be managed to a goal of <145 mg/dL.[10] SOR C
    - Children with fasting levels of TG between 200 to 499 mg/dL, non-HDL >145 mg/dL, after a trial of lifestyle/diet management, consider fish oil supplementation.[10] SOR C
    - Children ≥10 years with non-HDL-C levels ≥145 mg/dL after the LDL-C goal is achieved can be considered for further intensification of statin therapy or additional therapy with a fibrate or niacin, in conjunction with referral to a lipid specialist.[10] SOR C
- Statin therapy is recommended as the initial medication for treating children with elevated LDL-C or non–HDL-C levels as noted above. The efficacy and tolerability of statins has been demonstrated in number of well-designed, short-term trials in children and adolescents.[17–21] In addition to significantly lowering LDL-C levels, statins may increase HDL-C levels and lower TG modestly.
    - Begin the statin with the lowest available dose, given once daily. If LDL-C target levels are not achieved following at least 3 months of adherent use, the dose can be increased by one increment.
    - Adverse effects from statins are uncommon at standard doses but include myopathy and hepatic enzyme elevation. In a meta-analysis of statin use in children, evidence of hepatic enzyme elevation did not differ between the statin and placebo groups.[22] Myopathy (muscle pain and weakness with creatine kinase elevations more than 10 times the upper limits of normal range) typically occurs in less than 1 in 10,000 adult patients. Evidence of muscle toxicity did not differ between the statin and placebo groups in the meta-analysis of statin use in children.[22]
    - Drug interactions with statins occur primarily with drugs that are metabolized by the cytochrome P–450 system. Drugs that potentially interact with statins include fibrates, azole antifungals, macrolide antibiotics, antiarrhythmics, and protease inhibitors.
- Bile acid sequestrants were the first-line medications recommended in the original *NCEP Pediatric Guidelines*. Studies of bile acid sequestrants (cholestyramine, colestipol, or colesevelam) in children and adolescents with FH and hence more extreme elevations of LDL-C levels, show 10 to 20 percent reductions of LDL-C levels and sometimes a modest elevation in TG levels.[23–25]
    - The primary adverse effects of the bile acid sequestrants are gastrointestinal including bloating, nausea, diarrhea, and constipation; these significantly affect adherence.
    - The bile acid-binding sequestrants can be used in combination with a statin for patients who fail to meet LDL-C target levels with either medication alone. One pediatric study that assessed the efficacy of the two agents together found the combination to be additive without increasing adverse effects.[26]

COMPLEMENTARY AND ALTERNATIVE THERAPY

- Consumption of a plant stanol-enriched margarine compared with control margarine as replacement for 20 g/day of dietary fat intake was found to decrease TC and LDL-C levels by 5.4 and 7.5 percent, respectively, in subset of 81 children.[27] There was no effect on HDL-C or TG levels. Safety was judged to be excellent.
- It is not clear whether supplementing with omega-3 fatty acids reduces mortality when combined primary and secondary prevention data are analyzed. A 2006 metaanalysis failed to find a reduction in overall mortality or cardiovascular events in adults.[28]
- In a randomized crossover trial, consuming walnuts (42.5 g walnuts/10.1 mJ) and fatty fish (113 g salmon, twice a week) in a healthy diet significantly lowered serum cholesterol and triglyceride concentrations, respectively.[29] In a metaanalysis, nut consumption (67 g) reduced lipid levels.[30]

SURGICAL PROCEDURES

- Xanthelasma lesions can be treated for cosmetic purposes. Methods of treatment include surgery, electrosurgery, cryotherapy, and laser therapy. SOR C
- When standard therapy fails, LDL apheresis has lowered lipid levels with subsequent regression of tendon xanthomas in patients with FH.[31] SOR C

REFERRAL

- Referral for nutritional counseling should be considered, especially if initial attempts at dietary control fail. Dietary advice has been shown to result in modest improvements in cardiovascular risk factors, such as blood pressure and total and LDL-cholesterol levels.[32] SOR A

PREVENTION AND SCREENING

- Screening recommendations are provided by the Expert Panel on Integrated Guidelines for Cardiovascular Health and Risk

Reduction in Children and Adolescents, updated in 2012 by National Heart Lung Blood Institute.[33]

- Birth to 2 years—No lipid screening. SOR C
- Two to 8 years—No routine lipid screening. SOR B Measure fasting lipid profile twice (as previously discussed for an average level) if the family history is positive for elevated cardiovascular risk or the child has a high level risk factor or condition (see the section "Risk Factors").
- Nine to 11 years—Universal screening with non-fasting lipid profile and calculate non-HDL-C (TC-HDL-C). SOR B If non-HDL-C is ≥145 mg/dL and HDL <40 mg/dL, repeat fasting lipid profile twice as discussed above to obtain average level.
- Twelve to 16 years—No routine screening. SOR B If new knowledge of positive family history, new risk factor or new high risk condition is identified in the patient, obtain fasting lipid panel (twice and average).
- Seventeen years to 21 years—Universal screening once in this time period, obtain non-fasting lipid profile and calculate non–HDL-C; if non–HDL-C ≥145 mg/dL, HDL-C <40 mg/dL, obtain fasting lipid panel (twice and average). SOR B

- Studies are not available to assess the efficacy of screening children and adolescents for dyslipidemia for delaying the onset and reducing the incidence of CHD-related events.

PROGNOSIS

- Based on observational data, each 30 mg/dL increase in LDL increases the relative risk of CHD by 30 percent.
- Use of strategies to lower elevated lipid levels will likely reduce CHD events and possibly overall mortality.
- With medical (diet or drugs) treatment of hyperlipidemia, many xanthomas and about half of xanthelasma resolve or improve with surgical treatment, recurrence is uncommon.[34]

PATIENT EDUCATION

- Patients should be counseled about benefits and risks of screening.
- Lifestyle changes should be stressed as primary prevention for patients with hyperlipidemia. Working with a registered dietician can be helpful. In one study, a pediatric office-based nutritional education program was effective in decreasing total fat, saturated fat, and cholesterol intakes, with significant decreases in TC and LDL-C levels after 16 weeks.[35]
- If persistent elevations in lipids continue despite lifestyle change, those with high level risk factor or CHD should consider medications.
- Patients with hyperlipidemia and/or diabetes should be encouraged to establish and maintain good control of these diseases, as this often results in regression of xanthomas.

PATIENT RESOURCES

For general information, these sites are helpful:

- National Institute of Heart, Lung and Blood—**www.nhlbi.nih.gov/health/public/heart/chol/wyntk.htm**.
- National Library of Medicine—**www.nlm.nih.gov/medlineplus/cholesterol.html**.

PROVIDER RESOURCES

- Expert Panel on Integrated Guidelines for Cardiovascular Health and Risk Reduction in Children and Adolescents Summary Report. National Heart Lung and Blood Institute. NIH publication No. 12-7486A. October 2012, **http://www.nhlbi.nih.gov/guidelines/cvd_ped/peds_guidelines_sum.pdf**. Also available at: **http://www.nhlbi.nih.gov/guidelines/cvd_ped/index.htm**.
- NCEP Expert Panel of Blood Cholesterol Levels in Children and Adolescents. National Cholesterol Education Program (NCEP): Highlights of the report of the Expert Panel on Blood Cholesterol Levels in Children and Adolescents. *Pediatrics*. 1992;89:495-501. Updated and available online at: **http://www.nhlbi.nih.gov/guidelines/cvd_ped/chapter9.htm**.

REFERENCES

1. Prevalence of abnormal lipid levels among youths—United States, 1999-2006. *MMWR Morb Mortal Wkly Rep*. 2010; 59(02):29-33, http://www.cdc.gov/mmwr/preview/mmwrhtml/mm5902a1.htm, accessed April 2013.
2. Rader DJ, Hobbs HH. Disorders of lipoprotein metabolism. In: Kasper DL, Braunwald E, Fauci AS, Hauser SL, Longo DL, Jameson JL, eds. *Harrison's Principles of Internal Medicine*. New York, NY: McGraw-Hill; 2005:2286-2298.
3. Bao W, Srinivasan SR, Valdez R, et al. Longitudinal changes in cardiovascular risk from childhood to young adulthood in off spring of parents with coronary artery disease: Bogalusa Heart Study. *JAMA*. 1997;278 (21):1749-1754.
4. Schrott HG, Bucher KA, Clark WR, Lauer RM. The Muscatine hyperlipidemia family study program. *Prog Clin Biol Res*. 1979;32: 619-646.
5. Third report of the National Cholesterol Education Program (NCEP) Expert Panel on Detection, Evaluation, and Treatment of High Blood Cholesterol in Adults. (Adult Treatment Panel III), Executive Summary. (NCEP/NHLBI., 2004-07-13). http://www.nhlbi.nih.gov/guidelines/cholesterol/index.htm, accessed April 2013.
6. Kwiterovich PO Jr. Prevention of coronary disease starting in childhood: what risk factors should be identified and treated? *Coron Artery Dis*. 1993;4(7):611-630.
7. Pathological Determinants of Atherosclerosis in Youth (PDAY) Research Group. Relationship of atherosclerosis [in young men] to serum lipoprotein cholesterol concentrations and smoking. *JAMA*. 1990;264:3018-3024.
8. Szalat R, Arnulf B, Karlin L, et al. Pathogenesis and treatment of xanthomatosis associated with monoclonal gammopathy. *Blood*. 2011;118(14):3777-3784.
9. Kavey RE, Allada V, Daniels SR, et al. American Heart Association Expert Panel on Population and Prevention Science; American Heart Association Council on Cardiovascular Disease in the Young; American Heart Association Council on Epidemiology and Prevention; American Heart Association Council on Nutrition, Physical Activity and Metabolism; American Heart Association

Council on High Blood Pressure Research; American Heart Association Council on Cardiovascular Nursing; American Heart Association Council on the Kidney in Heart Disease; Interdisciplinary Working Group on Quality of Care and Outcomes Research. Cardiovascular risk reduction in high-risk pediatric patients: a scientific statement from the American Heart Association Expert Panel on Population and Prevention Science; the Councils on Cardiovascular Disease in the Young, Epidemiology and Prevention, Nutrition, Physical Activity and Metabolism, High Blood Pressure Research, Cardiovascular Nursing, and the Kidney in Heart Disease; and the Interdisciplinary Working Group on Quality of Care and Outcomes Research: endorsed by the American Academy of Pediatrics. *Circulation.* 2006;114(24):2710-2738.

10. NCEP Expert Panel of Blood Cholesterol Levels in Children and Adolescents. National Cholesterol Education Program (NCEP): Highlights of the report of the Expert Panel on Blood Cholesterol Levels in Children and Adolescents. *Pediatrics.* 1992;89:495-501.
11. Bachorik PS, Lovejoy KL, Carroll MD, Johnson CL. Apolipoprotein B and AI distributions in the United States, 1988-1991: results of the National Health and Nutrition Examination Survey III (NHANES III). *Clin Chem.* 1997;43(12):2364-2378.
12. Srinivasan SR, Myers L, Berenson GS. Distribution and correlates of non-high-density lipoprotein cholesterol in children: the Bogalusa Heart Study. *Pediatrics.* 2002;110(3):e29.
13. Bachorik PS, Lovejoy KL, Carroll MD, Johnson CL. Apolipoprotein B and AI distributions in the United States, 1988-1991: results of the National Health and Nutrition Examination Survey III (NHANES III). *Clin Chem.* 1997;43(12):2364-2378.
14. Epstein LH, Kuller LH, Wing RR, et al. The effect of weight control on lipid changes in obese children. *Am J Dis Child.* 1989; 143(4):454-457.
15. Nemet D, Barkan S, Epstein Y, et al. Short- and long-term beneficial effects of a combined dietary-behavioral-physical activity intervention for the treatment of childhood obesity. *Pediatrics.* 2005;115(4):e443-e449.
16. Becque MD, Katch VL, Rocchini AP, et al. Coronary risk incidence of obese adolescents: reduction by exercise plus diet intervention. *Pediatrics.* 1988;81(5):605-612.
17. Wiegman A, Hutten BA, de Groot E, et al. Efficacy and safety of statin therapy in children with familial hypercholesterolemia: a randomized controlled trial. *JAMA.* 2004;292(3):331-337.
18. van der Graaf A, Nierman MC, Firth JC, et al. Efficacy and safety of fluvastatin in children and adolescents with heterozygous familial hypercholesterolemia. *Acta Paediatrica.* 2006;95:1461-1466.
19. Clauss SB, Holmes KW, Hopkins P, et al. Efficacy and safety of lovastatin therapy in adolescent girls with heterozygous familial hypercholesterolemia. *Pediatrics.* 2005;116(3):682-688.
20. de Jongh S, Ose L, Szamosi T, et al. Simvastatin in Children Study Group. Efficacy and safety of statin therapy in children with familial hypercholesterolemia: a randomized, double-blind, placebo-controlled trial with simvastatin. *Circulation.* 2002;106(17):2231-2237.
21. Avis HJ, Hutten BA, Gagne C, et al. Efficacy and safety of rosuvastatin therapy for children with familial hypercholesterolemia. *J Am Coll Cardiol.* 2010;55:1121-1126.
22. Avis HJ, Vissers MN, Stein EA, et al. A systematic review and meta-analysis of statin therapy in children with familial hypercholesterolemia. *Arterioscle Thromb Vasc Biol.* 2007;27:1803-1810.
23. Tonstad S, Knudtzon J, Sivertsen M, Refsum H, Ose L. Efficacy and safety of cholestyramine therapy in peripubertal and prepubertal children with familial hypercholesterolemia. *J Pediatr.* 1996;129(1):42-49.
24. Tonstad S, Sivertsen M, Aksnes L, Ose L. Low dose colestipol in adolescents with familial hypercholesterolaemia. *Arch Dis Child.* 1996;74(2):157-160.
25. Stein EA, Marais AD, Szamosi T, et al. Colesevelam hydrochloride: efficacy and safety in pediatric subjects with heterozygous familial hypercholesterolemia. *J Pediatr.* 2010;156(2):231-236.
26. McCrindle BW, Helden E, Cullen-Dean G, Conner WT. A randomized crossover trial of combination pharmacologic therapy in children with familial hyperlipidemia. *Pediatr Res.* 2002;51(6): 715-721.
27. Tammi A, Rönnemaa T, Gylling H, et al. Plant stanol ester margarine lowers serum total and low-density lipoprotein cholesterol concentrations of healthy children: the STRIP project. Special Turku Coronary Risk Factors Intervention Project. *J Pediatr.* 2000;136(4):503-510.
28. Hooper L, Thompson RL, Harrison RA, et al. Risks and benefits of omega 3 fats for mortality, cardiovascular disease, and cancer: systematic review. *BMJ.* 2006;332:752-760.
29. Rajaram S, Haddad EH, Mejia A, Sabaté J. Walnuts and fatty fish influence different serum lipid fractions in normal to mildly hyperlipidemic individuals: a randomized controlled study. *Am J Clin Nutr.* 2009;89(5):1657S-1663S.
30. Sabaté J, Oda K, Ros E. Nut consumption and blood lipid levels: a pooled analysis of 25 intervention trials. *Arch Intern Med.* 2010; 170(9):821-827.
31. Scheel AK, Schettler V, Koziolek M, et al. Impact of chronic LDL apheresis treatment on Achilles tendon affection in patients with severe familial hypercholesterolemia: a clinical and ultrasonographic 3-year follow-up study. *Atherosclerosis.* 2004;174(1): 133-139.
32. Brunner E, Rees K, Ward K, Burke M, Thorogood M. Dietary advice for reducing cardiovascular risk. *Cochrane Database Syst Rev.* 2007;(4):CD002128.
33. Expert Panel on Integrated Guidelines for Cardiovascular Health and Risk Reduction in Children and Adolescents Summary Report. National Heart Lung and Blood Institute. NIH publication No. 12-7486A. October 2012, http://www.nhlbi.nih.gov/guidelines/cvd_ped/peds_guidelines_sum.pdf, accessed April 2013.
34. Fair KP. Xanthoma treatment and management. In: emedicine. Medscape. http://emedicine.medscape.com/article/1103971-treatment#a1128, accessed April 2013.34
35. Kuehl KS, Cockerham JT, Hitchings M, et al. Effective control of hypercholesterolemia in children with dietary interventions based in pediatric practice. *Prev Med.* 1993;22(2):154-166.

194 OBESITY

Stacy McConkey, MD, FAAP
Angela M. Fals, MD, FAAP

PATIENT STORY

A 13-year-old Hispanic female is brought to her pediatrician with various concerns, including that her neck always appearing dirty no matter how much she washes and scrubs it. The pediatrician notes that the child has acanthosis nigricans of the neck and axillae along with obesity (**Figure 194-1**). The mother is obese and admits to having type 2 diabetes. A diet history reveals that the mother cooks traditional Mexican cuisine and the daughter is very fond of tortillas. She also loves to eat pizza, french fries, and other fast food. The girl is a good student but does not like to exercise or play sports. The pediatrician is concerned that the girl may have insulin resistance or type 2 diabetes so she plans to send the patient for screening labs including hemoglobin A1c and fasting blood sugar. She also recommends a healthier diet with less calories and increased physical activity. A referral to a nutritionist is offered.

INTRODUCTION

Obesity in children is defined as a BMI greater than or equal to the age- and sex-specific 95th percentiles of the 2000 Centers for Disease Control (CDC) growth charts; a child is considered overweight at the 85th to 95th percentile.

EPIDEMIOLOGY

- Based on the National Health and Nutrition Examination Surveys (NHNS), 12.5 million children and adolescents (16.9%) are obese.[1] Slightly more boys (19.3%) were obese than girls (16.8%) of all included ages in the study. Since 1980, the prevalence of obesity in children has tripled.[1]

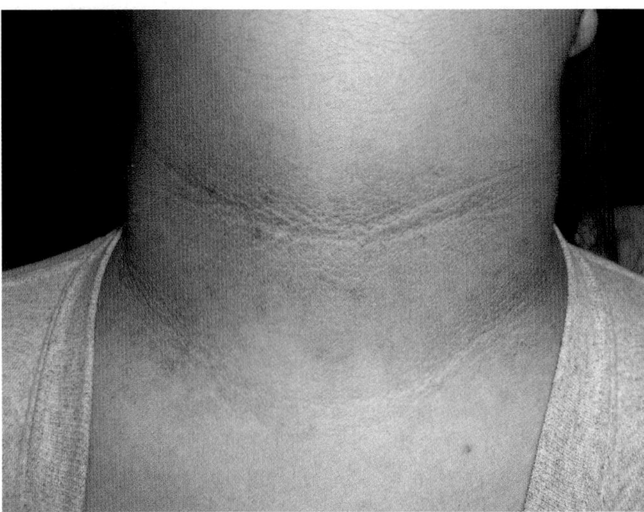

FIGURE 194-1 Acanthosis nigricans of the neck in a 13-year-old obese girl with a family history of obesity and type 2 diabetes. She eats a high-calorie high fat diet and gets little physical activity. (*Used with permission from Richard P. Usatine, MD.*)

- The direct medical care costs (prescriptions, outpatient visits, and ER visits) for children aged 6 to 19 years for complications of obesity are 14.1 billion dollars annually.[2]
- There is an overrepresentation of low-income children in the numbers of obese children, with 1 in 7 lowincome preschool children being obese.[3,4] The National Longitudinal Study of Adolescent Health showed that being obese (BMI > 95%) is highly associated with lower household income.[4]
- Race and ethnicity are also associated with obesity, with high rates present in American Indian/Eskimo children.[3] In the NHNS study (2007 to 2008), Hispanic boys, aged 2 to 19 years, were significantly more likely to be obese than non-Hispanic white males and non-Hispanic black girls aged 2 to 19 years were significantly more likely to be obese than non-Hispanic white girls.[5]
- Interestingly, the effect of ethnicity appears to be mediated by income; Caucasian teenage girls from the lowest income quintile had relative risks for obesity of 2.72 compared to teens in the highest quintile.[4]

ETIOLOGY AND PATHOPHYSIOLOGY

Obesity is a complex problem involving genetics, health behaviors (e.g., diet or exercise), environment, culture, and sometimes medical diseases (see differential diagnosis) or drugs (e.g., steroids or antidepressants). The simplest explanation of obesity is an imbalance between intake (calories eaten) and output (physical activity).

- Genetics—Studies on twins, nontwin siblings, and adopted siblings show that the genetic component of obesity is somewhere between 40 to 70 percent. Researchers using Genome Wide Association Studies have identified 42 different genes likely associated with obesity.[6] Most of these genes only make a small contribution to the overall elevation of BMI (around 0.17 kg/m^2). The cumulative risk for developing obesity not only relies on the individuals genotype, but also on the environment and a wide variety of other factors.[6]
- Diet—Many low-income families live in neighborhoods lacking supermarkets with fresh produce or healthy choices. Calorie dense "junk food" or fast food is more readily available and less expensive than healthier options. Daycares and schools are not regulated or monitored on their ability to provide healthy options for children. Exposure to sugary drinks and snack foods in school vending machines may lead to increased consumption of calorie dense foods.[7] In addition, portion size is commonly much larger than what typical serving sizes for children should be. This leads to overeating and the expectation for increased food consumption at meals and snacks.
- Television viewing—Sedentary TV viewing displaces physical play and exercise, and exposes children to targeted advertising.[8] Authors of a recent study of 1,638 hours of television found 9000 food ads of which only 165 promoted fitness and good nutrition.[9] TV viewing may lead to an increase in snacking behavior and interfere with normal sleep patterns; hours of TV watching predicts

higher BMI in adulthood.[8] In addition, having a bedroom TV set is an independent risk factor for obesity.[8]

- Physical activity—School programs have limited the amount of time devoted to exercise, which falls well below the recommended 60 minutes per day for a child. Access to safe and appealing play areas, parks, and recreation facilities may be limited, especially in urban and rural areas.

RISK FACTORS

- Family history of obesity—In a retrospective cohort study of 854 children, children aged 1 to 2 year olds with non-obese parents had an 8 percent chance of being obese adults while children aged 10 to 14 years with one obese parent had a 79 percent chance of being obese as adults.[10]
- Diet—High calorie, low in fruits and vegetables, high number of snack foods, and fast food consumption.
- Low levels of physical activity.
- Mother with gestational diabetes.
- Small-for-gestational-age at birth.
- Stressors—Investigators in the Fragile Families and Child Well Being Study found that cumulative social stressors between the ages of 1 to 3 years were associated with increased odds of early onset obesity among girls.[11] The greater the number of stressors at one time predicted a greater risk for obesity at the age of 5 years.

DIAGNOSIS

- Body mass index (BMI) is calculated by taking the child's weight in kilograms divided by the standing height in m^2. That number is highly variable over the child's growing years, and should be charted on the 2000 CDC growth chart for BMI to determine if the child is normal (<85th percentile), overweight (85 to 94th percentile), or obese (>95th percentile). As the child's age gets closer to 19 years, the adult definition for obesity of 30 kg/m^2 can be utilized. The 2007 expert committee of the American Academy of Pediatrics (AAP) on Child and Adolescent Obesity proposed a new category of severe obesity, defined as BMI of 30 to 32 kg/m^2 for 10 to 12 year olds and >34 kg/m^2 for 14 to 16 year olds.[12]
- Children grow very rapidly in the first 24 months and standards for BMI are not available for children <2 years of age. The BMI as a percentage usually peaks in the first 8 months and then falls to a nadir at around age 6 years. By around 8 years of age, most children are at the percentile that they will follow into adolescence. In general, the earlier a child reaches their nadir, the more likely the child will have an elevated BMI later.
- In adults, increased waist circumference (WC) confers additional morbidity risk for those who have elevated weight. For children, WC and skin fold measurement are not valid indicators of risk or predictors for obesity and are not followed routinely.

CLINICAL FEATURES

- Obese children (**Figure 194-1**) are more likely to have hypertension (2.9 times higher), high cholesterol (2.1 times higher), insulin resistance, and type 2 diabetes mellitus (2.9 times higher).
- Obese children have a higher incidence of increased severity asthma and may suffer from sleep apnea.
- There is an increased prevalence of non-alcoholic fatty liver disease (NAFLD) and gastro esophageal reflux among obese children.
- Acanthosis nigricans is a skin condition that is commonly present in obese children (**Figures 194-1** and **194-2**; see Chapter 190, Acanthosis Nigricans).
- Obese children can also develop striae (**Figure 194-3**).

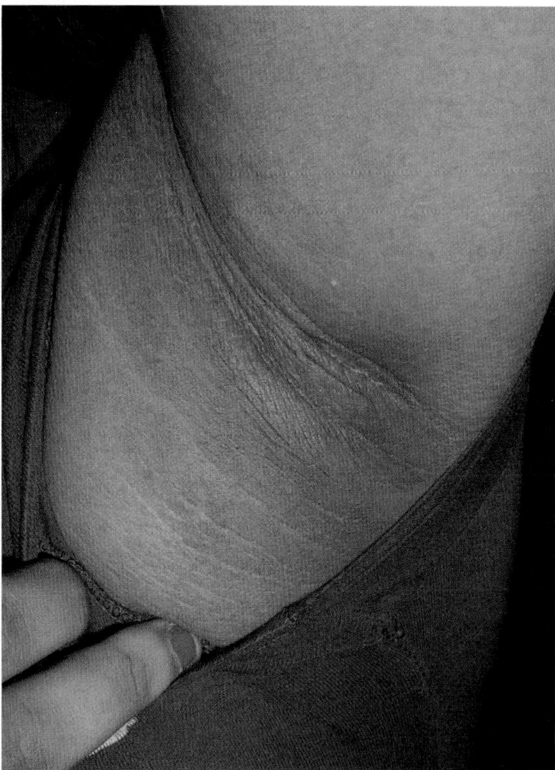

FIGURE 194-2 Acanthosis nigricans in the axilla of on obese Hispanic teenage girl. (*Used with permission from Richard P. Usatine, MD.*)

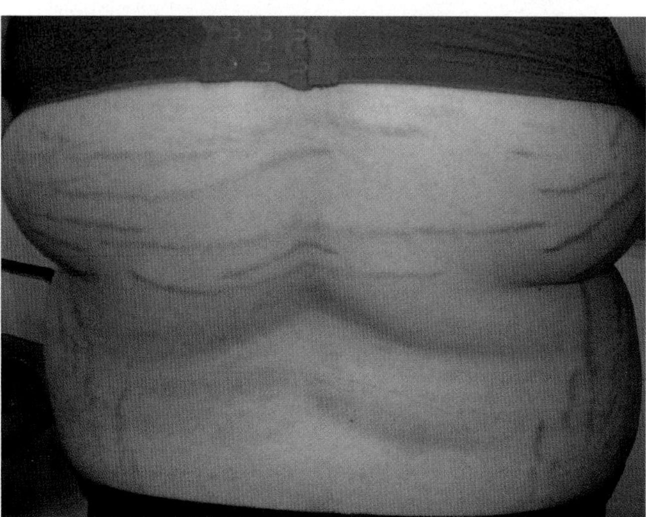

FIGURE 194-3 Striae caused by obesity in this growing teenager. (*Used with permission from Richard P. Usatine, MD.*)

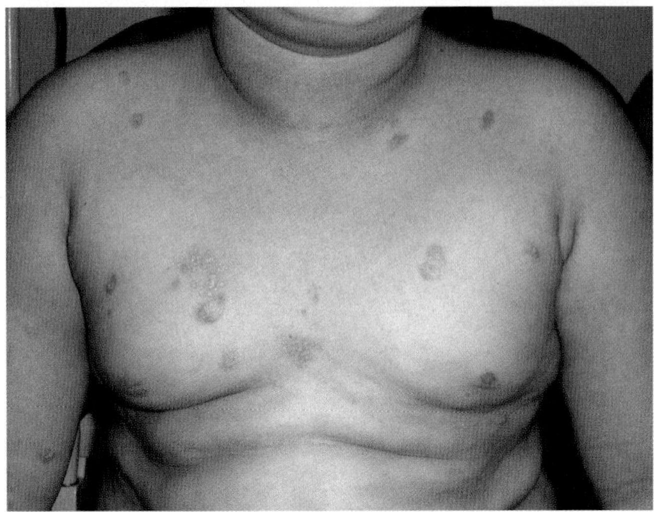

FIGURE 194-4 Pseudogynecomastia in an obese boy who also has guttate psoriasis. (*Used with permission from Richard P. Usatine, MD.*)

- Obese boys are more likely to have pseudogynecomastia (**Figures 194-4** and **194-5**). This appears similar to gynecomastia but this is not real breast development just increased adipose tissue.
- Slipped capital femoral epiphysis, joint problems, and muscle strain/pain often limit obese children's ability to exercise.
- It is common for obese children to experience depression, low self-esteem, discrimination, and bullying.

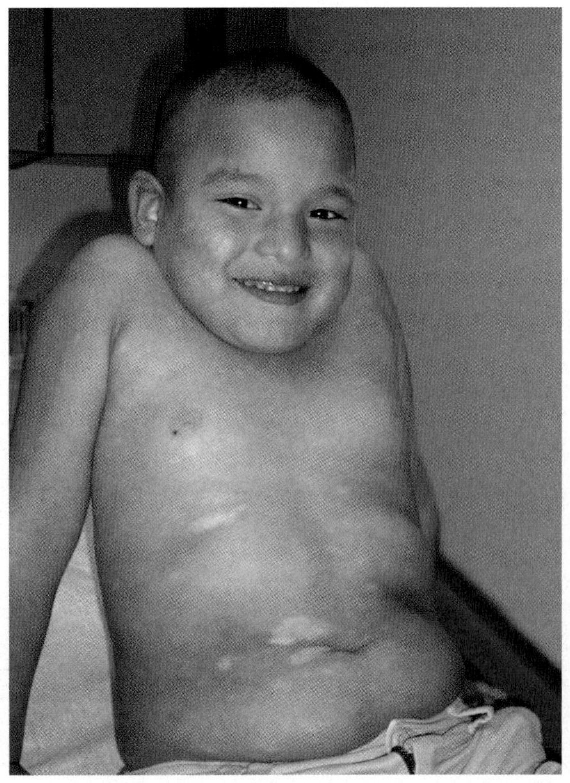

FIGURE 194-5 Pseudogynecomastia in this obese boy with pityriasis alba. (*Used with permission from Richard P. Usatine, MD.*)

LABORATORY TESTING

- Laboratory testing is performed to diagnose complications of obesity and recommendations are based on BMI percentile.[12]
- For children between the 5th and 84th percentile, no laboratory testing is recommended.
- For those in the 85th to 94th percentile who are ≥age 10 years and have other risk factors and children with a BMI >95th percentile, biannual fasting glucose, AST, and ALT levels are recommended. Fasting lipids should be checked on all children >10 years of age with a BMI >85 percent (baseline and every 2 years if BMI remains >85%).

DIFFERENTIAL DIAGNOSIS

The differential diagnosis of a patient with obesity includes the following medical conditions:

- Hypothyroidism—Uncommon and typically these children's growth has slowed or stopped; laboratory testing (thyroid stimulating hormone and free thyroxine) confirms the diagnosis (see Chapter 191, Hypothyroidism).
- Cushing syndrome—Uncommon in children; caused by prolonged exposure to endogenous or exogenous glucocorticoids. Findings include truncal obesity, purple striae, and linear growth cessation. Diagnosis is confirmed with inappropriately high serum or urine cortisol levels (see Chapter 195, Cushing Disease).
- Polycystic ovary syndrome—Criteria include 2 of 3 of oligo-ovulation or anovulation, hyperandrogenism, and polycystic ovaries.
- Genetic syndromes include Prader Willi, Lawrence-Moon-Bardet-Biedel syndrome, Albright Hereditary Osteodystrophy, Carpenter syndrome, Cohen syndrome; these obesity syndromes in children are frequently associated with developmental delay. Beckwith Wiedemann syndrome is associated with fasting hypoglycemia and Alstrom syndrome with blindness and deafness. If any of these syndromes are suspected, consult a geneticist.
- Medications—Antidepressants, antipsychotic medications, mood stabilizers, and glucocorticoids can cause weight gain.

MANAGEMENT

- The primary goal of obesity treatment in children and adolescents is improvement of long-term physical and mental health through permanent lifestyle and habit changes leading to and maintaining a healthy weight and BMI for life. Depending on age and starting BMI values, this may be accomplished through either gradual, steady weight loss or decreased weight velocity and maintenance of BMI as the child grows taller. Reduced BMI can improve conditions such as hypertension, diabetes, steatohepatitis, and metabolic syndrome.
- Currently, there are effective behavioral, pharmaceutical, and surgical methods for treatment. AAP identifies four stages for treatment of childhood obesity in children ages 2 to 19 years.[12] The first three involve nonpharmacologic approaches. Additional nutritional and activity recommendations by age group are displayed in

TABLE 194-1 Nutritional and Activity Recommendations by Age Group[1]

Age Group	Nutrition	Activity
Infants	Breastfeeding reduces the incidence of obesity and should be encouraged from birth through 6 months of age; ideally, continued through 1 year of life. Mothers should lead by example and model healthy eating habits to maximize her child's health.	N/A
Toddlers and preschool-aged children	Introduce a variety of foods and textures early in life (especially fruits and vegetables) as food preferences develop early. Allowing the child to stop eating when full, teach them to listen to their internal "hunger cues" to determine level of satiation as a means of portion-control.	Promote routines of eating more than 5 nights per week together as a family, obtaining at least 10.5 hours of sleep per night, and limiting screen time to less than 2 hours per day decreases obesity prevalence.
Older children	Children are encouraged to eat a balanced diet with emphasizing appropriate portions of fruits, vegetables, whole grains, low-fat dairy, and lean protein; Choose My Plate is a model that can be used to understand portion sizes.	Fun and engaging play is most effective for promoting exercise in children. Sleep 9 hours nightly and avoid disruption of the normal sleep cycle with overly busy schedules, eating prior to bedtime, and the use of electronics.

[1]Data from Information from American Academy of Pediatrics: The first year in A Parent's Guide to Childhood Obesity: A Roadmap to Health, edited by SG Hassink, USA, American Academy of Pediatrics, 2006 p.141; Hassink SG: Toddler in Pediatric Obesity—Prevention, Intervention, and Treatment Strategies for Primary Care. USA, American Academy of Pediatrics, 2007 p.53; Jakicic JM, Clark K, Coleman E, et al. American College of Sports Medicine position stand: appropriate intervention strategies for weight loss and prevention of weight regain for adults. *Med Sci Sports Exerc.* 2001;33(12):2145-2156; Anderson SE, Whitaker RC. Household routines and obesity in US preschool-aged children. *Pediatrics.* 2010;125(3):420-428.

Table 194-1. Tools available to assist primary-care providers in screening and basic strategies for addressing health and wellness are provided in the AAP guidelines.[12]

NONPHARMACOLOGIC

Stage 1—Prevention Plus-Primary Care Office. Initial management for obese children can be undertaken in the office setting by any appropriately-trained provider or clinical staff. It is important to involve the entire family in making permanent lifestyle changes. Changes may need to be slow and in a stepwise fashion, and should be tailored to family behaviors, cultural values, norms, and usual foods.

- Nutrition—Limit or eliminate consumption of sugar-sweetened beverages; encourage 5 to 9 daily servings of fruits and vegetables; provide a healthy daily breakfast; limit eating out (especially fast food), engage in meal planning and preparation at home; provide family meals 5 to 6 times weekly; allow the child to self-regulate meals, and avoid restrictive feeding behaviors.
- Activity—Moderate to vigorous physical activity for at least 60 minutes daily; 2 hour daily limit on TV/screen time (no TV for children <2 years); and removal of TVs and other screens from child's sleeping area. Regular exercise incorporated into the daily schedule is very important in long-term weight maintenance and helps avoid weight regain.[13,22]
- If no progress has been made after 3 to 6 months of attempted Stage 1 interventions, consider moving to Stage 2.

Stage 2—Structured Weight Management, Primary Care Office with Support. This stage combines Stage 1 recommendations for nutrition and activity education with added family support and accountability.

- Offer monthly visits and include other professionals as indicated: a dietician, staff trained in motivational interviewing for follow up care, a counselor, and/or physical therapist. Group sessions can be considered.
- Nutrition—In additional to Stage 1 nutritional recommendations, incorporate a daily eating plan with balanced macronutrients (fats, carbohydrates, and protein), planned snacks, and age-appropriate portions. In 2011, the well-known food pyramid was replaced by the US Department of Agriculture (USDA) with *Choose My Plate* as a way to simplify and facilitate healthy eating to the public.[14] The "plate" emphasizes appropriate portions for fruits, vegetables, whole grains, low-fat dairy, and lean protein.
- Activity—Moderate to vigorous physical activity for at least 60 minutes per day and limitation of TV and other screen time to <1 hour per day. Frequent self-monitoring of nutrition and activity behaviors such as through use of a journal is an effective means of regulating behavior change;[15] planned reinforcement is important for achieving goals and continued motivation.

- If no progress has been made after 3 to 6 months of attempted Stage 2 interventions, consider moving to Stage 3.

Stage 3—Comprehensive Multidisciplinary Team, Pediatric Weight Management Center. Continue Stage 1 and 2 recommendations for nutrition and activity education at a pediatric weight management center run by a trained multidisciplinary team. The team includes a physician, behavioral counselor, registered dietician, and exercise specialist. Implement a structured program with features of behavior modification, monitoring of nutrition and activity behaviors, short-term diet (if indicated), regular (weekly or monthly) visits, and goal setting. Systematic evaluation of body measurements should be performed at baseline and specified intervals.

- Nutrition—The recommended rate of weight loss for children ages 2 to 5 years is <1 pound per month and for children >5 years old, about 1 to 2 pounds per week. The US Preventive Services Task Force (USPSTF) recommends that clinicians screen children aged 6 years and older for obesity and offer them or refer them to comprehensive, intensive behavioral interventions to promote improvement in weight status.[16] This recommendation is based in part on data showing that moderate- to high-intensity programs (>25 hours of contact with the child and/or the family over a 6-month period) improve weight status primarily in children with obesity.[14]

Stage 4—Tertiary Care Center Intervention. For severely obese teens, intensive interventions are reserved for those who have repeatedly had unsuccessful attempts at medical weight management in the prior 3 stages, have the maturity to make life-altering decisions, and have reached skeletal maturity (for bariatric surgery).

MEDICATIONS

- There have been several medications approved for use in children and adolescents, but currently only Orlistat is available. Orlistat can be given to adolescents aged 12 to 18 years under the supervision of a physician and by prescription only. Orlistat prevents fat absorption. Daily exercise and healthy lifestyle must continue as medication alone has demonstrated only modest weight loss effects and discontinuing diet and exercise can result in a major setback with weight regain.
- Metformin is a commonly used medication for the treatment of diabetes and appears effective for decreasing BMI while preventing progression to diabetes in children.[17]

SURGERY

- Bariatric surgery, along with diet and exercise, provides about 25 to 75 kg of weight loss after 2 to 4 years in adults.[18] Long-term outcome data are not available in children, but short-term results appear to be similar to those in adults.[19]
- Specific criteria are used to determine eligibility of an adolescent for bariatric surgery (Roux-en-Y gastric bypass, laparoscopic adjustable gastric banding or sleeve).[20] These include being at Tanner Stage 4 or 5 and at final or near-final height with a BMI >50 or BMI >40 and having comorbidities. Surgery is best performed at one of a few Children's Hospitals and Bariatric Centers of Excellence.

OTHER INTERVENTIONS

- There are many co-morbid mental health issues associated with overweight and obesity in children including depression, low self-esteem, distorted body image, and bullying.
- Excessive caloric intake is linked to many eating habits/eating behaviors including the use of food for non-nutritive purposes (e.g., using food as a reward or punishment and using food for comfort).[21]
- Several techniques can be helpful as adjuncts to improve mental health and social function in children and adolescents struggling with obesity.
  - Mindful eating—It is important to be "in the moment" at mealtimes, not only savoring the food but also enjoying mealtime company. Family meals aid in family bonding and help children reach the goal of eating slowly to promote satiation, tune into internal cues of fullness, and minimize overeating.[22] Yoga has been shown to be an effective means to allay teen fears and help them to deal with anxiety.[23] Patient-centered communication and motivational interviewing describe a set of counseling techniques directed towards motivating families to make necessary changes towards healthy lifestyles. Key characteristics include: (1) nondirective questions; (2) reflective, nonjudgemental listening; (3) combining family values and current health practices; (4) assessing the patient's (or parent's) level of confidence that they will be successful.[12]

PREVENTION AND SCREENING

Obesity prevention should be a priority for the pediatrician since it is much more difficult to treat rather than prevent child and adolescent obesity. Active involvement and engagement of the entire family is key to successful obesity prevention. The basic approach to prevention and screening of childhood obesity is to identify particular challenges and barriers that a particular family has to changing lifestyles and assess level of readiness to change to tailor messages. Use of motivational interviewing helps patients achieve success.

- The Transtheoretical model for behavior change originally described by Prochaska and Diclemente is still widely used today.[24] There are six proposed stages: precontemplation, contemplation, preparation, action, maintenance, and termination. Depending on level of readiness to change, it may be appropriate to discuss the risks obesity and the benefits of maintaining a healthy weight.
- In order to help individuals work through these stages and frequently through ambivalence towards change, there are five general principles of effective motivational interviewing that can be used: (1) effective empathy, (2) developing discrepancy between present behavior and goals, (3) avoiding argumentation, (4) rolling with resistance, and (5) supporting self-efficacy.[25]
- Pediatricians should calculate the BMI, determine the corresponding percentile, and plot it on standard growth charts at every annual visit for well child checks.[9] In addition, blood pressures should be taken frequently as well as consideration of family history and medical risks assessment.

- Address parenting style—Studies have shown that between the four parenting styles (authoritarian, authoritative, permissive, and neglectful), authoritarian parenting was associated with the highest risk of overweight in children in the first grade.[26]
- Secretly cooking and baking with hidden vegetables and fruits in kids' favorite dishes is one way to improve nutrition until a taste preference develops for those foods. For example, adding cauliflower to macaroni and cheese.

PROGNOSIS

- Overweight adolescents are more susceptible than their leaner peers to hypertension, type 2 diabetes mellitus, dyslipidemia, lung problems (e.g., asthma or obstructive sleep apnea), orthopedic problems (e.g., genu varum or slipped capital femoral epiphysis) and nonalcoholic steatohepatitis. Obese adolescents may also suffer from depression and low self-esteem.
- The risk of being obese as an adult increases with obesity at different ages as follows:[2] infancy, 14 percent; preschool, 25 percent; age 7 years, 41 percent; age 12 years, 75 percent; adolescence, 90 percent. In addition, over half of obese adolescents remain overweight as young adults.[27]
- In adults, it has been shown that just a 5 to 10 percent weight loss can reduce or eliminate comorbidities such as hypertension, noninsulin-dependent diabetes, and coronary heart disease.[28] Similar results could be anticipated for children as well.

FOLLOW-UP

- Pediatricians should continue to calculate and plot BMI (or weight percentile) yearly and watch for excessive weight gain compared with linear growth, identify and track patients at risk of obesity based on risk factors, encourage and support breastfeeding, routinely promote healthy diets and levels of physical activity, and monitor changes in obesity-associated risk factors.[28]

PATIENT EDUCATION

- Pediatricians should regularly advise parents and families to strive for a healthy life style with a diet that is high in fruits and vegetables, fiber, and calcium while adhering to appropriate portion sizes, and to pursue daily physical activity in the form of different, engaging activities for children and adolescents. Maintaining normal weight and treating obesity-related comorbidities will not only maximize health but also improve quality of life.

PATIENT RESOURCES

- Medline Plus. National Library of Medicine—**www.nlm.nih.gov/medlineplus/obesity.html**.
- US Department of Agriculture—**www.choosemyplate.gov**.
- Let's Move—**www.letsmove.gov**.

PROVIDER RESOURCES

- Academy of Nutrition and Dietetics—**www.eatright.org**.
- Alliance for a Healthier Generation—**www.healthiergeneration.org**.
- American Academy of Pediatrics books—**www.aap.org**.
  - A Parent's Guide to Childhood Obesity: A Roadmap to Health
  - Pediatric Nutrition Handbook
  - Pediatric Obesity Clinical Decision Support Chart
  - Pediatric Obesity – Prevention, Intervention, and Treatment Strategies for Primary care
- American Academy of Sports Medicine—**www.acsm.org**.
- American Society of Bariatric Physicians—**www.asbp.org**.
- The Obesity Society—**www.obesity.org**.
- UCSD School of Medicine: The HOPE Obesity Project.
- Centers for Disease Control and Prevention. Overweight and Obesity—**www.cdc.gov/obesity/index.html**.

REFERENCES

1. Centers for Disease Control and Prevention. Prevalence of Obesity in the United States, 2009-2010. Available at http://www.cdc.gov/nchs/data/databriefs/db82.pdf, accessed March 2012.
2. Rome ES. Obesity prevention and treatment. *Pediatr Rev*. 2011; 32(9):363-373.
3. Centers for Disease Control. Overweight and Obesity. Available at http://www.cdc.gov/obesity/data/index.html, accessed March 2013.
4. Graham EA. Economic, racial, and cultural influences on the growth and maturation of children. *Pediatr Rev*. 2005;26(8): 290-294.
5. Ogden C, Carroll M. Prevalence of obesity among children and adolescents: United States, trends 1963-1965 through 2007-2008. National Health and Nutrition Examination Survey NHANES. Available at http://www.cdc.gov/nchs/data/hestat/obesity_child_07_08/obesity_child_07_09.htm, accessed March 2013.
6. Manco M, Dallapiccola B. Genetics of pediatric obesity. *Pediatrics*. 2012;130(1):123-133.
7. Centers for Disease Control. Children's Food Environment State Indicator Report, 2011. Available at http://www.cdc.gov/obesity/downloads/childrensfoodenvironment.pdf, accessed March 2013.
8. Strasburger VC. Children, adolescents, obesity, and the media. *Pediatrics*. 2011;128(1):201-208.
9. Gantz W, Schwartz N, Angelini JR, Rideout V. *Food for Thought: Television Food Advertising to Children in the United States.* Menlo Park, CA. Kaiser Family Foundation; 2007.
10. Witaker RC, Wright JA, Pepe MS, et al. Predicting obesity in young adulthood from childhood and parental obesity. *N Engl J Med*. 1997;337:869-873.
11. Suglia SF, Duarte CS, Chamber EC, Boynton-Jarrett R. Cumulative social risk and obesity in early childhood. *Pediatrics*. 2012;129(5): e1173-e1179.

12. Barlow SE, and Expert Committee. Expert committee recommendations regarding the prevention, assessment, and treatment of child and adolescent overweight and obesity: summary report. *Pediatrics*. 2007;120(4):s164-s192.

13. Jakicic JM, Clark K, Coleman E, et al. American College of Sports Medicine position stand: appropriate intervention strategies for weight loss and prevention of weight regain for adults. *Med Sci Sports Exerc*. 2001;33(12):2145-2156.

14. United States Department of Agriculture. Choose My Plate. Available at http://www.choosemyplate.gov, accessed March 2013.

15. Burke LE, Wang J, Sevick MA. Self-monitoring in weight loss: a systematic review of the literature. *J Am Diet Assoc*. 2011;111(1): 92-102.

16. US Preventive Services Task Force. Screening for obesity in children and adolescents: US Preventive Services Task Force recommendation statement. *Pediatrics*. 2010;125(2):361-367.

17. Kendall D, Vail A, Amin R, et al. Metformin in obese children and adolescents: the MOCA trial. *J Clin Endocrinol Metab*. 2013; 98(1):322-329.

18. Douketis JD, Macie C, Thabane L, Williamson DF. Systematic review of long-term weight loss studies in obese adults: clinical significance and applicability to clinical practice. *Int J Obes (Lond)*. 2005;29(10):1153-1167.

19. Ciangura C, Basdevant A. Bariatric surgery in young massively obese diabetic patients. *Diabetes Metab*. 2009;35(6 Pt 2):532-536.

20. Perez MK, Nield LS. When to consider surgery for an obese teen. *Consultant for Pediatricians*. 2009;8(12):430-431.

21. Pinto C. Book review: body image, eating disorders, and obesity in youth, 2nd edition. *Eur Eat Disord Rev*. 2010;18(3):244.

22. Hammons AJ, Fiese BH. Is frequency of shared family meals related to the nutritional health of children and adolescents? *Pediatrics*. 2011;127(6):e1565-e1574.

23. Browser D. Yoga good for teen anxiety. *J Dev Behav Pediatr*. 2012; 33:193-201.

24. Prochaska JO, Velicer WF. The transthoretical model of health behavior change. *Am J Health Promot*. 1997;12(1):38-48.

25. University of California San Diego School of Medicine: The HOPE obesity project. American Board of Pediatrics, 2010-2013.

26. Rhee KE, Lumeng JC, Appugliese DP, Kaciroti N, Bradley RH. Parenting styles and overweight status in first grade. *Pediatrics*. 2006;117(6):2047-2054.

27. Krebs NF, Jacobson MS, American Academy of Pediatrics Committee on Nutrition: Prevention of pediatric overweight and obesity. *Pediatrics*. 2003;112(2):424-430.

28. Blackburn G. Effect of degree weight loss on health benefits. *Obes. Res*. 1995;3(2):211s-216s.

195 CUSHING SYNDROME

Elumalai Appachi, MD, MRCP

PATIENT STORY

A 21-month-old girl is brought to the pediatrician for a routine physical examination. The mother notes that the child has recently gained an excessive amount of weight. Examination shows an obese toddler who has a blood pressure of 130/90 mm Hg. The linear growth is noted to be abnormal and her weight has jumped from the 50th percentile at the last visit 6 months ago to above the 90th percentile. The girl has hirsutism and acne on the forehead (**Figure 195-1**). Urinalysis shows glycosuria. The pediatrician is suspicious for hypercortisolism and refers the child to a pediatric endocrinologist. A dexamethasone suppression test reveals lack of suppression of cortisol, consistent with Cushing syndrome. A CT scan of the abdomen reveals an adrenal tumor, which is surgically resected and found to be an adrenal adenoma. The girl is maintained on glucocorticoid therapy and recovers.

INTRODUCTION

Cushing syndrome occurs as a result of cortisol or glucocorticoid excess from any cause. Excess plasma cortisol production in endogenous Cushing syndrome may be caused by either excess ACTH secretion from the pituitary gland (Cushing disease) or adrenal overproduction of plasma cortisol from adrenal tumors. Cushing syndrome can also be the result of exogenous administration of ACTH or glucocorticoids (iatrogenic).

SYNONYMS

Hypercortisolism.

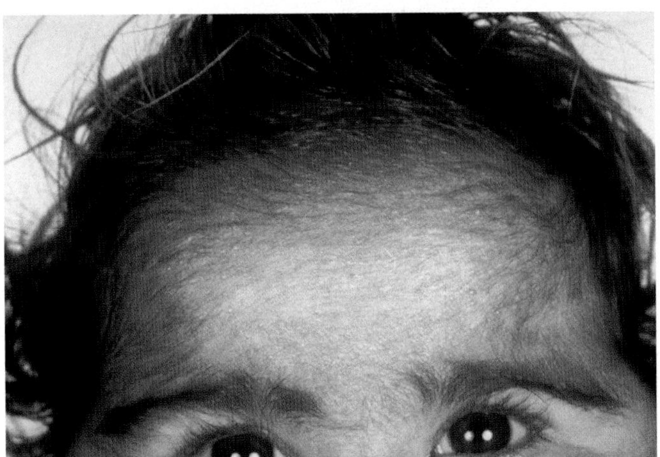

FIGURE 195-1 Acne, milia, and hirsutism on the forehead of a girl with Cushing syndrome caused by an adrenal adenoma. *(Used with permission from Elumalai Appachi, MD.)*

EPIDEMIOLOGY

- Non-iatrogenic Cushing syndrome is rare in children.
- Children with lymphoproliferative disorders, nephrotic syndrome, and autoimmune disorders are at risk for developing exogenous Cushing syndrome.
- The incidence of Cushing syndrome is higher in obese patients with type 2 diabetes, occurring in 2 to 5 percent of these patients.[1]
- Cushing syndrome is 2 to 3 times more common in girls than boys.

ETIOLOGY AND PATHOPHYSIOLOGY

- Cushing syndrome is most commonly caused by the administration of oral, parenteral, or topical glucocorticoids (exogenous or iatrogenic Cushing syndrome).
- In children over 7 years of age, true Cushing disease (hypersecretion of pituitary ACTH causing adrenal hyperplasia) is the most common cause of Cushing syndrome.[2]
- In infants and young children, Cushing syndrome is most often caused by a functioning adrenocortical tumor. Infants show signs of hypercortisolism along with signs of hypersecretion of other steroids such as androgens, estrogens, and aldosterone.[3–5]
- ACTH-dependent Cushing syndrome may also result from ectopic production of ACTH, although this is uncommon in children. Ectopic ACTH secretion in children has been associated with islet cell carcinoma of the pancreas, neuroblastoma, hemangiopericytoma, Wilms tumor, and thymic carcinoid.[6]

RISK FACTORS

- Lymphoproliferative disorders.
- Nephrotic syndrome.
- Autoimmune disorders.
- Obesity and type 2 Diabetes mellitus.

DIAGNOSIS

The diagnosis is made by the combination of clinical features and specific lab tests.

CLINICAL FEATURES

- Weight gain and growth arrest are the earliest and most reliable indicators of hypercortisolism in children (**Figure 195-2**).[3–5]
- The features of Cushing syndrome in children develop slowly and may take years before they are fully apparent.
- Rounded face with prominent and flushed cheeks **(Figure 195-3)**.
- Central obesity with "buffalo hump."
- Signs of abnormal masculinization.

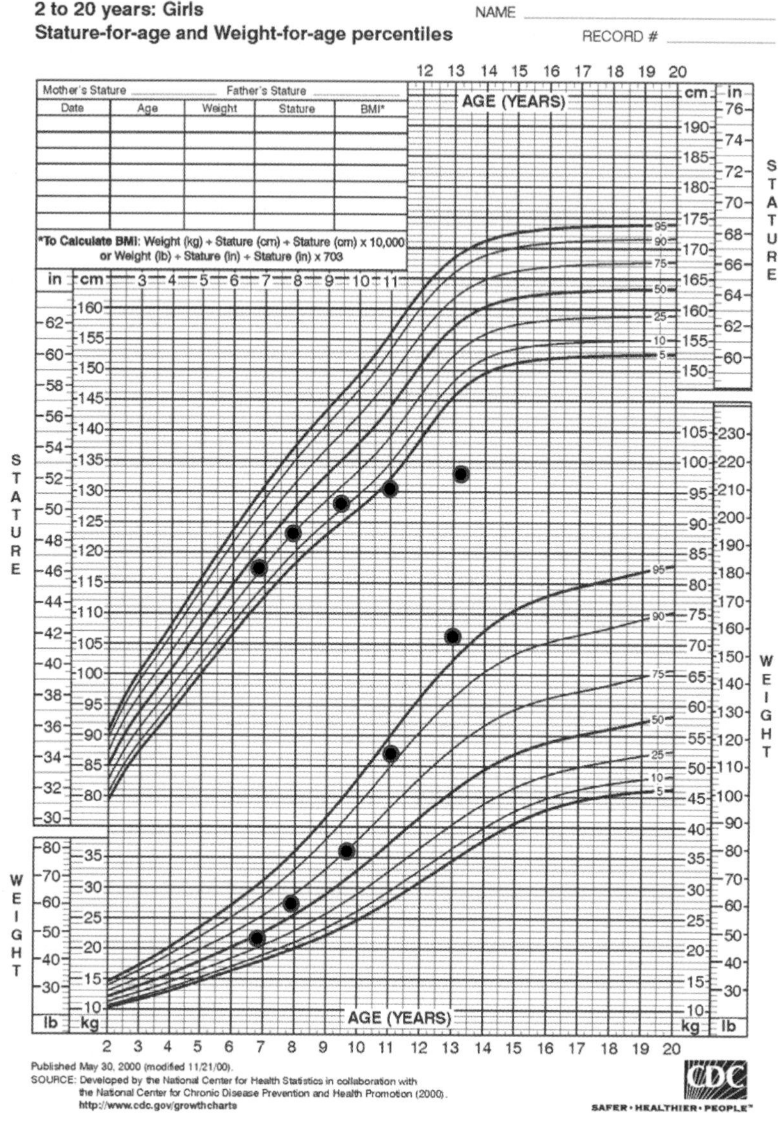

FIGURE 195-2 Growth chart of a girl with Cushing syndrome. Note the growth arrest in the face of significant weight gain, which is typical of Cushing syndrome. (*Used with permission from Camille Sabella, MD.*)

- Hirsutism on the face and trunk, pubic hair, acne, deepening of the voice, and enlargement of the clitoris in girls can occur (**Figure 195-1**).
- Hypertension is common and may occasionally lead to heart failure.
- An increased susceptibility to infection may lead to sepsis.
- Hyperglycemia and glucose intolerance is common.
- Purplish striae on the hips, abdomen, and thighs are common (**Figure 195-4**).
- Pubertal development may be delayed, or amenorrhea may occur in girls past menarche.
- Weakness, headache, and emotional lability may be prominent.
- Osteoporosis is common and may cause pathologic fractures.

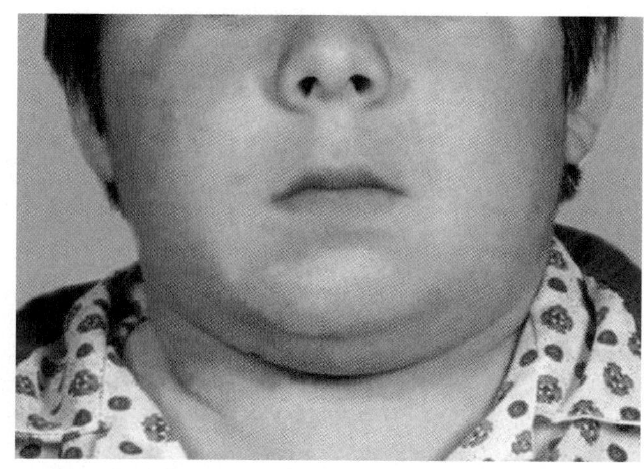

FIGURE 195-3 Rounded face and prominent cheeks in a boy with Cushing syndrome. (*Used with permission from Cleveland Clinic Children's Hospital Photo Files.*)

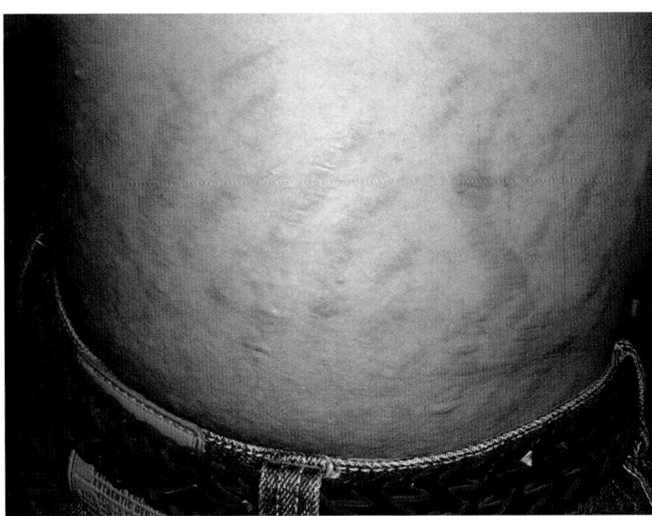

FIGURE 195-4 Striae due to Cushing syndrome caused by exogenous glucocorticoid administration in a 13-year-old boy. (*Used with permission from Richard P. Usatine, MD.*)

LABORATORY TESTING

- Loss of the normal diurnal variation of cortisol and ACTH are usually the first laboratory findings in Cushing disease.
- A midnight serum cortisol level greater than 4.4 ug/dL strongly suggests the diagnosis.
- Evening salivary cortisol levels are increased.
- Urinary excretion of free cortisol is increased. This is best measured in a 24-hr urine sample and is expressed as a ratio of micrograms of cortisol excreted per gram of creatinine.
- Dexamethasone suppression test can be done with a single dose of 25 to 30 μg/kg (maximum of 2 mg) given at 11 PM and the plasma cortisol level is measured the next day. In normal individuals, cortisol level will be suppressed to a level less than 5 μg/dL, but will not be suppressed in children who have Cushing syndrome.[7]
- Measurement of ACTH concentrations show suppressed levels in patients with cortisol-secreting tumors, but may be normal in patients with ACTH-secreting pituitary adenomas.[8]

IMAGING

- CT is the imaging of choice to detect adenomas of the adrenal glands and detects virtually all adrenal tumors larger than 1.5 cm in diameter.
- Contrast MRI may be needed to identify ACTH-secreting pituitary adenomas.

DIFFERENTIAL DIAGNOSIS

Children with simple dietary obesity may have similar clinical features, such as striae and hypertension, but do not have growth failure. These children grow more rapidly and are usually tall for their age (**Figure 195-5**). Furthermore, the urinary excretion of cortisol is also often elevated in simple obesity, but salivary nighttime levels of cortisol are normal and cortisol secretion is suppressed by oral administration of low doses of dexamethasone.

MANAGEMENT

- Treatment of Cushing syndrome should be directed at the primary cause of the excess corticosteroids.
- Tumors responsible for the hypercortisolism are generally surgically removed.
- The role of medications that inhibit steroidogenesis and irradiation in the management of Cushing disease in children is not well established.
- Corticosteroid replacement therapy is often necessary following removal of the source of corticosteroids until normal adrenal function returns.

MEDICATIONS

- Cyproheptadine, a centrally acting serotonin antagonist that blocks ACTH release, has been used to treat Cushing disease in adults but is rarely successful in children and has unacceptable adverse effects (weight gain, irritability, and hallucinations).
- Inhibitors of adrenal steroidogenesis (metyrapone, ketoconazole, aminoglutethimide, and etomidate) have been used preoperatively to normalize circulating cortisol levels, but there is very little experience using these agents in the treatment of Cushing disease in children.

SURGERY

- Transsphenoidal pituitary microsurgery is the treatment of choice for pituitary Cushing disease in children.[9,10]
- Complications of transsphenoidal surgery include transient diabetes insipidus and cerebrospinal fluid rhinorrhea.[11]
- Adrenalectomy is usually performed for adrenal tumors.[12]
- Adrenalectomy may lead to increased ACTH secretion by an unresected pituitary adenoma, which can expand and impinge on the optic nerves and produce melanocyte stimulating hormone to produce profound hyperpigmentation of the skin; this condition is termed Nelson Syndrome and is very rare in children.

REFERRAL

- Children suspected of having Cushing syndrome should be referred to a pediatric endocrinologist for work-up and close follow-up.

PREVENTION AND SCREENING

- Although there are no data supporting screening for Cushing syndrome in healthy asymptomatic patients, there may be a role for prudent screening in specific clinical situations as in patients with growth failure, osteoporosis, and easy bruising. Patients on long-term glucocorticoid therapy are at risk and should be closely monitored.

PROGNOSIS

- Prognosis after removal of an adrenal adenoma is good. Adrenal carcinomas are often metastatic and are characterized by a poor 5-year survival rate.

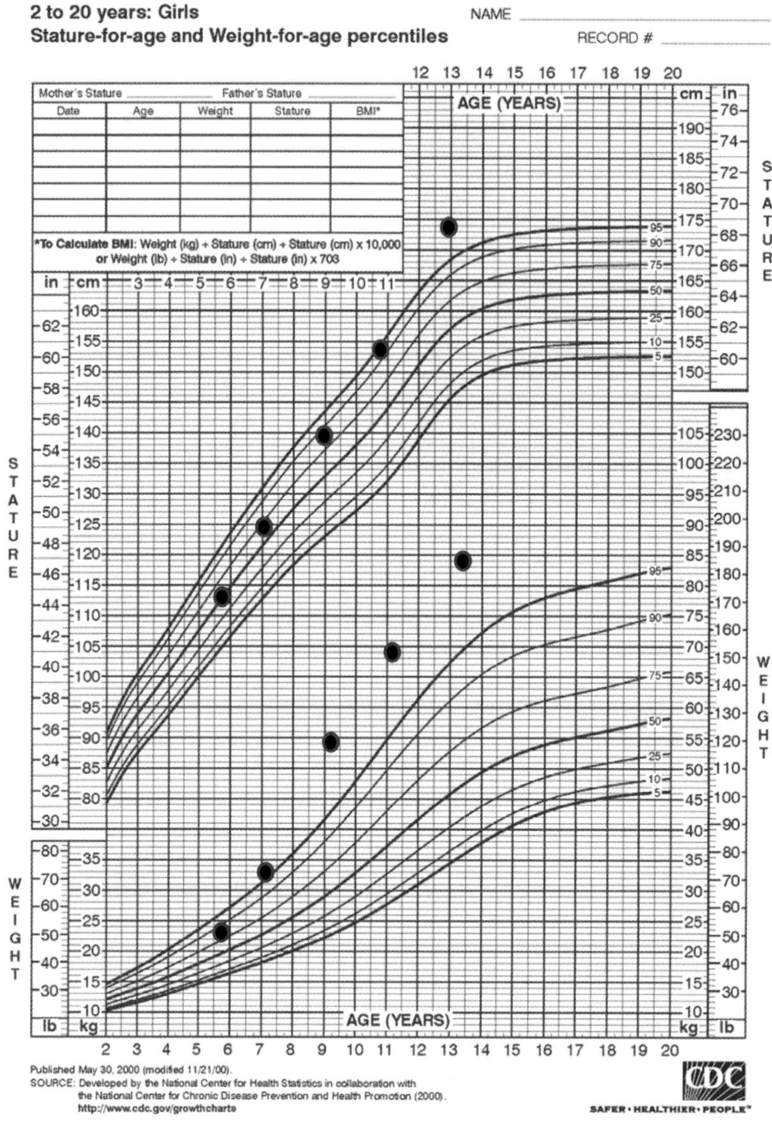

FIGURE 195-5 Growth chart of a girl with exogenous dietary obesity. Note the significant increase in growth velocity as well as weight, which distinguishes exogenous obesity from Cushing syndrome. (*Used with permission from Camille Sabella, MD.*)

- Initial remission rate after transsphenoidal surgery is 60 to 80 percent, but about 20 percent of children will have a relapse within 5 years.[13,14]

FOLLOW-UP

- Lifelong follow-up and hormone replacement therapy is usually required for nonexogenous causes of Cushing syndrome.

PATIENT EDUCATION

- Patients should be told that the features of Cushing syndrome, including hypertension, glucose intolerance and emotional disturbance may persist after treatment.
- Patients and parents should be educated about stress dose replacement therapy. These patients should wear medical alert labels and carry with them a prefilled glucocorticoid syringe for intramuscular injection when illness develops unexpectedly and oral medication administration is not an option.

PATIENT RESOURCES

- **www.cushingsdisease.com.**
- **www.nlm.nih.gov/medlineplus/ency/article/000348.htm.**

PROVIDER RESOURCES

- Cushing's Support and Research Foundation—**www.csrf.net/**.
- National Endocrine and Metabolic Disease Services—**http://endocrine.niddk.nih.gov/pubs/cushings/cushings.htm**.
- Pituitary Network Association—**http://www.pituitary.org/disorders/cushings_disease.aspx**.

REFERENCES

1. Catargi B, Rigalleau V, Poussin A, et al. Occult Cushing's syndrome in type-2 diabetes. *J Clin Endocrinol Metab*. 2003;88:5808-5813.
2. McArthur RG, Cloutier MD, Hayles AB, Sprague RG. Cushing's disease in children. Findings in 13 cases. *Mayo Clin Proc.* 1972;47:318-326.
3. Joshi SM, Hewitt RJ, Storr HL, et al. Cushing's disease in children and adolescents: 20 years of experience in a single neurosurgical center. *Neurosurgery*. 2005;57:281-285.
4. Kanter AS, Diallo AO, Jane JA Jr, et al. Single-center experience with pediatric Cushing's disease. *J Neurosurg*. 2005;103:413-420.
5. Devoe DJ, Miller WL, Conte FA, et al. Long-term outcome of children and adolescents following transsphenoidal surgery for Cushing disease. *J Clin Endocrinol Metab*. 1997;82:3196-3202.
6. Styne DM, Isaac R, Miller WL, et al. Endocrine, histological, and biochemical studies of adrenocorticotropin-producing islet cell carcinoma of the pancreas in childhood with characterization of proopiomelanocortin. *J Clin Endocrinol Metab*. 1983;57:723-731
7. Findling JW, Raff H, Aron DC. The low-dose dexamethasone suppression test: a reevaluation in patients with Cushing's syndrome. *J Clin Endocrinol Metab*. 2004;89:1222-1226.
8. Batista DL, Riar J, Keil M, Stratakis CA. Diagnostic tests for children who are referred for the investigation of Cushing syndrome. *Pediatrics*. 2007;120(3):e575-586.
9. Styne DM, Grumbach MM, Kaplan SL, Wilson CB, Conte FA. Treatment of Cushing's disease in childhood and adolescence by transcriptional microadenomectomy. *N Engl J Med.* 1984;310:889-894.
10. Magiakou MA, Mastorakos G, Oldfield EH, et al. Cushing's syndrome in children and adolescents. Presentation, diagnosis, and therapy. *N Engl J Med.* 1994;331:629-636.
11. Massoud AF, Powell M, Williams RA, Hindmarsh PC, Brook CG. Transsphenoidal surgery for pituitary tumors. *Arch Dis Child.* 1997;76:398-404.
12. Savage et al, 2008Savage MO, Chan LF, Grossman AB, et al. Operative management of Cushing syndrome secondary to micronodular adrenal hyperplasia. *Surgery*. 2008;143:750-758.
13. Leinung MC, Kane LA, Scheithauer BW, Carpenter PC, Laws ER Jr., Zimmerman D. Long term follow-up of transsphenoidal surgery for the treatment of Cushing's disease in childhood. *J Clin Endocrinol Metab*. 1995;80:2475-2479.
14. Storr HL, Afshar F, Matson M, et al. Factors influencing cure by transsphenoidal selective adenomectomy in paediatric Cushing's disease. Eur J Endocrinol. 2005;152:825-833.

196 ADDISON'S DISEASE

Swathi Appachi, BS
Elumalai Appachi, MD, MRCP

PATIENT STORY

A 14-year-old girl with a history of type I diabetes mellitus is brought to her pediatrician because of a 2-month history of fatigue, dizziness, and nausea. On physical exam, she is found to have orthostatic hypotension and the pediatrician notes that she has hyperpigmentation of dorsum of her hands and over her knees (**Figures 196-1** and **196-2**). The pediatrician is concerned about adrenal insufficiency and promptly refers the girl to an endocrinologist. The girl is found to have a low early morning serum cortisol, high serum adrenocorticotropin hormone level, and anti-adrenal antibodies, confirming the diagnosis of primary adrenal insufficiency.

INTRODUCTION

Addison's disease refers to dysfunction or hypofunction of the adrenal cortex which leads to primary adrenal insufficiency. The adrenal cortex is unable to produce and secrete glucocorticoids (cortisol) and mineralocorticoids (aldosterone), leading to an increase in adrenocorticotropin hormone (ACTH) and systemic effects in children, such as fatigue and gastrointestinal symptoms. Hyperpigmentation of the skin is a distinguishing feature. In children, congenital adrenal hyperplasia is the most common cause of Addison's disease (see Chapter 197, Congenital Adrenal Hyperplasia). The second most common cause of Addison's disease worldwide is tuberculosis and other granulomatous disorders. In developed countries, the second most common cause is autoimmune disease, which is the focus of this chapter.[1]

SYNONYMS

Primary adrenal insufficiency, adrenocortical hypofunction.

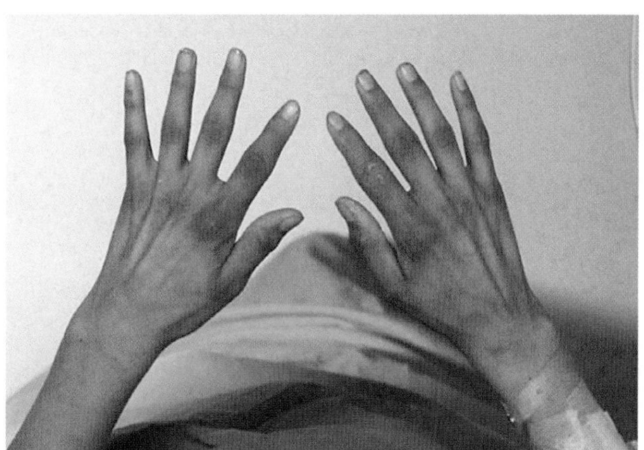

FIGURE 196-1 Hyperpigmentation over the dorsal aspect of the hands in a teenager with primary adrenal insufficiency. (*Used with permission from Cleveland Clinic Children's Hospital Photo Files.*)

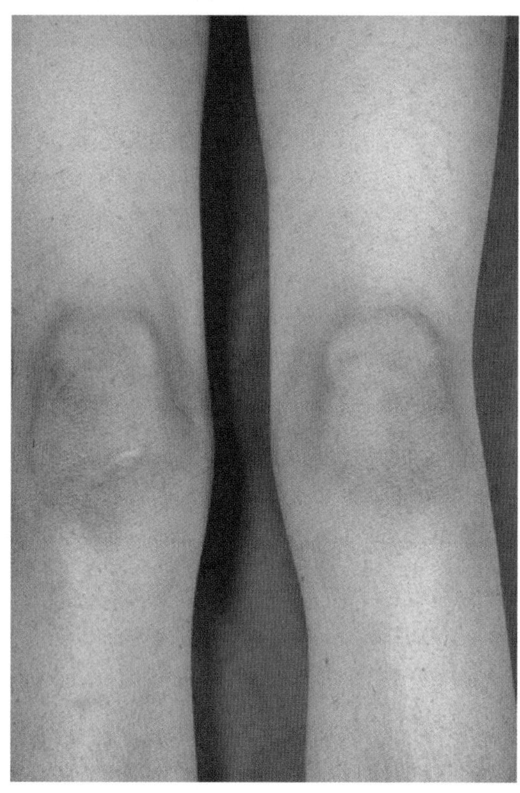

FIGURE 196-2 Hyperpigmentation of the skin overlying the knees in the same girl as in **Figure 196-1**. (*Used with permission from Cleveland Clinic Children's Hospital Photo Files.*)

EPIDEMIOLOGY

- Addison's disease is rare, with a prevalence of 140 per million.[1]
- Autoimmune Addison's disease constitutes 15 percent of all cases of primary adrenal insufficiency and usually presents during childhood.
  - Other causes include infection, adrenal hypoplasia congenital (congenital adrenal hypoplasia caused by a mutation in the DAX1 gene), and adrenoleukodystrophy.[2]
- Approximately 1/2 of patients with this disorder also have autoimmune disorders of other endocrine glands. This condition is known as autoimmune polyglandular syndrome (APS) and occurs more often in females (70%).
  - Isolated autoimmune disease is more prevalent in males (71%).[2]

ETIOLOGY AND PATHOPHYSIOLOGY

- Addison's disease is thought to result from autoimmune attack of the adrenal gland, leading to destruction of the cortical parenchyma.
  - There is evidence that both humoral and cell-mediated immunity are involved.[2]
- Autoimmune Addison's disease is often associated with other autoimmune phenomena, especially polyglandular syndromes.
  - APS1 (also known as autoimmune polyendocrinopathy-candidiasis-ectodermal dystrophy, or APECED)—This syndrome includes adrenal insufficiency, hypoparathyroidism, and chronic

mucocutaneous candidiasis. Autosomal recessive mutations in the autoimmune regulator (AIRE) gene are responsible.
  - APS2 (also known as Schmidt syndrome)—This entity consists of adrenal insufficiency, thyroiditis, and diabetes mellitus type 1. It is more prevalent than APS1.[3]
- Destruction of the adrenal cortex leads to low cortisol and low aldosterone, producing the symptoms of Addison's disease. Low cortisol also leads to increased synthesis of the prohormone pro-opiomelanocortin, which is cleaved to form ACTH and melanocyte stimulating hormone (MSH). Increased MSH levels in turn lead to increased melanin synthesis in melanocytes causing hyperpigmentation.[2]

RISK FACTORS

- Family history.[3]
- Other autoimmune diseases such as:
  - Diabetes mellitus type 1.
  - Graves disease.
  - Hypoparathyrodism.
  - Hypopituitarism.
  - Vitiligo.

DIAGNOSIS

CLINICAL FEATURES

- The most common presenting features of Addison's disease in children are fatigue, nausea, and vomiting. Clinical features of Addison's disease are due to hormonal deficiencies.[2–4]
- Low aldosterone leads to sodium wasting which in turn causes hypotension, dizziness, anorexia, weight loss, salt craving, electrolyte abnormalities, and dehydration.[2–4]
- Low cortisol leads to fatigue, weakness, morning headache, nausea, vomiting, diarrhea, and failure to thrive. Severe hypoglycemia can occur as well.[1,2,4]
- Hyperpigmentation from increased MSH is most apparent in areas exposed to sunlight or pressure, as well as the tongue, gingiva, axillary creases, and scars (**Figures 196-1** to **196-3**).
- It is important to remember that due to the autoimmune destruction of melanocytes that is sometimes seen in autoimmune Addison's disease, vitiligo and hypopigmentation may actually occur.[2]
- Amenorrhea can be seen in females.

LABORATORY TESTING

- Laboratory testing is essential for the diagnosis of Addison's disease. Adrenal insufficiency must be proven with tests of adrenocortical function.
- An early morning serum cortisol or ACTH stimulation test should be done to establish adrenal sufficiency. In the former, serum cortisol is measured at 8 AM, which corresponds with a peak in cortisol production. Low cortisol indicates adrenal insufficiency. In the latter test, serum cortisol is measured before and 60 minutes after administration of synthetic ACTH (cosyntropin). A low cortisol response demonstrates adrenal insufficiency.[4]

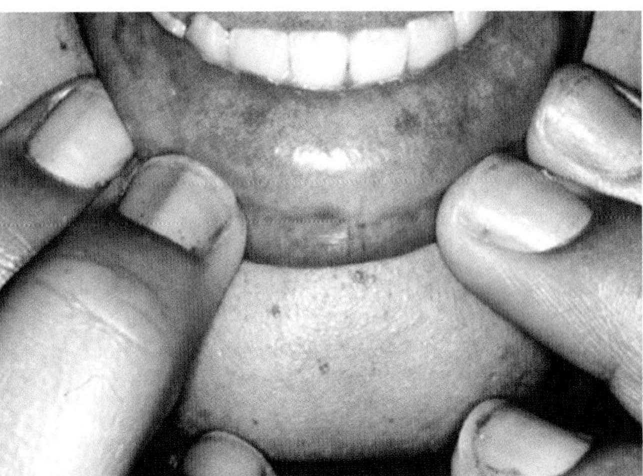

FIGURE 196-3 Hyperpigmentation of the lip, skin, and nails in a child with primary adrenal insufficiency. *(Used with permission from Strange GR, Ahrens WR, Schafermeyer RW, Wiebe RA: Pediatric Emergency Medicine, 3rd edition: http://www.accessemergencymedicine.com. Figure 77-2.)*

- Plasma ACTH levels should then be measured to differentiate between primary and secondary adrenal insufficiency. High ACTH levels indicate primary adrenal insufficiency.[4]
- To establish the diagnosis of autoimmune Addison's disease, levels of anti-adrenal antibodies, such as adrenal cortex autoantibody or 21-hydroxylase autoantibody, should be measured.[3,4]
  - If positive, antibodies against other glands (such as the parathyroid or thyroid) should be measured to test for APS.
  - If negative, the other causes of primary adrenal insufficiency, such as tuberculosis, adrenoleukodystrophy, or adrenal hypoplasia congenita, should be ruled out.

DIFFERENTIAL DIAGNOSIS

- If the patient's initial presentation is that of a salt-losing crisis with vomiting, hyponatremia, and hyperkalemia, these symptoms can also be seen in obstructive uropathy, pyelonephritis, or tubulointerstitial nephritis. These can especially occur in infants and occurs as a result of secondary aldosterone resistance in the kidneys.[4]
- The differential for autoimmune Addison's specifically includes other causes of primary adrenal insufficiency, such as congenital adrenal hyperplasia, infection, drugs, hemorrhage, adrenoleukodystrophy, or adrenal hypoplasia congenita.[2]

MANAGEMENT

- There is no cure for the autoimmune form of Addison's disease, but it can be managed by physiological replacement of cortisol and aldosterone.

MEDICATIONS

- Cortisol can be replaced with hydrocortisone, prednisone, or dexamethasone. In children, the former two are used more often. Hydrocortisone is less potent than prednisone and has a shorter

half-life, allowing for better titration. However, prednisone can be given less frequently. Normal cortisol secretion in children is estimated to be about 7 to 12 mg/m^2/day. Somatic growth should be followed closely.[3]
  - Doses must be increased in times of physiologic stress, such as illness or surgical procedures. Children may not be able to take the medication orally during these times, and thus injection of hydrocortisone is the preferred method of administration.
- Aldosterone is usually replaced with fludrocortisone at 0.05 to 0.2 mg/day. This dosage may need to be increased in infants, and infants younger than 1 year may require supplementation with sodium chloride. Again, somatic growth should be monitored.[3]

REFERRAL

- An endocrinologist should be involved in care of the patient.

PREVENTION AND SCREENING

- Addison's disease cannot be prevented. Physicians should retain a high index of suspicion in children presenting with nonspecific symptoms such as fatigue and gastrointestinal symptoms.

PROGNOSIS

- With appropriate replacement of glucocorticoids and mineralocorticoids, most patients with autoimmune Addison's disease can live normal lives.

FOLLOW-UP

- Follow-up is contingent on the affected systems. An endocrinologist should be involved with the patient's care.

PATIENT EDUCATION

- Patients and their families should carry prefilled syringes with steroids in case of emergency or sudden physiologic stress. A Medic Alert bracelet should also be considered.

PATIENT RESOURCES

- National Institutes of Health—**www.nlm.nih.gov/medlineplus/ency/article/000378.htm**.
- National Adrenal Diseases Foundation—**www.nadf.us/diseases/addisons.htm**.

PROVIDER RESOURCES

- **www.ncbi.nlm.nih.gov/pubmedhealth/PMH0001416/**.
- **http://emedicine.medscape.com/article/919077**.

REFERENCES

1. Ten S, New M, and Maclaren N. Clinical Review 130: Addison's Disease 2001. *J Clin Endocrinol Metab*. 2001;86(7):2909-2922.
2. Neiman LK, Chanco Turner ML. Addison's Disease. *Clinics in Dermatology*. 2006 Jul;24(4):276-280.
3. Neary N and Nieman. Adrenal insufficiency: etiology, diagnosis and treatment. *Curr Opin Endocrinol Diabetes Obes*. 2010;17(3): 217-223.
4. Simm PJ, McDonnell CM, Zacharin MR. Primary adrenal insufficiency in childhood and adolescence: advances in diagnosis and management. *J Pediatr Child Health*. 2004;40(11):596-599.

197 CONGENITAL ADRENAL HYPERPLASIA

Elumalai Appachi, MD, MRCP

PATIENT STORY

A 3400-gram infant is being evaluated by the pediatrician after an uncomplicated term gestation and vaginal delivery. The infant is noted to have ambiguous genitalia, characterized by clitoromegaly, enlarged labia, and no palpable testes. A single urethral/vaginal opening is present (**Figure 197-1**). A diagnosis of congenital adrenal hyperplasia is suspected based on these findings. A pediatric endocrinologist is consulted, who orders a serum 17-hydroxyprogesterone level, which is markedly elevated, and a rapid karyotype, which reveals a 46 XX karyotype, confirming the diagnosis of CAH caused by 21-hydroxylase deficiency. The infant is treated with glucocorticoids and the parents receive psychosocial and genetic counseling regarding the diagnosis.

INTRODUCTION

Congenital adrenal hyperplasia (CAH) is an autosomal-recessive disorder most commonly (95%) caused by 21-hydroxylase deficiency. Classic CAH refers to the salt wasting and simple virilizing form, while nonclassic, or late onset CAH, refers to a less severe form of the disorder and may not be apparent until later in life. This chapter will focus on classic CAH caused by 21-hydroxylase deficiency. Patients with the salt-wasting variety of congenital adrenal hyperplasia present with failure to thrive, dehydration, vomiting, and anorexia. In female infants, virilization of the external genitalia leads to an early diagnosis; the condition is often diagnosed later in male infants with the salt-wasting variety (2 to 3 weeks of life) because the external genitalia may appear normal.

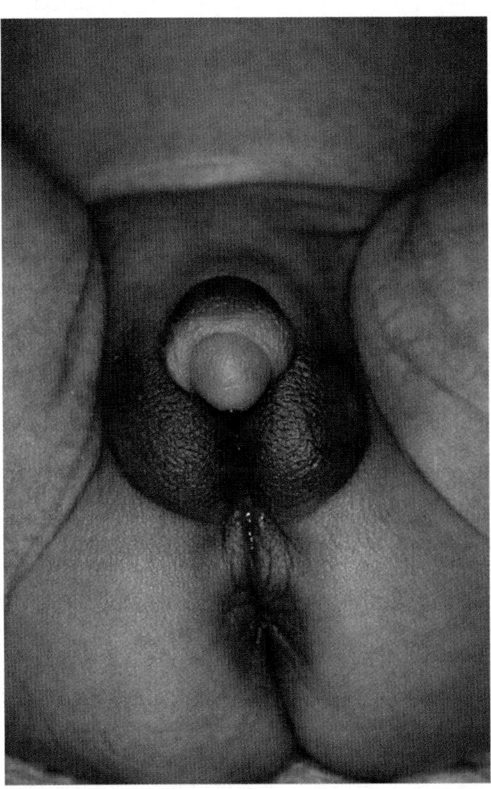

FIGURE 197-1 Ambiguous genitalia, manifested by clitoromegaly, enlarged and hyperpigmented labia, fused urogenital opening, in a female infant with congenital adrenal hyperplasia. (*Used with permission from Elumalai Appachi, MD.*)

SYNONYMS

Primary adrenal insufficiency, 21-hydroxylase deficiency, pseudohermaphroditism.

EPIDEMIOLOGY

- 21-hydroxylase deficiency accounts for 95 percent of all forms of CAH.
- The incidence of 21-hydroxylase deficiency is 1 in 15,000 live births and is one of the most common inborn errors of metabolism.[1–3]
- The incidence of CAH is equal among Caucasians and Hispanics and about fourfold less common in African Americans.[3]

ETIOLOGY AND PATHOPHYSIOLOGY

- Inherited defects in the enzymatic steps of cortisol biosynthesis (steroidogeneses) result in congenital adrenal hyperplasia.
- The resulting decrease in cortisol levels increases the secretion of adrenocorticotropic hormone (ACTH), thereby stimulating the production of adrenal steroids up to and including the substrate for the defective enzyme. This chronic ACTH stimulation results in hyperplasia of the adrenal cortex (**Figure 197-2**).

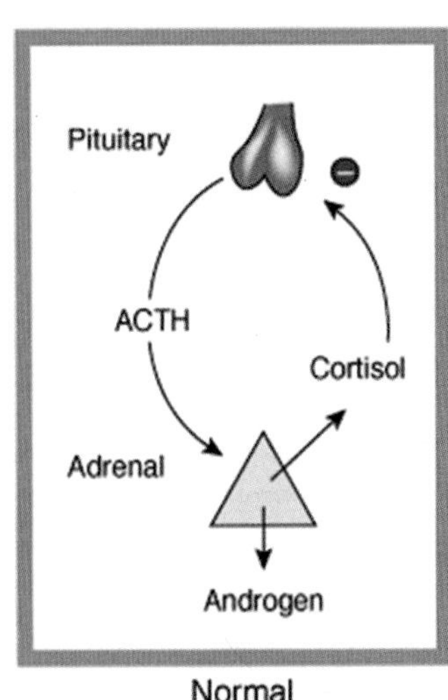

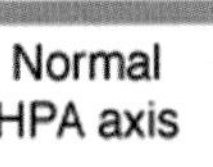

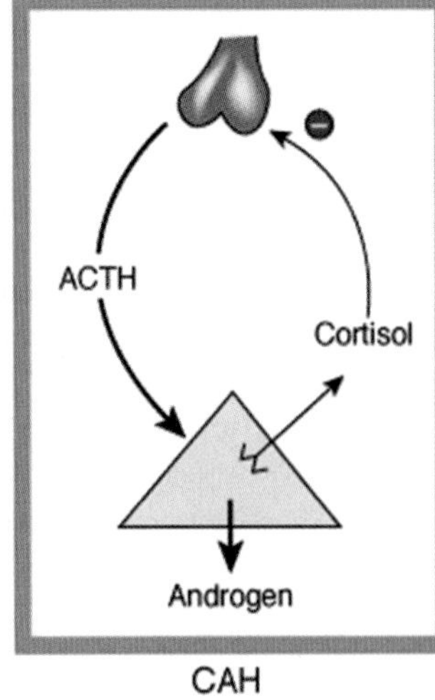

FIGURE 197-2 Classic adrenal hyperplasia (CAH) showing loss of the negative feedback loop caused by impaired glucocorticoid synthesis, resulting in adrenocorticotropic hormone (ACTH) excess resulting in androgen overproduction. HPA = hypothalamic-pituitary axis. (*Used with permission from Kappy, MD, Allen DB, Geffner ME: Pediatric Practice: Endocrinology: www.accesspediatrics.com. Figure 8-6.*)

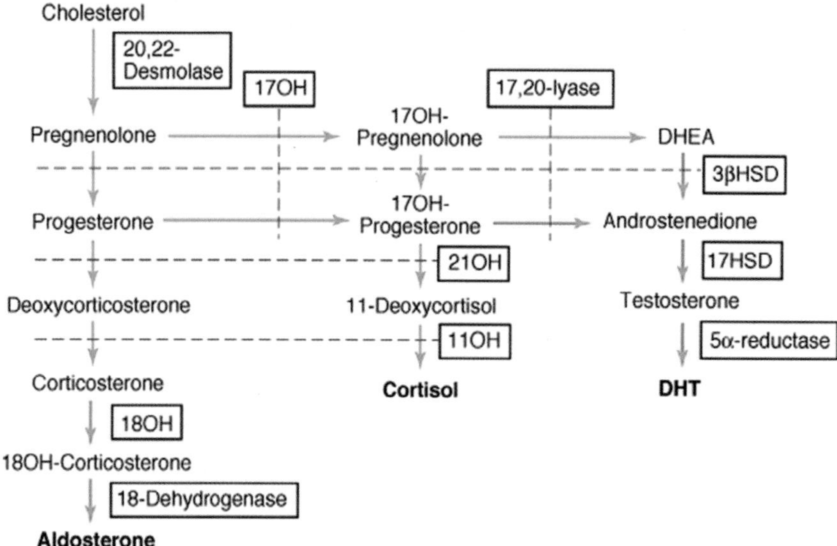

FIGURE 197-3 Adrenal steroidogenesis pathway. 21-hydroxylase enzyme deficiency leads to accumulation of 17-hydroxyprogesterone and other precursors causing overproduction of androstenedione and underproduction of aldosterone. Abbreviations: 11OH, 11-Hydroxylase; 17OH, 17-hydroxylase; 18OH, 18-hydroxylase; 21OH, 21-hydroxylase; 3βHSD, 3β-hydroxysteroid dehydrogenase; 17HSD, 17-hydroxysteroid dehydrogenase (17-ketosteroid reductase); DHEA, dehydroepiandrosterone; DHT, dihydrotestosterone. *(Used with permission from Cunningham MD, Eyal FG, Tuttle D: Neonatology: Management, Procedures, On-Call Problems, Diseases, and Drugs, 6th edition. www.accesspediatrics.com. Figure 82-1.)*

- Accumulation of 17-hydroxyprogesterone and other steroid precursors results in shunting into a pathway for androgen biosynthesis, leading to high levels of androstenedione that are converted outside the adrenal gland to testosterone. The effects of this shunting begin in affected fetuses by 8 to 10 weeks of gestation and leads to abnormal genital development in females (**Figure 197-3**).
- The clinical manifestations of these disorders are related to one or both of the following pathologic processes:
  - Impaired synthesis of cortisol—Results in increased ACTH secretion causing accumulation of 17-hydroxyprogesterone and other steroids that can be converted to testosterone. In the male fetus with 21 hydroxylase deficiency, the additional testosterone produced in the adrenals has no phenotypic effect. In a female fetus, the testosterone inappropriately produced by the adrenals of the affected female fetus causes varying degrees of virilization of the external genitalia.
  - Impaired synthesis of aldosterone—Resulting in severe hyponatremia, hyperkalemia, and acidosis with concomitant hypotension, shock, cardiovascular collapse, and death in an untreated newborn infant; this usually develops during the second week of life.
- In some forms of CAH (11-hydroxylase deficiency), there is excessive synthesis of mineralocorticoids such as deoxycorticosterone, which can cause hypertension.[1,2]
- 21-hydroxylase deficiency can be caused by a gene deletion, conversion or point mutation in *CYP21A2* (termed *21b*) gene. The severity of the manifestations is related to whether the genetic mutations are heterozygous or homozygous.[4]

RISK FACTORS

- Autosomal recessive inheritance.
- Consanguineous marriage.

DIAGNOSIS

- Neonatal screening for 21-hydroxylase deficiency has become a routine test in the neonatal screening program. This is performed by screening for 17-hydroxyprogesterone (17OHP), which is measured using a filter paper blood sample obtained by a heel puncture, preferably at 2 to 4 days of age.[5]
- Neonatal screening allows early diagnosis and treatment of infants who may be missed on clinical examination. This may prevent adrenal crisis and death and allows earlier gender assignment.

CLINICAL FEATURES

- Female infants usually present at birth with ambiguous genitalia (**Figures 197-1** and **197-4**). This is manifested by enlargement of the clitoris and by partial or complete labial fusion. The vagina usually has a common opening with the urethra (urogenital sinus). The clitoris may be so enlarged that it resembles a penis; because the urethra opens below this organ, some affected females may be mistakenly presumed to be males with hypospadias and cryptorchidism. Hyperpigmentation of the labioscrotal folds is common. The severity of virilization is usually greatest in females with the salt-losing form of 21-hydroxylase deficiency.

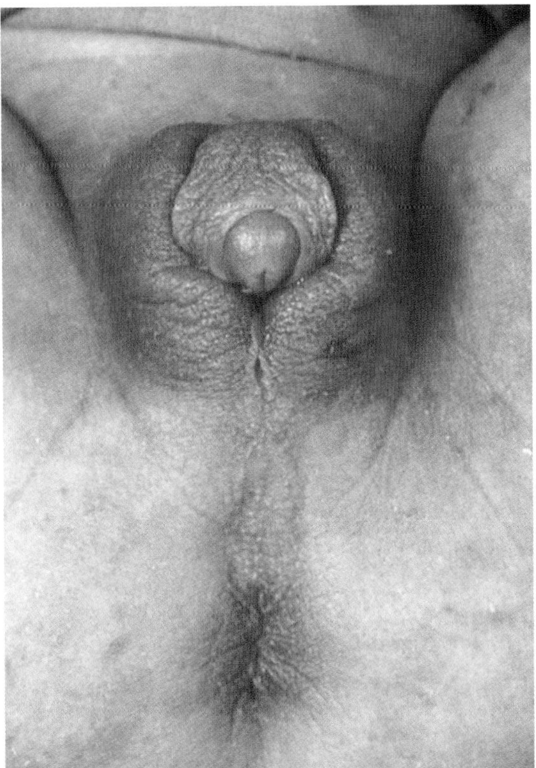

FIGURE 197-4 Clitoromegaly and enlarged labial folds in a girl with congenital adrenal hyperplasia. (*Used with permission from Cleveland Clinic Children's Hospital Photo Files.*)

The internal genital organs are normal, because affected females have normal ovaries and not testes and thus do not secrete anti-müllerian hormone.

- Male infants appear normal at birth. They present with weight loss, anorexia, vomiting, dehydration, shock, hyponatremia, hyperkalemia, and azotemia typically at 10 to 14 days of age. Thus, the diagnosis may not be made in boys until signs of adrenal insufficiency develop. Because patients with this condition can deteriorate quickly, male infants are more likely to die than female infants.

LABORATORY TESTING

- Infants with classic CAH have markedly elevated baseline adrenocortical hormones, due to a highly stimulated adrenal cortex. A very high serum concentration of 17-hydroxyprogesterone (random or ACTH-stimulated) is diagnostic of classic 21-hydroxylase deficiency.
- A rapid karyotype (such as fluorescence in situ hybridization of interphase nuclei for X and Y chromosomes) can quickly determine the genetic sex of the infant, and is an important first step in diagnosis and gender assignment.
- Blood levels of cortisol are usually low in patients with the salt-losing type of disease. They are often normal in patients with simple virilizing disease but inappropriately low in relation to the ACTH and 17-hydroxyprogesterone levels.
- In addition to 17-hydroxyprogesterone, levels of androstenedione and testosterone are elevated in affected females; although testosterone levels in affected males are high in relation to levels seen later in childhood, they are not elevated in relation to normal unaffected infants.
- Levels of urinary 17-ketosteroids and pregnanetriol are elevated in affected infants. Because these require 24-hour urine collections, they are rarely used in the diagnostic work-up.[5]

IMAGING

- Ultrasonography is helpful in demonstrating the presence or absence of a uterus and can often locate the gonads in infants with ambiguous genitalia.

DIFFERENTIAL DIAGNOSIS

- The first step in evaluating an infant with ambiguous genitals is a thorough physical examination to define the anatomy of the genitalia, locate the urethral meatus, and palpate the scrotum or labia and the inguinal regions for testes. Palpable gonads almost always indicate the presence of testicular tissue and thus a genetic male infant. Ultrasound and a rapid karyotype can help with gender assignment.
- Neonatal sepsis and infection can present with acidosis, dehydration, and abnormal electrolytes, and should be ruled out by obtaining appropriate cultures (see Chapter 187, Congenital and Perinatal Infections).
- Renal Dysplasia—Infants with renal dysplasia present with hyponatremia and acidosis and can be confused with CAH. Renal work up including renal ultrasound usually points towards the diagnosis.

MANAGEMENT

- The management of CAH in newborns requires consultation with a pediatric endocrinologist.[1,2,6,7]
- Cortisol deficiency is treated with glucocorticoids. Glucocorticoids also suppress excessive production of androgens by the adrenal cortex and will minimize problems such as excessive growth, skeletal maturation, and virilization.

MEDICATIONS

- Newly diagnosed newborns often require larger glucocorticoid doses than are needed in other forms of adrenal insufficiency.
- Infants with salt-wasting disease (i.e., aldosterone deficiency) require mineralocorticoid replacement with fludrocortisone. Infants may have very high mineralocorticoid requirements in the first few months of life, and often require sodium supplementation.[7]

SURGERY

- Significantly virilized females may undergo surgery between 2 to 6 months of age. If there is severe clitoromegaly, the clitoris is reduced in size, with partial excision of the corporal bodies and preservation of the neurovascular bundle; however, moderate clitoromegaly may become much less noticeable even without surgery as the patient grows.
- Vaginoplasty and correction of the urogenital sinus usually are performed at the time of clitoral surgery; revision in adolescence is often necessary.[8]

PREVENTION AND SCREENING

- Because 21-hydroxylase deficiency is often undiagnosed in affected males until they have severe adrenal insufficiency, all states in the US and many other countries have instituted newborn screening programs. These programs analyze 17-hydroxyprogesterone levels in dried blood obtained by heel-stick and absorbed on filter paper cards; the same cards are screened in parallel for other congenital conditions such as hypothyroidism and phenylketonuria. The parents of potentially affected infants are quickly contacted so the infant may receive additional testing (electrolytes and repeat 17-hydroxyprogesterone determination) at approximately 2 weeks of age.
- Prenatal diagnosis may help facilitate appropriate prenatal treatment of affected females. Mothers with pregnancies at risk (when both parents are known to be heterozygotes) may be given dexamethasone as soon as pregnancy is diagnosed, which can suppress secretion of steroids by the fetal adrenal, including secretion of adrenal androgens, and may ameliorate virilization of the external genitals in affected females.[9] Chorionic villus biopsy is then performed to determine the sex and genotype of the fetus; therapy is continued only if the fetus is an affected female.
- DNA analysis of fetal cells isolated from maternal plasma for sex determination and CYP21 gene analysis may permit earlier identification of the affected female fetus.

PROGNOSIS

- With proper treatment, the prognosis of CAH is good. Most infants will have minimal morbidity and normal longevity with appropriate medical therapy and surgical restoration, if needed.

FOLLOW-UP

- Infants and children with CAH require regular follow-up with a pediatric endocrinologist.
- Increasing doses of glucocorticoids are often required during times of stress.

PATIENT EDUCATION

- Parents should be offered psychosocial as well as genetic counseling on confirmation of diagnosis.
- Children should be informed of their condition in a manner appropriate to their age and development, by both their physicians and parents. Information should be communicated sensitively, simply, and should be repeated at appropriate intervals.
- Parents should receive anticipatory counseling about the possible tendency toward male gender role behavior in affected girls.
- Adolescent girls should receive independent psychosexual counseling.
- Patients must understand the importance of lifelong treatment and monitoring.
- Reduced fertility has been reported in females who have a history of CAH. This should be discussed with patients at the appropriate age.
- The need for increasing dosing of glucocorticoids during times of stress should be discussed with parents and patients.
- Injectable hydrocortisone should be kept in the home and parents should be able to administer this in emergency situations (e.g., if the patient is unconscious or has severe diarrhea).
- Patients with CAH should wear medical identification jewelry with details of their condition and medication.

PATIENT RESOURCES

- The Magic Foundation: Congenital adrenal hyperplasia—**www.magicfoundation.org/www/docs/100**.
- **www.congenitaladrenalhyperplasia.org**.
- National Adrenal Diseases Foundation—**www.nadf.us/diseases/cah.htm**.

PROVIDER RESOURCES

- **www.ncbi.nlm.nih.gov/pubmedhealth/PMH0001448/**.
- **www.ncbi.nlm.nih.gov/pmc/articles/PMC3329455/**.

REFERENCES

1. Speiser PW, White PC: Congenital adrenal hyperplasia. *N Engl J Med*. 2003;349:776-788.
2. Merke DP, Bornstein SR: Congenital adrenal hyperplasia. *Lancet*. 2005;365:2125-2136.
3. Therrell BL Jr, Berenbaum SA, Manter-Kapanke V, et al. Results of screening 1.9 million Texas newborns for 21-hydroxylase-deficient congenital adrenal hyperplasia. *Pediatrics*. 1998;101:583-590.
4. White PC, Tusie-Luna MT, New MI, Speiser PW: Mutations in steroid 21-hydroxylase (CYP21). *Hum Mutat*.1994;3:373-378.
5. Forest MG: Recent advances in the diagnosis and management of congenital adrenal hyperplasia due to 21-hydroxylase deficiency. *Hum Reprod Update*. 2004;10:469-485.
6. Van der Kamp HJ, Otten BJ, Buitenweg N, et al. Longitudinal analysis of growth and puberty in 21-hydroxylase deficiency patients. *Arch Dis Child*. 2002;87:139-144.
7. Mullis PE, Hindmarsh PC, Brook CG: Sodium chloride supplement at diagnosis and during infancy in children with salt-losing 21-hydroxylase deficiency. *Eur J Pediatr*. 1990;150:22-25.
8. Schnitzer HH, Donahoe PK: Surgical treatment of congenital adrenal hyperplasia. *Endocrinol Metab Clin North Am*. 2001;30:137-154.
9. Fernandez-Balsells MM, Muthusamy K, Smushkin G, et al. Prenatal dexamethasone use for the prevention of virilization in pregnancies at risk for classical congenital adrenal hyperplasia due to 21-hydroxylase (CYP21A2) deficiency: a systematic review and meta-analyses. *Clin Endocrinol (Oxf)*. 2010;73:436-444.

198 RICKETS

Di Sun, BS, MPH
Elumalai Appachi, MD, MRCP

PATIENT STORY

A 2-year-old boy is brought to the pediatrician by his mother, who reports that the boy appears more irritable lately and does not seem to be growing. After further questioning, the mother mentions that her child has also complained of leg pain and a "waddling" gait. On exam, the boy has widening of the wrists and bowing of his legs and prominence of the costochondral junctions (rachitic rosary; **Figures 198-1** and **198-2**). The pediatrician asks about the child's diet, and the mother reveals that the patient is a very picky eater and drinks only fruit juice that is not fortified with vitamin D. The pediatrician is concerned about rickets and orders a serum alkaline phosphatase, which is elevated, and vitamin D level (25-OH Vitamin D), which is low. X-ray of the tibia and femur demonstrated widening of the growth plate and metaphysis (**Figure 198-3**). The pediatrician prescribes vitamin D and calcium supplementation for the child. After 3 months of supplementation, the boy's symptoms have resolved and repeat x-ray showed a dense zone of calcification at the metaphysis with improvement in the widened growth plate.

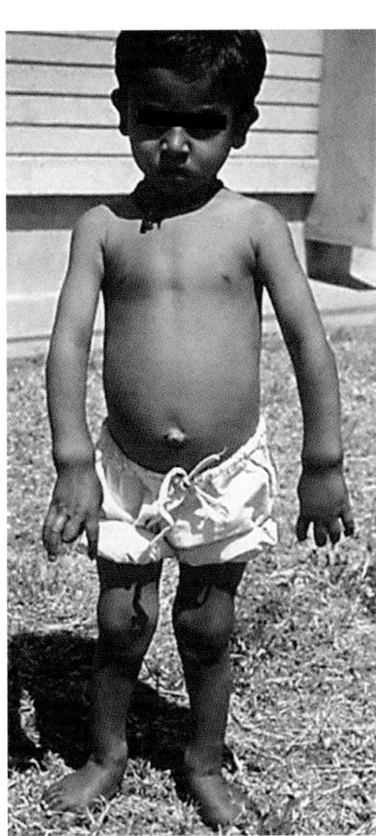

FIGURE 198-1 Widening of the wrists, bowed legs, bowing of the forearms, and frontal bossing in a young child with nutritional rickets. (*Used with permission from Cleveland Clinic Children's Hospital Photo Files.*)

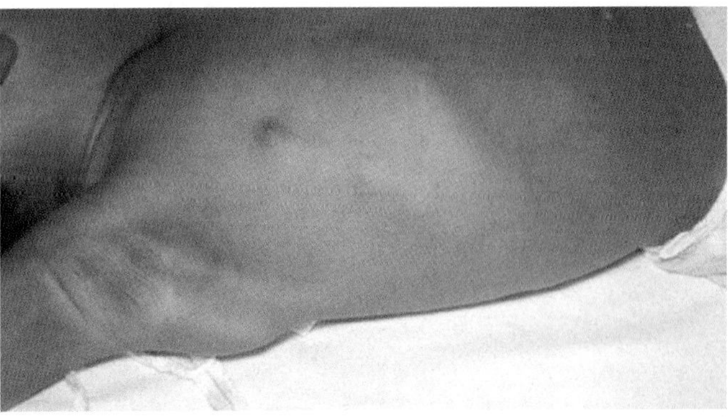

FIGURE 198-2 Prominence of the costochondral junction (rachitic rosary) in the same child as in **Figure 198-1**. (*Used with permission from Cleveland Clinic Children's Hospital Photo Files.*)

INTRODUCTION

- Rickets is a defect in bone mineralization that occurs in children prior to epiphyseal fusion, resulting in widening of the growth plates, bone pain, decreased strength of bone, bone deformities, and signs of hypocalcemia.[1–3] This condition is primarily due to nutritional deficiency, specifically vitamin D deficiency, but can also occur with calcium or phosphorus deficiency. There are also hereditary and secondary (renal losses of calcium and phosphate) causes of rickets. Management of rickets depends on the specific etiology. Nutritional deficiencies can be treated with supplementation.

SYNONYMS

Osteomalacia in children, Osteomalacia (Rickets in adults).

EPIDEMIOLOGY

- Nutritional rickets in the US is relatively uncommon; in case reports published between 1986 to 2003, there were 166 cases of documented rickets.[4]
- The prevalence of hypovitaminosis D in the US ranges from 1 to 78 percent with breastfed infants born in the winter being the most likely to be vitamin D-deficient. Vitamin D deficiency was associated with older age, winter season, higher body mass index, African-American race, and elevated parathyroid hormone as a result.[5]
- Hereditary causes of rickets are very rare, the most common being X-linked hypophosphatemic rickets (XLH), which has a prevalence of 1/20,000.[6]

ETIOLOGY AND PATHOPHYSIOLOGY

- Rickets is defined as a defect of bone mineralization of the osteoid, or protein matrix, of growing bone (prior to epiphyseal fusion). The mineral component of bone consists of calcium and phosphate hydroxyapatite crystals. When there is inadequate mineralization of growing bone, there is impaired growth at the metaphysis and a general decrease in bone strength.[1]

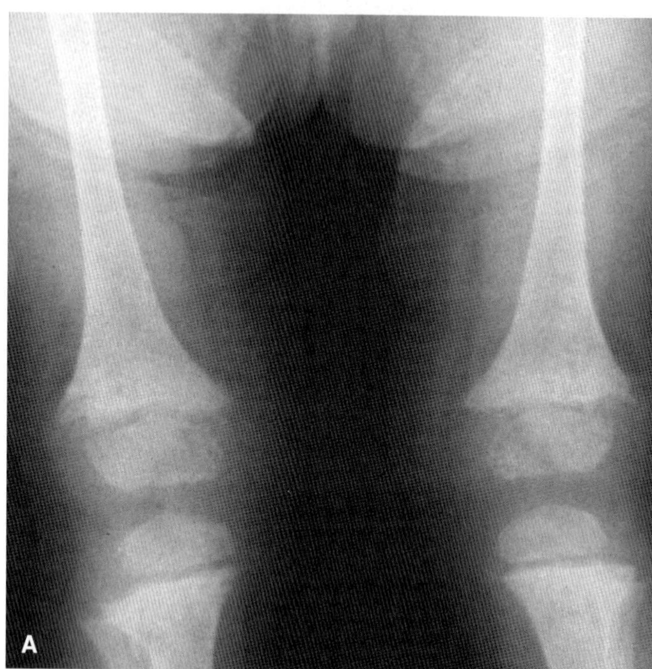

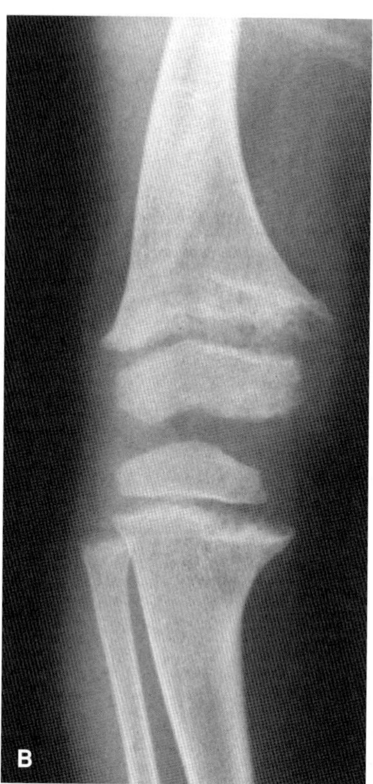

FIGURE 198-3 Cupping and fraying of the metaphyses and bowing of the tibia and femur on (**A**) bilateral and (**B**) unilateral views. (*Used with permission from Cleveland Clinic Children's Hospital Photo Files.*)

- The regulation of bone mineralization depends on the calcium*phosphorus product, which is modulated by vitamin D, parathyroid hormone (PTH), and phosphatonin.
  - The majority of vitamin D is generated from skin following ultraviolet B exposure. Vitamin D can also be obtained from vitamin D_2 found in plants and vitamin D_3 found in animal products such as milk. Vitamin D is converted to Calcidiol (25(OH)-D) via 25-hydroxylase in the liver. 25(OH)-D is then converted to Calcitriol (1,25$(OH)_2$-D) by 1-α-hydroxylase in the kidneys. 1,25$(OH)_2$-D is the active form of vitamin D and upregulates calcium and phosphorus absorption.[2]
  - Low ionized calcium stimulates PTH release. To maintain calcium homeostasis, PTH increases bone resorption to release calcium from bone, upregulates 1,25$(OH)_2$-D synthesis, and increases phosphorus excretion to decrease the calcium*phosphorus product to promote calcium release.[2]
  - Phosphatonins, specifically fibroblast growth factor-23 (FGF-23), are proteins secreted by osteocytes in bone that decrease renal tubular reabsorption of phosphate and 1-α-hydroxylase activity.[7]
- The etiology of rickets can be widely classified based on the defect in mineralization: vitamin D disorders, calcium deficiency, phosphorus deficiency, and defects in renal regulation.
- Vitamin D disorders can be further classified as nutritional (vitamin D deficiency), secondary (due to malabsorption or chronic kidney disease), or hereditary (vitamin D-dependent rickets type 1 and 2).
  - Nutritional vitamin D deficiencies are due to inadequate sun exposure; darker-skinned children, and those with decreased dietary intake, are more at risk.
  - Secondary vitamin D disorders can occur with gastrointestinal disorders such as Crohn disease or other disturbances impairing fat absorption and thus vitamin D absorption. Chronic kidney disease manifests with impaired synthesis of 1,25$(OH)_2$-D, resulting in vitamin D deficiency.
  - Vitamin D-dependent rickets type 1 is an autosomal recessive disorder resulting in a mutation in 1-α-hydroxylase that impairs 1,25$(OH)_2$-D synthesis. Vitamin D-dependent rickets type 2 is also an autosomal recessive disorder characterized by a defect in the vitamin D receptor preventing patients from responding appropriately to 1,25$(OH)_2$-D.[8]
- Deficiency in calcium, which is found in leafy vegetables and dairy products, typically arises in children who are on unconventional diet or have milk allergies. Phosphorus deficiency rarely occurs in healthy children, but can arise in anorexics and malabsorptive processes.
- Defects in renal regulation of calcium and phosphorus homeostasis can also be classified into hereditary (X-linked hypophosphatemic rickets, autosomal dominant hypophosphatemic rickets, autosomal recessive hypophosphatemic rickets, and hereditary hypophosphatemic rickets with hypercalciuria) and secondary causes (Fanconi Syndrome, renal tubular acidosis, or tumor-induced).
- XLH rickets occurs due to a gene mutation in *PHEX*, which inactivates the phosphatonin FGF-23. Consequently, there is an increase in FGF-23 expression, which normally inhibits phosphate reabsorption and 1-α-hydroxylase. This leads to decreased phosphate reabsorption and decreased 1,25$(OH)_2$-D production.

- Autosomal dominant hypophosphatemic rickets (ADHR) involves a mutation in FGF-23 that impairs degradation of the protein. Similar to XLH, increased FGF-23 levels results in decreased reabsorption of phosphate and decreased 1,25$(OH)_2$-D production.
- Autosomal recessive hypophosphatemic rickets is a very rare disorder due to a mutation in dentin matrix protein 1 that also leads to elevated FGF-23. This is characterized by decreased reabsorption of phosphate and decreased 1,25$(OH)_2$-D production.
- Hereditary hypophosphatemic rickets with hypercalciuria (HHRH) is an autosomal recessive disorder due to a mutation in the sodium-phosphate channel in the proximal tubule. The subsequent decrease in serum phosphate stimulates 1,25$(OH)_2$-D production, which suppresses PTH and increases calcium absorption in the gut resulting in hypercalciuria.
- Secondary losses of calcium and phosphate are due to defects in proximal tubule reabsorption. These disorders include Fanconi syndrome, characterized by generalized dysfunction of the proximal tubules that cause hypophosphatemia, and renal tubular acidosis, which can cause impaired calcium reabsorption.[1]
- Another secondary cause of rickets is tumor-induced rickets which can occur when mesenchymal tumors secrete phosphatonins leading to increased phosphate excretion and low 1,25$(OH)_2$-D.

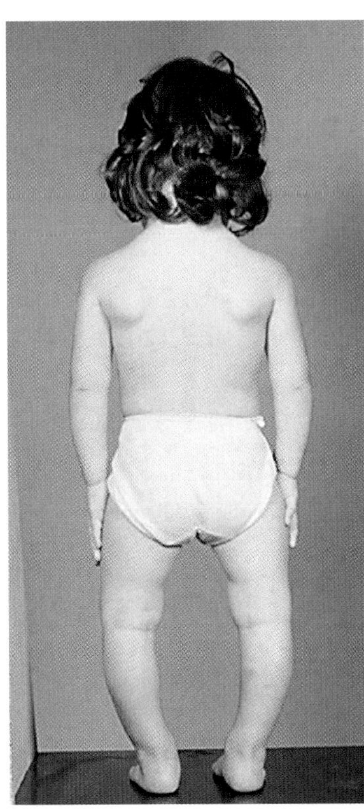

FIGURE 198-4 Bow-legged appearance of a child with rickets. (*Used with permission from Cleveland Clinic Children's Hospital Photo Files.*)

RISK FACTORS

- The most prevalent cause of rickets is nutritional deficiencies. Risk factors for developing vitamin D deficiency in children include being exclusively breastfed, living at higher latitudes (above 40°), darker skin, decreased sun exposure, older age (adolescence), and higher body mass index.[2,4,5]
- Calcium deficiency is uncommon in industrialized countries but can occur in children with milk allergies, malabsorptive disorders, or with unconventional diets.[1]
- Phosphate deficiency is very rare except in anorexia, malabsorptive disorders, or in children using aluminum-containing antacids.

DIAGNOSIS

CLINICAL FEATURES

- The general presentation of rickets is characterized by skeletal deformities such as prominence of the costochondral junction (rachitic rosary), delayed fontanelle closing, softening of cranial bones (craniotabes), bowing of the legs (genu varum), horizontal groove demarcating the diaphragmatic insertion (Harrison groove), waddling gait, and widening of the wrists and ankles (**Figures 198-1**, **198-2**, and **198-4** to **198-6**).
    - Children may complain of bone pain, weakness, or an inability to walk. Parents may notice failure to thrive or delayed teething.
    - If rickets is due to vitamin D deficiency, children may also be more irritable and present with signs of hypocalcemia. In infants, this can include seizures or tetany. In older children, hypocalcemia can manifest with apneic spells, hypotonia, hyperreflexia, cardiomyopathy, or stridor and wheezing.[2]

LABORATORY TESTING

- Laboratory findings vary depending on the etiology of rickets.
- The first step in laboratory analysis should be to evaluate alkaline phosphatase, a marker of bone turnover, which is increased in all forms of rickets.
- Next, 25(OH)-D should be evaluated. In children, 25(OH)-D should be ≥50 nmol/L. If the patient is vitamin D deficient, 25(OH)-D will be low while 1,25$(OH)_2$-D ranges from low to

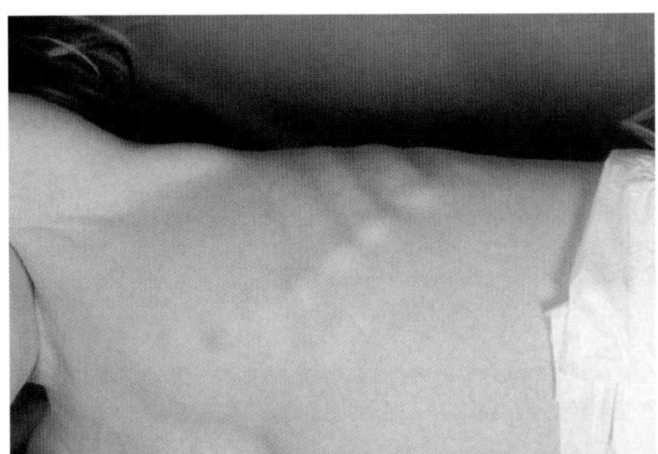

FIGURE 198-5 Prominence of the costochondral junction (rachitic rosary) and indentation of the lower anterior thoracic wall (Harrison groove) in a child with rickets. (*Used with permission from Cleveland Clinic Children's Hospital Photo Files.*)

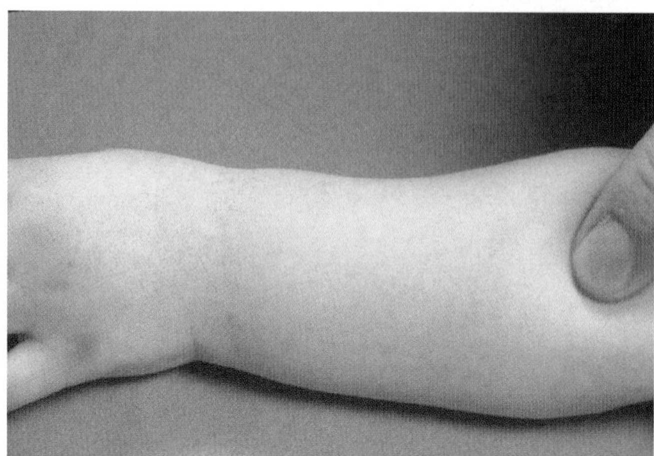

FIGURE 198-6 Widening of the wrist in the same child as in **Figure 198-5**. (*Used with permission from Cleveland Clinic Children's Hospital Photo Files.*)

elevated, phosphate is decreased, PTH is increased, and calcium can be normal to decreased.[2]

- If 25(OH)-D is normal, 1,25$(OH)_2$-D values should be obtained. This is elevated in vitamin D-dependent rickets type 2 and decreased in vitamin D-dependent rickets type 1.[2]
- Calcium, phosphate, and PTH levels should also be checked.
- In chronic kidney disease, there will be elevated phosphate, high PTH, and decreased 1,25$(OH)_2$-D.[2]
- In dietary calcium deficiency, there is decreased phosphate, elevated PTH, and a compensatory increase in 1,25$(OH)_2$-D. Calcium is normal to decreased. In phosphorus deficiency, there is normal calcium, decreased phosphate, decreased to normal PTH, and elevated 1,25$(OH)_2$-D.[2]
- In the hereditary forms of rickets arising from dysregulation of phosphate homeostasis, there is usually normal calcium, decreased phosphate with no compensatory increase in 1,25$(OH)_2$-D, normal PTH, and normal 25(OH)-D. To differentiate among these disorders, urinary phosphate and calcium can be obtained. Urinary phosphate will be elevated in all of these conditions and urinary calcium is elevated only in HHRH.[2]
- Secondary causes of rickets arising from defects in renal homeostasis are characterized by decreased phosphate with no compensatory increase in 1,25$(OH)_2$-D and increased urinary phosphate.[2]

IMAGING

- Initially, patients present with radiographic findings of osteopenia and blurring of the demarcation between the metaphysis and growth plate. As rickets progresses, there is widening of the growth plate and then of the metaphysis (**Figures 198-3** and **198-7**).[2]

DIFFERENTIAL DIAGNOSIS

- Juvenile idiopathic arthritis—May present with bone pain, weakness, and fracture. However, these patients have joint swelling and systemic features of disease (see Chapter 172, Juvenile Idiopathic Arthritis).

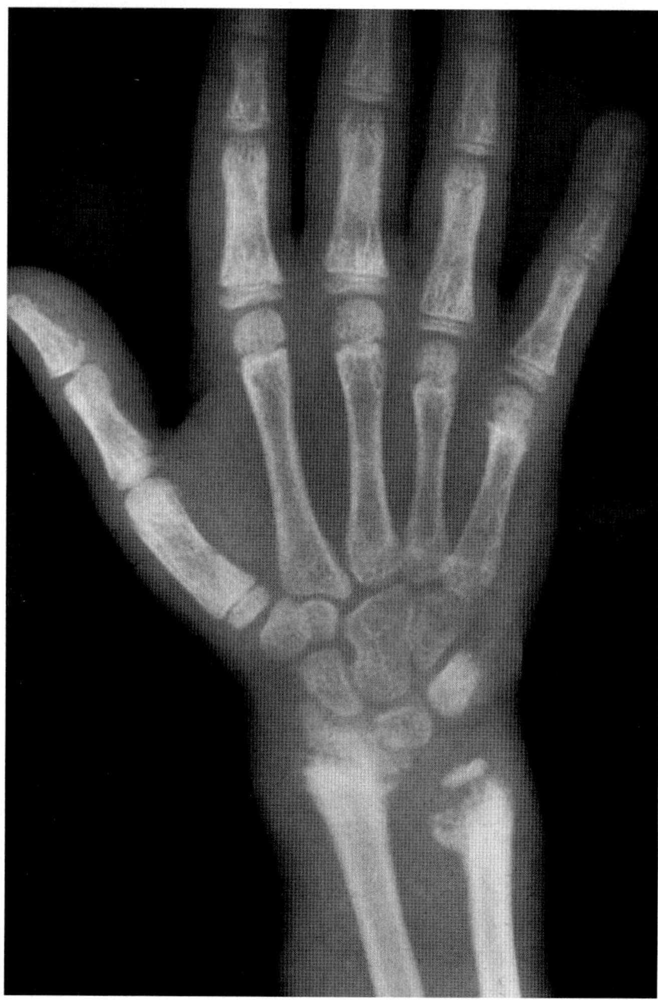

FIGURE 198-7 Diffuse demineralization of the hand bones and severe fraying of the metaphyses of the wrist bones in a child with rickets. (*Used with permission from Cleveland Clinic Children's Hospital Photo Files.*)

- Muscular dystrophy—Patients have proximal muscle weakness and elevated creatinine kinase levels (see Chapter 208, Duchenne Muscular Dystrophy).
- Hypothyroidism—Clinical features of hypothyroidism will be apparent, along with abnormal thyroid function tests (see Chapter 191, Hypothyroidism).
- Polymyositis—Muscle tenderness and typical lab studies will point towards the diagnosis.
- Malignancies (either primary of bone or secondary to bone infiltration)—Appropriate tissue study will reveal the diagnosis.

MANAGEMENT

- Management of the disease depends on the etiology and efforts should be made to educate the family regarding the cause.

NONPHARMACOLOGIC

- For vitamin D deficient rickets, moderate exposure to sunlight can help ameliorate the vitamin D deficiency. This needs to be balanced against the recommendation to keep young infants out of direct sunlight and using protective clothing to limit direct sunlight exposure.

MEDICATIONS

- Patients with vitamin D deficiency (≤37.5 nmol/L) should be treated with ergocalciferol and calcium supplementation as per American Academy of Pediatrics recommendations:[2]
    - Ergocalciferol (Vitamin D2).
        - <1 month—1000 IU/day followed by maintenance with 400 IU/day.
        - One month to 12 months—1000 to 5000 IU/day followed by maintenance with 400 IU/day.
        - >12 months—>5000 IU/day IU/day followed by maintenance with 400 IU/day.
        - In teenagers and adults, 50000 IU/week × 8 weeks.
        - Calcium
        - Thirty to 75 mg/kg per day calcium divided in 3 doses and wean toward lower dose of 30 mg/kg over 2 to 4 weeks.
- Cholecalciferol (vitamin D3), which is commonly used to treat vitamin D deficiency in adults, is three times more potent than ergocalciferol and has been suggested as an alternative for the treatment of vitamin D deficiency in children.[9] However, because of concerns regarding toxicity and the lack of safety data in infants and children, this is not the standard recommended formulation at this time.
- Patients with vitamin D–dependent rickets type 1 can be treated with calcitriol ($1,25(OH)_2$-D) supplementation (0.25 to 2 μg/day) to maintain a low-normal calcium and high-normal PTH (target urinary calcium <4 mg/kg/day).[10]
- Patients with vitamin D–dependent rickets type 2 can be treated with high doses of ergocalciferol, calcidiol, or calcitriol (2 μg/day). If there is no response to treatment, patients can be treated with IV calcium.[10]
- Patients with chronic kidney disease can be treated with calcitriol, a low-phosphate diet, and phosphate binders.[10]
- Dietary deficiency in calcium should be treated with a supplement—For ages 1 to 3: 700 mg/day; ages 4 to 8: 1000 mg/day; ages 9 to 18: 1300 mg/day [2]
- Patients with XLH, ADHR, and autosomal recessive hypophosphatemic rickets should be treated with calcitriol (30 to 70 ng/kg/day divided into two doses) and phosphorus supplementation (1 to 3 g divided into four to five doses).[11]

SURGERY

- If skeletal abnormalities progress without treatment, surgery may be necessary to correct these deformities (e.g., scoliosis).

REFERRAL

- For cases of vitamin D deficiency, refer to pediatric endocrinology if there is no radiographic evidence of healing with current therapy after 3 months of vitamin D and calcium supplementation. Always consider compliance with therapy, concurrent malabsorptive disease, or interactions with other medications (e.g., anticonvulsants, glucocorticoids).
- Refer to pediatric nephrology, if the cause of rickets is renal in nature.
- Refer to pediatric endocrinology, if the cause of rickets is due to a hereditary cause.
- Refer to pediatric gastroenterology, if a malabsorptive process is suspected.

PREVENTION AND SCREENING

- Physicians should have a low index of suspicion to screen for vitamin D deficiency, especially if children are at higher risk or are presenting with poor growth, irritability, and motor delays. Screening involves measurement of serum 25(OH)-D and alkaline phosphatase. If these return normal, but clinical suspicion is high, x-ray of distal ends of the radius and ulna and the tibia and femur should be obtained.[2]
- For exclusively breastfed infants and children not drinking 1L vitamin D–fortified milk daily, supplementation with 400 IU vitamin D should be initiated. Darker-skinned infants at higher latitudes (above 40°) may require 800 IU vitamin D/day.[3] SOR Ⓒ

PROGNOSIS

- In general, children with vitamin D deficiencies or dietary calcium deficiency will respond well to treatment with correction of radiographic abnormalities and clinical symptoms.
- For the hereditary and secondary causes of rickets, prognosis depends on the specific condition.

FOLLOW-UP

- Children with vitamin D deficiency should be monitored as follows:
    - One month—Calcium, phosphorus, and alkaline phosphatase.
    - Three months—Calcium, phosphorus, magnesium, alkaline phosphatase, 25(OH)-D, urine calcium/creatinine, and x-ray.
    - One year and annually—25(OH)-D.
- For all other causes of rickets, patients should follow-up as recommended by pediatric endocrinology or other specialist.

PATIENT EDUCATION

- For patients with vitamin D deficiency, education should be provided regarding the importance of a well-balanced diet with vitamin D fortified milk (including soy-milk), green leafy vegetables (calcium), and adequate dairy products.
- Parents should also be advised on the importance of balancing sun exposure with the risk of skin cancer. While children should be encouraged to play outdoors and participate in outdoor sports, sun protection can be sensibly applied with sunscreens and protective clothing. Sun is still the number one risk factor for skin cancer and photoaging. There are many foods and high quality vitamin

supplements for children that include vitamin D, so there is no reason to send children outside without sun protection to get vitamin D.

PATIENT RESOURCES

- Medline—**www.nlm.nih.gov/medlineplus/rickets.html**.
- **www.healthychildren.org/English/news/Pages/Preterm-Infants-Need-Vitamin-D-and-Calcium-Supplements-Says-AAP.aspx**.
- Vitamin D facts—**http://ods.od.nih.gov/factsheets/VitaminD-QuickFacts**.
- Calcium facts—**http://ods.od.nih.gov/factsheets/Calcium-QuickFacts**.
- Information for healthy diet—**www.choosemyplate.gov/food-groups/downloads/MyPlate/DG2010Brochure.pdf**.

PROVIDER RESOURCES

- **http://pediatrics.aappublications.org/content/122/2/398.long**.
- **http://pediatrics.aappublications.org/content/122/5/1142.long**.

REFERENCES

1. Wharton B, Bishop N. Rickets. *Lancet.* 2003;362:1389-1400.
2. Misra M, Pacaud D, Petryk A, Collett-Solberg PF, Kappy M. Drug and Therapeutics Committee of the Lawson Wilkins Pediatric Endocrine Society. Vitamin D deficiency in children and its management: review of current knowledge and recommendations. *Pediatrics.* 2008;122(2):398-417.
3. Wagner CL, Greer FR. American Academy of Pediatrics Section on Breastfeeding, American Academy of Pediatrics Committee on Nutrition. Prevention of rickets and vitamin D deficiency in infants, children, and adolescents. *Pediatrics.* 2008;122(5):1142-1152.
4. Weisberg P, Scanlon KS, Li R, Cogswell ME. Nutritional rickets among children in the United States: review of cases reported between 1986 and 2003. *Am J Clin Nutr.* 2004;80(6):1697S-705S.
5. Rovner AJ, O'Brien KO. Hypovitaminosis d among healthy children in the united states: A review of the current evidence. *Arch Pediatr Adolesc Med.* 2008;162(6):513-519.
6. Tenenhouse HS. X-linked hypophosphataemia: a homologous disorder in humans and mice. *Nephrol Dial Transplant.* 1999;14(2):333-341.
7. Renkema KY, Alexander RT, Bindels RJ, Hoenderop JG. Calcium and phosphate homeostasis: concerted interplay of new regulators. *Ann Med.* 2008;40(2):82-91.
8. Cheng JB, Levine MA, Bell NH, et al. Genetic evidence that human CYPR1 enzyme is a key vitamin D 25-hydroxylase. *Proc Natl Acad Sci.* 2004;101:7711-7715.
9. Gordon CM, Williams AL, Feldman HA, May J, Sinclari L, Vasquez A, Cox JE. Treatment of hypovitaminosis D in infants and toddlers. *J Clin Endocrinol Metab.* 2008;93(7):2716-2721.
10. Demay MB. Rickets caused by impaired vitamin D activation and hormone resistance: pseudovitamin D deficiency rickets and hereditary vitamin D-resistant rickets. In: Favus MJ, ed. *Primer on the Metabolic Bone Diseases and Disorders of Mineral Metabolism*, 6th ed. Washington, DC: American Society for Bone and Mineral Research; 2006:338-341.
11. Makitie O, Doria A, Kooh SW, et al. Early treatment improves growth and biochemical and radiographic outcome in X-linked hypophosphatemic rickets. *J Clin Endocrinol Metab.* 2003;88:3591-3597.

199 DELAYED PUBERTY

Elumalai Appachi, MD, MRCP

PATIENT STORY

A 14-year-old boy with an unremarkable medical history presents to his pediatrician with concerns about his short height and lack of pubertal development as compared to his peers. His father relates to the pediatrician that he was a "late bloomer." His height has been progressing along the 5th percentile and his weight has been at the 10th percentile. His physical exam reveals Tanner stage 1 and prepubertal sized testes, but is otherwise normal. The pediatrician makes the diagnosis of constitutional delay of growth and puberty, reviews the expected growth and development with the family, and recommends watchful waiting (**Figure 199-1**). The boy begins spontaneous sexual development at 15 years of age and his growth velocity increases shortly thereafter.

INTRODUCTION

Delayed puberty is defined as a lack of initiation of secondary sexual development in boys 14 years or older and in girls 13 years or older. The majority of boys with delayed puberty have constitutional delay of growth and puberty (CDGP), defined on the basis of a normal physical examination and a growth chart showing short stature but normal growth velocity. Pathologic delayed puberty may be due to primary endocrine disorders such as gonadal failure, isolated gonadotrophic deficiency, panhypopituitarism, or chronic underlying diseases.

EPIDEMIOLOGY

- CDGP is the single most common cause of delayed puberty in both sexes, but it can be diagnosed only after any underlying pathologic causes have been ruled out.[1]
- CDGP occurs more commonly in boys than in girls.
- Hypergonadotrophic hypogonadism, also known as primary gonadal failure, is more common in girls.
- Competitive swimmers, gymnasts, and ballet dancers are at high risk for functional hypogonadotrophic hypogonadism.

ETIOLOGY AND PATHOPHYSIOLOGY

- CDGP represents the single most common cause of delayed puberty in both sexes. The cause is unknown but a genetic predisposition with an autosomal dominant effect as well as environmental modifiers is likely.[1–3]
- Causes of hypergonadotrophic hypogonadism include Turner syndrome, gonadal dysgenesis, chemotherapy, or radiation therapy to testes or ovaries, and autoimmune ovarian function. The diagnosis is based on demonstrating very high levels of Follicle stimulating hormone (FSH).
- Functional hypogonadotrophic hypogonadism (FHH) occurs in 20 percent of boys and girls referred for delayed puberty. Underlying conditions include eating disorders (anorexia or bulimia) and other chronic systemic illnesses such as inflammatory bowel disease, celiac disease, cystic fibrosis, and hypothyroidism. Excessive exercise is a relatively common cause of delayed menarche in girls. Although body fat is decreased in those affected, BMI is often in the normal range because of an increase in muscle mass.
- Permanent hypogonadotrophic hypogonadism (PHH) is diagnosed in 10 percent of boys and 20 percent of girls with delayed puberty. Two types occur: (1) Isolated gonadotrophin deficiency (IGD) or (2) Multiple pituitary hormone deficiencies (MPHD).[2,3]
  - Most boys who have not had spontaneous pubertal development by 18 years or girls by 16 years have PHH, if they do not have risk factors for FHH.
  - About half of boys with delayed puberty due to PPH also have defective smell (anosmia or hyposmia), which is called Kallman syndrome. The most common form is due to a mutation in a gene on the X chromosome.
  - Acquired MPHD is caused by tumors of the hypothalamic-pituitary axis or a head and neck tumor requiring radiation therapy with the pituitary gland in field of radiation. Rarely an infiltrative process such as Langerhans cell histiocytosis can be a cause of acquired MPHD.

RISK FACTORS

- Genetic factors—Fifty to seventy-five percent of children with CDGP has at least one parent with pubertal delay and inheritance is often autosomal dominant.[1]
- Decreased body fat in girls is a common risk factor associated with pubertal delay.
- Excessive exercise.
- Chronic illness and obesity are implicated in some cases of pubertal delay.

DIAGNOSIS

- Health maintenance visits are opportunities to screen children and teenagers about eating habits, pubertal delay and chronic illnesses. A complete physical examination including Tanner staging of breast development in girls and genital development in boys must be done.
- Accurate measurement of plotting of height and weight during each visit is important.
- A diagnostic approach to the evaluation of delayed puberty is provided in **Figure 199-2**.
- Since CDGP is less common in girls, they may need more diagnostic testing, especially to rule out primary gonadal failure.

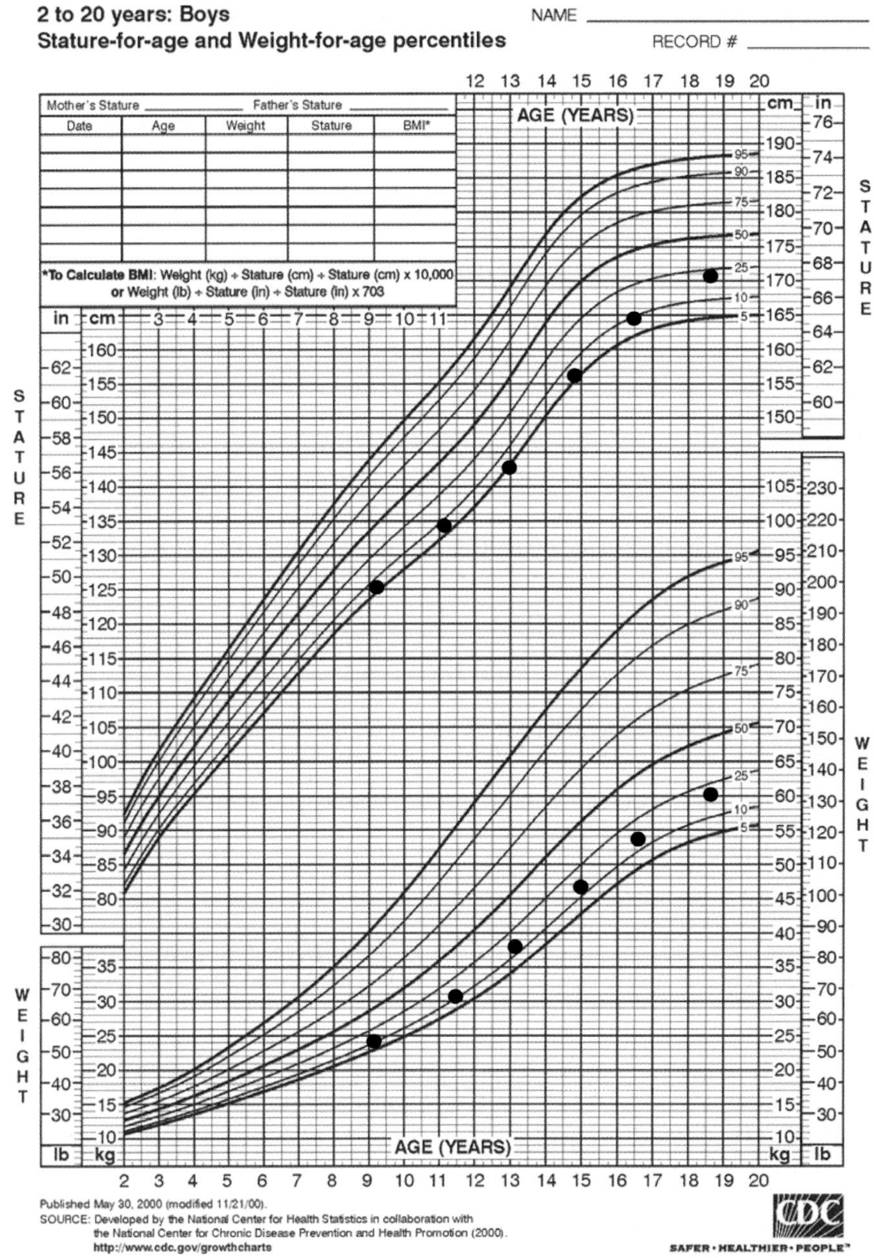

FIGURE 199-1 Growth chart of a boy with classic constitutional delay in growth and puberty (CDGP). (*Used with permission from Camille Sabella, MD.*)

CLINICAL FEATURES

- Most boys with CDGP grow below the 10th percentile on the growth chart but have normal growth velocity of 4 to 6 cm per year (**Figure 199-1**).
- Turner syndrome should be considered in girls who have decreased growth velocity and have delayed puberty (**Figure 199-3**). High arched palate, webbing of neck, shield-like chest, and wide spaced nipples are the most common associated findings (**Figure 199-4**).
- Presence of goiter in neck may indicate hypothyroidism.
- Absence of fat stores in abdomen may suggest chronic illness or an eating disorder or may be due to high level of exercise.
- Presence of pubic hair does not rule out delayed puberty as this reflects adrenal androgen secretion. Girls who have not had menarche within 3 years of breast development require an evaluation for delayed puberty.

LABORATORY TESTING

- Blood tests that assess the activity of pituitary-gonadal axis (luteinizing hormone [LH]), FSH for all and testosterone in boys and

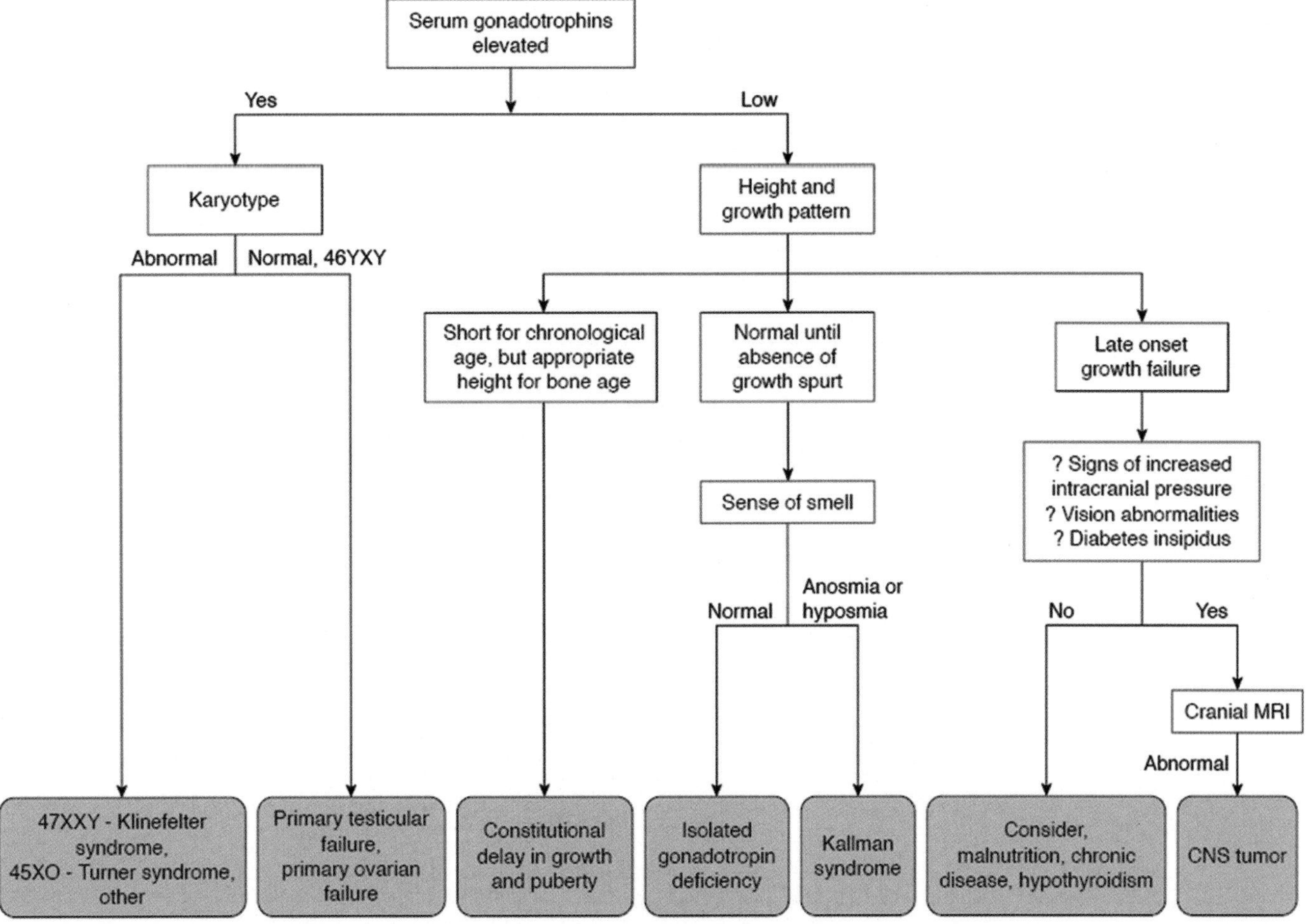

FIGURE 199-2 Diagnostic evaluation of delayed puberty among boys at 14 years and girls at 13 years. (*Used with permission from Rudolph CD, Rudolph AM, Lister GE, First LR, Gershon AA: Rudolph's Pediatrics, 22nd edition: www.accesspediatrics.com. Figure 541-4.*)

estradiol in girls) may be indicated depending on the specific clinical features.[3]

- CBC, CMP, Thyroid function tests and screening for celiac disease and cystic fibrosis are useful testing for children with underlying chronic illness.

IMAGING

- Bone age radiograph of left hand and wrist is often helpful to differentiate benign from pathologic short stature and to predict adult height.

DIFFERENTIAL DIAGNOSIS

- The causes and evaluation of delayed puberty are summarized in **Figure 199-2**.

MANAGEMENT

- Psychosocial support and reassurance should be provided for adolescents with CDGP.
- Expectant observation for puberty to start spontaneously is one option, especially if the child is not distressed about his or her delayed development or short stature.
- Many teenagers, particularly boys, are impatient for puberty to start and can be offered a brief course of sex steroids (intramuscular testosterone for boys and oral estradiol for girls) to trigger growth spurt and pubertal development. This is a safe and effective approach that appears to have no negative impact on adult height.[4,5]
    - The largest published randomized trial of testosterone for CDGP was done in Egypt and included 148 boys aged 14 to 18 years who were given monthly injections of testosterone enanthate for 6 months and a control group of 50 untreated patients. Both groups had a final evaluation at 12 months, at which time the treated group had a more advanced growth rate, more advanced genital development, and a larger mean testicular diameter, than the control group. All of the treated boys, but only 40 percent of the untreated boys, reported satisfaction with the result.[6]
    - A randomized, placebo-controlled trial involving 40 patients with constitutional delay of growth and puberty treated with placebo or oxandrolone for 1 year reported that the treated group grew an average of 9.5 cm versus 6.8 cm in the placebo group and gained 2.4 kg more weight.[7]
- Children with clinical and laboratory evidence of PHH, MPHD, or primary gonadal failure can be treated with long-term sex steroid replacement with escalation of doses over a 2 year period.[8]

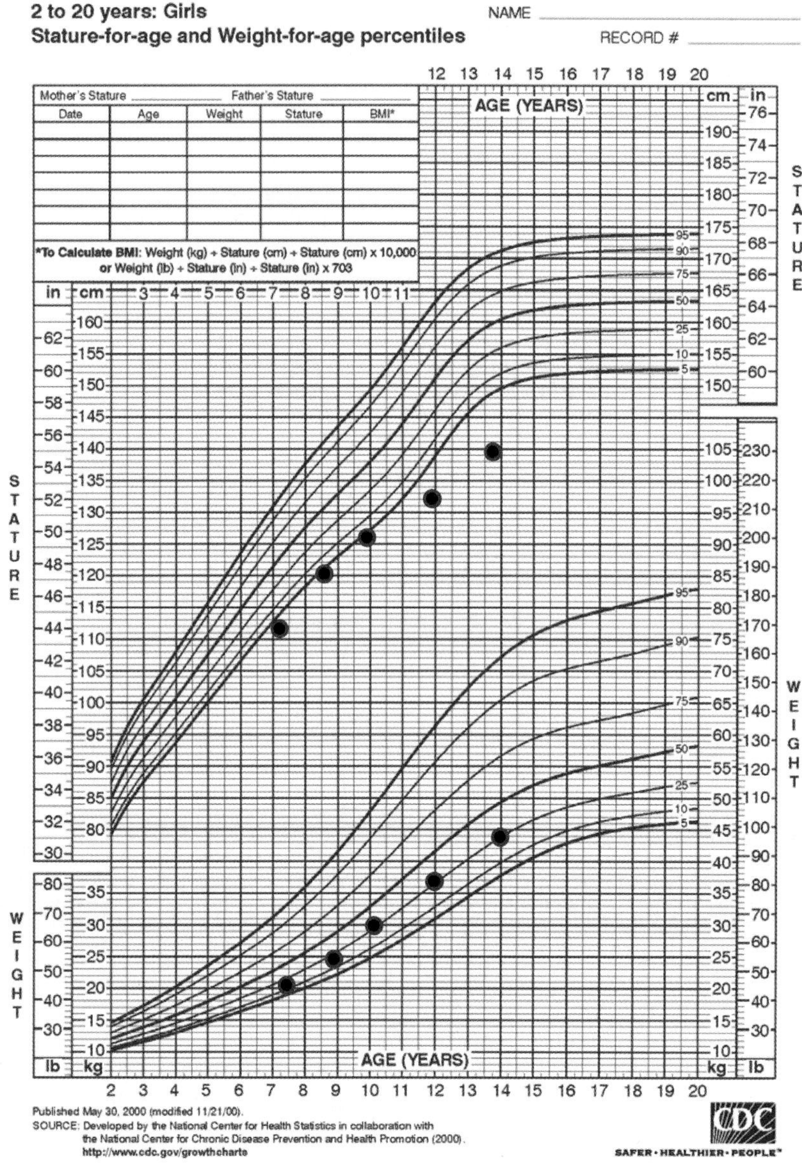

OK135S058

FIGURE 199-3 Growth chart of a girl with Turner syndrome who has delayed puberty. Note the decrease in growth velocity, which is characteristic of a pathologic etiology. (*Used with permission from Camille Sabella, MD.*)

- Patients with chronic illnesses causing pubertal delay may need ongoing treatment with sex steroids to maximize nutrition and development.

CONSULTATION

- Patients with the following clinical scenarios should be referred to an endocrinologist for further evaluation:
  - Boys who have not started puberty by age 16 to 17 years old, as they are less likely to have CDGP.
  - Boys who have CDGP but do not start puberty within 6 months of receiving testosterone therapy.
  - Girls who have not started puberty by age 14 or 15 years or who have gonadal failure or elevated FSH levels.
  - Boys and girls with pubertal delay and severe short stature or growth failure.

FOLLOW-UP

- Close monitoring of children who have CGDP and not on treatment, to make sure that they are still growing appropriately and to verify that puberty is progressing (breast enlargement in girl; penis and testicular enlargement in boys).
- Boys receiving testosterone injections should be monitored closely for pubertal changes.

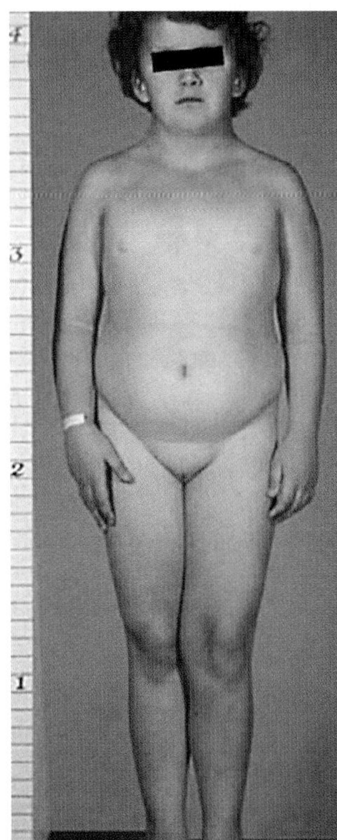

FIGURE 199-4 Delayed puberty in a girl with Turner syndrome. Note the short stature, broad shield like chest, wide spaced nipples, and mild webbing of the neck. (*Used with permission from Cleveland Clinic Children's Hospital Photo Files.*)

PROGNOSIS

- Children with CGDP will eventually attain puberty after prolonged follow-up or more quickly after a brief course of sex steroids.
- Boys and girls with primary gonadal failure based on absent gonads or history of gonadal failure and supported by increased FSH levels will generally need long term sex steroid replacement. They will usually grow well and develop appropriate secondary sexual characteristics but are unlikely to be fertile.

PATIENT EDUCATION

- Families of boys with delayed puberty likely due to CDGP should be reassured that the condition is a variation of normal development and that, in most cases, it resolves with time.
- If the child is healthy, diagnostic testing can be limited to bone age radiograph to reassure the family and patient that there is still ample time to grow.
- A brief course of testosterone injections can provide early boost in growth and jump start puberty for boys anxious to start growing and developing sooner.
- If the patient is very thin, athletic, anorexic or with chronic illness, the family may be advised that puberty is likely to progress if the child is able to gain significant weight.

PATIENT RESOURCES

- **www.healthychildren.org/English/ages-stages/gradeschool/puberty/Pages/Delayed-Puberty.aspx.**
- **http://children.webmd.com/growth-delay-constitutional.**
- **http://kidshealth.org/teen/sexual_health/changing_body/delayed_puberty.html.**

PROVIDER RESOURCES

- **www.nejm.org/doi/full/10.1056/NEJMcp1109290.**
- **www.ncbi.nlm.nih.gov/pubmed/11932291.**

REFERENCES

1. Sedlmeyer IL, Palmert MR: Delayed puberty: analysis of a large case series from an academic center. *J Clin Endocrinol Metab*. 2002;87:1613-1620.
2. Kaplowitz PB: Delayed puberty. *Pediatr Rev*. 2010;31:189-195.
3. Palmert MR, Dunkel L: Clinical practice. Delayed puberty. *N Engl J Med*. 2012;366:443-453.
4. Harrington J, Palmert MR: Clinical review: Distinguishing constitutional delay of growth and puberty from isolated hypogonadotropic hypogonadism: critical appraisal of available diagnostic tests. *J Clin Endocrinol Metab*. 2012;97:3056-3067.
5. Crowne EC, Shalet SM, Wallace WH, Eminson DM, Price DA: Final height in boys with untreated constitutional delay in growth and puberty. *Arch Dis Child*. 1990;65:1109-1112.
6. Soliman A, Abdul Khadir MM, Asfour M: Testosterone treatment in adolescent boys with constitutional delay of growth and puberty. *Metabolism*. 1995;44:1013-1015.
7. Wilson DM, McCauley E, Brown DR, et al. Oxandrolone therapy in constitutionally delayed growth and puberty. *Pediatrics* 1995; 96:1095-1100.
8. Richman RA, Kirsch LR: Testosterone treatment in adolescent boys with constitutional delay in growth and development. *N Engl J Med*. 1988;319:1563-1567.

200 PRECOCIOUS PUBERTY

Elumalai Appachi, MD, MRCP

PATIENT STORY

A 4-year-old Caucasian girl presents to her pediatrician because of early development of breast buds, pubic hair, and body odor. On exam, the girl is noted to have Tanner stage 3 breast buds and pubic hair. She is also noted to have clitoromegaly (**Figure 200-1**). The pediatrician refers the girl to a pediatric endocrinologist, who orders a bone age, estradiol levels, and an MRI of the brain. The girl is found to have an advanced bone age of 7 years, and levels of estradiol consistent with her stage of sexual development. An MRI of the brain is normal. She is diagnosed with idiopathic central precocious puberty. The options for management are discussed with the family.

INTRODUCTION

The age at which puberty begins in normal children varies among the different ethnic groups. Early, or precocious puberty, is defined as the onset of sexual development occurring before the age of 7 years in Caucasian girls, 6 years in African American girls, and 9 years for all boys. Central precocious puberty refers to gonadotropin-releasing hormone (GnRH)-dependent activation from the hypothalamic-pituitary-gonadal axis leading to secondary sexual characteristics. Peripheral precocious puberty refers to GnRH-independent activation.

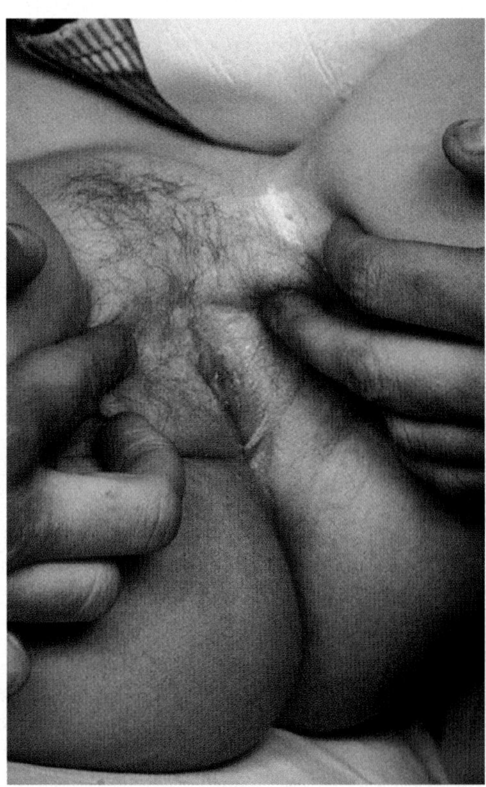

FIGURE 200-1 Pubic hair development and clitoromegaly in a 4-year-old girl with central idiopathic precocious puberty. (*Used with permission from Elumalai Appachi, MD.*)

SYNONYMS

Early puberty.

EPIDEMIOLOGY

- The incidence is estimated to be 15 to 30 per 100,000 girls and is 1- to 15-fold less common on boys.[1,2]
- Idiopathic precocious puberty is more common in girls than boys.
- African American girls develop secondary sexual characteristics at an earlier age than Caucasian girls. Thus, age of evaluation of precocious puberty in girls depends on ethnicity and race.
- Boys mature at comparable ages regardless of ethnicity and race.
- Age of onset of precocious puberty varies depending on the etiology; it can present as early as the first month of life.

ETIOLOGY AND PATHOPHYSIOLOGY

Central or GnRH-dependent precocious puberty may be idiopathic or may be caused by a central nervous system (CNS) abnormality.[3,4]

- Precocious puberty is idiopathic in more than 90 percent of girls. This diagnosis is one of exclusion, in that no clinical, biochemical, or radiologic abnormalities are present other than those of precocious puberty.
- Boys with precocious puberty have an idiopathic cause much less commonly than girls; CNS abnormalities are found in 25 to 75 percent of boys with precocious puberty.
- The most common CNS abnormality causing precocious puberty is a hypothalamic hamartoma. This is a GnRH-producing nonmalignant congenital mass that causes pulsatile secretion of gonadotropins leading to stimulation of the gonads during childhood.[5]
- Other structural CNS abnormalities include tumors such as pinealoma, astrocytoma, ganglioneuroma, ependymoma, and optic glioma, or congenital malformations such as ventricular and arachnoid cysts.
- Neurofibromatosis and tuberous sclerosis, as well as CNS insults such as acute head injury, hydrocephalus, CNS infection, or cranial radiation therapy can cause central precocious puberty.

Causes of GnRH-independent precocious puberty include:[6]

- McCune Albright syndrome—More common in girls. Caused by constitutive somatic activation mutations in the GNAS1 gene encoding the α-subunit of the stimulatory G-protein resulting in autonomous hypersecretion of hormones. It may be associated with other endocrine abnormalities including hyperthyroidism, hypercortisolism, hypersomatotropism, and hypophosphatemia.
- Ovarian tumors and cysts may cause isosexual (changes appropriate for same sex) or heterosexual (changes appropriate for opposite sex) pubertal changes.

- Testicular tumors, such as a testosterone secreting Leydig cell tumor, may manifest as isosexual precocious puberty in young boys.
- Familial male-limited GnRH-independent pseudoprecocious puberty Otherwise known as testotoxicosis. Caused by a luteinizing hormone receptor-activating mutation resulting in significant enlargement of penis without enlargement of testes.
- Congenital adrenal hyperplasia—Occurs in both boys and girls is caused by a deficiency of either CYP21A2 (21-hydroxylase), CYP11B1 (11β-hydroxylase), or 3β-HSD enzyme. Can presents in early childhood with bone age advancement; usually isosexual in boys and manifests as pubic hair development, acne, body odor, and increased penis size without testicular enlargement; usually heterosexual (virilizing features) in girls.
- Adrenocortical tumors—Occurs in both boys and girls; usually isosexual in boys and heterosexual (virilizing) in girls.
- Ectopic human chorionic gonadotropin (hCG)—Secreting tumors such as chorioblastoma, hepatoblastoma, germinoma of the pineal gland. Mainly occur in boys and result in testosterone production in the testes.
- Exogenous estrogen—Can result from oral (contraceptive pills or anabolic steroids) or topical agents. Estrogens are readily absorbed through the skin, so estrogens in cosmetics, hair creams, and breast-augmentation creams can cause breast development in girls and gynecomastia in boys.
- Severe long standing hypothyroidism can cause early puberty in boys and girls.

RISK FACTORS

- CNS insults.
- Positive family history.
- Obesity.
- Adopted child status from a developing country—Maybe due to early malnutrition followed by normal or excessive nutrition with resultant advancement of pubertal age.

DIAGNOSIS

- A careful history and physical examination should provide helpful clues as to the etiology and guide the evaluation. Tanner (sexual maturation rating) charts should be used to stage pubertal development.

CLINICAL FEATURES

- Breast buds or pubic hair development before the age of 7 years in Caucasian girls or age 6 years in African American girls, or the onset of menarche before age 9 years are the signs of early puberty.
  - The first sign of early puberty in girls is breast development; pubic hair may appear simultaneously, but more often appears later. Maturation of the external genitals, the appearance of axillary hair, and the onset of menstruation follow. Clitoromegaly may be present. The early menstrual cycles may be more irregular than with normal puberty (**Figure 200-1**).

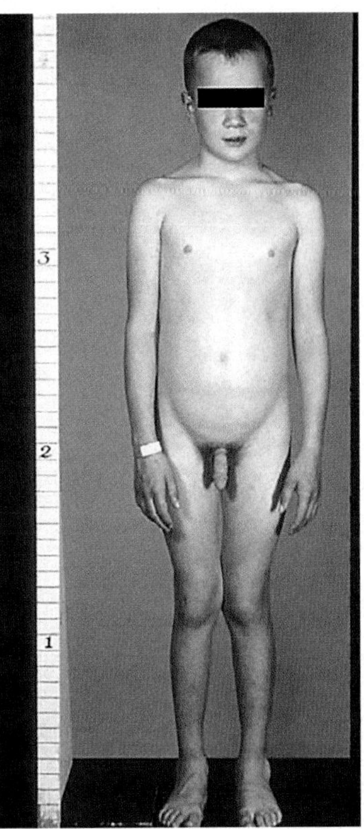

FIGURE 200-2 Enlargement of the penis and pubic hair development in a 5-year-old boy with precocious puberty. (*Used with permission from Cleveland Clinic Children's Hospital Photo Files.*)

- Testicular enlargement or pubic hair development before the age of 9 years are signs of early puberty in boys (**Figures 200-2** and **200-3**).
  - Enlargement of the testes is followed by enlargement of the penis, appearance of pubic hair, and acne. Erections are common and nocturnal emissions may occur. The voice deepens and linear growth is accelerated.
  - In boys with central precocious puberty testicular size is disproportionately greater than penile size. In peripheral precocious puberty penile dimensions are disproportionately greater than testicular size.
- Height velocity is increased during sexual maturation, but final adult height is reduced owing to premature fusion of epiphyses (tall child but short adult).
- Body odor, acne, and emotional lability may occur.
- Headaches and visual disturbances may accompany signs of puberty if a CNS abnormality is the cause.
- If hypothyroidism is the cause, intolerance of cold, fatigue, increased sleepiness, hair and skin changes, and constipation may be present.
- Signs of a specific etiology may be present:
  - Myxedema in hypothyroidism.
  - Café-au-lait spots in neurofibromatosis.
  - McCune Albright syndrome—Average age of onset of precocious puberty in affected girls is 3 years and may present with breast development and vaginal bleeding. Patients have café-au-lait macules and fibrous dysplasia of the skeletal system.

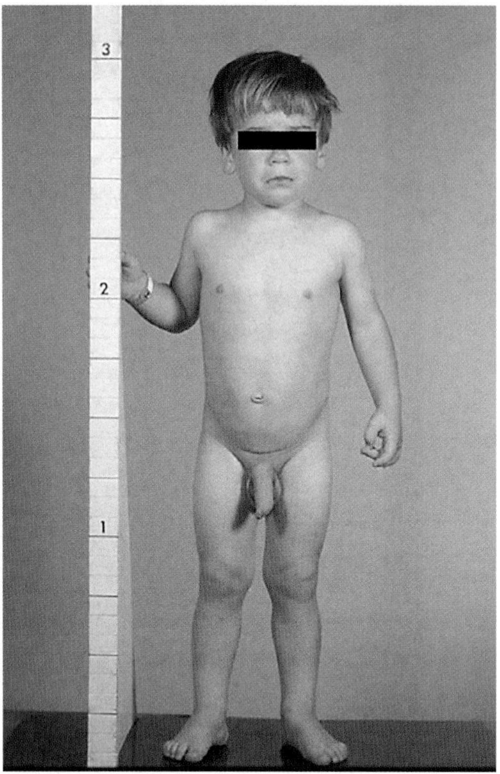

FIGURE 200-3 Enlarged penis and testes in a 2-year-old boy with precocious puberty. (*Used with permission from Cleveland Clinic Children's Hospital Photo Files.*)

LABORATORY TESTING

- Basal luteinizing hormone levels, follicle-stimulating hormone (FSH) levels, and sex hormone (serum testosterone in boys, serum estradiol in girls) levels are generally determined.
  - Luteinizing hormone and FSH measurements fluctuate and must be interpreted in relation to clinical findings, bone age, and sex hormone levels. Single determinations are usually inadequate.
  - Gonadotropin-releasing hormone (GnRH) stimulation test with measurement of gonadotropin (luteinizing hormone, FSH) and gonadal hormones (estradiol in girls; testosterone in boys) are generally more useful than single random measurements.
  - In precocious puberty, serum levels of testosterone and estradiol are appropriate for the child's level of sexual development but not appropriate for the chronological age.
- Thyroid hormone levels should be obtained if hypothyroidism is suspected.
- Dehydroepiandrostenedione sulfate, androstenedione, and 17-hydroxyprogesterone levels should be obtained if adrenal pathology is suspected.
- Serum hCG levels should be obtained if an hCG-producing tumor is suspected.

IMAGING

- Bone age radiographs should be obtained in cases of precocious puberty and will be advanced (usually by more than 2 years) for chronologic age in children who have true precocious puberty.
- MRI of the head is required to rule out organic causes of central precocious puberty. This should be done in all boys and girls less than 6 years of age.
- Pelvic and abdominal ultrasound or CT scan can be obtained to evaluate the adrenal glands and ovaries for tumors and cysts if non-central precocious puberty is suspected based on the physical exam.

DIFFERENTIAL DIAGNOSIS

Premature thelarche—A benign process in which there is early breast development, but without any other features of puberty such as pubic or axillary hair, or linear growth acceleration (**Figure 200-4**). Typically in girls aged 1to 4 years. Bone age is not advanced.

Premature adrenarche—A benign process in which there is isolated pubic or axillary hair and odor, but without any other evidence of virilization. Bone age may be slightly, but not significantly, advanced.

Premature menarche—Isolated menstruation (usually one or two periods) without any other manifestations of puberty. This is a benign process of unclear etiology.

- Transient condition of isolated breast development that most often appears in the first 2 years of life; in some girls breast development is present at birth and persists.
- Growth and osseous maturation are normal or slightly advanced.
- The genitals show no evidence of estrogenic stimulation.

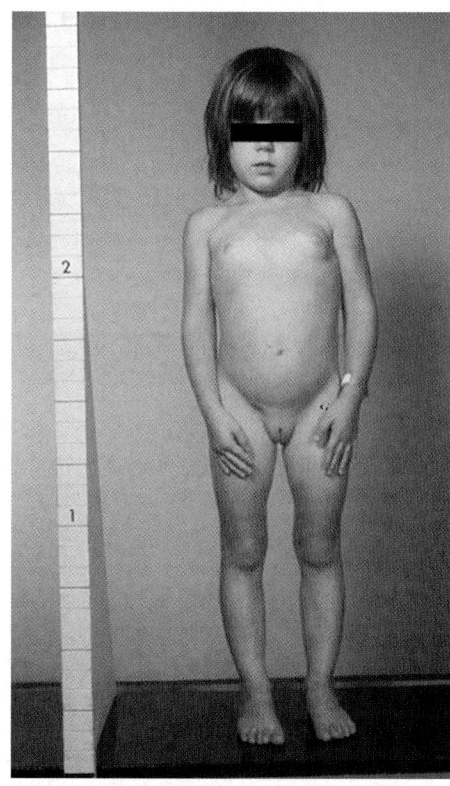

FIGURE 200-4 Premature thelarche (early breast buds) in a 2-year-old girl who has no other signs of sexual development or puberty. (*Used with permission from Cleveland Clinic Children's Hospital Photo Files.*)

- Breast development may regress after 2 years, although it often persists for 3 to 5 years and is rarely progressive.
- Menarche occurs at the expected age and reproduction is normal.
- The serum concentrations of FSH, luteinizing hormone, and estradiol are generally low and not diagnostic.
- Luteinizing hormone response to GnRHa stimulation is prepubertal.
- Ovarian and uterine volume on ultrasound is prepubertal.
- A benign condition, but 10 percent of cases progress to central precocious puberty, so continued observation is important.
- Isolated appearance of sexual hair and, less commonly, body odor or acne without other signs of puberty or virilization before the age of 7 years in white girls, 6 years in black girls, or 9 years in boys without other evidence of maturation.
- More frequent in girls than in boys and may occur more frequently in black girls than in other patients.
- Hair appears on the mons and labia majora in girls and on perineal and scrotal area in boys; axillary hair generally appears later. It is more frequent in children with CNS abnormalities.
- Independent of gonadal development.
- Affected children are slightly advanced in height and osseous maturation.
- Adrenal androgens (dehydroepiandrostenedione sulfate, androstenedione) level may be slightly elevated, but appropriate for pubic Tanner stage.
- A benign condition that requires no therapy; however, long-term follow-up suggests that girls with premature adrenarche are at a higher risk (20%) for hyperinsulinism, metabolic syndrome, hyperandrogenism, and polycystic ovarian syndrome as adults.

MANAGEMENT

- Management depends on the underlying cause and should focus on delaying sexual maturation until the normal age of onset of puberty, and prevent short stature in adulthood by delaying the premature epiphyseal fusion.
- Psychologic support is important for the child and family.
- Children with exogenous hormone intake usually respond well when the source is removed.
- Functional ovarian cysts are benign and usually regress spontaneously without treatment.

MEDICATIONS

- GnRH analogs are the mainstay of treatment for central precocious puberty. These drugs provide constant serum concentrations of GnRH activity, which in turn overrides the pulsatility of endogenous GnRH.[7–10] SOR Ⓐ
- The most widely used analog is Leuprolide acetate, which is administered by injection or subcutaneous implant. Injections are painful and a common complication is the development of sterile abscesses.
- The greatest height benefit of GnRH analog therapy has occurred in children who have been diagnosed before age 6 years. These patients achieved a mean height gain of 8.2 cm versus a gain of 4.2 cm in patients who were diagnosed and underwent treatment between ages 6 and 8 years. With GnRH analog treatment, the adult height of children with central precocious puberty is 8 to 12 cm greater than before the therapy was introduced.[8–10]
- GnRH agonists are also used to manage hypothalamic hamartomas, as these congenital lesions generally do not require surgery.[5]
- Children with Gonadotropin-independent peripheral precocious puberty do not respond to GnRH agonist therapy. Treatment of these children relies on eliminating the underlying cause of estrogen or androgen excess.
- Corticosteroids are indicated for congenital adrenal hyperplasia (see Chapter 197, Congenital Adrenal Hyperplasia).
- The treatment of McCune-Albright Syndrome is challenging. Trials using aromatase inhibition or partial estrogen receptor blockade have been conducted. Most of the agents have shown inadequate efficacy or have been associated with increased ovarian or uterine size.[10]
- Supplemental calcium and vitamin D to the treatment of central precocious puberty may help preserve bone mass density. SOR Ⓒ

SURGERY

- CNS tumors may require surgical removal depending on the location, size, and type of lesion.
- Testicular, adrenal, and ovarian tumors are generally removed surgically.
- hCG-secreting tumors may be treated with a combination of surgery, radiation and chemotherapy.

REFERRAL

- A pediatric endocrinologist should be involved in the evaluation and treatment of children with precocious puberty.

PREVENTION AND SCREENING

- Routine health maintenance visits with attention to growth and sexual maturation are important in detecting early puberty.

PROGNOSIS

- Prognosis depends on the primary etiology.
- Treatment of central precocious puberty results in enhancement of the predicted height, although the actual adult height of patients followed to epiphyseal closure is approximately one standard deviation below the midparental height.
- Therapeutic failure may occur if GnRH analog pulses are not adequately suppressed because of noncompliance, inappropriate dose, or frequency of administration.

FOLLOW-UP

- In the first few months of GnRH analog treatment, frequent follow-up is required to ensure suppression of the hypothalamic-pituitary-gonadal axis, tolerance to the medication, and adherence to the medication regimen.
- The frequency of follow-up depends on age, etiology, and progression of the problem.
- Hormonal assays and bone age need to be reviewed every 3 to 12 months.

PATIENT RESOURCES

- **http://kidshealth.org/PageManager.jsp?article_set=22543&lic=410&cat_id=10008**.
- **www.ncbi.nlm.nih.gov/pubmedhealth/PMH0002152**.
- **www.everydayhealth.com/kids-health/a-parents-guide-to-precocious-puberty.aspx**.

PROVIDER RESOURCES

- **http://emedicine.medscape.com/article/924002-overview**.
- **http://omim.org/entry/176400**.

REFERENCES

1. Muir A. Precocious puberty. *Pediatr Rev*. 2006;27:373-381.
2. Carel JC, Léger J. Clinical practice: Precocious puberty. *N Eng J Med.* 2008;358;2366-2377.
3. Kaplowitz P. Clinical characteristics of 104 children referred for evaluation of precocious puberty. *J Clin Endocrinol Metab*. 2004; 89:3644-3650.
4. Cesario SK, Hughes LA. Precocious puberty: a comprehensive review of literature. *J Obstet Gynecol Neonatal Nurs*. 2007;36: 263-274.
5. Maixner W. Hypothalamic hamartomas—Clinical, neuropathological and surgical aspects. *Childs Nerv Syst*. 2006;22:867-873.
6. Stephen MD, Zage PE, Waguespack SG. Gonadotropin dependent precocious puberty: neoplastic causes and endocrine considerations. *Int J Pediatr Endocrinol*. 2011;2011:184502.
7. Carel JC, Eugster EA, Rogol A, et al. Consensus statement on the use of gonadotropin-releasing hormone analogs in children. *Pediatrics*. 2009;123:e752-62.
8. Fuld K, Chi C, Neely EK. A randomized trial of 1- and 3-month depot leuprolide doses in the treatment of central precocious puberty. *J Pediatr*. 2011;159:982-987.
9. Eugster EA, Clarke W, Kletter GB, et al. Efficacy and safety of histrelin subdermal implant in children with precocious puberty: a multicenter trial. *J Clin Endocrinol Metab* 2007;92:1697-1704.
10. John SF. Treatment and outcomes of Precocious puberty. *J Clin Endocrinol Metab* 2013, 98(6):2198-2007.

PART 18

NEUROLOGY

Strength of Recommendation (SOR)	Definition
A	Recommendation based on consistent and good-quality patient-oriented evidence.*
B	Recommendation based on inconsistent or limited-quality patient-oriented evidence.*
C	Recommendation based on consensus, usual practice, opinion, disease-oriented evidence, or case series for studies of diagnosis, treatment, prevention, or screening.*

*See Appendix A on pages 1320–1322 for further information.

201 HEADACHE

Heidi Chumley, MD

PATIENT STORY

A 15-year-old girl presented to the office with her mother to discuss her migraines. She has episodic unilateral throbbing headaches accompanied by nausea, photophobia, and phonophobia. She also reports a visual prodrome, characterized by a jagged line pattern (**Figure 201-1**). She used to have a migraine about every 3 months, but is now having one almost every week. She misses a day of school with each migraine. She is not under any unusual stressors. Her mother has migraines and benefitted greatly from taking a prophylactic medication.

INTRODUCTION

More than 50 percent of children report a headache in the past year. Headaches are either primary or secondary and the presence or absence of red flags is useful to distinguish dangerous causes of secondary headaches. The most common primary headaches are tension and migraine headaches. Medication overuse can complicate headache therapy. Treatment and prognosis is dependent on type of headache.

EPIDEMIOLOGY

- Prevalence of headache in children increases during childhood, peaking between ages 11 and 13.
- Fifty-three percent of children have had a headache in the past year.[1]

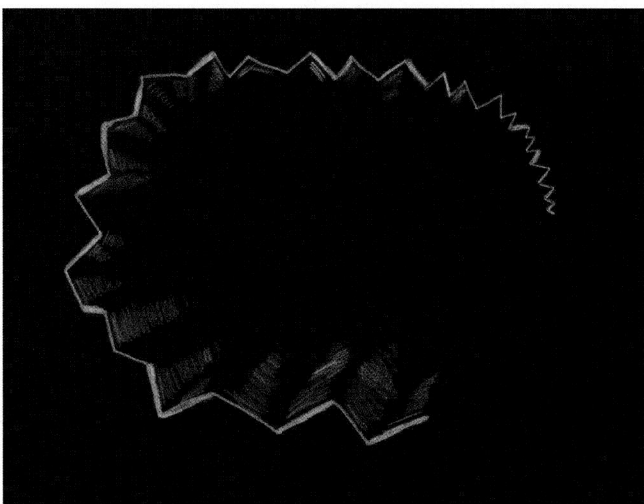

FIGURE 201-1 Jagged line pattern prodrome often described in patients with migraine headaches. This is called teichopsia and may resemble the fortification pattern of a medieval town. *(Used with permission from Richard P. Usatine, MD.)*

- Episodic tension-type headache (TTH) prevalence is 15.9 percent in children.[1]
- Chronic (>15 days per month) TTH has a prevalence of 0.9 percent in children.[1]
- Migraine has a prevalence of 9.2 percent in children.[1]
- Chronic daily headache has lifetime prevalence of 4 to 5 percent.[2]
- Cluster headache has a lifetime prevalence of 0.2 to 0.3 percent.[1]

ETIOLOGY AND PATHOPHYSIOLOGY

- The most common causes of headaches in children and adolescents are migraine and TTH.[3]
- TTH etiology is uncertain, but likely caused by activation of peripheral afferent neurons in head and neck muscles.[4]
- Migraine headache is thought to be caused by central sensory processing dysfunction, which is genetically influenced.[5] Nociceptive input from the meningeal vessels is abnormally modulated in the dorsal raphe nucleus, locus coeruleus, and nucleus raphe magnus. This activation can be seen on positron emission tomography (PET) scan during an acute attack.
- Cluster headache is caused by trigeminal activation with hypothalamic involvement, but the inciting mechanism is unknown.[6]

RISK FACTORS

- For migraines—Family history reported in over 60 percent.

DIAGNOSIS

A headache diary is helpful for diagnosis and follow-up.

CLINICAL FEATURES

- Red flags for dangerous secondary cause:[3]
  - Worst headache of life.
  - Recent onset of headache.
  - Increase in severity or frequency of headache.
  - Headache occurring only in the morning with severe vomiting.
  - Headache worsened with Valsalva.
  - Presence of focal neurological signs, seizures, or papilledema (**Figures 201-2** to **201-4**).
  - Headache located in the occipital region.
- Episodic TTH—At least 10 episodes of bilateral, mild to moderate, pressure (nonpulsating) type pain without nausea or vomiting, not aggravated by exertion, and rare photophobia or phonophobia, occurring less than 15 days per month.[7]
- Migraine headache—At least 5 episodes of unilateral, pulsating, moderate-to-severe headache, often with visual prodrome or visual field defects, lasting 1[3] to 72 hours, aggravated by physical activity, accompanied by nausea or emesis or photophobia and phonophobia.[7] Children may also have a bilateral headache, and symptoms of lightheadedness, difficulty thinking, or fatigue.[3]

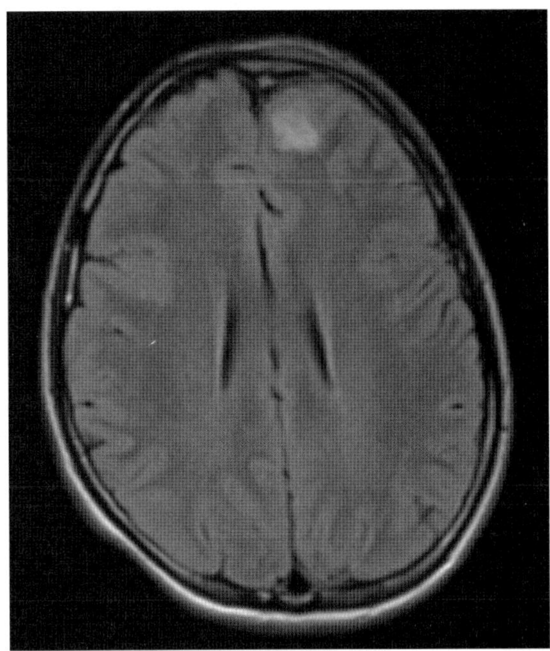

FIGURE 201-2 Intracranial abscess in the left frontal pole on brain MRI as a complication of sinusitis in a 14-year-old boy who presented with a severe headache and focal neurological signs. *(Used with permission from Camille Sabella, MD.)*

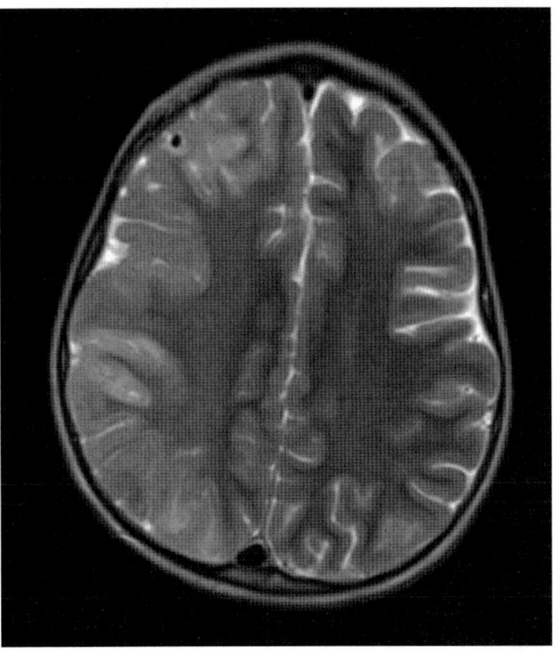

FIGURE 201-4 Diffuse ischemic changes in the right cerebral hemispheres with patchy areas of ischemia in the left frontal and temporal lobes on brain MRI in a young child with pneumococcal meningitis. This child presented with fever, severe headache and lethargy. *(Used with permission from Camille Sabella, MD.)*

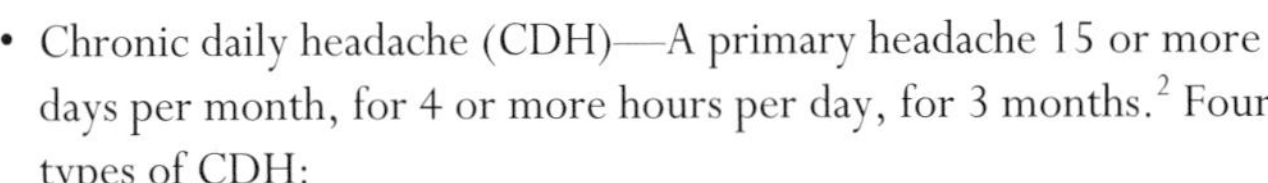

- Chronic daily headache (CDH)—A primary headache 15 or more days per month, for 4 or more hours per day, for 3 months.[2] Four types of CDH:
  - Chronic migraine—Episodic migraines increase in frequency while associated symptoms decrease; resembles tension headache with occasional typical migraine; often accompanied by medication overuse.[2]
  - Chronic TTH—Bilateral, nonpulsating, without nausea. Photophobia or phonophobia can be present.[2]

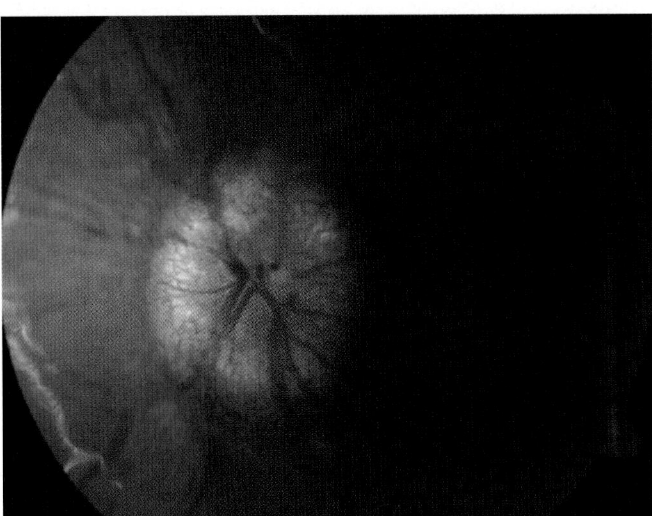

FIGURE 201-3 Papilledema on fundoscopic examination in an adolescent, signifying increased intracranial pressure. *(Used with permission from Paul Rychwalski, MD.)*

  - New daily persistent headache—Abrupt onset of daily headache in patient without a history of a headache disorder; patient often remembers exactly where and when the headaches started.[2]
  - Hemicrania continua—Chronic unilateral pain with exacerbations, often associated with ipsilateral autonomic features.[2]
- Medication overuse headache—Accompanies one of the CDHs; acute medications, such as triptans or opiates are taken more than 10 days a month, or analgesics more than 15 days a month, for more than 3 months.[7]
- Cluster headache—The most common type of trigeminal autonomic cephalgias; can be episodic or chronic; sharp stabbing unilateral pain in trigeminal distribution, lasting 15 minutes to 3 hours, with ipsilateral autonomic features.[2] Typically occurs in children over age 10 years, but has been reported in younger children.[3]
- Sinus headache—Purulent nasal discharge, co-onset of sinusitis, headache localized to facial and cranial areas.

TYPICAL DISTRIBUTION

- Tension headaches are typically bilateral.
- Migraine and cluster headaches are typically unilateral.

LABORATORY TESTING

- Generally not indicated.
- May be used when a secondary cause, such as infection is suspected.

IMAGING

- Generally not indicated.
- MRI when red flags are present (**Figures 201-2** to **201-4**).

DIFFERENTIAL DIAGNOSIS

- Common primary headaches include episodic TTH, migraine, and chronic daily headache.
- Secondary causes of headache include trauma, vascular disorders, substance use, systemic illnesses/infections, metabolic disorders, or sinus or eye disorders.
- Medication overuse headache is predominately seen with a primary headache, but may also accompany a secondary headache.

MANAGEMENT

General principles include:[8]

- Establish the diagnosis.
- Evaluate for somatic and psychiatric comorbidities.
- Use a headache diary to track progress.
- Educate the child and family.
- Set realistic goals.
- Identify triggers and reduce emotional mechanisms that promote stress.
- Maintain a normal daily schedule.

Episodic TTH

- Acute therapy.
  - NSAIDs, acetaminophen, and aspirin (over age 15 years) are effective treatments for acute episodes. [8]
  - Avoid opiates.
  - Limit acute medications to less than 3 times a week to reduce the risk of medication overuse headache.[4]
- Consider preventive therapy if headaches occur once a week.
  - Amitriptyline 1 mg/kg/day may be effective.
  - Biofeedback may be effective.[4]
  - Acupuncture may be helpful.[4]

Migraine Headache

- Use a stepped approach to treat acute migraine episodes.
  - Start with simple analgesics. Acetaminophen and ibuprofen are often effective.[8]
  - Consider an anti-emetic.[8]
  - Reserve migraine-specific agents such as triptans for patients who fail the preceding therapies.[9] Sumatriptan nasal spray, rizatriptan 5 mg tablets and wafers, and zolmitriptan have been shown to be effective.[8]
- Consider prophylaxis for patients whose migraines occur more than 3 times a month and have a negative impact on their lives or to decrease risk of developing medication overuse headache when frequency requires use of simple analgesics more than 15 days a month or use of opioids, triptans, or combination analgesics more than 10 days a month.
  - Amitriptyline 1 mg/kg/day, divalproex sodium 15 to 45 mg/kg/day, topiramate 2–3 mg/kg daily up to 100 mg daily have each demonstrated greater than 50 percent reduction in migraine frequency.[8] Propranolol has equivocal results and can activate asthma in children with atopic disorders.[8]
- Cognitive behavioral therapy, biofeedback, stress management, music therapy, and lifestyle modification may also be useful.[9]

Cluster Headache

- Acute episode:
  - Inhaled high-flow oxygen 10 to 15 L per minute.[6]
  - Sumatriptan nasal spray or subcutaneous is an off-label use in children, but may be effective.[8]
  - Prednisone is effective in adolescents.[8]
- Verapamil may be effective for prophylactic therapy.[8]
- Refer refractory patients for evaluations for other medical or surgical therapies.

Medication Overuse Headaches

- Educate patients that chronic medication use is contributing to their daily headaches.[10]
- Abruptly stop (when safe) or taper the overused medication.[10]

REFERRAL

- Refer patients when the diagnosis is unclear or response to therapy is inadequate.
- Consider referral for medication overuse headaches as these are difficult to treat.

PREVENTION

- Closely monitor use of medications for acute episodes. Advise patients to limit simple analgesics to less than 15 days per month; limit triptans and combination medications to less than 10 days per month.
- Appropriately prescribe preventive therapies to reduce frequency of headaches and avoid development of CDHs.

PROGNOSIS

- Migraine headaches—Tend to be recurrent; frequent migraines are often reduced with prophylactic treatment.
- Tension headaches—Unknown; tend to be at risk for chronic headaches as adults.
- Cluster headaches—Unknown; ranges from total remission to chronic form.[6]

FOLLOW-UP

- Dangerous causes of secondary headaches require immediate evaluation and management.
- Frequency of follow-up for primary headaches is determined by type and severity of headache and response to therapy.

PATIENT EDUCATION

Advise patients to limit frequency of acute medications to less than 2 to 3 times a week to reduce the risk of medication overuse headache.

PATIENT RESOURCES

National headache foundation has information for patients on many topics including:

- Migraine—**www.headaches.org/education/Headache_Topic_Sheets/Migraine**.
- Medication Overuse Headache—**www.headaches.org/education/Headache_Topic_Sheets/Analgesic_Rebound**.
- Cluster Headache—**www.headaches.org/education/Headache_Topic_Sheets/Cluster_Headaches.**
- New Daily Persistent Headache—**www.headaches.org/education/Headache_Topic_Sheets/New_Daily_Persistent_Headache**.

PROVIDER RESOURCES

- The Institute for Clinical Systems Improvement has a comprehensive guideline on the diagnosis and treatment of headache—**www.icsi.org/guidelines_and_more/gl_os_prot/other_health_care_conditions/headache/headache__diagnosis_and_treatment_of__guideline_.html**.
- The International Headache Society has a searchable website to assist with headache classification using ICHD-II criteria—**http://ihs-classification.org/en/02_klassifikation/**.

REFERENCES

1. Stovner LJ, Andree C. Prevalence of headache in Europe: a review for the Eurolight project. *J Headache Pain*. 2010;11(4):289-299.
2. Bigal ME, Lipton RB. The differential diagnosis of chronic daily headaches: an algorithmic-based approach. *J Headache Pain*. 2007;8(5):263-272.
3. Ozge A, Termine C, Antonaci F, Natriashvili S, Guidetti V, Wöber-Bingöl C. Overview of diagnosis and management of paediatric headache. Part 1: diagnosis. *J Headache Pain*. 2011;12(1):13-23.
4. Loder E, Rizzoli P. Tension-type headache. *BMJ*. 2008:336(7635):88-92.
5. Sprenger T, Goadsby PJ. Migraine pathogenesis and state of pharmacological treatment options. *BMC Med*. 2009;7:71.
6. Leroux E, Ducros A. Cluster headache. *Orphanet J Rare Dis*. 2008;3:20.
7. Headache Classification Subcommittee of the International Headache Society. The International Classification of Headache Disorders: 2nd edition. *Cephalalgia*. 2004;24(1):9-160.
8. Termine C, Ozge A, Antonaci F, Natriashvili S, Guidetti V, Wöber-Bingöl C. Overview of diagnosis and management of paediatric headache. Part II: therapeutic management. *J Headache Pain*. 2011;12(1):25-34.
9. Buse DC, Rupnow MFT, Lipton RB. Assessing and managing all aspects of migraine: migraine attacks, migraine-related functional impairment, common comorbidities, and quality of life. *Mayo Clin Proc*. 2009;84(5):422-435.
10. Evers S, Jensen R. Treatment of medication overuse headache—guideline of the EFNS headache panel. *Eur J Neurol*. 2011;18(9):1115-1121.

202 BELL'S PALSY

Heidi Chumley, MD

PATIENT STORY

A teenage girl was brought in by her parents because she was unable to move the left side of her face for the past 2 days. She had no history of trauma or recent ear infections and was otherwise well. On examination it was found that she had absent brow furrowing, weak eye closure, and dropping of the angle of her mouth (**Figure 202-1**). She had a normal complete blood count and serum glucose. She was diagnosed with Bell's palsy and was provided eye lubricants and guidance on keeping her left eye moist. Her physician discussed the available evidence about treatment with steroids and the excellent prognosis without treatment in children. She (with her parents in agreement) chose not to take the steroids. She had a full recovery over the next several weeks.

INTRODUCTION

Bell's palsy is an idiopathic paralysis of the facial nerve resulting in loss of brow furrowing, weak eye closure, and dropped angle of mouth. Treatment is eye protection. Treatment with oral steroids is standard of care in adults, but controversial in children. Prognosis for full recovery is excellent.

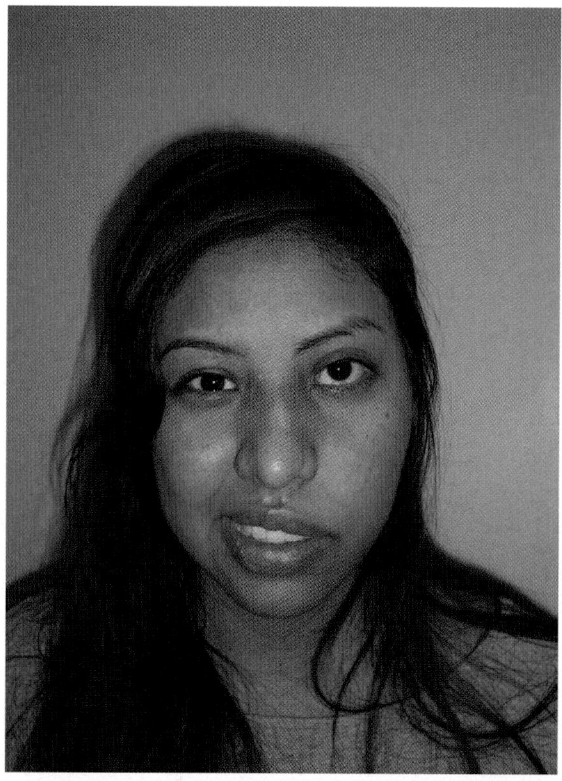

FIGURE 202-1 Bell's palsy for 2 days in a teenage girl. Note the loss of brow furrowing and dropped angle of the mouth on the affected left side of her face demonstrated during a request to smile and raise her eyebrows. (*Used with permission from Richard P. Usatine, MD.*)

SYNONYMS

Idiopathic facial paralysis.

EPIDEMIOLOGY

- In a population-based study, incidence was 18.8/100,000 children.[1]
- Incident rate increases by age and is higher is female children.[1]
- Seventy percent of cases of acute peripheral facial nerve palsy are idiopathic (Bell's palsy); 30 percent have known etiologic factors such as trauma, diabetes mellitus, polyneuritis, tumors, or infections such as herpes zoster, leprosy (**Figure 202-2**), or *Borrelia*.[2]

ETIOLOGY AND PATHOPHYSIOLOGY

- Etiology of Bell's palsy is currently unknown and under debate; the prevailing theory suggests a viral etiology from the herpes family.
- The facial nerve becomes inflamed, resulting in nerve compression.
- Compression of the facial nerve compromises muscles of facial expression, taste fibers to the anterior tongue, pain fibers, and secretory fibers to the salivary and lacrimal glands.
- This is a lower motor neuron lesion; the upper and lower portions of the face are affected (**Figure 202-1**). In upper motor neuron lesions (e.g., cortical stroke), the upper third of the face is spared,

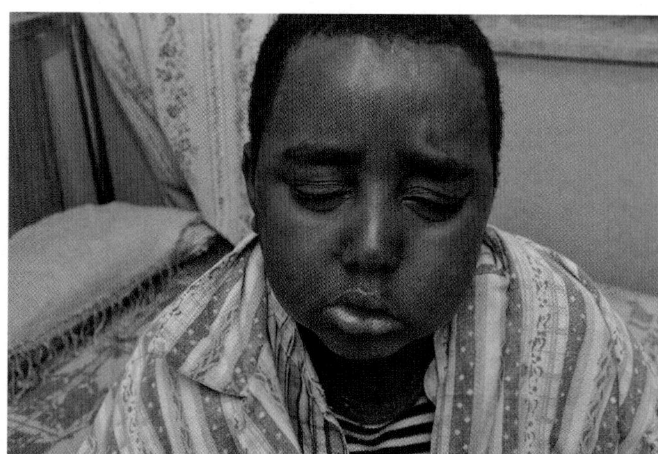

FIGURE 202-2 Bell's palsy secondary to leprosy. The hypopigmented patches on his face are further signs of the leprosy. He also is Cushingoid from the prednisolone being used to treat the immunological reaction to his leprosy treatment. (*Used with permission from Richard P. Usatine, MD.*)

while the lower 2/3 are affected as a result of the bilateral innervation of the orbicularis, frontalis, and corrugator muscles, which allows sparing of upper face movement.

DIAGNOSIS

CLINICAL FEATURES

- Weakness of all facial muscles on the affected side—Loss of brow furrowing, weak eye closure, and dropped angle of mouth.
- Postauricular pain.
- Dry eyes.
- Involuntary tearing.
- Hyperacusis.
- Altered tastes.

LABORATORY TESTING

Laboratory testing is not usually indicated:

- Consider complete blood count to rule out leukemia.
- Consider serologic tests for Lyme disease in endemic areas.
- Consider testing for diabetes mellitus in patients with risk factors.

IMAGING

- Consider MRI to look for a space-occupying lesion with atypical presentations.

DIFFERENTIAL DIAGNOSIS

- Facial nerve paralysis is most commonly Bell's palsy (40 to 70%), but can also be due to:
  - Infection (13 to 36%), including otitis media, herpes zoster, Lyme disease in endemic areas. Facial nerve paralysis is the most common neurologic manifestation of Lyme disease (see Chapter 183, Lyme Disease).
  - Trauma (19% to 21%), including facial injuries or trauma to middle ear.
  - Congenital condition (8% to 14%).
  - Neoplasm (2% to 3%), including cholesteatoma, leukemia, and facial nerve tumor.
- Upper motor neuron diseases including stroke—Normal brow furrowing, eye closure, and blinking.
- Facial nerve damage from microvascular disease—Most commonly in diabetes mellitus.
- Isolated third nerve palsy—Manifestations include diplopia and drooping of the upper eyelid (ptosis). The affected eye may deviate out and down in straight-ahead gaze; adduction is slow and cannot proceed past the midline. Upward gaze is impaired. When downward gaze is attempted, the superior oblique muscle causes the eye to adduct. The pupil may be normal or dilated; its response to direct or consensual light may be sluggish or absent (efferent defect). Pupil dilation (mydriasis) may be an early sign.

MANAGEMENT

NONPHARMACOLOGIC

- Provide eye protection with artificial tears, lubricants, or closing of the eyelid. SOR Ⓒ

MEDICATIONS

- A systematic review of steroid treatment for children with Bell's palsy found no controlled trials and recommended further trials to determine the role of steroids in children.[3]
- New data and a Cochrane systematic review supports treating adult patients with systemic corticosteroids. Steroids significantly decrease a patient's risk for incomplete recovery from 33 to 23 percent, risk ratio 0.71.[4] SOR Ⓐ
  - Dosing of steroids in the studies analyzed within the Cochrane review varied from oral methylprednisolone 1 mg/kg daily for 10 days, and then gradually withdrawn for another 3 to 5 days to prednisone given as a single dose of 60 mg daily for 5 days, followed by a dose reduced by 10 mg, per day, with a total treatment of 10 days. One trial used high-dose prednisolone given intravenously.
- A Cochrane systematic review does not support using antiviral medications. There is no significant benefit from acyclovir or valacyclovir when compared to placebo. Antivirals are less likely than steroids to produce complete recovery.[5] SOR Ⓐ

REFERRAL

- In longstanding facial paralysis, consider referral to an ear, nose, and throat (ENT) surgeon or plastic surgeon with experience in treating Bell's palsy with surgery. It is possible to restore some facial movement with specialized surgical procedures including regional muscle transfer and microvascular free tissue transfer.[6] SOR Ⓒ

PROGNOSIS

Prognosis for full recovery is excellent.

FOLLOW-UP

Consider seeing patients in 2 to 3 weeks to evaluate recovery and to reconsider diagnosis if there has been no recovery.

PATIENT EDUCATION

- Most patients recover spontaneously. Steroid treatment is indicated for adults but remains controversial in children.
- Ninety-five percent of children recover; 70 percent recover within 3 weeks.

PATIENT RESOURCES

- The American Academy of Family Physicians has written and auditory information in English and in Spanish—**www.familydoctor.org**.
- FamilyDoctor.org. *Bell's Palsy Overview*—**http://familydoctor.org/familydoctor/en/diseases-conditions/bells-palsy.html**.
- The National Institute of Neurologic Disorders and Stroke has written and auditory patient information in English and Spanish—**http://www.ninds.nih.gov/disorders/bells/bells.htm**.

PROVIDER RESOURCES

- The Cochrane Collaborative contains updated systematic reviews of steroid and/or antiviral treatment of Bell palsy at **http://onlinelibrary.wiley.com/doi/10.1002/14651858.CD001942.pub4/full**.
- **http://onlinelibrary.wiley.com/doi/10.1002/14651858.CD001869.pub4/full**.

REFERENCES

1. Rowhani-Rahbar A, Baxter R, Rasgon B, et al. Epidemiologic and clinical features of Bell's palsy among children in Northern California. *Neuroepidemiology*. 2012;38(4):252-258.
2. Berg T, Jonsson L, Engström M: Agreement between the Sunnybrook, House-Brackmann, and Yanagihara facial nerve grading systems in Bell's palsy. *Otol Neurotol*. 2004;25(6): 1020-1026.
3. Pitaro J, Waissbluth S, Daniel SJ: Do children with Bell's palsy benefit from steroid treatment? A systematic review. *Int J Pediatr Otorhinolaryngol*. 2012;76(7):921-926.
4. Salinas RA, Alvarez G, Daly F, Ferreira J: Corticosteroids for Bell's palsy (idiopathic facial paralysis). *Cochrane Database Syst Rev*. 2010;(3):CD001942.
5. Lockhart P, Daly F, Pitkethly M, et al. Antiviral treatment for Bell's palsy (idiopathic facial paralysis.) *Cochrane Database Syst Rev*. 2009;(4):CD001869.
6. Chuang DC: Free tissue transfer for the treatment of facial paralysis. *Facial Plast Surg*. 2008;24(2):194-203.

203 SUBDURAL HEMATOMA

Heidi Chumley, MD

PATIENT STORY

A 2-month-old previously healthy male infant was brought in by his mother after a seizure. She noted that he had seemed irritable and was not feeding well several hours prior to the seizure. She denied any trauma or fever. On examination, retinal hemorrhages were noted, but there were no other signs of trauma, and no signs of infection. The child was irritable, lethargic, and had poor tone. An emergent non-contrast CT was obtained and demonstrated a subdural hematoma (**Figure 203-1**). Neurosurgery was consulted and the infant underwent emergency craniectomy and evacuation of the subdural hematoma (**Figure 203-2**). An evaluation for child abuse was initiated.

INTRODUCTION

Subdural hematomas (SHs) can occur at any age, but are most common in infants. Most SHs are caused by trauma. Symptoms are generally nonspecific such as irritability or poor feeding in infants and confusion or headaches in older children. Treatment is prompt consultation with a neurosurgeon.

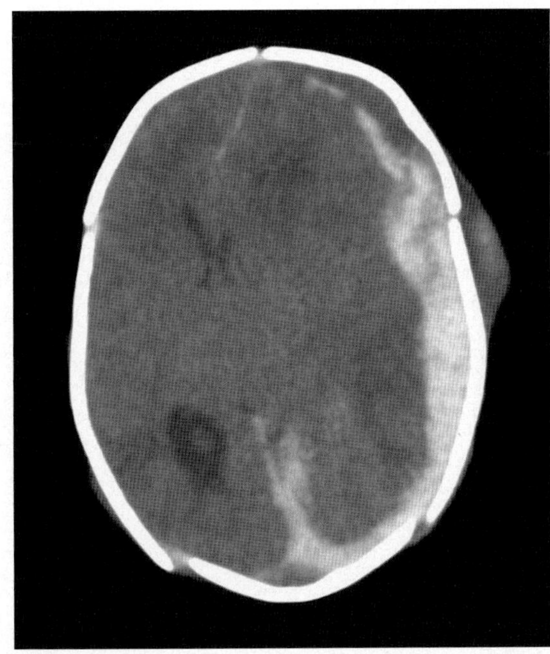

FIGURE 203-1 Large acute left hemispheric subdural hematoma with left to right midline shift on CT scan of the brain in a 2-month-old infant suspected of being the victim of child abuse. (*Used with permission from Camille Sabella, MD.*)

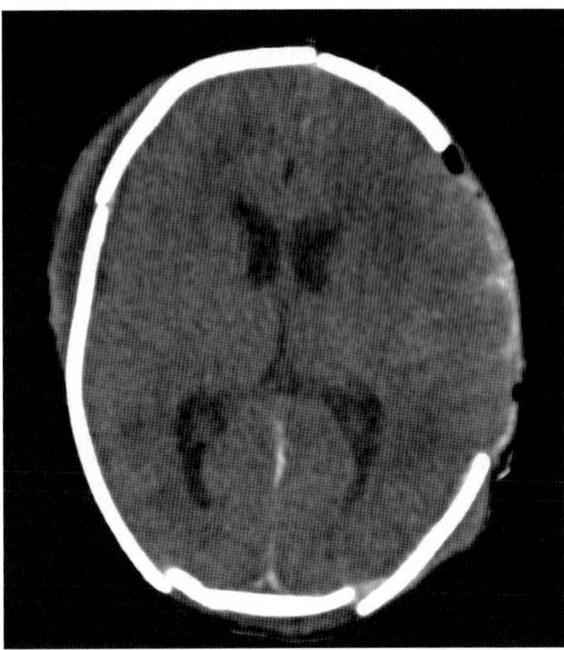

FIGURE 203-2 CT of the brain of the same 2-month-old infant as in **Figure 203-1** after craniectomy and evacuation of the subdural hematoma. Note the marked decrease in mass effect. (*Used with permission from Camille Sabella, MD.*)

EPIDEMIOLOGY

- SHs occur at all ages.
- Eight percent of asymptomatic newborns can have an SH.[1]
- Twenty-four of 100,000 infants ages 0 to 1 year in United Kingdom population studies.[2]
- Mortality rate of traumatic SH in treated children ages 0 to 17 is approximately 22 percent.[3]

ETIOLOGY AND PATHOPHYSIOLOGY

- Most SHs are caused by trauma, either accidental or intentional, from a direct injury to the head or shaking injury in an infant.
- Nonaccidental trauma, falls, and motor vehicle accidents are the most common causes of traumatic SH.
- SHs can occur during a nontraumatic birth.
- Motion of the brain within the skull causes a shearing force to the cortical surface and interhemispheric bridging veins.[2]
- This force tears the weakest bridging veins as they cross the subdural space, resulting in an acute SH as seen in **Figure 203-1**.[2]
- Three days to 3 weeks after the injury, the body breaks down the blood in an SH; water is drawn into the collection causing hemodilution, which appears less white and more gray on noncontrast CT.[2]
- If the hematoma fails to resolve, the collection has an even higher content of water and appears darker on a noncontrast CT; it may

have fresh bleeding or may calcify (chronic SH).[2] This is often of the same color as brain parenchyma on noncontrast CT.

- Nontraumatic causes reported in the literature include spontaneous bleeding because of bleeding disorders or anticoagulation, meningitis, and complications of neurologic procedures, including spinal anesthesia.

RISK FACTORS

Poor prognosis is seen in children with:[4]

- Early seizures.
- Apnea.
- Raised intracranial pressure and/or hypotension.
- Retinal hemorrhages
- Skull fractures
- Brain swelling

DIAGNOSIS

The clinical features are often nonspecific, making the diagnosis difficult in the absence of known trauma.

- Infants may present with drowsiness, irritability, poor tone, poor feeding, or new seizures.[2]
- Older children may present with vomiting, seizures, headaches, or confusion.

TYPICAL DISTRIBUTION

SHs by definition occur in the subdural space, most commonly seen in the parietal region.

IMAGING

Acute SHs are seen easily on a noncontrast CT scan (**Figure 203-1**). Subacute and chronic SHs can be similar in color to the brain parenchyma and may be easier to see on a contrast CT or an MRI.

DIFFERENTIAL DIAGNOSIS

Other causes of nonspecific symptoms seen with SH can be differentiated by neuroimaging and include the following:

- Infections such as sepsis or meningitis—Fever, elevated white blood cells, positive blood cultures, and cerebral spinal fluid consistent with meningitis.
- Hemorrhagic (**Figure 203-3**) or ischemic stroke or transient ischemic attacks—Consider risk factors for stroke such as congenital heart malformations, hemolytic anemias, collagen vascular diseases, and thrombophilia (see Chapter 204, Cerebral Vascular Accident).
- Primary or metastatic brain neoplasms—History of cancer and risk factors for cancer.

Other causes of intracranial bleeding can also be differentiated by neuroimaging and include the following:

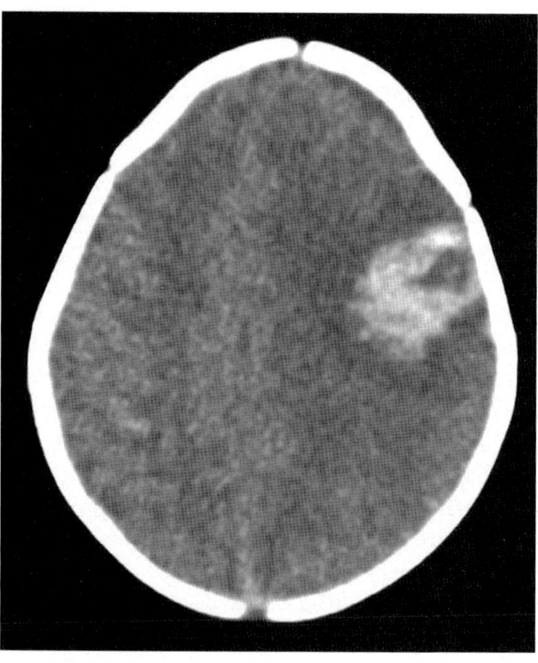

FIGURE 203-3 Hemorrhagic infarct on CT scan of the brain in a young infant with hemorrhagic disease of the newborn. (*Used with permission from Camille Sabella, MD.*)

- Epidural hematoma (**Figure 203-4**)—Well-defined biconvex bright white density that resembles the shape of the lens of the eye.
- Subarachnoid hemorrhage (**Figure 203-5**)—Bright white blood outlines cerebral sulci.
- Hemorrhage in brain parenchyma—Bright white lesion apart from dura.

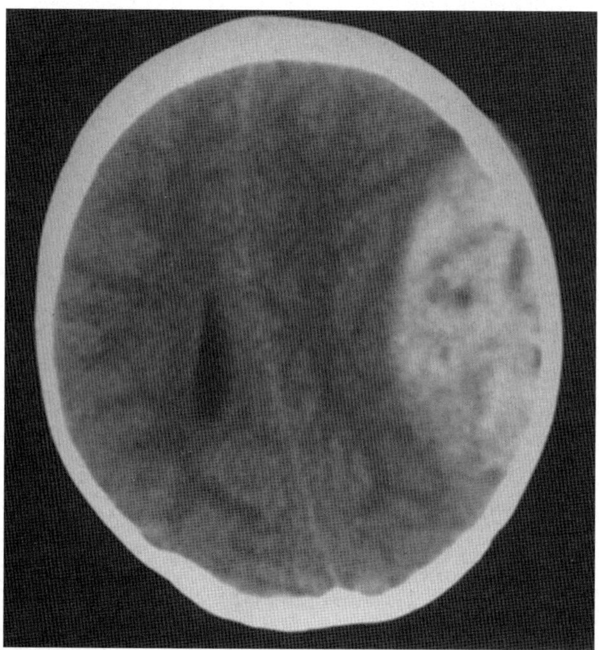

FIGURE 203-4 Epidural hematoma on MRI of the brain. Note the typical lenticular biconvex appearance. (*Used with permission from Strange GR, Ahrens WR, Schafermeyer RW, Wiebe RA. Pediatric Emergency Medicine, 3rd edition: http://www.accessemergencymedicine.com. Figure 29-2, with permission.*)

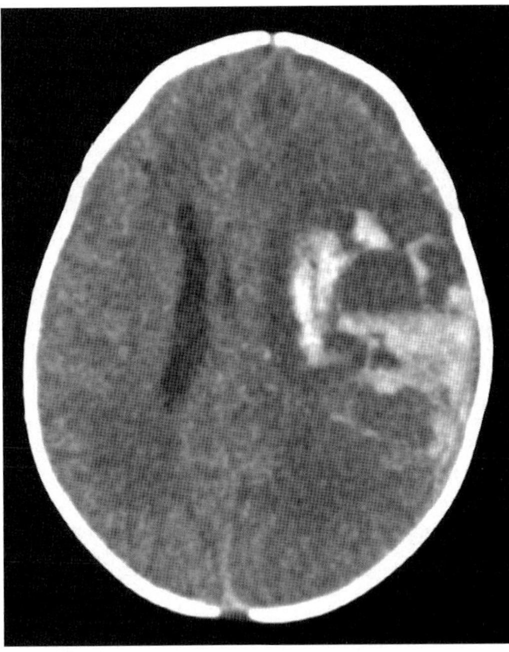

FIGURE 203-5 A subarachnoid hemorrhage appearing as an area of high density (more white like bone rather than the gray of brain tissue) in the same infant as in **Figure 203-3**. (*Used with permission from Camille Sabella, MD.*)

MANAGEMENT

Most SHs are managed surgically, and there is little evidence about conservative management (**Figure 203-2**).

- Determine the Glasgow Coma Scale in patients with serious head trauma and consider airway protection in patients with a score less than 12.
- Obtain an urgent noncontrast CT scan on any patient suspected of having an SH.
- If the noncontrast CT scan is nonrevealing, obtain a contrast CT or MRI, particularly if the traumatic event occurred 2 to 3 days prior.
- Emergently refer patients with an SH and deteriorating neurologic status or evidence of brain edema or midline shift to a hospital with neurosurgeons.
- Consult a neurosurgeon expediently in patients with an SH and stable focal neurologic signs.
- Evaluate any infant with an SH for child abuse or neglect.[2,4] SOR Ⓒ

PREVENTION

- Follow safety measures that reduce motor vehicle accidents.
- Use recommended protective gear for sports and recreational activities and follow guidelines for return to play after a head injury.

PROGNOSIS

- Traumatic SH in children ages 0 to 17 years has a mortality of 22 percent.[3]
- Infants with nonaccidental SH have a mortality of 11 to 36 percent. Infants who survive typically have long-term complications that range from learning difficulties to severe cognitive and physical impairment.[4]
- Children with SH from accidental trauma have a better prognosis and over half have a good outcome.[4]
- SH occurring from the birth process are typically asymptomatic and resolve without treatment within 4 weeks.[4]

FOLLOW-UP

- Follow-up is determined by severity of SH and type of treatment.
- Ideally, follow-up is conducted jointly between the neurosurgeon and primary care physician to ensure resolution of the SH and maximal return of function.

PATIENT EDUCATION

- Advise patients to seek medical care immediately for head trauma, which can cause several emergencies including an SH.
- Discuss with parents or guardians the need for a thorough evaluation for child abuse and neglect in infants with an SH.

PATIENT RESOURCES

- MedlinePlus. *Subdural Hematoma*—**www.nlm.nih.gov/medlineplus/ency/article/000713.htm**.

PROVIDER RESOURCES

- **http://emedicine.medscape.com/article/1137207**.
- Glasgow Coma Scale Calculator—**www.mdcalc.com/glasgow-coma-scale-score**.

REFERENCES

1. Whitby EH, Griffiths PD, Rutter S, et al. Frequency and natural history of subdural haemorrhages in babies and relation to obstetric factors. *Lancet*. 2004;363(9412):846-851.
2. Minns RA: Subdural haemorrhages, haematomas, and effusions in infancy. *Arch Dis Child*. 2005;90(9):883-884.
3. Kalanithi P, Schubert RD, Lad SP, Harris OA, Boakye M: Hospital costs, incidence, and inhospital mortality rates of traumatic subdural hematoma in the United States. *J Neurosurg*. 2011;115(5):1013-1018.
4. Jayawant S, Parr J: Oucome following subdural haemorrhages in infancy. *Arch Dis Child*. 2007;92(4):343-347.

204 CEREBRAL VASCULAR ACCIDENT

Heidi Chumley, MD

PATIENT STORY

A 16-year-old boy with a history of idiopathic dilated cardiomyopathy and severe ventricular dysfunction was admitted to the hospital for vomiting, confusion, involuntary movements, and slurred speech. On physical examination, he was found to be lethargic and to have dysmetria with the finger-to-nose test, ataxia, and incoordination of rapid alternating movements. He was found to have decreased biventricular systolic dysfunction and a large thrombus at the apex of the left ventricle on cardiac echocardiogram, and a left cerebellar stroke on CT scan of the brain (**Figure 204-1**). He was treated with anticoagulation and supportive care, with improvement of his neurologic symptoms. He eventually underwent a successful orthotopic heart transplant.

INTRODUCTION

Cerebral vascular accidents are uncommon in children. Ischemic and hemorrhagic strokes are often due to an underlying cause which should be identified and addressed. Acute treatment is largely supportive. Prevention of recurrence is critical.

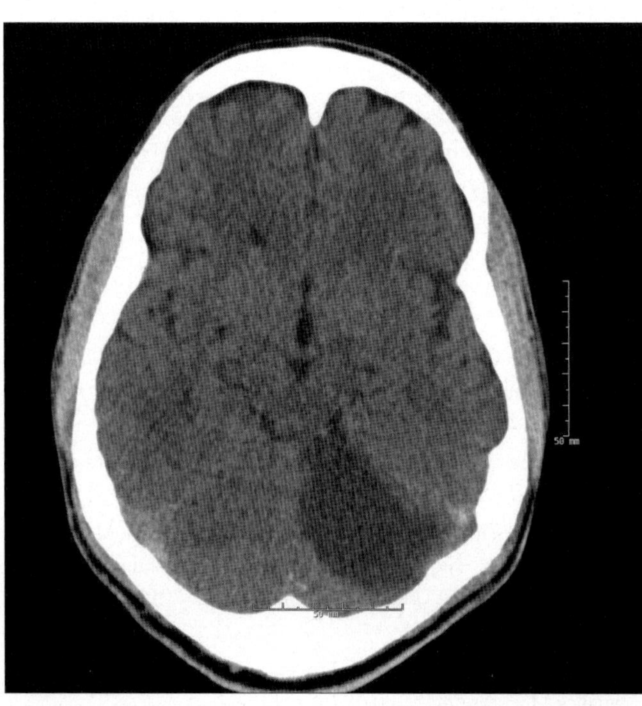

FIGURE 204-1 Acute/subacute left cerebellar infarct on brain CT of a 16-year-old with dilated cardiomyopathy and severe ventricular dysfunction. (*Used with permission from Camille Sabella, MD.*)

SYNONYMS

Stroke.

EPIDEMIOLOGY

- Approximately 2 CVAs per 100,000 person per year.[1]
- Approximately 50 percent of strokes are ischemic and 50 percent are hemorrhagic.[1]
- Ten percent of hemorrhagic strokes are due to central venous sinus thrombosis.[2]
- Fifty percent of patients presenting with a focal neurologic deficit have a previously identified risk factor for stroke.[3]

ETIOLOGY AND PATHOPHYSIOLOGY

- Ischemic CVAs can be secondary to a wide range of underlying causes.
  - The cause can be determined in approximately 2/3 of patients.[2]
  - Major causes include congenital heart disease, sickle cell disease, infections, and prothrombotic states.
  - Moyamoya is rare in the US, but the most common cause in Japan.
  - Fibromuscular dysplasia more commonly presents in young adults.
- Hemorrhagic CVAs occur when vessels bleed into the brain, usually as the result of a vascular abnormality or clotting disorder.

RISK FACTORS

Ischemic Stroke

- Congenital heart malformations (**Figure 204-1**).
- Cerebrovascular abnormalities.
- Sickle cell disease (10% have a clinically evident stroke by age 20 years; **Figure 204-2**).
- Collagen vascular diseases.
- Infection (meningitis and sepsis).
- Prothrombotic risk factors (elevated homocysteine, elevated lipoprotein (a), protein C and protein S deficiencies, Factor V Leiden, and anti-phospholipid antibodies).
- Migraine with aura, especially with smoking, pregnancy, or oral contraceptive use.
- Trauma.

Hemorrhagic Stroke

- Arteriovenous malformation or fistula or another vascular anomaly.
- Coagulation disorders (**Figure 204-3**).
- Sickle cell disease.
- Trauma.

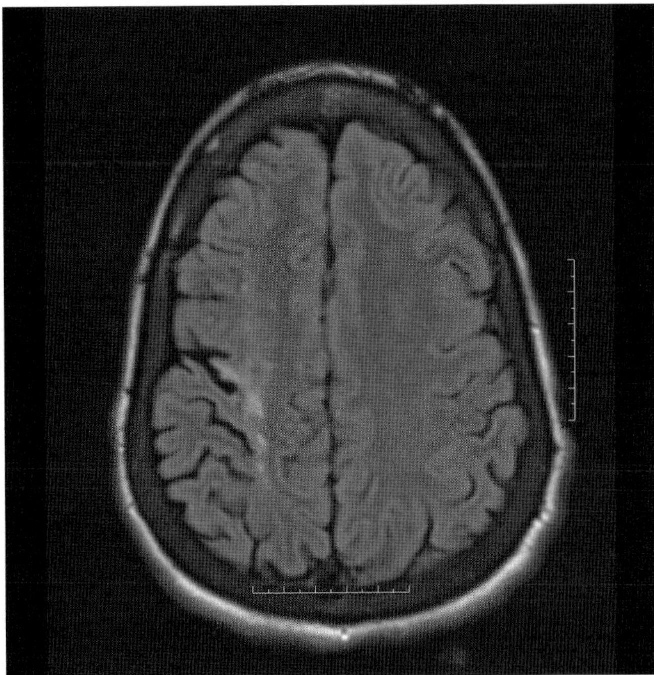

FIGURE 204-2 Brain MRI showing remote infarction in the distribution of the middle cerebral artery and volume loss at the right frontoparietal cortex in a patient with sickle cell disease. (*Used with permission from Stefanie Thomas, MD.*)

DIAGNOSIS

Diagnosis of CVA must be made expediently to minimize mortality and morbidity.

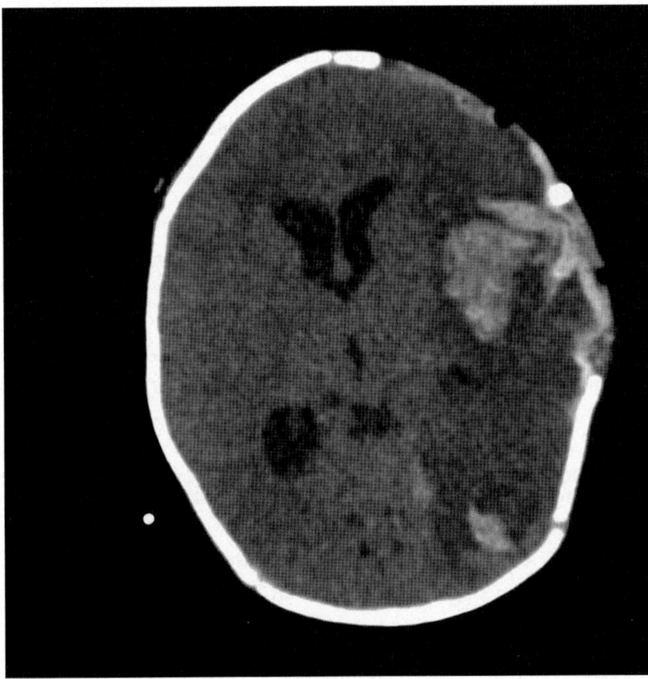

FIGURE 204-3 Left middle cerebral and posterior cerebral artery hemorrhagic infarct in a patient with hemorrhagic disease of the newborn. This CT was performed after craniectomy for evacuation of multifocal hemorrhages and mass affect. (*Used with permission from Camille Sabella, MD.*)

CLINICAL FEATURES

- History of risk factors or previous transient ischemic attack (TIA) or stroke.
- Acute onset of neurologic signs and symptoms based on the site of the CVA (see the following section "Typical Distribution").
- Hemorrhagic strokes present with headache and deteriorating neurological function. In younger children, headaches, emesis, and seizures with hemiparesis are less common.

TYPICAL DISTRIBUTION

TIA or stroke can occur in any area of the brain; common areas with typical symptoms include the following:

- Middle cerebral artery.
    - Superior branch occlusion causes contralateral hemiparesis and sensory deficit in face, hand, and arm, and an expressive aphasia if the lesion is in the dominant hemisphere.
    - Inferior branch occlusion causes a homonymous hemianopia, impairment of contralateral graphesthesia and stereognosis, anosognosia and neglect of the contralateral side, and a receptive aphasia if the lesion is in the dominant hemisphere.
- Internal carotid artery (approximately 20 percent of ischemic strokes) occlusion causes contralateral hemiplegia, hemisensory deficit, and homonymous hemianopia; aphasia is also present with dominant hemisphere involvement.
- Posterior cerebral artery occlusion causes a homonymous hemianopia affecting the contralateral visual field.

LABORATORY TESTING (INCLUDE ANCILLARY TESTING)

These tests may be helpful in the context of an acute stroke, particularly when the cause of the stroke is not immediately evident:

- Complete blood count (CBC) for thrombocytosis or polycythemia.
- Erythrocyte sedimentation rate (ESR) for collagen vascular diseases when suspected.
- Serum glucose to eliminate hypoglycemia as the cause of the neurologic symptoms.
- Sickle cell disease screen if status is unknown.
- Prothrombotic factors including elevated homocysteine, elevated lipoprotein (a), protein C and protein S deficiencies, Factor V Leiden, and antiphospholipid antibodies. Further testing of less common prothrombotic factors may be considered.

IMAGING

- Imaging should be completed as soon as possible. CT or MRI can distinguish ischemic from hemorrhagic and localize the lesion. MRA noninvasively identifies the majority of vascular lesions.[2]
- Cardiac echocardiography when an embolic event is suspected.

DIFFERENTIAL DIAGNOSIS

Other causes of acute neurologic dysfunction include the following:

- Brain mass—More common presentation is headache or seizure; however, may present with focal neurologic signs based on location. CT or MRI will help to diagnose a brain mass and differentiate this from stroke.

- Migraines—Throbbing, unilateral headache with photophobia, and nausea; hemiparesis or aphasia may be part of the aura.
- Hypoglycemia—Confused state is similar to large stroke syndromes but is easily differentiated by a blood glucose measurement.
- Multiple sclerosis—Multiple anatomically distinct neurologic signs and symptoms that occur over time and resolve; vision is often affected. MRI findings should help to distinguish multiple sclerosis from CVA.

MANAGEMENT

Acute Ischemic Stroke (AIS)

- Supportive therapy for AIS includes—Control fever if present, provide oxygen if hypoxic, correct systemic hypertension or hypotension, correct glucose levels, treat dehydration and anemia.[2] SOR C
- Prophylactic administration of antiepileptic medications is NOT necessary.[2]
- Consider anticoagulation with low molecular weight heparin or unfractionated heparin for up to 1 week while evaluating for underlying risk factors that would be mitigated by anticoagulation.[2]
- Evaluate children with one stroke risk factor for prothrombotic states.

Acute Hemorrhagic Stroke

- Optimize respiratory effort, control systemic hypertension, prevent epileptic seizures, medically manage increased intracranial pressure.
- Consult neurosurgery.
- Evaluate children with nontraumatic hemorrhagic stroke for vascular abnormalities and clotting disorders. An underlying treatable cause can be found in most cases.

Special Situations

- Sickle cell disease.
  - Order transcranial Doppler to identify patients with sickle cell disease at high risk for stroke. Children with cerebral blood flow velocity rates >/= 200 cm/s have a stroke rate of 10 percent per year.[4]
  - Refer patients with SCD and a high cerebral blood flow velocity for chronic transfusion to decrease the risk of stroke by 90 percent.[4] SOR A

PREVENTION

- Primary prevention for SCD (follow cerebral blood flow velocity and refer for exchange transfusion when indicated) and congenital heart disease (refer for repair).
- Secondary prevention.
  - Ischemic.
    - Anticoagulation for children with substantial risk of recurrent cardiac embolism, CVST, and hypercoagulable states.[2] SOR C
    - Three to 5 mg/kg per day aspirin can be considered win children without SCD with AIS without a high risk of recurrent embolism or severe hypercoagulable disorder.[2] SOR C
    - Lower homocysteine level in children with AIS through diet or supplementation of folate, B12, or B6.[2] SOR C
    - Avoid oral contraceptives in adolescents with history of acute ischemic stroke
- Hemorrhagic.
  - If a severe coagulation factor deficiency is present, provide appropriate factor replacement therapy.
  - Refer patients with congenital vascular anomalies to be evaluated for surgical correction.

PROGNOSIS

CVA prognosis varies based on size and location of ischemia or hemorrhage, time to recognition, and institution of appropriate management.

- Twenty percent mortality rate.[5]
- High recurrence rate.
- Over 50 percent with permanent cognitive or motor disability.[5]

FOLLOW-UP

- Patients with symptoms of an acute stroke should be hospitalized, evaluated immediately for treatment of reversible causes, and managed, if possible, in a stroke unit or using the "best practices" associated with these units.
- After a stroke and rehabilitation, patients should be followed at regular intervals based on appropriate strategies for secondary prevention.

PATIENT EDUCATION

Educate patients who have had a stroke about the need for a work-up to identify underlying causes, the high risk of having a second stroke, and the need for secondary prevention strategies to reduce this risk.

PATIENT RESOURCES

- The National Stroke Association has patient information on pediatric stroke—**www.stroke.org/site/PageServer?pagename=PEDSTROKE**.
- The Children's Hemiplegia and Stroke Association has an infant and child stroke fact sheet available—**www.chasa.org/wp-content/uploads/2011/06/chasa_pediatric_stroke_fact_sheet_2012.pdf**.

PROVIDER RESOURCES

- The American Heart Association and American Stoke Association have management guidelines—**http://stroke.ahajournals.org.proxy.kumc.edu:2048/content/39/9/2644.full.pdf+html**.

REFERENCES

1. Fullerton HJ, Wu YW, Zhao S, Johnston SC: Risk of stroke in children: ethnic and gender disparities. *Neurology*. 2003;61:189-194.
2. Roach ES, Golomb MR, Adams S, et al. Management of Stroke in Infants and Children: A Scientific Statement from a special writing group of the American Heart Association Stroke Council and the Council on Cardiovascular Disease in the Young. *Stroke*. 2008;39: 2644-2691.
3. Ganesan V, Prengler M, McShane MA, Wade AM, Kirkham FJ: Investigation of risk factors in children with arterial ischemic stroke. *Ann Neurol*. 2003;53:167-173.
4. Adams RJ, McKie VC, Hsu L, et al. Prevention of a first stroke by transfusions in children with sickle cell anemia and abnormal results on transcranial Doppler ultrasonography. *N Engl J Med*. 1998;339:5-11.
5. Pappachan J, Kirkham FJ: Cerebrovascular disease and stroke. *Arch Dis Child*. 2008;93:890-898.

205 TUBEROUS SCLEROSIS

Carla Torres-Zegarra, MD
Elumalai Appachi, MD, MRCP

PATIENT STORY

A 2-year-old girl was brought to her pediatrician for her well child visit. On exam, she was noted to have several hypomelanotic lesions over her trunk (**Figures 205-1** to **205-3**). Based on the presence of these lesions, the pediatrician orders an MRI of the brain, which revealed subependymal tubers, which also projected into the ventricles. She was diagnosed with Tuberous sclerosis, and a renal ultrasound and cardiac echocardiogram were obtained, which did not reveal any abnormalities. A multidisciplinary approach to her care was planned and included a pediatric neurologist, developmental pediatrician, and dermatologist.

INTRODUCTION

Tuberous sclerosis (also called Tuberous sclerosis complex-TSC) is an inherited neurocutaneous and multisystemic disorder characterized by hamartomas (sclerotic tubers), which most notably affect the skin, brain, kidneys, heart and eyes.[1,2] TSC results in a wide spectrum of clinical manifestations and neurologic sequelae.

SYNONYMS

- Bourneviller Pringle Syndrome, Epiloia, Phakomatosis TS, Tuberose sclerosis, Tuberous Sclerosis-1, and Tuberous Sclerosis Complex (TSC).

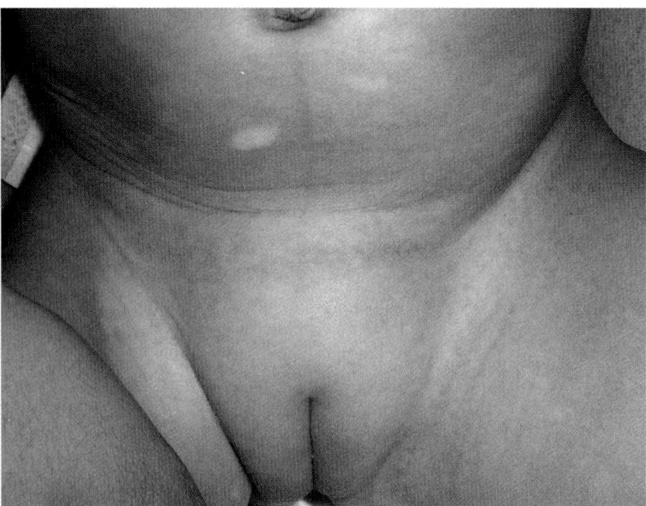

FIGURE 205-1 Hypomelanotic, or "ash leaf" lesion on the abdomen of a 2-year-old girl found to have tuberous sclerosis. She presented with over five hypomelanotic lesions on exam. This prompted the physician to order an MRI of the brain. Tubers were found to confirm the diagnosis. (*Used with permission from Richard P. Usatine, MD.*)

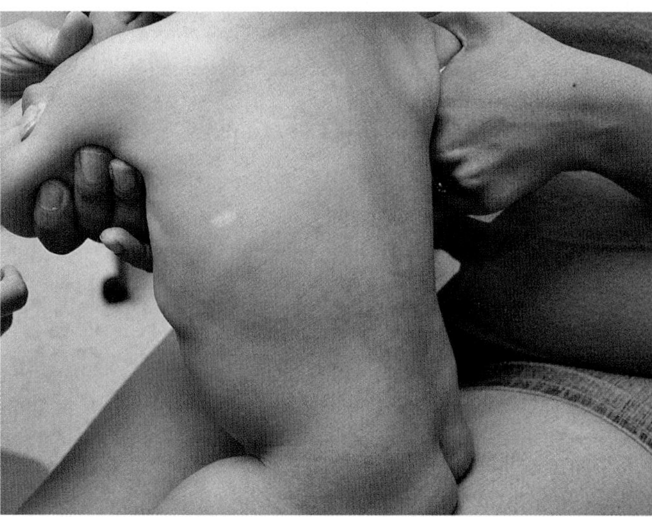

FIGURE 205-2 Hypomelanotic, or "ash leaf" lesion on the back of the same child as in **Figure 205-1**. (*Used with permission from Richard P. Usatine, MD.*)

EPIDEMIOLOGY

- TSC affects both sexes equally and all ethnic groups.
- The prevalence is estimated to be one per 6,000 to 10,000 individuals.[3]
- With one affected parent, the recurrence risk is 50 percent. When both parents appear to be unaffected, the recurrence risk is 1 in 22 after one affected offspring and 1 in 3 after two affected offspring.
- Only 7 to 37 percent of newly diagnosed cases have a family history of TSC.

ETIOLOGY AND PATHOPHYSIOLOGY

- TSC is caused by mutations on two genes, named TSC1 and TSC2. Only one of the genes needs to be affected for TSC to be present.

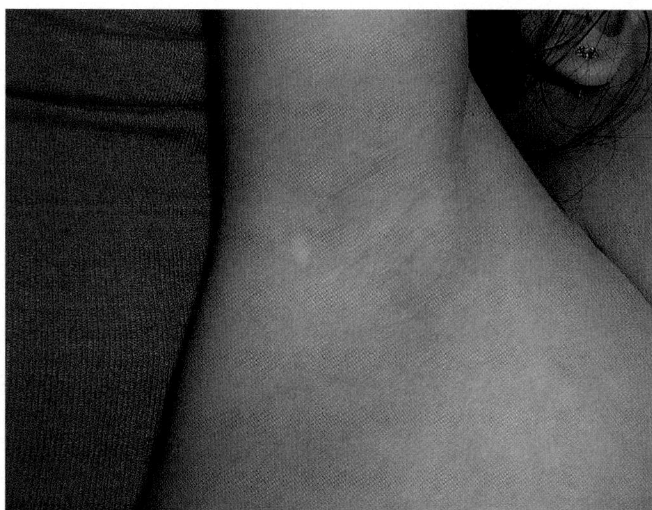

FIGURE 205-3 Hypomelanotic or "ash leaf" lesion in axilla of the child in **Figure 205-1**. (*Used with permission from Richard P. Usatine, MD.*)

- TSC has an autosomal dominant mode of inheritance with almost complete penetrance, but a variable expressivity range in terms of the age of onset, severity of disease, and different signs and symptoms that result from a specific genotype.
- The variability is due to multiple causes. These include somatic mosaicism, differences between TSC1 and TSC2 genes, a variety of mutation types found in each gene, and the requirement for a secondary somatic mutation in the wild-type copy of the gene for the development of many pathologic features of TSC.
- Approximately 65 percent of cases are caused by a spontaneous mutation.
- Molecular genetic studies have identified two loci for TSC—TSC1 is located on the long arm of chromosome 9 (9q34) and TSC2 is located on the short arm of chromosome 16 (16p13.3). These loci encode for hamartin and tuberin, respectively. Hamartin and tuberin are thought to function together as a protein complex or as adjacent steps within the same intracellular pathway, which may explain why the phenotypic expression of either mutation leads to almost identical disease.[2,4]
- Both TSC1 and TSC2 have tumor suppressor activity, which, when not activated, leads to uncontrolled cell cycle progression and the proliferation of hamartomas throughout the body.

RISK FACTORS

- Having an affected parent or sibling (autosomal dominant mode of inheritance).

DIAGNOSIS

CLINICAL FEATURES

- Dermatologic manifestations:
  - Hypomelanotic macules or "ash leaf" spots are found in more than 90 percent of patients with TSC, are evident within the first 2 years of life, and become more evident with age (**Figures 205-1** to **205-3**). In newborn infants and in fair-skinned individuals, these lesions often are difficult to visualize without the aid of an ultraviolet light (Wood's lamp).
  - Facial angiofibromas (adenoma sebaceum) are comprised of vascular and connective tissue elements and are found in approximately 75 percent of patients with TSC. The lesions typically appear during the preschool years in the malar area as small pink to red dome-shaped papules in a "butterfly distribution" (**Figures 205-4** to **205-6**).
  - A shagreen or "leather" patch is identified in 20 to 30 percent of patients with TSC. They result from accumulation of collagen, and are typically is found in the lumbosacral area. The lesion presents as an irregularly shaped, grayish-green, or light brown, unevenly thickened plaque with a cobblestone or orange-peel appearance (**Figure 205-7**).
  - Periungual and ungual fibromas are smooth, firm, nodular, or fleshy lesions that are adjacent to or underneath the nails. These usually appear later in life and are not typically apparent in the pediatric age-group (**Figures 205-8** to **205-10**).

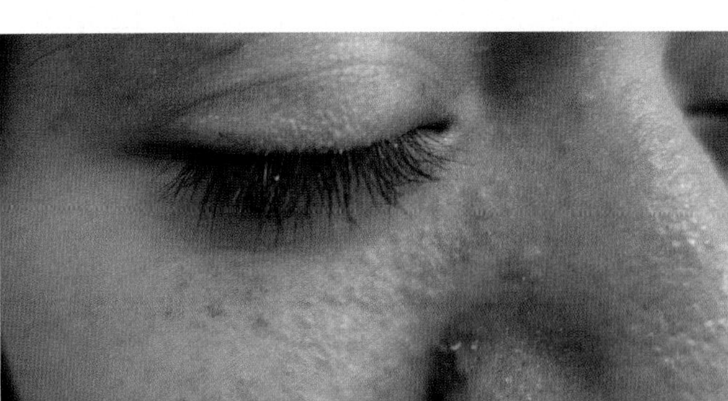

FIGURE 205-5 Angiofibromas on the nose and face of a teenager with tuberous sclerosis. These lesions can be easily confused with acne in adolescents. (*Used with permission from Emily Becker, MD.*)

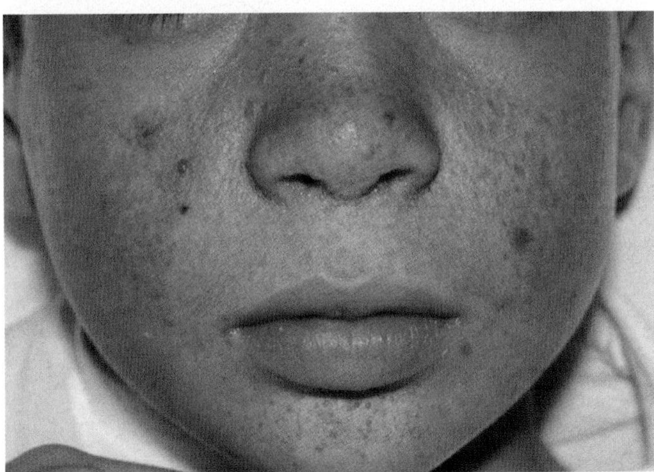

FIGURE 205-4 Facial angiofibromas (adenoma sebaceum) in a typical butterfly distribution in a child with tuberous sclerosis. (*Used with permission from Elumalai Appachi, MD.*)

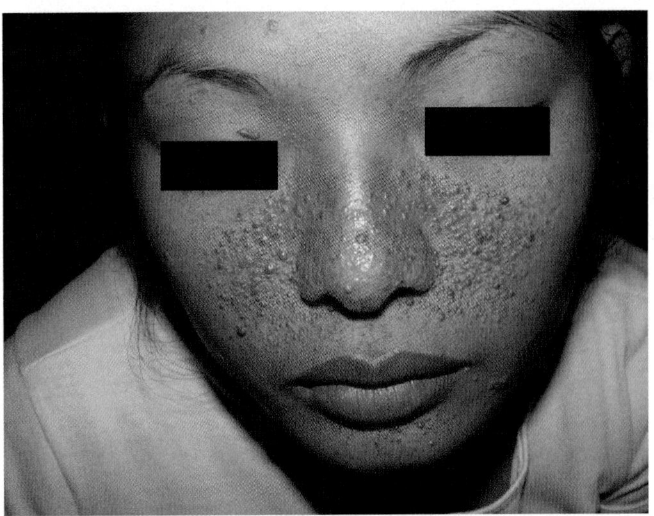

FIGURE 205-6 Angiofibromas on the nose and face of a teenager with tuberous sclerosis. This is also called adenoma sebaceum. (*Used with permission from Marisa Pongprutthipan, MD*)

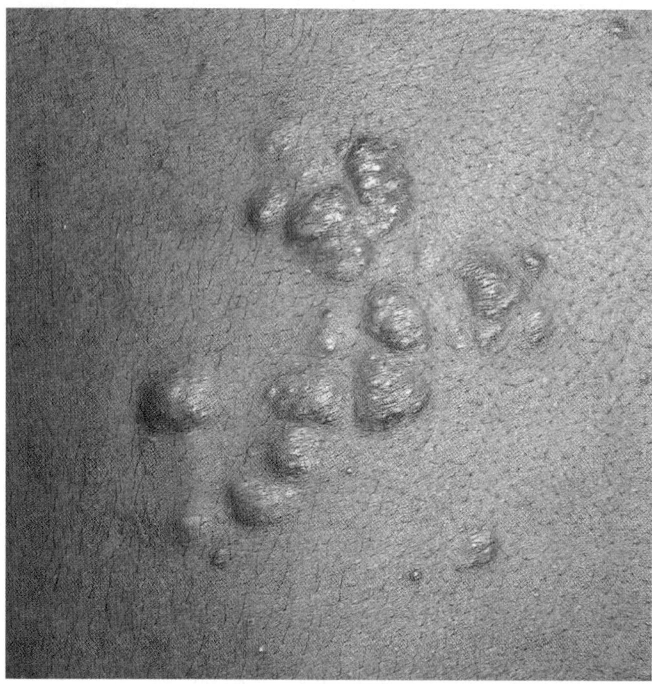

FIGURE 205-7 Shagreen patch (collagenoma) is a slightly elevated skin-colored connective tissue plaque found in tuberous sclerosis. These collagenomas are on the back of a young patient with tuberous sclerosis. (*Used with permission from Richard P. Usatine, MD.*)

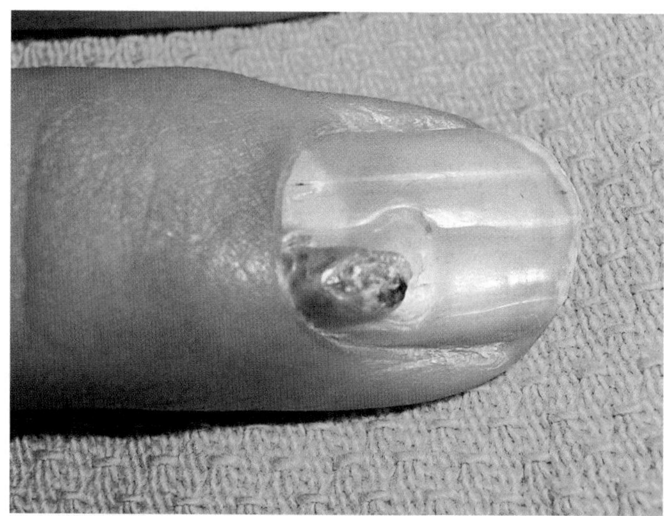

FIGURE 205-9 Periungual fibroma (Koenen tumor) in a young adult with tuberous sclerosis. (*Used with permission from Richard P. Usatine, MD.*)

- Café au lait spots are seen in up to 30 percent of patients with TSC. Most patients have fewer than six lesions whereas patients with neurofibromatosis usually have at least six (see Chapter 206, Neurofibromatosis).
- Neurologic manifestations:
  - There is a wide spectrum of neurological manifestations.
  - About half of persons with TSC will have normal intellect.
  - Neurologic complications, when present, are the most common causes of mortality and morbidity, and the most likely to affect the quality of life.
  - Seizures are the most common neurologic complication and are reported to occur in 75 to 90 percent of patients. These most commonly present as infantile spasms, partial motor seizures, and generalized tonic clonic seizures.[3,4]
  - Autism, attention deficit, hyperactivity, and sleep problems are the most frequent behavioral disorders.
  - Intracranial abnormalities include tubers, subependymal nodules, and subependymal giant cell astrocytomas (**Figure 205-11**).[5]
  - Patients with numerous cortical tubers tend to have more cognitive impairment and more difficulty with seizure control.
  - Subependymal giant cell astrocytomas develop in about 5 percent of patients and may lead to obstructive hydrocephalus.
- Renal manifestations:
  - Renal complications are the second most common cause of mortality.
  - The most common renal lesion is an angiomyolipoma, which occurs in approximately 75 to 80 percent of affected children and

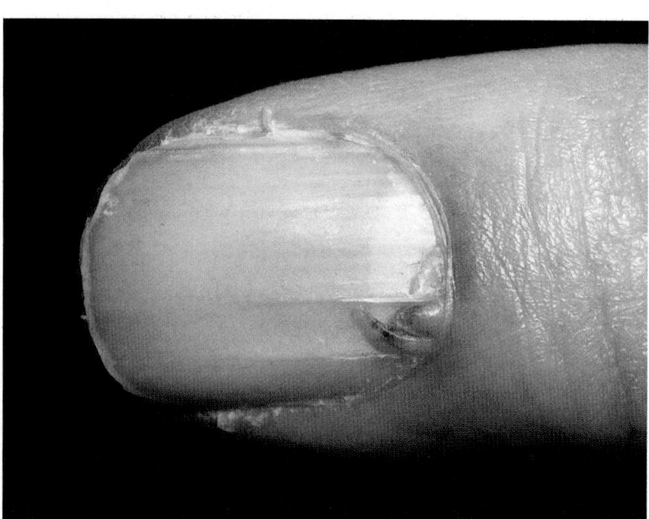

FIGURE 205-8 Periungual fibroma (Koenen tumor) in a patient with tuberous sclerosis. These appear later in life and are not typically seen in children. (*Used with permission from Richard P. Usatine, MD.*)

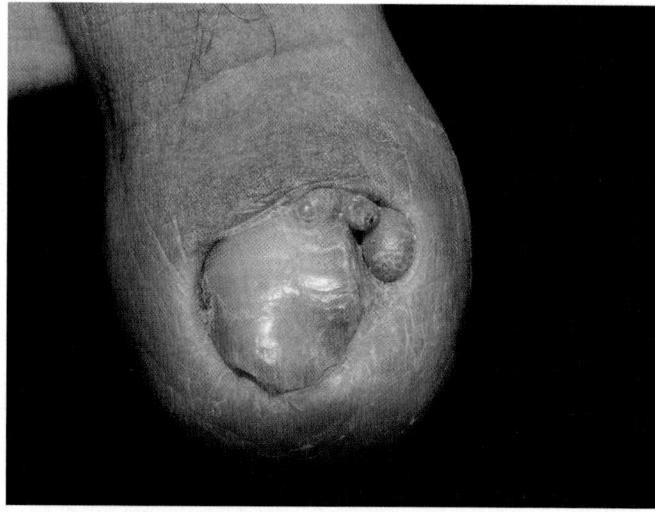

FIGURE 205-10 Periungual fibroma distorting the toe nail architecture of a teenager with tuberous sclerosis. (*Used with permission from Marisa Pongprutthipan, MD.*)

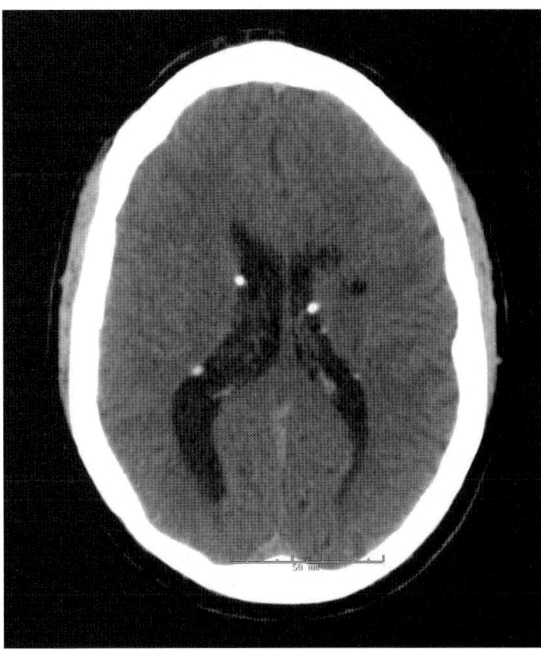

FIGURE 205-11 Bilateral subependymal calcified tubers on CT scan of a teenager with tuberous sclerosis. (*Used with permission from Elumalai Appachi, MD.*)

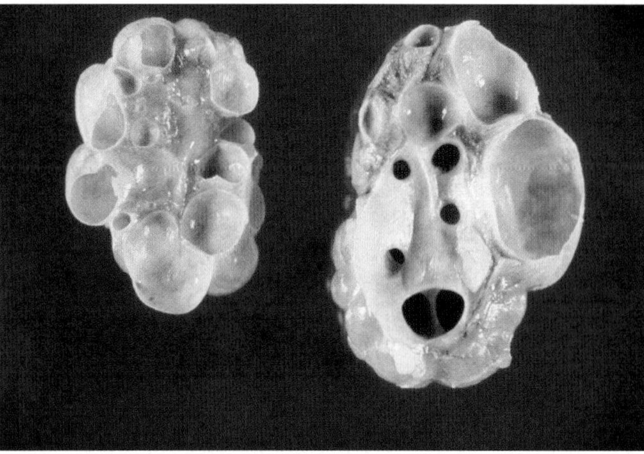

FIGURE 205-12 Multiple renal cysts found in both kidneys at autopsy from a teenager who succumbed to the complications of tuberous sclerosis. (*Used with permission from Elumalai Appachi, MD.*)

is usually present in older children and adults. These are benign vascular, smooth muscle, and adipose tissue tumors. The lesions are often multiple and bilateral, and increase in size and number with age.[6]

  - Renal cysts are the second most frequent renal manifestation (**Figure 205-12**). Cysts greater than 4 cm in diameter are more likely to be symptomatic. Presenting features may include flank pain, gross hematuria, or a tender mass.

- Cardiac manifestations:
  - Cardiac rhabdomyomas are usually asymptomatic but can result in outflow obstruction, valvular dysfunction, arrhythmias (especially Wolff-Parkinson-White syndrome), and cerebral thromboembolism.
  - The most common presentation of cardiac dysfunction is heart failure soon after birth. The lesions often regress over the first few years of life.
- Ophthalmologic manifestations:
  - Retinal hamartomas occur in 40 to 50 percent of patients with TSC and are bilateral in a third of cases. While these are mostly asymptomatic, visual impairment as a result of a large macular lesion do occur in some patients.
- Respiratory manifestations:
  - Pulmonary involvement, as lymphangioleiomyomatosis, occurs in only approximately 1 percent of patients with TSC. This can manifest as spontaneous pneumothorax and progressive lung disease seen mainly in adult females.

DIAGNOSTIC CRITERIA

The diagnostic criteria for TSC are based upon specific clinical features.[7]

- Major clinical features of TSC:
  - Facial angiofibromas or forehead plaques (**Figures 205-4** to **205-6**).
  - Shagreen patch (connective tissue nevus; **Figure 205-7**).
  - Three or more hypomelanotic macules (**Figures 205-1** to **205-3**).
  - Nontraumatic ungual or periungual fibromas (**Figures 205-8** to **205-10**).
  - Lymphangioleiomyomatosis (also known as lymphangiomyomatosis).
  - Renal angiomyolipoma.
  - Cardiac rhabdomyoma.
  - Multiple retinal nodular hamartomas.
  - Glioneuronal hamartomas (i.e., cortical tubers).
  - Subependymal nodules (**Figure 205-11**).
  - Subependymal giant cell astrocytoma.
- Minor clinical features of TSC:
  - Confetti skin lesions (multiple 1 to 2 mm hypomelanotic macules).
  - Gingival fibromas.
  - Multiple randomly-distributed pits in dental enamel.
  - Hamartomatous rectal polyps.
  - Multiple renal cysts (**Figure 205-12**).
  - Nonrenal hamartomas.
  - Bone cysts.
  - Retinal achromic patch.
  - Cerebral white matter radial migration lines.
- According to these criteria, the diagnostic certainty of TSC for any individual depends upon the number of major and minor features:
  - *Definite*—TSC requires two major features (excluding women with only renal angiomyolipoma and pulmonary lymphangioleiomyomatosis) or one major and two minor features.
  - *Probable*—TSC requires one major plus one minor feature.
  - *Suspected*—TSC requires one major feature only, or two or more minor features but no major features.

LABORATORY TESTING

- Molecular genetic testing for disease-causing mutations in the TSC1 and TSC2 genes is clinically available.
- A positive test for a TSC1 or TSC2 mutation is most helpful in confirming the diagnosis in any individual with probable or possible TSC who does not meet the criteria for definite TSC by clinical evaluation.

IMAGING

- Calcification is frequently seen in subependymal nodules and giant cell astrocytomas and is best detected on a CT scan (**Figure 205-11**).
- MRI is more sensitive for the detection of cortical and subcortical tubers, areas of heteropia, and small subependymal nodules, especially when they not calcified.
- An electroencephalogram (EEG) should be performed if seizures are present.
- Cardiac echocardiogram and renal ultrasound should be done all the patients with TSC to identify abnormalities.

DIFFERENTIAL DIAGNOSIS

- TSC should be considered in any child with epilepsy and cognitive impairment. Clinical evaluation will usually reveal the diagnosis based on the diagnostic criteria previously outlined.
- Infants with Infantile Spasm (West Syndrome) should be evaluated for TSC.
- Periventricular calcifications can be associated with congenital CMV infection. These infants will not have the cutaneous manifestations noted in children with TSC, and may have other manifestations of congenital infection.
- Renal cysts of TSC can be confused with polycystic kidney disease. In these cases, the common presence of neurologic manifestations will point to the diagnosis of TSC.

MANAGEMENT

NONPHARMACOLOGIC

- Treatment should be supportive and organ specific, depending on the specific organ(s) involved and the spectrum of the manifestations.
- A multidisciplinary approach is highly recommended and should be aimed at improving the patient's quality of life and outcome.
- Early intervention and special education is warranted when neurodevelopmental problems are evident.
- Control of seizures and cardiac dysrhythmias, when present, is paramount.

MEDICATIONS

- Seizures are managed with anticonvulsant medications. Specific recommendations depend on the specific seizure types.
- Vigabatrin has been shown to be effective for treating infantile spasms, and may help prevent more severe cases of cognitive dysfunction.[8] SOR Ⓑ
- Lamotrigine is effective in the treatment of generalized seizures.[9]

SURGICAL

- Neurosurgical intervention should be considered for intractable seizures, increased intracranial pressure, and giant cell astrocytomas. SOR Ⓒ
- Facial angiofibromas are potentially embarrassing cosmetic stigmata of TSC and can be treated with dermabrasion or laser surgery. SOR Ⓒ

REFERRAL

- A multidisciplinary approach to care is warranted; thus, consultations with a dermatologist, neurologist, nephrologist, cardiologist, and ophthalmologist should be strongly considered for patients who are diagnosed or suspected of having TSC.

PREVENTION AND SCREENING

- When a specific TSC mutation is identified, the family may elect to use preimplantation genetic diagnosis. This involves single cell analysis after biopsy of an embryo obtained through in vitro fertilization and subsequent implantation of embryos at low risk of carrying the mutation.
- Prenatal testing for TSC1 or TSC2 mutations of specimens obtained during pregnancy through either chorionic villus sampling or amniocentesis is also available.[9]
- Preimplantation or prenatal genetic testing with DNA analysis can be performed in families in which a specific mutation in the TSC1 or TSC2 gene has been identified in an affected family member.[10]
- Parents should be aware that TSC exhibits wide clinical variability within families and that establishing the diagnosis prenatally cannot predict the severity or outcome.
- When either parent is affected, fetal echocardiography should be performed in pregnancy. Echocardiography should be repeated in the neonatal period because it provides a better assessment than fetal echocardiography. An electrocardiogram should be performed to look for arrhythmias.
- When the diagnosis is made in a child with no family history of the disorder, both parents should be evaluated. This evaluation should include:
  - A thorough examination of the skin (in normal light and a Wood's lamp exam).
  - Ophthalmic examination.
  - Cranial CT or MRI.
  - Renal ultrasound.
- The importance of determining whether a parent is affected lies in providing appropriate follow-up for the parent, that is, screening for renal disease, and in providing an appropriate risk estimate of having a subsequent child with TSC.

PROGNOSIS

- Life expectancy historically was reduced mainly because of intercurrent infection, uncontrolled seizures, or other complications. Diagnostic imaging and treatment has improved both the quality of life and life expectancy of patients with TSC.

FOLLOW-UP

- Close follow-up by a multidisciplinary team, based on the manifestations of the condition and the organ systems involved is important.
- Ongoing screening for central nervous system, renal, and pulmonary tumors is recommended.

PATIENT RESOURCES

- The Tuberous Sclerosis Alliance Web Site—**www.tsalliance.org**.
- National Institute of Neurologic Disorders and Stroke: Tuberous Sclerosis Information Page—**www.ninds.nih.gov/disorders/tuberous_sclerosis/tuberous_sclerosis.htm**.
- Genetics Home Reference: Tuberous Sclerosis—**http://ghr.nlm.nih.gov/condition/tuberous-sclerosis-complex**.

PROVIDER RESOURCES

- **www.rarediseases.org**.
- **http://emedicine.medscape.com/article/1177711**.

REFERENCES

1. Stanley B., Vail E., Thiele E. Tuberous Sclerosis Complex: Diagnostic Challenges, Presenting Symptoms, and Commonly Missed Signs. *Pediatrics*. 2011;127(1):125-129.
2. Crino PB, Nathanson KL, Henske EP. The tuberous sclerosis complex. *N Engl J Med*. 2006;355:1345.
3. Osborne JP, Fryer A, Webb D. Epidemiology of tuberous sclerosis. *Ann N Y Acad Sci*. 1991;615:125.
4. Schwartz RA, Fernández G, Kotulska K, Jóźwiak S. Tuberous sclerosis complex: advances in diagnosis, genetics, and management. *J Am Acad Dermatol*. 2007;57:189.
5. Houser OW, Shepherd CW, Gomez MR. Imaging of intracranial tuberous sclerosis. *Ann N Y Acad Sci*. 1991;615:81-93.
6. O'Callaghan FJ, Noakes M, Martyn C, Osborne JP. An epidemiological study of renal pathology in tuberous sclerosis complex. *BJU Int*. 2004;94:853-857.
7. Roach ES, Sparagana SP. Diagnosis of tuberous sclerosis complex. *J Child Neurol*. 2004;19:643-649.
8. Parisi P, Bombardieri R, Curatolo P. Current role of vigabatrin in infantile spasms. *Eur J Paediatr Neurol*. 2007;11:331-336.
9. Curatolo P, Bombardieri R, Jozwiak S. Tuberous sclerosis. *Lancet*. 2008;372:657.
10. Hallett L, Foster T, Liu Z, et al. Burden of disease and unmet needs in tuberous sclerosis complex with neurological manifestations: systematic review. *Curr Med Res Opin*. 2011;27:1571.

206 NEUROFIBROMATOSIS

Heidi Chumley, MD

PATIENT STORY

A 12-year-old asymptomatic girl was noted to have six café-au-lait macules (**Figure 206-1A**) and axillary freckles (**Figure 206-1B**) during a general physical examination. No neurofibromas were noted at the time. Although neither parent had neurofibromatosis, that diagnosis was entertained. She was referred to an ophthalmologist and monitored closely for scoliosis. In time, she began to develop neurofibromas and was eventually diagnosed with sporadic neurofibromatosis type 1 (NF-1).

INTRODUCTION

NF-1 is a common autosomal dominant disorder that predisposes to tumor formation. Café-au-lait spots are often the first clinical sign. Other clinical signs include neurofibromas, axillary or inguinal freckling, optic gliomas, Lisch nodules, and sphenoid bone dysplasia. Treatment at present is early recognition and monitoring for complications such as cognitive dysfunction, scoliosis or other orthopedic problems, tumor pressure on vital structures, or malignant transformation.

SYNONYMS

Café-au-lait spots and café-au-lait macules are synonyms.

EPIDEMIOLOGY

- NF-1 is relatively common—Birth incidence is 1 in 3000 and prevalence in the general population is 1 in 5000.[1]
- Autosomal-dominant inheritance; however, up to 50 percent of cases are sporadic.[1]
- Diagnosis is typically made during childhood.

ETIOLOGY AND PATHOPHYSIOLOGY

- Mutations in the NF-1 gene (on the long arm of chromosome 17) result in loss of function of neurofibromin, which helps keep protooncogene ras (which increases tumorigenesis) in an inactive form.
- Loss of neurofibromin results in increased protooncogene ras activity in neurocutaneous tissues, leading to tumorigenesis.[1]

RISK FACTORS

A first-degree relative with NF-1.

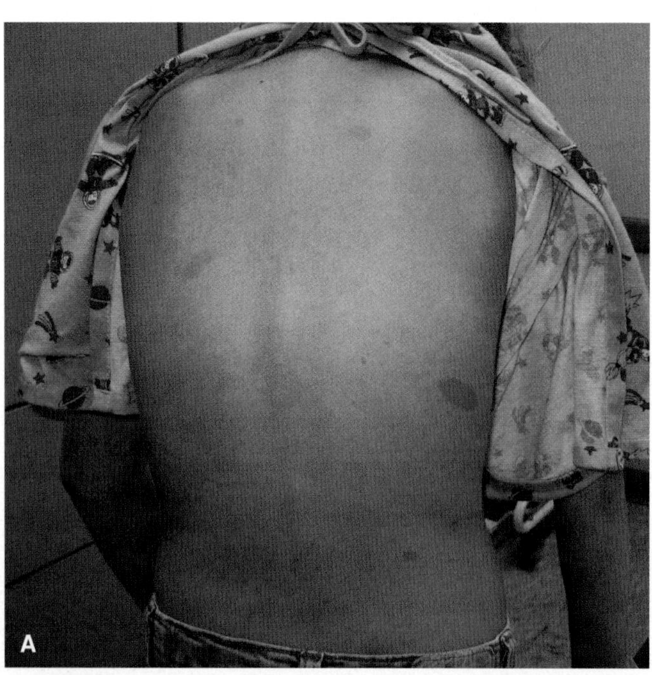

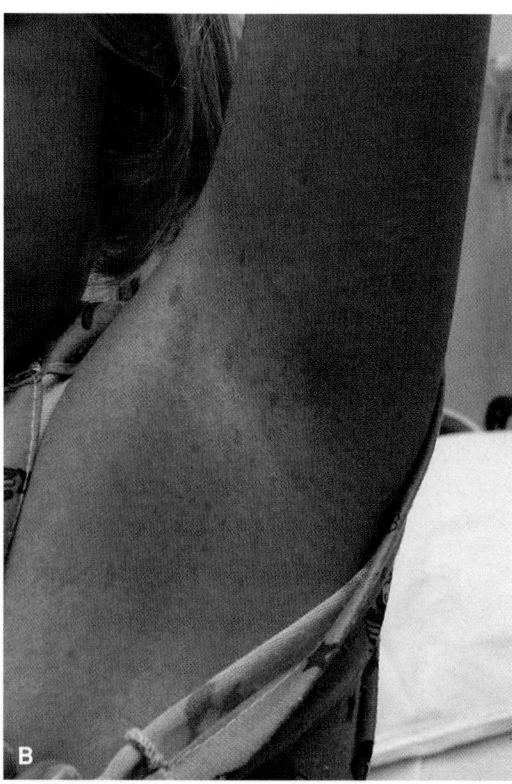

FIGURE 206-1 **A.** A 12-year-old girl presenting with over six café-au-lait macules (0.5 cm or larger) and **B.** axillary freckling (Crow sign). She does not have any neurofibromas visible but does meet criteria for neurofibromatosis. *(Used with permission from Emily Scott, MD.)*

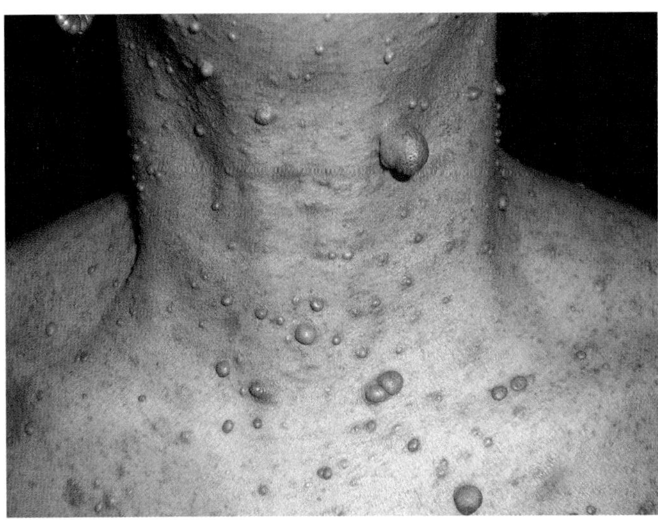

FIGURE 206-2 Close-up of neurofibromas on the neck and upper chest. These are soft and round. (*Used with permission from Richard P. Usatine, MD.*)

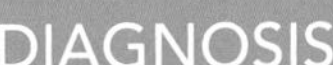

DIAGNOSIS

For a diagnosis of NF-1, patients need to have at least 2 of the following:[2]

- Two or more neurofibromas (**Figures 206-2** and **206-3**) or one or more plexiform neurofibromas (**Figures 206-4** and **206-5**).
- Six or more café-au-lait spots, 0.5 cm, or larger before puberty and 1.5 cm or larger after puberty (**Figures 206-6** to **206-9**).
- Axillary or inguinal freckling (**Figures 206-1** and **206-9**).
- Optic glioma.
- Two or more Lisch nodules (melanotic iris hamartomas; **Figure 206-10**).
- Dysplasia of the sphenoid bone or dysplasia/thinning of long bone cortex.
- A first-degree relative with NF-1.

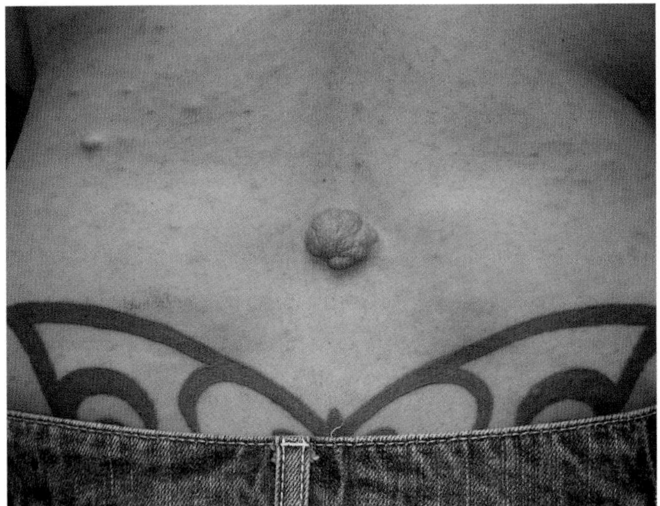

FIGURE 206-3 Large neurofibroma on the back of his teenage patient with neurofibromatosis. (*Used with permission from Richard P. Usatine, MD.*)

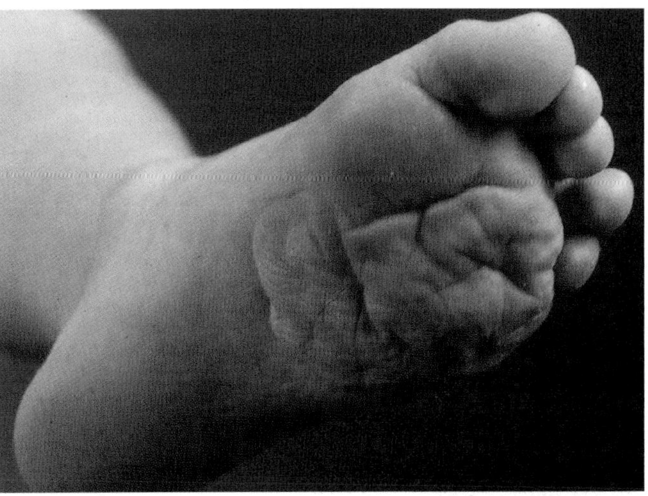

FIGURE 206-4 Neurofibromatosis (NF-1) in a child with a plexiform neuroma on the sole of the foot. This subcutaneous mass is soft and asymptomatic. The child also has café-au-lait macules and multiple neurofibromas. (*Used with permission from Fitzpatrick dermatology Atlas.*)

CLINICAL FEATURES

History and physical

- Ninety-five percent have café-au-lait macules, mostly before the age of 1 year.
- Ninety percent have axillary or inguinal freckling (**Figures 206-1** and **206-9**).
- Eighty-one percent have cognitive dysfunction manifest as learning disorder, attention deficit hyperactivity disorder, or mild cognitive impairment.[3]
- Nerve sheath, intracranial, or spinal tumors.
- Cutaneous or subcutaneous neurofibromas (**Figures 206-2** to **206-3**).
- Other bony pathology, including dysplasia of the sphenoid or long bones, scoliosis, or short stature (**Figure 206-9**).

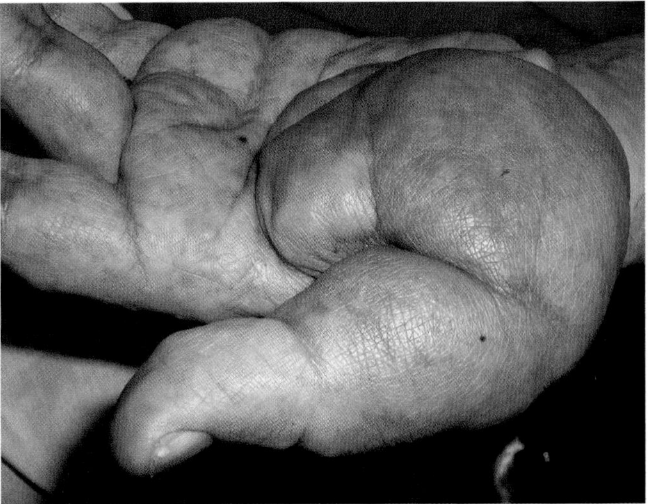

FIGURE 206-5 Plexiform neurofibroma on the thenar eminence feels like a bag of worms in this patient with neurofibromatosis. This is a benign tumor of the peripheral nerve sheath and is most often asymptomatic. (*Used with permission from Richard P. Usatine, MD.*)

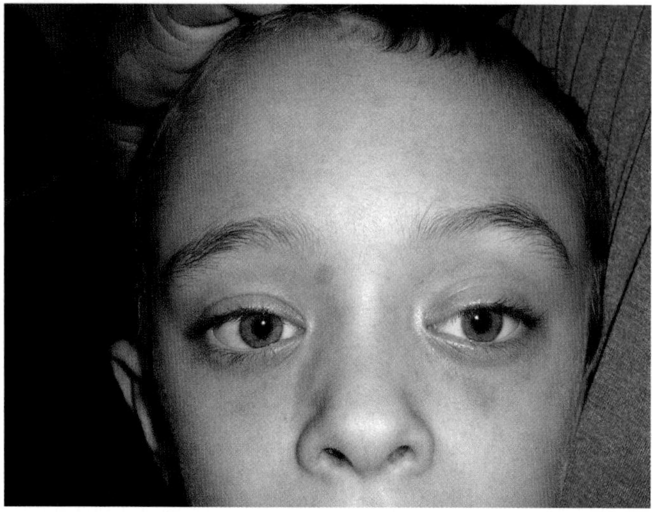

FIGURE 206-6 Neurofibromatosis in a 7-year-old boy with café-au-lait macules on the face. (*Used with permission from Richard P. Usatine, MD.*)

- Eye abnormalities, including Lisch nodules or early glaucoma (**Figure 206-10**).

LABORATORY TESTING

- Genetic testing for parents considering having other children.

IMAGING

- Although not typically used for diagnosis, imaging may be needed if tumor compression of vital structures is suspected.

DIFFERENTIAL DIAGNOSIS

NF-1 is the predominant cause of café-au-lait spots, which can also be seen in the following cases:

- Normal childhood—Thirteen percent to 27 percent of children younger than 10 years of age have at least 1 spot.

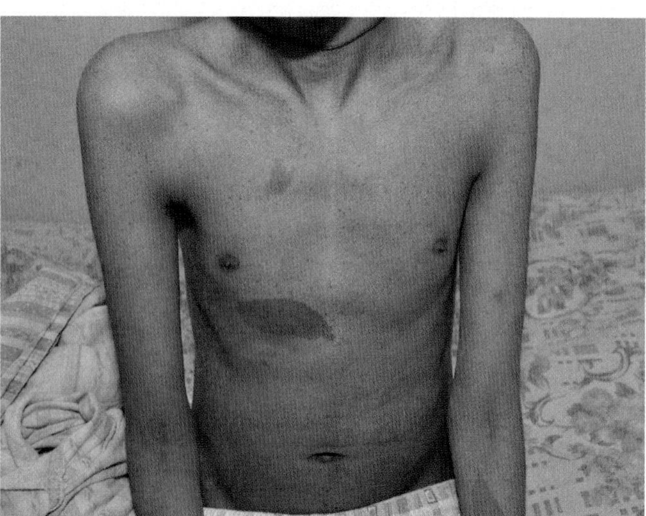

FIGURE 206-7 Neurofibromatosis with visible café-au-lait macule in a boy with leprosy in Africa. (*Used with permission from Richard P. Usatine, MD.*)

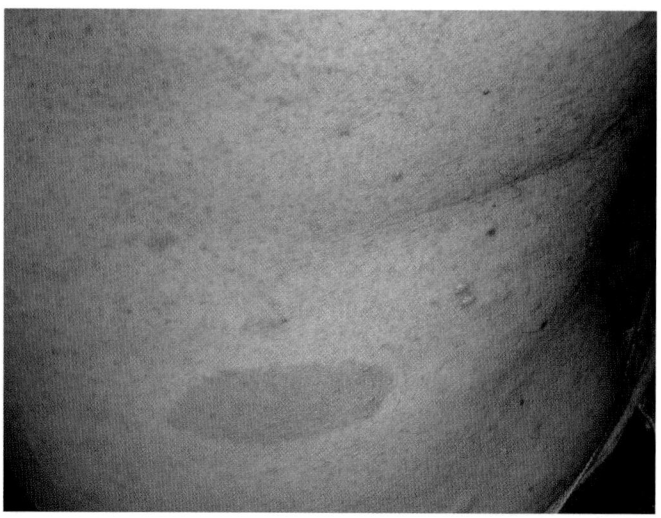

FIGURE 206-8 Neurofibromatosis with visible café-au-lait macule and small neurofibromas on the trunk. (*Used with permission from Richard P. Usatine, MD.*)

- Neurofibromatosis type 2 (NF-2)—Vestibular schwannomas, family history of NF-2, meningioma, glioma, schwannoma, juvenile posterior subcapsular lenticular opacities, or juvenile cortical cataracts.
- Tuberous sclerosis—Angiofibromas (skin-colored telangiectatic papules most commonly in the nasolabial folds, cheek, or chin; and hypopigmented ovoid or ash leaf-shaped macules (see Chapter 205, Tuberous Sclerosis).
- McCune-Albright syndrome—Fibrous dysplasia of bone and endocrine gland hyperactivity.
- Fanconi anemia—Decreased production of all blood cells, short stature, upper limb anomalies, genital changes, skeletal anomalies, eye/eyelid anomalies, kidney malformations, ear anomalies/deafness, and GI/cardiopulmonary malformations.
- Segmental NF—Cutaneous neurofibromas limited to specific dermatome(s); very rare.
- Bloom syndrome—Growth delay and short stature, increased risk of cancer, telangiectatic erythema on the face, cheilitis, narrow face, prominent nose, large ears, and long limbs.
- Ataxia telangiectasia—Progressive neurologic impairment, cerebellar ataxia, immunodeficiency, impaired organ maturation, ocular and cutaneous telangiectasia, and a predisposition to malignancy.
- Proteus syndrome—Very rare condition with hamartomatous and multisystem involvement. Joseph Merrick (also known as "the elephant man") is now, in retrospect, thought by clinical experts to have had Proteus syndrome and not NF.

MANAGEMENT

Management focuses on early recognition and treatment of manifestations.

- Evaluate children twice a year. SOR Ⓒ
- Screen for cognitive impairment and refer early for intervention. SOR Ⓒ
- Screen for scoliosis and treat accordingly.

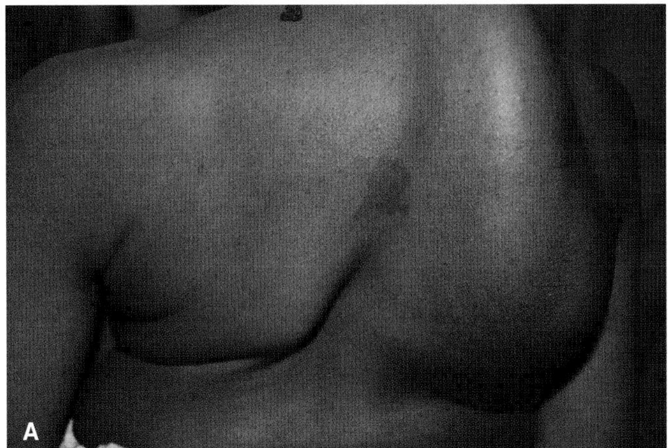

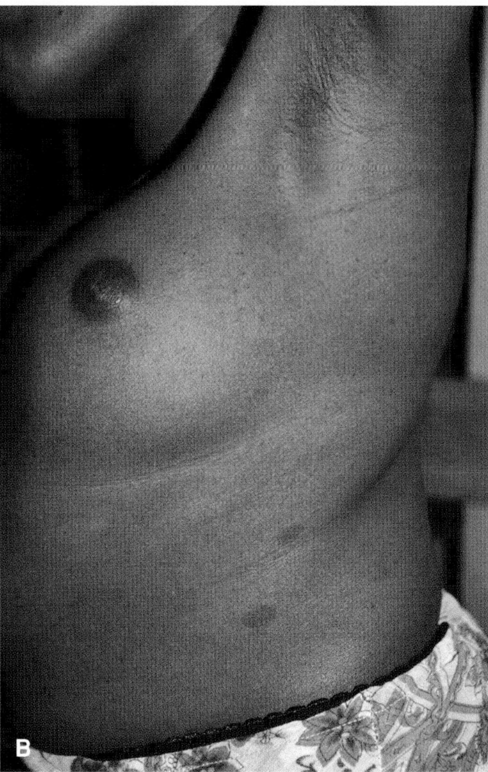

FIGURE 206-9 **A.** Neurofibromatosis in a teenage girl with severe scoliosis and a visible café-au-lait macule on the back. **B.** Axillary freckling (Crow sign) in the same teen with neurofibromatosis and scoliosis. (*Used with permission from Richard P. Usatine, MD.*)

- Refer patients annually for ophthalmologic evaluation.
- Consider treatment or referral for treatment of café-au-lait spots if desired by the patient. Topical vitamin D_3 analogs (calcipotriene [Dovonex]) and laser therapy independently may improve the appearance of café-au-lait spots.[4,5] SOR Ⓑ One small study suggests that intense pulsed light–radio frequency (IPL-RF) in combination with topical application of vitamin D_3 ointment may lighten small-pigmented lesions in patients with NF-1.[6] SOR Ⓑ Although calcipotriene is approved for use in psoriasis, it can be prescribed off-label to patients disturbed by their hyperpigmented macules.[4,6] SOR Ⓑ
- Examine other undiagnosed first-degree relatives. SOR Ⓒ
- Surgical excision of tumors is required for tumors pressing on vital structures (i.e., spinal cord impingement, and optic glioma) or when characteristics such as rapid enlargement are worrisome for malignant transformation.

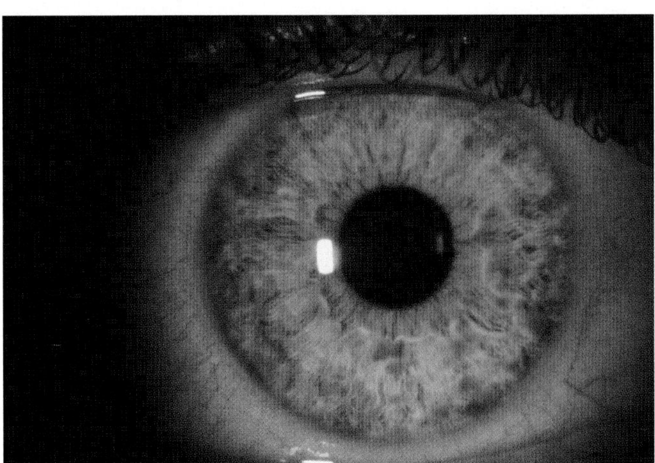

FIGURE 206-10 Lisch nodules (melanotic hamartomas of the iris) are clear yellow-to-brown, dome-shaped elevations that project from the surface of this blue iris. These hamartomas are the most common type of ocular involvement in neurofibromatosis type 1 and do not affect vision. (*Used with permission from Paul Comeau.*)

PROGNOSIS

- Clinical manifestations are variable leading to difficulty in prognosis.
- There is a 10 percent lifetime risk of developing a malignant peripheral nerve sheath tumor.

FOLLOW-UP

- Primary care evaluation biannually for children, including monitoring of blood pressure.
- Ophthalmologic examination annually for children for early detection of optic gliomas and glaucoma. Neurofibromas and plexiform neuromas can occur on the eyelids. Neurofibromas on the eyelids usually are not a problem (**Figure 206-10**) but a plexiform neuroma can present with ptosis and need surgical intervention.
- Genetic counseling for parents of a child with NF-1 considering having other children.

PROVIDER RESOURCE

- Neurofibromatosis, Inc. has a variety of resources including NF specialists by location—**www.nfinc.org**.

PATIENT RESOURCES

- Neurofibromatosis, Inc. has a variety of patient education materials, information about local support groups, ongoing clinical trials, and camp New Friends for children with NF—**www.nfinc.org**.
- The National Institute of Neurological Diseases and Stroke has patient information at its *Neurofibromatosis Information Page*—**www.ninds.nih.gov/disorders/NF/NF.htm**.

REFERENCES

1. Yohay K: Neurofibromatosis types 1 and 2. *Neurologist*. 2006; 12(2):86-93.
2. Hirsch NP, Murphy A, Radcliffe JJ: Neurofibromatosis: clinical presentations and anaesthetic implications. *Br J Anaesth*. 2001; 86(4):555-564.
3. Hyman SL, Shores A, North KN. The nature and frequency of cognitive deficits in children with neurofibromatosis type 1. *Neurology*. 2005;65(7):1037-1044.
4. Nakayama J, Kiryu H, Urabe K, et al. Vitamin D3 analogues improve café au lait spots in patients with von Recklinghausen's disease: experimental and clinical studies. *Eur J Dermatol*. 1999; 9(3):202-206.
5. Shimbashi T, Kamide R, Hashimoto T: Long-term follow-up in treatment of solar lentigo and café-au-lait macules with Q-switched ruby laser. *Aesthetic Plast Surg*. 1997;21(6):445-448.
6. Yoshida Y, Sato N, Furumura M, Nakayama J: Treatment of pigmented lesions of neurofibromatosis 1 with intense pulsed-radio frequency in combination with topical application of vitamin D_3 ointment. *J Dermatol*. 2007;34(4):227-230.

207 STURGE-WEBER SYNDROME

Swathi Appachi, BS
Elumalai Appachi, MD, MRCP

PATIENT STORY

A 3-year-old girl is referred to a pediatric neurologist because of a history of developmental delay and focal seizures since birth that are no longer being well controlled with two antiseizure medications. On physical exam, the neurologist notes a large bilateral port-wine stain on the face (**Figure 207-1**). The neurologist suspects that the child has Sturge-Weber syndrome and orders brain imaging and an ophthalmologic exam. The MRI reveals leptomeningeal angiomas and the ophthalmologist diagnoses glaucoma. The diagnosis of Sturge-Weber syndrome is confirmed and education is provided to the parents on this condition. The child's anti-epileptic medications are maximized and her glaucoma is treated by the ophthalmologist.

INTRODUCTION

Sturge-Weber syndrome (SWS) is a sporadic congenital neurocutaneous syndrome that is characterized by facial capillary malformation known as a port-wine stain, ocular abnormalities including glaucoma and choroidal hemangioma, and leptomeningeal angiomas. Seizures, developmental delay and glaucoma comprise the major clinical features. SWS is associated with mutations in the GNAQ gene.

SYNONYMS

Encephalotrigeminal angiomatosis and encephalofacial angiomatosis. Port-wine stains are also called nevus flammeus.

EPIDEMIOLOGY

- SWS occur sporadically at a rate of 1 per 20,000 to 50,000 newborns and in equal frequency in both genders.[1]

ETIOLOGY AND PATHOPHYSIOLOGY

- SWS is caused by somatic activating mutations in GNAQ gene, as confirmed by a whole-genome sequencing study that examined skin and brain tissue samples.[1]
- GNAQ encodes for G-alpha-q, a G-protein alpha subunit that acts as a mediator between G-protein coupled receptors and downstream signaling molecules.
- In fetal ectodermal tissue, this mutation is thought to cause inappropriate maturation of capillaries, thus leading to capillary malformations.[1] The port-wine stain is due to a dilation of capillaries and

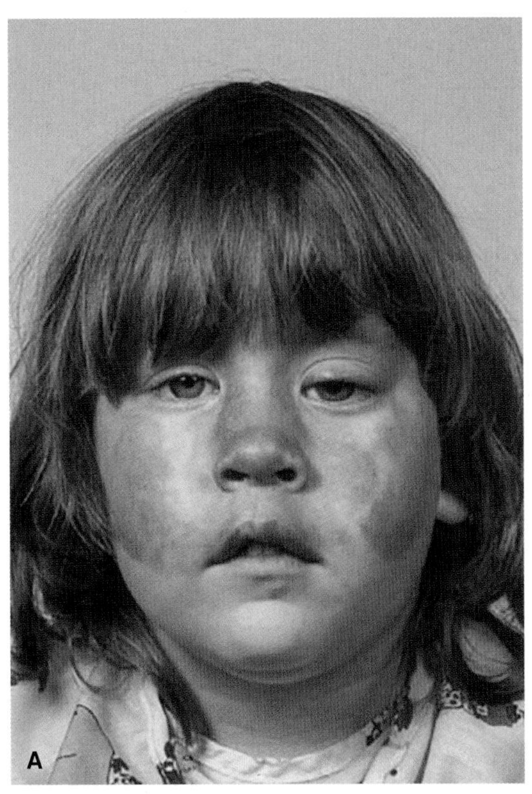

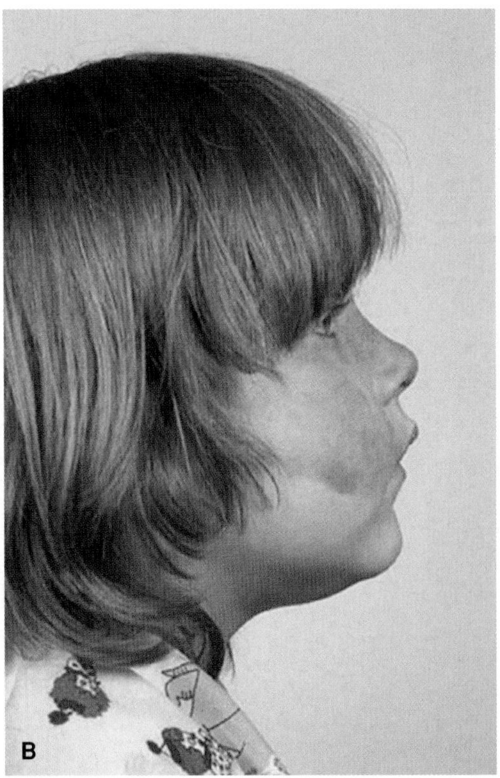

FIGURE 207-1 Port-wine stain on frontal (**A**) and right lateral (**B**) views in a young girl with Sturge-Weber syndrome. Although bilateral involvement is not common, it is associated with intracranial findings such as leptomeningeal angiomas. (*Used with permission from Cleveland Clinic Children's Hospital Photo Files.*)

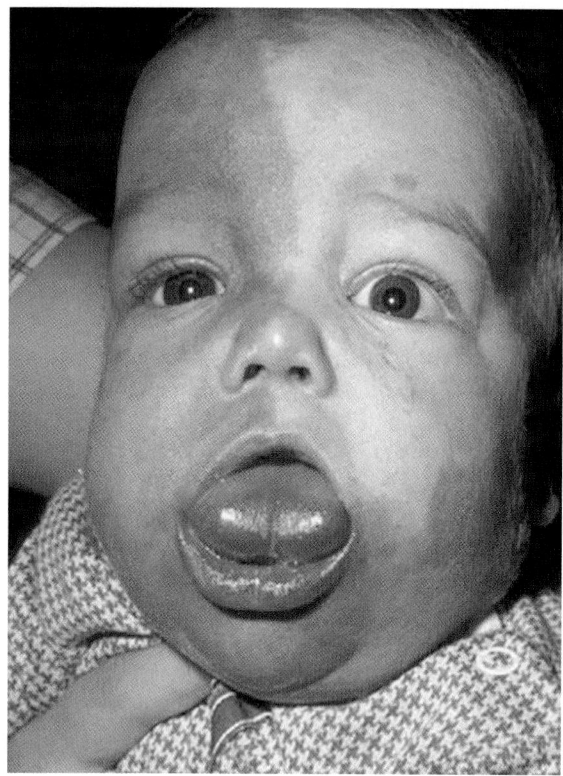

FIGURE 207-2 Port-wine stain in a young infant with seizures and developmental delay due to Sturge-Weber syndrome. (*Used with permission from Cleveland Clinic Children's Hospital Photo Files.*)

venous blood vessels in the dermis rather than a proliferation of the capillaries.[2]

DIAGNOSIS

CLINICAL FEATURES

- Physical manifestations of SWS can be divided into cutaneous, ocular, and neurologic. The diagnosis is usually made based on the presence of the facial capillary malformations and leptomeningeal angiomas.[2]
- Cutaneous:
  - The most obvious sign of SWS is the facial capillary malformation, known as a port-wine stain, due to its color (**Figures 207-1** to **207-3**).
  - Note that a capillary malformation is not the same as a cutaneous hemangioma even though these are often confused as the same entity. While there are ocular and CNS angiomas present in SWS, the port-wine stain is not a hemangioma.
  - It normally involves at least the distribution of the ophthalmic branch of the trigeminal nerve, overlying the forehead and the upper eyelid.
  - Although it usually does not cross the midline, those with bilateral port-wine stains are more likely to have cerebral involvement.[2,3]
- Neurological:
  - Leptomeningeal capillary-venous malformations, or angiomas can occur in children with SWS, usually ipsilaterally to the

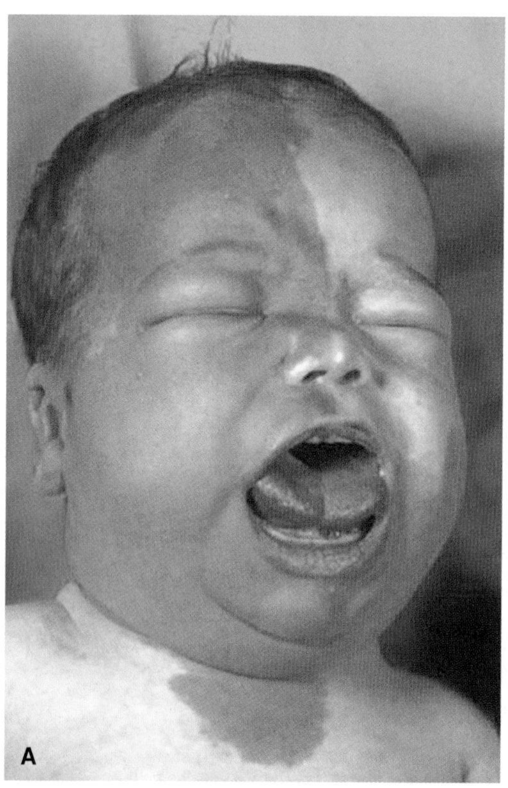

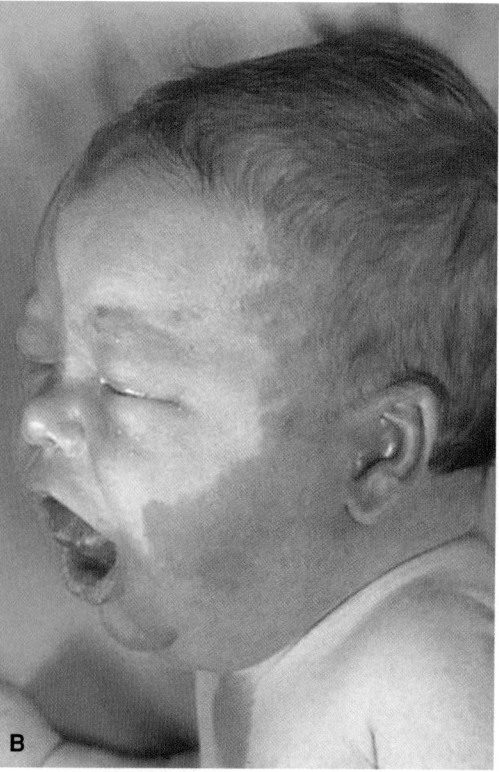

FIGURE 207-3 Bilateral port-wine stain on frontal (**A**) and lateral (**B**) views in a young child with Sturge-Weber syndrome. This is the same child as seen in **Figure 207-2** at an older age. (*Used with permission from Cleveland Clinic Children's Hospital Photo Files.*)

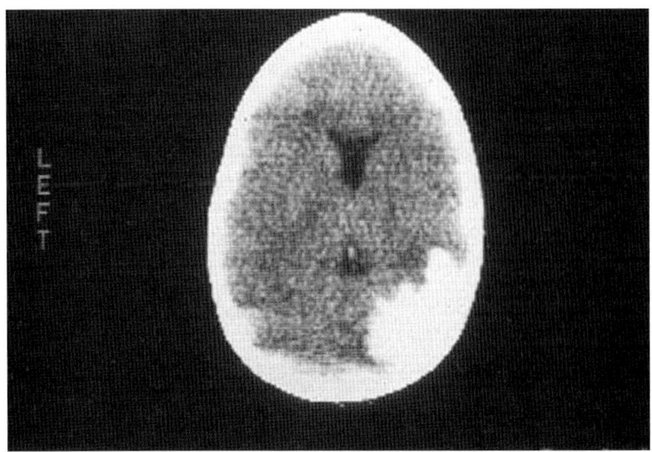

FIGURE 207-4 Leptomeningeal angioma on CT scan in a child with a port-wine stain, seizures, and developmental delay. (*Used with permission from Cleveland Clinic Children's Hospital Photo Files.*)

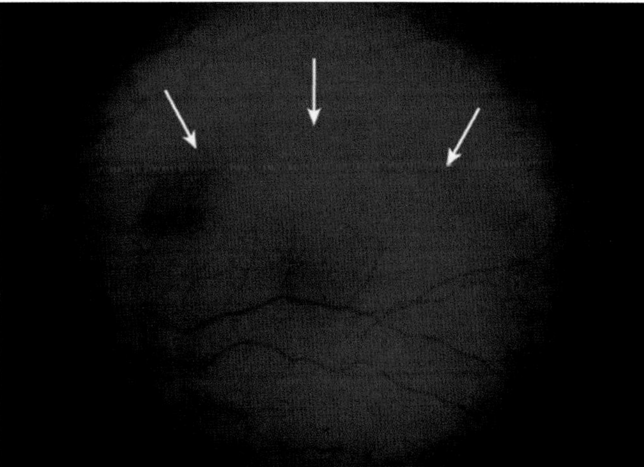

FIGURE 207-5 Choriodal hemangioma in a patient with Sturge-Weber syndrome. The arrows point to the superior border of the hemangioma. The posterior retina, including the fovea, is elevated. (*Used with permission from Lueder GT. Pediatric Practice Ophthalmology: Figure 32-19, and www.accesspediatrics.com.*)

port-wine stain in the parietal or occipital areas (**Figure 207-4**). Underlying brain parenchyma may be atrophic and calcified.[2]
  - Seizures are the usual presenting neurologic manifestation of this syndrome and can occur in 23 to 83 percent of patients. They can occur at any age but often manifest before 2 years of age. Seizures are typically focal motor seizures, but secondary generalization can occur. Infantile spasms are less common but can also occur. Seizures often present initially during a febrile episode. They can be more severe in patients with bilateral leptomeningeal angiomas.[2]
  - Developmental delay is present in approximately half of these patients. Degree of handicap is usually correlated with younger age at onset of seizures.
  - Recurrent headaches are also common in these patients.
  - Stroke-like episodes can occur, with hemiparesis or visual field defects.
- Ocular:
  - Glaucoma, the most common ocular manifestation of SWS, develops in 30 to 70 percent of patients with SWS in some studies, and is usually ipsilateral to the port-wine stain. It can occur early in childhood and has an insidious onset. For this reason, any newborn or child presenting with a port-wine stain in the V1 distribution of the trigeminal nerve should be referred for a complete ophthalmologic exam.[2]
  - Choroidal hemangioma occurs in many patients with SWS and is also usually ipsilateral to the port-wine stain (**Figure 207-5**). Over time, these lesions can cause retinal pigment epithelium degeneration, fibrous metaplasia, or cystic retinal degeneration, leading to vision loss. The presence of a choroid hemangioma almost always indicates presence of leptomeningeal hemangiomas.[2]

IMAGING

- In addition to an ophthalmologic exam, any infant with a port-wine stain in the V1 distribution should have neuroimaging, specifically a brain MRI with gadolinium contrast.
  - If neonatal imaging is negative, repeat scans at 1 or 2 years of life or with onset of symptoms such as seizure or glaucoma.[4]
- Intracranial calcifications (Railroad or tramline calcifications) may be found on plain film or on CT scan (**Figure 207-6**). These represent calcification of the cortex.
- Leptomeningeal angiomas are common and cause seizures (**Figure 207-4**).

DIFFERENTIAL DIAGNOSIS

- The presence of a port-wine stain is not enough to diagnose SWS as only 8 to 20 percent of patients with this lesion have manifestations of neurological symptoms. Many children with facial port-wine stains do not have SWS (**Figures 207-7** and **207-8**).
- Facial hemangiomas that appear dermatomal are often confused with port-wine stains (**Figure 207-9**). Port-wine stains are usually

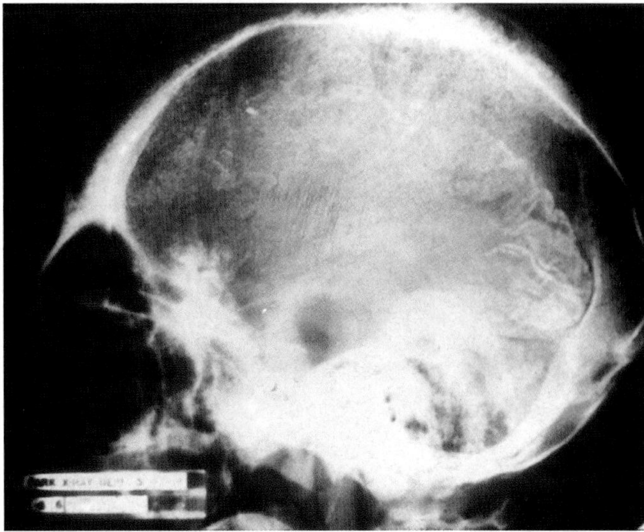

FIGURE 207-6 Intracranial calcifications on skull x-ray in a patient with Sturge-Weber syndrome. Note the tram track or railroad track pattern, signifying atrophic and calcified brain parenchyma, which is characteristic of this syndrome. (*Used with permission from Elumalai Appachi, MD.*)

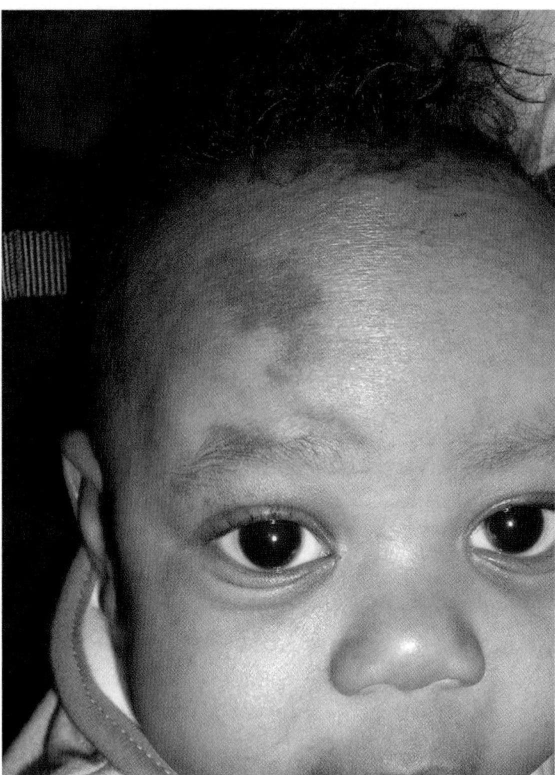

FIGURE 207-7 Port-wine stain in the V1 distribution in an infant without Sturge-Weber syndrome. The child has had no seizures and was developing normally. (*Used with permission from Richard P. Usatine MD.*)

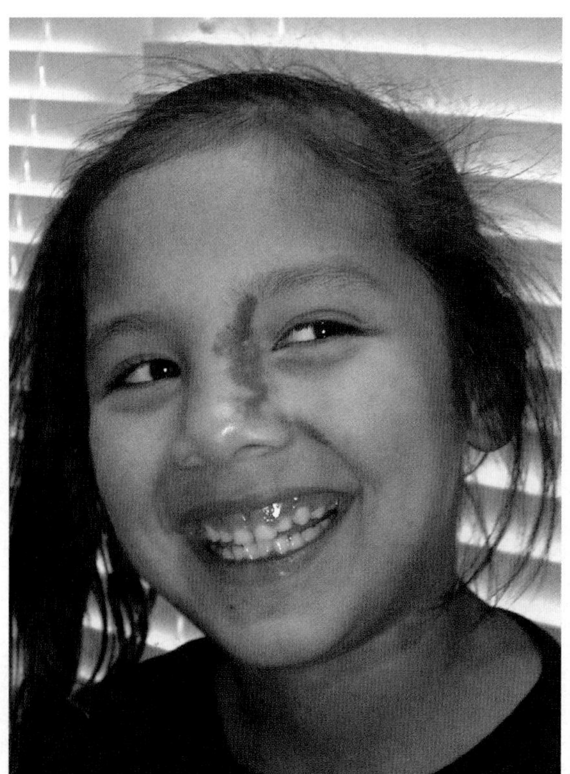

FIGURE 207-8 Port-wine stain on the face of a healthy young girl. She is doing well in school, has never had a seizure and has always had normal cognitive development. (*Used with permission from Richard P. Usatine MD.*)

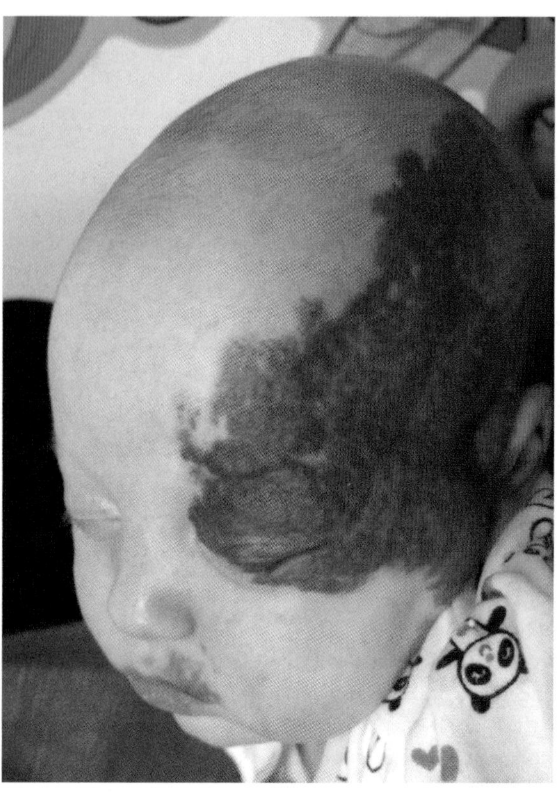

FIGURE 207-9 Large facial hemangioma in an infant without PHACE syndrome. Note that this is a hemangioma and not a port-wine stain. The hemangioma is not flat like a port-wine stain. This hemangioma resolved with propanolol and time. (*Used with permission from John Browning, MD.*)

flatter than hemangiomas and will not resolve over time as many hemangiomas do. Hemangiomas are benign vascular tumors that differ from capillary malformations (see Chapter 93, Childhood Hemangiomas and Vascular Malformations). Large facial hemangiomas may be seen with the PHACE syndrome (see Chapter 227, PHACE Syndrome).

- Patients with a port-wine stain, other extensive cutaneous capillary malformations, venous and lymphatic malformations, and limb hypertrophy have Klippel-Trenaunay syndrome.[3]

MANAGEMENT

- There is no cure for SWS. Management is aimed at controlling seizures and ocular manifestations such as glaucoma.

NONPHARMACOLOGIC

- A ketogenic diet has been shown in one study to be beneficial in stopping seizures refractory to pharmacological treatment.[3]

MEDICATIONS

- Managing epilepsy in patients with SWS is difficult and often requires more than one anti-epileptic drug (AED). However, management is crucial as increased seizure activity is thought to lead to neurocognitive deterioration.[3]

- Patients should be aggressively started on an AED to prevent seizure activity from occurring and have an AED prescribed as abortive therapy.
- If seizures are not controlled with a combination of 2 to 3 AEDs at their maximum doses, other routes of therapy, such as a ketogenic diet or surgery, should be considered.

SURGERY

- Surgery appears to be the treatment of choice for glaucoma in patients with SWS. Surgical treatments include cryocoagulation of the ciliary body, goniotomy, or trabeculotomy.[5,6]
- For refractory seizures, some small studies have shown that focal resection of the affected portion of the brain or hemispherectomy can achieve long-term seizure control. However, there is significant morbidity associated with these procedures, especially hemispherectomy (which is associated with hemiparesis and homonymous hemianopsia), and these should be discussed with the family.[3]
- The port-wine stain can be treated with pulsed dye laser.[2] This is a cosmetic procedure that is usually not covered by health insurance.

REFERRAL

- For any neonate with a port-wine stain, especially in the V1 distribution, an ophthalmologist should be consulted. Close monitoring of the child is necessary as onset of glaucoma can be insidious.[2]
- Similarly, in these children, a neurologist or epileptologist should be consulted for neuroimaging recommendations and possible management of seizures, especially if leptomeningeal angiomas are seen on imaging.
- In children with medically refractory seizures, a neurosurgeon should be consulted for surgical planning and decision-making.

PREVENTION AND SCREENING

- SWS cannot be prevented as it is sporadic.
- However, in any neonate or child with a port-wine stain on the face, a careful ophthalmologic exam with close follow-up is highly recommended.
- Neuroimaging is also necessary in children with a port-wine stain on the face, and should be repeated in 1 to 2 years if negative.

PROGNOSIS

- Prognosis depends directly on the severity and extent of the ocular manifestations and leptomeningeal angiomas.
- Screening for and surgical correction of glaucoma will be imperative for a good prognosis.
- Early onset of seizure activity and presence of leptomeningeal angiomas can cause developmental delay and neurocognitive decline. Thus careful control of seizure activity is necessary. However, cognitive deterioration can still occur as the patient ages.[3]

FOLLOW-UP

- Follow-up is contingent on the affected systems. An ophthalmologist and neurologist should be closely involved in care of the child with SWS.

PATIENT RESOURCES

- The Sturge-Weber Foundation—**www.sturge-weber.org**.
- National Institutes of Health NINDS—**www.ninds.nih.gov/disorders/sturge_weber/sturge_weber.htm**.

PROVIDER RESOURCES

- **www.rarediseases.org/**.
- **http://emedicine.medscape.com/article/1177523**.

REFERENCES

1. Shirley MD, Tang H, Gallione CJ, Baugher JD, Frelin LP, Cohen B, North PE, Marchuk DA, Comi AM, Pevsner J: Sturge-Weber syndrome and port-wine stains caused by somatic mutation in GNAQ. *N Engl J Med*. 2013;368(21):1971-1979.
2. Baselga E. Sturge: Weber Syndrome. Seminars in Cutaneous Medicine and Surgery. 2004;23(2):87-98.
3. Lo W, Marchuk DA, Ball KL, Juhasz C, Jordan LC, Ewen JB, Comi A: Brain Vascular Malformation Consortium National Sturge-Weber Syndrome Workgroup. Updates and future horizons on the understanding, diagnosis, and treatment of Sturge-Weber syndrome brain involvement. *Dev Med Child Neurol*. 2012;54(3):214-223.
4. Truhan AP, Filipek PA: Magnetic resonance imaging. Its role in the neuroradiologic evaluation of neurofibromatosis, tuberous sclerosis, and Sturge-Weber syndrome. *Arch Dermatol*. 1993 Feb;129(2):219-226.
5. van Emelen C, Goethals M, Dralands L, Casteels I: Treatment of glaucoma in children with Sturge-Weber syndrome. *J Pediatr Ophthalmol Strabismus*. 2000;37(1):29.
6. Olsen KE, Huang AS, Wright MM: The efficacy of goniotomy/trabeculotomy in early-onset glaucoma associated with the Sturge-Weber syndrome. *J AAPOS*. 1998;2(6):365.

208 DUCHENNE MUSCULAR DYSTROPHY

Neil Friedman, MBChB

PATIENT STORY

A 9-year-old boy with a history of Duchenne muscular dystrophy (DMD) is being seen by his pediatrician for a routine maintenance exam. He initially presented at 3 years of age for evaluation of toe walking and excessive falling, and was diagnosed with DMD. He started walking independently between 12 to 14 months of age. He had always been slower than his peers and has difficulty keeping up with them. At the time of diagnosis, the family reported increasing difficulty going up steps which he can only do one step at a time. He also had difficulty getting up from the floor, needing to push on his knee or use furniture for assistance (Gower sign), which has continued and is pronounced at the current visit (**Figure 208-1**). He also tends to be clumsy with excessive falling and has an awkward appearing waddling gait, exacerbated by running.

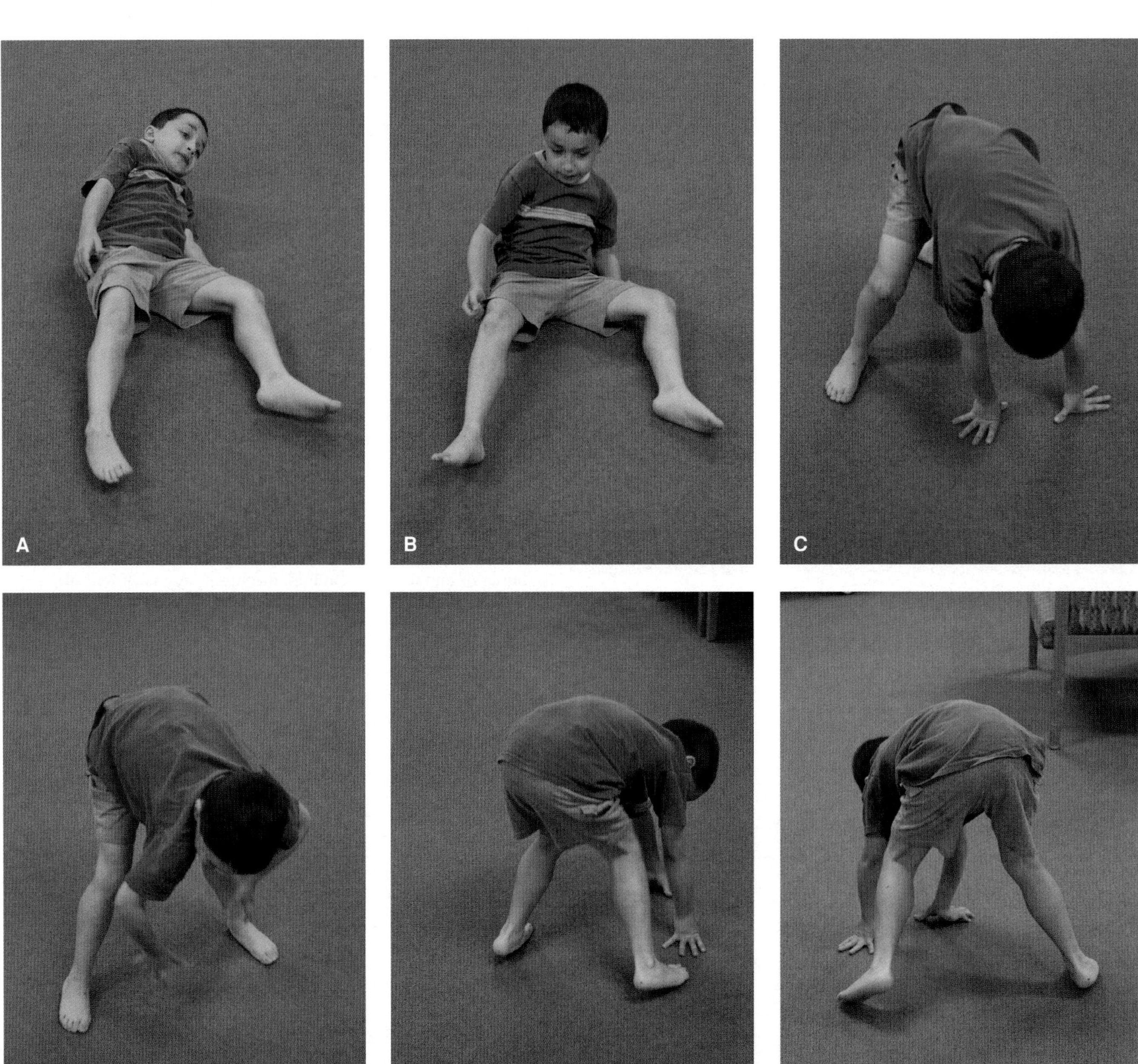

FIGURE 208-1 Gower sign. In order to stand up, the child gets into a prone crawl position with hands on the floor (**A**-**D**), extends and locks the legs in a widened stance (**E**-**F**), then using extended arms they shift their weight backwards and use their hands on their knees and thighs until they can achieve an upright position (**G**-**H**). (*Used with permission from Neil Friedman, MD.*) (*continued*)

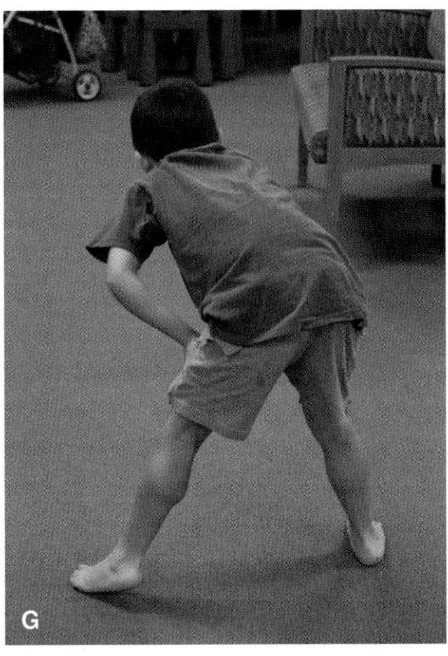

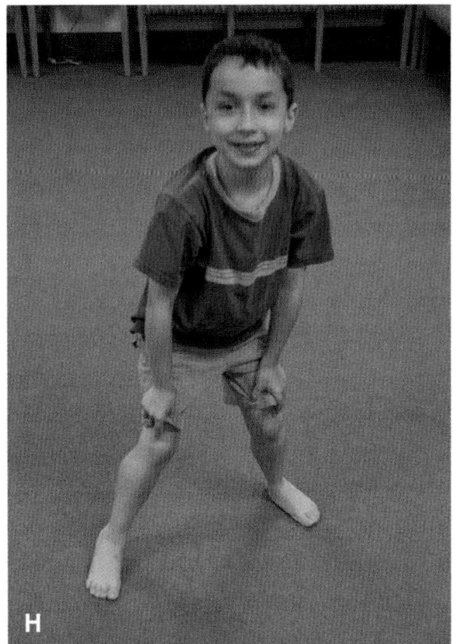

FIGURE 208-1 *(Continued)*

INTRODUCTION

- Most common form of muscular dystrophy.
- Presents between 2 to 5 years of with progressive, symmetric proximal weakness manifesting as difficulty getting up from the floor, difficulty climbing stairs, a waddling gait, and excessive tripping and falling.
- Loss of ambulation typically between 7 to 13 years of age.
- Early demise in 2nd or 3rd decade secondary to cardiomyopathy and progressive respiratory failure due to weakness.
- Results from mutation of the *DMD* gene; dystrophin is the gene product.
- X-linked recessive inheritance—Primarily affects males but female carriers may manifest disease characteristics due to skewed inactivation of the X-chromosome (Lyon hypothesis).
- Variable phenotype depending on the nature of the gene mutation.
  - Absence of dystrophin results in the severe Duchenne muscular dystrophy (DMD) phenotype.
  - Preservation of some dystrophin results in the allelic, milder Becker muscular dystrophy (BMD) phenotype or a dilated cardiomyopathy (DCM) in which the heart is primarily affected with little or no skeletal muscle involvement (**Table 208-1**).
- 1851—Edward Meryon reported first clinical cases of DMD in the medical literature.
- 1868—The French neurologist Duchenne de Boulogne describes a series of children with the disease that would later bear his name.

TABLE 208-1 Comparison of Duchenne and Becker Muscular Dystrophy

	Duchenne	Becker
Age of presentation	3–5 years	5–10 years, sometimes adolescence
Loss of ambulation	Before 13th birthday	Beyond 16th birthday
Death	Early 20's—from cardiopulmonary failure	Variable—long-term survival possible
CK	Massively elevated >10-100 × normal	Massively elevated >10–100 × normal
Cardiomyopathy	Late—end stage	Early, disproportionate to muscle weakness May be presenting feature
Dystrophin	Absent (<5%)	Reduced in quantity or quality (>10%)
Gene deletion	Large Deletions: about 2/3 of cases Small deletions, point mutations and duplications: about 1/3 of cases	Large Deletions: about 2/3 of cases Small deletions, point mutations and duplications: about 1/3 of cases

- 1954—Walton and Nattrass developed first classification of muscular dystrophies based on clinical and inheritance factors.
- 1986—*DMD* gene identified by Luis Kunkel (positional cloning or "reverse genetics").

SYNONYMS

- Dystophinopathies.
- Pseudo-hypertrophic muscular dystrophy.

EPIDEMIOLOGY[1]

- DMD is one of the more common genetic disorders affecting one in 3,500 live male births.
- BMD affects 1 in 30,000 to 35,000 live male births.
- Duchenne muscular dystrophy is the most frequent muscle disorder in childhood.

ETIOLOGY AND PATHOPHYSIOLOGY

- DMD is caused by an out-of-frame deletion, point mutation or duplication in the *DMD* gene leading to a complete absence of protein; whereas BMD results from an in-frame deletion or duplication in the *DMD* gene resulting in the expression of an altered size, but partially functional dystrophin protein.[2]
    - Deletions account for approximately 65 percent of cases of DMD and 85 percent of cases of BMD; the remainder due to point mutations or rarely duplications.
- *De novo* mutations occur in approximately 1/3 of cases, while 2/3 of cases are inherited from the mother.
- The *DMD* gene is the largest in the human genome (0.1% of the entire genome), encompassing 2.6 million base pairs of DNA and containing 79 exons.
- Dystrophin is a large, subsarcolemmal structural protein that has a major structural role in muscle as it links the internal actin cytoskeleton to the dystrophin-associated glycoproteins (DAG) in the sarcolemmal membrane (**Figure 208-2**).[3]
- Absence of dystrophin disrupts the muscle ultra structure resulting in muscle injury, inflammatory changes and ultimately degeneration of the muscle fibers with resultant replacement of muscle fibers by connective tissue and fatty infiltration, which is irreversible.[4]

RISK FACTORS

- Family history of DMD since it is a genetically inherited disease.
    - X-linked recessive inheritance.

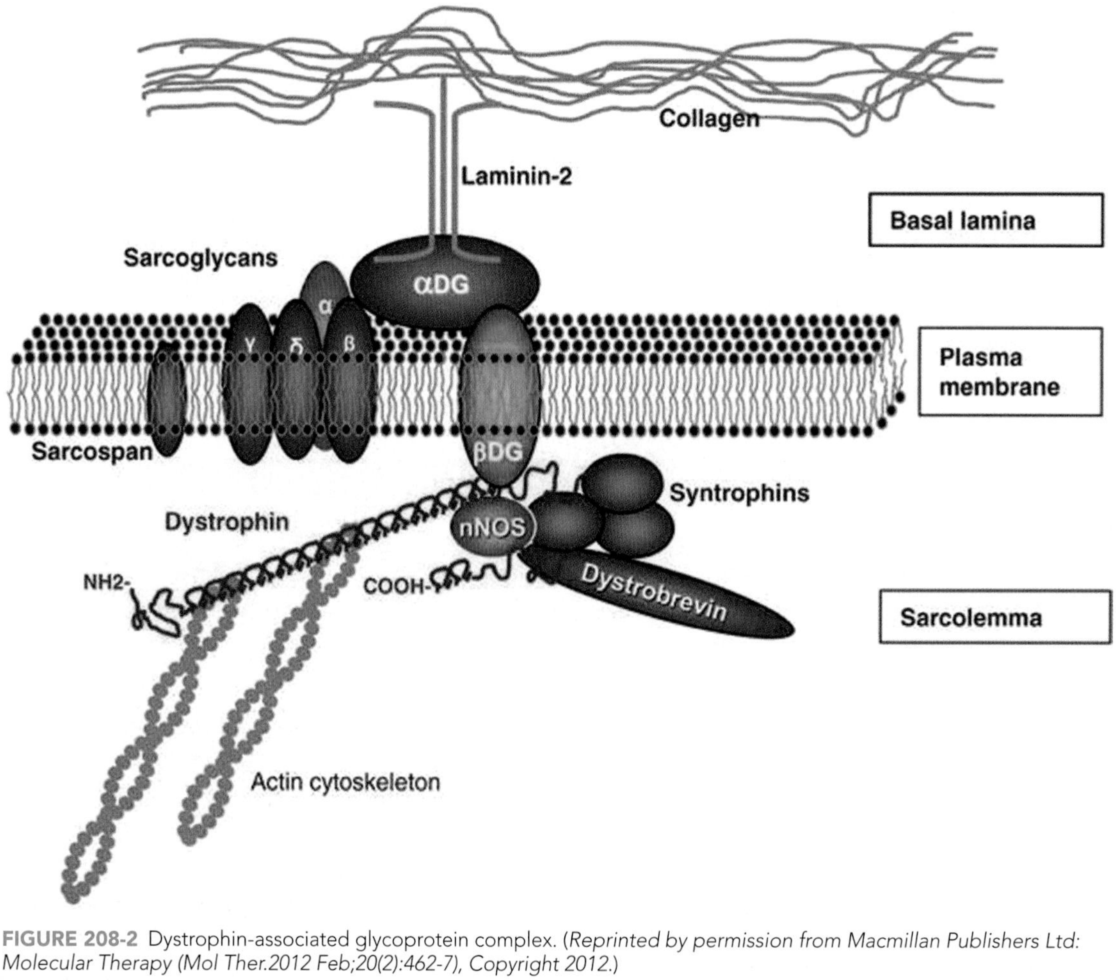

FIGURE 208-2 Dystrophin-associated glycoprotein complex. (*Reprinted by permission from Macmillan Publishers Ltd: Molecular Therapy (Mol Ther.2012 Feb;20(2):462-7), Copyright 2012.*)

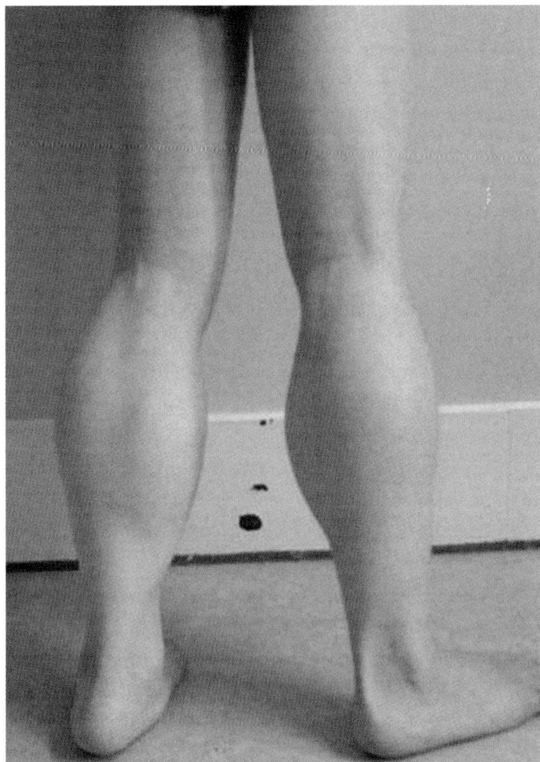

FIGURE 208-3 Calf hypertrophy in patient with Duchenne muscular dystrophy. (*Used with permission from Neil Friedman, MBChB.*)

- ◦ Mother is found to be a carrier in approximately 2/3 of cases; remaining cases due to spontaneous mutations.

DIAGNOSIS

CLINICAL FEATURES

- Progressive, symmetric proximal weakness initially affecting pelvic girdle muscles and later shoulder girdle muscles; with disease progression, neck muscles and distal muscles also become involved.
- Frequent calf hypertrophy (pseudohypertrophy; **Figure 208-3**).
- Gower sign (**Figure 208-1**)—While not pathognomonic for DMD, this is suggestive of proximal girdle muscle weakness.
- Waddling gait typically with toe walking.
- Hypo/areflexia.
- Contractures of Achilles tendons.
- Scoliosis usually later in the disease course.
- Becker muscular dystrophy is similar to DMD but has later onset and slower, more variable progression of symptoms.

DISTRIBUTION

- Initial proximal pelvic girdle weakness, which progresses over time to involve proximal shoulder girdle muscles, neck flexor and extensor muscles, and distal upper and lower extremity muscles.

LABORATORY TESTING

- Creatine kinase—Markedly elevated in all cases of DMD/BMD but is not discriminatory for DMD versus BMD or from other forms of neuromuscular disease.
- EMG/Neuroconductive studies—Rarely helpful but if performed will show a necrotizing myopathy. This is non-discriminatory for DMD versus BMD or from other forms of muscular dystrophy.
- Molecular diagnosis remains the testing of choice:
    - ◦ Initial screening includes either multiplex PCR of the exons most commonly deleted, which will pick up about 2/3 of cases but misses small deletions, point mutations and duplications; versus quantitative analysis of all exons using multiplex ligation-dependent probe amplification (MLPA) or oligonucleotide-based array comparative genomic hybridization (array-CGH).
    - ◦ If negative, reflex testing to full sequence analysis of genomic DNA.
- Muscle biopsy—Molecular testing has increasingly obviated the need for muscle biopsy, which shows dystrophic features including variation in muscle fiber size, increased internal nuclei, muscle replacement by fat and connective tissue, and whirling or splitting of muscle fibers.
    - ◦ Immunohistochemistry using antibodies directed against the dystrophin protein will be absent in DMD (rare revertent fibers may be seen) and show patchy and incomplete staining in BMD (**Figure 208-4**).

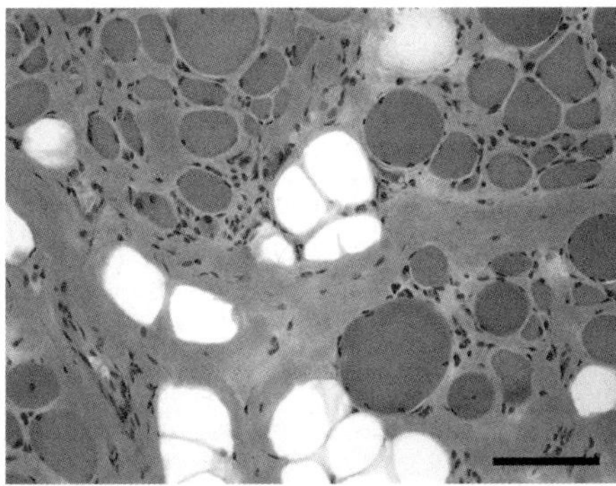
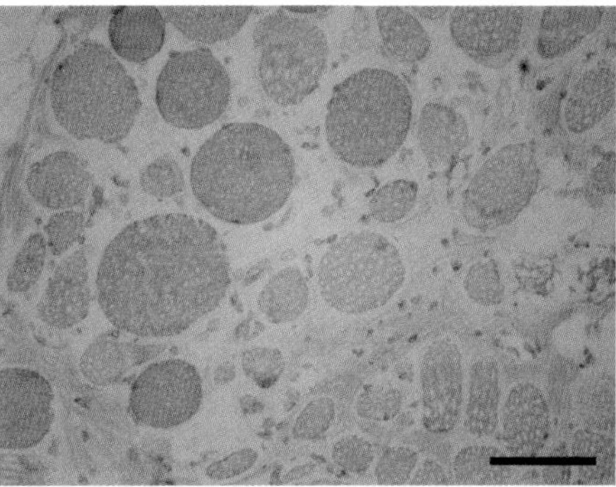
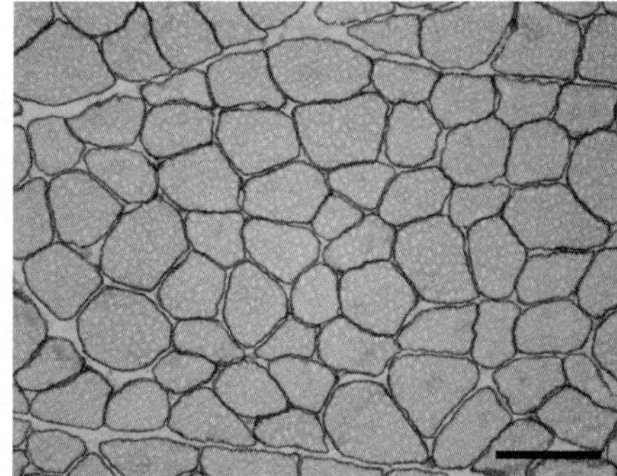

FIGURE 208-4 Duchenne muscular dystrophy. (Left) Hematoxylin and eosin stained section demonstrating dystrophic pattern of injury. There is a marked variation in fiber size and endomysial fibrosis and fat. Many large fibers are hyalinized consistent with early necrosis. Some have centrally located myocyte nuclei. Some small fibers are slightly basophilic and have plump nuclei consistent with fiber regeneration. (Center) Immunoperoxidase stain with antibody to dystrophin. There is no evidence of dystrophin expression. (Right) Positive control section demonstrating the normal pattern of dystrophin immunoreactivity. Scale bar = 100 μm. (*Used with permission from Susan M. Staugaitis, MD, PhD.*)

- Western blot analysis allows for quantitative measurement of dystrophin that is essentially absent (<10%) in DMD and reduced in quality and quantity in BMD.

IMAGING

- Not usually indicated but ultrasound and/or MRI can show fatty replacement of muscle and fibrosis

DIFFERENTIAL DIAGNOSIS

- Other forms of muscular dystrophy including limb-girdle muscular dystrophies, Emery-Dreifuss muscular dystrophy, or fascioscapular humeral muscular dystrophy—Age of onset, pattern of weakness, and involvement of joint contractures can help to differentiate this group of disorders.
- Spinal muscular atrophy—The presence of tongue fasciculations (anterior horn cell involvement), pattern of muscle involvement, and early age of onset differentiate this from DMD.
- Dermatomyositis—An inflammatory myopathy that often presents with lower extremity proximal weakness. The short duration of symptoms, presence of muscle pain or discomfort, and presence of heliotrope rash, capillary telangiectasias of nail folds or Gottron papules differentiates this from DMD (see Chapter 174, Juvenile Dermatomyositis).

MANAGEMENT

NONPHARMACOLOGIC

- Supportive care:[5–7]
  - Respiratory: SOR Ⓐ
  - Pulmonary function test monitoring.
  - Manual and mechanically assisted cough techniques as needed.
  - Obstructive sleep apnea and nocturnal ventilation resulting in early morning headache, fatigue, nausea is effectively treated with continuos positive airway pressure (CPAP).
  - Cardiac—Inevitable progression to dilated cardiomyopathy and heart failure in DMD. Early identification and treatment of heart failure and/or myocardial fibrosis with anti-failure medications can provide symptomatic relief and prolong life. SOR Ⓐ
  - Orthopedic—Surgical releases of contractures as appropriate and repair of scoliosis to preserve lung function and facilitate sitting posture and care. SOR Ⓐ
  - Bone health—Increased risk for osteopenia with loss of ambulation and/or use of corticosteroid therapy.
  - Measurement of serum concentrations of calcium and phosphorus, and activity of alkaline phosphatase.
  - 25-hydroxyvitamin D (25-OHD) level in springtime or biannually.
  - Magnesium and parathyroid hormone levels may be considered.
  - Urine (calcium, sodium, or creatinine).
  - Dual energy x-ray absorptiometry (DEXA) scanning.
    - At baseline (age ≥3 years) or at start of corticosteroid therapy.
    - Repeated annually in those at risk (history of fractures or chronic corticosteroid therapy) and those with DEXA Z score <−2.
  - Cognitive impairment and Learning difficulties—Frequent association with DMD and should be appropriately addressed when present, including individualized educational plans as needed; autism has also been reported in association with DMD in some instances and should be screened for in the appropriate clinical setting.
  - Non-specific strength treatment:
    - Physical and occupational therapy to promote mobility and prevent contractures.
    - Aquatherapy.

MEDICATIONS

- Drug therapy directed at disease pathogenesis:
  - Corticosteroids:[5,8,9] SOR Ⓐ
    - Early corticosteroid therapy is the only medication currently available that can slow the progression of the muscle weakness but cannot cure the disease.
    - Appears beneficial in reducing the risk of scoliosis, and may help to stabilize pulmonary and cardiac function.
    - No generally accepted guidelines about the best time to initiate corticosteroid therapy.
    - The recommended starting dose for prednisone in ambulatory boys is 0.75 mg/kg daily given in the morning; alternative intermittent dosing regimes include 0.75 mg/kg daily for 10 days each month or high dose weekend dosing of 5 mg/kg given each Friday and Saturday; the minimum effective dose that shows some benefit (albeit not to the maximum extent possible) is believed to be 0.3 mg/kg daily for prednisone.
- Experimental/Research Therapy:
  - Cell therapy to compensate for gene defect—Myoblast transplant.
  - Modify or regulate gene expression—Exon skipping strategies; mutation suppression.
  - Gene therapy—Gene transfer therapy via viral vectors.

REFERRAL

- Requires multi-specialty care including—Neurology, cardiology, pulmonology, orthopedic surgery, endocrinology, medical genetics, physical therapy, occupational therapy, nutrition, social worker, and/or case manager.
- Consider psychosocial support as indicated.

PREVENTION AND SCREENING

- Genetic counseling for affected individuals and family.
- Carrier testing is available for at-risk females.
- Prenatal testing and pre-implantation diagnosis of affected female carriers is possible, if the specific gene mutation is known.
- Currently study is underway to look at the feasibility of creatine kinase screening of the newborn blood screen to facilitate the diagnosis of DMC.

PROGNOSIS

- No cure currently exists for DMD or BMD.
- Life expectancy in DMD is typically the 2nd or 3rd decade with aggressive management and appropriate care.
- Long term survival possible in BMD but depends on disease severity.

- Cardiac involvement in BMD may be disproportionate to the muscle weakness and may occur early; may be amenable to heart transplantation.

FOLLOW-UP

- Chronic disease—Requires regular life-long medical care and follow up with multi-disciplinary team.

PATIENT RESOURCES

- Muscular dystrophy—**www.mda.org**.
- Muscular Dystrophy Campaign-UK—**www.muscular-dystrophy.org**.
- Parent Project Muscular Dystrophy—**www.parentprojectmd.org**.

PROVIDER RESOURCES

- Muscular dystrophy—**www.mda.org**.
- European Neuromuscular Centre (ENMC)—**www.enmc.org**.

REFERENCES

1. Emery AEH: Population frequencies of inherited neuromuscular diseases—a world survey. *Neuromuscul Disord.* 1991;1:19-29.
2. Koenig M, Beggs AH, Moyer, et al. The molecular basis for Duchenne versus Becker muscular dystrophy: correlation of severity with type of deletion. *Am J Hum Genet.* 1989;45:498-506.
3. Dalkilic I, Kunkel LM: Muscular dystrophies: genes to pathogenesis. *Curr Opin Genet Dev.* 2003;13:231-238.
4. Deconinck N, Dan B: Pathophysiology of Duchenne muscular dystrophy: current hypotheses. *Pediatr Neurol.* 2007;36:1-7.
5. Bushby K, Finkel R, Birnkrant DJ, et al: Diagnosis and management of Duchenne muscular dystrophy, part 1: diagnosis, and pharmacological and psychosocial management. *Lancet Neurol.* 2010;9:77-93.
6. Bushby K, Finkel R, Birnkrant DJ et al: Diagnosis and management of Duchenne muscular dystrophy, part 2: implementation of multidisciplinary care. *Lancet Neurol.* 2010;9:177-189.
7. American Academy of Pediatrics Section on Cardiology and Cardiac Surgery. Clinical Report: Cardiovascular health supervision for individuals affected by Duchenne or Becker muscular dystrophy. *Pediatrics.* 2005;116:1569-1573.
8. Moxley RT 3rd, Ashwal S, Pandya S, et al. Practice parameter: corticosteroid treatment of Duchenne dystrophy: report of the Quality Standards Subcommittee of the American Academy of Neurology and the Practice Committee of the Child Neurology Society. *Neurology.* 2005;64:13-20.
9. Manzur AY, Kuntzer T, Pike M, et al. Glucocorticoid corticosteroid therapy in Duchenne muscular dystrophy. *Cochrane Database Syst Rev.* 2008;(1):CD003725.

PART 19

HEMATOLOGY-ONCOLOGY

Strength of Recommendation (SOR)	Definition
A	Recommendation based on consistent and good-quality patient-oriented evidence.*
B	Recommendation based on inconsistent or limited-quality patient-oriented evidence.*
C	Recommendation based on consensus, usual practice, opinion, disease-oriented evidence, or case series for studies of diagnosis, treatment, prevention, or screening.*

*See Appendix A on pages 1320–1322 for further information.

209 IRON DEFICIENCY ANEMIA

Margaret C. Thompson, MD, PhD

PATIENT STORY

A 24-month-old well appearing girl who is at the 50th percentile for height and 95th percentile for weight is being evaluated by her pediatrician. Her vital signs reveal a heart rate of 150 per minute, blood pressure 85/50 mm Hg, and respiratory rate of 15 per minute. She is noted to be an active toddler sucking on a bottle and upon questioning the mother reveals that the girl drinks 38 ounces of whole milk a day. She is not jaundiced or icteric but the pediatrician notes that she has conjunctival pallor (**Figure 209-1**). No hepatosplenomegaly is appreciated. Because of the conjunctival pallor and the dietary history, the pediatrician obtains a complete blood count, which shows a white blood cell count of 5100/mm3, hemoglobin 6.1 g/dL, and platelet count of 499,000/mm3. The lab reports microcytosis, hypochromia, mild anisocytosis, and polychromasia. There is no basophilic stippling. A diagnosis of iron deficiency anemia is made and the girl is treated with oral ferrous sulfate. The pediatrician suggests that the amount of milk intake should be limited to 20 ounces per day. One month later, her hemoglobin increased to 8 g/dl and she is continued on iron supplementation for 3 months after her hemoglobin is normal for age.

INTRODUCTION

Iron deficiency is the most common cause of anemia in the United State and worldwide.[1] Although iron deficiency has decreased with the use of iron supplements and with iron fortification of foods, especially infant formula, it remains a common problem.

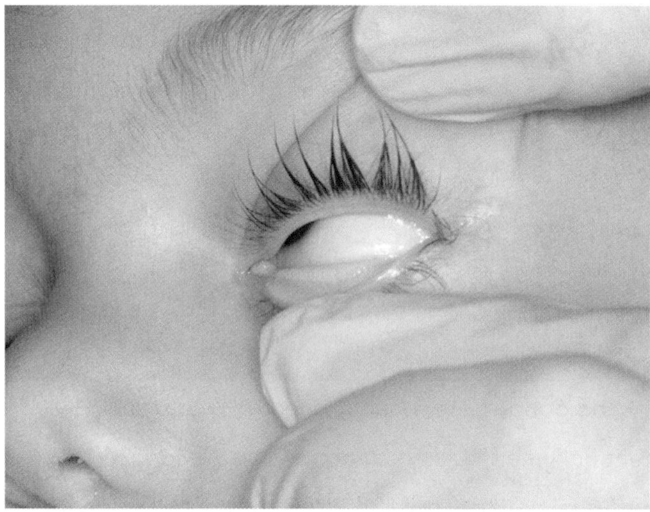

FIGURE 209-1 Conjunctival pallor in a toddler with severe anemia due to iron deficiency. (*Used with permission from Margaret C Thompson, MD PhD.*)

EPIDEMIOLOGY

- Iron deficiency is rare before 9 months of age in full term infants.
- Iron stores are usually high in the full-term newborn and sufficient until 4 to 6 months of age. Children between 9 and 18 months of age are at highest risk for developing iron deficiency due to rapid growth combined with insufficient intake.
- Iron deficiency anemia is present in 7 percent of toddlers aged 1 to 2 years and 9 percent of adolescent girls.[2]
- Risk factors include early introduction of cow's milk and consumption of more than 24 ounces of day of milk per day.
- Iron deficiency anemia is frequently seen in toddlers with excessive milk intake. The iron in milk is poorly absorbed. Further, the child may forego intake of other calorie sources because he or she is full from the milk. In addition, the child may develop mild blood loss from the gastrointestinal tract associated with the excessive milk.
- Preterm infants are at increased risk for iron deficiency anemia because of lower iron stores at birth and greater requirements due to faster growth rate.

ETIOLOGY AND PATHOPHYSIOLOGY

- Iron deficiency anemia occurs when iron is not available for the production of red blood cells. Most of the body's iron is found in the hemoglobin of circulating red blood cells.
- The remaining iron is stored in ferritin. Ferritin is an intracellular protein found in all cells but primarily in the bone marrow, liver, and spleen. The liver's stores of ferritin are the primary physiologic source of reserve iron in the body. A small amount of iron (0.1%) is found circulating and bound to transferrin.
- As red blood cells are destroyed and taken out of circulation, the iron is efficiently scavenged by macrophages and reused for production of new red cells. Only a small amount of iron is lost each day and is usually replaced by dietary absorption.
- When loss exceeds exogenous replacement (food or iron supplement), iron stores decrease and iron deficiency anemia may occur. This may occur in the following settings:
  - Blood loss.
    - Gastrointestinal loss as in Crohn disease, excessive milk intake, peptic ulcers, varices, or hookworm infection.
    - Uterine blood loss with menses.
    - Urinary loss.
  - Inadequate dietary intake.
  - Impaired absorption.
    - Celiac disease.
    - Crohn disease.
    - After surgery involving the duodenum.
    - Proton Pump Inhibitors and H2 blockers.
    - Regional Enteritis.
    - Consumption of foods such as calcium, phytate, and tannins.

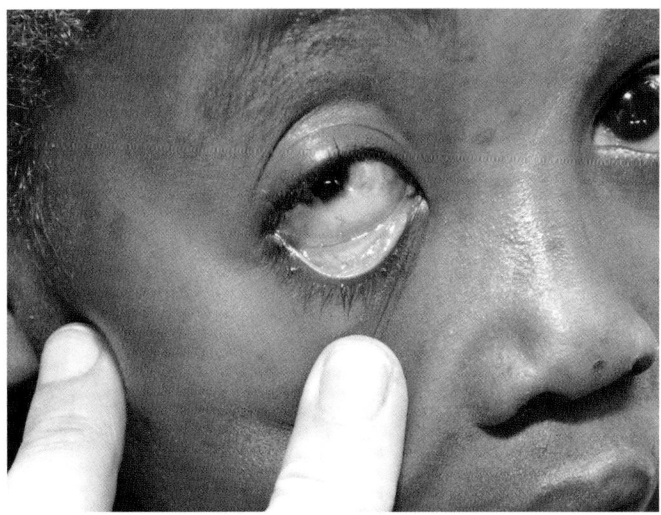

FIGURE 209-2 Conjunctival pallor in an African child with iron deficiency anemia. This child lives in extreme poverty in rural Africa with limited access to iron in her diet. (*Used with permission from Richard P. Usatine, MD.*)

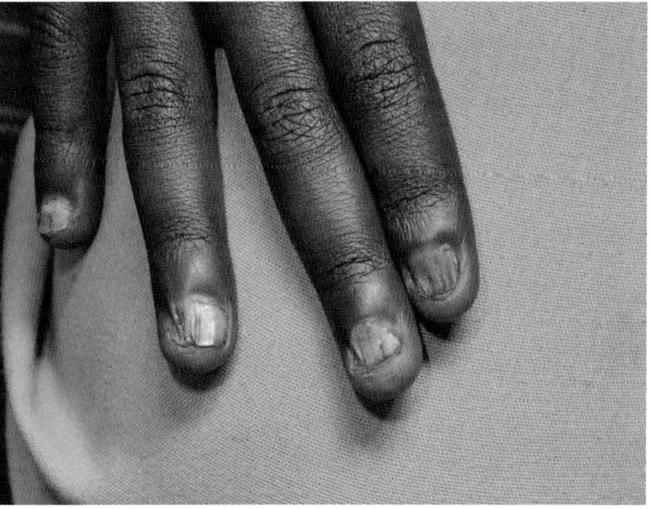

FIGURE 209-3 Koilonychia (spoon-shaped nails) in the same African child with iron deficiency anemia as in **Figure 209-2.** Children in her village may only have one to 2 meals per day and are lucky if they receive meat once a year in their diet. (*Used with permission from Richard P. Usatine, MD.*)

RISK FACTORS

- Socioeconomic risk factors include low income, minority ethnicity, and poor maternal iron status.[3,4]
- Early introduction of cow's milk into the diet of an infant (below the age of one year).
- Consumption of more than 24 ounces of milk per day.
- Pagophagia (craving and chewing ice) and pica (ingestion of non-food substances).

DIAGNOSIS

CLINICAL FEATURES

- Symptoms of iron deficiency anemia are the same as in all forms of anemia and depend on severity of the anemia as well as the rapidity of onset.
- These symptoms include fatigue, decreased stamina, tachycardia, and shortness of breath with exertion.
- Physical signs include pallor, mucosal pallor (conjunctiva and gums; **Figures 209-1** and **209-2**), and blue sclerae.
- Spooning of the fingernails (koilonychias; **Figure 209-3**) and atrophy of the papillae of the tongue are rare findings in children.

LABORATORY TESTING

- Iron deficiency anemia is characterized by microcytic, hypochromic red blood cells on peripheral smear (**Figure 209-4**). This is reflected by a low mean corpuscular volume (MCV) and low mean corpuscular hemoglobin (MCH).
- It also results in an uneven red blood cell size (anisocytosis), which is reflected by an increased red blood cell distribution width (RDW).
- The reticulocyte count is low or inappropriately normal for the degree of anemia.
- Serum ferritin reflects iron stores in the reticuloendothelial system and the liver. A low serum ferritin is the most specific laboratory test for iron deficiency anemia. Ferritin, however, is an acute phase reactant and may be increased in the settings of infection or chronic inflammation. As a result, its sensitivity is decreased, and a normal ferritin does not completely rule out iron deficiency anemia.
- Serum iron concentrations are generally low and serum total iron binding capacity (TIBC) is increased.
- Serum transferrin receptor, which reflects erythropoietic activity, is another nonspecific marker of the iron status and is elevated in iron deficiency, and can be used to help distinguish iron deficiency from anemia of chronic inflammation.[5]
- Initially, as iron stores decrease, iron deficiency erythropoiesis occurs. In this state, a very mild decrease in hemoglobin may be observed without a decrease in MCV. This decrease in hemoglobin

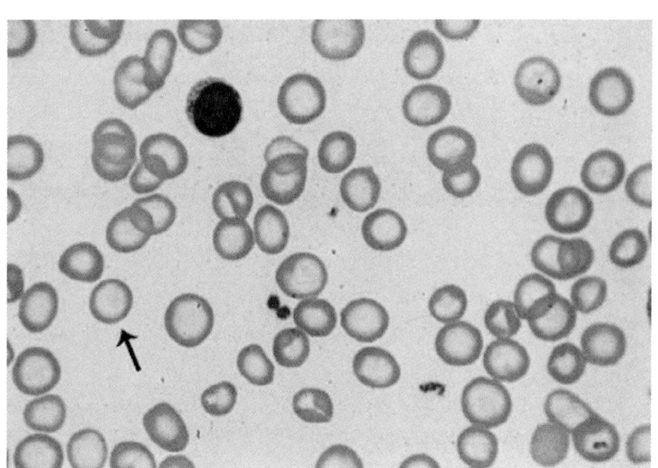

FIGURE 209-4 Microcytic, hypochromic red blood cells, which are characteristic of iron deficiency anemia, on peripheral smear. (*Used with permission from Lichtman MA, Shafer MS, Felgar RE, Wang N. Lichtman's Atlas of Hematology. http://www.accessmedicine.com.*)

TABLE 209-1 Laboratory Differentiation of the Causes of Microcytic Anemia

Study	Iron Deficiency	Thalassemia (including thalassemia trait)	Chronic Inflammation
Ferritin	Low	Normal	Low to Elevated
Serum Iron	Low	Normal to Increased	Low
Total iron binding capacity (TIBC)	High	Normal	Low
Transferrin-receptor	Increased	Normal to Increased	Normal
Mean corpuscular volume (MCV)	Low	Low and may be out or proportion to degree of anemia	
Red blood cell count	Low	Low to High (high if adequate compensation occurs)	Low

is generally asymptomatic. With continued decrease in iron availability, true iron deficiency anemia occurs, with concomitant abnormalities in the MCV and hemoglobin.

- It may help to order a urinalysis to look for urinary blood loss if the cause of iron deficiency is not readily available based on history and physical examination. If there are concerns for chronic illness, a comprehensive metabolic profile may show signs of liver or renal disease. If gastrointestinal blood loss is a concern, stool heme studies may be added to the workup.

DIFFERENTIAL DIAGNOSIS

- Thalassemia syndromes and anemia of chronic disease (anemia of inflammation) also cause a microcytic anemia. These can be distinguished from iron deficiency based on family and dietary history, current medical condition of the patient, and laboratory studies (**Table 209-1**).
- Congenital and acquired sideroblastic anemias are rare causes of microcytic anemia. The acquired form can be due to lead toxicity or isoniazid toxicity.
- Other rare causes of microcytic anemia include congenital absence of transferrin, copper deficiency, and lymphoid hamartoma syndrome (Castleman disease).

MANAGEMENT

NONPHARMACOLOGIC

- Sources of ongoing blood loss should be identified.
- Nutritional counseling may be beneficial in individuals with inadequate dietary intake of iron.
- Milk should be limited to 20 to 24 ounces per day in milk-associated iron deficiency anemia.
- Transfusion of red blood cells for iron-deficiency anemia is indicated only in the most severe cases such as extremely low serum hemoglobin, heart failure, or when ongoing blood losses exceed (or equal) bone marrow production after appropriate iron therapy.

MEDICATIONS

- Iron may be given orally, intravenously, or intramuscularly. Regardless of the route, an increase in peripheral reticulocytes is generally seen within 3 or 4 days.
- Oral iron salts are inexpensive and almost always sufficient to correct the anemia.
- There are many pharmacologic forms of iron available for oral therapy. For all forms, the dose is 3 to 6 mg/kg of elemental iron divided into 3 or 4 doses daily. This should be continued for at least 3 months after the hemoglobin has normalized. Iron supplements should be taken with vitamin C to increase absorption. Some experts recommend giving the iron between meals and with vitamin C juice, to increase absorption.[6] SOR Ⓒ
- Adverse effects of iron therapy, such as gastrointestinal upset and constipation are unusual in children. Temporary staining of the teeth can occur but is temporary and can be avoided by rinsing the mouth after the medication is given.
- Iron replacement may be given parenterally in patients who have impaired absorption, when there are concerns of adherence, and when rapid replacement therapy is required.[7] Three commonly used parenteral forms of iron are:
    - Iron dextran may be given intravenously and is also the only form of iron that may be given intramuscularly. The benefit of iron dextran is that a larger dose may be given at a time, and thus a patient may be able to receive a full replacement dose in a single infusion. Iron dextran, however, is associated with a significantly greater risk of allergic reaction including anaphylaxis. Intramuscular injection has become less common and requires experience with the Z-track method of administration. It is associated with pain, staining of the skin and inconsistent absorption of the iron.
- Sodium Ferric gluconate is a parenteral form, which is associated with a very low risk of allergic reaction. The maximum dose that may be given with this form is less than with iron dextran, and as a result, full replacement frequently requires several doses given weekly. Pediatric dosing is not fully established, but based on its use in hemodialysis patients is 0.12 mL/kg or 1.5 mg/kg of elemental iron with a single dose not to exceed 125 mg.

- Iron Sucrose is a parenteral form which also has associated with a low risk of allergic reaction. Pediatric dosing is not fully established but based on use in hemodialysis patients is 0.05 mg/kg, with a maximum 200 mg per infusion.

REFERRAL

- Depending on the degree of anemia, referral to a hematologist may be appropriate.
- Referral to gastroenterology or gynecology should be made, as needed to identify potential sources of blood loss.

PREVENTION AND SCREENING

- The committee on Nutrition of the American Academy of Pediatrics[8] has made the following recommendations for the prevention of iron deficiency anemia in term infants:
  - Breast milk should be given for at least 6 months, if possible. Iron supplementation (1 mg/kg/day) should be provided for infants who are exclusively breast-fed, starting at 4 months of age and continuing until appropriate iron containing complementary foods have been introduced.
  - Iron fortified formula, rather than cow's milk, should be given to infants who are weaned from breast milk before 12 months of age.
  - An iron-supplemented formula for the first year of life should be provided for infants who are not breast-fed.
  - Iron enriched cereals and other foods rich in iron should be introduced gradually to infants starting at 4 to 6 months of age.
  - All preterm infants who are fed human milk should receive an iron supplement of 2 mg/kg per day by one month of age and continued until the infant is weaned to iron fortified formula or begins eating complementary foods that supply the 2 mg/kg of iron.
- Universal screening for anemia, by determination of hemoglobin concentration and assessment of risk factors for iron deficiency, should be performed at 12 months of age.
- Consumption of more than 20 ounces of whole cow's milk per day in toddlers should be avoided.

PROGNOSIS

- The prognosis for complete resolution of iron deficiency anemia is excellent in otherwise healthy children.
- Effects of ongoing anemia include cardiomegaly, impaired growth and development in infants, poor school performance in older children, and decreased physical endurance.[9,10]

FOLLOW-UP

- A complete blood count of hemoglobin should be obtained after 4 weeks of treatment to assess response.
- An increase in hemoglobin of at least 1 g/dL after one month is diagnostic of iron deficiency.
- If the response is adequate, the complete blood count should be retested every 2 to 3 months until the hemoglobin is normal for age.
- Once the hemoglobin is normal, iron supplementation should be continued for 3 more months to replenish iron stores.

PATIENT EDUCATION

- Appropriate dietary education should be provided to parents and caregivers regarding the appropriate modalities of nutrition that will avoid iron deficiency in the first year of life.
- Families should be counseled regarding limiting milk and juice intake in the toddler years.

PATIENT RESOURCES

- **http://patiented.aap.org/content.aspx?aid=6578.**
- **http://emedicine.medscape.com/article/202333-overview.**
- **www.healthychildren.org/English/News/pages/AAP-Offers-Guidance-to-Boost-Iron-Levels-in-Children.aspx?nfstatus=401&nftoken.**

PROVIDER RESOURCES

- **http://pediatrics.aappublications.org/content/108/3/e56.full.**

REFERENCES

1. Cogswell et. al. Assessment of iron deficiency in US preschool children and nonpregnant females of childbearing age: National Health and Nutrition Examination Survey 2003–2006, The American Journal of Clinical Nutrition. *Am J Clin Nutr*. 2009;89(5):1334-1342.
2. Iron deficiency in the United States, 1999-2000. *MMWR Morb Mortal Wkly Rep*. 2002;51(40): 897-899.
3. Bogen DL, Duggan AK, Dover GJ, Wilson MH. Screening for iron deficiency anemia by dietary history in a high-risk population. *Pediatrics*. 2000;105(6):1254-1259.
4. Brotanek JM, Gosz J, Weitzman M, Flores G. Iron deficiency in early childhood in the United States: risk factors and racial/ethnic disparities. *Pediatrics*. 2007;120(3):568-575.
5. Punnonen K, Irjala K, Rajamaki A. Serum transferrin receptor and its ratio to serum ferritin in the diagnosis of iron deficiency. *Blood*. 1997;89(3):1052-1057.
6. Abrams SA, O'Brien KO, Wen J, et al. Absorption by 1-year old children of an iron supplement given with cow's milk or juice. *Pediatr Res*. 1996;39:171.
7. Silverstein S and Rodgers G. Parenteral Iron Therapy Options. *American Journal of Hematology*. 2004;76:74-78
8. Baker RD, Greer FR, and the Committee on Nutrition: Diagnosis and prevention of iron deficiency and iron deficiency anemia in infants and young children (0–3 months of age). *Pediatrics*. 2010; 126:1040-1050.
9. Eden AN. Iron deficiency and impaired cognition in toddlers: an underestimated and undertreated problem. *Paediatr Drugs*. 2005; 7(6):347-352.
10. Lozoff B, Jimenez E, Hagen J, Mollen E, Wolf AW. Poorer behavioral and developmental outcome more than 10 years after treatment for iron deficiency in infancy. *Pediatrics*. 2000;105(4):E51.

210 IMMUNE THROMBOCYTOPENIA PURPURA

Margaret C. Thompson, MD, PhD

PATIENT STORY

A 22-month-old boy is brought to his pediatrician by his parents because he has developed several dark purple bruises on his back and spine (**Figure 210-1**). He has additional bruises over both legs (**Figure 210-2**) along with smaller bruises over his neck and cheeks. He developed these over the past 2 to 3 days, and his mother reports that 3 weeks prior to this presentation, he had an illness characterized by vomiting, nausea, and diarrhea. The pediatrician suspects immune thrombocytopenic purpura (ITP) and orders a CBC, which shows a normal white blood cell count, differential count, and hemoglobin, but a platelet count of 7,000 microL. His liver function studies, prothrombin time (PT), and partial thromboplastin time (PTT) are all normal. A diagnosis of ITP is made and the child is admitted to the hospital, where his activity is restricted and he is treated with intravenous immunoglobulin. His platelet count increases rapidly over 3 days and he is discharged home with close follow-up.

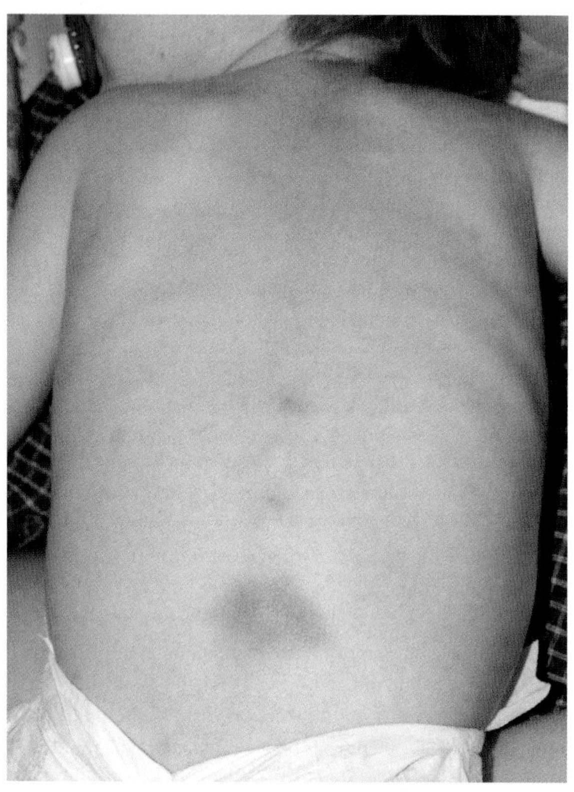

FIGURE 210-1 Purpuric and ecchymotic lesion over the back, and petechial lesions on the face of a child with immune thrombocytopenic purpura. (*Used with permission from Margaret C Thompson, MD, PhD.*)

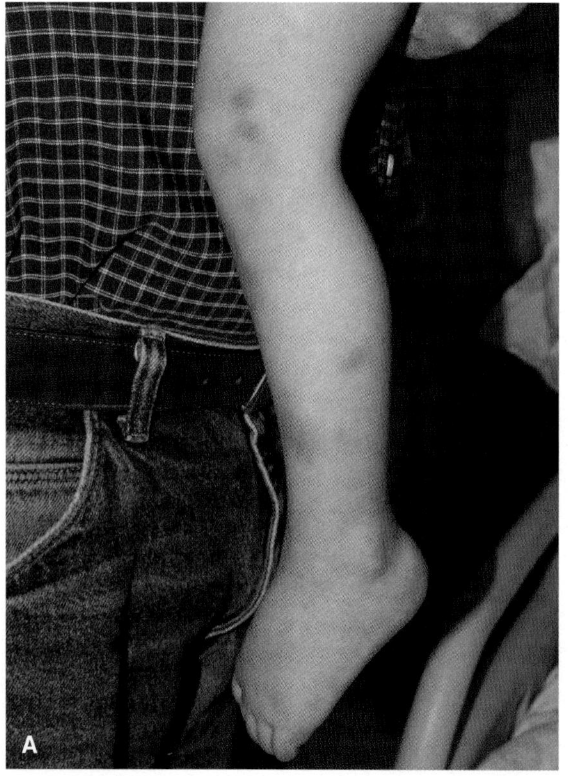

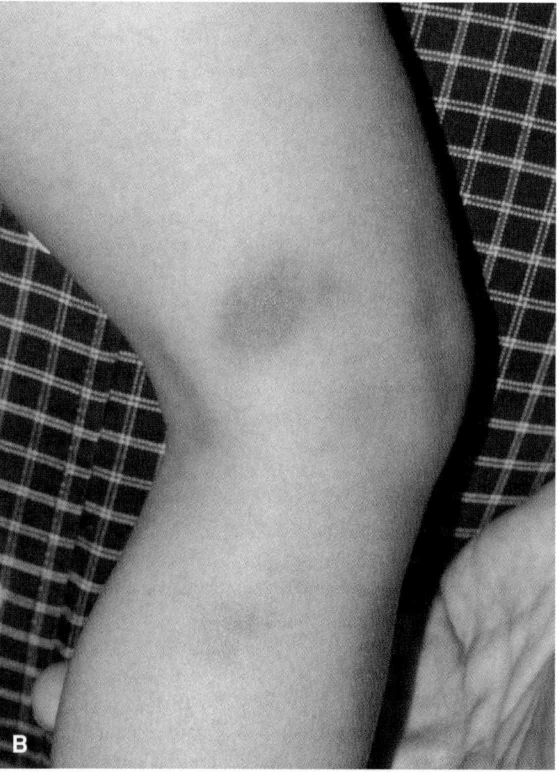

FIGURE 210-2 **A.** Large purpuric lesions on the legs of the child in **Figure 210-1**. **B.** Close-up of an ecchymotic lesion on the same child. (*Used with permission from Margaret C Thompson, MD, PhD.*)

INTRODUCTION

Immune thrombocytopenia purpura (ITP), formerly called idiopathic thrombocytopenic purpura, is an acquired disorder in which there is increased destruction of platelets causing thrombocytopenia (platelet count <100,000 microL). ITP may be divided into acute and chronic forms. Acute ITP is defined as having duration less than 6 months while chronic ITP is defined as lasting more than 6 months.

SYNONYMS

Idiopathic Thrombocytopenic Purpura.

EPIDEMIOLOGY

- The incidence of symptomatic disease is estimated to be 3 to 8 per 100,000 per year.[1–3]
- Acute ITP is the most common bleeding disorder in children.
- It is seen most frequently in children between the ages of 2 and 10 years with a peak occurring between 2 and 5 years of age.[2]
- It affects males more frequently among children younger than 8 years and equally among males and females beyond that age.[2]
- More common in winter and spring.
- In approximately 2/3 of cases, ITP in children occurs within 6 weeks of a recent viral illness.[4]
- Chronic ITP is defined as persistent thrombocytopenia that persists for longer than 6 months from the initial presentation. This occurs in 10 to 20 percent of children with ITP.
- Chronic ITP occurs more frequently in adolescents (and adults) than in young children. It affects females more than males and may be associated with underlying autoimmune disorders such as collagen-vascular diseases.

ETIOLOGY AND PATHOPHYSIOLOGY

- ITP is an immune mediated process whereby the body produces antibodies that attach to the glycoproteins expressed on platelet membranes.[5]
- The spleen and reticuloendothelial system then destroy the antibody coated platelets.
- There appears to be some differences between acute and chronic ITP with respect to pathophysiologic mechanisms. It is believed that acute ITP occurs when antibodies produced in response to a viral or bacterial infection cross-react with platelet antigens. On the other hand, chronic ITP may be the result of an underlying defect in immune regulation. There is also evidence of decreased thrombopoietin level in chronic ITP patients and megakaryocytes from patients with chronic ITP may demonstrate decreased growth in vitro.
- ITP may rarely follow measles-mumps-rubella (MMR) vaccination. Although mild thrombocytopenia after such vaccination is not uncommon, the incidence of clinically significant thrombocytopenia (<50,000 microL) is between 1:30,000 and 1:40,000 vaccinations. The onset is within 6 weeks of vaccination and the majority of cases resolve within 1 month and in 93 percent of the children, the thrombocytopenia resolves within 6 months.[6,7]
- Vaccination is not associated with a relapse of ITP in children with a history of non-vaccine associated ITP but revaccination may be associated with relapse in children with vaccination associated disease.
- ITP is felt to be unlikely after other early childhood vaccines.

DIAGNOSIS

The diagnosis is suggested by the finding of isolated thrombocytopenia in an otherwise healthy child. A history of a recent viral illness, especially in children under the age of 10 years, is common.

CLINICAL FEATURES

- Acute presentation of bruising, bleeding, and/or a petechial rash in an otherwise healthy child is the most common presentation.
- Mucosal bleeding, especially in the nares and gums, may be present.
- Physical examination reveals signs of bleeding, including petechiae, purpura and ecchymoses (**Figures 210-1** to **210-4**).
- Mucosal bleeding involving the nares, gingiva, gastrointestinal, genitourinary, or vaginal tract may be present.

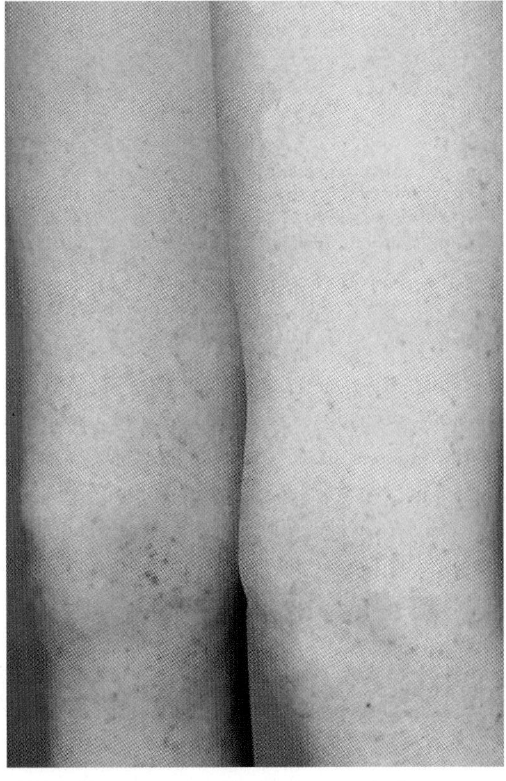

FIGURE 210-3 Numerous petechial lesions on the lower extremities of a young child with immune thrombocytopenic purpura. (*Used with permission from Cleveland Clinic Children's Hospital Photo Files.*)

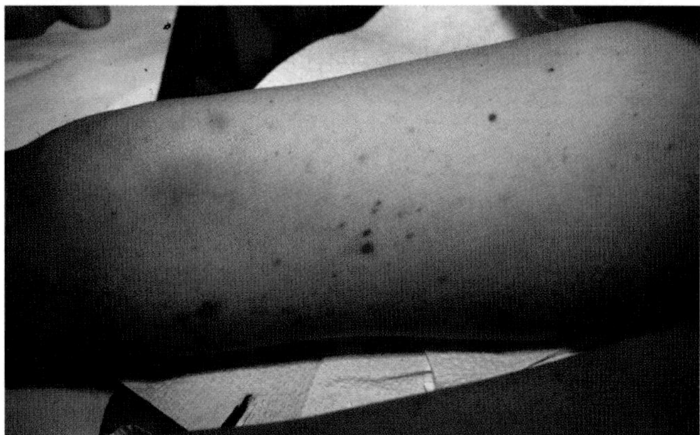

FIGURE 210-4 Petechial and purpuric lesions in a child with immune thrombocytopenic purpura following chickenpox infection. The platelet count dropped to 10,000 and the child was also bleeding from her gums. (*Used with permission from Richard P. Usatine, MD.*)

- Increased menstrual flow may be present.
- Amount of bleeding is usually related to the degree of thrombocytopenia.
- Except for signs of cutaneous and mucosal bleeding, the child usually appears well. Lymphadenopathy, hepatomegaly and splenomegaly are not present, although the spleen tip may be palpated in a minority of cases.
- Serious gastrointestinal or intracranial bleeding occurs in about 1 to 3 percent of patients. These are usually associated with platelet counts of less than 20,000/microL.
- Intracranial hemorrhage is the most serious consequence of ITP and occurs in 0.1 to 1.0 percent of patients.[2,8]

LABORATORY FEATURES

- A platelet count of less than 100,000 microL is used to make diagnosis but counts of less than 20,000 microL are frequently present at the time of clinical presentation.
- The white blood cell line is normal and anemia is not present unless there is significant hemorrhage.
- Peripheral blood smear may show scattered large platelets without hypogranulation and morphologically normal red and white blood cells.
- Bone marrow (not required for diagnosis) will show normal trilineage hematopoiesis with normal or increased megakaryocytes.
- Anti-platelet antibodies may be sought on testing but the sensitivity is poor and is not required for diagnosis.
- The mean platelet volume (MPV) may be elevated but this is neither a sensitive nor specific finding.
- The prothrombin time and partial thromboplastin time are normal.

DIFFERENTIAL DIAGNOSIS

- Thrombocytopenia may be the result of decreased production or increased destruction.
- Causes of decreased production include:
  - Infection—Mainly caused by viruses.
  - Bone marrow failure—Such as with aplastic anemia.
  - Bone marrow infiltration—Such as a neoplastic process such as leukemia.
  - Medications.
  - Nutritional deficiencies—Such as B12 and folic acid.
  - Liver failure that results in decreased thrombopoietin synthesis.
  - Genetic disorders that cause impaired thrombopoiesis—Such as Thrombocytopenia-Absent Radius (TAR) syndrome, giant platelet disorder, Bernard Soulier syndrome, congenital amegakaryocytic thrombocytopenia, and Wiskott-Aldrich syndrome.
  - Most causes of decreased production of platelets also result in decreased production of at least one other cell line and this helps to differentiate these disorders from ITP.
- Causes of increased destruction include:
  - Neonatal alloimmune thrombocytopenia (NAIT)—Occurs in neonates.
  - Drug induced (e.g., anti-epileptic agents).
  - Platelet consumption such as Hemolytic uremic syndrome (HUS), Disseminated intravascular coagulation (DIC), Thrombotic Thrombocytopenic Purpura (TTP), Kasabach-Merrit syndrome, thrombosis—These entities result in more systemic manifestations than seen with ITP.
  - Mechanical destruction.
  - Platelet sequestration associated with hypersplenism as in sickle cell, chronic liver disease, and type 2B and platelet-type von Willebrand disease.

TREATMENT AND MANAGEMENT

- The natural history of ITP is spontaneous remission, which occurs in 80 percent of children.
- Although thrombocytopenia is frequently severe at the time of diagnosis, platelet counts usually improve within 6 weeks.
- Restriction of activity, especially contact sports is recommended for all children with ITP.
- Medications with antiplatelet activity should also be avoided.
- While the goal of therapy is to increase platelets so that the risk of hemorrhage is decreased while waiting for spontaneous remission, it is unclear whether intervention actually prevents clinically significant bleeding, including intracranial hemorrhage.
- There are no randomized studies comparing treatment to observation in the management of ITP. Thus, management is highly physician dependent.
- Given the natural history, many pediatric hematologists will observe non-bleeding patients with close follow-up.
- Some pediatric hematologists will initiate treatment for platelet counts less than 20,000 microL or 10,000 microL.
- The American Society of Hematology recommends treatment in any child with ITP and either severe bleeding or platelet count of less than 10,000 microL.[9]

MEDICATIONS

- Although improvement and spontaneous resolution usually occurs regardless of treatment, there is some evidence that the duration of symptomatic thrombocytopenia is shortened by pharmacologic therapy, such as corticosteroids, intravenous immune globulin (IVIG), or intravenous anti-Rho(D) immune globulin.[10–16] SOR Ⓒ
- If pharmacologic management is felt necessary, the following treatments are commonly used:
  - Corticosteroids—Oral prednisone therapy can be administered and weaned over several weeks as the platelet count allows. Because of the risk of pretreating a patient with a missed diagnosis of acute leukemia, many pediatric hematologists will not use corticosteroids as a first line treatment or will perform a bone marrow evaluation prior to initiating steroids. However, current guidelines recommend performing a bone marrow examination only if the history, physical examination, complete blood count, and smear evaluation are not consistent with ITP or there are any findings suggestive of an alternative diagnosis. SOR Ⓒ
  - IVIG—One to two doses of IVIG may be used as first line treatment particularly in the setting of severe acute bleeding. The response is usually within 24 hours with a continued rise over the new few days. The response may be transient lasting only a few weeks or may be sufficient as a one-time treatment. Adverse effects include headache, nausea, and aseptic meningitis, which may mimic acute intracranial hemorrhage. SOR Ⓒ
  - Winrho or Anti D antibody—Use of this treatment is limited to patients who are Rh-positive and have a spleen. Administration of Winrho causes a hemolytic anemia competitively sparing some platelets. As a result, a patient receiving Winrho usually sees a drop in hemoglobin. While this is usually mild, it can be severe. Winrho should not be used in patients with evidence of hemolytic anemia, such as in patients with Evan's syndrome, or in patients with preexisting anemia.
  - Platelet transfusion is used only in the case of acute significant bleeding. The transfused platelets are quickly destroyed with the patient's own platelets and any benefit is usually short lived.

SURGERY

- Splenectomy is reserved for patients who are refractory to other treatments, whose thrombocytopenia lasts over a year, and whose baseline platelet count is at a level where there is significant bleeding risk or the child's quality of life is impaired.
- Immunization against encapsulated organisms, including *Haemophilus influenzae* type b, *Streptococcus pneumoniae*, and *Neisseria meningitidis*, should be completed prior to splenectomy.

REFERRAL

- Consultation with a hematologist is important in the diagnosis and management of ITP and in determining the need for admission, treatment, and follow-up.

PROGNOSIS

- Spontaneous remission occurs in about 90 percent of patients.
- Progression to chronic ITP occurs in about 10 percent of patients.
- Although approximately 20 percent of children present with mucous membrane bleeding, petechiae and bruising at the time of diagnosis, only 2.9 percent of patients will have severe hemorrhage.
- The most serious complication of ITP is intracranial hemorrhage and the incidence is very low (0.1 to 1%) with the greatest risk felt to be in patients with platelet counts less than 10,000 microL.

FOLLOW-UP

- Close monitoring for acute bleeding is critical in the management of ITP.
- Close follow-up of platelet counts is important in monitoring spontaneous resolution, response to therapy, and risk of severe bleeding.

PATIENT EDUCATION

- The risk of bleeding and measures to limit the risk of bleeding should be discussed at length with the family.
- Discussion of the activities in which the child can participate will depend on the platelet count and risk of bleeding.

PATIENT RESOURCES

- **www.nlm.nih.gov/medlineplus/ency/article/000535.htm**.
- **www.nhlbi.nih.gov/health/health-topics/topics/itp/**.
- **www.itpfoundation.org/**.
- **http://pdsa.org/about-itp/in-children.html**.

PROVIDER RESOURCES

- **http://emedicine.medscape.com/article/202158**.

REFERENCES

1. Fogarty PF, Segal JB. The epidemiology of immune thrombocytopenic purpura. *CurrOpinHematol.* 2007;14: 515-519. http://www.ncbi.nlm.nih.gov/pubmed/17934361.
2. Zeller B, Helgestad J, Hellebostad M, et al. Immune thrombocytopenic purpura in childhood in Norway: a prospective, population-based registration. *PediatrHematolOncol.* 2000;17(7):551-558. http://www.ncbi.nlm.nih.gov/pubmed/15981751.
3. Segal JB, Powe N. Prevalence of immune thrombocytopenia: analyses of administrative data. *J ThrombHaemost.* 2006;4(11):2377-2383. http://www.ncbi.nlm.nih.gov/pubmed/16869934
4. KühneT, Buchanan GR, Zimmerman S, et al. A prospective comparative study of 2540 infants and children with newly diagnosed idiopathic thrombocytopenic purpura (ITP) from the Intercontinental Childhood ITP Study Group. *J Pediatr.* 2003;143:605.
5. Cooper N, Bussel J. The pathogenesis of immune thrombocytopaenic purpura. *Br J Haematol.* 2006;133:364.

6. O'Leary ST, Glanz JM, McClure DL, et al. The risk of immune thrombocytopenicpurpura after vaccination in children and adolescents. *Pediatrics*. 2012;129(2):248-255.
7. Mantadakis E, Farmaki E, Buchanan GR. Thrombocytopenicpurpura after measles-mumps-rubella vaccination: a systematic review of the literature and guidance for management. *J Pediatr*. 2010;156(4):623-628.
8. Kühne T, Berchtold W, Michaels LA, et al. Newly diagnosed immune thrombocytopenia in children and adults: a comparative prospective observational registry of the Intercontinental Cooperative Immune Thrombocytopenia Study Group. *Haematologica*. 2011;96:1831.
9. Nunert C, Lim W, Crowther M, Cohen A, Solbert L, Crowther MA. The American Society of Hematology 2011 evidence-based practice guideline for immune thrombocytopenia. *Blood*. 2011;117:4190-4207.
10. Provan D, Stasi R, Newland AC, et al. International consensus report on the investigation and management of primary immune thrombocytopenia. *Blood*. 2010;115:168.
11. Kühne T. Update on the Intercontinental Cooperative ITP Study Group (ICIS) andon the Pediatric and Adult Registry on Chronic ITP (PARC ITP). *Pediatric Blood Cancer*. 2013;60(1):S15.
12. Buchanan GR, Holtkamp CA. Prednisone therapy for children with newly diagnosed idiopathic thrombocytopenic purpura. A randomized clinical trial. *Am J Pediatr Hematol Oncol*. 1984;6:355.
13. Imbach P, Wagner HP, Berchtold W, et al. Intravenous immunoglobulin versus oral corticosteroids in acute immune thrombocytopenic purpura in childhood. *Lancet*. 1985;2:464.
14. Tarantino MD, Madden Rm, Fennewald DL, et al. Treatment of childhood acute immune thrombocytopenic purpura with anti-D immune globulin or pooled immune globulin. *J Pediatr*. 1999;134:21.
15. Scaradavou A, Woo B, Woloski BM, et al. Intravenous anti-D treatment of immune thrombocytopenic purpura: experience in 272 patients. *Blood* 1997;89:2689.
16. Blanchette V, Carcao M. Approach to the investigation and management of immune thrombocytopenicpurpura in children. *Semin Hematol*. 2000;37(3):299-314.

211 SICKLE CELL DISEASE

Arunkumar Modi, MD, MPH
Margaret C. Thompson, MD, PhD

PATIENT STORY

A 4-year-old boy with known sickle cell disease is brought to the emergency department with worsening pain in his thighs, lower back, abdomen, and chest. He developed pain in both thighs 2 days ago, and was treated with ibuprofen without improvement. His chest pain began today and he refused to walk or eat. In the emergency department, he was tachypneic and had an oxygen saturation by pulse oximetry of 84 percent on room air, which increased to 95 percent on 2 liters oxygen by nasal canula. A chest x-ray showed bilateral infiltrates (**Figure 211-1**). He was diagnosed with acute chest syndrome and admitted to the pediatric intensive care unit, where he was treated with intravenous fluids, pain medications, and antibiotics, and made a full recovery.

INTRODUCTION

Sickle cell diseases (SCD) are a group of genetic disorders in which the affected individual has at least one copy of the genes that encode β-globin chains affected by the sickle cell mutation. This mutation causes sickling of red blood cells with resultant hypoxia and acidosis leading to a chronic progressive multisystem disorder. Sickle cell trait (SCT) is a condition in which affected individuals have one normal copy of the β chain gene and one sickle mutated copy. These individuals are generally unaffected. Hemoglobin SS disease (SCD-SS) is a condition in which affected individuals are homozygous for the sickle mutated β chain gene.[1]

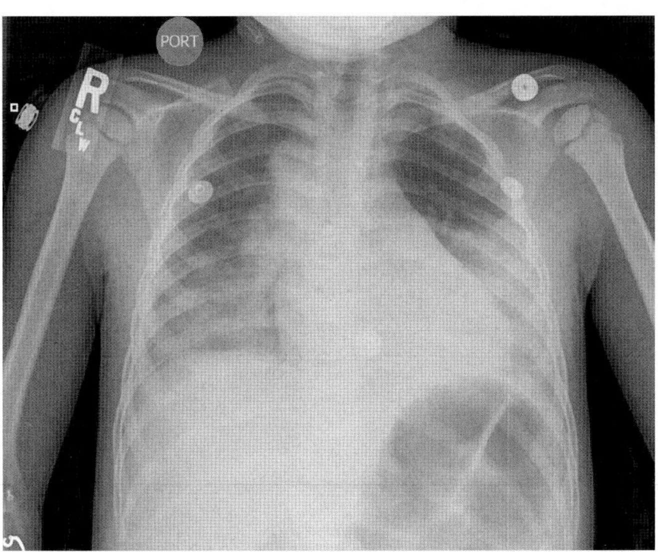

FIGURE 211-1 Acute chest syndrome on chest x-ray in a young child with sickle cell disease. (*Used with permission from Arunkumar Modi, MD, MPH.*)

SYNONYMS

- Sickle cell disease (SCD), Sickle cell anemia, Hemoglobin SS disease (SCD-SS).
- Hemoglobin SC disease (SCD-SC) and Hemoglobin *S β-thalassemia* (SCD-S-β Thalassemia) are types of sickle cell disease with different mutations than SCD-SS.

EPIDEMIOLOGY

- SCD affects 90,000 to 100,000 Americans.
- SCD occurs in approximately 1 out of every 500 Black or African-American births.
- SCD occurs in approximately 1 out of every 36,000 Hispanic-American births.
- SCT occurs in approximately 1 in 12 Blacks or African-Americans.[2]

ETIOLOGY AND PATHOPHYSIOLOGY

- Sickle cell disease is caused by a hemoglobin structural defect that results from the substitution of valine for glutamic acid at the 6th position on the gene coding for β globin.
- The mutation causes sickling in deoxygenated cells and leads to red cell membrane rigidity, increased red blood cell adhesion to the vascular endothelium, venous occlusion, and a decreased red cell life span of 10 to 20 days.
- The point mutation in Hemoglobin C disease results from a hemoglobin structural defect that results from the substitution of lysine for glutamic acid at the 6th position on the gene coding for β globin.
- This mutation results in persistent cellular potassium loss and cellular dehydration, causing increased blood viscosity and subsequent vaso-occlusion.
- The clinical problems associated with sickle cell diseases are a consequence of hypoxia and acidosis, which are caused by tissue ischemia that results from vaso-occlusion by irreversibly sickled red blood cells.

RISK FACTORS

- Hemoglobin S occurs frequently in areas previously exposed to falciparum malaria. This includes western coastal Africa, central Africa, India, Saudi Arabia, and the Mediterranean. It is also seen in South America.
- Hemoglobin C occurs more frequently in individuals of western African descent.
- In the US, SCD is found most commonly among African Americans.

DIAGNOSIS

CLINICAL FEATURES

Sickle cell diseases are chronic progressive multisystem disorders.[3] The acute clinical manifestations may be grouped into three categories:

- Vaso-occlusive events.
  - Vaso-occlusive crisis commonly affects bone, lung, liver, and spleen.
  - Bone infarction or ischemia of periarticular tissues is the most common form of acute pain crisis.
  - Diffuse or localized pain and tenderness, along with swelling and limited range of motion, is common.
  - Dactylitis (hand-foot syndrome) is a painful swelling of the metacarpals, metatarsals and phalanges and usually occurs in children under 2 years of age (**Figures 211-2** and **211-3**).
  - Cerebrovascular events include occlusive stroke in large vessels and aneurysms in small vessels.
  - Acute chest syndrome is defined as a new infiltrate on chest x-ray associated with one or more new symptoms including fever, cough, sputum production, dyspnea, or hypoxia and may be the result of sickling in the lungs with or without infection (**Figure 211-1**).[4]
  - Priapism is a painful and persistent erection secondary to sickling in the corpora cavernosa.
- Hemolytic events.
  - Hemolytic crises occur when the patient experiences an increase in their baseline level of hemolysis.
  - Aplastic crisis occurs when there is temporary suppression of the markedly increased production of reticulocytes in the marrow. It can be associated with many viral and bacterial infections, but is most frequently associated with parvovirus B19 infection (**Figure 211-4**).
  - Cholecystitis occurs due to gallstones and results from persistent hemolytic anemia.
  - Splenic sequestration is the acute pooling of blood within the spleen with a resultant precipitous drop in the hemoglobin level and/or platelet count.
- Infectious Events.
  - Patients with SCD are at increased risk for infection as a result of functional asplenia. They are particularly susceptible to infection with encapsulated organisms, such as *Streptococcus pneumoniae*, *Haemophilus influenzae*, and *Neisseria meningitides*.

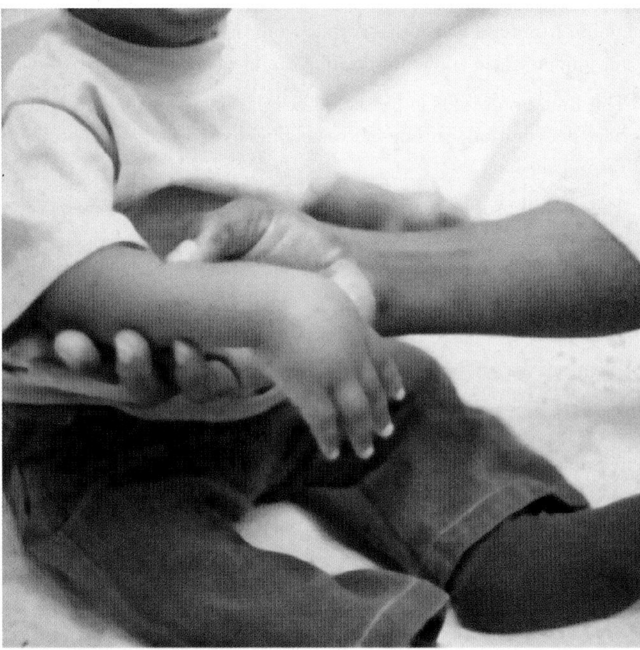

FIGURE 211-2 Dactylitis, characterized by painful swelling of the hands and fingers, in a toddler with sickle cell disease. (*Used with permission from http://www.accessemergencymedicine.com.*)

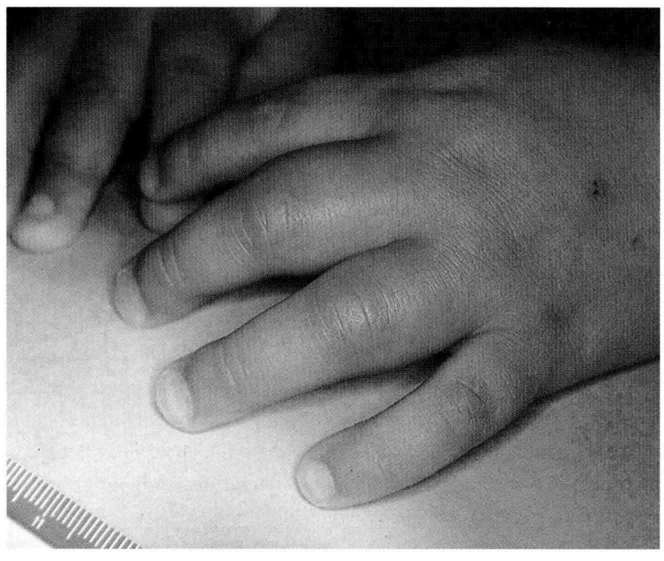

FIGURE 211-3 Acute sickle dactylitis caused by a vaso-occlusive crisis in a young child with sickle cell disease. (*Reproduced with permission from Knoop et al., The Atlas of Emergency Medicine, 3rd edition, McGraw-Hill, 2010, Figure 14-67.*)

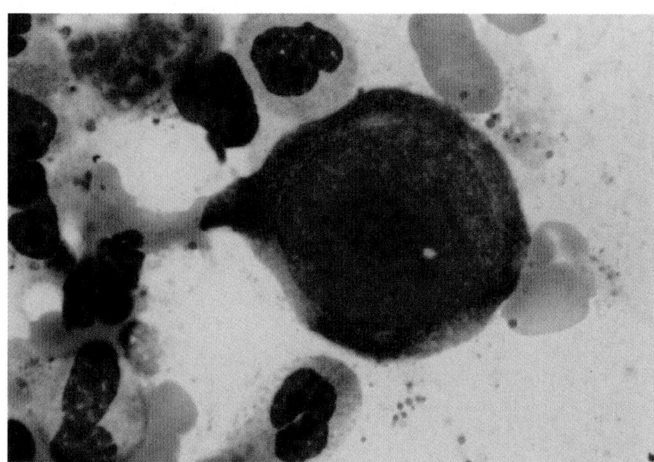

FIGURE 211-4 Giant pronormoblast seen on peripheral smear of a patient with aplastic crisis due to parvovirus B19. This represents an early erythroid cell that has been infected with this virus, which has a predilection to infect erythroid progenitor cells. (*Used with permission from Camille Sabella, MD.*)

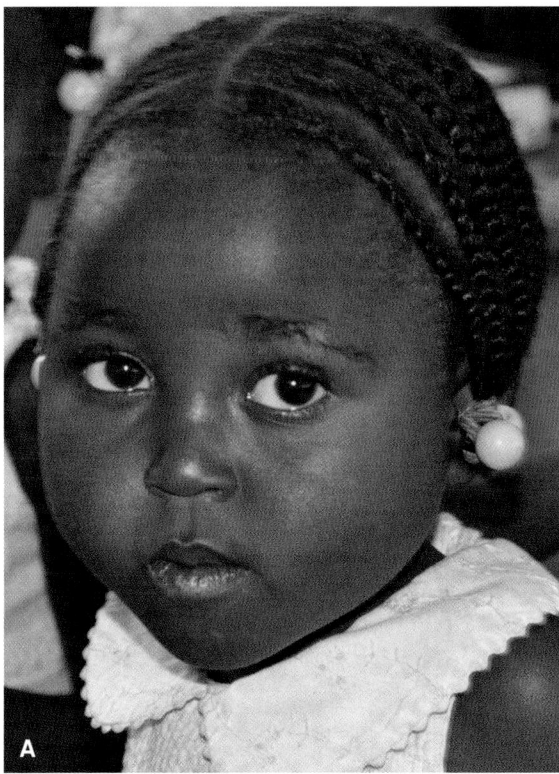

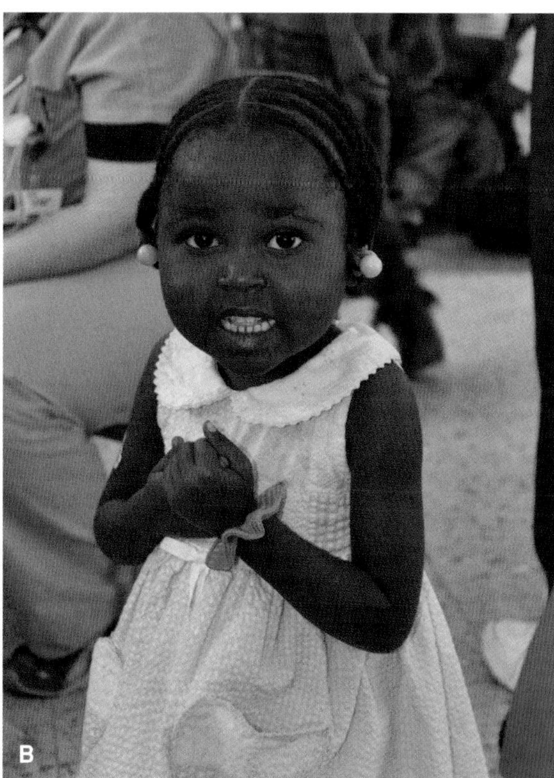

FIGURE 211-5 Frontal bossing (**A**) and stunted growth (**B**) in a young child from Haiti with untreated sickle cell disease. (*Used with permission from Richard P. Usatine, MD.*)

- Overwhelming sepsis from pneumococcal infection was especially common prior to universal antimicrobial prophylaxis in young children and a major cause of early death in young children with SCD.[5]
- Osteomyelitis most often occurs at the site of necrotic segments of bone, and is most frequently caused by *Salmonella* and *Staphylococcus aureus*.

- Chronic complications of sickle cell diseases are the result of persistent ischemic damage and include pulmonary, cardiac, renal, central nervous system, orthopedic, urinary, and ophthalmologic complications.
- Decreased growth, frontal bossing of the forehead (**Figure 211-5**), signs of chronic anemia (**Figure 211-6**), and delayed puberty are possible manifestations of long standing sickle cell disease.
- Patients who have received chronic red cell transfusions are at risk for organ damage from iron overload.

LABORATORY TESTING

- The diagnosis of SCD is confirmed by hemoglobin electrophoresis.
- As of May 1, 2006, in the US, all states provide universal newborn screening for sickle cell disease.[6]
- Thus, most patients in the US are diagnosed at birth by newborn screening, which shows the presence of hemoglobin S.
- Neonatal screening for sickle cell disease reports the level of expression of the different hemoglobins. In individuals without sickle cell, at birth, there is more fetal hemoglobin (Hb F) than

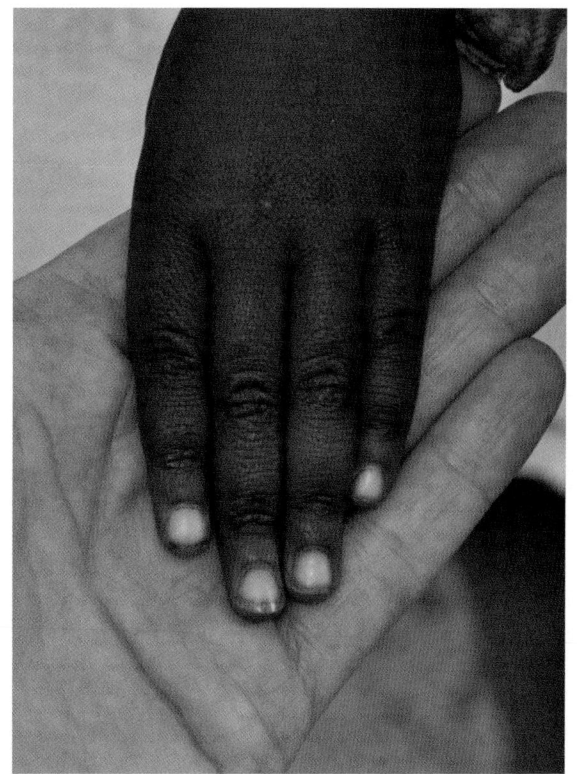

FIGURE 211-6 White nail beds in the same patient as in **Figure 211-5**. (*Used with permission from Richard P. Usatine, MD.*)

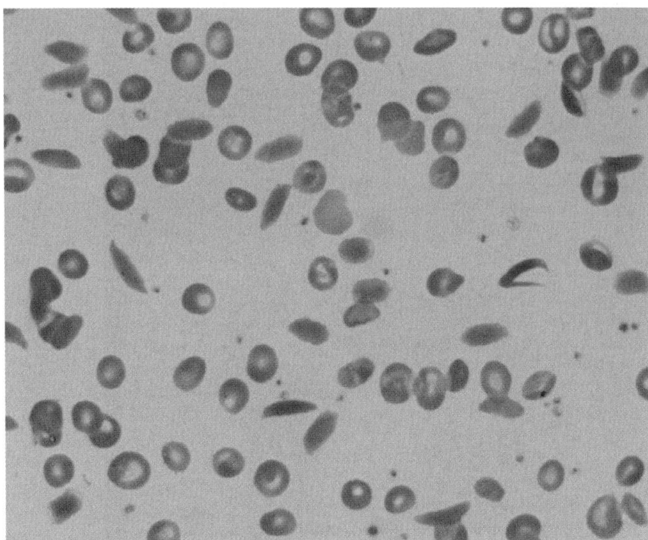

FIGURE 211-7 Numerous crescent shaped and sickled cells on a blood smear from a patient with sickle cell disease. (*Used with permission from Gary Ferenchick MD.*)

adult hemoglobin (Hb A) and the screening would report "FA." Individuals with sickle cell disease syndromes show hemoglobin S, hemoglobin F, and depending on the syndrome possibly hemoglobin A or hemoglobin C.[3]

- A simple peripheral smear of blood will demonstrate drepanocytes, which are the sickled red blood cells (**Figure 211-7**). Microcytosis and target cells are also seen in patients with SCD-Sβ Thalassemia.

IMAGING

- Plain bone x-rays are helpful in detecting bony infarcts or osteomyelitis (**Figure 211-8**). Differentiating infarct from osteomyelitis can be difficult.
- Chest x-ray is used to diagnose acute chest syndrome (**Figure 211-1**).
- Transcranial Doppler Studies (TCD) is used to measure vascular velocities and may be helpful in evaluating the risk for cerebral stroke. This study should be done annually.[1,3]
- MRI of bone should be performed when there is concern for avascular necrosis or osteomyelitis (**Figure 211-9**).
- Echocardiogram is used for monitoring cardiac complications related to chronic anemia.

DIFFERENTIAL DIAGNOSIS

- In addition to SCT and SCD-SS disease, there are three conditions with varying degrees of clinical severity associated with sickle mutated β-chain genes.
    - Two of these conditions involve a combination of sickle cell disease and β thalassemia. In these disorders, one copy of the β-chain gene contains the sickle cell mutation while the other copy contains a qualitative defect resulting in normal but decreased (or absent) β chains from that gene. These disorders are *Hemoglobin S β-thalassemia plus* (SCD-$S\beta^+$) where there is some normal Hemoglobin A produced in addition to the Hemoglobin S and *Hemoglobin S β-thalassemia null* (SCD-$S\beta^0$) where there is no normal Hemoglobin A.
    - *Hemoglobin SC* (SCD-SC) disease is a condition in which affected individuals have one sickle mutated copy of the β chain gene and one copy with a mutation with Hemoglobin C.
- The clinical manifestations of these disorders may be quite variable. In general, the higher the percentage of hemoglobin S, the more clinically severe the disease. Thus, SCD-SS and SCD-$S\beta^0$ tend to be clinically most severe while SCD-SC and SCD-Sβ+ tend to be less severe.

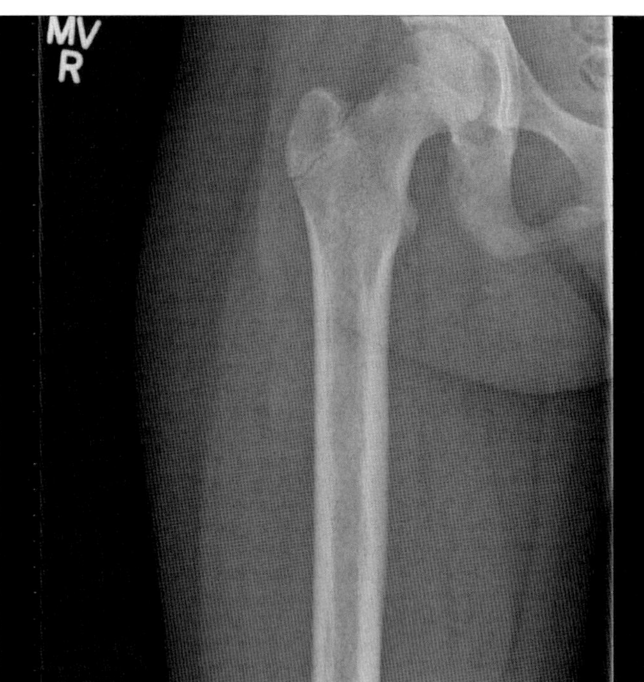

FIGURE 211-8 Femoral bone infarcts on plain x-ray in a 14-year-old girl with sickle cell disease. Note the "bone within bone" appearance present in the proximal and mid-femoral shaft. (*Used with permission from Margaret C. Thompson, MD, PhD.*)

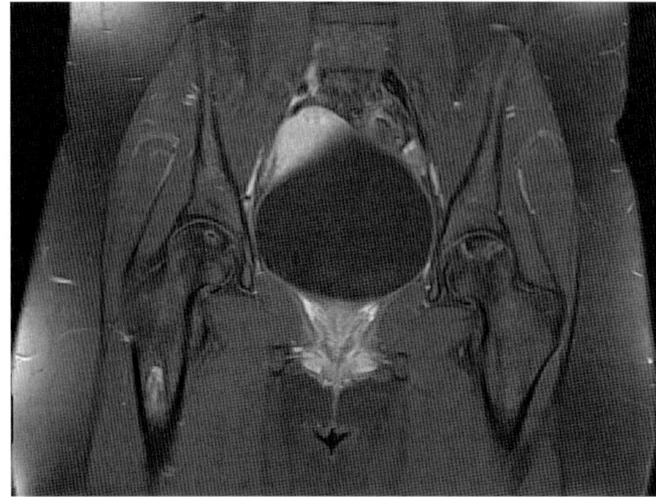

FIGURE 211-9 Bilateral femoral head osteonecrosis on MRI in a teenager with sickle cell disease. (*Used with permission from Arunkumar Modi, MD, MPH.*)

MANAGEMENT

- The only cure for SCD is hematopoietic stem cell transplant, which has been used successfully in patients with SCD. However, because of significant complications and limitations associated with this intervention, it is currently not the standard of care for all patients.[3]
- The screening of newborns for SCD has led to early diagnosis. Early medical intervention and education and care in specialty clinics have decreased morbidity and mortality in individuals with SCD.
- Routine health maintenance, with an emphasis on nutrition, education of families, infection prophylaxis, rapid response to signs of infection, and anticipatory guidance has significantly increased the lifespan of individuals with SCD.
- Individuals with sickle cell disease should receive care at a comprehensive sickle cell clinic under the guidance of a hematologist.[3]

NONPHARMACOLOGIC

- All patients with SCD should be vaccinated against *Haemophilus influenzae* type b, meningococcal, and 23-valent pneumococcal polysaccharide vaccines, in addition to routine age-appropriate vaccinations. They should also receive annual influenza vaccine.[3,7,8] SOR Ⓐ
- Simple blood transfusions and exchange transfusions may be required intermittently, especially for acute chest syndrome, stroke, splenic sequestration, and prior to anesthesia.[3] SOR Ⓑ
- Chronic simple transfusions, chronic exchange transfusions and apheresis are used in high-risk sickle cell patients to prevent or decrease the risk of long-term morbidity. SOR Ⓒ
- Patients on regular transfusion protocol are increased risk for acquiring transfusion related iron overload and the development of allo-antibodies.
- Patients with SCD should maintain good hydration and may require cautious hydration when admitted to the hospital.

MEDICATIONS

- Amoxicillin or penicillin prophylaxis prevents pneumococcal sepsis in young children with SCD and should be given to all patients starting at 2 months of age and continued until 5 years of age.[9–11] SOR Ⓐ
- Folic acid supplementation is needed to meet the demands of increased red cell production.[3] SOR Ⓑ
- Hydroxyurea increases the production of hemoglobin F and is beneficial in preventing complications of SCD.[12–14] SOR Ⓐ
- Patients with fever should be evaluated and treated empirically with intravenous antibiotics until infection has been ruled out.[3]
- Patients with acute pain crises and dactylitis may require non-steroidal anti-inflammatory agents and opioids. When possible, they should be treated at home, but frequently require admission for intravenous administration.

SURGERY

- Surgical intervention may be necessary for treatment of complication, such as avascular necrosis and cholecystitis.

REFERRAL

- Referral to a center specializing in blood disorders is recommended for all patients with SCD at the time of diagnosis.

PREVENTION AND SCREENING

- All infants are screened at birth for sickle cell disease.[6]
- Screening for complications should be followed as per national sickle cell guidelines.[3]

PROGNOSIS

- The median age at death for SCD-SS has improved greatly and is approximately 42 years for males and 48 years for females. For SCD-SC, median age at death for males is 60 years and for females is 68 years. Symptomatic patients are more likely to die early. Hemoglobin F percentage is a positive predictor for survival.[15]

FOLLOW-UP

Patients with SCD should be seen at least once per year by a hematologist and once a year by their primary care physicians.

PATIENT EDUCATION

- Families and patients should be counseled regarding the importance of follow-up care and seeking immediate care whenever there are signs of infection.

PATIENT RESOURCES

- Sickle cell disease homepage at CDC—**www.cdc.gov/ncbddd/sicklecell/index.html**.
- National heart, lung and blood institute at National Institute of Health—**www.nhlbi.nih.gov/health/health-topics/topics/sca/**.

PROVIDER RESOURCES

- **www.cdc.gov/NCBDDD/sicklecell/recommendations.html**.
- **http://pedsinreview.aappublications.org/content/28/7/259.extract**.
- **www.jpeds.com/article/S0022-3476(08)00861-5/abstract**.

REFERENCES

1. American Academy of Pediatrics Health Supervision for Children with Sickle Cell Disease, Section on Hematology/Oncology and Committee on Genetics. *Pediatrics*. 2002;109(3):526-535.
2. National Heart, Lung, and Blood Institute. Disease and conditions index. Sickle cell anemia: who is at risk? Bethesda, MD: US Department of Health and Human Services, National Institutes of

Health, National Heart, Lung, and Blood Institute; 2009. http://www.nhlbi.nih.gov/health/dci/Diseases/Sca/SCA_WhoIsAtRisk.html, accessed on February 3, 2014.

3. National Institutes of Health. The Management of Sickle Cell Disease, 4th Ed. revised June 2002. NIH National Heart, Lung and Blood Institute. NIH Publication No. 02-2117. http://www.nhlbi.nih.gov/health/prof/blood/sickle/sc_mngt.pdf, accessed on August 2, 2007.
4. Poncz M, Kane E, Gill FM. Acute chest syndrome in sickle cell disease: etiology and clinical correlates. *J Pediatr* 1985;107:861-866.
5. Leikin SL, Gallagher D, Kinney TR, et al. Mortality in children and adolescents with sickle cell disease. Cooperative Study of Sickle Cell Disease. *Pediatrics.* 1989;84:500-508.
6. U.S. Preventive Services Task Force. Screening for Sickle Cell Disease in Newborns: U.S. Preventive Services Task Force Recommendation Statement. AHRQ Publication No. 07-05104-EF-2, September 2007. http://www.uspreventiveservicestaskforce.org/uspstf07/sicklecell/sicklers.htm, accessed on December 1, 2013.
7. Committee on Infectious Diseases. American Academy of Pediatricts. Policy statement: recommendations for the prevention of pneumococcal infections, including the use of pneumococcal conjugate vaccine (Prevnar), pneumococcal polysaccharide vaccine, and antibiotic prophylaxis. *Pediatrics.* 2000;106:362-366.
8. Overturf GD, the American Academy of Pediatrics Committee on Infectious Disease. Technical report: prevention of pneumococcal infections, including the use of pneumococcal conjugate and polysaccharide vaccine, and antibiotic prophylaxis. *Pediatrics.* 2000;106(2 Pt 1):367-376.
9. Gaston MH, Verter JI, Woods G, et al. Prophylaxis with oral penicillin in children with sickle cell anemia. A randomized trial. *N Engl J Med* 1986;314:1593-9.
10. Powars D, Overturf G, Weiss J, et al. Pneumococcal septicemia in children with sickle cell anemia. Changing trend of survival. *JAMA.* 1981;245:1839-1842.
11. Falletta JM, Woods RM, Verter JI, et al. Discontinuing penicillin prophylaxis in children with sickle cell anemia. *J Pediatr.* 1995;127:685-690.
12. Heeney, MM, Ware, RE. An Update on Pediatric Oncology and Hematology Hydroxyurea for Children with Sickle Cell Disease. *Hematology/Oncology Clinics of North America* 2010;24(1):199-214.
13. Charache S, Terrin ML, Moore RD, et al. Multicenter Study of Hydroxyurea in Sickle Cell Anemia. Effect of hydroxyurea on the frequency of painful crises in sickle cell anemia. *N Engl J Med.* 1995;332:1317-1322.
14. Kinney TR, Helms RW, O'Branski EE, et al. Safety of hydroxyurea in children with sickle cell anemia: results of the HUG-KIDS study, a phase I/II trial. *Blood.* 1999;94:1550-1554.
15. Platt OS et al. Mortality in sickle cell disease. Life expectancy and risk factors for early death. *N Eng J Med.* 1994;330(23):1639-1644.

212 NEUROBLASTOMA

Meghan Drayton Jackson, DO
Margaret C. Thompson, MD, PhD

PATIENT STORY

A 3-year-old girl presents to the emergency department with decreased appetite, fatigue, and irritability for 1 month. She has periorbital ecchymoses (raccoon eyes) without a history of trauma (**Figure 212-1**). A CT scan is ordered to look for a neuroblastoma. The CT scan of her orbit shows bony erosions and periosteal reaction of her orbits. An MRI scan of her abdomen reveals a primary adrenal tumor. A biopsy is performed of the adrenal tumor confirming the diagnosis of neuroblastoma. She responds well to several courses of chemotherapy.

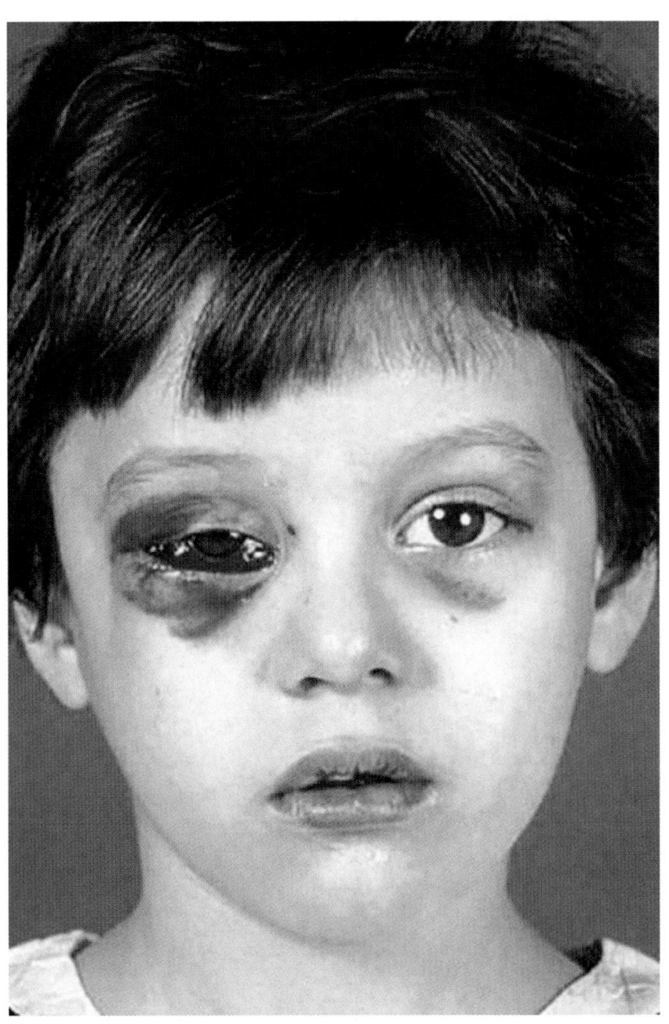

FIGURE 212-1 Neuroblastoma presenting with periorbital ecchymoses (raccoon eyes) in a 3-year-old girl. In this case, the eye tumor is metastatic disease from a primary neuroblastoma of the adrenal gland. *(Used with permission from Cleveland Clinic Children's Hospital Photo Files.)*

INTRODUCTION

Neuroblastoma is a malignant embryonal childhood tumor of the sympathetic nervous system derived from primordial neural crest cells.

EPIDEMIOLOGY

- Neuroblastoma is the most common malignant extracranial solid tumor of childhood and accounts for 8 to 10 percent of childhood cancers in children under 15 year of age.[1]
- There are between 600 to 650 cases each year in the US.
- Occurs in approximately 14/100,000 live births.
- Occurs in approximately 0.8 to 1/100,000 children under age 15 per year.
- It is the most common cancer of infancy (<12 months; 58/1,000,000 infants per year).
- Median age at diagnosis is 17 to 22 months. Ninety percent of cases are diagnosed by 5 years of age. It is rare after the age of 10 years.[1]
- Accounts for approximately 15 percent of all pediatric cancer fatalities.
- More common in Caucasians.
- Occurs slightly more frequently in boys that girls (1.2:1).[2]

ETIOLOGY AND PATHOPHYSIOLOGY

- Neuroblastic tumors arise from the primitive sympathetic ganglion cells and include neuroblastomas, ganglioneuroblastomas, and gangliomas. They may arise anywhere along the sympathetic ganglia and in the adrenal medulla. The etiology of neuroblastoma in most cases remains unknown, but certain recurrent molecular abnormalities have been found including amplification of the oncogene MYCN in approximately 20 percent of tumors, deletion of 1p36 and 11q, and in patients under 18 months of age.[3]
- Familial neuroblastoma accounts for 1 to 2 percent of all cases and demonstrates an autosomal dominant pattern of inheritance with incomplete penetrance. It is associated with an earlier presentation, and bilateral adrenal or multifocal disease. It has been linked to mutations in the *Phox2B* and *ALK* genes.[4]
- Mutations in Phox2B mutations are also associated with Haddad's syndrome, a rare congenital neurocristopathy that includes Hirschsprung disease, congenital central hypoventilation, and sympathetic ganglia tumors.
- Neuroblastoma may be detected in utero on prenatal ultrasound and often regresses or differentiates without intervention.

RISK FACTORS

- Epidemiologic studies have failed to show identifiable environmental etiologic risk factors.[1]
- The consistent rates of neuroblastoma suggest a major role of genetic factors.[4]

DIAGNOSIS

Clinical presentation depends on the site of the primary tumor, the extent of disease as well as the presence of a paraneoplastic syndrome. Approximately 65 percent of patients have metastatic disease at the time of diagnosis.

CLINICAL FEATURES

- Children with adrenal primary tumors may present with an asymptomatic palpable abdominal mass along with constipation, hypertension due to renal artery compression, and early satiety.
- Patients with neuroblastoma originating along the lower sympathetic chain may present with evidence of cord compression such as urinary incontinence and decreased lower extremity movement.
- Patients with a thoracic primary tumor may present with superior vena cava syndrome, and those with a tumor originating in the superior cervical ganglion with Horner's syndrome (**Figure 212-2**).
- Evidence of metastatic disease depends on the location and may include periorbital ecchymoses (raccoon eyes; **Figures 212-1** and **212-3**) and bone pain with bone metastasis, hepatomegaly, and "blueberry muffin" spots. Extensive bone marrow involvement may result in signs and symptoms of anemia and thrombocytopenia (**Figure 212-4**).
- Systemic symptoms include weight loss, irritability, and fever.
- Patients may also present with hypertension as a result of catecholamine production by the tumor and diarrhea as result of vaso-intestinal peptide production by the tumor.
- Opsoclonus/myoclonus is an autoimmune paraneoplastic syndrome associated with neuroblastoma. Opsoclonus is rapid, involuntary, multivectorial, unpredictable, and conjugate fast eye movements.
- Infants under a year of age may present with wide spread metastatic disease including subcutaneous tumor nodules and extensive liver involvement but with limited bone marrow disease and a small primary tumor. This presentation is termed stage "4S" and does not include patients with bone or other metastatic lesions. These

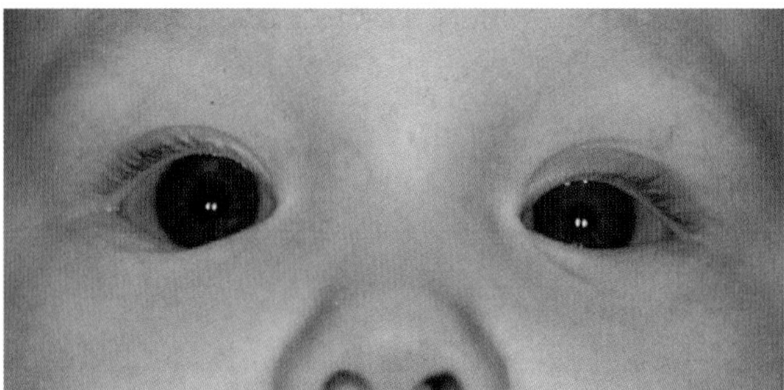

FIGURE 212-2 Horner syndrome in a patient with neuroblastoma. Note the smaller pupil and ptosis of the left eye. (*Used with permission from Access Pediatrics, Lueder, Pediatric Practice Ophthalmology, Figure 18-1, McGraw Hill.*)

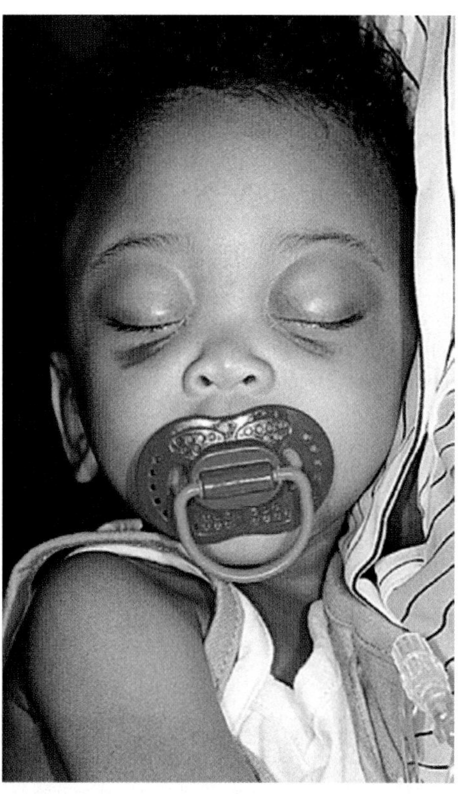

FIGURE 212-3 Bilateral periorbital ecchymoses (raccoon eyes) in an 11-month old infant with neuroblastoma. (*Used with permission from Binita R. Shah, MD, Atlas of Pediatric Emergency Medicine, Figure 8-4, www.accessemergencymedicine, McGraw Hill.*)

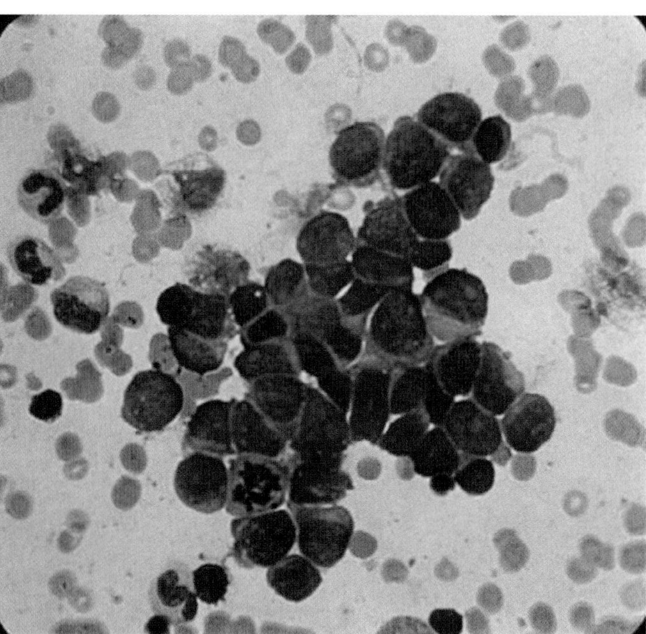

FIGURE 212-4 Neuroblasts in the bone marrow of a young child with metastatic neuroblastoma. (*Used with permission from Cleveland Clinic Children's Hospital Photo Files.*)

patients have a surprisingly good outcome despite extensive disease at diagnosis.

DISTRIBUTION

- Tumors can arise from any site along the sympathetic nervous system chain including the adrenal gland. Approximately 65 percent of neuroblastomas occur in the abdomen with 40 percent being in the adrenal and 25 percent occurring in the paraspinal ganglia. Fifteen percent of neuroblastomas occur in the thorax presenting as a posterior mediastinal mass; 5 percent present in the pelvic region; 3 percent present as cervical tumors; and 12 percent elsewhere.
- Infants are more likely to present with thoracic and cervical primary tumors while children over one year of age are more likely to present with abdominal primaries.
- Metastatic spread, which is more common in children older than one year of age at diagnosis, occurs through both lymphatic and hematogenous routes. The most common sites are regional or distant lymph nodes, bone (long bones and skull), bone marrow, liver, and skin.[2,4] Lung and brain metastases are rare and occur in less than 3 percent of cases.[4]

LABORATORY TESTING

- Urine should be sent for measurement of the urine catecholamines, vanillylmandelic acid (VMA), and homovanillic acid (HVA), which are secreted by the majority of neuroblastomas.
- Complete blood count should be evaluated for evidence of bone marrow involvement.
- Complete metabolic panel should be performed to evaluate for evidence of tumor lysis syndrome as well as liver and kidney function.
- Biopsy is necessary for definitive diagnosis and risk-based staging. It may be taken from the primary tumor or a metastatic site. Histology will show a small round blue cell tumor. The tumor will be graded as favorable or unfavorable based on degree of neuroblastic differentiation and mitotic index.[2,3]
- Bilateral bone marrow biopsies must be obtained to evaluate for evidence of metastatic disease in the bone marrow (**Figure 212-4**).

IMAGING

- CT and/or MRI are done to locate the primary site. Primary tumors are not encapsulated and often displace important structures (**Figure 212-5**).
- CT of the abdomen and pelvis to evaluate for evidence of metastatic disease if the adrenal is the primary site.
- Metaiodobenzylguanidine (MIBG) scan is a nuclear medicine study using the radio- isotope iodine-123-meta-iodobenzylguanidine. MIBG is specifically taken up by norepinephrine transporters on catecholamine producing tumors. MIBG is very sensitive and specific for catecholamine producing tumors and should be performed to evaluate for sites of metastatic disease and to evaluate the primary tumor for MIBG sensitivity.[5]
- Bone scan may be performed but is frequently replaced by the MIBG scan if the latter is positive.

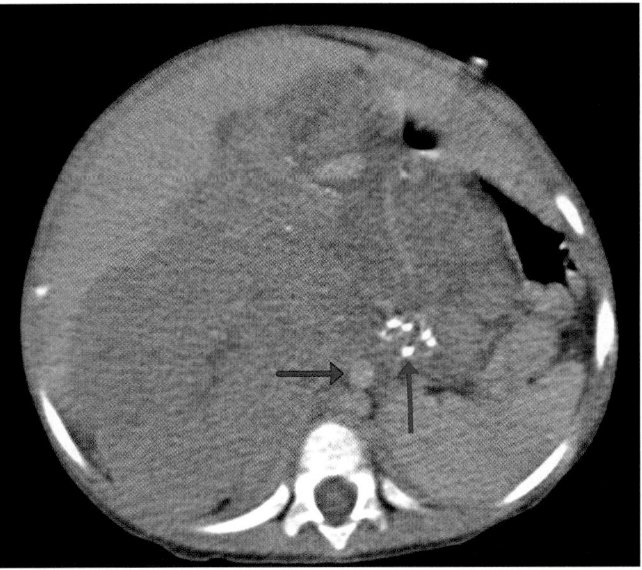

FIGURE 212-5 Large heterogenous upper abdominal mass on CT scan of a 2-year-old girl with neuroblastoma. The mass does not have well defined borders, displaces and encases the aorta (red arrow), compresses the kidneys, and has punctate calcifications (blue arrow), which are typical features of neuroblastoma. (*Used with permission from Margaret C. Thompson, MD, PhD.*)

DIFFERENTIAL DIAGNOSIS

- Wilm's Tumor—Usually presents as an asymptomatic flank mass in a well appearing child (see Chapter 213, Wilms Tumor).
- Adrenal hemorrhage—Usually associated with overwhelming sepsis or significant trauma.
- Rhabdomyosarcoma—Soft tissue malignant tumor of skeletal muscle. Biopsy of tissue will distinguish this from neuroblastoma.

MANAGEMENT

- Treatment is risk stratified based on the age of the patient at diagnosis, stage of disease at diagnosis, histology of the tumor prior to treatment, and presence or absence of recurrent cytogenetic changes including amplification of NMYC in all tumors and DNA ploidy for children under 18 months at diagnosis.
- Adrenal tumors are sometimes identified in utero and perinatally. These tumors may spontaneously regress and are frequently observed with resection performed only if they grow or the patient becomes symptomatic.
- Patients with 4S disease without MYCN amplification frequently have spontaneous regression of their disease. In cases where the patient is symptomatic, such as with large adrenal primary tumors causing hepatomegaly and respiratory compromise, chemotherapy, and/or low dose radiation may be used.[3]
- Low-risk patients include those with stage 1 disease regardless of biologic factors and those with stage 2 disease with favorable biologic factors. These patients may be treated with surgery alone with a low risk for relapsed. Those who do relapse are effectively

salvaged with chemotherapy. Survival for these patients is greater than 95 percent.[2,4]

- The intermediate risk group includes patients with non-metastatic disease but with <50 percent resection of the primary tumor (including biopsy only) and whose tumor is MYCN non-amplified. Patients with metastatic disease under 18 months of age whose tumor shows favorable biologics may also be treated as intermediate risk. Treatment includes surgical resection plus radiation to residual disease along with 2 to 8 cycles of chemotherapy. Outcomes for this group of patients is greater than 95 percent.[2]
- With the exception of children with stage 1 disease, any patients whose tumor is MYCN amplified is treated on a high-risk protocol and requires multimodality therapy including intensive induction chemotherapy, surgery, consolidation therapy with high dose chemotherapy and stem cell rescue, radiation, immune therapy, and cis-retinoic acid as a differentiating agent.[2,3] Despite such aggressive treatment, survival is only 40 to 50 percent with significant treatment associated morbidities.

SURGERY

Surgery for removal of the primary tumor is required in all but perinatal and disease classified as 4S.

PREVENTION AND SCREENING

- Several studies have evaluated the effectiveness of routine screening for neuroblastoma in infants. While these studies doubled the incidence, because they detect tumors with good prognosis, there was no reduction of mortality rates due to neuroblastoma. Thus, routine screening for neuroblastoma is not recommended.[2]

PROGNOSIS

- Low risk neuroblastoma—5 year survival >95 percent.
- Intermediate risk neuroblastoma—5 year survival rate >95 percent
- High risk neuroblastoma—Long-term survival rate 30 to 40 percent.

PATIENT RESOURCES

- **http://kidshealth.org/parent/medical/cancer/neuroblastoma.html**.
- **www.cancer.gov/cancertopics/types/neuroblastoma**.
- **www.childrensoncologygroup.org/index.php/neuroblastoma**.

PROVIDER RESOURCES

- **http://emedicine.medscape.com/article/988284**.

REFERENCES

1. Goodman MT, Gurney JG, Smith MA, Olshan, AF: Sympathetic Nervous System Tymors ICCC IV in Ries LAG, Smith MA, Gurney JG, Linet M, Tamra T, Young JL, Bunin GR, (eds). *Cancer Incidence and Survival among Children and Adolescents: United States SEER Program 1975-1995*, National Cancer Institute, SEER Program. NIH Pub. No. 99-4649. Bethesda, MD, 1999.
2. Park JR, Eggert A, Caron H: An Update on Pediatric Oncology and Hematology Neuroblastoma. *Biology, Prognosis, and Treatment, Hematology/Oncology Clinics of North America* 2010;24(1):65-86.
3. Øra I, Eggert, A: Progress in treatment and risk stratification of neuroblastoma: Impact on future clinical and basic research. *Seminars in Cancer Biology*. 2011;21:217-228.
4. Zage PE, Ater, JL. Neuroblastoma. In: Kliegman, RM, Stanton, BF, St. Geme, JW, Schor, NF, Behrman, RE, eds. *Nelson Textbook of Pediatrics, 19th ed*. Philadelphia: Saunders, Elsevier, Inc.; 2011:1753-1757.
5. Taggart et al. Comparison of Iodine-123 Metaiodobenzylguanidine (MIBG) Scan and [18F]Fluorodeoxyglucose Positron Emission Tomography to Evaluate Response After Iodine-131 MIBG Therapy for Relapsed Neuroblastoma. *JCO*. 2009;27(32): 5343-5349.

213 WILMS TUMOR

Stefanie Thomas, MD
Margaret C. Thompson, MD, PhD

PATIENT STORY

A 6-year-old previously healthy boy presented to his pediatrician with abdominal fullness for one month. The child had no abdominal or gastrointestinal complaints. On examination, he had left-sided abdominal firmness. An ultrasound revealed a mass that appeared to originate from the kidney. He was referred to pediatric oncology. CT scan of the abdomen confirmed a large kidney mass with displacement of the structures within the left abdomen, most consistent with a Wilms tumor (**Figure 213-1**). Work-up for metastatic disease, including a chest CT was negative. The patient underwent nephrectomy (**Figure 213-2**). Pathology of the mass revealed Wilms tumor with favorable histology. The child received chemotherapy and has been tumor-free.

INTRODUCTION

Renal cancer, including Wilms tumor, accounts for approximately 6.3 percent of cancer diagnosed in children under the age of 15 years and 4.4 percent of cancer diagnosed in children and young adults under the age of 20 years.[1] Treatment may include surgery, chemotherapy, and radiation. With multimodality therapy, long-term cure rates exceed 85 percent for children diagnosed with favorable histology, even in cases of higher stage disease.

SYNONYMS

Nephroblastoma.

EPIDEMIOLOGY

- Approximately 550 children and young adults under 20 years of age are diagnosed with renal tumors in the US each year and approximately 500 of these are Wilms tumor.[1]
- Wilms tumor accounts for approximately 95 percent of all renal cancers in children under 15 years of age.
- Wilms tumor occurs most commonly in children under age 5 years, with the highest incidence in the first 2 years of life.[1]

ETIOLOGY AND PATHOPHYSIOLOGY

- Wilms tumor is an embryonal malignancy of the kidney.
- It is believed to develop in retained nephrogenic rests which are foci of persistent embryonal kidney cells. Although nephrogenic

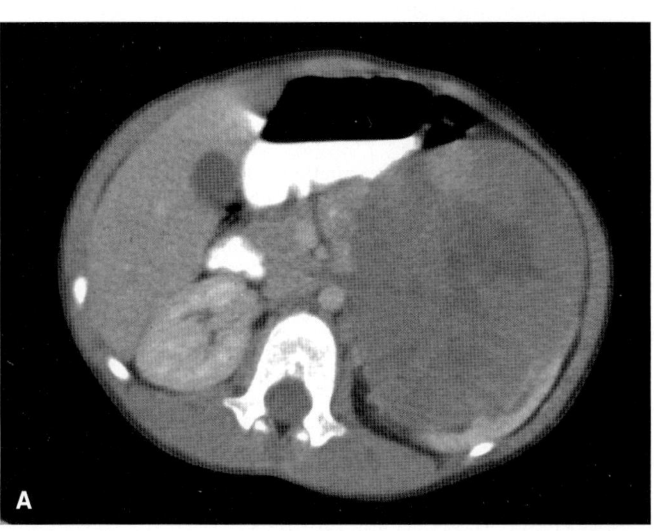

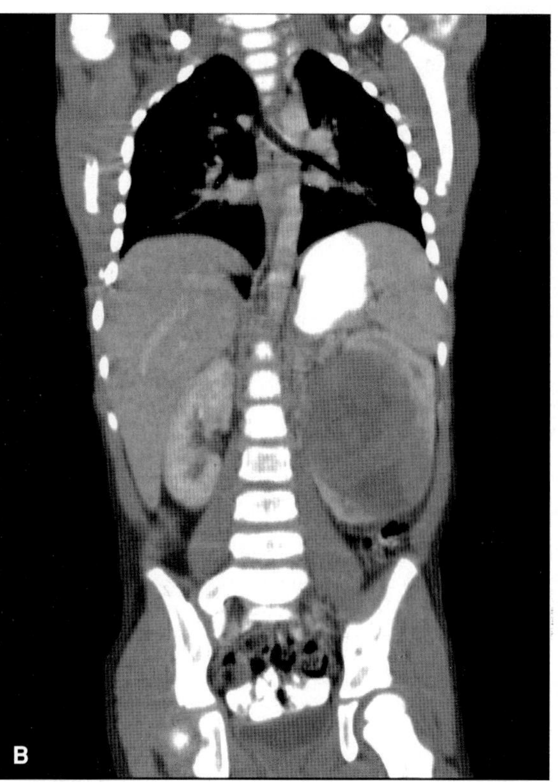

FIGURE 213-1 Large left-sided renal mass that is well circumscribed and without calcifications on transverse (**A**) and coronal (**B**) CT scan of the abdomen, in a 6-year-old boy with Wilms tumor. Note the normal appearing right kidney. (*Used with permission from Stefanie Thomas, MD.*)

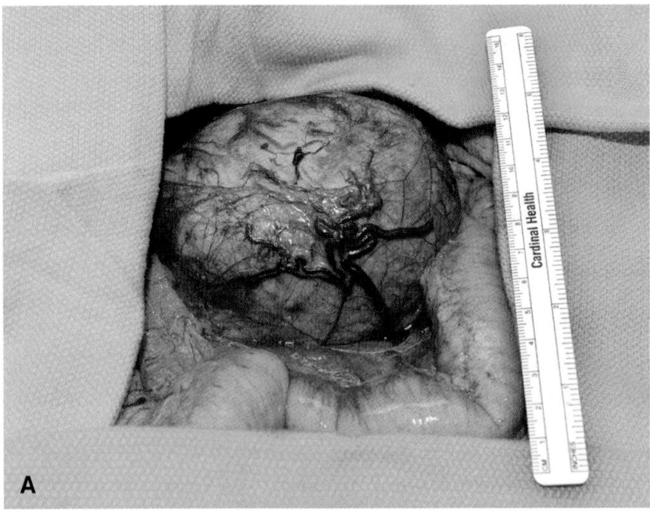

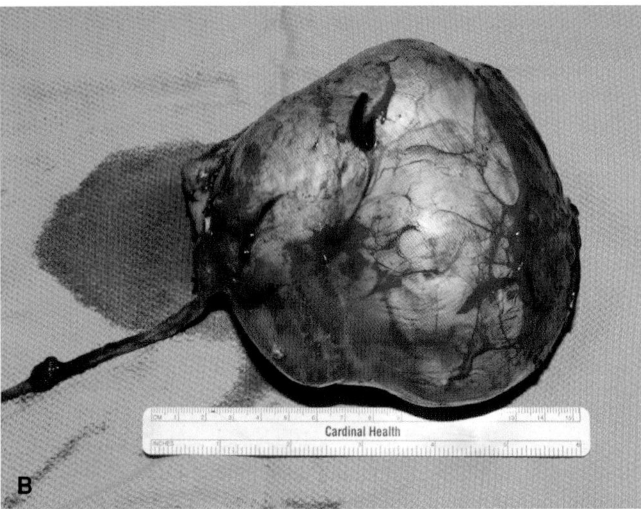

FIGURE 213-2 Gross appearance of the large renal mass in the abdomen (**A**) during laparotomy and following removal (**B**) from the child in **Figure 213-1**. This mass was well-demarcated from the renal parenchyma and well encapsulated, and was confirmed to be a Wilms tumor with favorable histology. *(Reprinted with permission, Cleveland Clinic Center for Medical Art & Photography © 2012-2013. All Rights Reserved.)*

rests may be seen in approximately 1 percent of kidneys at birth, they usually regress or differentiate early in life.[2]

- Persistent nephrogenic rests outside of the perinatal period are felt to be precancerous lesions.
- The majority of cases of Wilms tumor occur in healthy children who do not have any identifiable risk factors.
- Approximately 10 percent of cases of Wilms tumor are associated with congenital urinary tract anomalies and may be associated with an established phenotypic syndrome.
- Associated urinary tract anomalies include cryptorchidism and hypospadias.
- Associated syndromes may be divided into overgrowth syndromes and nonovergrowth syndromes.
  - Overgrowth syndromes include:
    - Beckwith-Wiedemann (Wilms tumor and other manifestations such as macrosomia, macroglossia, omphalocele, prominent eyes, ear creases, large kidneys, pancreatic hyperplasia, and hemihypertrophy).
    - Perlman syndrome (Wilms tumor, fetal gigantism, visceromegaly, unusual face, and bilateral renal hamartomas with nephroblastomatosis).
    - Isolated hemihypertrophy.
    - Sotos syndrome (cerebral gigantism).
    - Simpson-Golabi-Behemel syndrome (Wilms tumor, organomegaly, bulldog facies, congenital heart disease, and polydactyly).
  - Nonovergrowth syndromes include:
    - WAGR syndrome (Wilms tumor, aniridia, genitourinary anomalies, and mental retardation).
    - Isolated aniridia.
    - Denys-Drash syndrome (Wilms tumor, progressive renal disease, and male pseudohermaphroditism).
    - Li-Fraumeni syndrome (Familial Wilms tumor).
- Approximately 1 to 3 percent of cases of Wilms tumor are familial and are usually inherited in a dominant pattern with incomplete penetrance.[3]
- Several genes have been identified as involved in the pathogenesis of Wilms tumor for both the sporadic form and those involving inherited predispositions syndromes, including familial occurrences.
- Genetic changes in inherited syndromes involve germline mutations. These mutations may be inherited or de novo.
- In addition to mutations in tumor suppressor genes, epigenetic changes at several sites have been identified as involved in the development of Wilms.[4]

DIAGNOSIS

CLINICAL PRESENTATION

- The most common presentation is an asymptomatic upper abdominal mass that is detected by a caretaker.
- Other findings and their approximate frequency include:
  - Abdominal pain (20 to 30%).
  - Fever (20 to 30%)
  - Hematuria (20 to 30%).
  - Hypertension (25%).
  - Anemia (bleeding into the tumor).
- The median age at presentation is 42 to 47 months for unilateral disease and 30 to 33 months for bilateral disease.[5]
- Five to ten percent of patients present with multicentric or bilateral disease (stage V).
- Bilateral and multicentric disease is usually associated with predisposition syndromes, the presence of nephrogenic rests, congenital malformations, or may be familial.[6]
- Extrarenal primary tumors can occur in the abdomen or pelvis but are rare.[7]
- Spread may be local through the renal capsule and into the renal sinus, renal vasculature, and ureter.[8]
- Local spread to the lymph nodes occurs in approximately 15 to 20 percent of cases.[8]

- The most common site of hematogenous spread involves the lungs, and less commonly liver, bone, bone marrow, or brain.[7]

LABORATORY TESTING

- Initial laboratory studies should include—Renal function tests, electrolytes, urinalysis, complete blood count, and liver function tests.
- Tumor specimens are evaluated for histology—Favorable histology versus anaplastic, extent of the tumor, and completeness of resection.

IMAGING

- CT scan of the primary tumor.
  - Commonly indicates an encapsulated mass originating from within the kidney. Calcifications are usually absent. An encapsulated tumor without calcifications helps to differentiate Wilms tumor from neuroblastoma (**Figure 213-1**).[7]
  - CT scan of the abdomen and pelvis also helps to evaluate for lymph spread and for evidence of disease in the contralateral kidney.
- Kidney ultrasound is performed to evaluate renal artery and veins for evidence of thrombus.
- CT scan of the chest is performed to evaluate for evidence of pulmonary disease (**Figure 213-3**).
- A chest x-ray may show metastatic lesions but is not sufficiently sensitive to identify metastatic disease for staging purposes (**Figure 213-4**).
- An MRI of the primary tumor may be performed and can be helpful in distinguishing between Wilms tumor and nephrogenic rests.

DIFFERENTIAL DIAGNOSIS

- Benign lesions that may mimic Wilms tumor include:
  - Congenital mesoblasticnephroma, diffuse hyperplastic perilobarnephrogenic rests (pre-cancerous lesions), nephrogenic rests (pre-cancerous lesions), and polycystic kidney disease.

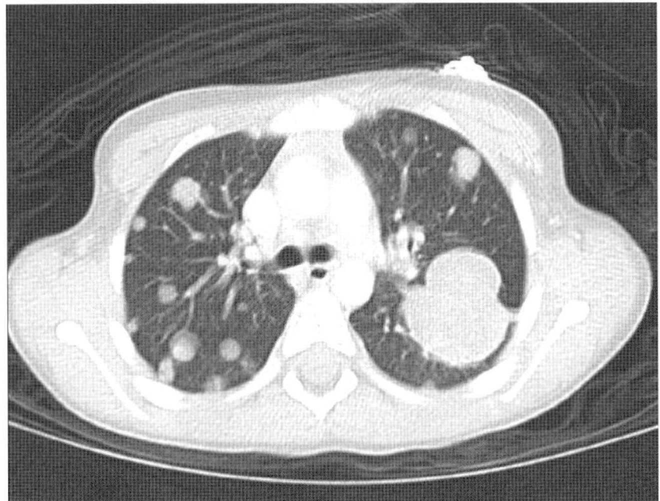

FIGURE 213-3 Extensive pulmonary metastatic disease on chest CT scan of a young child with Wilms tumor. *(Used with permission from Stefanie Thomas, MD.)*

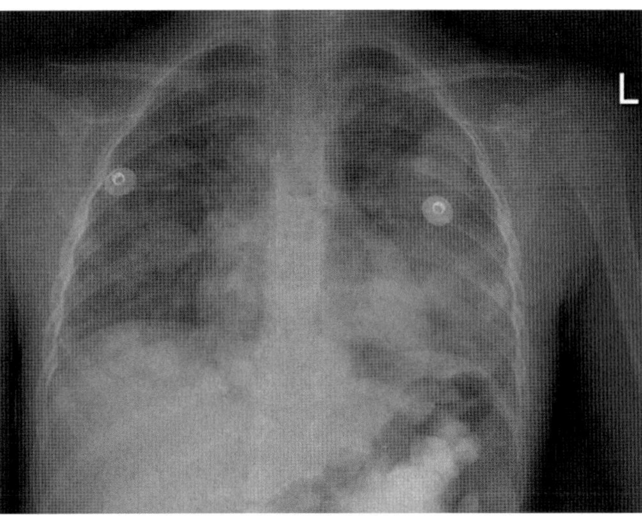

FIGURE 213-4 Bilateral pulmonary nodules, representing metastatic disease, on chest x-ray of the same child as in **Figure 213-3**. *(Used with permission from Stefanie Thomas, MD.)*

- Malignant Lesions that may mimic Wilms tumor on imaging include:
  - Clear cell sarcoma of the kidney, malignant rhabdoid tumor of the kidney, renal cell carcinoma, and neuroblastoma.
- Imaging studies read by experienced pediatric radiologists may help to distinguish these lesions from Wilms tumor but the ultimate diagnosis is based on pathology.

MANAGEMENT

- Treatment is risk stratified based on stage, histology (favorable or anaplastic), and completeness of resection.[9]
- Biopsy (including needle biopsy) upstages a patient and should be avoided in lieu of initial complete excision if possible.
- The more common approach in the US is up front resection followed by chemotherapy based on margins, tumor spill, and histology.
- In Europe, a more common approach is neoadjuvant chemotherapy based on presumed diagnosis followed by resection and subsequent further chemotherapy.
- Patients with evidence of regional lymph spread or tumor spillage either before or during surgery or those who had a biopsy of the tumor initially require abdominal or flank radiation.
- Radiation is directed to sites of metastasis including the lungs.
- Individuals with bilateral (stage V) disease are treated with a nephron sparing approach and may have partial nephrectomies for local control. These patients are frequently treated without biopsy. The need for radiation is based on the local stage of each primary kidney tumor.
- Standard chemotherapeutic agents include Vincristine, Dactinomycin, Doxorubicin, Cyclophosphamide, and Etoposide. Additional agents are used in patients with tumors with anaplastic histology or those whose tumor demonstrates chemotherapy resistance.

PREVENTION AND SCREENING

- Children with predisposition syndromes including Beckwith-Wiedemann, WAGR, Denys-Drash, idiopathic hemihypertrophy, or sporadic aniridia, and those with a family history of familial Wilms, should be screened with an ultrasound every 3 months until age 8 years.[10]

PROGNOSIS

- The overall survival rate for Wilms tumor is 90 percent.[11]
- For patients with favorable histology disease, 4-year overall survival is greater than 80 percent, including those with metastatic disease (stage 4) and/or bilateral disease at diagnosis.[11]
- Patients with anaplastic disease fare worse—Patients with low stage 1 or 2 disease have a 4-year overall survival rate of approximately 80 percent while those with stage 4 disease have a 4-year overall survival rate of only 33 percent.[11]
- Studies of long-term survivors of Wilms tumor show a cumulative incidence of 65 percent for all chronic conditions at 25 years after therapy with the cumulative incidence of severe chronic health conditions being 24 percent. The late effects include:[12]
  - Cardiomyopathy, arrhythmias, left ventricular dysfunction associated with doxorubicin, and whole lung radiation.
  - End-stage renal disease associated with surgery.
  - Secondary malignancies associated with doxorubicin, alkylating agents, and radiation.
  - Acute ovarian failure and premature menopause associated with pelvic radiation and exposure to alkylating agents.
  - Oligospermia/azoospermia associated with alkylating agents.
  - Linear growth changes associated with radiation affecting the spine.

PATIENT RESOURCES

- Children's Oncology Group—**www.curesearch.org/Wilms-Tumor-in-Children**.
- American Cancer Society—**www.cancer.org/cancer/wilmstumor/index**.

PROVIDER RESOURCES

- National Cancer Institute—**www.cancer.gov/cancertopics/pdq/treatment/wilms/HealthProfessional**.
- **http://emedicine.medscape.com/article/453076**.

REFERENCES

1. Bernstein L, Linet M, Smith MA, et al. Cancer incidence and survival among children and adolescents: United States SEER Program 1975–1995, SEER Program. Bethesda, MD, National Cancer Institute, 1999: 79.
2. Breslow, Alshan et al. Age distributions, birthweights, nephrogenics rests and heterogeneity in the pathogenesis of Wilms tumor. *Pediatric Blood Cancer*. 2006;47:260-267.
3. Rahman et al. Penetrance of Mutations in the Familial Wilms Tumor Gene FWT1, *JNCI J Natl Cancer Inst*. 2000;92(8):650-652.
4. Dome JS, Huff, V. Wilms Tumor Overview in GeneReviews™, Pagon RA, Adam MP, Bird RD et al, editors. NCBI Bookshelf. www.geneclinics.org; www.genetests.org.
5. Breslow N, Beckwith JB, Ciol M, Sharples K. Age distribution of Wilms' tumor: report from the National Wilms' Tumor Study. *Cancer Res*. 1988;48:1653.
6. Owens CM, Brisse HJ, Olsen OE, et al. Bilateral disease and new trends in Wilmstumour. *PediatrRadiol*. 2008;38:30-39.
7. Pizzo PA, Poplack DG. Principles and Practice of Pediatric Oncology, 6th edition. Philadelphia, PA. Lippincott Williams & Wilkins, 2010.
8. Breslow N, Sharples K, Beckwith JB, et al. Prognostic factors in nonmetastatic, favorable histology Wilms' tumor. Results of the Third National Wilms' Tumor Study. *Cancer* 1991;68:2345-2353.
9. Metzger ML, Dome JS. Current therapy for Wilms' tumor. *Oncologist*. 2005;10(10):815-826.
10. http://www.cancer.gov/cancertopics/pdq/treatment/wilms/HealthProfessional/page1#Section_558
11. Dome et al. Children's Oncology Group's 2013 blueprint for research: renal tumors. *Pediatric Blood Cancer*. 2013:60(6):994-1000.
12. Sadak, KT, Ritchey ML, Dome JS. Paediatric genitourinary cancers and late effects of treatment. *Nature Reviews Urology*. 2013;10:15-25.

214 LANGERHANS CELL HISTIOCYTOSIS

Stefanie Thomas, MD
Margaret C. Thompson, MD

PATIENT STORY

A 3-month-old female infant presented to her pediatrician with a history of a rash that had been present from birth. Her parents report that her rash initially involved her face and trunk, and the lesions had a red base. The rash seemed to slightly improve over the first 2 weeks of her life, but then progressed into red and brown, rough lesions involving her head, face, trunk, and spread to her back then bilateral lower extremities (**Figures 214-1** and **214-2**). They have also noted that her right eye has been watering and she has not been able to open it completely over the past few days. Based on the appearance and persistence of the rash, she was referred to a dermatologist, who performed a skin biopsy, which showed CD1 positive immuno-histochemical staining, consistent with the diagnosis of Langerhans Cell Histiocytosis. Further work-up included a skull film, which revealed an ocular bony lesion (**Figure 214-3**). She underwent treatment with a chemotherapy regimen and has done well without evidence of recurrence.

INTRODUCTION

Langerhans Cell Histiocytosis (LCH) is characterized by clonal proliferation of histiocytic cells that resemble Langerhans cells of the skin and can result in widely variable organ involvement and extent of disease.[1] Because of the wide spectrum of the disease, treatment depends on extent of disease.

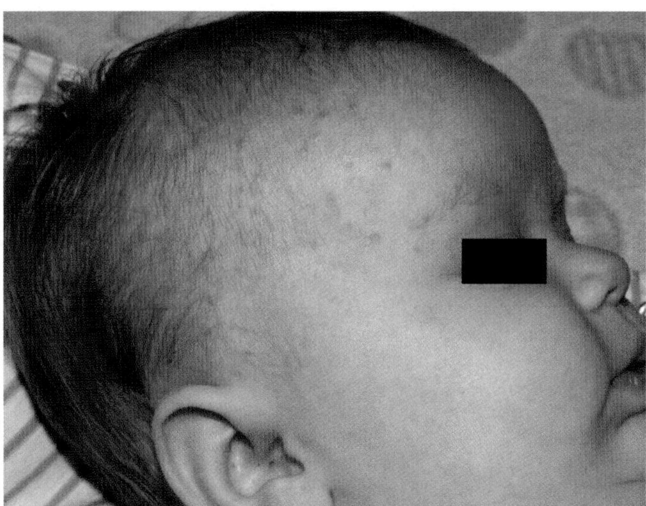

FIGURE 214-1 Multiple reddish- brown papules on the face and scalp of an infant with Langerhans cell histiocytosis. These lesions can be confused with chronic cradle cap (seborrheic dermatitis). (*Used with permission from Stefanie Thomas, MD.*)

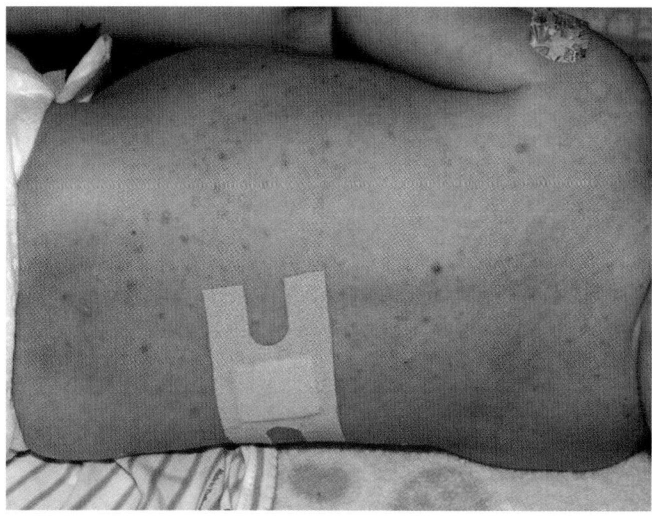

FIGURE 214-2 Multiple erythematous papules, vesicles and crusted papules on the back in the same infant as in **Figure 214-1**. Note the presence of some areas of postinflammatory hypopigmentation, where papules were previously present. (*Used with permission from Stefanie Thomas, MD.*)

SYNONYMS

- Eosinophilic granuloma of the bone—LCH with a single bone lesion.
- Hand-Schuller-Christian Disease—LCH with Exophthalmus, Diabetes Insipidus, and skull lesions.

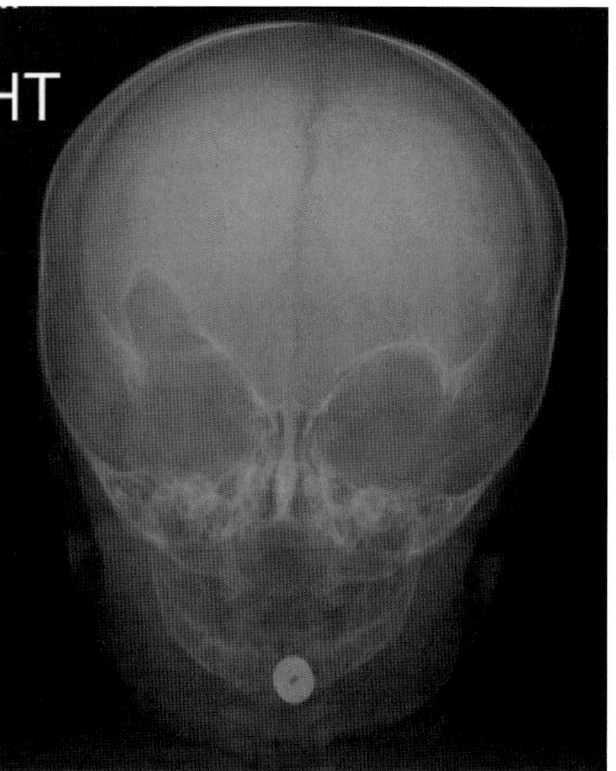

FIGURE 214-3 Lytic lesion of the lateral roof of the right orbit on skull x-ray in the same infant as in **Figure 214-1**. (*Used with permission from Stefanie Thomas, MD.*)

- Letterer-Siwe Disease—Multifocal-multisystem LCH.
- Hashimoto-Pritzker Disease—LCH rash in an infant which is usually self-resolving.
- Histiocytosis-X.

EPIDEMIOLOGY

- Incidence is approximately 2 to 10 cases per million children under age 15 years with a median age at presentation of 30 months.[2]
- 1:1—Male to Female ratio.[2]

ETIOLOGY AND PATHOPHYSIOLOGY

- Exact etiology remains unknown.
- Exhibits features of both malignant transformation (proliferation and clonality) and immune dysregulation.[1]
- Recently, recurrent mutations in BRAF gene have been identified.[3]

RISK FACTORS

- Weak associations but no known risk factors to developing LCH.

DIAGNOSIS

CLINICAL FEATURES

- Most typical presentation is skin rash or bone lesion, which may be painful or asymptomatic (**Figures 214-1** to **214-3**).
- Non-specific inflammatory response may be present including fever, weight loss, diarrhea, edema, and dyspnea.[1]
- Because of the frequent involvement of the pituitary gland, symptoms of diabetes insipidus, including polydipsia and polyuria, may also be present.[1]
- Other presenting features depend on which organs are involved.

DISTRIBUTION

- The distribution of the skin and bony lesions are wide and varied.
- May result in single system/organ involvement with single or multiple sites of involved system.
- Organs that may be involved are classified as high-risk or low-risk organs. High-risk organs include the bone marrow, liver, spleen, and lungs. Low-risk organs include skin, bones, lymph nodes, gastrointestinal system, and the pituitary gland. The prognosis is worse for children with involvement of any of the high-risk organs.
- Most frequent bone lesions occur in the skull (**Figure 214-3**), but can also include the femur, ribs, humerus, and vertebrae (**Figure 214-4**).

LABORATORY TESTING

- The diagnosis is primarily made on biopsy. If skin lesions are present, skin biopsy is typically the least invasive diagnostic procedure.

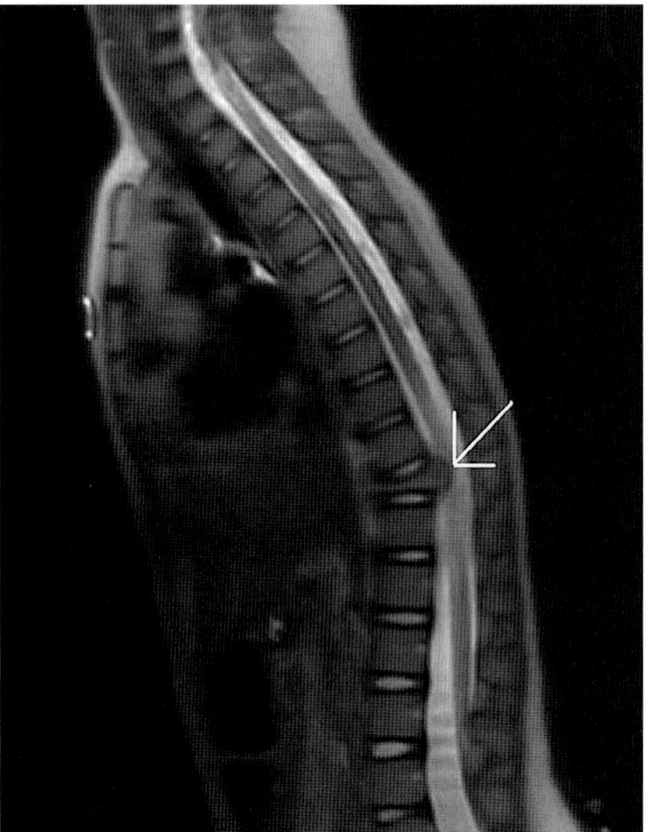

FIGURE 214-4 Vertebra Plana (flattening of the body of the vertebra), a feature of vertebral bone involvement in a patient with Langerhans cell histiocytosis. (*Used with permission from Margaret C. Thompson, MD.*)

- Positive immunohistochemical staining with CD207 (langerin) and CD1a are diagnostic.[1]
- Birbeck granules (tennis-racket shaped rods with handle appearance that are present in Langerhans cells) seen on electronic microscopy are pathognomonic for LCH but not required for diagnosis (**Figure 214-5**).
- Other laboratory testing is dependent on organ involvement.

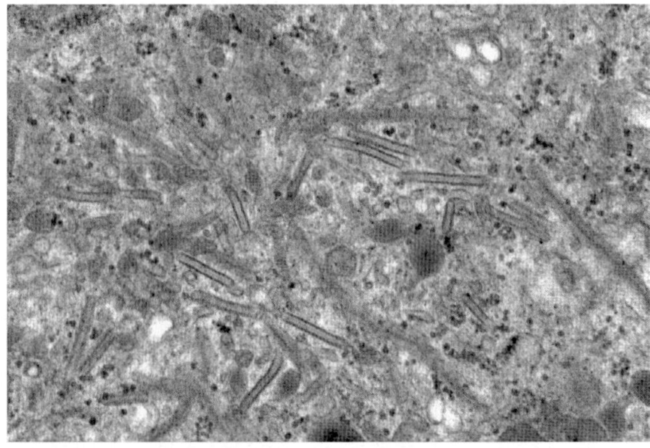

FIGURE 214-5 Birbeck granules seen on electron microscopy of a skin biopsy in a patient with Langerhans cell histiocytosis. (*Used with permission from Melissa Piliang, MD.*)

IMAGING

- Lytic lesions of the bone are best seen on plain x-ray (**Figure 214-3**).
- MRI of the head is typically done at diagnosis to assess for pituitary involvement.

DIFFERENTIAL DIAGNOSIS

- The differential diagnosis of cutaneous LCH includes seborrheic dermatitis, erythema toxicum neonatorum, mastocytosis, acrodermatitis enteropathica, acropustulosis of infancy, and benign cephalic histiocytosis (**Figure 140-7**). LCH should be considered when cutaneous manifestations do not resolve despite appropriate treatment or observation for these entities.
- Differential of vertebral LCH includes tuberculosis of the spine, which can be excluded with a good history and biopsy results.

MANAGEMENT

Management depends on location and extent of disease.

NONPHARMACOLOGIC

- For isolated cutaneous LCH, particularly in an infant, observation alone may be an appropriate option.

MEDICATIONS

- For isolated cutaneous LCH, topical corticosteroids can be tried but are rarely effective alone.[4] Oral methotrexate[5] may also be used in this setting.
- Isolated single site bone involvement has been treated with oral corticosteroids or injection of corticosteroids into the area that is involved.[6]
- Single site bone involvement in a high-risk location such as a vertebral body or skull should be treated with systemic chemotherapy.
- Treatment of a single system (i.e., bone) but in multiple sites should be treated with systemic chemotherapy to decrease the risk of recurrence, particularly in the pituitary gland.
- Multisystem disease or disease involving high-risk organs requires treatment with systemic chemotherapy. Such treatment usually includes vinblastine, oral corticosteroids, and 6-Mercaptopurine. Treatment duration is typically for 1 year.

SURGICAL

- For single site bone involvement, curettage alone by an orthopedic surgeon may be sufficient.

REFERRAL

- Referral to a hematologist/oncologist is recommended.

PROGNOSIS

- Infants with single system LCH without high-risk organ involvement have a very favorable outcome.[1]
- Infants less than two years of age, particularly those with multiorgan involvement, have poor outcomes. With intensified therapy, infants without high-risk organ involvement have had significant improvement in survival.[7]
- Children with high-risk organ involvement continue to have poor outcome although this has improved with intensified treatment with mortality decreasing from 44 to 27 percent.[7]
- Children with high-risk organ involvement who do not respond to treatment within 6 weeks have the highest mortality.[1]
- Infants with skin only LCH often progress to multisystem LCH and should be monitored closely for development of other organ involvement.[4]

PATIENT RESOURCES

- National Cancer Institute—**www.cancer.gov/cancertopics/pdq/treatment/lchistio/Patient**.

PROVIDER RESOURCES

- National Cancer Institute—**www.cancer.gov/cancertopics/pdq/treatment/lchistio/HealthProfessional**.
- Histiocyte Society—**www.histiocytesociety.org/sslpage.aspx?pid=707**.

REFERENCES

1. Pizzo PA, Poplack DG: *Principles and Practice of Pediatric Oncology (Sixth edition)*. Philadelphia, PA: Lippincott Williams & Wilkins; 2010.
2. Salotti JA, Nanduri V, Pearce MS, et al. Incidence and clinical features of Langerhans cell histiocytosis in the UK and Ireland. *Arch Dis Child*. 2009;94(5):376-380.
3. Badalain-Very G, Vergilio HA, et al. Recurrent BRAF mutations in Langerhans cell histiocytosis. *Blood*. 2010;116(11):1919-1923.
4. Lau L, Krafchik B, Trebo MM, et al. Cutaneous Langerhans cell histiocytosis in children under one year. *Pediatr Blood Cancer*. 2006;46(1):66-71.
5. Steen AE, Steen KH, Bauer R, et al. Successful treatment of cutaneous Langerhans cell histiocytosis with low-dose methotrexate. *Br J Dermatol*. 2001;145(1):137-140.
6. Baptista AM, Camargo AF, de Camargo OP, et al. Does adjunctive chemotherapy reduce remission rates compared to cortisone alone in unifocal or multifocal histiocytosis of bone? *Clin Orthop Relat Res*. 2012;470(3):663-669.
7. Gadner H, Grois N, Pötschger U, et al. Improved outcome in multisystem Langerhans cell histiocytosis is associated with therapy intensification. *Blood*. 2008;111(5):2556-2562.

PART 20

ALLERGY AND IMMUNOLOGY

Strength of Recommendation (SOR)	Definition
A	Recommendation based on consistent and good-quality patient-oriented evidence.*
B	Recommendation based on inconsistent or limited-quality patient-oriented evidence.*
C	Recommendation based on consensus, usual practice, opinion, disease-oriented evidence, or case series for studies of diagnosis, treatment, prevention, or screening.*

*See Appendix A on pages 1320–1322 for further information.

215 ALLERGIC RHINITIS

Brian Schroer, MD

PATIENT STORY

A 9-year-old girl presents to her pediatrician for constant nasal congestion, runny nose, and intermittent bouts of sneezing and itching. Her symptoms occur year-round with increased symptoms in the spring and fall. On examination she has dark circles under her eyes ("allergic shiners"; **Figure 215-1**), bilateral conjunctivitis (**Figure 215-2**), swollen, pale, inferior turbinates, and a copious clear watery nasal discharge (**Figure 215-3**). Over-the-counter antihistamines have helped minimally so she is given a prescription for a nasal steroid spray to use daily. This significantly improves but does not eliminate the symptoms. She is seen by an allergist who obtains a history that she sleeps on feather pillows, lives with two cats, and also has eye itching and redness when outside in the spring. Skin prick testing to local environmental allergens shows positive reactions to dust mites, cats, and grass and ragweed pollens (**Figures 215-4** and **215-5**). Recommendations for avoidance of the dust mites, cats, and the outdoor pollens were given. Her technique and adherence with the nasal steroids was discussed and she was given nasal antihistamines to treat breakthrough symptoms.

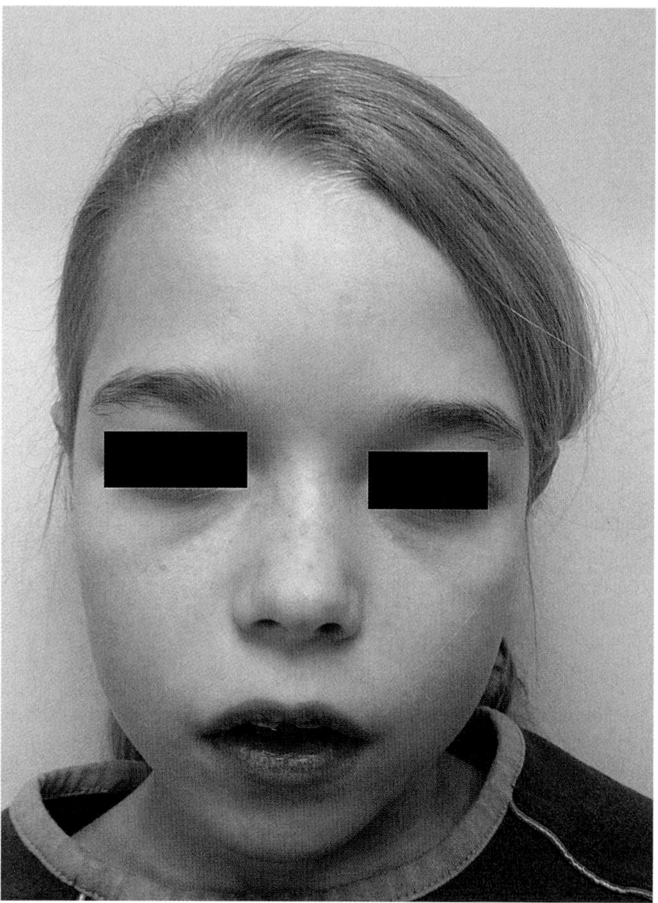

FIGURE 215-1 Mouth breathing and "allergic shiners" evident in a young child with allergic rhinitis. (*Used with permission from Brian Schroer, MD.*)

INTRODUCTION

Allergic rhinitis is a syndrome of upper airway symptoms in patients who are sensitive to aeroallergens including but not limited to animal dander, dust mites, mold spores, pollen, cockroaches, and rodents. Many patients have a history of atopic dermatitis, allergic rhinitis and asthma that together make up the "atopic triad." These symptoms may be present in a seasonal pattern or year-round with seasonal exacerbations.

SYNONYMS

Hay fever, Allergies, Pollinosis, the sniffles.

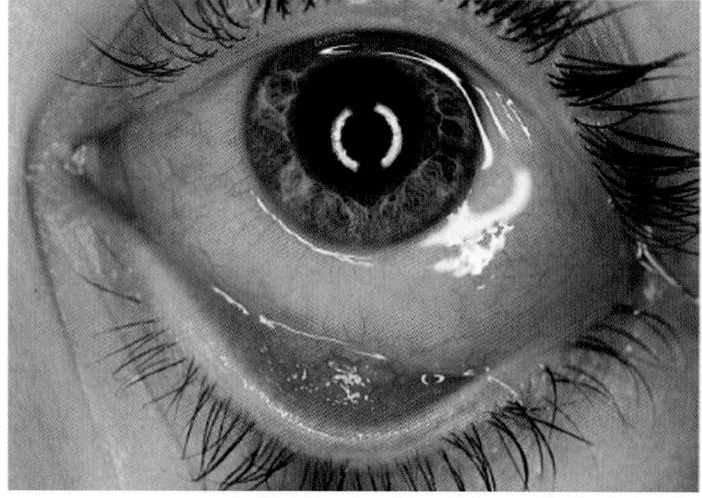

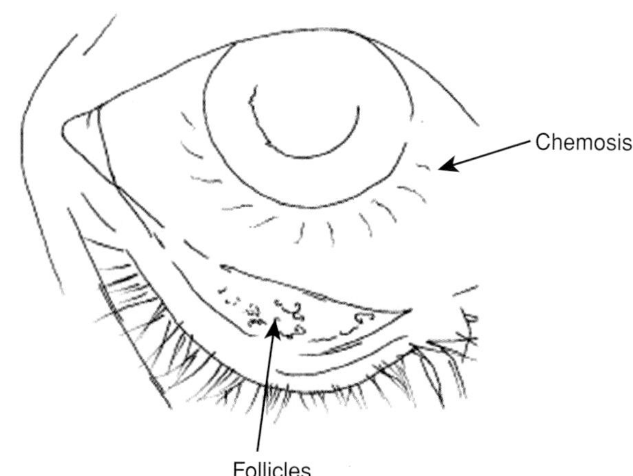

FIGURE 215-2 Conjunctival injection and chemosis in a patient with allergic conjunctivitis. (*Used with permission from Strange GR, Ahrens WH, Schafermeyer RW, Wiebe R. Pediatric Emergency Medicine 3rd edition. Figure 69-1, New York: McGraw-Hill; 2009.*)

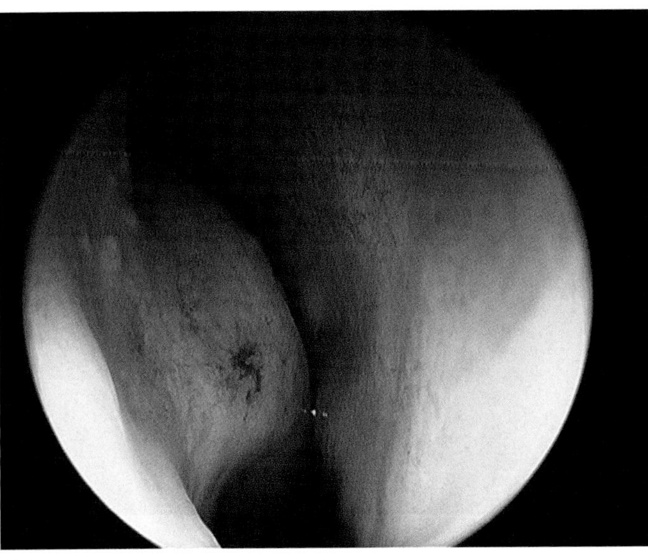

FIGURE 215-3 Right inferior turbinate hypertrophy with production of clear thin mucous typical of allergic rhinitis on nasal endoscopy in a young child. (*Used with permission from Prashant Malhotra, MD.*)

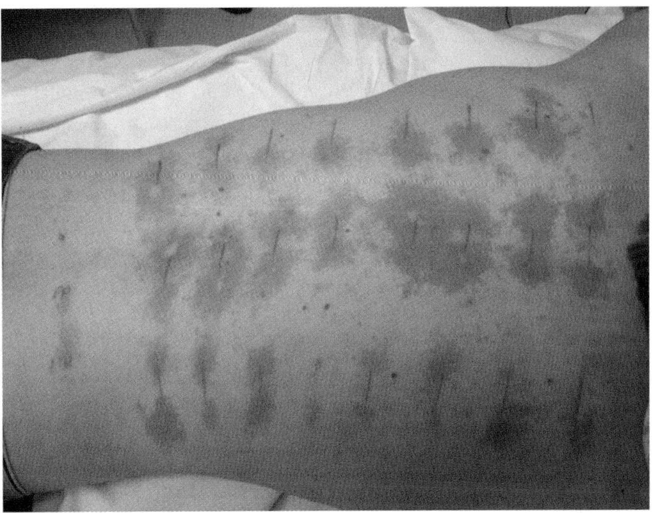

FIGURE 215-5 Positive wheal and flare reactions to multiple tested allergens on Skin Prick Testing in a young child. (*Used with permission from Brian Schroer, MD.*)

EPIDEMIOLOGY

- By 6 years of age, 42 percent of children will be diagnosed with allergic rhinitis by a physician.[1]
- Seasonal allergic rhinitis symptoms due to outdoor pollens rarely occur before the age of 2 years. However, sensitivity to indoor allergens can be present by the age of 1 year.
- The prevalence of allergic rhinitis increases throughout childhood and adolescence.
- Allergic rhinitis has been found in people from many different genetic backgrounds, but it tends to occur more often in people who have been raised in the urban/suburban areas of Westernized countries or in higher socioeconomic classes.[2]

RISK FACTORS

- Allergic rhinitis occurs in genetically predisposed individuals who are exposed to common aeroallergens.
- The prevalence of allergic rhinitis and all atopic disease is much higher in people who are raised in more modern/western communities and occurs in all ethnic groups.
- Most patients have a family history of atopic disease.

ETIOLOGY AND PATHOPHYSIOLOGY

- Genetically predisposed individuals can get allergic rhinitis symptoms when they are exposed to allergens, which float in the air,

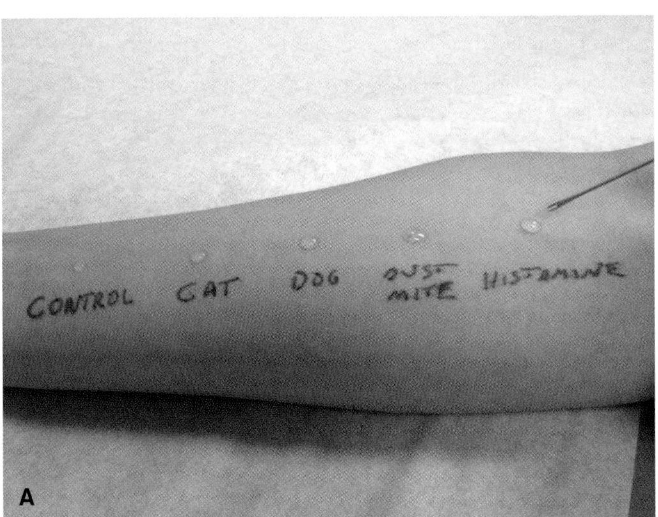

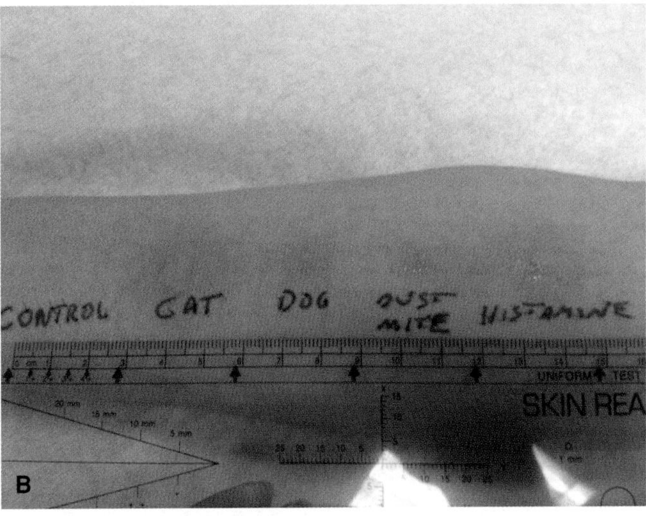

FIGURE 215-4 Skin prick testing showing wheal and flare reaction before prick (**A**) and after 15 minutes (**B**). (*Used with permission from Brian Schroer, MD.*)

enter the nasal mucosa, and bind specific allergic antibodies called IgE.

- When IgE recognizes an allergen, it leads to mast cell degranulation and intracellular signaling causing the cells to release preformed mediators such as histamine and start production of other inflammatory cytokines such as leukotrienes.
- Histamine and other preformed mediators cause sneezing and itching.
- Late phase inflammation leads to congestion and rhinorrhea.
- Indoor allergens from cats, dogs, cockroaches, and dust mites are present year-round and lead to perennial allergic rhinitis.
- Mold spores germinate when weather conditions are warm and wet.
- Tree pollen, grass pollen, and weed pollen are produced by the 10 percent of plants, which use the wind to disperse their pollen. The pollen is released into the air when these plants flower, leading to seasonal allergic rhinitis.
- Flowers, which are showy such as rose bushes, daisies, or cherry trees, do not cause allergic rhinitis as the pollen is too heavy to get into the nose or eyes. These flowers need the flowers to attract pollinators such as bees and insects to carry the pollen from one flower to the other.

DIAGNOSIS

The diagnosis of allergic rhinitis is based on a history of typical symptoms, which occur after exposure to known allergens. Response to treatment with over-the-counter oral antihistamines can be helpful but will not decrease symptoms of congestion and runny nose in patients with severe allergy. Physical exam findings may include enlarged, pale colored turbinates (**Figure 215-3**) with clear rhinorrhea, mouth breathing (**Figure 215-1**), conjunctivitis (**Figure 215-2**), allergic crease (**Figure 215-6**), Dennie Morgan lines (infraorbital folds; **Figure 215-7**), or a gothic arch palate. Positive history of physical exam findings support but do not confirm a diagnosis.[2]

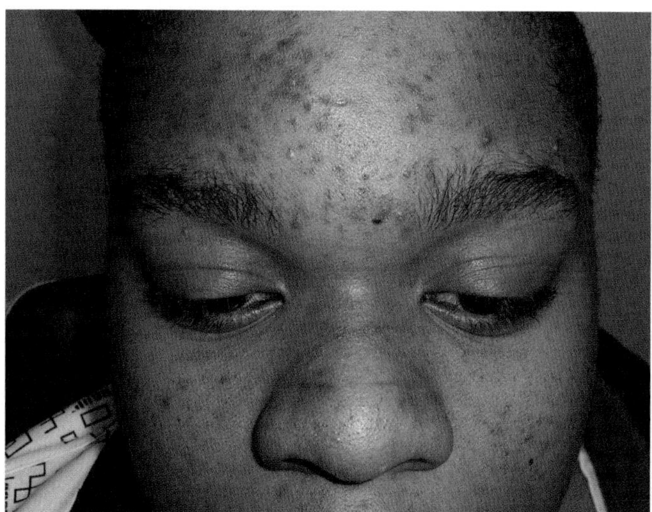

FIGURE 215-6 Allergic creases on the nose of a teenage boy with allergic rhinitis. He was observed performing the allergic salute in the office. (*Used with permission from Richard P. Usatine, MD.*)

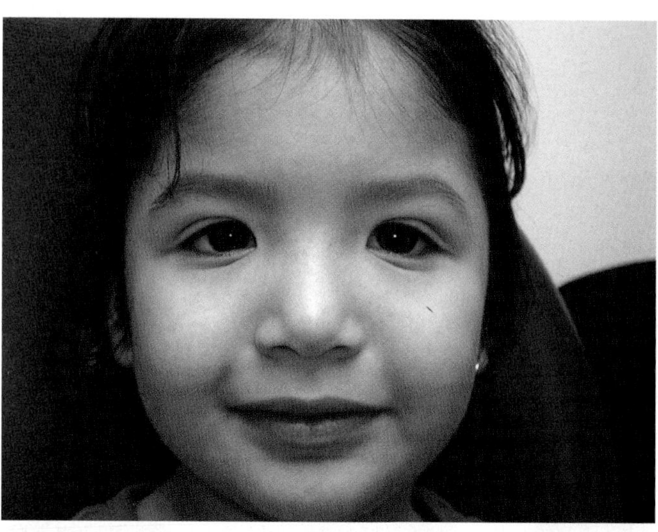

FIGURE 215-7 Dennie-Morgan lines (infraorbital lines) in a girl with the atopic triad. (*Used with permission from Richard P. Usatine, MD.*)

CLINICAL FEATURES

- Nasal congestion, stuffiness, inability to breath through the nose, or allergic shiners.
- Rhinorrhea—Clear watery mucous running out of the nose or down the throat.
- Sneezing—Fits of sneezing in the morning or when around an allergen.
- Itching—Allergic salute, rubbing the nose.
- Throat itching, ear itching.
- Associated with allergic conjunctivitis symptoms when outside—Eye redness, itching, swelling, watering, or asthma symptoms of coughing, chest tightness, shortness of breath, or wheezing.

LABORATORY TESTING

- Allergy skin prick or intradermal testing can be done in the office quickly and easily. Positive skin tests lead to a small hive for each allergen (**Figures 215-4** and **215-5**).
- Blood testing for serum specific IgE to relevant allergens can also be obtained, although it is less sensitive than skin prick testing.[3]
- Positive skin or blood allergy tests should be correlated with the clinical history.

IMAGING

- CT scans are helpful in further evaluating other causes of nasal congestion such as polyps (**Figures 215-8** and **215-9**), anatomic changes such as concha bullosa (middle turbinate pneumatization; **Figure 215-8**), or Haller cells (infraorbital ethmoidal air cells) and chronic rhinosinusitis.

DIFFERENTIAL DIAGNOSIS

- Nonallergic rhinitis—Very similar nasal symptoms when exposed to weather changes, cold air, perfumes, tobacco smoke, air pollution, or strong odors such as cleaning agents or chemicals. Thirty-four

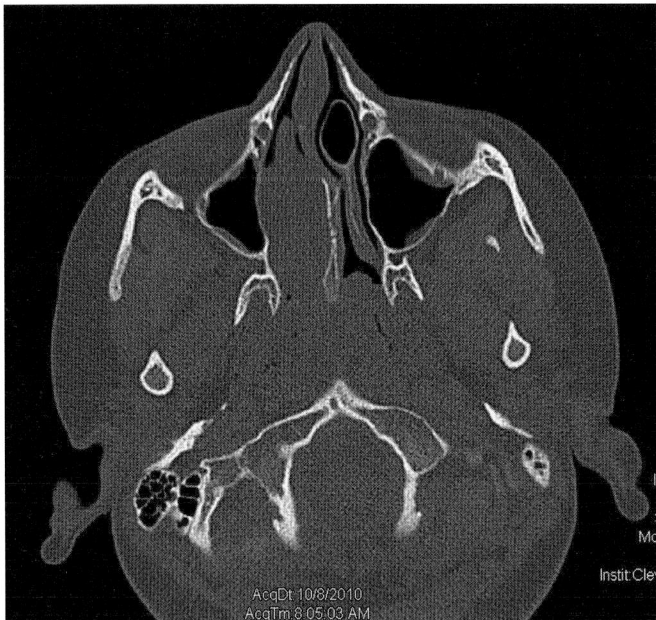

FIGURE 215-8 Right-sided nasal polyp and left-sided concha bullosa with deviated septum in a child with nasal congestion. (*Used with permission from Prashant Malhotra, MD.*)

percent of patients with allergic rhinitis also have nonallergic triggers and this can be called mixed rhinitis.[4] Various forms of nonallergic rhinitis include vasomotor rhinitis, gustatory rhinitis, occupational rhinitis, or drug induced rhinitis.[5]

- Infectious rhinosinusitis—Acute viral and bacterial infections often lead to acute nasal congestion and thick discolored discharge, which is different from the thin and watery mucous of allergic rhinitis. Chronic rhinosinusitis is diagnosed using a history of congestion, mucopurulent discharge, facial pain, or dysosmia, lasting over 12 weeks and confirmed with nasal endoscopy or imaging with CT or MRI (see Chapter 26, Sinusitis).[6]
- Nasal polyposis—Nasal polyps may occur as a consequence of allergic rhinitis or with no allergic sensitization. Characteristic symptoms include hyposmia or anosmia along with refractory nasal congestion (**Figures 215-8** and **215-9**).
- Adenoidal hypertrophy—Obstruction of the nasopharynx leads to nasal congestion, rhinorrhea, snoring, and allergic shiners but without sneezing and itching or other atopic diseases.
- Anatomic anomalies—Deviated septum, concha bullosa (**Figure 215-8**), or haller cells can cause obstruction leading to the symptom of congestion.

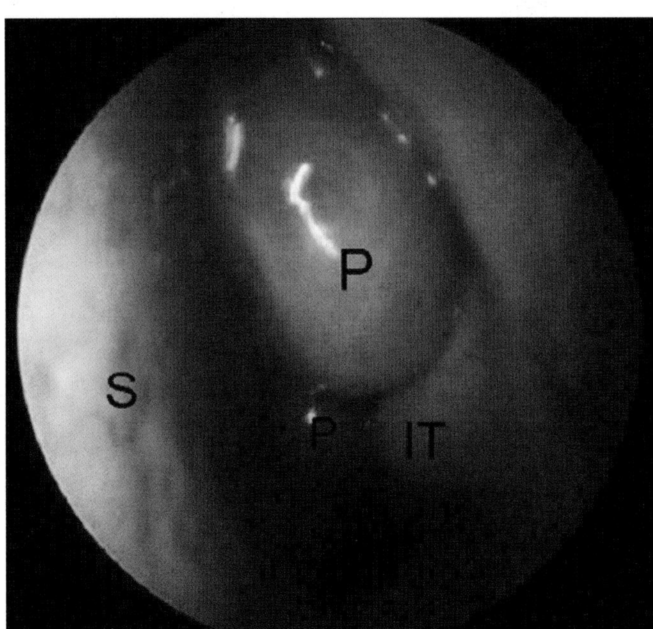

FIGURE 215-9 Nasal polyps seen on left sided nasal endoscopy in a young child. P=polyp; S=nasal septum; IT=inferior turbinate. (*Used with permission from Rudolph's Pediatrics 22nd edition, e-370-1, www.accesspediatrics.com.*)

MANAGEMENT

NONPHARMACOLOGIC

- Allergen avoidance—The primary treatment of allergic rhinitis should involve avoiding known triggers. Avoidance can be targeted based on the results of allergy testing to the aeroallergens including animal dander, dust mites, cockroaches and rodents, mold spores, and outdoor pollens from trees, grasses, and weeds.
- Avoidance of animal dander requires complete removal of the animal from the home as there is no evidence that any cats or dogs are "hypoallergenic."[7] SOR Ⓐ
- Cockroach and mouse allergen avoidance involves comprehensive pest control measures such as decreasing food sources or professional exterminator services.[2,3] SOR Ⓐ
- Dust mite allergens can be decreased by decreasing relative humidity levels, using special dust mite covers on the pillows, mattress, and any stuffed comforter on the bed, replacing carpeting with a solid surface floor, and frequent vacuuming/cleaning.[2,3] SOR Ⓐ
- Mold spores are ubiquitous both indoors and outdoors though central air conditioning can decrease exposure. SOR Ⓒ Spore levels are often dependant on outdoor spore production, which occurs when it is warm and wet.
- Avoidance of the outdoor pollens may require remaining indoors during the peak pollen seasons. These seasons are dependent on geography with trees typically pollinating in the spring, grasses in the spring/early summer and weeds in the fall.
- Central or portable HEPA air filters can significantly decrease outdoor allergens but are not as helpful for most indoor allergens. SOR Ⓑ
- Personal humidifiers are not recommended as they increase relative humidity levels allowing dust mites to survive and they may spread mold spores. SOR Ⓒ

MEDICATIONS

- If avoidance measures are not possible or effective, then medications such as short or long acting oral antihistamines, nasal steroids, or nasal antihistamines can be used. The nasal steroid medications give the most relief for all of the typical symptoms including sneezing, itching, rhinorrhea, and congestion. They can be used daily and have few side effects with nose bleeding being the most common.[2,3] SOR A

- Nasal antihistamines can be helpful for all of the nose symptoms, which occur despite the nasal steroids or if the symptoms are not frequent. Nasal antihistamines generally have a bad taste, which can be minimized by using good technique when spraying.[2,3] SOR A
- Second generation, long acting, nonsedating oral antihistamines are helpful for the symptoms of sneezing and itching but do not help for nasal congestion or rhinorrhea.
- **Allergy Immunotherapy**—If avoidance and medication use is not fully effective then allergy immunotherapy can be considered.
    - Allergy shots have long been proven to decrease symptoms and the need for medications for allergic rhinitis, conjunctivitis, and asthma.[2] SOR A
    - This therapy is done by giving frequent subcutaneous injections containing increasing amounts of the naturally occurring purified allergens specific to each patient.
    - After 3 to 5 years, this therapy changes the immune response to the allergens leading to decreased symptoms, which can last for years after discontinuation.[2] SOR A
    - The drawbacks include the time and expense of frequent visits to the doctor's office, injection site reactions, or rarely anaphylaxis.

COMPLIMENTARY/ALTERNATIVE THERAPY

- Bee pollen has been used as a folk remedy to improve allergic rhinitis symptoms. No randomized studies support its efficacy in allergic rhinitis and anaphylaxis has been reported when used to treat allergic patients.
- The pollens bees collect are not typically the pollens which cause allergic rhinitis. Therefore, ingesting these pollens regularly would not lead to desensitization as occurs in allergy immunotherapy. However some may cross react and large oral doses may lead to local or systemic allergic reactions in highly sensitive individuals. SOR C

SURGERY

- Surgery may help improve symptoms of nasal polyposis and chronic rhinosinusitis if present.

REFERRAL

- Further evaluation should be done by an allergist if the patient has not responded to typical therapies such as oral antihistamines or nasal steroid sprays.
- Surgical consultation to otolaryngology should be made if there is suspicion of adenoidal hypertrophy or other structural causes of the symptoms have been identified.

PREVENTION AND SCREENING

- There is no proven strategy for prevention of allergic sensitization.
- There is a controversy about whether having dogs or cats in the home prevent allergic rhinitis.
- Allergic rhinitis should be suspected in patients who present with typical symptoms, especially if they have a history of other atopic diseases such as atopic dermatitis, food allergy, or asthma.

PROGNOSIS

- Patients can outgrow their allergies, although this usually does not happen until the 4th or 5th decade of life. Some patients can continue to experience symptoms into old age.

FOLLOW-UP

- Follow-up can be based on the frequency and severity of symptoms or during evaluation of co-morbid conditions such as asthma.

PATIENT RESOURCES

- **www.AAAAI.org**.
- **www.ACAAI.org**.

PROVIDER RESOURCES

- Practice Parameters—**www.AAAAI.org**.
    - The diagnosis and management of rhinitis—An updated practice parameter (2008).
    - Allergen immunotherapy—A practice parameter third update (2011).
    - Allergy diagnostic testing—An updated practice parameter (2008).
    - The diagnosis and management of sinusitis—A practice parameter update (2005).

REFERENCES

1. Wright AL, Holberg CJ, Martinez FD, et al. Epidemiology of physician-diagnosed allergic rhinitis in childhood. *Pediatrics*. 1994; 94:895-901.
2. Joint Task Force on Practice Parameters, American Academy of Allergy, Asthma and Immunology, American College of Allergy, Asthma and Immunology, Joint Council of Allergy, Asthma and Immunology. Allergen immunotherapy: A practice parameter second update. *J Allergy Clin Immunol*. 2007;20(S):S25-85.
3. Wallace DV, Dykewicz MS, Bernstein DI, et al. The diagnosis and management of rhinitis: An updated practice parameter. *J Allergy Clin Immunol*. 2008;122(2):S1-84.
4. Settipane RA, Charnock DR: Epidemiology of rhinitis: Allergic and nonallergic. *Clin Allergy Immunol*. 2007;19:23-34.
5. Schroer B, Pien LC: Nonallergic rhinitis: Common problem, chronic symptoms. *Cleve Clin J Med*. 2012;79:285-93.
6. Bhattacharyya N: The role of CT and MRI in the diagnosis of chronic rhinosinusitis. *Curr Allergy Asthma Rep*. 2010;10:171-174.
7. Lockey RF: The myth of hypoallergenic dogs (and cats). *J Allergy Clin Immunol*. 2012;130:910-991.

216 DIGEORGE SYNDROME

Lisanne Newton, MD
Brian Schroer, MD

PATIENT STORY

A newborn infant is noted to have micrognathia, a bulbous nasal tip, a crumpled ear helix (**Figure 216-1**), hooded eyes, a high arched palate, and a submucosal cleft palate. She was diagnosed prenatally with Tetralogy of Fallot. Tetany due to hypocalcemia is noted in the first 48 hours of life and requires treatment. A chest x-ray obtained is notable for absence of a thymic shadow (**Figure 216-2**). Immunologic laboratory data reveal CD3+T cells are <500/mm^3. Chromosomal analysis is sent and reveals a deletion of chromosome 22q11.2. She undergoes surgical repair of her heart lesion at one week of age, and requires close follow-up of her cardiac, immunological, and metabolic problems.

INTRODUCTION

DiGeorge Syndrome (DGS), also known as 22.q11 deletion syndrome, or velocardiofacial syndrome (VCFS), describes patients with a distinct clinical phenotype. Patients classically present with a triad of conotruncal cardiac anomalies, hypoplastic thymus, and hypocalcemia. However, there is a wide variation in phenotypic presentations.

SYNONYMS

- Velocardiofacial syndrome (VCFS).
- Chromosome 22q11.2 deletion syndrome (22qDS).
- Congenital Thymic hypoplasia/aplasia.
- Conotruncal Anomaly Face syndrome.
- Shprintzen syndrome.
- Strong syndrome.

EPIDEMIOLOGY

- DGS is the most common microdeletion syndrome.
- Population studies in the US have found an incidence of approximately 1:3,000 to 1:6,000 births.[1]
- This incidence may be increasing due to affected parents having their own children, and the incidence may be underestimated because of under diagnosis of patients with mild phenotypic features, particularly in African Americans.[2]
- DGS has an equal distribution in males and females, races, and geographic location.[3]

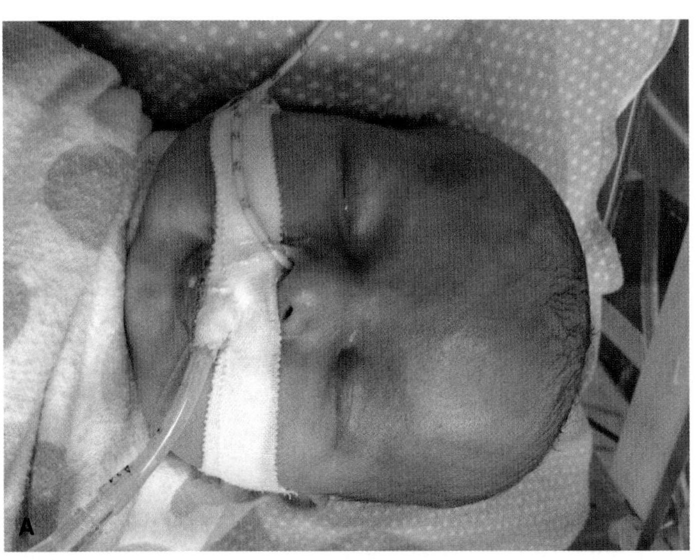

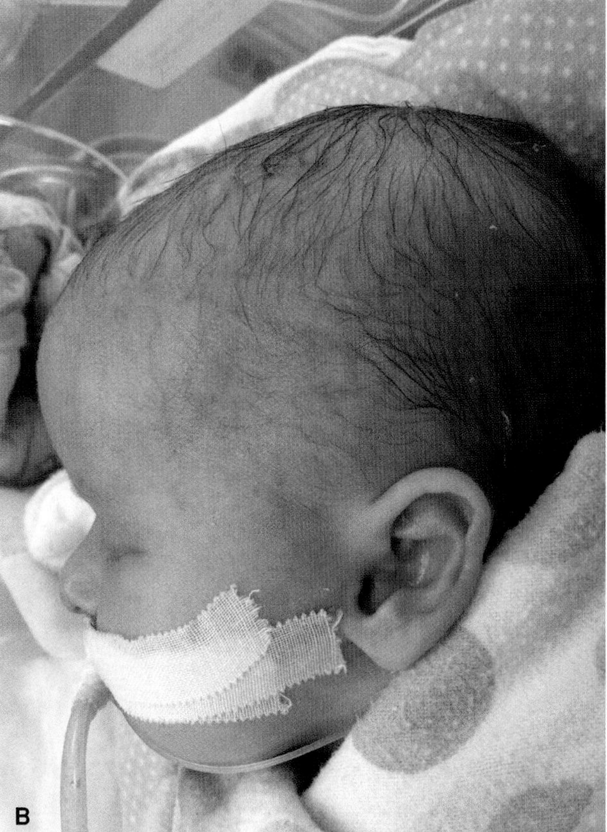

FIGURE 216-1 Dysmorphic facial features, including a small chin, crumpled ear helix, and bulbous nasal tip in a newborn girl with Di George syndrome on frontal (**A**) and lateral (**B**) view. (*Used with permission from Brian Schroer, MD.*)

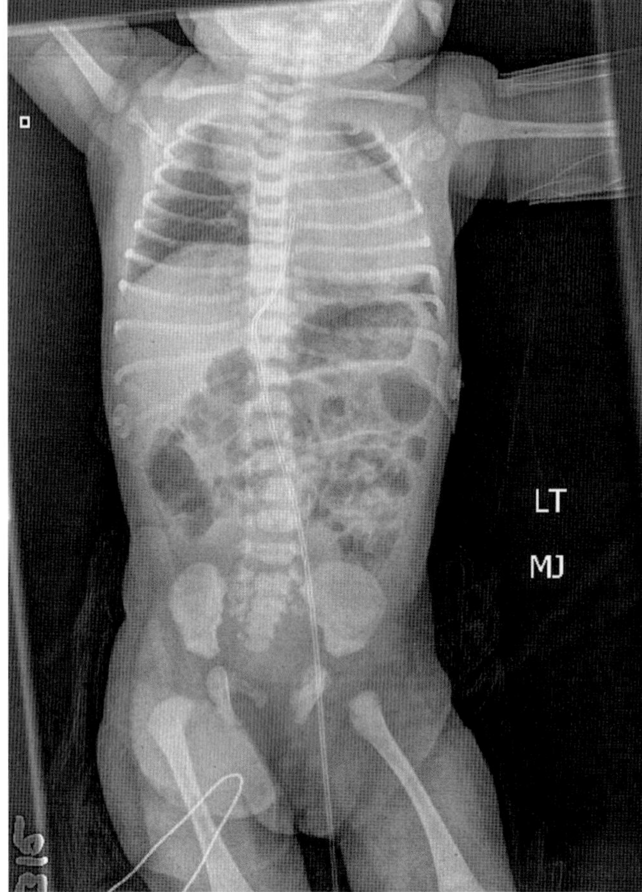

FIGURE 216-2 Decreased thymic shadow and cardiomegaly due to Tetralogy of Fallot in a newborn girl with DiGeorge syndrome. On operative repair of the cardiac defect, essentially no thymic tissue was noted. (*Used with permission from Brian Schroer, MD.*)

- The syndrome typically presents in infancy but diagnosis may be delayed in patients with partial DGS and mild phenotypes.

ETIOLOGY AND PATHOPHYSIOLOGY

- The features associated with DGS result from dysmorphogenesis of the 3rd and 4th pharyngeal pouches during embryogenesis, leading to thymus or parathyroid gland hypoplasia or aplasia. Related anomalies involve structures forming around the same time, including the great vessels, esophagus, uvula, heart, facial, and ear anomalies.[4]
- The most common genetic deletion is a hemizygous microdeletion from chromosome 22q11.2.[3] The size of the deletion does not appear to correlate with the clinical phenotype.
- Clinical features and are determined by which organs are affected and the degree to which they are affected.

RISK FACTORS

- Most cases (>90%) are spontaneous mutations and therefore are not inherited.
- Parents with 22q11 deletions can pass the deletion to their children in an autosomal dominant manner.[3]

DIAGNOSIS

CLINICAL FEATURES

- Diagnosis is made by identifying the clinical features and confirming the diagnosis with identification in the 22q11 deletion.
- Partial DGS is the most common phenotype and occurs if there is hypoplasia of the thymus and parathyroid glands. The severity of the immune disorder and hypocalcemia is determined by the level of hypoplasia but neonates with partial DGS typically present with non-life-threatening immunologic defects.
- Complete DGS is defined by total aplasia[4] and comprises <1 percent of patients. It is critical to confirm this diagnosis in a timely manner as they have a combined immunodeficiency similar to SCID and are susceptible to opportunistic pathogens. They will die within the first year of life without treatment.

DIAGNOSTIC CRITERIA FOR DIGEORGE SYNDROME

In general, if a patient has 2 or more of the following features, testing for chromosome 22q11.2 deletion should be sent:

- Hypocalcemia.
- Immunodeficiency (CD3+ T cells <1500/ml).
- Characteristic facial features.
  - Low set and posteriorly rotated ears, crumpled ear deformity (**Figures 216-1**, **216-3**, and **216-4**).
  - Tall nasal root and bridge (**Figures 216-1**, **216-3**, and **216-5**).
  - Bulbous nasal tip (**Figures 216-1**, **216-4**, and **216-5**).
  - Ocular hypertelorism (widely spaced eyes).
- Developmental or behavioral problems.
- Palatal problems, including overt and mucosal cleft palate and hyponasal speech.
- Conotruncal cardiac anomaly.

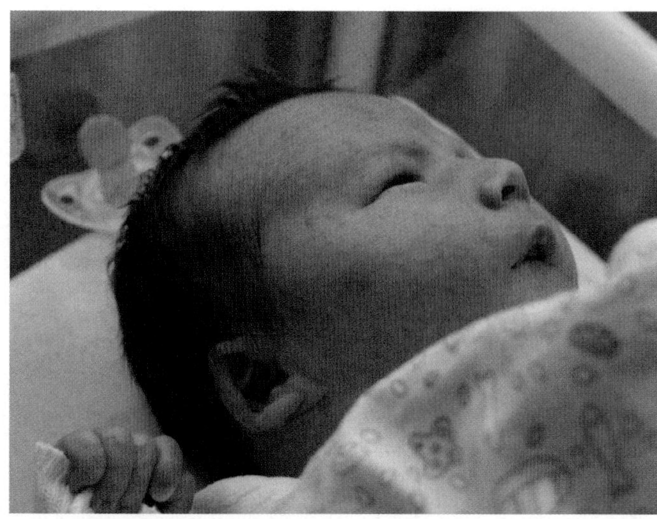

FIGURE 216-3 Posteriorly rotated, crumpled ear helix in a newborn boy with chromosome 22q11.2 deletion syndrome. (*Used with permission from Gregor Dueckers, MD and Tim Niehues, MD.*)

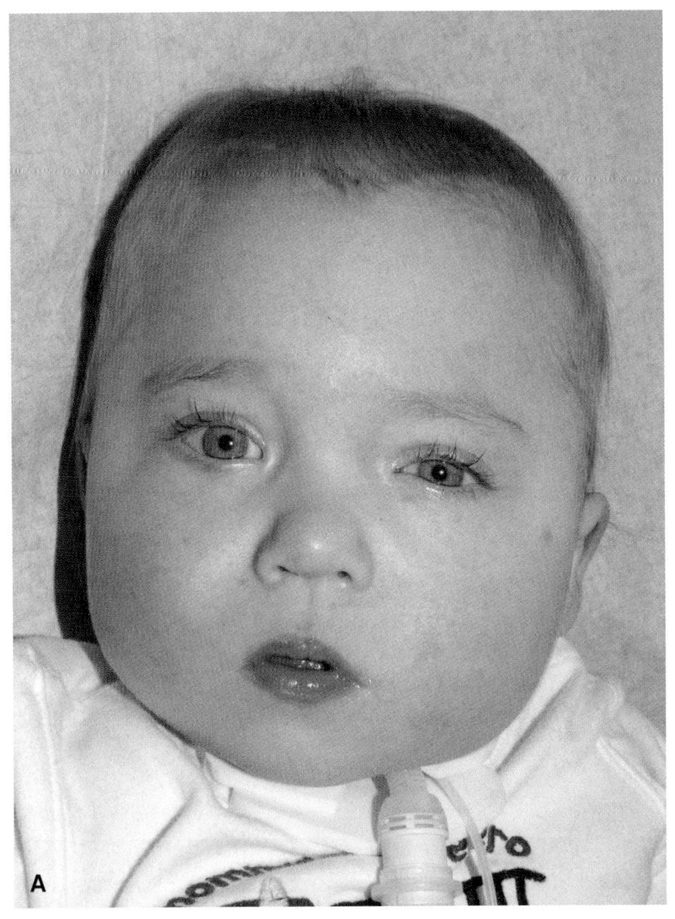

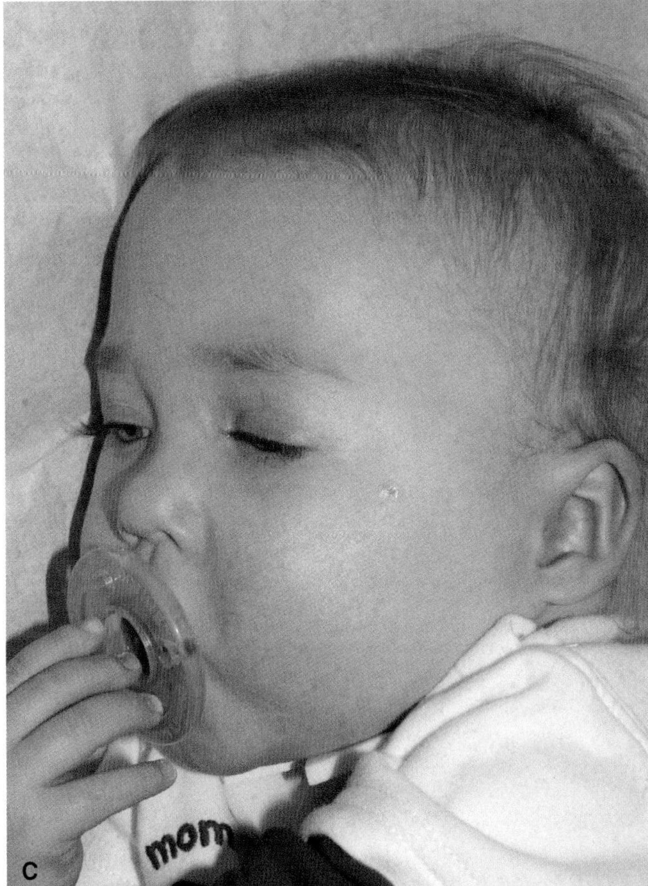

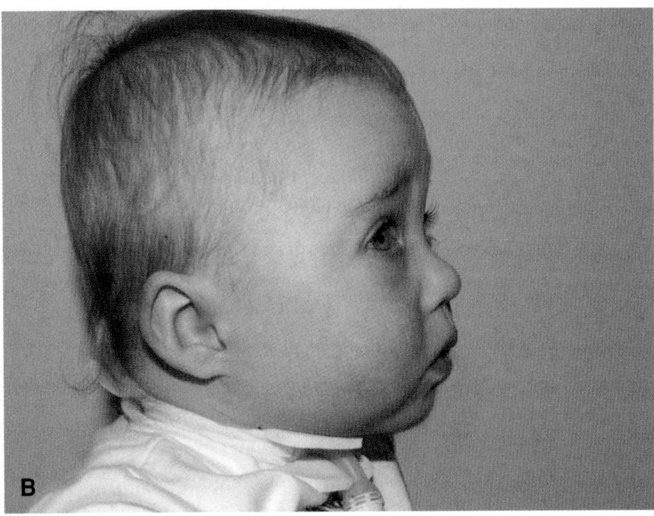

FIGURE 216-4 Hooded eyes, bulbous nasal tip, micrognathia, and posteriorly rotated ears on frontal (**A**), lateral (**B**), and oblique (**C**) view in a 13-month-old boy with DiGeorge syndrome. (*Used with permission from Brian Schroer, MD.*)

LABORATORY TESTING

- FISH (fluorescent in situ hybridization) method for chromosome 22q11.2 deletion.
- Chromosome SNP (single-nucleotide polymorphism) microarray, uses a "gene chip" to detect multiple micro-deletion and -duplication syndromes. It is more sensitive than FISH analysis.
- If 22q11.2 deletion testing is negative in a patient with a classic phenotype, consider sending testing for a point mutation in T-box 1 gene (TBX1), which is associated with 22q11.2 deletion.[1]
- Blood Testing for associated complications and immune function should include the following. The results will depend on the degree of thymic and parathyroid hypoplasia:
  - Calcium—Total and ionized.
  - Parathyroid hormone.
  - TSH.
  - CBC with differential.
  - Flow Cytometry for T and B cell Subsets (CD3, CD4, CD8, and CD19).
  - T and B cell Mitogen Stimulation panels, ATP assay.

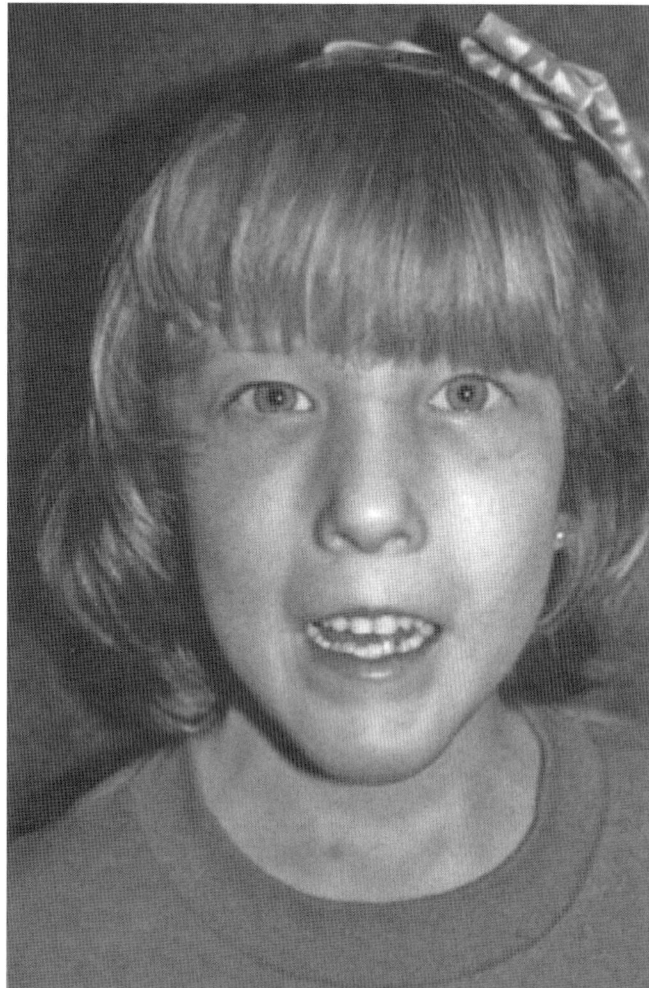

FIGURE 216-5 A 6-year-old girl with DiGeorge syndrome, illustrating the distinctive tall nasal root and bridge with a bulbous nasal tip and a small mouth. (*Used with permission from Jorde LB, Carey JC, Bamshad MJ, White RL. Medical Genetics. St. Louis, MO: Mosby; 2006. Rudolph's Pediatrics, 22nd edition. www.accesspediatrics.com. The McGraw Hill Companies.*)

- Total immunoglobulin levels and specific antibody levels to infant vaccines at diagnosis and again at 6 and 12 months old.

IMAGING

- A chest x-ray may show absence of a thymic shadow in complete DiGeorge Syndrome (**Figure 216-2**). Most infants have hypoplasia of the thymus and the thymus will be visualized on chest x-ray (**Figure 216-6**).
- Congenital heart disease may be identified on prenatal ultrasound or echocardiography in the neonate.
- Imaging studies to evaluate for intestinal malrotation should be obtained if there is abdominal distention, vomiting, or not passing stools or any other concerning clinical signs or symptoms.
- An MRI should be considered if there is microcephaly.
- Renal ultrasound will detect renal anomalies such as a structural anomaly, agenesis, dysplasia, hypoplasia, or hydronephrosis. A swallowing study may be needed if there are feeding difficulties.[2]

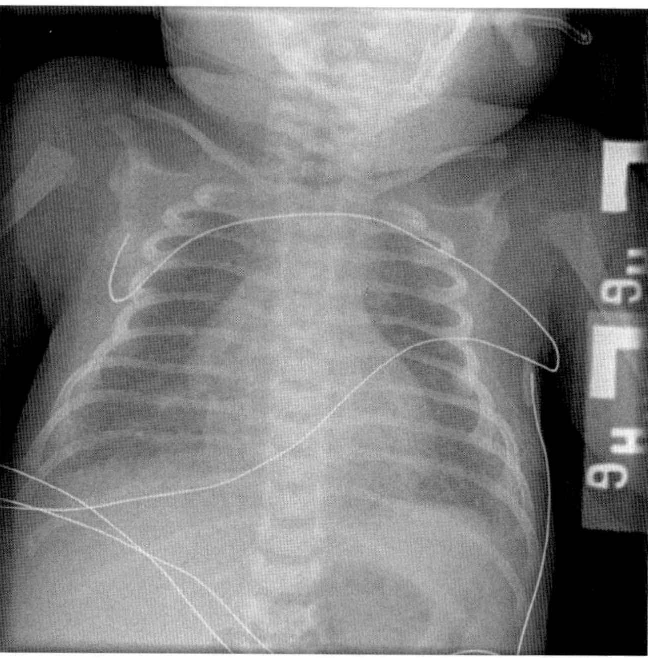

FIGURE 216-6 Normal thymic shadow on chest x-ray in a neonate with DiGeorge syndrome and Tetralogy of Fallot. (*Used with permission from Lisanne Newton, MD.*)

DIFFERENTIAL DIAGNOSIS

- CHARGE syndrome—Genetic disorder characterized by colobomas in the eye, heart defect, atresia of the choanae, retarded growth and development, genital abnormality, and ear abnormality.
- Zellweger syndrome—Genetic disorder caused by degeneration of myelin and characterized by central nervous system, cardiac, feeding, hearing, visual, and liver manifestations.
- Kabuki syndrome—Genetic disorder characterized by distinctive facial features (arched eyebrows, long eyelashes, long palpebral fissures, everted lids, flat, broadened tip of the nose, and large protruding earlobes), microcephaly, and hypotonia.
- Smith Lemli Opitz—Syndrome caused by a defect in cholesterol synthesis that results in multiple congenital malformations, dysmorphic facial features, and developmental delay.
- Goldenhar syndrome (Oculo-auricular-vertebral syndrome)—Genetic disorder resulting in malformations of the cheekbones, jaw, mouth, ears, eyes, and/or vertebrae (see Chapter 34, Congenital Malformations).
- Primary hypoparathyroidism—May manifest with severe hypocalcemia early in life but without the abnormal facial features and congenital heart disease.
- Fetal alcohol syndrome—Can manifest with dysmorphic facial features (widely set and narrow eyes, small upper jaw, and epicanthal folds), growth problems and nervous system abnormalities, and cardiac abnormalities (VSD and ASD; **Figure 216-7**).
- SCID in complete DGS—May manifest with severe immunosuppression in the neonatal period.

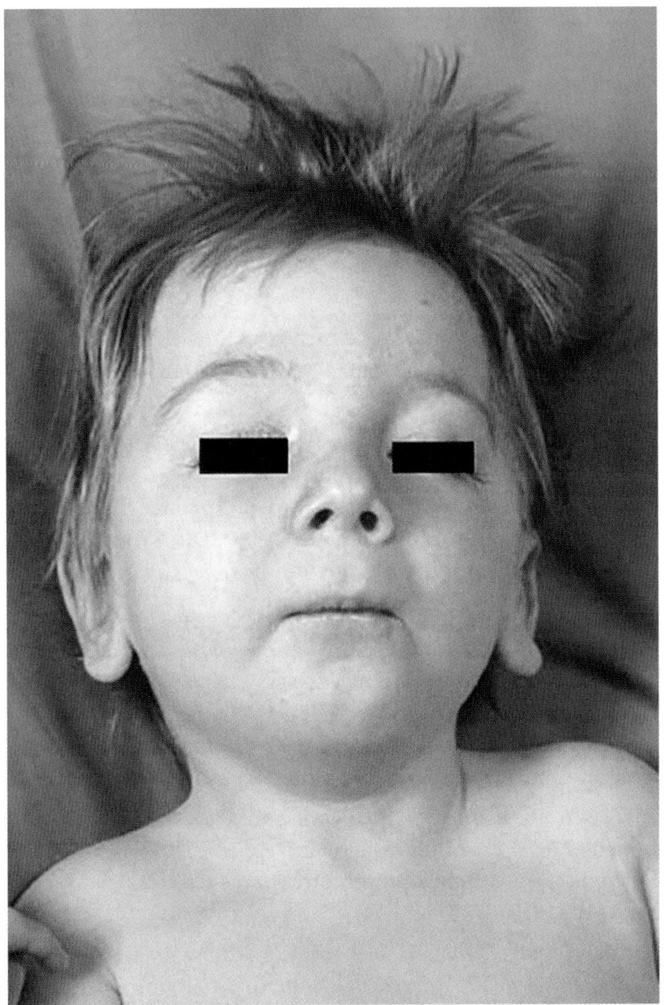

FIGURE 216-7 Wide-set and narrow eyes, small upper jaw, and epicanthal folds in an infant with characteristic features of fetal alcohol syndrome. (*Used with permission from Cleveland Clinic Children's Hospital Photo Files.*)

MANAGEMENT

- The management of DGS depends on the severity of the clinical phenotype and associated anomalies and the age of the patient.
- It requires a multidisciplinary approach including cardiology, genetics, immunology, otolaryngology, urology, or endocrinology based on clinical presentation.
- Life-threatening conditions should be evaluated without delay in neonates, including severe immune deficiency in patients with complete DGS, congenital heart disease if present, and significant hypocalcemia.

IMMUNOLOGIC

- Partial DGS—T cell function is largely intact in the majority of partial DGS patients. Most patients experience improvement in any abnormality in T cell production and function over time. In some DGS patients, there is a progressive decrease in T cell production, suggesting that patients may be at risk for increasing frequency of infections with age.[5]
- Increased risk for sinopulmonary infections is most common and should be treated with antibiotics as appropriate. Any deficiency in humoral immunity should be treated with immunoglobulin replacement if necessary.
- Complete DGS—These infants are similar to patients with severe combined immunodeficiency (SCID) and must be placed in isolation. Once identified, infants with complete DGS ideally should be promptly referred to a center capable of cultured unrelated thymic tissue transplants, or a center capable of bone marrow or hematopoietic cell transplants. Ideally, patients should be transplanted before the onset of significant infections, to optimize their chances for successful engraftment. Patients are at risk for opportunistic infections including fungi, viruses, and *Pneumocystis jiroveci* pneumonia (PJP) and should be on antimicrobial prophylaxis based on T cell number and function. However, stable infants may be observed for several weeks to monitor for T cell development.

CARDIAC

- Cardiac defects should be treated based on the specific defect and requires referral to cardiology/cardiothoracic surgery.

ENDOCRINE

- Hypocalcemia—Prompt identification and treatment of neonatal hypocalcemia may prevent complications such as seizures. This is especially important in patients with heart failure before or during surgery.

FEEDING

- Depending on associated palatal defects, feeding and swallowing problems can be extremely difficult in early infancy and can be distressing for parents. There can be poor coordination of pharyngeal muscles, tongue, and esophageal muscles.

NONPHARMACOLOGIC

- As previously described, much of the management of DGS is nonpharmacologic and medications vary greatly depending on the clinical phenotype and associated behavioral and psychiatric anomalies.

MEDICATIONS

- Hypocalcemia should be treated with calcium, vitamin D, or parathyroid hormone replacement.
- Prophylactic antibiotics should be used if the immune defect is severe. SOR Ⓒ Otherwise, antibiotics should be targeted to specific infections.
- IVIG should be given if immunoglobulin levels or function is low. SOR Ⓒ

SURGERY

- Surgery may be indicated for associated cardiac defects, thymus transplant for patients with complete DGS, and correction of palatal defects if present.

REFERRAL

- Referral to pediatric subspecialists again depends on the associated anomalies.
- Routine referral to cardiology, cardiothoracic surgery, endocrinology, genetics, immunology, and otolaryngology is indicated.

- Genetics is helpful at confirming diagnosis and discussing future reproductive issues.

PREVENTION AND SCREENING

SCREENING

- There is currently no available newborn screening for DGS.
- Complete DGS may be identified by newborn screening with T Cell Receptor Excision Circles (Trec) used to detect SCID, which is being done in some states.
- If an affected parent is found to have the same mutation as an affected offspring the risk of future children being affected is 50 percent, similar to an autosomal dominant condition.
- If the parents are not found to have the gene defect, then the risk of a future sibling of an affected child is low, less than 1 percent.
- Prenatal screening options include a level II ultrasound early in the 2nd trimester, a fetal echocardiogram, CVS sampling, and amniocentesis. FISH or SNP arrays can be performed on CVS or amniocentesis samples.[3]

VACCINATION

- The decision of whether to administer live vaccines (rotavirus, measles-mumps-rubella, varicella, and live attenuated influenza) depends on the degree of T cell dysfunction and should be made on a case-by-case basis.
- Generally, live vaccines should be withheld in patients with DGS until 1 year of age when immune function has been more firmly established and after referral to an immunologist.

PROGNOSIS

- Prognosis depends largely on the degree of immune deficiency and other associated anomalies, especially congenital heart disease.
- The overall mortality in childhood is approximately 4 percent.[1]
- Those infants who undergo thymic transplant have a survival rate of about 75 percent. Causes of death in the majority of these patients are infections.[6]

FOLLOW-UP

- It is important to continue regular follow-up with special attention paid to developmental delays, learning disabilities, speech delays, hearing, or vision difficulties.
- Adolescents with DGS are at higher risk for psychiatric disorders, including schizoaffective disorder, schizophrenia, and major depression.

PATIENT EDUCATION

- Each patient with DiGeorge Syndrome is treated individually depending on their unique features and the degree to which their organs are affected.
- The vast majority of patients have near-normal immune systems or only mild to moderate difficulty with infections that usually improves with age.
- The care of young infants with DGS will depend greatly on the presence and severity of heart disease.
- Most patients with DGS will need to be followed regularly by doctors in different specialties to ensure the best health and quality of life.

PATIENT RESOURCES

- Immune Deficiency Foundation—**http://primaryimmune.org**.
- Patient & Family Handbook for Primary Immunodeficiency Diseases, 5th edition, IDF- Immune Deficiency Foundation. Chapter 13 DiGeorge Syndrome—**http://primaryimmune.org/wp-content/uploads/2013/06/IDF_Patient_Family_Handbook_5th_Edition.pdf**.

PROVIDER RESOURCES

- AAAAI (American Academy of Allergy, Asthma and Immunology) on DiGeorge Syndrome—**http://www.aaaai.org/conditions-and-treatments/primary-immunodeficiency-disease/digeorge-syndrome.aspx**.
- Bassett AS, et al. Practical Guidelines for Managing Patients with 22q11.2. Deletion Syndrome. *J Pediatric*. 2011;159:2. **http://www.ncbi.nlm.nih.gov/pmc/articles/PMC3197829/**.
- Markert ML, Devlin BH, McCarthy EA: Thymus transplantation. *Clin Immunol*. 2010;135(2):236-246. **http://ncbi.nlm.nih.gov/pmc/articles/PMC3646264**.

REFERENCES

1. McDonald-McGinn DM, Sullivan KE: Chromosome 22q11.2 deletion syndrome (DiGeorge syndrome/velocardiofacial syndrome). *Medicine (Baltimore)*. 2011;90(1):1-18.
2. Kobrynski LJ, Sullivan KE: Velocardiofacial syndrome, DiGeorge syndrome: The chromosome 22q11.2 deletion syndromes. *Lancet*. 2007;370(9596):1443-1452.
3. Bassett AS, McDonald-McGinn DM, Devriendt K, Digilio MC, Goldenberg P, Habel A, et al. Practical guidelines for managing patients with 22q11.2 deletion syndrome. *J Pediatr*. 2011; 159(2):332,9.e1.
4. Buckley RH: Primary cellular immunodeficiencies. *J Allergy Clin Immunol*. 2002;109(5):747-757.
5. Chinen J, Rosenblatt HM, Smith EO, Shearer WT, Noroski LM: Long-term assessment of T-cell populations in DiGeorge syndrome. *J Allergy Clin Immunol*. 2003;111(3):573-579.
6. Ryan AK, Goodship JA, Wilson DI, Philip N, Levy A, Seidel H, et al. Spectrum of clinical features associated with interstitial chromosome 22q11 deletions: A european collaborative study. *J Med Genet*. 1997;34(10):798-804.

217 PRIMARY CILIARY DYSKINESIA

Timothy Campbell, MD
Brian Schroer, MD

PATIENT STORY

A 13-year-old boy presents for evaluation of a chronic productive cough and fever. Since birth, he has had persistent rhinitis, thick nasal drainage, and recurrent otitis media. He has been seen three times in the past year for pneumonia each time diagnosed and treated without a chest x-ray. On physical exam, heart sounds are greater on the right side and point of maximal impulse is felt in the right 5th intercostals space. A chest x-ray shows situs inversus totalis with dextrocardia (**Figure 217-1**). Computed tomography of the sinuses shows chronic sinusitis (**Figure 217-2**). The diagnosis of primary ciliary dyskinesia was considered and he underwent a biopsy of his nasal epithelium, which revealed abnormal ciliary structure and function. This confirmed the diagnosis and the physician explained the meaning of primary ciliary dyskinesia and the situs inversus to the patient and his parents. He was told that he will need aggressive treatments for all future infections.

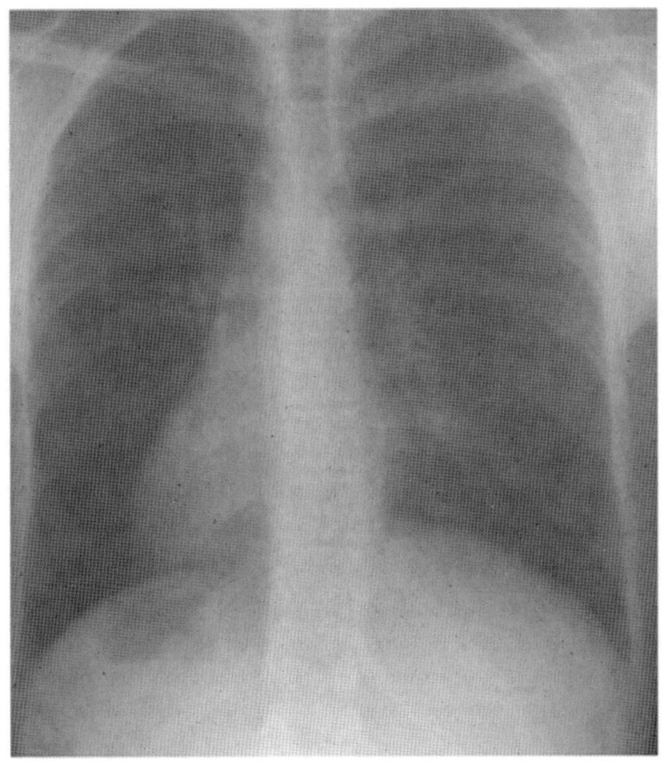

FIGURE 217-1 Dextrocardia on chest x-ray of a 13-year-old boy with Kartagener syndrome. (*Used with permission from McGraw-Hill Fig 30-6a . Clement P, Fisher BT. Chapter 30. Rhinosinusitis. In: Shah SS, ed. Pediatric Practice: Infectious Disease. New York: McGraw-Hill; 2009.*)

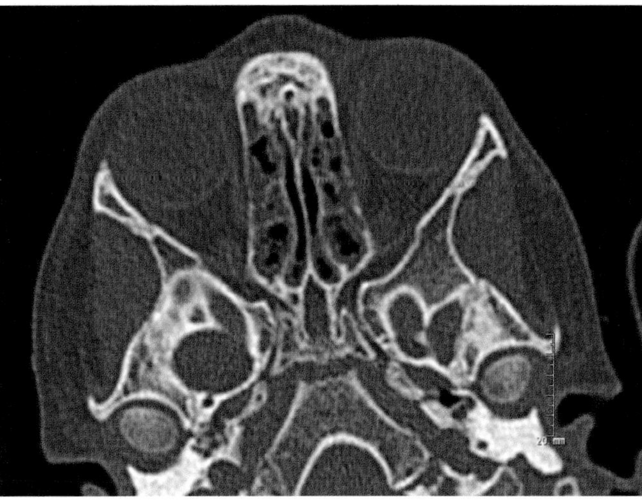

FIGURE 217-2 Soft tissue swelling of the sinuses on sinus CT scan in a patient with chronic sinusitis. (*Used with permission from Camille Sabella, MD.*)

INTRODUCTION

Primary Ciliary Dyskinesia (PCD) is a rare genetic disease associated with abnormal cilia structure and function causing impaired clearance of bacteria from the lungs, paranasal sinuses, and middle ear, which leads to recurrent infections. It can be associated with other developmental abnormalities such as situs inversus totalis, nasal polyposis, and frontal sinus agenesis. Clinical manifestations include chronic cough and chronic rhinosinusitis and recurrent sinopulmonary and ear infections.

SYNONYMS

- Primary Cilia Disorder.
- Immotile Cilia Syndrome (ICS).
- Kartagener syndrome—A triad consisting of situs inversus with bronchiectasis and paranasal sinusitis (secondary to PCD).

EPIDEMIOLOGY

- PCD is inherited in an autosomal recessive pattern and occurs in approximately 1 in 10,000 to 30,000 births.[1–3]

ETIOLOGY AND PATHOPHYSIOLOGY

PCD is caused by genetic mutations on genes which code for proteins found in the ciliary outer dynein arm which controls the cilia beat force and frequency.

- Motile cilia (**Figure 217-3**) contain a cylinder of 9 microtubule doublets, arranged around a central pair of microtubules in the characteristic "9 + 2" arrangement as viewed by cross-sectional views on electron microscopy.

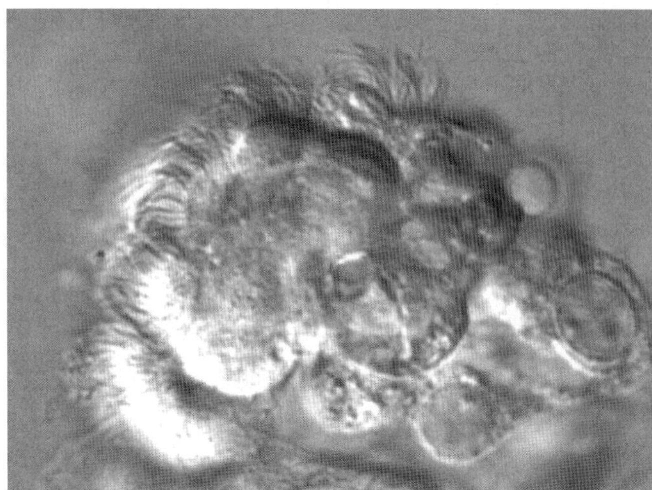

FIGURE 217-3 Electron micrograph of motile cilia. Notice the long curving cilia demonstrating active movement. (*Used with permission from Ian Myles MD, Steve Holland MD, and Harry Malech, MD. Scans were obtained for diagnostic and research purposes after informed consent under NIH IRB approved protocols.*)

- Defective cilia (**Figure 217-4**) resemble sensory or primary cilia, which lack a central microtubule doublet and outer dynein arms, thus creating a "9 + 0" arrangement and leaving these structures immotile.
- Defects in cilia during embryogenesis may result in left-right body orientation abnormalities, such as situs inversus or situs inversus totalis (**Figures 217-1** and **217-5**).
- Any disturbance in the coordinated movement of cilia can contribute to poor mucous clearance resulting in more frequent and severe infections. It can inhibit sperm motility leading to infertility in men or cause fallopian tube dysfunction and infertility in women.[4]

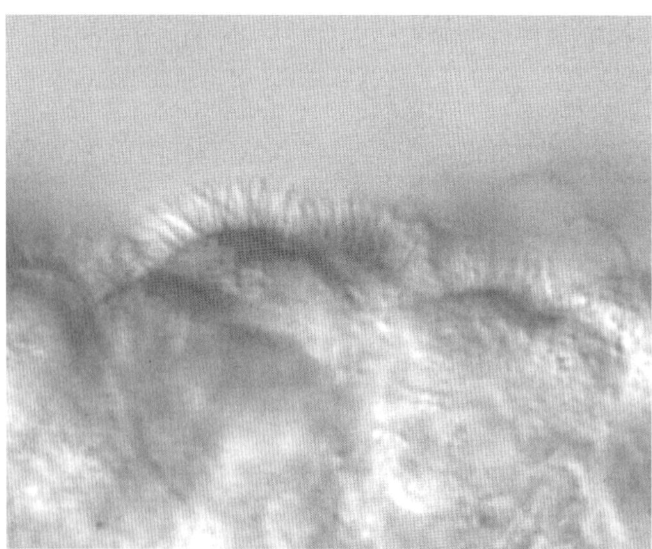

FIGURE 217-4 Electron micrograph of defective cilia. Notice the straight immotile cilia. (*Used with permission from Ian Myles MD, Steve Holland MD, and Harry Malech, MD. Scans were obtained for diagnostic and research purposes after informed consent under NIH IRB approved protocols.*)

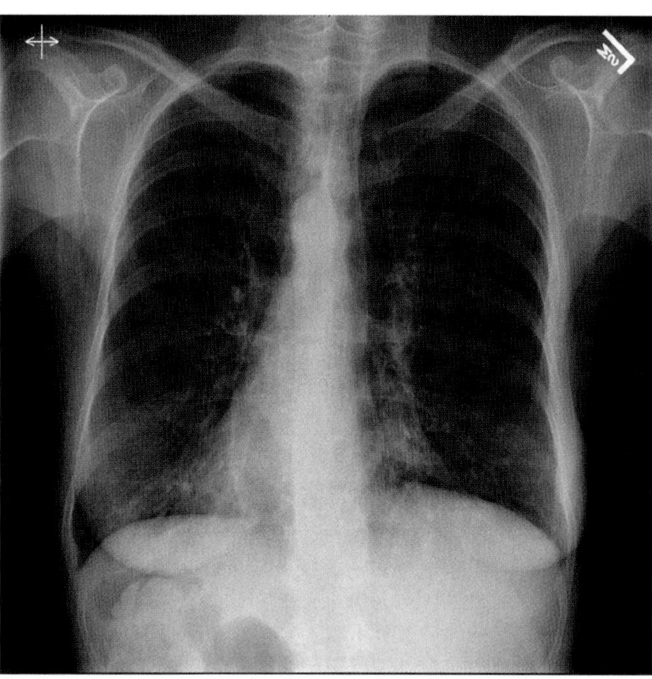

FIGURE 217-5 Situs inversus totalis on chest x-ray of a young woman. Note complete mirror image reversal of organs. (*Used with permission from Ian Myles MD, Steve Holland MD, and Harry Malech, MD. Scans were obtained for diagnostic and research purposes after informed consent under NIH IRB approved protocols.*)

DIAGNOSIS

- Patients must exhibit the characteristic clinical phenotype and specific ciliary ultrastructural defects identified by electron microscopy from biopsy samples of the respiratory epithelium such as from the mucosa of the nasal turbinates.
- Saccharin test—Assesses mucociliary function of nasal epithelium by depositing small particles of saccharin (or radiotracer dye particles) in the inferior nasal turbinate and measuring the time required for the patient to taste the sweet flavor or for the dye to become visible in the throat.[5]
- An exhaled nasal nitric oxide test is a useful screening test in patients with PCD. Patients with PCD will have low or absent exhaled nitric oxide.[6]

CLINICAL FEATURES

- Unexplained respiratory distress in the newborn period.[7]
- Chronic recurrent respiratory infections, including sinusitis, bronchitis, bronchiectasis (**Figure 217-6**), pneumonia, or otitis media. Bronchiectasis is the irreversible dilation of the bronchi secondary to repeated infections damaging the elastic tissue and smooth muscle within the bronchi.
- Conductive hearing loss due to damage of the middle ear from recurrent infections.[8]
- Situs inversus totalis (mirror-image reversal of all visceral organs with no apparent physiologic consequences) is present in 50 percent of individuals with PCD (**Figure 217-5**).[9]

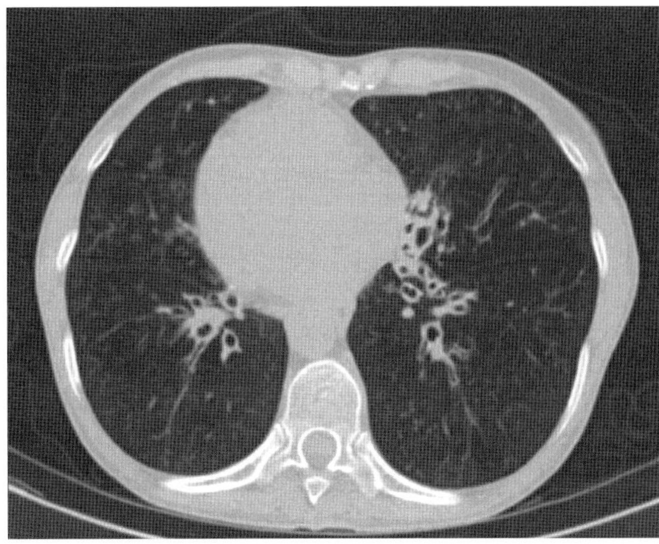

FIGURE 217-6 Bronchiectasis on coronal CT scan of the lungs. *(Used with permission from Ian Myles MD, Steve Holland MD, and Harry Malech, MD. Scans were obtained for diagnostic and research purposes after informed consent under NIH IRB approved protocols.)*

- Approximately 50 percent of males are infertile as a result of abnormal sperm motility. Female infertility has also been reported due to dysfunctional fallopian tubes.[4]

LABORATORY STUDIES

- Respiratory cultures (typically sputum cultures) are obtained to determine the etiology of infections in order to be more precise with antibiotic therapy.

IMAGING

- Chest radiographs and/or chest CT should be obtained to define distribution and severity of airway disease and bronchiectasis.
- Sinus imaging (sinus x-rays or preferably sinus CT) should be obtained when symptoms suggest sinus disease.

DIFFERENTIAL DIAGNOSIS

- Cystic fibrosis—May present in a similar manner and must be excluded (see Chapter 51, Cystic Fibrosis).
- Immunodeficiency—may have similar clinical features, but can be ruled out with measurement of serum immunoglobulins and B- and T-cell studies (see Chapters 218, B Cell Immunodeficiencies, 219, B and T Cell Immunodeficienies, and 220, Chronic Granulomatous Disease).
- Allergic rhinitis and asthma—may have similar clinical features, but usually responds well to standard therapies (see Chapters 49, Asthma, and 215, Allergic Rhinitis).
- Gastroesophageal reflux disease—Will often have symptoms specific for reflux and does not usually lead to chronic infections.
- Young syndrome—Male infertility (obstruction of the epididymis by inspissated secretions) with chronic sinopulmonary infection.[10]
- Wegener's granulomatosis—Upper- and lower-airway disease involvement may present with chronic lung and sinus disease.
- Situs inversus totalis or dextrocardia—May occur as isolated findings without ciliary dysfunction.

MANAGEMENT

- At present, no specific therapies can correct ciliary dysfunction. Therapies are empiric and aimed at treating consequences of dysfunctional cilia and are extrapolated from treatments of other lung diseases such as cystic fibrosis.
- Pulmonary disease.
    - Pulmonary function tests (spirometry) to define severity of obstructive impairment.
    - Chest percussion and postural drainage, oscillatory vest, and breathing maneuvers to enhance mucus clearance.
- Chronic/recurrent ear infections. Formal hearing evaluation with hearing aids and speech therapy when necessary.
- Prompt institution of antibiotic therapy for bacterial infections of the airways (bronchitis, sinusitis, and otitis media) is essential for preventing irreversible damage.
- Because cough is an effective clearance mechanism, patients should be encouraged to cough and engage in activities that promote deep breathing and cough (e.g., vigorous exercise).
- Routine immunizations to protect against respiratory pathogens including pertussis, *Haemophilus influenzae* type b, pneumococcus, and influenza (annually).
- Lung transplantation has been performed in persons with end-stage lung disease.
- Typically, situs abnormalities do not require intervention unless physiologic dysfunction requiring surgical intervention is present.
- Sperm harvesting and in vitro fertilization have been successful for male infertility.

FOLLOW-UP

The patient should be followed by his pulmonary, ENT, and/or cardiology specialists regularly and as the clinical presentation dictates.

PATIENT EDUCATION

- Patients should remain up-to-date on vaccinations, avoid the use of cough suppressants, avoid exposure to respiratory pathogens, tobacco smoke, and other pollutants that may damage airway mucosa and stimulate mucus secretion.
- Relatives with symptoms or findings suggestive of PCD including neonatal respiratory distress despite term gestation, chronic sinopulmonary disease, bronchiectasis, situs inversus totalis, other situs abnormalities, and male infertility should undergo diagnostic evaluation for PCD.

PATIENT RESOURCES

- **www.pcdfoundation.org**.
- **http://rarediseasesnetwork.epi.usf.edu/gdmcc/learnmore/faqs.htm**.

PROVIDER RESOURCES

- **www.nhlbi.nih.gov/health/health-topics/topics/pcd/**.
- **http://ghr.nlm.nih.gov/condition/primary-ciliary-dyskinesia**.

REFERENCES

1. Afzelius BA, Stenram U. Prevalence and genetics of immotile-cilia syndrome and left-handedness. *Int J Dev Biol*. 2006;50:571-573.
2. Ferkol T. Primary ciliary dyskinesia (immotile cilia syndrome). In: Kliegman R, Stanton B, St. Geme B, Schor N, Behrman R, eds. *Nelson Textbook of Pediatrics*, 19th ed. Philadelphia: Saunders; 2011:1497.
3. Seaton D. Bronchiectasis. In: Seaton A, Seaton D, Leitch AG, eds. Crofton and Douglas's Respiratory Diseases, 5th Ed. Oxford, UK: Blackwell Science Ltd.; 2008:794-828.
4. McComb P, Langley L, Villalon M, et al. The oviductal cilia and kartagener's syndrome. *Fertil Steril*. 1986;46:412-416.
5. Karja J, Nuutinen J. Immotile cilia syndrome in children. *Int J Pediatr Otorhinolaryngol*. 1983;5:275-279.
6. Corbelli R, Bringolf-Isler B, Amacher A, et al. Nasal nitric oxide measurements to screen children for primary ciliary dyskinesia. *Chest*. 2004;126:1054-1059.
7. Coren ME, Meeks M, Morrison I, et al. Primary ciliary dyskinesia: Age at diagnosis and symptom history. *Acta Paediatr*. 2002;91:667-669.
8. Pruliere-Escabasse V, Coste A, Chauvin P, et al. Otologic features in children with primary ciliary dyskinesia. *Arch Otolaryngol Head Neck Surg*. 2010;136:1121-1126.
9. Noone PG, Leigh MW, Sannuti A, et al. Primary ciliary dyskinesia: Diagnostic and phenotypic features. *Am J Respir Crit Care Med*. 2004;169:459-467.
10. Handelsman DJ, Conway AJ, Boylan LM, et al. Young's syndrome—Obstructive azoospermia and chronic sinopulmonary infections. *N Engl J Med*. 1984;310:3-9.

218 B CELL IMMUNODEFICIENCIES

Ahila Subramanian, MD, MPH
Brian Schroer, MD

PATIENT STORY

A 13-month-old boy is hospitalized with high fever, cough, and decreased oral intake. Diagnostic work up reveals pneumococcal pneumonia (**Figure 218-1**). He responds well to intravenous and oral antibiotic treatment with complete resolution of symptoms. His birth history is unremarkable with a normal full-term delivery and birth weight (3.3kg). At 4 months of age, he developed otitis media successfully treated with oral antibiotics. Since then he has had numerous upper respiratory and ear infections. At 8 months of age, he was hospitalized for treatment of *Staphylococcus aureus* cellulitis. Each infection responded well to short courses of antibiotic therapy. He has received all scheduled immunizations up to 12 months. Physical exam reveals a pale, thin child who is below the 3rd percentile for height and weight. He has normal features and developmental milestones. Further family history reveals a maternal uncle with similar symptoms in childhood. Immunologic work up is notable for severe hypogammaglobulinemia and low antibody vaccine titers. Genetic testing for BTK mutation confirms the diagnosis of X-Linked Agammaglobulinemia (XLA). Treatment with intravenous immunoglobulin replacement is started for management of antibody deficiency. Over the next 12 months, the boy has a significant decrease in infections and is noted to have improved growth.

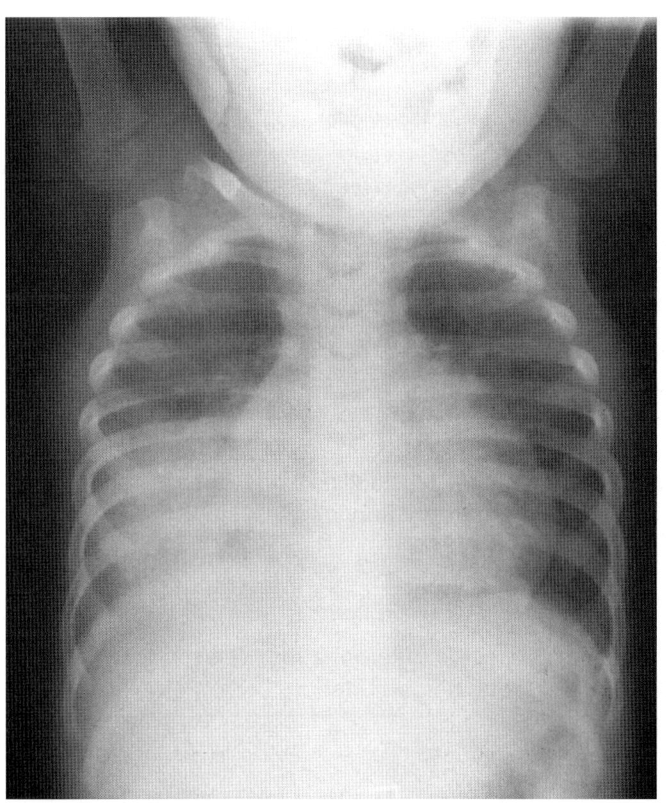

FIGURE 218-1 Right middle lobe consolidation on chest x-ray on an infant with X-linked agammaglobulinemia. Blood culture from this infant grew *Streptococcus pneumonia*. (*Used with permission from Camille Sabella, MD.*)

INTRODUCTION

Disorders of primary B cell immunodeficiency comprise approximately half of all primary immunodeficiencies. They are a group of heterogeneous disorders resulting from disruption of B cell maturation and function at various stages of development. The main role of B lymphocytes is production of antibodies for recognition and destruction of foreign antigens. Dysfunction of B lymphocytes results in impaired antibody production leading to illness characterized by unusual susceptibility to recurrent infections, particularly by encapsulated bacterial pathogens.

B cell immunodeficiencies are distinguished phenotypically by clinical severity, mode of inheritance, and age of onset. As a group, they share common clinical features and strategies for evaluation and management that will be discussed in this chapter.

SYNONYMS

- Humoral immune deficiency.
- Antibody deficiency syndrome.
- X-Linked Agammaglobulinemia (XLA)/Bruton's Agammaglobulinemia.
- Common Variable Immunodeficiency (CVID).
- Acquired Hypogammaglobulinemia.
- Transient Hypogammaglobulinemia of Infancy.
- Hyper IgM Syndrome.

EPIDEMIOLOGY

- B cell immunodeficiencies make up approximately 50 percent of primary immune deficiencies.[1]
- IgA deficiency is the most common B cell disorder (estimated incidence of 1 in 700 persons of European ancestry).[2]
- The second most common B cell disorder is CVID (estimated incidence of 1 in 30,000 ro 50,000 persons).[3]
- Early B cell defects such as X-linked Agammaglobulinemia (XLA) are rare (estimated incidence of XLA is 1 per 200,000 male births).[2]
- XLA accounts for approximately 85 percent of individuals with profound hypogammaglobulinemia and markedly reduced or absent B cells.[1]
- Age of onset is variable among primary B cell immunodeficiencies.
- The degree of immunoglobulin deficiency is a key determinant of disease severity and time of presentation. Individuals with more

severe hypogammaglobulinemia or agammaglobulinemia have clinical presentation earlier in life.

- Disorders with severe hypogammaglobulinemia present most commonly between 6 and 18 months of age. Their first infections can present as early as 4 months as protection from passive maternal IgG wanes.
- CVID can present as early as 4 years of age but is more commonly diagnosed as an adult with onset between the 2nd and 4th decade of life.
- Transient Hypogammaglobulinemia of infancy occurs in patients with low IgG, with or without low IgA or IgM, whose immunoglobulin levels are low but increase over time.

ETIOLOGY AND PATHOPHYSIOLOGY

- B cells originate in the bone marrow and undergo maturation in peripheral lymphoid organs including the lymph nodes, spleen, and mucosa-associated lymphoid tissue (MALT).
- B cell immunodeficiencies are caused by molecular defects leading to disruption of B cell development or the interactions between B and T cells required for B cell function.
- The etiologies of these defects are variable including genetic inheritance and spontaneous mutation.
- **Table 218-1** summarizes the modes of inheritance and known genetic mutations of the major disorders of B cell immunodeficiency.[4]

DIAGNOSIS

CLINICAL FEATURES

- Recurrent fever.
- Recurrent bacterial infections with encapsulated pyogenic organisms (i.e., *Haemophilus influenzae, Streptococcus pneumoniae, Staphylococcus aureus, Neisseria meningitides*).
- Chronic gastrointestinal infections (i.e., *Giardia lamblia, Campylobacter jejuni*)
- Enterovirus infections (i.e., Coxsackievirus, ECHOvirus, wild-type and vaccine-associated polio virus).
- Opportunistic viral infections are rare in pure B cell disorders but can be seen in subset of CVID involving T cell dysfunction (**Figure 218-2**).
- Poor growth, failure to thrive.
- Chronic diarrhea.
- Concomitant autoimmune conditions (i.e., diabetes mellitus, autoimmune hepatitis, autoimmune hemolytic anemia, idiopathic thrombocytopenic purpura, rheumatoid arthritis, interstitial lung disease, inflammatory bowel disease, or uveitis).
- Family history of immunodeficiency or frequent infections.

PHYSICAL FINDINGS

- Absent tonsils, small lymph nodes (seen only in early B cell defect disorders that result in severe hypogammaglobulinemia; **Figure 218-3**).

TABLE 218-1 Mode of Inheritance and Important Genetic Mutations of the Major B Cell Immunodeficiency Syndromes

B Cell Immunodeficiency	Mode of Inheritance	Genetic Mutation
Common Variable Immunodeficiency	Variable	Variable (TACI gene mutation - AD)
X-linked agammaglobulinemia[1]	XL	*BTK*
Autosomal recessive agammaglobulinemia	AR	*BLNK, LRRC8*, μ, λ5, Igα
Specific antibody deficiency	Unknown	Unknown
HyperIgM syndrome[1]	AR	*AID, UNG*
Selective Antibody deficiency • IgA • IgG subclass • IgE • IgM	Variable	For IgA deficiency: Failure of terminal differentiation in IgA-positive B cells
Transient hypogammaglobulinemia of infancy	Unknown	Defect in differentiation: delayed maturation of T helper function

[1]The X-linked mutations causing Hyper IgM syndrome involve cell mediated immune dysfunction and are classified under Combined Immunodeficiencies.

AD – autosomal dominant, XL – X-linked, AR – autosomal recessive, AID - activation-induced adenosine deaminase deficiency, UNG – uracil nucleoside glycosylase deficiency.

Used with permission from Chatila TA: Immunologic Disorders, in Rudolph's Pediatrics, 22nd edition, edited by C Rudolph, et al. McGraw-Hill, 2011. Section 13.

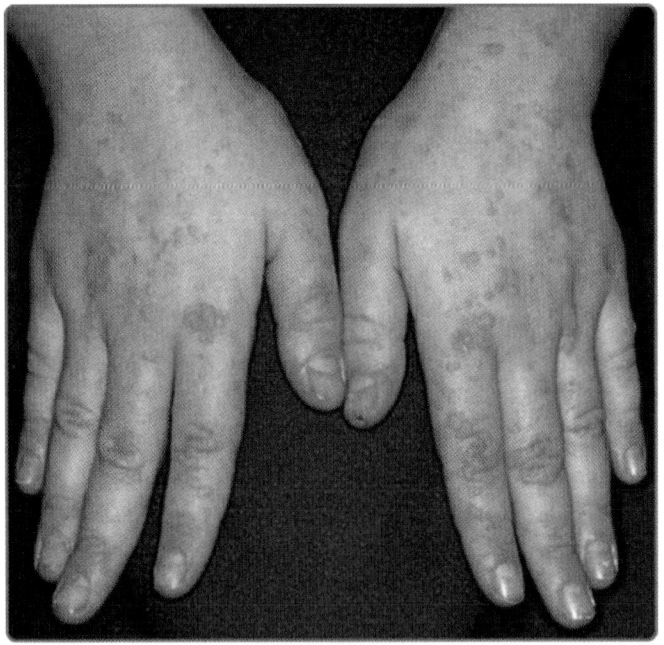

FIGURE 218-2 Recalcitrant verrucae vulgaris on the dorsal hands of a girl with common variable immunodeficiency. (*Used with permission from RL Fuleihan, AS Paller: Genetic Immunodeficiency Disease, in Fitzpatrick's Dermatology in General Medicine, 8th edition, edited by LA Goldsmith, et al. McGraw-Hill, 2012. Chapter 143*).

- Nodular lymphoid hyperplasia in peripheral lymph nodes, mesenteric lymph nodes, tonsils, liver, and spleen.
- Hepatomegaly, splenomegaly (**Figure 218-4**).
- Chronic inflammation and swelling of joints.
- Bronchiectasis (**Figure 218-5**).
- Granulomatous lesions on skin and internal organs (**Figures 218-6** and **218-7**).

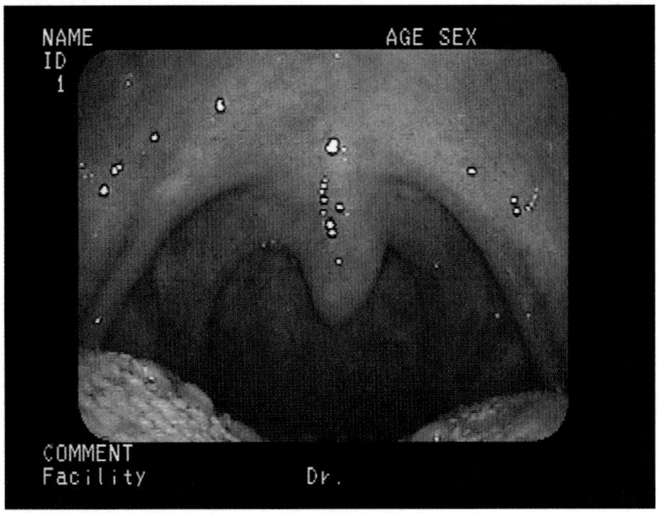

FIGURE 218-3 Oropharynx showing absence of tonsils in a patient with X-linked agammaglobulinemia. (*Used with permission from David Kosakowski, MD.*)

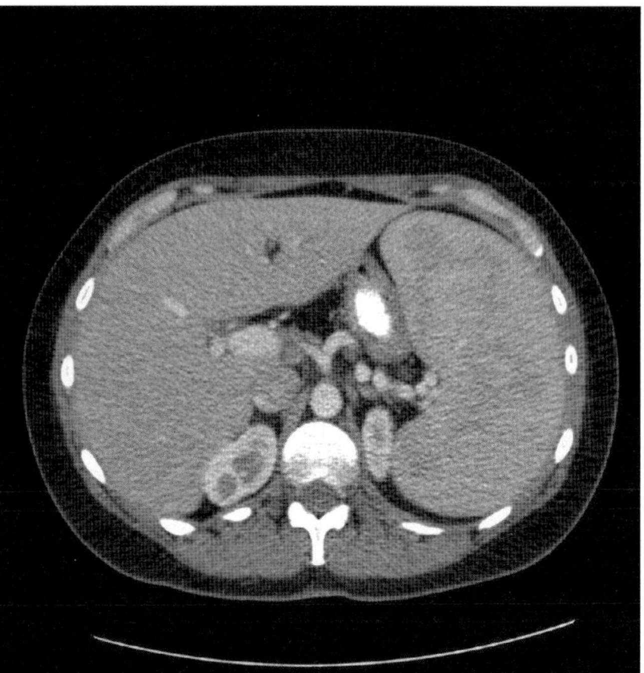

FIGURE 218-4 Splenomegaly in a woman with common variable immunodeficiency. (*Used with permission from James Fernandez, MD.*)

LABORATORY TESTING

- Total serum IgG, IgA, IgM, and IgE.
- Immunoglobulin vaccine titers:
  - Pneumococcal antigen serotypes (polysaccharide).
  - *H influenza* type B (polysaccharide).
  - Diphtheria (protein).
  - Tetanus (protein).
- If vaccine titers are low, individual should be challenged with the relevant vaccine followed by reevaluation of vaccine titers in 4 to 6 weeks to assess antibody response.
- Isohemagglutinins in infants who have not completed the primary immunization series.
- B cell enumeration using flow cytometry.
- B cell phenotypes, specific genetic mutation analysis.
- **Table 218-2** summarizes the common lab findings among B cell immunodeficiencies.

IMAGING

- CT imaging can be helpful in identification of chronic and acute sequelae of B cell immunodeficiencies including size of adenoid tissue, infection, granulomas, and bronchiectasis.
- MRI may be used in assessment of soft tissue infections.
- Imaging should be guided by localization of symptoms.

DIFFERENTIAL DIAGNOSIS

- Combined immunodeficiency- Primary and Acquired (HIV)—These children will have features of both B- and T-cell

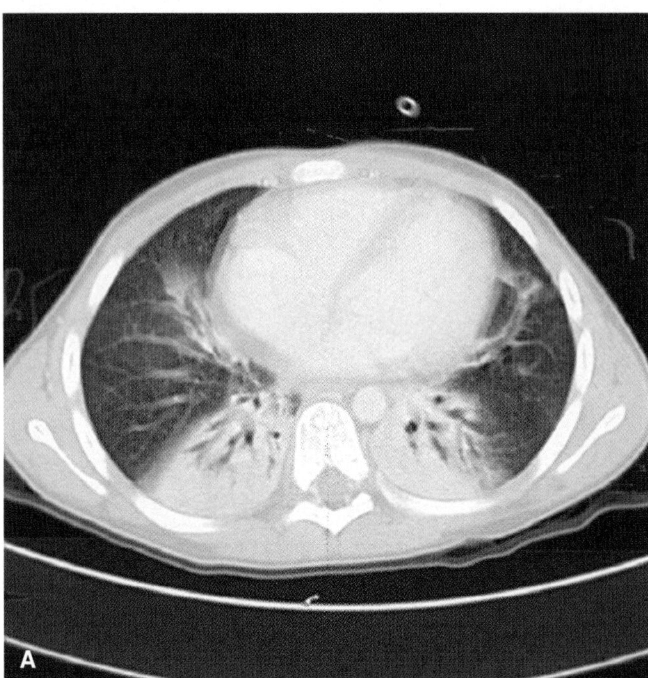

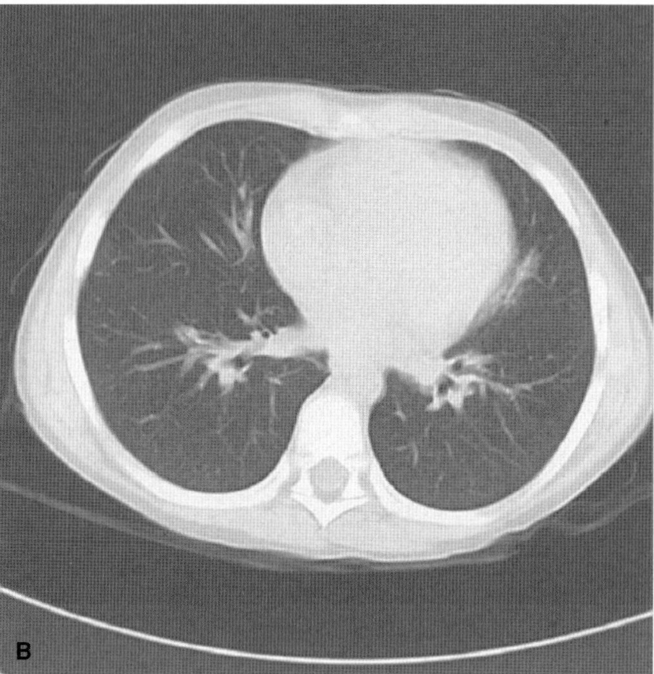

FIGURE 218-5 Initial and follow-up high resolution CTs of the chest of a 10-year-old boy with common variable immunodeficiency. **A.** Initial study demonstrating bilateral densities with areas of early bronchiectasis and tree-in-bud formations; **B.** Following 2 months of intravenous gamma globulin therapy and antibiotics, there is a resolution of parenchymal disease. (*Used with permission from Fiorino, EK, Panitch HB: Recurrent Pneumonia, in Pediatric Practice: Infectious Disease, edited by SS Shah, McGraw-Hill; 2009. Chapter 35.*)

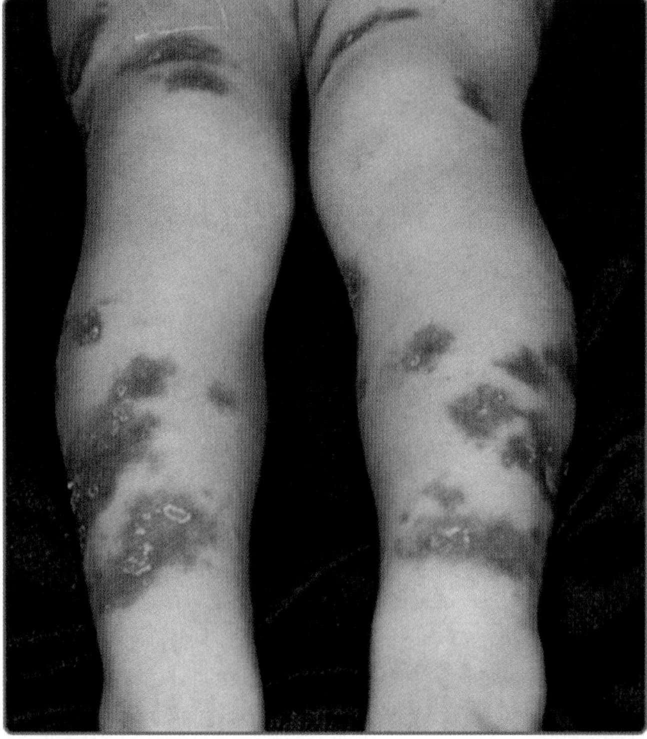

FIGURE 218-6 Non-caseating granulomas on the legs of a child with common variable immunodeficiency. Cultures and special stains showed no organisms. (*Used with permission from RL Fuleihan, AS Paller: Genetic Immunodeficiency Disease, in Fitzpatrick's Dermatology in General Medicine, 8th edition, edited by LA Goldsmith, et al. McGraw-Hill; 2012. Chapter 143*).

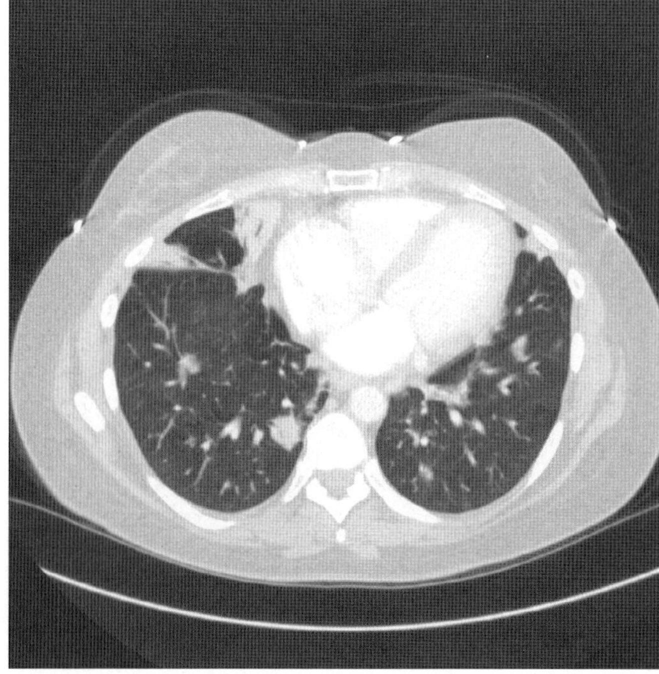

FIGURE 218-7 Bronchiectasis and lung granulomas in a patient with common variable immunodeficiency. (*Used with permission from James Fernandez, MD.*)

TABLE 218-2 Laboratory Features of the B Cell Immunodeficiency Syndromes

B Cell Immunodeficiency	B/T Cells	Serum Ig	Specific Antibody Response	
			Protein	Polysaccharide
Common Variable Immunodeficiency	Variable: normal or low B/T cells	• Decreased IgG • Decreased IgA or IgM	Usually low	Usually low
X-linked agammaglobulinemia	Very low or absent B cells	All isotypes very low or absent	None	None
Autosomal recessive agammaglobulinemia	Very low or absent B cells	All isotypes very low or absent	None	None
Specific antibody deficiency	Normal	Normal	Usually normal	Low
Hyper IgM syndrome	Normal	• Normal or high IgM • Decreased IgA, IgG	IgM only	IgM only
Selective Antibody deficiency • IgA • IgG subclass • IgE • IgM (rare)	Normal	• Very low or absent Ig for respective condition	Usually normal	Variable
Transient hypogammaglobulinemia of infancy	Normal	Low IgG	Usually normal	Usually normal

immunodeficiency, rather than just B cell deficiency manifestations (see Chapter 219, B and T cell Immunodeficiencies).

- Protein-losing enteropathy—Loss of immunoglobulins through the gut usually secondary to a chronic condition such as heart disease. Will generally not respond to immunoglobulin replacement.
- Nephrotic syndrome—Loss of function and quantity of immunoglobulins (see Chapter 67, Nephrotic Syndrome).
- Malnutrition or decreased protein production—Will be apparent on history and physical examination.
- Acquired humoral immune deficiency secondary to drugs (i.e., chronic steroids, immunosuppressants, and anti-B cell cytotoxic therapeutics) in children with chronic conditions.

MANAGEMENT

- Aim of treatment is to prevent future infections and minimize progression of chronic disease (i.e., bronchiectasis).

NONPHARMACOLOGIC

- Standard infection prevention measures including hand hygiene and avoidance of sick contacts may be helpful for mitigating pathogen exposure.

MEDICATIONS

- Replacement of immunoglobulin is the primary treatment in individuals with immunoglobulin deficiency and associated clinical symptoms.[5–9] SOR Ⓐ
- Replacement immunoglobulin is available in two forms:
  - Intravenous immunoglobulin (IVIG) given once every 3 to 4 weeks.
  - Subcutaneous immunoglobulin given once a week.
- Antibiotic treatment for acute infections should be started early and in conjunction with a diagnostic workup to identify the organism and its antibiotic susceptibilities if possible.
- Antibiotic prophylaxis may be helpful in prevention of chronic infections. While the risk of antibiotic resistance should be considered, prophylaxis may be indicated in individuals who continue to have clinical symptoms while on immunoglobulin replacement. SOR Ⓒ
- Antibiotic prophylaxis is recommended prior to dental and surgical procedures. SOR Ⓒ
- Killed vaccinations can be safely administered and have found to have some benefit. Patients as well as close household contacts should receive an annual influenza vaccine.[10] SOR Ⓒ
- Live virus vaccines are contraindicated in all individuals with B cell immunodeficiencies.[10] SOR Ⓒ

REFERRAL

- Refer patients with any of the clinical features mentioned above or following criteria to an immunologist:[11]
  - Four or more new ear infections within one year.
  - Two or more serious sinus infections within one year.
  - Two or more months on antibiotics with minimal effect or need for intravenous antibiotics for clearing infections.
  - Two or more pneumonias in lifetime.
  - Recurrent deep skin or organ abscesses.
  - Family history of primary immunodeficiency.
  - Two or more serious infections including septicemia.

PREVENTION AND SCREENING

- Routine assessment of growth parameters and frequency/severity of infections at well child visits.

PROGNOSIS

- Prognosis is variable depending on the severity of antibody deficiency. Overall, individuals with B cell immunodeficiencies who are treated with immunoglobulin replacement have a reasonably good prognosis.
- Early initiation of immunoglobulin replacement in patients with profound hypogammaglobulinemia is crucial for improved outcome.
- Individuals with B cell immunodeficiencies have an increased risk of malignancy and autoimmune disease that in turn increase morbidity and mortality.
- The presence of chronic disease sequelae is a predictor of poor outcomes.

FOLLOW-UP

- Patients with evidence of B cell immunodeficiency should have regular follow-up with an immunologist.
- Frequency of monitoring with labs and imaging is dependent on the degree of immunoglobulin impairment and clinical severity.

PATIENT RESOURCES

- Immune Deficiency Foundation—**http://primaryimmune.org**.
- Primary immunodeficiency resource center of Jeffrey Modell Foundation—**www.info4pi.org/jmf/**.

PROVIDER RESOURCES

- American Academy of Allergy, Asthma, & Immunology, practice parameters, position statements—**www.aaaai.org**.

REFERENCES

1. Hoernes, M, Reinhard S, Reichenbach, J. Modern management of primary B-cell immunodeficiencies. *Pediatr Allergy and Immunology*. 2011;22:758-769.
2. Hauk P, Johnston R, Lieu A. Immunodeficiency. In WH Hay, et al, eds. *Current Diagnosis & Treatment: Pediatrics 20th ed*, New York: McGraw-Hill; 2011. Chapter 31.
3. Bonilla, F. *Primary Humoral Immune Deficiencies: An Overview*. http://www.uptodate.com/contents/primary-humoral-immune-deficiencies.htm. 2012.
4. Chatila TA. Immunologic Disorders. In: C Rudolph, et al. *Rudolph's Pediatrics, 22nd ed.*, New York: McGraw-Hill; 2011. Section 13.
5. Cunningham-Rundles C, Siegal FP, Smithwick EM, et al. Efficacy of intravenous immunoglobulin in primary humoral immunodeficiency disease. *Ann Intern Med*. 1984;101:435-439.
6. Bernatowska E, Madalinski K, Janowicz W, et al. Results of a prospective controlled two-dose crossover study with intravenous immunoglobulin and comparison (retrospective) with plasma treatment. *Clin Immunol Immunopathol*. 1987;43:153-162.
7. Buckley RH, Schiff RI. The use of intravenous immune globulin in immunodeficiency diseases. *N Engl J Med*. 1991;325:110-117.
8. Schwartz SA. Intravenous immunoglobulin treatment of immunodeficiency disorders. *Pediatr Clin North Am*. 2000;47:1355-1369.
9. Steihm ER. Human intravenous immunoglobulin in primary and secondary antibody deficiencies. *Pediatr Infect Dis J*. 1997;16(7):696-707.
10. American Academy of Pediatrics. Immunization in Special Clinical Circumstances. In: Pickering LK, Baker CJ, Kimberlin DW, Long SS, eds. *Red Book: 2012 Report of the Committee on Infectious Diseases, 29th ed*. Elk Grove Village, IL: American Academy of Pediatrics; 2012:74-90.
11. Primary immunodeficiency resource center. Jeffrey Modell Foundation. *10 Warning Signs of Primary Immunodeficiency*. http://www.info4pi.org/aboutPI. 2009.

219 B AND T CELL IMMUNODEFICIENCIES—SEVERE COMBINED IMMUNODEFICIENCY (SCID) AND OTHER WELL DEFINED PRIMARY IMMUNODEFICIENCIES

Brian Schroer, MD
Tim Niehues, MD
Gregor Dückers, MD

PATIENT STORY

A 2.5-month-old-baby boy presented to his pediatrician because of a 10-day history of diarrhea, which began soon after his first series of immunizations, which included the oral rotavirus vaccine. He was born via uncomplicated vaginal delivery and his birth weight and height were at the 55 percent percentile. There were no known ill contacts. His weight and height, which had been 15 percent at two months, was now lower and he had a fever to 101F. Thrush was noted on his tongue and throat, and he was noted to have a diffuse scaling rash on the face and hands (**Figures 219-1** and **219-2**). A CBC with differential showed an absolute lymphocyte count of 1,200 cells/microliter. A chest x-ray was performed which showed diffuse infiltrates and the absence of a thymic shadow. He was referred to an immunologist for immediate evaluation and treatment. T and B cell subsets were obtained, which revealed that 90 percent of his lymphocytes are B cells and that he had very low numbers of T of maternal origin and NK cells. He was treated with intravenous immune globulin (IVIG), placed on trimethoprim-sulfamethoxazole for *Pneumocystis jirovecii* prophylaxis and referred to a specialized immunology center for a bone marrow transplant. His bone marrow transplantation was successful.

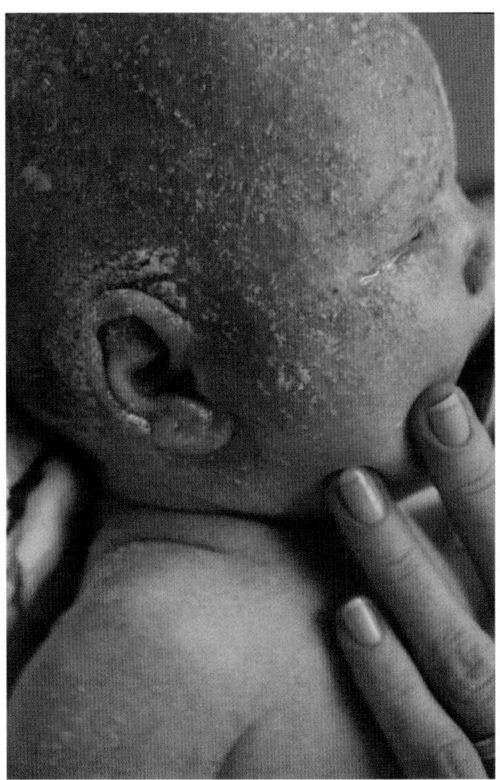

FIGURE 219-1 Exfoliative dermatitis caused by maternal T-cells in a young infant with severe combined immunodeficiency. (*Used with permission from Tim Niehues, MD and Gregor Dückers, MD.*)

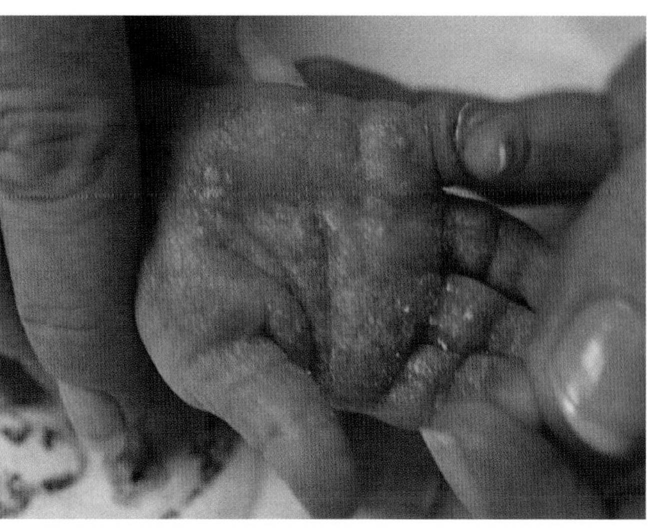

FIGURE 219-2 Exfoliative dermatitis on the palms of the same infant as in **Figure 219-1**. (*Used with permission from Tim Niehues, MD and Gregor Dückers, MD. Reprinted from Clinical Immunology, 2010, p. 187, with permission from Elsevier.*)

INTRODUCTION

Combined immunodeficiency syndromes arise from genetic defects leading to T lymphocyte dysfunction. Because B cells require T cells to produce antibodies, these patients are susceptible to opportunistic infections as well as skin and sinopulmonary infections due to bacterial, viral and fungal organisms. Immune dysregulation can lead to autoimmune disease and auto-inflammation in some syndromes. A diagnosis of a Severe Combined Immunodeficiency (SCID) is fatal before the age of 2 years if untreated and is a medical emergency. Some well-defined primary immunodeficiencies including Wiskott-Aldrich Syndrome, Hyper IgE syndrome, and Ataxia Telangiectasia may present in older patients.

SYNONYMS

- Primary or Congenital Immunodeficiency.
- Swiss type agammaglobulinemia.
- T-Cell Deficiency.
- Bubble Boy Disease.

TABLE 219-1 Representative Combined Immunodeficiency Syndromes with their Gene Defects, Mode of Inheritance, and the Types of Characteristic Infections the Patients are Susceptible to

Disease	Gene Defects	Mode of Inheritance-Gene	Infections
Severe Combined Immunodeficiency (SCID)			
T-B+NK-	Common gamma chain (Most common: 45 to 50% of cases)	XL-IL2RG	Mucocutaneous candidiasis, Pneumocystis, Chronic diarrhea, Severe Viral infections including from attenuated vaccines
	Janus Kinase 3	AR-JAK3	
T-B+NK+	Il-7 Receptor Alpha Chain	AR-IL-7RA	
	CD3 components	AR-CD3 Delta, Epsilon, Zeta	
T-B-NK+	Recombinase activating genes 1/2	AR-RAG1/RAG2	
	Artemis	AR-DCLER1C	
	DNA Ligase IV	AR-LIG4	
T-B-NK-	Adenosine Deaminase	AR-ADA	
	Reticular Dysgenesis	AR-AK2	
ZAP70 Deficiency	Zeta Chain Associated Protein Kinase 70kd	AR-ZAP70	Similar to SCID
T+B+NK+: CD8 Lymphopenia, CD4 Dysfunction	Defective T-cell receptor–associated tyrosine kinase	AR-P56lck	
Complete DiGeorge Syndrome	22q11 deletion	AD. Spontaneous- 22q11	Similar to SCID
Nijmegen Breakage Syndrome	DNA Repair Mechanisms	AR-NBN	Viral URI, UTI, Gastrointestinal infections.
DNA Ligase IV Deficiency	DNA Repair Mechanisms	AR-LIG	Variable severity- some similar to SCID, others less severe.
Hyper IgE Syndrome (HIES)	Signal transducer and Activator of Transcription- 3	AD-STAT3	Cold Abscesses, *Staphylococcus aureus*- Impetigo and lung abscesses, *Aspergillus, Pseudomonas, Pneumocystis,* Mucocutaneous Candidiasis (**Figure 219-3**), Sinopulmonary- *Haemophilus, Streptococcus pneumoniae*
	Dedicator of Cytokinesis- No skeletal anomalies	AR-DOCK8	Severe viral skin infections- (**Figures 219-4** and **219-5**) molluscum, warts. Bacterial and fungal infections. Do not form abscesses or pneumatoceles
	Tyrosine Kinase 2	AR-TYK2	Nontuberculous Mycobacteria Infections

TABLE 219-1 Representative Combined Immunodeficiency Syndromes with their Gene Defects, Mode of Inheritance, and the Types of Characteristic Infections the Patients are Susceptible to (*Continued*)

Disease	Gene Defects	Mode of Inheritance-Gene	Infections
Hyper IgM Syndromes	CD40 Ligand, and CD40	XL-CD40L, AR-CD40	Combined immune deficiency: Sinopulmonary infections (encapsulated bacteria), Pneumocystis, Cryptosporidium, Histoplasma
	AID- B cell class switching gene Uracil DNA Glycosylase	AR-AID AR-UNG	Humoral Immune deficiency: sinopulmonary infections, no opportunistic infections
Ataxia Telangiectasia	Ataxia Telangiectasia Mutated	AR-ATM	Sinopulmonary infections, rare opportunistic infections or infections outside of the respiratory tract.
Chronic Mucocutaneous Candidiasis	Autoimmune Regular Gene STAT1 Rare- Lyp, Dectin-1, TLR3	AR-AIRE AD-STAT1 AR	Invasive candidal infections in mucosal surfaces, skin, and nails.
Wiskott-Aldrich Syndrome	Wiskott-Aldrich Syndrome Protein	XL- WAS AD=Autosomal Dominant, AR=Autosomal Recessive XL=X-Linked	*S pneumoniae, Neisseria meningitidis, H influenzae, Pneumocystis,* Molluscum, Varicella, Fungal rare

EPIDEMIOLOGY

- SCID is very rare with an incidence reported at 1.8/100,000 live births per year.[1]
- Newborn screening with T cell receptor excision circles (Trec) has found a rate of 1.64/100,000 tests in Wisconsin. Trec screening does miss some atypical forms of SCID.[2]

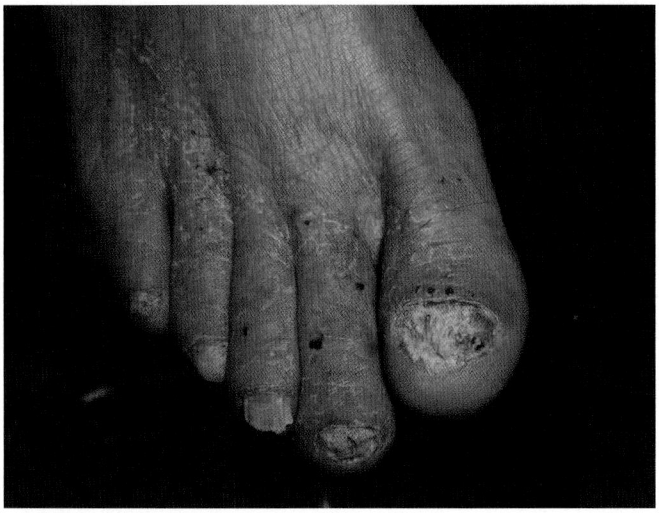

FIGURE 219-3 Onychomycosis of the toes and severe eczema of the skin in a patient with AD- Hyper IgE syndrome. (*Used with permission from Tim Niehues, MD and Gregor Dückers, MD.*)

- The etiologies of these defects are variable including genetic inheritance and spontaneous mutation.
- Modes of inheritance (**Table 219-1**).
  - Spontaneous mutations—All forms of congenital immune deficiency can occur as a spontaneous mutation.
  - The rate of all combined immunodeficiencies is likely an underestimate due to children who die at an early age before a diagnosis can be made.

ETIOLOGY AND PATHOPHYSIOLOGY

- **Table 219-1** describes the gene defects and infections, which occur with many primary immunodeficiencies. The table does not include every immunodeficiency but is meant to highlight representative examples.

RISK FACTORS

- Family history of recurrent infections or early unexplained death.
- Parents who have been previously diagnosed with a congenital immune deficiency.
- Consanguinity.

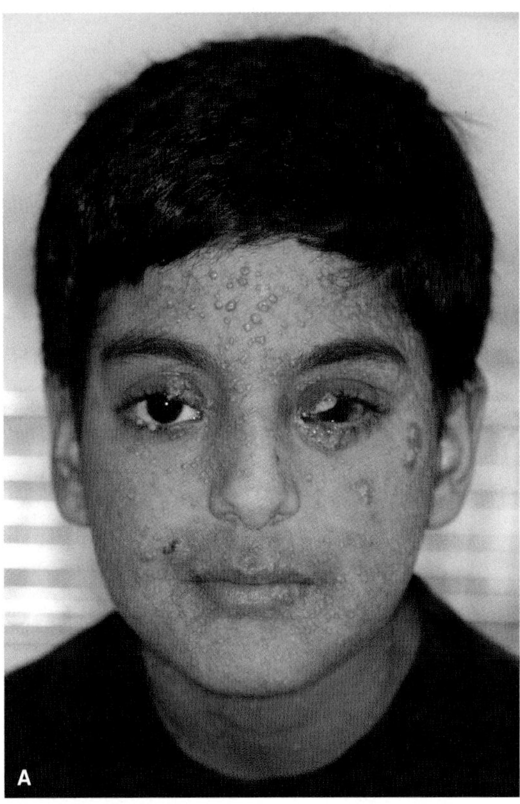

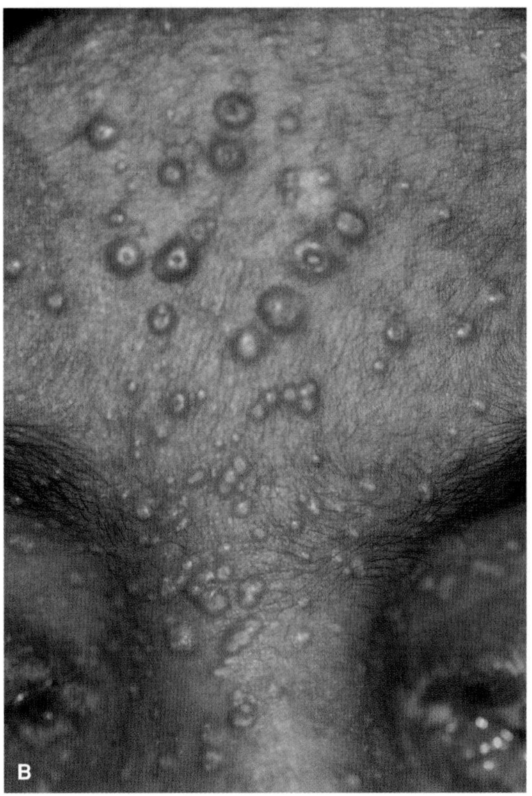

FIGURE 219-4 Disseminated molluscum viral infection and granulomas on upper eyelids bilaterally (**A**) and on close up view (**B**) in a young boy with AR-Hyper IgE syndrome. (*Used with permission from Tim Niehues, MD and Gregor Dückers, MD. Photo B is reprinted from Journal of Allergy and Clinical Immunology, 2009, p. 1296, with permission from Elsevier.*)

DIAGNOSIS

CLINICAL FEATURES (See Table 219-2)

- Most patients with immune deficiency present with failure to thrive as the first physical exam finding.
- SCID in infants is often not associated with specific physical exam findings.

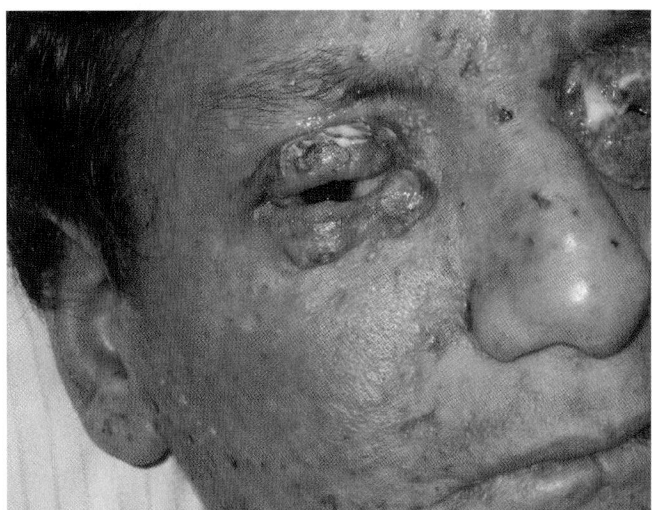

FIGURE 219-5 Severe viral infection of the eyelids in a patient with AR-Hyper IgE syndrome. (*Used with permission from Tim Niehues, MD and Gregor Dückers, MD.*)

- In toddlers and older children, immune deficiency syndromes have specific findings, which may help guide the diagnosis.
- Occurrence of atypical (opportunistic) infection, such as *Pneumocystis jirovecii* and mycobacteria, or unusually severe or complicated infections, may serve as clues to the underlying diagnosis.
- Neonatal eczema or Graft versus Host Disease (GvHD)—Skin rash may be present.

LABORATORY TESTING

- CBC and Fluorescence Activated Cell Sorting (FACS)—Combined deficiency should be immediately suspected if the total lymphocyte count is less than 2500/cubic mm or if the T cell percentage is <20 percent. Fluorescence Activated Cell Sorting (FACS) is a type of flow cytometry.
- A characteristic finding is the demonstration of highly activated (HLA DR^+/ $CD45^+$/ RO^+) maternal T-cells in the child's blood, that is, by HLA Typing
- Mitogen stimulation of lymphocytes showing a response of <10 percent of controls should prompt further evaluation.
- Specialized gene testing based on the clinical presentation should be done by a center, which specializes in congenital immune deficiencies.
- T cell receptor excision circles (Trec) newborn screening will detect many but not all combined immune deficiencies (see **Table 219-2**).

TABLE 219-2 Combined Immunodeficiencies, Their Characteristics, Clinical Findings, and Non-Infectious Complications

Syndrome	Special Physical Exam/Lab/ Radiology Findings	Serious Non-infectious Complications	Trec Newborn Screening
SCID	Failure to thrive Eczematous rash due to graft vs host disease from maternal immune cell engraftment	Malignancy Graft vs. host disease Exfoliative Dermatitis (**Figures 219-1**, **219-2**, **219-6** and **219-7**)	Will Detect
ZAP70 Deficiency	Normal Thymic Shadow, Normal or elevated lymphocyte count	Autoimmune disease such as colitis or cytopenias	Will Detect
Omenn Syndrome RAG1/ RAG2	Erythroderma Eosinophilia Lymphadenopathy Hepatosplenomegaly Expanded oligoclonal T cells	Malignancy	Will Detect
DNA Ligase IV Deficiency (**Figures 219-8**)	Microcephaly Narrow Bird like face Pancytopenia Photosensitivity Psoriasis	Developmental delay Radiosensitivity Photosensitivity Malignancy	Will Detect
Complete DiGeorge Syndrome	Low set and posteriorly rotated ears Ocular Hypertelorism Bulbous Nasal Tip Palate and Laryngeal defects	Conotruncal Cardiac Defects Hypocalcemia Autoimmunity	Will Detect
Nijmegen Breakage Syndrome	Microcephaly Narrow Bird like face Short Stature	Mild mental retardation Malignancy	Will Detect
AR HIES- DOCK8	No typical Physical exam findings as found in AD-HIES	Neurologic Complications Autoimmune disease	Will Detect
AD-HIES- STAT3 (**Figure 219-9)**	Broad nasal base and bridge Pneumatoceles Frontal bossing Coarse facies Retained primary teeth Scoliosis	Severe Atopic Dermatitis Bone fractures Vascular Abnormalities Lymphoma	Will Not Detect
Ataxia Telangiectasia (**Figures 219-10** and **219-11**)	Progressive cerebellar ataxia. Oculocutaneous telangiectasias	Radiosensitivity photosensitivity Diabetes Malignancy Bleeding	May Detect (3)
Hyper IgM Syndrome AID Deficiency	Lymphoid hyperplasia Varies based on defect May include Diarrhea, liver disease, cholangitis and cholangiocarcinoma	Autoimmune disease	Will Not Detect
Chronic Mucocutaneous Candidiasis (**Figure 121-8**)	Mucocutaneous fungal infection often extensive Onychomycosis Vitiligo Alopecia Areata	Autoimmune disease Endocrinopathy Malignancy	Will Not Detect
Wiskott-Aldrich Syndrome	Eczema Lymphadenopathy and Hepatospenomegaly Small Platelets	Autoimmune Disease Malignancy Bleeding	Will Not Detect

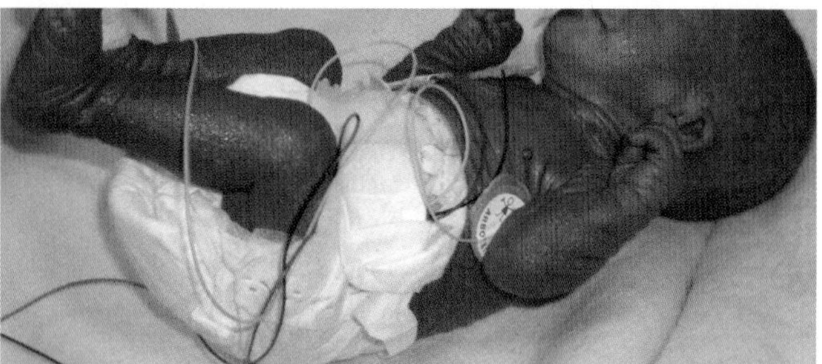

FIGURE 219-6 Severe exfoliative dermatitis in a 5-week-old infant highly suspected of having severe combined immunodeficiency in association with an unknown syndromatic disease. (*Used with permission from Tim Niehues, MD and Gregor Dückers, MD.*)

IMAGING

- Chest x-ray may show a lack of a thymus as an early sign of a T cell immune deficiency and may show evidence of atypical pneumonia.
- Facial and bone changes may be found with specific immunodeficiencies.
- Care must be taken with radiology studies as some forms of SCID demonstrate increased radiosensitivity. x-ray imaging poses more risk for malignancy in these patients.

DIFFERENTIAL DIAGNOSIS

- Recurrent infections in otherwise healthy children can be evaluated with a CBC and differential to identify the T and B lymphocyte subset pattern.

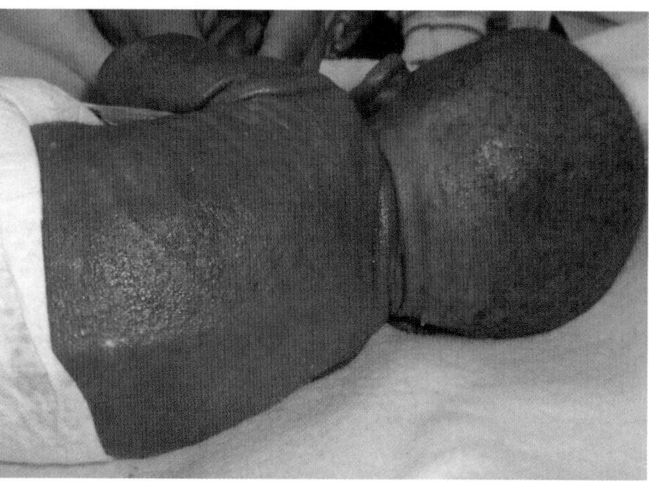

FIGURE 219-7 Exfoliative dermatitis on the back and scalp of the same infant as in **Figure 219-6**. (*Used with permission from Tim Niehues, MD and Gregor Dückers, MD.*)

- Serum Immunoglobulin levels are often helpful in determining the type and extent of involvement.
- Some diseases with chromosomal abnormalities (e.g., DiGeorge Syndrome or CHARGE) will show decreased but present numbers of T cells. These patients will have other characteristic congenital defects (e.g., skeletal and conotruncal abnormalities, or hypocalcemia. The diagnosis can be confirmed with appropriate genetic testing for 22q11 (see Chapter 216, DiGeorge Syndrome).

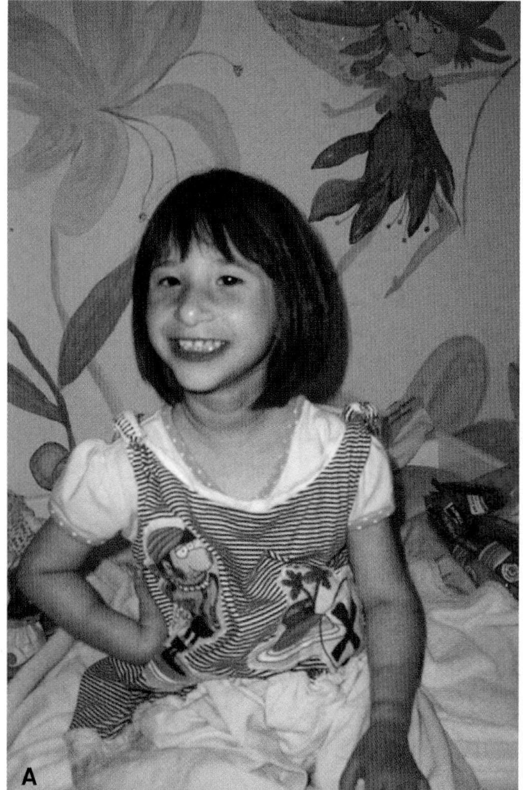

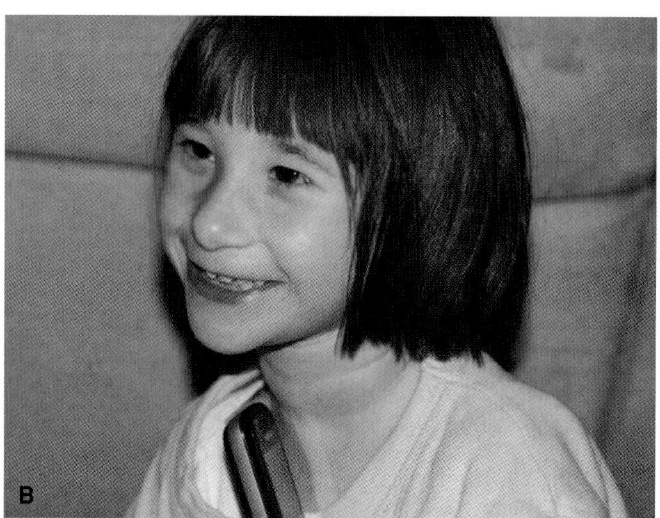

FIGURE 219-8 Microcephaly and narrow face in a patient with DNA Ligase IV deficiency on full (**A**) and close-up (**B**) views. (*Used with permission from Tim Niehues, MD and Gregor Dückers, MD. Reprinted from Wahn/Niehues Primäre Immundefekte, 2013, p. 22, with permission from Marseille Verlag.*)

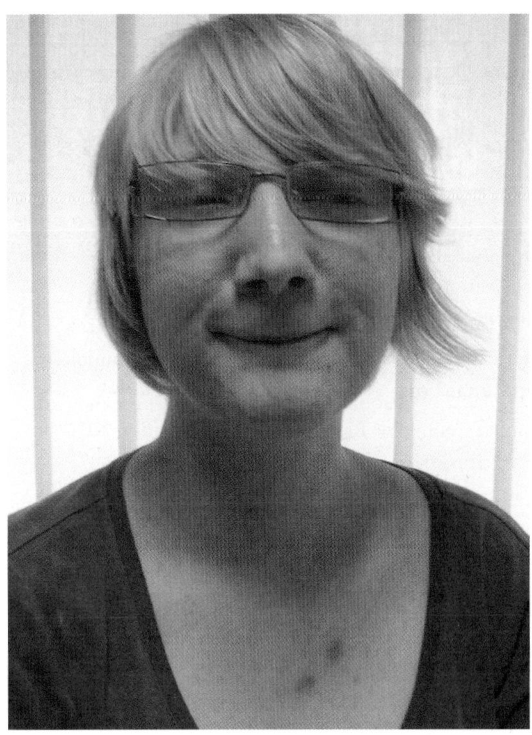

FIGURE 219-9 Characteristic facial features of broad nasal bridge, deep set eyes, eczematous lesions on the chest and coarsening of the facial skin in an 18-year-old woman with AD-Hyper IgE deficiency. *(Used with permission from Gregor Dückers, MD and Tim Niehues, MD.)*

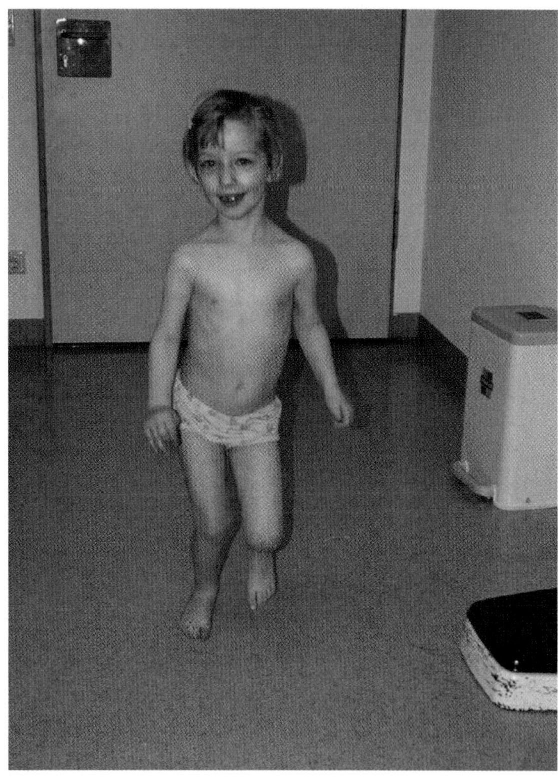

FIGURE 219-11 Gait changes in a young girl with Ataxia Telangiectasia. *(Used with permission from Tim Niehues, MD and Gregor Dückers, MD.)*

- Congenital humoral immune deficiency due to X-linked Agammaglobulinemia. These patients will have absent B cells and antibodies but normal T cell numbers, and usually present from 1to 2-years-old due to initial protection from maternal passively transferred antibodies (see Chapter 218, B Cell Immunodeficiencies).
- Failure to thrive and recurrent infections due to malnutrition or metabolic conditions (i.e., folate malabsorption; see Chapter 53, Failure to Thrive).
- HIV infection—These patients will have a normal thymic shadow and normal or increased immunoglobulin levels and usually a mother who is infected (see Chapter 182, Pediatric HIV Infection).
- Bone marrow failure due to secondary causes such as cancer.
- Intestinal lymphangiectasia—Can cause a severe protein losing enteropathy and loss of immunoglobulins.
- Congenital or acquired chylothorax with continuous drainage can lead to low immunoglobulins and lymphocyte counts.

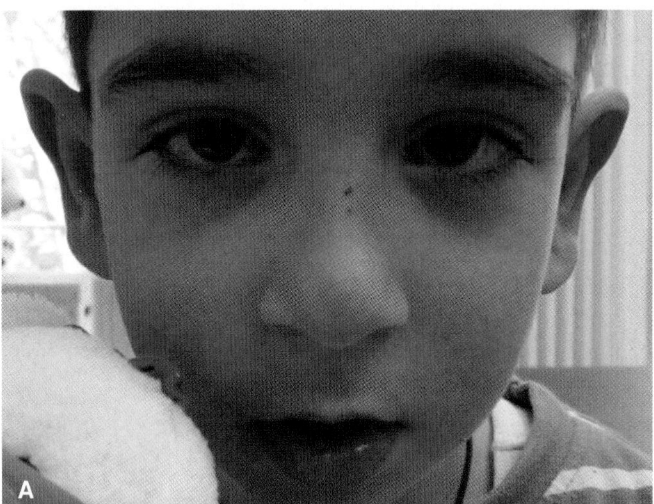

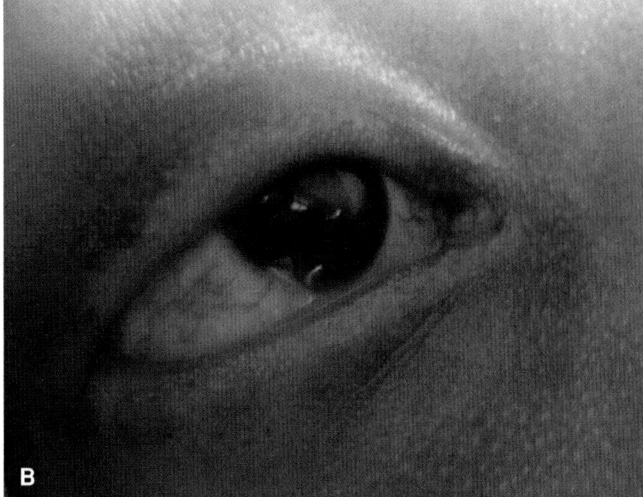

FIGURE 219-10 Characteristic bilateral (**A**) and right eye (**B**) conjunctival telangiectasias in a young boy with Ataxia Telangiectasia. *(Used with permission from Tim Niehues, MD and Gregor Dückers, MD.)*

MANAGEMENT

- Evaluation in a pediatric immunology center should occur immediately on suspicion of a combined immune deficiency.

NONPHARMACOLOGIC

- Protection of the patient from infections using contact and respiratory precautions should be considered.
- Avoid transfusion or if transfusion is indicated, use filter to delete residual lymphocytes entirely, because donor lymphocytes can cause fatal GvHD.
- Gene therapy has been tried in patients with certain types of immune defects (Adenosine Deaminase [ADA] deficiency, Il-2RG).[4,5] SOR Ⓐ
- Pegylated Adenosine Deaminase has been tried in ADA deficiency.[6] SOR Ⓐ

MEDICATIONS

- Early and aggressive diagnosis and treatment of infections.
- Based on the genetic defect, IVIG, *P jirovecii* prophylaxis, Stem cell transplant, and prophylactic antibiotics should be considered.
- Bone Marrow Transplantation is lifesaving and has been used successfully in many types of combined immunodeficiency.[7]

REFERRAL

Patients with combined immunodeficiencies should be immediately referred to an immunologist or a center specializing in immunodeficiency.

PREVENTION AND SCREENING

Many states and countries have begun universal newborn screening for combined and humoral immunodeficiencies using Trec and κ- deleting recombination excision circles (Krec) respectively. This allows for early diagnosis and intervention before infections can begin.

PROGNOSIS

- The prognosis is based on the specific gene defect and the individual clinical situation.
- Without prompt recognition many patients will die due to complications of infection and inflammation.

FOLLOW-UP

The patients should be followed in centers, which have experience dealing with primary immune deficiencies.

PATIENT RESOURCES

- Immune Deficiency Foundation—**http://primaryimmune.org**.
- Primary immunodeficiency resource center of Jeffrey Modell Foundation—**www.info4pi.org/jmf**.

PROVIDER RESOURCES

- NIH (National Institutes of Health) Genetics Home Reference—**http://ghr.nlm.nih.gov**.
- American Academy of Allergy, Asthma, & Immunology—**www.aaaai.org**.
- National Center for Biotechnology Information NIH—**www.ncbi.nlm.nih.gov**.
- European Society for primary immunodeficiencies—**www.esid.org**.
- Primary immunodeficiency diseases—An update on the classification from the internationalunion of immunological societies expert committee for primary immunodeficiency.[8]

REFERENCES

1. Yee A, DeRavin SS, Elliott E, Ziegler JB: Severe combined immunodeficiency: a national surveillance study. Pediatr Allergy Immunol. 2008;19(4):298-302.
2. Buckley RH: The long quest for neonatal screening for severe combined immunodeficiency. *J All Clin Immunol*. 2012;129(3): 597-604.
3. Mallott J, Kwan A, Church J, Gonzalez-Espinosa D, Lorey F, Tang LF, Sunderam U, Rana S, Srinivasan R, Brenner SE, Puck J. Newborn screening for SCID identifies patients with ataxia telangiectasia. *J Clin Immunol*. 2013;33(3):540-549.
4. Booth, C:. Gaspar ,H.B, .Thrasher ,A.J:. Gene therapy for primary immunodeficiency. Current opinion in pediatrics. *Curr Opin Pediatr*. 2011;23(6):659-666.
5. Aiuti A, Cattaneo F, Galimberti S, Benninghoff U, et al. Gene therapy for immunodeficiency due to adenosine deaminase deficiency. *The New England Journal of Medicine*. 2009;360(5):447-458.
6. Hershfield, M.S:. PEG-ADA: an alternative to haploidentical bone marrow transplantation and an adjunct to gene therapy for adenosine deaminase deficiency. *Hum Mutat*. 1995;5(2):107-112.
7. Slater MA, Gennery AR. Advances in hematopoietic stem cell transplantation for primary immunodeficiency. *Expert Rev Clin Immunol*. 2013;9(10):991-999.
8. Al-Herz W, et al. Primary immunodeficiency diseases: an update on the classification from the international union of immunological societies expert committee for primary immunodeficiency. *Front Immunol*. 2014;22(5):162.

220 CHRONIC GRANULOMATOUS DISEASE

Justin Greiwe, MD
Gregor Dückers, MD
Tim Niehues, MD
Brian Schroer, MD

PATIENT STORY

A 4-year-old boy presents with a recent history of persistent pneumonia. A detailed past medical history reveals several recurrent infections including pneumonia and lymph node abscesses growing *Staphylococcus aureus* and *Burkholderia cepacia*. His parents claim that he has been prescribed multiple courses of antibiotics over the last month with no improvement in his respiratory symptoms. There is no family history of immunodeficiency. Examination of the child revealed mild subcostal retractions and diffuse rales bilaterally. A chest x-ray demonstrated bilateral infiltrates of the upper and middle lung fields and a CT showed multifocal pneumonia (**Figure 220-1**). Diagnostic bronchoalveolar lavage and serological tests confirmed the presence of invasive pulmonary aspergillosis and the patient was placed on appropriate antifungal treatment. Because of the history and types of infection, a work-up for immunodeficiency was undertaken and the child was found to have chronic granulomatous disease.

INTRODUCTION

Chronic granulomatous disease (CGD) is the result of impaired intracellular microbial killing by phagocytes leading to formation of granulomata and recurrent infections with bacteria and fungi. Phagocytes are unable to kill the microbes they ingest secondary to a defect in a system of enzymes that produce reactive oxygen compounds. The most common and severe form of CGD is the X-linked type (~70% of all CGD cases) seen only in boys.

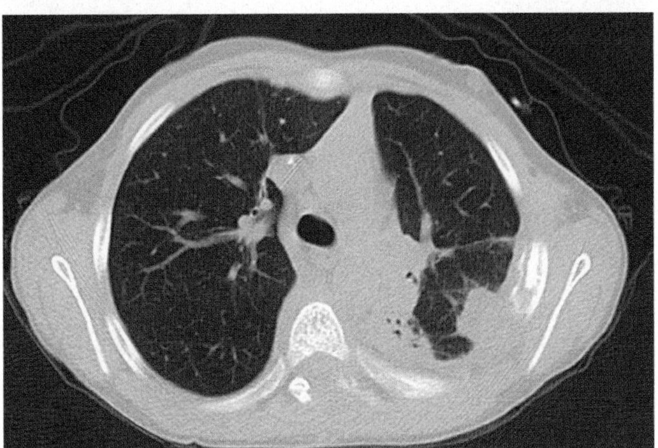

FIGURE 220-1 Multifocal pneumonia on CT scan in a young boy with chronic granulomatous disease. *(Used with permission from Alison Greiwe, MD.)*

SYNONYMS

CGD, Chronic Dysphagocytosis, Chronic Familial Granulomatosis, Septic Progressive Granulomatosis, Fatal Granulomatosis of Childhood, Impotent Neutrophil Syndrome, Congenital Dysphagocytosis, Bridges-Good syndrome, and Quie syndrome.

EPIDEMIOLOGY

- CGD affects around 1:200,000 people in the US.[1]
- The frequency of CGD is equal across ethnic and racial groups with disease presentation ranging from infancy into late adulthood.
- Most patients receive a diagnosis as toddlers.

ETIOLOGY AND PATHOPHYSIOLOGY

- Normal phagocytes utilize NADPH oxidase to generate reactive oxygen compounds like superoxide, which is essential for direct killing of certain catalase-positive bacteria and fungi.
- The enzyme that catalyzes the respiratory burst, NADPH oxidase, is a complex made up of subunits. One of 4 subunits may be defective in CGD.[2]
- Approximately 2/3 of CGD cases result from defects in the X-linked gene encoding the gp91phox subunit. The autosomal recessive forms of CGD are caused by mutations in the remaining subunits p22phox, p47phox, and p67phox. A recently discovered fifth subunit, p40phox, has been found to contribute to the autosomal recessive form of CGD as well.[3]
- Mutations leading to a loss or functional inactivation of one of these subunits leads to susceptibility of infection from any number of microorganisms (most commonly Staphylococci, *Aspergillus*, *Serratia*, *Nocardia*, and *Burkholderia*).

RISK FACTORS

The following factors increase the risk of developing CGD:

- Parents who are carriers of the recessive gene and thus can transmit the gene to their offspring in an autosomal recessive manner.
- Male gender, as most mutations are X-linked.
- A family history of unexplained recurrent or chronic infections.
- Rare cases may be due to spontaneous mutations.[4]

DIAGNOSIS

- Median age at diagnosis is 2.5 to 3 years.[5]
- Diagnosis may be delayed as a result of broad spectrum antibiotic use or if the manifestations are less severe (as in the autosomal recessive forms of the disease).
- Carrier females can exhibit some symptoms due to high degree of lyonization of the functional gene creating a mosaic pattern. This

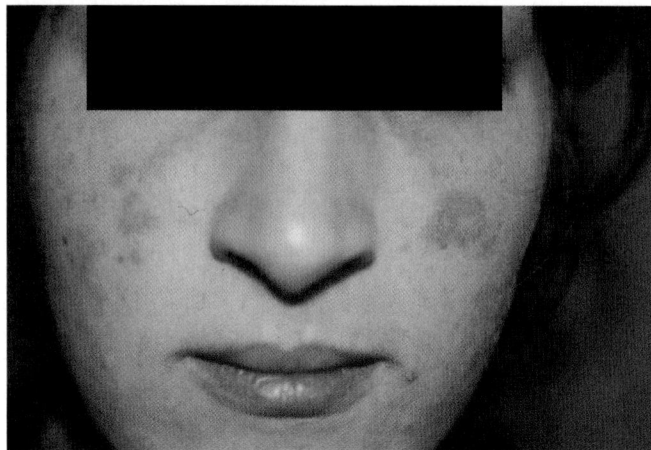

FIGURE 220-2 Lupus exanthema in the mother of a patient with chronic granulomatous disease, exemplifying the concept of lionization of the functional gene in carriers. (*Used with permission from Gregor Dückers, MD, and Tim Niehues, MD.*)

can create a discoid lupus appearance (**Figure 220-2**).[6] Most female carriers are asymptomatic.

CLINICAL FEATURES

Infection

- Recurrent or unusually severe bacterial and fungal infections most often manifesting as pneumonia, abscesses, suppurative adenitis (**Figure 220-3**), osteomyelitis (**Figure 220-4**), bacteremia/fungemia, superficial skin infections, and organ abscesses (liver, spleen, brain; **Figure 220-5**).
- Typical bacteria found in US and European patients include *S. aureus* and *Burkholderia*. Fungi isolated in CGD are *Aspergillus* and *Nocardia* species.[7]

Inflammation

- Recurrent fever or fever of unknown origin.

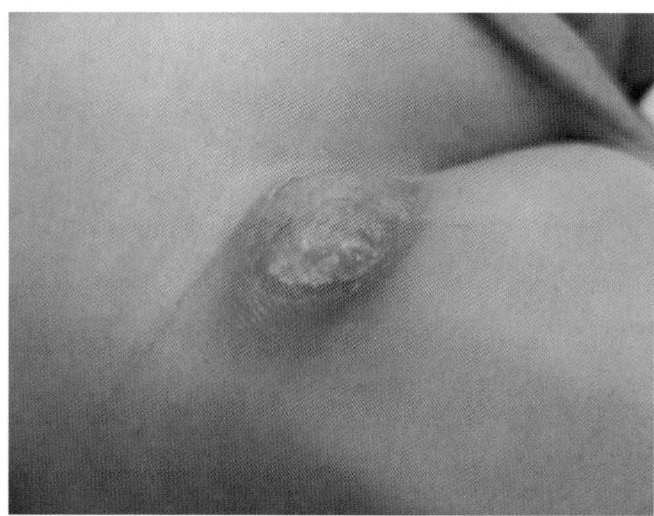

FIGURE 220-3 Fluctuant inguinal lymphadenitis in a young patient with chronic granulomatous disease. (*Used with permission from Gregor Dückers, MD and Tim Niehues, MD.*)

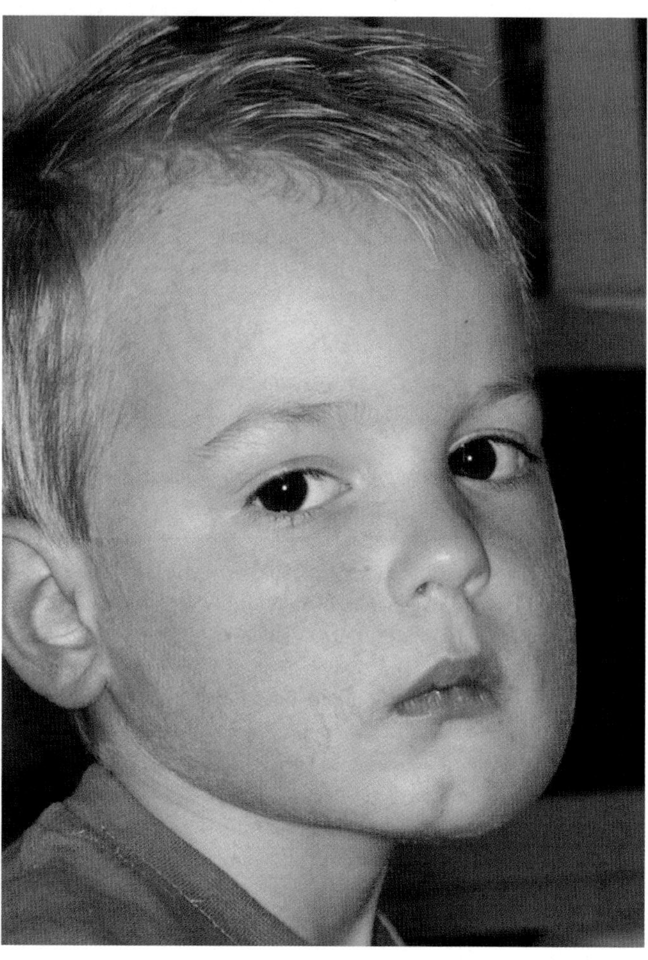

FIGURE 220-4 Osteomyelitis of the left mandible in a young boy with chronic granulomatous disease. (*Used with permission from Gregor Dückers, MD and Tim Niehues, MD.*)

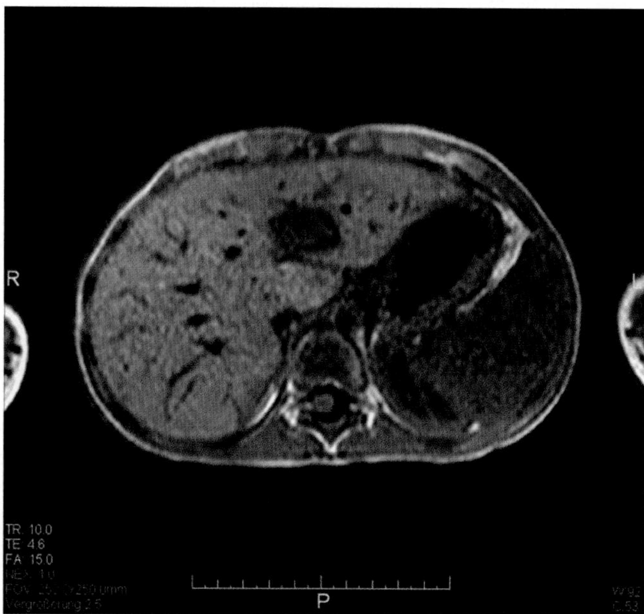

FIGURE 220-5 Hepatic abscess in liver, as a manifestation of chronic granulomatous disease in a young patient. (*Used with permission from Gregor Dückers, MD and Tim Niehues, MD.*)

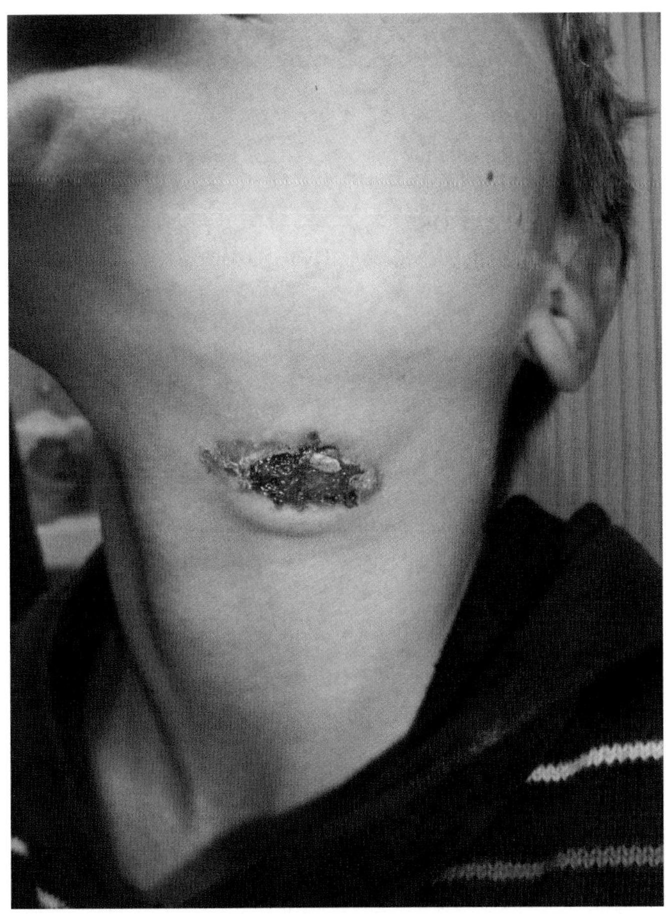

FIGURE 220-6 Impaired wound healing after incision and drainage of an infected lymph node in a child with chronic granulomatous disease. (*Used with permission from Gregor Dückers, MD and Tim Niehues, MD.*)

- Diffuse granulomas that affect a number of different systems including the gastrointestinal, genitourinary, pulmonary, and central nervous systems.
- Abnormal wound healing (**Figure 220-6**).
- Patients with CGD may have features that may mimic the clinical picture of inflammatory bowel disease.[8]

PHYSICAL FINDINGS

- Growth failure/short stature.
- Lymphadenopathy.
- Hepatosplenomegaly.
- Cutaneous abscesses.

LABORATORY TESTING

- Dihydrorhodamine (DHR) test—This has replaced Nitro blue tetrazolium as a more effective screening tool because it is easier to use, more objective and more accurate.[9]
- Genetic mutation analysis: This may help to verify the diagnosis, establish an inheritance pattern, and provide valuable information for family counseling.
- An aggressive search for unusual and rare pathogens is necessary (**Figure 220-7**). This requires help from an experienced microbiology lab.

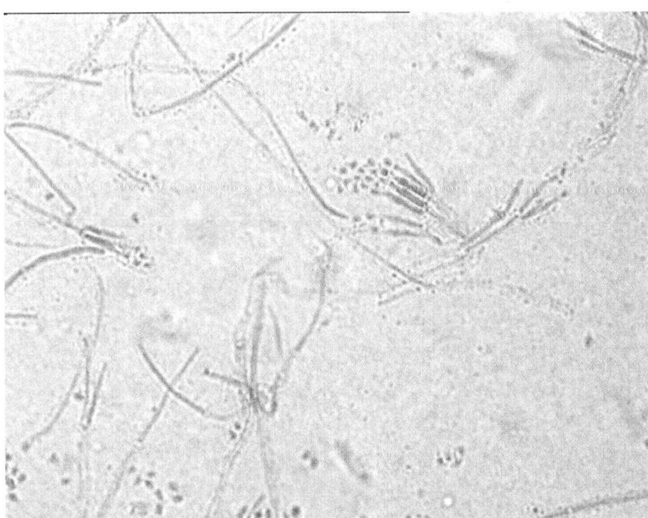

FIGURE 220-7 *Geosmithia* fungus isolated from a patient with osteomyelitis and chronic granulomatous disease. (*Used with permission from Gregor Dückers, MD, and Tim Niehues, MD.*)

IMAGING

- X-rays may be helpful in diagnosing pneumonia.
- CT imaging is useful at evaluating the size, number, and location of abscesses in the lung, spleen, or liver (**Figure 220-5**).

DIFFERENTIAL DIAGNOSIS

- Severe and/or recurrent infections with catalase-positive microorganisms can be caused by any of the following and should be considered when working up a child for CGD:
    - Other primary immunodeficiencies (B-cell deficiency, Hyperimmunoglobulin E syndrome (HIES), leukocyte adhesion deficiency, complement deficiencies, Myeloperoxidase deficiency)—See Chapters 218, B Cell Immunodeficiencies and 219, T- and B-cell Immunodeficiencies.
    - Secondary immunodeficiencies, that is, Human Immunodeficiency Virus (HIV/AIDS)—See Chapter 182, Pediatric HIV Infection.
    - Metabolic disorders (cystic fibrosis, G6PD deficiency)—See Chapter 51, Cystic Fibrosis.
    - Inflammatory disorders (Crohn disease)—See Chapter 59, Inflammatory Bowel Disease.

MANAGEMENT

- As with other primary immunodeficiencies, the diagnosis and treatment of infections in CGD must be early and aggressive.

NONPHARMACOLOGIC

- Standard infection prevention measures include good hand hygiene for the patient, family, and close contacts.
- Avoidance of sick contacts when possible.
- All immunizations are safe for these children and should be given on time as per the standard schedule. They may receive live virus vaccines.

- Experimental gene therapy trials for CGD are currently underway and may be appropriate in refractory or life-threatening infections. Gene therapy as a cure is still far from becoming a reality.[10]

MEDICATION

- Prophylactic regimens of antimicrobials and antifungals like trimethoprim-sulfamethoxazole and itraconazole remain first-line therapy and are commonly used.[10] SOR ©
- Immunomodulatory treatment. In one placebo trial, patient who received subcutaneous interferon (IFN)-gamma had significant reductions in the number of serious infections.[11] SOR Ⓑ The potential drawbacks for IFN-gamma include adverse side effects (fever/myalgias), time commitment (injections 3 times/week), and cost.

▶ Treatment of infections

- Starts with an aggressive diagnostic approach (cultures, open biopsies) and targeted treatment (parenteral, several weeks duration). SOR ©
- WBC transfusions during infections may be of benefit but should be performed only in specialized centers who are experienced with CGD. SOR ©

▶ Treatment of inflammation

- Obstructive or painful granulomas that impinge on nearby organs like the stomach, ureters, or urinary bladder can be relieved by short-term steroid therapy. SOR ©

SURGERY

- Liver and lymph node abscesses and obstructive or painful granulomas are very often drained or removed surgically, if steroid therapy fails. SOR ©

▶ Curative treatment

- Stem cell transplantation (SCT) results have improved significantly. SCT is a good option for children who suffer from serious infections despite prophylaxis.[12] SOR ©
- Gene therapy has been tried but the long-term efficacy and risks remain to be determined. SOR ©

REFERRAL

- Immunology referral should be made in all patients who are suspected to have an immunodeficiency.
- Referral to an infectious disease specialist is necessary to help with treatment for fungal or severe bacterial infections.
- Surgical referral should be made if there is pain or organ dysfunction as a result of granuloma formation.
- Referral to a geneticist is useful for the family of a newly diagnosed patient. Family members will receive counseling about the benefits and risks of testing for the carrier state. As the patient gets older, he or she may want to discuss the issues of childbearing and the risk of passing on CGD to their offspring.

PREVENTION AND SCREENING

- CGD is an inherited disease and therefore cannot be prevented.
- If there is a known family history of CGD, genetic counseling may be beneficial prior to conception.
- Patients with CGD should avoid construction sites and long-term travel in tunnels due to the risk of exposure to *Aspergillus* spores/conidia.

PROGNOSIS

- Patients with the more severe X-linked form of CGD suffer from increased morbidity and mortality in their early teen years.
- Mainly due to effective, intracellular active anti-bacterial and anti-fungal prophylaxis as well as more successful stem cell transplantation, prognosis of patients with CGD has significantly improved over the past two decades.

FOLLOW UP

- Frequent follow-up in a specialized institution is necessary for patients with CGD because early and aggressive treatment of infections and inflammation is essential to prevent severe complications.

PATIENT RESOURCES

Organizations Providing General Support

- Jeffrey Modell Foundation (JMF)—**www.info4pi.org/jmf**.
- Chronic Granulomatous Disorder Research Trust (CGD)—**www.cgd.org.uk**.
- Chronic Granulomatous Disease Association, Inc.—**www.cgdassociation.org**.
- Genetic Alliance—**www.geneticalliance.org**.
- National Organization for Rare Disorders (NORD)—**www.rarediseases.org**.

Social Networking Websites

- DNAandU.org is a web site and blog that collects firsthand stories from people facing issues, making tough decisions, and using genomic (DNA) information in their own health care—**www.dnaandu.org**.
- Madisons Foundation—**www.madisonsfoundation.org**.
- RareShare is an online social hub dedicated to patients, families and health care professionals affected by rare medical disorders—**www.rareshare.org**.

PROVIDER RESOURCES

- **www.aaaai.org/conditions-and-treatments/primary-immunodeficiency-disease/chronic-granulomatous-disease.aspx**.

- The American Society of Gene & Cell Therapy—**www.asgct.org/general-public/educational-resources/gene-therapy-and-cell-therapy-for-diseases/immunodeficiency-diseases**.
- Genetics Home Reference (GHR) contains information on chronic granulomatous disease—**http://ghr.nlm.nih.gov/condition/chronic-granulomatous-disease**.
- The National Institute of Allergy and Infectious Diseases (NIAID) supports scientists developing better ways to diagnose, treat, and prevent the many infectious, immunologic, and allergic diseases that afflict people worldwide—**www.niaid.nih.gov/topics/immuneDeficiency/Understanding/Pages/cgd.aspx**.
- The National Organization for Rare Disorders (NORD)—**www.rarediseases.org/rare-disease-information/rare-diseases/viewSearchResults?term=Granulomatous%20Disease,%20Chronic**.
- The Online Mendelian Inheritance in Man (OMIM)—**http://omim.org/entry/306400**.

REFERENCES

1. Winkelstein JA, Marino MC, Johnston RB Jr, et al. Chronic granulomatous disease. Report on a national registry of 368 patients. *Medicine (Baltimore)*. 2000;79(3):155-169.
2. Van den Berg JM, van Koppen E, Ahlin A, Belohradsky BH, Bernatowska E, et al. *Chronic Granulomatous Disease: The European Experience*. 2009;4(4):e5234.
3. Matute JD, Arias AA, et al. A new genetic subgroup of chronic granulomatous disease with autosomal recessive mutations in p40 phox and selective defects in neutrophil NADPH oxidase activity. *Blood*. 2009;114(15): 3309-3315.
4. Anderson-Cohen M, Holland SM, et al. Severe phenotype of chronic granulomatous disease presenting in a female with a de novo mutation in gp91-phox and a non-familial, extremely skewed X chromosome inactivation. *Clin Immunol*. 2003; 109(3):308-317.
5. Rosenzweig SD, Holland SM. Chronic granulomatous disease: Pathogenesis, clinical manifestations, and diagnosis. UpToDate http://www.uptodate.com/contents/chronic-granulomatous-disease-pathogenesis-clinical-manifestations-and-diagnosis?source=search_result&search=chronic+granulomatous+disease&selectedTitle=1%7E81.
6. Barton LL, Johnson CR. Discoid lupus erythematosus and X-linked chronic granulomatous disease. *Pediatr Dermatol*. 1986;3(5):376-369.
7. Johnston RB Jr: Clinical aspects of chronic granulomatous disease. *Curr Opin Hematol*. 2001;8(1):17-22.
8. Marciano BE, Rosenzweig SD, Kleiner DE, et al. Gastrointestinal involvement in chronic granulomatous disease. *Pediatrics*. 2004; 114(2):462-468.
9. N. Franklin Adkinson et al. *Middleton's Allergy: Principles and Practice, 7th Edition*. New York: Elsevier Mosby; 2009
10. Seger RA. Modern management of chronic granulomatous disease. *Br J Haematol*. 2008;140(3):255-266.
11. The International Chronic Granulomatous Disease Cooperative Study Group: A controlled trial of interferon gamma to prevent infection in chronic granulomatous disease. *N Engl J Med*. 1991; 324:509-516.
12. Kang EM, Marciano BE, et al. Chronic granulomatous disease: overview and hematopoietic stem cell transplantation. *J Allergy Clin Immunol*. 2011;127(6):1319-1326.

PART 21

GENETIC DISORDERS

Strength of Recommendation (SOR)	Definition
A	Recommendation based on consistent and good-quality patient-oriented evidence.*
B	Recommendation based on inconsistent or limited-quality patient-oriented evidence.*
C	Recommendation based on consensus, usual practice, opinion, disease-oriented evidence, or case series for studies of diagnosis, treatment, prevention, or screening.*

*See Appendix A on pages 1320–1322 for further information.

221 DOWN SYNDROME

Di Sun, BS, MPH
Elumalai Appachi, MD, MRCP

PATIENT STORY

A 2-day-old baby boy is brought to the emergency department for vomiting. The patient's mother is a 25 year-old single parent who did not receive prenatal care, and the baby was born at home via vaginal delivery at 39 weeks gestation. The mother reports that the baby vomits whenever she tries to breastfeed him and that the emesis appears green and thick. The infant is noted to have epicanthal folds, upward-slanting palpebral fissures, flat nasal bridge, a single transverse palmar (simian) crease, and small ears (**Figures 221-1** and **221-2**). The examining physician suspects the child has Down syndrome and orders an abdominal x-ray, which reveals a "double-bubble," consistent with duodenal atresia, and is associated with Down syndrome. (**Figure 221-3**). The baby undergoes surgical correction of the atresia and recovers completely. A chromosomal analysis confirms the diagnosis of Down syndrome.

INTRODUCTION

- Down syndrome (DS) is an aneuploidy that develops from excess genetic material on chromosome 21, and results in a distinctive phenotypic appearance.[1,2] Children commonly present with congenital cardiac, hematologic, musculoskeletal, visual, and/or auditory defects.[3] The incidence of DS increases with maternal age.[4]

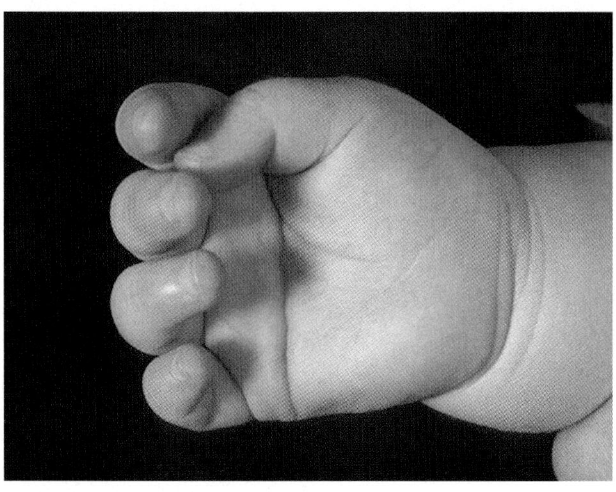

FIGURE 221-2 Single transverse palmar crease in an infant with Down syndrome (simian crease). This is seen in about 50 percent of infants with Down syndrome and can be seen in infants and children who do not have Down syndrome. (*Used with permission from Cleveland Clinic Children's Hospital Photo Files.*)

SYNONYMS

Trisomy 21.

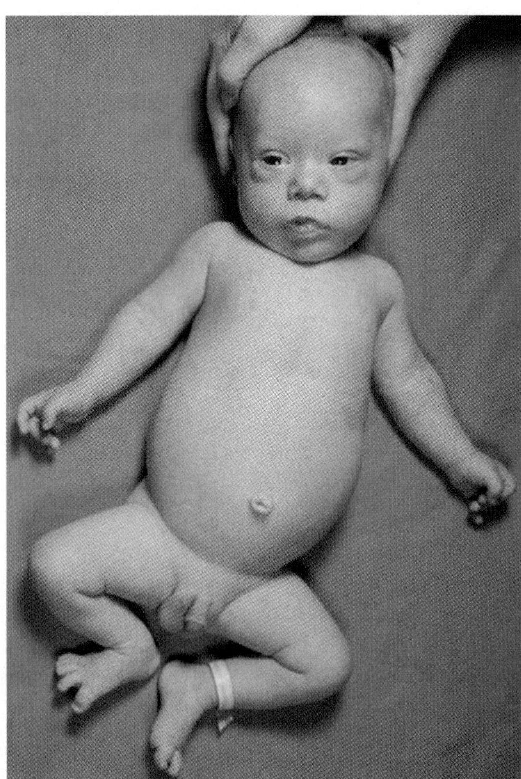

FIGURE 221-1 Epicanthal folds, upslanting palpebral fissures, flat nasal bridge, and wide gap between the first and second toe in an infant with Down syndrome. (*Used with permission from Cleveland Clinic Children's Hospital Photo Files.*)

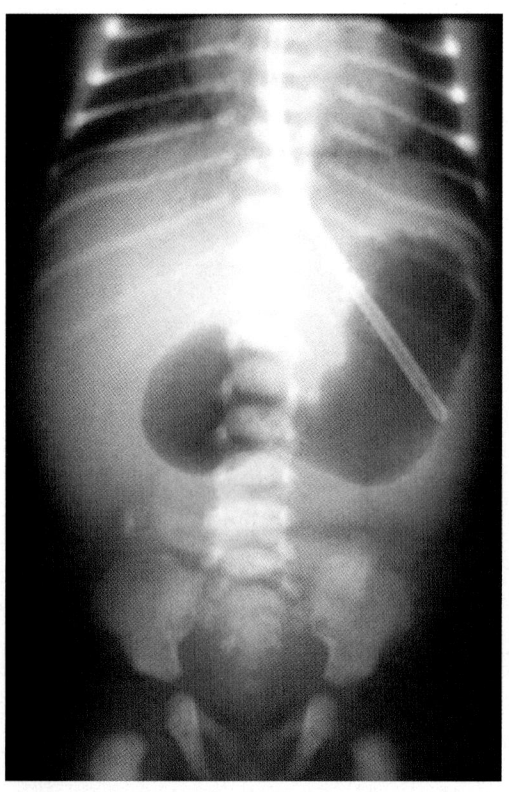

FIGURE 221-3 "Double bubble" sign of duodenal atresia on plain x-ray in a child with Down syndrome. Infants with Down syndrome have an increased incidence of intestinal atresias. (*Used with permission from Elumalai Appachi, MD.*)

EPIDEMIOLOGY

- DS is the most commonly occurring genetic disorder among live births, occurring in 1 in 691 of all live births in the US.[5]
- The risk of having a prenatal diagnosis for DS is thought to be higher since it is estimated that 67 percent women (range 61% to 93%) in the US with a fetus demonstrating trisomy 21 will terminate the pregnancy.[6]
- Compared to Caucasian mothers, the prevalence ratio of trisomy 21 live births was 0.77 among African American mothers and 1.12 among Hispanic mothers. These differences could reflect ethnic differences in accessibility to prenatal screening, variation in the decision to terminate the pregnancy, or reporting bias inherent to the design of the study.[7]
- Although the risk of DS increases with increasing maternal age, approximately 80 percent of babies with DS are born to women <35 years of age.[4]

ETIOLOGY AND PATHOPHYSIOLOGY

- Ninety-five percent of DS cases arise from nondisjunction of chromosome 21, resulting in 3 complete copies of chromosome 21.[2]
  - In 86 percent of these cases, the extra chromosome originated from the mother due to nondisjunction during meiosis II (75%) rather than meiosis I (25%). Nine percent of complete trisomy 21 is derived from the father. Less than 5 percent of complete trisomy 21 is due to mitotic errors.[1]
  - These nondisjunction events are associated with increasing maternal age, which is correlated with a decrease in genetic recombination.[1]
- Three to four percent of DS cases occur due to chromosome 21 translocations, including balanced Robertsonian translocations of chromosome 21q paired most commonly with chromosome 14q. In patients with balanced translocations, parents should be screened to ensure that one of them is not a phenotypically normal carrier of a balanced translocation.[1]
- One to two percent of DS cases are due to mosaicism in which two cell lines are expressed, one with trisomy 21 and the other with normal cytogenetics.[1]
- The extra genetic materials lead to the characteristic DS phenotype, the best studied of which being the central nervous system manifestations. On histopathological studies, DS patients have decreased numbers of cortical neurons, stagnation of dendritic tree development at 4 months of age, decreased number of synapses, and delayed myelination when compared to normal subjects.[1]

RISK FACTORS

- Increasing maternal age is the single risk factor most associated with nondisjunction errors hypothesized to be secondary to accumulation of environmental insults to the oocyte and/or gradual attrition of the meiotic machinery.[1]
- Altered recombination pattern during meiosis, characterized by decreased recombination or pericentromeric exchange, will increase risk of DS.[1]
- Other environmental factors implicated in DS include maternal alcohol use, maternal irradiation, and low socioeconomic status. However, these associations have not been confirmed.[7]

DIAGNOSIS

CLINICAL FEATURES

Typical physical findings characteristic of DS are:

- Hypotonia (**Figure 221-1**).
- Wide gap between first and second toes (**Figure 221-1**).
- Clinodactyly (bend or curvature of one finger toward the other fingers, most commonly the fifth finger toward the other four fingers; **Figure 221-4**).
- Simian crease (**Figure 221-2**).
- Craniofacial abnormalities such as brachycephaly.
- Small and low-set ears (**Figure 221-5**).
- Epicanthal folds, upward-slanting palpebral fissures (**Figures 221-6** and **221-7**).
- Flat nasal bridge (**Figures 221-6** and **221-7**).
- Brushfield spots (speckled white spots on the iris; **Figure 221-8**).

Patients can also have maxillary and pharyngeal hypoplasia, which can lead to hearing loss and nasal obstruction.[2,3]

In early development, children with DS will demonstrate achievement of normal milestones in the low-normal timeframe, but their cognitive function stops developing in adolescence. Alzheimer's is present in 75 percent patients with DS who are over 60 years of age.[3]

- DS is associated with many other medical conditions:
  - Hearing loss (75%).
  - Eye disease (60%) including cataracts, strabismus, and refractive errors.

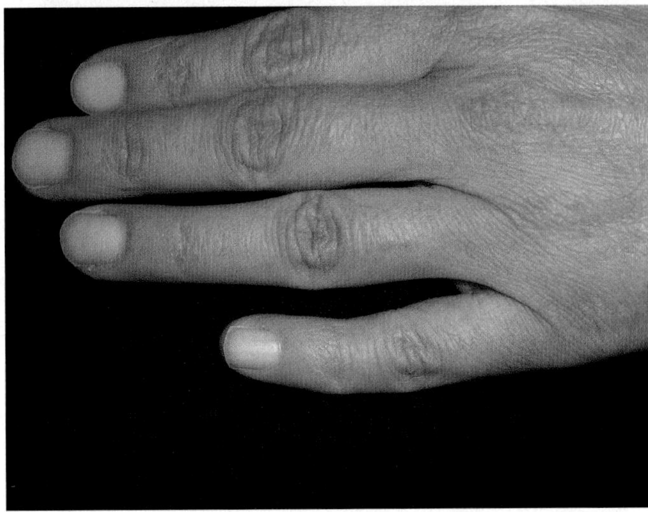

FIGURE 221-4 Clinodactyly (curvature of one finger toward the other fingers) is commonly seen in Down syndrome. (*Used with permission from Richard P. Usatine, MD.*)

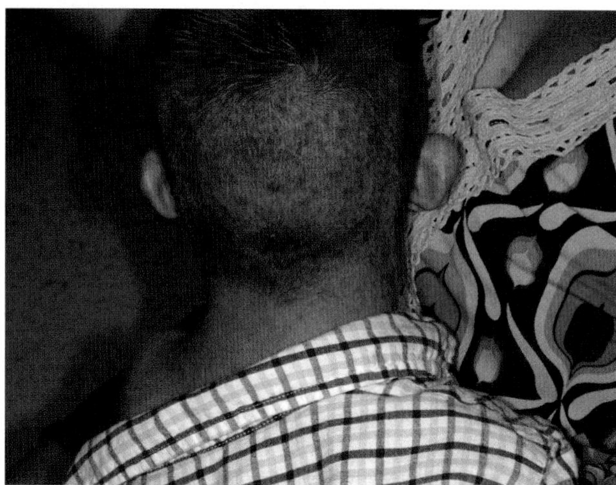

FIGURE 221-5 Small, low-set ears in a boy with Down syndrome. This boy also has crusted scabies, visible on his scalp and neck. (*Used with permission from Richard P. Usatine, MD.*)

- Congenital heart disease (50%) with the most common being atrioventricular septal defect (see Chapter 47, Syndrome Associated with Heart Disease).
- Gastrointestinal atresia (12%; **Figure 221-3**).
- Thyroid disease (4 to 18%).
- Polycythemia (18 to 64%).
- Seizures (1 to 13%).
- Transient myeloproliferative disorder (10%).
- Celiac disease (5%).
- Leukemia (1%).
- Atlantoaxial instability (1 to 2%).
- Autism (1%).
- Hirschsprung (<1%).[3]
- Behavioral disorders, including attention deficit hyperactivity disorder (6.1%), conduct disorder (5.4%), or aggressive behavior (6.5%). Many adults with DS will also have major depressive disorder (6.1%).[3]

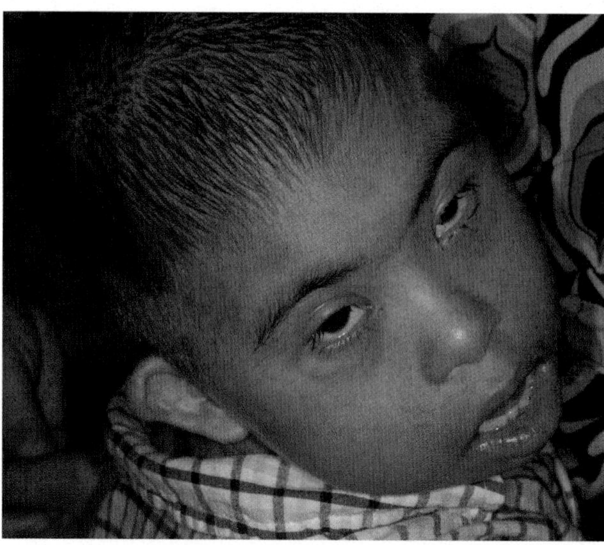

FIGURE 221-6 Epicanthal folds, upward slanting palpebral fissures and flat nasal bridge in the same boy as in **Figure 221-5**. (*Used with permission from Richard P. Usatine, MD.*)

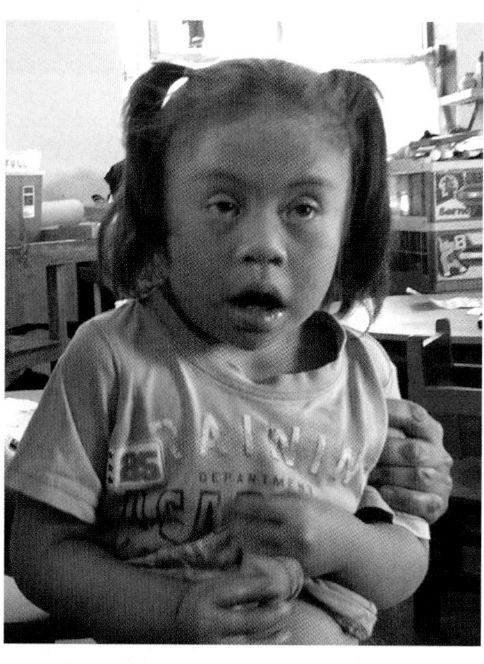

FIGURE 221-7 Epicanthal folds, upward-slanting palpebral fissures, and flat nasal bridge in a 3-year-old girl with Down syndrome. This girl was living in shelter for children with disabilities in a remote part of Peru and was found to have a grade 4 pansystolic murmur and signs of congestive heart failure, likely from an undiagnosed ventricular septal defect. (*Used with permission from Sangeeta Krishna, MD.*)

LABORATORY TESTING

- In a newborn with no prenatal testing, if clinical exam is suspicious for DS (hypotonia, craniofacial abnormalities, etc.), a blood sample should be sent for fluorescent in situ hybridization (FISH), which detects trisomy 21 and is available within 1 to 2 days. A positive test requires confirmation with a complete cytogenetic analysis which detects translocations.[2]
- Once the diagnosis of DS is established, the newborn should receive a thorough physical exam evaluating for duodenal and anorectal atresia, problems with feeding, stridor/wheezing, congenital cataracts using red reflex testing, and hearing loss via brainstem auditory evoked response.[2]
- A CBC should be obtained to assess for hematologic abnormalities including transient myeloproliferative disorder, which increases the risk for later development of leukemia and polycythemia. TSH and free thyroxine should also be drawn to screen for congenital hypothyroidism.[2]

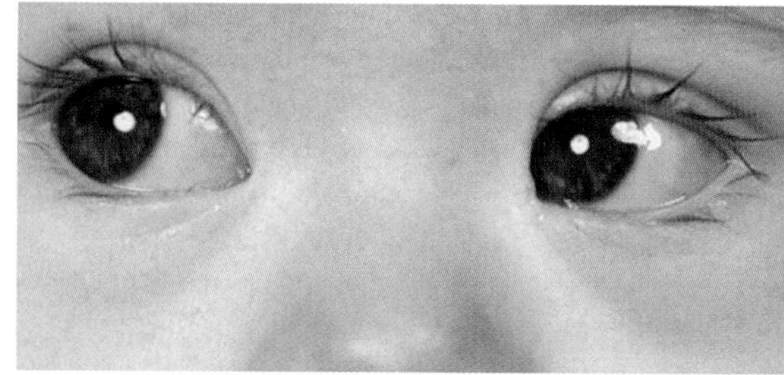

FIGURE 221-8 Speckled white spots on the iris (Brushfield spots) in an infant with Down syndrome. These are present in 90 percent of infants with Down syndrome but are also seen in infants without Down syndrome. (*Used with permission from Cleveland Clinic Children's Hospital Photo Files.*)

IMAGING

- All infants with DS should receive an echocardiogram to evaluate for congenital heart disease.[2]
- If clinically indicated, a swallow study can assess for feeding difficulties, laryngoscopy can assess for airway abnormalities, and abdominal x-ray can diagnose duodenal atresia (**Figure 221-3**).[2]

DIFFERENTIAL DIAGNOSIS

- Physical exam findings in isolation, such as simian crease, epicanthal folds, etc., may be variants of normal and may not indicate DS. Rely on clinical suspicion to judge whether or not cytogenetic testing may be useful.
- Other conditions to consider in the differential are trisomy 18 which presents with typical clinical features including rocker bottom feet and severe neurodevelopmental delay.
- Zellweger syndrome, a peroxisomal disorder, presents with hypotonia and abnormal elevation of very long chain fatty acids, especially those with 26 carbon atoms, and an increased ratio of C26 to C22 fatty acids in the plasma, as well as fibroblasts and amniocytes.

MANAGEMENT

- Management of a patient with DS should focus on education of the family, early screenings to allow for early interventions for any anomalies associated with DS, and routine follow-up at well-child visits to screen for conditions associated with DS.

NONPHARMACOLOGIC

- Parents should be educated about what to expect in their child. Children with DS are at risk for increased susceptibility for respiratory tract infections. Those with hemodynamically significant congenital heart lesions or comorbid conditions should receive respiratory syncytial virus prophylaxis between birth and 12 months old.[2] SOR Ⓐ
- All parents should be educated about atlantoaxial instability and should warn providers to avoid excessive extension or flexion of the cervical spine during procedures.[2]
- At annual appointments, parents should be asked whether their children have frequent ear infections, drainage from the ear, or hearing loss. Patients should be referred to otolaryngology as necessary.[2]
- Annually, parents should also be asked about presence of obstructive sleep apnea. A sleep study can be ordered for symptomatic patients but it is recommended that all patients undergo a sleep study by 4 years of age. Patients found to have obstructive sleep apnea should be referred to otolaryngology and/or pulmonology.[2]
- Parents should also be asked whether their child has seizures with referral to neurology as needed.[2]
- Refer children with DS to ophthalmology within 6 months of age to evaluate for strabismus or cataracts. Ensure that patients follow-up with ophthalmology since 50 percent patients will develop refractive errors leading to amblyopia at <5 years of age.[2]
- At well-child visits, patients should also be screened for any indications of heart failure including failure to thrive, feeding difficulties, or tachypnea and asked about seizures.[2]
- Annual labs should include TSH to screen for thyroid dysfunction and CBC and reticulocyte hemoglobin (CHr) concentrations to monitor for iron-deficiency anemia. In children with DS, mean corpuscular volume is elevated in up to 45 percent of patients, and serum ferritin may be elevated from chronic inflammation. Thus, neither of these are useful screening tools for iron deficiency.[2]
- Assess patients for behavioral or social issues. Refer to child psychiatry if there is high suspicion for autism or attention-deficit/hyperactivity disorder, for early intervention.[2]
- Parents should be referred to support groups and given resources to help with behavioral and neurocognitive development of the patient.[2]

MEDICATIONS

- There are no specific medications for DS. Treat associated conditions with medications specific to the condition.

SURGERY

- Children with cataracts may undergo cataract surgery; those with congenital heart disease may require surgical correction; those with intestinal atresia require abdominal surgeries.
- Atlantoaxial subluxation poses an extra anesthetic risk during elective surgeries, especially during intubations, and should be kept in mind.

REFERRAL

- By 6 months of age, all children with DS should be referred to ophthalmology for evaluation of strabismus, cataracts, and amblyopia.
- By 4 years of age, all children with DS should have obtained a sleep study to assess for obstructive sleep apnea.
- For abnormalities detected on echocardiogram, children with DS should be referred to cardiology.
- Children with elevated white blood cell count or hemoglobin/hematocrit should be referred to hematology/oncology.
- For children with stridor/wheezing or signs of obstructive sleep apnea, refer to pulmonology.
- Children with recurrent otitis media should be referred to otolaryngology.
- Children with gastrointestinal atresia should be referred to general surgery.
- Children who have difficulty swallowing or are suspected of having aspiration pneumonia should be referred to pulmonology and may require gastrostomy tube placement by surgery to maintain feeds.

PREVENTION AND SCREENING

- Screening for DS is routine in prenatal care and is offered to women of all ages.
- The first trimester screen examines—Nuchal translucency on ultrasound and maternal serum levels of β-hCG and pregnancy associated plasma protein (PAPP-A). Increased nuchal translucency, high β-hCG, and low PAPP-A are associated with DS. Taking these factors and maternal age into account, the risk of the fetus having DS is calculated. This screen has a sensitivity of 82 to 87 percent. False positive rates are higher with increasing maternal age.[6,8]

- Mothers at increased risk for having a child with DS can choose to have diagnostic testing via chorionic villus sampling in the first trimester or can proceed with the quad screen (maternal serum levels of β-hCG, unconjugated estriol, alpha-fetoprotein, and inhibin A) for a revised risk assessment.[6,8]
- Mothers who missed the first trimester screen or would like a final risk assessment can undergo the quad screen in the second trimester. DS fetuses tend to have decreased alpha-fetoprotein and estriol and increased inhibin A and β-hCG. Similar to the first trimester screen, the patient's risk of having a baby with DS is calculated based on this data and patient data. The quad screen alone has a sensitivity of 80 percent, but when combined with first semester screen, the two tests have a sensitivity of 95 percent with a 5 percent false positive rate.[6,8]
- Mothers with a risk of having a DS baby exceeding 1 in 270 (the risk of miscarriage with diagnostic testing) and who desire a definitive diagnosis can proceed with amniocentesis during the second trimester. Amniocentesis allows for definitive chromosomal analysis.[6,8]

PROGNOSIS

- With routine care and behavioral support, most individuals with DS without severe neurocognitive deficits can participate in normal activities of daily living.[9]
- Individuals with DS have a decreased lifespan (50 to 60 years) with an increased susceptibility for earlier development of Alzheimer's.[3]
- Through childhood (infancy to age 20 years), the risk for mortality was highest among patients with congenital heart disease both in the immediate post-natal period and through age 20 years.[9]
- Survival of non-Hispanic Caucasian children who have DS is higher than non-Hispanic African American children with DS in the post-natal period and through age 10 years.[9]

FOLLOW-UP

- Children with DS should follow routine well-child visits and see their pediatricians at least annually.
- Children with DS should follow-up with pediatric specialties as determined by the individual specialty depending on patient situation.

PATIENT EDUCATION

- Educate parents about what to expect with their child—Hypotonia, delayed teething, and lower intelligence quotients. All parents should understand the importance of warning other providers about possible atlantoaxial instability during procedures.
- Patients and their families should be educated on signs to watch out for that may indicate development of conditions associated with DS—Hypothyroidism, hearing loss, or middle ear disease, obstructive sleep apnea, heart failure, vision problems, and hematologic derangements including anemia and lymphoproliferative disorders.
- Taking care of a child with disabilities, while rewarding, can often be very taxing on the family. Ensure that the family is in touch with resources/support groups that can help parents.

PATIENT RESOURCES

- National Down Syndrome Society—**www.ndss.org**.
- National Down Syndrome Congress—**www.ndsccenter.org**.
- For families with a new diagnosis of DS—**www.brightertomorrows.org**.
- Pamphlet for new families—**www.ndss.org/PageFiles/2981/NDSS-NPP_English_LR.pdf**.
- Location of support groups—**www.ndss.org/Resources/Local-Support**.

PROVIDER RESOURCES

- Prenatal Diagnosis—**www.guideline.gov/content.aspx?id=10921**.
- **http://emedicine.medscape.com/article/943216**.
- Management of DS patient: Bull MJ, Committee on Genetics. Health supervision for children with Down syndrome. *Pediatrics*. 2011;128(2):393-406. **http://pediatrics.aappublications.org/content/128/2/393.full.pdf**.

REFERENCES

1. Hernandez D, Fisher EM: Down syndrome genetics: unravelling a multifactorial disorder. *Hum Mol Genet*. 1996;5:1411-1416.
2. Bull MJ: Committee on Genetics. Health supervision for children with Down syndrome. *Pediatrics*. 2011;128(2):393-406.
3. Roizen NJ, Patterson D: Down's syndrome. *Lancet*. 2003;361(9365):1281-1289.
4. Resta RG: Changing demographics of advanced maternal age (AMA) and the impact on the predicted incidence of Down syndrome in the US: Implications for prenatal screening and genetic counseling. *Am J Med Genet A*. 2005;133A(1):31-36.
5. Parker SE, Mai CT, Canfield MA, et al. Updated National Birth Prevalence estimates for selected birth defects in the United States, 2004-2006. *Birt Defects Res A Clin Mol Teratol*. 2010;88(12):1008-1016.
6. Natoli JL, Ackerman DL, McDermott S, Edwards JG: Prenatal diagnosis of Down syndrome: a systematic review of termination rates (1995–2011). *Prenat Diagn*. 2012;32(2):142-153.
7. Sherman SL, Allen EG, Bean LH, Freeman SB: Epidemiology of Down syndrome. *Ment Retard Dev Disabil Res Rev*. 2007;13(3):221-227.
8. Driscoll DA, Gross S: Prenatal Screening for Aneuploidy. *N Engl J Med*. 2009;360(24):2556-2562.
9. Kucik JE, Shin M, Siffel C, Marengo L, Correa A: Congenital Anomaly Multistate Prevalence and Survival Collaborative. Trends in survival among children with Down syndrome in 10 regions of the United States. *Pediatrics*. 2013;131(1):e27-36.

222 TURNER SYNDROME

Elumalai Appachi, MD, MRCP

PATIENT STORY

A 6-year-old girl is brought to the pediatrician because of swelling in her lower legs that was noted by her mother over the past few weeks. The child has otherwise been well. Review of the growth parameters showed the girl to be at less than the 5th percentile for height. The girl exhibited edema of the lower extremities (right > left), low set ears, ptosis, and mild micrognathia (**Figures 222-1** and **222-2**). The pediatrician suspected Turner syndrome and referred the child to a pediatric endocrinologist, who confirmed the diagnosis with a karyotype (45, XO pattern). The child and family received counseling and education, and the girl was treated with growth hormones and has done well. Screening tests for renal and cardiac abnormalities were normal.

INTRODUCTION

Turner syndrome is an absence of one of the X chromosome (partial or complete) with a resultant female phenotype of short stature, lack of normal sexual maturation, and diverse somatic findings.

SYNONYMS

Gonadal dysgenesis, Haploinsufficiency of the X chromosome (45, XO karyotype), Bonnevie-Ullrich syndrome, and monosomy X.

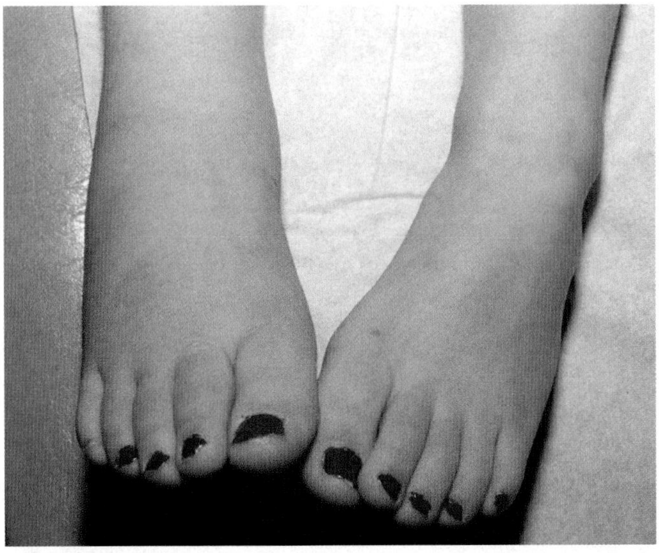

FIGURE 222-1 Lymphedema in the lower extremities, which is especially prominent on the right, in a 6-year-old girl with Turner syndrome. This was the presenting feature of this syndrome in this girl. (*Used with permission from Camille Sabella, MD.*)

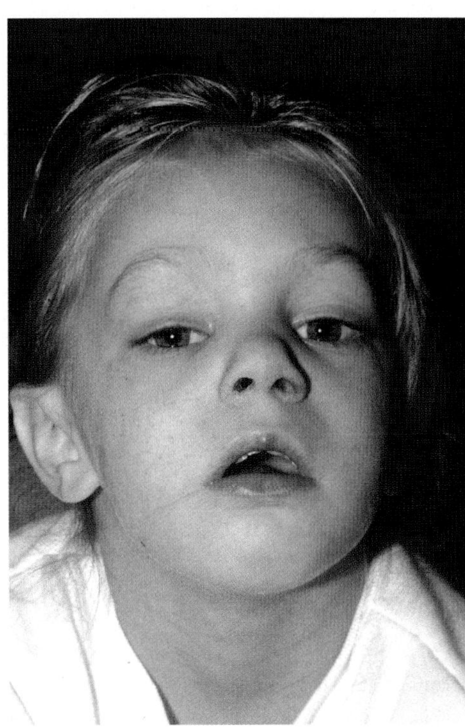

FIGURE 222-2 Low set ears, low hairline, mild ptosis, and small lower jaw in the same 6-year-old girl in **Figure 222-1**. (*Used with permission from Camille Sabella, MD.*)

EPIDEMIOLOGY

- Turner syndrome is the most common sex-linked chromosomal abnormality.
- Turner syndrome is a common cause of first-trimester spontaneous abortions, accounting for approximately 20 percent of the spontaneous abortions caused by chromosomal defects.
- Incidence is 1/2,500 to 1/5,000 live births; only 5 to 10 percent of affected fetuses survive to birth.[1]
- There are roughly 50,000 to 75,000 cases total in the US

ETIOLOGY AND PATHOPHYSIOLOGY

- Turner syndrome is a chromosomal abnormality caused by complete or partial absence of the second sex chromosome in a woman (most common karyotype is 45, XO) or mosaicism (e.g., karyotype 46, XX/45, XO or 46, XY/45, XO).
- Not related to maternal age.

DIAGNOSIS

The diagnosis of Turner syndrome is suspected on clinical features and confirmed by chromosomal analysis. Any girl with pathological short stature should have a karyotype performed to rule out Turner syndrome.[2,3]

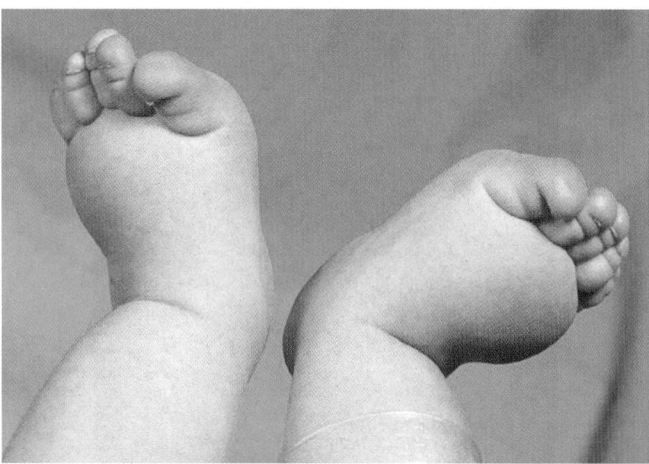

FIGURE 222-3 Lymphedema in a newborn infant who was found to have Turner syndrome. Thirty percent of infants with Turner syndrome will have lymphedema at birth. (*Used with permission from Cleveland Clinic Children's Hospital Photo Files.*)

CLINICAL FEATURES

- Can be identified at birth by the presence of lymphedema and excessive skin folds in the neck—Present in 30 percent of cases (**Figures 222-3** and **222-4**).[4]
- Growth failure and short stature.[2]
- Lymphedema of the limbs and neck usually occurs during infancy but may occur later, including during adolescence (**Figures 222-1**, **222-3**, and **222-4**).

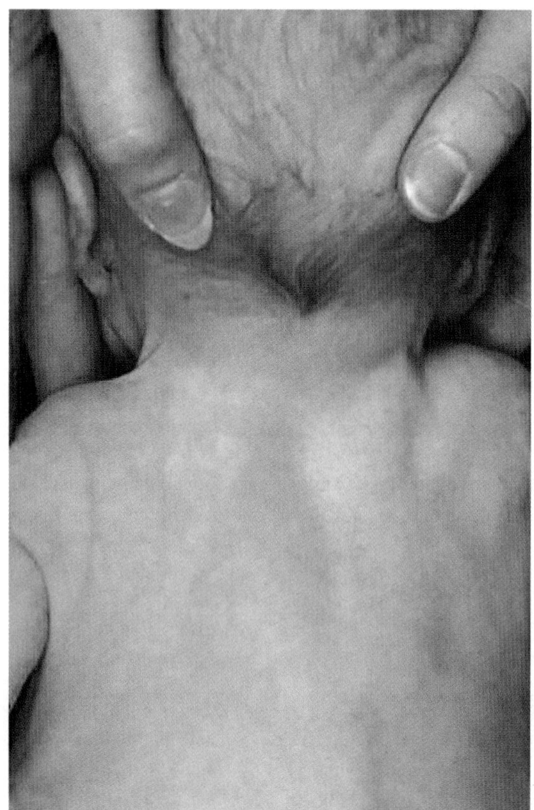

FIGURE 222-4 Loose skin folds and webbing of the neck in a newborn with Turner syndrome. (*Used with permission from Cleveland Clinic Children's Hospital Photo Files.*)

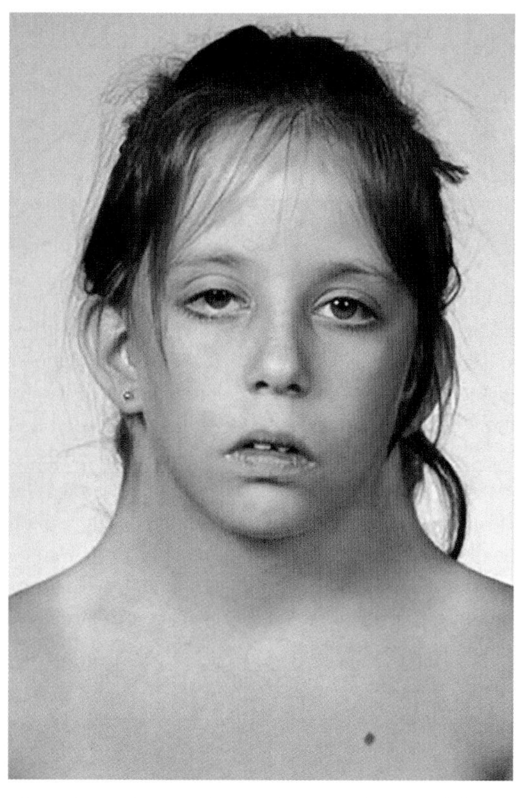

FIGURE 222-5 Prominent webbing of the neck in an adolescent with Turner syndrome. Also note the low set ears, low hairline, and mild ptosis. (*Used with permission from Cleveland Clinic Children's Hospital Photo Files.*)

- Loose skin folds and webbing of the neck (**Figure 222-5**).
- Broad, shield-like chest and wide spaced nipples (**Figures 222-6** and **222-7**).
- Shortened fourth and fifth metacarpals and metatarsals—Found in 50 percent of patients.
- Atypical facies that may include prominent or low-set ears, low hairline, ptosis, and hypertelorism (**Figures 222-2** and **222-5**).

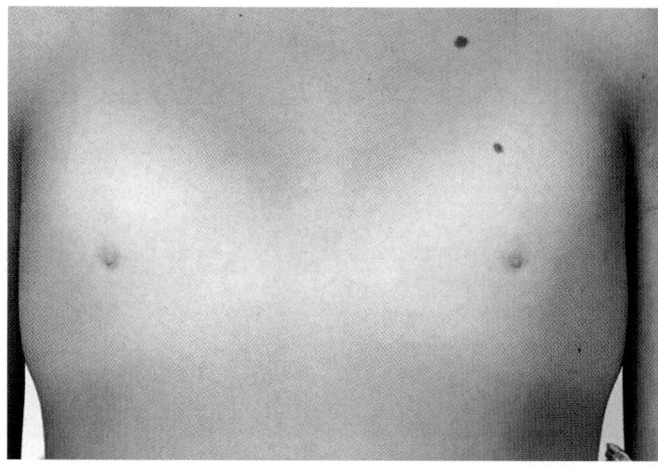

FIGURE 222-6 Wide spaced nipples and broad, shield-like chest, in the same girl with Turner syndrome in **Figure 222-5**. (*Used with permission from Cleveland Clinic Children's Hospital Photo Files.*)

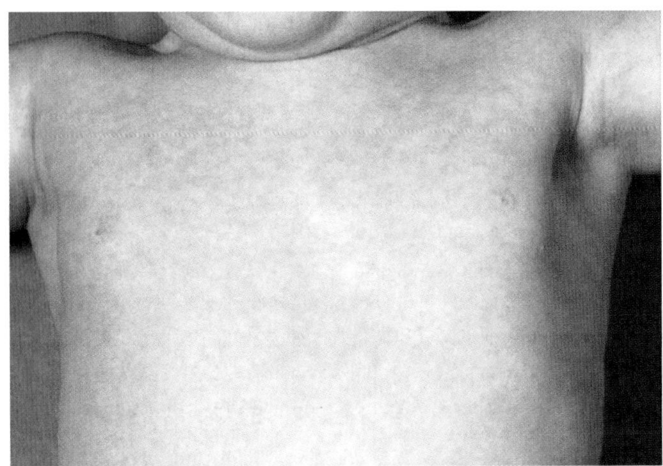

FIGURE 222-7 Wide-spaced nipples and loose skin folds in the neck visible in an infant with Turner syndrome. (*Used with permission from Cleveland Clinic Children's Hospital Photo Files.*)

- Cardiovascular abnormalities, such as bicuspid aortic valve, dilated aortic root, or coarctation of aorta (50%), especially if there is presence of webbed neck.[5]
- Early menopause.
- Renal anomalies, such as horseshoe kidneys, pelvic kidney, UPJ obstruction, idiopathic hypertension, and renal infections.
- Recurrent otitis media (75%) mild neurological problems.
- Hearing defects.[6]
- Bone abnormalities.
- Feeding problems.
- Hypothyroidism and thyroiditis.
- Delayed onset of menstruation.
- Infertility.
- Learning problems.

LABORATORY TESTING

- Karyotype should be performed to confirm the diagnosis.
- Thyroid function tests should be obtained to screen for thyroid dysfunction.
- Audiology screening should be performed in all patients with Turner syndrome.

IMAGING

- Echocardiogram should be done to screen for cardiovascular abnormalities.
- Renal ultrasound should be done to screen for renal anomalies.

DIFFERENTIAL DIAGNOSIS

- Noonan Syndrome—Mainly seen in males who have a similar phenotype to Turner syndrome. It can be seen in females (see Chapter 226, Noonan Syndrome).
- Congenital lymphedema—Findings present at birth, but not associated with other features of Turner syndrome and associated with a normal karyotype.

MANAGEMENT

NONPHARMACOLOGIC

- Audiology screening and subsequent hearing aids may be necessary for hearing defects.
- Counseling and monitoring of the child and the family is a vital part of the management.

MEDICATIONS

- Growth hormone therapy is indicated for all patients and should be instituted in early childhood to maximize growth potential.[7–12] SOR Ⓐ
- Hormone replacement therapy with estrogen should be started in adolescence when follicle-stimulating hormone and luteinizing hormone levels are increased; preferably, therapy should not begin until age 13 to 15 years of age to maximize the linear growth.[13–15] SOR Ⓐ
- During adolescence, estrogen is cycled with progesterone to achieve sexual maturity and to maximize bone development, including the prevention of osteoporosis.
- Treatment with thyroid hormone replacement may be required for hypothyroidism.
- Treatment for obesity may be required, and lifestyle education with advice on diet and exercise must be included to prevent complications such as diabetes, osteoporosis, and hypertension.

SURGERY

- Gonadectomy (gonadal ablation) may be indicated for patients with Turner syndrome who have Y chromosomal mosaicism, to eliminate the risk of malignancy in the streak gonad.
- Patients who have coarctation of the aorta or bicuspid aortic valve may need surgical repair.

REFERRAL

- A multidisciplinary team approach, including endocrinologists, geneticists, and nutritionists, is recommended for the management of patients with Turner syndrome.
- Appropriate referral is made based on the age at presentation.

PREVENTION AND SCREENING

- Turner syndrome may be suspected during prenatal ultrasound if there is a cystic hygroma or edema of the limbs.
- Prenatal diagnosis to confirm the diagnosis can be made by chorionic villus sampling or amniocentesis.

PROGNOSIS

- Normal life expectancy.
- Adult height is well below the average even with growth hormone therapy.[16,17]
- The majority of patients with Turner syndrome are infertile, although pregnancy has been achieved with the use of assisted reproductive techniques.

FOLLOW-UP

- Patients need speech evaluation especially when presented with hearing defects.
- Cardiology follow up with echocardiography should be done annually or twice a year.
- Thyroid function should be checked annually or twice a year.
- Regular follow up with endocrinologist and regular monitoring of follicle-stimulating hormone and luteinizing hormone levels should be performed at 10 years of age onward.
- Evaluate for secondary sexual development at adolescence.
- Discuss social adaptation, and provide support group contacts.

PATIENT RESOURCES

- Turner Syndrome Society of the US—**www.turner-syndrome-us.org**.
- Alliance of Genetic Support Groups—**http://www.geneticalliance.org**.

PROVIDER RESOURCES

- **http://ghr.nlm.nih.gov/condition/turner-syndrome**.
- **http://rarediseases.info.nih.gov/gard/7831/resources/resources/1**.

REFERENCES

1. Sybert VP. Turner syndrome. In: Cassiday SB, Allanson JA, eds. *Management of Genetic Syndromes*. Hoboken, NJ. John Wiley & Sons; 2005:589-606.
2. Styne DM. New aspects in the diagnosis and treatment of pubertal disorders. *Pediatr Clin North Am.* 1993;44:505.
3. Saenger P, Wikland KA, Conway GS, et al. Recommendations for the diagnosis and management of Turner syndrome. *J Clin Endocrinol Metab*. 2001;86:3061-3069.
4. Bellini C, Boccardo F, Campisi C, et al. Lymphatic dysplasias in newborns and children: the role of lymphoscintigraphy. *J Pediatr*. 2008;152:587-589.
5. Bondy CA. Congenital cardiovascular disease in Turner syndrome. *Congenit Heart Dis*. 2008;3:2-15.
6. Morimoto N, Tanaka T, Taiji H, et al. Hearing loss in Turner syndrome. *J Pediatr*. 2006;149:697-701.
7. Bondy CA. Turner Syndrome Study Group. Care of girls and women with Turner syndrome: a guideline of the Turner Syndrome Study Group. *J Clin Endocrinol Metab*. 2007;92:10-25.
8. Donaldson MD, Gault EJ, Tan KW, Dunger DB. Optimising management in Turner syndrome: from infancy to adult transfer. Arch Dis Child. 2006;91:513-520.
9. Reiter EO, Blethen SL, Baptista J, Price L. Early initiation of growth hormone treatment allows age-appropriate estrogen use in Turner's syndrome. *J Clin Endocrinol Metab*. 2001;86:1936-1941.
10. Davenport ML, Crowe BJ, Travers SH, et al. Growth hormone treatment of early growth failure in toddlers with Turner syndrome: a randomized, controlled, multicenter trial. *J Clin Endocrinol Metab*. 2007;92:3406-3416.
11. Bolar K, Hoffman AR, Maneatis T, Lippe B. Long-term safety of recombinant human growth hormone in Turner syndrome. *J Clin Endocrinol Metab*. 2008;93:344-351.
12. Carel JC. Growth hormone in Turner syndrome: twenty years after, what can we tell our patients? *J Clin Endocrinol Metab*. 2005;90:3793-3794.
13. Drobac S, Rubin K, Rogol AD, Rosenfield RL. A workshop on pubertal hormone replacement options in the United States. *J Pediatr Endocrinol Metab*. 2006;19:55-64.
14. Piippo S, Lenko H, Kainulainen P, Sipilä I. Use of percutaneous estrogen gel for induction of puberty in girls with Turner syndrome. *J Clin Endocrinol Metab*. 2004;89:3241-3247.
15. Ankarberg-Lindgren C, Elfving M, Wikland KA, Norjavaara E. Nocturnal application of transdermal estradiol patches produces levels of estradiol that mimic those seen at the onset of spontaneous puberty in girls. *J Clin Endocrinol Metab*. 2001;86:3039-3044.
16. Quigley CA. Growth hormone treatment of non-growth hormone-deficient growth disorders. *Endocrinol Metab Clin North Am*. 2007;36:131-186.
17. Plotnick L, Attie KM, Blethen SL, et al. Growth hormone treatment of girls with Turner syndrome: the National Cooperative Growth Study experience. *Pediatrics* 1998;102:479.

223 MARFAN SYNDROME

Elumalai Appachi, MD, MRCP

PATIENT STORY

A 14-year-old girl is brought to her pediatrician for a routine health maintenance visit. The pediatrician notes that she is tall for her age, has long, slender fingers, hypermobile joints, and that her arm span is longer than her body span (**Figures 223-1** to **223-3**). She also has a high arched palate and a systolic murmur. The pediatrician refers the girl to a cardiologist, who performs an echocardiogram, which reveals mitral valve prolapse without regurgitation, and dilatation of the aortic root. The pediatrician and cardiologist suspect that the child has Marfan syndrome and order a test for fibrillin 1 mutation, which confirms the diagnosis. Her pediatrician plans a multidisciplinary team for the girl, including baseline and follow-up ophthalmology examinations, and close follow-up visits with the cardiologist, orthopedist, and geneticist.

INTRODUCTION

Marfan syndrome (MFS) is a heritable disorder of connective tissue resulting from mutations in the gene encoding the extracellular matrix protein fibrillin 1(FBN1). Individuals with MFS manifest variable clinical features, which often involve the skeletal, cardiovascular, and ocular systems.

EPIDEMIOLOGY

- The incidence of this disorder is about 1 per 5,000 to 10,000 births.[1]
- MFS is inherited in an autosomal dominant manner; thus, there is a 50 percent chance of an offspring inheriting the condition from the affected parent.
- Approximately 1/3 of cases are sporadic due to *de novo* mutations; new mutations are often associated with advanced paternal age.

ETIOLOGY AND PATHOPHYSIOLOGY

- MFS is associated with abnormal biosynthesis of fibrillin-1, which is the major constituent of microfibrils. Mutations in FBN1 are found in about 95 percent of patients who meet the diagnostic criteria for Marfan syndrome.[2,3]
- The FBN1 locus resides on the long arm of chromosome 15 (15q21) and the gene is composed of 65 exons. More than 1,000 mutations distributed throughout FBN1 have been identified, many being unique to a given family.[4,5]
- The condition results from a structural deficiency of connective tissues. The decreased fibrillin-1 leads to a primary derangement of elastic fiber deposition, along with elastic fiber fragmentation. The decreased elastin in the aorta, skin, and other connective tissue is responsible for accelerated degeneration of tissue resulting in the clinical manifestations.
- Mutations in FBN1 are associated with a wide phenotypic spectrum ranging from severe rapidly progressing neonatal manifestations, manifestations that present in childhood and early adulthood, to isolated features such as ectopia lentis or skeletal manifestations.

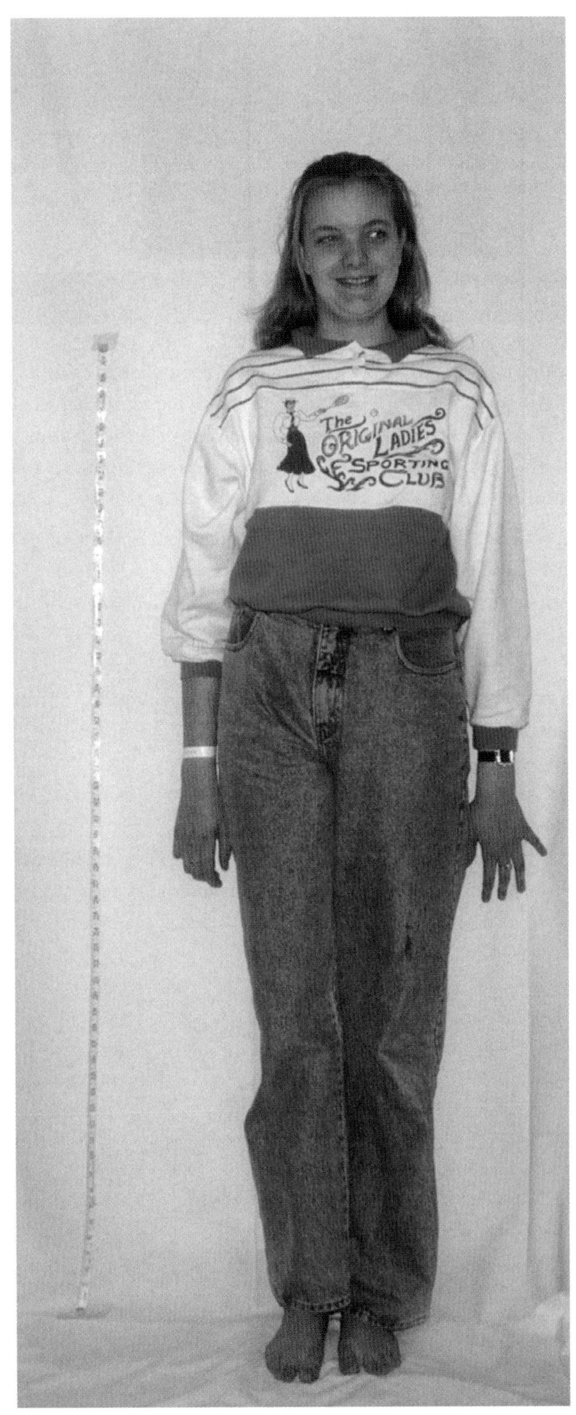

FIGURE 223-1 Tall stature, reduced upper to lower segment ratio, and increased arm-span-to-height ratio in a 14-year-old girl with Marfan syndrome. (*Used with permission from Elumalai Appachi, MD.*)

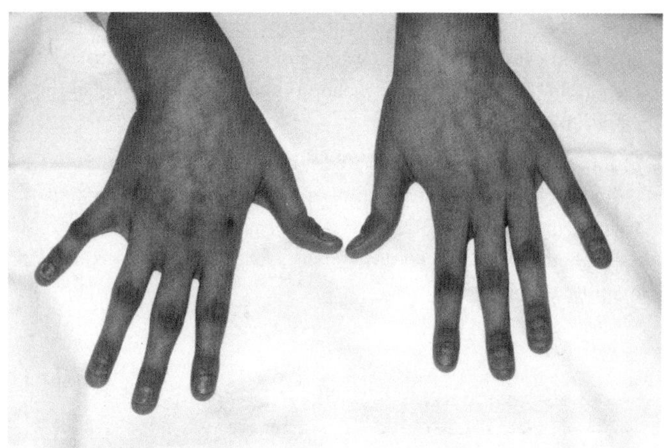

FIGURE 223-2 Arachnodactyly (long, slender fingers) in the same girl as in **Figure 223-1**. This is a non-specific feature of Marfan syndrome. *(Used with permission from Elumalai Appachi, MD.)*

DIAGNOSIS

- The diagnosis of MFS is based on well-defined clinical criteria. Genetic testing of FBN1 should be reserved for those patients in whom there is strong suspicion of the diagnosis, or for patients who are suspected of having the disorder but who may not meet full clinical criteria.[6]
- The revised Ghent diagnostic criteria[7] outlines a *definitive* diagnosis of MFS when any of the following are present:
  - Aortic root dilation (≥2 z score) and ectopia lentis (z score is a standard measure of aortic root diameter at the sinus of Valsalva based on body surface area).
  - Aortic root dilation (≥2 z score) and FBN1 mutation.
  - Aortic root dilation (≥2 z score) and systemic score ≥7 (see the following for scoring system).
  - Ectopia lentis and FBN1 mutation known to be associated with Marfan syndrome.
  - Positive family history of Marfan syndrome and ectopia lentis.
  - Positive family history of Marfan syndrome and systemic score ≥7.

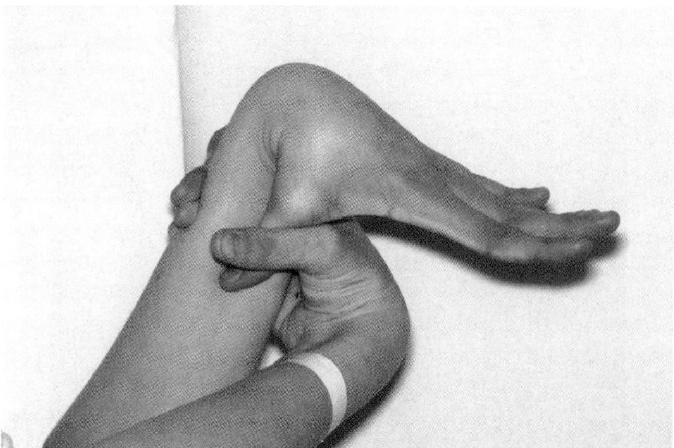

FIGURE 223-3 Hypermobility of the thumb joint in Marfan syndrome illustrated by the same girl as **Figures 223-1** and **223-2**. *(Used with permission from Elumalai Appachi, MD.)*

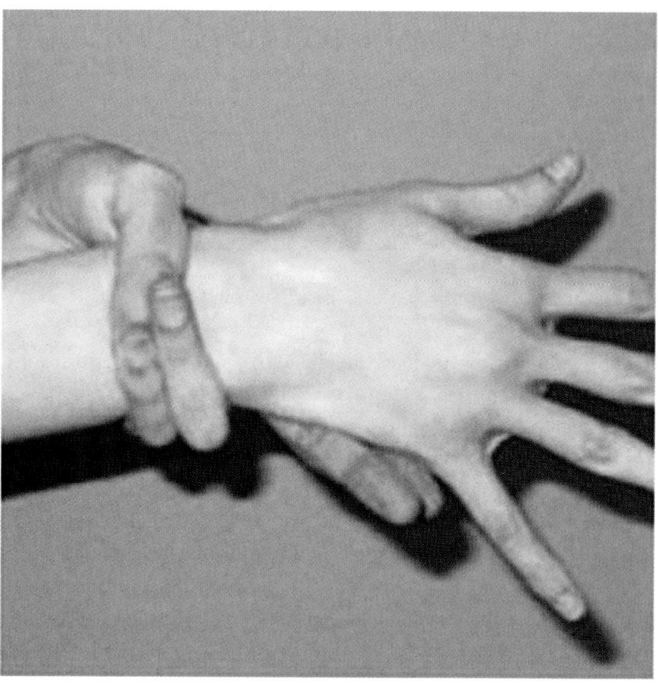

FIGURE 223-4 "Wrist" sign, which is a full overlap of the distal phalanges of the thumb and fifth finger when wrapped around the contralateral wrist, in a patient with Marfan syndrome. *(Used with permission from Rudolph CD, Rudolph AM, Lister G, First LR, Gershon AA: Rudolph's Pediatrics, 22nd edition. www.accesspediatrics.com. Figure 181-1B, New York: McGraw-Hill.)*

  - Positive family history of Marfan syndrome and aortic root dilation (≥3 z score) in those <20 y of age or ≥2 z score in those >20 y of age.
- A *potential* diagnosis is made when there is an FBN1 mutation with aortic root dilation with a z score <3 in those <20 years of age.
- The systemic scoring system used for the diagnosis of MFS includes:
  - Wrist and thumb sign (3 points; **Figures 223-4** and **223-5**).
  - Wrist or thumb sign (1 point).
  - Pectus carinatum (2 points; **Figure 223-6**).
  - Pectus excavatum (1 point; **Figure 223-6**).
  - Hindfoot deformity (2 points).
  - Pes planus (1 point; **Figure 223-7**).
  - Pneumothorax (2 points).
  - Dural ectasia (2 points).
  - Protrusio acetabulae (2 points).
  - Reduced upper to lower segment ratio and increased arm-span-to-height ratio (1 point; **Figure 223-1**).
  - Scoliosis or thoracolumbar kyphosis (1 point; **Figure 223-8**).
  - Reduced elbow extension (1 point).
  - Craniofacial features such as dolichoencephaly, downward-slanting palpebral fissures, endophthalmos, retrognathia, and malar hypoplasia (1 point if at least 3 of these are present).
  - Skin striae (1 point; **Figure 223-9**).
  - Myopia (1 point).
  - Mitral valve prolapse (1 point).

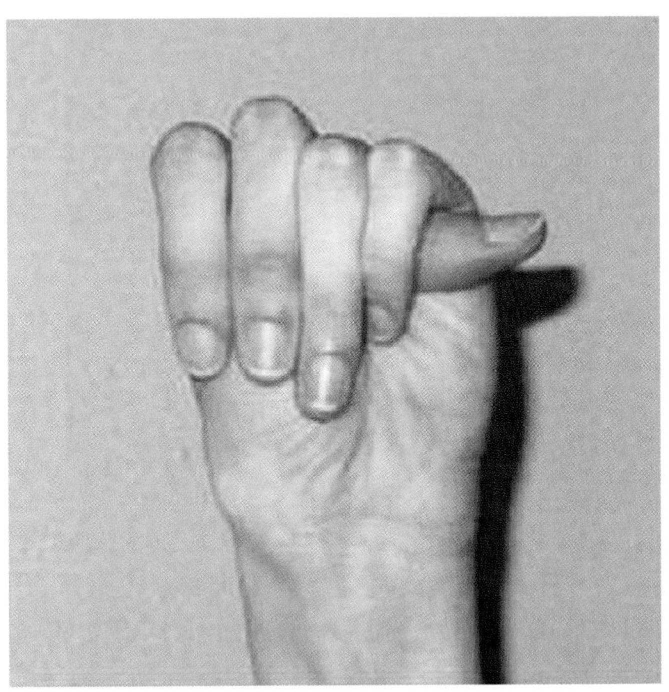

FIGURE 223-5 "Thumb" sign, the distal phalanx of the thumb fully extending beyond the ulnar border of the hand when folded across the palm, in a patient with Marfan syndrome. (*Used with permission from Rudolph CD, Rudolph AM, Lister G, First LR, Gershon AA: Rudolph's Pediatrics, 22nd edition. www.accesspediatrics.com. Figure 181-1C, New York: McGraw-Hill.*)

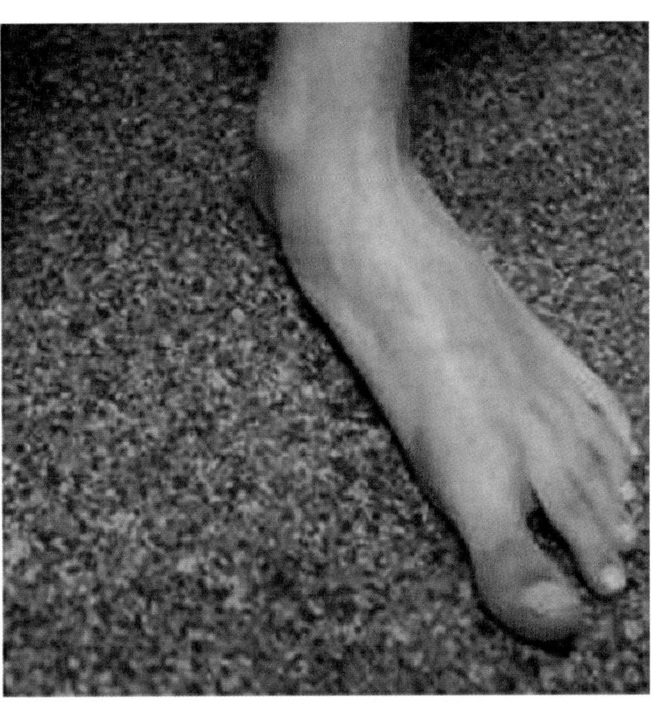

FIGURE 223-7 Pes planus (flat foot) in a patient with Marfan syndrome. (*Used with permission from Rudolph CD, Rudolph AM, Lister G, First LR, Gershon AA: Rudolph's Pediatrics, 22nd edition. www.accesspediatrics.com. Figure 181-1 F, New York: McGraw-Hill.*)

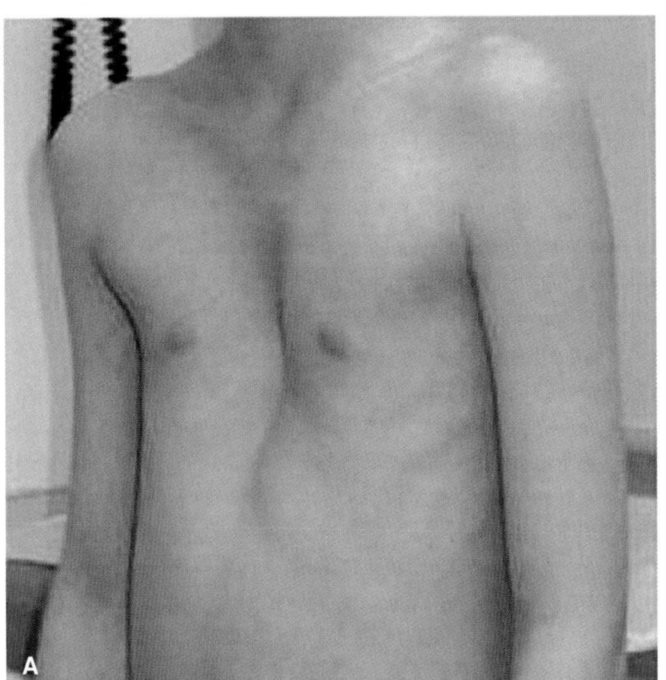

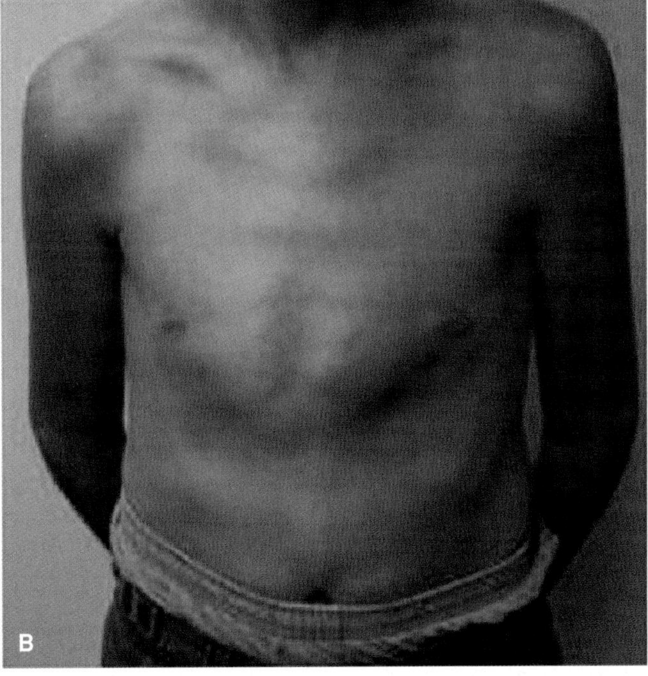

FIGURE 223-6 Pectus excavatum (**A**) and pectus carinatum (**B**) resulting from overgrowth of the ribs in two patients with Marfan syndrome. (*Used with permission from Rudolph CD, Rudolph AM, Lister G, First LR, Gershon AA: Rudolph's Pediatrics, 22nd edition. www.accesspediatrics.com. Figure 181-1 D and E, New York: McGraw-Hill.*)

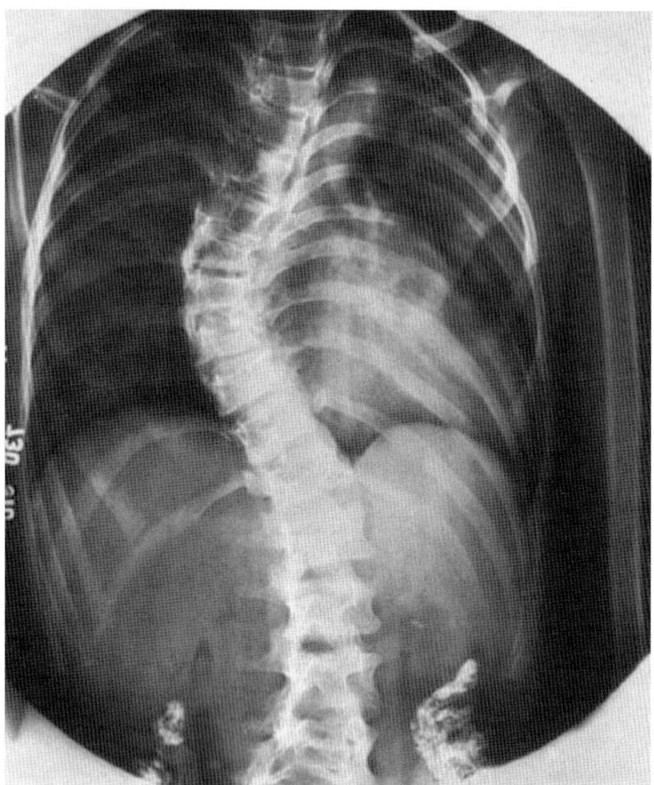

FIGURE 223-8 Severe scoliosis in a patient with Marfan syndrome. (*Used with permission from Cleveland Clinic Children's Hospital Photo Files.*)

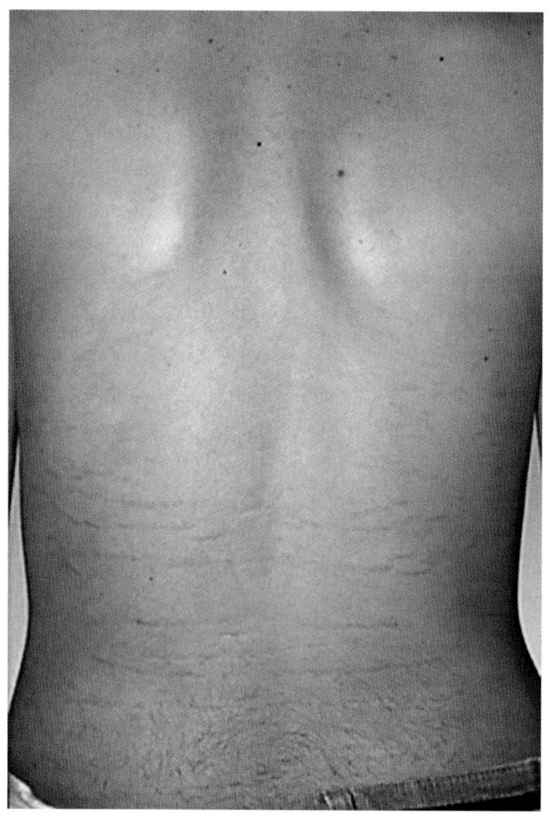

FIGURE 223-9 Horizontal skin striae in a patient with Marfan syndrome. These are a result of rapid growth and typically perpendicular to the growth axis. (*Used with permission from Cleveland Clinic Children's Hospital Photo Files.*)

CLINICAL FEATURES

▶ The skeletal system

- Excessive growth of long bones is common, typically resulting in tall stature.
- Disproportionate growth of skeletal systems results in an arm span >1.05 times the height, or a reduced upper to lower segment ratio (in the absence of severe scoliosis; **Figure 223-1**).
- Arachnodactyly (long spider like fingers) is generally a subjective finding (**Figure 223-2**). The combination of long fingers and loose joints leads to the characteristic:
    - Walker-Murdoch or "Wrist" sign—Full overlap of the distal phalanges of the thumb and fifth finger when wrapped around the contralateral wrist (**Figure 223-4**).
    - The Steinberg or "Thumb" sign—Distal phalanx of the thumb fully extends beyond the ulnar border of the hand when folded across the palm, with or without active assistance by the patient or examiner (**Figure 223-5**).
- Patients may have overgrowth of the ribs, pushing the sternum anteriorly (pectus carinatum) or posteriorly (pectus excavatum; **Figure 223-6**).
- Thoracolumbar scoliosis is present in about half of individuals with MFS and can range from mild to severe and can be progressive (**Figure 223-8**).
- Pes planus (flat feet) is commonly present and varies from mild and asymptomatic to severe deformity (**Figure 223-7**).

▶ Cardiac system

- Involvement of the cardiovascular system is the major cause of morbidity and mortality in MFS.
- Aortic aneurysm and dissection remain the most life-threatening manifestations. This finding is age dependent, prompting life-long monitoring by echocardiography or other imaging modalities.
- The aortic dilation is progressive over time, with the majority of cases becoming evident before 18 years of age.
- Aortic valve dysfunction is generally a late occurrence, attributed to stretching of the aortic annulus by an expanding root aneurysm.
- Atrioventricular (AV) valves are most often affected. Thickening of the AV valves is common and often associated with prolapse of the mitral and/or tricuspid valves. Variable degrees of regurgitation may be present.
- Other cardiovascular manifestations include ventricular and supraventricular arrhythmias and dilated cardiomyopathy. Patients may present with heart failure, pulmonary hypertension or sudden death.

▶ Ocular system

- Myopia is the most common ocular feature and can progress rapidly early during childhood.
- Ectopia lentis (dislocation of the lens) occurs in 70 percent of patients (**Figure 223-10**). This is often the presenting feature of MFS and occurs commonly before 10 years of age. A slit lamp

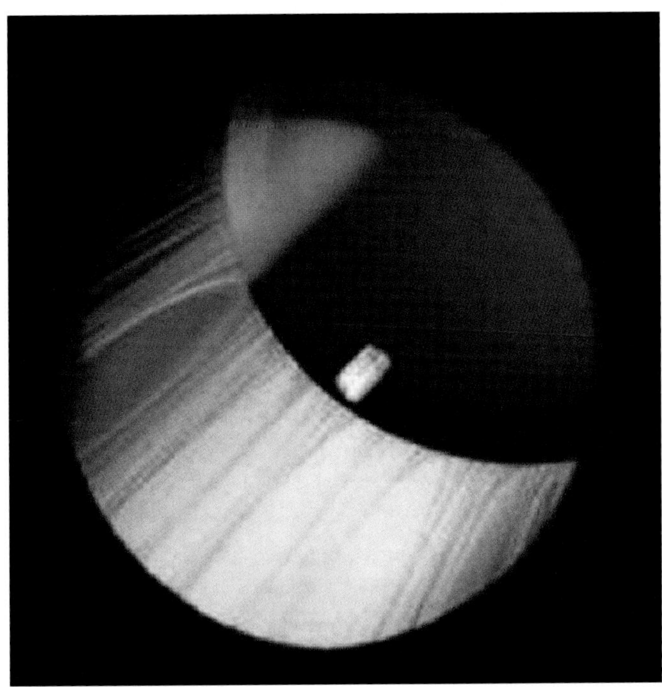

FIGURE 223-10 Ectopia lentis (dislocation of the lens) in a patient with Marfan syndrome. (*Used with permission from David Dreis, MD, in Rudolph CD, Rudolph AM, Lister LE, First LR, Gershon AA: Rudolph's Pediatrics, 22nd edition. www.accesspediatrics.com. Figure 181-1H, New York: McGraw-Hill.*)

examination after full pupillary dilation is the most reliable method to appreciate this finding.

- Other manifestations include a flat cornea, retinal detachment, and glaucoma.

▶ Pulmonary system

- Pectus and scoliosis can cause restrictive lung disease.
- Widening of the distal airspaces with or without discrete bullae or (often apical), blebs can predispose to spontaneous pneumothorax, which occurs in up to 15 percent of patients.

▶ Integument

- Skin striae, which are signs of rapid growth, are commonly apparent; these are typically horizontal and located across the lower back and inguinal and axillary regions (**Figure 223-9**).
- Patients with MS have an increased incidence of inguinal and other hernias, which may be apparent at birth or acquired during adolescence. These may be require surgical correction and may recur.

LABORATORY TESTING

- Molecular analysis for an identifiable FBN1 mutation is important in confirming the diagnosis.
- Echocardiogram of the heart to evaluate for cardiovascular manifestations should be performed in all patients at diagnosis.
- A urine cyanide nitroprusside test or a serum homocysteine level should be performed to exclude homocystinuria, which may have similar clinical findings.

DIFFERENTIAL DIAGNOSIS

- Ehlers-Danlos syndrome can have similar clinical features, such as mitral valve prolapse, thin atrophic scars, joint hypermobility, and rupture of hollow organs (see Chapter 223, Ehlers-Danlos Syndrome).
- Homocystinuria may have similar clinical features such as ectopia lentis and skeletal abnormalities. This entity is inherited in an autosomal recessive manner, associated with variable cognitive defects, and increased risk for thromboembolism. The plasma homocystine levels will be elevated.
- Loeys-Dietz syndrome—Affected patients show malar hypoplasia, arched palate, retrognathia, pectus deformity, scoliosis, joint laxity, dural ectasia, and aortic root aneurysms and dissection. Although their fingers tend to be long, overgrowth of the long bones is subtle or absent and ectopia lentis is not a feature.

MANAGEMENT

- A multidisciplinary team approach is required to screen and prevent complications and to provide ongoing support for the patient and the family.
- The aim of management is to diminish aortic complications. This can be accomplished by paying close attention to the need for activity restrictions, surgery, and pharmacologic therapy.

NONPHARMACOLOGIC

- Although physical activity is encouraged for all patients to promote overall health, skill development, coordination, musculoskeletal health, and socialization, these patients are at significant risk of physical injury and complications.[6]
- Limitations on strenuous exercise or sport activities to decrease the risk of aortic dissection or retinal detachment are often recommended.
- In general, patients with MFS who do not have aortic dilation or significant valvular problems are encouraged to participate in competitive and noncompetitive activities, as tolerated.

MEDICATIONS

- β-blockers, based on their ability to reduce hemodynamic stress on the aortic wall, have traditionally been considered the standard of care for patients with MFS. SOR C However, there is insufficient evidence to support their routine use.[8]
- Losartan, an angiotensin II receptor type 1 blocker, has been shown to prevent pathologic aortic root growth and to normalize both aortic wall thickness and architecture in a small group of patients.[9] Randomized controlled trials using losartan for MFS are ongoing.

SURGERY

- Successful surgical repair of aortic root aneurysms may be the single most important cause of improvement in life expectancy.
- Surgical repair of the aorta is indicated once:[10]
  - The maximal aortic root measurement exceeds 5 cm.
  - The rate of increase of the aortic diameter approaches 1 cm per year.
  - There is progressive aortic regurgitation.

REFERRAL

- A multidisciplinary team approach is important for the long-term management of these patients and should include a cardiologist, ophthalmologist, orthopedic surgeon, and geneticist.

PREVENTION AND SCREENING

- Prenatal diagnostic testing is available if a disease causing mutation has been identified in the family. As the severity of the condition is unpredictable, analyses and planning should ideally be done prior to conception.
- Prevention of cardiac morbidity is critical and patients require close monitoring by a cardiologist.
- Annual echocardiogram is recommended for all patients with MFS, as long as aortic dimensions are low and the rate of dilation is low.[6] More frequent studies are needed when abnormalities are noted.

PROGNOSIS

- The prognosis is variable based on the clinical manifestations and ongoing care.
- Aortic dissection is exceedingly rare in early children.
- Generally, a normal life expectancy is possible, especially after aortic root repair.

FOLLOW-UP

- It is important for these patients to have a medical home to assure that there coordination of care with the various specialists and to offer psychosocial support.
- Close follow-up with a cardiologist, along with annual echocardiography, is mandatory.
- Annual ophthalmology exam is recommended for all patients with MS.
- Screening for scoliosis is recommended yearly until 6 years of age, every 6 months between 6 to 18 years of age, and yearly after age 18 years.

PATIENT RESOURCES

- National Marfan Foundation—**www.marfan.org**.
- **www.webmd.com/heart-disease/guide/marfan-syndrome**.

PROVIDER RESOURCES

- **http://pediatrics.aappublications.org/content/132/4/e1059.full.html**.

REFERENCES

1. Dietz HC, Loeys B, Carta L, Ramirez F. Recent progress towards a molecular understanding of Marfan syndrome. *Am J Med Genet C Semin Med Genet*. 2005;139C(1):4-9.
2. Loeys BL, Dietz HC, Braverman AC, et al. The revised Ghent nosology for the Marfan syndrome. *J Med Genet*. 2010;47(7):476-485.
3. Attanasio M, Lapini I, Evangelisti L, et al. FBN1 mutation screening of patients with Marfan syndrome and related disorders:detection of 46 novel FBN1 mutations. *Clin Genet*. 2008;74(1):39-46.
4. Judge DP, Dietz HC. Marfan's syndrome. *Lancet*. 2005;366 (9501):1965.
5. Ramirez F, Godfrey M, Lee B, et al. Marfan syndrome and related disorders. In: Scriver CR, Beaudet AL, Sly WS, et al., eds. *The Metabolic and Molecular Basis of Inherited Disease*. New York: McGraw Hill; 1995:4079.
6. Tinkle BT, Saal HM and the Committee on Genetics: Health supervision for children with Marfan syndrome. *Pediatrics*. 2013;132:e1059.
7. Loeys BL, Dietz HC, Braverman AC, et al. The revised Ghent nosology for the Marfan syndrome. *J Med Genet*. 2010;47:476-485.
8. Yetman AT, Bornemeier RA, McCrindle BW, et al. Beta-blocker therapy does not alter the rate of aortic root dilation in pediatric patients with Marfan syndrome. *J Pediatr*. 2007;150: 77-82.
9. Brooke BS, Habashi JP, Judge DP, Patel N, Loeys B, Dietz HC III. Angiotensin II blockade and aortic-root dilation in Marfan's syndrome. *N Engl J Med*. 2008;358:2787-2795.
10. Gott VL, Cameron DE, Alejo DE, et al. Aortic root replacement in 271 Marfan patients: a 24-year experience. *Ann Thorac Surg*. 2002;73(2):438-443.

224 EHLERS–DANLOS SYNDROMES

Elumalai Appachi, MD, MRCP

PATIENT STORY

A 12-year-old boy presents to his pediatrician with pain in his knees while walking. On physical examination, he is noted to be short, has hyperextensibility of the skin, and hypermobile joints (**Figures 224-1** and **224-2**). His mother mentions that there are family members who have hypermobile joints, and who have had problems with dislocation and sprains of their joints. The pediatrician makes a clinical diagnosis of Ehlers-Danlos Syndrome and orders an echocardiogram, which is normal.

INTRODUCTION

The Ehlers–Danlos syndromes (EDS) constitute a genetically heterogeneous group of conditions, characterized by fragility of the connective tissues, resulting in skin, ligament, joint, blood vessels, and visceral organ manifestations. The clinical spectrum ranges from mild skin and joint hyperlaxity to severe physical disability and life-threatening vascular complications.

SYNONYMS

Hereditary collagen dysplasia.

EPIDEMIOLOGY

- The prevalence of EDS (all types) is estimated to be approximately one in 5,000 individuals.[1]

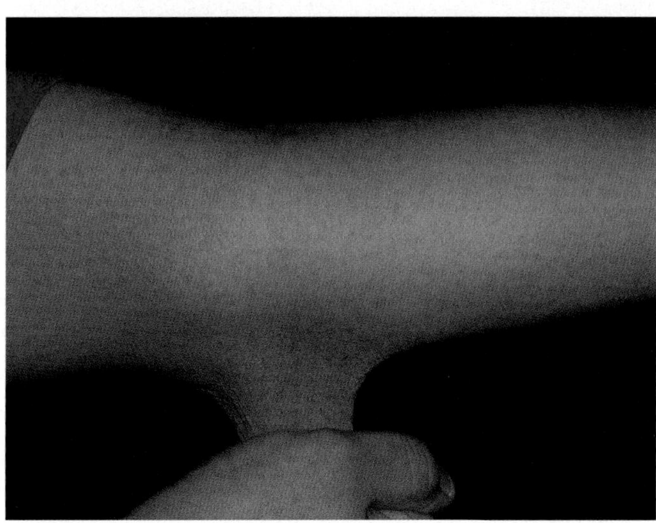

FIGURE 224-1 Hyperextensibility of the skin in a boy with proven Ehlers-Danlos syndrome. (*Used with permission from Richard P. Usatine, MD.*)

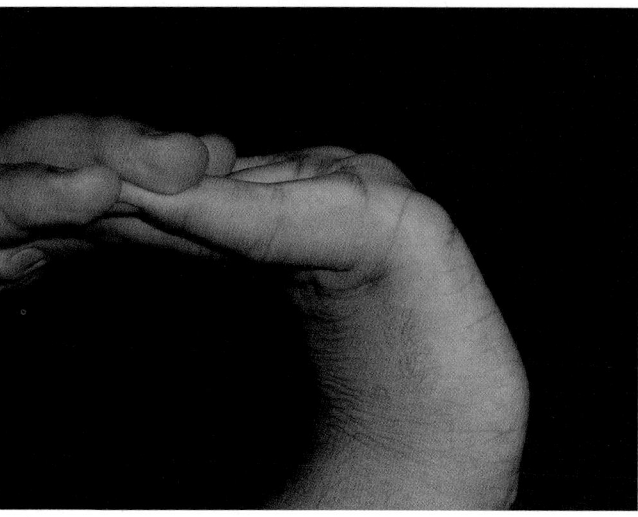

FIGURE 224-2 Hypermobility of the fingers in the same boy with Ehlers-Danlos syndrome. (*Used with permission from Richard P. Usatine, MD.*)

- The most recent classification of EDS relies on clinical and biochemical criteria.[2]
- Classification of the EDS types and prevalence:
  - Classic type—Affects 1 in 20,000 to 40,000 individuals.
  - Hypermobility type—Affects 1 in 10,000 to 15,000 individuals.
  - Vascular type—Affects 1 in 250,000 individuals. Accounts for about 5 percent of cases of EDS. Not often diagnosed until adulthood.
  - Kyphoscoliosis type—Very rare.
  - Arthrochalasia type—Very rare.
  - Dermatosparaxis type—Very rare
- The vascular form of EDS is the most dangerous, because it is associated with spontaneous rupture of medium and large-sized arteries and hollow organs, especially the large intestine and uterus; vascular events typically occur between the third and fifth decade.

ETIOLOGY AND PATHOPHYSIOLOGY

- Mode of inheritance is autosomal dominant for all forms of EDS except the kyphoscoliosis and dermatosparaxis types (recessive mode), and an unclassified X-linked form which is extremely rare.
- Abnormalities of mature collagen structure in extracellular matrices of multiple tissues (skin, tendons, blood vessels, and viscera) are common to all forms of EDS.
- Classic EDS is associated with defects in type V collagen, corresponding to mutations of COL5A genes, as well as type I collagen (COL1A1).
- The precise etiology for the hypermobility form has not been identified.
- Vascular EDS involves a deficiency in type III collagen and several studies suggest that mutations of gene COL3A1 lead to this deficiency.[3]
- The kyphoscoliotic type of EDS is caused by a deficiency of lysyl hydroxylase (PLOD), a collagen modifying illness.

- The arthrochalasia form of EDS results from a defect in type I collagen, caused by mutations in the COL1A2 genes.

RISK FACTORS

- Family history.

DIAGNOSIS

- The diagnosis of EDS is based solely on clinical criteria, which have been established for the six major types of EDS.
- Major and minor criteria have been established for each type; the presence of one or more major criteria is highly indicative and warrants laboratory confirmation if possible.
- A minor criterion is less specific, but the presence of one or more minor criteria contributes to the diagnosis of a specific type; in the absence of a major criterion, minor criteria are not sufficient to establish a diagnosis.
- Positive family history is a minor criterion for all forms.
- Skin hyperextensibility (**Figure 224-1**) should be tested at a site not subjected to mechanical forces or scarring, and measured by pulling up the skin until resistance is felt.
- Joint hypermobility should be assessed using the Beighton scale. A score of 5 or greater defines hypermobility:
  - Passive dorsiflexion of the fifth finger >90° (one point if present, 2 points if bilateral).
  - Passive flexion of thumb to the forearm (one point if present, 2 points if bilateral).
  - Hyperextension of the elbow beyond 10° (one point if present, 2 points if bilateral).
  - Hyperextension of the knee beyond 10° (one point if present, 2 points if bilateral).
  - Ability to place the palms on the floor with extension of the knees (one point if present).
- Easy bruising is defined as spontaneous ecchymosis, frequently located in the same areas, and causing a brownish discoloration.

CLINICAL FEATURES

- Classic EDS.
  - Skin hyperextensibility, widened atrophic scars (tissue fragility), and joint hypermobility are the major criteria (**Figures 224-1 to 224-3**).
  - Dermatologic features predominate, although the range of these manifestations varies greatly.
  - Minor criteria include:
    - Smooth, velvety skin.
    - Molluscoid pseudotumors—Fleshy lesions associated with scars (**Figure 224-4**).
    - Subcutaneous spheroids—Small, firm, cyst-like nodules along shins or forearms.
    - Muscle hypotonia, delayed gross motor development.
    - Easy bruising.
    - Complications of hypermobility (dislocations or sprains).

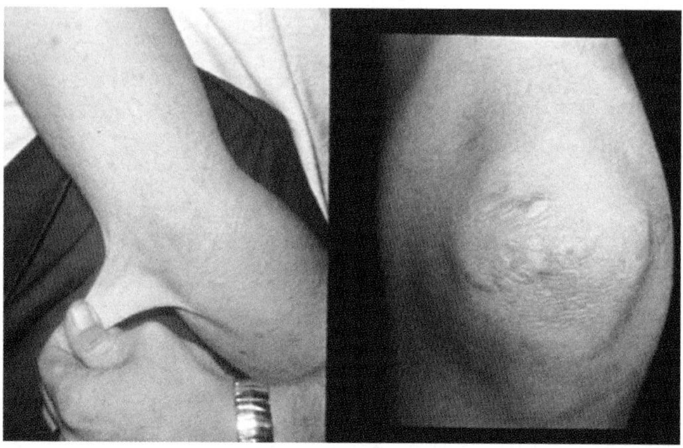

FIGURE 224-3 Hyperextensibility of the skin (left) and atrophic scarring of the knee in a patient with the classic form of Ehlers-Danlos syndrome. *(Used with permission from Cleveland Clinic Children's Photo Files.)*

    - Manifestations of tissue extensibility and fragility (hiatal hernia, prolapsed pelvic organ, premature arthritis, and cervical insufficiency).[4]
- Hypermobility EDS.
  - Often presents with joint pain, joint dislocations, and inability to walk. Skin manifestations are less prominent.
  - Major criteria include generalized joint hypermobility and skin involvement (hyperextensibility and/or smooth velvety skin).
  - Minor criteria include recurring joint dislocations as well as chronic joint and limb pain.
- Vascular EDS.
  - Most severe form of EDS.[4,5]
  - Major criteria for diagnosis include:
    - Arterial, intestinal, or uterine fragility or rupture.
    - Easy bruising.

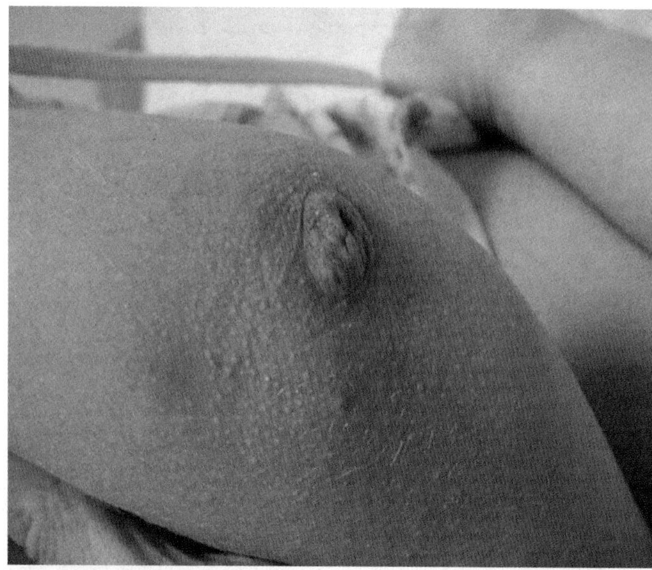

FIGURE 224-4 Small fleshy pseudotumor on the elbow of a girl with Ehlers-Danlos syndrome. These represent calcified herniations of fat through the dermis. *(Used with permission from Weinberg S, Prose NS, Kristal L: Color Atlas of Pediatric Dermatology, 4th edition: www.accesspediatrics.com. Figure 11-10. New York: McGraw-Hill, 2009.)*

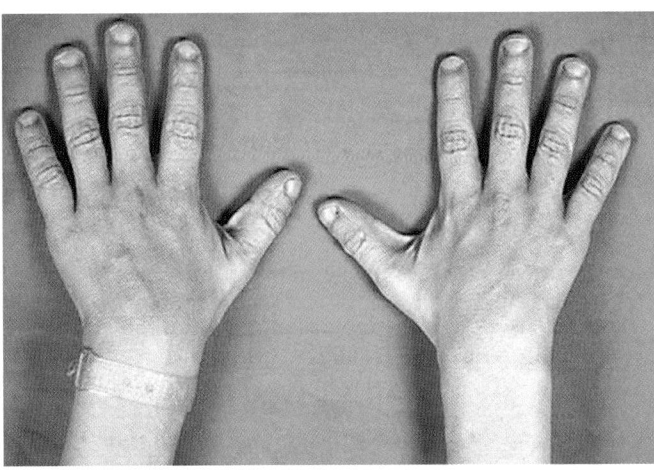

FIGURE 224-5 Acrogeria (fragile, thin, prematurely aging skin) in a child with the vascular form of Ehlers-Danlos syndrome. *(Used with permission from Cleveland Clinic Children's Hospital Photo Files.)*

- Thin, translucent skin.
- Characteristic facial features (thin, delicate, and pinched nose, hollow cheeks, prominent staring eyes).
- Occurs in <30 percent of patients and not prominent in children.

- Minor criteria:
  - Small joint hypermobility.
  - Gingival recession.
  - Spontaneous pneumothorax/hemothorax.
  - Tendon or muscle rupture.
  - Early-onset varicose veins.
  - Carotid-cavernous fistula.
  - Talipes equinovarus (clubfoot).
  - Acrogeria (**Figure 224-5**).
- The vascular form of EDS is severe and it is important to identify patients early for management.[3,6–8]
- Kyphoscoliotic EDS.
  - Characterized by marked muscular hypotonia at birth, joint hypermobility, progressive scoliosis, and optic globe fragility.
  - Vascular involvement, such as mitral valve prolapse and aortic root dilatation, has been described.
- Arthrochalasia EDS.
  - Characterized by severe general joint hypermobility with recurrent subluxations, congenital hip dislocation, skin hyperextensibility, and tissue fragility, including atrophic scars.
- Dermatosparaxis EDS.
  - Characterized by severe skin fragility, sagging and redundant skin, easy bruising, and large hernias.

LABORATORY TESTING

- Genetic and biochemical testing for collagen type V abnormalities may be performed to aid in the diagnosis of classic EDS.
- There is currently no molecular test to diagnose hypermobility EDS.
- Biochemical and gene testing for known molecular defects of type III collagen from cultured fibroblasts and/or identification of mutations in COL3A1 can confirm the diagnosis of vascular EDS.

IMAGING

- Plain radiographs may reveal calcified nodules along the shin or forearms corresponding to the subcutaneous spheroids.
- Echocardiogram should be performed to identify mitral valve prolapse and aortic dilatation.

DIFFERENTIAL DIAGNOSIS

- Marfan syndrome may present with similar cardiovascular manifestations. Other manifestations of Marfan are usually present and can serve to differentiate from EDS (see Chapter 223, Marfan Syndrome).
- Osteogenesis imperfecta—May manifest with similar features, but blue sclerae and bone fractures of osteogenesis imperfecta help to differentiate (see Chapter 225, Osteogenesis Imperfecta).
- Autosomal dominant cutis laxa—Usually characterized by abnormalities limited to the skin, although visceral organs may also be involved rarely.
- Familial joint hypermobility—Can be difficult to differentiate from the hypermobility form of EDS. The diagnostic criteria from hypermobility type of EDS can help in differentiating these.
- Non-accidental trauma—Should always be considered when there is easy bruising in early childhood (see Chapter 8, Child Physical Abuse)

MANAGEMENT

- All patients should receive genetic counseling about the mode of inheritance of their EDS.
- Management of most skin and joint problems should be conservative and preventive. Joint hypermobility and pain in EDS usually does not require surgical intervention.
- For patients with vascular EDS:
  - Special surgical care is required because of increased tissue friability.
  - Patients should be advised to avoid contact sports especially if they have cardiac problems.
  - Elevated blood pressure should be aggressively treated with beta-blockers, given the risk of arterial dissection.
  - Women with vascular EDS should be counseled about the risk of uterine, intestinal, and arterial rupture. Pregnancy is associated with up to a 25 percent mortality rate; however, successful childbirth is possible.[4,5,9]

NONPHARMACOLOGIC

Physical therapy to strengthen muscles is helpful.

MEDICATIONS

- Beta-blocker therapy for patients with cardiac complications, especially aortic root dilatation, is often prescribed. SOR Ⓒ

SURGERY

- Surgical intervention should be considered on an individual basis.
- The instability of joints, leading to subluxations and joint pain, often require surgical intervention in patients.

- Surgical repair and tightening of joint ligaments can be performed, but ligaments frequently will not hold sutures.
- Risk of complications in patients with EDS include decreased strength of the tissues, which makes the tissue less suitable for surgery; the fragility of the blood vessels, which can cause problems during surgery; and wound healing is often delayed or incomplete.
- Surgery requires careful tissue handling and a longer post-operative immobilization.
- Local anesthetics have less effect in EDS.
- Patients should generally be referred to specialized surgical centers who have experience with EDS. Wound healing and rupture of visceral organs during surgery is a concern.
- In the vascular form of EDS, arterial aneurysms are difficult to manage surgically as the vessels are often friable and not amenable to anastomosis.[3]

REFERRAL

- Referral to dermatology for skin biopsy to confirm the diagnosis of vascular EDS.
- Cardiology, orthopedic surgery, general surgery, and physical therapy as needed.

PROGNOSIS

- Prognosis varies according to type of EDS.
    - Vascular EDS is associated with a 25 percent risk of significant complication by the age of 25 years; >80 percent will have a complication by the age of 40 years. Most vascular complications consist of arterial dissections. Vascular events typically occur between the third and fifth decade. Median age of survival is 48 years. Most deaths are related to arterial rupture.

FOLLOW-UP

Close multispecialty follow-up is often required. This may include orthopedic surgery, general surgery, dermatology, and physiotherapy as needed.

PATIENT RESOURCES

- **www.medicinenet.com/ehlers-danlos_syndrome/article.htm**.
- **www.ncbi.nlm.nih.gov/pubmedhealth/PMH0002439/**.
- Ehlers-Danlos National Foundation—**www.ednf.org**.

PROVIDER RESOURCES

- **www.pathology.washington.edu/clinical/collagen/index.php/disorders/ehlers-danlos/**.
- **www.ncbi.nlm.nih.gov/books/NBK1494/**.
- **http://emedicine.medscape.com/article/1114004**.

REFERENCES

1. http://ghr.nlm.nih.gov/condition/ehlers-danlos-syndrome.
2. Beighton P, De Paepe A, Steinmann B, Tsipouras P, Wenstrup RJ: Ehlers-Danlos syndromes: revised nosology, Villefranche, 1997, for the Ehlers-Danlos National Foundation (USA) and Ehlers-Danlos Support Group (UK). *Am J Med Genet.* 1998;77:31-37.
3. Pepin M, Schwarze U, Superti-Furga A, Byers PH: Clinical and genetic features of Ehlers-Danlos syndrome type IV, the vascular type. *N Engl J Med.* 2000;342:673-680.
4. Pyeritz R: Ehlers-Danlos syndrome. *N Engl J Med.* 2000;342:730.
5. Oderich GS: Current concepts in the diagnosis and management of vascular Ehlers-Danlos syndrome. *Perspect Vasc Surg Endovasc Ther.* 2006;18:206.
6. Fernandes NF, Schwartz RA: A "hyperextensive" review of Ehlers-Danlos syndrome. *Ped Dermatol.* 2008;82:242.
7. Gawthrop G: Ehlers-Danlos syndrome. *BMJ.* 2008;335:448-450.
8. Parapia LA, Jackson C: Ehlers-Danlos syndrome–a historical review. *Br J Haematol.* 2008;141:32-35.
9. Prahlow JA: Death due to Ehlers-Danlos syndrome type IV. *Am J Forensic Med Pathol.* 2005;26:78.

225 OSTEOGENESIS IMPERFECTA

Elumalai Appachi, MD, MRCP

PATIENT STORY

A newborn infant is being evaluated by the pediatrician in the hospital. On physical exam, the infant is noted to have blue sclerae and deformities in the legs (**Figure 225-1**). X-rays of the long bones of the legs reveal multiple fractures (**Figure 225-2**). Prenatal ultrasound screening in the second trimester showed bowing of long bones, fractures, and shortened limbs, suspicious for osteogenesis imperfecta (OI). The infant is treated with supportive care and a referral to genetics and orthopedics is made. The diagnosis of OI is formally established by identifying mutations in type 1 collagen.

INTRODUCTION

Osteogenesis imperfecta (OI) is a genetic disorder characterized by fragility of the skeletal system, and resulting in frequent fractures. The four major types of OI are caused by structural or quantitative defects in type 1 collagen, which is the primary component of the extracellular matrix of bone and skin protein.

SYNONYMS

Brittle bone disease (type 1 OI), Osteogenesis imperfecta congenita (type 3 OI).

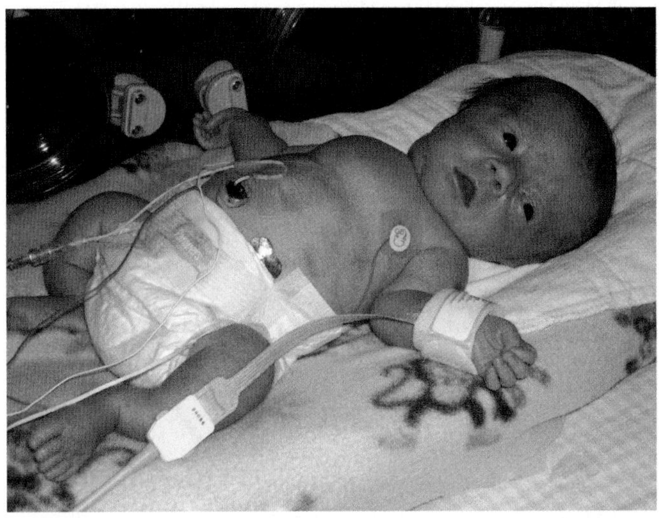

FIGURE 225-1 Blue sclerae and leg deformities in a 3-day-old infant with osteogenesis imperfecta. The diagnosis was suspected before birth based on bony abnormalities seen during prenatal ultrasound imaging. (*Used with permission from Betsy Tapani.*)

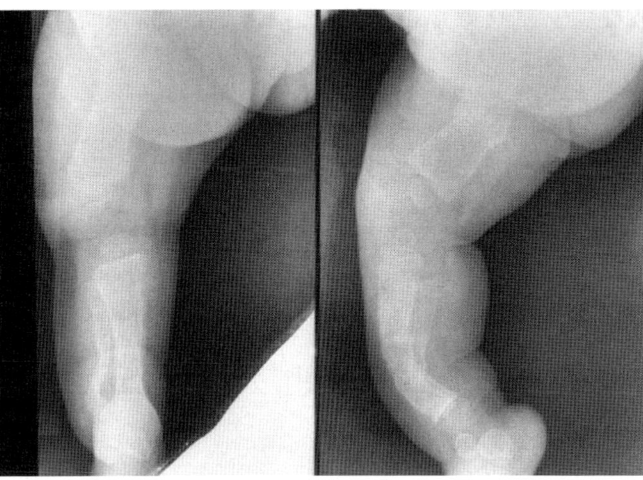

FIGURE 225-2 Multiple fractures present at birth in a newborn with osteogenesis imperfecta. (*Used with permission from Cleveland Clinic Children's Hospital Photo Files.*)

EPIDEMIOLOGY

- Overall incidence of OI is 1 in 20,000 births. The number of individuals affected by OI in the US is estimated to be between 20,000 and 50,000.[1]
- Eight types of OI have been described and are classified according to clinical presentation, radiographic findings, mode of inheritance, and molecular findings.
- Types 1 through 4 of OI are the most common; types 5 to 8 are very rare.[2]
- Type 1 is the most common form and is inherited in an autosomal dominant pattern. Type 4 is also inherited in an autosomal dominant pattern. Type 2 and Type 3 are usually the result of new mutations.
- Type 2 is the most severe form; 50 percent of cases are stillborn.
- The autosomal dominant forms of OI (types 1 and 4) occur equally in all racial and ethnic groups, and recessive forms (types 2 and 3) occur predominantly in ethnic groups with consanguineous marriages.

ETIOLOGY AND PATHOPHYSIOLOGY

- OI types 1 through 4 are the result of mutations of genes that code for type I collagen, while types 5 to 8 are caused by mutations of other less-well characterized genes.
- Types 1 and 4 are inherited in an autosomal dominant pattern and are caused by mutations in COL1A1 and COL1A2 genes that code for the alpha-1 and alpha-2 chains of type 1 collagen.
- Collagen structural defects are predominantly of two types:
  1. Eighty percent are point mutations causing substitutions of helical glycine residues or crucial residues in the C-propeptide by other amino acids.
  2. Twenty percent are single exon splicing defects.
- The clinically mild OI type 1 has a quantitative defect, with null mutations in one $\alpha 1(I)$ allele leading to a reduced amount of normal collagen.[3]

- Types 2 and 3 may be inherited in a recessive pattern and most cases are related to new point mutations of COL1A1 or COL1A2.
- The collagen structural mutations cause OI bone to be globally abnormal. The bone matrix contains abnormal type I collagen fibrils and relatively increased levels of types III and V collagen.

RISK FACTORS

- Affected parent for OI types 1 and 4.
- Consanguineous marriage for OI types 2 and 3.

DIAGNOSIS

- The diagnosis is made based on clinical grounds in most cases.
- Collagen and genetic testing are available to help to make the diagnosis in difficult cases.

CLINICAL FEATURES

- Fragile bones, blue sclerae, and early deafness are the hallmark features of OI (**Figure 225-1**).
- Common presenting features include bone fragility, repeated fractures with minimal trauma, and easy bruisability.
- Deafness may be a presenting feature of children with type 1 OI.
- Prenatal ultrasound screening in the second trimester may show bowing of long bones, fractures, shortened limbs, and other bone abnormalities.
- The majority of fractures occur during childhood.
- The blue sclerae is due to thinning of the sclera.
- Some patients have short stature and develop hearing loss later in life.
- Specific features are specific to the types of OI:
    - Osteogenesis Imperfecta Type 1 (Mild).
        - Major features include blue sclerae, recurrent fractures in childhood, easy bruising, joint laxity, and hearing loss (30 to 60%), which often develops in the 2nd or 3rd decade.
        - Fractures result from mild to moderate trauma, are uncommon at birth, and decrease after puberty.
        - Deformities of bones are uncommon.
        - Short stature, compared with family members, may or may not be present.
        - Differentiation from nonaccidental trauma can be challenging.
    - Osteogenesis Imperfecta Type 2 (Perinatal Lethal).
        - Most severe form of OI.
        - Lethal in utero or in the majority of newborns because of respiratory insufficiency.
        - Extreme fragility of the skeleton and other connective tissues.
        - Multiple intrauterine fractures of long bones are evident, which have a crumpled appearance on radiographs.
        - Limbs are short and bowed, and legs are held abducted at right angles to the body creating a frog-leg position.
        - Multiple rib fractures create a beaded appearance and the small thorax contributes to respiratory insufficiency.
        - A large, soft skull and open fontanelles are common.

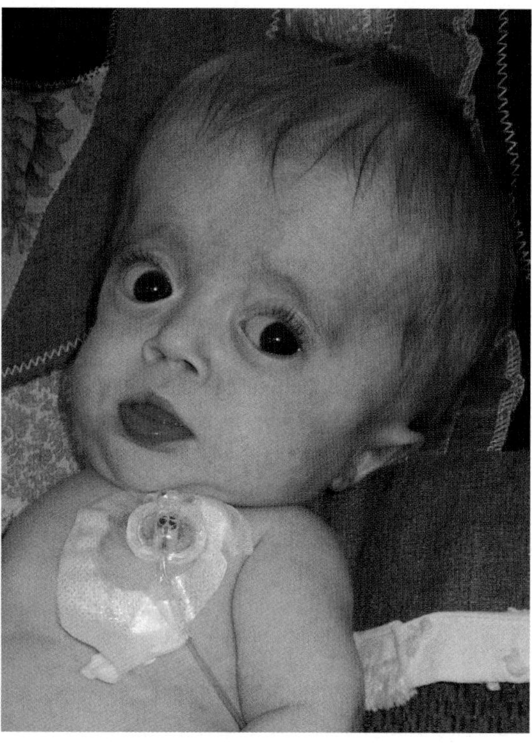

FIGURE 225-3 Blue sclerae, macrocephaly, and triangular facies in a 10-month-old infant with osteogenesis imperfecta type 3. (*Used with permission from Betsy Tapani.*)

- Osteogenesis Imperfecta Type 3 (Severe, Progressive Deforming).
    - Nonlethal form but patients have severe physical disability.
    - Usually presents in the newborn period with multiple fractures.
    - Infants have low birth weight and in utero fractures are common.
    - There is relative macrocephaly, triangular facies and blue sclera (**Figure 225-3**).
    - Postnatally, fractures occur from inconsequential trauma and heal with deformity.
    - Disorganization of the bone matrix results in a "popcorn" appearance at the metaphyses.
    - The rib cage has flaring at the base and pectal deformity is frequent.
    - Almost all patients have scoliosis and vertebral compression.
    - Pulmonary function can be affected due to associated scoliosis.
    - Extreme short stature is common (**Figure 225-4**).
- Osteogenesis Imperfecta Type 4 (Mild to Moderately Severe).
    - Marked variability in clinical findings.
    - In utero fractures can occur.
    - Bowing of the tibia is the hallmark of this type of OI and can occur even without fractures.
    - Children require orthopedic and rehabilitation intervention, but they are usually able to attain community ambulation skills.
    - Fracture rates decrease after puberty. X-ray findings show osteoporotic and have metaphyseal flaring and vertebral compressions.
    - Short stature is common, like in other types of OI.
- Osteogenesis Imperfecta Type 5 (Hyperplastic Callus) and Type 6 (Mineralization Defect).
    - These types of OI are similar clinically to type 4, but they have distinct findings on bone histology.

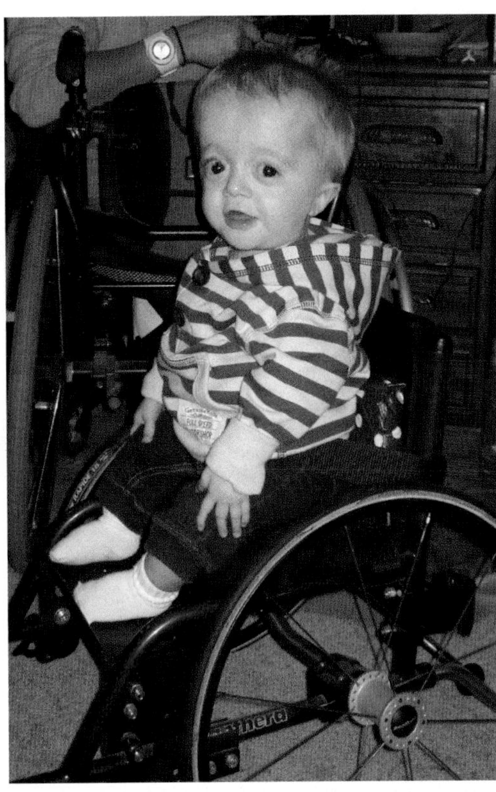

FIGURE 225-4 Happy 2-year-old boy with osteogenesis imperfecta type 3. His measured height is well below the normal for his age. He successfully uses a wheelchair for mobility. He is greatly loved by his family. (*Used with permission from Betsy Tapani.*)

   - Type 5 patients also have hyperplastic callus, calcification of the interosseous membrane of the forearm, and a radiodense metaphyseal band.
   - The absence of a collagen defect supports the distinct grouping; the genetic etiology is unknown.
- Osteogenesis Imperfecta Types 7 and 8 (Recessive Forms).
   - Caused by null mutations in proteins involved in posttranslational modifications of type I procollagen.
   - Clinically overlap types 2 and 3, but have distinct features including white sclerae, rhizomelia, and small to normal head circumference. Rhizomelia is a disproportion in the length of the most proximal segment of the limbs (upper arms and thighs).
   - Surviving children have severe osteochondrodysplasia with extreme short stature.

LABORATORY TESTING

- Collagen synthesis and DNA analyses can be obtained to identify mutations.

IMAGING

- Routine radiologic testing is done to identify fractures and bony deformities (**Figures 225-2** and **225-5**).
- Dual energy x-ray absorptiometry may offer more evidence for OI.

DIFFERENTIAL DIAGNOSIS

- Child Abuse—Nonaccidental trauma can be challenging to distinguish from OI. Examination of psychosocial factors, along with

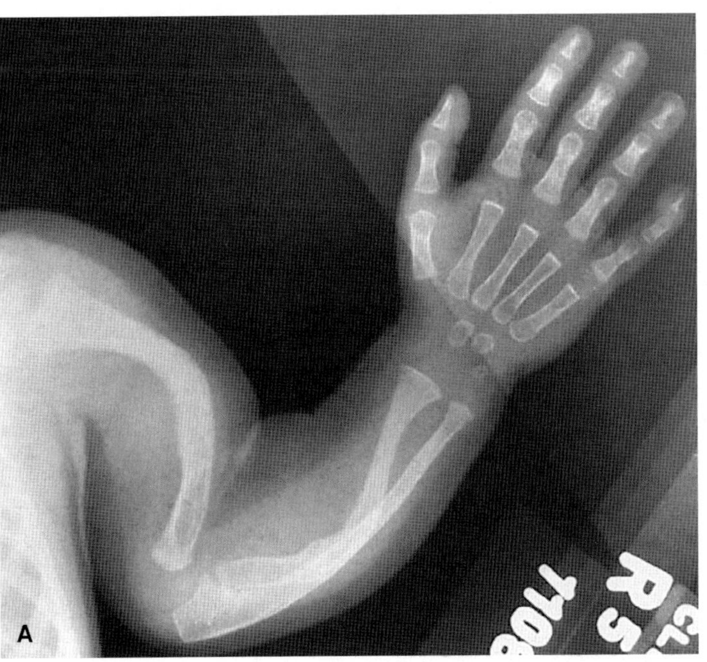

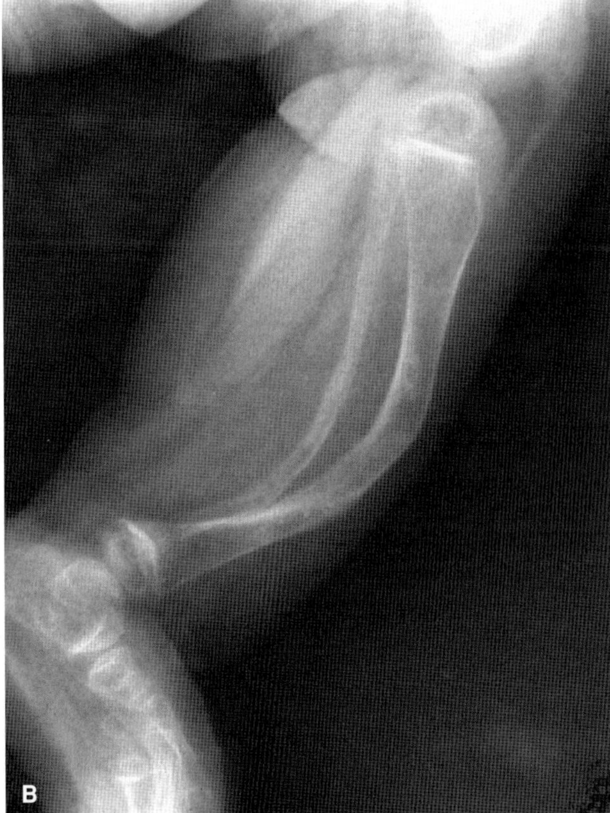

FIGURE 225-5 Severe deformities and multiple fractures of the long bones in a child with osteogenesis imperfecta before the advent of bisphosphonate therapy. **A.** Arms. **B.** Legs. (*Used with permission from Cleveland Clinic Children's Hospital Photo Files.*)

other evidence of nonaccidental trauma (retinal hemorrhage, intracranial hemorrhage) can help in distinguishing these entities from child abuse (see Chapter 8, Child Physical Abuse).

- Rickets—Can cause similar bone fractures. Rickets can be distinguished from OI based on history, characteristic investigations (elevated alkaline phosphatase and parathyroid hormone levels). Typical radiologic features are also helpful in distinguishing these entities (see Chapter 198, Rickets).
- Osteoporosis—Very rare in children.

MANAGEMENT

- There is no cure for OI, although gene therapy is under investigation.
- Management is directed toward improving joint mobility and muscle strength.

NONPHARMACOLOGIC

- Physical therapy, directed toward improvement of joint mobility and muscle strength development is critical (**Figure 225-6**).
- Occupational therapy should aim to improve function in daily living, social integration, and educational achievement.
- Caution should be taken with physical and occupational therapy to avoid causing fractures in more severe forms. Risks may outweigh potential benefits in some cases.
- Treatment may be required, as necessary and appropriate, for hearing loss and for neurological, and cardiorespiratory complications.

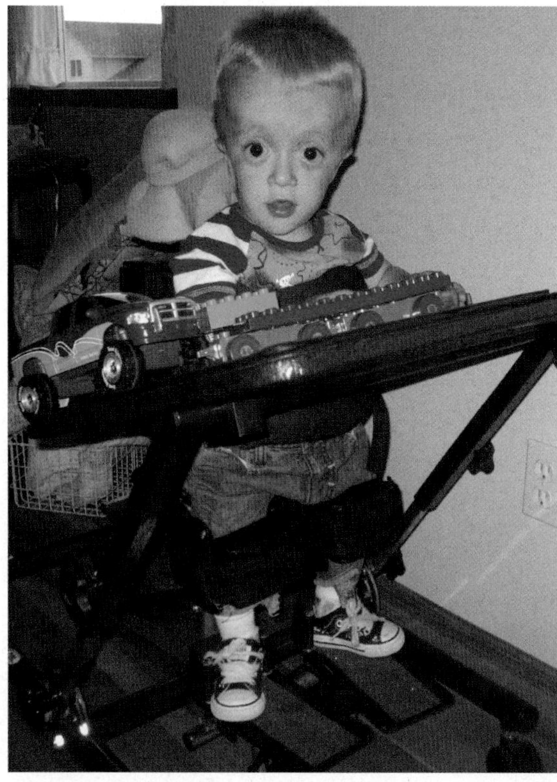

FIGURE 225-6 A 3-year-8-month-old boy with osteogenesis imperfecta is using a special device as part of his home physical therapy to improve his motor function and balance. (*Used with permission from Betsy Tapani.*)

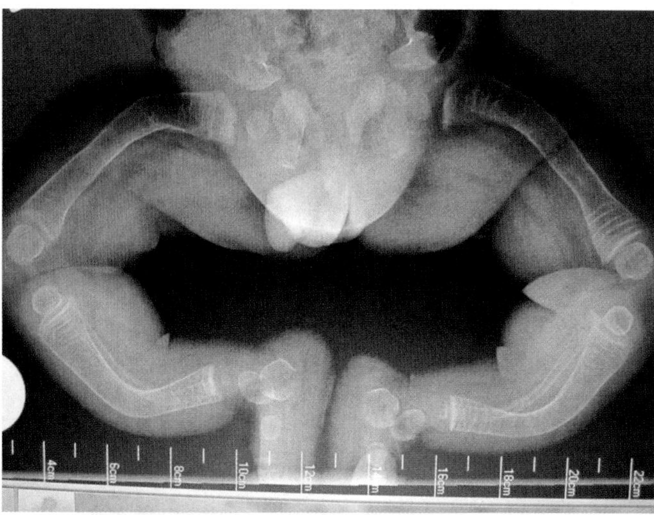

FIGURE 225-7 Leg bowing and metaphyseal bands in an 8-month-old child with osteogenesis imperfecta undergoing pamidronate therapy to prevent fragility fractures. This child received many cycles of pamidronate, resulting in metaphyseal bands, known as "zebra lines." (*Used with permission from Betsy Tapani.*)

MEDICATIONS

- Bisphosphonates are used in OI type 3 and in more severe presentations of other forms, to reduce the incidence of fractures and improve bone quality.[4]
- Intravenous and oral forms of bisphosphonates have been shown to result in improvement in clinical symptoms (less pain), increased mobility, and reduction in fracture frequency in children with OI.[5-7]
- The use of pamidronate (a bisphosphonate) can lead to metaphyseal bands, known as "zebra lines." These lines are not problematic but produce an interesting pattern on radiographs (**Figure 225-7**).
- A Cochrane review concluded that oral or intravenous bisphosphonates equally increase bone mineral density in children with OI; it is unclear whether either treatment decreases fractures.[8]
- Gene therapy and bone marrow transplantation are under investigation.[9]

SURGERY

- Surgical procedure that involves internally splinting the long bones by insertion of a metal rod is recommended to control repeated fractures and to improve bone deformities that interfere with function (**Figure 225-8**).
- Posterior spinal fusion— for severe scoliosis may be required.
- Limb lengthening procedures and correction of angular deformities may be required.[7,10,11]

REFERRAL

- Genetics referral may be required if the diagnosis is in doubt, to better classify the type of OI, and for genetic counseling.
- Orthopedic, pulmonary, and neurology referrals may be needed depending on the clinical spectrum of involvement and the severity of the findings.
- Audiology referral is important for patients with hearing deficits and for monitoring and screening.

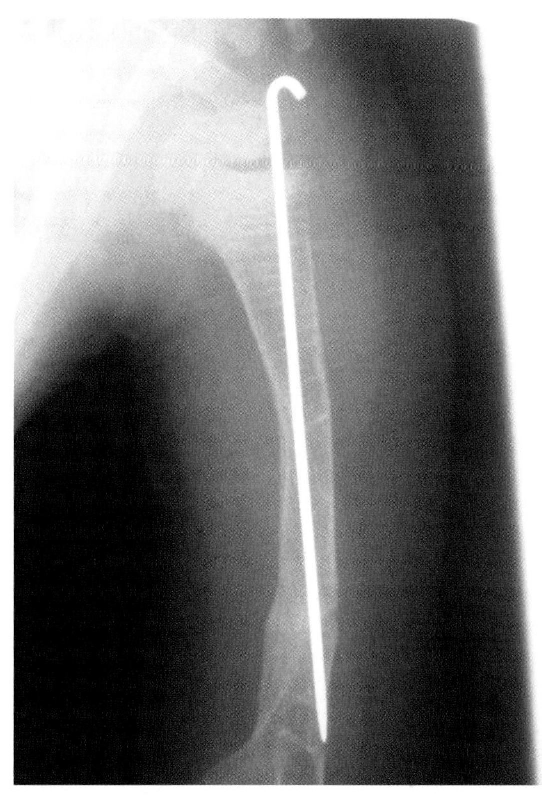

FIGURE 225-8 A metal rod has been inserted into the humerus of a 2-year-old boy with osteogenesis imperfecta to control repeated fractures and to improve bone deformities that interfere with function. (*Used with permission from Betsy Tapani.*)

PREVENTION AND SCREENING

- Genetic counseling is indicated for families with OI.
- Chorionic villous sampling may be analyzed for abnormal collagen or collagen mutations.

PROGNOSIS

- The prognosis for an individual with OI varies greatly, depending upon the type of OI and severity of symptoms. In general, the prognosis improves if the child survives beyond age 10 years.
- Type 1—Life expectancy similar to that of the general population.
- Type 2—Poor prognosis.
- Type 3—Life expectancy is reduced significantly as a result of concurrent problems such as respiratory infection and skull fractures.

FOLLOW-UP

- Audiological follow-up is important for children with OI.
- Orthopedic follow-up is indicated for most patients with OI.

PATIENT RESOURCES

- The Osteogenesis Imperfecta—**www.oif.org**.
- National Institutes of Health: Osteoporosis and Related Bone Diseases—**www.osteo.org**.
- The Osteogenesis Imperfecta Clinic at Kennedy Krieger Institute—**www.osteogenesisimperfecta.org**.

PROVIDER RESOURCES

- **http://emedicine.medscape.com/article/947588**.

ACKNOWLEDGEMENT

We greatly thank Betsy Tapani for the photographs and radiographs of her son with osteogenesis imperfecta (**Figures 225-1, 225-3, 225-4, 225-6** to **225-8**). One can learn more about their family story at http://www.oif.org/site/PageServer?pagename=meetbrennan.

The Osteogenesis Imperfecta Foundation has been of great help to Betsy and her family and she is committed to giving to those parents who face similar challenges.

REFERENCES

1. Marini JC. Osteogenesis imperfecta: comprehensive management. *Adv Pediatr*. 1988;35:391.
2. Glorieux FH, Rauch F, Plotkin H, Ward L, et al. Type V Osteogenesis Imperfecta: A New Form of Brittle Bone Disease. *J Bone Miner Res*. 2000;15:1650-1658.
3. Barnes AM, Chang W, Morello R, Cabral WA, et al. Deficiency of cartilage-associated protein in recessive lethal osteogenesis imperfecta. *N Engl J Med*. 2006;355:2757-2764.
4. Rauch F, Glorieux FH. Osteogenesis imperfecta, current and future medical treatment. *Am J Med Genet*. Part C. 2005;139C:31-37.
5. Zacharin M, Kanumakala S. Pamidronate treatment of less severe forms of osteogenesis imperfecta in children. *J Pediatr Endocrinol Metab*. 2004;17:1511-1517.
6. DiMeglio LA, Ford L, McClintock C, Peacock M. Intravenous pamidronate treatment of children under 36 months of age with osteogenesis imperfecta. *Bone* 2004;35:1038-1045.
7. Zeitlin A, Frassier F, Glorieux FH. Modern approach to children with osteogenesis imperfecta. *J Pediatr Orthop B*. 2003;12:77-87.
8. Phillipi CA, Remmington T, Steiner RD. Biphosphonate therary for osteogenesis imperfect. *Cochrane database syst Rev*. 2008;(4):CD005088.
9. Chamberlain JR, Schwarze U, Wang PR, et al. Gene targeting in stem cells from individuals with osteogenesis imperfecta. *Science*. 2004;303:1198-1201.
10. Saldanha KA, Saleh M, Bell MJ, Fernandes JA. Limb lengthening and correction of deformity in the lower limbs of children with osteogenesis imperfecta. *J Bone Joint Surg Br*. 2004;86:259-265.
11. Wilkinson JM, Scott BW, Clarke AM, Belle MJ. Surgical stabilisation of the lower limb in osteogenesis imperfecta using the Sheffield Telescopic Intramedullary Rod System. *J Bone Joint Surg Br*. 1998;80:999-1004.

226 NOONAN SYNDROME

Elumalai Appachi, MD, MRCP

PATIENT STORY

A 3-year-old boy is brought to see his pediatrician for a health maintenance visit. During the exam, the pediatrician notes that the child's face lacks expression, has a short neck with excessive skin, a low hairline, low set ears, and a short broad nose (**Figure 226-1**). The child is appropriate for weight but his height is well below the third percentile. An audible systolic ejection murmur is heard. The pediatrician refers the child to a pediatric cardiologist who makes the diagnosis of pulmonic stenosis from physical exam and echocardiogram. Based on these findings, the pediatrician and cardiologist make a clinical diagnosis of Noonan syndrome, which is confirmed by genetic testing. A multidisciplinary approach to the child's care is planned.

INTRODUCTION

Noonan syndrome is an autosomal dominant, variably expressed, multisystem disorder characterized by distinctive facial features, developmental delay, learning difficulties, short stature, congenital heart disease, renal anomalies, lymphatic malformations, and bleeding difficulties. Mutations that cause Noonan syndrome alter genes encoding proteins with roles in the RAS–MAPK pathway, leading to pathway dysregulation.

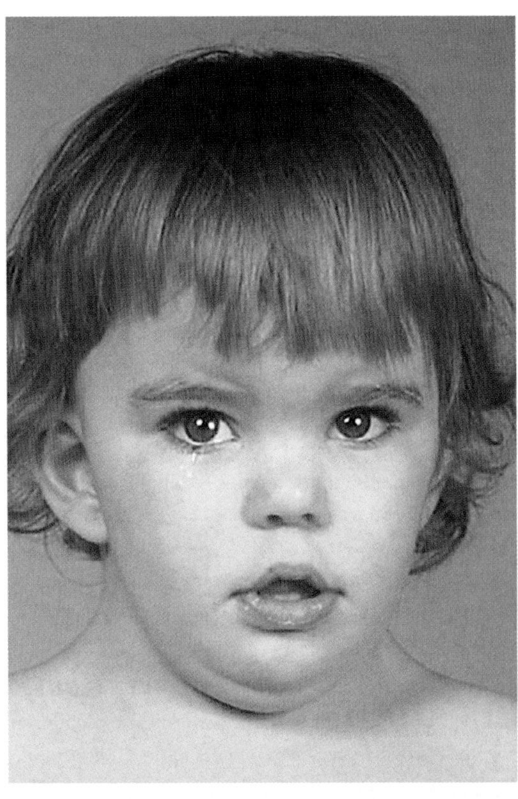

FIGURE 226-1 Distinctive facial features, including a short neck with excessive skin, a low hairline, low set ears, and a short broad nose, in a boy with Noonan syndrome. This child also has hypertelorism (widely spaced eyes). The lack of facial expression resembling a myopathy has also been described in these patients. (*Used with permission from Cleveland Clinic Children's Hospital Photo Files.*)

SYNONYMS

Male Turner syndrome.

EPIDEMIOLOGY

- First described by Jacqueline Noonan, who reported nine patients with pulmonary stenosis, short stature, chest deformities, and mild developmental delay.[1,2]
- Estimated prevalence is 1 in 1000 to 2500.[2]
- Although this syndrome was first described in males who had the Turner syndrome phenotype, it is now recognized in females as well.
- Autosomal dominant condition with complete penetrance but variable expressivity.
- Congenital heart disease present in 80 to 90 percent of patients.
- After trisomy 21, Noonan syndrome is the second most common syndromic cause of congenital heart disease.

ETIOLOGY AND PATHOPHYSIOLOGY

- Autosomal dominant inheritance.
- Eight genes in the RAS–MAPK signaling pathway cause Noonan syndrome or closely related conditions (*PTPN11*, *SOS1*, *KRAS*, *NRAS*, *RAF1*, *BRAF*, *SHOC2*, and *CBL*).
- The RAS–MAPK pathway is a well-studied, widely important signal transduction pathway through which extracellular ligands—such as some growth factors, cytokines, and hormones—stimulate cell proliferation, differentiation, survival, and metabolism.
- Noonan syndrome has been linked to the chromosomal band 12q24.1 and *PTPN11,* which encodes the protein SHP2. Because SHP2 has essential roles in signal transduction pathways that control several developmental processes, including cardiac semilunar valvulogenesis, *PTPN11* was deemed an excellent candidate gene.
- Studies suggest that 50 percent of cases of Noonan syndrome are caused by missense, gain of-function mutations in *PTPN11*.[3,4]

RISK FACTORS

- Autosomal dominant and the risk for having an affected child is 50 percent.

DIAGNOSIS

Diagnosis is made from the key clinical features and genetic testing.

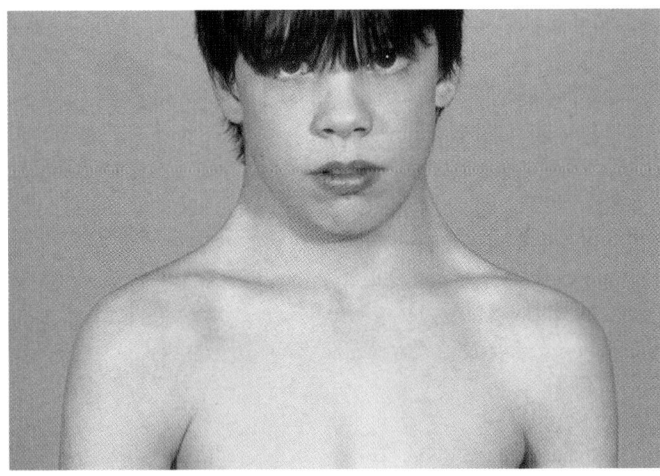

FIGURE 226-2 Hypertelorism, pointed chin, accentuation of skin webbing in the neck and prominence of the trapezius muscle in an adolescent boy with Noonan syndrome. *(Used with permission from Cleveland Clinic Children's Hospital Photo Files.)*

CLINICAL FEATURES

- Facial features, especially early in life, most often lead to the clinical diagnosis of Noonan syndrome. Wide-spaced and prominent eyes, epicanthal folds, ptosis, and down-slanting palpebral fissures are common. Other features include hypertelorism (widely spaced eyes), low set posteriorly rotated ears, distinctive upper lip, short neck with excessive skin, and low posterior hairline (**Figure 226-1**).[2]
- During adolescence, the face shape becomes an inverted triangle, wide at the forehead and tapered to a pointed chin. The eyes become less prominent, the neck is longer, and there is accentuation of skin webbing or prominence of the trapezius muscle (**Figures 226-2** and **226-3**).
- Multiple cardiovascular conditions occur in Noonan syndrome. The most common are pulmonary stenosis (often with dysplastic valves; 50 to 60%), hypertrophic cardiomyopathy (20%), and secundum atrial septal defect (6 to 10%).[5,6,7]
- Short stature is present in 50 to 75 percent of patients, who may have growth hormone deficiency, neurosecretory dysfunction, and growth hormone resistance. Mean age at puberty is delayed compared to general population.[8]

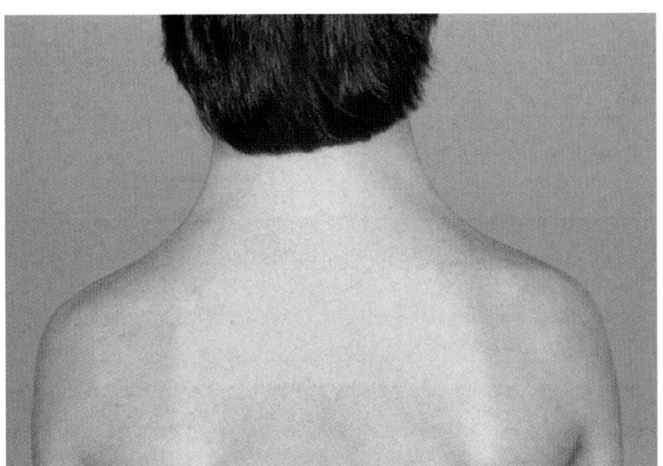

FIGURE 226-3 Prominence of the trapezius muscle and webbed neck in the same boy as in **Figure 226-2**. *(Used with permission from Cleveland Clinic Children's Hospital Photo Files.)*

- Most infants with Noonan syndrome have feeding difficulties that can lead to failure to thrive. Poor suck, prolonged feeding time, or recurrent vomiting have been reported and about 25 percent of infants need to be fed by tube for 2 weeks or longer. Gastroesophageal reflux is also common.[6,8]
- Up to 80 percent of boys diagnosed with Noonan syndrome have unilateral or bilateral cryptorchidism. Male gonadal dysfunction has been reported and is suggested to be caused by primary Sertoli cell dysfunction rather than cryptorchidism.
- An estimated 30 percent of children have a spinal deformity with surgical correction recommended in two thirds of cases. Chest deformity (superior pectus carinatum and inferior pectus excavatum), widely spaced nipples, cubitus valgus, and genu valgum have also been reported.
- Though several hematological abnormalities, including transient monocytosis, thrombocytopenia, and myeloproliferative disorders, have been seen, the most common hematologic disorders are abnormalities of bleeding caused by coagulation defects. Hematological cancers, including juvenile myelomonocytic leukemia, acute myelogenous leukemia, and B-cell acute lymphoblastic leukemia have been reported.
- Lymphatic abnormalities, most commonly peripheral lymphedema, are present in less than 20 percent of individuals but can cause substantial morbidity. Peripheral lymphedema can occur in infants and resolves in the first few years of life or it can develop in adolescence or adulthood.
- In most affected individuals, intelligence is within the normal range, with intelligence quotient generally varying between 70 and 120.
- Roughly 10 percent of affected individuals have auditory deficits in the low frequency range caused by sensorineural hearing loss and 25 percent have deficits in the high frequency range. Inner ear structural abnormalities, including temporal bone abnormalities, have been reported.
- Language impairments are more common in patients with the disease than in the general population and, when present, are associated with a high risk of reading and spelling difficulties.
- Up to 95 percent of affected individuals will have at least one characteristic eye finding including strabismus, refractive errors, amblyopia, or nystagmus. 2/3 of patients develop anterior chamber abnormalities including cataracts. Fundal changes, including optic head drusen, optic disk hypoplasia, colobomas, and myelinated nerves, occur in 20 percent of patients.
- Abnormal pigmentation can occur, including multiple pigmented nevi, café-au-lait spots, and lentigines. Keratosis pilaris of the upper arms and face is common and can impede hair and eyebrow growth. Hair is often thick and curly, although thin, sparse hair has also been reported.

LABORATORY TESTING

- Genetic testing is widely available and chip-based sequencing, which enables the simultaneous assessment of all genes related to diseases caused by changes in RAS, has reduced the cost compared with individual sequencing of each gene. Positive genetic testing can confirm the diagnosis but negative testing cannot exclude the diagnosis.

- Screening CBC with differential and prothrombin time/activated partial thromboplastin should be obtained at the time of diagnosis and after 6 to 12 months of age if the initial screen was performed in infancy.

IMAGING

- Echocardiogram and electrocardiogram should be obtained at the time of diagnosis.
- Renal ultrasound should be obtained on all patients at the time of diagnosis.

DIFFERENTIAL DIAGNOSIS

- Leopard Syndrome—Autosomal dominant disorder with lentigines, electrocardiogram abnormalities, hypertelorism, pulmonary stenosis, abnormal genitalia, retardation of growth, and deafness. Many affected individuals have hypertrophic cardiomyopathy. Is mainly caused by PTPN11 missense mutations and, less often, by RAF1 mutations.
- Cardiofaciocutaneous syndrome—Presents with multiple congenital anomalies and intellectual disability, failure to thrive and short stature, congenital heart defects, and a characteristic facial appearance. Patients have a rounder, more bulbous nasal tip, wider nasal base, fuller lips, and coarser facial features. They also often have follicular hyperkeratosis, sparse eyebrows and lashes, and ichthyosis (see Chapter 171, Ichthyosis). They also develop moderate intellectual disability.[9] Molecular gene testing will distinguish this from Noonan syndrome.
- Costello Syndrome—Infants with high birthweight and delayed growth, developmental delay, coarse facial features, wide nasal bridge, loose and soft skin, increased pigmentation over time, deep palmar and plantar creases, facial or perianal papillomata, premature ageing and hair loss, moderate intellectual disability, flexion or ulnar deviation of the wrist and fingers, and cardiac abnormalities (most commonly pulmonic stenosis and hypertrophic cardiomyopathy).
- Turner syndrome—Only girls are affected and chromosomal analysis helps in the diagnosis. Patients typically have left-sided heart lesions (compared with right-sided lesions in Noonan syndrome), have no or arrested pubertal development, and have gonadal dysgenesis.[10]
- Aarskog syndrome—X-linked disorder, which can cause similar phenotypic features as Noonan syndrome, but caused by FGD1 mutations. These patients do not have congenital heart disease and affected boys have a shawl scrotum (scrotum surrounds the penis like a shawl).

MANAGEMENT

- Multidisciplinary approach with many subspecialists involved in the care of these patients is essential.

NONPHARMACOLOGIC

- Developmental screening yearly.
- Cardiac evaluation by a cardiologist at the time of diagnosis, including an electrocardiogram and echocardiogram.
- Neuropsychological testing.
- Growth should be monitored closely. Children with growth failure and delayed puberty should be referred to a pediatric endocrinologist.
- Routine ophthalmological and auditory evaluations.
- Blood work including coagulation studies every 6 to 12 months and prior to surgical procedures.
- Spine exams yearly.

MEDICATIONS

- Therapeutic interventions for growth failure includes growth hormone therapy.[11] SOR Ⓒ
- Thyroid hormone replacement should be provided for hypothyroidism.
- Estrogen or testosterone therapy should be provided for pubertal delay.

SURGERY

- Orchiopexy by age 1 year for persistent cryptorchidism.
- Cardiac surgery for congenital heart defects when needed.

REFERRAL

- Genetics consultation and follow-up.
- Cardiac evaluation by a cardiologist.
- Children with evidence of delayed puberty (no breast development in girls by the age of 13 years or no testicular enlargement in boys by 14 years of age) should be referred to a pediatric endocrinologist.
- Pediatric gastroenterology/nutrition consultation for feeding difficulties/recurrent vomiting.
- Pediatric Surgery and preoperative evaluation of bleeding risk; hematology consultation as needed for management of bleeding risk.

PREVENTION AND SCREENING

- Prenatal screening is done when prenatal ultrasound shows features suggestive of Noonan syndrome.[12]

PROGNOSIS

- Prognosis depends on the severity of the cardiac lesions.

FOLLOW-UP

- Regular detailed follow-up with a multidisciplinary approach is often needed to address the medical and developmental complications of Noonan syndrome.

PATIENT RESOURCES

- **www.teamnoonan.org**.
- **http://www.teamnoonan.org/information/**.
- **www.teamrasopathies.org**.

PROVIDER RESOURCES

- **http://pediatrics.aappublications.org/content/126/4/746.full.pdf+html**.
- **http://www.teamnoonan.org/information/**.

REFERENCES

1. Noonan JA, Ehmke DA. Associated noncardiac malformations in children with congenital heart disease. *J Pediatr.* 1963;31:150-153.
2. Romano AA, Allanson JE, Dahlgren J et al. Noonan Syndrome: Clinical Features, Diagnosis, and Management Guidelines. *Pediatrics.* 2010;126:746-759.
3. Schubbert S, Zenker M, Rowe SL, et al. Germline KRAS mutations cause Noonan syndrome. *Nat Genet*. 2006;38(3):331-336.
4. Tartaglia M, Mehler EL, Goldberg R, et al. Mutations in *PTPN11*, encoding the protein tyrosine phosphatase *SHP-2*, cause Noonan syndrome. *Nat Genet.* 2001;29(4):465-468.
5. Patton MA. Noonan syndrome: a review. *Growth Genet Horm* 1994;33:1-3.
6. Shaw AC, Kalidas K, Crosby AH, Jeffery S, Patton MA. The natural history of Noonan syndrome: a long-term follow-up study. *Arch Dis Child* 2007;92:128-132.
7. Marino B, Digilio MC, Toscano A, Giannotti A, Dallapiccola B. Congenital heart diseases in children with Noonan syndrome: an expanded cardiac spectrum with high prevalence of atrioventricular canal. *J Pediatr.* 1999;135(6):703-706.
8. Sharland M, Burch M, McKenna WM, Patton MA. A clinical study of Noonan syndrome. *Arch Dis Child*. 1992;67(2):178-183.
9. Roberts A, Allanson J, Jadico SK, et al. The cardiofaciocutaneous syndrome. *J Med Genet*. 2006;43(11):833-842.
10. Loscalzo ML. Turner syndrome. *Pediatr Rev*. 2008;29(7):219-227.
11. Romano AA, Blethen SL, Dana K, Noto RA. Growth hormone treatment in Noonan syndrome: the National Cooperative Growth Study experience. *J Pediatr.* 1996;128:S18-21.
12. Lee K, Williams B, Roza K, et al. *PTPN11* analysis for the prenatal diagnosis of Noonan syndrome in fetuses with abnormal ultrasound findings. *Clin Genet*. 2009;75(2):190-194.

227 PHACE SYNDROME

Carla Torres-Zegarra, MD
Joan Tamburro, DO
Allison Vidimos, MD

PATIENT STORY

A 2.5-year-old girl who was diagnosed with PHACE syndrome at 5 months of age is brought to her dermatologist for a routine follow-up visit. She had presented with multiple hemangiomas on her face, chest, and right arm, microphthalmia, corneal hazing, and a sternal pit. The dermatologist recognized the associated findings as concerning for PHACE syndrome. Work-up at that time revealed moderate to severe dysgenesis of the anterior segment of her right eye and elevated intraocular pressure. An MRI/MRA of her brain showed hypoplasia of the right cerebellum and multiple arterial anomalies (**Figures 227-1** and **227-2**). The facial hemangiomas were treated locally with sequential laser treatments and eventually required removal of a hypertrophic scar on her upper lip. She is doing well clinically. She continues to have residual hemangiomas on her face and arm, microphthalmia, and a sternal pit (**Figures 227-3** and **227-4**).

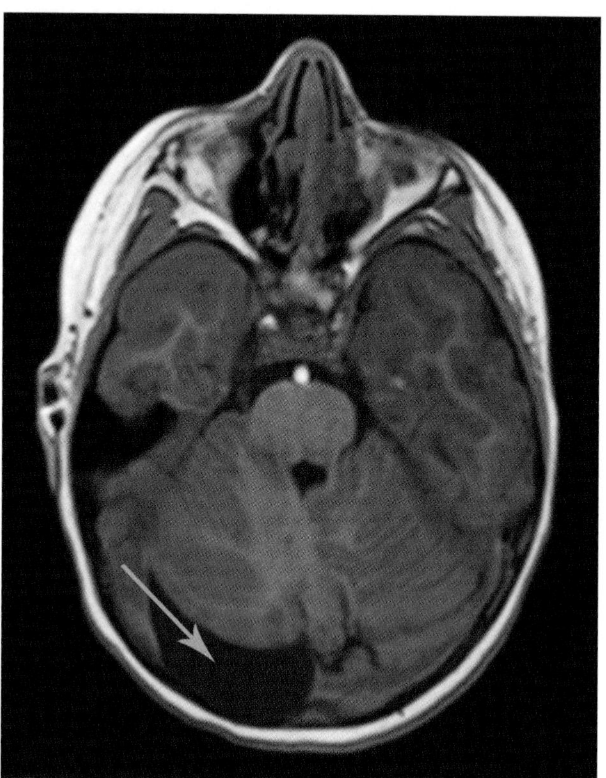

FIGURE 227-1 Hypoplasia of the right cerebellum and superior displacement of the hypoplastic right hemisphere due to an arachnoid cyst on MRI brain in a patient with PHACE syndrome. (*Used with permission from Carla Torres-Zegarra, MD.*)

INTRODUCTION

Hemangiomas are the most common benign tumor in infancy. Associations between infantile hemangiomas with anomalies in the brain, cerebral vasculature, cardiovascular system, eyes, and chest wall have led to the designation of PHACE syndrome, which is defined by the presence of a large, segmental hemangioma, more commonly found on the face or head, associated with one or more congenital malformations, most commonly structural or cerebrovascular anomalies of the brain and cardiovascular system. In 1996, Frieden proposed an acronym for this syndrome as shown in the following:[1]

P—Posterior fossa malformations, that is, Dandy Walker malformation (**Figure 227-1**).

H—Hemangiomas, usually large, segmental, "plaque-like" lesions (**Figure 227-5**).

A—Arterial anomalies (**Figure 227-2**).

C—Cardiac anomalies and coarctation of the aorta.

E—Eye abnormalities, that is, microphthalmos (**Figure 227-3**), exophthalmos, colobomas, retinal vascular abnormalities, optic nerve atrophy, iris hypertrophy, or hypoplasia. A coloboma is a hole in one of the structures of the eye that can cause blindness (**Figure 227-6**).

Ventral anomalies, such as sternal cleft or pits and supraumbilical raphe may also be associated (**Figure 227-4**).

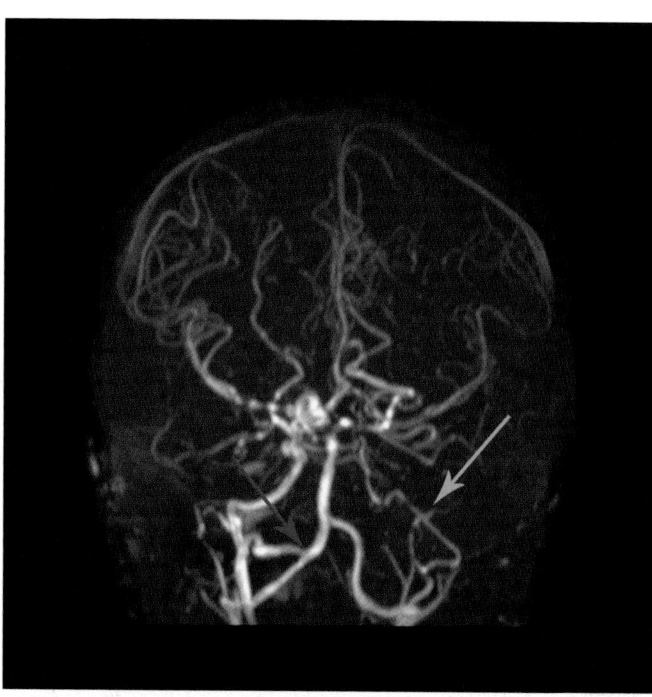

FIGURE 227-2 Left internal carotid hypoplasia (*blue arrow*) and duplicated right vertebral artery (*red arrow*) with marked hypoplasia on MRA of the brain in a patient with PHACE syndrome. (*Used with permission from Carla Torres-Zegarra, MD.*)

SYNONYMS

PHACES syndrome, PHACES association, Pascual Castroviejo type II syndrome, Sternal malformation/vascular dysplasia association, Cutaneous hemangioma: vascular anomaly complex.

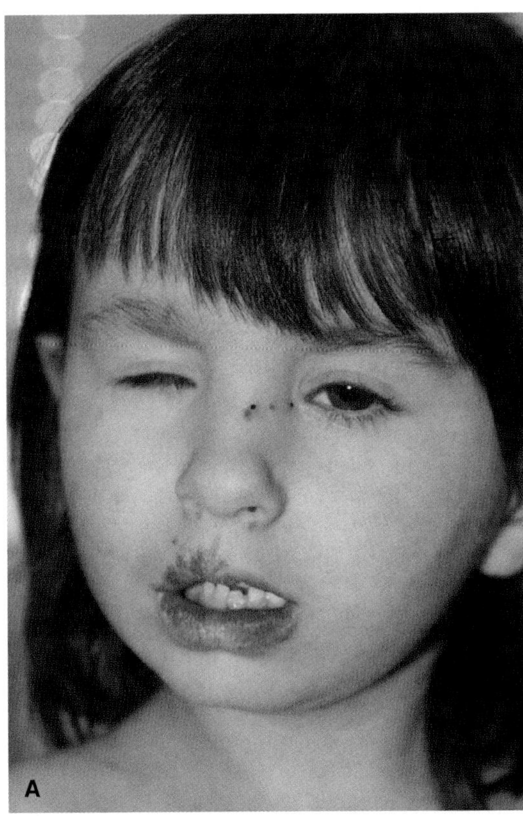

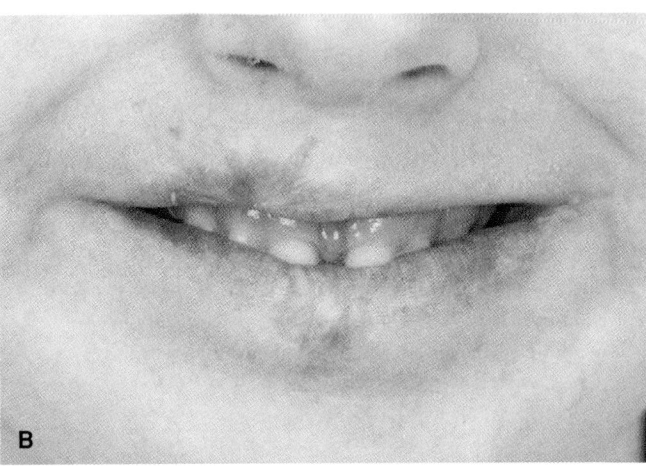

FIGURE 227-3 **A.** Multiple facial hemangiomas and microphthalmia of the right eye in a 2.5-year-old girl with PHACE syndrome. **B.** A hypertrophic scar is evident at the site of laser therapy for her lip hemangioma. (*Used with permission from Carla Torres-Zegarra, MD.*)

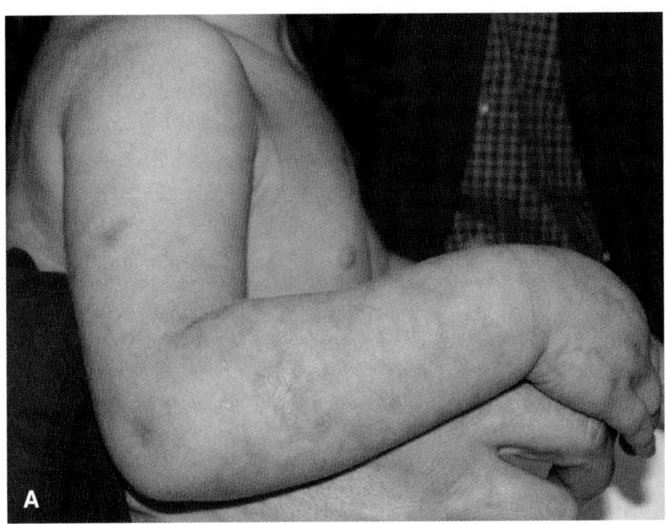

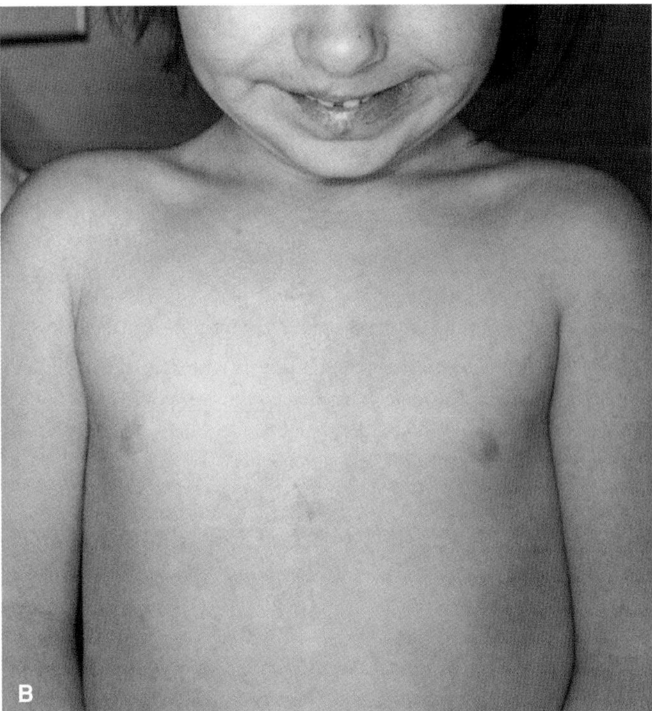

FIGURE 227-4 Residual hemangioma on the arm (**A**) and a sternal pit (**B**), representing evidence of a ventral developmental defect, of the 2.5-year-old girl in **Figure 227-3**. (*Used with permission from Carla Torres-Zegarra, MD.*)

EPIDEMIOLOGY

- There is significant female predominance in PHACE syndrome, with 80 percent of affected children being females.
- Seventy percent of cases only have one extracutaneous manifestation.
- Although uncommon, incidence probably exceeds that of Sturge Weber syndrome (SWS).[2]
- PHACE syndrome is probably still under-recognized since it rarely presents with all associated features.
- Most affected infants are born at term with normal birth weight, which is in contrast to infants with non-PHACE associated infantile hemangiomas, who have a greater incidence of prematurity and low birth weight.[3]

ETIOLOGY AND PATHOPHYSIOLOGY

- The precise pathogenesis of PHACE syndrome is unknown.
- Female predominance was thought to be due to an X-linked dominant condition, which is lethal in males, but this has recently been questioned.[4]
- The structural anomalies found in association with PHACE syndrome suggests that the timing of these errors in morphogenesis occurs early, probably between 6 to 8 weeks of gestation, prior to or during vasculogenesis.
- Both HOX and Eph genes have been linked to capillary, sternal, ocular, neural, and thyroid development and may have an important role in PHACE syndrome.
- The long-term outcome is unclear, mostly due to under diagnosis and lack of data.
- In patients with PHACE syndrome, there is an increase risk of stroke during the 1st year of life due to progressive vasculopathy.

RISK FACTORS

- Size and distribution of the facial hemangiomas appear to play an important role in the development of PHACE syndrome.
- Segmental infantile hemangiomas are more likely to be associated extracutaneous manifestations than localized infantile hemangiomas.[2,5]
- One study found that 2.3 percent of infants with a facial hemangioma developed at least one extracutaneous feature of PHACE, while 20 percent of those with segmental facial hemangiomas developed one or more PHACE anomalies.[2]

DIAGNOSIS

CLINICAL FEATURES

- The hallmark of PHACE syndrome is a large, segmental hemangioma, which is usually on the face or head (**Figure 227-5**). The hemangioma is likely to enlarge during the first year of life (**Figure 227-7**).
- Awareness of this entity and early recognition is crucial.

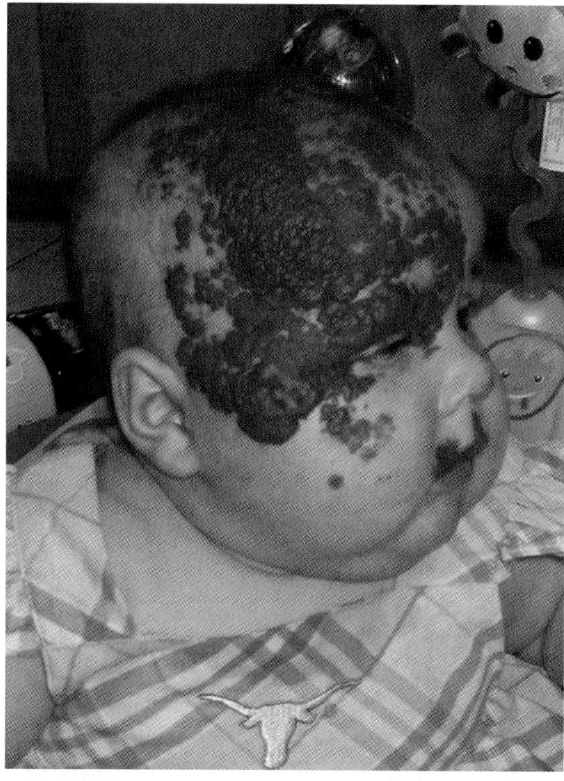

FIGURE 227-5 Large segmental hemangioma on the face of a 5-month-old girl with PHACE syndrome before onset of propranolol therapy. (*Used with permission from AngelPHACE.com.*)

- The diagnosis should be considered when large "plaque-like" segmental hemangiomas are present.
- There is a wide spectrum of features associated with PHACE syndrome which include:[1,6]
  - Large facial hemangiomas (**Figure 227-5**).
  - Posterior fossa malformations including Dandy Walker malformations (**Figure 227-1**).
  - Arterial anomalies (**Figure 227-2**).
  - Cardiac or aortic malformations.
  - Unusual ophthalmologic abnormalities (**Figures 227-3** and **227-6**).
  - Ventral defects such as sternal clefting, supraumbilical raphe, and sternal pits (**Figure 227-4**).
- Cerebral vascular malformations are the most common extracutaneous manifestations of PHACE syndrome; predominant involvement of the arterial system is unique and serves to distinguish this from other neurocutaneous syndromes.
- Most infants have a normal neurologic exam; thus screening for abnormalities should not be based on the presence of neurologic findings.
- Coarctation of the aorta is the most important cardiac finding in these patients.
- Commonly reported ophthalmologic anomalies include microphthalmia, optic nerve hypoplasia, persistent fetal vasculature, and morning glory disc abnormalities.
- Although sternal clefting and/or supraumbilical abdominal raphe are most commonly reported ventral developmental defects, subtle features such as sternal pits, dimples, and papules can be seen.

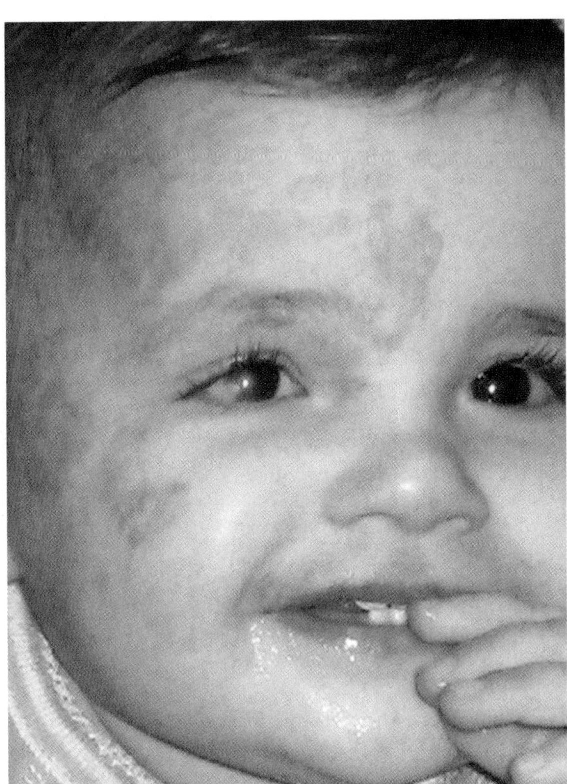

FIGURE 227-6 This infant girl from **Figure 227-5** has a coloboma (hole) of the cornea of the right eye. While she can detect some light she does not have useful vision in that eye. (*Used with permission from AngelPHACE.com.*)

IMAGING

- A variety of imaging studies are used for the evaluation of PHACE syndrome, including:
  - Magnetic resonance imaging and magnetic resonance angiography of the brain to evaluate for posterior fossa and arterial malformations.
  - Echocardiogram to evaluate cardiac anomalies.
  - Ultrasound and/or computed tomography to delineate internal organ involvement where indicated.

DIFFERENTIAL DIAGNOSIS

- Early in the course the hemangioma may be mistaken for a port-wine stain, concerning for SWS. However, a port-wine stain does not proliferate or regress like hemangiomas do (see Chapter 93, Childhood Hemangiomas and Vascular Malformations).

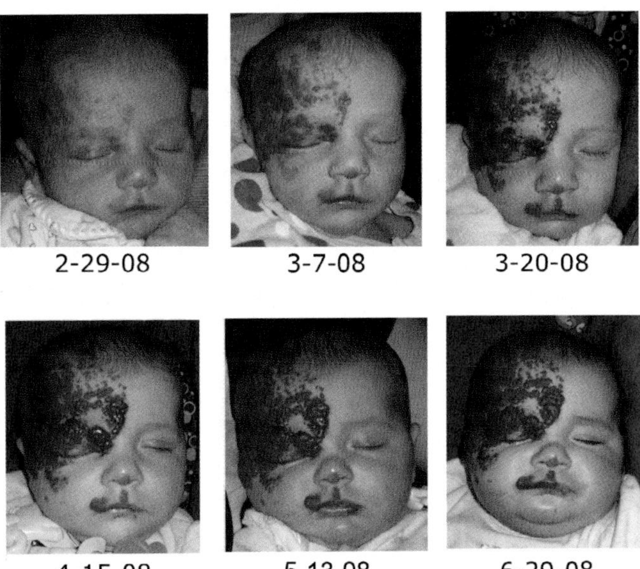

FIGURE 227-7 Progression of a large segmental hemangioma in an infant with PHACE syndrome. (*Used with permission from AngelPHACE.com.*)

- Differences between PHACE syndrome and SWS are listed in the **Table 227-1** (see Chapter 207, Sturge Weber).

MANAGEMENT

- Although it is recommended that all infants with characteristic features of segmental facial hemangiomas undergo thorough evaluation of the brain, heart, and eyes, there are little data to guide the management, risks, prognosis, or anticipatory guidance.[3]
- Infants and children suspected of having PHACE syndrome should undergo a thorough ophthalmologic examination for potential features.
- Brain imaging studies (MRI and MRA) are recommended for all infants with segmental facial hemangiomas.
- Echocardiography is recommended to rule out aortic arch and other abnormalities associated with this syndrome.
- Treatment of hemangiomas can include observation, propranolol, and laser, depending on the stage of the lesion and location. SOR C

TABLE 227-1 Differences in Features Between PHACE Syndrome and Sturge-Weber Syndrome

Feature	PHACES Syndrome	Sturge-Weber Syndrome
Vascular birthmark	Hemangioma	Port-wine stain
CNS vascular defects	Anomalous arteries	Leptomeningeal vascular malformation
Structural CNS defects	Dandy-Walker complex, posterior fossa malformations, cerebellar hypoplasia	Usually none
Eye abnormalities	Microphthalmia, optic nerve hypoplasia, cataracts, ↑ retinal vascularity, coloboma	Glaucoma, ↑ retinal vascularity, buphthalmos

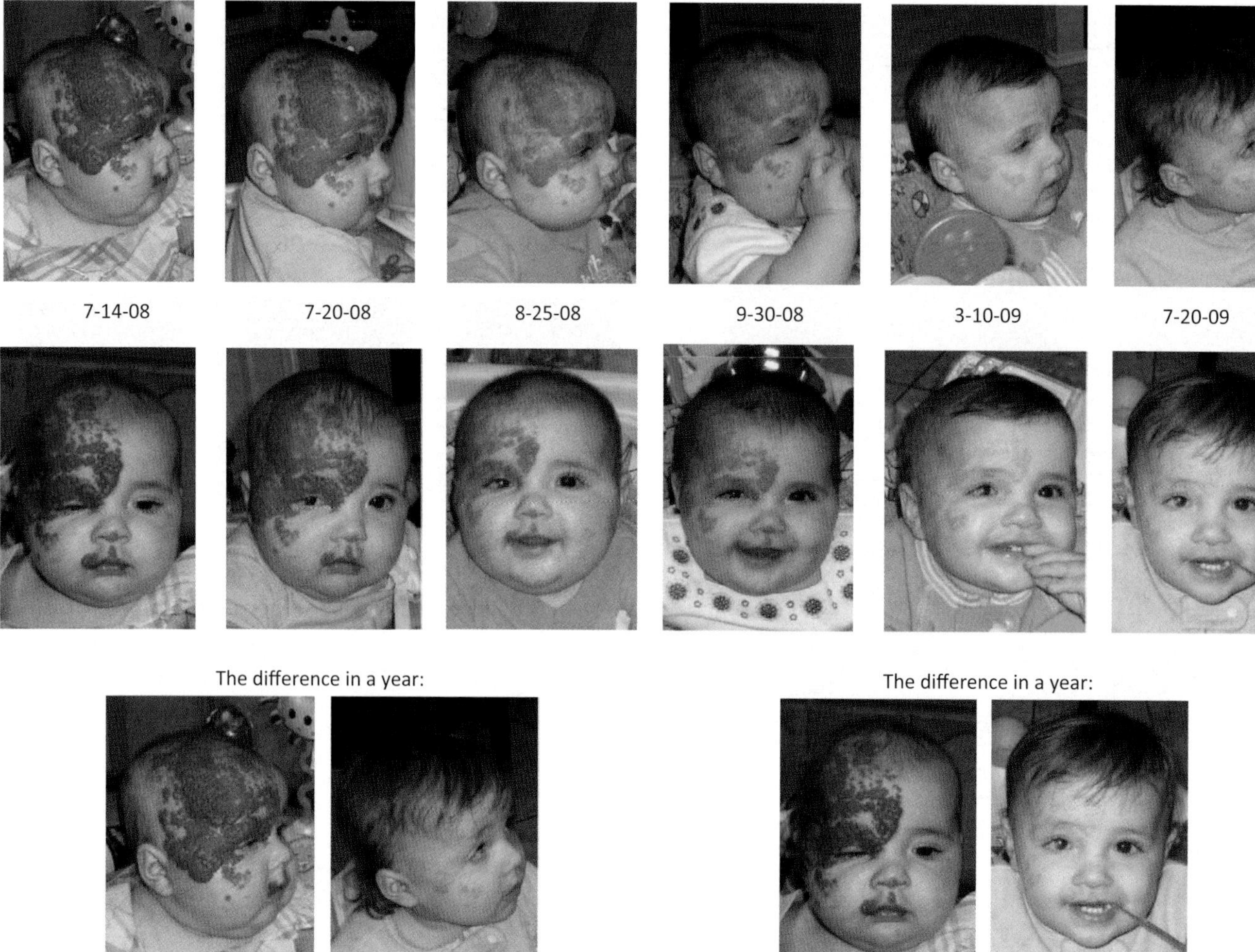

FIGURE 227-8 Regression of a large segmental hemangioma in an infant with PHACE syndrome after nearly 11 months of propranolol therapy. Initially prednisolone was being used simultaneously but that was stopped approximately halfway through the treatment with the propranolol. Note the presence of a coloboma of the right eye. *(Used with permission from AngelPHACE.com.)*

- Although propranolol is now the treatment of choice for large segmental hemangiomas (**Figure 227-8**), there is at least theoretical concern that this drug could cause infarcts if stenotic vessels are present as a part of this syndrome. Thus, it is recommended that cardiac and neuroimaging be completed before propranolol therapy is considered in an infant at risk for PHACE syndrome.[3] SOR Ⓒ
- Aspirin has been advocated for patients with PHACE due to increased risk of stroke during infancy. However, data regarding its benefits are lacking. SOR Ⓒ

REFERRAL

- Infants suspected of having PHACE syndrome should be referred to centers that have experience with the manifestations and are able to provide a multi-disciplinary approach to the diagnosis and management.
- If a PHACE center is not available, referrals to separate specialists can be made:
  - Pediatric dermatologists are likely to be experienced in the use of propranolol for hemangioma treatment. Other dermatologists especially in academic centers should be able to manage this therapy as well.
  - Referrals to neurologists, cardiologists, and ophthalmologists may be needed.

PROGNOSIS

- Long-term studies on neurologic or cardiac outcomes are not currently available.
- A PHACE registry has been established to promote further understanding of this disorder.
- Prognosis for the facial hemangioma is usually excellent, especially with propranolol therapy (**Figures 227-8** and **227-9**).

FOLLOW-UP

- Follow-up should be determined by the clinical features that are present after the initial work-up has been performed
- There are no standard recommendations for the need or frequency of reimaging if manifestations are detected.

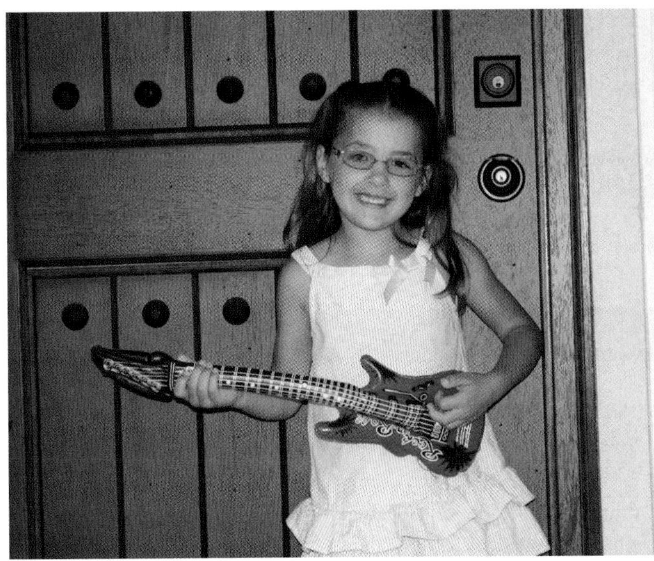

FIGURE 227-9 The girl from **Figures 227-5** to **227-8** on her first day of Kindergarten showing almost complete regression of the hemangioma. *(Used with permission from AngelPHACE.com.)*

PATIENT EDUCATION

The results of propanolol therapy for the facial hemangioma can be very impressive (**Figures 227-8** and **227-9**). Showing the photos in this chapter to the parents of affected children can provide hope for improvement. Continuity of care with appropriate medical providers is essential to the management of this syndrome.

PATIENT RESOURCES

- Information about the PHACE registry may be found on the Texas Children's Hospital Dermatology web site—**www.texaschildrens.org/Locate/Departments-and-Services/Dermatology/Research/**.
- PHACE syndrome community—**http://www.phacesyndromecommunity.org/**.
- National Organization of Vascular Anomalies—**www.novanews.org**.
- **AngelPHACE.com**—Web site started by the parents of the girl shown in **Figures 227-5** through **227-9**.

PROVIDER RESOURCES

- A prospective study of PHACE syndrome in infantile hemangiomas: demographic features, clinical findings, and complications. *Am J Med Genet A*. 2006;140:975-986. **www.ncbi.nlm.nih.gov/pubmed/16575892**.

ACKNOWLEDGEMENT

We greatly thank Mary Alice for the photographs of her daughter with PHACE syndrome (**Figures 227-5** to **227-9**). One can learn more about their family story at http://angelphace.com/. Also visit http://www.phacesyndromecommunity.org/ the site for the organization that supports individuals with PHACE and their families.

REFERENCES

1. Frieden IJ et al. PHACE syndrome: the association of posterior fossa malformations, hemangiomas, arterial anomalies, coarctation of aorta and cardiac defects, and eye abnormalities. *Arch Dermatol*. 1996;132:307-311.
2. Metry DW, Haggstrom AN, Drolet BA, et al. A prospective study of PHACE syndrome in infantile hemangiomas: demographic features, clinical findings, and complications. *Am J Med Genet*. 2006;140:975-986.
3. Metry DW, Garzon MC, Drolet BA, et al. PHACE syndrome: Current knowledge, future directions. *Pediatr Dermatol*. 2009; 26:381-389.
4. Metry DW, Siegel DH, Cordisco MR, et al. A comparison of disease severity among affected male versus female patients with PHACE syndrome. *J Am Acad Dermatol*. 2008;58:81-87.
5. Chiller KG, Passaro D, Frieden IJ: Hemangiomas of infancy: clinical characteristics, morphologica subtypes and their relationship to race, ethnicity and sex. *Arch Dermatol*. 2002;138:1567-1576.
6. Metry D et al. Consensus Statement on Diagnostic Criteria for PHACE Syndrome. *Pediatrics*. 2009;124:1447-1456.

228 INCONTINENTIA PIGMENTI

Carla Torres-Zegarra, MD
Elumalai Appachi, MD, MRCP

PATIENT STORY

A 6-day-old girl is brought by her parents to the emergency department for a rash on her arms and chest. The parents noted that over the past 3 days, the baby has had intermittent episodes of right eye deviation and upper extremity stiffening. These episodes lasted approximately 30 seconds, occurred approximately 3 times per day and were associated with cyanosis. The family history was notable for seizures in a maternal aunt. On physical examination the infant was quiet, seemingly withdrawn with stable vital signs. The infant had erythematous papules and vesicles, some of which had eroded with crusting on the arms and anterior chest (**Figure 228-1**). A direct fluorescent antibody test and culture from the lesions were negative for herpes simplex virus. Skin biopsy of the lesions showed spongiotic dermatitis with many eosinophils and large dyskeratotic cells. Based on the skin lesions and the neurological manifestations, the infant was diagnosed with incontinentia pigmenti. Genetic, neurologic, and ophthalmology consults were obtained.

INTRODUCTION

- Incontinentia pigmenti (IP) is an X-linked dominant systemic disease, usually lethal in males, and characterized by skin involvement at birth in 50 percent of cases. IP is a rare genodermatosis that presents in the neonatal period.

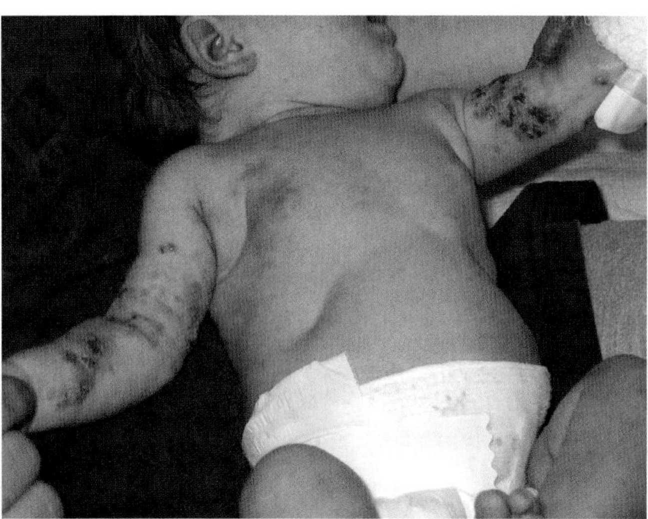

FIGURE 228-1 Papular and vesicular lesions, many of which are hyperkeratotic, on the upper extremities and trunk of a neonate with incontinentia pigmenti. (*Used with permission from Camille Sabella, MD.*)

- The disease involves tissues of ectodermic and mesodermic origin including cutaneous tissue, teeth, eyes and the central nervous system (CNS), amongst other organs.[1]

SYNONYMS

Bloch-Sulzberger syndrome.

EPIDEMIOLOGY

- The incidence of IP is 1 case per 40,000.[1] It is more common in Caucasians than other ethnicities.
- Because IP is an X-linked dominant disease, affected male fetuses usually do not survive, and therefore over 97 percent of living affected individuals are female.
- IP has high penetrance. Most persons with IP begin to express the phenotype within a few months of birth.[2]

ETIOLOGY AND PATHOPHYSIOLOGY

- This X-linked dominant disorder is caused by mutations in the gene known as NEMO (NF-kappa essential modulator, also known as IKK-gamma). The gene NEMO encodes a protein that regulates the function of various chemokines, cytokines, and adhesion molecules, and is essential for protection against tumor necrosis factor induced apoptosis, inflammatory, and immune response[3].
- With this mutated gene, endothelial cells and other cells throughout the body can overexpress chemotactic factors specific for eosinophils, explaining why serum eosinophilia is common in IP patients.
- The epidermal skin lesions also show extensive involvement of eosinophils. It appears that the eosinophils, combined with other factors, lead to extensive inflammation, affecting not only the skin, but also endothelial cells.
- It is believed that this inflammation leads to vaso-occlusion, which results in ischemia, causing both the retinal and neurologic manifestations of IP.

RISK FACTORS

- Family history appears to be the only known risk factor for IP.
- Living males are likely to be affected with Klinefelter syndrome, where an extra X chromosome is present (XXY).

DIAGNOSIS

CLINICAL FEATURES

- Skin manifestations are prominent and develop in four stages:[4]
  - Stage 1—Erythematous papules and vesicles (Bullous stage) that appear in crops in linear streaks along the lines of Blaschko (lines along which skin and appendages, such as hair, melanocytes, and

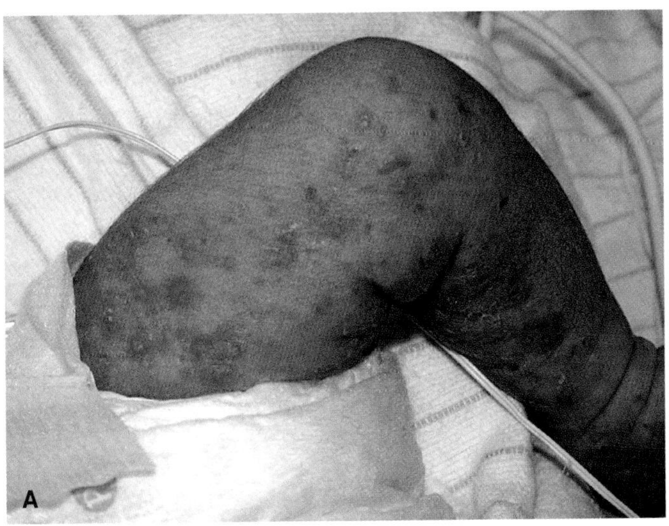

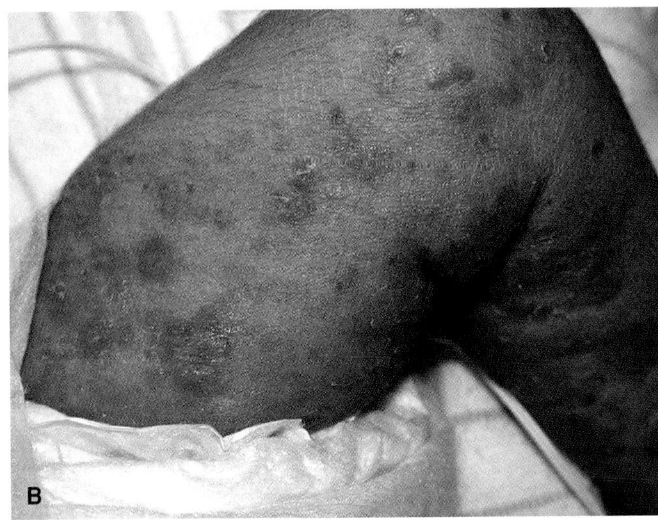

FIGURE 228-2 Erythematous papules and vesicles in a linear pattern in an infant with incontinentia pigmenti (**A**) and on close-up view (**B**). Hyperkeratotic papules and plaques are also evident. (*Used with permission from Eric Kraus, MD.*)

eccrine glands migrate during embryogenesis; **Figures 228-2** to **228-4**). Presentation is usually at birth or within the neonatal period. Each crop typically lasts 1 to 2 weeks.

- Stage 2—"Verrucous stage" that consists of hyperkeratotic warty papules or plaques in linear or swirling patterns (**Figures 228-1** and **228-2**). This stage usually last weeks to months.
- Stage 3—Streaks of hyperpigmentation develop in a "marble cake" or swirled pattern typically occuring at 3 to 6 months of age, often begins to fade in adolescents, but can persist into adulthood (**Figure 228-5**).
- Stage 4—By the second or third decade of life, the hyperpigmented streaks become hypopigmented and atrophic.

- All stages may be present simultaneously, and may also occur in utero. Additional cutaneous changes include patchy alopecia, woolly-hair nevus, and nail dystrophy.
- Systemic abnormalities occur in nearly 80 percent of patients and include:
  - Dental abnormalities (i.e., adontia or conical deformities of the teeth).
  - Ocular problems (strabismus, cataracts, and retinal vascular changes leading to blindness).
  - Neurologic abnormalities (seizures, intellectual disability, mental retardation, and spastic paralysis).
  - Structural malformations (less frequently).
- In 1993, Landy and Donnai proposed a set of clinical diagnostic criteria for IP.[5] The criteria focus on whether or not the suspected patient has a first-degree relative with IP. If this relative exists, then only one of the following is needed for diagnosis of IP:
  - History or evidence of typical skin lesions.
  - Pale, hairless, atrophic linear skin streaks.
  - Dental anomalies.
  - Retinal disease.
  - Multiple male miscarriages.
- If a first-degree relative with IP cannot be established, then diagnostic criteria are separated into major and minor categories.

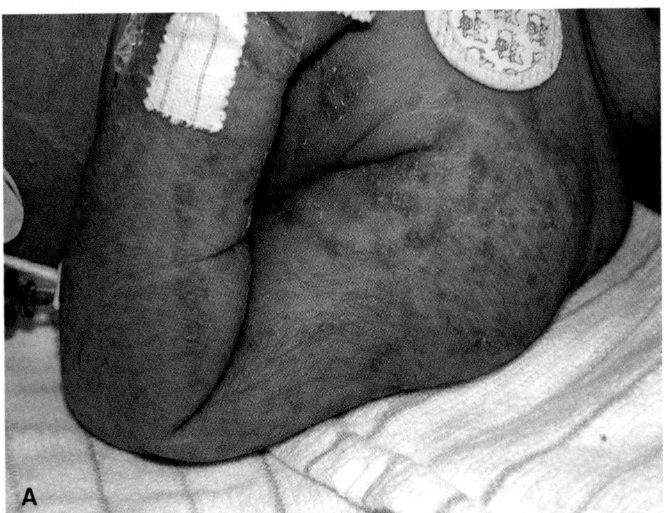

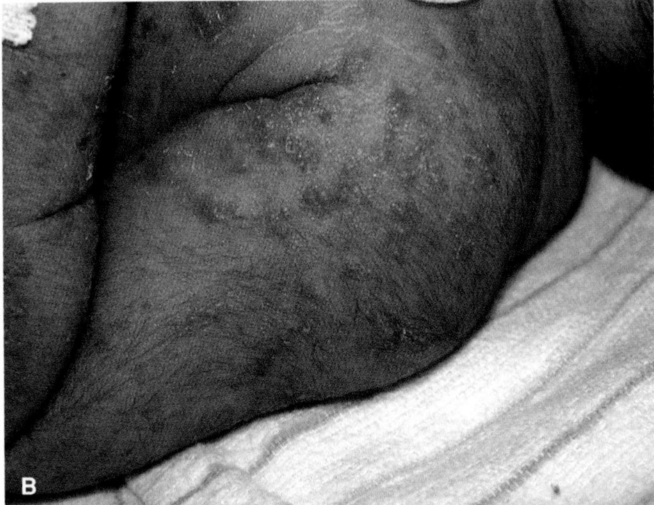

FIGURE 228-3 Crops of vesicular and crusted lesions on the upper extremity and chest of the same infant as in **Figure 228-2** (**A**) and on close-up view (**B**). Note the linear distribution of the lesions on the lower arm. (*Used with permission from Eric Kraus, MD.*)

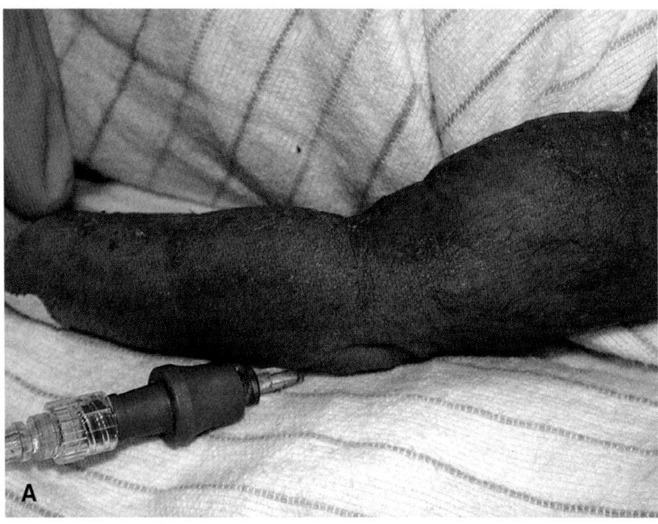

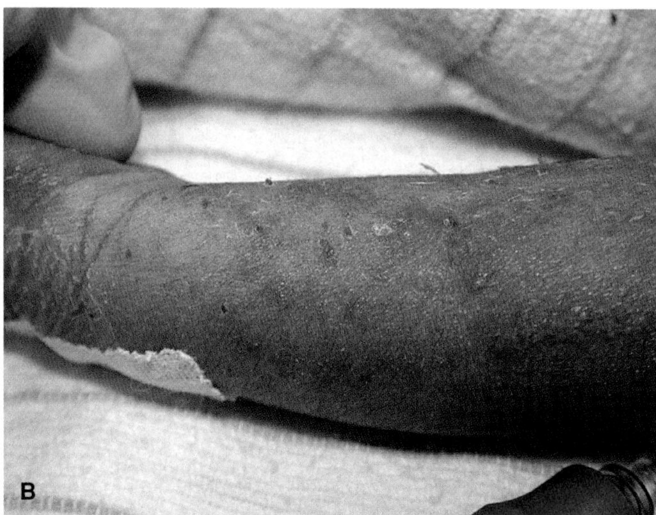

FIGURE 228-4 Linear erythematous papules and vesicles in the same infant (**A**). Note the vesicular and crusting appearance of some of the lesions on the close-up view (**B**). (*Used with permission from Eric Kraus, MD.*)

- Major criteria—Skin lesions that occur in stages from infancy to adulthood.
  - Erythematous lesions followed by vesicles anywhere on the body (sparing the face), usually in a linear distribution.
  - Hyperpigmented streaks and whorls respecting Blaschko lines, occurring mainly on the trunk and sparing the face, fading in adolescence.
  - Pale, hairless, atrophic linear streaks or patches.
- Minor criteria:
  - Hypodontia or anodontia (partial or complete absence of teeth), microdontia (small teeth), or abnormally shaped teeth.
  - Alopecia, wiry coarse hair.
  - Mild nail ridging or pitting, hypertrophied, or curved nails.
  - Retinal abnormalities.

- If a first-degree relative with IP cannot be established, one major criteria and two or more minor criteria are needed for diagnosis. If none of the minor criteria are present, then a diagnosis other than IP should be considered.

LABORATORY TESTING

- The clinical diagnosis is confirmed with skin biopsy that demonstrates spongiotic dermatitis with many eosinophils and large dyskeratotic cells during the vesicular stage.
- Peripheral eosinophilia typically is present in early infancy.[2,3]
- Molecular-based diagnosis is available to detect mutations in NEMO (NF-kappaB essential modulator) that occur in 85 percent of affected patients.[2,4]

IMAGING

- Generally, brain imaging, such as an MRI, should be obtained to investigate the vaso-occlusive consequences of IP in the brain.
- Electroencephalogram should be obtained if seizures are present.

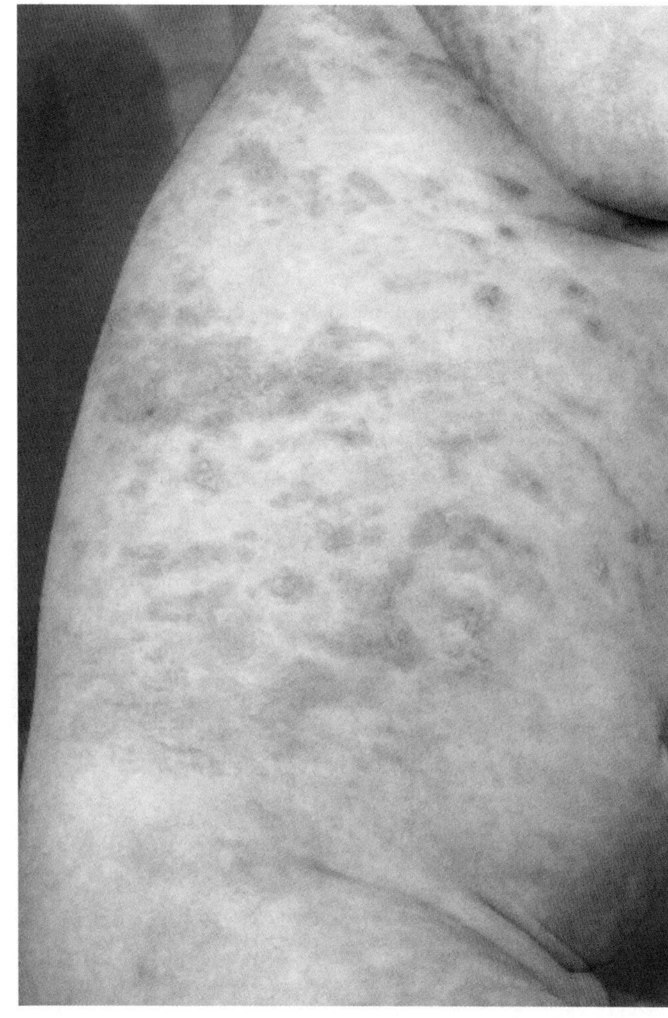

FIGURE 228-5 Hyperpigmentation plaques in a "marble cake" pattern in an infant with Incontinentia pigmenti. (*Used with permission from Cleveland Clinic Children's Photo Files.*)

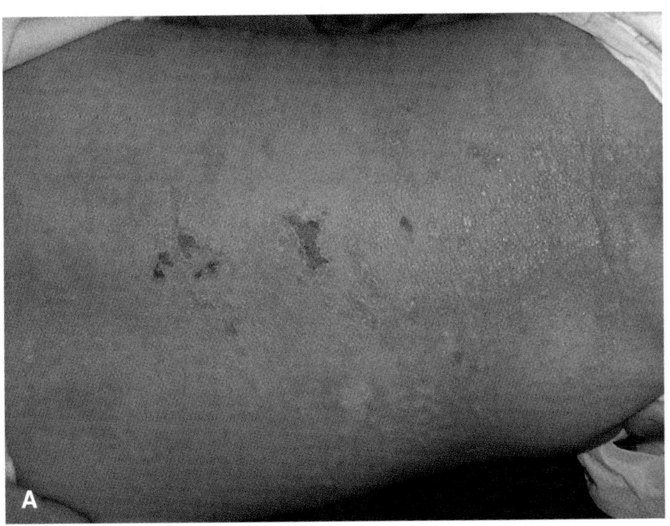

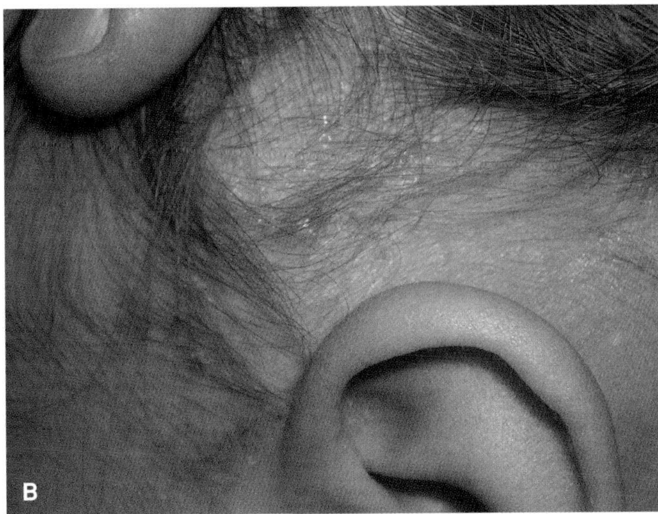

FIGURE 228-6 Bullous mastocytosis in a 9-month-old infant presenting with wheals, bullae, and crusts on the (**A**) back and (**B**) scalp. (*Used with permission from Richard P. Usatine, MD.*)

DIFFERENTIAL DIAGNOSIS

- Erythema toxicum neonatorum—A self-limited neonatal macular or papular rash usually appearing at 2 days of life (see Chapter 92, Normal Skin Changes [newborn]).
- Herpes simplex virus infection—Vesicular lesions on erythematous base often appearing in crops. Needs to be excluded in any infant who has vesicular lesions by direct testing of the lesions for the virus (see Chapter 114, Herpes Simplex and Chapter 187, Congenital and Perinatal Infections).
- Diffuse cutaneous mastocytosis—The affected infants develop urticaria when exposed to hot water or other physical stimuli (see Chapter 134, Urticaria and Angioedema). They may also get bullous mastocytosis, which can crust in a manner very similar to IP (**Figure 228-6**). A biopsy can differentiate between these 2 diagnoses.
- Hypomelanosis of Ito.[6] Lesions are hypopigmented, rather than hyperpigmented, macules arranged in sharply demarcated whorls, streaks, and patches over the body, extremities (**Figure 228-7**) and face that follow the lines of Blaschko. There are no papules, vesicles or crusts as seen in IP (see Chapter 167, Vitiligo and Hypopigmentation).

MANAGEMENT

- There is no cure or specific treatment. Genetic therapies are not currently available; management is aimed at managing the presenting signs and symptoms.
- Local care of the skin manifestations is needed to prevent infection or excessive scarring.
- The skin abnormalities of IP usually disappear by adolescence or adulthood without treatment.
- Diminished vision may be treated with corrective lenses, medication, or, in severe cases, surgery.
- A dental specialist may treat dental problems.
- Neurological symptoms such as seizures, muscle spasms, or mild paralysis may be controlled with medication and/or medical devices, and with the advice of a neurologist.
- Developmental therapy may be needed for those with developmental delay.

REFERRAL

- Because IP is a multisystemic disease, dermatologic, genetic, ophthalmic, neurologic, and dental consultations should be obtained upon diagnosis.

PREVENTION AND SCREENING

- If a proband is identified, clinical examination of family members and genetic testing of the mother is warranted.

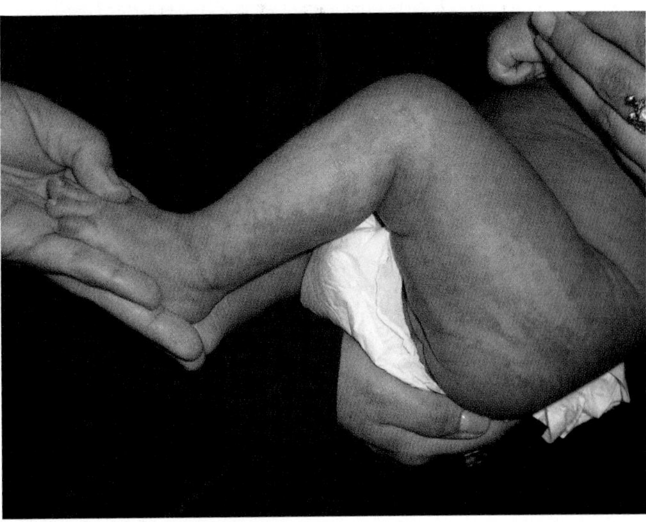

FIGURE 228-7 Hypomelanosis of Ito in a 2-month-old infant showing linear and whorled hypopigmentation from the buttocks down to the foot. These areas of hypopigmentation extend up the trunk and down the arm on the same side of the body. They follow Blaschko lines. (*Used with permission from Richard P. Usatine, MD.*)

- If a female has IP (IKBKG mutation), the risk of conceiving a fetus with IP is 50 percent. However, most affected males die in utero, meaning that an affected mother has a near 33 percent probability of giving birth to either an affected female, unaffected female, or unaffected male.
- In parents without IP or an IP-related IKBKG mutation that have had a child with IP, the risk of a subsequent child having IP is less than 1 percent.[7]
- Prenatal diagnosis of fetuses with a family history of IP is possible via DNA analysis obtained by amniocentesis or chorionic villus sampling.

PROGNOSIS

- Although the skin abnormalities usually regress, and sometimes disappear completely, the prognosis is dependent upon residual neurological impairment.
- Survival in male patients may be related to genetic heterogeneity or postzygotic mosaicism. In polymerase chain reaction analysis of samples from 18 boys with clinical and histologic features of IP, 15 had the normal NEMO allele in leukocyte DNA, whereas three had both the normal NEMO allele and the NEMO mutation that occurs in the majority of girls with IP, confirming postzygotic mosaicism.[4]

FOLLOW-UP

Follow-up is contingent on the affected systems.

PATIENT EDUCATION

- Families should be educated as to the genetics of the disorder and genetic counseling should be provided for all affected families.

PATIENT RESOURCES

- Incontinentia Pigmenti International Foundation—**www.ipif.org**.
- NINDS Incontinentia Pigmenti Information Page—**www.ninds.nih.gov/disorders/incontinentia_pigmenti/incontinentia_pigmenti.htm#What_is_the_prognosis**.

PROVIDER RESOURCES

- **http://emedicine.medscape.com/article/1114205**.
- **http://archderm.jamanetwork.com/article.aspx?articleid=479497**.

REFERENCES

1. Spallone A: Incontinentia pigmenti (Bloch-Sulzberger syndrome): seven case reports from one family. *British Journal of Ophthalmology*. 1987;(71):629-634.
2. Berlin A, Paller A, Chan L. Incontinentia pigmenti: A review and update on the molecular basis of pathophysiology. *J Am Acad Dermatol*. 2002;(47):169-187.
3. Kitakawa D, Campos Fontes P, Cintra Magalhães F, Dias Almeida J, Guimarães Cabral L: Incontinentia pigmenti presenting as hypodontia in a 3-year-old girl: a case report. *Journal of Medical Case Reports*. 2009;(3):1943-1947.
4. Hadj-Rabia S, Froidevaux D, Bodak N, Hamel-Teillac D, Smahi A, Touil J, Fraitag S, de Prost Y, Bodemer C: Clinical Study of 40 Cases of Incontinentia Pigmenti. *Arch Dermatol*. 2003;139:(9)1163-1170.
5. Landy SJ, Donnai D: Incontinentia pigmenti (bloch-sulzberger syndrome). *J Med Genet*. 1993;30(1):53-59.
6. Ciarallo L, Paller A: Two Cases of Incontinentia Pigmenti Simulating Child Abuse *Pediatrics*. 1997;100(4):1-5.
7. Scheuerle A, Ursini M: Incontinentia Pigmenti: Bloch-Sulzberger Syndrome. GeneReviews™ [Internet]. Pagon RA, Adam MP, Bird TD, et al., eds. University of Washington, Seattle; 1993-2013.

PART 22

SUBSTANCE ABUSE

Strength of Recommendation (SOR)	Definition
A	Recommendation based on consistent and good-quality patient-oriented evidence.*
B	Recommendation based on inconsistent or limited-quality patient-oriented evidence.*
C	Recommendation based on consensus, usual practice, opinion, disease-oriented evidence, or case series for studies of diagnosis, treatment, prevention, or screening.*

*See Appendix A on pages 1320–1322 for further information.

229 SUBSTANCE ABUSE DISORDER

Richard P. Usatine, MD
Heidi Chumley, MD
Kelli Hejl Foulkrod, MS

PATIENT STORY

A young mother and her four children are being seen in a free clinic within a homeless shelter for various health reasons (**Figure 229-1**). The woman is currently clean and sober, but has a long history of cocaine use and addiction (**Figure 229-2**). Her children span the ages of 3 months to 5 years. She was recently living with her mother after the birth of her youngest child, but was kicked out of her mother's home when she began to use cocaine once again. The patient gave written consent to the photograph and when she was shown the image on the digital camera she noted how depressed she looked. She asked for us to tell the viewers of this photograph that these can be the consequences of drug abuse—being depressed, homeless, and a single mom. Only time will reveal the effect of this situation on her four children. They are at risk for so many problems including neglect, abuse, behavioral issues and being placed in foster care. They are also at higher risk of developing substance abuse disorder. Being the health care provider for these children requires understanding the disease of addiction and the consequences of this on the family.

INTRODUCTION

Addiction occurs when substance use has altered brain function to an extent that an individual loses a degree of control over his or her behaviors. Addiction is an epigenetic phenomenon. Many genes influence the brain functions that affect behavior and genetic variants.

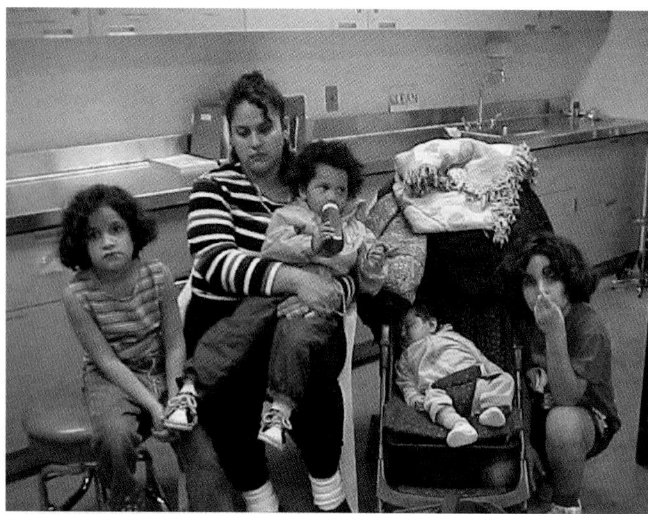

FIGURE 229-1 A cocaine-addicted mother with her children in a homeless shelter. Her drug addiction resulted in their homelessness. (*Used with permission from Richard P. Usatine, MD.*)

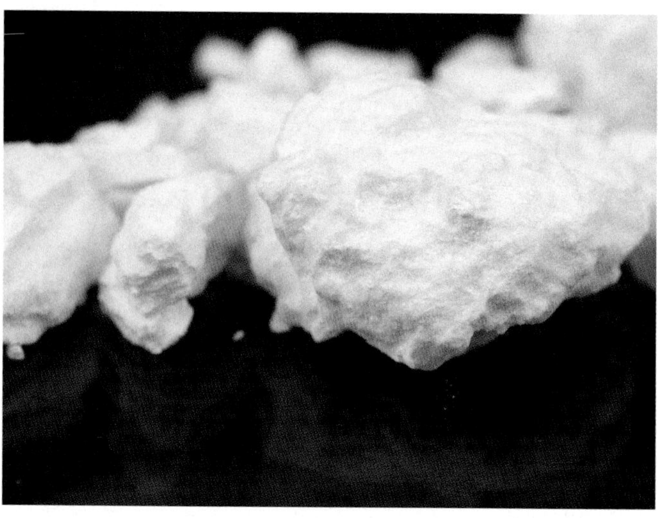

FIGURE 229-2 Purified cocaine. (*Used with permission from DEA.*)

These genes differ in their susceptibility to environmental conditions, which trigger the changes in brain circuitry, and contribute to the development of addiction. Addiction must be recognized and treated as a chronic illness with an interprofessional team and social support.

EPIDEMIOLOGY

- An estimated 69.6 million Americans age 12 years or older were current users of a tobacco product in 2010. This represents 27.4 percent of the population in that age range. In addition, 58.3 million persons (23% of the population) were current cigarette smokers, 13.2 million (5.2%) smoked cigars, 8.9 million (3.5%) used smokeless tobacco, and 2.2 million (0.8%) smoked tobacco in pipes.[1]
- An estimated 22.6 million Americans age 12 years or older were current illicit drug users in 2010. This represents 8.9 percent of the population in that age range.[1]
- Marijuana was the most commonly used illicit drug (17.4 million users; **Figures 229-3** and **229-4**). It was used by 76.8 percent of

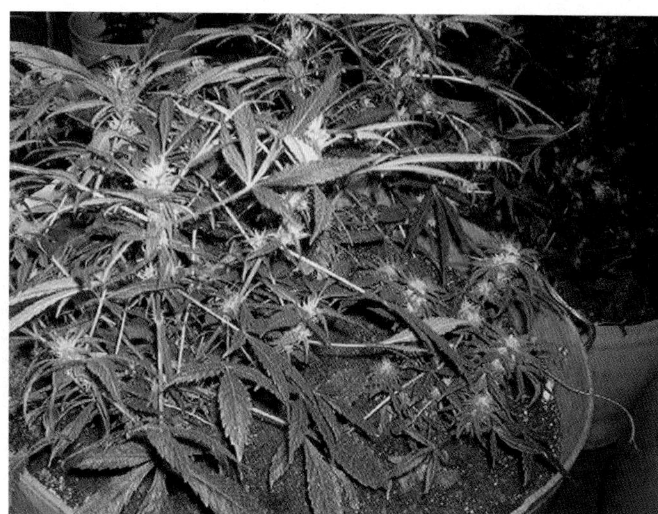

FIGURE 229-3 Home-grown marijuana plant. (*Used with permission from DEA.*)

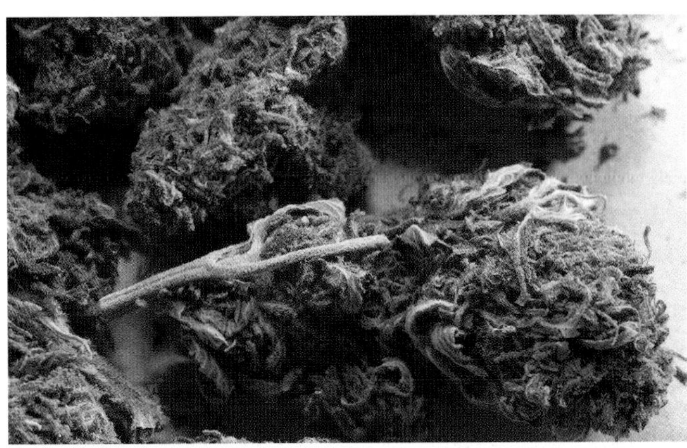

FIGURE 229-4 Marijuana ready to be smoked. (*Used with permission from DEA.*)

current illicit drug users. Among current illicit drug users, 60.1 percent used only marijuana, 16.7 percent used marijuana and another illicit drug, and the remaining 23.2 percent used only an illicit drug other than marijuana.[1]

- There were 1.5 million persons who were current cocaine users in 2010.[1]
- There were 353,000 persons who were current methamphetamine users in 2010 (**Figure 229-5**).[1]
- Hallucinogens were used by 1.2 million persons (0.5%) in 2010, including 695,000 (0.3%) who had used ecstasy (**Figure 229-6**).[1]
- In 2010, 140,000 persons used heroin for the first time (**Figure 229-7**).[1]
- There were 9 million people age 12 years or older (3.6%) who were current users of illicit drugs other than marijuana in 2010. Most (7 million, 2.7%) used psychotherapeutic drugs nonmedically (including prescription drugs). Of these, 5.1 million used pain relievers, 2.2 million used tranquilizers, 1.1 million used stimulants, and 374,000 used sedatives.[1]
- Among persons who used pain relievers nonmedically in the past 12 months, 55 percent reported that the source of the drug was from a friend or relative for free. Another 17.3 percent reported that they got the drug from a physician. Only 4.4 percent obtained the pain relievers from a drug dealer or other stranger, and only 0.4 percent reported buying the drug on the Internet.[1]

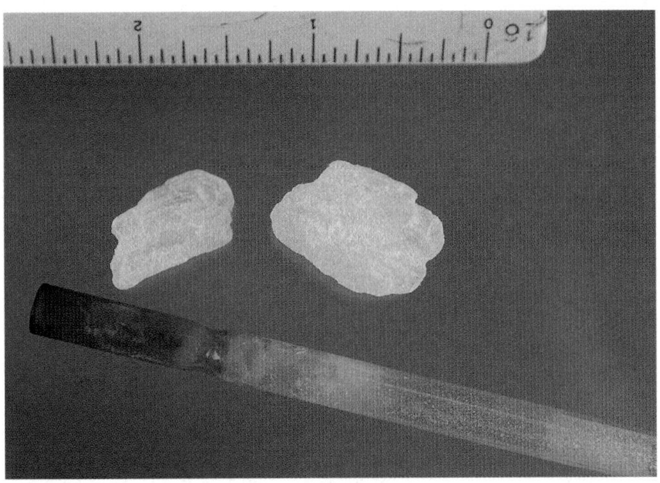

FIGURE 229-5 Methamphetamine ice with pipe. (*Used with permission from DEA.*)

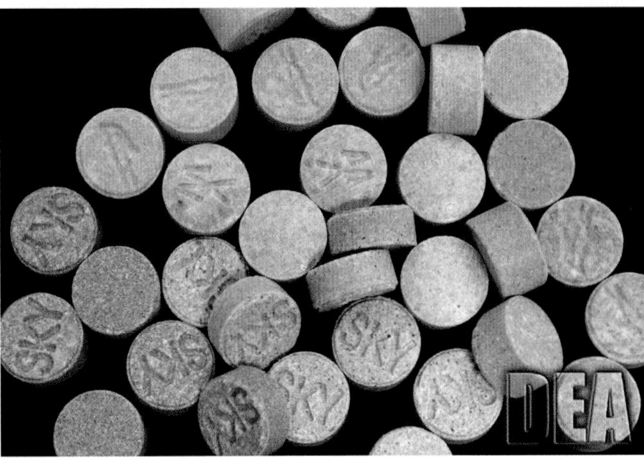

FIGURE 229-6 Ecstasy tablets used at raves where people dance all night long and some collapse in dehydration. (*Used with permission from DEA.*)

ASSOCIATION WITH CIGARETTE AND ALCOHOL USE

- In 2010, the rate of current illicit drug use was 8.5 times higher among youths age 12 to 17 years who smoked cigarettes in the past month (52.9%) than it was among youths who did not smoke cigarettes in the past month (6.2%).[1]
- Past month illicit drug use was also associated with the level of past month alcohol use. Among youths age 12 to 17 years in 2010 who were heavy drinkers (i.e., drank 5 or more drinks on the same

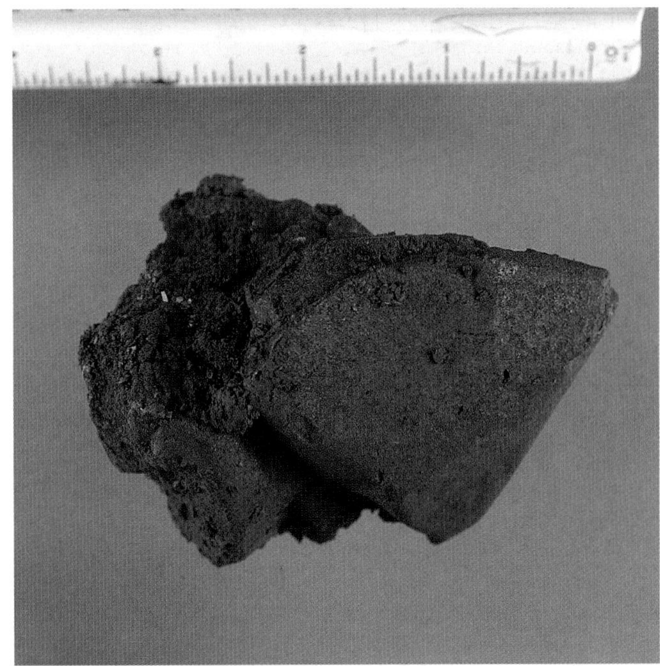

FIGURE 229-7 Black tar heroin for injection. (*Used with permission from DEA.*)

occasion [i.e., at the same time or within a couple of hours] on each of 5 or more days in the past 30 days), 70.6 percent were also current illicit drug users, which was higher than among nondrinkers (5.1%).[1]

ETIOLOGY AND PATHOPHYSIOLOGY

- "Drug addiction is a brain disease. Although initial drug use might be voluntary, drugs of abuse have been shown to alter gene expression and brain circuitry, which in turn affect human behavior. Once addiction develops, these brain changes interfere with an individual's ability to make voluntary decisions, leading to compulsive drug craving, seeking and use."[2]
- Addiction is a polygenic disorder. Many genes have direct or indirect influences on neurotransmitters, drug metabolic pathways, and behavioral patterns. For example, variants of receptors for dopamine or opiates influences perceived reward.[3]
- Epigenetic mechanisms, external influences that trigger changes in gene expression, are believed to play a role through modulation of reward and emotion.[3] As such, both genetics and environment/learned behaviors can increase a person's risk for substance abuse.
- Family, twin, and adoption studies convincingly demonstrate that genes play an important role in the development of alcohol dependence, with heritability estimates in the range of 50 to 60 percent for both men and women. Important genes include those involved in alcohol metabolism, and those involved in γ-aminobutyric acid (GABA), endogenous opioid, dopaminergic, cholinergic, and serotonergic transmission.[4]
- Several drinking behaviors, including alcohol dependence, history of blackouts, age at first drunkenness, and level of response to alcohol are associated with single-nucleotide polymorphisms (SNPs) within 1 of 4 GABA receptor genes on chromosome 5q.[5]
- Comorbid mental health issues and chronic pain disorders are highly prevalent among persons with substance abuse disorders. Commonly, a person begins using drugs to self-treat feelings of depression and symptoms of pain.
- The medical consequences of addiction are far reaching and very costly to society. Cardiovascular disease, stroke, cancer, HIV/AIDS, hepatitis, and lung disease can all be increased by drug abuse. Some of these effects occur when drugs are used at high doses or after prolonged use. Some consequences occur after just one use.[2]
- Classes of substances that are frequently abused and involved in addiction include:
    - Depressants—Alcohol, sedatives, hypnotics, opioids, and anxiolytics.
    - Stimulants—Cocaine, amphetamines, and nicotine.
    - Hallucinogens—Cannabis, phencyclidine (PCP), and lysergic acid diethylamide (LSD).
    - Toxic inhalants.
- The onset of drug effects is approximately:
    - Seven to ten seconds for inhaling or smoking.
    - Fifteen to thirty seconds for intravenous injection.
    - Three to five minutes for intramuscular or subcutaneous injection.
    - Three to five minutes for intranasal use (snorting).

RISK FACTORS

- Family history.
- Personal history of prior addiction.

DIAGNOSIS

The diagnosis of a substance use disorder is based on a pathological pattern of behaviors related to use of the substance.[6] The DSM V uses 11 criteria to make this diagnosis. One example of these criteria is the following 11 symptoms for alcohol abuse disorder. If one substitutes other substances like cannabis or cocaine the same criteria still apply.

Alcohol abuse disorder is diagnosed when there is a problematic pattern of alcohol use leading to clinically significant impairment or distress, manifested by at least two of the following, occurring within a 12-month period:

1. Alcohol is often taken in larger amounts or over a longer period than was intended.
2. There is a persistent desire or unsuccessful efforts to cut down or control alcohol use.
3. A great deal of time is spent in activities necessary to obtain alcohol, use alcohol, or recover from its effects.
4. Craving, or a strong desire or urge to use alcohol.
5. Recurrent alcohol use resulting in a failure to fulfill major role obligations at work, school, or home.
6. Continued alcohol use despite having persistent or recurrent social or interpersonal problems caused or exacerbated by the effects of alcohol.
7. Important social, occupational, or recreational activities are given up or reduced because of alcohol use.
8. Recurrent alcohol use in situations in which it is physically hazardous.
9. Alcohol use is continued despite knowledge of having a persistent or recurrent physical or psychological problem that is likely to have been caused or exacerbated by alcohol.
10. Tolerance, as defined by either of the following:
    - A need for markedly increased amounts of alcohol to achieve intoxication or desired effect.
    - A markedly diminished effect with continued use of the same amount of alcohol.
11. Withdrawal, as manifested by either of the following:
    - The characteristic withdrawal syndrome for alcohol (refer to Criteria A and B of the criteria set for alcohol withdrawal).
    - Alcohol (or a closely related substance, such as a benzodiazepine) is taken to relieve or avoid withdrawal symptoms.

Severity is graded based on the number of symptoms present:

Mild: Presence of 2–3 symptoms.

Moderate: Presence of 4–5 symptoms.

Severe: Presence of 6 or more symptoms.[6]

CLINICAL FEATURES VISIBLE WITH SUBSTANCE ABUSE

- With intoxication, the following signs may be visible:
  - Via stimulants—Dilated pupils and increase in blood pressure, respiratory rate, pulse, and body temperature.
  - Via depressants—Decrease in blood pressure, respiratory rate, pulse, and body temperature. Opioids produce pinpoint pupils. Alcohol intoxication produces dilated pupils.
  - Withdrawal develops with decline of substance in the central nervous system (CNS). Withdrawal reactions vary by the substance used. Alcohol withdrawal is one of the most deadly and dangerous types of withdrawal.

LABORATORY TESTING

- All injection-drug users and persons engaged in high-risk sexual activities should be screened for HIV (with consent), hepatitis B and hepatitis C, and syphilis (rapid plasma reagin [RPR]).
- Persons who have multiple sex partners or use sex to obtain drugs are at high risk for sexually transmitted infections (STIs) and should be tested.
- Urine screen for common drugs of abuse may reveal other drugs not admitted to in the history. Most laboratories can differentiate prescription from nonprescription drugs (i.e., opiates) upon request. Substances have different physiologic half-lives in the body and show up for varying amounts of time in the urine. Marijuana has a long excretion half-life and may be detectable for 1 month after its use. Other substances may last for only days.

DIFFERENTIAL DIAGNOSIS

Substance abuse disorders coexist with and complicate the course and treatment of numerous psychiatric conditions.

- Mood/anxiety disorders—Especially depression, bipolar affective disorder, panic disorder, and generalized anxiety disorder. Persons with addictions can develop the symptoms of these disorders from the drugs of abuse. However, mood and anxiety disorders can predate the use of drugs, and some of the motivation for drug use can stem from the desire to self-treat these psychological conditions. It is best to evaluate persons when they are off the drugs whenever possible.
- Schizophrenia—Although drugs can cause temporary psychosis and paranoia, if these symptoms persist after the drugs are stopped for some time, consider schizophrenia and other causes of psychosis.
- Personality disorders—These are a complicated set of disorders that can coexist and be confused with substance abuse disorder. A person in the midst of their addiction may appear to have an antisocial personality disorder when committing crimes to get money for expensive drugs. It is best to not use this diagnosis unless the behaviors continue when the person is off the drugs.

MANAGEMENT

- Recognize addiction (dependence). One simple mnemonic device is the "three C's of addiction":
  - **C**ompulsion to use.
  - Lack of **C**ontrol.
  - **C**ontinued use despite adverse consequences.
- Use the "5 *A*s"—Ask, Advise, Assess, Assist, and Arrange—to help smokers who are willing to quit. This model can be applied to any substance of abuse.[7]
- Offer counseling and pharmacotherapy to aid your patients to quit smoking.
- Use the CAGE[7] questionnaire when asking about alcohol use:
  - Cut down (Have you ever felt you should *cut* down on your drinking?).
  - Annoyed (Have people *annoyed* you by criticizing your drinking?).
  - Guilty (Have you ever felt bad or *guilty* about your drinking?).
  - Eye opener (Have you ever had a drink first thing in the morning to steady your nerves or get rid of a hangover?).

Interpreting the results: one positive suggests at risk, two positives suggest abuse, and three or four positives suggest dependence. This is just a screening tool, and further evaluation is always needed.

- Recommend 12-step programs. These have been very effective for millions of people worldwide.
- Refer to substance abuse programs. Such programs include hospital- and community-based programs. Some programs include detoxification and others require the patient to have gone through detoxification before starting the program. There are residential treatment units, outpatient programs, and ongoing self-help programs. Learn about the programs in your community and work with them.
- When prescribing opioid analgesics for chronic pain consider the outcomes in four domains, or the "4 *A*s." Is the patient:
  - Receiving adequate Analgesia?
  - Experiencing improvements in Activities of daily life?
  - Experiencing any Adverse effects?
  - Demonstrating Aberrant medication-taking behaviors that may be linked to addiction?[8]
- When patients are exhibiting aberrant drug-taking behaviors, consider the following:
  - They may have an addiction.
  - They may not be getting adequate pain relief taking the drug as prescribed.
  - They may have a comorbid mental illness.
  - They may intend to distribute pain medications illegally.[9]
- Help your patients acknowledge that they have a problem and offer them help in a nonjudgmental manner.
- Enlist parents and family members to help.
- Demonstrate genuine concern and care; suspend judgment and you will have a higher chance of succeeding to help your patients overcome addiction.
- Advanced brain imaging and genetic tests are helping us to understand the physiologic basis of addiction and will ultimately provide us with better treatments for the medical disease of addiction.

PERSONS IN RECOVERY

- Be careful how you prescribe medications to persons in recovery. A "simple" prescription for hydrocodone (Vicodin) postoperatively can start a recovered person down the road of active addiction.
- Avoid giving opioids and benzodiazepines whenever there are good alternatives. Use NSAIDs for pain if possible. Use selective serotonin reuptake inhibitors (SSRIs), other antidepressants, or buspirone for anxiety if a medication is needed.
- If an opioid is needed, work with the patient to monitor the amount and manner of use. Involving a third person or sponsor to help meter out the dose may prevent relapse.
- Be upfront and honest about a shared goal to avoid relapse.

FOLLOW-UP

- Follow-up is critical to the treatment of all types of substance abuse. Substance abuse is a chronic condition (similar to hypertension or diabetes mellitus) and requires ongoing intervention to maintain sobriety.
- The frequency and intensity of follow-up depends on the substance, the addiction, and the patient.
- Do not give up on patients who relapse because it often takes more than 1 attempt before long-term cessation can be achieved.

PATIENT EDUCATION

Explain to patients that addiction is a disease and not a failing of their moral character. Inform patients about the existing treatment programs in their community and offer them names and phone numbers so that they may get help. If your patient is not ready for help today, give the numbers and names for tomorrow. Speak about the value of 12-step programs because these are effective and everyone can afford a 12-step program (they are free). There are 12-step programs in the community for everyone, including nonsmokers and agnostics.

PATIENT RESOURCES

- Alcoholics Anonymous (AA)—Meetings and the Big Book are free. The Big Book is online for free in three languages. **www.alcoholics-anonymous.org/**.
- Narcotics Anonymous (NA)—Meetings are free. The *Basic Text* costs $10; it is similar to the AA big book, but the language is more up to date and readable. **http://www.na.org/**.
- Cocaine Anonymous (CA)—Meetings are free. Their first book *Hope, Faith and Courage: Stories from the Fellowship of Cocaine Anonymous* was published in 1994 and sells for $10. **www.ca.org**.
- Crystal Meth Anonymous (12-step meetings)—**www.crystalmeth.org**.

PROVIDER RESOURCES

- The National Institute on Drug Abuse (NIDA). *Medical Consequences of Drug Abuse*—**www.nida.nih.gov/consequences**.
- Substance Abuse and Mental Health Services Administration—**www.samhsa.gov**.
- Drug Enforcement Agency. *Multi-Media Library* (includes many images of illegal drugs)—**www.usdoj.gov/dea/multimedia.html**.

REFERENCES

1. Substance Abuse and Mental Health Services Administration, *Results from the 2010 National Survey on Drug Use and Health: Summary of National Findings*, NSDUH Series H-41, HHS Publication No. (SMA) 11-4658. Rockville, MD: Substance Abuse and Mental Health Services Administration; 2011. Report online at: http://www.samhsa.gov/data/NSDUH/2k10NSDUH/2k10Results.pdf.
2. The National Institute on Drug Abuse (NIDA). *Medical Consequences of Drug Abuse*. http://www.nida.nih.gov/consequences/, accessed April 24, 2012.
3. Baler RD, Volkow ND: Addiction as a systems failure: focus on adolescence and smoking. *J Am Acad Child Adolesc Psychiatry*. 2011;50(4):329-339.
4. Dick DM, Bierut LJ: The genetics of alcohol dependence. *Curr Psychiatry Rep*. 2006;8:151-157.
5. Dick DM, Plunkett J, Wetherill LF, et al. Association between GABRA1 and drinking behaviors in the collaborative study on the genetics of alcoholism sample. *Alcohol Clin Exp Res*. 2006;30(7):1101-1110.
6. The American Psychiatric Association. *Diagnostic and Statistical Manual of Mental Disorders*, 5th ed (DSM-V). Washington, DC: American Psychiatric Association, 2013.
7. Fiore MC, Bailey WC, Cohen SJ, et al. *Treating Tobacco Use and Dependence. Quick Reference Guide for Clinicians*. Rockville, MD: U.S. Department of Health and Human Services, Public Health Service; 2000.
8. Ewing JA: Detecting alcoholism: the CAGE questionnaire. *JAMA*. 1984;252(14):1905-1907.
9. Passik SD, Kirsh KL, Whitcomb L, et al. A new tool to assess and document pain outcomes in chronic pain patients receiving opioid therapy. *Clin Ther*. 2004;26(4):552-561.

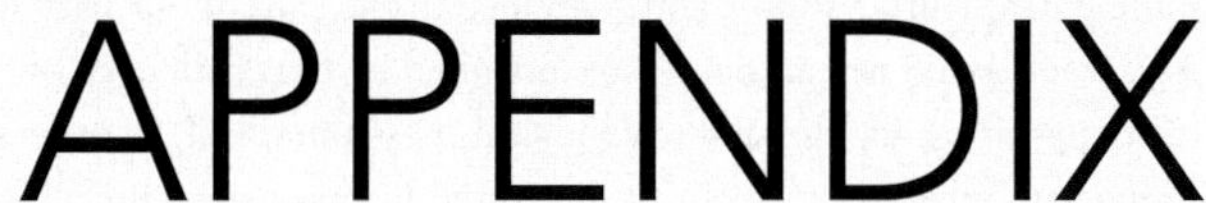

APPENDIX

Strength of Recommendation (SOR)	Definition
A	Recommendation based on consistent and good-quality patient-oriented evidence.*
B	Recommendation based on inconsistent or limited-quality patient-oriented evidence.*
C	Recommendation based on consensus, usual practice, opinion, disease-oriented evidence, or case series for studies of diagnosis, treatment, prevention, or screening.*

*See Appendix A on pages 1320–1322 for further information.

APPENDIX A INTERPRETING EVIDENCE-BASED MEDICINE

Mindy A. Smith, MD, MS

"Evidence-based medicine—is this something new?" asked my father, incredulously. "What were you practicing before?"

Like my father, our patients assume that we provide recommendations to them based on scientific evidence. The idea that there might not be relevant evidence or that we might not have access to that evidence has not even occurred to most of them. This is certainly not to imply that such evidence is the be-all and end-all of medical practice or that our patients would follow such recommendations blindly—rather, for me, it is a starting point from which to begin rational testing or outline a possible therapeutic plan.

The first time that I recall the term *evidence-based medicine* (EBM) being discussed was in the early 1990s.[1,2] It seemed that we would need to develop skills in evaluating the published literature and determining its quality, validity, and relevance to the care of our patients. As a teacher and researcher, I was intrigued by the challenges of critically appraising articles and teaching this newfound skill to others. As a clinician, however, I was most interested in answering clinical questions and doing so in a compressed time frame. I need rapid access to tools or sources that provided summary answers to those questions tagged to information about the quantity and quality of the evidence and the consistency of information across studies.

There seemed to be many systems for rating literature but few that met the needs of the busy practitioner trying to make sense of individual clinical trials and the hundreds of both evidence-based and consensus-based guidelines that seemed to spring up overnight. In 2004, the editors of the U.S. family medicine and primary care journals and the Family Practice Inquiries Network published a paper on a unified taxonomy called *Strength of Recommendation* (SOR) Taxonomy that seemed to fit the bill (**Figure A-1**).[3] This taxonomy made use of existing systems for judging study quality while incorporating the concept of patient-oriented (e.g., mortality, morbidity, symptom improvement) rather than disease-oriented (e.g., change in blood pressure, blood chemistry) outcomes as most relevant. SOR Ⓐ recommendation is one based on consistent, good-quality patient-oriented evidence; SOR Ⓑ is a recommendation based on inconsistent or limited-quality patient-oriented evidence; and SOR Ⓒ is a recommendation based on consensus, usual practice, opinion, disease-oriented evidence, or case series (**Figures A-1** and **A-2**).

In this book, we made a commitment to search for patient-oriented evidence to support the information that we provide in each of the chapter sections (i.e., epidemiology, etiology and pathophysiology, risk factors, diagnosis, differential diagnosis, management, prevention, prognosis, and follow-up) and to provide a SOR rating for that evidence whenever possible. The bulleted format within these divisions would allow the practitioner to quickly find answers to their clinical questions while providing some direction about how confident we were that a recommendation had high-quality patient-oriented evidence to support it.

For example, a parent of a child with suspected sinusitis asks about the need for treating with antibiotics rather than saline nose spray and decongestants? As noted in Chapter 26, Sinusitis, under Medications, there is strong data (SOR Ⓐ) that antihistamines and decongestants confer no benefit in symptom relief in children and are associated with significant toxicity. Data are absent with regard to saline nose spray for sinusitis in children. Using antibiotics, there is modest potential benefit (about 10% decrease in clinical failure rate) and risks of harm (primarily diarrhea in just under half [44%] but also skin rash, headache, dizziness, and fatigue; although few discontinue medications because of these).

The physician armed with this information can discuss the options with the parent and explore potential benefits and risks. Particularly in difficult cases where there are multiple options, the clinician's experience and the patient preferences are important aspects of shared decision-making. One definition of EBM is, "The integration of best research evidence with clinical expertise and patient values."

Several other concepts are used throughout the book that can assist practitioners in using evidence-based information and explaining that information to patients. Risk reductions from medical treatments are often presented in relative terms—the *relative risk reduction* (RRR) or the difference in the percentage of adverse outcomes between the intervention group and the control group divided by the percentage of adverse outcomes in the control group. These numbers are often large and use of them not only causes us to overestimate the importance of a treatment but misses its clinical relevance. A more meaningful term is the *absolute risk reduction* (ARR)—the risk difference between the two groups. This number can then be used to obtain a *number needed to treat* (NNT)—the number of patients that would need to be treated (over the same time as used in the treatment trial) to prevent 1 bad outcome or produce 1 good outcome. This is calculated as 100 percent divided by the ARR. NNT is more easily understood by us and our patients. See the NNT example in **Box A-1**.

Another term that is used in this book is the *likelihood ratio* (LR). This number, based on the sensitivity and specificity of a diagnostic test, is used to determine the probability of a patient with a positive test (LR+) having the disease or the probability of the patient with a negative test (LR+) not having the disease in question. The LR is defined as the likelihood that a given test result would be expected in a patient with the target disorder compared to the likelihood that the same result would be expected in a patient without the target disorder.[4] The number obtained for the LR+ [Sensitivity/(100 – Specificity)] or the LR– [(100 – Sensitivity)/Specificity] can be multiplied by

BOX A-1 NNT Example

If a new drug was released for the treatment of pain and a randomized controlled trial found that the 70 percent of the treated group reported significant pain control (based on the defined end point) and 20 percent of the placebo group reported significant pain control this would produce an absolute risk reduction (ARR) of 50 percent. In this case, the NNT would be 100%/50% = 2. On average, only 2 patients would need to be treated for 1 patient to receive the defined pain control benefit. If the ARR was only 10 percent (30% of the intervention group and 20 percent of the control group benefitted), then the NNT = 10 or 10 patients would need treatment on average for 1 to receive benefit.

How recommendations are graded for strength, and underlying individual studies are rated for quality

In general, only key recommendations for readers require a grade of the "Strength of Recommendation." Recommendations should be based on the highest quality evidence available. For example, vitamin E was found in some cohort studies (level 2 study quality) to have a benefit for cardiovascular protection, but good-quality randomized trials (level 1) have not confirmed this effect. Therefore, it is preferable to base clinical recommendations in a manuscript on the level 1 studies.

Strength of recommendation	Definition
A	Recommendation based on consistent and good-quality patient-oriented evidence.*
B	Recommendation based on inconsistent or limited-quality patient-oriented evidence.*
C	Recommendation based on consensus, usual practice, opinion, disease-oriented evidence,* or case series for studies of diagnosis, treatment, prevention, or screening

Use the following scheme to determine whether a study measuring patient-oriented outcomes is of good or limited quality, and whether the results are consistent or inconsistent between studies.

	Type of Study		
Study quality	**Diagnosis**	**Treatment/prevention/ screening**	**Prognosis**
Level 1— good-quality patient-oriented evidence	Validated clinical decision rule SR/meta-analysis of high-quality studies High-quality diagnostic cohort study†	SR/meta-analysis of RCTs with consistent findings High-quality individual RCT‡ All-or-none study§	SR/meta-analysis of good-quality cohort studies Prospective cohort study with good follow-up
Level 2— limited-quality patient-oriented evidence	Unvalidated clinical decision rule SR/meta-analysis of lower-quality studies or studies with inconsistent findings Lower-quality diagnostic cohort study or diagnostic case-control study§	SR/meta-analysis lower-quality clinical trials or of studies with inconsistent findings Lower-quality clinical trial‡ or prospective cohort study Cohort study Case-control study	SR/meta-analysis of lower-quality cohort studies or with inconsistent results Retrospective cohort study with poor follow-up Case-control study Case series
Level 3— other evidence	Consensus guidelines, extrapolations from bench research, usual practice, opinion, other evidence disease-oriented evidence (intermediate or physiologic outcomes only), or case series for studies of diagnosis, treatment, prevention, or screening		

Consistency across studies

Consistent	Most studies found similar or at least coherent conclusions (coherence means that differences are explainable); ***or*** If high-quality and up-to-date systematic reviews or meta-analyses exist, they support the recommendation
Inconsistent	Considerable variation among study findings and lack of coherence; ***or*** If high-quality and up-to-date systematic reviews or meta-analyses exist, they do not find consistent evidence in favor of the recommendation

*Patient-oriented evidence measures outcomes that matter to patients: morbidity, mortality, symptom improvement, cost reduction, and quality of life. Disease-oriented evidence measures intermediate, physiologic, or surrogate end points that may or may not reflect improvements in patient outcomes (ie, blood pressure, blood chemistry, physiologic function, and pathologic findings).

† High-quality diagnostic cohort study: cohort design, adequate size, adequate spectrum of patients, blinding, and a consistent, well-defined reference standard.

‡ High-quality RCT: allocation concealed, blinding if possible, intention-to-treat analysis, adequate statistical power, adequate follow-up (greater than 80 percent).

§ In an all-or-none study, the treatment causes a dramatic change in outcomes, such as antibiotics for meningitis or surgery for appendicitis, which precludes study in a controlled trial.

SR, systematic review; RCT, randomized controlled trial

FIGURE A-1 Used with permission from Ebell MH, Siwek J, Weiss BD, et al. Simplifying the language of evidence to improve patient care: Strength of recommendation taxonomy (SORT). *J. Fam Pract 2004;53(2):110-120. With permission from Frontline Medical Communications.*

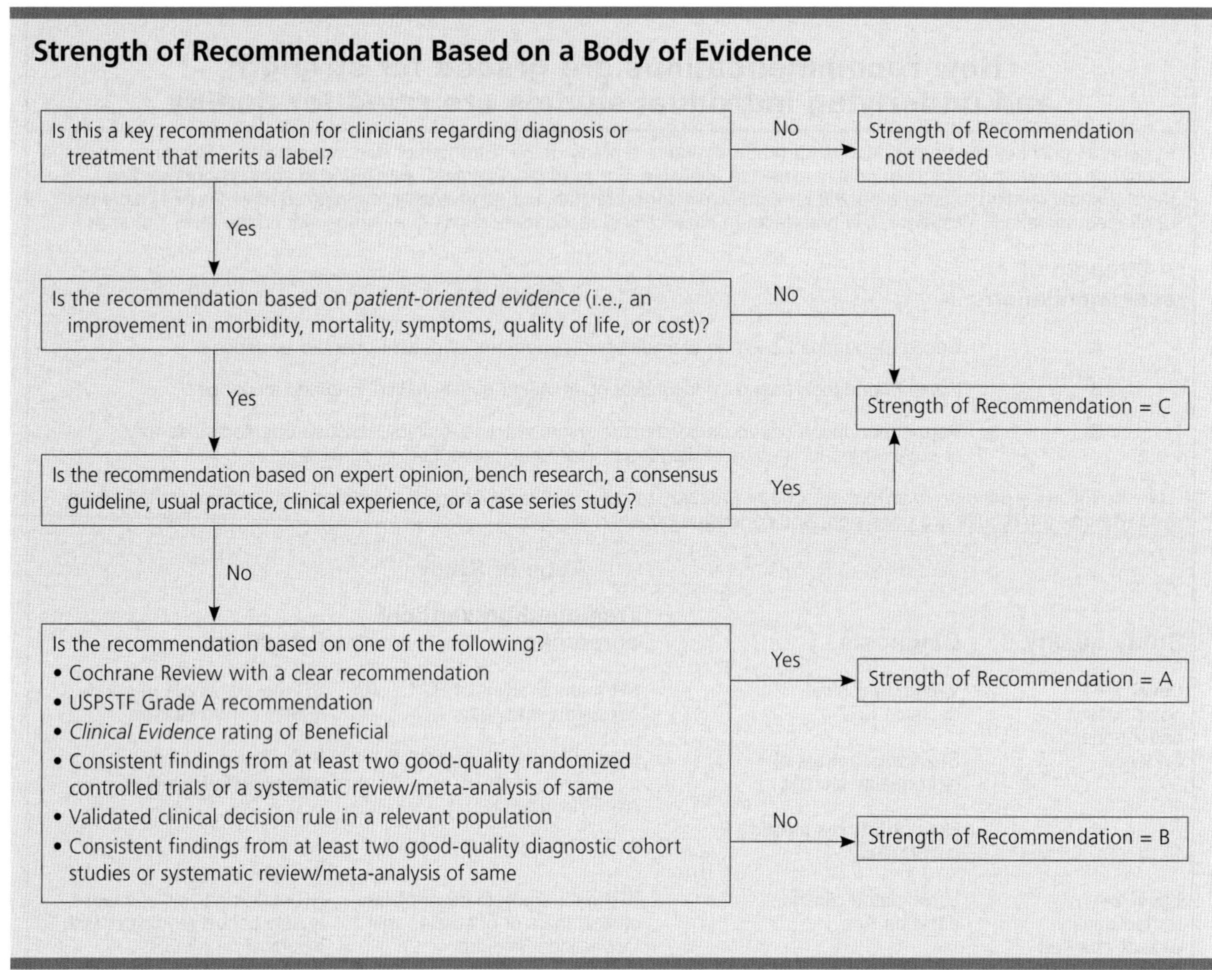

FIGURE A-2 Assigning a Strength-of-Recommendation grade based on a body of evidence. (USPSTF = US Preventive Services Task Force.) (*Used with permission from Ebell MH, Siwek J, Weiss BD, et al. Simplifying the language of evidence to improve patient care: Strength of recommendation taxonomy (SORT). J. Fam Pract 2004;53(2):110-120. With permission from Frontline Medical Communications.*)

the pretest probability of disease to determine the posttest probability of disease. A nomogram (one can be found by visiting the website mentioned in reference 6) can be used to more easily work with these numbers to convert a pretest probability into a posttest probability. A LR+ over 10 is considered strong evidence to rule in disease while a LR– of less than 0.1 is strong evidence to rule out disease.

We are both privileged and cursed with practicing medicine in an information-rich environment. We have designed our *Color Atlas* to link evidence to clinical recommendations so that we can provide our patients the best science available. When the evidence is lacking, we make that clear and encourage you to engage in frank and honest discussions that lead to the shared responsibility for decisions. Our patients are justified in expecting science along with humanism—can we give them anything less?

REFERENCES

1. Evidence-Based Medicine Working Group. Evidence-based medicine. A new approach to teaching the practice of medicine. *JAMA.* 1992;268:2420-2425.
2. Shaughnessy AF, Slawson DC, Bennett JH. Becoming an information master: a guidebook to the medical information jungle. *J Fam Pract.* 1994;39:489-499.
3. Ebell MA, Siwek J, Weiss BD, et al. Strength of Recommendation Taxonomy (SORT): a patient-centered approach to grading evidence in the medical literature. *J Fam Pract.* 2004;53(2): 111-120.
4. Center for Evidence-Based Medicine. http://www.cebm.net/index.aspx?o=1162, accessed May 12, 2014.

APPENDIX B USE OF TOPICAL AND INTRALESIONAL CORTICOSTEROIDS

TABLE B-1 Corticosteroid Potency Chart

Generic Name	Trade Name and Strength
Class 1—Superpotent	
Betamethasone dipropionate*	Diprolene ointment 0.05 percent
Diflorasone diacetate**	Psorcon ointment, 0.05 percent
Clobetasol propionate	Temovate cream, gel, ointment, shampoo, spray, or foam, 0.05 percent; also as Cormax, Clobex, Clarelux, Olux
Halobetasol propionate*	Ultravate cream/ointment, 0.05 percent
Class 2—Potent	
Amcinonide	Cyclocort cream/ointment/lotion, 0.1 percent
Betamethasone dipropionate	Diprosone ointment, 0.05 percent
Desoximetasone	Topicort cream 0.25 percent, gel 0.05 percent, and ointment 0.25 percent
Diflorasone diacetate**	Psorcon, ApexiCon ointment 0.05 percent
Fluocinonide	Lidex, Lidemol, Lyderm, Tiamol, Topactin, Topsyn, Vanos cream 0.05 percent, 0.1 percent/ointment/gel, 0.05 percent
Halcinonide	Halog cream/ointment/topical solution, 0.1 percent
Class 3—Upper mid-strength	
Betamethasone valerate*	Diprolene, Luxiq, Dermabet, Alphatrex, Diprolene AF, Diprolene Glycol, Diprosone, Valnac, BetaVal cream/lotion 0.05 percent or 0.1 percent, foam 0.12 percent
Diflorasone diacetate**	Psorcon, ApexiCon, ApexiCon E cream 0.05 percent
Mometasone furoate	Elocon cream/lotion/ointment, 0.1 percent
Triamcinolone acetonide	Kenalog topical, Pediaderm, Triacet, Trianex cream, 0.5 percent
Class 4—Mid-strength	
Desoximetasone	Topicort LP cream, 0.05 percent
Fluocinolone acetonide	Synalar-HP cream, 0.2 percent; Synalar ointment, 0.025 percent
Flurandrenolide	Cordran ointment, 0.05 percent
Triamcinolone acetonide	Aristocort, Kenalog ointments, 0.1 percent
Class 5—Lower mid-strength	
Betamethasone dipropionate	Diprosone lotion, 0.05 percent
Betamethasone valerate	Valisone cream, 0.1 percent; Betatrex 0.1 percent
Fluocinolone acetonide	Synalar cream, 0.025 percent
Flurandrenolide	Cordran cream, 0.05 percent
Hydrocortisone butyrate	Locoid cream, 0.1 percent
Hydrocortisone valerate	Westcort cream, 0.2 percent
Prednicarbate	Dermatop cream/ointment, 0.1 percent
Triamcinolone acetonide	Kenalog cream/lotion, 0.1 percent
Class 6—Mild	
Alclometasone dipropionate	Aclovate cream/ointment, 0.05 percent
Triamcinolone acetonide	Aristocort cream, 0.1 percent
Desonide	Desonate, DesOwen, Tridesilon, Verdeso cream/lotion/ointment 0.05 percent, foam 0.05 percent, gel, 0.05 percent, 0.05 percent
Fluocinolone acetonide	Synalar cream/solution, 0.01 percent; Capex shampoo, Dermasmooth, 0.01 percent
Betamethasone valerate	Valisone lotion, 0.1 percent
Class 7—Least potent	
Hydrocortisone	Hyton, Cortate, Unicort, other OTC cream/lotion/foam

*<12 years old: Not recommended.
**Safety and efficacy not established in pediatric patients.

TABLE B-2 Common Side Effects of Topical Corticosteroids

Skin atrophy	Most common adverse effect Epidermal thinning may begin after only a few days Dermal thinning usually takes several weeks to develop Usually reversible within 2 months after stopping the corticosteroid
Telangiectasia	Most often occurs on the face, neck, and upper chest Tends to decrease when steroid discontinued, but may be irreversible
Striae	Usually occur around flexures (groin, axillary, and inner thigh areas) Usually permanent, but may fade with time
Purpura	Frequently occurs after minimal trauma Attributed to loss of perivascular supporting tissue in the dermis
Hypopigmentation	Reversible upon discontinuing the corticosteroid
Acneform eruptions	Particularly common on the face, especially with the "potent" and "very potent" corticosteroids Usually reversible
Fine hair growth	Reversible upon discontinuation of the corticosteroid
Infections	May worsen viral, bacterial, or fungal skin infections May cause tinea incognito
Hypothalamic-pituitary-adrenal axis suppression	Rare with topicals >30 g/wk of "very potent" corticosteroids should be limited to 3–4 wk Children (>10 g/wk) and elderly are at higher risk because of thinner skin

TABLE B-3 Intralesional Steroids—Concentrations for Injection

Condition	Concentration of Triamcinolone Acetonide Solution (mg/mL)
Acne (**Figure B-1**)	2 to 2.5
Alopecia areata (**Figure B-2**)	5 to 10
Granuloma annulare	5 to 10
Psoriasis	5 to 10
Hypertrophic lichen planus	5 to 10
Prurigo nodularis	10
Hidradenitis suppurativa	10
Keloids and hypertrophic scars (**Figure B-3**)	10 to 40

Use a 27-gauge or 30-gauge needle when injecting intralesional steroids to minimize pain. Steroid dilutions can be made with sterile saline for injection. The injection hurts less than when diluting the steroid with lidocaine. A Luer-Lok syringe is helpful to avoid the needle from popping off during the injection. For further information on performing intralesional injections see Usatine R, Pfenninger J, Stulberg D, Small R. *Dermatologic and Cosmetic Procedures in Office Practice*. Philadelphia, PA: Elsevier; 2012. This text and accompanying videos can also be purchased as an electronic application at **http://www.usatinemedia.com**.

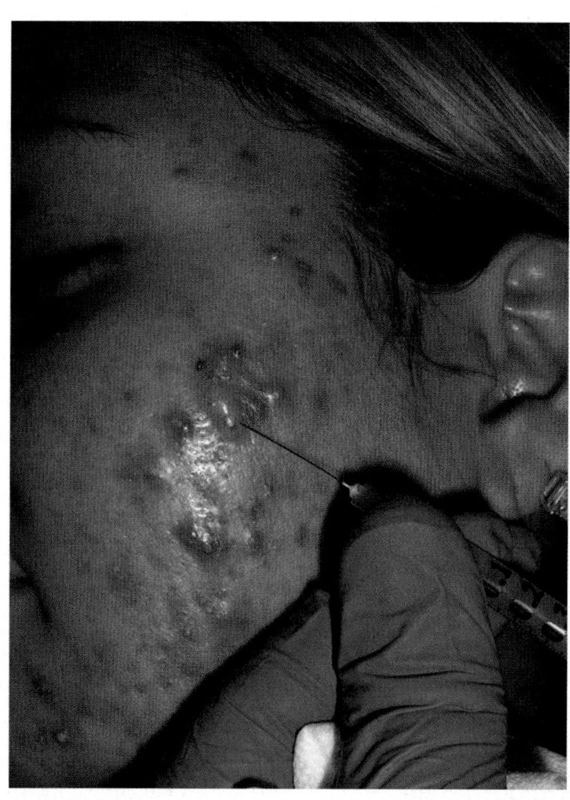

FIGURE B-1 Injecting painful cystic acne with 2 mg/mL triamcinolone using a 30-gauge needle. (*Used with permission from Richard P. Usatine, MD.*)

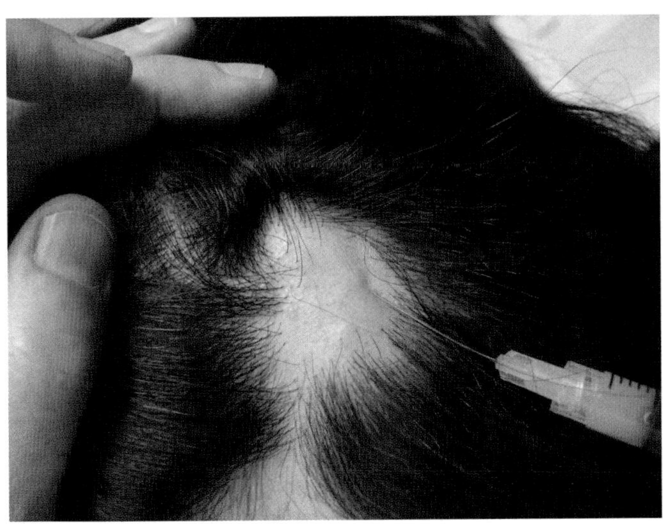

FIGURE B-2 Injecting alopecia areata with 5 mg/mL triamcinolone using a 27-gauge needle on a Luer-Lok syringe. (*Used with permission from Richard P. Usatine, MD.*)

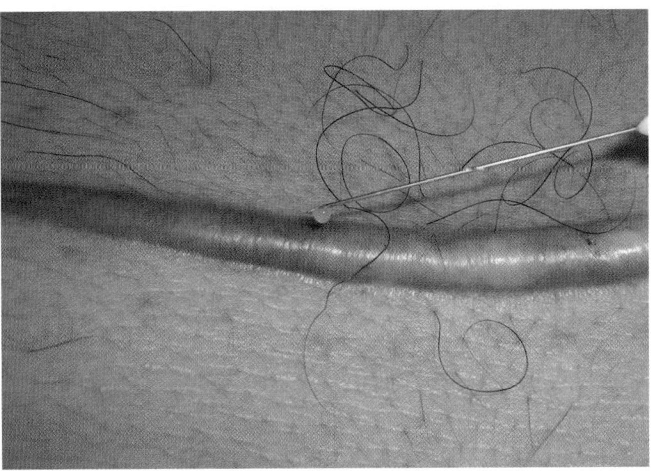

FIGURE B-3 Injecting a hypertrophic scar with 10 mg/mL triamcinolone using a 27-gauge needle on a Luer-Lok syringe. (*Used with permission from Richard P. Usatine, MD.*)

Note: In this index, the letters "f" and "t" denote figures and tables, respectively.

C

E

F

H

J

S

T

U